ENDOCRINOLOGY

ENDOCRINOLOGY

FOURTH EDITION

Edited by

LESLIE J. DeGROOT
J. LARRY JAMESON

Henry G. Burger
D. Lynn Loriaux
John C. Marshall
Shlomo Melmed
William D. Odell
John T. Potts, Jr.
Arthur H. Rubenstein

Volume

1

W.B. SAUNDERS COMPANY
A Harcourt Health Sciences Company
Philadelphia London New York St. Louis Toronto Sydney

W.B. SAUNDERS COMPANY
A Harcourt Health Sciences Company

The Curtis Center
Independence Square West
Philadelphia, Pennsylvania 19106

Library of Congress Cataloging-in-Publication Data

Endocrinology/edited by Leslie J. DeGroot, J. Larry Jameson [and] Henry Burger . . . [et al.]—4th ed.

p.   cm.

Includes bibliographical references and index.

ISBN 0–7216–7840–8 (set)

1. Endocrine glands—Diseases.   2. Endocrinology.   I. DeGroot, Leslie J.
II. Jameson, J. Larry.

[DNLM: 1. Endocrine Diseases.   2. Endocrine Glands.   3. Hormones.
WK 140 E5585 2001]

RC648.E458   2001   616.4—dc21

DNLM/DLC   00-030134

Acquisitions Editor: Richard Zorab
Developmental Editor: Hazel N. Hacker
Manuscript Editor: Deborah Thorp, Marjory Fraser
Production Manager: Norman Stellander
Illustration Specialist: Walter Verbitski
Book Designer: Steven Stave

ISBN 0–7216–7841–6 (vol. 1)
ISBN 0–7216–7842–4 (vol. 2)
ISBN 0–7216–7843–2 (vol. 3)
ISBN 0–7216–7840–8 (set)

ENDOCRINOLOGY

Printed in the United States of America.

Last digit is the print number: 9   8   7   6   5   4   3   2

Contributors

Rexford S. Ahima, MD, PhD
Assistant Professor of Medicine, Division of Endocrinology/Diabetes and Metabolism, Department of Medicine, University of Pennsylvania School of Medicine; Attending Endocrinologist, Hospital of the University of Pennsylvania; Director, Physiology Core Laboratory, Penn Diabetes Center, Philadelphia, Pennsylvania
Leptin

Nobuyuki Amino, MD
Professor of Medicine, Department of Laboratory Medicine, Osaka University Medical School, Osaka, Japan
Chronic (Hashimoto's) Thyroiditis

Marianne S. Anderson, MD
Assistant Professor, Department of Pediatrics, University of Colorado School of Medicine, Denver, Colorado
Fuel Homeostasis in the Fetus and Neonate

Josephine Arendt, BSc, PhD, FRCPath
Professor of Endocrinology, School of Biological Sciences, University of Surrey; Director, Centre for Chronobiology, Surrey, England
The Pineal Gland: Basic Physiology and Clinical Implications

Lora Armstrong, RPh, PharmD, BCPS
Clinical Pharmacist, Clinical Services Department, Caremark, Northbrook, Illinois
Drugs and Hormones Used in Endocrinology

David C. Aron, MD, MS
Professor of Medicine and Professor of Epidemiology and Biostatistics, Case Western Reserve University School of Medicine; Senior Scholar and Associate Chief of Staff for Education, Louis Stokes Cleveland Veterans Affairs Medical Center, Cleveland, Ohio
Diagnostic Implications of Adrenal Physiology and Clinical Epidemiology for Evaluation of Glucocorticoid Excess and Deficiency

Sylvia L. Asa, MD, PhD
Professor, Department of Laboratory Medicine and Pathobiology, University of Toronto; Consultant in Endocrine Pathology, Department of Pathology and Laboratory Medicine, Mount Sinai Hospital, Toronto, Ontario, Canada
Functional Pituitary Anatomy and Histology

Richard J. Auchus, MD, PhD
Assistant Professor, Division of Endocrinology and Metabolism, Department of Internal Medicine, University of Texas Southwestern Medical Center; Attending Physician, Parkland Memorial Hospital, VANTHCS, Dallas, Texas
The Principles, Pathways, and Enzymes of Human Steroidogenesis

Louis V. Avioli, MD
Schoenberg Professor of Medicine and Director, Division of Bone and Mineral Diseases, Washington University School of Medicine; Director, Division of Endocrinology and Metabolism, The Jewish Hospital of St. Louis, St. Louis, Missouri
Disorders of Calcification: Osteomalacia and Rickets

Joseph Avruch, MD
Professor of Medicine, Harvard Medical School; Physician and Chief, Diabetes Unit, Medical Services, and Member, Department of Molecular Biology, Massachusetts General Hospital, Boston, Massachusetts
Receptor Tyrosine Kinases

Lloyd Axelrod, MD
Associate Professor of Medicine, Harvard Medical School; Physician and Chief, James Howard Means Firm, Massachusetts General Hospital, Boston, Massachusetts
Glucocorticoid Therapy

Sami T. Azar, MD
Assistant Professor in Medicine, American University in Beirut, Beirut, Lebanon
Hypoaldosteronism and Mineralocorticoid Resistance

David T. Baird, MB, DSc
MCR Clinical Research Professor, Faculty of Medicine, University of Edinburgh; Director, Reproductive Medicine, Royal Infirmary, Edinburgh, Scotland
Amenorrhea, Anovulation, and Dysfunctional Uterine Bleeding

H. W. Gordon Baker, MD, PhD, FRACP
Principal Research Fellow, Department of Obstetrics and Gynaecology, University of Melbourne, Melbourne; Andrologist, The Royal Women's Hospital, Clayton, Victoria, Australia
Male Infertility

Giuseppe Barbesino, MD
Assistant Professor, Department of Endocrinology, University of Pisa Medical School, Pisa, Italy
Graves' Disease

Randall B. Barnes, MD
Associate Professor, Department of Obstetrics and Gynecology, University of Chicago Pritzker School of Medicine; Attending Physician, Chicago Lying-in Hospital, Chicago, Illinois
Hyperandrogenism, Hirsutism, and the Polycystic Ovary Syndrome

George B. Bartley, MD
Associate Professor of Ophthalmology, Mayo Medical School; Chair, Department of Ophthalmology, Mayo Clinic, Rochester, Minnesota
Ophthalmopathy

Etienne-Emile Baulieu, MD, PhD
Professor, Collège de France; Chef de Service de Biochimie
Hormonale, Hôpital de Bicêtre, Bicêtre, France
Nuclear Receptor Superfamily

Peter H. Baylis, BSc, MD, FRCP
Dean of Medicine and Professor of Experimental Medicine,
University of Newcastle Upon Tyne Medical School; Consultant
Endocrinologist, Royal Victoria Infirmary, Newcastle Upon Tyne,
England
*Vasopressin, Diabetes Insipidus, and Syndrome of
Inappropriate Antidiuresis*

Paolo Beck-Peccoz
Professor of Endocrinology, Institute of Endocrine Sciences,
University of Milan; Chief, Endocrine Unit, Ospedale Maggiore
IRCCS, Milan, Italy
TSH-Producing Adenomas; Resistance to Thyroid Hormone

Graeme I. Bell, PhD
Professor of Biochemistry and Molecular Biology, Medicine, and
Human Genetics, University of Chicago Pritzker School of
Medicine; Investigator, Howard Hughes Medical Institute,
Chicago, Illinois
*Chemistry and Biosynthesis of the Islet Hormones: Insulin, Islet
Amyloid Polypeptide (Amylin), Glucagon, Somatostatin, and
Pancreatic Polypeptide*

Eren Berber, MD
Fellow, Department of General Surgery, Cleveland Clinic Foundation,
Cleveland, Ohio
Adrenal Surgery

Richard M. Bergenstal, MD
Executive Director and Chief Medical Officer, International Diabetes
Center; Consultant in Endocrinology, Park Nicollet Clinic,
Minneapolis, Minnesota
*Management of Type 2 Diabetes: A Systematic Approach to
Meeting the Standards of Care, I: Self-Management Education,
Medical Nutrition Therapy, and Exercise; II: Oral Agents, Insulin,
and Management of Complications*

John P. Bilezikian, MD
Professor of Medicine and Pharmacology, Department of Medicine,
Columbia University College of Physicians and Surgeons;
Attending Physician, New York–Presbyterian Hospital, New York,
New York
Primary Hyperparathyroidism

Richard E. Blackwell, PhD, MD
Professor, Department of Obstetrics and Gynecology, University of
Alabama School of Medicine, Birmingham, Alabama
Female Infertility: Evaluation and Treatment

Stephen R. Bloom, MD, DSc, FRCP, FRCPath
Professor of Medicine, Imperial College School of Medicine; Chief,
Investigative Sciences, The Hammersmith Hospital, London,
England
Gastrointestinal Hormones and Tumor Syndromes

Jeffrey A. Bluestone, PhD
Daniel K. Ludwig Professor, University of Chicago Pritzker School
of Medicine; Director, Ben May Institute for Cancer Research,
Chicago, Illinois
*Immunologic Mechanisms Causing Autoimmune Endocrine
Disease*

Manfred Blum, MD
Professor of Clinical Medicine and Radiology, New York University
School of Medicine; Attending Physician and Director, Nuclear
Endocrine Laboratory, Tisch Hospital, New York, New York
Thyroid Imaging

Roger Bouillon, MD, PhD
Professor of Endocrinology, Faculty of Medicine, Katholieke
Universiteit Leuven; Chairman, Department of Endocrinology,
University Hospitals, Gasthuisberg, Leuven, Belgium
*Vitamin D: From Photosynthesis, Metabolism, and Action to
Clinical Applications*

Andrew J. M. Boulton, MD, FRCP
Professor of Medicine, Faculty of Medicine, University of
Manchester; Consultant Physician, Manchester Royal Infirmary,
Manchester, England
Diabetes Mellitus: Neuropathy

Glenn D. Braunstein, MD
Professor and Vice Chair, Department of Medicine, University of
California, Los Angeles, UCLA School of Medicine; Chairman,
Department of Medicine, Cedars-Sinai Medical Center, Los
Angeles, California
Hypothalamic Syndromes

F. Richard Bringhurst, MD
Associate Professor of Medicine, Harvard Medical School; Physician
and Chief of Staff, Medical Services, Massachusetts General
Hospital, Boston, Massachusetts
Regulation of Calcium and Phosphate Homeostasis

Arthur E. Broadus, MD, PhD
Professor of Medicine, Yale University School of Medicine; Chief of
Endocrinology, Yale–New Haven Hospital, New Haven,
Connecticut
Malignancy-Associated Hypercalcemia

Edward M. Brown, MD
Professor of Medicine, Harvard Medical School; Senior Physician,
Brigham and Women's Hospital, Boston, Massachusetts
*Parathyroid Hormone and Parathyroid Hormone–Related
Peptide in the Regulation of Calcium Homeostasis and Bone
Development; Familial Hypocalciuric Hypercalcemia and Other
Disorders Due to Calcium-Sensing Receptor Mutations*

Henry B. Burch, MD
Associate Professor of Medicine, Uniformed Services University of
the Health Sciences, Bethesda, Maryland; Assistant Chief,
Endocrine–Metabolic Service, Walter Reed Army Medical Center,
Washington, D.C.
Ophthalmopathy

Henry G. Burger, MD, FRACP
Honorary Professor of Medicine, Faculty of Medicine, Monash University; *formerly* Director, Prince Henry's Institute of Medical Research, Monash Medical Centre, Clayton, Victoria, Australia
Gonadal Peptides: Inhibins, Activins, Follistatin, Müllerian-Inhibiting Substance (Antimüllerian Hormone); Menopause and Hormone Replacement

Gerard N. Burrow, MD
David Paige Smith Professor of Medicine and Professor of Obstetrics and Gynecology, Yale University School of Medicine, New Haven, Connecticut
Diagnosis and Treatment of Thyroid Disease During Pregnancy

Jose F. Caro, MD
Professor of Medicine, Indiana University School of Medicine, Indianapolis, Indiana
Obesity

Don H. Catlin, MD
Associate Professor, Department of Medicine and Department of Molecular and Medical Pharmacology, University of California, Los Angeles, UCLA School of Medicine, Los Angeles, California
Use and Abuse of Anabolic Steroids

Ralph R. Cavalieri, MD
Professor Emeritus, Department of Medicine and Department of Radiology, University of California, San Francisco, School of Medicine; Consultant in Endocrinology and Nuclear Medicine, Veterans Administration Medical Center, San Francisco, California
Thyroid Imaging

Alan Chait, MD
Professor of Medicine and Head, Division of Metabolism, Endocrinology, and Nutrition, Department of Medicine, University of Washington School of Medicine, Seattle, Washington
Diabetes, Lipids, and Atherosclerosis

John R. G. Challis, PhD, DSc, FIBiol, FRCOG, FRSC
Ernest B. and Leonard B. Smith Professor and Chair, Department of Physiology, and Professor of Obstetrics and Gynecology, MRC Group in Fetal and Neonatal Health and Development, Faculty of Medicine, University of Toronto, Toronto; Affiliate Scientist, Samuel Lunenfeld Research Institute, Mount Sinai Hospital; Toronto Affiliate, Lawson Research Institute, London, Ontario, Canada
Endocrinology of Parturition

Shu J. Chan, PhD
Associate Professor of Biochemistry and Molecular Biology, University of Chicago Pritzker School of Medicine; Senior Research Associate, Howard Hughes Medical Institute, Chicago, Illinois
Chemistry and Biosynthesis of the Islet Hormones: Insulin, Islet Amyloid Polypeptide (Amylin), Glucagon, Somatostatin, and Pancreatic Polypeptide

Roland D. Chapurlat, MD
Assistant Professor, Department of Rheumatology and Bone Diseases and INSERM U403, Hôpital E. Herriot, Lyon, France
Osteoporosis

V. Krishna Chatterjee, MBChB, FRCP
Professor of Endocrinology, Department of Medicine, Faculty of Medicine, University of Cambridge; Honorary Consultant Physician, Addenbrooke's Hospital, Cambridge, England
Resistance to Thyroid Hormone

Qiao-Yi Chen, MD, PhD
Assistant Professor, Department of Pediatrics Louisiana State University School of Medicine in New Orleans, New Orleans; Research Institute for Children, Harahan, Louisiana
The Autoimmune Polyglandular Syndromes

Luca Chiovato, MD
Assistant Professor, Department of Endocrinology, University of Pisa Medical School, Pisa, Italy
Graves' Disease

George P. Chrousos, MD
Chief, Pediatric and Reproductive Endocrinology Branch, National Institute of Child Health and Human Development, National Institutes of Health, Bethesda, Maryland
Interactions of the Endocrine and Immune Systems

David R. Clemmons, MD
Chief, Division of Endocrinology, and Kenan Professor of Medicine, University of North Carolina at Chapel Hill School of Medicine; Attending Physician, UNC Hospitals, Chapel Hill, North Carolina
Insulin-Like Growth Factor-1 and Its Binding Proteins

Jack W. Coburn, MD
Adjunct Professor of Medicine, University of California, Los Angeles, UCLA School of Medicine; Staff Physician, VA West Los Angeles Medical Center, Los Angeles, California
The Renal Osteodystrophies

Georges Copinschi, MD, PhD
Professor of Endocrinology, Free University of Brussels Medical School; Consultant in Endocrinology, Erasme University Hospital, Brussels, Belgium
Endocrine and Other Biologic Rhythms

Gerald R. Cunha, PhD
Professor, Department of Anatomy, University of California, San Francisco, School of Medicine, San Francisco, California
Endocrinology of the Prostate and Benign Prostatic Hyperplasia

Leona Cuttler, MD
Professor of Pediatrics, Case Western Reserve University School of Medicine; Endocrinologist, Rainbow Babies and Children's Hospital, Cleveland, Ohio
Somatic Growth and Maturation

Jamie Dananberg, MD
Senior Physician-Scientist and Senior Clinical Research Physician, Lilly Research Laboratories, Eli Lilly and Company, Indianapolis, Indiana
Obesity

David L. Daniels, MD
Professor of Radiology, Medical College of Wisconsin; Froedtert Memorial Lutheran Hospital, Milwaukee, Wisconsin
Radiographic Evaluation of the Pituitary and Anterior Hypothalamus

Mario De Felice, MD
Associate Professor of Immunology, University of Messina Medical School, Messina; Scientist, Stazione Zoologica Anton Dohrn, Naples, Italy
Anatomy and Development

Ralph A. DeFronzo, MD
Professor of Medicine, University of Texas Health Sciences Center School of Medicine; Chief, Diabetes Division, South Texas Veterans' Health Care System, Audie Murphy Division, San Antonio, Texas
Regulation of Intermediary Metabolism During Fasting and Feeding

Leslie J. DeGroot, MD
Professor of Medicine, Thyroid Study Unit, University of Chicago Pritzker School of Medicine; Attending Physician, University of Chicago Hospitals, Chicago, Illinois
Nonthyroidal Illness Syndrome; Thyroid Neoplasia

David M. de Kretser
Professor and Director, Institute of Reproduction and Development, Monash University; Consultant, Reproductive Biology Unit, Monash Medical Centre, Clayton, Victoria, Australia
Functional Morphology

Pierre D. Delmas, MD, PhD
Professor of Medicine and Director, INSERM U403, Department of Rheumatology and Bone Diseases, Hôpital E. Herriot, Lyon, France
Osteoporosis

Ruben Diaz, MD, PhD
Instructor in Pediatrics, Harvard Medical School; Assistant in Medicine, Children's Hospital, Boston, Massachusetts
Familial Hypocalciuric Hypercalcemia and Other Disorders Due to Calcium-Sensing Receptor Mutations

Roberto Di Lauro, MD
Full Professor of Human Genetics, University of Naples Federico II Medical School; Head, Laboratory of Biochemistry and Molecular Biology, Stazione Zoologica Anton Dohrn, Naples, Italy
Anatomy and Development

Sean F. Dinneen, MD, FACP, FRCPI
Consultant Diabetologist, Addenbrooke's Hospital, Cambridge, England
Classification and Diagnosis of Diabetes Mellitus

Annemarie A. Donjacour, PhD
Assistant Researcher, Department of Anatomy, University of California, San Francisco, School of Medicine, San Francisco, California
Endocrinology of the Prostate and Benign Prostatic Hyperplasia

John L. Doppman, MD
Staff Radiologist, Department of Radiology, The Clinical Center, National Institutes of Health, Bethesda, Maryland
Adrenal Imaging

Daniel J. Drucker, MD
Professor, Department of Medicine, University of Toronto Faculty of Medicine; Staff Physician and University Division Director, Endocrinology, Toronto General Hospital, Toronto, Ontario, Canada
Glucagon Secretion, α Cell Metabolism, and Glucagon Action

Jacques E. Dumont, MD, PhD
Professor of Biochemistry, Free University of Brussels Medical School, Brussels, Belgium
Thyroid Regulatory Factors

John T. Dunn, MD
Professor, Division of Endocrinology, Department of Medicine, University of Virginia School of Medicine; Attending Physician, University of Virginia Hospital, Charlottesville, Virginia
Biosynthesis and Secretion of Thyroid Hormones

Christopher R. W. Edwards, MD
Professor of Clinical Medicine, Department of Medicine, University of Edinburgh; Honorary Consultant Physician, Western General Hospital, Edinburgh, Scotland
Primary Mineralocorticoid Excess Syndromes

David A. Ehrmann, MD
Associate Professor, Section of Endocrinology, Department of Medicine, University of Chicago Pritzker School of Medicine; Attending Physician, University of Chicago Hospitals, Chicago, Illinois
Hyperandrogenism, Hirsutism, and the Polycystic Ovary Syndrome

Ilia J. Elenkov, MD, PhD
Guest Researcher, Pediatric Endocrinology Section, Pediatric and Reproductive Endocrinology Branch, National Institute of Child Health and Human Development, and Inflammatory Joint Diseases Section, Arthritis and Rheumatism Branch, National Institute of Arthritis and Musculoskeletal and Skin Diseases, National Institutes of Health, Bethesda, Maryland
Interactions of the Endocrine and Immune Systems

Gregory F. Erickson, PhD
Professor, Department of Reproductive Medicine, University of California, San Diego, School of Medicine, La Jolla, California
Folliculogenesis, Ovulation, and Luteogenesis

Eric A. Espiner, MD, FRACP, FRS(NZ)
Professor in Medicine, Christchurch School of Medicine; Department of Endocrinology, Christchurch Hospital, Christchurch, New Zealand
Hormones of the Cardiovascular System

Erica A. Eugster, MD
Clinical Assistant Professor, Department of Pediatrics, Division of Endocrinology and Diabetes, Indiana University School of Medicine; Staff, James Whitcomb Riley Hospital for Children, Indianapolis, Indiana
Precocious Puberty; Delayed Puberty

Giovanni Faglia, MD
Professor of Endocrinology, School of Medicine, Faculty of
Medicine, and Postgraduate School of Endocrinology and
Metabolism, University of Milan; Chief, Division of
Endocrinology, Ospedale Maggiore IRCCS, Milan, Italy
Prolactinomas and Hyperprolactinemic Syndrome

Lisa A. Farah, MD
Courtesy Assistant Clinical Professor, University of Florida Medical
Center (Jacksonville); Physician, North Florida Gynecologic
Specialists, Jacksonville, Florida
Female Infertility: Evaluation and Treatment

Murray J. Favus, MD
Professor of Medicine, University of Chicago Pritzker School of
Medicine; Director, Bone Program, and Director, Clinical Research
Center, University of Chicago Hospitals, Chicago, Illinois
Clinical Approach to Metabolic Bone Disease

Eleuterio Ferrannini, MD
Professor of Internal Medicine, Department of Internal Medicine and
CNR Institute of Clinical Physiology, University of Pisa School of
Medicine, Pisa, Italy
*Regulation of Intermediary Metabolism During Fasting and
Feeding*

Joel S. Finkelstein, MD
Associate Professor of Medicine, Harvard Medical School; Associate
Physician, Endocrine Unit, Massachusetts General Hospital,
Boston, Massachusetts
Medical Management of Hypercalcemia

Delbert A. Fisher, MD
Professor Emeritus, Department of Pediatrics and Department of
Medicine, University of California, Los Angeles, UCLA School of
Medicine, Los Angeles; Vice President, Science and Innovation,
Quest Diagnostics, Nichols Institute, San Juan Capistrano,
California
Fetal and Neonatal Endocrinology; Endocrine Testing

Susan J. Fisher, PhD
Departments of Stomatology, Obstetrics and Gynecology and
Reproductive Sciences, Pharmaceutical Chemistry and Anatomy,
University of California at San Francisco, San Francisco,
California
*Implantation and Placental Physiology in Early Human
Pregnancy: The Role of the Maternal Decidua and the
Trophoblast*

Jeffrey S. Flier, MD
George C. Reisman Professor of Medicine, Harvard Medical School;
Vice Chair for Research, Department of Medicine, and Chief,
Division of Endocrinology, Beth Israel Deaconess Medical Center,
Boston, Massachusetts
Leptin; Syndromes of Insulin Resistance and Mutant Insulin

Maguelone G. Forest, MD, PhD
Hôpital Debrousse, Lyon, France
Diagnosis and Treatment of Disorders of Sexual Development

Daniel W. Foster, MD
Donald W. Seldin Distinguished Chair in Internal Medicine and
Chairman, Department of Internal Medicine, University of Texas
Southwestern Medical School, Dallas, Texas
*Acute Complications of Diabetes Mellitus: Ketoacidosis,
Hyperosmolar Coma, and Lactic Acidosis*

Jayne A. Franklyn, MBChB, MD, PhD, FRCP
Professor of Medicine, Division of Medical Sciences, University of
Birmingham; Consultant Physician, Queen Elizabeth Hospital,
Birmingham, England
Thyroid Function Tests

Marion J. Franz, MS, RD, CDE
Director of Nutrition and Professional Education, International
Diabetes Center, Minneapolis, Minnesota
*Management of Type 2 Diabetes: A Systematic Approach to
Meeting the Standards of Care, I: Self-Management Education,
Medical Nutrition Therapy, and Exercise; II: Oral Agents, Insulin,
and Management of Complications*

Aaron L. Friedman, MD
Professor and Chair, Department of Pediatrics, University of
Wisconsin School of Medicine, Madison, Wisconsin
Hormonal Regulation of Electrolyte and Water Metabolism

Eli A. Friedman, MD
Distinguished Teaching Professor and Chief, Renal Disease Division,
State University of New York Downstate Medical Center College
of Medicine, Brooklyn, New York
Nephropathy: A Major Diabetic Complication

Peter J. Fuller, MBBS, BMedSc, PhD, FRACP
Associate Professor, Monash University Department of Medicine;
NH&MRL Principal Research Fellow, Prince Henry's Institute of
Medical Research, Clayton, Victoria, Australia
Biochemistry of Mineralocorticoids

John W. Funder, BA, MDBS, PhD, FRACP
Professor, Monash University, Department of Medicine, Alfred
Hospital; Director, Baker Medical Research Institute, Victoria,
Australia
Biochemistry of Mineralocorticoids

Dana Gaddy-Kurten, MD
Associate Professor, Department of Medicine and Endocrinology,
University of Arkansas for Medical Sciences, Little Rock,
Arkansas
*Hormone Signaling via Cytokine Receptors and Receptor Serine
Kinases*

Robert F. Gagel, MD
Professor of Medicine and Chairman, Department of Internal
Medicine Specialties, University of Texas–Houston Medical
School; Chief, Section of Endocrine Neoplasia and Hormonal
Disorders, M. D. Anderson Cancer Center, Houston, Texas
Multiple Endocrine Neoplasia Type 2

Thomas J. Gardella, PhD
Assistant Professor in Medicine, Harvard Medical School; Assistant
Professor in Biochemistry, Massachusetts General Hospital,
Boston, Massachusetts
*Parathyroid Hormone and Parathyroid Hormone–Related
Peptide in the Regulation of Calcium Homeostasis and Bone
Development*

Bruce D. Gaylinn, PhD
Research Assistant Professor, Department of Internal Medicine,
University of Virginia School of Medicine, Charlottesville, Virginia
*Growth Hormone–Releasing Hormone and Growth Hormone
Secretagogues: Basic Physiology and Clinical Implications*

Harry K. Genant, MD
Professor of Radiology, Medicine, Epidemiology, and Orthopaedic
  Surgery, University of California, San Francisco, School of
  Medicine, San Francisco, California
  Bone Density and Imaging of Osteoporosis

Hans Gerber, MD
Privatdozent, University of Bern School of Medicine; Head of
  Division, Department of Clinical Chemistry, University Hospital,
  Inselspital, Bern, Switzerland
  Multinodular Goiter

John E. Gerich, MD
Professor of Medicine, University of Rochester School of Medicine,
  Rochester, New York
  Hypoglycemia

Marvin C. Gershengorn, MD
Abby Rockefeller Mauze Distinguished Professor of Endocrinology
  in Medicine, Weill Medical College and Graduate School of
  Medical Sciences of Cornell University, New York, New York
  *Second Messenger Signaling Pathways: Phospholipids and
  Calcium*

Mohammad A. Ghatei, PhD
Reader in Regulatory Peptides, Imperial College School of Medicine,
  London, England
  Gastrointestinal Hormones and Tumor Syndromes

Gary W. Gibbons, MD
Professor of Surgery, Boston University School of Medicine;
  Executive Director, Foot Care Specialists of Boston Medical
  Center, Boston, Massachusetts
  Management of the Diabetic Foot Complication

Neil J. L. Gittoes, BSc, MBChB, MRCP, PhD
Lecturer in Medicine, Division of Medical Sciences, University of
  Birmingham; Specialist Registrar in Endocrinology and Diabetes,
  Queen Elizabeth Hospital, Birmingham, England
  Thyroid Function Tests

Linda C. Giudice, MD, PhD
Department of Obstetrics and Gynecology, Division of Reproductive
  Endocrinology, Stanford University Medical Center, Stanford,
  California
  *Endometriosis; Implantation and Placental Physiology in Early
  Human Pregnancy: The Role of the Maternal Decidua and the
  Trophoblast*

Francis H. Glorieux, MD, PhD
Professor of Surgery and Pediatrics, McGill University Faculty of
  Medicine; Director of Research and Head, Genetics Unit, Shriners
  Hospital for Children, Montreal, Quebec, Canada
  Hereditary Defects in Vitamin D Metabolism and Action

Steven R. Goldring, MD
Associate Professor of Medicine, Harvard Medical School; Chief of
  Rheumatology, New England Deaconess Hospital; Clinical
  Associate, Massachusetts General Hospital, Boston, Massachusetts
  Disorders of Calcification: Osteomalacia and Rickets

Theodore L. Goodfriend, MD
Professor of Internal Medicine and Pharmacology, University of
  Wisconsin Medical School; Associate Chief of Staff, Research,
  Veterans Hospital, Madison, Wisconsin
  Hormonal Regulation of Electrolyte and Water Metabolism

William G. Goodman, MD
Professor of Medicine, University of California, Los Angeles, UCLA
  School of Medicine; UCLA Medical Center, Los Angeles,
  California
  The Renal Osteodystrophies

Louis J. G. Gooren, MD, PhD
Professor of Endocrinology, Hospital of the Vrije Universiteit,
  Amsterdam, The Netherlands
  Gender Identity and Sexual Behavior

Colum A. Gorman, MB, BCh, PhD
Professor of Medicine, Mayo Medical School; Consultant, Mayo
  Clinic, Rochester, Minnesota
  Ophthalmopathy

William J. Gradishar, MD
Associate Professor of Medicine, Department of Medicine,
  Northwestern University Medical School; Director, Breast Medical
  Oncology, Robert H. Lurie Comprehensive Cancer Center,
  Chicago, Illinois
  Breast Cancer and Hormonal Management

Mathis Grossmann, MD
Research Officer, The Walter and Eliza Hall Institute of Medical
  Research, Parkville, Victoria, Australia
  *Thyroid-Stimulating Hormone and Regulation of the Thyroid
  Axis*

Joel F. Habener, MD
Professor of Medicine, Harvard Medical School; Associate Physician,
  Massachusetts General Hospital; Investigator, Howard Hughes
  Medical Institute, Boston, Massachusetts
  The Cyclic AMP Second Messenger Signaling Pathway

Steven Haffner, MD
Professor of Medicine, University of Texas Health Science Center,
  San Antonio, Texas
  Diabetes, Lipids, and Atherosclerosis

Charles B. Hammond, MD
E. C. Hamblen Professor and Chairman, Department of Obstetrics
  and Gynecology, Duke University School of Medicine, Durham,
  North Carolina
  Gestational Trophoblastic Neoplasms

David J. Handelsman, MBBS, FRACP, PhD
Professor of Reproductive Endocrinology and Andrology, University
  of Sydney Faculty of Medicine; Director, ANZAC Research
  Institute and Department of Andrology, Concord Hospital, Sydney,
  New South Wales, Australia
  Androgen Action and Pharmacologic Uses; Male Contraception

Victor M. Haughton, MD
Professor of Radiology and Director of MRI Research, Medical
  College of Wisconsin; Radiologist, Milwaukee County Medical
  Complex, Froedtert Memorial Lutheran Hospital; Consultant in
  Radiology, Veterans Affairs Medical Center, Milwaukee,
  Wisconsin
  *Radiographic Evaluation of the Pituitary and Anterior
  Hypothalamus*

William W. Hay, Jr., MD
Professor, Department of Pediatrics, University of Colorado School of Medicine; Scientific Director, Perinatal Research Center; Director, Training Program in Neonatal Perinatal Medicine, University of Colorado Health Sciences Center, Denver, Colorado
Fuel Homeostasis in the Fetus and Neonate

Simon W. Hayward, PhD
Assistant Adjunct Professor, Department of Urology, University of California, San Francisco, School of Medicine, San Francisco, California
Endocrinology of the Prostate and Benign Prostatic Hyperplasia

David Heber, MD, PhD
Professor of Medicine and Chief, Division of Clinical Nutrition, Department of Medicine, University of California, Los Angeles, UCLA School of Medicine; Director, Clinical Nutrition Research Unit, UCLA Medical Center, Los Angeles, California
Starvation and Nutritional Therapy

Laszlo Hegedüs, MD
Department of Endocrinology, Odense University Hospital, Odense, Denmark
Multinodular Goiter

Georg Hennemann, MD, PhD, FRCP, FRCP(E)
Professor of Medicine and Endocrinology, Medical Faculty, Erasmus University, Rotterdam, The Netherlands
Autonomously Functioning Thyroid Nodules and Other Causes of Thyrotoxicosis

Kevan C. Herold, MD
Associate Professor of Clinical Medicine, Columbia University College of Physicians and Surgeons; Associate Attending Physician, New York–Presbyterian Hospital, New York, New York
Immunologic Mechanisms Causing Autoimmune Endocrine Disease

Yoh Hidaka, MD
Associate Professor, Department of Laboratory Medicine, Osaka University Medical School, Osaka, Japan
Chronic (Hashimoto's) Thyroiditis

Patricia M. Hinkle, PhD
Department of Pharmacology and Physiology, University of Rochester Medical Center, Rochester, New York
Second Messenger Signaling Pathways: Phospholipids and Calcium

Ken K. Y. Ho, MD, FRACP
Professor of Medicine, University of New South Wales Faculty of Medicine; Head, Pituitary Research Unit, The Garvan Institute of Medical Research, St. Vincent's Hospital, Sydney, New South Wales, Australia
Growth Hormone Deficiency in Adults

Joseph J. Hoet, MD*
Anatomy, Developmental Biology, and Pathology of the Pancreatic Islets

*Deceased.

Nelson D. Horseman, MS, PhD
Professor, Department of Molecular and Cellular Physiology and Department of Medicine, University of Cincinnati College of Medicine, Cincinnati, Ohio
Prolactin

Eva Horvath, PhD
Associate Professor, Department of Laboratory Medicine and Pathobiology, University of Toronto, Faculty of Medicine; Research Associate, Department of Laboratory Medicine, St. Michael's Hospital, Toronto, Ontario, Canada
Functional Pituitary Anatomy and Histology

Aaron J. W. Hsueh, PhD
Professor, Division of Reproductive Biology, Stanford University Medical School, Stanford, California
Ovarian Hormone Synthesis

John M. Hutson, MD(Monash), MD(Melb), FRACS
Professor and Director of Paediatric Surgery, Department of Paediatrics, Faculty of Medicine, University of Melbourne; Director of General Surgery, Royal Children's Hospital; Associate Director (Clinical Sciences), Murdoch Children's Research Institute, Melbourne, Victoria, Australia
Cryptorchidism and Hypospadias

J. Larry Jameson, MD, PhD
Irving S. Cutter Professor of Medicine and Chairman, Department of Medicine, Northwestern University Medical School; Physician-in-Chief, Northwestern Memorial Hospital, Chicago, Illinois
Applications of Molecular Biology and Genetics in Endocrinology; Mechanisms of Thyroid Hormone Action

Reza Jarrahy, MD
Resident, Department of Surgery, New York University Medical Center, New York, New York; Fellow, Division of Skull Base Surgery, Cedars-Sinai Medical Center, Los Angeles, California
Surgical Management of Pituitary Tumors

Michael Jergas, MD
Assistant Professor of Radiology, Teaching Hospital of the University of Cologne; Director, Department of Radiology, St. Katharinen-Hospital, Frechen, Germany
Bone Density and Imaging of Osteoporosis

V. Craig Jordan, PhD, DSc
Diana, Princess of Wales Professor of Cancer Research, Northwestern University Medical School; Director, Lyn Sage Breast Cancer Research Program, Robert H. Lurie Comprehensive Cancer Center, Chicago, Illinois
Breast Cancer and Hormonal Management

Nathalie Josso, MD
Research Director, École Normale Supérieure; Physician (Consultant), Hôpital St. Vincent de Paul, Paris, France
Anatomy and Endocrinology of Fetal Sex Differentiation

Harald W. Jüppner, MD
Associate Professor of Pediatrics, Harvard Medical School; Associate Biologist and Associate Pediatrician, Endocrine Unit, Department of Medicine and Pediatrics, Massachusetts General Hospital, Boston, Massachusetts
Parathyroid Hormone and Parathyroid Hormone–Related Peptide in the Regulation of Calcium Homeostasis and Bone Development; Genetic Disorders of Calcium Homeostasis Caused by Abnormal Regulation of Parathyroid Hormone Secretion or Responsiveness

Edwin L. Kaplan, MD
Professor of Surgery, University of Chicago Pritzker School of Medicine; University of Chicago Hospitals, Chicago, Illinois
Surgery of the Thyroid

Walter H. Kaye, MD
Professor of Psychiatry, University of Pittsburgh School of Medicine; Director, Center for Overcoming Problem Eating, Department of Psychiatry, Western Psychiatric Institute and Clinic, Pittsburgh, Pennsylvania
Anorexia Nervosa and Other Eating Disorders

Rasa Kazlauskaite, MD
Fellow, Division of Endocrinology, Diabetes and Nutrition, Department of Medicine, University of Maryland School of Medicine, Baltimore, Maryland
Thyroid-Stimulating Hormone and Regulation of the Thyroid Axis

Gary L. Keeney, MD
Assistant Professor, Mayo Medical School; Consultant, Department of Laboratory Medicine and Pathology, Division of Anatomic Pathology, Mayo Clinic, Rochester, Minnesota
Ovarian Tumors with Endocrine Manifestations

Harry R. Keiser, MD
Scientist Emeritus; Attending Physician, The Clinical Center, National Institutes of Health, Bethesda, Maryland
Pheochromocytoma and Related Tumors

David M. Kendall, MD
Medical Director, Adult Diabetes Services and Affiliate Program, International Diabetes Center; Consultant in Endocrinology, Park Nicollet Clinic, Minneapolis, Minnesota
Management of Type 2 Diabetes: A Systematic Approach to Meeting the Standards of Care, I: Self-Management Education, Medical Nutrition Therapy, and Exercise; II: Oral Agents, Insulin, and Management of Complications

Jeffrey B. Kerr, PhD
Associate Professor, Department of Anatomy, Monash University, Clayton, Victoria, Australia
Functional Morphology

Ronald Klein, MD, MPH
Professor, Department of Ophthalmology and Visual Sciences, University of Wisconsin Medical School, Madison, Wisconsin
Diabetes Mellitus: Oculopathy

David L. Kleinberg, MD
Professor of Medicine, New York University School of Medicine; Chief of Endocrinology, Department of Veterans Affairs, New York Harbor Health Care System, New York, New York
Endocrinology of Mammary Development, Lactation, and Galactorrhea

Christian A. Koch, MD
Senior Fellow, National Institutes of Health, National Institute of Child Health and Human Development, Bethesda, Maryland
Aging, Endocrinology, and the Elderly Patient

John J. Kopchick, MS, PhD
Department of Biomedical Sciences, College of Osteopathic Medicine, Ohio University; Edison Biotechnology Institute, Athens, Ohio
Growth Hormone

Stanley G. Korenman, MD
Professor of Medicine (Endocrinology) and Associate Dean, Ethics and Medical Sciences Training Program, University of California, Los Angeles, UCLA School of Medicine, Los Angeles, California
Erectile Dysfunction

Kenneth S. Korach, PhD
Professor of Endocrinology, University of North Carolina at Chapel Hill School of Medicine, Chapel Hill; Duke University School of Medicine, Durham; North Carolina State University, Raleigh; Program Director, Environmental Disease and Medicine Program, and Chief, Laboratory of Reproductive and Developmental Toxicology, National Institute of Environmental Health Science, National Institutes of Health, Research Triangle Park, North Carolina
Environmental Agents and the Reproductive System

Kalman Thomas Kovacs, MD, PhD
Professor, Department of Laboratory Medicine and Pathobiology, University of Toronto Faculty of Medicine; Pathologist, Department of Laboratory Medicine, St. Michael's Hospital, Toronto, Ontario, Canada
Functional Pituitary Anatomy and Histology

James M. Kozlowski, MD
Associate Professor, Department of Urology, Northwestern University Medical School, Chicago, Illinois
Prostate Cancer

Stephen M. Krane, MD
Persis, Cyrus and Marlow B. Harrison Professor of Medicine, Harvard Medical School; Physician and Chief of Arthritis Unit, Massachusetts General Hospital, Boston, Massachusetts
Disorders of Calcification: Osteomalacia and Rickets

Henry M. Kronenberg, MD
Professor of Medicine, Harvard Medical School; Chief, Endocrine Unit, Massachusetts General Hospital, Boston, Massachusetts
Parathyroid Hormone and Parathyroid Hormone–Related Peptide in the Regulation of Calcium Homeostasis and Bone Development

Yolanta T. Kruszynska, PhD, MRCP
Associate Professor of Medicine, University of California, San Diego, School of Medicine, La Jolla, California
Type 2 Diabetes Mellitus: Etiology, Pathogenesis, and Natural History

Anjli Kukreja, PhD
Research Associate, Department of Pediatrics, Weill Medical College of Cornell University, New York, New York
The Autoimmune Polyglandular Syndromes

Sandeep Kunwar, MD
Assistant Professor, Department of Neurological Surgery, University of California, San Francisco, School of Medicine; Principal Investigator, Brain Tumor Research Center, University of California at San Francisco, San Francisco, California
Sellar and Parasellar Tumors in Children

John M. Kyriakis, PhD
Associate Professor of Medicine, Department of Medicine, Harvard Medical School; Assistant Biochemist, Diabetes Unit, Department of Medicine, Massachusetts General Hospital, Boston, Massachusetts
Mitogen-Activated Protein Kinase and Growth Factor Signaling Pathways

Hop N. Le, MD
Research Fellow, Department of Surgery, University of California, San Francisco, School of Medicine, San Francisco, California
Surgical Management of Hyperparathyroidism

Harold E. Lebovitz, MD
State University of New York Downstate Medical Center College of Medicine, Brooklyn, New York
Hyperglycemia Secondary to Nondiabetic Conditions and Therapies

Chung Lee, PhD
Professor, Northwestern University Medical School, Chicago, Illinois
Prostate Cancer

Åke Lernmark, MD
Professor, Department of Medicine, University of Washington School of Medicine, Seattle, Washington
Type 1 (Insulin-Dependent) Diabetes Mellitus: Etiology, Pathogenesis, and Natural History

Michael A. Levine, MD
Professor of Pediatrics, Medicine, and Pathology, and Director, Division of Pediatric Endocrinology, Johns Hopkins University School of Medicine; Physician, Johns Hopkins Hospital, Baltimore, Maryland
Hypoparathyroidism and Pseudohypoparathyroidism

Stephen L. Lin, MD
Fellow in Endocrinology, Diabetes, and Nutrition and Assistant Clinical Instructor, Department of Medicine, University of Maryland School of Medicine, Baltimore, Maryland
Appetite Regulation

Jill S. Lindberg, MD
Evanston–Northwestern Hospital, Evanston, Illinois
Nephrolithiasis

Jonathan Lindzey, PhD
Assistant Professor, Department of Biology, University of South Florida, Tampa, Florida
Environmental Agents and the Reproductive System

Catherine Ann Lissett, MBChB, MRCP
Clinical Research Fellow, Department of Endocrinology, Christie Hospital, Manchester, England
Hypopituitarism

D. Lynn Loriaux, MD, PhD
Professor of Medicine and Head, Division of Endocrinology, Diabetes and Clinical Nutrition, Department of Medicine, Oregon Health Sciences University School of Medicine, Portland, Oregon
An Introduction to Endocrinology; Adrenal Insufficiency

Noel K. Maclaren, MD
Professor of Pediatrics, Weill College of Medicine of Cornell University; Director, Cornell Juvenile Diabetes Center, New York Hospitals, New York, New York
The Autoimmune Polyglandular Syndromes

Carl D. Malchoff, MD, PhD
Associate Professor, Department of Medicine, University of Connecticut School of Medicine, Farmington, Connecticut
Generalized Glucocorticoid Resistance

Diana M. Malchoff, PhD
Assistant Professor, Department of Medicine, University of Connecticut School of Medicine, Farmington, Connecticut
Generalized Glucocorticoid Resistance

Rayaz A. Malik, MD, PhD
Clinical Lecturer, Faculty of Medicine, University of Manchester; Senior Registrar, Manchester Royal Infirmary, Manchester, England
Diabetes Mellitus: Neuropathy

Susan J. Mandel, MD, MPH
Assistant Professor, Department of Medicine, University of Pennsylvania School of Medicine; Associate Chief for Clinical Affairs, Division of Endocrinology, Diabetes, and Metabolism, Hospital of the University of Pennsylvania, Philadelphia, Pennsylvania
Diagnosis and Treatment of Thyroid Disease During Pregnancy

Christos Mantzoros, MD, DSc
Assistant Professor, Department of Medicine, Division of Endocrinology, Harvard Medical School; Attending Endocrinologist, Beth Israel Deaconess Medical Center, Boston, Massachusetts
Syndromes of Insulin Resistance and Mutant Insulin

Leighton P. Mark, MD
Professor of Radiology, Medical College of Wisconsin; Froedtert Memorial Lutheran Hospital, Milwaukee, Wisconsin
Radiographic Evaluation of the Pituitary and Anterior Hypothalamus

John C. Marshall, MD, PhD
Arthur and Margaret Ebbert Professor of Medical Science Professor of Internal Medicine, University of Virginia School of Medicine; Director, Center for Research in Reproduction, University of Virginia Health Sciences Center, Charlottesville, Virginia
Regulation of Gonadotropin Synthesis and Secretion; Hormonal Regulation of the Menstrual Cycle and Mechanisms of Ovulation

T. John Martin, MD, DSc, FRACP
Director, St. Vincent's Institute of Medical Research, Melbourne, Victoria, Australia
Calcitonin

Thomas F. J. Martin, PhD
Department of Biochemistry, University of Wisconsin Medical School, Madison, Wisconsin
Control of Hormone Secretion

Lawrence S. Mathews, PhD
Department of Biochemistry, University of Michigan, Ann Arbor, Michigan
Hormone Signaling via Cytokine Receptors and Receptor Serine Kinases

Walter J. McDonald, MD
Associate Dean for Education, Oregon Health Sciences University; Active Staff, University Hospital, Portland, Oregon
Adrenal Insufficiency

Samy I. McFarlane, MD, FACE, CCD
Assistant Professor, Department of Medicine, Division of Endocrinology, Diabetes, and Hypertension, State University of New York, Health Science Center at Brooklyn, Brooklyn, New York
Hyperglycemia Secondary to Nondiabetic Conditions and Therapies

J. Denis McGarry, PhD
Clifton and Betsy Robinson Chair in Biomedical Research and Professor of Internal Medicine and Biochemistry, University of Texas Southwestern Medical School, Dallas, Texas
Acute Complications of Diabetes Mellitus: Ketoacidosis, Hyperosmolar Coma, and Lactic Acidosis

Michael J. McPhaul, MD
Professor of Internal Medicine, Division of Endocrinology and Metabolism, University of Texas Southwestern Medical Center, Dallas, Texas
Mutations That Alter Androgen Receptor Function

Geraldo Medeiros-Neto, MD, PhD
Professor of Endocrinology, Department of Clinical Medicine, University of São Paulo Medical School; Chief, Thyroid Unit, Hospital Das Clinicas FMUSP, São Paulo, Brazil
Iodine Deficiency Disorders

James C. Melby, MD
Professor of Medicine, Boston University School of Medicine, Boston, Massachusetts
Hypoaldosteronism and Mineralocorticoid Resistance

Shlomo Melmed, MD, FACP
Professor of Medicine and Associate Dean, University of California, Los Angeles, UCLA School of Medicine; Director, Research Institute, Cedars-Sinai Medical Center, Los Angeles, California
Evaluation of Pituitary Masses; Acromegaly

Jan Mester
Signalisation et Fonctions Cellulaires: Application au Diabete et aux Cancers Digestifs, INSERM, Paris, France
Nuclear Receptor Superfamily

Boyd E. Metzger, MD
Professor of Medicine, Northwestern University Medical School; Attending Physician, Northwestern Memorial Hospital, Chicago, Illinois
Diabetes Mellitus and Pregnancy

Roger L. Miesfeld, PhD
Professor of Biochemistry, University of Arizona College of Medicine, Tucson, Arizona
Glucocorticoid Action: Biochemistry

Robert Peter Millar BSc(Hons), MSc, PhD, FRCPath(Chem)
Professor, University of Edinburgh; Director, MRC Human Reproductive Sciences Unit, and Department of Medical Biochemistry, University of Cape Town, Cape Town, South Africa
Gonadotropin-Releasing Hormone (GnRH) and GnRH Receptors

Walter L. Miller, MD
Professor of Pediatrics, Chief of Endocrinology, and Director, Child Health Research Center, University of California, San Francisco; Director, Pediatric Endocrine Services, Moffit/Long Hospitals, San Francisco, California
The Principles, Pathways, and Enzymes of Human Steroidogenesis

Daniel R. Mishell, Jr., MD
Lyle G. McNeil Professor and Chairman, Department of Obstetrics-Gynecology, Keck School of Medicine, University of Southern California; Chief, Professional Services, Los Angeles County–University of Southern California Medical Center, Women's and Children's Hospital, Los Angeles, California
Contraception

Mark E. Molitch, MD
Professor of Medicine, Center for Endocrinology, Metabolism and Molecular Medicine, Northwestern University Medical School; Attending Physician, Northwestern Memorial Hospital, Chicago, Illinois
Hormonal Changes and Endocrine Testing in Pregnancy

Richard M. Mortensen, MD, PhD
Assistant Professor of Medicine, Harvard Medical School; Associate Physician, Brigham and Women's Hospital, Boston, Massachusetts
Aldosterone Action

Jane M. Moseley, PhD
Associate Professor of Medicine, University of Melbourne; Principal Research Fellow (NHMRC), St. Vincent's Institute of Medical Research, Melbourne, Victoria, Australia
Calcitonin

William R. Moyle, PhD
Professor of Obstetrics and Gynecology, University of Medicine and Dentistry of New Jersey–Robert Wood Johnson (Rutgers) Medical School, Piscataway, New Jersey
Gonadotropins

Allan Munck, PhD
Professor of Physiology, Dartmouth Medical School, Lebanon, New Hampshire
Glucocorticoid Action: Physiology

Martin G. Myers, Jr., MD, PhD
Assistant Professor in Medicine, Harvard Medical School; Assistant Investigator, Joslin Diabetes Center, Boston, Massachusetts
The Molecular Basis of Insulin Action

Anikó Náray-Fejes-Tóth, MD
Professor of Physiology, Dartmouth Medical School, Lebanon, New Hampshire
Glucocorticoid Action: Physiology

Ralf Nass, MD
Research Associate, University of Virginia School of Medicine, Charlottesville, Virginia
Growth Hormone–Releasing Hormone and Growth Hormone Secretagogues: Basic Physiology and Clinical Implications

Jerald C. Nelson, MD
Professor of Medicine and Pathology, Loma Linda University, School of Medicine, Loma Linda; Senior Medical Director, Quest Diagnostics, Nichols Institute, San Juan Capistrano, California
Endocrine Testing

Maria I. New, MD
Harold and Percy Uris Professor of Pediatric Endocrinology and Metabolism and Professor, Department of Pediatrics, Weill Medical College of Cornell University; Chairman, Department of Pediatrics, and Chief, Pediatric Endocrinology, New York–Presbyterian Hospital, New York, New York
Defects of Adrenal Steroidogenesis

Lynnette K. Nieman, MD
Chief, Unit on Reproductive Medicine, Developmental Endocrinology Branch, and Senior Staff Physician, National Institute of Child Health and Human Development, National Institutes of Health, Bethesda, Maryland
Cushing's Syndrome

John H. Nilson, PhD
John H. Hord Professor and Chair, Department of Pharmacology, and Director, Medical Scientist Training Program, Case Western Reserve University School of Medicine, Cleveland, Ohio; Editor-in-Chief, *Molecular Endocrinology*
Hormones and Gene Expression: Basic Principles

Christopher F. Njeh, BSc, MSc, PhD, CPhys
Assistant Adjunct Professor, Department of Radiology, University of California, San Francisco, School of Medicine, San Francisco, California
Bone Density and Imaging of Osteoporosis

Jeffrey A. Norton, MD, FACS
Vice Chairman, Department of Surgery, University of California, San Francisco, School of Medicine; Chief, Department of Surgery, San Francisco Veterans Affairs Medical Center, San Francisco, California
Surgical Management of Hyperparathyroidism

William D. Odell, MD, PhD, MACP
Emeritus Professor of Medicine and Physiology, University of Utah School of Medicine, Salt Lake City, Utah
Endocrinology of Sexual Maturation; Menopause and Hormone Replacement

Jerrold M. Olefsky, MD
Professor of Medicine and Chief, Endocrinology and Metabolism Division, University of California, San Diego, School of Medicine, La Jolla, California
Type 2 Diabetes Mellitus: Etiology, Pathogenesis, and Natural History

Niall M. O'Meara, MD
Consultant Physician/Endocrinologist, Department of Diabetes and Endocrinology, Mater Misericordiae Hospital, Dublin, Ireland
Secretion and Metabolism of Insulin, Proinsulin, and C Peptide

Furio Pacini, MD
Associate Professor, Department of Endocrinology, University of Pisa Medical School, Pisa, Italy
Thyroid Neoplasia

Lawrence N. Parker, MD
Professor of Medicine, Division of Endocrinology, University of California, Irvine, College of Medicine; Assistant Chief, Endocrinology Section, Veterans Affairs Medical Center, Long Beach, California
Adrenarche

Samuel Parry, MD
Assistant Professor, University of Pennsylvania School of Medicine, Philadelphia, Pennsylvania
Placental Hormones

Yogesh C. Patel, MD, PhD, FACP, FRCP(C), FRSC
Professor, Department of Medicine, Department of Neurology and Neurosurgery, and Department of Pharmacology and Therapeutics, McGill University Faculty of Medicine; Director, Division of Endocrinology and Metabolism, McGill University Health Center, Montreal, Quebec, Canada
Neurotransmitters and Hypothalamic Control of Anterior Pituitary Function

Luca Persani, MD, PhD
Senior Research Fellow, Institute of Endocrine Sciences, University of Milan; Senior Research Fellow, Istituto Auxilogico Italiano IRCCS, Milan, Italy
TSH-Producing Adenomas

Ora Hirsch Pescovitz, MD
Edwin Letzter Professor of Pediatrics and Professor of Physiology and Biophysics, Indiana University School of Medicine; Director of Pediatric Endocrinology and Diabetology, James Whitcomb Riley Hospital for Children, Indianapolis, Indiana
Precocious Puberty; Delayed Puberty

Richard L. Phelps, MD
Assistant Clinical Professor of Medicine, Northwestern University Medical School; Attending Physician, Northwestern Memorial Hospital, Chicago, Illinois
Diabetes Mellitus and Pregnancy

Aldo Pinchera, MD
Professor and Chairman, Department of Endocrinology, University of Pisa Medical School, Pisa, Italy
Graves' Disease

JoAnn Pinkerton, MD
Associate Professor, Department of Obstetrics and Gynecology; Director, Midlife Health University of Virginia Health Sciences Center, Charlottesville, Virginia
Benign Breast Disorders

Kenneth S. Polonsky, MD
Chairman, Department of Medicine, Washington University School of Medicine, St. Louis, Missouri
Secretion and Metabolism of Insulin, Proinsulin, and C Peptide

John T. Potts, Jr., MD
Jackson Distinguished Professor of Clinical Medicine, Harvard Medical School, Boston; Director of Research, Massachusetts General Hospital, Charlestown, Massachusetts
Parathyroid Hormone and Parathyroid Hormone–Related Peptide in the Regulation of Calcium Homeostasis and Bone Development

Lisa P. Purdy, MD, CM, MPH
Assistant Professor of Medicine, University of Rochester School of Medicine and Dentistry; Attending Physician, Genesee Hospital, Rochester General Hospital, and Strong Memorial Hospital, Rochester, New York
Diabetes Mellitus and Pregnancy

Charmian A. Quigley, MBBS
Assistant Professor, Indiana University School of Medicine; Clinical Research Physician, Department of Endocrinology, Lilly Research Laboratories, US Medical Division, Eli Lilly and Company, Indianapolis, Indiana
Genetic Basis of Sex Determination and Sex Differentiation

Christine Campion Quirk, PhD
NRSA Post-Doctoral Fellow, Department of Pharmacology, Case Western Reserve University School of Medicine, Cleveland, Ohio
Hormones and Gene Expression: Basic Principles

Miriam T. Rademaker, BSc, PhD
Research Fellow, Department of Medicine, Christchurch School of Medicine, Christchurch, New Zealand
Hormones of the Cardiovascular System

Ewa Rajpert-De Meyts, MD, PhD
Senior Scientist, Department of Growth and Reproduction, Copenhagen University Hospital (Rigshospitalet), Copenhagen, Denmark
Testicular Tumors with Endocrine Manifestations

Valerie Anne Randall, BSc, PhD
Senior Lecturer in Biomedical Sciences, Department of Biomedical Sciences, University of Bradford, Bradford, England
Physiology and Pathophysiology of Androgenetic Alopecia

David W. Ray, MD, PhD
Endocrine Science Research Group, School of Biological Sciences, University of Manchester, Manchester, England
Adrenocorticotropic Hormone

Nancy E. Reame, MSN, PhD
Professor, Center for Nursing Research, and Research Scientist, Reproductive Sciences Program, University of Michigan, Ann Arbor, Michigan
Premenstrual Syndrome

Gerald M. Reaven, MD
Professor of Medicine (Active Emeritus), Stanford University School of Medicine, Stanford, California
Syndrome X

Gézard Redeuilh
Signalisation et Fonctions Cellulaires: Application au Diabete et aux Cancers Digestifs, INSERM, Paris, France
Nuclear Receptor Superfamily

Samuel Refetoff, MD
Professor of Medicine and Pediatrics, University of Chicago Pritzker School of Medicine; Attending Physician, University of Chicago Hospitals, Chicago, Illinois
Thyroid Function Tests

Claude Remacle
Professor, Université Catholique de Louvain, Faculté des Sciences, Louvain-la-Neuve, Belgium
Anatomy, Developmental Biology, and Pathology of the Pancreatic Islets

Brigitte Reusens, DSc
Université Catholique de Louvain, Faculté des Sciences, Louvain-la-Neuve, Belgium
Anatomy, Developmental Biology, and Pathology of the Pancreatic Islets

Gail P. Risbridger, PhD
NH and MRC Senior Research Fellow, Institute of Reproduction and Development, Monash University, Melbourne, Australia
Functional Morphology

Robert A. Rizza, MD
Professor of Medicine, Mayo Medical School; Chair, Division of Endocrinology, Diabetes and Metabolism, Mayo Clinic, Rochester, Minnesota
Classification and Diagnosis of Diabetes Mellitus

R. Paul Robertson, MD
Affiliate Professor of Pharmacology, University of Washington
   School of Medicine; University of Washington Medical Center;
   CEO/Scientific Director, Pacific Northwest Research Institute,
   Seattle, Washington
Pancreas and Islet Transplantation

Gideon A. Rodan, MD, PhD
Adjunct Professor of Pathology, University of Pennsylvania School
   of Medicine, Philadelphia; Research Vice President, Bone Biology
   and Osteoporosis, Merck Research Laboratories, West Point,
   Pennsylvania
Bone Development and Remodeling

Ron G. Rosenfeld, MD
Professor and Chair, Department of Pediatrics, and Professor,
   Department of Cell and Developmental Biology, Oregon Health
   Sciences University School of Medicine; Physician-in-Chief,
   Doernbecher Memorial Hospital for Children, Portland, Oregon
Growth Hormone Deficiency in Children

Robert L. Rosenfield, MD
Professor of Pediatrics and Medicine, University of Chicago Pritzker
   School of Medicine; Head, Section of Pediatric Endocrinology,
   University of Chicago Children's Hospital, Chicago, Illinois
*Somatic Growth and Maturation; Hyperandrogenism,
   Hirsutism, and the Polycystic Ovary Syndrome*

Jesse Roth, MD
Raymond and Anna Lublin Professor of Medicine, Division of
   Geriatric Medicine and Gerontology, Johns Hopkins University
   School of Medicine, Baltimore, Maryland
Aging, Endocrinology, and the Elderly Patient

Kristina I. Rother, MD
Clinical Investigator, Diabetes Branch, NIDDK, National Institutes of
   Health, Bethesda, Maryland
Aging, Endocrinology, and the Elderly Patient

Peter S. Rotwein, MD
Professor of Medicine, Molecular Medicine Division, Department of
   Medicine, Oregon Health Sciences University School of Medicine,
   Portland, Oregon
*Peptide Growth Factors Other Than Insulin-Like Growth Factors
   or Cytokines*

Brian G. Rowan, PhD
Postdoctoral Fellow, Department of Molecular and Cellular Biology,
   Baylor College of Medicine, Houston, Texas
Estrogen and Progesterone Action

Arthur H. Rubenstein, MB, BCh
Dean and Gustave L. Levy Distinguished Professor, Mount Sinai
   School of Medicine of New York University, New York, New
   York
*Chemistry and Biosynthesis of the Islet Hormones: Insulin, Islet
   Amyloid Polypeptide (Amylin), Glucagon, Somatostatin, and
   Pancreatic Polypeptide; Management of Type 2 Diabetes: A
   Systematic Approach to Meeting the Standards of Care, I: Self-
   Management Education, Medical Nutrition Therapy, and
   Exercise; II: Oral Agents, Insulin, and Management of
   Complications*

Robert T. Rubin, MD, PhD
Professor of Neurosciences and Psychiatry, MCP Hahnemann
   University School of Medicine; Director, Center for Neurosciences
   Research, Allegheny General Hospital, Pittsburgh, Pennsylvania
Anorexia Nervosa and Other Eating Disorders

Irma M. Russo, MD
Professor, Jefferson Medical College of Thomas Jefferson University;
   Director, Molecular Endocrinology, Breast Cancer Research, Fox
   Chase Cancer Center, Philadelphia, Pennsylvania
Hormonal Control of Breast Development

Jose Russo, MD
Professor, Jefferson Medical College of Thomas Jefferson University;
   Director, Breast Cancer Research, Fox Chase Cancer Center,
   Philadelphia, Pennsylvania
Hormonal Control of Breast Development

Isidro B. Salusky, MD
Professor of Pediatrics, University of California, Los Angeles, UCLA
   School of Medicine; Director, Pediatric Dialysis Program, and
   Director, General Clinical Research Center, UCLA Medical Center,
   Los Angeles, California
The Renal Osteodystrophies

Richard J. Santen, MD
Professor of Medicine, University of Virginia School of Medicine,
   Charlottesville, Virginia
*Hormonal Control of Breast Development; Benign Breast
   Disorders; Gynecomastia*

David H. Sarne, MRCP, PhD
Associate Professor of Medicine and Director, Endocrine Clinic,
   Department of Medicine, University of Illinois, Chicago, Illinois
Thyroid Function Tests

Maurice F. Scanlon, BSc, MD, FRCP
Professor of Endocrinology, University of Wales College of
   Medicine; Honorary Consultant Physician, University Hospital of
   Wales, Cardiff, Wales
*Thyrotropin-Releasing Hormone and Thyroid-Stimulating
   Hormone*

Agnes Schonbrunn, PhD
Professor, Department of Integrative Biology and Pharmacology,
   University of Texas–Houston School of Medicine, Houston, Texas
Somatostatin

David E. Schteingart, MD
Professor of Internal Medicine and Associate Division Chief for
   Faculty Affairs, University of Michigan Medical School, Ann
   Arbor, Michigan
Adrenal Cancer

Machelle M. Seibel
Medical Director, Faulkner Center for Reproductive Medicine,
   Boston, Massachusetts
Ovulation Induction and Assisted Reproduction

Patrick M. Sexton, PhD
National Health and Medical Research Council Fellow, Molecular Pharmacology Laboratory, Department of Pharmacology, University of Melbourne, Melbourne, Victoria, Australia
Calcitonin

Hrayr K. Shahinian, MD
Director, Division of Skull Base Surgery, Department of Surgery, Cedars-Sinai Medical Center, Los Angeles, California
Surgical Management of Pituitary Tumors

Stephen Michael Shalet, MD, FRCP
Professor of Medicine (Endocrinology), Faculty of Medicine, University of Manchester; Attending Physician, Christie Hospital, Manchester, England
Hypopituitarism

Andrew Shenker, MD, PhD
Assistant Professor of Pediatrics, Molecular Pharmacology and Biological Chemistry, Northwestern University Medical School; Crown Family Young Investigator in Developmental Systems Biology, Children's Memorial Institute for Education and Research, Children's Memorial Hospital, Chicago, Illinois
Hormone Signaling via G Protein–Coupled Receptors

Yoram Shenker, MD
Associate Professor of Medicine and Interim Section Head, Endocrinology, Diabetes, and Metabolism, Department of Medicine, University of Wisconsin Medical School; Chief, Section of Endocrinology, William S. Middleton Memorial VA Hospital, Madison, Wisconsin
Hormonal Regulation of Electrolyte and Water Metabolism

Michael C. Sheppard, MBChB, PhD, FRCP
Professor of Medicine and Head, Division of Medical Sciences, University of Birmingham; Consultant Physician, Queen Elizabeth Hospital, Birmingham, England
Thyroid Function Tests

Shonni J. Silverberg, MD
Associate Professor, Department of Medicine, Columbia University College of Physicians and Surgeons; Associate Attending Physician, New York–Presbyterian Hospital, New York, New York
Primary Hyperparathyroidism

Frederick R. Singer, MD
Clinical Professor of Medicine, University of California, Los Angeles, UCLA School of Medicine, Los Angeles; Director, Endocrine/Bone Disease Program, John Wayne Cancer Institute, St. John's Health Center, Santa Monica, California
Paget's Disease of Bone

Allan E. Siperstein, MD
Staff Surgeon and Head, Section of Endocrine Surgery, Cleveland Clinic Foundation, Cleveland, Ohio
Adrenal Surgery

Niels E. Skakkebaek, MD, DSc
Professor, University of Copenhagen; Head, Department of Growth and Reproduction, Copenhagen University Hospital (Rigshospitalet), Copenhagen, Denmark
Testicular Tumors with Endocrine Manifestations

Peter J. Snyder, MD
Professor of Medicine, University of Pennsylvania School of Medicine, Philadelphia, Pennsylvania
Gonadotroph Adenomas

John T. Soper, MD
Professor, Department of Obstetrics and Gynecology, Duke University School of Medicine, Durham, North Carolina
Gestational Trophoblastic Neoplasms

Stuart M. Sprague, DO
Associate Professor of Medicine, Northwestern University Medical School, Chicago; Director, Metabolic Bone and Stone Disease Program, Evanston Northwestern Healthcare, Evanston, Illinois
Nephrolithiasis

René St-Arnaud, PhD
Associate Professor of Surgery and Human Genetics, McGill University Faculty of Medicine; Senior Staff Scientist, Genetics Unit, Shriners Hospital for Children, Montreal, Quebec, Canada
Hereditary Defects in Vitamin D Metabolism and Action

Donald L. St. Germain, MD
Professor of Medicine and Physiology, Dartmouth Medical School, Lebanon, New Hampshire
Thyroid Hormone Binding and Metabolism: Thyroid Hormone Metabolism

Donald F. Steiner, MD
Professor of Biochemistry and Molecular Biology and Medicine, University of Chicago Pritzker School of Medicine; Senior Investigator, Howard Hughes Medical Institute, Chicago, Illinois
Chemistry and Biosynthesis of the Islet Hormones: Insulin, Islet Amyloid Polypeptide (Amylin), Glucagon, Somatostatin, and Pancreatic Polypeptide

Andrew F. Stewart, MD
Professor of Medicine, University of Pittsburgh School of Medicine; Chief of Endocrinology, University of Pittsburgh Medical Center, Pittsburgh, Pennsylvania
Malignancy-Associated Hypercalcemia

Jan R. Stockigt, MD, FRACP, FRCPA
Professor of Medicine, Monash University; Senior Endocrinologist, Ewen Downie Metabolic Unit, Alfred Hospital, Melbourne, Victoria, Australia
Thyroid Hormone Binding and Metabolism: Thyroid Hormone Binding; Transport Protein Variants

Jerome F. Strauss III, MD, PhD
Luigi Mastroianni, Jr. Professor and Director, Center for Research and Reproduction and Women's Health, and Associate Chairman, Department of Obstetrics and Gynecology, University of Pennsylvania School of Medicine; Staff Physician, Hospital of the University of Pennsylvania, Philadelphia, Pennsylvania
Ovarian Hormone Synthesis; Placental Hormones

David H.P. Streeten, MBBCh, DPhil, FRCP, FACP
Professor Emeritus of Medicine and *former* Head, Section of Endocrinology, State University of New York Upstate Medical University, Syracuse, New York
Orthostatic Hypotension

Sonia L. Sugg, MD
Assistant Professor of Surgery, University of Chicago Medical
  Center, Chicago, Illinois
  Surgery of the Thyroid

Mariusz W. Szkudlinski, MD, PhD
Assistant Professor, Division of Endocrinology, Diabetes and
  Nutrition, Department of Medicine, University of Maryland School
  of Medicine; Chief, Section of Protein Engineering, Laboratory of
  Molecular Endocrinology, Institute of Human Virology, University
  of Maryland Biotechnology Institute, Baltimore, Maryland
  *Thyroid-Stimulating Hormone and Regulation of the Thyroid
  Axis*

Hisato Tada, MD
Assistant Professor, Department of Laboratory Medicine, Osaka
  University Medical School, Osaka, Japan
  Chronic (Hashimoto's) Thyroiditis

Shahrad Taheri, BSc, MSc, MBBS, MRCP
Wellcome Trust Research Fellow, Imperial College School of
  Medicine and The Hammersmith Hospital, London, England
  Gastrointestinal Hormones and Tumor Syndromes

Robert B. Tattersall, MD, FRCP
Retired; former Professor of Clinical Diabetes, University of
  Nottingham, Nottingham, England
  The Relationship of Diabetic Control to Complications

Rajesh V. Thakker, MD, FRCP, FRCPath, FMedSc
May Professor of Medicine, University of Oxford; Consultant
  Physician and Endocrinologist, Nuffield Department of Medicine,
  John Radcliffe Hospital, Oxford, England
  *Genetic Disorders of Calcium Homeostasis Caused by Abnormal
  Regulation of Parathyroid Hormone Secretion or
  Responsiveness; Multiple Endocrine Neoplasia Type 1*

Axel A. Thomson, PhD
Group Leader, MRC Reproductive Biology Unit, Edinburgh, England
  Endocrinology of the Prostate and Benign Prostatic Hyperplasia

Michael O. Thorner, MB, BS, DSc
Henry B. Mulholland Professor of Medicine and Chair, Department
  of Medicine, University of Virginia School of Medicine,
  Charlottesville, Virginia
  *Growth Hormone–Releasing Hormone and Growth Hormone
  Secretagogues: Basic Physiology and Clinical Implications*

Andrew A. Toogood, MB, ChB, MRCP
Lecturer in Medicine, Department of Medicine, Division of Medical
  Sciences, Queen Elizabeth Hospital, Birmingham, England
  *Growth Hormone–Releasing Hormone and Growth Hormone
  Secretagogues: Basic Physiology and Clinical Implications*

Jorma Toppari, MD, PhD
Senior Scientist of the Academy of Finland, Department of Pediatrics
  and Department of Physiology, University of Turku, Turku,
  Finland
  Testicular Tumors with Endocrine Manifestations

Fred W. Turek, PhD
Charles E. and Emma H. Morrison Professor of Biology and
  Director, Center for Circadian Biology and Medicine, Professor of
  Neurobiology and Physiology, Northwestern University, Evanston,
  Illinois
  Endocrine and Other Biologic Rhythms

Helen E. Turner, MA, MBChB, MRCP
Senior Registrar, Department of Endocrinology, Radcliffe Infirmary,
  Oxford, England
  Ectopic Hormone Syndromes

Eve Van Cauter, PhD
Professor of Medicine, University of Chicago Pritzker School of
  Medicine, Chicago, Illinois
  Endocrine and Other Biologic Rhythms

Gilbert Vassart, MD, PhD
Professor of Genetics, Faculty of Medicine, Institute of
  Interdisciplinary Research, University of Brussels; Head, Medical
  Genetics, Erasme Hospital, Brussels, Belgium
  *Thyroid Regulatory Factors; Thyroid-Stimulating Hormone
  Receptor Mutations*

Jan J. M. de Vijlder, MSc, PhD
Professor of Biochemistry, University of Amsterdam; Emma
  Children's Hospital, Academic Medical Center, Amsterdam, The
  Netherlands
  *Genetic Defects in Thyroid Hormone Synthesis and Action:
  Defects in Thyroid Hormone Synthesis*

Aaron I. Vinik, MD
Professor of Internal Medicine and Anatomy/Neurobiology and
  Director, Diabetes Research Institute, Eastern Virginia Medical
  School, Norfolk, Virginia
  Carcinoid Tumors

**Robert Volpé, MD, FRCP(C), MACP, FRCP(Edin and
Lond)**
Professor Emeritus, Division of Endocrinology and Metabolism,
  Department of Medicine, University of Toronto Faculty of
  Medicine; Active Staff, Division of Endocrinology and
  Metabolism, Wellesley Division, St. Michael's Hospital, Toronto,
  Ontario, Canada
  Infectious, Subacute, and Sclerosing Thyroiditis

Thomas Vulsma, MD, PhD, MSc
Associate Professor of Pediatric Endocrinology, University of
  Amsterdam; Pediatric Endocrinologist, Emma Children's Hospital,
  Academic Medical Center, Amsterdam, The Netherlands
  *Genetic Defects in Thyroid Hormone Synthesis and Action:
  Defects in Thyroid Hormone Synthesis*

Michael P. Wajnrajch, MD
Assistant Professor of Pediatrics, Department of Pediatrics, Division
  of Pediatric Endocrinology, Weill Medical College of Cornell
  University; Visiting Associate Research Scientist, Department of
  Pediatrics, Division of Molecular Genetics, Columbia University
  College of Physicians and Surgeons, New York, New York
  Defects of Adrenal Steroidogenesis

John A. H. Wass, MA, MD, FRCP
Professor of Endocrinology, University of Oxford; Consultant Physician, Department of Endocrinology, Radcliffe Infirmary, Oxford, England
Ectopic Hormone Syndromes

Anthony P. Weetman, MD, DSc
Professor of Medicine and Dean, Medical School, University of Sheffield; Honorary Consultant Physician, Northern General Hospital, Sheffield, England
Autoimmune Thyroid Disease

Nancy L. Weigel, PhD
Associate Professor, Department of Molecular and Cellular Biology, Baylor College of Medicine, Houston, Texas
Estrogen and Progesterone Action

Bruce D. Weintraub, MD
Professor, Department of Medicine, University of Maryland School of Medicine; Chief, Laboratory of Molecular Endocrinology, Institute of Human Virology, University of Maryland Biotechnology Institute, Baltimore, Maryland
Thyroid-Stimulating Hormone and Regulation of the Thyroid Axis

Anne White, PhD
Professor of Endocrine Sciences, School of Biological Sciences and Faculty of Medicine, University of Manchester, Manchester, England
Adrenocorticotropic Hormone

Morris F. White, PhD
Harvard Medical School; Principal Investigator, Joslin Diabetes Center, Boston, Massachusetts
The Molecular Basis of Insulin Action

Wilmar M. Wiersinga, MD, PhD
Professor of Endocrinology, Department of Medicine, University of Amsterdam; Chief, Department of Endocrinology and Metabolism, Academic Medical Center, Amsterdam, The Netherlands
Hypothyroidism and Myxedema Coma

John F. Wilber, MD
Professor, Department of Medicine, University of Maryland School of Medicine, Baltimore, Maryland
Appetite Regulation

Gordon H. Williams, MD
Professor of Medicine, Harvard Medical School; Senior Physician and Chief, Endocrine-Hypertension Service, Brigham and Women's Hospital, Boston, Massachusetts
Aldosterone Action

Charles B. Wilson, MD, MSHA, DSc
Professor, Department of Neurological Surgery, University of California, San Francisco, School of Medicine; Principal Investigator, Brain Tumor Research Center, University of California at San Francisco, San Francisco, California
Sellar and Parasellar Tumors in Children

Stephen J. Winters, MD
Professor of Medicine and Chief, Division of Endocrinology and Metabolism, University of Louisville School of Medicine, Louisville, Kentucky
Clinical Disorders of the Testis

Robert J. Witte, MD
Assistant Professor of Radiology, Mayo Medical School, Rochester, Minnesota; Consultant, Mayo Clinic, Diagnostic Radiology, Jacksonville, Florida
Radiographic Evaluation of the Pituitary and Anterior Hypothalamus

Hans H. Zingg, MD, PhD
Professor, Department of Medicine, McGill University Faculty of Medicine; Director, Laboratory of Molecular Endocrinology, Royal Victoria Hospital, Montreal, Quebec, Canada
Oxytocin

Preface

The changes buffeting endocrinology have accelerated in the 5 years between the third edition and this, the fourth edition of *Endocrinology*. New hormones and factors abound. The discovery of leptin and agouti protein, along with their receptors, provides just one example. Whole groups of factors—interleukins, chemokines, and others—have been characterized but are yet to be fully integrated into the structure of endocrinology as it is generally conceived. Genetic approaches to endocrine diseases bring new discoveries almost weekly, and several hundred endocrine diseases are now understood at the genetic level. These include disorders such as the multiple endocrine neoplasia syndromes, the various forms of "maturity-onset diabetes of the young," numerous hormone resistance syndromes, and myriad defects in transcription factors and enzymes that control glandular development and hormone synthesis. The instrumentation available for bone density measurements, imaging techniques, minimally invasive surgery, and noninvasive continuous monitoring glucose is changing the way in which we practice endocrinology. Development of specialization in assisted fertility, breast disease, and prostate disease has wrested out of our hands certain illnesses that were long considered to be part of endocrinology. The care of diabetic patients is shifting to teams of doctors, nutritionists, and educators; increasingly, daily management is transferred to the patient, while we attempt to attain a level of glycemic control that was previously thought impossible. Paperwork engulfs us and detracts from patient care, while we attempt to survive economically.

However, despite all of this, the practice of endocrinology remains the same cottage industry that it has always been. One patient pours out his or her troubles and his or her heart to one physician, who does his or her best to provide scientifically based care in a humanistic manner. The physician must often be wise enough to do this in a setting complicated by rampant "anti-scientism," much poorly digested information gleaned from the Internet, and a host of practitioners who offer cures by diet therapy, holistic medicine, acupuncture, and the numerous "natural" herbal remedies.

Perhaps the newly board-certified endocrinologist can get by on the material that he or she learned in training for a few months or a year. But beyond that time, the endocrinologist must again become a student, seeking continuing education at meetings and in journals and textbooks, if he or she is to remain abreast of this field. The reality of our rapidly changing field is that we are students for life—a role that is challenging but rewarding. It is these students of endocrinology who want to, and must, continuously refresh their knowledge to whom we dedicate *Endocrinology*. We believe that this book can serve as an invaluable resource for the busy practitioner who encounters an unfamiliar endocrine problem, as well as the investigator who wishes to find an updated and scholarly review of a topic. It is our intention to provide a complete, current review and analysis of all aspects of endocrinology, both basic and clinical. We hope to provide a source that will answer any endocrine question, which is perhaps at least a laudable goal, even if it is not always reached. We strive to integrate the lessons learned from basic research into the practice of clinical endocrinology. We have provided both the traditional gland-by-gland analysis of disease processes and sections that integrate the hormonal systems and the immune and hormonal systems.

The current edition consists of 194 chapters. About one third of these are completely new, and the remainder have been completely rewritten and brought up to date. There are new sections on Growth and Maturation, Immunology and Endocrinology, Obesity and Nutrition, and Endocrinology of the Breast and two additional "minibooks" on Endocrine Testing and Drugs and Hormones used in Endocrinology. Some readers describe our book as the "Bible of Endocrinology." Whether that is appropriate or not, we are certain that readers will find many of the chapters to be absolutely the best presentation of the topic that has ever been put together. We are very proud of the scholarship that is evident throughout.

With more than 300 authors, it is not possible to give individual credit for outstanding contributions. But here the Editors offer their thanks and appreciation to all of the authors who have contributed such outstanding chapters. Their erudition and ability to make science and practice readable make *Endocrinology* a special book. We also owe thanks to Hazel Hacker and Richard Zorab at W.B. Saunders for their commitment to quality publishing and for expeditiously preparing this book to keep the information current.

We are very pleased that Shlomo Melmed has joined our group as the editor of the neuroendocrine section, and we wish to acknowledge the important contributions of Michael Besser to this section in previous editions. The wisdom, hard work, and friendship of our co-editors—Henry G. Burger, D. Lynn Loriaux, John C. Marshall, Shlomo Melmed, William D. Odell, John T. Potts, Jr., and Arthur H. Rubenstein—have made this experience pleasurable, as well as enlightening. Last, we note with special pleasure the contribution of Dr. J. Larry Jameson as co-editor in chief.

LESLIE J. DEGROOT, MD
J. LARRY JAMESON, MD, PHD

Contents

Color Plates follow frontmatter.

Volume *1*

PART III **Growth and Maturation, 389**

Editor: Shlomo Melmed

BASIC PHYSIOLOGY, 389

CLINICAL DISORDERS, 477

PART IV **Immunology and Endocrinology, 556**

Editor: Leslie J. DeGroot

PART V **Obesity, Anorexia Nervosa, and Nutrition in Endocrinology, 600**

Editor: John C. Marshall

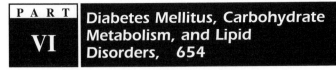

PART **VI** Diabetes Mellitus, Carbohydrate Metabolism, and Lipid Disorders, 654

Editor: Arthur H. Rubenstein

Volume 2

CLINICAL DISORDERS, 1409

P A R T IX Adrenal Gland and Glucocorticoids, 1616

Editor: D. Lynn Loriaux

BASIC PHYSIOLOGY, 1616

CLINICAL DISORDERS, 1671

ENDOCRINOLOGY

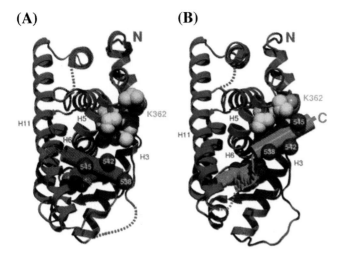

(A)   **(B)**

FIGURE 10–6. Structure of ER LBD as a function of the ligand. The ligand is estradiol in *A*, raloxifene in *B*. The position of the helix H12, drawn as a *blue* (E2-complex) or *green* (raloxifene complex), is radically different in the two complexes. In the E2-liganded complex, it forms a "lid" of the binding cavity, whereas raloxifene prevents this alignment. *Dotted lines* indicate unmodeled regions. (From Brzozowski AM, Pike AC, Dauter Z, et al: Molecular basis of agonism and antagonism in the oestrogen receptor. Nature 389:756, 1997.)

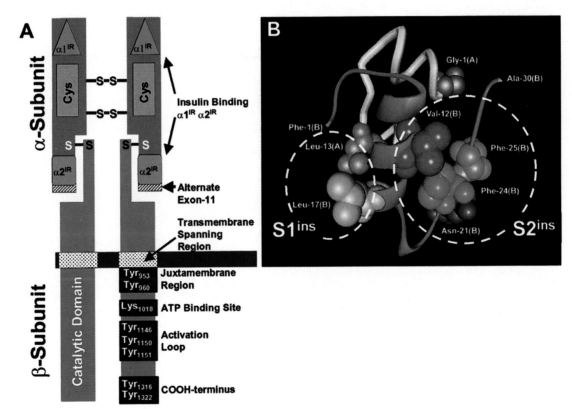

FIGURE 50–3. Structure of insulin and the insulin receptor. *A*, Insulin receptor functional domains. Shown is a cartoon of the insulin receptor with its functional domains. The mature insulin receptor consists of a heterotetramer of two extracellular α subunits linked to two β subunits that contain extracellular, transmembrane, and intracellular components. The holoreceptor is joined by disulfide bonds between cysteine residues in the extracellular α and β subunits, as well as by noncovalent interactions. The α subunit contains the insulin binding regions α1^{IR} and α2^{IR} in addition to a cysteine-rich region and a 12-amino acid alternatively spliced region encoded by exon 11. The β subunit contains a tyrosine kinase catalytic domain with an ATP-binding site and a number of tyrosine phosphorylation sites, including those in the juxtamembrane, activation loop, and COOH-terminal regions. *B*, Structure of insulin. Shown is a ribbon diagram of the mature insulin molecule in which the α chain is light in color and the β chain is dark. Also shown are the side chains of specific amino acids, which form the contact regions for the insulin receptor (S1^{ins} and S2^{ins}).

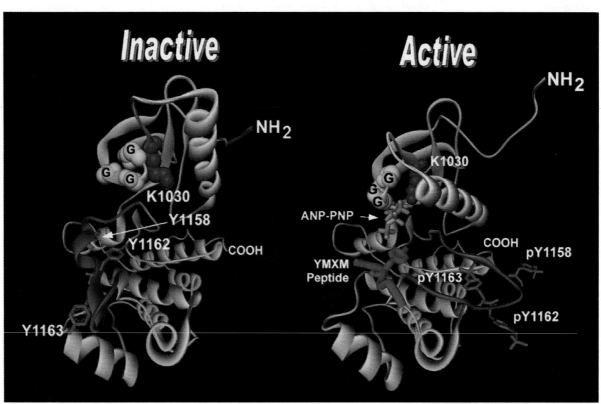

FIGURE 50–4. Structure of the insulin receptor activation loop. Shown are ribbon diagrams of the active site of the insulin receptor tyrosine kinase along with the side chains of important amino acids, including the three glycine residues and K1030 that form the ATP-binding site. The activation loop is shown in *red*; the three activation loop tyrosine residues (Y1158, Y1162, and Y1163) are shown with their side chains. In the inactive, unphosphorylated state *(left panel)*, the activation loop blocks access by potential substrates. After phosphorylation *(right panel)*, however, the activation loop moves and thus allows substrates such as YMXM peptides (shown in *green*) to access the active site. ANP-PNP, nonhydrolyzable ATP analogue.

Chapter 1

An Introduction to Endocrinology

D. Lynn Loriaux

Endocrinology is the study of cell-to-cell communication by messenger molecules traversing an extracellular space. In this way cells communicate with themselves, with nearest neighbors, with distant cells via a circulatory system, and with separate organisms across an intervening "environment." These types of cell-to-cell communication are designated as autocrine, paracrine, endocrine, and "pherocrine," respectively. The biologic beginnings of these processes probably occurred with the transition from unicellular to multicellular organisms having sufficient size to prohibit direct communication between all constituent cells. The process, in its generic sense, provided the framework that permitted cooperation among cells and ultimately the striking biologic diversity inherent in the natural tendency of cells to differentiate toward specialized function. Because of this early deployment in the process of evolution, endocrine systems play important roles in many of the most basic biologic activities of complex organisms—food seeking and satiety, metabolism and caloric economy, growth and differentiation, reproduction, homeostasis, response to environmental change, arousal, defense, flight, and secluding behaviors.

As cell-to-cell communication provided survival advantage, evolutionary pressure across the last billion years layered complexity upon complexity in extant endocrine systems. Old systems were scrapped and new ones invented. Old hormones took on new functions as new receptor molecules evolved, and new ligands were devised for old receptors. Systems began to subserve different specialized functions in different species.

Attempts to unravel this tangled skein began a mere 2500 years ago with the beginning of free inquiry in the city-states of Greece. The development of our understanding of the endocrine system closely parallels the evolution of the physical and biologic sciences across the intervening years. The earliest allusions to an endocrine system came from Aristotle who, in 400 BC, described the effects of castration on the songbird.[1] Galen, more than 500 years later, described and named the thyroid gland in dissections of great apes and, perhaps, of humans.[2] Galen's monumental contributions to medicine and biology were unchallenged across the 1000 years of the Middle Ages, an incubation that culminated in the Renaissance and its efflorescence of art and science. Attention to anatomic detail, heightened by artists like Leonardo and Michelangelo, proved to be a focus that energized the landmark collaboration of Vesalius and Kalkar and its product, *De humani corporis fabrica libri septum*.[3] Published in 1543, this work, one of the true inflection points in biologic science, provided the first accurate account of human anatomy and, along with it, descriptions of many human endocrine organs. More importantly, *De fabrica* lifted the cloak of infallibility from the teachings of Galen and set the trajectory of modern scientific inquiry as no other single event has done.

In short order anatomists such as Eustachius and Fallopius,[4] primarily of the Paduan school, precisely described the structure of the endocrine system in humans. The physiologists followed. Bernard demonstrated the process of "internal secretion,"[5] and Bayliss and Starling[6] showed that the epithelium of the small intestine contained a substance that could, when injected into the blood stream of dogs, stimulate the exocrine secretion of the pancreas. They called the substance *secretin*. Molecules with this property, stimulating a response in a distant organ via the blood stream, were first referred to as *hormones*, from the Greek *hormao* (to rouse), by Professor Starling in 1905 in his Croonian Lectures to the Royal College, "The Chemical Correlation of the Functions of the Body."

The work of the physiologists was vested with clinical relevance by the observations of the great physicians: Addison on adrenal insufficiency,[7] Graves and von Basedow on goiter and hyperthyroidism,[8, 9] Minkowski and von Mering on diabetes,[10] Marie on acromegaly,[11] Cushing on glucocorticoid excess,[12] and Albright on hyperparathyroidism.[13] These "untreatable diseases" energized the efforts of the biochemists who followed to isolate and purify the hormones; thyroxine by Harrington,[14] cortisone by Kendall[15] and Reichstein,[16] insulin and parathormone by Collip,[17, 18] growth hormone and adrenocorticotropic hormone (ACTH) by Li,[19] and the hypothalamic-releasing hormones by Guillemin and Schally.[20] Medicine was advanced by these discoveries. Examples include the successful treatment of hypothyroidism by Murray,[21] adrenal insufficiency by Thorn,[22] growth hormone deficiency by Raben,[23] and diabetes mellitus by Joslin. In addition, the purification of the various hormones permitted the development of measurements for them, culminating in the development of radioimmunoassay by Berson and Yalow in 1969.[24] This advance greatly stimulated the study of endocrine physiology, particularly "feedback regulation" of hormone secretion. Our understanding of endocrine pathophysiology was also enhanced by this advance, as was the clinical management of diseases of the endocrine system. Finally, the "receptor" concept was advanced in endocrinology, primarily by the example of the syndrome of pseudohypoparathyroidism, a receptor-mediated resistance to the effects of parathormone described by Fuller Albright and colleagues in 1942.[25] This finding ushered in the current era of investigation in endocrinology, including the cell biology of hormone action, receptor structure and function, signal transduction, gene regulation, peptide processing, and the mechanisms of hormone secretion.

From this accumulated body of knowledge our current concept of the basic attributes of the "endocrine system" has emerged. There are nine classic glands (hypothalamus, pineal, pituitary, thyroid, parathyroid, pancreas, adrenal, testis, and ovary) and an ever-increasing number of nonclassic glands (thymus, heart, gut, kidney, placenta, skin) that secrete hormones. These hormones can be divided into two categories: lipid-soluble and water-soluble. Examples of lipid-soluble hormones are steroids and iodothyronines. Examples of water-soluble hormones are glycoprotein hormones (luteinizing hormone, follicle-stimulating hormone, and human chorionic gonadotropin) and the catecholamines (epinephrine and norepinephrine).

The synthesis and secretion of hormones is not different from that of other molecules in the same general class. The peptide hormones, for example, are generally derived from larger precursor molecules that are the first products of translation. These large molecules are sequentially processed by "cleavage" enzymes, often yielding a number of biologically active products. A good example of this is the biosynthesis of ACTH. In the anterior pituitary gland, the precursor molecule, proopiomelanocortin (POMC), is first cleaved to β-lipotropic hormone (β-LPH), ACTH, a "junction peptide" (JP), and an inactive C-terminal peptide, POMC 1–74. In the intermediate lobe, further processing cleaves β-LPH into γ-LPH and β-endorphin, and ACTH is cleaved into corticotropin-like intermediate lobe peptide (CLIP) and ACTH 1–13. Several of these products are biologically active. Prohormones exist for insulin, somatostatin, glucagon, enkephalin, antidiuretic hormone, gastrin, parathyroid hormone, and calcitonin, among others. The steroid hormones are metabolic products of cholesterol, and both the iodothyronines and catecholamines are derived from tyrosine.

Water-soluble hormones, such as insulin, can be transported in plasma as is, whereas the lipid-soluble hormones must be "solubilized" by noncovalent binding to transport proteins. Testosterone, dihydrotestosterone, and estradiol circulate in a bound complex with sex hormone–binding globulin (SHBG), a 90-kDa glycoprotein. Cortisol, progesterone, and aldosterone circulate largely bound to cortisol-binding globulin (CBG), a 52-kDa α_2-globulin. Thyroxine, and to a much lesser extent, triiodothyronine circulate bound to thyroxine-binding globulin, a 54-kDa glycoprotein. In addition to permitting vascular transport in an aqueous medium, the "binding proteins" retard the metabolic clearance of the bound hormones and serve as a reservoir of bound hormone that can defend the circulating free, and presumably biologically active, hormone concentration.

Lipid-soluble hormones gain entry into cells passively by virtue of miscibility with the lipid component of the cell membrane. These hormones interact with cytosol or nuclear receptors that recognize and interact with specific gene regulatory sequences. This interaction leads to a "hormone action" mediated by new protein synthesis. Water-soluble hormones are, by themselves, excluded from the interior of the cell and must interact with cell surface or "membrane-bound" receptors. These hormones must interact with the nucleus through the medium of a "second messenger." Second messengers are not single entities but represent a cascade of events set in motion by a hormone-receptor interaction that leads to an alteration in the concentration of molecular species interacting with "hormone-responsive" gene regulatory elements (GREs). The best understood of the second messengers is the adenylate cyclase system. In this system the hormone receptor is linked to adenylate cyclase and, hence, cyclic adenosine monophosphate (cAMP) production. This linkage is effected by two G proteins, one that can suppress and one that can enhance adenylate cyclase activity. In this way, cAMP alone can mediate more than one hormone response in a given cell. cAMP activates a protein "kinase" by altering its heteromeric structure. This enzyme, in turn, catalyzes the activation of a cAMP response element-binding protein (CREB) that is the effector of hormone action in this particular second messenger system. Other second messengers depend on the modulation of guanylate cyclase, tyrosine kinase, phosphoinositol turnover, calcium flux, and, in some cases, ion channel activity.

In the classic endocrine system, one or more consequences of hormone action are "sensed" at some level, and the hormone secretory process is modulated to preserve a given "normal" level of hormone action. This is the phenomenon of *negative feedback*. It can be conceptualized most readily in the form of a home heating system. The typical home heating system consists of fuel source, furnace, and thermostat. The temperature set on the thermostat is the independent variable in the system. As the temperature in the house falls below that set on the thermostat, the furnace is switched on, consuming fuel and heating the house until the temperature exceeds that set on the thermostat. Thus, the actual temperature oscillates around a mean temperature that approximates that set on the thermostat. The furnace will burn more or less depending upon open windows and people coming and going through the various portals to the outside. Most endocrine systems function in an analogous way. The plasma concentration of calcium, for example, is tightly regulated in the human. As the calcium concentration falls, parathormone is secreted to raise it; as the calcium concentration rises, parathormone secretion is curtailed and the calcium concentration falls. The "thermostat" for this system resides in the parathyroid glands where parathormone is synthesized

and secreted. The "fuel source" is the skeletal reserve of calcium, and the furnace is the parathormone-responsive cadre of bone cells—osteoclasts and osteocytes. Feedback systems are inherently rhythmic. There is a basal fluctuation around the independent variable, but more complicated rhythms can be superimposed, as in a house that has the thermostat turned down for the night. The endocrine rhythms have been named for the duration of the period. *Circhoral* rhythms occur about once an hour; *circadian* rhythms have a cycle of about 24 hours (*circa*, about; *dies*, day); *circatrigantan* rhythms, about once a month; and *circannual* rhythms, about once a year. Examples are the 90-minute periods of basal gonadotropin secretion, the daily rhythm of plasma cortisol concentration, the monthly period of the reproductive cycle in women, and the annual period of seasonal breeding in ungulates.

Gland, hormone, transport, action, and feedback—these are the fundamental attributes of the endocrine system. This book attempts to distill into a single-source reference work the accumulated understanding of these processes in the human endocrine system, as well as the diseases that emanate from their disordered function. The authors have attempted to walk the fine line that separates "encyclopedic from pedantic" and "comprehensive from irrelevant." This necessitates selectivity; everything cannot be presented. The book is current as of the time of publishing. This means that considerable material of a "research" nature will be found here. It is well to remember that medicine is differentiated from the other healing arts primarily by its scientific base, and endocrinology is foremost in this regard. The inclusion of this material is necessary to round out the picture of "where we are now." Nonetheless, the reader is advised to keep in mind the current pace of discovery. The most recent material in this book is the least likely to stand the test of time. Fuller Albright said it best: "Hypotheses are subject to change without notice!" This is the essence of endocrinology.

REFERENCES

1. Aristotle: Historia animalium, book 9, vol 4.
2. Sarton G: Galen of Pergamon. Lawrence, University of Kansas Press, 1954.
3. Vesalius A: De humani corporis fabrica libri septum, Basel, 1543.
4. Eustachius B: Opuscula anatomica, Venice, 1563.
5. Loriaux DL: Claude Bernard. Endocrinologist 1:362–363, 1991.
6. Bayliss WM, Starling EH: The mechanism of pancreatic secretion. J Physiol (Lond) 28:325–353, 1902.
7. Addison T: On the Constitutional and Local Effects of Disease of the Suprarenal Glands. London, Highly, 1855.
8. Graves RJ: Clinical Lectures. Lond Med Surg J (Renshaws) 7:599, 1835.
9. von Basedow K: Exophthalmos durch Hypertrophie des Zellegewebes in der Augenhöhle. Wochenschr Gesamte Heilkd 6:197–204, 1840.
10. von Mering J, Minkowski O: Arch Exp Pathol Pharmakol 26:371–387, 1890.
11. Marie P, de Souza-Leite JD: Essays on Acromegaly. London, New Sydenham Society, 1891.
12. Cushing H: The basophil adenomas of the pituitary body and their clinical manifestations (pituitary basophilism). Bull Johns Hopkins Hosp 50:137–195, 1932.
13. Albright F, Aub J, Bauer W: Hyperparathyroidism—a common and polymorphic condition as illustrated by seventeen proven cases from one clinic. JAMA 102:1276–1287, 1934.
14. Sawin CT, Kendall EC: Endocrinologist 1:291–293, 1991.
15. Kendall EC, Mason HL, McKenzie BF, et al: Proc Mayo Clin 9:245–250, 1934.
16. Grollman A: Physiological and chemical studies on the adrenal cortical hormone. Symp Quant Biol 5:313, 1937.
17. Collip JB: The original method as used for the isolation of insulin in semi-pure form for the treatment of the first clinical cases. J Biol Chem 55:50–51, 1923.
18. Collip JB: The extraction of a parathyroid hormone that will prevent or control parathyroid tetany and which regulates the level of blood calcium. J Biol Chem 63:395–438, 1925.
19. Li CH, Evans HM, Simpson ME: Isolation and properties of the anterior hypophyseal growth hormone. J Biol Chem 159:353–366, 1945.
20. Burgus R, Guillemin R, et al: Structure moléculaire du facteur hypothalamique hypophysiotrope TRF d'origine ovine: Mise en évidence par spectrometrie de masse de la séquence PCA-His-Pro-NH$_2$. CR Seances Soc Biol Fil 269:226–228, 1969.
21. Murray GR: Note on the treatment of myxedema by hypodermic injections of an extract of the thyroid gland of sheep. BMJ 2:796–797, 1891.
22. Thorn GW, Firor WM: Desoxycorticosterone acetate therapy in Addison's disease: Clinical consideration. JAMA 231:76, 1940.
23. Raben MS: Recent Prog Horm Res 15:71, 1959.
24. Berson SA, Yalow RS: Radioimmunoassays of peptide hormones in plasma. N Engl J Med 277:640–647, 1967.
25. Albright F, Burnett CH, Smith PH, Parson W: Pseudohypoparathyroidism: An example of the "Seabright-Bantam" syndrome. Endocrinology 30:922–932, 1942.

Chapter 2

Hormones and Gene Expression: Basic Principles

Christine Campion Quirk ▪ John H. Nilson

Synthesis of hormones and other biologically active substances requires gene expression. Peptide and polypeptide hormones are encoded directly by one or more genes, whereas biogenic amines and steroid hormones are indirect products of several genes that provide enzymes necessary for their biosynthesis. In some instances, more than one peptide hormone can be derived from the expression of a single gene, which further underscores the complexity of their synthesis. Furthermore, ensuring synthesis of the right amount of hormone at the right time requires that gene expression be regulated. Finally, all hormones also regulate gene expression, including expression of non–hormone-encoding genes as well as genes that encode hormones. Some hormones even exert autologous feedback on their own cognate gene. Because regulating gene expression plays such a pivotal role in the synthesis of hormones and their subsequent action, it is fitting that this chapter focus largely on exploring the basic principles underlying this process. We would, however, be remiss were we to omit a brief description of the effects that polypeptide and peptide hormones have on protein secretion. Thus in considering both the synthesis and action of hormones, we propose extending the term "gene expression" to include the entire process required for production of a biologically active substance that acts at a distance.

THE CENTRAL DOGMA OF MOLECULAR BIOLOGY REVISITED

Expression of genes encoding proteins follows the central dogma of molecular biology first outlined by Francis Crick.[1–3] This dogma states that genetic information is stored in the cell as DNA, a macromolecule that serves as a template for its own replication. When this genetic information is expressed in a cell, it flows unidirectionally from DNA to messenger RNA (mRNA) (transcription) to protein (translation). Within the last several years, however, it has become clear that the scope of this process is far more complicated than envisioned by its early proponents.

As will be described in more detail later (see Transcription: Creating the Template for Protein Synthesis), the first transfer of genetic information occurs in the nucleus, where a gene residing within the chromatin mass undergoes transcription and yields a large precursor RNA historically referred to as heteronuclear RNA (hnRNA).[3] This large precursor undergoes 5′, 3′, and internal modifications to generate the mature form of mRNA that is transported from the nucleus to the cytoplasm (see Post-transcriptional Modification of mRNA). The second transfer of genetic information takes place in the cytoplasm, where the mature mRNA interacts with ribosomes and other protein synthetic machinery to encode a protein through the process of translation (see Translation: Regulated Protein Biosynthesis). During translation, several ribosomes, composed of structural RNA and associated proteins, produce a convoy of nascent polypeptide chains as they move in the 5′ to 3′ direction along the mRNA template. This complex structure, designated polyribosome, either resides free in the cytoplasm or is tightly attached to a specialized membrane, the endoplasmic reticulum (ER), that vectors the nascent polypeptide chains down a path typically leading to their secretion from the cell. For polypeptide hormones, this vectored transport is an essential component of their synthetic life cycle.

In short, expression of genes begins with activation of structural changes in chromatin that allow for initiation of gene transcription, processing of the emergent RNA transcript, transport of mature RNA to the cytoplasm, and translation of the encoded polypeptide. Of course, one must not forget that a translated protein may require major post-translational modifications before it acquires the biologic activity underlying the phenotype determined by its cognate gene (see Post-translational Modifications). In the ensuing sections we will highlight additional conceptual details for each of these aspects of gene expression and protein biosynthesis and summarize how hormones function to regulate each stage.

CHEMICAL NATURE OF DNA AND ITS RELATIONSHIP TO CHROMATIN

Although DNA was first discovered to be a component of chromosomes in 1869,[3] the simple composition of nucleic acids actually misled investigators into believing that they were a purely structural component of the chromosome and that proteins accounted for cell specificity. The idea that DNA may be the genetic material was spawned by studies performed by Griffith in 1928.[1, 3, 4] Griffith observed that heat-killed pathogenic bacteria had the capacity to transform live nonpathogenic bacteria into pathogenic organisms. Upon transformation, the once nonvirulent bacteria acquired the appearance of pathogenic bacteria. In 1944, Avery and colleagues chemically identified this "transforming factor" as DNA.[1, 3, 4] However, this information was not well received by the entire scientific community inasmuch as many believed that the "genetic protein" was overlooked in the experiments. It was not until 1952 that Hershey and Chase firmly identified DNA as the genetic material,[1, 3, 4] which they accomplished by infecting *Escherichia coli* with a bacteriophage in which DNA was radiolabeled with ^{32}P and protein with ^{35}S. They found that only radioactive DNA entered the infected *E. coli*. Additionally, the radiolabeled parental DNA was identified in the progeny phage expelled from the infected cells.

Even before DNA was determined to be the genetic material, scientists had begun to characterize the chemical makeup of the molecule. Each polynucleotide chain contains a "random" array of four different nitrogenous bases representing two chemical classes, pyrimidines (cytosine [C] and thymine [T]) and purines (adenine [A] and guanine [G]) (Fig. 2–1). Each base contains a pentose sugar moiety (deoxyri-

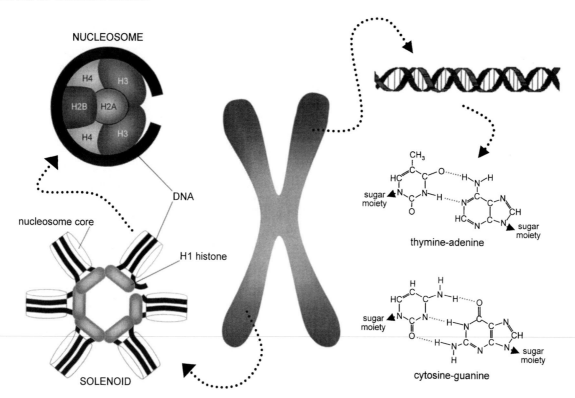

FIGURE 2–1. *Chemical structure of DNA and its relationship to chromatin. The most basic unit of the chromosome is DNA, which is composed of polynucleotide chains made up of four different nitrogenous bases—thymine, adenine, cytosine, and guanine—found in an apparently random array. Each polynucleotide chain runs in an opposite direction to form a right-handed double helical structure, with hydrogen bonding between complementary base pairs and adenine always pairing with thymine and guanine always pairing with cytosine. This double helix is compacted by its being wrapped around a protein octamer consisting of two copies each of four core histone proteins (H3, H4, H2A, and H2B) to form a nucleosome. Nucleosomes are further condensed via another histone (H1), which complexes with flanking DNA entering or leaving the core particle and functions to pack nucleosomes upon each other to form solenoid structures.*

bose) and a phosphate group and links to the deoxyribose through an N1 glycosidic bond to form a nucleoside. The 5′ carbon of the pentose ring of the deoxyribonucleoside links to the phosphate through a phosphodiester bond to form a deoxyribonucleotide. The backbone of a polynucleotide chain forms by linking the 5′ phosphate group of one nucleotide to the 3′ hydroxyl of the deoxyribose ring of the adjacent nucleotide, with the nitrogenous bases allowed to protrude. Two polynucleotide chains run in opposite directions to form a right-handed double helix structure with hydrogen bonding between complementary nitrogenous base pairs in which A always pairs with T and G with C.[1-4]

The DNA from an individual haploid human cell contains approximately 3×10^9 base pairs,[1] which would be 2 m long if extended end to end. Because the nucleus of a eukaryotic cell is less than 10 μm in diameter, fitting long linear DNA into this small space requires several ordered steps of compaction. In a sense, compaction is initially achieved through segmentation of DNA into a series of discrete fragments, with each length of DNA forming the backbone of the chromosome, the ultimate compacted form of DNA. The second level of compaction occurs as the long fragmented strands of DNA begin to wrap around a class of highly basic proteins referred to as histones. DNA wraps around a protein octamer consisting of two copies each of four core histone proteins[1-5] (H3, H4, H2A, and H2B) (see Fig. 2–1). The surface of the histone octamer contains two left-hand turns of DNA that span 146 bp.[2, 4, 6] This complex of DNA and histones defines a nucleosome that is flanked by DNA entering or leaving the core particle. The length of DNA that links two nucleosomes varies between 8 and 114 bp and is itself complexed with another histone (H1).[1, 4, 5, 7] The ordered periodicity of histone octamers that underlies the nucleosomal structure can be visualized by electron microscopy and yields a classic "beads on a string" appearance. Ultimately, nucleosomes become covered by nonhistone chromosomal proteins, the largest and best characterized group of which are the high-mobility

group proteins.[4, 5, 8, 9] This ternary complex of DNA, histone proteins, and nonhistone proteins defines chromatin, which is the basic unit of genetic material found in transcriptionally active, nondividing cells.

Although chromatin is essential for compaction of the eukaryotic genome, it creates a formidable obstacle between the gene expression machinery and DNA regulatory elements. In fact, the topologic problem becomes even more complex as the nucleosome structure of chromatin that forms the so-called beads on a string becomes even more compacted. Histone H1 proteins are responsible for packing nucleosomes upon each other to form solenoid structures (see Fig. 2–1),[2, 4, 7] which are higher-order arrays where DNA is further condensed to form euchromatin. Heterochromatin is the highly compacted form of chromatin that makes DNA sequences structurally inaccessible to the transcription machinery and results in functionally inactive genes. In fact, chromosomes represent the culminating form of compaction. These transcriptionally inactive, transient structures occur only during a unique temporal period of the cell cycle that leads ultimately to DNA replication and cell division.[10]

One of the most striking examples of heterochromatinization that correlates with gene inactivation is the nuclear structure called the Barr body. All female mammals have evolved a mechanism to permanently inactivate one of the two X chromosomes present in virtually all somatic cells to achieve dosage equivalence of gene products of the X chromosome between males and females.[11] One of the X chromosomes is randomly chosen and highly condensed to form a distinct structure known as the Barr body.[2] Hypoacetylation of histone H4 moieties is necessary for maintenance of X inactivation. Additionally, it appears that hypermethylation stabilizes the inactive X chromosome. Studies have shown that genes on the inactive X chromosome can be reactivated by preventing methylation of the DNA.

In sum, nucleosomes, which may be randomly or very specifically located over the bulk of chromosomal DNA, provide an important conceptual framework for fully understanding how hormones regulate

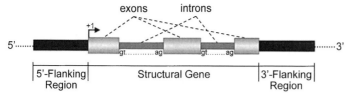

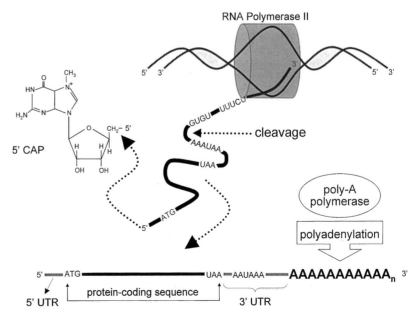

FIGURE 2–2. *Functional anatomy of a gene. Regions of the structural gene that are retained in mature mRNA are known as exons, whereas the intervening sequences that are excised are called introns. The 5' and 3' sequences of all introns are conserved in that they encode the splice donor (gt) and splice acceptor (ag), respectively. The region immediately upstream of the first transcribed nucleotide is referred to as the 5' flanking region, whereas the portion of the gene that is located downstream of the structural gene is referred to as the 3' flanking region. The gene promoter is typically located in the 5' flanking region to allow for correct initiation and efficiency of transcription. The nucleotide where transcription begins is designated +1.*

gene transcription. The structure of chromatin is dynamic, with the state of the nucleosome core playing a pivotal role in governing the transcriptional competence of the targeted genes. Consequently, acetylation (associated with activation) and deacetylation (associated with repression) of histone proteins represent important steps that must be accommodated in a mechanistic model that defines hormone action.[4] We will explore this issue in greater detail in a subsequent section (see Hormonal Control of Gene Expression and Protein Biosynthesis).

FUNCTIONAL ANATOMY OF A GENE

Within the vast amount of DNA from each eukaryotic cell, approximately 80,000 genes can be found per haploid genome. Although Mendel called them particulate factors instead of genes in 1865,[1] he clearly characterized their essential attributes. Strictly defined, a gene is the region of DNA transcribed by RNA polymerase.[1, 4] This definition holds for both prokaryotes and eukaryotes. In prokaryotes, however, the gene is colinear with respect to the transcribed mRNA, whereas in eukaryotes, colinearity is often lacking. Regions of the transcribed gene found in mature mRNA are referred to as exons, short for expressed regions of DNA (Fig. 2–2). The precursor hnRNA exons are interrupted by intervening sequences (introns) that are excised as the nascent transcript is processed to its mature form. Steps involved in RNA processing will be explored in more detail below.

The region immediately upstream of the first transcribed nucleotide is referred to as the 5' flanking region[1, 2, 4] (see Fig. 2–2). Within this

region lies the promoter, functionally defined as containing all the information necessary for specifying the correct initiation of transcription and for regulating the efficiency of transcription. Typically, the nucleotide where transcription begins is designated +1. Consequently, most portions of a promoter are denoted by a negative numbering system of nucleotides indicating the upstream positioning of the domain. Achieving accurate initiation of transcription is essential for ensuring constancy of the reading frame used for translation of the transcribed mRNA. Modulating the efficiency of transcription gives cells the capacity to produce more or less protein as the need arises.

Because a gene is typically defined as that region transcribed by RNA polymerase, it follows that all transcribed regions downstream of the +1 nucleotide fall within this functional domain. Most genes encoding mRNA (those transcribed by RNA polymerase II) begin with a purine, either A or G (Fig. 2–3). Defining the end of a gene transcribed by RNA polymerase II, however, is more problematic. Unlike prokaryotic genes, no fixed site specifies termination of transcription.[1] Instead, a post-transcriptional processing event, the addition of a homopolymeric tail of adenine nucleotides (poly A), signifies the end of the precursor hnRNA that will be further processed to generate mature mRNA.[1–4, 12] The enzyme that specifies polyadenylation, poly A polymerase, recognizes a specific hexameric sequence (AATAAA) and then cleaves the precursor mRNA approximately 29 bp downstream, with the resulting 3'-OH group used as a substrate for the subsequent addition of approximately 200 to 250 adenine deoxyribonucleotides.[1, 3, 12] The region of the gene that extends beyond the site of polyadenylation is referred to as the 3' flanking region.

In most mRNAs transcribed by RNA polymerase II, the start codon that specifies the beginning of the translation reading frame (ATG) is located between 5 and 100 bp downstream from the 5' end of the transcribed mRNA.[1, 3] Thus the region between the 5' end of the mRNA and the translation start site is referred to as the 5' untranslated region. Similarly, the codon that defines the end of the translation reading frame (UAG, UAA, or UGA) is usually followed by a relatively long run of nucleotides before reaching the hexanucleotide sequence that defines the site for polyadenylation (see Fig. 2–3). This region is referred to as the 3' untranslated region.

Processing of the precursor mRNA (hnRNA) will be described in more detail in a subsequent section (see Post-transcriptional Modification of mRNA). Before treating this subject, however, it bears mentioning that the functional significance of introns remains unclear. One important clue stems from the observation that some mRNAs can undergo alternative processing. When such processing occurs, a specific transcribed segment can either be retained and act as an exon or be excised and act as an intron. Introns that can act as exons when retained contain long open reading frames that encode a polypeptide

FIGURE 2–3. *Transcription by RNA polymerase II creates the template for protein synthesis. Messenger RNA is the single-stranded molecule that transfers the genetic information from DNA in the nucleus to the cytoplasm, where proteins are translated. Mature mRNA is "capped" by the addition of 7-methylguanosine to the 5' end through a triphosphate linkage formed between its 5' hydroxyl and the 5' hydroxyl of the terminal residue in the untranslated region (5' UTR) of the initial transcript. The 3' ends of growing transcripts are cleaved between the polyadenylation sequence and sequences rich in guanine and uracil found in the 3' untranslated region (3' UTR). After this cleavage event, poly A polymerase enzyme adds 200 to 250 adenine residues. Both modifications of the mRNA confer mRNA stability and translational efficiency and play a role in exportation of mature mRNA from the nucleus to the cytoplasm.*

fragment. The unique duality of this type of intron (the capacity to act as a translation reading frame when retained) may allow for the shuffling of functional units to create families of related products from a single gene.[1, 3] Additionally, certain intronic sequences in lower eukaryotes have been shown to contain open reading frames that encode proteins involved in either DNA or RNA metabolism, including endonucleases, reverse transcriptases, and maturases.[1] These "parasitic genes" have the intrinsic capacity to remove themselves from the nascent host transcript that surrounds them. This excision process is known as self-splicing or autosplicing.[1]

FUNCTIONAL ANATOMY OF THE PROMOTER-REGULATORY REGION

In general, a promoter contains two functional domains. The core region of the promoter is defined as the minimal 5′ flanking region required for accurate initiation of transcription. The second promoter domain usually resides immediately upstream and contains from one to several regulatory elements that modulate the efficiency of transcription. Because these elements are physically linked to the gene they regulate, they are referred to as *cis*-acting regulatory elements. The functionality of these elements, however, emerges only upon the binding of a specific transcription factor that is inevitably encoded by a different gene. Hence, *cis*-acting elements bind *trans*-acting factors.

All transcription factors that bind *cis*-acting elements are modular and contain at least two functional domains: one that binds specifically to a given *cis*-acting element and another domain that directly or indirectly either influences correct initiation or modulates the efficiency of transcription. The boundaries of *cis*-acting elements reflect the region of DNA actually contacted by the DNA-binding domain of a specific *trans*-acting factor and are usually less than 20 bp in length.[1, 2] Frequently, they contain a core recognition sequence of 8 to 10 bp that is often palindromic,[1, 2] which means that most *trans*-acting factors are dimers composed of the same subunit (homodimers) or different subunits (heterodimers).

The core promoter usually consists of an initiator element (Inr) that encompasses the transcription start site and a TATA box that is typically located 25 to 35 bp upstream of the transcription start site in higher eukaryotes and binds TATA-binding protein (TBP)[13, 14] (Fig. 2–4). TBP is a key component of the transcription factor TFIID, the first general transcription factor to recognize and the only to bind DNA in a sequence-specific manner.[3, 4, 13] TBP binds in the minor groove of the DNA double helix and forms the foundation of the pre-initiation complex. Native TFIID is a large multi-subunit protein (>700 kDa) consisting of TBP and at least eight TATA-associated factors.[13, 14]

Once TFIID binds, several other general transcription factors bind in an ordered succession to form an extremely large core transcription complex (see Fig. 2–4). TFIIA, which is composed of three subunits (14, 19, and 34 kDa), binds TFIID and DNA upstream of TBP, although this event is not DNA sequence specific.[2, 4, 13] TFIIA stabilizes TFIID and causes a conformational change in TBP that may displace a negative component in the native TFIID.[13] TFIIB, a single 35-kDa subunit, binds to and stabilizes the TFIID-TFIIA complex. TFIIF, which is made up of two polypeptides (30 and 74 kDa), forms a molecular bridge with TFIIB between RNA polymerase II and TBP.[4, 13] Both TFIIB and TFIIF appear to function in start site selection. RNA polymerase II consists of 10 polypeptides ranging in size from 10 to 240 kDa, the largest of which contains an unusual C-terminal domain that is extensively phosphorylated.[13, 15] It is the unphosphorylated form of RNA polymerase II (Pol IIA) that preferentially associates with the committed complex over the phosphorylated form (Pol IIO). TFIIE, which functions as a tetramer (two copies each of 34- and 56-kDa subunits), binds TBP, TFIIF, Pol IIA, and TFIIH, the next protein to bind the growing complex.[16] TFIIH (at least eight subunits totaling 200–300 kDa) is the only general transcription factor to show catalytic activity, including C-terminal domain kinase activity that is regulated by TFIIE.[13, 16] Additionally, TFIIH appears to function as a helicase and a DNA-dependent ATPase.[13, 16] TFIIJ is the last factor to enter the preinitiation complex. Although it is known that

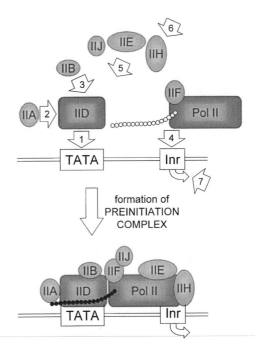

FIGURE 2–4. *Assembly of the basal transcription machinery. The first step in formation of the preinitiation complex is recognition and binding of the transcription factor TFIID (TBP [TATA-binding protein] plus eight TAFs [TATA-associated factors]) to the TATA box. The second step consists of coupling of TFIIA to TFIID to stimulate and stabilize TFIID binding. The third step involves TFIIB binding to either TFIID or the TFIID/TFIIA complex. Fourth is association of the unphosphorylated form of RNA polymerase II (Pol IIA) with the growing complex. The fifth step consists of sequential binding of TFIIE, TFIIH, and TFIIJ to form the pre-initiation complex. The sixth step involves the enzymatic activities of TFIIH, which allows for phosphorylation of RNA polymerase II (Pol IIO), melting of the DNA duplex at the transcription start site, and the release of TFIIE, TFIIB, and two subunits of TFIIH. Finally, TFIIA and TFIID remain bound to the promoter whereas Pol IIO, TFIIF, and one subunit of TFIIH move to form the elongation complex.*

TFIIJ is required, the function of this factor has not been characterized. It is the formation of this core transcription complex that determines the accurate initiation of transcription.

Although TFIID is capable of recognizing several nonconsensus TATA sequences, some promoters clearly lack a TATA box.[2, 17] This observation is especially true of the promoters in some housekeeping genes, such as the gene encoding an enzyme that catalyzes the formation of adenosine monophosphate from adenine and phosphoribosylpyrophosphate.[1] This protein acts as a salvage enzyme for recycling of adenine into nucleic acids. Preinitiation complex assembly on these TATA-less promoters is mediated through the Inr, the consensus sequence of which is pyrimidine-pyrimidine-A-N-T/A-pyrimidine-pyrimidine, with **A** being the transcription start site at +1.[17] In these cases, RNA polymerase II recognizes and binds the Inr directly and nucleates binding of the other factors during formation of the preinitiation complex.[18]

From one to several *cis*-acting elements are located in close proximity and 5′ to the TATA box (Fig. 2–5). These accessory elements set the basal transcriptional tone of the promoter by increasing the efficiency of transcription. The *trans*-acting factors that bind these elements are generally ubiquitous and include Sp1 and NF-Y, which bind GC-rich regions and CCAAT boxes, respectively.[1, 2, 19] Binding of these factors to DNA generally results in protein-protein interactions with the basal transcription machinery to increase or decrease transcription in a non–tissue-specific manner. Given the ubiquitous presence of factors such as Sp1 and NF-Y, it is not surprising that their corresponding *cis* elements are located on the promoters of many genes, including housekeeping genes that provide the basic functions needed for maintenance of all cell types.

In view of their close proximity and direct interaction with the

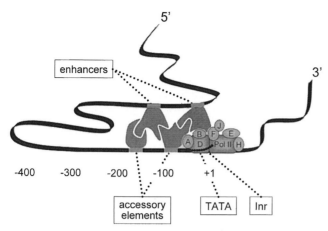

FIGURE 2–5. *Functional anatomy of the promoter-regulatory region. The core region of the promoter, defined as the minimal 5′ flanking region required for accurate initiation of transcription, is typically made up of the initiator element (Inr), which encompasses the transcription start site, and a TATA box. The second domain resides in close proximity to the core promoter and contains one to several accessory elements that modulate the efficiency of transcription. Enhancers, another class of promoter regulatory elements, are usually located further upstream from the gene that they regulate. Contact between trans-acting factors that bind enhancers, accessory elements, and the basal transcription machinery occurs through looping of the DNA. All transcription factors that bind regulatory elements contain a domain that binds specifically to a given cis-acting element and another domain that directly or indirectly influences transcription.*

core transcriptional machinery, accessory elements are position and orientation dependent, as opposed to enhancers, another class of promoter-regulatory elements (see Fig. 2–5) that are located much further upstream, from 100 bp to several thousand bp or even within or 3′ to the gene that they regulate.[1-4] When assayed for activity by attachment to a heterologous core promoter, activities of enhancers display considerable distance, orientation, and position independence. Nevertheless, the *trans*-acting factors that bind this class of regulatory element must also make contact with the core transcriptional machinery. Although the distance between an enhancer and the TATA box may be considerable, it is thought that this contact may occur through looping of the DNA.[1-3]

Enhancers represent a broad class of elements capable of binding a variety of transcriptional factors. Some of them are tissue- or cell-specific and thus confer this property to the promoter that they regulate. In addition to increasing transcription, enhancers can also repress transcription, depending on the nature of the protein that they bind. Whereas some enhancers act alone, others are represented by tightly packed arrays of *cis*-acting elements and are hence designated as composite enhancers.[1] In fact, it is not uncommon to find that tissue- or cell-specific expression is determined by the concerted action of composite enhancers that bind both ubiquitous and tissue- or cell-specific proteins.

In addition to housing elements that determine basal transcriptional tone and spatially restricted expression, promoter-regulatory regions also contain *cis*-acting elements that confer responsiveness in the presence of a wide variety of homeostatic agents such as hormones and after an equally wide array of environmental cues and insults. Such elements can be referred to generically as response elements. Like the elements noted above, response elements can bind proteins that are either ubiquitous or relatively cell type–specific. One such inducible factor, presumably activated by stress, is the heat shock transcription factor that binds heat shock elements.[1] Normally this factor exists in cells but is inactive. When cells are insulted by a sudden increase in temperature, heat shock transcription factor is converted to an active form that binds the heat shock elements located in the promoters of genes encoding proteins that aid in cell survival at higher temperatures. Later we will explore in greater detail how

hormones bind response elements and either induce or repress transcription of the genes that they regulate (see Hormonal Control of Gene Expression and Protein Biosynthesis).

TRANSCRIPTION: CREATING THE TEMPLATE FOR PROTEIN SYNTHESIS

DNA, although the genetic material, does not function as the scaffold for protein synthesis. mRNA is the single-stranded intermediate molecule that transfers the genetic information from DNA in the nucleus to the cytoplasm, where it serves as a template for the formation of polypeptides. RNA is quite similar in structure to DNA; in fact, a single strand of RNA can even form a double-stranded hybrid helix with a DNA strand. One minor difference between RNA and DNA involves the pentose sugar of RNA.[1, 2] It contains an additional hydroxyl group (ribose as opposed to deoxyribose). In addition, uracil (U) replaces T in RNA. Despite these subtle differences, organisms have evolved mechanisms allowing for a smooth transition from DNA to RNA through transcription.

Transcription is the first step in conversion of the genetic information in DNA into RNA and proteins. It is also the major point at which gene expression is regulated. A eukaryotic gene can be classified on the basis of the enzyme that serves to drive its transcription. RNA polymerases are multi-subunit enzymes that synthesize RNA by using a DNA template. The most active of the RNA polymerases is RNA polymerase I, which resides in the nucleolus and is responsible for transcribing genes encoding ribosomal RNA (rRNA), a major component of ribosomes.[1, 3, 4] RNA polymerase II, as mentioned previously, is also a highly active nuclear enzyme that is responsible for synthesizing hnRNA, a precursor to mRNA.[1, 3, 4] The final RNA polymerase, RNA polymerase III, transcribes transfer RNA (tRNA), an adapter molecule involved in translation. For the purposes of this chapter, we will remain focused on genes whose expression is transcribed by RNA polymerase II.

POST-TRANSCRIPTIONAL MODIFICATION OF mRNA

As they are being synthesized, immature mRNA molecules are covalently modified at both their 5′ and 3′ ends (see Fig. 2–3). Almost immediately after initiation of precursor mRNA synthesis, the 5′ end of the molecule is "capped" by the addition of a methylated guanosine.[1, 3, 4] 7-Methylguanosine is attached through a triphosphate linkage formed between its 5′ hydroxyl and the 5′ hydroxyl of the terminal residue in the initial transcript. This cap plays a role in nuclear transport of the mRNA. Additionally, the 5′ cap is essential for the translation of most mRNA because it facilitates binding of the translation machinery to the 5′ end of the mRNA.[1, 3] This modification also protects the fragile mRNA from degradation in that the unique 5′-to-5′ phosphodiester bond of the cap makes it intrinsically resistant to general ribonucleases.[20]

The 3′ ends of growing transcripts are cleaved at a point 10 to 30 bases downstream from the polyadenylation signal sequence AAU-AAA (see Fig. 2–3). This sequence is found in nearly all eukaryotic mRNA and is one of the most conserved elements known.[1, 3, 4, 12, 21] Other elements containing GUGU and UUUCU sequences are located 20 to 40 bases downstream of the cleavage site.[12, 21] Immediately after cleavage of the nascent transcript, the poly A polymerase enzyme adds 200 to 250 adenylate residues.[1, 21] Like the 5′ cap, this modification confers mRNA stability, promotes mRNA translational efficiency, and plays a role in exportation of the mature mRNA from the nucleus to the cytoplasm.[1, 3, 21]

Many mRNA precursors in the nucleus are much larger than their cytoplasmic mRNA counterparts associated with ribosomes. The most important modification that mRNA undergoes before the mature form is transported to the cytoplasm is excision of the intronic, or noncoding, sequences (Fig. 2–6). Each intron contains conserved sequences at the 5′ and 3′ ends, known as the splice donor (GU) and acceptor

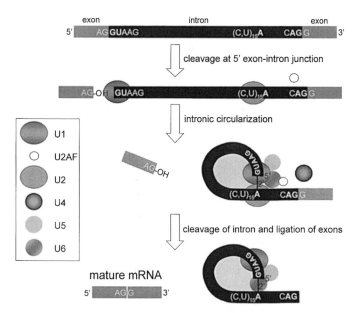

FIGURE 2–6. Splicing is a post-transcriptional modification of mRNA. Splicing involves the excision of intronic sequences from the mRNA before the mature form is transported to the cytoplasm. Immature mRNA is cleaved immediately upstream of the splice donor (GU) at the 5′ end of the intron, and the terminal G nucleotide covalently links to an A residue found near a pyrimidine-rich region around the 3′ end of the intron to form a lariat structure. A large array of small ribonucleoproteins and associated nuclear proteins identified in the box to the left form a complex known as a spliceosome, which recognizes the ends of the intron and brings them together. This lariat is cleaved immediately downstream of the splice acceptor (AG), and the adjacent two exons are joined together while the intron is degraded.

(AG), respectively.[1, 3, 4] A large array of small ribonucleoproteins and associated nuclear proteins form a complex known as the spliceosome, which recognizes the ends of the intron and brings them together.[1, 3, 4] The immature mRNA is cleaved immediately upstream of the splice donor at the 5′ end of the intron, and the terminal G covalently links to an A found near a pyrimidine-rich region that precedes the splice acceptor to form a lariat structure.[1, 3, 4] The lariat is cleaved immediately downstream of the splice acceptor, and the intron is rapidly degraded while the adjacent two exons are joined together.

Alternative splicing of precursor mRNA is a common mechanism whereby cells exploit the splicing mechanism to generate multiple related proteins from a single gene.[22] Once thought to be an exception to the rule (one gene, one protein), alternative splicing is now estimated to occur in at least 1 of every 20 genes.[22] One example of a single gene that is alternatively spliced is α-tropomyosin, which encodes seven tissue-specific variants of the muscle protein that associates with actin in the rat.[3, 4] This gene consists of "constitutive" exons that are found in all transcripts of the gene, "cell-specific" exons that appear only in transcripts produced in certain tissues, and exons that show variable expression. The mechanism of splice site selection and the interaction between multiple *cis*-acting elements and corresponding protein factors during these alternative splicing events remain to be determined. Another type of alternative processing involves the inclusion or removal of various intronic sequences. Such is the case for the bovine growth hormone gene, in which the last intronic sequence may be retained in a fraction of mRNA and transported to the nucleus, thereby allowing for production of a variant form of the hormone.[23–26] Additionally, the use of alternative polyadenylation signals from a single transcript also increases the diversity of its biologic responses, as with the hormone calcitonin, which is produced in the thyroid gland, and calcitonin gene–related peptide, which is produced in the hypothalamus.[2, 21, 24, 27, 28] Both hormones are the products of a single gene that undergoes alternative processing and polyadenylation of its RNA transcript.

TRANSLATION: REGULATED PROTEIN BIOSYNTHESIS

Once a mature mRNA molecule is transported from the nucleus to the cytoplasm by unknown mechanisms, it becomes an integral part of protein synthesis because it now carries the genetic message, in the form of nucleotides, that determines the specific amino acid sequence composing a protein. Each amino acid is represented in the mRNA by a sequence of triplet nucleotides called codons that are arranged in a contiguous reading frame. The first codon in mRNA, known as the start codon, is usually AUG, which encodes methionine and is most often used to initiate translation. The 3′ end of the reading frame contains one or more specific "stop" codons that serve as signals to terminate extension of the polypeptide chain.[2]

Amino acids are delivered to the mRNA via an adapter molecule, the cloverleaf-shaped tRNA. Each tRNA contains a trinucleotide sequence, an anticodon complementary to the codon sequence of the amino acid to which it is covalently linked. The anticodon allows each tRNA to recognize the appropriate codon sequence in the mRNA through the complementary base pairing that occurs in conjunction with ribosomes. Ribosomes are compact ribonucleoproteins composed of two subunits (40S and 60S) whose mass consists primarily of rRNAs that control recognition between a codon of mRNA and the anticodon of tRNA.[1] Protein synthesis requires synchronized involvement of all the above-listed RNA species and is generally considered in three stages—initiation, elongation, and termination—each of which will be considered further.

To initiate eukaryotic protein synthesis, the ribosome must first bind to the mRNA to form the initiation complex and deliver the first amino acid. This step usually determines the rate of synthesis of a given protein.[1, 3] Binding of the ribosome 40S subunit to the mRNA requires the presence of methionine-tRNA, as well as several initiation factors, including proteins that recognize the 5′ methylated cap on mRNA. Once bound, the 40S subunit migrates along the mRNA until it identifies the start codon, as well as a conserved sequence around the initiation codon GCC(A/G)CC**AUG**G.[1, 3, 4] Binding of the ribosome is stabilized at the initiation site as the 40S subunit is joined by the 60S subunit.

Once the complete ribosome is formed at the start codon, the elongation phase of protein synthesis can begin. Ribosomes have two sites for binding of tRNA: peptidyl-tRNA, which is the most recent amino acid to have been added to the nascent polypeptide chain, occupies the P, or donor, site, and aminoacyl-tRNA, which is the next amino acid to be added, enters the A, or acceptor, site.[1, 4] Constituents of the ribosomal 60S subunit catalyze peptide bond formation when the polypeptide chain carried by peptidyl-tRNA is transferred to the amino acid carried by aminoacyl-tRNA. After the bond forms, a deacetylated tRNA devoid of an amino acid occupies the P site and a peptidyl-tRNA now occupies the A site, and the peptide chain has increased in length by one amino acid. The ribosome translocates by advancing three nucleotides and moving the deacetylated tRNA out of the ribosome by expelling it directly into the cytosol, and the new peptidyl-tRNA moves into the P site while the next codon lies in the A site and waits for the appropriate aminoacyl-tRNA to enter. An elongation factor mediates entry of the next aminoacyl-tRNA to the A site.[1, 4]

The final stage of translation is termination, which encompasses the steps needed to release the completed polypeptide chain from tRNA and allow for dissociation of the ribosome from mRNA. Three stop or termination codons—UAG, UAA, and UGA, known as amber, ochre, and opal, respectively—do not encode an amino acid but rather function to end protein synthesis.[3, 4] These codons are recognized directly by protein factors that signal the termination of protein synthesis, which involves release of the completed polypeptide from the last tRNA. This reaction is analogous to peptidyl-tRNA transfer, except that water enters instead of aminoacyl-tRNA. The ribosome is also released from mRNA by an unknown mechanism that includes dissociation resulting from a conformational change, but the complex set of accessory factors involved has not yet been identified.[1]

POST-TRANSLATIONAL MODIFICATIONS

Many secreted peptide hormones are biosynthesized as larger precursor species.[4, 28] These precursor species are converted by proteolytic processing to a final hormone. Such is the case for the biosynthesis of parathyroid hormone (PTH). Pre-pro-PTH, an initial product of synthesis on the ribosomes, is converted to pro-PTH during transport of the polypeptide into the cisterna of the rough ER. The function of the "pre-" sequence that is cleaved is to facilitate insertion of the nascent peptide into the membrane of the rough ER. The resulting pro-PTH is further cleaved by another specific peptidase to form PTH, the mature form of the hormone, which is packaged into secretory granules in the parathyroid gland.[24]

We have already mentioned that alternative splicing in which more than one transcript can be derived from a single gene allows an exception to the "one gene, one protein" rule that is part of the central dogma of molecular biology. Another exception to this rule can be found later in the pathway of gene expression and protein biosynthesis, specifically, alternative protein processing, a process by which a single gene is transcribed into a single mRNA and translated into a large precursor protein molecule that is fragmented into several functional units. Proopiomelanocortin (POMC) undergoes this type of post-translational processing.

Corticotroph cells of the anterior lobe and melanotroph cells of the intermediate lobe of the pituitary gland, as well as specific loci of the brain, synthesize the precursor glycoprotein molecule known as POMC. However, processing of the propolyhormone varies depending on its cellular site. In the anterior lobe most POMC is processed to adrenocorticotropic hormone (ACTH), β-lipotropin, γ-lipotropin, and β-endorphin.[24, 28] Processing of POMC is different in the intermediate lobe of the pituitary gland, where peptide bonds in the ACTH sequence are broken to produce mainly α-melanocyte–stimulating hormone (α-MSH) and a corticotropin-like intermediate lobe peptide called CLIP. In the brain, the major products are ACTH, β-endorphin, and α-MSH.[24, 28]

Many newly synthesized polypeptides undergo major modifications as they mature to functional proteins: formation of disulfide bonds; protein folding, including the possible formation of multichain proteins; proteolytic cleavage; and the addition and modification of carbohydrates, phosphates, and lipids. All these events may be regulated functions, although the magnitude of their importance may be variable.[28]

REGULATED SECRETION OF PROTEINS

Translation occurs free in the cytosol unless a signal sequence directs its synthesis elsewhere. The sequence of many proteins begins with approximately 20 amino acids that function as a signal sequence in that it directs the protein to its proper destination within the cell. For example, the signal sequence of secretory proteins, which is made up mostly of hydrophobic amino acids, is bound by a complex of ribonucleoproteins called the signal recognition particle (SRP) that directs ribosome attachment to an SRP receptor site on the cytosolic face of the ER. As the newly synthesized protein enters the cisternal space of the ER, a complex of five proteins called the signal peptidase cleaves off this signal sequence as translation of the rest of the protein continues. In essence, the cell uses signal sequences as a general mechanism to dispatch proteins to specific sites.[1, 4, 24, 28]

Many proteins leave the ER wrapped in transport vesicles budded from a specialized region termed transitional ER to the *cis* face of the Golgi apparatus, which functions to modify and/or store proteins until they are eventually shipped to the cell surface or other destinations. Mature proteins exit the *trans* faces of Golgi within the lumen of budding membranous vesicles; these vesicles eventually fuse with the plasma membrane to allow for secretion of the proteins.[1, 28] The stored polypeptides remain in these vesicles, known as secretory granules, until the appropriate extracellular signals, such as interaction of a hormone with cellular membrane receptors, produce secondary and tertiary messengers that trigger the release of such stored proteins. Such signals may activate specific intracellular kinases that phosphorylate other proteins within the cell, which then interact with the secretory granules to participate in the release of their stored contents.[1, 24, 28] These intracellular signals will be discussed in the following section and in detail in many subsequent chapters, including Chapters 4 through 9.

HORMONAL CONTROL OF GENE EXPRESSION AND PROTEIN BIOSYNTHESIS

From this rather general overview of the flow of information from the gene to the secretory granule in terms of the biosynthesis of a polypeptide, it is clear that multiple potential sites are available for regulation by factors such as hormones. Of these, however, only regulation of the initiation of transcription is common to all hormones. For example, polypeptide hormones regulate transcription and secretion of stored proteins. In contrast, steroid hormones regulate transcription but not protein secretion. Therefore this section will focus on this one property that is common to the action of all hormones. Furthermore, even though all hormones regulate transcription, both common and unique mechanisms are involved in the action of steroid and polypeptide hormones. Many of these details will be covered in subsequent chapters, including Chapters 4 through 10. Consequently, here we will focus on a conceptual model that unifies their mechanism of action, as well as highlight a few of the important differences.

All hormones act on distant cellular targets,[28] and as will be seen, all hormones basically function by the same ultimate mechanism to regulate transcription, although the paths that they take for this purpose may be vastly different. To regulate transcription, hormones must transduce their signals from outside the cell to the nucleus and ultimately to a set of specific gene targets (Fig. 2–7). All hormone-responsive cells must harbor a receptor specific for the incoming hormone. Additionally, all hormone-responsive genes must contain a specific hormone response element that binds a cognate DNA-binding protein. Transcriptional factors that interpret the hormone signal can be regarded as a subclass of DNA-binding proteins that regulate transcription. As such, they contain at least two modular domains shared by all transcriptional factors: a DNA-binding domain and a domain required for transcriptional activation.

All polypeptide and peptide hormones, along with some biogenic amines such as epinephrine and norepinephrine, bind receptors that reside on the cell surface[28] (see Fig. 2–7). Because these hormones cannot enter cells to initiate their biologic actions, they rely instead on an indirect mechanism for communicating with their hormone-responsive DNA-binding proteins. The signal transduction event begins when this class of hormones binds their cell-surface receptors with great specificity and high affinity. Binding induces a conformational change in the receptor that converts it from an inactive to an active state.[1, 2, 4] The activated receptor directly or indirectly activates or inhibits a cascade of molecular effectors that culminates in the post-transcriptional activation of a specific hormone-responsive DNA-binding protein.

Cell-surface hormone receptors can be divided into three general classes, which will be referred to in more detail in Chapters 4 through 6. The first types of cell-surface receptors are themselves effectors, in that binding of agonists directly activates the effector function.[28] These receptors may be ion channels or have enzymatic function upon ligand binding and activation of the receptor, as is the case with some γ-aminobutyric acid receptors, which are chloride channels, and epidermal growth factor receptors, which are tyrosine kinases.[28] Some activated receptors also couple through guanosine triphosphate–binding regulatory proteins to activate effectors. These receptors, known as G protein–coupled receptors, include receptors for epinephrine, dopamine, and thyroid-stimulating hormone.[28] The last class of membrane-bound receptors consists of those that associate with and thereby activate cytosolic effector molecules without a coupling protein.[28]

Generally, DNA-binding proteins that transduce signals from polypeptide hormones retain their binding specificity in the absence of hormone. Thus signal transduction along this pathway generally involves a series of kinases that ultimately lead to phosphorylation and

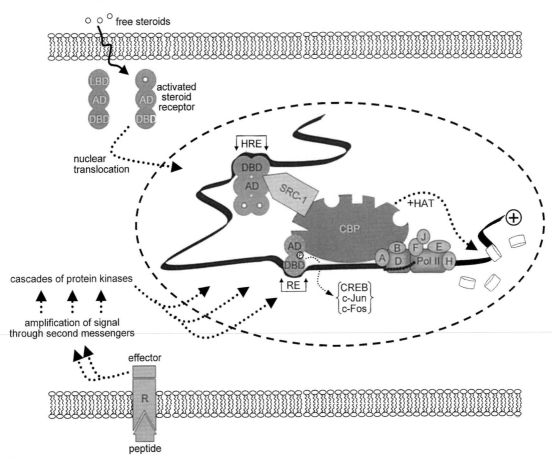

FIGURE 2–7. *Steroid and peptide hormone control of gene expression. Free steroid hormones diffuse easily through the cellular membrane and associate with the ligand-binding domain (LBD) of intracellular nuclear receptors found in the cytoplasm, which causes phosphorylation of the receptor, dissociation of several receptor-associated proteins, and exposure of a cysteine-rich zinc finger DNA-binding domain (DBD). This "activated" receptor, which is itself a transcription factor, translocates to the nucleus and binds specifically to its cognate hormone response element (HRE). The transcription factor typically associates with the CBP (CREB [cAMP response element–binding protein]-binding protein) integrator indirectly via an additional coactivator, such as steroid coactivator-1 (SRC-1), that binds both the activation domain (AD) of the steroid receptor and a glutamine-rich region in CBP. In contrast, some steroid hormones function through the binding of corepressors, which interact with extrinsic factors, including histone deacetylases, that function to tighten the chromatin structure and provide a barrier to transcription by making nucleosomes more stable. Peptide hormones, on the other hand, bind receptors (R) located on the cell surface and induce a conformational change in the receptor that converts it to an active state. This activity starts a signal transduction cascade culminating in the post-transcriptional activation of a specific hormone-responsive DNA-binding protein that binds to specific response elements (REs) in the 5′ flanking region of the promoter from the hormonally responsive gene. The CBP integrator, which has intrinsic histone acetyltransferase (HAT) activity that acts to relieve the nucleosome barrier to transcription, provides the bridge that serves to functionally integrate the signal from the transcription factor to the basal transcription complex.*

subsequent activation of the target transcription factor. Prime examples of hormone-responsive DNA-binding proteins that serve in this capacity include members of the b-Zip family of transcription factors: cAMP response element–binding protein (CREB) and c-Jun/c-Fos in the protein kinase A and C signaling systems, respectively.[4, 29, 30]

Although necessary, activation of the transcription factor is often not sufficient for subsequent transduction of a signal that requires communication with components of the downstream core transcription complex. A large nuclear "integrator" provides the bridge that serves to functionally integrate the signal from the hormone-responsive transcription factor into the basal transcription complex (see Fig. 2–7). This integrator, known as CREB-binding protein (CBP), belongs to a distinct subclass of transcription factors known as coactivators that do not bind directly to DNA but instead to proteins that bind DNA.[31] CBP was originally identified as a coactivator of the transcription factor CREB. However, CBP and its homologue p300 have multiple domains capable of interacting with the transactivation domains from several different hormone-responsive DNA-binding proteins. In fact, an array of transcription factors are able to form stable physical complexes with and respond to the coactivating properties of CBP/

p300, including CREB, MyoD, c-Jun, c-Fos, c-Myb, nuclear factor κB, nuclear receptors, and numerous others.[31, 32] The p300 and CBP integrators bind multiple factors simultaneously with their protein-binding domains and assist in "recruitment" of basal transcription machinery, as well as other coactivators. The integrator also has domains required for interacting with members of the core transcription complex.

Multiple coactivators, including the integrator, have been identified that fit the definition of a protein that interacts with DNA-bound transcription factors and the basal transcription machinery; such proteins form a functional connection between the two to enhance transcription.[32–34] Besides this bridging function, CBP/p300 has intrinsic histone acetyltransferase activity and the capacity to interact with extrinsic histone acetyltransferases.[6, 31–33, 35] As histones become hyperacetylated, they fall off of DNA and as a consequence open up chromatin for increased transcription by unraveling nucleosomes.[4, 6, 36] In addition to these critical roles, CBP/p300 can also acetylate transcription factors directly, which may result in stimulation of their DNA-binding activity. Indeed, a rich network of communication encompassing various signaling pathways results in abundant molecular crosstalk. Additionally, increasing evidence indicates that this integrator molecule appears to transduce signals from virtually all steroid and polypeptide hormones studied to date.

In contrast to polypeptide hormones, steroids are hydrophobic molecules that usually circulate in the serum bound with low affinity to nonspecific carrier proteins. Because steroid hormones are lipophilic, free hormone can easily diffuse through the cellular membrane and bind with high affinity to intracellular nuclear receptors, which are themselves transcription factors[28, 32] (see Fig. 2–7). These nuclear receptors are members of a superfamily of functionally and structurally related transcription factors that have a third domain required for ligand-specific binding. Indeed, steroid hormone receptors were among the first transcription factors to be cloned and characterized. Members of this superfamily include receptors for steroid hormones, such as estrogen, androgens, progesterone, glucocorticoids, and aldosterone, as well as hormonal forms of vitamins A and D, thyroid hormone, and others, many for which ligands have not yet been identified.[28, 32]

Unlike the DNA-binding proteins that transduce the signal from polypeptide hormones, most of the members of the nuclear receptor family reside in the cytosol in the absence of hormone (see Fig. 2–7). Initiation of the hormone response is triggered upon the noncovalent, reversible association of the steroid receptor with its ligand.[4, 28, 34, 37] In general, when such an association occurs, steroid receptors become phosphorylated and several receptor-associated proteins, including heat shock protein 90, are dissociated. This "activated" receptor translocates to the nucleus via a nuclear localization signal.[4, 28] Hormone activation also exposes a cysteine-rich zinc finger DNA-binding domain that permits the ligand-occupied steroid receptor to bind specifically to its cognate hormone response element.[4, 28, 37]

As will be discussed in more detail in a subsequent chapter (see Chapter 10), nuclear receptors can be subclassified according to the sequence and spatial relationship of the *cis*-acting elements to which they bind. These steroid hormone response elements are organized as two partially palindromic half-sites separated by a specific number of nucleotides[32, 37]; for example, the consensus glucocorticoid response element (GRE) is AGAACAnnnTGTTCT, where the three "n" bases can be any nucleotide but the spacing is invariant. The configuration of other hormone response elements is quite similar to that of the GRE, but slight variations in sequence, orientation, and spacing between the half-sites allow for specificity of hormone binding. Alteration of any of these sequences may result in loss of hormonal responsiveness.

In contrast to the hormone-responsive DNA-binding proteins that mediate the action of polypeptide hormones, ligand-occupied steroid receptors, although capable of interacting directly with the integrator CBP molecule, typically exhibit an indirect interaction through the bridging of additional cofactors[32, 33] (see Fig. 2–7). These nuclear receptor coactivator proteins, which functionally link the hormone-responsive DNA-binding protein to the integrator, do not bind directly to DNA but instead bind specifically to the transactivation domains of the hormone-responsive DNA-binding proteins and to specific domains found within CBP.[32, 34] The yeast two-hybrid system and Far Western blotting have been used to identify several cofactor proteins that interact with members of the nuclear receptor superfamily.[33, 34] The first functional coactivator that was identified was termed steroid receptor coactivator-1 (SRC-1) and appears to be a general enhancer of transactivation of steroid hormone–dependent target genes.[32, 34] Subsequently, many more coactivators have been identified, including TIF1, TIF2, and RIP140.[34] CBP functionally interacts with steroid hormone receptor coactivators to synergistically enhance the transcription of steroid hormone–dependent genes.

The activity of some members of the nuclear receptor superfamily is not regulated by coactivators, but rather through relief of tonic inhibition by corepressors.[33] Such is the case for thyroid hormone receptors; in the absence of thyroid hormone, thyroid hormone receptors repress the transcription of many genes, and in the presence of thyroid hormone, thyroid hormone receptors activate the transcription of those same genes.[34, 38, 39] In the unliganded state, thyroid hormone receptors interact with one of several corepressor proteins. These proteins interact with extrinsic factors, including histone deacetylases, that function to tighten the chromatin structure; thus nucleosomes

become more stable and provide a barrier to transcription. Binding of thyroid hormone to the thyroid hormone receptor elicits a conformational change that causes release of the corepressor and recruitment of coactivator proteins.

Although the mechanism by which steroid and peptide hormones ultimately regulate transcription is the same, polypeptides work through second messengers whereas steroid hormones directly activate the target DNA-binding protein, in this case its receptor (see Fig. 2–7). This difference means that much higher concentrations of steroid hormones are required to achieve a transcriptional response because of the absence of amplification of the hormonal signal. For example, a single polypeptide hormone can interact with a receptor on the cell surface. Each activated receptor can in turn interact with several downstream effectors. Each activated effector generates a large number of second messengers that activate protein kinases. Each protein kinase may phosphorylate and thereby activate other enzymes and produce a large number of product molecules, each of which contributes to the cellular response. In contrast, each steroid receptor must be bound by ligand to elicit the active conformation of each individual *trans*-acting factor.

Although we have focused our attention on events occurring at the gene transcriptional level, it is evident that other sites of the protein synthesis pathway may be points at which regulation by hormones may occur. For example, estrogen has been shown to stabilize chicken liver vitellogenin mRNA, and prolactin can increase the half-life of casein mRNA in breast tissue. RNA splicing may also be hormonally regulated. In addition to the tissue-specific RNA-splicing events that have already been described, it is possible that such processes are hormonally regulated not only to yield different mRNA species by alternative exon and polyadenylation site choice but also to alter the expression of one vs. another mRNA by alternative promoter choice. In addition, it is possible that transcription elongation and termination may be other foci for hormonal regulation. Furthermore, translation and protein processing are also likely to be hormonally regulated.

FUNCTIONAL GENOMICS

It has been said that we have entered the third technologic revolution. Great advances have been made with the passing of the Industrial and Computer Revolutions. The next great era, the Genomics Revolution, is upon us.[40] The term "genome," first used by Winkler in 1920, was created by merging the words *genes* and *chromosomes* and refers to an organism's complete set of chromosomes and genes.[41] The term "genomics" was coined much later, in 1986, by Roderick to describe the scientific discipline of mapping, sequencing, and analyzing genomes and was consequently the namesake of a scientific journal that was initiated at that time, *Genomics*.[41, 42] In essence, the goal of genomics is to make biologic and functional sense of raw genetic information.

Structural genomics represents an initial phase of genomic analysis, that is, the construction of a high-resolution genetic map of an organism. These efforts have produced a wealth of sequence information since emergence of the Human Genome Project (HGP) in 1990, which is a coordinated effort to characterize all human genetic material by determining the complete sequence of the 3 billion base pairs of DNA in the human genome. By the completion of the HGP, estimated to occur by the year 2003, 80,000 human genes are likely to have been identified.[43] Further information pertaining to the HGP can be accessed via the National Human Genome Research Institute website at http://www.nhgri.nih.gov/HGP/.

Already, the field of genomics is beginning to undergo expansion from mapping and sequencing of the human and other genomes to include an emphasis on genome function.[42] With this further amplification we will develop a better understanding of the function of human genes and their roles in health and disease.[44] In fact, the technology and resources promoted by the HGP are starting to have a profound impact on biomedical research and promise to revolutionize the wider spectrum of biologic research and clinical medicine. Increasingly detailed genome maps have aided researchers seeking genes associated with many genetic conditions, including myotonic dystrophy, fragile X syndrome, neurofibromatosis types 1 and 2, inherited colon cancer, Alzheimer's disease, and familial breast cancer.

A substantial fraction of the genome (approximately 20%) is dedicated to genes that encode transcription factors.[25] Mutations in transcription factors have been associated with numerous genetic endocrine disorders. Hence it is not surprising that the HGP, by identifying thousands of new genes, many of which encode transcription factors, will ultimately provide the building blocks needed to identify the causes of many genetic diseases. Additionally, in connection with the shift to functional genomics, study of the gene expression involved in genetic disorders has become invaluable because important therapeutic strategies are based on an understanding of how the promoter-regulatory elements drive or inhibit the expression of specific genes.

Although complete sequencing of an organism's genome is no doubt an amazing accomplishment, it pales by comparison to the task that awaits scientists who must put meaning to these base pairs.[41] Functional genomics makes use of the vast amount of information provided by structural genomics to develop experimental approaches to assess gene function and has been defined as the continuum from a gene's physical structure to its role in the context of the biology of the whole organism.[44, 45] The "new science," that is, functional or physiologic genomics, has actually been among us for many years, although its name was coined only a few years ago in connection with the HGP initiative.

The field of functional genomics has focused on elucidating the function of proteins encoded by genes that have been identified and to understand the pathways in which these genes participate.[46] The concept of one gene causing one phenotype is rapidly giving way to the appreciation that many human diseases are genetically complex, with the phenotype reflecting the combined contribution of many genes. In fact, it is increasingly being appreciated that any perturbation of a cell has a global impact that affects the expression of many genes that ultimately define the homeostatic response. To approach analysis of this complex biology the field of functional genomics can be subdivided into two complementary approaches: measurement of transcriptomes and measurement of proteomes. Transcriptome refers to all the mRNA expressed by a specific cell in a given physiologic state. This type of measurement is accomplished by using a genome-wide array of specific DNA probes.[47–50] Similarly, a proteome describes all the proteins associated with a specific physiologic state.[51–53] Resolving these complex mixtures of proteins can be accomplished via two-dimensional gel electrophoresis and mass spectrometry using a procedure known as "mass profiling."[51–54] Even with these emerging subdisciplines, there is a growing awareness of the need for development of mathematic models and other bioinformatic tools that will allow contributions of kinetic parameters that govern biologic processes to be included in the analysis of transcriptomes and proteomes. In short, phenotypes are the net result of complex interactions and rate processes that occur among members of a specific pathway.

Rapid progress in genome science and a glimpse into its potential applications have spurred observers to predict that mathematically based biology will be the foremost science of the 21st century.[55] The technology and resources generated by the HGP and other genomics research are already having a major impact on research across the life sciences. On the horizon is a new era of molecular medicine characterized less by treating symptoms and more by looking for the most fundamental causes of disease.[55] Rapid and more specific diagnostic tests will make possible earlier treatment of countless maladies. Medical researchers will also be able to devise novel therapeutic regimens based on new classes of drugs, immunotherapy techniques, avoidance of environmental conditions that may trigger disease, and possibly augmentation or even replacement of defective genes through gene therapy.[45, 55]

REFERENCES

1. Lewin BM: Genes VI. New York, Oxford University Press, 1997.
2. Darnell J, Lodish H, Baltimore D: Molecular Cell Biology, ed 2. New York, Scientific American, 1990.
3. Watson JD, Gilman M, Witkowski J, Zoller M: Recombinant DNA, ed 2. New York, Scientific American, 1992.
4. Zubay G: Biochemistry, ed 3. Dubuque, IA, WC Brown, 1993.
5. Wolffe AP, Kurumizaka H: The nucleosome: A powerful regulator of transcription. Prog Nucleic Acid Res Mol Biol 61:379–422, 1998.
6. Workman JL, Kingston RE: Alteration of nucleosome structure as a mechanism of transcriptional regulation. Annu Rev Biochem 67:545–579, 1998.
7. Laybourn PJ, Kadonaga JT: Role of nucleosomal cores and histone H1 in regulation of transcription by RNA polymerase II. Science 254:238–245, 1991.
8. Bustin M, Reeves R: High-mobility-group chromosomal proteins: Architectural components that facilitate chromatin function. Prog Nucleic Acid Res Mol Biol 54:35–100, 1996.
9. Goodwin G: The high mobility group protein, HMGI-C. Int J Biochem Cell Biol 30:761–766, 1998.
10. Wolffe AP: Packaging principle: How DNA methylation and histone acetylation control the transcriptional activity of chromatin. J Exp Zool 282:239–244, 1998.
11. Kay GF: Xist and X chromosome inactivation. Mol Cell Endocrinol 140:71–76, 1998.
12. Barabino SM, Keller W: Last but not least: Regulated poly(A) tail formation. Cell 99:9–11, 1999.
13. Orphanides G, Lagrange T, Reinberg D: The general transcription factors of RNA polymerase II. Genes Dev 10:2657–2683, 1996.
14. Barberis A, Gaudreau L: Recruitment of the RNA polymerase II holoenzyme and its implications in gene regulation. Biol Chem 379:1397–1405, 1998.
15. Corden JL: Tails of RNA polymerase II. Trends Biochem Sci 15:383–387, 1990.
16. Goodrich JA, Tjian R: Transcription factors IIE and IIH and ATP hydrolysis direct promoter clearance by RNA polymerase II. Cell 77:145–156, 1994.
17. Zenzie-Gregory B, Khachi A, Garraway IP, Smale ST: Mechanism of initiator-mediated transcription: Evidence for a functional interaction between the TATA-binding protein and DNA in the absence of a specific recognition sequence. Mol Cell Biol 13:3841–3849, 1993.
18. Colgan J, Manley JL: TFIID can be rate limiting in vivo for TATA-containing, but not TATA-lacking, RNA polymerase II promoters. Genes Dev 6:304–315, 1992.
19. Maity SN, de Crombrugghe B: Role of the CCAAT-binding protein CBF/NF-Y in transcription. Trends Biochem Sci 23:174–178, 1998.
20. Sachs AB: Messenger RNA degradation in eukaryotes. Cell 74:413–421, 1993.
21. Colgan DF, Manley JL: Mechanism and regulation of mRNA polyadenylation. Genes Dev 11:2755–2766, 1997.
22. Sharp PA: Split genes and RNA splicing. Cell 77:805–815, 1994.
23. Edens A, Talamantes F: Alternative processing of growth hormone receptor transcripts. Endocr Rev 19:559–582, 1998.
24. Norman AW, Litwack G: Hormones, ed 2. San Diego, CA, Academic, 1997.
25. Stallings-Mann ML, Ludwiczak RL, Klinger KW, Rottman F: Alternative splicing of exon 3 of the human growth hormone receptor is the result of an unusual genetic polymorphism. Proc Natl Acad Sci U S A 93:12394–12399, 1996.
26. Hampson RK, Rottman FM: Alternative processing of bovine growth hormone mRNA: Nonsplicing of the final intron predicts a high molecular weight variant of bovine growth hormone. Proc Natl Acad Sci U S A 84:2673–2677, 1987.
27. Lou H, Gagel RF: Alternative RNA processing—its role in regulating expression of calcitonin/calcitonin gene–related peptide. J Endocrinol 156:401–405, 1998.
28. Baulieu E-E, Kelley P: Hormones, from Molecules to Disease. New York, Chapman & Hall, 1990.
29. Habener JF: Cyclic AMP response element binding proteins: A cornucopia of transcription factors. Mol Endocrinol 4:1087–1094, 1990.
30. Tamai KT, Monaco L, Nantel F, et al: Coupling signalling pathways to transcriptional control: Nuclear factors responsive to cAMP. Recent Prog Horm Res 52:121–139, 1997.
31. Goldman PS, Tran VK, Goodman RH: The multifunctional role of the co-activator CBP in transcriptional regulation. Recent Prog Horm Res 52:103–119, 1997.
32. Giguere V: Orphan nuclear receptors: From gene to function. Endocr Rev 20:689–725, 1999.
33. Jenster G: Coactivators and corepressors as mediators of nuclear receptor function: An update. Mol Cell Endocrinol 143:1–7, 1998.
34. Shibata H, Spencer TE, Onate SA, et al: Role of co-activators and co-repressors in the mechanism of steroid/thyroid receptor action. Recent Prog Horm Res 52:141–164, 1997.
35. Utley RT, Ikeda K, Grant PA, et al: Transcriptional activators direct histone acetyltransferase complexes to nucleosomes. Nature 394:498–502, 1998.
36. Kadonaga JT: Eukaryotic transcription: An interlaced network of transcription factors and chromatin-modifying machines. Cell 92:307–313, 1998.
37. Freedman LP: Anatomy of the steroid receptor zinc finger region. Endocr Rev 13:129–145, 1992.
38. Koenig RJ: Thyroid hormone receptor coactivators and corepressors. Thyroid 8:703–713, 1998.
39. Apriletti JW, Ribeiro RC, Wagner RL, et al: Molecular and structural biology of thyroid hormone receptors. Clin Exp Pharmacol Physiol Suppl 25:2–11, 1998.
40. Abelson PH: A third technological revolution (editorial). Science 279:2019, 1998.
41. McKusick VA: Genomics: Structural and functional studies of genomes. Genomics 45:244–249, 1997.
42. Hieter P, Boguski M: Functional genomics: It's all how you read it. Science 278:601–602, 1997.
43. Cowley AW Jr: The emergence of physiological genomics. J Vasc Res 36:83–90, 1999.
44. Woychik RP, Klebig ML, Justice MJ, et al: Functional genomics in the post-genome era [published erratum appears in Mutat Res: 1998 Dec 3;422(2):367]. Mutat Res 400:3–14, 1998.
45. Cowley AW Jr: The Banbury Conference. Genomics to physiology and beyond: How do we get there? Physiologist 40:205–211, 1997.
46. Borrebaeck CA: Tapping the potential of molecular libraries in functional genomics. Immunol Today 19:524–527, 1998.
47. Kozian DH, Kirschbaum BJ: Comparative gene-expression analysis. Trends Biotechnol 17:73–78, 1999.

48. Brent R: Functional genomics: Learning to think about gene expression data. Curr Biol 9:R338–R341, 1999.
49. Lipshutz RJ, Fodor SP, Gingeras TR, Lockhart DJ: High density synthetic oligonucleotide arrays. Nat Genet 21:20–24, 1999.
50. Schena M, Heller RA, Theriault TP, et al: Microarrays: Biotechnology's discovery platform for functional genomics. Trends Biotechnol 16:301–306, 1998.
51. Dove A: Proteomics: Translating genomics into products? Nat Biotechnol 17:233–236, 1999.
52. Hochstrasser DF: Proteome in perspective. Clin Chem Lab Med 36:825–836, 1998.
53. Blackstock WP, Weir MP: Proteomics: Quantitative and physical mapping of cellular proteins. Trends Biotechnol 17:121–127, 1999.
54. Lopez MF: Proteome analysis. I. Gene products are where the biological action is. J Chromatogr B Biomed Sci Appl 722:191–202, 1999.
55. Bailey JE: Lessons from metabolic engineering for functional genomics and drug discovery. Nat Biotechnol 17:616–618, 1999.

Chapter 3

Control of Hormone Secretion

Thomas F. J. Martin

MORPHOLOGY OF PEPTIDE HORMONE–SECRETING ENDOCRINE CELLS AND THE REGULATED SECRETORY PATHWAY
SYNTHESIS, PROCESSING, AND SORTING OF PREPROHORMONE PRECURSORS

COMPOSITION OF MATURE SECRETORY GRANULES
SEQUENTIAL STAGES OF THE REGULATED SECRETORY PATHWAY
ESSENTIAL PROTEIN MACHINERY FOR DENSE-CORE GRANULE EXOCYTOSIS

REGULATION OF EXOCYTOSIS BY CALCIUM
MODULATION OF CALCIUM-DEPENDENT HORMONE SECRETION BY PROTEIN KINASE C

MORPHOLOGY OF PEPTIDE HORMONE–SECRETING ENDOCRINE CELLS AND THE REGULATED SECRETORY PATHWAY

Like other cell types (e.g., acinar pancreatic) dedicated to the synthesis of secretory proteins, peptide hormone–secreting endocrine cells are endowed with an abundant rough endoplasmic reticulum (ER), a stack of Golgi cisternae, and an array of dense-core secretory granules, all of which are components of an anterograde pathway for conveying secretory proteins to the extracellular space (Fig. 3–1). Classic mor-

phologic and autoradiographic studies established the sequence for trafficking of secretory proteins, which consists of their initial synthesis in the ER, segregation into the ER cisternal space, intracellular transport to the Golgi stacks, concentration in Golgi-derived secretory granules, intracellular storage of granules, and finally, granule discharge and protein secretion by exocytosis upon cellular activation.[1] Proteins synthesized on bound polyribosomes in the ER have several cellular destinations, with critical protein-targeting events occurring in late Golgi cisternae or the *trans*-Golgi network (TGN), where proteins are sorted to the endosome-lysosomal system or to the cell surface.[2] Multiple post-Golgi pathways mediate protein transport from the Golgi to the plasma membrane and extracellular space.[3, 4] All cells continu-

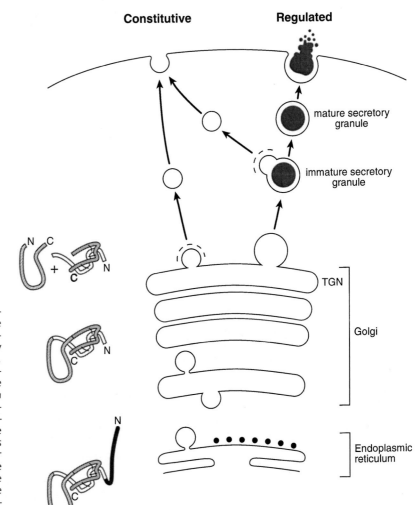

FIGURE 3–1. Schematic diagram of the anterograde secretory pathway in a peptide hormone–secreting endocrine cell. Secretory proteins synthesized in the endoplasmic reticulum (ER) are transported to and through Golgi stacks by vesicular transport. Within the *trans*-Golgi network (TGN), proteins are sorted to either constitutive or regulated secretory pathways. Immature secretory granules formed in the TGN are subject to additional sorting events during which clathrin-coated vesicles *(dashes)* divert constitutive membrane and soluble proteins back into the constitutive pathway. During exocytosis, mature secretory granules fuse with the plasma membrane, which is activated by increases in cytoplasmic calcium levels. Processing intermediates for a prepropeptide (such as preproinsulin) secreted by the regulated pathway are shown on the left and include cleavage of the N-terminal signal sequence *(filled)* in the ER and cleavage of the pro-region *(stippled)* in the TGN–immature secretory granule stage.

ously replenish plasma membrane proteins and export proteins to the extracellular space via constitutive secretory pathways with the use of several types of small (40–100 nm) clear Golgi-derived transport vesicles that translocate to and fuse with the plasma membrane.[4] Delivery of secreted proteins to the extracellular space by the constitutive pathway is rapid[5] (half-life of about 20 minutes), and protein secretion is rate-limited by the biosynthetic rates of the proteins rather than by regulated trafficking steps within the pathway.

In contrast, specialized secretory cells such as peptide hormone–secreting endocrine cells contain an additional pathway from the TGN to the cell surface, known as the regulated secretory pathway (see Fig. 3–1), that allows the acute regulated export of high concentrations of secretory proteins.[5] In this pathway, proteins are sorted to dense-core secretory granules that form by budding from the TGN with condensed luminal contents.[5, 6] The immature secretory granules that form undergo further maturation during which clathrin-coated vesicles bud from the immature granule and sort out excess membrane and soluble contents for constitutive-like secretion[7–9] (see Fig. 3–1). Immature secretory granules may also fuse with each other during maturation.[10] Mature granules are stored in the cytoplasm for considerable periods ($t_{1/2} > 10$ hours) in the absence of stimulation,[5, 6] which enables endocrine cells to accumulate secretory products over an integrated period of biosynthetic activity. Endocrine cells accumulate a large number of secretory granules (Fig. 3–2), which can constitute 10% to 20% of the cellular volume, that are filled with high (millimolar) peptide concentrations.[11] Secretory granules discharge their contents only when an appropriate physiologic stimulus to the cell activates exocytotic fusion of the granule with the plasma membrane (see below), a process that is rapid (seconds to minutes) and mediated through rises in cytoplasmic calcium levels initiated through signal transduction events.[12] Thus an accumulated biosynthetic cargo can be rapidly discharged into the blood stream at relatively high concentrations. The large size and condensed state of the contents of dense-core secretory granules are probably features of a specialized branch of the secretory pathway that coevolved with the development of an expanded circulatory system and the need to deliver adequate concentrations of signaling peptides into the blood stream.

SYNTHESIS, PROCESSING, AND SORTING OF PREPROHORMONE PRECURSORS

Secretory peptide precursors contain an N-terminal leader or signal peptide sequence to direct their synthesis in the ER and vectorial transfer into the cisternae of the ER-Golgi pathway[13] (see Fig. 3–1).

After transfer from the ER to the Golgi, most peptide hormone and neuropeptide precursors exist as prohormones from which multiple peptides are excised by proteolytic processing at sites usually marked by pairs of basic amino acid residues.[14–16] The endoproteases responsible for precursor maturation belong to a prohormone convertase (PC) family of serine proteases related to bacterial subtilisin that currently has seven members[16] (furin, PACE4, PC1/3, PC2, PC4, PC5/6, and PC7/8). PC1/3 and PC2, whose expression is restricted to tissues of neuroendocrine lineage, undergo sorting to dense-core granules formed in the TGN and are considered to be the proteases essential for the initial proteolytic maturation of neuropeptide and peptide hormone precursors.[14–16] Although proteolytic cleavage of hormonal precursors may be initiated in the TGN,[17] most of the cleavage occurs after entry into immature granules[18] in the low-pH, high-calcium environment required for optimal PC activity (see Fig. 3–1). Mature secretory granules contain a "cocktail" of multiple peptides derived from a prohormone precursor that is discharged upon exocytosis, and the multiple bioactive peptides can exert concerted physiologic regulation.[15, 17, 19] Sorting events in the immature granule also result in constitutive-like secretion of some of the peptide products (such as the C peptide of proinsulin).[8] In some instances, mature peptides from a common precursor are segregated into distinct secretory granules, which may involve initial proteolysis before sorting in the TGN.[17] Production of distinct dense-core granules (e.g., those for prolactin and growth hormone in mammosomatotrophs) can also occur for proteins that are separate gene products.[20]

The biogenesis of immature secretory granules is closely linked to the condensation and sorting of prohormones in the TGN.[1, 2, 6, 7, 15, 17] Cellular mechanisms used for sorting to the regulated pathway appear to be common to neural, endocrine, and probably exocrine cell types as inferred from the finding that peptide hormone precursors, as well as pancreatic prozymogens expressed by DNA transfection, are properly sorted to the regulated pathway in neuroendocrine and exocrine cells.[5, 6] Because expressed protein chimeras containing prohormone sequences are in many cases properly targeted to the regulated secretory pathway in neuroendocrine cells, it is thought that prohormonal precursors share consensual features that provide sorting information. The nature of the putative sorting signal is not entirely clear.[5–7, 15, 21–24] Recent studies have indicated that precursors for adrenocorticotropic hormone, enkephalins, and insulin may contain a sorting signal that consists of similarly spaced acidic and hydrophobic residues on the surface of an amphipathic loop.[25, 26] This region was reported to interact with carboxypeptidase E, a hormone-processing enzyme that is membrane associated in regulated granules, and was proposed to be a sorting signal receptor.[25, 26] Controversial aspects of this model have recently been discussed.[27] An alternative, sorting-by-condensation model proposes that sorting in the TGN is mediated by the protein

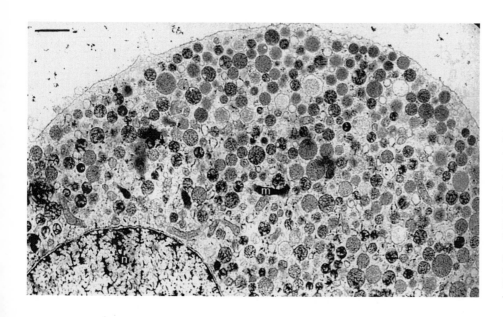

FIGURE 3–2. Transmission electron micrograph of a bovine adrenal medullary chromaffin cell prepared by cryofixation. Pleomorphic dense-core secretory granules with a mean diameter of 356 +/− 91 (SD) nm are dispersed throughout the cytoplasm. Of the approximately 22,000 granules per cell, very few (~500) are in close proximity to the plasma membrane, possibly in a docked state. The scale bar corresponds to 1 μm. (From Plattner H, Artalejo AR, Neher E: Ultrastructural organization of bovine chromaffin cell cortex—analysis by cryofixation and morphometry of aspects pertinent to exocytosis. J Cell Biol 139:1709–1717, 1997.)

aggregation that is promoted at the low-pH and high-calcium concentration present within the TGN cisternae.[5, 6, 28, 29] Chromogranin B, an acidic granule protein ubiquitously expressed in neuroendocrine cells, aggregates under these conditions and also associates with membranes via a disulfide-bonded loop region of the protein that is required for proper targeting to regulated granules.[22, 23] The general property of regulated (e.g., growth hormone, prolactin, follicle-stimulating hormone, PC2) but not constitutive (e.g., IgGs, albumin) secretory proteins to self-aggregate, as well as to aggregate heterophilically[30] and to associate with membranes[16, 31] under TGN luminal conditions, provides the basis for the sorting-by-condensation model, which envisions prohormonal aggregates sorting away from constitutive secretory proteins by associating with specific membrane domains in the TGN.[29] An alternative version of this model suggests that these features of regulated secretory proteins dictate their retention in immature granules during post-Golgi sorting events that remove constitutive proteins from immature granules.[7, 8] Targeting of transmembrane proteins to regulated granules, in contrast, appears to require the cytoplasmic regions of these proteins, which interact with cytosolic protein factors.[32, 33]

For vesicle budding at several sites in the anterograde secretory pathway, transmembrane proteins link cargo in the vesicle lumen to the cytosolic components (e.g., coat proteins) required for vesicle formation, which provides a mechanism for coupling vesicle generation with contents filling.[34–36] It is unclear whether similar events occur during the formation of secretory granules in the TGN because potential cargo receptors and protein coats have not been identified. However, aspects of immature granule biogenesis in the TGN have been elucidated by studies of cell-free budding reactions.[37–44] Granule formation in vitro requires ATP and cytosolic protein factors. One of the required cytosolic factors is phosphatidylinositol transfer protein (PITP), which interacts with membrane phosphatidylinositol and to a lesser extent with phosphatidylcholine. PITP may alter the phospholipid composition of the Golgi membrane to facilitate budding[45] or may alternatively promote the phosphorylation of phosphatidylinositol by a lipid kinase.[39, 46] The latter could account for the ATP dependence of vesicle formation. Phosphorylated inositides such as phosphatidylinositol bisphosphate (PIP_2) are known to regulate membrane events by promoting protein (e.g., coat or cytoskeletal) recruitment to membranes[47] or by serving as essential cofactors for membrane enzymes such as phospholipase D,[48] which converts phosphatidylcholine to phosphatidic acid (see Chapter 8). The small guanosine triphosphate (GTP)-binding protein ARF (ADP [adenosine diphosphate] ribosylation factor), which is required for coat protein recruitment for generating other Golgi-derived transport vesicles,[35] is also required for secretory granule formation.[41] ARF may function by recruiting an unidentified coat protein or cytoskeletal constituents or by regulating the activity of a PIP_2-dependent phospholipase D.[42–44] Overall, the TGN-budding process that generates immature granules resembles other vesicle-budding events in their requirement for GTP-binding proteins and factors that alter membrane phospholipids.[48]

COMPOSITION OF MATURE SECRETORY GRANULES

Mature secretory granules in endocrine and neural cells consist of a membrane bilayer surrounding an electron-opaque dense core that consists of condensed secretory materials such as peptide hormones, granin proteins, and processing enzymes. In some endocrine cells such as β cells in the islets of Langerhans, the contents are crystalline and consist of insulin hexamers chelated by zinc.[49] Proteolytic processing of proinsulin in the immature granule is required for the formation of this crystalline deposit.[50] Dense-core granules vary widely in properties from one endocrine cell type to another and range in size from 50 nm in the sympathetic nervous system, to 200 nm in pituitary corticotrophs or gonadotrophs, and up to 1000 nm in pituitary mammotrophs or neurohypophyseal cells.

Mature secretory granules engage in multiple cellular functions, including vectorial transport of small molecules into the luminal space (nucleotides, divalent cations, protons, and neurotransmitters), translo-

cation of the granules through the cytoplasm and their anchorage to cytoskeletal elements, docking of the granules at the plasma membrane, and their calcium-dependent exocytotic fusion at the plasma membrane. These functions would require an array of organelle-specific proteins exposed on the cytoplasmic face of the granule. Analyses of purified secretory granules have been undertaken to identify proteins that participate in aspects of the granule life cycle. The chromaffin granules of adrenal medullary tissue are best studied (see Fig. 3–2), although granules purified from anterior and posterior pituitary or from pancreatic islet cells have also been analyzed to a lesser extent.[51, 52] Individual adrenal chromaffin cells contain 10 to 30,000 granules with a mean diameter of 350 nm,[53–55] which has enabled extensive purification at yields of 2 to 3 mg per bovine adrenal gland.[54]

The adrenal chromaffin granule possesses a number of general features likely to be representative of other secretory granules. Chromaffin granules consist of approximately 20% lipid and about 42% protein (percent dry weight). The membrane of the chromaffin granule exhibits a lipid composition similar to that of other cellular membranes but is notable for its relatively high cholesterol content, which is characteristic of late Golgi-derived membranes.[56] In addition, a surprisingly high concentration of lysophosphatidylcholine is present, which has also been reported for exocrine tissue granules but not for pituitary granules and synaptic vesicles.[56] Thus a high lysophospholipid content does not appear to be essential for a common granule function such as exocytotic fusion, but the precise role of lysophospholipids in granules is not known. Chromaffin (and other) granules contain, like many cellular membranes, 2% to 5% phosphatidylinositol, a phospholipid that is an essential precursor for the formation of PIP_2, which is required in membrane fusion mechanisms (see below).

Although the characterization of chromaffin granule proteins was anticipated to identify constituents that mediate general functions of dense-core granules, including exocytosis, it instead revealed specialized constituents unique to the function of these catecholaminergic and peptidergic granules.[55] Chromaffin granule protein composition is dominated by abundant proteins that catalyze catecholamine synthesis or the posttranslational processing of neuropeptides. About 75% of the protein is soluble in the lumen. Luminal contents are dominated by a family of acidic, heat-stable glycoproteins, the granins (chromogranin A and secretogranins I and II) and their proteolytic products. Granins may function in the aggregative sorting of peptide hormone precursors to the regulated pathway (see above) and are general constituents of neuroendocrine secretory granules from the parathyroid, pituitary, thyroid, and pancreas, as well as sympathetic neurons.[57] Granins are also precursors for a variety of bioactive peptides such as pancreastatin, vasostatin, parastatin (derived from chromogranin A), and secretoneurin (derived from secretogranin II).[29, 53–55] Other chromaffin granule luminal proteins are glycoproteins (glycoprotein III), neuropeptides (enkephalins and neuropeptide Y), and enzymes for catecholamine synthesis (dopamine β-monooxygenase), neuropeptide proteolytic cleavage (carboxypeptidase E/H, PC1, and PC2), or peptide amidation (peptidylglycine α-monooxygenase). The dense core of chromaffin granules observed by transmission electron microscopy is attributed to the high luminal content of granin proteins and neuropeptides present in the millimolar concentration range.[53–55] Small-molecular-weight constituents are also abundant and consist of catecholamines (~0.6 M), ATP (~0.15 M), ascorbic acid (~0.02 M), and calcium (~0.02 M). Other endocrine dense-core vesicles contain high concentrations of ATP and calcium.[58]

The membrane protein composition of chromaffin granules is dominated by membrane-bound dopamine β-monooxygenase and cytochrome b_{561}, both dedicated constituents that function in the oxidation of dopamine to norepinephrine.[55] Other membrane proteins found in lesser abundance are the subunits of the chromaffin granule proton pump (H+-ATPase), lysosome-associated membrane proteins (LAMP-1 and LAMP-2), and neuropeptide-processing enzymes that are present in soluble and membrane-anchored forms (PC1, PC2, carboxypeptidase E/H, peptidylglycine α-monooxygenase).[53] Molecular cloning with subsequent immunochemical detection also identified catecholamine transporters (VMAT1 and VMAT2) as chromaffin granule membrane constituents.[59]

A large number of more minor but functionally important membrane

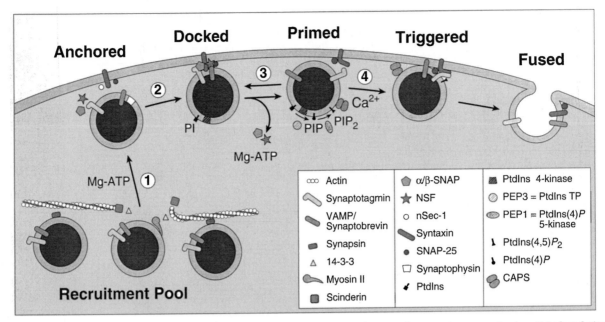

FIGURE 3–3. Late stages of dense-core vesicle exocytosis. The diagram depicts several stages that secretory granules transit before fusion with the plasma membrane. *1,* A recruitment pool of granules associated with cytoskeletal elements is recruited to the plasma membrane. *2,* Granules are anchored close to and docked at the plasma membrane by mechanisms that remain to be clarified. *3,* An ATP-dependent priming process involving the action of NSF on SNARE proteins and the synthesis of phosphatidylinositol 4,5-bisphosphonate (PIP$_2$) is required for granules to attain competence for calcium-triggered fusion. *4,* Calcium elevations to the 1 to 30 μM range trigger fusion in a process that requires SNARE proteins, synaptotagmin, and CAPS. Inset and symbols refer to several proteins essential at these stages of dense-core vesicle exocytosis (see Martin[67]). (From Martin TFJ: Stages of regulated exocytosis. Trends Cell Biol 7:271–276, 1997.)

protein constituents have been identified immunochemically on chromaffin granules by using antibodies to proteins initially discovered on the compositionally simpler neuronal small clear synaptic vesicles (see Fig. 3–6). Several of these proteins, which are also found on other neural and endocrine dense-core granules,[60] function in regulated exocytosis (synaptotagmin, synaptobrevin/VAMP [vesicle-associated membrane protein], Rab3A, cysteine string proteins). Proteins with putative regulatory roles (G$_o$ and ARF-6) or of unknown function (SV2, synaptophysin) have also been identified.[61, 62] Additional membrane constituents detected by activity include K$^+$ channels,[63] N-type Ca^{2+} channels,[64] and a phosphatidylinositol 4-kinase.[65]

SEQUENTIAL STAGES OF THE REGULATED SECRETORY PATHWAY

In most endocrine cells, the majority of dense-core granules are cytoplasmic, with only a small portion in direct contact with the plasma membrane in a docked state (see Fig. 3–2). Peptide hormone secretion upon cellular activation is believed to proceed by the rapid exocytotic fusion of a portion of the docked granules (release-ready pool), which are subsequently replenished by recruitment of granules to the plasma membrane from a cytoplasmic recruitment pool.[66, 67] Thus current views suggest a sequential pathway in which granules transit through recruitment, docking, and exocytotic fusion steps (Fig. 3–3). Evidence for the sequential model is provided by rapid kinetic studies of exocytosis by patch clamp electrophysiologic methods, in which increases in membrane capacitance reflect expansion of the surface membrane area after exocytosis,[68, 69] and from amperometry studies, which use carbon fiber electrodes to detect secreted oxidizable granule constituents such as catecholamines.[70] Capacitance increases and amperometric spikes from single granule fusion events have been detected in adrenal chromaffin and other secretory cell types.[68–71] Combining these techniques in a single pipette revealed that content release can occur during transient reversible fusion of the granule with the plasma membrane.[71] Cellular activation to elevate cytoplasmic calcium levels results in multiphasic increases in secretion (Fig. 3–4)

that consist of at least two components, an ultrafast (or exocytotic burst) component within the first 100 msec, followed by a slower component over the ensuing 1 to 10 seconds. These components of exocytosis are interpreted to represent the sequential fusion of secretory granules in a docked release-ready state, followed by fusion of

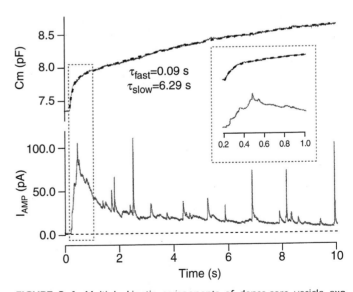

FIGURE 3–4. Multiple kinetic components of dense-core vesicle exocytosis in chromaffin cells. Capacitance measurements with a patch clamp pipette in the whole-cell configuration *(upper trace)* and amperometric current determinations with a carbon fiber electrode *(lower trace)* were obtained simultaneously from a bovine adrenal medullary cell that was stimulated by elevating calcium levels to 27 μM by flash photolysis with a photolabile calcium chelator. A rapid (exocytotic burst) component exhibiting a time constant of 0.09 seconds and a slow component with a time constant of 6.29 seconds were detected. (From Xu T, Binz T, Niemann H, Neher E: Multiple kinetic components of exocytosis distinguished by neurotoxin sensitivity. Nat Neurosci 1:192–200, 1998.)

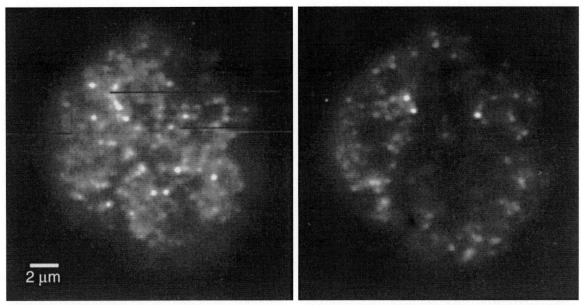

FIGURE 3–5. Exocytosis of chromaffin granules recorded by evanescent-wave fluorescence microscopy. Bovine adrenal medullary cells were loaded with acridine orange, an acidophilic dye, to render chromaffin granules fluorescent. Total internal reflection fluorescence microscopy was used to visualize granules in an optical section representing about 300 nm from the cell surface. Images were captured before *(left)* and after *(right)* 2 minutes of depolarization with high K+, during which numerous granules close to the cell surface underwent exocytosis. (Reprinted by permission from Steyer JA, Horstmann H, Almers W: Transport, docking and exocytosis of single secretory granules in live chromaffin cells. Nature 388:474–478, 1997. Copyright © MacMillan Magazines Ltd.)

granules that require recruitment into the release-ready pool.[68–72] The size of the exocytotic burst or release-ready pool (corresponding to 100–300 granules in chromaffin cells) is smaller than the number of morphologically detected docked granules (500–1000 granules in chromaffin cells, see Fig. 3–2), thus indicating that docked granules may exist in several functional states.[68, 73, 74] The release-ready pool represents a very small fraction of the cellular granule complement of 10 to 30,000.[54] Under physiologic stimulation conditions (i.e., splanchnic nerve stimulation), catecholamine secretion corresponding to 1% to 2% of the adrenal pool is mobilized, which indicates that the docked pool of granules in a release-ready pool is sufficient to mediate physiologic responses with short latency.[75] Similar fractional release during physiologic stimulation is commonly observed in other endocrine tissues.[76]

Recent technical developments have allowed the study of secretory granule movement in living neuroendocrine cells (Fig. 3–5). Fusion proteins consisting of prohormone peptides with green fluorescent protein at the carboxyl terminus undergo proper sorting to dense-core vesicles when expressed in neuroendocrine cells.[77–78] Confocal fluorescence or evanescent-wave microscopy has enabled the tracking of individual granules during their cytoplasmic translocation, docking at the plasma membrane, and exocytosis.[74, 77–79] Granule movement to the plasma membrane is a directed process that occurs at speeds of approximately 50 nm/second, followed by immobilization at the plasma membrane by a presumed docking process that either occasionally reverses or culminates in exocytosis if calcium levels are elevated.[74, 78, 79] New granules move to the plasma membrane and replenish the pool of docked granules within several minutes.[79] Sustained stimulated secretion entails a cytoplasmic pool of mobile granules.[77] Previous biochemical studies had implicated an actin cytoskeleton as a barrier to the plasma membrane recruitment of granules, but mediation of granule recruitment to the plasma membrane by motor proteins and cytoskeletal elements remains poorly understood.[67, 80]

ESSENTIAL PROTEIN MACHINERY FOR DENSE-CORE GRANULE EXOCYTOSIS

Regulated dense-core vesicle exocytosis is mediated by protein machinery that is the neuroendocrine counterpart of a universal core

apparatus generally involved in membrane fusion events.[81–84] The key neuroendocrine proteins are the SNARE (*s*oluble *N*SF [*N*-ethylmaleimide–sensitive factor] *a*ttachment protein *re*ceptor, or SNAP receptor) proteins syntaxin 1, SNAP-25, and synaptobrevin/VAMP2. Synaptobrevin/VAMP was initially identified[83, 84] as a brain synaptic vesicle and *Torpedo* cholinergic vesicle protein of approximately 18 kDa that spans the vesicle membrane with a short luminal C-terminal tail (Fig. 3–6). It is ubiquitously expressed in endocrine secretory tissues and localizes to large dense-core and small clear synaptic vesicles.[60] Syntaxin 1 was identified as a plasma membrane protein of around 35

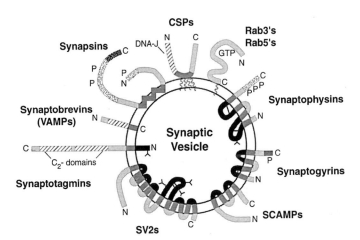

FIGURE 3–6. Membrane proteins associated with brain synaptic vesicles. Some of the characterized organelle-specific membrane proteins associated with synaptic vesicles are summarized in the figure. P indicates phosphorylation sites, and N or C refers to the N- or C-terminus of the proteins. Synaptic vesicles are compositionally simpler than dense-core vesicles. Many of these proteins have also been identified on dense-core vesicles with the exception of synapsins and synaptogyrins. (Reprinted by permission from Sudhof TC: The synaptic vesicle cycle: A cascade of protein-protein interactions. Nature 375:645–653, 1995. Copyright © MacMillan Magazines Ltd.)

kDa in a complex with synaptic vesicle proteins, and it has a membrane topology similar to that of synaptobrevin/VAMP.[83] SNAP-25 (synapse-associated protein of ~25 kDa) was discovered as a synapse-specific protein of 25 kDa by subtractive screening for brain-specific cDNAs.[85] The plasma membrane association of SNAP-25 is mediated by palmitoylation at four central cysteine residues. The central importance of SNARE proteins for calcium-dependent synaptic vesicle exocytosis is indicated by the finding that these three proteins constitute the major, if not exclusive substrates for clostridial neurotoxins,[86, 87] which are highly specific proteases that enter nerve cells by receptor-mediated endocytosis. Eight members of this bacterial neurotoxin family act to proteolytically cleave the three SNARE proteins at seven distinct cleavage sites (Table 3–1), which results in strong inhibition of neurotransmitter release. The neuroendocrine SNARE proteins were also identified as components of a 20S protein complex isolated by affinity chromatography of brain detergent extracts on immobilized NSF plus SNAP.[88] This observation linked the general role of NSF and SNAP proteins in constitutive membrane fusion to the function of neural proteins involved in synaptic vesicle exocytosis.[82]

The neuronal SNARE proteins exhibit an expression pattern that is not restricted to neurons, and virtually all peptide hormone–secreting endocrine tissues that have been examined express syntaxin 1, SNAP-25, and synaptobrevin/VAMP2.[60] Importantly, regulated peptide hormone secretion in all instances in which it has been examined is strongly inhibited by clostridial neurotoxins.[72, 81, 89] The neurotoxins need to be introduced into endocrine cells by cell permeabilization, microinjection, patch clamp pipette, or transfection methods because endocrine cells lack receptors that mediate endocytic uptake of the toxins.[86, 87] Inhibition of stimulated peptide hormone secretion by clostridial neurotoxins provides compelling evidence that regulated exocytosis in endocrine cells is a SNARE protein–dependent process.

SNARE proteins self-assemble into heterotrimeric complexes that are extremely stable.[90, 91] Structural studies of the central portion of the SNARE complex (Fig. 3–7) revealed that it consists of a four-helix bundle containing α-helical regions in parallel register contributed by each of the SNARE proteins, one each from the C-terminal segment of syntaxin 1 and the central region of synaptobrevin/VAMP and one each from the N- and C-terminal regions of SNAP-25.[92] Although this complex of SNARE proteins, as well as its individual constituents, is considered to be central to regulated exocytosis, their precise roles remain to be clarified (Fig. 3–8).

The self-assembly properties of the SNARE proteins in vitro,[90, 91] the specificity of their binding interactions,[83, 93] and their distribution on either vesicles or the plasma membrane originally led to a proposed role in vesicle–plasma membrane docking interactions,[82, 83, 88, 90] but this hypothesis has not been supported by subsequent toxin inhibition or genetic SNARE deletion studies.[94] More recently, a direct role for SNARE complexes in membrane fusion reactions has been suggested.[95-99] The formation of SNARE helix bundles contributed by the proteins in *trans* would be anticipated to mediate the close apposition of vesicle and plasma membranes that could drive bilayer mixing and fusion. There is direct experimental support in neuroendocrine cells for an essential role of SNARE proteins after secretory granule dock-

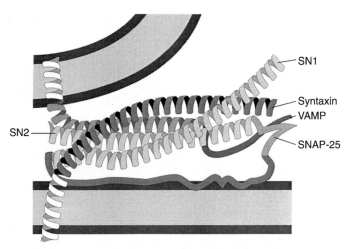

FIGURE 3–7. Structure of the neuronal SNARE protein complex. The structure of a protease-resistant core derived from heterotrimeric complexes of syntaxin 1, SNAP-25, and synaptobrevin/VAMP was solved by x-ray crystallography.[92] The figure reproduced here with modification from Sutton et al.[92] provides a hypothetic structure of the membrane-associated complex. The structure is a four-helix bundle consisting of helical regions in parallel register. Whereas syntaxin and synaptobrevin/VAMP each contribute a helical region, SNAP-25 contributes N-terminal (SN1) and C-terminal (SN2) regions connected by a linker region.

ing.[67, 89] However, it remains unclear whether SNARE protein interactions directly drive membrane fusion (as indicated in Fig. 3–8) or, alternatively, mediate essential steps required for membrane fusion.[95-97]

An additional set of biochemical reactions are essential for late steps in regulated dense-core vesicle exocytosis (see Fig. 3–3). ATP is required for the regulated secretion of hormones,[67, 68, 72] and multiple roles for ATP-dependent processes in the secretory granule exocytotic pathway have been described.[67] Granules proceed through an ATP-dependent priming step before calcium-triggered exocytosis.[100] Although this step involves in part the action of ATPase NSF on SNARE complexes,[101] it has also been found to involve ATP acting as a substrate for phospholipid phosphorylation reactions.[102, 103] Phosphatidylinositol on the secretory granule membrane undergoes conversion to PI-4-P and PI-4,5-P_2 catalyzed sequentially by granule phosphatidylinositol 4-kinase and by a soluble PIP 5-kinase[67, 103] (see Chapter 8). PI-4,5-P_2 may be synthesized to serve a signaling role on the granule for recruitment or activation of proteins for calcium-triggered fusion reactions.[47] One potential mechanism by which PIP_2 has been proposed to act is by activating CAPS, a neural/endocrine-specific PIP_2-binding protein that is required for the calcium-triggered exocytosis of dense-core granules.[104, 105] ATP-dependent priming involving the synthesis of PIP_2 may be a process that is restricted to dense-core vesicles and may not be essential for synaptic vesicle exocytosis.[106, 107] CAPS is required for dense-core vesicle but not synaptic vesicle exocytosis,[105, 108, 109] and this protein may play a role in mediating contact between the larger dense-core granules and the plasma membrane.[67]

REGULATION OF EXOCYTOSIS BY CALCIUM

The neuronal SNARE proteins that are essential for regulated exocytosis are the neuroendocrine counterparts of a protein superfamily whose members are required for membrane trafficking and fusion reactions in the constitutive secretory pathway.[82, 83] Unregulated constitutive secretion in the yeast *Saccharomyces cerevisiae* uses homologues of synaptobrevin/VAMP (SNC1/2), syntaxin 1 (SSO1/2), and SNAP-25 (SEC9).[83] A unique feature of neural synaptic vesicle and endocrine dense-core vesicle exocytosis is its regulation mediated by cytoplasmic calcium increases[66, 67, 84, 110] (see Chapter 8).

As studied in permeable neuroendocrine cells, regulated dense-core vesicle exocytosis is completely calcium dependent and activated by

TABLE 3–1. Clostridial Neurotoxin Substrates

Toxin	Substrate	Cleavage Site
Tetanus	Synaptobrevin/VAMP	Gln76-Phe77
Botulinum serotype B	Synaptobrevin/VAMP	Gln76-Phe77
Botulinum serotype D	Synaptobrevin/VAMP	Lys59-Leu60
Botulinum serotype F	Synaptobrevin/VAMP	Gln58-Lys59
Botulinum serotype G	Synaptobrevin/VAMP	Ala81-Ala82
Botulinum serotype A	SNAP-25	Gln197-Arg198
Botulinum serotype E	SNAP-25	Arg180-Ile181
Botulinum serotype C	Syntaxin	Lys253-Ala254
	SNAP-25	Arg198-Ala199

SNAP, soluble NSF (*N*-ethylmaleimide–sensitive factor) attachment protein; VAMP, vesicle-associated membrane protein.

Data from Montecucco and Schiavo[86] and Niemann et al.[87]

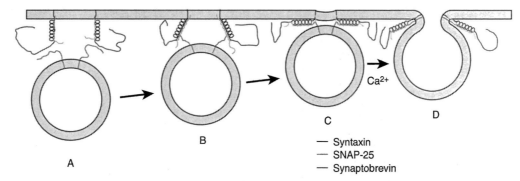

FIGURE 3–8. Hypothetic model of SNARE protein–mediated fusion. Although the SNARE protein complexes shown in Figure 3–7 are thought to be essential for an aspect of vesicle docking or fusion, their role remains to be elucidated. One hypothesis for the essential role of SNARE complexes is depicted in this figure. Heterodimers of syntaxin and SNAP-25 on the plasma membrane are shown progressively "zippering" with synaptobrevin/VAMP on the vesicle to form a four-helix bundle. In this model, SNARE complex formation is shown to promote the close apposition of membrane bilayers such that calcium, acting through a component not depicted, triggers the final transition to bilayer fusion. (Reprinted by permission from Jahn R, Hanson PI: SNAREs line up in a new environment. Nature 393:14–15, 1998. Copyright © MacMillan Magazines Ltd.)

calcium ion concentrations in the micromolar range.[110] The basal hormone secretion in intact endocrine cells that is detected in the absence of secretagogues, which is mediated by exocytosis of dense-core granules rather than by constitutive vesicles,[111] probably arises from cytoplasmic calcium that exceeds the threshold for activating exocytosis.

Although numerous mechanistic similarities can be found between the dense-core vesicle–mediated release of peptide hormones and biogenic amines in neuroendocrine cells and the synaptic vesicle–mediated release of neurotransmitters such as acetylcholine and glutamate in nerve cells, these two processes have significant differences in their physiologic regulation.[81, 108, 109] Dense-core vesicle exocytosis exhibits a longer latency (~10 msec) between calcium entry and fusion than does synaptic vesicle exocytosis, in which latencies of less than 1 msec have been reported.[66, 70] Most of the delay between calcium entry through calcium channels and hormone release has been attributed to the diffusion delay for calcium because of a lack of colocalization of dense-core granules with calcium channels.[112] Conversely, the short latency observed for evoked neurotransmitter release is thought to involve SNARE protein–mediated tethering of synaptic vesicles to N-type calcium channels.[113, 114] In addition to differences in latencies, dense-core granule exocytosis is triggered by calcium concentrations that are considerably lower (1–30 μM) than those reached in close proximity to open calcium channels that trigger synaptic vesicle exocytosis, which is estimated to occur with a median effective concentration of about 200 μM.[66, 81, 94, 109, 110, 115] Dense-core vesicle exocytosis is also triggered by cytoplasmic calcium rises resulting from inositol triphosphate–induced mobilization from the ER, which have been estimated to be lower than 5 μM even at cisternal sites that are located close to granules.[116]

Regulation of the dense-core granule exocytotic pathway by calcium, including granule recruitment, exocytosis, fusion pore dilation, and endocytic membrane retrieval, occurs at multiple sites. Release-ready granules are depleted by strong stimulation, and replenishment of the release-ready pool occurs within approximately 1 minute after depletion.[66, 117] Rates of pool replenishment depend on cytoplasmic calcium at concentrations lower than the threshold for exocytosis.[118] Although the molecular basis for calcium-dependent pool replenishment is unknown, it may be mediated in part through calcium activation of protein kinase C.[117, 119]

Calcium regulation of exocytosis has been proposed to be mediated by the synaptotagmins, a protein family not expressed in yeast whose members are abundant secretory vesicle C2 domain–containing proteins that bind three calcium ions.[84, 120] Genetic studies in *Drosophila*, *Caenorhabditis elegans*, and mice have demonstrated an essential role for synaptotagmins in evoked neurotransmitter release, but direct evidence that they mediate calcium sensing for exocytosis is lacking.[83, 94] Synaptotagmins exhibit calcium-dependent interactions with the plasma membrane SNARE proteins syntaxin 1 and SNAP-25 and

are found in biochemically isolated heterotrimeric SNARE complexes,[90] so it has been suggested that these proteins could directly mediate the calcium triggering of SNARE complex–dependent membrane fusion.[84]

The molecular basis for differences in the calcium sensitivity of dense-core and synaptic vesicle exocytosis is unclear. Multiple synaptotagmin isoforms are present on both vesicle classes, and it has been suggested that distinct isoforms may dictate differing calcium sensitivities for exocytosis. Synaptotagmin I and II exhibit low-affinity calcium binding characteristics of synaptic vesicle exocytosis, whereas synaptotagmin III and VII exhibit calcium sensitivities similar to that of dense-core vesicle exocytosis.[120] Alternatively, other calcium-binding proteins such as rabphilin,[121] CAPS,[104] or the SNARE complex itself[92] may mediate aspects of the calcium regulation of exocytosis.

After fusion, the rate of dilation of the fusion pore is regulated by calcium levels, but the molecular basis for this process is unknown.[122] Beyond fusion, retrieval of the dense-core granule membrane by endocytosis is stimulated by calcium in a calmodulin-dependent process.[123] In synaptic vesicle endocytosis, calcineurin, a calcium-activated, calmodulin-dependent protein phosphatase that dephosphorylates several proteins (dynamin, amphiphysin, synaptojanin) involved in endocytosis, is a major locus for calcium regulation.[124, 125] A similar mechanism may underlie calcium regulation of endocytic retrieval of the dense-core granule membrane, whose components are trafficked back to the Golgi.[2]

MODULATION OF CALCIUM-DEPENDENT HORMONE SECRETION BY PROTEIN KINASE C

Because the proximal regulator of dense-core granule exocytosis is cytoplasmic calcium, receptor mechanisms that mobilize intracellular calcium through inositol triphosphate generation or that promote calcium influx will correspondingly influence the rates of hormone secretion (see Chapter 8). However, other signal transduction pathways exert significant modulatory effects on calcium-dependent hormone secretion. In virtually all endocrine cells that have been examined, phorbol ester activators of protein kinase C enhance hormone secretion.[126] In some cases, phorbol ester stimulation of hormone secretion may be indirect and mediated through ion channel regulation that alters calcium entry.[127] However, stimulatory effects of phorbol esters are also seen at sites distal to calcium entry. In some cases, phorbol ester stimulation is observed at a low resting cytoplasmic calcium concentration,[128, 129] whereas in other cases, phorbol ester treatment synergistically enhances the stimulation of secretion by cytoplasmic calcium elevation.[130, 131] Although some phorbol ester–binding proteins other than protein kinase C (e.g, mUNC-13 protein) may mediate some of the actions of phorbol esters in the nervous system, a stimulatory role for protein kinase C on exocytosis has been directly demonstrated in studies of calcium-dependent hormone secretion in permeable neuroendocrine cells.[132, 133]

Protein kinase C regulates hormone secretion at several sites in the exocytotic pathway. Strong enhancing effects of phorbol esters on constitutive secretion have been reported and attributed to steps in the secretory pathway between the ER and Golgi or at vesicle-budding reactions in the TGN.[134–136] Stimulation of rate-limiting steps early in the secretory pathway will alter the transit of proteins to both the regulated and constitutive secretory pathways (see Fig. 3–1). In addition, protein kinase C activation stimulates steps in regulated secretion close to exocytosis. As inferred from phorbol ester treatment, replenishment of release-ready granules at the plasma membrane is enhanced by protein kinase C activation.[119] Direct stimulation of calcium-dependent exocytosis by protein kinase C at a postdocking step has also been observed in permeable neuroendocrine cells.[132]

Many protein substrates for protein kinase C have been identified in endocrine cells, but protein substrates that mediate the stimulatory effects of protein kinase C on hormone secretion or exocytosis have remained elusive.[137–139] Of identified proteins that function at a late step in regulated exocytosis, two (mUNC-18 and SNAP-25) have been shown to be direct substrates for protein kinase C–mediated phosphorylation.[140, 141] Although enhanced phosphorylation has been correlated with increases in regulated secretion, no direct evidence has shown that these proteins are essential mediators of the activating effects of protein kinase C on exocytosis. The search for a specific protein(s) substrate that mediates the ubiquitous stimulation of calcium-dependent hormone secretion by protein kinase C is ongoing.

REFERENCES

1. Palade G: Intracellular aspects of the process of protein synthesis. Science 189:347–358, 1975.
2. Farquhar MG: Multiple pathways of exocytosis, endocytosis, and membrane recycling: Validation of a Golgi route. Fed Proc 42:2407–2413, 1983.
3. Griffiths G, Simons K: The trans-Golgi network: Sorting at the exit site of the Golgi complex. Science 234:438–443, 1986.
4. Traub LM, Kornfeld S: The trans-Golgi network: A late secretory sorting station. Curr Opin Cell Biol 9:527–533, 1997.
5. Kelly RB: Pathways of protein secretion in eukaryotes. Science 230:25–32, 1985.
6. Burgess TL, Kelly RB: Constitutive and regulated secretion of proteins. Annu Rev Cell Biol 3:243–293, 1987.
7. Arvan P, Castle D: Sorting and storage during secretory granule biogenesis: Looking backward and looking forward. Biochem J 332:593–610, 1998.
8. Arvan P, Kuliawat R, Prabakaran D, et al: Protein discharge from immature secretory granules displays both regulated and constitutive characteristics. J Biol Chem 266:14171–14174, 1991.
9. Dittie A, Thomas L, Thomas G, Tooze SA: Interaction of furin in immature secretory granules from neuroendocrine cells with AP-1 adaptor complex is modulated by casein kinase II phosphorylation. EMBO J 16:4859–4870, 1997.
10. Tooze SA, Flatmark T, Tooze J, Huttner WB: Characterization of the immature secretory granule, an intermediate in granule biogenesis. J Cell Biol 115:1491–1503, 1991.
11. Phillips JH, Pryde JG: The chromaffin granule: A model system for the study of hormone and neurotransmitters. Ann N Y Acad Sci 493:27–42, 1987.
12. Rubin RP: Calcium and Cellular Secretion. New York, Plenum, 1982.
13. Schatz G, Dobberstein B: Common principles of protein translocation across membranes. Science 271:1519–1526, 1996.
14. Rouille Y, Duguay SJ, Lund K, et al: Proteolytic processing mechanisms in the biosynthesis of neuroendocrine peptides: The subtilisin-like proprotein convertases. Front Neuroendocrinol 16:322–361, 1995.
15. Halban PA, Irminger J-C: Sorting and processing of secretory proteins. Biochem J 299:1–18, 1994.
16. Creemers JWM, Jackson RS, Hutton JC: Molecular and cellular regulation of prohormone processing. Semin Cell Dev Biol 9:3–10, 1998.
17. Jung LJ, Scheller RH: Peptide processing and targeting in the neuronal secretory pathway. Science 251:1330–1335, 1991.
18. Orci L, Ravazzola M, Storch MJ, et al: Proteolytic maturation of insulin is a post-Golgi event which occurs in acidifying clathrin-coated secretory vesicles. Cell 49:865–868, 1987.
19. Eipper BA, Mains RE: Structure and biosynthesis of pro-adrenocorticotropin/endorphin and related peptides. Endocr Rev 1:1–27, 1980.
20. Hashimoto S, Fumagalli G, Zanini A, Meldolesi J: Sorting of three secretory proteins to distinct secretory granules in acidophilic cells of cow anterior pituitary. J Cell Biol 105:1579–1586, 1987.
21. Natori S, Huttner WB: Chromogranin B promotes sorting to the regulated secretory pathway of processing intermediates derived from a peptide hormone precursor. Proc Natl Acad Sci U S A 93:4431–4436, 1996.
22. Thiele C, Huttner WB: The disulfide-bonded loop of chromogranins, which is essential for sorting to secretory granules, mediates homodimerization. J Biol Chem 273:1223–1231, 1998.

23. Kromer A, Glombik MM, Huttner WB, Gerdes HH: Essential role of the disulfide-bonded loop of chromogranin B for sorting to secretory granules is revealed by expression of a deletion mutant in the absence of endogenous granin synthesis. J Cell Biol 140:1331–1346, 1998.
24. Kelly RB: Storage and release of neurotransmitters. Cell 72:43–53, 1993.
25. Cool DR, Normant E, Shen F-S, et al: Carboxypeptidase E is a regulated secretory pathway sorting receptor: Genetic obliteration leads to endocrine disorders in Cpe^fat mice. Cell 88:73–83, 1997.
26. Cool DR, Loh PY: Carboxypeptidase E is a sorting receptor for prohormones: Binding and kinetic studies. Mol Cell Endocrinol 139:7–13, 1998.
27. Thiele C, Gerdes HH, Huttner WB: Protein secretion: Puzzling receptors. Curr Biol 7:R496–R500, 1997.
28. Chanat E, Huttner WB: Milieu-induced selective aggregation of regulated secretory proteins in the trans-Golgi network. J Cell Biol 115:1505–1519, 1991.
29. Huttner WB, Natori S: Helper proteins for neuroendocrine secretion. Curr Biol 5:242–245, 1995.
30. Colomer V, Kicska GA, Rindler MJ: Secretory granule content proteins and the luminal domains of granule membrane proteins aggregate in vitro at mildly acidic pH. J Biol Chem 271:48–55, 1996.
31. Sheenan KIJ, Taylor NA, Docherty K: Calcium- and pH-dependent aggregation and membrane association of the precursor of the prohormone convertase PC2. J Biol Chem 269:18646–18650, 1994.
32. Alam MR, Johnson RC, Darlington DN, et al: Kalirin, a cytosolic protein with spectrin-like and GDP/GTP exchange factor–like domains that interacts with peptidylglycine alpha-amidating monooxygenase, an integral membrane peptide-processing enzyme. J Biol Chem 272:12667–12675, 1997.
33. Disdier M, Morrissey JH, Fugate RD, et al: Cytoplasmic domain of P selectin contains the signal for sorting into the regulated secretory pathway. Mol Biol Cell 3:309–321, 1992.
34. Marcusson EG, Horazdovsky BF, Cereghino JL, et al: The sorting receptor for yeast vacuolar carboxypeptidase Y is encoded by the VPS10 gene. Cell 77:579–586, 1994.
35. Rothman JE, Wieland FT: Protein sorting by transport vesicles. Science 272:227–234, 1996.
36. Kuehn MJ, Herrmann JM, Schekman R: COPII-cargo interactions direct protein sorting into ER-derived transport vesicles. Nature 391:187–190, 1998.
37. Tooze SA, Huttner WB: Cell-free protein sorting to the regulated and constitutive secretory pathways. Cell 60:837–847, 1990.
38. Tooze SA, Weiss U, Huttner WB: Requirement for GTP hydrolysis in the formation of secretory vesicles. Nature 347:207–208, 1990.
39. Ohashi M, DeVries KJ, Frank R, et al: A role for the phosphatidylinositol transfer protein in secretory vesicle formation. Nature 377:544–547, 1995.
40. Chen Y-G, Shields D: ADP-ribosylation factor-1 stimulates formation of nascent secretory vesicles from the trans-Golgi network of endocrine cells. J Biol Chem 271:297–300, 1996.
41. Barr FA, Huttner WB: A role for ADP-ribosylation factor 1, but not COP I, in secretory vesicle biogenesis from the trans-Golgi network. FEBS Lett 384:65–70, 1996.
42. Chen Y-G, Siddhanta A, Austin CD, et al: Phospholipase D stimulates release of nascent secretory vesicles from the trans-Golgi network. J Cell Biol 138:495–504, 1997.
43. Siddhanta A, Shields D: Secretory vesicle budding from the trans-Golgi network is mediated by phosphatidic acid levels. J Biol Chem 273:17995–17998, 1998.
44. Tuscher O, Lorra C, Bouma B, et al: Cooperativity of phosphatidylinositol transfer protein and phospholipase D in secretory vesicle formation from the TGN-phosphoinositides as a common denominator? FEBS Lett 419:271–275, 1997.
45. Simon J-P, Morimoto T, Bankaitis VA, et al: An essential role for the phosphatidylinositol transfer protein in the scission of coatomer-coated vesicles from the trans-Golgi network. Proc Natl Acad Sci U S A 95:11181–11186, 1998.
46. Martin TFJ: New directions for phosphatidylinositol transfer. Curr Biol 5:990–992, 1995.
47. Martin TFJ: Phosphoinositide lipids as signaling molecules: Common themes for signal transduction, cytoskeletal regulation and membrane trafficking. Annu Rev Cell Dev Biol 14:231–264, 1998.
48. Roth MG, Sternweis PC: The role of lipid signaling in constitutive membrane traffic. Curr Opin Cell Biol 9:519–526, 1997.
49. Greider MH, Howell SL, Lacy PE: Isolation and properties of secretory granules from rat islets of Langerhans. Ultrastructure of the beta granule. J Cell Biol 41:162–168, 1969.
50. Naggert JK, Fricker LD, Varlamov O, et al: Hyperproinsulinemia in obese fat/fat mice associated with a carboxypeptidase E mutation which reduces enzyme activity. Nat Genet 10:135–142, 1995.
51. Pelletier G, Labrie F: Anterior pituitary secretory granules. In Poisner AM, Trifaro JM (eds): The Secretory Granule. New York, Elsevier, 1982, pp 173–209.
52. Howell SL, Tyhurst M: The insulin storage granule. In Poisner AM, Trifaro JM (eds): The Secretory Granule. New York, Elsevier, 1982, pp 155–172.
53. Apps DK: Membrane and soluble proteins of adrenal chromaffin granules. Semin Cell Dev Biol 8:121–131, 1997.
54. Winkler H, Carmichael SW: The chromaffin granule. In Poisner L, Trifaro JM (eds): The Secretory Granule. New York, Elsevier, 1982, pp 3–79.
55. Winkler H: Membrane composition of adrenergic large and small dense core vesicles and of synaptic vesicles: Consequences for their biogenesis. Neurochem Res 8:921–932, 1997.
56. Westhead EW: Lipid composition and orientation in secretory vesicles. Ann N Y Acad Sci 493:92–100, 1987.
57. Wiedenmann B, Huttner WB: Synaptophysin and chromogranins/secretogranins—widespread constituents of distinct types of neuroendocrine vesicles and new tools in tumor diagnosis. Virchows Arch 58:95–121, 1989.

58. Howell SL, Montague W, Tyhurst M: Calcium distribution in islets of Langerhans: A study of calcium concentrations and of calcium accumulation in B cell organelles. J Cell Sci 19:395–409, 1975.
59. Liu Y, Schweitzer ES, Nirenberg MJ, et al: Preferential localization of vesicular monoamine transporter to dense core vesicles in PC12 cells. J Cell Biol 127:1419–1433, 1994.
60. Martin TFJ: Mechanisms of protein secretion in endocrine and exocrine cells. Vitam Horm 54:207–226, 1998.
61. Gasman S, Chasserot-Golaz S, Hubert P, et al: Identification of a potential effector pathway for the trimeric G₀ protein associated with secretory granules. J Biol Chem 273:16913–16920, 1998.
62. Caumont A-S, Galas M-C, Vitale N, et al: Regulated exocytosis in chromaffin cells—translocation of ARF6 stimulates a plasma membrane-associated phospholipase D. J Biol Chem 273:1373–1379, 1998.
63. Arispe N, De Mazancourt P, Rojas E: Direct control of a large conductance K⁺-selective channel by G proteins in adrenal chromaffin granule membranes. J Membr Biol 147:109–119, 1995.
64. Passafaro M, Rosa P, Sala C, et al: N-type Ca²⁺ channels are present in secretory granules and are transiently translocated to the plasma membrane during regulated exocytosis. J Biol Chem 271:30096–30104, 1996.
65. Phillips JH: Phosphatidylinositol kinase—a component of the chromaffin granule membrane. Biochem J 136:579–587, 1973.
66. Neher E: Vesicle pools and calcium microdomains: New tools for understanding their roles in neurotransmitter release. Neuron 20:389–399, 1998.
67. Martin TFJ: Stages of regulated exocytosis. Trends Cell Biol 7:271–276, 1997.
68. Parsons TD, Coorssen JR, Horstmann H, Almers W: Docked granules, the exocytic burst, and the need for ATP hydrolysis in endocrine cells. Neuron 15:1085–1096, 1995.
69. Neher E, Zucker RS: Multiple calcium-dependent processes related to secretion in bovine chromaffin cells. Neuron 10:21–30, 1993.
70. Chow RH, von Ruden L, Neher E: Delay in vesicle fusion revealed by electrochemical monitoring of single secretory events in adrenal chromaffin cells. Nature 356:60–63, 1992.
71. Albillos A, Dernick G, Horstmann H, et al: The exocytotic event in chromaffin cells revealed by patch amperometry. Nature 389:509–512, 1997.
72. Xu T, Binz T, Niemann H, Neher E: Multiple kinetic components of exocytosis distinguished by neurotoxin sensitivity. Nat Neurosci 1:192–200, 1998.
73. Plattner H, Artalejo AR, Neher E: Ultrastructural organization of bovine chromaffin cell cortex—analysis by cryofixation and morphometry of aspects pertinent to exocytosis. J Cell Biol 139:1709–1717, 1997.
74. Steyer JA, Horstmann H, Almers W: Transport, docking and exocytosis of single secretory granules in live chromaffin cells. Nature 388:474–478, 1997.
75. Blaschko H, Comline RS, Schneider FH, et al: Secretion of a chromaffin granule protein chromogranin from the adrenal gland after splanchnic stimulation. Nature 215:58–59, 1967.
76. Levine R: Mechanisms of insulin secretion. N Engl J Med 283:522–526, 1970.
77. Burke NV, Han W, Li D, et al: Neuronal peptide release is limited by secretory granule mobility. Neuron 19:1095–1102, 1997.
78. Lang T, Wacker I, Steyer J, et al: Ca²⁺-triggered peptide secretion in single cells imaged with green fluorescent protein and evanescent-wave microscopy. Neuron 18:857–863, 1997.
79. Oheim M, Loerke D, Stuhmer W, Chow RH: The last few seconds in the life of a secretory granule: Docking, dynamics and fusion visualized by total internal reflection fluorescence microscopy (TIRFM). Eur Biophys J 27:83–98, 1998.
80. Burgoyne RD: Control of exocytosis in adrenal chromaffin cells. Biochim Biophys Acta 1071:174–202, 1991.
81. Martin TFJ: The molecular machinery for fast and slow neurosecretion. Curr Opin Neurobiol 4:626–632, 1994.
82. Rothman JE: Mechanisms of intracellular protein transport. Nature 372:55–63, 1994.
83. Bennett MK, Scheller RH: A molecular description of synaptic vesicle membrane trafficking. Annu Rev Biochem 63:63–100, 1994.
84. Sudhof TC: The synaptic vesicle cycle: A cascade of protein-protein interactions. Nature 375:645–653, 1995.
85. Bark IC, Wilson MC: Regulated vesicular fusion in neurons: Snapping together the details. Proc Natl Acad Sci U S A 91:4621–4624, 1994.
86. Montecucco C, Schiavo G: Tetanus and botulism neurotoxins: A new group of zinc proteases. Trends Biochem Sci 18:324–329, 1993.
87. Niemann H, Blasi J, Jahn R: Clostridial neurotoxins: New tools for dissecting exocytosis. Trends Cell Biol 4:179–185, 1994.
88. Sollner T, Whiteheart SW, Brunner M, et al: SNAP receptors implicated in vesicle targeting and fusion. Nature 362:318–324, 1993.
89. Banerjee J, Kowalchyk JA, DasGupta BR, Martin TFJ: SNAP-25 is required for a late postdocking step in calcium-dependent exocytosis. J Biol Chem 271:20227–20230, 1996.
90. Sollner T, Bennett MK, Whiteheart SW et al: A protein assembly-disassembly pathway in vitro that may correspond to sequential steps of synaptic vesicle docking, activation and fusion. Cell 75:409–418, 1993.
91. Hayashi T, McMahon H, Yamasaki S, et al: Synaptic vesicle membrane fusion complex: Action of clostridial neurotoxins on assembly. EMBO J 13:5051–5061, 1994.
92. Sutton RB, Fasshauer D, Jahn R, Brunger AT: Crystal structure of a SNARE complex involved in synaptic exocytosis at 2.4A resolution. Nature 395:347–353, 1998.
93. Bennett MK: SNAREs and the specificity of transport vesicle targeting. Curr Opin Cell Biol 7:581–586, 1995.
94. Augustine GJ, Burns ME, DeBello WM, et al: Exocytosis: Proteins and perturbations. Annu Rev Pharmacol Toxicol 36:659–701, 1996.
95. Hanson P, Heuser J, Jahn R: Neurotransmitter release—four years of SNARE complexes. Curr Opin Neurobiol 7:310–315, 1997.
96. Jahn R, Hanson PI: SNAREs line up in a new environment. Nature 393:14–15, 1998.
97. Weis WI, Scheller RH: SNARE the rod, coil the complex. Nature 395:328–329, 1998.
98. Rizo J, Sudhof TC: Mechanics of membrane fusion. Nat Struct Biol 5:839–842, 1998.
99. Weber T, Zemelman, McNew JA, et al: SNAREpins: Minimal machinery for membrane fusion. Cell 92:759–772, 1998.
100. Hay JC, Martin TFJ: Resolution of regulated secretion into sequential MgATP-dependent and calcium-dependent stages mediated by distinct cytosolic proteins. J Cell Biol 119:139–151, 1992.
101. Banerjee J, Barry VA, DasGupta BR, Martin TFJ: N-ethylmaleimide–sensitive factor acts at a prefusion ATP-dependent step in calcium-activated exocytosis. J Biol Chem 271:20223–20226, 1996.
102. Hay JC, Martin TFJ: Phosphatidylinositol transfer protein required for ATP-dependent priming of calcium-activated secretion. Nature 366:572–575, 1993.
103. Hay JC, Fisette PL, Jenkins GH, et al: ATP-dependent inositide phosphorylation required for calcium-activated secretion. Nature 374:173–177, 1995.
104. Ann K, Kowalchyk JA, Loyet KM, Martin TFJ: Novel calcium binding protein (CAPS) related to UNC-31 required for calcium-activated exocytosis. J Biol Chem 272:19637–19640, 1997.
105. Loyet KM, Kowalchyk JA, Chaudhary A, et al: Specific binding of PIP₂ to CAPS, a potential phosphoinositide effector protein for regulated exocytosis. J Biol Chem 273:8337–8343, 1998.
106. Khvotchev M, Sudhof TC: Newly synthesized phosphatidylinositol phosphates are required for synaptic norepinephrine but not glutamate or γ-aminobutyric acid release. J Biol Chem 273:21451–21454, 1998.
107. Wiedemann C, Schafer T, Burger MM, Sihra TS: An essential role for a small synaptic vesicle–associated phosphatidylinositol 4-kinase in neurotransmitter release. J Neurosci 18:5594–5602, 1998.
108. Berwin B, Floor E, Martin TFJ: CAPS (mammalian UNC-31) protein localizes to membranes involved in dense-core vesicle exocytosis. Neuron 21:137–145, 1998.
109. Tandon A, Bannykh S, Kowalchyk JA, et al: Differential regulation of exocytosis by calcium and CAPS in semi-intact synaptosomes. Neuron 21:147–154, 1998.
110. Burgoyne RD, Morgan A: Calcium and secretory-vesicle dynamics. Trends Neurosci 18:191–196, 1995.
111. Varro A, Nemeth J, Dickinson CJ, et al: Discrimination between constitutive secretion and basal secretion from the regulated secretory pathway in GH3 cells. Biochim Biophys Acta 1313:101–105, 1996.
112. Chow RH, Klingauf J, Heinemann C, et al: Mechanisms determining the time course of secretion in neuroendocrine cells. Neuron 16:369–376, 1996.
113. Sheng Z-H, Rettig J, Cook T, Catterall WA: Calcium-dependent interaction of N-type calcium channels with the synaptic core complex. Nature 379:451–454, 1996.
114. Mochida S, Sheng Z-H, Baker C, et al: Inhibition of neurotransmission by peptides containing the synaptic protein interaction site of N-type calcium channels. Neuron 17:781–788, 1996.
115. Heidelberger R, Heinemann C, Neher E, Matthews G: Calcium dependence of the rate of exocytosis in a synaptic terminal. Nature 371:513–515, 1994.
116. Tse FW, Tse A, Hille B, et al: Local calcium release from internal stores controls exocytosis in pituitary gonadotrophs. Neuron 18:121–132, 1997.
117. Smith C, Moser T, Xu T, Neher E: Cytosolic calcium acts by two separate pathways to modulate the supply of release-competent vesicles in chromaffin cells. Neuron 20:1243–1253, 1998.
118. von Ruden L, Neher E: A Ca²⁺-dependent early step in the release of catecholamines from adrenal chromaffin cells. Science 262:1061–1065, 1993.
119. Gills KD, Mossner R, Neher E: Protein kinase enhances exocytosis from chromaffin cells by increasing the size of the readily releasable pool of secretory granules. Neuron 16:1209–1220, 1996.
120. Sudhof TC, Rizo J: Synaptotagmins: C2-domain proteins that regulate membrane traffic. Neuron 17:379–388, 1996.
121. Chung S-H, Takai Y, Holz RW: Evidence that the Rab3a-binding protein Rabphilin enhances regulated secretion. J Biol Chem 270:16714–16718, 1995.
122. Scepek S, Coorssen J, Lindau M: Fusion pore expansion in horse eosinophils is modulated by calcium and protein kinase C via distinct mechanisms. EMBO J 17:4340–4345, 1998.
123. Artalejo CR, Elhamdani A, Palfrey HC: Calmodulin is the divalent cation receptor for rapid endocytosis, but not exocytosis, in adrenal chromaffin cells. Neuron 16:195–205, 1996.
124. Marks B, McMahon HT: Calcium triggers calcineurin-dependent synaptic vesicle recycling in mammalian nerve terminals. Curr Biol 8:740–749, 1998.
125. Slepnev VI, Ochoa G-C, Butler MH, et al: Role of phosphorylation in regulation of the assembly of endocytic coat complexes. Science 281:821–824, 1998.
126. Nishizuka Y: Intracellular signaling by hydrolysis of phospholipids and activation of protein kinase C. Science 258:607–614, 1992.
127. Conn PJ, Sweatt JD: Protein kinase C in the nervous system. *In* Kuo JF (ed): Protein Kinase C. Oxford, Oxford University Press, 1994, pp 199–235.
128. Knight DE, Baker PF: The phorbol ester TPA increases the affinity of exocytosis for calcium ions in "leaky" adrenal medullary cells. FEBS Lett 160:98–100, 1983.
129. Billiard J, Koh D-S, Babcock DF, Hille B: Protein kinase C as a signal for exocytosis. Proc Natl Acad Sci U S A 94:12192–12197, 1997.
130. Yamanishi J, Takai K, Kaibuchi K, et al: Synergistic functions of phorbol ester and calcium in serotonin release from human platelets. Biochem Biophys Res Commun 112:778–786, 1983.
131. Ronning SA, Martin TFJ: Characterization of phorbol ester– and diacylglycerol-stimulated secretion in permeable GH₃ pituitary cells. J Biol Chem 261:7840–7845, 1986.
132. Nishizaki T, Walent JH, Kowalchyk JA, Martin TFJ: A key role for a 145 kD cytosolic protein in the stimulation of calcium-dependent secretion by protein kinase C. J Biol Chem 267:23972–23981, 1992.

133. Naor Z, Dan-Cohen H, Hermon J, Limor R: Induction of exocytosis in permeabilized pituitary cells by alpha- and beta-type protein kinase C. Proc Natl Acad Sci U S A 86:4501–4504, 1989.
134. Luini A, DeMatteis MA: Receptor-mediated regulation of constitutive secretion. Trends Cell Biol 3:290–292, 1993.
135. Westermann P, Knoblich M, Maier O, et al: Protein kinase C bound to the Golgi apparatus supports the formation of constitutive transport vesicles. J Biol Chem 320:651–658, 1996.
136. Simon JP, Ivanov IE, Shopsin B, et al: The in vitro generation of post-Golgi vesicles carrying viral envelope glycoproteins requires an ARF-like GTP-binding protein and a protein kinase C associated with the Golgi apparatus. J Biol Chem 271:16952–16961, 1996.
137. Pocotte SL, Frye RA, Senter RA, et al: Effects of phorbol ester on catecholamine secretion and protein phosphorylation in adrenal medullary cell cultures. Proc Natl Acad Sci U S A 82:930–934, 1985.
138. Drust DS, Martin TFJ: Thyrotropin-releasing hormone rapidly activates protein phosphorylation in GH_3 pituitary cells by a lipid-linked, protein kinase C–mediated pathway. J Biol Chem 259:14520–14530, 1984.
139. Morgan A, Burgoyne RD: Interaction between protein kinase C and exo I and its relevance to exocytosis in permeabilized adrenal chromaffin cells. Biochem J 286:807–811, 1992.
140. Fujita Y, Sasaki T, Fukui, et al: Phosphorylation of Munc-18/n-Sec1/rbSec1 by protein kinase C. J Biol Chem 271:7265–7268, 1996.
141. Shimazaki Y, Nishiki T, Omori A, et al: Phosphorylation of 25 kD synaptosome–associated protein. J Biol Chem 271:14548–14553, 1996.

Receptor Tyrosine Kinases

Joseph Avruch

Protein phosphorylation, reciprocally regulated by protein kinases and protein phosphatases, is the dominant posttranslational modification used for rapid reversible control of intracellular protein function. The vast majority of protein phosphorylation occurs on the hydroxyl amino acid residues serine and threonine, with less than 1% recovered on tyrosine. Despite this low abundance, protein tyrosine phosphorylation plays a crucial role in cellular regulation. Phosphotyrosine does not occur in prokaryotes, and tyrosine-specific protein kinases are not evident in the *Saccharomyces cerevisiae* (a fungal) genome. Yeast protein tyrosine–specific phosphatases do exist, however; these enzymes apparently act to reverse tyrosine phosphorylations catalyzed by so-called dual-specificity kinases, a minor class of protein kinases (e.g., mitogen-activated protein [MAP] kinase kinases [MKKs]; see below and Chapter 9) capable of phosphorylating both Ser/Thr and tyrosine residues concomitantly on their substrates. The earliest evidence of tyrosine-specific protein phosphorylation is in the cellular slime mold *Dictyostelium discoideum*, a probable precursor of the animal and fungal phyla. Protein kinase catalytic domain sequences clearly recognizable as protein tyrosine kinases are first observed in the earliest multicellular forms of the animal phyla, such as sponges and hydra. These observations, together with the pivotal role of tyrosine phosphorylation in mammalian cellular differentiation, point to the probable emergence of tyrosine-specific protein kinases at the dawn of metazoan evolution, concomitant with the development of multicellular animals containing differentiated cell types.

Tyrosine-specific protein kinases are classified into two major groups, the receptor tyrosine kinases (RTKs) and the nonreceptor tyrosine kinases (Table 4–1). The former are transmembrane proteins whose extracellular segment contains a ligand-binding domain, a single transmembrane segment followed by an intracellular extension that contains the tyrosine kinase catalytic domain (Fig. 4–1). Catalytic activity is normally controlled by occupancy of the extracellular ligand-binding domain, with activation resulting from ligand-induced apposition of the RTK polypeptides as homodimers or heterodimers. The nonreceptor tyrosine kinases are entirely intracellular, mostly cytoplasmic proteins whose catalytic activity is regulated through protein-protein interactions, usually at the plasma membrane (Fig. 4–2). Both classes of protein tyrosine kinases participate in signal transduction pathways that specify cell differentiation and/or proliferation, with the former outcome predominant in vivo and proliferation most evident when examined in a tissue culture setting using immortalized cells. An exception is the insulin receptor (IR), which acts primarily to control cellular fuel metabolism on a minute-to-minute basis.

The RTKs, by virtue of their regulation by extracellular ligands such as insulin, polypeptide growth factors, and other cell surface and extracellular matrix proteins, are perched at the apex of cellular signaling pathways, whereas the intracellular tyrosine kinases act as one of several signal generators downstream of these and other receptors. This chapter will focus on the RTKs, with emphasis placed on their structure, general mechanism of activation/deactivation, the signal

transduction pathways most relevant to their action, their reciprocal interactions with other signaling pathways, mechanisms of downregulation/desensitization, and their role in disease, particularly disease of the endocrine system.

HISTORY

The work that led to the discovery of RTKs arose from the effort to understand the biochemical basis for the transforming activity of acutely transforming oncogenic retroviruses such as the Rous sarcoma virus, a tumor virus of chickens. Earlier work had shown that Rous sarcoma virus encoded just a few genes,[4, 5] only one of which, named v-Src, appeared to be both indispensable to cellular transformation and lacking other known function (e.g., envelope protein, reverse transcriptase). This viral gene came to be considered the oncogene, and the protein product, pp60 v-Src, the transforming agent. In 1978, Collett and Erikson, having succeeded in obtaining a polyclonal antibody to pp60 v-Src, showed that immunoprecipitates of this antigen, incubated in vitro in the presence of γ-^{32}P-ATP, catalyzed the transfer of ^{32}P onto the immunoglobulin heavy chain,[1] thus indicating that protein kinase activity had been precipitated by this antibody, which was perhaps attributable to the pp60 v-Src itself. Subsequently, a subset of transforming antigens were shown to possess such protein kinase activity. This finding immediately implied that transformation could be due to inappropriate phosphorylation of cellular proteins. This view was strongly supported by the discovery that pp60 v-Src catalyzed the phosphorylation of a novel target, specifically, protein tyrosine residues. In 1979, Hunter and colleagues,[2] while characterizing the amino acid residue phosphorylated in vitro on polyomavirus middle T antigen, noted that the ^{32}P-amino acid recovered in acid hydrolysates of ^{32}P-labeled middle T antigen did not migrate on electrophoresis exactly with a phosphothreonine standard, as had previously been reported for pp60 v-Src; by changing the pH of the electrophoresis buffer from 1.9 to 3.5, an entirely clean separation of the ^{32}P-amino acid from the phosphothreonine standard was obtained, thus indicating that the residue phosphorylated on polyoma middle T antigen was novel. The identity of the novel phosphoamino acid generated in vitro on middle T antigen, as well as by the Rous sarcoma virus[3] and Abl[4] oncoproteins, was rapidly shown to be phosphotyrosine, a known but uncharacterized amino acid derivative. Thus these transforming proteins were associated with a tyrosine-specific protein kinase activity.

Contemporaneously, Stanley Cohen, the first to purify the polypeptide, epidermal growth factor (EGF), was attempting to detect and isolate the EGF receptor (EGFR). Using radioiodinated EGF polypeptide, Cohen surveyed cell lines for receptor abundance and identified a human epidermoid carcinoma cell line (A431) that expressed more than 10^6 EGFRs per cell; the addition of EGF to membrane vesicles from these cells stimulated overall ^{32}P incorporation from γ-^{32}P-ATP into the membrane proteins severalfold. Further work showed that

TABLE 4–1. Protein Tyrosine Kinases

Receptor tyrosine kinases

Epidermal growth factor receptor family	Fibroblast growth factor receptor family
EGF receptor c-ErbB	FGF receptor-1 (Flg/Cek1)
ErbB2 Neu HER2	FGF receptor-2 (Bek/K-Sam Cek3)
ErbB3 HER3	FGF receptor-3
ErbB4 HER4 Tyro2	FGF receptor-4
Insulin receptor family	
Insulin receptor	Nerve growth factor receptor family
IGF-1 receptor	NGF receptor (Trk)
Insulin receptor–related kinase	BDNF/NT-3/NT-4/5 receptor (TrkB)
IRR	NT-3 receptor (TrkC)
c-Ros	
Ltk	
Alk	
	Platelet-derived growth factor receptor family
Hepatic growth factor (HGF) receptor family	PDGF receptor α *patch* locus
HGF receptor Met	PDGF receptor β
Ron	CSF-1 receptor (c-Fms)
c-Sea	SCF receptor (c-Kit) (*W* locus)
	Flk2/Flt3
Vascular endothelial growth factor receptor family	Ror family
	Ror1
VEGF receptor (Flt1)	Ror2
VEGF receptor (Flk1)	DDr family
KDR	DDR (Nep/Cak)
Flt4	TKT/Tyro10
Eph family	Axl family
EphA1 (Eph)	Axl (UFO/Ark/Tyro7)
EphA2 (Eck/Sek2/Myk2)	Rse (Brt/Sky/Tif/Tyro3)
EphA3 (Hek/Cek4/Mek4/ Tyro4)	Dtk/Etk2)
EphA4 (Sek1/Cek8/Hek8/ Tyro1)	Mer (c-Eyk/Nyk/Tyr12)
	Tie family
EphA5 (Cek7/Bsk/Hek7/Ehk1/ Rek7)	Tie
	Tek/Tie2
EphA6 (Ehk2)	Ret family
EphA7 (Hek11/Mdk1/Ehk3/ Ebk)	Klg
	Ryk (Nyk-r/Voik)
EphA8 (Eek/Ptk4)	MuSK (Nsk2)
EphB1 (Elk/Cek6/Net)	
EphB2 (Cek5/Nuk/Erk/Sek3/ Tyro5/Hek5)	
EphB3 (Hek2/Cek10/Sek4/ Mdk5/Tyro6)	
EphB4 (Myk1/Htk/Hek5)	
EphB5 (Cek9)	
EphB6 (Mep)	

Nonreceptor tyrosine kinases

Src family	Src family related
c-Src	Frk/Rak (Mkk3)
c-Yes	Brk (Sik)
Fyn	Srm
Yrk	Sad
Lck	Lyk
Lyn	Btk family
c-Fgr	Btk (Atk/Bpk/Emb)
Blk	Itk (Tsk/Emt)
Hck	Tec
Csk family	Bmx (Etk)
Csk (Cyl)	Txk (Rlk)
Ctk (Hyl/Matk/Ntk/Lsk/Batk)	
Abl family	Janus kinase family
c-Abl	JAK1
Arg	JAK2
Fes/Fps family	JAK3
c-Fes/Fps	Tyk2
Fer	Fak family
Twin SH2 domain family	Fak
Zap 70	Pyk2
Syk	Ack family
	Ack
	AckII

the EGF-binding activity and EGF-stimulated autokinase activities exhibited copurification. The EGFR, purified as a 180-kDa polypeptide, proved to be the dominant substrate for the EGF-stimulated membrane phosphorylation reaction. Moreover, using the newly modified conditions for phosphoamino acid separation, Cohen showed that the amino acid modified by EGF-stimulated phosphorylation was not threonine, as originally concluded, but tyrosine.[5]

These findings established EGFR as the first RTK and provided the first linkage between the biochemical function of retroviral transforming proteins and human growth factor receptors. In 1982, the receptors for insulin,[6] insulin-like growth factor-1 (IGF-1), and platelet-derived growth factor[7] (PDGF) were shown to possess analogous ligand-activated tyrosine kinase activity. The identification in 1983 of the v-*sis* oncogene as a transduced form of the PDGF (B) gene[8, 9] and the discovery in 1984 that the molecular sequence of the v-*Erb*-B oncogene[10] and the EGFR were closely related served to reinforce the conceptual link between RTKs and cellular growth regulation. By 1990, a large number of RTKs assignable to several subfamilies had been identified.

RECEPTOR TYROSINE KINASE SUBFAMILIES

The RTKs are all type 1 membrane proteins, with large N-terminal extracellular ligand-binding domains, a single membrane-spanning segment, and an intracellular extension encompassing the catalytic domain (see Fig. 4–1). The RTK extracellular domains vary greatly in structure across subfamilies, which is a reflection of the broad diversity of interacting ligands. RTK polypeptides are monomeric proteins, with the exception of the insulin and hepatic growth factor receptor (HGFR) subfamilies; here the receptors are synthesized as a single polypeptide chain and cotranslationally cleaved into two subunits that become covalently linked through disulfide bonds. The IR-α/β heterodimer then undergoes further oligomerization through the formation of disulfide bonds between two α subunits, which represents the N-terminal, extracellular, ligand-binding component, to form a covalent βααβ tetramer; only the β subunit spans the membrane and contains the tyrosine kinase domain. RTK catalytic domains, approximately 260 amino acids in length, all exhibit nearly 30% amino acid sequence identity and in turn exhibit the conserved features of the protein kinase superfamily. The number of human RTKs known has grown to nearly 60, and despite the overall similarities in catalytic domain sequence, at least 16 subfamilies can be identified based on the alignment of catalytic domain amino acid sequences.

LIGAND BINDING

Very little definitive structural information is available regarding the interaction of an RTK ligand with its receptor-binding site. Nevertheless, for those ligand-receptor pairs whose interaction has been studied in depth, a large and compelling body of data indicate that ligand binding causes dimerization of two RTK polypeptides, or in the case of the preassembled IR (βααβ) structure, ligand promotes an even more intimate coupling between the two αβ half-receptors.[11–15] Importantly, this ligand-induced dimerization is indispensable to the ability of ligand to activate the kinase catalytic function. Mutations in the RTK or ligand that inhibit dimerization prevent ligand-dependent kinase activation, and a variety of mutations or gene translocations that cause ligand-independent dimerization of the kinase domain are sufficient to cause ligand-independent kinase activation. Ligand-induced RTK dimerization may be achieved because the ligand itself is a dimer (e.g., PDGF and CSF-1 are disulfide linked dimers, whereas c-kit ligand/stem cell factor is a noncovalent dimer), because a monomeric ligand has two binding surfaces (e.g., EGF and probably insulin), or because a monomeric ligand is bridged to a second ligand by an accessory molecule (e.g., fibroblast growth factor [FGF]) (Fig. 4–3).

PDGF occurs as a homodimer or heterodimer of A and/or B chains; the PDGF A chain binds only to the α isoform of the PDGF receptor (PDGFR), whereas the PDGF B chain binds with high affinity to both

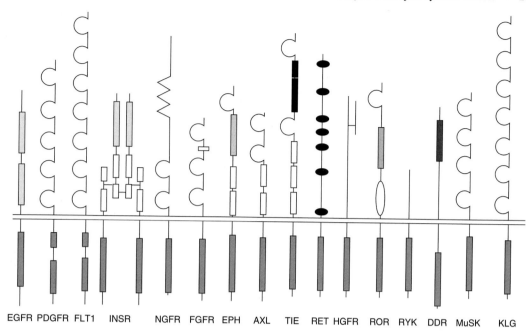

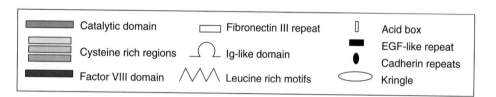

FIGURE 4–1. *Schematic structures of receptor protein-tyrosine kinase families. (From Hunter T: The Croonian Lecture, 1997. Phil Trans Roy Soc Lond B 353:587, 1997.)*

the α and β isoforms of PDGFR. Thus PDGF AA will dimerize and activate only PDGFR αα dimers, PDGF AB activates αα and αβ PDGFR dimers, and PDGF BB dimerizes and activates all three possible PDGFR dimers.[14]

An even more diverse array of ligand-receptor dimers is available in the EGF/EGFR (ErbB) family[16, 17] (Fig. 4–4). Invertebrates, such as *Drosophila* or *Caenorhabditis elegans,* exhibit one ErbB homologue, and four ligands are known for the *Drosophila* EGFR homologue (DER); three are activating ligands and include one membrane-bound transforming growth factor-α (TGF-α) homologue (Gurken), a second TGF-α homologue that acts as a soluble ligand after proteolytic cleavage from a membrane precursor (Spitz), and a third, conventional secreted polypeptide (Vein), homologous to the mammalian ErbB[3/4] ligands, termed neuregulin.[18, 19] A fourth ligand, Argos, appears to be a diffusible inhibitory DER ligand whose expression is activated by DER signaling. Four ErbB RTK isoforms have been identified in mammalian systems and at least a dozen high-affinity ligands with a dissociation constant (K_d) in the nanomolar range. The expanded mammalian ErbB family consists of ErbB[1], the EGFR, which binds at least six distinct ligands with high affinity (EGF, TGF-α, amphiregulin, β-cellulin, heparin-binding EGF, and epiregulin); ErbB[2], for which no high-affinity ligand (i.e., K_d in the nanomolar range) is known; ErbB[3], which binds strongly to the neuregulins and less avidly to EGF, β-cellulin, and epiregulin but completely lacks kinase activity because of amino acid sequence variation at a number of catalytic domain residues otherwise highly conserved among the protein kinase superfamily; and ErbB[4], which has ligand-binding properties similar to those of ErbB[3] but contains a catalytically competent kinase domain. Among ligands for which the question of valency has been examined, specifically, EGF and neuregulin, considerable evidence indicates that these ligand polypeptides each contain two topologically distinct binding sites that bind to different regions on the RTK surface. EGF is thus bivalent, and therefore a single EGF polypeptide can dimerize a pair of EGFRs. ErbB[2], although lacking high-affinity binding sites for any known ligand, is readily coprecipitated as a heterodimer with the other ErbB isoforms in a ligand-dependent manner and often in prefer-

ence to the generation of ErbB[1], ErbB[3], or ErbB[4] homodimers. This behavior is probably explained by the existence of low-affinity (K_d in the micromolar range) binding sites on ErbB[2] for many EGF-like ligands. In turn, the ligand surfaces that participate in this low-affinity interaction with ErbB[2] are probably different from those involved in the high-affinity interactions with other ErbB isoforms and are therefore probably available, in a noncompetitive manner, for binding to unoccupied ErbB[2] after initial ligand binding to the high-affinity site on the other ErbB isoforms (Fig. 4–5). In this manner, ErbB[2], despite its lack of a high-affinity binding site, functions as a potent and preferred coreceptor.[16] The ErbB[2/3] heterodimer, for example, generates a very potent and prolonged signal even though the ErbB[3] dimer half is catalytically inactive. It is likely that all the EGF-like ligands are bivalent (except perhaps the inhibitory ligand Argos) and thereby engender a combinatorial array of ErbB homodimers and heterodimers. The ErbB family members are important proproliferative elements in many human cancers through either activating mutations, overexpression, or autocrine autostimulation.

Recent evidence suggests that insulin is also a bivalent ligand for the IR and provides two surfaces that each bind to a distinct site on the IR-α subunit, one with high affinity and the other with low affinity. Optimal apposition (i.e., for kinase activation) of the two IR-αβ halves is achieved when a single insulin molecule is bound to the high-affinity site on one α subunit and to the low-affinity site on the other α subunit, that is, a stoichiometry of one insulin per βααβ receptor assembly. This model explains some long-standing anomalies in insulin action, such as the occurrence of diminished IR signaling at very high insulin concentrations. Presumably, large excesses of insulin ($\geq 10^{-7}$ mol/L, never achieved in vivo) enable binding of two insulins per βααβ assembly, each to the high-affinity site, which results in a receptor configuration that is less productive for kinase activation.[20] Interestingly, despite the 49% identity in amino acid sequence and great similarity in three-dimensional structures between insulin and IGF-1,[21] as well as the considerable amino acid sequence identity in the α subunits of the IR and IGF-1 receptor (IGF-1R) and particularly the very high conservation in the placement of cysteine residues and

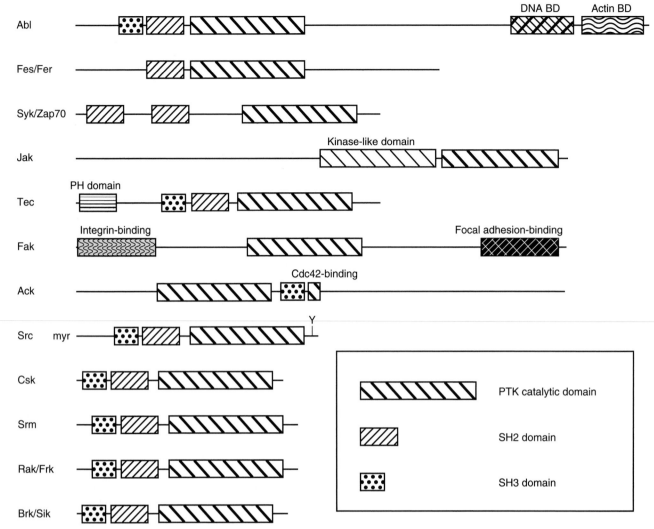

FIGURE 4–2. Schematic structures of nonreceptor protein tyrosine kinase (PTK) families. (From Hunter T: The Croonian Lecture, 1997. Phil Trans Roy Soc Lond B 353:586, 1997.)

N-linked glycosylation sites in the two α subunits, each receptor nevertheless binds the cognate ligand with about 100-fold higher affinity than it binds the other ligand. Moreover, insulin binding to the IR exhibits negative cooperativity (i.e., binding of the first insulin to

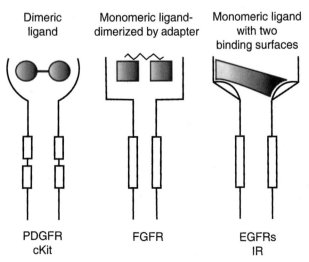

FIGURE 4–3. Differing modes of ligand-induced dimerization of receptor protein-tyrosine kinases.

the α₂β₂ receptor inhibits the binding of a second insulin molecule to the same receptor), whereas IGF-1 binding to the IGF-1R exhibits no cooperativity. In view of these differences, the finding that insulin and IGF-1 bind to very different sites on their respective receptors, in part through different ligand surface domains, is not entirely surprising.[22] High-affinity IGF-1 binding to the IGF-1R is crucially dependent on the integrity of the IGF-1R cysteine-rich domain; swapping this segment from the IGF-1R into the IR confers high affinity for IGF-1 but does not abrogate high-affinity insulin binding, whereas the reciprocal swap (IR cysteine-rich domain into the IGF-1R) gives a chimera incapable of high-affinity binding to either ligand. In contrast, high-affinity insulin binding requires specific IR-α residues N-terminal to the cysteine-rich domain (IR amino acids 38–68), and if amino acids found at these IR sites crucial to high-affinity insulin binding are introduced into the homologous sites on the IGF-1R, high-affinity binding of insulin is conferred without the loss of high-affinity IGF-1 binding. Heterodimers of the IR and IGF1 receptors (IR-βα–αβ-IGF-1R) occur; these chimeric receptors show highly preferential activation by IGF-1 as compared with insulin, comparable to the IGF-1R. The in vivo abundance and physiologic relevance of such obligate IR/IGF-1R heterodimers is unclear.

It should be mentioned that the most secure example of ligand bivalency and existence of two structurally distinct ligand-binding surfaces is provided by x-ray analysis of growth hormone–growth hormone receptor cocrystals, discussed in Chapter 5.

Another mechanism of ligand-induced RTK heterodimerization is presented by the FGF receptor (FGFR) family.[23] Early work had established that heparin or heparan sulfate proteoglycans were critical for FGF signaling; FGF freed of traces of heparin-like molecules is unable to activate FGFRs. Heparin is a linear, highly sulfated polysaccharide that binds FGF through a minimum tetrasaccharide unit; a heparin decasaccharide unit will bind two FGF molecules and is thus the minimal unit capable of "dimerizing" the FGF ligand (see Fig. 4–3). Conventional heparin and heparan sulfate proteoglycans can bind many molecules of FGF but do not interact directly with the FGFRs themselves. Heparin analogues that bind a single FGF molecule (e.g., tetrasaccharide units) block FGF signaling, presumably by preventing FGFR dimerization, whereas heparin decasaccharide will enable FGF-induced receptor activation.[24, 25] At least 12 FGF variants are known, each capable of binding heparin; thus the diversification of ligand pairs created by heparin is very substantial.

Four FGFR isoforms are known. The sufficiency of FGFR dimeriza-

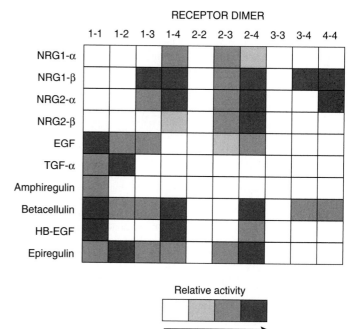

FIGURE 4–5. ErbB specificity of EGF-like ligands. Each column represents one of ten possible dimeric complexes of ErbB proteins. The extent of response to various ligands (horizontal rows) is shown by boxes: *black* indicates a potent response, and *white* stands for no response. Responses that are either detectable at high ligand concentration, or require extreme receptor overexpression, are shown as *light gray or dark gray* boxes. Note that ErbB-3 homodimers bind all forms of neuregulin (NRG), but their response is defective due to an inactive kinase domain. The abbreviations used are: NRG, neuregulin; EGF, epidermal growth factor; TGFα, transforming growth factor α; HB-EGF, heparin binding EGF-like growth factor. (From Tzahar E, Yarden Y: The ErbB-2/HER2 oncogenic receptor of adenocarcinomas: From orphanhood to multiple stromal ligands. Biochim Biophys Acta 1377:M25–M37, 1998.)

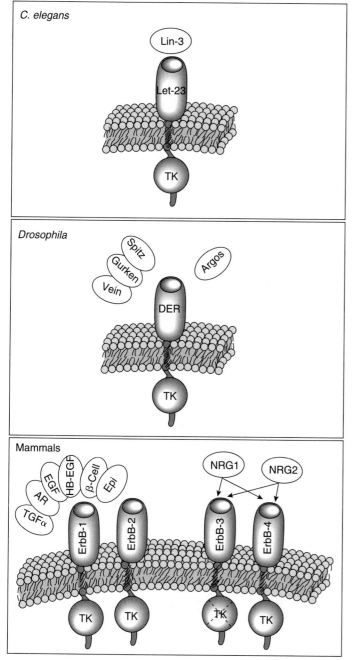

FIGURE 4–4. The evolution of EGF-related ligands and receptors. (From Tzahar E, Yarden Y: The ErbB-2/HER2 oncogenic receptor of adenocarcinomas: From orphanhood to multiple stromal ligands. Biochim Biophys Acta 1377:M25–M37, 1998.)

tion for signaling is graphically illustrated by a variety of autosomal dominant human chondrodysplasias, skeletal dysplasias, and craniostenosis disorders that are caused by activating mutations of FGFRs. These disorders include the Crouzon, Pfeiffer, Jackson-Weiss, and Apert syndromes, each attributable to mutations in FGFR2,[26–28] and achondroplasia, hypochondroplasia, and thanatophoric dysplasia, each caused by mutations in FGFR3.[29] Most of these mutations are found in the Cys-rich Ig-like region of the receptor extracellular domain and result in the creation of an unpaired Cys residue (either by mutational loss or gain of a Cys residue). The generation of an extracellular unpaired Cys promotes intermolecular disulfide formation and ligand-independent receptor dimerization.[30] A few mutations appear to cause intermolecular disulfide formation without altering the number of Cys residues, presumably by reconfiguring the Cys-rich domain to interfere with normal intramolecular disulfide formation.

The RET (*re*arrangement during *t*ransfection) tyrosine kinase is an important regulator of the differentiation of a subset of cells of neural crest origin. Targeted disruption of the murine *RET* gene causes a severe defect in development of the enteric nervous system and absent or rudimentary kidneys and ureters.[31] The RET extracellular domain contains two centrally located cadherin-like repeats and a Cys-rich region immediately before the transmembrane segment.[32] The ligands known to activate RET are the secreted proteins glial-derived neurotrophic factor (GDNF), bitemin, neurturin, and persephin, members of the TGF-β superfamily. As with *RET* deletion, *GDNF* knockout results in the absence of enteric neurons and renal agenesis. These ligands activate RET indirectly, through their binding to one of a family of glycosylphosphatidylinositol (GPI)-linked membrane proteins known as GDNF receptor-α (GFR-$α_{1-4}$); the GRF-α–ligand–RET complex is the active signaling unit.[33, 34] Encoding of a ligand-binding subunit on a different gene from that encoding the tyrosine kinase domain is exceptional among the transmembrane tyrosine kinases, but it is the usual situation with the hematopoietic growth factor (including, for example, growth hormone, prolactin) and cytokine (e.g., interleukin-2 [IL-2], interferons) receptors; the latter classes of receptor generally consist of a transmembrane ligand-binding subunit with a short, noncatalytic intracellular segment encoded by genes distinct from those that encode the intracellular tyrosine kinase polypeptides, which are entirely cytoplasmic, "nonreceptor" tyrosine kinases, mostly of the Janus kinase (JAK) or Src subfamilies.

RET is of special interest in endocrinology because germline activating mutations in *RET* account for multiple endocrine neoplasia syndrome type 2A (MEN-2A, medullary thyroid carcinoma, pheochromocytoma, and parathyroid hyperplasia)[35, 36] and type 2B (MEN-2B, medullary thyroid carcinoma, pheochromocytoma, buccal neuromas, and hyperganglionosis of the hindgut) and the familial medullary thyroid cancer (FMTC) syndrome,[36–38] whereas inactivating mutations of *RET* cause 15% to 20% of familial colonic aganglionosis (Hirschsprung's disease)[39, 40] (see Chapter 189). In addition, sporadic cases of thyroid cancer containing rearranged *RET* oncogenes have been reported.[41–43] RET is encoded by a large (approximately 60 kb) gene composed of at least 21 exons expressing a large variety of alternatively spliced mRNAs specifying at least 10 different polypeptides (Fig. 4–6). The mutations that underlie aganglionosis (i.e., loss of function) are missense, nonsense, and frameshift mutations (nearly 50 thus far) that are distributed randomly all along the gene. By contrast, the activating mutations of MEN-2A/FMTC are overwhelmingly (>85%) clustered in exons 10 and 11, which encode the Cys-rich region of the extracellular domain, and nearly all are missense mutations that result in the elimination of a Cys, thereby creating an unpaired extracellular Cys, intermolecular disulfide formation, and RET dimerization and activation. The clinical syndrome correlates with the specific Cys residue mutated; 80% of cases of MEN-2A involve the loss of Cys634, with the remainder attributable to loss of Cys609, Cys611, and scattered other residues. Approximately 50% of families with FMTC exhibit mutations at Cys618 or Cys620. The basis for this correlation appears to arise primarily from the proclivity of each of these mutations to promote intermolecular disulfide formation, which determines the abundance of RET dimers and thus the extent of RET activation. The Cys634 mutation (MEN-2A) generates more kinase activation than do the Cys618/Cys620 mutations (FMTC) when the mutant recombinant RET is examined at comparable polypeptide expression on the same cellular background.[44, 45] A few MEN-2A families with loss-of-Cys mutations (e.g., at 609, 618, or 620) also exhibit colonic aganglionosis; conversely, some families with aganglionosis resulting from *RET* mutations typical of MEN-2A fail to show any clinical features of MEN-2A. How the same *RET* mutation

results in the activation of endocrine cells and involution of enteric ganglion cells is not currently understood. Conceivably, in addition to promoting dimerization, these Cys mutations may also impair RET maturation and delivery to the surface, and relative expression of the mutant RET may differ in the two cell backgrounds.[46]

Interestingly, *RET* was originally discovered as a rearranged oncogene through the transfection of DNA from a human T cell lymphoma into murine fibroblasts. Subsequent studies, however, revealed that *RET* had been activated by rearrangement during transfection rather than in the original tumor DNA. Nevertheless, spontaneous or radiation-induced *RET* gene translocations are identified in about 10% to 40% of cases of human papillary thyroid carcinoma (*RET/PTC* genes) and illustrate another mechanism of aberrant RET dimerization. These translocations fuse new open reading frames to the region on Chr10 upstream of the RET tyrosine kinase domain. The three different fusion partners (*PTC* genes) identified thus far include the gene encoding the R1α regulatory (cyclic adenosine monophosphate [cAMP] binding) subunit of the cAMP-dependent protein kinase (*PTC2*) and the genes encoding proteins of unknown function, H4 (*PTC1*) and ELL1 (*PTC3*). The R1α sequences fused N-terminal to the RET tyrosine kinase domain include the R1α dimerization domain, which provides a ready explanation for kinase activation.[42] The MEN-2B syndrome is *not* due to mutations in the RET Cys-rich domain and is not associated with RET dimerization, but instead is due to a novel mutation in the RET catalytic domain that increases intrinsic activity and probably alters substrate specificity (see below).[47]

The largest RTK subfamily, the EPH receptors,[48] is involved in axonal guidance in development and interacts with a family of membrane protein ligands called ephrins that are expressed either as GPI-linked membrane proteins or as transmembrane polypeptides with short intracellular tails. Membrane-attached RTK ligands are not susceptible to internalization by the target cell bearing the RTK and consequently produce sustained and potent RTK activation when compared with the cleaved, soluble form of the same ligand. Regarding the functional importance of prolonged RTK stimulation, a variety of experiments indicate that several-hour engagement of RTK by ligand is important to entrain DNA synthesis. The greater mitogenic potency of cell-associated ligand over the soluble ligand has also been well shown for the c-kit ligand (stem cell factor), CSF-1, and several of the Erb ligands. The mitogenic potency of various mutant insulins, for example, correlates closely with their rate of dissociation (K_d) from the IR (slower dissociation is more mitogenic) rather than the rate of association or overall affinity.[20] As regards the biologic importance of membrane-bound ligands for the EPH RTKs, soluble versions of ephrins appear completely incapable of EPH RTK activation. The

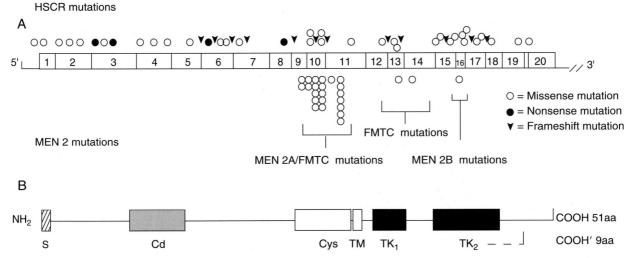

FIGURE 4–6. *A,* Different types of mutations of the RET proto-oncogene found in HSCR *(above diagram)* and in MEN 2 syndromes *(below diagram),* represented with respect to the RET exons. *B,* The corresponding structural features of the RET receptor tyrosine kinase are indicated: S, signal sequence; Cd, cadherin-like domain; TM, transmembrane domain; Cys, cysteine-rich domain; TK1 and TK2, tyrosine kinase domains. (From Edery P, Eng C, Munnick A, et al: RET in human development and oncogenesis. Bioessays 19:389–395, 1997. Copyright © 1997. Reprinted by permission of John Wiley & Sons, Inc.)

sustained nature of the ephrin-EPH interaction is probably critical for spatial localization and continuous axonal guidance during axon or cell migration. In addition, the EPH RTKs appear to be capable of transmitting a signal through the ephrin ligand into the cytoplasm of the ligand-bearing cell; thus a soluble form of the extracellular domain of the EphB2 RTK is capable of inducing tyrosine phosphorylation of the intracellular tail of the ephrin B1 or B2 transmembrane ligands. Moreover, deletion of the entire EphB2 RTK gene produces substantial defects in axonal connections that are not reproduced by deletion of only the tyrosine kinase domain.[48]

Among the other RTK subfamilies listed in Table 4–1, few have been subjected to extensive analysis of their ligand-binding properties and ligand-binding domains. It can be anticipated that a variety of novel ligand-RTK pairs remain to be uncovered, some of which may introduce paradigms not yet encountered in the several well-studied subfamilies reviewed above. In addition, structural analysis of ligand-RTK domains is eagerly anticipated because this information should provide a great impetus to drug development.

Kinase Activation

Immediately after the transmembrane segment, the intracellular extension of RTKs contains a noncatalytic segment of 50 to 100 amino acids followed by the tyrosine kinase domain (usually 250–280 amino acids), which in some subfamilies (e.g., PDGFR, Flt1) is interrupted by a short nonconserved noncatalytic segment of variable length; the catalytic domain is followed by a noncatalytic C-terminal tail that usually contains several tyrosine autophosphorylation sites (see Fig. 4–1). Given that receptor dimerization is indispensable for ligand activation of kinase function, how precisely is activation brought about? The solution of several protein kinase catalytic domain crystal structures has revealed that the three-dimensional organization of these enzymes shares a common framework, as would be expected from 11 clusters (subdomains) of highly conserved amino acid sequence distributed through the catalytic domains, first described by Hanks and Hunter.[49] All Ser/Thr and Tyr protein kinases examined thus far exhibit a bilobed architecture,[50] with a smaller upper lobe, primarily responsible for binding ATP, connected by a single polypeptide strand to a larger lower lobe, which is primarily responsible for peptide substrate binding. Catalysis (phosphotransfer) occurs in the cleft between the lobes; ATP is bound with its base moiety lodged deeply in the cleft, and the (poly)peptide substrate is bound along the surface of the lower lobe, with the substrate phosphoacceptor site positioned toward the cleft. An active kinase conformation requires an optimal degree of apposition between the two lobes, as well as access of ATP and the protein substrate to the crucial kinase residues lining the cleft between the lobes. Both factors (i.e., lobe apposition and substrate access) are strongly determined by the position of a peptide segment in the lower lobe located between catalytic subdomains VII and VIII and flanked by the conserved residues DFG and APE; this segment, generally called the "activation loop" or "A" loop, forms part of the border between the lower and upper lobes. Many, but not all kinases require phosphorylation of one or more residues on this loop to attain optimal positioning of the two lobes and/or enable substrate access. In some instances, as with the kinase A catalytic subunit, activation loop phosphorylation occurs in a constitutive manner immediately post-translation and is an unregulated step in the structural maturation of kinase polypeptide.[50] In most instances, however, phosphorylation of the activation loop occurs posttranslationally in a regulated manner and provides a major mechanism for control of the activity of both Ser/Thr and tyrosine-specific protein kinases. Among the RTKs, the regulatory role of "A" loop phosphorylation was first demonstrated for the IR[51] and is now known to occur in response to ligand binding and dimerization for many RTK subfamilies, for example, the FGFRs, HGFR, Trks, and so on.[52] In the case of the IR, binding of insulin promotes a concerted phosphorylation of at least 6 of the 13 tyrosine residues on the IR-β subunit intracellular extension, including a set of three tyrosines (1146/1150/1151) situated on the activation loop[51, 53]; phosphorylation of these 3 tyrosines closely corresponds with acquisition of the capacity of the IR to phosphorylate exogenous peptide/

protein substrates.[54, 55] The other tyrosine autophosphorylation sites, one in the juxtamembrane segment (Tyr960) and two in the C-terminal tail (Tyr1314, Tyr1322), although not concerned with activation of kinase catalytic function, play an important role in signaling through different mechanisms (see below). Once phosphorylation of the activation loop occurs, kinase activity persists despite removal of insulin from the ligand-binding site, and RTK deactivation requires "A" loop tyrosine dephosphorylation. Mutagenesis of the A loop tyrosines shows that in addition to the importance of their phosphorylation in insulin-induced kinase activation, these tyrosine residues in their unphosphorylated state are also crucial to maintenance of the basal, inactive state of the kinase inasmuch as mutation to Phe also produces a significant increase in ligand-independent kinase activity.[56] The molecular basis for these features was revealed by comparison of the structures of the IR catalytic domain in the unphosphorylated[57] and in the triply phosphorylated[58] active state, as solved by x-ray crystallography. The unphosphorylated IR kinase exhibits a relatively open bilobed structure, with the side chain of A loop Tyr1150 lodged in the active site much as a "*pseudo*substrate" and hydrogen bonded to the catalytic base Asp1120. Nevertheless, although positioned in the active site, IR Tyr1150 fails to undergo *cis*-autophosphorylation because the ATP site is occluded both by the proximal portion of the unphosphorylated activation loop (G1140, M1141) and by the side chain of Tyr1150, which extends into the hydrophobic pocket usually occupied by the adenine ring of ATP. Phosphorylation of Tyr1146/1150/1151 results in a major rearrangement of the A loop that disoccludes both the ATP-binding site and the active site. Moreover, the specificity of the IR for tyrosine was illuminated, in part, by a cocrystal of triply phosphorylated active IR kinase with a synthetic tyrosine peptide substrate that clearly showed that the hydroxyl group of a serine or threonine inserted into the peptide in place of the substrate tyrosine would be unable to reach the active site. The FGFR also undergoes activation through ligand-dependent phosphorylation at the tandem tyrosines (Tyr653/654) within the activation loop and illustrates a second, perhaps more general mechanism of RTK activation (see Fig. 4–2). In contrast to the IR, the unphosphorylated FGFR activation loop does not obstruct ATP binding or the active sites, but rather appears to preempt peptide substrate binding by the presence of FGFR residues Arg661 and Pro663 near the putative substrate-binding pocket.[59]

How does ligand binding promote "A" loop phosphorylation?[52] Abundant evidence indicates that ligand-induced dimerization enables one kinase domain to catalyze phosphorylation of the opposing kinase domain A loop. Although certain genetically engineered RTK mutants can be shown to catalyze dimer-independent *cis*-autophosphorylation, this activity does not occur in the context of ligand-induced RTK autophosphorylation. It is entirely clear, for example, that an IR-αβ half-receptor, despite well-preserved insulin-binding capacity, is unable to catalyze insulin-stimulated tyrosine autophosphorylation if reassembly into an (αβ)$_2$ structure is prevented. Moreover, the ability of one receptor dimeric assembly (e.g., an IR-α$_2$β$_2$) to catalyze the intermolecular phosphorylation of another receptor dimer appears negligible. The significance of this intradimer transphosphorylation mechanism to the signaling capacity of RTKs is heavily dependent on whether the RTK forms a fixed, covalent dimer (i.e., the IR subfamily) and whether the ability of the RTK to signal arises primarily from its ability to phosphorylate exogenous protein substrates (also true of the IR subfamily) or from its ability to catalyze its own autophosphorylation (as is the case for EGFR/PDGFR and most RTKs). In the case of the IR, dimers that contain one catalytically active RTK with a kinase-dead RTK mutant exhibit greatly inhibited signaling ability because the normal RTK peptide will fail to undergo transphosphorylation by the inactive partner (and thus will remain unable to phosphorylate exogenous substrates), and the kinase-inactive RTK, despite tyrosine phosphorylation by the nonmutant partner, is unable to signal. This "dominant inhibitory" phenotype may be ameliorated by diminished expression of the mutant receptor (e.g., because of accelerated degradation) as compared with wild-type receptor. Nevertheless, clinically evident insulin resistance has been observed in the setting of heterozygous inactivating mutations of the IR.[60] Conversely, RTKs whose kinase activation does not require A loop phosphorylation are not covalent dimers and, most importantly, signal primarily through tyrosine autophosphorylation rather than by substrate phosphorylation (see below); they experience little or no impairment in signaling potency when coexpressed with kinase-inactive EGFRs. This point is well illustrated by ErbB$_3$, an RTK isoform whose wild-type polypeptide is intrinsically kinase inactive but that nevertheless functions as a potent signal generator when coexpressed with a compatible dimer partner whose kinase domain is active[16] (see Fig. 4–5). Other examples are RTKs related to the avian RTK Klg, such as the human colon carcinoma kinase-4 (CCK-4).[61] The catalytic domain of these RTKs contains an Ala in place of an indispensable Asp in a highly conserved catalytic motif, a substitution known to render the kinase catalytically inactive. Whether CCK-4 acts as a coreceptor capable of unique signal generation or as a signal attenuator is not yet known. This assignment will require examination of these "inactive" kinases in their native contexts because the experimental format used and the impact of potential dimer partners can strongly bias the conclusion reached. For example, overexpression of kinase-dead EGFRs in the absence of any detectable active Erb isoform is still able to confer a weak, partial response to added EGF (e.g., activation of MAP kinase [MAPK]) where none was evident before overexpression of recombinant, kinase-dead EGFRs. This finding appears to be attributable to the association of kinase-dead EGFRs with nonreceptor tyrosine kinases; when RTKs are dimerized by ligand, the nonreceptor tyrosine kinases catalyze modest tyrosine phosphorylation of the kinase-negative EGFR polypeptide.

Regarding the mechanism of ligand-induced kinase activation for RTKs that do not require activation loop autophosphorylation, little direct information is available. It is clear from the structures of the unphosphorylated IR and FGFR tyrosine kinase domains that the activation loops are relatively mobile and that a distribution of different "A" loop conformations exists, among which are some that would allow access of polypeptide substrate and consequent substrate Tyr phosphorylation. It is suggested that for RTKs activated by dimerization without A loop phosphorylation, such as the EGFR, the conformation of the A loop is sufficient to prevent significant autophosphorylation unless a substrate is imposed through the ligand-induced dimerization. Presumably these RTKs, monomers in the absence of ligand, experience few random collisions and may therefore tolerate a somewhat more open kinase domain configuration and a rather modest autoinhibitory mechanism, whereas the IR is a preassembled, covalent dimer in the absence of ligand and requires an extensive autoinhibitory apparatus to prevent autophosphorylation of the A loop.[52]

The critical importance of protein tyrosine phosphatases (PTPs) in maintaining the low RTK activity of the ligand-free state should be emphasized. The addition of general tyrosine phosphatase inhibitors (such as vanadate) to cells in the absence of ligand will allow a slow accumulation of RTK tyrosine phosphorylation that over several hours will cause substantial and ultimately full RTK activation. Thus PTPs are constitutively active at a level sufficient to overcome the ligand-free activity of RTKs (and in general, nonreceptor protein tyrosine kinases). Conversely, overexpression of RTKs, as is easily accomplished experimentally or as occurs spontaneously with the RTK gene amplification seen in malignancies such as breast cancer, readily results in significant signaling in the absence of ligand, thus demonstrating the intrinsic leakiness of the RTK autoinhibitory mechanisms and the importance of the balance between basal cellular PTPase and total RTK abundance in signal generation.[16, 17, 62] The impact of RTK overexpression is greatly enhanced if it is also associated with even a small increase in ligand-independent activity. Thus a mutant, truncated EGFR is found to be amplified in many cases of glioblastoma multiforme. The truncation deletes the ligand-binding domain, thereby abrogating ligand-induced activation and resulting in a kinase whose activity is greatly diminished in comparison to the ligand-activated wild-type EGFR. Nevertheless, truncation also results in a small increase in ligand-independent activity, which is constitutive and when combined with substantial overexpression results in the creation of a potent oncogene.

Mutations within the kinase catalytic domain are most often associated with loss of function caused by either premature termination or major structural disorganization resulting in misfolding and accelerated degradation. Missense mutations that are relatively conservative may nevertheless still disrupt the structure necessary for optimal binding of ATP or polypeptide substrate or for optimal alignment of these substrates at the active site in an arrangement that permits phosphotransfer. Occasionally, however, catalytic domain mutations may disrupt the autoinhibitory mechanisms and promote activation and/or alter the determinants for protein substrate binding. Thus a patient with the fatal skeletal disorder thanatophoric dysplasia exhibited a mutation in FGFR3 that substituted an acidic residue (Lys660→Glu) immediately after the double tyrosine autophosphorylation sites in the FGFR3 "A" loop and resulted in ligand-independent activation. Activating A loop mutations have also been observed in c-kit (in a mast cell leukemia) and HGFR (in a human renal papillary carcinoma). The activating mutation of *RET* (Met918→Thr, ATG→ACG) seen in 95% of cases of MEN-2B and in 30% to 40% of sporadic medullary thyroid cancers involves a residue situated in catalytic subdomain VIII, distal to the activation loop, in a region that in protein (Ser/Thr) kinases is known to influence substrate selectivity (see Fig. 4–6). Although Met918 is well conserved among RTKs, the homologous site in most nonreceptor tyrosine kinases is usually Thr. Studies using synthetic peptide substrates have shown that the wild-type RET favors peptides resembling those optimal for the EGFR and other RTKs, whereas the mutant RET (Thr918) selects peptide substrates more like those chosen by the nonreceptor tyrosine kinases Src and Abl.[47] It is tempting to relate this change in RET substrate specificity to the different clinical picture engendered by RET (Met918→Thr) in MEN-2B as compared with that seen with RET activation by dimerization in MEN-2A.

MECHANISM OF RECEPTOR TYROSINE KINASE SIGNALING

Identification of RTK Targets

Progress in understanding the signaling mechanisms used by this receptor family advanced only slightly during the 1980s.[11] Although the RTKs showed vigorous phosphotransferase activity in vitro, the abundance of phosphotyrosine in intact cells was very low and endogenous RTK substrates were hard to find. Even in Rous sarcoma virus–transformed cells containing a mutant, constitutively active retroviral tyrosine kinase–transforming protein, the abundance of phosphotyrosine was less than 0.1% that of phosphoserine plus phosphothreonine. In such cells many of the proteins found to have phosphotyrosine proved to be abundant proteins (e.g., enolase or lactate dehydrogenase) phosphorylated incidentally to a trivial stoichiometry (<0.1 mol P per mole protein). The development of polyclonal[63] and subsequently monoclonal antibodies selectively reactive with phosphotyrosine greatly accelerated the detection and isolation of physiologic RTK substrates. With the use of immunoblotting and immunoprecipitation it was shown that the phosphotyrosine content of an array of proteins was increased by activation of the RTK. Subsequently, it was shown that receptors lacking intrinsic protein tyrosine kinase activity but that were capable of promoting cell proliferation or differentiation also promoted protein tyrosine phosphorylation in the "appropriate" cell backgrounds. Nevertheless, it was repeatedly observed that the RTK polypeptides themselves were among the most prominent tyrosine-phosphorylated (TyrP) proteins detected in such experiments. This observation presented a paradox—namely, how was signal transmission occurring if the dominant substrate for the RTK was the RTK itself.

Complementary experiments using immunoprecipitation of the RTKs (EGFR, PDGFR, CSF-1R) from ligand-stimulated cells showed that many of the same polypeptide bands detected in antiphosphotyrosine immunoprecipitates were also recovered in anti-RTK immunoprecipitates. Labeling of cells with ^{35}S-methionine to tag the polypeptide backbones rather than phosphate groups revealed that many of the proteins that coprecipitated with the RTKs were seen only after ligand stimulation. Thus it emerged that ligand activation of many RTKs (but not all, e.g., not IR or IGF-1R) resulted in the assembly on the receptor of a set of polypeptides, most of which exhibited some tyrosine phosphorylation. Several of these polypeptides were isolated, cloned, and functionally identified; among the first was a phospholipase C enzyme, the γ isoform (PLC-γ)[64, 65] (see Chapter 8). Inasmuch as products of the PLC-γ reaction (i.e., diacylglycerol and inositol trisphosphate) were already well recognized as signaling molecules, the identification of PLC-γ as one of the proteins recruited to (at least some) RTKs consequent to receptor activation supported the view that activated RTKs were capable of recruiting intracellular signal generators.[66] PLC-γ was subsequently shown to undergo receptor-catalyzed tyrosine phosphorylation with a further increase in catalytic activity, thus providing one of the first examples of positive regulation of enzyme catalytic activity through tyrosine phosphorylation in *trans* (as distinct from the IR and c-Src autoactivating tyrosine autophosphorylations). Other RTK-associated polypeptides identified were a 120-kDa polypeptide that contained a guanosine triphosphatase (GTPase)-activating domain (GAP) for Ras near its C terminus, the c-Src kinase polypeptide, and several noncatalytic polypeptides, most notably, an 85-kDa protein later shown to be a noncatalytic subunit of the lipid kinase phosphatidylinositol-3′-OH kinase (PI-3-kinase). This enzyme had been discovered as a phosphatidylinositide kinase of novel specificity (3′-OH) associated with the polyoma middle T antigen, a viral transforming protein.[67] The Ptd Ins-3,4,5-P₃ product is now known to be a membrane lipid signaling molecule (see later).

Recruitment of RTK Targets

How do the ligand-activated RTKs recruit these candidate signaling molecules to associate with the receptor? The first important clue was provided by experiments directed at understanding the functional significance of a novel feature of the PDGFR kinase domain whose structure is interrupted by a noncatalytic segment ("kinase insert") that contains several candidate tyrosine autophosphorylation sites and that is not conserved among other RTKs (Fig. 4–7). Deletion of this segment or conversion of two of these Tyr residues to Phe abolished the mitogenic function of the PDGFR as effectively as did inactivation

of the PDGFR kinase ATP-binding site. In contrast to the PDGFR kinase-negative mutant, the PDGFR kinase-insert deletion (KI) mutant exhibited vigorous tyrosine phosphotransferase activity, continued autophosphorylation at other tyrosine residues, and an unimpaired ability to activate PLC-γ in response to PDGF. Most importantly, after PDGF binding, the immunoprecipitates of the PDGFR KI mutant lacked one of the major receptor-associated polypeptides; the p85 polypeptide, or the noncatalytic subunit of PI-3-kinase, was selectively absent, which correlated with a lack of receptor-associated PI-3-kinase activity.[68] These observations, in addition to indicating the importance of PI-3-kinase activity to the mitogenic action of the PDGFR, provided the first evidence that specific receptor-associated signaling proteins bound to the receptor in a manner that was dependent on specific, individual receptor phosphotyrosine residues.[69, 70] Conclusive evidence for this idea was the demonstration that synthetic peptides as short as five amino acids with a sequence based on the PDGFR KI segment were capable of selectively displacing the p85 polypeptide from activated receptors; such displacement depended on the presence of phosphotyrosine on the peptide and on preservation of the specific amino acid sequence immediately surrounding the phosphotyrosine, especially to the C-terminal side.[70, 71] The PDGFR is somewhat unique in that its various phosphotyrosine sites show little overlap in their ability to bind different polypeptide targets; other RTKs, such as the EGFR, exhibit substantial overlap in the specificity of their phosphotyrosine sites with regard to the binding of receptor-associated signaling polypeptides. Nevertheless, conversion of five to six EGFR Tyr autophosphorylation sites to Phe results in marked impairment in the signaling function of the EGFR, as well as the PDGFR, despite well-maintained RTK activity.

SH2 Domains

Given that signaling proteins assemble on active RTKs by binding at or near specific TyrP autophosphorylation sites and that this assem-

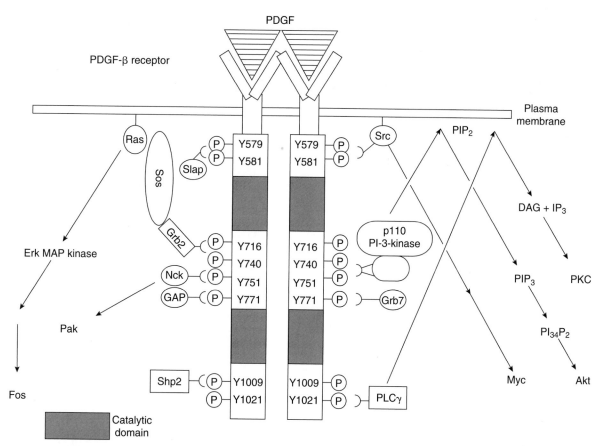

FIGURE 4–7. Platelet-derived growth factor (PDGF) receptor protein-tyrosine kinase signaling pathways. (From Hunter T: The Croonian Lecture, 1997. Phil Trans Roy Soc Lond B 353:588, 1997.)

blage is important in the efficiency of signaling to downstream targets (at least for PDGFR/EGFR/CSF-1R), what enables phosphotyrosine-specific binding of the RTK-associated signaling proteins? It is now known that these polypeptides each contain domains capable of specifically binding to short peptide segments that contain a TyrP residue (Fig. 4–8). The first of these domains to be identified was characterized by Pawson and colleagues, who analyzed a set of mutations of the v-Fps tyrosine kinase located outside the catalytic domain that markedly impaired or rendered temperature sensitive the transforming activity or altered the host range of v-Fps without much effect on its catalytic activity measured in vitro.[72] They noted that these mutations tended to cluster in regions that like the catalytic domain, were well conserved in amino acid sequence among all the Src family kinases. They identified two such conserved domains that they named Src homology (SH) domains 2 and 3 (with the catalytic domain representing SH domain 1) and suggested that the SH2 and SH3 domains might function in vivo to assist in substrate selection and/or direct the kinases to specific locations within the cells. Molecular cloning of PLC-γ[66] and p120 Ras-GAP,[73] two RTK-associated signaling proteins, provided the first examples of enzymes other than nonreceptor tyrosine kinases that contained SH2 and SH3 domains. Cloning of the retroviral oncogene v-*Crk* revealed the first example of a polypeptide that was composed entirely of SH2 and SH3 domains, without any catalytic domain.[74] Nonetheless, immunoprecipitates of the v-Crk polypeptide from transformed cells were heavily decorated by phosphotyrosine-containing proteins and by associated tyrosine kinase activity. It was soon appreciated that essentially all the RTK-associated proteins, p120 Ras-GAP, PLC-γ, c-Src, the p85 subunit of PI-3-kinase, and so on,

contained at least one SH2 domain and often an SH3 domain.[75] Expression cloning with the multiply (tyrosine) phosphorylated, non-catalytic C-terminal tail of the EGFR as a hybridization probe yielded more than a dozen polypeptides that bound only to the phosphotyrosine-containing form of the EGFR tail; these polypeptides, named "growth factor receptor–binding" (Grb) proteins, each contained one or more SH2 domains. The specific biochemical function of SH2 domains was established by the demonstration that recombinant SH2 domains per se were capable of binding directly to activated, phosphotyrosine-containing receptors in a manner entirely dependent on prior RTK tyrosine autophosphorylation, as well as binding to short phosphotyrosine-containing synthetic peptide modeled on the sequence surrounding RTK tyrosine around autophosphorylation sites.[76, 77] Peptide binding to SH2 domains absolutely requires phosphotyrosine and is strongly influenced by the identity of the four to five amino acids immediately C-terminal to the phosphotyrosine.[78]

Proteins that contain SH2 domains can be classified into two groups, depending on the presence of a catalytic domain; those lacking catalytic function are presumed to serve as adaptors. A catalog of SH2 adaptor proteins is shown in Table 4–2; the mode of action of two important examples, the p85 subunit of the PI-3-kinases and Grb2, is discussed below.

PTB/PID Domains

A second type of phosphotyrosine-binding domain was identified through analysis of the proto-oncogene *Shc*, which contains a single C-terminal SH2 domain and is phosphorylated at a single tyrosine by

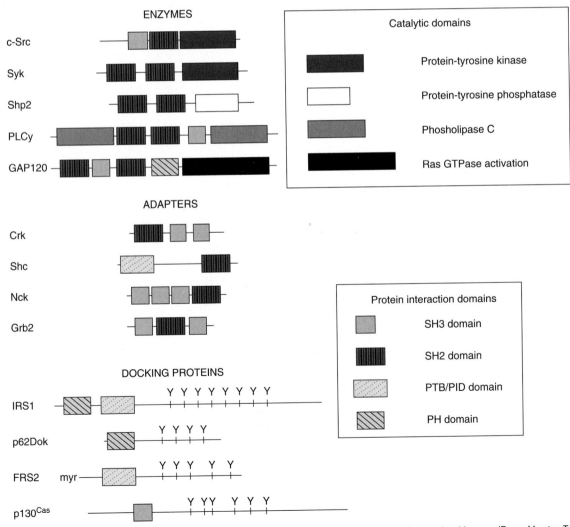

FIGURE 4–8. Schematic structures of representative enzyme and adapter targets for signaling protein tyrosine kinases. (From Hunter T: The Croonian Lecture, 1997. Phil Trans Roy Soc Lond B 353:589, 1997.)

TABLE 4–2. Representative SH2 Domain–Containing Proteins

Substrates	Targets
Enzymes	
PLC-γ_1 and PLC-γ_2 (PI-specific phospholipase)	SH2 (2), SH3, split PHD
GAP 120 (Ras GTPase activator)	SH2, SH3, PHD
Src family PTKs	SH2, SH3
Zap 70/Syk family PTKs	SH2 (2)
Shp1 (PTP1c/SH-PTP1/HC-PTP)	SH2 (2)
Shp2 (PTP1D/SH-PTP2/SYP)	SH2 (2)
PI-3 kinase p85 (p110 regulatory subunit)	SH2 (2), SH3
Ship (inositol polyphosphate-5′-phosphatase)	SH2
Vav (and Vav2) (Rho/Rac/Cdc42 GEF)	SH2, SH3, PHD
Adaptors	
Shc and (ShcB and ShcC) Shb	SH2, PTB
Nck	SH2, SH3 (3)
Crk (and CrkL)	SH2, SH3 (2)
Lnk	SH2
Slp76	SH2
Slap (negative regulator)	SH3, SH2
Grb2 (and Grap)	SH2, SH3 (2) (not phosphorylated)
Structural proteins	
Talin (focal adhesion)	SH2
Others	
STAT1–STAT5 (transcription factors)	SH2, SH3
Grb7 (Ras GAP related)	SH2, PHD
Grb10	SH2, PHD

GAP, guanosine triphosphatase (GTPase)-activating protein; GEF, guanine nucleotide exchange factor; Grb2, growth factor receptor–binding protein-2; PHD, pleckstrin homology domain; PI, phosphatidylinositol; PLC, phospholipase C; PTK, protein tyrosine kinase; PTP, protein tyrosine phosphatase; SH2, Src homology-2; STAT, signal transducer and activator of transcription.

many RTKs; this arrangement creates an excellent binding site for the adaptor Grb2 (see Fig. 4–9). Thus Shc can bind through its SH2 domain to an activated RTK, undergo tyrosine phosphorylation, recruit Grb2/SOS (son of sevenless), and promote Ras activation (see below). Surprisingly, it was observed that despite deletion of its SH2 domain, Shc still bound to some proteins in a phosphotyrosine-dependent manner.[79, 80] The novel Shc phosphotyrosine-specific binding was mediated by an N-terminal segment whose primary sequence proved to be conserved among several other proteins, such as insulin receptor substrate-1 (IRS-1); these segments are now known as the phosphotyrosine-binding (PTB) or phosphotyrosine-interacting domains (PID). Like the SH2 domain, the PTB/PID domains exhibit the ability to bind to phosphotyrosine-containing peptides, but with a specificity distinct from SH2 domains in that the PTB/PID domains bind the motif NPXY(P), with additional specificity provided by hydrophobic residues situated five to eight residues N-terminal to the phosphotyrosine.[81] The NPXY sequence, which is found in IR, EGFR, Trk, and polyoma middle T antigen, among others, can also serve as a protein-interacting surface in the absence of phosphorylation for a different set of polypeptides that function primarily in membrane protein sorting and localization.

Phosphotyrosine Docking Proteins: The IR/IGF-1R System

The paradigms developed from study of the PDGFR and EGFR did not appear to be directly relevant to signaling from the IR and IGF-1R because despite robust autophosphorylation, few signaling molecules coprecipitate with these receptors, save for a modest and inconsistent recovery of PI-3-kinase activity. Mutation of the IR "A" loop Tyr residues abolishes insulin-regulated signaling but does not completely abolish IR signaling inasmuch as these mutations somewhat increase

the basal, insulin-independent receptor kinase activity.[56] However, mutation of IR-Tyr960, an NPXY motif situated in the juxtamembrane segment N-terminal to the IR catalytic domain, essentially abolishes the IR signaling function in vivo, although causing no impairment in IR kinase activity in vitro or in IR autophosphorylation at other sites.[82] This null phenotype was accompanied by the in vivo disappearance of insulin-stimulated tyrosine phosphorylation of a 180-kDa polypeptide, the dominant insulin-stimulated phosphotyrosine-containing polypeptide in all cell backgrounds. This protein was molecularly cloned and named IRS-1; the structure of IRS-1 suggested a specific model for IR signaling[83] (see Fig. 4–8). The N-terminal third of IRS-1 contains a pleckstrin homology (PH) domain followed by a PTB domain, which together mediate the binding of IRS-1 to the activated IR at the NPEY(P) 960 site. The C-terminal two-thirds of IRS-1 contains at least 16 tyrosine phosphorylation sites, most of which can be phosphorylated by the IR in vivo and in vitro and provide an array of phosphotyrosine-containing motifs that enable the binding of SH2 domain–containing proteins such as p85, Grb2, Nck, and others, proteins that bind directly to other RTKs such as the EGFR. The identification of IRS-1 was followed by IRS-2 (similar in size and overall structure to IRS-1), IRS-3 (about 60 kDa), and IRS-4.[84] Evidence that these IR substrates are critical for IR/IGF-1R signaling in vivo is provided by the phenotypes of mice whose IRS genes have been deleted. Mice with a homozygous deletion of both IRS-1 alleles are about half the size of wild-type mice and are moderately insulin resistant, but rarely hyperglycemic.[85] IRS-2 "knockout" mice are 80% of wild-type size and insulin resistant; hyperglycemia ultimately develops at a high frequency because the compensatory β cell hyperplasia that occurs in IRS-1 knockout mice does not occur in IRS-2 knockouts, who instead exhibit reduced β cell mass.[86] Interestingly, whereas heterozygous deletion of either IR or IRS-1 has no specific phenotype, profound insulin resistance and hyperglycemia develop in the double-heterozygote IR$^-$/IRS-1$^-$ mouse.[87] These features establish the crucial role of the IRS family in the signaling function of IR and IGF-1R in vivo.

Although initially considered to be relatively specific substrates for IR and IGF-1R, it is now clear that a variety of hematopoietic and cytokine receptors (including the receptors for interferons, IL-4, and growth hormone), acting through recruitment of the Janus family of nonreceptor tyrosine kinases (JAKs), can also cause IRS tyrosine phosphorylation and therefore signal via insulin-like, RTK-activated pathways.[84] Moreover, although the EGFR has no ability to phosphorylate IRS-1 to IRS-4, an analogous protein called GAB-1 can be multiply phosphorylated by both the IR and EGFR to provide a platform apart from the EGFR polypeptide for multiple SH2-containing proteins.[88] *Drosophila* genetics first identified "daughter of sevenless" (DOS), a PH domain–containing protein that like IRS-1 and GAB-1 has many tyrosine phosphorylation sites but, unlike IRS and GAB-1, is a substrate for EGFR but not (apparently) for IR. Other docking proteins are shown in Figure 4–8. Thus it appears that most RTKs will use substrate docking proteins analogous in function to the IRS polypeptides, although the specific contribution of these docking proteins to signal generation, as compared with the RTK autophosphorylation sites, remains to be determined. Docking proteins presumably allow for great diversification and wide cellular localization of the RTK signal, comparable to that available to diffusible ligands such as cAMP and Ca^{2+}. Interestingly, the *Drosophila* and *C. elegans* IR homologues exhibit C-terminal extensions that encode multiple additional tyrosine phosphorylation sites not observed in the mammalian counterparts, which may therefore enable the invertebrate IRs to function as docking sites, whereas this role has evolved to a separate function in mammals. This evolution may reflect some further divergence in function, not as yet elucidated. Nevertheless, as is true of the mammalian IR, the *Drosophila* IR expressed in mammalian cells will not support insulin-stimulated mitogenesis without the coexpression of IRS-1 despite the presence of additional C-terminal TyrP sites.[89]

Specificity Determinants in RTK Signaling

The structure of several SH2 domains has been solved, both unliganded and complexed with TyrP-containing peptides; the SH2 domain is a compact globular structure that contains a bipartite binding site for the tyrosine phosphopeptide.[77] The phosphotyrosine residue itself sits in a pocket lined by basic residues, including an invariant Arg conserved in all SH2 domains. The crucial binding energy is provided by this site inasmuch as unphosphorylated peptides of the same sequence exhibit a 2-log lower affinity. In addition, a second, immediately adjacent binding surface enables specific accommodation of the amino acids immediately C-terminal to the phosphotyrosine. Studies with synthetic peptides indicate that the binding site for these C-terminal sequences falls into several broad categories.[90] The most common SH2 subtype, found in nearly all nonreceptor tyrosine kinases, preferentially accommodates amino acids with hydrophilic side chains at the (TyrP) +1 and +2 positions and a small hydrophobic residue at +3. Another common type of SH2 exhibits a long hydrophobic groove extending from the Tyr(P)-binding pocket that can accommodate up to five hydrophobic amino acids. The disparate preferences of various SH2 domains for the +1 residue is determined largely by a single amino acid on the fourth β strand of the SH2 domain; a Tyr or Phe at the fifth residue on this strand confers a preference for smaller hydrophilic residues at the Tyr(P) +1 position, whereas an Ile or Cys at this site in the SH2 domain leads to a preference for hydrophobic residues at the Tyr(P) +1 position (Table 4–3). A comparison of the binding preferences of SH2 domains to the specificity determinants of tyrosine kinases reveals several informative patterns (Table 4–4). Although each tyrosine kinase exhibits a relatively distinct amino acid sequence preference for synthetic peptide substrates, all protein tyrosine kinases select peptides with hydrophobic residues at +3; this tendency is in turn consistent with the binding preferences of all SH2 domains. In addition, the nonreceptor tyrosine kinases (e.g., Src, Lck), all of which contain SH2 domains themselves, prefer to phosphorylate peptides that contain, at the Tyr(P) positions +1 and +2, amino acids with small neutral (Gly, Ala) or acidic (Glu) side chains at +1 and +2. Thus the specificity of these kinases closely corresponds with the binding preferences of their endogenous SH2 domains. In contrast, the RTKs prefer to phosphorylate peptides that contain multiple hydrophobic amino acids at +1 through +4, as well as multiple acidic residues at the −1 to −3 positions. This pattern corresponds best with the binding specificity of the SH2 domains found on p85, PLC-γ, and SH-PTP2, targets known to bind consistently to activated RTKs. These general correlations accommodate exceptions and considerable variation. Thus the binding specificity of the Grb2 SH2 domain is determined primarily by a preference for N at the +2 residue, thereby allowing Grb2 to accommodate a wide range of amino acids at +1 and +3, which probably accounts in part for the ubiquitous recruitment of Grb2. Moreover, many activated RTKs recruit nonreceptor tyrosine kinases, which bind through their SH2 domains to RTK autophosphorylation sites whose sequence matches more closely the binding specificity of the nonreceptor tyrosine kinase SH2 domain than the RTK specificity toward peptide substrates. This arrangement reflects a broadening of RTK specificity when catalyzing autophosphorylation, presumably because of the imposed proximity of an intramolecular substrate. The effect of proximity on RTK substrate selection is re-created when protein substrate becomes bound to the autophosphorylated RTK through its SH2, PTB, or perhaps PH domains; the RTK is then capable of catalyzing a multiple, processive substrate phosphorylation, including the phosphorylation of sites that would be unfavorable in a conventional bimolecular reaction. Thus in contrast to most Ser/Thr protein kinases, the intrinsic specificity of the RTK domain is greatly modified by associations imposed by the high-affinity binding of proteins through their SH2 and PTB domains.

Signal Transmission through the Cell

The net output of RTK-mediated tyrosine phosphorylation and SH2/PTB domain recruitment is to activate a set of secondary intracellular signal generators, among which four major types are well understood. These signal generators include the STAT (signal transducer and activator of transcription) transcriptional regulatory proteins[91] and three enzymatic proteins: PLC-γ, PI-3-kinase, and the guanyl nucleotide

TABLE 4–3. Phosphopeptide Motifs for SH2 Domains*

Group	SH2 Domain	Y(P) + 1	Y(P) + 2	Y(P) + 3	βD5
1A	Src	E	E	I	Y
	Fyn	E	E	I	Y
	Lck	E	E	I	Y
	Fgr	E	E	I/V	Y
	Lyn				Y
	Yes				Y
	Hck				Y
	D-Src				Y
1B	Syk C	Q/T/E	E/Q/T	L	Y
	Syk N	T	T	I/L/M	Y
	ZAP70 C				Y
	Tec				Y
	Atk				Y
	Itk				Y
	Abl	E	N	P	Y
	Arg				Y
	Csk	T	N	M/R	Y
	Crk	D	H	P	Y
	Nck	D	E	P	F
	Fes/Fps	E	-	V/I	F
	ZAP70 N				
	Sem5	L/V	N	V/P	F
	D-Grb2	Y	N		F
	Grb2	QY	N	Y	F
	GAP C				F
	GAP N				F
	Tensin	E	N	F/I/V	F
	3BP2	E	N	-	Y
2	Vav	M	E	P	T
3	P85α N	M/I/V/E	-	M	I
	p85β N				I
	p85α C	M/L/I		M	C
	p85β C				C
	PLC-γ₁ C	V/I	I/L	P/I/V	C
	PLC-γ₂ C				C
	PLC-γ₁ N	L/I/V	E/D	L/I/V	C
	PLC-γ₂ N				C
	SHPTP1 N	F	-	F	I
	SHPTP2 N	I/V	-	V/I	I
	Csw N				I
	SHPTP1 C				I
	Shc	E/I	-	I/L/M	L
4	Shb	T	T	L	M
	SHPTP2 C				V
	Csw C				V
	STATs				A?S?

*Columns Y(P) + 1, 2, and 3 comprise the first, second, and third residues C-terminal to phosphotyrosine of the optimal phosphopeptide selected by each SH2 domain (e.g., Y(P)YEEI for Src SH2). The far-right column indicates the residue at the βD5 position of the SH2 domain. Strength of selection varies; see original for details. A hyphen indicates no selection. Motifs not yet determined or not submitted for publication are left blank. C or N in the first column designates the C- or N-terminal SH2 domain.

SH2, Src homology-2.

Adapted from Songyang Z, Cantley LC: Recognition and specificity in protein tyrosine kinase–mediated signaling. TIBS 20:470–475, 1995.

exchangers for small GTPases, especially those acting on Ras. Each of these elements generates one or more secondary signals that each entrain multiple separate signal transduction pathways extending to all compartments of the cell. Clearly, SH2 domain proteins of still uncharacterized function are known that may yet be shown to regulate novel signaling pathways; a plausible working hypothesis is that each of the already known, but uncharacterized RTK targets, as well as those yet to be uncovered, will be found to function in a critical manner in vivo downstream of one or more RTKs in one or more cells at one or more times in development or during adult life. Nevertheless, based on a variety of genetic and biochemical data, it is possible at present to identify several of the known secondary signals, specifically, the small GTP-binding protein Ras and the products of PI-3-kinase, as indispensable outputs for cellular differentiation and mitogenesis. This conclusion is strongly supported by identification of the apical two members of each of these two pathways, namely, Ras/

TABLE 4–4. *Optimal Substrate Sequences Recognized by Different Protein Tyrosine Kinases*

	Substrate Sequence at Position								
	−4	−3	−2	−1	0	+1	+2	+3	+4
Tyrosine kinases									
c-Fps/Fes	E	E	E	I	Y	E	E	I	E
Middle T antigen/c-Src	D	E	E	I	Y	G/E	E	F	F
v-Src	E	E	E	I	Y	G/E	E	F	D
Lck	X	E	X	I	Y	G	V	L	F
c-Abl	A†	X	V	I	Y	A	A	P	F
EGF receptor	E	E	E	E	Y	F	E	L	V
PDGF receptor	E	E	E	E	Y	V	F	I	X
FGF receptor	A†	E	E	E	Y	F	F	L	F
Insulin receptor	X	E	E	E	Y	M	M	M	M

*Relative importance of substrate residues for selection by the protein tyrosine kinases varies; see original for details. Consistent with known phosphorylation sites of receptor protein tyrosine kinases (PTKs), these kinases favorably phosphorylated peptides with the general motif Tyr-hydrophobic-x-hydrophobic. This motif, once phosphorylated, is predicted to bind proteins in group III SH2 (Src homology-2) domains (see Table 4–3). In contrast, the SH2-containing PTKs preferentially phosphorylate peptides with the motif Tyr-hydrophilic-hydrophilic-hydrophobic. Sites phosphorylated by these PTKs are predicted to bind proteins with group I SH2 domains (see Table 4–3). These results suggest that the binding sites of individual SH2 domains and PTKs have converged upon overlapping selectivities to maintain specificity in downstream signalling.

†Partially caused by lag from the previous sequencing cycle.

EGF, epidermal growth factor; FGF, fibroblast growth factor; PDGF, platelet-derived growth factor.

Adapted from Songyang Z, Cantley LC: Recognition and specificity in protein tyrosine kinase–mediated signaling. TIBS 20:470–475, 1995.

Raf[92] and PI-3-kinase/Akt,[93–95] as spontaneously occurring, dominant transforming oncogenes. Thus any of these four elements, converted to a constitutively active state, is sufficient to drive "susceptible," but otherwise normal cells into a state that exhibits at least some of the properties of an oncogenically transformed cell, such as immortality, increased growth rate, loss of growth inhibition on cell-cell contact, loss of dependence on matrix attachment for survival and growth, and others. In addition, the tumor suppressor gene PTEN/MMAC, inactivated in many breast cancers as well as in 60% to 70% of advanced prostate cancers and glioblastoma multiforme,[96] has been identified as a PI-3′-phosphatase, that is, the key degradative enzyme for 3′-OH phosphorylated phosphatidylinositides.[97] In addition to their capacity for promoting mitogenesis, the genes encoding each of these polypeptides have been identified as crucial determinants in a variety of developmental programs in *C. elegans* and *Drosophila*. Thus the ability of RTKs to promote the accumulation of Ras-GTP and Ptd Ins 3, 4, 5 P$_3$ is central to their characteristic biologic actions. Both these responses are initiated by the recruitment of an enzyme polypeptide (i.e., a Ras-specific guanyl nucleotide exchanger or a PI-3′-OH-kinase) to an RTK-generated phosphotyrosine motif through an SH2 domain–containing adaptor protein (i.e., Grb2 or p85, respectively). The Ras-GTP and Ptd Ins 3, 4, 5 P$_3$ signals, although chemically different, function in an analogous manner; they, like the RTKs themselves, represent membrane-bound signals that attract an array of effectors through specific, high-affinity binding. Once recruited to the membrane, these effectors, which are mostly protein (Ser/Thr) kinases and guanyl nucleotide exchangers for other small GTPases, become activated and convey the message downstream into all cellular compartments to the proteins that mediate the ultimate enzymatic, structural, synthetic, and degradative functions required for the final biologic response.

RTK-Ras Signal Transduction Pathway

The first RTK-initiated pathway to be unraveled was that underlying the activation of Ras and the mechanism of Ras action. Ras is the progenitor of a superfamily of small GTPase proteins that now number more than 60 and encompass four subfamilies: Ras, Rho, Rabs, and Arfs.[98] These proteins serve as GTP-dependent timers that interact with and initiate the activation of target proteins in a GTP-dependent

reaction. The three Ras genes (giving four polypeptides: Harvey, Kirsten-a, Kirsten-b, and N-Ras) encode very similar polypeptides of approximately 190 amino acids that must be anchored to the inner surface of the plasma membrane for biologic activity. Membrane localization is initiated by the attachment of a hydrophobic C-15 farnesyl (Ha-Ras, N-Ras) or C-20 geranylgeranyl group (Ki-Ras4b) to a cysteine, four amino acids from the Ras C terminus, through a thioether linkage. This prenylation reaction is followed by cleavage of the C-terminal three amino acids and methylation of the C-terminal carboxyl group. These modifications greatly increase the hydrophobicity of the Ras polypeptide. Ki-Ras contains a polybasic segment (six lysines) just N-terminal to the prenylation site. Prenylation is sufficient to confer constitutive binding to the inner surface of the plasma membrane. Ha-Ras, which lacks a C-terminal polybasic segment, requires further hydrophobic modification that is accomplished by the attachment of two palmitate thioesters to each of two cysteines just upstream of the prenylation.

Ras is a GTPase that operates in a cyclic fashion: binding GTP (whose cytoplasmic concentration is 10-fold higher than that of guanosine diphosphate [GDP]), hydrolyzing GTP to GDP, releasing GDP, and rebinding GTP. The intrinsic Ras GTPase activity is very low but can be accelerated over 1000-fold by Ras-specific GTPase activating proteins (GAPs), which thereby deactivate Ras. In the presence of a GAP, dissociation of GDP becomes the rate-limiting step in the overall GTPase cycle, and some catalytic proteins, first identified in yeast, accelerate the release of bound guanyl nucleotide and are thus guanyl nucleotide exchange factors (GNEFs). Given the much higher cytosolic concentrations of GTP over GDP, GNEF action favors Ras occupancy by GTP in vivo. Although first encountered in mutant form as a retroviral transforming gene, Ras gained wide notice from its discovery in mutant form as the first human dominant oncogene, that is, the gene responsible for the transformation of cultured murine fibroblasts as a result of the introduction of DNA from human tumors. The mutations in Ras found to confer oncogenic capacity are generally those that inactivate intrinsic GTPase and its ability to be stimulated by GAPs; a few activating mutations result from an increase in the rate of spontaneous guanyl nucleotide dissociation, thus mimicking the effect of GNEF action. The oncogenic behavior of such mutations established that Ras is active, or promitogenic, when bound to GTP.

Identification of the link between RTK and Ras activation required elucidation of the TyrP adaptor protein Grb2, a 25-kDa polypeptide composed of an SH2 domain flanked by two SH3 domains[77, 99] (Figs. 4–8 and 4–9). Mutations in the gene encoding the *C. elegans* homologue of Grb2 (called SEM-5) inhibit cellular (vulval) differentiation downstream of the gene encoding an EGFR homologue (Let23); this defect can be overcome by an activated Ras gene. *Drosophila* photoreceptor cell development, a process known to be regulated by an RTK (sevenless), is also dependent on Drk, the fly homologue of SEM-5 and Grb2, and on Ras. Another *Drosophila* gene named SOS (son of sevenless) is necessary for photoreceptor development and by genetic epistasis appears to function downstream of the sevenless RTK but upstream of Ras; SOS encodes a polypeptide that contains an N-terminal PH domain, a centrally located catalytic domain homologous to the Ras guanyl nucleotide exchange enzymes first characterized in yeast, and a proline-rich C-terminal segment. Thus genetic evidence provided the first indication that cellular development was directed by the ability of an RTK to promote GTP charging (i.e., activation) of the Ras GTPase. The biochemical operation of the steps between the RTK and Ras was established by work in both insect and mammalian cells showing that Grb2, through its SH3 domains (see below), associates with the C-terminal proline-rich segment of the SOS protein, and the Grb2/mammalian SOS (mSOS) complex is recruited to the activated, tyrosine-phosphorylated RTK through the Grb2 SH2 domain; however, the SOS PH domain is also necessary for effective membrane association and Ras activation. Together, these N- and C-terminal noncatalytic segments ensure that SOS is positioned to enable Ras-GTP charging. Recruitment of Grb2 directly to the RTK is only one of several pathways by which Grb2/mSOS is recruited to the plasma membrane. The proto-oncogene *Shc* is a particularly versatile TyrP adaptor that contains an N-terminal PTB domain and a C-terminal SH2 domain. The Shc SH2 domain is recruited to the vast majority of

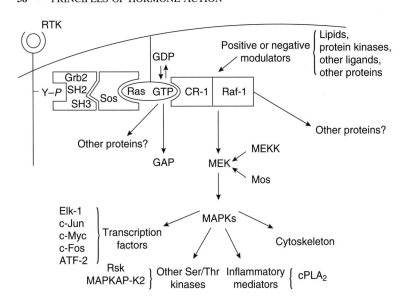

FIGURE 4–9. Model for receptor tyrosine kinase signal transduction through the Ras-activated protein kinase cascade. Activation of an RTK leads to its phosphorylation on tyrosine residues (Y-P), which allows the receptor to interact with SH2-domain–containing proteins, such as Grb2. In turn, Grb2 binds to an adapter protein, SOS (son of sevenless), which recruits Ras to the receptor. Ras recruits Raf to the complex, allowing Raf activation and providing a means of activating the MAPK cascade. MAPKAP-K2, MAPK-activated protein kinase 2; cPLA₂, cytoplasmic phospholipase A₂. (From Avruch J, Zhang ZF, Kyriakis J: Raf meets Ras: Completing the framework of a signal transduction pathway. Trends Biochem Sci 19:279–283, 1994.)

activated RTKs and nonreceptor tyrosine kinases, which thereupon catalyze Shc tyrosine phosphorylation and create an excellent binding site for the Grb2 SH2 domain. Another Grb2 partner is the SH2 domain–containing intracellular tyrosine phosphatase SH-PTP2; once recruited to an RTK, SH-PTP2, like Shc, undergoes tyrosine phosphorylation to create an effective Grb2-binding site. Although it is counterintuitive for a PTPase to serve as a positive element in RTK signaling, genetic evidence indicates that loss of the *Drosophila* SH-PTP2 homologue Corkscrew (CSW) impairs DER signaling in a manner that can be bypassed by active Ras. Thus numerous pathways have evolved to enable RTKs to recruit Ras to an active state. In addition, SOS is only one of several types of Ras-specific guanyl nucleotide exchangers; some Ras-specific RTK-independent guanyl nucleotide exchangers (primarily expressed in the central nervous system) are directly regulated by Ca^{2+} and diacylglycerol and indirectly by heterotrimeric GTPases acting through nonreceptor tyrosine kinases.

A comparison of the crystal structures of Ras bound to GDP or to GTP shows that only two Ras loops adopt a different configuration, depending on which nucleotide is bound—one loop involves amino acids 32 to 40, and the second, amino acids 60 to 72; these segments are therefore named switch 1 and 2, respectively. An extensive analysis of the effect of site-specific mutations on the ability of mutant active (GTPase deficient) Ras to transform fibroblasts revealed that alterations in the switch 1 loop greatly impaired transforming ability. The importance of the switch 1 loop for transformation, together with its selective GTP-dependent reconfiguration, strongly suggested that the switch 1 loop is (part of) the Ras "effector" domain, that is, the Ras segment that mediates GTP-dependent interaction with the proteins that act as "effectors" of Ras transforming action.[100] This prediction was verified with the discovery that c-Raf-1, a proto-oncogene protein (Ser/Thr) kinase, selectively binds to Ras in a GTP-dependent manner through the Ras effector loop.[101] The Raf kinase contains an N-terminal noncatalytic regulatory domain and a C-terminal kinase catalytic domain; deletion of the Raf regulatory domain produces an oncogenic, constitutively active kinase. Because Raf is an RTK-regulated protein kinase, the Raf regulatory domain must have two functions: in unstimulated cells it must act to suppress the kinase domain, whereas with RTK stimulation, the Raf regulatory domain must serve as the receptor for the activating upstream signal. This activating signal is the Ras-GTP complex itself. The Raf N-terminal regulatory domain contains a segment of about 100 amino acids that bind directly to the Ras effector loop with high affinity (K_d in the nanomolar range) in a reaction that is essentially completely GTP dependent.[102] Immediately C-terminal to this Raf segment is a Cys-His-rich, zinc-binding (so-called zinc finger) structure (homologous to those found in protein kinase C [PKC] isozymes) that mediates a second, lower-affinity, GTP-independent binding interaction with a second Ras epitope distinct from the effector loop.[103, 104] This second binding step between the Raf zinc finger and Ras is absolutely required to convert Raf to an active state,[105] a process that also requires the active participation of 14-3-3 proteins and the (serine) phosphorylation of Raf by a still unknown protein kinase.[106] This second-site Ras-Raf binding interaction confers a crucial additional specificity inasmuch as other Ras-like proteins contain an effector loop sequence identical to that of Ras to enable binding of Raf; however, because they fail to engage in a productive second-site interaction, they are unable to support c-Raf activation in vivo. Once activated, Raf then serves as the immediate upstream activator of the MAPKK[107] and thus the MAPK pathway (see Chapter 9).

Several proteins other than Raf are known to bind to Ras in a GTP-dependent manner and are thus candidates to serve as Ras effectors, like Raf. The best supported among these candidates are the three p110 polypeptides that serve as the type 1A PI-3-kinase catalytic subunits and a family of three guanyl nucleotide exchangers that act on the Ras-related small GTPase known as Ral.[108] Little is known at present concerning the biologic consequences of Ral activation. As regards PI-3-kinase, the importance of Ras-GTP for full activation of the type 1A subfamily is now well established. Mutations in p110 polypeptides that impair their ability to bind to Ras-GTP substantially decrease their activation in vivo by RTKs;[109] conversely, RTK mutations that diminish activation of Ras also impair the activation of PI-3-kinase to some degree.[110] Nevertheless, Ras-GTP plays only a secondary role in the regulation of PI-3-kinase. The affinity of p110 for Ras-GTP is 100-fold lower than for Raf[111]; whereas Raf is recruited to the membrane entirely through its high-affinity binding to Ras-GTP, p110 PI-3-kinase polypeptides are recruited to the membrane through their p85 adaptor subunits, independent of Ras-GTP, and interact with Ras effectively only after p85-mediated recruitment. The contribution of other candidate Ras-GTP effectors, such as MEKK1, NORE 1, AF-6, and others, to the biologic responses caused by activated Ras is not yet known. It is presumed that elucidation of the biochemical function of the substantial number of candidate Ras effectors will ultimately be required to achieve full understanding of the mechanism of Ras action.

RTK–PI-3-Kinase Signal Transduction Pathway

PI-3-kinases were first encountered as PI kinases of novel specificity that coprecipitated with polyoma middle T antigen (a viral transforming protein) and appeared to copurify with an 85-kDa polypeptide.[67] A similar p85 polypeptide and PI kinase activity were found to coprecipitate with a variety of activated RTKs,[112] and p85 was ultimately isolated and cloned from this source. Independently, purification of a hepatic PI-3-kinase yielded a p85/p110 heterodimer, and the p85 polypeptide was shown to be the noncatalytic adaptor subunit of

PI-3-kinase (Figs. 4–10 and 4–11). This adaptor protein (p85α) has an N-terminal SH3 domain, followed by a segment with substantial homology to the C-terminal portion of the breakpoint cluster region *(Bcr)* gene product (a GAP for Rho family GTPases) that is flanked by proline-rich sequences on both sides. The C-terminal half of p85α contains two SH2 domains separated by a segment that binds tightly to the N terminus of a p110 PI kinase catalytic subunit. Three other splice variants of this gene are described: p85α1, p55α, and p50α. The p85α1 variant is nearly identical to p85α, whereas the shorter isoforms lack SH3, the first proline-rich sequence, and the BCR domain; p55α contains a novel 32–amino acid N terminus immediately before the second proline-rich segment that is lacking in p50α, which is otherwise identical. Two related genes encode p85β and p55γ, which are architecturally identical to p85α and p55α, respectively. Each of these SH2 adaptor proteins contains a functional inter-SH2 segment that binds to a p110 catalytic subunit. PI-3-kinase catalytic subunits that bind to this family of adapters have been classified as type 1A, and three closely related type 1A p110s are known: α, β, and δ; each contains an N-terminal segment that binds to the adaptor protein, a Ras-binding domain, a noncatalytic domain conserved among all PI-4- and PI-3-kinases (the PIK domain), and a C-terminal lipid kinase catalytic domain. When TyrP-containing synthetic peptides bind to a p85/p110 heterodimer, lipid kinase activity is increased severalfold. However, if both SH2 domains are simultaneously ligated, either by a multiply phosphorylated receptor polypeptide or by a single synthetic peptide containing two TyrP motifs, the catalytic activity of the p110 lipid kinase is activated to an extent that greatly exceeds that caused by a peptide containing a single phosphotyrosine. Thus binding of the p85 subunit to the RTK brings the p85/p110 lipid kinase to the membrane in contiguity to its PI substrate, and simultaneous engagement of the two SH2 domains (per se, without p85 tyrosine phosphorylation) strongly activates PI-3-kinase catalytic function. Recruitment of the p85/p110 heterodimer to the membrane contributes in one further way to activation of the lipid kinase: membrane association facilitates a relatively low-affinity, but specific interaction of p110 with Ras-GTP as described above. This interaction enables optimal activation of the p110 lipid kinase inasmuch as mutations in the p110 Ras-binding domain or in the RTK sites critical to Ras activation substantially diminish the ability of the RTK to activate PI-3-kinase despite the integrity of the RTK sites that mediate p85 SH2 binding.

Type 1A PI-3-kinases can phosphorylate PI, PI-4-P, and PI-4,5-P_2 comparably in vitro but appear to use PI-4,5-P_2 preferentially in vivo[113–115] (Fig. 4–12). PI-4-P and PI-4,5-P_2 are minor but constitutive components of cell membranes; the PI-4,5-P_2 content is regulated by the activity of PLC isozymes (which catalyze hydrolysis to inositol-

1,4,5-P_3 and diacylglycerol) and by PI-4-kinases, which convert PI to PI-4-P and PI-4,5-P_2. The 3′-OH phosphorylated phosphatidylinositides appear only with activation of PI-3-kinase and are maximally present at no more than 10% the level of PI-4,5-P_2; 3′-OH phosphorylated phosphatidylinositide derivatives are not susceptible to phospholipase (PLC/PLD) action and are catabolized by 5′-OH– and 3′-OH–specific phosphatases. The catalytic function of type 1A PI-3-kinases is inhibited somewhat specifically by low concentrations of the drugs wortmannin (≤0.1 μmol/L) and Ly294002 (<10 μmol/L), which are therefore useful probes. The class 1B PI-3-kinase catalytic subunits have similar substrate specificity, but different regulatory properties; thus p110γ does not bind to the p85/p50/p55 class of SH2 domain–containing adaptors, but rather to a p101 adaptor. The p101-p110γ complex is activated by the βγ subunits of heterotrimeric GTPases. The class II PI-3-kinases are 170-kDa polypeptides distinguished by a C-terminal C2 domain, homologous to the sequences in PKCs that mediate Ca^{2+}-sensitive phospholipid (phosphatidylserine and PI) binding. In contrast to class 1A and 1B enzymes, class II PI-3-kinases are not known to be recruited to receptors or GTPases and are insensitive to the inhibitors wortmannin and LY294002. Class III PI-3-kinases exhibit a substrate specificity distinct from that of the class 1A, 1B, and II enzymes acting only on phosphatidylinositide and not on PI-4-P or PI-4,5-P_2. Class III enzymes are homologous in structure and specificity to the yeast PI-3-kinase VPS 34p, which functions in vesicle trafficking, osmoregulation, and endocytosis; no evidence for RTK regulation exists for the mammalian class III PI-3-kinases. The downstream effectors of PI-3,4,5-P_3 include a subset of the many proteins that contain PH domains (discussed below) or other polyphosphatidylinositide-binding domains such as atypical PKC. Genetic evidence points to the PI-3,4,5-P_3–binding protein (Ser/Thr) kinases, protein kinase B (PKB), and its "A" loop kinase PDK1 as central effectors, as well as a large family of GNEFs (the Dbl family) for the Rho subfamily (RHO, Rac, Cdc42) of small GTPases. Moreover, genetic evidence identifies PI-3-kinase, PDK1, and PKB as crucial downstream targets of the *C. elegans* IR/IGF-1R homologue.[116, 117] Further discussion of the PI-3,4,5-P_3–regulated protein kinases (i.e., PDK1, PKBs, p70 S6 kinase, GSK3) can be found in Chapter 9.

Other Protein-Protein Interaction Domains Relevant to RTK Signaling

Pleckstrin Homology Domains

PH domains, named after pleckstrin, the major PKC substrate of platelets, are found in both catalytic and noncatalytic proteins and are

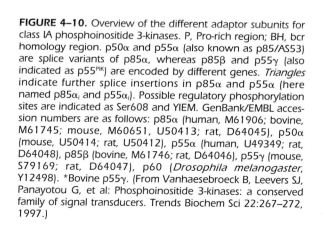

FIGURE 4–10. *Overview of the different adaptor subunits for class IA phosphoinositide 3-kinases. P, Pro-rich region; BH, bcr homology region. p50α and p55α (also known as p85/AS53) are splice variants of p85α, whereas p85β and p55γ (also indicated as p55^{PIK}) are encoded by different genes. Triangles indicate further splice insertions in p85α and p55α (here named p85α$_i$ and p55α$_i$). Possible regulatory phosphorylation sites are indicated as Ser608 and YIEM. GenBank/EMBL accession numbers are as follows: p85α (human, M61906; bovine, M61745; mouse, M60651, U50413; rat, D64045), p50α (mouse, U50414; rat, U50412), p55α (human, U49349; rat, D64048), p85β (bovine, M61746; rat, D64046), p55γ (mouse, S79169; rat, D64047), p60 (Drosophila melanogaster, Y12498). *Bovine p55γ. (From Vanhaesebroeck B, Leevers SJ, Panayotou G, et al: Phosphoinositide 3-kinases: a conserved family of signal transducers. Trends Biochem Sci 22:267–272, 1997.)*

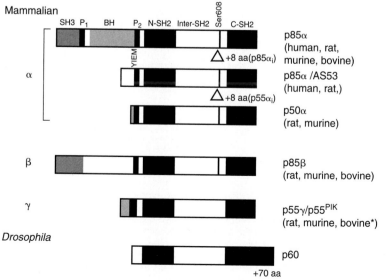

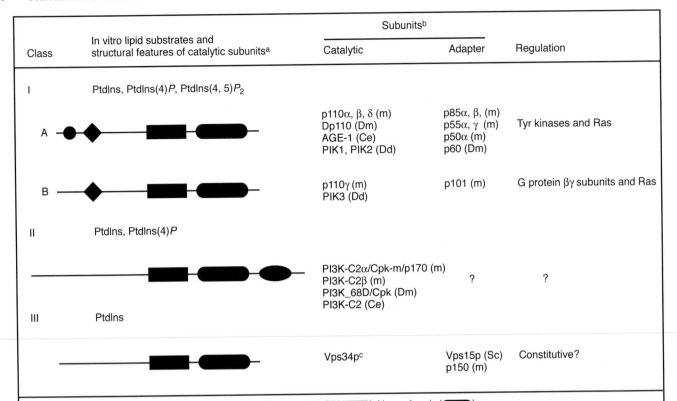

Class	In vitro lipid substrates and structural features of catalytic subunits[a]	Subunits[b]		Regulation
		Catalytic	Adapter	
I	PtdIns, PtdIns(4)P, PtdIns(4, 5)P$_2$			
A		p110α, β, δ (m) Dp110 (Dm) AGE-1 (Ce) PIK1, PIK2 (Dd)	p85α, β, (m) p55α, γ (m) p50α (m) p60 (Dm)	Tyr kinases and Ras
B		p110γ (m) PIK3 (Dd)	p101 (m)	G protein βγ subunits and Ras
II	PtdIns, PtdIns(4)P			
		PI3K-C2α/Cpk-m/p170 (m) PI3K-C2β (m) PI3K_68D/Cpk (Dm) PI3K-C2 (Ce)	?	?
III	PtdIns			
		Vps34p[c]	Vps15p (Sc) p150 (m)	Constitutive?

[a]Key of structural motifs: adapter-binding (●); Ras-binding (◆); C2 (⬬); PIK (▬); kinase domain (⬭).
[b]For the proteins other than those derived from yeast, fruit fly and mammals, no biochemical proof of PI3K lipid kinase activity is available. These enzymes have been allocated to a particular class of PI3K mainly based on primary sequence homology of the core kinase domain[5]. The abbreviations used are: m, mammalian; Ce, *Caenorhabditis elegans*; Dd, *Dictyostelium discoideum*; Dm, *Drosophila melanogaster*; Sc, *Saccharomyces cerevisiae*. The GenBank/EMBL accession numbers for class I and II catalytic subunits are: *mammalia*: p110α (human: Z29090, HSU79143; mouse: U03279; bovine: M93252), p110β (human: S67334), p110γ (human: X83368; pig Y10743), p110δ (human: Y10055, U57843, U86587; mouse, U86453), PI3K-C2α (human: Y13367), Cpk-m (also known as p170) (mouse: U52193; U55772), PI3K-C2β (Y13892, Y11312) - *D. melanogaster*: Dp110 (Y09070), PI3K_68D (also known as Cpk) (X92892; U52192)—*C. elegans*: age-1 (U56101), putative C2-domain containing PI3K (on cosmid Z69660)—*D. discoideum*: PIK1 (U23476), PIK2 (U23477) and PIK3
[c]The prototype of the class III PI3Ks is the *S. cerevisiae* protein Vps34p (X53531). Vps34p homologues from other species are not shown individually. They are: human PI3K (Z46973); *D. melanogaster*, PI3K_59F (X99912); *D. discoideum*, PIK5 (U23480); and the Vps34p-related PI3Ks from *Schizosaccharomyces pombe* (U32583), Soybean (L29770), *Arabidopsis thaliana* (U10669) and *C. elegans* (Y12543).

FIGURE 4–11. A classification of phosphoinosotide 3-kinase (PI-3-K) family members. (From Vanhaesebroeck B, Leevers SJ, Panayotou G, et al: Phosphoinositide 3-kinases: a conserved family of signal transducers. Trends Biochem Sci 22:267–272, 1997.)

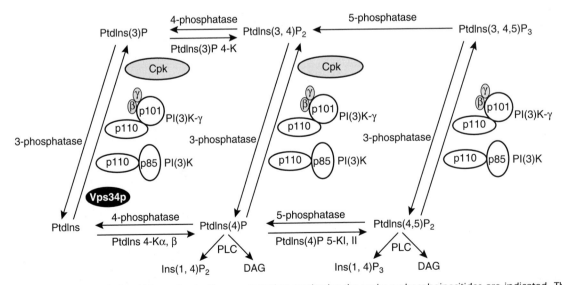

FIGURE 4–12. Pathways for phosphoinositide synthesis. The enzymes that synthesize the various phosphoinositides are indicated. Three classes of PI-3-K enzymes exist: the class I enzymes (p110) can use phosphatidylinositol (PtdIns), PtdIns(4)P, or PtdIns(4,5)P$_2$ as substrates; class II enzymes (Cpk) phosphorylate PtdIns and PtdIns(4)P; and class III enzymes (Vps34p) can only phosphorylate PtdIns. PtdIns(4,5)P$_2$ is of particular importance: hydrolysis by phosphoinositide-specific phospholipase C (PLC) generates the two second messengers, diacylglycerol (DAG) and Ins(1,4,5)P$_3$, and phosphorylation by PI-3-K generates the putative second messenger PtdIns(3,4,5)P$_3$. PtdIns(3,4)P$_2$ can be generated through the phosphorylation of PtdIns(4)P by a PI-3-K (Cpk, C2-domain–containing PI-3-K), as well as by dephosphorylation of PtdIns(3,4,5)P$_3$. In mammalian cells, D3 phosphoinositides are degraded by phosphatases that convert them back to PtdIns, PtdIns(4)P, or PtdIns(4,5)P$_2$. (From Toker A, Cantley LC: Signalling through the lipid products of phosphoinositide-3-OH kinase. Nature 387:673, 1997.)

among the most ubiquitous motifs encountered in signal transduction proteins[118, 119] (Table 4–5). PH domains are roughly 100 to 120 amino acids in length and, although relatively divergent in primary sequence, exhibit a well-conserved three-dimensional architecture that is very similar to the PTB/PID domains.[120, 121] A similar domain detected in a noncatalytic region of the β-adrenergic receptor kinase (β-ARK) was shown to mediate membrane binding of the kinase to the βγ subunits of heterotrimeric G proteins; the optimal βγ-binding region of β-ARK, however, extends C-terminal to the borders of a canonic PH domain.[122, 123] Isolated recombinant PH domains of the two guanyl nucleotide exchangers mSOS and Dbl (specific for Ras and the Rho subfamily, respectively), as well as from IRS-1, also bind directly to βγ with high affinity (K_d of 20–45 nmol/L); nevertheless, little evidence exists for βγ as a physiologic ligand except for β-ARK.[124] Much more evidence favors the likelihood that polyphosphorylated inositides (i.e., PI-4,5-P_2; PI-3,4,5-P_3; PI-3,4-P_2), as well as the free inositol polyphosphates (inositol-1,4,5-P_3; inositol-1,3,4,5-P_4), are physiologic ligands for PH domains.[125, 126] Some PH domains (e.g., from β-spectrin, gelsolin, and others) bind PI-4,5-P_2 and PI-3,4,5-P_3 with comparable avidity, whereas the PH domains of other proteins exhibit a substantial preference for PI-3,4,5-P_3 over PI-4,5-P_2; examples of the latter include the nonreceptor B cell tyrosine kinase BTK, the serine kinase PKB/Akt, the guanyl nucleotide exchange proteins SOS (Ras specific), and T cell lymphoma invasion and metastasis protein (TIAM, a Rac-specific member of the Db1 family). These polypeptides are likely to be specifically recruited to the membrane by the activation of PI-3-kinase and synthesis of PI-3,4,5-P_3, whereas proteins whose PH domains exhibit comparable affinity for PI-4,5-P_2 and PI-3,4,5-P_3 are likely to be associated primarily with the more abundant PI-4,5-P_2. Such proteins may be constitutively membrane associated and perhaps released or untethered by activation of PLC, both because of a local decrease in PI-4,5-P_2 content and by generation of the competing soluble ligands inositol-1,4,5-P_3, especially by the higher polyphosphoinositols such as inositol-P_4 or inositol-P_5. The very similar structure of the PH and PTB domains suggested that PTB domains might represent a subclass of PH domains capable of phosphotyrosine as well as phospholipid binding. The ability of PI-4,5-P_2 to displace the autophosphorylated EGFR from the PTB domain of Shc is consistent with this idea.

Perhaps the most striking evidence for the functional importance of PH domains in signaling is Bruton's X-linked agammaglobulinemia, where a point mutation of the B cell tyrosine kinase BTK in a conserved PH domain Arg residue involved in PI-phosphate binding is the mutation responsible for a substantial subset of families.[115] The ability of IRS-1 to undergo insulin-stimulated tyrosine phosphorylation in vivo is abolished by mutation or deletion of the IRS-1 PH domain despite the presence of an intact IRS PTB domain.[127] Mutation in the PH domain of the *Dbl* oncogene abolishes its transforming activity despite unimpaired Rac guanylnucleotide exchange factor (GNEF) activity.[128] Thus PH domains are major targets for the signals generated by PI-3-kinase and are regulated as well by the PLC hydrolysis of PI-4,5-P_2.

SH3, WW, and EVH-1, Polyproline-Binding Domains

SH3 domains are compact globular domains of about 60 amino acids that bind with a K_d in the micromolar range to short, proline-rich motifs of the minimal type, XPXXPX; this motif, which binds as a left-handed helix with three amino acids per turn, can bind to the SH3 domain in either direction (i.e., N→C or C→N) by fitting into two adjacent hydrophobic pockets, one for each XP pair.[77, 129, 130] Further specificity is conferred by interaction between the amino acids flanking the PXXP with adjacent SH3 domain residues (Fig. 4–13). The relatively low affinity of these domains for ligands points to their operation primarily in intramolecular interactions, as illustrated by the role of the Src SH3 domain in maintaining Src in an inactive state through an intramolecular interaction. The ability of SH3 domains to couple effectively in intermolecular interactions probably depends on the presence of multiple SH3 domains on a single polypeptide (e.g., as in Grb2, Nck, Crk) or on the forced proximity to a polyproline

sequence induced by a higher-affinity protein-protein interaction mediated by, for example, an SH2 domain on the same protein.

WW domains contain 38 to 40 amino acids and are named for the conserved tryptophans located 20 to 22 amino acids apart. Initial studies defined two general core binding motifs, PPXY and PPLP, with additional N- and C-terminal flanking residues on the peptide providing further affinity and specificity. WW domains are not *pseudo*-symmetric like SH3 domains, but they do exhibit overlap with SH3 domains in their ability to bind PPLP-containing substrates. More recent studies of the WW domains of the prolyl isomerase PIN1 and the ubiquitin ligase Nedd4 have clearly shown that these WW domains bind preferentially to phosphoserine/phosphothreonine-containing sequences, probably involving (Ser/Thr) Pro motifs.[131] Thus by analogy with SH2 and PTB domains in phosphotyrosine binding, WW domains (and 14-3-3 proteins) bind to short peptide segments containing phosphoserine/phosphothreonine with a specificity yet to be fully defined. The actin-binding protein profilin also contains a polyproline-binding domain, and the profilin-binding proteins VASP and Mena exhibit a conserved domain called EVH1 that binds another polyproline motif. The SH3, EVH1, and profilin polyproline-binding domains are not recruited in a regulated manner as occurs with SH2 domains; however, phosphorylation within the polyproline regions, either by tyrosine kinases (e.g., at PPXY) or by proline-directed Ser/Thr kinases (at [S/T] P motifs), as well as competition with polyphosphoinositides, may negatively regulate these protein-protein interactions. Conversely, proline-directed (Ser/Thr) kinases may generate binding sites for proteins containing WW domains.

PDZ Domains

These domains were first identified in the postsynaptic density protein *PSD-95*, the *Drosophila* Discs large septate protein, and the tight junction protein ZO-1 and thus labeled PDZ. Such domains are now known to be present in more than 100 proteins.[132] PDZ domains bind other proteins through a specific sequence at the protein C terminus that end in Leu, Ile, or Val (see Fig. 4–13). These partners are thus available either to be modified by the catalytic domain of the PDZ-containing protein or to act selectively at the cellular locus bearing the PDZ proteins. An example of the latter is InaD, a *Drosophila* noncatalytic protein containing multiple PDZ domains, each capable of binding a protein involved in phototransduction, for example, the Ca^{2+} channel Trp, PLC-β, and PKC. Loss of InaD greatly impairs light-induced responses despite unimpaired expression of all the catalytic elements required for this process.

The picture of the early steps in RTK signaling developed above emphasizes the importance of phosphotyrosine-initiated protein-protein interactions in collecting multiple effectors, colocalizing them with their activators and substrates, and thereby initiating wide distribution of the RTK signal down multiple independent pathways. The ability of protein-protein associations to speed up and/or spatially restrict signaling events should also be considered; however, the features of these assemblies most important under physiologic circumstances remain largely conjectural at present.

TERMINATION OF THE RTK SIGNAL

A variety of mechanisms exist for termination of the signal initiated by ligand binding to the RTK, such as (1) ligand dissociation from the cell surface receptor; (2) internalization of the ligand-receptor complex into an endosomal compartment, endosomal acidification, and ligand dissociation followed by ligand degradation; the RTK can be recycled to the cell surface or may undergo degradation in parallel with the ligand; (3) tyrosine-specific dephosphorylation of the RTK and other early mediators; and (4) Ser/Thr phosphorylation of the RTK and other early mediators in a feedback manner by downstream Ser/Thr kinases or by "crosstalk" from antagonistic signal transduction pathways. The contribution of RTK/target serine phosphorylations to the termination and downregulation of RTK-activated tyrosine phosphorylation under physiologic conditions remains to be established. By contrast, the ability of pharmacologic inhibition of PTPases and noninternalizable

TABLE 4–5.   Mammalian Proteins Containing Pleckstrin Homology Domains

Serine/threonine kinases	
β-ARK1	β-Adrenergic receptor kinase type 1
β-ARK2	β-Adrenergic receptor kinase type 2
Aktl/Rac-α/PKB	AKT8 retrovirus proto-oncogene, related to A and C kinase, protein kinase B
AktII/Rac-β/PKB	AKT8 retrovirus proto-oncogene, related to A and C kinase, protein kinase B
PKCμ	Protein kinase C, unique isoform
Bcr	Breakpoint cluster region gene
Tyrosine kinases	
Tec	Tyrosine kinase expressed in hepatocellular carcinoma
BTK (Atk, Bpk, Emb)	B cell tyrosine kinase, a.k.a. Bruton's tyrosine kinase for Bruton's XLA (see text)
Itk (Tsk, Emt)	Interleukin-2–inducible T cell tyrosine kinase
Bmx	Bone marrow–expressed tyrosine kinase
Regulators of small G proteins	
Ras-GAP	GTPase activator protein for the Ras family of small G proteins
Ras-GRF (2)	Guanine nucleotide–releasing factor for the Ras family of small G proteins
GAP1^{IP4BP}	GTPase activator protein for the Ras family, inositol (1,3,4,5) tetraphosphate–binding protein
SOS1	Son of sevenless is required for development of the seventh ommatidial cell in *Drosophila* retina
SOS2	Grb2 binding, Ras and probably also Rac/Rho activating
HUMORF3_1	Human open reading frame. Hypothetical Ras-GAP protein
Vav	DNA from human esophageal carcinomas*
Dbl	Diffuse B cell lymphoma
Dbs	Dbl's big sister; close relative of Dbl (see above)
Ect2	Epithelial cell transforming
Ost	Truncated protein associated with osteosarcoma
Bcr	Breakpoint cluster region gene in Philadelphia chromosome
Abr	Active Bcr (see above) related gene
Lbc	Lymphoid blast crisis gene
Lfc	Lbc's first cousin; very close relative of Lbc (see above)
Tim	Transforming immortalized mammary gene
Tiam-1 (2)†	T lymphocyte invasion and metastasis; mRNA upregulated in metastatic cells
FGD-1 (2)	Faciogenital dysplasia causative gene
Endocytotic GTPases	
Dynamin-1	GTPase involved in endocytotic vesicle formation, brain
Dynamin-2	GTPase involved in endocytotic vesicle formation, general
Dynamin T	GTPase involved in endocytotic vesicle formation, testes
Adaptors	
IRS-1	Insulin receptor substrate-1, tyrosine-phosphorylated by the insulin receptor
IRS-2	Insulin receptor substrate-2, tyrosine-phosphorylated by the insulin receptor
Grb7	Growth factor receptor–binding protein-7
Grb10	Growth factor receptor–binding protein-10
3BP2	SH3 domain binding protein, binds certain SH3 domains in vitro
Cytoskeletal-associated molecules	
Spectrin βIεII	Major component of erythrocyte membranous cytoskeleton
Fodrin/spectrin βIIεII	Major component of neuron membranous cytoskeleton
Kif1a/Unc104	Neuronal kinesin family homologue
hSEC7	Human homologue of yeast protein involved in vascular secretion
Syntrophin-α/DAP59 (2)	Dystrophin associated protein, molecular weight of 59 kDa
Synthrophin-β (2)	Syntrophin = protein neighbor of dystrophin
AFAP-110, AFAP-120 (2)	Actin filament–associated proteins, 110 and 120 kDa
Pleckstrin (2)	Platelet and leukocyte C-kinase substrate; major platelet PKC substrate
Lipid-associated enzymes	
Phospholipase C-β$_1$	Isotype of PLC, N-terminal PH domain
Phospholipase C-β$_2$	Isotype of PLC, N-terminal PH domain
Phospholipase C-β$_3$	Isotype of PLC, N-terminal PH domain
Phospholipase C-β$_4$	Isotype of PLC, N-terminal PH domain
Phospholipase C-γ$_1$ (2)	Isotypes contain 2 PH domains, 2 SH2 domains, and 1 SH3 domain
Phospholipase C-γ$_2$ (2)	Isotypes contain 2 PH domains, 2 SH2 domains, and 1 SH3 domain
Phospholipase C-δ$_1$	PIP$_2$, IP$_3$, and membrane binding mediated by N-terminal PH domain
Phospholipase C-δ$_2$	PIP$_2$, IP$_3$, and membrane binding mediated by N-terminal PH domain
Phospholipase C-δ$_3$	PIP$_2$, IP$_3$, and membrane binding mediated by N-terminal PH domain
PI-3 kinase-γ	Adds 3-phosphate to phosphoinositides
PI-4 kinase	Adds 4-phosphate to phosphoinositides
Unknown	
IGBP	Interferon-γ–binding protein
Eps8	EGF receptor pathway substrate protein
Mig2	Migration–inducing gene
OSBP	Oxysterol-binding protein; involved in cellular response to oxysterols
HUMORFV_1	Human open reading frame, hypothetic protein
HUMORA5_1	Human open reading frame, hypothetic protein
LL5	Named after discoverer, ubiquitous protein

In some cases, alternative transcripts of these proteins do not contain PH domains (e.g., βIεII and βIεI spectrin, respectively). Many proteins with PH domains (e.g., Tec/Btk-family, β-ARK family, Kif1a/Unc104, PKCμ, dynamins) are closely related to proteins lacking PH domains (e.g., Src family, rhodopsin kinase, Kif1b, other PKCs, Mx proteins, respectively). PH domains have been described in a PI-4 kinase and somewhat less convincing examples have been claimed for eps8, an epidermal growth factor receptor tyrosine kinase substrate, and GAP1^{IP4BP}, a human Ras-GAP protein that also binds PI-3,4,5-P. Allocation of proteins to particular classes is in many cases tentative. Proteins with (2) after their name contain two PH domains. In many cases the acronyms contain useful information about the source or properties of the protein and are therefore given here.

*An exception is Vav, which is Hebrew for 6. The *Vav* gene was the sixth oncogene isolated by Katzav and colleagues.

†The C-terminal PH domain in Tiam-1 is the only one thus known that lacks the conserved Trp residue in the C-terminal (presumably α-helical) region, instead having a Phe. Assuming that this substitution has no functional consequence, we can conclude that no single amino acid in the PH domain is absolutely conserved.

EGF, epidermal growth factor; IP$_3$, inositol 1,4,5-triphosphate; PIP$_2$, phosphatidylinositol 4,5-bisphosphate; XLA, X-linked agammaglobulinemia.

From Shaw G: The pleckstrin homology domain: An intriguing multifunctional protein module. Bioessays 18:35–46, 1996. Copyright © 1996. Reprinted by permission of John Wiley & Sons, Inc.

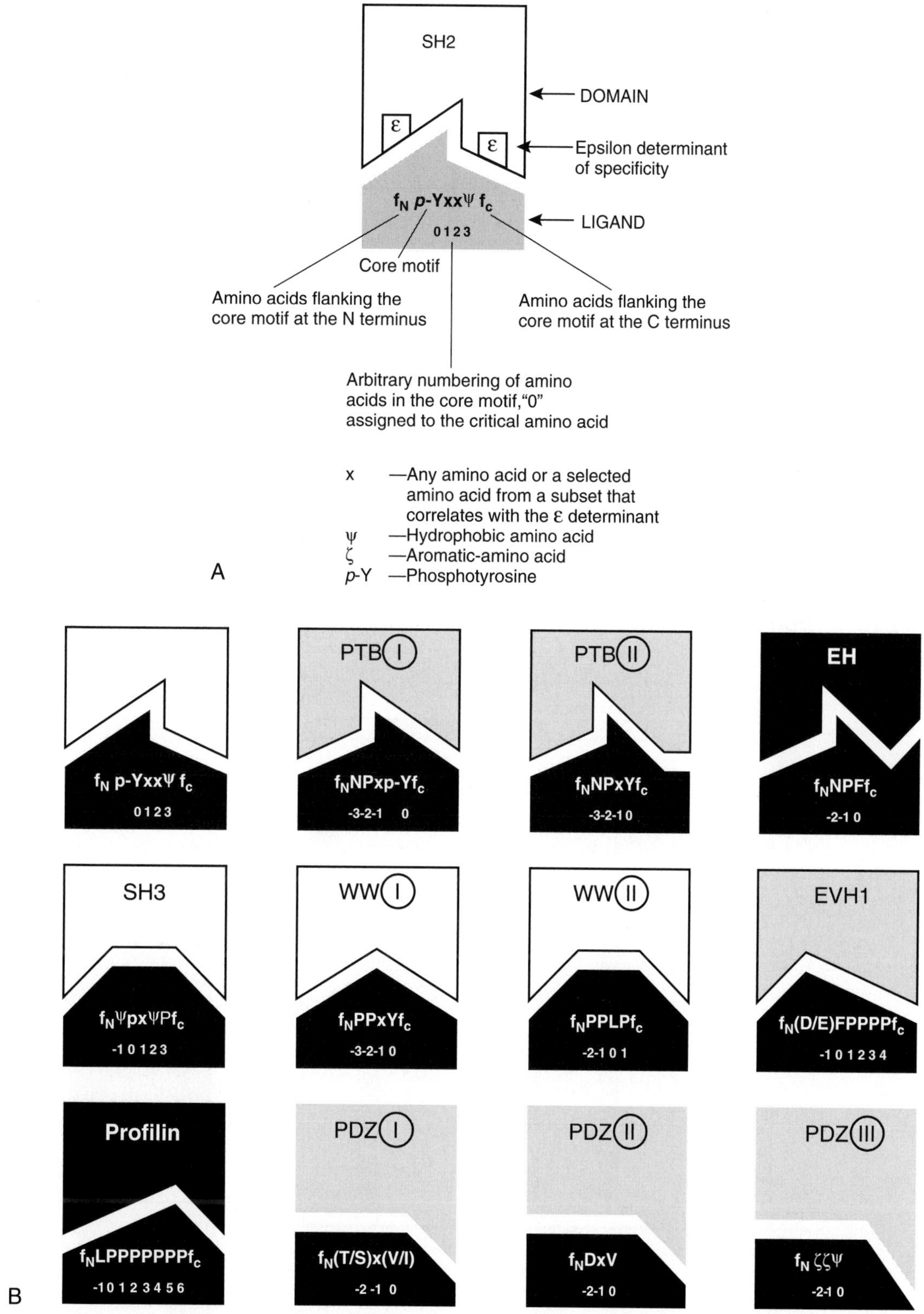

FIGURE 4–13. *A,* Formalization of terms to describe protein-protein interaction mediated by modules using the SH2 domain and its ligand as an example. *B,* Modular protein domains and core sequences of their dognate ligands. SH2 and a subgroup of PTB domains recognize phosphotyrosine in the context of specific sequences. Another subgroup of PT domains, and the EH domain, bind ligands with NP × Y and NPF cores, respectively. SH3, WW, and EVH1 domains, and EVH1 domains bind proline-rich sequences. Profilin also recognizes polyprolines (a minimum of six to eight prolines). Profilin is both a protein domain and an independent, functional protein of 13 to 15 kDa molecular mass. PDZ domains evolved to recognize motifs at the C-terminal ends of proteins. Many more intracellular and extracellular modular protein domains have been identified. However, their ligands are as yet unknown, and significant portions of the newly described modules so far seem to be confined to a limited number of specialized proteins. (From Sudol M: From Src homology domains to other signaling modules: Proposal of the 'protein recognition code'. Oncogene 17:1469–1474, 1998.)

RTK ligands to greatly increase RTK signal intensity and duration has established beyond question the importance of tyrosine phosphatase– and receptor-mediated endocytosis in signal termination.

Protein Tyrosine Phosphatases

First discovered in 1988,[133] PTPs are now nearly as numerous as the protein tyrosine kinases, and like the tyrosine kinases, PTPs can also be classified into transmembrane and intracellular types[134, 135] (Fig. 4–14). The type 1 transmembrane (receptor-like) PTPases (RPTPases) can be classified into seven or more subfamilies that, like the RTKs, display widely divergent extracellular extensions but more uniform intracellular domains. A distinctive feature of all but one RPTPase subfamily is the presence of two tandem catalytic domains, with the membrane-proximal domain contributing all or nearly all the catalytic activity. As purified from cells, both RPTPases and intracellular PTPases exhibit very high catalytic activity, with turnover numbers (using model phosphotyrosine peptide as protein substrates) that far exceed those of the tyrosine kinases. Although some RPTP subfamilies

have been show to form homotypic transcellular associations, the identification of RPTP ligands has proceeded slowly. Consequently, characterization of the effects of native ligands on PTP activity is largely unknown. Replacement of the extracellular and transmembrane domains of the T cell PTP CD45 with those of the EGFR does not impair the measured PTP activity; however, the addition of EGF and consequent dimerization result in a marked inhibition of PTP activity.[15] The crystal structure of the membrane-proximal PTP domain of RPTP-α shows the domains to adopt a symmetric dimeric configuration wherein a wedge-shaped loop just N-terminal to the phosphatase domain is inserted into the catalytic site of the other PTP monomer. Based on these observations, a reasonable inference is that RPTP activity may be negatively regulated by ligand in a manner precisely opposite that of the ligand activation of RTKs; that is, ligand-induced dimerization of RPTP induces inhibition of the catalytic function. CD45 activity is crucial to T cell receptor signaling by virtue of its ability to dephosphorylate the C-terminal autoinhibitory tyrosine phosphorylation site of the c-Src family PTKs, for example, fyn, lyn, and others. The extracellular domain of CD45 is known to undergo extensive modification by alternative mRNA splicing during T cell

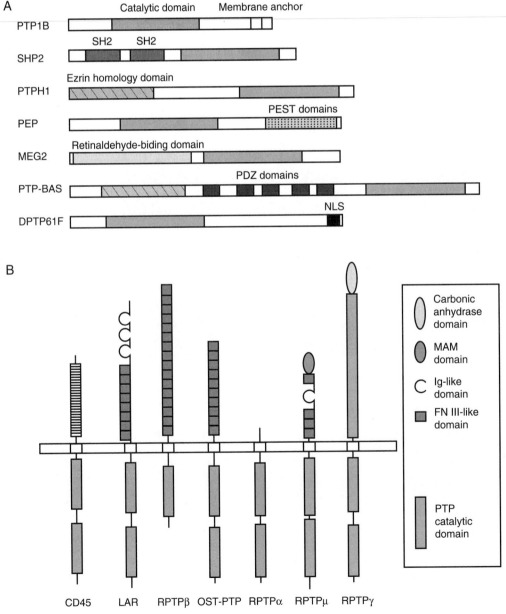

FIGURE 4–14. Schematic structures of non–receptor- (A) and receptor-like (B) protein tyrosine phosphatase families. (From Hunter T: The Croonian Lecture, 1997. Phil Trans Roy Soc Lond B 353:597, 1997.)

development, a process that may substantially alter the binding specificity and/or affinity of the extracellular domain and thereby modify RPTP activity, even without changes in ligand availability. In turn, changes in the CD45 extracellular domain may greatly modify the sensitivity, intensity, and duration of T cell receptor signaling.

The nonreceptor PTPases contain a variety of noncatalytic targeting domains that tether them to the nucleus, cytoskeleton, endoplasmic reticulum, and other structures. Of particular interest are intracellular PTPases that contain protein-protein interaction domains such as SH2 domains.[135] Thus the intracellular PTP, SH-PTP1, and SH-PTP2 each contain a pair of SH2 domains in their N-terminal half, followed by a single C-terminal PTP domain. These PTPs are recruited to activated RTKs/nonreceptor tyrosine kinases through the PTP SH2 domains. Genetic evidence indicates that as expected, SH-PTP1 is a negative regulatory element in the hematopoietic system. Surprisingly however, SH-PTP2 (and its *Drosophila* homologue CSW) appears to function as a positive regulator in RTK signaling; loss of CSW gene function impairs RTK signaling. The basis for this apparently paradoxic response is uncertain, although once recruited to the RTK, SH-PTP2 can undergo RTK-catalyzed phosphorylation to create a strong site for the Grb2 SH2 domain and enable recruitment of SOS and activation of Ras. Phosphotyrosine-containing synthetic peptides stimulate SH-PTP2 catalytic activity, and a structural explanation is provided by the finding that in unliganded SH-PTPase, a segment of the N-terminal SH2 domain is wedged into the catalytic site; binding of a TyrP–containing substrate to the SH2 domain may therefore disocclude the catalytic site. Whether the catalytic activity of other intracellular PTPs is subject to dynamic regulation or is constitutively available at crucial intracellular sites remains uncertain. A frequent mechanism for the pathologic inactivation of tyrosine phosphatase in vivo arises from the presence of a critical, highly reactive cysteine residue at the catalytic site of all PTPs. This residue is especially susceptible to oxidation by reactive oxygen intermediates, with subsequent PTP inactivation. Such a mechanism has been claimed to underlie the increase in RTK-mediated tyrosine phosphorylation engendered by ultraviolet irradiation and ionizing radiation because these responses can be suppressed by antioxidants.[136] Surprisingly, identification of PTPs as tumor suppressor genes in the context of human tumors has not emerged, perhaps reflecting the substantial redundancy and high catalytic efficiency of these enzymes. Similarly, it is not yet possible to state for any RTK which RPTP or intracellular PTPs are primarily responsible for their tyrosine dephosphorylation. The RTK most extensively studied in this regard is the IR, and suggestive, but not conclusive evidence points to the RPTP known as LAR and to SH-PTP2 as the strongest candidate negative regulators.

Receptor Internalization

Receptor-mediated endocytosis is a complex process of general importance in the biology of all surface receptors, and its mechanisms and regulation continue to be under active investigation. RTK internalization plus recycling is a constitutive process that depending on RTK, is accelerated by ligand to a varying extent and is the major route for ligand removal in vivo.[137, 138] This process is best shown for the insulin/IR interaction, where abundant evidence indicates that receptor-mediated endocytosis is the primary and dominant physiologic pathway for insulin clearance in vivo. Internalization of IR is considerably accelerated by insulin; the insulin is largely degraded, but the bulk of IR recycles to the plasma membrane freed of ligand, so the ligand-induced fall in steady-state surface IR content is modest. By contrast, high levels of EGF can promote nearly complete clearance of EGFR from the cell surface, partly because of the relative resistance of EGF to acid-induced dissociation from the EGFR, which results in diversion of the EGFR from recycling endosomes into late endosomes and lysosomes and subsequent EGFR degradation. TGF-α, in contrast, dissociates readily from EGFR at low pH and is associated with much less EGFR degradation. Receptor internalization occurs through clathrin-coated pits, and ligand strongly promotes clustering in the pits. The signals for RTK internalization reside on the intracellular segment of the RTK and are predominantly tyrosine-based motifs,

either NPXY or YXX φ (hydrophobic); internalization involves interaction of the tyrosine motif with one or more adaptor protein complexes. After entry into an early endosome, the decision regarding receptor recycling vs. degradation involves a complex interplay between the pH-dependent dissociation of ligand, interaction of the RTK with a variety of other proteins such as epsin (which bind through Epsin Homology domains to asparagine proline phenylalanine motifs), and RTK targets.[139] Among the latter is the proto-oncogene c-*Cbl*, an RTK substrate that associates with the EGFR in endosomes and promotes EGFR ubiquitination and degradation by proteosomal and lysosomal pathways.[140]

REFERENCES

1. Collett MS, Erikson RL: Protein kinase activity associated with the avian sarcoma virus src gene product. Proc Natl Acad Sci U S A 75:2021–2024, 1978.
2. Echkart W, Hutchinson MA, Hunter T: An activity phosphorylating tyrosine in polyoma T antigen immunoprecipitates. Cell 18:925–933, 1979.
3. Collett MS, Purchio AF, Erikson RL: An activity phosphorylating tyrosine in polyoma T antigen immunoprecipitates. Nature 285:167–169, 1980.
4. Witte ON, Dasgupta A, Baltimore D: Abelson murine leukaemia virus protein is phosphorylated in vitro to form phosphotyrosine. Nature 283:826–831, 1980.
5. Ushiro H, Cohen S: Identification of phosphotyrosine as a product of epidermal growth factor–activated protein kinase in A-431 cell membranes. J Biol Chem 255:8363–8365, 1980.
6. Kasuga M, Karlsson FA, Kahn CR: Insulin stimulates the phosphorylation of the 95,000-dalton subunit of its own receptor. Science 215:185–187, 1982.
7. Ek B, Westermork B, Warteson A, Heldin CH: Stimulation of tyrosine-specific phosphorylation by platelet-derived growth factor. Nature 295:419–420, 1982.
8. Doolittle RF, Hinkapillar MW, Hood LE, et al: Simian sarcoma virus onc gene, v-sis, is derived from the gene (or genes) encoding a platelet-derived growth factor. Science 221:275–277, 1983.
9. Waterfield MD, Scrace GT, Whittle N, et al: Platelet-derived growth factor is structurally related to the putative transforming protein p28sis of simian sarcoma virus. Nature 304:35–39, 1983.
10. Ullrich A, Coussens L, Hayflick JS, et al: Human epidermal growth factor receptor cDNA sequence and aberrant expression of the amplified gene in A431 epidermoid carcinoma cells. Nature 309:418–425, 1984.
11. Ullrich A, Schlessinger J: Signal transduction by receptors with tyrosine kinase activity. Cell 61:203–212, 1990.
12. Fantl WJ, Johnson DE, Williams LT: Signalling by receptor tyrosine kinases. Annu Rev Biochem 62:453–481, 1993.
13. van der Geer P, Hunter T, Lundberg RA: Receptor protein-tyrosine kinases and their signal transduction pathways. Annu Rev Cell Biol 10:251–337, 1994.
14. Heldin C-H: Dimerization of cell surface receptors in signal transduction. Cell 80:213–223, 1995.
15. Weiss A, Schlessinger J: Switching signals on or off by receptor dimerization. Cell 94:277–280, 1998.
16. Tzahar E, Yarden Y: The ErbB-2/HER2 oncogenic receptor of adenocarcinomas: From orphanhood to multiple stromal ligands. Biochim Biophys Acta 1377:25–37, 1988.
17. Alroy I, Yarden Y: The ErbB signaling network in embryogenesis and oncogenesis: Signal diversification through combinatorial ligand-receptor interactions. FEBS Lett 410:83–86, 1997.
18. Perrimon N, Perkins LA: There must be 50 ways to rule the signal: The case of the *Drosophila* EGF receptor. Cell 89:13–16, 1997.
19. Edery P, Eng C, Munnich A, Lyonnet S: RET in human development and oncogenesis. Bioessays 19:389–395, 1997.
20. DeMeyts P, Urso B, Christofferson CT, Shymko RM: Mechanism of insulin and IGF-1 activation and signal transduction specificity. Ann N Y Acad Sci 766:388–401, 1995.
21. McInnes C, Sykes BD: Growth factor receptors: Structure, mechanism, and drug discovery. Biopolymers 43:339–366, 1997.
22. Blakesley VA, Scrimgeour A, Esposito D, LeRoith D: Signaling via the insulin-like growth factor-I receptor: Does it differ from insulin receptor signaling. Cytokine Growth Factor Rev 7:153–159, 1996.
23. Schlessinger J: Direct binding and activation of receptor tyrosine kinases by collagen. Cell 91:869–872, 1997.
24. Moy FJ, Safran M, Seddon AP, et al: Properly oriented heparin-decasaccharide–induced dimers are the biologically active form of basic fibroblast growth factor. Biochemistry 36:4782–4791, 1997.
25. DiGabriele AD, Lax I, Chen DI, et al: Structure of a heparin-linked biologically active dimer of fibroblast growth factor. Nature 393:812–817, 1998.
26. Mangasarian K, Li Y, Mansukhani A, Basilico C: Mutation associated with Crouzon syndrome causes ligand-independent dimerization and activation of FGF receptor-2. J Cell Physiol 172:117–125, 1997.
27. Steinberger D, Vriend G, Mulliken JB, Muller U: The mutations in FGFR2-associated craniosynostoses are clustered in five structural elements of immunoglobulin-like domain III of the receptor. Hum Genet 102:145–150, 1998.
28. Robertson SC, Meyer AN, Hart KC, et al: Activating mutations in the extracellular domain in the fibroblast growth factor receptor 2 function by disruption of the disulfide bond in the third immunoglobulin-like domain. Proc Natl Acad Sci U S A 95:4567–4572, 1998.
29. Horton WA: Fibroblast growth factor receptor 3 and the human chondrodysplasias. Curr Opin Pediatr 9:437–442, 1997.

30. Neilson KM, Friesel R: Ligand-independent activation of fibroblast growth factor receptors by point mutations in the extracellular, transmembrane, and kinase domain. J Biol Chem 271:25049–25057, 1996.
31. Schucahrdt A, D'Agati V, Larsson-Blomberg L, et al: Defects in the kidney and enteric nervous system of mice lacking the tyrosine kinase receptor Ret. Nature 367:380–383, 1994.
32. Edery P, Eng C, Munnich A, Lyonnet S: RET in human development and oncogenesis. Bioessays 19:389–395, 1997.
33. Jing S, Wen D, Yu Y, et al: GDNF induced activation of the Ret protein tyrosine kinase is mediated by GDNFR-alpha, a novel receptor for GDNF. Cell 85:1113–1124, 1996.
34. Enokido Y, de Sauvage F, Hongo J-A, et al: GFRα-4 and the tyrosine kinase Ret form a functional receptor complex for persephin. Curr Biol 8:1019–1022, 1998.
35. Mulligan LM, Kwok JB, Healey CS, et al: Germ-line mutations of the RET proto-oncogene in multiple endocrine neoplasia type 2A. Nature 363:458–460, 1993.
36. Donis-Keller H, Dou S, Chi D, et al: Mutations in the RET proto-oncogene are associated with MEN 2A and FMTC. Hum Mol Genet 7:851–856, 1993.
37. Hofstra RM, Landsvater RM, Ceccherini I, et al: A mutation in the RET proto-oncogene associated with endocrine neoplasia type 2B and sporadic medullary thyroid carcinoma. Nature 367:375–376, 1994.
38. Carlson KM, Dou S, Chi D, et al: Single missense mutation in the tyrosine kinase catalytic domain of the RET proto-oncogene is associated with multiple endocrine neoplasia type 2B. Proc Natl Acad Sci U S A 91:1579–1583, 1994.
39. Romeo G, Ronchetto P, Luo Y, et al: Point mutations affecting the tyrosine kinase domain of the Ret proto-oncogene in Hirschsprung's disease. Nature 367:377–378, 1994.
40. Edery P, Lyonnet S, Mulligan LM, et al: Mutations of the Ret proto-oncogene in Hirschprung's disease. Nature 367:378–380, 1994.
41. Grieco M, Santoro M, Berlingieri MT, et al: PTC is a novel rearranged form of the Ret proto-oncogene and is frequently detected in vivo in human thyroid papillary carcinomas. Cell 60:557–563, 1990.
42. Bongarzone I, Monzini N, Borrello MG, et al: Molecular characterization of a thyroid tumor–specific transforming sequence formed by the fusion of Ret tyrosine-kinase and the regulatory subunit RI alpha of cyclic AMP protein kinase A. Mol Cell Biol 13:358–366, 1993.
43. Santoro M, Dathan NA, Berlingieri MT, et al: Molecular characterization of Ret/PTC3: A novel rearranged version of the Ret proto-oncogene in a human thyroid papillary carcinoma. Oncogene 9:509–516, 1994.
44. Eng C, Clayton D, Schuffenecker I, et al: The relationship between specific RET proto-oncogene mutations and disease phenotype in multiple endocrine neoplasia Type 2. JAMA 276:1575–1578, 1996.
45. Takahashi M, Asai N, Iwashita T, et al: Molecular mechanisms of development of multiple endocrine neoplasia 2 by RET mutations. J Intern Med 243:509–513, 1998.
46. Pelet A, Geneste O, Edery P, et al: Various mechanisms cause RET-mediated signaling defects in Hirschsprung's disease. J Clin Invest 101:1415–1423, 1998.
47. Songyang Z, Carraway KL III, Eck MJ, et al: Catalytic specificity of protein tyrosine kinases is critical for selective signalling. Nature 373:536–539, 1995.
48. Chang HW, Aoki M, Fruman D, et al: Transformation of chicken cells by the gene encoding the catalytic subunit of PI 3-kinase. Science 276:1848–1850, 1997.
49. Hanks SK, Hunter T: Protein kinases 6. The eukaryotic protein kinase superfamily: Kinase (catalytic) domain structure and classification. FASEB J 9:576–596, 1995.
50. Knighton DR, Zheng J, Ten Eyck LF, et al: Crystal structure of the catalytic subunit of cyclic adenosine monophosphate–dependent protein kinase. Science 253:407–414, 1991.
51. Tornqvist HE, Pierce MW, Frackelton AR, et al: Identification of insulin receptor tyrosine residues autophosphorylated in vitro. J Biol Chem 262:10212–10219, 1987.
52. Hubbard SR, Mohammadi M, Schlessinger J: Autoregulatory mechanisms in protein-tyrosine kinases. J Biol Chem 273:11987–11990, 1998.
53. Tornqvist HE, Gunsalus JR, Nemenoff RA, et al: Identification of the insulin receptor tyrosine residues undergoing insulin-stimulated phosphorylation in intact rat hepatoma cells. J Biol Chem 263:350–359, 1988.
54. Rosen OM, Herrera R, Olowe Y, et al: Phosphorylation activates the insulin receptor tyrosine protein kinase. Proc Natl Acad Sci U S A 80:3237–3240, 1983.
55. Tornqvist HE, Avruch J: Relationship of site-specific beta subunit tyrosine autophosphorylation to insulin activation of the insulin receptor (tyrosine) protein kinase activity. J Biol Chem 263:4593–4601, 1988.
56. Ellis L, Clauser E, Morgan DO, et al: Replacement of insulin receptor tyrosine residues 1162 and 1163 compromises insulin-stimulated kinase activity and uptake of 2-deoxyglucose. Cell 45:721–732, 1986.
57. Hubbard SR, Wei L, Ellis L, Hendrickson WA: Crystal structure of the tyrosine kinase domain of the human insulin receptor. Nature 372:746–754, 1994.
58. Hubbard SR: Crystal structure of the activated insulin receptor tyrosine kinase in complex with peptide substrate and ATP analog. EMBO J 16:5572–5581, 1997.
59. Mohammadi M, Schlessinger J, Hubbard SR: Structure of the FGF receptor tyrosine kinase domain reveals a novel autoinhibitory mechanism. Cell 86:577–587, 1996.
60. Taylor SI: Molecular mechanisms of insulin resistance. Diabetes 41:1473–1490, 1992.
61. Mossie K, Jallal B, Alves F, et al: Colon carcinoma kinase-4 defines a new subclass of the receptor tyrosine kinase family. Oncogene 11:2179–2184, 1995.
62. Kolibaba KS, Druker BJ: Protein tyrosine kinases and cancer. Biochim Biophys Acta 1333:217–248, 1997.
63. Ross AH, Baltimore D, Eisen HN: Phosphotyrosine-containing proteins isolated by affinity chromatography with antibodies to a synthetic hapten. Nature 294:654–656, 1981.
64. Margolis B, Rhee SG, Felder S, et al: EGF induces tyrosine phosphorylation of phospholipase C-II: A potential mechanism for EGF receptor signaling. Cell 57:1101–1107, 1989.
65. Meisenhelder J, Suh PG, Rhee SG, Hunter T: Phospholipase C-gamma is a substrate for the PDGF and EGF receptor protein-tyrosine kinases in vivo and in vitro. Cell 57:1109–1122, 1989.
66. Rhee SG, Choi KD: Regulation of inositol phospholipid–specific phospholipase C isozymes. J Biol Chem 267:12393–12396, 1992.
67. Whitman M, Downes CP, Keeler M, et al: Type I phosphatidylinositol kinase makes a novel inositol phospholipid, phosphatidylinositol-3-phosphate. Nature 332:644–646, 1988.
68. Coughlin SR, Escobedo JA, Williams LT: Role of phosphatidylinositol kinase in PDGF receptor signal transduction. Science 243:1191–1194, 1989.
69. Kazlauskas A, Cooper JA: Phosphorylation of the PDGF receptor beta subunit creates a tight binding site for phosphatidylinositol 3 kinase. EMBO J 9:3279–3286, 1990.
70. Fantl WJ, Escobedo JA, Martin GA, et al: Distinct phosphotyrosines on a growth factor receptor bind to specific molecules that mediate different signaling pathways. Cell 69:413–423, 1992.
71. Escobedo JA, Kaplan DR, Kavanaugh WM, et al: A phosphatidylinositol-3 kinase binds to platelet-derived growth factor receptors through a specific receptor sequence containing phosphotyrosine. Mol Cell Biol 11:1125–1132, 1991.
72. Sadowski I, Stone JC, Pawson T: A noncatalytic domain conserved among cytoplasmic protein-tyrosine kinases modifies the kinase function and transforming activity of Fujinami sarcoma virus P130gag-fps. Mol Cell Biol 6:4396–4408, 1986.
73. Bollag G, McCormick F: Regulators and effectors of ras proteins. Annu Rev Cell Biol 7:601–632, 1991.
74. Mayer BJ, Hamaguchi M, Hanafusa H: A novel viral oncogene with structural similarity to phospholipase C. Nature 332:272–275, 1988.
75. Matsuda M, Mayer BJ, Fukui Y, Hanafusa H: Binding of transforming protein, P47gag-crk, to a broad range of phosphotyrosine-containing proteins. Science 248:1537–1539, 1990.
76. Koch CA, Anderson D, Moran MF, et al: SH2 and SH3 domains: Elements that control interactions of cytoplasmic signalling proteins. Science 252:668–674, 1991.
77. Pawson T: Protein modules and signalling networks. Nature 373:573–580, 1995.
78. Songyang Z, Shoelson SE, Chaudhurl M, et al: SH2 domains recognize specific phosphopeptide sequences. Cell 72:767–778, 1993.
79. Kavanaugh WM, Williams LT: An alternative to SH2 domains for binding tyrosine-phosphorylated proteins. Science 266:1862–1865, 1994.
80. Blaikie P, Immanuel D, Wu J, et al: A region in Shc distinct from the SH2 domain can bind tyrosine-phosphorylated growth factor receptors. J Biol Chem 269:32031–32034, 1994.
81. van der Geer P, Pawson T: The PTB domain. TIBS 20:277–280, 1995.
82. White MF, Livingston JN, Backer JM, et al: Mutation of the insulin receptor at tyrosine 960 inhibits signal transmission but does not affect its tyrosine kinase activity. Cell 54:641–649, 1988.
83. Sun XJ, Rothenberg P, Kahn CR, et al: Structure of the insulin receptor substrate IRS-1 defines a unique signal transduction protein. Nature 382:73–77, 1991.
84. Yenush L, White MF: The IRS-signalling system during insulin and cytokine action. Bioessays 19:491–500, 1997.
85. Araki E, Lipes MA, Patti ME, et al: Alternative pathway of insulin signalling in mice with targeted disruption of the IRS-1 gene. Nature 372:186–190, 1994.
86. Withers DJ, Gutierrez JS, Towery H, et al: Disruption of IRS-2 causes type 2 diabetes in mice. Nature 391:900–904, 1998.
87. Bruning JC, Winnay J, Bonner-Weir S, et al: Development of a novel polygenic model of NIDDM in mice heterozygous for IR and IRS-1 null alleles. Cell 88:561–572, 1997.
88. Holgado-Madruga M, Emlet DR, Moscatello DK, et al: A Grb2-associated docking protein in EGF- and insulin-receptor signalling. Nature 379:560–556, 1996.
89. Yenush L, Fernandez R, Myers MG Jr, et al: The *Drosophila* insulin receptor activates multiple signaling pathways but requires insulin receptor substrate proteins for DNA synthesis. Mol Cell Biol 16:2509–2517, 1996.
90. Songyang Z, Cantley L: Recognition and specificity in protein tyrosine kinase–mediated signalling. TIBS 20:470–475, 1995.
91. Darnell JE Jr: STATs and gene regulation. Science 277:1630–1635, 1997.
92. Bos JL: ras oncogenes in human cancer: A review [published erratum appears in Cancer Res 1990 Feb 15;50(4):1352]. Cancer Res 49:4682–4689, 1989.
93. Jiminez C, Jones DR, Rodriquez-Viciana P, et al: Identification and characterization of a new oncogene derived from the regulatory subunit of phosphoinositide 3-kinase. EMBO J 17:743–753, 1998.
94. Chang HW, Aoki M, Fruman D, et al: Transformation of chicken cells by the gene encoding the catalytic subunit of PI 3-kinase. Science 276:1848–1850, 1997.
95. Staal SP: Molecular cloning of the akt oncogene and its human homologues AKT1 and AKT2: Amplification of AKT1 in a primary human gastric adenocarcinoma. Proc Natl Acad Sci U S A 84:5034–5037, 1987.
96. Li J, Yen C, Liaw D, et al: *PTEN,* a putative protein tyrosine phosphatase gene mutated in human brain, breast, and prostate cancer. Science 275:1943–1947, 1997.
97. Maehama T, Dixon JE: The tumor suppressor, PTEN/MMAC1, dephosphorylates the lipid second messenger, phosphatidylinositol 3,4,5-trisphosphate. J Biol Chem 273:13375–13378, 1998.
98. Bos JL: Ras-like GTPases. Biochim Biophys Acta 1333:19–31, 1997.
99. Schlessinger J: How receptor tyrosine kinases activate Ras. TIBS 18:273–275, 1993.
100. Marshall MS: The effector interactions of p21ras. TIBS 18:250–255, 1993.
101. Avruch J, Zhang X-F, Kyriakis JM: Ras meets Raf. TIBS 19:279–283, 1994.
102. Chuang E, Barnard D, Hettich L, et al: Critical binding and regulatory interactions between Ras and Raf occur through a small, stable N-terminal domain of Raf and specific Ras effector residues. Mol Cell Biol 14:5318–5325, 1994.
103. Hu CD, Kariya K, Tamada M, et al: Cysteine-rich region of Raf-1 interacts with activator domain of post-translationally modified Ha-Ras. J Biol Chem 270:30274–30277, 1995.
104. Luo Z, Diaz B, Marshall MS, Avruch J: An intact raf zinc finger is required for optimal binding to processed ras and for ras-dependent raf activation in situ. Mol Cell Biol 17:46–53, 1997.

105. Mineo C, Anderson RG, White M: Physical association with Ras enhances activation of membrane-bound Raf (Raf CAAX). J Biol Chem 272:10345–10348, 1997.

106. Tzivion G, Luo Z, Avruch J: A dimeric 14-3-3 protein is an essential cofactor for Raf kinase activity. Nature 394:88–92, 1998.

107. Kyriakis JM, App H, Zhang XF, et al: Raf-1 activates MAP kinase-kinase. Nature 358:417–421, 1992.

108. Malumbreas M, Pellicer A: Ras pathways to cell cycle control and cell transformation. Front Biosci 3:887–912, 1998.

109. Rodriquez-Viciana, Warne PH, Vanhaesebroeck B, et al: Activation of phosphoinositide 3-kinase by interaction with Ras and by point mutation. EMBO J 15:2442–2451, 1996.

110. Klinghoffer RA, Duckworth B, Valius M, et al: Platelet-derived growth factor–dependent activation of phosphatidylinositol 3-kinase is regulated by receptor binding of SH2-domain–containing proteins which influence Ras activity. Mol Cell Biol 16:5905–5914, 1996.

111. Rodriquez-Viciana P, Warne PH, Dhand R, et al: Phosphatidylinositol-3-OH kinase as a direct target of Ras. Nature 370:527–532, 1994.

112. Courtneidge SA, Heber A: An 85 kd protein complexed with middle T antigen and pp60c-src: A possible phosphatidylinositol kinase. Cell 50:1031–1037, 1987.

113. Vanhaesebroeck B, Leevers SJ, Panayotou G, Waterfield MD: Phosphoinositide 3-kinases: A conserved family of signal transducers. TIBS 22:267–272, 1997.

114. Shepherd PR, Withers DJ, Siddle K: Phosphoinositide 3-kinase: The key switch mechanism in insulin signalling. Biochem J 333:471–490, 1998.

115. Toker A, Cantley L: Signalling through the lipid products of phosphoinositide-3-OH kinase. Nature 387:673–676, 1997.

116. Morris JZ, Tissenbaum HA, Ruvkun G: A phosphatidylinositol-3-OH kinase family member regulating longevity and diapause in *Caenorhabditis elegans*. Nature 382:536–539, 1996.

117. Kimura KD, Tissenbaum HA, Liu Y, Ruvkun G: daf-2, an insulin receptor–like gene that regulates longevity and diapause in *Caenorhabditis elegans*. Science 277:942–946, 1997.

118. Mayer BJ, Ren R, Clark KL, Baltimore D: A putative modular domain present in diverse signaling proteins. Cell 73:629–630, 1993.

119. Haslam RJ, Koide HB, Hemmings BA: Pleckstrin domain homology. Nature 363:309–310, 1993.

120. Lemmon MA, Ferguson KM, Schlessinger J: PH domains: Diverse sequences with a common fold recruit signaling molecules to the cell surface. Cell 85:621–624, 1996.

121. Shaw S: The pleckstrin homology domain: An intriguing multifunctional protein module. Bioessays 18:35–46, 1996.

122. Touhara K, Inglese J, Pitcher JA, et al: Binding of G protein βγ-subunits to pleckstrin homology domains. J Biol Chem 269:10217–10220, 1994.

123. Pitcher JA, Touhara K, Payne SE, Lefkowitz RJ: Pleckstrin homology domain–mediated membrane association and activation of the β-adrenergic receptor kinase requires coordinate interaction with Gβγ subunits and lipid. J Biol Chem 270:11707–11710, 1995.

124. Mahadevan D, Thanki N, Singh J, et al: Structural studies on the PH domains of Dbl, Sos1, IRS-1, and βARK1 and their differential binding to Gβγ subunits. Biochemistry 34:9111–9117, 1995.

125. Harlan JE, Hajduk PH, Yoon H-S, Feslk SW: Pleckstrin homology domains bind to phosphatidylinositol-4,5-bisphosphate. Nature 371:168–170, 1994.

126. Rameh LE, Arvidsson A-K, Carraway KL III, et al: A comparative analysis of the phosphoinositide binding specificity of pleckstrin homology domains. J Biol Chem 272:22059–22066, 1997.

127. Voliovitch H, Schindler DG, Hadari YR, et al: Tyrosine phosphorylation of insulin receptor substrate-1 in vivo depends upon the presence of its pleckstrin homology region. J Biol Chem 270:18083–18087, 1995.

128. Zheng Y, Zangrilli D, Cerione RA, Eva A: The pleckstrin homology domain mediates transformation by oncogenic Dbl through specific intracellular targeting. J Biol Chem 271:19017–19020, 1996.

129. Pawson T, Scott JD: Signaling through scaffold, anchoring, and adaptor proteins. Science 278:2075–2080, 1997.

130. Sudol M: From Src homology domains to other signaling modules: Proposal of the "protein recognition code." Oncogene 17:1469–1474, 1998.

131. Lu P-J, Zhou XZ, Shen M, KP Lu: Function of WW domains as phosphoserine- or phosphothreonine-binding modules. Science 283:1325–1328, 1999.

132. Ponting CP, Phillips C, Davies KE, Blake DJ: PDZ domains: Targeting signalling molecules to sub-membranous sites. Bioessays 19:469–479, 1997.

133. Tonks NK, Diltz CD, Fischer EH: Purification of the major protein-tyrosine-phosphatases of human placenta. J Biol Chem 263:6722–6730, 1988.

134. Denu JM, Stuckey JA, Saper MA, Dixon JE: Form and function in protein dephosphorylation. Cell 87:361–364, 1996.

135. Streuli M: Protein tyrosine phosphatases in signaling. Curr Opin Cell Biol 8:182–188, 1996.

136. Weiss UF, Daub H, Ullrich A: novel mechanisms of RTK signal generation. Curr Opin Genet Dev 7:80–86, 1997.

137. Vieira AV, Lamaze C, Schmid SL: Control of EGF receptor signaling by clathrin-mediated endocytosis. Science 274:2086–2089, 1996.

138. Mukherjee S, Ghosh RN, Maxfield FR: Endocytosis. Physiol Rev 77:759–803, 1997.

139. Sorkin A: Endocytosis and intracellular sorting of receptor tyrosine kinases. Front Biosci 3:729–738, 1998.

140. Levkowitz G, Waterman H, Zamir E, et al: c-Cbl/Sli-1 regulates endocytic sorting and ubiquitination of the epidermal growth factor receptor. Genes Dev 12:3663–3674, 1998.

Hormone Signaling via Cytokine Receptors and Receptor Serine Kinases

Lawrence S. Mathews ▪ Dana Gaddy-Kurten

Numerous hormones and growth factors initiate cellular signaling by direct stimulation of protein kinase activity, as discussed in Chapters 4 and 6. The cytokine receptors and the receptor serine kinases (RSKs) represent the two most recently characterized classes of transmembrane signaling systems that use membrane-associated kinases. Together with the receptor tyrosine kinases (RTKs), these systems represent all the known ways in which binding of an extracellular factor at the cell membrane directly activates protein kinases. The similarities and differences between these different systems are summarized at the end of this chapter.

CYTOKINE RECEPTOR SIGNALING

A large number of extracellular agents, including growth hormone (GH), prolactin, eythropoietin, interferons (IFNs), and numerous interleukins (ILs), bind to cell surface receptors that do not have intrinsic enzymatic activity.[1] The GH receptor (GHR) was among the first of these agents to be cloned,[2] and the lack of any obvious signaling motif in the receptor was surprising given that changes in tyrosine phosphorylation of the receptor had been detected in response to GH stimulation.[3] Resolution of that paradox came with the realization that ligand binding stimulated the activity of a receptor-associated tyrosine kinase.[4] That mode of action is now known to be widespread.

Ligands and Biologic Effects

Factors that signal through members of the cytokine receptor family exhibit a wide variety of biologic activities, including classic hormonal effects (GH, prolactin), regulation of hematopoietic cell development and differentiation (ILs, erythropoietin), and antiviral activity (IFNs). Two key issues concerning cytokine action (pleiotropy and redundancy) have been at least partly addressed by studies of cell signaling. Pleiotropy refers to the diverse actions of individual factors on many different cell types in the body; redundancy refers to the observation that in any given cell, many different agents can elicit the same set of responses. Where appropriate, this section emphasizes signaling by GH because it is the best-studied endocrine agent of this group. Additional information can be found in several comprehensive recent reviews of these and other cytokines.[5–8]

Receptors

Analysis in this section focuses on the class I (hematopoietin) and class II (IFN) cytokine receptor families. Members of these classes have an amino-terminal extracellular domain, a single transmembrane domain, and a carboxy-terminal signaling domain. These receptors share conserved sequences in the extracellular domain that are related to the fibronectin type III repeat; in the intracellular domain they have only localized regions of sequence identity that couple the receptors to signaling proteins (Fig. 5–1). The intracellular domains have no known catalytic activity. Sequence features that define membership in this family include a set of four conserved cysteine residues and the motif WSXWS (tryptophan-serine-X-tryptophan-serine) in the extracellular domain. Receptor proteins that directly transmit downstream signals (e.g., gp130), as opposed to those involved solely in ligand binding (e.g., IL-6Rα), also have either one or two copies of a conserved motif (termed box 1 and box 2) in the intracellular juxtamembrane region that is required for coupling to downstream kinases.

Several patterns of holoreceptor complex formation are known for the cytokine receptor family (Fig. 5–2). The simplest pattern (used by a minority of ligands) is the formation of a receptor homodimer in response to ligand binding. In addition, some groups of ligands activate shared sets of receptor subunits, in varied combinations, by inducing the formation of receptor heteromers. The cytokines IL-6, IL-11, leukemia inhibitory factor (LIF), cardiotrophin-1, ciliary neurotrophic factor, and oncostatin M all have receptor complexes that contain the receptor protein gp130. Within this group, however, different arrangements are used (see Fig. 5–2). Although IL-6 does not bind to gp130 alone,[9] it binds with low affinity to an IL-6–specific receptor subunit (IL-6Rα) that does not contain an intracellular signaling domain; it binds with high affinity to a complex containing one IL-6Rα and two molecules of gp130.[10] As discussed below, oligomerization of the gp130 intracellular domains initiates subsequent signaling events. In contrast, LIF also binds a LIF-specific receptor subunit with low affinity and a LIF receptor–gp130 complex with high affinity; however, the LIF receptor, like gp130, has an intracellular domain that participates directly in signaling (see Fig. 5–2).

Using a similar theme, IL-3, IL-5, and granulocyte-macrophage colony-stimulating factor all have specific low-affinity receptor subunits that lack signaling domains, and each binds to high-affinity receptor complexes that contain the specific receptor subunit in combination with a shared receptor component[11] (see Fig. 5–2). IL-2, IL-4, IL-7, IL-9 and IL-13 also signal via a shared receptor subunit.[11] This common feature of sharing a signaling receptor monomer accounts in part for the redundant biologic actions displayed by many of these factors.

The GHR can be considered a prototype of the single-chain, homomeric receptors.[6] Both structural and biochemical studies indicate that the ligand-bound GHR is a dimer; interestingly, that receptor dimer

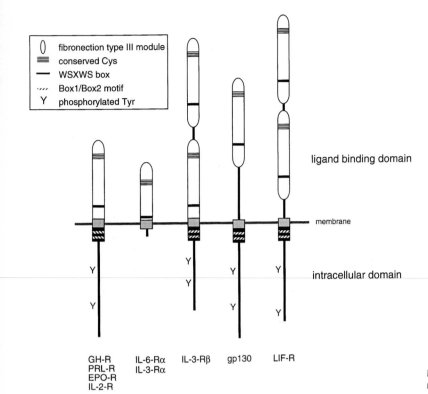

FIGURE 5–1. Schematic diagram of members of the cytokine receptor family. Specific features of the receptors are indicated.

FIGURE 5–2. Modes of ligand binding by cytokine receptors. The growth hormone receptor binds ligand as a homodimer. The interleukin-6 (IL-6) receptor contains an IL-6–specific receptor subunit and two monomers of the signaling protein gp 130; conversely, the leukocyte-inhibitory factor (LIF) receptor contains gp 130 with a LIF-specific subunit. The IL-3 receptor contains an IL-3–specific α subunit and a β subunit shared by IL-5 and granulocyte-macrophage colony-stimulating factor (GM-CSF).

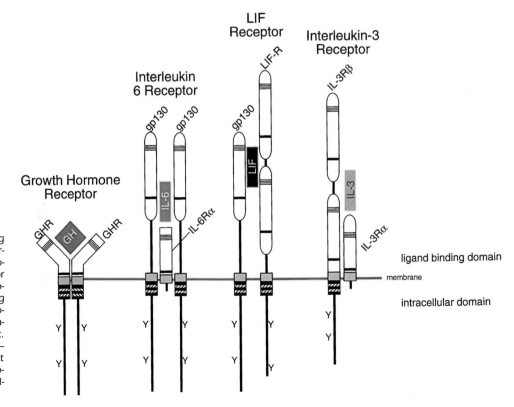

binds a single molecule of GH.[12] Formation of the GH-GHR complex is thus the direct mechanism through which receptor dimers arise. As discussed below, receptor dimerization is an essential event in transmitting an intracellular signal. Ligand-induced receptor dimerization is both necessary and sufficient for signal transmission, evidence for which comes from three sources. (1) Rational mutagenesis of growth hormone, based on analysis of the 3-dimensional structure, yielded altered ligands that can bind receptor but cannot form receptor dimers and do not produce cellular responses.[13] (2) Study of the GHR gene from patients with Laron-type dwarfism (in which circulating GH is normal but cells are nonresponsive[14]) identified receptor mutants that can bind ligand but cannot dimerize and do not signal.[15] (3) Erythropoietin receptor mutants, which are always dimerized because of the presence of an interchain disulfide bond, are constitutively active.[16]

JAKs

Although several ligands with receptors in the cytokine receptor family—including GH[17] and erythropoietin[18]—increase the tyrosine phosphorylation of intracellular proteins, unlike the epidermal growth factor (EGF) receptor tyrosine kinase, those cytokine receptors do not contain an intrinsic kinase domain. The cytokine receptors all associate with and signal through members of the JAK group of cytoplasmic protein tyrosine kinases. Although JAK originally stood for *just an-other kinase*, it now stands for Janus kinase (after the two-faced Roman god) because these molecules contain a pseudokinase domain in addition to the canonical protein kinase motif. Four members of the JAK family are known—JAK1, JAK2, JAK3, and Tyk2. In addition to substantial sequence similarity in the kinase and pseudokinase domains, these proteins have several other regions of high sequence conservation termed JAK homology (JH) domains (Fig. 5–3). Those regions participate in JAK-receptor, JAK-JAK, or JAK-substrate interactions.

The JAKs were initially implicated in cytokine receptor signaling via two routes. In the first line of research, investigators using somatic cell genetics to identify proteins required for IFN signaling found several JAKs to be essential for the generation of IFN responses.[19, 20] This powerful approach involved the selection of cell mutants that could no longer undergo transcriptional activation after IFN treatment and was central to elucidating key details of the pathway. In addition, direct biochemical analysis implicated JAKs as the kinases responsible for tyrosine phosphorylation of both the GH and erythropoietin receptors after ligand binding.[17, 18] Notably, different receptors activate different combinations of JAKs. The homomeric receptor complexes generally activate only a single JAK, usually JAK2; however, in the heteromeric receptor complexes, each receptor subunit can bind a different JAK and hence multiple kinases can be simultaneously activated by a single ligand to create a unique signal. For example, IFN-α activates JAK1 and Tyk2, whereas IFN-γ activates JAK1 and JAK2 and IL-6 activates JAK1, JAK2, and Tyk2. Interestingly, in such cases each kinase requires the presence of the other for activation, thus implying concomitant, reciprocal phosphorylation of the two JAKs in the complex.

Events after cytokine receptor dimerization closely parallel those resulting from RTK activation (Fig. 5–4). JAKs bind to the receptors through the two conserved membrane-proximal motifs. Ligand binding brings two receptor-associated JAKs in proximity to form a very stable holoreceptor complex, after which the JAKs *trans*-phosphorylate each other to increase enzymatic activity and thereby cause extensive tyrosine phosphorylation of both receptors and JAKs. Phosphotyrosines on all those molecules then potentially serve as docking sites for the

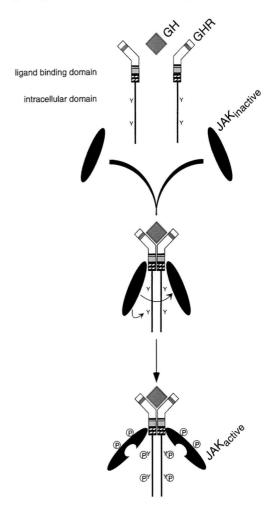

FIGURE 5–4. Activation of cytokine receptor–associated tyrosine kinases, the Janus kinases (JAKs) by growth hormone (GH) binding. A single molecule of GH dimerizes two GH receptors which lead to JAK recruitment and *trans*-phosphorylation and consequent phosphorylation of the receptors.

binding of intracellular signaling proteins. A number of Src homology-2 (SH2) domain–containing proteins interact with phosphorylated cytokine receptor–JAK complexes to mediate the ligand-initiated signal. Many pathways known to be used by RTKs are also stimulated by activation of cytokine receptors, including activation of ras and the mitogen-activated protein kinase (MAPK) pathway and phosphorylation of IRS-1.[6]

Intracellular Signal Mediators

STATs

One well-characterized class of signal mediators for the cytokine receptors, as well as for other RTKs, is the STATs (*signal transducers and activators of transcription*). STATs were originally purified biochemically as components of IFN-induced transcriptional complexes[21]; a total of seven members of the family were identified through various means, including genetic screens and sequence similarity.[22] Like many other signaling proteins, STATs are modular and contain a DNA-binding domain, a transcriptional activation domain, and an SH2 domain[22] (Fig. 5–5). The SH2 domain participates in two features of STAT function. It is required for initial binding of STATs to phosphotyrosines on the activated JAK-receptor complex[23]; as with other SH2 interactions, the specificity of which phosphotyrosine different STATs bind depends on the sequence of the STAT SH2. The SH2 domain is also required for a unique feature of STAT activation;

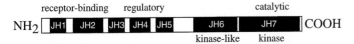

FIGURE 5–3. Schematic diagram of Janus kinases (JAKs). Domains associated with functional features are indicated. JH, JAK homology domain.

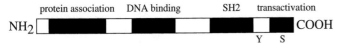

$$NH_2 \quad \blacksquare\quad COOH$$

protein association   DNA binding   SH2   transactivation

Y   S

FIGURE 5–5. *Schematic diagram of STATs (signal transducers and activators of transcription). Domains associated with functional features are indicated. Y, site of activating tyrosine phosphorylation; S, site of regulatory serine phosphorylation; SH2, Src homology domain.*

STATs themselves become tyrosine-phosphorylated by JAKs, with the subsequent formation of STAT dimers (both homodimers and heterodimers have been demonstrated).[24] These dimers arise through interaction of the phosphotyrosine on one STAT with the SH2 domain on another; mutation of either the tyrosine or key residues within the SH2 domain abolishes the interaction and results in complete loss of function.[24] Such data demonstrate that STAT dimerization is required for nuclear entry and DNA binding. The three-dimensional structures of the STAT1 and STAT3β DNA-binding domains reveal that STATs bind DNA through an immunoglobulin-like fold similar to that used by p53.[25, 26] The transcriptional activating domain of some STATs, although not all, is modulated by specific serine phosphorylation.[27]

STATs exist in a latent form in the cytoplasm. After ligand binding, they translocate to the nucleus where they can directly bind to DNA in target genes and activate transcription[22] (Fig. 5–6). Different STAT complexes form in response to the activation of different JAK combinations. Some of these complexes contain only STAT proteins, whereas others, such as the IFN-α–stimulated gene factor, also contain other IFN-regulated proteins.[24] These different STAT-containing complexes recognize different DNA sequences and hence stimulate transcription from different sets of promoters, thereby providing an expla-

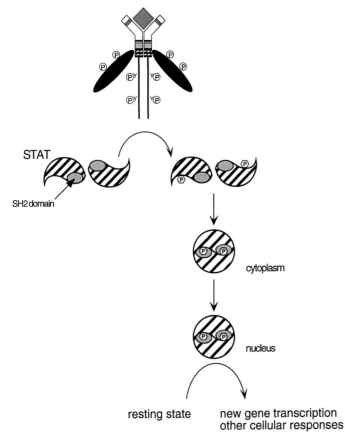

STAT

SH2 domain

cytoplasm

nucleus

resting state   new gene transcription
other cellular responses

FIGURE 5–6. *Activation of STATs (signal transducers and activators of transcription) by JAKs (Janus kinases). Active JAK phosphorylation of STATs on specific tyrosine residues leads to the formation of STAT dimers via binding of the phosphotyrosine to the SH2 (Src homology-2) domain of another STAT molecule. Dimerized STATs translocate to the nucleus and bind DNA.*

nation for how various ligands elicit diverse cellular responses. Detailed analysis of STAT-inducible promoters suggests that cooperative transcription factor interactions are important for STAT function. In some promoters, multiple STAT-binding sites are found in tandem, which implies STAT multimer formation; in other promoters, STAT-binding sites are found immediately adjacent to sites for other factors, including C/EBPβ (CAAT/enhancer/binding protein β), nuclear factor κB (NF-κB), activator protein-1 (AP-1) and the glucocorticoid receptor.[5]

Other Signal Mediators

In addition to activating STATs, cytokine receptor–JAK complexes also use other signaling pathways. Prominent among these is the MAPK pathway; GH and other factors stimulate the Shc, Grb2 (growth factor receptor–binding protein-2), ras, raf, ERK (extracellular signal–related kinase), and MEK (MAPK/ERK kinase) series of proteins,[28] as outlined in Chapter 9. Furthermore, GH can also activate MAPK indirectly by affecting the EGF receptor via JAK2-dependent phosphorylation.[29] Various cytokines also exert their effects in part through activation of insulin receptor substrate-1 (IRS-1) and IRS-2, phosphatidylinositol 3-kinase, and protein kinase C,[28] through mechanisms described in Chapters 4 and 9.

Regulation of Cytokine Receptor Signaling

As with other hormonally activated signaling systems, the output of cytokine receptor pathways is subject to regulation at several levels, and STAT activation is a transient phenomenon. At the receptor level, ligand-receptor complexes are internalized and, in some cases, subject to ubiquitin-dependent proteolysis.[30] At the JAK level, proteins known as suppressors of cytokine signaling (SOCS) bind to JAKs and inhibit their activity.[31] At the STAT level, proteins in the PIAS (protein inhibitor of activated STATs) family bind STATs and prevent DNA binding.[32] In addition, protein tyrosine phosphatases are also implicated in signal attenuation. Two SH2 domain–containing phosphatases bind to phosphorylated tyrosines in the receptor-JAK complex; genetic data demonstrate that these enzymes limit signal transmission.[33] Analysis of the kinetics of STAT phosphorylation and subcellular redistribution suggests that a nuclear tyrosine phosphatase rapidly dephosphorylates STATs, after which they return to the cytoplasm.[34]

RECEPTOR SERINE KINASE SIGNALING

The final class of kinases activated by binding of extracellular ligands at the plasma membrane encompasses receptors for transforming growth factor-β (TGF-β) and related proteins. TGF-β and related factors signal through a heteromeric complex of transmembrane receptors with intrinsic protein serine/threonine kinase activity. Conceptually, the design of this RSK signaling system shares substantial similarity with both the RTK and JAK/STAT signaling systems.

Ligands and Biologic Effects

Like the cytokine family, the TGF-β family includes peptide growth factors that regulate a broad range of cellular functions, including proliferation, cell differentiation, immune surveillance, extracellular matrix secretion and cell adhesion, apoptosis, and specification of developmental fate[35–37]; detailed discussion of the functions of inhibin and activin is found in Chapter 140. These ligands are disulfide-linked dimers; both homodimers and heterodimers are known. In mammals, the study of TGF-β-related molecules has focused on control of sexual development and function (meiosis-inducing substance [MIS], inhibin, and activin), pituitary hormone production (activin and inhibin), and the creation and maintenance of bones and cartilage (activin, bone morphogenetic proteins [BMPs], and GDFs [growth and differentiation

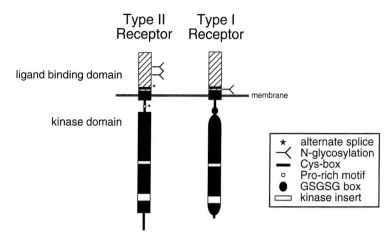

FIGURE 5–7. Schematic diagram of type I and type II receptor serine kinases. Specific features are indicated.

factors]). These activities can be exerted by classic delivery of the factor to its target tissue from a distant site of production via the circulation (endocrine), by local action on neighboring cells (paracrine), or by stimulation of the same cell that produced and secreted the factor (autocrine). As with the cytokines discussed above, insight into the mechanisms of pleiotropy and redundancy for TGF-β-related factors has been gained through signal transduction studies in a variety of cell types.

Receptors

Structures and Binding Properties

The holoreceptor complex for TGF-β-related factors contains proteins from each of the two subfamilies of RSKs. In mammals, five type II receptors and eight type I receptors have been identified that transduce signals for activin, TGF-β, BMP2/4, BMP7/OP-1 (osteogenic, protein-1) MIS, and GDF-5.[38–41] Most receptor complexes bind several ligands, and several type I receptors form combinatorial interactions with type II receptors, thus creating signal diversity.

The RSKs contain an extracellular ligand-binding domain, a single membrane-spanning region, and a cytoplasmic kinase domain with serine-threonine phosphorylation specificity (Fig. 5–7). Several structural features distinguish the type I and type II receptors. They share conserved cysteine residues in their extracellular domains; the three-dimensional structure of the extracellular domain of a type II activin receptor indicates that these cysteines probably direct all the members of this family to adopt a common fold.[42] Type I and type II receptors possess distinct kinase domain sequences with less than 50% sequence identity. In general, the type II receptor confers ligand-binding specificity, whereas the type I receptor, in combination with the type II receptor, transmits the phosphorylation signal. The type I receptors contain a unique, approximately 30–amino acid juxtamembrane sequence called the glycine/serin–rich (GS) domain that contains serine and threonine residues whose phosphorylation by type II receptors is essential for signal propagation.[43, 44] The three-dimensional structure of the kinase domain of the type I TGF-β receptor suggests that phosphorylation of GS domain residues places the kinase in an enzymatically active conformation.[45]

For TGF-β and activin signaling, ligands bind to type II receptors in the absence of type I receptors; however, type I receptors bind ligands only in the presence of type II receptors. In contrast to the receptor requirements for activin and TGF-β binding, BMPs bind with low affinity to BMP type I or type II receptors individually. High-affinity BMP binding and signaling are observed only when both receptor types are presented together.[39, 46, 47] Several different combinations of type I and type II receptors are possible for each ligand (Table 5–1), some of which result in signal diversity for each ligand. For example, BMP2 can stimulate the differentiation of pluripotent stromal cells to an adipogenic lineage by signaling through BMPRII-BMPRIA and can stimulate differentiation to an osteoblastic lineage through BMPRII-BMPRIB signaling.[48]

Receptors I and II are both necessary and sufficient to generate a transmembrane signal; however, other cell surface binding proteins have been described. TGF-β binds to a type III receptor called betaglycan with a core size of 130 kDa, which can either facilitate or modulate TGF-β (and possibly activin) binding to type I/II receptors.[49, 50] A related proteoglycan, endoglin, a dimer of disulfide-linked 95-kDa subunits,[51, 52] also binds TGF-β as well as activin and BMPs.[53] Although its role in signaling remains unclear, mutations in endoglin are associated with hereditary hemorrhagic telangiectasia type 1.[54]

Two receptors for TGF-β-related ligands may not be RSKs. The receptor for glial-derived neurotrophic factor, a protein distantly related to TGF-β, is a dimer containing the RTK RET and a specific glycosyl-phosphoinositol (GPI)–linked binding protein.[55] Conversely, the receptor for inhibin remains undefined. Inhibin and activin share a common subunit, but inhibin exerts antagonizing effects on most, but not all activin functions[56–59] (see Chapter 138). At least some of that inhibin antagonism is based in part on dominant negative interaction of the shared β-subunit of inhibin with activin receptors[59]; however, both binding[60] and preliminary purification data[61] suggest that inhibin also binds a unique cell surface receptor. The identification and functional characterization of inhibin receptors await further study.

Biochemical Activation

The mechanism of activation of RSKs has been characterized for TGF-β and activin signaling (Fig. 5–8). Signaling is initiated by high-affinity binding of the ligand to the constitutively phosphorylated type

TABLE 5–1. Mammalian Transforming Growth Factor-β Family Members, Their Receptors, and Their Signaling Molecules

Ligands	Receptors		Pathway-Restricted Smads	Common-Mediator Smad
	Type II	*Type I*		
TGF-β	TβRII	TβRI	Smad2 Smad3	Smad4
Activin	ActRII ActRIIB	ActRI ActRIB	Smad2 Smad3	Smad4
BMP2/4	BMPRII ActRII	BMPRIA BMPRIB ActRI	Smad1 Smad5 Smad8	Smad4
BMP7 (OP-1)	BMPRII ActRII ActRIIB	ActRI BMPRIB BMPRIA	Smad1 Smad5 Smad8	Smad4
GDF5	BMPRII ActRII ActRIIB	BMPRIB	Smad1 Smad5 Smad8	Smad4

BMP, bone morphogenetic protein; GDF, growth and differentiation factor; OP-1, osteogenic protein-1; TGFB, transforming growth factor-β.

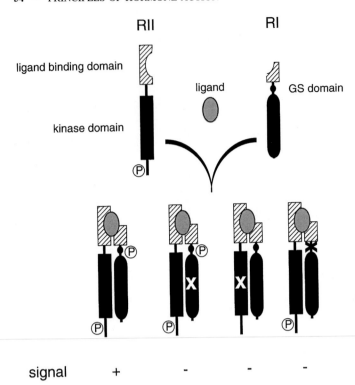

FIGURE 5–8. Activation of receptor serine kinases by ligand binding. Ligand brings about the formation of a RI:RII heteromer, which results in phosphorylation of receptor I by receptor II. "X"s represent inactivating mutations, either in the kinase domain to abrogate enzymatic activity or in the GS domain to prevent receptor II–mediated phosphorylation.

II receptor and formation of the ligand–RI-RII complex. The type II receptor kinase then phosphorylates the type I receptor cytoplasmic domain, at least in part at the GS site. Once phosphorylated and activated, the type I receptor phosphorylates substrate proteins, which transmit the signal to the nucleus. Although several type I–interacting proteins have been described, only the Smads (see below) are known to be activated by type I receptor–mediated phosphorylation and transmit the ligand-dependent signal to the nucleus to alter gene transcription.

The RSK model resembles the JAK/STAT signal transduction pathway for cytokine receptors described in the previous section. In RSK signaling, the type I receptor corresponds to the JAK, and the Smads correspond to the STATs. As with cytokine signaling, these proteins manifest diversity through different combinatorial associations between type II–type I receptors, as well as through different type I–Smad interactions. Pathway redundancy can be achieved by multiple ligands using similar receptors or activating similar Smads.

Intracellular Signal Mediators

Smads

Activation of the Smads is a central cytoplasmic event in TGF-β signaling.[62] The Smads are so named as a contraction of the first identified members of this class of signaling proteins, Sma (from *Caenorhabditis elegans*[63]) and Mad (from *Drosophila melanogaster*[64]). Alignment of Smad sequences reveals strongly conserved domains in the amino- and carboxy-termini (termed Mad homology [MH] domains), separated by a central linker region (Fig. 5–9). Such analysis suggests a division into three subgroups of Smads. The pathway-restricted or receptor-activated Smads include members that are phosphorylated by TGF-β and activin receptors (Smads 2 and 3) or BMP (types 2, 4, and 7) receptors (Smads 1, 5, and 8).[62] Specific sequences in the carboxyl domain serve to restrict Smad interaction with the type I receptors.[65] Once phosphorylated in the C-terminal SSXS motif, the pathway-restricted Smad then associates with a member of the second

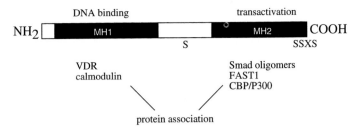

FIGURE 5–9. Schematic diagram of Smads. Domains associated with functional features are indicated. SSXS, site of receptor serine kinase type I receptor–activating phosphorylation; S, site of mitogen-activated protein kinase regulatory phosphorylation.

group, the common mediator Smad4, to allow nuclear translocation and facilitation of TGF-β, activin, or BMP responses.[66, 67] The third group includes the inhibitory or antagonistic Smad6 and Smad7. These inhibitory Smads act as competitors for binding of the pathway-restricted Smads to activated receptors[68, 69] or to Smad4.[70] A summary of Smad activation and function is shown in Figure 5–10. The expression of cell-specific repertoires of receptors, Smads, and transcription factors can thus underlie both the pleiotropic and the redundant effects of ligands within the TGF-β superfamily.

Smads directly bind DNA and induce transcriptional responses through cooperative binding with other transcription factors.[62] A consensus Smad recognition core element, AGAC, is found in several TGF-β- and activin-inducible promoters that bind to Smad complexes.[62] Smads activate transcription in response to ligand either alone or through functional cooperation with other transcription factors, which themselves also bind to DNA. Interaction of Smad2 with FAST-

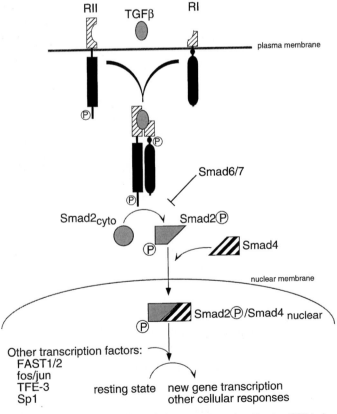

FIGURE 5–10. Activation of Smads by receptor serine kinases (RSKs). An active, phosphorylated RSK complex phosphorylates specific Smads, in this case Smad2 by the TβRs. Phosphorylated Smad2 can dimerize with Smad4, translocate to the nucleus, and either directly or indirectly influence transcription. Smad6 and Smad7 inhibit this signaling pathway either at the level of Smad phosphorylation or at the level of Smad association.

1 (forkload action signal transducer) or FAST-2 is required for activin-dependent Smad2/4-mediated transcription from the Mix.2 (mesoderm inducer) and goosecoid promoters, respectively.[48, 71, 72] Similarly, Smads 3 and 4 cooperate with TFE3 (transcription factor mu E3) to induce TGF-β-dependent transcription from the plasminogen activator inhibitor-1 (PAI-1) promoter.[73] Finally, TGF-β inducible transcription via AP-1 sites can be achieved through Smad3 interaction with c-Jun and c-Fos to form a multiprotein complex with Smad4.[62, 74] Interaction of Smads and members of the AP-1 transcription factor family provides one example of converging signaling pathways. Others are described below.

Interestingly, these studies demonstrate that Smad2 and Smad3 are not functionally equivalent. Smad3, but not Smad2 participates in ligand-dependent DNA binding to Smad-binding elements (SBEs) in both the PAI-1[75] and JunB[76] promoters. The lack of Smad2 binding to DNA is due to a sequence insert in the DNA-binding region of Smad2 that is not present in Smad3; this insert probably interferes with DNA recognition.[77, 78] Conversely, Smad2 and Smad3 have opposing functions in transcriptional activation of the goosecoid promoter.[72]

Smads also interact with transcriptional regulators from other signaling pathways and induce either enhancement or inhibition of Smad-dependent responses. Of particular note, the transcriptional coactivators CBP (cyclic adenosine monophosphate [cAMP] response element [CREB] binding protein) and p300 interact with and enhance the transcriptional activity of Smads after Smad phosphorylation.[79–82] CBP and p300 modify chromatin organization and may serve to bridge specific transcription factors, such as CREB, AP-1, STATs, NF-κB, p53, and steroid/nuclear receptors, with components of the basal transcriptional apparatus.[80] Thus the identification of Smads as transcription factors that bind p300/CBP provides a site whereby integration of signals from multiple ligands can occur. Smads also cooperate with activated vitamin D receptors to enhance the transcription of vitamin D–regulated genes,[83] which explains the known crosstalk between the TGF-β and vitamin D signaling pathways.[84]

Other Signal Mediators

Several proteins have been identified that mediate downstream aspects of RSK-initiated signaling. TAK1 (TGF-β-activated kinase-1), a protein involved in the JNK (c-Jun NH2-terminal kinase) and p38/RK pathways,[85] is a TGF-β or BMP-activated MAPK kinase kinase that can regulate a TGF-β-responsive promoter.[86, 87] TRIP-1 (TGF-β receptor–interacting protein-1) appears to inhibit TGF-β signaling[88, 89] through interaction with the type II TGF-β receptor.

Regulation of Receptor Serine Kinase Signaling

The magnitude of the RSK signal is subject to extensive regulation, similar to the cytokine receptors. One notable difference is the characterization of several soluble, extracellular ligand-binding proteins that block signaling through RSKs. Local expression of these modulators provides an additional level of control.

Ligand Antagonists

Follistatin suppresses several activin-induced functions[90, 91] (see Chapter 138 for more information). Follistatin also antagonizes the effects of inhibin, BMP7 (OP-1),[92] and BMP11,[93] although at higher concentrations than needed to neutralize activin. This result is consistent with the ability of BMP7 and inhibin to bind to and potentially signal through both type II and type I activin receptors.[94] However, follistatin has not been reported to directly bind BMP2/4, and it does not neutralize the effects of TGF-β1, even at 3000-fold molar excess.[92]

In contrast to follistatin, other secreted proteins bind and neutralize BMPs but not activin. Noggin binds with high affinity (K_d of 19 pM) to BMP2/4 and prevents interaction with cognate receptors; noggin binds to BMP7 less tightly and not at all to TGF-β or activin, even at nanomolar concentrations.[95] A second BMP4-binding antagonist, chordin, binds specifically to BMP4 (K_d of 3 pM) but not to activin

or TGF-β.[96] Other more recently identified antagonists include gremlin and cerberus.[97] Cerberus blocks signaling by BMPs, as well as by activin- and nodal-like members of the TGF-β superfamily.[97] In addition, cerberus functions as a multivalent growth factor antagonist in the extracellular space; it binds to nodal, BMP, and Wnt proteins via independent sites.[98] The fact that these antagonists are usually expressed in the same local environment as the ligands that they antagonize suggests a mechanism whereby ligand-dependent effects can be limited by the secretion of a specific antagonist that can act to sequester extracellular ligand in the absence of receptor signaling.

Receptors

At the receptor level, the immunophilin FKBP12 (FK506-binding protein-12) binds to all type I receptors tested and inhibits RSK signaling in the absence of ligand.[99, 100] Furthermore, during TGF-β signaling, clathrin-dependent internalization of an activated type I–type II TGF-β receptor complex occurs within minutes of ligand stimulation.[101] Optimal endocytosis and subsequent downregulation of the heteromeric TGF-β receptor requires kinase activity of the type II but not the type I receptor.[101] Studies of TGF-β receptor downregulation in murine osteoblastic cells have also implicated focal adhesion kinase (FAK) activation and its diverse downstream signals in this process.[102] Thus additional levels of limiting or extending TGF-β signaling may be achieved through modulation of receptor downregulation in response to ligand stimulation.

Smads

Accumulating evidence supports the presence of a negative feedback loop through which activation of Smad-dependent signaling induces expression of the inhibitory Smads Smad6 and Smad7.[68–70, 103] The inhibitory Smads block TGF-β–, activin-, and BMP-dependent responses either by inactivating ligand-bound receptors or by interfering with intracellular Smad-dependent reactions.[68–70, 104, 105] Crosstalk with the JAK-STAT pathway may be achieved by a similar mechanism. IFN-γ also induces Smad7 expression, which opposes TGF-β signaling.[106] These data provide a transmodulation mechanism between the JAK/STAT and the Smad signaling pathways whereby a cell can integrate signals from cytokines as well as TGF-β ligands.

A membrane-anchored Smad-binding protein, SARA (smad anchor for receptor activation) serves to bind quiescent Smads. SARA localizes Smad2 to specific subcellular regions in the cell that are near TGF-β receptors for ligand-dependent activation.[107] Ligand binding results in the formation of a receptor-SARA-Smad complex, presumably increasing the efficiency of Smad phosphorylation. Phosphorylated Smads no longer bind SARA and are released to the cytoplasm for complex formation with Smad4 and subsequent signaling.[107] Thus an additional level of regulation of TGF-β signaling can be achieved through the control of SARA protein expression, localization, or interactions with Smad2 or Smad3. Because SARA specifically binds the TGF-β- and activin-activated Smads 2 and 3, it is likely that BMP-activated Smads may use other SARA-like molecules.

Two additional routes to regulation of Smad activity have been described. RTK activation by EGF and hepatocyte growth factor modulates the activation of Smad-dependent signaling.[108–110] Additional crosstalk between TGF-β and other signaling pathways was demonstrated by the finding that EGF induced the expression of inhibitory Smad6 and Smad7 mRNA.[110] Finally, the calcium-binding protein calmodulin has been found to bind Smads and to potentially inhibit their activity.[111] These observations demonstrate that Smad proteins interact with calmodulin in a calcium-dependent way through conserved N-terminal amino acids and suggest a role for calmodulin in regulating Smad function.

COMMON THEMES

The Importance of Oligomerization

For the two pathways under discussion, as well as for the RTKs and other signaling systems, the formation of dimers or higher-order oligomers is a key feature for activation at different steps of the pathway. For both the cytokine receptors and the RSKs, such formation is seen at the level of receptors, where the formation of a receptor heteromer is an obligate step in receptor activation, as well as at the level of receptor targets, the STATs and the Smads. Conceptually, dimerization of receptors provides an efficient way to transmit information across the cell membrane. The process of bringing together the extracellular domains of two receptors places two kinase domains, either intrinsic or extrinsic, in proximity and allows for initiation of signaling via receptor trans-phosphorylation. The dimerization of signaling proteins in response to receptor-mediated phosphorylation allows those proteins to acquire distinct functional properties. For both STATs and Smads, the nonoligomerized proteins remain in the cytoplasm whereas the oligomerized forms localize in the nucleus where they can participate in transcriptional induction.

Direct Signaling to the Nucleus

A notable aspect of each of these systems is the activation of latent cytoplasmic transcription factors via direct phosphorylation by growth factor receptors at the cell membrane. Other well-characterized transcription factors that become activated in response to extracellular factors—for example, CREB and AP-1—do so as the end result of a multiple-step pathway. In contrast, for both STATs and Smads, it appears that the flow of information from the receptor to the nucleus is brief and direct. It is not currently clear what benefits accrue from the use of a simple as opposed to a complex pathway.

SUMMARY

Although the two signaling networks discussed herein both involve direct activation of protein kinases at the cell membrane, virtually all the components of those pathways are distinct. Nevertheless, the pathways have striking similarities in the kinds of reactions involved and in the manner in which they are organized. Of particular note is the characteristic of pleiotropy and redundancy present in both systems. Each pathway is used by a large number of extracellular factors that influence a diverse set of biologic responses, but that diversity is achieved through the use of a relatively limited number of receptors and signaling molecules. Utilization of multimeric components allows cells to greatly increase the repertoire of responses stimulated by a small group of factors as a result of different combinatorial possibilities. Significant challenges remain in understanding the codes through which distinct combinations of proteins form and signal.

REFERENCES

1. Bazan JF: Structural design and molecular evolution of a cytokine receptor superfamily. Proc Natl Acad Sci U S A 87:6934–6938, 1990.
2. Leung DW, Spencer SA, Cachianes G, et al: Growth hormone receptor and serum binding protein: Purification, cloning and expression. Nature 330:537–543, 1987.
3. Foster CM, Shafer JA, Rozsa FW, et al: Growth hormone promoted tyrosyl phosphorylation of growth hormone receptors in murine 3T3-F442A fibroblasts and adipocytes. Biochemistry 27:326–334, 1988.
4. Carter-Su C, Stubbart JR, Wang XY, et al: Phosphorylation of highly purified growth hormone receptors by a growth hormone receptor–associated tyrosine kinase. J Biol Chem 264:18654–18661, 1989.
5. Heinrich PC, Behrmann I, Muller-Newen G, et al: Interleukin-6-type cytokine signalling through the gp130/Jak/STAT pathway. Biochem J 334:297–314, 1998.
6. Moutoussamy S, Kelly PA, Finidori J: Growth-hormone-receptor and cytokine-receptor-family signaling. Eur J Biochem 255:1–11, 1998.
7. Thomson AW (ed): The Cytokine Handbook. San Diego, CA, Academic Press, 1998.
8. Nicola NA (ed): Cytokines and Their Receptors. Oxford, Oxford University Press, 1994.
9. Hibi M, Murakami M, Saito M, et al: Molecular cloning and expression of an IL-6 signal transducer, gp130. Cell 63:1149–1157, 1990.
10. Murakami M, Hibi M, Nakagawa N, et al: IL-6–induced homodimerization of gp130 and associated activation of a tyrosine kinase. Science 260:1808–1810, 1993.
11. Kishimoto T, Taga T, Akira S: Cytokine signal transduction. Cell 76:253–262, 1994.
12. de Vos AM, Ultsch M, Kossiakoff AA: Human growth hormone and extracellular domain of its receptor: Crystal structure of the complex. Science 255:306–312, 1992.
13. Fuh G, Cunningham BC, Fukunaga R, et al: Rational design of potent antagonists to the human growth hormone receptor. Science 256:1677–1680, 1992.
14. Amselem S, Duquesnoy P, Attree O, et al: Laron dwarfism and mutations of the growth hormone–receptor gene. N Engl J Med 321:989–995, 1989.
15. Duquesnoy P, Sobrier ML, Duriez B, et al: A single amino acid substitution in the exoplasmic domain of the human growth hormone (GH) receptor confers familial GH resistance (Laron syndrome) with positive GH-binding activity by abolishing receptor homodimerization. EMBO J 13:1386–1395, 1994.
16. Watowich SS, Yoshimura A, Longmore GD, et al: Homodimerization and constitutive activation of the erythropoietin receptor. Proc Natl Acad Sci U S A 89:2140–2144, 1992.
17. Argetsinger LS, Campbell GS, Yang X, et al: Identification of JAK2 as a growth hormone receptor–associated tyrosine kinase. Cell 74:237–244, 1993.
18. Witthuhn BA, Quelle FW, Silvennoinen O, et al: JAK2 associates with the erythropoietin receptor and is tyrosine phosphorylated and activated following stimulation with erythropoietin. Cell 74:227–236, 1993.
19. Watling D, Guschin D, Muller M, et al: Complementation by the protein tyrosine kinase JAK2 of a mutant cell line defective in the interferon-gamma signal transduction pathway. Nature 366:166–170, 1993.
20. Muller M, Briscoe J, Laxton C, et al: The protein tyrosine kinase JAK1 complements defects in interferon-alpha/beta and -gamma signal transduction. Nature 366:129–135, 1993.
21. Darnell JE Jr, Kerr IM, Stark GR: Jak-STAT pathways and transcriptional activation in response to IFNs and other extracellular signaling proteins. Science 264:1415–1421, 1994.
22. Horvath CM, Darnell JE: The state of the STATs: Recent developments in the study of signal transduction to the nucleus. Curr Opin Cell Biol 9:233–239, 1997.
23. Stahl N, Farruggella TJ, Boulton TG, et al: Choice of STATs and other substrates specified by modular tyrosine-based motifs in cytokine receptors. Science 267:1349–1353, 1995.
24. Shuai K, Horvath CM, Huang LH, et al: Interferon activation of the transcription factor Stat91 involves dimerization through SH2-phosphotyrosyl peptide interactions. Cell 76:821–828, 1994.
25. Chen X, Vinkemeier U, Zhao Y, et al: Crystal structure of a tyrosine phosphorylated STAT-1 dimer bound to DNA. Cell 93:827–839, 1998.
26. Becker S, Groner B, Muller CW: Three-dimensional structure of the Stat3beta homodimer bound to DNA. Nature 394:145–151, 1998.
27. Wen Z, Zhong Z, Darnell JE Jr: Maximal activation of transcription by Stat1 and Stat3 requires both tyrosine and serine phosphorylation. Cell 82:241–250, 1995.
28. Argetsinger LS, Carter-Su C: Mechanism of signaling by growth hormone receptor. Physiol Rev 76:1089–1107, 1996.
29. Yamauchi T, Ueki K, Tobe K, et al: Tyrosine phosphorylation of the EGF receptor by the kinase Jak2 is induced by growth hormone. Nature 390:91–96, 1997.
30. Strous GJ, van Kerkhof P, Govers R, et al: The ubiquitin conjugation system is required for ligand-induced endocytosis and degradation of the growth hormone receptor. EMBO J 15:3806–3812, 1996.
31. Nicholson SE, Hilton DJ: The SOCS proteins: A new family of negative regulators of signal transduction. J Leukoc Biol 63:665–668, 1998.
32. Chung CD, Liao J, Liu B, et al: Specific inhibition of Stat3 signal transduction by PIAS3. Science 278:1803–1805, 1997.
33. Klingmuller U, Lorenz U, Cantley LC, et al: Specific recruitment of SH-PTP1 to the erythropoietin receptor causes inactivation of JAK2 and termination of proliferative signals. Cell 80:729–738, 1995.
34. Haspel RL, Salditt-Georgieff M, Darnell JE Jr: The rapid inactivation of nuclear tyrosine phosphorylated Stat1 depends upon a protein tyrosine phosphatase. EMBO J 15:6262–6268, 1996.
35. Roberts AB, Sporn MB: Physiological actions and clinical applications of transforming growth factor-beta (TGF-beta). Growth Factors 8:1–9, 1993.
36. Wall NA, Hogan BL: TGF-beta related genes in development. Curr Opin Genet Dev 4:517–522, 1994.
37. Moses HL, Serra R: Regulation of differentiation by TGF-beta. Curr Opin Genet Dev 6:581–586, 1996.
38. Massagué J: TGF-beta signal transduction. Annu Rev Biochem 67:753–791, 1998.
39. Yamashita H, Ten Dijke P, Heldin CH, et al: Bone morphogenetic protein receptors. Bone 19:569–574, 1996.
40. Mathews LS: Activin receptors and cellular signaling by the receptor serine kinase family. Endoc Rev 15:310–325, 1994.
41. Josso N, di Clemente N: Serine/threonine kinase receptors and ligands. Curr Opin Genet Dev 7:371–377, 1997.
42. Greenwald J, Fischer WH, Vale WW, et al: Three-finger toxin fold for the extracellular ligand–binding domain of the type II activin receptor serine kinase. Nat Struct Biol 6:18–22, 1999.
43. Wrana JL, Attisano L, Wieser R, et al: Mechanism of activation of the TGF-beta receptor. Nature 370:341–347, 1994.
44. Willis SA, Zimmerman CM, Li L, et al: Formation and activation by phosphorylation of activin receptor complexes. Mol Endocrinol 10:367–379, 1996.
45. Huse M, Chen YG, Massagué J, et al: Crystal structure of the cytoplasmic domain of the type I TGFbeta receptor in complex with FKBP12. Cell 96:425–436, 1999.
46. Koenig BB, Cook JS, Wolsing DH, et al: Characterization and cloning of a receptor for BMP-2 and BMP-4 from NIH 3T3 cells. Mol Cell Biol 14:5961–5974, 1994.
47. ten Dijke P, Yamashita H, Sampath TK, et al: Identification of type I receptors for osteogenic protein-1 and bone morphogenetic protein-4. J Biol Chem 269:16985–16988, 1994.
48. Chen D, Ji X, Harris MA, et al: Differential roles for bone morphogenetic protein (BMP) receptor type IB and IA in differentiation and specification of mesenchymal precursor cells to osteoblast and adipocyte lineages. J Cell Biol 142:295–305, 1998.
49. López-Casillas F, Payne HM, Andres JL, et al: Betaglycan can act as a dual modulator of TGF-beta access to signaling receptors: Mapping of ligand binding and GAG attachment sites. J Cell Biol 124:557–568, 1994.
50. López-Casillas F, Wrana JL, Massagué J: Betaglycan presents ligand to the TGF-β signaling receptor. Cell 73:1435–1444, 1993.

51. Yamashita H, Ichijo H, Grimsby S, et al: Endoglin forms a heteromeric complex with the signaling receptors for transforming growth factor-beta. J Biol Chem 269:1995–2001, 1994.

52. Cheifetz S, Bellon T, Cales C, et al: Endoglin is a component of the transforming growth factor-β receptor system in human endothelial cells. J Biol Chem 267:19027–19030, 1992.

53. Barbara NP, Wrana JL, Letarte M: Endoglin is an accessory protein that interacts with the signaling receptor complex of multiple members of the transforming growth factor-beta superfamily. J Biol Chem 274:584–594, 1999.

54. Pece N, Vera S, Cymerman U, et al: Mutant endoglin in hereditary hemorrhagic telangiectasia type 1 is transiently expressed intracellularly and is not a dominant negative. J Clin Invest 100:2568–2579, 1997.

55. Robertson K, Mason I: The GDNF-RET signalling partnership. Trends Genet 13:1–3, 1997.

56. Mather JP, Moore A, Li RH: Activins, inhibins, and follistatins: Further thoughts on a growing family of regulators. Proc Soc Exp Biol Med 215:209–222, 1997.

57. Yu J, Dolter KE: Production of activin A and its roles in inflammation and hematopoiesis. Cytokines Cell Mol Ther 3:169–177, 1997.

58. Gaddy-Kurten D, Coker JK: Activin substitutes for the BMP2/4 requirement for, and the noggin inhibition of, osteoblastogenesis and osteoclastogenesis in adult murine bone marrow cultures. Bone 23(suppl 5):166, 1998.

59. Xu J, McKeehan K, Matsuzaki K, et al: Inhibin antagonizes inhibition of liver cell growth by activin by a dominant-negative mechanism. J Biol Chem 270:6308–6313, 1995.

60. Lebrun JJ, Vale WW: Activin and inhibin have antagonistic effects on ligand-dependent heteromerization of the type I and type II activin receptors and human erythroid differentiation. Mol Cell Biol 17:1682–1691, 1997.

61. Draper LB, Matzuk MM, Roberts VJ, et al: Identification of an inhibin receptor in gonadal tumors from inhibin alpha-subunit knockout mice. J Biol Chem 273:398–403, 1998.

62. Derynck R, Zhang Y, Feng XH: Smads: Transcriptional activators of TGF-beta responses. Cell 95:737–740, 1998.

63. Savage C, Das P, Finelli AL, et al: *Caenorhabditis elegans* genes sma2, sma-3, and sma-4 define a conserved family of transforming growth factor beta pathway components. Proc Natl Acad Sci U S A 93:790–794, 1996.

64. Sekelsky JJ, Newfeld SJ, Raftery LA, et al: Genetic characterization and cloning of mothers against *dpp*, a gene required for decapentaplegic function in *Drosophila melanogaster.* Genetics 139:1347–1358, 1995.

65. Lo RS, Chen YG, Shi YG, et al: The L3 loop: A structural motif determining specific interactions between SMAD proteins and TGF-beta receptors. EMBO J 17:996–1005, 1998.

66. Lagna G, Hata A, Hemmati-Brivanlou A, et al: Partnership between DPC4 and SMAD proteins in TGF-beta signalling pathways. Nature 383:832–836, 1996.

67. Zhang Y, Feng XH, Wu RY, et al: Receptor-associated Mad homologues synergize as effectors of the TGF-beta response. Nature 383:168–172, 1996.

68. Hayashi H, Abdollah S, Qiu YB, et al: The MAD-related protein Smad7 associates with the TGF-β receptor and functions as an antagonist of TGF-β signaling. Cell 89:1165–1173, 1997.

69. Nakao A, Afrakhte M, Morén A, et al: Identification of Smad7, a TGF-β-inducible antagonist of TGF-β signaling. Nature 389:631–635, 1997.

70. Hata A, Lagna G, Massagué J, et al: Smad6 inhibits BMP/Smad1 signaling by specifically competing with the Smad4 tumor suppressor. Genes Dev 12:186–197, 1998.

71. Liu F, Pouponnot C, Massagué J: Dual role of the Smad4/DPC4 tumor suppressor in TGF-β-inducible transcriptional complexes. Genes Dev 11:3157–3167, 1997.

72. Labbe E, Silvestri C, Hoodless PA, et al: Smad2 and Smad3 positively and negatively regulate TGF-β-dependent transcription through the forkhead DNA-binding protein FAST2. Mol Cell 2:109–120, 1998.

73. Hua XX, Liu XD, Ansari DO, et al: Synergistic cooperation of TFE3 and Smad proteins in TGF-beta–induced transcription of the plasminogen activator inhibitor-1 gene. Genes Dev 12:3084–3095, 1998.

74. Zhang Y, Feng XH, Derynck R: Smad3 and Smad4 cooperate with c-Jun/c-Fos to mediate TGF-beta–induced transcription. Nature 394:909–913, 1998.

75. Dennler S, Itoh S, Vivien D, et al: Direct binding of Smad3 and Smad4 to critical TGF-β-inducible elements in the promoter of human plasminogen activator inhibitor-type 1 gene. EMBO J 17:3091–3100, 1998.

76. Jonk L, Itoh S, Heldin CH, et al: Identification and functional characterization of a Smad binding element (SBE) in the JunB promoter that acts as a transforming growth factor-beta, activin, and bone morphogenetic protein–inducible enhancer. J Biol Chem 273:21145–21152, 1998.

77. Shi YG, Wang YF, Jayaraman L, et al: Crystal structure of a Smad MH1 domain bound to DNA: Insights on DNA binding in TGF-beta signaling. Cell 94:585–594, 1998.

78. Yagi K, Goto D, Hamamoto T, et al: Alternatively spliced variant of Smad2 lacking exon 3—comparison with wild-type Smad2 and Smad3. J Biol Chem 274:703–709, 1999.

79. Shen X, Hu PP, Liberati NT, et al: TGF-beta–induced phosphorylation of Smad3 regulates its interaction with coactivator p300/CREB-binding protein. Mol Biol Cell 9:3309–3319, 1998.

80. Janknecht R, Wells NJ, Hunter T: TGF-beta–stimulated cooperation of Smad proteins with the coactivators CBP/p300. Genes Dev 12:2114–2119, 1998.

81. Nishihara A, Hanai JI, Okamoto N, et al: Role of p300, a transcriptional coactivator, in signalling of TGF-beta. Genes Cells 3:613–623, 1998.

82. Pouponnot C, Jayaraman L, Massagué J: Physical and functional interaction of SMADs and p300/CBP. J Biol Chem 273:22865–22868, 1998.

83. Yanagisawa J, Yanagi Y, Masuhiro Y, et al: Convergence of transforming growth factor-beta and vitamin D signaling pathways on SMAD transcriptional coactivators. Science 283:1317–1321, 1999.

84. Takeshita A, Imai K, Kato S, et al: 1alpha,25-dehydroxyvitamin D₃ synergism toward transforming growth factor-beta–induced AP-1 transcriptional activity in mouse osteoblastic cells via its nuclear receptor. J Biol Chem 273:14738–14744, 1998.

85. Moriguchi T, Kuroyanagi N, Yamaguchi K, et al: A novel kinase cascade mediated by mitogen-activated protein kinase kinase 6 and MKK3. J Biol Chem 271:13675–13679, 1996.

86. Yamaguchi K, Shirakabe T, Shibuya H, et al: Identification of a member of the MAPKKK family as a potential mediator of TGF-beta signal transduction. Science 270:2008–2011, 1995.

87. Shibuya H, Iwata H, Masuyama N, et al: Role of TAK1 and TAB1 in BMP signaling in early *Xenopus* development. EMBO J 17:1019–1028, 1998.

88. Chen RH, Miettinen PJ, Maruoka EM, et al: A WD-domain protein that is associated with and phosphorylated by the type II TGF-beta receptor. Nature 377:548–552, 1995.

89. Choy L, Derynck R: The type II transforming growth factor (TGF)-beta receptor–interacting protein TRIP-1 acts as a modulator of the TGF-beta response. J Biol Chem 273:31455–31462, 1998.

90. DePaolo LV, Bicsak TA, Erickson GF, et al: Follistatin and activin: A potential intrinsic regulatory system within diverse tissues. Proc Soc Exp Biol Med 198:500–512, 1991.

91. Mather JP, Moore A, Li RH: Activins, inhibins, and follistatins: Further thoughts on a growing family of regulators. Proc Soc Exp Biol Med 215:209–222, 1997.

92. Yamashita H, Ten Dijke P, Huylebroeck D, et al: Osteogenic protein-1 binds to activin type II receptors and induces certain activin-like effects. J Cell Biol 130:217–226, 1995.

93. Gamer LW, Wolfman NM, Celeste AJ, et al: A novel BMP expressed in developing mouse limb, spinal cord, and tail bud is a potent mesoderm inducer in *Xenopus* embryos. Dev Biol 208:222–232, 1999.

94. Macías-Silva M, Hoodless PA, Tang SJ, et al: Specific activation of Smad1 signaling pathways by the BMP7 type I receptor, ALK2. J Biol Chem 273:25628–25636, 1998.

95. Zimmerman LB, De Jesús-Escobar JM, Harland RM: The Spemann organizer signal noggin binds and inactivates bone morphogenetic protein 4. Cell 86:599–606, 1996.

96. Piccolo S, Sasai Y, Lu B, et al: Dorsoventral patterning in *Xenopus*: Inhibition of ventral signals by direct binding of Chordin to BMP-4. Cell 86:589–598, 1996.

97. Hsu DR, Economides AN, Wang X, et al: The *Xenopus* dorsalizing factor Gremlin identifies a novel family of secreted proteins that antagonize BMP activities. Mol Cell 1:673–683, 1998.

98. Piccolo S, Agius E, Leyns L, et al: The head inducer Cerberus is a multifunctional antagonist of Nodal, BMP and Wnt signals. Nature 397:707–710, 1999.

99. Wang T, Li B-Y, Danielson PD, et al: The immunophilin FKBP12 functions as a common inhibitor of the TGF-β family type I receptors. Cell 86:435–444, 1996.

100. Chen YG, Liu F, Massagué J: Mechanism of TGF-β receptor inhibition by FKBP12. EMBO J 16:3866–3876, 1997.

101. Anders RA, Doré J Jr, Arline SL, et al: Differential requirement for type I and type II transforming growth factor beta receptor kinase activity in ligand-mediated receptor endocytosis. J Biol Chem 273:23118–23125, 1998.

102. Takeuchi Y, Suzawa M, Kikuchi T, et al: Differentiation and transforming growth factor-beta receptor down-regulation by collagen–α2β1 integrin interaction is mediated by focal adhesion kinase and its downstream signals in murine osteoblastic cells. J Biol Chem 272:29309–29316, 1997.

103. Imamura T, Takase M, Nishihara A, et al: Smad6 inhibits signaling by the TGF-β superfamily. Nature 389:622–626, 1997.

104. Whitman M: Smads and early developmental signaling by the TGFbeta superfamily. Genes Dev 12:2445–2462, 1998.

105. Lebrun JJ, Takabe K, Chen Y, et al: Roles of pathway-specific and inhibitory Smads in activin receptor signaling. Mol Endocrinol 13:15–23, 1999.

106. Ulloa L, Doody J, Massagué J: Inhibition of transforming growth factor-beta/SMAD signalling by the interferon-gamma/STAT pathway. Nature 397:710–713, 1999.

107. Tsukazaki T, Chiang TA, Davison AF, et al: SARA, a FYVE domain protein that recruits Smad2 to the TGF-β receptor. Cell 95:779–791, 1998.

108. De Caestecker MP, Parks WT, Frank CJ, et al: Smad2 transduces common signals from receptor serine-threonine and tyrosine kinases. Genes Dev 12:1587–1592, 1998.

109. Kretzschmar M, Doody J, Massagué J: Opposing BMP and EGF signalling pathways converge on the TGF-beta family mediator Smad1. Nature 389:618–622, 1997.

110. Afrakhte M, Morén A, Jossan S, et al: Induction of inhibitory Smad6 and Smad7 mRNA by TGF-beta family members. Biochem Biophys Res Commun 249:505–511, 1998.

111. Zimmerman CM, Kariapper M, Mathews LS: Smad proteins physically interact with calmodulin. J Biol Chem 273:677–680, 1998.

▲▲▲▲

Hormone Signaling via G Protein–Coupled Receptors

Andrew Shenker

Heptahelical membrane-spanning receptors and the heterotrimeric guanine nucleotide regulatory (G) proteins that they activate represent a major mechanism used by cells to respond to their extracellular environment. Extracellular stimuli, including photons, hormones, neurotransmitters, odorants, nucleotides, eicosanoids, proteases, and ions, trigger a conformational change that is relayed from the transmembrane helices of the receptor to its cytoplasmic surface. This agonist-induced conformational change leads to G protein activation. G protein α and βγ subunits modulate the activity of one or more effectors, including adenylyl cyclases, phospholipases, ion channels for potassium or calcium, and components of the mitogen-activated protein kinase (MAPK) cascade. The activity of these effector enzymes and channels determines the intracellular concentration of the "second messenger" molecules, ions, and transcription factors that drive additional cellular responses. A fundamental grasp of G protein–coupled receptor (GPCR) pathways is necessary not only for understanding normal hormone signaling mechanisms but also for gaining insight into the pathogenesis of a variety of human endocrine diseases that have been shown to be caused by naturally occurring mutations in G protein signaling pathway genes. Because of the scope of this topic, citation of the literature is not comprehensive but concentrates on the most recent references and relevant reviews.

RECEPTORS

GPCRs represent the largest known superfamily of signal transduction proteins, with more than a thousand already defined.[1–7] It has been estimated that more than 60% of modern pharmaceuticals are targeted to GPCRs. The ligands that act through GPCRs and the physiologic responses that they trigger are remarkably diverse, as are associated regulatory mechanisms. The first two GPCRs to be purified, cloned, and characterized in detail were rhodopsin, the retinal photoreceptor, and the β2-adrenergic receptor (β2AR). In many regards these remain the best model systems for understanding GPCR–G protein coupling. Although it is tempting to extrapolate insights from these receptors to all others, important functional variations have been shown to exist.

Classification

Despite the number of receptor subtypes, all GPCRs share significant structural homology, and they are predicted to exhibit a common "serpentine" structure: seven hydrophobic regions that form transmembrane α-helices (TM1–TM7), connected by alternating extracellular (e1–e3) and intracellular (i1–i3) loops. The seven helices span the membrane and form a relatively compact bundle with a central, elongated cavity. GPCRs are heterogeneously *N*-glycosylated at residues in the N-terminal domain, a modification that appears to be necessary

for the normal expression of some GPCRs at the plasma membrane. A highly conserved disulfide bond between a Cys residue in e2 and a Cys at the junction of e1 and TM3 appears to play a key structural role in some receptors. Many GPCRs have Ser and Thr residues in i3 and the C-terminal tail; these residues are substrates for GPCR kinases involved in the desensitization process.

Based on sequence similarity, GPCRs can be classified into four families (Table 6–1). The largest group of receptors consists of rhodopsin-like GPCRs (family A), whose ligands include the biogenic amines, glycoprotein hormones, a variety of peptides, adenosine, and thrombin. Sequence alignment reveals that almost all GPCRs in this group share certain highly conserved amino acids within their transmembrane domains[2, 3, 7, 8] (Fig. 6–1). Some of these residues have been

TABLE 6–1.　G Protein–Coupled Receptor Classification

Family A
　Biogenic amine receptors (catecholamines, serotonin, histamine,
　　acetylcholine)
　Angiotensin, chemokine, conopressin, C3a, C5a, eicosanoid, fMLP, galanin,
　　glycoprotein hormone (LH/hCG, TSH, FSH), GnRH, leukotriene,
　　nucleotide, opioid, oxytocin, PAF, and protease-activated, somatostatin,
　　vasopressin, and vasotocin receptors
　Adenosine, cannabinoid, melanocortin, and olfactory receptors
　Bombesin, CCK, endothelin, growth hormone secretagogues,
　　neuropeptide Y, neurotensin, tachykinin, TRH, and vertebrate opsins
　Bradykinin receptors and invertebrate opsins
　Melanocortin receptors

Family B
　Calcitonin, CGRP, CRF, and diuretic hormone receptors
　Glucagon, glucagon-like peptide, GIP, GHRH, PACAP, secretin, and VIP
　　receptors
　PTH/PTHrP receptors
　Latrotoxin receptors

Family C
　Calcium receptors
　GABA_B receptors
　Metabotropic glutamate receptors
　Vomeronasal pheromone receptors (G_o coupled)
　Putative taste receptors

Family D
　Vomeronasal pheromone receptors (G_i coupled)

CCK, cholecystokinin; CGRP, calcitonin gene–related peptide; CRF, corticotropin-releasing factor; fMLP, formyl-methionyleucyl-phenylalanine; FSH, follicle-stimulating hormone; GABA, γ-aminobutyric acid; GHRH, growth hormone–releasing hormone; GIP, gastric inhibitory peptide; GnRH, gonadotropin-releasing hormone; hCG, human chorionic gonadotropin; LH, luteinizing hormone; PACAP, pituitary adenylyl cyclase–activating polypeptide; PAF, platelet-activating factor; PTH, parathyroid hormone; PTHrP, PTH-related peptide; TRH, thyrotropin-releasing hormone; VIP, vasoactive intestinal polypeptide.

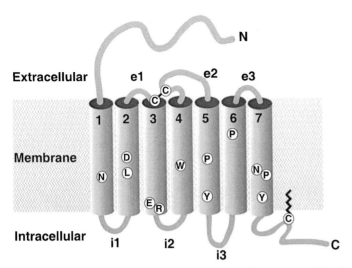

FIGURE 6–1. Two-dimensional diagram of a generic member of the G protein–coupled receptor family A. Seven membrane-spanning α-helices (TM1–TM7) are connected by alternating extracellular (e1, e2, e3) and intracellular (i1, i2, i3) loops. Palmitoylation of a conserved Cys residue may act to anchor the C-terminal tail to the membrane and thereby form a fourth intracellular loop. A highly conserved disulfide bond connects e2 to the junction of e1 and TM3. The residues shown in each helix are those that are highly conserved. (Adapted from Shenker A: G Protein–Coupled Receptors. *In* Introduction to Molecular and Cellular Research (syllabus). Bethesda, MD, The Endocrine Society, 1998.)

shown to play key roles in receptor expression, structure, or function. For example, an Arg residue at the TM3/i2 junction and a Pro residue at the cytoplasmic end of TM7 are invariant, and site-directed mutagenesis has implicated both in the process of receptor activation. The Asp/Glu-Arg motif at the cytoplasmic end of TM3 is characteristic, and a conserved Asn side chain in TM1 is predicted to form a hydrogen bond with a conserved Asp side chain in TM2. A conserved Cys residue in the C-terminal tail of many family A GPCRs serves as a potential site for palmitoylation, and this modification may serve to anchor the tail to the plasma membrane and form a short, fourth intracellular loop.

Family B includes the receptors for calcitonin, secretin, glucagon and other related peptides, parathyroid hormone (PTH), growth hormone-releasing factor, and corticotropin-releasing hormone. These receptors share several structural features, including a relatively large N-terminal domain with six conserved Cys residues and other conserved amino acids within their transmembrane domains.[9–11] Family C contains the metabotropic glutamate receptors, the Ca²⁺ sensor, the γ-aminobutyric acid type B (GABA_B) receptor, certain pheromone receptors, and putative taste receptors. These receptors are characterized by a very large N-terminal extracellular domain with conserved cysteine residues whose structure resembles that of a group of bilobed periplasmic binding proteins that are involved in amino acid uptake by bacteria.[12–15] The fourth class of GPCRs is composed of another group of putative pheromone receptors that are expressed in apical neurons of the vomeronasal organ.[16] Other varieties of seven-transmembrane–spanning signaling bundles that have been described include proteins known as *frizzled* and *smoothened*. Direct coupling of these receptors to G proteins[17] or other types of signaling molecules[18] remains to be explored.

Genome sequencing and homology-based molecular cloning with the use of degenerate polymerase chain reaction primers have resulted in the discovery of a large number of genes encoding GPCRs of unknown function, termed "orphan receptors." Deducing the physiologic and potential pathophysiologic roles of such receptors involves studying their expression patterns and similarity to known receptors, identifying natural or surrogate agonists, and determining their G protein–coupling preferences and downstream effects.[19–22]

Three-Dimensional Models

The fact that GPCRs are low-abundance, membrane-embedded proteins has thwarted high-resolution crystallographic analysis of their structure. Sequence alignment of multiple GPCRs, analysis of the pattern of conserved, polar, and hydrophobic residues in the α-helical transmembrane domains, consideration of the restraints imposed by the relatively short length of some connecting loops, and a low-resolution structure of rhodopsin obtained by electron cryomicroscopy have therefore been used to construct three-dimensional GPCR models.[23] Additional sequence analysis and a refined, three-dimensional map of frog rhodopsin[24, 25] have allowed Baldwin and colleagues to more accurately predict the relative position of residues in the transmembrane helices of this family of proteins.[8] One of the notable features of the new rhodopsin projection map is that TM3 is dramatically tilted so that its cytoplasmic end is in proximity to the ends of TM5, TM6, and the i3 loop, a configuration that is likely to have functional significance (Fig. 6–2). The Baldwin structure is consistent with results from experimental studies using various techniques on many different GPCRs. For example, almost all the amino acids thought to be involved in binding small ligands are located on transmembrane helices 3, 5, 6, and 7 and are oriented toward the central, hydrophilic receptor cleft. Potential spatial relationships between residues on different helices are revealed that would not be evident otherwise. Furthermore, the Baldwin model provides a generic residue numbering scheme with which helices from different types of class A receptors can be aligned by virtue of certain highly conserved, "signature" residues (see Fig. 6–1). This and similar alignments[3] are necessary for interpreting the daunting amount of mutagenesis data currently being generated on GPCRs.

Available GPCR models are oversimplified and likely to be incorrect in many of their details, but they are nevertheless useful in designing experiments and provide a valuable framework for understanding the process of ligand binding and receptor activation.[23, 26–29] Although the

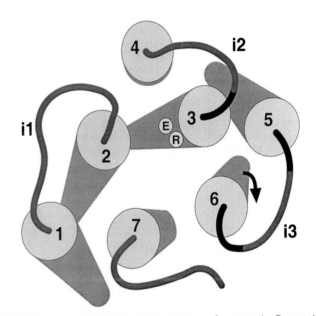

FIGURE 6–2. Three-dimensional diagram of a generic G protein–coupled receptor based on a projection map of rhodopsin. A view from the cytoplasmic surface of the cell shows that the seven helical domains are packed in a compact bundle with a central, elongated cavity. The tilt of TM3 results in narrowing of the receptor cavity at the intracellular surface and puts the TM3/i2 junction in proximity to the cytoplasmic ends of TM5 and TM6 and the i3 loop. Photoisomerization of retinal or agonist binding is predicted to cause a conformational change in the bundle that includes protonation of the conserved acidic residue (E) at the base of TM3 and a tilting movement of TM6 away from TM3 *(arrow)*. Regions of i2 and i3 implicated in G protein binding are shown in black. (Adapted from Shenker A: G Protein–Coupled Receptors. *In* Introduction to Molecular and Cellular Research (syllabus). Bethesda, MD, The Endocrine Society, 1998.)

vast majority of modeling work has concentrated on the rhodopsin-like GPCRs, the predicted helical arrangement of members of family B is also available now.[10, 11, 30]

Ligand Binding

GPCRs differ dramatically in the way that they interact with their ligands[4, 31] (Fig. 6–3). The best-studied GPCR ligand pocket is that of rhodopsin.[32] The chromophore retinal is covalently bound via a protonated Schiff base that involves a Lys residue in TM7, and a negatively charged Glu residue in TM3 serves as a counterion. This Lys-Glu salt bridge and the 11-*cis* conformation of bound retinal help stabilize rhodopsin in an inactive state. Exposure to light converts retinal to an all-*trans* conformation and triggers additional changes in receptor structure that allow productive coupling to the retinal rod G protein transducin.

The ligand-binding domain of receptors for biogenic amines has also been shown to be located in the hydrophilic pocket formed by the bundle of membrane-spanning helices, close to the top of the membrane bilayer. The positively charged amine group of this class of agonists binds to an Asp in TM3, and substituents at the other end of the ligand interact, probably indirectly, with residues on TM5 and TM6. Although there is evidence that some agonists and competitive antagonists have spatially overlapping binding pockets, the actual residues involved in agonist and antagonist contacts are clearly not the same.

The binding pocket for the tripeptide thyrotropin-releasing hormone also appears to lie within the transmembrane core, but for many other peptide receptors, both transmembrane residues and residues in the extracellular domains have been implicated in agonist binding. Glycoprotein hormone receptors have extended N-terminal extracellular domains (>300 amino acids) that can independently determine agonist binding affinity and specificity. The hybrid character of these receptors

and receptors in family C suggests that each group may have originated as the result of recombination between a gene encoding a basic heptahelical membrane bundle and one encoding some type of binding protein. This evolutionary mechanism could obviously promote the creation of chimeric GPCRs with novel signaling functions.

Several receptors with the ability to respond to proteases have evolved a novel activation strategy that involves cleavage of the distal N-terminal domain and resultant exposure of a tethered peptide ligand. As with the traditional peptide receptors, extracellular domains of the thrombin receptor (proximal N-terminus and e2) have been shown to play a role in agonist recognition.

Mechanism of Activation

STERIC AND ELECTROSTATIC FACTORS. In rhodopsin, light-induced isomerization of retinal acts as a steric trigger that forces the Lys in TM7 away from its Glu counterion and thereby disrupts the TM3–TM7 interhelical salt bridge and causes deprotonation of the Schiff base.[32, 33] A major conformational change ensues that is associated with an increase in free volume, or lateral "expansion," of the protein. Subsequently, the side chains of at least two other residues in rhodopsin must become protonated to achieve transition to the fully active receptor conformation. One of these residues appears to be Glu134, the acidic residue that is part of the highly conserved "Glu-Arg" peptide sequence at the base of TM3. Studies of normal and mutant rhodopsin suggest that this residue is directly involved in binding and activating transducin when it becomes protonated.

Some features of the rhodopsin activation mechanism are probably conserved throughout the entire family of transmembrane heptahelical bundles, but it is likely that there will also be significant variation in the details.[5, 31] Indeed, one of the reasons that evolution may have favored the heptahelical structure for conformational signaling is its tolerance for change in the residues lining the receptor cavity and its ability to provide a similar cytoplasmic effect in response to variable input. In the case of retinal, a change in shape of the chromophore upon light-driven isomerization apparently imposes a strain on the protein-binding pocket that drives structural rearrangement of other parts of the receptor. Residues in TM5 and TM6 have been implicated in the binding of biogenic amines, which has led to speculation that simultaneous binding of residues in these two helices causes a conformational change that affects the i3 loop connecting their cytoplasmic ends. Unlike rhodopsin or the amine receptors, where a rearrangement of side chains in the transmembrane-binding pocket is probably the primary event, it is possible that the activation of receptors for large peptides, glycoprotein hormones, glutamate, and Ca^{2+} may be triggered wholly or partially by forces imposed on the extracellular surface of the receptor.

The precise events that link agonist binding to G protein coupling remain unknown.[5, 34, 35] In some receptors, a highly conserved Asp residue in TM2 has been shown to mediate the inhibitory effect of Na^+ on agonist affinity and on G protein coupling, although it seems clear that it does not play a direct role in ligand binding. Substitution of this Asp with Asn has been made in many different receptors, and the effect is usually a decrease in agonist (but not antagonist) affinity and a decrease in agonist efficacy. This result suggests that the normal role of this residue is to facilitate the conformational change that leads to G protein activation.

As with rhodopsin, site-directed mutagenesis of different GPCRs indicates that the conserved polar sequence at the cytoplasmic end of TM3 is critically involved in G protein activation. Given that an acidic residue is found at the end of TM3 in many GPCRs, it is plausible that protonation of this side chain is important not only for activation of rhodopsin but also as part of a general mechanism for GPCR activation. Mutations analogous to the one that causes enhanced activation of rhodopsin produce an equivalent phenotype in some, but not all other GPCRs.[27] It has been proposed that the side chain of the invariant TM3 Arg residue might act as a general molecular "switch" for GPCRs by rearranging its position in the receptor pocket in response to agonist binding. The precise structural role of this side chain is unclear, however.[36, 37] General models of G protein activation

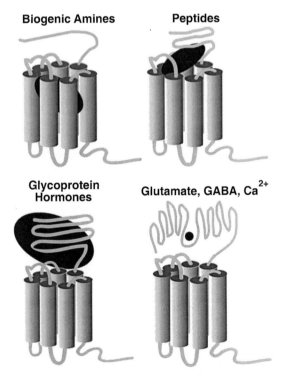

FIGURE 6–3. Comparison of agonist binding domains in four different types of G protein–coupled receptor. Biogenic amines and many other small ligands bind to residues in the TM cavity, peptides bind to both TM residues and residues in the N-terminus and/or extracellular loops, glycoprotein hormones bind exclusively to a large N-terminal receptor domain, and the small agonists glutamate, γ-aminobutyric acid (GABA), and Ca^{2+} bind to an extremely large N-terminal domain characteristic of family C receptors.

will ultimately have to address the fact that the secretin and metabotropic glutamate receptor families lack the conserved Asp/Glu-Arg motif at the TM3-i2 junction.

It has been suggested that the propagation of agonist signal down the transmembrane bundle involves conserved aromatic side chains or critical "irregularities" in the secondary structure, such as proline kinks or short stretches that do not form a stable α-helix. Proline kinks have the potential to participate in key conformational transitions. Molecular dynamics simulations of the effect of agonist docking in a GPCR model may suggest the types of side chain rearrangements and helix movements that normally occur during activation and may be correlated with experimentally derived data.[27, 29]

Although GPCRs were traditionally believed to function as monomeric units, recent biochemical evidence suggests that GPCRs can also form oligomers.[38, 39] It remains to be seen how universally this process is involved in receptor activation or regulation. For some receptors in family A, dimerization occurs between transmembrane segments, but the metabotropic glutamate receptor[40] and Ca^{2+} receptor each form dimers via disulfide linkages of their extracellular domains.[41] Other members of family C, the $GABA_B$ receptors, have been shown to function only as heterodimers.[42-45] In some contexts, GPCRs apparently require accessory proteins to be correctly folded and targeted to the membrane.[39] In the case of the calcitonin receptor–like receptor, association with a single transmembrane domain protein designated RAMP (receptor activity–modifying protein) also affects critical pharmacologic properties.[46]

ROLE OF THE INTRACELLULAR DOMAINS. Analysis of the effects of (1) chimeric receptors, (2) receptors with deletions or point mutations, (3) naturally expressed receptor splice variants, and (4) synthetic peptides or expressed cDNAs that correspond to portions of the receptor loop sequence has been used to map potential sites of interaction between receptor and G protein and to gain insight into activation mechanisms.[6, 8, 35, 47-49] It has become evident that the concerted action of several noncontiguous intracellular domains, including part of i2 and the N- and C-terminal ends of i3, are involved in determining the receptor's affinity for different G proteins and for transmitting the signal produced by agonist binding. There is good evidence that the amphiphilic, α-helical nature of the N-terminal segment of i3 is critical for G protein interaction, with the hydrophobic surface of that helix providing residues important for coupling. Detailed comparison of i3 sequences from many different GPCRs fails to reveal consensus sequences or similarities that segregate according to G protein–coupling preference, however, which suggests that the function of i3 may depend on its three-dimensional conformation in the context of other loop domains, especially i2. Recent studies of spin-labeled rhodopsin indicate that the N- and C-terminal portions of i3 may actually exist as cytoplasmic, α-helical extensions of TM5 and TM6, respectively.[50] It is not possible to predict the G protein–coupling specificity of a receptor simply by looking at its primary structure, and it is likely that loop sequences from distantly related receptors have undergone convergent evolution to generate three-dimensional shapes that are able to activate the same G protein.[48] For example, both the β_2AR receptor (family A) and the PTH/PTH-related peptide (PTHrP) receptor (family B) preferentially couple to the stimulatory G protein G_s, and the α_1AR (family A) and calcium receptor (family C) share coupling to members of the G_q family.

Analysis of spectra from double spin–labeled mutant rhodopsin suggests that during receptor activation, the cytoplasmic end of TM6 rotates by 30 degrees (clockwise as viewed from the cytoplasm) and tilts away from TM3 (see Fig. 6–2).[50] Further evidence for the importance of this type of motion in rhodopsin is provided by site-specific chemical and fluorescent labeling[51] and by studies in which transducin activation is blocked by the formation of artificial disulfide links or Zn^{2+}/His bridges[50, 52] between residues in TM3 and TM6. Recent studies of β_2AR also provide an indication that TM6 moves as a consequence of receptor activation.[5, 29, 53] Structural changes in the vicinity of the cytoplasmic ends of TM3 and TM7 also appear to accompany rhodopsin activation.[37]

CONSTITUTIVELY ACTIVATING MUTANTS. In the course of performing extensive site-directed mutagenesis of $\alpha_{1B}AR$, it was discovered that substitution of an Ala residue located at the junction of i3 and TM6 with any other amino acid caused increased agonist affinity, increased sensitivity to agonist, and increased activation of G proteins in the absence of agonist (i.e., constitutive activation).[54] Substitutions of corresponding or nearby amino acids in a variety of other GPCRs have subsequently been found to produce constitutive activation as well. For example, activating mutations in TM6 or at the i3-TM6 junction have been discovered or created in other adrenergic receptors,[55] the luteinizing hormone receptor,[28, 56] the thyroid-stimulating hormone receptor,[57, 58] muscarinic receptors,[59-61] and the PTH/PTHrP receptor.[62] The ability of some of these substitutions to cause constitutive G protein coupling has been attributed to changes in charge or the relative positioning of critical residues at the i3-TM6 junction, a concept that is consistent with the recent biophysical data on rhodopsin discussed above. Activating mutations are certainly not restricted to the i3/TM6 region. In addition to the TM3–TM7 interhelical salt bridge in rhodopsin, convincing evidence has now emerged from a number of different GPCRs that a stabilizing network of interhelical bonds is involved in maintaining the delicate balance between inactive and active receptor conformations.[5, 33, 63] The pattern and identity of activating mutations can help define hydrophobic or polar packing surfaces on α-helical domains that are important for supporting the inactive receptor state.[28, 49]

The function of the inactive, constrained GPCR conformation (R) may be to conceal key cytoplasmic peptide sequences and thus prevent them from interacting with G proteins.[55, 64] According to this model, agonists act to disrupt the constraints and stabilize the receptor in an active conformation (R*) in which the newly exposed cytoplasmic residues are able to bind and activate the relevant G proteins. This extended ternary complex model for GPCR signaling includes the assumption that some unoccupied receptors occasionally undergo spontaneous isomerization to the activated conformation, thereby producing some low level of "basal" activity. The intrinsic tendency for a receptor to undergo isomerization and activate G proteins in the absence of agonist is variable. For example, wild-type $\alpha_{1B}AR$ and the luteinizing hormone receptor are apparently silent in the absence of agonist, but β_2AR and the thyroid-stimulating hormone receptor are not. The proportion of receptor that exists as R* can be increased either by agonist binding or by mutational events that disrupt key constraints. The activating effect of certain disease-causing amino acid substitutions can thus be viewed as augmenting the receptor's intrinsic ability to adapt an activated conformation in the absence of agonist.

It is likely that even the extended ternary complex model is an oversimplification and that the GPCR actually has multiple, distinct, activated states, some of which may differ in their G protein–coupling abilities or preferences.[65-69] Furthermore, it has become clear that the cytoplasmic conformation that drives downstream signaling is not necessarily equivalent to those that serve as substrates for the cellular machinery involved in receptor desensitization and internalization.[70, 71]

Activating mutations of GPCRs have been shown to cause a number of endocrine and nonendocrine diseases.[33, 34, 62, 72, 73] In addition to their importance for understanding and diagnosing human disease, spontaneously occurring activating mutations have highlighted the significance of several structural determinants in the GPCR activation process that would have been difficult to identify otherwise. Some of the mutations may be relevant only to the receptor in which they were discovered, but others provide more general insights.

Although the classic definition of an antagonist is a drug that binds to a receptor and has no intrinsic activity, it has become clear that many antagonists have the ability to inhibit basal GPCR activity; specifically, they have negative intrinsic activity. These so-called negative antagonists (or inverse agonists) are characterized by their ability to preferentially bind and stabilize the inactive conformation of the receptor, thereby decreasing the ratio of R* to R.[74, 75] Negative antagonists may represent a novel therapeutic option for diseases caused by increased agonist-independent GPCR activity.

G PROTEINS

Classification

Unlike the integral membrane protein GPCRs, G protein heterotrimers are attached to the inner surface of the plasma membrane and

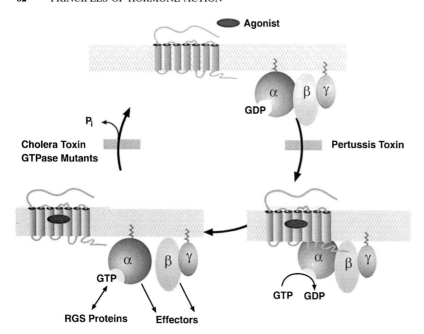

FIGURE 6–4. G protein activation cycle. G proteins are inactive in their guanosine diphosphate (GDP)-bound state, and interaction with activated receptor is necessary to promote release of the nucleotide from Gα. Binding of guanosine triphosphate (GTP) leads to a change in conformation of the G protein and effector activation by the dissociated Gα and Gβγ subunits. Effector activation is terminated when the γ-phosphate of GTP is hydrolyzed by the GTPase intrinsic to Gα; GTP hydrolysis liberates inorganic phosphate (Pᵢ) and leads to reassociation of Gα-GDP and Gβγ. RGS (regulator of G protein signaling) proteins can interact with Gα-GTP to enhance GTPase activity and may be regulated themselves. Modifications of Gα subunits by bacterial toxins and mutations interfere with the cycle. Pertussis toxin prevents members of the Gαᵢ family from interacting with receptors, thereby blocking Gᵢ-mediated signals. Modification of a conserved Arg residue by cholera toxin or certain mutational substitutions that inhibit GTPase activity lead to persistent signaling.

poised to relay signals to a variety of other membrane-associated and cytoplasmic signaling components[76–80] (Fig. 6–4). Historically, G proteins are defined by the identity of their α subunits. According to similarities in structural and functional properties, G protein α subunits have been grouped into four families: $G\alpha_s$, $G\alpha_i$, $G\alpha_q$, and $G\alpha_{12}$ (Table 6–2). At least 20 Gα subunits (encoded by 16 distinct genes) have been characterized, as well as 5 Gβ subunits and 12 Gγ subunits, but it is difficult to enumerate functionally distinct G proteins because the heterogeneity offered by all possible combinations of these subunits is not yet understood. Gα subunits range between 39 and 52 kDa in size, Gβ subunits are 35 to 39 kDa, and Gγ subunits are 5 to 10 kDa. Complexes between Gβ and Gγ are extremely stable and are typically regarded as one functional unit.

Different G proteins subserve different signaling functions. Direct stimulation of adenylyl cyclases by GPCRs involves the G protein G_s, which is expressed ubiquitously. The $G\alpha_s$ gene gives rise to four splice variants that are functionally indistinguishable. G_{olf} is a member of the G_s family localized to olfactory epithelium. The broadly expressed

$G\alpha_{i2}$ and its close relatives $G\alpha_{i1}$ and $G\alpha_{i3}$ mediate inhibition of adenylyl cyclases. Because of their relatively high abundance, G_i proteins also represent the most important source for liberation of free βγ complexes. G_o is a related family member and is predominately expressed in neuronal and neuroendocrine cells and in the heart. It represents 0.2% to 0.5% of brain particulate protein and helps mediate inhibition of Ca^{2+} channels, although direct targets of activated $G\alpha_o$ have not been well described. G_i family members involved in sensory perception include rod transducin, cone transducin, and gustducin. The transducins are localized in specialized retinal photoreceptor cells and regulate cyclic guanosine monophosphate (cGMP) phosphodiesterase activity. All members of the $G\alpha_i$ family, except $G\alpha_z$, are sensitive to modification by pertussis toxin. $G\alpha_z$ is found predominantly in neuronal tissue and platelets and can subserve some of the same functions played by other members of the $G\alpha_i$ family, but its physiologic roles in vivo remain unclear.[81]

The four members of the G_q family are involved in pertussis toxin–insensitive coupling of GPCRs to activate phospholipase Cβ (PLCβ) isoforms; such activation results in the hydrolysis of phosphatidylinositol 4,5–bisphosphate and generation of diacylglycerol and inositol 1,4,5–triphosphate (see Chapter 8). These second messengers mediate activation of protein kinase C (PKC) and mobilization of intracellular Ca^{2+}, respectively. $G\alpha_q$ and $G\alpha_{11}$ are expressed ubiquitously, human $G\alpha_{16}$ (and its murine counterpart $G\alpha_{15}$) is expressed in only a subset of hematopoietic cells, and localization of $G\alpha_{14}$ is restricted to the kidney, lung, and spleen. $G\alpha_{12}$ and $G\alpha_{13}$ are ubiquitously expressed, closely related pertussis toxin–insensitive proteins for which a number of biologic functions related to activation of the small G protein Rho have only recently been defined.

Structure and Function

Heterotrimeric G proteins are inactive in their guanosine diphosphate (GDP)-bound state. The rate of spontaneous GDP dissociation is very slow ($k \sim 0.01$/min), and interaction with an activated receptor is necessary to promote release of the nucleotide (see Fig. 6–4). GTP is in 10-fold molar excess to GDP in the cytosol, and binding of ambient guanosine triphosphate (GTP) to the vacated site on the G protein α subunit leads to a change in conformation of the Gα "switch regions," dissociation of the complex, and effector activation by the free α and βγ subunits. Once freed, the activated receptor can promote GDP dissociation from multiple other G protein molecules, thus providing signal amplification. Effector activation is terminated when the γ-phosphate of GTP is hydrolyzed by a GTPase that is intrinsic to the

TABLE 6–2. G Protein α Subunit Classification

Family	Subunit	Tissue Expression	Effector
G_s	α_s	Ubiquitous	↑ Adenylyl cyclase
	α_{olf}	Olfactory cells	↑ Adenylyl cyclase
G_i	α_{t1}	Rod photoreceptors	↑ cGMP phosphodiesterase
	α_{t2}	Cone photoreceptors	↑ cGMP phosphodiesterase
	α_{i1}	Neuronal more than other tissues	↓ Adenylyl cyclase
	α_{i2}	Ubiquitous	↓ Adenylyl cyclase
	α_{i3}	Other tissues more than neuronal	↓ Adenylyl cyclase
	α_o	Neuronal, neuroendocrine, heart	↓ Ca^{2+} channel
	α_z	Neuronal, platelets	?
	α_{gust}	Taste cells	?
G_q	α_q	Ubiquitous	↑ Phospholipase Cβ
	α_{11}	Most cells	↑ Phospholipase Cβ
	α_{14}	Kidney, lung, spleen	↑ Phospholipase Cβ
	$\alpha_{15/16}$	Hematopoietic cells	↑ Phospholipase Cβ
G_{12}	α_{12}	Ubiquitous	RhoGEF
	α_{13}	Ubiquitous	RhoGEF

cGMP, cyclic guanosine monophosphate; RhoGEF, Rho guanine nucleotide exchange factor.

α subunit (k_{cat} ~4/min). Thus GTP/GDP exchange is the rate-limiting step in the cycle, and GTPase serves as the critical timing mechanism that helps determine the longevity of the response. The rate of GTP hydrolysis by Gα is accelerated by interaction with certain effector molecules or with members of a newly discovered family of proteins known as regulators of G protein signaling (RGS) proteins. Synthetic, nonhydrolyzable analogues of GTP, such as GTPγS, can lead to persistent G protein activation in the absence of receptor stimulation. The combination of GDP and aluminum fluoride in the guanine nucleotide–binding pocket produces a similar effect because of fluoride's mimicry of the γ-phosphate of GTP. These reagents have proved valuable in biochemical, pharmacologic, and structural studies of G protein function.

Crystal structures of transducin, G_i, and G_s have revealed the shapes of active α subunits, inactive heterotrimers, and the surface-exposed residues that can potentially interact with receptor, effector, and other proteins[82–88] (Fig. 6–5). Gα subunits contain two structural domains. The domain involved in binding and hydrolyzing GTP is structurally similar to the superfamily of GTPases that includes small G proteins (e.g., Ras, Rho) and elongation factors. This domain contains three mobile polypeptide segments bordering the catalytic site (switch I, II, and III) that undergo dramatic remodeling when GTP is hydrolyzed or when GDP is replaced with GTP. The second domain is an α-helical structure not found in other GTPases that helps bury the guanine nucleotide in the core of the protein.

The Gβ subunit consists of an N-terminal helix and a circular β-propeller structure with seven blades that is a reflection of a repeating amino acid sequence motif called a WD-repeat. Gβ interacts with Gγ through an N-terminal coiled coil and additional contact sites to form a stable functional unit that is not dissociable unless denatured. The variable regions of the WD-repeats form a ring around the outer surface of the propeller, in a location likely to be important for protein-protein contacts. $Gβ_1$, $Gβ_2$, $Gβ_3$, and $Gβ_4$ are 80% identical, but $Gβ_5$ differs significantly from the others in its N-terminus, undoubtedly related to its ability to associate in a tight complex with proteins other than Gγ.[89, 90] Most potential combinations of Gβ and Gγ subunits can form, but a variety of experimental approaches have demonstrated selectivity in dimerization between different subtypes that is attributable to their varying affinities for one another.[91, 92]

The N-terminal region of the α subunit and the C-terminal region of the γ subunit are close together in the heterotrimeric structure (see Fig. 6–5) and provide a site for membrane attachment via lipid modifications.[93] Certain α subunits require N-terminal myristoylation for membrane association, and Gγ subunits contain a conserved C-terminal sequence that is the site of posttranslational modification with a farnesyl or geranylgeranyl moiety, which is critical for membrane binding of the βγ complex. Although the extreme C-terminus of Gγ is not visualized in the x-ray structures of G protein heterotrimers, prenylation of the γ subunit tail has been shown to be important for interaction with GPCRs.[69, 92] Yet another lipid modification of G pro-

teins consists of palmitoylation of a conserved N-terminal cysteine residue in Gα subunits. This modification is reversible and appears to be regulated during G protein activation and deactivation.[93, 94]

Regions of the G protein that have been implicated in receptor contact include the C-terminus of the α subunit, including the tail and α4-β6 loop, and C-terminal regions of the β and γ subunits.[48, 69, 86, 92, 95] Exactly how an activated receptor catalyzes the release of GDP remains unknown. The tail domains of Gα and Gγ both appear to play a direct role at the receptor cytoplasmic surface, with the tail of Gα predicted to project into a crevice between TM3, TM6, and TM7. Conformational changes in the receptor must be propagated to the distant guanine nucleotide–binding pocket via intervening structural elements in Gα, and residues in Gβ that contact Gα are also likely to be involved. One of the known functions of Gβγ in the inactive heterotrimer is to lock GDP into the nucleotide-binding site on Gα. The membrane face of the heterotrimer contains a prominent cavity between Gα and Gβγ, and activated loops of the receptor may use this cavity to tilt Gβγ away from Gα and open an escape route for GDP.[95] Identifying the configuration of the molecular interface between GPCR and G protein remains an important goal for future investigation. Nuclear magnetic resonance–imaged structures of the cytoplasmic loops of rhodopsin have recently become available and may provide additional insight.[96]

GDP release leads to a transient complex of agonist, receptor, and empty G protein. The affinity of agonist for this complex is much higher than for the receptor alone. Subsequent GTP binding to the α subunit produces a change in the conformation of switches I, II, and III. This change leads to a profoundly altered Gα surface with decreased affinity for Gβγ (causing subunit dissociation) and increased affinity for effectors. The concept that rapid depalmitoylation of Gα accompanying activation triggers translocation of this subunit from the membrane into the cytoplasm[93] has not been confirmed by all investigators,[97] although removal of palmitate may modulate important interactions of Gα with other proteins.[98] Hydrolysis of GTP to GDP terminates signaling by Gα and leads to reassociation of the Gα and Gβγ subunits (see Fig. 6–4).

Alterations Caused by Toxins and Mutations

Two bacterial toxins that interact with G protein α subunits have been tremendously helpful as pharmacologic tools and have increased our basic knowledge of the biochemistry and structure of these proteins. Pertussis toxin derived from *Bordetella pertussis* causes ADP ribosylation of a cysteine residue near the C-terminus of most members of the $Gα_i$ family. This modification prevents Gα from interacting with receptor and is one of the key pieces of evidence that implicates the C-terminus of Gα in receptor coupling (see Figs. 6–4 and 6–5). Cholera toxin also catalyzes ADP ribosylation, in this case a conserved

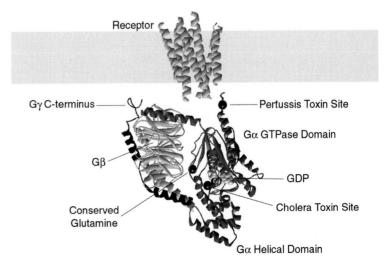

FIGURE 6–5. The predicted orientation of a G protein–coupled receptor (GPCR) transmembrane bundle and a generic heterotrimeric G protein. Receptor loops are not pictured. Guanosine diphosphate (GDP) is buried between the Ras-like guanosine triphosphatase (GTPase) domain and the helical domain of Gα. The N-terminus of Gα and the C-terminus of Gγ are close together and provide sites for the lipid modifications involved in membrane attachment. The C-terminal tail domains of Gα and Gγ have been implicated as key receptor contact sites. Conformational changes in the receptor may be propagated to the distant guanine nucleotide binding pocket via structural elements in Gα and a reorientation of Gβγ and lead to GDP release. Pertussis toxin modification of a C-terminal Cys residue in $Gα_i$ members blocks receptor interaction. Modification of a conserved Arg side chain by cholera toxin or mutational substitution of this site or a nearby conserved Gln residue (Arg201 and Gln227 in $Gα_s$) inhibits GTPase activity and causes constitutive activation. The G protein structure is based on that of transducin, and the GPCR bundle is based on a model of rhodopsin.

Receptor

Gγ C-terminus

Pertussis Toxin Site

Gα GTPase Domain

Gβ

GDP

Cholera Toxin Site

Conserved Glutamine

Gα Helical Domain

arginine residue in the $G\alpha_s$ subunit that points toward the γ-phosphate of GTP and is involved in stabilizing the transition state of the G protein (see Figs. 6–4 and 6–5). Covalent modification of Arg201 in $G\alpha_s$ in intestinal cells infected by *Vibrio cholerae* inhibits GTPase activity, leads to persistent production of cyclic adenosine monophosphate (cAMP) in the presence of little or no hormone, and causes severe secretory diarrhea.

Naturally occurring and artificial mutations of G protein subunits that lead to deficient or inappropriate activation have also provided important insight into G protein structure and function.[72, 73, 99] Amino acid substitutions in $G\alpha$ have been described that block receptor activation or interfere with GTP binding or GTP-triggered conformational changes. The pattern of hormone resistance that typifies patients with pseudohypoparathyroidism type Ia (diminished response to PTH and certain other hormones that act through G_s-coupled receptors) is usually caused by mutations that lead to decreased protein expression, but some of these cases are attributable to specific and informative functional defects in the $G\alpha_s$ subunit.

The first example of an activating mutation in a G protein α subunit gene was the discovery of somatic heterozygous mutations of $G\alpha_s$ (*gsp* mutations) in a subset of growth hormone–secreting tumors of the human pituitary and in thyroid adenomas. One set of mutations involved Arg201 (the cholera toxin target), and another affected the nearby Gln227 residue. Substitutions for either of these residues in $G\alpha_s$ results in impaired GTPase activity and prolonged signaling through adenylyl cyclase in the absence of receptor stimulation. The pathology associated with *gsp* mutations is consistent with the known effects of cAMP in mediating increased cell proliferation and function in somatotrophs, thyroid follicular cells, and certain other types of cells.[100] For example, early embryologic mutations of Arg201 result in McCune-Albright syndrome, a rare sporadic disease defined by polyostotic fibrous dysplasia, café au lait spots, sexual precocity, and other hyperfunctional endocrinopathies.[101] Mutations that block GTPase activity of the α subunit of G_{i2} have been described in only a very small number of ovarian and adrenocortical tumors, and their general significance is questionable.[102, 103] The use of constitutively active forms of different $G\alpha$ subunits has proved indispensable in defining the function of G protein–coupled signaling pathways in vitro.

Two other G protein gene alterations appear to mimic or augment the effects of receptor.[95, 99, 104] A rare condition characterized by a combination of gonadotropin-independent male precocious puberty (gain of function) and pseudohypoparathyroidism type Ia (loss of

function) has been shown to be due to a unique mutation of $G\alpha_s$ in the nucleotide-binding pocket that allows spontaneous release of GDP in the absence of receptor. At testis temperature (34°C) the mutant protein is constitutively active, but at normal body temperature (37°C) it is rapidly degraded, thus explaining the paradoxical phenotype. A polymorphism in the human $G\beta_3$ gene has recently been detected that results in loss of an internal stretch of 41 amino acids (corresponding to one propeller blade) and a gain of function in G protein signaling.[104] The enhanced sensitivity of G_i proteins containing this variant $G\beta$ to receptor stimulation is presumably due to the role of $\beta\gamma$ subunits in facilitating the release of GDP, as discussed above.[95] This polymorphism is found more frequently in hypertensive subjects than in normal controls, which suggests that variation in $G\beta$ function may also be associated with human disease.

Effector Pathways

$G\alpha$ TARGETS. The classic effector enzymes are directly regulated by the GTP-bound form of α subunits.[105, 106] For example, $G\alpha_s$ stimulates adenylyl cyclase, $G\alpha_i$ inhibits adenylyl cyclase, $G\alpha_t$ activates photoreceptor cGMP phosphodiesterase, and $G\alpha_q$ activates PLCβ. Recent crystallization of a complex of the adenylyl cyclase catalytic core with active $G\alpha_s$ has provided the first glimpse of the structural features involved in regulation of enzymatic activity by a $G\alpha$ subunit.[107] $G\alpha_s$ binds at a distance from the catalytic site and may therefore impart its stimulatory effect indirectly by reorienting the two homologous cyclase cytoplasmic domains. It is hypothesized that inhibitory $G\alpha_i$ subunits bind to adenylyl cyclase in a position directly opposite that of $G\alpha_s$, much closer to the substrate binding site. $G\alpha_s$ evokes its intracellular effects primarily through cAMP-mediated activation of protein kinase A (PKA) and the subsequent phosphorylation of substrates involved in metabolism, gene transcription, and secretion, although novel alternative pathways have also been described[108–110] (see Chapter 7).

Activation of $G\alpha_{12}$ family members has been associated with a variety of cellular effects, including Na^+/H^+ exchanger stimulation, regulation of tyrosine kinase activity, cell transformation, platelet shape change, and formation of actin stress fibers through the small GTPase Rho.[111–114] The phenotype of $G\alpha_{13}$ knockout mice suggests that this protein plays an important role in angiogenesis and chemotaxis.[113] Only of late have effectors directly regulated by $G\alpha_{12}$ been

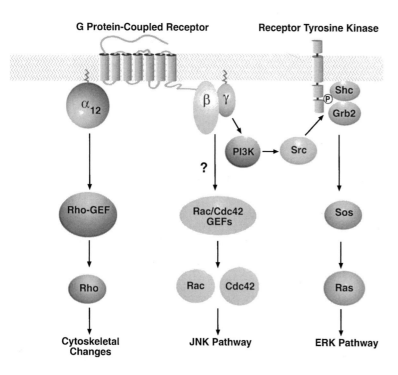

FIGURE 6–6. Pathways linking G protein–coupled receptors (GPCRs) to small G proteins (Rho, Rac, Cdc42, Ras) and mitogen-activated protein kinase (MAPK) cascades. Members of the $G\alpha_{12}$ family have recently been shown to activate proteins that serve as guanine nucleotide exchange factors (GEF) for Rho. Many GPCRs stimulate the extracellular signal–regulated kinase (ERK) cascade via release of $\beta\gamma$ subunits and activation of some of the same signaling machinery used by classic receptor kinases, including the adapter proteins Shc and Grb2, the guanine nucleotide exchange factor Sos, and Ras. The lipid kinase phosphatidylinositol 3-kinase (PI-3-K) and the nonreceptor kinase Src are likely intermediates. A distinct pathway that remains to be defined leads from GPCR activation to the c-Jun N-terminal kinase (JNK) cascade via the small G proteins Rac and Cdc42. (Modified from Murga C, Fukuhara S, Gutkind JS: Novel molecular mediators in the pathway connecting G-protein–coupled receptors to MAP kinase cascades. Trends Endocrinol Metab 10:122–127, 1999. With permission from Elsevier Science.)

identified, including a Ras GTPase-activating protein (GAP) and Bruton's tyrosine kinase.[115] Bruton's tyrosine kinase, identified as the defective protein in an X-linked form of human immunodeficiency, is also reported to be stimulated by $G\alpha_q$[116] and by $\beta\gamma$ subunits.[117] The recent discovery that members of the $G\alpha_{12}$ family activate two proteins that serve as guanine nucleotide exchange factors for Rho, p115-RhoGEF[118] and PDZ-RhoGEF,[119] establishes the first firm link between heterotrimeric G proteins and monomeric GTP-binding proteins of the Rho family (Fig. 6–6). Other putative targets for α subunits whose physiologic significance has not yet been defined include nucleobindin[120] and a novel LGN (Leu-Gly-Asn) repeat protein.[121]

G$\beta\gamma$ TARGETS. The original concept that regulation of different effectors by G proteins was mediated only by Gα and that $\beta\gamma$ served merely as a passive binding partner for the inactive form of Gα was repudiated several years ago. It is now clear that once Gα-GTP has dissociated from G$\beta\gamma$, free $\beta\gamma$ can also serve as an activator of numerous downstream targets[80, 91, 92] (Table 6–3). In some cases, Gα and G$\beta\gamma$ bind to the same effectors to mediate synergistic or opposing effects, but effectors activated exclusively by G$\beta\gamma$ have also been identified. The conformation of free $\beta\gamma$ is identical to that of $\beta\gamma$ in the heterotrimer, which suggests that the effector-binding site on $\beta\gamma$ is normally occluded by interaction with Gα.[122] Mutating residues on Gβ known to contact Gα can in fact impair G$\beta\gamma$ activation of certain effectors,[123] but other regions of G$\beta\gamma$ have also been implicated in effector activation, and G$\beta\gamma$ may interact with different effectors through distinct domains on its surface.[80, 91, 92, 124–126] G$\beta\gamma$ activates certain isoforms of classic second messenger enzymes, including the β_2 and β_3 isoforms of PLC and the $G\alpha_s$-activated forms of adenylyl cyclase II, IV, and VII, but it inhibits the production of cAMP by adenylyl cyclase I.

It is now firmly established that $\beta\gamma$ is the physiologic activator of G protein–activated inward rectifier K$^+$ (GIRK) channels in cardiac myocytes, neurons, and endocrine cells.[91, 127–129] Similar K$^+$ channels activated by somatostatin and dopamine receptors in the anterior pituitary may play a role in inhibitory regulation of hormone secretion. G$\beta\gamma$ binding to the C-terminal intracellular domain of one of the GIRK subunits that forms the heterotetrameric channel in myocytes is critical for channel activation.[129, 130] G$\beta\gamma$ also inhibits voltage-gated N- and P/Q-type Ca^{2+} channels by binding to specific regions on the channel α_1 subunit[128, 131, 132] and directly modulates activity of a brain Na$^+$ channel.[133] G$\beta\gamma$ activates isoforms of phosphatidylinositol 3-kinase (PI-3-K), including P110γ.[134, 135] PI-3-K is a lipid kinase that serves as an important mediator of intracellular signal transduction[136, 137] and may normally inhibit morphologic and functional differentiation of endocrine cells.[138]

G$\beta\gamma$ also stimulates receptor desensitization by binding and activating members of the GPCR kinase (GRK) family, a process that will be discussed in more detail below. Several targets for G$\beta\gamma$, including PLCβ, receptor kinases, and members of the Bruton tyrosine kinase family, contain pleckstrin homology domains, but it is unclear whether the pleckstrin homology domain is the functionally important binding site.[91] Although G$\beta\gamma$ subunits do not bind directly to small GTP-binding proteins, they do influence their activity indirectly and result in stimulation of key protein kinase cascades.

MITOGEN-ACTIVATED PROTEIN KINASE CASCADES. The MAPK cascades help transduce signals at the cell surface into changes in gene transcription[139] (see Chapter 9). They have been implicated in the control of cell growth and differentiation by an assortment of growth factor receptors and, more recently, by GPCRs.[112, 140, 141] Eukaryotes contain several distinct types of MAPKs, including the extracellular signal–regulated kinase (ERK) subgroup, the c-Jun NH$_2$-terminal kinase (JNK) subgroup (also known as stress-activated protein kinases), and the p38 MAPK subgroup. Each MAPK is a Ser/Thr kinase that is activated by a conserved multistep kinase cascade in response to extracellular stimuli. The components that lead from GPCR activation to these kinase cascades are currently topics of intense investigation. Although it is difficult to generalize about a common scheme by which GPCRs activate MAPKs, it now seems that GPCRs share some of the same signaling machinery used by the classic receptor kinases.

In the case of the ERK cascade, receptors signaling either via pertussis toxin–sensitive G$_{i/o}$ proteins or pertussis toxin–insensitive G$_{q/11}$ proteins may activate the ERK cascade primarily through a mechanism involving the release of $\beta\gamma$ subunits, tyrosine phosphorylation of the adapter proteins Shc (Src homologous and collagen-like protein) and Grb2 (growth factor receptor–binding protein-2), recruitment of the guanine nucleotide exchange factor Sos (son of sevenless), and activation of Ras[140] (see Fig. 6–6). In certain cellular settings, however, GPCRs may stimulate ERKs by biochemical routes that bypass the requirement for Ras.

At least three types of GPCR-directed scaffolds leading to ERK activation have been identified[140]: one involving phosphorylation and *trans*-activation of the classic receptor tyrosine kinases (such as the epidermal growth factor receptor),[142] another using integrin-based focal adhesion complexes (FAK family kinases Pyk2 and p125FAK),[143] and one consisting of the desensitized GPCRs themselves.[144] The relative contribution of each of these mechanisms, or yet to be discovered components, remains to be determined for a variety of GPCRs in different cell types. Regardless of the type of scaffold used, recruitment and activation of the nonreceptor tyrosine kinase Src seem to be critical steps in GPCR-triggered Ras-dependent ERK signaling.[140, 143, 144] Identification of PI-3-Kγ as a component that acts downstream of $\beta\gamma$ subunits and upstream of Src-like kinases and Ras suggests one potential mechanism by which heterotrimeric G proteins can regulate nonreceptor tyrosine kinases and, in turn, control MAPK pathways.[145] Ras-GRF, a novel Ras guanine nucleotide exchange factor stimulated by GPCR-mediated signaling, represents another molecule that may connect G$\beta\gamma$ to MAPK pathways.[146]

In addition to the ERK pathway, a distinct signaling cascade leads from GPCRs to the JNK pathway (see Fig. 6–6). The small GTP-binding proteins Rac1 and Cdc42, rather than Ras, play an integral part in initiating the JNK cascade. Free $\beta\gamma$ dimers or α_{12} may convey the initial signal, but the precise mechanisms by which different GPCRs stimulate JNK, p38 MAPK, and other newly described MAPKs remain to be determined.[112, 147–149]

Although GPCR-mediated activation of MAPKs does not primarily involve the regulation of G protein effectors such as adenylyl cyclase and PLC, many examples in which classic second messengers affect MAPK stimulation have been presented.[112] Changes in intracellular Ca^{2+} levels can facilitate MAPK activity via several mechanisms.[112, 140] Experiments using selective PKC inhibitors or PKC depletion indicate that activation of ERK or JNK by extracellular stimuli may be fully PKC dependent,[150–152] partially PKC dependent,[152, 153] PKC independent,[112, 154–156] or actually inhibited[152,156] by PKC activation. In most systems, signaling by G$_s$-coupled receptors and accumulation of cAMP leads to the inhibition of ERK pathways, but important exceptions include stimulatory effects in neuronal and endocrine cells.[157–160]

It is important to realize that closely related receptor subtypes in the same cell[161]—or even the same subtype expressed in different cells[160, 162, 163]—have been shown to promote similar MAPK responses via different intervening pathways. Interactions between G protein–coupled components and downstream protein kinase cascades have

TABLE 6–3. G$\beta\gamma$ Effectors

Target	Effect
Adenylyl cyclase	
Type I	Inhibition
Type II, IV, VII	Stimulation
Phospholipase Cβ	Stimulation
Ion channels	
Potassium channels (GIRK)	Stimulation
Calcium channels (N, P/Q)	Inhibition
Phosphatidylinositol 3-kinase	Stimulation
G protein–coupled receptor kinase	Stimulation
Bruton's tyrosine kinase	Stimulation

GIRK, G protein–activated inward rectifier K$^+$ channel.

already been shown to be very intricate, and additional signaling molecules probably remain to be identified. It is clear that activation of transcription factors and other mitogenic signals by GPCRs is best viewed as a complex integrative process rather than resulting from stimulation of a single, linear cascade.[149]

REGULATORY MECHANISMS

Receptor Desensitization

Adaptation to persistent stimulation (desensitization) is a characteristic of many biologic systems. In the case of G protein–coupled signaling pathways, the immediate compensatory response involves diminishing the receptor's ability to activate its G protein.[164–168] This process occurs rapidly over seconds to minutes and involves phosphorylation of one or more intracellular receptor domains, especially the C-terminus and i3 loop. Binding of adapter proteins to the phosphorylated receptor is often involved in uncoupling receptor from G protein. A second event that occurs on a slightly slower time course (minutes to hours) is sequestration or internalization of receptors away from the cell surface. This event may be phosphorylation dependent or independent. Internalized receptors are frequently recycled to the cell surface, although in some cases, such as with the thrombin receptor,[169] receptors are targeted for degradation. After hours of agonist exposure, additional mechanisms may contribute to downregulation of the total number of receptors expressed in the cell.[168, 170] This physiologic process may allow cells to adjust to long-lasting changes in the concentration of agonists in their environment. GPCR downregulation may involve a decrease in synthesis, an increase in degradation, or both.

GPCR phosphorylation is primarily carried out by members of the GRK family, serine/threonine protein kinases that specifically recognize an agonist-bound receptor conformation.[164, 167] GPCRs can also be phosphorylated by PKA and PKC.[168, 171–173] Six mammalian members of the GRK family have been cloned: GRK1 (rhodopsin kinase) and GRK4 have localized tissue distributions in the retina and testis, respectively, but the other GRKs are widely distributed. The activity of GRKs is regulated by charged membrane phospholipids and by binding to Gβγ subunits.[164, 167] Gβγ subunits mediate agonist-dependent recruitment of cytosolic GRKs by translocating them to the plasma membrane environment where their receptor substrates reside.

Our current model of GPCR desensitization is based primarily on studies of β₂AR (Fig. 6–7). This model suggests that a receptor phosphorylated by a GRK subsequently binds to a member of the family of cytoplasmic proteins known as arrestins.[165, 167] Binding to arrestin serves at least two purposes: it sterically prevents the phosphorylated receptor from further coupling to G proteins, and it initiates a process of internalization via binding to clathrin-coated pits.[174] The crystal structure of arrestin has recently been solved and has provided new insight into its activation and preferential binding to phosphorylated receptors.[175, 176] Inactive arrestin is shown to consist of two domains whose relative position is maintained in part by a hydrogen-bonded network of buried, charged side chains. Insertion of a phosphorylated receptor polypeptide into this critical region is predicted to disrupt the interactions and promote an altered conformation of arrestin with high affinity for receptor.[177]

Internalization of receptors has also been shown to involve dynamin, a motor protein that surrounds the necks of clathrin-coated pits and drives vesicle formation. Internalization of GPCRs through the clathrin/dynamin endocytic pathway is thought to be a prerequisite for dephosphorylation and resensitization of certain receptor types (see Fig. 6–7) and may also be necessary for targeting receptors destined for destruction in the lysosomes.[170] Additional proteins may also be involved in regulating clathrin coat–mediated GPCR endocytosis.[178, 179]

Recent data suggest that in at least three cases the very processes involved in β₂AR desensitization and internalization can also initiate a secondary wave of cell signaling events.[140, 144] For example, phosphorylation of the i3 loop of β₂-ARs by PKA not only uncouples the receptor from G_s but also enhances its ability to activate pertussis-insensitive G_i proteins.[163] Second, for some receptors, agents that inhibit GPCR internalization have been shown to impair activation of the ERK pathway, thus suggesting that endocytosis may be involved in relaying signals from the plasma membrane to cytoplasmic kinases.[180] Internalization is not universally essential for activation of ERK by other GPCRs, however.[181] Finally, it seems that β-arrestin can serve as an adapter protein for the recruitment and activation of Src protein kinase to a signaling complex that includes GRK-phosphorylated β₂AR, a process that may be also be required for subsequent activation of ERK.[144]

Although desensitization of β₂AR has been thoroughly studied and is the most widely accepted model system, additional data suggest that a variety of different signals and modes of regulation may be operative with other types of GPCRs and in different cell types.[168, 182, 183] For example, alternative internalization pathways that are independent of arrestin and/or dynamin have been described.[168, 184] In the case of the PTH/PTHrP receptor and glycoprotein hormone receptors, inhibition of G protein coupling[185, 186] and receptor endocytosis[173, 187] can occur independently of phosphorylation.

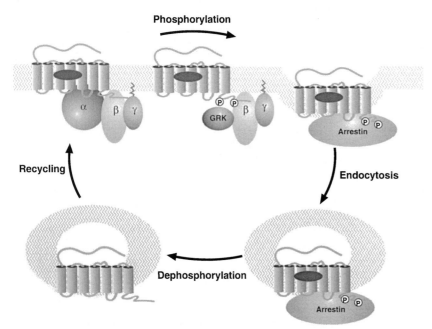

FIGURE 6–7. Desensitization of a prototypic G protein–coupled receptor. Agonist-bound receptor is phosphorylated on Ser residues in its C-terminal tail by a specific receptor kinase (G protein–coupled receptor kinase [GRK]). The phosphorylated receptor subsequently binds arrestin, which prevents further G protein coupling and initiates the process of endocytosis via clathrin-coated pits. Internalization is a prerequisite for dephosphorylation and recycling of some receptors.

RGS Proteins

In many signaling pathways the duration of a response under physiologic conditions is much shorter than would be predicted from the intrinsic rate of $G\alpha$-GTP hydrolysis in vitro. An explanation for these discrepancies has been provided by the recognition that some effectors can accelerate the GTPase activities of their $G\alpha$ subunit–binding partners[188, 189] and by the discovery of an important new family of proteins that act as GAPs (RGS proteins).[190–193]

RGS proteins were first identified by genetic techniques as inhibitors of G protein signaling and in a two-hybrid screen for $G\alpha_i$-interacting proteins. Over 20 mammalian proteins containing the conserved RGS domain have now been identified. RGS proteins have been shown to have GTPase-enhancing activity toward $G\alpha$ subunits from the G_i, G_q, and G_{12} families, but not toward $G\alpha_s$. GTPase hydrolysis rates are increased as much as 100-fold, and several types of G protein–mediated signaling are blunted when RGS proteins are overexpressed in cells.

The crystal structure of the core domain of RGS4 complexed with activated $G\alpha_{i1}$ suggests that RGS proteins act as GAPs by stabilizing the flexible switch regions of $G\alpha$ in conformations resembling those found in the transition state, thus lowering the energy barrier for GTP hydrolysis.[194] The simplest scenario predicts that RGS would rapidly deactivate $G\alpha$-GTP, facilitate $G\alpha$-GDP reassociation with $\beta\gamma$ subunits, and block downstream interactions by both α and $\beta\gamma$. It is also seems likely, however, that some RGS proteins can function by competing for binding of effector or $\beta\gamma$ to the $G\alpha$ switch regions. For example, in the case of $\beta\gamma$-regulated potassium and N-type Ca^{2+} channels, expression of RGS proteins appears to augment $\beta\gamma$-mediated signaling by sequestering $G\alpha$ subunits and thereby increasing the concentration of free $\beta\gamma$.[195]

Our biochemical understanding of RGS proteins has grown enormously in the last few years, but little is known about their physiologic roles. The activity and selectivity of different RGS proteins in vivo will probably be shown to depend on their relative affinities for the different conformations of $G\alpha$, their subcellular targeting, their transcriptional regulation, and their interaction with other proteins. For example, the fact that in some cases RGS proteins are able to influence the initiation of signaling and that they differentially inhibit the same $G\alpha$ subunit, depending on which particular receptor is stimulated, suggests that RGS proteins may be capable of binding to the GPCR–G protein complex itself.[192, 196] Reversible, receptor-driven modification of the N-terminus of $G\alpha$ subunits with palmitate has also been shown to affect RGS activity,[98] thus suggesting yet another way in which GPCR-mediated signal amplitude and duration may be controlled.

Many members of the RGS family with key additional functional domains have been identified.[193] One of these members is an RGS isoform containing an N-terminal PDZ domain, a structural feature that is capable of directly binding to motifs found in the C-termini of certain GPCRs.[197] Other RGS proteins contain $G\gamma$-like sequences and have been shown to form tight, functional complexes with $G\beta_5$,[89, 90] a stunning observation that invalidates the classic concept that $G\beta$ subunits can only perform in the cell by binding to $G\gamma$ subunits. The recently described $G\alpha_{13}$-activated RhoGEF mentioned earlier in this chapter is in fact a multidomain RGS protein with selectivity toward members of the $G\alpha_{12}$ family, thus providing a direct regulatory link between two important classes of cellular GTPases.[118, 198] Other domains found in RGS proteins predict interactions with Rap GTPases, PKA, and components of the Wnt signaling pathway.[193] In summary, it is becoming evident that RGS proteins do more than just enhance the GTPase activity of $G\alpha$ subunits and that many of them are positioned to regulate the activity of other important cell signaling pathways and to be regulated themselves.

Other Regulatory Mechanisms

Another protein that interacts with $G\beta\gamma$ is phosducin, a cytosolic protein found in the retina, pineal gland, and other tissues that downregulates signaling by controlling the availability of $\beta\gamma$. $G\beta\gamma$ bound to phosducin is unable to reassociate with $G\alpha$ and receptor. A crystal-

lographic study of transducin $\beta\gamma$ shows that phosducin allosterically generates a crevice on the surface of $G\beta$ that sequesters the $G\gamma$ farnesyl group, thereby releasing the complex from the membrane.[199] cAMP-dependent phosphorylation of a serine residue in phosducin reverses this process.

Recent studies suggest other novel mechanisms by which GPCR-mediated signaling might be physiologically regulated. Posttranscriptional editing of 5-hydroxytryptamine 2C ($5HT_{2C}$) receptor mRNA has been shown to generate receptor isoforms that differ in their i2 loop sequences and vary in basal activity and G protein–coupling efficiency.[200, 201] Deamidation of Asn residues in the C-terminal tail of a $G\alpha_o$ isoform has the potential to affect receptor recognition and activation.[202]

NONTRADITIONAL INTERACTIONS

It is possible that some GPCRs coordinate cellular responses by physically associating with proteins other than heterotrimeric G proteins or that guanine nucleotide exchange by G proteins is influenced by proteins other than heptahelical receptors.[18] Direct, agonist-dependent interaction of GPCRs with GRKs and arrestin has already been discussed. In addition, activated angiotensin II type 1 receptor has been shown to directly bind the tyrosine kinase Janus kinase-2 (JAK2),[203] and activated β_2AR associates with the Na^+/H^+ exchanger regulatory factor (NHERF), a PDZ domain protein that regulates the activity of the type 3 Na^+/H^+ exchanger.[204] The PDZ domain of NHERF interacts with residues in the C-terminus of β_2AR that are distinct from those involved in coupling to G_s. Other examples of GPCRs that interact with PDZ domain–containing proteins via residues in their C-termini are the metabotropic glutamate receptor, which binds to a protein known as Homer,[39, 205] and the $5HT_{2C}$ receptor, which binds to MUPP1 (multi-PDZ-domain protein 1).[206] The C-terminal tails of several subtypes of adrenergic receptor also associate with the α subunit of eukaryotic initiation factor 2B in discrete regions of the plasma membrane, although the physiologic significance of this interaction remains to be defined.[207] The ζ isoform of 14-3-3 proteins, a protein family known to form signaling scaffolds, has recently been shown to interact with the i3 loop of α_2ARs.[208] Finally, some GPCRs seem to form agonist-dependent complexes with the small G proteins ARF and RhoA and cause enhanced activation of phospholipase D, although it is possible that unidentified adapter proteins mediate this association.[209]

Nontraditional activators of G proteins that have been described include a neuronal growth cone–associated protein known as GAP43,[210] β-amyloid precursor protein,[211] Purkinje cell protein-2,[212] and a partially characterized membrane-associated protein from NG108-15 cells.[213] Apoptosis induced by the mutant forms of amyloid precursor protein and presenilin 2 that are associated with familial Alzheimer's disease appears to involve activation of pertussis toxin–sensitive G proteins.[211, 214] Identification of novel accessory proteins that act by influencing nucleotide exchange, GTP hydrolysis, and/or localization of G protein–coupled signaling components may reveal new levels of regulatory control.

In addition to their well-established role in transmembrane signal transduction, heterotrimeric G protein subunits are also found attached to intracellular membranes, including secretory granules, the endoplasmic reticulum, and the Golgi complex. This distinctive distribution and the observed effects of reagents that act on the G protein cycle suggest that G proteins may play a role in vesicular transport and intracellular membrane trafficking.[215–219]

SPECIFICITY OF COUPLING

Versatility in the pattern of interactions at the both the GPCR–G protein and G protein–effector level provides a regulatory network of remarkable complexity. All cells contain a variety of homologous GPCRs, G proteins, and effector proteins, and delineating coupling specificity is often difficult. Activation of even a single G protein is now known to give rise to a two-pronged signal resulting from the independent effector roles of Gα and Gβγ. Multiple receptors can converge on a single G protein, and a single hormone receptor may activate several types of G proteins. For example, several receptors that couple primarily to G_s (including glycoprotein hormone receptors and some family B members) have also been found to activate PLC through secondary coupling to G_i or G_q.

A variety of approaches have been used to help define the specificity of GPCR-coupling preferences. These methods include the use of bacterial toxins, reconstitution of purified proteins, cotransfection of receptor and G protein subunit cDNAs, the use of selective antibodies directed against the C-termini of Gα subunits, the use of minigenes that encode Gα C-termini, solubilization of native receptor–G protein complexes, and agonist-dependent radiolabeling of G proteins.[6, 65, 220] In most cases, coupling is found to be neither absolutely specific nor totally promiscuous. Although reconstitution and transfection experiments are ideal for exploring the mechanistic basis of G protein–mediated signaling, different approaches are needed to identify physiologically relevant couplings in situ. For example, a series of studies using microinjection of antisense oligonucleotides that suppress expression of specific G protein subunits in cultured pituitary cells have revealed a surprisingly high level of specificity: different Gβγ pairs seem to combine with different alternatively spliced forms of $Gα_o$ to couple muscarinic and somatostatin receptors to the same cellular response.[65]

Specificity in intact cells is often greater than that seen in vitro, and it is possible that compartmentalization mechanisms for G protein–coupled signaling components furnish a level of organization in vivo that is lost when cells are disrupted.[80] In intact cells, particular groups of GPCRs, G proteins, and effectors may have a restricted localization that limits their interaction with some groups of proteins or facilitates their contact with others.[221] Organizing components for G protein–mediated signaling may include cytoskeletal proteins, scaffolding proteins, clathrin-coated pits, or specialized membrane microdomains known as caveolae.[221–223]

GENE TARGETING AND DISEASE MUTATIONS

Because many receptors are capable of coupling to several types of G proteins, it is obviously difficult to selectively study the cellular signaling processes regulated by a single G protein subtype in vivo. A recent experimental strategy that has been useful in this regard involves the generation of "knockout" mice that are deficient in specific G protein subunits. Gene targeting techniques permit the study of G protein–mediated signaling in the context of the development and biologic functions of tissues in an intact organism.[113] Most Gα genes have now been inactivated; the result has been mostly unforeseen phenotypes that have provided important insight into the physiologic roles of these Gα genes.[113, 224–227] Knockout of GPCR genes has also been used to shed light on the normal function of GPCRs in vivo.[228–232] Deficient GPCR or G protein function can result in embryonic lethality, tissue hypoplasia, or other specific developmental or behavioral disorders. The generation of transgenic mice overexpressing either wild-type GPCRs, constitutively active mutant GPCRs, or GRKs has also been extremely helpful in understanding complicated pathophysiologic processes, including myocardial hypertrophy[232, 233] and thyroid neoplasia.[234]

Naturally occurring mutations in G protein signaling pathway genes cause a variety of human diseases, many of which are discussed in detail elsewhere in this text. Endocrine diseases caused by mutations in GPCR and G protein genes are listed in Table 6–4. Studying the molecular mechanisms responsible for these dysfunctional phenotypes has provided significant clues regarding activation and deactivation of GPCRs and G proteins.[72, 95, 99] Although many natural mutations cause loss of function by interfering with proper protein synthesis, others are associated with more informative structural alterations in targeting, ligand recognition, or conformational signaling. In addition to GPCR gene mutations that serve as the primary basis of disease, common polymorphic variations in GPCR sequences that affect receptor function may have subtle influences on disease phenotype or drug response.[73, 235–238] The potential range of GPCR-related human pathology is underscored by the discoveries that certain chemokine receptors serve as cofactors for HIV infection[239] and that a constitutively active chemokine receptor encoded by Kaposi's sarcoma–associated herpesvirus may act as an oncogene in AIDS-related malignancies.[240]

FUTURE PROSPECTS

Because of their vast importance in understanding and treating human disease, GPCRs will continue to be prime targets for drug discovery by the pharmaceutical and biotechnology industries. These efforts involve identification of novel, selective ligands for both known and orphan GPCRs by using high-throughput strategies to screen natural extracts, combinatorial chemical libraries, and plasmid-based peptide libraries.[19, 20, 241] The development of peptides and other small ligands that act on G proteins or at the GPCR–G protein interface represents another avenue with possible therapeutic applications.[220, 242, 243] Determining the high-resolution crystal structure of a GPCR and a GPCR–G protein complex remains an important goal for future research.

TABLE 6–4. Endocrine Diseases Caused by G Protein–Coupled Receptor and G Protein Gene Mutations

Gene	Inactivating Mutations	Activating Mutations
Receptors		
V2 vasopressin	X-linked nephrogenic diabetes insipidus	—
ACTH	Hereditary isolated glucocorticoid deficiency	—
Ca^{2+}	Familial hypocalciuric hypercalcemia and neonatal severe hyperparathyroidism	Autosomal dominant hypocalcemia
TSH	Thyrotropin resistance	Hyperfunctional thyroid adenomas and autosomal dominant thyroid hyperplasia
LH	Familial Leydig cell hypoplasia and amenorrhea	Gonadotropin-independent male-limited precocious puberty
FSH	Hypergonadotropic ovarian dysgenesis	—
PTH/PTHrP	Blomstrand's chondrodysplasia	Jansen's metaphyseal chondrodysplasia
GHRH	Familial growth hormone deficiency	—
TRH	Isolated central hypothyroidism	—
GnRH	Familial hypogonadotropic hypogonadism	—
G protein		
$Gα_s$	Pseudohypoparathyroidism type Ia	Somatotroph adenomas, thyroid adenomas, and McCune-Albright syndrome
	Combined pseudohypoparathyroidism type Ia (loss of function) and gonadotropin-independent male precocious puberty (gain of function)	

ACTH, adrenocorticotropic hormone; FSH, follicle-stimulating hormone; GnRH, gonadotropin-releasing hormone; LH, luteinizing hormone; PTH, parathyroid hormone; PTHrP, PTH-related peptide; TRH, thyrotropin-releasing hormone; TSH, thyroid-stimulating hormone.

It is becoming increasingly clear that GPCR and G protein genes not only play key roles in differentiated cellular function but are also critically involved in the processes of cell proliferation, differentiation, and migration necessary for normal tissue development and embryogenesis. The potent oncogenic potential of mutations that lead to inappropriate activation of GPCRs or α subunits from several different G protein families has been demonstrated in cultured fibroblasts and in certain types of human tumors.[100, 112, 244] Signaling cascades triggered by the release of βγ subunits have been shown to be important for mitogenic signaling, although the downstream biochemical mechanisms by which GPCRs stimulate DNA synthesis and cell division under either normal or abnormal conditions are not yet understood.

The diversity of G proteins and downstream effector molecules located in different cells means that predicting the pattern and significance of biochemical, cytoskeletal, electrophysiologic, and transcriptional responses to activation of even a single GPCR subtype can be a daunting task. In addition to the identity, affinities, and relative concentrations of the various signaling pathway components, it is now evident that other factors are involved in determining the magnitude and time course of the cellular response. The trajectories of hormone signals can converge or diverge at each level of a GPCR-mediated signal transduction cascade, and a simple linear model is inadequate to explain most experimental findings.[18, 65, 112, 245, 246] The recent awareness that GPCR-mediated cascades are highly interconnected with pathways triggered by small GTPases and traditional receptor tyrosine kinases introduces additional degrees of complexity. Unraveling the roles of RGS proteins, PDZ domain proteins, scaffolding proteins, and other novel components that participate in G protein–coupled signaling networks will undoubtedly provide challenges for years to come.

REFERENCES

1. Strader CD, Fong TM, Tota MR, et al: Structure and function of G protein–coupled receptors. Annu Rev Biochem 63:101–132, 1994.
2. Watson S, Arkinstall S: The G-Protein Linked Receptor Facts Book. New York, Harcourt Brace, 1994.
3. van Rhee AM, Jacobson KA: Molecular architecture of G protein–coupled receptors. Drug Dev Res 37:1–38, 1996.
4. Ji TH, Grossmann M, Ji I: G protein–coupled receptors I. Diversity of receptor-ligand interactions. J Biol Chem 273:17299–17302, 1998.
5. Gether U, Kobilka BK: G protein–coupled receptors II. Mechanism of agonist activation. J Biol Chem 273:17979–17982, 1998.
6. Wess J: Molecular basis of receptor/G-protein–coupling selectivity. Pharmacol Ther 80:231–364, 1998.
7. Horn F, Weare J, Beukers MW, et al: GPCRDB: An information system for G protein–coupled receptors. Nucleic Acids Res 26:275–279, 1998. (http://www.gpcr.org/7tm)
8. Baldwin JM, Schertler GFX, Unger VM: An alpha-carbon template for the transmembrane helices in the rhodopsin family of G-protein–coupled receptors. J Mol Biol 272:144–164, 1997.
9. Segre GV, Goldring SR: Receptors for secretin, calcitonin, parathyroid hormone (PTH)/PTH-related peptide, vasoactive intestinal peptide, glucagon-like peptide 1, growth hormone–releasing hormone and glucagon belong to a newly discovered G-protein–linked family. Trends Endocrinol Metab 4:309–314, 1993.
10. Horn F, Bywater R, Krause G, et al: The interaction of class B G protein–coupled receptors with their hormones. Receptors Channels 5:305–314, 1998.
11. Tams J, Knudsen S, Fahrenkrug J: Proposed arrangement of the seven transmembrane helices in the secretin receptor family. Receptors Channels 5:79–90, 1998.
12. Conklin BR, Bourne HR: Marriage of the flytrap and the serpent. Nature 367:22, 1994.
13. Conn PJ, Pin J-P: Pharmacology and functions of metabotropic glutamate receptors. Annu Rev Pharmacol Toxicol 37:205–237, 1997.
14. Brown EM, Chattopadhyay N, Vassilev PM, et al: The calcium-sensing receptor (CaR) permits Ca^{2+} to function as a versatile extracellular first messenger. Recent Prog Horm Res 53:257–281, 1998.
15. Hoon MA, Adler E, Lindemeier J, et al: Putative mammalian taste receptors: A class of taste-specific GPCRs with distinct topographic selectivity. Cell 96:541–551, 1999.
16. Bargmann CI: Olfactory receptors, vomeronasal receptors, and the organization of olfactory information. Cell 90:585–587, 1997.
17. Slusarski DC, Corces VG, Moon RT: Interaction of Wnt and Frizzled homologue triggers G-protein–linked phosphatidylinositol signalling. Nature 390:410–413, 1997.
18. Hall RA, Premont RT, Lefkowitz RJ: Heptahelical receptor signaling: Beyond the G protein paradigm. J Cell Biol 145:927–932, 1999.
19. Wilson S, Bergsma DJ, Chambers JK, et al: Orphan G-protein–coupled receptors: The next generation of drug targets? Br J Pharmacol 125:1387–1392, 1998.
20. Klein C, Paul JI, Sauve K, et al: Identification of surrogate agonists for the human FPRL-1 receptor by autocrine selection in yeast. Nat Biotechnol 16:1334–1337, 1998.
21. McDonald T, Wang R, Bailey W, et al: Identification and cloning of an orphan G protein–coupled receptor of the glycoprotein hormone receptor subfamily. Biochem Biophys Res Commun 247:266–270, 1998.
22. Hsu SY, Liang SG, Hsueh AJ: Characterization of two *LGR* genes homologous to

23. Bikker JA, Trumpp-Kallmeyer S, Humblet C: G-protein coupled receptors: Models, mutagenesis, and drug design. J Med Chem 41:2911–2927, 1998.
24. Unger VM, Hargrave PA, Baldwin JM, et al: Arrangement of rhodopsin transmembrane α-helices. Nature 389:203–206, 1997.
25. Krebs A, Villa C, Edwards PC, et al: Characterisation of an improved two-dimensional p22121 crystal from bovine rhodopsin. J Mol Biol 282:991–1003, 1998.
26. Laakkonen LJ, Guarnieri F, Perlman JH, et al: A refined model of the thyrotropin-releasing hormone (TRH) receptor binding pocket. Novel mixed mode Monte Carlo/stochastic dynamics simulations of the complex between TRH and TRH receptor. Biochemistry 35:7651–7663, 1996.
27. Scheer A, Fanelli F, Costa T, et al: The activation process of the $α_{1B}$-adrenergic receptor: Potential role of protonation and hydrophobicity of a highly conserved aspartate. Proc Natl Acad Sci U S A 94:808–813, 1997.
28. Lin Z, Shenker A, Pearlstein R: A model of the lutropin/choriogonadotropin receptor: Insights into the structural and functional effects of constitutively activating mutations. Protein Eng 10:501–510, 1997.
29. Gether U, Lin S, Ghanouni P, et al: Agonists induce conformational changes in transmembrane domains III and VI of the $β_2$ adrenoceptor. EMBO J 16:6737–6747, 1997.
30. Donnelly D: The arrangement of the transmembrane helices in the secretin receptor family of G-protein–coupled receptors. FEBS Lett 409:431–436, 1997.
31. Schwartz TW, Rosenkilde MM: Is there a 'lock' for all agonist 'keys' in 7TM receptors? Trends Pharmacol Sci 17:213–216, 1996.
32. Shieh T, Han M, Sakmar TP, et al: The steric trigger in rhodopsin activation. J Mol Biol 269:373–384, 1997.
33. Rao VR, Oprian DD: Activating mutations of rhodopsin and other G protein–coupled receptors. Annu Rev Biophys Biomol Struct 25:287–314, 1996.
34. Shenker A: G protein–coupled receptor structure and function: The impact of disease-causing mutations. Baillieres Clin Endocrinol Metab 9:427–451, 1995.
35. Wess J: G-protein–coupled receptors: Molecular mechanisms involved in receptor activation and selectivity of G-protein recognition. FASEB J 11:346–354, 1997.
36. Ballesteros J, Kitanovic S, Guarnieri F, et al: Functional microdomains in G-protein–coupled receptors. The conserved arginine-cage motif in the gonadotropin-releasing hormone receptor. J Biol Chem 273:10445–10453, 1998.
37. Kim JM, Altenbach C, Thurmond RL, et al: Structure and function in rhodopsin: Rhodopsin mutants with a neutral amino acid at E134 have a partially activated conformation in the dark state. Proc Natl Acad Sci U S A 94:14273–14278, 1997.
38. Hébert TE, Bouvier M: Structural and functional aspects of G protein–coupled receptor oligomerization. Biochem Cell Biol 76:1–11, 1998.
39. Bockaert J, Pin JP: Molecular tinkering of G protein–coupled receptors: An evolutionary success. EMBO J 18:1723–1729, 1999.
40. Romano C, Yang WL, O'Malley KL: Metabotropic glutamate receptor 5 is a disulfide-linked dimer. J Biol Chem 271:28612–28616, 1996.
41. Bai M, Trivedi S, Kifor O, et al: Intermolecular interactions between dimeric calcium-sensing receptor monomers are important for its normal function. Proc Natl Acad Sci U S A 96:2834–2839, 1999.
42. Jones KA, Borowsky B, Tamm JA, et al: $GABA_B$ receptors function as a heteromeric assembly of the subunits $GABA_BR1$ and $GABA_BR2$. Nature 396:674–679, 1998.
43. White JH, Wise A, Main MJ, et al: Heterodimerization is required for the formation of a functional $GABA_B$ receptor. Nature 396:679–682, 1998.
44. Kaupmann K, Malitschek B, Schuler V, et al: $GABA_B$-receptor subtypes assemble into functional heteromeric complexes. Nature 396:683–687, 1998.
45. Kuner R, Köhr G, Grünewald S, et al: Role of heteromer formation in $GABA_B$ receptor function. Science 283:74–77, 1999.
46. McLatchie LM, Fraser NJ, Main MJ, et al: RAMPs regulate the transport and ligand specificity of the calcitonin-receptor–like receptor. Nature 393:333–339, 1998.
47. Hedin KE, Duerson K, Clapham DE: Specificity of receptor–G protein interactions: Searching for the structure behind the signal. Cell Signal 5:505–518, 1993.
48. Bourne HR: How receptors talk to trimeric G proteins. Curr Opin Cell Biol 9:134–142, 1997.
49. Burstein ES, Spalding TA, Brann MR: The second intracellular loop of the m5 muscarinic receptor is the switch which enables G-protein coupling. J Biol Chem 273:24322–24327, 1998.
50. Farrens DL, Altenbach C, Yang K, et al: Light activation of rhodopsin requires rigid body motion of transmembrane helices. Science 274:768–770, 1996.
51. Dunham TD, Farrens DL: Conformational changes in rhodopsin. J Biol Chem 274:1683–1690, 1999.
52. Sheikh SP, Zvyaga TA, Lichtarge O, et al: Rhodopsin activation blocked by metal-ion–binding sites linking transmembrane helices C and F. Nature 383:347–350, 1996.
53. Javitch JA, Fu D, Liapakis G, et al: Constitutive activation of the $β_2$ adrenergic receptor alters the orientation of its sixth membrane-spanning segment. J Biol Chem 272:18546–18549, 1997.
54. Kjelsberg MA, Cotecchia S, Ostrowski J, et al: Constitutive activation of the $α_{1B}$-adrenergic receptor by all amino acid substitutions at a single site: Evidence for a region which constrains receptor activation. J Biol Chem 267:1430–1433, 1992.
55. Lefkowitz RJ, Cotecchia S, Samama P, et al: Constitutive activity of receptors coupled to guanine nucleotide regulatory proteins. Trends Pharmacol Sci 14:303–307, 1993.
56. Kosugi S, Mori T, Shenker A: An anionic residue at position 564 is important for maintaining the inactive conformation of the human lutropin/choriogonadotropin receptor. Mol Pharmacol 53:894–901, 1998.
57. Van Sande J, Parma J, Tonacchera M, et al: Somatic and germline mutations of the TSH receptor gene in thyroid tissues. J Clin Endocrinol Metab 80:2577–2585, 1995.
58. Wonerow P, Schöneberg T, Schultz G, et al: Deletions in the third intracellular loop of the thyrotropin receptor. A new mechanism for constitutive activation. J Biol Chem 273:7900–7905, 1998.

59. Högger P, Shockley MS, Lameh J, et al: Activating and inactivating mutations in N- and C-terminal i3 loop junctions of muscarinic acetylcholine Hm1 receptors. J Biol Chem 270:7405–7410, 1995.

60. Spalding TA, Burstein ES, Brauner-Osborne H, et al: Pharmacology of a constitutively active muscarinic receptor generated by random mutagenesis. J Pharmacol Exp Ther 275:1274–1279, 1995.

61. Liu J, Blin N, Conklin BR, et al: Molecular mechanisms involved in muscarinic acetylcholine receptor–mediated G protein activation studied by insertion mutagenesis. J Biol Chem 271:6172–6178, 1996.

62. Schipani E, Langman CB, Parfitt AM, et al: Constitutively activated receptors for parathyroid hormone and parathyroid hormone–related peptide in Jansen's metaphyseal chondrodysplasia. N Engl J Med 335:736–738, 1996.

63. Porter JE, Hwa J, Perez DM: Activation of the α_{1b}-adrenergic receptor is initiated by disruption of an interhelical salt bridge constraint. J Biol Chem 271:28318–28323, 1996.

64. Samama P, Cotecchia S, Costa T, et al: A mutation-induced activated state of the β_2-adrenergic receptor: Extending the ternary complex model. J Biol Chem 268:4625–4636, 1993.

65. Gudermann T, Kalkbrenner F, Schultz G: Diversity and selectivity of receptor–G protein interaction. Annu Rev Pharmacol Toxicol 36:429–459, 1996.

66. Onaran HO, Costa T: Agonist efficacy and allosteric models of receptor action. Ann N Y Acad Sci 812:98–115, 1997.

67. Kenakin T: Agonist-specific receptor conformations. Trends Pharmacol Sci 18:416–417, 1997.

68. Zuscik MJ, Porter JE, Gaivin R, et al: Identification of a conserved switch residue responsible for selective constitutive activation of the β_2-adrenergic receptor. J Biol Chem 273:3401–3407, 1998.

69. Kisselev OG, Meyer CK, Heck M, et al: Signal transfer from rhodopsin to the G-protein: Evidence for a two-site sequential fit mechanism. Proc Natl Acad Sci U S A 96:4898–4903, 1999.

70. Min K-S, Liu X, Fabritz J, et al: Mutations that induce constitutive activation and mutations that impair signal transduction modulate the basal and/or agonist-stimulated internalization of the lutropin/choriogonadotropin receptor. J Biol Chem 273:34911–34919, 1998.

71. Mhaouty-Kodja S, Barak LS, Scheer A, et al: Constitutively active *alpha*-1b adrenergic receptor mutants display different phosphorylation and internalization features. Mol Pharmacol 55:339–347, 1999.

72. Spiegel AM: Mutations in G proteins and G protein–coupled receptors in endocrine disease. J Clin Endocrinol Metab 81:2434–2442, 1997.

73. Spiegel AM (ed): Contemporary Endocrinology: G Proteins, Receptors, and Disease. Totowa, NJ, Humana Press, 1998.

74. Schütz W, Freissmuth M: Reverse intrinsic activity of antagonists on G protein–coupled receptors. Trends Pharmacol Sci 13:376–380, 1992.

75. Costa T, Ogino Y, Munson PJ, et al: Drug efficacy at guanine nucleotide–binding regulatory protein–linked receptors: Thermodynamic interpretation of negative antagonism and of receptor activity in the absence of ligand. Mol Pharmacol 41:549–560, 1992.

76. Simon MI, Strathmann MP, Gautum N: Diversity of G proteins in signal transduction. Science 252:802–808, 1991.

77. Hepler JR, Gilman AG: G proteins. Trends Biochem Sci 17:383–387, 1992.

78. Neer EJ: Heterotrimeric G proteins: Organizers of transmembrane signals. Cell 80:249–257, 1995.

79. Spiegel AM, Jones TLZ, Simonds WF, et al: G Proteins. Austin, TX, RG Landes, 1994.

80. Hamm HE: The many faces of G-protein signaling. J Biol Chem 273:669–672, 1998.

81. Jeong SW, Ikeda SR: G protein alpha subunit $G\alpha_z$ couples neurotransmitter receptors to ion channels in sympathetic neurons. Neuron 21:1201–1212, 1998.

82. Noel JP, Hamm HE, Sigler PB: The 2.2 Å crystal structure of transducin-α complexed with GTPγS. Nature 366:654–663, 1993.

83. Coleman DE, Berghuis AM, Lee E, et al: Structures of active conformations of $G_{i\alpha1}$ and the mechanism of GTP hydrolysis. Science 265:1405–1412, 1994.

84. Wall MA, Coleman DE, Lee E, et al: The structure of the G protein heterotrimer $G_{i\alpha1}\beta1\gamma2$. Cell 83:1047–1058, 1995.

85. Lambright DG, Sondek J, Bohm A, et al: The 2.0 Å crystal structure of a heterotrimeric G protein. Nature 379:311–319, 1996.

86. Sprang SR: G protein mechanisms: Insights from structural analysis. Annu Rev Biochem 66:639–678, 1997.

87. Sunahara RK, Tesmer JJG, Gilman AG, et al: Crystal structure of the adenylyl cyclase activator $G_s\alpha$. Science 278:1943–1947, 1997.

88. Wall MA, Posner BA, Sprang SR: Structural basis of activity and subunit recognition on G protein heterotrimers. Structure 6:1169–1183, 1998.

89. Snow BE, Krumins AM, Brothers GM, et al: A G protein γ subunit–like domain shared between RGS11 and other RGS proteins specifies binding to Gβ5 subunits. Proc Natl Acad Sci U S A 95:13307–13312, 1998.

90. Makino ER, Handy JW, Li T, et al: The GTPase activating factor for transducin in rod photoreceptors is the complex between RGS9 and type 5 G protein β subunit. Proc Natl Acad Sci U S A 96:1947–1952, 1999.

91. Clapham DE, Neer EJ: G protein βγ subunits. Annu Rev Pharmacol Toxicol 37:167–203, 1997.

92. Gautam N, Downes GB, Yan K, et al: The G-protein βγ complex. Cell Signal 10:447–455, 1998.

93. Wedegaertner PB: Lipid modifications and membrane targeting of G_α. Biol Signals Recept 7:125–135, 1998.

94. Degtyarev MY, Spiegel AM, Jones TLZ: Increased palmitoylation of the G_s protein α subunit after activation by the α-adrenergic receptor or cholera toxin. J Biol Chem 268:23769–23772, 1993.

95. Iiri T, Farfel Z, Bourne HR: G-protein diseases furnish a model for the turn-on switch. Nature 394:35–38, 1998.

96. Yeagle PL, Alderfer JL, Albert AD: Three-dimensional structure of the cytoplasmic face of the G protein receptor rhodopsin. Biochemistry 36:9649–9654, 1997.

97. Huang C, Duncan JA, Gilman AG, et al: Persistent membrane association of activated and depalmitoylated G protein α subunits. Proc Natl Acad Sci U S A 96:412–417, 1999.

98. Tu Y, Wang J, Ross EM: Inhibition of brain G_z GAP and other RGS proteins by palmitoylation of G protein α subunits. Science 178:1132–1135, 1997.

99. Farfel Z, Bourne HR, Iiri T: The expanding spectrum of G protein diseases. N Engl J Med 340:1012–1020, 1999.

100. Roger PP, Reuse S, Maenhaut C, et al: Multiple facets of the modulation of growth by cAMP. Vitam Horm 51:59–191, 1995.

101. Collins MT, Shenker A: McCune-Albright syndrome: New insights. Curr Opin Endocrinol Diabetes 6:119–125, 1999.

102. Shen Y, Mamers P, Jobling T, et al: Absence of the previously reported G protein oncogene (gip2) in ovarian granulosa cell tumors. J Clin Endocrinol Metab 81:4159–4161, 1996.

103. Demeure MJ, Doffek KM, Komorowski RA, et al: Gip–2 codon 179 oncogene mutations: Absent in adrenal cortical tumors. World J Surg 20:928–932, 1996.

104. Siffert W, Rosskopf D, Siffert G, et al: Association of a human G-protein beta3 subunit variant with hypertension. Nat Genet 18:45–48, 1998.

105. Sunahara RK, Dessauer CW, Gilman AG: Complexity and diversity of mammalian adenylyl cyclases. Annu Rev Pharmacol Toxicol 36:461–480, 1996.

106. Exton JH: Regulation of phosphoinositide phospholipases by hormones, neurotransmitters, and other agonists linked to G proteins. Annu Rev Pharmacol Toxicol 36:481–509, 1996.

107. Tesmer JJG, Sunahara RK, Gilman AG, et al: Crystal structure of the catalytic domains of adenylyl cyclase in a complex with $G_s\alpha\cdot GTP\gamma S$. Science 278:1907–1916, 1997.

108. Lader AS, Xiao Y-F, Ishikawa Y, et al: Cardiac Gsα overexpression enhanced L-type calcium channels through an adenylyl cyclase independent pathway. Proc Natl Acad Sci U S A 95:9669–9674, 1998.

109. Kawasaki H, Springett GM, Mochizuki N, et al: A family of cAMP-binding proteins that directly activate Rap1. Science 282:2275–2279, 1998.

110. de Rooij J, Zwartkruis FJT, Verheijen MHG, et al: Epac is a Rap1 guanine-nucleotide-exchange factor directly activated by cyclic AMP. Nature 396:474–477, 1998.

111. Hooley R, Yu CY, Symons M, et al: G alpha 13 stimulates Na^+-H^+ exchange through distinct Cdc42-dependent and RhoA-dependent pathways. J Biol Chem 271:6152–6158, 1996.

112. Gutkind S: Cell growth control by G protein–coupled receptors: From signal transduction to signal integration. Oncogene 17:1331–1342, 1998.

113. Offermanns S, Simon MI: Genetic analysis of mammalian G-protein signalling. Oncogene 17:1375–1381, 1998.

114. Klages B, Brandt U, Simon MI, et al: Activation of G_{12}/G_{13} results in shape change and Rho/Rho-kinase–mediated myosin light chain phosphorylation in mouse platelets. J Cell Biol 144:745–754, 1999.

115. Jiang Y, Ma W, Wan Y, et al: The G protein Gα12 stimulates Bruton's tyrosine kinase and a rasGAP through a conserved PH/BM domain. Nature 395:808–813, 1998.

116. Bence K, Ma W, Kozasa T, et al: Direct stimulation of Bruton's tyrosine kinase by G_q-protein α-subunit. Nature 389:296–299, 1997.

117. Langehans-Rajasekaran SA, Wan Y, Huang XY: Activation of Tsk and Btk tyrosine kinases by G protein βγ subunits. Proc Natl Acad Sci U S A 92:8601–8605, 1995.

118. Hart MJ, Jiang X, Kozasa T, et al: Direct stimulation of the guanine nucleotide exchange activity of p115 RhoGEF by Gα13. Science 280:2112–2114, 1998.

119. Fukuhara S, Murga C, Zohar M, et al: A novel PDZ domain containing guanine nucleotide exchange factor links heterotrimeric G proteins to Rho. J Biol Chem 274:5868–5879, 1999.

120. Mochizuki N, Hibi M, Kanai Y, et al: Interaction of the protein nucleobindin with G alpha i2, as revealed by the two-hybrid system. FEBS Lett 373:155–158, 1995.

121. Mochizuki N, Cho G, Wen B, et al: Identification and cDNA cloning of a novel human mosaic protein, LGN, based on interaction with G alpha i2. Gene 181:39–43, 1996.

122. Chen Y, Weng G, Li J, et al: A surface of the G protein β-subunit involved in interactions with adenylyl cyclases. Proc Natl Acad Sci U S A 94:2711–2714, 1997.

123. Ford CE, Skiba NP, Bae H, et al: Molecular basis for interactions of G protein βγ subunits with effectors. Science 280:1271–1274, 1998.

124. Pellegrino S, Zhang S, Garritsen A, et al: The coiled-coil region of the G protein β subunit. Mutational analysis of Gγ and effector interactions. J Biol Chem 272:25360–25366, 1997.

125. Yamauchi J, Kaziro Y, Itoh H: C-terminal mutation of G protein β subunit affects differentially extracellular signal–regulated kinase and c-Jun N-terminal kinase pathways in human embryonal kidney 293 cells. J Biol Chem 272:7602–7607, 1997.

126. Panchenko MP, Saxena K, Li Y, et al: Sites important for $PLC\beta_2$ activation by the G protein βγ subunit map to the sides of the β propeller structure. J Biol Chem 273:28298–28304, 1998.

127. Yamada M, Inanobe A, Kurachi Y: G protein regulation of potassium ion channels. Pharmacol Rev 50:723–757, 1998.

128. Schneider T, Igelmund P, Hescheler J: G protein interaction with K^+ and Ca^{2+} channels. Trends Pharmacol Sci 18:8–11, 1997.

129. Jan LY, Jan YN: Receptor-regulated ion channels. Curr Opin Cell Biol 9:155–160, 1997.

130. Krapivinsky G, Kennedy ME, Nemec J, et al: Gβ binding to GIRK4 subunit is critical for G protein–gated K^+ channel activation. J Biol Chem 273:16946–16952, 1998.

131. Qin N, Platano D, Olcese R, et al: Direct interaction of Gβγ with a C-terminal Gβγ-binding domain of the Ca^{2+} channel α1 subunit is responsible for channel inhibition by G protein–coupled receptors. Proc Natl Acad Sci U S A 94:8866–8871, 1997.

132. Page KM, Canti C, Stephens GJ, et al: Identification of the amino terminus of neuronal Ca^{2+} channel alpha1 subunits alpha1B and alpha1E as an essential determinant of G-protein modulation. J Neurosci 18:4815–4824, 1998.

133. Ma JY, Catterall WA, Scheuer T: Persistent sodium currents through brain sodium channels induced by G protein βγ subunits. Neuron 19:443–452, 1997.
134. Stoyanov B, Volinia S, Hanck T, et al: Cloning and characterization of a G protein–activated human phosphoinositide-3 kinase. Science 269:690–693, 1995.
135. Stephens LR, Eguinoa A, Erdjument-Bromage H, et al: The Gβγ sensitivity of a PI3K is dependent upon a tightly associated adaptor, p101. Cell 89:105–114, 1997.
136. Carpenter CL, Cantley LC: Phosphoinositide 3-kinase and the regulation of cell growth. Biochim Biophys Acta 1288:M11–M16, 1996.
137. Leevers SJ, Vanhaesebroeck B, Waterfield MD: Signalling through phosphoinositide 3-kinases: The lipids take center stage. Curr Opin Cell Biol 11:219–225, 1999.
138. Ptasznik A, Beattie GM, Mally MI, et al: Phosphatidylinositol 3-kinase is a negative regulator of cellular differentiation. J Cell Biol 137:1127–1136, 1997.
139. Robinson MJ, Cobb MH: Mitogen-activated protein kinase pathways. Curr Opin Cell Biol 9:180–186, 1997.
140. Luttrell LM, Daaka Y, Lefkowitz RJ: Regulation of tyrosine kinase cascades by G-protein–coupled receptors. Curr Opin Cell Biol 11:177–183, 1999.
141. Murga C, Fukuhara S, Gutkind JS: Novel molecular mediators in the pathway connecting G-protein–coupled receptors to MAP kinase cascades. Trends Endocrinol Metab 10:122–127, 1999.
142. Daub H, Wallasch C, Lankenau A, et al: Signal characteristics of G protein–transactivated EGF receptor. EMBO J 16:7032–7044, 1997.
143. Della Rocca GJ, Maudsley S, Daaka Y, et al: Pleiotropic coupling of G protein–coupled receptors to the mitogen-activated protein kinase cascade. Role of focal adhesions and receptor tyrosine kinases. J Biol Chem 274:13978–13984, 1999.
144. Luttrell LM, Ferguson SSG, Daaka Y, et al: β-Arrestin–dependent formation of β_2 adrenergic receptor–Src protein kinase complexes. Science 283:655–661, 1999.
145. Lopez-Ilasaca M, Crespo P, Pellici PG, et al: Linkage of G protein–coupled receptors to the MAPK signaling pathway through PI 3-kinase γ. Science 275:394–397, 1997.
146. Mattingly RR, Macara IG: Phosphorylation-dependent activation of the Ras-GRF/CDC25Mm exchange factor by muscarinic receptors and G-protein beta gamma subunits. Nature 382:268–272, 1996.
147. Voyno-Yasenetskaya TA, Faure MP, Ahn NG, et al: Gα12 and Gα13 regulate extracellular signal–regulated kinase and c-Jun kinase pathways by different mechanisms in COS-7 cells. J Biol Chem 271:21081–21087, 1996.
148. Nagao M, Yamauchi J, Kaziro Y, et al: Involvement of protein kinase C and the Src family tyrosine kinase in $G\alpha_{q/11}$-induced activation of c-Jun N-terminal kinase and p38 mitogen-activated protein kinase. J Biol Chem 274:22892–22898, 1998.
149. Marinissen MJ, Chiariello M, Pallante M, et al: A network of mitogen-activated protein kinases links G protein–coupled receptors to the *c-jun* promoter: A role for c-Jun NH_2-terminal kinase, p38s, and extracellular signal–regulated kinase 5. Mol Cell Biol 39:4289–4301, 1999.
150. Hawes BE, van Biesen T, Koch WJ, et al: Distinct pathways of G_i- and G_q-mediated mitogen-activated protein kinase activation. J Biol Chem 270:17148–17153, 1995.
151. Levi NL, Hanoch T, Benard O, et al: Stimulation of Jun N-terminal kinase (JNK) by gonadotropin-releasing hormone in pituitary αT3-1 cell line is mediated by protein kinase C, c-Src, and CDC42. Mol Endocrinol 12:815–824, 1998.
152. Wylie PG, Challiss RAJ, Blank JL: Regulation of extracellular-signal regulated kinase and c-Jun N-terminal by G-protein–linked muscarinic acetylcholine receptors. Biochem J 338:619–628, 1999.
153. Crespo P, Xu N, Daniotti JL, et al: Signaling through transforming G protein–coupled receptors in NIH 3T3 cells involves c-Raf activation. Evidence for a protein kinase C–independent pathway. J Biol Chem 269:21103–21109, 1994.
154. Charlesworth A, Rozengurt E: Bombesin and neuromedin B stimulate the activation of p42 (MAPK) and p74 (Raf-1) via a protein kinase C–independent pathway in Rat-1 cells. Oncogene 14:2323–2329, 1997.
155. Zohn IE, Yu H, Li X, et al: Angiotensin II stimulates calcium-dependent activation of c-Jun N-terminal kinase. Mol Cell Biol 15:6160–6168, 1995.
156. Cadwallader K, Beltman J, McCormick F, et al: Differential regulation of extracellular signal–regulated protein kinase 1 and Jun N-terminal kinase 1 by Ca^{2+} and protein kinase C in endothelin-stimulated Rat-1 cells. Biochem J 321:795–804, 1997.
157. Faure M, Voyno-Yasenetskaya TA, Bourne HR: cAMP and beta gamma subunits of heterotrimeric G proteins stimulate the mitogen-activated protein kinase pathway in COS-7 cells. J Biol Chem 269:7851–7854, 1994.
158. Das S, Maizels ET, DeManno D, et al: A stimulatory role of cyclic adenosine 3′,5′-monophosphate in follicle-stimulating hormone–activated mitogen-activated protein kinase signaling pathway in rat ovarian granulosa cells. Endocrinology 137:967–974, 1996.
159. Vossler M, Yao H, York RD, et al: cAMP activates MAP kinase and Elk-1 through a B-Raf– and Rap1-dependent pathway. Cell 89:73–82, 1997.
160. Wan Y, Huang XY: Analysis of the G_s/mitogen-activated protein kinase pathway in mutant S49 cells. J Biol Chem 273:14533–14537, 1998.
161. Hu ZW, Shi XY, Lin RZ, et al: Contrasting signaling pathways of alpha1A- and alpha1B-adrenergic receptor subtype activation of phosphatidylinositol 3-kinase and Ras in transfected NIH3T3 cells. Mol Endocrinol 13:3–14, 1999.
162. Crespo P, Cachero TG, Xu N, et al: Dual effect of β-adrenergic receptors on mitogen-activated protein kinase. Evidence for a βγ-dependent activation and a $G\alpha_s$-cAMP–mediated inhibition. J Biol Chem 270:25259–25265, 1995.
163. Daaka Y, Luttrell LM, Lefkowitz RJ: Switching of coupling of the β_2-adrenergic receptor to different G proteins by protein kinase A. Nature 390:88–91, 1997.
164. Krupnick JG, Benovic JL: The role of receptor kinases and arrestins in G protein–coupled receptor regulation. Annu Rev Pharmacol Toxicol 38:289–319, 1998.
165. Lefkowitz RJ: G protein–coupled receptors III. New roles for receptor kinases and β-arrestins in receptor signaling and desensitization. J Biol Chem 273:18677–18680, 1998.
166. Carman CV, Benovic JL: G-protein–coupled receptors: Turn-ons and turn-offs. Curr Opin Neurobiol 8:335–344, 1998.
167. Pitcher JA, Freedman NJ, Lefkowitz RJ: G protein–coupled receptor kinases. Annu Rev Biochem 67:653–692, 1998.
168. Bunemann M, Lee KB, Pals-Rylaarsdam R, et al: Desensitization of G-protein–coupled receptors in the cardiovascular system. Annu Rev Physiol 61:169–192, 1999.
169. Hein L, Ishii K, Coughlin SR, et al: Intracellular targeting and trafficking of thrombin receptors. A novel mechanism for resensitization of a G protein–coupled receptor. J Biol Chem 269:27719–27726, 1994.
170. Gagnon AW, Kallal L, Benovic JL: Role of clathrin-mediated endocytosis in agonist-induced down-regulation of the β_2-adrenergic receptor. J Biol Chem 273:6976–6981, 1998.
171. Hausdorff WP, Caron MG, Lefkowitz RJ: Turning off the signal: Desensitization of beta-adrenergic receptor function. FASEB J 4:2881–2889, 1990.
172. Oppermann M, Freedman NJ, Alexander RW, et al: Phosphorylation of the type 1A angiotensin II receptor by G protein–coupled receptor kinases and protein kinase C. J Biol Chem 271:13266–13272, 1996.
173. Nakamura K, Krupnick JG, Benovic JL, et al: Signaling and phosphorylation-impaired mutants of the rat follitropin receptor reveal an activation- and phosphorylation-independent but arrestin-dependent pathway for internalization. J Biol Chem 273:24346–24354, 1998.
174. Goodman OB Jr, Krupnick JG, Santini F, et al: Role of arrestins in G-protein–coupled receptor endocytosis. Adv Pharmacol 42:429–433, 1998.
175. Granzin J, Wilden U, Choe HW, et al: X-ray crystal structure of arrestin from bovine rod outer segments. Nature 391:918–921, 1998.
176. Hirsch JA, Schubert C, Gurevich VV, et al: The 2.8 A crystal structure of visual arrestin: A model for arrestin's regulation. Cell 97:257–269, 1999.
177. Vishnivetskiy SA, Paz CL, Schubert C, et al: How does arrestin respond to the phosphorylated state of rhodopsin? J Biol Chem 274:11451–11454, 1999.
178. McDonald PH, Cote NL, Lin FT, et al: Identification of NSF as a β-arrestin1–binding protein. J Biol Chem 274:10677–10680, 1999.
179. Laporte SA, Oakley RH, Zhang J, et al: The β2-adrenergic receptor/βarrestin complex recruits the clathrin adaptor AP-2 during endocytosis. Proc Natl Acad Sci U S A 96:3712–3717, 1999.
180. Daaka Y, Luttrell LM, Ahn S, et al: Essential role for G protein–coupled receptor endocytosis in the activation of mitogen-acted protein kinase. J Biol Chem 273:685–688, 1998.
181. Budd DC, Rae A, Tobin AB: Activation of the mitogen-activated protein kinase pathway by a $G_{q/11}$-coupled muscarinic receptor is independent of receptor internalization. J Biol Chem 274:12355–12360, 1999.
182. Mundell SJ, Kelly E: The effect of inhibitors of receptor internalization on the desensitization and resensitization of three G_s-coupled receptor responses. Br J Pharmacol 125:1594–1600, 1998.
183. Beaumont V, Hepworth MB, Luty JS, et al: Somatostatin receptor desensitization in NG108-15 cells. J Biol Chem 273:33174–33183, 1998.
184. Zhang J, Ferguson SSG, Barak LS, et al: Dynamin and β-arrestin reveal distinct mechanisms for G protein–coupled receptor internalization. J Biol Chem 271:18302–18305, 1996.
185. Dicker F, Quitterer U, Winstel R, et al: Phosphorylation-independent inhibition of parathyroid hormone receptor signaling by G protein–coupled receptor kinases. Proc Natl Acad Sci U S A 96:5476–5481, 1999.
186. Mukherjee S, Palczewski K, Gurevich V, et al: A direct role for arrestins in desensitization of the luteinizing hormone/choriogonadotropin receptor in porcine ovarian follicular membranes. Proc Natl Acad Sci U S A 96:493–498, 1999.
187. Malecz N, Bambino T, Bencsik M, et al: Identification of phosphorylation sites in the G protein–coupled receptor for parathyroid hormone. Receptor phosphorylation is not required for agonist-induced internalization. Mol Endocrinol 12:1846–1856, 1998.
188. Arshavsky VY, Bownds MD: Regulation of deactivation of photoreceptor G protein by its target enzyme and cGMP. Nature 357:416–417, 1992.
189. Berstein G, Blank JL, Jhon DY, et al: Phospholipase C-β1 is a GTPase-activating protein for Gq/11, its physiologic regulator. Cell 70:411–418, 1992.
190. Berman DM, Gilman AG: Mammalian RGS proteins: Barbarians at the gate. J Biol Chem 273:1269–1272, 1998.
191. Arshavsky VY, Pugh EN: Lifetime regulation of G protein–effector complex: Emerging importance of RGS proteins. Neuron 20:11–14, 1998.
192. Zerangue N, Jan LY: G-protein signaling: Fine-tuning signaling kinetics. Curr Biol 8:R313–R316, 1998.
193. De Vries L, Farquhar MG: RGS proteins: More than just GAPs for heterotrimeric G proteins. Trends Cell Biol 9:138–144, 1999.
194. Tesmer JJ, Berman DM, Gilman AG, et al: Structure of RGS4 bound to AlF_4^--activated Giα1: Stabilization of the transition state for GTP hydrolysis. Cell 89:251–261, 1997.
195. Bunemann M, Hosey MM: Regulators of G protein signaling (RGS) proteins constitutively activate Gβγ-gated potassium channels. J Biol Chem 273:31186–31190, 1998.
196. Xu X, Zeng W, Popov S, et al: RGS proteins determine signaling specificity of G_q-coupled receptors. J Biol Chem 274:3549–3556, 1999.
197. Snow BE, Hall RA, Krumins AM, et al: GTPase activating specificity of RGS12 and binding specificity of an alternatively spliced PDZ (PSD-95/Dlg/ZO-1) domain. J Biol Chem 273:17749–17755, 1998.
198. Kozasa T, Jiang X, Hart MJ, et al: p115 RhoGEF, a GTPase activating protein for Gα12 and Gα13. Science 280:2109–2111, 1998.
199. Loew A, Ho YK, Blundell T, et al: Phosducin induces a structural change in transducin beta gamma. Structure 6:1007–1019, 1998.
200. Burns CM, Chu H, Rueter SM, et al: Regulation of serotonin-2C receptor G-protein coupling by RNA editing. Nature 387:303–308, 1997.
201. Miswender CM, Copeland SC, Herrick-Davis K, et al: RNA editing of the human serotonin 5-hydroxytryptamine 2C receptor silences constitutive activity. J Biol Chem 274:9472–9478, 1999.
202. McIntire WE, Schey KL, Knapp DR, et al: A major G protein α_o isoform in bovine brain is deamidated at Asn346 and Asn347, residues involved in receptor coupling. Biochemistry 37:14651–14658, 1998.

203. Ali MS, Sayeski PP, Dirksen LB, et al: Dependence on the motif YIPP for the physical association of Jak2 kinase with the intracellular carboxyl tail of the angiotensin II AT1 receptor. J Biol Chem 272:23382–23388, 1997.

204. Hall RA, Premont RT, Chow EW, et al: The β2-adrenergic receptor interacts with the Na+/H+-exchanger regulatory factor to control Na+/H+ exchange. Nature 392:626–630, 1998.

205. Brakeman PR, Lanahan AA, O'Brien R, et al: Homer: A protein that selectively binds metabotropic glutamate receptors. Nature 386:284–288, 1997.

206. Ullmer C, Schmuck K, Figge A, et al: Cloning and characterization of MUPP1, a novel PDZ domain protein. FEBS Lett 424:63–68, 1998.

207. Klein U, Ramirez TM, Kobilka BK, et al: A novel interaction between adrenergic receptors and the α-subunit of eukaryotic initiation factor 2B. J Biol Chem 272:19099–19102, 1997.

208. Prezeau L, Richman JG, Edwards SW, et al: The zeta isoform of 14-3-3 interacts with the third intracellular loop of different α2-adrenergic receptor subtypes. J Biol Chem 274:13462–13469, 1999.

209. Mitchell R, McCulloch D, Lutz E, et al: Rhodopsin-family receptors associate with small G proteins to activate phospholipase D. Nature 392:411–414, 1998.

210. Strittmatter SM: GAP-43 as a modulator of G protein transduction in the growth cone. Perspect Dev Neurobiol 1:13–19, 1992.

211. Giambarella U, Yamatsuji T, Okamoto T, et al: G protein βγ complex–mediated apoptosis by familial Alzheimer's disease mutant of APP. EMBO J 16:4897–4907, 1997.

212. Luo Y, Denker BM: Interaction of heterotrimeric G protein Gα₀ with Purkinje cell protein-2. J Biol Chem 274:10685–10688, 1999.

213. Sato M, Ribas C, Hildebrandt JD, et al: Characterization of a G-protein activator in the neuroblastoma-glioma cell hybrid NG108-15. J Biol Chem 271:30052–30060, 1996.

214. Lolozin B, Iwasaki K, Vito MP, et al: Participation of presenilin 2 in apoptosis: Enhanced basal activity conferred by an Alzheimer mutation. Science 274:1710–1713, 1996.

215. Bomsel M, Mostov K: Role of heterotrimeric G proteins in membrane traffic. Mol Biol Cell 3:1317–1328, 1992.

216. Pimplikar SW, Simons K: Regulation of apical transport in epithelial cells by a Gₛ class of heterotrimeric G protein. Nature 362:456–458, 1993.

217. Wilson BS, Komuro M, Farquhar MG: Cellular variations in heterotrimeric G protein localization and expression in rat pituitary. Endocrinology 134:233–244, 1994.

218. Helms JB: Role of heterotrimeric GTP binding proteins in vesicular protein transport: Indications for both classical and alternative G protein cycles. FEBS Lett 369:84–88, 1995.

219. Denker SP, McCaffery JM, Palade GE, et al: Differential distribution of α subunits and βγ subunits of heterotrimeric G proteins on Golgi membranes of the exocrine pancreas. J Cell Biol 133:1027–1040, 1996.

220. Gilchrist A, Mazzoni MR, Dineen B, et al: Antagonists of the receptor–G protein interface block Gᵢ-coupled signal transduction. J Biol Chem 273:14912–14919, 1998.

221. Neubig RR: Membrane organization in G-protein mechanisms. FASEB J 8:939–946, 1994.

222. Li S, Okamoto T, Chun M, et al: Evidence for a regulated interaction between heterotrimeric G proteins and caveolin. J Biol Chem 270:15693–15701, 1995.

223. Anderson RG: The caveolae membrane system. Annu Rev Biochem 67:199–225, 1998.

224. Rudolph U, Finegold MJ, Rich SS, et al: Ulcerative colitis and adenocarcinoma of the colon in Gα₁₂-deficient mice. Nat Genet 10:143–150, 1995.

225. Offermanns S, Zhao L-P, Gohla A, et al: Embryonic cardiomyocyte hypoplasia and craniofacial defects in Gα_q/Gα₁₁-mutant mice. EMBO J 17:4304–4312, 1998.

226. Jiang M, Gold MS, Boulay G, et al: Multiple neurological abnormalities in mice deficient in the G protein G₀. Proc Natl Acad Sci U S A 95:3269–3274, 1998.

227. Yu S, Yu D, Lee E, et al: Variable and tissue-specific hormone resistance in heterotrimeric Gₛ protein α-subunit (Gₛα) knockout mice is due to tissue-specific imprinting of the Gₛα gene. Proc Natl Acad Sci U S A 95:8715–8720, 1998.

228. Brunner D, Hen R: Insights into the neurobiology of impulsive behavior from serotonin receptor knockout mice. Ann N Y Acad Sci 836:81–105, 1997.

229. Drago J, Padungchaichot P, Acili D, et al: Dopamine receptors and dopamine transporter in brain function and addictive behaviors: Insights from targeted mouse mutants. Dev Neurosci 20:188–203, 1998.

230. Kronenberg HM, Lanske B, Kovacs CS, et al: Functional analysis of the PTH/PTHrP network of ligands and receptors. Recent Prog Horm Res 53:283–301, 1998.

231. Rohrer DK: Physiological consequences of β-adrenergic receptor disruption. J Mol Med 76:764–772, 1998.

232. Rohrer DK, Kobilka BK: Insights from in vivo modification of adrenergic receptor gene expression. Annu Rev Pharmacol Toxicol 38:351–373, 1998.

233. Koch WJ, Lefkowitz RJ, Milano CA, et al: Myocardial overexpression of adrenergic receptors and receptor kinases. Adv Pharmacol 42:502–506, 1998.

234. Ledent C, Denef J-F, Cottecchia S, et al: Costimulation of adenylyl cyclase and phospholipase C by a mutant α₁B-adrenergic receptor transgene promotes malignant transformation of thyroid follicular cells. Endocrinology 138:369–378, 1997.

235. Hager J, Hansen L, Vaisse C, et al: A missense mutation in the glucagon receptor gene is associated with non–insulin-dependent diabetes. Nat Genet 9:299–304, 1995.

236. Fujisawa T, Ikegami H, Yamato E, et al: A mutation in the glucagon receptor gene (Gly40Ser): Heterogeneity in the association with diabetes mellitus. Diabetologia 38:983–985, 1995.

237. Liggett SB, Wagoner LE, Craft LL, et al: The Ile164 β₂-adrenergic receptor polymorphism adversely affects the outcome of congestive heart failure. J Clin Invest 102:1534–1539, 1998.

238. Mason DA, Moore JD, Green SA, et al: A gain-of-function polymorphism in a G-protein coupling domain of the human β₁-adrenergic receptor. J Biol Chem 274:12670–12674, 1999.

239. Berger EA, Murphy PM, Farber JM: Chemokine receptors as HIV-coreceptors: Roles in viral entry, tropism, and disease. Annu Rev Immunol 17:657–700, 1999.

240. Arvanitakis L, Geras-Raaka E, Varma A, et al: Human herpesvirus KSHV encodes a constitutively active G-protein–coupled receptor linked to cell proliferation. Nature 385:347–350, 1997.

241. Rohrer SP, Birzin ET, Mosley RT, et al: Rapid identification of subtype-selective agonists of the somatostatin receptor through combinatorial chemistry. Science 282:737–740, 1998.

242. Höller C, Freissmuth M, Nanoff C: G proteins as drug targets. Cell Mol Life Sci 55:257–270, 1999.

243. Akhter SA, Luttrell LM, Rockman HA, et al: Targeting the receptor-G_q interface to inhibit in vivo pressure overload myocardial hypertrophy. Science 280:574–577, 1998.

244. Dhanasekaran N, Tsim ST, Dermott JM, et al: Regulation of cell proliferation by G proteins. Oncogene 17:1383–1394, 1998.

245. Selbie LA, Hill SJ: G protein-coupled-receptor cross-talk: The fine-tuning of multiple receptor-signalling pathways. Trends Pharmacol Sci 19:87–93, 1998.

246. Weng G, Bhalla US, Iyengar R: Complexity in biological signaling systems. Science 284:92–96, 1999.

Chapter 7

The Cyclic AMP Second Messenger Signaling Pathway

Joel F. Habener

The discovery of the cyclic adenosine monophosphate (cAMP) second messenger signaling pathway made a major impact in understanding how growth, development, and metabolism of cells are regulated in response to environmental cues. Studies that led to the elucidation of the mechanisms involved in the important cAMP-directed signaling pathway have spanned over five decades. The historical aspects of the key research discoveries are reviewed briefly. Lessons can be learned by appreciating the conceptualization and experimentation that systematically led to further conclusions, modifications of hypotheses, and additional experimentation carried out successively by Cori and Cori,[1] Rall and Sutherland,[2] Fischer,[3] and Krebs,[4] all of whom were awarded the Nobel Prize in physiology and medicine. Several excellent reviews of various aspects of the cAMP-dependent signaling system have appeared.[5-15]

HISTORICAL PERSPECTIVES

In the early 1940s, Cori and Cori established the basic biochemistry of glycogenolysis by identification of the key enzymes of glycogen metabolism, namely, glycogen phosphorylase, phosphoglucomutase, and glucose-6-phosphatase.[16] Most importantly, they demonstrated that glycogen breakdown is stimulated by the hormones glucagon and epinephrine. A key finding was that glycogen phosphorylase was interconvertible from an inactive form (phosphorylase *b*) to an active form (phosphorylase *a*), a discovery for which the Cori's were jointly awarded the Nobel Prize in 1951.[1] These pioneering studies were further pursued by Sutherland and coworkers, who used broken liver cell preparations to show that glucagon and epinephrine stimulated the activity of glycogen phosphorylase, a rate-limiting step in the conversion of glycogen to glucose.[2] Furthermore, they demonstrated that although the hormonally responsive enzymatic activity resided in the particulate fraction, generation of activity required re-addition of the soluble fraction contained in the broken cell preparation.[17] These seminal observations assisted Sutherland in isolating and identifying the essential factor in the soluble fraction as an adenine ribonucleotide, subsequently established to be adenosine 3',5'-cyclic monophosphate, otherwise known as cAMP.[18] The work of this group of investigators culminated in the isolation and characterization of adenylyl cyclase and phosphodiesterase, the two key enzymes responsible for the synthesis and degradation of cAMP, respectively. Identification of cAMP was an essential step in the consequent conceptualization of the "second messenger" hypothesis by which hormones, acting on receptors located on the cell surface, lead to the synthesis of the second messenger (cAMP), which in turn regulates cellular activity. This concept provided a model to explain how extracellular signals, such as hormones, can transduce their informational cues to the interior of the

cell. For this series of brilliant discoveries, Sutherland was awarded the Nobel Prize in 1971.

During the time that Sutherland and coworkers were characterizing adenylyl cyclase and phosphodiesterase, Fischer and Krebs pursued the further identification of targets in the signal transduction pathway on which cAMP exerts its effects. In the late 1950s they discovered that the activity of glycogen phosphorylase is altered by a reversible phosphorylation mediated by phosphorylase kinase and opposing phosphatases and that the phosphorylation required cAMP.[10, 19, 20] In 1968, the laboratories of Krebs and Greengard independently isolated the enzyme responsible for activation of phosphorylase kinase.[21, 22] The enzyme was called *phosphorylase kinase kinase* because it phosphorylated phosphorylase kinase; however, it was soon discovered to be the key enzyme activated by cAMP and was renamed *cAMP-dependent protein kinase A* (PKA) because of its widespread importance in the phosphorylation of many substrate proteins other than phosphorylase kinase.[10] As discussed below, PKA is a heterotetrameric protein consisting of two regulatory and two catalytic subunits. cAMP binds to the regulatory subunit and thereby relieves inhibition of the catalytic subunit by releasing the activated catalytic subunit from an inactive complex with the regulatory subunit. The catalytic subunit is then free to specifically phosphorylate certain serine and threonine residues in proteins whose functions are regulated by PKA. Krebs and Fischer shared the Nobel Prize in 1992 for their seminal work on this critically important pathway of phosphorylation (and dephosphorylation) initiated by cAMP-dependent PKA.[3, 4]

THE PLEIOTROPIC ACTIONS OF cAMP

The cellular actions of cAMP are numerous (Fig. 7–1). Notably, with few exceptions, all the actions of cAMP are mediated by PKA. One exception appears to be that cAMP binds to and directly regulates the activity of olfactory and brain receptor–regulated ion channels.[23-25] cAMP, via its actions on PKA, activates certain enzymes and inactivates others. For example, phosphorylase kinase[10] and type II PKA[6, 7] are activated and glycogen synthase is inactivated by PKA[10] (see below). Certain receptors, such as β-adrenergic receptors (βARs),[26, 27] and ion channels, such as cystic fibrosis transmembrane conductance regulator (CFTR),[28] are regulated via phosphorylation by PKA. In addition, the structural proteins tubulin[29] and microtubule-associated proteins[30] are modified by PKA-induced phosphorylation. An important function of PKA is the phosphorylation and consequent activation of nuclear transcription factors that bind to the cAMP response enhancer elements of many genes. These proteins are known variously as cAMP response element (CRE)-binding proteins (CREBs) or activating transcription factors (ATFs).[31-33] PKA also stimulates glucocor-

Pleiotropic Actions of cAMP Second Messenger

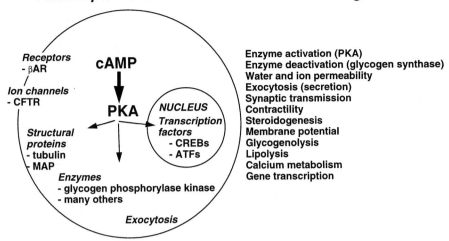

Enzyme activation (PKA)
Enzyme deactivation (glycogen synthase)
Water and ion permeability
Exocytosis (secretion)
Synaptic transmission
Contractility
Steroidogenesis
Membrane potential
Glycogenolysis
Lipolysis
Calcium metabolism
Gene transcription

FIGURE 7–1. The cyclic adenosine monophosphate (cAMP)-dependent second messenger pathway modifies many different cellular functions. Almost all functions of cAMP are mediated by activation of protein kinase A (PKA). Some of the known functions modulated by PKA are shown on the right. Representative proteins whose functions are regulated by PKA-directed phosphorylation are depicted in the diagram of the cell shown on the left. βAR, β-adrenergic receptor; ATF, activating transcription factor; CFTR, cystic fibrosis transmembrane conductance regulator; CREB, cAMP response element–binding protein; MAP, microtubule-associated protein.

ticoid receptor–mediated gene transcription, but this effect of PKA may be indirect via phosphorylation of an intermediate factor.[34] The regulatory subunit of PKA is a homologue of the prokaryotic catabolite activating protein,[35] and the regulatory subunit has been shown by fluorescence assays to bind DNA in vitro.[26] As yet, however, no clear evidence supports a functional role for the regulatory subunit in animal cells apart from its important actions as an inhibitor of the catalytic subunit.

The mechanism by which phosphorylation activates or inactivates the biologic functions of a protein most often involves a change in the conformation or folding of the protein.[36, 37] The change in conformation is considered to be allosteric when the change in shape of the protein occurs at a distance from the site that is phosphorylated by a specific protein kinase, for example, by PKA. Examples of the involvement of PKA in the allosteric regulation of protein activities are discussed in more detail later in this chapter.

COMPONENTS OF THE cAMP-DEPENDENT CELLULAR SIGNALING PATHWAY

The cAMP-dependent signaling pathway consists of several intermolecular interactions leading to the generation of an active catalytic subunit of PKA capable of phosphorylating target sites on protein substrates. A generalized overall schematic illustration of this pathway is given in Figure 7–2. The detailed molecular mechanisms at work in

the cascade of molecular interactions have yet to be completely elucidated. However, some interpretations can be made regarding how the individual components of the pathway are linked together.

Model of Activation of PKA by cAMP

The initiating event in the pathway of cAMP-dependent signaling is the binding of a hormone (ligand) to its receptor. This type of interaction appears to be a crucial first step in the signaling cascade that results in the eventual formation of cAMP. Binding of the hormone ligand to its receptor, which occurs specifically and with high affinity (in the range of nanomolar concentrations of ligand), results in a change in conformation of the receptor reflected within the transmembrane and cytoplasmic domains. The second step in the signaling cascade is the receptor-directed conversion of an associated guanine-binding protein (G protein) from an inactive to an active form. The cycling of G protein from an inactive to an active state and back to the inactive form is described in greater detail below in reference to the model shown in Figure 7–3. The activated G protein, the guanosine triphosphate (GTP)-bound derivative of the G protein α subunit, activates the enzyme adenylyl cyclase, referred to earlier, which leads to the conversion of ATP to 3′,5′-cAMP. Degradation of cAMP to 5′-AMP is accomplished by the enzyme phosphodiesterase (see Fig. 7–2). The key role of cAMP is to bind to the regulatory subunit of the inactive heterotetrameric complex of PKA, thereby eliciting an allosteric change in the complex that results in liberation of the active

Cyclic AMP -Dependent Signal Transduction Pathway

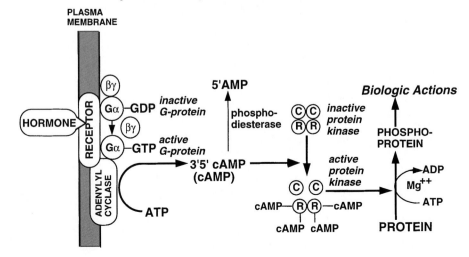

FIGURE 7–2. Cyclic adenosine monophosphate (cAMP)-dependent signal transduction pathway. The diagram depicts the essential components of the cellular signaling pathway mediated by the second messenger cAMP. The "first" messenger or activator is the hormone/receptor/G protein complex. The "second" messenger effector is cAMP. The "third" messenger is a protein kinase A that phosphorylates critical protein substrates to generate the final bioactive "fourth" messenger. See the text for a more detailed explanation. ADP, adenosine diphosphate; GDP, guanosine diphosphate; GTP, guanosine triphosphate.

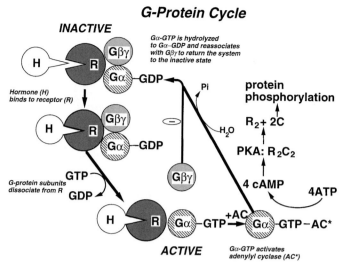

FIGURE 7–3. *The guanine nucleotide–binding protein (G protein) cycle. The diagram is a more detailed depiction of the G protein function shown in Figure 7–2. The G_α subunit can be either stimulatory (G_s) or inhibitory (G_i), depending on the isotype of the subunit involved. The activated G_α–guanosine triphosphate (GTP) complex modulates the activity of adenylyl cyclase, which leads to the activation of protein kinase A (PKA) and the resultant phosphorylation of key protein substrates that manifest the cellular response. G_α-GTP is inactivated by hydrolysis of GTP to guanosine diphosphate (GDP) by the intrinsic GTPase activities of the G_α subunit. cAMP, cyclic adenosine monophosphate.*

catalytic subunit from the inactive complex. The catalytic subunits, once freed from their regulatory subunits, are available to phosphorylate sites on protein substrates, thereby resulting in modification of the biologic actions of the proteins (see Fig. 7–2). A more detailed explanation of cAMP-stimulated activation of PKA is given later in this chapter.

The G Protein Cycle

The coupling of G proteins is of critical importance in transmitting the signal generated by hormone receptor interactions to the formation of cAMP (see Fig. 7–3). G proteins consist of complex families of α, β, and γ subunits that in the inactive state form heterotrimeric complexes with guanosine diphosphate (GDP) bound to the α subunit. Much attention has been focused on the regulatory functions of the α subunit, various isotypes of which can be either stimulatory (G_s) or inhibitory ($G_{\alpha i}$).

Binding of a ligand to its receptor causes a conformational change in the receptor and its associated G protein that leads to the exchange of GTP for GDP and concomitant dissociation of the GTP-bound α subunit from the βγ subunit dimeric complex. This GTP-activated G_α then binds to adenylyl cyclase to either activate or inhibit the enzyme, depending on whether the type of G_α is stimulatory ($G_{\alpha s}$) or inhibitory ($G_{\alpha i}$). The quantity of activated adenylyl cyclase formed depends on the relative amounts of stimulatory or inhibitory G_α subunits present in a given location within the cell at a given time. Pharmacologic distinction between the actions of stimulatory and inhibitory G_α proteins has been facilitated by the use of two bacterial toxins that result in ribosylation of G_α subunits by adenosine diphosphate (ADP). Cholera toxin activates $G_{\alpha s}$ and pertussis toxin inhibits $G_{\alpha i}$ and $G_{\alpha o}$ ("other"), a G protein enriched in brain but whose functions are poorly understood. The use of nonhydrolyzable analogues of GTP, such as GPP(NH)P and GTPγS, has also been of great value in dissecting the G protein pathways. These GTP analogues constitutively activate G_α proteins because they cannot be hydrolyzed to GDP.

After activation of adenylyl cyclase, the G proteins return to the inactive state. GTP is hydrolyzed to GDP by the intrinsic GTPase activity contained in the G_α subunit. G_α dissociates from adenylyl cyclase and the βγ subunits reassociate with the α subunit. It is

unknown to what extent the inactivation of G protein is due to hydrolysis of GTP to GDP or to reassociation of the α and βγ subunits. It appears that the βγ complex may control certain effectors directly. It has been proposed that βγ can inhibit adenylate cyclase directly or indirectly through interactions with calmodulin. Studies in vitro have shown that βγ inhibits type I adenylyl cyclase and stimulates the type II enzyme whereas G_s stimulates both enzyme isotypes.[42] In addition, βγ may regulate the activities of K^+ channels and certain isotypes of phospholipase C. The inhibitory or stimulatory actions of βγ appear to reside in the particular isotype of the γ subunit involved, a minimum of eight of which have been identified so far. Unraveling of the complex interactions of the G protein subunits is at the forefront of molecular and cellular research.

Investigators are just now beginning to understand the complex nature of G proteins. In addition to the G_s and G_i heterotrimeric complexes, G_q and G_o complexes also exist and are coupled to phospholipid/Ca^{2+} and brain-specific pathways of signal transduction, respectively. Specific G protein isotypes are found in the retina (G_t) and the olfactory epithelium (G_{olf}). Twenty or more isotypes of G and at least a dozen isotypes of the G_β (4) and G_γ (8) subunits have been identified by sequencing of cloned recombinant cDNA.[11] Many of the primary transcripts derived from the subunit genes are alternatively spliced and result in the formation of mRNAs that encode yet additional isoforms of the subunit proteins.[11] The precise functions of most of the large number of G protein subunit isoforms are unknown because at present they are proteins identified only by recombinant DNA cloning technology; investigators are in search of their cellular functions. An additional important function, however, of the class of G proteins that has been shown to couple to receptors is to regulate ion channels. G_s directly modulates the activity of voltage-dependent calcium channels,[43] and evidence has been presented in support of a role for pertussis-sensitive G_i and G_o in the coupling of receptors of a variety of hormones and neurotransmitters to potassium and calcium channels; such receptor coupling results in either stimulatory or inhibitory control, depending on the type of channel affected.[44, 45] Furthermore, the receptor-coupled and channel-coupled G proteins represent merely a subfamily of a much larger family of GTP-binding proteins involved in such diverse functions as control of protein synthesis (e.g., elongation factor), protein translocation across membranes, and ADP ribosylation (ADP ribosylation factors, or ARFs).[38] In addition, an entire complex family of small GTP-binding proteins known as the Ras proteins are involved in growth and differentiation, regulation of adenylyl cyclase, vesicular transport, and many other functions that have yet to be defined.[38]

The Adenylyl Cyclases

The adenylyl cyclases consist of a diverse family of membrane-associated enzymes, at least nine distinct isotypes of which have been identified.[46–48] The distribution of the various enzyme isotypes among different tissues is highly variable. Most tissues contain several different isotypes, but in many tissues one or more of the isotypes are absent.

The structure of adenylyl cyclases consists of two alternating hydrophobic and hydrophilic domains[47, 49] (Fig. 7–4). The hydrophobic domains contain six membrane-spanning domains, and the cytoplasmic hydrophilic domains each contain 250 residues that are homologous to the putative catalytic domains of the guanylyl cyclases. This overall structure of adenylyl cyclase is similar to that of the glucose transporters and P glycoprotein, the product of the multidrug resistance gene. This structure suggests that in addition to its catalytic function of converting ATP to cAMP, the enzyme serves as the transporter that exports cAMP from the cell. Disposal of cAMP appears to involve two mechanisms: degradation by phosphodiesterase in the cell and transport out of the cell. Both mechanisms may in turn be regulated as a means of titrating the amount of cAMP available in the cell during the time that the catalytic activity of the enzyme is turned on by the active G protein G_α-GTP. The differences in functions of the various isoforms of the adenylyl cyclases have not yet been completely determined. However, it is now appreciated that most, if not all, of the

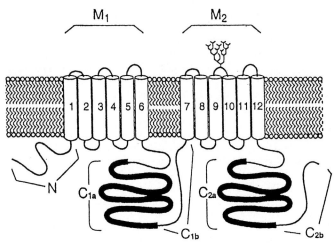

FIGURE 7–4. Diagram of the cellular location and orientation of adenylyl cyclase predicted from its primary amino acid sequence. The cyclase contains two symmetric regions that span the plasma membrane six times (M_1 and M_2). Two large cytoplasmic loops (C_{1a}/C_{1b} and C_{2a}/C_{2b}) share sequence similarities with guanylyl cyclase *(black)*.

nine different adenylyl cyclases are multiply regulated.[50] Both Ca^{2+} and the phospholipase C signaling pathways are implicated in the regulation of adenylyl cyclase activity.[47, 50] For example, Ca^{2+}-calmodulin kinases II and IV inhibit adenylyl cyclase types III and I, respectively. Ca^{2+}-calmodulin activates type II adenylyl cyclase.[47] In general, Mn^{2+} activates and Ca^{2+} inhibits the activity of all the adenylyl cyclase isotypes. The G protein subunits also regulate the adenylyl cyclases. $G_{s\alpha}$ activates all isotypes (I–IX), whereas $G_{i\alpha}$ specifically inhibits isotypes V and VI. The G protein $\beta\gamma$ subunit activates several of the adenylyl cyclases, but it is relatively specific in activation of the type II isotype.

Structures of the Regulatory and Catalytic Subunits of PKA

The heterotetrameric complex that constitutes the holoenzyme of PKA consists of two catalytic and two regulatory subunits.[5–8] Thus far, three isotypes have been identified for the catalytic subunit (C_α, C_β, C_γ), with apparent molecular weights of 40,800, and two types for the regulatory subunit (RI, RII), each of which has two isotypes (RI$_\alpha$, RI$_\beta$ and RII$_\alpha$, RII$_\beta$) and molecular weights of 92,000 to 108,000 (Table 7–1). The sequences of both the catalytic and the regulatory subunits are highly conserved. For example, the amino acid sequences of C_α and C_β are 93% identical. The C_γ subunit is somewhat less well conserved: 79% and 83% identical to C_α and C_β, respectively.[6] Conservation of the sequences among the four regulatory subunits is likewise quite high. As discussed below in more detail, certain of the various types and isotypes of subunits have distinct subcellular distributions and functions.

The Catalytic Subunits

The catalytic subunit contains a region that is highly conserved in the catalytic core of many different protein kinases. This region contains several motifs involved in ATP-Mg^{2+} binding, substrate recogni-

TABLE 7–1. Cyclic Adenosine Monophosphate–Dependent Protein Kinase A Heterotetrameric Complex

Subunits	2 Regulatory (R)
	2 Catalytic (C)
Isoforms	R: RI$_\alpha$, RI$_\beta$, RII$_\alpha$, RII$_\beta$
	C: C_α, C_β, C_γ

tion, and phosphotransfer (Fig. 7–5). The structure of C_α has been partially solved by x-ray crystallography both with and without a bound pseudosubstrate, so the relevant contacts between ATP, Mg^{2+}, and substrate are relatively well understood.[51, 52]

The ATP-binding fold resides in the N-terminal region and contains a glycine loop motif GXGXXG followed proximal to the C terminus by a lysine (K-72) and an acidic residue, glutamic acid (E-91), common to a variety of proteins that bind nucleotides. The glycine loop, lysine 72, glutamic acid 91, and aspartic acid 184 are all involved in the coordinate binding of Mg^{2+}-ATP. For reasons as yet unknown, Mg^{2+}-ATP binds more tightly to the catalytic subunit when complexed with type I as opposed to the type II regulatory subunit.

The catalytic subunit of PKA phosphorylates serines or threonines in protein substrates when the serine or threonine is located in a motif RRXS/TY (where X and Y are usually hydrophobic amino acids) that is accessible to the kinase on the surface of the protein substrate. The catalytic subunit can also bind to (but cannot phosphorylate) pseudosubstrate motifs in which the serine or threonine is replaced by any other amino acid. Both phosphorylatable (RII) substrates and pseudosubstrates (RI) are present in the regulatory subunits and serve as so-called autoinhibitory domains[53] (Fig. 7–5 and Table 7–2). In addition to the regulatory subunits, the catalytic subunits can be inhibited by endogenous cellular proteins known as *protein kinase inhibitors* (PKIs). At least four isoforms of PKI have been cloned from skeletal muscle and testis, all of which contain a pseudosubstrate site for interaction with the catalytic subunits of PKA.[54] PKIs are described in more detail later in this chapter.

The substrate recognition domain overlaps the Mg^{2+}-ATP– and

Subunits of Protein Kinase-A

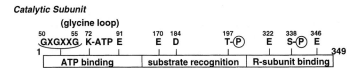

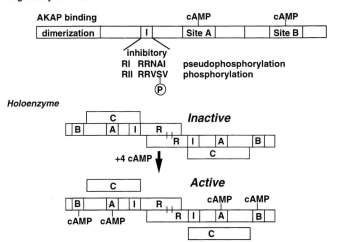

FIGURE 7–5. Diagrammatic representations of the catalytic and regulatory subunits of protein kinase A. Shown are the catalytic subunit *(upper)*, regulatory subunit *(middle)*, and the holoenzyme consisting of the heterotetrameric complex of catalytic and regulatory subunits *(lower)*. The holoenzyme is depicted in both the inactive, fully complexed form and the active, dissociated form. As described in detail in the text, the catalytic subunit consists of three (overlapping) domains responsible for the binding of Mg^{2+}-ATP, recognition of and binding to substrate, and binding to dimerization domains with the regulatory (R) subunit. The regulatory subunits consist of dimerization domains that also function as sites for binding to A-kinase anchoring proteins (AKAPs), domains that serve as inhibitory domains, and two cyclic adenosine monophosphate (cAMP)-binding sites designated as sites A and B.

TABLE 7–2. *Pseudosubstrate and Autoinhibitor Sequences in Protein Kinase A*

						R	R	G	A	I	S	A	E	V
atRIα	K	G	R	R	—	R	R	G	A	I	S	A	E	V
RIβ	K	A	R	R	—	R	R	G	C	V	S	A	E	V
RIIα	P	G	R	F	D	R	R	V	S*	V	C	A	E	T
RIIβ	I	N	R	F	T	R	R	A	S*	V	C	A	E	A
PKI	S	G	R	T	G	R	R	N	A	I	H	D	I	L
Consensus	X	X	R	X	X	R	R	X	X	X	X	A	E	X
Phosphorylation motif						R	R	X	S*/T*	Y				

*Serines or threonines phosphorylated by protein kinase A.
PKI, protein kinase inhibitor.

the regulatory subunit–binding regions and appears to consist of a hydrophobic pocket in which key acidic residues such as glutamic acids 170, 322, and 346 (E-170, E-322, E-346) form ionic interactions with one of the arginines in the substrate recognition motif RRXS/TY. Threonine 197 is phosphorylated and the negatively charged phosphothreonine seems to likewise potentiate interaction with the positively charged arginines in substrate recognition motifs. The regulatory subunit–binding domain is not yet clearly delineated but appears to involve the C-terminal region of the catalytic subunit as well as an inhibitory region. The catalytic subunits undergo at least two types of posttranslational modification, phosphorylation[55] and myristylation[56] at the N terminus, the functional consequences of which are entirely unknown.

The Regulatory Subunits

The regulatory subunits are highly asymmetric proteins of apparent molecular weights ranging from 92,000 to 108,000 and consist of functionally distinct domains (see Fig. 7–5). The N-terminal domain is responsible for protein-protein interactions, that is, dimerization of the two regulatory subunits, binding to the catalytic subunit, and binding to anchoring proteins that target the inactive holoenzyme to specific subcellular locations. The C-terminal domain consists of two tandem repeated sequences that bind cAMP and thereby allosterically regulate the affinity of association of the regulatory with the catalytic subunit (see below).

The two regulatory subunits form antiparallel dimers through binding interactions at the N-terminal regions of the proteins. The RI subunits are covalently cross-linked by two disulfide linkages between Cys16 and Cys37. Dimerization of the RII subunits, however, does not involve covalent linkage. Rather, dimerization of RII involves strong noncovalent interactions of the β sheet–like secondary structure contained within the first 30 amino acids of the RII subunits. The contrast in the biochemical mechanisms of dimer formation between RI and RII subunits may reflect important differences in biologic function of the RI and RII subunit isotypes. The type II regulatory subunit differs from the type I subunit in several respects. Autophosphorylation of RII by the catalytic subunits facilitates its release from the catalytic subunit. The phosphorylated type II holoenzyme dissociates at a lower concentration of cAMP than does dephosphorylated holoenzyme. Unlike RI, RII is located in particulate fractions of cells and readily binds to membrane-located anchoring proteins (A-kinase anchor protein [AKAPs]). In addition, RII associates much more tightly with the catalytic subunits than does RI, and much higher concentrations of cAMP are required to effect the allosteric change in conformation necessary to release the catalytic from the regulatory subunits.

In addition to "autophosphorylation" of the type II regulatory subunit by the catalytic subunit of PKA, both type I and II regulatory subunits are phosphorylated by protein kinases other than PKA. The biologic relevance, however, of such phosphorylation is unknown. RIα is phosphorylated by cyclic guanosine monophosphate–dependent protein kinase but requires the presence of cAMP. Both isotypes of the RII subunit (RIIα and RIIβ) are phosphorylated by the synergistic actions of the processive protein kinases glycogen synthase kinase-3 (GSK3) and casein kinase II (CKII).[61] Although the functional signifi-

cance of these multiple phosphorylations is unclear, it seems certain that they represent important posttranslational modification of the subunits that in some way alters their biologic functions.

Allosteric Regulation of the Activation of PKA by cAMP

Each regulatory subunit monomer contains two high-affinity cAMP-binding sites termed A and B that are located in the C-terminal region of the subunit.[6, 7] The domain A and B regions share sequence similarities and probably arose by gene duplication. Analysis of the kinetics of dissociation of the catalytic subunit from the regulatory subunit in response to cAMP indicates that binding of cAMP to sites A and B of the holoenzyme involves positive cooperative interaction. cAMP first binds to site B on the regulatory subunit, which leads to a partial conformational change in the regulatory subunit that loosens its association with the catalytic subunit and thereby renders site A more accessible for binding of a second molecule of cAMP. Occupancy of both sites A and B by cAMP results in complete dissociation of the catalytic subunits from the heterotetrameric enzyme complex.

The A and B sites have different exchange rates for cAMP: site A has a faster rate of cAMP dissociation than does site B. Furthermore, sites A and B have different binding preferences for cAMP analogues. Site A preferentially binds N-6 and C-6 substituted cAMP analogues such as dibutyl-cAMP, whereas site B prefers C-8–substituted analogues such as 8-bromo-cAMP or 8-chlorophenylthio-cAMP.[60] In addition, cAMP analogues differ in preferential selectivity between the type I and type II regulatory subunits.[60] Certain of the analogues bind more tightly to sites A or B of RI than RII and vice versa. These differences in the relative potency and selectivity of cAMP analogues for RI vs. RII further indicate that the biologic roles of the subunits must differ significantly.

Two particularly useful analogues of cAMP have been developed, one of which is an agonist (Sp-cAMPS) and the other is an antagonist (Rp-cAMPS) for the activation of PKA.[62] The analogues contain alterations of the two exocyclic oxygen molecules. The two chiral isomers of 3′,5′-monophosphothioate contain sulfur at either the equatorial (Rp) or axial (Sp) position. Rp-cAMPS is the first bona fide cAMP antagonist, and its actions can be compared directly with those of the Sp-cAMPS agonist.

Functions of the Isotypes of the Regulatory and Catalytic Subunits of PKA

As discussed earlier, when compared with the extensive complexity of the isotypes of the G proteins and adenylyl cyclases, isoforms of the PKA subunits appear to be relatively limited in number. The two major types of regulatory subunit are RI and RII, each of which has two subtypes: RIα, RIβ and RIIα, RIIβ. Three isotypes of the catalytic subunit have been identified thus far: Cα, Cβ, and Cγ. The differences in function of the various isotypes of the subunits are not fully understood. Their relative expression, however, appears to depend on the type of tissue involved, and they vary in their distributions among different subcellular compartments. In general, the α isotypes, RI_α, RII_α, and C_α, are expressed uniformly in a wide variety of tissues, whereas expression of the β isotypes, RI_β, RII_β, and C_β, is more restricted to the brain and neuroendocrine and endocrine tissues.[6] The RI_α and RI_β subunits are located in the cytoplasm and soluble fractions of broken cell preparations, in contrast to RII_β and RII_β, which are in the particulate, membranous fraction. A substantial fraction of RII has been localized to the nucleus and perinuclear regions, which suggests a special role for this subunit in targeting of the associated catalytic subunit close to substrate sites for phosphorylation in the nucleus.[63]

In particular, the RII subunits associate with high affinity with AKAPs that are located at specific sites within the cell and are proposed to target the PKA holoenzyme to specific subcellular locations by binding to the RII subunits.[58, 64] No distinctions have been made between the substrate recognition properties or actions of C_α and C_β. However, the catalytic subunits apparently have a higher affinity for histone than for kemptide, LRRASLG, the high-affinity standard substrate for phosphorylation by C_α and C_β.[65] Furthermore, the activity of C_γ is not inhibited by the PKI peptide (5–24 amide), which is widely used as a PKA-specific inhibitor. Expression of C_γ appears to be restricted to the testis, from which a unique testis inhibitor isoform has been cloned.[66] It is possible that C_γ may have novel kinase activities distinct from those of C_α and C_β and that by analogy, subtle differences in the functions of C_α and C_β also exist but have not yet been discovered. For example, certain AKAPs target PKA next to ion channels to facilitate phosphorylation and modulation of various ion channels.[67]

Regulation of Subunit Gene Expression, Stability, Translocation, and Reassociation

The complexities of the interactions, regulation, and even autoregulation of the expression of PKA subunits are only now beginning to be understood. Regulation of the expression of many of the subunits in a specific phenotype of cell under a certain circumstance can involve changes in gene transcription, RNA processing and export from the nucleus, mRNA stability, translocation, and protein stability. In spite of the complexities of regulation, some generalizations can be made. First, free subunits are less stable than subunits in the intact holoenzyme complex; that is, free subunits are more susceptible to proteolysis than bound subunits are. Second, RII binds catalytic subunits more tightly than RI does. Higher cellular levels of cAMP are required to dissociate RII than RI from catalytic subunits. Thus at relatively low levels of cAMP, RI will preferentially dissociate and be susceptible to degradation. Third, in certain cells such as Sertoli cells of the testis, sustained high levels of cAMP increase RII_β subunit by increasing the half-lives of both RII_β mRNA and protein, whereas mRNA for RI_α, RII_α, and C_α is increased only twofold to fourfold.[68] Fourth, it is likely that the induction of mRNA for certain of the subunits, for instance, RI_α, involves increased gene transcription mediated by activation of cAMP-responsive transcription factors such as CREB, whose transcriptional transactivational activity is stimulated by phosphorylation by C_α or C_β (see below). Phospho-CREB stimulates the transcription of many genes by binding to CREs located in their promoters.[31–33]

Increased RII_β can serve as a "trap" to inactivate catalytic subunits. For example, overexpression of C_α programmed by an expression plasmid transfected into rat pheochromocytoma cells results in 50-fold–enhanced stimulation of a cotransfected reporter plasmid consisting of the vasoactive intestinal polypeptide promoter containing a CRE and the chloramphenicol acetyltransferase gene.[69] Cotransfection, however, with an expression plasmid encoding the RII_β subunit inhibits stimulation by the C_α subunit to 10% of control levels.[69] Because RII_β associates more tightly with catalytic subunits than does RI_β or RI_α, all free catalytic subunits will be complexed with RII_β, which results in the liberation of RI subunits and their subsequent degradation. Thus increased RII_β not only lowers levels of catalytic subunits but also lowers levels of RI subunits.

Paradoxically, in some circumstances RII can also stimulate or restore cAMP-dependent gene transcription.[70] The cAMP-unresponsive pheochromocytoma cell line A126-1B2 is incapable of activating a transfected somatostatin gene promoter containing a CRE. However, cotransfection of a vector expressing the RII_β but not the RII_α or RI_α subunit restores cAMP responsiveness to transcription driven by the somatostatin gene promoter. Although the role of RII_β in the restoration of cAMP-responsive transcription is unknown, it is possible that RII_β may target the catalytic subunit in a holoenzyme complex to the nucleus or to a perinuclear location. Activation of PKA by cAMP releases catalytic subunit, which phosphorylates and activates the nuclear transcription factor CREB. Localization of RII to the perinuclear Golgi apparatus has been demonstrated by immunocytochemical techniques.[63] It seems unlikely that RII has a direct role in the activation of transcription, but such a possibility cannot be totally discarded. Evidence has been presented that RII can bind to CREs.[71]

The type I regulatory subunit of PKA can also inhibit the transcription of cAMP-responsive genes.[72] Several liver-specific genes are transcriptionally regulated by cAMP-dependent mechanisms probably involving CREBs. In the course of carrying out studies of cell fusion between hepatocytes and fibroblasts, extinction of the transcription of hepatic genes was observed.[72] By genetic and recombinant DNA approaches, the gene encoding the tissue-specific extinguisher was isolated and shown to be RI_α.[72] Further analysis revealed that in hepatic cells, RI_α levels are unusually low but are at normal levels in most other tissues, including fibroblasts. Thus fusion of fibroblasts to hepatocytes introduced RI_α into the hepatocyte, thereby binding catalytic subunit and preventing phosphorylation of the CREBs necessary for the activation of transcription of the liver-specific genes. It appears that regulation of both the translocation and activity of PKA subunit isotypes plays a major role in the cAMP-dependent signal transduction pathway.

The Protein Kinase Inhibitors

In addition to the inhibitory actions of the regulatory subunits, the catalytic subunits are also inhibited by the actions of PKIs, a family of endogenous cellular proteins distinct in structure from the regulatory subunits. PKIs are increasingly being recognized as important components in regulation of the cAMP signaling pathway. PKIs are unique novel molecules inasmuch as they are small (71–76 amino acids) and thus resemble peptide ligands and inhibit cAMP signaling by at least two mechanisms: by direct pseudosubstrate inhibition, a mechanism similar to that of the RI_α and RI_β subunits, and by active export of catalytic subunit from the nucleus to the cytoplasm.

PKI was first reported in 1965 as a heat stable, protease-sensitive component of rabbit skeletal muscle extracts.[73] Subsequently, cloning and structural characterization revealed at least three isoforms of PKI: $PKI\alpha$, $PKI\beta1$, and $PKI\gamma$.[74] The α, β, and γ isoforms are encoded by separate genes in the mouse. The evolutionary duplication and maintenance of the expression of different isoforms of PKI attest to the potential importance of their functions in cellular metabolism (Fig. 7–6).

The tissue distributions of the three PKI isoforms are quite different.

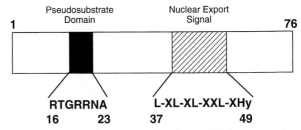

FIGURE 7–6. Diagram of a protein kinase A inhibitor showing the locations of the two known functional domains, pseudosubstrate and nuclear export signal. Numbers indicate amino acid sequence positions. The amino acids are given in single-letter designations: X, any amino acid; Hy, hydrophobic amino acid.

At the mRNA level, PKIα is expressed predominantly in brain, heart, and skeletal muscle; PKIβ expression is mostly restricted to the testis, and PKIγ is widely expressed at relatively high levels in all tissues tested. PKIγ was discovered only recently.[74] Before the discovery of PKIγ it was estimated that the amount of PKIα in the heart was only sufficient to inhibit 20% of the total catalytic subunits.[75] The contribution of the newly discovered, widely distributed γ isoform of PKI can now account for inhibition of approximately 50% of the catalytic subunits.

Structural-functional studies of the PKIs have established two distinct mechanisms by which they inhibit steps in the cAMP signaling pathway. A pseudosubstrate domain consisting of the sequence RTGRRNA is located at residues 16 to 23 in the N-terminal region of the PKIs, and a demonstrated nuclear export signal sequence (NES) L-XL-XXL-XHy is highly conserved at residues 37 to 49.[76, 77]

The pseudosubstrate and NES domains act together in the attenuation phase of the burst-attenuation kinetics of cAMP signaling responses within cells and the partitioning of catalytic subunit between the cytoplasm and the nucleus. On activation of a cell, such as by a ligand binding to a cAMP-coupled receptor, the catalytic subunit is released from the inhibitory regulatory subunit (burst phase). Although the catalytic subunit is 40 kDa, just at the upper size limit for passing through nuclear pores, it is generally believed that after release from the regulatory subunit, the catalytic subunit can passively diffuse into the nucleus where it phosphorylates and activates transcription factors such as CREB, specifically stimulating gene transcription.[78] PKI is freely capable of entering the nucleus, where it tethers to the catalytic subunit via its pseudosubstrate domain to form a catalytic subunit–PKI complex (Fig. 7–7). The NES domain of PKI is then activated by ATP via a temperature-dependent mechanism[79] involving the formation of a complex among PKI, the catalytic subunit, and the proteins CRMI[80] (exportin) and Ran.[81] Such activation results in the shuttling of catalytic subunit–PKI out of the nucleus back into the cytoplasm, where GTPase-activating proteins bind and stimulate the hydrolysis of Ran-bound GTP and thereby cause the complex to dissociate. Then the catalytic subunit recombines with regulatory subunits to form inactive holoenzyme and restore cAMP regulation to the cell. Thus with respect to its nuclear functions, the burst of cAMP signaling activity within the nucleus is attenuated by the export of catalytic subunit back into the cytoplasm. Further attenuation of the nuclear cAMP response is accomplished by phosphatases that dephosphorylate CREB and other cAMP-responsive transcription factors (see Fig. 7–7).

Notably, the NES is not essential per se for the inhibition of cAMP-mediated gene expression. In experiments in which the catalytic subunit was epitope-tagged and transfected to cells, the catalytic subunit was distributed evenly between the cytoplasm and nucleus. Cotransfection of either PKI or the regulatory subunit inhibited nuclear localization and gene expression. A mutated PKI lacking the NES still inhibited gene expression but not the nuclear accumulation of catalytic subunit, thus indicating that the NES and nuclear export are not essential for inhibition of gene expression. These findings suggest that the function of the NES to export catalytic subunit out of the nucleus back into the cytoplasm may not be so much to inhibit catalytic activity but rather to recycle the catalytic subunit back into the holoenzyme in the cytoplasm. By this means the catalytic subunit is available to phosphorylate cytoplasmic as well as nuclear proteins on initiation of another cycle of cAMP signaling.

Crosstalk of cAMP with Other Signaling Pathways

The cAMP-dependent signaling pathway is frequently coupled to and works in concert with other cellular signaling pathways. Such pathways include (1) phospholipase C–mediated production of the second messengers diacylglycerol (DAG) and inositol triphosphate, which activate protein kinase C and the intracellular receptors responsible for the mobilization of ionic calcium from intracellular stores, respectively[82, 83] (see Chapter 8); (2) calcium-calmodulin kinases[84]; and (3) receptor kinases, including the insulin, epidermal growth factor, insulin-like growth factor type 1, and platelet-derived growth factor receptors,[85, 86] among others[87, 88] (see Chapter 4).

Crosstalk among the different signaling pathways can occur by at least two mechanisms involving either intermolecular or intramolecular phosphorylation cascades. A classic example of an intermolecular cascade is the activation of an isoform of type II PKA in which the catalytic subunit "autophosphorylates" the regulatory subunit and is thereby at least partially responsible for activation of the catalytic subunit (discussed below). Active PKA then phosphorylates and activates phosphorylase kinase, which in turn phosphorylates and activates glycogen phosphorylase, the key enzyme in converting glycogen to glucose 1-phosphate. Intramolecular phosphorylation cascades involve multisite and hierarchic protein phosphorylation by the participation of several so-called processive kinases that act synergistically with other kinases by successive phosphorylation of closely adjacent sites on the same protein.[61, 89] For example, glycogen synthase is regulated (inactivated) by such a cascade in which an initial phosphorylation by PKA (the primary kinase) is required for phosphorylation on a close-by

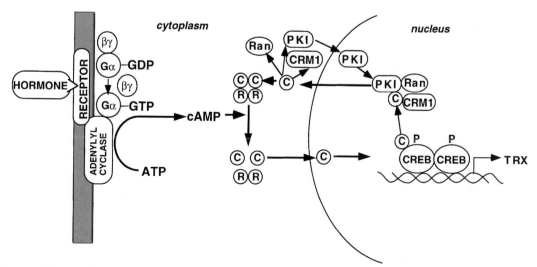

FIGURE 7–7. *Schematic diagram of a cell showing cycling of protein kinase A (PKA) inhibitor (PKI) and the catalytic subunit of PKA (C) between the cytoplasm and nucleus. PKI and C enter the nucleus by passive diffusion and form an inhibitory complex along with Ran and CRM1 that prevents phosphorylation (P) and activation of cyclic adenosine monophosphate (cAMP) response element–binding protein (CREB). The PKI/C/Ran/CRM1 complex is actively exported out of the nucleus to the cytoplasm. Such export is dependent on the presence of the nuclear export signal in PKI (see Fig. 7–6). After re-entering the cytoplasm, PKI is liberated from the complex by the actions of guanosine triphosphatase (GTPase) on Ran, thereby allowing PKI to enter the nucleus and begin another cycle of translocation. GDP, guanosine diphosphate; TRX, transcription.*

serine or threonine by CKI. Types I and II casein kinase preferentially phosphorylate serines or threonines in proteins that contain acidic amino acids within two to three residues that are N-terminal proximal (CKI) or C-terminal proximal (CKII) to the serine or threonine being phosphorylated. Phosphorylation of a serine or threonine (or tyrosine) converts a neutral or hydrophobic amino acid to a negatively charged amino acid because of the highly negative charge imparted by the phosphate. To fully inactivate glycogen synthase, yet another intramolecular processive phosphorylation by CKII is required, followed by secondary phosphorylation by GSK3. The intricacies of the signaling pathways involved in the activation of these multiple kinases are not fully understood. However, a potent activator of CKII is the activated (ligand-bound) epidermal growth factor receptor kinase, a finding pointing to crosstalk of signaling pathways between a receptor tyrosine kinase and cAMP-dependent protein kinase.[91]

The actions of cAMP on cellular proliferation and differentiation are diverse.[13, 92] In some cell culture systems, cAMP signaling inhibits proliferation and promotes differentiation.[93] In other types of cells, cAMP stimulates proliferation.[94] Although the mechanisms involved in the control of cell proliferation and differentiation are highly complex, the mitogen-activated protein kinase (MAPK) signaling pathway is generally believed to be a critical determinant in governing the cell division cycle[95] (see Chapter 9). Activation of the MAPK pathway promotes cellular proliferation, and conversely, inhibition of the MAPK pathway slows down or arrests proliferation. The MAPK pathway consists of a wide variety of factors that are only partially understood. A working model of this complex MAPK pathway includes, in order of signaling, a growth factor ligand, a receptor (typically a tyrosine kinase receptor), guanine nucleotide–binding protein (Ras), a MAP kinase kinase kinase (Raf), a MAP kinase kinase, MAPK, and a transcription factor (Fos, Myc, CREB) that activates the promoter of genes involved in control of the cell division cycle.[96, 97] Until recently, the reasons for these differing actions of cAMP signaling in different cell types cultured in different environments of growth factors have been largely unknown.

It now appears likely that the cAMP signaling pathway "crosstalks" with the MAPK signaling pathway by at least two distinct mechanisms: one mechanism inhibits and another mechanism stimulates the MAPK pathway (Fig. 7–8). Both inhibitory and stimulatory cAMP signaling act on Ras in the MAPK pathway, although by quite different mechanisms. Phosphorylation of Raf-1 by PKA inhibits its translocation and consequent activation by Ras.[93] In contrast, PKA is not involved in the activation of MAPK signaling. Rather, cAMP binds to and activates a cAMP-regulated guanine nucleotide exchange factor (cAMP-GEF).[98] Ras is a member of an extensive family of so-called small G proteins that serve as signal switches early in the MAPK and other signaling pathways.[99–102] In the GTP-bound form, Ras is active, and in the GDP form, it is inactive. GEFs, including cAMP-GEF, convert GDP to GTP on Ras and thus activate Ras. Ras is then inactivated by the actions of GTPases.[103]

The discovery of cAMP-GEFs was made only recently.[98] Two distinct gene products have been identified, and probably many more are awaiting discovery. Notably, GEFs with binding sites for DAG and for calcium (CalDAG-GEF) have been detected.[98, 104] Thus at least three major second messenger systems (cAMP, DAG, and calcium) are coupled to Ras and Ras-like protein signaling, thereby providing direct mechanisms for transducing second messenger input to GEF output.

REPRESENTATIVE CELLULAR ACTIONS OF cAMP-DEPENDENT PKA

Targets for the biologic actions of cAMP mediated by PKA are multiple. In almost every instance, phosphorylation of a protein substrate results in a change in the biologic activity of the protein, either stimulatory or inhibitory. Phosphorylation evokes crucial changes in conformation of the proteins, often by allosteric mechanisms. Four representative examples of how PKA-directed phosphorylation regulates the activity of proteins are given below: an enzyme, glycogen phosphorylase; a receptor, βAR; an ion channel, CFTR, which is a chloride channel; and a DNA-binding transcription factor, CREB.

Glycogen Phosphorylase

As discussed earlier, glycogen phosphorylase was important historically as the model protein for investigations that led to defining the essential roles of cAMP and phosphorylation in the transmission of hormone action to modulate the biologic activity of a protein.[2, 10] In the 1940s it was recognized that glycogen phosphorylase existed in both active (phosphorylase *a*) and inactive (phosphorylase *b*) forms.[1] Subsequent studies of the phosphorylation of glycogen phosphorylase in both skeletal muscle and liver showed that phosphorylase *b* was activated to phosphorylase *a* by a phosphorylase kinase and inactivated by a phosphorylase phosphatase (see later).

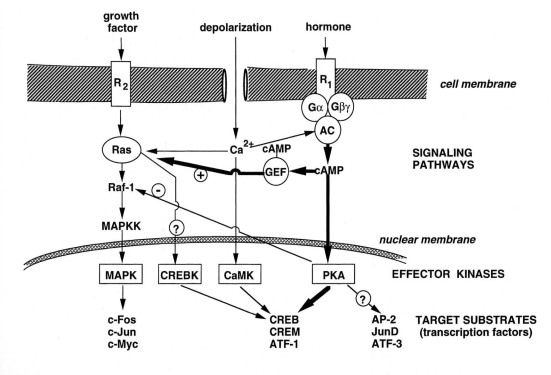

FIGURE 7–8. Model diagram depicting the newly discovered potential signal transduction pathway by which cyclic adenosine monophosphate (cAMP) not only activates protein kinase A (PKA) but also binds to the cAMP family of guanine nucleotide exchange factor proteins (GEF) and thereby activates Ras-like proteins in the mitogen-activated pathways (MAP). Thus the cAMP signaling pathway is more versatile than previously considered. Activation of PKA by cAMP leads to cellular differentiation, whereas activation of cAMP-binding proteins, such as GEFs, leads to the stimulation of cell proliferation. AC, adenylyl cyclase; ATF, activating transcription factor; CaMK, calcium calmodulin kinase; CREB, cAMP response element (CRB)-binding protein; CREM, CRE modulator.

Enzymatic Cycle of Glycogen Breakdown

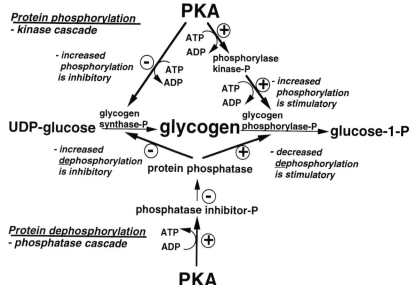

FIGURE 7–9. The enzymatic cycle of glycogen breakdown (conversion of glycogen to glucose). Phosphorylation of key enzymes in the cycle by cyclic adenosine monophosphate–dependent protein kinase A (PKA) regulates the formation of glucose (glucose 1-phosphate) by the breakdown of glycogen in muscle tissue. By phosphorylation PKA stimulates the activity of the enzyme phosphorylase kinase, which in turn phosphorylates and activates glycogen phosphorylase. At the same time, PKA phosphorylates and thereby inactivates the glycogen synthetic enzyme glycogen synthase. Protein phosphatases provide counterregulatory influences imposed by the protein kinases. Furthermore, phosphatase inhibitor proteins and PKA inhibitor proteins modulate the phosphorylation-dependent cascade of regulation and counter regulation of the enzymes involved in glycogen breakdown. ADP, adenosine diphosphate, UDP, uridine diphosphate.

$$\text{Phosphorylase b} \underset{\substack{\text{phosphatase} \\ Pi \leftarrow H_2O}}{\overset{\substack{ATP \rightarrow ADP \\ \text{kinase}}}{\rightleftharpoons}} \text{Phosphorylase a}$$
Phosphorylase b (inactive) — Phosphorylase a (active)

Next, it was demonstrated that the activity of phosphorylase kinase was reversible, and although the kinase was capable of autophosphorylation, its activation was mediated by phosphorylation by yet another kinase, phosphorylase kinase kinase, subsequently renamed cAMP-dependent PKA[10] (Fig. 7–9).

The enzymatic cycle of glycogen breakdown represents a classic example of regulation by successive phosphorylations, a so-called kinase cascade. PKA activates phosphorylase kinase, which then activates glycogen phosphorylase. In addition, both negative and positive counterregulatory phosphorylation is effected by PKA. Phosphorylations initiated by PKA but followed by an additional phosphorylation by the processive kinase CKI inhibit glycogen synthase, the biosynthetic enzyme in the cycle (see Fig. 7–9). Phosphorylation by PKA activates a phosphatase inhibitor protein that results in inhibition of protein phosphatase, thereby enhancing the PKA-mediated phosphorylation.[105]

β-Adrenergic Receptor

The mechanism of the rapid agonist-induced desensitization of βAR appears to involve phosphorylations by PKA and an additional cAMP-independent protein kinase known as βAR kinase (βARK)[26, 27] (Fig. 7–10). These phosphorylations are essential for the rapid desensitization that occurs within 30 minutes after the receptor is occupied by ligand. The rapid phase of receptor desensitization is to be distinguished from the slow desensitization that takes place during longer (several hours) periods of exposure to ligand.[26] The rapid desensitization is reversible, does not require ongoing protein synthesis, and almost certainly involves an "uncoupling" of the receptor to G protein (see below). In contrast, slow desensitization results from sequestration and internalization of the receptor and recovery requires new protein synthesis.

The mechanisms of the desensitization appear to be distinct for the two different kinases: phosphorylation by PKA occurs at low (nanomolar) concentrations of ligand and phosphorylation by βARK occurs at high (micromolar) concentrations. βARK was discovered by analysis of the βAR expressed in two distinct mutant S49 mouse lymphosar-coma cell lines.[26] The CYC⁻ mutant line lacks G protein (G_{sα}), and the Kin⁻ mutant line lacks PKA. In both cell lines, rapid desensitization occurred (albeit somewhat less than in wild-type cells), which points to the existence of a relevant kinase other than PKA. The agonist-induced desensitization of receptors can be either homologous or heterologous. In the former, the agonist specifically desensitizes the distinct receptors that are occupied. In the latter, a ligand-bound receptor desensitizes other distinctly different receptors on the cell surface.

βARK appears to induce homologous and PKA to induce heterolo-

Human β₂-Adrenergic Receptor

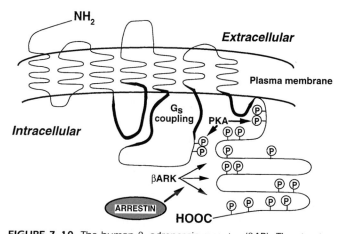

FIGURE 7–10. The human β₂-adrenergic receptor (βAR). The structure of the amino acid sequence or βAR was determined by cloning the cDNA encoding the receptor. The model shown has been deduced from the structure of the receptor, as well as from analysis of the perturbations in function induced by mutations introduced into the receptor. The βAR is a member of a large family of receptors that are coupled to G proteins. It consists of seven membrane-spanning segments and three cytoplasmic domains that are believed to be involved in interactions of the receptor with G proteins (highlighted by the *thickened lines*). The cytoplasmic domains are phosphorylated by both protein kinase A (PKA) and a β-adrenergic receptor kinase (βARK). The phosphorylations in some way mediate desensitization or uncoupling of the receptor from the G proteins (see the text). Arrestin is a protein that is involved in the modulation of phosphorylations by PKA and βARK.

gous desensitization of βAR.[26] Although the reasons for the dependence of these two kinases on different concentrations of agonist are not known, it appears that a functionally significant level of phosphorylation of the receptor by βARK occurs only when a substantial number of receptors in a cell are occupied by agonist. The physiologic implications of this circumstance are unknown. It has been proposed that PKA-mediated desensitization may be tuned to receptors that respond to low concentrations of circulating hormones whereas βARK-induced desensitization occurs in locally acting paracrine or autocrine systems such as receptors located at nerve synapses where concentrations of agonist are relatively high.[26]

That agonist-induced rapid desensitization of βAR involves phosphorylation by either PKA or βARK was shown in reconstitution experiments using isolated receptors incorporated into phospholipid vesicles.[106] Receptors prepared from desensitized cells or from cells that had not been treated with agonist and were phosphorylated in vitro with either PKA or βARK were all resistant to desensitization. Evidence that phosphorylation of the receptor uncouples it from Gₛ was likewise shown in reconstitution experiments in which phosphorylation of the receptor by PKA or βARK attenuated agonist-induced GTPase activity.[107] Cloning of βAR has allowed analysis of the effects of mutations in the receptor on its function. The serines and threonines that are phosphorylated by PKA and βARK reside in the third cytoplasmic loop and the cytoplasmic C-terminal tail of the receptor (see Fig. 7–10). PKA phosphorylates at least two sites, one in the cytoplasmic loop and the other in the tail, whereas βARK phosphorylates several sites, all of which reside in the tail. The integrity of both the loop and the tail have been shown to be important in coupling of the G protein to the receptor. Mutations of the sites for PKA or βARK phosphorylation reduced the level of phosphorylation of the receptor and agonist-induced desensitization by 50% of that of the wild-type receptor.[26] Mutations of both PKA and βARK sites extinguished phosphorylation and markedly attenuated desensitization.

The mechanisms by which phosphorylation of βAR results in uncoupling of the G protein from the receptor are not yet understood. At least two mechanisms have been proposed, however, and are under investigation: phosphorylation-induced modification of amphipathic α helixes in the receptor and inhibition of G protein–receptor coupling by an effector protein, arrestin.[26] Amphipathic α helixes are well known to be structured motifs in proteins that are used in protein-protein interactions. Introduction of a highly negatively charged phosphoserine in place of a neutral serine residue may in some way perturb the helicity and/or amphipathy of the helix, thereby impairing interaction with the G protein. Arrestin is a protein that has been proposed to competitively inhibit the interaction of G protein with the receptor.[108] It was first identified as an inhibitor of the interaction of transducin, a retinal G protein, with phosphorylated rhodopsin.[109] Later, a cDNA encoding a homologue of retinal arrestin was cloned from a bovine brain library. The brain and retinal arrestins are 59% identical in their amino acid sequences. Furthermore, when the brain and retinal arrestins, prepared by cDNA-directed expression and isolation from COS-7 cells, were tested in a reconstitution assay containing Gₛ and βAR phosphorylated by βARK, brain arrestin was much more effective than retinal arrestin in facilitating desensitization. Conversely, retinal arrestin was more effective than brain arrestin in reversing light activation of the rhodopsin receptor.[26] Thus it seems likely that the arrestins are important regulatory effectors whose actions are integrated with both PKA and βARK phosphorylation of the receptors and with interactions of G proteins with the receptors.

The Cystic Fibrosis Transmembrane Conductance Regulator

The CFTR is a regulated chloride channel located in the apical membranes of secretory epithelia.[28] The channel regulates the transepithelial secretion of chloride. cDNAs and genes encoding the channel have been cloned.[110] It has now been determined that mutations in the gene impair normal functioning of the channel and cause the inborn error of metabolism known as cystic fibrosis.[111] Defective secretion of chloride and accompanying water leads to an increased viscosity of epithelial cell secretions that culminates in the development of impaired airway and gastrointestinal function. Mutations in the *CFTR* gene result in the synthesis of defective CFTR chloride channels that do not open in response to intracellular signaling pathways.

Activation of the CFTR (opening of the channel) is mediated by phosphorylation by PKA and is enhanced by the binding of ATP at two sites located on the cytoplasmic face of the channel. cAMP-dependent signaling is crucial for activation (opening) of the CFTR channel. It has been shown that cAMP agonists increase the chloride permeability of the apical membranes of normal epithelia but not the epithelia of patients with cystic fibrosis.[112]

The CFTR chloride channel is composed of five distinct domains: two transmembrane-spanning domains, each of which spans the membrane six times and forms the pore that conducts the chloride ions; two nucleotide-binding domains that regulate the channel by binding and/or hydrolysis of ATP; and a regulatory domain phosphorylated on at least four serines by PKA[28, 110] (Fig. 7–11). These serines in the regulatory domain are phosphorylated by PKA in vitro and by cAMP agonists in vivo.[111] Furthermore, mutation of the serines to alanines results in a loss of channel activation, and mutational deletion of the regulatory domain results in a constitutively active channel that is only partially responsive to increases in cAMP. Dephosphorylation of the serines phosphorylated by PKA appears to involve protein phosphatase 2A and not phosphatases 1 or 2B.[113] Evidence has been presented that the regulatory domain may also be phosphorylated by both calcium-dependent and calcium-independent isotypes of protein kinase C.

Activation of CFTR chloride channels also requires ATP; once phosphorylated by PKA, the channels require cytosolic ATP to open. The ATP binds to single sites on each of the nucleotide-binding domains (see Fig. 7–8). Notably, ATPγS, the nonhydrolyzable analogue of ATP, does not open CFTR channels, whereas the hydrolyzable analogues (ATP > GTP > cytosine triphosphate [CTP], in order of potency) reversibly open the channels phosphorylated by PKA. Thus both phosphorylation of the regulatory domain and binding of ATP to the nucleotide-binding domains are required to fully activate (open) the channels.

These observations on the effects of phosphorylation and ATP binding on the function of the CFTR have led to the proposal of a model to explain how the channel might work.[28, 110] The membrane-spanning domains constitute a hollow cylinder with a central pore or channel created by 12 α helical structures inserted transversely through the membrane (see Fig. 7–8). The nucleotide-binding domains, located on the cytoplasmic face adjacent to the opening of the channel, change conformation on binding of ATP to enlarge the "diameter" of the pore. In the unphosphorylated state, the regulatory domain, presumed to be globular in shape, "plugs" the pore and, when phosphorylated (by PKA), is repelled from the region of the opening (perhaps by electrostatic forces), thereby opening the pore to allow passage of chloride ions through the channel.

Phosphorylation by cAMP-dependent PKA is clearly an important step in regulation of the activity of the CFTR chloride channel. It is highly likely that PKA is of tantamount importance in the regulation of many other ion channels as well. Evidence has been presented that suggests a role for PKA in modulation of the activity of ATP-sensitive potassium channels on pancreatic β cells, again in concert with the binding and/or hydrolysis of ATP.[114, 115]

Activation of Gene Transcription by PKA

A major discovery during the past several years has been the identification of DNA-binding proteins whose transcriptional functions are activated by phosphorylation by PKA.[31–33, 116] These proteins bind specific DNA elements located in the promoters of many genes. These elements and the DNA-binding proteins that interact with them are referred to as CREs and CREBs, respectively.[31–33] The term *activating transcription factor* is also used to describe proteins that bind to CREs because the nomenclature was derived from virologic research in which viral proteins activate cellular proteins that bind to CREs.[31] Not all ATFs mediate cAMP responses. A representative example of the

Cystic Fibrosis Transmembrane Conductance Regulator

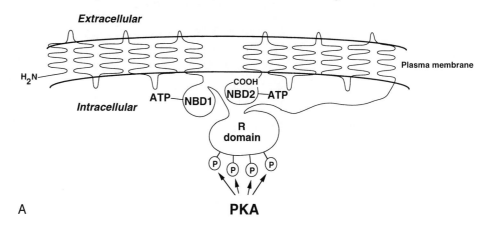

A

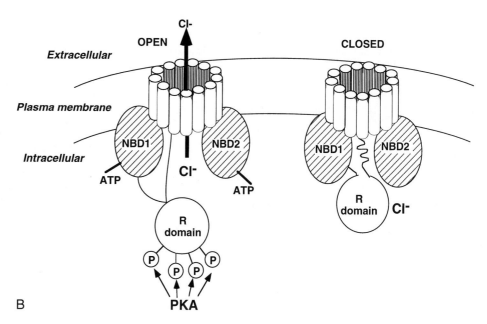

B

FIGURE 7–11. Models of the cystic fibrosis transmembrane conductance regulator (CFTR), a chloride channel in which defective functioning causes the disease cystic fibrosis. *A,* Overall topography of the CFTR. The channel spans the plasma membrane 12 times and thereby forms a 12-sided cylinder creating the pore through which chloride ions flow as shown schematically in *B.* The two nucleotide-binding domains (NBD1 and NBD2) located on the cytoplasmic face of the channel bind ATP and as such are believed to conformationally widen the channel opening. The globular regulatory domain (R domain) is phosphorylated on at least four sites by cyclic adenosine monophosphate–dependent protein kinase A (PKA). It has been proposed that in the unphosphorylated state the R domain plugs the pore of the channel and thereby closes the channel. When phosphorylated, the R domain is repelled by electrostatic forces away from the channel pore and thereby opens the channel to allow export of chloride ions from the inside to the outside of the cell.

role of PKA and CREB in the regulation of proinsulin gene transcription in pancreatic β cells is shown in Figure 7–12.[117]

The CREB DNA-binding protein and its structurally closely related homologues CRE modulator (CREM) and ATF-1 have all been cloned. Numerous isoforms of CREB and CREM exist that arise by way of the alternative splicing of exons.[118–121] The structural components responsible for the functions of CREB and CREM have been characterized in considerable detail. These proteins are members of a subfamily of a large superfamily of DNA-binding proteins known collectively as the bZIP proteins, so named because of similar structures of their DNA-binding domains that consist of a basic region (b) involved in recognition and binding to DNA and a leucine zipper (ZIP), a coiled-coil structure with heptad repeats of leucines responsible for dimerization[33] (Fig. 7–13). Additional information is contained in several reviews on CREB and bZIP proteins.[31–33, 122]

The transcriptional activities of CREB and the proteins that most closely resemble it in structure are intensely regulated by the cAMP-dependent signaling pathway and appear to be unique in this regard. Given that the bZIP transcriptional proteins now identified constitute a large family, members of which compete for binding to their enhancer DNAs, it is understandable that only a limited set of these proteins are used for activation by cAMP-dependent PKA, with the other proteins responsive to other non–cAMP-directed pathways. Thus as far as known, CREB, CREM, and ATF-1 represent the final communicative link in the regulation of gene expression in response to the activation of cAMP-dependent signaling systems.[33]

The primary amino acid sequences of the bZIP proteins diverge considerably outside their DNA-binding and dimerization domains—that is, their domains that activate transcription (transactivation) have evolved to mediate signal transduction, each factor in response to distinct stimuli. For example, of the known bZIP transcription factors, only CREB, CREM, and ATF-1 are activated upon phosphorylation by cAMP-dependent PKA; in some circumstances, CREB is also activated by calcium-calmodulin kinase.[123, 124] By contrast, the protein kinase C signal transduction pathway regulates phosphorylation of the Jun-Fos (activator protein-1) complex.[88] Consistent with the role of CREB in the cAMP pathway, a consensus site, RRPSY (A-kinase box), for phosphorylation by PKA is located at serine 119 in CREB-327 and at the corresponding serine 133 in CREB-341 (see Fig. 7–10). The two CREB isoforms differ by an alternatively spliced exon of 14 amino acids. The identical A-kinase box, RRPSY, is present in the corresponding location in CREM and ATF-1. The PKA site in CREB is surrounded by a cluster of potential phosphorylated serine and threonine residues (kinase-inducible domain of phosphorylation [P-Box]) over a stretch of about 50 residues. Consensus sites for potential phosphorylations by PKC, CKII, and GSK3 reside in the P-Box. The protein kinases CKII and GSK3 are known to be processive or hierarchic kinases inasmuch as phosphorylation of one site facilitates the successive phosphorylation of adjacent sites.[61] Phosphorylation of the PKA site may trigger a cascade of phosphorylations by the other kinases (Fig. 7–10B). Studies have shown that phosphorylation of the PKA site (serine 119) is essential for the activation of CREB.[125] However, phosphorylation of serine 119 of CREB-327 or the corresponding serine 133 in CREB-341 is necessary, but not sufficient to

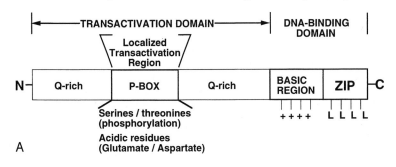

FIGURE 7–12. Hypothetic model of a pancreatic β cell showing opposing actions of the hormones glucagon-like peptide-1(7–37) (GLP-I) and galanin in regulation of the cyclic adenosine monophosphate (cAMP)-dependent signalling pathway. The receptor for GLP-1(7–37) is coupled to a stimulatory G protein (G$_s$), whereas the receptor for galanin is coupled to an inhibitory G protein (G$_i$, see Fig. 7–3). Thus the extent of activation of adenylyl cyclase (AC) is a result of the relative levels of G$_s$ and G$_i$. The final response in the signaling pathway is activation of the DNA-binding transcription factor CREB, which binds to cAMP response elements (CREs) located in the promoters of genes such as the proinsulin gene and thereby stimulates transcription of the gene. The pharmacologic agents cholera toxin (CT) and pertussis toxin (PT) activate G$_s$ and G$_i$, respectively. Forskolin directly stimulates the activity of adenyl cyclase. Isobutylmethylxanthine (IBMX) inhibits phosphodiesterase (PDE) and 8-br-cAMP is a cell-permeable cAMP agonist. AKAP, A-kinase anchoring protein (see the text).

generate the transactivation functions of CREB. Sequences located C terminus proximal to serine 119 are required to confer the transcriptional transactivation functions of CREB.[126] Phosphorylation of the P-Box may allosterically alter CREB to reveal the protein conformational structure required for transcriptional transactivation.[126] It has been proposed that the regions involved in transactivation are the glutamine-rich regions that flank the kinase-inducible domain.[126, 127] Furthermore, this model predicts that this allosteric effect would be potentiated by insertion of the alternatively spliced 14 amino acids that constitute the difference between CREB-327 and CREB-341.[128] Whether these extra 14 amino acids enhance the transactivation of CREB-341 over CREB-327, however, is uncertain. In addition to the kinase-inducible domain that is crucial for transcriptional transactivation, evidence has been presented that the additional spliced 14 amino acids are important for transactivation in some but not all cell lines.[125–128]

The importance in vivo of the requirement for phosphorylation of CREB by PKA to generate its transactivational functions was shown by Struthers et al., who produced dwarfism in transgenic mice expressing a CREB with a serine-to-alanine substitution mutation at the site

(residue serine 133) phosphorylated by PKA.[129] The transgene consisted of the promoter of the rat growth hormone gene fused to the coding sequence of the point-mutated CREB. Thus expression of the mutated CREB was directed to the somatotrophs of the pituitary during development. Because the mutated CREB still dimerized with wild-type CREB and bound to CREs but could not transactivate gene transcription, the mutated CREB completed the actions of wild-type CREB and produced atrophied pituitary glands deficient in somatotrophs and growth hormone production. Because CREB proteins are expressed at relatively high levels in the testis,[122] it would be interesting to learn the effects on mice that have been rendered transgenic with mutated CREB Ser133Ala under the regulation of testis-specific promoters.

Notably, in certain circumstances CREB appears to activate gene transcription independent of its phosphorylation by PKA. In the pancreatic islet cell line Tu6, both wild-type CREB and CREB with a mutation in the PKA-regulated Ser133 phosphorylation site of a somatostatin CRE reporter plasmid activate transcription equally in the presence of cAMP-activated PKA.[130] In this case, activation of

cAMP Response Element Binding Protein (CREB)

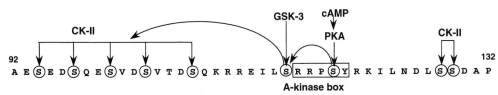

FIGURE 7–13. Diagram of the structure of CREB, the cyclic adenosine monophosphate (cAMP) response element–binding protein. *A*, CREB belongs to the superfamily of transcription factors known as the bZIP proteins, so named because the DNA-binding region consists of a basic region (b) responsible for DNA recognition and a leucine zipper–coiled coil (ZIP) involved in dimerization. *B*, The transcriptional transactivation domain of CREB consists of a region of approximately 50 residues and contains multiple sites that are phosphorylated by protein kinases, among the most important of which is cAMP-dependent protein kinase A. CK-II, casein kinase-II; GSK-3, glycogen synthase kinase-3.

CRE transcription required a second promoter element that appears to bind an islet cell factor called Isl-1. Thus in the absence of phosphorylation by PKA, CREB may activate transcription via other non-phosphorylation-dependent mechanisms. CREB has also been reported to lack transactivational activity on somatostatin and vasoactive intestinal polypeptide–CRE reporters in undifferentiated F9 embryonal carcinoma cells, but in differentiated cells, such is not the case.[131] Both undifferentiated and differentiated cells appeared to contain equivalent amounts of functionally active PKA, which suggests the possibility that an inhibitor of CREB transactivation is present in the undifferentiated cells. Because the state of phosphorylation of CREB in undifferentiated vs. differentiated cells was not examined in these studies, the mechanism or mechanisms for the inhibition remain unknown.

Whereas most research on the regulation of CREB transactivation has been directed toward mechanisms involving protein kinases, relatively little is known about phosphatase-mediated inactivation of CREB. Recently, however, Hagiwara et al. have provided compelling evidence that protein phosphatase-1 (PP-1) selectively dephosphorylates serine 133 in CREB-341 (serine 119 in CREB-327) and correspondingly attenuates the transactivational activity of CREB.[132] Although both PP-1 and PP-2A will dephosphorylate this site in CREB, examination of the relative inhibition constants of PP-1 and PP-2A for the phosphatase inhibitor okadaic acid (50% inhibitory concentration of 20 and 0.2 nM, respectively) strongly suggests that PP-1 is the relevant phosphatase in vivo. Furthermore, the PP-1–specific phosphatase inhibitor protein-1 (IP-1) abrogated the activity of PP-1. Thus an interesting model for regulation is proposed because the activity of IP-1 depends on phosphorylation by either PKA or calcium-calmodulin kinase. In this model, activation of PKA by cAMP would result in the phosphorylation and activation of CREB and IP-1, the latter leading to inhibition of PP-1.

The effects of phosphorylation on the dimerization and DNA binding of CREB are less certain than are the effects on transactivation. Yamamoto et al. originally reported that phosphorylation of a partially purified CREB or CREB-like protein by protein kinase C, but not PKA, enhanced dimerization and binding to a CRE.[133] The studies, however, relied on analysis of the effects of phosphorylation on the transition of CREB from a monomer to a dimer as assessed by binding to a CRE-containing oligonucleotide in an electrophoretic mobility shift assay. Because it is now generally believed that bZIP proteins, including CREB, bind to DNA only as dimers and not as monomers, these observations of Yamamoto et al. may have to be reinterpreted in a different light.[133] Recently, Nichols et al. provided evidence that phosphorylation of CREB by PKA enhances binding to asymmetric CREs, such as the CRE in the tyrosine aminotransferase gene (TGACGCAG), but not to symmetric CREs such as those found in the promoters of the somatostatin (TGACGTCA) gene.[134] These observations are interesting because they indicate that phosphorylation of a site approximately 150 amino acids distant from the bZIP DNA-binding domain can influence binding. Such a mechanism must involve phosphorylation-induced folding or stabilization of CREB. Such effects of phosphorylation on distant sites have also been observed for the transcription factors jun, myb, and SRF (serum response factor). The binding of CREB to CREs may also be enhanced by phosphorylation through a non–cAMP-dependent signaling pathway. Transforming growth factor-β induces phosphorylation of CREB or a CREB-like protein that results in increased binding to a fibronectin gene CRE and collagenase gene tetraphorbol acetate response element.[135] The studies suggest that the CREB-like protein binds to these DNA elements as a heterodimer with a Fos-like protein, but the identity of the DNA-binding complex remains to be determined.

It has been proposed that negatively charged amphipathic helixes of the DNA-binding proteins GAL4 and GCN4 interact with the basal transcriptional machinery to stimulate transcription.[136–138] It is likely that the negatively charged residues and phosphorylation of the CREB P-Box serve to transactivate transcription in a manner similar to the way in which the yeast GAL4 and GCN4 transcription factors transactivate RNA polymerase II.

SUMMARY

The cAMP-dependent signal transduction pathway is one of several such signaling pathways whose function is to convey information from the environment outside cells to the complex metabolic activities that take place within the cell. Essentially all of the many actions of cAMP are conveyed by way of its activation of the enzyme cAMP-dependent PKA. The inactive holoenzyme is a heterotetrameric complex consisting of two regulatory and two catalytic subunits. The allosteric regulator cAMP binds to two sites on each of the two regulatory subunits, thereby dissociating the two catalytic subunits from the complex. The free catalytic subunits bind Mg^{2+}-ATP and are phosphotransferases that phosphorylate protein substrates on serines and threonines in the sequence motif RRXS/TY. Two isoforms of the regulatory subunit have been identified (RI and RII), each of which has two isotypes (RI_α, RI_β and RII_α, RII_β). Three isotypes of the catalytic subunit are known (C_α, C_β, C_γ). The RI and RII isoforms are either located predominantly in the cytoplasm or are associated with membranous organelles, respectively. The α isotypes are distributed ubiquitously in most tissue types, whereas the β isotypes appears to be restricted to the brain, endocrine glands, and testes. The RII subunits are targeted to specific subcellular locations by binding to AKAPs, perhaps to bring the catalytic subunits in close proximity to their substrates. Functional differences among the three catalytic subunits have not yet been found, except that C_γ is enriched in the testis and phosphorylates substrates with other than the standard motif. The relative cellular levels of subunits of PKA are autoregulated in a complex manner at levels of gene transcription, subunit mRNA and protein stability, and subunit interactions. PKA phosphorylation of substrate proteins such as enzymes, receptors, ion channels, and DNA-binding transcription factors alters the conformation and thereby the functional activities of the proteins.

Acknowledgments

I thank George Holz IV, Mario Vallejo, and Christopher Miller for helpful suggestions and Townley Budde for preparation of the manuscript.

REFERENCES

1. Cori CF, Cori GT: Polysaccharite phosphorylase. *In* Nobel Lectures: Physiology or Medicine 1942–1962. Amsterdam, Elsevier Publishing Company, 1964, p 186.
2. Sutherland EW: Studies on the mechanism of hormone action. Science 177:401–408, 1972.
3. Krebs EG: Nobel Lecture: Protein phosphorylation and cellular regulation: I. Biosci Rep 13:127–142, 1993.
4. Deleted in proof.
5. Edelman AM, Blumerthal DK, Krebs EG: Protein serine/threonine kinases. Annu Rev Biochem 56:567–613, 1987.
6. Scott JK: Cyclic nucleotide–dependent protein kinases. Pharmacol Ther 50:123–145, 1991.
7. Taylor ST, Buechler JA, Yonemoto W: cAMP-dependent protein kinase: Framework for a diverse family of regulatory enzymes. Annu Rev Biochem 59:971–1005, 1990.
8. Taylor SS: cAMP-dependent protein kinase: Model for an enzyme family. J Biol Chem 264:8443–8446, 1989.
9. Harper JF, Haddox MK, Johanson RA, et al: Compartmentation of second messenger action: Immunocytochemical and biochemical evidence. Vitam Horm 42:197–252, 1985.
10. Krebs EG: Role of the cyclic AMP–dependent protein kinase in signal transduction. JAMA 262:1815–1818, 1989.
11. Gilman AG: G Proteins and regulation of adenylyl cyclase. JAMA 262:1819–1825, 1989.
12. Hanks SK, Quinn AM, Hunter T: The protein kinase family: Conserved features and deduced phylogeny of the catalytic domains. Science 241:42–52, 1988.
13. Walsh DA, Van Patten SM: Multiple pathway signal transduction by the cAMP-dependent protein kinase. FASEB J 8:1227–1236, 1994.
14. Daniel PB, Walker WH, Habener JF: Cyclic AMP signaling and gene regulation. Annu Rev Nutr 18:353–383, 1998.
15. Sassone-Corsi P: Coupling gene expression to cAMP signalling: Role of CREB and CREM. Int J Biochem Cell Biol 30:27–38, 1998.
16. Cori CF, Cori CT: The enzymatic conversion of phosphorylase *a* to *b*. J Biol Chem 158:321–345, 1945.
17. Rall TW, Sutherland EW, Berthet J: The relationship of epinephrine and glucagon to liver phosphorylase IV. J Biol Chem 224:463–475, 1957.
18. Sutherland EW, Rall TW: Fractionation and characterization of a cyclic adenine ribonucleotide formed by tissue particles. J Biol Chem 232:1077–1091, 1958.
19. Fischer EH, Krebs EG: Conversion of phosphorylase *b* to phosphorylase *a* in muscle extracts. J Biol Chem 216:121–132, 1955.
20. Krebs EG, Graves DJ, Fischer EH: Factors affecting the activity of phosphorylase *b* kinase. J Biol Chem 234:2867–2873, 1959.
21. Kuo EG, Greengard P: An adenosine 3′, 5′-monophosphate–dependent protein kinase from *E. coli*. J Biol Chem 244:3417–3419, 1969.

22. Walsh DA, Perkins JP, Krebs EG: An adenosine 3', 5'-monophosphate–dependent protein kinase from rabbit skeletal muscle. J Biol Chem 243:3763–3765, 1968.

23. Nakamura T, Gold GH: A cyclic nucleotide–gated conductance in olfactory receptor cilia. Nature 325:442–444, 1987.

24. Zufall F, Shepherd GM, Barnstable CJ: Cyclic nucleotide gated channels as regulators of CNS development and plasticity. Curr Opin Neurobiol 7:404–412, 1997.

25. Pedarzani P, Storm JF: Protein kinase A–independent modulation of ion channels in the brain by cyclic AMP. Proc Natl Acad Sci U S A 92:11716–11720, 1995.

26. Hausdorff WP, Caron MG, Lefkowitz RJ: Turning off the signal: Desensitization of β-adrenergic receptor function. FASEB J 4:2881–2889, 1990.

27. Okamoto T, Murayama Y, Hayashi Y, et al: Identification of a Gₛ activator region of the β-adrenergic receptor that is autoregulated via protein kinase A–dependent phosphorylation. Cell 67:723–730, 1991.

28. Collins FS: Cystic fibrosis: Molecular biology and therapeutic implications. Science 256:774–779, 1992.

29. Sandoval IV, Cuatrecasas P: Opposing effects of cyclic AMP and cyclic GMP on protein phosphorylation in tubulin preparations. Nature 262:511–514, 1976.

30. Lohmann SM, DeCamilli P, Einig I, Walter U: High-affinity binding of the regulatory subunit (RII) of cAMP-dependent protein kinase to microtubule-associated and other cellular proteins. Proc Natl Acad Sci U S A 81:6723–6727, 1984.

31. Habener JF: Cyclic AMP response element binding proteins: A cornucopia of transcription factors. Mol Endocrinol 4:1087–1093, 1990.

32. Meyer TE, Habener JF: Cyclic AMP–dependent transactivation of gene transcription mediated by the CREB phosphoprotein. In Mond JJ, Cambier JC, Weiss A (eds): Advances in Regulation of Cell Growth, vol 2. New York, Raven, 1991, pp 61–81.

33. Meyer TE, Habener JF: Cyclic AMP response element binding protein (CREB) and related transcription-activating DNA-binding proteins. Endocr Rev 14:269–290, 1993.

34. Rangarajan PN, Umesono K, Evans RM: Modulation of glucocorticoid receptor function by protein kinase A. Mol Endocrinol 6:1451–1457, 1992.

35. Weber IT, Steitz TA, Bubis J, Taylor SS: Predicted structures of cAMP binding domains of type I and type II regulatory subunits of cAMP-dependent protein kinase. Biochemistry 26:343–351, 1987.

36. Johnson LN, Barford D: The structural basis of the allosteric response and comparison with other allosteric proteins. J Biol Chem 265:2409–2412, 1990.

37. Sprang SR, Acharya KR, Goldsmith EJ, et al: Structural changes in glycogen phosphorylase induced by phosphorylation. Nature 336:215–221, 1988.

38. Bourne HR, Sanders DA, McCormick F: The GTPase superfamily: Conserved structure and molecular mechanism. Nature 349:117–127, 1991.

39. Johnson GL, Dhanasekaran N: The G-protein family and their interaction with receptors. Endocr Rev 10:317–331, 1989.

40. Neer EJ, Clapham DE: Roles of G protein subunits in transmembrane signalling. Nature 333:129–134, 1988.

41. Birnbaumer L: Transduction of receptor signal into modulation of effector activity by G proteins: The first 20 years or so. FASEB J 4:3068–3078, 1990.

42. Taussig R, Quarmby LM, Gilman AG: Regulation of purified type I and type II adenylyl cyclases by G protein β subunits. J Biol Chem 268:9–12, 1993.

43. Holz GG, Rane SG, Dunlop K: GTP-binding proteins mediate transmitter inhibition of voltage-dependent calcium channels. Nature 319:670–672, 1986.

44. Yatani A, Codina J, Brown AM, Birnbaumer L: Direct activation of mammalian muscarinic potassium channel by GTP regulatory protein Gₖ. Science 235:207–211, 1987.

45. Hescheler J, Rosenthal W, Trautwein W, Shultz G: The GTP-binding protein, Gₒ, regulates neuronal calcium channels. Nature 325:445–447, 1987.

46. Krupinski J, Lehman TC, Frankenfield CD, et al: Molecular diversity in the adenylyl cyclase family. J Biol Chem 267:24858–24862, 1992.

47. Hurley JH: Structure, mechanism, and regulation of mammalian adenylyl cyclase. J Biol Chem 274:7599–602, 1999.

48. Leech CA, Castonguay MA, Habener JF: Expression of adenylyl cyclase subtypes in pancreatic beta-cells. Biochem Biophys Res Commun 254:703–706, 1999.

49. Taussig R, Gilman AG: Mammalian membrane-bound adenylyl cyclases. J Biol Chem 270:1–4, 1995.

50. Cooper DM, Mons N, Karpen JW: Adenylyl cyclases and the interaction between calcium and cAMP signalling. Nature 374:421–424, 1995.

51. Knighton DR, Zheng J, Eyck LFT, et al: Crystal structure of the catalytic subunit of cyclic adenosine monophosphate–dependent protein kinase. Science 253:407–414, 1991.

52. Knighton DR, Zheng J, Eyck LFT, et al: Structure of a peptide inhibitor bound to the catalytic subunit of cyclic adenosine monophosphate–dependent protein kinase. Science 253:414–420, 1991.

53. Soderling TH: Regulation by autoinhibitory domains. J Biol Chem 265:1823–1826, 1990.

54. Van Patten SM, Howard P, Walsh DA, Maurer RA: The α- and β-isoforms of the inhibitor protein of the 3',5'-cyclic adenosine monophosphate–dependent protein kinase: Characteristics and tissue- and developmental-specific expression. Mol Endocrinol 6:2114–2122, 1992.

55. Toner-Webb J, Van Patten SM, Walsh DA, Taylor SC: Autophosphorylation of the catalytic subunit of cAMP-dependent protein kinase. J Biol Chem 267:25174–25180, 1992.

56. Clegg CH, Ran W, Uhler MD, McKnight GS: A mutation in the catalytic subunit of protein kinase A prevents myristylation but does not inhibit biological activity. J Biol Chem 264:20140–20146, 1989.

57. Scott JD, Stofko RE, McDonald JR, et al: Type II regulatory subunit dimerization determines the subcellular localization of the cAMP-dependent protein kinase. J Biol Chem 265:21561–21566, 1990.

58. Carr DW, Stofko-Hahn RE, Fraser IDC, et al: Interaction of the regulatory subunit (RII) of cAMP-dependent protein kinase with RII-anchoring proteins occurs through an amphipathic helix binding motif. J Biol Chem 266:14188–14192, 1991.

59. Hirsch AH, Glantz SB, Ki Y, et al: Cloning and expression of an intron-less gene for ADAP75, an anchor protein for the regulatory subunit of cAMP-dependent protein kinase II beta. J Biol Chem 267:2131–2134, 1992.

60. Ally S, Tortora G, Clair T, et al: Selective modulation of protein kinase isozymes by the site-selective analog 8-chloroadenosine 3',5'-cyclic monophosphate provides a biologic means for control of human colon cancer cell growth. Proc Natl Acad Sci U S A 85:6319–6322, 1988.

61. Roach PJ: Multisite and hierarchical protein phosphorylation. J Biol Chem 266:14139–14142, 1991.

62. Rothermel JD, Stec WJ, Baronisk J, et al: Inhibition of glycogenolysis in isolated rat hepatocytes by the Rp diastereomer of adenosine cyclic 3',5'-phosphorothioate. J Biol Chem 258:12125–12128, 1983.

63. Nigg EA, Schafer G, Hilz H, Eppenberger HM: Cyclic-AMP–dependent protein kinase type II is associated with the Golgi complex and with centrosomes. Cell 41:1039–1051, 1985.

64. Colledge M, Scott JD: AKAPs: From structure to function. Trends Cell Biol 9:216–221, 1999.

65. Beeb SJ, Salomonsky P, Jahnsen T, Li Y: The C subunit is a unique isozyme of the cAMP-dependent protein kinase. J Biol Chem 267:25505–25512, 1992.

66. Van Patten SM, Ng DC, Th'ng JPH, et al: Molecular cloning of a rat testis form of the inhibitor protein of the cAMP-dependent protein kinase. Proc Natl Acad Sci U S A 88:5383–5387, 1991.

67. Gray PC, Scott JD, Catterall WA: Regulation of ion channels by cAMP-dependent protein kinase and A-kinase anchoring proteins. Curr Opin Neurobiol 8:330–334, 1998.

68. Knutsen HK, Tasken KA, Eskild W, Hansson V: Inhibitors of RNA and protein synthesis stabilize messenger RNA for the RII subunit of protein kinase A in different cellular compartments. Biochem Biophys Res Commun 183:632–639, 1992.

69. Buchler W, Meinicke M, Chakraborty T, et al: Regulation of gene expression by transfected subunits. Eur J Biochem 188:253–259, 1990.

70. Tortora G, Cho-Chung YS: Type II regulatory subunit of protein kinases restores cAMP-dependent transcription in a cAMP-unresponsive cell line. J Biol Chem 265:18067–18070, 1990.

71. Wu JC, Wang JH: Sequence-selective DNA binding to the regulatory subunit of cAMP-dependent protein kinase. J Biol Chem 264:9989–9993, 1989.

72. Jones KW, Shapero MH, Chevrette M, Fournier REK: Subtractive hybridization cloning of a tissue-specific extinguisher: TSE1 encodes a regulatory subunit of protein kinase A. Cell 66:861–872, 1991.

73. Posner JB, Hammermeister KE, Bratvold GE, Krebs EG: The assay of adenosine-3', 5'-phosphate in skeletal muscle. Biochemistry 3:1040–1044, 1964.

74. Collins SP, Uhler MD: Characterization of PKIγ, a novel isoform of the protein kinase inhibitor of cAMP-dependent protein kinase. J Biol Chem 272:18169–18178, 1997.

75. Walsh DA, Ashby CD: Protein kinases: Aspects of their regulation and diversity. Recent Prog Horm Res 29:329–359, 1973.

76. Wiley JC, Wailes LA, Idzerda RL, McKnight GS: Role of regulatory subunits and protein kinase inhibitor (PKI) in determining nuclear localization and activity of the catalytic subunit of a protein kinase A. J Biol Chem 274:6381–6387, 1999.

77. Wen W, Meinkoth JL, Tsien RY, Taylor SS: Identification of a signal for rapid export of proteins from the nucleus. Cell 82:463–473, 1995.

78. Harootunian AT, Adams SR, Wen W, et al: Movement of the free catalytic subunit of cAMP-dependent protein kinase into and out of the nucleus can be explained by diffusion. Mol Biol Cell 4:993–1002, 1993.

79. Fantozzi DA, Harootunian AT, Wen W, et al: Thermostable inhibitor of cAMP-dependent protein kinase enhances the rate of export of the kinase catalytic subunit from the nucleus. J Biol Chem 269:2676–2686, 1994.

80. Fornerod M, Ohno M, Yoshida M, Mattaj IW: CRM1 is an export receptor for leucine-rich nuclear export signals. Cell 90:1051–1060, 1997.

81. Ohno M, Fornerod M, Mattaj IW: Nucleocytoplasmic transport: The last 200 nanometers. Cell 92:327–336, 1998.

82. Berridge MJ: Inositol trisphosphate and calcium signaling. Nature 361:315–325, 1988.

83. Nishizuka Y: The role of protein kinase C in cell surface signal transduction and tumour promotion. Nature 308:693–698, 1984.

84. Schulman H, Lou LL: Multifunctional C²⁺/calmodulin-dependent protein kinase: Domain structure and regulation. Trends Biol Sci 14:62–66, 1989.

85. Hunter T, Cooper JA: Protein-tyrosine kinases. Annu Rev Biochem 54:897–930, 1985.

86. Blackshear PJ, Nairn AC, Kuo JF: Protein kinases 1988: A current perspective. FASEB J 2:2957–2969, 1988.

87. Karin M: Signal transduction from cell surface to nucleus in development and disease. FASEB J 6:2581–2590, 1992.

88. Hunter T, Karin M: The regulation of transcription by phosphorylation. Cell 70:375–387, 1992.

89. Roach PJ: Control of glycogen synthase by hierarchal protein phosphorylation. FASEB J 4:2961–2968, 1990.

90. Woodgett JR: A common denominator linking glycogen metabolism, nuclear oncogenes, and development. Trends Biol Sci 16:177–181, 1991.

91. Ackerman P, Glover CVC, Osheroff N: Stimulation of casein kinase II by epidermal growth factor: Relationship between the physiological activity of the kinase and the phosphorylation state of its subunit. Proc Natl Acad Sci U S A 1990.

92. Dumont JE, Jauniaux JC, Roger PP: The cyclic AMP-mediated stimulation of cell proliferation. Trends Biochem Sci 14:67–71, 1989.

93. Burgering BM, Bos JL: Regulation of Ras-mediated signaling: More than one way to skin a cat. Trends Biol Sci 20:18–22, 1995.

94. Cook SJ, McCormick F: Inhibition by cAMP of Ras-dependent activation of Raf. Science 262:1069–1072, 1993.

95. Cobb MH, Goldsmith EJ: How MAP kinases are regulated. J Biol Chem 270:14843–14846, 1995.

96. Pierrat B, Correia JS, Mary JL, et al: RSK-B, a novel ribosomal S6 kinase family member, is a CREB kinase under dominant control of p38alpha mitogen-activated protein kinase (p38alphaMAPK). J Biol Chem 273:29661–29671, 1998.

97. Tan Y, Rouse J, Zhang A, et al: FGF and stress regulate CREB and ATF-1 via a pathway involving p38 MAP kinase and MAPKAP kinase-2. EMBO J 15:4629–4642, 1996.

98. Kawasaki H, Springett GM, Mochizuki N, et al: A family of cAMP-binding proteins that directly activate Rap1. Science 282:2275–2279, 1998.

99. Boguski MS, McCormick F: Proteins regulating Ras and its relatives. Nature 366:643–654, 1993.

100. Singh LP, Aroor AR, Wahba AJ: Translational control of eukaryotic gene expression. Role of the guanine nucleotide exchange factor and chain initiation factor-2. Enzyme Protein 48:61–80, 1994.

101. Quilliam LA, Khosravi-Far R, Huff SY, Der CJ: Guanine nucleotide exchange factors: Activators of the Ras superfamily of proteins. Bioessays 17:395–404, 1995.

102. Overbeck AF, Brtva TR, Cox AD, et al: Guanine nucleotide exchange factors: Activators of Ras superfamily proteins. Mol Reprod Dev 42:468–476, 1995.

103. Franke B, Akkerman JW, Bos JL: Rapid Ca²⁺-mediated activation of Rap1 in human platelets. EMBO J 16:252–259, 1997.

104. Ebinu JO, Bottorff DA, Chan EY, et al: RasGRP, a Ras guanyl nucleotide–releasing protein with calcium- and diacylglycerol-binding motifs. Science 280:1082–1086, 1998.

105. Cohen P, Cohen PTW: Protein phosphatases come of age. J Biol Chem 264:21435–21438, 1989.

106. Hausdorff WP, Vouvier M, O'Dowd BF, et al: Phosphorylation sites on two domains of the 2 adrenergic receptor are involved in distinct pathways of receptor desensitization. J Biol Chem 264:12657–12665, 1989.

107. Sibley DR, Benovic JL, Caron MG, Lefkowitz RJ: Regulation of transmembrane signalling by receptor phosphorylation. Cell 48:913–922, 1987.

108. Benovic JL, Kuhn H, Weyand I, et al: Functional desensitization of the isolated beta-adrenergic receptor kinase: Potential role of an analog for the retinal protein arrestin (48-kDa protein). Proc Natl Acad Sci U S A 84:8879–8882, 1987.

109. Wilden U, Hall SW, Kuhn H: Phosphodiesterase activation by photoexcited rhodopsin is quenched when rhodopsin is phosphorylated and binds the intrinsic 48-kDa protein of rod outer segments. Proc Natl Acad Sci U S A 83:1174–1178, 1986.

110. Cheng SH, Rich DP, Marshall J, et al: Phosphorylation of the R domain by cAMP-dependent protein kinase regulates the CFTR chloride channel. Cell 66:1027–1036, 1991.

111. Anderson MP, Berger HA, Rich DP, et al: Nucleotide triphosphates are required to open the CFTR chloride channel. Cell 67:775–784, 1991.

112. Riordan JR, Tommens JM, Kerem B-S, et al: Identification of the cystic fibrosis gene: Cloning and characterization of complementary DNA. Science 245:1066–1073, 1989.

113. Berger HA, Travis SM, Welsh MJ: Regulation of the cystic fibrosis transmembrane conductance regulator Cl⁻ channel by specific protein kinases and protein phosphatases. J Biol Chem 268:2037–2047, 1993.

114. Holz GG, Kühtreiber WM, Habener JF: Pancreatic beta cells are rendered glucose-competent by the insulinotropic hormone glucagon-like peptide-1(7–37). Nature 361:362–365, 1993.

115. Holz GG, Habener JF: Signal transduction crosstalk in the endocrine system: Pancreatic β-cells and the glucose competence concept. Trends Biol Sci 17:388–393, 1992.

116. Montminy MR, Gonzalez GA, Yamamoto KK: Regulation of cAMP-inducible genes by CREB. Trends Neurosci 13:184–188, 1990.

117. Fehmann H-C, Habener JF: Galanin inhibits proinsulin gene expression stimulated by the insulinotropic hormone glucagon-like peptide-I(7–37) in mouse insulinoma αTC-1 cells. Endocrinology 130:2890–2896, 1992.

118. Hoeffler JP, Meyer TE, Yun Y, et al: Cyclic AMP–responsive DNA-binding protein: Structure based on a cloned placental cDNA. Science 242:1430–1433, 1988.

119. Gonzalez GA, Yamamoto KK, Fischer WH, et al: A cluster of phosphorylation sites on the cyclic AMP–regulated nuclear factor CREB predicted by its sequence. Nature 337:746–752, 1989.

120. Foulkes NS, Mellstrom B, Benusiglio E, Sassone-Corsi P: Developmental switch of CREM function during spermatogenesis: From antagonist to activator. Nature 355:80–84, 1992.

121. Meyer TE, Habener JF: Cyclic AMP response element binding protein CREB and modulator protein CREM are products of distinct genes. Nucleic Acids Res 20:6106, 1992.

122. DeGroot RP, Sassone-Corsi P: Hormonal control of gene expression: Multiplicity and versatility of cAMP-responsive nuclear regulators. Mol Endocrinol 7:145–153, 1993.

123. Dash PK, Karl KA, Colicos MA, et al: cAMP response element–binding protein is activated by Ca²⁺/calmodulin—as well as cAMP-dependent protein kinase. Proc Natl Acad Sci U S A 88:5061–5065, 1991.

124. Sheng M, Thompson MA, Greenberg ME: CREB: A Ca²⁺-regulated transcription factor phosphorylated by calmodulin-dependent kinases. Science 252:1427–1430, 1991.

125. Gonzalez GA, Montminy RM: Cyclic AMP stimulates somatostatin gene transcription by phosphorylation of CREB at serine 133. Cell 59:675–680, 1989.

126. Gonzalez GA, Menzel P, Leonard J, et al: Characterization of a bipartite activator domain in transcription factor CREB. Mol Cell Biol 11:1306–1312, 1991.

127. Lamph WW, Dwarki VJ, Ofir R, et al: Negative and positive regulation by transcription factor cAMP response element binding protein is modulated by phosphorylation. Proc Natl Acad Sci U S A 37:4320–4324, 1990.

128. Yamamoto KK, Gonzalez GA, Menzel P, et al: Characterization of a bipartite activator domain in transcription factor CREB. Cell 60:611–617, 1990.

129. Struthers RS, Vale WW, Arias C, et al: Somatotroph hypoplasia and dwarfism in transgenic mice expressing a non-phosphorylatable CREB mutant. Nature 350:622–625, 1991.

130. Leonard J, Serup P, Gonzalez G, et al: The LIM family transcription factor Isl-1 requires cAMP response element binding protein to promote somatostatin expression in pancreatic islet cells. Proc Natl Acad Sci U S A 89:6247–6251, 1992.

131. Masson N, Ellis M, Goodbourn S, Lee KAW: Cyclic AMP response element–binding protein and the catalytic subunit of protein kinase A are present in F9 embryonal carcinoma cells but are unable to activate the somatostatin promoter. Mol Cell Biol 12:1096–1106, 1992.

132. Hagiwara M, Alberts A, Brindle P, et al: Transcriptional attenuation following cAMP induction requires PP-1–mediated dephosphorylation of CREB. Cell 70:105–113, 1992.

133. Yamamoto KK, Gonzalez GA, Biggs WHI, Montminy MR: Phosphorylation-induced binding and transcriptional efficacy of nuclear factor CREB. Nature 334:494–498, 1988.

134. Nichols M, Weih F, Schmid W, et al: Phosphorylation of CREB affects its binding to high and low affinity sites: Implications for cAMP-induced gene transcription. EMBO J 11:3337–3346, 1992.

135. Kramer IM, Koornneef I, de Laat W, van den Eljnden-van Raaij AFM: TGF-β₁ induces phosphorylation of the cyclic AMP responsive element binding protein in ML-CC164 cells. EMBO J 10:1083–1089, 1991.

136. Weinmann R: The basic RNA polymerase II transcriptional machinery. Gene Expr 2:81–91, 1992.

137. Pugh BF, Tjian R: Diverse transcriptional functions of the multisubunit eukaryotic TFIID complex. J Biol Chem 267:679–682, 1992.

138. Rigby PWJ: Three in one and one in three: It all depends on TBP. Cell 72:7–10, 1993.

Chapter 8

Second Messenger Signaling Pathways: Phospholipids and Calcium

Marvin C. Gershengorn ▪ Patricia M. Hinkle

Extracellular regulatory molecules, such as hormones, neurotransmitters, and growth factors, interact with cells by binding to specific cell surface receptors. As a result of this interaction, the receptor may be activated to lead to the generation of second messenger molecules intracellularly. A ubiquitous second messenger system entails the hydrolysis of phosphoinositides (PPIs), or phospholipids that contain the sugar *myo*-inositol as the polar head group. The primary PPI hydrolyzed is phosphatidylinositol 4,5-bisphosphate (PI-4,5-P_2) to generate two molecules that serve as second messengers, inositol 1,4,5-triphosphate (I-1,4,5-P_3) and 1,2-diacylglycerol (1,2-DAG).[1, 2] In addition, PI-4,5-P_2 is a substrate for phosphatidylinositoinositide 3-kinase (PI-3-kinase), an activator of phospholipase D (PLD) and a docking site for proteins with lipid-binding motifs. Closely related to the actions of these messengers are changes in the concentration of free (or ionized) calcium in the cytoplasm ($[Ca^{2+}]_i$). Because the same signaling pathway is used in many different cell types to stimulate distinct responses, for example, secretion from endocrine cells and contraction of smooth muscle cells, it is evident that cell-specific factors are required to elicit the final responses. The major aim of this chapter is to discuss the mechanisms by which these second messengers are generated, regulated, and metabolized, as well as their proximate effects. (The more distal steps that lead to specific cellular responses will not be discussed.) It has become apparent that other membrane phospholipids, such as phosphatidylcholines (PCs), can be hydrolyzed by specific phospholipases to generate 1,2-DAG; these systems, as well as interactions between second messenger systems, are described also.

PHOSPHOINOSITIDES

PPIs, or inositol lipids, are composed of a glycerol backbone containing fatty acyl groups at the 1- and 2-positions and a phosphate group coupled via a phosphodiester linkage at the 3-position to *myo*-inositol (Fig. 8–1). The *myo*-inositol head group may have additional phosphates, usually at the 4-position or the 4- and 5-positions. A subclass of PPIs has been described that contains a phosphate at the 3-position of *myo*-inositol (see 3-Phosphoinositides). PPIs are minor lipids in cells and constitute on average 5% to 10% of the total phospholipid. Phosphatidylinositol (PI) is the parent lipid and is phosphorylated by a specific enzyme, PI-4-kinase, to yield PI-4-monophosphate (PI-4-P), which is in turn phosphorylated by PI-4-P 5-kinase to PI-4,5-P_2 (Fig. 8–2). PI, PI-4-P, and PI-4,5-P_2 can be phosphorylated at the 3-position by PI-3-kinase. Certain lipid phosphatases within cells dephosphorylate PI-4-P and PI-4,5-P_2 to PI. Specific enzymes that dephosphorylate 3-phosphoinositides at the 3-position are present

also. These phosphatases are active and limit the levels of polyphosphorylated PIs in unstimulated cells. PI accounts for 85% to 95% of PPIs, whereas PI-4,5-P_2, which is the primary PPI substrate in cells for second messenger generation, constitutes only 2% to 3%. An agonist such as a hormone binds to its receptor, which in turn activates a PPI-specific phospholipase C (PPI-PLC) to hydrolyze PI-4,5-P_2 to I-1,4,5-P_3 and 1,2-DAG. I-1,4,5-P_3 is water soluble; it is released into the cytoplasm and diffuses away from the membrane, whereas 1,2-DAG remains membrane bound. I-1,4,5-P_3 leads to the release of Ca^{2+}

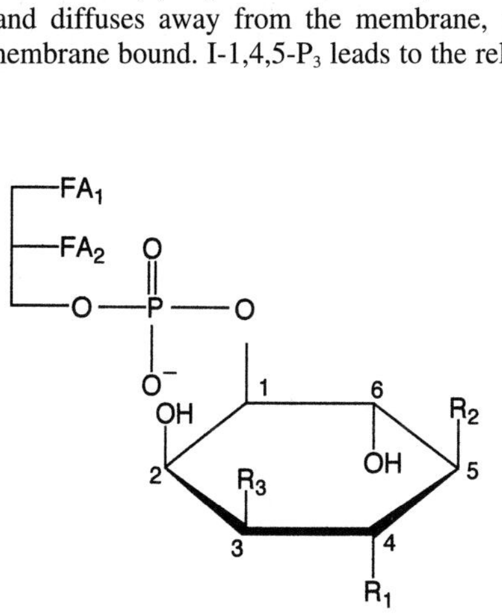

	R_1	R_2	R_3
PI	OH	OH	OH
PI-4-P	OPO_3^-	OH	OH
PI-4,5-P_2	OPO_3^-	OPO_3^-	OH
PI-3-P	OH	OH	OPO_3^-
PI-3,4-P_2	OPO_3^-	OH	OPO_3^-
PI-3,4,5-P_3	OPO_3^-	OPO_3^-	OPO_3^-

FIGURE 8–1. Structures of the major phosphoinositides. The glycerol backbone is esterified at positions 1 and 2 to fatty acids FA_1 and FA_2, respectively. FA_1 is usually a saturated fatty acid, whereas FA_2 may be arachidonic acid. The phosphate head group is coupled to *myo*-inositol at the 3-position of glycerol. PI, phosphatidylinositol; PI-4-P, phosphatidylinositol 4-monophosphate; PI-4,5-P_2, phosphatidylinositol 4,5-bisphosphate; PI-3-P, phosphatidylinositol 3-monophosphate; PI-3,4-P_2, phosphatidylinositol 3,4-bisphosphate; PI-3,4,5-P_3, phosphatidylinositol 3,4,5-triphosphate.

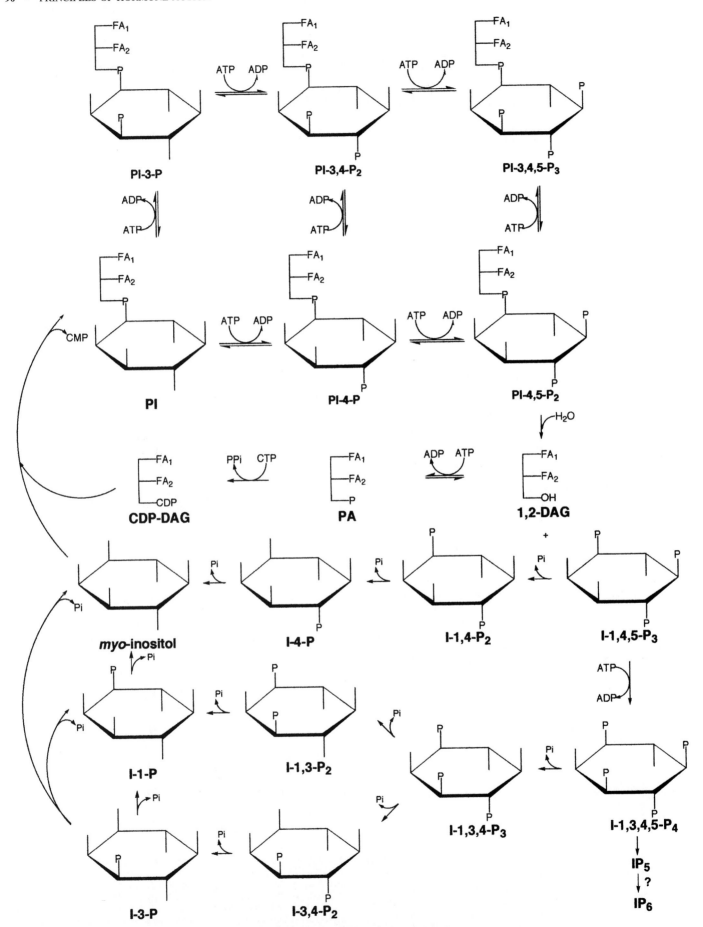

FIGURE 8–2 *See legend on opposite page.*

from intracellular stores into the cytoplasm and elevates $[Ca^{2+}]_i$, and 1,2-DAG activates protein kinase C (PKC).

3-Phosphoinositides are not substrates for PPI-PLC but are important in signal transduction because they serve to anchor signaling proteins to cellular membranes (see 3-Phosphoinositides). In this regard, it is noteworthy that PI-4,5-P$_2$ has been found to bind to AKAP79, a multivalent anchoring protein that binds several protein kinases and phosphatases,[3] and to several cytoskeletal proteins, such as ezrin.[4] Therefore, PI-4,5-P$_2$ appears to play a role in signal transduction as an anchoring protein in addition to being a substrate for second messenger generation.

Phosphoinositide-Specific Phospholipase C

Enzymes that hydrolyze phospholipids at the 3-position phosphodiester bond of the glycerol backbone are phospholipases C (PLCs). When PI-4,5-P$_2$ is the substrate, PLC action leads to the formation of I-1,4,5-P$_3$ and 1,2-DAG (Fig. 8–3). Because of its well-established role in signaling, I-1,4,5-P$_3$ is often referred to simply as IP$_3$. PPI-PLC is a subfamily of PLC that acts specifically on inositol-containing lipids and does not hydrolyze other phospholipids such as PC. Three families of PPI-specific PLCs are recognized and generally referred to as PLCβ, PLCγ, and PLCδ.[5, 6] Each PLC family comprises several closely related members, encoded by distinct genes, that share a high degree of sequence identity: PLCβ$_1$, β$_2$, β$_3$, and β$_4$; PLCδ$_1$, δ$_2$, δ$_3$, and δ$_4$; and PLCγ$_1$ and γ$_2$. The PLCs are single polypeptide chains with molecular weights between 85 kDa (PLCδs) and 140 to 155 kDa (PLCβs and PLCγs) without separate regulatory subunits. PLCβ, PLCδ, and PLCγ carry out the same enzymatic reaction and share high sequence homology in their catalytic domains. Each of the enzymes also contains a pleckstrin homology (PH) domain[7] and a C2 domain[8] involved in phospholipid binding. Other regions of the various PLCs differ markedly in structure, and there are important differences in how PLCβ, PLCδ, and PLCγ are regulated.

PI-4,5-P$_2$ is the primary substrate for the PPI-PLCs in vivo, although these enzymes also catalyze the hydrolysis of PI and PI-4-P in vitro and may do so in vivo in some cell types. PPIs that are phosphorylated at the 3-position of the *myo*-inositol head group, such as PI-3,4,5-P$_3$, the product of PI-3-kinase, are not substrates for PPI-PLCs. In cells, enzymes in the PLCβ and PLCγ families are regulated by activation of G protein–coupled receptors and tyrosine kinase pathways, respectively, whereas the PLCδs are not known to be hormonally regulated. PLCγs contain two Src homology domains, SH2 and SH3, that mediate binding to certain phosphorylated tyrosine residues and proline-rich regions, respectively. The binding of PLCγs to phosphotyrosines docks them at activated tyrosine kinases, where they are subsequently phosphorylated on key tyrosine residues and thereby activated. PLCβs lack SH2 domains and are not activated by tyrosine phosphorylation, but they interact with and are activated by either the activated α subunits of the G$_q$ family or with G protein βγ subunits.

Receptor Activation of Phosphoinositide-Specific Phospholipase C

The general features of signal transduction by G protein–coupled receptors, as well as the heterotrimeric G proteins, are discussed in

Chapter 6. In most cell types, hormones that activate the "PPI pathway" via G protein–coupled receptors activate members of the G$_q$ family, and the responses are not blocked by prior treatment with pertussis toxin.[9] An exception to this generalization, as discussed below, occurs with cells of hematopoietic lineage. Figure 8–4 illustrates the two mechanisms by which G protein–coupled receptors activate PPI-PLCs. Members of the G$_q$ family, including G$_q$, G$_{11}$, G$_{14}$, and G$_{16}$, activate PLCβs. The active α subunits of each of these G proteins can stimulate PLCβ activity in vitro, and the α subunits are believed to be primarily responsible for PLC activation in vivo, although the possible importance of βγ in signaling by G$_q$ remains controversial. PLCβ$_1$ and PLCβ$_3$, which are widely expressed, and PLCβ$_4$, which is present at high levels in some neuronal tissues and retina, are strongly stimulated by the activated α subunits of G$_q$ family members. PLCβ$_2$, which is found primarily in hematopoietic cells, is only weakly activated by Gα$_q$ or guanine nucleotides such as GTPγS, a poorly hydrolyzable analogue of guanosine triphosphate (GTP) that activates α subunits. Gβγ has been shown to activate several of the PLCβs in the order PLCβ$_3$ > PLCβ$_2$ > PLCβ$_1$. In hematopoietic cells, activation of PPI turnover usually results from the activation of receptors coupled to G$_i$ and G$_o$ and is blocked by pertussis toxin, which adenosine diphosphate (ADP)-ribosylates the α subunits of G$_i$ and G$_o$ and inhibits interaction with receptors. The α subunits of G$_i$ and G$_o$ do not affect the activity of any PLC, but the βγ subunits activate PLCβ$_2$. Although concentrations of Gβγ needed to activate PLCβ$_2$ are quite high, G$_i$ and G$_o$ are generally present at high enough concentrations to account for responses via pertussis toxin–sensitive pathways. Gβγ also activates PLCβ$_3$, and increased hydrolysis of PI-4,5-P$_2$ is sometimes observed in nonhematopoietic cells, such as fibroblasts and smooth muscle cells, after activation of receptors coupled to G$_i$ and G$_o$.

PLCγs, in contrast to PLCβs, have been shown to associate with and be activated by activated tyrosine kinases. As discussed in Chapter 4, receptors for numerous growth factors, including epidermal growth factor, platelet-derived growth factor, and fibroblast growth factor, are themselves tyrosine kinases that carry out autophosphorylation or *trans*-phosphorylation after agonist binding. Once phosphorylated, specific tyrosines in these growth factor receptors serve as binding sites for the SH2 domains of PLCγ. PLCγ is itself a substrate for the tyrosine kinase. Once it has docked at the kinase, PLCγ becomes phosphorylated on specific tyrosines, which increases its enzyme activity. Activation of nonreceptor (intracellular) tyrosine kinases can lead to activation of PLCγ by a similar mechanism. In this way, PLCγ can be activated by cytokines that activate kinases in the JAK/STAT (Janus kinase/signal transducer and activator of transcription) pathway and by hormones that activate tyrosine kinases such as src. Once PLCγ is activated, it carries out the same reaction as PLCβ and activates the same downstream pathways, although the extent of PI-4,5-P$_2$ hydrolysis is usually less when PLCγ is activated.

Phosphoinositide Metabolism

After hydrolysis of PI-4,5-P$_2$, both I-1,4,5-P$_3$ and 1,2-DAG serve as intracellular messengers and are then rapidly metabolized. I-1,4,5-P$_3$ undergoes a series of metabolic conversions that generate a large number of inositol phosphate derivatives. I-1,4,5-P$_3$ can be hydrolyzed by a series of phosphatases to *myo*-inositol, or it can be phosphorylated by a specific kinase to inositol 1,3,4,5-tetrakisphosphate (I-1,3,4,5-P$_4$). Although it has not been proved, some investigators think that I-

FIGURE 8–2. Phosphoinositide metabolism. The major products and pathways of phosphoinositide metabolism in animal cells are shown. Functional groups on *myo*-inositol are hydroxyl groups unless otherwise indicated as P (phosphate). I, *myo*-inositol; PI, phosphatidylinositol; PI-4-P, phosphatidylinositol 4-monophosphate; PI-4,5-P$_2$, phosphatidylinositol 4,5-bisphosphate; PI-3-P, phosphatidylinositol 3-monophosphate; PI-3,4-P$_2$, phosphatidylinositol 3,4-bisphosphate; PI-3,4,5-P$_3$, phosphatidylinositol 3,4,5-triphosphate; FA$_1$, fatty acid at the 1-position; FA$_2$, fatty acid at the 2-position; 1,2-DAG, 1,2-diacylglycerol; PA, phosphatidic acid; I-1,4,5-P$_3$, inositol 1,4,5-triphosphate; I-1,3,4-P$_3$, inositol 1,3,4-triphosphate; I-1,3,4,5-P$_4$, inositol 1,3,4,5-tetrakisphosphate; IP$_5$, inositol pentakisphosphate; IP$_6$, inositol hexakisphosphate; I-1,4-P$_2$, inositol 1,4-bisphosphate; I-1,3-P$_2$, inositol 1,3-bisphosphate; I-3,4-P$_2$, inositol 3,4-bisphosphate; I-4-P, inositol 4-monophosphate; I-1-P, inositol 1-monophosphate; I-3-P, inositol 3-monophosphate; ATP, adenosine 5'-triphosphate; ADP, adenosine 5'-diphosphate; CTP, cytidine 5'-triphosphate; CMP, cytidine 5'-monophosphate; PP$_i$, pyrophosphate; P$_i$, inorganic phosphate.

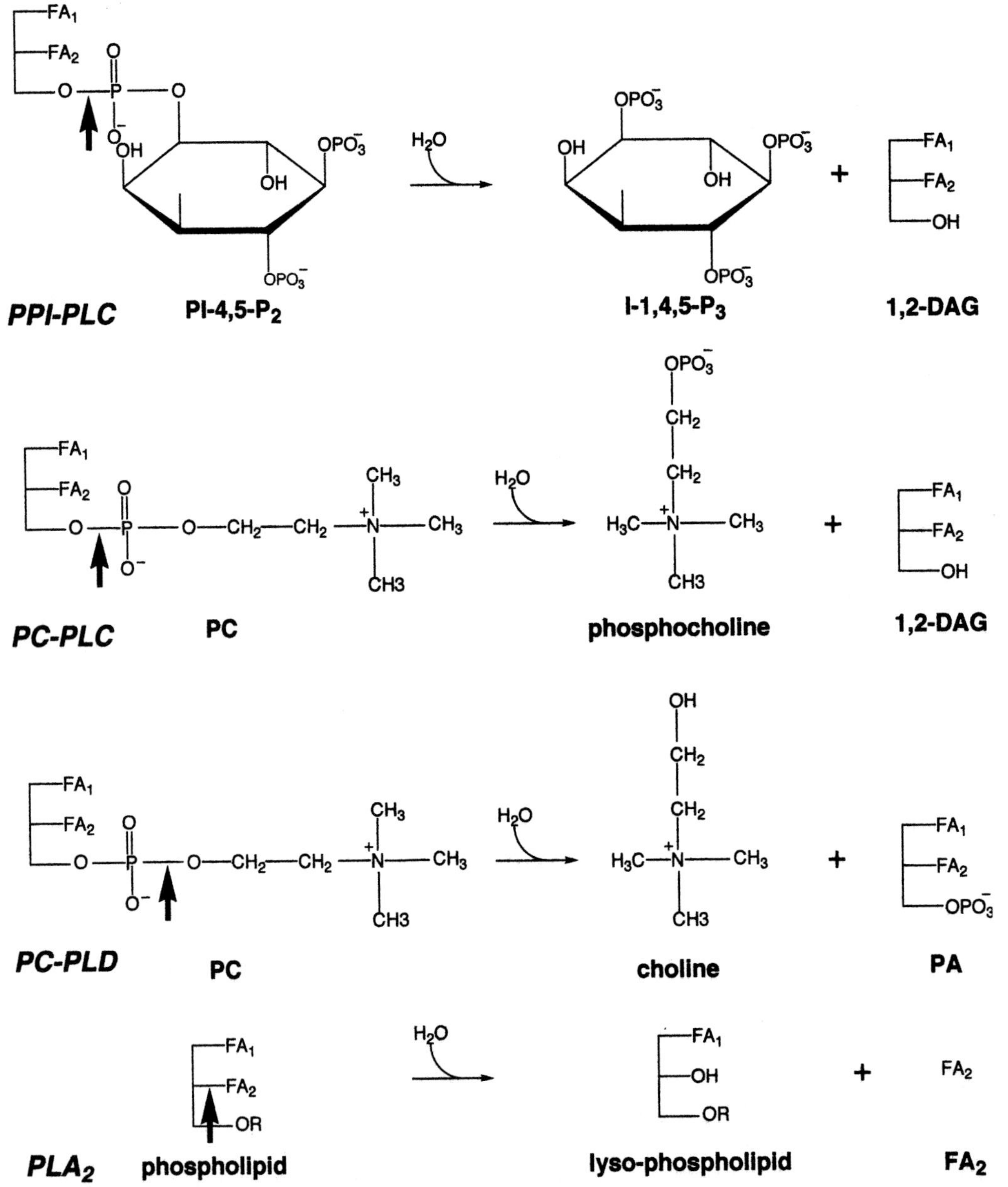

FIGURE 8–3. Enzymatic hydrolysis of phospholipids. The sites of hydrolysis are indicated by *arrows*. PPI-PLC, phosphoinositide-specific phospholipase C; PC-PLC, phosphatidylcholine-specific phospholipase C; PC-PLD, phosphatidylcholine-specific phospholipase D; PLA_2, phospholipase A_2; $PI-4,5-P_2$, phosphatidylinositol 4,5-bisphosphate; $I-1,4,5-P_3$, inositol 1,4,5-triphosphate; 1,2-DAG, 1,2-diacylglycerol; PL, phospholipid; *lyso*-PL, lysophospholipid; FA_2, fatty acid at position 2.

$1,3,4,5-P_4$ is biologically active and can influence cellular Ca^{2+} homeostasis. $I-1,3,4,5-P_4$ can be dephosphorylated to inositol 1,3,4-triphosphate ($I-1,3,4-P_3$), which does not affect Ca^{2+} fluxes, and can be converted by successive dephosphorylation to *myo*-inositol. Alternatively, $I-1,3,4,5-P_4$ can be phosphorylated to inositol pentakisphosphate (IP_5) and possibly to inositol hexakisphosphate (IP_6). It is not known whether IP_5 or IP_6 has second messenger activity. Thus $I-1,4,5-P_3$ is metabolized in a series of dephosphorylation reactions that constitute a degradative pathway, whereas phosphorylation of $I-1,4,5-P_3$ may be an activating pathway.

1,2-DAG may be phosphorylated by 1,2-DAG kinase to phosphatidic acid (PA). 1,2-DAG and PA are central intermediates in the synthesis of many cellular phospholipids. PA, which may be an important signaling molecule itself, as discussed below, can be condensed with cytidine triphosphate to form cytidine diphosphate-diacylglycerol (CDP-DAG), a reaction catalyzed by PA: cytidylyl transferase. CDP-DAG and *myo*-inositol are used by PI synthase to form PI; cytidine monophosphate is a by-product of this reaction. PI synthase is the only enzyme specific for the synthesis of PI. PI may then be successively

phosphorylated to PI-4-P and $PI-4,5-P_2$ by PI-4-kinase and PI-4-P 5-kinase, respectively.

During stimulation of PPI hydrolysis, synthesis of PI, PI-4-P, and $PI-4,5-P_2$ is increased to replenish the pool of $PI-4,5-P_2$ that would otherwise be rapidly depleted.[10] For example, the amount of inositol phosphates formed in cells during a 15-minute stimulation by agonist can be the equivalent of 10 times the original content of $PI-4,5-P_2$. Therefore, during agonist stimulation, PI synthase, PI-4-kinase, and PI-4-P 5-kinase are markedly activated. The mechanism(s) through which synthesis of these lipids is increased has not been conclusively demonstrated. No evidence has been presented of direct activation of the synthetic enzymes by the receptor or by the second messengers generated. A mechanism for activation of PI synthase has been proposed[11]; however, data supporting it have been obtained in only a few cell types. This hypothesis is based on the observation that PI inhibits the activity of PI synthase, a phenomenon that has been termed product inhibition. It was proposed that during agonist-stimulated hydrolysis of PPIs and synthesis of PI-4-P and $PI-4,5-P_2$, the decrease in the level of PI releases the PI synthase from product inhibition and increases

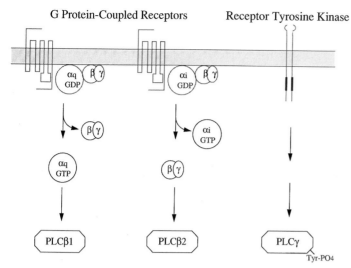

FIGURE 8–4. *Receptor activation of phosphoinositide-specific phospholipase C (PPI-PLC). G protein–coupled receptor activation of PI-4,5-P$_2$ hydrolysis may proceed via two pathways. Receptor may couple to a member of the G$_q$ subfamily of G proteins and lead to exchange of guanosine triphosphate (GTP) for guanosine diphosphate (GDP) on the α_q subunit, and α_q-GTP in turn activates PPI-PLCβ$_1$. Another receptor may couple to a member of the G$_i$ subfamily and result in exchange of GTP for GDP on the α_i subunit and release of βγ, which in turn activates PPI-PLC β$_2$. Receptor tyrosine kinase autophosphorylates, binds PPI-PLC γ$_1$ via an SH2 domain, and phosphorylates PPI-PLCγ$_1$, thereby activating PPI-PLCγ$_1$.*

fore, it is clear that events that lead to changes in $[Ca^{2+}]_i$ constitute an important signaling mechanism for diverse cellular functions. The $[Ca^{2+}]_i$ in unstimulated cells is approximately 100 nM (1×10^{-7} M), which is about 10,000-fold lower than the ambient extracellular free Ca^{2+} concentration (Fig. 8–5). The low concentration of Ca^{2+} in the cytoplasm is maintained by the concerted effects of a number of cellular processes that limit the influx of extracellular Ca^{2+} and cause active removal of Ca^{2+} into the extracellular space or into cellular organelles. Cellular membranes are highly impermeable to Ca^{2+}. Ca^{2+} can flow into the cell through ion channels in the plasma membrane; these channels are predominantly inactive (or "closed") in unstimulated cells. In some cells, especially excitable cells such as neurons and neuroendocrine cells, voltage-operated Ca^{2+} channels (VOCCs) can exhibit brief spontaneous activation leading to "Ca^{2+} spikes" that allow significant basal Ca^{2+} influx. VOCCs in the plasma membrane can be activated (or "opened") by depolarization to permit a large Ca^{2+} influx as Ca^{2+} flows down its electrochemical gradient. Ca^{2+} is pumped out of the cell, against a gradient, by two energy-dependent processes. The plasma membrane contains a Ca^{2+} pump, a Ca^{2+},Mg^{2+}-ATPase that uses ATP directly to move Ca^{2+} across the plasma membrane. Four plasma membrane Ca^{2+} pumps are known, as well as multiple splice variants of these pumps, and they differ in their modes of regulation and tissue expression.[19] Cytoplasmic Ca^{2+} can also be moved across the plasma membrane by the Na^+-Ca^{2+} exchanger, which is dependent on the Na^+ gradient established by Na^+,K^+-ATPase and can operate in either direction.

Within the cell, several organelles sequester Ca^{2+} from the cytoplasm and thereby contribute to the maintenance of a low $[Ca^{2+}]_i$. The major organelles involved in this process are the endoplasmic reticu-

its activity. A similar mechanism does not account for the increase in activity of the PPI kinases because PI-4-P or PI-4,5-P$_2$ is only transiently decreased during stimulation. Another circumstance in which PI synthesis can be diminished in some cell types in tissue culture is when they are deprived of the precursor *myo*-inositol. This situation does not seem to be operative in intact animals or humans because the levels of *myo*-inositol in blood do not vary widely enough to affect PI synthesis under normal physiologic conditions. It has been suggested, however, that *myo*-inositol depletion may occur in patients with diabetes mellitus[12] or that intracellular *myo*-inositol depletion could occur in cells of the central nervous system in patients who are receiving lithium therapy for manic-depressive illness.[13] Lithium may deplete cellular *myo*-inositol by inhibiting several of the phosphatases that dephosphorylate the inositol polyphosphates.

The principal cellular site of synthesis of PI appears to be within the endoplasmic reticulum, but some evidence demonstrates that it also occurs in the plasma membrane.[14] Phosphorylation of PI to PI-4-P and then to PI-4,5-P$_2$ occurs predominantly in the plasma membrane. Because most PPI hydrolysis occurs at the cell surface membrane, PI synthesized within the endoplasmic reticulum would have to be transferred to the plasma membrane. Transport proteins for phospholipids have been found, and recent evidence is consistent with a role for these proteins in PPI signaling.[15] However, it is not clear whether these proteins bind and transfer PI from the endoplasmic reticulum to the plasma membrane or participate in membrane cycling from the endoplasmic reticulum to the plasma membrane. Receptor activation stimulates internalization (or endocytosis) and recycling (or retroendocytosis) of receptors[16] and may stimulate exocytosis in secretory cells. It is noteworthy that PI transfer proteins are involved in exocytosis also.[17] These movements of membrane-delimited vesicles from within the cell to the cell surface could serve to replenish some of the PI lost secondary to PPI hydrolysis. PI synthesis within the plasma membrane could be activated also.

CALCIUM SIGNALING

Regulated changes in intracellular calcium mediate many critical processes, including secretion, contraction, and transcription.[18] There-

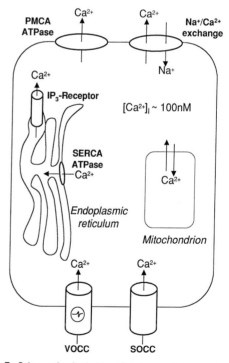

FIGURE 8–5. *Schematic depiction of a cell illustrating mechanisms of regulation of intracellular ionized calcium. The concentration of ionized, or free, intracellular Ca^{2+} ($[Ca^{2+}]_i$) in the unstimulated cell is approximately 100 nM. The plasma membrane contains Ca^{2+}/Mg^{2+} ATPases, or plasma membrane "Ca^{2+} pumps," and Na^+/Ca^{2+} antiporters that extrude Ca^{2+} from the cell, as well as voltage-operated calcium channels (VOCCs) and store-operated Ca^{2+} channels (SOCCs), through which Ca^{2+} can enter the cell. VOCCs are present in excitable cells. The endoplasmic or sarcoplasmic reticulum contains Ca^{2+}/Mg^{2+} ATPases, which are different from those present in the plasma membrane and allow sequestration of Ca^{2+}, as well as I-1,4,5-P$_3$–sensitive (I-1,4,5-P$_3$ receptor, IP$_3$-R) and I-1,4,5-P$_3$–insensitive mechanisms to allow for mobilization of Ca^{2+}. The mitochondria sequester calcium by less well defined mechanisms.*

lum[20] and mitochondria.[21] The lumen of the endoplasmic reticulum maintains a much higher Ca^{2+} concentration than does the cytoplasm. The concentration of free Ca^{2+} in the endoplasmic reticulum is not known with certainty but is estimated at 10 to 1000 μM, far above the typical cytoplasmic level of 0.1 μM. The ATP-driven Ca^{2+} pump SERCA (for sarcoplasmic/endoplasmic reticulum Ca^{2+}-ATPase) sequesters Ca^{2+} in the endoplasmic reticulum. SERCA pumps in the endoplasmic reticulum are distinct from Ca^{2+} pumps in the plasma membrane and can be selectively inhibited by drugs such as thapsigargin. Ca^{2+} in the endoplasmic reticulum can be released into the cytoplasm in response to I-1,4,5-P_3 when hormones activate PPI-PLCs, as described below. The I-1,4,5-P_3–sensitive Ca^{2+} stores can also be depleted experimentally by thapsigargin. Because Ca^{2+} spontaneously "leaks" from the endoplasmic reticulum, blockade of the SERCA pump leads to gradual depletion of Ca^{2+} stores and prevents agonist-activated responses. Mitochondria also contain a high total concentration of Ca^{2+}. Mitochondria have traditionally been viewed as low-affinity, high-capacity buffers for Ca^{2+} that protect the cell against very large increases in $[Ca^{2+}]_i$. However, recent work has shown that mitochondrial Ca^{2+} concentrations change in response to agonists that mobilize Ca^{2+} from the endoplasmic reticulum and that mitochondrial Ca^{2+} oscillates along with cytoplasmic Ca^{2+}.[21, 22] These results suggest that mitochondria may play a much more active role in Ca^{2+} homeostasis than previously appreciated. Thus $[Ca^{2+}]_i$ can rise either through entry of extracellular Ca^{2+} via the plasma membrane or through release of Ca^{2+} from intracellular stores. Elevations from either source are usually from 0.1 to 10 μM (1×10^{-7} to 10^{-5} M) and may take the form of oscillations or sustained changes (see below).

A central aspect of Ca^{2+} signaling is that changes in $[Ca^{2+}]_i$ are translated into changes in cellular function through a number of specific, Ca^{2+}-binding regulatory proteins or protein subunits. Upon binding Ca^{2+}, these proteins undergo conformational changes that regulate their activity. For example, in skeletal muscle cells, Ca^{2+} binds to troponin C and stimulates contraction. Calmodulin is a ubiquitous Ca^{2+}-binding protein[23] that regulates a number of processes, including macromolecular synthesis, secretion, cytoskeletal function, carbohydrate metabolism, and ion transport. The activity of a calmodulin target protein is altered when Ca^{2+}-calmodulin binds to its calmodulin-binding domain or, much less often, when free calmodulin binds to an IQ domain. Ca^{2+}-calmodulin complexes bind to and activate several enzymes. Activation of some enzymes by the Ca^{2+}-calmodulin complexes leads directly to the response, for example, activation of Ca^{2+},Mg^{2+}-ATPase leads to Ca^{2+} transport. Ca^{2+}-calmodulin complexes also activate a number of protein kinases that in turn phosphorylate other regulatory proteins on serine and threonine residues.[24] Some of these Ca^{2+}-calmodulin–dependent protein kinases, such as myosin light chain kinase (which regulates cytoskeletal function) and phosphorylase kinase (which regulates carbohydrate metabolism), phosphorylate a limited number of proteins and regulate specific processes. In contrast, Ca^{2+}-calmodulin–dependent multifunctional protein kinases phosphorylate a broad array of proteins and may mediate many of the more diverse actions caused by elevation of $[Ca^{2+}]_i$, for example, regulation of gene transcription, protein synthesis, and secretion in many different cells. Thus, subsequent to the elevation of $[Ca^{2+}]_i$, Ca^{2+} binds to regulatory proteins, which in turn amplify and propagate the signal by activating a number of enzymes that activate other distal steps in the signaling cascade.

Inositol 1,4,5-Triphosphate Mobilization of Calcium

Agonist stimulation of PI-4,5-P_2 hydrolysis leads to the rapid formation of I-1,4,5-P_3, which causes an elevation in $[Ca^{2+}]_i$ within seconds.[25] I-1,4,5-P_3 is generated on the intracellular side of the plasma membrane and very rapidly diffuses in the cytoplasm to bind to receptors on localized regions of the endoplasmic reticulum. The I-1,4,5-P_3 receptors, called simply IP_3 receptors, are Ca^{2+} channels.[26] When I-1,4,5-P_3 binds to an IP_3 receptor, the IP_3 receptor undergoes a conformational change that causes the channel to open and allows the

"downhill" flow of Ca^{2+} from the lumen of the endoplasmic reticulum into the cytoplasm.[27]

The IP_3 receptor is a glycosylated homotetramer composed of four noncovalently bound subunits with single-subunit molecular weights of over 300,000.[28] Three different genes encoding IP_3 receptors have been identified to date, and splice variants exist.[29] Type I IP_3 receptor is ubiquitously expressed, whereas type II and III receptors are less widely distributed. It has been postulated that each of the subunits contains six membrane-spanning segments such that both the amino- and carboxyl-termini are facing the cytoplasm. The four subunits form a single central transmembrane pore through which Ca^{2+} flows.

I-1,4,5-P_3 binding to the IP_3 receptor results in opening of the calcium channel. The kinetics of channel regulation are complex, and the number of I-1,4,5-P_3 molecules binding to the tetrameric receptor and the rate of binding are both important. It is also well documented that the concentration of Ca^{2+} on the cytoplasmic side of the membrane regulates channel opening by I-1,4,5-P_3.[30] The type I IP_3 receptor exhibits a biphasic dependence on Ca^{2+} such that I-1,4,5-P_3 becomes more effective at opening the channel as the cytoplasmic Ca^{2+} concentration rises and then becomes less effective as cytoplasmic Ca^{2+} reaches high micromolar concentrations. This regulation is thought to underlie oscillatory Ca^{2+} responses in nonexcitable cells.[31] Unfortunately, specific, effective, membrane-permeable inhibitors of I-1,4,5-P_3 receptor function are not available. Heparin, which must be introduced into cells by microinjection or permeabilization, does block I-1,4,5-P_3 binding and receptor activation.

Sequence homology is shared between IP_3 receptors and the skeletal muscle ryanodine receptor, a calcium channel in the muscle sarcoplasmic reticulum that is involved in stimulus-contraction coupling.[32] The ryanodine receptor appears to be responsible for calcium-induced calcium release in muscle cells. Calcium-induced calcium release may also occur in nonmuscle cells and could sustain a Ca^{2+} response or generate Ca^{2+} oscillations stimulated by agonists that signal via PPI hydrolysis (see below).

Receptor Activation of Calcium Influx

Cell surface calcium channels can be viewed as pores in the plasma membrane that when opened permit the rapid influx of a large number of Ca^{2+} ions down an electrochemical gradient. Ca^{2+} channels have been divided into two large classes: VOCCs and non–voltage-operated Ca^{2+} channels.[33] The latter class includes channels regulated by depletion of intracellular Ca^{2+} stores, termed "store-operated Ca^{2+} channels" (SOCCs).[34, 35]

Much more is known about the structures and pharmacology of VOCCs than SOCCs. Multiple subtypes of VOCCs have been described in different tissues, including L, T, N, P, Q, and R channels. In general, the different types of VOCCs display differences in the membrane potential (or voltage) at which they are activated and in the magnitude and duration of their conductance. The names of several of the major subtypes of VOCCs have been based on these properties, including the L-type (long-lasting) and T-type (transient) channels. Important pharmacologic tools for the study of these channels are antagonists that block Ca^{2+} flux. Dihydropyridine drugs such as nifedipine, benzodiazepines such as diltiazem, and diphenylalkylamines such as verapamil are three classes of highly effective and relatively selective inhibitors of L-type calcium channels. L channels play an important role in regulating the function of excitable endocrine tissues. For example, in the anterior pituitary gland, agonists that act via G protein–coupled receptors, such as thyrotropin-releasing hormone (TRH) and gonadotropin-releasing hormone (GnRH), cause a gradual membrane depolarization that leads to an influx of Ca^{2+} through L channels.[36] Ca^{2+} influx through these VOCCs is important in hormone secretion and transcriptional activation. In the β cells of the pancreas, glucose metabolism leads to increased concentrations of ATP. ATP inhibits an ATP-regulated potassium channel and thereby depolarizes the cell, also leading to increased influx of Ca^{2+} through L-type Ca^{2+} channels. Conversely, L channels can play an important role in inhibitory regulation of endocrine cells. Hormones such as somatostatin and dopamine can hyperpolarize pituitary cells by activating certain potassium channels, with subsequent reduced influx of extracellular Ca^{2+}. VOCCs can also be regulated as a consequence of second messenger formation. For example, in cardiac myocytes, activation of the β-adrenergic receptor leads to the generation of cyclic adenosine monophosphate (cAMP), which activates cAMP-dependent protein kinase (protein kinase A) (see Chapter 7), which in turn phosphorylates the L-type Ca^{2+} channel. Phosphorylation of the L channel does not in itself activate the channel; rather, it increases Ca^{2+} flux when the channel is activated by depolarization.

It has been recognized for some time that Ca^{2+} influx across the plasma membrane increases when Ca^{2+} stores in the endoplasmic reticulum become depleted. This phenomenon is often referred to as "capacitative Ca^{2+} entry."[37] This Ca^{2+} influx does not occur through either VOCCs or the Na^{+}-Ca^{2+} exchanger, but instead through distinct Ca^{2+} channels that are not regulated by voltage. SOCCs are not activated directly by agonists or by second messenger pathways. Instead, these channels are activated in response to severe depletion of intracellular Ca^{2+} pools, which can be brought about by either high concentrations of an agonist that depletes stores by activating IP_3 receptors or by drugs such as thapsigargin that deplete stores by preventing Ca^{2+} sequestration.[38] It is not known how a decline in Ca^{2+} in the lumen of the endoplasmic reticulum signals the plasma membrane to activate SOCCs. Much active research is attempting to identify this mechanism, which may involve anything from a diffusible messenger to a physical coupling. Ca^{2+} currents that are activated by depletion of intracellular Ca^{2+} stores have been characterized in electrophysiologic experiments. Although the identity of the proteins responsible for store-operated Ca^{2+} influx is unknown, several of the mammalian homologues of the *Drosophila melanogaster* trp and trpl proteins have some of the characteristics expected of SOCCs.[39] These proteins may be some of the Ca^{2+} channels, or subunits of such channels, responsible for capacitative Ca^{2+} influx. In fact, it has been suggested that store-operated trp channels may interact with and be "activated" by I-1,4,5-P_3–occupied I-1,4,5-P_3 receptors.[40]

Regulated Ca^{2+} influx can occur not only through the VOCCs and SOCCs described above but also through several cell surface receptors that are themselves cation channels. Gating of these receptor-operated channels with influx of cations is activated by agonist binding. The nicotinic acetylcholine receptor and the *N*-methyl-D-aspartate glutamate receptor, for example, are cation channels that allow monovalent cation influx, but Ca^{2+} transits through these channels also.

Receptor-Mediated Changes in [Ca²⁺]ᵢ

This section describes the changes in $[Ca^{2+}]_i$ that result from agonist action. Techniques for monitoring $[Ca^{2+}]_i$ that use intracellularly trapped, fluorescent Ca^{2+}-sensing dyes such as fura2, indo1, and fluo3 allow $[Ca^{2+}]_i$ in individual cells to be measured on a rapid time scale. Scores of receptors couple to PPI-PLCs. Many G protein–coupled receptors signal predominantly or exclusively via PLCβ, including receptors for TRH and GnRH. Other receptors are what are called "dual couplers," and these receptors can couple to several effectors. For example, thyroid-stimulating hormone (TSH), parathyroid hormone, and calcitonin all stimulate the activity of both adenylyl cyclase and PLCβ. The physiologic significance of dual coupling is unclear inasmuch as one pathway is usually activated at much lower agonist concentrations than the other. Agonist activation of PLC leads to an increase in I-1,4,5-P_3, and I-1,4,5-P_3 releases Ca^{2+} from intracellular stores via the IP_3 receptors. In many cell types, Ca^{2+} spikes, or waves, are initiated in specific parts of the cell. Such subcellular specificity in Ca^{2+} signaling can occur if either plasma membrane receptors or I-1,4,5-P_3 receptors are spatially restricted. When G protein–coupled receptors linked to PLCβ are activated with high concentrations of agonist, $[Ca^{2+}]_i$ often increases in a spike/plateau pattern in which $[Ca^{2+}]_i$ rises to a high level but quickly declines to a lower plateau phase (Fig. 8–6). The initial $[Ca^{2+}]_i$ response, which is due to I-1,4,5-P_3–induced release of Ca^{2+}, is independent of extracellular Ca^{2+}. In some cell types that contain both I-1,4,5-P_3 and ryanodine receptors, Ca^{2+}-induced Ca^{2+} release may follow I-1,4,5-P_3–induced Ca^{2+} release and amplify the early $[Ca^{2+}]_i$ response. Many factors combine

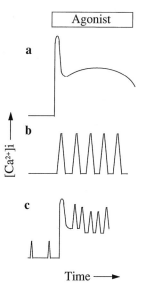

FIGURE 8–6. *Examples of calcium responses to an agonist for a receptor coupled to PPI-PLC activation. A, Response to a high dose of agonist. B, Response to a low dose of agonist. C, Response of an excitable cell that displays spontaneous $[Ca^{2+}]_i$ spikes and a complex response to agonist.*

to limit the duration of the initial $[Ca^{2+}]_i$ spike, including desensitization of receptor signaling, depletion of intracellular Ca^{2+} stores, and active extrusion of Ca^{2+} from the cytoplasm by the plasma membrane Ca^{2+} pump and uptake into the endoplasmic reticulum and mitochondria. The plateau phase of a spike/plateau response often results from the influx of Ca^{2+} through SOCCs and/or VOCCs, and it is dependent on extracellular Ca^{2+}. Both the spike and sustained increases in $[Ca^{2+}]_i$ may be critical for cellular responses such as changes in secretion or transcription.

When receptors coupled to PLC are activated with low concentrations of agonist, oscillatory $[Ca^{2+}]_i$ responses often result (see Fig. 8–6). In this case, transient, moderate increases in $[Ca^{2+}]_i$ are seen anywhere from every few seconds to every few minutes. The elevations in $[Ca^{2+}]_i$ are limited in magnitude and duration. At low concentrations of agonist, great heterogeneity is usually seen in the response patterns of individual cells. Oscillatory changes in $[Ca^{2+}]_i$ can occur in both excitable and nonexcitable cells. $[Ca^{2+}]_i$ oscillations can occur as a result of the cyclic release of Ca^{2+} from intracellular stores and have been termed cytosolic oscillations. In many cases, extracellular Ca^{2+} does not seem to be needed for sustained oscillations except to maintain intracellular stores. Many models have been proposed to explain oscillatory $[Ca^{2+}]_i$ increases in cells. In most of these models, a key feature is the ability of low $[Ca^{2+}]_i$ to potentiate and high $[Ca^{2+}]_i$ to inhibit I-1,4,5-P_3–induced release of Ca^{2+} from internal stores. In excitable cells, agonists may initiate an I-1,4,5-P_3–induced release of intracellular Ca^{2+} and also lead to an increase in action potential frequency. During depolarizations, Ca^{2+} enters via VOCCs and spikes in $[Ca^{2+}]_i$ result. Evidence is growing that both the amplitude and the frequency of $[Ca^{2+}]_i$ oscillations can be important in controlling intracellular, Ca^{2+}-dependent processes. One of the calmodulin-dependent kinases, CaM kinase II, has properties that make it a strong candidate for a protein that responds to the frequency of $[Ca^{2+}]_i$ transients.[41] In most cases, however, it is not known how the information encoded by the frequency and amplitude of $[Ca^{2+}]_i$ transients is translated into downstream responses.[42]

1,2-Diacylglycerol and Protein Kinase C

The other limb of the PPI pathway is activated by 1,2-DAG. 1,2-DAG, in combination with phosphatidylserine and, depending on the isoenzyme subtype (see below), with or without an elevation in $[Ca^{2+}]_i$, activates the phospholipid-dependent PKC.[43] PKC in turn phosphorylates a number of regulatory proteins that cause more distal effects such as stimulation of secretion (see Chapter 3) and stimulation of transcription (see Chapter 2). In unstimulated cells, the level of 1,2-DAG in membranes is very low, but 1,2-DAG accumulates transiently in response to an agonist. Agonists that activate PI-4,5-P_2 hydrolysis cause a transient translocation of some isoforms of PKC to the plasma membrane within seconds.

PKC is a serine and threonine kinase, that is, it phosphorylates serine and threonine residues in protein substrates but does not phosphorylate tyrosine residues. The PKC family contains multiple structurally related isoenzymes divided into what are called conventional, novel, and atypical PKCs.[44] Conventional PKCs have in their N-terminal regions a C2 domain that binds both Ca^{2+} and phospholipids,[8] and these enzymes (PKC α, β, and γ) are activated by Ca^{2+} and by phorbol esters in vitro. Phorbol esters, such as phorbol myristate acetate (12-O-tetradecanoylphorbol-13-acetate), are potent tumor promoters that can mimic 1,2-DAG. The novel PKCs (PKC ϵ, η, δ, and θ) lack a typical C2 domain and are activated by phorbol esters but not by Ca^{2+}. The atypical PKCs (PKC ζ and τ) are not activated by Ca^{2+} or by phorbol esters. The Ca^{2+}-dependent PKC isoenzymes may require involvement of both limbs of the PPI pathway for activation in vivo, whereas the Ca^{2+}-independent isoenzymes apparently require 1,2-DAG alone. As discussed later, some receptor-activated phospholipases can hydrolyze phospholipids other than PPIs to generate 1,2-DAG without forming I-1,4,5-P_3 or stimulating increases in $[Ca^{2+}]_i$. It has been suggested that activation of different PKC isoenzymes in vivo may lead to distinct cellular responses. The basis for such specificity is not certain and is the subject of intensive investigation. The different isoenzymes of PKC do not appear to differ much in their substrate specificity, but they have been shown to differ in their intracellular localization. PKCs are soluble enzymes activated by membrane lipids, and most of them undergo translocation when activated by either receptor agonists or pharmacologic agents. PKCs are often found in association with cytoskeletal elements, and localization of individual types of PKC is thought to occur because they bind to specific targeting proteins. Good evidence has been presented for association of individual isoenzymes of PKC to anchoring proteins (RACKs, or receptors for activated C kinase) that are not phosphorylated by activated PKC.[45]

An important proximate effect of activation of PKC is one of negative feedback to inhibit PPI signaling, which has been observed in several cell types.[46] This effect, which can be mediated by phosphorylation of a receptor or PPI-PLC, can inhibit continued activation of the PPI-PLC and thereby limit the response. Activation of PKC has also been found to inhibit Ca^{2+} influx by phosphorylation of Ca^{2+} channels. The more distal effects of activation of PKC, which are primarily mediated by phosphorylation of regulatory proteins, include stimulation of secretion from endocrine, exocrine, and blood cells; steroidogenesis in adrenal and Leydig cells; lipogenesis in adipocytes; glycogenolysis in hepatocytes; and contraction of smooth muscle cells. PKC is also a mediator of cellular growth and proliferation and may be abnormally activated in some forms of tumorigenesis.[47]

Activation of Phospholipase D

The major substrate for PLD is PC,[48] and as shown in Figure 8–3, hydrolysis of PC by PLD leads to the formation of choline and PA. Activation of PLD is complex, and many agonists that activate PLCs also activate PLD.[49] Interestingly, PI-4,5-P_2 strongly activates PLD. In addition, PLD is activated by some G proteins acting through a member of the Rho family of small monomeric G proteins, by another small monomeric G protein ARF (adenosine diphosphate ribosylation factor), and by PKC in a manner that does not depend on its kinase activity. Activation of PLD changes the localized lipid milieu by decreasing the localized concentration of neutral PC while increasing the localized concentration of acidic PA. Because choline is abundant, it seems unlikely that it plays a signaling role. Evidence is growing that changes in the lipid composition caused by PLD may have important localized effects on processes such as vesicle budding.[49, 50]

Activation of Phospholipase A₂

As shown in Figure 8–3, phospholipase A_2 (PLA$_2$)[51, 52] releases the fatty acyl group from the sn-2 position of the glycerol backbone. The PLA$_2$ family contains secreted, low-molecular-weight forms that are not thought to be hormonally regulated and two classes of cytoplasmic PLA$_2$, the Ca^{2+}-dependent forms (cPLA$_2$s), which are widely expressed, and the Ca^{2+}-independent forms, which are more restricted.[52] The well-studied Ca^{2+}-sensitive PLA$_2$s require Ca^{2+} for binding to membranes rather than for catalysis. These cPLA$_2$s are activated by many of the same agonists that stimulate PI-4,5-P_2 hydrolysis. Because PI-4,5-P_2 is the preferred substrate of cPLA$_2$, arachidonic acid is released when the enzyme is activated. Arachidonic acid has signaling activity by itself and serves as a precursor for eicosanoids, including those made via the cyclooxygenase pathway (prostaglandins, prostacyclins, and thromboxanes) and those made by the lipoxygenase pathway (leukotrienes).

Formation of 1,2-Diacylglycerol without Inositol 1,4,5-Triphosphate

Other phospholipases also appear to be involved in signal transduction, although they are not as well understood as the pathway activated by PPI-PLC. Activation of a PC-specific PLC (PC-PLC) that hydrolyzes PC to yield 1,2-DAG and phosphocholine (see Fig. 8–3) has been implicated in signaling in several cell types. A number of agonists that appear to activate PC-PLC may also activate PPI hydrolysis. However, it has often been difficult to distinguish between hydrolysis of PC caused by a PLC to yield 1,2-DAG and phosphocholine directly and PC hydrolysis by a PLD to yield PA and choline followed by rapid hydrolysis of PA to yield 1,2-DAG and inorganic phosphate by a PA phosphohydrolase. (These reactions therefore not only produce 1,2-DAG but also PA, which may have separate effects in signal transduction.[50]) Several differences between the signals generated by PC hydrolysis and PI-4,5-P_2 hydrolysis may be noted. PC-PLC activation does not lead to a second messenger that can elevate $[Ca^{2+}]_i$ because phosphocholine does not affect cellular Ca^{2+} homeostasis. Because $[Ca^{2+}]_i$ does not increase, Ca^{2+}-dependent processes are not activated and the Ca^{2+}-independent PKC isoenzymes may be activated specifically (see above). Different PKC isoenzymes may also be more activated during PC hydrolysis than during PPI hydrolysis because the fatty acid composition of PCs and PPIs is different[53] and 1,2-DAGs with different fatty acyl groups may activate PKC isoenzymes differently. Furthermore, the magnitude and duration of formation of 1,2-DAG are markedly greater with activation of PC-PLC than with PPI-PLC, apparently because the cell content of PC (35% to 40% of phospholipids) is greater than that of PPIs and negative feedback to inhibit PC hydrolysis is not as marked as with PI-4,5-P_2 hydrolysis. This property suggests that stimulation of PC hydrolysis may be involved in processes that are dependent on persistent activation of PKC, such as cell growth and differentiation.

3-PHOSPHOINOSITIDES

An enzyme activity that adds a phosphate group to the D-3 position of PI (PI-3-kinase) was discovered in 1988.[54] At approximately the same time, 3-phosphoinositides (PI-3-P, PI-3,4-P_2, and PI-3,4,5-P_3) were identified in mammalian cells and shown to constitute only a small fraction of the total PPIs.[55] 3-Phosphoinositides are not substrates for PPI-PLC and are therefore not precursors for second messenger formation. Nevertheless, they appear to play important roles in the regulation of many cellular processes, including vesicle trafficking, adhesion, actin rearrangement, proliferation, and survival.[56] Rapid activation of PI-3-kinase leading to the synthesis of, in particular, PI-3,4,5-P_3 occurs after cell stimulation by a number of extracellular regulatory factors, including growth factors that signal via tyrosine kinase receptors (see Chapter 4) and hormones that signal via G proteins (see Chapter 6).[57]

PI-3-kinases make up a family of enzymes that exhibit different activities to phosphorylate PI, PI-4-P, or PI-4,5-P$_2$ and that exhibit different modes of regulation.[58] Class I enzymes can phosphorylate PI, PI-4-P, and PI-4,5-P$_2$, class II enzymes phosphorylate PI and PI-4-P, and class III enzymes phosphorylate PI only. PI-3-kinases are heterodimers composed of an adapter/regulatory subunit and a catalytic subunit. Class Ia PI-3-kinases contain adapter subunits that have SH2 domains that bind phosphorylated Tyr residues and are thereby linked to Tyr kinase signaling pathways. Class Ib PI-3-kinases are activated by βγ subunits of heterotrimeric G proteins and are thereby linked to G protein signaling pathways. Both type 1a and 1b enzymes also interact with Ras proteins in a GTP-dependent manner, and this interaction may contribute to regulation of PI-3-kinase activity, localize the enzyme to the plasma membrane, or both. Class II PI-3-kinases bind lipid in a calcium-dependent manner, but whether this enzyme is activated in an extracellular regulatory factor–mediated pathway is not known. Class III PI-3-kinase appears to be primarily involved in intracellular membrane trafficking and vesicle morphogenesis.

Accumulating evidence has led to the idea that phospholipid products of PI-3-kinases, in particular, PI-3,4,5-P$_3$, are involved in signal transduction pathways because these lipids interact with proteins of these cascades. It has been postulated that 3-phosphoinositides localize proteins to the macromolecular complexes that are needed to propagate a signal along the transduction pathway, affect the activities of these proteins, or both. Two domains within some of these proteins, the PH[7] and C2[8] domains, bind D-3 PPIs and appear responsible for these interactions. A number of proteins bind to 3-phosphoinositides and appear to function downstream of PI-3-kinases in signaling pathways. Three pathways appear to have PI-3-kinase upstream of different Ser/Thr protein kinases: Akt/protein kinase B, which appears to be important for cell survival and gluconeogenesis; p70[S6k], which plays a role in the progression of cells through the cell cycle; and PKC, which is important in signal transduction through the PI-4,5-P$_2$ pathway (see above). However, the physiologic relevance of activating PKC through PI-3-kinases has not been established.

As with other intracellular mediators of signal transduction, the levels of 3-phosphoinositides are tightly controlled not only by the activities of their synthetic enzymes but also by degradative enzymes. Specific phosphatases catalyze the dephosphorylation of these lipids. One of these enzymes that specifically dephosphorylates at the D-3 position is PTEN (MMAC1).[59] This lipid phosphatase was first discovered as a candidate tumor suppressor gene and has been shown to mediate cell survival in a PI-3,4,5-P$_3$–dependent manner.[60]

Thus 3-phosphoinositides, in particular, PI-3,4,5-P$_3$, are important intracellular mediators of proliferation and programmed death (apoptosis) in mammalian cells.

INTERACTIONS BETWEEN SIGNALING PATHWAYS

It is important to consider that agonist stimulation of the PPI signaling cascade often occurs in a physiologic setting in which the cell is receiving input from multiple extracellular regulatory factors. The cell integrates these several stimuli, and different responses are elicited depending on the number and types of agonists and their respective signaling mechanisms. One type of interaction at the PPI signaling cascade may involve activation of two G protein–coupled receptors. Both receptors may use the same G protein and activate the same PPI-PLC, or one receptor may signal through G$_q$ so that the α$_q$ subunit would activate PPI-PLCβ$_1$, and the other may signal via G$_i$ so that the βγ subunit would activate PPI-PLCβ$_2$ or PPI-PLCβ$_3$. Another type of interaction may occur when a G protein–coupled receptor activates PPI-PLCβ, and a receptor for a growth factor (see Chapter 6) that contains intrinsic protein tyrosine kinase activity activates PPI hydrolysis by phosphorylating PPI-PLCγ.[61]

In another circumstance, several signaling pathways may be activated simultaneously by the same agonist or by different agonists. It is now clear that several of the hormones, neurotransmitters, and growth factors that activate the I-1,4,5-P$_3$/1,2-DAG/Ca^{2+} signaling pathway activate other pathways concomitantly. Such concomitant

activation may occur because a cell expresses more than one receptor (or receptor subtype) that can bind a given agonist (see Chapter 6). For example, adrenergic agonists can bind to different G protein–coupled receptors to activate PPI hydrolysis (α$_1$-receptors) or stimulate (β-receptors) or inhibit (α$_2$-receptors) adenylyl cyclase, depending on the G protein.[62] Alternatively, a single receptor can couple to two different G proteins and regulate two different signaling pathways.[63] The advent of molecular cloning techniques has made it possible to transfect a cell with a specific receptor and distinguish whether a single receptor can activate more than one G protein. For example, activation of the M$_2$ muscarinic receptor causes marked inhibition of adenylyl cyclase and weak stimulation of PPI hydrolysis[64] by interacting with G$_i$ and G$_q$, respectively, whereas binding of agonist to the receptor for TSH (thyrotropin) simultaneously stimulates adenylyl cyclase and PPI hydrolysis, apparently by activating G$_s$ and G$_q$, respectively.[65]

When the same signaling pathway is activated by two or more receptors or when two or more transduction cascades are activated simultaneously, cellular response(s) to a single pathway can be varied. Two (or more) distinct pathways can affect the same response in an additive, synergistic, or antagonistic fashion as a result of interactions at one or several steps in the signaling cascade. For example, secretion from the anterior pituitary gland can be stimulated by elevations of either [Ca^{2+}]$_i$ or cAMP[66] (see Chapter 7). In prolactin-secreting cells, TRH stimulates prolactin secretion by activating the PPI signaling cascade, whereas vasoactive intestinal polypeptide (VIP) stimulates prolactin secretion by elevating cAMP. When TRH and VIP are added simultaneously, stimulation of prolactin secretion is approximately additive. Angiotensin II (AII), like TRH, stimulates prolactin secretion by activating the PPI signaling cascade. When both TRH and AII are added simultaneously, stimulation of prolactin secretion is not fully additive. If cells are exposed to TRH before the addition of AII, stimulation of prolactin secretion by AII is attenuated. This diminished response to AII may be the result of feedback inhibition caused by TRH, which might be mediated by PKC-mediated phosphorylation of the AII receptor or G protein (see Chapter 6) or by PPI-PLC (see above). Attenuation of the response to TRH is also observed when pituitary cells are stimulated persistently by TRH.[67, 68] This attenuation of response to agonist has been termed *desensitization*.[69] Desensitization caused during persistent or repeated stimulation by the same agonist is called homologous desensitization, whereas desensitization of the response to one agonist caused by a different agonist is called heterologous desensitization. The molecular mechanisms of homologous and heterologous desensitization are different.

Thus variation in cellular response is a result of not only the agonists that are acting at a given time but also the regulatory factors to which a cell has been previously exposed. These interactions, for example, among hormones, neurotransmitters, and growth factors, are common and are responsible for the differences observed in the actions of these extracellular regulatory factors under different physiologic and pathophysiologic conditions.

CONCLUDING REMARKS

A fundamental aspect of cell regulation is that different extracellular regulatory molecules in a single cell can elicit specific responses by using the same signal transduction pathway. For receptors that signal through phospholipid hydrolysis, specificity is in part the result of interactions among the three intracellular messengers—I-1,4,5-P$_3$, 1,2-DAG, and Ca^{2+}—and the effects of PI-4,5-P$_2$ and PI-3,4,5-P$_3$ serving as anchoring proteins. These molecules interact in positive and negative ways to modulate initiation and propagation of the signaling cascade. Because different receptors cause distinct patterns of generation of second messengers, distinct interactions occur and varied responses are elicited. This situation contrasts with another ubiquitous signaling system, adenylyl cyclase–cAMP, in which a single messenger is generated. Thus signaling via phospholipid hydrolysis appears to generate a broader range of specific responses than can be elicited by receptors that signal via cAMP. Moreover, the variety of cellular responses elicited through the PPI-PLC signal transduction pathway is greatly expanded through interactions with other signaling pathways.

REFERENCES

1. Berridge MJ, Irvine RF: Inositol phosphates and cell signalling. Nature 341:197–205, 1989.
2. Majerus PW, Ross TS, Cunningham TW, et al: Recent insights in phosphatidylinositol signaling. Cell 63:459–465, 1990.
3. Lester LB, Scott JD: Anchoring and scaffold proteins for kinases and phosphatases. Recent Prog Horm Res 52:409–429, 1997.
4. Heiska L, Alfthan K, Gronholm M, et al: Association of ezrin with intercellular adhesion molecule-1 and -2 (ICAM-1 and ICAM-2): Regulation by phosphatidylinositol-4,5-bisphosphate. J Biol Chem 273:21893–21900, 1998.
5. Rhee SG, Bae YS: Regulation of phosphoinositide-specific phospholipase C isozymes. J Biol Chem 272:15045–15048, 1997.
6. Singer WD, Brown HA, Sternweis PC: Regulation of eukaryotic phosphatidylinositol-specific phospholipase C and phospholipase D. Annu Rev Biochem 66:475–509, 1997.
7. Lemmon MA, Ferguson KA: Pleckstrin homology domains. Curr Top Microbiol Immunol 228:39–74, 1998.
8. Rizo J, Sudhof TC: C$_2$-domains, structure and function of a universal Ca^{2+}-binding domain. J Biol Chem 273:15879–15882, 1998.
9. Exton JH: Cell signalling through guanine-nucleotide–binding regulatory proteins (G proteins) and phospholipases. Eur J Biochem 243:10–20, 1997.
10. Monaco ME, Gershengorn MC: Subcellular organization of receptor-mediated phosphoinositide turnover. Endocr Rev 13:707–718, 1992.
11. Imai A, Gershengorn MC: Regulation by phosphatidylinositol of rat pituitary plasma membrane and endoplasmic reticulum phosphatidylinositol synthase activities: A mechanism for activation of phosphoinositide resynthesis during cell stimulation. J Biol Chem 262:6457–6459, 1987.
12. Zhu X, Eichberg J: A myo-inositol pool utilized for phosphatidylinositol synthesis is depleted in sciatic nerve from rats with streptozotocin-induced diabetes. Proc Natl Acad Sci U S A 87:9818–9822, 1990.
13. Berridge MJ, Downes CP, Hanley MR: Neural and developmental actions of lithium: A unifying hypothesis. Cell 59:411–419, 1989.
14. Imai A, Gershengorn MC: Independent phosphatidylinositol synthesis in pituitary plasma membrane and endoplasmic reticulum. Nature 325:726–728, 1987.
15. Cockcroft S: Phosphatidylinositol transfer proteins: A requirement in signal transduction and vesicle traffic. Bioessays 20:423–432, 1998.
16. Goldstein JL, Brown MS, Anderson RGW, et al: Receptor-mediated endocytosis: Concepts emerging from the LDL receptor system. Annu Rev Cell Biol 1:1–39, 1985.
17. Hay JC, Fisette PL, Jenkins GH, et al: ATP-dependent inositide phosphorylation required for Ca^{2+}-activated secretion. Nature 374:173–177, 1995.
18. Berridge MJ: Elementary and global aspects of calcium signalling. J Physiol (Lond) 499:291–306, 1997.
19. Carafoli E: Plasma membrane calcium pump: Structure, function and relationships. Basic Res Cardiol 92(suppl 1):59–61, 1997.
20. Meldolesi J, Pozzan T: The endoplasmic reticulum Ca^{2+} store: A view from the lumen. Trends Biochem Sci 23:10–14, 1998.
21. Gunter TE, Buntinas L, Sparagna GC, et al: The Ca^{2+} transport mechanisms of mitochondria and Ca^{2+} uptake from physiological-type Ca^{2+} transients. Biochim Biophys Acta 1366:5–15, 1998.
22. Rizzuto R, Simpson AW, Brini M, et al: Rapid changes of mitochondrial Ca^{2+} revealed by specifically targeted recombinant aequorin. Nature 358:325–327, 1992.
23. Klee CB, Crouch TH, Richman PG: Calmodulin. Annu Rev Biochem 49:489–515, 1980.
24. Heist EK, Schulman H: The role of Ca^{2+}/calmodulin-dependent protein kinases within the nucleus. Cell Calcium 23:103–114, 1998.
25. Berridge MJ: Inositol trisphosphate as a second messenger in signal transduction. Ann N Y Acad Sci 494:39–51, 1987.
26. Joseph SK: The inositol triphosphate receptor family. Cell Signal 8:1–7, 1996.
27. Ferris CD, Snyder SH: Inositol 1,4,5-trisphosphate–activated calcium channels. Annu Rev Physiol 54:469–488, 1992.
28. Wilcox RA, Primrose WU, Nahorski SR, et al: New developments in the molecular pharmacology of the myo-inositol 1,4,5-trisphosphate receptor. Trends Pharmacol Sci 19:467–475, 1998.
29. Taylor CW, Traynor D: Calcium and inositol trisphosphate receptors. J Membr Biol 145:109–118, 1995.
30. Ehrlich BE, Kaftan E, Bezprozvannaya S, et al: The pharmacology of intracellular Ca^{2+}-release channels. Trends Pharmacol Sci 15:145–149, 1994.
31. Berridge MJ: Inositol trisphosphate and calcium signaling. Ann N Y Acad Sci 66:31–43, 1995.
32. Franzini-Armstrong C, Protasi F: Ryanodine receptors of striated muscles: A complex channel capable of multiple interactions. Physiol Rev 77:699–729, 1997.
33. Jones SW: Overview of voltage-dependent calcium channels. J Bioenerg Biomembr 30:299–312, 1998.
34. Thomas D, Kim HY, Hanley MR: Capacitative calcium influx. Vitam Horm 54:97–119, 1998.
35. Bootman MD, Berridge MJ: The elemental principles of calcium signaling. Cell 83:675–678, 1995.
36. Stojilkovic SS, Catt KJ: Calcium oscillations in anterior pituitary cells. Endocr Rev 13:256–280, 1992.
37. Putney JW Jr: "Kissin' cousins": Intimate plasma membrane–ER interactions underlie capacitative calcium entry. Cell 99:5–8, 1999.
38. Parekh AB, Penner R: Store depletion and calcium influx. Physiol Rev 77:901–930, 1997.
39. Zhu X, Birnbaumer L: Calcium channels formed by mammalian Trp homologues. News Physiol Sci 13:211–217, 1998.
40. Kiselyov K, Xu X, Mozhayeva G, et al: Functional interaction between InsP3 receptors and store-operated Htrp3 channels. Nature 396:478–482, 1998.
41. De Koninck P, Schulman H: Sensitivity of CaM kinase II to the frequency of Ca^{2+} oscillations. Science 279:227–230, 1998.
42. Berridge MJ: Calcium signalling and cell proliferation. Bioessays 17:491–500, 1995.
43. Nishizuka Y: Protein kinase C and lipid signaling for sustained cellular responses. FASEB J 9:484–496, 1995.
44. Mellor H, Parker PJ: The extended protein kinase C superfamily. Biochem J 332:281–292, 1998.
45. Mochly-Rosen D, Gordon AS: Anchoring proteins for protein kinase C: A means for isozyme selectivity. FASEB J 12:35–42, 1998.
46. Chuang TT, Iacovelli L, Sallese M, et al: G protein–coupled receptors: Heterologous regulation of homologous desensitization and its implications. Trends Pharmacol Sci 17:416–421, 1996.
47. Weinstein IB, Kahn SM, O'Drscoll K, et al: The role of protein kinase C in signal transduction, growth control and lipid metabolism. Adv Exp Med Biol 400A:313–321, 1997.
48. Cockcroft S: Phospholipase D: Regulation by GTPases and protein kinase C and physiological relevance. Prog Lipid Res 35:345–370, 1997.
49. Exton JH: New developments in phospholipase D. J Biol Chem 272:15579–15582, 1997.
50. Hodgkin MN, Pettitt TR, Martin A, et al: Diacylglycerols and phosphatidates: Which molecular species are intracellular messengers? Trends Biochem Sci 23:200–204, 1998.
51. Balsinde J, Dennis EA: Function and inhibition of intracellular calcium–independent phospholipase A$_2$. J Biol Chem 272:16069–16072, 1997.
52. Leslie CC: Properties and regulation of cytosolic phospholipase A$_2$. J Biol Chem 272:16709–16712, 1997.
53. Holub BJ, Kuksis A: Metabolism of molecular species of diacylglycerophospholipids. Adv Lipid Res 16:1–125, 1978.
54. Whitman M, Downes CP, Keeler M, et al: Type I phosphatidylinositol kinase makes a novel inositol phospholipid, phosphatidylinositol-3-phosphate. Nature 332:644–646, 1988.
55. Traynor-Kaplan AE, Harris AL, Thompson BL, et al: An inositol tetrakisphosphate–containing phospholipid in activated neutrophils. Nature 334:353–356, 1988.
56. Toker A, Cantley LC: Signalling through the lipid products of phosphoinositide-3-OH kinase. Nature 387:673–676, 1997.
57. Shepherd PR, Withers DJ, Siddle K: Phosphoinositide 3-kinase: The key switch mechanism in insulin signalling. Biochem J 333:471–490, 1998.
58. Vanhaesebroeck B, Leevers SJ, Panayotou G, et al: Phosphoinositide 3-kinases: A conserved family of signal transducers. Trends Biochem Sci 22:267–272, 1997.
59. Maehama T, Dixon JE: The tumor suppressor, PTEN/MMAC1, dephosphorylates the lipid second messenger phosphatidylinositol 3,4,5-trisphosphate. J Biol Chem 273:13375–13378, 1998.
60. Stambolic V, Suzuki A, de la Pompa JL, et al: Negative regulation of PKB/Akt-dependent cell survival by the tumor suppressor PTEN. Cell 95:29–39, 1998.
61. Selbie LA, Hill SJ: G protein–coupled-receptor cross-talk: The fine-tuning of multiple receptor-signalling pathways. Trends Pharmacol Sci 19:87–93, 1998.
62. Dohlman HG, Thorner J, Caron MG, et al: Model systems for the study of seven-transmembrane-segment receptors. Annu Rev Biochem 60:653–688, 1991.
63. Strader CD, Fong TM, Tota MR, et al: Structure and function of G protein–coupled receptors. Annu Rev Biochem 63:101–132, 1994.
64. Hosey MM: Diversity of structure, signaling and regulation within the family of muscarinic cholinergic receptors. FASEB J 6:845–852, 1992.
65. Vassart G, Desarnaud F, Duprez L, et al: The G protein–coupled receptor family and one of its members, the TSH receptor. Ann N Y Acad Sci 766:23–30, 1995.
66. Mason WT, Rawlings SR, Cobbett P, et al: Control of secretion in anterior pituitary cells—linking ion channels, messengers and exocytosis. J Exp Biol 139:287–316, 1988.
67. Perlman JH, Gershengorn MC: Thyrotropin-releasing hormone stimulation of phosphoinositide hydrolysis desensitizes. Evidence against mediation by protein kinase C or calcium. Endocrinology 129:2679–2686, 1991.
68. Yu R, Hinkle PM: Desensitization of thyrotropin-releasing hormone receptor–mediated responses involves multiple steps. J Biol Chem 272:28301–28307, 1997.
69. Lefkowitz RJ, Cotecchia S, Kjelsberg MA, et al: Adrenergic receptors: Recent insights into their mechanism of activation and desensitization. Adv Second Messenger Phosphoprotein Res 28:1–9, 1993.

Chapter 9

Mitogen-Activated Protein Kinase and Growth Factor Signaling Pathways

John M. Kyriakis

Since the discovery of protein phosphorylation over 40 years ago, the mechanisms by which extracellular stimuli regulate protein phosphorylation have been the subject of intense interest. Protein phosphorylation, the covalent addition of phosphate groups to proteins at Ser, Thr, or Tyr residues, is catalyzed by protein kinases, and protein kinases are pivotal to cellular signal transduction. From the vantage point of the endocrinologist, protein kinase signaling pathways represent the primary means by which hormones such as insulin, which act at the cell surface, can generate pleiotropic intracellular responses. Protein tyrosine kinases and their mechanisms of signal transduction have been discussed in Chapter 4. This chapter will focus on protein serine/threonine kinase cascades, the phosphatidylinositol-3′-OH-kinase (PI-3-kinase) and Ras mitogen–activated protein kinase (MAPK) pathway in particular, that are activated by receptors coupled to tyrosine kinases. Recent studies of protein kinase signaling mediated by stress and inflammatory cytokines of the tumor necrosis factor (TNF) family will also be discussed.

GENERAL THEMES

It is often an initial impression that protein phosphorylation, catalyzed by protein tyrosine (Tyr) or serine/threonine (Ser/Thr) kinases, activates biochemical processes whereas dephosphorylation, catalyzed by protein Tyr or Ser/Thr phosphatases, inactivates these processes. This assumption is an erroneous oversimplification. Regulation of

cellular processes by protein phosphorylation can take two forms; although many biochemical processes are activated by phosphorylation, protein translation and some transcriptional responses being examples, many are activated by dephosphorylation, insulin activation of glycogen synthase (GS) being a major example. Many protein kinase signaling pathways are complex and involve several protein kinases arrayed in a multitiered manner. Often, these pathways have considerable apparent redundancy, and conversely, individual component elements often participate in several signaling pathways.

This chapter will deal with a subset of insulin-, mitogen-, and stress-activated Ser/Thr kinases and their regulation of cellular physiology. Accordingly, a few words on protein Ser/Thr kinase structure are warranted. The overall structure of all protein kinases (Ser/Thr, Tyr, or dual specificity) is well conserved, and in 1987, Hanks et al. aligned the sequences of all known protein kinases and identified 11 protein kinase subdomains (referred to with the roman numerals I–XI).[1] Of note, subdomain VIII is critically important to the regulation of many protein kinases. This domain, referred to as the activation loop, often contains sites of regulatory phosphorylation, catalyzed by upstream protein kinases.[2]

All protein kinases share a bilobed structure. The two lobes are oriented such that protein kinase catalysis occurs in the cleft between the two protein kinase lobes. For protein kinases that are activated by phosphorylation (the MAPKs are examples), the regulatory phosphorylation is thought to reorient the two lobes so that they are brought into a conformation optimal for catalyzing the phosphotransfer reaction.[2, 3]

INITIAL STEPS IN INSULIN AND MITOGEN SIGNALING

The receptors for insulin, as well as many mitogens and hormones, are either ligand-activated protein tyrosine kinases or are functionally coupled to tyrosine kinases. This insulin/mitogen-activated Tyr phosphorylation is followed by a quantitatively much larger wave of Ser/Thr phosphorylation,[4, 5] and recent research has begun to dissect the mechanisms by which receptor tyrosine kinases couple to Ser/Thr kinases. Activation of insulin, as well as other Tyr kinase receptors, is discussed in further detail in Chapter 4, as is the recruitment of insulin receptor substrate (IRS) proteins by the insulin receptor. Regulation and function of the plekstrin homology (PH), Src homology-2 (SH2), phosphotyrosine binding, and SH3 domains are also discussed in Chapter 4. With regard to activation of Ser/Thr protein kinase pathways by mitogen receptors, among the most important SH2-containing polypeptides that bind to Tyr-phosphorylated mitogen receptors and IRSs are the 85-kDa regulatory subunit of PI-3-kinase (p85) and growth factor receptor–binding protein-2 (Grb2).[5]

PI-3-KINASE. PI-3-kinases are a family of heterodimeric lipid kinases that phosphorylate the 3'-hydroxyl group of inositol phospholipids, including phosphatidylinositol 4,5-bisphosphate (PI-4,5-P_2) and phosphatidylinositol 4-phosphate (PI-4-P_2), thereby generating PI-3,4,5-P_3 and PI-3,4-P_2, respectively[6] (Fig. 9–1). The triphosphorylated phosphatidylinositol is thought to be the most biologically active 3'-phosphoinositide. 3'-Phosphorylated inositol lipids are believed to serve as second messengers; however, their functions are not completely understood (see Chapter 8).

Accumulating evidence suggests that at least one function of 3'-phosphorylated inositol lipids is to bind proteins containing certain PH domain subsets (see Chapter 4) thereby recruiting or tethering such proteins to the plasma membrane. Such binding may serve to nucleate proteins at the membrane and allow for the regulation of signaling.[6] This sort of lipid-dependent protein recruitment is thought to be critical for regulation of the protein kinase B (PKB)/Akt and p70 S6 kinase pathways (discussed below).

The PI-3-kinases regulated by insulin and mitogens consist of an 85-kDa regulatory subunit (p85) and a 110-kDa catalytic subunit (p110). A related 60-kDa regulatory subunit has also been identified. p85 is an adapter molecule that couples p110 to phosphotyrosine-containing polypeptides (see Chapter 4).[6]

Grb2. Grb2 is another adapter molecule with the configuration SH3-SH2-SH3 (see Chapter 4). Perhaps the best characterized effector for Grb2 is mammalian son of sevenless (mSOS), a guanine nucleotide exchange factor (GEF) required for activation of the Ras proto-oncoprotein.[4] Regulation of Ras and Ras regulation of MAPKs will be discussed below and are also discussed in Chapter 4.

INSULIN/MITOGEN ACTIVATION OF Ser/Thr PHOSPHORYLATION-I: SIGNALING THROUGH PI-3-KINASE

General Considerations: Early Studies of Insulin Regulation of Glycogen Synthase

Activation of Ser/Thr kinases by insulin was initially unexpected because among the first polypeptides shown to be regulated by insulin in a phosphorylation-dependent manner was GS, and this regulation involved dephosphorylation. Inactive GS is phosphorylated at up to seven sites: 1, 2, 3a, 3b, 3c, 4, and 5. Sites 3a to 3c and 4 reside near the GS carboxyl-terminus. Insulin stimulates glucose-6-phosphate–independent activation of GS by fostering GS dephosphorylation—primarily of sites 2, 3a to 3c, and to a lesser extent, 4. GS is phosphorylated and inactivated by protein kinases that are active in the resting cell, such as casein kinase-II and glycogen synthase kinase-3 (GSK3, see Figs. 9–2A and 9–7; also see below), which phosphorylate sites 2, 3a to 3c, and 4.[4, 7, 8]

GS is also inactivated, albeit to a slightly lesser extent, by agonists that elevate levels of cyclic adenosine monophosphate (cAMP) and activate the cAMP-dependent protein kinase (PKA) cascade, which culminates in the phosphorylation of sites 1 and 2 (Fig. 9–2A; see Chapter 7). The PKA pathway can be antagonized by insulin, and the opposing effects of insulin and cAMP agonists on GS phosphorylation led to the view that insulin's primary effect on Ser/Thr phosphorylation would be to promote dephosphorylation.[4, 7–9] This view came into question with the identification of several polypeptides that undergo rapid insulin-stimulated Ser/Thr phosphorylation in vivo. Most prominent among these was S6, a protein of the 40S small ribosomal subunit.[10, 11] Identification of insulin-stimulated Ser/Thr phosphorylation led to reassessment of the effect of insulin and other receptor Tyr kinases on protein phosphorylation, and it is now accepted that the major mode of insulin action is to promote protein phosphorylation. The next two sections will focus on two of the major mechanisms of insulin and mitogen-stimulated protein Ser/Thr phosphorylation: (1) protein Ser/Thr kinases activated by PI-3-kinase and (2) the Ras-MAPK pathway.

PKB/Akt, a Major PI-3-Kinase Effector

The effectors of PI-3-kinase are likely to be important in insulin regulation of metabolism. For example, insulin-resistant Native American (Pima) individuals manifest defective insulin activation of the protein kinase signaling pathways that are regulated through PI-3-

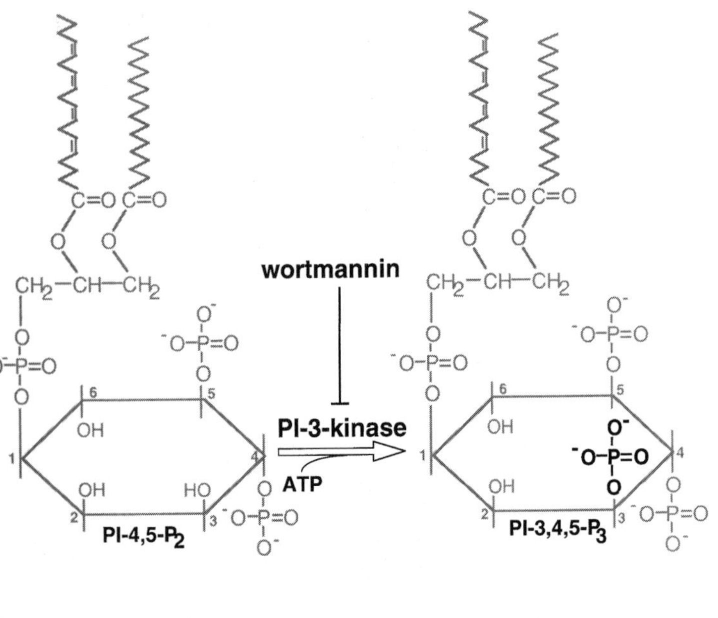

FIGURE 9–1. Reaction catalyzed by PI-3-kinase. Only phosphorylation of PI-4,5-P_2 is shown, although PI-4-P is also a substrate. Inhibition by the fungal toxin wortmannin is indicated.

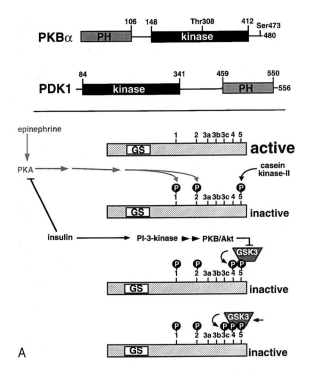

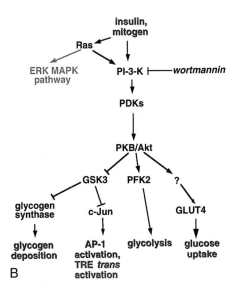

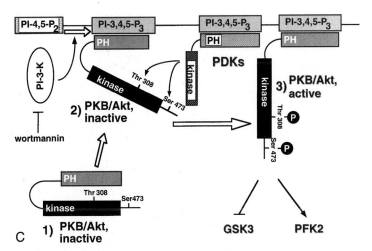

FIGURE 9–2. Regulation and function of PKB/Akt. *A, Top,* Structure of PKBα and PDK1. The critical residues of regulatory phosphorylation on PKBα (Thr308 and Ser473) are shown. PH, plekstrin homology. *Bottom,* Processive regulation of GS by phosphorylation and dephosphorylation. Input by the PKA pathway is in gray. Insulin inhibition of GSK3 is indicated. *B,* Signaling cascades regulated by PI-3-kinase through PKB/Akt. The parallel MAPK pathway emanating from Ras is also shown in gray. *C,* Three-step, substrate-directed activation of PKB/Akt by PDK1. Wortmannin inhibits this process by preventing the generation of PI-3,4,5-P₃, to which PKB/Akt must bind to permit phosphorylation of Thr308. The black P indicates phosphorylation.

kinase, specifically, GS activation and activation of p70 S6 kinase (see below).[5]

The Ser/Thr kinase PKB/Akt is a critical element that links PI-3-kinase with several downstream effectors. PKB/Akt is the normal cellular homologue of the oncoprotein encoded by v-akt of the acutely transforming retrovirus AKT8. PKB/Akt is activated by a wide variety of stimuli, including insulin, mitogens, and stress. Activation of PKB/Akt by insulin and mitogens (but not stress) requires PI-3-kinase inasmuch as blocking PI-3-kinase with the fungal toxin wortmannin, a potent inhibitor of PI-3-kinase, completely abrogates recruitment of PKB/Akt by these stimuli. In addition, dominant inhibitory mutants of the p85 adapter subunit of PI-3-kinase can block mitogen activation of PKB/Akt, and constitutively active mutants of the p110 subunit of PI-3-kinase are sufficient to induce activation of PKB/Akt in the absence of extracellular stimuli.[12]

Four PKB family members (α, $\beta1$, $\beta2$, and γ) have been identified. All are composed of an N-terminal regulatory region containing a PH domain, as well as a C-terminal kinase domain; the structure of PKBα is shown in Figure 9–2A. The role of the PH domain in the in vivo activation of PKB has recently been characterized. The products of PI-3-kinase activity, PI-3,4,5-P_3 and PI-3,4,-P_2, bind with high affinity to the PH domain of PKB/Akt. Binding of PI-3,4,5-P_3 does not activate PKB/Akt directly. Instead, the function of phosphatidylinositol lipid binding is to mediate the translocation of PKB/Akt from the cytosol to the membrane. This translocation/lipid binding appears to be necessary to present PKB/Akt to upstream activating kinases (see below).[12]

PKB/Akt Substrates Reveal a Role in Metabolic Regulation and Gene Expression

With regard to hormone action, the two best characterized substrates of PKB/Akt are GSK3 and the cardiac isoform of 6-phosphofructo-2-kinase (PFK2). The consequences of PKB/Akt-mediated phosphorylation of these substrates, as well as recent studies implicating PI-3-kinase and PKB/Akt in insulin regulation of glucose uptake, indicate that PKB/Akt is important in both insulin's metabolic functions and the regulation of gene expression (see Fig. 9–2A and B).

GSK3. As noted earlier (see Fig. 9–2A), inactive GS is phosphorylated at up to seven sites. Sites 2, 3a to 3c, and 4 are dephosphorylated in response to insulin.[4, 7, 8] The GSK3s constitute a highly conserved family of Ser/Thr kinases that are among the major protein kinases involved in the phosphorylation and inactivation of GS.[5, 13–15] In the absence of insulin, GSK3 is active and phosphorylates 3a to 3c and 4 on the GS polypeptide (but not site 2, which is phosphorylated by many kinases, including PKA and phosphorylase b kinase), thereby contributing to GS inactivation (see Fig. 9–2A). GSK3 phosphorylation of GS is described as processive or hierarchic (see Fig. 9–2A). Thus phosphorylation of GS by GSK3 requires prior phosphorylation of site 5 by casein kinase-2, which creates a GSK3 docking site for recruitment of GSK3 to the GS polypeptide. GSK3 then phosphorylates GS at a Ser residue amino-terminal to site 5, thereby creating a new GSK3-binding motif with the sequence Ser-X-X-X-Ser(P) (X is any amino acid and P indicates phosphorylation). This step enables the next phosphorylation, and another Ser-X-X-X-Ser(P) motif is created.[14, 15]

GSK3 has several additional physiologic functions. In particular, GSK3 can phosphorylate c-Jun, a component of the activator protein-1 (AP-1) transcription factor, at a site just amino-terminal to the c-Jun DNA binding domain (at Thr231, Thr239, Ser243, and Ser249). This phosphorylation inhibits DNA binding and inactivates AP-1 activity[16] (see below and Figs. 9–2B, 9–12A, and 9–13A).

GSK3 is phosphorylated at a single Ser residue (Ser21 in the GSK3-α isoform and Ser9 in GSK3-β) and inactivated in response to mitogens and insulin.[5, 17] By this process, proteins that are phosphorylated by GSK3 in resting cells, such as GS and c-Jun, are rapidly dephosphorylated by constitutively active Ser/Thr phosphatases. Several kinases, most notably p70 S6 kinase and MAPK-activated protein kinase-1 (MAPKAPK-1)/ribosomal S6 kinase (Rsk) (discussed below), have been implicated as GSK3 kinases in vitro; however, PKB/Akt is

probably the most physiologically relevant insulin-activated GSK3 kinase[5, 17] (see Fig. 9–2B).

PFK2. Insulin rapidly stimulates glycolysis in cardiomyocytes via activation of cardiac PFK2.[18] This process involves phosphorylation of the PFK2 polypeptide at Ser466 and Ser483. Phosphorylation of these sites can be catalyzed by several insulin-stimulated kinases, including PKB/Akt (see Fig. 9–2B) and p70 S6 kinase, which are effectors of PI-3-kinase, and MAPKAP-K1/Rsk, which is a Ras-MAPK effector.

Finally, insulin stimulation of glucose transport appears to require PI-3-kinase inasmuch as this process can be inhibited with the PI-3-kinase inhibitor wortmannin.[5, 12] Some evidence suggests that PKB/Akt may relay signals from PI-3-kinase to the glucose transport machinery; thus, dominant inhibitory PKB/Akt constructs can also inhibit insulin activation of glucose transport, and constitutively active PKB/Akt constructs can activate glucose uptake in the absence of insulin.[5, 12] However, a role for PKB/Akt in insulin activation of glucose transport has not been definitively established, nor is any mechanistic information yet available regarding how PKB/Akt might couple to glucose uptake.

Regulation of PKB/Akt by PDK Enzymes

In response to mitogen or insulin treatment, PKB/Akt undergoes rapid phosphorylation at two key sites. In PKBα these sites are Thr308 in the protein kinase domain activation loop (subdomain VIII) and Ser473 in the C-terminal tail. Phosphorylation of both sites is necessary for full activation (see Fig. 9–2A and C). In vivo, phosphorylation of both sites requires the activity of PI-3-kinase and can be blocked by PI-3-kinase inhibitors such as wortmannin[12, 19] (see Fig. 9–2C). In vitro, biochemical dissection of the mechanism of activation of PKB/Akt by phosphorylation indicates that the role of PI-3-kinase–derived phosphatidylinositol lipids in PKB/Akt activation is complex.

3-Phosphoinositide–dependent kinase-1 (PDK1) was originally identified as a Ser/Thr kinase that could specifically phosphorylate Thr308 of PKB/Akt. PDK1 contains an N-terminal protein kinase domain that is in the same general protein kinase family as that of PKB/Akt itself. At the PDK1 C-terminus is a PH domain that can bind 3′-inositol lipids (see Fig. 9–2A). PDK1 alone can catalyze a 30-fold activation of recombinant PKB/Akt in vitro in a reaction that absolutely requires 3′-phosphorylated inositol lipids and PI-3,4,5-P_3 in particular[12, 20, 21] (see Fig. 9–2C).

It appears that a major component of 3′-phosphoinositide-dependent activation of PKB/Akt by PDK1 is substrate directed; in other words, PDK1 intrinsic activity does not appear to increase upon binding phosphatidylinositol lipids. Instead, the binding of phosphatidylinositol lipids to PKB/Akt renders Thr308 of PKB/Akt available for PDK1-dependent phosphorylation (see Fig. 9–2C). Thus deletion of the PKB/Akt PH domain results in a modest elevation of PKB/Akt activity and permits lipid-independent PDK1 activation of PKB/Akt, which suggests that the PH domain restricts access of Thr308 and lipid binding reverses this inhibition and makes PKB/Akt a better PDK1 substrate. Moreover, PDK1, when purified or immunoprecipitated from resting or stimulated cells, appears to be constitutively active and does not undergo further activation in response to mitogens or insulin, thus suggesting that much of the regulation of PDK1 involves gating access to PKB/Akt phosphoacceptor sites rather than alterations in PDK1 activity per se.[12, 20, 21]

The identity of the kinase responsible for PKB/Akt Ser473 phosphorylation has yet to be established. This kinase plus PDK1 is necessary for full activation of PKB/Akt. Inasmuch as phosphorylation of Ser473 in vivo requires PI-3-kinase products, it has been proposed that the Ser473 kinase, although possessing a substrate selectivity targeted toward Ser473, is at least superficially similar to PDK1.[12, 22] Indeed, the sequences of several protein kinases similar to PDK1 have been deposited in various databases,[12, 22] and accordingly, the Ser473 kinase has been tentatively designated PDK2.

The p70 S6 Kinase: A Putative Regulator of Protein Translation

As noted above, phosphorylation of the 40S small ribosomal subunit protein S6 was among the first insulin- and mitogen-stimulated Ser/Thr phosphorylation events to be identified.[10, 11] Although the physiologic significance of this phosphorylation was initially unclear, S6 phosphorylation served as a distal marker that could be used as a means of dissecting signal transduction pathways recruited by insulin and growth factors.

MAPKAP-K1/Rsk, the first enzyme with S6 kinase activity to be purified and cloned was isolated from *Xenopus* oocytes arrested in the first meiotic prophase after treatment of the oocytes with insulin or progesterone.[4, 5, 23, 24] Subsequent analysis revealed that MAPKAP-K1/Rsk, although representing the dominant S6 kinase in oocytes, was not the major S6 kinase activated by insulin or mitogens in somatic cells even though MAPKAP-K1/Rsk is expressed in these cells.[5, 24, 25] MAPKAP-K1/Rsk is a component of the Ras-MAPK pathway and will be discussed below.

Purification of the major mammalian somatic cell S6 kinase revealed an enzyme with an apparent molecular weight of 70 kDa upon sodium dodecyl sulfate (SDS)–polyacrylamide gel electrophoresis, hence the name p70 S6 kinase (p70). Copurifying with the 70-kDa polypeptide was an 85-kDa species.[4, 5, 26] Molecular cloning has identified two p70 genes: p70α and p70β.[4, 5, 27, 28] The mRNAs transcribed from either the α or β gene contain two alternative translational start sites. The more 5′ start sites give rise to the 85-kDa polypeptides, whereas the more 3′ sites give rise to the 70-kDa polypeptides. The 85-kDa polypeptides each contain an amino-terminal nuclear localization signal. Consequently, these longer p70 polypeptides reside exclusively in the nucleus. Sequence analysis of p70α and p70β cDNAs predicts proteins of 55 to 60 kDa; therefore, the 70- and 85-kDa apparent molecular weights indicate that these proteins migrate aberrantly on SDS gels.[4, 5, 27, 28]

p70 S6 Kinase Substrates

The best characterized substrates for p70 (Fig. 9–3A) suggest that p70 is intimately involved in the regulation of protein synthesis and, possibly, gene expression. In addition, p70 may participate in the regulation of key metabolic pathways in response to insulin.

RIBOSOMAL S6. The S6 protein of the 40S small ribosomal subunit is the best characterized p70 substrate. The sites phosphorylated on rat S6 reside in a cluster at the C-terminus of the polypeptide (Ser235, Ser236, Ser240, Ser244, and Ser247). Both purified and recombinant p70 can phosphorylate all five sites on ribosomal S6. Importantly, p70 preferentially phosphorylates these sites when S6 is in the context of 40S ribosomal subunits. By contrast, other kinases such as PKC and PKA, although able to phosphorylate synthetic peptides containing the phosphoacceptor sites of S6, cannot appreciably phosphorylate S6 as part of an intact 40S subunit.[4, 5]

The physiologic role of p70 was obscure until it was observed that the immunosuppressant macrolide rapamycin, a potent inhibitor of p70 activation in vivo (discussed below), could selectively block the insulin- and mitogen-stimulated translation of 5′terminal oligopyrimidine tract (5′TOP) mRNAs—a subset of mRNAs containing a polypyrimidine tract immediately C-terminal to the N^7-methylguanosine cap.[5, 29, 30] Serum-stimulated increases in protein synthesis usually occur at the level of initiation and correlate with rapid recruitment of 80S ribosomes onto actively translating polysomes. Thus upon serum stimulation, a relative increase is observed in the number of actively translating polysomes. Most mRNAs redistribute to polysomes of the same size after insulin or mitogen stimulation; in other words, simply more of the same-size polysomes are present upon stimulation with insulin or mitogen. However, 5′TOP mRNAs redistribute to larger polysomes (i.e., ones with more ribosomes) after insulin or mitogen stimulation; thus initiation of translation from 5′TOP mRNAs is markedly enhanced by insulin or growth factors, even against an overall agonist-stimulated increase in protein translation. Most 5′TOP mRNAs encode proteins that are involved in the translation process itself, such as the

translational elongation factor eEF-1α, as well as most ribosomal proteins, and insulin is known to preferentially increase the translation of these polypeptides. Thus increased translation of these mRNAs in response to insulin and mitogen serves to further increase protein synthesis in response to extracellular stimuli[29–31] (Fig. 9–4A).

As we shall see, rapamycin does not act directly on p70, but acts instead to inhibit p70 activation by upstream components. The mechanism by which p70 might regulate translation of 5′TOP mRNAs remains unclear. It has been proposed that S6 phosphorylation allows for enhanced binding of the 40S subunit to 5′TOP mRNAs, perhaps through a process involving additional cytosolic polypeptides.[29–31] The ability of p70 to influence 5′TOP mRNA translation coincides in vivo with an additional insulin- and mitogen-regulated signaling pathway that acts on the general translational mechanism to enhance overall protein synthesis (discussed below).

CREM. Transcriptional mechanisms activated by cAMP, mitogen, and stress pathways are mediated in part by the cAMP-responsive element (CRE)-binding proteins (CREB)/activating transcription factors (ATFs), a subgroup of the bZIP family of leucine zipper–containing transcription factors. In response to elevations in cAMP, CREB/ATFs can *trans*-activate genes containing a CRE[32, 33] (see Chapter 7). In partnership with c-Jun, some ATFs can also *trans*-activate CREs and 12-*o*-tetradecanoyl phorbol acetate (TPA) response elements (TREs) in response to stress or other stimuli (see below). CRE modulator (CREM) is a CREB/ATF family member that is important to the regulation of gene expression in response to mitogenic and neuroendocrine stimuli.[32–36] The *crem* gene encodes a large number of polypeptides that arise from alternative promoter usage, differential heterogeneous nuclear RNA splicing, and the presence of alternate translational start sites on several of the resulting mRNAs. The heterogeneous population of CREM proteins includes transcriptional repressors such as CREMα, CREMβ, and CREMγ, which arise from alternative splicing to remove glutamine-rich *trans*-activation domains, and S-CREM, which is generated from an alternative initiation codon and gives rise to a protein lacking phosphoacceptor sites.[36, 37] mRNAs encoding additional CREM repressors can also be transcribed from an alternative, intronic, cAMP-inducible promoter. These transcripts, referred to as inducible cAMP early repressors (ICERs), encode truncated CREM polypeptides containing only the bZIP domains and are potent repressors of cAMP- and CREB-mediated gene expression[38] (see Chapter 7).

The *crem* gene also encodes transcriptional activators containing one (CREMτ1 or CREMτ2) or both (CREMτ) glutamine-rich *trans*-activation domains.[38] Expression of CREMτ is particularly prevalent in male germ cells. There, expression is developmentally regulated by follicle-stimulating hormone during spermatogenesis.[39] CREMτ is rapidly phosphorylated at Ser117 by PKA, a reaction that activates CREMτ *trans*-activation function, thus implicating CREMτ in cAMP-mediated gene expression. CREMτ Ser117 is also a target for Ca/calmodulin-dependent kinases and PKC, which suggests that multiple signaling pathways can activate CREMτ.[40]

Mitogens and serum can also stimulate CREMτ phosphorylation at Ser117 under conditions wherein p70 is activated (Fig. 9–3A). This phosphorylation is completely inhibited by rapamycin and can be recapitulated in vitro with purified p70. From these results it can be concluded that p70 represents the major mechanism by which insulin and mitogens regulate CREMτ. p70 phosphorylation of CREMτ has no effect on DNA binding. Coexpression of a GAL4-CAT reporter, p70, and a GAL4-CREM fusion protein indicates that p70 enhances the *trans*-activating activity of CREMτ.[41]

PFK2. The insulin-stimulated phosphorylation of cardiac PFK2 and the ramifications of this phosphorylation to metabolic regulation have been discussed earlier. In addition to PKB/Akt, p70 can phosphorylate PFK2 at the activating sites[18] (see Fig. 9–3A).

Regulation of p70 S6 Kinase: Requirement for PI-3-Kinase Activity through PDK Enzymes

That p70 was regulated by Ser/Thr phosphorylation was evident when it was observed that the kinase undergoes rapid Ser/Thr phos-

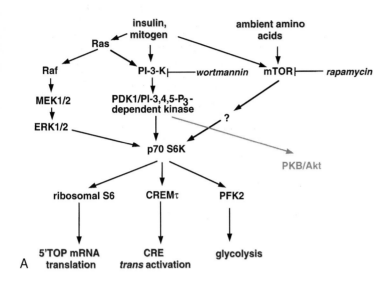

A

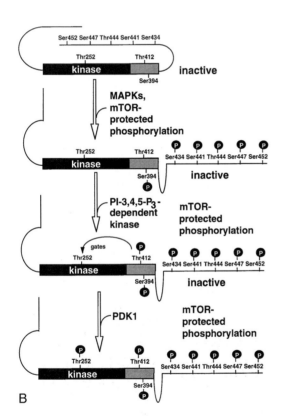

B

FIGURE 9–3. Regulation and function of p70 S6 kinase. *A,* Signaling pathways regulated by Ras, PI-3-kinase, and mTOR through the p70 S6 kinase. The parallel PKB/Akt pathway is indicated in gray. *B,* Multistep regulation of p70 S6 kinase. MAPKs and proline-directed kinases mediate initial phosphorylations that permit phosphorylation of Thr412 by an unknown kinase. As indicated, phosphorylation of Thr412 gates the phosphorylation of Thr252 by PDK1. The white P in the black circle indicates phosphorylation. The function of mTOR in p70 regulation is unclear. mTOR-protected phosphorylation indicates that mTOR probably does not directly phosphorylate p70 but is instead necessary for preventing dephosphorylation of key regulatory sites on p70.

phorylation upon insulin and mitogen stimulation and that this phosphorylation correlates with activation. Moreover, treatment of p70 with Ser/Thr-specific phosphatases rapidly deactivates p70 in a reaction accompanied by dephosphorylation of the p70 polypeptide.[4, 26]

The mechanism by which p70 is activated by upstream phosphorylation is exceedingly complex and still incompletely understood. p70 undergoes regulatory phosphorylation in three domains: (1) several sites in a C-terminal pseudosubstrate autoinhibitory domain (Ser434, Ser441, Thr444, Ser447, Ser452); (2) two sites in a short motif immediately C-terminal to the catalytic domain, the catalytic domain extension (Ser394, Thr412); and (3) a site in the activating loop of the kinase domain[5] (Thr252) (see Fig. 9–3B). Phosphorylation of these sites is hierarchic, with phosphorylation of some sites gating the phosphorylation of other sites. Moreover, these phosphorylations are subject to regulation by several different pathways.

Phosphorylation of the pseudosubstrate autoinhibitory domain of

p70 in response to insulin and mitogens is probably mediated primarily by proline-directed Ser/Thr kinases, including MAPKs, insofar as these kinases represent the major peaks of ΔCT104 kinase activity detectable upon fractionation, over several chromatographic steps, of insulin-stimulated cell extracts.[5, 42] However, phosphorylation of these sites alone is insufficient to activate p70 in vitro. Moreover, deletion of the pseudosubstrate autoinhibitory domain (ΔCT104 deletion) does not result in a constitutively active p70 mutant, and in fact, the pseudosubstrate autoinhibitory domain construct can still be activated by mitogen and insulin in vivo. Current evidence suggests that phosphorylation of the MAPK sites is necessary to render p70 capable of undergoing additional activating phosphorylation events at the sites within the catalytic domain and the catalytic domain extension[5] (see Fig. 9–3B).

Activation of p70 in vivo can be inhibited by wortmannin and rapamycin. Phosphorylation of Thr412 and Thr252 is wortmannin

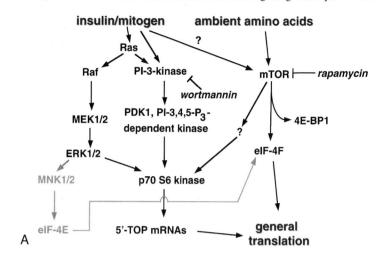

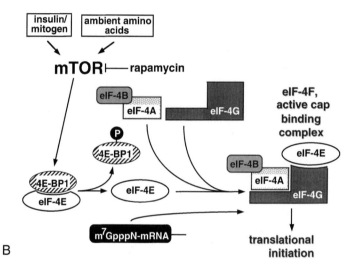

FIGURE 9–4. *Regulation of protein translation by p70 S6 kinase and mTOR. A, Protein kinase cascades signaling to p70 S6 kinase and activation of eIF-4F, mediated by PI-3-kinase, MAPK, and mTOR. Sites of inhibition by wortmannin and rapamycin are indicated. The regulation of eIF-4E by MNKs is shown in gray. B, Mechanism of disinhibition of eIF-4E by mTOR. Phosphorylation of 4E-BP1 causes dissociation from eIF-4E and permits formation of the eIF-4F complex consisting of eIF-4E, eIF-4A, and eIF-4F. This complex binds to the 5'-N7-methylguanosine cap (m7GpppN) and permits translational initiation.*

sensitive, which indicates that these sites are phosphorylated by a PI-3-kinase–dependent mechanism.[5] PDK1 can phosphorylate Thr252 and probably contributes to the activation of p70 in vivo inasmuch as coexpression of PDK1 and p70ΔCT104 results in a substantial elevation in basal p70 activity and dominant inhibitory mutant constructs of PDK1 can block the activation of p70 by mitogen. However, PDK1 phosphorylation of p70 requires prior phosphorylation of the p70 polypeptide by additional upstream kinases. Thus PDK1 cannot phosphorylate inactive, unphosphorylated full-length p70 in vitro. Deletion of the pseudosubstrate autoinhibitory domain results in a p70 construct that can still be activated in vivo by coexpressed PDK1; however, this construct also cannot be activated by PDK1 in vitro[5, 43] (see Fig. 9–3B).

Phosphorylation of Thr252 by PDK1 requires prior phosphorylation of Thr412. Thus mutagenesis of p70ΔCT104 Thr412 to an acidic residue (Asp), a mutation that mimics the charge of phosphorylation, results in a modest (5- to 10-fold) elevation in basal p70 activity and renders the mutant construct capable of being activated in vitro by PDK1.[5, 43] To summarize thus far, p70 is regulated by MAPK-catalyzed phosphorylation of the pseudosubstrate autoinhibitory domain.[5, 42, 43] This phosphorylation is then thought to permit PI-3-kinase–dependent phosphorylation of Thr412. Once these sites are phosphorylated, PDK1 phosphorylates Thr252. Whereas phosphorylation of Thr252 alone by PDK1 (on the p70ΔCT104/Asp412 mutant) results in 15-fold activation of p70, dual Thr412 and Thr252 phosphorylation of wild-type p70 results in synergistic (>200-fold) activation of p70. The identity of the Thr412 kinase is unknown[5, 42, 43] (see Fig. 9–3B).

Although phosphorylation of the Thr412 and Thr252 of p70 is wortmannin sensitive, the specific role of phosphatidylinositol lipids

in the regulation of p38 is uncertain. In contrast to activation of PKB/Akt by PDK1, activation of P70ΔCT104/Asp412 by PDK1 is unaffected by PI-3,4,5,P₃ in vitro. It is possible that p70 phosphorylation by Thr412 kinase is phosphatidylinositol lipid dependent, a situation that would, by virtue of the gating function of Thr412 phosphorylation, make PDK1 phosphorylation of Thr252 phosphatidylinositol lipid dependent in vivo[43] (see Fig. 9–3B).

Regulation of p70 S6 Kinase by mTOR: The Role of Ambient Amino Acids

Rapamycin is a macrolide immunosuppressant that potently inhibits T cell activation and can block eukaryotic cell cycle progression at G₁/S. Rapamycin strongly and selectively inhibits the activation of p70 in vivo and has no effect on the MAPK → MAPKAP-K1/Rsk or PI-3-kinase → PKB/Akt pathways. Rapamycin does not directly bind or inhibit p70 in vitro.[25, 44–46]

Rapamycin exerts its effects by binding to a small polypeptide, FK506-binding protein-12 (FKBP12). Interestingly, as its name suggests, FKBP12 is also a target for another immunosuppressant, FK506. Complexes of FKBP12-FK506 can bind and inhibit the calcium-dependent protein phosphatase calcineurin, and this inhibition accounts for most of the biologic effects of FK506.[44]

Rapamycin and FK506 are structurally related—they share a similar FKBP12-binding interface. Outside this interface, however, the structures differ. Therefore, whereas FKBP12 can bind both FK506 and rapamycin, FKBP12-rapamycin complexes neither bind nor inhibit calcineurin.[44] Potential targets of rapamycin (TORs) were first identified in the budding yeast *Saccharomyces cerevisiae* as mutant alleles that conferred rapamycin resistance. Yeast *TOR1* and *TOR2* encode proteins that consist of a kinase domain that is distantly related to the PI-3-kinase p110 subunit; however, it is still unclear whether Tor1p and Tor2p are lipid or protein kinases. The kinase domain is preceded by a very large amino-terminal domain that may serve a regulatory function.[47]

Mammalian TOR (mTOR, also called rapamycin and FKBP12 target [RAFT] and FKBP-rapamycin–associated protein [FRAP]) was identified by biochemical purification as a polypeptide that could bind immobilized FKBP12-rapamycin. mTOR cannot bind FKBP12 in the absence of rapamycin, nor can rapamycin directly bind mTOR. mTOR contains a kinase domain that is strikingly homologous to those of Tor1p and Tor2p and is also distantly related to PI-3-kinase p110. Like Tor1p and Tor2p, mTOR also possesses an extensive amino-terminal domain. Deletion and truncation studies have shown that the rapamycin-binding site lies within this amino-terminal domain.[47, 48]

mTOR is presumed to be active in resting cells; nevertheless, co-expression of mTOR and p70 results in little or no p70 activation in vivo.[49, 50] However, if the cell culture medium is depleted of amino acids, mTOR activity is dramatically inhibited. In addition, p70 is no longer responsive to mitogen and no longer undergoes phosphorylation at Thr412—a site whose phosphorylation is repressed both by wortmannin and rapamycin[50] (see Figs. 9–3B and 9–4A). Thus it appears that mTOR is a sensor for ambient amino acids—a role fitting for a pathway implicated in the regulation of protein synthesis.

The exact function of mTOR in the regulation of p70 remains to be established unambiguously. Rapamycin blocks phosphorylation of Thr252 and Thr412, sites that are phosphorylated in a PI-3-kinase–dependent manner[5, 43] (see Fig. 9–3B). The mechanism of this inhibition is unclear. Immunoprecipitates of mTOR can catalyze the phosphorylation of p70 in vitro at Thr412, one of the rapamycin-sensitive sites[50, 51]; however, the stoichiometry of this phosphorylation is unknown, and it remains to be determined whether this phosphorylation is catalyzed directly or by an mTOR-associated kinase. In particular, a p70 mutant, Δ2-46/ΔCT104, is entirely resistant to rapamycin yet remains mitogen responsive and inhibited by wortmannin. Moreover, insulin stimulates the phosphorylation of Δ2-46/ΔCT104 at Thr412 in the presence of rapamycin, thus indicating that inhibition of mTOR by rapamycin does not result in inhibition of Thr412 kinase activity.[5, 50] For now it is plausible to propose that Thr412 is phosphorylated by a phosphatidylinositol lipid–dependent kinase distinct from mTOR and that mTOR inhibits a phosphatase selective for phosphorylated Thr412.[5] Inhibition of Thr412 phosphorylation prevents Thr252 phosphorylation because of the gating function of Thr412 phosphorylation (see Fig. 9–3B).

mTOR and General Protein Synthesis: Phosphorylation of 4E-BP1

As mentioned above, insulin and mitogens stimulate an increase in the synthesis of proteins required for progression through the cell cycle. The p70 pathway contributes to this increase by enhancing the translation of 5'TOP mRNAs. In addition to regulating the p70 pathway (and therefore 5'TOP mRNA translation), mTOR directly regulates general protein synthesis through disinhibition of the eukaryotic initiation factor-4E (eIF-4E), a component of the multisubunit translational initiating complex eIF-4F[52–54] (see Fig. 9–4A and B).

Cellular mRNAs contain a 5' cap structure, the N^7-methylguanosine cap. Efficient translation of proteins is dependent on the binding of eIF-4F to the methylguanosine cap. Binding of eIF-4F to mRNA is thought to result in relaxation of mRNA secondary structure, thereby facilitating binding of the 40S small ribosomal subunit. eIF-4F is a hetero-oligomer that consists of eIF-4A, which is an RNA helicase that acts in collaboration with eIF-4B, an RNA-binding protein, to unwind mRNA and thereby allow for ribosome binding. The eIF-4F complex also contains eIF-4G, a multifunctional scaffolding protein that binds eIF-4A, eIF-4B, and the final eIF-4F component, eIF-4E. The ability of eIF-4F to bind to the 5' cap is dictated by the association between eIF-4E and eIF-4G. This association is thought to recruit the remaining eIF-4F subunits and foster the formation of a complete eIF-4F complex capable of binding to the 5' cap[53, 54] (see Fig. 9–4B).

The eIF-4E–eIF-4G interaction is negatively regulated by the translational repressor protein 4E–binding protein-1 (4E-BP1, also called phosphorylated heat- and acid-stable protein regulated by insulin [PHAS-I]). 4E-BP1 is rapidly phosphorylated at Ser64 in response to insulin and mitogens, and this phosphorylation results in the dissociation of 4E-BP1 from eIF-4E.[52-54] In vivo, phosphorylation of 4E-BP1 is completely inhibited by rapamycin, and immunoprecipitates of mTOR can directly phosphorylate 4E-BP1 at Ser64, when 4E-BP1 is bound to eIF-4E, and promote dissociation of the 4E-BP1–eIF4E complex. This dissociation in turn fosters formation of the eIF-4F complex[52] (see Fig. 9–4B). One remaining conundrum is the observation that mTOR is constitutively active in resting cells maintained in medium replete with amino acids whereas 4E-BP1 phosphorylation is clearly insulin stimulated. It is conceivable that a 4E-BP1 kinase, activated by insulin through mTOR-dependent and mTOR-independent mechanisms, coimmunoprecipitates with mTOR.

Inasmuch as rapamycin can completely block insulin/mitogen activation of protein translation, mTOR regulation of translation represents a key step in translational control. However, the mTOR → 4E-BP1 mechanism is not the only way in which eIF-4F is regulated by insulin and mitogens. eIF-4E itself is also directly phosphorylated by insulin/mitogen- and stress-activated MAP kinases.

INSULIN/MITOGEN ACTIVATION OF Ser/Thr PHOSPHORYLATION-II: SIGNALING THROUGH Ras AND THE MAP KINASES

The MAP3K → MEK → MAPK Core Signaling Module, an Emerging Paradigm

MAPK signal transduction pathways are among the most widespread mechanisms of cellular regulation. All eukaryotic cells possess multiple MAPK pathways, each of which is preferentially recruited by distinct sets of stimuli, thereby allowing the cell to respond in parallel to multiple divergent inputs. Mammalian MAPK pathways can be recruited by a wide variety of different stimuli ranging from hormones such as insulin and growth hormone to mitogens (i.e., epidermal growth factor [EGF], platelet-derived growth factor [PDGF], fibroblast growth factor [FGF]), vasoactive peptides (angiotensin II, endothelin), inflammatory cytokines of the TNF family, and environmental stresses such as osmotic shock, ionizing radiation, and ischemic injury.[55–59]

All MAPK pathways consist of a central three-tiered "core signaling module" wherein MAPKs are activated by concomitant Thr and Tyr phosphorylation catalyzed by a family of dual-specificity kinases referred to as MAPK/extracellular signal–regulated kinase (ERK) kinases (MEKs or MKKs). MEKs, in turn, are regulated by Ser/Thr phosphorylation catalyzed by several protein kinases collectively referred to as MAPK kinase kinases (MAP3Ks) (Fig. 9–5A). The core signaling modules are themselves regulated by a divergent variety of upstream activators and inhibitors, including guanosine triphosphatases (GTPases) of the Ras superfamily and adapter proteins coupled to cytokine receptors.[55–59]

The notion of multiple parallel MAPK signaling cascades was first appreciated from studies of simple eukaryotes such as the budding yeast *S. cerevisiae*. To date, six *S. cerevisiae* MAPK signaling pathways have been identified.[55] Several features of yeast signaling pathways are relevant to an understanding of mammalian signaling, and these features illustrate general properties of MAPK signaling modules (see Fig. 9–5B).

SIGNALING COMPONENTS WITH MORE THAN ONE BIOLOGIC FUNCTION. In some cases, individual elements can function in more than one pathway; for example, MAP3K Ste11p functions as part of the mating pheromone response pathway and the osmosensing pathway[60] (see Fig. 9–5B).

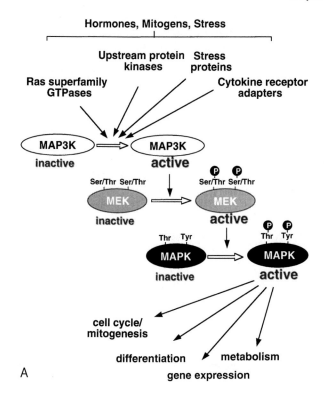

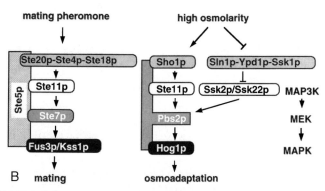

A

B mating   osmoadaptation

FIGURE 9–5. *General themes of MAPK pathway regulation and function. A, Canonical MAPK core signaling module (MAP3K → MEK → MAPK). MAP3Ks are subject to divergent regulatory mechanisms whereas MAPKs can phosphorylate divergent targets and regulate numerous cellular processes. B, Yeast pheromone response and osmosensing pathways of Saccharomyces cerevisiae illustrate important points about MAPK pathways: regulation of signaling components by multiple upstream activators (regulation of Pbs2p by Ste11p, Ssk2p, and Ssk22p), signaling components with multiple functions (Ste11p), and scaffolding proteins (Ste5p and Pbs2p). Sho1p is an osmosensing receptor. Sln1p-Ypd1p-Ssk1p are three elements in a histidine-aspartate phosphotransferase mechanism that forms a second osmosensor. Inactivation of this pathway by high osmolarity relieves inhibition of Ssk2p and Ssk22p. Ste20p, Ste4p, and Ste18p represent a protein kinase and trimeric Gβ and γ subunits, respectively, that are genetically upstream of Ste11p in the pheromone response pathway (reviewed by Herskowitz[55]).*

PATHWAY SEGREGATION BY SCAFFOLDING PROTEINS.

Some yeast signaling pathways include distinct scaffolding proteins that act to segregate signaling components and maintain pathway integrity. Alternatively, in some MAPK pathways, the signaling components themselves possess intrinsic scaffolding properties. Thus, Ste5p of the yeast mating pheromone pathway is a scaffolding protein that selectively binds a MAP3K (Ste11p), a MEK (Ste7p), and a MAPK (Fus3p) and couples them to upstream activators.[55, 61] There-

fore, although Ste11p can function in both the mating and osmosensing pathways, it selectively activates different MEKs in each pathway: Ste7p for the mating pathway and Pbs2p for the osmosensing pathway. This selectivity is due in part to the fact that Ste5p maintains signaling pathway specificity by binding Ste7p selectively and not Pbs2p.[54] Conversely, Pbs2p, in addition to serving as a MEK, acts as a scaffold protein that selectively binds Ste11p and the osmosensing MAPK Hog1p. Pbs2p does not bind Fus3p, and thus Pbs2p maintains signaling pathway integrity by interacting specifically with Hog1p and not with Fus3p or Kss1p[60] (see Fig 9–5B).

REDUNDANCY OF SIGNALING COMPONENTS. Some signaling elements in yeast MAPK pathways can be activated by several upstream components, often in response to the same class of stimulus. Thus as part of the osmosensing pathway, not only can MEK Pbs2p be activated by MAP3K Ste11p, but it can also be activated by two additional osmosensing MAP3Ks: Ssk2p and Ssk22p (see Fig. 9–5B).[55, 60]

The Ras → MAPK Pathway, a MAPK Pathway in Mammalian Cells that Is Activated by Insulin and Mitogens—General Considerations

The first mammalian MAPK was detected as an insulin-stimulated 40- to 44-kDa Ser/Thr kinase that could phosphorylate microtubule-associated protein-2 (MAP2). The name MAPK stemmed from the observation that this kinase was activated not only by insulin but also by a wide variety of mitogens that couple to Tyr kinases. Activation of the insulin-stimulated MAPK was rapid—preceding activation of other known mitogen-activated Ser/Thr kinases—thus suggesting a proximal role in signal transduction. Subsequently, it was shown that this MAPK could in fact phosphorylate and activate another insulin-activated kinase, MAPKAP-K1/Rsk[4, 5] (Fig. 9–6A and B).

Molecular cloning of the insulin- and mitogen-stimulated MAPKs revealed 44- and 42-kDa protein Ser/Thr kinases. These cDNAs were designated, respectively, ERK1 and ERK2 (Table 9–1). Structural analysis of the ERK1 and ERK2 sequences revealed a striking homology to *S. cerevisiae* Fus3p and Kss1p, kinases of the yeast mating pheromone pathway[4, 55] (see Fig. 9–5B). This finding was the first indication of the conservation of MAPK pathways.

Substrates of ERK1 and ERK2 Include Other Protein Kinases as well as Transcription Factors

ERK1 and ERK2 phosphorylate and activate both transcription factors and other protein kinases. These physiologic substrates serve to illustrate the importance of MAPKs in cellular physiology (see Fig. 9–6A).

MAPKAP-K1/Rsk. MAPKAP-K1/Rsk was the first insulin-stimulated protein kinase with S6 phosphorylating activity to be purified and cloned.[4, 23, 24] As we have seen, however, MAPKAP-K1/Rsk does not represent the physiologic S6 kinase activated by insulin and mitogens in somatic cells.[25] At least three MAPKAP-K1/Rsk isoforms have been cloned, and they have a distinct molecular structure in that each possesses two complete protein kinase domains[4, 24] (see Fig. 9–6B). Both domains are necessary for MAPKAP-K1/Rsk regulation and function.

MAPKAP-K1/Rsk is thought to be important in insulin and mitogen regulation of glycogen metabolism. GSK3 can phosphorylate GS at sites 3a to 3c and 4; however, site 2 is not phosphorylated by GSK3, and insulin-stimulated dephosphorylation of GS involves dephosphorylation of site 2, sites 3a to 3c, and to a lesser extent, site 4. Thus, insulin-mediated inhibition of GSK3 cannot account for all of insulin's action on GS.

MAPKAP-K1/Rsk phosphorylation of the G subunit of phosphatase-1 (PP1-G) represents a mechanism by which MAPK pathways, in conjunction with the PI-3-kinase → GSK3 pathway, can regulate skeletal muscle GS activation (Fig. 9–7). PP1-G is a skeletal muscle

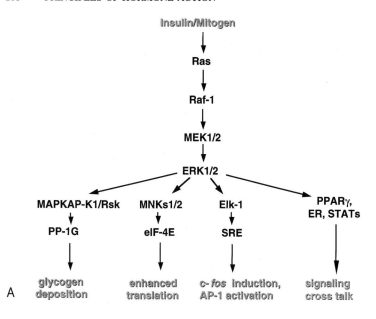

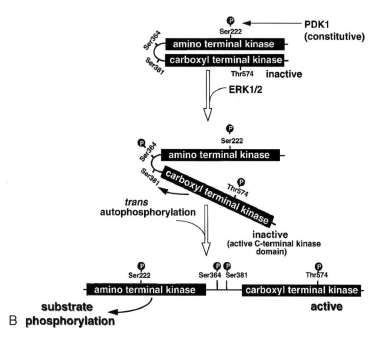

FIGURE 9–6. Major signaling pathways activated via ERK1 and ERK2. *A,* Activation of MAPKAP-K1, MNKs, Elk-1, and crosstalk mechanisms (PPARγ, the estrogen receptor [ER], and the STATs) by ERK-dependent mechanisms. *B,* Mechanism of activation of MAPKAP-K1/ Rsk by ERK1/ERK2. ERK phosphorylation of the C-terminal catalytic domain at Thr574 and the N-terminal catalytic domain at Ser364 is followed by *trans*-autophosphorylation (the C-terminal catalytic domain phosphorylates Ser381 of the N-terminal catalytic domain) and *cis*-autophosphorylation (the N-terminal catalytic domain autophosphorylates Ser222).

polypeptide that binds phosphatase-1 (PP1) in a reversible fashion and interacts constitutively with the glycogen granule (see Fig. 9–7). Of note, GS is constitutively associated with skeletal muscle glycogen granules. PP1-G can be phosphorylated at two sites referred to, somewhat confusingly, as sites 1 and 2. PP1-G site 2 is a substrate for cAMP-dependent protein kinase. Dephosphorylation of PP1-G site 2, which occurs under conditions wherein PKA is inactive, promotes the association of PP1 with PP1-G.[4, 14] Phosphorylation of PP1-G site 1 by MAPKAP-K1/Rsk substantially enhances the rate at which PP1 dephosphorylates GS. By these processes, PP1 is targeted, in an insulin-stimulated manner, to GS and can efficiently dephosphorylate (at sites 2 and 3a–3c, but not site 4) and contribute to the activation of GS[4, 62] (see Fig. 9–7). It should be noted that this mechanism is specific for skeletal muscle inasmuch as PP1-G is a muscle-specific protein. Whether analogous mechanisms exist in other tissues is unclear.

Thus in response to insulin and mitogens, both the PI-3-kinase and MAPK pathways can potentially regulate GS, and from the preceding discussion, it would seem that both mechanisms acting in concert are in fact necessary for GS activation. However, studies using blockers of the MAPK pathway (the Parke-Davis compound PD98059) or the PI-3-kinase pathway (wortmannin) suggest that depending on the stimulus used, the MAPK or PI-3-kinase pathway may exert a more dominant effect on GS activation. Thus inhibition of the PI-3-kinase pathway strongly blocks insulin activation of GS, which suggests that the PI-3-kinase → GSK3 mechanism is the predominant pathway for GS activation by insulin; indeed, insulin comparatively modestly activates the MAPKs in many cell types, including muscle, whereas the PI-3-kinase pathway is robustly activated by insulin. By contrast, EGF activation of GS is substantially blocked upon inhibition of the MAPK → MAPKAP-K1/Rsk mechanism, thus suggesting that the MAPKs are more important in EGF regulation of GS.[4, 5]

MAPKAP-K1/Rsk, once activated by insulin or mitogens, can be completely inactivated with protein Ser/Thr phosphatases. Both ERK1 and ERK2 can phosphorylate and activate phosphatase-inactivated MAPKAP-K1/Rsk. That ERK1 and ERK2 are physiologically relevant MAPKAP-K1/Rsk kinases is evidenced by the observation that the ERKs are activated in vivo before MAPKAP-K1/Rsk activation, and

TABLE 9–1. Nomenclature

Name	Alternative Names*
MAPKs	
ERK1	p44-MAPK
ERK2	p42-MAPK
SAPK-α	JNK2, SAPK1a
SAPK-β	JNK3, SAPK1b
SAPK-γ	JNK1, SAPK1c
p38α	SAPK2a, CSBP1
p38β	SAPK2b
p38γ	SAPK3, ERK6
p38δ	SAPK4
MEKs	
MEK1	MAPKK1, MKK1
MEK2	MAPKK2, MKK2
SEK1	MKK4, JNK kinase (JNKK)-1, MEK4, SAPK-kinase (SKK)-1
MKK7	JNKK2, MEK7, SKK4
MKK3	MEK3, SKK2
MKK6	MEK6, SKK3
MAP3Ks	
MEKK4	MTK1
MLK32	MKN28 cell-derived Ser/Thr kinase (MST)
MLK3	SH3 domain–containing proline-rich kinase (SPRK), protein Tyr kinase-1 (PTK1)
DLK	MAPK upstream kinase (MUK), zipper-containing protein kinase (ZPK)

*Alternative nomenclature for mammalian MAPK pathway components. Only enzymes with multiple names are shown. Included are all accepted nomenclatures commonly used in the primary literature; however, not all of these are included in the text.

CSBP, cytokine-suppressive anti-inflammatory drug (CSAID)-binding protein; ERK, extracellular signal–regulated kinase; JNK, c-Jun NH₂-terminal kinase; MAPK, mitogen-activated protein kinase; MAP3K, MAPK kinase kinase; MAPKK, MAPK kinase; MLK, mixed-lineage kinase; MNK, MAPK-interacting kinase; MTK1, MAP three kinase-1; SAPK, stress-activated protein kinase; SH, Src homology.

high-resolution column chromatography and other methods have revealed that ERK1 and ERK2 represent the dominant, indeed the only insulin- and mitogen-activated MAPKAP-K1/Rsk kinases.[4, 5]

The mechanism by which ERK1 and ERK2 activate MAPKAP-K1/Rsk is complex (see Fig. 9–6B). Rsk requires a preliminary phosphorylation in the amino terminal catalytic domain (Ser222 of the subdomain VIII activation loop), which is probably catalyzed by PDK1. This phosphorylation is constitutive, occurring in resting cells, but is necessary for subsequent activation triggered by extracellular stimuli. The actual activating phosphorylations are catalyzed by the ERKs.[62a] MAPKs activate the carboxyl-terminal catalytic domain by phosphorylating Thr574 and participate in activation of the amino-terminal catalytic domain by phosphorylating Ser364 in the hinge region between the two kinase domains. The activated carboxyl-terminal catalytic domain then phosphorylates Ser381, also in the hinge region (trans-autophosphorylation), which together with phosphorylation of Ser364, fully activates the amino-terminal catalytic domain. Activation requires phosphorylation of Ser222 in the activation loop of the amino-terminal kinase domain which is catalyzed by PDK1 and occurs constitutively in resting cells, as noted previously. It is the amino-terminal kinase domain that is responsible for phosphorylation of MAPKAP-K1/Rsk substrates. Thr574, Ser364, and Ser381 all lie within the subdomain VIII activation loops.[63]

MNKs. Although dissociation of 4E-BP1 is probably the rate-limiting step in the regulation of formation of a functional eIF-4F complex (discussed above), eIF-4E itself also undergoes regulatory phosphorylation at Ser209 in response to both insulin/mitogen and environmental stress.[54, 64] This phosphorylation is thought to increase the affinity of eIF-4E for the 5′ cap, and both crystallographic and biochemical data indicate that phosphorylated eIF-4E is preferentially associated with the 5′ cap. The MAPK-interacting kinases (MNK1 and MNK2) are two closely related kinases that are the physiologically relevant eIF-4E Ser209 kinases. As the name implies, MNKs associate in vivo with MAPKs and are in vitro and in vivo MAPK substrates. MNKs are phosphorylated and activated both by ERK1 and ERK2 (in response to insulin and mitogens) and by the p38 MAPKs[64] (in response to stress, see below). The sites on the MNKs that are phosphorylated by MAPKs have not yet been determined.

Elk-1. One of the earliest transcriptional events known to occur in response to mitogen is the induction of c-*fos* expression. c-Fos is a bZIP transcription factor that together with c-Jun represents one form of the AP-1 transcription factor (discussed below).[65] AP-1 regulation is quite complex, and serum or growth factor induction of c-*fos* is one mechanism for AP-1 activation. Elevated levels of c-Fos polypeptide correlate well with elevations in AP-1 *trans*-activating activity.[65, 66]

The *fos* promoter contains a *cis*-acting element, the serum response element (SRE), that mediates the recruitment of transcription factors that induce *fos* expression. The SRE binds a heterodimeric transcription factor containing two polypeptides, serum response factor (SRF) and ternary complex factor (TCF).

TCFs comprise a family of Ets domain (related to avian leukemia virus oncogene *E t*wenty-*six*) transcription factors that includes Elk-1 and Sap-1. Regulation of Elk-1 by MAPKs has been characterized extensively. Activation of ERK1 and ERK2 (and, indeed, all MAPKs) coincides with the translocation of a portion of the ERK1/ERK2 pool to the nucleus (Fig. 9–8), thereby enabling phosphorylation of nuclear substrates.[4, 5, 65, 66] ERK1 and ERK2, as well as SAPKs/c-Jun NH₂-terminal kinases (JNKs), and at least one of the p38 MAPKs (discussed below), can phosphorylate two critical residues in the Elk-1 C-terminus (Ser383, Ser389). This activity enhances the binding of Elk-1 to the SRF and thereby elevates *trans*-activation at the SRE. By this process, both stress- and mitogen-regulated MAPKs contribute to c-*fos* induction[65] (see Fig. 9–8).

Crosstalk between the ERK and Other Signaling Pathways that Regulate Transcription: Phosphorylation by ERK1/ERK2 of PPARγ, the Estrogen Receptor, and STATs

Several important nuclear hormone receptors and transcription factors activated predominantly by signaling pathways outside the insulin/

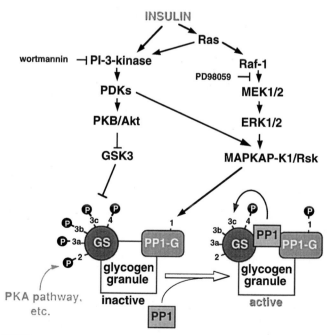

FIGURE 9–7. Insulin regulation of dephosphorylation and activation of skeletal muscle GS by the PKB/Akt → GSK3 and MAPK → MAPKAP-K1/Rsk mechanisms. PKB/Akt inhibits GSK3, thereby preventing its inhibitory phosphorylation of GS sites 3a to 3c and 4. MAPKAP-K1 phosphorylates site 1 of the PP1 glycogen targeting subunit (PP1-G), which accelerates the rate at which it dephosphorylates GS at sites 2 and 3a to 3c.

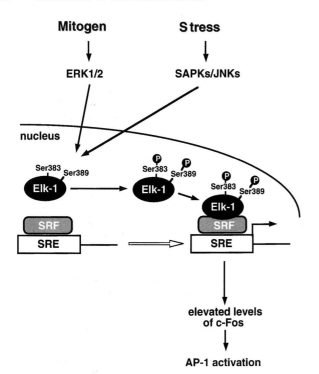

FIGURE 9–8. Coordinate regulation of Elk-1 and the SRE by MAPKs (ERKs and SAPKs/JNKs). MAPKs phosphorylate Elk-1 at Ser383 and Ser389. This reaction fosters enhanced binding to SRF, which in turn promotes *trans*-activation of the SRE. The resulting elevations in c-fos expression contribute to AP-1 activation.

mitogen pathways discussed herein are also substrates of the ERK pathway. Phosphorylation by the ERKs influences the activity of these transcription factors and allows for modulation of nuclear hormone receptors and other transcription factors not normally recruited by insulin or mitogen.

PPARγ. Peroxisome proliferator–activated receptor-γ (PPARγ) is a member of the nuclear hormone receptor family that includes the steroid hormone receptors (see Chapter 10). PPARγ is expressed primarily in adipose tissue and binds several compounds, including synthetic antidiabetic thiazolidinediones and 15-deoxy-$\Delta^{12,\ 14}$prostaglandin J_2. Binding of these compounds activates the *trans*-activating function of PPARγ and results in a powerful adipogenic response. PPARγ-mediated adipogenesis can be inhibited by contemporaneous administration of serum or growth factors such as PDGF. Insulin has a more complicated role in the development of adipose cells in that it serves as either a growth or differentiation factor, depending on the specific cell type. Preadipocytes express few insulin receptors, but they generally undergo adipogenesis in response to insulin or insulin-like growth factor type I (IGF-I) and growth in response to mitogens such as PDGF. By contrast, mature, differentiated adipocytes express large numbers of insulin receptors and undergo lipogenesis in response to insulin (as a result of the ability of insulin to activate lipogenic enzymes and stimulate glucose transporter-4 (GLUT4)-mediated glucose transport).

Rat fibroblasts programmed to express large numbers of insulin receptors respond to insulin with cell growth; however, expression of PPARγ in National Institutes of Health (NIH) 3T3 fibroblasts (NIH PPARγ cells) will result in insulin stimulation of adipogenesis. Accordingly, mitogen but not insulin treatment of NIH PPARγ cells stimulates the phosphorylation of Ser112 of PPARγ and results in inhibition of PPARγ *trans*-activating activity and adipogenesis. ERK1 and ERK2 are poorly activated by insulin but strongly activated by mitogens (EGF, PDGF) in NIH 3T3 cells. ERK1 and ERK2 can phosphorylate the Ser112 of PPARγ, and inhibition of ERK activity blocks mitogenic inhibition of PPARγ-induced adipogenesis.[67]

ESTROGEN RECEPTOR. The estrogen receptor is a member of the nuclear hormone receptor superfamily (see Chapter 10). Maximal

activation of the estrogen receptor requires not only the binding of estrogen but also phosphorylation of Ser118 in the amino-terminal transcriptional activation function-1 (AF-1) domain (see Chapter 10). This phosphorylation is catalyzed by ERK1 and ERK2 and is stimulated in vivo by EGF, IGF-I, and transforming alleles of *ras*.[68] From a clinical standpoint, this finding is particularly important inasmuch as physiologic responses to estrogen and other steroid hormones often require the collaboration of polypeptide growth factors; moreover, regulation of the estrogen receptor by the ERKs indicates a convergence of steroid hormone and mitogen action. In addition, many breast cancers that require estrogen for viability also manifest genetic amplification of the *ras* proto-oncogene.

STATs. The signal transducers and activators of transcription (STATs) are a family of SH2 domain–containing transcription factors that are activated by a wide variety of mitogens and cytokines, including EGF, PDGF, interleukin-6 (IL-6), interferon-γ, growth hormone, and the antilipogenic hormone leptin. Many of these agonists (IL-6, growth hormone, and leptin, in particular) act through a common signaling receptor subunit, gp130, that couples to specific agonist binding receptor subunits. Recruitment of the STATs requires agonist activation of the Janus kinase (JAK) family of Tyr kinases. JAKs phosphorylate the STATs at Tyr residues. Tyr phosphorylation of STATs results in dimerization mediated by the binding of P-Tyr on one STAT to the SH2 domain on its partner. STAT dimerization is followed by nuclear translocation and *trans*-activation of STAT-responsive genes that contain a consensus interferon-γ activation site (consensus ATTTCCCCGAAAT). In addition to Tyr phosphorylation, STATs also require ERK-catalyzed Ser phosphorylation for maximal *trans*-activating function.[69]

Regulation of ERK1 and ERK2 by MEK1 and MEK2

Partial purification of ERK2 from ^{32}P-labeled, mitogen-stimulated cells revealed that upon insulin stimulation, ERK1 underwent concomitant Tyr and Thr phosphorylation. It was subsequently demonstrated that ERK2 could be inactivated with Tyr-specific protein phosphatases, which selectively dephosphorylate the P-Tyr, and with Ser/Thr-specific phosphatases, which selectively dephosphorylate the P-Thr. These results indicated that ERK2 requires both Tyr and Thr phosphorylation for activity. The sites of phosphorylation of ERK2 were mapped to Thr185 and Tyr187, sites located in the activation loop of subdomain VIII of the catalytic domain[4, 5] (Fig. 9–9).

The existence of a MAPK "activator" was first demonstrated by fractionating cytosolic extracts of EGF-treated cells on ion-exchange columns and assaying the fractions for an activity that could activate ERK1 and/or ERK2 in vitro. It was observed that a single peak of activity could catalyze Tyr and Thr phosphorylation and activation of ERK1 and ERK2. Purification and molecular cloning of this activity revealed a family of novel dual-specificity (Thr/Tyr) protein kinases

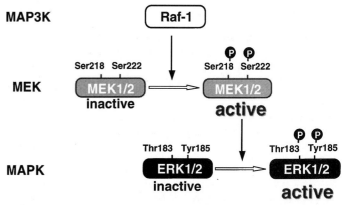

FIGURE 9–9. The Raf → ERK three-tiered MAPK core signaling module. Phosphorylation is indicated with the white P in the black circle.

variously termed MAPK kinase-1 and MAPK kinase-2 (MAPKK1/MAPKK2) or MEK1/MEK2.[4, 5]

As with ERK1 and ERK2, MEK1 and MEK2 share a remarkable homology with kinases from lower eukaryotes. Thus Fus3p and Kss1p, MAPKs of the *S. cerevisiae* mating pheromone response pathway, are regulated in vivo by a MEK homologue, Ste7p. Likewise, Hog1p, a MAPK of the *S. cerevisiae* osmosensing pathway, is activated by the MEK Pbs2p (see Fig. 9–5B).[4, 5, 55]

MEK1 and MEK2 Are Substrates of the Raf-1 Proto-oncoprotein

Any notions of a swift completion of the characterization of the ERK pathway were dashed when it was shown that MEK1 and MEK2 were inactivated not by Tyr phosphatases but by Ser/Thr phosphatases. Thus at least one Ser/Thr kinase lay between MEK1 and MEK2 and receptor Tyr kinases.[4, 5]

Raf-1 is the normal cellular homologue of v-*raf*, an acutely transforming oncogene that encodes a Ser/Thr protein kinase (see Fig. 9–11A). Raf-1 is one of a small family of related Ser/Thr kinases, A-Raf, B-Raf, and Raf-1, all of which share similar properties.[4, 5] Several observations pointed to the possibility that Raf-1 was upstream of ERK1 and ERK2. First, some v-*raf*–transformed cells manifest constitutively active ERK1 and ERK2. Second, expression of dominant inhibitory constructs of Raf-1 could block induction of AP-1 in response to mitogens. As noted above, AP-1 can be regulated in part by the ERK pathway via Elk-1/SRF induction of c-*fos*.[4, 5, 65] However, there remained the possibility that Raf-1 was not upstream of the ERKs, a hypothesis based on the observation that not all *raf*-transformed cells displayed constitutive MAPK activation. Moreover, yeast studies had identified protein kinases homologous to *STE11* as MEK activators[4, 5, 55] (see Fig. 9–5B). Although mammalian kinases homologous to *STE11* have been identified (e.g., MEK kinase-1 [MEKK1], see below), the sequence of Raf-1 has no significant homology to *STE11* outside the regions shared by all protein kinases.[4, 5, 55]

The placement of Raf-1 as a direct upstream activator of MEK1 and MEK2 was established with the observation that upon phosphatase inactivation, purified MEK could be phosphorylated and reactivated by purified oncogenic Raf-1.[4, 5, 70] It was subsequently shown that endogenous Raf-1 activity toward MEK1 was stably activated by insulin and mitogens. Detailed analysis of Raf-1 phosphorylation of MEK1 indicated that MEK1 was phosphorylated at Ser218 and Ser222. Again, these residues lie within the activation loop of subdomain VIII of the catalytic domain[4, 5] (see Fig. 9–9).

Ras, a Molecular Switch that Couples Tyrosine Kinases to Raf-1 and the ERK Pathway

Activating mutations in one or more of the *ras* proto-oncogenes are present in at least 30% of human cancers. Accordingly, the role of Ras proteins in mitogenic signaling has attracted widespread interest. Three *ras* proteins have been identified, Ha-Ras, Ki-Ras and N-Ras. These proteins constitute a subfamily, the Ras subfamily, of a large superfamily of small monomeric GTPases referred to as the Ras superfamily.[4, 5, 56, 71]

Ras superfamily proteins are molecular switches that relay signals from receptor complexes to downstream effectors. All Ras proteins bind the guanine nucleotides guanosine triphosphate (GTP) and guanosine diphosphate (GDP) and possess a slow, intrinsic GTPase activity. Ras proteins are competent to signal downstream when they have GTP bound. GDP-bound Ras proteins are inactive[4, 5, 56, 71] (Fig. 9–10A and B).

Members of the Ras superfamily also share a common structural configuration (see Fig. 9–10A). At the N-terminus is a GTP-binding domain, followed by the effector loop, a domain that binds downstream effector proteins. Two switch domains (switch-I and switch-II) are also present and undergo conformational changes when Ras pro-

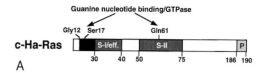

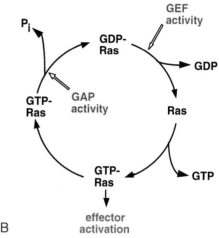

FIGURE 9–10. *Regulation of signaling by Ras superfamily GTPases. The Ras subfamily is shown here as a canonical example. A, Schematic structure of Ha-Ras. Residues essential to guanine nucleotide binding and GTPase activity (Gly12, Ser17, and Gln61) are indicated. S1, switch-I domain; S2, switch-II domain; P, prenylation/palmitoylation domain. Amino acid numbers are indicated. B, The cycle of activation/inactivation of Ras superfamily proteins.*

teins exchange GDP for GTP. The switch-I domain overlaps considerably with the effector loop, whereas the switch-II domain contains residues important to Ras GTPase activity. Crystallographic studies indicate that GTP binding causes conformational changes that render switch-I accessible to effector proteins. At the extreme C-terminus of mature Ras family proteins is the CAAX domain, a region of posttranslational modification: prenylation (farnesylation in the case of the Ras subfamily and geranylgeranylation in the case of the Rho subfamily) and palmitoylation. These lipid modifications localize Ras proteins to the inner leaflet of the plasma membrane and are essential for Ras protein function—one of the major roles of Ras superfamily proteins is to recruit effector proteins to the plasma membrane.[4, 5, 56, 71]

Activation of Ras superfamily proteins is catalyzed by GEFs (see Chapter 4). These proteins act to accelerate the dissociation of GDP (see Fig. 9–10B). Inasmuch as GTP is in excess in the cytosol, GDP dissociation is quickly followed by GTP binding and activation of the Ras protein signaling capacity.[4, 6, 56, 71] Inactivation of Ras superfamily proteins is catalyzed by GTPase-activating proteins (GAPs). These proteins act to accelerate the rate of Ras protein GTPase activity (see Fig. 9–10B). By extension, then, GTPase-deficient mutants of Ras proteins, such as Val12-Ras, are constitutively active and oncogenic. Conversely, Ras superfamily proteins, such as Asn17-Ras, that cannot exchange GDP for GTP if overexpressed, can titer out or sequester GEFs and prevent activation of endogenous, wild-type Ras proteins.[4, 5, 56, 71]

That proteins of the Ras subfamily of the Ras superfamily were involved in insulin and mitogen signaling and, in particular, activation of the ERKs became clear as a consequence of several independent lines of investigation. First, treatment of cells with insulin or mitogen was shown to stimulate the GTP loading of Ras. Moreover, either ectopic expression or scrape loading of cells with Val12–Ha-Ras resulted in activation of the ERKs. Furthermore, the addition of active, GTP-loaded Val12–Ha-Ras to cell extracts could trigger ERK activation. In addition, several genetic models of tyrosine kinase signaling, in particular, the *sevenless* Tyr kinase pathway of *Drosophila* photoreceptor development and the vulval induction pathway in the nematode worm *Caenorhabditis elegans*, implicated Ras as a downstream effector of receptor Tyr kinases. Finally, ectopic overexpression of dominant inhibitory Asn17–Ha-Ras could effectively block activation of the ERKs by mitogens and insulin, thus suggesting that Ras was downstream of mitogen receptors in mammalian cells.[4, 5, 56, 71]

GTP-loaded Ras activates the ERK pathway by directly binding and promoting activation of Raf family kinases (see Fig. 9–11B). The identification of Raf-1 as a direct effector for GTP-loaded Ras came from biochemical and genetic studies which showed that the two polypeptides could interact in vivo and in vitro.[4, 5, 72] The Raf-1 polypeptide consists of three domains conserved among Raf family members: a carboxyl-terminal kinase domain (conserved region-3 [CR-3]); CR-2, a Ser/Thr-rich hinge domain; and CR-1, an amino-terminal regulatory domain that contains a canonical Ras-binding domain (RBD) and a cysteine-rich zinc finger motif (the CRD, Fig. 9–11A). The interaction of Ras and Raf-1 is mediated in large part by interactions between the Raf-1 RBD and the Ras effector loop and between the Ras CAAX motif and the CRD of Raf-1 CR-1 (see Fig. 9–11B).[5]

Binding of Raf-1 to Ras is insufficient for Raf-1 activation, and the exact mechanism of Raf-1 activation has not been elucidated completely. It is apparent that Ras fosters Raf-1 phosphorylation and oligomerization, both of which appear necessary for Raf-1 activation.[4,]

[5, 73] Current evidence suggests that Raf-1 is maintained in an inactive state by interactions with a dimeric form of the protein 14-3-3ζ.[5, 74] 14-3-3 proteins represent a large class of abundant cytosolic polypeptides that can simultaneously homodimerize and heterodimerize with several signaling proteins in a regulatory manner. 14-3-3 proteins require prior phosphorylation of their target proteins within the consensus motif Arg-P-Ser-X-X-Ser-Pro (X is any amino acid and P indicates phosphorylation) for binding.[75] Inactive Raf-1 residues P-Ser259 and P-Ser621 bind a homodimer of 14-3-3ζ. GTP-loaded Ras is thought to displace the 14-3-3ζ dimer from P-Ser259, leaving the 14-3-3ζ bound only to P-Ser621. GTP-loaded Ras also unmasks a set of as yet incompletely characterized phosphorylation sites in the Raf-1 CR-2 hinge region. These sites are then phosphorylated by upstream kinases, which have also yet to be identified. The free end of the 14-3-3 dimer, which had dissociated from Ser259, then binds to one of these newly phosphorylated sites to generate a stable, active Raf-1 conformation[5, 74] (see Fig. 9–11B).

Collaborative Activation of PI-3-Kinase by p85 and Ras

As mentioned above (see also Chapter 4), the activity of PI-3-kinase can be increased in vitro and in vivo upon binding of the p85 subunit SH2 domains to P-Tyr residues on receptor Tyr kinases, nonreceptor Tyr kinases, or IRS proteins. Although this activation is significant, full activation of PI-3-kinase by mitogens also requires GTP-loaded Ras.[76] Thus coexpression of Val12-Ras and PI-3-kinase results in substantial PI-3-kinase activation in the absence of mitogen. GTP-loaded Ras binds to the p110 catalytic subunit of PI-3-kinase in a manner that is independent of the p85 subunit. Lysine 227 of the α isoform of p110 appears to be critical for Ras–PI-3-kinase interaction, and mutation of this residue results in a construct that can no longer be activated by Ras. This construct can still be activated by the P-Tyr–p85 interaction, however.[76, 77] Therefore, Ras is a crucial regulator not only of the MAPK pathway but also of signaling to PI-3-kinase.

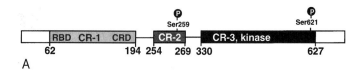

A

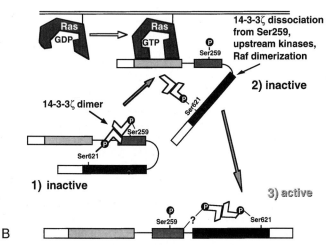

B

FIGURE 9–11. *Structure and regulation of Raf-1. A, Structure of c-Raf-1. Constitutively phosphorylated residues are indicated with the white P in the black circle. CR, conserved region; RBD, canonical Ras-binding domain—this region binds the Ras effector loop; CRD, cysteine-rich Zn finger domain, which contributes to binding the Ras C-terminus. B, Hypothetical model of Raf-1 regulation based on current evidence. In resting cells Raf-1 is held in an inactive conformation by a dimer of 14-3-3ζ that interacts with phosphorylated Ser621 and Ser259. Binding of Ras displaces the 14-3-3ζ dimer from Ser259 and exposes additional phosphorylation sites. These sites are phosphorylated by unidentified kinases. Ras also fosters Raf-1 dimerization, which is, in addition to phosphorylation, important to Raf regulation. Phosphorylation of Raf reorients the binding of the 14-3-3ζ such that it now interacts with one of the newly phosphorylated sites (indicated with ?). This interaction results in a stable, active conformation.*

THE SAPK/JNK, p38, AND NF-κB PATHWAYS: MAMMALIAN SIGNALING PATHWAYS ACTIVATED BY ENVIRONMENTAL STRESS AND INFLAMMATORY CYTOKINES

General Considerations

The cellular and physiologic responses to inflammation are central to the pathology of a number of important conditions, including ischemic injury, endotoxin shock, arthritis, inflammatory bowel disease, and diabetic nephropathy. From the point of view of the endocrinologist, an understanding of these mechanisms is critical inasmuch as many inflammatory conditions are treated with steroids or steroid analogues. It has become clear that parallel mammalian MAPK pathways exist and that these, in conjunction with the nuclear factor κB (NF-κB) pathway (discussed below), are pivotal to the inflammatory response. A subset of the targets of these stress-activated MAPK pathways, transcription factors, can interact antagonistically with the targets of steroidal anti-inflammatory pharmaceuticals, and mutual antagonism of these steroids and the stress signaling pathways forms the basis of steroidal anti-inflammatory action. As mammalian stress-activated signaling pathways are elucidated, it is becoming clear that these pathways will be important novel targets for anti-inflammatory therapies.

Mammalian Stress-Activated MAPKs

The existence of multiple MAPK pathways in yeast (see Fig. 9–5B) was an indication that mammalian cells possessed analogous signaling mechanisms. Indeed, indications that mammalian cells had several

MAPK pathways came shortly after identification of the ERKs during the search for potential regulators of p70 S6 kinase.[55, 57, 58] The protein synthesis inhibitor cycloheximide, when administrated to rats, can elicit the in vivo activation of ribosomal S6 phosphorylation, and in fact, this strategy was used to activate p70 S6 kinase in vivo before purification.[4, 26] Although no p70 activators were uncovered with this strategy, the idea that cycloheximide could recruit p70 led to the notion that several protein kinase signaling pathways might be activated by cycloheximide.

This hypothesis was proved correct when it was demonstrated that injection of cycloheximide into rats activated a Ser/Thr kinase activity that could be inactivated with Tyr or Ser/Thr phosphatases, thus indicating that like the ERKs, this kinase required concomitant Tyr and Ser/Thr phosphorylation for activity. This novel MAPK was initially referred to as p54 because the purified kinase was observed to migrate at 54 kDa on SDS polyacrylamide gels.[4, 5, 57, 58, 78, 79]

The substrate specificity of this kinase differed from that of the ERKs. In particular, p54 was unable to activate MAPKAP-K1/Rsk in vitro under conditions wherein ERK-mediated activation of MAPKAP-K1/Rsk was observed. More importantly, p54 was able to phosphorylate the c-Jun transcription factor at two sites (Ser63 and Ser73) implicated in the regulation of c-Jun and AP-1 *trans*-activation function[4, 78–80] (see below).

Immunoprecipitation of endogenous p54 from extracts of cells subjected to various treatments revealed that in most cells, p54 was not strongly activated by mitogens such as insulin, EGF, PDGF, or FGF. By contrast, p54 was vigorously activated by environmental stresses such as heat shock, ionizing radiation, oxidant stress, DNA-damaging chemicals such as topoisomerase inhibitors and alkylating agents, reperfusion injury, mechanical shear stress, and of course, protein synthesis inhibitors. In addition, p54 could be activated by vasoactive peptides (endothelin and angiotensin II) and inflammatory cytokines of the TNF family (TNF, IL-1, CD40 ligand, CD27 ligand, Fas ligand, etc.).[57–59, 81, 82] p54 has since been renamed, and the nomenclature of this family of kinases is somewhat confusing (see Table 9–1). Two systems are generally accepted: SAPK in reference to regulation of these kinases by environmental stress and inflammation and JNK in reference to phosphorylation of the c-Jun amino-terminal *trans*-activation domain by these kinases (see below).

Molecular cloning of SAPK/JNK revealed a family of at least three genes (see Table 9–1): SAPKα/JNK2, SAPKβ/JNK3, and SAPKγ/JNK1. Like the ERKs, each of these genes contains a characteristic phosphoacceptor loop in subdomain VIII of the protein kinase catalytic domain. The ERK sequence is Thr-Glu-Tyr, whereas that of the SAPKs/JNKs is Thr-Pro-Tyr. The SAPK/JNK genes are further diversified into up to 12 polypeptides by differential mRNA splicing.[57, 58, 81, 82]

The p38 MAPKs represent a third mammalian MAPK family. p38 was originally described as a 38-kDa polypeptide that underwent Tyr phosphorylation in response to endotoxin treatment and osmotic shock. p38 was purified by antiphosphotyrosine immunoaffinity chromatography, and cDNA cloning revealed that p38 was the mammalian MAPK homologue most closely related to *HOG1*, the osmosensing MAPK of *S. cerevisiae* (see Fig. 9–5B). Most notably, the p38s, like Hog1p, contain the phosphoacceptor sequence Thr-Gly-Tyr.[55, 83]

Of particular interest, p38 was also independently purified as a polypeptide that could bind to a class of experimental pyridinylimidazole anti-inflammatory drugs, the cytokine-suppressive anti-inflammatory drugs (CSAIDs). CSAIDs were originally characterized as compounds that could inhibit the transcriptional induction of TNF and IL-1 during endotoxin shock. As we shall see, the basis for these compounds' efficacy as anti-inflammatory agents was their ability to bind and directly inhibit a subset of the p38s, thereby blocking p38-mediated activation of AP-1, a *trans*-acting factor crucial to TNF and IL-1 induction.[84]

Like the SAPKs/JNKs, p38 is one of a family of kinases. Four p38 genes have been described thus far (see Table 9–1): p38α (also called CSAID-binding protein [CSBP] and, somewhat confusingly, SAPK2a), p38β (also called SAPK2b), p38γ (also called SAPK3 and ERK6), and p38δ (also called SAPK4). Interestingly, only p38α/CSBP/SAPK2a and p38β/SAPK2b are inhibited by CSAIDs; p38γ/SAPK3/

ERK6 and p38δ/SAPK4 are completely unaffected by these drugs in vitro or in transfected cells.[83–86]

In further similarity with the SAPKs/JNKs, p38s are activated in vivo by environmental stresses and inflammatory cytokines and are only poorly activated by insulin and growth factors. In almost all instances, the same stimuli that recruit the SAPKs/JNKs also recruit the p38s. One important exception is ischemia-reperfusion. SAPKs/JNKs are selectively activated during reperfusion, whereas the p38s are activated during ischemia and remain active during reperfusion. The basis for this difference is unknown.[57, 58, 83–86]

SAPK/JNK and p38 Substrates

As with the ERKs, the SAPKs/JNKs and p38s phosphorylate both transcription factors and other protein kinases (Fig. 9–12). These reactions are important to the inflammatory response.

MAPKAP-K2 and MAPKAP-K3. In addition to transcription factors, p38 can phosphorylate other protein kinases. MAPKAP-K2 and the highly related MAPKAP-K3, which are structurally unrelated to MAPKAP-K1/Rsk, are Ser/Thr kinases that are responsible for phosphorylation of the small heat shock protein Hsp27. Nonphosphorylated Hsp27 normally exists in multimers that serve as molecular chaperones by assisting in maintaining protein conformation. Phosphorylation of Hsp27 by MAPKAP-K2 at residues Ser15, Ser78, and Ser82 correlates with the redistribution of Hsp27 to the actin cytoskeleton, where it may mediate the isolation of F-actin, thereby regulating cell motility.[57, 87, 88] MAPKAP-K2 is itself phosphorylated at residues Thr25, Thr222, and Ser272 by p38α/CSBP/SAPK2a and p38β/SAPK2b (but not p38γ/SAPK3 or p38δ/SAPK4) (see Fig. 9–12A). Phosphorylation of Thr25 gates the phosphorylation of Thr222 and Ser272, which reside in the kinase activation loop (see Fig. 9–12A). Together, these phosphorylations result in the activation of MAPKAP-K2, accompanied by an additional autophosphorylation at Thr334. Consistent with regulation by p38α/CSBP/SAPK2a and p38β/SAPK2b, MAPKAP-K2 activation and Hsp27 phosphorylation are inhibited by CSAIDs[89] (see Fig. 9–12A).

MNKs. The p38s can phosphorylate and activate MNK1 and MNK2 in response to stress and cytokines.[64] Thus the MNKs, as with AP-1 (see below), are a site of integration of stress and mitogenic signaling. MNK regulation and function are discussed above.

CHOP/GADD153. CREB homologous protein (CHOP)/growth arrest and DNA damage-153 (GADD153) is a CREB/ATF family member that is transcriptionally induced in response to genotoxic and inflammatory stresses (see Chapter 7). These stimuli can also activate the transcriptional regulatory functions of CHOP/GADD153 through agonist-induced phosphorylation of Ser78 and Ser81. CHOP/GADD153 acts as a transcriptional repressor of certain cAMP-regulated genes and a transcriptional activator of stress-induced genes. Recruitment of CHOP/GADD153 correlates with cell cycle arrest at G_1/S. This cell cycle arrest is an important consequence of DNA damage inasmuch as it allows for DNA repair before DNA replication, thereby preserving genomic integrity. p38α/CSBP/SAPK2a can phosphorylate CHOP/GADD153 at Ser78 and Ser81 in vivo and in vitro and is a likely regulator of CHOP/GADD153 function[90] (see Fig. 9–12B).

AP-1. The SAPKs/JNKs and p38s are the dominant Ser/Thr kinases responsible for recruitment, in response to environmental stresses and inflammatory stimuli, of the AP-1 transcription factor[4, 5, 57, 58] (see Fig. 9–12B). AP-1 is composed of bZIP transcription factors—typically c-Jun and JunD, along with members of the c-*fos* (usually c-Fos) and ATF (usually ATF2) families. ATFs are a subgroup of the CREB family[32, 33] (see Chapter 7). All bZIP transcription factors contain leucine zippers that enable homodimerization and heterodimerization, and AP-1 components are organized into Jun-Jun, Jun-Fos, or Jun-ATF dimers.[66]

The presence of Jun family members enables AP-1 to bind to *cis*-acting elements containing TRE (consensus sequence: TGA$^C/_G$TCA).[32, 33, 70] AP-1 heterodimers containing ATF transcription factors can also bind to CRE (consensus sequence: TGACGTCA; see Chapter 7). AP-1 is an important *trans*-activator of a number of stress-responsive

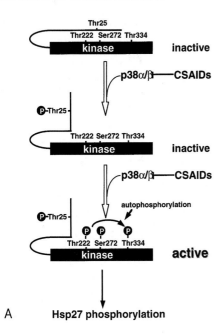

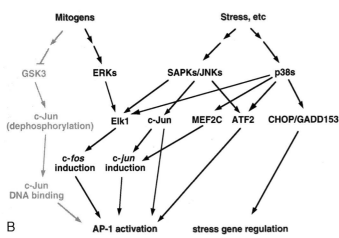

FIGURE 9–12. Functions of the p38 and SAPK/JNK pathways. *A,* Regulation of MAPKAP-K2 by p38α/SAPK2α/CSBP1 or p38β/SAPK2β. Phosphorylation of Thr25 gates phosphorylation of sites in the kinase domain activation loop (Thr222, Ser272). The site of action of CSAIDs is indicated. *B,* Regulation of transcription factors by MAPKs, including the complex regulation of AP-1. ERKs, SAPKs/JNKs, and p38s phosphorylate Elk-1, which elevates c-Fos levels. p38 activates MEF2C, which contributes to c-*jun* induction. Elevations in the levels of c-Fos and c-Jun contribute to AP-1 activation. In addition, SAPKs/JNKs phosphorylate and activate the *trans*-activating activity of c-Jun and ATF2. p38 can also activate the *trans*-activating activity of ATF2, which also results in AP-1 activation. AP-1 binding to a TRE in the c-*jun* promoter contributes (along with MEF2C) to further c-*jun* induction and even greater AP-1 activation. The PKB/Akt GSK3 mechanism contributes to AP-1 activation by inhibiting c-Jun phosphorylation in the C-terminal sites. This activity fosters enhanced c-Jun DNA binding. p38 can also activate CHOP/GADD153, another member of the CREB/ATF family.

genes, including the genes for IL-1, IL-2, and TNF. In addition, AP-1 participates in the transcriptional induction of cell adhesion proteins important to inflammation, including E-selectin.[66]

Activation of AP-1 involves both the direct phosphorylation/dephosphorylation of AP-1 components and the phosphorylation and activation of transcription factors that induce elevated expression of c-*jun* or c-*fos*. Both events can be activated independently by several

pathways.[66] Phosphorylation of c-Jun or ATF2 within their *trans*-activation domains correlates well with enhanced *trans*-activating activity[66] (see Figs. 9–12B and 9–13). The SAPKs/JNKs can phosphorylate the c-Jun *trans*-activating domain at Ser63 and Ser73. These residues are phosphorylated in vivo under conditions wherein the SAPKs are activated, and depletion of SAPK/JNK from cell extracts removes all stress-activated c-Jun kinase. Thus the SAPKs/JNKs appear to be the dominant kinases responsible for c-Jun phosphorylation.[81, 91] JunD is also phosphorylated by SAPKs, albeit less effectively than c-Jun. This phosphorylation occurs at Ser90 and Ser100, a region of the JunD *trans*-activation domain similar to the phosphoacceptor domain of c-Jun[92] (Fig. 9–13A and B).

Both the SAPKs and p38s can phosphorylate ATF2 at Thr69 and Ser71 in the *trans*-activation domain. Again, these residues are phosphorylated under circumstances in which the SAPKs/JNKs and/or the p38s are activated (see Figs. 9–12A and 9–13D), and phosphorylation of ATF2 activates its *trans*-activating activity. Whether the SAPKs/JNKs or p38s represent the dominant ATF2 kinases depends on the cell type and stimulus used. During reperfusion of ischemic kidney, for example, the SAPKs/JNKs are the only detectable ATF2 kinases. By contrast, in response to IL-1, the p38s are the major ATF2 kinases activated in KB keratinocytes.[85, 86, 93]

The SAPKs/JNKs and p38s also contribute to AP-1 activation by stimulating the transcription of genes encoding AP-1 components. Thus the SAPKs/JNKs and p38α can phosphorylate Elk-1 at Ser383 and Ser389, the same sites phosphorylated by the ERKs. This phosphorylation results in activation of the SRF and induction of c-*fos* expression. The p38s can also phosphorylate at Thr293 and Thr300 and activate the *trans*-activating activity of the transcription factor myocyte enhancer factor-2C (MEF2C). A *cis*-element for MEF2C resides in the promoter for c-Jun; thus p38 activation can contribute to induction of c-*jun* expression. The c-Jun promoter also contains a consensus AP-1 site and can therefore be autoregulated by elements that activate AP-1.[65, 66, 94]

MAPK Substrates Often Possess MAPK-Binding Sites that Confer MAPK Substrate Specificity: The SAPK/JNK–c-Jun Interaction

Phosphorylation of c-Jun by the SAPKs/JNKs illustrates an important point about the mechanism of substrate recognition by members of the MAPK family. All MAPKs are "proline directed" in that they phosphorylate Ser/Thr residues only if followed immediately by proline.[4, 5, 42] However, the specificity of MAPKs for their physiologic substrates is often dictated in large part by the presence of binding sites, often distal from the phosphoacceptor sites, that are specific for distinct MAPK subgroups. These MAPK-binding sites allow for the selective interaction between MAPKs and their true in vivo substrates.[4, 5, 57, 66, 92] Phosphorylation of Jun family transcription factors by the SAPKs/JNKs is an excellent example. Thus the SAPKs/JNKs, but not the ERKs or p38s, bind c-Jun quite strongly.[91, 92] The SAPK/JNK-binding site on c-Jun lies between residues 30 and 50, well away from Ser63 and Ser73, the sites of phosphorylation. This binding site lies within the so-called δ domain (amino acids 30–57), a hydrophobic region initially implicated in the regulation of c-Jun oncogenicity because of its deletion in oncogenic v-Jun[4, 5, 91, 92] (for this reason, v-Jun is not a SAPK/JNK substrate) (see Figs. 9–13A–C).

The presence of the SAPK/JNK-binding site coupled with the ability of c-Jun to heterodimerize with other members of the Jun family enables the SAPKs/JNKs to phosphorylate other AP-1 constituents in vivo and in vitro that as monomers or homodimers are ordinarily poor SAPK/JNK substrates (see Fig. 9–13C). Thus although JunD possesses a phosphoacceptor region and even a SAPK/JNK-binding pocket homologous to those of c-Jun (see Fig. 9–13B), JunD binds SAPK/JNK poorly. Accordingly, JunD is not ordinarily a SAPK/JNK substrate in vitro; however, when heterodimerized with c-Jun, JunD can undergo SAPK/JNK-catalyzed phosphorylation and activation in vivo and in vitro (see Fig. 9–13B and C). JunB, by contrast, possesses a SAPK/

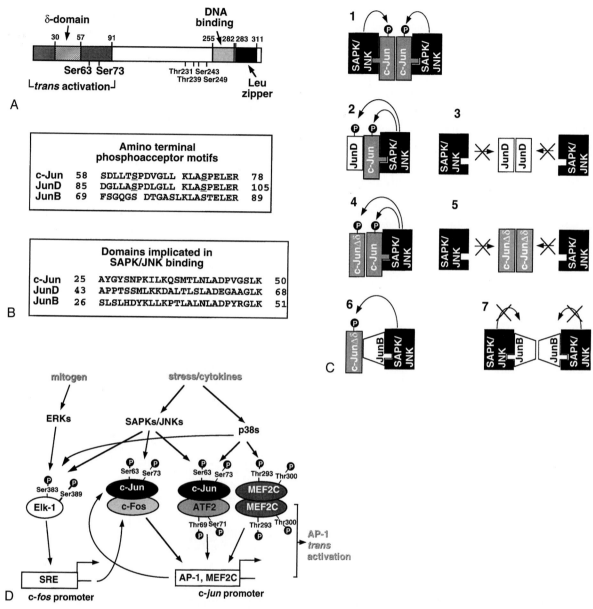

FIGURE 9–13. Mechanistic characteristics of the regulation of AP-1 by MAPKs. *A,* Schematic structure of c-Jun. Note that the SAPK/JNK-binding pocket (amino acids [AAs] 30–50, which lie within the δ domain [AAs 30–57]) is considerably distal from the sites of phosphorylation (Ser63 and Ser73). The C-terminal GSK3 phosphorylation sites near the DNA-binding domain are indicated. *B,* Comparison of phosphoacceptor and SAPK/JNK-binding motifs among members of the Jun family. Phosphorylated residues are underlined, and a single-letter amino acid code is used; gaps are introduced to optimize alignment. Note that JunB contains two protential phosphorylation sites; however, these sites are not followed by Pro. MAPKs are proline directed, and therefore JunB cannot undergo SAPK/JNK-catalyzed phosphorylation. Noe also that JunD contains a putative SAPK/JNK-binding pocket that is significantly similar to that of c-Jun and JunB. In spite of this similarity, JunD cannot interact strongly with SAPK/JNK. *C,* Phosphorylation of Jun family members by SAPKs/JNKs involves both the presence of a SAPK/JNK-binding site and SAPK/JNK proline-directed phosphorylation sites and the ability of Jun family members to dimerize. Thus in *(1),* SAPK/JNK binds c-Jun dimers, and can phosphorylate the canonical proline-directed sites. In *(2),* JunD heterodimerizes with c-Jun, which in turn binds SAPK/JNK. in this scheme, both proteins, which have phosphoacceptor sites for SAPK/JNK, are phosphorylated, whereas in *(3),* JunD homodimers cannot bind SAPK/JNK and undergo SAPK/JNK-catalyzed phosphorylation in spite of the presence of phosphoacceptor sites. Similarly, in *(5),* deletion of the δ domain (c-JunΔδ) from c-Jun abrogates SAPK/JNK binding and, accordingly, phosphorylation; however, if c-JunΔδ heterodimerizes with a Jun partner with an intact SAPK/JNK-binding pocket (such as wild-type c-Jun in *(4)* or JunB in *(6),* it can be phosphorylated by SAPK/JNK bound to the wild-type c-Jun or JunB. Finally, in *(7),* although JunB can bind SAPK/JNK, it cannot be phosphorylated because of a lack of suitable phosphoacceptor sites. *D,* Induction of AP-1 components plus direct phosphorylation of AP-1 components contributes to activation of AP-1 by MAPK pathways.

JNK-binding pocket and binds SAPK/JNK well, but it does not possess the proline-directed phosphoacceptor sites that are prerequisite for SAPK/JNK phosphorylation. Thus JunB can bind SAPK/JNK, but it is not phosphorylated in vivo or in vitro by SAPK/JNK. However, JunB can heterodimerize with c-Jun mutants missing the δ domain and foster SAPK/JNK phosphorylation of these mutants. Interestingly, JunB can function as a negative regulator of c-Jun[91, 92] (see Fig. 9–13A and C).

Regulation of AP-1 Involves the Integration of Several MAPK Pathways and Is Mediated by Divergent AP-1 Component Transcription Factor Subunits

How does the complex regulation of AP-1 constituent transcription factors translate into the recruitment of AP-1 by extracellular stimuli? The various aspects of AP-1 regulation, activation of constituent transcription factor expression and direct phosphorylation/activation of constituent transcription factors, can be independently regulated by several pathways.[66] Thus mitogenic stimuli, which preferentially recruit the ERKs and inhibit GSK3 (via PKB/Akt), will preferentially activate AP-1, respectively, through enhancement of expression of AP-1 components (via ERK phosphorylation of Elk-1, which results in c-*fos* expression, for example) and through the relief of GSK3-mediated inhibition of c-Jun DNA binding[4, 5, 16, 65, 66, 81] (see Fig. 9–13D).

By contrast, stresses and inflammatory cytokines such as TNF, which preferentially activate the SAPKs/JNKs and p38s, can recruit AP-1 through direct phosphorylation of AP-1 components (c-Jun by SAPKs/JNKs and ATF2 by both SAPKs/JNKs and p38s). However, stress pathways can also promote enhanced expression of AP-1 components through recruitment of Elk-1 (mediated by SAPK/JNK and p38α phosphorylation), which results in elevated c-*fos* expression, and through p38-catalyzed phosphorylation of MEF2C. Both MEF2C and AP-1 itself can bind and *trans*-activate the promoter for c-Jun.[4, 5, 65, 66, 81, 82, 93, 94] Stresses can also modestly recruit PKB/Akt, which in turn can inhibit GSK3 and thereby block its negative regulation of c-Jun DNA binding[12, 16] (see Fig. 9–13D).

Finally, the c-Jun promoter contains an AP-1 site; thus c-*jun* expression can be autoregulated by any pathway that activates AP-1[66] (see Fig. 9–13D).

MEKs and MAP3Ks Upstream of the SAPKs/JNKs and p38s

As with the ERK pathway and all MAPK pathways, the p38 and SAPK/JNK pathways are organized into three-tiered MAP3K → MEK → MAPK core signaling modules.[55, 57, 58] At least two MEKs have been identified as activators of p38, MAPK kinase-3 (MKK3) and MKK6.[57, 58, 95, 96] Likewise, the SAPKs/JNKs are activated by at least two MEKs, SAPK/ERK-kinase-1 (SEK1, also called MKK4) and MKK7 (see Table 9–1 and Fig. 9–14A).[57, 58, 95–99] Biochemical and genetic studies indicate that in spite of the fact that the SAPKs/JNKs and p38s are each activated by multiple MEKs, the functions of these MEKs are not entirely redundant. SEK1/MKK4 and MKK7 have considerably overlapping substrate specificity with regard to the different SAPK/JNK isoforms; however, MKK7 is significantly more sensitive to activation by inflammatory cytokines whereas SEK1/MKK4 is preferentially recruited by physical stresses such as hyperosmolar stress and protein synthesis inhibition.[97–100] MKK3 and MKK6 differ more substantially in their substrate selectivity. MKK3 preferentially activates p38α/CSBP/SAPK2a and p38β/SAPK2b, whereas MKK6 can strongly activate all known p38 isoforms. Similarly, MKK3 appears to be more restricted with regard to activation by upstream stimuli. Whereas MKK6 is activated by all known p38 activators, MKK3, like SEK1/MKK4, is more strongly activated by physical and chemical stresses.[101, 102]

A somewhat daunting array of diverse MAP3Ks have been impli-

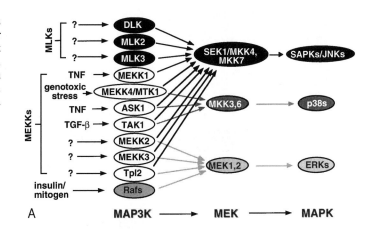

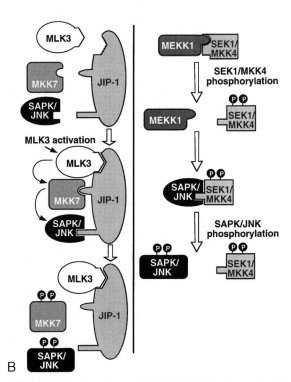

FIGURE 9–14. Mammalian stress-activated MAPK pathways illustrate the basic principles of MAPK pathways. *A*, Complexity of SAPK/JNK and p38 core signaling modules. Note the very large and diverse number of MAP3Ks upstream of p38-specific and, especially, SAPK/JNK-specific MEKs. Note also that many of these MAP3Ks have several MEK substrates. *B*, Scaffolding proteins in SAPK/JNK signaling. *Left*, JIP-1 is a distinct scaffold protein that nucleates a core signaling module consisting specifically of MLK3, MKK7, and SAPK/JNK. *Right*, SEK1/MKK4 has both kinase and scaffolding properties. The N-terminus (amino acids 1–77) of inactive, dephosphorylated SEK1/MKK4 can form a specific complex with the SAPK/JNK-specific MAP3K MEKK1. Upon phosphorylation and activation of SEK1/MKK4, this complex dissociates and the N-terminus of SEK1/MKK4 forms a new complex with inactive, dephosphorylated SAPK/JNK. Upon phosphorylation and activation of SAPK/JNK, this second complex dissociates. Thus the SEK scaffolding function is dynamic and ensures specific, coordinated, and sequential association with both upstream activators and downstream targets.

cated in regulation of the SAPKs/JNKs and p38s (see Fig. 9–14A). This diversity is consistent with the heterogeneous nature of the stimuli that recruit the SAPKs/JNKs and p38s. The MEKKs (see Table 9–1) are mammalian homologues of *S. cerevisiae* Ste11p, a MAP3K that regulates both the yeast mating pheromone and osmosensing pathways (see Figs. 9–5B and 9–14A). Mammalian MEKKs include MEKK1 to

MEKK4, apoptosis signal–regulating kinase-1 (ASK1), transforming growth factor-β (TGF-β)-activated kinase-1 (TAK1), Tpl-2 (the product of the *cot* proto-oncogene), and NF-κB–inducing kinase (NIK), which is an activator of the NF-κB pathway (discussed below).[55, 57, 103-113] MEKK1 can directly and strongly activate SEK1/MKK4 and MKK7 and is predominantly SAPK specific; however, under certain circumstances it weakly activates MEK1 and the mitogenic MAPK pathway. MEKK1 cannot recruit the p38 pathway.[57, 103, 111] MEKK4 (also called MAP three kinase-1 [MTK1]), ASK1, and TAK1 can each activate both the SAPK and p38 pathways with equal potency in vivo and can activate SEK1, MKK3, and MKK6 in vitro and in vivo.[57, 106-109, 113] MEKK2 and MEKK3, as well as Tpl-2, can activate both the SAPK pathway (via SEK1) and the mitogenic MAPK pathway[57, 105, 113] (via MEK1) (see Fig. 9–14A).

The mixed-lineage kinases (MLKs, see Table 9–1) are another family of MAP3Ks. These kinases bear structural homology to both Ser/Thr and Tyr kinases and also contain leucine zippers and SH3-binding sites, as well as, in the case of MLK2 and MLK3, SH3 domains. MLK2, MLK3, and dual-lineage kinase (DLK) are SAPK-specific MAP3Ks and can activate SEK1/MKK4 and MKK7 in vivo and in vitro.[57, 114-116] (see Fig. 9–14A).

Extracellular stimuli that recruit stress-responsive MAP3Ks have been identified in only a few cases. Thus TNF can activate ASK1 and, possibly, MEKK1 and NIK, whereas TGF-β can activate TAK1.[108-110, 112, 117] MEKK4/MTK1 appears to be a major MAP3K recruited by genotoxic stresses. These stresses induce the expression of a family of small polypeptides, the growth arrest and DNA damage-45 (GADD45) family. At least a subset of GADD45 proteins may bind and directly activate MEKK4/MTK1 in vivo and in vitro[118] (see Fig. 9–14A).

Stress-Activated MAPK Core Signaling Modules Illustrate General Principles of Eukaryotic Cell MAPK Signaling Modules

Three overarching principles of MAPK pathways are apparent from an examination of yeast signaling: (1) many MAPK signaling components have more than one biochemical/biologic function; (2) MAPK pathway components are often segregated by proteins with scaffolding properties, and these scaffold proteins may either be distinct or be intrinsic to the signaling kinases themselves; and (3) individual MAPK pathway elements are often subject to regulation by several divergent upstream activators[55] (see Fig. 9–5B). Mammalian stress signaling pathways possess all these properties.

With regard to signaling components with more than one function (or target), as we have seen, several MAP3Ks can impinge on more than one MAPK pathway. Thus, for example, ASK1 can activate both the SAPKs/JNKs and p38s whereas MEKK2 can activate both the ERK and SAPK/JNK pathways. Similarly, elements in mammalian stress-activated MAPK pathways can be activated by multiple mechanisms. Thus SEK1 is a substrate for several MAP3Ks, including the MLKs, and all of the MEKKs except for NIK. Similarly, p38 is a substrate for MKK3 and MKK6, whereas SAPKs/JNKs are activated by MKK7 and SEK1/MKK4[57, 93, 116] (see Fig. 9–14A).

Mammalian MAPK pathway scaffold proteins are only beginning to be identified. JNK-interacting protein-1 (JIP1) is a novel mammalian scaffold protein that forms a complex with MLK3, MKK7, and SAPK/JNK. MEKK1 and SEK1/MKK4 cannot bind JIP1 (see Fig. 9–14B). JIP1 consists of a C-terminal SH3 domain (amino acids 491–600), an N-terminal SAPK-binding site (amino acids 143–163), and an intermediate domain with several SH3-binding motifs. The MLK3-JIP1 interaction is mediated by the JIP1 SH3 domain and any of several SH3-binding sites on MLK3. MKK7 interacts with the middle segment of JIP1 (amino acids 283–571).[119, 120] The physiologic function of JIP1 is unclear; however, it is plausible to propose that as with the *S. cerevisiae* scaffold protein Ste5p (see Fig. 9–5B), JIP1 segregates individual SAPK/JNK core signaling modules and thereby allows for specific regulation and function.

As with the *S. cerevisiae* MEK Pbs2p (see Fig. 9–5B), SEK1/MKK4 possesses intrinsic scaffold properties. Thus the N-terminus (amino acids 1–77) of inactive, dephosphorylated SEK1/MKK4 can

specifically bind one of its upstream activators, MEKK1. Upon phosphorylation and activation of SEK1/MKK4, the SEK1/MKK4-MEKK1 complex dissociates and SEK1/MKK4 forms a second specific complex with SAPK/JNK, again mediated by the SEK1/MKK4 amino-terminal MEKK1-binding domain. Upon activation of SAPK/JNK, this second complex dissociates. The intrinsic scaffold properties of SEK1/MKK4 therefore enable it to form specific, sequential dynamic complexes with both an upstream activator and a substrate.[121]

Regulation of the SAPKs/JNKs and p38s by Rho Family GTPases

Although considerable progress has been made in the identification of MEKs and MAP3Ks that recruit the SAPKs/JNKs and p38s, elucidation of the molecular mechanisms of MAP3K regulation has been difficult and little is known of the physiologic function and coupling to cell surface receptors of stress-regulated MAP3Ks. However, as with the Ras-ERK pathway, evidence is accumulating that Ras superfamily GTPases may couple the SAPKs/JNKs and p38s to selective upstream activators.

Thus GTPases of the Rho subfamily of the Ras superfamily have been implicated in SAPK/JNK and p38 regulation. The Rho subfamily in mammals is composed of the Rho (RhoA to RhoE), Rac (Rac1 and Rac2), and Cdc42 (Cdc42Hs, G25K, and Tc10) subgroups. As with other members of the Ras superfamily, Rho subfamily GTPases are active in the GTP-bound state and inactive in the GDP-bound state (see Fig. 9–10B). Activation of Rho subfamily GTPases is mediated by GEFs homologous to the proto-oncogene *dbl*. GAPs selective for the Rho subfamily have also been identified.[122] Constitutively active, GTPase-deficient forms of Rac1 and Cdc42Hs can activate both the SAPKs/JNKs and p38s in cotransfection experiments. Ras itself can, in some instances, recruit the SAPKs/JNKs, and it appears that Rac1 mediates the relatively modest activation of SAPK/JNK incurred by transforming alleles of *ras* and in response to mitogens such as EGF.[123-129] Aside from these findings, few stimuli that selectively recruit Rac1 and Cdc42Hs have been identified.

Most but not all effectors for Rac1 and Cdc42Hs contain a Cdc42-Rac interaction and binding (CRIB) domain to which the GTP-loaded Rac and Cdc42 bind. Several potent SAPK/p38 activators can also bind Rac1 and Cdc42Hs in a GTP-dependent manner, including MEKK1 and MLK2 and MLK3, and MLK2 and MLK3 possess CRIB domains. However, the role of Rac1 or Cdc42Hs in the regulation of these MAP3Ks is unclear.[106, 126-128]

The NF-κB Pathway, an Additional Mechanism whereby Stress and Inflammatory Cytokines Regulate Gene Expression

The transcription factor NF-κB, like AP-1, the SAPKs, and p38s, is regulated by environmental stresses and inflammatory cytokines of the TNF family. In most cell types, NF-κB is composed of a heterodimer of the Rel family transcription factor subunits p50 (50 kDa) and p65 (65 kDa) that is sequestered in the cytosol by inhibitory polypeptides of the inhibitor of κB (IκB) family (IκBα, IκBβ, IκBε) (Fig. 9–15B). IκBs mask the nuclear localization signals of Rel proteins, thereby preventing NF-κB nuclear translocation. Activation of NF-κB requires the signal-induced phosphorylation of Ser residues on IκB proteins (Ser32 and Ser36 of IκBα or Ser19 and Ser23 of IκBβ). This phosphorylation in turn results in the polyubiquitination (primarily at Lys21 in IκBα) and proteolytic degradation of IκB through a 26S proteasome–dependent mechanism (see Fig. 9–15B). NF-κB is then free to migrate to the nucleus, where it *trans*-activates genes that contain the κB enhancer *cis*-acting element (consensus: GGGACTTCC). NF-κB is a pivotal transcription factor in the inflammatory response. Thus, for example, in addition to its important role in *trans*-activation of the immunoglobulin κ light chain, NF-κB is required for full induction of IL-2 and E-selectin in response to inflammatory signals.[129]

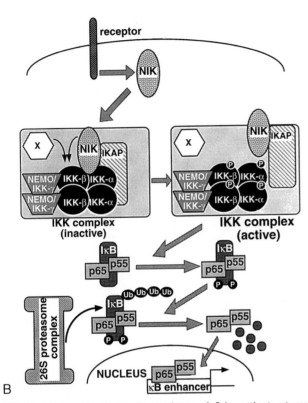

FIGURE 9–15. The NF-κB signaling pathway. *A,* Schematic structures of the IKK catalytic core. LZ, leucine zipper; HLH, helix-loop-helix domain. Amino acid numbers are indicated. *B,* Regulation of IκB phosphorylation by signaling pathways that use NIK and IKAP. Receptor activation of NIK results in NIK association with the IKK complex, probably via binding to both IKAP and IKK-α and IKK-β. IKAP is also associated with IKK-α. Activation of IKK-α and IKK-β kinase activity ensues coincident with phosphorylation of IKK polypeptides and, possibly, other mechanisms (indicated by "X"). IκB is then phosphorylated. IκB phosphorylation promotes proteasome-dependent polyubiquitination (Ub) and proteolytic degradation of the IκB polypeptide. The nuclear localization signals of the p65 and p55 subunits of NF-κB are then unmasked and the NF-κB migrates into the nucleus and *trans*-activates the appropriate target genes.

Initial gel filtration isolates of a protein complex with IκB kinase (IKK) activity selective for Ser32/36 of IκBα suggested a massive oligomer (700–900 kDa).[130, 131] Present evidence indicates that the catalytic nucleus of the IKK complex consists of at least three and possibly four subunits. IκB phosphorylation is catalyzed by either of two protein kinase subunits: IKK-α and IKK-β. Both kinases are highly selective for the phosphoacceptor sites on IκBα and IκBβ, and even substitution of Thr for the Ser residues is not tolerated.[130–134] A third subunit, NF-κB essential modulator (NEMO, also called IKK-γ), is devoid of apparent catalytic activity but can interact in vivo with IKK-β and is required for proper regulation of the IKK complex in vivo.[135, 136] IKK complex–associated protein (IKAP) is a putative fourth IKK subunit. IKAP copurifies with the high-molecular-weight IKK

complex activated by IL-1. IKAP can also associate with the IKK upstream activating MAP3K NIK[137] (see Fig. 9–15).

The IKK subunits can form higher-order oligomers in vivo. IKAP can bind IKK-α and IKK-β, as well as NIK (see Fig. 9–15B). The amino-terminus of IKAP is required for binding NIK, whereas the carboxyl-terminus binds IKKs. In addition to binding IKAP and NEMO/IKK-γ, IKK-β can interact in vivo and in vitro with itself and with IKK-α. IKK-α can also homodimerize[132–136] (see Fig. 9–15B). IKK-α and IKK-β share 50% homology; both consist of an amino-terminal kinase domain, a leucine (Leu) zipper, and a C-terminal helix-loop-helix (HLH) motif.[130–134] Likewise, the NEMO/IKK-γ primary sequence contains an N-terminal HLH domain and a C-terminal leucine zipper[135, 136] (see Fig. 9–15A). Deletion of the Leu zipper from either kinase subunit abrogates IKK-α/β homodimerization or heterodimerization.[131–134] Thus it appears that the Leu zippers are critical for dimerization of the IKK kinase subunits. NEMO/IKK-γ itself can form homodimers and can heterodimerize with IKK-β, and the Leu zipper appears necessary for both functions, as well as for NEMO/IKK-γ biologic activity.[135, 136] Functionally speaking, the entire IKK complex may consist of an oligomer of IKK-α/β, NEMO/IKK-γ, and possibly IKAP; however, the exact makeup of the IKK complex has yet to be established (see Fig. 9–15B).

The likeliest known candidate for a proximal upstream activator of IKK is NIK. Interestingly, NIK is a Ser/Thr kinase that is significantly homologous to the MEKKs (see above).[109, 130, 131, 138] IKK-α and IKK-β are both strongly activated in vivo upon coexpression with NIK, and both IKK kinase subunits bind NIK and are NIK substrates.[130, 133, 138] The mechanism by which NIK activates IKK is unclear; direct phosphorylation by NIK appears unlikely,[138] although IKK is regulated by phosphorylation.[131] Interestingly, IKAP dissociates from IKK-α/β but not NIK upon stimulation of cells with IL-1. Thus in vivo, IKAP may direct activation and deactivation of the IKK complex by specific upstream stimuli[137] (see Fig. 9–15B).

Signaling through the TNFR Family: Activation of the SAPKs/JNKs, p38s, and NF-κB

The TNF receptor (TNFR) family includes TNFR1, TNFR2, the IL-1 and lymphotoxin-β receptors, CD27, CD30, CD40, Fas, receptor activator of NF-κB (RANKL, also called osteoprotegerin or TNF-related activation-induced cytokine receptor [TRANCE receptor]), Ox40, the p75 neurotrophin receptor, and others.[59, 139] Upon binding ligand, these receptors can elicit a wide variety of inflammatory responses and are critical to immune cell development, innate and acquired immunity, and the pathogenesis of a number of diseases such as arthritis, inflammatory bowel disease, septic shock, and possibly, type II diabetes. Accordingly, this family of receptors is among the most important activators of the SAPKs/JNKs, p38s, and NF-κB. Many ligands of the TNF family are homotrimeric and initiate responses by binding to cell surface receptors, a process that results in receptor homotrimerization or, in some cases, hetero-oligomerization with receptor accessory proteins (Fig. 9–16). Some, but not all of these receptors contain an intracellular death domain. Death domains, so named for their role in promoting programmed cell death (apoptosis), mediate homotypic and heterotypic protein-protein interactions and are critical for nucleating receptor-effector complexes and implementing several signaling programs.[59]

Signal transduction by TNF has been characterized in some detail, although the picture is far from complete. TNF homotrimers bind to one of two receptors, TNFR1 (55–60 kDa) or TNFR2 (75–80 kDa) (see Fig. 9–16). Ligand binding induces receptor trimerization and the initiation of signal transduction. TNFR1 contains a death domain.[59] Upon ligand-induced trimerization, the TNFR1 death domain binds the adapter protein TNFR-associated death domain protein (TRADD). Overexpression of TRADD activates NF-κB but, curiously, not SAPK/JNK. TRADD in turn associates with TNFR-associated factor-2 (TRAF2), a member of the TRAF family, and with receptor-interacting protein (RIP), a death domain–containing Ser/Thr kinase. RIP can also

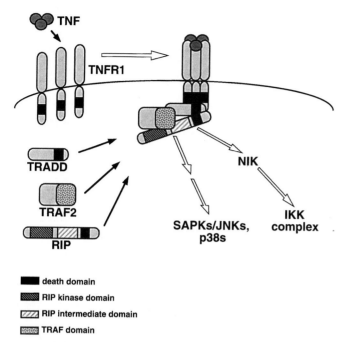

FIGURE 9–16. *TNF receptor-1 (TNFR1) signaling is initiated by protein recruitment. TNF promotes TNFR1 trimerization, which in turn fosters binding of the TRADD death domain to the TNFR1 death domain. TRAF2 binds TRADD via the TRAF domains of TRAF2, whereas RIP associates with TRADD via the death domains of both proteins. RIP also binds TRAF2 via an interaction between the TRAF2 TRAF domains and the RIP kinase and intermediate domains. Formation of this receptor complex then recruits the SAPKs/JNKs and p38s (through TRAF2) and the IKK complex (through RIP and, possibly, TRAF2 or other TRAFs).*

bind TRAF2, and accordingly, TNF treatment is thought to result in the formation of a TRADD-RIP-TRAF2 complex[59, 140–145] (see Fig. 9–16).

The TRAFs and RIP represent key adapter proteins in regulation of the SAPKs/JNKs, p38s, and NF-κB. Six TRAFs (TRAF1 to TRAF6) have been identified. Transient expression of TRAFs 2, 5, and 6 results in potent activation of NF-κB and SAPK/JNK.[59, 146, 147] Gene disruption studies indicate that TRAF2 is essential for SAPK but not NF-κB activation by TNF; thus TRAF5 and TRAF6 may mediate signaling to SAPK/JNK by other TNF family receptors.[148] Similarly, TRAF2 may couple TNFR family members other than TNFR1 to NF-κB. Notably, NIK, a regulator of NF-κB, was isolated by virtue of its interaction with TRAF2 in a yeast two-hybrid system, thus supporting a role for TRAF2 in some aspect of NF-κB regulation.[110] RIP overexpression can activate the SAPKs/JNKs, p38s, and NF-κB; however, gene deletion studies indicate that RIP is not required for SAPK/JNK activation. On the other hand, deletion of *rip* completely abrogates TNF activation of NF-κB, which suggests that RIP is critical for coupling TNFR1 and, possibly, NIK to NF-κB.[117, 142–145, 149] Little is known of how TRAFs and RIP signal to their effectors; however, recent studies indicate that these adapter proteins associate directly in vivo with MAP3Ks or with proximal protein kinases, which in turn couple directly to MAP3Ks.[117]

Antagonism between Glucocorticoid Receptors and AP-1

It has been known for some time that glucocorticoids are potent anti-inflammatory agents. Similarly, the ability of inflammatory mediators to inhibit the actions of glucocorticoids is well known and is discussed in Chapter 10 and Part IX. The glucocorticoid receptor (GR) is a member of the steroid receptor superfamily (see Chapter 10). The basis for the mutual antagonism of glucocorticoids and inflammation was unclear until it was observed that AP-1 and the GR could block each other's transcriptional activity.[150–152] The presence of c-Jun pre-

vents association of the GR with the glucocorticoid response element (GRE); similarly, the presence of GR blocks AP-1 association with the TRE. This antagonism is not due to a dislodging of GR or AP-1 already bound to DNA, nor is it due to covalent modifications of either the GR or Fos-Jun per se (notably, glucocorticoids do not affect Jun phosphorylation). Instead, this inhibitory activity is due to a direct interaction between the DNA-binding domain of c-Jun and the DNA-binding domain of the GR that prevents *subsequent* DNA binding by either transcription factor.[150–152] This phenomenon indicates that stress-regulated MAPK pathways and steroid receptor pathways share intimate crosstalk at the molecular level and should not be considered independent entities when contemplating existing therapeutic options or designing new ones.

SOME UNIFYING THEMES AND CONCLUDING REMARKS

This chapter has discussed some of what is known about how polypeptide hormones such as insulin, as well as environmental and physiologic stress mechanisms, recruit protein Ser/Thr kinases to effect changes in cellular function. Several general themes emerge from the findings covered.

Subdomain VIII of the kinase domain is often critical to regulation. PKB/Akt, MAPKAP-K1/Rsk, p70, MAPKAP-K2, all of the MAPKs, and all of the MEKs are regulated at least in part by phosphorylation within the kinase domain activation loop in subdomain VIII. Thus phosphorylation within this region is a common theme in Ser/Thr kinase regulation.

Ras superfamily GTPases are critical signaling intermediates. It is clear that the ERK pathway (through Ras) and the SAPK/JNK and p38 pathways (through Rac1 and Cdc42Hs, as well as Ras in some instances) rely heavily on Ras family proteins to relay signals from activated receptors to MAP3Ks. In addition, PI-3-kinase also requires Ras for optimal activation by insulin and mitogens.

Signaling pathways are often multitiered. All MAPK pathways proceed through three-tiered core signaling pathways. In addition, the PKB/Akt and p70 S6 kinase pathways require multiple upstream protein kinases for regulation. In the case of the MAPK pathways, the core signaling modules can activate additional distal protein kinases (MAPKAP-K1/Rsk and MAPKAP-K2). Moreover, each tier in the MAPK pathways is apparently occupied by multiple homologues (especially at the MEK and MAP3K level). The significance of this complexity is unclear; however, it probably permits regulation of these pathways by multiple, often divergent inputs (for example, stimuli as varied as TNF and hyperosmolarity can activate SAPK/JNK). In addition, this complexity permits kinases at each level to influence multiple effectors (thus PKB/Akt can regulate both GSK3 and p70 S6 kinase). Multitiered protein kinase cascades also allow for catalytic amplification at each level and render these pathways exquisitely sensitive to external stimuli.

Pathway crosstalk requires consideration of signal integration. As we have seen, individual effectors can be influenced by divergent agonistic and antagonistic stimuli. Thus the ERKs can influence non-mitogenic signaling pathways such as those involving PPARγ, the estrogen receptor, and the STATs. AP-1 can be activated through mitogen–Elk-1 induction of c-*fos* expression, TNF or stress activation of c-Jun *trans*-activation function (as well as c-Jun and p38-MEF2C induction of c-*jun* expression), and antagonism by glucocorticoids and GSK3. Similarly, insulin and cAMP agonists can, through p70 S6 kinase and PKA, respectively, activate CREMτ function. Conversely, insulin and cAMP are antagonistic regulators of GS. Thus as more of these signaling pathways are elucidated, conventional treatment strategies will have to consider the effects of novel therapeutics on multiple pathways that could be affected by drugs that "apparently" target a single signaling constituent.

REFERENCES

1. Hanks SK, Quinn MA, Hunter T: The protein kinase family: Conserved features and deduced phylogeny of the catalytic domains. Science 241:42–52, 1988.

2. Knighton DR, Zheng J, Ten Eyck LF, et al: Crystal structure of the catalytic subunit of cyclic adenosine monophosphate–dependent protein kinase. Science 253:407–414, 1991.

3. Zhang F, Strand A, Robbins D, et al: Atomic structure of the MAP kinase ERK2 at 2.3 ÅA resolution. Nature 367:704–711, 1994.

4. Kyriakis JM, Avruch J: S6 kinases and MAP kinases: Sequential intermediates in insulin/mitogen-activated protein kinase cascades. In Woodgett JR (ed): Protein Kinases: Frontiers in Molecular Biology. Oxford, Oxford University Press, 1994, p 85.

5. Avruch J: Insulin signal transduction through protein kinase cascades. Mol Cell Biochem 182:31–48, 1998.

6. Carpenter CL, Cantley LC: Phosphoinositide kinases. Curr Opin Cell Biol 8:153–158, 1996.

7. Cohen P: Muscle glycogen synthase. In Boyer P, Krebs EG (eds): The Enzymes. New York, Academic Press, 1988, p 461.

8. Larner J: Insulin signalling mechanisms—lessons from the old testament of glycogen metabolism and from the new testament of molecular biology. Diabetes 37:262–282, 1988.

9. Krebs EG: Protein kinases. Curr Top Cell Regul 5:99–120, 1972.

10. Avruch J, Witters LA, Alexander MC, et al: The effect of insulin and glucagon on the phosphorylation of hepatic cytoplasmic peptides. J Biol Chem 253:4754–4762, 1978.

11. Haselbacher GK, Humbel RE, Thomas G: Insulin-like growth factors, insulin or serum increase phosphorylation of ribosomal S6 during transition of stationary chick embryo fibroblasts in early G$_1$ phase of the cell cycle. FEBS Lett 100:185–191, 1979.

12. Downward J: Mechanisms and consequences of activation of protein kinase B/Akt. Curr Opin Cell Biol 10:262–267, 1998.

13. Embi N, Rylatt DB, Cohen P: Glycogen synthase kinase-3 from rabbit skeletal muscle. Separation from cyclic-AMP–dependent protein kinase and phosphorylase kinase. Eur J Biochem 107:519–527, 1980.

14. Parker PJ, Embi N, Caudwell FB, et al: Glycogen synthase from rabbit skeletal muscle. State of phosphorylation of the seven phosphoserine residues in vivo in the presence and absence of adrenaline. Eur J Biochem 124:47–55, 1982.

15. Roach PJ: Multisite and hierarchical protein phosphorylation. J Biol Chem 266:14139–14142, 1991.

16. Boyle WJ, Smeal T, Defize LHK, et al: Activation of protein kinase C decreases phosphorylation of c-jun at sites that negatively regulate its DNA binding activity. Cell 64:573–584, 1991.

17. Cross DAE, Alessi DR, Cohen P, et al: Inhibition of glycogen synthase kinase-3 by insulin mediated by protein kinase B. Nature 378:785–789, 1995.

18. Deprez J, Vertommen D, Alessi DR, et al: Phosphorylation and activation of heart phosphofructo-2-kinase by protein kinase B and other protein kinases of the insulin signaling cascades. J Biol Chem 272:17269–17275, 1997.

19. Alessi DR, Andjelkovic M, Caudwell B, et al: Mechanism of activation of protein kinase B by insulin and IGF-1. EMBO J 15:6541–6551, 1996.

20. Alessi DR, James SR, Downes CP, et al: Characterization of a 3-phosphoinositide–dependent protein kinase which phosphorylates and activates protein kinase Bα. Curr Biol 7:261–269, 1997.

21. Alessi DR, Deak M, Casamayor A, et al: 3-Phosphoinositide–dependent protein kinase-1 (PDK1): Structural and functional homology with the Drosophila DSTPK61 kinase. Curr Biol 7:776–789, 1997.

22. Stephens L, Anderson K, Stokoe D, et al: Protein kinase B kinases that mediate phosphatidylinositol 3,4,5-trisphosphate–dependent activation of protein kinase B. Science 279:710–714, 1998.

23. Erikson E, Maller JL: Purification and characterization of a protein kinase from Xenopus eggs highly specific for ribosomal protein S6. J Biol Chem 261:350–355, 1986.

24. Alcorta DA, Crews CM, Sweet LJ, et al: Homologs of Xenopus laevis ribosomal S6 kinase. Mol Cell Biol 9:3850–3859, 1989.

25. Calvo V, Crews CM, Vik TA, et al: Interleukin 2 stimulation of p70 S6 kinase activity is inhibited by the immunosuppressant rapamycin. Proc Natl Acad Sci U S A 89:7571–7575, 1992.

26. Price DJ, Nemenoff RA, Avruch J: Purification of a hepatic S6 kinase from cycloheximide-treated rats. J Biol Chem 264:13825–13833, 1989.

27. Banerjee P, Ahmad MF, Grove JR, et al: Molecular structure of a major insulin/mitogen-activated 70-kDa S6 protein kinase. Proc Natl Acad Sci U S A 87:8550–8554, 1990.

28. Gout I, Minami T, Hara K, et al: Molecular cloning and characterization of a novel p70 S6 kinase, p70 S6 kinase-β, containing a proline-rich region. J Biol Chem 273:30061–30064, 1998.

29. Jeffries HBJ, Reinhard C, Kozma SC, et al: Rapamycin selectively represses translation of the "polypyrimidine tract" mRNA family. Proc Natl Acad Sci U S A 91:4441–4445, 1994.

30. Jeffries HBJ, Fumagalli S, Dennis PB, et al: Rapamycin suppresses 5′TOP mRNA translation through inhibition of p70 S6k. EMBO J 16:3693–3704, 1997.

31. Jeffries HBJ, Thomas G: Ribosomal protein S6 phosphorylation and signal transduction. In Hershey JWB, Mathews MB, Sonenberg N (eds): Translational Control. Cold Spring Harbor, NY, Cold Spring Harbor Press, 1996, p 389.

32. Habener JF: Cyclic AMP-response element binding proteins: A cornucopia of transcription factors. Mol Endocrinol 4:1087–1094, 1990.

33. de Groot RP, Sassone-Corsi P: Hormonal control of gene expression: Multiplicity and versatility of cyclic adenosine 3′,5′-monophosphate–responsive nuclear regulators. Mol Endocrinol 7:145–153, 1993.

34. Foulkes NS, Borelli E, Sassone-Corsi P: CREM gene: Use of alternative DNA binding domains generates multiple antagonists of cAMP-induced transcription. Cell 64:739–749, 1991.

35. Foulkes NS, Mellström B, Benusiglio E, et al: Developmental switch of CREM function during spermatogenesis from antagonist to activator. Nature 355:80–84, 1992.

36. Laoide BM, Foulkes NS, Schlotter F, et al: The functional diversity of CREM is determined by its modular structure. EMBO J 12:1179–1191, 1993.

37. Delmas V, Laoide BM, Masquilier D, et al: Alternative usage of initiation codons in mRNA encoding the cAMP-responsive element modulator (CREM) gene generates regulators with opposite functions. Proc Natl Acad Sci U S A 89:4226–4230, 1992.

38. Molina CA, Foulkes NS, Lalli E, et al: Inducibility and negative autoregulation of CREM: An alternative promoter directs the expression of ICER, an early response repressor. Cell 75:875–886, 1993.

39. Foulkes NS, Schlotter F, Pevet P, et al: Pituitary hormone FSH directs the CREM functional switch during spermatogenesis. Nature 362:264–267, 1993.

40. de Groot RP, den Hertog J, Vandenheede JR, et al: Multiple and cooperative phosphorylation events regulate the CREM activator function. EMBO J 12:3903–3911, 1993.

41. de Groot RP, Ballou LM, Sassone-Corsi P: Positive regulation of the cAMP-responsive activator CREM by the p70 S6 kinase: An alternative route to mitogen-induced gene expression. Cell 79:81–91, 1994.

42. Mukhopadhyay NK, Price DJ, Kyriakis JM, et al: An array of insulin-activated, proline-directed (Ser/Thr) protein kinases phosphorylate the p70 S6 kinase. J Biol Chem 267:3325–3335, 1992.

43. Alessi DR, Kozlowski MT, Weng QP, et al: 3-phosphoinositide–dependent protein kinase 1 (PDK1) phosphorylates and activates the p70 S6 kinase in vivo and in vitro. Curr Biol 8:69–81, 1997.

44. Schreiber SL, Crabtree GR: The mechanism of action of cyclosporin A and FK506. Immunol Today 13:136–142, 1992.

45. Chung J, Kuo CJ, Crabtree GR, et al: Rapamycin FKBP specifically blocks growth-dependent activation of signaling by the 70 kd S6 protein kinase. Cell 69:1227–1236, 1992.

46. Kuo CJ, Chung J, Fiorentino DF, et al: Rapamycin selectively inhibits interleukin-2 activation of p70 S6 kinase. Nature 358:70–73, 1992.

47. Heitman J, Movva NR, Hall MN: Targets for cell cycle arrest by the immunosuppressive agent rapamycin in yeast. Science 253:905–909, 1991.

48. Brown EJ, Alberts MW, Shin TB, et al: A mammalian protein targeted by G$_1$-arresting rapamycin-receptor complex. Nature 369:756–758, 1994.

49. Brown EJ, Beal PA, Keith CT, et al: Control of p70 S6 kinase by kinase activity of FRAP in vivo. Nature 377:441–446, 1995.

50. Hara K, Yonezawa K, Weng QP, et al: Amino acid sufficiency and mTOR regulate p70 S6 kinase and eIF-4E BP1 through a common effector mechanism. J Biol Chem 273:14484–14494, 1998.

51. Burnett PE, Barrow RK, Cohen NA, et al: RAFT1 phosphorylation of the translational regulators p70 S6 kinase and 4E-BP1. Proc Natl Acad Sci U S A 95:1432–1437, 1998.

52. Brunn GJ, Hudson CC, Sekulic A, et al: Phosphorylation of the translational repressor PHAS-I by the mammalian target of rapamycin. Science 277:99–101, 1997.

53. Pause A, Belsham GJ, Gingras A-C, et al: Insulin-dependent stimulation of protein synthesis by phosphorylation of a regulator of 5′-cap function. Nature 371:762–767, 1994.

54. Sonenberg N, Gingras A-C: The mRNA 5′ cap-binding protein eIF4E and control of cell growth. Curr Opin Cell Biol 10:268–275, 1998.

55. Herskowitz I: MAP kinase pathways in yeast: For mating and more. Cell 80:187–197, 1995.

56. Marshall CJ: Specificity of receptor tyrosine kinase signaling: Transient versus sustained extracellular signal regulated kinase activation. Cell 80:179–185, 1995.

57. Kyriakis JM, Avruch J: Sounding the alarm: Protein kinase cascades activated by stress and inflammation. J Biol Chem 271:24313–24316, 1996.

58. Kyriakis JM, Avruch J: Protein kinase cascades activated by stress and inflammatory cytokines. Bioessays 18:567–577, 1996.

59. Arch RH, Gedrich RW, Thompson CB: Tumor necrosis factor receptor–associated factors (TRAFs)—a family of adapter proteins that regulates life and death. Genes Dev 12:2821–2830, 1998.

60. Posas F, Saito H: Osmotic activation of the HOG MAPK pathway via Ste11p MAPKKK: Scaffold role of Pbs2p MAPKK. Science 276:1702–1705, 1997.

61. Choi K-Y, Satterberg B, Lyons DM, et al: Ste5 tethers multiple protein kinases in the MAP kinase cascade required for mating in S. cerevisiae. Cell 78:499–512, 1994.

62. Dent P, Lavoinne A, Nakielny S, et al: The molecular mechanism by which insulin stimulates glycogen synthesis in mammalian skeletal muscle. Nature 348:302–308, 1990.

62a. Richards SA, Fu J, Romanelli A, et al: Ribosomal S6 kinase 1 (RSK1) activation requires signals dependent on and independent of the MAP kinase ERK. Curr Biol 9:810–820, 1999.

63. Dalby KN, Morrice N, Caudwell FB, et al: Identification of regulatory phosphorylation sites in mitogen-activated protein kinase (MAPK)-activated protein kinase-1a/p90rsk that are inducible by MAPK. J Biol Chem 273:1496–1505, 1998.

64. Waskiewicz AJ, Flynn A, Proud CG, et al: Mitogen-activated protein kinases activate the serine/threonine kinases Mnk1 and Mnk2. EMBO J 16:1909–1920, 1997.

65. Treisman R: Regulation of transcription by MAP kinase cascades. Curr Opin Cell Biol 8:205–215, 1996.

66. Karin M, Liu Z-G, Zandi E: AP-1 function and regulation. Curr Opin Cell Biol 9:240–246, 1997.

67. Hu E, Kim JB, Sarraf P: Inhibition of adipogenesis through MAP kinase–mediated phosphorylation of PPARγ. Science 274:2100–2103, 1996.

68. Kato S, Endo H, Matsuhiro Y, et al: Activation of the estrogen receptor through phosphorylation by mitogen-activated protein kinase. Science 270:1491–1494, 1995.

69. Zhang X, Blenis J, Li H-C, et al: Requirement of serine phosphorylation for formation of STAT promoter complexes. Science 267:1900–1994, 1995.

70. Kyriakis JM, App H, Zhang X-F, et al: Raf-1 activates MAP kinase-kinase. Nature 358:417–421, 1992.

71. Avruch J, Zhang X-F, Kyriakis JM: Raf meets Ras: Completing the framework of a signal transduction pathway. Trends Biochem Sci 19:279–283, 1994.

72. Zhang XF, Settleman J, Kyriakis JM, et al: Normal and oncogenic p21ras bind to the amino-terminal regulatory domain of c-Raf-1. Nature 364:308–313, 1993.

73. Luo Z, Tzivion G, Belshaw PJ, et al: Oligomerization activates c-Raf-1 through a Ras-dependent mechanism. Nature 383:181–184, 1996.

74. Tzivion G, Luo Z, Avruch J: A dimeric 14-3-3 protein is an essential cofactor for Raf kinase activity. Nature 394:88–92, 1998.

75. Muslin AJ, Tanner JW, Allen PM, et al: Interaction of 14-3-3 with signaling proteins is mediated by the recognition of phosphoserine. Cell 84:889–897, 1996.

76. Rodriguez-Viciana P, Warne PH, Dhand R, et al: Phosphatidyl-3-OH kinase as a direct target for Ras. Nature 370:527–532, 1994.

77. Rodriguez-Viciana P, Warne PH, Vanhaesebroeck B, et al: Activation of phosphoinositide 3-kinase by interaction with Ras and by point mutation. EMBO J 15:2442–2451, 1996.

78. Kyriakis JM, Avruch J: pp54 MAP-2 kinase. A novel serine/threonine protein kinase regulated by phosphorylation and stimulated by poly-L-lysine. J Biol Chem 265:17355–17363, 1990.

79. Kyriakis JM, Brautigan DL, Ingebritsen TS, et al: pp54 microtubule-associated protein-2 kinase requires both tyrosine and serine/threonine phosphorylation for activity. J Biol Chem 266:10043–10046, 1991.

80. Pulverer BJ, Kyriakis JM, Avruch J, et al: Phosphorylation of c-jun mediated by MAP kinases. Nature 353:670–674, 1991.

81. Kyriakis JM, Banerjee P, Nikolakaki E, et al: The stress-activated protein kinase subfamily of c-Jun kinases. Nature 369:156–160, 1994.

82. Dérijard B, Hibi M, Wu I-H, et al: JNK1: A protein kinase stimulated by UV light and Ha-Ras that binds and phosphorylates the c-Jun transactivation domain. Cell 76:1025–1037, 1994.

83. Han J, Lee J-D, Bibbs L, et al: A MAP kinase targeted by endotoxin and hyperosmolarity in mammalian cells. Science 265:808–811, 1994.

84. Lee JC, Laydon JT, McDonnell PC, et al: A protein kinase involved in the regulation of inflammatory cytokine biosynthesis. Nature 273:739–746, 1994.

85. Mertens S, Craxton M, Goedert M: SAP kinase-3, a new member of the family of mammalian stress-activated protein kinases. FEBS Lett 383:273–276, 1996.

86. Goedert M, Cuenda A, Craxton M, et al: Activation of the novel stress-activated protein kinase SAPK4 by cytokines and cellular stresses is mediated by SKK3 (MKK6); comparison of its substrate specificity with that of other SAP kinases. EMBO J 16:3563–3571, 1997.

87. Stokoe D, Campbell DG, Nakielny S, et al: MAPKAP kinase-2; a novel protein kinase activated by mitogen-activated protein kinase. EMBO J 11:3985–3994, 1992.

88. Stokoe D, Engel K, Campbell DG, et al: Identification of MAPKAP kinase 2 as a major enzyme responsible for the phosphorylation of the small mammalian heat shock proteins. FEBS Lett 313:307–313, 1992.

89. Ben-Levy R, Leighton IA, Doza YN, et al: Identification of novel phosphorylation sites required for activation of MAPKAP kinase-2. EMBO J 14:5920–5930, 1995.

90. Wang XZ, Ron D: Stress-induced phosphorylation and activation of the transcription factor CHOP (GADD153) by p38 MAP kinase. Science 272:1347–1349, 1996.

91. Dai T, Rubie E, Franklin CC, et al: Stress-activated protein kinases bind directly to the delta domain of c-jun in resting cells: Implications for repression of c-jun function. Oncogene 10:849–855, 1995.

92. Kallunki T, Deng T, Hibi M, et al: c-Jun can recruit JNK to phosphorylate dimerization partners via specific docking interactions. Cell 87:929–939, 1996.

93. Gupta S, Campbell D, Dérijard B, et al: Transcription factor ATF2 regulation by the JNK signal transduction pathway. Science 267:389–393, 1995.

94. Han J, Jiang Y, Li Z, et al: MEF2C participates in inflammatory responses via p38-mediated activation. Nature 386:563–566, 1997.

95. Dérijard B, Raingeaud J, Barrett T, et al: Independent human MAP kinase signal transduction pathways defined by MEK and MKK isoforms. Science 267:682–685, 1995.

96. Raingeaud J, Whitmarsh AJ, Barett T, et al: MKK3- and MKK6-regulated gene expression is mediated by the p38 mitogen-activated protein kinase signal transduction pathway. Mol Cell Biol 16:1247–1255, 1996.

97. Sánchez I, Hughes RT, Mayer BJ, et al: Role of SAPK/ERK kinase-1 in the stress-activated pathway regulating transcription factor c-Jun. Nature 372:794–798, 1994.

98. Tournier C, Whitmarsh AJ, Cavanagh J, et al: Mitogen-activated protein kinase kinase 7 is an activator of the c-Jun NH₂-terminal kinase. Proc Natl Acad Sci U S A 94:7337–7342, 1997.

99. Holland PM, Suzanne M, Campbell JS, et al: MKK7 is a stress-activated mitogen-activated protein kinase kinase functionally related to hemopterous. J Biol Chem 272:24994–24998, 1997.

100. Nishina H, Fischer KD, Radvanyi L, et al: Stress signalling kinase Sek1 protects thymocytes from apoptosis mediated by CD95 and CD3. Nature 385:350–353, 1997.

101. Cuenda A, Alonso G, Morrice N, et al: Purification and cDNA cloning of SAPKK3, the major activator of RK/p38 in stress- and cytokine-stimulated monocytes and epithelial cells. EMBO J 15:4156–4164, 1996.

102. Meier R, Rouse J, Cuenda A, et al: Cellular stresses and cytokines activate multiple mitogen-activated-protein kinase kinase homologues in PC12 and KB cells. Eur J Biochem 236:796–805, 1996.

103. Lange-Carter CA, Pleiman C, Gardner AM, et al: A divergence in the MAP kinase regulatory network defined by MEK kinase and Raf. Science 260:315–319, 1993.

104. Xu S, Robbins DJ, Christerson LB, et al: Cloning of Rat MEK kinase 1 cDNA reveals an endogenous membrane-associated 195-kDa protein with a large regulatory domain. Proc Natl Acad Sci U S A 93:5291–5295, 1996.

105. Blank JL, Gerwins P, Elliot EM, et al: Molecular cloning of mitogen activated protein/ERK kinase kinases (MEKK) 2 and 3. J Biol Chem 271:5361–5368, 1996.

106. Gerwins P, Blank JL, Johnson GL: Cloning of a novel mitogen-activated protein kinase-kinase-kinase, MEKK4, that selectively regulates the c-Jun amino terminal kinase pathway. J Biol Chem 272:8288–8295, 1997.

107. Takekawa M, Posas F, Saito H: A human homolog of the yeast Ssk2/Ssk22 MAP kinase kinase kinases, MTK1, mediates stress-induced activation of the p38 and JNK pathways. EMBO J 16:4973–4982, 1997.

108. Ichijo H, Nishida E, Irie K, et al: Induction of apoptosis by ASK1, a mammalian MAPKKK that activates SAPK/JNK and p38 signaling pathways. Science 275:90–94, 1997.

109. Yamaguchi K, Shirakabi K, Shibuya H, et al: Identification of a member of the MAPKKK family as a potential mediator of TGF-β signal transduction. Science 270:2008–2011, 1995.

110. Malinin NL, Boldin MP, Kovalenko AV, et al: MAP3K-related kinase involved in NF-κB induction by TNF, CD-95 and IL-1. Nature 385:540–544, 1997.

111. Yan M, Dai T, Deak JC, et al: Activation of stress-activated protein kinase by MEKK1 phosphorylation of its activator SEK1. Nature 372:798–800, 1994.

112. Moriguchi T, Kuroyanagi N, Yamaguchi K, et al: A novel kinase cascade mediated by mitogen-activated protein kinase kinase 6 and MKK3. J Biol Chem 271:13675–13679, 1996.

113. Salmerón A, Ahmad TB, Carlile GW, et al: Activation of MEK-1 and SEK-1 by Tpl-2 proto oncoprotein, a novel MAP kinase kinase kinase. EMBO J 15:817–826, 1996.

114. Rana A, Gallo K, Godowski P, et al: The mixed lineage protein kinase SPRK phosphorylates and activates the stress-activated protein kinase activator, SEK1. J Biol Chem 271:19025–19028, 1996.

115. Hirai S-I, Katoh M, Terada M, et al: MST/MLK2, a member of the mixed lineage kinase family, directly phosphorylates and activates SEK1, an activator of c-Jun N-terminal kinase/stress-activated protein kinase. J Biol Chem 272:15167–15173, 1997.

116. Fan G, Merritt SE, Kortenjann M, et al: Dual leucine zipper-bearing kinase (DLK) activates p46SAPK and p38mapk but not ERK2. J Biol Chem 271:24788–24793, 1996.

117. Yuasa T, Ohno S, Kehrl JH, et al: Tumor necrosis factor signaling to stress-activated protein kinase (SAPK)/Jun NH₂-terminal kinase (JNK) and p38. J Biol Chem 273:22681–22692, 1998.

118. Takekawa M, Saito H: A family of stress-inducible GADD45-like proteins mediate activation of the stress-responsive MTK1/MEKK4 MAPKKK. Cell 95:521–530, 1998.

119. Dickens M, Rogers JS, Cavanagh J, et al: A cytoplasmic inhibitor of the JNK signal transduction pathway. Science 277:693–696, 1997.

120. Whitmarsh AJ, Cavanagh J, Tournier C, et al: A mammalian scaffold complex that selectively mediates MAP kinase activation. Science 281:1671–1674, 1998.

121. Xia Y, Wu Z, Su B, et al: JNKK1 organizes a MAP kinase module through specific and sequential interactions with upstream and downstream components mediated by its amino-terminal extension. Genes Dev 12:3369–3381, 1998.

122. Van Aelst L, D'souza-Schorey C: Rho GTPases and signaling networks. Genes Dev 11:2295–2322, 1997.

123. Coso OA, Chiarello M, Yu J-C, et al: The small GTP binding proteins Rac1 and Cdc42 regulated the activity of the JNK/SAPK signaling pathway. Cell 81:1137–1146, 1995.

124. Minden A, Lin A, Claret F-X, et al: Selective activation of the JNK signaling cascade and c-Jun transcriptional activity by the small GTPases Rac and Cdc42Hs. Cell 81:1147–1157, 1995.

125. Bagrodia S, Dérijard B, Davis RJ, et al: Cdc42 and PAK-mediated signaling leads to Jun kinase and p38 mitogen-activated protein kinase activation. J Biol Chem 270:27995–27998, 1995.

126. Burbelo PD, Drechsel D, Hall A: A conserved binding motif defines numerous candidate target proteins for both Cdc42 and Rac GTPases. J Biol Chem 270:29071–29074, 1995.

127. Tapon N, Nagata K, Lamarche N, et al: A new Rac target POSH is an SH3-containing scaffold protein involved in the JNK and NF-κB signalling pathways. EMBO J 17:1395–1404, 1998.

128. Nagata K, Puls A, Futter C, et al: The MAP kinase kinase kinase MLK2 co-localizes with activated JNK along microtubules and associates with kinesin superfamily motor KIF3. EMBO J 17:149–158, 1998.

129. Verma IM, Stevenson JK, Schwartz EM, et al: Rel/NF-κB/IκB family: Intimate tales of association and dissociation. Genes Dev 9:2723–2735, 1995.

130. Régnier CH, Song HY, Gao X, et al: Identification and characterization of an IκB kinase. Cell 90:373–383, 1997.

131. DiDonato JA, Mayakawa M, Rothwarf DM, et al: A cytokine-responsive IκB kinase that activates the transcription factor NF-κB. Nature 388:548–554, 1997.

132. Zandi E, Rothwarf DM, Delhase M, et al: The IκB kinase complex (IKK) contains two kinase subunits, IKK-α and IKK-β, necessary for IκB phosphorylation and NF-κB activation. Cell 91:243–252, 1997.

133. Woronicz JD, Gao X, Cao Z, et al: IκB kinase-β–NF-κB activation and complex formation with IκB kinase-α and NIK. Science 278:866–869, 1997.

134. Mercurio F, Zhu HY, Murray BW, et al: IKK-1 and IKK-2-cytokine–activated IκB kinases essential for NF-κB activation. Science 278:860–866, 1997.

135. Yamaoka S, Courtois G, Bessia C, et al: Complementation cloning of NEMO, a component of the IκB kinase complex essential for NF-κB activation. Cell 93:1231–1240, 1998.

136. Rothwarf DM, Zandi E, Natoli G, et al: IKK-γ is an essential regulatory subunit of the IκB kinase complex. Nature 395:297–300, 1998.

137. Cohen L, Henzel WJ, Baeuerle PA: IKAP is a scaffold protein of the IκB kinase complex. Nature 395:292–296, 1998.

138. Rothwarf DM, Karin M: The NF-κB activation pathway: A paradigm in information transfer from membrane to nucleus. Science (STKE) www.stke.org/cgi/content/full/OC_sigtrans;1999/5/re1

139. Smith CA, Farrah T, Goodwin RG: The TNF receptor superfamily of cellular and viral proteins: Activation, costimulation and death. Cell 76:959–962, 1994.

140. Hsu H, Xiong J, Goeddel DV: The TNF receptor-1–associated protein TRADD signals cell death and NF-κB activation. Cell 81:495–504, 1995.

141. Hsu H, Shu H-B, Pan M-G, et al: TRADD-TRAF2 and TRADD-FADD interactions define two distinct TNF receptor 1 signal transduction pathways. Cell 84:299–308, 1996.

142. Hsu H, Huang J, Shu H-B, et al: TNF-dependent recruitment of the protein kinase RIP to the TNF receptor-1 signaling complex. Immunity 4:387–396, 1996.

143. Takeuchi M, Rothe M, Goeddel DV: Anatomy of TRAF2. J Biol Chem 271:19935–19942, 1996.

144. Rothe M, Wong SC, Henzel WJ, et al: A novel family of putative signal transducers associated with the cytoplasmic domain of the 75-kDa tumor necrosis factor receptor. Cell 78:681–692, 1994.

145. Stanger BZ, Leder P, Lee T-H, et al: RIP: A novel protein containing a death domain that interacts with Fas/APO-1 (CD95) in yeast and causes cell death. Cell 81:513–523, 1995.

146. Liu Z-G, Hsu H, Goeddel DV, et al: Dissection of TNF receptor-1 effector functions: JNK activation is not linked to apoptosis while NF-κB activation prevents cell death. Cell 87:565–576, 1996.

147. Natoli G, Costanzo A, Ianni A, et al: Activation of SAPK/JNK by TNF receptor-1 through a noncytotoxic TRAF2-dependent pathway. Science 275:200–203, 1997.

148. Yeh W-C, Shahinian A, Speiser D, et al: Early lethality, functional NF-κB activation, and increased sensitivity to TNF-induced cell death in TRAF2-deficient mice. Immunity 7:715–725, 1997.

149. Kelliher MA, Grimm S, Ishida Y, et al: The death domain kinase RIP mediates the TNF-induced NF-κB signal. Immunity 8:297–303, 1998.

150. Jonat C, Rahnsdorf HJ, Park K-K, et al: Antitumor promotion and antiinflammation: Down-modulation of AP-1 (Fos/Jun) activity by glucocorticoid hormone. Cell 62:1189–1204, 1990.

151. Yang-Yen H-F, Chambard J-C, Sun Y-L, et al: Transcription interference between c-Jun and the glucocorticoid receptor: Mutual inhibition of DNA binding due to direct protein-protein interaction. Cell 62:1205–1215, 1990.

152. Schüle R, Rangarajan P, Kliewer S, et al: Functional antagonism between oncoprotein c-Jun and the glucocorticoid receptor. Cell 62:1217–1226, 1990.

Chapter 10

Nuclear Receptor Superfamily

Etienne-Emile Baulieu ▪ Jan Mester ▪ Gézard Redeuilh

The external signals that regulate the behavior of eukaryotic cells are recognized by specific "receptor" molecules. Signal transduction mechanisms initiated by activation of the receptor then lead to a given cellular response via changes in transcription factors and induction (or inhibition) of the expression of specific genes. In the case of nuclear receptors (NRs), the regulatory molecules (ligands) enter the cell, usually by passive diffusion, and interact directly with their receptors to form active complexes in the nucleus. This interaction induces structural changes in the receptor molecule, which in turn initiates its transcription regulatory activity. Members of the NR superfamily therefore represent a unique category of proteins that act as both receptors and transcription factors.

Compiling a succinct description of NRs has required several decades of research. Recently, the Nuclear Receptors Nomenclature Committee adopted a unified nomenclature of the NR superfamily members.[1] Although the breadth of the current chapter does not allow for a review of all NR superfamily members, we intend to focus in some detail on receptors that are activated by signaling molecules secreted into the circulation. Additional information concerning the actions of specific NRs can be found in Chapters 72, 95, 114, 117, 129, 140, 149, and 165.

The existence of cellular receptors activated by small lipophilic molecules was first demonstrated nearly 40 years ago. Confirmation came to fruition after identification of the selective retention of tritium-labeled estradiol in its target organ the uterus, in vivo, and in uterine proteins capable of binding estradiol with high affinity (K_d on the order of 0.1 nmol/L) and specificity. The definition of the estradiol-binding protein as the receptor—that is, as the molecule actually involved in transduction of the estrogen signal in the uterine cell—was initially based on indirect evidence involving a correlation between binding characteristics and estrogen-induced responses. The discovery of specific antagonists bound by the presumed estrogen receptor (ER) supported this evidence. Changes in physicochemical properties (size, binding characteristics) and in the apparent subcellular distribution (soluble when ligand-free, nuclear bound when complexed) provided further corroboration.

Similar experimental approaches and reasoning greatly facilitated the detection and characterization of receptors for several types of steroid hormones and other structurally related signaling molecules (vitamin D, retinoids, thyroid hormones).[2–4] These types of receptor ligands share general structural features such as small size and lipophilic characteristics (Fig. 10–1).

Intensive efforts by many laboratories have greatly enhanced our understanding of how these small lipophilic molecules signal through their receptors. This information has been derived from purification of the receptors for estrogens,*[5–7] progesterone,[8, 9] and glucocorticosteroids[10, 11] and the use of specific antibodies to allow molecular cloning of the corresponding cDNAs. Hybridization under low-stringency conditions has also accelerated the identification of additional cDNA clones coding for the numerous members of the NR superfamily (for representative references see elsewhere[12–20]).

Results from these studies revealed a transcription factor–like molecule (an *active* receptor) with a central portion characterized by two zinc finger structures that bind to DNA and by transcription-promoting activity in the C-terminal domain, which is obstructed by its association with the chaperone molecule heat shock protein-90 (hsp90). The transactivating function of the receptor is induced by agonist ligands after conformational changes in the structure of the ligand-binding domain (LBD) of the molecule and the simultaneous or subsequent dissociation of hsp90.

RESEARCH METHODS USED FOR STUDIES OF NUCLEAR RECEPTORS

Evolving technology has greatly enhanced our understanding of the structure-function relationships of NRs. The first chapter in this success story involved the synthesis of *radioactively labeled steroids* with high specific activity,[3] which led to identification of the first receptors. Synthesis of materials with appropriate affinity resulted in their *purification* (in conjunction with ligand and DNA affinity chromatography), whereas the *antibodies* raised against such receptors permitted cloning of the corresponding cDNA. *Recombinant DNA technology,* as well as methods that study protein/DNA interactions (*electrophoretic mobility shift assay*; *DNA footprinting*) and transcription regulation under in vitro and *transient transfection* conditions, was then used to analyze the functional domains of the receptors. These seminal studies have been complemented by recent experiments involving protein-protein interactions ("*supershift*" in the electrophoretic mobility shift assay, immunoprecipitation, "*far-Western*" blotting, which involves interaction of labeled DNA probes with proteins immobilized on a filter after electrophoretic fractionation and transfer) and by pull-down experiments using in vitro translated ^{35}S-labeled proteins. In addition, the advent of *targeted gene disruption* methods has led to the production of laboratory animals with lack of efficient genes coding for NRs and attempts to determine their role in the entire organism. Examination of conditional, cell type–specific gene inactivation methods appears to be an important new phase of NR research.

---

*By "estrogen receptor" we mean the α isotype, unless otherwise indicated.

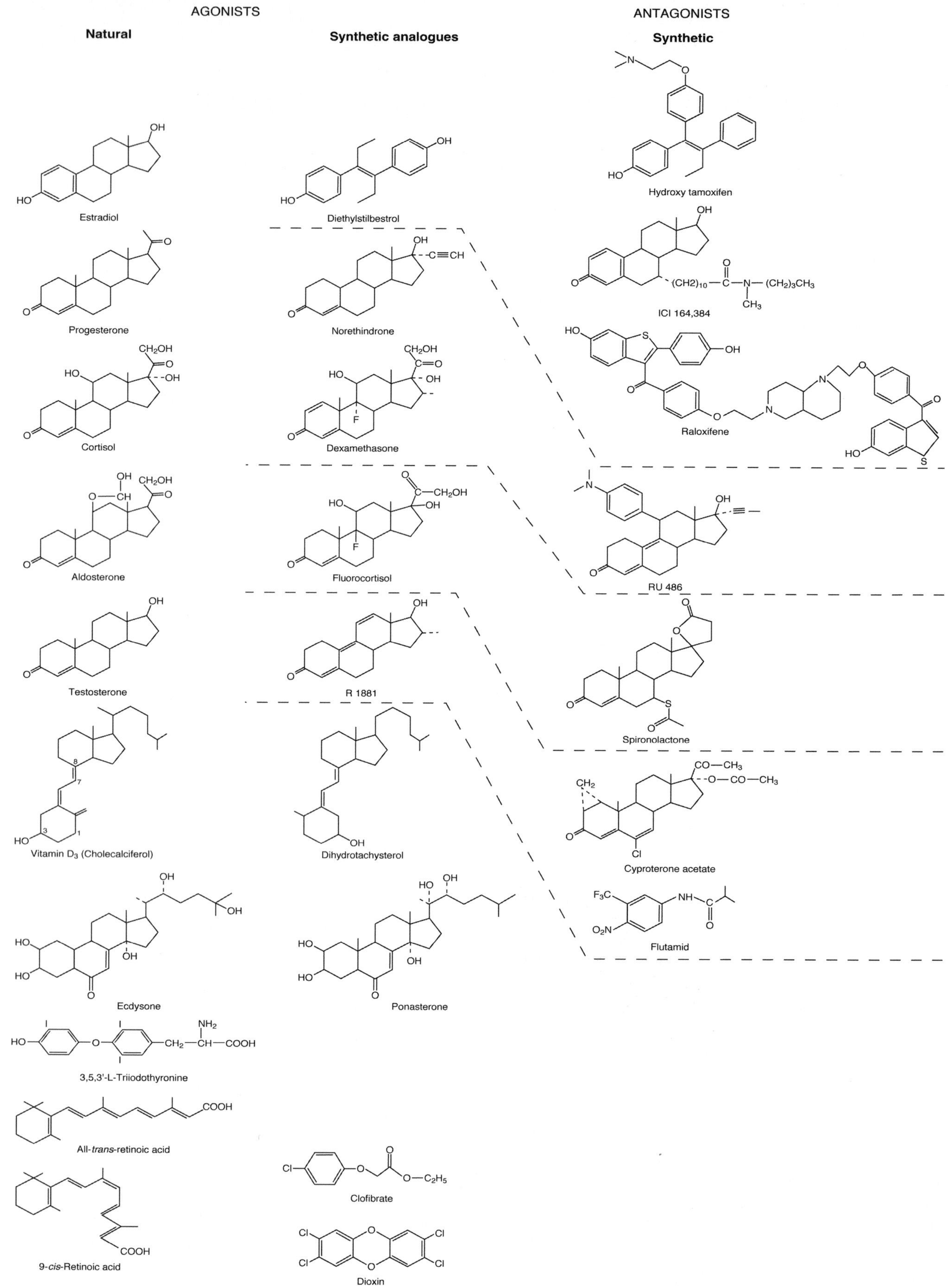

FIGURE 10–1. Chemical structures of ligands of different families of nuclear receptors. The most important *natural agonists* are represented. In most animals, there are five categories of steroidal ligands, each activating its appropriate receptor. In rodents, the most important glucocorticosteroid is corticosterone instead of cortisol. The most active androgen is 5α-dihydrotestosterone, a metabolite produced intracellularly from the secreted testosterone. Similarly, 1,25-dihydroxycholecalciferol and β-ecdysone are the active metabolites, respectively, of vitamin D₃ and ecdysone. The two retinoic acids shown (metabolites of vitamin A) bind to different receptor isoforms. Among *synthetic agonists*, representative examples have been selected. There exist also a few natural antihormonal activities, such as that of progesterone displaying anti-mineralocorticosteroid action.

OLIGOMERIC STRUCTURE AND SUBCELLULAR LOCALIZATION OF NATIVE STEROID HORMONE RECEPTORS

In the absence of ligand, steroid hormone receptors are present in target tissues as large protein complexes. Such is the case, for example, in the uterus of an immature or ovariectomized female. Binding the ligand at a low temperature does not modify the general characteristics of this form of the receptor. In contrast, exposure to the ligand at physiologic temperatures, either in vivo or in vitro, leads to marked changes in the apparent subcellular distribution (the receptor becomes tightly associated with the nucleus) and physicochemical characteristics (smaller size, altered pI, altered rate of dissociation of the ligand) (see elsewhere for further references[10, 21–28]).

Successful efforts to purify different receptor forms have brought considerable clarity to the aforementioned observations. The large receptor form, denoted as "native" receptor, contains at least two different proteins: the ligand-binding subunit and hsp90.[29, 30] As a rule, the latter is present as a dimer, and the resulting structure is that of a hetero-oligomer.[31, 32] All steroid hormone receptors and some other members of the NR superfamily conform to this type of "native" structure. The role of the hsp90 component has been unclear for some time; however, a generally accepted idea is that hsp90 prevents the hormone-binding component from binding to DNA. The negative regulatory role of hsp90 is passive, but it can actively detach the hormone-binding subunit from DNA.[33] Hsp90 also exercises a protective function (particularly for the receptor of glucocorticosteroids and mineralocorticosteroids) consistent with the "chaperone" role that it plays with numerous other cellular proteins.[34, 35] Disruption of this chaperone activity by the ansamycin antibiotic geldanamycin leads to rapid loss of the hormone-binding and/or transactivation function of receptors that form hsp90-containing oligomers.[36–38] Henceforth the term *receptor* will be used to denote the *hormone- and DNA-binding subunit* of the oligomeric complex or the intracellular protein complexes that interact directly with the ligand and mediate hormone action.

Additional proteins are also associated with native receptors, although generally via the hsp90 component. Among these proteins are (1) p59 immunophilin (FKBP52 [FK506–binding protein-52]), which is capable of binding the immunosuppressors FK506 and rapamycin[39, 40]; (2) Cyp40,[41] the cyclosporine-binding protein; (3) hsp70; and (4) p23. The role that these proteins play in the action of steroid hormones has yet to be demonstrated. However, p59 and hsp70, in conjunction with hsp90, appear to participate in the folding of the glucocorticosteroid receptor (GR) that converts the LBD from the non–steroid-binding to the steroid-binding conformation. Although p23 is not required for the maturation of newly synthesized receptors,[42] it does stabilize the hetero-oligomeric, ligand-binding complex.[35]

Unlike steroid hormone receptors, other members of the NR family were detected in the nuclear compartment (irrespective of cell exposure to the ligand). When appropriate methods were applied to determine the subcellular localization of ER, they refuted the view of the cyto-plasmic receptor (which binds the hormone and subsequently translocates in the nucleus). In fact, native (unliganded) steroid hormone receptors are generally (although weakly) associated with the nuclear compartment.[43–45] The GR is an exception, and the cytoplasmic localization and nuclear translocation after steroid binding have been verified in living cells of this receptor (e.g., after being tagged with green fluorescent protein).[46] The observed subcellular distribution reflects the dynamic equilibrium produced by nucleocytoplasmic exchange or shuttling. Structural analysis of several NRs revealed the presence of nuclear localization sequences. Some were constitutive, whereas others were liberated after the structural modifications induced by hormone binding. The latter nuclear localization signals are responsible for the receptor molecule's entry into and exit from the nucleus.[47–50]

Although ligand-free receptors can bind to their cognate DNA sequences, their transactivating function is not functional under these conditions.[33, 51] The association between the nonliganded receptor and the hormone response element (HRE) is partially responsible for the suppression of promoter activity. This observation is particularly true of receptors that do not bind steroid hormones.[52] Nuclear localization can be prevented by occupying the receptor-binding site with an antagonistic ligand (which has been demonstrated for ER bound to RU 58668[53]). Evidently the situation is different for "true orphan" receptors, or those lacking an activating ligand. Their activity may be constitutive or regulated by posttranslational mechanisms or simply be dependent on the presence of appropriate transcription coactivators. Of course, it is conceivable that such "true" orphan receptors do not exist and that ultimately a ligand will be found for every member of the NR superfamily.

STRUCTURE-FUNCTION RELATIONSHIPS

Modular Structure of Nuclear Receptors

Initial characterization of the primary sequences of NRs was based on the degree of conservation observed in six different segments (A through F from the N to the C termini)[54–56] (Fig. 10–2). It has been increasingly recognized that each of these regions subserves several distinct functional purposes. The LBD, for example, covers a large C-terminal portion of the molecule that corresponds to the original E segment. The weakly conserved F segment has no known function. The LBD also carries one of the two transcription-transactivating functions, AF-2, which is strictly dependent on hormone binding. The other transactivating function, AF-1, is situated in the N-terminal domain (segments A and B) and is much less dependent on ligand binding. AF-1 is largely inactive in the intact unliganded receptor molecule, but it may become active when separated from the rest of the receptor sequence. The length of the N-terminal portion of the molecule is highly variable. The middle portion contains the DNA-binding domain (DBD; original segment C). An important feature of this portion of the receptor molecule is the presence of two zinc finger structures, that is, two loops, each containing four cysteines stabilized by coordination bonds with Zn^{2+} ions (Fig. 10–3). The junction between the DBD and the adjoining C-terminal sequences is denoted as

FIGURE 10–2. Modular structure of NRs. Based on sequence homologies and on functional studies, the NR molecule contains six segments, A through F, with an ill-defined A/B frontier. The C and E domains are best conserved across different species, in contrast with the poorly conserved A/B domain. The F domain is absent in many receptors and has no known function. The functional domains identified in the different receptors are indicated in the figure. NLS are nuclear localization sequences; AF-1, AF-2 are the transcription transactivating functions 1 and 2, respectively.

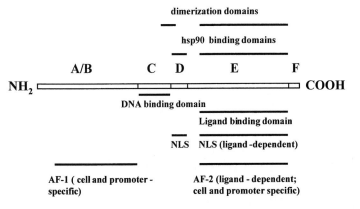

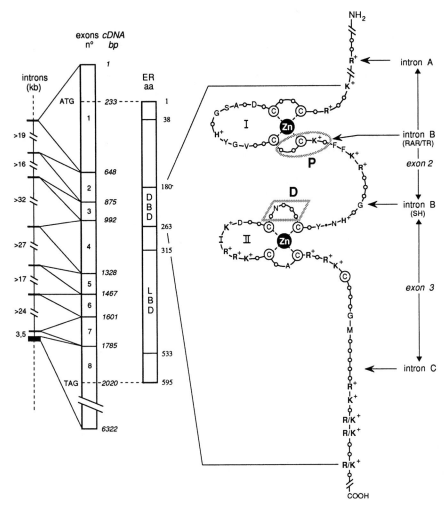

FIGURE 10–3. Genomic organization and DNA-binding region. The genomic organization is shown using ER as an example. The first in-frame ATG is situated at the base pair 233. The two characteristic zinc fingers of the DNA-binding domain of steroid hormone (SH) receptors are represented; they are encoded by separate exons 2 and 3. The intervening introns (denoted A, B, and C) are indicated for the receptors of SH, retinoids and thyroid hormones; the position of the B intron differs between SH receptors and RAR/TR. Coordination bonds with four cysteine residues attach the zinc atoms; a fifth conserved cysteine is situated in the C-terminal extremity of the second zinc finger. Conserved amino acids are shown, and the proximal (P) and distal (D) domains involved in the DNA sequence recognition are boxed.

the "hinge" and corresponds to the original segment D. This flexible segment may be important for spatial configuration of the protein. The distribution of tasks between the different functional domains of the receptor molecule has been verified in numerous laboratories that have produced various sorts of chimeric molecules. The DBD is crucial in recognizing DNA sequences regulated by the receptors, whereas the LBD is decisive in discrimination between the respective ligand molecules.

Other functional features of the different segments coincide with the aforementioned domains (see Fig. 10–2). For example, the LBD contains sequences involved in hsp90 binding, dimerization, and the ligand-dependent nuclear localization sequences. Other sequences required for dimerization, hsp90 binding, and the constitutive nuclear localization sequences are situated within the DBD and adjoining sequences of the hinge segment.[54]

Apart from the receptors involved in hormone signaling (and similar molecules such as steroids, ecdysteroids, vitamin D, retinoids, and thyroid hormones), sequence homologies have extended the NR superfamily beyond the term "receptor" to include DNA-binding proteins for which no ligand is known (and may not exist). The number of these "orphan receptors" is still increasing, and for many, no specific biologic function has been identified to date[52] (Fig. 10–4). Besides, some ligand-activated transcription factors do not display any significant homology with NRs and are not considered superfamily members. These factors include the arylhydrocarbon receptor, whose structure is more similar to a basic helix-loop-helix rather than a zinc finger protein.

The modular structure of NRs outlined above represents only a general framework. Individual proteins, such as the progesterone receptor (PR), possess additional specific features. For example, PR exists as two isoforms encoded by two different mRNAs transcribed

from a single gene. As we shall discuss, receptor isoforms encoded by different genes are quite common. These two PR isoforms, A and B, differ in length of the N-terminal domain: the human PR-A isoform lacks the first 164 amino acids present in PR-B. Both are active as modulators of transcription but display important functional differences that in turn vary among species. Unlike PR-B, for example, human PR-A has been reported to act predominantly as a *trans*-dominant repressor of transcription activated not only by PR-B but also by the receptors of androgens, glucocorticosteroids, and estrogens. In contrast, the chicken PR-A isoform acts as a transcriptional transactivator and lacks repressor activity.[57] In the mouse, overexpression of the PR-A form has led to abnormalities in development of the mammary gland; in the rabbit, however, only PR-B is expressed.[58, 59]

Conservation of the structure of NRs suggests that they are derived from a single ancestral gene that presumably coded for a ligand-independent transcription factor.[60] Comparisons of primary sequences form the basis of the evolutionary tree[61] (see Fig. 10–4).

Activation of Steroid Hormone Receptors

Binding of the ligand induces important changes in the spatial structure of the LBD. In the case of steroid hormone receptors, these changes cause the receptor to dissociate from its partner constituents of the hetero-oligomeric native complex. Similarly, all ligand-activated NRs liberate the transcription-activating functions (Fig. 10–5). X-ray crystallography of the cloned LBD of several receptors (some in the unliganded form and others complexed with the ligand) has shed considerable light on these changes. Molecular modeling of the three-dimensional structure of different LBDs suggests a remarkable degree

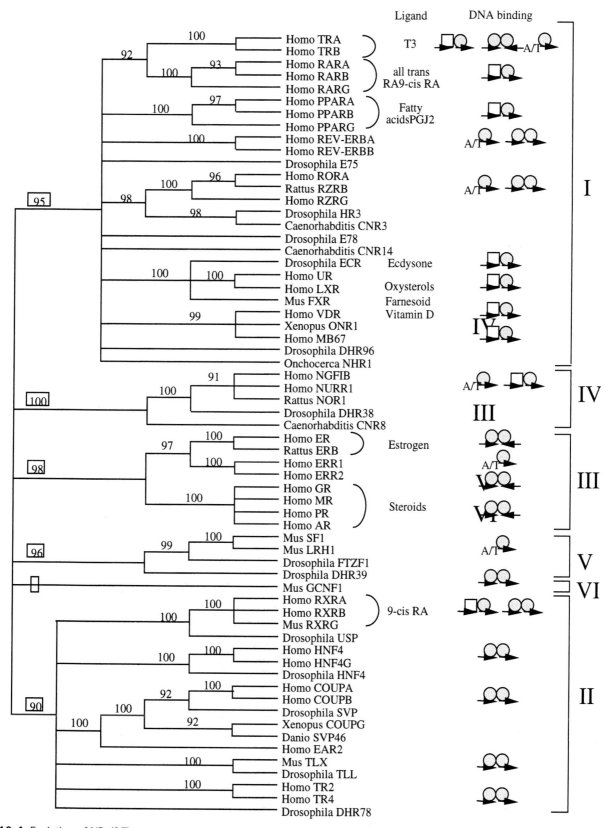

FIGURE 10–4. Evolution of NRs.[60] The consensus tree, based on the comparisons of amino acid sequences (evaluated in terms of "bootstrap values" reflecting the robustness of the homologies), is shown. Bootstrap values above 90% allow the definition of six subfamilies (I–VI). The ligand binding and dimerization/HRE binding is schematized at the right of the figure. The *arrows* represent the PuGGTCA core motifs, which can be a single unit preceded by an A/T rich sequence, a palindrome, or a direct repeat. *Gray circles* represent the receptors; *white squares*, RXR in the heterodimeric complexes.

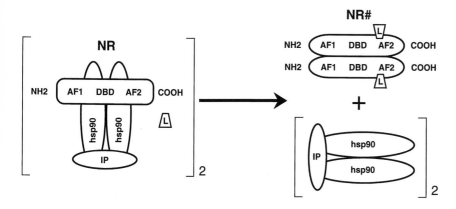

NR - nuclear receptor
NR# - activated nuclear receptor
IP - immunophilin
L - ligand
AF1, AF2 - transactivation domain
DBD-DNA-binding domain

FIGURE 10-5. Activation of steroid hormone receptors. Nontransformed complexes between NR and hsp90 dimer associated with an immunophilin (IP) binding ligand (L), undergo structural changes, release hsp90/IP complexes, and form homodimers able to assume their transactivating function.

of similarity, although important differences still exist between the primary structures.[62, 63] The LBD contains 12 α helixes (H1 to H12), the first 11 of which are organized in an antiparallel "sandwich" of three α helix layers (Fig. 10-6A; see also color plate) with a central cavity fitted to accommodate the ligand. The C-terminal helix (H12) of the ER extends out from the LBD, and after binding of the agonistic ligand, it moves to close the cavity. The subsequent surface formed is then able to interact with coactivator proteins and components of the transcription preinitiation complex.[62] Remarkably, when the binding site is occupied by the antagonist raloxifene, the positioning of helix H12 is altered (see Fig. 10-6B; see also color plate); instead of closing the ligand-binding pocket, H12 interacts with H5 and the C-terminal end of H3 to occlude the conserved Lys362 required for the recruitment of certain coactivators[64] (see below). This observation may explain the partial antiestrogenic activity of raloxifene. Moreover, given that the spatial configuration of LBD is apparently conserved between different NRs, the design of antagonists and partial agonists will probably be facilitated by these structural studies.

In vitro, release of the steroid hormone receptor from the native oligomeric protein complex takes place after binding the ligand under conditions that resemble those of the living cell. This process is temperature dependent; that is, it is very slow at 4°C and quite rapid above 25°C. In contrast, exposure of the native complex to conditions that interfere with electrostatic bonds (high ionic strength) disrupts the native complex even at low temperatures. Similarly, the receptor is released from native complexes by treatments such as polyanions (heparin), chaotropic agents (NaSCN), or ATP. Although the resulting receptor can bind to DNA, its transcription transactivation capacity has not been verified. In this context it is interesting that mutation of a conserved Tyr of the ER (537 in the α, 443 in the β isotype) to Ser or Asn results in a constitutively active molecule whose activity is inhibited by antiestrogens.[65]

Receptor molecules, in the absence of ligand, often bind to their regulatory elements in vivo without activation of transcription. The pattern of ligand-activated receptors not interacting with hsp90 is common and plays an important role in extinction of the expression of regulated genes in the absence of ligand. Within the steroid receptor subfamily, unliganded PR and ER have also been shown to bind to their respective DNA sequences.[33, 51] It is possible that such interactions, always nonproductive, are a part of the negative regulation of gene expression. Because hsp90 efficiently prevents receptor-DNA interaction,[33, 66] hormone-independent mechanisms that dissociate the native oligomeric complexes may be responsible for the availability of free, unliganded receptor molecules that can occupy the regulatory element in the absence of hormone.

Apart from "natural" activation by the agonist ligand, it has been observed that several steroid hormone receptors can be activated by phosphorylation. In the case of orphan receptors, activation by such posttranslational modifications can occur through physiologic mechanisms; it is not clear whether the same is true for steroid hormone receptors. However, signaling pathways triggered by peptide growth factors (insulin-like growth factor-1 [IGF-1], epidermal growth factor [EGF], transforming growth factor-α [TGF-α]) or by small molecules that bind to membrane receptors (e.g., dopamine) have been shown to lead to activation of the transactivating function of PR and ER. This type of signaling is mediated via serine/threonine protein kinases (PKA, PKC).[67-70] It is interesting that treatment of ER-containing cells with agonist or antagonist ligands induces the same type of phosphorylation.[71]

The effects of the steroid ligand- and kinase-mediated signals are additive, and both are inhibited by antagonist ligands. It is possible that the cellular protein kinase–mediated type of activation may enhance the action of steroid hormones and that its deregulation may be responsible for certain pathologies.

Modulation of transactivation by mechanisms linked to the state of phosphorylation has also been observed in the receptor for vitamin D_2, for several subtypes of retinoic acid receptor (RAR) and retinoid X receptor (RXR) (for example, see Matkovits and Christakos,[72] and for review see Weigel and Zhang[73]), as well as for ER[74] and GR.[75, 76]

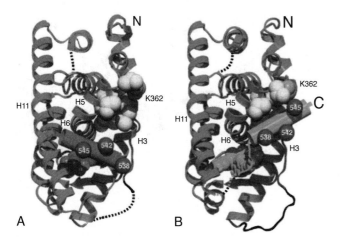

FIGURE 10-6. Structure of ER LBD as a function of the ligand. The ligand is estradiol in A, raloxifene in B. The position of the helix H12, drawn as A (E2-complex) or B (raloxifene complex), is radically different in the two complexes. In the E2-liganded complex, it forms a "lid" of the binding cavity, whereas raloxifene prevents this alignment. Dotted lines indicate unmodeled regions. (From Brzozowski AM, Pike AC, Dauter Z, et al: Molecular basis of agonism and antagonism in the oestrogen receptor. Nature 389:756, 1997.)

Interactions with DNA

Analysis of promoters of hormone-regulated genes by transient transfection, electrophoretic mobility shift assay, and DNA-footprinting methods has led to identification of the sequence elements recognized by their respective receptors. These HREs, which act as DNA-binding sites for the receptor, consist of two hexanucleotides or pentanucleotides ("half-sites") organized as direct or inverted (imperfect) repeats separated by a shorter or longer spacer (Table 10–1). Each half-site interacts with one molecule of the receptor, and the two receptor molecules form a dimer, either before or after binding to the half-sites.[77, 78]

Receptor specificity at this level is much less marked than that of the hormonal ligand-receptor interaction. As a result, the consensus element is identical for the receptors of glucocorticosteroids, mineralocorticosteroids, progestogens, and androgens; receptors for retinoid, thyroid hormone, and vitamin D also recognize similar response elements. Conversely, several if not all receptors interact with more than one type of HRE. Retinoid receptors, for example, regulate transcription of genes that contain either the appropriate inverted repeat or direct repeat sequences (see Table 10–1).

When extended to orphan receptors, similar studies have shown that apart from the mechanism relying on receptor dimers, monomer-activated response elements also exist. Mangelsdorf and collaborators propose that NRs be divided into four classes based on their type of interaction with DNA: class I functions as homodimers that recognize half-sites organized as inverted repeats (steroid receptors), class II uses RXR to form heterodimers (see the next section) and interacts with half-sites that are organized as either direct or inverted repeats (all remaining ligand-activated receptors), and orphan receptors are grouped in classes III (homodimers binding to direct repeats) and IV (monomer-activated core sites).[52, 79] This classification is useful for understanding certain aspects of their structure-function relationships, and in spite of several deviations from standard rules, overall it is very applicable. "Homodimers" of class I receptors can in fact be heterodimeric in that they may have two different isoforms, such as forms A and B of the PR (see Dimerization), as well as the α and β forms of the ER and their splice variants.[80, 81]

Detailed analysis has been performed on how several types of NRs interact with DNA. Two short amino acid elements, proximal (P-box) and distal (D-box),[82] are situated respectively at the C-terminal portion of the first zinc finger and at the N-terminal portion of the second zinc finger. Both elements are important to the specificity of this interaction (see Fig. 10–3; Table 10–1). The P-box appears to be crucial for sequence recognition, whereas the D-box plays an important role in positioning the two receptor molecules that interact with the half-sites, that is, for the length of the spacer DNA. These conclusions are a result of mutagenesis experiments and have been verified by x-ray crystallography and nuclear magnetic resonance[83, 84] (Fig. 10–7).

At this point we wish to stress the complexity of the receptor-DNA interactions. Earlier studies led to discovery of the simplest of these interactions and to definition of the consensus sequence elements for the respective members of the superfamily. Over time, the spectrum of sequences that any given receptor recognized became progressively larger and, consequently, less well defined. Thus although the simple scheme shown in the Table 10–1 is essentially correct, it does not encompass all the receptor-DNA interactions that may take place in different cells and on different promoters. In addition, indirect and secondary modes of transcriptional regulation by NRs lead to the involvement of HRE-unrelated regulatory DNA sequences.

It is clear that to ensure correct regulation of gene expression, mechanisms other than the simple HRE-receptor interaction must be involved. These mechanisms rely on the presence of cellular proteins that modulate transcriptional activation by NRs. The tridimensional structure of the ER molecule has been shown to be influenced by its interaction with DNA.[85] According to the estrogen response element (ERE) sequence (originated from different gene promoters), the accessibility of specific antibodies to their epitopes is different. As a result, EREs can be considered allosteric modulators of the receptor and, consequently, can regulate receptor interactions with different transcriptional cofactors.

Dimerization

As discussed above, dimer formation is essential for transcriptional activation of gene expression by NRs. Association with DNA favors the formation and stability of receptor dimers. Still, several receptors are dimeric when not bound to DNA. The native form of the ER, for instance, contains two hormone-binding subunits associated with an hsp90 dimer.[32] Its transformation after ligand binding releases a stable receptor dimer.[86, 87] Unliganded ER also binds to DNA as a dimer. This process appears to involve the Ser residue at position 236 in that its mutation to glutamic acid prevents both DNA binding and dimerization.[88] Cyclic adenosine monophosphate (cAMP)-dependent PKA phosphorylates Ser236 and inhibits dimerization in the absence of ligand. This inhibition is overcome by the addition of estradiol or the partial agonist 4-hydroxytamoxifen. Interestingly, treatment with the complete antagonist ICI 182,780 does not overcome the inhibitory effect of PKA. In the absence of ligand, ER dimerization involves interactions between DBDs. Dimerization mediated by the LBD occurs only upon ligand binding but is prevented by ICI 182,780.

Only one PR subunit is associated with the hsp90 dimer in the native form.[31] However, its release upon hormone binding also leads to the formation of dimers, although they are much less stable in solution than are ER dimers. Two isoforms of the PR (A and B) exist in most species, and both homodimers and heterodimers have been observed.

The subgroup of receptors for retinoid, thyroid hormone, and vitamin D presents a unique case of regulation of gene expression in

TABLE 10–1. Receptor-DNA Interactions: Constraints on Specificity

| Receptor | Structural Features of the Receptor | | Consensus HRE Sequence | |
	P-Box	D-Box	Direct Repeats	Inverted Repeats
"GR subfamily"				
GR, PR, MR, AR	GSCKV	AGRND		AGAACA(n_3)TGTTCT
"ER/TR subfamily"				
ER	EGCKA	PATNQ		AGGTCA(n_3)TGACCT
TR-α	EGCKG	KYDSC	AGGTCA(n_4)AGGTCA	AGGTCATGACCT
TR-β	EGCKG	KYEGK	AGGTCA(n_4)AGGTCA	AGGTCATGACCT
RAR-α, RAR-β	EGCKG	HRDKN	AGGTCA(n_5)AGGTCA	
VDR	EGCKG	PFNGD	AGGTCA(n_3)AGGTCA	
RXR	EGCKG	RDNKD	AGGTCA(n)AGGTCA	

Only some selected examples are shown. Note that the HRE sequences present in the promoters of the different nuclear receptor–regulated genes often present considerable deviations from the "consensus" shown in this table. The same is true for the length of spacers of the response elements for RAR/TR/VDR.

AR, androgen receptor; ER, estrogen receptor; GR, glucocorticoid receptor; HRE, hormone response element; MR, mineralocorticoid receptor; PR, progesterone receptor; RAR, retinoic acid receptor; RXR, retinoid X receptor; TR, thyroid hormone receptor; VDR, vitamin D_3 receptor.

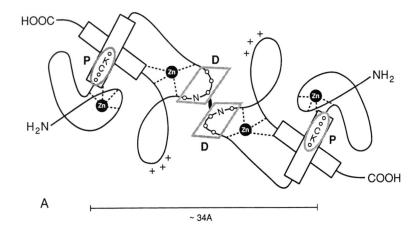

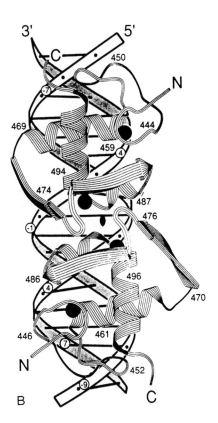

FIGURE 10–7. DBD dimerization and interaction with HRE.[83, 242] *A,* Relative orientation of the ER DBD monomer subunits as indicated by two-dimensional ¹H NMR. Each monomer contains two helixes perpendicular to each other (rectangles). The zinc atoms are coordinated by four cysteines *(dashed lines).* The positions of P- and D-box sequences are shown; the dimerization sequences overlap the D-box. In this orientation, the recognition helixes of the monomers are antiparallel, to fit in successive major grooves separated by 34Å. *B,* Interaction with DNA. The DBD subunits bind to successive major grooves, whereas the dimerization surfaces are positioned over the minor grooves. This model is based on a crystallographic analysis using the GR DBD and an artificial GRE where the two half-sites are separated by four (instead of three) nucleotides. As a consequence, only one subunit faces the target half-site, and the second subunit faces a noncognate DNA sequence, shifted by one base pair.

which the formation of dimers helps ensure the specificity of action. For instance, six different receptor subtypes—α, β, and γ RAR receptors and α, β, and γ RXR receptors—have been identified, each of which is able to bind retinoids. Several isoforms of the different RAR and RXR subtypes are known.[89] RAR is activated by the all-*trans* and 9-*cis* isomers of retinoic acid, whereas RXR is bound and activated only by the 9-*cis* isomer. Transcriptional activation requires heterodimers composed of one RAR and one RXR subunit. The particular heterodimer formed appears to depend on cellular expression of the appropriate isotypes and on the type of ligand.[90] Remarkably, RXR serves as a "coactivator" for RARs and other members of this subgroup, such as thyroid hormone receptor (TR), vitamin D receptors (VDRs), and peroxisome proliferator–activated receptors (PPARs), several subtypes of which have been identified.

Structure and Expression of Genes Coding for Nuclear Receptors

A hormonally regulated cell requires expression of the appropriate set of receptors. For other proteins that characterize the state of cell differentiation, however, it is still unclear exactly how this expression is acquired and maintained. Still, the mechanisms behind this expression are known to share the following properties: (1) remodeling of the chromatin structure in the vicinity of the genes, (2) establishment and maintenance of chemical modifications such as DNA methylation, and (3) expression of the appropriate transcription regulatory factors whose promoters are subject to the same structural constraints. Understanding regulation of the activity of the promoters of genes coding for the receptors is necessary (but clearly not sufficient) for elucidation of these differentiation-related processes. In the differentiated cell, the structure of the promoter of a given receptor gene will ensure its appropriate expression (according to the organ [cell type] and given physiologic situation).

Study of the promoters of the genes coding for NRs has attracted surprisingly little attention in recent years. One possible reason is that the genes themselves are extremely large (>140 kb for the human ER-α gene,[91] >90 kb for the human PR gene[92]). In addition, these genes are transcribed from multiple promoters, some of which are situated far upstream from the first coding exon.[55] Nevertheless, there are several reasons to believe that the complex structure of the 5′ flanking region of these genes is precisely what underlies many of the cell-specific mechanisms that regulate expression of these genes. In the case of human ER (hER; apart from a proximal promoter [promoter A]), analysis of hER mRNA from different cell types has led to the identification of two distal promoters, B and C (reviewed by Grandien et al.[55]). All these promoters display relatively low transcriptional activity corresponding to low mRNA cellular levels. Different isoforms of hER mRNA (i.e., transcribed from different promoters of the ER-α gene) are present in varying ratios according to the cell type. For example, the A and B isoforms are present in the uterus and the mammary gland, whereas the C isoform is predominant in the liver, where a low amount of the B isoform is also found. Additionally, a disproportionally high level of the A isoform is present in cell lines derived from hormone-dependent cancers.[55] The presence of multiple promoters also characterizes other genes coding for the NR superfamily members, although detailed studies have yet to be performed.[55]

Finally, apart from transcriptional regulation, the cellular concentration of the receptor gene product depends on the following posttranscriptional mechanisms: (1) processing of the RNA transcript, (2) mRNA stability, (3) translation, (4) posttranscriptional modifications, and (5) mechanisms leading to inactivation/degradation of the receptor. Posttranscriptional processes at the RNA level will be influenced by the structure of the 5′ untranslated sequences and, consequently, will depend on the alternative promoter usage discussed previously.

At least six modes of regulation of the expression of steroid hormone receptors can be distinguished:

1. *Constitutive expression,* which requires non–hormone-dependent transcription factors. This type of "regulation" involves the basal expression evident in the ERs of immature female reproductive organs, as well as in the androgen receptors (ARs) of immature males. GRs are constitutively expressed in most, if not all mammalian tissues and cell types, but their expression may not be independent of external (hormonal or nonhormonal) factors (see below).

2. *Homologous induction* (i.e., induction of expression of the recep-

tor by the ligand). This type of regulation is the case, for example, with ERs and ARs. Molecular analysis of androgen-induced AR upregulation reveals that it relies on transcriptional regulation mediated by two androgen recognition half-sites, separated by 182 bp, that are situated in the coding region.

3. *Homologous downregulation.* Temporary or lasting downregulation can be caused by both transcriptional and posttranscriptional mechanisms, depending on the receptor and cell type.

4. *Heterologous induction.* One example involves induction of the PR by estrogens and appears to be mediated by non–consensus response elements present as a set of half-sites separated by long intervening sequences.[93]

5. *Heterologous downregulation.* Exposure to progestagens frequently leads to a decrease in the content of ER. This phenomenon is undoubtedly of physiologic importance, particularly with regard to reducing the sensitivity of target tissues to circulating estrogens. In breast cancer T47D cells, incubation with ORG 2058 results in rapid downregulation of ER mRNA levels to a nadir of 35% to 40% of control by 6 hours, apparently by reducing transcription of the ER gene. Similar effects have been observed with respect to the level of the ER protein, which is consistent with earlier reports concerning the effects of progesterone in vivo on the ER of the rat uterus and chicken oviduct.[94–96]

6. *Induction or downregulation by nonsteroidal stimuli*, such as the actions of peptide hormones or other signaling molecules. One example that may have physiopathologic implications is inhibition of expression of the ER gene in the hormone-dependent breast cancer cell line MCF7 by TGF-β.[97] Activation of PKC by phorbol esters has been reported to downregulate ER, apparently by posttranscriptional destabilization of ER mRNA.[98]

Several different mechanisms can be observed for any given receptor (also see the section Signaling Crosstalk). For instance, ER is transiently downregulated by estrogens in the rat uterus (during the first 4–6 hours) but is induced in the long term (12–24 hours). In other organs such as the chick liver or oviduct, only the induction is observed. In tissue culture cells it has been shown that incubation with the "pure" antiestrogen ICI 164,384 causes ER downregulation by shortening the half-life of the ER protein from 5 to less than 1 hour.[99] Similarly, progesterone downregulates its own receptors in a quasipermanent manner in the rodent uterus, but only transiently in the chicken oviduct. PR is induced by estrogens in many estrogen target tissues (e.g., rodent uterus, chicken oviduct, human breast cancer cells) but not all (absent from the liver under any condition). This diversity is ensured, in part, by the fact that the promoters of the receptor genes can be differentially regulated. Such differential regulation has been observed in the ER gene, which is transcribed from three alternative promoters; transcripts are produced with different 5′ noncoding sequences and thus have unique coding sequences.[55]

REGULATION OF GENE EXPRESSION BY NUCLEAR RECEPTORS

Since the discovery of NRs it has been hypothesized that they act as regulators of gene expression. The effects of steroid hormones on the accumulation of specific mRNAs was described in the 1970s. At that time both transcriptional and translational modes of action were considered, although the latter (e.g., see Pennequin et al.[100]) did not lead to conclusive data capable of accounting for the rapid and powerful induction of specific gene expression observed in the target cells. Overall, the experimental data pointed to the role of NRs as regulators of transcription. As knowledge concerning transcription advanced, it became clear that the mechanisms involved were more complex than initially thought.

Regulation of transcription of chromosomal genes operates on at least three levels: (1) recognition of specific DNA sequences ("enhancer elements") proximal to the site of initiation of transcription by the appropriate proteins ("enhancer-binding proteins"), (2) association of cofactors/modulators, and (3) formation of the preinitiation complex, which includes general transcription factors and RNA polymer-

ase II. At present, consensus has been reached concerning the role of NRs as members of the category of enhancer-binding proteins that bind to their cognate DNA sequences (HRE); on occasion, however, they can also exercise other modes of transcriptional regulation and act as cofactors (coactivators or co-repressors) (cyclin D1, AP-1 [activator protein-1]). In addition, NRs display indirect modes of action: among the genes induced by their direct action, some code for other transcriptional regulators (e.g., see Dean et al.[101]) and cellular signaling proteins (e.g., cyclin-dependent kinase inhibitory protein p21[102]).

During the last decade most of the general transcription factors involved in formation of the preinitiation complex have been characterized and cloned.[103–105] It was natural to assume that interactions between NRs and one or more basal transcription factors mediate their transcriptional effects. A class of chromatin-remodeling proteins dependent on ATP hydrolysis and recruited by NRs to the nucleosome core has recently emerged. The architectural DNA-binding proteins such as high-mobility group protein-1 (HMG-1) and the highly related HMG-2 have been reported to stimulate DNA binding of ER, PR, AR, and GR[106–108] (although the physiologic relevance of this observation is unproved). The concept that NRs may require the participation of cellular factors named coactivators/adapters/transcription intermediary factors (TIFs) available in limited quantities was derived from the squelching phenomenon—that is, a reduction in transcription observed when the receptor is overexpressed and presumably competes with the promoter for TIFs.[109] A large and growing family of coactivators has been discovered in the last several years. These discoveries are largely due to recent technologic advances in protein-protein interaction screening strategies.

Interactions with General Transcription Factors

Promoter-specific initiation of mRNA synthesis in eukaryotic cells requires the assembly of RNA polymerase II and a set of general transcription initiation factors, TFIIA, TFIID, TFIIB, TFIIE, TFIIF, and TFIIH, at the core promoter elements.[110] Biochemical dissection of TFIID has revealed that this transcription factor consists of TATA box–binding protein (TBP) and as many as 13 bound subunits (the TBP-associated factors, called TAFIIs, ranging in size from 18 to 250 kDa[111, 112]). Formation of the preinitiation complex at the core promoter elements begins with the binding of TFIID at the TATA box. It is then followed by the binding of TFIIA, TFIIB, TFIIF–RNA polymerase II, TFIIE, and TFIIH, either in an ordered stepwise fashion[110] or as part of an RNA polymerase II holoenzyme whose exact composition remains to be established.[113, 114] Similar to many other sequence-specific transcription factors, NRs interact directly with several components of the general transcription machinery. For example, ER transactivation is increased in response to overexpression of TBP, and the two proteins interact directly in vitro.[115] The yeast two-hybrid screening technique detects a specific ligand-dependent interaction between TBP and RXR that requires integrity of the transcription activation domains.[116] It has been proposed that TAFIIs act as coactivators of upstream enhancer-binding factors.[117] Indeed, a new TBP-associated factor, TAFII30, is required for transactivation by ER.[118] Human TAFII28 promotes strong ligand-dependent activity of RXR-α on a minimal promoter and potentiates transactivation by ER and VDR; other classes of activators are not affected.[119] *Drosophila* TAFII110 (corresponding to human TAFII135) interacts with regions situated outside the transcription activation domains of PR, RAR, and TR-α and TR-β, but it does not affect the AF-2 domains of ER or RXR.[120] These observations led to the hypothesis that NRs might recruit a functionally distinct subpopulation of TFIID complexes composed of common TAFIIs and unique TAFII subunits. Several members of the NR superfamily, such as ER, PR, TR, VDR, and the orphan receptors chick ovalbumin upstream promoter transcription factor (COUP-TF) and hepatocyte nuclear factor-4 (HNF-4), have been reported to interact directly with TFIIB.[121–126] However, the domains of the receptors involved in TFIIB binding differ. It has been suggested that ER does not increase the recruitment or stabilization of TFIIB binding to the promoter, but rather it induces a qualitative conformational change in the TBP/TFIID-TFIIB-promoter complex, thereby enhancing the binding of subsequent components of the preinitiation complex.[126] The physiologic significance of these interactions remains to be established.

Phosphorylation on a specific amino acid residue is also a mechanism of regulation of activity. For instance, the AF-1 domain of RAR-α_1 is phosphorylated and activated by cdk7 (cyclin-dependent kinase-7) associated with the general transcription factor TFIIH. It has also been shown that RAR-α is associated with TFIIH in HeLa cells.[127] Phosphorylation of specific amino acid residues of the GR by cellular enzymes can either activate or inhibit its transcriptional activity.[76]

As a rule, the binding of NRs to components of the general transcription machinery is not dependent on the presence of a functional receptor activation domain. Therefore, interactions between NRs and general transcription initiation factors are necessary, but not sufficient for effective mediation of the transcriptional activity of receptors.

Interaction with Chromatin Factors

Before describing the interactions of NRs with chromatin factors, we shall briefly summarize the role of chromatin structure in gene regulation. Eukaryotic nuclear DNA is organized by association with histones and nonhistone proteins into nucleosomes and higher-order chromatin structures. DNA is packaged as a polynucleosome string (the 10-nm fiber) that is further folded into a solenoidal array to form the 30-nm fiber.[128–130] Active genes are located within the region of chromatin exhibiting increased sensitivity to digestion with DNase I. It is commonly assumed that the 10-nm fiber is the template for transcription of DNA by RNA polymerase II.[128]

A critical step in activation of a eukaryotic gene is the generation of an active conformation at promoters. Previous studies have demonstrated correlations between the availability of promoters for the induction of transcription by hormones and their pattern of accessibility to nuclease digestion, thus indicating the role of chromatin organization in the regulation of gene expression by NRs. Such findings suggest that the basal repression of gene promoters before hormone induction is due to their organization in chromatin.[131, 132] These findings have been obtained primarily from functional studies concerning regulation by GR of the mouse mammary tumor virus (MMTV) promoter in cell lines carrying stable minichromosomes and in nucleosome reconstitution systems. The hormone receptors are able to bind their cognate sequences within positioned nucleosomes and induce a rearrangement of nucleosomes that facilitates the access of other transcription factors, such as NF-1 and Oct-1.[133, 134] Thus the nucleosomal organization of the promoter plays a dual role, both in constitutive repression and in synergy between receptors NF-1 and Oct-1 (essential for optimal transcription after hormone induction).

Several in vitro studies have shown that binding of GR, ER, and PR to their response elements in a nucleosome is insufficient for nucleosome rearrangement. Genetic and biochemical studies in yeast have identified a set of genes, *SWI/SNF*, whose products remodel the nucleosome structure in an ATP-dependent manner.[135] The exact nature of this remodeling has not been determined. Human homologues of these proteins, termed hbrm and BRG-1, enhance the activity of ER, RAR, and GR in transfected cells. As a result, it is postulated that NRs functionally target the SWI/SNF complex to the promoter and thereby trigger nucleosome remodeling. Recently, the SWI/SNF complex has been identified as an integral component of the polymerase II holoenzyme. Although alterations in chromatin structure are usually limited to the region involved in the regulation of initiation, it remains possible that the SWI/SNF complex may facilitate the elongation process.[136]

Recently, the chromatin nonhistone HMG-1 and the highly related HMG-2 have been reported to stimulate DNA binding of steroid receptors (e.g., ER, PR, AR, and GR) while having no effect on DNA binding by several nonsteroid NRs (e.g., RAR, RXR, and VDR[106]). In transient transfection assays, coexpression of HMG-1/HMG-2 increased steroid receptor–mediated transcription in mammalian cells without altering the basal promoter activity of target genes. HMG-1 and HMG-2 themselves do not bind to the HRE in the absence of steroid hormone receptors. Thus, HMG-1/HMG-2 recruited to the

receptor-DNA complex may contribute to modification of chromatin structure and/or establish the three-dimensional structure at the promoter required for the assembly of higher-order nucleoprotein complexes.[105] However, the physiologic relevance of these observations remains to be verified.

Most of the studies concerning the mechanism of transcriptional regulation by NRs have been performed on transiently transfected cells. Under such conditions, the transfected DNA does not seem to be organized along correctly positioned nucleosomes. Consequently, the extent to which transiently expressed reporter genes reproduce the mechanisms involving chromatin remodeling are unclear.

Interactions with Coactivators

Evidence that NRs may require additional factors, termed coactivators/adapters/transcription intermediary factors, for optimal transcriptional activity was derived from the squelching phenomenon. In transiently transfected cells, both the AF-1 and AF-2 domains of several NRs activate transcription in a promoter and cell-dependent manner, thus suggesting that different coactivators are present in different target tissues and in limited quantities.[54] It should be stressed that the definition of a coactivator is not yet clear. In this chapter we consider a coactivator to be any protein that (1) enhances the transcriptional activity of an NR without affecting the basal transcription level and (2) can relieve autoreceptor or interreceptor squelching when overexpressed in transiently transfected mammalian cells.

Coactivators can function by relaying the AF signals of NRs to stimulate several processes involved in the initiation of transcription, including (1) recruitment of polymerase II and general transcription factors to the promoter, (2) covalent modifications of polymerase II and/or general transcription factors, and (3) allosteric effects on configuration of the preinitiation complex.

Several proteins that interact with NRs have been identified and characterized by biochemical strategies such as the two-hybrid screening system and genetic screens. Some of these proteins belong to the family termed steroid receptor coactivators (SRCs), which includes SRC-1[137] (NCoA-1[138] [nuclear receptor coactivator-1]), SRC-2 (TIF-2,[139] GRIP1 [GR-interacting protein-1],[140] and NCoA-2[141]), and SRC-3 (AIB1,[142] RAC3,[143] p/CIP,[141] and ACTR[144]). Several other proteins that interact with NRs in a ligand-dependent manner have also been identified, such as RIP140,[115] RIP160,[115] ERAP140,[145] TIF-1α and TIF-1β,[146, 147] TRIP1/SUG1,[148, 149] TRIP230,[150] ARA70,[151] and CBP [CREB-binding protein]/p300[138, 152] (the last originally identified as coactivators of the transcription factor CREB [cAMP response element–binding protein]). Recruitment of these proteins to activate NRs depends on the integrity of a short α helical sequence LXXLL.[153] SRCs, the CBP/p300 family, and the androgen receptor coactivator ARA70 have been unequivocally shown to enhance AF-2 activity in transient transfection assays, whereas TIF-1 and RIP140 have only a minor effect. However, TIF-1α is both a phosphoprotein and protein kinase that undergoes ligand-dependent hyperphosphorylation as a consequence of binding NRs (ER-α and RXR-α). In addition, recombinant TIF-1α selectively phosphorylates the transcription factors TFIIEα, TAFII28, and TAFII55 in vitro. These findings suggest that TIF-1α may act by modulating the activity of the transcriptional machinery.[154] Moreover, although targeted disruption of the gene coding for SRC-1 caused partial hormone resistance,[155] expression of this coactivator has been found to be neither necessary nor sufficient for induction of expression of the PR gene by the estrogen-activated ER in the rat mammary gland.[156] Although it is virtually certain that coactivators are involved in transcriptional transactivation by NRs, it is difficult to establish the identity of such coactivators and their relevance to physiologic regulatory mechanisms. Data obtained from experimental models, by methods that lead to artificial overexpression of the supposed actors, do not necessarily correspond to the situation in an ordinary living cell.

The SRC family and CBP/p300 have been shown to interact directly with each other and with general transcription factors such as TBP and TFIIB, as well as with another coactivator p/CAF (p300 and CBP-associated factor). Furthermore, SRCs and CBP/p300 have been found to possess intrinsic histone acetyltransferase activity,[157] consistent with the contention that transcriptional activators stimulate remodeling of chromatin. It remains to be determined, however, whether histones complexed in the nucleosome are unique substrates for acetylation in vivo. Several other proteins may be substrates of histone acetyltransferase: HMG proteins, as well as TFIIF and TFIIE, have been reported to be acetylated by CBP/p300 in vitro. Acetylation of the transcriptional regulator and anti-oncoprotein p53 has also been observed.[158] SRC-1, which harbors two distinct activation domains, interacts with the AF-1 and AF-2 domains of steroid receptors. These interactions concern multiple regions of SRC-1. Thus coactivators provide a mechanism by which the two independent transactivation domains of the steroid receptors, AF-1 and AF-2, communicate to achieve full transcriptional activity.[159] Recently, p300 has been reported, in vitro, to enhance the efficiency of transcription initiation of ER in a cooperative manner. When transcription reinitiation was allowed to occur, ER, but not p300 was able to increase the number of rounds of transcription. Therefore, ER displays a dual function in transactivation initiation and reinitiation.[160]

A large, multisubunit complex of TR-associated proteins (TRAPs)—which interact with and facilitate TR function on natural DNA templates in conjunction with general transcription factors and upstream-factor stimulatory activity components—has also been identified.[161] The TRAPs were initially isolated from cell lines expressing epitope-tagged TR. It is significant that the TRAP complexes closely resemble hSMCC (human SRB/MED-containing cofactor complex),[161, 162] both with respect to the presence of the same polypeptide subunits and with respect to its coactivator function. TRAP and hSMCC complexes possess a set of at least 10 proteins but do not contain any of the known NR coactivators, such as CBP, p300, and SRC.

A complex of vitamin D_3 receptor–associated proteins (DRIP) has also been described.[163] The DRIP complex binds to the AF-2 domain of the VDR LBD in a ligand-dependent manner. It has been reported that the DRIP complex strongly stimulates synergistic activation of the promoter of the low-density lipoprotein (LDL) receptor gene by SREBP (steroid receptor element–binding protein)-1a/Sp1 on a chromatin template.[164] Affinity chromatography of SREBP-1a has allowed for purification of a complex denoted as "activation-recruited cofactor" (ARC), at least 11 constituent polypeptides of which are identical to those present in DRIP; 3 of them are also subunits of TRAP. ARC interacts directly with several different activators, including SREBP-1a, VP16, and the p65 subunit of the nuclear factor NF-κB.[164] These data indicate that distinct activators may use common associated subunits to mediate their different functions.

Interactions with Co-repressors

Co-repressors were postulated to antagonize liganded steroid receptors and to contribute to the silencing function of unliganded TR and RAR. Two such factors that interact with TR and RAR, referred to as N-CoR (NR co-repressor) and SMRT (silencing mediator for retinoid and thyroid hormone receptors),[165] were identified by the two-hybrid screening approach. N-CoR,[166, 167] SMRT/TRAC-2, and their splice variants—thyroid hormone and retinoic acid–associated co-repressors type 1 (TRAC-1), RIP13, and retinoic X receptor interacting protein (RIP)13Δ1—belong to a family of silencing mediators (co-repressors). These co-repressors interact with a critical region within the hinge domain of TR and RAR, as well as with a portion of the N-terminal part of the LBD. Ligand-dependent activation is associated with displacement of co-repressors and recruitment of coactivators.[168]

Binding of N-CoR to TR and RAR is not ligand regulated in solution. When the receptor is bound to its cognate DNA sequences, two types of regulation are observed. In the case of RAR-RXR interaction with a direct repeat element containing a five-nucleotide spacer (DR5), ligand binding and activation of transcription involve the release of N-CoR and coactivator recruitment. In contrast, on the inverse repeat element with a one-nucleotide spacer (DR1 element), where the polarity of the heterodimer is reversed (Fig. 10–8), N-CoR cannot be dissociated by the binding of ligand and remains tethered to the complex, thus making it unable to activate transcription. These results

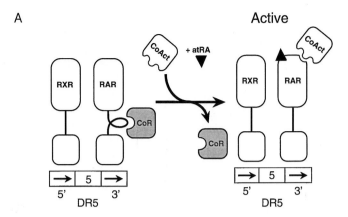

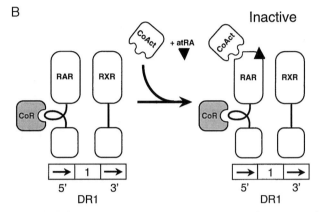

FIGURE 10–8. DNA sequence-dependent regulation of receptor activity. The negative regulation of transcription by NR co-repressors is illustrated for promoters containing RAR/RXR response elements. *A,* On DR5 direct repeat (five spacer nucleotides), RXR binds 5′ of RAR. In the absence of agonist ligand (all-*trans*-retinoic acid; atRA), co-repressor (CoR) is associated with the complex and blocks basal transcription. On binding of atRA, co-repressor dissociates from the DNA-bound RAR/RXR complex and coactivator (CoAct) binding permits gene activation. *B,* On DR1 element, the orientation RAR/RXR is reversed so that RAR is 5′ of RXR. Both in the absence and presence of atRA, co-repressor remains bound to the complex and prevents transcriptional activation.

indicate that DNA-binding sequences can allosterically regulate RAR-co-repressor interactions and thus determine positive or negative regulation of gene expression.[167]

It has recently been shown that N-CoR and SMRT directly interact with Sin3 and histone deacetylase-1, two mammalian homologues of yeast general transcriptional repressors, to form a multisubunit repressor complex.[169, 170] Moreover, N-CoR interacts directly with TFIIB, TAFII32, and TAFII70 in a noncompetitive manner. These findings suggest that TR and RAR bind to N-CoR or SMRT that target histone deacetylase, thereby repressing transcription, and that N-CoR and SMRT can also interact with the basal transcription machinery to induce a nonfunctional complex for transcription.[171]

Evidence that co-repressors are involved in the inhibitory action of antagonist-bound steroid receptors is growing. One such argument comes from the study of transcriptional transactivation by the PR. PR-B, when complexed with the antiprogestin RU 486, can function as a transactivator of transcription, although only in the presence of ER complexed with the antiestrogen 4-hydroxytamoxifen. This effect is absent if ER is complexed with an agonist ligand. Because RU 486–PR-B interacts directly with N-CoR in vitro, it can be hypothesized that the complex ER-antagonist competes for N-CoR and releases the transactivation potential of the PR-B–RU 486 complex.[172] In addition, SAP30, a component of the Sin3 multiprotein complex, is required for N-CoR–mediated repression by antagonist-bound ER, but not for N-CoR–mediated repression by unliganded TR and RAR.[170] The different processes leading to transcriptional activation by NRs are illustrated in Figure 10–9.

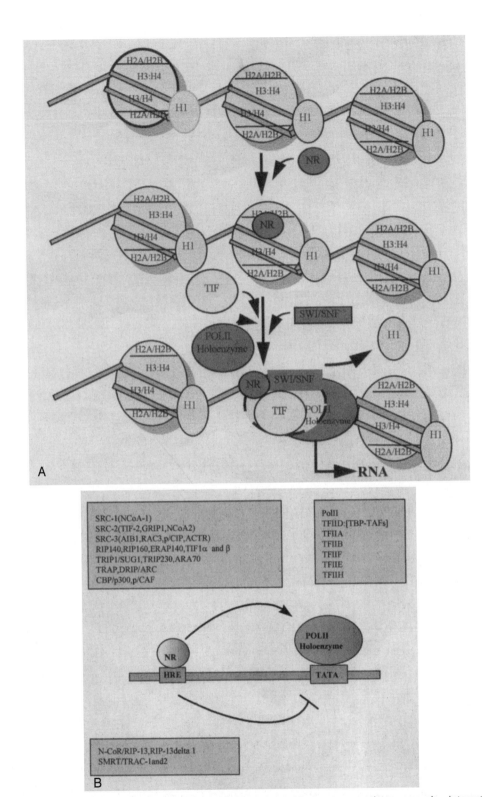

FIGURE 10–9. Transcription activation by nuclear receptors. *A,* Models of steroid receptor-coactivator complex interactions. Receptor acts in a multistep process. In the first step, the ligand-receptor complex (NR) binds to its cognate DNA binding site on the surface of a nucleosome. In a second step, NR interacts with a series of coactivators possessing intrinsic histone acetyltransferase activity; their action produces a local modification of chromatin structure. NR may then interact with other coactivators (such as TRAP, DRIP, ARE) whose role probably involves targeting the PolII holoenzyme to the promoter, along with the SWI/SNF chromatin remodeling complex, which may facilitate the RNA elongation. For other receptors, the first step is short-circuited, as the complex with the response element exists prior to the binding of the ligand. Co-repressors are associated with the NR/DNA complex, and can be displaced after ligand binding. *B,* Nuclear partners of NRs. *Top right,* General transcription initiation factors. *Top left,* Coactivators/adapters/transcription intermediary factors. *Bottom,* Co-repressors. For each category, several representative examples (nonexhaustive) are indicated.

SIGNALING CROSSTALK

The functions of a cell are regulated by a multitude of external stimuli: signaling molecules (endocrine, paracrine, autocrine), nutrients, and environmental signals (e.g., temperature, toxins). The signaling pathways triggered by any of these stimuli interact to produce a coherent outcome. The NRs, in essence transcription modulators, are subject to the effects of different regulatory mechanisms on the level of their expression, activation/inactivation (posttranslational mechanisms), and activity (transactivation of transcription); on the other hand, they intervene by modulating the transcription of other factors and indirectly regulate the expression of proteins, which in turn exercise their effects of cell regulation.

Effects of Steroid Hormones on Cell Contents and Activities of Their Receptors

As discussed above, steroid hormones modulate the expression of their receptors in both homologous and heterologous fashion. Estrogens and androgens generally induce expression of the genes coding for their respective receptors. In mammalian cells, progesterone generally causes a decrease in the expression of its receptor; this decrease can be dramatic, such as in the guinea pig uterus.[173] Similarly, glucocorticosteroids downregulate their receptors.[174] PRs are usually induced by estrogens; in contrast, progesterone often downregulates ER,[94-96] which is partially responsible for the "antiestrogenic" activity of progestagens. In addition, some evidence indicates that liganded PR represses ER-mediated transcriptional activity, apparently by interfering with ER's ability to interact productively with the transcriptional machinery.[175]

One question that demands further examination is what happens to the receptor after it has bound its ligand, performed its function (transcriptional activation), and undergone ligand dissociation. Experience with cell surface receptors shows that they are generally internalized after use and then frequently degraded (although recycling to the membrane is sometimes observed). In the case of NRs, dissociation of the ligand does not appear to direct the receptor for degradation. For instance, after the hormone dissociates from GR, the unliganded receptor is inactive but remains bound to chromatin. Its recycling can be accomplished by rebinding the hormone through a process requiring hsp90 and ATP.[176] The half-life of the liganded receptor, however, is often shorter than that of the free receptor. In the absence of dexamethasone, GR protein half-life is approximately 25 hours, whereas in the presence of hormone it decreases to approximately 11 hours.[177] In addition, negative feedback by the ligand operates at the gene expression level. The type of ligand (agonist vs. antagonist) here is of importance.[178] Agonists of GR are effective at downregulating GR at both the mRNA and protein levels. Although the antagonist RU 38486 is also capable of downregulating GR protein levels by shortening the half-life of the receptor, it appears to be incapable of altering the rate of transcription of the GR gene. Glucocorticoid target tissue sensitivity may therefore be decreased via multiple independent mechanisms, such as agonist-induced repression of GR gene transcription and/or ligand-induced degradation of total cellular GR protein levels. Moreover, it has been reported that GR recognizes several segments of its coding cDNA,[179] which suggests that it may interact with GR mRNA and direct it for degradation. Homologous downregulation is also observed for the PR, both in vivo[173, 180] and in cultured cells (see below). In T47D cells exposed to the synthetic progestagen R5020, both PR half-life and the rate of synthesis of PR were found to be reduced.[181] The accelerated half-life of liganded receptors may be the result of ubiquitinylation and degradation by proteasome[174, 182]; this mechanism has also been described for VDR.[183] However, acceleration of the half-life of NRs by ligand binding is not a general phenomenon and does not seem to be the case for the ER[184] (although transient downregulation of ERs by estradiol has been observed in some target tissues such as the rodent uterus[3, 185]). Transcriptional repression of the genes coding for PR[186] and GR[187] is probably involved in the long-term inhibition of expression of the receptor gene.

Interactions with Membrane-Initiated Signaling Pathways

Ligand-activated NRs trigger a multitude of complex cellular responses, and consequently, interactions with other signaling pathways are inevitable. Membrane-initiated signaling pathways can lead to posttranslational modifications (phosphorylation) of NRs that modulate their transactivation functions (see the section Activation of Steroid Hormone Receptors). Examples of interactions important for endocrine regulation include crosstalk between the actions of steroid hormones and the calcium- and/or PKC-dependent signaling pathways on the sensitivity to gonadotropin-releasing hormone in the pituitary[188] and the involvement of NO signaling in estrogen-induced luteinizing hormone secretion.[189] Phosphorylation of NRs on specific sites is probably a common mechanism by which membrane-initiated signaling cascades (under the action of growth factors, cytokines, etc.) affect transcriptional transactivation. One example concerning nonsteroidal receptors involves PPARγ, whose phosphorylation in the A/B region by a mitogen-activated protein (MAP) kinase site inhibits both ligand-independent and ligand-dependent transactivation functions.[190]

Breast epithelial cells and estrogen-dependent breast cancer cells require estrogen stimulation for their proliferation, but they also secrete the peptide growth factors TGF-α (acting via the epidermal growth factor receptor [EGFR]),[191, 192] IGF-1, and IGF-2 and express their receptors.[193-195] Secretion of these growth factors is often estrogen inducible. Their role as possible autocrine growth factors has been suggested by the observation that the polyanionic compound suramin is a potent in vitro growth inhibitor of breast cancer cells that are both hormone-insensitive, ER-negative and hormone-responsive, ER-positive.[195]

An inverse relationship appears to exist between the expression of EGF and ERs in breast cancer cell lines.[196] Sustained activation of PKC represses the expression of ER while inducing the expression of EGF.[197] Reduction of endogenous ER by antisense RNA has led to increased expression of EGFR, which supports the contention that loss of steroid sensitivity may be related to the expression of EGFR.[198]

It is somewhat surprising that breast cancer cell receptors for both estrogens and progestins appear to activate the ras/MAP kinase pathway via interaction with the src protein tyrosine kinase[199, 200] independent of their interaction with DNA. This mechanism could be important for the growth-promoting effect of estrogens, although it is paradoxical for progestins, which exercise antiproliferative activity.

Apart from positive regulation of cell proliferation, estrogens also induce the secretion of IGF-binding proteins whose function appears to be the sequestration of IGFs. The apparent conflicting actions of estrogens may in fact be related to paracrine signaling between the breast (cancer) epithelial cells and the stroma. Another example of negative regulation of breast cancer cell proliferation is transcriptional repression by estrogens of the gene coding for the *neu* proto-oncogene protein product p185neu, a homologue of the EGFR.[201] The repression appears to be a consequence of an alteration in the nuclear factor(s) binding to this promoter region in estradiol-stimulated vs. estradiol-deprived breast cancer cells (see the next section). It is remarkable that when ER was stably introduced into ER-negative cells—originated from breast cancer or not—instead of mediating estrogen-induced cell proliferation, it conferred inhibition of the cell cycle by the ligand.[202-204] The molecular mechanisms underlying the proliferation inhibitory effects of estrogens remain unknown.

Interactions with Sequence-Specific Transcription Factors

With regard to natural promoters, NR binding is necessary, although not sufficient for gene regulation. Mutation analysis has shown that in addition to the HRE, other sequence elements in the regulated promoters can also play an essential role in the modulation of promoter efficiency. On artificial promoters, HREs can synergize with binding sites for several transcription factors, such as NF-1 or Sp1. In addition, it is known that the presence of two HREs, when tandemly linked or appropriately spaced in the 5′ flanking sequence of a promoter, can result in transcriptional synergy.[205] Similarly, repression of transcription by NRs, as well as by other DNA-bound transcription factors, may be explained by competition between binding sites on the promoter or by mechanisms that do not depend on DNA binding but rather on protein-protein interactions (e.g., squelching, surface saturation).

Induction of transcription by steroid hormones can be partially or totally dependent on additional transcription factors. The latter situation is particularly striking in the case of the ovalbumin promoter, which is responsible for one of the most powerful estrogen-induced activities. In fact, activation of this promoter by estrogens is mediated, in part, by interaction of the ER with the AP-1–binding transcription factor (c-Jun/c-Fos complex) and does not require the binding of ER to DNA.[206]

Interactions between NRs and the transcriptional machinery have been studied almost exclusively with simple synthetic promoters containing one or multiple copies of DNA-binding sites. Natural promoters are generally complex and contain DNA-binding sites for several distinct transcription factors. The arrangement of these sites, with respect to nucleosomal organization of the promoter and the presence or absence of corresponding transcription factors, will determine the selective and synergistic modulation of target genes in response to extracellular signals. Experiments with the MMTV promoter show that positioned nucleosomes not only account for constitutive repression (absence of inducer) but also participate in induction by mediating cooperative binding and functional synergism between GR, NF-1, and Oct-1[133, 134] (see above). Transcriptional activation of the MMTV promoter by receptor-hormone complexes can be reproduced on naked DNA, although much less efficiently, independent of the NF-1 transcription factor.[207] Similar observations were reported for the TAT (tyrosine aminotransferase) promoter,[208] where activated GR binds to its target sequence, modifies the local chromatin structure, and renders the chromatin accessible to the liver-specific transcription factor HNF-3.

A different role for positioned nucleosome has been postulated for the *Xenopus* vitellogenin B1 gene, where a nucleosome-mediated static loop potentiates transcriptional stimulation by bringing the ERE-bound ER into juxtaposition with the proximal promoter element binding the NF-1 transcription factor. Thus positioned nucleosomes can facilitate transcription by providing a scaffold on which transcription factors bound to distal sites are assembled.[133, 134]

Steroid hormone receptors can also repress transcription of specific genes via direct interaction with other transcription factors; inhibition of the expression of AP-1–dependent genes by GR is one example. Consistent with the proposed mechanism (direct binding between GR and AP-1), this inhibition is reciprocal.[209] Genomic footprinting experiments on the endogenous collagenase promoter have demonstrated that the interfering factor does not bind to DNA whereas the repressed factor remains attached to its specific element.[210] Interactions between GR and AP-1, however, are not exclusively negative. c-Jun (component of AP-1) enhances GR-dependent expression of the proliferin gene, whereas overexpression of c-Fos (c-Jun partner in the AP-1 heterodimer) leads to inhibition.[211] Direct interactions between GR and the p65 subunit of NF-κB also form the basis of their mutual antagonism. Gel shift experiments have shown that GR prevents NF-κB binding to DNA. In addition, a part of the inhibition of NF-κB activity is probably a consequence of induction of the inhibitory subunit, IF-κB, by GR agonists.[212, 213] Inhibition of the transcriptional activity of NF-κB is likely to play a role in the anti-inflammatory properties of glucocorticosteroids.

Under transient transfection conditions, another mechanism of transcriptional interference has been encountered: competition between different transcription factors for limiting the cellular components necessary for transcription (coactivators), or "squelching."[109] No solid evidence has been presented that this sort of inhibition ever occurs under physiologic or pathologic conditions.

PHYSIOLOGY, PATHOLOGY, AND CLINICAL ASPECTS

The different members of the NR superfamily cover virtually all aspects of cell development and function. Only the receptors activated by circulating ligands involve aspects of endocrinology. In addition, paracrine/autocrine mechanisms overlap with true endocrine regulation. These modes of regulation of cell development and function are ensured by (1) steroid hormones (receptors of class I) and (2) thyroid hormones, vitamin D, retinoids, and certain prostaglandins and aliphatic chain lipids (receptors of class II). In this section we shall resume our discussion of the essential physiologic situations in which NRs are involved. Specific chapters in this book will deal with the relevant details.

Steroid Hormone Actions

The actions of the five classes of hormonal steroids cover the functions of virtually all organs and cell types. Activation of any given steroid receptor can lead to a variety of cellular responses. For example, estrogens are powerful inducers of proliferation of certain target cells, particularly those of organs implicated in reproductive functions, such as the mammalian uterus, the mammary gland, and the avian oviduct. In other target cells (pituitary gland, hypothalamus, chicken liver), induction of cell proliferation is weak or absent. The diverse actions of estrogens in different target organs are conveyed by the presence of different coactivators/co-repressors. Besides, certain differences are apparently related to expression of the α or β ER isotype. The physiologic impact of the expression of these isotypes, however, is not yet clear. In an immature animal, estrogens will induce the development and differentiation of organs required for reproductive function; a good example is the mammary gland. The development of muscle is favored by androgens; the synthesis of androgen analogues that carry out this function has recently led to some spectacular, if undesirable improvements in the performance of many men and women athletes. In differentiated cells, estrogens induce the expression of specific proteins according to the particular cell type. Examples include egg proteins, mainly in birds (egg white by the oviduct, yolk vitellogenin by the liver) and lower vertebrates, but also in mammals; secreted signaling polypeptides in the hypothalamus and the pituitary gland; and intracellular signaling molecules (PR in the uterus). It is important to note that synthetic estrogens can mimic specific actions of hormones in a manner that depends on the target cells. It is well known that tamoxifen (as well as several other structurally related nonsteroidal antiestrogens) binds to the ER in hormone-dependent breast cancer cells, where it antagonizes the growth-promoting action of estrogens while at the same time mimicking their estrogenic activity by inducing the accumulation of PR (see, for example, Reddel et al.[214] and Borgna and Rochefort[215]). Transient transfection experiments have shown that tamoxifen can activate AF-1 activity in spite of lacking the capacity to activate AF-2; AF-1 is sufficient to promote transcription of the PR gene (and probably some other estrogen-inducible genes) in certain cell types. In addition, certain ligands can produce different effects via the α and β isotypes of the ER (see Paich et al.,[216] for example).

Hormone-Dependent Cancer: Role of Receptors

Among common types of cancer, breast cancer (estrogen dependent) and cancer of the prostate (androgen dependent) frequently express the feature of dependence on sex hormone. Logically, hormone dependence requires expression of the appropriate receptors in the tumor cells. For many patients, treatment by surgical removal of the gonads leads to remission of the disease. This fact has prompted a search for pharmacologic means to eliminate the need for surgery. Tamoxifen has been the first antiestrogen with a powerful cytostatic effect in estrogen-responsive breast cancer patients. The fact that it not only inhibited tumor growth but also caused regression in a significant proportion of patients could not be explained solely by its inhibition of cell proliferation. An additional apparent effect of the suppression of estrogen stimulation of breast cancer cells is apoptosis, which suggests an additional role of estrogen as an antiapoptotic molecule. However, the response of breast cancer is nearly always of a transient character. The same situation occurs in prostate cancer, the masculine variant of hormone-dependent cancer (efficiently, if transiently treated by the antiandrogens flutamide or nilutamide). Total suppression of endogenous secretion of the agonist estrogen (by aromatase inhibitors) leads to a second, usually short-lasting response in only a small proportion of relapsed patients. Therefore, two problems are posed: first, how does it happen that an initially hormone-dependent tumor becomes hormone independent, and second, is it realistic to attempt to prevent or to overcome this secondary—or possibly primary—hormone independence?

To the first question, several answers have been proposed. First, certain mutations or splicing abnormalities can produce constitutively active (hormone-independent, antagonist-insensitive) proteins.[217–219] One may include mutations that render receptor complexes transcriptionally active (i.e., antihormone acting as an agonist[220–222]) in the same category. Second, activation of alternative pathways of mitogenic signaling can relieve the cancer cell of its need for estrogenic stimulation (which requires that the cell concomitantly lose its need for the antiapoptotic action of estrogens or androgens). Third, activation of the receptor can be ensured by a mechanism different from ligand binding (see above). In principle, any of these explanations can occur in a patient. However, the first explanation appears to be rare and the third not very likely because cancers that have become hormone independent frequently lose their expression of ER. We presume that the genetic instability of cancer cells will favor the second explanation: activation of an oncogene (or loss of the expression of a tumor suppressor gene) will offer a growth advantage to a cell, which can then repopulate the regressed tumor. Such cells are generally already present in the patient at the moment of the diagnosis (in a total of $>10^9$ tumor cells, an absolute minimum to be detected by any available physical method).

Another type of hormonal therapy for breast cancer is based on the administration of progestagens. Such therapy is applied to patients with PR-positive tumors, either simultaneously with antiestrogen (particularly tamoxifen, whose partial agonist activity maintains a high level of PR) or, more commonly, after the tumor fails to respond. Progesterone acts by inhibiting (residual) estrogen-dependent growth, although it has its own cell proliferation inhibitory action that results from induction of the cdk inhibitor p21WAF1/CIP1 and inhibition of cyclin D– and cyclin E–dependent kinase activities.[223, 224]

Prostate cancer responds to hormonal treatment (surgical or chemical castration, combined or without antiandrogens) in a high proportion of patients. As in breast cancer, however, remissions are usually transient (for analogous reasons).

With regard to preventing the escape of tumor cells from hormonal control, the best strategy seems to be the development of new estrogen or androgen antagonists with higher capacity to induce apoptosis in their target cells to efficiently eliminate the hormone-dependent cells. The presence of a subpopulation of hormone-independent cells at the time of initiation of therapy is an observable limit to this strategy. It is of interest in this context that ER-negative cells stably transfected with ER do not respond to estradiol by accelerated growth but, on the contrary, demonstrate inhibited proliferation.[202–204] The underlying mechanism is unknown; it is not excluded that ER-hormone complexes may interfere with cell physiology by competing for general transcription factors.

Estrogen Analogues and Osteoporosis

ER-dependent cellular signaling is involved in skeletal maturation at puberty. Such is apparently the case in both males and females, as evidenced by the fact that an adult male with the unique null-allele ER-α suffered from severe osteoporosis at only age 28. In addition, the epiphyses of his bones were unfused.[225] ER-α knockout mice (both sexes) are sterile and their bone density is markedly lower than normal (see Grandien et al.[55] and references therein). In the human female, the need for estrogen-dependent signaling persists throughout life, and postmenopausal osteoporosis is a physiopathologic aspect of importance for public health. Hormone replacement therapy by estrogens is burdened by side effects (in particular, increased risk of breast cancer).

Tamoxifen has a certain activity in the prevention of bone demineralization, but it is insufficient and has side effects of its own in the endometrium. Intensive search for more specific molecules able to deal with these problems has led to the development of raloxifene, which has an estrogen-like effect in preventing bone loss while lacking estrogenic activity in tissues such as the endometrium and breast (including breast cancer). The effects of estrogens and raloxifene appear to be mediated by induction of expression of the gene coding for TGF-β via noncanonic promoter sequences (i.e., without the palindromic ERE). For promoters containing such "classic" ERE, raloxifene acts as an antagonist of estrogen action.[226]

Actions of Thyroid Hormones, Retinoids, Vitamin D, and Peroxisome Proliferator–Activated Receptor

Thyroid hormones and retinoids are involved in the embryonal development and regulation of cell function (see Chapter 95) This conclusion relies on data from studies based on deprivation of the ligand rather than gene inactivation. This latter approach is rendered difficult by the complexity of the receptor systems, which leads to complementation as well as mutual interference between the different gene products.

Thyroid hormones are bound by receptors of the classes TR-α and TR-β and their isoforms, which transmit the specific signals according to the cellular environment. Besides the well-known pathologies that result from inappropriate activity of the thyroid gland, genetic defects linked to mutations of TR have also been identified. They are denoted as the syndrome of "general resistance to thyroid hormone." This syndrome is inherited in a dominant fashion, thus demonstrating that a single mutated allele confers resistance to the thyroid hormone (see Chapter 114).

Retinoids are indispensable for normal prenatal and postnatal development, as well as for numerous functions of the adult organism such as reproduction and vision; lasting deprivation of retinoids leads to death. Numerous studies have been carried out with animals bearing null mutations of different RAR/RXR subtypes or isoforms. Single knockouts of receptor genes generally have only mild or no consequences, probably because of functional redundancy of the individual receptor subtypes/isoforms. When paired receptors are inactivated, specific developmental defects are observed. The deficiencies observed in such animals reproduce some of those seen in retinoid deprivation and allow for the allocation of specific roles to the respective receptor gene products. However, different double mutants frequently lead to the same defects. Any conclusions based on these studies are to be taken with caution because subtle survival/reproduction handicaps and minor alterations in cellular function and behavior are difficult to appreciate in laboratory conditions (for review see Chen et al.[88]).

The numerous physiologic functions of VDRs are dealt with elsewhere (see Chapter 72). First, besides the direct role of VDR, interactions with other signaling pathways that involve NRs appear to be important in bone formation and homeostasis via the induction of cytochrome P450 aromatase activity by vitamin D.[227] Second, unlike retinoids and in spite of its role in cell differentiation, vitamin D–dependent signaling is not indispensable for prenatal development, as indicated by the fact that VDR null mutant mice are apparently normal until weaning. The defects observed later in life coincided with those produced by vitamin D deprivation (impaired bone formation, infertility); alopecia and uterine hypoplasia were also observed. These additional defects probably reflect functions in which heterodimers between VDR and other transcription modulators are implicated. Finally, different vitamin D analogues have been shown to inhibit the proliferation of cancer cells; the underlying mechanism may involve an action of VDR on cell differentiation.

NRs activated by compounds that activate peroxisome proliferation, PPARα, PPARβ, and PPARγ, respond to a variety of natural ligands (essentially fatty acids and eicosanoids) to transmit different physiologic signals (see, for example, Desvergne et al.[228] for review). Synthetic compounds such as the antidiabetic thiazolidinediones can also bind to and activate PPARs, particularly the γ isotype.[229–231] PPARα is strongly expressed in the liver, and its activity is involved in lipid oxidation; it is this isotype that is specifically activated by fibrates, drugs used to treat patients with hypertriglyceridemia. Expression of the different PPAR isotypes underlies the specific pharmacologic effects of the different families of medications.[232] On the other hand, the γ isotype is critical for the differentiation and function of adipocytes. The β isotype is ubiquitous but its physiologic role remains unknown. The activity of PPARγ in adipocytes is regulated by prostaglandins: the derivatives of PGJ$_2$ bind to PPARγ and have a positive effect on its activity, whereas PGG$_{2\alpha}$ activates the MAP kinase pathway, which results in an inhibiting phosphorylation of PPARγ.[233]

NONGENOMIC ACTIONS OF NUCLEAR RECEPTORS?

Although it seems paradoxical, localization of NRs (ER, PR) in the membranes of the guinea pig hypothalamus has been observed by electron microscopic analysis.[234] Using antibodies directed against a peptide representing the hinge region of the intracellular ER, another group has observed the presence of a membrane ER in rat pituitary tumor cells.[235] In functional studies, activation of the ras/MAP kinase pathway by estrogens and progestins has also been reported.[199, 200]

These observations suggest the possible involvement of "true" NRs in the nongenomic action of steroids and other ligands. Extremely rapid actions of such molecules have been known since the early period of research on steroid hormone action (e.g., the effect of progesterone on the maturation of *Xenopus* oocytes,[236, 237] although they generally require "receptor" molecules that appear different from their "NR" counterparts in affinity and specificity criteria[238, 239]). In vascular tissue, the effect of estrogen on the vessel wall also has a rapid nongenomic component involving membrane phenomena, such as alteration of membrane ionic permeability and activation of membrane-bound enzymes,[240] suggestive of actions mediated by "receptors" situated at the cell membrane (see Baulieu et al.[237] for a review of the nongenomic actions of steroids).

The question of the mechanisms involved in the rapid, nongenomic actions of estrogens was addressed recently.[241] Researchers observed that estradiol rapidly (<20 minutes) attenuated the ability of μ opioids to hyperpolarize guinea pig hypothalamic (β-endorphin) neurons. Apparently, estrogen binds to a specific receptor that activates PKA and rapidly uncouples the μ opioid receptor from its K$^+$ channel. Diethylstilbestrol, a powerful agonist of the nuclear ER, acted as an inhibitor of these effects of estradiol by a mechanism that did not require protein synthesis. These results suggest that estrogenic uncoupling of the μ opioid receptor from its K$^+$ channel results from a nongenomic mechanism of action mediated by a receptor different from the "true" nuclear ER. The action of estradiol involves crosstalk with other membrane signaling pathways and depends on activation of PKA.

REFERENCES

1. A unified nomenclature for the nuclear receptor superfamily (letter). Cell 97:161–163, 1999.
2. Baulieu EE, Alberga A, Jung I, et al: Metabolism and protein binding of sex steroids in target organs: An approach to the mechanism of hormone action. Recent Prog Horm Res 27:351–419, 1971.
3. Jensen EV, DeSombre ER: Mechanism of action of the female sex hormones. Annu Rev Biochem 41:203–230, 1972.
4. Baulieu EE, Atger M, Best-Belpomme M, et al: Steroid hormone receptors. Vitam Horm 33:649–736, 1975.
5. Secco C, Redeuilh G, Radanyi C, et al: Two-step purification of estradiol calf uterine cytosol receptor. C R Seances Acad Sci D 289:907–910, 1979.
6. Greene GL, Nolan C, Engler JP, Jensen EV: Monoclonal antibodies to human estrogen receptor. Proc Natl Acad Sci U S A 77:5115–5119, 1980.
7. Redeuilh G, Secco C, Baulieu EE: The use of the biotinyl estradiol-avidin system for the purification of "nontransformed" estrogen receptor by biohormonal affinity chromatography. J Biol Chem 260:3996–4002, 1985.
8. Renoir JM, Yang CR, Formstecher P, et al: Progesterone receptor from chick oviduct: Purification of molybdate-stabilized form and preliminary characterization. Eur J Biochem 127:71–79, 1982.
9. Renoir JM, Mester J, Buchou T, et al: Purification by affinity chromatography and immunological characterization of a 110kDa component of the chick oviduct progesterone receptor. Biochem J 217:685–692, 1984.
10. Denis M, Poellinger L, Wikstom AC, Gustafsson JA: Requirement of hormone for thermal conversion of the glucocorticoid receptor to a DNA-binding state. Nature 333:686–688, 1988.
11. Gustafsson JA, Carlstedt-Duke J, Wrange O, et al: Functional analysis of the purified glucocorticoid receptor. J Steroid Biochem 24:63–68, 1986.
12. Walter P, Green S, Greene G, et al: Cloning of the human estrogen receptor cDNA. Proc Natl Acad Sci U S A 82:7889–7893, 1985.
13. Green S, Walter P, Kumar V, et al: Human oestrogen receptor cDNA: Sequence, expression and homology to v-erb-A. Nature 320:134–139, 1986.
14. Jeltsch JM, Krozowski Z, Quirin-Stricker C, et al: Cloning of the chicken progesterone receptor. Proc Natl Acad Sci U S A 83:5424–5428, 1986.
15. Conneely OM, Sullivan WP, Toft DO, et al: Molecular cloning of the chicken progesterone receptor. Science 233:767–770, 1986.
16. Giguere V, Yang N, Segui P, Evans RM: Identification of a new class of steroid hormone receptors. Nature 331:91–94, 1988.
17. Misrahi M, Loosfelt H, Atger M, et al: Organisation of the entire rabbit progesterone receptor mRNA and of the promoter and 5′ flanking region of the gene. Nucleic Acids Res 16:5459–5472, 1988.
18. Chang C, Kokontis J, Liao SS, Chang Y: Isolation and characterization of human TR3 receptor: A member of steroid receptor superfamily. J Steroid Biochem 34:391–395, 1989.
19. Tora L, Mullick A, Metzger D, et al: The cloned human oestrogen receptor contains a mutation which alters its hormone binding properties. EMBO J 8:1981–1986, 1989.
20. Showers MO, Darling DS, Kieffer GD, Chin WW: Isolation and characterization of a cDNA encoding a chicken beta thyroid hormone receptor. DNA Cell Biol 10:211–221, 1991.
21. Moudgil VK, Eessalu TE, Buchou T, et al: Transformation of chick oviduct progesterone receptor in vitro: Effects of hormone, salt, heat, and adenosine triphosphate. Endocrinology 116:1267–1274, 1985.
22. Notides AC, Hamilton DE, Auer HE: A kinetic analysis of the estrogen receptor transformation. J Biol Chem 250:3945–3950, 1975.
23. Notides AC, Weichman BM, Lerner N, de Boer W: The role of ligand-binding as a determinant of the structure and activation of the estrogen receptor. Adv Exp Med Biol 117:297–307, 1979.
24. Wrange O, Carlstedt-Duke J, Gustafsson JA: Purification of the glucocorticoid receptor from rat liver cytosol. J Biol Chem 254:9284–9290, 1979.
25. Mester J, Renoir JM, Yang CR, et al: Characterisation of "native" and "activated" progesterone and oestrogen receptors from chick oviduct. In Lewis GP, Ginsburg M (eds): Mechanisms of Steroid Action. London, Macmillan Press, 1981, pp 15–38.
26. de Boer W, Notides AC: Dissociation kinetics of the nuclear estrogen receptor. Biochemistry 20:1290–1294, 1981.
27. Wrange O, Okret S, Radojcic M, et al: Characterization of the purified activated glucocorticoid receptor from rat liver cytosol. J Biol Chem 259:4534–4541, 1984.
28. Nemoto T, Ohara-Nemoto Y, Denis M, Gustafsson JA: The transformed glucocorticoid receptor has a lower steroid-binding affinity than the nontransformed receptor. Biochemistry 29:1880–1886, 1990.
29. Joab I, Radanyi C, Renoir M, et al: Common non-hormone binding component in non-transformed chick oviduct receptors of four steroid hormones. Nature 308:850–853, 1984.
30. Catelli MG, Binart N, Jung-Testas I, et al: The common 90-kd protein component of non-transformed '8S' steroid receptors is a heat-shock protein. EMBO J 4:3131–3135, 1985.
31. Renoir JM, Buchou T, Mester J, et al: Oligomeric structure of the molybdate-stabilized, non-transformed "8S" progesterone receptor from chicken oviduct cytosol. Biochemistry 23:6016–6023, 1984.
32. Redeuilh G, Moncharmont B, Secco C, Baulieu EE: Subunit composition of the molybdate-stabilized "8–9 S" nontransformed estradiol receptor purified from calf uterus. J Biol Chem 262:6969–6975, 1987.
33. Sabbah M, Radanyi C, Redeuilh G, Baulieu EE: The 90 kDa heat-shock protein (hsp90) modulates the binding of the oestrogen receptor to its cognate DNA. Biochem J 314:205–213, 1996.
34. Binart N, Lombes M, Baulieu EE: Distinct functions of the 90 kDa heat-shock protein (hsp90) in oestrogen and mineralocorticosteroid receptor activity: Effects of hsp90 deletion mutants. Biochem J 311:797–804, 1995.
35. Ditmar KD, Demady DR, Stancato LF, et al: Folding of the glucocorticoid receptor by the heat shock protein (hsp) 90–based chaperone machinery. The role of p23 is to stabilize receptor.hsp90 heterocomplexes formed by hsp90.p60.hsp70. J Biol Chem 272:21213–21220, 1997.
36. Whitesell L, Cook P: Stable and specific binding of heat shock protein 90 by geldanamycin disrupts glucocorticoid receptor function in intact cells. Mol Endocrinol 10:705–712, 1996.
37. Segnitz B, Gehring U: The function of steroid hormone receptors is inhibited by the hsp90-specific compound geldanamycin. J Biol Chem 272:18694–18701, 1997.
38. Bamberger CM, Wald M, Bamberger AM, Schulte HM: Inhibition of mineralocorticoid and glucocorticoid receptor function by the heat shock protein 90–binding agent geldanamycin. Mol Cell Endocrinol 131:233–240, 1997.
39. Lebeau MC, Massol N, Herrick J, et al: P59, an hsp 90–binding protein. Cloning and sequencing of its cDNA and preparation of a peptide-directed polyclonal antibody. J Biol Chem 267:4281–4284, 1992.
40. Callebaut I, Renoir JM, Lebeau MC, et al: An immunophilin that binds M(r) 90,000 heat shock protein: Main structural features of a mammalian p59 protein. Proc Natl Acad Sci U S A 89:6270–6274, 1992.
41. Pratt WB, Toft DO: Steroid receptor interactions with heat shock protein and immunophilin chaperones. Endocr Rev 18:306–360, 1997.
42. Bohen SP: Genetic and biochemical analysis of p23 and ansamycin antibiotics in the function of Hsp90-dependent signaling proteins. Mol Cell Biol 18:3330–3339, 1998.
43. King WJ, Greene GL: Monoclonal antibodies localize oestrogen receptor in the nuclei of target cells. Nature 307:745–747, 1984.

44. Welshons WV, Lieberman ME, Gorski J: Nuclear localization of unoccupied oestrogen receptors. Nature 307:747–749, 1984.

45. Welshons WV, Krummel BM, Gorski J: Nuclear localization of unoccupied receptors for glucocorticoids, estrogens, and progesterone in GH3 cells. Endocrinology 117:2140–2147, 1985.

46. Leclerc P, Jibard N, Meng X, et al: Quantification of the nucleocytoplasmic distribution of wild type and modified proteins using confocal microscopy: Interaction between 90-kDa heat shock protein (Hsp90 alpha) and glucocorticosteroid receptor (GR). Exp Cell Res 242:255–264, 1998.

47. Guiochon-Mantel A, Lescop P, Christin-Maitre S, et al: Nucleocytoplasmic shuttling of the progesterone receptor. EMBO J 10:3851–3859, 1991.

48. Ylikomi T, Bocquel MT, Berry M, et al: Cooperation of proto-signals for nuclear accumulation of estrogen and progesterone receptors. EMBO J 11:3681–3694, 1992.

49. Guiochon-Mantel A, Delabre K, Lescop P, Milgrom E: Nuclear localization signals also mediate the outward movement of proteins from the nucleus. Proc Natl Acad Sci U S A 91:7179–7183, 1994.

50. Tyagi RK, Amazit L, Lescop P, et al: Mechanisms of progesterone receptor export from nuclei: Role of nuclear localization signal, nuclear export signal, and ran guanosine triphosphate. Mol Endocrinol 12:1684–1695, 1998.

51. Mymryk JS, Archer TK: Dissection of progesterone receptor–mediated chromatin remodeling and transcriptional activation in vivo. Genes Dev 9:1366–1376, 1995.

52. Mangelsdorf DJ, Evans RM: The RXR heterodimers and orphan receptors. Cell 83:841–850, 1995.

53. Devin-Leclerc J, Meng X, Delahaye F, et al: Interaction and dissociation by ligands of estrogen receptor and Hsp90: The antiestrogen RU 58668 induces a protein synthesis-dependent clustering of the receptor in the cytoplasm. Mol Endocrinol 12:842–854, 1998.

54. Gronemeyer H: Transcription activation by estrogen and progesterone receptors. Annu Rev Genet 25:89–123, 1991.

55. Grandien K, Berkenstam A, Gustafsson JA: The estrogen receptor gene: Promoter organization and expression. Int J Biochem Cell Biol 29:1343–1369, 1997.

56. Parker MG: Transcriptional activation by oestrogen receptors. Biochem Soc Symp 63:45–50, 1998.

57. Giangrande PH, Pollio G, McDonnell DP: Mapping and characterization of the functional domains responsible for the differential activity of the A and B isoforms of the human progesterone receptor. J Biol Chem 272:32889–32900, 1997.

58. Loosfelt H, Atger M, Misrahi M, et al: Cloning and sequence analysis of rabbit progesterone-receptor complementary DNA. Proc Natl Acad Sci U S A 83:9045–9049, 1986.

59. Shyamala G, Yang X, Silberstein G, et al: Transgenic mice carrying an imbalance in the native ratio of A to B forms of progesterone receptor exhibit developmental abnormalities in mammary glands. Proc Natl Acad Sci U S A 95:696–701, 1998.

60. Escriva H, Safi R, Hanni C, et al: Ligand binding was acquired during evolution of nuclear receptors. Proc Natl Acad Sci U S A 94:6803–6808, 1997.

61. Laudet V: Evolution of the nuclear receptor superfamily: Early diversification from an ancestral orphan receptor. J Mol Endocrinol 19:207–226, 1997.

62. Brzozowski AM, Pike AC, Dauter Z, et al: Molecular basis of agonism and antagonism in the oestrogen receptor. Nature 389:753–758, 1997.

63. Maalouf GJ, Xu W, Smith TF, Mohr SC: Homology model for the ligand-binding domain of the human estrogen receptor. J Biomol Struct Dyn 15:841–851, 1998.

64. Henttu PM, Kalkhoven E, Parker MG: AF-2 activity and recruitment of steroid receptor coactivator 1 to the estrogen receptor depend on a lysine residue conserved in nuclear receptors. Mol Cell Biol 17:1832–1839, 1997.

65. Tremblay GB, Tremblay A, Labrie F, Giguere V: Ligand-independent activation of the estrogen receptors alpha and beta by mutations of a conserved tyrosine can be abolished by antiestrogens. Cancer Res 58:877–881, 1998.

66. Kang KI, Meng X, Devin-Leclerc J, et al: The molecular chaperone Hsp90 can negatively regulate the activity of a glucocorticosteroid-dependent promoter. Proc Natl Acad Sci U S A 96:1439–1444, 1999.

67. Power RF, Conneely OM, O'Malley BW: New insights into activation of the steroid hormone receptor superfamily. Trends Pharmacol Sci 13:318–323, 1992.

68. Aronica SM, Katzenellenbogen BS: Stimulation of estrogen receptor–mediated transcription and alteration in the phosphorylation state of the rat uterine estrogen receptor by estrogen, cyclic adenosine monophosphate, and insulin-like growth factor-I. Mol Endocrinol 7:743–752, 1993.

69. Ignar-Trowbridge DM, Pimentel M, Teng CT, et al: Cross talk between peptide growth factor and estrogen receptor signaling systems. Environ Health Perspect 103(suppl 7):35–38, 1995.

70. Ignar-Trowbridge DM, Pimentel M, Parker MG, et al: Peptide growth factor cross-talk with the estrogen receptor requires the A/B domain and occurs independently of protein kinase C or estradiol. Endocrinology 137:1735–1744, 1996.

71. Le Goff P, Montano MM, Schodin DJ, Katzenellenbogen BS: Phosphorylation of the human estrogen receptor. Identification of hormone-regulated sites and examination of their influence on transcriptional activity. J Biol Chem 269:4458–4466, 1994.

72. Matkovits T, Christakos S: Ligand occupancy is not required for vitamin D receptor and retinoid receptor–mediated transcriptional activation. Mol Endocrinol 9:232–242, 1995.

73. Weigel NL, Zhang Y: Ligand-independent activation of steroid hormone receptor. J Mol Med 76:469–479, 1998.

74. Trowbridge JM, Rogatsky I, Garabedian MJ: Regulation of estrogen receptor transcriptional enhancement by the cyclin A/Cdk2 complex. Proc Natl Acad Sci U S A 94:10132–10137, 1997.

75. Rogatsky I, Trowbridge JM, Garabedian MJ: Glucocorticoid receptor–mediated cell cycle arrest is achieved through distinct cell-specific transcriptional regulatory mechanisms. Mol Cell Biol 17:3181–3193, 1997.

76. Krstic MD, Rogatsky I, Yamamoto KR, Garabedian MJ: Mitogen-activated and cyclin-dependent protein kinases selectively and differentially modulate transcriptional enhancement by the glucocorticoid receptor. Mol Cell Biol 17:3947–3954, 1997.

77. Tsai SY, Carlstedt-Duke J, Weigel NL, et al: Molecular interactions of steroid hormone receptor with its enhancer element: Evidence for receptor dimer formation. Cell 55:361–369, 1988.

78. Naar AM, Boutin JM, Lipkin SM, et al: The orientation and spacing of core DNA-binding motifs dictate selective transcriptional responses to three nuclear receptors. Cell 65:1267–1279, 1991.

79. Mangelsdorf DJ, Thummel C, Beato M, et al: The nuclear receptor superfamily: The second decade. Cell 83:835–839, 1995.

80. Pace P, Taylor J, Suntharalingam S, et al: Human estrogen receptor beta binds DNA in a manner similar to and dimerizes with estrogen receptor alpha. J Biol Chem 272:25832–25838, 1997.

81. Moore JT, McKee DD, Slentz-Kesler K, et al: Cloning and characterization of human estrogen receptor beta isoforms. Biochem Biophys Res Commun 247:75–78, 1998.

82. Umesono K, Evans RM: Determinants of target gene specificity for steroid/thyroid hormone receptors. Cell 57:1139–1146, 1989.

83. Luisi BF, Xu WX, Otwinowski Z, et al: Crystallographic analysis of the interaction of the glucocorticoid receptor with DNA. Nature 352:497–505, 1991.

84. Schwabe JW, Neuhaus D, Rhodes D: Solution structure of the DNA-binding domain of the oestrogen receptor. Nature 348:458–461, 1990.

85. Wood JR, Greene GL, Nardulli AM: Estrogen response elements function as allosteric modulators of estrogen receptor conformation. Mol Cell Biol 18:1927–1934, 1998.

86. Kumar V, Chambon P: The estrogen receptor binds tightly to its responsive element as a ligand-induced homodimer. Cell 55:145–156, 1988.

87. Sabbah M, Redeuilh G, Baulieu EE: Subunit composition of the estrogen receptor. Involvement of the hormone-binding domain in the dimeric state. J Biol Chem 264:2397–2400, 1989.

88. Chen D, Pace PE, Coombes RC, Ali S: Phosphorylation of human estrogen receptor alpha by protein kinase A regulates dimerization. Mol Cell Biol 19:1002–1015, 1999.

89. Kastner P, Mark M, Chambon P: Nonsteroid nuclear receptors: What are genetic studies telling us about their role in real life? Cell 83:859–869, 1995.

90. Kersten S, Gronemeyer H, Noy N: The DNA binding pattern of the retinoid X receptor is regulated by ligand-dependent modulation of its oligomeric state. J Biol Chem 272:12771–12777, 1997.

91. Ponglikitmongkol M, Green S, Chambon P: Genomic organization of the human oestrogen receptor gene. EMBO J 7:3385–3388, 1988.

92. Misrahi M, Venencie PY, Saugier-Veber P, et al: Structure of the human progesterone receptor gene. Biochim Biophys Acta 1216:289–292, 1993.

93. Kraus WL, Montano MM, Katzenellenbogen BS: Identification of multiple, widely spaced estrogen-responsive regions in the rat progesterone receptor gene. Mol Endocrinol 8:952–969, 1994.

94. Mester I, Martel D, Psychoyos A, Baulieu EE: Hormonal control of oestrogen receptor in uterus and receptivity for ovoimplantation in the rat. Nature 250:776–778, 1974.

95. Hsueh AJ, Peck EJ Jr, Clark JH: Progesterone antagonism of the oestrogen receptor and oestrogen-induced uterine growth. Nature 254:337–339, 1975.

96. Sutherland RL, Geynet C, Binart N, et al: Steroid receptors and effects of oestradiol and progesterone on chick oviduct proteins. Eur J Biochem 107:155–164, 1980.

97. Stoica A, Saceda M, Fakhro A, et al: The role of transforming growth factor-beta in the regulation of estrogen receptor expression in the MCF-7 breast cancer cell line. Endocrinology 138:1498–1508, 1997.

98. Saceda M, Knabbe C, Dickson RB, et al: Post-transcriptional destabilization of estrogen receptor mRNA in MCF-7 cells by 12-O-tetradecanoylphorbol-13-acetate. J Biol Chem 266:17809–17814, 1991.

99. Dauvois S, Danielian PS, White R, Parker MG: Antiestrogen ICI 164,384 reduces cellular estrogen receptor content by increasing its turnover. Proc Natl Acad Sci U S A 89:4037–4041, 1992.

100. Pennequin P, Robins DM, Schimke RT: Regulation of translation of ovalbumin messenger RNA by estrogens and progesterone in oviduct of withdrawn chicks. Eur J Biochem 90:51–58, 1978.

101. Dean DM, Jones PS, Sanders MM: Regulation of the chicken ovalbumin gene by estrogen and corticosterone requires a novel DNA element that binds a labile protein, Chirp-1. Mol Cell Biol 16:2015–2024, 1996.

102. Cha HH, Cram EJ, Wang EC, et al: Glucocorticoids stimulate p21 gene expression by targeting multiple transcriptional elements within a steroid responsive region of the p21waf1/cip1 promoter in rat hepatoma cells. J Biol Chem 273:1998–2007, 1998.

103. Zawel L, Kumar KP, Reinberg D: Recycling of the general transcription factors during RNA polymerase II transcription. Genes Dev 9:1479–1490, 1995.

104. Burley SK, Roeder RG: Biochemistry and structural biology of transcription factor IID (TFIID). Annu Rev Biochem 65:769–799, 1996.

105. Svejstrup JQ, Vichi P, Egly JM: The multiple roles of transcription/repair factor TFIIH. Trends Biochem Sci 21:346–350, 1996.

106. Boonyaratanakornkit V, Melvin V, Prendergast P, et al: High-mobility group chromatin proteins 1 and 2 functionally interact with steroid hormone receptors to enhance their DNA binding in vitro and transcriptional activity in mammalian cells. Mol Cell Biol 18:4471–4487, 1998.

107. Onate SA, Prendergast P, Wagner JP, et al: The DNA-bending protein HMG-1 enhances progesterone receptor binding to its target DNA sequences. Mol Cell Biol 14:3376–3391, 1994.

108. Verrier CS, Roodi N, Yee CJ, et al: High-mobility group (HMG) protein HMG-1 and TATA-binding protein–associated factor TAF(II)30 affect estrogen receptor–mediated transcriptional activation. Mol Endocrinol 11:1009–1019, 1997.

109. Bocquel MT, Kumar V, Stricker C, et al: The contribution of the N- and C-terminal regions of steroid receptors to activation of transcription is both receptor and cell-specific. Nucleic Acids Res 17:2581–2595, 1989.

110. Roeder RG: The role of general initiation factors in transcription by RNA polymerase II. Trends Biochem Sci 21:327–335, 1996.

111. Verrijzer CP, Tjian R: TAFs mediate transcriptional activation and promoter selectivity. Trends Biochem Sci 21:338–342, 1996.

112. Dubrovskaya V, Lavigne AC, Davidson I, et al: Distinct domains of hTAFII100 are required for functional interaction with transcription factor TFIIF beta (RAP30) and incorporation into the TFIID complex. EMBO J 15:3702–3712, 1996.

113. Ossipow V, Tassan JP, Nigg EA, Schibler U: A mammalian RNA polymerase II holoenzyme containing all components required for promoter-specific transcription initiation. Cell 83:137–146, 1995.

114. Koleske AJ, Young RA: The RNA polymerase II holoenzyme and its implications for gene regulation. Trends Biochem Sci 20:113–116, 1995.

115. Cavailles V, Dauvois S, L'Horset F, et al: Nuclear factor RIP140 modulates transcriptional activation by the estrogen receptor. EMBO J 14:3741–3751, 1995.

116. Schulman IG, Chakravarti D, Juguilon H, et al: Interactions between the retinoid X receptor and a conserved region of the TATA-binding protein mediate hormone-dependent transactivation. Proc Natl Acad Sci U S A 92:8288–8292, 1995.

117. Goodrich JA, Tjian R: TBP-TAF complexes: Selectivity factors for eukaryotic transcription. Curr Opin Cell Biol 6:403–409, 1994.

118. Jacq X, Brou C, Lutz Y, et al: Human TAFII30 is present in a distinct TFIID complex and is required for transcriptional activation by the estrogen receptor. Cell 79:107–117, 1994.

119. May M, Mengus G, Lavigne AC, et al: Human TAF(II)28 promotes transcriptional stimulation by activation function 2 of the retinoid X receptors. EMBO J 15:3093–3104, 1996.

120. Mengus G, May M, Carre L, et al: Human TAF(II)135 potentiates transcriptional activation by the AF-2s of the retinoic acid, vitamin D_3, and thyroid hormone receptors in mammalian cells. Genes Dev 11:1381–1395, 1997.

121. Ing NH, Beekman JM, Tsai SY, et al: Members of the steroid hormone receptor superfamily interact with TFIIB (S300–II). J Biol Chem 267:17617–17623, 1992.

122. Baniahmad A, Ha I, Reinberg D, et al: Interaction of human thyroid hormone receptor beta with transcription factor TFIIB may mediate target gene derepression and activation by thyroid hormone. Proc Natl Acad Sci U S A 90:8832–8836, 1993.

123. Hadzic E, Desai-Yajnik V, Helmer E, et al: A 10-amino-acid sequence in the N-terminal A/B domain of thyroid hormone receptor alpha is essential for transcriptional activation and interaction with the general transcription factor TFIIB. Mol Cell Biol 15:4507–4517, 1995.

124. Malik S, Karathanasis SK: TFIIB-directed transcriptional activation by the orphan nuclear receptor hepatocyte nuclear factor 4. Mol Cell Biol 16:1824–1831, 1996.

125. Blanco JC, Wang IM, Tsai SY, et al: Transcription factor TFIIB and the vitamin D receptor cooperatively activate ligand-dependent transcription. Proc Natl Acad Sci U S A 92:1535–1539, 1995.

126. Sabbah M, Kang KI, Tora L, Redeuilh G: Oestrogen receptor facilitates the formation of preinitiation complex assembly: Involvement of the general transcription factor TFIIB. Biochem J 336:639–646, 1998.

127. Rochette-Egly C, Adam S, Rossignol M, et al: Stimulation of RAR alpha activation function AF-1 through binding to the general transcription factor TFIIH and phosphorylation by CDK7. Cell 90:97–107, 1997.

128. Wolffe AP, Hayes JJ: Chromatin disruption and modification. Nucleic Acids Res 27:711–720, 1999.

129. Luger K, Mader AW, Richmond RK, et al: Crystal structure of the nucleosome core particle at 2.8 Å resolution. Nature 389:251–260, 1997.

130. Arents G, Moudrianakis EN: The histone fold: A ubiquitous architectural motif utilized in DNA compaction and protein dimerization. Proc Natl Acad Sci U S A 92:11170–11174, 1995.

131. Richard-Foy H, Hager GL: Sequence-specific positioning of nucleosomes over the steroid-inducible MMTV promoter. EMBO J 6:2321–2328, 1987.

132. Krude T, Elgin SCR: Pushing nucleosomes around. Chromatin. Curr Biol 6:511–515, 1996.

133. Truss M, Candau R, Chavez S, Beato M: Transcriptional control by steroid hormones: The role of chromatin. Ciba Found Symp 191:7–17, 1995.

134. Truss M, Bartsch J, Schelbert A, et al: Hormone induces binding of receptors and transcription factors to a rearranged nucleosome on the MMTV promoter in vivo. EMBO J 14:1737–1751, 1995.

135. Pazin MJ, Kadonaga JT: SWI2/SNF2 and related proteins: ATP-driven motors that disrupt protein-DNA interactions? Cell 88:737–740, 1997.

136. Wu C: Chromatin remodeling and the control of gene expression. J Biol Chem 272:28171–28174, 1997.

137. Onate SA, Tsai SY, Tsai MJ, O'Malley BW: Sequence and characterization of a coactivator for the steroid hormone receptor superfamily. Science 270:1354–1357, 1995.

138. Kamei Y, Xu L, Heinzel T, et al: A CBP integrator complex mediates transcriptional activation and AP-1 inhibition by nuclear receptors. Cell 85:403–414, 1996.

139. Voegel JJ, Heine MJ, Zechel C, et al: TIF2, a 160 kDa transcriptional mediator for the ligand-dependent activation function AF-2 of nuclear receptors. EMBO J 15:3667–3675, 1996.

140. Hong H, Kohli K, Trivedi A, et al: GRIP1, a novel mouse protein that serves as a transcriptional coactivator in yeast for the hormone binding domains of steroid receptors. Proc Natl Acad Sci U S A 93:4948–4952, 1996.

141. Torchia J, Rose DW, Inostroza J, et al: The transcriptional co-activator p/CIP binds CBP and mediates nuclear-receptor function. Nature 387:677–684, 1997.

142. Anzick SL, Kononen J, Walker RL, et al: AIB1, a steroid receptor coactivator amplified in breast and ovarian cancer. Science 277:965–968, 1997.

143. Li H, Gomes PJ, Chen JD: RAC3, a steroid/nuclear receptor–associated coactivator that is related to SRC-1 and TIF2. Proc Natl Acad Sci U S A 94:8479–8484, 1997.

144. Chen H, Lin RJ, Schiltz RL, et al: Nuclear receptor coactivator ACTR is a novel histone acetyltransferase and forms a multimeric activation complex with P/CAF and CBP/p300. Cell 90:569–580, 1997.

145. Halachmi S, Marden E, Martin G, et al: Estrogen receptor–associated proteins: Possible mediators of hormone-induced transcription. Science 264:1455–1458, 1994.

146. Le Douarin B, Zechel C, Garnier JM, et al: The N-terminal part of TIF1, a putative mediator of the ligand-dependent activation function (AF-2) of nuclear receptors, is fused to B-raf in the oncogenic protein T18. EMBO J 14:2020–2033, 1995.

147. Le Douarin B, Nielsen AL, Garnier JM, et al: A possible involvement of TIF1 alpha and TIF1 beta in the epigenetic control of transcription by nuclear receptors. EMBO J 15:6701–6715, 1996.

148. Lee JW, Ryan F, Swaffield JC, et al: Interaction of thyroid-hormone receptor with a conserved transcriptional mediator. Nature 374:91–94, 1995.

149. vom Baur E, Zechel C, Heery D, et al: Differential ligand-dependent interactions between the AF-2 activating domain of nuclear receptors and the putative transcriptional intermediary factors mSUG1 and TIF1. EMBO J 15:110–124, 1996.

150. Chang KH, Chen Y, Chen TT, et al: A thyroid hormone receptor coactivator negatively regulated by the retinoblastoma protein. Proc Natl Acad Sci U S A 94:9040–9045, 1997.

151. Yeh S, Chang C: Cloning and characterization of a specific coactivator, ARA70, for the androgen receptor in human prostate cells. Proc Natl Acad Sci U S A 93:5517–5521, 1996.

152. Yao TP, Ku G, Zhou N, et al: The nuclear hormone receptor coactivator SRC-1 is a specific target of p300. Proc Natl Acad Sci U S A 93:10626–10631, 1996.

153. Heery DM, Kalkhoven E, Hoare S, Parker MG: A signature motif in transcriptional co-activators mediates binding to nuclear receptors. Nature 387:733–736, 1997.

154. Fraser RA, Heard DJ, Adam S, et al: The putative cofactor TIF1alpha is a protein kinase that is hyperphosphorylated upon interaction with liganded nuclear receptors. J Biol Chem 273:16199–16204, 1998.

155. Xu J, Qiu Y, DeMayo FJ, et al: Partial hormone resistance in mice with disruption of the steroid receptor coactivator-1 (SRC-1) gene. Science 279:1922–1925, 1998.

156. Shim WS, DiRenzo J, DeCaprio JA, et al: Segregation of steroid receptor coactivator-1 from steroid receptors in mammary epithelium. Proc Natl Acad Sci U S A 96:208–213, 1999.

157. Spencer TE, Jenster G, Burcin MM, et al: Steroid receptor coactivator-1 is a histone acetyltransferase. Nature 389:194–198, 1997.

158. Gu W, Roeder RG: Activation of p53 sequence-specific DNA binding by acetylation of the p53 C-terminal domain. Cell 90:595–606, 1997.

159. Onate SA, Boonyaratanakornkit V, Spencer TE, et al: The steroid receptor coactivator-1 contains multiple receptor interacting and activation domains that cooperatively enhance the activation function 1 (AF1) and AF2 domains of steroid receptors. J Biol Chem 273:12101–12108, 1998.

160. Kraus WL, Kadonaga JT: P300 and estrogen receptor cooperatively activate transcription via differential enhancement of initiation and reinitiation. Genes Dev 12:331–342, 1998.

161. Ito M, Yuan CX, Malik S, et al: Identity between TRAP and SMCC complexes indicates novel pathways for the function of nuclear receptors and diverse mammalian activators. Mol Cell 3:361–370, 1999.

162. Gu W, Malik S, Ito M, et al: A novel human SRB/MED-containing cofactor complex, SMCC, involved in transcription regulation. Mol Cell 3:97–108, 1999.

163. Rachez C, Lemon BD, Suldan Z, et al: Ligand-dependent transcription activation by nuclear receptors requires the DRIP complex. Nature 398:824–828, 1999.

164. Naar AM, Beaurang PA, Zhou S, et al: Composite co-activator ARC mediates chromatin-directed transcriptional activation. Nature 398:828–832, 1999.

165. Chen JD, Evans RM: A transcriptional co-repressor that interacts with nuclear hormone receptors. Nature 377:454–457, 1995.

166. Horlein AJ, Naar AM, Heinzel T, et al: Ligand-independent repression by the thyroid hormone receptor mediated by a nuclear receptor co-repressor. Nature 377:397–404, 1995.

167. Kurokawa R, Soderstrom M, Horlein A, et al: Polarity-specific activities of retinoic acid receptors determined by a co-repressor. Nature 377:451–454, 1995.

168. Baniahmad A, Köhne AC, Renkawith R: A transferable silencing domain is present in the thyroid hormone receptor, in the v-erbA oncogene product and in the retinoic acid receptor. EMBO J 11:1015–1023, 1992.

169. Nagy L, Kao HY, Chakravarti D, et al: Nuclear receptor repression mediated by a complex containing SMRT, mSin3A, and histone deacetylase. Cell 89:373–380, 1997.

170. Laherty CD, Billin AN, Lavinsky RM, et al: SAP30, a component of the mSin3 corepressor complex involved in N-CoR–mediated repression by specific transcription factors. Mol Cell 2:33–42, 1998.

171. Muscat GE, Burke LJ, Downes M: The corepressor N-CoR and its variants RIP13a and RIP13Δ1 directly interact with the basal transcription factors TFIIB, TAFII32 and TAFII70. Nucleic Acids Res 26:2899–2907, 1998.

172. Zhang X, Jeyakumar M, Petukhov S, Bagchi MK: A nuclear receptor corepressor modulates transcriptional activity of antagonist-occupied steroid hormone receptor. Mol Endocrinol 12:513–524, 1998.

173. Milgrom E, Luu Thi M, Atger M, Baulieu EE: Mechanisms regulating the concentration and the conformation of progesterone receptor(s) in uterus. J Biol Chem 248:6366–6374, 1973.

174. Vedeckis WV, Ali M, Allen HR: Regulation of glucocorticoid receptor protein and mRNA levels. Cancer Res 49(suppl):2295–2302, 1989.

175. Kraus WL, Weis KE, Katzenellenbogen BS: Inhibitory cross-talk between steroid hormone receptors: Differential targeting of estrogen receptor in the repression of its transcriptional activity by agonist- and antagonist-occupied progestin receptors. Mol Cell Biol 15:1847–1857, 1995.

176. Liu J, DeFranco DB: Chromatin recycling of glucocorticoid receptors: Implications for multiple roles of heat shock protein 90. Mol Endocrinol 13:355–365, 1999.

177. Dong Y, Poellinger L, Gustafsson JA, Okret S: Regulation of glucocorticoid receptor expression: Evidence for transcriptional and posttranslational mechanisms. Mol Endocrinol 2:1256–1264, 1988.

178. Meyer AS, Schmidt TJ: Differential effects of agonist and antagonists on autoregulation of glucocorticoid receptors in a rat colonic adenocarcinoma cell line. J Steroid Biochem Mol Biol 62:97–105, 1997.

179. Okret S, Poellinger L, Dong Y, Gustafsson JA: Down-regulation of glucocorticoid receptor mRNA by glucocorticoid hormones and recognition by the receptor of a specific binding sequence within a receptor cDNA clone. Proc Natl Acad Sci U S A 83:5899–5903, 1986.

180. Mester J, Baulieu EE: Progesterone receptors in the chick oviduct. Determination of the total concentration of binding sites in the cytosol and nuclear fraction and effect of progesterone on their distribution. Eur J Biochem 72:405–414, 1977.

181. Nardulli AM, Katzenellenbogen BS: Progesterone receptor regulation in T47D human breast cancer cells: Analysis by density labeling of progesterone receptor synthesis and degradation and their modulation by progestin. Endocrinology 122:1532–1540, 1988.

182. Syvala H, Vienonen A, Zhuang YH, et al: Evidence for enhanced ubiquitin-mediated proteolysis of the chicken progesterone receptor by progesterone. Life Sci 63:1505–1512, 1998.

183. Masuyama H, MacDonald PN: Proteasome-mediated degradation of the vitamin D receptor (VDR) and a putative role for SUG1 interaction with the AF-2 domain of VDR. J Cell Biochem 71:429–440, 1998.

184. Campen CA, Gorski J: Anomalous behavior of protein synthesis inhibitors on the turnover of the estrogen receptor as measured by density labeling. Endocrinology 119:1454–1461, 1986.

185. Mester J, Baulieu EE: Dynamics of oestrogen-receptor distribution between the cytosol and nuclear fractions of immature rat uterus after oestradiol administration. Biochem J 146:617–623, 1975.

186. Alexander IE, Shine J, Sutherland RL: Progestin regulation of estrogen receptor messenger RNA in human breast cancer cells. Mol Endocrinol 4:821–828, 1990.

187. Vig E, Barrett TJ, Vedeckis WV: Coordinate regulation of glucocorticoid receptor and c-jun mRNA levels: Evidence for cross-talk between two signaling pathways at the transcriptional level. Mol Endocrinol 8:1336–1346, 1994.

188. Colin IM, Jameson JL: Estradiol sensitization of rat pituitary cells to gonadotropin-releasing hormone: Involvement of protein kinase C– and calcium-dependent signaling pathways. Endocrinology 139:3796–3802, 1998.

189. Bonavera JJ, Kalra PS, Kalra SP: L-Arginine/nitric oxide amplifies the magnitude and duration of the luteinizing hormone surge induced by estrogen: Involvement of neuropeptide Y. Endocrinology 137:1956–1962, 1996.

190. Adams M, Reginato MJ, Shao D, et al: Transcriptional activation by peroxisome proliferator–activated receptor gamma is inhibited by phosphorylation at a consensus mitogen-activated protein kinase site. J Biol Chem 272:5128–5132, 1997.

191. Lippman ME, Dickson RB, Gelmann EP, et al: Growth regulatory peptide production by human breast carcinoma cells. J Steroid Biochem 30:53–61, 1988.

192. Clarke R, Brunner N, Katz D, et al: The effects of a constitutive expression of transforming growth factor-alpha on the growth of MCF-7 human breast cancer cells in vitro and in vivo. Mol Endocrinol 3:372–380, 1989.

193. Dickson RB, Huff KK, Spencer EM, Lippman ME: Induction of epidermal growth factor–related polypeptides by 17 beta-estradiol in MCF-7 human breast cancer cells. Endocrinology 118:138–142, 1986.

194. Yee D, Rosen N, Favoni RE, Cullen KJ: The insulin-like growth factors, their receptors, and their binding proteins in human breast cancer. Cancer Treat Res 53:93–106, 1991.

195. Vignon F, Prebois C, Rochefort H: Inhibition of breast cancer growth by suramin. J Natl Cancer Inst 84:38–42, 1992.

196. Lee CS, Hall RE, Alexander IE, et al: Inverse relationship between estrogen receptor and epidermal growth factor receptor mRNA levels in human breast cancer cell lines. Growth Factors 3:97–103, 1990.

197. Lee CS, deFazio A, Ormandy CJ, Sutherland RL: Inverse regulation of oestrogen receptor and epidermal growth factor receptor gene expression in MCF-7 breast cancer cells treated with phorbol ester. J Steroid Biochem Mol Biol 58:267–275, 1996.

198. deFazio A, Chiew YE, McEvoy M, et al: Antisense estrogen receptor RNA expression increases epidermal growth factor receptor gene expression in breast cancer cells. Cell Growth Differ 8:903–911, 1997.

199. Migliaccio A, Di Domenico M, Castoria G, et al: Tyrosine kinase/p21ras/MAP-kinase pathway activation by estradiol-receptor complex in MCF-7 cells. EMBO J 15:1292–1300, 1996.

200. Migliaccio A, Piccolo D, Castoria G, et al: Activation of the Src/p21ras/Erk pathway by progesterone receptor via cross-talk with estrogen receptor. EMBO J 17:2008-2018, 1998.

201. Russell KS, Hung MC: Transcriptional repression of the neu protooncogene by estrogen stimulated estrogen receptor. Cancer Res 52:6624-6629, 1992.

202. Kushner PJ, Hort E, Shine J, et al: Construction of cell lines that express high levels of the human estrogen receptor and are killed by estrogens. Mol Endocrinol 4:1465–1473, 1990.

203. Gaben AM, Mester J: BALB/c mouse 3T3 fibroblasts expressing human estrogen receptor: Effect of estradiol on cell growth. Biochem Biophys Res Commun 176:1473–1481, 1991.

204. Garcia M, Derocq D, Freiss G, Rochefort H: Activation of estrogen receptor transfected into a receptor-negative breast cancer cell line decreases the metastatic and invasive potential of the cells. Proc Natl Acad Sci U S A 89:11538–11542, 1992.

205. Tsai SY, Tsai MJ, O'Malley BW: Cooperative binding of steroid hormone receptors contributes to transcriptional synergism at target enhancer elements. Cell 57:443–448, 1989.

206. Gaub MP, Bellard M, Scheuer I, et al: Activation of the ovalbumin gene by the estrogen receptor involves the fos-jun complex. Cell 63:1267–1276, 1990.

207. Kalff M, Gross B, Beato M: Progesterone receptor stimulates transcription of mouse mammary tumour virus in a cell-free system. Nature 344:360–362, 1990.

208. Rigaud G, Roux J, Pictet R, Grange T: In vivo footprinting of rat TAT gene: Dynamic interplay between the glucocorticoid receptor and a liver-specific factor. Cell 67:977–986, 1991.

209. Yang-Yen HF, Chambard JC, Sun YL, et al: Transcriptional interference between c-Jun and the glucocorticoid receptor: Mutual inhibition of DNA binding due to direct protein-protein interaction. Cell 62:1205–1215, 1990.

210. Konig H, Ponta H, Rahmsdorf HJ, Herrlich P: Interference between pathway-specific

211. Diamond MI, Miner JN, Yoshinaga SK, Yamamoto KR: Transcription factor interactions: Selectors of positive or negative regulation from a single DNA element. Science 249:1266–1272, 1990.

212. Scheinman RI, Cogswell PC, Lofquist AK, Baldwin AS Jr: Role of transcriptional activation of I kappa B alpha in mediation of immunosuppression by glucocorticoids. Science 270:283–286, 1995.

213. Auphan N, DiDonato JA, Rosette C, et al: Immunosuppression by glucocorticoids: Inhibition of NF-kappa B activity through induction of I kappa B synthesis. Science 270:286–290, 1995.

214. Reddel RR, Alexander IE, Koga M, et al: Genetic instability and the development of steroid hormone insensitivity in cultured T 47D human breast cancer cells. Cancer Res 48:4340–4347, 1988.

215. Borgna JL, Rochefort H: Effects and mechanism of action of antiestrogens in breast cancer. Semin Hop 60:703–709, 1984.

216. Paech K, Webb P, Kuiper GG, et al: Differential ligand activation of estrogen receptors ERα and ERβ at AP1 sites. Science 277:1508–1510, 1997.

217. Potthoff SJ, Romine LE, Nardulli AM: Effects of wild type and mutant estrogen receptors on DNA flexibility, DNA bending, and transcription activation. Mol Endocrinol 10:1095–1106, 1996.

218. Zhang QX, Hilsenbeck SG, Fuqua SA, Borg A: Multiple splicing variants of the estrogen receptor are present in individual human breast tumors. J Steroid Biochem Mol Biol 59:251–260, 1996.

219. Fanelli MA, Vargas-Roig LM, Gago FE, et al: Estrogen receptors, progesterone receptors, and cell proliferation in human breast cancer. Breast Cancer Res Treat 37:217–228, 1996.

220. Suzuki H, Akakura K, Komiya A, et al: Codon 877 mutation in the androgen receptor gene in advanced prostate cancer: Relation to antiandrogen withdrawal syndrome. Prostate 29:153–158, 1996.

221. Fenton MA, Shuster TD, Fertig AM, et al: Functional characterization of mutant androgen receptors from androgen-independent prostate cancer. Clin Cancer Res 3:1383–1388, 1997.

222. Mahfoudi A, Roulet E, Dauvois S, et al: Specific mutations in the estrogen receptor change the properties of antiestrogens to full agonists. Proc Natl Acad Sci U S A 92:4206–4210, 1995.

223. Musgrove EA, Lee CS, Cornish AL, et al: Antiprogestin inhibition of cell cycle progression in T-47D breast cancer cells is accompanied by induction of the cyclin-dependent kinase inhibitor p21. Mol Endocrinol 11:54–66, 1997.

224. Musgrove EA, Swarbrick A, Lee CS, et al: Mechanisms of cyclin-dependent kinase inactivation by progestins. Mol Cell Biol 18:1812–1825, 1998.

225. Smith EP, Boyd J, Frank GR, et al: Estrogen resistance caused by a mutation in the estrogen-receptor gene in a man. N Engl J Med 331:1056–1061, 1994.

226. Yang NN, Bryant HU, Hardikar S, et al: Estrogen and raloxifene stimulate transforming growth factor-beta 3 gene expression in rat bone: A potential mechanism for estrogen or raloxifene-mediated bone maintenance. Endocrinology 137:2075–2084, 1996.

227. Tanaka S, Haji M, Takayanagi R, et al: 1,25-Dihydroxyvitamin D$_3$ enhances the enzymatic activity and expression of the messenger ribonucleic acid for aromatase cytochrome P450 synergistically with dexamethasone depending on the vitamin D receptor level in cultured human osteoblasts. Endocrinology 137:1860–1869, 1996.

228. Desvergne B, Ijpenberg A, Devchand PR, Wahli W: The peroxisome proliferator–activated receptors at the cross-road of diet and hormonal signalling. J Steroid Biochem Mol Biol 65:65–74, 1998.

229. Forman BM, Tontonoz P, Chen J, et al: 15-Deoxy-delta 12, 14-prostaglandin J$_2$ is a ligand for the adipocyte determination factor PPAR gamma. Cell 83:803–12, 1995.

230. Lehmann JM, Moore LB, Smith-Oliver TA, et al: An antidiabetic thiazolidinedione is a high affinity ligand for peroxisome proliferator–activated receptor gamma (PPAR gamma). J Biol Chem 270:12953–12956, 1995.

231. Spiegelman BM: PPAR-gamma: Adipogenic regulator and thiazolidinedione receptor. Diabetes 47:507–514, 1998.

232. Auwerx J, Schoonjans K, Fruchart JC, Staels B: Regulation of triglyceride metabolism by PPARs: Fibrates and thiazolidinediones have distinct effects. J Atheroscler Thromb 3:81–89, 1996.

233. Reginato MJ, Krakow SL, Bailey ST, Lazar MA: Prostaglandins promote and block adipogenesis through opposing effects on peroxisome proliferator–activated receptor gamma. J Biol Chem 273:1855–1858, 1998.

234. Blaustein JD, Lehman MN, Turcotte JC, Greene G: Estrogen receptors in dendrites and axon terminals in the guinea pig hypothalamus. Endocrinology 131:281–290, 1992.

235. Pappas TC, Gametchu B, Watson CS: Membrane estrogen receptors identified by multiple antibody labeling and impeded-ligand binding. FASEB J 9:404–410, 1995.

236. Godeau F, Schorderet-Slatkine S, Boquet P, et al: Involvement of cAMP in the cytoplasmic control of meiotic cell division in Xenopus laevis oocytes. Adv Cyclic Nucleotide Res 14:421–428, 1981.

237. Baulieu EE, Godeau F, Schorderet M, Schorderet-Slatkine S: Steroid-induced meiotic division in Xenopus laevis oocytes: Surface and calcium. Nature 275:593–598, 1978.

238. Baulieu EE, Robel P: Non-genomic mechanisms of action of steroid hormones. Ciba Found Symp 191:24–42, 1995.

239. Andresson T, Ruderman JV: The kinase Eg2 is a component of the Xenopus oocyte progesterone-activated signaling pathway. EMBO J 17:5627–5637, 1998.

240. Farhat MY, Lavigne MC, Ramwell PW: The vascular protective effects of estrogen. FASEB J 10:615–624, 1996.

241. Lagrange AH, Ronnekleiv OK, Kelly MJ: Modulation of G protein–coupled receptors by an estrogen receptor that activates protein kinase A. Mol Pharmacol 51:605–612, 1997.

242. Rastinejad F, Perlmann T, Evans RM, Sigler PB: Structural determinants of nuclear receptor assembly on DNA direct repeats. Nature 375:203–211, 1995.

▲▲▲▲

Applications of Molecular Biology and Genetics in Endocrinology

J. Larry Jameson

Recombinant DNA technology is revolutionizing our understanding of genetics, physiology, cell biology, and biochemistry. Because many recent advances rely on the use of recombinant DNA methods, a basic understanding of these approaches is relevant for clinicians as well as scientists engaged in laboratory investigation. A recurring theme throughout this book is the synergism derived by combining information from traditional studies of pathophysiology with new insights from molecular biology. Nowhere is this more apparent than in studies of inherited endocrine disorders like MEN1 and 2 (see Chapters 188 and 189).

In addition to providing a new means for the diagnosis of inherited disorders, the identification of mutations in endocrine genes also enhances our understanding of pathophysiology.[1] Mutations have been described at multiple different steps in the pathways of hormone action. There are now examples of mutations in hormones themselves, hormone receptors, second messenger signaling pathways, and the transcription factors that transduce hormone signals. One can predict continued rapid advances in this field with the transfer of genetic testing into clinical practice in the near future.

In the first half of this chapter, fundamental methods in molecular genetics are reviewed to provide a brief overview of recombinant DNA terminology and the experimental approaches that are used elsewhere in the book. In the second half of the chapter, genetic principles are reviewed and a selected group of well-characterized disorders are used as examples of how genetics is impacting our understanding of endocrine diseases.

CLONING AND SEQUENCING GENES

Preparation and Screening of DNA Libraries

A first step in the analysis of endocrine gene expression is to obtain a cDNA clone for the gene in question. The first step in the cloning of a cDNA is to prepare a library (Fig. 11–1). This involves making a complementary copy of mRNA using the enzyme reverse transcriptase. This complementary DNA or cDNA is then replicated to create a double-stranded sequence that can be inserted into λ phage vectors[2] or occasionally into plasmid cloning vectors.[3, 4] Ideally, the entire population of cDNAs is inserted into the cloning vector. In this manner, the library contains a population of cDNAs that reflects the composition of mRNA in a given tissue or cell type. Thus, mRNAs that are more abundant will be represented more frequently in the library. A critical aspect of cDNA cloning is to prepare libraries from tissues that either have abundant levels of a given mRNA or have been treated to induce expression of a specific mRNA. For example, pituitary mRNA is the appropriate tissue source for cloning the GH cDNA whereas pancreatic islet mRNA would be used to isolate the insulin cDNA.

Having created a library, the next step is to screen it for a specific clone (see Fig. 11–1). Library screening is typically performed in one of two fashions, although alternative strategies are available. In one approach, the phage is used to infect a lawn of *Escherichia coli* to create phage plaques from which DNA can be transferred to replicate filters to allow screening with radioactive hybridization probes.[5] This strategy requires knowledge of the DNA sequence that is being sought, either from information derived from protein sequence or perhaps gleaned from a homologous gene sequence in a related species. A second strategy for library screening uses antibodies to detect the protein that is being sought. In this approach, the phage library is created in such a manner that the cDNAs are linked to a β-galactosidase fusion gene that can be induced after the phage has infected *E. coli*. The infected *E. coli* can be used to express large quantities of proteins encoded by the cDNA and expressed as fusion proteins. Analogous to screening by DNA hybridization, these fusion proteins can be transferred to replicate membranes, and are then screened using specific antibodies raised against the protein in question.[6] The goal of the screening process is to identify the one λ phage out of perhaps 100,000 that contains the clone of interest. Once identified, this phage can be recovered, purified, and amplified to provide a renewable source of the cDNA. The cDNA insert from the phage can be excised and subcloned into a plasmid for further analyses.[7]

This work was supported in part by Public Health Service grants DK42144, HD23519, and HD29164.

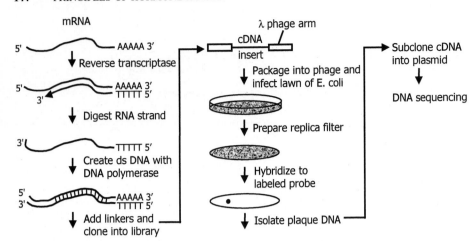

FIGURE 11–1. Preparation and screening of DNA libraries. Libraries are used for cloning genes or cDNAs. In the example shown for a cDNA library, a series of enzymatic steps are used to prepare double-stranded cDNA from mRNA. The cDNAs are inserted into a modified λ phage that can be used to infect a lawn of E. coli. After phage-induced lysis of the E. coli, DNA from the lytic plaques is transferred to a membrane and hybridized with radiolabeled probes. Identified plaques are rescreened and DNA from positive clones is subcloned into plasmids for further characterization. See text for details and for variations on the procedure.

DNA Sequencing

A great advantage of transferring cDNAs into plasmids is that it allows rapid and large-scale amplification of cloned DNA in E. coli.[8] It is then possible to perform recombinant DNA manipulations with larger quantities of DNA and to rapidly analyze the DNA sequence of the cDNA insert. A variety of methods are available for DNA sequencing. Initially, the Maxam-Gilbert procedure was used for most DNA sequencing.[9] It is based on selective chemical derivatization of the different nucleotides (G,A,T,C) followed by cleavage and electrophoresis on a gel that allows DNA fragments to be resolved at a single base level. This procedure for DNA sequencing has been supplanted by protocols derived from the Sanger method for chain termination.[10] Chain termination protocols are based on the principle that dideoxynucleotides can be used to terminate DNA polymerization (Fig. 11–2). By establishing four different reactions, each containing a dideoxynucleotide for each base, the DNA sequence can be randomly terminated at specific nucleotides (e.g., T). When the four reactions are run in parallel on a DNA sequencing gel, the sequence can be determined by "reading" the base that terminates the sequence at each new position. DNA sequencing is readily amenable to automation. There are now protocols that allow robotic handling of the sequencing reactions as well as automated reading of the sequencing gels. With the DNA sequence in hand, computer programs are used to convert DNA sequence into predicted amino acid codons and to identify characteristic restriction enzyme sites and other structural features that are useful for further studies of the clone.

Uses of Cloned cDNAs and Genes

A cDNA clone is a critical first step for a number of subsequent studies. For example, the cloned cDNA can be used to isolate the gene that encodes it. In a manner somewhat analogous to cDNA library screening, genomic libraries can be screened using radiolabeled cDNAs.[11] Isolation of genes allows detailed analyses of genomic organization and promoter structure. The promoters of endocrine genes are of particular interest because they often contain regulatory elements that allow modulation by hormonal and second messenger signaling systems. For example, regulatory elements for glucocorticoid receptors and transcription factors that respond to cAMP (via protein kinase A) often reside in the promoter regions of genes (see Chapters 7 and 10). The availability of a cDNA also provides a radioactive probe that can be used to analyze patterns and levels of mRNA expression by Northern blot. Cloned cDNAs also allow detailed structure-function analyses of hormones or their receptors. The cDNAs can be translated in vitro using reticulocyte lysates[12] or overexpressed in E. coli,[13] baculovirus,[14] or tissue culture cells[15] to allow analyses of structure by physical methods or by mutagenesis.

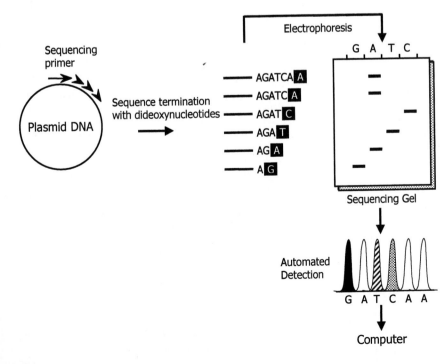

FIGURE 11–2. DNA sequencing. A variety of methods are available for sequencing DNA. In the example shown, the chain termination procedure[10] is illustrated schematically. Single stranded DNA is first prepared either by denaturing the double stranded plasmid or by using M13 phage that infect E. coli. A sequencing primer complementary to the DNA is used to synthesize radiolabeled DNA. By establishing four separate reactions that contain dideoxynucleotides for each base (G,A,T,C), the sequences are terminated randomly. Electrophoresis and autoradiography of each of the reactions run in parallel create a "sequencing ladder." In the example shown, the sequence reads G-A-T-C-A-A from the bottom to the top of gel (5' to 3'). Currently, most DNA sequencing is performed using automated sequencers. In this case, fluorescent nucleotides are incorporated into the sequencing reactions, either in the sequencing primer or in the nucleotides. A laser-mediated device detects the fluorescent fragments and inputs the information into a computer, where the data can be manipulated further.

METHODS USED TO ANALYZE GENE EXPRESSION

Perhaps the most widespread use of cloned cDNAs is to analyze patterns of gene expression in different tissues and in response to various hormonal manipulations. The Northern blot is the most common procedure used for analyses of mRNA expression[16] (Table 11–1). In this technique, total messenger RNA is extracted from a tissue or cell line and subjected to electrophoresis to fractionate the mRNA according to size. The fractionated mRNA is then transferred and bound to a membrane followed by hybridization to a radiolabeled cDNA probe. Because the radioactive probe is complementary to its corresponding mRNA, a radioactive hybridization signal is seen only for this specific mRNA and in proportion to its abundance.

A number of other methods are available for analyzing mRNA expression. RNase protection is a particularly sensitive method that relies on solution hybridization of the mRNA to a specific radiolabeled cRNA.[17] Hybridization of the mRNA to the probe allows it to be protected from digestion by RNase, an enzyme that destroys single stranded RNA, but not the double-stranded product of the hybridization probe annealed to the mRNA. Although RNase protection is very sensitive, it is technically difficult and does not allow repeated analyses of the same mRNA sample as is possible with a Northern blot membrane.

The advent of the polymerase chain reaction (PCR) has impacted a wide array of molecular biology protocols. A reaction combining reverse transcriptase and the polymerase chain reaction (RT-PCR) has gained favor as a highly sensitive method for measuring mRNA.[18] In this procedure, mRNA is first copied into cDNA by reverse transcriptase, a step that is analogous to the method used for producing a cDNA library. Subsequently, the polymerase chain reaction (PCR) is used to amplify the cDNA product (see below). If PCR is carried out under carefully controlled conditions, the amount of amplified product will reflect the amount of a specific mRNA that was present in the starting material. By using radiolabeled primers or nucleotides in the PCR reaction, the method is amenable to quantitation. RT-PCR is remarkably sensitive, allowing the detection of even a few mRNA transcripts per cell. In addition, it can be readily adapted for measurement of virtually any mRNA, since one only needs to know the DNA sequence to design specific PCR primers.

In situ hybridization is a procedure that combines analyses of mRNA expression with histology.[19] Tissue samples are hybridized with radiolabeled probes, allowing determination of patterns as well as levels of gene expression. In situ hybridization is particularly useful for tissues with complex or heterogeneous arrangements of cell types (e.g., ovary, brain) because it allows identification of which cells are producing a given mRNA transcript (Fig. 11–3).

TRANSCRIPTIONAL AND POST-TRANSCRIPTIONAL REGULATION OF GENES

Nuclear Run-On Assays

Having demonstrated regulation of a given mRNA, it is often important to know whether steady state mRNA levels are altered

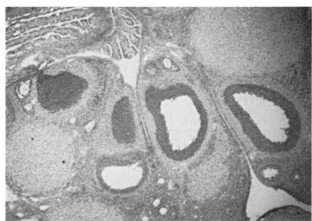
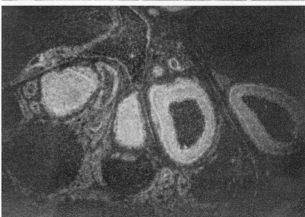

FIGURE 11–3. In situ hybridization. Expression of inhibin α-subunit mRNA in the rat ovary on the day of proestrus. The top panel shows an hematoxylin-eosin stained section, and the bottom panel shows the paired darkfield micrograph of silver grains produced by the radioactive probe that hybridizes to α-inhibin mRNA. Expression of α-inhibin is seen in the granulosa cells of healthy follicles, and there is little or no expression in interstitial cells, the corpus luteum, or atretic follicles. Photographs are ×40 magnification. (Adapted with permission from Woodruff TK, D'Agostino J, Schwartz NB, Mayo KE: Dynamic changes in inhibin messenger RNAs in rat ovarian follicles during the reproductive cycle. Science 239, 1296, 1988. Copyright 1988 by the American Association for the Advancement of Science.)

because of changes in transcription of the gene, or as a consequence of changes in mRNA stability. A classic approach for studies of transcriptional regulation involves the nuclear "run-on assay."[20] In this procedure, nuclei are isolated after a specific stimulus and allowed to carry out mRNA synthesis in vitro. Because the amount of mRNA synthesis under these conditions reflects the number of transcripts initiated prior to isolation of nuclei, one can estimate the transcription rate by determining the amount of elongated mRNA. Radiolabeled mRNA is hybridized to immobilized DNA to allow quantitation. Although a classic procedure, this technique is used rarely because it is technically demanding, and most laboratories now analyze transcriptional control using transient gene expression assays (see below).

Post-transcriptional Regulation

Messenger RNA stability can be assessed in a number of ways. Actinomycin D, which inhibits RNA synthesis, is often used to assess whether a specific treatment alters the stability of mRNA. Although widely used, actinomycin D is toxic to cells and may block the synthesis of proteins that are involved in mRNA stabilization or degradation, thereby confounding the results. Pulse-chase analyses provide an alternative procedure for studies of mRNA stability.[21] In this technique, RNA is labeled with a pulse of radioactive uridine

TABLE 11–1. Summary of Blotting Procedures

Procedure	Substance Detected	Probe	Major Application
Southern blot	DNA	Nucleic acid	Gene structure
Northern blot	RNA	Nucleic acid	Gene expression
Western blot	Protein	Antibody	Protein levels
Southwestern blot	Protein	DNA	DNA-protein interactions
Farwestern blot	Protein	Protein	Protein-protein interactions

followed by a prolonged incubation (chase) with nonradioactive ribonucleotides. The nonradioactive chase prevents further incorporation of radioactive uridine into newly transcribed mRNA. Thus, the length of retention of the radioactive pulse in a specific mRNA reflects its half-life. The amount of labeled RNA is quantitated by hybridization to DNA immobilized on filters analogous to the procedure used in nuclear run-on assays.

Transient Gene Expression Studies in Transfected Cells

Transient gene expression studies provide an alternative technique for examining transcriptional control (Fig. 11–4). In addition, this method allows detailed mutagenesis of cloned promoter sequences before their introduction into cells.[22] In this procedure, the promoter sequences of genes are typically fused to a reporter gene that can be assayed readily.[23] Common reporter genes include *chloramphenicol acetyltransferase (CAT), luciferase (LUC),* and *β-galactosidase (β-GAL).* In each case, the reporter genes are enzymes whose activities are not normally found in eukaryotic cells. Thus, in the absence of gene transfer, the background activity of these reporter enzymes is negligible.

The promoter-reporter fusion gene constructs are introduced into cells using a process referred to as "transfection."[22] Transfected genes are transcriptionally active over 24 to 72 hours, allowing relatively rapid analyses of promoter function. Alternatively, transfected genes can be stably introduced into cells by selecting for a resistance marker such as neomycin or dihydrofolate reductase. The principal goal of transfection experiments is to define DNA sequences that are required for promoter function and mediate a specific hormone signal or second messenger pathway. A variety of methods are now available to allow deletion or site-directed mutagenesis of promoter elements.[24] This approach has been critical for defining DNA sequences that regulate tissue-specific expression, basal promoter activity, and a variety of

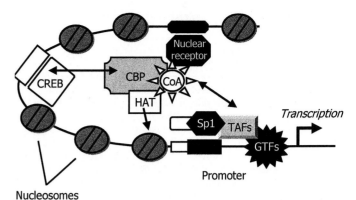

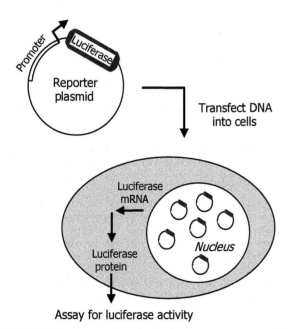

FIGURE 11–4. Transient gene expression using reporter genes. Plasmids are transfected into mammalian cell lines for transient expression studies. The transfected plasmids are transcribed for several days, after which the DNA is either degraded or becomes integrated into the host cell genome. If a selectable marker (e.g., neomycin resistance) is included in the transfection, it is possible to isolate stably transfected clones of cells. A common experimental paradigm uses transient expression to measure the activity and regulation of a promoter. In the example shown, the promoter drives expression of a luciferase reporter gene. The amount of luciferase enzyme produced is proportionate to the transcriptional activity of the promoter.

FIGURE 11–5. Formation of an active transcription complex. Interactions between enhancer-binding proteins and components of the basal transcription complex are illustrated schematically. There is evidence that many enhancer binding proteins, like nuclear receptors and cAMP response element binding protein (CREB), interact with the basal transcription machinery via coactivator (CoA) proteins, including CREB-binding protein (CBP). This protein complex contains histone acetyl transferase (HAT) activity that modifies the acetylation status of histones and other transcription factors, thereby altering nucleosome structure and converting chromatin into a more open configuration that allows access of additional transcription factors. Other transcription factors, such as selective promoter factor 1 (Sp1), make contacts with transcriptional activating factors (TAFs) that interact with the TATA binding protein (TBP) and a large group of general transcriptions factors (GTFs). Implicit in this model is the idea that specific protein-protein contacts as well as protein-DNA contacts are involved in the assembly of active transcription complexes.

hormone response elements such as cAMP response elements (CREs) and regulatory sequences for steroid and thyroid hormone receptors. Identification of these DNA regulatory sequences is often a first step toward characterization of the transcription factors that interact with these elements.

Analyses of Transcription Factor Interactions with DNA

The regulatory DNA sequences in genes function by binding transcription factors (see Chapter 2). These proteins are generally classified into three groups: general transcription factors, enhancer binding proteins, and transcriptional activating factors (Fig. 11–5). Because this is a relatively nascent area of research, our understanding of these proteins and their classification are changing rapidly. General transcription factors include proteins that bind to the proximal regions of genes near the start site of transcription. These proteins include the TATA binding protein (TBP), as well as series of other general transcriptions factors (GTF) such as TFIIA, B, E, etc., that comprise a complex group of proteins that regulate transcriptional initiation.[25, 26] Enhancer binding proteins typically interact with DNA sequences located upstream of the basal transcription complex. Enhancer binding proteins are usually bipartite, having a DNA binding domain and a separate domain involved in protein-protein contacts and transcriptional activation. This group of proteins includes transcription factors with a broad range of regulatory functions. For example, proteins such as Pit1 are involved in cell-specific expression. Pit1 is a homeodomain class (related to homeobox genes involved in *Drosophila* embryonic development) of transcription factor that is expressed specifically in somatotropes, lactotropes, and thyrotropes where it controls expression of the *growth hormone* and *prolactin* genes.[27, 28] As described below, mutations in the *Pit1* gene cause deficiencies of GH, Prl, and TSH.[29–31] Other enhancer proteins bind to second messenger signal response elements such as cAMP response elements (CREs). cAMP response elements bind a large family of transcription factors referred to as CRE-binding (CREB) proteins or activating transcription factors (ATF) (see Chapter 7).[32] Structurally related DNA sequences bind members of the Jun/Fos family of transcription factors that are involved in cell signaling by protein kinase C and a variety of growth factor signaling pathways.[33] Other enhancer proteins include nuclear receptors such as the glucocorticoid, estrogen, and thyroid hormone receptors (see Chapters 10 and 94). These receptors bind to hormone response elements in target genes to activate or repress transcription. Enhancer proteins in each of these groups typically bind to DNA with high affinity (e.g., K_d less than 10^{-9} M).

The mechanism by which transcription factors alter the rate of RNA synthesis is an area of active investigation that has brought studies of transcriptional coactivators (CoAs) and corepressors (CoRs) to the forefront.[34] In some cases, DNA-bound transcription factors form direct protein-protein contacts with components of the basal transcription complex such as TBP or TFIIB.[35–37] Perhaps more commonly, there are interactions between DNA-bound transcription factors and an intermediary group of proteins that include the transcription activating factors (TAFs),[38, 39] coactivators, and corepressors to form large complexes that interface with the general transcriptional machinery. Because these adaptor proteins do not bind to DNA with high affinity, their identification and characterization have lagged behind those of other groups of transcription factors. Biochemical purification and yeast two-hybrid approaches (see below) have been used to identify many of these proteins. Studies of the nuclear receptor superfamily have provided an important paradigm for the identification of CoAs and CoRs and for understanding basic principles of transcriptional regulation.[34] For any given gene, the array of different transcription factors bound to the promoter is relatively large (usually more than 20). And this group of proteins, in turn, interacts with an equally complex group of adaptor proteins and general transcription factors.

This large repertoire of proteins provides an important means for regulatory control at the level of transcription. Consequently, when considering the role of any given regulatory DNA element and its cognate transcription factor, it is important to recognize that specific combinations of transcription factors may result in unique properties that are not necessarily applicable to another gene. Ultimately, the assembly of transcription complexes appears to alter transcription by a series of coordinated steps that are used to varying degrees in different genes. One step involves the modification of chromatin structure by shifting nucleosome phasing to allow access of additional transcription factors.[40] Another step involves the assembly of a committed transcription complex that recruits basal transcription factors from the initiator region of the promoter.[41] Finally, RNA polymerase is activated to initiate RNA synthesis for one or more rounds of transcription.[42] These aspects of transcriptional control are particularly relevant in endocrinology where many genes are expressed in a tissue-specific manner, and are dynamically regulated by hormonal signals. Moreover, as discussed below, a surprising number of endocrine disorders involve defects in transcription factors.

Two techniques have been particularly useful for identifying protein interactions with DNA. DNase 1 footprinting is a method that relies on the ability of bound protein to protect DNA from digestion by the enzyme DNase 1[43] (Fig. 11–6). Consequently, protein-bound regions

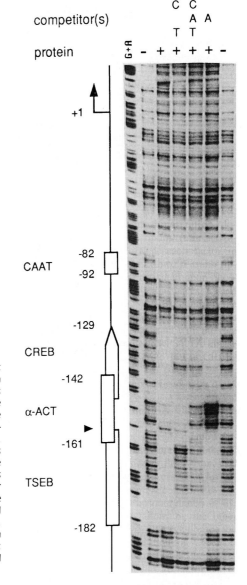

FIGURE 11–6. DNase 1 footprinting of protein-DNA interactions. Proteins that bind to specific DNA sites with high affinity can be detected as a "footprint" by exposing the DNA-protein complex to DNase1, an enzyme that digests DNA. When DNA fragments are radiolabeled, areas bound by proteins are protected from DNase 1 digestion and appear as footprints when the partially digested DNA is subjected to denaturing electrophoresis. In the example shown, the glycoprotein hormone α-subunit gene promoter has been footprinted by nuclear proteins extracted from a placental cell line (JEG-3) that expresses the α and β subunit genes of hCG. Distinct protein binding sites can be detected by the presence of separate footprints as well as the ability to compete for protein binding with short oligonucleotides that correspond to the DNA recognition sequence. Labeled DNA was incubated without (-) or with (+) nuclear extracts from JEG-3 cells before partial digestion with DNase 1. A G+A Maxam-Gilbert sequencing ladder is shown on the left. Sequences protected from Dnase1 digestion are indicated by boxes on the left. Competitor oligonucleotides (~1000-fold excess) that correspond to the individual protected regions are indicated above the lanes. The competitors are: C, cAMP response element (CRE); A, α-activating element (α-ACT); T, trophoblast specific element (TSE). (Adapted with permission from Steger DJ, Altschmied J, Buscher M, Mellon PL: Evolution of placenta-specific gene expression: Comparison of the equine and human gonadotropin alpha-subunit genes. *Mol Endocrinol* 5:243, 1991.)

of DNA appear as a "footprint" on the DNA sequence ladder that is created after partial digestion of radiolabeled DNA with the enzyme. DNase 1 footprinting is most useful for screening 100 to 300 bp regions of DNA for the locations of protein binding sites. After identification of protein-binding sites by footprinting or functional studies, in which promoter mutations have localized a regulatory element, the electrophoretic gel mobility shift assay (EMSA) is useful for more detailed analyses of protein-DNA interactions.[44] The EMSA is based on the fact that the mobility of short DNA fragments (usually 15 to 50 bp) is markedly reduced during nondenaturing gel electrophoresis when protein is bound[45] (Fig. 11–7). The degree of mobility shift is roughly proportional to the size of the bound protein complex. Therefore, the EMSA is also useful for detecting the presence of proteins as monomers, homodimers, and heterodimers. EMSA is a sensitive measure of protein-DNA interactions, and it allows detection of specific binding proteins, even in crude nuclear extracts. The method is also relatively simple to perform from a technical perspective, and it is amenable to competition assays to demonstrate specificity and binding affinity. The addition of antibodies can be used to "supershift" protein-DNA complexes and is valuable for identifying a specific protein within a complex mixture of shift complexes.

The yeast two-hybrid assay has been used to identify and clone

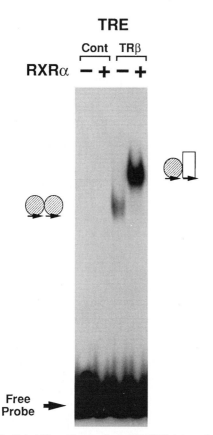

TRE

Cont   TRβ

RXRα   − +   − +

Free Probe →

FIGURE 11–7. Gel shift analyses of protein-DNA interactions. Protein interactions with DNA can be detected by analyzing the ability of DNA-bound proteins to shift (decrease) the mobility of radiolabeled DNA during nondenaturing gel electrophoresis. The gel shift technique is very sensitive and is particularly useful for detailed analyses of the DNA sequence determinants for specific protein binding. In the example shown, binding of the thyroid hormone receptor β (TRβ) to a thyroid hormone response element (TRE) is demonstrated. The thyroid hormone receptor binds to this element as homodimer or as a heterodimer with the retinoic acid X receptor α (RXRα). The mobility of the unbound DNA is very rapid, whereas the mobility of the TRβ-TRE complex is shifted upward in the gel. The TRβ/RXRα heterodimers cause an even greater mobility shift of the DNA, probably because of the increased molecular mass of the heterodimeric protein complex. (Adapted with permission from Nagaya T, Jameson JL: Thyroid hormone receptor dimerization is required for dominant negative inhibition by mutations that cause thyroid hormone resistance. J Biol Chem 268:15766, 1993.)

proteins that interact directly, as opposed to proteins that bind to DNA.[46, 47] Plasmids are constructed to encode the two different components of the hybrid proteins. One hybrid consists of the DNA-binding domain of the yeast transcriptional activator protein GAL4 fused to a known protein; the other hybrid consists of the GAL4 activation domain fused to protein sequences encoded by a library of yeast genomic DNA fragments. Interaction between the known protein and a protein encoded by one of the plasmids in the library leads to transcriptional activation of a reporter gene containing a binding site for GAL4. This strategy is very powerful because it selects proteins based on protein-protein interactions. Specificity can be confirmed using additional in vitro studies of protein interaction, as well as the ability of proteins to interact functionally in mammalian cells.

APPLICATIONS OF TRANSGENIC MODELS

Expression of Endocrine Genes in Transgenic Animals

Transgenic mice provide an opportunity to examine developmental and hormonal regulation of transferred genes in vivo. Transgenic mice are produced most commonly by a technique that involves microinjection of genes into one of the pronuclei of a fertilized mouse egg[48–50] (Fig. 11–8). The microinjected eggs are then implanted into a pseudopregnant foster mother. The next step is to identify progeny that have actually incorporated the transgene. Typically, this involves Southern blot or PCR analyses of tail DNA to determine whether the transgene has been incorporated. Transgenic models have been used widely in endocrinology to define the function of promoter sequences, as well as to assess the physiologic effects of hormone or growth factor expression.[51]

The selection of promoter sequences used to drive expression of the transgene is a critical aspect of the transgenic strategy. For studies that are primarily used to address regulation of a given promoter, these sequences are often linked to reporter genes such as β-galactosidase to allow rapid histologic analyses based on expression of β-galactosidase. Promoter mutagenesis studies can be used to delineate functional regulatory elements in vivo. For example, some of the regulatory elements required for cell-specific expression of the pro-opiomelanocortin (POMC) promoter have been defined using transgenic approaches.[52, 53] Alternatively, when the goal is to overexpress a hormone or enzyme, it is sometimes preferable to use a widely expressed and strong promoter such as the metallothionein or actin promoters. A dramatic example of the effects of hormone expression in transgenic mice is provided by overexpression of growth hormone resulting in a model of gigantism.[54] It is frequently necessary to use relatively long fragments of promoter sequences or additional intronic or 3′ gene sequences to obtain appropriate developmental and tissue-specific expression. An example of using transgenes that function in a manner that recapitulates physiology is illustrated by insertion of the normal GnRH gene into a strain of hypogonadal mouse (hpg/hpg) that contains a deletion of the native GnRH gene.[55, 56] The GnRH transgene is expressed in the hypothalamus and corrects the hypogonadotropic hypogonadism, providing a model of "gene therapy" in which both the pattern of expression and the physiologic function of the abnormal gene are replicated.

Targeted Oncogenesis and Development of Endocrine Tumors

There has been great interest in using transgenic animals to ablate specific cell lineages or to perform targeted oncogenesis by expressing strong transforming genes in specific cell types.[57] Each of these techniques requires that a promoter drive expression of the transgene in selected cell types in a very specific manner. For ablation experiments, reagents such as diphtheria toxin or other agents have been used to eliminate specific cell types.[58, 59] Targeted oncogenesis has been per-

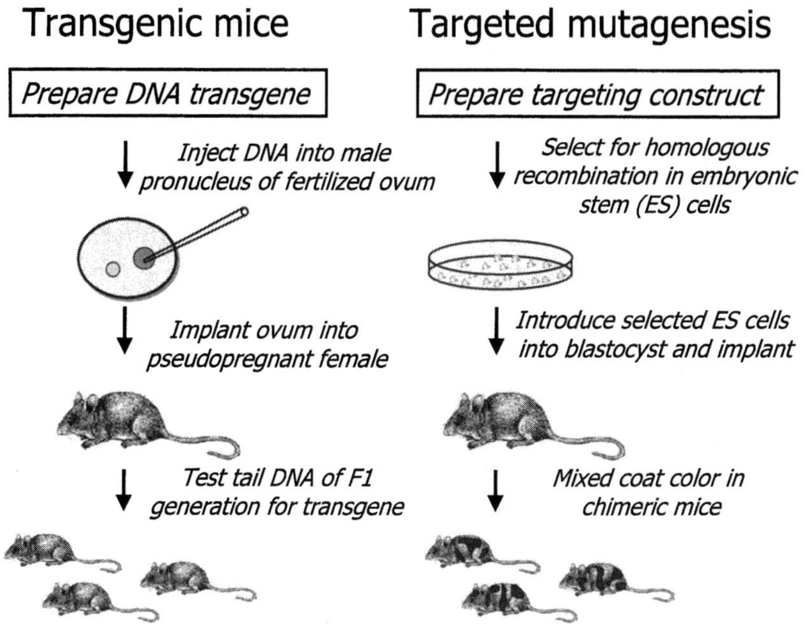

Transgenic mice

Targeted mutagenesis

| Prepare DNA transgene | | Prepare targeting construct |

FIGURE 11–8. Transgenic models. Transgenic mice allow studies of recombinant genes in vivo. On the left, a strategy is shown for introducing transgenes into fertilized eggs with subsequent implantation into surrogate females. In this approach, the purpose of the transgenes may be to overexpress a hormone (e.g., growth hormone) from an active promoter (e.g., metallothionein). Alternatively, the transgene may use a specific promoter (e.g., insulin) to target expression of a different gene (e.g., large T antigen) in specific cells (β cells of the islets). On the right, a strategy for targeted mutagenesis or "gene knockout" is illustrated. In this approach, homologous recombination is used to mutate the endogenous gene in embryonic stem (ES) cells. After selection of ES cells containing the altered gene, the cells are injected into blastocysts, which are introduced into a surrogate female. Mixed coat color identifies progeny that contain the ES cells. Additional breeding of mice heterozygous for the gene knockout allows production of mice that are homozygous for the gene knockout.

formed using several oncogenes, most frequently the SV40 large T antigen.[60–62] In several instances, tumors from transgenic mice have been adapted to cell culture to provide new cell lines for detailed studies in vitro.[62]

Homologous Recombination and Gene Knockout Approaches

More recently, it has been possible to perform "gene knockout" experiments to generate null mutations in transgenic mice.[63] This strategy uses homologous recombination in embryonic stem (ES) cells in culture to mutagenize a specific target gene (see Fig. 11–8). Homologous recombination implies that the exogenous mutant form of a gene recognizes homologous genomic sequences and undergoes recombination at a rate that greatly exceeds that of a random insertion. Selectable markers attached to the exogenous gene are used to efficiently identify cells that have undergone homologous recombination. After selection of cells containing a mutated, nonfunctional target gene, the ES cells are injected into mouse blastocysts where they are incorporated into a variety of normal tissues, including the germ line. Mice can subsequently be bred such that the gene knockout is carried in a heterozygous or homozygous form. In principle, this approach allows the null phenotype to be analyzed for essentially any gene. An example in endocrinology of information derived from a gene knockout experiment is illustrated by the developmental and physiologic consequences of eliminating the gene encoding the α-subunit of inhibin.[64] Deletion of the *inhibin α-subunit* gene caused a high incidence of gonadal tumors, suggesting an important role for inhibin as a biologic repressor of gonadal cell proliferation and transformation. Gene knockout experiments such as this create biologic models that would occur rarely in nature and allow detailed analyses of the physiologic role of deleted genes.

It is also possible to "knock in" mutations. In this approach, a point mutation is inserted into the gene in the targeting vector. After homologous recombination, the normal gene is replaced with a copy that contains the point mutation. This approach is particularly useful for dominant diseases or for examining the genotype-phenotype correlations of specific mutations.

IMPACT OF THE HUMAN GENOME PROJECT

The Human Genome Project (HGP) was launched in 1990 and has already had a tremendous impact on biomedical research.[65, 66] The

ultimate goal of this project is to characterize the sequence of the entire human genome. Inherent in this goal is the need to develop new technologies for gene mapping, cloning, DNA sequencing, and bioinformatics. The HGP will, therefore, impact endocrinology in the same manner that it affects all areas of medicine. It has already speeded the process of gene discovery and characterization. The number of identified genes that cause endocrine disorders has nearly doubled since the last edition of this book.

The scope of the HGP provides a useful perspective for the complexity of studying genetic endocrine disorders. The 23 pairs of human chromosomes are thought to encode approximately 70,000 genes. The total length of DNA is about 3 billion bp. Much of this DNA does not encode expressed genes. For this reason, initial emphasis was placed on gene mapping and on the development of new sequencing and computer database technologies. The genetic map (ordered array of heritable traits or markers) now exists at about 1 cM resolution using a large array of short tandem repeat (STR) markers. A goal for the near term is to add about 100,000 single nucleotide polymorphisms (SNPs) to this map. The addition of SNPs will facilitate automation (using DNA chips) and enhance the ability to perform linkage studies of complex genetic diseases. The construction of a physical map (ordered array of cloned genes or markers) has paralleled determination of the genetic map. The goal of achieving a high-resolution physical map of the human genome has essentially been achieved; almost all of the genome has been cloned into libraries as overlapping fragments. The physical map provides the substrate for DNA sequencing and also allows the rapid physical retrieval of genes from libraries, since their locations are known.

Completion of the human genome sequence is anticipated by the year 2003. The sequences of model organisms like *E. coli, Saccharomyces cerevisiae,* and *Caenorhabditis elegans* have already been completed. And, there is interest in sequencing the genomes of *Drosophila melanogaster* and the laboratory mouse as well.

The development of ethical guidelines is an important component of the HGP. The remarkably rapid discovery of new disease-causing genes and the advances in genetic testing have raised many ethical, social, and financial questions concerning the use of genetic techniques in medicine. For example, the discovery of the *BRCA1* and *BRCA2* genes, which predispose to breast and ovarian cancer, have enhanced our understanding of familial forms of these cancers. However, it remains unclear how to use genetic testing in potentially affected individuals and family members. Breast cancer is a common disease, and mutations in the *BRCA* genes account for relatively few cases. Thus, the absence of mutation does not eliminate the risk of breast cancer. And, it is unclear, at present, how the presence of a mutation should be used in patient management. Should prophylactic mastectomy be performed, or should genetically susceptible individuals only undergo more intensive screening? What are the implications for insurability, employment, childbearing, and interpersonal relationships? The answers to these questions will require additional clinical investigation, legislative policy to prevent discrimination, and greater availability of genetic counseling. On the other hand, the discovery of the *MEN2* gene has provided a useful strategy for identifying affected individuals with this highly penetrant autosomal dominant disorder. In this case, unaffected individuals can be spared screening for pheochromocytoma, medullary thyroid cancer, and hyperparathyroidism. Prophylactic thyroidectomy has been advocated in affected individuals because it is highly penetrant and it is hoped that early removal of the thyroid will prevent later development of the disease. Thus, the discoveries resulting from the HGP are only the beginning of a much larger effort to apply this new information.

CATEGORIES OF GENETIC DISORDERS

Although many disorders are transmitted according to traditional mendelian rules, it is now clear that a variety of different mechanisms can lead to genetic diseases (Table 11–2). Fundamental principles of genetic transmission are summarized briefly here, and additional information is available in other sources.[67, 68]

Disorders of chromosome number or structure were among the first to be recognized because they can be detected using cytogenetic techniques. In endocrinology, disorders of the sex chromosomes are particularly relevant, including Klinefelter's syndrome (XXY) and Turner's syndrome (XO).

Mendelian disorders are caused by mutations in single genes. Information about many of these genetic disorders is updated continuously in a compendium that is accessible on-line (OMIM: On-line Mendelian Inheritance in Man, http://www3.ncbi.nlm.nih.gov/Omim). The patterns of mendelian transmission are now part of classical genetic teaching and include autosomal recessive, autosomal dominant, and X-linked disorders (Fig. 11–9). The transmission of genes or traits is typically depicted in family trees or pedigrees. Analysis of the pattern of transmission, particularly in large families with multiple generations, can be very valuable for predicting the mode of inheritance. This information is useful for genetic counseling, and it often narrows the differential diagnosis, particularly when mutations in several different genes can give rise to similar phenotypes (nonallelic heterogeneity). For example, diabetes insipidus can be transmitted in an autosomal dominant manner (neurohypophyseal DI), in a recessive manner (nephrogenic DI secondary to mutations in aquaporin 2), or as an X-linked disorder (nephrogenic DI secondary to mutations in the V2 receptor). For this reason, when dealing with a genetic disorder, it is

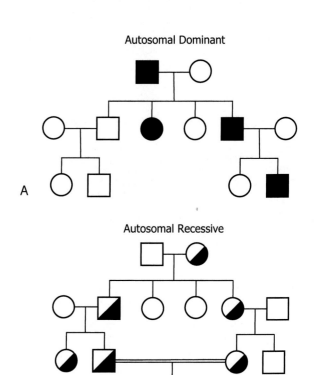

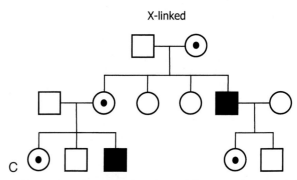

FIGURE 11–9. Classic patterns of mendelian genetic transmission. *A,* Autosomal dominant transmission. *B,* Autosomal recessive transmission. *C,* X-linked transmission. Males are depicted by squares, and females are depicted by circles. Double lines linking parents indicate consanguinity. Affected individuals are shown by filled symbols. Half-filled symbols indicate heterozygous individuals. Dot-filled symbols indicate female carriers of X-linked traits.

important to obtain a detailed family history, often from several different family members. This information can then be combined with laboratory and genetic testing to arrive at an accurate diagnosis.

Autosomal Dominant Disorders

Diseases inherited in an autosomal dominant manner are characterized by the presence of one mutant allele and a normal allele on the other chromosome. A single mutant allele is sufficient to cause the disorder. In some instances, such as male-limited precious puberty, the gene is dominant because the mutations in the LH receptor are constitutively active[69] (see Chapter 6). In other cases, like thyroid hormone resistance, the mutant gene acts in a dominant negative manner to antagonize the function of the normal, wild-type gene[70, 71] (see Chapter 114). In MEN1, the mutant tumor suppressor gene is transmitted in a dominant manner, but secondary, somatic mutations

TABLE 11–2. Mechanisms of Transmission of Genetic Endocrine Diseases

Transmission	Example of Endocrine Disorder	
	Gene	*Disorder*
Chromosomal	XXY multiple genes	Klinefelter's syndrome
Autosomal recessive	CYP21 (21-hydroxylase)	Congenital adrenal hyperplasia
Autosomal dominant	MEN1 (menin)	Multiple endocrine neoplasia type 1
X-linked	KAL1 (Kallmann)	Kallmann's syndrome
Y-linked	SRY (testis determining factor)	XY sex-reversal
Mitochondrial	tRNA (Leu-UUR)	Diabetes-deafness syndrome
Mosaic	GNAS1 (Gsα)	McCune-Albright syndrome
Somatic	TSHR (TSH receptor)	Autonomous thyroid nodules
Imprinting	GNAS1 (Gsα)	Albright hereditary osteodystrophy
Multigenic	Multiple genes	Type II diabetes mellitus

occur in the remaining copy of the normal gene during the process of tumorigenesis[72] (see Chapter 188). Thus, the mechanisms by which genes act in a dominant manner are highly variable, even though they share similar features of transmission. In dominant disorders, the probability that an offspring will inherit the mutant gene is 50% and individuals can be affected in each generation (Fig. 11–9A). The disease does not occur in the offspring of unaffected individuals. Males and females are affected with equal frequency.

Autosomal Recessive Disorders

In an autosomal recessive disease, both parents of an affected individual are obligate heterozygotes (Fig. 11–9B). The affected individual, who can be of either sex, can be homozygous (inherit two copies of the same mutation) or inherit distinct mutations in each copy of the gene (compound heterozygote). Heterozygous carriers of a defective gene do not usually display phenotypic features of the disease. When both parents are heterozygous for a mutation, the genotypes of their offspring are predicted to be as follows: a 25% chance of a normal genotype, a 50% probability of a heterozygous state, and a 25% risk of disease. If one parent is heterozygous and one is homozygous, the probability of disease increases to 50% for each child and the pedigree analysis may mimic that of autosomal dominant inheritance. Most cases of homozygous mutations occur in situations of parental consanguinity or in isolated populations in which the gene pool is small. The likelihood of compound heterozygous mutations depends on the gene frequency in the population for each of the mutations, which is usually very low. Congenital adrenal hyperplasia, caused by mutations in 21-hydroxylase, is representative of autosomal recessive disorders. There are many distinct mutations in the *21-hydroxylase* gene (*CYP21*), and the prevalence of these mutations is high enough (1/100 in most populations) that it is not unlikely for unrelated parents to be heterozygous. As a result, a child that inherits two distinct mutations in 21-hydroxylase will be affected with the disorder. Depending on the degree to which the mutation affects enzyme function, a range of phenotypic severity can be seen in different individuals.

X-Linked Disorders

A daughter always inherits her father's X chromosome together with one of the two maternal X chromosomes. A son inherits one of the maternal X chromosomes and the Y chromosome from his father. Thus, there is no father-to-son transmission in X-linked inheritance and all daughters of an affected male are obligate carriers of the mutant allele (Fig. 11–9C). Because males have only one X chromosome, they are hemizygous for a mutant allele and are therefore more likely to develop the mutant phenotype. Several endocrine disorders are transmitted in an X-linked manner, including Kallmann's syndrome, adrenal hypoplasia congenita, adrenal leukodystrophy, nephrogenic diabetes insipidus, androgen insensitivity, and hypophosphatemic vitamin D–resistant rickets. As expected from the aforementioned mechanism of X-linked transmission, these disorders are much more common in males than females.

Y-Linked Disorders

Only a few genes are known on the Y chromosome, and there are few Y-linked disorders. One of the Y chromosome genes, the sex-region determining Y gene (*SRY*), which encodes the testis-determining factor (TDF), can cause XY sex reversal when mutated.[73] Alternatively, translocation of the *SRY* gene to the X chromosome can cause an XX male phenotype. Another group of genes on the Y chromosome includes the highly repetitive *DAZ* genes that are important for spermatogenesis. Deletions of these genes, often transmitted as a new germline mutation, are an important cause of azoospermia and male infertility.[74]

Nonmendelian Forms of Inheritance

For many diseases that appear to have some genetic component, there is no clear pattern of classical mendelian inheritance. In recent years, other forms of genetic transmission have been identified (see Table 11–2). Perhaps most common among these are multigenic disorders like type 2 diabetes mellitus, hypertension, obesity, and most hyperlipidemias. These disorders are generally thought to involve multiple different genes, each of which contributes partially to a disease phenotype. Because the contribution of any one of these genes is relatively weak, they are difficult to localize using classical genetic linkage approaches in large pedigrees. Rather, population-based genetic studies are required. In this approach, one can search for genetic variants that occur with increased frequency in affected individuals. Or, one can search for genetic variants that occur more often in affected sib-pairs versus the population at large. These types of linkage analyses are challenging because of the large number of individuals who need to be studied (usually several hundred). In addition, the entire genome must be searched for candidate genetic markers associated with the disease. Because many different genes (and environmental events) can cause these diseases, this type of gene search is most successful when one can identify specific sub-phenotypes that are likely to be caused by a relatively small number of genes. The sib-pair approach has been used successfully to identify genetic loci associated with type 1 diabetes mellitus. Although several different genes confer some degree of risk, the major histocompatibility locus on chromosome 6 is a particularly strong risk factor that predisposes to the disease.[75]

The circular mitochondrial genome is transmitted exclusively through the maternal line, as all mitochondria reside within the oocyte cytoplasm. Thus, mitochondrial disorders are transmitted only from mother to offspring, and males and females are affected equally. Mitochondrial DNA predominantly encodes proteins that are components of the respiratory chain. Certain forms of diabetes, associated with deafness, can be caused by mutations in mitochondrial DNA.[76]

Genomic imprinting can also influence the expression of certain genetic diseases. This refers to the preferential expression of an allele depending on its parental origin. A classic example involves the Prader-Willi syndrome and the Angelman syndrome, which are caused by genes located on the short arm of chromosome 15. Gene deletions in the Prader-Willi syndrome occur exclusively on the paternally derived chromosome. In contrast, patients with the Angelman syndrome have deletions in the same region of chromosome 15, but they occur only on the maternally derived chromosome. Genomic imprinting is also likely to be involved in the expression of Albright hereditary osteodystrophy (AHO).[77] This disorder is transmitted in an autosomal dominant manner, and it is linked to the *Gs* (*GNAS*) gene on chromosome 20q13. However, AHO individuals only inherit the disorder from an affected mother because the normal copy of the gene is imprinted and not actively expressed from the paternal chromosome.

Mosaicism refers to the presence of two or more cell lines in an individual that differ in their genotype. Mosaicism can result from a mutation that occurs during embryogenesis or later in development. The developmental stage at which the defect arises will determine whether germ cells or only somatic cells are involved. Somatic mosaicism is characterized by a patchy distribution of somatic cells containing a mutation. For example, activating mutations that occur in the Gs subunit early in development cause the McCune-Albright syndrome. The clinical phenotype, which can include ovarian cysts that secrete sex steroids and cause precocious puberty, polyostotic fibrous dysplasia, café au lait skin pigmentation, pituitary adenomas, and hypersecreting autonomous thyroid nodules, varies depending on the tissue distribution of the mutation.

Somatic mutations also play an important role in various forms of neoplasia. When somatic mutations enhance cell proliferation or prolong cell survival, they can be associated with the clonal expansion of the cell population and the development of tumors. Activating mutations in the TSH-R or Gs can cause autonomously functioning thyroid nodules (see below). Somatic, inactivating mutations in tumor suppressor genes play an important role in inherited cancer syndromes in which the "first hit" has already been transmitted in the germline.

Multiple endocrine neoplasia type I provides an example of such a disorder.

Trinucleotide repeats are found in several genes, and their number varies among healthy individuals (polymorphic variants). For example, the number of CAG repeats found in the first exon of the androgen receptor (AR) gene is lowest in blacks, intermediate in whites, and highest in Asians. However, an increase in the number of repeats above a certain critical threshold is associated with the X-linked form of spinal and bulbar muscular atrophy (SBMA, Kennedy's syndrome).

PRINCIPLES OF GENETIC LINKAGE

Genetic linkage refers to the fact that genes are physically attached to one another along the length of the chromosome. Consequently, two genes that are close together on a chromosome are usually transmitted together, unless a recombination event separates them. Recombination, which occurs during meiosis, is useful for purposes of mapping genes, because it provides a landmark that delineates borders for the location of a gene. The odds of a cross-over, or recombination event, are proportionate to the distance that separates them. Thus, genes that are far apart are more likely to be separated by a recombination event than genes that are close together. These features make it possible, given large pedigrees or populations, to calculate the genetic distance between two genes. A centiMorgan (cM) is defined as a recombination frequency between two loci of 1% and corresponds to about 1 Mb of DNA.

Linkage is usually expressed as a logarithm of the odds (lod) score, which is a ratio that reflects the probability that the disease and marker loci are linked rather than unlinked.[78] Positive numbers favor linkage, and negative scores support nonlinkage. Lod scores of +3 are generally accepted as supporting linkage, whereas a score of −2 is consistent with the absence of linkage. When candidate genetic regions have been identified by linkage, more detailed analyses can be performed using additional markers, or if the region is small enough, one can attempt to identify the disease gene among the many genes present within a particular locus.

The presence of polymorphic variation in DNA is essential for linkage studies. Genetic variation provides a means to distinguish the maternal and paternal chromosomes in an individual, as well as providing markers of different regions along the chromosomes. Historically,

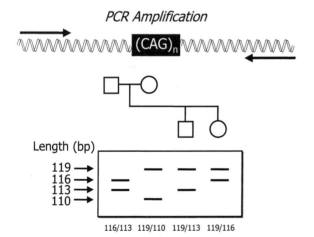

FIGURE 11–10. PCR amplification of polymorphic short tandem repeat markers. Polymorphic di-, tri-, and tetra-nucleotide short tandem repeats, or microsatellites, are common in the human genome. These regions are very useful for tracking chromosomal segregation within pedigrees and for mapping genes. If PCR primers are placed on either side of these repeats, the resulting fragments will vary in length depending on the number of copies of the repeats. When an individual is heterozygous (the allele on each chromosome harbors a different number of repeats), two distinct PCR products are generated that can be resolved by electrophoresis. The genotype, at this locus, of each individual in the pedigree can therefore be determined based on the length of the marker that it inherits.

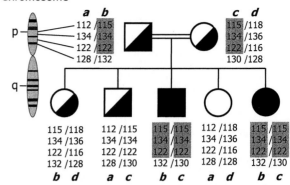

FIGURE 11–11. Linkage analysis using short tandem repeat markers. Short tandem repeats (STRs) can be used to track the transmission of genes within a pedigree (see Fig. 11–10). In the pedigree shown, two heterozygous parents, who are first cousins, have transmitted a disease gene to several progeny. A series of STR markers, located on the short arm (p) of a chromosome, are used to determine the haplotype of various members of the family. Note that the parents are heterozygous for most of the markers, but are homozygous for others (e.g., 134/134). Nevertheless, because a panel of markers is used, one can readily ascertain the pattern of chromosomal segregation. In addition, recombination events on the parental chromosome b and the maternal chromosome c are apparent because their haplotypes differ between the 3rd and 4th markers. Shaded regions indicate homozygous, shared haplotypes in the affected children. Although these data are not sufficient to prove linkage, they are consistent with this region of the genome being involved in the disease. Additional studies of this region in other pedigrees could be used to support, or refute, the possibility of linkage. Studies of additional families might also identify recombination events that would narrow the disease locus further, ultimately allowing the cloning of a responsible gene.

these polymorphisms consisted of restriction fragment length polymorphisms (RFLPs), in which nucleotide sequence variation altered the presence of specific restriction sites in DNA. Thus, when combined with Southern blot analysis, RFLPs allow one to track the transmission of genes within a pedigree. Although principles of RFLP analysis are useful for understanding disease transmission and gene mapping, the technique has been supplanted by other means of polymorphic analysis. In particular, short tandem repeats (STRs), consisting of highly repetitive 2, 3, or 4 bp sequences, are now used for linkage studies. The HGP has generated high-density maps of STRs throughout the entire genome. The technique is performed using PCR and can be automated (Fig. 11–10). In a similar manner, maps of single nucleotide polymorphisms (SNPs) are also being generated. In addition to their greater frequency (1 in 1000 bp), the SNPs are amenable to analyses using DNA chips, providing a promising means for rapid analysis of genetic variation and linkage.

An example of using STRs to examine linkage within a pedigree is shown in Figure 11–11. In this case, two heterozygous, related parents have transmitted an autosomal recessive disorder. A series of STRs on the short arm of the chromosome are used to track transmission of this chromosomal region within the family. Note that a recombination event distinguishes the shared chromosomes (b and c) of the parents. Two of their children are affected with the disorder. A group of closely linked markers that are inherited together is referred to as a haplotype. They each inherit the b/c haplotype and are homozygous for the markers 115-134-122. Although this pattern does not prove linkage, it is consistent with a disease gene within this region of the chromosome. Additional studies would be necessary to confirm linkage in an expanded version of the pedigree or using other families with the same disorder.

METHODS USED TO DETECT GENE DELETIONS AND POINT MUTATIONS

Recombinant DNA approaches that are used to investigate a particular disorder are usually based on clues derived from its clinical and

TABLE 11–3. Approach to Patient with a Suspected Genetic Disease

Detailed clinical characterization
    Establish phenotypes and heterogeneity
    Consider possible candidate genes based on phenotype
Are there major deletions or rearrangements?
    Cytogenetics or FISH
    Southern blot analyses
Disorders caused by an unknown gene
    Linkage by short tandem repeats (STRs) or single nucleotide
        polymorphisms (SNPs)
    Cloning of candidate genes
Small deletions or point mutations
    Screen for mutations by SSCP or DGGE
    Screen for mutations by direct DNA sequencing
Does the mutation alter a known function of the protein?
    In vitro analyses of mutant proteins
    In vivo and transgenic analyses of mutant proteins
Therapeutic implications
    Genetic counseling
    Other interventions based on nature of the mutation

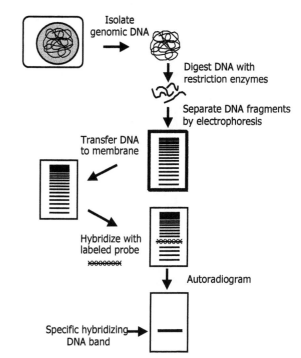

FIGURE 11–12. *Southern blot method. The Southern blot is used to analyze gene structure. Genomic DNA is isolated and digested into an array of fragments using restriction enzymes. The DNA is separated according to length by agarose gel electrophoresis and transferred to a membrane. The immobilized DNA is hybridized with a radiolabeled probe, which binds only to its complementary sequence. Specific hybridizing bands are detected by autoradiography.*

pathophysiologic characteristics, which in some cases allow one to predict the gene that harbors a defect (Table 11–3). For example, it is reasonable to postulate that selective GH deficiency in several members of a family might be due to a defect in the gene encoding GH, GHRH, or the GHRH receptor. In other cases, however, there are no obvious candidate genes. For example, in the multiple endocrine neoplasia syndromes, it was difficult to predict a gene that causes proliferation of selected lineages of endocrine cells. In this case, the most expeditious approach was to localize chromosomal regions carrying markers associated with the disease phenotype (see above). After candidate genes were identified, they could be analyzed for mutations in affected patients to verify that they cause the disorder. A summary of techniques that are used to identify different types of mutations are listed in Table 11–4.

Use of Southern Blots to Analyze Gene Structure

After identification of a disease gene, a number of different types of molecular techniques are available for defining specific mutations. To define the gross structure of the gene, a useful first approach is to use Southern blot analyses to detect large gene deletions or rearrangements (Fig. 11–12).[79] In this method, genomic DNA is digested with one or more restriction endonucleases, creating an array of DNA fragments that are separated according to length using agarose gel electrophoresis. After transfer of the DNA fragments to a membrane, a radiolabeled probe that is specific for the gene of interest is hybridized to the DNA on the membrane. Under appropriate conditions of hybridization stringency, the probe will only detect the few DNA

fragments that are complementary in sequence. Gene deletions would be detected as absent fragments or by fragments with reduced size. Gene rearrangements result in complex patterns of DNA fragments with increased and/or decreased lengths. If the gene appears to be intact when analyzed using multiple restriction enzymes, a single base mutation or a small deletion that alters the final protein product is more likely than a gross alteration in gene structure.

The Polymerase Chain Reaction (PCR) and Detection of Point Mutations

The PCR has greatly improved the efficiency of detecting single base changes by allowing rapid amplification and analyses of a particular gene or a portion of the gene (Fig. 11–13).[80] The PCR technique is a very powerful tool for molecular diagnostics for the following reasons. First, the dramatic amplification of DNA allows diagnostic analyses using very small amounts of initial starting tissue. Sufficient

TABLE 11–4. Molecular Genetic Diagnostic Procedures

Method	Gene Deletions	Gene Rearrangements	Loss of Heterozygosity	Linkage	Point Mutations
Cytogenetics		+	+		
FISH	+	+	+		
Southern blot	+	+			
RFLP			+	+	
VNTR			+	+	
PCR	+	+	+	+	+
Direct DNA sequencing					+
RNase cleavage					+
OSH					+
DGGE					+
SSCP					+

FISH, fluorescent in situ hybridization; RFLP, restriction fragment length polymorphism; VNTR, variable number tandem repeat; PCR, polymerase chain reaction; OSH, oligonucleotide specific hybridization; DGGE, denaturing gradient gel electrophoresis; SSCP, single-stranded conformational polymorphism.

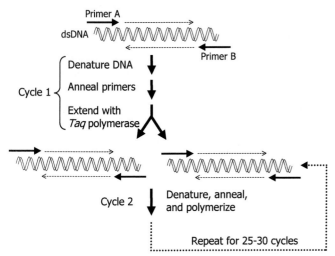

FIGURE 11–13. The polymerase chain reaction (PCR). In the initial cycle of PCR, the double-stranded DNA template is heat-denatured to allow primers A and B to anneal and initiate synthesis of a new copy of each strand of DNA. Because Taq polymerase is heat-stable, the reaction mixture can be immediately subjected to another round of denaturation and new DNA synthesis. In each cycle of PCR, the number of DNA molecules is doubled, resulting in a rapid expansion in the amount of DNA as the cycle number progresses. In a typical reaction of 25 to 30 cycles, the amount of DNA is theoretically amplified by several million-fold. PCR has broad applications including DNA diagnostics from small amounts of tissue, quantitative mRNA analysis, cloning, construction of plasmids, and site-directed mutagenesis.

DNA for PCR is routinely extracted from lymphocytes or from cells present in saliva, hair, amniotic fluid, chorionic villi, or other accessible tissue sources. Second, because PCR uses short synthetic oligonucleotides to prime the reaction, it can be readily applied to any gene as long as the DNA sequence is known. Even when the gene sequence is not known, PCR is useful for linkage studies because highly polymorphic sequences (short tandem repeats, STRs) occurring near the gene can be amplified.[81] Finally, the PCR technique is straightforward enough that it can be readily transferred to different medical centers and laboratories.

In many cases, the PCR is the starting point for more detailed characterization of a mutation. In early studies to identify a specific mutation, the PCR product is often used for DNA sequencing to establish the location and base change that is present in the gene. Because the amount of DNA provided by PCR is relatively large, it is usually not difficult to subclone the amplified DNA fragment into a plasmid to allow subsequent DNA sequencing. Alternatively, automated DNA sequencing methods allow direct sequencing of the DNA fragment without an intervening subcloning step.[82] In addition to efficiency, direct sequencing has the advantage that the sequence analysis is based on a large population of amplified DNA molecules rather than individual clones that may contain PCR generated sequence errors (occur in approximately 1/3000 bases). Direct DNA sequencing of the PCR product also has the advantage that a heterozygous mutation can be detected by the presence of two different nucleotides at the mutant position.

After characterization of specific mutations, several techniques allow more rapid screening for the mutation in other family members or patients. In some methods, the critical regions of a gene can be screened for mutations by detecting altered mobility during gel electrophoresis. In denaturing gradient gel electrophoresis (DGGE), the PCR primers contain a long stretch of Gs and Cs that anneal to create a "GC clamp."[83] In this manner, the double stranded DNA can be partially melted during electrophoresis, but will be clamped at the end because of the relatively high melting temperature of G-C bonds (three hydrogen bonds for G-C versus two for A-T). Consequently, the GC clamp emphasizes differences in melting temperatures that result from sequence mismatches caused by mutations. If a mutation is present, a mismatch with the wild type sequence lowers the melting point of the DNA hybrid resulting in strand separation and altered mobility in the gel. A similar technique, referred to as single stranded conformational polymorphism (SSCP), is based on the property that mutations will cause altered conformation and mobility of single stranded DNA during nondenaturing electrophoresis.[84] Both DGGE and SSCP can be applied to PCR products to screen large regions of a gene for mutations or to screen large numbers of patients in separate reactions. At present, SSCP appears to be more readily applied to a wide array of sequences. Both of these methods require that the reaction conditions be established rigorously to avoid false negative results. It should also be noted that polymorphisms appear as mutations until further characterized.

After a particular mutation has been identified, oligonucleotide specific hybridization (OSH) can be useful to establish whether this nucleotide change is present in other family members or in other unrelated patients.[85] For example, specific mutations have been identified that cause constitutive activation of the GTP-binding *ras* and Gs proteins that are involved in cellular signaling. These mutations prevent GTP hydrolysis, which is necessary to inactivate signaling by these proteins. In the case of the *ras* genes (*H-ras, K-ras, N-ras*), mutations in two different regions of the proteins (codons 12/13 or codon 61) cause constitutive activation. Because the number of nucleotide changes at these positions is limited, it is possible to use oligonucleotides that are complementary to the mutant allele to screen for specific mutations. In this case, it is practical to amplify DNA samples from a large number of specimens and apply them to a membrane to screen for different mutations. This technique is based upon the principle that single base pair mismatches cause alterations in hybridization efficiency when short oligonucleotides are used as probes. Consequently, hybridization conditions and control specimens have to be established for each mutant sequence. Oligonucleotide specific hybridization is most useful when the number of potential mutations is small and when it is necessary to screen large numbers of specimens for mutations.

Mutations often eliminate, or generate, restriction enzyme sites. Thus, another useful strategy for screening for specific mutations is to amplify the relevant region of a gene by PCR and then test the pattern of restriction enzyme digestion. If a mutation does not create a new restriction site, it is usually possible to generate a new site by inserting a base pair change in the PCR primer, near the mutation site, to create a unique digestion pattern. Because restriction enzymes are very specific and easy to use, this strategy is a powerful and inexpensive means to screen for known mutations.

Functional Studies of Mutant Hormones and Receptors

Identification of a DNA sequence alteration is not sufficient to establish that it is responsible for the disease phenotype. First, nucleotide substitutions could represent polymorphisms or DNA sequence variations that occur in the population as a whole. If the base change occurs in the coding sequence, but does not alter an amino acid, it is most likely a polymorphism. However, even if the amino acid sequence is changed, it is still possible that the amino acid substitution is "physiologically silent" and doesn't significantly alter protein function. One approach for addressing the issue of polymorphisms is to screen a large number of normal individuals (e.g., 100) for the putative mutation. If the amino acid substitution is found in normals, it is by definition, a polymorphism. Substitution of codons that are highly conserved across species (presumably implying functional importance) have a higher chance of being mutations than amino acids that are more variable in different species. Finally, mutations tend to be "linked" to the disease phenotype when examined in several family members, whereas polymorphisms should sort randomly unless they are located close to the disease locus. Although these determinations of polymorphisms are not entirely reliable, they are of practical importance because the next steps of assessing the functional importance of a "candidate mutation" can require significant experimental effort.

Assuming there is evidence against a polymorphism, it is almost always possible using recombinant techniques to assess the effect of a mutation in a functional assay. As illustrated in Figure 11–14, recombinant mutant and wild type proteins can be expressed and subjected to a variety of functional assays. In the example shown, expression of mutant LHβ allows it to be assessed for its ability to form an α-β heterodimer, to undergo glycosylation, to bind to its receptor, and to activate receptor signaling pathways.[86] Mutant enzymes such as 21-hydroxylase can be analyzed for their ability to bind substrate or to carry out catalysis.[87] Mutant receptors like the insulin receptor have been subjected to an array of functional tests including insulin binding, receptor autophosphorylation, receptor internalization, and receptor stability.[88] Likewise, G protein–coupled receptors containing activating, or inactivating mutations, can be tested for their abilities to bind hormones and to signal through second messenger pathways.[69, 89] Nuclear receptors, such as the thyroid hormone receptor, can be analyzed not only for their ability to bind thyroid hormone and DNA target sequences, but also for their capacity to function as transcription factors in transient gene expression assays.[90] These types of studies not only establish whether a given mutation is of functional importance, but also provide insight into protein structure-function and hormone action. In many instances, these "experiments of nature" provide rapid identification of critical functional domains because identification of the mutations is biased by the presence of a recognizable clinical phenotype.

OVERVIEW OF INHERITED ENDOCRINE DISORDERS

The technical aspects of the foregoing discussion of recombinant DNA methodology may raise questions concerning how such techniques will be useful to the practicing endocrinologist. In large measure, molecular biology is already transforming the practice of endocrinology and will continue to do so for the near term.[1] In addition to improving our understanding of hormone and receptor structure-function, these techniques have allowed the production of large quantities of recombinant insulin, growth hormone, and gonadotropins. There is also an increasing reliance on recombinant DNA methods to identify new growth factors, cytokines, and hormones as well as their physiologic functions. The presentation of a few "case studies" in the use of these procedures coupled with an overview of recent progress in the molecular basis of endocrine diseases foreshadows the future role of these methods in clinical practice.

Several hundred endocrine disorders exhibit an inheritance pattern suggestive of a primary gene defect.[91] Gene mutations have now been identified in many of these disorders (Table 11–5). Some common themes emerge even from the relatively small number of mutations that have been described to date. First, the phenotypic variability that characterizes many endocrine diseases is often reflected in genetic heterogeneity. Some clinical phenotypes that were thought previously to represent distinct diseases can now be interpreted as manifestations of different types of mutations within a single gene. For example, the clinical variants of congenital adrenal hyperplasia can be attributed to distinct mutations in 21-hydroxylase or other enzymes involved in steroid biosynthesis.[87] Second, the propensity of certain genes to be frequent targets for mutations may be explained in part by gene structure and organization. Genes such as *growth hormone* that have been duplicated to form gene clusters are predisposed to undergo recombination and deletion.[92, 93] Third, although many of the mutations reported initially have been associated with severely affected patients, it is likely that mutations with less severe consequences will also be identified. For example, the phenotype of androgen insensitivity includes a spectrum of disorders that ranges from severe resistance in the case of testicular feminization to milder resistance in Reifenstein's syndrome and other syndromes of mild androgen resistance associated with gynecomastia and infertility.[94] These disorders are each caused by mutations in the androgen receptor, but the mutations result in different degrees of receptor dysfunction. In some cases, the receptor is deleted or mutated in a manner that it is completely inactive. In other examples, mutations perturb the amount or stability of the receptor, causing partial resistance. An extension of this concept is that genetic polymorphisms (DNA sequence variants) in the normal population could also cause subtle differences in hormone or receptor activity, thereby constituting part of the basis for the variability that is seen in the normal range of hormone levels and activity.

Because a staggering number of mutations in different endocrine genes has already been reached,[1] it is not practical to describe each of these disorders in a comprehensive manner. The interested reader is referred to individual chapters and to the references in Table 11–5. In addition, many of these disorders can be found online in the Mendelian Inheritance in Man database (http://www3.ncbi.nlm.nih.gov/Omim) or at the human gene mutation database (http://www.uwcm.ac.uk/uwcm/mg/hgmd0.html). It is, nevertheless, useful to provide an overview of mutations that occur at different steps in endocrine pathways, if for no other reason than to illustrate the breadth and heterogeneous nature of disorders caused by gene defects.

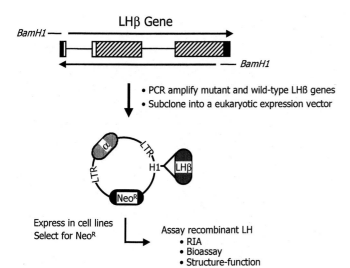

FIGURE 11–14. Expression of recombinant hormones to verify the biological effect of a mutation. The ability to express recombinant hormones or receptors is an important strategy for testing the effects of putative disease-causing mutations. A variety of expression systems are available, including *E. coli*, baculovirus, vaccinia virus, and mammalian cells. The choice of expression system is dictated by a variety of issues including characteristics of the protein, desired production level, and the nature of the bioassay that will be used. A strategy for producing recombinant LH is illustrated for the purpose of analyzing the functional consequences of mutations in the *LHβ* gene.[86] The *LHβ* gene is amplified by PCR from genomic DNA and inserted into a eukaryotic expression vector. The presence of a viral long terminal repeat (LTR) provides a strong promoter to drive expression in transfected mammalian cell lines. Because LH is a heterodimer containing an α and β subunit, the vector is designed to contain a copy of the α gene to allow the genes to be coexpressed from the same plasmid. A third gene encoding neomycin resistance (Neo^R) allows selection and isolation of clonal cell lines that have been successfully transfected with the expression vector. Secreted LH can be analyzed by structural methods and for its functional properties. This approach allows delineation of hormone domains important for α-β subunit dimerization, receptor binding, and receptor activation.

Hormone Mutations

One might have expected that mutations in hormones would represent a common molecular basis for endocrine disorders. However, this does not appear to be the case. For the most part, causes of hormone deficiency syndromes remain enigmatic. For example, growth hormone deficiency rarely involves deletions or mutations in the *growth hormone* gene.[95] Rather, most cases can be attributed to an inherited or acquired hypothalamic defect that could involve GHRH, the GHRH producing neuron, the GHRH receptor, or one of the regulatory pathways that control GHRH secretion. Attempts to attribute GH deficiency to GHRH mutations have not been successful, and most patients respond to exogenous GHRH, implying that GHRH and GHRH receptor mutations[96] may also be uncommon. In some respects, GH defi-

TABLE 11–5. Examples of Genetic Endocrine Diseases

Endocrine Mutation	Disorder	Mode of Inheritance	Chromosome Location	Types of Mutation	Reference
Hormone Mutations					
Insulin	Hyperproinsulinemia	AR	11p15.5	P	101
Growth hormone	Dwarfism	AR, AD	17q22–q24	D, P	93
POMC	Adrenal insufficiency; obesity	AR	2p23.3	P	113
Parathyroid hormone	Hypoparathyroidism	AD	11p15.3–15.1	P	102
Thyroid stimulating hormone	TSH deficiency; hypothyroidism	AR	1p22	D, P	107
Thyroglobulin	Hypothyroidism; goiter	AR	8q24.2–q24.3	P	236
Luteinizing hormone	LH deficiency; hypogonadism	AR	19q13.32	P	86
Follicle-stimulating hormone	FSH deficiency; hypogonadism	AR	11p13	P	109
Vasopressin/neurophysin II	Neurohypophyseal DI	AD	20p12.21	P	103
Anti-müllerian hormone	Retained müllerian ducts	AR	19p13.3–p13.2	P	237
Leptin	Obesity	AR	7q31.3	P	112
Binding Protein Mutations					
Thyroxine binding globulin	Euthyroid hypothyroxinemia	XL	Xq21–22	D, P	115
Transthyretin	Euthyroid hyperthyroxinemia	AD	18q11.2–12.1	P	120
Albumin	Euthyroid hyperthyroxinemia	AD	4q11–q13	P	117
Membrane Receptor Mutations					
Insulin-receptor	Insulin resistance	AR, AD	19p13.3–13	P	88
GnRH receptor	Hypogonadotropic hypogonadism	AR	4q21.2	P	129
GHRH receptor	GH deficiency	AR	7p15–p14	P	96
TRH receptor	Hypothalamic hypothyroidism	AR	8q23	P	238
Growth hormone receptor	Laron dwarfism	AR	5p13–p12	P	121
TSH receptor (inactive)	TSH resistance	AR	14q31	P	137
TSH receptor (activating)	Hyperthyroidism	AD, S	14q31	P	89
LH receptor (inactive)	Hypogonadism	AR	2p21	P	239
LH receptor (activating)	Male precocious puberty	AD, S	2p21	P	69
FSH receptor (inactivating)	Ovarian failure; ↓ spermatog.	AR	2p21–p16	P	142
PTH receptor (inactivating)	Blomstrand chondrodysplasia	AR	3p22–p21.1	P	240
PTH receptor (activating)	Jansen chondrodysplasia	AD	3p22–p21.1	P	132
ACTH receptor	Adrenal insufficiency	AR	18p11.2	P	241
Vasopressin V2 receptor	Nephrogenic DI	XL	Xq27–q28	P	126
Calcium receptor (inactive)	Hypocalciuric hypercalcemia	AD, AR	3q21–q24	P	144
Calcium receptor (activating)	Hypoparathyroidism	AD	3q21–q24	P	133
AMH receptor	Retained müllerian ducts	AR	12q13	P	242
Leptin receptor	Obesity	AR	1p31	P	243
Melanocortin 4 receptor	Obesity	AD	18q22	P	244
Nuclear Receptor Mutations					
Vitamin D	Type II vitamin D–resistant rickets	AR	12q12–q14	P	162
Thyroid hormone	Thyroid hormone resistance	AD	3p24.3	P, D	245
Glucocorticoid	Glucocorticoid resistance	AR	5q31	P	164
Mineralocorticoid	Pseudohypoaldosteronism type 1	AD	4q31.1	P	246
Androgen	Androgen resistance	XL, S	Xcen–q13	P, D	247
Estrogen	Estrogen resistance	AR, S	6p25.1	P	165
PPAR γ2	Obesity; insulin resistance	AD	3p25	P	248
Steroidogenic factor 1	XY sex-reversal; adrenal insuffic.	AD	9q33	P	170
DAX1	Adrenal hypoplasia congenita	XL	Xp21.3–p21.2	P, D	172
HNF4α	MODY 1	AD	20q12–q13.1	P	249
Signal Pathway Mutations					
Ras P21	Tumorigenesis	S	20q12–13.2	P	250
Gsα	Acromegaly	S	20q13.2–13.3	P	145
Gsα	Albright osteodystrophy	AD; imprinting	20q13.2–13.3	P	150
Gsα	McCune-Albright	Mosaic	20q13.2–13.3	P	148
Giα	Tumorigenesis	S	3p21	P	145
PTTG (Pit tumor transf. gene)	Pituitary tumors	S	5q33	Overexpression	251
p53	Tumorigenesis	S	17p13	D, P	252
Retinoblastoma	Tumorigenesis	S	13q14	D, P	253
PRAD1 (cyclin D1)	Tumorigenesis	S	11q13	Translocation	153
PTC (papillary thyroid carcin.)	Tumorigenesis	S	10q11–q12	Translocation	197
BRCA1	Breast, ovarian Ca.	AD, S	17q21	P, D	254
BRCA2	Breast, ovarian Ca.	AD, S	13q12.3	P, D	255

TABLE 11–5. Examples of Genetic Endocrine Diseases *Continued*

Endocrine Mutation	Disorder	Mode of Inheritance	Chromosome Location	Types of Mutation	Reference
Transcription Factor Mutations					
HNF α	MODY 3	AD	12q24.2	P	256
HNF β	MODY 5	AD	17cen–q21.3	P	257
Insulin promoter factor 1	MODY 4	AD	13q12.1	P	187
Pit1	GH, PRL, TSH deficiency	AR, AD	3p11	D, P	30
Prop1	GH, PRL, TSH, LH, FSH deficiency	AR	5q	P	182
Thyroid transcription factor 1	Congenital hypothyroidism	Unknown	14q13	Underexpression	184
Thyroid transcription factor 2	Congenital hypothyroidism	AR	9q22	P	185
PAX-8	Congenital hypothyroidism	AR	2q12–q14	P	186
SRY translocation	XX male	XL	Ypter	Translocation	178
SRY mutation	XY female	YL	Ypter	P	258
SOX-9	XY female; campomelic dysplasia	AD	17q24.3–q25.1	P	175
Wilm tumor	Frasier syndrome; Denys-Drash	AD	11p13	P	176
DAZ (RNA-binding protein)	Azoospermia	YL	Yq11	D	74
Endocrine Syndromes					
Kallmann	Hypogonadotropic hypogonadism	XL, AR, AD	Xp22.3	D, P, translocation	259
Prader-Willi	Hypogonadism, obesity	AD; imprinting	15q11	D	260
Von Hippel–Lindau	Pheochromocytoma; renal Ca.	AD	3p26–p25	D, P	261
MEN1	Neoplasia: Pit., pancreas, parathy.	AD	11q13	P	72
MEN2 (*ret* mutations)	Neoplasia: parathy., pheo., MTC	AD	10q11.2	P	195
MEN2b	MEN II and neurofibromas	AD	10q11.2	P	196
Carney complex	Cushing's; acromegaly, myxomas	AD	2p16	Unknown	216
Pendred syndrome	Goiter; deafness	AR	7q31	P, D	213
DiGeorge syndrome	Hypoparathyroidism; cardiac abn.	AD	22q11	D	262
Prohormone convertase 1	ACTH, GnRH, insulin deficiency	AR	5q15–q21	P	263
Polyglandular failure type 1	Polyglandular failure	AR	21q22.3	P	215
Enzyme and Channel Mutations					
Glucokinase	MODY 2	AD	7p15–p13	P	188
Sulfonylurea receptor	Nesidioblastosis	AR	11p15.1–p14	P	234
Potassium channel KCNJ11	Nesidioblastosis	AR	11p15.1	P	235
Sodium iodide symporter	Goiter, hypothyroidism	AR	19p12–13.2	P	230
Thyroid peroxidase	Goiter, hypothyroidism	AR	2pter–12	P	229
21-Hydroxylase	CAH, androgen excess	AR	6p21	P, D	87
17α-Hydroxylase	Androgen deficiency, HTN	AR	10q24.3	P	221
17, 20-Lyase activity	XY ambiguous genitalia	AR	10q24.3	P	222
11β-Hydroxylase	Androgen excess, HTN	AR	8q21	P	220
3β-Hydroxysteroid dehydrog.	CAH; androgen deficiency	AR	1p13.1	P	223
Steroidogenic acute regulatory	Lipoid CAH	AR	8p11.2	P	225
5α-Reductase type 2	Male pseudohermaphroditism	AR	2p23	D, P	227
Aldosterone synthase	Glucocorticoid, remediable HTN	AD	8q21	D; translocation	231
Amiloride sensitive Na channel	Liddle syndrome; HTN	AD	16p13–p12	P	264
Aquaporin 2	Nephrogenic DI	AR	12q13	P	128
PEX	Hypophos. vitamin D–resistant rickets	XL	Xp22.2–p22.1	P	233
1α-Hydroxylase	Type 1 vitamin D–resistant rickets	AR	12q14	P	232

AD, autosomal dominant; AR, autosomal recessive; S, somatic cell mutation; XL, X-linked; YL, Y-linked; P, point mutation. Representative references are provided. Many endocrine disorders are not listed, including a large number of metabolic disorders. The interested reader is referred to additional references (Jameson[1]; Scriver et al.[265]).

ciency is reminiscent of idiopathic hypogonadotropic hypogonadism, which is not due to a *GnRH* gene defect, but rather to a defect in a gene *(KAL1)* that controls migration of the GnRH producing neurons.[97] A relatively rare form of GH deficiency involves a deletion of the *GH* gene (~35 cases),[92] and it represents one of the few well-studied hormone mutations. In early studies, Southern blot analyses of DNA from affected children demonstrated a homozygous deletion of the *GH* gene, consistent with the autosomal recessive inheritance pattern for transmission. More recently, autosomal dominant mutations in the *GH* gene have been described. In these cases, it is proposed that the mutation generates a misfolded protein that aggregates with the normal GH protein.[98, 99] These complexes may also be toxic to somatotrope cells.

The *GH* gene is a member of a large gene cluster that also includes a growth hormone variant gene as well as several structurally related *chorionic somatomammotropin* genes and pseudogenes (highly homologous but functionally inactive relatives of a normal gene). Because such gene clusters contain multiple homologous DNA sequences arranged in tandem, they are particularly prone to undergo recombination, leading to gene duplication or deletion. It has been proposed that mispairing of areas with sequence homology can lead to unequal

crossover during meiosis with resultant gene duplication on one chromosome and gene deletion on the other chromosome.[93, 100]

Other mutations that have been described in hormones are listed in Table 11–5. The mutations in pre-proinsulin prevent processing of the pre-proinsulin precursor molecule, causing secretion of biologically inactive insulin molecules.[101] A mutation in the signal sequence of PTH causes hypoparathyroidism, even when only one of the two *PTH* genes is affected.[102] It has been shown that this mutation interferes with hormone transport and processing, leading to the hypothesis that the mutant molecule could interfere with the transport of other cellular proteins, including the normal PTH protein. Mutations in the *vasopressin* gene appear to be somewhat analogous to the PTH mutation. An autosomal dominant form of diabetes insipidus is caused by heterozygous mutations in neurophysin, the precursor protein for vasopressin.[103] The fact that the amino acid changes occur in the signal sequence and carboxyterminal vasopressin carrier protein, neurophysin, suggests that abnormalities in protein processing may prevent vasopressin synthesis or result in cellular toxicity. In vitro studies demonstrate abnormal processing and cellular toxicity of the mutant forms of vasopressin,[104, 105] likely accounting for the delayed onset of the disease.[106]

Homozygous mutations in the *TSH* gene cause hypothyroidism. One

TSHβ-subunit mutation defines a region of the molecule that is required for heterodimerization with the α subunit,[107] whereas others either truncate the protein or interfere with its biological activity.[108] An LHβ-subunit mutation defines a region that is critical for binding to the LH receptor.[86] Interestingly, FSHβ mutations have different phenotypes in males and females. They cause primary ovarian failure in females because of a defect in follicular maturation and estrogen synthesis.[109, 110] In males, FSHβ mutations do not impair virilization or testosterone production, but they cause variable impairment of spermatogenesis.[111] *Leptin* mutations, initially described in murine models of obesity, have now been identified in humans.[112] Unexpectedly, mutations in *POMC* not only cause adrenal insufficiency, but also lead to obesity, apparently because of a role for α-MSH in appetite control.[113] In these and other autosomal recessive disorders, there is an opportunity to examine the effect of a "gene knockout" in humans. Thus, elimination of functional hormones such as growth hormone, LH, FSH, or TSH allows one to attribute specific physiologic roles to the hormone that may be difficult to discern in normal individuals. For example, complete elimination of LH, with retention of normal FSH, allows the functions of these hormones to be discriminated. As described above, creation of gene knockouts by homologous recombination in transgenic mice is an active area of research that allows the creation of animal models for studying hormone and receptor function.

Binding Protein Mutations

The binding protein mutations cause little in the way of clinical disease, but if not recognized, often lead to unnecessary treatment. As shown in Table 11–5, these defects are confined largely to proteins that bind thyroid hormone (see Chapter 113). Thyroxine binding globulin (TBG) is the major thyroid hormone transport protein in the serum. Abnormalities in its production are not rare, occurring in approximately 1/2500 male births.[114] Complete TBG deficiency is X-linked and is clinically apparent in males who are euthyroid but have very low levels of thyroid hormone in the serum. They are often mistakenly treated for hypothyroidism. Although large deletions of the *TBG* gene have not been found,[115] a number of different point mutations can cause functional loss of TBG, either by alterations in protein structure or glycosylation.[114]

In addition to TBG, thyroid hormone binds to albumin and transthyretin (thyroxine binding prealbumin). Euthyroid hyperthyroxinemia can result from an altered form of binding protein or from excess production of one of the binding proteins. TBG excess is most commonly due to effects of drugs or hormones, although familial examples have been described. Familial dysalbuminemic hyperthyroxinemia (FDH) is an autosomal dominant condition in which albumin has an increased affinity for thyroid hormone.[116] Most cases are caused by a mutation in codon 218, in which there is replacement of Arg by His[117] or Pro.[118] It is characterized by elevated levels of total T_4 and normal levels of free T_4 and TSH. Another form of the disorder causes a selective increase in T_3 binding.[119] The presence of abnormal binding proteins can be detected using electrophoretic analyses of serum thyroid hormone binding proteins, or now, by mutational analyses. Transthyretin (thyroid hormone binding prealbumin, TBPA) can be overproduced, usually in patients with pancreatic endocrine tumors, or there are mutant forms that have increased affinity for thyroxine.[120] The mutant forms of transthyretin also cause dysalbuminemic hyperthyroxinemia, resulting in elevated total T_4 without apparent clinical consequences. Patients with this and similar thyroid hormone binding protein disorders need to be distinguished from individuals who are truly hyperthyroid.

Membrane Receptor Mutations

In Laron-type dwarfism, a receptor or post-receptor defect had been proposed because growth hormone levels were high, IGF levels were low, and patients failed to respond to growth hormone therapy. A number of different point mutations have now been identified in the growth hormone receptor.[121, 122] Such hormone resistance is characteristic of many receptor mutations,[123] although alterations in signaling pathways can result in a similar phenotype (e.g., pseudohypoparathyroidism).

Mutations in the insulin receptor have been characterized extensively in patients with severe insulin resistance. Multiple missense and nonsense mutations have been described in different regions of the receptor, causing different insulin resistance phenotypes such as leprechaunism, the Rabson-Mendenhall syndrome, and type A insulin resistance.[88, 124] The mechanisms of insulin receptor inactivation and their relationship to the preceding syndromes and others are summarized in Chapter 43.

An X-linked form of vasopressin resistance has now been attributed to mutations in the *vasopressin 2 (V2)* receptor gene on the long arm of the X chromosome.[125-127] There are many different vasopressin receptor mutations, reflecting allelic heterogeneity. However, a similar phenotype (nephrogenic diabetes insipidus) can be caused by mutations in the *aquaporin 2* gene,[128] providing an example of nonallelic heterogeneity.

In recent years, mutations have been defined in most peptide hormone receptors. For the most part, the phenotypes are predictable based on the known function of the hormone pathway. However, several exceptions warrant emphasis. Some GnRH receptor mutations only partially alter its function.[129] Consequently, patients may exhibit an LH response to pharmacologic doses of exogenous GnRH, whereas they do not respond normally to lower levels of endogenous GnRH. These patients usually present with idiopathic hypogonadism. GHRH-R mutations cause severe GH deficiency, even though other releasing factors theoretically might compensate for the defect.[130]

Among the most important revelations in recent years is the finding that a subset of mutations in G-protein coupled receptors (GPCRs) can cause constitutive activation of receptor function, whereas other mutations cause loss of function. This phenomenon was first recognized in adrenergic receptors, in which certain mutations in the sixth transmembrane domain were found to cause constitutive activation of cAMP signaling, in the absence of added ligand.[131] The ability of mutations to activate GPCR has had a tremendous impact in the field of endocrinology. Based on the idea that activating mutations of GPCR could mimic the effects of hormone excess, phenotypes for activating mutations have now been identified in the TSH-R,[89] LH-R,[69] PTH-R,[132] and Ca-R.[133]

Constitutively active mutations in the TSH-R are characteristic of this class of mutations. The activating mutations in the TSH-R were first identified in autonomously functioning thyroid nodules. In this case, they are somatic mutations that occur in the thyroid follicular cell but are not present in the germline. These mutations cause an increase in basal production of cAMP by the receptor, indicating that it couples to Gs in the absence of TSH. Because the TSH-R mediates thyroid cell growth as well as function, the mutant receptor leads to the clonal expansion of cells harboring the mutation, ultimately resulting in a clinically apparent "hot" nodule. In addition to somatic mutations, activating TSH-R mutations can also occur as de novo germline mutations causing congenital hyperthyroidism.[134] Or, they can be transmitted as an autosomal dominant disorder, since a mutation in one allele is sufficient to cause hyperfunction.[135] The locations of these activating mutations delineate residues in the TSH-R that play a critical role in G-protein coupling, either because they are involved directly, or, more likely, because they play a structural role to maintain the receptor in an inactive state.[136] Homozygous inactivating mutations in the TSH receptor cause resistance to TSH.[137]

Activating mutations in the LH-R cause familial male-limited precocious puberty.[69] The autonomous function of the LH-R induces testosterone production in the absence of LH (prepubertally), causing virilization in boys. Interestingly, females with the mutations exhibit no phenotypic abnormalities, presumably because autonomous function of the LH-R in the ovary does not significantly alter steroidogenesis since the receptor is only expressed as follicles mature and are normally exposed to high levels of LH. For this reason, pedigrees with LH-R mutations exhibit an autosomal dominant pattern of transmission, but only males are affected. Analogous mutations in the FSH-R appear to be rare,[138] or perhaps do not cause a phenotype that is readily recognized. Homozygous inactivating mutations in the LH-R cause Leydig cell hypoplasia and pseudohermaphroditism in males[139, 140] and primary amenorrhea in females.[141] Homozygous inactivating mutations in the FSH receptor cause primary ovarian failure in females[142] and impaired spermatogenesis in males.[142]

The cloning of a GPCR that binds calcium was quite unexpected.[143] However, identification of this receptor led to a molecular basis for familial hypocalciuric hypercalcemia, which is caused by inactivating mutations,[144] as well as one of the familial causes of hypoparathyroidism.[133] The heterozygous inactivating mutations cause calcium resistance, resulting in increased PTH and a new setpoint for calcium feedback. On the other hand, activating mutations of the calcium receptor mimic the effects of calcium, leading to suppression of PTH and low calcium levels. Activating mutations in the PTH-R cause severe skeletal abnormalities (Jansen syndrome), as well as hypercalcemia, because autonomous function of the receptor is present from early development.[132]

Signaling Pathway Mutations

Mutations at several steps along signaling pathways can alter hormone action or contribute to tumorigenesis. As noted above, there is now evidence that somatic mutations in membrane receptors, such as the TSH receptor, can lead to constitutive activation of downstream signaling pathways resulting in altered cell growth.[89] Mutations in G proteins have been described in several different types of endocrine neoplasia.[145] For example, mutations in the Gs subunit have been identified in somatotroph adenomas, either at codon 201 or 227.[146] Both of these mutations inhibit GTP hydrolysis and thereby cause constitutive activation of the Gs subunit. Activation of Gs in this cell type stimulates adenylyl cyclase, leading to elevated cAMP levels, a situation that mimics GHRH stimulation. As a result, the Gs mutation causes excess GH secretion and contributes to abnormal cell growth as well. Gs mutations are found in approximately 30 to 40% of somatotrope adenomas.[147] Importantly, these mutations are somatic rather than inherited, as evidenced by the fact that G proteins from other tissues do not contain the amino acid substitution. Gs mutations have also been identified in autonomous thyroid adenomas.[145] It is interesting to note that Gs mutations identical to those described in somatotroph adenomas also occur in McCune-Albright syndrome.[148] In McCune-Albright, the mutations occur early in development such that the tissue distribution of the mutation is broad rather than being restricted to somatotroph cells.

Albright hereditary osteodystrophy (AHO) is also caused by a Gs mutation, although in this case the mutation eliminates Gs function rather than causing constitutive activity.[149] AHO is characterized by short stature, obesity, and skeletal abnormalities. Resistance to several Gs protein coupled hormones such as PTH, TSH, LH, and FSH is characteristic. Different Gs mutations have been described in several families with AHO.[150, 151] As noted above, the disease is inherited in an autosomal dominant manner, but imprinting causes an unusual inheritance pattern through the maternal line.

A novel mechanism for tumorigenesis has been provided by studies of parathyroid adenomas. A subset of parathyroid tumors were found to contain rearrangements of the PTH gene.[152] Analysis of the translocation revealed that the PTH promoter was fused to a member of the cyclin D family.[153] The translocation involved an intrachromosomal rearrangement on chromosome 11. The fusion gene is referred to as *PRAD,* for parathyroid adenomatosis. Because cyclins regulate progression through the cell cycle, it is likely that overexpression of cyclin D1 from the PTH promoter, rather than from its native promoter, causes abnormal regulation of the parathyroid cell.

Endocrine neoplasms, although not necessarily representing the most aggressive forms of cancer, are providing important models for the identification of new oncogenes as well as the steps involved in the progression of tumors from the benign to the malignant phenotype. Because many oncogenes involve alterations of cellular signaling pathways that have been well characterized in hormone-secreting cells, it is likely endocrine tumors will continue to provide important models for the pathophysiology of neoplasia.

Nuclear Receptor Mutations

In addition to the mutations in membrane receptors (e.g., LH resistance), hormone resistance syndromes also occur as a consequence of defects in nuclear receptors (i.e., resistance to thyroid hormone). The syndrome of resistance to thyroid hormone (RTH) is representative of nuclear receptor resistance syndromes, but it also illustrates some unique aspects of a disease that is inherited in a dominant manner (see Chapters 95 and 114). RTH was first described by Refetoff and colleagues[154] and is characterized by elevated circulating levels of free thyroid hormone, inappropriately normal or increased levels of TSH, and the absence of clinical manifestations of thyrotoxicosis. Two thyroid hormone receptor genes, designated *TR* and *TR,* encode highly homologous proteins with different tissue distributions. Genetic analyses show linkage between the RTH syndrome and the *TR* receptor gene locus.[70, 155] This observation has been confirmed by sequencing receptor genes in multiple different families with this disorder. In the families that have a dominant mode of transmission, affected individuals have mutations in one allele of the *TR* receptor together with a second normal allele.[156, 157] Interestingly, these and additional mutations are clustered in three discrete regions of the receptor carboxy-terminal, ligand binding domain. The mutant receptors bind hormone with reduced affinity or they have defects in hormone-dependent transcriptional activation. Consequently, their ability to modulate target gene expression is impaired.[158] Because the affected individuals possess a second normal receptor allele and two normal receptor alleles, the mutant receptor has been proposed to inhibit the activity of normal receptors. In support of this concept, the receptor mutants have been shown to block the action of the wild type receptors in transient gene expression assays, probably by binding to DNA target sites where the mutant receptors function as antagonists.[159] It is also notable that the mutant receptors retain the ability to bind transcriptional corepressors.[160] Thus, once bound to DNA target sites, they act as repressors of these target genes.

Mutations have also been identified in several other members of the nuclear hormone receptor family. Syndromes of androgen resistance represent one of the more common and well-studied receptor defects.[94] These disorders exhibit sex-linked transmission, consistent with the location of the androgen receptor on the X chromosome. The *androgen receptor* gene has now been sequenced in a relatively large number of affected individuals, although primarily those with severe forms of resistance.[94] Many mutations result in premature termination codons, although gene deletions and single amino acid substitutions have also been found. No clinical effects of the heterozygous condition have been noted in females with androgen receptor mutations. In female carriers of the mutation, X inactivation would likely allow expression of only one of the receptor alleles within a given cell and the dominant negative activity seen with the thyroid hormone receptor may not be possible.

Hypocalcemic vitamin D–resistant rickets (HVDRR) is a rare inherited form of rickets that is unresponsive to treatment with 1,25-dihydroxyvitamin D.[161, 162] The disease has a recessive pattern of inheritance, and most cases have involved consanguineous families. A variety of mutations have been identified in different kindreds, including amino acid substitutions in the zinc-finger DNA binding domains, as well as nonsense mutations that cause premature termination. The naturally occurring mutations in the vitamin D receptor have been useful for providing insights into the biologic role of vitamin D in skin differentiation, hair growth, and lymphocyte function.[162, 163]

In familial glucocorticoid resistance, serum concentrations of cortisol and cortisol production rates are elevated without the characteristic clinical manifestations of glucocorticoid excess. ACTH levels are inappropriately increased, indicating reduced feedback inhibition at the level of the hypothalamic-pituitary axis. Because ACTH also stimulates adrenal androgens and mineralocorticoids, precocious puberty and hypertension can comprise features of this syndrome. An autosomal codominant mode of inheritance has been suggested in view of the fact that heterozygotes are mildly affected.[164] Mutations in the mineralocorticoid receptor cause a form of pseudohypoaldosteronism type I, which is characterized by neonatal renal salt wasting with dehydration, hypotension, hyperkalemia, and metabolic acidosis, despite elevated aldosterone levels. It is transmitted in an autosomal dominant manner and it is less severe than the homozygous form of pseudohypoaldosteronism, which is caused by homozygous mutations in the amiloride-sensitive epithelial sodium channel.

A homozygous estrogen receptor mutation has been described in a male.[165] In addition to reduced estrogen action on the hypothalamic-pituitary-gonadal axis, it impaired fusion of the epiphyses, leading to increased linear growth. Estrogen receptor variants and mutations have been described in breast cancers, although a role in pathogenesis has not been clearly defined.[166, 167]

Mutations in orphan nuclear receptors also cause endocrine disorders. Steroidogenic factor 1 (SF1) controls adrenal and gonadal development and it is expressed in the ventromedial hypothalamus and pituitary gonadotropes.[168] SF1 also regulates the expression of a wide array of steroidogenic enzyme genes.[169] A heterozygous mutation in *SF1* has been demonstrated in an XY individual with adrenal insufficiency and complete male-to-female sex reversal.[170] The orphan nuclear receptor, DAX1, is expressed in the same distribution as SF1 and inhibits its transcriptional activity.[171] *DAX1* is located on the X chromosome and mutations cause X-linked adrenal hypoplasia congenita (AHC), which is characterized by adrenal insufficiency and hypogonadotropic hypogonadism.[172]

Transcription Factor Mutations

One of the final steps in hormone action involves effects on gene expression, mediated via transcription factors. In principle, the nuclear hormone receptors could be classified as transcription factors and described under this category. Not surprisingly, some of the other transcription factor mutations have involved developmental pathways. Elucidation of mutations in the *SRY* gene provides a dramatic example of one of these developmental mutations.[73] The Y chromosome determines male sex by virtue of encoding the testis determining factor (TDF). In the absence of a Y chromosome, ovaries form, and the female gender develops. The *SRY* gene was located by examining rare cases of phenotypic females with an XY genotype. It was hypothesized that these individuals might have deleted or mutated *SRY* genes on the Y chromosome. The sex-determining region on the short arm of the Y chromosome was delineated by mapping large deletions or translocations of the Y chromosome that were associated with a female phenotype. Three lines of evidence support the view that *SRY* is the primary testis-determining gene. First, in XY females who do not have a large deletion of the Y chromosome, mutations are found in *SRY* that are not present in their fathers.[73] Second, there is a deletion in the mouse homolog of *SRY* in sex-reversed mice.[173] Third, expression of *SRY* in transgenic mice is sufficient to induce testis development in females.[174] Although these data indicate that *SRY* is the critical gene for an early step in male sex determination, it is likely that *SRY* is only one of several developmental switches that initiate a cascade of sex-specific gene expression. As noted above, mutations in *SF1* also preclude normal testis development in XY individuals. *SOX9*[175] and *WT1*[176] mutations also impair testis development.

XX males have been shown to have translocations of Y chromosome–specific sequences onto the pseudoautosomal region of the X chromosome.[177, 178] These translocated Y chromosome sequences contain *SRY*. Sterility in XX males may reflect the presence of two X chromosomes (analogous to Klinefelter's syndrome) or the absence of additional Y chromosome sequences that are required for fertility.

The transcription factor, Pit1, was first identified based upon its binding to multiple sites in the growth hormone and prolactin promoters.[27, 28] Pit1 expression is restricted to the pituitary gland and the protein is found only in somatotropes, lactotropes, and thyrotropes.[179] Pit1 mutations have been identified in several strains of mice that have specific deficits of GH, Prl, and TSH.[180] These data confirm a central role for Pit1 in the development of these cell types and/or the expression of these genes. Similar patterns of pituitary hormone deficiencies have been described in humans[181] with mutations in Pit1. Interestingly, different *Pit1* mutations result in autosomal recessive[29, 31] and autosomal dominant[30] inheritance patterns, suggesting that the distinct mutations have different effects on Pit1 function. The recessive mutation

inactivates Pit1, whereas the dominant disorder involves a dominant negative mutation analogous to that for the thyroid hormone receptor. Another pituitary transcription factor, Prop1, which acts upstream of Pit1 during pituitary development, causes a more severe form of pituitary hormone deficiency that includes GH, Prl, and TSH, as well as ACTH.[182]

Like transcription factors involved in pituitary development, the discovery of factors involved in thyroid gland development has provided insight into genetic causes of thyroid dysfunction. Thyroid transcription factor 1 (TTF1), thyroid transcription factor 2 (TTF2), and paired homeobox 8 (PAX8) each play a key role in thyroid gland development.[183] These factors are therefore candidates for genetic causes of thyroid agenesis. Although several cases of mutations have been reported, the incidence of mutations in these developmental transcription factors appears to be relatively low.[184–186]

A genetic pathway that involves transcription factors causes several forms of maturity-onset diabetes of the young (MODY). At present, five different types of MODY are recognized. They share in common an autosomal dominant mode of transmission and late-onset nonketotic form of diabetes mellitus of variable severity. MODY 1 is caused by mutations in *hepatocyte nuclear receptor 4α (HNF4α)*, which is a member of the steroid/thyroid nuclear receptor superfamily. It is expressed in the liver, but also in the kidney, intestine, and pancreatic islets. HNF-4α controls the expression of a wide variety of genes, including *HNF1α* (which causes MODY 3). As noted above, HNF1α, a homeodomain transcription factor, is regulated by HNF-4α. It is involved in the expression of hepatocyte genes as well as certain islet genes, including insulin. Mutations have also been described in HNF1β, which is structurally related to HNF1α. HNF1β can form homodimers or heterodimers with HNF1α. MODY 4 is caused by mutations in insulin promoter factor 1 (IPF1), which is a homeobox transcription factor, also referred to as STF1 or IDX1. It controls development of the pancreas. Homozygous mutations cause pancreatic agenesis, whereas heterozygous mutations cause diabetes.[187] MODY 2 was the first form of MODY to be characterized at the genetic level. In contrast to the other forms of MODY, it is not caused by a transcription factor mutation. Rather, it results from mutations in glucokinase, an enzyme that phosphorylates glucose to glucose-6-phosphate.[188] This reaction plays a key role in glucose sensing by the pancreatic β-cell. As a result of glucokinase mutations, increased glucose levels are required to elicit insulin secretory responses.

Endocrine Syndromes

Multiple endocrine neoplasia (MEN) syndromes have long been recognized as autosomal dominant disorders that predispose to endocrine tumor development. Both syndromes are associated with hyperplasia and adenomas of the parathyroid glands. However, MEN1 is also characterized by adenomas of the pituitary and pancreas (see Chapter 188), whereas MEN2 is associated with adrenal (pheochromocytomas) and thyroid C cell (medullary carcinoma) neoplasia (see chapter by Gagel).

The MEN syndromes represent good examples of the experimental approaches that are required to identify and characterize unknown genes that cause well-characterized syndromes. A critical first step is to determine the chromosome on which a candidate *MEN* gene resides. Subsequently, the position of the disease-causing gene can be more precisely mapped in relation to known genes and other DNA markers on that chromosome. For MEN1 and 2, candidate genes were mapped to chromosomes 11 and 10, respectively, using linkage analyses.[189, 190] The *MEN1* locus was found to be near *PYGM*, the muscle phosphorylase gene, which is known to be located on chromosome 11, band q13.[189, 191] After a long search, and a tribute to the power of modern genomics, the gene for *MEN1* was identified within this locus.[72] The protein, menin, is localized in the nucleus, although its function is not well understood at present. It appears to act like a classic tumor suppressor gene, as inactivating mutations are found in the germline of most families with the disorder. And, the second copy of the gene is deleted or mutated in tumor tissue, apparently because of acquired "second hits" or somatic mutations.[192] This scenario is analogous to the two-hit model for loss of *retinoblastoma* gene function, a well-characterized example of a tumor suppressor gene.[193]

Unlike MEN1, loss of heterozygosity is not seen at the *MEN2* locus on chromosome 10, suggesting a different pathophysiology for MEN2.[194] In the case of MEN2, affected individuals often have thyroid C-cell hyperplasia in childhood before the development of medullary thyroid carcinoma. This observation is consistent with a model in which the *MEN2* gene predisposes to hyperplastic growth with a second and perhaps distinct somatic mutation leading to tumorigenesis and clonal proliferation. Mutations in the *ret* proto-oncogene, a putative tyrosine kinase receptor, have been identified as the cause of MEN2a.[195] In several MEN2 kindreds, distinct *ret* mutations were found in a cluster of cysteines located at the juncture of the extracellular and transmembrane domains of the protein. These mutations appear to induce receptor dimerization, leading to constitutive function. Distinct mutations, in the tyrosine kinase domain of the Ret receptor, cause MEN2b.[196] Interestingly, rearrangements of *ret* had previously been identified in papillary thyroid carcinoma, leading to its designation as a "PTC" oncogene.[197, 198] Identification of *MEN2* gene carriers is particularly important because of the consequences of allowing medullary thyroid carcinoma or pheochromocytoma to go unrecognized. Screening for *ret* mutations allows at-risk individuals to undergo prophylactic thyroidectomy and more intense endocrine screening, whereas low-risk individuals do not require further hormone testing (see Chapter 189).

Kallmann's syndrome, or idiopathic hypogonadotropic hypogonadism (IHH) associated with anosmia, is an inherited disorder that is caused by GnRH deficiency. Several different inheritance patterns have been described, including autosomal recessive, X-linked, and autosomal dominant with incomplete penetrance.[199–201] In contrast to an animal model of this disorder (the hypogonadal mouse) in which there is a *GnRH* gene deletion,[202] all IHH patients examined to date appear to have an intact *GnRH* gene.[203] Furthermore, the sequence of the GnRH gene in several different individuals with IHH has been shown to be normal.[204, 205] Thus, it appears that IHH in the human, unlike the hypogonadal mouse model, may involve defects in the processes that regulate development of GnRH producing neurons or expression of the *GnRH* gene, rather than defects in the gene itself.[206, 207] Genetic linkage studies provided evidence for a candidate gene on the short arm of the X chromosome (Xp22.3) in patients with the X-linked form of Kallmann's syndrome,[208, 209] and mutations in the *KAL* gene were found in several individuals with the syndrome.[206, 207] Coupled with the finding that GnRH neurons migrate into the hypothalamus from the olfactory placode,[206, 210] the *KAL* gene appears to be involved in the migration of the GnRH neurons, as well as development of the olfactory tract.[211] These observations are consistent with a model in which a defect in this gene causes Kallmann's syndrome and might account for some of its phenotypic variants in that different degrees of developmental aberrations in neuronal migration could lead to isolated anosmia, IHH, or both. Causes of other forms of idiopathic hypogonadotropic hypogonadism, including autosomal recessive and dominant forms, remain to be described.[201]

Pendred's syndrome is an autosomal recessive syndrome characterized by goiter, defective organification of iodine, and deafness that is caused by a malformation of the cochlea. The genetic defect in Pendred's syndrome was determined by genetic linkage studies in consanguineous families.[212, 213] The use of short tandem repeat markers throughout the genome identified a region on chromosome 7q31 in which affected individuals were homozygous for a series of the microsatellite markers. Because the same region was localized in several different pedigrees, genes within this locus were cloned and screened for mutations. Ultimately, the Pendred syndrome gene, which encodes a putative iodine and chloride transporter protein (pendrin), was cloned.[213, 214]

Autoimmune polyendocrinopathy–candidiasis–ectodermal dystrophy (APECED) is an autosomal recessive syndrome that causes polyglandular failure syndrome type I. The disorder usually presents in childhood and is characterized by autoimmune destruction of several glands including the parathyroids, adrenal cortex, gonads, pancreatic cells, gastric parietal cells, and the thyroid gland. As implied by its name, other features include chronic mucocutaneous candidiasis, dystrophy

of the dental enamel and nails, alopecia, vitiligo, and keratinopathy. Although the spectrum of clinical features is variable, the most common presentation includes hypoparathyroidism, adrenal insufficiency, and mucocutaneous candidiasis. Linkage analysis localized the gene for *APECED* to chromosome 21 q22.3. Subsequently, the gene was cloned and found to encode a 545-amino-acid putative transcription factor that is expressed in the thymus, lymph nodes, and fetal liver.[215] Although the exact function of the APECED gene product remains unknown, its pattern of expression is consistent with a primary defect of immune function.

Carney's complex is an autosomal dominant syndrome characterized by multiple neoplasias, including myxomas at various sites, endocrine tumors, and lentiginosis. Common endocrine manifestations include Cushing's syndrome caused by pigmented nodular adrenal hyperplasia and acromegaly caused by pituitary tumors. Linkage analysis using short tandem repeat markers has localized a candidate region to chromosome 2p16.[216] The gene that causes Carney's complex remains to be identified.

Steroidogenic Enzyme Mutations

Because a number of enzymatic steps are required for steroid hormone biosynthesis and metabolism, it is not surprising that defects occur in multiple different enzymes, giving rise to distinct clinical syndromes. Deficiency of 21-hydroxylase is the most common cause of congenital adrenal hyperplasia (CAH).[217] 21-Hydroxylase is responsible for conversion of progesterone to corticosterone in the mineralocorticoid pathway and for conversion of 17-hydroxyprogesterone to 11-deoxycortisol in the glucocorticoid pathway. Because of decreased cortisol production, excess ACTH is secreted, leading to stimulation of the adrenal gland and the overproduction of precursor steroids, including adrenal androgens.

Deficiency of 21-hydroxylase encompasses a broad phenotypic spectrum. The severe classic form occurs in approximately 1/5,000 to 1/20,000 births; less severe nonclassic forms occur as frequently as 1/30 to 1/100 births in certain genetic populations. In females affected with the classic form of the disease, hypersecretion of adrenal androgens during fetal development causes ambiguous external genitalia, whereas in males the classic form is usually recognized because of severe salt wasting and glucocorticoid deficiency. In the nonclassic form, prenatal virilization does not occur, but virilization of variable severity occurs postnatally.

Many of the earlier clinical observations regarding CAH are now well explained by the molecular basis for the disease.[87] The 21-hydroxylase locus is on the short arm of chromosome 6, adjacent to the HLA locus, explaining previous findings that HLA typing was useful for predicting disease risk (the HLA locus is linked to the *21 hydroxylase* locus). There are two *21-hydroxylase* genes, A and B. The *21A* gene is a functionally inactive pseudogene, whereas the adjacent *21B* gene is the active copy. The *21-hydroxylase* genes appear to have been duplicated along with the adjacent *C4A* and *C4B* complement genes. A large number of different types of deletions and point mutations of the *21B* gene have been described. Large deletions and rearrangements probably occur in 10 to 20% of cases. On the other hand, small deletions and point mutations are relatively common. Interestingly, many of the mutations in the *21B* gene correspond to sequences in the inactive *21A* gene. These data have been interpreted as evidence for gene conversion in which sequences from the adjacent *21A* gene are substituted for sequences in 21B, probably as a consequence of chromatid mispairing coupled with a DNA repair mechanism. The inheritance of CAH is autosomal recessive. Heterozygotes are typically unaffected clinically and are detected only by hormonal testing. The classic form of the disease is due to large deletions or severe mutations of both 21B alleles, whereas the nonclassic form of the disease is caused by one of several combinations of severe and mildly affected 21B alleles. Thus, the variability in clinical phenotype is partly the consequence of a high degree of heterogeneity at the genetic level. Prenatal testing for CAH is now possible using either HLA typing or DNA analyses.[218, 219] It is important to recognize the disorder during the first trimester for glucocorticoids to ameliorate prenatal virilization in females.

Mutations in the *11β-hydroxylase* and *17α-hydroxylase* genes are also classified under congenital adrenal hyperplasia because impaired production of cortisol causes elevation of ACTH and consequently, adrenal stimulation. Mutations in 11β-hydroxylase cause androgen excess and virilization, but are distinguished clinically from 21 hydroxylase mutations by mineralocorticoid excess, which causes hypertension in about two-thirds of patients.[220] In contrast, defects in 17-hydroxylase cause sex steroid deficiency with overproduction of mineralocorticoids, resulting in hypertension and hypokalemia. Recognition of mutations in the *P450c17* gene led to the finding that a single protein had two different enzymatic activities (17α-hydroxylase and 17,20-lyase) that were previously thought to represent different proteins.[221, 222] Mutations in 3β-hydroxysteroid dehydrogenase are a relatively rare cause of CAH.[223] Because the block in steroid synthesis occurs early in the pathway of steroid synthesis, it is also associated with androgen deficiency.

A critical step in steroid synthesis actually involves the transport of cholesterol into the mitochondrion by steroidogenic acute regulatory protein (StAR).[224] Mutations in StAR cause lipoid CAH, which is characterized by large, lipid-filled adrenal glands and gonads.[225] The discovery of this protein has provided important new insights into how steroidogenesis is rapidly modulated by hormones like ACTH and LH.

Defects in the enzyme 5α-reductase result in a complex phenotype of male pseudohermaphroditism.[226] 5α-reductase converts testosterone to dihydrotestosterone, an androgen that plays an important role in the development of male external genitalia. These individuals have an XY karyotype and are born with ambiguous genitalia characterized as pseudovaginal perineoscrotal hypospadias. At puberty, there is masculinization with good muscle development, enlargement of the phallus, but the prostate remains small and beard growth is scanty. In some cultures where the prevalence of the disease is high, affected individuals are raised as girls, but change gender identity at puberty.[226] 5α-Reductase is encoded by two enzymes designated 1 and 2. 5α-Reductase 2 is the major enzyme in genital tissue and is the site of mutations that cause male pseudohermaphroditism. As with 21 hydroxylase deficiency, a number of different sites in the enzyme are mutated in different families and many affected individuals are compound heterozygotes.[227, 228]

Defects in thyroid peroxidase are characterized by hypothyroidism and goiter, presumably as a result of prolonged thyroid gland stimulation by TSH. The disorder is manifest in the homozygous state. In one individual, there is a short insertion in the eighth exon of the *thyroid peroxidase* gene.[229] Based on previous biochemical studies, defects in thyroid peroxidase may represent a relatively common cause of inborn errors of thyroid hormone metabolism. The transport of iodine into the thyroid gland is mediated by the sodium-iodide symporter (NIS). Homozygous mutations in NIS also cause congenital hypothyroidism and goiter.[230]

Glucocorticoid remediable hypertension (GRA) is characterized by high levels of abnormal adrenal steroids, 18-oxocortisol and 18-hydroxycortisol, and a variable degree of hyperaldosteronism. Because production of these steroids occurs in a region of the adrenal cortex that is under the control of ACTH, their production is reduced by administration of glucocorticoids. This disorder is caused by an unusual gene rearrangement.[231] The genes encoding aldosterone synthetase and steroid 11β-hydroxylase are arranged in tandem on chromosome 8q. Aldosterone synthetase is expressed in the zona glomerulosa where it is involved in aldosterone production, whereas 11β-hydroxylase is expressed in the ACTH-dependent fasciculata, as well as in the glomerulosa. These two genes are 95% identical, predisposing to gene duplication by unequal crossing over. Because the fusion gene contains the regulatory regions of 11β-hydroxylase and the coding sequence of aldosterone synthetase, the latter enzyme is subjected to an abnormal pattern of expression in the ACTH-dependent zone of the adrenal gland, resulting in overproduction of mineralocorticoids.

Type I vitamin D–dependent rickets (also known as pseudovitamin D–deficient rickets) is caused by mutations in the enzyme 1α-hydroxylase, which converts 25-vitamin D_3 to its more active metabolite 1α,25-hydroxyvitamin D_3.[232] In this disorder, patients have low concentrations of 1,25-hydroxyvitamin D_3 and normal or elevated concentrations of the precursor, 25-vitamin D_3. They can be treated with physiologic doses of 1α,25-hydroxyvitamin D_3. An X-linked form of rickets is referred to as hypophosphatemic vitamin D–resistant rickets, in which the *PEX* gene (a phosphate-regulating gene) is mutated.[233]

Closure of ATP-sensitive potassium channels in pancreatic islet β-cells initiates a cascade of events that leads to insulin secretion. Potassium currents are reconstituted by the inward rectifier Kir6.2 and the sulfonylurea receptor (SUR), a member of the ATP-binding cassette superfamily. Homozygous mutations in either SUR[234] or Kir6.2 can cause PHHI.[235]

REFERENCES

1. Jameson JL: Principles of Molecular Medicine. Totowa, Humana Press, 1998, p 1–1123.
2. Okayama H, Berg P: Bacteriophage lambda vector for transducing a cDNA clone library into mammalian cells. Mol Cell Biol 5:1136–1142, 1985.
3. Okayama H, Berg P: High-efficiency cloning of full-length cDNA. Mol Cell Biol 2:161–170, 1982.
4. Okayama H, Berg P: A cDNA cloning vector that permits expression of cDNA inserts in mammalian cells. Mol Cell Biol 3:280–289, 1983.
5. Benton WD, Davis RW: Screening gt recombinant clones by hybridization to single plaques in situ. Science 196:180, 1977.
6. Huynh TV, Young RA, Davis RW: Constructing and screening cDNA libraries in gt10 and gt11. In DNA Cloning Techniques: A Practical Approach. Oxford, IRL Press, 1984, pp 49–78.
7. Dugaiczyk A, Boyer HW, Goodman HM: Ligation of *Eco*RI endonuclease-generated DNA fragments into linear and circular structures. J Mol Biol 96:174–184, 1975.
8. Birnboim HC, Doly J: A rapid alkaline extraction method for screening recombinant plasmid DNA. Nucl Acids Res 7:1513–1523, 1979.
9. Maxam AM, Gilbert W: A new method for sequencing DNA. Proc Natl Acad Sci USA 74:560–564, 1977.
10. Sanger F, Nicklen S, Coulson AR: DNA sequencing with chain-terminating inhibitors. Proc Natl Acad Sci USA 74:5463–5467, 1977.
11. Maniatis T, Hardison RC, Lacy E, et al: The isolation of structural genes from libraries of eucaryotic DNA. Cell 15:687–701, 1978.
12. Lodish HF, Rose JK: Relative importance of 7-methylguanosine in ribosome binding and translation of vesicular stomatitis virus mRNA in wheat germ and reticulocyte cell-free systems. J Biol Chem 252:1181–1188, 1977.
13. Studier FW, Moffatt BA: Use of bacteriophage T7 RNA polymerase to direct selective high-level expression of cloned genes. J Mol Biol 189:113–130, 1986.
14. Smith GE, Summers MD, Fraser MJ: Production of human beta interferon in insect cells infected with a baculovirus expression vector. Mol Cell Biol 3:2156–2165, 1983.
15. Mulligan RC, Berg P: Expression of a bacterial gene in mammalian cells. Science 209:1422–1427, 1980.
16. Alwine JC, Kemps DJ, Stark GR: Method for detection of specific RNAs in agarose gels by transfer to diazobenzyloxymethyl-paper and hybridization with DNA probes. Proc Natl Acad Sci USA 74:5350–5354, 1977.
17. Melton DA, Krieg PA, Rebagliati MR, et al: Efficient in vitro synthesis of biologically active RNA and RNA hybridization probes from plasmids containing a bacteriophage SP6 promoter. Nucleic Acids Res 12:7035–7056, 1984.
18. Wang AM, Doyle MV, Mark DF: Quantitation of mRNA by the polymerase chain reaction. Proc Natl Acad Sci USA 86:9717–9721, 1989.
19. Pardue ML. In situ hybridization. In Nucleic Acid Hybridization: A Practical Approach. Oxford, IRL Press, 1985, pp 179–202.
20. McKnight GS, Palmiter RD: Transcriptional regulation of the ovalbumin and conalbumin genes by steroid hormones in chick oviduct. J Biol Chem 254:9050–9058, 1979.
21. Rodgers JR, Johnson ML, Rosen JM: Measurement of mRNA concentration and mRNA half-life as a function of hormonal treatment. Methods Enzymol 109:572–592, 1985.
22. Graham FL, van der Eb AJ: A new technique for the assay of infectivity of human adenovirus 5 DNA. Virology 52:456, 1973.
23. Gorman CM, Moffat LF, Howard BH: Recombinant genomes which express chloramphenicol acetyltransferase in mammalian cells. Mol Cell Biol 2:1044–1051, 1982.
24. Kunkel TA: Rapid and efficient site-specific mutagenesis without phenotypic selection. Proc Natl Acad Sci USA 82:488–492, 1985.
25. Rigby PW: Three in one and one in three: It all depends on TBP. Cell 72:7–10, 1993.
26. Zawel L, Reinberg D: Initiation of transcription by RNA polymerase II: A multistep process. Prog Nucleic Acid Res Mol Biol 44:67–108, 1993.
27. Ingraham HA, Chen RP, Mangalam HJ, et al: A tissue-specific transcription factor containing a homeodomain specifies a pituitary phenotype. Cell 55:519–529, 1988.
28. Castrillo JL, Bodner M, Karin M: Purification of growth hormone-specific transcription factor GHF-1 containing homeobox. Science 243:814–817, 1989.
29. Pfaffle RW, DiMattia GE, Parks JS, et al: Mutation of the POU-specific domain of Pit-1 and hypopituitarism without pituitary hypoplasia. Science 257:1118–1121, 1992.
30. Radovick S, Nations M, Du Y, et al: A mutation in the POU-homeodomain of Pit-1 responsible for combined pituitary hormone deficiency. Science 257:1115–1118, 1992.
31. Tatsumi K, Miyai K, Notomi T, et al: Cretinism with combined hormone deficiency caused by a mutation in the PIT1 gene. Nat Genet 1:56–58, 1992.
32. Habener JF: Cyclic AMP response element binding proteins: A cornucopia of transcription factors. Mol Endocrinol 4:1087–1094, 1990.

33. Hunter T, Karin M: The regulation of transcription by phosphorylation. Cell 70:375–387, 1992.

34. McKenna NJ, Lanz RB, O'Malley BW: Nuclear receptor coregulators: Cellular and molecular biology. Endocr Rev 20:321–344, 1999.

35. Ing NH, Beekman JM, Tsai SY, et al: Members of the steroid hormone receptor superfamily interact with TFIIB (S300–II). J Biol Chem 267:17617–17623, 1992.

36. Lin YS, Ha I, Maldonado E, et al: Binding of general transcription factor TFIIB to an acidic activating region. Nature 353:569–571, 1991.

37. Hagemeier C, Bannister AJ, Cook A, et al: The activation domain of transcription factor PU.1 binds the retinoblastoma (RB) protein and the transcription factor TFIID in vitro: RB shows sequence similarity to TFIID and TFIIB. Proc Natl Acad Sci USA 90:1580–1584, 1993.

38. Ruppert S, Wang EH, Tjian R: Cloning and expression of human TAFII250: A TBP-associated factor implicated in cell-cycle regulation. Nature 362:175–179, 1993.

39. Hoey T, Weinzierl RO, Gill G, et al: Molecular cloning and functional analysis of Drosophila TAF110 reveal properties expected of coactivators. Cell 72:247–260, 1993.

40. Struhl K: Histone acetylation and transcriptional regulatory mechanisms. Genes Dev 12:599–606, 1998.

41. Roeder RG: Role of general and gene-specific cofactors in the regulation of eukaryotic transcription. Cold Spring Harb Symp Quant Biol 63:201–218, 1998.

42. Hampsey M, Reinberg D: RNA polymerase II as a control panel for multiple coactivator complexes. Curr Opin Genet Dev 9:132–139, 1999.

43. Galas D, Schmitz A: DNase footprinting: A simple method for the detection of protein-DNA binding specificity. Nucl Acids Res 5:3157–3170, 1978.

44. Singh H, Sen R, Baltimore D, et al: A nuclear factor that binds to a conserved sequence motif in transcriptional control elements of immunoglobulin genes. Nature 319:154–158, 1986.

45. Fried M, Crothers DM: Equilibria and kinetics of *lac* repressor-operator interactions by polyacrylamide gel electrophoresis. Nucl Acids Res 9:6505–6525, 1981.

46. Fields S, Song O: A novel genetic system to detect protein-protein interactions. Nature 340:245–246, 1989.

47. Fields S, Sternglanz R: The two-hybrid system: An assay for protein-protein interactions. Trends Genet 10:286–292, 1994.

48. Erickson RP: Creating animal models of genetic disease. Am J Hum Genet 43:582–586, 1988.

49. Hanahan D: Transgenic mice as probes into complex systems. Science 246:1265–1275, 1989.

50. Lipes MA, Eisenbarth GS: Transgenic mouse models of type I diabetes. Diabetes 39:879–884, 1990.

51. Kumar TR, Matzuk MM. Transgenic mice as models of disease. In Jameson JL (ed): Principles of Molecular Medicine. Totowa, Humana Press, 1998, pp 97–112.

52. Tremblay Y, Tretjakoff I, Peterson A, et al: Pituitary-specific expression and glucocorticoid regulation of a proopiomelanocortin fusion gene in transgenic mice. Proc Natl Acad Sci USA 85:8890–8894, 1988.

53. Liu B, Hammer GD, Rubinstein M, et al: Identification of DNA elements cooperatively activating proopiomelanocortin gene expression in the pituitary glands of transgenic mice. Mol Cell Biol 12:3978–3990, 1992.

54. Palmiter RD, Brinster RL, Hammer RE, et al: Dramatic growth of mice that develop from eggs microinjected with metallothionein–growth hormone fusion genes. Nature 300:611–615, 1982.

55. Mason AJ, Pitts SL, Nikolics K, et al: The hypogonadal mouse: Reproductive functions restored by gene therapy. Science 234:1372–1378, 1986.

56. Mason AJ, Hayflick JS, Zoeller RT, et al: A deletion truncating the gonadotropin-releasing hormone gene is responsible for hypogonadism in the hpg mouse. Science 234:1366–1371, 1986.

57. Hanahan D: Oncogenes in transgenic mice. Nature 312:503–504, 1984.

58. Palmiter RD, Behringer RR, Quaife CJ, et al: Cell lineage ablation in transgenic mice by cell-specific expression of a toxin gene [published erratum appears in Cell 1990 Aug 10;62(3):following 608]. Cell 50:435–443, 1987.

59. Kendall SK, Saunders TL, Jin L, et al: Targeted ablation of pituitary gonadotropes in transgenic mice. Mol Endocrinol 5:2025–2036, 1991.

60. Hanahan D: Heritable formation of pancreatic beta-cell tumours in transgenic mice expressing recombinant insulin/simian virus 40 oncogenes. Nature 315:115–122, 1985.

61. Mellon PL, Windle JJ, Goldsmith PC, et al: Immortalization of hypothalamic GnRH neurons by genetically targeted tumorigenesis. Neuron 5:1–10, 1990.

62. Windle JJ, Weiner RI, Mellon PL: Cell lines of the pituitary gonadotrope lineage derived by targeted oncogenesis in transgenic mice. Mol Endocrinol 4:597–603, 1990.

63. Mansour SL, Thomas KR, Capecchi MR: Disruption of the proto-oncogene int-2 in mouse embryo-derived stem cells: A general strategy for targeting mutations to non-selectable genes. Nature 336:348–352, 1988.

64. Matzuk MM, Finegold MJ, Su JG, et al: Alpha-inhibin is a tumour-suppressor gene with gonadal specificity in mice. Nature 360:313–319, 1992.

65. Collins FS, Patrinos A, Jordan E, et al: New goals for the U.S. Human Genome Project: 1998–2003. Science 282:682–689, 1998.

66. Jameson JL. The human genome project. In Jameson JL (ed): Principles of Molecular Medicine. Totowa, Humana Press, 1998, pp 59–64.

67. Beaudet AL. Genetics and disease. In Fauci AS, Braunwald E, Isselbacher KJ, et al (eds): Harrison's Principles of Internal Medicine, ed 14. New York, McGraw-Hill, 1998, pp 365–394.

68. Kopp P, Jameson JL: Transmission of human genetic disease. In Jameson JL (ed): Principles of Molecular Medicine. Totowa, Humana Press, 1998, pp 43–58.

69. Shenker A, Laue L, Kosugi S, et al: A constitutively activating mutation of the luteinizing hormone receptor in familial male precocious puberty. Nature 365:652–654, 1993.

70. Refetoff S, Weiss RE, Usala SJ: The syndromes of resistance to thyroid hormone. Endocr Rev 14:348–399, 1993.

71. Chatterjee VKK, Clifton-Bligh RJ, Gurnell M. Thyroid hormone resistance. *In* Jameson JL (ed): Hormone Resistance Syndromes. Totowa, Humana Press, 1999, pp 145–164.

72. Chandrasekharappa SC, Guru SC, Manickam P, et al: Positional cloning of the gene for multiple endocrine neoplasia–type 1. Science 276:404–407, 1997.

73. Berta P, Hawkins JR, Sinclair AH, et al: Genetic evidence equating SRY and the testis-determining factor. Nature 348:448–450, 1990.

74. Reijo R, Lee TY, Salo P, et al: Diverse spermatogenic defects in humans caused by Y chromosome deletions encompassing a novel RNA-binding protein gene. Nat Genet 10:383–393, 1995.

75. Davies JL, Kawaguchi Y, Bennett ST, et al: A genome-wide search for human type 1 diabetes susceptibility genes. Nature 371:130–136, 1994.

76. van den Ouweland JM, Lemkes HH, Trembath RC, et al: Maternally inherited diabetes and deafness is a distinct subtype of diabetes and associates with a single point mutation in the mitochondrial tRNA(Leu(UUR)) gene. Diabetes 43:746–751, 1994.

77. Peters J, Wroe SF, Wells CA, et al: A cluster of oppositely imprinted transcripts at the Gnas locus in the distal imprinting region of mouse chromosome 2. Proc Natl Acad Sci USA 96:3830–3835, 1999.

78. Ott J: Estimation of the recombination fraction in human pedigrees: Efficient computation of the likelihood for human linkage studies. Am J Hum Genet 26:588–597, 1974.

79. Southern EM: Detection of specific sequences among DNA fragments separated by gel electrophoresis. J Mol Biol 98:503–517, 1975.

80. Saiki RK, Gelfand DH, Stoffel S, et al: Primer-directed enzymatic amplification of DNA with a thermostable DNA polymerase. Science 239:487–491, 1988.

81. Nakamura Y, Leppert M, O'Connell P, et al: Variable number of tandem repeat (VNTR) markers for human gene mapping. Science 235:1616–1622, 1987.

82. Zhang X, Kousoulas KG: Direct sequencing of PCR-amplified high GC DNA. Biotechniques 14:376–377, 1993.

83. Top B: A simple method to attach a universal 50-bp GC-clamp to PCR fragments used for mutation analysis by DGGE. Pcr Methods Appl 2:83–85, 1992.

84. Poduslo SE, Dean M, Kolch U, et al: Detecting high-resolution polymorphisms in human coding loci by combining PCR and single-strand conformation polymorphism (SSCP) analysis. Am J Hum Genet 49:106–111, 1991.

85. Verlaan-de Vries M, Bogaard ME, van den Elst H, et al: A dot-blot screening procedure for mutated ras oncogenes using synthetic oligodeoxynucleotides. Gene 50:313–320, 1986.

86. Weiss J, Axelrod L, Whitcomb RW, et al: Hypogonadism caused by a single amino acid substitution in the β-subunit of luteinizing hormone. N Engl J Med 326:179–183, 1991.

87. White PC, New MI: Genetic basis of endocrine disease 2: Congenital adrenal hyperplasia due to 21-hydroxylase deficiency. J Clin Endocrinol Metab 74:6–11, 1992.

88. Taylor SI, Cama A, Accili D, et al: Genetic basis of endocrine disease. 1. Molecular genetics of insulin resistant diabetes mellitus. J Clin Endocrinol Metab 73:1158–1163, 1991.

89. Parma J, Duprez L, Van Sande J, et al: Somatic mutations in the thyrotropin receptor gene cause hyperfunctioning thyroid adenomas. Nature 365:649–651, 1993.

90. Jameson JL: Thyroid hormone resistance: Pathophysiology at the molecular level. J Clin Endocrinol Metab 74:708–711, 1992.

91. McKusick VA: Mendelian Inheritance in Man. Baltimore, Johns Hopkins University Press, 1988, pp 1–1626.

92. Vnencak JCL, Phillips JAD, Chen EY, et al: Molecular basis of human growth hormone gene deletions. Proc Natl Acad Sci USA 85:5615–5619, 1988.

93. Vnencak JCL, Phillips JA: Hot spots for growth hormone gene deletions in homologous regions outside of Alu repeats. Science 250:1745–1748, 1990.

94. McPhaul MJ, Marcelli M, Zoppi S, et al: Genetic basis of endocrine disease. 4. The spectrum of mutations in the androgen receptor gene that causes androgen resistance. J Clin Endocrinol Metab 76:17–23, 1993.

95. Rogol AD, Blizzard RM, Foley T Jr, et al: Growth hormone releasing hormone and growth hormone: Genetic studies in familial growth hormone deficiency. Pediatr Res 19:489–492, 1985.

96. Wajnrajch MP, Gertner JM, Harbison MD, et al: Nonsense mutation in the human growth hormone–releasing hormone receptor causes growth failure analogous to the little (lit) mouse. Nat Genet 12:88–90, 1996.

97. Franco B, Guioli S, Pragliola A, et al: A gene deleted in Kallmann's syndrome shares homology with neural cell adhesion and axonal path-finding molecules. Nature 353:529–536, 1991.

98. Cogan JD, Prince MA, Lekhakula S, et al: A novel mechanism of aberrant pre-mRNA splicing in humans. Hum Mol Genet 6:909–912, 1997.

99. Cogan JD, Ramel B, Lehto M, et al: A recurring dominant negative mutation causes autosomal dominant growth hormone deficiency—a clinical research center study. J Clin Endocrinol Metab 80:3591–3595, 1995.

100. Vnencak JCL, Phillips JAD, Wang DF: Use of polymerase chain reaction in detection of growth hormone gene deletions. J Clin Endocrinol Metab 70:1550–1553, 1990.

101. Steiner DF, Tager HS, Chan SJ, et al: Lessons learned from molecular biology of insulin-gene mutations. Diabetes Care 13:600–609, 1990.

102. Arnold A, Horst SA, Gardella TJ, et al: Mutation of the signal peptide–encoding region of the preproparathyroid hormone gene in familial isolated hypoparathyroidism. J Clin Invest 86:1084–1087, 1990.

103. Ito M, Mori Y, Oiso Y, et al: A single base substitution in the coding region for neurophysin II associated with familial central diabetes insipidus. J Clin Invest 87:725–728, 1991.

104. Ito M, Yu RN, Ito M, et al: Mutant vasopressin precursors that cause autosomal dominant neurohypophyseal diabetes insipidus retain dimerization and impair the secretion of wild-type proteins. J Biol Chem 274:9029–9037, 1999.

105. Ito M, Jameson JL: Molecular basis of autosomal dominant neurohypophyseal diabe-

tes insipidus. Cellular toxicity caused by the accumulation of mutant vasopressin precursors within the endoplasmic reticulum. J Clin Invest 99:1897–1905, 1997.

106. McLeod JF, Kovacs L, Gaskill MB, et al: Familial neurohypophyseal diabetes insipidus associated with a signal peptide mutation. J Clin Endocrinol Metab 77:599A–599G, 1993.

107. Hayashizaki Y, Hiraoka Y, Endo Y, et al: Thyroid-stimulating hormone (TSH) deficiency caused by a single base substitution in the CAGYC region of the beta-subunit. EMBO J 8:2291–2296, 1989.

108. Dacou-Voutetakis C, Feltquate DM, Drakopoulou M, et al: Familial hypothyroidism caused by a nonsense mutation in the thyroid-stimulating hormone beta-subunit gene. Am J Hum Genet 46:988–993, 1990.

109. Matthews CH, Borgato S, Beck-Peccoz P, et al: Primary amenorrhoea and infertility due to a mutation in the beta-subunit of follicle-stimulating hormone. Nat Genet 5:83–86, 1993.

110. Layman LC, Lee EJ, Peak DB, et al: Delayed puberty and hypogonadism caused by mutations in the follicle-stimulating hormone beta-subunit gene. N Engl J Med 337:607–611, 1997.

111. Phillip M, Arbelle JE, Segev Y, et al: Male hypogonadism due to a mutation in the gene for the beta-subunit of follicle-stimulating hormone. N Engl J Med 338:1729–1732, 1998.

112. Montague CT, Farooqi IS, Whitehead JP, et al: Congenital leptin deficiency is associated with severe early-onset obesity in humans. Nature 387:903–908, 1997.

113. Krude H, Biebermann H, Luck W, et al: Severe early-onset obesity, adrenal insufficiency and red hair pigmentation caused by POMC mutations in humans. Nat Genet 19:155–157, 1998.

114. Mori Y, Seino S, Takeda K, et al: A mutation causing reduced biological activity and stability of thyroxine-binding globulin probably as a result of abnormal glycosylation of the molecule. Mol Endocrinol 3:575–579, 1989.

115. Mori Y, Refetoff S, Flink IL, et al: Detection of the thyroxine-binding globulin (TBG) gene in six unrelated families with complete TBG deficiency. J Clin Endocrinol Metab 67:727–733, 1988.

116. Yeo PP, Yabu Y, Etzkorn JR, et al: A four generation study of familial dysalbuminemic hyperthyroxinemia: Diagnosis in the presence of an acquired excess of thyroxine-binding globulin. J Endocrinol Invest 10:33–38, 1987.

117. Sunthornthepvarakul T, Angkeow P, Weiss RE, et al: An identical missense mutation in the albumin gene results in familial dysalbuminemic hyperthyroxinemia in 8 unrelated families. Biochem Biophys Res Commun 202:781–787, 1994.

118. Wada N, Chiba H, Shimizu C, et al: A novel missense mutation in codon 218 of the albumin gene in a distinct phenotype of familial dysalbuminemic hyperthyroxinemia in a Japanese kindred. J Clin Endocrinol Metab 82:3246–3250, 1997.

119. Sunthornthepvarakul T, Likitmaskul S, Ngowngarmratana S, et al: Familial dysalbuminemic hypertriiodothyroninemia: A new, dominantly inherited albumin defect. J Clin Endocrinol Metab 83:1448–1454, 1998.

120. Moses AC, Rosen HN, Moller DE, et al: A point mutation in transthyretin increases affinity for thyroxine and produces euthyroid hyperthyroxinemia. J Clin Invest 86:2025–2033, 1990.

121. Amselem S, Sobrier ML, Duquesnoy P, et al: Recurrent nonsense mutations in the growth hormone receptor from patients with Laron dwarfism. J Clin Invest 87:1098–1102, 1991.

122. Laron Z: Laron syndrome: Primary growth hormone resistance. In Jameson JL (ed): Hormone Resistance Syndromes. Totowa, Humana Press, 1999, pp 17–38.

123. Jameson JL (ed): Hormone Resistance Syndromes. Totowa, Humana Press, 1999.

124. Taylor SI, Arioglu E: Diabetes mellitus: Insulin resistance. In Jameson JL (ed): Hormone Resistance Syndromes. Totowa, Humana Press, 1999, pp 165–184.

125. Merendino J Jr, Speigel AM, Crawford JD, et al: Brief report: A mutation in the vasopressin V2-receptor gene in a kindred with X-linked nephrogenic diabetes insipidus. N Engl J Med 328:1538–1541, 1993.

126. Holtzman EJ, Harris H Jr, Kolakowski L, Jr, et al: Brief report: A molecular defect in the vasopressin V2-receptor gene causing nephrogenic diabetes insipidus. N Engl J Med 328:1534–1537, 1993.

127. Lightman SL: Molecular insights into diabetes insipidus. N Engl J Med 328:1562–1563, 1993.

128. Deen PM, Verdijk MA, Knoers NV, et al: Requirement of human renal water channel aquaporin-2 for vasopressin dependent concentration of urine. Science 264:92–95, 1994.

129. de Roux N, Young J, Misrahi M, et al: A family with hypogonadotropic hypogonadism and mutations in the gonadotropin-releasing hormone receptor. N Engl J Med 337:1597–1602, 1997.

130. Baumann G: Dwarfism: GHRH resistance. In Jameson JL (ed): Hormone Resistance Syndromes. Totowa, Humana Press, 1999, pp 1–16.

131. Kjelsberg MA, Cotecchia S, Ostrowski J, et al: Constitutive activation of the alpha 1B-adrenergic receptor by all amino acid substitutions at a single site. Evidence for a region which constrains receptor activation. J Biol Chem 267:1430–1433, 1992.

132. Schipani E, Kruse K, Juppner H: A constitutively active mutant PTH-PTHrP receptor in Jansen-type metaphyseal chondrodysplasia. Science 268:98–100, 1995.

133. Pollak MR, Brown EM, Estep HL, et al: Autosomal dominant hypocalcaemia caused by a Ca(2+)-sensing receptor gene mutation. Nat Genet 8:303–307, 1994.

134. Kopp P, van Sande J, Parma J, et al: Brief report: Congenital hyperthyroidism caused by a mutation in the thyrotropin-receptor gene. N Engl J Med 332:150–154, 1995.

135. Duprez L, Parma J, Van Sande J, et al: Germline mutations in the thyrotropin receptor gene cause non-autoimmune autosomal dominant hyperthyroidism. Nat Genet 7:396–401, 1994.

136. Vassart G: New pathophysiological mechanisms for hyperthyroidism. Horm Res 48:47–50, 1997.

137. Sunthornthepvarakul T, Gottschalk ME, Hayashi Y, et al: Brief report: Resistance to thyrotropin caused by mutations in the thyrotropin-receptor gene. N Engl J Med 332:155–160, 1995.

138. Gromoll J, Simoni M, Nieschlag E: An activating mutation of the follicle-stimulating

139. Kremer H, Kraaij R, Toledo SP, et al: Male pseudohermaphroditism due to a homozygous missense mutation of the luteinizing hormone receptor gene. Nat Genet 9:160–164, 1995.

140. Latronico AC, Anasti J, Arnhold IJ, et al: Brief report: Testicular and ovarian resistance to luteinizing hormone caused by inactivating mutations of the luteinizing hormone-receptor gene. N Engl J Med 334:507–512, 1996.

141. Toledo SP, Brunner HG, Kraaij R, et al: An inactivating mutation of the luteinizing hormone receptor causes amenorrhea in a 46,XX female. J Clin Endocrinol Metab 81:3850–3854, 1996.

142. Aittomaki K, Lucena JL, Pakarinen P, et al: Mutation in the follicle-stimulating hormone receptor gene causes hereditary hypergonadotropic ovarian failure. Cell 82:959–968, 1995.

143. Brown EM, Gamba G, Riccardi D, et al: Cloning and characterization of an extracellular Ca(2+)-sensing receptor from bovine parathyroid. Nature 366:575–580, 1993.

144. Pollak MR, Brown EM, Chou YH, et al: Mutations in the human Ca(2+)-sensing receptor gene cause familial hypocalciuric hypercalcemia and neonatal severe hyperparathyroidism. Cell 75:1297–1303, 1993.

145. Lyons J, Landis CA, Harsh G, et al: Two G protein oncogenes in human endocrine tumors. Science 249:655–659, 1990.

146. Landis CA, Masters SB, Spada A, et al: GTPase inhibiting mutations activate the alpha chain of Gs and stimulate adenylyl cyclase in human pituitary tumours. Nature 340:692–696, 1989.

147. Spada A, Arosio M, Bochicchio D, et al: Clinical, biochemical, and morphological correlates in patients bearing growth hormone–secreting pituitary tumors with or without constitutively active adenylyl cyclase. J Clin Endocrinol Metab 71:1421–1426, 1990.

148. Weinstein LS, Shenker A, Gejman PV, et al: Activating mutations of the stimulatory G protein in the McCune-Albright syndrome. N Engl J Med 325:1688–1695, 1991.

149. Al-Zahrani A, Levine MA, Schwindinger WF: Pseudohypoparathyroidism. In Jameson JL (ed): Hormone Resistance Syndromes. Totowa, Humana Press, 1999, pp 39–58.

150. Patten JL, Johns DR, Valle D, et al: Mutation in the gene encoding the stimulatory G protein of adenylate cyclase in Albright's hereditary osteodystrophy. N Engl J Med 322:1412–1419, 1990.

151. Weinstein LS, Gejman PV, Friedman E, et al: Mutations of the Gs alpha-subunit gene in Albright hereditary osteodystrophy detected by denaturing gradient gel electrophoresis. Proc Natl Acad Sci USA 87:8287–8290, 1990.

152. Arnold A, Kim HG, Gaz RD, et al: Molecular cloning and chromosomal mapping of DNA rearranged with the parathyroid hormone gene in a parathyroid adenoma. J Clin Invest 83:2034–2040, 1989.

153. Motokura T, Bloom T, Kim HG, et al: A novel cyclin encoded by a bcl1-linked candidate oncogene. Nature 350:512–515, 1991.

154. Refetoff S, DeWind LT, DeGroot LJ: Familial syndrome combining deaf-mutism, stuppled epiphyses, goiter and abnormally high PBI: Possible target organ refractoriness to thyroid hormone. J Clin Endocrinol Metab 27:279–294, 1967.

155. Usala SJ, Weintraub BD: Thyroid hormone resistance syndromes. Trends Endocrinol Metab 2:140–144, 1991.

156. Sakurai A, Takeda K, Ain K, et al: Generalized resistance to thyroid hormone associated with a mutation in the ligand-binding domain of the human thyroid hormone receptor beta. Proc Natl Acad Sci USA 86:8977–8981, 1989.

157. Usala SJ, Tennyson GE, Bale AE, et al: A base mutation of the C-erbA beta thyroid hormone receptor in a kindred with generalized thyroid hormone resistance. Molecular heterogeneity in two other kindreds. J Clin Invest 85:93–100, 1990.

158. Chatterjee VK, Nagaya T, Madison LD, et al: Thyroid hormone resistance syndrome. Inhibition of normal receptor function by mutant thyroid hormone receptors. J Clin Invest 87:1977–1984, 1991.

159. Nagaya T, Madison LD, Jameson JL: Thyroid hormone receptor mutants that cause resistance to thyroid hormone. Evidence for receptor competition for DNA sequences in target genes. J Biol Chem 267:13014–13019, 1992.

160. Tagami T, Jameson JL: Nuclear corepressors enhance the dominant negative activity of mutant receptors that cause resistance to thyroid hormone. Endocrinology 139:640–650, 1998.

161. Hughes MR, Malloy PJ, Kieback DG, et al: Point mutations in the human vitamin D receptor gene associated with hypocalcemic rickets. Science 242:1702–1705, 1988.

162. Malloy PJ, Hochberg Z, Tiosano D, et al: The molecular basis of hereditary 1,25-dihydroxyvitamin D3 resistant rickets in seven related families. J Clin Invest 86:2071–2079, 1990.

163. Feldman D, Malloy PJ: Hereditary 1,25-dihydroxyvitamin D resistant rickets: Molecular basis and implications for the role of 1,25(OH) 2D3 in normal physiology. Mol Cell Endocrinol 72:57–62, 1990.

164. Hurley DM, Accili D, Stratakis CA, et al: Point mutation causing a single amino acid substitution in the hormone binding domain of the glucocorticoid receptor in familial glucocorticoid resistance. J Clin Invest 87:680–686, 1991.

165. Smith EP, Boyd J, Frank GR, et al: Estrogen resistance caused by a mutation in the estrogen-receptor gene in a man. N Engl J Med 331:1056–1061, 1994.

166. McGuire WL, Chamness GC, Fuqua SA: The importance of normal and abnormal oestrogen receptor in breast cancer. Cancer Surv 14:31–40, 1992.

167. Fuqua SA, Chamness GC, McGuire WL: Estrogen receptor mutations in breast cancer. J Cell Biochem 51:135–139, 1993.

168. Luo X, Ikeda Y, Parker KL: A cell-specific nuclear receptor is essential for adrenal and gonadal development and sexual differentiation. Cell 77:481–490, 1994.

169. Parker KL, Schimmer BP: Steroidogenic factor 1: a key determinant of endocrine development and function. Endocr Rev 18:361–377, 1997.

170. Achermann JC, Ito M, Hindmarsh PC, et al: A mutation in the gene encoding steroidogenic factor–1 causes XY sex reversal and adrenal failure in humans. Nat Genet 22:125–126, 1999.

171. Ito M, Yu R, Jameson JL: DAX-1 inhibits SF-1-mediated transactivation via a carboxy-terminal domain that is deleted in adrenal hypoplasia congenita. Mol Cell Biol 17:1476–1483, 1997.

172. Muscatelli F, Strom TM, Walker AP, et al: Mutations in the DAX-1 gene give rise to both X-linked adrenal hypoplasia congenita and hypogonadotropic hypogonadism. Nature 372:672–676, 1994.

173. Gubbay J, Collignon J, Koopman P, et al: A gene mapping to the sex-determining region of the mouse Y chromosome is a member of a novel family of embryonically expressed genes. Nature 346:245–250, 1990.

174. Koopman P, Gubbay J, Vivian N, et al: Male development of chromosomally female mice transgenic for Sry. Nature 351:117–121, 1991.

175. Foster JW, Dominguez-Steglich MA, Guioli S, et al: Campomelic dysplasia and autosomal sex reversal caused by mutations in an SRY-related gene. Nature 372:525–530, 1994.

176. Pelletier J, Bruening W, Kashtan CE, et al: Germline mutations in the Wilms' tumor suppressor gene are associated with abnormal urogenital development in Denys-Drash syndrome. Cell 67:437–447, 1991.

177. Petit C, de la Chapelle A, Levilliers J, et al: An abnormal terminal X-Y interchange accounts for most but not all cases of human XX maleness. Cell 49:595–602, 1987.

178. Page DC, Brown LG, de la Chappelle A: Exchange of terminal portions of X- and Y-chromosomal short arms in human XX males. Nature 328:437–440, 1987.

179. Simmons DM, Voss JW, Ingraham HA, et al: Pituitary cell phenotypes involve cell-specific Pit-1 mRNA translation and synergistic interactions with other classes of transcription factors. Genes Dev 4:695–711, 1990.

180. Li S, Crenshaw EBd, Rawson EJ, et al: Dwarf locus mutants lacking three pituitary cell types result from mutations in the POU-domain gene pit–1. Nature 347:528–533, 1990.

181. Wit JM, Drayer NM, Jansen M, et al: Total deficiency of growth hormone and prolactin, and partial deficiency of thyroid stimulating hormone in two Dutch families: A new variant of hereditary pituitary deficiency. Horm Res 32:170–177, 1989.

182. Wu W, Cogan JD, Pfaffle RW, et al: Mutations in PROP1 cause familial combined pituitary hormone deficiency. Nat Genet 18:147–149, 1998.

183. Missero C, Cobellis G, De Felice M, et al: Molecular events involved in differentiation of thyroid follicular cells. Mol Cell Endocrinol 140:37–43, 1998.

184. Acebron A, Aza-Blanc P, Rossi DL, et al: Congenital human thyroglobulin defect due to low expression of the thyroid-specific transcription factor TTF-1. J Clin Invest 96:781–785, 1995.

185. Clifton-Bligh RJ, Wentworth JM, Heinz P, et al: Mutation of the gene encoding human TTF-2 associated with thyroid agenesis, cleft palate and choanal atresia. Nat Genet 19:399–401, 1998.

186. Macchia PE, Lapi P, Krude H, et al: PAX8 mutations associated with congenital hypothyroidism caused by thyroid dysgenesis. Nat Genet 19:83–86, 1998.

187. Stoffers DA, Ferrer J, Clarke WL, et al: Early-onset type-II diabetes mellitus (MODY4) linked to IPF1. Nat Genet 17:138–139, 1997.

188. Froguel P, Zouali H, Vionnet N, et al: Familial hyperglycemia due to mutations in glucokinase. Definition of a subtype of diabetes mellitus. N Engl J Med 328:697–702, 1993.

189. Larsson C, Skogseid B, Oberg K, et al: Multiple endocrine neoplasia type 1 gene maps to chromosome 11 and is lost in insulinoma. Nature 332:85–87, 1988.

190. Mathew CG, Chin KS, Easton DF, et al: A linked genetic marker for multiple endocrine neoplasia type 2A on chromosome 10. Nature 328:527–528, 1987.

191. Bystrom C, Larsson C, Blomberg C, et al: Localization of the MEN1 gene to a small region within chromosome 11q13 by deletion mapping in tumors. Proc Natl Acad Sci USA 87:1968–1972, 1990.

192. Marx S, Spiegel AM, Skarulis MC, et al: Multiple endocrine neoplasia type 1: Clinical and genetic topics. Ann Intern Med 129:484–494, 1998.

193. Friend SH, Bernards R, Rogelj S, et al: A human DNA segment with properties of the gene that predisposes to retinoblastoma and osteosarcoma. Nature 323:643–646, 1986.

194. Kidd KK, Simpson NE: Search for the gene for multiple endocrine neoplasia type 2A. Recent Prog Horm Res 46:305–341, 1990.

195. Mulligan LM, Kwok JBJ, Healey CS, et al: Germ-line mutations of the *RET* proto-oncogene in multiple endocrine neoplasia type 2A. Nature 363:458–460, 1993.

196. Carlson KM, Dou S, Chi D, et al: Single missense mutation in the tyrosine kinase catalytic domain of the RET protooncogene is associated with multiple endocrine neoplasia type 2B. Proc Natl Acad Sci USA 91:1579–1583, 1994.

197. Fusco A, Grieco M, Santoro M, et al: A new oncogene in human thyroid papillary carcinomas and their lymph-nodal metastases. Nature 328:170–172, 1987.

198. Grieco M, Santoro M, Berlingieri MT, et al: PTC is a novel rearranged form of the ret proto-oncogene and is frequently detected in vivo in human thyroid papillary carcinomas. Cell 60:557–563, 1990.

199. Santen RJ, Paulsen CA: Hypogonadotropic eunuchoidism. I. Clinical study of the mode of inheritance. J Clin Endocrinol Metab 36:47–54, 1973.

200. White BJ, Rogol AD, Brown KS, et al: The syndrome of anosmia with hypogonadotropic hypogonadism: A genetic study of 18 new families and a review. Am J Med Genet 15:417–435, 1983.

201. Waldstreicher J, Seminara SB, Jameson JL, et al: The genetic and clinical heterogeneity of gonadotropin-releasing hormone deficiency in the human. J Clin Endocrinol Metab 81:4388–4395, 1996.

202. Capecchi MR: Mouse genetics. YACs to the rescue. Nature 362:205–206, 1993.

203. Weiss J, Crowley WF, Jameson JL: Structure of the GnRH gene in patients with idiopathic hypogonadotropic hypogonadism. J Clin Endocrinol Metab 69:299–303, 1989.

204. Nakayama Y, Wondisford FE, Lash RW, et al: Analysis of gonadotropin-releasing hormone gene structure in families with familial central precocious puberty and idiopathic hypogonadotropic hypogonadism. J Clin Endocrinol Metab 70:1233–1238, 1990.

205. Weiss J, Adams E, Whitcomb RW, et al: Normal sequence of the GnRH gene in

206. Schwanzel-Fukuda M, Bick D, Pfaff DW: Luteinizing hormone releasing hormone (LHRH)–expressing cells do not migrate normally in an inherited hypogonadal (Kallmann) syndrome. Brain Res Mol Brain Res 6:311–326, 1989.

207. Crowley WF, Jameson JL: Clinical counterpoint: Gonadotropin-releasing hormone deficiency: Perspectives from clinical investigation. Endocr Rev 13:635–640, 1993.

208. Ballabio A, Bardoni B, Carrozzo R, et al: Contiguous gene syndromes due to deletions in the distal short arm of the human X chromosome. Proc Natl Acad Sci USA 86:10001–10005, 1989.

209. Meitinger T, Heye B, Petit C, et al: Definitive localization of X-linked Kallman syndrome (hypogonadotropic hypogonadism and anosmia) to Xp22.3: Close linkage to the hypervariable repeat sequence CRI-S232. Am J Hum Genet 47:664–669, 1990.

210. Wray S, Nieburgs A, Elkabes S: Spatiotemporal cell expression of luteinizing hormone–releasing hormone in the prenatal mouse: Evidence for an embryonic origin in the olfactory placode. Brain Res Dev Brain Res 46:309–318, 1989.

211. Bick D, Curry CJ, McGill JR, et al: Male infant with ichthyosis, Kallmann syndrome, chondrodysplasia punctata, and an Xp chromosome deletion. Am J Med Genet 33:100–107, 1989.

212. Gausden E, Coyle B, Armour JA, et al: Pendred syndrome: Evidence for genetic homogeneity and further refinement of linkage. J Med Genet 34:126–129, 1997.

213. Everett LA, Glaser B, Beck JC, et al: Pendred syndrome is caused by mutations in a putative sulphate transporter gene (PDS). Nat Genet 17:411–422, 1997.

214. Scott DA, Wang R, Kreman TM, et al: The Pendred syndrome gene encodes a chloride-iodide transport protein. Nat Genet 21:440–443, 1999.

215. Nagamine K, Peterson P, Scott HS, et al: Positional cloning of the APECED gene. Nat Genet 17:393–398, 1997.

216. Stratakis CA, Carney JA, Lin JP, et al: Carney complex, a familial multiple neoplasia and lentiginosis syndrome. Analysis of 11 kindreds and linkage to the short arm of chromosome 2. J Clin Invest 97:699–705, 1996.

217. New MI: Basic and clinical aspects of congenital adrenal hyperplasia. J Steroid Biochem 27:1–7, 1987.

218. Speiser PW, Laforgia N, Kato K, et al: First trimester prenatal treatment and molecular genetic diagnosis of congenital adrenal hyperplasia (21-hydroxylase deficiency). J Clin Endocrinol Metab 70:838–848, 1990.

219. Pang S, Pollack MS, Marshall RN, et al: Prenatal treatment of congenital adrenal hyperplasia due to 21-hydroxylase deficiency. N Engl J Med 322:111–115, 1990.

220. White PC, Dupont J, New MI, et al: A mutation in CYP11B1 (Arg-448-His) associated with steroid 11 beta-hydroxylase deficiency in Jews of Moroccan origin. J Clin Invest 87:1664–1667, 1991.

221. Kagimoto K, Waterman MR, Kagimoto M, et al: Identification of a common molecular basis for combined 17 alpha-hydroxylase/17,20-lyase deficiency in two Mennonite families. Hum Genet 82:285–286, 1989.

222. Geller DH, Auchus RJ, Mendonca BB, et al: The genetic and functional basis of isolated 17,20-lyase deficiency. Nat Genet 17:201–205, 1997.

223. Rheaume E, Simard J, Morel Y, et al: Congenital adrenal hyperplasia due to point mutations in the type II 3 beta-hydroxysteroid dehydrogenase gene. Nat Genet 1:239–245, 1992.

224. Stocco DM: A review of the characteristics of the protein required for the acute regulation of steroid hormone biosynthesis: The case for the steroidogenic acute regulatory (StAR) protein. Proc Soc Exp Biol Med 217:123–129, 1998.

225. Bose HS, Sugawara T, Strauss JF 3rd, et al: The pathophysiology and genetics of congenital lipoid adrenal hyperplasia. International Congenital Lipoid Adrenal Hyperplasia Consortium. N Engl J Med 335:1870–1878, 1996.

226. Imperato-McGinley J, Gautier T, Peterson RE, et al: The prevalence of 5 alpha-reductase deficiency in children with ambiguous genitalia in the Dominican Republic. J Urol 136:867–873, 1986.

227. Thigpen AE, Davis DL, Milatovich A, et al: Molecular genetics of steroid 5 alpha-reductase 2 deficiency. J Clin Invest 90:799–809, 1992.

228. Thigpen AE, Davis DL, Gautier T, et al: Brief report: The molecular basis of steroid 5 alpha-reductase deficiency in a large Dominican kindred. N Engl J Med 327:1216–1219, 1992.

229. Abramowicz MJ, Targovnik HM, Varela V, et al: Identification of a mutation in the coding sequence of the human thyroid peroxidase gene causing congenital goiter. J Clin Invest 90:1200–1204, 1992.

230. Fujiwara H, Tatsumi K, Miki K, et al: Congenital hypothyroidism caused by a mutation in the Na+/I-symporter. Nat Genet 16:124–125, 1997.

231. Lifton RP, Dluhy RG, Powers M, et al: A chimaeric 11 beta-hydroxylase/aldosterone synthase gene causes glucocorticoid-remediable aldosteronism and human hypertension. Nature 355:262–265, 1992.

232. Kitanaka S, Takeyama K, Murayama A, et al: Inactivating mutations in the 25-hydroxyvitamin D3 1alpha-hydroxylase gene in patients with pseudovitamin D–deficiency rickets. N Engl J Med 338:653–661, 1998.

233. A gene (PEX) with homologies to endopeptidases is mutated in patients with X-linked hypophosphatemic rickets. The HYP Consortium. Nat Genet 11:130–136, 1995.

234. Thomas PM, Cote GJ, Wohllk N, et al: Mutations in the sulfonylurea receptor gene in familial persistent hyperinsulinemic hypoglycemia of infancy. Science 268:426–429, 1995.

235. Thomas P, Ye Y, Lightner E: Mutation of the pancreatic islet inward rectifier Kir6.2 also leads to familial persistent hyperinsulinemic hypoglycemia of infancy. Hum Mol Genet 5:1809–1812, 1996.

236. Ieiri T, Cochaux P, Targovnik HM, et al: A 3' splice site mutation in the thyroglobulin gene responsible for congenital goiter with hypothyroidism. J Clin Invest 88:1901–1905, 1991.

237. Knebelmann B, Boussin L, Guerrier D, et al: Anti-Mullerian hormone Bruxelles: A nonsense mutation associated with the persistent Mullerian duct syndrome. Proc Natl Acad Sci USA 88:3767–3771, 1991.

238. Collu R, Tang J, Castagne J, et al: A novel mechanism for isolated central hypothyroidism: Inactivating mutations in the thyrotropin-releasing hormone receptor gene. J Clin Endocrinol Metab 82:1561–1565, 1997.

239. Laue L, Wu SM, Kudo M, et al: A nonsense mutation of the human luteinizing hormone receptor gene in Leydig cell hypoplasia. Hum Mol Genet 4:1429–1433, 1995.

240. Zhang P, Jobert AS, Couvineau A, et al: A homozygous inactivating mutation in the parathyroid hormone/parathyroid hormone-related peptide receptor causing Blomstrand chondrodysplasia. J Clin Endocrinol Metab 83:3365–3368, 1998.

241. Clark AJ, McLoughlin L, Grossman A: Familial glucocorticoid deficiency associated with point mutation in the adrenocorticotropin receptor. Lancet 341:461–462, 1993.

242. Imbeaud S, Faure E, Lamarre I, et al: Insensitivity to anti-mullerian hormone due to a mutation in the human anti-mullerian hormone receptor. Nat Genet 11:382–388, 1995.

243. Clement K, Vaisse C, Lahlou N, et al: A mutation in the human leptin receptor gene causes obesity and pituitary dysfunction. Nature 392:398–401, 1998.

244. Yeo GS, Farooqi IS, Aminian S, et al: A frameshift mutation in MC4R associated with dominantly inherited human obesity. Nat Genet 20:111–112, 1998.

245. Weiss RE, Refetoff S: Thyroid hormone resistance. Annu Rev Med 43:363–375, 1992.

246. Geller DS, Rodriguez-Soriano J, Vallo Boado A, et al: Mutations in the mineralocorticoid receptor gene cause autosomal dominant pseudohypoaldosteronism type I. Nat Genet 19:279–281, 1998.

247. Zoppi S, Marcelli M, Deslypere JP, et al: Amino acid substitutions in the DNA-binding domain of the human androgen receptor are a frequent cause of receptor-binding positive androgen resistance. Mol Endocrinol 6:409–415, 1992.

248. Deeb SS, Fajas L, Nemoto M, et al: A Pro12Ala substitution in PPARgamma2 associated with decreased receptor activity, lower body mass index and improved insulin sensitivity. Nat Genet 20:284–287, 1998.

249. Yamagata K, Furuta H, Oda N, et al: Mutations in the hepatocyte nuclear factor-4alpha gene in maturity-onset diabetes of the young (MODY1). Nature 384:458–460, 1996.

250. Bos JL: ras oncogenes in human cancer: A review. Cancer Res 49:4682–4689, 1989.

251. Zhang X, Horwitz GA, Heaney AP, et al: Pituitary tumor transforming gene (PTTG) expression in pituitary adenomas. J Clin Endocrinol Metab 84:761–767, 1999.

252. Vogelstein B, Kinzler KW: p53 function and dysfunction. Cell 70:523–526, 1992.

253. Weinberg RA: Tumor suppressor genes. Science 254:1138–1146, 1991.

254. Castilla LH, Couch FJ, Erdos MR, et al: Mutations in the BRCA1 gene in families with early-onset breast and ovarian cancer. Nat Genet 8:387–391, 1994.

255. Weber BH, Brohm M, Stec I, et al: A somatic truncating mutation in BRCA2 in a sporadic breast tumor. Am J Hum Genet 59:962–964, 1996.

256. Yamagata K, Oda N, Kaisaki PJ, et al: Mutations in the hepatocyte nuclear factor-1alpha gene in maturity-onset diabetes of the young (MODY3). Nature 384:455–458, 1996.

257. Horikawa Y, Iwasaki N, Hara M, et al: Mutation in hepatocyte nuclear factor–1 beta gene (TCF2) associated with MODY. Nat Genet 17:384–385, 1997.

258. Jager RJ, Anvret M, Hall K, et al: A human XY female with a frame shift mutation in the candidate testis-determining gene SRY. Nature 348:452–454, 1990.

259. Bick D, Franco B, Sherins RJ, et al: Brief report: Intragenic deletion of the KALIG-1 gene in Kallmann's syndrome. N Engl J Med 326:1752–1755, 1992.

260. Nicholls RD, Knoll JH, Butler MG, et al: Genetic imprinting suggested by maternal heterodisomy in nondeletion Prader-Willi syndrome. Nature 342:281–285, 1989.

261. Latif F, Tory K, Gnarra J, et al: Identification of the von Hippel–Lindau disease tumor suppressor gene. Science 260:1317–1320, 1993.

262. Wilson DI, Cross IE, Goodship JA, et al: DiGeorge syndrome with isolated aortic coarctation and isolated ventricular septal defect in three sibs with a 22q11 deletion of maternal origin. Br Heart J 66:308–312, 1991.

263. Jackson RS, Creemers JW, Ohagi S, et al: Obesity and impaired prohormone processing associated with mutations in the human prohormone convertase 1 gene. Nat Genet 16:303–306, 1997.

264. Hansson JH, Schild L, Lu Y, et al: A de novo missense mutation of the beta subunit of the epithelial sodium channel causes hypertension and Liddle syndrome, identifying a proline-rich segment critical for regulation of channel activity. Proc Natl Acad Sci USA 92:11495–11499, 1995.

265. Scriver CR, Beaudet AL, Sly WS, et al: The Metabolic and Molecular Basis of Inherited Disease. New York, McGraw-Hill, 1995.

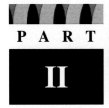

BASIC PHYSIOLOGY

Chapter 12

Functional Pituitary Anatomy and Histology

Sylvia L. Asa ▪ Eva Horvath ▪ Kalman Thomas Kovacs

ANATOMY AND HISTOLOGY OF THE NORMAL GLAND

The pituitary, surrounded by the sphenoid bone and covered with the sellar diaphragm, lies in the sella turcica, near the hypothalamus and optic chiasm.[1] The adult pituitary measures $12 \times 9 \times 6$ mm in diameter and weighs about 0.6 g; it enlarges during pregnancy[2] and although it regresses after cessation of lactation, the enlargement is not completely reversible and the gland may weigh 1 g or even more in multiparous women. The pituitary is capable of producing hormones at quite an early phase of fetal life. At about the end of the third month of gestation the pituitary is grossly apparent, and acidophil and basophil cells can be detected in the anterior lobe.[3] From the sixth week of pregnancy, electron microscopy detects the presence of secretory granules in the cytoplasm of some adenohypophysial cells, and storage of hormones can be demonstrated by using immunocytologic techniques.[4, 5] During embryologic development, the process of adenohypophysial cell differentiation follows a highly specific pattern and temporal sequence.[6] Insights into the molecular basis of cell differentiation and phenotype expression have been advanced by the identification of transcription-regulating proteins that have been implicated as key elements in the definition of cell-specific phenotypes and the regulation of hormone gene expression.

The human pituitary is divided into two parts: (1) the adenohypophysis, which derives from the evagination of the stomodeal ectoderm, known as Rathke's pouch, and (2) the neurohypophysis, which arises from the neural ectoderm of the floor of the forebrain. It has been suggested that the adenohypophysis also is of neuroectodermal derivation, arising from the neural ridge; experimental evidence, obtained in

quail chick chimeras, supports this hypothesis, but data are not yet available in mammalian embryos.[7] Novel transcription factors that play a role in anterior primordial development are implicated in early pituitary organogenesis.[8] These include the bicoid-related pituitary homeobox factor Ptx1, pituitary homeobox factor 2 (Ptx2), *Lhx3* and *Lhx4*, two members of the *Lhx* group of LIM homeobox genes, P-LIM, another LIM homeobox protein, and Rathke's pouch homeobox *(Rpx)* protein. The Prophet of Pit-1 (PROP-1) is a paired-like homeodomain protein that is expressed early in pituitary development. Inactivating mutations of PROP-1 have been identified as the cause of Pit-1 deficiency in Ames dwarf mice[9] and in humans with combined pituitary hormone deficiency.[10, 11]

The adenohypophysis (lobus glandularis), which constitutes approximately 80% of the entire pituitary, consists of the pars distalis (pars anterior, anterior lobe), the pars intermedia (intermediate lobe, intermediate zone), and the pars tuberalis (pars infundibularis, pars proximalis). The pars distalis is the largest and, from the functional point of view, the most important part of the adenohypophysis.

The pars intermedia in the human pituitary[12, 13] is a poorly developed, rudimentary structure with no apparent endocrine significance. It lies between the anterior and posterior lobes and consists of a few cystic cavities lined by cuboidal epithelium and filled with colloid material.

The pars tuberalis is the upward extension of the pars distalis along the pituitary stalk. It is composed of a few layers of chromophobe cells interspersed with occasional acidophil and basophil cells. Although immunocytologic techniques reveal the presence of hormones, mainly follicle-stimulating hormone (FSH) and luteinizing hormone (LH) in the cytoplasm of the pars tuberalis cells,[14] this part of the pituitary is assumed to play no major role in adenohypophysial secretion.

Adenohypophysial cells can be found in two regions outside the adenohypophysis: (1) in the posterior lobe and (2) in the pharyngeal pituitary. Accumulation of basophil cells in the posterior lobe is known as basophil cell invasion[12, 13] and is noted in more than 50% of adult autopsies. It is not apparent before puberty, and it occurs more frequently in men and with advancing age. The cells are periodic–acid schiff (PAS) positive but smaller and less granular than those of the anterior lobe. In some cases, they are numerous and spread deeply into the posterior lobe. Basophil cell invasion is not associated with any specific endocrine abnormality, disease, or therapy. Although immunocytologic techniques have revealed the presence of adrenocorticotropic hormone (ACTH) and other proopiomelanocortin (POMC)-derived peptides in these cells, their principal function is unknown.

The pharyngeal hypophysis,[15, 16] usually less than 4 mm in diameter, is embedded in the sphenoid bone and consists of small clusters of poorly differentiated chromophobe cells and occasional acidophil and basophil cells. Unlike the pars distalis, it has a rich innervation but no portal blood supply; that is, the blood flowing through the pharyngeal hypophysis contains no hypothalamic-regulating hormones. Although immunocytologic techniques have detected the presence of adenohypophysial hormones in the cytoplasm of these cells[17, 18] and although it has been claimed that it can take over some of the functions of the anterior pituitary in cases of hypophysectomy or hypopituitarism, no direct evidence indicates that the pharyngeal hypophysis plays a major role in endocrine secretion.

A substantial knowledge of pituitary circulation[19, 20] is of fundamental importance if one wishes to understand the functional correlations between the hypothalamus and pituitary and the details of how adenohypophysial secretory activity is regulated by the hypophysiotropic area of the hypothalamus. The pituitary receives its blood supply from the superior and inferior hypophysial arteries. The superior hypophysial arteries arise from the internal carotid arteries. Some of their branches penetrate the infundibulum (the funnel-shaped upper end of the neural stalk attached to the bottom surface of the hypothalamus) and terminate either in gomitoli or in the capillary network around the gomitoli. The gomitoli lie in large numbers in the infundibulum and upper part of the neural stalk. They are about 1 to 2 mm long and 50 to 100 μm wide and consist of a long central artery with a strong muscular coat surrounded by a dense capillary plexus. Their function is not clearly understood, but they appear to regulate blood flow to the anterior lobe and also to the adjacent capillary network, thereby affecting the entry of hypothalamic-regulating hormones into the blood stream. The hypothalamic-regulating hormones produced in various parts of the hypothalamus flow downward along the nerve fibers to the infundibulum. The perigomitolar capillary network is the site at which they enter the circulation. Larger parallel veins are formed from these capillaries. These are the long portal vessels that run down the pituitary stalk and terminate in the capillaries of the anterior lobe, carrying with them in high concentration the hypothalamic-regulating hormones. The short portal vessels, originating in the distal part of the stalk and in the posterior lobe, also penetrate the anterior lobe and transport susbstances from the posterior pituitary to the pars distalis.

The question of whether the anterior lobe receives blood exclusively from the portal circulation or has some additional direct arterial blood supply is not fully resolved. Some data[20] seem to indicate that 70% to 90% of adenohypophysial blood comes from the large portal vessels and the remainder from the short portal vessels. Early morphologic studies showed that the loral artery not only supplies the infundibulum and upper part of the stalk with blood but also gives rise to the artery of the fibrous core, which penetrates the anterior lobe without passing through the infundibulum and carries arterial blood to the adenohypophysial cells. Conflicting evidence has been published by Bergland and Page[21] denying the role of the loral artery in the blood supply of the pars distalis. Other sources of direct arterial blood to the adenohypophysis are the capsular arteries. These arteries arise from the inferior hypophysial arteries and not only supply blood to the pituitary capsule but also penetrate the superficial portions of the adenohypophysis, transporting arterial blood to a few cell rows beneath the capsule. Recent studies of 182 human pituitaries, performed by Gorczyca and Hardy,[22] confirm the roles of the middle hypophysial artery and small capsular arteries in supplying direct arterial blood to

the anterior lobe. The inferior hypophysial arteries, originating in the internal carotid arteries, supply blood to the posterior lobe and do not participate in adenohypophysial circulation outside the capsular arteries. Venous blood is transported from the pituitary via the adjacent venous sinuses into the internal jugular vein. Observations[21] on vascular casts have led to the revelation that the volume of venous drainage from the pars distalis is considerably smaller than that of portal blood reaching the gland. This discrepancy prompted Bergland and Page[21] to postulate that the direction of blood flow within the common neurohypophysial vascular bed may be reversed, causing the short portal vessels to serve as both afferent and efferent channels. Such a mechanism would indeed be of utmost importance in hypothalamic regulatory functions.

Electron microscopic studies revealed that the capillaries of the anterior lobe consist of fenestrated endothelium, subendothelial space, and a distinct basal lamina.[12] Hormones released from adenohypophysial cells first have to pass through their own basal lamina and subsequently all the layers of the capillary walls before entering the circulation. Secretory granules, which contain the hormone within the adenohypophysial cells, become invisible following their release. Thus, the process of hormone transport between the cell and the capillary lumen cannot be studied currently by morphologic techniques, nor is sufficient information available on various factors that may affect this process.

Despite its close proximity to the brain, the anterior lobe contains no nerves except for a few sympathetic fibers that enter the adenohypophysis along the vessels. These fibers may influence blood flow to the anterior lobe, but innervation has no significance in regulating adenohypophysial secretory activity. The hypothalamus influences adenohypophysial function by the releasing and inhibiting hormones that are transported to the anterior lobe via the portal vessels. The posterior lobe,[13, 19] which consists histologically of nerve fibers, nerve endings with neurosecretory granules containing vasopressin, oxytocin, and neurophysins, and glial cells (pituicytes), has a rich arterial blood supply independent of the anterior lobe. The inferior hypophysial arteries, which arise in the internal carotid arteries, supply the posterior lobe with blood. The posterior lobe is richly innervated by the supraopticohypophysial and the tuberohypophysial tracts. The supraopticohypophysial tract arises in the supraoptic and paraventricular nuclei, located in the anterior part of the hypothalamus.[19] The tuberohypophysial tract originates in the central and posterior parts of the hypothalamus. Both tracts reach the posterior lobe via the pituitary stalk. The integrity of the neurohypophysial structure depends upon its innervation: the posterior lobe undergoes marked atrophy following destruction of the pituitary stalk or from various hypothalamic lesions interfering with the integrity of supraopticohypophysial or tuberohypophysial tracts.[19] The neurons of the supraoptic and paraventricular nuclei also atrophy if their axons are damaged.[23]

Cytology of Normal and Abnormal Gland

Currently, six distinct cell types are believed to exist in the human adenohypophysis, distinguished by their distribution, histology, ultrastructure, and hormone content.[12, 13] It was once believed that one cell could make only one hormone. However, it was recognized long ago that pituitary adenomas were often plurihormonal.[24] The concept of plurihormonality in pituitary adenomas was controversial and poorly understood. A number of elegant techniques such as multiple labeling ultrastructural immunocytochemistry, the sequential reverse hemolytic plaque assay (RHPA) or the RHPA combined with immunocytochemistry, and combined in situ hybridization with immunohistochemistry, all were applied to prove that one cell is capable of producing more than one hormone.

Advances in our recognition of the factors that regulate cell differentiation in the adenohypophysis have led to a more sophisticated understanding of the mechanisms that determine the patterns of hormone production in adenohypophysial cells and pituitary adenomas. The molecular factors that determine hormone production have now been identified as transcription factors that target specific hormone genes.

These factors have clarified three main pathways of cell differentiation.[25] The complex family of Pit-1-expressing cells can mature into somatotrophs, mammosomatotrophs, lactotrophs, or thyrotrophs with the additional expression of estrogen receptor α (ER-α), which enhances prolactin (PRL) secretion, or thyrotroph embryonic factor (TEF) which stimulates TSH-β production. ACTH-producing corticotrophs are determined by corticotropin upstream transcription-binding element (CUTE) proteins, including neuroD1/beta2. Bihormonal gonadotrophs require expression of steroidogenic factor-1 (SF-1). The recognition of these molecular determinants of adenohypophysial cytodifferentiation has clarified the patterns of plurihormonality which have been recognized in pituitary adenomas, and provide a framework for classification of these tumors.

Somatotrophs

Somatotrophs, or growth hormone (GH)–producing cells, constitute approximately 50% of the adenohypophysial cell population. The middle-sized ovoid cells, residing chiefly in the lateral wings of the anterior lobe, stain with acid dyes (acidophils) and show strong cytoplasmic immunoreactivity for GH. A subset of GH cells contains and probably secretes glycoprotein hormone α subunit. These cells have strong nuclear positivity for Pit-1.

By electron microscopy, the majority of the somatotrophs are spherical or oval cells with a spherical nucleus; well-developed, lamellar, rough-surfaced endoplasmic reticulum (RER) located at the periphery of the cells; and a prominent Golgi complex, usually containing a few immature secretory granules (Fig. 12–1). Many GH cells are densely granulated, possessing a large number of spherical, evenly dense secretory granules measuring between 250 and 500 nm, the majority between 350 and 450 nm. Less densely granulated cells with lucent cytoplasm also occur.

The number, immunoreactivity, and ultrastructure of GH cells appear remarkably stable throughout life and in various pathologic conditions. No distinct morphologic appearance is recognized for the functionally suppressed somatotroph. Some cases of hyposomatotropism are associated with a reduction or absence of somatotrophs, such as in

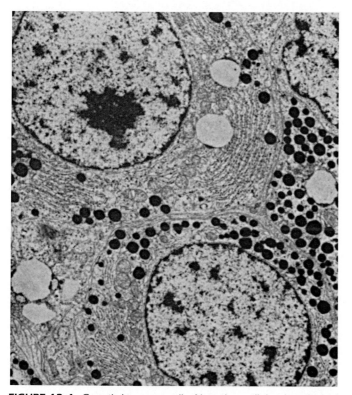

FIGURE 12–1. *Growth hormone cells. Note the well-developed rough endoplasmic reticulum and the numerous dense secretory granules (×7900).*

association with Pit-1 deficiency,[8] but most patients with pituitary dwarfism seem to have a nearly normal GH and somatotroph content,[26] and respond appropriately to GH-releasing hormone (GHRH),[27] suggesting that the primary lesion resides outside of the pituitary.

Mammosomatotrophs

A contingent of the GH cell population is capable of producing PRL as well.[28] These dual secretors, called mammosomatotrophs, are considered transitional cells with potential for alternating between somatotroph and lactotroph functions.[29] These large acidophilic cells are difficult to detect using conventional histology or even immunohistochemistry, but the application of double staining techniques, particularly at the level of the electron microscope using immunogold,[28] allows recognition of their bihormonal nature.

Their ultrastructural appearance resembles that of densely granulated somatotrophs but is distinguished by pleomorphic and unusually large secretory granules that often have a mottled rather than a homogeneous core. These cells also exhibit the hallmark of PRL secretion, the presence of granule extrusions along the lateral cell membrane known as "misplaced exocytosis."

Lactotrophs

Lactotrophs, the PRL-producing cells also called mammotrophs, belong to the acidophil cell series and are less numerous than the somatotrophs, constituting 10% to 30% of the total cell population. This cell type, scattered throughout the pars distalis and showing focal accumulation within the posterolateral areas, can be demonstrated by their strong PRL immunoreactivity, localized chiefly in the Golgi region. Only a small minority of PRL cells are granulated densely enough to display diffuse cytoplasmic staining. They also have strong nuclear Pit-1 reactivity and stain for ER-α.

By electron microscopy, the uncommon densely granulated PRL cell is ovoid and contains parallel arrays of well-developed RER and a prominent Golgi complex. The spherical or ovoid secretory granules are numerous and measure in the range of 400 to 700 nm. The majority of PRL cells have a middle-sized or small polyhedral cell body with long processes. The lucent cytoplasm contains abundant RER, a well-developed Golgi complex, and small (200 to 350 nm), sparse secretory granules (Fig. 12–2). The fine-structural marker of the PRL cell is misplaced exocytosis, that is, extrusion of secretory granules on the lateral cell membranes, distant from the capillaries.

A sharp increase in the number of PRL cells (hyperplasia) occurs in pregnancy and lactation[2, 30] and as a result of estrogen treatment.[31] During development of gestational PRL cell hyperplasia (Fig. 12–3), some of the PRL-producing cells appear to be recruited from the bihormonal mammosomatotroph population.[29]

PRL cells show signs of suppression in glands harboring PRL cell adenoma or in cases of dopamine agonist treatment. Such cells are decreased in size, have dark heterochromatic nucleus, have lost most of their RER and Golgi membranes, but still show signs of exocytosis.[31]

Thyrotrophs

Thyrotrophs, or TSH-producing cells, constitute approximately 5% of adenohypophysial cells. Their cytoplasm stains with the PAS technique, aldehyde fuchsin, and aldehyde thionin. TSH cells, however, are best identified with the immunoperoxidase technique using specific monoclonal antibodies raised against TSH-β.[13] They also contain α subunit and Pit-1 immunoreactivity, but these markers are not specific for thyrotrophs.

Electron microscopy reveals that the elongated, characteristically angular cells possess short profiles of slightly dilated RER and globular Golgi complex with numerous Golgi vesicles. The small secretory granules measure 100 to 300 nm, are mostly spherical, vary in electron opacity, and, especially in sparsely granulated cells, are often positioned near the plasmalemma.

Thyrotrophs undergo hypertrophy and hyperplasia in various forms of primary hypothyroidism, such as chronic thyroiditis, surgical or radiation thyroidectomy, or prolonged treatment with goitrogens.[31, 32]

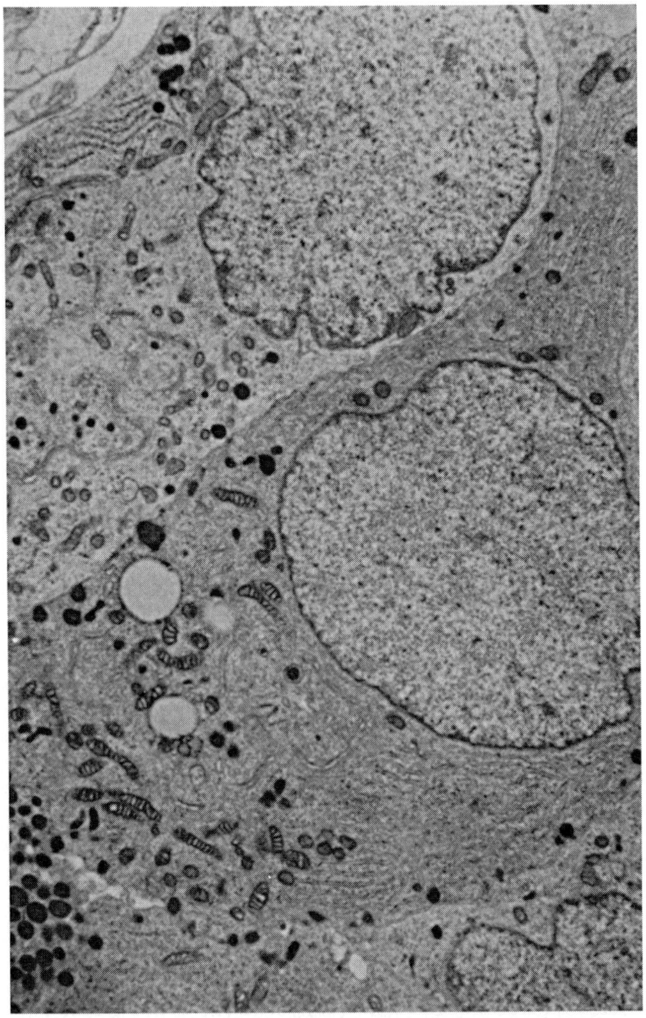

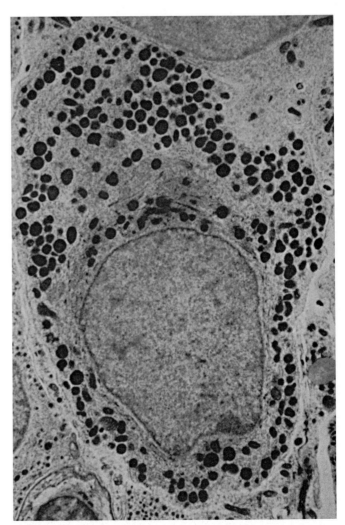

FIGURE 12–2. Sparsely granulated prolactin cell. The Golgi complex is prominent with numerous developing secretory granules (×7100).

The markedly enlarged "thyroidectomy" cells contain immunoreactive TSH. The stimulated thyrotrophs possess extensively developed, dilated RER and prominent Golgi apparatus containing developing secretory granules. The number of secretory granules in the cytoplasm may be reduced. Accumulation of lysosomes, appearing as coarse PAS-

and aldehyde thionin–positive globules in histologic specimens, is common. Thyrotrophs regress following treatment with thyroxine (T_4) or in cases of Graves' disease.[33] The fine structure of suppressed thyrotrophs in the human pituitary has not been sufficiently explored.

Corticotrophs

Corticotrophs, or ACTH-producing cells, constitute approximately 20% of adenohypophysial cells and are basophilic and PAS positive. Corticotrophs can also be identified with the immunoperoxidase technique by using specific antisera raised against 1–39 ACTH and some other derivatives of the POMC molecule such as β-lipotropin (β-lipotropic pituitary hormone, β-LPH) and endorphins.

By electron microscopy, the elongated, angular cells have round or slightly irregular nuclei. The well-developed RER usually appears in the form of widely dispersed, slightly dilated profiles. The prominent Golgi complex may contain immature secretory granules. The cytoplasm usually harbors a large number of spherical or irregular, slightly dented, or heart-shaped secretory granules having different electron density and measuring 250 to 400 nm in diameter (Fig. 12–4). Features facilitating the recognition of this cell type are the morphology of secretory granules, the frequent occurrence of large lysosomal bodies, and the presence of filaments that measure about 70 Å in width and represent cytokeratins.[34, 35]

Untreated primary adrenal insufficiency is rarely seen today. In such cases, the enlarged pituitary corticotrophs contain little granulation.[31] Massive diffuse nodular hyperplasia or adenoma may develop in situations of prolonged glucocorticoid deficiency.[36]

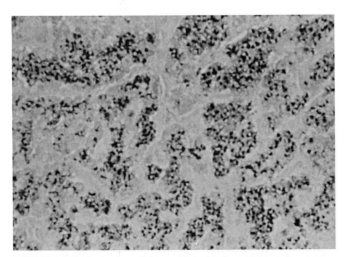

FIGURE 12–3. Prolactin cell hyperplasia in the pituitary of a woman who died during the third trimester of pregnancy (Immunoperoxidase method for prolactin, ×100).

FIGURE 12–4. Corticotroph cell. Note the often indented or irregular secretory granules and bundles of type 1 microfilaments adjacent to the nucleus, the morphologic markers of this cell type (×9400).

The most common morphologic abnormality of human corticotrophs is Crooke's hyalinization (Fig. 12–5), constituted by the perinuclear accumulation of a faintly eosinophilic, glassy, homogeneous substance displacing the cytoplasmic granules to the cell periphery. This phenomenon is seen in conditions of endogenous or exogenous hypercortisolism. Crooke's hyaline material is composed of keratin filaments that are immunoreactive with antibodies against low-molecular-weight cytokeratins,[34] and contains no ACTH.

Gonadotrophs

According to current views, one cell type secretes both gonadotropic hormones (FSH and LH). FSH and LH cells, or gonadotropin-producing cells, constitute approximately 15% of the adenohypophysial cell population. They are PAS positive and contain cytoplasmic immunoreactivity for β subunits of FSH and LH, as well as α subunit. They exhibit nuclear staining for SF-1. By electron microscopy, the middle-sized or small ovoid cells always have a considerable surface area adjoining the capillaries. The cells possess uniform spherical or ovoid nuclei. The well-developed RER consists of slightly dilated meandering cisternae containing a fine granular substance of low electron density. The RER may occupy as much as 15% of the cytoplasmic area. The mitochondria are rod-shaped and moderately dense, with numerous lamellar cristae. The large ring-shaped Golgi complex may contain immature secretory granules. The majority of the secretory granules measure between 250 and 300 nm, but larger granules with a diameter of 400 to 450 nm occur regularly as well. Following removal of the ovaries or testes and in various other forms of primary hypogonadism, gonadotrophs enlarge and become vacuolated (castration cells)[31] (Fig. 12–6). By electron microscopy, the marked changes consist of a sharp increase in volume density of the dilated RER (up to 50%) and hypertrophy of the Golgi complex. Many of these castration cells become sparsely granulated, with margination of remaining secretory granules along the cell membrane.

An interesting finding is the juxtaposition of gonadotrophs and PRL cells[31] in the human as well as rodent pituitary, suggesting a paracrine relationship between the two cell types.[37]

Follicular Cells and Folliculostellate Cells

Follicular cells are epithelial cells joined by terminal bars and forming follicle- or acinus-like structures, but they are not delimited by basement membrane as are true follicles.[31, 38] Most of them are practically agranular. The function of follicles is unclear. They may be formed by different types of granulated cells, undergoing degranulation and other marked cytologic changes, around the foci of ruptured glandular cells.[38]

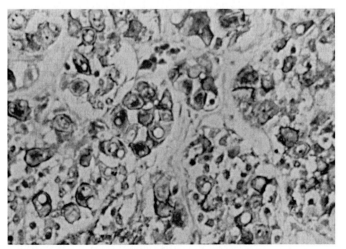

FIGURE 12–5. Crooke's hyalinization of corticotrophs. Note the unstained ringlike accumulation of Crooke's hyalin in a case of ectopic ACTH syndrome. (Lead hematoxylin, ×250.)

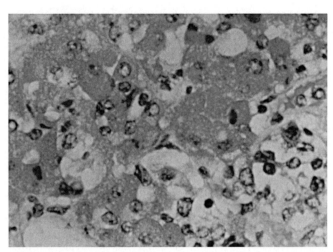

FIGURE 12–6. This large group of hypertrophied cells with finely vacuolated cytoplasm (positive for anti-FSH-β and anti-LH-β) represents gonadotroph cell hyperplasia in the pituitary of an elderly man with Klinefelter's syndrome. (PAS technique, ×400.)

Folliculostellate cells, also known as stellate cells to avoid confusion with follicular cells, are agranular cells that are immunoreactive for S100 protein; some also contain immunoreactivity for glial fibrillary acidic protein (GFAP).[39, 40] They are believed to have a supportive role similar to that of the sustentacular cells of the adrenal medulla and paraganglia. Experimental evidence suggests that these cells produce a number of cytokines and play a role in the paracrine regulation of adjacent hormone-secreting cells.[41]

ANATOMY AND HISTOLOGY OF THE ABNORMAL GLAND

Although the pathologic anatomy of the anterior lobe is not dealt with here in detail, it is pertinent to give a brief account of some abnormalities that affect the structure of the anterior lobe and can be associated with changes in adenohypophysial secretory activity and clinical symptoms. These lesions are not limited to a specific cell type; nevertheless, they have considerable importance in endocrine pathology.

Vascular Lesions

Lesions caused by circulatory disturbances constitute an important portion of adenohypophysial pathology. Hemorrhages in the anterior lobe are uncommon. They are found in association with head injuries or with rapidly growing pituitary neoplasms. Proliferation of tumor cells may alter intrahypophysial pressure, resulting in the compression of vascular walls and the redistribution of blood, and the vessels may undergo hypoxic injury. In cases of severe vascular damage, the vessel walls may be impaired to such an extent that they can no longer withstand rises in blood pressure and rupture. Pituitary apoplexy is the extreme variant of this process.[42] Occasionally, almost the entire tumor can undergo destruction. In cases of hormone-secreting adenomas, massive hemorrhage may cause striking amelioration of the clinical symptoms, even hypopituitarism.

Infarcts are due to interruption of blood supply to the anterior lobe. Smaller necrotic foci in the adenohypophysis are not an uncommon finding at autopsy[43, 44] and occur in approximately 1% to 6% of unselected autopsy material. Smaller infarcts remain unrecognized clinically and can be noted only by histologic investigation. Severe hypopituitarism occurs only if more than 90% of functional adenohypophysial parenchyma is destroyed.

Adenohypophysial infarcts can be found in association with various diseases.[43, 44] They can be detected more frequently in patients with diabetes mellitus, after head injury, and in association with cerebrovascular accidents, increased intracranial pressure, and epidemic hemorrhagic fever. Adenohypophysial infarction develops following transection or destruction of the pituitary stalk, which interrupts blood flow to the anterior lobe. Frequent occurrences of adenohypophysial necrosis have been reported in patients who, as a result of various diseases, are maintained on mechanical ventilators or respirators before they die.[45, 46] Histologically, the lesions correspond to coagulative infarcts and are frequently, but not always, accompanied by severe hypoxic lesions of the brain ("respirator brain").

A special form of pituitary infarction, rarely seen today in developed countries, is postpartum pituitary necrosis, which is found in women who die during the puerperium after a complicated labor.[47] These women usually suffer severe blood loss and are in shock around the time of delivery, the most common obstetric factors being retained placenta and postpartum hemorrhage. At the end of gestation, the enlarged anterior lobe appears to be unusually susceptible to ischemic necrosis because shock in men and in nonpregnant women is only rarely accompanied by pituitary infarction. Fibrous atrophy is the final phase of ischemic necrosis of the anterior lobe. The necrotic areas are gradually replaced by fibrous tissue. Adenohypophysial cells are not capable of sufficient regeneration, so permanent hypopituitarism may develop in cases of extensive infarction. Postpartum hypopituitarism due to massive adenohypophysial ischemic infarction is called Sheehan's syndrome, after the Liverpool pathologist who described numerous details of this intriguing disease entity.

Hyperplasias

Stimulation by GHRH, produced by various endocrine neoplasms, leads to a potentially massive GH cell hyperplasia causing acromegaly or gigantism.[48, 49] Such lesions usually are strongly acidophilic, consisting of densely granulated somatotrophs distinguished only by unusually prominent Golgi apparatus. Rarely, patients may go on to develop adenomas.[25] Patients with McCune-Albright syndrome develop mammosomatotroph hyperplasia[50]; a similar lesion has been described as idiopathic hyperplasia, inducing gigantism.[51] Both forms of hyperplasia may eventually lead to formation of adenoma.

PRL cell hyperplasia may accompany neoplastic or non-neoplastic pituitary lesions, such as corticotroph adenomas, thyrotroph hyperplasia, or any suprasellar mass of pituitary or nonpituitary origin impinging upon the pituitary stalk. The association of PRL cell adenoma and hyperplasia seldom occurs. Idiopathic PRL cell hyperplasia as a sole pathologic lesion accounting for clinically evident hyperprolactinemia and its sequelae is exceptionally rare.[52, 53] By morphology, it consists of enlarged, stimulated cells with excessively developed RER and Golgi membranes, sparse secretory granules, and exocytosis similar to PRL cell hyperplasia caused by estrogen excess or loss of dopamine inhibition.

Thyrotroph hyperplasia in patients with untreated hypothyroidism may be associated with significant enlargement of the pituitary gland and sometimes with elevation of serum PRL levels, thereby mimicking PRL-producing adenoma.[54, 55] Such a combination of signs is known to have led to unwarranted surgical exploration of the pituitary. Treatment with physiologic doses of thyroid hormone results in regression of the hyperplasia.

Idiopathic corticotroph hyperplasia is an uncommon cause of Cushing's disease.[56, 57] The proliferation of corticotrophs may be dispersed, not leading to changes in tissue architecture, or nodular, associated with expansion and distortion of reticulin network. Massive nodular corticotroph hyperplasia may be seen in cases of ectopic production of corticotropin-releasing hormone (CRH).[58]

Inflammatory Lesions

Massive destruction of the adenohypophysis may occur in various inflammatory lesions. Infectious causes include tuberculosis and syphilis, as well as the opportunistic infections seen in patients with acquired immunodeficiency syndrome (AIDS).[59]

An autoimmune mechanism has been postulated as the cause of lymphocytic hypophysitis.[60] This chronic inflammatory disorder occurs most often in women, usually late in pregnancy or in the postpartum period. It is frequently associated with hyperprolactinemia and mimics prolactinoma; the inflamed gland is enlarged and may even extend beyond the sella with symptoms of suprasellar involvement. Inflammatory destruction may cause hypopituitarism, but it can be transient with full recovery. Rarely, the disease has been associated with isolated pituitary hormone deficiency, suggesting selective destruction by targeted antibodies.

Inflammatory lesions characterized by granulomatous inflammation, including sarcoidosis and the idiopathic giant cell granuloma, may cause extensive damage to the anterior lobe with resultant hypopituitarism. They may present as mass lesions and mimic adenoma. The cause of localized giant cell granuloma may be autoimmune and some investigators have suggested that it is related to lymphocytic hypophysitis.[61, 62]

Cysts

Non-neoplastic cysts in the sellar region[13] can cause tissue destruction by compression with resulting hypopituitarism. When they interfere with the pituitary portal vascular supply and hypothalamic regulation, they can cause hypopituitarism with hyperprolactinemia.

Rathke's cleft cysts are mucus-containing remnants of Rathke's pouch lined by ciliated cuboidal or columnar epithelium; they usually occur within the sella but suprasellar extension is not uncommon. Arachnoid, dermoid, and epidermoid cysts can form within or above the sella.

PITUITARY NEOPLASMS

Pituitary neoplasms, which constitute approximately 10% of all intracranial tumors, can be primary or secondary, benign or malignant, hormone-producing or functionally inactive. Only the most important forms are dealt with here.

Pituitary Adenomas

Pituitary adenomas, the most frequent primary tumors of this gland, are benign neoplasms arising in adenohypophysial cells[12, 13, 63] (Fig. 12–7). They used to be divided into chromophobe, acidophil, and basophil tumors, but this classification is misleading when correlation of structure is made with secretory activity. Chromophobe adenomas are highly active tumors in some cases, capable of secreting various

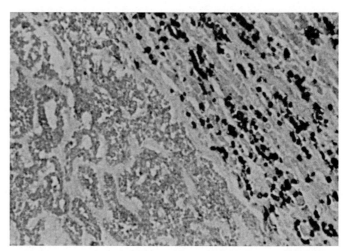

FIGURE 12–7. Border of a "chromophobe" adenoma and of surrounding nontumorous gland. The tumor contains no immunoreactive hormones. (Immunoperoxidase technique for growth hormone, ×100.)

pituitary hormones, such as GH, PRL, and ACTH. Acidophil adenomas can produce GH or PRL or can be functionless. Basophil adenomas may secrete ACTH or may be inactive endocrinologically. Thus, the distinction of chromophobe, acidophil, and basophil adenomas discloses only the tinctorial characteristics of the cytoplasm of adenoma cells; it fails to shed light on their functional activity or on the hormones they produce.

According to current classification, based primarily on immunocytochemistry and electron microscopy, pituitary adenomas can be divided into the following morphologic entities:

1. Somatotroph adenomas
2. Mammosomatotroph and mixed somatotroph-lactotroph adenomas
3. Lactotroph adenomas
4. Acidophil stem-cell adenomas
5. Thyrotroph adenomas
6. Corticotroph adenomas
7. Gonadotroph adenomas
8. Null cell adenomas and oncocytomas
9. Plurihormonal adenomas

Many of these tumor types are associated with clinical syndromes of hormone excess; however, approximately one third of pituitary adenomas are classified clinically as nonfunctioning adenomas because they are unassociated with clinical or biochemical evidence of hormone hypersecretion. These clinically silent adenomas may have immunohistochemical and ultrastructural evidence of differentiation and can be morphologically classified as one of the above entities.

Somatotroph Adenomas

GH-producing tumors of the pituitary are usually clinically associated with acromegaly or gigantism. Two morphologic variants are known to exist. In our surgical material, the incidence of the two types of GH cell adenomas is very close. Contrary to earlier claims, we have found no correlation between serum GH level and morphologic type of pituitary adenoma.

The acidophilic, densely granulated GH cell adenoma is a highly differentiated tumor that usually exhibits a slow growth rate, often not expanding beyond the boundaries of the sella. The cytoplasm of adenoma cells shows a strong overall positivity for immunoreactive GH (Fig. 12–8) and often contains α subunit as well as nuclear Pit-1 reactivity. Ultrastructurally, the adenoma cells display a strong resemblance to nontumorous somatotrophs, possessing regular nuclei with light chromatin, prominent nucleolus, and well-developed cytoplasm (Fig. 12–9). The RER, arranged in parallel cisternae at the cell periphery, is prominent. The sacculi of the conspicuous Golgi apparatus consistently harbor developing secretory granules. The mitochondria

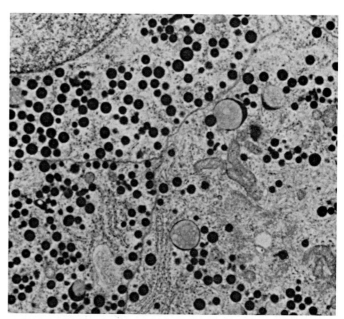

FIGURE 12–9. *Densely granulated growth hormone cell adenoma (×9300). (From Horvath E. Kovacs K: Ultrastructural classification of pituitary adenomas. Can J Neurol Sci 3:9–21, 1976.)*

show regular features. In the rest of the cytoplasm, the secretory granules are numerous and have closely fitted, limiting membrane and high electron opacity. They measure mostly 300 to 500 nm, but considerably larger granules may be noted as well as an anomaly of granule formation; elongated, pointed, or rhomboid granules may be present occasionally.

The sparsely granulated GH cell adenomas are mostly chromophobic, often displaying nuclear pleomorphism. These tumors are more likely to run an aggressive course characterized by faster growth rate, sellar erosion, and parasellar extension. At the time of pituitary surgery, the average age of patients harboring sparsely granulated GH cell adenoma is lower than the age of those with the densely granulated variant. Immunocytochemistry reveals Pit-1 in the pleomorphic nucleus and GH in the cytoplasm of adenoma cells. The positivity for GH, however, is usually limited to the Golgi region owing to the sparsity of secretory granules. In contrast to the densely granulated variant, sparsely granulated somatotroph adenomas are decorated by antibodies to low-molecular-weight cytokeratins with a characteristic juxtanuclear globular positivity that indicates the presence of fibrous bodies.[64] Sparsely granulated adenomatous GH cells have a highly distinctive ultrastructure that has little in common with the well-differentiated, densely granulated type. They are irregular with strikingly pleomorphic, often crescent-shaped or multiple nuclei. The RER is fairly well developed in randomly scattered profiles. Sparsely granulated GH cell adenomas regularly contain smooth-surfaced endoplasmic reticulum (SER) in association with the fibrous bodies. The Golgi apparatus is well developed. The most distinguishing diagnostic feature of this adenoma type is the occurrence of spherical fibrous bodies (Fig. 12–10). They are composed of concentrically arranged type 2 cytokeratin filaments (average width 115 Å) or tubular SER, or both, and are invariably located in the Golgi region, often displacing the Golgi apparatus. Various cytoplasmic components may be engulfed within the fibrous bodies. The incidence of these structures varies from case to case, but they are usually numerous. Another characteristic mark of sparsely granulated GH cell adenomas is the frequent occurrence of supernumerary centrioles, which are usually located near or within the fibrous bodies. The reason for the accumulation of centrioles, which occurs selectively in sparsely granulated GH cell adenomas and acidophilic stem-cell adenomas, is unknown. The secretory granules are spherical and sparse and usually measure no more than 250 nm. Deposition of endocrine amyloid may be an additional feature in both densely and sparsely granulated GH cell tumors.[65]

The medical treatment of GH-producing adenomas, often in a form

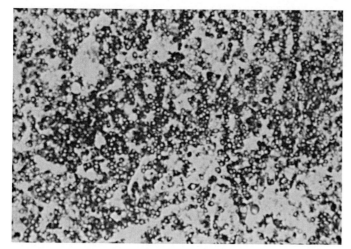

FIGURE 12–8. *Densely granulated growth hormone cell adenoma exhibiting strong cytoplasmic immunostaining for human growth hormone. (Immunoperoxidase technique, ×100.)*

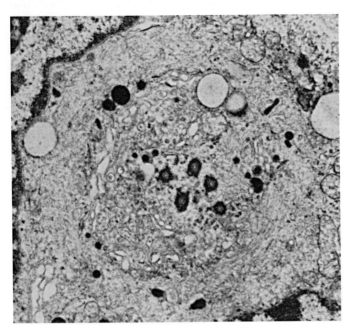

FIGURE 12–10. *Sparsely granulated growth hormone cell adenoma. Group of five centrioles encircled by type 2 microfilaments of a fibrous body (×17,300). (From Kovacs K. Horvath E, Strattman IE, Ezrin C: Cytoplasmic microfilaments in the anterior lobe of the human pituitary gland. Acta Anat 87:414–426, 1974.)*

of preoperative medication, is becoming increasingly common. At present, a long-acting analogue of somatostatin (Sandostatin, octreotide acetate, SMS 201-995) is the most frequently used compound[66]; the morphologic effects of the drug are variable[67] and show no close correlations with the clinical effects of treatment. Varying degrees of perivascular or interstitial fibrosis are the most common change. A significant reduction in the volume of tumor or the number of tumor cells is infrequent. If it occurs, it is usually associated with increased size and volume density of secretory granules. Other morphologic alterations, such as lysosomal accumulation with crinophagy or onco-cytic change, are not consistently present either.

Mammosomatotroph and Mixed Somatotroph-Lactotroph Adenomas

In about 40% of acromegalic patients, hypersecretion of GH is accompanied by simultaneous elevation of serum PRL levels. In a number of cases, this finding signifies that the growing tumor, imping-ing upon the stalk, median eminence, and hypophysiotropic area of the hypothalamus, interferes with the production, release, or transport of PRL-inhibiting factor(s) (PIFs), resulting in increased PRL secretion from the nontumorous part of the pituitary. In other cases, hyperprolac-tinemia is caused by a bihormonal pituitary neoplasm.[68] The morpho-logic, especially fine-structural analysis, is the only reliable way to reveal the exact nature of pituitary lesions in such cases.

Mammosomatotroph adenomas are monomorphous, bihormonal ad-enomas that are well differentiated, slowly growing lesions. The ade-noma cells are acidophilic by histology; they show intense cytoplasmic positivity for immunoreactive GH and strong nuclear staining for Pit-1. Immunostaining for PRL, present in the same cells, is usually less diffuse. These tumors often have cytoplasmic positivity for α subunit and may occasionally contain scattered cells with TSH-β reactivity. The fine-structural appearance of the tumor bears strong resemblance to that of highly differentiated, densely granulated GH cell adenomas but the secretory granules are more pleomorphic and unusually large, measuring up to 2000 nm. Large, irregular secretory granules with a mottled core and extrusions of large granules, with permanence of extruded secretory material in the intercellular spaces, are the fine-structural markers of this adenoma type (Fig. 12–11). Some of these tumors, beginning in childhood, may have less typical features.[69]

The bimorphous mixed GH cell–PRL cell adenomas are associated clinically with acromegaly or gigantism and varying degrees of hyper-prolactinemia. By histology, they are acidophilic to chromophobic, depending on the number of cytoplasmic granules. The immunoperoxi-dase technique reveals GH and PRL in different cell populations. The distribution of the two cell types may be uneven in some tumors. The ultrastructural details of GH cells and PRL cells are identical to those described earlier in this chapter as either densely or sparsely granulated forms. Although every variant may occur in mixed adenomas, the combination of densely granulated GH cells and sparsely granulated PRL cells appears to be the most frequent (Fig. 12–12). It should be noted that some mixed tumors, especially those of children and adolescents, may contain some bihormonal cells, chiefly mammosoma-totrophs, as well.[70]

Lactotroph Adenomas

PRL cell adenoma is the most common endocrinologically active tumor type, accounting for about 25% of symptomatic pituitary tumors in adult surgical material. In recent years, the number of surgical cases has noticeably declined, owing to the wider use of dopaminergic agonists (bromocriptine, lisuride, quinagolide) in the management of PRL-producing tumors.

As with GH-producing tumors, two morphologic variants of PRL cell adenomas are recognized, but, in the case of lactotroph adenomas, there is a marked predominance of the sparsely granulated variant. The two adenoma types cannot be distinguished clinically, as both forms are associated with signs and symptoms of hyperprolactinemia.

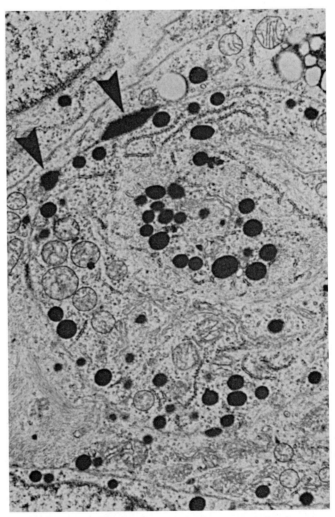

FIGURE 12–11. *Mammosomatotroph adenoma possessing large secre-tory granules and deposits of secretory material in the intercellular space (arrowheads) (×11,900).*

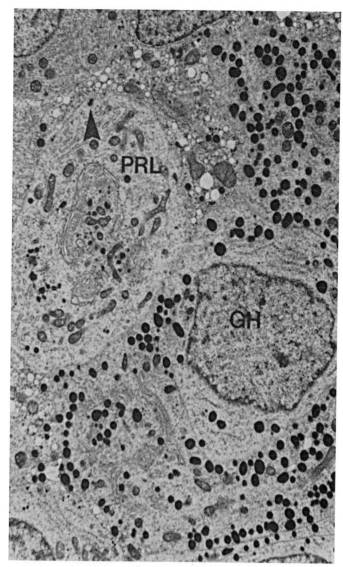

FIGURE 12-12. *Mixed adenoma composed of densely granulated growth hormone cells (GH) and sparsely granulated prolactin cells (PRL). Note granule extrusion in the prolactin cell (arrowhead) (×6900).*

The very rare, densely granulated PRL cell adenoma is intensely acidophilic by histology and shows a strong all-over cytoplasmic positivity for immunoreactive PRL, as well as nuclear staining for Pit-1. The fine-structural appearance of adenoma cells displays a resemblance to those of nontumorous, densely granulated PRL cells, as well as to some of the adenomatous mammosomatotroph cells. The oval or elongated, well-differentiated cells possess prominent RER and Golgi apparatus and numerous spherical or pleomorphic, evenly electron-dense secretory granules in the range of 500 to 700 nm. Granule extrusions are noted regularly.

Nearly all PRL cell adenomas are sparsely granulated and chromophobic or slightly acidophilic by histology. They consistently give a strong positivity for immunoreactive PRL with highly characteristic globular staining in the juxtanuclear Golgi region. The positivity of sparse and small secretory granules may not be readily apparent at the resolution of the optical microscope. Nuclear Pit-1 staining is usually strong. The fine structure of the tumor is very characteristic. The closely apposed polyhedral cells have oval or slightly irregular nuclei with light, finely dispersed chromatin and a dense, prominent nucleolus. The RER is extensively developed and often organized in parallel rows and concentric whorls called nebenkerns. The Golgi complex occupies a large area of the cytoplasm and regularly contains numerous developing secretory granules (Fig. 12-13). The sparse secretory granules are spherical or pleomorphic, are evenly electron dense, and

measure 130 to 300 nm, the majority between 200 and 250 nm. The most characteristic feature of this tumor type is the extrusion of secretory granules on the lateral cell membranes, distant from the perivascular spaces and intercellular extensions of the basal lamina (misplaced exocytosis). It should be stressed that this form of secretion is the normal means of hormone discharge from PRL cells. Misplaced exocytosis is diagnostic of PRL production in both nontumorous and neoplastic human pituitary.

Two additional features that occur relatively often in these tumors are calcification (about 15%) and deposition of endocrine amyloid (5% to 6%).

With the advent of medical treatment for PRL-producing adenomas, it must be kept in mind that the dopaminergic agonist bromocriptine, while reducing the volume of prolactinomas, exerts a profound effect on the morphology of these tumors, including their ultrastructure.[71] The changes, which appear to be reversible in the majority of cases, are the reduction in the size of the cell, cytoplasmic area, nucleus, and nucleolus; increase in the nuclear-cytoplasmic ratio; decrease in the volume of the cytoplasmic area, nucleus, and nucleolus; and decrease in the volume density of the RER and Golgi complex. The degree of change depends on the dose of bromocriptine, length of treatment, length of drug-free periods (if any) before surgery, and individual response to the drug. All these variables make the histologic and fine-structural appearance of treated PRL-producing tumors quite incalculable and difficult to interpret without knowledge of relevant clinical data.

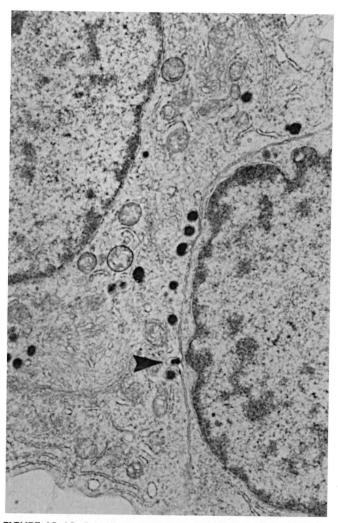

FIGURE 12-13. *Sparsely granulated prolactin cell adenoma. The cells contain abundant rough endoplasmic reticulum and a large Golgi complex but relatively few and small secretory granules. Note granule extrusion (arrowhead) on lateral cell membrane (×16,100).*

Acidophil Stem-Cell Adenomas

Acidophil stem-cell adenomas, monomorphous, bihormonal tumors, are likely to show a fast growth rate and invasion of parasellar, especially infrasellar areas.[72] They are associated clinically with signs and symptoms of hyperprolactinemia, although serum PRL levels are usually much lower than the values expected with well-differentiated PRL cell adenomas of comparable sizes. Occasionally, physical stigmata of acromegaly may develop, usually without any apparent elevation of serum GH levels ("fugitive acromegaly"). These lesions show a female preponderance and are often resistant to bromocriptine therapy.

Histologically, the tumor may be chromophobic but more often, owing to mitochondrial accumulation, the tumor cells are acidophilic. Immunocytochemistry detects PRL and, in some cases, also GH in the tumors. The two hormones may be present in the same cells. Staining for low-molecular-weight cytokeratins reveals scattered round cytoplasmic fibrous bodies. Electron microscopy of the adenoma cells documents some fine-structural markers of both adenomatous PRL cells (granule extrusions) and adenomatous, sparsely granulated GH cells (fibrous bodies, tubular SER, multiple centrioles) coupled, in most cases, with oncocytic change and an unusual form of mitochondrial gigantism (Fig. 12–14). The last appears to be specific and thus diagnostic of this tumor type.

The importance of recognizing this lesion cannot be overemphasized. Unlike the more common lactotroph adenoma, these lesions are aggressive lesions with a high rate of recurrence.

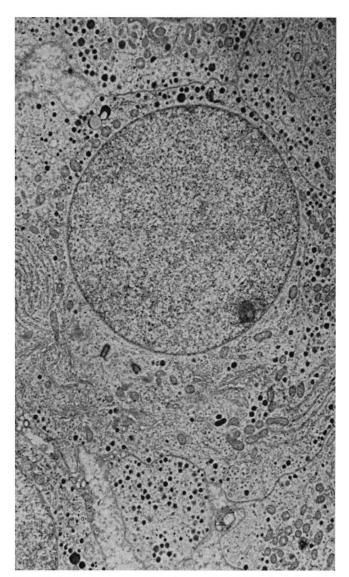

FIGURE 12–15. Thyrotroph adenoma associated with hyperthyroidism. The well-differentiated cells harbor prominent rough endoplasmic reticulum and Golgi apparatus, as well as numerous small (~200 nm) secretory granules (×8500).

Thyrotroph Adenomas

The rare thyrotroph adenoma may be associated with long-standing untreated or insufficiently treated primary hypothyroidism or with hyperthyroidism characterized by high T_4 and triiodothyronine (T_3) values, as well as elevated serum TSH levels.[73] In some cases, for reasons not understood at present, morphologically typical thyrotroph tumors may appear clinically silent in euthyroid patients.[73] By histology, thyrotroph adenomas are chromophobic with a sinusoidal pattern. Immunostaining using highly specific monoclonal antibodies demonstrates TSH-β in most of these tumors. They also contain α subunit and nuclear Pit-1 positivity. Electron microscopy may reveal well-differentiated middle-sized or large angular cells with uniform nuclei; prominent, slightly dilated RER; large Golgi area; and a varying number of small (100 to 350 nm) granules accumulating mainly in the cell processes (Fig. 12–15). Some tumors appear to be less differentiated, with irregular nuclei, small cytoplasm containing poorly or moderately developed RER, inconspicuous Golgi complex, and small, sparse, secretory granules, resembling the null cell adenoma. No close correlation exists between fine-structural features and hormonal activity of the tumors.

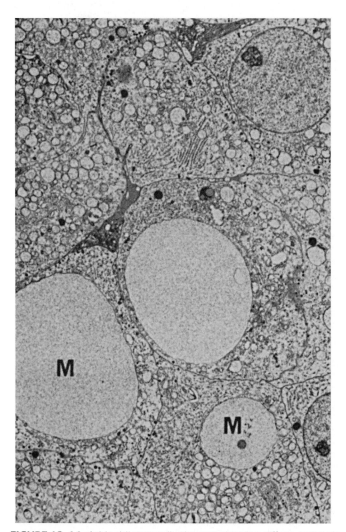

FIGURE 12–14. Acidophil stem-cell adenoma showing diffuse oncocytic change and mitochondrial gigantism (M) (×4600).

Corticotroph Adenomas

Clinically functioning corticotroph adenomas are either associated with Cushing's disease or occur in paients who have had bilaterally adrenalectomy to cure their hypercorticism (Nelson's syndrome). Owing to the increased use of greatly improved imaging and neurosurgical techniques for operative removal of pituitary corticotroph cell microadenomas, the frequency of Nelson's syndrome is now rare.

The majority of corticotroph cell tumors are basophilic microadenomas, showing a characteristic sinusoidal pattern. The adenoma cells exhibit strong PAS positivity and contain, as demonstrated by the immunoperoxidase technique, ACTH and related peptides, β-LPH, and endorphins. They characteristically are positive for low-molecular-weight cytokeratins. The ultrastructural features of tumor cells resemble those of nontumorous corticotrophs. The often angular cells have ovoid nuclei and relatively electron-dense cytoplasm. The well-developed, slightly dilated RER is randomly distributed in the cytoplasm; free ribosomes are numerous. The prominent Golgi complex regularly harbors developing secretory granules. The secretory granules are numerous, may be spherical or irregular (indented or heart-shaped), and exhibit varying electron density. They measure 250 to 450 nm, the majority being 300 to 350 nm. The diagnostic marker of corticotroph cell adenomas is the presence of fine (70 Å width) cytokeratin filaments that form bundles (Fig. 12–16), and their location is mainly perinuclear. The filaments are identical to those seen in normal corticotrophs and those forming Crooke's hyaline material in corticotrophs

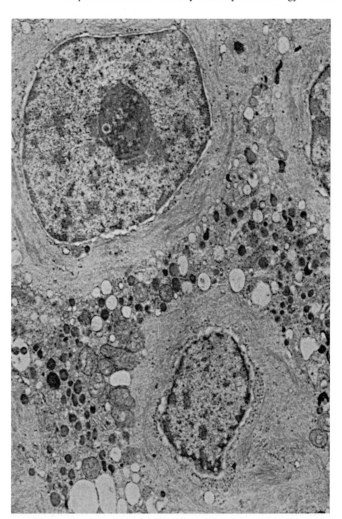

FIGURE 12–17. Corticotroph adenoma in Cushing's disease, showing extensive Crooke's hyalinization. The accumulating type 1 microfilaments displace secretory granules and other cytoplasmic components to the cell periphery. The cell membranes are not discernible, a common but unexplained finding in Crooke's cells (×9700).

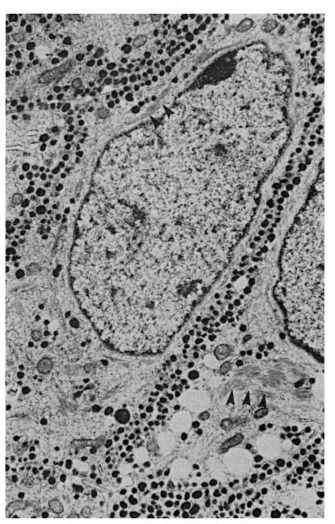

FIGURE 12–16. Corticotroph adenoma associated with Cushing's disease. The elongated, angular cells often have indented, irregular secretory granules with varying electron opacity and bundles of type 1 microfilaments *(arrowheads)* (×11,800).

of patients with hypercortisolism. Tumors in Nelson's syndrome contain few or no filaments.

Rarely, patients with Cushing's disease have macroadenomas at the time of presentation. It is not clear whether this is due to a faster tumor growth rate or relatively low hormonal activity, allowing the tumors to remain undetected for a longer time. These lesions are almost always chromophobic and PAS negative, or contain only a few PAS-positive granules. These tumors have a diffuse rather than sinusoidal pattern, and immunopositivity for ACTH and related peptides is scanty. Electron microscopy reveals considerably less differentiated tumors than the basophilic variant. The RER and Golgi apparatus are poorly developed, and the secretory granules are uncharacteristic, sparse, and small, measuring around 200 nm. A few keratin filaments are usually present, aiding the pathologic diagnosis.

In a minority of corticotroph cell adenomas, excessive accumulation of keratin filaments takes place, endowing the adenoma cells with the appearance of Crooke's cells[74–76] (Fig. 12–17). In view of the variations in clinical presentation and morphologic features, Crooke's hyalinization cannot be explained satisfactorily in these cases.

Gonadotroph Adenomas

The diagnosis of gonadotroph adenoma may prove to be very difficult, requiring the aid of hormone assays as well as immunocytochemistry and electron microscopy.[77, 78] Most clinically diagnosed cases so far occur in men, as elevated serum FSH (and rarely LH) levels are detected in a large percentage of male patients with gonadotroph tumors. On the other hand, in women with gonadotroph cell adenomas, serum FSH and LH levels rarely exceed the upper limit of the normal range for the patient's age.

By histology, gonadotroph tumors are chromophobic lesions with a sinusoidal structure that exhibits characteristic perivascular pseudo-rosette formation. Cells showing basophilic staining and intense PAS positivity occur only rarely. Immunohistochemical detection of gonadotropin subunits has improved with better tissue fixation techniques and the availability of highly specific monoclonal antibodies against α subunit, FSH-β, and LH-β. In addition, these adenomas exhibit specific nuclear positivity for SF-1. Most gonadotroph adenomas have subtle electron microscopic features that may be hard to distinguish from null cell adenomas. Some tumors may be well-differentiated, displaying some similarity to normal gonadotrophs. They are composed of elongated cells with nuclear localization at one pole of the cell. The cytoplasm harbors short profiles of slightly dilated RER that often contains flocculent material. The Golgi complexes are prominent and well developed (Fig. 12–18) but secretory granules are sparse and small, usually less than 200 nm. A subset of gonadotroph adenomas in women have unusual features that characterize a sex-linked dichotomy unparalleled so far in any other tumor type.[79] These highly differentiated tumors have abundant, slightly dilated RER and a prominent Golgi complex that exhibits a highly characteristic and unique vesicular dilation of the Golgi sacculi ("honeycomb Golgi") (Fig. 12–19). The reason for the unique sex-related fine-structural variance in gonadotroph adenomas is unexplained.

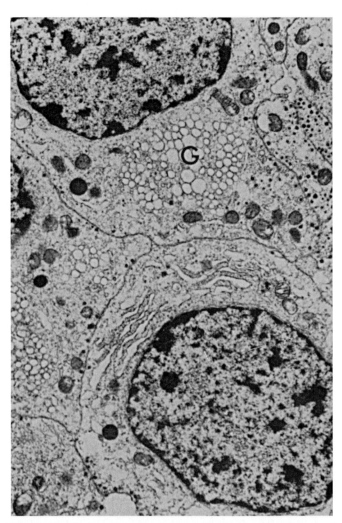

FIGURE 12–19. Gonadotroph adenoma, female type. The uniform cells possess abundant dilated rough endoplasmic reticulum and small (150 nm) secretory granules accumulating in the cell processes. Note the vesicular transformation of the Golgi complex (G, "honeycomb Golgi"), the hallmark of this tumor type (×10,000).

Null Cell Adenomas and Oncocytomas

The term *null cell adenoma*[80] denotes pituitary tumors that consist of cells provided with the general characteristics of endocrine secretory cells but lacking distinctive fine-structural or immunocytochemical markers that could assign them to a specific cell type. Clinically, these neoplasms appear to be nonfunctional. They are chromophobic by histology, with a sinusoidal or diffuse pattern. By immunocytology, they are negative for all pituitary hormones or contain only scattered cells staining positively for one or more hormones, mainly glycoprotein hormones and their α subunit. Electron microscopy reveals tumors consisting of closely apposed, small polyhedral cells with irregular nuclei. The small cytoplasm contains short, scattered profiles of poorly developed RER, clusters of free ribosomes, and a variable number of small, rod-shaped mitochondria (Fig. 12–20). The Golgi apparatus may be more prominent than the rest of the cytoplasmic organelles. The secretory granules are sparse and small, measuring 100 to 250 nm. They often have an irregular dense core and a halo under the limiting membrane.

Oncocytic transformation—that is, the increase in number and volume density of mitochondria—may be evident in a variable proportion of cells of null cell adenomas. If oncocytic change is very extensive, involving practically every adenoma cell, we label the tumor pituitary oncocytoma. By histology, these tumors are either chromophobic or, owing to the accumulation of mitochondria, show various degrees of acidophilia over the coarsely granular cytoplasm. By immunohisto-

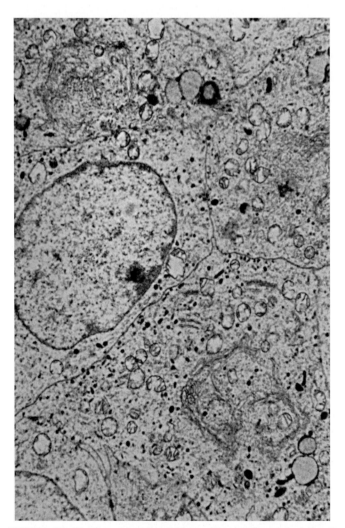

FIGURE 12–18. Gonadotroph adenoma. The small, polyhedral cells possess prominent Golgi complexes but only moderately developed rough endoplasmic reticulum and sparse secretory granules (×10,400).

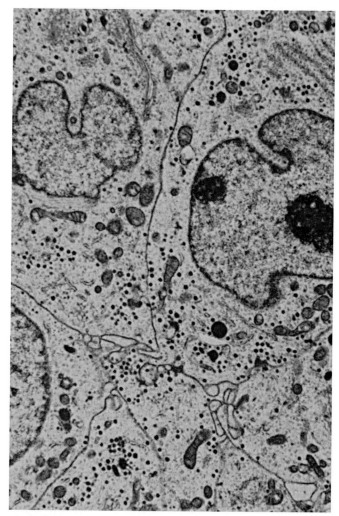

FIGURE 12–20. Null cell adenoma. The small cells have irregular nuclei and poorly developed cytoplasmic organelles (×10,400).

chemistry, oncocytomas behave in the same manner as null cell adenomas, and the ultrastructure of cellular organelles is essentially the same in the two variants, with the exception of mitochondrial abundance, which is the sole fine-structural marker of oncocytomas (Fig. 12–21). The mitochondria, occupying up to 55% of the cytoplasmic area, are either small and rod-shaped with numerous cristae ("dark" oncocytes, acidophilic by histology) or large and ovoid or spherical and rarefied with loss of cristae ("light" oncocytes, chromophobic by histology).[81]

Null cell adenomas and oncocytomas are grouped together on the basis of absence or paucity of morphologic markers. They most probably represent a heterogeneous group, although the majority of clinically nonfunctioning adenomas secrete and express the genes for α and β subunits of gonadotropic hormones[82, 83] and express SF-1.[13]

It is important to note that oncocytic transformation may also occur in any type of clinically functioning adenoma, especially in older patients. In these tumors, however, the immunohistochemical and fine-structural markers of that particular adenoma type are retained, and these neoplasms should be classified according to their cytogenesis and hormonal function.

Plurihormonal Adenomas

The term *plurihormonal adenoma* designates pituitary tumors producing more than one hormone. Plurihormonal adenomas may consist of one cell type (monomorphous) or more cell types (plurimorphous) by electron microscopy.[24] The most common bihormonal adenomas, producing GH and PRL, are discussed earlier in this chapter. These

plurihormonal adenomas often produce α subunit, frequently associated with scattered immunoreactivity for TSH-β. These profiles of hormone immunoreactivity are now understood on the basis of the common regulatory impact of Pit-1 on the expression of these hormones. Discrepancies between the immunohistochemical profile, ultrastructure, and clinical presentation of these adenomas are not unusual because some of the hormones produced by the tumor are unassociated with clinical and biochemical abnormalities. GH is almost invariably symptomatic. Apart from the frequent simultaneous occurrence of increased GH and PRL levels, the most common association of endocrine disorders caused by the same pituitary adenoma is acromegaly and hyperthyroidism.

Other unusual combinations of hormones expressed in rare plurihormonal adenomas (e.g., ACTH + PRL, ACTH + α subunit, ACTH + LH, PRL + FSH, TSH + PRL, PRL + α subunit + endorphin, ACTH + PRL) are not yet well understood. Some of these are plurimorphous lesions in which each pattern of hormone production is identified in appropriately differentiated cells; these may represent "collision" tumors or intermingled synchronous adenomas.[84]

Others, such as the silent subtype 3 adenoma, are monomorphous lesions. These rare tumors[85] are generally unassociated with evidence of hormone excess in men, whereas in young women they are usually associated with oligomenorrhea, amenorrhea, galactorrhea, and mild to moderate hyperprolactinemia, thus mimicking PRL-producing tumors. These fast-growing tumors are chromophobic or slightly acidophilic and may exhibit light PAS positivity. They may show positive immunostaining in a minority of cells with antisera raised against ACTH and endorphins and, in some cases, with antisera generated against

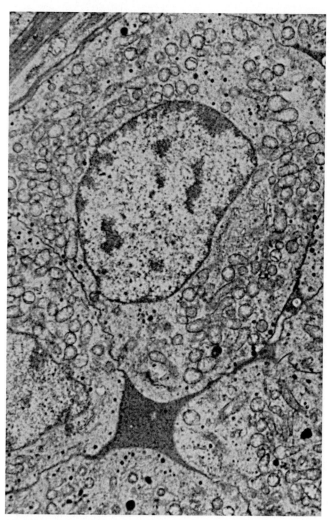

FIGURE 12–21. Pituitary oncocytoma showing marked abundance of mitochondria (×9900).

other pituitary hormones as well, whereas the majority of cells remain negative. The highly differentiated fine-structural features of these tumors bear similarity to those of glycoprotein hormone-producing adenomas. The tumor cells, however, are often unusually large, containing well-developed RER, SER, and Golgi apparatus in the abundant cytoplasm. The small, chiefly spherical secretory granules measure up to 250 nm (Fig. 12–22).

Clinically Nonfunctioning (Silent) Adenomas

Any morphologic tumor type may be unassociated with clinical evidence of hormone hypersecretion.[13] These lesions usually present with symptoms of a sellar mass, most often with extrasellar involvement, and varying degrees of hypopituitarism. The vast majority of clinically nonfunctioning adenomas are gonadotroph adenomas, null cell adenomas, or oncocytomas. However, silent somatotroph adenomas, lactotroph adenomas, and thyrotroph adenomas occur.

Silent corticotroph adenomas are worthy of special note since they may have an unusually aggressive clinical course. Subtype 1 silent corticotroph adenomas are basophilic, contain immunoreactive ACTH, β-LPH, and endorphins, and possess an ultrastructural appearance indistinguishable from that of basophilic corticotroph cell adenomas in cases of Cushing's disease. Subtype 2 tumors show a striking male preponderance. By histology, they are chromophobic or contain a modest amount of basophilic and PAS-positive granulation. Immunopositivity for ACTH and related peptides is invariably present. By

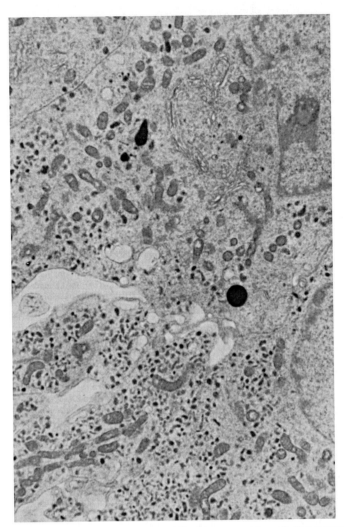

FIGURE 12–23. Silent "corticotroph" adenoma, subtype 2. The tumor contains immunoreactive ACTH and related peptides, but the only endocrine sign in the young male patient is hyperprolactinemia (×10,300).

electron microscopy, the usually well-differentiated, angular cells possess well-developed RER and Golgi complex and a varying number of spherical, oval, or distinctly teardrop-shaped secretory granules measuring up to 450 nm, the majority being around 250 nm (Fig. 12–23). Microfilaments are not present. Both variants of silent corticotroph adenomas express POMC messenger RNA (mRNA) but it is thought that they process the protein product differently, accounting for the lack of clinical evidence of ACTH excess.[86–88]

Silent subtype 3 adenomas[85] are also important to recognize because they are notoriously aggressive and invasive lesions with a high rate of recurrence.

Pituitary Carcinoma

Primary carcinomas[12, 13, 89] of the anterior lobe are rare and originate in adenohypophysial cells. They may produce GH, ACTH, or PRL, resulting in clinical symptomatology, or they may be clinically nonfunctioning.

The histologic features of these lesions are not consistently different from usual pituitary adenomas. They may exhibit a high MIB-1 labeling index indicating rapid proliferation,[90] but the values are not diagnostic because there is overlap with pituitary adenomas. The diagnosis can only be established when the lesion metastasizes, proving its biologic behavior.

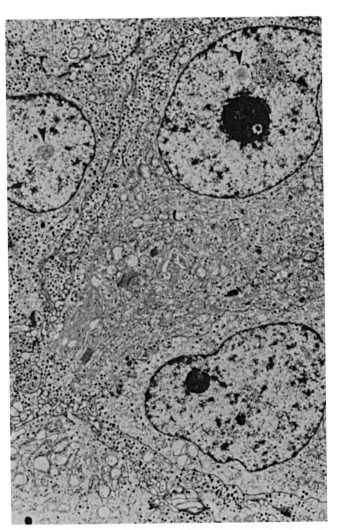

FIGURE 12–22. Silent subtype 3 adenoma. The large cells have extensively developed endoplasmic reticulum, a Golgi complex, and a varying number of small secretory granules. Note nuclear spheridia *(arrowheads)* (×5400).

Craniopharyngioma

Craniopharyngiomas are thought to arise from remnants of Rathke's pouch[12, 13, 19, 91]; they account for approximately 3% of all intracranial neoplasms. They are almost always benign, but are frequently locally infiltrative, are more commonly suprasellar than intrasellar in location, and often show calcification, which enables them to be diagnosed by imaging techniques. They never produce pituitary hormones, but the presence of immunoreactive human chorionic gonadotropin (hCG) has been reported in the cyst fluid of these neoplasms.[92] Craniopharyngiomas may cause hypopituitarism by compressing or destroying adenohypophysial tissue or the hypophysiotropic area of the hypothalamus. They can compress the pituitary stalk and interfere with portal circulation and can affect pituitary function either by reducing the blood supply to the anterior lobe or by blocking the synthesis or flow of hypothalamic-regulating hormones to the adenohypophysis, in some cases causing hyperprolactinemia.

Other Pituitary Neoplasms

The pituitary can be involved with a wide range of primary lesions that arise from brain, including neuronal and glial tumors, meningiomas, germinomas, granular cell tumors, and chordomas.[13] While any of these lesions can result in hypopituitarism and hyperprolactinemia, only the rare hypothalamic gangliocytomas that produce GHRH or CRH have been implicated as hormonally active lesions.[93–95] The sella turcica is also the site of germ cell tumors that occasionally produce hCG, with resulting symptoms of gonadotropin excess.[13] Hematologic, vascular, and mesenchymal tumors occur at this site, as they do throughout the body[13]; some of these, especially sarcomas, have been attributed to previous irradiation for aggressive pituitary tumors.

Secondary tumors in the pituitary gland are infrequently found at autopsy and are rarely recognized clinically.[13] In general, they are not accompanied by overt clinical symptoms except occasionally by diabetes insipidus, which may develop in patients with metastases to the posterior lobe. Hypopituitarism is extremely rare because a large part of the anterior lobe has to be replaced by tumor tissue before a decrease in secretion of adenohypophysial hormones becomes clinically evident. Suprasellar metastases may produce clinical hypopituitarism by interfering with the production or transport of hypothalamic-regulating hormones to the portal circulation; in such cases, there may be little or no ischemic necrosis of the adenohypophysis. Pituitary metastases usually occur in the advanced phase of neoplastic disease, when several other organs are also affected by disseminated cancer. These patients usually do not survive long enough to develop hypopituitarism.

Studies on autopsy material indicate that secondary tumor deposits occur in the hypophysis in approximately 1% to 3% of all cancer patients.[96] This figure is presumably somewhat lower than the real incidence because small foci of cancer metastases can easily be overlooked unless numerous sections are made from the gland. The breast is the most frequent site of primary neoplasm. Pituitary metastases, however, may also arise in patients with primary tumors in other locations, such as bronchus, prostate, and colon. The cause of increased incidence of pituitary metastases in breast cancer patients is not known.

REFERENCES

1. Bergland RM, Ray BS, Torack RM: Anatomical variations in the pituitary gland and adjacent structures in 225 human autopsy cases. J Neurosurg 28:93–99, 1968.
2. Scheithauer BW, Sano T, Kovacs KT, et al: The pituitary gland in pregnancy: A clinicopathologic and immunohistochemical study of 69 cases. Mayo Clin Proc 65:461–474, 1990.
3. Asa SL, Kovacs K: Functional morphology of the human fetal pituitary. Pathol Annu 19(pt 1):275–315, 1984.
4. Asa SL, Kovacs K, Laszlo FA, et al: C. Human fetal adenohypophysis. Histologic and immunocytochemical analysis. Neuroendocrinology 43:308–316, 1986.
5. Asa SL, Kovacs K, Horvath E, et al: Human fetal adenohypophysis. Electron microscopic and ultrastructural immunocytochemical analysis. Neuroendocrinology 48:423–431, 1988.
6. Asa SL, Kovacs K, Singer W: Human fetal adenohypophysis: Morphologic and functional analysis in vitro. Neuroendocrinology 53:562–572, 1991.
7. Pearse AGE, Takor T: Embryology of the diffuse neuroendocrine system and its relationship to the common peptides. Fed Proc 38:2288–2294, 1979.
8. Asa SL, Ezzat S. Molecular determinants of pituitary cytodifferentiation. Pituitary 1:159–168, 1999.
9. Sornson MW, Wu W, Dasen JS, et al: Pituitary lineage determination by the Prophet of Pit-1 homeodomain factor defective in Ames dwarfism. Nature 384:327–333, 1996.
10. Wu W, Cogan JD, Pfäffle RW, Dasen JS, et al: Mutations in PROP1 cause familial combined pituitary hormone deficiency. Nature Genet 18:147–149, 1998.
11. Fofanova O, Takmura N, Kinoshita E, et al: Compound heterozygous deletion of the prop-1 gene in children with combined pituitary hormone deficiency. J Clin Endocrinol Metab 83:2601–2604, 1998.
12. Kovacs K, Horvath E: Tumors of the Pituitary Gland. Atlas of Tumor Pathology, 2nd ser. Washington, DC, Armed Forces Institute of Pathology, fascicle 22, 1986.
13. Asa SL: Tumors of the Pituitary Gland. Atlas of Tumor Pathology, 3rd ser. Washington, DC, Armed Forces Institute of Pathology, 1998.
14. Asa SL, Kovacs K, Bilbao JM. The pars tuberalis of the human pituitary. A histologic, immunohistochemical, ultrastructural and immunoelectron microscopic analysis. Virchows Arch 399:49–59, 1983.
15. Melchionna RH, Moore RA: The pharyngeal pituitary gland. Am J Pathol 14:763–771, 1938.
16. Boyd JD: Observations of the human pharyngeal hypophysis. J Endocrinol 14:66–77, 1956.
17. Ciocca DR, Puy LA, Stati AO: Identification of seven hormone-producing cell types in the human pharyngeal hypophysis. J Clin Endocrinol Metab 60:212–216, 1985.
18. Puy LA, Ciocca DR: Human pharyngeal and sellar pituitary glands: Differences and similarities revealed by an immunocytochemical study. J Endocrinol 108:231–238, 1986.
19. Scheithauer BW: The hypothalamus and neurohypophysis. In Kovacs K, Asa SL (eds): Functional Endocrine Pathology. Boston, Blackwell Scientific, 1991, pp 170–244.
20. Stanfield JP: The blood supply of the human pituitary gland. J Anat 94:257–273, 1960.
21. Bergland RM, Page RB. Pituitary-brain vascular relations: A new paradigm. Science 204:18–24, 1979.
22. Gorczyca W, Hardy J: Arterial supply of the human anterior pituitary gland. Neurosurgery 20:369–368, 1987.
23. Sheehan HL, Kovacs K: The subventricular nucleus of the human hypothalamus. Brain 89:589–614, 1966.
24. Kovacs K, Horvath E, Asa SL, et al: Pituitary cells producing more than one hormone. Human pituitary adenomas. Trends Endocrinol Metab 1:104–107, 1989.
25. Asa SL, Ezzat S: The cytogenesis and pathogenesis of pituitary adenomas. Endocr Rev 19:798–827, 1998.
26. Schechter J, Kovacs K, Rimoin D: Isolated growth hormone deficiency: Immunocytochemistry. J Clin Endocrinol Metab 59:798–800, 1984.
27. Borges JLC, Blizzard RM, Evans WS, et al: Stimulation of growth hormone (GH) and somatomedin C in idiopathic GH-deficient subjects by intermittent pulsatile administration of synthetic human pancreatic tumor GH-releasing factor. J Clin Endocrinol Metab 59:1–6, 1984.
28. Losinski NE, Horvath E, Kovacs K, Asa SL: Immunoelectron microscopic evidence of mammosomatotrophs in human adult and fetal adenohypophyses, rat adenohypophyses and human and rat pituitary adenomas. Anat Anz 172:11–16, 1991.
29. Frawley LS, Boockfor FR: Mammosomatotropes: Presence and functions in normal and neoplastic pituitary tissue. Endocr Rev 12:337–355, 1991.
30. Asa SL, Penz G, Kovacs K, Ezrin C: Prolactin cells in the human pituitary. A quantitative immunocytochemical analysis. Arch Pathol Lab Med 106:360–363, 1982.
31. Horvath E, Kovacs K: Fine structural cytology of the adenohypophysis in rat and man. J Electron Microsc Tech 8:401–432, 1988.
32. Scheithauer BW, Kovacs K, Randall RV, Ryan N: Pituitary gland in hypothyroidism. Histologic and immunocytologic study. Arch Pathol Lab Med 109:499–504, 1985.
33. Scheithauer BW, Kovacs K, Young WF Jr, Randall RV: The pituitary in hyperthyroidism. Mayo Clin Proc 67:22–26, 1992.
34. Neumann PE, Horoupian DS, Goldman JE, Hess MA: Cytoplasmic filaments of Crooke's hyaline change belong to the cytokeratin class. An immunochemical and ultrastructural study. Am J Pathol 116:214–222, 1984.
35. Halliday WC, Asa SL, Kovacs K, Scheithauer BW: Intermediate filaments in the human pituitary gland: An immunohistochemical study. Can J Neurol Sci 17:131–136, 1990.
36. Scheithauer BW, Kovacs K, Randall RV: The pituitary gland in untreated Addison's disease. A histologic and immunocytologic study of 18 adenohypophyses. Arch Pathol Lab Med 107:484–487, 1983.
37. Denef C: Paracrine interaction in anterior pituitary. In MacLeod RM, Thorner MO, Scapagnini U (eds): Prolactin, Basic and Clinical Correlates. Padva, Italy, Liviana Press, 1985, pp 53–57.
38. Horvath E, Kovacs K, Penz G, Ezrin C: Origin, possible function and fate of "follicular cells" in the anterior lobe of the human pituitary. Am J Pathol 77:199–212, 1974.
39. Höfler H, Walter GF, Denk H: Immunohistochemistry of folliculo-stellate cells in normal human adenohypophyses and in pituitary adenomas. Acta Neuropathol (Berl) 65:35–40, 1984.
40. Girod C, Trouillas J, Dubois MP: Immunocytochemical localization of S-100 protein in stellate cells (folliculo-stellate cells) of the anterior lobe of the normal human pituitary. Cell Tissue Res 241:505–511, 1985.
41. Baes M, Allaerts W, Denef C: Evidence for functional communication between folliculo-stellate cells and hormone-secreting cells in perifused anterior pituitary aggregates. Endocrinology 120:685–691, 1987.
42. Cardoso ER, Peterson EW: Pituitary apoplexy: A review. Neurosurgery 14:363–373, 1984.
43. Kovacs K. Necrosis of anterior pituitary in humans. Neuroendocrinology 4:179–199, 1969.

44. Kovacs K: Adenohypophysial necrosis in routine autopsies. Endokrinologie 60:309–316, 1972.
45. McCormick WF, Halmi NS: The hypophysis in patients with coma dépasse ("respirator brain"). Am J Clin Pathol 54:374–383, 1970.
46. Kovacs K, Bilbao JM: Adenohypophysial necrosis in respirator maintained patients. Pathol Microbiol 41:275–282, 1974.
47. Sheehan HL: Post-partum necrosis of the anterior pituitary. J Pathol Bacteriol 45:189–214, 1937.
48. Sano T, Asa SL, Kovacs K: Growth hormone–releasing hormone-producing tumors: Clinical, biochemical, and morphological manifestations. Endocr Rev 9:357–373, 1988.
49. Ezzat S, Asa SL, Stefaneanu L, et al: Somatotroph hyperplasia without pituitary adenoma associated with a long standing growth hormone-releasing hormone-producing bronchial carcinoid. J Clin Endocrinol Metab 78:555–560, 1994.
50. Kovacs K, Horvath E, Thorner MO, Rogol AD: Mammosomatotroph hyperplasia associated with acromegaly and hyperprolactinemia in a patient with the McCune-Albright syndrome. Virchows Arch 403:77–86, 1984.
51. Moran A, Asa SL, Kovacs K, et al: Gigantism due to pituitary mammosomatotroph hyperplasia. N Engl J Med 323:322–327, 1990.
52. Jay V, Kovacs K, Horvath E, et al: Idiopathic prolactin cell hyperplasia of the pituitary mimicking prolactin cell adenoma: A morphological study including immunocytochemistry, electron microscopy, and in situ hybridization. Acta Neuropathol (Berl) 82:147–151, 1991.
53. Peillon F, Dupuy M, Li JY, et al: Pituitary enlargement with suprasellar extension in functional hyperprolactinemia due to lactotroph hyperplasia: A pseudotumoral disease. J Clin Endocrinol Metab 73:1008–1015, 1991.
54. Khalil A, Kovacs K, Sima AAF, et al: Pituitary thyrotroph hyperplasia mimicking prolactin-secreting adenoma. J Endocrinol Invest 7:399–404, 1984.
55. Grubb MR, Chakeres D, Malarkey WB: Patients with primary hypothyroidism presenting as prolactinomas. Am J Med 43:765–769, 1987.
56. McKeever PE, Koppelman MCS, Metcalf D, et al: Refractory Cushing's disease caused by multinodular ACTH-cell hyperplasia. J Neuropathol Exp Neurol 41:490–499, 1982.
57. McNicol AM: Patterns of corticotropic cells in the adult human pituitary in Cushing's disease. Diagn Histopathol 4:335–341, 1981.
58. Carey RM, Varma SK, Drake CR Jr, et al: Ectopic secretion of corticotropin-releasing factor as a cause of Cushing's syndrome. A clinical, morphologic, and biochemical study. N Engl J Med 311:13–20, 1984.
59. Sano T, Kovacs K, Scheithauer BW, et al: Pituitary pathology in acquired immunodeficiency syndrome. Arch Pathol Lab Med 113:1066–1070, 1989.
60. Thodou E, Asa SL, Kontogeorgos G, et al: Lymphocytic hypophysitis: Clinicopathological findings. J Clin Endocrinol Metab 80:2302–2311, 1995.
61. Hassoun P, Anayssi E, Salti I: A case of granulomatous hypophysitis with hypopituitarism and minimal pituitary enlargement. J Neurol Neurosurg Psychiatry 48:949–951, 1985.
62. Klaer W, Nørgaard JOR: Granulomatous hypophysitis and thyroiditis with lymphocytic adrenalitis. Acta Pathol Microbiol Scand 76:229–238, 1969.
63. Horvath E, Kovacs K: The adenohypophysis. In Kovacs K, Asa SL (eds): Functional Endocrine Pathology. Boston, Blackwell Scientific 1991, pp 245–281.
64. Neumann PE, Goldman JE, Horoupian DS, Hess MA: Fibrous bodies in growth hormone–secreting adenomas contain cytokeratin filaments. Arch Pathol Lab Med 109:505–508, 1985.
65. Landolt AM, Kleihues P, Heitz PhU: Amyloid deposits in pituitary adenomas. Differentiation of two types. Arch Pathol Lab Med 111:453–458, 1987.
66. Ezzat S, Snyder PJ, Young WF, et al: Octreotide treatment of acromegaly. A randomized, multicenter study. Ann Intern Med 117:711–718, 1992.
67. Ezzat S, Horvath E, Harris AG, Kovacs K: Morphological effects of octreotide on growth hormone-producing pituitary adenomas. J Clin Endocrinol Metab 79:113–118, 1994.
68. Horvath E, Kovacs K, Killinger DW, et al: C. Mammosomatotroph cell adenoma of the human pituitary: A morphologic entity. Virchows Arch 398:277–289, 1983.
69. Black VH, Russo JJ: Stereological analysis of the guinea pig adrenal: Effects of dexamethasone and ACTH treatment with emphasis on the inner cortex. Am J Anat 159:85–120, 1980.
70. Li J, Stefaneanu L, Kovacs K, et al: Growth hormone (GH) and prolactin (PRL) gene expression and immunoreactivity in GH- and PRL-producing human pituitary adenomas. Virchows Arch 422:193–201, 1993.
71. Kovacs K, Stefaneanu L, Horvath E, et al: Effect of dopamine agonist medication on prolactin producing pituitary adenomas. A morphological study including immunocytochemistry, electron microscopy and in situ hybridization. Virchows Arch 418:439–446, 1991.
72. Horvath E, Kovacs K, Singer W, et al: Acidophil stem cell adenoma of the human pituitary: Clinicopathologic analysis of 15 cases. Cancer 47:761–771, 1981.
73. Beck-Peccoz P, Brucker-Davis F, Persani L, et al: Thyrotropin–secreting pituitary tumors. Endocr Rev 17:610–638, 1996.
74. Felix IA, Horvath E, Kovacs K: Massive Crooke's hyalinization in corticotroph cell adenomas of the human pituitary. A histological, immunocytological and electron microscopic study of three cases. Acta Neurochir 58:235–243, 1981.
75. Horvath E, Kovacs K, Josse R: Pituitary corticotroph cell adenoma with marked abundance of microfilaments. Ultrastruct Pathol 5:249–255, 1983.
76. Franscella S, Favod-Coune C-A, Pizzolato G, et al: Pituitary corticotroph adenoma with Crooke's hyalinization. Endocr Pathol 2:111–116, 1991.
77. Snyder PJ: Gonadotroph cell adenomas of the pituitary. Endocr Rev 6:552–563, 1985.
78. Snyder PJ: Gonadotroph cell pituitary adenomas. Endocrinol Metab Clin North Am 16:755–764, 1987.
79. Horvath E, Kovacs K: Gonadotroph adenomas of the human pituitary: Sex-related fine-structural dichotomy. A histologic, immunocytochemical, and electron-microscopic study of 30 tumors. Am J Pathol 117:429–440, 1984.
80. Kovacs K, Horvath E, Ryan N, Ezrin C: Null cell adenoma of the human pituitary. Virchows Arch 387:165–174, 1980.
81. Yamada S, Asa SL, Kovacs K: Oncocytomas and null cell adenomas of the human pituitary: Morphometric and in vitro functional comparison. Virchows Arch 413:333–339, 1988.
82. Asa SL, Cheng Z, Ramyar L, et al: Human pituitary null cell adenomas and oncocytomas in vitro: Effects of adenohypophysiotropic hormones and gonadal steroids on hormone secretion and tumor cell morphology. J Clin Endocrinol Metab 74:1128–1134, 1992.
83. Jameson JL, Klibanski A, Black PM, et al: Glycoprotein hormone genesare expressed in clinically nonfunctioning pituitary adenomas. J Clin Invest 80:1472–1478, 1987.
84. Apel RL, Wilson RJ, Asa SL: A composite somatotroph-corticotroph pituitary adenoma. Endocr Pathol 5:240–246, 1994.
85. Horvath E, Kovacs K, Smyth HS, et al: A novel type of pituitary adenoma: Morphological feature and clinical correlations. J Clin Endocrinol Metab 66:1111–1118, 1988.
86. Lloyd RV, Fields K, Jin L, et al: Analysis of endocrine active and clinically silent corticotropic adenomas by in situ hybridization. Am J Pathol 137:479–488, 1990.
87. Stefaneanu L, Kovacs K, Horvath E, Lloyd RV: In situ hybridization study of proopiomelanocortin (POMC) gene expression in human pituitary corticotrophs and their adenomas. Virchows Arch 419:107–113, 1991.
88. Chabre O, Martinie M, Vivier J, et al: A clinically silent corticotrophic pituitary adenoma (CSCPA) secreting a biologically inactive but immunoreactive assayable ACTH J Endocrinol Invest 14 (suppl. 1):87, 1991 (abstract).
89. Beauchesne P, Trouillas J, Barral F, Brunon J: Gonadotropic pituitary carcinoma: Case report. Neurosurgery 37:810–815, 1995.
90. Thapar K, Kovacs K, Scheithauer BW, et al: Proliferative activity and invasiveness among pituitary adenomas and carcinomas: An analysis using the MIB-1 antibody. Neurosurgery 38:99–107, 1996.
91. Laws ER Jr: Craniopharyngioma: Diagnosis and treatment. Endocrinologist 2:184–188, 1992.
92. Harris PE, Perry L, Chard T, et al: Immunoreactive human chorionic gonadotropin from the cyst fluid and CSF of patients with craniopharyngioma. Clin Endocrinol (Oxf) 29:503–508, 1988.
93. Asa SL, Scheithauer BW, Bilbao JM, et al: A case for hypothalamic acromegaly: A clinicopathological study of six patients with hypothalamic gangliocytomas producing growth hormone–releasing factor. J Clin Endocrinol Metab 58:796–803, 1984.
94. Asa SL, Kovacs K, Tindall GT, et al: Cushing's disease associated with an intrasellar gangliocytoma producing corticotrophin-releasing factor. Ann Intern Med 101:789–793, 1984.
95. Puchner MJA, Lüdecke DK, Saeger W, et al: Gangliocytomas of the sellar region—a review. Exp Clin Endocrinol Diabetes 103:129–149, 1995.
96. Kovacs K: Metastatic cancer of the pituitary gland. Oncology 27:533–542, 1973.

Chapter 13

▲▲▲

Neurotransmitters and Hypothalamic Control of Anterior Pituitary Function

Yogesh C. Patel

The function of anterior pituitary cells is regulated by stimulatory and inhibitory hormones that are synthesized by parvocellular neurons in the hypothalamus, are released from axon terminals in the external zone of the median eminence into the hypophysial portal blood, and are transported to the anterior pituitary for binding and activation of specific target cell receptors. Since the 1960s, the hypophysiotropic function of a number of these hormones has been defined.[1] They include thyrotropin-releasing hormone (TRH), dopamine (DA), gonadotropin-releasing hormone (GnRH) somatostatin (SST), corticotropin-releasing hormone (CRH) and growth hormone–releasing hormone (GHRH).[1] The functional activity of the hypothalamic hypophysiotropic neurons is in turn modulated by a large number of neurotransmitters and neuropeptides via afferent input from the rest of the brain as well as from local hypothalamic circuits.[1–4] In addition to DA, several other transmitters such as acetylcholine (Ach), γ-aminobutyric acid (GABA), and epinephrine (Epi) have been detected in portal blood and may serve a dual role as both a central transmitter and a neurohormone with hypophysiotropic functions. This chapter focuses on the role of classic and key peptidergic neurotransmitters in regulating anterior pituitary cell function through their effects on the hypothalamus. It provides an overview of neurotransmitters and neurotransmitter pathways impinging on the hypothalamus as necessary background toward a detailed understanding of the transmitter control of the individual pituitary hormones.

NEUROTRANSMITTERS AND NEUROMODULATORS: GENERAL PRINCIPLES

A classic neurotransmitter is defined as a chemical substance that is synthesized in a neuron, is stored in presynaptic terminals, is released in response to nerve activation, and acts on specific postsynaptic receptors to produce changes such as ionic conductance or activation of intracellular second messenger systems in target cells.[5] The actions of the transmitter are terminated by its removal from the synapse by diffusion, enzymatic modification, or reuptake via transporter molecules into the presynaptic terminal. Classic neurotransmitters are small molecules that are synthesized by specialized enzyme systems and are expressed in neural tissue in nanograms per milligram of protein (Fig. 13–1). They include Ach; the biogenic amines (norepinephrine [NE], Epi, DA, serotonin—5-hydroxytryptamine [5-HT], and histamine); amino acids, both excitatory (glutamate [GLU], aspartate [ASP]) and inhibitory (GABA, glycine); and nitric oxide (NO) and carbon monoxide, which only recently have been recognized as an important class of diffusible, gaseous neurotransmitter substances.[1, 5–11] Amino acids form the main group of central transmitters released at an estimated 25 to 40% of brain synapses.[5] Cholinergic transmission occurs at approximately 5 to 10% of brain synapses, whereas the monoamines are released at only 1 to 2% of brain synapses.[5] In addition to these classic transmitters, an important and expanding group of regulatory molecules synthesized by neurons are neuropeptides, the first of which—oxytocin and vasopressin—were isolated from the posterior pituitary in the early 1950s.[12] Since then, more than 50 neuropeptides have been isolated either from the hypothalamus as hypophysiotropic substances (TRH, GnRH, SST, CRH) or from peripheral tissues (GHRH, substance P, vasoactive intestinal polypeptide [VIP], cholecystokinin [CCK]) and shown subsequently to be localized in neurons.[12, 13] In contrast to the enzymatic synthesis of the classic neurotransmitters, neuropeptides are synthesized in the rough endoplasmic reticulum as part of a large precursor molecule that is proteolytically cleaved to generate the bioactive peptide molecules that are also stored in nanograms per milligram of protein tissue concentration.[14] Furthermore, unlike the classic transmitters that have a reuptake mechanism for replenishing terminal stores, peptide molecules are not recycled after release and must be replaced by new synthesis. Neuropeptides allow both diverse and overlapping functions. Many of the precursor molecules generate more than one bioactive form that interacts with different classes of receptors, for example, pro-opiomelanocortin (POMC).[14] Another property of neuropeptides is their occur-

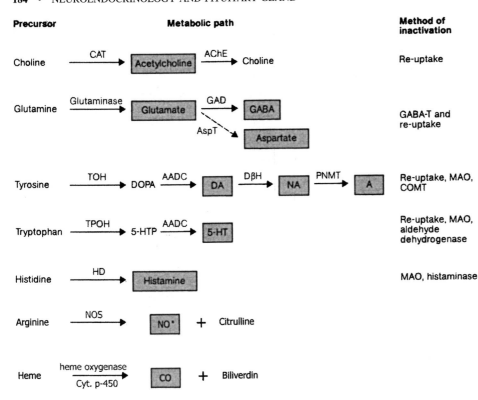

FIGURE 13–1. *Steps in the synthesis of classic neurotransmitters. A, adrenaline; AADC, amino acid decarboxylase; AchE, acetylcholinesterase; AspT, mitochondrial aspartate transaminase; CAT, choline acetyltransferase; COMT, catechol-O-methyltransferase; DβH, dopamine β-hydroxylase; DA, dopamine; DOPA, dihydroxyphenylalanine; GABA-T, γ-aminobutyric acid transaminase; GAD, glutamic acid decarboxylase; HD, histamine decarboxylase; 5-HT, 5-hydroxytryptamine; 5-HTP, 5-hydroxytryptophan; MAO, monoamine oxidase; NA, noradrenaline; PNMT, phenylethanolamine-N-methyltransferase; TOH, tyrosine hydroxylase; TPOH, tryptophan hydroxylase; NOS, nitric oxide synthase; NO, nitric oxide; CO, carbon monoxide.*

rence as structurally related gene families, for example, opioids.[14] Although some of the peptides such as substance P and the opioids have been shown to fulfill the criteria for classic neurotransmitters, the majority of neuropeptides display a slower course of action and are thought to be neuromodulators, defined as chemical messengers that have no effect on postsynaptic excitability but that can alter the responsiveness of classic neurotransmitters by influencing their release, binding, or other actions.[5] Neuropeptides are produced not only in neurons but also in peripheral neuroendocrine cells and function in different ways as neurohormones, local paracrine-autocrine regulators, and circulating hormones that act systemically on distant targets.[12–14] Many peptides coexist with classic transmitters in the same neuron, for example, NE with neuropeptide Y (NPY); Ach with VIP in autonomic nerves; GABA and CCK in cortical neurons; SST, NPY, and NO in NADPH-diaphorase–positive cortical and striatal neurons; and TRH with 5-HT in the spinal cord.[15, 16] The functional significance of such co-localizations is unclear. It may provide synergy, for example, VIP and Ach in salivary glands, or a mechanism for modulating receptor functions such as agonist-dependent regulatory responses or signaling through molecular crosstalk.

FUNCTIONAL ANATOMY OF TRANSMITTER PATHWAYS

Acetylcholine

Ach, the first substance to be established as a neurotransmitter, is synthesized from dietary choline by the action of the enzyme choline acetyl transferase (CAT) (see Fig. 13–1). Cell bodies of cholinergic neurons are located in the septum, diagonal band, nucleus basalis magnocellularis, and pontine nuclei (Fig. 13–2). Axons from these nuclei project to the hippocampus and throughout the cortex. The hypothalamus is rich in Ach (measured as CAT), which is localized predominantly in the median eminence (ME), the paraventricular nucleus (PVN), the arcuate nucleus (ARC), the ventromedial nucleus (VMN), and the dorsomedial nucleus (DMN).[17] Surgical isolation of the medial basal hypothalamus does not change CAT activity in the ME but causes a significant decrease in the DMN.[17, 18] There thus appears to be a tuberoinfundibular cholinergic system of neurons

probably in the ARC or VMN projecting to the ME. Cholinergic neurons outside the hypothalamus terminate mainly in the DMN. Released Ach binds to both nicotinic and muscarinic receptors and acts predominantly as an excitatory neurotransmitter.[19, 20] Nicotinic receptors are made of pentameric subunits, each possessing four-transmembrane domains.[19, 21] There are four distinct subtypes that are expressed at neuromuscular junctions in autonomic ganglia and throughout the brain. In contrast, muscarinic receptors comprise a family of five G protein–coupled receptors designated M_1 to M_5 that are found throughout the brain, including the hypothalamus.[20] The pituitary itself synthesizes Ach, and M receptors have been identified in several of the pituitary cell subsets, suggesting the existence of an intrapituitary cholinergic paracrine-autocrine regulatory system.[22]

Norepinephrine and Epinephrine

Noradrenergic pathways play an important role in facilitating luteinizing hormone (LH), adrenocorticotropic hormone (ACTH), prolactin (PRL), growth hormone (GH), and thyroid-stimulating hormone (TSH) secretion (Table 13–1). The hypothalamus does not have an intrinsic NE system, but nevertheless is rich in NE localized in axons and nerve terminals that arise from cell bodies outside the hypothalamus. Dense NE networks are found in the PVN, VMN, ARC, and retrochiasmatic nucleus; lower densities of NE occur in the supraoptic nucleus (SON), the preoptic area (POA), and the periventricular nucleus (PeVN).[17, 23–25] NE terminals have also been identified in the inner layer of the ME, where they likely modulate presynaptic transmission. This is in contrast to DA, which is secreted into the portal vessels and localized in the external zone of the ME. Noradrenergic neurons in the brain comprise a few hundred cells confined to the lower brain stem that send extensive ascending and descending projections to the cortex, hypothalamus, limbic system, and spinal cord[5, 23–28] (see Fig. 13–2). Projections from this nucleus reach the hypothalamus via the ventral ascending noradrenergic bundle, which carries noradrenergic afferents from the lateral reticular nucleus of the medulla (A1 cell group), nucleus of the solitary tract (A2 group), locus coeruleus (A6), ventrolateral pons (A5), and mesencephalic reticular formation (A7), as well as adrenergic fibers from C1 to C3 cells.[27] Noradrenergic projections from the A2 and A6 cell groups are directed primarily

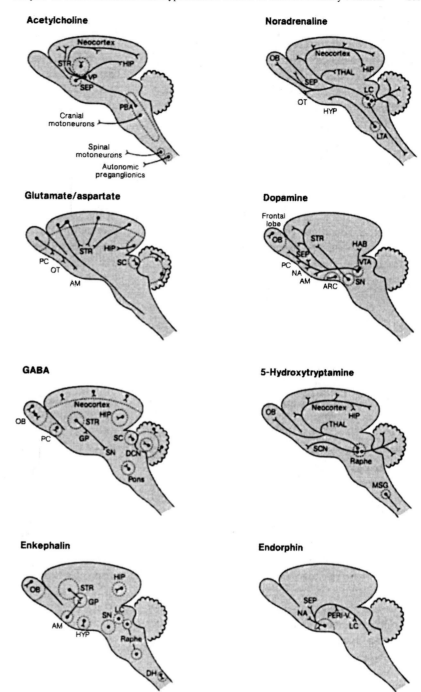

FIGURE 13–2. Principal locations of neurotransmitter pathways in the brain. AM, amygdala; ARC, arcuate nucleus; DCN, deep cerebellar nuclei; DH, dorsal horn; DRG, dorsal root ganglion; EPN, entopeduncular nucleus; GP, globus pallidus; HAB, habenula; HIP, hippocampus; HYP, hypothalamus; LC, locus coerulus; LTA, lateral tegmental area; MED, medulla; MSG, medullary serotonin group; NA, nucleus accumbens; OB, olfactory bulb; OT, olfactory tubercle; PBA, parabrachial area; PC, piriform cortex; PERI-V, periventricular gray matter; SC, superior colliculus; SCN, suprachiasmatic nucleus; SEP, septum; SN, substantia nigra; STR, striatum; THAL, thalamus; VP, ventral pallidum; VTA, ventral tegmental area. (Modified from McQueen JK: Classic transmitters and neuromodulators. *In* Fluckiger E, Muller EE, Thorner MO (eds): Transmitter Molecules in the Brain: Basic and Clinical Aspects of Neuroscience, vol 2: Springer Sandoz Advanced Texts. Heidelberg, Springer-Verlag, 1987, p 7.)

toward the parvocellular neurons that regulate the anterior pituitary, whereas the A1 group is involved mainly with posterior pituitary regulation and thus projects to the magnocellular neurons.[27] Many of the aminergic fibers in the ventral ascending bundle co-stain for NPY.[28]

Adrenergic pathways in the brain are more restricted than NE.[17] Neuronal cell bodies positive for phenylethinyl-*n*-methyltransferase, (PNMT), the enzyme that synthesizes Epi from NE, are found in the medulla and lower pons.[29] Ascending projections from these cells reach the central gray, the ME, and the hypothalamus (ME, ARC, PVN, and DMN). The pathway through which the fibers reach the hypothalamus has not been determined but appears to be separate from the ventral noradrenergic bundle.[25] Descending pathways project to the spinal cord. Deafferentation of the hypothalamus causes a substantial decrease in PNMT activity in the ME and ARC, confirming that the adrenergic input to these regions comes from an extrahypothalamic source.[18] Noradrenergic and adrenergic transmission is mediated via a large family of G protein–coupled receptors that fall into three distinct

classes: α_1, α_2, and β-adrenergic receptors, each with three separate subtypes (α_{1A}, α_{1B}, α_{1D}, α_{2A}, α_{2B}, α_{2C}; β_1, β_2, β_3).[19]

Dopamine

Dopaminergic neurons are concentrated in four discrete regions of the brain: the substantia nigra, ventral tegmentum, olfactory bulb, and hypothalamus[5] (see Fig. 13–2). The nigral dopaminergic neurons play a major role in extrapyramidal movement control, whereas the ventral tegmental DA neurons influence behavior and affect. Dopamine exerts a key role in the neuroendocrine regulation of PRL secretion and may play a part in the modulation of GH, LH, and TSH from the adenohypophysis and of POMC peptides from intermediate lobe melanotrophs (see Table 13–1). The hypothalamus has an intrinsic tuberoinfundibular dopaminergic (TIDA) system with cell bodies in the ARC and axons that terminate in the zona externa of the ME, where DA is

TABLE 13–1. Effect of Neurotransmitters on Pituitary Hormone Secretion

	Gonadotropins		Corticotropins		Prolactin		Growth Hormone		Thyrotropin	
	Ht	*Pit*	*Ht*	*Pit*	*Ht*	*Pit*	*Ht*	*Pit*	*Ht*	*Pit*
Norepinephrine	↑		↑	↑	↑		↑↓		↑	
Dopamine	↑↓		—			↓	↑↓		↓	↓
Acetylcholine	—		↑	—			↑			
Serotonin	↑↓				↑	—	↑			
EAAs	↑	↑	↑	—				↑	↑	
GABA	↓	↑	↓	↑↓		↑	↓	↓	↑	

Ht, effect at hypothalamic level; Pit, direct pituitary action; ↑, stimulation (arrows in boldface type signify important reproducible effects); ↓, inhibition; —, no effect.

directly released into the portal vessels.[17, 25, 26] Lower amounts of DA are present in the suprachiasmatic nucleus (SCN), PVN, VMN, and DMN.[17, 25] Some of the projections of the TIDA neurons continue down the stalk to the pituitary intermediate lobe, where axons make synaptic contacts with melanotrophs.[27] Deafferentation of the basal hypothalamus has no effect on hypothalamic DA content, suggesting that extrahypothalamic cell bodies do not contribute to hypothalamic DA.[18] TIDA neurons thus likely represent the main source of DA found in other regions of the hypothalamus. The effects of DA result from interaction with a family of G protein–coupled receptors with five subtypes termed D_1 to D_5.[19, 31, 32] In addition, the D_2 receptor exists as two splice variants termed D_{2s} and D_{2L} (short and long forms). Pharmacologically, the receptor family can be further subdivided into the D_1-like receptors (D_1 and D_5), which interact with G_s and stimulate adenylyl cyclase, and the D_2-like receptors (D_2, D_3, D_4), which couple to Gi/o and inhibit adenylyl cyclase.[31, 32] The hypothalamus expresses several DA receptor subtypes of which D_1 and D_2 are the most abundant, with relatively weak expression of D_4 and D_5.[31, 33] mRNA for the D_1 receptor is expressed in the SCN, SON, and PVN. In the case of the D_2 receptor, both the long and short forms are expressed in the hypothalamus.[31] However, cell bodies of the ARC DA neurons and their axonal projections express principally the D_{2s} isoform, which therefore likely functions as a DA autoreceptor for presynaptic inhibition, whereas the D_{2L} form is targeted to dopaminergic fibers and is primarily a postsynaptic receptor.[34] The D_5 receptor is weakly expressed in the SON and PVN of primates and humans.[35] The pituitary expresses predominantly the D_2 receptor subtype localized on lactotrophs, thyrotrophs, somatotrophs, and melanotrophs.[28] mRNA for both the long and short forms has been identified in both melanotroph and lactotroph cells, in which the longer form is predominant.[31, 36] The D_4 receptor has also been identified in the anterior pituitary, but its cellular localization and function in hormone regulation remains to be defined.[37]

Serotonin

5-HT exerts an important influence on the secretion of LH, ACTH, PRL, and GH (see Table 13–1). Networks of serotoninergic fibers are found throughout the brain and can be traced to cell bodies in the raphe nucleus in the midbrain and in the medulla[5, 16, 38] (see Fig. 13–2). In addition, 5-HT–containing cell bodies have been identified in the hypothalamus, substantia nigra, and spinal cord.[5, 38] Projections from the raphe nucleus to the hypothalamus form a compact bundle in the mesencephalon just above the interpeduncular nucleus before entering the hypothalamus, where they terminate in the ARC, VMN, and ME.[39] Intrinsic hypothalamic neurons that synthesize 5-HT (identified by the presence of tryptophan hydroxylase) have been demonstrated in several areas, especially the SCN, ARC, and VMN.[17, 24] 5-HT is also synthesized in the pituitary, where it is localized mainly in secretory granules of gonadotrophs.[40] There are at least 16 distinct subtypes of 5-HT receptors that have been cloned so far from mammalian tissues.[19] The majority are seven–transmembrane domain G protein–coupled receptors that have been divided into three major subclasses: 5-HT₁ (types 1ₐ, 1ᵦ, 1ᴅ, 1ᴇ, 1ꜰ), 5-HT₂ (types 2ₐ, 2ᵦ, 2c), and miscellaneous (5-HT₃, 5-HT₄, 5-HT₅ₐ, 5-HT₅ᵦ, 5-HT₆, and 5-HT₇).[19, 41, 42] The 5-HT₃ receptor is a pentameric ligand-gated ion channel. The first 5-HT

receptors appeared in evolution more than 750 million years ago before muscarinic, dopamine, and adrenergic receptors, and all biogenic amine receptors can be considered to be direct descendants of the primordial 5-HT receptor.[42] High-affinity binding sites for 5-HT have been identified in the anterior pituitary,[43] and several of the 5-HT receptor subtypes have been mapped to distinct hypothalamic loci that play a role in a number of autonomic functions and behavior. 5-HT₁ₐ is expressed at moderate levels in the preoptic area (POA) and VMN of the monkey hypothalamus.[40] 5-HT₂ₐ is confined to the PVN, SON, and mammillary nuclei.[44] 5-HT₂c is extensively distributed in the POA, anterior hypothalamic area, PeVN, VMN, ARC, DMN, and choroid plexus. 5-HT₃ receptors have been identified in the rat VMN.[45]

Histamine

Although histamine has been detected in discrete hypothalamic regions such as the ME and posterior hypothalamic nuclei, it was not clear whether the amine was produced in nerve cells or whether it was derived from mast cells that are present in regions such as the ME. Histamine-secreting neurons have now been identified with certainty in the posterior hypothalamus, from where they project to the magnocellular and parvicellular nuclei and play an important role in the control of the neurohypophysis.[46, 47] There are three pharmacologic classes of histamine receptor subtypes—H₁, H₂, and H₃—two of which (H₁ and H₂) have been identified by molecular cloning as typical seven transmembrane–domain receptors.[19] Dehydration-induced activation of the magnocellular vasopressinergic neuron is produced in part through activation of the central histaminergic system. Histamine also stimulates the secretion of oxytocin and induces ACTH release by stimulating CRH-containing neurons via activation of both H₁- and H₂-receptors.[48]

Aminergic Transmitters

Excitatory Amino Acids

GLU is the major endogenous excitatory amino acid (EAA) in the central nervous system (CNS) that mediates excitatory synaptic transmission through EAA receptors.[5] It has long been known to be an important mediator of neuronal plasticity, long-term potentiation, and neurotoxicity,[6, 50] but it is now recognized as a prominent transmitter in the hypothalamus with an important role in the regulation of, especially, gonadotropin secretion, but also regulation of ACTH and GH[49, 50] (see Table 13–1). GLU is synthesized from glutamine mainly by the mitochondrial enzyme phosphate-activated glutaminase (see Fig. 13–1) present in both neurons and glia and exists as four different pools: a transmitter pool, metabolic pool, glial pool, and GABA precursor pool.[49, 51] Because of its ability to induce excitotoxic cell death, the extracellular concentration of GLU is kept low (0.3 μm) compared with that in synaptic vesicles (100 mM).[49, 51] Released GLU is rapidly cleared by high-affinity transporters on neurons and glia and is either used directly by neurons or recycled through glia. Glutamine synthetase, an enzyme found only in glial cells, converts GLU to glutamine, which is then released into the extracellular space for uptake by neurons for use as a substrate for the phosphate-activated glutaminase–driven neuronal production of GLU. GLU-positive neurons are extensively distributed throughout the brain, principally in the neocortex, hippocampus, olfactory bulb, and cerebellum[5] (see Fig. 13–2). GLU immunostaining has been localized in most of the principal hypothalamic nuclei: SON, PVN, SCN, ARC, VMN; the lateral hypothalamic area; the infundibular stalk; and the ME.[52] Most of the immunoreactivity is concentrated in presynaptic terminals, with lesser amounts in astrocytic processes.[52] GLU receptors are heterogeneous and can be classified into two major categories: (1) ionotropic receptors comprising *N*-methyl-D-aspartate (NMDA) receptors, kainate (KA) receptors, and α-amino-3-hydroxy-5-methyl-4-isoxazole propionate (AMPA) receptors, which are ligand-gated, cation-specific channels with different permeabilities for Ca^{2+}, Na^+, and K^+ ions, and (2) metabotropic (MGlu) receptors, which signal via G proteins to modulate second messenger systems such as adenylyl cyclase and inositol triphosphate.[53] GLU receptor ion channels are made of multiple subunits with different configurations. The NMDA receptor comprises five separate subunit genes termed *NMDAR-1 (NR1),* the common subunit, and *NR2A-D.* The NR1 subunits assemble either as homomeric structures or heteromeric complexes with NR2A to D subunits to form a diverse array of functional receptor channels.[53] A similar complexity applies for the AMPA-KA receptors. There are at least six MGlu receptor subtypes that can be divided into three subclasses. Binding studies have shown a rich expression of GLU receptors throughout the rat hypothalamus, with the following relative densities: NMDA receptor > MGlu receptor > KA receptor > AMPA receptor.[54] mRNA for NR1 has been localized to the SON, PVN, POA, ARC, VMN, and the ME.[55] NR1 has also been localized in the anterior pituitary to LH, follicle-stimulating hormone (FSH), GH, and PRL cells.[56] AMPA receptors also occur throughout the hypothalamus in virtually the same regions as do NMDA receptors.[49] KA receptors have been less well characterized but have been described in the ARC and ME.[49] Metabotropic receptors have been identified in the POA, SCN, SON, the lateral hypothalamus, and the anterior pituitary.[49]

Inhibitory Amino Acids

GABA is the principal inhibitory neurotransmitter in the brain. It inhibits virtually all tuberohypophysial neurons, including SST and CRH neurons, and exerts a direct effect on PRL release from the pituitary (see Table 13–1). Glycine is also an inhibitory transmitter in spinal interneurons but does not appear to affect neurons above the brain stem. GABA is synthesized from GLU by the enzyme glutamic acid decarboxylase (GAD) and is secreted by many neurons throughout the brain, including those in the hypothalamus[17] (see Fig. 13–1). Immunohistochemical studies using antibodies to GAD have mapped GABA-containing neurons throughout the forebrain, in the cerebellum and pons, and in small interneurons in the dorsal horn of the spinal cord[57] (see Fig. 13–2). Dense networks of GAD immunoreactive fibers occur throughout the hypothalamus, especially in the posterior hypothalamus and ME.[57, 58] Deafferentation studies have indicated that many of the GABA-ergic terminals arise from cell bodies located outside the hypothalamus.[17] A tuberoinfundibular GABA-ergic system also exists, with perikarya located in the ARC and projections to the ME that release GABA directly into the portal blood.[59, 60] There are two main classes of GABA receptors, $GABA_A$ and $GABA_B$, both with complex structures.[19] $GABA_A$ receptors are ligand-gated oligomeric ion channels, typically organized in a pentameric configuration, which regulate chloride ion permeability.[19] Benzodiazepine, barbiturates, and muscimol act as agonists at these receptors, and bicuculline is a selective antagonist. $GABA_B$ receptors have been characterized as G protein–coupled receptor heterodimers made up of two seven transmembrane–domain proteins that associate in the endoplasmic reticulum via the receptor C-tail and are targeted to the plasma as a functional dimeric receptor complex.[61] Binding of $GABA_B$ receptor agonists such as baclofen activates adenylyl cyclase, K^+, and Ca^{2+} ion channels via Gi/Go proteins. Both $GABA_A$ and $GABA_B$ receptors have been demonstrated in the dorsomedial hypothalamus.[62] GABA receptors are also present in the pituitary and mediate inhibition of LH, GH, and PRL release.[63]

Gaseous Neurotransmitters: Nitric Oxide and Carbon Monoxide

NO is a diffusible intercellular and intracellular messenger that is synthesized from L-arginine by the action of nitric oxide synthase (NOS) (see Fig. 13–1), a heme protein enzyme that exists in at least three isoforms, neuronal (nNOS), endothelial (eNOS), and macrophage (mNOS) forms.[8, 9] NO activates soluble guanylate cyclase to generate cyclic guanosine monophosphate and subserves a wide variety of physiologic functions, including vasodilatation, immune cell regulation, and neural effects.[8, 9] In the brain, NO influences learning and memory through long-term potentiation, sex drive, aggression, and ingestive behaviors; mediates hypothalamic portal blood flow; and is involved in the secretion of GnRH, oxytocin, vasopressin, CRH, GH, and PRL.[9, 64] nNOS is highly concentrated in the olfactory bulb, the pontine tegmental nucleus, the superior and inferior colliculi, the islands of Calleja, the striatum, and the hippocampus.[9] Within the hypothalamic-pituitary unit, nNOS-containing neurons are densely expressed in the SON and PVN, where they frequently coexist with oxytocin and vasopressin in magnocellular neurons.[65] The axonal projections of the paraventricular neurons show intense nNOS staining as they traverse the inner layer of the ME and into the neurohypophysis. nNOS also colocalizes with a proportion of parvicellular CRH-producing neurons in the anterior hypothalamus as well as in neurons in the medial POA, VMN, SCN, and lateral hypothalamus. Some of the anterior pituitary cells have also been shown to colocalize nNOS. Carbon monoxide formed by heme oxygenase is an inhibitory neurotransmitter involved in the regulation of GnRH and CRH release.[49]

Peptides

Both the magnocellular and parvocellular hypothalamic tuberoinfundibular neurons that regulate the pituitary are themselves regulated by other neuropeptides, both from within the hypothalamus and from outside. Peptides found in the hypothalamus may either be produced locally in hypothalamic neurons or derived from transport from neurons located in other brain regions such as the brain stem, for example, NPY.[67] Most of the peptides are distributed both in the hypothalamus and in the extrahypothalamic brain, with the hypothalamus typically expressing the highest concentrations, the exceptions being VIP, CCK, and NPY.[1, 5, 12, 13] Prominent neuropeptide systems such as SST, TRH, CRH, VIP, CCK, NPY, substance P, and neurotensin are distributed in nerve cell bodies and fibers both in the hypothalamus and in other CNS regions; they influence appetite, thirst, pain perception, body temperature, memory, and learning, in addition to neuroendocrine functions such as growth, reproduction, and stress responses.[1] Neurons that secrete these peptides are distributed throughout the various hypothalamic nuclei and form a network of local feedback circuits, for example, between SST- and GHRH-producing neurons; they also send ascending and descending projections to the rest of the brain. A description of all the hypothalamic peptide networks is outside the scope of this chapter, and only POMC, NPY, and galanin, which feature prominently in neuroendocrine control, are mentioned.

Opioid Peptides

Opioid peptides and their synthetic agonists exert broad effects on pituitary hormone secretion, stimulating the release of PRL, GH, and ACTH and inhibiting the release of LH, oxytocin, and arginine vasopressin (AVP).[69] Met- and leu-enkephalin were the first endogenous opioids to be isolated from brain.[14] Since then, a number of larger neuropeptides containing enkephalin sequences have been identified, including β-endorphin (contains the met-enkephalin sequence) and the dynorphins (contains the leu-enkephalin sequence). In mammals, the opioid peptides are synthesized from three separate precursors—POMC, preproenkephalin A, and preproenkephalin B (preprodynorphin)—that arise from a single ancestral gene.[1, 12–14] POMC yields the opioid β-endorphin and the nonopioid peptides ACTH and α-melanocyte–stimulating hormone (α-MSH).[14] Within the hypothalamus, POMC neurons are localized exclusively in the ARC and innervate the VMN, PVN, DMN, and other areas of the hypothalamus as well as the amygdala and the periaqueductal gray of the midbrain[69] (see Fig. 13–2). Preproenkephalin A and preproenkephalin B show an overlapping and more extensive distribution in the hypothalamus, hippocampus, nucleus accumbens, and spinal cord[70] (see Fig. 13–2). Leu- and met-enkephalin–producing neurons occur in the ARC, VMN, DMN, and PVN.[70] Dynorphin-producing neurons are concentrated mainly in the ARC and PVN.[69] There are three pharmacologic subtypes of the opioid receptors referred to as μ, δ, and κ.[69] All three have been structurally characterized by molecular cloning and shown to consist of seven transmembrane–domain proteins that signal via Gi/Go.[17] β-Endorphin binds to both μ- and δ-receptors, whereas leu- and met-enkephalin show selectivity for the δ opioid receptor, and dynorphin A binds preferentially to the κ-receptor.[19, 69] Preproenkephalin B contains three leu-enkephalin sequences, but the most significant products of its processing may be larger opioid peptides, the dynorphins and neoendorphins.[14] Binding studies as well as mRNA distribution suggest that μ- and κ-receptors predominate in the hypothalamus, the expression of δ-receptors being relatively sparse.[69] κ-receptors are predominantly localized in the SON, PVN, ME, and posterior pituitary, suggesting that this isoform mediates the inhibition of AVP and oxytocin. Expression of μ- and κ-receptors in the medial POA and the ARC suggests that both these isotypes are involved in inhibiting LH release and augmenting PRL, GH, and ACTH.[69]

Melanocortins

The hypothalamic melanocortin system comprises peptides such as α-MSH derived from neuronal POMC processing in the hypothalamic ARC and the brain stem.[14] α-MSH induces satiety, hypothermia, and behavioral and cardiovascular effects, in addition to neuroendocrine actions such as the inhibition of PRL and LH secretion. There are five melanocortin receptors (MCRs) that belong to a subfamily of G protein–coupled receptors.[19, 71] MC1R is the peripheral MSH receptor that controls skin color in some species. MC2R is the ACTH receptor in the adrenal cortex. MC3R and MC4R are primarily expressed in the brain. MC3R is localized in the ARC, whereas MC4R is widely distributed in many sites throughout the brain (including several in the hypothalamus, e.g., PVN, VMN, and DMN) that are involved in anterior pituitary regulation.[72]

Neuropeptide Y

NPY, a 36–amino acid peptide, is a member of the pancreatic polypeptide (PP) family that includes peptide YY (PYY) and PP. It is the most abundant neuropeptide in the central and peripheral nervous system and has been shown to exert powerful and complex effects on feeding, reproduction, anxiety, circadian rhythms, memory retention, thermoregulation, pituitary adrenal function, and cardiovascular and gastrointestinal regulation.[73] There are two main sites of NPY-producing neurons in the brain, one in the hypothalamus in the ARC and another in the brain stem in the locus coeruleus.[74, 75] Arcuate NPY neurons project along two distinct pathways, the reproductive axis—ARC-ME and medial preoptic area (MPOA)—and the orexigenic axis—ARC-PVN and neighboring regions.[73–75] Transection studies have shown that 40% to 50% of hypothalamic NPY is derived from the brain stem via ascending pathways that overlap with the ascending catecholaminergic system and is involved in the regulation of feeding behavior.[67] NPY activates a heterogeneous group of at least six G protein–coupled receptors termed Y1 to Y6, all of which except the Y3 receptor have been cloned.[76] The Y1 and Y5 receptors are localized in the ARC, lateral hypothalamus, and PVN and appear to be the subtypes that mediate appetite regulation by NPY.[76] The Y2 receptor is also localized in the ARC and may be an autoreceptor regulating NPY release.[76] The Y4 receptors are PP-preferring and the Y6 receptor is either absent or inactive in rats and humans.[76] NPY stimulates LH release by acting on GnRH neurons via Y1 receptors[77] as well as through a direct action on pituitary gonadotrophs to potentiate the LH response to GnRH.[78]

Galanin

Galanin is a 29–amino acid peptide that is widely distributed in the brain.[79] In the hypothalamus, it is found mainly in arcuate neurons where it colocalizes with GHRH and GnRH as well as with GABA and TIDA neurons.[80] It is coreleased with GnRH in the portal circulation and potentiates GnRH action on the pituitary.[81] Galanin also colocalizes with PRL,[82, 83] GH, and TSH[84] in the pituitary. Galanin acts through two receptors, GALR1 and GALR2, both of which occur in the hypothalamus.[85]

TRANSMITTER CONTROL OF PITUITARY HORMONES

Gonadotropins

GnRH is the principal hypothalamic regulator of LH and FSH secretion.[1, 2, 49, 86–90] Cell bodies of GnRH neurons are located in the MPOA and SCN and send projections that terminate in the external zone of the ME, especially in the anterolateral portion.[89–91] Some axons project to the brain stem and may be involved in mating behavior.[90] In most species, there is a second collection of GnRH perikarya in the arcuate nucleus, whose axons also project to the ME.[89, 90] Release of GnRH occurs either in a pulsatile manner with a characteristic 90-minute ultradian variation or as a preovulatory surge.[2, 92] Both types of secretion are profoundly influenced by gonadal steroids, with superimposed neural control mediated by biogenic amines, neuropeptides, excitatory amino acids, and NO.[86–88] Basal release of GnRH occurs in a pulsatile manner in both sexes through the action of the hypothalamic GnRH pulse generator.[86–88, 92, 93] Castration increases pulsatile secretion but with a differential effect in males and females.[2, 88, 92, 93] In female rats and in humans, both the pulse amplitude and frequency are affected, whereas in male rats there is a change in frequency but not in amplitude of the GnRH–induced LH pulses.[88, 93–95] Administration of testosterone or estradiol-17β inhibits pulsatile GnRH release. The preovulatory LH surge that causes ovulation is triggered by a surge of GnRH induced as a result of positive feedback by rising preovulatory estrogen levels.[88] In addition to increased GnRH release, there is a 20- to 50-fold increase in pituitary GnRH responsiveness that occurs between the diestrous stage and the late afternoon of the proestrous stage in the rat and between the early follicular and ovulatory phases of the cycle in humans.[93, 96] The pulsatile mode of GnRH release prevents downregulation of the GnRH receptor and indeed may be responsible for the upregulated receptor function, which is responsible for pituitary GnRH sensitization because exposure of the pituitary to small exogenous pulses of GnRH can also produce a massive LH surge.[97, 98] Despite the fact that GnRH neurons are subject to such tight control by estrogen, remarkably these neurons have been found by autoradiography and immunocytochemistry essentially to be devoid of estrogen receptors.[99] The rapid negative feedback effect of estrogen on the GnRH-LH release system does not require new protein synthesis and seems to be due to a direct nongenomic action on membrane ion channels and other transmembrane effectors.[88] The effects of estrogen that involve a genomic mechanism such as the positive feedback effect on the midcycle GnRH surge must therefore be mediated indirectly by estrogen receptor–positive non-GnRH neurons that terminate on GnRH neurons.[88, 100, 101] The likely candidates are noradrenergic, glutamatergic, and NO-producing transmitter neurons and NPY-, galanin-, neurotensin-, and tachykinin-producing peptidergic neurons (all of which are facilitatory) and opioid-, dopaminergic, and CRH-producing neurons (which are inhibitory).[2, 4, 49, 86–88]

Norepinephrine

There is good evidence that noradrenergic neurons facilitate both pulsatile and preovulatory LH release. For instance, inhibition of NE synthesis,[92, 103] blockade of α-adrenergic receptors,[104] or destruction of the ventral noradrenergic bundle with 6-hydroxy-dopamine[105] results in suppression of pulsatile LH release in the castrated rat. Other studies, however, have found inhibition of pulsatile LH release by intraventricular infusion of NE[92] or by electrical stimulation of the ascending NE bundle.[106] Furthermore, hypothalamic deafferentation does not affect pulsatile LH release in the monkey.[107] Although these findings clearly suggest the involvement of adrenergic receptors in regulating pulsatile LH release, the mechanism of action remains unclear and the site of action is likely extrahypothalamic, at least in primates. The role of NE pathways in stimulating the preovulatory LH surge is more definite. The MPOA is innervated by ascending noradrenergic fibers from the locus coeruleus, and these fibers stimulate GnRH and LH release.[87, 92, 98, 102, 103] As in the case of pulsatile LH release, drugs that block NE synthesis or α-adrenergic receptors interrupt ovulation.[87, 88] Estrogen treatment increases NE turnover in the MPOA,[108] and lesions of the ventral noradrenergic tract inhibit the ovulatory surge of LH.[109]

Dopamine

The nature of the interaction between DA and GnRH neurons is less clear.[4] DA nerve terminals overlap with those of GnRH in the external layer of the ME[110] and D_1- and D_2-receptor expression has been localized in the ARC and SCN, which contain GnRH neurons. Some studies have suggested that DA inhibits both pulsatile and phasic GnRH secretion and that the amenorrhea that occurs in prolactinomas may be explained by this mechanism through short-loop feedback stimulation of hypothalamic DA by PRL.[3, 87] Dopamine, however, has also been shown to augment GnRH release from rat ME fragments in vitro,[111] and intraventricular injections of DA stimulate LH release.[112] High doses of DA or DA agonists given peripherally inhibit GnRH and LH release.[2, 92]

γ-Aminobutyric Acid

GABA exerts an inhibitory effect on both the pulsatile and preovulatory LH surge.[87] For instance, the infusion of GABA or the GABA agonists muscimol or baclofen inhibit both pulsatile and steroid-induced LH surges in rats.[113] Conversely, the administration of $GABA_A$ and $GABA_B$ receptor antagonists potentiate basal and NE-induced LH release.[114] A functional relationship between GABA and GnRH is suggested by the finding of GABA-containing synapses on GnRH neurons[116] as well as an inverse correlation between LH pulses and GABA release in the POA measured by a push-pull cannula.[116] Direct studies of GnRH release from ME fragments in vitro or from the GnRH neuronal cell line GT1 have shown a biphasic effect of GABA characterized by transient stimulation mediated via $GABA_A$ receptors and a more potent inhibitory action via $GABA_B$ receptors.[87, 117] Finally, a direct stimulatory effect of GABA on LH release from the pituitary, mediated via $GABA_A$ receptors,[118] has been proposed. However, the effect of GABA in this system is small and of doubtful significance.

Acetylcholine and Serotonin

Cholinergic innervation does not appear to play a significant role in gonadotrophin secretion. Likewise, the role of the 5-HT system in GnRH regulation remains controversial.[3, 119] 5-HT exerts both a stimulatory and inhibitory effect on pulsatile LH release in ovariectomized rats, with no clear effect in male rats. Like DA, 5-HT stimulates in vitro GnRH release from ME fragments, and the preovulatory LH surge is accompanied by increased 5-HT turnover in the ME, suggesting a facilitatory role of the amine on phasic GnRH discharge.[119]

Excitatory Amino Acids

Although recognized for many years as a major transmitter system in the brain, it is only since the late 1980s that GLU has assumed a pre-eminent role in the hypothalamus.[5, 49, 50] Both GLU and GLU receptors are localized in a variety of hypothalamic nuclei involved in reproduction and other neuroendocrine functions. The first demonstration of an effect of GLU on the reproductive axis came from the work of Olney and colleagues[120] and Ondo and coworkers[121] who showed that GLU administered either systemically or into the third ventricle stimulated LH release in male rats. Subsequent studies showed a

similar effect of NMDA.[122] The non-NMDA agonists KA and AMPA also induce gonadotropin secretion but to a lesser extent than do the NMDA agonists.[49] Antagonists of the NMDA and non-NMDA receptors block both pulsatile GnRH release and the estradiol-induced preovulatory LH surge.[49, 123] The effect of GLU on LH secretion is steroid dependent. Both estradiol and progesterone enhance LH response to EAAs through mechanisms that remain unclear but could involve enhanced hypothalamic release or pituitary sensitivity to GnRH or induction of GLU receptors by, for example, steroids.[49, 124, 125] The effect of GLU on LH secretion is targeted primarily at the hypothalamic level because central administration of GLU induces LH secretion and GnRH antagonists block the ability of GLU to stimulate LH, providing indirect evidence for GLU-induced hypothalamic GnRH release.[49, 126] A pituitary effect of GLU has not been entirely excluded because ionotropic receptors have been described in anterior pituitary cells, and some but not all studies have shown an effect of GLU agonists on LH release from anterior pituitary cells in culture.[56, 127, 128] Direct studies have shown that all three classes of ionotropic EAA receptors (NMDA, AMPA, and KA) stimulate GnRH release from hypothalamic fragments.[129, 130] The site of action of GLU in the hypothalamus has been determined by measurement of c-fos immunoreactivity as a marker of neuronal activity after GLU administration. These studies have shown that NMDA induces an increase in c-fos in the POA and ARC-ME as well as in noradrenergic cells of the locus coeruleus.[131, 132] They suggest that the POA is the major site of action of NMDA in the regulation of GnRH and LH release and that the ARC and extrahypothalamic nuclei such as the locus coeruleus may be important contributing sites. Although the induction of c-fos in GnRH neurons by NMDA argues for a direct effect of the transmitter, other lines of evidence suggest that the action of GLU on GnRH neurons is indirect via interneurons.[49] The most compelling evidence is the finding that less than 5% of GnRH neurons express NMDA receptors.[133] Furthermore, induction of c-fos by NMDA has been reported to involve not GnRH neurons but adjacent neurons. If the effect of GLU on GnRH neurons is indirect, what are the intermediary connections? The findings that NMDA induces c-fos in noradrenergic neurons of the locus coeruleus and that EAAs can stimulate NE release from the hypothalamus[134] have led to the suggestion that catecholamines may mediate the effects of EAAs on GnRH release. A similar though lesser role has also been proposed for DA.[135]

Other potential mediators include galanin, NO, opioids, and NPY. Galanin is a potent stimulator of GnRH secretion.[81] Blockade of the midcycle LH surge by NMDA receptor antagonists reduces galanin mRNA levels in the hypothalamus, implicating galanin as a mediator of GLU effects on GnRH neurons.[136] NPY is coreleased with galanin and GnRH in the ME and, in concert with galanin, amplifies the pituitary sensitivity to GnRH.[87] NO activates guanylate cyclase in the POA and elevates cyclic guanosine monophosphate levels, which stimulate GnRH secretion.[137] NO also stimulates GnRH release from GT1 to GT7 GnRH neurons that have undergone immortalization.[138] Furthermore, the NMDA-induced LH increase as well as the steroid-induced preovulatory LH surge has been shown to be blocked by NOS inhibitors.[139] Likewise, central administration of nNOS antisense oligonucleotides attenuates the steroid-induced LH surge.[140] All this evidence supports a key role for NO as an important regulator of GnRH neurons.

There is considerable evidence that the hypothalamic opioid system exerts a potent inhibitory effect on GnRH secretion, both in humans and in experimental animals.[86, 87, 93, 98] After the initial observation by Barraclough and colleagues in 1955 that morphine blunts the preovulatory LH surge,[141] subsequent studies showed that the endogenous opioid peptides β-endorphin and dynorphin inhibit LH secretion and that naloxone injection to block μ opioid–receptors augments LH secretion.[142, 143] The functional relationship between the opioid system and GnRH secretion is modulated by ovarian steroids, with maximal sensitization by high estrogen–high progesterone feedback, resulting in opioid inhibitory effects on both pulsatile and phasic GnRH secretion.[143, 144] Studies suggest that GLU- and NO-producing neurons in the MPOA and medial basal hypothalamus of the rat are tonically inhibited by the opioid system because the administration of naloxone leads to enhanced NOS activity in these regions.[49] Treatment with

GLU receptor antagonists blocks both the naloxone-induced LH surge and the naloxone-induced increase in hypothalamic NOS activity, suggesting that opioid inhibition may be exerted on GLU neurons and that release of this inhibition facilitates hypothalamic GLU release and activation of NOS.[49, 145]

The overall model that emerges suggests a central role for GLU in triggering the preovulatory LH surge.[49] According to this model, GnRH secretion is under the influence of both excitatory and inhibitory neurotransmitters, which are regulated by steroid hormones. GLU, NO, NPY, galanin, and catecholamines provide the stimulatory effect, and opioid neurons, along with contributions from GABA and neuropeptide K, serve as the inhibitory components.[49, 86] Under basal conditions, opioids tonically restrain GnRH secretion by inhibiting GLU, catecholamine, and NPY neurons. The preovulatory LH surge is induced by rising steroid hormone levels in the blood, which turn off the opioid neurons and thereby activate the stimulatory transmitter components.

Role of Neurotransmitters in Puberty

GnRH neurons are capable of normal responses in fetal life and postnatally but display only low basal GnRH secretion up to the time of puberty.[1] The fundamental change at the time of puberty is the onset of pulsatile GnRH secretion and has led to the concept that GnRH secretion is under tonic inhibition because of increased sensitivity to steroid hormone feedback and that puberty represents a resetting of gonadal steroid feedback and release from inhibition. Given the central role of GLU neurons in GnRH control, it is not surprising that the establishment of excitatory GLU input to GnRH neurons may play a fundamental role in initiating puberty.[49] Pulsatile or prolonged intermittent administration of NMDA to rats and monkeys has been shown to advance puberty.[146, 147] Likewise, treatment with NMDA antagonists delays puberty in female rats.[148] The administration of KA has no effect on the timing of puberty, and the role of AMPA and metabotropic GLU receptors has not been adequately investigated. Consistent with the effect of exogenous NMDA in advancing puberty, the levels of endogenous GLU increase in the POA in female rats at the time of puberty.[149] Thus, GLU acting through NMDA receptors appears to be an important mediator of the onset of pulsatile and phasic GnRH secretion that characterizes puberty.

Corticotropin

Although a variety of substances secreted into the portal blood are known to influence ACTH secretion, it is CRH that sets the tone for the dynamic control of the synthesis and release of ACTH and β-endorphin from the anterior pituitary, both normally and in response to a variety of stressors.[150–152] Normal ACTH secretion displays a circadian rhythm with superimposed ultradian peaks and reflects a pulsatile as well as phasic CRH release pattern.[1] The parvocellular division of the PVN contains the majority of CRF-positive neurons whose axonal projections terminate in the ME.[153] The PVN CRH neurons receive afferent input from the SCN, amygdala, hippocampus, locus coeruleus, and raphe nucleus of the brain stem.[27, 154, 155] AVP, which is synergistic with CRH in stimulating ACTH release,[150–152] is colocalized in approximately 50% of CRH neurons and is cosecreted with ACTH in the ME.[156] The relative proportion of CRH neurons that colocalize AVP is regulated by glucocorticoid feedback and increases dramatically after adrenalectomy.[157] Many of the PVN CRH neurons also co-stain for other peptides, including dynorphin and enkephalin.[158, 159] Scattered CRH-positive cells are also found in other regions of the hypothalamus such as the POA, PeVN, SCN, premammillary nucleus, and the dorsal and lateral hypothalamic areas.[89, 153] CRH is also produced in many extrahypothalamic structures such as the cerebral cortex, the limbic system (particularly the amygdala and the nucleus of the striae terminalis), locus coeruleus, cerebellum, and spinal cord, and in a number of peripheral tissues including the gut, adrenals, testes, placenta, and immune cells.[160]

Acetylcholine

There is general agreement that stimulation of cholinergic transmission activates the hypothalamic-pituitary-adrenal (HPA) axis in both animals and humans. Early studies in rats showed that the peripheral administration of cholinesterase inhibitors such as physostigmine, as well as intracerebroventricular injection or ME implantation of cholinergic agonists, stimulated corticosterone secretion in rats.[161] The administration of physostigmine has also been shown to stimulate ACTH, β-endorphin, and cortisol secretion in humans,[162] although other studies have attributed cholinergic stimulation of the HPA to nonspecific side effects of the drugs used.[163, 164] Atropine implanted in the ME inhibits plasma ACTH responses to surgical stress, ether anesthesia, and intravenous injection of AVP.[165] Unfortunately, these types of experiments do not discriminate between the effects of CRH or AVP released in the ME and whether the cholinergic agents act directly on PVN CRH neurons or on the pituitary. Other studies, however, have shown that cholinergic agents do not stimulate ACTH release from the pituitary in vitro and that Ach stimulates CRH release directly from rat hypothalamus in vitro.[165, 166] Both muscarinic and nicotinic receptors are involved in the control of CRH, the predominant effect being muscarinic.[165, 166]

Catecholamines

The PVN CRH neurons receive a rich catecholaminergic innervation from brain stem noradrenergic and adrenergic neurons. Light and electron microscopic immunocytochemical studies have identified the presence of synaptic contacts between CRH and both NE and Epi terminals.[27, 167–170] These afferents convey visceral sensory information from the vagus and glossopharyngeal nerves and thus may mediate ACTH responses to hypovolemia. Although an anatomic link between the central catecholaminergic system and CRH has been clearly established, the nature of the pharmacologic and functional interaction between the two systems is controversial.[171] Several studies have suggested a facilitatory role of central catecholamines on CRH and ACTH secretion, whereas others have found an inhibitory effect.[171] Analysis of the stimulatory activity of catecholamines in in vivo studies is complicated by the fact that catecholamines possess weak ACTH-stimulating activity at the pituitary level.[172, 173] Direct sampling of portal blood for CRH after electrical stimulation of the ventral noradrenergic ascending bundle, or after intracerebroventricular administration of NE, has shown a predominantly stimulatory effect of NE on hypothalamic CRH secretion.[155] Pretreatment with the α1-adrenergic antagonist coryanthine blocked the facilitatory effect of electrical stimulation on portal vein CRH levels.[156] The effect of NE was dose dependent, low doses stimulating CRH via α1-adrenergic receptors and high doses inhibiting CRH via β2-adrenergic receptors.[155] In vitro studies with cultured rat hypothalami have consistently shown a stimulatory effect of catecholamines.[174, 175] Human studies have also shown that the HPA can be stimulated by the α1-adrenergic agonist methoxamine and that this α-adrenergic pathway is involved in food-stimulated ACTH release but not in circadian rhythmicity.[171, 176] In contrast to the catecholamines, DA is thought to play only a minor role in the regulation of CRH secretion or ACTH release from the anterior pituitary.[4, 177] However, the ACTH that is produced in the intermediate lobe in rodents, and that produced in humans during pregnancy and fetal development, is under tonic hypothalamic dopaminergic inhibition.

Serotonin

There is considerable evidence to suggest the involvement of 5-HT in regulating pituitary-adrenal function in experimental animals and humans.[178] CRF-containing PVN neurons receive synaptic input from ascending serotoninergic projections from the midbrain raphe nuclei.[39] Serotoninergic neurotransmission appears to be profoundly involved in the circadian periodicity of the HPA. Lesions of the raphe nuclei or limbic pathways or blockade of 5-HT synthesis abolishes circadian rhythm of plasma corticosterone in rats.[3] Drugs that enhance 5-HT function, including 5-HT precursors, 5-HT uptake inhibitors, 5-HT releasers, and direct 5-HT receptor agonists, stimulate CRF, ACTH, and corticosterone release in vivo in the rat.[178] This effect is mediated at the hypothalamic level because 5-HT stimulates the release of bio- or immunoassayable CRF from isolated rat hypothalami in vitro.[179] ACTH elevation in rats by the 5-HT agonists, 8-hydroxy-2-(di-*n*-propyl) aminotetralin (8-OH-DPAT), *m*-chlorophenylpiperazine, and 1-(2,5-dimethoxy-4-iodophenyl)-2-amino propane (DOI) is blocked by antibody to CRF, suggesting that stimulation of CRF release is the primary mechanism for the effect of the agonists in vivo.[180] Among the multiple 5-HT receptor subtypes that have been identified in brain, 5-HT$_{1A}$, and 5-HT$_2$/5-HT$_{1C}$ receptors have been shown to mediate activation of pituitary-adrenal function.[178] Uncertainty remains about the involvement of the other 5-HT subtypes, in large part because of the absence of subtype-selective antagonists.

γ-Aminobutyric Acid

GABA exerts an inhibitory effect on resting and stimulated ACTH secretion.[1, 3, 152] The PVN CRH neurons are innervated by a rich network of GABA-ergic fibers, and GABA may also be cosynthesized and coreleased from CRH neurons in the ME.[152] GABA agonists inhibit stress-induced ACTH responses, and GABA antagonists have been shown to stimulate ACTH under basal conditions.[181] The actions of GABA are mediated by both the GABA$_A$ and GABA$_B$ receptor subtypes.[182] GABA and GABA$_A$ receptor agonists such as the benzodiazepines inhibit CRH release from rat hypothalamus in vitro.[182] Additionally, however, both GABA$_A$ and GABA$_B$ receptors are expressed on corticotrophs where they exert stimulatory (GABA$_A$) or inhibitory (GABA$_B$) effects.[183] The effect of GABA agonists on ACTH inhibition in humans is relatively mild but forms the basis for the medical treatment of some patients with Cushing's disease with sodium valproate.

Excitatory Amino Acids

EAAs play a major role in regulating the HPA.[49, 184] NMDA, KA, and quisqualate all evoke ACTH secretion through a central effect.[184] Dual-label in situ hybridization studies have colocalized NMDA, AMPA, and KA receptors in 30 to 70% of PVN CRH neurons, suggesting a direct influence of GLU on CRH release through NMDA, as well as non-NMDA, receptors.[185] EAAs do not stimulate ACTH release from rat pituitaries incubated in vitro, thereby excluding a direct pituitary level of action.[186] The injection of GLU into the PVN has been shown to stimulate ACTH release.[187] Likewise, EAAs have been reported to stimulate CRH release from hypothalamic fragments incubated in vitro.[49] Other studies, however, found that EAAs stimulate AVP and had no effect on CRH in this system.[188] Both GLU and NMDA facilitate CRH release when incubated with hypothalamic slices instead of whole hypothalamic fragments.[189] Furthermore, in vivo immunoneutralization experiments in the rat have shown that CRF antiserum, but not AVP antiserum, blocks NMDA- and KA-induced ACTH release, providing firm evidence for a facilitatory role of EAAs on CRH regulation.[186] Besides the hypothalamus, GLU has been shown to be capable of acting at other CNS sites, notably the amygdala and locus coeruleus, to stimulate ACTH release. The latter effect likely involves GLU-induced activation of noradrenergic afferents to the PVN CRH neurons.[189]

Nitric Oxide

NO is intimately involved in the regulation of the HPA axis.[64] NOS is colocalized with a proportion of PVN CRH–containing neurons. However, whether NO acts directly on these cells or indirectly through other neuromodulators remains unclear. Cytokines are capable of activating NOS as well as CRH secretion and appear to influence the HPA axis by modulating NOS activity. For instance, interleukins 1β (IL-1β), IL-2, and IL-6 stimulate CRH release from incubated hypothalami.[192, 193] IL-2–mediated release of CRH is augmented by L-arginine (the precursor for NO),[192] whereas inhibitors of NOS such as N(G)-monomethyl-L-arginine suppress IL-2–induced release of CRH.[192] Like the interleukins, there is evidence that neurotransmitters

such as Ach and neurohormones such as oxytocin and AVP influence CRH secretion by affecting NOS activity.[191] Overall then, these results imply a key role for NO as a mediator of the neuroendocrine-immune effects on the HPA axis.

Opioids

Opioids such as morphine and β-endorphin inhibit ACTH secretion via inhibition of hypothalamic CRH release.[194, 195] This effect is mediated via μ- and κ- but not δ–opioid receptors. The likely endogenous regulators are the dynorphins, which are cosynthesized by CRH neurons and act at κ-receptors,[196] as well as proenkephalin products such as adrenorphin, which act at both μ and κ sites. Although met-enkephalin has been reported to be produced in parallel with CRH in the hypothalamus in response to stress, it is a weak agonist of the μ- and κ-receptors, and its role as an endogenous inhibitory regulator of CRH release is thus uncertain.[197]

Prolactin

PRL is secreted in a pulsatile manner and displays a circadian rhythm as well as increases in response to stress, sexual intercourse, breast stimulation, and suckling.[1, 87, 198, 199] Neuroendocrine control of PRL is unique compared with the other adenohypophysial hormones in that it is under tonic inhibition by the hypothalamus and the mediator is not a peptide but an amine—DA acting as a neurohormone. DA is produced by ARC TIDA neurons and secreted into the portal capillaries. From there it is transported to the lactotrophs and interacts with D$_2$-receptors to inhibit both the synthesis and release of PRL, which, in turn, feeds back on the hypothalamus to increase the release and turnover of DA via PRL receptors on the TIDA neurons. The action of DA on the pituitary is opposed by estrogens that stimulate PRL synthesis directly. Furthermore, a long list of PRL-releasing factors (PRFs) have been identified, of which VIP, TRH, and galanin appear to be physiologically important. Secretion of DA and PRFs is in turn controlled by extrahypothalamic influences. Central dopaminergic pathways inhibit PRL release, whereas central serotoninergic and possibly noradrenergic pathways are excitatory.

Dopamine

There is substantial evidence that DA is the principal physiologic regulator of PRL secretion in animals and humans.[87, 198, 199] The in vivo secretion of PRL is severely restrained by hypothalamic DA because lesions of the ME or pituitary stalk or isolation of the pituitary in vitro increases basal PRL output. Drugs such as reserpine, which deplete catecholamines, and α-methyl-*p*-tyrosine, which blocks DA synthesis, augment PRL secretion. Dopamine has been identified in portal blood at concentrations ($\sim 10^{-8}$M) that are 5- to 10-fold higher than levels found in the peripheral circulation and sufficient to inhibit PRL secretion from the pituitary.[200] Stimuli such as cervical stimulation or electrical stimulation of the mammary nerve that produce an acute increase in PRL levels are temporally associated with decreased portal blood concentrations of DA, suggesting that inhibition of DA is the physiologic trigger for PRL release.[201] The degree of PRL stimulation in these experiments cannot be explained by a decline in DA concentration alone, however, and has led to the view that both a reduction in DA and a priming effect of a PRF are required for the full PRL stimulatory response. Infusions of DA in humans to achieve peripheral blood concentrations that mimic those in the rat or monkey portal blood are capable of suppressing basal PRL levels.[202, 203] Dopamine and D$_2$-receptor agonists like bromocriptine block PRL responses to provocative stimuli such as hypoglycemia,[204] arginine,[205] and TRH,[206] and drugs such as phenothiazines, butyrophenones, metoclopramide, and domperidone that antagonize D$_2$R stimulate PRL secretion.[198, 199, 206]

The pre-eminent role of the DA-D$_2$R pathway in regulating PRL secretion has been confirmed by gene knockout experiments.[208–210] Mice lacking the DA transporter display increased extracellular concentrations of DA and increased DA turnover in the hypothalamus and pituitary associated with downregulation of the lactotroph D_2-receptors.[208] The knockout mice fail to lactate and display a profound depletion of pituitary PRL stores as well as lactotroph hypoplasia, consistent with the impact of DA not only on PRL secretion but also on lactotroph proliferation. Alternatively, removal of DA action at the pituitary by D_2-receptor knockout in mice resulted in chronic hyperprolactinemia, more marked in females than in males, associated with lactotroph hyperplasia.[209, 210] Lactotroph proliferation was also more marked in females than in males and in one study,[210] but not another study, ultimately led to the development of prolactinomas in aged animals. Maintenance of the normal sexual dimorphism in PRL secretion in these animals highlights the important independent role of estrogen on PRL synthesis. These results demonstrate both an antisecretory and an antiproliferative effect of DA on lactotrophs, and overall they reveal a pivotal role of DA and the D_2-receptor in the physiologic regulation of PRL secretion and lactotroph cell growth.

Norepinephrine

The role of central noradrenergic neurons in the regulation of basal PRL secretion is unclear. Drugs that inhibit NE synthesis inhibit pulsatile PRL release in ovariectomized but not in intact male rats,[211, 212] and blockade of α_2-adrenergic receptors increases basal PRL secretion.[213] The administration of clonidine in humans fails to affect plasma PRL levels.[214] A noradrenergic pathway does not appear to be involved in the suckling-induced release of PRL. Hypothalamic NE turnover does not change in response to suckling,[215] and the suckling-induced release of PRL is unaffected by blockade of NE synthesis.[216] These findings are consistent with the results of hypothalamic deafferentation, which also does not affect PRL levels.[217] The role of NE innervation on stress-induced PRL secretion has not been well characterized. Available evidence based on blockade of stress-induced PRL release in rats by drugs that inhibit NE synthesis suggests a facilitatory role of noradrenergic neurons in the stress-induced PRL response.[87]

Serotonin

Serotoninergic neurons appear to be important in modulating the circadian variations in PRL secretion as well as suckling and stress-induced PRL responses. Central or systemic administration of 5-hydroxytryptophan increases PRL release.[218] A similar stimulatory effect is obtained by fenfluramine (5-HT–releasing agent) and fluoxetine (5-HT uptake inhibitor) in humans.[219, 220] By contrast, depletion of 5-HT stores or destruction of 5-HT nerve terminals decreases basal as well as stimulated PRL release.[221, 222] Lesions of the dorsal raphe nucleus abolish the nocturnal PRL surges that characterize the circadian PRL rhythm, and stimulation of the dorsal raphe nucleus increases PRL release.[223] Suckling-induced PRL release is accompanied by a rapid fall in hypothalamic 5-HT levels, and blockade of 5-HT synthesis with p-chlorophenylalanine or 5-HT receptors with methysergide inhibits the suckling-induced PRL surge, suggesting the involvement of 5-HT neurons in mediating the suckling response.[224–226] Finally, stress-induced PRL release appears to be under serotoninergic control and is blocked by pretreatment with 5-HT receptor antagonists.[227] All these effects of 5-HT are mediated by activation of $5-HT_1$, $5-HT_2$, and $5-HT_3$ receptors.[227] The site of action of 5-HT in mediating PRL secretion is unclear. A direct pituitary level of action is excluded by the absence of an effect of 5-HT on PRL release from the pituitary in vitro.[228] One possibility is that 5-HT may influence PRL release by modulating hypothalamic TIDA neurons. This is supported by the presence of a dense serotoninergic innervation of dopaminergic cell bodies in the arcuate nucleus[38, 229] as well as the finding that intraventricular administration of 5-HT inhibits DA levels in rat hypophysial stalk blood.[230]

γ-Aminobutyric Acid

GABA is present in portal blood and exerts an overall inhibitory influence on PRL secretion in both rodents and humans.[3, 60, 87, 198] GABA and muscimol inhibit PRL synthesis and secretion from human and rat pituitaries in vitro because of a direct action via pituitary GABA receptors.[231–233] Besides this inhibitory component of GABA

action, there is evidence that GABA and GABA agonists stimulate PRL secretion centrally via inhibition of the activity of TIDA neurons.[234] The intravenous administration of GABA to normal women elicits a biphasic response characterized by a transient increase followed by a sustained inhibition of PRL secretion.[235] A similar biphasic pattern of peripherally administered muscimol on PRL secretion has been described in the rat. Activation of the endogenous GABAergic system with sodium valproate inhibits the PRL response to mechanical breast stimulation in lactating women[236] but has no effect on PRL secretion in prolactinomas.[237] Overall, these results suggest a dual effect of systemically administered GABA on PRL secretion, an initial centrally mediated stimulatory phase followed by direct pituitary inhibition.

Peptides

Of the large number of peptides with PRF activity that have been identified, only VIP, galanin, and possibly TRH appear to be physiologically important. VIP, a 28–amino acid peptide originally purified from the duodenum, is widely distributed throughout the CNS.[12, 13] An intrinsic VIPergic system exists in the hypothalamus, with perikarya located in the parvocellular region of the PVN whose axons terminate in the external zone of the ME.[238] VIP stimulates PRL synthesis and release in rats, monkeys, and humans both in vivo and in vitro through a direct action on VIP receptors found in anterior pituitary cells.[198, 199] The peptide is released into the portal blood stream in concentrations (~1 ng/mL) sufficient to stimulate PRL release from anterior pituitary cells, consistent with its role as a physiologic mediator of PRL release.[239] VIP is also produced by the anterior pituitary cells and plays a role as a paracrine factor.[199, 240] Passive immunization with antiserum to VIP has been shown to partially block stress-induced PRL release and to attenuate the suckling-induced PRL response consistent with a physiologic role of the peptide in mediating these responses.[241, 242] Like VIP, TRH is a potent stimulator of PRL secretion and mRNA, but its physiologic role as a PRF is less clear.[198, 199] Although suckling has been reported to increase portal blood levels of TRH,[201] and immunoneutralization with TRH antiserum has been shown to suppress basal PRL levels in some studies,[243] other studies have failed to detect any effect of TRH antibodies on PRL levels basally and in response to stress and suckling stimuli.[244] More importantly, although TRH is equipotent in stimulating TSH and PRL, the two hormones are regulated independently and show dissociated release during stress and suckling, the two most important neurogenic stimuli for PRL release.[198, 199] Overall, TRH qualifies as a putative physiologic mediator of PRL release, although its role appears to be relatively minor. In contrast to TRH, galanin has emerged as an important physiologic regulator of PRL release and lactotroph proliferation. Galanin influences PRL secretion in two ways—as a hypophysiotropic substance that is released in the ME and inhibits DA release from TIDA neurons[245] and as a paracrine regulator that is colocalized with PRL in the same secretory granule in lactotrophs.[82, 83, 245] Mice lacking the endogenous galanin gene grow normally but fail to lactate because of a marked reduction in pituitary and circulating PRL levels.[246] Lactotrophs in these mice are hypoplastic and show a complete absence of the normal proliferative response to estrogen.[246] These findings clearly establish galanin as an important physiologic regulator of PRL secretion and as a lactotroph growth factor.

Growth Hormone

Secretion of GH is regulated by a complex interaction of stimulatory and inhibitory hypothalamic influences mediated largely by SST and GHRH.[1, 247–249] Within the hypothalamus, SST perikarya are concentrated in the anterior PeVN region close to the third ventricle.[247, 250] Axons from these cells sweep caudally through the hypothalamus to form a discrete pathway that enters the ME as a compact band throughout the zona externa. The anterior hypothalamic PeVN SST pathway to the ME accounts for approximately 80% of SST immunoreactivity in the hypothalamus.[247] SST perikarya in low to moderate densities occur in several other hypothalamic regions, notably the

PVN, SCN, ARC, and VMN.[250] The heaviest concentration of GHRH-positive perikarya is located in the ARC, with fibers projecting to the external zone of the ME.[251] Small numbers of GHRH-staining cells have also been identified in the anterior and lateral hypothalamus in the PVN and VMN, especially in the rat and monkey. GHRH and SST neurons are anatomically coupled and influence each other reciprocally, SST inhibiting GHRH and GHRH possibly stimulating SST release.[248, 249] The GH regulatory system receives input from dopaminergic, noradrenergic, serotoninergic, cholinergic, and GABAergic pathways and is itself subject to feedback control by GH and insulin-like growth factor-I, which stimulate SST and likely inhibit GHRH.[248, 249] Basal secretion of GH occurs in a pulsatile manner in all species that have been examined.[248, 249] In the rat in particular, GH secretion is characterized by an endogenous ultradian rhythm with high-amplitude GH secretory bursts occurring at 3.3-hour intervals followed by trough periods mediated by episodic release of GHRH and SST.[252] This intrinsic GH rhythm is modified by a number of external and metabolic signals such as sleep, exercise, physical and emotional stress, hypoglycemia, and nutrient ingestion.[1, 248, 249] The GH system is further modified hormonally by gonadal steroids and thyroid hormone, which are stimulatory, and glucocorticoids, which are inhibitory.[1, 248, 249]

Norepinephrine and Epinephrine

Biogenic amines play a major role as predominantly excitatory agents in the neuroregulation of GH secretion. Early classic neuroendocrine studies in the rat showed that direct stimulation of brain stem monoaminergic neurons in the rat caused GH release and that inhibition of catecholamine synthesis by α-methyl-*p*-tyrosine blocked GH release induced by stimulation of the hippocampus and basolateral amygdala.[253, 254] GH release is stimulated by intraventricular injection of NE or Epi in rats or by microinjections of NE into the VMN in baboons.[255, 256] In humans, GH release induced by a variety of stimuli such as insulin-induced hypoglycemia, exercise, stress, arginine, levodopa, and GHRH is blocked by the nonselective α₁, α₂–antagonist phentolamine.[249, 257, 258] The administration of the α₂-receptor agonist clonidine stimulates GH secretions in humans and animals,[249, 259] whereas α₁-agonists do not influence basal or insulin-stimulated GH secretion in humans and, unlike phentolamine, the α₁-selective blocker prazosin does not inhibit GH effectively, suggesting the predominant involvement of α₂-receptor pathways in facilitating GH secretion.[249, 259, 260] Interference with adrenergic neurotransmission abolishes the spontaneous GH surges in rats.[261] Passive immunization of rats with antibody to GHRH or arcuate lesion experiments with monosodium glutamate to destroy GHRH neurons block the GH response to α₂-receptor agonists, suggesting that GH secretion induced by α₂-receptor agonists is mediated by GHRH release from the ME.[262, 263] Other studies, especially in humans, have suggested a role for non-GHRH mechanisms, such as reduced SST secretion as the basis for α₂-receptor–induced GH secretion.[249, 264] Direct studies, however, have generally found a stimulatory effect of NE on SST release from cultured hypothalamic cells, suggesting that a role of SST in mediating the GH response to α₂-adrenergic stimulation is complex and may differ among species.[247, 265, 266]

In contrast to the stimulatory effect of α₂-adrenergic receptors on GH release, β-adrenergic pathways inhibit GH. Evidence in support of this hypothesis comes from the finding that β-receptor antagonists such as propranolol enhance GH responses to a variety of stimuli such as hypoglycemia, exercise, and GHRH.[267] Although rat somatotrophs express β-adrenergic receptors, β-agonists stimulate GH secretion from rat pituitary cells in vitro, suggesting that β-adrenergic inhibition of GH release in vivo probably occurs through a central mechanism.[263] A likely mediator for this effect is SST, as indicated by the finding that propranolol inhibits SST release from hypothalamic slices in vitro[269] and that β-adrenergic antagonists disrupt the GH autofeedback loop, which requires induction of SST.[270] Thus, catecholamines regulate GH secretion through two different pathways: stimulation by α₂-receptors mediated via GHRH release and inhibition by β-adrenergic receptors through stimulation of SST.

Dopamine

Dopamine is an important regulator of GH secretion but its effects are complex, involving both stimulation and inhibition, and are targeted at the pituitary as well as the hypothalamus. In normal individuals, the acute administration of DA and DA agonists such as L-dopa, apomorphine, and bromocriptine stimulates GH release.[249, 271] Treatment with DA or bromocriptine augments the GH response to GHRH.[249, 271] Although DA stimulates basal GH secretion in vivo, it inhibits GH secretion by cultured normal rat and human pituitary cells and somatotroph adenomas.[271, 272] Furthermore, GH secretion stimulated in vivo by arginine or exercise and insulin-induced hypoglycemia is also inhibited by DA.[273, 274] Thus, DA acts directly on the pituitary to inhibit GH secretion. The precise manner in which DA stimulates basal GH secretion or inhibits stimulated GH secretion in vivo remains unclear but is likely mediated at the hypothalamic level. DA agonists stimulate both GHRH and SST release from the hypothalamus in vitro, which adds further difficulty in interpreting the mode of action of the hypothalamic mediators of DA effects on GH secretion.[247, 265, 266, 275]

Acetylcholine

Cholinergic muscarinic pathways play an important role in modulating GH secretion in animals and humans.[249, 276] For instance, drugs that potentiate cholinergic transmission increase pulsatile GH secretion as well as the GH response to GHRH in humans.[277] Conversely, blockade of muscarinic receptors with drugs such as atropine or pirenzepine reduces or abolishes GH secretory responses to sleep, arginine, exercise, and GHRH.[276, 278] The underlying mechanism has not been well defined, although some but not all evidence points to cholinergic inhibition of hypothalamic SST release. Direct evidence in support of this hypothesis comes from the finding that passive immunization of rats with SST antiserum abolishes the inhibitory effect of atropine on GH response to GHRH.[279] Ach has been reported to inhibit SST release from rat hypothalamic fragments in vitro,[280] but other studies using cultured rat fetal hypothalamic cells or portal blood measurements have found Ach to have a stimulatory effect.[265, 281] In the sheep, neostigmine, an indirect cholinergic agonist, stimulates GHRH release in portal blood without inhibiting SST.[282] Although species differences may explain some of this confusion, the overall picture suggests at best only partial mediation by SST of cholinergic stimulation of GH secretion.

Serotonin

5-HT pathways stimulate GH release in the rat. Electrical stimulation of the raphe nucleus results in GH release.[254] Conversely, blockade of 5-HT synthesis with *P*-chlorophenylalanine prevents GH release after stimulation of the amygdala.[253] Pharmacologic activation of the 5-HT system induces GH secretion, possibly through stimulation of GHRH release, since pretreatment with GHRH antiserum inhibits the GH secretory response to 5-HT agonists.[283] In contrast to the rat, the effects of 5-HT in human studies have produced variable results. For instance, the administration of 5-hydroxytryptophan increases GH secretion, whereas fenfluramine, which releases 5-HT from 5-HT terminals, has no effect on basal GH concentration but abolishes GH release stimulated by levodopa and propranolol.[249] Likewise, the administration of the 5-HT receptor antagonists cyproheptadine and methysurgide inhibit GH responses to hypoglycemia, levodopa, and clonidine.[284] It should be noted that several of the drugs used in these clinical studies, for example, fenfluramine and cyproheptidine, are not completely specific for 5-HT receptors and may interfere with dopaminergic (fenfluramine) and cholinergic (cyproheptidine) pathways.[3] In this respect, it is of interest that sumatriptan, a pure agonist for the 5-HT₁D receptor, increases basal GH release in normal individuals.[285] The availability of selective agonists and antagonists for the other 5-HT receptor subtypes should help clarify the role of the different 5-HT receptor pathways in regulating GH secretion.

γ-Aminobutyric Acid

Pharmacologic manipulation of the GABA system evokes both stimulatory and inhibitory GH responses. Activation of the GABA pathway with drugs such as sodium valproate, muscimol, or baclofen facilitates basal GH secretion in the rat, sheep, and human.[1, 3, 249] Baclofen, which stimulates basal GH release, inhibits the GH responses to L-arginine and hypoglycemia.[286] Stimulation of basal GH secretion by GABA agonists does not appear to be mediated through GHRH release from the hypothalamus, at least in the rat, since GH stimulation is not blocked by passive immunization with GHRH antiserum.[287] Conversely, GABA is a potent inhibitor of SST release from cultured hypothalamic neurons, suggesting a potential role of a GABA-induced decrease in hypothalamic SST tone in mediating basal GH stimulation.[281] GABA is also capable of stimulating GH release directly from neonatal rat pituitary cells in vitro.[288] Overall, therefore, GABA acting via $GABA_A$ and $GABA_B$ receptors inhibits stimulated GH secretion and enhances basal GH secretion through either a direct pituitary effect or via inhibition of hypothalamic SST release.

Excitatory Amino Acids

Peripheral or intrahypothalamic injections of NMDA or KA stimulate GH release in the rat, sheep, and monkey.[49] This effect is mediated via stimulation of GHRH release from the ARC because (1) NMDA-induced GH release is blocked by administration of GHRH antibodies, (2) lesions of the ARC abolish the ability of NMDA to induce GH release, and (3) NMDA receptor antagonists reduce hypothalamic GHRH peptide and mRNA levels in the rat hypothalamus without altering SST mRNA.[289] In addition to a hypothalamic site of action, EAAs also stimulate GH secretion directly from somatotrophs in vitro.[290] Thus, EAAs facilitate GH secretion primarily through regulation of GHRH release from the ARC and possibly through a direct pituitary action. The potential additional role of SST, whose release from incubated hypothalami has been reported to be increased by NMDA agonists, needs to be determined.[290]

Peptides

In addition to GHRH and SST, there are a number of other peptides that occur endogenously in the hypothalamus and that have been shown to influence GH secretion either directly at the pituitary level or through modulation of the two principal regulators SST and GHRH. The group comprises galanin, calcitonin, pituitary adenylate cyclase–activating polypeptide, opioid peptides, TRH, NPY, substance P, bombesin, and putative as yet unidentified peptide or nonpeptide endogenous ligands for the orphan growth hormone–releasing peptide receptor.[249] A complete description of the GH-regulating properties of these compounds is outside the scope of this chapter. Comparable to its effect on GnRH, galanin coexists with GHRH neurons in the arcuate nucleus,[291] stimulates GH release when given alone, and facilitates the action of GHRH. Immunoneutralization of endogenous galanin attenuates the normal GH secretory pattern in male rats, suggesting an important physiologic role for the peptide in pulsatile GH secretion.[292] Opioid peptides stimulate GH secretion in both rodents and humans, possibly through inhibition of hypothalamic SST release or stimulation of GHRH release.[249] They may participate in some forms of stress-induced GH secretion. NPY inhibits GH secretion, possibly by stimulating hypothalamic SST release, and may participate in GH autonegative feedback as well as in mediating nutritional effects on the GH axis.[293]

Thyrotropin

TSH secretion from the anterior pituitary is governed by two interacting elements: negative feedback control by thyroid hormone and neural input from the hypothalamus, which determines the set point for thyroid hormone feedback.[1-3, 294] The dominant hypothalamic influence is stimulatory via TRH, since disconnection of the pituitary by stalk section or hypothalamic lesions results in reduced TSH output

and hypothyroidism.[1, 294] The hypothalamus also exerts negative control through SST and DA, which act directly through their respective receptors on thyrotrophs. The main inhibitory regulator of long-term TSH secretion, however, is thyroid hormone, with SST and DA playing ancillary roles in modulating short-term changes. TRH immunoreactivity is widely distributed throughout the brain and gut, with the highest concentration in the ME. Within the hypothalamus, cell bodies of tuberoinfundibular TRH-producing neurons are concentrated in the parvocellular division of the PVN, with axonal projections that terminate in the zona externa of the ME. Lower densities of TRH-positive neurons occur in the SCN, POA, VMN, and DMN.[295] The PVN TRH neurons receive aminergic and peptidergic input from the brain stem and forebrain, which likely mediates the TSH response to various physiologic stimuli such as circadian rhythm, acute cold exposure, and stress.[1] Basal TSH secretion in rats and humans displays a circadian periodicity characterized in humans by a maximum between 9 PM and 6 AM and a minimum between 4 PM and 7 PM.[296] Superimposed on the circadian rhythm are smaller TSH oscillations occurring every 2 to 4 hours. Deafferentation of the hypothalamus in rats abolishes the circadian rhythm, suggesting the requirement for extrahypothalamic input.[296] Acute cold exposure stimulates TSH release in animals and in the human neonate by activating the central ascending noradrenergic pathway.[297] Various forms of stress such as immobilization or ether inhalation in rats inhibits TSH (as well as GH) through release of SST from the hypothalamus.[247, 248]

Norepinephrine

In general, NE has been found to be a stimulatory regulator of TSH release in rats but with variable effects in humans. Systemic administration of the α-receptor agonist clonidine or the intraventricular injection of NE or Epi stimulates TSH release in rats.[2, 255] Conversely, α-receptor antagonists or catecholamine-depleting drugs block TSH secretion in response to cold exposure.[298, 299] An inhibitory effect of α-adrenergic agonists, however, has also been described,[300] and other studies have found that the adrenergic influence on TSH secretion involves Epi rather than NE.[301] Both Epi and NE stimulate TSH release from the rat pituitary in vitro, suggesting that Epi at least, which is secreted into the portal blood, may exert a direct hypophysiotropic effect on the pituitary to influence TSH release.[302] NE, which has been shown to stimulate TRH release from the hypothalamus in vitro, could act at the hypothalamic level.[203] In humans, a role of the adrenergic system in regulating TSH secretion is even more hazy. Blockade of α-adrenergic receptors with phentolamine diminishes the serum TSH response to TRH, and blockade of NE synthesis with fusaric acid reduces serum TSH levels in hypothyroid patients.[294, 304] Numerous other studies, however, have failed to show any effect of adrenergic agonists or antagonists on either basal or TRH-stimulated TSH levels.[2, 294, 298]

Dopamine

In contrast to the adrenergic system, there is firm evidence that DA is an important inhibitory regulator in the maintenance of thyrotroph function. Infusion of DA at concentrations that exist in the rat portal blood, or the administration of L-dopa or the D_2-receptor agonist bromocriptine inhibit basal and TRH-stimulated TSH secretion in vivo and in vitro.[305-307] In humans, DA infusions rapidly suppress short-term TSH fluctuations and abolish the nocturnal TSH surge.[308] The administration of D_2-receptor antagonists elevates circulating TSH.[309] The inhibitory effect of DA on TSH secretion is seen only acutely, since continued administration of D_2-receptor agonists such as bromocriptine does not lead to persistent TSH suppression or hypothyroidism, probably because of receptor escape from the initial acute inhibitory effects of the drug similar to the maintenance of normal thyroid function that has been observed during long-term pharmacotherapy with SST analogues like octreotide.[271] The effect of DA is more pronounced in female than in male subjects[307] and in hypothyroid patients than in euthyroid patients.[310] The action of DA is targeted directly on the pituitary based on evidence that DA is released into the portal blood, that DA and DA receptor agonists such as bromocriptine inhibit TSH secretion from dispersed pituitary cells in vitro, and that thyrotroph cells express the D_2-receptor subtype.[26, 311] A direct action of DA on the hypothalamus is also conceivable, although such an effect is difficult to rationalize given that DA stimulates both SST and TRH release from the rat hypothalamus in vitro.[265, 266, 312] DA inhibits not only TSH secretion but also TSH subunit gene transcription.[313] Mice lacking D_2-receptors show an increased number of thyrotrophs (along with lactotroph hyperplasia and lactotroph cell tumors), suggesting that DA not only acts as an inhibitory regulator of TSH secretion and synthesis but also is involved in the maintenance of thyrotroph cell growth.[210]

Serotonin

The role, if any, of 5-HT on TSH regulation has remained a contentious issue over the years. Pharmacologic manipulations that activate the 5-HT system in humans have produced either increased or decreased TSH levels or no effect,[2, 314] whereas blockade of 5-HT receptors has been reported to blunt the TSH response to TRH in some studies[315] but had no effect in others.[2, 316] Similar conflicting results have been obtained in the rat. The reasons for these discordant results remain unclear. They do not appear to be species-related and can be best explained by a minor role of the 5-HT system in TSH regulation.

Acknowledgment

The author acknowledges with gratitude the assistance of Mrs. M. Correia in preparing this chapter.

REFERENCES

1. Reichlin S: Neuroendocrinology. *In* Wilson JD, Foster DW (eds): Williams Textbook of Endocrinology, 9th ed. Philadelphia, WB Saunders, 1998, p 165.
2. McCann SM, Krulich L: Role of transmitters in control of anterior pituitary hormone release. *In* DeGroot LJ (ed): Endocrinology, 2nd ed. Philadelphia, WB Saunders, 1989, pp 117–130.
3. Muller EE: Role of neurotransmitters and neuromodulators in the control of anterior pituitary hormone secretion. *In* DeGroot LJ (ed): Endocrinology, 3rd ed. Philadelphia, WB Saunders, 1995, pp 178–191.
4. Weiner RI, Ganong WI: Role of brain monoamines and histamine in regulation of anterior pituitary secretion. Physiol Rev 58:905–976, 1978.
5. McQueen JK: Classic transmitters and neuromodulators. *In* Fluckiger E, Muller EE, Thorner MO (eds): Transmitter Molecules in the Brain: Basic and Clinical Aspects of Neuroscience, vol 2. Springer Sandoz Advanced Texts, Heidelberg, Springer-Verlag, 1987, p 7.
6. Monaghan DT, Bridges RJ, Cotman CW: The excitatory amino acid receptors: Their classes, pharmacology and distinct properties in the function of the central nervous system. Annu Rev Pharmacol Toxicol 29:365–402, 1989.
7. Fogg GE, Foster AC: Amino acid neurotransmitters and their pathways in the mammalian central nervous system. Neuroscience 9:701, 1983.
8. Moncada S, Higgs A: The L-arginine-nitric oxide pathway. N Engl J Med 329:2002–2012, 1993.
9. Bredt DS, Snyder SH: Nitric oxide, a novel neuronal messenger. Neuron 8:3, 1992.
10. Bowker RM, Westlund KN, Sullivan MC, et al: Descending serotonergic, peptidergic, and cholinergic pathways from the raphe nuclei: A multiple transmitter complex. Brain Res 288:33, 1983.
11. Verma A, Hirsch DJ, Glatt CA, et al: Carbon monoxide: A putative neuronal messenger. Science 259:381, 1993.
12. Krieger DT: Brain peptides: What, where, and why. Science 222:975, 1983.
13. Krieger DT, Bronstein MJ, Martin JB (eds): Brain Peptides. New York, John Wiley & Sons, 1983.
14. Harmar AJ: Neuropeptides. *In* Fluckiger E, Muller EE, Thorner MO (eds): Transmitter Molecules in the Brain: Basic and Clinical Aspects of Neuroscience, vol 2. Springer Sandoz Advanced Texts, Heidelberg, Springer-Verlag, 1987, p 17.
15. Lundberg JM, Hokfelt T: Coexistence of peptides and classical neurotransmitters. *In* Bousfield D (ed): Neurotransmitters in Action. Amsterdam, Elsevier, 1985, pp 104–119.
16. Bowker RM, Westlund KN, Sullivan MC, et al: Descending serotonergic peptidergic and cholinergic pathways from the raphe nuclei: A multiple transmitter complex. Brain Res 288:33–48, 1983.
17. Brownstein MJ, Palkovits M, Saavedra JM, Kizer JS: Distribution of hypothalamic hormones and neurotransmitters within the diencephalon. Frontiers Neuroendocrinol 4:1, 1976.
18. Brownstein M, Palkovits M, Tappaz M, et al: Effect of surgical isolation of the hypothalamus on its neurotransmitter content. Brain Res 117:287, 1976.
19. Alexander SPH, Peters JA: Receptor and ion channel nomenclature supplement compiled in association with the IUPHAR, 9th ed. Trends Pharmacol Sci Cambridge, 1998, pp 1–98.
20. Wess J: Molecular basis of muscarinic acetylcholine receptor function. Trends Pharmacol Sci 14:308, 1993.
21. Lindstrom J, Schaeffer R, Whiting P: Molecular studies of the neuronal nicotinic acetylcholine receptor family. Mol Neurobiol 1:281, 1987.
22. Carmeliet P, Denef C: Synthesis and release of acetylcholine by normal and tumoral pituitary corticotroph. Endocrinology 124:2218, 1989.
23. Dahlstrom A, Fuxe K: Evidence for the existence of monoamine containing neurons in the central nervous system: I. Demonstration of monoamine in cell bodies of brain stem neurons. Acta Physiol Scand (suppl) 232:1, 1964.
24. Ajika K: Relationship between catecholaminergic neurons and hypothalamic hormone-containing neurons in the hypothalamus. Frontiers Neuroendocrinol 6:1, 1980.
25. Palkovits M: Catecholamines in the hypothalamus: An anatomical review. Neuroendocrinology 33:123, 1981.
26. Ben Jonathan N, Oliver C, Weiner H, et al: Dopamine in hypophysial portal plasma of the rat during the estrous cycle and throughout pregnancy. Endocrinology 100:452, 1997.
27. Sawchenko PE, Swanson LW: The organization of noradrenergic pathways from the brain stem to the paraventricular and supraoptic nuclei in the rat. Brain Res Rev 4:275, 1982.
28. Sawchenko PE, Swanson LW, Grzanna R, et al: Colocalization of neuropeptide Y immunoreactivity in brain stem catecholaminergic neurons that project to the paraventricular and supraoptic nuclei in the rat. Comp Neurol 241:138, 1985.
29. Hokfelt T, Fuxe K, Goldstein M, Johnsson O: Evidence for adrenaline neurons in the rat brain. Acta Physiol Scand 89:286, 1973.
30. Chronwall BM, Millington WR, Griffin ST, et al: Histological evolution of the dopaminergic regulation of proopiomelanocortin gene expression in the intermediate lobe of the rat pituitary following in situ hybridization and [^{3}H] thymidine uptake measurement. Endocrinology 120:1201, 1987.
31. Missala C, Nach SR, Robinson SW, et al: Dopamine receptors: From structure to function. Physiol Rev 78:189, 1998.
32. Seeman P, Van Tol HHM: Dopamine receptor. Pharmacol Trends Pharmacol Sci 15:264, 1994.
33. Weiner DM, Levey AI, Sunahara RK, et al: Dopamine D_1 and D_2 receptor mRNA expression in rat brain. Proc Natl Acad Sci USA 88:1859, 1991.
34. Khan ZU, Mvzljak L, Gutierrez A, et al: Prominence of the dopamine D_2 short isoform in dopaminergic pathways. Proc Natl Acad Sci USA 95:7731, 1998.
35. Rivkees SA, Lachowicz JE: Functional D_1 and D_5 receptors are expressed in the suprachiasmatic, supraoptic, and paraventricular nuclei of primates. Synapse 26:1, 1997.
36. Dal Toso R, Sommer B, Ewart M, et al: The dopamine receptor: Two molecular forms generated by alternative splicing. EMBO J 8:4025, 1989.
37. Valerio A, Belloni M, Gorro ML, et al: Dopamine D_2, D_3, D_4 receptor mRNA levels in rat brain and pituitary during aging. Neurobiol Aging 15:713, 1994.
38. Steinbusch HWM: Distribution of serotonin immunoreactivity in the central nervous system of the rat—cell bodies and terminals. Neuroscience 6:557, 1981.
39. Azmita EC, Segal M: An autoradiographic analysis of the differential ascending projections of the dorsal and median raphe nuclei in the rat. J Comp Neurol 179:641, 1970.
40. Payette RF, Gershon MD, Nunez EA: Serotonergic elements of the mammalian pituitary. Endocrinology 116:1933, 1985.
41. Hartig P: Serotoninergic neurons and 5-HT receptors in the CNS. *In* Baumgarten HG, Gothert M (eds): Handbook of Experimental Pharmacology, vol 129. New York, Springer-Verlag, 1997, p 175.
42. Peroutka SJ: 5-HT receptors: Past, present, and future. Trends Neurosci 18:68–69, 1995.
43. De Souza EB: Serotonin and dopamine receptors in the rat pituitary gland: Autoradiographic identification, characterization and localization. Endocrinology 119:1534, 1986.
44. Gundlah C, Pecins-Thompson M, Shutzer WE, Bethea CL: Ovarian steroid effects on serotonin 1A, 2A, 2C receptor mRNA in macaque hypothalamus. Brain Res Mol Brain Res 63:325, 1999.
45. Maswood N, Caldarola-Pastuszka M, Uphouse L: 5-HT$_3$ receptors in the ventromedial nucleus of the hypothalamus and female sexual behaviour. Brain Res 769:13, 1997.
46. Kjaer A, Larsen PJ, Knigge U, et al: Histamine stimulates c-fos expression in hypothalamic vasopressin, oxytocin, and corticotropin-releasing hormone containing neurons. Endocrinology 134:482, 1994.
47. Kjaer A, Larsen PJ, Knigge U, et al: Dehydration stimulates hypothalamic gene expression of histamine synthesis enzyme: Importance for neuroendocrine regulation of vasopressin and oxytocin secretion. Endocrinology 136:189, 1995.
48. Kjaer A, Larsen PJ, Knigge U, et al: Neuronal histamine and expression of corticotropin releasing hormone, vasopressin and oxytocin in the hypothalamus: Relative importance of H1 and H2 receptors. Eur J Endocrinol 139:238, 1998.
49. Brann DW, Mahesh VB: Excitatory amino acids: Evidence for a role in the control of reproduction and anterior pituitary hormone secretion. Endocr Rev 18:678–700, 1997.
50. Van Den Pol AN, Wuarin JP, Dudek FE: Glutamate neurotransmission in the neuroendocrine hypothalamus. *In* Brann DW, Mahesh VB (eds): Excitatory Amino Acids: Their Role in Neuroendocrine Function. Boca Raton, FL, CRC Press, 1996, p 1.
51. Fonnum F, Hassel B: Glutamate synthesis, metabolism, and uptake. *In* Stone TW (ed): CNS Neurotransmitters and Neuromodulators: Glutamate. Boca Raton, FL, CRC Press, 1995, p 19.
52. Van Den Pol AN: Glutamate and aspartate immunoreactivity in hypothalamic presynaptic axons. J Neurosci 11:2087, 1991.
53. Nakanishi S: Molecular diversity of glutamate receptors and implications for brain function. Science 258:597–603, 1992.
54. Meeker RB, Greenwood RS, Hayward JN: Glutamate receptors in the rat hypothalamus and pituitary. Endocrinology 134:621–629, 1994.
55. Kus S, Handa R, Sanderson J, Kerr J, Beitz A: Distribution of NMDAR1 receptor subunit mRNA and [^{125}I] MK-801 binding in the hypothalamus of intact, castrate, and castrate-DHTP treated male rats. Mol Brain Res 28:55–60, 1995.

56. Bhat GK, Mahesh VB, Chu ZW, et al: Localization of the *N*-methyl-*D*-aspartate R1 receptor subunit in specific anterior hormone cell types of the female rat. Neuroendocrinology 62:178–186, 1995.

57. Mugnaini E, Oertel WH: An atlas of the distribution of GABAergic neurons and terminals in the rat CNS as revealed by GAD administration. *In* Bjorklund A, Hokfelt T (eds): Handbook of Chemical Neuroanatomy: GABA and Neuropeptides in the CNS: Part I. Amsterdam, Elsevier Science, vol 4. 1986, pp 436–595.

58. Tappaz ML, Wassef M, Oertel WH, et al: Light- and electron-microscopic immunocytochemistry of glutamic acid decarboxylase (GAD) in the basal hypothalamus: Morphological evidence for neuroendocrine γ-aminobutyrate (GABA). Neuroscience 9:271–287, 1983.

59. Vincent SR, Hokfelt T, WU JY: GABA neuron system in hypothalamus and the pituitary gland. Neuroendocrinology 34:117–125, 1982.

60. Mulcahey JJ, Neill JD: γ-Amino butyric acid (GABA) levels in hypophysial stalk plasma of rats. Life Sci 32:453–456, 1982.

61. Mohler H, Fritschy J-M: GABA_B receptors make it to the top—as dimers? Trends Pharmacol Sci 20:87–89, 1999.

62. Di Micco JA, Monroe AJ: GABA_B receptors in the dorsomedial hypothalamus and heart rate in anaesthetized rats. Brain Res 788:245–250, 1998.

63. Anderson RA, Mitchell R: Effects of GABA agonists on the secretion of GH, LH, ACTH, and TSH from the rat pituitary gland in vitro. J Endocrinol 108:1–8, 1986.

64. Grossman A, Costa A, Forsling ML, et al: Gaseous neurotransmitters in the hypothalamus: The roles of nitric oxide and carbon monoxide in neuroendocrinology. Horm Metab Res 29:477–482, 1997.

65. Bernstein HE, Stanarius A, Baumann B, et al: Nitric oxide synthase–containing neurons in the human hypothalamus: Reduced number of immunoreactive cells in the paraventricular nucleus of depressive patients and schizophrenics. Neuroscience 83:867–875, 1998.

66. Parkes D, Kasckoiw J, Vale W: Carbon monoxide modulates secretion of corticotropin releasing factor from rat hypothalamic cell cultures. Brain Res 646:315–318, 1994.

67. Kalra SP, Sahu A, Kalra PS, Crowley WR: Hypothalamic neuropeptide Y: A circuit in the regulation of gonadotropin secretion and feeding behaviour. Ann NY Acad Sci 611:273–283, 1990.

68. Mansour A, Fox CA, Akil A, Watson SJ: Opioid-receptor mRNA expression in the rat CNS: Anatomical and functional implications. Trends Neurosci 18:22–29, 1995.

69. Khachaturian H, Lewis ME, Shafer MKH, Watson SJ: Anatomy of CNS opioid system. Trends Neurosci 8:111–119, 1985.

70. Finley JA, Maderdrut JL, Petrusz P: The immunocytochemical localization of enkephalin in the central nervous system of the rat. J Comp Neurol 198:541–565, 1981.

71. Mountjoy KG, Robbins LS, Mortrud MT, Cone RD: The cloning of a family of genes that encode the melanocortin receptors. Science 257:1248–1251, 1992.

72. Mountjoy KG, Mortrud MT, Low MJ, et al: Localization of the melanocortin-4 receptor (MC4-R) in neuroendocrine and autonomic control circuits in the brain. Mol Endocrinol 8:1298–1308, 1994.

73. Kalra SP, Dube MG, Pu S, et al: Interacting appetite-regulating pathways in the hypothalamic regulation of body weight. Endocr Rev 20:68–100, 1999.

74. Chronwall BB: Anatomical distribution of NPY and NPY messenger RNA in the brain. *In* Mutt V, Fuxe K, Hokfelt T, Lundberg JD (eds): Neuropeptide Y. New York, Raven Press 1988, pp 51–60.

75. Kalra SP: Appetite and body weight regulation: Is it all in the brain? Neuron 19:227–230, 1997.

76. Inui A: Neuropeptide Y feeding receptors: Are multiple subtypes involved? Trends Pharmacol Sci 20:43–46, 1999.

77. Pau K-YF, Kaynard AH, Hess DL, Spies HG: Effects of neuropeptide Y on the in vitro release of gonadotropin releasing hormone, leutinizing hormone, and β-endorphin and pituitary responsiveness to gonadotropin releasing hormone in female macaques. Neuroendocrinology 53:396–403, 1991.

78. Crowley WR, Hassid A, Kalra SP: Neuropeptide Y enhances the release of leutinizing hormone (LH) induced by LH releasing hormone. Endocrinology 120:941–945, 1987.

79. Melander T, Hokfelt T, Rokaeus A: Distribution of galanin-like immunoreactivity in the rat central nervous system. J Comp Neurol 248:475–517, 1986.

80. Melander T, Hokfelt T, Rokaeus A, et al: Coexistence of galanin-like immunoreactivity with catecholamines, 5-hydroxytryptamine, GABA, and neuropeptides in the rat CNS. J Neurosci 6:3640–3654, 1986.

81. Lopez FJ, Merchenthaler I, Ching M, et al: Galanin: A hypothalamic-hypophysiotropic hormone modulating reproductive functions. Proc Natl Acad Sci USA 88:4508–4512, 1991.

82. Steel JH, Gon G, O'Halloran DJ, et al: Galanin and vasoactive intestinal peptide are colocalized with classical pituitary hormones and show plasticity of expression. Histochemistry 93:183–189, 1989.

83. Hyde JF, Engle MG, Maley BE: Colocalization of galanin and prolactin within secretory granules of anterior pituitary cells in estrogen-treated Fischer 344 rats. Endocrinology 129:270–276, 1991.

84. Hyde JF, Keller BK: Galanin secretion from anterior pituitary cells in vitro is regulated by dopamine, somatostatin and thyrotropin releasing hormone. Endocrinology 128:917–922, 1991.

85. Howard AD, Tan C, Shiao LL et al: Molecular cloning and characterization of a new receptor for galanin. FEBS Lett 405:285–290, 1997.

86. Kalra SP, Kalra PS: Regulation of gonadotropin secretion: Emerging new concepts. *In* Imura H (ed): The Pituitary Gland, 2nd ed. New York, Raven Press, 1994, pp 285–307.

87. Kordon C, Drouva SV, Martinez de la Escalera G, Weiner RI: Role of classic and peptide neuromediators in the neuroendocrine regulation of luteinizing hormone and prolactin. *In* Knobil E, Neill JT (eds): The Physiology of Reproduction, 2nd ed. New York, Raven Press, 1994, pp 1621–1681.

88. Fink G: Normal and disordered central neurotransmitter function studied through the

neuroendocrine window of the brain. *In* Fluckiger E, Muller EE, Thorner MO (eds): Transmitter Molecules in the Brain. Basic and Clinical Aspects of Neuroscience, vol 2. Springer-Sandoz Advanced Texts, Heidelberg, Springer-Verlag, 1987, pp 55–74.

89. Riskind PN, Martin JB: Functional anatomy of the hypothalamic anterior pituitary complex. *In* DeGroot LJ (ed): Endocrinology, 3rd ed. Philadelphia, WB Saunders, 1995, pp 151–159.

90. Sternberger LA, Hoffman GE: Immunocytology of luteinizing hormone–releasing hormone. Neuroendocrinology 25:111–128, 1978.

91. King JL, Anthony ELP, Fitzgerald DM, Stopa EG: Luteinizing hormone–releasing hormone neurons in human preoptic/hypothalamus: Differential intraneuronal localization of immunoreactive forms. J Clin Endocrinol Metab 60:88–97, 1985.

92. Gallo RV: Neuroendocrine regulation of pulsatile luteinizing hormone release in the rat. Neuroendocrinology 30:122–131, 1980.

93. Yen SSC, Lasley BL, Wang CF, et al: The operating characteristics of the hypothalamic pituitary system during the menstrual cycle and observations of biological action of somatostatin. Recent Prog Horm Res 31:321–357, 1975.

94. Fox SR, Smith MS: Changes in the pulsatile pattern of leutinizing hormone secretion during the rat oestrous cycle. Endocrinology 116:1485–1492, 1985.

95. Plant TM, Dubey AK: Evidence from the rhesus monkey (Macaca mulatta) for the view that negative-feedback control of luteinizing hormone secretion by the testis is mediated by a deceleration of hypothalamic gonadotropin releasing hormone pulse frequency. Endocrinology 115:2145–2153, 1984.

96. Aiyer MS, Fink G, Greig F: Changes in sensitivity of the pituitary gland to luteinizing hormone releasing factor during the oestrous cycle of the rat. J Endocrinol 60:47–64, 1974.

97. Naor Z, Amsterdam A, Catt KJ: Binding and activation of gonadotropin-releasing hormone receptors in pituitary gonadotrophs. *In* Saxena BB, Birnbaumber KJ, Lutz L, Martini L (eds): Hormone Receptors in Growth and Reproduction. New York, Raven Press, 1984.

98. Fink G, Chiappa SA, Aiyer MS: Priming effect of luteinizing hormone releasing factor elicited by preoptic stimulation and by intravenous infusion and multiple injections of the synthetic decapeptide. J Endocrinol 69:359–372, 1976.

99. Shivers BD, Harlan RE, Morell JI, Pfaff DW: Immunocytochemical localization of luteinizing hormone releasing hormone in male and female rat brains. Neuroendocrinology 36:1–12, 1983.

100. Jackson GL: Effect of actinomycin D on estrogen-induced release of luteinizing hormone in ovariectomized rats. Endocrinology 91:1284–1287, 1972.

101. Jackson GL: Time interval between injection of estradiol, benzoate and LH release in the rat and effect of actinomycin D or cycloheximide. Endocrinology 93:887–892, 1973.

102. Day T, Blessing W, Willoughby J: Noradrenergic and dopaminergic projections to the medial preoptic area of the rat. A combined horseradish peroxidase/catecholamine fluorescence study. Brain Res 193:543–548, 1980.

103. Negro-Vilar A, Advis J, Ojeda S, McCann S: Pulsatile luteinizing hormone (LH) patterns in ovariectomized rats: Involvement of norepinephrine and dopamine in the release of LH-releasing hormone and LH. Endocrinology 111:932–938, 1982.

104. Weick R: Acute effects of adrenergic receptor blocking drugs and neuroleptic agents on pulsatile discharges of luteinizing hormone in the ovariectomized rat. Neuroendocrinology 26:108–117, 1978.

105. Hancke J, Berk W, Baumgarten H, et al: Modulatory effect of noradrenaline and serotonin on circhoral LH release in adult ovariectomized rats. Acta Endocrinol suppl 208:22–23, 1977.

106. Leung P, Arendash G, Whitmoyer D, et al: Electrical stimulation of mesencephalic noradrenergic pathway: Effects on luteinizing hormone levels in blood of ovariectomized and ovariectomized steroid-primed rats. Endocrinology 109:720–728, 1981.

107. Krey L, Buttler W, Knobil E: Surgical disconnection of the medial basal hypothalamus and pituitary function in the rhesus monkey: I. Gonadotropin secretion. Endocrinology 96:1073–1087, 1975.

108. Wise P, Rance N, Barraclough C: Effects of estradiol and progesterone on catecholamine turnover rates in discrete hypothalamic regions in ovariectomized rats. Endocrinology 108:2186–2193, 1981.

109. Nicholson G, Greeley G, Humm J, et al: Lack of effect of noradrenergic denervation of the hypothalamus and medial preoptic area on the feedback regulation of gonadotropin secretion and the oestrous cycle. Endocrinology 103:539–566, 1978.

110. Selmanoff M: The lateral and medial median eminence distribution of dopamine, norepinephrine, and luteinizing hormone releasing hormone and the effect of prolactin on catecholamine turnover. Endocrinology 108:1716–1722, 1981.

111. Negro-Vilar A, Ojeda SR, McCann SM: Catecholaminergic modulation of luteinizing hormone–releasing hormone release by median eminence terminals in vitro. Endocrinology 104:1749–1757, 1979.

112. Vijayan E, McCann SM: Re-evaluation of the role of catecholamines in control of gonadotropin and prolactin release. Neuroendocrinology 25:150–165, 1978.

113. Adler B, Crowley W: Evidence for γ-aminobutyric acid modulation of ovarian hormonal effects on luteinizing hormone secretion and hypothalamic catecholamine activity in the female rat. Endocrinology 118:91–97, 1986.

114. Hartman RD, He JR, Barraclough CA: γ-Amino butyric acid-a and -b receptor antagonists increase LHRH neuronal responsiveness to intracerebral ventricular norepinephrine in ovariectomized estrogen treated rats. Endocrinology 127:1336–1345, 1990.

115. Leranth C, Maclusky N, Salamoto H, et al: Glutamic acid decarboxylase–containing axons synapse on LHRH neurons in the rat medial preoptic area. Neuroendocrinology 40:536–539, 1985.

116. Demling J, Fuchs E, Baumet M, Wuttke W: Preoptic catecholamine, GABA, and glutamate release in ovariectomized and ovariectomized-estrogen primed rats utilizing a push-pull cannula technique. Neuroendocrinology 41:212–218, 1985.

117. Nikolarakis KE, Loeffler JP, Almeida OFX, Herz A: Pre- and post-synaptic actions of GABA on the release of hypothalamic GnRH. Brain Res Bull 21:677–683, 1988.

118. Anderson RA, Mitchell R: Effects of GABA agonists on the secretion of GH, LH, ACTH, and TSH from the rat pituitary gland in vitro. J Endocrinol 108:1–8, 1986.

119. Vitale ML, Chiocchio SR: Serotonin, a neurotransmitter involved in the regulation of leutinizing hormone release. Endocr Rev 14:480–493, 1993.
120. Olney JW, Cicero TJ, Meyer E, De Gubareff T: Acute glutamate-induced elevations in serum testosterone and luteinizing hormone. Brain Res 112:420–424, 1976.
121. Ondo JG, Pass KA, Baldwin R: The effects of neurally active amino acids on pituitary gonadotropin secretion. Neuroendocrinology 21:79–87, 1976.
122. Price M, Olney J, Cicero T: Acute elevations of serum luteinizing hormone induced by kainic acid, N-methylaspartic acid or homocysteic acid. Neuroendocrinology 26:352–358, 1978.
123. Lopez F, Donoso AO, Negro-Vilar A: Endogenous excitatory amino acid neurotransmission regulates the estradiol-induced LH surge in ovariectomized rats. Endocrinology 126:1771–1773, 1990.
124. Arias P, Jarry H, Leonhardt S, et al: Estradiol modulates the LH release response to N-methyl-D-aspartate in adult female rats: Studies on hypothalamic luteinizing hormone releasing hormone and neurotransmitter release. Neuroendocrinology 57:710–715, 1993.
125. Brann DW, Mahesh VB: Excitatory amino acid regulation of gonadotropin secretion: Modulation by steroid hormones. J Steroid Biochem Molec Biol 41:847–850, 1992.
126. Strobl FJ, Luderer U, Besecke L, et al: Differential gonadotropin responses to *N*-methyl-D-L-aspartate in intact and castrated male rats. Biol Reprod 48:867–873, 1993.
127. Ondo JG, Pass KA, Baldwin R: The effects of neurally active amino acids on pituitary gonadotropin secretion. Neuroendocrinology 21:79–87, 1976.
128. Zanisi M, Messi E: Sex steroids and the control of LHRH secretion. J Steroid Biochem Mol Biol 40:155–163, 1991.
129. Lopez FJ, Donoso AO, Negro-Vilar A: Endogenous excitatory amino acids and glutamate receptor subtypes involved in the control of hypothalamic luteinizing hormone–releasing hormone secretion. Endocrinology 130:1986–1992, 1992.
130. Roberts JL, Gore A: Regulation of gonadotropin releasing hormone gene expression by the excitatory amino acids, kainic acid and *N*-methyl-D,L-aspartate in the male rat. Endocrinology 134:2026–2031, 1994.
131. Lee W, Abbud R, Hoffman GE, Smith MS: Effects of *N*-methyl-D-aspartate receptor activation on c-fos expression in luteinizing hormone–releasing hormone neurons in female rats. Endocrinology 133:2248–2254, 1993.
132. Saitoh Y, Silverman A, Gibson M: Norepinephrine neurons in mouse locus coeruleus express c-fos protein after *N*-methyl-D,L-aspartic acid (NMDA) treatment: Relation to LH release. Brain Res 561:11–19, 1991.
133. Abbud R, Smith MS: Do GnRH neurons express the gene for the NMDA receptor? Brain Res 690:117–120, 1995.
134. Blandina P, Johnson D, Walcott J, Goldfarb J: Release of endogenous norepinephrine from rat hypothalamus by stimulation of N-methyl-D-aspartic acid receptors. J Pharmacol Exp Ther 263:61–68, 1992.
135. Price MT, Olney JW, Mitchell MV, et al: Luteinizing hormone releasing action of N-methyl-aspartate is blocked by GABA or tyrine but not by dopamine antagonists. Brain Res 158:461–465, 1978.
136. Rossmanith WG, Marks DL, Steiner RA, Clifton DK: Inhibition of steroid-induced galanin mRNA expression in GnRH neurons by specific NMDA-receptor blockade. J Neuroendocrinol 8:179–184, 1996.
137. Moretto M, Lopez FJ, Negro-Vilar A: Nitric oxide regulates luteinizing hormone–releasing hormone secretion. Endocrinology 133:2399–2402, 1993.
138. Mahachoklertwattana P, Black SM, Kaplan SL, et al: Nitric oxide synthesized by gonadotropin-releasing hormone neurons is a mediator of *N*-methyl-D-aspartate (NMDA)-induced GnRH secretion. Endocrinology 135:1709–1712, 1994.
139. Bonavera JJ, Sahu A, Kalra PS, Kalra SP: Evidence in support of nitric oxide (NO) involvement in the cyclic release of prolactin and LH surges. Brain Res 660:175–179, 1994.
140. Aguan K, Mahesh VB, Ping L, et al: Evidence for a physiological role for nitric oxide in the regulation of the LH surge: Effect of central administration of antisense oligonucleotides to nitric oxide synthase. Neuroendocrinology 64:449–455, 1997.
141. Barraclough CA, Sawyer CH: Inhibition of the release of pituitary ovulatory hormone in the rat by morphine. Endocrinology 57:329–336, 1955.
142. Bruni JF, Van Vugt D, Marshall S, Meites J: Effects of naloxone morphine and methionine enkephalin of serum prolactin luteinizing hormone, follicle stimulating hormone, thyroid stimulating hormone and growth hormone. Life Sci 21:461–466, 1977.
143. Shultz R, Wilhelm A, Pirke KM, et al: Endorphin and dynorphin control serum luteinizing hormone level in immature female rats. Nature 294:757–759, 1981.
144. Ferin M, Van Vugt D, Wardlaw S: The hypothalamic control of the menstrual cycle and the role of endogenous opioid peptides. Recent Prog Horm Res 39:46, 1984.
145. Chiba A, Kema A, Nagami Y, et al: Differential inhibition of NMDA- and naloxone-induced LH release by an NMDA receptor antagonist and CRH in ovariectomized estrogen-primed rats. Neuroendocrinology 65:141–146, 1997.
146. Urbanski HF, Ojeda SR: Activation of luteinizing hormone–releasing hormone release advances the onset of female puberty. Neuroendocrinology 46:273–276, 1987.
147. Plant TM, Gay VL, Marshall GR, Arslan M: Puberty in monkey is triggered by chemical stimulation of the hypothalamus. Proc Natl Acad Sci USA 86:2506–2510, 1989.
148. Urbanski H, Ojeda S: A role for *N*-methyl-D-aspartate (NMDA) receptors in the control of LH secretion and initiation of female puberty. Endocrinology 126:1774–1776, 1990.
149. Goroll D, Arias P, Wuttke W: Preoptic release of amino acid neurotransmitters evaluated in peripubertal and young adult female rats by push-pull perfusion. Neuroendocrinology 58:11–15, 1993.
150. Rivier CL, Plotsky PM: Mediation by corticotropin releasing factor (CRF) of adenohypophysial hormone secretion. Ann Rev Physiol 48:475–494, 1986.
151. Antoni FA: Hypothalamic control of adrenocorticotropin secretion: Advances since the discovery of 41-residue corticotropin releasing factor. Endocr Rev 7:351, 1986.
152. Grossman A: Corticotropin releasing hormone: Basic physiology and clinical applications. *In* DeGroot LJ (ed): Endocrinology, 3rd ed. Philadelphia, WB Saunders, 1995, pp 341–354.
153. Bloom FE, Battenberg ELF, Rivier J, Vale WW: Corticotropin releasing factor (CRF): Immunoreactive neurons and fibers in rat hypothalamus. Regul Pept 4:43–83, 1982.
154. Makara GB, Antoni FA, Stark E, Karteszi M: Hypothalamic organization of corticotropin releasing factor (CRF) producing structures. *In* Muller EE, MacLeod RM (eds): Neuroendocrine Perspectives, vol 4. New York, Elsevier, 1984, pp 71–119.
155. Plotsky PM: Facilitation of immunoreactive corticotropin releasing factor secretion into the hypophysial-portal circulation after activation of catecholaminergic pathways or central norepinephrine injection. Endocrinology 121:924–930, 1987.
156. Engler D, Liu J-P, Clarke IJ: Corticotropin release inhibitory factor: Evidence for dual stimulatory and inhibitory hypothalamic regulation over adrenocorticotropin secretion and biosynthesis. Trends Endocrinol Metab 5:272–283, 1994.
157. Kiss JZ, Mezey E, Skirboll L: Corticotropin-releasing factor-immunoreactive neurons of the paraventricular nucleus become vasopressin positive after adrenalectomy. Proc Natl Acad Sci USA 81:1854–1858, 1984.
158. Roth KA, Weber E, Barchas JD, et al: Immunoreactive dynorphin-(1–8) and corticotropin releasing factor in a subpopulation of hypothalamic neurons. Science 219:189–191, 1982.
159. Hokfelt T, Kahrenkrug J, Tatemoto K, et al: The PH1 (PH1–27)/corticotropin releasing factor/enkephalin immunoreactive hypothalamic neuron: Possible morphological basis for integrated control of prolactin, corticotropin, and growth hormone secretion. Proc Natl Acad Sci USA 80:895–898, 1983.
160. Olschowka JA, O'Donahue TL, Muller JP, Jacobowitz DM: Hypothalamic and extrahypothalamic distribution of CRF-like immunoreactive neurons in the rat brain. Neuroendocrinology 35:305–308, 1982.
161. Jones MT, Hillhouse EW: Neurotransmitter regulation of corticotropin-release factor in vitro. Ann NY Acad Sci 297:536–560, 1977.
162. Raskind MA, Peskind ER, Veith RC, et al: Differential effects of aging on neuroendocrine responses to physostigmine in normal men. J Clin Endocrinol Metab 70:1420–1425, 1990.
163. Lewis DA, Sherman BM, Kathol ORG: Analysis of the specificity of physostigmine stimulation of adrenocorticotropin in man. J Clin Endocrinol Metab 58:570–573, 1984.
164. Freeman E, Touzel R, Grossman A, et al: Pyridostigmine, an acetylcholinesterase inhibitor, stimulates growth hormone release but has no effect on basal TSH or ACTH levels or on the TSH response to TRH. J Neuroendocrinol 2:429–432, 1990.
165. Calogero EA, Gallucci WT, Bernadini R, et al: Effect of cholinergic agonists and antagonists on rat hypothalamic corticotropin-releasing hormone secretion in vitro. Neuroendocrinology 47:303–308, 1988.
166. Tsagarakis S, Holly JMP, Rees LH, Grossman A: Acetylcholine and norepinephrine stimulate the release of corticotropin releasing factor-41 from the rat hypothalamus in vitro. Endocrinology 123:1962, 1988.
167. Liposits ZS, Phelix C, Paull WK: Adrenergic innervation of corticotropin releasing factor (CRF)-synthesizing neurons in the hypothalamic paraventricular nucleus of the rat. Histochemistry 84:201, 1986.
168. Liposits ZS, Phelix C, Paull WK: Electronmicroscopic analysis of tyrosine hydroxylase, dopamine-β-hydroxylase and phenylethanolamine-*N*-methyl transferase immunoreactive innervation of the hypothalamic paraventricular nucleus in the rat. Histochemistry 84:105, 1986.
169. Liposits ZS, Sherman D, Phelix C, Paull WK: A combined light and electronmicroscopic immunocytochemical method for the simultaneous localization of multiple tissue antigens. Histochemistry 85:95, 1986.
170. Olchowska JA, Molliver NE, Grzanna R, et al: Ultrastructural demonstration of noradrenergic synapses in the rat central nervous system by dopamine-β-hydroxylase immunocytochemistry. J Histochem Cytochem 29:271, 1981.
171. Al-Damluiji S: Review: Adrenergic mechanisms in the control of corticotropin secretion. J Endocrinol 119:5, 1988.
172. Vale W, Vaughn J, Smith M, et al: Effects of synthetic ovine corticotropin-releasing factor, glucocorticoids, catecholamines, neurohypophysial peptides, and other substances on cultured corticotropic cells. Endocrinology 113:1121, 1983.
173. Giguere V, Cote J, Labrie F: Characteristics of the α-adrenergic stimulation of adrenocorticotropin secretion in rat anterior pituitary cells. Endocrinology 109:757, 1981.
174. Calogero AE, Galluci WT, Chrousos GP, et al: Catecholamine effect upon rat hypothalamus corticotropin releasing hormone secretion in vitro. J Clin Invest 82:839, 1988.
175. Hillhouse EW, Milton NGF: Effect of noradrenalin and γ-aminobutyric acid on the secretion of corticotropin releasing factor-41 and arginine vasopressin from the rat hypothalamus in vitro. J Endocrinol 122:719, 1989.
176. Al-Damluiji S, Iveson T, Thomas JM, et al: Food-induced cortisol secretion is mediated by central α1-adrenoceptor modulation of pituitary ACTH secretion. Clin Endocrinol (Oxf) 26:629–636, 1987.
177. Fehm HL, Voight KH, Lang RE, Pfeiffer EF: Effects of neurotransmitters on the release of corticotropin releasing hormone (CRH) by rat hypothalamic tissue in vitro. Exp Brain Res 39:229, 1980.
178. Fuller RW: The involvement of serotonin in regulation of pituitary-adrenocortical function. Frontiers Neuroendocrinol 13:250–270, 1992.
179. Calogero AE, Bernadini R, Margioris AN, et al: Effects of serotoninergic agonists and antagonists on corticotropin-releasing hormone secretion by explanted rat hypothalami. Peptides 10:189–200, 1989.
180. Calogero AE, Bagdy G, Szemeredi K, et al: Mechanisms of serotonin receptor agonist-induced activation of the hypothalamic-pituitary-adrenal axis in the rat. Endocrinology 126:1888–1894, 1990.
181. Makara JB, Stard E: Effect of γ-aminobutyric acid (GABA) and GABA antagonistic drugs on ACTH release. Neuroendocrinology 16:178, 1974.
182. Calogero AE, Gallucci WT, Chrousos GP, Gold PW: Interaction between GABAergic neurotransmission and rat hypothalamic corticotropin-releasing hormone secretion in vitro. Brain Res 463:28–36, 1988.

183. Anderson RA, Mitchell R: Effects of γ-aminobutyric acid receptor agonists on the secretion of growth hormone, luteinizing hormone, adrenocorticotrophic hormone and thyroid stimulating hormone from the rat pituitary gland in vitro. J Endocrinol 108:1–8, 1986.

184. Oliver C, Jezova D, Grino M, et al: Excitatory amino acids and the hypothalamic pituitary-adrenal axis. In Brann DW, Mahesh VB (eds): Excitatory Amino Acids: Their Role in Neuroendocrine Regulation. Boca Raton, FL, CRC Press, 1996, pp 167–183.

185. Aubry JM, Bartanusz V, Pagliusi S, et al: Expression of ionotropic glutamate receptor subunit mRNAs by paraventricular corticotropin releasing factor (CRF) neurons. Neurosci Lett 205:95–98, 1996.

186. Chautard T, Boudouresque F, Guillaume V, Oliver C: Effect of excitatory amino acids on the hypothalamic pituitary-adrenal axis in the rat during the stress-hyporesponsive period. Neuroendocrinology 57:70–78, 1993.

187. Darlington DN, Miyamoto M, Keil L, Dallman MF: Paraventricular stimulation with glutamate elicits bradycardia and pituitary responses. Am J Physiol 256:R112–R119, 1989.

188. Patchev V, Karalis K, Chrousos GP: Effects of excitatory amino acid transmitters on hypothalamic corticotropin-releasing hormone (CRH) and arginine vasopressin (AVP) release in vitro: Implications in pituitary adrenal regulation. Brain Res 633:312–318, 1994.

189. Joanny P, Steinberg J, Oliver C, Grino M: Glutamate and N-methyl-D-aspartate stimulate rat hypothalamic corticotropin releasing factor secretion in vitro. J Neuroendocrinol 9:93–97, 1997.

190. Carlson WE, Gann DS: Response of plasma adrenocorticotropin to injections of glutamate or norepinephrine in the dorsal rostral pons of cats. Endocrinology 128:3021–3031, 1991.

191. Nelson RJ, Kriegsfeld LJ, Dorson VL, Dorson TM: Effects of nitric oxide on neuroendocrine function and behaviour. Frontiers Neuroendocrinol 18:463–491, 1997.

192. Karanth S, Lyson K, McCann SM: Role of nitric oxide in interleukin 2-induced corticotropin releasing factor release from incubated hypothalami. Proc Natl Acad Sci USA 90:3383–3387, 1993.

193. Costa A, Trainer P, Besser M, Grossman A: Nitric oxide modulates the release of corticotropin releasing hormone from the rat hypothalamus in vitro. Brain Res 605:187–192, 1993.

194. Pittman QJ, Hatton JD, Bloom FE: Morphine and opioid peptides reduce paraventricular neuronal activity: Studies on the rat hypothalamic slice preparation. Proc Natl Acad Sci USA 77:5527–5531, 1980.

195. Plotsky PM: Opioid inhibition of immunoreactive corticotropin releasing factor secretion into hypophysial portal circulation of rats. Regul Pept 15:235, 1986.

196. Roth KA, Weber E, Barchas JD, et al: Immunoreactive dynorphin (1–8) and corticotropin-releasing factor in subpopulation of hypothalamic neurons. Science 219:189, 1983.

197. Lightman SL, Young S: Changes in hypothalamic preproenkephalin A mRNA following stress and opiate withdrawal. Nature 238:263, 1987.

198. Molitch ME: Prolactin. In Melmed S (ed): The Pituitary. Cambridge, Blackwell, 1995, pp 136–186.

199. Neill JD, Nagy GM: Prolactin secretion and its control. In Knobil E, Neill JT (eds): The Physiology of Reproduction, 2nd ed. New York, Raven Press, 1994, pp 1833–1860.

200. Gibbs DM, Neill JD: Dopamine levels in hypophysial stalk blood in the rat are sufficient to inhibit prolactin secretion in vivo. Endocrinology 102:1895–1900, 1978.

201. De Greef WJ, Plotsky PM, Neill JD: Dopamine levels in hypophysial stalk plasma and prolactin levels in peripheral plasma of the lactating rat: Effects of a simulated stimulus. Neuroendocrinology 32:229–233, 1981.

202. Mogg RJ, Samson WK: Interactions of dopaminergic and peptidergic factors in the control of prolactin release. Endocrinology 126:728–735, 1990.

203. Leblanc H, Lachelin CL, Abu-Fadil S, Yen SSC: Effects of dopamine infusion on pituitary hormone secretion in humans. J Clin Endocrinol Metab 43:668–674, 1976.

204. Leebaw WF, Lee LA, Woolf PD: Dopamine affects basal and augmented pituitary hormone secretion. J Clin Endocrinol Metab 47:480–487, 1978.

205. Bansal S, Lee LA, Woolf PD: Dopaminergic modulation of arginine-mediated growth hormone and prolactin release in man. Metabolism 30:649–653, 1981.

206. Burrow GN, May PB, Spaulding SW, Donabedian RK: TRH and dopamine interactions affecting pituitary hormone secretion. J Clin Endocrinol Metab 45:65–72, 1977.

207. Langer G, Sachar EJ: Dopaminergic factors in human prolactin regulation: Effects of neuroleptics and dopamine. Psychoneuroendocrinology 2:373–378, 1977.

208. Bosse R, Fumagalli F, Jaber M: Anterior pituitary hypoplasia and dwarfism in mice lacking the dopamine transporter. Neuron 19:127–138, 1997.

209. Kelly MA, Rubinstein M, Asa SL, et al: Pituitary lactotroph hyperplasia and chronic hyperprolactinemia in dopamine D₂ receptor–deficient mice. Neuron 19:103–113, 1997.

210. Saiardi A, Bozzi Y, Baik J-H: Antiproliferative role of dopamine: Loss of D₂ receptors causes hormonal dysfunction and pituitary hyperplasia. Neuron 19:115–126, 1997.

211. Negro-Vilar A, Ojeda S, Advis J, McCann S: Evidence for noradrenergic involvement in episodic prolactin and growth hormone release in ovariectomized rats. Endocrinology 105:86, 1979.

212. Terry L, Martin J: Evidence for α-adrenergic regulation of episodic growth hormone and prolactin secretion in the undisturbed male rat. Endocrinology 108:1869–1873, 1981.

213. Lawson D, Gala R: The influence of adrenergic, dopaminergic, cholinergic and serotoninergic drugs on plasma prolactin levels in ovariectomized, estrogen treated rats. Endocrinology 96:313–318, 1975.

214. Lal S, Tolis G, Martin JB, et al: Effect of clonidine on growth hormone, prolactin, luteinizing hormone, follicle stimulating hormone, and thyroid stimulating hormone in the serum of normal men. J Clin Endocrinol Metab 37:719–724, 1975.

215. Voogt J, Carr L: Plasma prolactin levels and hypothalamic catecholamine synthesis during suckling. Neuroendocrinology 16:108–118, 1974.

216. Carr L, Conway P, Voogt J: Role of norepinephrine in the release of prolactin induced by suckling and estrogen. Brain Res 133:305–314, 1977.

217. Langelier P, McCann S: The effects of interruption of the ventral noradrenergic pathway on the proestrous discharge of prolactin in the rat. Proc Soc Exp Biol Med 154:553–557, 1977.

218. Lancranjan I, Wirz-Justice A, Puhringer W, et al: Effect of 1–5 hydroxytryptophan infusion on growth hormone and prolactin secretion in man. J Clin Endocrinol Metab 45:588–593, 1977.

219. Lewis DA, Sherman BM: Serotonergic regulation of prolactin and growth hormone secretion in man. Acta Endocrinol 110:152–157, 1985.

220. Urban RJ, Veldhuis JD: A selective serotonin reuptake inhibitor fluoxitine hydrochloride modulates the pulsatile release of prolactin in post menopausal women. Am J Obstet Gynecol 164:147–152, 1991.

221. Gil-Ad I, Zambotti F, Carruba MO, et al: Stimulatory role of brain serotoninergic system on prolactin secretion in male rat. Proc Soc Exp Biol Med 151:512–518, 1976.

222. Advis JP, Simpkins JW, Bennett J, Meites J: Serotoninergic control of prolactin release in male rats. Life Sci 24:359–366, 1979.

223. Mulloy AL, Moberg GP: Effects of p-chlorophenylalanine and raphe lesions on diurnal prolactin release in the rat. Fed Proc Fed Am Soc Exp Biol 34:251, 1975.

224. Gallo RV, Rabii J, Moberg GP: Effect of methysurgide, a blocker of serotonin receptors on plasma prolactin levels in lactating and ovariectomized rats. Endocrinology 97:1096–1105, 1975.

225. Kordon C, Blake CA, Terkel J, Sawyer CH: Participation of serotonin-containing neurons in the suckling-induced rise in plasma prolactin levels in lactating rats. Neuroendocrinology 13:213–223, 1973.

226. Mena F, Enjalbert A, Carbonell A, et al: Effect of suckling on plasma prolactin and hypothalamic monoamine levels in the rat. Endocrinology 99:445–452, 1976.

227. Jorgensen H, Knigge U, Warberg J: Effect of serotonin 5-HT₁, 5-HT₂ and 5-HT₃ receptor antagonists on the prolactin response to restraint and ether stress. Neuroendocrinology 56:371–377, 1992.

228. Lamberts SWJ, MacLeod RM: The interaction of the serotonergic and dopaminergic systems on prolactin secretion in the rat. Endocrinology 105:287–295, 1978.

229. Descarries L, Beaudet A: The serotonin innervation of adult rat hypothalamus. In Vincent JD, Kordon C (eds): Cell Biology of Hypothalamic Neurosecretion. Paris: CNRS, 1978, pp 135–153.

230. Pilotte NS, Porter JC: Dopamine in hypophysial portal plasma and prolactin in systemic plasma of rats treated with 5-hydroxytryptamine. Endocrinology 108:2137–2141, 1981.

231. Grandison L, Guidotti A: γ-Aminobutyric acid receptor functions in rat anterior pituitary: Evidence for control of prolactin release. Endocrinology 105:754–759, 1979.

232. Loeffler J, Kley N, Pittius C, et al: In vivo and in vitro studies of GABAergic inhibition of prolactin biosynthesis. Neuroendocrinology 43:504–510, 1986.

233. Grandison L, Cavagnini F, Schmid R, et al: γ-Aminobutyric acid- and benzodiazepine-binding sites in human anterior pituitary tissue. J Clin Endocrinol Metab 54:597–601, 1982.

234. Apud JA, Cocchi D, Mosotto C, et al: Prolactin control by the tuberoinfundibular GABAergic system: Role of anterior pituitary GABA receptors. Psychoneuroendocrinology 9:125–133, 1984.

235. Melis GB, Paoletti AM, Mais V, Fioretti P: Interference of dopamine infusion on γ-aminobutyric acid (GABA)-stimulated prolactin increase. J Endocrinol Invest 4:445–448, 1980.

236. Melis GB, Fruzzetti F, Paoletti AM, et al: Pharmacological activation of γ-aminobutyric acid–system blunts prolactin response to mechanical breast stimulation in puerperal women. J Clin Endocrinol Metab 58:201–205, 1984.

237. Melis GB, Paoletti AM, Mais V, et al: The effects of the GABAergic drug sodium valproate on prolactin secretion in normal and hyperprolactinemic subjects. J Clin Endocrinol Metab 54:485–489, 1982.

238. Mezey E, Kiss JZ: Vasoactive intestinal peptide–containing neurons in the paraventricular nucleus may participate in regulating prolactin secretion. Proc Natl Acad Sci USA 82:245–247, 1985.

239. Shimatsu A, Kato Y, Matsushita N: Immunoreactive vasoactive intestinal polypeptide in rat hypophysial portal blood. Endocrinology 108:395–398, 1981.

240. Arnaout MA, Garthwaite TL, Martinson DR: Vasoactive intestinal polypeptide is synthesized in anterior pituitary tissue. Endocrinology 181:2052–2057, 1986.

241. Kaji H, Chihara K, Kita T, et al: Administration of antisera to vasoactive intestinal polypeptide and polypeptide histidine isoleucine attenuates ether-induced prolactin secretion in rats. Neuroendocrinology 41:529–531, 1985.

242. Abe H, Engler D, Molitch ME, et al: Vasoactive intestinal peptide is a physiological mediator of prolactin release in the rat. Endocrinology 116:1383–1390, 1985.

243. Koch Y, Goldhaber G, Fireman I, et al: Suppression of prolactin and thyrotropin secretion in the rat by antiserum to thyrotropin releasing hormone. Endocrinology 100:1476–1478, 1977.

244. Harris ARC, Christianson D, Smith MS, et al: The physiological role of thyrotropin releasing hormone in the regulation of thyroid stimulating hormone and prolactin secretion in the rat. J Clin Invest 61:441–448, 1978.

245. Nordstrom O, Melander T, Hokfelt T, et al: Evidence for an inhibitory effect of the peptide galanin on dopamine release from the rat median eminence. Neurosci Lett 73:21–26, 1987.

246. Wynick D, Small CJ, Bacon A, et al: Galanin regulates prolactin release and lactotroph proliferation. Proc Natl Acad Sci USA 95:12671–12676, 1998.

247. Patel YC, Srikant CB: Somatostatin mediation of adenohypophysial secretion. Annu Rev Physiol 48:551–567, 1986.

248. Tannenbaum GS, Eppelbaum J: Somatostatin. In Costio JL (ed): Handbook of Physiology, section VII, The Endocrine System, vol 5, Hormonal Control of Growth. New York, Oxford, 1999, pp 221–266.

249. Giustina A, Veldhuis JD: Pathophysiology of the neural regulation of growth hormone secretion in experimental animals and the human. Endocr Rev 19:717–797, 1998.
250. Finley JCW, Maderdrut JL, Roger LJ, et al: The immunocytochemical localization of somatostatin containing neurons in the rat central nervous system. Neuroscience 6:2173–2192, 1981.
251. Bloch B, Brazeau P, Ling N, et al: Immunocytochemical detection of growth hormone releasing factor in brain. Nature 301:607–608, 1983.
252. Tannenbaum GS, Ling N: The interrelationship of growth hormone (GH)–releasing factor and somatostatin in generation of the ultradian rhythm of GH secretion. Endocrinology 115:1952–1957, 1984.
253. Martin JB: The role of hypothalamic and extrahypothalamic structures in the control of GH secretion. *In* Raiti S (ed): Advances in Human Growth Hormone Research, DHEW Publication No. NIH 74–612. Washington DC, 1974.
254. Martin JB: Brain regulation of growth hormone secretion. *In* Martini L, Ganong WF (eds): Frontiers in Neuroendocrinology, vol 4. New York, Raven Press, 1976, p 129.
255. Vijayan E, Krulich L, McCann SM: Catecholaminergic regulation of TSH and growth hormone release in ovariectomized and ovariectomized steroid-primed rats. Neuroendocrinology 26:174–185, 1978.
256. Toivola PTK, Gale CC: Stimulation of growth hormone release by microinjection of norepinephrine into hypothalamus of baboons. Endocrinology 90:895–902, 1972.
257. Martin JB: Neural regulation of growth hormone secretion. N Engl J Med 228:1384, 1973.
258. Ghigo E, Bellone J, Arvat E, et al: Effect of α and β-adrenergic agonists and antagonists on growth hormone secretion in men. J Neuroendocrinol 2:157–159, 1990.
259. McWilliam JR, Melldrum BS: Noradrenergic regulation of growth hormone secretion in the baboon. Endocrinology 112:254–259, 1983.
260. Tatar P, Vigas M: Role of α_1- and α_2-adrenergic receptors in the GH and prolactin response to insulin-induced hypoglycemia in man. Neuroendocrinology 39:275–281, 1980.
261. Terry CL, Martin JB: Evidence for α-adrenergic regulation of episodic growth hormone and prolactin secretion in the undisturbed male rat. Endocrinology 108:1869–1873, 1981.
262. Miki N, Ono M, Shizume K: Evidence that opioidergic and α-adrenergic mechanisms stimulate rat growth hormone release via growth hormone releasing factor (GRF). Endocrinology 114:1950–1952, 1984.
263. Katakami H, Kaito Y, Matsushita N, Imura H: Effects of neonatal treatment with monosodium glutamate on growth hormone release induced by clonidine and prostaglandin E1 in conscious male rats. Neuroendocrinology 38:1–5, 1984.
264. Valcavi R, Dieguez C, Page MD: α_2-Adrenergic pathways release growth hormone via a non–GRF-dependent mechanism in normal human subjects. Clin Endocrinol 29:309–316, 1988.
265. Chihara K, Arimura A, Schally AV: Effect of intraventricular injection of dopamine, norepinephrine, acetylcholine, and 5-hydroxytryptamine on immunoreactive somatostatin release into rat hypophysial portal blood. Endocrinology 104:1656–1662, 1979.
266. Negro-Vilar A, Ojeda SR, Arimura A, McCann SM: Dopamine and norepinephrine stimulate somatostatin release by median eminence fragments in vitro. Life Sci 23:1493–1498, 1978.
267. Chihara K, Kodama H, Kaji H, et al: Augmentation by propranolol of growth hormone releasing hormone (1–44) NH_2-induced growth hormone release in normal short and normal children. J Clin Endocrinol Metab 61:229–233, 1985.
268. Perkins SN, Evans WS, Thorner MO, Cronin MJ: β-Adrenergic stimulation of growth hormone release from perfused rat anterior pituitary cells. Neuroendocrinology 37:473–475, 1983.
269. Richardson SB, Twente S: Inhibition of hypothalamic somatostatin release by β-adrenergic antagonist. Endocrinology 126:1043–1046, 1990.
270. Kelijman M, Frohman LA: β-Adrenergic modulation of growth hormone (GH)-autofeedback on sleep-associated and pharmacologically induced GH secretion. J Clin Endocrinol Metab 69:1187–1193, 1989.
271. Thorner MO, Vance ML: Clinical aspects of dopamine in the regulation of human anterior pituitary function. *In* Fluckiger E, Muller EE, Thorner MO (eds): The Role of Brain Dopamine. Basic and Clinical Aspects of Neuroscience, vol 3: Springer-Sandoz Advanced Texts. Heidelberg, Springer-Verlag, 1989, pp 19–29.
272. Tallo D, Malarkey WB: Adrenergic and dopaminergic modulation of growth hormone and prolactin secretion in normal and tumour bearing human pituitaries in monolayer culture. J Clin Endocrinol Metab 53:1279–1284, 1981.
273. Schwinn G, Schwarck H, MacIntosh C, et al: Effect of the dopamine receptor blocking agent pimozide on the growth hormone response to arginine and exercise and on the spontaneous growth hormone fluctuations. J Clin Endocrinol Metab 43:1183–1185, 1987.
274. Bansal SA, Lee LA, Woolf PD: Dopaminergic stimulation and inhibition of growth hormone secretion in normal man: Studies of the pharmacological specificity. J Clin Endocrinol Metab 53:1273–1277, 1981.
275. Kitajima N, Chihara K, Abe K, et al: Effects of dopamine on immunoreactive growth hormone releasing factor and somatostatin secretion from rat hypothalamic slices perfused in vitro. Endocrinology 124:69–76, 1989.
276. Casanueva FF, Villanueva L, Cabranes JA, et al: Cholinergic mediation of growth hormone secretion elicited by arginine, clonidine, and physical exercise in man. J Clin Endocrinol Metab 59:526–530, 1984.
277. Friend K, Iranmanesh A, Login IS, Veldhuis JD: Peridostigmine treatment selectively amplifies the mass of GH secreted per burst without altering the GH burst frequency, half-life, basal GH secretion, or the orderliness of the GH release process. Eur J Endocrinol 137:377–386, 1997.
278. Peters JR, Evans PJ, Page MD, et al: Cholinergic muscarinic receptor blockade with pirenzepine abolishes slow wave sleep-related growth hormone release in normal adult males. Clin Endocrinol (Oxf) 25:213–217, 1986.
279. Locatelli V, Torsello A, Redaelli M, et al: Cholinergic agonist and antagonist drugs modulate the growth hormone response to growth hormone-releasing hormone in the rat: Evidence for mediation by somatostatin. J Endocrinol 111:271–278, 1987.
280. Richardson SB, Hollender CS, De'Eletto R: Acetylcholine inhibits the release of somatostatin from rat hypothalamus in vitro. Endocrinology 107:1837–1842, 1980.
281. Peterfreund RA, Vale WW: Muscarinic cholinergic stimulation of somatostatin secretion from longterm dispersed cell cultures of fetal rat hypothalamus: Inhibition by γ-aminobutyric acid and serotonin. Endocrinology 112:526–534, 1983.
282. Magnan E, Cataldi M, Guillaume V, et al: Neostigmine stimulates growth hormone releasing hormone release into hypophysial portal blood of conscious sheep. Endocrinology 132:1247–1251, 1993.
283. Murakami Y, Kato KY, Tojo K, et al: Involvement of growth hormone releasing factor in GH secretion induced by serotoninergic mechanism in conscious rat. Endocrinology 119:1089–1092, 1986.
284. Biwens CH, Lebovitz HE, Feldman JM: Inhibition of hypoglycemia induced GH secretion by the serotonin antagonists cyproheptadine and methysergide. N Engl J Med 289:236–238, 1973.
285. Rolandi E, Franceschini R, Cataldi A, Barreca T: Endocrine effects of sumatryptan. Lancet 339:1365–1368, 1992.
286. Cavagnini F, Invitti C, Di Landro A: Effects of a GABA derivative, baclofen, on growth hormone and prolactin secretion in man. J Clin Endocrinol Metab 45:579–584, 1977.
287. Acs Z, Lonart G, Makara GB: Role of hypothalamic factors (growth hormone releasing hormone and γ-aminobutyric acid) in the regulation of growth hormone secretion in the neonatal and adult rat. Neuroendocrinology 52:156–160, 1990.
288. Acs Z, Szabo B, Kapocs G, Makara GB: γ-Aminobutyric acid stimulates pituitary growth hormone secretion in the neonatal rat: A superfusion study. Endocrinology 120:1790–1798, 1987.
289. Cocilovo L, Colonna V, Zoli M: Central mechanisms subserving the impaired growth hormone secretion induced by persistent blockade of NMDA receptors in immature male rats. Neuroendocrinology 55:416–421, 1992.
290. Lindstrom P, Ohlsson L: Effect of *N*-methyl-D-aspartate on isolated rat somatotrophs. Endocrinology 131:1903–1907, 1992.
291. Niimi M, Takhara J, Saito M, Kawanishi K: Immunohistochemical identification of galanin and growth hormone releasing factor containing neurons projecting to the median eminence in the rat. Neuroendocrinology 51:572–575, 1990.
292. Maiter DM, Hooi SC, Koenig JI, Martin JB: Galanin is a physiological regulator of spontaneous pulsatile secretion of growth hormone in the male rat. Endocrinology 126:1216–1222, 1990.
293. Rettori V, Milenkovic L, Aguila MC, McCann SM: Physiologically significant effect of neuropeptide Y to suppress growth hormone release by stimulating somatostatin discharge. Endocrinology 126:2296–2301, 1990.
294. Sarapura VD, Samuels MH, Ridgway C: Thyroid stimulating hormone. *In* Melmed S (ed): The Pituitary. Boston, Blackwell Science, 1995, pp 187–229.
295. Lechan RM, Jackson IMD: Immunohistochemical localization of thyrotropin releasing hormone in the rat hypothalamus and pituitary. Endocrinology 111:55–65, 1982.
296. Burger HG, Patel YC: TSH and TRH: Their physiological regulation and the clinical applications of TRH. *In* Martini L, Besser GM (eds): Clinical Neuroendocrinology. New York Academic, 1977, pp 67–131.
297. Krulich L: Central neurotransmitters and the secretion of prolactin, GH, LH, and TSH. Ann Rev Physiol 41:603–615, 1979.
298. Molley JE: Neuroendocrine control of thyrotropin secretion. Endocr Rev 2:396–436, 1981.
299. Krulich L, Mayfield MA, Steele MK, et al: Differential effects of pharmacological manipulations of central α_1- and α_2-adrenergic receptors on the secretion of thyrotropin and growth hormone in male rats. Endocrinology 35:139–145, 1982.
300. Mannisto PT, Mattila J, Tuomisto J: Further evidence of the dual role of noradrenaline in regulation of thyrotropin secretion in male rats. Acta Endocrinol 97:213–220, 1981.
301. Terry LC: Regulation of thyrotropin secretion by the central epinephrine system. Neuroendocrinology 42:102–108, 1986.
302. Dieguez C, Foord SM, Peters JR, et al: Interactions among epinephrine, thyrotropin (TSH)-releasing hormone, dopamine and somatostatin in the control of TSH secretion in vitro. Endocrinology 114:957–963, 1984.
303. Tapia-Arancibia L, Arancibia S, Astier H: Evidence for α_1-adrenergic stimulatory control of in vitro release of immunoreactive thyrotropin releasing hormone from rat median eminence: In vivo corroboration. Endocrinology 116:2314–2319, 1985.
304. Yoshimura M, Hachiya T, Ochi Y, et al: Suppression of elevated serum TSH levels in hypothyroidism by fusaric acid. J Clin Endocrinol Metab 45:95–98, 1997.
305. Spaulding SW, Burrow GN, Donabedian R, Van Woert M: L-Dopa suppression of thyrotropin releasing hormone in man. J Clin Endocrinol Metab 35:182–185, 1972.
306. Miyai K, Onishi T, Hosokava M, et al: Inhibition of thyrotropin and prolactin secretion in primary hypothyroidism by 2-Br-α-urgocryptine. J Clin Endocrinol Metab 39:391–394, 1979.
307. Scanlon MF, Weightman DR, Shale DJ, et al: Dopamine is a physiological regulator of thyrotropin (TSH) secretion in normal man. Clin Endocrinol 10:7–15, 1979.
308. Samuels MH, Henry P, Ridgway EC: Effects of dopamine and somatostatin on pulsatile pituitary glycoprotein secretion. J Clin Endocrinol Metab 74:217–222, 1992.
309. Pourmand M, Rodriguez-Arnao MD, Weightman DR, et al: Domperidone: A novel agent for the investigation of anterior pituitary function and control in man. Clin Endocrinol 12:211–215, 1980.
310. Scanlon MF, Chan V, Heith M, et al: Dopaminergic control of thyrotropin, α-subunit and prolactin in euthyroidism and hypothyroidism: Dissociated responses to dopamine receptor blockade with metochlopramide in euthyroid and hypothyroid subjects. J Clin Endocrinol Metab 53:360–365, 1981.
311. Foord SM, Peters JR, Dieguez C, et al: Hypothyroid pituitary cells in culture: An analysis of thyrotropin and prolactin responses to dopamine (DA) and DA receptor binding. Endocrinology 115:407–415, 1984.
312. Lewis BM, Dieguez C, Lewis MD, Scanlon MF: Dopamine stimulates release of

thyrotrophin releasing hormone from perfused intact rat hypothalamus via hypothalamic D_2 receptors. J Endocrinol 115:419–424, 1987.

313. Shupnik MA, Ridgway EC, Chin WW: Molecular biology of thyrotropin. Endocr Rev 10:459–475, 1989.

314. Woolf PD, Lee L: Effect of serotonin precursor tryptophan on pituitary hormone secretion. J Clin Endocrinol Metab 45:123–133, 1977.

315. Ferrari C, Paracchi A, Rodena M, et al: Effect of two serotonin antagonists on prolactin and thyrotropin secretion in man. Clin Endocrinol 5:575–578, 1976.

316. O'Malley BP, Janning PE, Cook N, et al: The role of serotonin (5-HT) in the control of TSH and prolactin in euthyroid subjects as assessed by the administration of ketanserin (5-HT$_2$ antagonist) and zimelidine (5-HT reuptake inhibitor). Psychoneuroendocrinology 9:13–19, 1984.

Chapter 14

Oxytocin

Hans H. Zingg

Oxytocin (OT) derives its name from the Greek *okytokos,* quick birth. Indeed, this neurohypophysial nonapeptide is the strongest uterotonic substance known and is widely used in clinical practice for induction and augmentation of labor, as well as for prevention and treatment of postpartum hemorrhage. The accidental discovery by Henry Dale of the uterus-contracting effects of pituitary extracts dates back to the beginning of the 20th century.[1] With the subsequent discovery of the milk-ejecting effect of pituitary extracts by Ott and Scott[2] in 1910, the two most prominent biologic actions of OT were defined. Purified preparations of the "active principles" of the posterior pituitary were commercially available in the late 1920s,[3] but only the pioneering work of Vincent of du Vigneaud in the early 1950s established the structure of the active principle by isolating and sequencing the nonapeptide OT. In fact, OT and the structurally related peptide vasopressin were the first peptides to be sequenced and subsequently synthesized, an achievement that led to the award of the Nobel Prize for chemistry to du Vigneaud in 1955.

In ensuing decades, the hypothalamo-neurohypophysial system of OT and vasopressin neurons has served as a classic model system for the development of the concepts of neurosecretion and stimulus-secretion coupling. With the cloning of the genes encoding vasopressin and OT and the cloning of the family of the receptors that mediate the actions of vasopressin and OT, new insights into the mechanisms of biosynthesis and action of these peptides have been gained.

Whereas recent evidence clearly supports an essential role for OT in lactation,[4, 5] it is still a matter of debate to what extent OT fulfills a critical role in the process of labor and parturition. Yet, the well-established tocolytic effects of OT antagonists in humans[6] and experimental animals[7, 8] argue for a physiologic and possibly pathophysiologic role of OT in normal and preterm labor, respectively. Moreover, they form the basis for novel pharmacotherapeutic approaches to the treatment of premature labor. The spectrum of proposed biologic functions of OT has recently been considerably expanded and now includes roles in cardiovascular, behavioral, central nervous system, renal, immune, pituitary, and male reproductive functions (Table 14–1). Two recent monographs contain detailed accounts of advances in the field of oxytocin.[9, 10] This chapter reviews first the basic knowledge of OT production, release, and action, and then focuses on current views on OT's role in the physiology and pathophysiology of several key functions.

MECHANISMS OF BIOSYNTHESIS

Peptide Structure and Processing

The structures of vasopressin and OT are shown in Table 14–2. Both peptides share with their ancestral molecules a disulfide linkage

TABLE 14–1. Location and Established or Proposed Functions of Oxytocin Receptors

Organ	Cell Type	Established or Proposed Functions	References*
Uterus	Myometrial cells	Uterine contractions	89, 90
	Endometrium, decidua	Prostaglandin $F_{2\alpha}$ release	52, 178
Mammary gland	Myoepithelial cells	Milk ejection	53, 41
Pituitary gland	Lactotrophs	Prolactin release	54, 102
Brain	Neurons	Social and reproductive behaviors, ↓ anxiety, ↓ stress response, ↓ memory storage, ↑ short-term olfactive memory	55, 179
	Astrocytes		56
Spinal cord	Neurons, specifically dorsal horn	↓ Nociception, ↑ erection	57, 159, 180
Kidney	Macula densa cells, tubular and collecting duct cells	Natriuresis	58, 181
Thymus	T cells	T-cell maturation	59
Ovary	Granulosa cells	Luteinization, luteolysis	60
Amnion	Amnion cells	Prostaglandin E_2 production	182
Testes	Leydig cells, Sertoli cells	Steroidogenesis, sperm transport	61, 183
Heart	Myocardial cells	Atrial natriuretic factor release, ↓ heart rate	62
Blood vessels	Endothelial cells	Vasodilation, proliferation	63
Neoplasms	Breast cancer cells, neuroblastoma cells, glioma cells, leiomyoma cells	Antiproliferative	172–175

*For recent reviews, see Zingg HH, Bourque CW, Bichet DG (eds): Vasopressin and oxytocin. Molecular, cellular and clinical advances. Adv Exp Med Biol 449:1998; and Zingg HH: Vasopressin and oxytocin receptors. Ballières Clin Endocrinol Metab 10:75–96, 1996.

TABLE 14–2. Sequences of Oxytocin and Related Molecules

Molecule	Position								
	1	*2*	*3*	*4*	*5*	*6*	*7*	*8*	*9*
					S-S				
OT	Cys-	Tyr-	Ile-	Gln-	Asn-	Cys-	Pro-	Leu-	Gly-NH$_2$
AVP	=	=	Phe-	=	=	=	=	Arg-	=
VT	=	=	Ile-	=	=	=	=	Arg-	=
MT	=	=	Ile-	=	=	=	=	Ile-	=
Atosiban	dCys-D-Tyr(OEt)-		Ile-	Thr	=	=	=	Orn-	=

OT, oxytocin; AVP, arginine vasopressin: VT, vasotocin; MT, mesotocin; atosiban, 1-deamino-2-D-tyr(OEt)-4-thr-8-orn-oxytocin; =, same residue as oxytocin; dCys, desamino cysteine; Orn, ornithine.

between residues 1 and 6 and consist of a six-residue cyclic part and a three-residue, amidated C-terminal part. The two molecules differ only in positions 3 and 8. Thus, these two residues mediate the differential affinity of these peptides for the different members of the vasopressin-OT receptor family.

OT, as well as vasopressin, is produced as part of a precursor molecule that contains, in addition to the biologically active nonapeptide, a 10-kDa peptide called neurophysin, of unclear biologic function. Following packaging into neurosecretory granules, the precursor molecule is enzymatically processed and transported along the axon toward the nerve terminals in the posterior pituitary. Processing involves cleavage of the lysine-arginine pair of basic amino acids between OT and its neurophysin and amidation of the C-terminal of OT.

Gene Structure and Regulation

The closely related neurohypophysial nonapeptides OT and vasopressin are the offsprings of a long phylogenetic evolution that can be traced to mollusks and insects.[11, 12] Vasotocin and mesotocin (see Table 14–2) are two examples of ancestral molecules that are distributed among nonmammalian species.[11] The genes encoding OT and vasopressin are in close proximity on the same chromosome in all mammalian species studied, and arose by gene duplication of an ancestral gene.[12] The two genes are positioned tail to tail and are thus transcribed from opposite strands. In all species studied, the OT and vasopressin genes consist of three exons that are separated by relatively small introns. In each gene, the nonapeptide is encoded by exon 1. Studies on the human, rat, and bovine OT gene revealed that the OT gene is under positive and negative control by a composite hormone regulatory region that is able to interact with several members of the nuclear receptor superfamily. This element is located about 160 nucleotides upstream of the site of transcriptional initiation and mediates positive transcriptional regulation by interacting with the estrogen,[13, 14] retinoic acid,[15] and thyroid hormone receptors,[16] as well as with the nuclear orphan receptor SF1.[17] Negative control is exerted by the nuclear orphan receptors COUP-TF I and II, involving competition with stimulatory factors,[17–19] as well as active silencing.[20] In vivo, hypothalamic OT gene expression is stimulated during pregnancy and lactation,[21] in response to dehydration,[22] and following a combination of estrogen stimulation and progesterone withdrawal.[23] By contrast, uterine OT expression is highly stimulated by combined estrogen-progesterone application,[24] as well as shortly before term.[25]

SITES OF BIOSYNTHESIS

Central Biosynthesis

The neural lobe of the pituitary gland represents the main site of OT and vasopressin storage and release. Both peptides are, however, produced in distinct hypothalamic neurons whose cell bodies are located mainly in two distinct areas, the supraoptic and the paraventricular nuclei of the hypothalamus. Owing to their relative size, the hypothalamic neurons projecting to the neural lobe have been termed *magnocellular neurons*. Together with their axonal processes, these neurons form the hypothalamo-neurohypophysial tract. On their way to the neural lobe, the axons transverse the internal zone of the median eminence and continue down the nervous part of the pituitary stalk (infundibular stem) to end on basement membranes of capillaries in the neural lobe, where the neurohormones are released into the general circulation. As detailed below, the axons of the neurohypophysial complex assume a dual role: transport of matter (the secretory material) and transport of information (the stimulus for release).

OT, as well as vasopressin, is also produced in smaller neurons, so-called parvicellular neurons, in the paraventricular nucleus of the hypothalamus. Axons emanating from these neurons project to different brain areas as well as to the spinal cord, where OT exerts neurotransmitter functions. Moreover, some OT neurons project to the external zone of the median eminence, giving OT access to the anterior pituitary gland via the pituitary portal system.

Peripheral Biosynthesis

Peripheral sites of OT production include ovarian granulosa cells,[26, 27] uterine epithelial cells,[25] uterine decidua,[28] placenta,[29] amnion,[30] testicular Leydig cells,[31] and thymic epithelium.[32] As discussed below, OT released from these sites is likely to have a role as a paracrine mediator.

MECHANISMS OF RELEASE

The Concept of Neurosecretion

OT release from neurons occurs in response to membrane depolarization consequent to the arrival of action potentials that originate from the neuronal cell bodies. Membrane depolarization, in turn, opens voltage-gated calcium channels. The resulting increase in intracellular calcium mediates the process of exocytosis, whereby secretory granules move to, and fuse with, the outer cell membrane and release their contents into the surrounding extracellular space.[33–35] The process by which neurons release their secretory content in response to action has been termed *neurosecretion*. Indeed, the magnocellular neurons of the hypothalamo-neurohypophysial OT and vasopressin system have long served as a model system for the development and refinement of this concept. The concept that neurons are capable of releasing secretory materials was first put forth by Carl Speidel in 1919.[36] This concept was revolutionary at the time. Over a decade later, Scharrer[37] and Bargman[38] provided evidence that the hypothalamo-neurohypophysial system is such a neurosecretory system and initiated decades of ongoing fruitful research, in which the synergistic application of electrophysiologic, biochemical, and histologic techniques led the way to a molecular definition of the concepts of neurosecretion and stimulus-secretion coupling.[33–35]

The Milk-Ejection Reflex

The molecular and cellular mechanisms by which hypothalamic OT neurons are activated have been, and still are, the subject of detailed electrophysiologic investigations.[39–41] The milk-ejection reflex, a classic neuroendocrine reflex, has been studied preferentially in the rat.[41] Stimulation of the nipple by the suckling infant activates, via a complex central gating mechanism, the quasi-totality of hypothalamic OT neurons for a brief 4- to 12-second period every 5 to 10 minutes. This highly synchronized burst of electrical activity of OT neurons leads to a short but massive peak of circulating OT, resulting in milk ejection from the mammary gland. The transmitters involved in modulating this complex pulsatile reflex mechanism include acetylcholine, dopamine, norepinephrine, and opioids.[39] The specific bursting pattern appears to be controlled by local, patterned γ-aminobutyric acid (GABA)ergic and glutamatergic inputs.[42] OT itself, released from dendrites and somata of OT neurons, is part of a positive feedback loop and exerts a facilitating effect on OT neurons.[43]

Other Stimuli of Release

In all placental mammals thus far studied, parturition is associated with an increase in circulating OT levels[44, 45] and a strong increase in electrical activity of OT neurons, specifically prior to the delivery of a fetus or the placenta.[46] It has remained unclear, however, whether this increased neuronal and secretory activity initiates, or is stimulated by, parturition. On the one hand, electrical stimulation of the neurohypophysis can bring about parturition.[47] On the other hand, parturition-induced distention of cervix and vagina represent a stimulus for OT release.[48] In reality, both views may be correct, because OT forms part of a positive, self-sustaining feedback loop that, once set in motion, promotes a cascade of events that culminate in parturition. Detailed measurements revealed that OT secretion in women occurs in short pulses. Pulse frequency increases during spontaneous labor from 1.2 per 30 minutes to 6.7 per 30 minutes and pulse duration increases from 1.2 to 2.0 minutes.[49]

Additional stimuli that affect, seemingly indiscriminately, the activity of both OT and vasopressin neurons include increased serum osmolality, a decrease in blood pressure, mating, and certain kinds of stress, including fever.[39] Whereas suckling induces short bursts of activation that are punctuated by relative silence, the above stimuli lead to a more continuous activation of OT neurons.

MECHANISMS OF ACTION

Oxytocin Receptors

The diverse physiologic actions of OT all appear to be mediated by a single OT receptor (OTR). Despite arguments for the existence of OTR subtypes,[50] only one OTR type has so far been structurally identified. Initially, OTRs were characterized by binding studies, using a highly specific iodinated OT antagonist.[51] Specific OT binding sites are present within the uterus at the level of the myometrium, as well as the uterine epithelium or decidua.[52] Whereas myometrial receptors mediate uterine contractions directly, activation of decidual receptors elicits prostaglandin $F_{2α}$ release,[52] which, in turn, not only enhances uterine contractions but also promotes cervical ripening and luteolysis. Additional OT binding sites have been characterized in mammary gland,[53] pituitary,[54] brain,[55] astrocytes,[56] spinal cord,[57] kidney,[58] thymic T cells,[59] ovary,[60] testes,[61] heart,[62] and vascular endothelial cells.[63]

The vasopressin-OTR family comprises four members, which include, in addition to the OTR, the V_{1a}, V_{1b}, and V_2 subtypes of vasopressin receptors.[64] Whereas vasopressin binds to all four receptors, including the OTR, OT interacts preferentially with the OTR and weakly with the V1b receptor.[64] The structures of the human,[65] rat,[66] pig,[67] sheep,[68] cow,[69] and mouse[70] OTRs have been elucidated by molecular cloning. The deduced amino acid sequences indicate that the OTR forms part of the family of G protein–coupled receptors consisting of seven hydrophobic transmembrane α helixes. Compared to other members of the OT-vasopressin receptor family, relatively little is known of the specific regions of the OTR involved in ligand binding and signaling. We assume that the cyclic part of the OT molecule is lodged in the upper third of the receptor binding pocket and interacts with transmembrane domains 3, 4, and 6, whereas the linear C-terminal part of the OT molecule remains closer to the surface and interacts with transmembrane domains 2 and 3, as well as with the connecting first extracellular loop.[71] This hypothesis is supported by studies employing site-directed mutagenesis,[71–74] as well as by experiments involving domain swapping between the V2 vasopressin receptor and the OTR.[75, 76]

Activation of the OTR leads to phospholipase C–mediated phosphoinositide hydrolysis, followed by activation of protein kinase C and intracellular calcium mobilization.[77–79] The rise in intracellular calcium is greatly attenuated in the absence of extracellular calcium, indicating that OTR activation also stimulates calcium influx, probably via calcium-induced (or capacitative) calcium entry.[79] Experiments with antibodies against different G proteins demonstrated that coupling to phospholipase C occurs mainly via a G protein of the $G_{q/11}$ family.[78] However, evidence for coupling to other G proteins, including G_i,[77, 80] and/or G_{ha}[81, 82] has also been presented. The regions of the OTR implicated in G protein interactions have been delineated by examining the inhibitory effect of co-expression of different intracellular domains of the receptor. The studies indicate that all four intracellular domains are involved in coupling to $G_{q/α11}$.[79, 83]

Additional proposed effector mechanisms involve coupling to phospholipase A_2[80, 84] and phosphorylation and activation of mitogen-activated protein kinase.[85, 86] These two pathways may be relevant to the stimulation of prostaglandin $F_{2α}$[84] and prostaglandin E_2 synthesis,[86] respectively. The precise mechanisms by which OTR activation induces smooth muscle contractions and prostaglandin synthesis remain to be defined. In myometrial cells, a calcium-induced activation of the calcium-calmodulin complex leading to activation of myosin light chain kinase is involved in initiating the contraction process. In decidual cells, stimulation of prostaglandin synthesis is the consequence of an OT-induced activation of cyclooxygenase II expression.[87] In vascular endothelial cells and renal macula densa cells, OTR activation leads to a calcium-dependent activation of nitric oxide synthase, inducing vasodilation or natriuresis, respectively.[63, 88]

Oxytocin Receptor Regulation

An outstanding feature of the OTR gene is the dramatic change in the expression of this gene in different tissues. This highly regulated expression sets the OTR apart from the majority of other G protein–coupled receptors in general and from the closely related vasopressin receptors in particular. During gestation, uterine OT (but not vasopressin) receptors are upregulated by one to two orders of magnitude in all mammalian species studied,[44, 89] including the human.[90] This phenomenon induces a strong increase in uterine sensitivity toward OT[91] and is due to a dramatic increase in uterine OTR gene expression just prior to parturition.[65, 92] Indeed, the increase in uterine OTRs is much more striking than, and precedes, the increase in circulating OT. Therefore, it has been proposed that OTR upregulation represents the trigger for parturition.[89] Whereas the number of *uterine* OT binding sites decreases quickly following parturition, *mammary gland* OT binding sites reach a maximum shortly after parturition and remain elevated throughout lactation.[89] This differential, tissue-specific regulation of OTR expression enables a switch in target organs and allows circulating OT to assume a dual role: uterine contractions during labor and milk ejection during lactation. The same OTR gene is expressed in both tissues; the molecular basis underlying this tissue-specific differential regulation of OTR gene expression remains to be elucidated.

Hormonal Factors

Several studies have shown that uterine OTRs are upregulated by estrogens and downregulated by progesterone.[93–95] Indeed, in most mammals, the situation before term is characterized by high estrogen levels (involving placental conversion of fetally produced dehydroepiandrogen and androstenedione to estradiol) and a sharp decline of progesterone (induced by luteolysis; exceptions include the humans and primates, in which no fall in progesterone occurs). The sudden drop in the progesterone-estrogen ratio is thought to be causally involved in triggering parturition. This idea is further supported by findings in the knockout mouse lacking the prostaglandin F receptor[96, 97]: in this mouse model, preterm luteolysis and the ensuing fall in progesterone are prevented. This leads to complete suppression of parturition and suppression of OTR gene expression. However, both OTR expression and parturition are restored if a fall in progesterone is induced by ovariectomy.

We have recently determined that the estrogen-induced upregulation is due to a genomic estrogen-mediated increase in OTR gene expression.[92, 98] On the other hand, progesterone may act to decrease OT binding via both a genomic effect[99] and a nongenomic effect, involving a direct interaction with the OTR that leads to inhibition of OTR binding and signaling functions.[100, 101] Moreover, the effect of estrogens on OTR expression is tissue-specific: whereas estrogens stimulate OTR gene expression in uterus,[92] pituitary,[102] kidney,[103] and hypothalamus,[104, 105] OTR expression in mammary gland[106] and nonhypothalamic brain sites such as the subiculum or the olfactory lobe[104, 105] remains unaffected by steroid treatment. Although the rat and human OTR genes contain potential estrogen-responsive sites in their promoter regions,[66, 107] none of these sites turns out to be estrogen responsive when analyzed at the original distance from the transcriptional initiation site.[107] Cell-specific estrogen responsiveness may be mediated indirectly or via other functional OTR promoter elements, including AP1 sites and a cyclic adenosine monophosphate (cAMP)–response element.[108, 109] Interleukins (ILs), specifically IL-1β and IL-6, represent additional potential regulators of OTR expression. They are present in high concentrations in amniotic fluid at term labor and are mediators of infection-induced preterm labor.[110] Indeed, the rat and human OTR genes contain potential interleukin-response elements in their promoter regions; however, proofs of their functionality have not been provided yet.

Local Factors

There is good evidence that local humoral and mechanical factors play an important role in the control of uterine OTR expression. In the tammar wallaby, an Australian marsupial, in which unilateral pregnancy occurs naturally, only the gravid horn exhibits an upregulation of OTR expression at term.[111] Similarly, in unilaterally pregnant rats, only the gravid horn exhibits increased OTR expression at term.[99] However, OTR expression in the nongravid horn reaches the levels present in the gravid horn if it is mechanically stretched by a Silastic implant.[99] In ruminants, the trophoblast of the developing blastocyst produces a characteristic type I interferon, named interferon-τ, which completely suppresses endometrial OTR expression.[112, 113] In unilaterally pregnant ewes, shortly after implantation, the gravid uterus contains high levels of interferon-τ, but low levels of OTRs. By contrast, the nongravid uterus exhibits over 10 times higher OTR levels due to the absence of interferon-mediated suppression.[114] Thus blastocyst-derived interferon ensures uterine quiescence necessary for implantation and fetal development. It also suppresses OTR-induced prostaglandin $F_{2\alpha}$ release and, therefore, suppresses luteolysis. Thus, this mechanism forms part of the ruminant system for the maternal recognition of pregnancy. It remains to be determined to what extent this mechanism may apply to nonruminant species as well.

PHYSIOLOGIC ROLES OF OXYTOCIN

Lactation

OTRs are present on myoepithelial cells of the mammary gland. These cells form a meshlike arrangement around the alveoli and, upon contraction, squeeze the milk out of the alveoli into the milk ducts and out through the nipple. Mice in which the OT gene was ablated by gene targeting were unable to lactate.[4, 5] Lactation could be restored by OT injection, indicating that milk production was not grossly affected. This finding attests to a critical, nonredundant functional role of OT in lactation. In addition to their inability to lactate, OT knockout mice had impaired postpartum alveolar proliferation and lacked expansion of the lobulo-alveolar units,[115] compatible with the observation of a trophic effect of OT on myoepithelial cell development.[116]

Parturition

Induction and progression of labor involves a complex network of signaling pathways, integrating signals originating from the mother, the fetus, and the placenta. Although many signaling mechanisms are common to most mammalian species, the relative importance of each and their individual roles in the overall balance of forces vary greatly among species. Moreover, none of them act in isolation; rather they are intertwined in a network of interconnected negative and positive feedback loops. Thus it is difficult to define a single mechanism as *the* trigger for parturition. It is more appropriate to describe the events leading up to labor as a shift in the balance between signals inducing uterine relaxation and those inducing uterine contractions. In this view, OT, and specifically the OTR, forms part of a gene "cassette"[117] that is induced prior to labor and promotes "tipping of the balance." The precise signaling mechanisms that bring about the dramatic upregulation of uterine OTR expression immediately prior to parturition remain to be determined. As discussed above, both hormonal and local factors are involved in a species-specific fashion.

There are strong arguments both for and against the importance of OT in the processes of labor and parturition. Mice in which the gene for OT has been inactivated are able to deliver normally. This indicates that, at least in the mouse, OT is not essential to normal parturition.[4, 5, 44, 118] Considering the multiplicity of interconnected mechanisms that are mediating the important function of parturition, it is not surprising that there is redundancy in this system, and that knocking out one of its components does not necessarily lead to the breakdown of the entire process. More important, this finding does not rule out that premature overactivation of the OT system may be a determining factor in cases of idiopathic premature labor. Support for this idea stems primarily from the large number of studies that attest to the effectiveness of OT antagonists in inducing uterine quiescence in normal labor as well as in cases of naturally occurring or experimentally induced premature labor.

The group of Nathanielsz demonstrated that, in pregnant monkeys, the administration of androstenedione (an estrogen precursor produced by the fetal adrenal) induces a condition of premature labor that exhibits biochemical, hormonal, and physiologic hallmarks of normal labor.[119] In this condition, co-administration of the OT antagonist atosiban[120] led to complete abolishment of uterine contractions, indicating that OT is a necessary part of the mechanisms mediating androstenedione-induced myometrial contractions.[121] The tocolytic effects of atosiban have been demonstrated in others species, including marsupials,[8] the baboon,[7] and the guinea pig.[122]

How efficient is atosiban in the human? Indeed, atosiban is the most studied tocolytic agent besides the β-agonist ritodrine, which represents the only currently Food and Drug Administration (FDA)–approved tocolytic agent.[6] The first European trials in the late 1980s showed that, in patients with uncomplicated premature labor, atosiban led in all cases to inhibition of uterine contractions without any relevant side effects.[123] After several years, clinical trials were also performed in the United States.[124] The most recent published randomized double-blind placebo-controlled trials[125, 126] showed that the proportion of patients who remained undelivered and had not used another tocolytic agent at 1 to 7 days after start of therapy was significantly higher in the atosiban group than in the placebo group, specifically in patients at a higher gestational age. The delay achieved by atosiban was comparable to that reported for ritodrine, but atosiban treatment was associated with significantly fewer side effects. However, the lack of improvement of infant outcomes and a question about adverse infant outcomes at lower gestational ages (which may be attributable to an uneven randomization of very premature infants to the atosiban group), prompted an FDA decision (April 1998) not to approve atosiban for use in the United States. Despite this negative decision, the development of OT antagonists remains an active field.[127–130] Owing to its additional V1a-antagonistic properties, atosiban is also effective against dysmenorrhea, a condition that involves vasopressin–V1a receptor interactions.[131, 132]

Roles in the Central Nervous System

Reproductive Behaviors

As a central neurotransmitter, OT modulates complex social behaviors, including parental care, mating behavior, and pair bond formation (see references[133–137] for review). In addition, central OT has effects on mood, feeding behavior, memory, and nociception. These effects are mediated through broadly distributed projections of OT neurons throughout the brain,[138] paralleled by an equally broad distribution of central OTRs.[139, 140] Most effects of OT on affiliative and social behavior depend on prior steroid hormone exposure that modulates receptor expression, ligand synthesis, and synaptic morphology.

Intracerebral injection of OT facilitates in the female rat the so-called lordosis reflex, a typical behavioral response that indicates sexual responsiveness.[141] Interestingly, there is also one anecdotal report of increased sexual receptivity in a human female in response to OT administration by nasal spray.[142] Intrahypothalamic infusion of antisense oligonucleotides directed against OTR messenger RNA (mRNA) or OTR antagonist administration is effective in reducing lordosis behavior in rats.[143, 144]

Maternal behavior is another typical behavioral response that is facilitated by central OT administration in estrogen-primed virgin or pregnant rats, mice, and ewes.[145] This behavior includes nest building and retrieval of the pups to the nest. The natural occurrence of the behavior can be blocked by intracerebroventricular (ICV) administration of OTR antagonists or OT antiserum.[146]

Oxytocin Effects on Other Behaviors

A wide group of affiliative behaviors involving social encounters, pair bonding, and attachment are facilitated by OT. Studies by Insel's group showed that a monogamous mammal, the prairie vole, shows strong partner preference and pair bonding following mating. This behavior can be induced in the absence of mating by central OT administration, and the natural occurrence of it can be blocked by ICV application of an OT antagonist prior to mating.[136, 137, 147] Thus it is thought that OT released during intercourse reinforces partnership bonding. To what extent this mechanism applies to the human and to what extent OT may be truly deserving of its nickname, "the love hormone," belong so far to the realm of speculation.

Reduction of anxiety represents an additional central OT effect. Using a maze with open and closed sections as a standard means of anxiety measurement, an anxiolytic effect of central OT administration to estrogen-primed rats or mice was demonstrated.[148, 149] These effects are likely mediated via estrogen-inducible OT binding sites in the limbic system.

Finally, OT may also modulate memory functions. Enhancing effects on short-term olfactory memory[150] and inhibitory effects on memory storage in avoidance task tests have been described.[151]

Unexpectedly, OT knockout mice did not exhibit any deficits in sexual or maternal behaviors.[152, 153] The only behavioral difference noted was that OT knockout mice were significantly more aggressive than wild-type mice,[152, 153] but only if they were born to homozygous OT knockout parents,[153] implying a potential role of in utero OT exposure. Moreover, they appeared to have impaired social memory.[153]

Role of Oxytocin in Male Reproductive Functions

In males, as well as females, including humans, OT secretion is stimulated during sexual activity.[154] OT has been ascribed essentially three functions in male reproductive physiology: a role in testicular steroidogenesis, a role in sperm transport via contraction of seminiferous tubules, and a role in erection.

OT is produced in Leydig cells, and Leydig cells are also endowed

with OTRs.[155] Whereas the effect of OT on Leydig cell testosterone production has remained controversial, a stimulatory effect on 5α-dehydrogenase has been described that results in increased production of the active metabolite dihydrotestosterone.[156] OTRs have been pharmacologically characterized in the epididymis and vas deferens,[157] and OTR immunoreactivity has been observed in smooth muscle cells of the epididymis.[155] Thus, OT released during ejaculation is thought to assist sperm transport. Intracerebral injection of OT, specifically into the area of the paraventricular nucleus, induces penile erection in rats.[158] This mechanism appears to involve NO as it can be inhibited by NO synthase inhibitors.[158, 159]

Pituitary Functions of Oxytocin

OT released from nerve terminals at the median eminence reaches the anterior pituitary via the pituitary–portal system where it acts as a releasing factor, potentiating the release of corticotropin, prolactin, and gonadotropins. Whereas the effect on corticotropin release is mediated via V1b receptors,[160] OTRs have been specifically located on lactotrophs[102] and likely mediate the demonstrated enhancing effects of OT on prolactin release.[161, 162] Since pituitary OTRs are strongly upregulated toward the end of pregnancy and in response to estrogens,[102] the functional role of OT as a prolactin-releasing factor may be enhanced during specific reproductive periods. Preovulatory OT administration also promotes the onset of the luteinizing hormone (LH) surge in human females.[163] Although no OTRs have been demonstrated on pituitary gonadotrophs in situ,[102] the gonadotroph-derived cell line alpha T3–1 responds to OT application with activation of phospholipase C and elevation of cytosolic calcium.[164]

Renal Functions of Oxytocin

Several lines of evidence support a role for OT as a natriuretic hormone. Neurohypophysectomy in rats leads to sodium retention that is corrected by OT administration.[165] OT levels within the physiologic range induce natriuresis.[166] This effect may be mediated by OTRs located at the basal pole of macula densa cells[167, 168] and suggests a role of OT in modulation of the tubuloglomerular feedback. Since renal OTR expression is upregulated by estrogens,[103, 168] OT may have a role as a regulator of sodium homeostasis, specifically during high-estrogen states.

Oxytocin in the Thymus

It appears that OT is involved as an intrathymic messenger in T-cell maturation and function. OT-like and vasopressin-like immunoreactivity has been detected in thymic nurse cells, a thymic epithelial cell population that is involved in facilitating T-cell maturation.[169] OTRs and vasopressin receptors have been identified on thymocytes. These receptors are functional, since addition of OT or vasopressin stimulates inositol phosphate production, DNA synthesis, and tyrosine phosphorylation.[170] Studies with different T-cell lines suggest that, during T-cell maturation, there is a switch from the expression of vasopressin receptors in immature cells to expression of the OTR in maturing cells.[169]

Novel Cardiovascular Functions of Oxytocin

The discovery that OT mediates cardiovascular functions is novel and is due to the recent detection of OTRs in endothelial cells and cardiocytes.[62] Although the vasodilating effects of neurohypophysial hormones have been known for some time, the nature of the receptor(s) mediating this process had remained controversial. By saturation binding and reverse transcriptase–polymerase chain reaction (RT-PCR) experiments, Thibonnier et al.[63] demonstrated the presence of specific

OTRs in endothelial cells of human umbilical vein, aorta, and pulmonary artery. None of the vasopressin receptor subtypes were detectable in these same tissues. The authors further demonstrated that OT application to endothelial cells led to intracellular calcium mobilization, NO production, and a calcium- and protein kinase C–dependent proliferation response.[63] Thus, vascular OTRs mediate NO-mediated vasodilation, as well as a trophic action on endothelium.

An additional novel pathway by which OT exerts a cardiovascular action has been defined by the recent detection of OTRs and OT biosynthesis in atria and ventricles of the heart.[62, 171] The addition of OT to the perfusate of the rat heart stimulates atrial natriuretic factor (ANF) release and slows down the heart rate, probably as a result of ANF release.[62] The OT-induced ANF release may also act as a mediator of OT's natriuretic action.

Oxytocin and Neoplasia

OTRs have been detected in breast cancer,[172, 173] leiomyomas,[174] and in neuroblastoma and glioma cells.[175] One study found that over 80% of breast cancers were OTR positive, but there was no apparent relationship between OTR expression and other clinical parameters.[172] OTR expression was also found in four different breast carcinoma cell lines.[172] Reports of OT effects on cell growth are conflicting. Whereas one group observed no effect on cell growth in mammary cancer lines,[172] another group reported cAMP-mediated growth-inhibitory effects in vitro and in vivo on mammary cancer cells,[176] as well as on different neuroblastoma cell lines and one astrocytoma line.[175, 177]

REFERENCES

1. Dale HH: On some physiological actions of ergot. J Physiol 34:163–206, 1906.
2. Ott I, Scott JC: The action of infundibulin upon the mammary secretion. Proc Soc Exp Biol Med 8:48–49, 1910.
3. Kamm O, Aldrich TB, Grote IW: The active principles of the posterior lobe of the pituitary gland. J Am Chem Soc 50:573–601, 1928.
4. Nishimori K, Young LJ, Guo Q, et al: Oxytocin is required for nursing but is not essential for parturition or reproductive behavior. Proc Natl Acad Sci USA 93:11699–11704, 1996.
5. Young WS III, Shepard E, Amico J, et al: Deficiency in mouse oxytocin prevents milk ejection, but not fertility or parturition. J Neuroendocrinol 8:847–853, 1996.
6. Goodwin TM, Zograbyan A: Oxytocin receptor antagonists—update. Clin Perinatol 25:859–871, 1998.
7. Nathanielsz PW, Honnebier MB, Mecenas C, et al: Effect of the oxytocin antagonist atosiban (1-deamino-2-D-tyr(OET)-4-thr-8-orn-vasotocin/oxytocin) on nocturnal myometrial contractions, maternal cardiovascular function, transplacental passage, and fetal oxygenation in the pregnant baboon during the last third of gestation. Biol Reprod 57:320–324, 1997.
8. Renfree MB, Parry LJ, Shaw G: Infusion with an oxytocin receptor antagonist delays parturition in a marsupial. J Reprod Fertil 108:131–137, 1996.
9. Zingg HH, Bourque CW, Bichet DG (eds): Vasopressin and oxytocin: Molecular, cellular and clinical advances. Adv Exp Med Biol 449:1998.
10. Ivell R, Russell JA (eds): Oxytocin: Cellular and molecular approaches in medicine and research. Adv Exp Med Biol 395:1995.
11. Acher R: Molecular evolution of biologically active polypeptides. Proc R Soc Lond B Biol Sci 210:21–43, 1980.
12. Gainer H, Wray S: Cellular and molecular biology of oxytocin and vasopressin. In Knobil E, Neill J (eds): The Physiology of Reproduction. New York, Raven Press, 1994, pp 1099–1129.
13. Richard S, Zingg HH: The human oxytocin gene promoter is regulated by estrogens. J Biol Chem 265:6098–6103, 1990.
14. Adan RA, Cox JJ, Beischlag TV, et al: A composite hormone response element mediates the transactivation of the rat oxytocin gene by different classes of nuclear hormone receptors. Mol Endocrinol 7:47–57, 1993.
15. Richard S, Zingg HH: Identification of a retinoic acid response element in the human oxytocin promoter. J Biol Chem 266:21428–21433, 1991.
16. Adan RA, Cox JJ, van Kats JP, et al: Thyroid hormone regulates the oxytocin gene. J Biol Chem 267:3771–3777, 1992.
17. Wehrenberg U, Ivell R, Jansen M, et al: Two orphan receptors binding to a common site are involved in the regulation of the oxytocin gene in the bovine ovary. Proc Natl Acad Sci U S A 91:1440–1444, 1994.
18. Chu K, Boutin J-M, Breton C, et al: Nuclear orphan receptors COUP-TFII and Ear-2: Presence in oxytocin-producing uterine cells and functional interaction with the oxytocin gene promoter. Mol Cell Endocrinol 137:145–154, 1997.
19. Burbach JP, Lopes da Silva S, Cox JJ, et al: Repression of estrogen-dependent stimulation of the oxytocin gene by chicken ovalbumin upstream promoter transcription factor I. J Biol Chem 269:15046–15053, 1994.
20. Chu K, Zingg HH: The nuclear orphan receptors COUP-TFII and Ear-2 act as silencers of the human oxytocin gene promoter. J Mol Endocrinol 19:163–172, 1997.
21. Zingg HH, Lefebvre DL: Oxytocin and vasopressin gene expression during gestation and lactation. Brain Res 464:1–6, 1988.
22. Burbach JPH, Van Tol HHM, Bakkus MHC, et al: Quantitation of vasopressin mRNA and oxytocin mRNA in hypothalamic nuclei by solution hybridization assays. J Neurochem 47:1814–1921, 1986.
23. Thomas A, Amico JA: Sequential estrogen and progesterone (P) followed by P withdrawal increases the level of oxytocin messenger ribonucleic acid in the hypothalamic paraventricular nucleus of the male rat. Life Sci 58:1615–1620, 1996.
24. Lefebvre DL, Farookhi R, Giaid A, et al: Uterine oxytocin gene expression: II. Induction by exogenous steroid administration. Endocrinology 134:2562–2566, 1994.
25. Lefebvre DL, Giaid A, Bennett H, et al: Oxytocin gene expression in rat uterus. Science 256:1553–1555, 1992.
26. Guldenaar SEF, Wathes DC, Pickering BT: Immunocytochemical evidence for the presence of oxytocin and neurophysin in the large cells of the bovine corpus luteum. Cell Tissue Res 237:349–352, 1984.
27. Ivell R, Bathgate RA, Walther N, et al: The molecular basis of oxytocin and oxytocin receptor gene expression in reproductive tissues. Adv Exp Med Biol 449:297–306, 1998.
28. Mitchell BF, Fang X, Wong S: Oxytocin: A paracrine hormone in the regulation of parturition? Rev Reprod 3:113–122, 1998.
29. Lefebvre DL, Giaid A, Zingg HH: Expression of the oxytocin gene in rat placenta. Endocrinology 130:1185–1192, 1992.
30. Lefebvre DL, Lariviere R, Zingg HH: Rat amnion: A novel site of oxytocin production. Biol Reprod 48:632–639, 1993.
31. Guldenaar SEF, Pickering BT: Immunocytochemical evidence for the presence of oxytocin in rat testis. Cell Tissue Res 240:485–487, 1985.
32. Wiemann M, Ehret G: Subcellular localization of immunoreactive oxytocin within thymic epithelial cells of the male mouse. Cell Tissue Res 273:79, 1993.
33. Hatton GI: Emerging concepts of structure-function dynamics in adult brain: The hypothalamo-neurohypophysial system. Prog Neurobiol 34:437–504, 190.
34. Renaud LP, Bourque CW: Neurophysiology and neuropharmacology of hypothalamic magnocellular neurons secreting vasopressin and oxytocin. Prog Neurobiol 36:131–169, 1991.
35. Hatton GI, Zhenhui L: Mechanisms of neuroendocrine cell excitability. In Zingg H, Bourque C, Bichet D (eds): Vasopressin and Oxytocin: Molecular, Cellular and Clinical Advances. New York, Plenum Press, 1998, pp 79–95.
36. Speidel C: Gland cells of internal secretion in the spinal cord of the skates. Carnegie Inst (Washington) 13:1–13, 1919.
37. Scharrer E: Die Lichtempfindlichkeit blinder Elritzen: Untersuchungen über das Zwischenhirn der Fische I. Z Vergleichende Physiol 7:1–38, 1928.
38. Bargman W: Über die neurosekretorische Verknüpfung von Hypothalamus und Neurohypophyse. Z Zellforschung Mikrosk Anat 34:610–634, 1949.
39. Poulain DA, Wakerley JB: Electrophysiology of hypothalamic magnocellular neurons secreting oxytocin and vasopressin. Neuroscience 7:773–808, 1982.
40. Crowley WR, Armstrong WE: Neurochemical regulation of oxytocin secretion in lactation. Endocr Rev 13:33–65, 1992.
41. Lincoln DW, Paisley AC: Neuroendocrine control of milk ejection. J Reprod Fertil 65:571–586, 1982.
42. Jourdain P, Dupouy B, Bonhomme R, et al: Electrophysiological studies of oxytocin neurons in organotypic slice cultures. Adv Exp Med Biol 449:135–145, 1998.
43. Moos F, Gouzenes L, Brown D, et al: New aspects of firing pattern autocontrol in oxytocin and vasopressin neurons. Adv Exp Med Biol 449:153–162, 1998.
44. Russell JA, Leng G: Sex, parturition and motherhood without oxytocin? J Endocrinol 157:343–359, 1998.
45. Fuchs A-R, Fuchs F: The endocrinology of human parturition: A review. Br J Obstet Gynaecol 91:948–967, 1984.
46. Summerlee AJS: Extracellular recordings from oxytocin neurones during the expulsive phase of birth in unanaesthetised rats. J Physiol (Lond) 321:1–9, 1981.
47. Boer K, Lincoln DW, Swaag DF: Effect of electrical stimulation of the neurohypophysis on labour in the rat. J Endocrinol 65:163–176, 1975.
48. Flint APF, Forsling ML, Mitchell MD, et al: Temporal relationship between changes in oxytocin and prostaglandin F levels in response to vaginal distention in the pregnant and puerpural ewe. J Reprod Fertil 43:551–554, 1975.
49. Fuchs AR, Romero R, Keefe D, et al: Oxytocin secretion and human parturition: Pulse frequency and duration increase during spontaneous labor in women. Am J Obstet Gynecol 165:1515–1523, 1991.
50. Chen DC, Chan WY, Manning M: Agonist and antagonist specificities of decidual prostaglandin-releasing and myometrial uterotonic oxytocin receptors in pregnant rats. J Reprod Fertil 102:337–343, 1994.
51. Elands J, Barberis C, Jard S, et al: ^{125}I-labelled d(CH2)5[Tyr(Me)2,Thr4,Tyr-NH2(9)]OVT: A selective oxytocin receptor ligand. Eur J Pharmacol 147:197–207, 1988.
52. Fuchs AR, Fuchs F, Husslein P, et al: Oxytocin receptors and human parturition: A dual role for oxytocin in the initiation of labor. Science 215:1396–1398, 1984.
53. Soloff MS, Fernstrom MA, Fernstrom MJ: Vasopressin and oxytocin receptors in rat mammary gland. Demonstration of vasopressin receptor by stimulation of inositol phosphate formation and oxytocin receptors by binding of a specific ^{125}I-labeled oxytocin antagonist, d(CH2)5[Tyr(Me)2,Thr4,Tyr-NH2(9)]OVT. Biochem Cell Biol 67:152–162, 1989.
54. Antoni F: Oxytocin receptors in rat adenohypophysis: Evidence from radioligand binding studies. Endocrinology 119:2393–2395, 1986.
55. Tribollet E, Barberis C, Jard S: Localization and pharmacological characterization of high affinity binding sites for vasopressin and oxytocin in the rat brain by light microscopic autoradiography. Brain Res 442:105–118, 1988.
56. Di Scala-Guenot D, Strosser MT: Oxytocin receptors on cultured astroglial cells. Kinetic and pharmacological characterization of oxytocin-binding sites on intact hypothalamic and hippocampic cells from foetal rat brain. Biochem J 284:491–497, 1992.
57. Tribollet E, Barberis C, Arsenijevic Y: Distribution of vasopressin and oxytocin receptors in the rat spinal cord: Sex-related differences and effect of castration in pudendal motor nuclei. Neuroscience 78:499–509, 1997.

58. Tribollet E, Barberis C, Dreifuss JJ: Autoradiographic localization of vasopressin and oxytocin binding sites in rat kidney. Kidney Int 33:959–965, 1988.
59. Elands J, Resink A, De Kloet ER: Oxytocin receptors in the rat thymic gland. Eur J Pharmacol 151:345–346, 1988.
60. Fuchs A-R, Behrens O, Helmer H: Oxytocin and vasopressin binding sites in human and bovine ovaries. Am J Obstet Gynecol 163:1961–1967, 1990.
61. Bathgate RAD, Sernia C: Characterization and localization of oxytocin receptors in the rat testis. J Endocrinol 141:343–352, 1994.
62. Gutkowska J, Jankowski M, Lambert C, et al: Oxytocin releases atrial natriuretic peptide by combining with oxytocin receptors in the heart. Proc Natl Acad Sci U S A 94:11704–11709, 1997.
63. Thibonnier M, Conarty DM, Preston JA, et al: Human vascular endothelial cells express oxytocin receptors. Endocrinology 140:1301–1309, 1999.
64. Zingg HH: Vasopressin and oxytocin receptors. Baillieres Clin Endocrinol Metab 10:75–96, 1996.
65. Kimura T, Tanizawa O, Mori K, et al: Structure and expression of a human oxytocin receptor. Nature 356:526–529, 1992.
66. Rozen F, Russo C, Banville D, et al: Structure, characterization, and expression of the rat oxytocin receptor gene. Proc Natl Acad Sci USA 92:200–204, 1995.
67. Gorbulev V: Molecular cloning and functional characterization of V2 [8-lysine] vasopressin and oxytocin receptors from a pig kidney cell line. Eur J Biochem 215:1–7, 1993.
68. Riley PR, Flint AP, Abayasekara DR, et al: Structure and expression of an ovine endometrial oxytocin receptor cDNA. J Mol Endocrinol 15:195–202, 1995.
69. Bathgate R, Rust W, Balvers M, et al: Structure and expression of the bovine oxytocin receptor gene. DNA Cell Biol 14:1037–1048, 1995.
70. Kubota Y, Kimura T, Hashimoto K, et al: Structure and expression of the mouse oxytocin receptor gene. Mol Cell Endocrinol 124:25–32, 1996.
71. Barberis C, Mouillac B, Durroux T: Structural basis of vasopressin/oxytocin receptor function. J Endocrinol 156:223–229, 1998.
72. Chini B, Mouillac B, Ala Y, et al: Tyr115 is the key residue for determining agonist selectivity in the V1a vasopressin receptor. EMBO J 14:2176–2182, 1995.
73. Chini B, Mouillac B, Balestre MN, et al: Two aromatic residues regulate the response of the human oxytocin receptor to the partial agonist arginine vasopressin. FEBS Lett 397:201–206, 1996.
74. Wheatley M, Hawtin SR, Yarwood NJ: Structure/function studies on receptors for vasopressin and oxytocin. Adv Exp Med Biol 449:363–365, 1998.
75. Postina R, Kojro E, Fahrenholz F: Separate agonist and peptide antagonist binding sites of the oxytocin receptor defined by their transfer into the V2 vasopressin receptor. J Biol Chem 271:31593–31601, 1996.
76. Postina R, Kojro E, Fahrenholz F: Identification of neurohypophysial hormone receptor domains involved in ligand binding and G protein coupling. Adv Exp Med Biol 449:371–385, 1998.
77. Phaneuf S, Carrasco MP, Europe-Finner GN, et al: Multiple G proteins and phospholipase C isoforms in human myometrial cells: Implication for oxytocin action. J Clin Endocrinol Metab 81:2098–2103, 1996.
78. Ku CY, Qian A, Wen Y, et al: Oxytocin stimulates myometrial guanosine triphosphatase and phospholipase-C activities via coupling to G alpha q/11. Endocrinology 136:1509–1515, 1995.
79. Sanborn BM, Dodge K, Monga M, et al: Molecular mechanisms regulating the effects of oxytocin on myometrial intracellular calcium. Adv Exp Med Biol 449:277–286, 1998.
80. Strakova Z, Soloff MS: Coupling of oxytocin receptor to G proteins in rat myometrium during labor: Gi receptor interaction. Am J Physiol 272:E870–876, 1997.
81. Baek KJ, Kwon NS, Lee HS, et al: Oxytocin receptor couples to the 80 kDa Gh alpha family protein in human myometrium. Biochem J 315:739–744, 1996.
82. Park ES, Won JH, Han KJ, et al: Phospholipase C-delta1 and oxytocin receptor signaling: Evidence of its role as an effector. Biochem J 331:283–289, 1998.
83. Qian A, Wang W, Sanborn BM: Evidence for the involvement of several intracellular domains in the coupling of oxytocin receptor to G alpha(q/11). Cell Signal 10:101–105, 1998.
84. Burns PD, Graf GA, Hayes SH, et al: Cellular mechanisms by which oxytocin stimulates uterine PGF2 alpha synthesis in bovine endometrium: Roles of phospholipases C and A2. Domest Anim Endocrinol 14:181–191, 1997.
85. Ohmichi M, Koike K, Nohara A, et al: Oxytocin stimulates mitogen-activated protein kinase activity in cultured human puerperal uterine myometrial cells. Endocrinology 136:2082–2087, 1995.
86. Strakova Z, Copland JA, Lolait SJ, et al: ERK2 mediates oxytocin-stimulated PGE2 synthesis. Am J Physiol 274:E634–641, 1998.
87. Burns PD, Tsai SJ, Wiltbank MC, et al: Effect of oxytocin on concentrations of prostaglandin H synthase-2 mRNA in ovine endometrial tissue in vivo. Endocrinology 138:5637–5640, 1997.
88. Conrad KP, Gellai M, North WG, et al: Influence of oxytocin on renal hemodynamics and sodium excretion. Ann NY Acad Sci 689:346–362, 1993.
89. Soloff MS, Alexandrova M, Fernstrom MJ: Oxytocin receptors: Triggers for parturition and lactation? Science 204:1313–1315, 1979.
90. Fuchs AR, Fuchs F, Husslein P, et al: Oxytocin receptors in the human uterus during pregnancy and parturition. Am J Obstet Gynecol 150:734–741, 1984.
91. Takahashi K, Diamond F, Bieniarz J, et al: Uterine contractility and oxytocin sensitivity in preterm, term, and postterm pregnancy. Am J Obstet Gynecol 136:774–779, 1980.
92. Larcher A, Neculcea J, Breton C, et al: Oxytocin receptor gene expression in the rat uterus during pregnancy and the estrous cycle and in response to gonadal steroid treatment. Endocrinology 136:5350–5356, 1995.
93. Fuchs AR, Periyasamy S, Alexandrova M, et al: Correlation between oxytocin receptor concentration and responsiveness to oxytocin in pregnant rat myometrium: Effects of ovarian steroids. Endocrinology 113:742–749, 1983.
94. Soloff MS, Fernstrom MA, Periyasamy S, et al: Regulation of oxytocin receptor concentration in rat uterine explants by estrogen and progesterone. Can J Biochem Cell Biol 61:625–630, 1983.
95. Maggi M, Magini A, Fiscella A, et al: Sex steroid modulation of neurohypophyseal hormone receptors in human nonpregnant myometrium. J Clin Endocrinol Metab 74:385–392, 1992.
96. Sugimoto Y, Yamasaki A, Segi E, et al: Failure of parturition in mice lacking the prostaglandin F receptor. Science 277:681–683, 1997.
97. Sugimoto Y, Segi E, Tsuboi K, et al: Female reproduction in mice lacking the prostaglandin F receptor. Roles of prostaglandin and oxytocin receptors in parturition. Adv Exp Med Biol 449:317–321, 1998.
98. Zingg HH, Rozen F, Breton C, et al: Gonadal steroid regulation of oxytocin and oxytocin receptor gene expression. Adv Exp Med Biol 395:395–404, 1995.
99. Ou CW, Chen ZQ, Qi SG, et al: Increased expression of the rat myometrial oxytocin receptor messenger ribonucleic acid during labor requires both mechanical and hormonal signals. Biol Reprod 59:1055–1061, 1998.
100. Grazzini E, Guillon G, Mouillac B, et al: Inhibition of oxytocin receptor function by direct binding of progesterone. Nature 392:509–512, 1998.
101. Zingg HH, Grazzini E, Breton C, et al: Genomic and non-genomic mechanisms of oxytocin receptor regulation. Adv Exp Med Biol 449:287–295, 1998.
102. Breton C, Pechoux C, Morel G, et al: Oxytocin receptor messenger ribonucleic acid: Characterization, regulation, and cellular localization in the rat pituitary gland. Endocrinology 136:2928–2936, 1995.
103. Breton C, Neculcea J, Zingg HH: Renal oxytocin receptor messenger ribonucleic acid: Characterization and regulation during pregnancy and in response to ovarian steroid treatment. Endocrinology 137:2711–2717, 1996.
104. Breton C, Zingg HH: Expression and region-specific regulation of the oxytocin receptor in rat brain. Endocrinology 138:1857–1862, 1997.
105. Tribollet E, Audigier S, Dubois-Dauphin M, et al: Gonadal steroids regulate oxytocin receptors but not vasopressin receptors in the brain of male and female rats. An autoradiographical study. Brain Res 511:129–140, 1990.
106. Breton C, Zingg HH: Expression and regulation of the oxytocin receptor gene in rat mammary gland. *In* Proceedings of the 1997 World Congress of Neurohypophysial Hormones, Montreal, 1997, abstract 137.
107. Bale TL, Dorsa DM: Cloning, novel promoter sequence, and estrogen regulation of a rat oxytocin receptor gene. Endocrinology 138:1151–1158, 1997.
108. Bale TL, Dorsa DM: NGF, cyclic AMP, and phorbol esters regulate oxytocin receptor gene transcription in SK-N-SH and MCF7 cells. Brain Res Mol Brain Res 53:130–137, 1998.
109. Grazzini E, Russo C, Zingg HH: Oxytocin receptor promoter: Induction by protein kinase C. *In* Abstracts 80th Annual Meeting of the Endocrine Society, New Orleans, 1998, p 394.
110. Romero R, Tartakovsky B: The natural interleukin-1 receptor antagonist prevents interleukin-1-induced preterm delivery in mice. Am J Obstet Gynecol 167:1041–1045, 1992.
111. Parry LJ, Bathgate RA, Shaw G, et al: Evidence for a local fetal influence on myometrial oxytocin receptors during pregnancy in the tammar wallaby (*Macropus eugenii*). Biol Reprod 56:200–207, 1997.
112. Flint AP: Interferon, the oxytocin receptor and the maternal recognition of pregnancy in ruminants and non-ruminants: A comparative approach. Reprod Fertil Devel 7:313–318, 1995.
113. Bazer FW, Spencer TE, Ott TL: Interferon tau: A novel pregnancy recognition signal [review]. Am J Reprod Immunol 37:412–420, 1997.
114. Lamming GE, Wathes DC, Flint AP, et al: Local action of trophoblast interferons in suppression of the development of oxytocin and oestradiol receptors in ovine endometrium. J Reprod Fertil 105:165–175, 1995.
115. Wagner KU, Young WS III, Liu X, et al: Oxytocin and milk removal are required for post-partum mammary-gland development. Genes Function 1:233–244, 1997.
116. Sapino A, Macri L, Tonda L, et al: Oxytocin enhances myoepithelial cell differentiation and proliferation in the mouse mammary gland. Endocrinology 133:838–842, 1993.
117. Lefebvre DL, Piersanti M, Bai XH, et al: Myometrial transcriptional regulation of the gap junction gene, connexin-43. Reprod Fertil Dev 7:603–611, 1995.
118. Young WS III, Shepard E, DeVries AC, et al: Targeted reduction of oxytocin expression provides insights into its physiological roles. Adv Exp Med Biol 449:231–240, 1998.
119. Mecenas CA, Giussani DA, Owiny JR, et al: Production of premature delivery in pregnant rhesus monkeys by androstenedione infusion. Nat Med 2:443–448, 1996.
120. Melin P, Trojnar J, Johansson B, et al: Synthetic antagonists of the myometrial response to vasopressin and oxytocin. J Endocrinol 111:125–131, 1986.
121. Giussani DA, Jenkins SL, Mecenas CA, et al: The oxytocin antagonist atosiban prevents androstenedione-induced myometrial contractions in the chronically instrumented, pregnant rhesus monkey. Endocrinology 137:3302–3307, 1996.
122. Schellenberg JC: The effect of oxytocin receptor blockade on parturition in guinea pigs. J Clin Invest 95:13–19, 1995.
123. Akerlund M, Stromberg P, Hauksson A, et al: Inhibition of uterine contractions of premature labour with an oxytocin analogue. Results from a pilot study. Br J Obstet Gynaecol 94:1040–1044, 1987.
124. Goodwin TM, Paul R, Silver H, et al: The effect of the oxytocin antagonist atosiban on preterm uterine activity in the human. Am J Obstet Gynecol 170:474–478, 1994.
125. The Antocin PTL096 Study Group, Sibai BM, Romero R, et al: A double-blind placebo-controlled trial of an oxytocin-receptor antagonist (antocin) in the treatment of preterm labor. Am J Obstet Gynecol 176:S2, 1997.
126. The Antocin PTL098 Study Group, Sanchez-Ramos L, Valenzuela M, et al: A double-blind placebo-controlled trial of oxytocin receptor antagonist (antocin) maintenance therapy in patients with preterm labor. Am J Obstet Gynecol 176:S30, 1997.
127. Manning M, Miteva K, Pancheva S, et al: Design and synthesis of highly selective in vitro and in vivo uterine receptor antagonists of oxytocin: Comparisons with atosiban. Int J Pept Protein Res 46:244–252, 1995.

128. Kuo MS, Bock MG, Freidinger RM, et al: Nonpeptide oxytocin antagonists—potent, orally bioavailable analogs of 1-371,257 containing a 1-*r*-(pyridyl)ethyl ether terminus. Bioorg Med Chem Lett 8:3081–3086, 1998.

129. Williams PD, Bock MG, Evans BE, et al: Progress in the development of oxytocin antagonists for use in preterm labor. Adv Exp Med Biol 449:473–479, 1998.

130. Chiu SH, Thompson KA, Vincent SH, et al: The role of drug metabolism in drug discovery: A case study in the selection of an oxytocin receptor antagonist for development. Toxicol Pathol 23:124–130, 1995.

131. Akerlund M: Can primary dysmenorrhea be alleviated by a vasopressin antagonist? Results of a pilot study. Acta Obstet Gynecol Scand 66:459–461, 1987.

132. Akerlund M, Melin P, Maggi M: Potential use of oxytocin and vasopressin V1a antagonists in the treatment of preterm labour and primary dysmenorrhoea. Adv Exp Med Biol 395:595–600, 1995.

133. Pedersen CA, Caldwell JD, Peterson G, et al: Oxytocin activation of maternal behavior in the rat. Ann NY Acad Sci 652:58–69, 1992.

134. Insel TR: Oxytocin—a neuropeptide for affiliation: Evidence from behavioral, receptor autoradiographic, and comparative studies. Psychoneuroendocrinology 17:3–35, 1992.

135. Witt DM: Oxytocin and rodent sociosexual responses: From behavior to gene expression. Neurosci Biobehav Rev 19:315–324, 1995.

136. Insel TR: A neurobiological basis of social attachment. Am J Psychiatry 154:726–735, 1997.

137. Insel TR, Winslow JT, Wang Z, et al: Oxytocin, vasopressin, and the neuroendocrine basis of pair bond formation. Adv Exp Med Biol 449:215–224, 1998.

138. Sawchenko PE, Swanson LW: Hypothalamic integration: Organization of the paraventricular and supraoptic nuclei. Annu Rev Neurosci 6:269–324, 1983.

139. Tribollet E: Vasopressin and oxytocin receptors in the rat brain. Handbook Chem Neuroanat 11:289–320, 1992.

140. Barberis C, Tribollet E: Vasopressin and oxytocin receptors in the central nervous system. Crit Rev Neurobiol 10:119–154, 1996.

141. Caldwell JD, Prange AJJ, Pedersen CA: Oxytocin facilitates the sexual receptivity of estrogen-treated female rats. Neuropeptides 7:175–189, 1986.

142. Anderson-Hunt M, Dennerstein L: Increased female sexual response after oxytocin. Br Med J 309:929, 1994.

143. McCarthy MM, Kleopoulos SP, Mobbs CV, et al: Infusion of antisense oligodeoxynucleotides to the oxytocin receptor in the ventromedial hypothalamus reduces estrogen-induced sexual receptivity and oxytocin receptor binding in the female rat. Neuroendocrinology 59:432–440, 1994.

144. Caldwell JD, Barakat AS, Smith DD, et al: A uterotonic antagonist blocks the oxytocin-induced facilitation of female sexual receptivity. Brain Res 512:291–296, 1990.

145. McCarthy MM, Kow L-M, Pfaff DW: Speculations concerning the physiological significance of central oxytocin in maternal behavior. Ann N Y Acad Sci 652:70–82, 1992.

146. Pedersen CA, Caldwell JD, Johnson MF, et al: Oxytocin antiserum delays onset of ovarian steroid-induced maternal behavior. Neuropeptides 6:175–182, 1985.

147. Insel TR, Hulihan TJ: A gender-specific mechanism for pair bonding—oxytocin and partner preference formation in monogamous voles. Behav Neurosci 109:782–789, 1995.

148. McCarthy MM, McDonald CH, Brooks PJ, et al: An anxiolytic action of oxytocin is enhanced by estrogen in the mouse. Physiol Behav 60:1209–1215, 1996.

149. Uvnas-Moberg K, Ahlenius S, Hillegaart V, et al: High doses of oxytocin cause sedation and low doses cause an anxiolytic-like effect in male rats. Pharmacol Biochem Behav 49:101–106, 1994.

150. Engelmann M, Ebner K, Wotjak CT, et al: Endogenous oxytocin is involved in short-term olfactory memory in female rats. Behav Brain Res 90:89–94, 1998.

151. Boccia MM, Kopf SR, Baratti CM: Effects of a single administration of oxytocin or vasopressin and their interactions with two selective receptor antagonists on memory storage in mice. Neurobiol Learn Mem 69:136–146, 1998.

152. DeVries AC, Young WS III, Nelson RJ: Reduced aggressive behaviour in mice with targeted disruption of the oxytocin gene. J Neuroendocrinol 9:363–368, 1997.

153. Winslow JT, Young LJ, Hearn E, et al: Phenotypic expression of an oxytocin peptide null mutation in mice. Adv Exp Med Biol 449:241–243, 1998.

154. Murphy MR, Seckl JR, Burton S, et al: Changes in oxytocin and vasopressin secretion during sexual activity in men. J Clin Endocrinol Metab 65:738–741, 1987.

155. Einspanier A, Ivell R: Oxytocin and oxytocin receptor expression in reproductive tissues of the male marmoset monkey. Biol Reprod 56:416–422, 1997.

156. Nicholson HD, Jenkin L: Oxytocin and prostatic function. Adv Exp Med Biol 395:529–538, 1995.

157. Maggi M, Malozowski S, Kassis S, et al: Identification and characterization of two classes of receptors for oxytocin and vasopressin in porcine tunica albuginea, epididymis, and vas deferens. Endocrinology 120:986–994, 1987.

158. Argiolas A: Oxytocin-induced penile erection: Pharmacology, site and mechanisms of action. Ann N Y Acad Sci 652:194–203, 1992.

159. Argiolas A, Melis MR: Oxytocin-induced penile erection. Adv Exp Med Biol 395:247–254, 1995.

160. Schlosser SF, Almeida OFX, Patchev VK, et al: Oxytocin-stimulated release of adrenocorticotropin from the rat pituitary is mediated by arginine vasopressin receptors of the V1b type. Endocrinology 135:2058–2063, 1994.

161. Chiodera P, Volpi R, Capretti L, et al: Oxytocin enhances the prolactin response to vasoactive intestinal polypeptide in healthy women. Fertil Steril 70:541–543, 1998.

162. Coiro V, Gnudi A, Volpi R, et al: Oxytocin enhances thyrotropin-releasing hormone–induced prolactin release in normal menstruating women. Fertil Steril 47:565–569, 1987.

163. Hull ML, Reid RA, Evans JJ, et al: Pre-ovulatory oxytocin administration promotes the onset of the luteinizing hormone surge in human females. Hum Reprod 10:2266–2269, 1995.

164. Evans JJ, Forrest-Owen W, McArdle CA: Oxytocin receptor-mediated activation of phosphoinositidase C and elevation of cytosolic calcium in the gonadotrope-derived alphaT3-1 cell line. Endocrinology 138:2049–2055, 1997.

165. Brimble MJ, Balment RJ, Smith CP, et al: Influence of oxytocin on sodium excretion in the anaesthetized Brattleboro rat. J Endocrinol 129:49–54, 1991.

166. Verbalis JG, Mangione MP, Stricker EM: Oxytocin produces natriuresis in rats at physiological plasma concentration. Endocrinology 128:1317–1322, 1991.

167. Stoeckel ME, Freund-Mercier MJ: Autoradiographic demonstration of oxytocin binding sites in the macula densa. Am J Physiol 257:F310–314, 1989.

168. Ostrowski NL, Young WS, Lolait SJ: Estrogen increases renal oxytocin receptor gene expression. Endocrinology 136:1801–1804, 1995.

169. Martens H, Robert F, Legros JJ, et al: Expression of functional neurohypophysial peptides receptors by murine immature and cytotoxic T-cell lines. Prog Neuroendocrin Immunol 5:31–39, 1992.

170. Martens H, Kecha O, Charlet-Renard C, et al: Phosphorylation of proteins induced in a murine pre-T cell line by neurohypophysial peptides. Adv Exp Med Biol 449:247–249, 1998.

171. Jankowski M, Hajjar F, Kawas SA, et al: Rat heart—a site of oxytocin production and action. Proc Natl Acad Sci USA 95:14558–14563, 1998.

172. Ito Y, Kobayashi T, Kimura T, et al: Investigation of the oxytocin receptor expression in human breast cancer tissue using newly established monoclonal antibodies. Endocrinology 137:773–779, 1996.

173. Sapino A, Cassoni P, Stella A, et al: Oxytocin receptor within the breast: Biological function and distribution. Anticancer Res 18:2181–2186, 1998.

174. Lee KH, Khan-Dawood FS, Dawood MY: Oxytocin receptor and its messenger ribonucleic acid in human leiomyoma and myometrium. Am J Obstet Gynecol 179:620–627, 1998.

175. Cassoni P, Sapino A, Stella A, et al: Presence and significance of oxytocin receptors in human neuroblastomas and glial tumors. Int J Cancer 77:695–700, 1998.

176. Cassoni P, Sapino A, Fortunati N, et al: Oxytocin inhibits the proliferation of MDA-MB231 human breast-cancer cells via cyclic adenosine monophosphate and protein kinase A. Int J Cancer 72:340–344, 1997.

177. Cassoni P, Sapino A, Stella A, et al: Antiproliferative effect of oxytocin through specific oxytocin receptors in human neuroblastoma and astrocytoma cell lines. Adv Exp Med Biol 449:245–246, 1998.

178. Fuchs AR, Fuchs F, Husslein P, et al: Oxytocin receptors and human parturition: A dual role for oxytocin in the initiation of labor. Science 215:1396–1398, 1982.

179. Insel TR, Young L, Wang Z: Central oxytocin and reproductive behaviours. Rev Reprod 2:28–37, 1997.

180. Jo Y-H, Stoeckel M-E, Freund-Mercier M-J, et al: Oxytocin modulates glutamatergic synaptic transmission between cultured neonatal spinal cord dorsal horn neurons. J Neurosci 18:2377–2386, 1998.

181. Teitelbaum I: Vasopressin-stimulated phosphoinositide hydrolysis in cultured rat inner medullary collecting duct cells is mediated by the oxytocin receptor. J Clin Invest 87:2122–2126, 1991.

182. Hinko A, Soloff MS: Up-regulation of oxytocin receptors in rabbit amnion by adenosine 3′,5′-monophosphate. Endocrinology 132:126–132, 1993.

183. Frayne J, Nicholson HD: Localization of oxytocin receptors in the human and macaque monkey male reproductive tracts: Evidence for a physiological role of oxytocin in the male. Mol Hum Reprod 4:527–532, 1998.

Chapter 15

▼▼▼
Prolactin

Nelson D. Horseman

Prolactin (PRL) was the first of the pituitary hormones to be biochemically identified and purified,[1,2] and hyperprolactinemia caused by hormone-secreting tumors is the most common human pituitary disease. Only recently, however, have the physiology and biochemistry of prolactin actions yielded to contemporary analytic methods to reveal a biology that is at once elegantly simple, and sublimely complex. PRL has been identified in the pituitary glands of members of all vertebrate classes, and it has diverse effects on osmoregulation, metabolism, reproduction, metamorphosis, migratory behavior, parental behavior, and lactation.[3–6] In most species, and especially in mammals, PRL has a specialized role in the postmating phase of reproduction. The predominant mammalian actions of PRL are stimulation of lactation and maternal behavior, and inhibition of reproductive function. Associated with the specialization of PRL in mammals, novel genes that encode placentally derived lactogens have evolved. PRL does not perform any indispensable function for the life of the individual, but gestation and lactation lie at the core of the mammalian life cycle, and they place extreme demands on physiology. Adaptations in the control of PRL secretion and its physiologic actions have, therefore, been integral to the biology of all mammals, and abnormalities of PRL secretion are a relatively common cause of endocrine disease. Prolactin receptors (PRL-Rs) are closely related to those for growth hormone (GH) and a wide variety of hematopoietic cytokines. Each of these receptors transduces intracellular signals by causing the activation of one or more protein tyrosine kinases, which, in turn, phosphorylate latent transcription factors, leading to gene activation. A conserved family of transcription factors, called "STAT" (signal transducer and activation of transcription) proteins, which are activated as a consequence of hormone binding, are specialized mediators of hormone action.[7,8] The deepening understanding of PRL actions on both physiologic and molecular levels has facilitated improved therapeutic approaches to diseases of PRL secretion, and opened opportunities to use the physiology of PRL and lactation in new ways.

THE EVOLUTIONARY BIOLOGY OF PROLACTIN

It has long been recognized that PRL and GH are related at the primary amino acid sequence level.[9] PRL has been identified in all of the vertebrate classes, and it has been inferred that the PRL and GH genes arose from a duplication of an ancestral gene at least 400 million years ago, at about the time of the origin of vertebrates.[10] Deeper relationships with other hormones are less certain, but erythropoietin shares substantial primary sequence similarity, as well as three-dimensional structural features with PRL and GH, suggesting that all three of these hormones share an ancient common ancestry. In addition to PRL and GH, which have been conserved in all vertebrate lineages, a wide variety of derivative genes have appeared in specific vertebrate

groups by duplication of either the PRL or GH gene. The most familiar of these are the various mammalian placental lactogens (PLs).[11,12]

Placental Lactogens

PLs are synthesized during pregnancy in most, but not all, eutherian mammals. Species which apparently do not produce any placental lactogens are distributed among many mammalian families, and include familiar species such as pigs, horses, and dogs.[13] Primates (including humans) synthesize a PL that is encoded by a gene duplicated within the GH locus.[10] The GH locus in humans encompasses five genes spanning a region of about 50 kb on the long arm (q22-24) of chromosome 17. This locus includes two PL, or, preferably, chorionic somatomammotropin (CS) genes (*hCS-A* and *hCS-B*). The *CS-A* and *CS-B* genes, though slightly divergent at the nucleotide sequence level, encode identical proteins, and the genes are coexpressed in the placenta during gestation. In nonprimates (e.g., rodents, ruminants) the PLs have descended evolutionarily from duplications of the PRL gene.[10] Multiple PL genes, and nonlactogenic PRL-like genes, have evolved from PRL. In mice, placental lactogen-I (PL-I) is synthesized early during gestation, appearing immediately post implantation. PL-I expression is extinguished at about midgestation and replaced by predominant secretion of PL-II. Both of the mouse PL genes are synthesized in trophoblast giant cells. In species that synthesize PLs, including humans, the major stimulus to mammary gland development during pregnancy is presumably from PLs, rather than pituitary PRL. PL levels generally rise in correlation with placental growth, and their secretion is controlled by both positive and negative regulators.[14] The loss of PLs and placental steroids at parturition is followed by elevation of PRL secretion, and a corresponding shift to pituitary-dominated regulation of mammary gland function during lactation. The importance of this shift is that pituitary PRL is strongly regulated by a suckling-induced neuroendocrine reflex, which allows nursing activity to determine directly the lactational stimulus to the mammary glands.

Nonlactogenic Prolactin Relatives

Nonlactogenic members of the PRL gene family are synthesized by the placenta. Although the physiologic activities of these PRL-related proteins have not yet been established, the expression patterns for some of these proteins are tightly regulated during gestation,[12] and this has been interpreted to indicate that the proteins are functionally important. In mice and rats there are at least five nonlactogenic PRL-like proteins (PLP-A through PLP-E). In addition, mice synthesize two proteins, named proliferin and proliferin-related protein, which have been proposed to act as regulators of angiogenesis.[15] Nonlactogenic PRL-like protein genes have also been extensively characterized in cattle.[16] One curious feature of the PRL-like gene family is the apparently rapid evolutionary divergence of members of this family. These proteins generally share less than 25% sequence identity with PRL, but all share two pairs of cysteine residues that are conserved throughout the PRL and GH superfamily.[12] Information regarding receptors for the nonlactogenic PRL-related proteins is scant. Proliferin binds to the mannose-6-phosphate–insulin-like growth factor-2 (IGF-2) receptor.[17]

THE BIOCHEMISTRY OF PROLACTIN

Human PRL is synthesized as a prehormone that is encoded by a messenger RNA (mRNA) with an open reading frame of 684 bases. The native gene for PRL is divided into five exons and the initiation site for translation is in exon 1[18] (Fig. 15–1). Preprolactin (pre-PRL) is 227 amino acids in length, with a deduced molecular weight of nearly 26,000. Cleaving the signal peptide from the N-terminus of pre-PRL results in a mature polypeptide that is 199 residues in length, and has a molecular weight of nearly 23,000 (23k PRL). Based on the fact that the bacterially synthesized recombinant 23k PRL monomer binds to the PRL-R and transduces functional signals, it is clear that no additional modifications are essential for the core functions of PRL. PRL folds itself into a tertiary structure that includes three intrachain disulfide bridges, two of which are conserved in all members of the PRL-GH family, and one, linking residues 4 and 11 in the N-terminus, which is unique to PRL and its closest relatives.[9] Four α-helical domains in PRL are arranged so that helixes 1 and 2 run antiparallel to helixes 3 and 4. The general molecular architecture of PRL is not only conserved with GH and other homologous proteins but also has evolved independently in several families of cytokines.[7] The convergent evolution of hormone and cytokine ligand architecture has apparently been driven by the properties of receptors that bind these hormones and transduce signals to the intracellular space.

A variety of biochemical variants of 23k PRL, which appear to have altered functions, have been identified. PRL has a tendency to aggregate and form intermolecular disulfide bridges spontaneously when in solution at high concentrations. High-molecular-weight variants (sometimes referred to as "big" PRLs) may arise by virtue of multimerization, glycosylation, or cross-linking with other proteins. Only a small fraction of human PRL is glycosylated, whereas in some other species, such as swine, glycosylated PRL represents a large portion of both pituitary and plasma hormone.[19] Glycosylation may alter the relative potency of PRL by either changing its receptor binding characteristics or by modifying its pharmacokinetic properties in the animal (plasma half-life, partitioning between plasma and interstitial compartments, etc.). PRL is metabolized by tissue uptake, and by proteolysis in the circulation or in cells. Proteolysis also produces a 16-kDa PRL fragment that has been proposed to have antiangiogenic bioactivity.[20]

Phosphorylated PRL has reduced potency in standard bioassays, and it antagonizes the actions of the predominant unphosphorylated form.[21] Actions of kinases or phosphatases in either the pituitary or individual target tissues may have an important effect on the bioactivity of PRL in vivo.

THE ONTOGENY, PHYSIOLOGY, AND PATHOLOGY OF PROLACTIN SECRETION

Development of the Pituitary Gland

PRL is synthesized by lactotrophs, which are acidophilic cells that represent 20% to 50% of the anterior pituitary cell population. The lactotrophs are the last of the pituitary cell types to fully differentiate, and, coincidentally, the most likely to give rise to pituitary adenomas. Pituitary PRL mRNA synthesis begins at 12 weeks in human gestation, and is preceded by GH synthesis by at least 4 weeks.[10, 22] In rodents the pattern is similar, with the GH gene being expressed several days before PRL, and dual-functioning somatolactotrophs being observed before fully differentiated lactotrophs.[23] The control of pituitary development and lactotroph differentiation depends on the orchestrated expression of a series of intrinsic, tissue-specific regulatory molecules that act as "molecular switches" to induce the sequence of developmental changes leading up to full pituitary differentiation. Many of the intrinsic factors that have been implicated in pituitary development

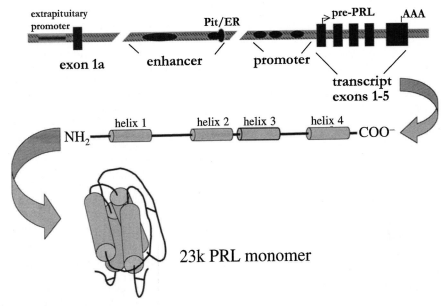

FIGURE 15–1. Biosynthesis of prolactin (PRL). The PRL gene is depicted at the top of the Figure as consisting of five exons (black rectangles) encoding the structural gene for preprolactin (pre-PRL). The translation start site in exon 1 is marked by an *arrow* and the polyadenylation site in exon 5 is marked AAA. The region labeled promoter includes multiple binding sites for the pituitary-specific transcription factor-1 (Pit-1, black ellipses), but only three are depicted in the diagram. The line that depicts the DNA sequence is broken by two interruptions to indicate that the upstream regulatory regions are separated from the promoter by several thousand base pairs. A distal regulatory region (enhancer) includes binding sites for Pit-1 and other factors, including a complex site that binds both Pit-1 and the estrogen receptor (Pit/ER). Exon 1a is transcribed in extrapituitary tissues, and is controlled by a distinct "extrapituitary promoter." After transcription and translation the PRL protein consists of four α-helical regions, that are labeled helix 1 through 4, and intervening β-strand regions. The protein spontaneously folds into a globular structure in which three disulfide bridges connect β-strand regions, and this mature structure is depicted as the 23k PRL monomer.

are evolutionarily related to "homeotic mutation" genes, which were first identified by their dramatic effects on development in fruit flies.[22] Some genetic diseases of the pituitary, pituitary tumors, and physiologic states of hormone deficiency or excess can be attributed to dysfunctions of these regulatory molecules.

The homeobox transcription factors are a diverse class of developmental regulatory proteins that share sequence similarities in their DNA binding regions, and are sequentially activated during organogenesis. Two pituitary homeobox proteins (Ptx1 and Ptx2) are expressed in multiple anterior (head and face) tissues prior to the development of Rathke's pouch, and continue to be expressed in some differentiated pituitary cells. Rathke's pouch homeobox protein (Rpx) is expressed first in neural structures associated with the head region, and then in Rathke's pouch. During the formation of Rathke's pouch a subgroup of LIM-related homeobox proteins are synthesized (P-LIM, Lhx3, and Lhx4), and these genes continue to be expressed in specific regions of the pituitary throughout life. Properly timed extinction of expression is, for certain genes, as important during development as is their appropriate induction. Rpx must be turned off after Rathke's pouch has been formed so that genes specific to later stages of pituitary differentiation can be turned on. The transcription factor that downregulates Rpx expression is PROP-1 (Prophet of Pit-1). PROP-1 turns off Rpx and turns on Pit-1, leading to differentiation of some of the hormone-producing cells of the pituitary gland, including lactotrophs.[24]

Pit-1 is essential for differentiation of both PRL- and GH-secreting cells, hence its alternative name, GH factor-1 (GHF-1).[25] An early-developing subpopulation of thyrotrophs is also dependent on Pit-1. The Pit-1 protein shares close sequence similarity with two other transcription factors within regions referred to as the POU (*Pit*, *Oct*, *Unc*)-specific domain, and the POU-homeo domain.[26] Pit-1 expression in the developing pituitary gland precedes the synthesis of hormones, and is necessary for the expression of GH, PRL, and thyroid-stimulating hormone (TSH) in fetal pituitaries. Variant forms of Pit-1 are encoded by alternatively spliced mRNAs, and may differentially control expression of individual hormones. Pit-1 binds not only to DNA sequences in the GH, PRL, and TSH genes but also to autoregulatory sites in the Pit-1 promoter. Autoactivation of Pit-1 transcription is one means of preserving phenotypic stability in differentiated pituitary cells. The factors that act after Pit-1 to drive the differentiation of lactotrophs from somatotroph progenitors are not known. Estrogen receptors synergize with Pit-1 to induce PRL, but not GH, gene expression. Estrogen may, therefore, be one of the factors that drives the ultimate differentiation of lactotrophs.[27–30]

Estrogen is one of several extrinsic factors that are apparently involved in lactotroph differentiation. Estrogen is an important positive effector of lactotroph function over the long term. Lactotrophs are greater in number, and contain more PRL per cell in females during their reproductive years. Estrogen acts directly on lactotrophs, as well as indirectly through the hypothalamus, posterior pituitary, and anterior pituitary, to stimulate PRL synthesis and secretion. Estrogen-induced galanin secretion is an important mediator of estrogen actions on lactotrophs.[31] Basic fibroblast growth factor (B-FGF or FGF-2) has a specific positive stimulatory effect on lactotrophs. Likewise, epidermal growth factor (EGF) stimulates lactotrophs, and may act as an extrinsic developmental regulatory factor, as well as a physiologic stimulator of PRL secretion.[32, 33] As will be presented in subsequent sections, the same factors that drive vectorial differentiation of pituitary cells can participate in regulating the tides of hormone biosynthesis that change on a physiologic time scale, and in disorders of hormone secretion.

Regulation of Pituitary Prolactin Synthesis and Secretion

In mammals PRL secretion is normally restrained by the action of dopamine (DA), which is secreted from the hypothalamus.[34] While the levels of other pituitary hormones are influenced by inhibitory secretagogues such as somatostatin, PRL is the only such hormone that is secreted at unrestrained high levels when completely isolated from the positive trophic influences of the hypothalamus. This uncon-

ventional situation is unique to mammals. The control of PRL secretion in birds and other nonmammals is more conventional in the sense that positively acting secretagogues are the predominant regulators of PRL secretion.[35, 36] Lactotrophs are similar to neurons in that they display spontaneous action potentials, and their resting membrane potential is influenced by neurotransmitters and peptide neuromodulators.

The normal secretory pattern of PRL is a series of daily pulses, occurring every 2 to 3 hours, which vary in amplitude so that the bulk of the hormone is secreted during rapid eye movement (REM) sleep. In the human REM sleep occurs mostly during the latter half of the sleep phase, so highest levels of PRL generally occur during the night.[37] In nocturnal rodents the pattern is reversed, so that PRL secretion occurs during the daytime, which is the inactive phase. REM sleep is the dominant organizer in men and nonparous women. It is unclear how REM and PRL secretion are linked. Infusion of PRL increases REM activity in the electroencephalogram (EEG),[38, 39] suggesting some causal relationship, which is likely to be very indirect. In lactating women the reflex elevation of PRL and oxytocin secretion caused by nipple stimulation during nursing is the dominant controller. To date, the precise pathway(s) that accounts for the nursing stimulus for PRL has not been worked out, and the relative importance of PRL-releasing (PRF) and PRL-inhibiting factors during the nursing stimulus remains controversial.

Dopamine

The primary PRL-regulating DA neurons are the tuberoinfundibular dopaminergic (TIDA) cells, which have their cell bodies in the arcuate nucleus of the hypothalamus, and they release DA in the median eminence and pituitary stalk (Fig. 15–2). A secondary tuberohypophysial dopaminergic (THDA) system has cell bodies in the rostral caudate and paraventricular nuclei, and these release DA in the posterior pituitary. The THDA neurons may play a secondary role in PRL regulation, but the primary system for inhibiting PRL secretion is the TIDA pathway.[34] The only isoform of DA receptor on lactotrophs is the type 2(D$_2$) receptor, and these receptors mediate the direct inhibitory action on PRL secretion and synthesis. Targeted disruption of the D$_2$ receptor of mice leads to a phenotype of PRL hypersecretion and lactotroph proliferation.[40]

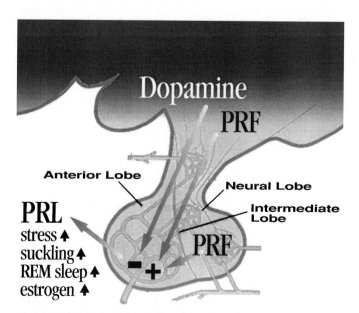

FIGURE 15–2. *Control of pituitary secretion of prolactin (PRL). Dopamine from the hypothalamus is the predominant inhibitory regulator of pituitary PRL secretion. Multiple factors act as PRL-releasing factors (PRF; see text), and these come from both the hypothalamus and the posterior pituitary. Physiologic states that stimulate PRL release are listed on the figure. REM, rapid eye movement.*

DA is synthesized by a two-step reaction in which tyrosine conversion to levodopa is catalyzed by tyrosine hydroxylase, and levodopa is converted to DA by the action of dopa decarboxylase. As is the case for catecholamine synthesis in other cells, the momentary rate of DA synthesis in the TIDA neurons is determined by the activity of tyrosine hydroxylase. The negative feedback mechanism for controlling PRL release is to increase tyrosine hydroxylase activity in the TIDA neurons, thereby increasing the amount of DA available for release from the median eminence. PRL may act by a short-loop feedback mechanism, being transported directly to the hypothalamus from the pituitary, or systemic PRL may enter the cerebrospinal fluid via the choroid plexus, which has high levels of a short isoform of the PRL-R. Systemically derived PRL then acts as a long-loop feedback regulator of DA synthesis. Isolated PRL deficiency resulting from targeted gene disruption in the mouse results in decreased DA in the median eminence, but does not affect DA levels in other regions of the hypothalamus.[41]

D_2 receptor activation in lactotrophs has at least two main actions that result in inhibition of PRL. D_2 receptors are members of the heptahelical G protein–coupled receptor superfamily, and they activate the α_i subunits, which leads to inhibition of cyclic adenosine monophosphate (cAMP) synthesis.[34] In addition, D_2 receptors activate a G protein–coupled, inwardly rectifying potassium channel (GIRK), which instantaneously causes hyperpolarization of the lactotroph membrane and closes voltage-gated calcium channels.[42] Cytoplasmic calcium levels fall because of decreased influx of extracellular calcium, and decreased release of calcium from intracellular stores. The reduction of cytosolic free calcium decreases the exocytosis of secretory vesicles.

cAMP inhibition by DA apparently influences PRL secretion through two mechanisms. First, inhibition of cAMP by DA opposes the actions of stimulatory factors such as vasoactive intestinal peptide (VIP), which acts via a positive effect on cAMP. This action decreases PRL release in the short to intermediate term. Second, because cAMP is mitogenic in lactotrophs, as well as other pituitary cells, activation of G_i signaling by DA is antimitogenic. Lactotroph proliferation is important for physiologic elevation of PRL release during lactation. The proliferative action of cAMP on lactotrophs is understood to be an important promoter of pituitary tumor growth, thereby contributing to pathologic hyperprolactinemia.[24]

Local pituitary peptides, as well as hypothalamic DA, can inhibit PRL secretion. Endothelin-1 is produced by lactotrophs and inhibits PRL secretion and transforming growth factor-β1 can act as a paracrine inhibitor of PRL.[43, 44] Calcitonin has also been shown to inhibit PRL secretion, and may be secreted from the hypothalamus.[45] The biologic significance of these factors in pituitary development and physiology is not yet established.

Prolactin-Releasing Factors

A wide variety of stimulatory PRL secretagogues have been identified over the years, and it is likely that additional PRFs will be identified in the future. The known stimulators of PRL secretion include steroids (estrogen[46]), hypothalamic peptides (thyrotropin-releasing hormone [TRH], VIP, and oxytocin[47, 48]), and growth factors such as EGF[49] and FGF-2.[50]

TRH is a potent and rapid stimulator of PRL release via a set of calcium-mediated pathways. However, physiologic states in which TRH is elevated, such as primary hypothyroidism, do not lead consistently to hyperprolactinemia, so it is unlikely that TRH has a primary role in stimulating PRL release in vivo. VIP acts through cAMP to stimulate PRL synthesis and release on an intermediate to long-term basis. The importance of VIP as a positive lactotrophic factor is supported by two types of evidence. Using antibodies against VIP the secretion of PRL can be inhibited to a very low level.[34] In addition, VIP appears to be the primary PRF in birds,[51, 52] suggesting that this positive mechanism may have been in place before the evolution of the dopaminergic inhibitory system in mammals. Oxytocin secretion is tightly coupled with PRL secretion during lactation, and both are secreted in response to nipple stimulation. The potential role of oxyto-

cin as a PRF, given that it can reach the anterior pituitary through the short portal system, has remained controversial. Oxytocin antagonism partially suppresses PRL secretion,[34] so this peptide is likely to provide some portion of the physiologic stimulus for PRL release. Pituitary adenylate cyclase activating protein (PACAP) stimulates PRL synthesis and release. Galanin is synthesized in both the pituitary and the hypothalamus. In the pituitary it colocalizes with PRL in lactotroph secretory granules, and acts by autocrine and paracrine mechanisms to stimulate lactotrophs.[31, 48]

There is physiologic evidence of a PRF that is synthesized in and secreted from the intermediate lobe of the pituitary.[34] However, biochemical identification of this factor has not yet been possible. A putative PRL-releasing peptide (PrRP) from the hypothalamus was identified by searching for ligands that activate an orphan pituitary G protein–coupled receptor. The mature peptide that was identified from bovine hypothalamus is a 20–amino acid molecule that caused rapid secretion of PRL from isolated pituitary cells. While this novel peptide might fulfill the criteria for a physiologic PRF, further evaluation of its functions will be necessary before the identity of this putative factor is confirmed.[53] Antagonists of serotonin or opioid receptors inhibit PRL secretion under physiologically meaningful stimuli. Conversely, antidepressants that inhibit serotonin reuptake (fluoxetine [Prozac], etc.) increase PRL secretion in humans and laboratory animals. Serotonin and opioids are important indirect regulators of PRL by virtue of their actions on DA and releasing factor secretion in the hypothalamus.

Lactotrophs display a large degree of functional heterogeneity within the anterior pituitary. This heterogeneity is manifested in differences of morphology (i.e., secretory granule size and density), basal hormone release, electrical activity, and response to releasing and inhibiting factors. Assay of hormone release from single cells has revealed not only substantial cell-to-cell variations in function but also marked temporal variations in a single cell.[54]

Transcription regulators that control the development of the anterior pituitary lactotrophs also participate in controlling PRL synthesis during adult life. Prominent among these factors is the Pit-1 protein. Pit-1 binds to two regions of the human PRL gene, the proximal promoter (within 250 bp of the transcription start) and a distal enhancer (beyond −1300 bp) (see Fig. 15–1). There are multiple Pit-1 binding sites in each of these regions. Transcription regulators such as cAMP and estrogen receptors can control PRL gene expression by influencing Pit-1 activity.[27, 46]

PATHOPHYSIOLOGY OF PROLACTIN SECRETION

Normal plasma PRL concentrations in women who are neither pregnant nor lactating range from 4 to less than 20 ng/mL. In men the values are, on average, several units lower. Late pregnancy and lactational levels are normally in the range of 100 to 200 ng/mL, with the highest levels that occur following active bouts of nursing. PRL is normally measured by radioimmunoassay (RIA). Although glycosylation and other chemical modifications of PRL can affect its immunoreactivity, and therefore lead to aberrant RIA results,[19] pathologic levels are generally readily detected by RIA. The original method for bioassay of PRL was by measuring the growth of the pigeon crop sac mucosal epithelium.[55] This method is still occasionally used, and is the basis of the international standardization of PRL bioactivity. However, the method has largely been supplanted by a simpler bioassay that takes advantage of the ability of PRL to stimulate the growth of Nb2 lymphoma cells in culture.[56]

Prolactin Deficiency

When PRL deficiency occurs it is normally one component of a combined pituitary hormone deficiency. However, a few cases of PRL deficiency without evidence of other pituitary defects have been reported in women. Isolated PRL deficiency resulted in lactational failure and reproductive difficulty, but no other obvious problems.[57, 58]

No cases of isolated PRL deficiency have been reported in men. These results in a few humans are consistent with the phenotype of mice in which the PRL gene has been disrupted by a targeted mutation. In the case of mice the mammary gland development was defective and the females failed to reproduce, but the males did not have any symptoms that would be overt.[41, 59] The concordance of these results from humans and mice is remarkable, given the well-known differences between PRL physiology in humans and rodents. In particular, humans secrete a lactogenic GH as well as PRL, and the rodent corpus luteum requires PRL, but the human does not. The difference in luteal control probably explains why the women who reportedly had PRL deficiency were merely subfertile, whereas mouse females were completely infertile.

Mice with a targeted mutation of the PRL gene develop pituitary hyperplasia[41] and adenomas (unpublished observation). The loss of PRL decreases hypothalamic DA, and the deficiency of DA presumably leads to unrestrained pituitary growth. It is possible that some "nonfunctional" pituitary adenomas in humans arise by virtue of mutations in the PRL gene, although there is currently no direct evidence of this. Some forms of combined pituitary hormone deficiency have been identified in which PRL, GH, and TSH are hyposecreted as a consequence of mutations in important developmental factors. Familial inheritance of defects in either the Pit-1 gene or PROP-1 results in individuals who fail to develop lactotrophs, somatotrophs, and thyrotrophs, and consequently are dwarfed and hypothyroid, as well as PRL-deficient. Two spontaneous mutations that cause dwarfism in mice have been shown to correspond to these human conditions. In Snell dwarf mice there is a mutation of the Pit-1 gene, and in Ames dwarfs the PROP-1 gene is mutated.[24, 60, 61]

Hyperprolactinemia

Hypersecretion of PRL is among the most common of pituitary disorders (see Chapter 25). Medications that elevate PRL secretion, and may cause hyperprolactinemia, include commonly used antiemetics, antidepressants, and narcotics. These medications alter PRL secretion by antagonizing DA action, or by elevating serotonin or endorphin bioactivity. Reserpine and methyldopa increase PRL secretion due to DA depletion. DA receptor antagonists, such as haloperidol and phenylthiazines, increase PRL secretion. Serotonin reuptake inhibitors, such as fluoxetine, elevate serum PRL.[34] It is uncommon for any of these medications to cause clinical signs of hyperprolactinemia because the levels of PRL seldom reach more than 30 to 50 ng/mL with these drugs. One could imagine that there might be subtle hormonal effects after long-term treatments.

Hyperprolactinemia that manifests clinical symptoms is most commonly a consequence of a lactotroph adenoma (see Chapter 25). These tumors may secrete high levels of PRL alone, or both PRL and GH. Any intracranial mass or trauma that causes compression or disruption of the pituitary stalk can cause hyperprolactinemia due to the loss of dopaminergic tone from the hypothalamus. Pituitary adenomas have been discovered to be much more common than once believed, with more than 20% of individuals harboring tumors of at least 3 mm at autopsy.[24] Tumors that do not hypersecrete hormones are usually of gonadotroph or lactotroph origin. Some symptoms of prolactinomas may be caused by tumor mass effects. These include visual field defects, associated with pressure on the medial aspect of the optic chiasm, and alterations in temperature regulation, feeding patterns, or other effects secondary to hypothalamic compression. However, effects associated with the physiologic actions of the hormone are the more common presenting symptoms.

Galactorrhea (breast milk secretion in an individual who is not postpartum) and amenorrhea are the result of PRL actions directly on the breast and hypothalamus-pituitary-ovarian axis. In men, galactorrhea and impotence are the most common presenting symptoms of a hypersecreting prolactinoma. The causes of impotence in hyperprolactinemia, whether hormonal or neurogenic, are unclear. Hyperprolactinemia is treated medically by administration of DA agonists, including bromocriptine and cabergoline, or surgically by resection of the tumor tissue.

Nonpituitary Prolactin

Many mammalian tissues, including the human mammary gland, brain, and uterine decidua, express the PRL gene (Fig. 15–3). Adding to the potential plasticity of the PRL regulatory system, various tissues alternatively process PRL in a variety of ways. PRL is synthesized by both the decidua and the uterine myometrium in humans.[62] High concentrations of PRL are present in the amniotic fluid, and this can be traced to both decidually synthesized hormone and plasma PRL that is translocated across the placenta into the amniotic fluid. The synthesis of human PRL in extrapituitary sites is controlled by a promoter that is distinct from the pituitary PRL promoter. Human extrapituitary PRL mRNA has a distinct 5′ untranslated (UTR) sequence corresponding to an additional exon (exon 1A)[63] (see Fig. 15–1). Exon 1A and the promoter elements associated with it are located about 8000 bp distal to the initiation site for pituitary PRL transcription. The factors that control extrapituitary PRL synthesis and secretion are not the same as those that control pituitary PRL. In the decidua, progesterone is an important regulator of PRL secretion. Unlike the pituitary, where cAMP inhibits PRL transcription, in the decidua cAMP is stimulatory.[62] In rodents the evidence for a distinct extrapituitary PRL promoter is less certain than in the human. It is conceivable that rodents use other mechanisms, such as growth factors that control the conventional pituitary PRL promoter, to provide for regulation of PRL synthesis in extrapituitary tissues. The mammary gland is an important site of PRL synthesis and secretion. PRL is present in significant concentrations in milk, and milk PRL is absorbed by the neonatal gut and causes changes in the maturation of the hypothalamic neuroendocrine system.[64] Pituitary PRL is transported

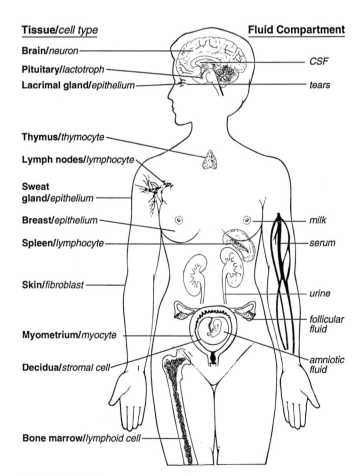

Tissue/*cell type*	Fluid Compartment
Brain/*neuron*	
Pituitary/*lactotroph*	*CSF*
Lacrimal gland/*epithelium*	*tears*
Thymus/*thymocyte*	
Lymph nodes/*lymphocyte*	
Sweat gland/*epithelium*	
Breast/*epithelium*	*milk*
Spleen/*lymphocyte*	*serum*
Skin/*fibroblast*	*urine*
	follicular fluid
Myometrium/*myocyte*	*amniotic fluid*
Decidua/*stromal cell*	
Bone marrow/*lymphoid cell*	

FIGURE 15–3. Sources of extrapituitary prolactin in the human. The tissues in which prolactin is synthesized are listed in the left column, and the fluid compartments where prolactin circulates are in the right column. (From Ben-Jonathan N, Merson JL, Allen DL, et al: Extrapituitary prolactin: Distribution, regulation, functions, and clinical aspects. Endocr Rev 17:639, 1997. © The Endocrine Society.)

out of the circulation, across the mammary epithelium, and into the alveolar lumen, and locally synthesized PRL is secreted into milk.[62] To date there are no disease states that have been connected to dysregulation of extrapituitary PRL secretion. The lack of any clear proofs that there are symptoms caused by either hypersecretion of extrapituitary PRL, say from a PRL-secreting ectopic tumor, or from loss of extrapituitary PRL gene expression, makes it difficult to surmise the normal functional roles of extrapituitary PRL in humans. It has been suggested that locally synthesized PRL in the mammary gland might act as a growth factor for both normal breast epithelium and breast cancer cells.[65]

PROLACTIN RECEPTORS AND SIGNAL TRANSDUCTION

Receptors

The PRL-R is a member of the type 1 cytokine receptor family,[66] and its nearest relative is the GH receptor. Several hematopoietic cytokine receptors, such as those for erythropoietin, most interleukins, and granulocyte-macrophage colony-stimulating factor (GM-CSF) are also very similar to PRL and GH receptors. Other receptors, such as those for the interferons, are members of a broader superfamily of proteins that also includes cell adhesion proteins. The features that define the type 1 cytokine receptor family include two signature motifs in the extracellular domain and one in the intracellular domain. Four cysteine residues in the extracellular domain are absolutely conserved among all of the type 1 cytokine receptors, and they form two disulfide bridges that are essential for the proper tertiary folding of the ligand binding domain. A short sequence, which includes a tandem repeat of tryptophan-serine interrupted by a single amino acid (the WSXWS motif), is the second signature motif in the extracellular domain. This sequence is highly conserved near the base of the extracellular domain, but the function of these residues has not yet been proved with any degree of certainty. The structure of the PRL-R extracellular domain, like that of the GH and other cytokine receptors, has been extensively analyzed by x-ray crystallography, as well as by biochemical methods.[67] This domain is comprised of two 100 amino acid subdomains, which are structurally related to the type III repeats of fibronectin. Each of the type III subdomains includes a conserved series of seven β-strands folded into two β-sheets that run in an antiparallel orientation. These type III subdomains are connected by a short, flexible

hinge peptide, and residues that contact the ligand span this connector to include amino acids in each of the type III subdomains.

Across the vertebrate lineages there is substantial conservation of the major features of the PRL-Rs, with some notable exceptions. In birds (pigeons, chickens) the extracellular domain has duplicated and diverged, and in cattle the distal C-terminus has been truncated, eliminating a tyrosine residue that is conserved in other lineages (Fig. 15–4). Neither of these evolutionary changes appears to have functional significance.[68, 69] Within the intracellular region of the PRL-R an 8–amino acid proline-rich motif, referred to as "box 1," is the third conserved signature motif that characterizes type 1 cytokine receptors. These amino acids interact directly with the tyrosine kinases that are activated upon ligand binding to the extracellular domain, and mutations in box 1 completely disable PRL-R signaling.[5] There are multiple PRL-R isoforms that vary in the length and amino acid sequence of the intracellular domain. The long isoform, which has been identified in all species to date, has an intracellular domain that is about 350 amino acids in length. Short isoforms (<100 intracellular residues) have been identified in rodents and several other mammalian species. The short forms of the PRL-R include box 1, but lack other regions of the intracellular domain that are required for signal transduction. In particular, there are conserved tyrosine residues in the distal portion of the long form of the receptor that are phosphorylated after ligand binding, and these tyrosines are required for normal signal transduction.

Mutations of the conserved tyrosines indicate that there is some degree of functional redundancy among these residues, but at least one of the conserved tyrosines must be present to allow normal receptor signal transduction. A mutant PRL-R isoform in rat Nb2 lymphoma cells has a large deletion between box 1 and the distal conserved tyrosines, and this receptor is able to transduce all of the known signaling functions of the long form. Whereas multiple short isoforms of the PRL-R have been discovered in some species (especially rodents), the occurrence of these short isoforms appears not to be universal.[5] The functional significance of the short isoforms is not completely known. Although these could provide for signaling diversity, they may also act as transport molecules. The possibility that the short PRL-R isoforms act as PRL transporters is supported by the observation that the choroid plexus and liver have a preponderance of short-form receptors. The most likely function of the receptors in these tissues is for transporting PRL across membranes.

Ligand binding appears to facilitate dimerization of the PRL-Rs as the first step toward signal transduction. The first evidence favoring receptor dimerization as a physiologically important step in PRL

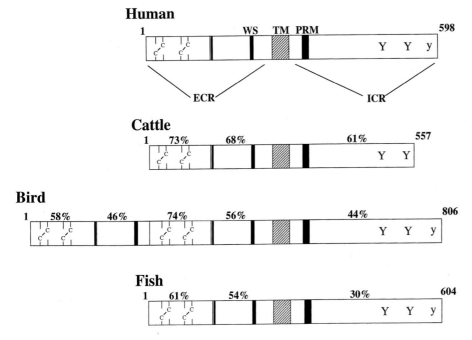

FIGURE 15–4. Prolactin receptor structure and function. Schematic diagram of the linear sequences of representative prolactin receptors. Pertinent structural features are two pairs of cysteines, the flexible hinge (double line), and the WSxWS repeat in the extracellular region (ECR). The transmembrane-spanning sequence (TM) marks the separation between the ECR and the intracellular region (ICR). In the ICR the conserved motifs are the proline rich box-1 motif (PRM), and conserved tyrosine residues. The uppercase Y indicates ubiquitously conserved tyrosines, and the lowercase y is a tyrosine that is conserved in all known species except cattle. The percentage of identical amino acid residues in each region, compared with the human receptor, is labeled above each receptor.

signaling was derived from experiments in which antibodies were used to artificially induce receptor dimerization and consequent signaling in PRL-responsive cells. The results from this creative experimental approach were ultimately proved to be correct when hormone-receptor complexes for human GH and PRL receptors were biochemically and crystallographically mapped.[5, 67, 70, 71] The formation of 1:2 complexes of the hormone with its receptor (Fig. 15–5) appears to be the essential first step in the transmission of the biologic signal within target cells. Transcriptional activation requires homodimerization of the long-form PRL-R. Heterodimers of short and long receptors, or short homodimers, do not mediate normal signal transduction.[72]

The PRL-R gene, which is located on the long arm of human chromosome 5 (p13-14), is comprised of at least 10 coding exons. Multiple transcripts, reflecting alternative splicing variants and transcription start sites, account for some of the variability in PRL-R structure and tissue distribution.[5]

Tyrosine Kinase Activation

JAK2 (Janus Kinase-2) is a protein kinase that is associated with the PRL-R through binding to the 'box 1' motif. Its activation is the first intracellular event in a complex, and incompletely understood, web of interactions that mediate PRL effects within its target cells (Fig. 15–6). JAK2 has been shown to be the essential PRL-regulated protein kinase by both biochemical and genetic experiments,[73, 74] but this kinase is also essential for signaling by other cytokines.[75] Although it is presumed today that JAK2 binds directly to the PRL-R, it remains possible that another protein could mediate this association. This possibility is raised by the observation that JAK2 is associated with unliganded PRL-Rs, whereas in the case of the GH signaling, where JAK2 is also the important receptor-activated kinase, ligand binding is necessary before the kinase can bind to GH receptor. Upon ligand-induced dimerization of PRL-Rs, JAK2 phosphorylates specific tyrosine residues on the receptor intracellular domain, and autophosphorylates residues within the kinase. These phosphotyrosines serve as docking sites for additional signal transduction proteins. The actions of the kinase are counteracted by multiple tyrosine phosphatases, which rapidly dephosphorylate specific proteins, and maintain the steady-state level of tyrosine phosphorylation at a very low level in the absence of hormonal stimulation.

In addition to the STAT-dependent events triggered by JAK2 activation, there are other STAT-independent signaling pathways that can be activated when PRL binds to its receptor, as shown in Figure 15–6. Src-family kinases may be involved in PRL signaling by virtue of their ability to couple to multiple signaling intermediates. Phosphotidylinositol-3'-kinase, mitogen-activated protein kinases (MAPKs), and protein kinase C have each been observed to be activated by PRL in some systems.[5] The tyrosine phosphatase SHP-2 is essential for PRL signaling.[76]

STAT-independent pathways have been proposed for PRL signaling, but the physiologic relevance of such mechanisms is not yet clear. It has been suggested that STAT-independent signaling mediates the mitogenic actions of PRl.[65] This would be consistent with findings in other cytokine signaling systems, where STAT activation determines certain differentiation-related effector functions, whereas other pathways, such as MAPK activation, are involved in mitogenic signal transduction. However, it is unclear whether this analogy can be extended to PRL. In tissues where PRL has a growth-stimulating action, such as mammary gland or pigeon crop sac, it is not established whether the growth stimulus is direct or is mediated by local synthesis of growth factors other than PRL. The rat Nb2 lymphoma cell line, for which PRL acts as a direct mitogen, expresses a mutated form of the PRL-R, which may transduce an unbalanced set of intracellular signals. The role of specific signal transducers in the proliferative response of Nb2 cells has not yet been established.

Transcriptional Regulation

Analysis of PRL-induced genes led, in 1994, to the identification of *cis*-acting elements that bind members of the STAT family of transcription factors.[7, 8] PRL-regulated genes were shown to include conserved DNA motifs in their promoter regions, and these sequences bound to STAT proteins.[77] A novel STAT protein (STAT5) was cloned from lactating sheep mammary glands.[78] Mammals synthesize two STAT5 proteins encoded by closely related genes. Genetic studies, making use of targeted gene disruption in mice, have made it clear that both STAT5a and STAT5b are partially responsible for mediating the primary PRL effects in the ovaries and mammary glands. STAT5a is more important in the mammary glands, whereas STAT5b is more important in the ovaries.[79–81] The mouse genetic studies also have revealed a remarkable degree of concordance of the characteristics of animals that lack genes for either the ligand (PRL), its receptor, or the PRL-regulated STAT5 transcription factors.[82, 83] The concordance among these studies convincingly demonstrates that the known PRL-R and STAT5 proteins are the primary mediators of the physiologic actions of PRL. There are, however, subtle differences among the various animal models that suggest that the STAT5-dependent mechanism may not be the only component of PRL signaling in mammalian cells. STAT5 is phosphorylated by JAK2 on an essential tyrosine residue in its C-terminus.[84] Following its tyrosine phosphorylation, STAT5 dimerizes through interactions between phosphotyrosine and src homology 2 (SH2) domains. Dimeric STAT complexes translocate into the nucleus, where they interact with specific sites in the promoters of PRL-regulated genes, leading to an increase in the rate of transcription of those genes (Fig. 15–7). The exact mechanism by which STAT5 is transported into the nucleus is not known, nor is it known how this inducible transcription factor interacts with the basal transcription machinery during activation of gene expression. There is good evidence that the glucocorticoid receptor (GR) collaborates with STAT5 during milk protein gene induction.[85] This positive interaction depends on occupancy of the GR by its ligand.

STAT activation by PRL is regulated inside the cell by a negative feedback mechanism. CIS (cytokine-inducible SH2 protein), and SOCS (suppressor of cytokine signaling) are members of a class of proteins that are transcriptionally regulated by activated STAT proteins. These proteins feed back on the receptor complex to inhibit the coupling of JAK to either receptor or to STAT.[86]

Whereas STAT5 appears to be the exclusive mediator of the primary physiologic PRL actions in mammals, other STAT proteins, such as STAT1, may be activated in response to PRL in certain pathophysiologic or pharmacologic conditions. In a rat T lymphoma cell line (Nb2) PRL induces the expression of the interferon response factor-1 (IRF-1) gene. This effect of PRL is mediated by STAT1 and, paradoxically, inhibited by STAT5.[87] Although IRF-1 gene regulation is probably not involved in the normal functions of PRL, the regulation of this gene through STAT1 in Nb2 cells provides important lessons regarding

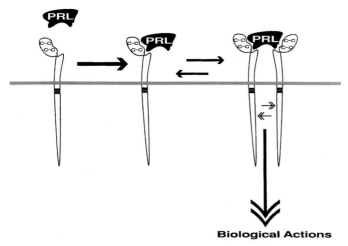

Biological Actions

FIGURE 15–5. *Dimerization of the prolactin (PRL) receptor causes activation. Based on studies described in the text, PRL is understood to cause receptor dimerization, and interaction between the receptors and associated proteins lead to activation of appropriate biologic actions.*

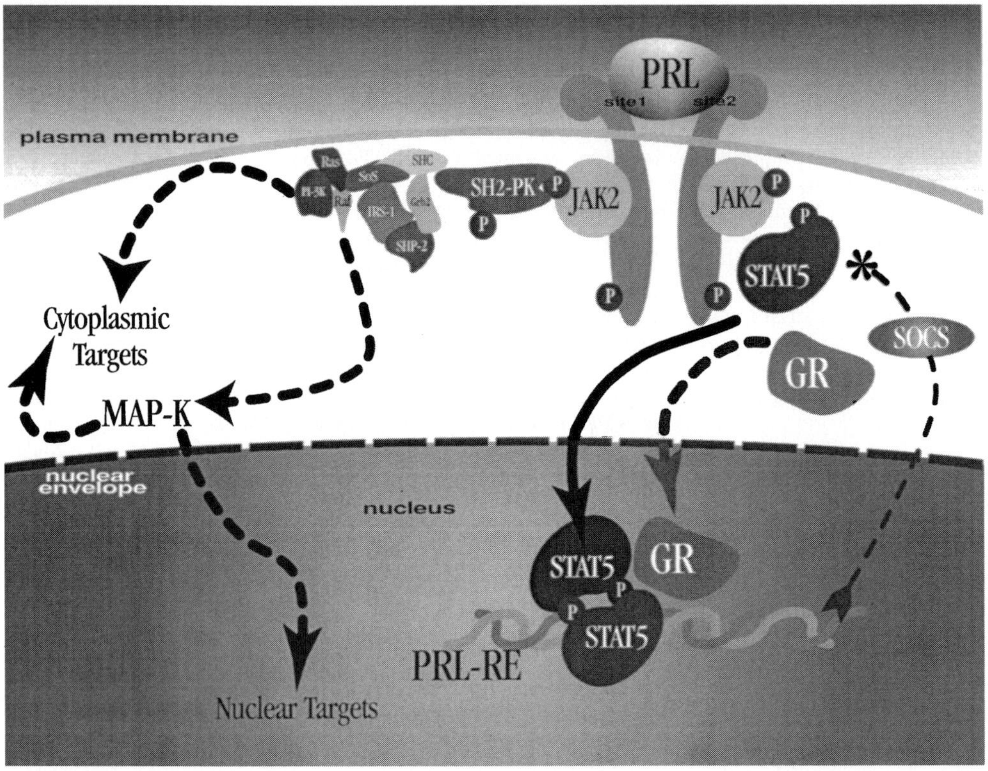

FIGURE 15-6. Intracellular signal transduction by prolactin (PRL). Janus kinase 2 (JAK2) is associated with the PRL receptor and becomes active after receptor dimerization. A signal transducer and activator of transcription protein (STAT5) is phosphorylated (P), dimerizes, associates with the glucocorticoid receptor (GR), and binds to appropriate genes through prolactin response elements (PRL-RE). Activation of the JAK2-STAT5 pathway is inhibited *(asterisk)* by suppressors of cytokine signaling proteins (SOCS). JAK2 also activates other Src-related protein kinases (SH2-PK), and these couple with an array of signaling molecules that can activate cytoplasmic or nuclear target molecules, including mitogen-activated protein kinases (MAP-K).

the potential derangements in PRL signaling that can mediate pathologic changes. Other experimental models in which the normal pathways of PRL signaling are subverted will provide additional important insights.

THE PHYSIOLOGY AND PATHOPHYSIOLOGY OF PROLACTIN ACTIONS IN MAMMALS

Mammary Glands

PRL is essential to lactation in all mammals, though the precise temporal dimensions of its actions vary among species. The first step

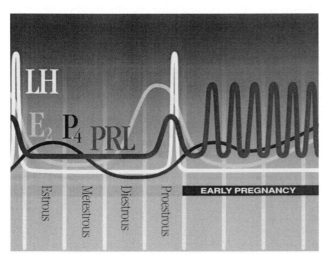

FIGURE 15-7. Prolactin (PRL) secretion in the estrous cycle and early pregnancy of the rodent. PRL, luteinizing hormone (LH), estradiol (E₂), and progesterone (P₄) profiles are schematized. PRL undergoes a modest elevation around the time of the ovulatory LH surge in the estrous cycle. If mating occurs, the coital stimulus to the cervix induces a pattern of twice-daily PRL surges that are required to maintain pregnancy.

in mammary gland organogenesis is the prenatal establishment of the mammary ductal rudiment. Parathyroid hormone–related peptide (PTH-rP) is essential at this first stage of mammary gland development, but PRL is not.[59, 83, 88] The epithelial rudiment and fat pad grow isometrically until puberty, at which time the epithelial ductal system expands rapidly under the influence of estrogen, GH, and IGF-1.[89, 90] During the latter stages of puberty lobular buds branch off from the ductal system under the influence of PRL and progesterone. As a consequence of the regular cycles of estrous or menstrual hormone surges, the complexity of the mammary ductal branching increases progressively, and the epithelial cells undergo cyclic changes. If the female becomes pregnant before lobule budding and maturation are complete, these processes occur during the first pregnancy. As a general rule, progesterone induces ductal arborization, whereas PRL induces the formation of alveolar progenitors. However, the relative roles of progesterone and PRL in the pubertal development of the mammary glands have not been completely resolved at the organ level, and the genes that are induced by each of these hormones during development are completely unknown.

During pregnancy the lobuloalveolar epithelium undergoes extensive proliferation under the influence of PRL, PLs, progesterone, and local growth factors. During and after parturition both progesterone and PLs fall precipitously, and PRL rises. This combination of hormone changes leads to functional lactogenesis and lactation. The lobuloalveolar epithelium is converted to a secretory phenotype and the full complement of milk proteins and lactogenic enzymes is synthesized. At the end of lactation involution of the lobuloalveolar system occurs in response to milk stasis and falling systemic lactogens.[91] According to this scheme of development, PRL and PLs, each of which bind to the PRL-R, act during three stages of mammary gland development: lobule budding during organogenesis, lobuloalveolar expansion during pregnancy, and lactational differentiation after parturition.

Pioneering studies using surgical ablation of endocrine glands and hormone replacement established specific roles for estrogen and GH in ductal development, and for PRL, progesterone, and corticosteroids in lobuloalveolar development and lactogenesis.[92] Transgenic and gene disruption techniques have recently added to our knowledge of hormone actions in mammary gland development in vivo. In laboratory mice, complete PRL deficiency results in the arrest of mammary organogenesis at an immature pubertal state. In this arrested developmental state the epithelial component of the gland consists of a basic ductal system, and terminal end buds, but none of the structures that are progenitors of the lobuloalveolar system.

PRL apparently induces the differentiation and growth of uncommitted alveolar progenitor cells from the ductal epithelium. Chepko and Smith, using transplantation techniques, described cells that have the characteristics of alveolar progenitors.[93, 94] The specialized features of hormonal responses in this population of cells are not yet known. The development of alveoli from precursor cells in the ductal epithelium may involve both clonal growth from committed precursors, and induction of phenotypic changes in cells that are near specialized "organizer" cells. During lactation PRL regulates several secreted milk proteins, including the caseins, lactoglobulin (except in rodents), lactalbumin, and whey acidic protein. Enzymes such as lactose synthetase, lipoprotein lipase, and fatty acid synthase, which are essential for milk synthesis, are induced by PRL in the mammary gland.

Female Reproductive Tissues

PRL has two general types of actions on female reproduction in mammals. First, PRL inhibits gonadal activity by means of actions at the hypothalamus, pituitary, and ovarian levels. Second, PRL is an essential luteotropic hormone in rodents, although not so in humans or most other mammals.

PRL inhibits reproductive function by decreasing the hypothalamic drive for pulsatile luteinizing hormone (LH) secretion,[95, 96] inhibiting ovarian folliculogenesis,[97] and inhibiting granulosa cell aromatase activity, which leads to lower estradiol synthesis.[98, 99] Elevated DA levels in the hypothalamus, secondary to high PRL levels, is one mechanism for the antigonadal effects of PRL. PRL contributes to the breakdown of the corpus luteum in many mammalian species, including humans. In rodents, however, PRL is essential to corpus luteum maintenance in early pregnancy. One of the well-characterized mechanisms of the luteotropic action of PRL is inhibition of 20α-hydroxysteroid dehydrogenase activity.[100] This action prevents the conversion of progesterone to 20α-hydroxyprogesterone, and therefore increases progesterone secretion from the corpus luteum.

The maintenance of early pregnancy in rodents depends on the establishment of a stereotypic pattern of twice-daily surges of PRL (see Fig. 15–7), which are established after coital stimulation of the cervix. In laboratory rodents the luteal phase of the estrous cycle is transient, and implantation cannot occur unless the corpus luteum is maintained by high levels of PRL. The cervical stimulus drives a hypothalamic reflex which alters the secretion of a variety of regulatory factors, including DA, opioids, and various putative PRFs. While it is clear that the diurnal and nocturnal PRL surges in early pregnancy are controlled by different sets of factors,[101] neither the exact circuitry nor the essential hypophysiotropic factors that are responsible for each of the surges are yet known.

Lactational infertility is one consequence of high PRL secretion in women who are breast-feeding. Suckling-induced elevation of PRL can decrease gonadotropin-releasing hormone (GnRH), LH, and estrogen secretion, and cause persistent amenorrhea. If ovulatory cycles occur in women who are breast-feeding, the luteal phase defect caused by luteolytic actions of PRL can prevent conception. Although breast-feeding has been promoted as a natural means of contraception, it is very unreliable for most women. Most studies have pointed out that frequent bouts of nursing, especially during the nighttime, are essential to successful lactational contraception. In some societies, where children sleep with the mother for many months, birth spacing has been strongly influenced by lactational infertility.

Male Reproductive Tissues

High levels of PRL are inhibitory to male reproductive function, much the same as they are to female function. A common presenting symptom of human hyperprolactinemia in males is loss of libido and impotence. These symptoms may or may not be associated with galactorrhea. PRL inhibits GnRH and LH secretion in males, as well

as in females.[102] The antigonadal actions of PRL are the most widely conserved PRL actions among a wide variety of mammals and non-mammalian vertebrates. Male mice with a targeted disruption of either the PRL gene itself, or the PRL-R gene, are completely fertile.[82, 83] Consistent with this, there are no reports in the literature of human males with isolated PRL deficiency.

The prostate gland of PRL-deficient mice was smaller (by about 30%) than that of normal mice, and high levels of PRL caused prostate hyperplasia in mice.[103] PRL secretion may, therefore, be a contributing factor in human prostate disease, but no data specifically addressing this possibility are yet available. PRL increases LH and follicle-stimulating hormone (FSH) receptors in the testis, as well as androgen receptors in the prostate.[104]

Ion Balance and Calcium Metabolism

PRL is an essential freshwater survival hormone in many species of fish and amphibians, and it has effects on all of the osmoregulatory epithelia in these species. Its actions include decreasing water permeability in the gills and skin, and increasing salt reabsorption in the kidney and urinary bladder (which is evolutionarily homologous with the collecting ducts of the mammalian kidney).[3] Similar actions have not been proved in mammals, which is not surprising since the osmoregulatory challenges facing terrestrial mammals are not at all similar to those confronted by freshwater fishes. PRL does increase the absorption of a variety of minerals in the intestine of mammals[105] and this effect may be physiologically important during pregnancy and breast-feeding, which place large demands on water and solute homeostasis.

PRL may have important physiologic actions on calcium metabolism in mammals, and these actions directly relate to changes of calcium balance during pregnancy and lactation. In the mammary gland PRL induces the secretion of PTH-rP, which can act as either a local or systemic effector of calcium homeostasis.[106]

Hyperprolactinemia in humans has been associated with decreased bone density, which is normalized when the elevated PRL levels are treated medically. Decreased estrogen, due to the antigonadal effects of PRL, may explain part of the loss of bone in hyperprolactinemia, but there appears to be a component of bone loss that is due to direct actions of PRL rather than estrogen loss.[107, 108] Recent genetic evidence has shown that the PRL-R is essential to normal bone formation and calcium homeostasis.[108] PRL-R-deficient mice displayed reductions in bone mineral density and bone mineral content, as well as a deceleration in the apposition rate for new bone. Plasma total calcium and parathyroid hormone (PTH) were each higher in the receptor-deficient mice. The phenotypic characteristics of bone growth and calcium homeostasis in PRL-R-deficient mice argue that there must be multiple sites of PRL action that influence calcium metabolism, including both direct effects on bone cells, and systemic actions on other hormones or carriers. PRL-R mRNA levels are very high in bone during development,[110] and PLs, as well as PRL per se, could contribute to prenatal control of bone growth.

Brain and Behavior

The vertebrate brain is a target tissue for numerous PRL actions, many of which are directly related to the parental care of offspring. The first evidence that PRL is a brain-regulating hormone was in birds, where systemic or intracranial PRL infusion stimulates behaviors associated with brooding and migration.[3, 52] In rats PRL infusions increase the intensity of parental attendance to offspring, or shorten the time required for inexperienced adults to begin showing parental behaviors.[111] Mice that lack the PRL-R were profoundly deficient in maternal behaviors,[112] although PRL-deficient mice were not.[82] The discrepancy between these strains requires further study to resolve. The neuroanatomic and neurochemical substrates that mediate the PRL-regulated parental behaviors in mammals are not yet known.

Whereas stereotypic maternal behavior patterns in animals such as birds, mice, and rats have been quantified and studied objectively, it has not been possible to characterize such behaviors in humans in a way that would allow one to determine whether PRL has a similar role in human parenting. Human PRL increases DA turnover in the nucleus accumbens, corpus striatum, and median eminence, but it decreases DA turnover in the substantia nigra, ventral tegmentum, and cingulate nucleus. It has been proposed that human hyperprolactinemia can be one component of an organic response to psychological traumas (particularly deprivation from parental attention), and that the behavior patterns associated with high PRL levels (a "maternal subroutine") may be an adaptive psychological response.[113]

Behavioral actions of PRL that are not directly related to parenting, but may be indirectly supportive, include stimulation of appetite (orexia) and analgesia, and increases in REM sleep activity.[39] The orexigenic effect of PRL may depend on interactions with leptin signaling. Leptin, which is a major hormonal regulator of appetite, acts through a cytokine-family receptor and JAK-STAT signal transduction pathway that is closely related to that used by PRL.[114] The analgesia caused by PRL is blocked by naloxone, indicating that the effect is through an opioid pathway.

Hematopoiesis and Immunoregulation

A strong case for an important immunoregulatory role of PRL has been made by several laboratories. PRL-Rs are found on a majority of immune precursor and effector cells in each of the major hematopoietic organs (bone marrow, spleen, thymus). PRL can potentiate the growth and effector functions of lymphoid and myeloid cells, and hematopoietic cytokine receptors and signal transducers are closely related to those used by PRL. The Nb2 cell line, grown from an estrogenized male rat lymphoma, is exquisitely sensitive to growth-promoting and antiapoptotic effects of PRL, and has been widely used as a model of PRL actions on immune cells.

In humans, PRL secretion is correlated with disease severity in systemic lupus erythematosus, an autoimmune disease that affects primarily women of childbearing age.[115] In a rat model of immunodepression following acute hemorrhagic shock, PRL stimulated immune effector cell functions, as well as normal cytokine secretion.[116] Whereas PRL can act as a positive stimulus for immune cells when given to animals by injection, or to cells in culture, PRL deficiency does not significantly impair immune function or hematopoiesis.[82] It is conceivable that the higher level of PRL secretion in females compared with males is one factor that contributes to a sexual difference in immune responses.

Metabolism

PRL-Rs are present in the liver, gut, and pancreas.[5] PRL causes splanchnomegaly (gut growth) and accelerates liver regrowth after partial hepatectomy.[117, 118] Bile acid secretion and taurocholate transport in liver are elevated by PRL during lactation.[119] PRL stimulates growth of pancreatic β cells in vivo and in vitro. During pregnancy and lactation the β cells proliferate. β cell proliferation may be both an adaptive response mediated by PLs and PRL,[120] and a direct response to gestational insulin resistance. In general, the actions of PRL on organs that control whole-body metabolism are consistent with the metabolic alterations that support successful gestation and lactation. Many hormones in addition to PRL contribute to these metabolic adjustments.

SUMMARY

PRL, along with PLs in many species, plays a central role in assuring successful reproduction by acting after fertilization to promote a variety of developmental, metabolic, and behavioral adaptations. DA, secreted from the hypothalamic arcuate nucleus, inhibits PRL secretion, and is the dominant PRL regulator in mammals, but not in other species. The specialization of the mammalian life cycle to include not only maternal gestation but also postpartum nurturing of

offspring has been accompanied by a wide range of physiologic adaptations. Breast milk secretion in mammals, as well as milk-like secretions that occur in certain nonmammalian vertebrates, are direct responses to PRL. Suppression of gonadal development and sexual drive in both males and females is mediated both centrally and peripherally. The physiologic actions of PRL are pathologically exaggerated in human hyperprolactinemia.

REFERENCES

1. Riddle O, Bates RW, Dykshorn SW: The preparation, identification and assay of prolactin—a hormone of the anterior pituitary. Am J Physiol 105:191, 1933.
2. Stricker P, Grueter F: Action du lobe antérior de l'hypophyse sur la montée laiteuse. C R Seances Soc Biol Fil 99:1978, 1928.
3. Horseman ND: Models of prolactin action in nonmammalian vertebrates. In Rillema JA (ed): Actions of Prolactin on Molecular Processes. Boca Raton, FL, CRC Press, 1987, p 41.
4. Bern HA, Nicoll CS: The comparative endocrinology of prolactin. Recent Prog Horm Res 24:681, 1968.
5. Bole-Feysot C, Goffin V, Edery M, et al: Prolactin (PRL) and its receptor: Actions, signal transduction pathways and phenotypes observed in PRL receptor knockout mice. Endocr Rev 19:225, 1998.
6. Nicoll CS: Physiological actions of prolactin. In Knobil E, Sawyer WH (eds): Handbook of Physiology. Section 7: Endocrinology, Washington, DC, American Physiology Society, 1974, p q253.
7. Horseman ND, Yu-Lee L-Y: Transcriptional regulation by the helix bundle peptide hormones: GH, PRL, and hematopoietic cytokines. Endocr Rev 15:627, 1994.
8. Darnell JE Jr, Kerr IM, Stark GR: Jak-Stat pathways and transcriptional activation in response to IFNs and other extracellular signaling proteins. Science 264:1415, 1994.
9. Li CH: The chemistry of prolactin. In Li CH (ed): Hormonal Proteins and Peptides, vol 8. New York, Academic Press, 1980, p 2.
10. Cooke NE, Liebhaber SA: Molecular biology of the growth hormone–prolactin gene system. Vitam Horm 50:385, 1995.
11. Soares MJ, Faria TN, Roby KF, et al: Pregnancy and the prolactin family of hormones: Coordination of anterior pituitary, uterine, and placental expression. Endocr Rev 12:402, 1991.
12. Soares MJ, Muller H, Orwig KE, et al: Uteroplacental prolactin family and pregnancy. Biol Reprod 58:273, 1998.
13. Talamantes F, Ogren L, Markoff E, et al: Phylogenetic distribution, regulation of secretion, and prolactin-like effects of placental lactogens. Fed Proc 39:2582, 1980.
14. Handwerger S: Clinical counterpoint: The physiology of placental lactogen in human pregnancy. Endocr Rev 12:329, 1991.
15. Jackson D, Volpert OV, Bouck N, et al: Stimulation and inhibition of angiogenesis by placental proliferin and proliferin-related protein. Science 266:1581, 1994.
16. Kessler MA, Schuler LA: Purification and properties of placental prolactin-related protein-I. Placenta 18:29, 1996.
17. Lee SJ, Nathans D: Proliferin secreted by cultured cells binds to mannose 6-phosphate receptors. J Biol Chem 263:3521, 1988.
18. Miller WL, Baxter JD, Eberhardt NL: Peptide hormone genes: Structure and evolution. In Krieger DT, Brownstein MJ, Martin JB (eds): Brain Peptides, vol 21, New York, John Wiley & Sons, 1983, p 16.
19. Sinha YN: Structural variants of prolactin: Occurrence and physiological significance. Endocr Rev 16:354, 1995.
20. Lee H, Struman I, Clapp C, et al: Inhibition of urokinase activity by the antiangiogenic factor 16K prolactin: Activation of plasminogen activator inhibitor 1 expression. Endocrinology 139:3696, 1998.
21. Wang Y-F, Walker AM: Dephosphorylation of standard prolactin produces a more biologically active molecule: Evidence for antagonism between nonphosphorylated and phosphorylated prolactin in the stimulation of Nb2 cell proliferation. Endocrinology 133:2156, 1993.
22. Kenyon C: If birds can fly, why can't we? Homeotic genes and evolution. Cell 78:175, 1994.
23. Frawley SL: Mammosomatotropes: Current status and possible functions. Trends Endocrinol Metab 1:31, 1989.
24. Asa SL, Ezzat S: The cytogenesis and pathogenesis of pituitary adenomas. Endocr Rev 19:798, 1998.
25. Theill LE, Castrillo J-L, Wu D, et al: Dissection of functional domains of the pituitary-specific transcription factor GHF-1. Nature 342:945, 1989.
26. He X, Treacy MN, Simmons DM, et al: Expression of a large family of POU-domain regulatory genes in mammalian brain development. Nature 340:35, 1989.
27. Ingraham HA, Chen R, Mangalam HJ, et al: A tissue-specific transcription factor containing a homeodomain specifies a pituitary phenotype. Cell 55:519, 1988.
28. Simmons DM, Voss JW, Ingraham HA, et al: Pituitary cell phenotypes involve cell-specific Pit-1 mRNA translation and synergistic interactions with other classes of transcription factors. Genes Dev 4:695, 1990.
29. Morris AE, Kloss B, McChesney RE, et al: An alternatively spliced Pit-1 isoform altered in its ability to trans-activate. Nucleic Acids Res 20:1355, 1992.
30. Seyfred MA, Kladde MP, Gorski J: Transcriptional regulation by estrogen of episomal prolactin gene regulatory elements. Mol Endocrinol 3:305, 1989.
31. Cai A, Bowers RC, Moore JPJ, et al: Function of galanin in the anterior pituitary of estrogen-treated fischer 344 rats: Autocrine and paracrine regulation of prolactin secretion. Endocrinology 139:2452, 1998.
32. Schweppe RE, Frazer-Abel AA, Gutierrez-Hartmann A, et al: Functional components of fibroblast growth factor (FGF) signal transduction in pituitary cells. Identification of FGF response elements in the prolaction gene. J Biol Chem 272:30852, 1997.

33. Zhang K, Kulig E, Jin L, et al: Effects of estrogen and epidermal growth factor on prolactin and Pit-1 mRNA in GH3 cells. Proc Soc Exp Biol Med 202:193, 1993.
34. Ben-Jonathan N: Regulation of prolactin secretion. *In* Imura H (ed): The Pituitary Gland, ed 2. New York, Raven Press, 1994, p 261.
35. Lea RW, Vowles DM: Vasoactive intestinal polypeptide stimulates prolactin release *in vivo* in the ring dove *(Streptopelia risoria)*. Experentia 42:420, 1986.
36. Lea RW, Talbot RT, Sharp PJ: Passive immunization against chicken vasoactive intestinal polypeptide suppresses plasma prolactin and crop sac development in incubating ring doves. Horm Behav 25:283, 1991.
37. Sassin JF, Frantz AG, Kapen S, et al: The nocturnal rise of human prolactin is dependent upon sleep. J Clin Endocrinol Metab 37:436, 1973.
38. Obál F Jr, Payne L, Kacsoh B, et al: Involvement of prolactin in the REM sleep–promoting activity of systemic vasoactive intestinal peptide (VIP). Brain Res 645:143, 1994.
39. Roky R, Obal F, Valatx J-L, et al: Prolactin and rapid eye movement sleep regulation. Sleep 18:536, 1995.
40. Kelly M, Rubinstein M, Asa S, et al: Pituitary lactotroph hyperplasia and chronic hyperprolactinemia in dopamine D2 receptor–deficient mice. Neuron 19:103, 1997.
41. Steger RW, Chandrashekar V, Zhao W, et al: Neuroendocrine and reproductive functions in male mice with targeted disruption of the prolactin gene. Endocrinology 139:3691, 1998.
42. Gregerson K, Flagg T, Anderson M, et al: Identification of the G-protein–coupled, inward rectifying potassium channel gene products in rat anterior pituitary gland. Endocrinology (in press).
43. Kanyicska B, Lerant A, Freeman ME: Endothelin is an autocrine regulator of prolactin secretion. Endocrinology 139:5164, 1998.
44. Sarkar DK, Kim KH, Minami S: Transforming growth factor β-1 messenger RNA and protein expression in the pituitary gland: Its action on prolactin secretion and lactotropic growth. Mol Endocrinol 6:1825, 1992.
45. Shah GV, Pedchenko V, Stanley S, et al: Calcitonin is a physiological inhibitor of prolactin secretion in ovariectomized female rats. Endocrinology 137:1814, 1996.
46. Seyfred MA, Gorski J: An interaction between the 5′ flanking distal and proximal regulatory domains of the rat prolactin gene is required for transcriptional activation by estrogens. Mol Endocrinol 4:1226, 1990.
47. Yan G-Z, Pan WT, Bancroft C: Thyrotropin-releasing hormone action on the prolactin promoter is mediated by the POU protein Pit-1. Mol Endocrinol 5:535, 1991.
48. Bredow S, Kacsóh B, Obál F Jr, et al: Increase of prolactin mRNA in the rat hypothalamus after intracerebroventricular injection of VIP or PACAP. Brain Res 660:301, 1994.
49. Pickett CA, Gutierrez-Hartmann A: Ras mediates Src but not epidermal growth factor-receptor tyrosine kinase signaling pathways in GH_4 neuroendocrine cells. Proc Natl Acad Sci U S A 91:8612, 1994.
50. Porter TE, Wiles CD, Frawley LS: Stimulation of lactotrope differentiation in vitro by fibroblast growth factor. Endocrinology 134:164, 1994.
51. El Halawani ME, Burke WH, Millam JR, et al: Regulation of prolactin and its role in gallinaceous bird reproduction. J Exp Zool 232:521, 1984.
52. Horseman ND, Buntin JD: Regulation of pigeon crop milk secretions and parental behaviors by prolactin. Annu Rev Nutr 15:213, 1995.
53. Hinuma S, Habata Y, Fujii R, et al: Prolactin-releasing peptide in the brain. Nature 393:272, 1998.
54. Castano JP, Kineman RD, Frawley LS: Dynamic fluctuations in the secretory activity of individual lactotropes as demonstrated by a modified sequential plaque assay. Endocrinology 135:1747, 1994.
55. Nicoll CS: Bioassay of prolactin. Analysis of the pigeon crop-sac response to local protein injection by objective and quantitative methods. Endocrinology 80:641, 1967.
56. Gout PW, Beer CT, Noble RL: Prolactin-stimulated growth of cell cultures established from malignant Nb rat lymphomas. Cancer Res 40:2433, 1980.
57. Kauppila A, Chatelain P, Kirkinen P, et al: Isolated prolactin deficiency in a woman with puerperal alactogenesis. J Clin Endocrinol Metab 64:309, 1987.
58. Falk RJ: Isolated prolactin deficiency: A case report. Fertil Steril 58:1060, 1992.
59. Vomachka AJ, Pratt SL, Lockefeer JA, et al: Prolactin gene-disruption arrests mammary gland development and retards T-antigen-induced tumor growth. Oncogene 19:1077, 2000.
60. Radovick S, Nations M, Du Y, et al: A mutation in the POU-homeodomain of Pit-1 responsible for combined pituitary hormone deficiency. Science 257:1115, 1992.
61. Voss JW, Rosenfeld MG: Anterior pituitary development: Short tales from dwarf mice. Cell 70:527, 1992.
62. Ben-Jonathan N, Mershon JL, Allen DL, et al: Extrapituitary prolactin: Distribution, regulation, functions, and clinical aspects. Endocr Rev 17:639, 1997.
63. Gellerson B, Dimattia GE, Friesen HG, et al: Prolactin (PRL) mRNA from human decidua differs from pituitary PP mRNA but resembles the IM-9-P3 lymphoblast PRL transcript. Mol Cell Endocrinol 64:127, 1989.
64. Kacsóh B, Veress Z, Tóth BE, et al: Bioactive and immunoreactive variants of prolactin in milk and serum of lactating rats and their pups. J Endocrinol 138:243, 1993.
65. Das R, Vonderhaar BK: Prolactin as a mitogen in mammary cells. J Mammary Gland Biol Neoplasia 2:29, 1997.
66. Cosman D, Lyman SD, Idzerda RL, et al: A new cytokine receptor superfamily. Trends Biochem Sci 15:265, 1990.
67. Somers W, Ultsh M, De Vos AM, et al: The x-ray structure of a growth hormone–prolactin receptor complex. Nature 372:478, 1994.
68. Chen X, Horseman ND: Cloning, expression, and mutational analysis of the pigeon prolactin receptor. Endocrinology 135:269, 1994.
69. Schuler LA, Nagel RJ, Gao J, et al: Prolactin receptor heterogeneity in bovine fetal and maternal tissues. Endocrinology 138:3187–3194, 1997.
70. de Vos AM, Ultsch M, Kossiakoff AA: Human growth hormone and extracellular domain of its receptor: Crystal structure of the complex. Science 255:306, 1992.
71. Gertler A, Grosclaude J, and Djiane J: Interaction of lactogenic hormones with prolactin receptors. Ann N Y Acad Sci 839:177, 1998.
72. Chang W-P, Clevenger CV: Modulation of growth factor receptor function by isoform heterodimerization. Proc Natl Acad Sci U S A, 93:5947, 1996.
73. Campbell GS, Argentsinger LS, Ihle JN, et al: Activation of JAK2 tyrosine kinase by prolactin receptors in Nb2 cells and mouse mammary gland explants. Proc Natl Acad Sci U S A 91:5232, 1994.
74. Gao J, Hughes JP, Auperin B, et al: Interaction among JANUS kinases and the prolactin (PRL) receptor in the regulation of a PRL response element. Mol Endocrinol 10:847, 1995.
75. Parganas E, Wang D, Stravopodis D, et al: Jak2 is essential for signaling through a variety of cytokine receptors. Cell 93:385, 1998.
76. Berchtold S, Volarevic S, Moriggl R, et al: Dominant negative variants of the SHP-2 tyrosine phosphatase inhibit prolactin activation of Jak2 (janus kinase 2) and induction of Stat5 (signal transducer and activator of transcription 5)–dependent transcription. Mol Endocrinol 12:556, 1998.
77. Sidis Y, Horseman ND: Prolactin induces rapid p95/p70 tyrosine phosphorylation, and protein binding to GAS-like sites in the *anx* I_{cp35} and *c-fos* genes. Endocrinology 134:1979, 1994.
78. Wakao H, Gouilleux F, Groner B: Mammary gland factor (MGF) is a novel member of the cytokine regulated transcription factor gene family and confers the prolactin response. EMBO J 13:2182, 1994.
79. Liu X, Robinson GW, Wagner K-U, et al: Stat5a is mandatory for adult mammary gland development and lactogenesis. Genes Dev 11:179, 1997.
80. Udy GB, Towers RP, Snell RG, et al: Requirement of STAT5b for sexual dimorphism of body growth rates and liver gene expression. Proc Natl Acad Sci U S A 94:7239, 1997.
81. Teglund S, McKay C, Schuetz E, et al. Stat5a and Stat5b proteins have essential and nonessential, or redundnat, roles in cytokine responses. Cell 93:841, 1998.
82. Horseman ND, Zhao W, Montecino-Rodriguez E, et al: Defective mammopoiesis, but normal hematopoiesis, in mice with a targeted disruption of the prolactin gene. EMBO J 16:6926, 1997.
83. Ormandy C, J., Camus A, Barra J, et al: Null mutation of the prolactin receptor gene produces multiple reproductive defects in the mouse. Genes Dev 11:167, 1997.
84. Gouilleux F, Wakao H, Mundt M, et al: Prolactin induces phosphorylation of tyr694 of Stat5 (MGF), a prerequisite for DNA binding and induction of transcription. EMBO J 13:4361, 1994.
85. Stocklin E, Wissler M, Gouilleux, et al: Functional interactions between Stat5 and the glucocorticoid receptor. Nature 383:726, 1996.
86. Helman D, Sandowski Y, Cohen Y, et al: Cytokine-inducible SH2 protein (CIS3) and Jak2 binding protein (JAB) abolish prolactin receptor–mediated Stat5 signaling. FEBS Lett 441:287, 1998.
87. Luo G, Yu-Lee L-Y: Transcriptional inhibition by Stat5. J Biol Chem 272:26841, 1997.
88. Wysolmerski JJ, Stewart AF: The physiology of parathyroid hormone–related protein: An emerging role as a developmental factor. Annu Rev Physiol 60:431, 1998.
89. Topper YJ, Freeman CS: Multiple hormone interactions in the developmental biology of the mammary gland. Physiol Rev 60:1049, 1980.
90. Kleinberg DL: Early mammary development: Growth hormone and IGF-1. J Mammary Gland Biol Neoplasms 2:49, 1997.
91. Schmitt-Ney M, Happ B, Hofer P, et al: Mammary gland–specific nuclear factor activity is positively regulated by lactogenic hormones and negatively by milk stasis. Mol Endocrinol 6:1988, 1992.
92. Lyons W, Li CH, Johnson RE: Hormonal control of mammary growth and lactation. Recent Prog Horm Res 14:219, 1958.
93. Chepko G, Smith GH: Three division-competent, structurally-distinct cell populations contribute to murine mammary epithelial renewal. Tissue Cell 29:239, 1997.
94. Smith GH: Experimental mammary epithelial morphogenesis in an *in vivo* model: Evidence for distinct cellular progenitors of the ductal and lobular phenotype. Breast Cancer Res Treat 39:21, 1996.
95. Sarkar D, Yen S: Hyperprolactinemia decreases the luteinizing hormone releasing hormone concentration in pituitary portal plasma: A possible role for β-endorphin as a mediator. Endocrinology 116:2080, 1985.
96. Cohen-Becker I, Selmanoff M, Wise P: Hyperprolactinemia alters the frequency and ampitude of pulsatile lutenizing hormone secretion in the ovariectomized rat. Neuroendocrinol 42:328, 1986.
97. Larsen J, Bhanu A, Odell W: Prolactin inhibition of pregnant mare's serum stimulated follicle development in the rat ovary. Endocr Res 16:449, 1990.
98. Tsai-Morris C, Ghosh M, Hirshfield A, et al: Inhibition of ovarian aromatase by prolactin in vivo. Biol Reprod 29:342, 1983.
99. Krasnow J, Hickey G, Richards J: Regulation of aromatase mRNA and estradiol biosynthesis in rat ovarian granulosa and luteal cells by prolactin. Mol Endocrinol 4:13, 1990.
100. Albarracin CT, Parmer TG, Duan WR, et al: Identification of a major prolactin-regulated protein as 20α-hydroxysteroid dehydrogenase: Coordinate regulation of its activity, protein content, and messenger ribonucleic acid expression. Endocrinology 134:2453, 1994.
101. Freeman ME, Smith MS, Nazian SJ, et al: Ovarian and hypothalamic control of the daily surges of prolactin secretion during pseudopregnancy. Endocrinology 94:875, 1974.
102. Voogt JL, de Greef WJ, Visser TJ, et al: In vivo release of dopamine, luteinizing hormone–releasing hormone and thyrotropin-releasing hormone in male rats bearing a prolactin-secreting tumor. Neuroendocrinol 46:110, 1987.
103. Wennbo H, Kindblom J, Isaksson OG, et al: Transgenic mice overexpressing the prolactin gene develop dramatic enlargement of the prostate gland. Endocrinology 138:4410, 1997.
104. Bex FJ, Bartke A: Testicular LH binding in the hamster: Modification by photoperiod and prolactin. Endocrinology 100:1223, 1977.
105. Mainoya JR, Bern HA, Regan JW: Influence of ovine prolactin on transport of fluid and sodium chloride by the mammalian intestine and gall bladder. J Endocrinol 63:311, 1974.

106. Ferrari SL, Rizzoli R, Bonjour JP: Parathyroid hormone–related protein production by primary cultures of mammary epithelial cells. J Cell Physiol 150:304, 1992.

107. Klibanski A, Neer RM, Beitins IZ, et al: Decreased bone density in hyperprolactinemic women. N Engl J Med 303:1511, 1980.

108. Klibanski A, Greenspan SL: Increase in bone mass after treatment of hyperprolactinemic amenorrhea. N Engl J Med 315:542, 1986.

109. Clément-Lacroix P, Ormandy C, Lepescheux L, et al: Osteoblasts are a new target for prolactin: Analysis of bone formation in prolactin receptor knockout mice. Endocrinology 140:96, 1999.

110. Freemark M, Nagano M, Edery M, et al: Prolactin receptor gene expression in the fetal rat. J Endocrinol 144:285, 1995.

111. Bridges RS: The role of lactogenic hormones in maternal behavior in female rats. Acta Paediatr Suppl 397:33, 1994.

112. Lucas BK, Ormandy CJ, Binart N, et al: Null mutation of the prolactin receptor gene produces a defect in maternal behavior. Endocrinology 139:4102, 1998.

113. Sobrinho LG: The psychogenic effects of prolactin. Acta Endocrinol 129:38, 1993.

114. Ghilardi N, Zeigler S, Weistner A, et al: Defective STAT signaling by the leptin receptor in diabetic mice. Proc Natl Acad Sci U S A 93:6231, 1996.

115. Walker SE, Allen SH, McMurray RW: Prolactin and autoimmune disease. Trends Endocrinol Metab 4:147, 1993.

116. Zellweger R, Zhu X-H, Wichmann MW, et al. Prolactin administration following hemorrhagic shock improves macrophage cytokine release capacity and decreases mortality from subsequent sepsis. J Immunol 157:5748, 1996.

117. Bates RW, Riddle O, Lahr EL, et al: Aspects of splanchnomegaly associated with the action of prolactin. Am J Physiol 119:603, 1937.

118. Buckley AR, Crowe PD, Russell DR: Rapid activation of protein kinase C in isolated rat liver nuclei by prolactin, a known hepatic mitogen. Proc Natl Acad Sci U S A 85:8649, 1988.

119. Liu Y, Hyde JF, Vore M: Prolactin regulates maternal bile secretory function post partum. J Pharmacol Exp Ther 261:560, 1992.

120. Brelje TC, Sorenson RL: Role of prolactin versus growth hormone on islet B-cell proliferation in vitro: Implications for pregnancy. Endocrinology 128:45, 1991.

Chapter 16

Adrenocorticotropic Hormone

Anne White ▪ David W. Ray

Adrenocorticotropic hormone (ACTH) is synthesized as part of the precursor proopiomelanocortin (POMC) and as such represents a challenge to endocrinologists in understanding how ACTH is cleaved from the precursor to produce the peptide that acts on the adrenal gland to stimulate the release of adrenal steroids.

This chapter focuses on ACTH in humans and aims to describe the structure, expression, and regulation of the *POMC* gene, with an emphasis on the difference between POMC in the pituitary and POMC in other tissues and tumors.

The second section covers ACTH and related peptides and examines the structure of the precursor, how it is processed, and the biologic activity of the different peptides derived from POMC. It is important to understand which peptides are present in the circulation and how differential processing of POMC produces an alternative spectrum of peptides (including precursors and fragments) in different tissues. The impact of the host of factors and mechanisms known to regulate ACTH and related peptides is considered in the context of biologic activity.

The hypothalamic-pituitary-adrenal (HPA) axis (Fig. 16–1) is well recognized for its role in the homeostatic mechanisms regulating the stress response. The hypothalamic secretion of corticotropin-releasing factor stimulates ACTH in the anterior pituitary, which in turn regulates the synthesis of glucocorticoids in the adrenal cortex.

The many important contributions made to the understanding of ACTH physiology make it difficult to provide a synopsis. However, the following events are some of the major milestones:

- 1930—Discovery by Smith that ACTH is a factor produced by the pituitary that maintains the weight of the adrenal cortex
- 1954—Primary structure of ACTH[1]
- 1964—Isolation of β-lipotropic pituitary hormone (β-lipotropin)[2]
- 1975—Peptide with opioid activity isolated from the pituitary and named β-endorphin
- 1978—Proof that POMC is the common precursor[4]
- 1979—Nucleotide sequence of POMC[5]
- 1981—Isolation and sequencing of corticotropin-releasing hormone (CRH)[6]
- 1992—Cloning of the ACTH receptor[7]
- 1998—Inherited mutations in POMC associated with early-onset obesity, adrenal insufficiency, and red hair pigmentation[8]

PROOPIOMELANOCORTIN GENE

Structure of the *POMC* Gene

Humans have a single *POMC* gene located on the short arm of chromosome 2 at 2p23 (the mouse and pig have two copies of the gene). The structure of the gene is well conserved and has been characterized in humans,[9–11] as well as in other species.[12] The *POMC* gene consists of three exons interspersed with two large introns (Fig. 16–2). The first exon, which consists of 87 base pairs (bp), contains no coding sequence, and its RNA transcript is thought to act as a leader sequence that binds the ribosome at the start of translation. Exon 2 (152 bp) contains the initiation sequence, a signal sequence that translocates the nascent peptide into the endoplasmic reticulum, and then the N-terminal part of the coding sequence for the POMC peptide. The third exon (835 bp) encodes most of the mature protein, including ACTH,[9–11] the termination codon, and the signal for addition of the poly A tail.

POMC Promoters

POMC contains three identified promoter regions (P1, P2, and P3 in Fig. 16–3) that give rise to RNA transcripts of 1150, 800, and 1350 nucleotides respectively.

- The pituitary promoter P1, which is near the 5′ boundary of exon 1, generates an RNA transcript consisting of exon 1, exon 2, and part of exon 3 after splicing out of the introns. This arrangement would be predicted to give a transcript of 1100 to 1200 nucleotides and concurs with the size of POMC mRNA from the pituitary, as detected by Northern blotting.
- The upstream promoter P3, which lies upstream of the pituitary promoter. Both these promoters should generate the same peptide product because the only relevant translation initiation site is in exon 1.
- The downstream promoter P2, which produces an 800-nucleotide RNA transcript, has been shown in humans and rats to arise from transcription initiation at the 5′ end of exon 3.[13, 14] This finding suggests that the promoter is located at the 3′ end of intron 2.[12] The smaller POMC transcript is found primarily in peripheral tissues, which indicates that there may be switching to the downstream promoter in peripheral tissues.

Regulatory Sites for Transcription

The *POMC* promoter has a number of common elements found in other genes that may contribute to regulation of *POMC* gene transcription.

TATA BOX. The TATA box is located 27 nucleotides upstream of

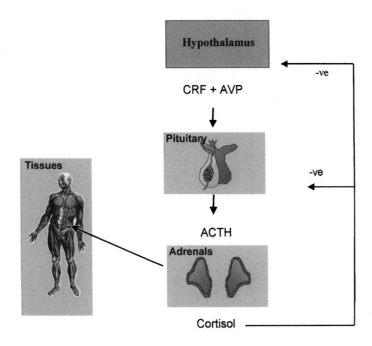

FIGURE 16–1. Schematic representation of the hypothalamic-pituitary-adrenal axis representing sites of glucocorticoid negative feedback. ACTH, adrenocorticotropic hormone; AVP, arginine vasopressin; CRF, corticotropin-releasing factor.

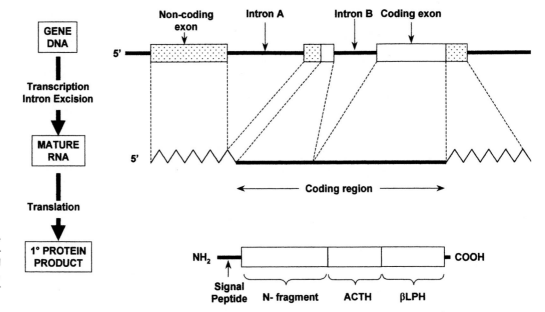

FIGURE 16–2. Genomic structure of human proopiomelanocortin with the major spliced product and preprohormone. ACTH, adrenocorticotropic hormone; βLPH, β-lipotropin.

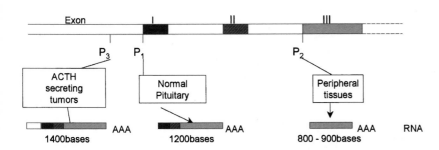

FIGURE 16–3. Tissue-specific promoter utilization of the human proopiomelanocortin (POMC) gene. P1 gives high-level expression of POMC in pituitary tissue. P2 gives low-level expression in numerous extrapituitary tissues. P3 is used in some extrapituitary tumors causing the ectopic adrenocorticotropic hormone (ACTH) syndrome. AAA, polyA tail.

the initiation site and binds a protein that positions RNA polymerase II on the gene to initiate transcription.

TISSUE-SPECIFIC ELEMENTS. Very little information is available for human *POMC*, but two regions in the rat *POMC* gene[15] confer tissue specificity on the promoter.[14, 16–18] These regions are between −320 and −478 bp and between −34 and −166 bp in the rat *POMC* gene. The factors that bind to these regions have not been characterized, but presumably they would be specific to corticotroph cells of the pituitary and binding would be required for *POMC* gene expression.

Expression of the *POMC* Gene

Expression in the Pituitary

In humans, expression of POMC is most abundant in the corticotroph cells of the anterior pituitary, and in healthy subjects, these cells are the only ones that express the gene at high levels.[19, 20] POMC mRNA expressed in the pituitary has a size of 1100 to 1200 nucleotides, which indicates that it is transcribed under control of the P1 promoter. POMC mRNA is also detected in the intermediate lobe of the pituitary, which is present during fetal life in humans and is found in other species such as the mouse and rat.

Expression in Other Tissues

POMC is also expressed, but at a much lower level, in other tissues such as the arcuate nucleus of the hypothalamus, testis, ovary, placenta, duodenum, liver, kidney, adrenal medulla, lung, thymus, and lymphocytes.[13, 21–24] POMC mRNA expressed in the hypothalamus has a size of 1100 to 1200 nucleotides, which is similar to that in the pituitary. However, POMC mRNA from extracranial tissues has a size of 800 nucleotides, which suggests that it is derived from transcription initiation at the downstream promoter (P2 in Fig. 16–3) 5′ to exon 3 and thus only includes the coding sequence for exon 3.[22] Therefore this transcript could not give rise to a mature POMC molecule and would lack a signal peptide, so its physiologic role is unclear.

Expression in Pituitary Tumors

Expression of the *POMC* gene in corticotroph adenomas giving rise to Cushing's disease appears to be similar to that in the normal pituitary.[25]

Expression in Nonpituitary Tumors

Tumors giving rise to the ectopic ACTH syndrome produce an mRNA transcript of 1200 bp, similar to that found in the pituitary, and approximately 20% of tumors express a larger transcript of 1400 to 1500 bp.[25] This larger transcript seems to be initiated from a promoter located at −392 and −432 bp relative to the conventional start site.[26–29] The larger transcript[29] would still initiate translation from the same site as that used by the pituitary promoter, and thus the POMC peptide would be identical to the pituitary product.

Some nonneuroendocrine tumors not associated with the ectopic ACTH syndrome express the smaller POMC mRNA transcript of 800 nucleotides that is found in many normal tissues.[22, 28, 30] It is probable that these tumors arose from cells that expressed the short mRNA transcript, and because this short transcript does not give rise to a peptide that is secreted, these tumors would not be expected to release POMC peptides.

Regulation of *POMC* Gene Expression

Regulation in Normal Tissues

POMC gene expression in the pituitary requires acute regulation and is subject to control from a number of factors. Expression of the *POMC* gene appears to be predominantly controlled at the level of gene transcription.[31] The rat *POMC* gene has been most extensively studied, and pituitary expression is conferred by the 5′ flanking region of the gene.[14, 16–18] There does not appear to be a specific element sufficient to direct high-level transcription, as for example, in the prolactin gene, where the pituitary-specific transcription factor Pit-1 binds to multiple sites to direct transcription. Rather, in the case of the *POMC* gene, there appears to be a requirement for integrity of the promoter. One sequence of DNA within the distal promoter, a "footprint" identified by DNase digestion, appears to be particularly important for corticotroph-specific transcription.[18]

CORTICOTROPIN-RELEASING HORMONE STIMULATION OF THE *POMC* GENE. CRH binds transmembrane receptors on corticotroph cells and stimulates cyclic adenosine monophosphate (cAMP) generation and thereby serine phosphorylation of the CREB (cAMP response element–binding protein) transcription factor (Fig. 16–4). Distally, this cascade appears to enhance gene transcription, but the rat *POMC* gene does not harbor a consensus cAMP response element. Further analysis of the *POMC* promoter has identified two DNA elements that appear capable of conferring CRH responsiveness

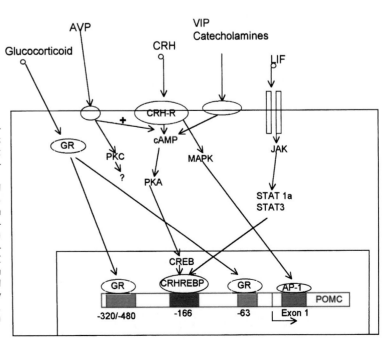

FIGURE 16–4. Intracellular signaling pathways regulating transcription of the proopiomelanocortin *(POMC)* gene. Through its receptor, corticotropin-releasing hormone (CRH) induces cyclic adenosine monophosphate (cAMP), which activates protein kinase A (PKA) and thereby phosphorylation of cAMP response, element–binding protein (CREB) and results in binding of CRH response element–binding protein (CRHREBP) to a motif at −166 on the *POMC* gene. cAMP is also activated by arginine vasopressin (AVP), vasoactive intestinal polypeptide (VIP), and catecholamines. CRH also activates mitogen-activated protein kinase (MAPK) pathways, which ultimately induce activator protein-1 (AP-1) binding to an exon 1 response element. AVP activates protein kinase C (PKC) pathways, which may also feed into this pathway. Leukemia inhibitory factor (LIF) signals via the JAK/STAT (Janus Kinase/signal transducer and activator of transcription) pathway and ultimately uses a DNA recognition site close to the CRHREBP binding site. Glucocorticoids acting through the glucocorticoid receptor (GR) can repress transcription through two cooperative binding sites.

to the gene. One element centered 166 nucleotides upstream from the transcription start site binds a protein termed the CRH response element–binding protein.[32] The second element reported to be CRH responsive is found in the noncoding exon 1 of the rat *POMC* gene.[33] This element shares close homology with a consensus activator protein-1 (AP-1) transcription factor–binding site and indeed appears to bind recombinant AP-1 protein in a sequence-specific manner. Because CRH treatment of the mouse pituitary corticotroph cell line AtT20 causes activation of mitogen-activated protein kinase (MAPK) and induction of the DNA-binding activity of AP-1 and because the *POMC* exon 1 element confers both phorbol ester and CRH responsiveness to a heterologous promoter, there is considerable evidence for a physiologic role of the MAPK/AP-1 cascade in mediating some actions of CRH.[33, 34]

GLUCOCORTICOID INHIBITION OF THE *POMC* GENE. Glucocorticoids are known to decrease ACTH levels, partly as a result of inhibition of POMC mRNA, although they also act at the level of translation and antagonize actions of CRH (Fig. 16–5). Considerable evidence indicates that glucocorticoids suppress transcription.[35–39] The binding sites for glucocorticoid receptors on the human *POMC* gene have not been identified. However, the rat gene has four sites, although only two of them, at −63 and between −480 and −320,[40] are needed in vivo. The −63-negative glucocorticoid-regulated element overlaps the putative COUP (chicken albumin upstream promoter) box, and it has been suggested that the inhibitory effect may occur by displacement of a stimulatory factor.

The more proximal element, an imperfect palindrome 63 nucleotides upstream of the transcription start site, is thought to bind three glucocorticoid receptor molecules in an unusual trimer formation.[41] It is thought that this conformation of receptors on DNA directs repression of transcription rather than enhancement. The glucocorticoid-regulated element further upstream between nucleotides −480 and −320, which is required to interact for the full effect of glucocorticoid to be manifested, has not been fully defined.[40]

STIMULATION OF THE *POMC* GENE BY ARGININE VASOPRESSIN. A number of other hypothalamic factors act on the pituitary corticotroph to influence *POMC* expression; however, their modes of action are less well defined. In particular, arginine vasopressin (AVP) augments the effect of CRH and, independently, rather weakly stimulates *POMC* expression.[19, 42, 43] It is less clear how AVP acts independently to stimulate *POMC* transcription. The intracellular pathways activated by AVP appear to be protein kinase C dependent, but AVP also potentiates the action of CRH on cAMP generation.

LEUKEMIA INHIBITORY FACTOR STIMULATION OF THE *POMC* GENE. A number of lines of evidence point to intrapituitary factors as important modulators of corticotroph function. One such factor is the proinflammatory cytokine leukemia inhibitory factor (LIF). This factor has been shown to stimulate the *POMC* gene through a specific response element that overlaps with the −166-nucleotide CRH response element.[34]

Regulation in Tumors

CORTICOTROPIN-RELEASING HORMONE REGULATION OF THE *POMC* GENE IN TUMORS. In general, CRH stimulates *POMC* expression only in pituitary corticotrophs, but exceptions do occur.[44–46]

GLUCOCORTICOID REGULATION OF THE *POMC* GENE IN TUMORS. In contrast to expression of the *POMC* gene in pituitary corticotroph cells, which is repressed by glucocorticoids, it has been known for a long time that ACTH in extrapituitary tumors is characteristically resistant to glucocorticoids.[47] This concept is the basis of the high-dose glucocorticoid suppression test used to distinguish eutopic from ectopic sources of ACTH in Cushing's syndrome. It is intriguing that most extrapituitary tumors are resistant to glucocorticoid inhibition of *POMC* expression. Receptors for glucocorticoids are present in most cells, including malignant cells, and thus exploration of the mechanisms of glucocorticoid resistance is of importance. To this end, a panel of human small cell lung carcinoma cell lines have been established as a model of the ectopic ACTH syndrome.[20, 48] These cell lines express the *POMC* gene, and expression is resistant to glucocorticoid suppression. Expression of the glucocorticoid receptor was identified both by Western blotting with a polyclonal anti–glucocorticoid receptor antibody and by ligand-binding assays using tritiated dexamethasone.[12, 20, 49]

To determine whether glucocorticoid signaling was present, a synthetic, glucocorticoid-responsive (mouse mammary tumor virus) gene linked to a chloramphenicol acetyltransferase reporter gene was transfected into the cells. In contrast to the brisk induction of expression seen in control pituitary cells, none of the human small cell lung carcinoma cells responded to either natural or synthetic glucocorticoids.[49] Thus resistance of the *POMC* gene to glucocorticoids is only part of the global resistance of malignant cells to glucocorticoid action. Expression of high concentrations of wild-type receptor in the cells was found to be sufficient to restore glucocorticoid signaling, thereby suggesting that resistance lay at the level of the endogenous receptor.[49] However, in one cell line studied, COR L103, even overexpression of wild-type receptor was insufficient to restore glucocorticoid signaling, which points to the possibility that multiple molecular mechanisms have been developed to evade glucocorticoid action.[49] Because one of the actions of glucocorticoids on pituitary corticotrophs is to inhibit proliferation and because in the developing lung glucocorticoids act to promote differentiation, it is possible that evasion of glucocorticoid signaling confers a survival advantage to the malignant cells. As yet,

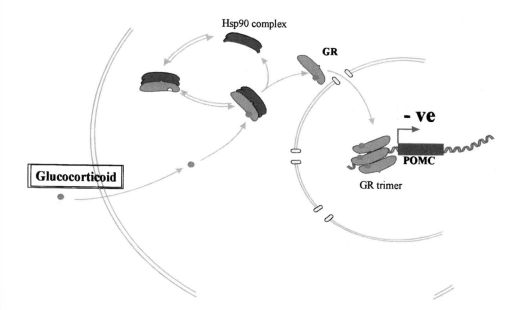

FIGURE 16–5. Glucocorticoid regulation of proopiomelanocortin (POMC). Glucocorticoids activate their receptor (GR) and release it from the heat shock protein (Hsp90) complex, thereby allowing translocation of the GR to the nucleus and binding to the *POMC* gene.

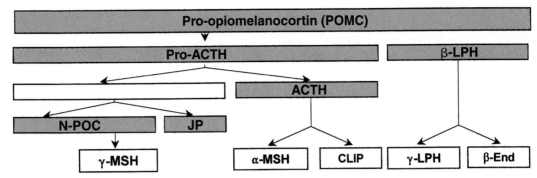

FIGURE 16–6. *Processing of proopiomelanocortin (POMC). POMC is cleaved into pro-adrenocorticotropic hormone (pro-ACTH) and β-lipotropin (βLPH). Further processing of pro-ACTH yields ACTH, joining peptide, and N-proopiomelanocortin (N-POC), all of which are found in human plasma. Cleavage to smaller fragments occurs in a tissue- and species-specific manner. Shaded boxes represent peptides found in the human circulation. CLIP, corticotropin-like intermediate lobe peptide; End, endorphin; JP, joining peptide; LPH, lipotropin; MSH, melanocyte-stimulating hormone.*

a single, unifying molecular mechanism of glucocorticoid resistance in the human small cell lung cancer cell lines remains to be defined.

ADRENOCORTICOTROPIC HORMONE AND RELATED PEPTIDES

Structure and Processing of POMC and Related Peptides

Many bioactive peptides are synthesized from large precursor molecules, and a number of techniques have been used to elucidate the structures of these peptides. Studies have used pulse chase analysis whereby labeled amino acids are incubated with cells to detect the labeled precursors and the peptides derived from them. Subsequently, sequence analysis and cDNA cloning have been important approaches to determine peptide structures. Discovery of the structure and biosynthesis of POMC and ACTH-related peptides and the differences between species is reviewed extensively by Eipper and Mains.[50]

POMC

The recognition that ACTH is synthesized as part of a precursor came in 1973 with the characterization of high-molecular-weight forms of ACTH in human plasma,[51] in mouse pituitary cells,[52, 53] and in human tumors.[54]

Processing of POMC to its constituent peptides varies in a tissue-specific fashion in terms of both the nature and the degree of processing, with the result that different groups of peptides are secreted from different tissues, although the exact details are still not fully understood.

Expression of the *POMC* gene leads to synthesis of the preprohormone POMC. This protein undergoes proteolytic cleavage at dibasic amino acid residues, which generates a series of small molecules, including ACTH[55] (Fig. 16–6).

ACTH

The ACTH peptide consists of 39 amino acids, is a single polypeptide chain, and has a molecular weight of 4.5 kDa (Fig. 16–7). The

N-terminal 12 amino acids are highly conserved between species, thus reflecting the importance of this region for biologic activity. In comparison with the human sequence, ACTH in other mammals has only one or two substitutions, which are in the region of amino acids 24 to 39. In birds, amphibians, and fish, although the N-terminal sequence is conserved, the ACTH sequence is more variable, particularly between amino acids 24 and 39. The melanocyte-stimulating hormone (MSH) sequence His-Phe-Arg-Trp is found at ACTH 6–9, and although this sequence is present in β-lipotropin (as β-MSH) and N-proopiomelanocortin (N-POC) (as γ-MSH), it is thought that the surrounding amino acids influence its specific activity.

α-MELANOCYTE–STIMULATING HORMONE. α-MSH consists of ACTH 1–13, which is N-terminally acetylated and C-terminally amidated. It is derived from ACTH 1–39 by proteolysis. α-MSH is produced by melanotroph cells in the intermediate lobe of the pituitary, particularly in species such as the rat and mouse, but the adult human pituitary does not have a distinct intermediate lobe and α-MSH immunoreactivity in the anterior lobe is quite variable.[56] In addition, it is not clear whether α-MSH circulates in humans under normal circumstances.[57, 58]

CLIP. Corticotropin-like intermediate lobe peptide (CLIP) consists of ACTH 18–39 and is produced during the cleavage that generates α-MSH. Because this process occurs primarily in the intermediate lobe of the pituitary, which is not present in humans, CLIP is not thought to circulate in humans under normal circumstances.

N-Proopiomelanocortin

Also called N-proopiocortin, N-POC (see Fig. 16–6) comes from the N-terminal sequence of POMC, and in humans, it is a 76–amino acid peptide with an MSH sequence in the midregion.[59] The peptide has a tryptophan residue at the N terminus and two disulfide bridges linking cysteines 2 to 24 and 8 to 20, which are thought to be important for the sorting signal that directs POMC to the regulated pathway.[60] N-POC can also undergo N-glycosylation at Asn65 and O-glycosylation at Thr45.

γ-MELANOCYTE–STIMULATING HORMONE. γ₁-MSH comes from position 51 to γ₂ 62 of human N-POC and has sequence homology with α-MSH. γ₂-MSH and γ₃-MSH are C-terminally extended forms of γ₁-MSH.

JOINING PEPTIDE. Joining peptide is found between N-POC

ACTH sequence

	1					6	7	8	9	10			13				17	18			20
	Ser-Tyr-Ser-Met-Glu-His-Phe-Arg-Trp-Gly-Lys-Pro-Val-Gly-Lys-Lys-Arg-Arg-Pro-Val-																				

FIGURE 16–7. *Sequence of human adrenocorticotropic hormone (ACTH).*

					30										39
Lys-Val-Tyr-Pro-Asn-Gly-Ala-Glu-Asp-Glu-Ser-Ala-Glu-Ala-Phe-Pro-Leu-Glu-Phe-OH															

and ACTH and was isolated from human pituitaries in 1981.[59] It is a 30–amino acid peptide and is amidated at the C terminus. Joining peptide has been shown to circulate in humans and is thought to form homodimers.[61]

β-Lipotropin

β-Lipotropin lies at the C terminus of POMC and can be cleaved to γ-lipotropin (which contains the β-MSH sequence at its C terminus) and β-endorphin (see Fig. 16–6). In the human anterior pituitary, cleavage appears to be limited inasmuch as the main form of this peptide in the human circulation is β-lipotropin with very little β-endorphin.[62, 63]

β-ENDORPHIN. This 31–amino acid peptide contains the sequence for met-enkephalin in the first five amino acids at its N terminus. β-Endorphin can undergo *N*-acetylation, which is thought to be a tissue-specific effect, and C-terminally truncated peptides have been found such as α-endorphin (β-endorphin 1–16), γ-endorphin (β-endorphin 1–17), and δ-endorphin (β-endorphin 1–27).

The Processing Pathway and Processing Enzymes

PROCESSING. After translation of the mRNA into peptide, a series of processing stages are needed to achieve release of the constituent peptides.[64] The N-terminal signal sequence that is involved in movement of the peptide into the endoplasmic reticulum is no longer required and is removed at an early phase of posttranslational modification. Subsequently, POMC undergoes glycosylation and phosphorylation in the Golgi apparatus before transport to secretory vesicles, where it undergoes cleavage into its constituent peptides. The ACTH-related peptides are stored in dense core secretory granules and released from the cell in the regulated secretory pathway.

N-GLYCOSYLATION AND PHOSPHORYLATION. These events occur in the Golgi apparatus before cleavage of the peptides. γ-MSH has the sequence Asn-X-Ser, which can be glycosylated on the Asn residue, and in mouse POMC, *N*-glycosylation of the CLIP sequence can occur. Some evidence indicates phosphorylation of the serine[31] in ACTH, although the significance of this finding is unclear.[65]

PROCESSING ENZYMES. POMC is cleaved to its constituent peptides by limited proteolysis at pairs of basic amino acids, primarily Lys-Arg and Arg-Arg. The mammalian convertases responsible for this endoproteolytic cleavage are precursor converting enzymes from the subtilisin/Kex2 serine proteases, which include furin, a protease known to cleave peptides in the constitutive pathway of secretion.[66] Prohormone convertase, or PC1 (also called PC3[67]), cleaves POMC preferentially at two pairs of basic residues and produces ACTH, β-lipotropin, N-POC, and joining peptide, a pattern similar to that found in the anterior pituitary. PC2 cleaves at five pairs of basic residues and releases smaller peptides such as β-endorphin and α-MSH,[68] as observed in the neurointermediate lobe. This arrangement suggests that these convertases work in a tissue-specific fashion. In addition, they are coregulated with POMC in that PC1 mRNA is regulated by CRH and glucocorticoids in mouse AtT20 cells[69] and bromocriptine decreases PC1 and PC2 mRNA in rat neurointermediate lobe cells.[70]

After cleavage at the dibasic amino acids, several peptides (e.g., ACTH 1–17) have amino acids removed from the C terminus by carboxypeptidase E. Subsequently, α-amidation is catalyzed by peptidylglycine α-amidating monooxygenase, an enzyme that has multiple molecular forms, and/or acetylation occurs by the action of specific acetyltransferases.[71]

Processing in Different Tissues

POMC processing varies depending on the species and the tissue. Although POMC is expressed primarily in the pituitary, POMC mRNA has been detected in many extrapituitary tissues. However, such detection does not provide evidence that the peptides are synthesized or secreted there. POMC peptides have been detected by immunocytochemistry or radioimmunoassay of human[22] and rat[72] tissue extracts.

Whether these peptides reach the circulation is debatable, and it is more likely that they act in an autocrine or paracrine role.

Anterior Pituitary

In the human anterior pituitary, POMC is cleaved to give pro-ACTH, which is then cleaved to ACTH, N-POC, and joining peptide (see Fig. 16–6). Interestingly, the ACTH precursors POMC and pro-ACTH are found in the human circulation with ACTH, N-POC, joining peptide, and β-lipotropin.[73] That very little β-endorphin appears to be present indicates that processing of β-lipotropin is minimal (Fig. 16–8). However, reports can be confounded by the fact that in some β-endorphin assays the antibodies also detect β-lipotropin. In the rat and sheep anterior pituitary, some ACTH is processed to des-acetyl-α-MSH and α-MSH.[71]

Studies in mouse pituitary tumor AtT20 cells suggest that cleavage is sequential, starting with the C terminus of ACTH.[50] However, the same pair of basic amino acids is found between ACTH and β-lipotropin, joining peptide and ACTH, ACTH 1–16 and ACTH 17–39, and γ-lipotropin and β-endorphin. Therefore the adjacent amino acids and peptide folding must influence the sequential processing.

Intermediate Lobe

In the rodent intermediate lobe, POMC is found in melanotroph cells and undergoes more comprehensive digestion to give the smaller fragments α-, β-, and γ-MSH, CLIP, and β-endorphin. The protease responsible for this cleavage is PC2. After endopeptidase cleavage, ACTH 1–17 is further modified by an exopeptidase that removes amino acids from the C terminus to give ACTH 1–13. Subsequently, ACTH 1–13 undergoes *N*-acetylation and C-terminal amidation.

Central Nervous System

POMC is produced primarily in the neurons of the hypothalamic arcuate nucleus, median eminence, and ventromedial border of the third ventricle and much smaller amounts in the tractus solitarius. Processing is different in the anterior pituitary, which produces smaller peptides characteristic of the neurointermediate lobe. However, most of the studies are limited to the rat hypothalamus. In these extracts,

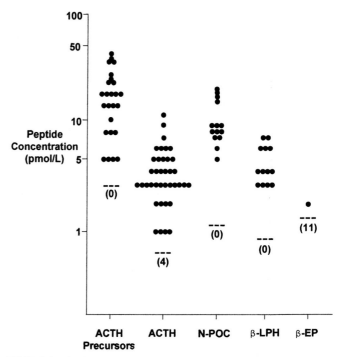

FIGURE 16–8. Concentrations of adrenocorticotropic hormone (ACTH) precursors and derived peptides in the circulation of normal subjects. EP, endorphin; LPH, lipotropin; N-POC, *N*-proopiomelanocortin.

high-performance liquid chromatographic separation of peptides suggests that ACTH is processed to CLIP and that des-acetyl-α-MSH is detected rather than α-MSH, thus indicating that N-terminal acetylation is limited. β-Endorphin 1–31 is the predominant form in the rat hypothalamus, again suggesting more extensive processing.[71, 74]

POMC peptides have also been detected in cerebrospinal fluid (CSF), although whether they originate from the pituitary or hypothalamus is uncertain. In human CSF, the POMC precursor peptide has been shown to occur at high concentrations and predominates over ACTH when molar ratios are compared.[75] However, several of the POMC peptides can be detected in CSF.[76, 77]

Other Tissues

In comparison to the pituitary, other tissues produce very low levels of POMC peptides, with reports in rat tissue extracts of 0.00003% of the levels in the pituitary and no mature ACTH.[22] POMC peptides have been detected in the thyroid, pancreas, gastrointestinal tract, placenta, testis, ovary, adrenal gland, and immune system.[71] POMC peptides are also produced in the skin. α-MSH, the first peptide to be detected, was found by immunostaining to predominate in human melanocytes, but ACTH has also been detected in human keratinocytes.[78] A role for POMC peptides in hair pigmentation is also suggested by two patients with inherited mutations in POMC that prevented synthesis of the ACTH/α-MSH region; both patients had red hair pigmentation.[8]

Pituitary Tumors

In patients with pituitary-dependent Cushing's syndrome, the processing of precursors to ACTH appears to be relatively normal as judged by the molar ratios of these peptides in plasma.[63] However, the molar ratio of precursors to ACTH is much higher for corticotroph macroadenomas, thus suggesting that processing is impaired.[79]

Extrapituitary Tumors

Data on tumor extracts suggest that most extrapituitary tumors causing the ectopic ACTH syndrome do not process the prohormone efficiently. In an early study, analysis of tumor tissue suggested the presence of immunoreactive ACTH, even in the absence of clinical features of hormone excess.[80] The ACTH was present predominantly in a high-molecular-weight form of approximately 20 kDa, but this purified material could be cleaved to mature ACTH (4.5 kDa) by the action of trypsin. Further work identified the presence of immunoreactive ACTH-like peptide in a variety of normal tissues, which suggested that extrapituitary ACTH expression was less "ectopic" than inappropriately regulated. The ACTH immunoreactivity was found to have no biologic activity and was assumed to be due to ACTH precursors.[80]

Evidence that processing is impaired in tumors from patients with the ectopic ACTH syndrome also comes from the elevated levels of ACTH precursors in plasma and the high ratio of precursors to ACTH.[63] Identification of ACTH precursors predominating in the circulation of patients with clinically apparent Cushing's syndrome suggests that these precursors may have some activity at the ACTH receptor or are processed at the adrenal. Most of these patients had clinically obvious small cell carcinoma of the lung. However, patients with highly differentiated, slowly growing tumors, typically bronchial carcinoids, have lower, but nevertheless elevated levels of ACTH precursors.[81] Interestingly, these types of tumors can also give rise to small fragments in the circulation, such as CLIP,[82] thus suggesting that some tumors may process POMC in the manner of the neurointermediate lobe. It is not yet clear whether the same tumors give rise to increased precursors and smaller fragments or whether processing varies in different tumors.

Biologic Activity of ACTH-Related Peptides

ACTH

The major role of ACTH is to stimulate steroidogenesis in the adrenal cortex, which results in the synthesis and release of cortisol in humans and corticosterone in rodents. In pathologic conditions it is evident that ACTH can increase the production of adrenal androgens and aldosterone; however, under physiologic situations these pathways are regulated by other factors. Long-term overexpression of ACTH can cause adrenal cell proliferation,[83, 84] although other POMC-derived peptides have also been implicated in this process. In situations with prolonged ACTH excess such as Nelson's syndrome, Addison's disease, and ectopic ACTH syndrome, skin pigmentation can occur and is thought to be due to ACTH binding through its MSH sequence to melanocortin receptors in the skin, although whether the skin pigmentation results from cleavage of ACTH to MSH peptides is unclear.

ACTH RECEPTORS AND SIGNALING. The ACTH 1–39 sequence is most potent in stimulating steroidogenesis, but ACTH 1–24 is also known to have full agonist activity in certain systems. It is clear that the ACTH 1–13 sequence is involved in binding and activation, but ACTH 6–24 has been shown to have some steroidogenic activity, so the exact role of the N-terminal peptides is less well defined.

ACTH binds to the melanocortin-2 receptor, which has been identified in human adrenal glands,[85, 86] although in rat and ovine adrenocortical cells, high- and low-affinity ACTH binding has been described. Binding of ACTH to human receptors requires calcium[85] and occurs with a K_d of approximately 2.0 nmol/L. However, ACTH at 10 pmol/L causes maximal steroidogenesis, and therefore only a small number of the predicted 3500 sites per cell need to be occupied to achieve this activity.

ACTH receptors are also present on human mononuclear leukocytes and have been identified on other rat and mouse immune cells, which suggests that ACTH may have a role in immune function.

The ACTH receptor is a member of the melanocortin receptor family. The members of this family of receptors all have similar seven-membrane-spanning domains and are G protein coupled.[86] On binding to its receptor, ACTH stimulates cAMP production,[85] and cAMP in turn stimulates a cAMP-dependent protein kinase that activates the steroidogenic pathway. Calcium is also involved in ACTH stimulation of cAMP in human adrenal cells.

Corticostatins, low-molecular-weight inhibitors of ACTH-induced steroidogenesis, are thought to act by preventing ACTH binding to its receptor, although their physiologic role is unclear.

ACTH EFFECTS ON THE ADRENAL. ACTH acts at a number of levels to increase cortisol production. On binding to its receptor, it stimulates lipoprotein uptake, activates hydrolysis of cholesterol, and increases transport of cholesterol to mitochondria. Importantly, ACTH also regulates cholesterol side chain cleavage, which is the rate-limiting step in steroidogenesis and results in the production of pregnenolone. This activity takes place in the inner membrane of the mitochondria and is catalyzed by cytochrome P450 side chain cleavage enzyme.[87]

Longer stimulation by ACTH will eventually result in downregulation of the ACTH receptor, but it is known to cause increased transcription of enzymes in the steroidogenic pathway and can result in adrenal cell proliferation.

α-MELANOCYTE–STIMULATING PEPTIDES. In most mammals, α-MSH is produced in the melanotroph cells of the neurointermediate lobe, but because these cells are absent from the human pituitary, it is unlikely that this peptide has a role as a secreted peptide in humans. In mice, α-MSH causes changes in coat color, and it is known for its ability to affect pigmentation in frog skin. It is also thought that locally produced α-MSH peptides stimulate melanogenesis in human skin.[78]

Des-acetyl-α-MSH is produced in the brain, and α-MSH–related peptides are known to be important in the regulation of energy balance by affecting food intake. However, different peptides may have opposing effects, and most of the studies have been performed in rodents. Reports that an inherited *POMC* deletion is associated with obesity[8] would suggest that POMC-derived peptides do have an important role in body weight regulation.

N-Proopiomelanocortin and Joining Peptide

N-POC has been reported to potentiate ACTH-induced steroidogenesis in human and rat adrenocortical cells, and it is thought that the

γ_3-MSH region may be responsible for this activity. N-POC also stimulates the release of aldosterone from human adrenal tumor cells.[88, 89] In addition, it has been shown that N-POC 1–48 stimulates adrenal growth after unilateral adrenalectomy in the rat, and this demonstration led to the proposal that N-POC 1–48 is an adrenal mitogenic hormone and that cleavage of N-POC occurs at the adrenal gland.[90]

The role of joining peptide is unclear. It has been suggested that it is the adrenal androgen-stimulating hormone, but subsequently, several reports have shown that joining peptide lacks the ability to increase adrenal androgens.[91]

β-Lipotropin and β-Endorphin

β-Lipotropin was named because of its lipolytic activity, and it was suggested that the β-MSH sequence in the midregion was responsible for this activity. Subsequently, most studies have concentrated on this peptide as a precursor of β-endorphin.

Data are conflicting regarding whether β-endorphin circulates in human plasma.[62, 73] It may have a more important role when released locally in the brain because when administered it has opiate-like analgesic activity associated with the met-enkephalin sequence at its N terminus and mice lacking β-endorphin exhibit absence of stress-induced analgesia.[92] β-Endorphin has also been shown to affect sexual behavior and learning.

ACTH Precursors

It has proved difficult to get a clear indication of ACTH precursor bioactivity because of problems in obtaining pure preparations of the peptides and the limitations of available bioassays. POMC itself is thought to have little biologic activity,[80] whereas pro-ACTH was shown to be equipotent with ACTH in a rat adrenal cell bioassay or 8% to 33% as potent in a cytochemical ACTH bioassay.[93] Nothing is currently known about the binding of POMC and pro-ACTH to the ACTH receptor (MC2-R) and the MSH receptors (MC1-R, MC3-R, MC4-R, MC5-R) (see Cone et al.[86]). Because ACTH precursors are present in the circulation at concentrations greater than those of ACTH,[73] it would be valuable to examine the agonist/antagonist activity of the precursors at the human receptors. In patients with pigmentation related to postadrenalectomy Cushing's disease, concentrations of both ACTH and ACTH precursors correlated with pigmentation scores.[94] The interaction of ACTH precursor peptides with the recently cloned receptor MC4-R found exclusively in the brain may also be of interest inasmuch as concentrations of ACTH precursors in CSF are 100-fold those of ACTH (414 vs. 3.2 pmol/L).[75]

Some information regarding in vivo POMC bioactivity can be gained from clinical studies. If patients with the ectopic ACTH syndrome produce ACTH precursors in preference to ACTH,[63] it must either have biologic activity when present at very high levels or be cleaved to ACTH at the level of the adrenal as previously suggested.[90]

Factors Regulating Secretion of ACTH and Related Peptides

Glucocorticoids

Glucocorticoids act in multiple ways to negatively regulate the activity of the HPA axis. These interactions have been grouped into fast, intermediate, and slow feedback, based on the timing of the phenomena.

FAST FEEDBACK. Fast feedback occurs over minutes and is linked to the rate of increase in glucocorticoid concentration. An acute reduction in ACTH release takes place, but fast feedback has no impact on gene expression or peptide synthesis. It appears that the targets of glucocorticoid action are hypothalamic CRH secretion and direct action on the pituitary corticotroph to reduce ACTH release.

INTERMEDIATE FEEDBACK. Intermediate feedback occurs over a few hours (typically maximal at 2 hours in vivo) and again appears to be due to acute inhibition of ACTH and CRH release, with no discernible effect on gene transcription or peptide synthesis.

SLOW FEEDBACK. The slow component is dependent on the concentration and time of exposure and occurs over days. *POMC* gene transcription and POMC peptide synthesis are reduced, but changes in CRH expression are uncertain. Glucocorticoids may also inhibit hypothalamic AVP levels, with an impact on urinary concentrating ability. In addition, glucocorticoids may act at the hippocampus, where their actions are mediated by both the type I receptor (mineralocorticoid receptor) and the type II receptor (glucocorticoid receptor). It appears that the type I receptor, which has higher affinity for cortisol, is important for mediating feedback at basal cortisol concentrations and that the lower-affinity type II receptor mediates feedback by stress levels of cortisol.

Corticotropin-Releasing Hormone

CRH stimulates ACTH secretion from dispersed pituitary cells in a sustained manner, initially causing the release of preformed peptide but simultaneously stimulating peptide synthesis (Fig. 16–9). In humans, a biphasic response to exogenous CRH reflects these two mechanisms of action.[95]

The effects of CRH on the levels of ACTH precursors in the human circulation have been examined only during the petrosal sinus sampling diagnostic test in patients with suspected Cushing's syndrome. In this test, CRH is given intravenously and ACTH peptides are measured in the petrosal sinuses draining the pituitary. In this situation, the increase in ACTH is much greater than the increase in precursors, which suggests that CRH is stimulating release of processed ACTH from secretory granules.[73]

Hypothalamic CRH is subject to regulation by multiple afferent signals and will in turn influence ACTH release. These signals include upregulation by catecholamines via β- and α_1-adrenoceptors, serotonin acting via the 1a and 2 receptors, acetylcholine acting through both muscarinic and nicotinic receptors, and the cytokines interleukin-1 (IL-1) and IL-6, possibly acting by generation of prostaglandins. In addition, CRH expression may be inhibited by glucocorticoids, catecholamines via α_2-receptors, and γ-aminobutyric acid (GABA) released by neuronal input from the hippocampus and amygdala.

Vasopressin

AVP is synthesized in the same cells of the paraventricular nucleus of the hypothalamus as CRH is (see Fig. 16–9). The two peptides are

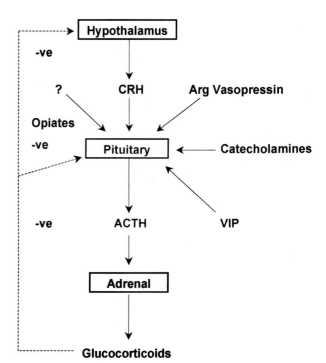

FIGURE 16–9. Factors regulating pituitary secretion of adrenocorticotropic hormone (ACTH)-related peptides. CRH, corticotropin-releasing hormone; VIP, vasoactive intestinal polypeptide.

released from the median eminence into the hypophysial portal system concurrently. In addition, AVP reaches portal blood from the supraoptic nucleus. AVP exerts weak, direct stimulation on ACTH release but powerfully synergizes with CRH. In vivo evidence indicates a role for AVP in stress-induced ACTH secretion.[96, 97] In contrast to CRH, which acts via protein kinase A, AVP acts by stimulation of protein kinase C. AVP also increases the cAMP response to CRH in isolated pituicytes, which suggests multiple sites of interaction between the two signaling cascades.

Neurotransmitters

L-Dopa and serotonin both increase ACTH secretion by means of neuronal release into the paraventricular nucleus of the hypothalamus.[98–100] In contrast, GABA inhibits ACTH when released from hippocampal afferents to the hypothalamus.[101]

Both atrial natriuretic peptide (ANP) and opiate receptor agonists inhibit ACTH release under certain circumstances. ANP has been shown to both increase ACTH secretion from isolated pituicytes and inhibit CRH gene expression. The opiate effects are probably mediated at the hypothalamic or hippocampal level, although it has been reported that met-enkephalin can directly inhibit corticotroph ACTH release.

Cytokines and Growth Factors

INTERLEUKIN-1. IL-1, α and β, are endogenous pyrogenic proteins induced by bacterial endotoxin. The two forms bind to the same receptor, the IL-1 receptor type 1, and display identical biologic activities. IL-1β is released by several cell types, including activated macrophages and monocytes.

The specifics of the action of IL-1 on ACTH release are controversial. Primary cultures of rat pituitary cells responded to IL-1β by increasing secretion of ACTH.[102] However, in the intact rat, although infusion of human IL-1 induced circulating levels of ACTH, this effect appeared to be due to action of the cytokine at the hypothalamus in stimulation of CRH release.[103] In another study using primary rat pituitary cultures, no effects of acute IL-I administration on *POMC* gene transcription or ACTH peptide release were observed. Interestingly, chronic treatment of these cultures with either IL-1α or IL-1β exerted weak induction of ACTH release with no effect on POMC mRNA accumulation.[104] An explanation for these divergent results may be that IL-1 modulates the actions of other ACTH secretogogues, including catecholamines.

INTERLEUKIN-2. IL-2 is a potent immunoregulatory T cell–derived cytokine important in T cell growth and differentiation.[105] Expression of IL-2 mRNA was detected in human corticotroph adenoma cells and in mouse pituitary AtT20 cells.[106] Both human pituitary adenoma cells and AtT20 cells express IL-2 receptor mRNA, and further studies in the rat showed colocalization of the IL-2 receptor with ACTH in primary pituitary cultures.[106]

IL-2 enhances *POMC* gene expression in the pituitary and also enhances ACTH secretion in AtT20 cells and in primary rat pituitary cultures. IL-2, when administered to human subjects during cancer therapy trials, was found to increase circulating β-endorphin and ACTH levels,[107, 108] thus demonstrating a role for IL-2 in activating the HPA axis in vivo.

INTERLEUKIN-6. IL-6 is involved in the terminal differentiation of B cells to antibody-secreting plasma cells, the activation of T cells, and the hepatic synthesis of acute phase proteins.[109, 110] IL-6 is synthesized and secreted by the bovine pituitary folliculostellate cell, which does not express pituitary trophic hormones or their precursors in vitro.[111] In addition, cultured primary rat pituitary cells release IL-6 relatively abundantly,[112] and IL-6 is synthesized by both normal human and neoplastic anterior pituitary tissue.[113–115]

In vivo, IL-6 is a potent stimulus of the HPA axis in humans and probably acts at the hypothalamus to stimulate AVP release and subsequent ACTH induction.[116] Because IL-6 is also present in the circulation, especially during inflammatory stress, the relative importance of locally derived vs. systemically available IL-6 in pituitary function remains to be determined.[117] The potent induction of ACTH

by IL-6 may in fact be of future utility as a diagnostic test for HPA axis function.

LEUKEMIA INHIBITORY FACTOR. LIF was originally isolated as a factor inducing differentiation and suppressing proliferation of the murine monocytic leukemia cell line M1.[118] Specific binding sites for LIF are present in murine AtT20 pituicytes.[119] LIF surface receptors (LIF-Rs) are present in human fetal corticotrophs and somatotrophs, as well as in other functional hormone-producing cells.[119] Pituitary LIF-R mRNA was induced by lipopolysaccharide (LPS) in vivo, although the changes were less pronounced than those observed for LIF mRNA.[120]

LIF action appears to occur principally on the pituitary corticotroph. Primary cultures of mouse pituitary cells respond to added LIF by enhanced ACTH secretion,[121] as do AtT20 murine corticotroph cells.[119, 122] In addition, LIF potentiates the action of CRH to induce ACTH secretion in AtT20 cells.[122] Oncostatin M, a related cytokine with similar receptor signaling, also induces ACTH.[122] LIF action on the corticotroph is blocked by antibodies directed against the gp130 receptor subunit and is also attenuated by dexamethasone. Because the addition of either LIF antiserum, gp130 antiserum, or LIF-R antiserum to AtT20 cultures attenuates endogenous ACTH secretion in the absence of added LIF, it would appear that autocrine or paracrine LIF regulates ACTH expression.[122]

LIF stimulates the JAK/STAT (Janus kinase/signal transducer and activator of transcription) pathway,[122] induces transcription of the *POMC* gene, and very potently synergizes with CRH to enhance POMC expression.[122] Unlike CRH, LIF does not induce cAMP or c-fos; thus it is likely that their synergy occurs distally. It is as yet unclear where the CRH and LIF intracellular signaling pathways interact. Both signaling cascades involve distal *POMC* promoter response elements apposed between −190 and −130 nucleotides upstream from the *POMC* transcription start site. Deletion studies of the *POMC* promoter and specific competitive gel shift assays confirm that the two *POMC* inducers interact directly on the *POMC* gene.[34]

Studies of the HPA axis in mice harboring a disrupted *LIF* transgene (LIF knockout) revealed a defect in activation of the axis in response to stress. Circulating ACTH levels are attenuated after fasting in the knockout animals, and chronic replacement by LIF infusion restores HPA responses to levels seen in wild-type littermates.[123]

Mechanisms Regulating Secretion of ACTH and Related Peptides

Circadian Rhythmicity

The primary "clock" is located in the suprachiasmatic nucleus (Fig. 16–10). Neuronal afferents from this nucleus feed into the paraventricular nucleus of the hypothalamus and regulate CRH expression. The circadian rhythm of ACTH is generated by variation in the amplitude of the pulses rather than variation in pulse frequency. Therefore, the amplitude of ACTH pulses during peak secretion is fourfold higher than during the ACTH nadir. Peak levels of ACTH, and concordantly cortisol, are reached at 6 AM, decline during the day to 4 PM, and then further decline to a nadir between 11 PM and 3 AM. The 6 AM peak is reached after an abrupt increase in ACTH secretion. Although all the circulating POMC peptides show a diurnal variation and peak at the same time, their decline occurs at different rates, probably conferred by different circulatory half-lives and/or variation in extrapituitary processing.

The Stress Response

In response to stress, peripheral and central signals are integrated by the pituitary to modulate adrenal glucocorticoid production. Several lines of evidence suggest a unifying hypothesis linking activation of peripheral cytokine cascades, hypothalamic releasing factors, and intrapituitary cytokine expression with pituitary-mediated modulation of the systemic inflammatory response.

An acute septic insult provokes a local inflammatory response, with coordinated and sequential activation of a series of proinflammatory

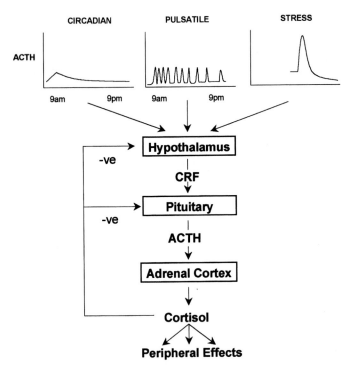

FIGURE 16–10. Mechanisms regulating pituitary secretion of adrenocorticotropic hormone (ACTH) and related peptides. CRF, corticotropin-releasing factor.

cytokines[117, 124, 125] and neural and bacterial toxin signals that activate the HPA axis.[126] Initially, peripheral activation of local and distal tumor necrosis factor (TNF) expression is followed by IL-1, IL-6, and LIF.[117] A number of the proinflammatory cytokines exert most, if not all their activities at the hypothalamus, notably IL-6 acting on hypothalamic AVP[116] and IL-1 and TNF acting on CRH.[103] Others clearly act at the pituitary, notably LIF.[122, 127]

At the hypothalamic level, both circulating and locally derived cytokines enhance expression of the powerful corticotropin-releasing factors CRH and AVP. Hypothalamic LIF mRNA is also upregulated by LPS treatment, especially the diffusible isoform,[120] which suggests regulation of corticotroph function by a hypothalamically released factor.

The pituitary is also a site of de novo cytokine synthesis, and thus in addition to the circulating, peripherally derived cytokines, an intrapituitary network of cytokines is established in the acute phase of septic shock. IL-1β and LIF are upregulated by LPS[120, 128] (a model for gram-negative septic shock), and macrophage migration inhibitory factor is acutely released from pituicytes in vitro and in vivo in response to LPS.[129] Intrapituitary IL-6 is upregulated by IL-1.[117, 130]

Two opposing pituitary responses to septic shock take place. The first involves cytokines such as IL-6 and LIF, which limit the inflammatory response, whereas the second group is associated with enhanced release of proinflammatory factors and increases the lethality of experimental endotoxemia (macrophage migration inhibitory factor[129]). The former group of cytokines causes activation of the HPA axis and increased glucocorticoid production, thus limiting the extent of the inflammatory response and protecting against lethality. The increase in intrapituitary LIF stimulates POMC expression and strongly potentiates CRH action on the corticotroph.[122] The LIF knockout mouse exhibits defective activation of the HPA axis in response to stress,[123] and it is tempting to speculate that the protective action of LIF may in part be mediated by activation of the HPA axis. The key role of HPA activation in conferring resistance to the lethal effects of unrestrained activation of proinflammatory cytokine cascades is underscored by the poor performance of the CRH knockout mouse exposed to endotoxin.[131] IL-1, TNF, and IL-6 have also been shown by some, but not all studies to exert direct effects on pituitary ACTH secretion.[102, 132, 133]

A further level of action of the cytokines is to antagonize the

negative feedback loop of adrenal glucocorticoids on hypothalamic CRH expression and pituitary POMC secretion.[126] The pattern of acute proinflammatory cytokines induced by septic shock opposes effective glucocorticoid signaling,[134, 135] in part by activation of the NF-κB nuclear transcription factor, which inhibits glucocorticoid receptor action.[136–138]

Integrated Control of ACTH Secretion

Three tiers of control subserve the regulation of anterior pituitary hormone secretion (see Figs. 16–9 and 16–10).

TIER 1. Tier 1 consists of central signals from the brain and hypothalamus and includes the hypothalamic release and inhibiting hormones, neurotransmitters, and brain peptides. These molecules traverse the portal venous system in classic endocrine fashion to impinge on their respective distal receptors located on the corticotroph cell surface. These highly differentiated receptors transduce their signals to the cell nucleus, thus determining biosynthesis and ultimate secretion of POMC peptides. The hypothalamic hormones also determine pituitary cell mitotic activity, and clinically, pathologic oversecretion of these hormones results in pituitary hyperplasia and adenoma formation.

TIER II. The second tier of pituitary control consists of an intrapituitary network of cytokines. These molecules provide highly specific unique signals to the pituicyte (e.g., epidermal growth factor regulation of prolactin) or an overlapping redundancy (e.g., interleukin regulation of ACTH). Furthermore, they may often synergize with hypothalamic hormones (e.g., LIF and CRH).

The pituitary factors invariably have dual functions—regulating cell development and replication and controlling differentiated gene expression. These two functions are often subserved independently and may in fact be discordant (e.g., LIF induces *POMC* transcription while blocking corticotroph cell proliferation).

TIER III. The third tier of pituitary control is the peripheral target hormone. Clinically, loss of negative feedback inhibition by target hormones results in pituitary trophic hormone hypersecretion, hyperplasia, and sometimes adenoma formation, as may be encountered in hypoadrenalism. Peripheral hormones may also directly induce pituitary hormone genes.

Measurement of ACTH and Related Peptides

ACTH was one of the first peptides to be measured by radioimmunoassay and presented a significant challenge because of the difficulty in generating high-affinity antisera and in labeling ACTH. The development of sensitive immunoradiometric assays for ACTH has improved the reliability of ACTH measurement.[81, 139] The assays are based on a labeled monoclonal antibody that usually binds within the N-terminal region of ACTH and a solid-phase antibody that recognizes a different sequence in ACTH. Because binding of both antibodies is required to generate a signal, the assay does not recognize MSH or CLIP. However, it is not always clear whether current ACTH assays recognize the ACTH precursors.

Recent years have seen a shift toward the measurement of ACTH by two-site immunometric assays in preference to radioimmunoassay. This change provides many benefits, including improved sensitivity, speed, reproducibility, and parallel results. The high sample throughput and wide working range of these assays make them ideal for measuring samples taken during inferior petrosal sinus sampling, a test that is fast becoming an important component in the diagnosis of pituitary tumors secreting ACTH.

However, we must recognize that in some clinical situations the use of an assay that is highly specific for ACTH 1–39 may be insufficient or misleading. In one patient with the ectopic ACTH syndrome shown by chromatography to be producing high-molecular-weight ACTH precursors, the ACTH concentration was very low when measured by immunoradiometric assay.[139] To ensure that patients with the ectopic ACTH syndrome are flagged by an ACTH assay, it is important that the ACTH precursors have a high degree of cross-reactivity in the

ACTH assay or that a separate specific assay for ACTH precursors be available.

Detection of ACTH precursors in plasma was first demonstrated in normal subjects after stimulation with metyrapone,[140] and it was later observed after insulin-induced hypoglycemia.[141] However, complex chromatographic techniques were required to separate ACTH precursors from ACTH. Clearly, this approach cannot be used for large numbers of patient samples and would not provide a quantitative assessment of the concentrations of ACTH precursors in plasma.

Direct measurement of ACTH precursors was made possible by the development of a two-site immunoradiometric assay for the ACTH precursors POMC and pro-ACTH.[142] The assay is based on a labeled monoclonal antibody that binds within the ACTH region of POMC and a solid-phase antibody that recognizes N-POC (see Fig. 16–1). Because binding of both antibodies is required to generate a signal, the assay does not detect ACTH. With this assay, the concentrations of ACTH precursors in normal subjects were found to be 5 to 40 pmol/L, which is equivalent to or greater than the concentrations of ACTH, N-POC, β-lipotropin, and β-endorphin.[73] Measurement of ACTH precursors in patients with ectopic ACTH syndrome has indicated that the precursors are present at much higher concentrations than is ACTH.[81] A similar approach has been used to measure POMC in aggressive ACTH-secreting tumors.[143]

OTHER POMC-DERIVED PEPTIDES. The development of radioimmunoassays and/or immunoradiometric assay for N-POC, γ-MSH, α-MSH, β-lipotropin, and β-endorphin has proved extremely valuable in understanding the production and action of POMC peptides. The development of specific immunometric assays that distinguish circulating levels of β-lipotropin and β-endorphin has shown that β-lipotropin is the main form in human plasma and that relatively little β-endorphin is secreted.[62] Nevertheless, questions relating to the relative molar ratios of the family of POMC peptides are still unanswered. The relative concentrations of ACTH precursors and ACTH in the circulation will depend not only on regulatory mechanisms influencing expression of the *POMC* gene but also on precursor processing and mechanisms of secretion from the corticotroph cells. Evidence from studies with the mouse corticotroph adenoma cell line AtT20 suggests that in the absence of stimulation, corticotroph cells "leak" newly synthesized POMC.[144] Therefore, the levels of ACTH precursors and constituent peptides in the circulation at any given time could well vary because of the differing regulatory mechanisms.

REFERENCES

1. Bell PH: Purification and structure of beta-corticotropin. J Am Chem Soc 76:5565–5567, 1954.
2. Li CH: Lipotropin, a new active peptide from pituitary glands. Nature 201:924, 1964.
3. Li CH: Isolation, characterization and opiate activity of beta-endorphin from human pituitary glands. Biochem Biophys Res Commun 72:1542–1547, 1976.
4. Eipper BA, Mains RE: Analysis of the common precursor to corticotropin and endorphin. J Biol Chem 253:5732–5744, 1978.
5. Inoue A, Kita T, Nakamura M, et al: Nucleotide sequence of cloned cDNA for bovine corticotropin– β-lipotropin precursor. Nature 278:423–427, 1979.
6. Vale W, Spiess J, Rivier C, Rivier J: Characterization of a 41-residue ovine hypothalamic peptide that stimulates secretion of corticotropin and beta endorphin. Science 213:1394–1397, 1981.
7. Mountjoy KG, Robbins LS, Mortrud MT, Cone RD: The cloning of a family of genes that encode the melanocortin receptors. Science 257:1248–1251, 1992.
8. Krude H, Biebermann H, Luck W, et al: Severe early-onset obesity, adrenal insufficiency and red hair pigmentation caused by POMC mutations in humans. Nat Genet 19:155–157, 1998.
9. Takahashi H, Teranishi Y, Nakanishi S, Numa S: Isolation and structural organisation of the human corticotropin–beta-lipotropin precursor gene. FEBS Lett 135:97–102, 1981.
10. Cochet M, Chang ACY, Cohen SN: Characterisation of the structural gene and putative 5′ regulatory sequences for human proopiomelanocortin. Nature 297:335–339, 1982.
11. Whitfield PL, Shire J: The human proopiomelanocortin gene: Organisation sequence and interspersion with repetitive DNA. DNA 1:133–143, 1982.
12. White A, Clark AJL, Stewart MF: The synthesis of ACTH and related peptides by tumours. Baillieres Clin Endocrinol Metab 4:1–27, 1990.
13. Jingami H, Nakanishi S, Numa S: Tissue distribution of messenger RNAs coding for opioid peptide precursors and related RNA. Eur J Biochem 142:441–447, 1984.
14. Jeannotte L, Trifiro MA, Plante RK, et al: Tissue specific activity of the pro-opiomelanocortin gene promoter. Mol Biol Cell 7:4058–4064, 1987.
15. Roberts JL, Lundblad JR, Eberwine JH: Hormonal regulation of *POMC* gene expression in the pituitary. Ann N Y Acad Sci 512:275–285, 1988.

16. Tremblay Y, Tretjakoff I, Peterson A, et al: Pituitary specific expression and glucocorticoid regulation of a proopiomelanocortin fusion gene in transgenic mice. Proc Natl Acad Sci U S A 85:8890–8894, 1988.
17. Hammer GD, Fairchild-Huntress V, Low MJ: Pituitary specific and hormonally regulated gene expression directed by the rat proopiomelanocortin promoter in transgenic mice. Mol Endocrinol 4:1689–1697, 1990.
18. Therrien M, Drouin J: Cell-specific helix-loop-helix factor required for pituitary expression of the proopiomelanocortin gene. Mol Cell Biol 13:2342–2353, 1993.
19. Lundblad JR, Roberts JL: Regulation of proopiomelanocortin gene expression in pituitary. Endocr Rev 9:135–158, 1988.
20. White A, Clark AJL: The cellular and molecular basis of the ectopic ACTH syndrome. Clin Endocrinol 39:131–141, 1993.
21. Chen C-LC, Chang AC, Krieger DT, Bardin CW: Expression and regulation of pro-opiomelanocortin–like gene in the ovary and placenta: Comparison with the testis. Endocrinology 118:2382–2389, 1986.
22. DeBold CR, Menefee JK, Nicholson WE, Orth DN: Pro-opiomelanocortin gene is expressed in many normal human tissues and in tumours not associated with ectopic ACTH syndrome. Mol Endocrinol 2:862–870, 1988.
23. Lacaze-Masmonteil T, de Keyzer Y, Luton JP, Kahn A: Characterization of POMC transcripts in human non-pituitary tissues. Proc Natl Acad Sci U S A 84:7261–7265, 1987.
24. Buzzetti R, McLoughlin L, Lavender PM, et al: Expression of proopiomelanocortin gene and quantification of adrenocorticotrophic hormone–like immunoreactivity in human normal peripheral mononuclear cells and lymphoid and myeloid malignancies. J Clin Invest 83:733–737, 1989.
25. de Keyzer Y, Lenne F, Girard F, et al: Altered proopiomelanocortin gene expression in ACTH-producing non-pituitary tumours. J Clin Invest 76:1892–1898, 1985.
26. de Keyzer Y, Kahn A: Variable modes of proopiomelanocortin gene transcription in human tumours. Mol Endocrinol 3:215–223, 1989.
27. de Keyzer Y, Rousseau-Merck M-F, Girard F, Kahn A: Proopiomelanocortin gene expression in human phaeochromocytomas. J Mol Endocrinol 2:175–181, 1989.
28. Texier PL, de Keyzer Y, Lacave R, et al: Pro-opiomelanocortin gene expression in normal tumoral human lung. J Clin Endocrinol Metab 73:414–420, 1991.
29. Nakai Y, Nakao K: Adrenocorticotropic hormone and related peptides in human tissue. In Black PM (ed): Secretory Tumours of the Pituitary Gland. New York, Raven, 1984, pp 227–243.
30. De Bold AC, Nicholson WE: Immunoreactive proopiomelanocortin (POMC) peptides and POMC-like messenger ribonucleic acid are present in many rat nonpituitary tissues. Endocrinology 66:6:2648, 1988.
31. Birnberg NC, Lissitsky J-C, Hinman M, Herbert E: Glucocorticoids regulate proopiomelanocortin gene expression in vivo at the levels of transcription and secretion. Proc Natl Acad Sci U S A 80:6982–6986, 1983.
32. Boutellier AL, Sassone-Corsi P, Loeffler JP: The protooncogene c-fos is induced by CRF and stimulates POMC gene transcription in pituitary cells. Mol Endocrinol 5:1301–1310, 1991.
33. Jin WD, Boutellier AL, Glucksman MJ, et al: Characterization of a CRH-responsive element in the rat proopiomelanocortin gene promoter and molecular cloning of its binding protein. Mol Endocrinol 8:1377–1399, 1994.
34. Bousquet C, Ray DW, Melmed S: A common proopiomelanocortin binding element mediates leukemia inhibitory factor and corticotrophin releasing hormone transcriptional synergy. J Biol Chem 272:10551–10557, 1997.
35. Eberwine JH, Roberts JL: Glucocorticoid regulation of pro-opiomelanocortin gene transcription in the rat pituitary. J Biol Chem 259:2166–2170, 1984.
36. Gagner JP, Drouin J: Opposite regulation of pro-opiomelanocortin gene transcription by glucocorticoids and CRH. Mol Cell Endocrinol 40:25–32, 1985.
37. Israel A, Cohen SN: Hormonally mediated negative regulation of human pro-opiomelanocortin gene expression after transfection into mouse L-cells. Mol Cell Biol 5:2443–2453, 1985.
38. Fremeau RT, Lundblad JR, Pritchett DB, et al: Regulation of pro-opiomelanocortin gene transcription in individual cell nuclei. Science 234:1265–1269, 1986.
39. Eberwine JH, Jonassen JA, Evinger MJQY, Roberts JL: Complex transcriptional regulation by glucocorticoid and corticotropin-releasing hormones of pro-opiomelanocortin gene expression in rat pituitary cultures. DNA 6:483–492, 1987.
40. Riegel AT, Ly Y, Remenick J, et al: Proopiomelanocortin gene promoter elements required for constitutive and glucocorticoid repressed transcription. Mol Endocrinol 5:1973–1982, 1991.
41. Drouin J, Sun YL, Chamberland M, et al: Novel glucocorticoid receptor complex with DNA element of the hormone-repressed POMC gene. EMBO J 12:145–156, 1993.
42. Smoak B, Deuster P, Rabin D, Chrousos G: Corticotropin releasing hormone is not the sole factor mediating exercise induced adrenocorticotropin release in humans. J Clin Endocrinol Metab 73:320–306, 1991.
43. Abou-Samra AB, Harwood JP, Manganiello VC, et al: Phorbol 12-myristate-13-acetate and vasopressin potentiate the effect of corticotropin-releasing factor on cyclic AMP production in rat anterior pituitary cells. J Biol Chem 262:1129–1136, 1987.
44. Malchoff D, Abboud C, Carney JA, et al: Ectopic ACTH syndrome caused by a bronchial carcinoid tumour responsive to dexamethasone, metyrapone, and corticotrophin-releasing factor. Am J Med 84:760–764, 1988.
45. Kubo M, Nakagawa K, Akikawa K, et al: In vivo and in vitro ACTH response to ovine corticotropin releasing factor in a bronchial carcinoid from a patient with ectopic ACTH. Endocrinol Jpn 42:577–581, 1985.
46. Suda T, Tozawa F, Dobashi I, et al: Corticotropin-releasing hormone, proopiomelanocortin, and glucocorticoid receptor gene expression in adrenocorticotropin-producing tumours in vitro. J Clin Invest 92:2790–2795, 1993.
47. Liddle GW, Nicholson WF, Island DP, et al: Clinical and laboratory studies of ectopic tumoral syndromes. Recent Prog Horm Res 25:283–305, 1969.
48. Gaitan D, DeBold CR, Turney M, et al: Glucocorticoid receptor structure and function in an adrenocorticotropin-secreting small cell lung cancer. Mol Endocrinol 9:1193–1201, 1995.

49. Ray DW, Littlewood AC, Clark AJL, et al: Human small cell lung carcinoma cell lines expressing the proopiomelanocortin gene have aberrant glucocorticoid receptor function. J Clin Invest 93:1625–1630, 1994.

50. Eipper BA, Mains RE: Structure and biosynthesis of pro-adrenocorticotropin/endorphin and related peptides. Endocr Rev 1:1–27, 1980.

51. Yalow RS, Berson SA: Characteristics of "big ACTH" in human plasma and pituitary extracts. J Clin Endocrinol Metab 36:415–423, 1973.

52. Orth DN, Nicholson WE, Mitchell WM, et al: ACTH and MSH production by a single cloned mouse pituitary tumour cell line. Endocrinology 92:385, 1973.

53. Eipper BA, Mains RE: High molecular weight forms of adrenocorticotropic hormone in the mouse pituitary and in a mouse pituitary cell line. Biochemistry 14:3836, 1975.

54. Lowry PJ, Rees LH, Tomlin S, et al: Chemical characterization of ectopic ACTH purified from a malignant thymic carcinoid tumour. J Clin Endocrinol Metab 43:831, 1976.

55. Daughaday WH, Rotwein P: Insulin-like growth factors I and II. Peptide, messenger ribonucleic acid and gene structures, serum, and tissue concentrations. Endocr Rev 10:68–91, 1989.

56. Coates PJ, Doniach I, Hale AC, Rees LH: The distribution of immunoreactive alpha-melanocyte–stimulating hormone cells in the adult human pituitary gland. J Endocrinol 111:335–342, 1986.

57. Croughs RJM, Thijssen JHH, Mol JA: Absence of detectable immunoreactive alpha melanocyte stimulating hormone in plasma in various types of Cushing's disease. J Endocrinol Invest 14:197–200, 1991.

58. Kortlandt W, De Rotte AA, Arts CJM, et al: Characterization of alpha-MSH–like immunoreactivity in human plasma. Acta Endocrinol (Copenh) 113:175–180, 1986.

59. Seidah NG, Chretien M: Complete amino acid sequence of a human pituitary glycopeptide: An important maturation product of proopiomelanocortin. Proc Natl Acad Sci U S A 78:4236, 1981.

60. Cool DR, Fenger M, Snell CR, Loh YP: Identification of the sorting signal motif within pro-opiomelanocortin for the regulated secretory pathway. J Biol Chem 270:8723–8729, 1995.

61. Camus F, Lenne F, Girard F, Luton JP: Human joining peptide: A proopiomelanocortin product secreted as a homodimer. Mol Endocrinol 2:1108–1114, 1988.

62. Gibson S, Crosby SR, White A: Discrimination between beta-endorphin and beta-lipotrophin in human plasma using two-site immunoradiometric assays. Clin Endocrinol 39:445–453, 1993.

63. Stewart PM, Gibson S, Crosby SR, et al: ACTH precursors characterize the ectopic ACTH syndrome. Clin Endocrinol 40:199–204, 1994.

64. Wilson H, White A: Prohormones: Their clinical relevance. Trends Endocrinol Metab 9:396–402, 1998.

65. Mountjoy KG, Wong J: Obesity, diabetes and functions for proopiomelanocortin-derived peptides. Mol Cell Endocrinol 128:171–177, 1996.

66. Steiner DF: The proprotein convertases. Curr Opin Chem Biol 2:31–39, 1998.

67. Thomas L, Leduc R, Thorne BA, et al: Kex2-like endoproteases PC2 and PC3 accurately cleave a model prohormone in mammalian cells: Evidence for a common core of neuroendocrine processing enzymes. Proc Natl Acad Sci U S A 88:5297–5301, 1991.

68. Benjannet S, Rondeau N, Day R: PC1 and PC2 are proprotein convertases capable of cleaving proopiomelanocortin at distinct pairs of basic residues. Proc Natl Acad Sci U S A 88:3564–3568, 1991.

69. Bloomquist BT, Eipper BA, Mains RE: Prohormone converting enzymes: Regulation and evaluation of function using antisense RNA. Mol Endocrinol 91:2014–2024, 1991.

70. Day R, Schafer MKH, Watson SJ, Seidah NG: Distribution and regulation of the prohormone convertases PC1 and PC2 in the rat pituitary. Mol Endocrinol 92:484–497, 1992.

71. Smith AI, Funder JW: Proopiomelanocortin processing in the pituitary, central nervous system, and peripheral tissues. Endocr Rev 9:159–179, 1988.

72. Saito E, Odell WD: Corticotropin/lipotropin common precursor-like material in normal rat extrapituitary tissues. Proc Natl Acad Sci U S A 80:3792–3796, 1983.

73. Gibson S, Crosby SR, Stewart MF, et al: Differential release of proopiomelanocortin-derived peptides from the human pituitary: Evidence from a panel of two-site immunoradiometric assays. J Clin Endocrinol Metab 78:835–841, 1994.

74. Castro MG, Morrison E: Post-translational processing of proopiomelanocortin in the pituitary and in the brain. Crit Rev Neurobiol 11:35–57, 1997.

75. Tsigos C, Crosby SR, Gibson S, et al: Proopiomelanocortin is the predominant adrenocorticotropin-related peptide in human cerebrospinal fluid. J Clin Endocrinol Metab 76:620–624, 1993.

76. Nakao K, Oki S, Tanaka I: Immunoreactive beta-endorphin and adrenocorticotropin in human cerebrospinal fluid. J Clin Invest 66:1383–1390, 1980.

77. McLoughlin L, Lowry PJ, Ratter SJ, et al: Characterisation of the proopiocortin family of peptides in human cerebrospinal fluid. Neuroendocrinology 32:209–212, 1981.

78. Thody AJ, Graham A: Does alpha-MSH have a role in regulating skin pigmentation in humans? Pigment Cell Res 11:265–274, 1998.

79. Gibson S, Crosby SR, Dornan TL, et al: Impaired processing of proopiomelanocortin in corticotroph macroadenomas. J Clin Endocrinol Metab 81:497–502, 1996.

80. Odell WD: Ectopic ACTH syndrome: A misnomer. Endocrinol Metab Clin North Am 20:371–379, 1991.

81. White A, Gibson S: ACTH precursors: Biological significance and clinical relevance. Clin Endocrinol 48:251–255, 1998.

82. Vieau D, Massias JF, Girard F, Bertagna X: Corticotrophin-like intermediary lobe peptide as a marker of alternate pro-opiomelanocortin processing in ACTH-producing non-pituitary tumours. Clin Endocrinol 31:691–700, 1989.

83. Dallman MF, Akana SF, Cascio CS, et al: Regulation of ACTH secretion: Variations on a theme of B. Recent Prog Horm Res 43:113–173, 1987.

84. Dallman MF, Makara GB, Roberts JL, et al: Corticotrope response to removal of releasing factors and corticosteroids in vivo. Endocrinology 117:2190–2197, 1985.

85. Catalano RD, Stuve L, Ramachandran J: Characterization of corticotrophin receptors in human adrenocortical cells. J Clin Endocrinol Metab 62:300–304, 1986.

86. Cone RD, Ly D, Koppula S, et al: The melanocortin receptors: Agonists, antagonists, and the hormonal control of pigmentation. Recent Prog Horm Res 51:287–317, 1996.

87. Miller WL: Molecular biology of steroid hormone synthesis. Endocr Rev 9:295–318, 1988.

88. Al-Dujaili EAS, Hope J, Estivariz FE, et al: Circulating human pituitary pro-γ-melanotropin enhances the adrenal response to ACTH. Nature 291:156–159, 1981.

89. Rochemont J, Hamelin J: The missing fragment of the pro-sequence of human pro-opiomelanocortin: Sequence and evidence for C-terminal amidation. Biochem Biophys Res Commun 102:710–716, 1981.

90. Lowry PJ, Silas L, McLean C, et al: Pro-γ-melanocyte–stimulating hormone cleavage in adrenal gland undergoing compensatory growth. Nature 306:70–73, 1983.

91. Robinson P, Bateman A, Mulay S, et al: Isolation and characterization of three forms of joining peptide from adult human pituitaries: Lack of adrenal androgen-stimulating activity. Endocrinology 129:859–867, 1991.

92. Rubinstein M, Mogil JS, Japon M, et al: Absence of opioid stress-induced analgesia in mice lacking beta-endorphin by site-directed mutagenesis. Proc Natl Acad Sci U S A 93:3995–4000, 1996.

93. Ratter SJ, Gillies G, Hope J, et al: Pro-opiomelanocortin related peptides in human pituitary and ectopic ACTH secreting tumours. Clin Endocrinol 18:211–218, 1983.

94. Gibson S, Crosby SR, Davies D, et al: Elevated levels of adrenocorticotropin (ACTH) precursors in post-adrenalectomy Cushing's disease and their regulation by glucocorticoids. J Clin Endocrinol Metab 80:2430–2436, 1995.

95. DeBold CR, Decherney GS, Jackson RV: Effect of synthetic ovine corticotropin-releasing factor: Prolonged duration of action and biphasic response of plasma adrenocorticotropin and cortisol. J Clin Endocrinol Metab 57:294–298, 1983.

96. Whitnall MH: Regulation of the hypothalamic corticotropin-releasing hormone neurosecretory system. Prog Neurobiol 40:573–629, 1993.

97. Guillaume V, Conte-Devolx B, Magnan E: Effect of chronic active immunization with antiarginine vasopressin on pituitary-adrenal function in sheep. Endocrinology 130:3007–3014, 1992.

98. Elias AN, Valenta LJ, Szekeres AV, Grossman MK: Regulatory role of gamma-aminobutyric acid in pituitary hormone secretion. Psychoneuroendocrinology 7:15–30, 1982.

99. Hornby PJ, Piekut DT: Opiocortin and catecholamine input to CRF-immunoreactive neurons in rat forebrain. Peptides 10:1139–1146, 1989.

100. Fish HR, Chernow B, O'Brian JT: Endocrine and neurophysiologic responses of the pituitary to insulin-induced hypoglycemia: A review. Metabolism 35:763–780, 1986.

101. Koenig JI: Pituitary gland: Neuropeptides, neurotransmitters and growth factors. Toxicol Pathol 17:256–265, 1989.

102. Bernton EW, Beach JE, Holaday JW, et al: Release of multiple hormones by a direct action of interleukin-1 on pituitary cells. Science 238:652–654, 1987.

103. Sapolsky R, Rivier C, Yamamoto G, et al: Interleukin-I stimulates the secretion of hypothalamic corticotropin-releasing factor. Science 238:522–524, 1987.

104. Suda T, Tozawa F, Ushiyama T: Effects of protein kinase C related adrenocorticotrophin secretogogues and interleukin-I on proopiomelanocortin gene expression in rat anterior pituitary cells. Endocrinology 124:1444–1449, 1989.

105. Roberts JL: Interleukin-2: The molecule and its function. Immunol Today 5:203–209, 1984.

106. Arzt E, Stelzer G, Renner U, et al: Interleukin-2 and interleukin-receptor expression in human corticotrophic adenoma and mouse pituitary cell cultures. J Clin Invest 90:1944–1951, 1992.

107. Lotze MT, Frana LW, Sharrow SO, et al: In vivo administration of purified human interleukin 2. I. Half-life and immunologic effects of the Jurkat cell line derived–interleukin 2. J Immunol 134:157–166, 1985.

108. Denicoff KD, Durkin TM, Lotze MT: The neuroendocrine effects of interleukin 2 treatment. Clin Endocrinol Metab 69:402–410, 1989.

109. Kishimoto T, Hirano T: Molecular regulation of B lymphocyte response. Annu Rev Immunol 6:485, 1988.

110. Snick JV: Interleukin-6: An overview. Annu Rev Immunol 8:253–278, 1990.

111. Vankelecom H, Carmeliet P, Van Damme J, et al: Production of interleukin-6 by folliculostellate cells of the anterior pituitary gland in a histiotypic cell aggregate culture system. Neuroendocrinology 49:102–106, 1989.

112. Spangelo BL, MacLeod RM, Isakson PC: Production of interleukin-6 by anterior pituitary cells in-vitro. Endocrinology 126:582, 1990.

113. Jones TH, Justice S, Price A, Chapman K: Interleukin-6 secreting human pituitary adenomas in vitro. J Clin Endocrinol Metab 73:207–209, 1991.

114. Tsagarakis S, Kontogeorgos G, Giannou P: Interleukin-6, a growth promoting cytokine, is present in human pituitary adenomas: An immunocytochemical study. Clin Endocrinol 37:163–167, 1992.

115. Jones TH, Daniels M, James RA, et al: Production of bioactive and immunoreactive interleukin-6 (IL-6) and expression of IL-6 messenger ribonucleic acid by human pituitary adenomas. J Clin Endocrinol Metab 78:180–187, 1994.

116. Mastorakos G, Weber JS, Magiakou MA, et al: Hypothalamic-pituitary-adrenal axis activation and stimulation of systemic vasopressin secretion by recombinant interleukin-6 in humans: Potential implications for the syndrome of inappropriate vasopressin secretion. J Clin Endocrinol Metab 79:934–939, 1994.

117. Fong Y, Moldawer LL, Marano M: Endotoxemia elicits increased circulating beta2-IFN/IL-6 in man. J Immunol 142:2321–2324, 1989.

118. Tomida M, Yamamoto-Yamaguchi M, Hozumi M: Purification of a factor inducing differentiation of mouse myeloid leukemic M1 cells from conditioned medium of mouse fibroblast L929 cells. J Biol Chem 259:10978–10982, 1984.

119. Akita S, Webster J, Ren SG, et al: Human and murine pituitary expression of leukemia inhibitory factor: Novel intrapituitary regulation of adrenocorticotrophin synthesis and secretion. J Clin Invest 95:1288–1298, 1995.

120. Wang Z, Ren SG, Melmed S: Hypothalamic and pituitary leukemia inhibitory factor gene expression in vivo: A novel endotoxin-inducible neuro-endocrine interface. Endocrinology 137:2947–2953, 1996.

121. Stefana B, Ray DW, Melmed S: Leukemia inhibitory factor (LIF) induces differentiation of pituitary corticotroph function: A neuro-endocrine phenotypic switch. Proc Natl Acad Sci U S A 93:12502–12506, 1996.

122. Ray DW, Ren SG, Melmed S: Leukemia inhibitory factor (LIF) stimulates proopiomelanocortin (POMC) expression in a corticotroph cell line. J Clin Invest 97:1852–1859, 1996.

123. Akita S, Malkin J, Melmed S: Disrupted murine leukemia inhibitory factor (LIF) gene attenuates adrenocorticotropic hormone (ACTH) secretion. Endocrinology 137:3140–3143, 1996.

124. Hesse DG, Tracey KJ, Fong Y: Cytokine appearance in human endotoxemia and primate bacteremia. Surg Gynecol Obstet 166:147–153, 1988.

125. Van Deveter SJH, Buller HR, ten Cate JW, et al: Experimental endotoxemia in humans: Analysis of cytokine release and coagulation, fibrolytic and complement pathways. Blood 76:2500–2526, 1990.

126. Chrousos GP: The hypothalamic-pituitary-adrenal axis and immune-mediated inflammation. N Engl J Med 332:1351–1362, 1995.

127. Ray DW, Stefana B, Zand O, Melmed S: Leukemia inhibitory factor: A potent modulator of CRH action on pituitary corticotroph cells. *In* Proceedings of the Annual Meeting of the Endocrine Society. San Francisco, 1996, p 3:532.

128. Takao T, Culp SG, De Souza EB: Reciprocol modulation of interleukin 1 beta and interleukin-I receptors by lipopolysaccharide (endotoxin) treatment in the mouse brain-endocrine-immune axis. Endocrinology 132:1497–1504, 1993.

129. Bernhagen J, Calandra T, Mitchell RA, et al: MIF is a pituitary-derived cytokine that potentiates lethal endotoxaemia. Nature 365:756–959, 1993.

130. Yamaguchi M, Matsuzaki N, Hirota K, et al: Interleukin-6 possibly induced by interleukin-1 in the pituitary gland stimulates the release of gonadotrophins and prolactin. Acta Endocrinol (Copenh) 122:201–205, 1990.

131. Muglia L, Jacobson L, Dikkes P, Majzoub JA: Corticotrophin-releasing hormone deficiency reveals major fetal but not adult glucocorticoid need. Nature 373:427–432, 1995.

132. Spangelo BL, Judd AM, Isakson PC, MacLeod RM: Interleukin-6 stimulates anterior pituitary hormone release in vitro. Endocrinology 125:575–577, 1989.

133. Milenkovic L, Rettori V, Snyder GD, et al: Cachectin alters pituitary hormone release by a direct action in vitro. Proc Natl Acad Sci U S A 86:2418–2422, 1989.

134. Almawi WY, Lupman ML, Stevens AR, et al: Abrogation of glucocorticoid-mediated inhibition of T cell proliferation by the synergistic actions of IL-6 and IFN-gamma. J Immunol 146:3523–3527, 1991.

135. Kam JC, Szeffer SJ, Surs W, et al: Combination IL-2 and IL-4 reduces glucocorticoid receptor-binding affinity and T cell response to glucocorticoids. J Immunol 151:3460–3466, 1993.

136. Scheinman RI, Gualberto A, Jewell CM, et al: Characterization of mechanisms involved in transrepression of NF-kappa B by activated glucocorticoid receptors. Mol Cell Biol 15:943–953, 1995.

137. Caldenhoven E, Liden J, Wissink S, et al: Negative cross-talk between Re1A and the glucocorticoid receptor: A possible mechanism for the anti-inflammatory action of glucocorticoids. Mol Endocrinol 9:401–412, 1995.

138. Ray A, Prefontaine KE: Physical association and functional antagonism between the p65 subunit of transcription factor NK-kappa B and the glucocorticoid receptor. Proc Natl Acad Sci U S A 91:752–756, 1994.

139. Raff H, Findling JW: A new immunoradiometric assay for corticotrophin evaluated in normal subjects and patients with Cushing's syndrome. Clin Chem 35:596–600, 1989.

140. Yalow RS, Berson SA: Size heterogeneity of immunoreactive human ACTH in plasma and in extracts of pituitary glands and ACTH-producing thymomas. Biochem Biophys Res Commun 44:439–445, 1971.

141. Hale AC, Besser GM: Characterisation of proopiomelanocortin-derived peptides in pituitary and ectopic adrenocorticotrophin-secreting tumours. J Endocrinol 108:49–56, 1986.

142. Crosby SR, Stewart MF, Ratcliffe JG, White A: Direct measurement of the precursors of adrenocorticotrophin in human plasma by two-site immunoradiometric assay. J Clin Endocrinol Metab 67:1271–1277, 1988.

143. Raffin-Sanson M-L, Massias J-F, Dumont C, et al: High plasma proopiomelanocortin in aggressive adrenocorticotrophin-secreting tumours. J Clin Endocrinol Metab 81:4272–4277, 1996.

144. Kelly RB: Pathways of protein secretion in eukaryotes. Science 230:25–32, 1985.

Chapter 17

Endocrine and Other Biologic Rhythms

Eve Van Cauter ▪ Georges Copinschi ▪ Fred W. Turek

MAJOR MECHANISMS CONTROLLING ENDOCRINE RHYTHMS

A prominent feature of the endocrine system is its high degree of temporal organization. Indeed, far from obeying the concept of "constancy of the internal milieu," circulating hormonal levels undergo pronounced temporal oscillations ranging in period from a few minutes to a year. This intricate temporal organization provides the endocrine system with remarkable flexibility. Not only can specific physiologic processes be turned on and off depending on the presence or absence of a particular hormone but the precise pattern of hormonal release may provide specific signaling information.

Hormonal variations in the circadian (i.e., approximately once per 24 hours) and ultradian (i.e., once per 1 to 2 hours) ranges are ubiquitous in endocrine systems. However, the whole spectrum of endocrine rhythms includes both higher and lower frequency ranges. Indeed, secretory oscillations with periods in the 5- to 15-minute range have been observed for a number of hormones. The menstrual cycle and seasonal rhythms belong to the so-called infradian range, corresponding to periods longer than the circadian range.

As schematically illustrated in Figure 17–1, the temporal variability and organization of hormonal concentrations during the 24-hour cycle ultimately result from the activity of two interacting timekeeping mechanisms in the central nervous system: endogenous circadian rhythmicity and sleep-wake homeostasis. While this dual control was first demonstrated for hormones of the hypothalamic-pituitary axis, a similar regulation appears to apply to other endocrine subsystems. In mammals, endogenous circadian rhythmicity is generated by a pacemaker located in the paired suprachiasmatic nucleus (SCN) of the hypothalamus.[1] Sleep-wake homeostasis is an hourglass-like mechanism relating the amount and quality of sleep to the duration of prior wakefulness.[2]

The first two sections of this chapter provide an overview of current concepts and recent advances in the fields of circadian and ultradian

rhythms. General properties, physiologic significance, and medical implications are presented in a broad context. Methodologic aspects specific to the study of hormonal rhythms in human subjects are described in the third section. The last section summarizes the present state of knowledge on circadian and ultradian endocrine rhythms in

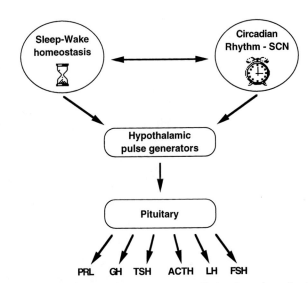

FIGURE 17–1. Schematic representation of the central mechanisms involved in the control of temporal variations in pituitary hormone secretions over the 24-hour cycle. Sleep-wake homeostasis is an hourglass-like mechanism relating the propensity for deep non–rapid eye movement (NREM) sleep to the amount of prior wakefulness. Circadian rhythmicity is an endogenous near–24-hour oscillation generated in the suprachiasmatic nuclei (SCN) of the hypothalamus and transmitted via neural as well as humoral mechanisms.

health and disease for some of the major endocrine axes. Owing to limitations on the length and scope of this chapter, this review is limited to findings in adults.

CIRCADIAN RHYTHMS

General Characteristics

Endogenous Nature

One of the most obvious characteristics of life on earth is the ability of almost all species to change their behavior on a daily or 24-hour basis. A remarkable feature of these daily rhythms is that they are not simply a response to the 24-hour changes in the physical environment imposed by the principles of celestial mechanics, but instead arise from an internal timekeeping system.[1] Under laboratory conditions devoid of any external time-giving cues, it has indeed been found that nearly all 24-hour rhythms continue to be expressed. However, under such constant conditions, the period of the rhythm rarely remains exactly 24 hours but instead is "about" 24 hours and this is why these rhythms are referred to as "circadian," from the Latin *circa dies*, meaning "about a day." When a circadian rhythm is expressed in the absence of any 24-hour signals in the external environment, it is said to be "free-running." Figure 17–2 provides an example of the circadian rhythm of locomotor activity in a male golden hamster held under free-running conditions for 100 days. Strictly speaking, a diurnal rhythm should not be referred to as "circadian" until it has been demonstrated that such a rhythm persists under constant environmental conditions. The purpose of this distinction is to separate out those rhythms that are simply a response to 24-hour changes in the environment from those that are endogenous. However, for practical purposes, there is little reason to make a distinction between "diurnal" and "circadian" rhythms since almost all diurnal rhythms are largely endogenous. In this chapter, we therefore extend the use of the term "circadian rhythm" to all diurnal variations recurring regularly at a time interval of approximately 24 hours.

An immense variety of circadian rhythms have been observed in humans. They include blood constituents such as white blood cells; amino acids; phosphorus; innumerable physiologic variables, such as body temperature, heart rate, blood pressure, and urine volume; as well as behavioral parameters such as mood, vigilance and cognitive performance. There are also rhythms in response to various challenges such as drugs and stress. Circadian rhythmicity is maintained when subjects are sleep-deprived, when they are starved, or when they receive equal amounts of food at short intervals over the day. The

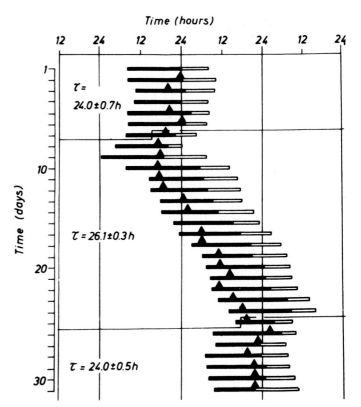

FIGURE 17–3. Circadian rhythms of wakefulness *(black bars)*, sleep *(white bars)*, and maximum rectal temperature *(triangles)* in a human subject who was exposed to the external synchronizing agents for the first and last 7 days and was isolated from all time cues in an underground bunker between days 8 and 24.

timing of single meals, however, can have effects on the pattern of at least some variables, including hormones, and the effects of sleep-wake homeostasis can alter the expression of many rhythms, especially those of the endocrine system.

The endogenous nature of human circadian rhythms has been established by experiments in which subjects were isolated with no access to the natural light-dark (LD) cycle and no time cues. Such experiments were first performed in natural caves, then in underground bunkers, and finally in specially designed windowless soundproof apartments. The results of such an experiment conducted in an artificial underground unit in Germany, are shown in Figure 17–3.[3, 4] The rest-activity cycle of the subject is plotted horizontally, day by day, and the times of occurrence of the daily maximum of the body temperature cycle are indicated by closed triangles. During the first 7 days of the experiment, the door of the isolation unit was left open and the subjects knew the time of day. The average period (τ) of the rest-activity cycle and of the rhythm of body temperature was 24 hours. When, thereafter, the subject lived in complete isolation, both rhythms free-ran but with a mean period of about 26 hours. The free-running period varies from one individual to another. In humans, free-running periods around 25 hours have been commonly observed under conditions of prolonged temporal isolation.

Synchronizing Agents and Entrainment

The fact that the endogenous circadian period observed under constant conditions is not exactly equal to 24 hours implies that changes in the physical environment must synchronize or entrain the internal clock. Otherwise, a clock with a period only a few minutes shorter or longer than 24 hours would soon be totally out of synchrony with the environmental day. An agent that is capable of entraining or synchronizing circadian rhythms is often called a "zeitgeber," a German neologism meaning "time giver."

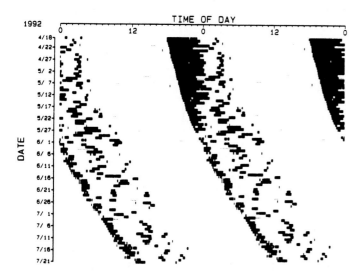

FIGURE 17–2. Continuous record of running wheel activity in a single golden hamster maintained in constant light for 100 days. The record has been double-plotted over a 48-hour scale to facilitate visual examination.

PHOTIC ZEITGEBERS. The LD cycle is the primary agent that synchronizes most circadian rhythms. Thus, in the presence of a 24-hour LD cycle, the period of circadian rhythms exactly matches the period of the LD cycle. In addition to establishing "period control," an entraining LD cycle establishes "phase control" such that specific phases of the circadian rhythm occur at the same time in each cycle. Entrainment is restricted to cycles with periods that are "close" to 24 hours in duration and, in general, is not possible for LD cycles that are more than a few hours shorter or longer than the endogenous circadian period. If the period of the LD cycle is too short or long for entrainment to occur, the circadian rhythm free-runs. This rigidity of the circadian pacemaker has been used in so-called forced desynchrony studies where the subjects are maintained on an LD and sleep-wake cycle with a period outside of the range of entrainment, such as 20 hours or 28 hours.[5, 6] Such protocols have recently provided newer estimations of the endogenous period of the human circadian system which are closer to 24 hours (i.e., averaging 24.2 hours) than those obtained in prolonged studies of temporal isolation.[6]

To examine how a zeitgeber such as light influences the circadian system, the organism is maintained in constant conditions and then briefly exposed to the zeitgeber before being returned to constant conditions.[7] The effects of zeitgeber exposure on a phase reference point of an overt circadian rhythm (e.g., onset of locomotor activity, minimum of body temperature) in subsequent cycles is then determined. A plot of the direction and magnitude of the phase shift as a function of the circadian time of zeitgeber exposure is called a "phase response curve" (PRC). In the human, light exposure during the late evening and first half of the usual sleep period results in phase delays, while light exposure at the end of the usual sleep period and in the early morning results in phase advances. The transition from phase delays to phase advances occurs around the time of the minimum body temperature, that is, between 4 AM and 6 AM in most subjects. Light during the usual daytime period causes little or no phase shift. While differences in amplitude may exist, the general shape and characteristics of the PRC to light pulses are similar for all species. Based on this PRC, appropriately, exposure to bright light can accelerate adaptation to shifts such as those occurring in jet lag and shift work. The amplitude of the phase shifts depends on light intensity and duration and on the number of consecutive exposures.[8] Exposure to single 3- to 5-hour light pulses, even of bright intensity (i.e., >3000 lux), results in immediate phase shifts on the order of 1 to 2 hours.[9, 10] Repeated exposure for 2 to 3 consecutive days may cause much larger (6- to 12-hour) shifts.[11, 12] The possible role of the intervening periods of dark and sleep exposure could play a role in enhancing the phase-shifting effects of repeated exposure to light.

There is indeed increasing evidence to indicate that exposure to dark (and to the associated increases in activity in nocturnal animals and decreases in activity or sleep induction in diurnal animals) is also able to phase-shift mammalian circadian rhythms. A PRC to dark has been described both in the nocturnal hamster[13] and in the *Octodon degus*, a diurnal rodent.[14] In humans, two studies have shown that abrupt 8-hour advances or 8-hour delays of the sleep-wake cycle result in immediate 2-hour phase shifts in the same direction.[15, 16] A recent study demonstrated that daytime naps of 6 hours' duration in total darkness presented over a background of very dim light cause delay shifts when initiated in the morning and advance shifts when initiated in the evening.[17] Naps initiated in the afternoon cause no significant phase shifts, consistent with the classic concept of a PRC.

NONPHOTIC ZEITGEBERS. Nonphotic cues, for example, social or behavioral cues, were long thought to be ineffective as zeitgebers in rodents and other mammals, but evidence to the contrary has accumulated over the last decade. Specifically, stimuli which cause an alteration of the rest-activity cycle, either by eliciting activity during the normal rest period or by preventing activity during the normal active period, result in phase shifts of circadian rhythms of activity and of other behavioral, physiologic, and endocrine markers.[18, 19] In nocturnal rodents, the PRC to activity-inducing stimuli is about 12 hours out of phase with the PRC to light pulses.

There is only limited evidence to indicate that nonphotic stimuli may affect human circadian rhythms. Exposure to a single session of 3 hours of moderate-intensity exercise during the usual nighttime period was found to result in phase shifts of markers of circadian phase on the next day, with the direction and magnitude of the phase shifts being dependent on the timing of exercise.[20] Similar findings were obtained with nocturnal exposure to high intensity 1-hour exercise sessions.[21] Supporting evidence for a zeitgeber effect of exercise was obtained in a field study which found that adaptation to night work could be facilitated by nocturnal exercise.[22] Finally, the fact that some totally blind subjects can entrain to 24-hour as well as non–24-hour cycles also supports the existence of a nonphotic control of the human circadian system.[23]

Another nonphotic agent that has been shown to induce phase shifts in human circadian rhythms is melatonin.[24] There are specific neural connections between the master circadian pacemaker and the pineal gland, and the diurnal variation of plasma melatonin levels is driven by the circadian clock.[25] Phase shifts of the central circadian signal induced by changes in the LD cycle will be faithfully reflected in the synchronization of the onset of nocturnal melatonin secretion.[10, 24, 26] There is evidence that, in turn, the melatonin rhythm feeds back on the clock (where melatonin receptors have been identified) and exerts synchronizing effects.[25] A PRC to repeated (on 4 consecutive days) oral administration of low-dose melatonin (0.5 mg) has been described.[27] Melatonin in the late afternoon or evening causes small (± 30 minutes) phase advances, whereas melatonin in the early morning causes phase delays.

The Organization of the Mammalian Circadian System

The Suprachiasmatic Nucleus: A Master Circadian Pacemaker

In mammals, the SCN, two small bilaterally paired nuclei in the anterior hypothalamus immediately above the optic chiasm, functions as the master clock. Under both free-running and entrained conditions, destruction of the SCN in a variety of species leads to abolishment or severe disruption of many behavioral and physiologic rhythms. The role of the SCN as the control center for the circadian system, first suggested by lesion studies, was confirmed by studies involving transplantation of the SCN from one animal to another. Indeed, circadian rhythmicity can be restored in adult arrhythmic SCN-lesioned rodents by transplanting fetal SCN tissue into the region of the SCN.[28, 29] Such transplant experiments were also conducted using fetal tissues from so-called tau mutant hamsters, who have an endogenous circadian period of about 20 hours.[30] In all cases in which rhythmicity was restored, the periods of the restored rhythms were similar to those of the donor genotype. A number of SCN rhythms persist in vitro, including those of neural firing, vasopressin release, and glucose metabolism.[31, 32] Finally, immortalized SCN cells can generate robust rhythms in both glucose uptake and in their content of neurotrophins.[33] It is now clear that the ability of SCN cells to generate a circadian signal does not rely on some inherent network property of many cells acting together: single SCN cells in culture can generate circadian neural signals.[34]

Photic Input Pathways to the Suprachiasmatic Nucleus

The eyes are involved in relaying entraining information from the LD cycle to the circadian timing system in mammals via a unique pathway, separate from the visual system, and referred to as the retinohypothalamic tract (RHT).[35] At the level of the optic chiasm, retinal projections first enter the brain in the region of the SCN and surrounding hypothalamic areas.[35] The primary visual centers of the brain or the "perception" of light is not necessary for entrainment of circadian rhythms by the LD cycle. In addition to the RHT, the SCN also receives retinal information indirectly from the lateral geniculate nucleus (LGN), which receives a direct projection from the retina.[35]

The novel and surprising finding that very bright light shone on the back of the knee can influence human circadian phase[36] raised the possibility that nonretinal photoreceptors may play a role in relaying

LD information to the circadian clock. This interesting observation awaits confirmation.

A substantial body of evidence indicates that circadian photoreceptors may be different from the image-forming rods and cones of the retina. Indeed, transgenic mice without cones, or without both rods and cones, respond normally to the phase-shifting and entraining effects of light. Recent studies indicate that the cryptochrome blue-light photoreceptors may mediate the effects of light on the mammalian circadian clock.[37] In some totally blind humans, light exposure is capable of suppressing melatonin, indicating that visual blindness should not be equated with circadian blindness.[38]

Nonphotic Input Pathways to the Suprachiasmatic Nucleus

How nonphotic information reaches the SCN is still not known, although there is evidence from lesion studies to suggest that a distinct subdivision of the LGN, the intergeniculate leaflet (IGL), may be involved in mediating the effects of activity on the clock.[39] Furthermore, the IGL is the source of the neuropeptide Y (NPY) innervation of the SCN, and the administration of NPY into the SCN area, as well as electrical stimulation of the geniculohypothalamic tract, induces phase shifts in the hamster locomotor activity rhythm that are similar to those induced by activity-inducing stimuli.[39] The LGN/IGL may be a common pathway by which information about the lighting environment and the activity-rest state reach the circadian clock, and may be involved in integrating information from both the external and internal environment. Both the LGN/IGL and the SCN receive a dense serotoninergic projection from the midbrain raphe nuclei, and there is now substantial evidence that these projections play a role in both the photic and nonphotic regulation of the mammalian circadian clock.[40, 41]

Genetic and Molecular Basis of Circadian Rhythms

The last few years have witnessed an explosion of new discoveries that have led to the identification of a number of genes, and their protein products, that form the core of the molecular circadian clock in mammals.[42, 43] Early studies demonstrating differences in circadian rhythm variables between various inbred strains of rodents indicated that the genetic background influences the expression of circadian rhythms in mammals.[44, 45] However, it was not until the late 1980s that it was demonstrated that a basic property of the mammalian circadian clock (period) could be influenced by a single gene.[30] The serendipitous discovery of the "*tau* mutant" hamster demonstrated that a single autosomal mutant gene could change the free-running period of the hamster circadian clock to about 22 hours in the heterozygous state, and to 20 hours in the homozygous condition. However, the paucity of genetic resources in the hamster has not allowed, even today, the identification of the gene involved in this altered phenotypic expression of circadian period. The breakthrough in the molecular genetics of the circadian clock system in mammals came with the discovery of a "mutant" mouse showing an abnormally long circadian period.[46] The gene responsible for the mutant circadian phenotype, called *Clock*, was eventually identified and cloned and was found to be a gene with approximately 100,000 bp coding for a protein that had the properties of a transcription factor.[47] In a remarkably short period of time after the discovery of the *Clock* gene, a number of other circadian clock genes were identified in mice (*bmel, tim,* and the three forms of the *per* gene, which was first found in fruit flies), and the nature of the interactions between these genes and their protein products was elucidated.[42, 43] Based on a series of converging studies, it now appears that plant photopigment-like molecules known as "cryptochromes" may also play a role in the circadian molecular machinery of mammals.[48]

Interactions between the Human Circadian Pacemaker and Sleep

There are several features of the interaction between sleep and circadian rhythmicity that appear to be unique to the human species.

First, human sleep is generally consolidated in a single 6- to 9-hour period, whereas fragmentation of the sleep period in several bouts is the rule in the majority of other mammals. Possibly as a result of this consolidation of the sleep period, the wake-sleep transition in man is associated with physiologic changes which are usually more marked than those observed in animals. For example, the secretion of growth hormone (GH) in normal adults is tightly associated with the beginning of the sleep period, whereas the relationship between GH secretory pulses and sleep stages is much less evident in rodents, primates, and dogs. Second, humans are also unique in their capacity to ignore circadian signals and to maintain wakefulness despite an increased pressure to go to sleep. Finally, approximately 25% of human subjects maintained for prolonged periods of time in temporal isolation have shown behavioral modifications that have not been observed in laboratory animals under constant conditions. These modifications consist of a desynchronization between the sleep-wake cycle and other rhythms, such as those of body temperature and cortisol secretion, which continue to free-run with a circadian period. Under conditions of so-called internal desynchronization, the sleep-wake cycle may be suddenly lengthened to 30 hours and more, while the rhythm of body temperature continues to free-run with a circadian period.[3, 4] Wakefulness may last more than 30 hours. Remarkably, the subjects are not aware of these drastic changes in their way of living. Instead, most of them believe they are living on a more or less regular 24-hour schedule. This can be explained by the observation that time perception is profoundly altered: estimations of 1-hour intervals are positively correlated with the duration of wakefulness.[49] Of particular interest is that the subjects continue to have three meals per "day," irrespective of the actual number of hours they are awake.[50] The intervals between meals as well as those between waking up and breakfast, or between dinner and bedtime, are stretched or compressed in strong proportionality to the duration of wakefulness.[51] The mechanisms causing spontaneous internal desynchronization are not completely understood.

Detailed analyses of data obtained during temporal isolation and forced desynchrony protocols showed that the timing, duration, and architecture of sleep are partially regulated by circadian rhythmicity.[5, 52] Thus, the duration of sleep episodes is correlated with the phase of the circadian rhythm of body temperature and not with the duration of prior wakefulness. Short (i.e., 7 to 8 hours) sleep episodes occur in free-running conditions when the subject goes to sleep at around the minimum of body temperature, whereas long (i.e., 12 to 14 hours) sleep episodes occur when sleep starts around the maximum of body temperature. Moreover, the distribution of REM (rapid eye movement) sleep and sleep spindle activity are also markedly modulated by circadian timing. In contrast, the hourglass-like mechanism of sleep-wake homeostasis is thought to be largely independent of the circadian system and to involve one or several putative neural sleep factors (factor S) which rise during waking and decay exponentially during sleep.[2] This homeostatic mechanism regulates the timing, amount, and intensity of the deeper stages of sleep, that is, stages III and IV of non-REM (NREM) sleep, usually referred to as slow-wave (SW) sleep because of the appearance of well-defined slow waves in the frequency range of 0.5 to 4.0 Hz in the electroencephalogram (EEG). The neuroanatomic and neurochemical basis of sleep-wake homeostasis has not been entirely elucidated but appears to involve the basal forebrain cholinergic region and adenosine, a neuromodulator whose extracellular concentrations in this region increase during sustained wakefulness and decrease during sleep.[53] The dual control of sleep by circadian and homeostatic mechanisms extends to the control of objective and subjective measures of sleep tendency, mood, and vigilance.[54–56] Figure 17–4 shows representative profiles of body temperature, subjective sleepiness, positive affect, and performance on a vigilance task in normal young men studied during 40 consecutive hours of continuous wakefulness. Maximum subjective sleepiness coincides with the minimum of body temperature, mood, and performance. Remarkably, despite continued sleep deprivation, subjective fatigue decreased, and mood and performance partially recovered during the daytime hours following nocturnal sleep deprivation, reflecting an interaction of circadian timing with the accumulation of waking time.[54–58] It is currently thought that the circadian clock generates a waking signal which increases from morning to evening and is maxi-

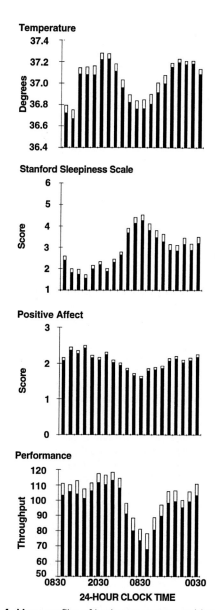

FIGURE 17–4. Mean profiles of body temperature, subjective sleepiness (using the Stanford Sleepiness Score), positive affect (using the Positive and Negative Affect Scale), and performance on a vigilance task in normal young men studied during 40 consecutive hours of continuous wakefulness at bedrest. Data are represented as mean *(black bar)* and SEM *(open bar)* for each 2-hour interval.

mally expressed in the early evening hours, 1 to 2 hours prior to the onset of nocturnal melatonin secretion.[55, 59] This circadian waking signal counteracts the build-up of the putative factor S underlying the homeostatic process, allowing maintenance of a high level of alertness throughout the usual waking period. In support of this theory, detailed studies have indicated that rodents with SCN lesions have an increased sleep duration.[59] Current data from human studies are also compatible with the hypothesis that the SCN also generates a "sleep" signal in the early morning hours.[60]

Circadian rhythmicity and sleep-wake homeostasis also interact to regulate hormonal secretion. These modulatory effects were long thought to be present only in hormones directly dependent on the hypothalamic-pituitary axis. However, it is now clear that modulation by circadian rhythmicity and sleep is also present in other endocrine systems, such as glucose regulation and the renin-angiotensin system.[61, 62] The pathways by which circadian rhythmicity, sleep-wake homeostasis, and their interaction modulate hormonal release are largely unknown. As illustrated in Figure 17–1, humoral or neural signals originating from the hypothalamic circadian pacemaker and

from brain regions involved in sleep regulation affect the activity of the hypothalamic structures responsible for the pulsatile release of neuroendocrine factors which stimulate or inhibit intermittent secretion of pituitary hormones. It appears that stimulatory or inhibitory effects of sleep on endocrine release are primarily associated with SW sleep, rather than REM sleep.[63–67] Theoretically, the modulation of neuroendocrine release by sleep and circadian rhythmicity could be achieved either by modulation of pulse amplitude, by modulation of pulse frequency, or by a combination of both. The data available so far seem to indicate that circadian rhythmicity of pituitary hormonal release is achieved primarily by modulation of pulse amplitude without changes in pulse frequency, whereas sleep-wake and REM-NREM transitions affect pulse frequency. Pituitary hormones that influence endocrine systems not directly controlled by hypothalamic factors, probably mediate, at least partially, the modulatory effects of sleep and circadian rhythmicity on these systems (e.g., counterregulatory effects of GH and cortisol on glucose regulation).[62]

To delineate the relative roles of circadian and sleep effects in the temporal organization of hormonal secretion, strategies based on the fact that circadian rhythmicity needs several days to adapt to abrupt shifts of the sleep-wake cycle have been used. Thus, by shifting the sleep times by 8 to 12 hours, the masking effects of sleep on circadian inputs are removed and the effects of sleep at an abnormal circadian time are revealed. Figure 17–5 illustrates mean profiles of plasma cortisol, plasma GH, plasma prolactin (PRL), and plasma thyrotropin (TSH) observed in normal subjects who were studied before and during an abrupt 12-hour shift of the sleep-wake and LD cycle. The study period extended over a 53-hour span and included an 8-hour period of nocturnal sleep, a 28-hour period of continuous wakefulness, and a daytime period of recovery sleep.

To eliminate the effects of feeding, fasting, and postural changes, the subjects remained recumbent throughout the study and the normal meal schedule was replaced by intravenous glucose infusion at a constant rate. As shown in Figure 17–6, this drastic manipulation of sleep had only modest effects on the wave shape of the cortisol profile, in sharp contrast with the immediate shift of the GH and PRL rhythms which followed the shift of the sleep-wake cycle. As reviewed in subsequent sections, numerous studies have indicated that the control of diurnal rhythms of corticotropic activity is primarily dependent on circadian timing, whereas sleep-wake homeostasis appears to be an important factor in the control of the 24-hour profiles of GH and PRL.[68] Nevertheless, small modulatory effects of sleep-wake homeostasis on cortisol secretion and, conversely, influences of circadian timing on somatotropic function have been clearly demonstrated.[69] The diurnal variation of TSH levels includes an evening elevation thought to be under circadian control and nocturnal inhibition by sleep-dependent processes which is clearly demonstrated during sleep deprivation, when a large increase in nocturnal TSH levels is apparent, as shown in the lower panel of Figure 17–6.[68]

Hormonal profiles are thus easily measurable reflections of central mechanisms of biologic timekeeping. In clinical investigations of conditions of abnormal circadian rhythmicity, such as jet lag, and in human studies of the effects of exposure to natural or artificial zeitgebers, they are commonly used as markers of the status of the circadian clock and of its interactions with sleep.

Impact of Age on Circadian Rhythms

Age-related changes in endocrine, metabolic, and behavioral circadian rhythms have been reported in a variety of species, including humans.[70–72] One of the most prominent changes is a reduction in rhythm amplitude. The overall findings of a study which examined age-related differences in 24-hour endocrine rhythms and sleep in healthy subjects are shown in Figure 17–6.[70] A decrease by at least 50% in the nocturnal release of both GH and melatonin was observed in the older volunteers and SW sleep was drastically diminished. Other studies have shown that these deficits in the maintenance and depth of nocturnal sleep[73] are paralleled by decreased alertness during the daytime. In both rodents and humans, many circadian rhythms are also advanced under entrained conditions such that specific phase

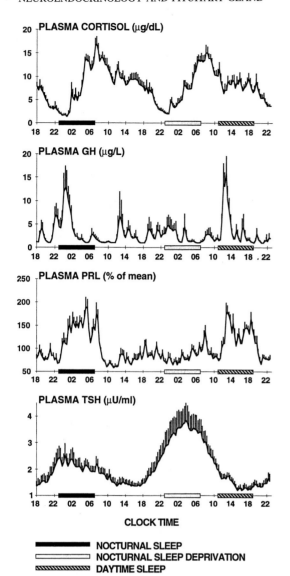

NOCTURNAL SLEEP
NOCTURNAL SLEEP DEPRIVATION
DAYTIME SLEEP

FIGURE 17–5. From top to bottom: Mean 24-hour profiles of plasma cortisol, growth hormone, prolactin, and thyrotropin in a group of eight normal young men (20 to 27 years old) studied during a 53-hour period, including 8 hours of nocturnal sleep, 28 hours of sleep deprivation, and 8 hours of daytime sleep. The *vertical lines* at each time point represent the SEM. The *black bars* represent the sleep periods. The *open bars* represent the period of nocturnal sleep deprivation. The *dashed bars* represent the period of daytime sleep. Data were sampled at 20-minute intervals. (From Van Cauter E, Spiegel K: Circadian and sleep control of endocrine secretions. *In* Turek FW, Zee PC (eds): Neurobiology of Sleep and Circadian Rhythms, vol 133. New York, Marcel Dekker, 1999, pp 397–426.)

points of the rhythms occur earlier than in young subjects.[70, 74] Both amplitude reduction and phase advance of the rhythm of body temperature have been observed in elderly subjects and these alterations in circadian regulation were closely associated with changes in sleep-wake habits, that is, earlier bedtimes and waketimes.[71]

Age-related changes in the amplitude or phase of circadian rhythms could be due to changes in the inner workings of the master clock, to alterations in the input pathways to the clock, or to factors "downstream" between the circadian clock and the system expressing the rhythm. Some,[75] but not all,[76] studies have reported that the free-running period of various rhythms in rodents is systematically shortened with age, suggesting that the circadian clock itself is altered in advanced age. Age-related phase advances of a number of different behavioral and endocrine rhythms are consistent with the hypothesis that the period of the human circadian clock is shorter in the elderly. However, a recent study which measured the free-running period in

healthy young and older adults using the forced desynchrony protocol has found no age difference.[6] It should be noted that the older subjects who participated in this demanding protocol passed extremely stringent exclusion criteria and may have been more representative of "successful aging" than "normal aging." Moreover, "after effects" of entrainment to the environmental 24-hour period may have obscured the expression of endogenous circadian rhythmicity and the demonstration of age differences. Nevertheless, these very healthy older subjects had marked decreases in sleep consolidation and had greater difficulties sleeping at adverse circadian phases than young subjects. These alterations and the clear advance of the propensity to awaken from sleep are thought to be related to both a reduction in the homeostatic drive to sleep and a reduction in the strength of the circadian signal.[60]

Studies in rodents indicate that aging is also associated with a decreased responsiveness to the phase-shifting effects of both photic and nonphotic stimuli. Old hamsters show a decreased response to the phase-shifting effects of low-intensity light pulses.[77] This observation raises the possibility that in old age there is either decreased signal transmission of light information to the SCN or that the SCN itself is less responsive to photic stimulation. Similarly, while induction of locomotor activity during a time of normal inactivity can induce pronounced phase shifts in the circadian rhythm of locomotor activity in young animals, in old animals the response is greatly diminished or completely abolished.[78, 79] Interestingly, transplantation of fetal SCN tissue into the SCN region of old hamsters with an intact SCN can restore the response to the phase-shifting effects of triazolam on the activity rhythm.[80]

Behavioral changes in the elderly may also lead to changes in environmental inputs to the clock. In older adults, exposure to bright light and social cues, both potential entraining agents, is markedly diminished when compared with young adults.[81–83] Absence of professional constraints, decreased mobility due to illness, and reduced socialization and outdoor activities are all hallmarks of old age. Thus, decreased exposure to environmental stimuli that entrain circadian rhythms could contribute to disruptions in circadian rhythmicity. The use of exposure to bright light to reinforce circadian rhythms in older adults and improve nighttime sleep and daytime alertness has proved beneficial.[84]

Conditions of Abnormal Circadian Rhythmicity

Circadian rhythms provide synchronization with the pronounced periodic fluctuations in the external environment and organize the internal milieu so that there is coordination and synchronization of internal processes. "External synchronization" is of obvious importance for the survival of the species and ensures that the organism does the "right thing" at the right time of the day. Of equal, but perhaps less appreciated, importance is the fact that the circadian clock system provides internal temporal organization between the myriad of biochemical and physiologic systems in the body. Lack of synchrony within the internal environment may lead to chronic difficulties, with serious consequences for the health and well-being of the organism. The physical and mental malaise occurring following rapid travel across time zones (i.e., the jet-lag syndrome), and the pathologic changes associated with long-term shift work are assumed to be due in part to an alteration in the normal phase relationships among various internal rhythms. In addition, it has been speculated that alterations of internal phase relationships among rhythms underlie certain forms of affective illness.

Transmeridian Flights (Jet Lag)

People who travel rapidly across time zones are confronted with a desynchronization between their internal circadian rhythms and the periodicity of the new external environment. Upon arrival, the timings of the LD cycle, social schedule, and meals are abnormally matched to the phase of the physiologic rhythms of the traveler. Associated with this lack of synchronization are symptoms of fatigue, subjective

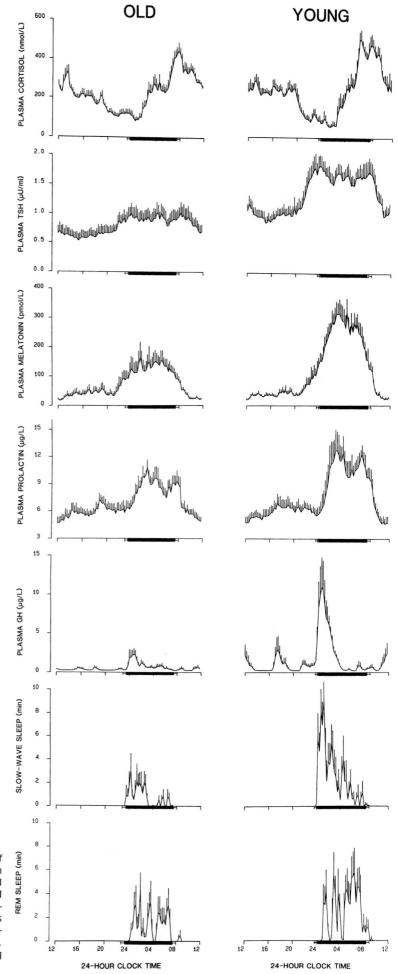

FIGURE 17–6. From top to bottom: Mean 24-hour profiles of plasma cortisol, thyrotropin, melatonin, prolactin, and growth hormone levels, and amounts of slow-wave (SW) sleep and rapid eye movement (REM) sleep in old (67 to 84 years) and young (20 to 27 years) subjects. Data were sampled at 15-minute intervals. At each time point, the *vertical line* represents the standard error for the group (n = 8). The *black bars* represent the mean sleep period. (From van Coevorden A, Mockel J, Laurent E, et al: Neuroendocrine rhythms and sleep in aging men. Am J Physiol 260:E651–E661, 1991.)

discomfort, sleep disturbances, reduced mental and psychomotor performance, and gastrointestinal disorders.

The rate of adaptation is generally slower for overt rhythms that are strongly dependent on the circadian system, such as those of cortisol and melatonin secretions, than for those that are markedly modulated by sleep-wake homeostasis, such as PRL and GH secretions. As a result, during the period of adaptation, abnormal phase relationships between overt rhythms occur. Thus, the jet-lag syndrome involves not only desynchronization between internal and external rhythms but also a perturbation of internal temporal organization of physiologic functions. Depending on the strength of the zeitgebers, the rate of adaptation can be as low as half an hour a day or as high as 3 hours a day. The rate of adaptation is not constant: adaptation to a large shift occurs at a faster rate during the first few days and progresses at a slower pace thereafter.[85] The rate of adaptation is also dependent on the direction of the shift, with adaptation occurring generally faster after a delay (i.e., westward) shift than after an advance (i.e., eastward) shift.[85] This eastward-westward difference in rate of adaptation is believed to be due to the fact that the endogenous circadian period of the human is longer than 24 hours and thus adjustment by delays is more easily achieved than adjustment by advances. There is strong evidence to suggest that reentrainment after a transmeridian flight is facilitated by exposure to bright light at appropriate circadian phases. It is widely believed that adherence to the local social and meal schedule upon arrival will accelerate adaptation to jet lag, but this has not been rigorously demonstrated. Laboratory studies suggest that physical exercise scheduled during the period corresponding to the nighttime prior to travel will facilitate adaptation to a delay (i.e., westward) shift.[20, 21]

Shift Work

Shift work, which is voluntarily accepted by millions of workers, is a major health hazard, involving an increased risk of cardiovascular illness, gastrointestinal disorders, infertility, and insomnia.[86–88] The medical consequences of shift work are associated with chronic misalignment of physiologic circadian rhythms and the activity-rest cycle. Shift work usually creates conditions in which some zeitgebers (e.g., an artificial LD cycle) and additional phase-setting factors such as the rest-activity cycle, are shifted while others remain unaltered, for example, the natural LD cycle and the routines of family life. Shift workers thus live in a situation of conflicting zeitgebers that almost never allow a complete shift of the circadian system. Indeed, several studies have shown that workers on permanent or rotating night shifts do not adapt to these schedules, even after several years.[89–91] Besides its health implications, this misalignment with the circadian system has important social and economic implications, because night work is associated with substantial decrements in performance and vigilance, resulting in diminished productivity and increased accident rates. A number of studies have demonstrated that scheduled exposure to bright light during night work and complete darkness during daytime sleep following night work are capable of accelerating the adjustment to the new schedule and improve nighttime alertness and performance.[92–97]

Blindness

Several studies have shown that some totally blind persons have abnormal sleep-wake cycles and rhythms of melatonin secretion.[98, 99] These disturbances reflect a lack of entrainment to the 24-hour environmental periodicity, similar to that seen in sighted people living in isolation units under free-running conditions. The free-running periods recorded in blind subjects have typically been in the range of 24.5 to 30 hours, that is, markedly longer than the recent evaluations obtained in sighted subjects under conditions of forced desynchrony. The abnormalities of circadian rhythms in blindness may be of diagnostic importance to the endocrinologist. For example, low morning or high evening levels of cortisol in this condition may reflect a lack of synchronization of the circadian rhythm rather than a disorder of the pituitary-adrenal axis. Interestingly, some totally blind persons who do not suppress melatonin secretion when exposed to light are able to

entrain to the 24-hour cycle,[23] indicating that nonphotic cues or light perception via extraretinal receptors may be operating.

Therapeutic strategies to treat circadian-related insomnias in the blind critically depend on the development of nonphotic methods of entrainment. Appropriately timed administration of oral melatonin in blind subjects has been reported to restore normal entrainment to a 24-hour cycle in several studies.[100, 101]

Sleep Disorders and Sleep Loss

Certain forms of sleep disorders seem to originate from a disturbance in the circadian system.[102] Delayed sleep phase insomnia is characterized by a chronic inability to fall asleep at a normal bedtime and to awake in the morning. Nonpharmacologic chronotherapy involving repeated scheduled exposure to bright light is the treatment of choice for this disorder. In contrast, in the advanced sleep phase syndrome, the timing of the major sleep episode is advanced in relation to normal bedtime, resulting in symptoms of extreme evening sleepiness and early morning awakening. Recent studies have indicated that familial forms of this syndrome could reflect an autosomal dominant mutation.[103]

A few studies have examined nocturnal hormonal release in patients with obstructive apnea before and after treatment.[104–107] As expected, the nocturnal release of the two pituitary hormones that are markedly dependent on sleep, that is, GH and PRL, is decreased in untreated apneic subjects. As illustrated in Figure 17–7, treatment with continuous positive airway pressure (CPAP) results in a clear increase in the amount of GH secreted during the first few hours of sleep.[104, 106] The effects of CPAP treatment on overnight PRL secretion are less clear than those seen for GH.[107] Indeed, the total amount of PRL secreted during the sleep period is not modified, but the frequency of PRL pulses is restored to values similar to those observed in normal subjects.

Chronic sleep loss is a hallmark of modern society. "Normal" sleep duration has decreased from approximately 9.0 hours in 1910 to an average of 7.5 hours today. Many people voluntarily choose to curtail their sleep to the shortest amount tolerable to maximize the time available for work and leisure activities. To meet the demands of

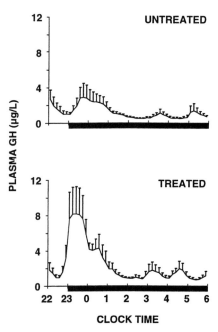

FIGURE 17–7. Mean profiles of plasma GH in patients with sleep apnea studied before *(top)* and after *(bottom)* treatment with continuous positive airway pressure *(CPAP)*. The *vertical line* at each time point represents the SEM. (Data from Saini et al.[106] Adapted from Van Cauter E, Spiegel K: Circadian and sleep control of endocrine secretions. *In* Turek FW, Zee PC [eds]: Neurobiology of Sleep and Circadian Rhythms. *In* Lenfant C: Lung Biology in Health and Disease, vol 133. New York, Marcel Dekker, 1999, pp 397–426.)

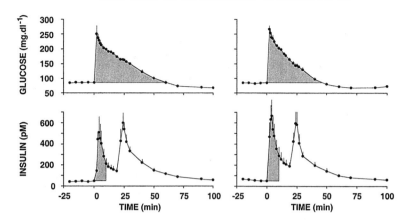

FIGURE 17–8. Upper panels: Impact of a sleep debt (4 hours in bed for 6 nights) on mean (+ SEM) profiles of blood glucose and serum insulin during an intravenous glucose tolerance test (IVGTT). In the sleep debt condition, the duration of the glucose response was longer *(shaded area)* and the acute insulin response to glucose *(shaded area)* was lower than after sleep recovery. The rate of disappearance of glucose post injection was nearly 40% slower in the sleep debt condition than after recovery, indicating a marked decrease in glucose tolerance. Lower panels: Impact of a sleep debt on the normal afternoon decrease of cortisol levels, estimated from total plasma concentrations or free saliva levels. The rate of decrease of free cortisol concentrations between 4 and 9 PM was approximately six times slower in the sleep debt condition than in the fully rested state. (Adapted from Spiegel K, Leproult R, Van Cauter E: Impact of sleep debt on metabolic and endocrine function. Lancet 354:1435–1439, 1999. © The Lancet Ltd., 1999.)

around-the-clock operations, millions of shift workers sleep on average less than 6 hours per day. Despite the fact that sleep is a major modulator of metabolic and endocrine regulation, the consensus which prevailed until recently is that sleep loss results in increased sleepiness and decreased cognitive performance but has little or no effect on peripheral function. A recent study that measured metabolic and hormonal values in subjects studied during 1 week of sleep restriction (4 hours in bed) and after 1 week of sleep recovery (12 hours in bed) provided evidence to the contrary.[108] The upper panels of Figure 17–8 show the mean glucose and insulin responses to an intravenous glucose tolerance test performed on the fifth day of both conditions. The values of glucose tolerance measured at the end of the recovery period were in the normal range for young healthy men, but the values measured in the state of sleep debt were consistent with a clinically significant impairment of carbohydrate tolerance. Thus, the rate of disappearance of glucose post injection was nearly 40% slower in the sleep debt condition than after recovery and the acute insulin response to glucose was reduced by 30%. The lower glucose tolerance appeared to partly reflect diminished non–insulin-dependent glucose utilization, consistent with findings of decreased cerebral glucose utilization in positron emission tomography (PET) studies of sleep-deprived subjects. When compared with the fully rested condition, the state of sleep debt was also associated with alterations of cortisol secretion, whether estimated by total cortisol levels in plasma or free cortisol levels in saliva. The

primary alteration was an elevation of cortisol concentrations in the afternoon and early evening (lower panels of Figure 17–8). This latter disturbance, which had been previously observed in conditions of acute total and partial sleep loss,[109] may reflect decreased efficacy of the negative feedback regulation of the hypothalamic-pituitary-adrenal (HPA) axis. An elevation of plasma cortisol levels in the afternoon and early evening similar to that observed in our subjects under the sleep debt condition has been previously reported in several studies of normal aging[70, 110, 111] and could promote the development of insulin resistance and memory impairments.[112, 113]

Affective Disorders

Early timing of a number of circadian rhythms, including hormonal rhythms, has been observed in acutely ill patients with endogenous depression. The most robust finding has been an advance and elevation of the nadir of the 24-hour rhythm of cortisol secretion. These findings provide the basis for the so-called phase-advance hypothesis for affective illness which proposes that abnormalities in circadian timekeeping are involved in the pathophysiology of depression.[114, 115] However, in view of the sleep disturbances that invariably accompany severe depression, it is also possible that the higher nocturnal cortisol levels partly reflect the impact of sleep loss.

ULTRADIAN RHYTHMS

Range of Ultradian Rhythms

The term "ultradian" is primarily used to designate rhythmicities with periods ranging from fractions of hours to several hours. Ultradian oscillations are often less regular and less reproducible than circadian rhythms. In most cases, they appear to represent an optimal functional status within the system where they occur rather than serve the primary function of a "clock", that is, an accurate time-measuring device. There is a wide variety of ultradian rhythms. The most prominent are pulsatile hormonal release and the alternation of REM and NREM stages in sleep. In the human, the approximately 90-minute REM-NREM cycle is accompanied by similar periodicity of dreaming, penile erections, sympathovagal balance, and breathing. Kleitman[116] suggested that this ultradian rhythm during sleep is a reflection of a "basic rest-activity cycle" (BRAC) which would occur during wakefulness as well. This concept has received some experimental support from a recent study demonstrating the existence of an ultradian rhythm of brain electrical activity in the frequency range of 13 to 35 Hz, an index of central alertness, during waking.[117] Interestingly, pulses of cortisol release were significantly associated with ultradian oscillations in alertness.[117]

Oscillations at frequencies higher than the hourly (i.e., circhoral) range characterizing pulsatile release have been observed for a variety of hormones. In particular, rapid oscillations of insulin secretion with periods in the 10- to 15-minute range have been well characterized in humans,[118] monkeys,[119] and dogs.[120]

Properties and Diagnostic Implications of Pulsatile Hormonal Release

In the endocrine system, ultradian variations have been observed for anterior and posterior pituitary hormones, for hormones under direct pituitary control, and for other endocrine variables such as parathyroid hormone, norepinephrine, plasma renin activity, leptin, and insulin secretion. The interval of recurrence of pulses varies from hormone to hormone and from species to species. In normal young men in whom blood was sampled every 15 minutes, the average number of pulses per 24-hour span was 12 for PRL, 15 for adrenocorticotropic hormone (ACTH), 18 for TSH, but only 4 for GH. The relative importance of pulsatile or oscillatory secretory activity vs. tonic release also varies from one axis to the other. For some hormones, secretory activity appears to be entirely pulsatile, with no detectable secretion between pulses. In normal men, evidence suggestive of intermittent secretion without tonic release has been obtained for luteinizing hormone (LH), follicle-stimulating hormone (FSH), GH, and ACTH.[121–123] For some hormones, pulsatile release is superimposed on a tonic level of secretion, or secretion occurs continuously but is increased and decreased in an oscillatory fashion. Pancreatic insulin secretion is a well-established example of this type of ultradian oscillations.[124, 125] Recent studies have also indicated the existence of tonic secretion for pituitary PRL and TSH release.[121, 122]

The pulsatile nature of hormonal release implies that changes well in excess of 100% may occur within 1 hour. Therefore, it is necessary to obtain multiple samples to estimate the mean circulating level of many hormones and determine the presence or absence of a circadian rhythm. Measurement of the cortisol level on only two blood samples taken in the morning (i.e., between 8 and 10 AM) and in the late afternoon (i.e., between 4 and 6 PM) is routinely used to assess the normality of the diurnal variation and is part of the diagnostic workup of Cushing's syndrome. However, this procedure may provide inaccurate results because of the highly pulsatile nature of cortisol secretion.

The physiologic significance of pulsatile hormone secretion became clear when the essential role of the episodic nature of gonadotropin-releasing hormone (GnRH) release for the normal functioning of the pituitary-ovarian axis was demonstrated.[126] Landmark studies showed that continuous infusions of exogenous GnRH in rhesus monkeys with lesions of the arcuate nucleus, which abolished endogenous GnRH production, inhibited the secretion of LH and FSH. In contrast, the pulsatile administration of the synthetic hypothalamic hormone at a rate of one 6-minute pulse per hour restored normal LH and FSH levels.[126] Furthermore, if the rate of pulse delivery was increased to three pulses per hour or decreased to one pulse every 2 hours, serum LH and FSH levels were decreased below the normal range. The findings from the early studies on GnRH pulsatility were rapidly applied to the treatment of a variety of disorders of the pituitary-gonadal axis[127] and led the way to the discovery of the functional significance of pulsatility in other endocrine systems. For example, it was found that oscillatory administration of insulin with a period matching that of the normal pulsatility of insulin secretion is more effective in lowering glucose levels than constant infusion.[128]

METHODOLOGIC ASPECTS OF ENDOCRINE RHYTHMS

Experimental Protocols

The majority of investigations of circadian rhythms of hormonal release are based on a "transversal" design, that is, a group of individuals are studied for a minimum of 24 hours each, following the same experimental protocol. The demonstration of circadian rhythmicity is then based on the observation of consistently reproducible characteristics in the observed set of temporal profiles. The group of subjects should be as homogeneous as possible not only in terms of physical variables such as age and sex but also in terms of living habits such as sleep-wake cycles, exercise habits, and meal schedules. Subjects who have regular social habits and describe themselves as "good sleepers" should be preferred. Shift workers or subjects having made a transmeridian flight less than 2 months before the experiment should be excluded. Prior to the beginning of the experiment, the volunteers should be asked to adhere to a standardized schedule of meals and bedtimes for several days in order to maximize interindividual synchronization. At least 1 night of habituation to the laboratory environment and recording procedures should be included.

To avoid disruptions of sleep due to the sampling procedure, the catheter should be connected to tubing extending to an adjoining room during the night. Because of the modulatory effects exerted by sleep stages on hormonal release, it is important to obtain polygraphic sleep recordings using standardized methods for recording and scoring. If polygraphic monitoring is not possible, the timings of sleep onset and awakenings should be carefully recorded and subjective estimations of sleep quality obtained upon awakening. Daytime naps should be avoided. The catheter should be inserted at least 2 hours before the collection of the first sample to avoid possible artifactual effects related to the venipuncture stress. To obtain valid estimations of the circadian variables, it is necessary to sample at intervals not exceeding 1 hour.

If hormonal profiles are measured as markers of the output of the central circadian oscillator, as is often the case for the 24-hour cortisol profile, direct effects of other factors need to be minimized. Sleep-wake transitions, meals, stressful activity, and postural changes may all be reflected in increases or decreases of hormonal secretion. To eliminate these "masking" effects, experimental protocols usually referred to as "constant routines" have been developed to reliably derive estimates of circadian amplitude and phase from temporal patterns of peripheral hormones and other physiologic variables, such as body temperature. Constant routine conditions generally involve a regimen of continuous wakefulness, constant recumbent posture, constant illumination, and constant caloric intake, either under the form of hourly identical aliquots of liquid diet or solid food, or under the form of a constant glucose infusion. While such constant routine conditions have been extensively used in basic studies of human circadian rhythmicity, the sleep deprivation inherent to this protocol is an obvious limitation. The use of circadian markers that are not masked by sleep, meals, and other factors, such as the 24-hour profile of melatonin, has therefore been advocated. Finally, if only circadian phase, and not amplitude, is of interest, measurements of both free cortisol and melatonin levels in saliva during the evening and first half of the night (therefore minimizing the period of sleep deprivation) provide a noninvasive way to observe the timings of two neuroendocrine events timed by the circadian clock: the onset of nocturnal melatonin secretion and the onset of the circadian rise of cortisol release.

To characterize episodic hormonal fluctuations, considerations of the total amount of blood withdrawn and the amount of plasma needed to assay the hormones under study are obviously essential to the definition of an adequate sampling protocol. The definition of an optimal sampling protocol depends thus on the type of phenomenon under study. Sampling rates of 1 and 2 minutes will uncover high-frequency, low-amplitude episodic variations superimposed on the slower pulsatile release at intervals of 1 to 2 hours. Sampling rates of 20 and 30 minutes will only detect major pulses lasting more than 1 hour.

Procedures to Quantify Circadian Variations

To determine rhythm parameters in biologic time series, mathematical procedures are necessary. Among the methods proposed for and applied to 24-hour profiles of blood components, the oldest is the cosinor test.[129] The major disadvantage of this test and of its derivatives is its assumption that the observed profile may be adequately described by a single sinusoidal curve. This assumption is practically never met for biologic rhythms which are asymmetrical in nature (e.g., the sleep-wake cycle is an 8:16 alternation, not 12:12). Therefore, the cosinor test generally provides unreliable estimations of rhythm parameters.

Other procedures for the detection and estimation of circadian variation have been based on periodogram calculations or on nonlinear regression procedures.[130, 131] These methods provide an adequate description of asymmetrical waveshapes. The times of occurrence of the maximum and the minimum of the best-fit curve are often referred to as the acrophase and the nadir, respectively. The amplitude of the rhythm may be estimated as 50% of the difference between the maximum and the minimum of the best-fit curve. With the periodogram procedure, confidence intervals for the amplitude, acrophase, and nadir may be calculated.

Procedures to Quantify Pulsatile Hormonal Secretion

The analysis of pulsatile variations may be considered at two levels.[132] One may wish to define and characterize significant variations in peripheral levels based on estimations of the size of the measurement error (i.e., primarily assay error). However, under certain circumstances, it is possible to mathematically derive secretory rates from the peripheral concentrations.[133–135] This procedure, often referred to as "deconvolution," will often reveal more pulses of secretion than the analysis of peripheral concentrations. It will also more accurately define the temporal limits of each pulse. However, deconvolution involves an amplification of measurement error, with increased risk of false-positive error.

A number of computer algorithms for identification of pulses of hormonal concentration have been proposed. A detailed presentation of the operating principles of each of these procedures is beyond the scope of this chapter. Review articles[136, 137] have provided comparisons of performance of several pulse detection algorithms. A comparative experimental study of the performance of various pulse detection algorithms indicated that ULTRA, CLUSTER, and DETECT perform similarly when used with appropriate choices of parameters.[137]

The regularity of pulsatile behavior may be quantified by examining the distribution of interpulse intervals. Alternatively, the issue of regularity of pulsatile behavior may be approached by examining the

distribution of spectral power in a frequency domain analysis.[138] Finally, another analytic tool, the "approximate entropy" (ApEn), has been introduced to quantify regularity of oscillatory behavior in endocrine and other physiologic time series.[139]

ENDOCRINE RHYTHMS IN HEALTH AND DISEASE

Diurnal or ultradian oscillations, or both, have been observed in essentially all endocrine systems. An exhaustive review of all such observations is not possible. The following summary of the findings is therefore limited to the hypothalamic-pituitary axis, leptin, and glucose regulation. Melatonin rhythmicity is reviewed in Chapter 29. The reader should be aware that there are also prominent rhythms in other hormonal secretions, for example, the parathyroid system and the renin-angiotensin-aldosterone system, and that these rhythms are likely to have important medical implications.

The Corticotropic Axis

Normal Rhythms of ACTH and Adrenal Secretions

The temporal organization of the corticotropic axis may be measured peripherally via plasma levels of ACTH and cortisol. The 24-hour profiles of ACTH and cortisol show an early morning maximum, declining levels throughout daytime, a quiescent period of minimal secretory activity centered around midnight, and an abrupt elevation during late sleep resulting in an early morning maximum. Mathematical derivations of secretory rates from plasma concentrations have suggested that the 24-hour profile of plasma cortisol reflects a succession of secretory pulses of magnitude modulated by a circadian rhythm with no evidence of tonic secretion.[123, 140] In normal conditions, the acrophase of the pituitary-adrenal periodicity occurs between 6 and 10 AM. With a 15-minute sampling interval, 12 to 18 significant pulses of plasma ACTH and cortisol per 24-hour span can be detected.[141] There appears to be a temporal coupling between pulses of cortisol secretion and ultradian variations in an EEG marker of alertness.[117]

The 24-hour rhythm of adrenal secretion is primarily dependent on the circadian pattern of ACTH release, which is amplified by a daily variation in adrenal responsiveness to ACTH. The rhythm in ACTH release results, in turn, from periodic changes in level of stimulation by corticotropin-releasing-hormone (CRH). Circadian and pulsatile variations parallel to that of cortisol have been demonstrated for the plasma levels of several other adrenal steroids, in particular dehydroepiandrosterone (DHEA)[142] (Fig. 17–9).

The profiles shown in the upper panels of Figure 17–5 illustrate the remarkable persistence of the cortisol—and by inference, ACTH—secretory rhythm when sleep is manipulated. Indeed, the overall waveshape of the profile was not markedly affected by the absence of sleep or the presence of sleep at an abnormal time of day. Thus, this rhythm is primarily controlled by the circadian pacemaker. Modulatory effects of sleep-wake homeostasis have, however, been clearly demonstrated. Sleep onset is consistently associated with a short-term inhibition of cortisol secretion (which may not be detectable when sleep is initiated in the morning, that is, at the peak of corticotropic activity.[143–146] This inhibitory effect of sleep appears to be related to SW sleep stages.[147] Conversely, during the second part of the sleep period, awakenings, and in particular the final awakening, are consistently followed by secretory cortisol pulses.[148, 149] Thus, in normal conditions, the sleep-wake transitions amplify the effects of circadian rhythmicity. Studies of the 24-hour cortisol profile in the course of adaptation to shifts of the sleep-wake cycle have demonstrated that the end of the quiescent period, which coincides with the onset of the early morning rise, takes longer to adjust and appears to be a robust marker of circadian timing. Twin studies have demonstrated that the timing of the nadir is influenced by genetic factors,[150] providing evidence for a genetic control of human circadian phase. In contrast, the

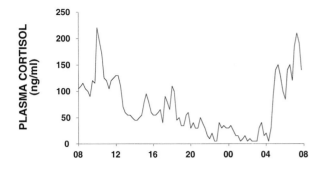

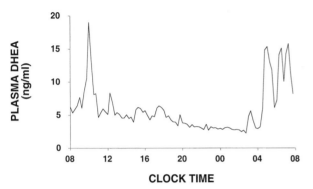

FIGURE 17–9. Twenty-four-hour profile of plasma cortisol and dehydroepiandrosterone levels sampled at 15-minute intervals in a healthy young man. Note the temporal concomitance of circadian and pulsatile variations of the two hormones. (Data from Lejeune-Lenain C, Van Cauter E, Desir D, et al: Control of circadian and episodic variations of adrenal androgens secretion in man. J Endocrinal Invest 10:267–276, 1987.)

timing of the morning acrophase is more labile, and may be influenced by the timing of sleep offset,[149] the transition from dark to bright light,[151] and breakfast intake.[152] Finally, anticipation of the expected time of waking has been reported to be associated with a rise in ACTH, but not cortisol, levels during the end of the sleep period.[153]

In addition to the immediate modulatory effects of sleep-wake transitions on ACTH and cortisol levels, nocturnal sleep deprivation, whether partial or total, acute (1 night) or chronic (1 week), results in elevated cortisol concentrations on the following evening[108, 109] (see Fig. 17–8). Thus, sleep loss appears to delay the return to quiescence of the HPA axis normally occurring in the evening. This suggests that sleep loss, similar to aging, may slow down the rate of recovery of the HPA axis response following a challenge and could therefore facilitate the development of central and peripheral disturbances associated with glucocorticoid excess—in particular with elevated cortisol concentrations at the time of the normal daily nadir, such as memory deficits, insulin resistance, and osteoporosis.[112, 154–156]

The circadian rhythm of cortisol persists throughout adulthood and has been observed through the ninth decade.[70, 111] In young adults, 24-hour cortisol levels are slightly lower in women than in men, primarily because of lower morning maxima. With aging, evening cortisol levels increase progressively, both in men and women, so that the cortisol nadir is three- to fourfold higher in healthy subjects over 70 years of age than in young adults. As a result, older subjects have elevated 24-hour mean cortisol levels and a reduced amplitude of cortisol variations. In addition, the timing of the nadir is advanced by 1 to 2 hours, indicating that aging is associated with an advance of circadian phase.[70, 111]

In pregnancy, total and, to a much lesser extent, free cortisol levels are elevated but the circadian pattern of secretion persists, albeit set at a higher level.[157] Interestingly, placental CRH is secreted into the maternal circulation in a pulsatile but not in a circadian fashion, and there is no correlation between maternal levels of CRH and ACTH.

Remarkably, ACTH and cortisol concentrations remain strongly correlated with each other over time, suggesting that maternal ACTH is probably driven by another ACTH secretagogue, most likely arginine vasopressin.[158]

Alterations in Disease States

The 24-hour profile of pituitary-adrenal secretion remains largely unaltered in a wide variety of pathologic states. Disease states in which pronounced alterations of the cortisol rhythm have been observed include primarily (1) disorders involving abnormalities in binding or metabolism of cortisol; (2) the various forms of Cushing's syndrome; and (3) severe depression.

The relative amplitude of the circadian rhythm and of the episodic fluctuations of cortisol is blunted in patients with liver disease[159] and in patients with anorexia nervosa,[160] primarily because of the decreased metabolic clearance of cortisol. In hypothyroid patients, the mean level is markedly elevated, and the relative amplitude of the rhythm is therefore dampened.[161] These alterations are thought to be due to both diminished clearance and decreased efficiency of the feedback control. In contrast, in hyperthyroidism, where cortisol production and peripheral metabolism are increased, episodic pulses are enhanced.[162]

In patients with Cushing's syndrome secondary to adrenal adenoma or ectopic ACTH secretion, the circadian variation of plasma cortisol is invariably absent.[163] In contrast, a low-amplitude circadian variation may persist in pituitary-dependent Cushing's disease. Cortisol pulsatility is blunted in about 70% of patients with Cushing's disease, suggesting autonomous tonic secretion of ACTH by a pituitary tumor. However, in about 30% of these patients, the magnitude of the pulses is instead enhanced.[164] These ''hyperpulsatile'' patterns could be caused by enhanced hypothalamic release of CRH or persistent pituitary responsiveness to CRH.[164, 165] It has also been shown that patients with Cushing's disease secrete ACTH and cortisol jointly more asynchronously than healthy subjects.[166] The left and middle panels of Figure 17–10 compare representative and mean 24-hour cortisol profiles in normal subjects and in patients with Cushing's disease.

The absence or even the dampening of cortisol circadian variations in Cushing's syndrome has obvious implications for clinical diagnosis, as the times of day when plasma samples are obtained have to be taken into account in the evaluation of the result. For example, a plasma cortisol level of 15 μg/dL (414 nmol/L) at 8 AM is perfectly normal while the same value obtained 12 hours later is indicative of some form of hypercortisolism. Differentiation between normal and pathologic levels may actually be greatly improved by adequately selecting the sampling time because the overlap between normal values and values in patients with Cushing's syndrome is minimal during a 4-hour interval centered around midnight.

Hypercortisolism with persistent circadian rhythmicity and increased pulsatility is found in a majority of severely depressed patients.[167, 168] This is illustrated in the right panel of Figure 17–10. In these patients, who do not develop the clinical signs of Cushing's syndrome despite the high circulating cortisol levels, the quiescent period of cortisol secretion is shorter and more fragmented, and often starts later and ends earlier than in normal subjects of comparable age. As discussed earlier, these alterations could reflect the impact of sleep disturbances, as well as an advance of circadian phase. When a clinical remission of the depressed state is obtained, the hypercortisolism and the alterations in quiescent period disappear, indicating that these disturbances are ''state''- rather than ''trait''-dependent.[169] Contrasting with the increased cortisol pulsatility frequently observed in major depression, a few studies have found decreased cortisol pulsatility in chronic fatigue syndrome and in post-traumatic stress disorder.[170, 171] In chronic fatigue syndrome, cortisol levels have been reported to be low, normal, or elevated.[171, 172]

The Somatotropic Axis

The 24-Hour Profile of Growth Hormone in Normal Subjects

In normal adult subjects, the 24-hour profile of plasma GH levels consists of stable low levels abruptly interrupted by bursts of secretion.

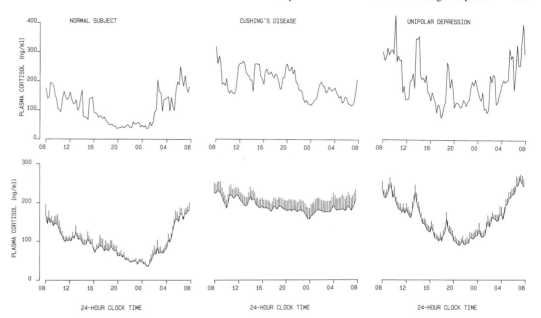

FIGURE 17–10. Twenty-four-hour profiles of plasma cortisol in normal subjects *(left)*, patients with pituitary Cushing's disease *(middle)*, and patients with major endogenous depression of the unipolar subtype *(right)*. For each condition, a representative example is shown in the top panel and mean profiles from 8 to 10 subjects are shown in the lower panel. In the lower panel, the vertical lines at each time point represent the SEM. (From Van Cauter E: Physiology and pathology of circadian rhythms. *In* Edwards CW, Lincoln DW (eds): Recent Advances in Endocrinology and Metabolism. Edinburgh, Churchill Livingstone, 1989, vol 3, pp 109–134.)

The most reproducible pulse occurs shortly after sleep onset, in association with the first phase of SW sleep.[173] Other secretory pulses may occur in later sleep and during wakefulness, in the absence of any identifiable stimulus. Studies in young male twins have evidenced a major genetic effect on GH secretion.[174] In adult men, the sleep-onset GH pulse is generally the largest, and often the only, pulse observed over the 24-hour span. In normally cycling women, the 24-hour GH levels are higher than in age-matched men, daytime pulses are more frequent, and the sleep-associated pulse, while still present in most cases, does not generally account for the majority of the 24-hour GH release.[175] Typical profiles of young men and women are shown in Figure 17–11. Well-documented studies have demonstrated that in women the amplitude of GH secretory pulses is correlated with the circulating level of estradiol.[175, 176] In addition, preliminary data indicate that in normally cycling young women, GH secretion during waking hours—but not during the sleep period—increases during the luteal phase as compared to the follicular phase and that this elevation correlates positively with plasma levels of progesterone but not estradiol.[177]

Sleep onset will elicit a GH secretory pulse whether sleep is advanced, delayed, interrupted, or fragmented.[173] Thus, as illustrated in Figure 17–5, shifts of the sleep-wake cycle are immediately followed by parallel shifts of the GH rhythm.[173] The release of GH in early sleep is temporally and quantitatively associated with the amount of SW sleep.[178, 179] The mechanisms underlying the relationship between SW sleep and GH release are thought to involve synchronous activity of growth hormone–releasing hormone (GHRH) neurons in the arcuate nucleus—resulting in stimulation of pituitary GH release—and of GHRH neurons in other hypothalamic areas which project to areas involved in the regulation of SW sleep.[180] Indeed, inhibition of endogenous GHRH, either by administration of a specific antagonist or by immunoneutralization, inhibits sleep as well as GH secretion,[181] indicating that GHRH plays a major role in the control of nocturnal GH secretion. However, while sleep is clearly the major determinant of GH secretion in man, there is also evidence for the existence of a circadian modulation of the occurrence and amplitude of GH pulses, reflecting decreased somatostatin inhibitory activity in the evening and during the night.[182] Thus, the major sleep onset–associated GH pulse is caused by a surge of hypothalamic GHRH coincident with a circadian period of relative somatostatin disinhibition.[173, 181]

Recent studies have indicated that compounds which promote SW sleep could represent a novel class of GH secretagogues. Indeed, enhancement of SW sleep by oral administration of low doses of γ-hydroxybutyrate, a natural metabolite of γ-aminobutyric acid (GABA) used in the treatment of narcolepsy,[183] or of ritanserin, a selective serotonin S_2 antagonist,[64] results in simultaneous and highly correlated increases in nocturnal GH secretion.

Aging is associated with dramatic decreases in circulating levels of GH.[70, 175] This reduction is achieved by a decrease in amplitude, rather than in frequency, of GH pulses.[70, 184, 185] However, it has recently been suggested that the orderliness of GH secretion is decreased in the elderly.[186] This age-related GH decrease occurs in an exponential fashion between young adulthood and midlife and follows the same chronology as the decrease in SW sleep. Despite the persistence of high levels of sex steroids, plasma concentrations and pulsatile secretion rates of GH fall in midlife to less than half the values achieved in young adulthood. Thereafter, smaller and more progressive decrements occur from midlife to old age.[187] In the elderly, GH secretory profiles are similar in men and in women.[175] The age-related reduction of GH secretion appears to result from increased somatostatin secretion and diminished GHRH responsiveness.[188]

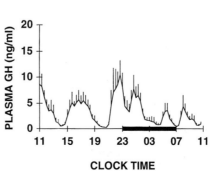
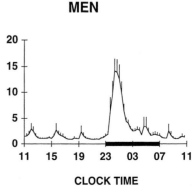

FIGURE 17–11. Mean (+SEM) 24-hour plasma growth hormone profiles in nine men, age 18 to 30 years, and in seven women, age 21 to 33 years, during the follicular phase. The *black bars* represent the sleep periods. (Adapted from Van Cauter E, Plat L, Copinschi G: Interrelations between sleep and the somatotropic axis. Sleep 21:533–566, 1998.)

Interestingly, during pregnancy a placental GH variant, which substitutes for pituitary GH to regulate maternal insulin-like growth factor-1 (IGF-1) levels,[189] is released in a tonic rather than pulsatile fashion.[190]

Alterations in Disease States

Abnormalities in the 24-hour profile of plasma GH have been reported in a variety of metabolic, endocrine, neurologic, and psychiatric conditions. We shall briefly describe the major alterations found in those conditions for which the temporal pattern has been defined in detail.

There is an inverse relationship between adiposity and GH release which results in a marked suppression of GH levels throughout the 24-hour span in obese subjects. A reduction in pulse frequency, as well as a decrease in GH half-life, has been suggested to underlie the hyposomatotropism of obesity.[191] A normal pattern can be restored after prolonged fasting.[192] In subjects of normal weight, fasting, even for only 1 day, enhances GH secretion via an increase in both pulse amplitude and pulse frequency.[193] Nonobese juvenile- or maturity-onset diabetic patients hypersecrete GH during wakefulness, as well as during sleep, primarily because of an increase in amplitude of pulses.[194] This abnormality may disappear when glycemia is strictly controlled.

In functional hypothalamic amenorrhea, the 24-hour mean GH levels are normal, but the pattern of pulsatile GH release is distinctly altered, with a decrease in pulse amplitude, a 40% increase in pulse frequency, and a twofold increase in interpulse GH concentrations.[195] In lean women with the polycystic ovary syndrome (PCOS), the amplitude—but not the frequency—of GH pulses is increased as compared with body mass index–matched normally cycling controls. In contrast, pulse amplitude is similarly reduced in both obese women with PCOS and obese controls.[196] Diurnal and nocturnal episodes of GH secretion are more frequent and of higher amplitude in adult subjects with hyperthyroidism, who have an overall daily GH production rate fourfold greater than normal.[197] Patients with major depression often have the major nocturnal GH pulse before, rather than after, sleep onset.[198]

In acromegaly, GH is hypersecreted throughout the 24-hour span, with a highly irregular pulsatile pattern superimposed on elevated basal levels, indicative of the presence of tonic secretion.[199] After pituitary surgery, a normal 24-hour pattern of GH release can be restored in most, but not all, patients.[199, 200]

The Lactotropic Axis

The 24-Hour Profile of Prolactin in Normal Subjects

Under normal conditions, the 24-hour profile of PRL levels exhibits a major nocturnal elevation starting shortly after sleep onset and culminating around midsleep (see Figure 17–5). Episodic pulses occur throughout the 24-hour span, but their amplitude and their frequency are higher during the night than during the day. Mean PRL levels, pulse amplitude, and pulse frequency are all higher in normally cycling women than in either postmenopausal women or normal young men.[201] These data indicate that endogenous estrogens play a critical role in the differential regulation of PRL secretion associated with sex and age. Deconvolution analysis has shown that the PRL profile reflects both tonic and intermittent release.[122] Twin studies have revealed that genetic factors determine partially the temporal organization of PRL secretion.[202]

Diurnal PRL variations are primarily regulated by sleep-wake homeostasis. Sleep onset is invariably associated with an increase in PRL secretion, irrespective of the time of the day, but the amplitude of the PRL rise may be dampened when associated with daytime sleep as compared to nocturnal sleep. Conversely, modest elevations of PRL levels may occur during waking around the time of the usual sleep onset, particularly in women. Thus, PRL secretion appears to be modulated by circadian rhythmicity and maximal secretion occurs when sleep and circadian effects are superimposed, that is, at the usual

bedtime.[203–205] Benzodiazepine (e.g., triazolam) and imidazopyridine (e.g., zolpidem) hypnotics taken at bedtime generally cause an increase in the nocturnal PRL elevation, resulting transiently in concentrations in the pathologic range.[206, 207]

A close temporal relationship has been evidenced between increased PRL secretion and SW activity when sleep structure is characterized by power spectral analysis of the EEG.[67] Conversely, prolonged awakenings interrupting sleep are consistently associated with decreasing PRL concentrations.[67] Thus, shallow and fragmented sleep will generally be associated with a dampening of the nocturnal PRL rise. This is indeed observed in elderly subjects who have a decreased amplitude of nocturnal PRL pulses.[70, 208] No sex difference in PRL pattern is observed between men and postmenopausal women, consistent with an absence of modulatory effects of the role of estrogens in older women.

During pregnancy, serum PRL levels rise, but the 24-hour pattern of secretion is maintained, albeit at a higher level. During the postpartum period, PRL secretory pulses follow suckling episodes and the nocturnal rise, independent of suckling, is only evident once breast-feeding has ceased.[209]

Alterations in Disease States

Absence or blunting of the nocturnal increase of plasma PRL has been reported in a variety of pathologic states, including uremia and breast cancer in postmenopausal women. In Cushing's disease, PRL levels are elevated throughout the 24-hour cycle and the relative amplitude of the nighttime rise is reduced.[210] In subjects with insulin-dependent diabetes, the circadian and sleep modulation of PRL secretion is preserved, but overall levels are markedly diminished.[211]

In hyperprolactinemia associated with prolactinomas, the number of PRL pulses is increased and the regularity of the pulsatile pattern is decreased. The nocturnal elevation of PRL may be preserved.[212, 213] Selective removal of PRL-secreting adenomas generally results in the normalization of the circadian pattern.

Abnormal PRL profiles have also been reported in a variety of neurologic and psychiatric disorders, including narcolepsy, depression, and schizophrenia.

The Gonadotropic Axis

Normal Diurnal Profiles of Luteinizing Hormone, Follicle-Stimulating Hormone, and Sex Steroids

Rhythms in the gonadotropic axis cover a wide range of frequencies, from episodic release in the ultradian range, to diurnal rhythmicity and monthly and seasonal cycles. These various rhythms interact to provide a coordinated temporal program governing the development of the reproductive axis and its operation at every stage of maturation. The following description of the current state of knowledge in this area will be limited to 24-hour rhythms and their interaction with pulsatile release during adulthood.

Patterns of LH release in adult men exhibit large interindividual variability.[214] The diurnal variation is dampened and may become undetectable. During the sleep period, LH pulses appear to be temporally related to the REM-NREM cycle.[215] In contrast, a marked diurnal rhythm in circulating testosterone levels is present in young normal men, with minimal levels in the late evening and maximal levels in the early morning.[142, 216] In young adult men, the amplitude of the testosterone rhythm averages 25%.[142] With a 15-minute sampling interval, 17 to 18 testosterone pulses per 24-hour span can be detected.[142] Thus, the robust circadian rhythm of plasma testosterone may be partially controlled by factors other than LH, such as sleep-associated variations in testicular blood flow, diurnal changes in Leydig cell response to LH, or circadian fluctuations in other hormones, singly or in combination. Diurnal profiles of testosterone are paralleled by inhibin B variations, with peak values in the early morning and nadirs in the late afternoon, and significant cross-correlations between inhibin B and testosterone or estradiol, but not between inhibin B and FSH, have been detected.[217] In older men, the amplitude of LH pulses is decreased,[218, 219] but their frequency is increased[220] and no significant diurnal pattern can be detected.[221] The circadian variation of testosterone is still present, although markedly dampened,[216, 221] but pulsatile testosterone secretion is attenuated, suggesting a partial desensitization of Leydig cells to LH.[220] In addition, older males secrete LH and testosterone more irregularly, and jointly more asynchronously, than younger men.[222]

In adult women, the 24-hour variation in plasma LH is markedly modulated by the menstrual cycle.[223, 224] Representative profiles are shown in Figure 17–12. In the early follicular phase, LH pulses are large and infrequent and a slowing of the frequency of secretory pulses occurs during sleep. In the midfollicular phase, pulse amplitude is decreased, pulse frequency increased, and the frequency modulation of LH pulsatility by sleep is less apparent. Pulse amplitude increases again by the late follicular phase. In the early luteal phase, the pulse amplitude is markedly increased, the pulse frequency is decreased, and nocturnal slowing of pulsatility is again evident. In the midluteal phase, pulse amplitude and frequency are decreased and there is no modulation by sleep. Both pulse amplitude and frequency further decrease in the late luteal phase. During the luteal-follicular transition, there is a four- to fivefold increase in LH pulse frequency, which accompanies the selective FSH rise necessary for normal folliculogenesis.[225] The apparent inhibitory effect of sleep during the early follicular phase is particularly intriguing, as this effect is in the opposite direction from that observed in pubertal girls, in whom the sleep period is associated with an increase in LH pulse amplitude and an elevation of overall LH levels. Circulating levels of LH and FSH and LH pulse frequency increase with aging and are higher in normal women over 40 years of age with regular menstrual cycles than in

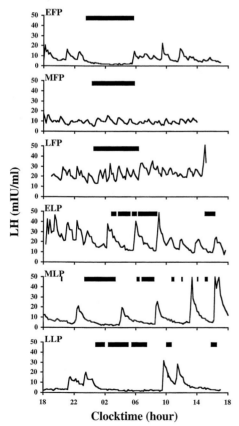

FIGURE 17–12. *Representative 24-hour profiles of plasma luteinizing hormone in healthy women studied in the early follicular phase (EFP), midfollicular phase (MFP), late follicular phase (LFP), early luteal phase (ELP), midluteal phase (MLP), and late luteal phase (LLP). Sleep periods are indicated by black bars.* (Adapted from Filicori M, Santoro N, Merriam GR, Crowley WFJ: Characterization of the physiological pattern of episodic gonadotropin secretion throughout the menstrual cycle. J Clin Endocrinol Metab 62:1136–1144, 1986.)

women under age 35.[226] After menopause, gonadotropin levels are elevated, but show no consistent circadian pattern.[227]

Alterations in Disease States

Early studies on the 24-hour profile of plasma LH in anorexia nervosa have established the importance of an adequate temporal secretory program in the maintenance of normal reproductive function. In women with amenorrhea secondary to anorexia nervosa, the secretory pattern of LH regresses to the pubertal or prepubertal pattern, with low daytime pulsatility and increased secretion at night.[227] Following weight gain and clinical remission, normal secretory profiles of LH are usually observed. Short-term fasting was recently shown to suppress pulsatile LH secretion while enhancing its regularity in young, but not older, men.[228]

The slowing or absence of pulsatile hypothalamic GnRH release is the underlying cause of ovarian acyclicity in women with functional hypothalamic amenorrhea (FHA).[227, 229] The reduction appears more marked during the daytime than during sleep, suggesting that the mechanisms involved in this pathologic suppression of pulsatile GnRH release are partially inhibited during sleep.[229] Women afflicted with FHA show an approximate 50% reduction in LH pulse frequency and an increase in the LH pulse interval, while the integrated plasma LH and FSH concentrations are reduced by 30% to 45%.[195] Decreased LH pulse frequency and amplitude may also be observed in women runners who are normally menstruating,[230] suggesting that exercise-associated amenorrhea is a further development of the alterations in the pattern of GnRH activity seen in eumenorrheic women runners.

Different forms of abnormal temporal organization of the GnRH signal seem involved in the PCOS. In pubertal girls with recent-onset PCOS,[231] the circadian rhythm of LH secretion was found to be out of phase with the sleep-wake cycle so that, in normal pubertal children, LH increased during the night, whereas in PCOS patients, the LH augmentation occurred during the day. Similar alterations were found in anovulatory healthy adolescent girls at early gynecologic age. Interestingly, these alterations persisted in those of the girls who were still amenorrheic at late gynecologic age, while the diurnal LH variations disappeared in the girls who became ovulatory.[232] Thus, the abnormal circadian timing of the LH rhythm in PCOS patients might not allow normal ovulatory cycles to develop. In adult PCOS patients, the amplitude and the frequency of LH pulses was consistently found to be increased and overall levels of FSH to be depressed,[196, 233, 234] suggesting that the excessively rapid GnRH pulsations selectively suppress FSH secretion. A similar defect of abnormally high GnRH frequency seems to underly luteal phase deficiency. Indeed, studies have shown that, in this condition, LH pulse frequency is increased during the follicular phase, indicating that this temporal alteration may be implicated in the etiology of the condition.[235]

Increased LH pulse frequency and decreased pulse amplitude have also been observed in patients suffering from premenstrual syndrome (PMS) and these findings have suggested the possible involvement of opioidergic dysfunction in this condition.[236] Alterations in circadian rhythmicity, consisting of advances in circadian rhythms relative to the timing of the sleep-wake cycle, as well as reduced melatonin levels, have also been found in PMS patients.[237] These abnormalities may contribute to pathologic conditions associated with PMS, and correcting such circadian disturbances may lead to clinical remission.[237] Patients with late luteal phase dysphoric disorders have abnormally phase-advanced rhythms, and exposure to bright light in the evening, but not in the morning, was effective in inducing a significant reduction in the depression score.[237] Since evening bright light can cause phase delays of circadian rhythms, these results raise the possibility that circadian dysregulation, whether induced by life-style, the environment, or the reproductive system itself, may be a common pathogenic factor in mood disorders observed in women.[237]

In the majority of men with idiopathic hypogonadotropic hypogonadism, LH pulses are undetectable.[238] In a small number of patients, an early pubertal pattern, with enhanced pulse amplitude during the nighttime, may be observed.[238] States of hyperprolactinemia are also associated with suppression of LH pulse amplitude and frequency.[239]

An attenuation of pulsatile LH secretion has been evidenced in men, but not in women, during both hypo- and hypercortisolism. The authors speculated that this sex difference could be due to a higher level of hypothalamic opioid activity in men.[240]

The Thyrotropic Axis

The 24-Hour Profile of Thyrotropin in Normal Subjects

The 24-hour pattern of TSH levels appears to be generated by frequency as well as amplitude modulation of thyrotropin releasing hormone (TRH)-driven secretory pulses.[241] In normal adult men and women, TSH levels are low throughout the daytime and begin to increase in the late afternoon or early evening. Maximal levels occur shortly before sleep.[241] During sleep, TSH levels generally decline slowly. Studies involving sleep deprivation and shifts of the sleep-wake cycle have consistently indicated that an inhibitory influence is exerted on TSH secretion during sleep. Interestingly, when sleep occurs during daytime, TSH secretion is not suppressed significantly below normal daytime levels. Profiles of plasma TSH during normal nocturnal sleep, nocturnal sleep deprivation, and daytime sleep are illustrated in the lower panel of Figure 17–5. Conversely, when the depth of sleep is enhanced by prior sleep deprivation, the inhibition of the nocturnal TSH rise is more pronounced than in basal conditions. The modulation of TSH secretion by sleep appears to be exerted by amplitude modulation of TRH pulses via dopaminergic mechanisms.[241] Descending slopes of TSH concentrations during sleep are consistently associated with SW stages.[242] Conversely, awakenings are frequently associated with TSH increments.[243] The timing of the TSH evening rise seems to be controlled by circadian rhythmicity and shifts in concordance with the melatonin rhythm following exposure to light or nocturnal exercise.[21]

Circadian or sleep-related variations in thyroid hormones are difficult to detect.[244, 245] It has been suggested that the nocturnal TSH surge could involve variant TSH molecules with reduced bioactivity. Under conditions of sleep deprivation, the increased amplitude of the TSH rhythm may result in a detectable increase in plasma triiodothyronine (T_3) levels, paralleling the nocturnal TSH rise,[246] although negative findings have been also reported.[247] If sleep deprivation is prolonged for a second night, the nocturnal rise of TSH is markedly diminished compared to that occurring during the first night.[246, 247] It is likely that, following the first night of sleep deprivation, the elevated thyroid hormone levels, which persist during the daytime period because of the prolonged half-life of these hormones, limit the subsequent TSH rise. A well-documented study involving 64 hours of sleep deprivation demonstrated a more than 50% increase in the T_3 level measured at 11 PM across the study period without significant change in the concomitant thyroxine (T_4) concentration.[248] During the second night of sleep deprivation, a nocturnal increase in both T_3 and T_4 levels was observed, contrasting with the decreases seen during normal sleep.[248] These data suggest that prolonged sleep loss may be associated with an upregulation of the thyroid axis. Consistent findings have been reported in a recent study of 1 week of partial sleep loss (4 hours in bed per night) where the nocturnal TSH rise was strikingly decreased, probably secondary to increased levels of thyroid hormones resulting from an initial TSH elevation at the beginning of sleep curtailment.[108]

Because inhibitory effects of sleep on TSH secretion are time-dependent, elevations of plasma TSH levels may occur in conditions of misalignment of sleep and circadian timing. This is illustrated in Figure 17–13 which shows the mean profiles of plasma TSH observed in a group of normal young men in the course of adaptation to a simulated jet lag involving an abrupt 8-hour advance of the sleep-wake cycle and the dark period, following a 24-hour baseline period. In the course of adaptation, TSH levels increased progressively because nighttime wakefulness was associated with large circadian-dependent TSH elevations while daytime sleep failed to inhibit TSH. This study indicates that the subjective discomfort and fatigue associated with jet lag may involve a prolonged elevation of a hormonal concentration in the peripheral circulation.

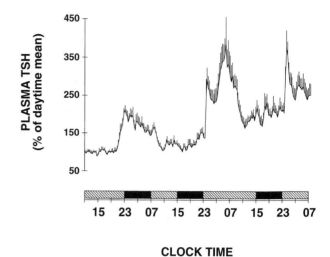

FIGURE 17–13. Mean (and SEM) profiles of plasma thyrotropin from eight normal young men who were submitted to an 8-hour advance of the sleep-wake and light-dark cycles. *Black bars* indicate bedtime periods. (Data from Hirschfeld U, Moreno-Reyes R, Akseki E, et al: Progressive elevation of plasma thyrotropin during adaptation to simulated jet lag: Effects of treatment with bright light or zolpidem. J Clin Endocrinol Metab 81:3270–3277, 1996.)

Aging is associated with a progressive decrease in overall TSH secretion (which is achieved by a decrease in amplitude, rather than in frequency, of secretory pulses) and in circulating TSH levels, and with a damping of the amplitude of the circadian variation.[70] In subjects in the seventh and eighth decades, TSH levels are lower than in young adults throughout the 24-hour span, although the difference is more marked during sleep than during the daytime period. In middle-aged subjects, age-related decreases in TSH levels may be evidenced only in response to nocturnal sleep deprivation. Thus, it appears that the TSH secretory capacity declines progressively with aging.

Alterations in Disease States

A decreased or absent nocturnal rise of TSH has been observed in a wide variety of nonthyroidal illnesses,[249] suggesting that hypothalamic dysregulation will generally affect the circadian TSH surge. This is in contrast to the circadian variation of plasma cortisol, which persists in a wide variety of disease states. The nocturnal TSH surge is diminished or absent in various conditions of hypercortisolism,[250] as well as in primary and secondary hypothyroidism[251] and hyperthyroidism. It has been reported that the lack of nocturnal TSH surge in patients with nontoxic nodular goiter may predict the subsequent occurrence of hyperthyroidism.[252] In poorly controlled diabetic states, whether insulin-dependent or non–insulin-dependent, the surge also disappears.[253] Correction of hyperglycemia is associated with a reappearance of the nocturnal elevation.[253] Interestingly, morning TSH values in the hyperglycemic patients do not differ from those of control subjects, and the TSH response to TRH is only marginally reduced.[253]

Glucose Tolerance and Insulin Secretion

Diurnal and Ultradian Variations in Normal Subjects

In normal humans, glucose tolerance varies with the time of day. Figure 17–14 shows circadian variations in glucose tolerance to oral glucose, identical meals, intravenous glucose, and constant glucose infusion. In all four conditions, plasma glucose levels are markedly higher in the evening than in the morning.[62] Studies of fasting during nocturnal sleep have consistently observed that, despite the prolonged fasting condition, glucose levels remain stable or fall only minimally across the night, contrasting with a clear decrease during daytime fasting. Thus, a number of mechanisms operative during nocturnal sleep are likely to maintain stable glucose levels during the overnight fast. Experimental protocols involving intravenous glucose infusion or enteral nutrition, while allowing for normal nocturnal sleep, have shown that glucose tolerance deteriorates further as the evening progresses, reaches a minimum around midsleep, and then improves to return to morning levels.[145, 254] There is evidence that this diurnal variation in glucose tolerance is partly driven by the wide and highly reproducible diurnal rhythm of plasma cortisol, an important counter-regulatory hormone.[62, 112, 255] Indeed, the diurnal variation in insulin secretion was found to be inversely related to the cortisol rhythm, with a significant correlation of the magnitudes of their morning-to-

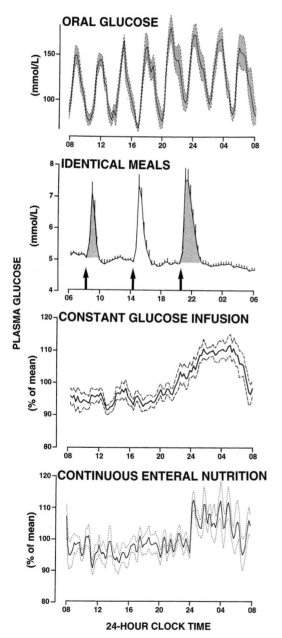

FIGURE 17–14. *Twenty-four-hour pattern of plasma glucose changes in response to oral glucose 50 g every 3 hours (top panel), identical meals (second panel from the top), constant glucose infusion (third panel from the top), and continuous enteral nutrition (bottom panel) in normal young adults. At each time point, the mean glucose level is shown with the SEM. (From Van Cauter E, Polonsky KS, Scheen AJ: Roles of circadian rhythmicity and sleep in human glucose regulation. Endocr Rev 18:716–738, 1997.)*

evening excursions. Rises in plasma levels of glucose and insulin following short-term elevations of plasma cortisol are more pronounced in the evening than in the morning.[112] Diminished insulin sensitivity and decreased β cell responsiveness are also involved in reduced glucose tolerance later in the day. Under conditions of constant glucose infusion, sleep-associated rises in glucose were found to correlate with the amount of concomitant GH secreted. Thus, during the first part of the night, decreased glucose tolerance is due to decreased glucose utilization both by peripheral tissues—resulting from muscle relaxation and rapid insulin-like effects of sleep-onset GH secretion—and by the brain—as assessed by imaging studies demonstrating a reduction in glucose uptake during SW sleep.[256] During the second part of the night, these effects subside as sleep becomes shallow and more fragmented and GH is no longer secreted. Thus, complex interactions of circadian and sleep effects, possibly partly mediated by cortisol and GH, result in a consistent pattern of changes of set-point of glucose regulation over the 24-hour period. Consistent with the important modulatory effects of sleep on glucose regulation, chronic sleep loss is associated with marked alterations of levels of glucose tolerance, as described above under Conditions of Abnormal Circadian Rhythmicity.[108]

Human insulin secretion is a complex oscillatory process involving rapid pulses of small amplitude recurring every 10 to 15 minutes superimposed on slower ultradian oscillations with periods in the 90- to 120-minute range.[124] The ultradian oscillations are tightly coupled to glucose, with a tendency for glucose pulses to lead insulin pulses by 10 minutes, and have been shown to promote more efficient glucose utilization.[128] They are best seen in conditions where insulin secretion is stimulated, including ingestion of a meal, continuous enteral nutrition, or constant intravenous glucose infusion.[124, 254] Under these conditions, their relative amplitude is about 50% to 70% for insulin secretory pulses and 20% for plasma glucose. Their amplitude is maximal immediately after a meal, then decreases progressively. Moreover, the periodicity of the insulin secretory oscillations can be entrained to the period of an oscillatory glucose infusion,[257] supporting the concept that these ultradian oscillations are generated by the glucose-insulin feedback mechanism.[258] However, ultradian oscillations, but less regular and of smaller amplitude, are still present in fasting conditions. Stimulatory effects of sleep on insulin secretion are mediated by an increase in the amplitude of the oscillation.[254] During constant glucose infusion, REM sleep and wake episodes coincide significantly with decreasing levels of glucose and insulin, while increasing glucose levels occur during the deeper stages of NREM sleep.[256] The rapid 10- to 15-minute pulsations seem to have a different origin than do the ultradian oscillations. Indeed, they may appear independently of glucose, since they were observed in the isolated perfused pancreas and in perfused islets.[124]

Alterations in Metabolic Disorders

In obese and diabetic subjects, the diurnal and ultradian variations in glucose regulation are abnormal. In obesity, the morning vs. evening difference in glucose tolerance is abolished. Obese adult subjects show no diurnal variation in glucose tolerance, no decline in insulin sensitivity in the afternoon, and only a marginally significant decline in β cell responsiveness to glucose in the later part of the day.[259] In insulin-dependent diabetic patients, an increase in glucose levels or insulin requirements occurs in a prebreakfast period ranging from 5 to 9 AM and has been called the "dawn phenomenon."[260] A role for nocturnal GH secretion in the pathogenesis of the dawn phenomenon was demonstrated.[261] The observation of a dawn phenomenon in non–insulin-dependent diabetes mellitus (NIDDM) patients under normal dietary conditions has been less consistent. However, prominent late night and early morning elevations in glucose levels and insulin secretion in both normal subjects and diabetic patients become apparent during prolonged fasting.[262]

The rapid and ultradian oscillations of insulin secretion are perturbed in NIDDM and impaired glucose tolerance without hyperglycemia.[124, 263] The ultradian oscillations, which have an exaggerated amplitude in obese subjects without apparent changes in frequency or pattern of recurrence, are also more irregular and of lower amplitude in subjects with established NIDDM.[124]

Leptin

Diurnal and Ultradian Variations in Normal Subjects

In normal lean men and women, plasma leptin levels show a robust circadian variation, with minimum values during the daytime, and a nocturnal rise with maximum values during early to midsleep.[264] It has been speculated that the nocturnal rise in leptin serves to suppress appetite during the overnight period of fast and sleep. The amplitude of the circadian variation averages 25% to 30% of the mean level and is slightly higher in men than in women.[265] There are marked sex differences in 24-hour mean leptin levels which are 2- to 10-fold higher in women than in men, regardless of fat mass.[265, 266] Studies involving shifts of the meal schedule have shown that the timing of the daily maximum of plasma leptin levels is markedly dependent on the timing of meals.[267] However, the 24-hour rhythm of leptin concentrations is not simply a response to the feeding pattern. Indeed, the rhythm persists, albeit with a smaller amplitude, in subjects who receive continuous enteral nutrition.[268] Following an abrupt shift of the sleep period, nocturnal leptin levels rise despite the absence of sleep and a second rise is observed following the onset of daytime recovery sleep,[268] indicating that both intrinsic circadian rhythmicity and sleep-wake homeostasis influence the release of leptin. Studies in middle-aged and older adults have indicated that aging is associated with a damping of the amplitude of the 24-hour rhythm of plasma leptin and an advance of the nocturnal acrophase.[269]

In addition to the diurnal variation, several studies have reported that human leptin levels are pulsatile. Studies which have used a 7-minute sampling interval in subjects receiving four meals per 24 hours have detected 30 to 35 pulses of plasma leptin in both men and women, suggesting the existence of a negative correlation between instantaneous changes in leptin on the one hand, and ACTH and cortisol on the other.[266, 270] In contrast, in subjects receiving continuous enteral nutrition who were sampled at 10-minute intervals, only 13 to 14 pulses per 24-hour period were detected, and peak leptin levels were found to coincide with troughs of glucose and insulin oscillations.[268] Yet another study using a 20-minute sampling interval found only an average of 3.6 leptin pulses per 24-hour span.[265]

Alterations in Obesity and Weight Loss

Leptin levels are inversely related to body mass index and fat mass, and are thus higher in obese—with and without NIDDM—than in lean subjects. The circadian pattern is preserved in obese subjects, but the relative amplitude is lower than in normal-weight controls.[265] In women, the amplitude is larger in patients with lower body obesity than in patients with upper body obesity.[271] Leptin levels are increased by insulin administration, regardless of glucose levels and it has been speculated that the positive correlation between body fat and leptin could be partially mediated by insulin.[272] Elevations in glucocorticoid levels consistently result in increased leptin levels,[273] but the 24-hour rhythm in cortisol secretion does not appear to be responsible for the diurnal pattern of leptin levels.[274] In anorexia nervosa, as in amenorrheic female athletes, leptin levels are low and diurnal variations are abolished.[275, 276]

Acknowledgments

We thank Ms. R. Leproult for assistance with the preparation of the illustrations. We were partially supported by grants DK-41814 (Eve Van Cauter), AG-11412 (Eve Van Cauter and Fred W. Turek), HD-09885, HD-21921, HL-96015 (Fred W. Turek), and a grant from the Belgian Fonds de la Recherche Scientifique Médicale (Georges Copinschi).

REFERENCES

1. Turek FW: Circadian rhythms. Horm Res 49:103–113, 1998.
2. Borbely AA: Processes underlying sleep regulation. Horm Res 49:114–117, 1998.
3. Aschoff J: Circadian rhythms: General features and endocrinological aspects. In Krieger DT (ed): Endocrine Rhythms. New York, Raven Press, 1979, pp 1–61.
4. Wever RA: The Circadian System of Man: Results of Experiments under Temporal Isolation. New York, Springer Verlag, 1979.
5. Dijk DJ, Czeisler CA: Contribution of the circadian pacemaker and the sleep homeostat to sleep propensity, sleep structure, electroencephalographic slow waves, and sleep spindle activity in humans. J Neurosci 15:3526–3538, 1995.
6. Czeisler CA, Duffy JF, Shanahan TL, et al: Stability, precision, and near-24-hour period of the human circadian pacemaker. Science 284:2177–2181, 1999.
7. Turek FW: Pharmacological probes of the mammalian circadian clock: Use of the phase response curve approach. Trends Pharmacol Sci 8:212–217, 1987.
8. Boivin DB, Duffy JF, Kronauer RE, Czeisler CA: Dose-response relationships for resetting of human circadian clock by light. Nature 379:540–542, 1996.
9. Minors DS, Waterhouse JM, Wirz-Justice A: A human phase-response curve to light. Neurosci Lett 13:36–40, 1991.
10. Van Cauter E, Sturis J, Byrne MM, et al: Demonstration of rapid light-induced advances and delays of the human circadian clock using hormonal phase markers. Am J Physiol 266:E953–E963, 1994.
11. Czeisler CA, Kronauer RE, Allan JS, et al: Bright light induction of strong (type 0) resetting of the human circadian pacemaker. Science 244:1328–1333, 1989.
12. Jewett M, Kronauer RE, Czeisler CA: Light-induced suppression of endogenous circadian amplitude in humans. Nature 350:59–62, 1991.
13. Ellis GB, McKlveen RE, Turek FW: Dark pulses affect the circadian rhythm of activity in hamsters kept in constant light. Am J Physiol 242:RR44–RR50, 1982.
14. Lee TM, Labyak SE: Free-running rhythms and light- and dark-pulse phase response curves for diurnal Octodon degus (Rodentia). Am J Physiol 273:R278–R286, 1997.
15. Van Cauter E, Moreno-Reyes R, Akseki E, et al: Rapid phase advance of the 24-h melatonin profile in response to afternoon dark exposure. Am J Physiol 275:E48–E54, 1998.
16. Goichot B, Weibel L, Chapotot F, et al: Effect of the shift of the sleep-wake cycle on three robust endocrine markers of the circadian clock. Am J Physiol 275:E243–E248, 1998.
17. Buxton OM, L'Hermite-Balériaux M, Turek FW, Van Cauter E: Daytime naps in darkness phase shift the human circadian rhythms of melatonin and thyrotropin secretion. Am J Physiol 278:R373–R382, 2000.
18. Mrosovsky N: Locomotor activity and non-photic influences on the circadian clock. Biol Rev 71:343–372, 1996.
19. Turek FW, Smith R, Van Reeth O, Wickland C: Disturbances of the activity rest cycle alter the circadian clock of mammals. In Inouye S, Krieger JM (eds): Endogenous Sleep Factors. The Hague, Netherlands, SPB Academic Publishing, 1990, pp 277–283.
20. Van Reeth O, Sturis J, Byrne MM, et al: Nocturnal exercise phase delays circadian rhythms of melatonin and thyrotropin in normal men. Am J Physiol 266:E964–E974, 1994.
21. Buxton OM, Frank SA, L'Hermite-Baleriaux M, et al: Roles of intensity and duration of nocturnal exercise in causing phase-shifts of human circadian rhythms. Am J Physiol 273:E536–E542, 1997.
22. Eastman CI, Hoese EK, Youngstedt SD, Liu L: Phase-shifting human circadian rhythms with exercise during the night shift. Physiol Behav 58:1287–1291, 1995.
23. Klerman EB, Rimmer DW, Dijk DJ, et al: Non photic entrainment of the human circadian pacemaker. Am J Physiol 274:R991–E996, 1998.
24. Lewy AJ, Sack RL, Blood ML, et al: Melatonin marks circadian phase position and resets the endogenous circadian pacemaker in humans. In Chadwick DJ, Ackrill K (eds): CIBA Foundation Symposium 183. Circadian Clocks and Their Adjustment. Chichester, UK, Wiley, 1995, pp 303–321.
25. Geoffriau M, Brun J, Chazot G, Claustrat B: The physiology and pharmacology of melatonin in humans. Horm Res 49:136–141, 1998.
26. Shanahan TL, Czeisler CA: Light exposure induces equivalent phase shifts of the endogenous circadian rhythms of circulating plasma melatonin and core body temperature in men. J Clin Endocrinol Metab 73:227–235, 1991.
27. Lewy AJ, Bauer VK, Ahmed S, et al: The human phase response curve (PRC) to melatonin is about 12 hours out of phase with the PRC to light. Chronobiol Int 15:71–83, 1998.
28. Lehman MN, Silver R, Bittman EL: Anatomy of suprachiasmatic nucleus grafts. In Klein DC, Moore RY, Reppert SM (eds): Suprachiasmatic Nucleus: The Mind's Clock. New York, Oxford University Press, 1991, pp 349–374.
29. Ralph M, Foster RG, Davis FC, Menaker M: Transplanted suprachiasmatic nucleus determines circadian period. Science 247:975–978, 1990.
30. Ralph MR, Menaker M: A mutation in the circadian system of the golden hamster. Science 241:1225–1227, 1988.
31. Earnest DJ, Sladek CD: Circadian vasopressin release from perifused rat suprachiasmatic explants in vitro: Effects of acute stimulation. Brain Res 422:398–402, 1987.
32. Gillette MU: SCN electrophysiology in vitro: Rhythmic activity and endogenous clock properties. In Klein DC, Moore RY, Reppert SM (eds): Suprachiasmatic Nucleus: The Mind's Clock. New York, Oxford University Press, 1991.
33. Earnest DJ, Liang FQ, Ratcliff M, Cassone VM: Immortal time: Circadian clock properties of rat suprachiasmatic cell lines. Science 283:693–695, 1999.
34. Welsh DK, Logothetis DE, Meister M, Reppert SM: Individual neurons dissociated from rat suprachiasmatic nucleus express independently phased circadian firing rhythms. Neuron 14:697–706, 1995.
35. Card JP, Moore RY: The organization of visual circuits influencing the circadian activity of suprachiasmatic nucleus. In Klein DC, Moore RY, Reppert SM (eds): Suprachiasmatic Nucleus: The Mind's Clock. New York, Oxford University Press, 1991, pp 51–76.

36. Campbell SS, Murphy PJ: Extraocular circadian phototransduction in humans. Science 279:396–399, 1998.

37. van den Horst GT, Muijtiens M, Kobayashi K, et al: Mammalian Cry1 and Cry2 are essential for maintenance of circadian rhythms. Nature 398:627–630, 1999.

38. Czeisler CA, Shanahan TL, Klerman EB, et al: Suppression of melatonin in some blind subjects by exposure to light. N Engl J Med 332:6–11, 1995.

39. Zlomanczuk P, Schwartz WJ: Cellular and molecular mechanisms of circadian rhythms in mammals. *In* Turek FW, Zee PC (eds): Regulation of Sleep and Circadian Rhythms, vol 133. New York, Marcel Dekker, 1999, pp 309–342.

40. Penev PD, Zee PC, Turek FW: Serotonin in the spotlight. Nature 385:123, 1997.

41. Morin LP: Serotonin and the regulation of mammalian circadian rhythmicity. Ann Med 31:12–33, 1999.

42. Dunlap JC: Molecular bases for circadian clocks. Cell 96:271–290, 1999.

43. Wisor JP, Takahashi JS: Molecular genetic approaches to the identity and function of circadian clock genes. *In* Turek FW, Zee PC (eds): Regulation of Sleep and Circadian Rhythms, vol 133. New York, Marcel Dekker, 1999, pp 369–396.

44. Schwartz WJ, Zimmerman P: Circadian timekeeping in BALB/c and C57 BL/6 inbred mouse strains. J Neurosci 10:3685–3694, 1990.

45. Turek FW, Pinto LH, Vitaterna MH, et al: Pharmacological and genetic approaches for the study of circadian rhythms in mammals. Front Neuroendocrinol 16:191–223, 1995.

46. Vitaterna MH, King DP, Chang AM, et al: Mutagenesis and mapping of a mouse gene, Clock, essential for circadian behavior. Science 264:719–725, 1994.

47. King DP, Zhao Y, Sangoram AM, et al: Positional cloning of the mouse circadian Clock gene. Cell 89:641–653, 1997.

48. Whitmore D, Sassone-Corsi P: Cryptic clues to clock function. Nature 398:557–558, 1999.

49. Aschoff J: On the perception of time during prolonged temporal isolation. Hum Neurobiol 4:41–52, 1985.

50. Aschoff J, von Goetz C, Wildgruber C, Wever RA: Meal timing in humans during isolation without time cues. J Biol Rhythms 1:151–162, 1986.

51. Aschoff J: On the dilatability of subjective time. Perspect Biol Med 35:276–280, 1992.

52. Czeisler CA, Weitzman ED, Moore-Ede MC, et al: Human sleep: Its duration and organization depends on its circadian phase. Science 210:1264–1267, 1980.

53. Porkka-Heiskanen T, Strecker RE, Thakkar M, et al: Adenosine: A mediator of the sleep-inducing effects of prolonged wakefulness. Science 276:1255–1258, 1997.

54. Monk TH, Buysse DJ, Reynolds CF, et al: Circadian rhythms in human performance and mood under constant conditions. J Sleep Res 6:9–18, 1997.

55. Dijk DJ, Czeisler CA: Paradoxical timing of the circadian rhythm of sleep propensity serves to consolidate sleep and wakefulness in humans. Neurosci Lett 166:63–68, 1994.

56. Boivin DB, Czeisler CA, Dijk DJ, et al: Complex interaction of the sleep-wake cycle and circadian phase modulates mood in healthy subjects. Arch Gen Psychiatry 54:145–152, 1997.

57. Akerstedt T, Folkard S: Validation of the S and C components of the three-process model of alertness regulation. Sleep 18:1–6, 1995.

58. Leproult R, Van Reeth O, Byrne MM, et al: Sleepiness, performance and neuroendocrine function during sleep deprivation: Effects of exposure to bright light or exercise. J Biol Rhythms 12:245–258, 1997.

59. Edgar DM, Dement WC, Fuller CA: Effects of SCN lesions on sleep in squirrel monkeys: Evidence for opponent processes in sleep-wake regulation. J Neurosci 13:1065–1079, 1993.

60. Dijk DJ, Duffy JF, Riel E, et al: Ageing and the circadian and homeostaic regulation of human sleep during forced desynchrony of rest, melatonin and temperature rhythms. J Physiol (Lond) 516:611–627, 1999.

61. Brandenberger G, Follenius M, Goichot B, et al: Twenty-four hour profiles of plasma renin activity in relation to the sleep-wake cycle. J Hypertens 12:277–283, 1994.

62. Van Cauter E, Polonsky KS, Scheen AJ: Roles of circadian rhythmicity and sleep in human glucose regulation. Endocr Rev 18:716–738, 1997.

63. Follenius M, Brandenberger G, Simon C, Schlienger JL: REM sleep in humans begins during decreased secretory activity of the anterior pituitary. Sleep 11:546–555, 1988.

64. Gronfier C, Luthringer R, Follenius M, et al: A quantitative evaluation of the relationships between growth hormone secretion and delta wave electroencephalographic activity during normal sleep and after enrichment in delta waves. Sleep 19:817–824, 1996.

65. Gronfier C, Luthringer R, Follenius M, et al: Temporal link between plasma thyrotropin levels and electroencephalographic activity in man. Neurosci Lett 200:97–100, 1995.

66. Gronfier C, Luthringer R, Follenius M, et al: Temporal relationships between pulsatile cortisol secretion and electroencephalographic activity during sleep in man. Electroencephalogr Clin Neurophysiol 103:405–408, 1997.

67. Spiegel K, Luthringer R, Follenius M, et al: Temporal relationship between prolactin secretion and slow-wave electroencephalographic activity during sleep. Sleep 18:543–548, 1995.

68. Van Cauter E, Spiegel K: Circadian and sleep control of endocrine secretions. *In* Turek FW, Zee PC (eds): Neurobiology of Sleep and Circadian Rhythms. *In* Lenfant C (series ed): Lung Biology in Health and Disease, vol 133. New York, Marcel Dekker, 1999, pp 397–426.

69. Van Cauter E, Copinschi G: Interactions between growth hormone secretion and sleep. *In* Smith RG, Thorner MO (eds): Human Growth Hormone Secretion: Basic and Clinical Practice. *In* Conn PM (series ed): Contemporary Endocrinology, vol 19. Totowa, NJ, Humana Press, 1999, pp 261–283.

70. van Coevorden A, Mockel J, Laurent E, et al: Neuroendocrine rhythms and sleep in aging men. Am J Physiol 260:E651–E661, 1991.

71. Czeisler CA, Dumont M, Duffy JF, et al: Association of sleep-wake habits in older people with changes in output of circadian pacemaker. Lancet 340:933–936, 1992.

72. Van Cauter E, Plat L, Leproult R, Copinschi G: Alterations of circadian rhythmicity and sleep in aging: Endocrine consequences. Horm Res 49:147–152, 1998.

73. Prinz PN: Sleep and sleep disorders in older adults. J Clin Neurophysiol 12:139–146, 1995.

74. Zee PC, Rosenberg RS, Turek FW: Effects of aging on entrainment and rate of resynchronization of the circadian locomotor activity. Am J Physiol 263:1099–1103, 1992.

75. Morin LP: Age-related changes in hamster circadian period, entrainment and rhythm splitting. J Biol Rhythms 3:237–248, 1988.

76. Duffy JF, Viswanathan N, Davis FC: Free-running circadian period does not shorten with age in female Syrian hamsters. Neurosci Lett 271:77–80, 1999.

77. Zhang Y, Kornhauser JM, Zee PC, et al: Effects of aging on light-induced phase-shifting of circadian behavioral rhythms, Fos expression, and Creb phosphorylation in the hamster suprachiasmatic nucleus. Neuroscience 70:951–961, 1996.

78. Van Reeth O, Zhang Y, Zee PC, Turek FW: Aging alters feedback effects of the activity-rest cycle in the circadian clock. Am J Physiol 263:R981–R986, 1992.

79. Van Reeth O, Zhang Y, Reddy A, et al: Aging alters the entraining effects of an activity-inducing stimulus on the circadian clock. Brain Res 607:286–292, 1993.

80. Van Reeth O, Zhang Y, Zee PC, Turek FW: Grafting fetal suprachiasmatic nuclei in the hypothalamus of old hamsters restores responsiveness of the circadian clock to a phase shifting stimulus. Brain Res 643:338–342, 1994.

81. Campbell SS, Kripke DF, Gillin JC, Hrubovcak JC: Exposure to light in healthy elderly subjects and Alzheimer's patients. Physiol Behav 42:141–144, 1988.

82. Ehlers CL, Frank E, Kupfer DJ: Social zeitgebers and biological rhythms. Arch Gen Psychiatry 45:948–952, 1988.

83. Ancoli-Israel S, Kripke DF, Jones DW, et al: 24-hour sleep and light rhythms in nursing home patients (abstract). Sleep Res 20A:410, 1991.

84. Campbell SS, Dawson D, Anderson MW: Alleviation of sleep maintenance insomnia with timed exposure to bright light. J Am Geriatr Soc 41:829–836, 1993.

85. Aschoff J, Hoffmann K, Pohl H, Wever RA: Re-entrainment of circadian rhythms after phase-shifts of the zeitgeber. Chronobiologia 28:119–133, 1975.

86. Knutsson A, Akerstedt T, Orth-Gomer K, Jonsson BG: Increased risk of ischaemic heart disease in shift workers. Lancet 89–92, 1986.

87. Czeisler CA, Johnson MP, Duffy JF, et al: Exposure to bright light and darkness to treat physiologic maladaptation to night work. N Engl J Med 322:1253–1259, 1990.

88. Rosa RR: Extended workshifts and excessive fatigue. J Sleep Res 4:51–56, 1995.

89. Roden M, Koller M, Pirich K, et al: The circadian melatonin and cortisol secretion pattern in permanent night shift workers. Am J Physiol 265:R261–R267, 1993.

90. Weibel L, Spiegel K, Follenius M, et al: Internal dissociation of the circadian markers of the cortisol rhythm in night workers. Am J Physiol 270:E608–E613, 1996.

91. Weibel L, Spiegel K, Gronfier C, et al: Twenty-four-hour melatonin and core body temperature rhythms: Their adaptation in night workers. Am J Physiol 272:R948–R954, 1997.

92. Dawson D, Encel N, Lushington K: Improving adaptation to stimulated night shift: Timed exposure to bright light versus daytime melatonin administration. Sleep 18:11–21, 1995.

93. Campbell SS, Dawson D: Enhancement of nighttime alertness and performance with bright ambient light. Physiol Behav 48:317–320, 1990.

94. Campbell SS: Effects of timed bright light exposure on shift work adaptation in middle-aged subjects. Sleep 18:408–416, 1995.

95. Eastman CI. High-intensity light for circadian adaptation to a 12-h shift of the sleep schedule. Am J Physiol 263:R428–R436, 1992.

96. Eastman CI, Steward KT, Mahoney MP, Fogg LF: Dark goggles and bright light improve circadian rhythm adaptation to night shift work. Sleep 17:535–543, 1994.

97. Eastman CI, Martin S: How to use light and dark to produce circadian adaptation to night shift work. Ann Med 31:87–98, 1999.

98. Sack RL, Lewy AJ, Blood ML, et al: Circadian rhythm abnormalities in totally blind people: Incidence and clinical significance. J Clin Endocrinol Metab 75:127–134, 1992.

99. Miles LEM, Raynal DM, Wilson MA: Blind man living in normal society has circadian rhythms of 24.9 hours. Science 198:421–423, 1977.

100. Arendt J, Deacon S: Treatment of circadian rhythm disorders—Melatonin. Chronobiol Int 14:185–204, 1997.

101. Sack RL, Lewy AJ, Blood ML, Stevenson J: Melatonin administration to blind people: Phase advances and entrainment. J Biol Rhythms 6:249–261, 1991.

102. American Sleep Disorders Association (ASD): The International Classification of Sleep Disorders. Lawrence, KS, Allen Press, 1990.

103. Jones CR, Campbell SS, Zone SE, et al: Familial advance sleep phase syndrome: A short-period circadian rhythm variant in humans. Nat Med 5:1062–1065, 1999.

104. Cooper BG, White JES, Ashworth LA, et al: Hormonal and metabolic profiles in subjects with obstructive sleep apnea syndrome and the effects of nasal continuous positive airway pressure (CPAP) treatment. Sleep 18:172–179, 1995.

105. Goldstein SJ, Wu RHK, Thorpy MJ, et al: Reversibility of deficient sleep entrained growth hormone secretion in a boy with achondroplasia and obstructive sleep apnea. Acta Endocrinol 116:95–101, 1987.

106. Saini J, Krieger J, Brandenberger G, et al: Continuous positive airway pressure treatment: Effects on growth hormone, insulin and glucose profiles in obstructive sleep apnea patients. Horm Metab Res 25:375–381, 1993.

107. Spiegel K, Follenius M, Krieger J, et al: Prolactin secretion during sleep in obstructive sleep apnea patients. J Sleep Res 4:56–62, 1995.

108. Spiegel K, Leproult R, Van Cauter E: Impact of sleep debt on metabolic and endocrine function. Lancet 354:1435–1439, 1999.

109. Leproult R, Copinschi G, Buxton O, Van Cauter E: Sleep loss results in an elevation of cortisol levels the next evening. Sleep 20:865–870, 1997.

110. Sherman B, Wysham C, Pfohl B: Age-related changes in the circadian rhythm of plasma cortisol in man. J Clin Endocrinol Metab 61:439–443, 1985.

111. Van Cauter E, Leproult R, Kupfer DJ: Effects of gender and age on the levels and circadian rhythmicity of plasma cortisol. J Clin Endocrinol Metab 81:2468–2473, 1996.

112. Plat L, Féry F, L'Hermite-Balériaux M, et al: Metabolic effects of short-term physiological elevations of plasma cortisol are more pronounced in the evening than in the morning. J Clin Endocrinol Metab 84:3082–3092, 1999.

113. McEwen BS: Stress, adaptation, and disease. Allostasis and allostatic load. Ann N Y Acad Sci 840:33–44, 1998.

114. Van Cauter E, Turek FW: Depression: A disorder of timekeeping? Perspect Biol Med 29:510–519, 1986.

115. Wehr TA, Wirz-Justice AA: Circadian rhythm mechanisms in affective illness and in antidepressant drug action. Pharmacopsychiatry 15:31–39, 1982.

116. Kleitman N: Basic rest activity cycle: 22 years later. Sleep 5:311–317, 1982.

117. Chapotot F, Gronfier C, Jouny C, et al: Cortisol secretion is related to electroencephalographic alertness in human subjects during daytime wakefulness. J Clin Endocrinol Metab 83:4263–4268, 1998.

118. Lang DA, Matthews DR, Peto J, Turner RC: Cyclic oscillations of basal plasma glucose and insulin concentrations in human beings. N Engl J Med 301:1023–1027, 1979.

119. Goodner C, Walike B, Koerker D, et al: Insulin, glucagon, and glucose exhibit synchronous, sustained oscillations in fasting monkeys. Science 195:177–179, 1977.

120. Jaspan JB, Lever E, Polonsky KS, Van Cauter E: In vivo pulsatility of pancreatic islet peptides. Am J Physiol 251:E215–E226, 1986.

121. Veldhuis JD, Iranmanesh A, Johnson ML, Lizarralde G: Twenty-four-hour rhythms in plasma concentrations of adenohypophyseal hormones are generated by distinct amplitude and/or frequency modulation of underlying pituitary secretory bursts. J Clin Endocrinol Metab 71:1616–1623, 1990.

122. Veldhuis JD, Johnson ML, Lizarralde G, Iranmanesh A: Rhythmic and nonrhythmic modes of anterior pituitary gland secretion. Chronobiol Int 9:371–379, 1992.

123. Van Cauter E, van Coevorden A, Blackman JD: Modulation of neuroendocrine release by sleep and circadian rhythmicity. In Yen S, Vale W (eds): Advances in Neuroendocrine Regulation of Reproduction. Norwell, MA, Serono Symposia USA, 1990, pp 113–122.

124. Polonsky KS, Sturis J, Van Cauter E: Temporal profiles and clinical significance of pulsatile insulin secretion. Horm Res 49:178–184, 1998.

125. Simon C, Brandenberger G, Saini J, et al: Slow oscillations of plasma glucose and insulin secretion rate are amplified during sleep in humans under continuous enteral nutrition. Sleep 17:333–338, 1994.

126. Knobil E, Hotchkiss J: The menstrual cycle and its neuroendocrine control. In Knobil E, Neill JD (eds): The Physiology of Reproduction. New York, Raven Press, 1988, pp 1971–1994.

127. Conn PM, Crowley WF: Gonadotropin-releasing hormone and its analogues. N Engl J Med 324:93–103, 1991.

128. Sturis J, Scheen AJ, Leproult R, et al: 24-hour glucose profiles during continuous or oscillatory insulin infusion. J Clin Invest 95:1464–1471, 1995.

129. Halberg F, Tong YL, Johson EA: Circadian System Phase: An Aspect of Temporal Morphology; Procedures and Illustrative Examples. In Cellular Aspects of Biorhythms. Berlin, Springer-Verlag, 1967, pp 20–48.

130. Cleveland WS: Robust locally weighted regression and smoothing scatterplots. J Am Stat Assoc 74:829–836, 1979.

131. Van Cauter E: Method for characterization of 24-h temporal variation of blood constituents. Am J Physiol 237:E255–E264, 1979.

132. Van Cauter E: Computer-assisted analysis of endocrine rhythms. In Rodbard D, Forti G (eds): Computers in Endocrinology. New York, Raven Press, 1990, pp 59–70.

133. Polonsky KS, Licinio-Paixao J, Given BD, et al: Use of biosynthetic human C-peptide in the measurement of insulin secretion rates in normal volunteers and type I diabetic patients. J Clin Invest 77:98–105, 1986.

134. De Nicolao G, Rocchetti M: Stable and efficient techniques for the deconvolution of hormone time series. In Guardabasso V, Rodbard D, Forti G (eds): Computers in Endocrinology: Recent Advances, vol. 72. New York, Raven Press, 1990, pp 83–91.

135. Veldhuis JD, Johnson ML: A review and appraisal of deconvolution methods to evaluate in vivo neuroendocrine secretory events. J Neuroendocrinol 2:755–771, 1990.

136. Urban RJ, Evans WS, Rogol AD, et al: Contemporary aspects of discrete peak-detection algorithms. I. The paradigm of the luteinizing hormone pulse signal in men. Endocr Rev 9:3–37, 1988.

137. Urban RJ, Kaiser DL, Van Cauter E, et al: Comparative assessment of objective pulse detection algorithms. II. Studies in men. Am J Physiol 254:E113–E119, 1988.

138. Sturis J, Polonsky KS, Shapiro ET, et al: Abnormalities in the ultradian oscillations of insulin secretion and glucose levels in type 2 (non–insulin-dependent) diabetic patients. Diabetologia 35:681–689, 1992.

139. Pincus SM, Keefe DL: Quantification of hormone pulsatility via an approximate entropy algorithm. Am J Physiol 262:E741–E754, 1992.

140. Veldhuis JD, Iranmanesh A, Johnson ML, Lizarralde G: Amplitude, but not frequency, modulation of adrenocorticotropin secretory bursts gives rise to the nyctohemeral rhythm of the corticotropic axis in man. J Clin Endocrinol Metab 71:452–463, 1989.

141. Van Cauter E, Honinckx E: Pulsatility of pituitary hormones. Exp Brain Res 12(suppl):41–60, 1985.

142. Lejeune-Lenain C, Van Cauter E, Desir D, et al: Control of circadian and episodic variations of adrenal androgens secretion in man. J Endocrinol Invest 10:267–276, 1987.

143. Weitzman ED, Zimmerman JC, Czeisler CA, Ronda JM: Cortisol secretion is inhibited during sleep in normal man. J Clin Endocrinol Metab 56:352–358, 1983.

144. Born J, Muth S, Fehm HL: The significance of sleep onset and slow wave sleep for nocturnal release of growth hormone (GH) and cortisol. Psychoneuroendocrinology 13:233–243, 1988.

145. Van Cauter E, Blackman JD, Roland D, et al: Modulation of glucose regulation and insulin secretion by circadian rhythmicity and sleep. J Clin Invest 88:934–942, 1991.

146. Weibel L, Follenius M, Spiegel K, et al: Comparative effect of night and daytime sleep on the 24-hour cortisol secretory profile. Sleep 18:549–556, 1995.

147. Follenius M, Brandenberger G, Bardasept J, et al: Nocturnal cortisol release in relation to sleep structure. Sleep 15:21–27, 1992.

148. Spath-Schwalbe E, Gofferje M, Kern W, et al: Sleep disruption alters nocturnal ACTH and cortisol secretory patterns. Biol Psychiatry 29:575–584, 1991.

149. Pruessner JC, Wolf OT, Hellhammer DH, et al: Free cortisol levels after awakening: A reliable biological marker for the assessment of adrenocortical activity. Life Sci 61:2539–2549, 1997.

150. Linkowski P, Van Onderbergen A, Kerkhofs M, et al: Twin study of the 24-h cortisol profile: Evidence for genetic control of the human circadian clock. Am J Physiol 264:E173–E181, 1993.

151. Scheer FA, Buijs RM: Light affects morning salivary cortisol in humans. J Clin Endocrinol Metab 84:3395–3398, 1999.

152. Van Cauter E, Shapiro ET, Tillil H, Polonsky KS: Circadian modulation of glucose and insulin responses to meals: Relationship to cortisol rhythm. Am J Physiol 262:E467–E475, 1992.

153. Born J, Hansen K, Marshall L, et al: Timing the end of nocturnal sleep. Nature 397:29–30, 1999.

154. McEwen B: Protective and damaging effects of stress mediators. N Engl J Med 338:171–179, 1998.

155. Dallman MF, Strack AL, Akana SF, et al: Feast and famine: Critical role of glucocorticoids with insulin in daily energy flow. Front Neuroendocrinol 14:303–347, 1993.

156. Dennison E, Hindmarsh P, Fall C, et al: Profiles of endogenous circulating cortisol and bone mineral density in healthy elderly men. J Clin Endocrinol Metab 84:3058–3063, 1999.

157. Nolten WE, Lindheimer MD, Rueckert PA, et al: Diurnal patterns and regulation of cortisol secretion in pregnancy. J Clin Endocrinol Metab 51:466–472, 1980.

158. Magiakou MA, Mastorakos G, Rabin D, et al: The maternal hypothalamic-pituitary-adrenal axis in the third trimester of human pregnancy. Clin Endocrinol (Oxf) 44:419–428, 1996.

159. Rosman PM, Farag A, Benn R, et al: Modulation of pituitary-adrenal function: Decreased secretory episodes and blunted circadian rhythmicity in patients with alcoholic liver disease. J Clin Endocrinol Metab 55:709–717, 1981.

160. Boyar RM, Hellman LD, Roffwarg H, et al: Cortisol secretion and metabolism in anorexia nervosa. N Engl J Med 296:190–193, 1977.

161. Iranmanesh A, Lizarralde G, Johnson ML, Veldhuis JD: Dynamics of 24-hour endogenous cortisol secretion and clearance in primary hypothyroidism assessed before and after partial thyroid hormone replacement. J Clin Endocrinol Metab 70:155–161, 1990.

162. Gallagher TF, Hellman L, Finkelstein J, et al: Hyperthyroidism and cortisol secretion in man. J Clin Endocrinol Metab 34:919–927, 1972.

163. Refetoff S, Van Cauter E, Fang V, et al: The effect of dexamethasone on the 24-hour profiles of adrenocorticotropin and cortisol in Cushing's Syndrome. J Clin Endocrinol Metab 60:527–535, 1985.

164. Van Cauter E, Refetoff S: Evidence for two subtypes of Cushing's disease based on the analysis of episodic cortisol secretion. N Engl J Med 312:1343–1344, 1985.

165. van Waveren Hogervorst CO, Koppeschaar HPF, Zelissen PMJ, et al: Cortisol secretory patterns in Cushing's disease and response to cyproheptadine treatment. J Clin Endocrinol Metab 81:652–655, 1996.

166. Roelfsema F, Pincus SM, Veldhuis JD: Patients with Cushing's disease secrete adrenocorticotropin and cortisol jointly more asynchronously than healthy subjects. J Clin Endocrinol Metab 83:688–692, 1998.

167. Linkowski P, Mendlewicz J, Leclercq R, et al: The 24-hour profile of adrenocorticotropin and cortisol in major depressive illness. J Clin Endocrinol Metab 61:429–438, 1985.

168. Rubin RT, Poland RE, Lesser IM, et al: Neuroendocrine aspects of primary endogenous depression: I. Cortisol secretory dynamics in patients and matched controls. Arch Gen Psychiatry 44:328–336, 1987.

169. Linkowski P, Mendlewicz J, Kerkhofs M, et al: 24-hour profiles of adrenocorticotropin, cortisol, and growth hormone in major depressive illness: Effect of antidepressant treatment. J Clin Endocrinol Metab 65:141–152, 1987.

170. Yehuda R, Teicher MH, Trestman RL, et al: Cortisol regulation in posttraumatic stress disorder and major depression: A chronobiological analysis. Biol Psychiatry 15:79–88, 1996.

171. MacHale SM, Cavanagh JT, Bennie J, et al: Diurnal variation of adrenocortical activity in chronic fatigue syndrome. Neuropsychobiology 38:213–217, 1998.

172. Wood B, Wessely S, Papadopoulos A, et al: Salivary cortisol profiles in chronic fatigue syndrome. Neuropsychobiology 37:1–4, 1998.

173. Van Cauter E, Plat L, Copinschi G: Interrelations between sleep and the somatotropic axis. Sleep 21:553–566, 1998.

174. Mendlewicz J, Linkowski P, Kerkhofs M, et al: Genetic control of 24-hour growth hormone secretion in man: A twin study. J Clin Endocrinol Metab 84:856–862, 1999.

175. Ho KY, Evans WS, Blizzard RM, et al: Effects of sex and age on the 24-hour profile of growth hormone secretion in man: Importance of endogenous estradiol concentrations. J Clin Endocrinol Metab 64:51–58, 1987.

176. Shah N, Evans WS, Veldhuis JD: Actions of estrogen on pulsatile, nyctohemeral, and entropic modes of growth hormone secretion. Am J Physiol 276:R1351–R1358, 1999.

177. Caufriez A, L'Hermite-Baleriaux M, Moreno-Reyes R, et al: Effects of the menstrual cycle on 24-hour hormonal profiles in normally cycling young women: Progesterone related elevation of growth hormone during luteal phase. In preparation.

178. Van Cauter E, Kerkhofs M, Caufriez A, et al: A quantitative estimation of GH secretion in normal man: Reproducibility and relation to sleep and time of day. J Clin Endocrinol Metab 74:1441–1450, 1992.

179. Holl RW, Hartmann ML, Veldhuis JD, et al: Thirty-second sampling of plasma growth hormone in man: Correlation with sleep stages. J Clin Endocrinol Metab 72:854–861, 1991.

180. Krueger J, Obal FJ: Growth hormone-releasing hormone and interleukin-1 in sleep regulation. FASEB J 7:645–652, 1993.

181. Ocampo-Lim B, Guo W, DeMott Friberg R, et al: Nocturnal growth hormone (GH)

secretion is eliminated by infusion of GH-releasing hormone antagonist. J Clin Endocrinol Metab 81:4396–4399, 1996.

182. Jaffe C, Turgeon D, DeMott Friberg R, et al: Nocturnal augmentation of growth hormone (GH) secretion is preserved during repetitive bolus administration of GH-releasing hormone: Potential involvement of endogenous somatostatin—A clinical research center study. J Clin Endocrinol Metab 80:3321–3326, 1995.
183. Van Cauter E, Plat L, Scharf M, et al: Simultaneous stimulation of slow-wave sleep and growth hormone secretion by gamma-hydroxybutyrate in normal young men. J Clin Invest 100:745–753, 1997.
184. Vermeulen A: Nyctohemeral growth hormone profiles in young and aged men: Correlation with somatomedin-C levels. J Clin Endocrinol Metab 64:884–888, 1987.
185. Veldhuis J, Liem A, South S, et al: Differential impact of age, sex steroid hormones, and obesity on basal versus pulsatile growth hormone secretion in men as assessed in an ultrasensitive chemiluminescence assay. J Clin Endocrinol Metab 80:3209–3222, 1995.
186. Veldhuis JD, Iranmanesh A, Weltman A: Elements in the pathophysiology of diminished growth hormone (GH) secretion in aging humans. Endocrine 7:41–48, 1997.
187. Van Cauter E, Leproult R, Plat L: Differential rates of aging of slow-wave sleep and REM sleep: Impact on growth hormone and cortisol levels. JAMA 2000. In press.
188. Martin FC, Yeo AL, Sonksen PH: Growth hormone secretion in the elderly: Aging and the somatopause. Baillieres Clin Endocrinol Metab 11:223–250, 1997.
189. Caufriez A, Frankenne F, Hennen G, Copinschi G: Regulation of maternal IGF-I by placental GH in normal and abnormal human pregnancies. Am J Physiol 265:E572–E577, 1993.
190. Eriksson L, Frankenne F, Eden S, et al: Growth hormone 24-h serum profiles during pregnancy—lack of pulsatility for the secretion of the placental variant. Br J Obstet Gynaecol 96:949–953, 1989.
191. Veldhuis JD, Iranmanesh A, Ho KKY, et al: Dual defects in pulsatile growth hormone secretion and clearance subserve the hyposomatotropism of obesity in man. J Clin Endocrinol Metab 72:51–59, 1991.
192. Copinschi G, De Laet MH, Brion JP, et al: Simultaneous study of cortisol, GH and PRL circadian variations of hourly integrated concentrations in normal and obese subjects. Clin Endocrinol 9:15–26, 1978.
193. Ho KY, Veldhuis JD, Johnson ML, et al: Fasting enhances growth hormone secretion and amplifies the complex rhythms of growth hormone secretion in man. J Clin Invest 81:968–975, 1988.
194. Edge JA, Dunger DB, Matthews DR, et al: Increased overnight growth hormone concentrations in diabetic compared with normal adolescents. J Clin Endocrinol Metab 71:1356–1362, 1990.
195. Laughlin GA, Dominguez CE, Yen SS: Nutritional and endocrine-metabolic aberrations in women with functional hypothalamic amenorrhea. J Clin Endocrinol Metab 83:25–32, 1998.
196. Morales AJ, Laughlin GA, Butzow T, et al: Insulin, somatotropic, and luteinizing hormone axes in lean and obese women with polycystic ovary syndrome: Common and distinct features. J Clin Endocrinol Metab 81:2854–2864, 1996.
197. Iranmanesh A, Lizarralde G, Johnson ML, Veldhuis JD: Nature of altered growth hormone secretion in hyperthyroidism. J Clin Endocrinol Metab 72:108–115, 1991.
198. Mendlewicz J, Linkowski P, Kerkhofs M, et al: Diurnal hypersecretion of growth hormone in depression. J Clin Endocrinol Metab 60:505–512, 1986.
199. Hartman ML, Veldhuis JD, Vance ML, et al: Somatotropin pulse frequency and basal concentrations are increased in acromegaly and are reduced by successful therapy. J Clin Endocrinol Metab 70:1375–1384, 1990.
200. van den Berg G, Pincus SM, Frolich M, et al: Reduced disorderliness of growth hormone release in biochemically inactive acromegaly after pituitary surgery. Eur J Endocrinol 138:164–169, 1998.
201. Katznelson L, Riskind PN, Saxe VC, Klibanski A: Prolactin pulsatile characteristics in postmenopausal women. J Clin Endocrinol Metab 83:761–764, 1998.
202. Linkowski P, Spiegel K, Kerkhofs M, et al: Genetic and environmental influences on prolactin secretion during wake and during sleep. Am J Physiol 274:E909–E919, 1998.
203. Désir D, Van Cauter E, L'Hermite M, et al: Effects of "jet lag" on hormonal patterns. III. Demonstration of an intrinsic circadian rhythmicity in plasma prolactin. J Clin Endocrinol Metab 55:849–857, 1982.
204. Spiegel K, Follenius M, Simon C, et al: Prolactin secretion and sleep. Sleep 17:20–27, 1994.
205. Waldstreicher J, Duffy JF, Brown EN, et al: Gender differences in the temporal organization of prolactin (PRL) secretion: Evidence for a sleep-independent circadian rhythm of circulating PRL levels—A clinical research center study. J Clin Endocrinol Metab 81:1483–1487, 1996.
206. Copinschi G, Van Onderbergen A, L'Hermite-Balériaux M, et al: Effects of the short-acting benzodiazepine triazolam, taken at bedtime, on circadian and sleep-related hormonal profiles in normal men. Sleep 13:232–244, 1990.
207. Copinschi G, Akseki E, Moreno-Reyes R, et al: Effects of bedtime administration of zolpidem on circadian and sleep-related hormonal profiles in normal women. Sleep 18:417–424, 1995.
208. Greenspan SL, Klibanski A, Rowe JW, Elahi D: Age alters pulsatile prolactin release: Influence of dopaminergic inhibition. Am J Physiol 258:E799–E804, 1990.
209. Tay CC, Glasier AF, McNeilly AS: Twenty-four hour patterns of prolactin secretion during lactation and the relationship to suckling and the resumption of fertility in breast-feeding women. Hum Reprod 11:950–955, 1996.
210. Caufriez A, Désir D, Szyper M, et al: Prolactin secretion in Cushing's disease. J Clin Endocrinol Metab 53:843–846, 1981.
211. Iranmanesh A, Veldhuis JD, Carlsen EC, et al: Attenuated pulsatile release of prolactin in men with insulin-dependent diabetes mellitus. J Clin Endocrinol Metab 71:73–78, 1990.
212. Boyar RM, Kapen S, Finkelstein JW, et al: Hypothalamic-pituitary function in diverse hyperprolactinemic states. J Clin Invest 53:1588–1598, 1974.
213. Groote Veldman R, van den Berg G, Pincus SM, et al: Increased episodic release and disorderliness of prolactin secretion in both micro- and macroprolactinomas. Eur J Endocrinol 140:192–200, 1999.
214. Spratt DI, O'Dea LL, Schoenfeld D, et al: Neuroendocrine-gonadal axis in men: Frequent sampling of LH, FSH and testosterone. Am J Physiol 254:E658–E666, 1988.
215. Fehm HL, Clausing J, Kern W, et al: Sleep-associated augmentation and synchronization of luteinizing hormone pulses in adult men. Neuroendocrinology 54:192–195, 1991.
216. Bremner WJ, Vitiello MV, Prinz PN: Loss of circadian rhythmicity in blood testosterone levels with aging in normal men. J Clin Endocrinol Metab 56:1278–1280, 1983.
217. Carlsen E, Olsson C, Petersen JH, et al: Diurnal rhythm in serum levels of inhibin B in normal men: Relation to testicular steroids and gonadotropins. J Clin Endocrinol Metab 84:1664–1669, 1999.
218. Vermeulen A, Deslypere JP, Kaukman JM: Influence of antiopioids on luteinizing hormone pulsatility in aging men. J Clin Endocrinol Metab 68:68–72, 1989.
219. Veldhuis JD, Urban RJ, Lizarralde G, et al: Attenuation of luteinizing hormone secretory burst amplitude as a proximate basis for the hypoandrogenism of healthy aging in men. J Clin Endocrinol Metab 75:52–58, 1992.
220. Mulligan T, Iranmanesh A, Gheorghiu S, et al: Amplified nocturnal luteinizing hormone (LH) secretory burst frequency with selective attenuation of pulsatile (but not basal) testosterone secretion in healthy aged men: Possible Leydig cell desensitization to endogenous LH signaling—a clinical research center study. J Clin Endocrinol Metab 80:3025–3031, 1995.
221. Tenover JS, Matsumoto AM, Clifton DK, Bremner WJ: Age-related alterations in the circadian rhythms of pulsatile luteinizing hormone and testosterone secretion in healthy men. J Gerontol 43:M163–169, 1988.
222. Pincus SM, Mulligan T, Iranmanesh A, et al: Older males secrete luteinizing hormone and testosterone more irregularly, and jointly more asynchronously, than younger males. Proc Natl Acad Sci U S A 93:14100–14105, 1996.
223. Reame N, Sauder SE, Kelch RP, Marshall JC: Pulsatile gonadotropin secretion during the human menstrual cycle: Evidence for altered frequency of gonadotropin-releasing hormone secretion. J Clin Endocrinol Metab 59:328–337, 1984.
224. Filicori M, Santoro N, Merriam GR, Crowley WFJ: Characterization of the physiological pattern of episodic gonadotropin secretion throughout the menstrual cycle. J Clin Endocrinol Metab 62:1136–1144, 1986.
225. Hall JE, Schoenfeld DA, Martin KA, Crowley WFJ: Hypothalamic gonadotropin-releasing hormone secretion and follicle-stimulating hormone dynamics during the luteal-follicular transition. J Clin Endocrinol Metab 74:600–607, 1992.
226. Reame NE, Kelch RP, Beitins IZ, et al: Age effects of follicle-stimulating hormone and pulsatile luteinizing hormone secretion across the menstrual cycle of premenopausal women. J Clin Endocrinol Metab 81:1512–1518, 1996.
227. Turek FW, Van Cauter E: Rhythms in Reproduction. *In* Knobil E, Neill JD (eds): The Physiology of Reproduction. New York, Raven Press, 1993, pp 1789–1830.
228. Bergendahl M, Aloi JA, Iranmanesh A, et al: Fasting suppresses pulsatile luteinizing hormone (LH) secretion and enhances orderliness of LH release in young but not older men. J Clin Endocrinol Metab 83:1967–1975, 1998.
229. Khoury SA, Reame NE, Kelch RP, Marshall JC: Diurnal patterns of pulsatile luteinizing hormone secretion in hypothalamic amenorrhea: Reproducibility and responses to opiate blockade and an alpha-adrenergic agonist. J Clin Endocrinol Metab 64:755–762, 1987.
230. Fumming DC, Vickovic MM, Fluker MR: Defects in pulsatile LH release in normally menstruating runners. J Clin Endocrinol Metab 60:810–812, 1985.
231. Zumoff B, Freeman R, Coupey S, et al: A chronobiologic abnormality in luteinizing secretion in teenage girls with the polycystic-ovary syndrome. N Engl J Med 309:1206–1209, 1983.
232. Porcu E, Venturoli S, Longhi M, et al: Chronobiologic evolution of luteinizing hormone secretion in adolescence: Developmental patterns and speculations on the onset of the polycystic ovary syndrome. Fertil Steril 67:842–848, 1997.
233. Venturoli S, Porcu E, Fabbri R, et al: Episodic pulsatile secretion of FSH, prolactin, oestradiol, oestrone, and LH circadian variations in polycystic ovary syndrome. Clin Endocrinol (Oxf) 28:93–107, 1988.
234. Waldstreicher J, Santoro NF, Hall JE, et al: Hyperfunction of the hypothalamo-pituitary axis in women with polycystic ovarian disease: Indirect evidence for partial gonadotroph desensitization. J Clin Endocrinol Metab 66:165–172, 1988.
235. Blomquist CH, Holt JPJ: Chronobiology of the hypothalamo-pituitary-gonadal axis in men and women. *In* Touitou Y, Haus E (eds): Biological Rhythms in Clinical and Laboratory Medicine. Berlin, Springer-Verlag, 1992, pp 315–329.
236. Fachinetti F, Genazzani AD, Martignoni E, et al: Neuroendocrine correlates of premenstrual syndrome: Changes in the pulsatile pattern of plasma LH. Psychoneuroendocrinology 15:269–277, 1990.
237. Parry BL: Sleep, mood, and the menstrual cycle. Semin Reprod Med 8:81–88, 1990.
238. Spratt DI, Carr DB, Merriam GR, et al: The spectrum of abnormal patterns of gonadotropin-releasing hormone secretion in men with idiopathic hypogonadotropic hypogonadism: Clinical and laboratory correlations. J Clin Endcrinol Metab 64:283–291, 1987.
239. Klibanski A, Beitins IZ, Merriam GR, et al: Gonadotropin and prolactin pulsations in hyperprolactinemic women before and during bromocriptine therapy. J Clin Endocrinol Metab 58:1141–1147, 1984.
240. Hangaard J, Andersen M, Grodum E, et al: Pulsatile luteinizing hormone secretion in patients with Addison's disease. Impact of glucocorticoid substitution. J Clin Endocrinol Metab 83:736–743, 1998.
241. Behrends J, Prank K, Dogu E, Brabant G: Central nervous system control of thyrotropin secretion during sleep and wakefulness. Horm Res 49:173–177, 1998.
242. Goichot B, Brandenberger G, Saini J, et al: Nocturnal plasma thyrotropin variations are related to slow-wave sleep. J Sleep Res 1:186–190, 1992.
243. Hirschfeld U, Moreno-Reyes R, Akseki E, et al: Progressive elevation of plasma thyrotropin during adaptation to simulated jet lag: Effects of treatment with bright light or zolpidem. J Clin Endocrinol Metab 81:3270–3277, 1996.

244. Greenspan SL, Klibanski A, Schoenfeld D, Ridgway EC: Pulsatile secretion of thyrotropin in man. J Clin Endocrinol Metab 63:661–668, 1986.
245. Brabant G, Brabant A, Ranft U, et al: Circadian and pulsatile thyrotropin secretion in euthyroid man under influence of thyroid hormone and glucocorticoid administration. J Clin Endocrinol Metab 65:83–88, 1987.
246. Van Cauter E, Turek FW: Endocrine and other biological rhythms. In DeGroot LJ (ed): Endocrinology, ed 3. Philadelphia, WB Saunders, 1995, pp 2487–2548.
247. Allan JS, Czeisler CA: Persistence of the circadian thyrotropin rhythm under constant conditions and after light-induced shifts of circadian phase. J Clin Endocrinol Metab 79:508–512, 1994.
248. Gary KA, Winokur A, Douglas SD, et al: Total sleep deprivation and the thyroid axis: Effects of sleep and waking activity. Aviat Space Environ Med 67:513–519, 1996.
249. Romijn JA, Wiersinga WM: Decreased nocturnal surge of thyrotropin in nonthyroidal illness. J Clin Endocrinol Metab 70:35–42, 1990.
250. Bartalena F, Martino E, Petrini L, et al: The nocturnal serum thyrotropin surge is abolished in patients with ACTH-dependent or ACTH-independent Cushing's syndrome. J Clin Endocrinol Metab 72:1195–1199, 1991.
251. Samuels MH, Lillehei K, Kleinschmidt-Demasters BK, et al: Patterns of pulsatile pituitary glycoprotein secretion in central hypothyroidism and hypogonadism. J Clin Endocrinol Metab 70:391–395, 1990.
252. Bartalena L, Martino E, Velluzzi F, et al: The lack of nocturnal serum thyrotropin surge in patients with non-toxic nodular goiter may predict the subsequent occurrence of hyperthyroidism. J Clin Endocrinol Metab 73:604–608, 1991.
253. Bartalena L, Cossu E, Grasso L, et al: Relationship between nocturnal serum thyrotropin peak and metabolic control in diabetic patients. J Clin Endocrinol Metab 76:983–987, 1993.
254. Simon C: Ultradian pulsatility of plasma glucose and insulin secretion rate: Circadian and sleep modulation. Horm Res 49:185–190, 1998.
255. Plat L, Byrne MM, Sturis J, et al: Effects of morning cortisol elevation on insulin secretion and glucose regulation in humans. Am J Physiol 270:E36–E42, 1996.
256. Scheen AJ, Byrne MM, Plat L, Van Cauter E: Relationships between sleep quality and glucose regulation in normal humans. Am J Physiol 271:E261–E270, 1996.
257. Sturis J, Van Cauter E, Blackman JD, Polonsky KS: Entrainment of pulsatile insulin secretion by oscillatory glucose infusion. J Clin Invest 87:439–445, 1991.
258. Sturis J, Polonsky KS, Mosekilde E, Van Cauter E: Computer model for mechanisms underlying ultradian oscillations of insulin and glucose. Am J Physiol 260:E801–E809, 1991.
259. Van Cauter E, Polonsky KS, Blackman JD, et al: Abnormal temporal patterns of glucose tolerance in obesity: Relationship to sleep-related growth hormone and circadian cortisol rhythmicity. J Clin Endocrinol Metab 79:1797–1805, 1994.
260. Bolli GB, Gerich JE: The "dawn phenomenon"—a common occurrence in both non–insulin-dependent and insulin-dependent diabetes mellitus. N Engl J Med 310:746–750, 1984.
261. Campbell PJ, Bolli GB, Cryer PE, Gerich JE: Pathogenesis of the dawn phenomenon in patients with insulin-dependent diabetes mellitus. N Engl J Med 312:1473–1479, 1985.
262. Shapiro ET, Polonsky KS, Copinschi G, et al: Nocturnal elevation of glucose levels during fasting in noninsulin-dependent diabetes. J Clin Endocrinol Metab 72:444–454, 1991.
263. O'Meara NM, Sturis J, Van Cauter E, Polonsky KS: Lack of control by glucose of ultradian insulin secretory oscillations in impaired glucose tolerance and in non–insulin-dependent diabetes mellitus. J Clin Invest 92:262–271, 1993.
264. Sinha MK, Ohannesian JP, Heiman ML, et al: Nocturnal rise of leptin in lean, obese and non-insulin-dependent diabetes mellitus subjects. J Clin Invest 97:1344–1347, 1996.
265. Saad MF, Riad-Gabriel MG, Khan A, et al: Diurnal and ultradian rhythmicity of plasma leptin: Effects of gender and adiposity. J Clin Endocrinol Metab 83:453–459, 1998.
266. Licino J, Negrao AB, Mantzoros C, et al: Sex differences in circulating human leptin pulse amplitude: Clinical implications. J Clin Endocrinol Metab 83:4140–4147, 1998.
267. Schoeller DA, Cella LK, Sinha MK, Caro JF: Entrainment of the diurnal rhythm of plasma leptin to meal timing. J Clin Invest 100:1882–1887, 1997.
268. Simon C, Gronfier C, Schlienger JL, Brandenberger G: Circadian and ultradian variations of leptin in normal man under continuous enteral nutrition: Relationship to sleep and body temperature. J Clin Endocrinol Metab 83:1893–1899, 1998.
269. Franceschini R, Corsini G, Cataldi A, et al: Twenty-four-hour variation in serum leptin in the elderly. Metabolism 48:1011–1014, 1999.
270. Licino J, Mantzoros C, Negrao AB, et al: Human leptin levels are pulsatile and inversely related to pituitary-adrenal function. Nat Med 3:575–579, 1997.
271. Langendonk JG, Pijl H, Toornvliet AC, et al: Circadian rhythm of plasma leptin levels in upper and lower body obese women: Influence of body fat distribution and weight loss. J Clin Endocrinol Metab 83:1706–1712, 1998.
272. Boden G, Chen X, Kolaczynski JW, Polansky M: Effects of prolonged hyperinsulinemia on serum leptin levels in normal human subjects. J Clin Invest 100:1107–1113, 1997.
273. Eliman A, Knutsson U, Bronnegard M, et al: Variations in glucocorticoid levels within the physiological range affect plasma leptin levels. Eur J Endocrinol 139:615–620, 1998.
274. Purnell JQ, Samuels MH: Levels of leptin during hydrocortisone infusions that mimic normal and reversed diurnal cortisol levels in subjects with adrenal insufficiency. J Clin Endocrinol Metab 84:3125–3128, 1999.
275. Laughlin GA, Yen SS: Hypoleptinemia in women athletes: Absence of a diurnal rhythm with amenorrhea. J Clin Endocrinol Metab 82:318–321, 1997.
276. Balligand JL, Brichard SM, Brichard V, et al: Hypoleptinemia in patients with anorexia nervosa: Loss of circadian rhythm and unresponsiveness to short-term refeeding. Eur J Endocrinol 138:415–420, 1998.

CLINICAL DISORDERS

Chapter **18**

Radiographic Evaluation of the Pituitary and Anterior Hypothalamus

Robert J. Witte ▪ Leighton P. Mark ▪ David L. Daniels ▪ Victor M. Haughton

Methods of imaging the pituitary gland and hypothalamus have continually evolved. Computed tomography (CT) provided the first imaging technique that directly visualized the pituitary gland and still best demonstrates the osseous structure of the sella and calcification within sellar lesions.[1–6] The superior soft tissue contrast of magnetic resonance imaging (MRI) has made it the preferred imaging modality to study the pituitary gland and hypothalamus.[7–10] MRI also provides an angiographic capability useful for demonstrating the cavernous carotid arteries and possible aneurysms. The purpose of this chapter is to describe CT and MRI of the pituitary fossa and to discuss the detection and differential diagnosis of intrasellar processes.

IMAGING TECHNIQUES

Computed Tomography

CT scanning can occasionally play an important role in imaging of the pituitary fossa, primarily in patients who have a contraindication to MRI (i.e., severe claustrophobia, cardiac pacemaker, large body habitus), and to identify and characterize lesion calcification.

The coronal plane provides the most efficient diagnosis of processes affecting the infundibulum, hypothalamus, cavernous sinuses, and pituitary gland.[11, 12] The best spatial resolution is provided by direct coronal images obtained by positioning the patient so the gantry is perpendicular to the sella floor. If a patient is unable to tolerate direct coronal imaging, reformatted thin coronal sections can be obtained from direct axial images (Fig. 18–1). Intravenous contrast is routinely used.

Magnetic Resonance Imaging

MRI has replaced CT as the primary modality for imaging the pituitary fossa.[13–15] Because of its multiplanar capabilities, MRI obviates the need for hyperextension of the head, which may be uncomfortable for some patients. MRI also has better tissue contrast resolution than CT does, which improves sensitivity for lesion detection. The risks associated with the large doses of intravenous iodinated contrast needed in CT (i.e., nausea, renal toxicity, anaphylaxis) are avoided in MRI. Reactions to the small doses (approximately 10 mL) of MRI paramagnetic contrast used in sellar imaging are extremely rare. Unlike CT, the patient is not exposed to ionizing radiation during MRI.

Typically, T1-weighted spin-echo images are obtained in the sagittal and coronal planes before and after contrast administration. T2-weighted coronal images and magnetic resonance angiography may occasionally be useful as supplementary sequences. Dynamic MRI of the sella can at times be valuable for identifying small microadenomas. T1-weighted coronal images are usually acquired at 15- to 20-second intervals after contrast bolus injection.

NORMAL ANATOMY

The osseous landmarks of the pituitary fossa have a characteristic high density on CT and low signal intensity on MRI. These landmarks include the tuberculum sellae, lamina dura, planum sphenoidale, and chiasmatic sulcus. Air in the sphenoid sinus just below the floor of the sella has no signal on either CT or MRI. The cerebrospinal fluid (CSF) in the chiasmatic cistern above the pituitary gland contrasts with the pituitary gland in both CT and MRI. The contents of the pituitary fossa include the anterior and posterior lobes of the pituitary gland and the pars intermedia. A small amount of fat in paramidline locations and small venous channels that connect the sphenoid sinuses is also present in the sella. The intercavernous veins and a small tuft of capillaries within the gland may be visualized, especially when dynamic techniques are used.

The pituitary gland is normally homogeneous on CT but may be mildly heterogeneous on MRI. In MRI or CT studies the gland shows nearly homogeneous contrast enhancement. After intravenous administration of MRI paramagnetic contrast medium, the signal intensity of the pituitary gland increases markedly and nearly homogeneously to nearly the same degree as the cavernous sinuses. The carotid arteries within the cavernous sinus, however, do not enhance in MRI as a result of time-of-flight effects. In CT, the gland enhances with iodinated contrast medium so that it is at or slightly below the density of the enhanced cavernous sinuses. Both the carotid arteries and the venous channels in the cavernous sinuses enhance with CT contrast medium. The cranial nerves in the cavernous sinuses, which do not enhance to the same degree, may be resolved as filling defects in a contrast-enhanced study.

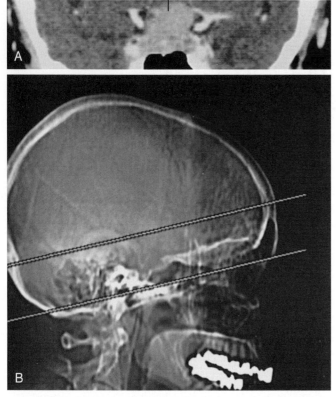

FIGURE 18–1. Coronal reformatted images (A), obtained from axial computed tomographic image locations shown in B. A macroadenoma is adequately demonstrated in this patient unable to be positioned for direct coronal imaging.

The upper surface of the pituitary is usually flat or slightly concave, but it may be mildly convex in adolescents and pregnant or menstruating women.[16] The gland homogeneously enhances and is often larger in women, measuring from 2 to 9 mm (Figs. 18–2 and 18–3). Within the posterior lobe of normal individuals may be identified a region of high signal intensity that appears to be related to phospholipid structures in vacuoles in the neurohypophysis.[17] This region of high signal intensity is absent in patients with diabetes insipidus and in some normal individuals.[18] In cases of an ectopic posterior lobe or transected infundibulum, the region of high signal intensity may be found in the residual stalk or inferior of the hypothalamus[19] (Fig. 18–4).

DIFFERENTIAL DIAGNOSIS OF PITUITARY AND ANTERIOR HYPOTHALAMIC PROCESSES

Pituitary Adenoma

The most common intrasellar tumor is a pituitary adenoma, and they are usually divided into microadenomas (<1 cm) and macroadenomas.[20–22] The most common microadenoma is a prolactin-secreting adenoma. Adenomas have a density slightly lower than that of the normal pituitary gland or cavernous sinuses on unenhanced CT.[23] They have slightly lower signal intensity on T1-weighted images and slightly greater signal intensity on T2-weighted images than the normal gland does.[7–10] Adenomas usually enhance to a lesser degree than the surrounding pituitary (Fig. 18–5).

Upward extension of the tumor appears as a mass with a curvilinear margin effacing the chiasmatic cistern (Fig. 18–6). Inferior extension results in a mass in the sphenoid sinus. Necrosis and cyst formation produce regions of diminished CT density and decreased T1-weighted and increased T2-weighted signal on MRI (Fig. 18–7). T2-Weighted sequences have been used with large suprasellar tumors to predict successful transsphenoidal removal.[24] Neoplasms in the cavernous sinuses enhance slightly less intensely than do normal cavernous sinuses. Carotid artery encasement is the most reliable sign of cavernous invasion.[25] Hemorrhage within an adenoma produces a characteristic high signal on T1-weighted images, which may occasionally be seen after treatment (Fig. 18–8). Pituitary apoplexy syndrome may be associated.[26] Calcification is uncommon, but best seen with CT.

CT and MRI are less sensitive and specific in diagnosing adrenocorticotropic hormone– and human growth hormone–secreting microadenomas. Rapid imaging during contrast delivery has been particularly useful in identifying these often subtle tumors[27] (Fig. 18–9).

Meningioma

Meningiomas that arise from the surface of the diaphragma sellae, from the cavernous sinus, or rarely from within the pituitary fossa are less common than pituitary adenomas are. Like pituitary adenomas, they may have a homogeneous density or signal intensity before contrast enhancement. They often contain calcification and enhance markedly with intravenous contrast medium (Fig. 18–10). Hyperostotic bone adjacent to the meningioma in the tuberculum sellae and anterior

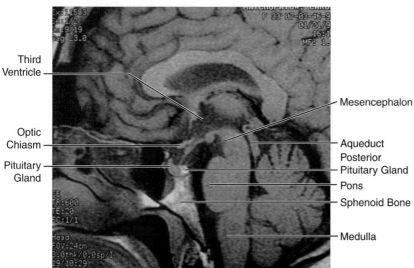

FIGURE 18–2. Normal appearance of the sella in a sagittal T1-weighted magnetic resonance image. The pituitary gland, optic chiasm, third ventricle, aqueduct, mesencephalon, pons, and medulla have been labeled. Note the high signal intensity in bone marrow within the sphenoid bone. High signal intensity is also evident in the posterior lobe of the pituitary gland.

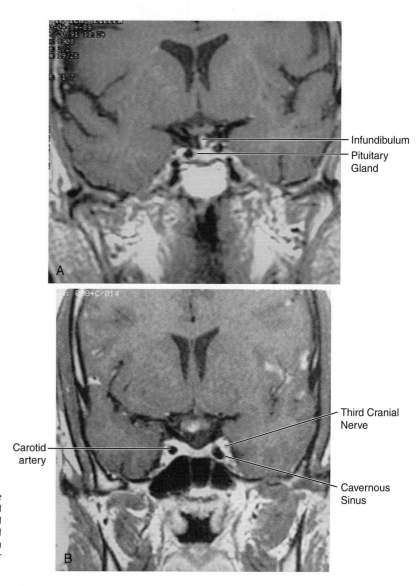

FIGURE 18-3. Coronal T1-weighted magnetic resonance images after intravenous contrast medium. The brain and optic chiasm do not show contrast enhancement. Marked enhancement is noted, however, in the infundibulum and the pituitary gland. *A,* The carotid arteries are evident as a region of very low or negligible signal intensity. *B,* The upper surface of the pituitary gland is concave.

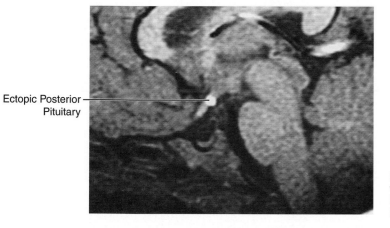

FIGURE 18-4. An ectopic posterior pituitary on a sagittal T1-weighted magnetic resonance image. The ectopic infundibular location in the median eminence is easily seen in this 4-year-old boy with hypopituitarism.

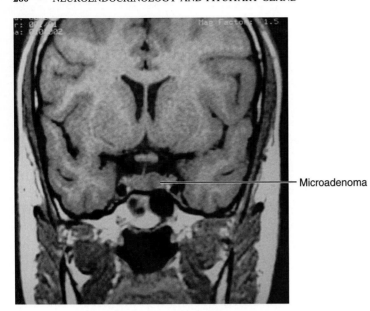

— Microadenoma

FIGURE 18–5. A coronal T1-weighted magnetic resonance image without contrast enhancement demonstrates a microadenoma. The tumor appears as a region of diminished signal intensity in the left portion of the gland. It causes very little distortion of the gland.

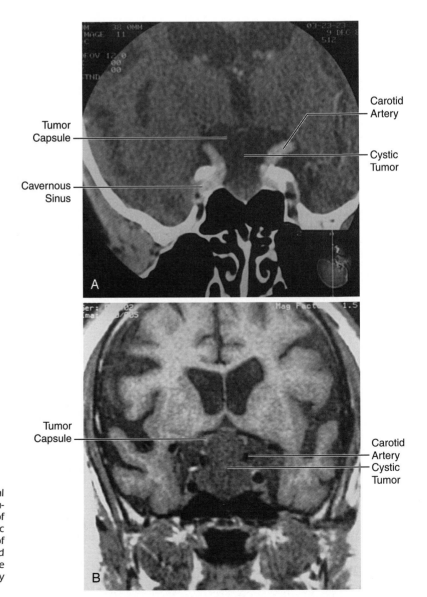

FIGURE 18–6. Cystic pituitary adenoma shown on coronal computed tomography (CT) *(A)* and magnetic resonance imaging (MRI) *(B)*. In the CT study the margin of the capsule of the tumor is barely visible in the chiasmatic cistern. The cystic tumor is differentiated from an empty sella by the absence of a pituitary stalk visible in the sella. The carotid arteries and cavernous sinuses appear normal. In T1-weighted MRI the capsule is somewhat better defined and the tumor has slightly different signal from that of cerebrospinal fluid.

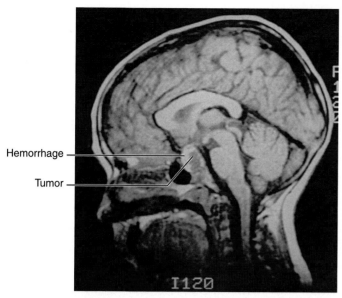

FIGURE 18–7. *Sagittal magnetic resonance image showing a large pituitary adenoma that fills the pituitary fossa and obliterates the chiasmatic cistern. Note the rim of high signal intensity indicating hemorrhage in the tumor in this patient with pituitary apoplexy.*

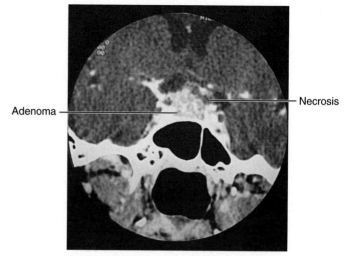

FIGURE 18–8. *Coronal computed tomography of a partially necrotic pituitary adenoma that extends into the chiasmatic cistern.*

or posterior clinoid processes may be demonstrated by CT.[28] Spread of tumor along the petroclinoid ligament or dura is more characteristic of meningioma than pituitary adenoma. Necrotic and cystic areas are rarer than in adenomas. With the exception of the rare intrasellar meningioma, they can usually be differentiated from pituitary adenomas by identifying their origin outside the pituitary fossa.

Craniopharyngioma

Although they are uncommon tumors of the chiasmatic region, craniopharyngiomas are benign tumors of squamous epithelium that arise from embryonic squamous cell rests of the involuted hypophysial-pharyngeal duct. They can occur at any age but peak in the second and fifth decades. Craniopharyngiomas are particularly important in the differential diagnosis in pediatric patients and have characteristic radiographic findings. Cysts and dense globular calcifications are easily seen on CT (Fig. 18–11). The cystic regions may have variable

signal intensity on MRI because of varying amounts of blood, cholesterol, and protein.[29] The solid portions of the tumor enhance markedly. The rarer homogeneously enhancing craniopharyngioma is difficult to distinguish radiographically from an adenoma.

Metastases

Tumors of the nasopharynx, lung, breast, kidney, or gastrointestinal tract may metastasize to the hypothalamus or sella. These tumors typically enhance homogeneously (Fig. 18–12). Bone destruction is frequent, and calcification and cyst formation are rare.

Aneurysm

A carotid aneurysm may rarely mimic an intrasellar or parasellar mass (Fig. 18–13). In an unenhanced CT image, an intrasellar aneurysm appears slightly denser than cerebral tissue or, if a large clot is present, substantially denser than cerebral tissue. The intensity of enhancement varies with the presence and extent of the clot. In MRI, flowing blood within the aneurysm usually has a characteristic signal void. The presence of clot or turbulent flow within the aneurysm

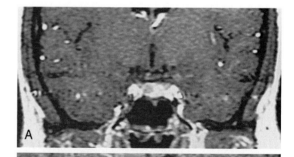

FIGURE 18–9. *Dynamic contrast-enhanced imaging demonstrating a small microadenoma. A small adrenocorticotropic hormone–secreting microadenoma located on the right side of the gland is better seen on images obtained during contrast administration (A) than on conventional delayed contrast-enhanced images (B).*

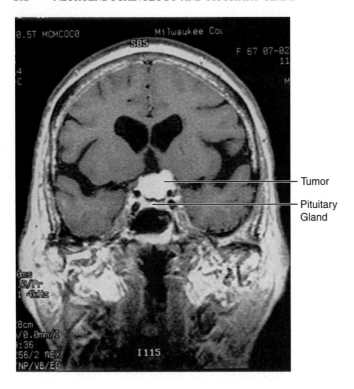

Tumor

Pituitary Gland

FIGURE 18–10. Coronal T1-weighted contrast-enhanced magnetic resonance image demonstrating a suprasellar meningioma. The tumor shows marked contrast enhancement. A thin line of low signal intensity, probably representing the diaphragma sellae, separates the tumor from the pituitary gland.

may create a variety of different patterns. Conventional or digital angiography must be used to document or exclude an aneurysm in questionable cases.

Lymphocytic Hypophysitis

Lymphocytic hypophysitis is a rare inflammatory disease of the pituitary gland that results in partial hypopituitarism or panhypopituitarism. Although originally thought to affect pregnant or postpartum women, it is now known to occur in all ages and in both sexes. It is considered one of the causes of idiopathic diabetes insipidus. Imaging often shows an enlarged pituitary gland and stalk. The enlargement may regress spontaneously or with glucocorticoids. Dynamic MRI may demonstrate a delay in pituitary enhancement (>90 seconds) when conventional MRI studies are normal.[30]

Empty Sella

Empty sella is usually an incidental finding, more common in women. It is generally due to incompetence of the diaphragma sellae, although it sometimes results from regression of a pituitary tumor. Imaging shows enlargement of the pituitary fossa and displacement of the remaining pituitary gland inferiorly (Fig. 18–14). Identification of the infundibulum is important in differentiation from an intrasellar cyst.[31]

Hypothalamic/Chiasmatic Glioma

The typical hypothalamic/chiasmatic gliomas found in children and young adults are usually benign pilocytic astrocytomas (malignant astrocytomas are more common in adults).[32] They usually occur in the first decade of life (generally in children younger than 5 years of age) and may be associated with neurofibromatosis type I.[33] These tumors appear as a lobulated mass with increased signal intensity on T2-weighted images (Fig. 18–15). They usually enhance and may contain cystic or necrotic areas. Because they are in a suprachiasmatic location, they are not normally confused with pituitary adenomas.

Hamartoma of the Tuber Cinereum

Hamartomas of the tuber cinereum contain cells similar to those normally found in the hypothalamus. These tumors are seen in children and are associated with central precocious puberty. The usual appearance is a pedunculated nonenhancing soft tissue mass at the posterior hypothalamus.[34]

Infundibular Tumors

Tumors of the infundibulum include metastases, glioma, and lymphoma. Other conditions that cause enlargement of the infundibulum include histiocytosis X and sarcoid. Patients with these tumors often have diabetes insipidus and variable degrees of hypopituitarism. CT and MRI show an enhancing, thickened (>4.5 mm) infundibulum.

Germ Cell Tumors

Germ cell tumors can be classified as germinomas or nongerminomas. Nongerminomas include teratomas (benign and malignant), embryonal carcinomas, and choriocarcinomas. Whereas males have a greater tendency for germ cell tumors to develop in the pineal region, a distinct predilection for a suprasellar location is seen in females (particularly germinomas)[35] (Fig. 18–16). Suprasellar germ cell tumors have a variable appearance on MRI and CT. Germinomas and teratocarcinomas that spread via CSF pathways characteristically appear as linear or nodular enhancing regions on the surface of the brain. Suprasellar germ cell tumors may appear similar to glial tumors. The suprasellar location distinguishes these tumors from pituitary adenomas.

Epidermoid and Dermoid Cysts

The appearance of intrasellar dermoid or epidermoid cysts will vary depending on the dermal elements of the tumor.[36] On CT, these tumors often have the density of CSF (5 to 15 Hounsfield units [HU]). Fat and calcium in the dermoid may be distinguished in the mass as low (−40 HU) and high (>100 HU) densities, respectively. In MRI,

Text continued on page 267

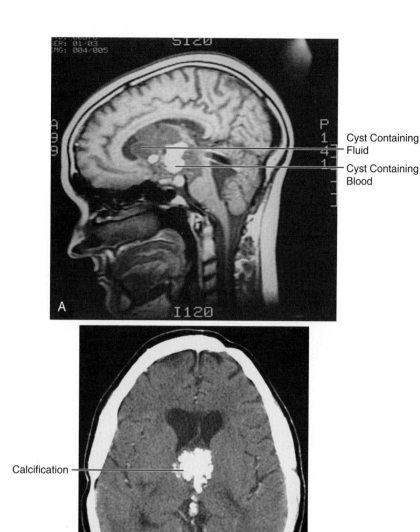

FIGURE 18–11. Sagittal T1-weighted magnetic resonance imaging (MRI) *(A)* and axial computed tomography (CT) without intravenous contrast *(B)* demonstrate a craniopharyngioma. In MRI the lobulated mass in the suprasellar region distorts the third and lateral ventricles and contains a mixture of high and low signal intensity. The low signal intensity regions represent cyst. In the CT scan the foci of increased density represent calcification.

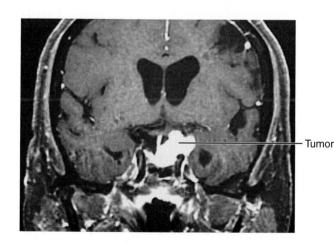

FIGURE 18–12. Suprasellar metastatic adenocarcinoma on a contrast-enhanced T1-weighted coronal magnetic resonance image. The tumor enhances homogeneously.

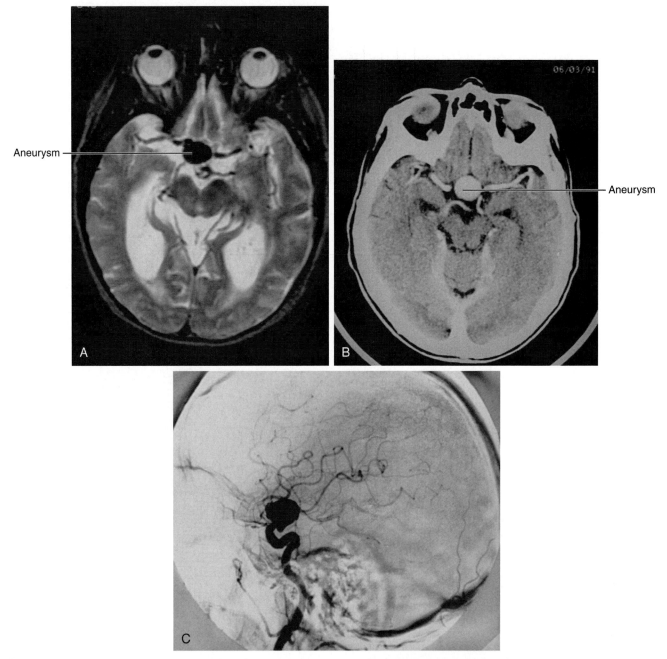

FIGURE 18–13. Axial magnetic resonance imaging *(A)*, computed tomography *(B)*, and lateral angiography *(C)* of a suprasellar carotid aneurysm.

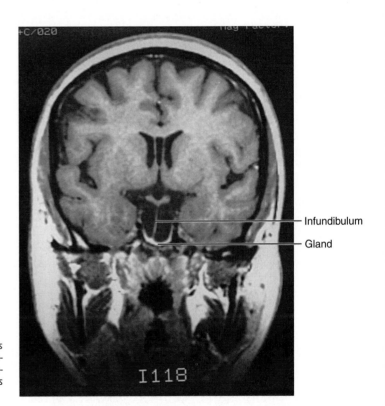

FIGURE 18–14. Coronal magnetic resonance image with intravenous contrast medium demonstrating an empty sella. Note that the infundibulum and pituitary gland are enhanced. Identification of the infundibulum connecting the pituitary gland directly with the hypothalamus excludes a cystic tumor.

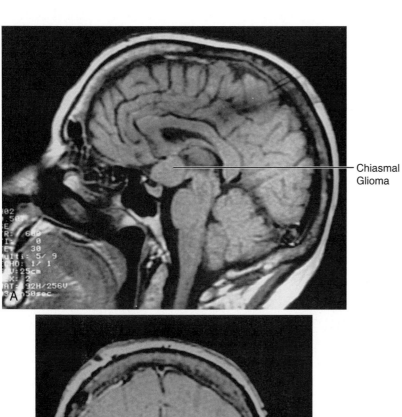

Chiasmal
Glioma

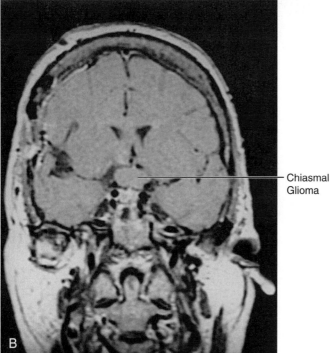

Chiasmal
Glioma

FIGURE 18–15. Sagittal (A) and coronal (B) magnetic resonance images demonstrating a chiasmal glioma. Note that the mass enlarges the optic chiasm. On the contrast-enhanced coronal image (B), it fails to enhance, unlike the adjacent pituitary gland and cavernous sinuses.

dermoid and epidermoid tumors appear as cysts with signal intensities consistent with a mixture of fluid, strands of tissue, calcium, or fat.

Arachnoid Cyst

The rare suprasellar arachnoid cysts are often manifested as visual impairment and endocrine dysfunction or hydrocephalus.[37] They may also be seen in adults evaluated for hypopituitarism and/or visual defects. Arachnoid cysts have a density on CT and signal intensity on MRI similar to that of CSF and do not enhance.

Rathke Cleft Cyst

Rathke cleft cysts are epithelial cysts derived from Rathke's cleft. They account for most sellar or parasellar cysts and are usually asymptomatic. Symptomatic enlargement is most common in adults. The T1- and T2-weighted signals will vary depending on the content of the cyst.[38]

Granulomatous Disease of the Hypothalamus

Sarcoidosis, eosinophilic granuloma, or histiocytosis X may involve the hypothalamus or infundibulum. Involvement appears on MRI as

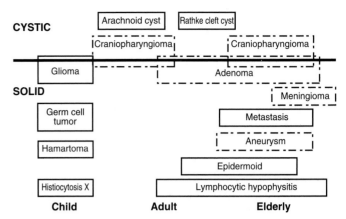

FIGURE 18–17. *Sellar/parasellar and hypothalamic lesions based on their most common imaging appearance and age of the patient at presentation of symptoms. Lesions surrounded by* dashed lines *may demonstrate calcification.*

enlargement of the infundibulum or a coating of abnormal tissue along the pial surface of the hypothalamus, brain stem, and optic chiasm. These changes are detected most effectively on MRI obtained after the administration of intravenous contrast medium. The radiologic differential diagnosis includes leptomeningeal carcinomatosis, basal meningitis, tuberculous meningitis, and cryptococcal meningitis.

CONCLUSION

The differential diagnosis of symptomatic sellar and hypothalamic lesions can often be narrowed by the imaging appearance and patient age. Figure 18–17 reviews the most common imaging appearance and age of occurrence of the symptomatic lesions discussed.

REFERENCES

1. Reich NE, Zelch JV, Alfidi RJ, et al: Computed tomography in the detection of juxtasellar lesions. Radiology 118:333–335, 1976.
2. Gyldensted C, Karle A: Computed tomography of infra- and juxtasellar lesions. A radiological study of 108 cases. Neuroradiology 14:5–13, 1977.
3. Belloni G, Baciocco A, Burelli P, et al: The value of CT for the diagnosis of pituitary microadenomas in children. Neuroradiology 15:179–181, 1978.
4. Wolpert SM, Pool KD, Biller BJ, et al: The value of computed tomography in evaluating patients with prolactinomas. Radiology 131:117–119, 1979.
5. Gardeur D, Naidich TP, Metzger J: CT analysis of intrasellar pituitary adenomas with emphasis on patterns of contrast enhancement. Neuroradiology 20:241–247, 1981.
6. Daniels DL: The sella and juxtasellar region. *In* Williams AL, Haughton VM (eds): Cranial Computed Tomography: A Comprehensive Text. St Louis, Mosby, 1985.
7. Macpherson P, Hadley DM, Teasdale G, et al: Pituitary microadenomas: Does gadolinium enhance their demonstration? Neuroradiology 31:293–298, 1991.
8. Stadnik TW, Stevenaert P, Beckers A, et al: Pituitary microadenomas: Diagnosis with two and three dimensional MR imaging at 1.5T before and after gadolinium. Radiology 176:419–423, 1990.
9. Miki Y, Matsuo M, Nishizawa S, et al: Pituitary adenomas and normal pituitary tissue: Enhancement patterns on gadopentetate enhanced MR imaging. Radiology 177:35–41, 1990.
10. Sakamoto Y, Takahashi M, Korogi Y, et al: Normal and abnormal pituitary glands. Gadopentetate enhanced MR imaging. Radiology 178:441–448, 1991.
11. Earnest FIV, McCullough EC, Frank DA: Fact or artifact: An analysis of artifact in high-resolution computed tomographic scanning of the sella. Radiology 140:109–114, 1981.
12. Taylor S: High resolution computed tomography of the sella. Radiol Clin North Am 20:207–236, 1982.
13. Mark L, Pech P, Daniels D, et al: The pituitary fossa: A correlative anatomic and MR study. Radiology 153:453–457, 1984.
14. Pojunas K, Daniels D, Williams A, Haughton V: MRI of prolactin-secreting microadenomas. AJNR Am J Neuroradiol 7:209–213, 1986.
15. Wolpert SM, Molitch ME, Goldman JA, et al: Size, shape and appearance of the normal female pituitary gland. AJNR Am J Neuroradiol 5:263–267, 1984.
16. Elster AD, Chen MY, Williams DW, Key LL. Pituitary gland: MR imaging of physiologic hypertrophy in adolescence. Radiology 174:681–685, 1990.
17. Holder CA, Elster AD: Magnetization transfer imaging of the pituitary: Further insights into the nature of the posterior "bright spot." J Comput Assist Tomogr 21:171–174, 1997.
18. Kurokawa H, Fujisawa I, Nakano Y, et al: Posterior lobe of the pituitary gland:

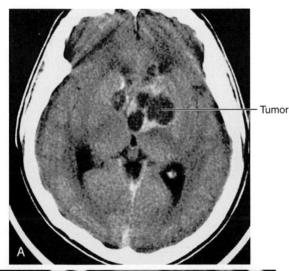

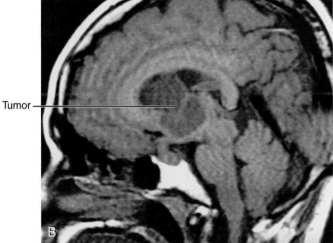

FIGURE 18–16. *Predominantly suprasellar germinoma. A heterogeneous suprasellar cystic germinoma is demonstrated on computed tomographic* (A) *and sagittal T2-weighted magnetic resonance images* (B). *Sellar invasion is better demonstrated on the magnetic resonance study.*

Correlation between signal intensity on T1-weighted MR images and vasopressin concentration. Radiology 207:79–83, 1998.

19. Kornreich L, Horev G, Lazar L, et al: MR findings in hereditary isolated growth hormone deficiency. AJNR Am J Neuroradiol 18:1743–1747, 1997.

20. Chason JL: Nervous system and skeletal muscle. *In* Anderson WAD (ed): Pathology. St Louis, Mosby, 1971, pp 1403–1428, 1796–1799, 1838–1842.

21. Post MJD, David NJ, Glasen JS, et al: Pituitary apoplexy: Diagnosis by computed tomography. Radiology 143:665–670, 1980.

22. Daniels DL, Williams AL, Thornton RS, et al: Differential diagnosis of intrasellar tumors by computed tomography. Radiology 141:697–701, 1981.

23. Critin GM, Davis DO: Computed tomography in the evaluation of pituitary adenomas. Invest Radiol 12:27–35, 1977.

24. Snow R, Johnson C, Morgello S, et al: Is magnetic resonance imaging useful in guiding the operative approach to large pituitary tumors? Neurosurgery 26:801–803, 1990.

25. Scotti G, Yu C, Dillon W, et al: MR imaging of cavernous sinus involvement by pituitary adenomas. AJNR Am J Neuroradiol 9:657–664, 1988.

26. Ostrov SG, Quencer RM, Hoffman JC, et al: Hemorrhage within pituitary adenomas: How often associated with pituitary apoplexy syndrome? AJNR Am J Neuroradiol 10:503–510, 1989.

27. Kucharczyk W, Bishop J, Plewes D, et al: Detection of pituitary microadenomas: Comparison of dynamic keyhole fast spin-echo, unenhanced, conventional contrast-enhanced MR imaging. AJR 163:671–679, 1994.

28. Lee KL: The diagnostic value of hyperostosis in midline subfrontal meningioma. Radiology 119:121–130, 1976.

29. Pusey E, Kortman K, Flannigan B, et al: MR of craniopharyngiomas: Tumor delineation and characterization. AJNR Am J Neuroradiol 8:439–444, 1987.

30. Sato N, Sze G, Endo K: Hypophysitis: Endocrinologic and dynamic MR findings. AJNR Am J Neuroradiol 19:439–444, 1998.

31. Haughton VM, Rosenbaum AE, Williams AL, et al: Recognizing the empty sella by CT: The infundibulum sign. AJNR Am J Neuroradiol 1:527–529, 1980.

32. Miller JH, Pena AM, Segall HD: Radiological investigation of sellar region masses in children. Radiology 134:81–87, 1980.

33. Rutka J, Hoffman H, Drake J, Humphreys R: Suprasellar and sellar tumors in childhood and adolescence. Neurosurg Clin North Am 3:803–820, 1992.

34. Burton E, Ball W, Crone K, Dolan L: Hamartoma of the tuber cinereum: A comparison of MR and CT findings in four cases. AJNR Am J Neuroradiol 10:497–501, 1989.

35. Legido A, Packer RJ, Sutton LN, et al: Suprasellar germinomas in childhood: A reappraisal. Cancer 63:340–344, 1989.

36. Paul LW, John H: The Essentials of Roentgen Interpretation. Hagerstown, MD, Harper & Row, 1972, pp 366–372, 375.

37. Armstrong EA, Harwood-Nash DCF, Hoffman H, et al: Benign suprasellar cysts: The CT approach. AJNR Am J Neuroradiol 4:163–166, 1983.

38. Kucharczyk W, Peck W, Kelly W, et al: Rathke cleft cysts: CT, MR imaging, and pathologic features. Radiology 165:491–495, 1987.

Hypothalamic Syndromes

Glenn D. Braunstein

The hypothalamus houses multiple nuclei along with afferent and efferent nerve fibers that connect the hypothalamus to the various portions of the brain and brain stem. It is divided into four regions: from anterior to posterior, the preoptic, supraoptic, tuberal, and mamillary regions; and three zones: laterally from the third ventricle, the periventricular, medial, and lateral[1–4] zones (Table 19–1, Figs. 19–1 and 19–2).

The hypothalamus is responsible for many of the body's homeostatic mechanisms, including water metabolism, temperature regulation, appetite control, the sleep-wake cycle, circadian rhythms, and control of the sympathetic and parasympathetic nervous system. In addition, this area has activity in regard to emotional expression, behavior, and memory. Finally, the hypothalamus is essential to the neuroendocrine control of anterior pituitary function. Table 19–2 lists the various functions along with the hypothalamic nuclei or hypothalamic regions that have been identified as being responsible for these functions and the disorders that result from either destructive or stimulatory lesions in or around the nuclei or region.[1, 4–23]

HYPOTHALAMIC DISORDERS: PATHOPHYSIOLOGIC PRINCIPLES

First, the small overall size of the hypothalamus and the close association of the nuclei and nerve tracts mean that a variety of different pathologic processes may give rise to the same signs and symptoms of neurologic and hypothalamic dysfunction.[4] The spectrum of disorders that can affect the hypothalamus is shown in Table 19–3. Tumors, infiltrative disorders, and infections, among other conditions,

frequently give rise to headaches, neuro-ophthalmologic disorders, pyramidal tract or sensory nerve dysfunction, extrapyramidal cerebellar signs, and recurrent vomiting.[9, 10] Other common manifestations include gonadal dysfunction, either hypogonadism or precocious puberty; diabetes insipidus; somnolence; dysthermia; and evidence of a caloric imbalance either with hyperphagia and obesity or anorexia with emaciation.[9, 10]

Second, although exceptions exist, most patients who have a systemic disorder, such as Langerhans' cell histiocytosis, sarcoidosis, tuberculosis, or leukemia, will exhibit manifestations of the disease outside of the hypothalamus and central nervous system.

Third, a lesion may disrupt a function that is subserved by a hypothalamic nucleus distant from the lesion. Since the afferent and efferent tracts to and from the hypothalamic nuclei traverse other areas of the hypothalamus and brain distant from the nuclei, lesions that affect those tracts may result in dysfunction of several hypothalamic nuclei.

Fourth, most lesions that result in chronic hypothalamic syndromes involve more than one nucleus. As can be seen in Table 19–2, most of the hypothalamic functions are controlled by more than one nucleus and this redundancy allows for some degree of compensation, should one nucleus be affected. In addition, most of the nuclei are paired and destruction of a single nucleus may not be sufficient to result in a clinical syndrome. Thus, lesions that affect the basal tuberal region of the hypothalamus (pituitary adenomas with suprasellar extension, optic gliomas, and craniopharyngiomas), or are multiple (granulomatous disorders, metastatic tumors, infiltrative disease), or cause enlargement of the third ventricle (aqueductal stenosis, colloid cysts, pinealomas, germ cell tumors, midbrain gliomas) will more likely result in clinical

TABLE 19–1. Major Hypothalamic Nuclei

Region	Zone		
	Periventricular	*Medial*	*Lateral*
Preoptic	Preoptic periventricular nucleus Anterior periventricular nucleus	Medial preoptic nucleus	Lateral preoptic nucleus
Supraoptic	Suprachiasmatic nucleus Paraventricular nucleus	Anterior hypothalamic nucleus Medial portion of supraoptic nucleus	Lateral portion of supraoptic nucleus
Tuberal	Arcuate (infundibular) nucleus	Dorsomedial hypothalamic nucleus Ventromedial hypothalamic nucleus	Lateral hypothalamic nucleus
Mamillary	Posterior hypothalamic nucleus	Premamillary nucleus Medial mamillary nucleus	Lateral mamillary nucleus Intercalatus nucleus

From Braunstein GD: The hypothalamus. *In* Melmed S (ed): The Pituitary. Cambridge, MA, Blackwell Scientific, 1994. Reprinted by permission of Blackwell Science, Inc.

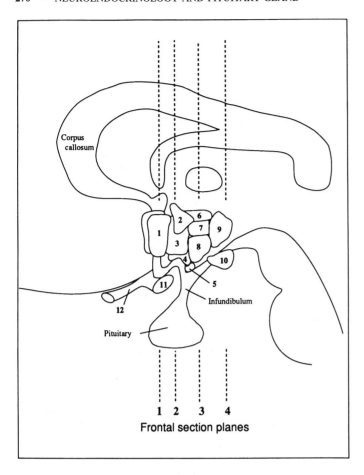

FIGURE 19–1. Schematic representation of lateral brain section demonstrating hypothalamic nuclei. *Dashed lines* represent the frontal (coronal) section planes illustrated in Figures 19–2 and 19–3. *1,* preoptic nucleus; *2,* paraventricular nucleus; *3,* anterior hypothalamic areas; *4,* supraoptic nucleus; *5,* arcuate nucleus; *6,* dorsal hypothalamic area; *7,* dorsomedial nucleus; *8,* ventromedial nucleus; *9,* posterior hypothalamic area; *10,* mamillary body; *11,* optic chiasm; *12,* optic nerve. (From Braunstein GD: The hypothalamus. *In* Melmed S [ed]: The Pituitary. Cambridge, MA, Blackwell Scientific, 1994, pp 309–340. Reprinted by permission of Blackwell Science, Inc.)

hypothalamic dysfunction than will disorders affecting the more lateral portions of the hypothalamus.

Fifth, the rate of progression of the pathologic process affects the patient's clinical manifestations. Slowly progressive lesions may give few or no symptoms until they achieve a large size, at which time altered endocrine function and deterioration of cognitive ability may be present, while small acute lesions may result in profound clinical manifestations such as alterations in consciousness, thermal dysregulation, and diabetes insipidus.

Sixth, the clinical syndrome due to involvement of a hypothalamic nucleus or tract may differ depending on whether the pathologic lesion is destructive or stimulatory. As an example, chronic, destructive lesions of the preoptic region may result in hypothermia and insomnia, while hyperthermia and lethargy may be seen with acute stimulatory lesions.

Finally, the clinical manifestations of the hypothalamic disease depend in part on the age of the patient. Thus, prepubertal gonadotropin deficiency results in sexual infantilism, while in the postpubertal state, there is regression, but not disappearance of, secondary sexual characteristics. Similarly, prepubertal growth hormone deficiency because of a hypothalamic lesion disturbing growth hormone–releasing hormone (GHRH) function results in short stature, while a similar lesion occurring in an adult may only be manifest by the adult growth hormone deficiency syndrome.

MANIFESTATIONS OF HYPOTHALAMIC DISEASE (Fig. 19–3)

Disorders of Water Metabolism

Central Diabetes Insipidus

Complete or partial central diabetes insipidus results from destruction of the antidiuretic hormone (ADH)–producing magnocellular neurons in the supraoptic and paraventricular nuclei, or interruption of the transport of ADH through their axons, which terminate in the pituitary stalk and posterior pituitary. Diabetes insipidus is relatively common in patients with chronic hypothalamic disorders, being found in approximately 35% of such patients.[9, 10] It is also frequently found in patients with acute insults to the hypothalamus or pituitary stalk as is seen in vascular accidents and neurosurgical trauma. Obesity and hypogonadism frequently are present in patients with diabetes insipidus due to tumors or infiltrative disorders.

The majority of patients with diabetes insipidus have idiopathic or familial diabetes insipidus associated with gliosis of the supraoptic and paraventricular nuclei.[24] Approximately one third of patients with idiopathic diabetes insipidus have detectable anti-ADH producing cell antibodies suggesting an autoimmune cause.[25] Both sex-linked recessive and autosomal dominant forms of familial diabetes insipidus have been described. In the more common autosomal dominant form, nucleotide deletions or substitutions in the ADH gene have been identified.[26] Wolfram's syndrome represents a rare autosomal recessive form of central diabetes insipidus associated with type 1 diabetes mellitus, optic atrophy, bilateral sensorineural deafness, and occasionally ataxia and autonomic neurogenic bladder.[27] Diabetes insipidus is a frequent manifestation of suprasellar and pineal germinomas, sarcoidosis, and the chronic disseminated form of Langerhans' cell histiocytosis.[28–35]

Adipsic or Essential Hypernatremia

Adipsic hypernatremia, also known as the cerebral salt retention syndrome, occurs when the osmoreceptors that are present in the anterior medial and anterior lateral preoptic regions are damaged. The affected patients have an impaired thirst mechanism, which results in insufficient fluid intake despite the hypernatremia. Although most of the affected patients have partial diabetes insipidus, their extracellular fluid volume remains normal and they are not dehydrated. Therefore, they exhibit chronic elevations of serum sodium, but normal blood pressure, pulse rate, serum creatinine, and creatinine clearance and can

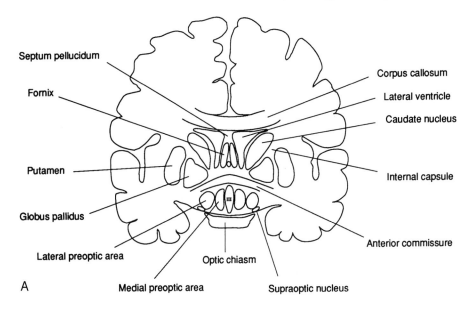

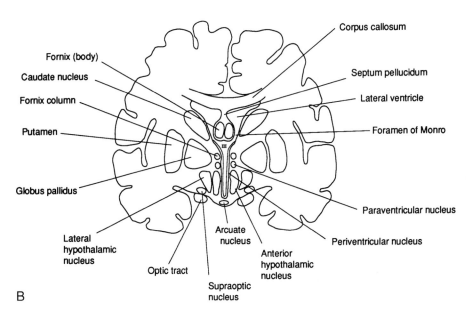

FIGURE 19–2. Frontal (coronal) sections of the hypothalamic regions. *A,* Preoptic region (frontal section plane 1 in Fig. 19–1). *B,* Supraoptic region (frontal section plane 2 in Fig. 19–1).

Illustration continued on following page

release ADH and concentrate their urine during fluid deprivation. When serum sodium concentrations are below 160 mmol/L, few symptoms are present. However, between 160 and 180 mmol/L patients may have fatigue, weakness, lethargy, muscle tenderness, cramps, anorexia, depression, and irritability, and above 180 mmol/L stupor and coma may be present. Close to half of these patients have hypothalamic obesity and almost three fourths demonstrate some degree of anterior pituitary hormone deficiency.[6, 9, 10, 12, 36, 37]

Essential hyponatremia has been described with a variety of lesions, including craniopharyngiomas, suprasellar germinomas, optic nerve gliomas, pineal tumors, Langerhans' cell histiocytosis, sarcoidosis, trauma, hydrocephalus, cysts, inflammatory conditions, ruptured aneurysms, and toluene exposure.[36–38] The Hayek-Peake syndrome is the association of essential hypernatremia with hypodipsia, obesity, lethargy, increased perspiration, central hypoventilation, hyperprolactinemia, hypothyroidism, and hyperlipidemia without an identifiable structural hypothalamic defect.[39, 40]

Syndrome of Inappropriate Secretion of Antidiuretic Hormone (SIADH)

SIADH is characterized by serum hyponatremia and hypo-osmolarity with an inappropriately elevated urine osmolarity in a patient with normal renal, adrenal, and thyroid function without evidence of intravascular or extracellular fluid volume expansion. The clinical symptoms depend upon the rate of fall of serum sodium, as well as the absolute serum sodium concentration. At serum sodium levels above 120 mmol/L, symptoms are generally mild and nonspecific and include anorexia, nausea, headache, weakness, and lethargy. Below 120 mmol/L, the above symptoms are accompanied by nausea, vomiting, and mental confusion, and at very low levels, by seizure and coma. The syndrome is found with a variety of intracranial abnormalities, including head trauma, intracranial bleeding, meningitis, encephalitis, neurosurgery, hydrocephalus, acute intermittent prophyria, craniopharyngiomas, germinomas, and pinealomas.[6, 12, 28] An idiopathic form has been described in young women who exhibit menstrual irregularities and have enlarged lateral ventricles and develop SIADH cyclically. No structural defect has been described in these patients.[4]

Dysthermia

Hyperthermia

The warm receptors present in the preoptic anterior hypothalamus are stimulated by an increase in the temperature of the blood. Together

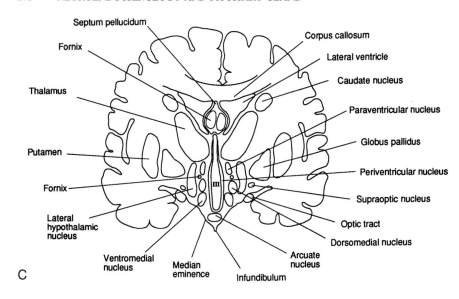

C

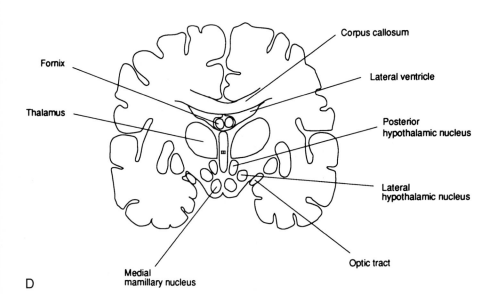

D

FIGURE 19–2 *Continued. C,* Tuberal region (frontal section plane 3 in Fig. 19–1). *D,* Mamillary region (frontal section plane 4 in Fig. 19–1). (From Braunstein GD: The hypothalamus. *In* Melmed S (ed): The Pituitary. Cambridge, MA, Blackwell Scientific, 1994, pp 309–340. Reprinted by permission of Blackwell Science, Inc.)

with signals from peripheral warm receptors that respond to a rise in external temperature, the afferent signals travel through the median forebrain bundle to the lateral portion of the posterior hypothalamus, which leads to vasodilation and sweating to dissipate heat. Conversely, stimulation of the preoptic anterior hypothalamic cold receptors through a decrease in temperature of the blood, or stimulation of the peripheral cold receptors through a decrease in ambient temperature, results in medial neurons in the posterior hypothalamus activating heat production through muscular shivering and heat conservation through vasoconstriction.[5, 6]

Acute injury to the anterior hypothalamic and preoptic areas may result in a rapid temperature elevation as high as 41°C associated with tachycardia and unconsciousness from failure of the heat-dissipating mechanisms to function while heat production continues. Chronic hyperthermia may be found with lesions in the tuberoinfundibular region, and in contrast to patients with elevated temperature from inflammation of infections, these patients generally do not experience malaise and paradoxically may have peripheral vasoconstriction.[1, 5, 6, 9, 10]

Wolff et al.[42] described a syndrome of hyperthermia associated with shaking chills, fever, hypertension, vomiting, and peripheral vasoconstriction that occurred cyclically at 3-week intervals, without a pathologic lesion in the hypothalamus being found. Similar paroxysms of

hyperthermia have been noted in other patients without the cyclicity, and together these episodes may represent a variant of diencephalic epilepsy.[6, 41, 42]

Approximately 0.2% of patients receiving neuroleptic drugs develop the neuroleptic malignant syndrome (NMS), which is characterized by hyperthermia to 41°C or higher; severe extrapyramidal signs, including "lead-pipe" muscle rigidity and tremor; signs of autonomic nervous system dysfunction such as pallor, tachycardia, arrhythmias, blood pressure lability, and diaphoresis; and changes in mental status, including mutism, delirium, and coma.[43, 44] All antipsychotic medications have been reported to cause NMS and most evidence suggests that disruption of the dopamine neurotransmission by neuroleptic-induced dopamine receptor blockade is the major pathophysiologic abnormality in susceptible individuals. Indeed, the greater the potency of the neuroleptic in regards to its dopamine D_2-receptor antagonism activity, the greater the frequency of NMS occurrence.[44] NMS is successfully treated with a variety of dopamine agonists. Injury to the preoptic medial and tuberal nuclei have been demonstrated at autopsy, as has a depletion of hypothalamic norepinephrine concentrations.[45] The syndrome generally begins within 2 weeks of initiating the neuroleptic and evolves over a 24- to 72-hour period. The most common complication is rhabdomyolysis, which may result in myoglobinuria and acute

TABLE 19–2. Hypothalamic Functions, the Nuclei or Regions Involved with the Specific Functions, and the Disorders Resulting from Stimulatory or Destructive Lesions in the Regions

Function	Nuclei [n] or Region Involved [r]	Disorders
Water metabolism	Supraoptic [n]; paraventricular [n]	Diabetes insipidus Essential hypernatremia SIADH
Temperature regulation	Preoptic anterior hypothalamic [r] Posterior hypothalamus [r]	Hyperthermia Hypothermia Poikilothermia
Appetite control	Ventromedial [n] (satiety center) Lateral hypothalamic [r] (feeding center)	Hypothalamic obesity Cachexia Anorexia nervosa Diencephalic syndrome Diencephalic glycosuria
Sleep-wake cycle and circadian rhythm	Anterior hypothalamic [r] (sleep center) Posterior hypothalamic [r] (arousal center) Suprachiasmatic [n]	Somnolence Reversal of sleep-wake cycle Alkinetic mutism Coma
Visceral (autonomic) fraction	Posterior medial [r] (sympathetic region) Preoptic anterior hypothalamus [r] (parasympathetic region)	Sympathetic activation Parasympathetic activation
Emotional expression and behavior	Ventromedial [n] Medial and posterior hypothalamus [r] Caudal hypothalamic [r]	Sham rage Fear or horror Apathy Hypersexual behavior
Memory	Ventromedial [n] Mamillary bodies	Short-term memory loss
Control of anterior pituitary function	Arcuate [n] Preoptic [n] Suprachiasmatic [n] Paraventricular [n] Neovascular zone (median eminence)	Hyperfunction syndromes Hypofunction syndromes

SIADH, syndrome of inappropriate secretion of antidiuretic hormone.

renal failure. The mortality of this syndrome is currently under 10%, which reflects the increasing recognition and the initiation of prompt therapy of the disorder.[44]

Hypothermia

Large destructive lesions of the anterior or posterior hypothalamus may result in inability to generate heat through vasoconstriction and muscular shivering. This occurs in 10% to 15% of patients with a variety of hypothalamic lesions, especially neoplasms, infiltrative disorders, and infections.[9, 10, 12] It has also been noted in patients with Parkinson's disease and Wernicke's encephalopathy, which are associated with lesions in the posterior hypothalamus and mamillary bodies, respectively.[46, 47]

Diencephalic autonomic epilepsy refers to episodic or paroxysmal hypothermia during which the body temperature decreases to 32°C or less over minutes to days along with evidence of autonomic nervous system dysfunction, including flushing, sweating, hypotension, bradycardia, salivation, lacrimation, pupillary dilation, Cheyne-Stokes respiration, nausea, vomiting, asterixis, ataxia, and obtundation.[6, 14, 48–51] Electroencephalographic (EEG) abnormalities occur during the episodes. Autopsy studies have shown gliosis and loss of the arcuate nucleus and premamillary area in some patients, while others have been found to have tumors involving the floor and lower portion of the third ventricle.[14, 48] The corpus callosum has been found to be absent in approximately half of the patients with episodic hypothermia and these individuals may also exhibit diabetes insipidus, reset osmostat, growth hormone deficiency, hypogonadism, or precocious puberty (Shapiro's syndrome).[52–54]

Poikilothermia

When both the heat loss and heat-conserving homeostatic mechanisms are impaired, wide fluctuations of body temperature might take place, without the patients experiencing thermal discomfort. This condition, known as poikilothermia, is found with both anterior and posterior hypothalamic destruction, as well as in patients with large lesions that may involve the posterior hypothalamus and rostal mesen-

cephalon.[6, 9, 10] Rarely, patients with Wernicke's encephalopathy may experience poikilothermia.[6]

Disorders of Appetite Control and Caloric Balance

Hypothalamic Obesity

Approximately 25% of patients with structural hypothalamic lesions exhibit hyperphagia and obesity.[9, 10] Usually the patients have lesions involving a large portion of the hypothalamus, although bilateral destruction of only the ventromedial nucleus may lead to hypothalamic obesity.[1, 9, 10, 16, 17, 21, 55] The majority of patients harbor a neoplasm, especially craniopharyngioma, with a minority having inflammatory or granulomatous processes, a history of trauma, or infiltrative disorders.[55] Common clinical findings in these patients include headaches, visual abnormalities, hypogonadism, diabetes insipidus, and somnolence. Less commonly, behavioral abnormalities, such as antisocial behavior or sham rage, and seizures may be present.[55]

Diencephalic Syndrome of Infancy

Infants harboring a low-grade hypothalamic or optic nerve glioma, or rarely ependymomas, gangliogliomas, or dysgerminomas that destroy the ventromedial nuclei, may develop an unusual syndrome at approximately 1 year of age, in which they begin to lose weight and subcutaneous fat, while maintaining an apparently good food intake and normal growth. They exhibit hyperactivity and a cheerful affect and often demonstrate nystagmus, pallor, vomiting, tremor, and optic atrophy. Endocrine evaluation is generally normal or may show nonspecific abnormalities. If the patients live beyond 2 years of age, they begin to gain weight and become obese. Their euphoria and cheerful affect disappear and are replaced by rage and irritability. Somnolence and precocious puberty also may be present.[5, 56, 57]

Hypothalamic Cachexia in Adults

Patients with destructive lesions of the lateral hypothalamus may develop rapid weight loss, decreased activity, hypophagia, muscle

TABLE 19–3. Causes of Hypothalamic Dysfunction

Congenital	*Nutritional, Metabolic*
Acquired	Anorexia nervosa
Developmental malformations	Kernicterus
Anencephaly	Wernicke-Korsakoff syndrome
Porencephaly	Weight loss
Agenesis of the corpus callosum	*Degenerative*
Septo-optic dysplasia	Glial scarring
Suprasellar arachnoid cyst	Parkinson's disease
Colloid cyst of the third ventricle	
Hamartoma	*Infectious*
Aqueductal stenosis	Bacterial
Trauma	Meningitis
Intraventricular hemorrhage	Mycobacterial
Genetic (familial or sporadic cases)	Tuberculosis
Hypothalamic hypopituitarism	Spirochetal
Familial diabetes insipidus	Syphilis
Prader-Willi syndrome	Viral
Bardet-Biedl and associated	Encephalitis
syndromes	Jakob-Creutzfeldt disease
Wolfram's syndrome	Kuru
Pallister-Hall syndrome	Poliomyelitis
	Varicella
Tumors	Cytomegalovirus infection
Primary intracranial tumors	*Vascular*
Angioma of the third ventricle	Aneurysm
Craniopharyngioma	Arteriovenous malformation
Ependymoma	Pituitary apoplexy
Ganglioneuroma	Subarachnoid hemorrhage
Germ cell tumors	
Glioblastoma multiforme	*Trauma*
Glioma	Birth injury
Hamartoma	Head injury
Hemangioma	Postneurosurgical
Lipoma	
Lymphoma	*Functional*
Medulloblastoma	Diencephalic epilepsy
Meningioma	Drugs
Neuroblastoma	Hayek-Peake syndrome
Pinealomas	Idiopathic syndrome of inappropriate
Pituitary tumors	secretion of antidiuretic hormone
Plasmacytoma	(SIADH)
Sarcoma	Kleine-Levin syndrome
Metastatic tumors	Periodic syndrome of Wolff
	Psychosocial deprivation syndrome
Infiltrative	
Histiocytosis	*Other*
Leukemia	
Sarcoidosis	Radiation
	Porphyria
Immunologic	Toluene exposure
Idiopathic diabetes insipidus	
Paraneoplastic syndrome	

Modified from Braunstein GD: The hypothalamus. *In* Melmed S (ed): The Pituitary. Cambridge, MA, Blackwell Scientific, 1994. Reprinted by permission of Blackwell Science, Inc.

wasting, cachexia, and death, usually due to a neoplasm.[9, 10, 16, 17, 20] Malignant multiple sclerosis also may cause the lateral hypothalamic syndrome.[16, 20]

Anorexia Nervosa

Anorexia nervosa is a common disorder, usually seen in young women beginning before the age of 25 years. Although it is not associated with a structural hypothalamic defect, functional hypothalamic abnormalities are present. These patients, with their distorted body image, exercise excessively, may induce vomiting, and develop amenorrhea with a prepubertal pattern of gonadotropin release.[58] Elevations of basal serum growth hormone with reduction of insulin-like growth factor I (IGF-I) concentrations are found and the patients may demonstrate abnormalities in hypothalamic-pituitary-adrenal activity with elevated plasma cortisol concentrations, decreased adrenocorticotropic hormone (ACTH) levels, and an attenuated ACTH response to

corticotropin-releasing hormone (CRH). Low concentrations of thyroxine (T_4) and triiodothyronine (T_3) with elevated reverse T_3 and a thyroid-stimulating hormone (TSH) response to thyrotropin-releasing hormone (TRH) that is either normal or demonstrates a delayed peak consistent with hypothalamic hypothyroidism are found.[59] Additionally, these patients may have hyperprolactinemia with galactorrhea, evidence of thermal dysregulation, and a partial diabetes insipidus.[60] The neuroendocrine and functional hypothalamic abnormalities remit when the patients regain their weight.

Diencephalic Glycosuria

Acute injuries to the tuberoinfundibular region from basal skull fractures, intracranial hemorrhage, or neurosurgical intervention around the third ventricle may lead to transient hyperglycemia and glycosuria.[1, 61] Although many of the "stress hormones" with glucose contraregulatory activity are elevated in these patients, they do not appear to be responsible for the glucose abnormality.

Sleep-Wake Cycle and Circadian Abnormalities

Approximately 10% of patients with hypothalamic disease will present with somnolence, and this condition is found in 30% of such patients at some time during the course of their illness.[9, 10] Somnolence is commonly seen in lesions involving the posterior hypothalamus, often in association with hypothermia.[1, 6, 62] Approximately 40% of patients with hypersomnolence also have hypothalamic obesity.[55] Most patients with these manifestations have neoplasms, especially craniopharyngiomas, epithelial pineal tumors, and suprasellar germinomas.[30, 63] Encephalitis and Wernicke's nutritional encephalopathy are other causes of hypothalamic hypersomnia.[1, 5, 6] As previously noted, acute hypothalamic injury may lead to a transient coma. Narcolepsy, which represents sudden episodes of sleep that last minutes to hours, may in some instances, have a hypothalamic cause as the syndrome has been found in patients with third ventricular tumors, multiple sclerosis, following head injuries, and encephalitis.[1]

Patients with lesions of the anterior and preoptic hypothalamic nuclei may exhibit hyperactivity and insomnia, or more commonly, alterations in the sleep-wake cycle, with daytime sleepiness and nighttime hyperactivity.[6, 22, 64] This is characteristically seen in patients with cystic craniopharyngiomas. Anterior tuberal lesions may also lead to alterations in the sleep-wake cycle, as well as an akinetic mutism type of syndrome in which the patient appears awake but does not respond to verbal stimuli and demonstrates little spontaneous movement.[64]

The suprachiasmatic nuclei are responsible for the maintenance of many of our circadian rhythms, and lesions involving this region will alter the sleep-wake cycle, temperature control, and cognitive function.[65]

Abnormalities of Emotional Expression or Behavior

Sham rage reactions with emotional lability, marked agitation, and aggressive, destructive behavior are found in patients with lesions involving the ventromedial nuclei.[6, 22, 62] Activation of the sympathetic nervous system is present during the episodes. In contrast, apathy, somnolence, and hypoactivity, as well as vocal and auditory unresponsiveness and akinetic mutism, have been found in patients with destruction of the mamillary bodies or lesions in the medial posterior hypothalamus.[1, 6]

Hypersexual behavior is seen in individuals with lesions involving the caudal hypothalamus.[66] The Kleine-Levin syndrome is believed to represent a functional abnormality of the hypothalamus. It generally affects adolescent boys, who have recurrent episodes of somnolence, with periodic arousal that is associated with irritability, abnormal speech, forgetfulness, food gorging, and masturbation and other sexual activity. The episodes may occur at 3- to 6-month intervals and

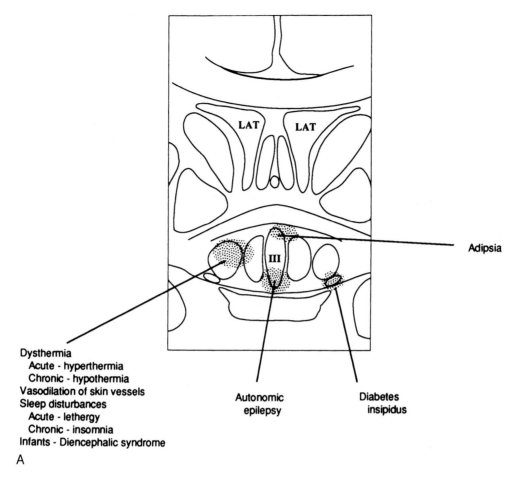

Adipsia

Dysthermia
    Acute - hyperthermia
    Chronic - hypothermia
Vasodilation of skin vessels
Sleep disturbances
    Acute - lethergy
    Chronic - insomnia
Infants - Diencephalic syndrome

Autonomic
epilepsy

Diabetes
insipidus

A

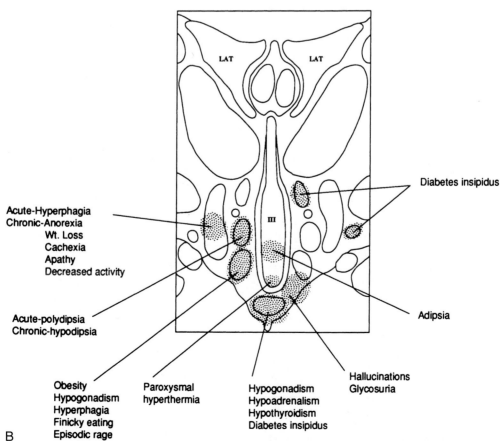

Diabetes insipidus

Acute-Hyperphagia
Chronic-Anorexia
    Wt. Loss
    Cachexia
    Apathy
    Decreased activity

Acute-polydipsia
Chronic-hypodipsia

Adipsia

Obesity
Hypogonadism
Hyperphagia
Finicky eating
Episodic rage

Paroxysmal
hyperthermia

Hypogonadism
Hypoadrenalism
Hypothyroidism
Diabetes insipidus

Hallucinations
Glycosuria

B

FIGURE 19–3. Clinical findings associated with hypothalamic lesions located at various anatomic sites. Clinicopathologic correlation based upon multiple studies.[14–23] *A,* Corresponds to region depicted in Figure 19–2A. *B,* Corresponds to region depicted in Figure 19–2C.

Illustration continued on following page

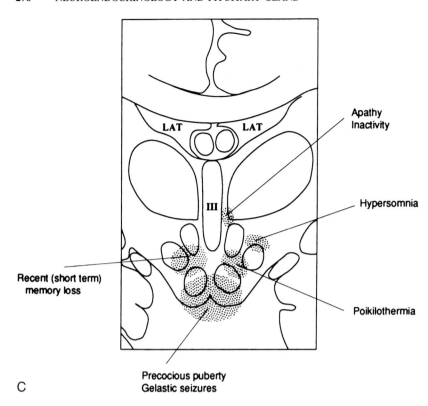

C

FIGURE 19–3 *Continued. C,* Corresponds to section depicted in Figure 19–2D. (From Braunstein GD: The hypothalamus. *In* Melmed S (ed): The Pituitary. Cambridge, MA, Blackwell Scientific, 1994, pp 309–340. Reprinted by permission of Blackwell Science, Inc.)

generally last 5 to 7 days. The disorder usually remits spontaneously in late adolescence or early adulthood.[67, 68]

Gelastic or laughing seizures are a form of diencephalic epilepsy due to lesions involving the floor of the third ventricle and mamillary area, especially hamartomas of the tuber cinereum.[69] The affected child does not lose consciousness, but stops his or her activity and begins to laugh or giggle or make bubbling noises, associated with a grimace from tightening of the facial muscles.[70, 71] EEG abnormalities are present during the seizure.

Disordered Control of Anterior Pituitary Function

Hyperfunction Syndromes

PRECOCIOUS PUBERTY. Isosexual pubertal development in girls below the age of 8 or boys below the age of 9 years represents sexual precocity, which most often is due to premature activation of the hypothalamic-pituitary-gonadal axis. The majority of girls have no discernible lesion and are therefore classified as having idiopathic central precocious puberty, while only 10% of boys have idiopathic precocious puberty.[72] In the latter, close to half have hypothalamic hamartomas and a third have other benign or malignant neoplasms that are located in the posterior hypothalamus or near the mamillary bodies.[72] The spectrum of pathologic conditions that can cause central precocious puberty are listed in Table 19–4.[4, 72–80] Some of these lesions may bring about early activation of the hypothalamic-pituitary-gonadal axis through increased intracranial pressure or irritation of the basal hypothalamus. Hypothalamic hamartomas involving the tuber cinereum are often associated with precocious puberty through premature activation of the normal hypothalamic gonadotropin-releasing hormone (GnRH) secretory mechanisms or through direct secretion of GnRH by the hamartoma, since GnRH has been located immunohistochemically within hamartomatous neurons.[81, 82] In addition to pressure effects, germ cell tumors may result in precocious puberty through the secretion of human chorionic gonadotropin (hCG), which may stimulate the child's gonads to secrete sex steroid hormones, bringing about precocious sexual development. Finally, premature activation of the normal hypothalamic-pituitary-gonadal axis has been described in

some patients who have had incomplete sexual precocity from congenital adrenal hyperplasia or polyostotic fibrous dysplasia (McCune-Albright) syndrome, in which the hypothalamus is exposed to elevated sex steroid hormones at an early age, and in patients with primary hypothyroidism who may also exhibit galactorrhea with elevated prolactin levels (Van Wyk-Grumbach syndrome) in which the mechanism for the premature activation is unknown, but usually ceases with correction of the hypothyroidism.

ACROMEGALY. Acromegaly due to the ectopic secretion of GHRH is rare and in most instances the source of the ectopic GHRH is a bronchial carcinoid, islet cell neoplasm, adrenal tumor, or lung carcinoma.[83, 84] However, acromegaly has also been found in patients with hypothalamic hamartomas, gangliocytomas, gliomas, and choristomas.[83–86] Some of these tumors have been shown to contain GHRH and they presumably secrete the releasing factor, which in turn stimulates the somatotrophs to hypersecrete growth hormone.

CUSHING'S DISEASE. There are several lines of evidence suggesting that Cushing's disease has a hypothalamic component to its pathophysiology.[87] First, it has been noted that the onset of the disease often follows an emotionally stressful event.[88] Since depression may

TABLE 19–4. Causes of Central Precocious Puberty

Idiopathic	Neurofibroma
Congenital Abnormalities	Astrocytoma
	Ependymoma
Hypothalamic hamartoma	Infundibuloma
Arachnoid cyst	Pinealoma
Myelomeningocele	Neuroblastoma
Aqueductal stenosis with hydrocephalus	Germinoma
Tuberous sclerosis	Craniopharyngioma
Congenital optic nerve hypoplasia	
Congenital adrenal hyperplasia	*Inflammatory Conditions*
McCune-Albright syndrome	Tuberculosis
Septo-optic dysplasia	Sarcoidosis
	Meningoencephalitis
Neoplasms	
	Subdural Hematoma
Optic nerve glioma	
Hypothalamic glioma	*Primary Hypothyroidism*

From Braunstein GD: The hypothalamus. *In* Melmed S (ed): The Pituitary. Cambridge, MA, Blackwell Scientific, 1994. Reprinted by permission of Blackwell Science, Inc.

be associated with pseudo-Cushing's syndrome with hypersecretion of glucocorticoids, it is conceivable that chronic corticotroph stimulation by hypothalamic CRH could lead to the development of a corticotroph adenoma and Cushing's disease, and may account for the recurrence of Cushing's disease following apparently successful removal of an ACTH-secreting corticotroph adenoma.[89, 90] Second, most patients with Cushing's disease, when given exogenous glucocorticoids in sufficient quantities, are able to suppress their ACTH secretion, a fact that has been known for some time and forms the basis for the high-dose portion of the dexamethasone suppression test.[87] Presumably this phenomenon reflects an increased set-point for negative feedback of glucocorticoids at the hypothalamic level. Third, some patients with Cushing's disease exhibit a reduction in ACTH and cortisol secretion and amelioration of symptoms following the administration of cyproheptadine, bromocriptine, or sodium valproate, which may work through the hypothalamus.[91–94] Nevertheless, most, if not all, corticotroph adenomas are of clonal origin rather than polyclonal as would be anticipated if CRH hypersecretion were responsible for the pituitary abnormality.[97] Hypothalamic factors such as CRH may promote clonal expansion of corticotroph cells that have become intrinsically abnormal.[96] An unusual cause of pituitary-dependent Cushing's disease is the secretion of CRH by an intracranial neoplasm, as had been demonstrated with an intrasellar gangliocytoma.[97]

HYPERPROLACTINEMIA. Since prolactin secretion by the lactotrophs is under hypothalamic dopamine inhibitory control, it is not surprising that patients with a variety of hypothalamic disorders may exhibit hyperprolactinemia. This is seen in 79% of patients with supersellar germinomas, 36% of patients with craniopharyngiomas, and 14% of patients with pineal germinomas.[30] Most patients have a prolactin concentration under 70 ng/mL and galactorrhea is infrequently seen, probably because of the coexistence of hypogonadism.[98] Nevertheless, amenorrhea and galactorrhea may be present in women and impotence in men.

Idiopathic hyperprolactinemia in patients without any demonstrable structural abnormality in the pituitary or hypothalamus is presumably due to a hypothalamic dopamine deficiency. The prolactin secretory dynamics of these patients in response to various stimulatory and inhibitory agents is similar to that seen in patients with prolactin-secreting pituitary adenomas. Indeed, some patients with idiopathic hyperprolactinemia when followed for a long period of time will eventually be found to have a prolactin-secreting pituitary microadenoma. Additional evidence supporting a hypothalamic cause for the pituitary adenoma is the finding of lactotroph hyperplasia in some patients who have had documented adenomas, as well as the recurrence of prolactin-secreting pituitary adenoma following successful removal of a microadenoma and an interval of normal prolactin-secretory dynamics.[99, 100]

Hypofunction Syndromes

HYPOTHALAMIC HYPOGONADISM. Kallmann's syndrome (olfactory-genital dysplasia) is the most common form of congenital isolated gonadotropin deficiency, and can occur sporadically or in a familial setting as an X-linked dominant or autosomal dominant trait with incomplete penetrance.[101] The disorder is due to a defect in the KAL gene whose product normally directs the migration of GnRH neurons from the olfactory placode to the hypothalamus. This results in a deficiency or absence of GnRH-secreting neurons in the hypothalamus, as well as agenesis or hypoplasia of the olfactory bulb, the latter defect being responsible for the hyposmia or anosmia seen in this syndrome. Males are affected more commonly than females and often exhibit cryptorchidism and microphallus at birth, reflecting the lack of fetal gonadotropins which stimulate testosterone secretion from the fetal testes. At the time of expected puberty, there is a failure of gonadotropins to rise, of testicular enlargement, or of development of secondary sexual characteristics. Following a single bolus injection of GnRH there is little or no rise in gonadotropins. However, if GnRH is given in a pulsatile fashion every 90 minutes, an increase in luteinizing hormone (LH) and follicle-stimulating hormone (FSH) will occur, reflecting the fact that the gonadotrophes are normal, but understimulated in this syndrome. Indeed, pulsatile GnRH therapy may result in full virilization.[101] Other components of this syndrome include color

blindness, nerve deafness, cleft palate, exostosis, and renal abnormalities.

Isolated LH deficiency with normal FSH production (fertile eunuch syndrome) results in decreased androgenization and poor development of secondary sexual characteristics at puberty. Because of the lack of gonadal steroid-induced epiphyseal closure of the long bones, the affected patients develop eunuchoid proportions. However, they exhibit testicular enlargement and spermatogenesis, reflecting the normal FSH secretion.[101] Congenital gonadotropin deficiency is also seen as a manifestation of panhypopituitarism, which may be on a hypothalamic basis, as well as with several complex hypothalamic disorders, including the Prader-Willi, Bardet-Biedl, and Laurence-Moon syndromes.

Hypogonadism is a relatively common manifestation of hypothalamic tumors and infiltrative disease, especially those that involve the floor of the third ventricle and median eminence. Obesity, diabetes insipidus, and neuro-ophthalmologic abnormalities often accompany the hypogonadism.[9, 10]

GROWTH HORMONE DEFICIENCY. A variety of congenital structural defects involving the hypothalamus, such as anencephaly, holoprosencephaly, encephalocele, and septo-optic dysplasia, may result in growth hormone deficiency either alone or with other anterior pituitary hormone deficiencies.[27] Monotropic growth hormone deficiency may occur sporadically or on a familial basis due to a deficient production or secretion of GHRH. Such patients will demonstrate an increase in growth hormone secretion following multiple injections of GHRH. Growth hormone deficiency also occurs as a manifestation of panhypopituitarism and is the hormone that is most frequently absent in these patients. As in patients with isolated growth hormone deficiency, those with panhypopituitarism generally have a hypothalamic basis for the abnormality with deficiencies of multiple hypothalamic releasing hormones.[102]

At birth, patients with congenital growth hormone deficiency have a normal length and weight, but may exhibit microphallus. During the first year, growth retardation is seen with a delay in both height and bone ages. Hypoglycemia may be found, because of the loss of the glucose contraregulation effect of growth hormone; during childhood there is an increase in subcutaneous fat along with proportional short stature. Even in the presence of normal gonadotrophs, puberty is often delayed in these patients. Treatment with growth hormone increases linear growth, reduces subcutaneous fat and glucose intolerance, and stimulates pubertal progression.[51]

Growth hormone deficiency is generally the earliest endocrine manifestation of a hypothalamic tumor or infiltrative process and results in growth retardation. Even in patients with structural hypothalamic disease who have no clinical evidence of growth retardation, provocative testing reveals a high frequency of inadequate growth hormone secretion.[101, 103]

HYPOTHALAMIC HYPOADRENALISM. Congenital or acquired isolated ACTH deficiency is quite rare. However, ACTH deficiency does occur commonly in association with deficiencies of other anterior pituitary hormones due to craniopharyngiomas, suprasellar germinomas, and septo-optic dysplasia.[29, 73, 74, 101, 103–106] Clinical manifestations include nausea, vomiting, hypotension, and hypoglycemia without the hyperpigmentation and electrolyte abnormalities from aldosterone deficiency seen in primary adrenocortical insufficiency.

HYPOTHALAMIC HYPOTHYROIDISM. Isolated TSH deficiency also is quite rare. However, TSH deficiency is found in approximately a third of the patients with craniopharyngiomas, suprasellar germinomas, and in patients with septo-optic dysplasia.[28, 29, 73, 74, 101, 103, 105] Clinically, the patients may exhibit dry skin, puffiness, pallor, lethargy, bradycardia, hypothermia, and weight gain with evidence of an atrophic thyroid gland. Serum free T_4 levels are low and the serum TSH may be low or slightly elevated, the latter reflecting abnormal glycoslyation of the TSH molecule, which results in decreased biologic activity.[107] Following an injection of TRH, there is a delayed and prolonged rise in TSH in patients with hypothalamic hypothyroidism.[28, 29, 67, 68]

SPECIFIC HYPOTHALAMIC DISORDERS
Prader-Willi Syndrome

Prader-Willi syndrome, first described in 1956, occurs in approximately 1 in 10,000 to 15,000 live births.[108, 109] The major clinical manifestations include infantile hypotonia; feeding problems; failure to thrive; rapid weight gain occurring between ages 1 and 6 years; a characteristic dysmorphic facial appearance with a narrow bitemporal diameter, almond-shaped eyes, palpebral fissues, down-turned mouth; developmental delay and mental retardation; and hypogonadism, which may be present at birth with cryptorchidism, scrotal hypoplasia, and a small penis in males, poor development of the labia minora and clitoris in females, and dalayed onset of puberty associated with low sex steroid hormones, low gonadotropins, and blunting of the gonadotropin response to GnRH. In addition, these patients have short stature, associated with growth hormone deficiency, and behavioral problems that appear during childhood and are characterized by temper tantrums, aggressive behavior, and obsessive-compulsiveness. One of the major characteristics of these patients is marked, indiscriminate hyperphagia and central obesity. These patients will exhibit abnormal food-seeking behavior, often eating discarded or spoiled food or pet food. Sleep disturbances and abnormalities in temperature control and heat generation also suggest a hypothalamic cause, despite the fact that no anatomic abnormalities have been found in this syndrome.[108–111]

Prader-Willi syndrome is a disorder of genetic (genomic) imprinting due to a microdeletion of the paternally contributed chromosome 15q11-q13.[109, 112] Thus, since only the paternal genes are normally expressed in this region, a mutation of the paternal gene results in absence of expression. A minority of patients have maternal uniparental disomy (both members of the chromosome pair inherited from the same parent). An even rarer cause is a translocation involving chromosome 15.[109, 112]

Bardet-Biedl and Related Syndromes

The Bardet-Biedl syndrome represents an autosomal recessive disorder characterized by retinal pigmentary dystrophy (retinitis pigmentosa), mental retardation, central obesity, polydactyly, a variety of renal abnormalities, and hypogonadotropic hypogonadism.[113] The Laurence-Moon syndrome also exhibits retinal pigmentary dystrophy, mental retardation, and hypogonadotropic hypogonadism. These patients also have progressive spastic paraparesis and distal muscle weakness, but do not exhibit polydactyly.[114] The Biemond syndrome is another autosomal recessive condition with mental retardation, polydactyly or brachydactyly, obesity, and hypogonadotropic hypogonadism. Retinal pigmentary dystrophy does not occur in this condition; rather, these patients have iris coloboma. The autosomal recessive Alström-Hallgren syndrome is associated with atypical retinal pigmentary dystrophy, obesity, nerve deafness, diabetes mellitus, and acanthosis nigricans. The affected patients have hypogonadism due to primary gonadal failure rather than hypothalamic dysfunction.[114, 115] The overlapping features of these different syndromes raise the possibility that they are due to a similar genetic abnormality.

Septo-optic Pituitary Dysplasia

The anatomic features of septo-optic pituitary dysplasia, a midline developmental abnormality, are an absence of the septum pellucidum, agenesis of the corpus callosum, unilateral or bilateral hypoplasia of the optic nerves, and absence of the supraoptic and paraventricular nuclei with posterior pituitary hypoplasia.[73, 74, 104, 105, 116–118] The nonendocrine manifestations of this disease include visual abnormalities, mental retardation, nystagmus, seizures, and various forms of cerebral palsy.[73] Approximately two thirds of affected patients have short stature associated with growth hormone deficiency; approximately 40% have ACTH deficiency; 20% TSH, deficiency; and one fourth exhibit gonadotropin deficiency. Close to one fourth of the patients exhibit diabetes insipidus and approximately 20% have hyperprolactinemia.[73, 74, 104, 105, 116–118] This disorder is caused by recessive mutation in the homeobox gene, HESX1.[118a]

Environmental Deprivation Syndrome (Psychosocial Dwarfism)

Environmental deprivation syndrome, a rare syndrome, which has its onset before the age of 2 years, occurs in some children exposed to a disturbed parent-child home environment. The clinical manifestations include short stature with delayed bone age associated with abnormal growth hormone response to provocative tests; low body weight despite an enormous appetite that is associated with gorging, vomiting, and production of foul-smelling stools; polydipsia; bizarre behavior; emotional or mental retardation; and a protuberant abdomen. In addition to the abnormal growth hormone responses, these patients may have an inadequate ACTH response to provocative testing, although thyroid function and urine concentrating ability are normal. The clinical findings are reversible and disappear when the children are placed in a nurturing environment.[119, 120]

Pseudocyesis

An extreme example of a functional hypothalamic disorder is seen in women who develop a conversion reaction in which they think they are pregnant, but, in fact, are not. Amenorrhea, morning nausea, breast enlargement and engorgement, and abdominal distention due to retained colonic gas are present in these women. Hyperprolactinemia is found and some women exhibit galactorrhea.[121, 122] Elevated levels of LH may account for the persistent corpus luteum activity that is seen in this syndrome.[123] When these women are informed of the diagnosis, the clinical manifestations rapidly disappear.

Hypothalamic Hamartoma

These benign hyperplastic malformations contain ganglion cells, myelinated nerve fibers, and glial matrix, and are generally located between the tuber cinereum and mamillary bodies.[70, 124] Most patients exhibit onset of clinical symptoms below the age of 2 years with the major endocrine abnormality being isosexual precocious puberty. Other common manifestations include gelastic seizures, emotional lability, hyperactivity, and neurodevelopmental delay.[69, 71, 81, 124–128] During late childhood or adolescence, many of these patients develop obesity. The precocious puberty in these patients responds to long-acting GnRH agonists that downregulate GnRH receptors. Neurosurgical removal of the hamartomas is generally not recommended unless there are signs of increased intracranial pressure or progressive growth with neurologic deterioration.[81]

The Pallister-Hall syndrome consists of hypothalamic hamartomas, panhypopituitarism, polydactyly, imperforate anus, and multiple craniofacial and limb abnormalities.[129–132] This may occur sporadically or be transmitted as an autosomal dominant trait. An abnormality on chromosome 7 has been identified in some patients affected with the familial syndrome.[133]

Germ Cell Tumors

Approximately 65% of intracranial germ cell tumors are germinomas, most of which occur in the suprasellar region, while 35% are nongerminomatous germ cell tumors, including teratomas, embryonal cell carcinomas, endodermal sinus tumors, and choriocarcinomas, most of which are located in the pineal region.[25, 30]

Patients with suprasellar germ cell tumors generally present in childhood or adolescence with diabetes insipidus, hypopituitarism, and visual field defects due to involvement of the optic chiasm. Headaches, emaciation, growth failure, hypogonadism, and hypernatremia also occur commonly.[28, 29, 134–138]

Patients with nongerminomatous germ cell tumors primarily exhibit neurologic abnormalities, including hydrocephalus, paralysis of upward gaze (Parinaud's sign), obtundation, pyramidal tract signs, and ataxia. Less than 20% develop diabetes insipidus or hypothalamic-pituitary abnormalities in contrast to patients with suprasellar germinomas, of whom 90% and 80% have those manifestations, respectively.[30] Precocious puberty may also be found with suprasellar germ cell tumors and nongerminomatous germ cell tumors.[28–30, 135, 136] Germinomas tend to be radiosensitive and have the best prognosis, while nongerminomatous germ cell tumors are treated with radiation therapy or cisplatin-based chemotherapy or both.[55]

Hypothalamic Glioma

Low-grade gliomas that involve the optic chiasm, optic tract, or hypothalamus present during childhood with visual field abnormalities, hydrocephalus, diabetes insipidus, the diencephalic syndrome of infancy, optic atrophy, and anterior pituitary dysfunction.[139–144] Neurofibromatosis is present in approximately 20% of the patients.[76, 140, 142] Since growth of these tumors tends to be slow and the course is variable, close observation is often warranted. Radiation therapy is indicated for progressive lesions.[139, 141, 144]

Craniopharyngioma

Approximately one half of the tumors involving the pituitary and chiasmatic region in childhood are craniopharyngiomas—benign neoplasms of Rathke's pouch origin. Most of the tumors are located in the suprasellar region, but may occur anywhere between the pharynx and sella turcica. The tumors generally grow slowly and are densely adherent to the surrounding structures.[78] In children the predominant clinical findings are due to increased intracranial pressure and include nausea, vomiting, headache, papilledema, and hydrocephalus, as well as decreased visual acuity, and visual field defects. Somnolence, abnormalities of the sleep-wake cycle, and growth hormone deficiency and diabetes insipidus are also frequently found in these children.[28, 78, 101, 103, 106, 145–150] The childhood tumors tend to have both cystic and solid components and the majority contain calcifications.[78]

Neurologic symptoms are the predominant presenting finding in adults and include visual abnormalities and visual field defects, headache, cognitive deterioration, personality change, obesity, and hypogonadism. Multiple anterior pituitary hormone deficiency is commonly present. Most of these tumors are solid, and fewer than one fourth are calcified in adults.[78, 146, 150]

The optimal treatment of these tumors has been very controversial, with strong advocates for radical surgery, subtotal resection combined with radiation therapy, or radiation therapy alone.[145, 150–152] Radical resection using microsurgical techniques is the procedure most commonly performed on these tumors.

Suprasellar Meningioma

Meningiomas of the planum sphenoidale or tuberculum sellae may compress the hypothalamus. Most patients present with neuro-ophthalmologic abnormalities and headache.[153] Memory impairment, confusion, and decreased cognition, along with hypogonadism, hypothyroidism, and rarely diabetes insipidus, also may be present. Surgical resection is the optimal treatment for these lesions.[153]

Suprasellar Arachnoid Cyst

Suprasellar arachnoid cyst, an uncommon developmental anomaly of the arachnoid membrane, leads to a cerebrospinal fluid (CSF)–filled cyst that obstructs CSF flow through the foramen of Monro, leading to hydrocephalus and increased intracranial pressure. Thus, headache, vomiting, lethargy, and increased head size are commonly found in these patients. The cysts may also compress the brain stem and optic nerve and optic chiasm leading to spasticity, ataxia, tremor, decreased visual acuity, and visual field defects. Endocrine abnormalities include growth hormone and ACTH deficiency, as well as precocious puberty.[154] Surgical decompression or percutaneous ventriculocystostomy are used to drain the cyst and reduce intracranial pressure.[155]

Infiltrative Disorders

Sarcoidosis may involve the basal hypothalamus and floor of the third ventricle and lead to diminished visual acuity, visual field abnor-malities, diabetes insipidus, thermal dysregulation, somnolence, personality changes, obesity, and hypothalamic hypopituitarism. Most patients with hypothalamic sarcoidosis also have involvement outside of the central nervous system.[32, 33, 35, 156–158]

The chronic disseminated form of Langerhans' cell histiocytosis (Hand-Schüller-Christian disease) is classically composed of the triad of membranous bone lesions, exophthalmos, and diabetes insipidus. Growth retardation, hyperprolactinemia, hypogonadism, and hypodipsia or adipsia may also be found in these patients.[31, 159]

Hypothalamic Dysfunction Following Brain Irradiation

Both whole-brain irradiation and localized radiotherapy for brain or head or neck neoplasms are associated with a delayed onset of hypothalamic dysfunction most often manifest by progressive loss of growth hormone secretion and hyperprolactinemia. ACTH and gonadotropin deficiency are also found, as are changes in personality and abnormalities in thirst, sleep-wake cycle, and appetite regulation. Children are more susceptible to hypothalamic damage than adults, and the incidence of hypothalamic abnormality increases with increasing radiation dose and decreasing intervals over which the radiation is administered.[160–162]

REFERENCES

1. Boshes B: Syndromes of the diencephalon. The hypothalamus and the hypophysis. *In* Vinken PJ, Bruyn GW (eds): Localization in Clinical Neurology. Handbook of Clinical Neurology, vol 2. Amsterdam, North-Holland, 1969, pp 432–468.
2. Kirgis HD, Locke W: Anatomy and embryology. *In* Locke W, Schally AV (eds): The Hypothalamus and Pituitary in Health and Disease. Springfield, IL, Charles C Thomas, 1972, pp 3–21.
3. Bruesch SR: Anatomy of the human hypothalamus. *In* Givens JR, Kitabchi AE, Robertson JT (eds): The Hypothalamus. St Louis, Mosby–Year Book, 1984, pp 1–16.
4. Braunstein GD: The Hypothalamus. *In* Melmed S (ed): The Pituitary. Cambridge, MA, Blackwell Scientific, 1994, pp 309–340.
5. Carmel PW: Surgical syndromes of the hypothalamus. Clin Neurosurg 27:133–159, 1980.
6. Plum F, Van Uitert R: Nonendocrine diseases and disorders of the hypothalamus. *In* Reichlin S, Baldessarini RJ, Martin JB (eds): The Hypothalamus. New York, Raven Press, 1978, pp 415–473.
7. Sano K, Mayanagi Y, Sekino H, et al: Results of stimulation and destruction of the posterior hypothalamus in man. J Neurosurg 33:689–707, 1970.
8. Garnica AD, Netzloff ML, Rosenbloom AL: Clinical manifestations of hypothalamic tumors. Ann Clin Lab Sci 10:474–485, 1980.
9. Bauer HG: Endocrine and other clinical manifestations of hypothalamic disease. A survey of 60 cases, with autopsies. J Clin Endocrinol Metab 14:13–31, 1954.
10. Bauer HG: Endocrine and metabolic conditions related to pathology in the hypothalamus: A review. J Nerv Ment Dis 128:323–338, 1959.
11. Dott NM: Surgical aspects of the hypothalamus. *In* Le Gros Clark WE, Beattie J, Riddoch G, Dott NM (eds): The Hypothalamus. Morphological, Functional, Clinical and Surgical Aspects. London, Oliver & Boyd, 1938, pp 131–185.
12. Frohman LA: Clinical aspects of hypothalamic disease. *In* Motta M (ed): The Endocrine Functions of the Brain. New York, Raven Press, 1980, pp 419–446.
13. Riddoch G: Clinical aspects of hypothalamic derangement. *In* Le Gros Clark WE, Beattie J, Riddoch G, Dott NM (eds): The Hypothalamus. Morphological, Functional, Clinical and Surgical Aspects. London, Oliver & Boyd, 1938, pp 101–130.
14. McLean AJ: Autonomic epilepsy. Arch Neurol 32:189–197, 1934.
15. Rothballer AB, Dugger GS: Hypothalamic tumor. Correlation between symptomatology, regional anatomy, and neurosecretion. Neurology 5:160–177, 1955.
16. White LE, Hain RF: Anorexia in association with a destructive lesion of the hypothalamus. Arch Pathol Lab Med 68:275–281, 1959.
17. Reeves AG, Plum F: Hyperphagia, rage, and dementia accompanying a ventromedial hypothalamic neoplasm. Arch Neurol 20:616–624, 1969.
18. Fox RH, Davies TW, Marsh FP, et al: Hypothermia in a young man with an anterior hypothalamic lesion. Lancet 2:185–188, 1970.
19. Lewin K, Mattingly D, Millis RR: Anorexia nervosa associated with hypothalamic tumour. BMJ 2:629–630, 1972.
20. Kamalian N, Keesey RE, Zurhein GM: Lateral hypothalamic demyelination and cachexia in a case of "malignant" multiple sclerosis. Neurology 25:25–30, 1975.
21. Celesia GG, Archer CR, Chung HD: Hyperphagia and obesity: Relationship to medial hypothalamic lesions. JAMA 246:151–153, 1981.
22. Haugh RM, Markesbery WR: Hypothalamic astrocytoma. Syndrome of hyperphagia, obesity, and disturbances of behavior and endocrine and autonomic function. Arch Neurol 40:560–563, 1983.
23. Schwartz WJ, Busis NA, Hedley-Whyte ET: A discrete lesion of ventral hypothalamus and optic chiasm that disturbed the daily temperature rhythm. J Neurol 233:1–4, 1986.
24. Bergeron C, Kovacs K, Ezrin C, et al: Hereditary diabetes insipidus: An immunohistochemical study of the hypothalamus and pituitary gland. Acta Neuropathol 81:345–348, 1991.

25. Scherbaum WA: Autoimmune hypothalamic diabetes insipidus ("autoimmune hypothalamitis"). Prog Brain Res 93:283–293, 1992.

26. McLeod JF, Kouvacs L, Gaskill MB, et al: Familial neurohypophyseal diabetes insipidus associated with a signal peptide mutation. J Clin Endocrinol Metab 77:599A–599G, 1997.

27. Rimon DL, Phillips JA III: Genetic disorders of the pituitary gland. In Rimoin DL, Connor JM, Pyeritz RI (eds): Emery and Rimoin's Principles and Practice of Medical Genetics, ed 3, vol 1. New York, Churchill Livingstone, 1996, pp 1331–1364.

28. Imura H, Kato Y, Nakai Y: Endocrine aspects of tumors arising from suprasellar, third ventricular regions. Prog Exp Tumor Res 30:313–324, 1987.

29. Buchfelder M, Fahlbusch R, Walther M, Mann K: Endocrine disturbances in suprasellar germinomas. Acta Endocrinol 120:337–342, 1989.

30. Jennings MT, Gelman R, Hochberg F: Intracranial germ-cell tumors: Natural history and pathogenesis. J Neurosurg 63:155–167, 1985.

31. Stosel H, Braunstein GD: Endocrine abnormalities associated with Langerhans' cell histiocytosis. Endocrinologist 1:393–397, 1991.

32. Delaney P: Neurologic manifestations in sarcoidosis. Review of the literature, with a report of 23 cases. Ann Intern Med 87:336–345, 1977.

33. Stuart CA, Neelon FA, Lebovitz HE: Hypothalamic insufficiency: The cause of hypopituitarism in sarcoidosis. Ann Intern Med 88:589–594, 1978.

34. Jawadi MH, Hanson TJ, Schemmel JE, et al: Hypothalamic sarcoidosis and hypopituitarism. Horm Res 12:1–9, 1980.

35. Vesely DL, Maldonado A, Levey GS: Partial hypopituitarism and possible hypothalamic involvement in sarcoidosis. Am J Med 62:425–431, 1977.

36. De Rubertis FR, Michelis MF, Davis BB: "Essential" hypernatremia. Report of three cases and review of the literature. Arch Intern Med 134:889–895, 1974.

37. Ball SG, Vaidja B, Baylis PH: Hypothalamic adipsic syndrome: Diagnosis and management. Clin Endocrinol 47:405–409, 1997.

38. Teelucksingh S, Steer CR, Thompson CJ, et al: Hypothalamic syndrome and central sleep apnoea associated with toluene exposure. Q J Med 78:185–190, 1991.

39. Hayek A, Peake GT: Hypothalamic adipsia without demonstrable structural lesion. Pediatrics 70:275–278, 1982.

40. Du Rivage SK, Winter RJ, Brouillette RT, et al: Idiopathic hypothalamic dysfunction and impaired control of breathing. Pediatrics 75:896–898, 1985.

41. Martin JB, Reichlin S: Clinical Neuroendocrinology. Philadelphia, FA Davis, 1987, p 393.

42. Wolff SM, Adler RC, Buskirk ER, et al: A syndrome of periodic hypothalamic discharge. Am J Med 36:956–967, 1964.

43. Guze BH, Baxter LR Jr: Neuroleptic malignant syndrome. N Engl J Med 313:163–166, 1985.

44. Keck PE Jr, Caroff SN, McElroy SL: Neuroleptic malignant syndrome and malignant hyperthermia: End of a controversy? J Neuropsychiatry Clin Neurosci 7:135–144, 1995.

45. Horn E, Lach B, Lapierre Y, et al: Hypothalamic pathology in the neuroleptic malignant syndrome. Am J Psychiatry 145:617–620, 1988.

46. Sandyk R, Iacono RP, Bamford CR: The hypothalamus in Parkinson disease. Ital J Neurol Sci 8:227–234, 1987.

47. Haak HR, van Hilten JJ, Roos RAC, et al: Functional hypothalamic derangement in a case of Wernicke's encephalopathy. Netherlands J Med 36:291–296, 1990.

48. Penfield W: Diencephalic autonomic epilepsy. Arch Neurol Psychiatry 22:358–369, 1929.

49. Fox RH, Wilkins DC, Bell JA, et al: Spontaneous periodic hypothermia: Diencephalic epilepsy. BMJ 2:693–695, 1973.

50. Mooradian AD, Morley GK, McGeachie R, et al: Spontaneous periodic hypothermia. Neurology 34:79–82, 1984.

51. Flynn MD, Sandeman DD, Mawson DM, et al: Cyclical hypothermia: Successful treatment with ephedrine. J R Soc Med 84:752–753, 1991.

52. Shapiro WR, Williams GH, Plum F: Spontaneous recurrent hypothermia accompanying agenesis of the corpus callosum. Brain 92:423–436, 1969.

53. Bannister P, Sheridan P, Penney MD: Chronic reset osmoreceptor response, agenesis of the corpus callosum, and hypothalamic cyst. J Pediatr 104:97–99, 1984.

54. Page SR, Nussey SS, Jenkins JS, et al: Hypothalamic disease in association with dysgenesis of the corpus callosum. Postgrad Med J 65:163–167, 1989.

55. Bray GA, Gallagher TF Jr: Manifestations of hypothalamic obesity in man: A comprehensive investigation of eight patients and a review of the literature. Medicine (Baltimore) 54:301–330, 1975.

56. Russell A: A diencephalic syndrome of emaciation in infancy and childhood. Arch Dis Child 26:274, 1951.

57. Burr IM, Slonim AE, Danish RK, et al: Diencephalic syndrome revisted. J Pediatr 88:439–444, 1976.

58. Bhasin S, Swerdloff RS: Hypothalamic hypogonadism. Special Topics Endocrinol Metab 7:237–266, 1985.

59. Newman MM, Halmi KA: The endocrinology of anorexia nervosa and bulimia nervosa. Neurol Clin 6:195–212, 1988.

60. Mecklenberg RS, Loriaux DL, Thompson RH, et al: Hypothalamic dysfunction in patients with anorexia. Medicine (Baltimore) 53:147–159, 1974.

61. Clark LG: The hypothalamus in man. In Le Gros, Clark WE, Beattie J, Riddoch G, et al (eds): The Hypothalamus. Morphological, Functional, Clinical and Surgical Aspects. London, Oliver & Boyd, 1938, pp 59–68.

62. Carpenter MB, Sutin J: Human Neuroanatomy. Baltimore, Williams & Wilkins, 1983, pp 552–578.

63. Locke W, Schally AV: The Hypothalamus and Pituitary in Health and Disease. Springfield, IL, Charles C Thomas, 1972, pp 427–432.

64. Martin JB, Reichlin S: Clinical Neuroendocrinology. Philadelphia, FA Davis, 1987, p 411.

65. Cohen RA, Albers HE: Disruption of human circadian and cognitive regulation following a discrete hypothalamic lesion: A case study. Neurology 41:726–729, 1991.

66. Fenzi F, Simonati A, Crosato F, et al: Clinical features of Kleine-Levin syndrome with localized encephalitis. Neuropediatrics 24:292–295, 1993.

67. Chesson AL Jr, Levine SN, Kong L-S, et al: Neuroendocrine evaluation in Kleine-Levin syndrome: Evidence of reduced dopaminergic tone during periods of hypersomnolence. Sleep 14:226–232, 1991.

68. Critchley M: Periodic hypersomnia and megaphagia in adolescent males. Brain 85:627–656, 1962.

69. Breningstall GN: Gelastic seizures, precocious puberty, and hypothalamic hamartoma. Neurology 35:1180–1183, 1985.

70. Sharma RR: Hamartoma of the hypothalamus and tuber cinereum: A brief review of the literature. J Postgrad Med 33:1–13, 1987.

71. Takeuchi J, Handa H: Pubertas praecox and hypothalamic hamartoma. Neurosurg Rev 8:225–231, 1985.

72. Shankar RR, Pescovitz OH. Precocious puberty. Adv Endocrinol Metab 6:55–89, 1995.

73. Margalith D, Jan JE, McCormick AQ, et al: Clinical spectrum of congenital optic nerve hypoplasia: Review of 51 patients. Dev Med Child Neurol 26:311–322, 1984.

74. Margalith D, Tze WJ, Jan JE: Congenital optic nerve hypoplasia with hypothalamic-pituitary dysplasia. Am J Dis Child 139:361–366, 1985.

75. Gross RE: Neoplasms producing endocrine disturbances in childhood. Am J Dis Child 59:579–628, 1940.

76. Laue L, Comite F, Hench K, et al: Precocious puberty associated with neurofibromatosis and optic gliomas. Am J Dis Child 139:1097–1100, 1985.

77. Gillett GR, Symon L: Hypothalamic glioma. Surg Neurol 28:291–300, 1987.

78. Banna M: Pathology and clinical manifestations. In Hankinson J, Banna M (eds): Pituitary and Parapituitary Tumours. London, WB Saunders, 1976, pp 13–58.

79. Weinberger LM, Grant FC: Precocious puberty and tumors of the hypothalamus. Arch Intern Med 67:762–792, 1941.

80. Balagura S, Shulman K, Sobel EH: Precocious puberty of cerebral origin. Surg Neurol 11:315–326, 1979.

81. Hochman HI, Judge DM, Reichlin S: Precocious puberty and hypothalamic hamartoma. Pediatrics 67:236–244, 1981.

82. Judge DM, Kulin HE, Page R, et al: Hypothalamic hamartoma: A source of luteinizing hormone–releasing factor in precocious puberty. N Engl J Med 296:7–10, 1977.

83. Losa M, von Werder K: Pathophysiology and clinical aspects of the ectopic GH-releasing hormone syndrome. Clin Endocrinol 47:123–135, 1997.

84. Saeger W, Puchner MJA, Ludecke DK: Combined sellar gangliocytomas and pituitary adenoma in acromegaly or Cushing's disease. Virchows Arch 425:93–99, 1994.

85. Asa SL, Bilbao JM, Kovacks K, et al: Hypothalamic neuronal hamartoma associated with pituitary growth hormone cell adenoma and acromegaly. Acta Neuropathol 52:231–234, 1980.

86. Asa SL, Scheithauer BW, Bilbao JM, et al: A case for hypothalamic acromegaly: A clinicopathological study of six patients with hypothalamic gangliocytomas producing growth hormone releasing factor. J Clin Endocrinol Metab 58:796–803, 1984.

87. Biller BMK. Pathogenesis of pituitary Cushing's syndrome. Pituitary versus hypothalamic. Endocrinol Clin North Am 23:547–554, 1994.

88. Gifford S, Gunderson JG: Cushing's disease as a psychosomatic disorder: A selective review of the clinical and experimental literature and a report of ten cases. Perspect Biol Med 13:169–221, 1970.

89. Bigos ST, Somma M, Rasio E, et al: Cushing's disease: Management by transsphenoidal pituitary microsurgery. J Clin Endocrinol Metab 50:348–354, 1980.

90. Lamberts SW, Stefanko SZ, DeLang SE, et al: Failure of clinical remission after transsphenoidal removal of a microadenoma in a patient with Cushing's disease: Multiple hyperplastic and adenomatous cell nests in surrounding pituitary tissues. J Clin Endocrinol Metab 50:793–795, 1980.

91. Krieger DT, Amorosa L, Linick F: Cyproheptadine-induced remission of Cushing's disease. N Engl J Med 293:893–896, 1975.

92. Lankford HU, Tucker HS, Blackard WG: A cyproheptadine-reversible defect in ACTH control persisting after removal of the pituitary tumor in Cushing's disease. N Engl J Med 305:1244–1248, 1981.

93. Cavagnini F, Invitti C, Polli EE: Sodium valproate in Cushing's disease. Lancet 2:162–163, 1984.

94. Lamberts SWJ, Klijn JG, deQuijada M, et al: The mechanism of the suppressive action of bromocriptine on adrenocorticotropin secretion in patients with Cushing's disease and Nelson's syndrome. J Clin Endocrinol Metab 51:307–311, 1980.

95. Biller BMK, Alexander JM, Zervas NT, et al: Clonal origins of adrenocorticotropin-secreting pituitary tissue in Cushing's disease. J Clin Endocrinol Metab 75:1303–1309, 1992.

96. Faglia G, Spada A: The role of hypothalamus in pituitary neoplasia. Clin Endocrinol 9:225–242, 1995.

97. Asa SL, Kovacs K. Tindall GT, et al: Cushing's disease associated with an intrasellar gangliocytoma producing corticotrophin-releasing factor. Ann Intern Med 101:789–793, 1984.

98. Kapcala LP, Molitch ME, Post KD, et al: Galactorrhea, oligo/amenorrhea, and hyperprolactinemia in patients with craniopharyngiomas. J Clin Endocrinol Metab 51:798–800, 1980.

99. McKeel DW Jr, Fowler M, Jacobs LS: The high prevalence of prolactin cell hyperplasia in the human adenohypophysis. In Proceedings of the Endocrine Society 60th Annual Meeting, Miami Beach, 1978, abstract 353.

100. Feigenbaum SL, Downey DE, Wilson CB, et al: Transsphenoidal pituitary resection for preoperative diagnosis of prolactin-secreting pituitary adenoma in women: Long term follow-up. J Clin Endocrinol Metab 81:1711–1719, 1996.

101. Post KD, McCormick PC, Bello JA: Differential diagnosis of pituitary tumors. Endocrinol Metab Clin North Am 16:609–645, 1987.

102. Borges JLC, Blizzard RM, Gelato MC, et al: Effects of human pancreatic tumour growth hormone releasing factor on growth hormone and somatomedin C levels in patients with idiopathic growth hormone deficiency. Lancet 2:119–124, 1983.

103. Fahlbusch R, Muller OA, Werder KV: Functional endocrinological disturbances in parasellar processes. Acta Neurochir 28(suppl):456–460, 1979.

104. Arslanian SA, Rothfus WE, Foley TP Jr, et al: Hormonal, metabolic, and neuroradio-

logic abnormalities associated with septo-optic dysplasia. Acta Endocrinol 107:282–288, 1984.

105. Izenberg N, Rosenblum M, Parks JS: The endocrine spectrum of septo-optic dysplasia. Clin Pediatr 23:632–636, 1984.

106. Korsgaard O, Lindholm J, Rasmussen P: Endocrine function in patients with suprasellar and hypothalamic tumours. Acta Endocrinol 83:1–8, 1976.

107. Beck-Peccoz P, Amr S, Menezes-Ferreira M, et al: Decreased receptor binding of biologically inactive thyrotropin in central hypothyroidism. N Engl J Med 312:1085–1090, 1985.

108. Bray GA, Dahms WT, Swerdloff RS, et al: The Prader-Willi syndrome: A study of 40 patients and a review of the literature. Medicine (Baltimore) 62:59–80, 1983.

109. Cassidy SB: Prader-Willi syndrome. J Med Genet 34:917–923, 1997.

110. Sapienza C. Hall JG. Genetic imprinting in human disease. *In* Scriver CR, Beaudet AR, Sly WS, Valle D (eds): The Metabolic and Molecular Basis of Inherited Diseases, vol 1. New York, McGraw-Hill, 1995, pp 437–458.

111. Rimoin DL, Schimke RN: Genetic Disorders of the Endocrine Glands, 1. St Louis, Mosby–Year Book; 1971, pp 189–191.

112. Cassidy SB, Schwartz S: Prader-Willi and Angelman syndromes: Disorders of genomic imprinting. Medicine (Baltimore) 77:140–151, 1998.

113. Klein D, Ammann F: The syndrome of Laurence-Moon-Bardet-Biedl and allied diseases in Switzerland. Clinical, genetic and epidemiological studies. J Neurol Sci 9:479–513, 1969.

114. Beales PL, Warner AM, Hitman GA, et al: Bardet-Biedl syndrome: A molecular and phenotypic study of 18 families. J Med Gent 34:922–928, 1997.

115. Edwards JA, Sethi PK, Scoma AJ, et al: A new familial syndrome characterized by pigmentary retinopathy, hypogonadism, mental retardation, nerve deafness and glucose intolerance. Am J Med 60:23–32, 1976.

116. Morishima A, Aranoff GS: Syndrome of septo-optic-pituitary dysplasia: The clinical spectrum. Brain Dev 8:233–239, 1986.

117. Roessmann U, Velasco ME, Small EJ, et al: Neuropathology of "septo-optic dysplasia" (de Morsier syndrome) with immunohistochemical studies of the hypothalamus and pituitary gland. J Neuropathol Exp Neurol 46:597–608, 1987.

118. Yukizane S, Kimura Y, Yamashita Y, et al: Growth hormone deficiency of hypothalamic origin in septo-optic dysplasia. Eur J Pediatr 150:30–33, 1990.

118a. Dattani MT, Martinez-Barbera JP, Thomas PQ, et al: Mutations in the homeobox gene HESX1/Hesx1 associated with septo-optic dysplasia in human and mouse. Nat Genet 19:125–133, 1998.

119. Powell GF, Brasel JA, Blizzard RM: Emotional deprivation and growth retardation simulating idiopathic hypopituitarism. I. Clinical evaluation of the syndrome. N Engl J Med 276:1271–1278, 1967.

120. Powell GF, Brasel JA, Raiti S, Blizzard RM: Emotional deprivation and growth retardation simulating idiopathic hypopituitarism. II. Endocrinologic evaluation of the syndrome. N Engl J Med 276:1279–1283, 1967.

121. Zuber T, Kelly J: Pseudocyesis. Am Fam Physician 30:131–134, 1984.

122. Bray MA, Muneyyirci-Delale A, Kofinas GD, et al: Circadian, ultradian, and episodic gonadotropin and prolactin secretion in human pseudocyesis. Acta Endocrinol 124:501–509, 1991.

123. Yen SSC, Rebar RW, Quesenberry W: Pituitary function in pseudocyesis. J Clin Endocrinol Metab 43:132–136, 1976.

124. List CF, Dowman CE, Bagchi BS, et al: Posterior hypothalamic hamartomas and gangliogliomas causing precocious puberty. Neurology 8:164–174, 1958.

125. Diebler C, Ponsot G: Hamartomas of the tuber cinereum. Neuroradiology 25:93–101, 1983.

126. Comite F, Psescovitz OH, Rieth KG: Luteinizing hormone-releasing hormone analog treatment of boys with hypothalamic hamartoma and true precocious puberty. J Clin Endocrinol Metab 59:888–892, 1984.

127. Sato M, Ushio Y, Arita N, et al: Hypothalamic hamartoma: Report of two cases. Neurosurgery 16:198–206, 1985.

128. Valdueza JM, Cristante L, Dammann O, et al: Hypothalamic hamartomas: With special reference to gelastic epilepsy and surgery. Neurosurgery 34:949–958, 1994.

129. Hall JG, Pallister PD, Clarren SK, et al: Congenital hypothalamic hamartoblastoma, hypopituitarism, imperforate anus, and postaxial polydactyly—a new syndrome? Part I: Clinical, causal, and pathogenetic considerations. Am J Med Genet 7:47–74, 1980.

130. Clarren SK, Alvord EC Jr, Hall JG: Congenital hypothalamic hamartoblastoma, hypopituitarism, imperforate anus, and postaxial polydactyly—a new syndrome? Part II: Neuropathological considerations. Am J Med Genet 7:75–83, 1980.

131. Biesecker LG, Abbott M, Allen J, et al: Report from the workshop on Pallister-Hall syndrome and related phenotypes. Am J Med Genet 65:76–81, 1996.

132. Biesecker LG, Graham JM Jr: Pallister-Hall syndrome. J Med Genet 33:585–589, 1996.

133. Kang S, Allen J, Graham JM Jr, et al: Linkage mapping and phenotypic analysis of autosomal dominant Pallister-Hall syndrome. J Med Genet 34:441–446, 1997.

134. Takeuchi J, Handa H, Nagata I: Suprasellar germinoma. J Neurosurg 49:41–48, 1978.

135. Sklar CA, Grumbach MM, Kaplan SL, et al: Hormonal and metabolic abnormalities associated with central nervous system germinoma in children and adolescents and the effect of therapy: Report of 10 patients. J Clin Endocrinol Metab 52:9–16, 1981.

136. Simson LR, Lampe I, Abell MR: Suprasellar germinomas. Cancer 22:533–544, 1968.

137. Aida T, Abe H, Fujieda K, et al: Endocrine functions in children with suprasellar germinoma. Neurol Med Chir 33:152–157, 1993.

138. Nishio S, Inamura T, Takeshita I, et al: Germ cell tumor in the hypothalamo-neurohypophysial region: Clinical features and treatment. Neurosurg Rev 16:221–227, 1993.

139. Roberson C, Till K: Hypothalamic gliomas in children. J Neurol Neurosurg Psychiatry 37:1047–1052, 1974.

140. Borit A, Richardson EP Jr: The biological and clinical behaviour of pilocytic astrocytomas of the optic pathways. Brain 105:161–187, 1982.

141. Garvey M, Packer RJ: An integrated approach to the treatment of chiasmatic-hypothalamic gliomas. J Neurooncol 28:167–183, 1996.

142. Rush JA, Younge BR, Campbell RJ, et al: Optic glioma. Long-term follow up of 85 histopathologically verified cases. Ophthalmology 89:1213–1219, 1982.

143. Alshail E, Rutka JJ, Becker LE, et al: Optic chiasmatic-hypothalamic glioma. Brain Pathol 7:799–806, 1997.

144. Rodriguez LA, Edwards MSB, Levin VA: Management of hypothalamic gliomas in children: An analysis of 33 cases. Neurosurgery 26:242–277, 1990.

145. Kjellberg RN: Craniopharyngiomas. *In* Tindall GT, Collins WF (eds): Clinical Management of Pituitary Disorders. New York, Raven Press, 1979, pp 373–388.

146. Wen B-C, Hussey DH, Staples J, et al: A comparison of the roles of surgery and radiation therapy in the management of craniopharyngiomas. Int J Radiat Oncol Biol Phys 16:17–24, 1989.

147. Randall RV, Laws ER Jr, Abboud CF: Clinical presentation of craniopharyngiomas. A brief review of 300 cases. *In* Givens JR, Kitabchi AE, Robertson JT (eds): The Hypothalamus. St Louis, Mosby–Year Book, 1984, pp 321–333.

148. Sanford RA, Muhlbauer MS: Craniopharyngioma in children. Neurol Clin 9:453–465, 1991.

149. Sklar CA: Craniopharyngioma: Endocrine abnormalities at presentation. Pediatr Neurosurg 21(suppl 1):18–20, 1994.

150. Yasargil MG, Curcic M, Kis M, et al: Total removal of craniopharyngiomas. Approaches and long-term results in 144 patients. J Neurosurg 73:3–11, 1990.

151. Laws ER Jr, Randall RV, Abboud CR, et al: Craniopharyngioma. The transsphenoidal microsurgical approach. *In* Givens JR, Kitabchi AE, Robertson JT (eds): The Hypothalamus. St Louis, Mosbry–Year Book, 1984, pp 335–347.

152. Samii M, Tatagiba M: Surgical management of craniopharyngiomas: A review. Neurol Med Chir 37:141–149, 1997.

153. Finn JE, Mount LA: Meningiomas of the tuberculum sellae and planum sphenoidale. A review of 83 cases. Arch Ophthalmol 74:23–27, 1974.

154. Pierre-Kahn A, Capelle L, Brauner R, et al: Presentation and management of suprasellar arachnoid cysts. Review of 20 cases. J Neurosurg 73:355–359, 1990.

155. Rappaport ZH: Suprasellar arachnoid cysts: Options in operative management. Acta Neurochir 122:71–75, 1993.

156. Winnacker JL, Becker KL, Katz S: Endocrine aspects of sarcoidosis. N Engl J Med 278:427–434, 1968.

157. Winnacker JL, Becker KL, Katz S: Endocrine aspects of sarcoidosis (concluded). N Engl J Med 278:483–492, 1968.

158. Bell NH: Endocrine complications of sarcoidosis. Endocrinol Metab Clin North Am 20:645–654, 1991.

159. Braunstein GD, Kohler PO: Pituitary function in Hand-Schüller-Christian disease. Evidence for deficient growth-hormone release in patients with short stature. N Engl J Med 286:1225–1229, 1972.

160. Samaaan NA, Schultz PN, Yang K-PP, et al: Endocrine complications after radiotherapy for tumors of the head and neck. J Lab Clin Med 109:364–372, 1987.

161. Littley MD, Shalet SM, Beardwell CG: Radiation and hypothalamic-pituitary function. Baillieres Clin Endocrinol Metab 4:147–175, 1990.

162. Constine LS, Woolf PD, Cann D, et al: Hypothalamic-pituitary dysfunction after radiation for brain tumors. N Engl J Med 328:87–94, 1993.

Chapter 20

▲▲▲▲

Evaluation of Pituitary Masses

Shlomo Melmed

NATURAL HISTORY OF A PITUITARY OR
    PARASELLAR MASS
LOCAL MASS EFFECTS OF AN ENLARGING
    SELLAR MASS

METABOLIC SEQUELAE OF
    HYPOTHALAMIC LESIONS
PARASELLAR MASSES
SECONDARY METASTASES TO THE
    PITUITARY REGION

MISCELLANEOUS PARASELLAR MASSES
APPROACH TO THE PATIENT WITH A
    SELLAR MASS

Both neoplastic and nonneoplastic sellar masses may arise from regions within and adjacent to the hypothalamus and pituitary. They are manifested either as a result of their local pressure effects on surrounding vital structures or as a result of distant metabolic or hormonal derangements. Rarely, sellar masses may be the initial feature of a previously undiagnosed systemic disorder.

This chapter outlines the natural history and local and metabolic sequelae of mass lesions arising in the parasellar region; the characteristics of the specific lesions causing these sequelae are described. Although the functional anatomy of the hypothalamic regions has been well demarcated, the relatively close contiguity of these vital centers results in manifestations of distant metabolic derangements that are not necessarily dependent on the nature or the exact localization of the parasellar mass lesion. In fact, similar hypothalamic "syndromes" may be caused by a large number of different pathologic processes, all of which arise in the general parasellar region.[1–3] Consequently, the natural history and long-term prognosis of a hypothalamic mass are important in managing the specific lesion, whose exact microanatomic localization in and of itself may not necessarily be clinically precise.

NATURAL HISTORY OF A PITUITARY OR PARASELLAR MASS

Before the advent of sensitive pituitary imaging techniques, a wide spectrum of clinical sequelae were evident from the effects of an enlarging mass arising from within the pituitary or its adjacent structures (Table 20–1). Although it is relatively uncommon today for such a mass to be invasive at the time of diagnosis, the relative subtlety of clinical features may delay the anatomic imaging of such a mass.

Most pituitary and hypothalamic masses are benign neoplasms, with the very rare occurrence of a true primary malignancy with proven distant metastases. Nevertheless, these benign lesions may be aggressively invasive locally into contiguous structures and result in clinical features that depend on the anatomic location of the impinging mass. Hemorrhage and infarction, which may often be coincidental, may occur in these masses, especially during pregnancy, when the normal pituitary and its surrounding soft tissue structures are edematous and swollen. Diabetes mellitus and hypertension have also been associated with pituitary infarction. Hemorrhage and infarction of the pituitary and hypothalamus are true endocrine emergencies. Acute pituitary failure may lead to hypoglycemia, hypothermia, hypotension, apoplexy, and death.

Clearly, many pituitary masses undergo silent infarction as evidenced by histologic proof of old infarct tissue in patients with other-wise normal pituitary function. Large infarcts may lead to the development of a partial or totally empty pituitary sella. Most of these patients exhibit normal pituitary reserve, which implies that the surrounding rim of pituitary tissue is fully functional. Large cysts associated with the hypothalamic-pituitary unit will also give the radiologic appearance of an empty sella. Rarely, functional pituitary adenomas may arise within the remnant pituitary tissue, and these tumors, although their presence is indicated by classic endocrine hyperactivity, may not be visible by sensitive magnetic resonance imaging (MRI) (i.e., <2 mm in diameter). Acute or chronic infection with abscess formation may be an extremely rare occurrence in the pituitary or hypothalamic mass. Finally, many of these mass lesions lead to clinically evident hormonal derangements caused by hormone hypersecretion or, more commonly, by failure of pituitary trophic hormone reserve.

Pituitary hormone hyposecretion may be due to the direct pressure effects of the expanding mass on the anterior pituitary hormone-secreting cells. Alternatively, parasellar pressure effects may directly attenuate the synthesis or secretion of hypothalamic hormones, with resultant pituitary failure. In contrast, a not uncommon association of hypothalamic masses is overproduction of a specific hypothalamic hormone with resultant hyperfunctioning of a specific hypothalamic-pituitary-target hormone axis.

The important diagnostic dilemma facing the clinician is to effectively distinguish an adenoma arising from the anterior pituitary gland from other parasellar masses. The compelling reason for this diagnosis is the fact that the management and prognosis of true anterior pituitary neoplasms differ so markedly from those of other nonpituitary masses. Most masses arising from within the sella are benign, hormonally functional or nonfunctional adenomas, with relatively good prognosis after appropriate therapy. Their invasiveness is relatively limited, and only rarely will local vital structures be compromised. In contrast, parasellar masses arising from structures contiguous with the pituitary are often malignant or invasive and usually portend a less favorable prognosis.

MAGNETIC RESONANCE IMAGING. Safe and sensitive pituitary visualization is obtained by high-resolution MRI. The anterior pituitary is isodense with white matter, and the posterior pituitary exhibits a characteristic bright spot caused by neurosecretory phospholipid signals. Microadenomas can be detected by T1-weighted coronal spin echo MRI before and after gadolinium administration in approximately 90% of patients, when the mass does not enhance. Most clinically nonfunctioning pituitary masses are, however, macroadenomas at the time of clinical diagnosis and are readily detectable by imaging. MRI is invaluable in visualizing the optic tracts and evaluating the degree of soft tissue changes caused by the tumor. MRI cannot readily distinguish a pituitary adenoma from other intrasellar masses, unless other characteristic signs (e.g., invasiveness, hemorrhage, suprasellar involvement) are considered. MRI may also be useful in the preoperative differential diagnosis of carotid artery aneurysms.

COMPUTED TOMOGRAPHY. Pituitary computed tomography (CT) offers the advantage of visualizing invasion of bony structures, including the sellar floor and clinoid bones. CT can also detect small calcifications characteristic of craniopharyngiomas, meningiomas, chordomas, and rarely aneurysms that would otherwise remain undiagnosed by MRI.

TABLE 20–1. Complications of a Pituitary or Parasellar Mass

Local invasion	Empty sella
Malignant transformation	Infection (abscess)
Hemorrhage	Hormonal derangement
Infarction	

TABLE 20–2. Local Neurologic Effects of an Impinging Pituitary or Hypothalamic Mass

Impacted Structure	Clinical Effect
Optic tract	Loss of red perception, bitemporal hemianopia, superior or bitemporal field defect, scotoma, blindness
Hypothalamus	Temperature dysregulation, appetite disorders, obesity, thirst disorders, diabetes insipidus, sleep disorders, behavioral dysfunction, autonomic nervous system dysfunction
Cavernous sinus	Ptosis, diplopia, ophthalmoplegia, facial numbness
Temporal lobe	Uncinate seizures
Frontal lobe	Personality disorder, anosmia
Central	Headache, hydrocephalus, psychosis, dementia, laughing seizures

SOMATOSTATIN RECEPTOR SCINTIGRAPHY. The radiolabeled somatostatin analogue ^{111}In-pentetreotide may be used for in vivo imaging of pituitary tumors expressing somatostatin receptors. Although growth hormone cell adenomas are the most abundant expressors of SRIF (somatostatin release–inhibiting factor) receptors, all other pituitary tumor types also express the SRIF receptor to a varying degree. Single-photon emission CT detects lesions approximately 1 cm in diameter. SRIF receptors that bind to the labeled analogue with high affinity have also been demonstrated in some nonfunctioning pituitary tumors, and variable positive scan imaging of nonfunctioning tumors has been reported. Scintigraphy has been proposed as an imaging technique to predict the response of these tumors to octreotide therapy, but this approach has proved disappointing.[3]

DOPAMINE RECEPTOR SCINTIGRAPHY. Prolactinomas may be imaged with a labeled D_2 receptor antagonist via ^{123}I-iodobenzamine single-photon emission CT. Nonfunctioning pituitary tumors have not been successfully identified with this imaging technique despite the fact that they possess membrane-bound dopamine receptors. This failure to image nonfunctioning tumors is probably due to the lower density of dopamine receptors found in these tumors in comparison to prolactinomas.[4]

LOCAL MASS EFFECTS OF AN ENLARGING SELLAR MASS

The anatomic location of the pituitary sella results in several possible local functional derangements caused by a mass in the midline region of the base of the brain (Table 20–2). The intrasellar mass may invade either soft tissue or bony surrounding structures. Because of its anatomic location, the dorsal roof of the sella presents the least resistance to expansion from within the confines of the bony sella. Nevertheless, both suprasellar and parasellar invasion inexorably occurs with an enlarging mass, with resultant clinical manifestations.

GENERAL EFFECTS. Headaches are common features of intrasellar tumors, even without demonstrable suprasellar extension. Because of the confined nature of the pituitary gland within the sella, small changes in intrasellar pressure presumably caused by a microadenoma are sufficient to increase pressure and stretching of the dural plate with resultant headache. Complaints of headache do not appear to correlate with the size of the adenoma or the presence of suprasellar extension.[5] In fact, relatively minor distortions of the sellar diaphragm or dural impingement are accompanied by persistent headache. Furthermore, medical management of small functional pituitary tumors with bromocriptine or octreotide is often accompanied by a remarkable disappearance of headache.

OPTIC TRACT. Pressure on the optic chiasm as a result of upward compression may result in visual defects ranging from small field defects to blindness.[5] The advent and refinement of sensitive pituitary imaging techniques during the past decade have resulted in earlier diagnosis of parasellar masses than previously feasible. Therefore, the incidence of optic tract compression by a large mass is certainly diminishing. Nevertheless, through 1972, 40% of 1000 patients with pituitary tumors had either bitemporal hemianopia or superior bitemporal defects.[5] One-third of patients had evidence of blindness, scotomas, or other visual disturbances.[6]

Reproducible assessment of visual fields with perimetry techniques should be performed on all patients with an intrapituitary or extrapituitary mass lesion. Loss of red perception appears to be an early sign of optic tract pressure, and red-colored visual signals should preferably be used.[6] Anterior frontal mass lesions may cause unilateral visual loss, whereas chiasmic or posterior pressure by the mass will usually result in bilateral defects. Classically, elevation and distortion of the optic chiasm result in bitemporal hemianopia, whereas dorsal chiasmic compression also results in field cuts. Homonymous hemianopia may result from tumor or vascular pressure on the regions of the optic tract lying anterior to the chiasm. Transient visual disorders, asymmetric deficits, or enlargement of the blind spot may all indicate the presence of a parasellar mass. If the mass causes an internal hydrocephalus by obstructing the flow of cerebrospinal fluid (CSF), secondary visual disturbances and papilledema may ensue.

Pituitary Stalk. Compression of the stalk by an expanding intrasellar or parasellar mass may result in pituitary failure caused by encroachment of the portal vessels that normally provide pituitary access to the hypothalamic hormones. Stalk compression usually leads to hyperprolactinemia and failure of the other pituitary trophic hormones.

CAVERNOUS SINUS. Lateral invasion of pituitary lesions or ventrolateral encroachment by parasellar or hypothalamic masses may impinge on the cavernous sinus and its neural contents. This invasion may lead to lesions of the third, fourth, and sixth cranial nerves, as well as the ophthalmic and maxillary branches of the fifth cranial nerve. Varying degrees of diplopia, ptosis, ophthalmoplegia, and decreased facial sensation occur, depending on the extent of neural involvement by the cavernous sinus mass.

SPHENOID SINUS. Dorsal extension into the sphenoid sinus implies that the parasellar mass has already eroded the bony sellar floor.

Although no vital structures are located in the sinus, aggressive tumors may invade the roof of the palate and cause severe nasopharyngeal obstruction, infection, and even CSF leakage.

BRAIN. Both the temporal and frontal brain lobes may be invaded by the expanding parasellar mass. Uncinate seizures, personality disorders, and anosmia may result from localized tumor involvement.

METABOLIC SEQUELAE OF HYPOTHALAMIC LESIONS

In addition to the anatomic lesions caused by the expanding mass just described, direct hypothalamic involvement of the encroaching mass may lead to important nonendocrine sequelae[7, 8] (Table 20–3). Clinical features associated with hypothalamic masses depend to a large extent on the site of the lesion rather than the nature of the pathologic process. The enlarging hypothalamic mass, regardless of its etiology, will usually result in local pressure effects, including headaches and recurrent vomiting with or without associated extrapyrami-

TABLE 20–3. Metabolic Sequelae of Hypothalamic Mass Lesions

Temperature dysregulation	Sleep disorders
Hyperthermia	Reversal of sleep-wake cycle
Hypothermia	Akinetic mutism
Appetite disorders	Somnolence and coma
Obesity	Behavioral dysfunction
Hyperphagia	Hyperkinesis
Anorexia and emaciation	Rage
Aphagia	Autonomic dysfunction
Thirst disorders	Cardiac arrhythmias
Adipsia	Loss of sphincter control
Compulsive drinking	Cardiac failure
Hypernatremia	

Adapted from Martin JB, Reichlin S: Clinical Neuroendocrinology. Copyright © 1987 by Oxford University Press, Inc. Used by permission of Oxford University Press, Inc.

dal or pyramidal tract involvement. Common metabolic clinical sequelae, which occur in about one-third of these patients, include precocious puberty or hypogonadism, diabetes insipidus, sleep disturbances, dysthermia, and appetite disorders (see Table 20–3). Because of the very close microanatomic contiguity of several highly specialized hypothalamic cells, precise site-function effects of an expanding mass are rarely documented. Most patients therefore exhibit a spectrum of metabolic sequelae that occur regardless of the etiology or site of the pathologic process.

Temperature dysregulation, appetite and thirst disorders, sleep disorders, and behavioral and autonomic dysfunction[9–16] caused by hypothalamic lesions are more fully considered in Chapter 19.

PARASELLAR MASSES

A list of pituitary and nonpituitary masses is contained in Table 20–4.

RATHKE'S CYST. During early embryogenesis, the anterior and intermediate lobes of the pituitary gland arise from Rathke's pouch. If the pouch fails to obliterate, cystic remnants remain at the interface between the anterior and posterior pituitary lobes. These small cysts (<5 mm) are found in about 20% of pituitary glands at autopsy.[17] Occasionally, a pituitary adenoma may also contain small cleft cysts.[18] Imaging of these cysts on MRI reveals hyperdense or hypodense masses on either T1- or T2-weighted images. CT scanning reveals the presence of homogeneous hypodense areas that may allow differentiation from pituitary adenomas.[19] Other sellar cysts include arachnoid, epidermoid, and dermoid cysts. Although these lesions develop mainly in the cerebellopontine angle, they may also occur in the suprasellar region. Clinical features of compression include internal hydrocephalus, visual disturbances, and rarely growth hormone or adrenocorticotropic hormone (ACTH) deficiency, hyperprolactinemia, and diabetes insipidus.[20–23] Rarely, a squamous cell carcinoma may develop in the cyst.[24]

GRANULAR CELL TUMORS. Pituitary choristomas, or schwannomas, usually occur only after the age of 20 and are probably acquired lesions.[25, 26] Their abundant cytoplasmic granules do not contain any of the known pituitary hormones, nor are these tumors associated with endocrine syndromes. However, several pituitary adenomas have been coincidentally associated with these tumors.

TABLE 20–4. Pituitary and Nonpituitary Sellar Masses

Cysts
  Rathke's
  Arachnoid
  Epidermoid
  Dermoid
Tumors
  Hormone-secreting or nonfunctional pituitary adenoma
  Granular cell tumor
  Craniopharyngioma
  Chordoma
  Meningioma
  Sarcomas
  Glioma
  Schwannoma
  Germ cell tumor
  Vascular tumor
  Solid or hematologic metastases
Malformation and hamartomas
  Ectopic pituitary, neurohypophysial, or salivary tissue
  Hypothalamic hamartoma
  Gangliocytoma
Miscellaneous lesions
  Aneurysms
  Lymphocytic hypophysitis
  Infections
  Sarcoidosis
  Giant cell granuloma
  Langerhans' histiocytosis

CHORDOMAS. These midline tumors arise from remnants of the notochord, are slowly growing and locally invasive, and may metastasize.[27, 28] Most arise from the vertebrae, but about one-third involve the clivus region. Characteristically, they contain a mucin-rich matrix that allows for histologic diagnosis by fine-needle aspiration. On imaging, the tissue mass is associated with osteolytic bony erosion and calcification. MRI may allow the normal pituitary gland to be visualized distinct from the very heterogeneous and often flocculent tumor mass. Nasopharyngeal obstruction may rarely occur, in addition to the more commonly encountered headaches and asymmetric visual disturbances. At surgery, these tumors appear rough and have a heterogeneous lobular appearance. Histologically, they exhibit markers for epithelial cells, including cytokeratin and vimentin. After surgical excision, local invasion and recurrence commonly occur, with mean patient survival of about 5 years. Rarely, chordomas become sarcomatous, with an aggressive natural history.

CRANIOPHARYNGIOMAS. These common parasellar tumors constitute about 3% of all intracranial tumors and up to 10% of childhood brain tumors.[12] Although the tumor may occur at any age, it is commonly diagnosed during childhood and adolescence. The mass may arise from embryonic squamous remnants of Rathke's pouch extending dorsally toward the diencephalon. These tumors may be large (>10 cm in diameter) and invade the third ventricle and associated brain structures. About two-thirds arise from within the sella, whereas the remaining tumors arise from cell rests situated in the parasellar region.[29] The cystic mass is usually filled with cholesterol-rich viscous fluid, and calcification may be present. Histologic analysis shows these tumors to consist of two cell populations: lining the cyst is squamous epithelium containing islands characterized by columnar cells; a mixed inflammatory reaction may also occur with calcification. Although craniopharyngiomas may be quite large and obstruct CSF flow, they rarely undergo malignant transformation.[30] Interestingly, cyst fluid contains immunoreactive human chorionic gonadotropin, which may actually leak into the CSF.[31] Features of increased intracranial pressure, including headache, projectile vomiting, papilledema, and somnolence, are usually encountered in children. Only about one-third of patients are older than 40 years, and they commonly have asymmetric visual disturbances, including papilledema, optic atrophy, and field deficits. Other cranial nerves may also be involved, especially those situated within the cavernous sinus.

On CT imaging, most children and about half of all adults have a characteristic flocculent or convex calcification pattern of the tumor. Rarely, however, pituitary adenomas, other parasellar tumors, and even vascular sellar lesions are also calcified.

The endocrine manifestations of craniopharyngioma usually result from partial or complete pituitary deficiency. Growth hormone deficiency, with resultant short stature and diabetes insipidus, and gonadal failure are common. Compression of the pituitary stalk or damage to the dopaminergic neurons in the hypothalamus results in hyperprolactinemia. This latter feature is especially important in the differential diagnosis of prolactinoma. Management of these common latter adenomas differs markedly from that of a craniopharyngioma, and careful imaging techniques may not easily distinguish the two lesions.[32] Certainly, a highly asymmetric mass (especially with preferential posterior or dorsal extension) that does not shrink after bromocriptine therapy should arouse suspicion of craniopharyngioma. The hyperprolactinemia associated with a craniopharyngioma will also respond quite effectively to bromocriptine. This favorable biochemical response to the dopamine agonist therefore does not rule out the presence of a craniopharyngioma. Thus craniopharyngioma may mimic a prolactinoma in terms of intrapituitary imaging, presence of hyperprolactinemia, and biochemical response to bromocriptine.

Treatment of these lesions consists of radical surgery, radiotherapy, or a combination of these modalities.[33, 34] In selected centers, stereotactic irradiation of the mass has been performed with some success. Nevertheless, regardless of which form of therapy is chosen, ablation of the mass invariably results in anterior and/or posterior pituitary hormone deficits. Postoperative recurrence may occur in about a fifth of patients who undergo radical surgical excision,[35] whereas no appreciable difference is noted in the outcome of those who undergo subtotal surgical excision followed by radiotherapy. The presence of pure papillary squamous cellular elements may portend a higher surgical recurrence rate.[36] The long-term effects of childhood irradiation for these tumors are considered elsewhere (Chapter 21).

MENINGIOMAS. Meningiomas account for about one-quarter of all intracranial tumors.[37] These tumors arise from arachnoid and meningoendothelial cells, and those occurring in the sellar and parasellar region account for about one-fifth of all meningiomas.[38] They are usually well circumscribed and do not achieve the size of craniopharyngiomas. Suprasellar meningiomas may invade the pituitary ventrally, whereas an intrasellar tumor origin is extremely rare. Several patients with functional pituitary adenomas have also been described who harbored coincidental parasellar meningiomas.[39] These tumors are not hormonally active, although secondary hyperprolactinemia has been reported in up to 50% of patients. They usually cause local mass effects, including headache and progressive visual disturbances accompanied by optic atrophy. Diagnosis by imaging is difficult because the differential radiologic diagnosis of a suprasellar meningioma with ventral extension from a pituitary adenoma with dorsal extension may be difficult. Improved MRI techniques have been used in attempts to distinguish the borders of meningiomas from adenomas, but the radiologic diagnosis remains difficult.[40] Typically, meningiomas are isodense on both T1- and T2-weighted imaging, in contrast to other parasellar lesions, which are usually hyperdense on T2-weighted imaging. Dural calcification may occasionally be discerned on CT scanning. Because of their rich vascularization, these tumors pose an increased intraoperative risk that results in a higher surgical mortality rate than usually encountered for pituitary tumor resection.[41]

GLIOMAS. Optic gliomas and low-grade astrocytomas may cause optic atrophy, papilledema, visual loss, and pituitary failure in children; in adults they may be more aggressively invasive. Most of these tumors actually arise from within the optic chiasm or optic tracts, and fewer than one-third are intraorbital.[42, 43] Von Recklinghausen's disease is present in about one-third of all patients with these tumors. Occasionally, these tumors may actually accompany growth retardation and delayed or precocious puberty,[44] and some may be malignant.[45] Mass effects include visual field disturbances, diencephalic syndrome, diabetes insipidus, and hydrocephalus.[46] Gliomas arising within the pituitary sella are exceedingly rare but, if present, may be associated with hyperprolactinemia and should be considered an uncommon mimicker of a prolactin-secreting pituitary adenoma. Important distinguishing features include the young age of these patients (80% <10 years old), relatively intact pituitary function, gross visual disturbances, and imaging localization of the mass. The tumor usually involves the optic chiasm, and optic nerve infiltration is also characteristic. Gliomas usually enhance after contrast injection, unlike hamartomas, which remain isodense.

HYPOTHALAMIC MASSES. Hypothalamic hamartomas are benign tumors composed of a mixture of neurons, astrocytes, and oligodendrocytes. These cell types are organized in varying degrees of differentiation, and they may express peptides released from the hypothalamus. Most commonly these tumors occur before the age of 2 years and have been shown to express gonadotropin-releasing hormone (GnRH) with associated precocious puberty.[47] In tumors in which GnRH immunoreactivity could not be demonstrated, hypothalamic dysfunction was postulated as causing the precocious puberty because injection of GnRH results in a pubertal gonadotropin response.[48] Most of these patients have psychomotor delay and seizures. Curiously, these tumors may also be associated with laughing seizures, emotional lability, and rage.[49–53] The Pallister-Hall syndrome consists of hypothalamic hamartoblastoma; abnormalities of the craniofacial area, heart, kidneys, and lungs; imperforate anus; and hypopituitarism.[53] Although surgical excision was usually advocated for hamartomas, long-acting GnRH analogues have been effectively used to downregulate gonadotropin secretion and control precocious puberty. Hypothalamic hamartomas are slowly growing tumors and rarely invasive. In contrast, gangliocytomas arising in the hypothalamic or intrasellar area do grow progressively. These tumors may be associated with pituitary tumors, and ganglion cells present with the pituitary adenoma may stain positively for hormones released from the hypothalamus. Although MRI distinction may be difficult,[54] when these tumors occur in association with concurrent pituitary adenomas, it has been tempting to speculate that the hypothalamic hormone expressed by the tumor is implicated in the pathogenesis of the pituitary adenoma.

In fact, besides GnRH, these tumors have been shown to express growth hormone–releasing hormone[55–61] and corticotropin-releasing hormone[62, 63] and to be associated with acromegaly and Cushing's syndrome, respectively.

Suprasellar germ cell tumors may be histologically indistinguishable from germinomas, teratomas, embryonal carcinomas, and choriocarcinomas.[64–68] Some of these tumors express immunoreactive β-human chorionic gonadotropin, human placental lactogen, or other placental peptides. These tumors may be manifested by precocious puberty in addition to diabetes insipidus and visual field abnormalities. Thirst disorders, with associated hypernatremia, emaciation, or even obesity, may also occur. Suppressed growth hormone secretion with growth delay is found in over 95% of these patients. After biopsy diagnosis, high-dose radiotherapy has proved to be very effective therapy, with about a 70% long-term survival rate.

Hypothalamic astrocytomas (gliomas), often arising in the anterior hypothalamus and associated with hypophagia of infancy, are rare tumors that may be malignant.

SECONDARY METASTASES TO THE PITUITARY REGION

Pituitary metastases occur quite commonly and are found in up to 3.5% of cancer patients (Table 20–5). The posterior pituitary is the preferred site for bloodborne metastatic spread. This preference may be explained by the vascular supply to the posterior pituitary; blood flows into it directly from the systemic circulation via the internal carotid arteries. The predominant blood supply to the anterior pituitary, in contrast, is by way of the hypothalamic portal system. Common primary carcinomas that metastasize to the pituitary include those of the lung, gastrointestinal tract, and breast. Up to one-quarter of patients with metastatic breast cancer have pituitary metastases. Interestingly, symptomatic pituitary metastases may be the initial sign of previously undiscovered malignancy and even of malignancy of unknown origin. Although anterior pituitary failure is rare, an isolated metastatic deposit in the pituitary stalk without involvement of the anterior lobe may also be seen as pituitary failure (Table 20–6). Metastases to the posterior pituitary lobe are far more common. About 15% of patients with diabetes insipidus harbor metastases from extrapituitary sources. Unfortunately, imaging of the pituitary mass does not distinguish these deposits from a pituitary adenoma unless extensive bony erosion is present. In fact, metastatic pituitary lesions may masquerade as a pituitary adenoma. In several instances the diagnosis of pituitary me-

TABLE 20–5. Neoplastic Source of Pituitary Metastases in 238 Patients*

Primary Neoplasm	Percentage of Patients
Breast	47
Lung	19
Gastrointestinal tract	6
Prostate	6
Leukemia	3
Pancreas	3
Unknown origin	2
Nasopharynx	<2
Melanoma	<2
Thyroid	<2
Plasmacytoma	<2
Endometrium	<1
Renal	<1
Ovary	<1
Liver	<1
Penis	<1

*Included are data from Post et al.,[69] Duchen,[70] Palladino and Andrioli,[71] Max et al.,[72] and Juneau et al.[73]

TABLE 20–6. Initial Clinical Findings in Patients with Pituitary Metastases

Disorder	Percentage
Diabetes insipidus	70
Visual disturbances	20
Cranial nerve palsy	15
Anterior pituitary failure	15

tastasis will be made only by histologic study of a specimen removed at transsphenoidal surgery.

MISCELLANEOUS PARASELLAR MASSES

Acute lymphoblastic leukemia may be associated with periglandular pituitary infiltrates with minimal pituitary dysfunction. Rarely, the syndrome of inappropriate antidiuretic hormone secretion has been reported in this condition. Primary lymphoma may also involve the hypothalamus and pituitary stalk, and these patients may have resultant hypopituitarism. Isolated patients with solitary pituitary plasmacytomas in whom classic multiple myeloma does not develop have been reported, as have patients with primary lymphomas.[74] Rarely, Langerhans' histiocytosis (histiocytosis X) lesions may be confined to the hypothalamic-pituitary axis. These patients usually have diabetes insipidus and occasionally hyperprolactinemia caused by destruction of the hypothalamic portal tract.

HISTIOCYTOSIS X. Histiocytosis X lesions are composed of eosinophilic proliferative infiltrates that may be local or generalized. Although the form of the disorder may depend on the location of the granulomatous infiltrate, most patients will exhibit disordered hypothalamic pituitary function, including diabetes insipidus and growth disorders. Exophthalmos and focally lytic bone lesions are also characteristic. On MRI, the suprasellar mass may be associated with signs of pituitary stalk and posterior pituitary involvement.

LYMPHOCYTIC HYPOPHYSITIS. Although more extensively described in Chapter 21, lymphocytic hypophysitis is an important cause of a sellar mass. This diffuse inflammatory process occurs predominantly in postpartum women and is characterized by a pituitary mass, pituitary failure, hyperprolactinemia, headache, and visual disturbances.[75] The natural history of the disorder is benign, with most intrasellar processes resolving with time. On MRI, the mass enhances after contrast injection, often rendering it indistinguishable from an adenoma.[76] Pituitary failure should be treated, and some patients demonstrate mass resolution after steroid therapy.[77]

MUCOCELE. Expanding accumulations of fluid in the sphenoid sinus may result in the formation of a mucocele, which may grow and compress parasellar structures. Severe headaches, visual disturbances (usually unilateral), and exophthalmos are characteristic features.[78] On MRI, the homogeneous sphenoid mass may be quite prominent, but occasionally it can be distinguished from the pituitary gland dorsally.

ANEURYSM. Aneurysms arising from within or adjacent to the parasellar vasculature may mimic a pituitary adenoma. Preoperative or intraoperative rupture is a potentially catastrophic complication, thus underscoring the absolute need for early diagnosis. The differentiating features from other pituitary masses may be subtle, including eye pain, very intense headaches, and relatively sudden onset of cranial nerve palsies. Although CT and MRI techniques can distinguish blood and hemorrhage from solid tumor or tissue, a highly vascular meningioma may be confused with an aneurysm.[79]

OTHER MASSES. Other rare parasellar masses include granulomas, sarcoidosis, and tuberculosis. Although evidence for systemic tuberculosis is usually present, isolated *sellar tuberculoma* may be encountered,[80, 81] as may isolated sarcoid lesions. Infiltrative *sarcoidosis* of the hypothalamic-pituitary unit occurs in most patients with central nervous system sarcoid involvement.[82] Typically, these patients have varying degrees of anterior pituitary failure with or without diabetes insipidus.

ABSCESS. Primary pituitary abscesses[83] may arise in immunocompromised subjects and may be caused by fungi (*Aspergillus, Nocardia,* or *Candida albicans*) or *Pneumocystis carinii*.

Usually these conditions are manifested as diabetes insipidus, with or without anterior pituitary dysfunction, and hyperprolactinemia. Gonadal dysfunction may be an early peripheral endocrine sign in adults with these sellar masses.

APPROACH TO THE PATIENT WITH A SELLAR MASS

The clinical approach to a patient harboring a pituitary mass is compounded by the observation that the incidence of incidental silent pituitary microadenomas discovered at autopsy is between 10% and 20%. Pituitary cysts, hemorrhage, and infarctions are also not uncommonly discovered at autopsy. With the widespread sensitive imaging techniques, asymptomatic pituitary lesions are being identified with increasing frequency.[84] Pituitary abnormalities compatible with the diagnosis of pituitary microadenoma are detectable in about 10% of the normal adult population. In view of the differential diagnosis of the intrasellar mass discussed above and in recognition of the fact that most lesions observed represent pituitary adenomas, several issues should be considered in the management of these masses. Of particular concern is whether the mass is hormonally functional and whether local mass effects are apparent at the time of diagnosis or develop in the future.[84]

Evaluation of pituitary mass function is important because the onset of symptoms and signs related to disordered hormone secretion is often insidious and may remain unnoticed for years. Clinical evaluation for changes compatible with ACTH, growth hormone, or prolactin hypersecretion or hyposecretion may reveal long-term serious systematic complications, and each may require distinct therapeutic approaches.[85] In the absence of clinical features of a humoral hypersecretory syndrome, recommendations for cost-effective laboratory screening are debatable. The incidence of hormone-secreting tumors in asymptomatic subjects with incidental pituitary masses is low, and low-grade asymptomatic hormone hypersecretion (e.g., for prolactin or α subunits) carries questionable long-term risk.

In the absence of evidence of hormone oversecretion, the presence of or the potential for local compressive effects must be considered. The risk for macroadenoma enlargement to a compressive macroadenoma is low, so a decision to operate may be confidently postponed. For hypothalamic or parasellar masses of uncertain origin, histologic tissue examination may be the only direct approach to yield an accurate diagnosis. Although distinguishing MRI or CT features may be helpful in the differential diagnosis of a nonpituitary sellar mass, the final diagnosis usually remains elusive until pathologic confirmation is obtained. The benefits of pituitary surgery must also be weighed carefully against the potential side effects,[86] although endoscopic approaches may now facilitate safer access to sellar tissue for histologic diagnosis or resection.[87] If surgery is not indicated, subsequent imaging studies can determine the lesion's slow growth rate, if any. In the absence of tumor growth, the interval between scans may be prolonged, and surgery should not be recommended in these asymptomatic cases. When an incidentally asymptomatic macroadenoma is diagnosed, visual field and pituitary function should be comprehensively evaluated. If the findings are normal, imaging follow-up should be conducted, with the awareness that evidence of progressive enlargement or impingement of vital structures will indicate a need for surgical intervention.

REFERENCES

1. Lechan RM: Neuroendocrinology of pituitary hormone regulation. Endocrinol Metab Clin 16:475–501, 1987.
2. Garnica AD, Netzloff NIL, Rosenbloom AL: Clinical manifestations of hypothalamic tumors. Ann Clin Lab Sci 10:474–485, 1980.

3. Maroldo TV, Dillon WP, Wilson CB: Advances in diagnostic techniques of pituitary tumors and prolactinomas. Oncology 4:105–115, 1992.
4. de Herder WW, Reijst AEM, Kwekkeboom DJ, et al: In vivo imaging of pituitary tumours using a radiolabelled dopamine D2 receptor radioligand. Clin Endocrinol 45:755–767, 1996.
5. Hollenhorst RW, Younge BR: Ocular manifestations produced by adenomas of the pituitary gland: Analysis of 1000 cases. *In* Kohler PO, Ross GT (eds): Diagnosis and Treatment of Pituitary Tumors. Amsterdam, Excerpta Medica, 1973, pp 53–64.
6. Melan 0: Neuro-ophthalmologic features of pituitary tumors. Endocrinol Metab Clin North Am 16:585–608, 1987.
7. Marques PR, Illner P, Williams DD: Hypothalamic control of endocrine thermogenesis. Am J Physiol 241:E420, 1981.
8. Bauer HG: Endocrine and other clinical manifestations of hypothalamic disease. J Clin Endocrinol Metab 14:13–31, 1954.
9. Mooradian AD, Morley GK, McGeachie R, et al: Spontaneous periodic hypothermia. Neurology 34:79–82, 1984.
10. Newman MM, Halmi KA: The endocrinology of anorexia nervosa and bulimia nervosa. Neurol Clin 6:195–212, 1988.
11. Bray GA, Gallagher TJ Jr: Manifestations of hypothalamic obesity in man: A comprehensive investigation of eight patients and a review of the literature. Medicine (Baltimore) 54:301–330, 1975.
12. Burr IM, Slonim AE, Danish RK, et al: Diencephalic syndrome revisited. J Pediatr 88:439–444, 1976.
13. Scherbaum WA, Wass KAJ, Besser GM, et al: Autoimmune cranial diabetes insipidus: Its association with other endocrine diseases and with histiocytosis X. Clin Endocrinol 25:411–420, 1986.
14. DeRubertis FR, Michelis ME, Davis BB: "Essential" hypernatremia. Report of three cases and review of the literature. Arch Intern Med 134:889–895, 1974.
15. Hayek A, Peake GT: Hypothalamic adipsia without demonstrable structural lesion. Pediatrics 70:275–278, 1982.
16. Imura H, Kato Y, Nakai Y: Endocrine aspects of tumors arising from suprasellar, third ventricular regions. Prog Exp Tumor Res 30:313–324, 1987.
17. El-Mahdy W, Powell M: Transsphenoidal management of 28 symptomatic Rathke's cleft cysts, with special reference to visual and hormonal recovery. Neurosurgery 42:7–17, 1998.
18. Nishio S, Mizuno J, Barrow DL, et al: Pituitary tumors composed of adenohypophysial adenoma and Rathke's cleft cyst elements: A clinicopathological study. Neurosurgery 21:371–377, 1987.
19. Mukherjee JJ, Islam N, Kaltsas G, et al: Clinical, radiological and pathological features of patients with Rathke's cleft cysts: Tumors that may recur. J Clin Endocrinol Metab 82:2357, 1997.
20. Baskin DS, Wilson CB: Transsphenoidal treatment of non-neoplastic intrasellar cysts. Report of 38 cases. J Neurosurg 60:8–13, 1984.
21. Yamakawa K, Shitara N, Genka S, et al: Clinical course and surgical prognosis of 33 cases of intracranial epidermoid tumors. Neurosurgery 24:568–573, 1989.
22. Lewis AJ, Cooper PW, Kassel EE, Schwartz ML: Squamous cell carcinoma arising in a suprasellar epidermoid cyst. Case report. J Neurosurg 59:538–541, 1983.
23. Voelker JL, Campbell RL, Muller J: Clinical radiographic and pathological features of symptomatic Rathke's cleft cysts. J Neurosurg 74:535, 1991.
24. Schlachter LB, Tindall GT, Pearl GS: Granular cell tumor of the pituitary gland associated with diabetes insipidus. Neurosurgery 6:418–421, 1980.
25. Morrison JG, Gray GF, Dao AH, Adkins RB: Granular cell tumors. Am Surg 53:156–160, 1987.
26. Perzin KH, Pushparaj N: Nonepithelial tumors of the nasal cavity, paranasal sinuses, and nasopharynx. A clinicopathological study. XIV: Chordomas. Cancer 57:784–796, 1986.
27. Meyer JE, Oot RF, Lindfors KK: CT appearance of clival chordomas. J Comput Assist Tomogr 10:34–36, 1986.
28. Volpe R, Mazabraud A: A clinicopathologic review of 25 cases of chordoma (a pleomorphic and metastasizing neoplasm). Am J Surg Pathol 7:161–170, 1983.
29. Ogilvy-Stuart AL, Shalet SM: Tumour of the endocrine glands in children. Endocr Relat Cancer 1:27–41, 1994.
30. Petito CK, DeGirolami U, Earle KM: Craniopharyngiomas: A clinical and pathological review. Cancer 37:1944–1952, 1976.
31. Harris PE, Perry L, Chard T, et al: Immunoreactive human chorionic gonadotrophin from the cyst fluid and CSF of patients with craniopharyngioma. Clin Endocrinol 29:503–508, 1988.
32. Pigeau I, Sigal R, Halimi P, et al: MRI features of craniopharyngiomas at 1.5 tesla. J Neuroradiol 15:276–287, 1988.
33. Yasargil MG, Curcic M, Kis M, et al: Total removal of craniopharyngiomas. Approaches and long term-results in 144 patients. J Neurosurg 73:3–11, 1990.
34. Wen BC, Hussey DH, Staples J, et al: A comparison of the roles of surgery and radiation therapy in the management of craniopharyngiomas. Int J Radiat Oncol Biol Phys 16:17–24, 1989.
35. Adamson TE, Wiestler OD, Kleihues P, Yasargil MG: Correlation of clinical and pathological features in surgically treated craniopharyngiomas. J Neurosurg 73:12–17, 1990.
36. Honegger J, Buchfelder M, Fahlbusch R: Surgical treatment of craniopharyngiomas: Endocrinological results. J Neurosurg 90:251–257, 1999.
37. Rohringer M, Sutherland GR, Louw DE, Sima AAF: Incidence and clinicopathological features of meningioma. J Neurosurg 71:665–672, 1989.
38. Grisoli F, Vincentelli F, Raybaud C, et al: Intrasellar meningioma. Surg Neurol 20:36–41, 1983.
39. Yamada K, Hatayama T, Ohta M, et al: Coincidental pituitary adenoma and parasellar meningioma: Case report. Neurosurgery 19:267–270, 1986.
40. Michael AS, Paige ML: MR imaging of intrasellar meningiomas simulating pituitary adenomas. J Comput Assist Tomogr 12:944–946, 1988.
41. Andrews BT, Wilson CB: Suprasellar meningiomas: The effect of tumor location on postoperative visual outcome. J Neurosurg 69:523–528, 1988.
42. Alvord EC, Lofton S: Gliomas of the optic nerve or chiasm. Outcome by patient's age, tumor site, and treatment. J Neurosurg 68:85–98, 1988.
43. Rush JA, Younge BR, Campbell RJ, MacCarty CS: Optic glioma. Long term followup of 85 histopathologically verified cases. Ophthalmology 89:1213–1219, 1982.
44. Flickinger JC, Torres C, Deutsch M: Management of low-grade gliomas of optic nerve and chiasm. Cancer 61:635–642, 1988.
45. Rudd A, Rees JE, Kennedy P, et al: Malignant optic nerve gliomas in adults. J Clin Neuroophthalmol 5:238–243, 1985.
46. Albers GW, Hoyt WF, Forno LS, Shratter LA: Treatment response in malignant optic glioma of adulthood. Neurology 38:1071–1074, 1988.
47. Judge DM, Kulin HE, Page R, et al: Hypothalamic hamartoma. A source of luteinizing-hormone releasing factor in precocious puberty. N Engl J Med 296:7–10, 1977.
48. Hirsch-Pescovitz 0, Comite F, Hench K, et al: The NIH experience with precocious puberty: Diagnostic subgroups and response to short term luteinizing hormone releasing hormone analogue therapy. J Pediatr 108:47–54, 1986.
49. Curatolo P, Cismai R, Fitiocchi G, Boscherini B: Gelactic epilepsy and true precocious puberty, due to hypothalamic hamartoma. Dev Med Child Neurol 26:509–514, 1984.
50. Nishio S, Fujiwara S, Aiko N, et al: Hypothalamic hamartoma. Report of two cases. J Neurosurg 70:640–645, 1989.
51. Berkovic SF, Andermanii F, Melanson D, et al: Hypothalamic hamartomas and ictal laughter: Evolution of a characteristic epileptic syndrome and diagnostic value of magnetic resonance imaging. Ann Neurol 23:429–239, 1989.
52. Breningstall GN: Gelactic seizures, precocious puberty and hypothalamic hamartoma. Neurology 35:1180–1183, 1985.
53. Iafolla K, Fratkin JD, Spiegel PK, et al: Case report and delineation of the congenital hypothalamic hamartoblastoma syndrome (Pallister-Hall syndrome). Am J Med Genet 33:489–499, 1989.
54. Hubbard AM, Egelhoff JC: MR imaging of large hypothalamic hamartomas in two infants. Am J Neuroradiol 10:1277, 1989.
55. Bevan JS, Asa SL, Rossi ML, et al: Intrasellar gangliocytoma containing gastrin and growth hormone–releasing hormone associated with a growth hormone–secreting pituitary adenoma. Clin Endocrinol 30:213–224, 1989.
56. Markin RS, Leibrock LG, Huseman CA, McComb RD: Hypothalamic hamartoma: A report of two cases. Pediatr Neurosci 13:19–26, 1987.
57. Asa SL, Scheithauer BW, Bilbao JM, et al: A case for hypothalamic acromegaly: A clinicopathological study of six patients with hypothalamic gangliocytomas producing growth hormone–releasing factor. J Clin Endocrinol Metab 58:796–803, 1984.
58. Kamel OM, Horoupian DS, Silverberg GD: Mixed gangliocytoma-adenoma: A distinct neuroendocrine tumor of the pituitary fossa. Hum Pathol 20:1198–1203, 1989.
59. Li JY, Racadot O, Kujas M, et al: Immunocytochemistry of four mixed pituitary adenomas and intrasellar gangliocytomas associated with different clinical syndromes: Acromegaly, amenorrhea-galactorrhea, Cushing's disease and isolated tumoral syndrome. Acta Neuropathol 77:320–328, 1989.
60. Yamada S, Stefaneanu I, Kovacs K, et al: Intrasellar gangliocytoma with multiple immunoreactivities. Endocr Pathol 1:58–63, 1990.
61. Freda PU, Wardlaw SL, Post KD: Unusual causes of sellar/parasellar masses in a large transsphenoidal surgery series. J Clin Endocrinol Metab 81:3455–3459, 1996.
62. Pelletier G, Desy L, Cote J, et al: Light microscope immunohistochemical localization of growth hormone–releasing factor (GRF) in the human hypothalamus. Cell Tissue Res 245:461–464, 1986.
63. Asa SL, Kovacs K, Tindall GT, et al: Cushing's disease associated with an intrasellar gangliocytoma producing corticotrophin-releasing factor. Ann Intern Med 101:789–793, 1984.
64. Jennings MT, Gelman R, Hochberg F: Intracranial germ cell tumors: Natural history and pathogenesis. J Neurosurg 63:155–167, 1985.
65. Marsden HB, Birch IM, Swindell R: Germ cell tumours of childhood: A review of 137 cases. J Clin Pathol 34:879–883, 1981.
66. Furukawa F, Haebara H, Hamashima Y: Primary intracranial choriocarcinoma arising from the pituitary fossa. Report of an autopsy case with literature review. Acta Pathol 36:773–781, 1986.
67. Poon W, Ng HK, Wong K, South JR: Primary intrasellar germinoma presenting with cavernous sinus syndrome. Surg Neurol 30:402–405, 1988.
68. Kageyama N, Kobayashi T, Kida Y, et al: Intracranial germinal tumors. Prog Exp Tumor Res 30:255–2267, 1987.
69. Post KD, McCormick PC, Kandji AD, Hays AP: Metastatic carcinoma to pituitary adenoma: Report of two cases. Surg Neurol 30:286–292, 1988.
70. Duchen LW: Metastatic carcinoma in the pituitary gland and hypothalamus. J Pathol Bacteriol 91:247–355, 1966.
71. Palladino AR, Andrioli GC: Pituitary metastases as presenting lesions of malignancy. J Neurosurg Sci 36:51–54, 1992.
72. Max MB, Deck MDF, Rottenberg DA: Pituitary metastasis: Incidence in cancer patients and clinical differentiation from pituitary adenoma. Neurology 31:998–1002, 1981.
73. Juneau P, Schoene WC, Black P: Malignant tumors in the pituitary gland. Arch Neurol 49:555–558, 1992.
74. Gottfredsson M, Oury TD, Bernstein C, et al: Lymphoma of the pituitary gland: An unusual presentation of central nervous system lymphoma in AIDS. Am J Med 5:563–564, 1996.
75. Honeggar J, Fahlbusch R, Bonnerman A, et al: Lymphocytic and granulomatous hypophysitis: Nine new cases. Neurosurgery 40:713, 1997.
76. Ahmadi J, Meyers GS, Segall HD: Lymphocytic adenohypophysitis: Contrast-enhanced MR imaging in five cases. Radiology 195:30, 1995.
77. Thodou E, Asa SL, Kontogeorgos G, et al: Clinical case seminar: Lymphocytic hypophysitis. Clinicopathological findings. J Clin Endocrinol Metab 80:2302, 1995.
78. Lanzieri CF, Shah M, Krauss D, et al: Use of gadolinium-enhanced MR imaging for differentiating mucoceles from neoplasms in the paranasal sinuses. Radiology 178:425, 1991.

79. Kayath MJ, Lengyel AMJ, Nogueira R, et al: Giant aneurysms of the sellar region simulating pituitary adenomas: A diagnosis to be considered. J Endocrinol Invest 14:975–979, 1991.

80. Ashkan K, Papadopoulos MC, Casey AT, et al: Sellar tuberculoma: Report of two cases. Acta Neurochir 139:523, 1997.

81. Taylor SL, Barakos JA, Harsh GR, et al: Magnetic resonance imaging of tuberculum sellae meningiomas: Preventing preoperative misdiagnosis as pituitary macroadenoma. Neurosurgery 31:621, 1992.

82. Cannavo S, Romano C, Buffa R, Faglia G: Granulomatous sarcoidotic lesion of hypothalamic-pituitary region associated with Rathke's cleft cyst. J Endocrinol Invest 20:77–81, 1997.

83. Jain KC, Varma A, Mahapatra AK: Pituitary abscess: A series of six cases. Br J Neurosurg Psychiatry 41:972, 1978.

84. Greenman Y, Melmed S: Diagnosis and management of nonfunctioning pituitary tumors. Annu Rev Med 47:95–106, 1996.

85. Shimon I, Melmed S: Management of pituitary tumors. Ann Intern Med 129:472–483, 1998.

86. Ciric I, Ragin A, Baumgartner C, Pierce D: Complications of transsphenoidal surgery: Results of a national survey, review of the literature, and personal experience. Neurosurgery 40:225–237, 1997.

87. Jho HD, Carrau RL: Endoscopic endonasal transsphenoidal surgery: Experience with 50 patients. J Neurosurg 87:44–51, 1997.

Chapter 21

Hypopituitarism

Catherine Ann Lissett ▪ Stephen Michael Shalet

Hypopituitarism is the deficiency of one or more pituitary hormones. It is relatively rare, with an incidence in adulthood of eight to ten new cases per million.[1, 2] It is, however, seen commonly in endocrine practice and, importantly, is associated with increased morbidity and mortality. Clinical manifestations are influenced by the etiology, severity, and rate of onset of pituitary hormone deficiency.

MORTALITY IN HYPOPITUITARISM

There is now overwhelming evidence to support the view that hypopituitary patients have an excess mortality compared with the normal population. The first study to demonstrate this was from Göteborg, Sweden.[1] Of 333 subjects diagnosed between 1956 and 1987 as having partial or complete hypopituitarism, 104 died during follow-up, representing a 1.8-fold higher mortality than the normal population. Patients with acromegaly and Cushing's disease were excluded, as these patients are known to have higher mortality. The principle cause of the twofold increase in mortality in both men and women was vascular disease. Deaths from malignancy were lower than expected in men but not in women. Neither the type nor degree of pituitary insufficiency influenced the excess mortality.

Two other studies, one from the United Kingdom[2] and the other from Lund, Sweden,[3] confirmed that hypopituitary patients have excess mortality ranging from 1.75- to 2.2-fold greater than the normal population. Again, vascular disease was responsible for the majority of excess deaths, although this figure was not statistically significant in the U.K. cohort. The epidemiologic studies are supported by the work of Markussis et al.[4] and Lehmann et al.[5] who demonstrated that even symptom-free adults with hypopituitarism show an increased prevalence of atherosclerosis and reduced aortic distensibility.

Many believe that growth hormone (GH) deficiency is likely to be responsible for this excess vascular mortality. The adverse changes in body composition, lipid profile, and insulin sensitivity associated with severe GH deficiency may predispose to the development of atherosclerosis. The severity of GH deficiency is known to increase if two or three additional pituitary hormone deficits are present. However, mortality does not increase with additional pituitary hormone deficits, which by definition implies that increasing severity of GH deficiency does not influence mortality risk. This paradoxical observation casts some doubt on the etiologic role of GH deficiency, and definitive evidence is awaited. Other potential causative factors include long-standing under- or oversubstitution of other pituitary hormones.

CAUSES

The causes of hypopituitarism are varied (Table 21–1). In adulthood, however, the most common cause is a pituitary adenoma or treatment with pituitary surgery or radiotherapy.

Pituitary and Hypothalamic Mass Lesions

Pituitary adenomas account for the vast majority of pituitary mass lesions, although secondary tumors do occur, with metastasis to the pituitary gland reported from carcinomas of the breast, lung, colon, and prostate. Pituitary microadenomas are surprisingly common, being found in between 1.5% and 27% of patients at autopsy[6]; these tumors are very rarely, if at all, associated with hypopituitarism. Macroadenomas are less common, but are more frequently associated with pituitary hormone deficiencies; some 30% of patients with pituitary macroadenomas have one or more anterior pituitary hormone deficiencies. Evidence suggests the causative mechanism of hypopituitarism in these patients is compression of the portal vessels in the pituitary stalk, either secondary to the expanding tumor mass directly or to raised intrasellar pressure.[7, 8]

Craniopharyngiomas are the third most common intracranial tumor and account for the majority of parapituitary tumors. They are thought to arise from Rathke's pouch and may be cystic or solid, commonly showing calcification. Fifty percent occur in children less than 15 years old. Patients commonly present with GH deficiency and diabetes insipidus, with or without a visual field defect.

Derangement of central endocrine regulation also occurs with other parapituitary space-occupying lesions such as chondromas, chordomas, suprasellar meningiomas, astrocytomas of the optic nerve, and primary tumors of the third ventricle.

Pituitary Surgery

Hypopituitarism is a common consequence of pituitary surgery. The incidence and degree of hypopituitarism depend on a number of

TABLE 21–1. Causes of Hypopituitarism

Pituitary and parapituitary tumors
Radiotherapy
Surgery
Trauma, including perinatal
Infarction, including apoplexy and Sheehan's syndrome
Infiltration, including sarcoidosis, Langerhans' cell histiocytosis,
   hemochromatosis
Lymphocytic hypophysitis
Infection, including tuberculosis
Genetic/embryologic disorders
Idiopathic

factors, including the size of the original tumor, the degree of infiltration, and the experience of the surgeon. Prompt postoperative assessment of pituitary function should be performed and the patient warned of a possible deterioration of pituitary function postoperatively. However, a decline in pituitary function postoperatively is not universal. Paradoxically, surgery for nonfunctioning pituitary adenomas may be associated with a significant recovery of pituitary function. Arafah[9] reported endocrine recovery in 57%, 38%, 32%, and 15% of patients with preoperative thyroid-stimulating hormone (TSH), adrenocorticotropic hormone (ACTH), gonadotropin, and GH deficiency, respectively. Prognostic indicators for recovery were smaller tumors and less severe hypopituitarism before the operation. The pituitary hormone least likely to recover was GH; this may reflect the fact that severe GH deficiency was more common preoperatively than other pituitary hormones. There is evidence that in those patients in whom recovery of pituitary function occurs, the process begins immediately after surgery.[7]

Radiotherapy

Deficiency of one or more anterior pituitary hormones may follow treatment with external radiation when the hypothalamic-pituitary axis lies within the fields of radiation. Hypopituitarism has been described in patients who received radiation therapy for nasopharyngeal carcinoma, tumors of the pituitary gland or nearby structures, and primary brain tumors, as well as in children who underwent prophylactic cranial irradiation for acute lymphoblastic leukemia or total body irradiation (TBI) for a variety of tumors and other diseases.[10]

The radiobiologic impact of an irradiation schedule is dependent on the total dose, number of fractions, and duration. The same total dose given in fewer fractions over a shorter time period is likely to cause a greater incidence of pituitary hormone deficiency than if the schedule is spread over a longer time interval with a greater number of fractions.

The degree of pituitary hormonal deficit is related to the radiation dose received by the hypothalamic-pituitary axis. Thus, after lower radiation doses, isolated GH deficiency ensues, while higher doses may produce panhypopituitarism (Fig. 21–1) Radiation dose also determines the speed of onset of hormonal deficiency. The greater the

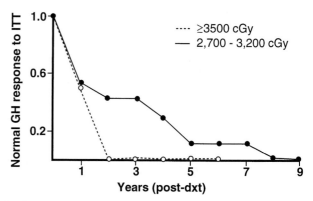

FIGURE 21–2. The incidence of growth hormone (GH) deficiency in children receiving 27 to 32 Gy or 35 Gy of cranial irradiation for a brain tumor in relation to time from irradiation (dxt). This illustrates that the speed at which individual pituitary hormone deficits develop is dose-dependent; the higher the radiation dose, the earlier GH deficiency occurs. (Courtesy of the Department of Medical Illustrations, Wilkington Hospital, Manchester, England.)

radiation dose, the earlier GH deficiency will occur after treatment, so that between 2 and 5 years after irradiation 100% of children receiving more than 30 Gy (over 3 weeks) to the hypothalamic-pituitary axis showed subnormal GH responses to an insulin tolerance test (ITT) while 35% of those receiving less than 30 Gy (over 3 weeks) still showed a normal GH response[11] (Fig. 21–2).

Another factor affecting the impact of irradiation of the hypothalamic-pituitary axis is age. In the human, investigations of GH secretion after cranial irradiation support the experimental animal data, which show the central nervous system (CNS) of young animals to be more radiosensitive than that of older animals.

Paradoxically, while high doses of cranial irradiation may render a child gonadotropin-deficient, lesser doses of irradiation may be associated with early puberty. The mechanism for early puberty after irradiation is likely to be related to disinhibition of cortical influences on the hypothalamus.

With increased longevity of survival, follow-up evaluation of patients irradiated for tumors of the brain and surrounding structures will need to focus less on the possibility of tumor recurrence and more on the delayed effects of therapy, including the endocrine effects.

Genetic Causes

Genetic or familial causes of hypopituitarism are rare, but over recent years, study of these conditions and their diverse pathophysiologic mechanisms has increased our understanding of anterior pituitary gland development and gene regulation in normal and disease states.

Isolated Growth Hormone Deficiency

Two broad types of genetic defect have been identified which cause isolated GH deficiency. These are mutations of the GH gene and of the growth hormone–releasing hormone (GHRH) receptor gene. The human GH (hGH) gene is located on chromosome 17 in a cluster of five genes: hGH-N encodes the gene for pituitary GH, hGH-V encodes the gene for placental GH and three genes for human chorionic somatotropin (hCS). Children with gene mutations or deletions of hGH-N present with severe short stature and, in males, microgenitalia. They have the characteristic phenotypic features of GH deficiency. Four mendelian disorders have been identified to date: two with autosomal recessive inheritance and an autosomal dominant, as well as an X-linked form.[12]

The gene encoding the GHRH receptor (GHRH-R) is expressed in pituitary somatotroph cells and belongs to a family of G protein–coupled receptors. A mutation in this gene has been identified in a number of kindreds which results in a severely truncated receptor lacking the seven membrane spanning domains.[13]

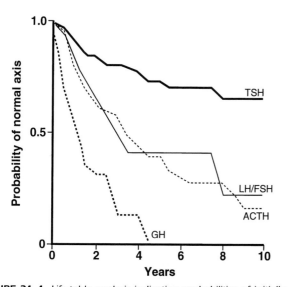

FIGURE 21–1. Life-table analysis indicating probabilities of initially normal hypothalamic-pituitary-target gland axes remaining normal after radiotherapy (3750 to 4250 cGy). Growth hormone (GH) secretion is the most sensitive of the anterior pituitary hormones to the effects of external radiotherapy, and thyroid-stimulating hormone (TSH) secretion is the most resistant. In two thirds of patients, gonadotropin deficiency develops before adrenocorticotropic hormone (ACTH) deficiency. The reverse occurs in the remaining third. LH, luteinizing hormone; FSH, follicle-stimulating hormone. (From Littley MD, Shalet SM, Beardwell CG, et al: Hypopituitarism following external radiotherapy for pituitary tumors in adults. QJM 70:145–160, 1989.)

Gonadotropin-Releasing Hormone Deficiency

Isolated gonadotropin-releasing hormone (GnRH) deficiency is a genetic defect characterized by a functional deficit in hypothalamic GnRH production or secretion. Patients with accompanying anosmia or hyposmia are referred to as having Kallmann's syndrome, whereas those without other associated abnormalities are described as having idiopathic hypogonadotropic hypogonadism (IHH). The hypogonadotropic state results from deficient hypothalamic secretion of GnRH and may be explained by a defect in the migration of GnRH neurons from their origin in the olfactory placode to the hypothalamus, whereas anosmia is due to agenesis of the olfactory bulbs. Whether IHH and Kallmann's syndrome represent a spectrum of manifestations of GnRH deficiency remains controversial. X-linked (*Kal* 1 gene), autosomal recessive, and autosomal dominant patterns of inheritance have been described.[14]

ACTH and TSH Deficiencies

Isolated deficiencies of TSH or ACTH are very rare; however, in a number of cases a genetic abnormality has been described or proposed. Mutations of the coding region of the TSH-β subunit gene resulting in TSH deficiency have been identified in a number of different families.[15] While a genetic basis for ACTH deficiency has not yet been elucidated, kindred studies suggest that abnormalities of the corticotropin-releasing hormone (CRH) gene may result in this rare phenomenon.[16]

Transcription Factor Defects (Table 21–2)

PIT-1. Pit-1, also termed growth hormone factor-1 (GHF-1) and POU1F1, is a pituitary-specific transcription factor responsible for pituitary development and hormone expression in mammals. It is a member of the POU family of transcription factors, which play a fundamental role in mammalian development. POU is an acronym for Pit-1; Oct-1, which is widely expressed; Oct-2, which is expressed in B lymphocytes and in certain areas of the brain; and Unc-86, which functions in *Caenorhabditis elegans* neuronal cell development.[17] Pit-1 (pituitary-specific transcription factor-1) contains two protein domains, termed *POU-specific* and *POU-homeo*, which are both necessary for high-affinity DNA binding of the GH and prolactin genes. Pit-1 is also important for hormonal regulation of the prolactin and thyrotropin-β subunit genes by thyrotropin-releasing hormone (TRH) and cyclic adenosine monophosphate (cAMP). Mutations of the Pit-1 gene have been found in dwarf mice strains (Snell mouse) displaying hypoplasia of GH, prolactin, and TSH-secreting cells of the anterior pituitary, demonstrating the importance of Pit-1 for the development of certain anterior pituitary cells. Humans with Pit-1 deficiency resemble Snell mice in that they lack GH and prolactin, have variable degrees of TSH deficiency, and often exhibit pituitary hypoplasia. Several of the human mutations, like the mouse *Trp261Cys* mutation, result in complete loss of DNA binding and transcriptional activation function. Others retain some DNA-binding properties but do not activate transcription. The dominant mutation altering arginine to tryptophan at codon 271, which accounts for over 50% of reported cases, owes its dominance to enhanced promoter binding affinity and hence a dominant negative effect.[17] At a clinical level Pit-1 abnormalities account for only a small minority of the total number of cases of hypopituitarism worldwide.

Pit-1 gene mutations have also been discovered in patients with idiopathic GH deficiency associated with preserved basal prolactin and TSH secretion.[18] This illustrates the variability of phenotypic presentation among these patients.

PROP1. A further, more recent discovery is a novel pituitary paired-like homeodomain factor which seems to be an important prerequisite of the expression of Pit-1. This has been named Prophet of Pit-1 (PROP1).[19] Individuals with a mutation of the PROP1 gene, which results in a product with reduced DNA-binding and transcriptional activation activity, are deficient in gonadotropin, GH, TSH, and prolactin.[20] They may also have pituitary hyperplasia followed by degeneration and the late appearance of partial ACTH deficiency. One or two base-pair deletions in codon 50 and 100 of the PROP1 gene are proving to be very common.[21] They account for the majority of cases of familial hypopituitarism in several reported series. There are as yet no examples of dominantly inherited mutations in the PROP1 gene. Molecular diagnosis of PROP1 gene abnormalities during early childhood will be of great assistance in developing strategies for comprehensive management as early as possible.

HESX1. HESX1 is a member of the paired-like class of homeobox genes and is first expressed during mouse embryogenesis in a small patch of cells in the anterior midline visceral ectoderm, which are destined to give rise to the ventral prosencephalon. Mice lacking HESX1 have variable anterior CNS defects and pituitary dysplasia. A comparable and equally variable phenotype in humans is septo-optic dysplasia (SOD) which is associated with hypopituitarism.[22] Dattani et al.[22] have now cloned the human HESX1 gene and demonstrated mutations in affected individuals. There is some interaction between HESX1 and PROP1, which may be the mechanism through which abnormalities of the HESX1 gene produce hypopituitarism. These data provide further insight into the pathophysiology of human development and potential causes of hypopituitarism.

Other Causes

Post-traumatic dysfunction of the hypothalamic-pituitary axis is uncommon, but well described. In particular, the pituitary stalk may be severed in deceleration injuries, leading to diabetes insipidus. Isolated pituitary hormone deficiencies, particularly GH (1 in 3000 to 6000 live births)[23, 24] or gonadotropin deficiency, have also been attributed to trauma, including perinatal trauma.

Pituitary apoplexy is the abrupt destruction of pituitary tissue resulting from infarction or hemorrhage into the pituitary, usually into an underlying pituitary tumor. Severe headache accompanies a variable degree of visual loss or cranial nerve palsies. The consequent pituitary hormone deficiencies may develop rapidly. In Sheehan's syndrome pituitary infarction occurs secondary to severe postpartum hemorrhage and ensuing circulatory failure. Once common, this complication is now mainly confined to areas where obstetric services are less well developed.

Granulomatous diseases, including sarcoidosis, tuberculosis, and Langerhans' cell histiocytosis, can affect the hypothalamic-pituitary axis and cause hypopituitarism, including diabetes insipidus. Diabetes insipidus complicates sarcoidosis rarely (1%). It is more common, however, in Langerhans' cell histiocytosis, with 15% of childhood cases developing diabetes insipidus, but it may also occur in patients presenting in adulthood. Lymphocytic hypophysitis, an immune-medi-

TABLE 21–2. Transcription Factor Defects Associated with Multiple Pituitary Hormone Deficits

Transcription Factor	Pituitary Hormone Deficiencies	Pituitary Size	Inheritance
Pit-1	GH, PRL, TSH	Normal or small	Dominant and recessive
PROP1	GH, PRL, TSH, LH, FSH (sometimes ACTH occurs later)	Normal or hyperplastic	Recessive
HESX1	Variable (GH, TSH, ACTH, FSH, LH, ADH) in association with midline brain abnormalities and optic nerve hypoplasia	Hypoplastic	Sporadic and autosomal recessive

GH, growth hormone; PRL, prolactin; TSH, thyroid-stimulating hormone; FSH, follicle-stimulating hormone; ACTH, adrenocorticotropic hormone; LH, luteinizing hormone; ADH, antidiuretic hormone.

ated diffuse infiltration of the anterior pituitary with lymphocytes and plasma cells, occurs predominantly in women and is often first evident in pregnancy or after delivery. The classic presentation is peripartum hypopituitarism, often with a pituitary mass and visual failure. Secondary adrenal failure is an almost universal feature which, when undiagnosed, has proved fatal. At an early stage the pituitary gland is enlarged and cannot be distinguished from a pituitary tumor by computed tomography (CT) or magnetic resonance imaging (MRI), while in the latter stages the gland may atrophy, leaving an empty sella. Lymphocytic hypophysitis is more common in patients with another autoimmune endocrine disease. Cytosolic autoantigens against the pituitary can be demonstrated in some cases, but are also present in patients whose hypopituitarism is secondary to other causes, and in normal patients, and thus the definitive diagnosis of this condition remains difficult without pituitary biopsy.[25] Spontaneous resolution of both the mass and the hypopituitarism have been reported and, in some cases, neurosurgical intervention has led to irreversible pituitary failure. Therefore, conservative management is appropriate in the majority of patients. Lastly, iron overload states, that is, hemochromatosis and patients with β-thalassemia receiving frequent blood transfusions, are associated with pituitary hyposecretion secondary to siderosis and a reduction of pituitary cell number. The gonadotrophs are particularly vulnerable to this mode of damage; however, as affected patients live longer owing to improved medical care, other pituitary hormone deficits, including deficits of GH and ACTH, are becoming more common.

CLINICAL FEATURES

The clinical features of hypopituitarism are affected principally by the degree, type, and speed of onset of the pituitary hormone deficiency. Local pressure effects or hormonal hypersecretion can, however, complicate the clinical picture.

In many forms of hypopituitarism, for example, secondary to a pituitary adenoma and following irradiation, a characteristic evolution of pituitary failure is apparent. Secretion of GH fails first, followed by luteinizing hormone (LH), follicle-stimulating hormone (FSH), and finally by failure of ACTH and TSH secretion. Prolactin deficiency is rare except as a component of Sheehan's syndrome. Hyperprolactinemia is much more common, either secondary to interference with the secretion or delivery of dopamine to the pituitary, releasing the normal lactotrophs from tonic inhibition, or because of hypersecretion from a prolactinoma. Diabetes insipidus is not generally a feature of pituitary disease, and the presence of diabetes insipidus usually denotes a hypothalamic or stalk disorder, except when occurring following hypothalamic or pituitary surgery. The symptoms and signs of individual hormone deficiencies are listed in Table 21–3.

TABLE 21–3. *Symptoms and Signs of Hormone Deficiencies*

Hormone Deficiency	Symptoms and Signs
Growth hormone	Short stature in children, abnormal body composition, increased fracture rate, reduced well-being and performance
Gonadotropins	In men: poor libido/impotence, infertility, small soft testes, reduced facial/body hair
	In women: amenorrhea/oligomenorrhea dyspareunia, infertility, breast atrophy
Thyroid-stimulating hormone	Growth retardation in children, decrease in energy, constipation, sensitivity to cold, dry skin, weight gain
ACTH	Weakness, tiredness, dizziness on standing, pallor, hypoglycemia
Prolactin	Failure of lactation
Antidiuretic hormone	Polyuria, polydipsia, nocturia, hypotension

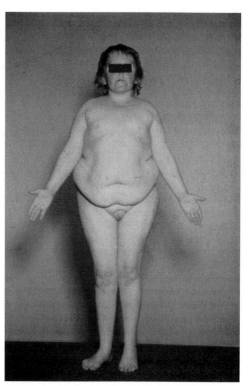

FIGURE 21–3. A 27-year-old individual with combined congenital growth hormone (GH) and gonadotropin deficiency who presented in adult life with extreme short stature (3 ft 9 in.), obesity with particular excess of truncal fat, immature face with depressed midfacial development, and microgenitalia.

Growth Hormone Deficiency

GH secretion is a continuous variable and a spectrum therefore exists from severe GH deficiency to mild GH insufficiency. Typically, the GH-deficient child has increased subcutaneous fat, especially around the trunk. The face is immature with a prominent forehead and depressed midfacial development; this is related to the lack of GH effect on endochondral growth at the base of the skull, occiput, and the sphenoid bone. Dentition is delayed. In males the phallus may be small, and the average age of pubertal onset is delayed in both boys and girls (Fig. 21–3).

GH continues to have significant functions in adult life. Severe GH deficiency in adults is associated with adverse changes in body composition, lipid profile, insulin sensitivity, exercise capacity, bone mineral density (BMD), and quality of life.[26] Adults with GH deficiency have a higher proportion of body fat than matched controls and a high ratio of waist-to-hip measurements, reflecting the predominantly central distribution of fat. On average, BMD in adults with GH deficiency is about 1 to 2 SD below the age-matched normal mean.[27] Correspondingly, a questionnaire-based study has estimated that the fracture rate in GH-deficient patients is increased twofold compared with that of an age-matched group.[28] Studies in adults with varying degrees of hypopituitarism indicate that GH deficiency per se, rather than the associated gonadotropin deficiency or overtreatment with glucocorticoid or thyroxine (T4) replacement, is responsible for the osteopenia. GH-deficient adults report more perceived health problems and a lower perceived quality of life than controls. The conclusions from studies of the lipid profiles in GH-deficient adult patients are not in complete agreement. Nonetheless, a significant number of authors have reported a modest increase in total plasma cholesterol and a rise in the ratio of low-density (LDL) to high-density lipoprotein (HDL). In contrast to the pediatric experience, adults with hypopituitarism show elevated fasting and postprandial plasma insulin levels in comparison with controls, and data from euglycemic-hyperinsulinemic clamp studies confirm that these patients are insulin-resistant.[29] These changes, associated with increased fibrinogen levels and plasminogen activator inhibitor levels,[30] underlie the suggestion that GH deficiency is responsible for the increased cardiovascular mortality in hypopituitarism.

Gonadotropin Deficiency

Gonadotropin deficiency may result from deficient secretion of pituitary gonadotropins, faulty secretion of GnRH, and hyperprolactinemia, which impairs the pulsatile release of GnRH and thus causes secondary hypogonadism. Gonadotropin secretion can also be reduced in some functional disorders, most commonly in women, for example, with excessive weight loss or exercise. The clinical features of secondary or hypogonadotropic hypogonadism are similar to those of primary gonadal failure.

In males the clinical features of gonadotropin deficiency differ according to whether the deficiency was acquired before or after pubertal age. If acquired before pubertal age, clinical examination reveals a small penis and testes, and eunuchoid proportions (span exceeds height by greater than 5 cm) (Fig. 21–4). Hypogonadism acquired postpubertally is associated with a reduction is testicular size, loss of facial and body hair, and thinning of the skin, leading to the characteristic finely wrinkled facial skin of the "aging youth." Other effects include a decrease in skeletal muscle mass, BMD, sexual function, libido, and general well-being. Azoospermia is an almost inevitable consequence of hypogonadotropic hypogonadism, but there are exceptions. In "the fertile eunuch," partial LH deficiency may result in low circulating testosterone levels and gynecomastia but preserved fertility; presumably, intratesticular testosterone levels remain high enough to maintain spermatogenesis. In the female child, hypogonadotropic hypogonadism is associated with primary amenorrhea and absent breast development. In the adult woman, amenorrhea or oligomenorrhea, infertility, breast atrophy, vaginal dryness, and dyspareunia are the result. Pubic and axillary hair remain unless ACTH deficiency is also present.

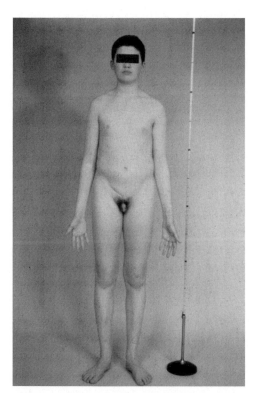

FIGURE 21–4. *An 18-year-old man with Kallmann's syndrome presenting in adult life. Note tall stature, eunuchoid proportions, lack of body hair, poor virilization, and an orchiopexy scar consistent with severe gonadotropin deficiency of very early onset.*

ACTH Deficiency

ACTH deficiency is the most life-threatening feature of hypopituitarism. In addition to the other causes of pituitary failure discussed earlier, functional ACTH deficiency may occur following discontinuation of exogenous glucocorticoids or ACTH, even when these agents have only been administered for a few weeks. Isolated acquired ACTH deficiency has also been well documented, although its occurrence is rare.[16] The features of glucocorticoid deficiency due to ACTH deficiency are similar to those of Addison's disease. Weakness, tiredness, nausea, vomiting, and orthostatic hypotension are common. Weight loss and anorexia may mimic anorexia nervosa or an underlying malignancy. Examination may reveal pallor of the skin, in contrast to the hyperpigmentation of Addison's disease, and in females particularly, there is loss of secondary sexual hair. In severe ACTH deficiency, particularly in childhood, hypoglycemia can occur: cortisol deficiency results in increased insulin sensitivity and a decrease in hepatic glycogen reserves. Hyponatremia, although less commonly seen than in Addison's disease due to preservation of aldosterone secretion, may be the presenting feature of ACTH deficiency, particularly in the elderly. Acute cortisol insufficiency should be considered in the differential diagnosis of a patient with a history of anorexia and weight loss, increasing fatigue and weakness, and nausea and vomiting. The clinical features may include hypovolemic shock, fever, and an acute abdomen. A history of an acute headache, pituitary surgery, or irradiation may provide important pointers to the diagnosis.

Thyroid-Stimulating Hormone Deficiency

TSH deficiency occurs late in most pituitary disorders. Symptoms include fatigue, weakness, inability to lose weight, constipation, and cold intolerance, in keeping with the symptoms of primary hypothyroidism. Symptoms are, however, generally milder than in primary hypothyroidism. This is because the hypothyroidism is usually less severe, as on the whole there is some residual TSH secretion.

Antidiuretic Hormone Deficiency

Polyuria and polydipsia with nocturia are the classic features of diabetes insipidus resulting from ADH deficiency. If the patient is unable to keep up with the fluid loss, hypotension and hypovolemia ensue. The features of diabetes insipidus may be masked in the presence of ACTH deficiency, due to the consequent hypovolemia and reduced glomerular filtration rate. Only when cortisol replacement therapy is commenced may the polyuria and polydipsia of diabetes insipidus be revealed.

DIAGNOSIS AND ENDOCRINE ASSESSMENT

Clinical examination can provide important clues to the cause and duration of hypopituitarism, and the physician must not neglect an assessment of height, weight, and pubertal status.

Examination of the visual fields clinically is essential, and should be supported by either Goldmann or computer-assisted perimetry. The latter is more sensitive, detecting visual field defects that other techniques are unable to demonstrate.

Imaging of the Pituitary Fossa

Imaging of the pituitary fossa is indicated when there is clinical evidence of a visual field defect or biochemical evidence of hypopituitarism. CT and MRI scanning have superseded the plain radiograph. MRI is the scanning technique of choice, as it offers higher resolution than CT scanning and is able to demonstrate microadenomas as small as 3 mm in diameter. If a pituitary adenoma is demonstrated, careful note should be taken of any extension of the tumor outside the pituitary fossa. In diabetes insipidus the normal high-intensity posterior pituitary signal may be absent and other causes of hypopituitarism may show classic CT or MRI findings, for example, craniopharyngioma.

An empty sella is a not uncommon finding. It refers to a cerebrospinal fluid–filled pituitary fossa, resulting from herniation of the arachnoid mater through an incomplete sellar diaphragm. The pituitary fossa may be enlarged or normal in size. An empty sella may be secondary to a congenital diaphragmatic defect (primary) or damage to the diaphragm by surgery, radiation, or infarction of a pituitary tumor (secondary). The pituitary gland is usually flattened against the floor of the sella and the pituitary stalk may be laterally deviated. The majority of patients with primary empty sella have normal pituitary function, but 15% have mild hyperprolactinemia,[31] and it has been described in association with headache, endocrine dysfunction (particularly GH deficiency in children), and visual disturbances. Patients with secondary empty sella more commonly have endocrine disturbances related to the underlying pathogenesis of the condition.

Endocrine Testing

The endocrine assessment of a patient with suspected hypopituitarism usually involves measurement of both baseline and stimulated hormone levels. Basal hormone levels yield much useful information, and therefore serum concentrations of prolactin, TSH, T_4, cortisol, LH, FSH, testosterone in men, and estradiol in women, should be measured. As a general rule, suspected anterior pituitary hormone deficiency should be confirmed and corrected before possible ADH deficiency is investigated, as ACTH deficiency can disguise the presence of ADH deficiency. Another important principle is that of retesting. This is important in two broad clinical contexts. The first is in young adults who received GH replacement in childhood. Over the last 10 years there have been a number of studies in which the status of children who received GH replacement during childhood was reassessed after completion of growth and puberty. At reassessment, GH status was considered normal in 20% to 87%.[32] The original childhood etiologic classification in the vast majority of the latter subjects was isolated idiopathic GH deficiency, while those young adults diagnosed as having organic GH deficiency in childhood as a consequence of either a mass lesion, pituitary surgery, or irradiation to the hypothalamic-pituitary axis rarely reverted to normal GH secretory status. Hence the etiology of the childhood diagnosis of GH deficiency should logically affect the strategy of retesting. Patients with isolated GH deficiency should undergo two tests of GH secretory status, whereas those with additional anterior pituitary hormone deficits require only one test at reassessment. The second cohort in whom retesting is indicated are those patients in whom progression of the hypopituitarism may be expected. This includes patients who were subject to irradiation of the hypothalamic-pituitary axis, following surgery, and in patients with an evolving pituitary or hypothalamic lesion. Following irradiation, endocrine testing should be performed on a yearly basis for at least 10 years, and again at 15 years. This is of particular importance because although the classic sequence of pituitary hormone deficits (GH, gonadotropins, ACTH, and TSH) occurs in the majority of patients, other patterns may occur, most notably ACTH deficiency before gonadotropin deficiency.[33]

Growth Hormone Deficiency

GH replacement therapy has been offered to GH-deficient children for more than 30 years, but it only became a licensed indication for GH-deficient adults in the United States, in a number of European countries, and in New Zealand in 1996. Thus, in contrast to the long-standing pediatric literature and interest in the biochemical diagnosis of GH deficiency, the concerns of the endocrinologist treating adults have been addressed only recently.

The underlying pathophysiology differs in childhood-onset compared with adult-onset GH deficiency, with isolated idiopathic GH deficiency predominating in childhood, while in adulthood, GH deficiency is most frequently due to a pituitary adenoma or treatment with

surgery or radiotherapy; isolated idiopathic GH deficiency acquired in adulthood has never been reported. In childhood, the differential diagnosis is dominated by alternative causes of poor growth, whereas difficulties in the diagnosis of adult-onset GH deficiency exist in the obese and elderly.

GH secretion is a spectrum between normality and abnormality and therefore with rare exceptions, the diagnosis of GH deficiency must be made on arbitrary grounds. The more severe the GH deficiency, the less arbitrary the diagnosis, whereas the "lesser degrees of GH deficiency" merge into normality. Today, in certain countries, children with all forms of GH insufficiency from mild to severe are considered for GH replacement, whereas in other countries only those with severe GH deficiency receive GH replacement. In adulthood, however, it is only severe GH deficiency that has been proved to be associated with any benefit from GH replacement and thus in adulthood the purpose of investigation is to diagnose severe GH deficiency.

GH secretion is pulsatile and serum levels are low during many hours of the day. Therefore a single basal GH estimation provides little useful information about GH secretory status. Twenty-four-hour GH profiles with 20-minute sampling are time-consuming, expensive, and there is controversy as to their scientific and practical value; thus in reality a 24-hour GH profile remains a research investigation. Provocative tests are the most popular method of determining GH secretory status.[32]

At present the ITT is the "gold standard" for the biochemical diagnosis of severe GH deficiency. The ITT provokes a pronounced GH response in normals, it allows the pituitary adrenal axis to be tested at the same time, and the morbidity associated with the performance of the test is low in experienced units.[34] For the diagnosis of severe GH deficiency in adults, a diagnostic cutoff of either 3 or 5 ng/mL has been evaluated by pooling the ITT data available from the literature, albeit with the necessary assumptions required when GH values from different centers are considered together. Nonetheless, based on a cutoff of 5 ng/mL, the ITT provides a specificity of 97%, a sensitivity of 100%, a positive predictive value of 99%, and a negative predictive value of 100%.[35] Nevertheless, each laboratory must establish its own diagnostic threshold values due to lack of standardization of GH assays rather than simply accepting the recommended cutoff level of 3 or 5 ng/mL.

A number of other GH provocative tests are available, including the arginine stimulation test and glucagon stimulation test, among others. Each has advantages and disadvantages, either as an alternative to the ITT in patients in whom this test is contraindicated or as an adjunct in patients requiring a second provocative test. Clonidine is, however, unsuitable in adulthood and the GHRH-pyridostigmine test would be more attractive if the physician could be certain he was dealing with a pituitary rather than a hypothalamic defect. It remains crucial that the results of each provocative test be interpreted in the context of normative values and local assays, as the "cutoff" used for the ITT is not broadly applicable to all other provocative tests, which may be more or less potent stimulators of GH secretion.

The pathophysiologic state of obesity is difficult to distinguish from organic GH deficiency in an adult. There is substantial evidence that morbid obesity is accompanied by suppression of GH release and that substantial weight loss may restore spontaneous and stimulated GH secretion. Even in clinically nonobese healthy adults, relative adiposity, in the abdominal region in particular, is a major negative determinant of stimulated GH secretion.[36] A recent study of age- and sex-matched subjects, however, suggested a much more profound reduction in total GH secretion in a group of individuals with organic GH deficiency compared with obese subjects.[37] Nonetheless, in the obese individual with pituitary disease and no other pituitary deficit, a reduced GH response to any of the standard provocative tests may reflect organic GH deficiency or obesity itself and distinction between the two is not easy at the present time.

GH secretion in healthy elderly adults is reduced compared with that in young adults. GH secretion declines by approximately 14% per decade from young adult life. Normal aging is associated with changes in body composition similar to those seen in patients with GH deficiency. In the clinical setting this raises the question, Can the GH status of elderly patients with organic pituitary disease be distinguished from that of the normal elderly? Toogood et al.[38] have now established that GH secretion is significantly reduced in the elderly with pituitary disease compared with normal controls of similar age. This work suggested that the arginine stimulation test is a reasonable choice to assess GH status in elderly patients with two or three additional pituitary hormone deficits, particularly in an age group in which an ITT carries an increased theoretical risk of morbidity or mortality. In an elderly patient with pituitary disease and with one or no additional pituitary hormone deficits, the distinction between GH deficiency and normality remains a challenge.

Serum insulin-like growth factor-1 (IGF-1) levels are stable throughout the day, mainly due to the complexing of IGF-1 with a family of IGF-binding proteins. Thus the potential for assessing GH status with a single estimation of the circulating IGF-1 level, which is known to be GH-dependent, proved attractive and led to the hope that dynamic GH provocation tests would prove unnecessary. However, IGF-1 levels are affected by a number of other variables, including nutritional status, hepatic function, hypothyroidism, age, and pubertal status, and thus matched values must be used. Even then, there is considerable overlap between the values in GH-deficient and normal persons, particularly in those patients who developed GH deficiency in adulthood or who were rendered GH-deficient by irradiation. Thus, an IGF-1 Standard Deviation Score (SDS) estimation is extremely useful for retesting young adults with a diagnosis of childhood-onset GH deficiency, moderately helpful (~30% to 50% positive predictive value) in middle-aged adults (25 to 55 years old), and rarely helpful in the elderly (>60 years).

Within the limitations of the tests we suggest that it is reasonable to perform only one provocative test of GH release in adult patients with two or three additional pituitary hormone deficiencies, as these patients are almost inevitably severely GH-deficient. In the patient with pituitary disease and a possible diagnosis of adult-onset isolated GH deficiency or GH deficiency plus one additional pituitary hormone deficit, two provocative tests of GH release would be appropriate. The same strategy can be applied to reassessing the GH secretory status of young adults who received GH replacement for childhood GH deficiency as has been utilized for establishing a diagnosis of adult-onset GH deficiency. However, IGF-1 SDS estimation itself should be considered adequate in those in whom multiple pituitary hormone deficits exist, and should serve as one of the two tests of GH status in the much larger cohort of patients with a putative diagnosis of isolated GH deficiency in whom retesting is required.

Gonadotropin Deficiency

In women gonadotropin deficiency is relatively easy to diagnose: in those of postmenopausal age gonadotropin levels are clearly low or undetectable, while in premenopausal women amenorrhea (or less commonly oligomenorrhea), in addition to low estradiol levels and low or normal gonadotropin levels, provides sufficient evidence of the diagnosis.

In men a similar picture of low testosterone levels and low or normal gonadotropin levels is seen. The most difficult distinction is between isolated gonadotropin deficiency and constitutional delay of puberty in the male of peripubertal age. Clinically delayed puberty is defined by failure to develop signs of puberty by the age of 14 years. Over 90% of boys 14 years old or older with delayed puberty have no endocrine abnormality, and will go through puberty spontaneously at a later date. No biochemical tests reliably improve this epidemiologic prediction. The key clinical response is to deal with the pubertal needs of the child and then return to the diagnosis later. Furthermore, if during androgen therapy testicular volumes increase, the diagnosis of constitutional delay in growth and puberty rather than gonadotropin deficiency is confirmed.

ACTH Deficiency

In normal people, the highest plasma cortisol levels are found between 6 AM and 8 AM, and the lowest before midnight. Plasma cortisol and ACTH concentrations are elevated in physical and emotional stress, including acute illness, trauma, surgery, infection, and starvation.

If a 9 AM cortisol level is below 100 nmol/L, particularly in an unwell patient, cortisol deficiency is highly likely and many authors suggest that dynamic assessment of the hypothalamic-pituitary axis is not necessary. A paired plasma ACTH level will help distinguish between primary and secondary glucocorticoid deficiency: in primary cortisol deficiency, that is, Addison's disease, the ACTH level will be high; correspondingly, in secondary glucocorticoid deficiency, the ACTH level will be normal or low.

If cortisol deficiency is suspected in an unwell patient, baseline cortisol and ACTH samples should be taken, but, replacement therapy should be commenced immediately and provocative testing performed at a later date if necessary. Clearly, in a patient with known pituitary disease, the ACTH estimation is unnecessary.

The ITT is the gold standard for the assessment of the hypothalamic-pituitary-adrenal (HPA) axis and pituitary GH reserve. Neuroglycopenia occurs when the blood glucose is less than 2.2 mmol/L resulting in the release of ACTH, cortisol, and GH. A serum cortisol response of greater than 550 nmol/L and a cortisol increment of greater than 170 nmol/L is considered to indicate a normal response. The test is not without risk, and loss of consciousness and seizures are recognized complications. Thus it is contraindicated in those with known ischemic heart disease or a history of seizures; extreme age is a relative contraindication. However, when performed in an experienced endocrine unit it is associated with a low risk of complications.[34]

Other provocative tests useful for assessment of the HPA axis include the short Synacthen test and the (intramuscular, IM) glucagon stimulation test. Each test has advantages and disadvantages, with some groups favoring the ITT and others the short Synacthen test. Of principle importance, however, is that the peak cortisol level (cutoff) achieved must be interpreted in light of the provocative test used. When the short Synacthen test is used, false-positive cortisol responses are common, and stringent criteria (a 30-minute serum cortisol >600 nmol/L in response to 250 μg of Synacthen[39]) are necessary to define normality. Even using these criteria, approximately 1 in 20 tests will produce misleading results. When glucagon is used as the provocative agent, the peak cortisol response occurs later (the test should be continued for 180 minutes) and it is smaller in magnitude than that seen in response to an ITT, and in a number (up to 10%) of normal persons a response is not seen.

As a consequence, while some patients can be classified as having "barn door" ACTH deficiency requiring glucocorticoid replacement therapy (i.e., cortisol response of <450 mmol to an ITT), a proportion fall into a gray zone where the results of testing must be interpreted in the light of clinical features; for example, patients with a cortisol response of between 450 and 550 mmol to an ITT may be advised only to take glucocorticoid replacement during an intercurrent illness or surgery. Lastly, tests of the HPA axis are not infallible, and consideration should be given to repeating a test if the results are at odds with the clinical picture.

Thyroid-Stimulating Hormone Deficiency

In secondary hypothyroidism one might expect to find reduced concentrations of free or total T[4] in association with a serum TSH concentration below the normal range, analogous to the biochemical findings in secondary hypogonadism. This picture is, however, only found in the minority of patients, the majority having normal or occasionally elevated TSH levels. The mechanism behind this apparent contradiction is poorly understood, and a number of different explanations have been explored. One such is that secondary hypothyroidism may be associated with TSH of reduced bioactivity. This hypothesis has been investigated in a number of ways: in 1979 Faglia et al.[40] used a cytochemical assay to demonstrate that in five patients with idiopathic hypopituitarism TSH bioactivity in both basal and TRH-stimulated samples was considerably lower than TSH immunoreactivity. In view of potential limitations of such cytochemical bioassays, a similar group of investigators[41] measured the adenylate cyclase–stimulating bioactivity (B) and receptor-binding (R) activity of purified immunoreactive serum TSH (I) from seven patients with hypothalamic hypothyroidism. Beck-Peccoz and colleagues[41] reported a strikingly decreased R/I ratio (<0.15) in patients compared with controls (0.6 to 2.7) and a similarly decreased B/I ratio (<0.2 vs. 2.8 to 5.6). After administration of TRH for 20 to 30 days, an increase in immunoreactive serum TSH was observed in all patients. Moreover, both ratios returned to normal in all but one patient. The authors concluded that in certain cases of hypothalamic hypothyroidism, secreted TSH lacks biologic activity because of impaired binding to its receptor and that TRH treatment can correct both defects.[41] These data suggest that TRH regulates not only the secretion of TSH but also its specific molecular and conformational features required for hormone action.

The TSH response to TRH (TRH test) has been proposed as a tool to help differentiate between hypothalamic and pituitary hypothyroidism. Classically, in hypothyroidism secondary to a hypothalamic lesion and hence TRH deficiency, the TSH response is delayed (the 60-minute response is greater than the 20-minute response), while in hypothyroidism of pituitary origin, damage to the thyrotrophs results in an absent or impaired TSH response. Studies have revealed no clear-cut differences between patients with hypothyroidism of pituitary and hypothalamic origin, and as such the test cannot be used as the sole criterion to differentiate between these lesions. Furthermore, the information gained has no therapeutic implications.

Antidiuretic Hormone Deficiency

The diagnosis of ADH deficiency first requires confirmation of excess urine output. *Polyuria* is defined as the excretion of greater than 3 L of urine per 24 hours (40 mL/kg/24 hours). Any patient with normal serum sodium and plasma osmolality who has a fluid output of less than 2 L/24 hours is likely to be normal and does not warrant further investigation.

Once excess urine output is confirmed, the usual first-line investigation is an 8-hour fluid deprivation test. The basis for this test is the rise in plasma osmolality resulting from a lack of fluid intake for several hours, stimulating ADH secretion. The test should be performed under strict observation because severe fluid and electrolyte depletion can occur. Plasma osmolality, urine volume, and osmolarity are measured hourly for 8 hours following which a synthetic analogue of ADH (desmopressin) is given IM. The urine osmolality is then remeasured. In a patient without diabetes insipidus, ADH is secreted throughout the test, water is normally absorbed, and there is a subsequent elevation of urine osmolality. In diabetes insipidus the urine fails to concentrate (normals achieve a urine osmolality at least twice the plasma osmolality) due to a lack of ADH, hence plasma osmolality rises. Urine concentrates adequately only after administration of des-

mopressin. Sometimes in cases where there has been long-standing polyuria, failure of urine concentration in response to desmopressin occurs not because of nephrogenic diabetes insipidus but because of a wash-out of interstitial solutes, including urea. This may lead to diagnostic difficulties. In cases where the results of a water deprivation test are inconclusive, the introduction of specific and sensitive radioimmunoassays for ADH has provided a further diagnostic avenue. Infusion of hypertonic saline (5%, 850 mmol) to increase plasma osmolality above 300 mOsmol/kg appears to be a better osmotic stimulus for ADH release than water deprivation. A definitive diagnosis of ADH deficiency can therefore be established by infusing hypertonic saline for 2 hours, with regular 20- to 30-minute blood sampling to estimate plasma osmolality and ADH.

The relationship between ADH level and urinary osmolality following a period of fluid restriction also provides useful information about the cause of diabetes insipidus. In nephrogenic diabetes insipidus ADH values are above the normal reference range while in cranial diabetes insipidus values are in the lower end or below the normal reference range.

TREATMENT OF HYPOPITUITARISM

The treatment of hypopituitarism can be separated into those therapies directed at the underlying disease process and endocrine replacement therapy (Table 21–4). Therapies directed at the underlying cause of hypopituitarism are discussed in the relevant chapters of this book.

Endocrine replacement therapy should aim to mimic the normal hormonal milieu as far as possible, thus improving symptoms while avoiding overtreatment. It remains to be seen whether present regimens normalize the excess mortality in hypopituitary patients.

Growth Hormone Deficiency

Until 1989, the sole indication for GH therapy was in children with GH deficiency. With the availability of recombinant DNA–derived GH, the situation has gradually changed as the biologic features of GH deficiency in adult life have been appreciated.

GH replacement therapy in adulthood induces favorable changes in body composition, with studies demonstrating a 15.5% reduction in fat mass and a 6% increase in lean body mass following 12 months of therapy. Correspondingly, there is an improvement in indices of physical performance and maximal oxygen uptake. In response to GH therapy the initial change in BMD over the first 3 to 6 months is a

TABLE 21–4. Endocrine Replacement Therapy for Hormone Deficiencies

Hormone Deficiency	Replacement	Usual Daily Dose Range
Growth hormone	Growth hormone	Subcutaneous: 0.27–0.7 mg during evening
Gonadotropins		
Women	Estradiol valerate	Oral: 1–2 mg/day
	or	
	Conjugated equine estrogens	Transdermal: 0.625–1.25 mg/day
	plus	
	Progesterone	Progesterone dose depends on preparation
		Sex steroids may be administered transdermally: estradiol 25–100 µg/24 hr
Men	Intramuscular:	
	Testosterone ester, i.e., testosterone propionate, phenylpropionate, and isocaproate (Sustanon)	250 mg IM, every 2–3 wk
	Transdermal:	
	Testosterone	5.0–7.5 mg/24 hr
	Implant:	
	Testosterone	600–800 mg every 4–6 mo
Thyroid-stimulating hormone	Thyroxine	75–150 µg/day
ACTH	Hydrocortisone	10 mg morning, 5 mg noon, 5 mg evening to 10 mg t.i.d.
Prolactin	Nil	—
Antidiuretic hormone	Desmopressin (DDAVP)	Intranasal: 10–40 µg/day in 2 or 3 divided doses
		Oral: 300–600 µg/day in 2 or 3 divided doses

decrease, believed to be due to increased bone remodeling activity. Markers of bone formation and resorption are increased early and remain elevated at 1 year. The subsequent response of bone differs in childhood-onset and adult-onset GH deficiency. By 6 months of treatment the BMD is significantly increased in childhood-onset GH deficiency and continues to rise over 18 months of GH replacement. In adult-onset GH deficiency BMD is not increased at 12 months, although there is a significant increase at 24 months which is more prominent in those with lower baseline BMD scores. There is evidence from placebo-controlled randomized studies that significant improvement in vitality, well-being, and overall quality of life occurs in GH-deficient adults in response to GH replacement. The exact mechanism for the improved sense of well-being remains controversial: possible explanations include increased exercise capacity, improved hydration status with normalization of extracellular volume, and a direct CNS effect. The effects of GH on the lipid profile are less clear. It appears that GH therapy is associated with a decrease in serum total cholesterol, triglycerides, and LDL levels. A complicating factor is the apparent increase in lipoprotein(a), an independent cardiovascular risk factor with GH replacement. While it is well established that earlier regimens using high-dose GH replacement (>0.7 mg/day) were associated with either a worsening of the insulin-resistant state or no change, the data on more physiologic dose regimens are not available. This raises the question as to whether the insulin resistance described in hypopituitary patients is solely secondary to GH deficiency or whether supraphysiologic glucocorticoid replacement therapy may play a role.

Practically, GH replacement still remains the remit of the specialist. Current practice in our department is to consider GH replacement therapy only in severely GH-deficient patients who describe symptoms of fatigue, reduced vitality, and poor quality of life or who have significant osteopenia or osteoporosis. Elsewhere, particularly in Scandinavia, GH replacement therapy is offered to all severely GH-deficient adults. The majority of modern regimens recommend a low starting dose, that is, 0.27 mg/day as a single subcutaneous (SC) injection. This should then be increased every 4 to 6 weeks, based on clinical response and the IGF-1 SDS, until a steady replacement dose is reached. Since improvements in physiologic well-being and quality of life do not occur in all GH-deficient patients on replacement therapy, it is suggested that patients started on GH primarily for a quality-of-life indication should have an initial trial period of therapy; only those with definite improvement should continue treatment thereafter. Improvements in quality of life and body composition often only occur after several months of maintenance therapy and therefore a trial of 6 months of GH at the correct maintenance dose is necessary to determine if treatment is beneficial. At the end of this trial, patients should be reassessed using a disease-specific questionnaire and with measurements of body composition and lipids. In patients started on GH for osteoporosis or osteopenia, therapy is reassessed following BMD estimation at 2 years. This regimen is rarely associated with the side effects such as peripheral edema, arthralgia, and myalgia described when higher doses of GH replacement, particularly weight-based dosing regimens, were used. Monitoring of GH replacement should include regular measurement of weight, blood pressure, hemoglobin A$_{1c}$, lipid profile, IGF-1, fat distribution (waist-hip ratio), and assessment of quality of life by disease-specific questionnaire and patient interview.

Gonadotropin Deficiency

In both sexes, sex steroid replacement therapy is important for the maintenance of normal body composition, BMD, and sexual function. In patients not desirous of fertility the most appropriate form of replacement therapy is sex steroid therapy. In women this can be provided by many standard hormone replacement therapy preparations. Progesterone must be given either cyclically or continuously in all women with a uterus to prevent the possible effect of unopposed estrogen on the endometrium, that is, dysfunctional bleeding or endometrial cancer. The dose of estrogen used should not be supraphysiologic (as in the oral contraceptive pill) unless there is a clear indication, such as significant patient preference or in a patient with partial

gonadotropin deficiency still having occasional menstrual cycles, with a desire for contraception. Estrogen can be delivered as a tablet, patch, gel, or implant. While estrogen replacement therapy started early can minimize the risk of osteoporosis, its long-term effects on the cardiovascular system remain contentious. Estrogen replacement therapy should ideally be continued at least until the age of 50. Continuation after this time should be based on a discussion of the risks and benefits between the patient and physician, supported by BMD measurement.

Androgen replacement therapy for men is available in many modalities. The choice of preparation depends on local availability and the wishes of the patient. IM injection of testosterone 17α-hydroxyl esters every 2 to 3 weeks is probably the most commonly used preparation. In some men, however, this mode of administration is associated with disturbing fluctuations in sexual function, energy level, and mood, mirroring the changes in testosterone concentrations. Changing to smaller doses on a more frequent basis or another preparation can be helpful. Transdermal testosterone systems have been recently developed: scrotal and nonscrotal patch systems are available. Both maintain physiologic testosterone profiles but have some drawbacks: the scrotal patch requires adequate hairless scrotal skin to apply the patch, while the nonscrotal patch causes local irritation in at least 25% of patients. In some patients adequate testosterone levels are not achieved and therefore testosterone levels must be monitored with both patch systems.

Testosterone pellets can also be implanted SC: three to six 200-mg pellets can maintain normal testosterone levels for up to 6 months. The implantation of the pellets requires minor surgery and may be complicated in a minority of patients by local infection, extrusion, and scarring.

Oral androgen replacement therapy is available using testosterone undecenoate, a 17α-hydroxyl ester of testosterone. However, this requires frequent dosing (two to four times daily) and often subnormal testosterone levels are achieved due to variable absorption. It is not, therefore, the preparation of choice in most men. 17α-methyltestosterone is another orally active testosterone preparation. It is, however, associated with serious hepatotoxicity due to the alkyl group in the 17α position, and thus it is not recommended.

In the hypogonadotropic hypogonadal patient fertility can be achieved with gonadotropin therapy. In males excellent success rates can be achieved, provided primary testicular dysfunction does not coexist. Testosterone replacement should be discontinued before initiating therapy. The choice of therapy lies between gonadotropin replacement or GnRH. The former is the traditional therapeutic approach; initially LH "activity" is provided by human chorionic gonadotropin (hCG) administered SC or IM at a dose of between 1000 and 2000 IU two to three times weekly. Spermatogenesis is unlikely within the first 3 months of therapy. Treatment with hCG alone is continued for 6 months with sperm counts being performed six to eight times weekly. If adequate spermatogenesis is not achieved, then FSH in the form of human menopausal gonadotropin (hMG), or a more purified preparation of FSH, is added. Side effects, usually from the LH component of the hMG, include acne, weight gain, and gynecomastia. The dose of FSH is increased if adequate spermatogenesis is not achieved following 6 months of combination therapy. The alternative regimen in patients with idiopathic hypogonadotropic hypogonadism and Kallmann's syndrome is pulsatile GnRH therapy. GnRH is administered SC via a catheter attached to a minipump. Its use implies a hypothalamic defect with essentially normal pituitary gonadotrophs. This regimen appears to have few advantages over gonadotropin therapy in males, but may cause less gynecomastia and be slightly more effective. Both regimens may take up to 2 years to achieve adequate spermatogenesis, and thus once effective, consideration should be given to storing several samples of frozen sperm for any future attempts at pregnancy.

In women with hypogonadotropic hypogonadism, pregnancy rates of 83% following therapy with either pulsatile GnRH or gonadotropins are reported. These are better than rates achieved in women undergoing ovulation induction for other pathologic conditions. Again, the choice of therapy lies between gonadotropin therapy or pulsatile GnRH, but in women there are obvious advantages to GnRH therapy should the patient have enough residual gonadotroph function to make a trial of GnRH a reasonable option.

Pulsatile GnRH therapy is more likely than hMG to result in development and ovulation of a single follicle, thereby reducing the risks of ovarian hyperstimulation and multiple gestation. However, in practice, GnRH therapy may not be practicable, and in more than 50% of women with organic pituitary disease, residual gonadotroph function is not sufficient to support this method.

Lastly, an area of debate at present is the therapeutic use of testosterone in women. In postmenopausal women, particularly those who have undergone bilateral oophorectomy, there is evidence in those who complain of loss of libido and impaired sexual function despite adequate estrogen replacement, that combined estrogen and testosterone replacement results in substantial benefits. The rationale behind such therapy is that following bilateral oophorectomy circulating testosterone levels fall by 50%. Patients with hypogonadotropic hypogonadism have a similar hormonal milieu and thus symptomatic patients may benefit from low-dose testosterone replacement therapy. Regimens using a 50-mg testosterone implant every 6 months have been employed. This practice is, however, not universal, and not well researched in the hypogonadotropic hypogonadal woman. Testosterone replacement regimens are not approved for the latter indication by most regulatory authorities.

ACTH Deficiency

As mentioned earlier, the decision to begin cortisol replacement therapy relies not only on the results of dynamic testing but also on clinical assessment. The next decision is the choice of glucocorticoid to use. Hydrocortisone is the logical choice, as it directly replaces the missing hormone. Alternatives include cortisone acetate, which is metabolized to cortisol to achieve glucocorticoid activity, and therefore can be monitored in the same way as hydrocortisone. Its onset of action is slower and its biologic activity is slightly longer, providing relative disadvantages and advantages over hydrocortisone, respectively. Other synthetic glucocorticoids, that is, prednisolone and dexamethasone, have significant disadvantages; monitoring is difficult and in the case of dexamethasone the limited number of pharmaceutical preparations available make dose titration impossible and thus overdosage is likely.

There is now growing evidence that the traditional hydrocortisone regimen of 20 mg in the morning and 10 mg in the evening is suboptimal. First, this regimen is not physiologic, as the plasma half-life of cortisol is less than 2 hours. Thus twice-daily dosing regimens are associated with very low cortisol levels in the late afternoon, and studies of a twice-daily regimen have demonstrated that quality-of-life scores are lower at this time. Thus dosing three times daily (on rising, at noon, and in the early evening) is recommended. The total dose of hydrocortisone used in traditional regimens is also likely to be supraphysiologic as recent evidence demonstrates that production rates in the normal individual are significantly lower than previously believed.[42] Thus a total daily dose of 20 mg, as 10 mg in the morning, 5 mg at noon, and 5 mg in the evening, is likely to be the best-guess starting dose. Monitoring of therapy usually involves the use of an 8-hour hydrocortisone day curve or a modified three-point day curve, aiming to normalize cortisol levels. Such monitoring allows the detection of minor degrees of over- or underreplacement which are unlikely to be clinically obvious. Minor overreplacement is proved to be associated with reduced BMD[42] and it is likely that other factors, including blood pressure, insulin sensitivity, and body composition, may also be adversely affected.

Thyroid-Stimulating Hormone Deficiency

Secondary hypothyroidism is treated in the same way as primary hypothyroidism, with T_4 replacement therapy. The normal starting dose in a young patient without evidence of cardiac disease is 100 μg/day. In the elderly or in a patient with evidence of ischemic heart disease, therapy should be started at lower doses, that is, 25 to 50 μg/day.

A complicating factor in this situation, however, is that measurement of serum TSH is obviously unhelpful in the monitoring of T_4 replacement therapy. Thus the objective, biochemically, should be to restore the serum free T_4 concentration to the normal range. TSH-deficient female patients will commonly also be on estrogen replacement therapy, with a consequent increase in T_4-binding globulin levels, and thus total T_4 levels may be misleading. Overreplacement with T_4 over long periods may be associated with reduced BMD, an increased risk of osteoporotic fracture, and an increase in the rate of development of atrial fibrillation; thus excessive doses of T_4 should be avoided. In a patient with suspected hypopituitarism, T_4 therapy should be delayed until ACTH deficiency has been excluded or treated, as there is a risk of worsening the features of cortisol deficiency.

Antidiuretic Hormone Deficiency

Desmopressin is the drug of choice for the treatment of ADH deficiency. It is a synthetic analog of arginine vasopressin with two minor alterations in its molecular structure: a switch of arginine from the L- to the D- form in position 8, and deamination of cysteine in position 1. This results in a two- to fourfold increase in antidiuretic activity, prolongation of the biologic half-life to 6 to 8 hours, and elimination of pressor activity. This last effect results in an absence of the side effects noted with arginine vasopressin, including hypertension, renal colic, coronary artery spasm, and abdominal colic.

Desmopressin is available in a number of preparations, including oral, intranasal, and parenteral. Dosages vary widely, up to 10-fold between individuals, with no apparent relationship to age, sex, weight, or degree of polyuria. The drug should be started at low dose and increased gradually until urine output is controlled. Overdosage carries a risk of hyponatremia and sodium levels should be checked after commencing therapy and dosage changes.

STRATEGIES TO PREVENT HYPOPITUITARISM

Hypopituitarism increases morbidity and mortality in affected patients, requires therapy with complex drug regimens, and incurs significant cost to the healthcare provider. The development of GH replacement therapy has exacerbated the problem, with a yearly cost in U.S. dollars of $4500 to $6000 per patient. Thus attention has turned to strategies that might reduce the incidence of hypopituitarism.

Pituitary tumors are treated by surgery, radiotherapy, and medically. Given that two modalities of therapy may achieve the same cure rate of the primary disorder, it is possible that the modality of therapy associated with the least risk of inducing hypopituitarism may be chosen for cost-benefit reasons.

One area worthy of consideration is the routine use of radiotherapy following surgery for nonsecreting pituitary adenomas. This is based on data suggesting that recurrence rates following craniotomy are as high as 25% to 75%.[43] However, these data cannot be extrapolated to transsphenoidal surgery. Using this modality, recurrence rates are reported to be between 12% and 22%. Data from Bradley et al[44] suggest that in the subgroup of patients with complete tumor removal as judged by the surgeon, without radiologic and surgical evidence of spread into the parapituitary structures or evidence of rapid tumor growth, there is a 90% recurrence-free survival at 5 years. It should be pointed out, however, that surgical results are highly operator-dependent in terms of tumor recurrence and that regular clinical and radiologic surveillance is mandatory. Nonetheless, by avoiding radiotherapy as a routine procedure, the incidence of long-term hypopituitarism will be significantly reduced.

Medical therapy offers an alternative to radiotherapy or surgery in patients with prolactinomas and now in patients with acromegaly. Dopamine agonist drug therapy can shrink prolactinomas in size and restore normoprolactinemia in many patients, 70% of macroadenomas shrinking by 25% or more, and restoration of normoprolactinemia and normal gonadal function in at least 75% of patients with prolactin-secreting microadenomas or macroadenomas. Whether these agents are also associated with a restoration of other aspects of pituitary function is less clear. Variable recovery from both ACTH and TSH deficiency has been described, but the data regarding GH status, particularly in adults, are scanty. Somatostatin analog as adjunct therapy following surgery for acromegaly have potential advantages over radiotherapy, as they are unlikely to be associated with a further deterioration in pituitary function. Few data are available as yet to confirm the effects of this modality of treatment on recurrence rates, and furthermore it is unknown whether acromegalic patients "cured by" somatostatin analogs are rendered functionally GH-deficient.

Increasingly, in the years to come, the ratio of benefit vs. side effects will influence the choice of treatment for patients with pituitary disease.

REFERENCES

1. Rosen T, Bengtsson BA: Premature mortality due to cardiovascular disease in hypopituitarism. Lancet 336:285–288, 1990.
2. Bates AS, Van't Hoff W, Jones PJ, et al: The effect of hypopituitarism on life expectancy. J Clin Endocrinol Metab 81:1169–1172, 1996.
3. Bulow B, Hagmar L, Mikoczy Z, et al: Increased cerebrovascular mortality in patients with hypopituitarism. Clin Endocrinol (Oxf) 46:75–81, 1997.
4. Markussis V, Beshyah SA, Fisher C, et al: Detection of premature atherosclerosis by high-resolution ultrasonography in symptom-free hypopituitary adults [see comments]. Lancet 340:1188–1192, 1992.
5. Lehmann ED, Hopkins KD, Weissberger AJ, et al: Aortic distensibility in growth hormone deficient adults (letter; comment). Lancet 341:309, 1993.
6. Molitch ME: Pituitary incidentalomas. Endocrinol Metab Clin North Am 26:725–740, 1997.
7. Arafah BM, Kailani SH, Nekl KE, et al: Immediate recovery of pituitary function after transsphenoidal resection of pituitary macroadenomas. J Clin Endocrinol Metab 79:348–354, 1994.
8. Lees PD, Pickard JD: Hyperprolactinemia, intrasellar pituitary tissue pressure, and the pituitary stalk compression syndrome. J Neurosurg 67:192–196, 1987.
9. Arafah BM: Reversible hypopituitarism in patients with large nonfunctioning pituitary adenomas. J Clin Endocrinol Metab 62:1173–1179, 1986.
10. Littley MD, Shalet SM, Beardwell CG: Radiation and hypothalamic-pituitary function. Baillieres Clin Endocrinol Metab 4:147–175, 1990.
11. Shalet SM, Beardwell CG, Pearson D, et al: The effect of varying doses of cerebral irradiation on growth hormone production in childhood. Clin Endocrinol (Oxf) 5:287–290, 1976.
12. Phillips JA III, Cogan JD: Genetic basis of endocrine disease. 6. Molecular basis of familial human growth hormone deficiency. J Clin Endocrinol Metab 78:11–16, 1994.
13. Netchine I, Talon F, Dastot F, et al: Extensive phenotypic analysis of a family with growth hormone (GH) deficiency caused by a mutation in the GH-releasing hormone receptor gene. J Clin Endocrinol Metab 83:432–436, 1998.
14. Waldstreicher J, Seminara SB, Jameson JL, et al: The genetic and clinical heterogeneity of gonadotropin-releasing hormone deficiency in the human. J Clin Endocrinol Metab 81:4388–4395, 1996.
15. Doeker BM, Pfaffle RW, Pohlenz J, et al: Congenital central hypothyroidism due to a homozygous mutation in the thyrotropin beta-subunit gene follows an autosomal recessive inheritance. J Clin Endocrinol Metab 83:1762–1765, 1998.
16. de Luis DA, Aller R, Romero E: Isolated ACTH deficiency. Horm Res 49:247–249, 1998.
17. Cohen LE, Wondisford FE, Radovick S: Role of Pit-1 in the gene expression of growth hormone, prolactin, and thyrotropin. Endocrinol Metab Clin North Am 25:523–540, 1996.
18. Radovick S, Cohen LE, Wondisford FE: The molecular basis of hypopituitarism. Horm Res 49(suppl 1):30–36, 1998.
19. Sornson MW, Wu W, Dasen JS, et al: Pituitary lineage determination by the Prophet of Pit-1 homeodomain factor defective in Ames dwarfism. Nature 384:327–333, 1996.
20. Dutour A: A new step understood in the cascade of tissue-specific regulators orchestrating pituitary lineage determination: The Prophet of Pit-1 (Prop-1). Eur J Endocrinol 137:616–617, 1997.
21. Deladoey J, Fluck C, Buyukgebiz A, et al: "Hot spot" in the PROP1 gene responsible for combined pituitary hormone deficiency. J Clin Endocrinol Metab 84:1645–1650, 1999.
22. Dattani MT, Martinez Barbera JP, Thomas PQ, et al: Mutations in the homeobox gene HESX1/Hesx1 associated with septo-optic dysplasia in human and mouse. Nat Genet 19:125–133, 1998.
23. Parkin JM: Incidence of growth hormone deficiency. Arch Dis Child 49:904–905, 1974.
24. Rona RJ, Tanner JM: Aetiology of idiopathic growth hormone deficiency in England and Wales. Arch Dis Child 52:197–208, 1977.
25. Crock PA: Cytosolic autoantigens in lymphocytic hypophysitis. J Clin Endocrinol Metab 83:609–618, 1998.
26. Shalet SM, Rahim A, Toogood AA: Growth hormone therapy for adult growth hormone deficiency. Trends Endocrinol Metab 7:287–290, 1996.
27. Holmes SJ, Economou G, Whitehouse RW, et al: Reduced bone mineral density in patients with adult onset growth hormone deficiency. J Clin Endocrinol Metab 78:669–674, 1994.
28. Rosen T, Wilhelmsen L, Landin Wilhelmsen L, et al: Increased fracture frequency in adult patients with hypopituitarism and GH deficiency. Eur J Endocrinol 137:240–245, 1997.
29. Beshyah SA, Gelding SV, Andres C, et al: Beta-cell function in hypopituitary adults before and during growth hormone treatment. Clin Sci (Colch) 89:321–328, 1995.
30. de Boer H, Blok GJ, Van der Veen EA: Clinical aspects of growth hormone deficiency in adults. Endocr Rev 16:63–86, 1995.
31. Vance ML: Hypopituitarism [erratum appears in N Engl J Med 18;331:487, 1994]. N Engl J Med 330:1651–1662, 1994.
32. Shalet SM, Toogood AA, Rahim A, et al: The diagnosis of growth hormone deficiency in children and adults. Endocr Rev 19:203–223, 1998.
33. Littley MD, Shalet SM, Beardwell CG, et al: Hypopituitarism following external radiotherapy for pituitary tumours in adults. QJM 70:145–160, 1989.
34. Jones SL, Trainer PJ, Perry L, et al: An audit of the insulin tolerance test in adult subjects in an acute investigation unit over one year [see comments]. Clin Endocrinol (Oxf) 41:123–128, 1994.
35. Hoffman DM, Ho KKY: Diagnosis of GH deficiency in adults. In Juul A, Jorgenson JOL (eds): Growth Hormone In Adults, Cambridge, UK, Cambridge University Press, 1996, pp 168–185.
36. Bjorntorp P: Endocrine abnormalities of obesity. Metabolism 44(suppl 3):21–23, 1995.
37. Salomon F, Cuneo RC, Umpleby AM, et al: Interactions of body fat and muscle mass with substrate concentrations and fasting insulin levels in adults with growth hormone deficiency. Clin Sci (Colch) 87:201–206, 1994.
38. Toogood AA, O' Neill PA, Shalet SM: Beyond the somatopause: Growth hormone deficiency in adults over the age of 60 years. J Clin Endocrinol Metab 81:460–465, 1996.
39. Hurel SJ, Thompson CJ, Watson MJ, et al: The short Synacthen and insulin stress tests in the assessment of the hypothalamic-pituitary-adrenal axis [see comments]. Clin Endocrinol (Oxf) 44:141–146, 1996.
40. Faglia G, Bitensky L, Pinchera A, et al: Thyrotropin secretion in patients with central hypothyroidism: Evidence for reduced biological activity of immunoreactive thyrotropin. J Clin Endocrinol Metab 48:989–998, 1979.
41. Beck-Peccoz P, Amr S, Menezes Ferreira MM, et al: Decreased receptor binding of biologically inactive thyrotropin in central hypothyroidism. Effect of treatment with thyrotropin-releasing hormone. N Engl J Med 312:1085–1090, 1985.
42. Peacey SR, Guo CY, Robinson AM, et al: Glucocorticoid replacement therapy: Are patients overtreated and does it matter? [see comments]. Clin Endocrinol (Oxf) 46:255–261, 1997.
43. Shalet SM, Peacey SR: Treatment strategies in the prevention of growth hormone deficiency. In Lamberts SWJ (ed): The diagnosis and treatment of pituitary insufficiency. Bristol, UK, BioScientifica, 1997, pp 263–277.
44. Bradley KM, Adams CB, Potter CP, et al: An audit of selected patients with nonfunctioning pituitary adenoma treated by transsphenoidal surgery without irradiation. Clin Endocrinol (Oxf) 41:655–659, 1994.

Acromegaly

Shlomo Melmed

Acromegaly is a disease of spectacular growth and metabolic disorders that has fascinated physicians for centuries. The natural history of the disorder, if left untreated, results in gross acral and facial disfigurement, musculoskeletal disability, cardiac failure, respiratory dysfunction, diabetes, and accelerated mortality.[1-3] If the disease occurs before epiphyseal closure, gigantism results.[1] After the first modern description of the disease in 1886 by Marie,[4] it was subsequently recognized that the disorder is associated with a growth hormone (GH)-secreting adenohypophysial adenoma resulting in both a central mass lesion and the protean peripheral effects of sustained tissue exposure to high GH levels.[1, 5-7]

PATHOGENESIS

The pathogenetic events that underlie the etiology of pituitary acromegaly include excessive pituitary somatotroph cell proliferation and unrestrained GH hypersecretion. GH is secreted by somatotroph cells, the largest differentiated compartment of the anterior pituitary. GH secretion is under dual hypothalamic inhibitory control: somatotropin release–inhibiting factor (SRIF) inhibits secretion and GH-releasing hormone (GHRH) stimulates both GH synthesis and secretion.[8, 9] Insulin-like growth factor-1 (IGF-1), the peripheral target molecule for GH action, also participates in negative GH feedback inhibition by acting both at the hypothalamus to induce SRIF and directly at the pituitary to inhibit GH gene transcription.[10-12] Peripheral sex and adrenal steroids also regulate GH secretion.[8, 13] GH itself binds to peripheral GH receptors that elicit signaling by JAK/STAT (Janus kinase/signal transducer and activator of transcription) intracellular phosphorylation cascades.[14] GH acts directly to attenuate insulin action and induce lipolysis.[15] The growth-promoting actions of GH are indirectly mediated by IGF-1, which is synthesized in the liver, kidney, pituitary, gastrointestinal tract, muscle, and cartilage.[12, 16, 17] GH actions mediated by IGF-1 include protein synthesis; amino acid transportation; muscle, cartilage, and bone growth; DNA and RNA synthesis; and cell proliferation.[18, 19] Local production of IGF-1 may be under autocrine and paracrine regulation[3, 20, 21] acting in concert with circulating IGF-1 and GH to elicit a final tissue impact.

Excess Growth Hormone Secretion

Tumors may arise from clonal expansion of one or more of the anterior pituitary differentiated cell types[22, 23] and thereby result in specific hormone hypersecretory syndromes. The most common cause of acromegaly is a somatotroph (GH-secreting) adenoma of the anterior pituitary, which accounts for 30% of all hormone-secreting pituitary adenomas[1] (Table 22–1).

GH-secreting adenomas arise from differentiated cells secreting GH gene products[1, 23, 24] (Table 22–2). These cells include somatotrophs, mixed mammosomatotrophs (secreting both GH and prolactin [PRL]), or more primitive acidophilic stem cells. Regardless of their cellular origin, transformation and subsequent replication of these cells result in adenoma formation, as well as unrestrained GH secretion.[1] Most patients harbor densely granulated GH cell adenomas, which are commonly encountered in older patients with indolent disease progression. Sparsely granulated GH cell adenomas, however, occur in younger patients with more aggressive disease onset and higher GH levels.[1, 2] Mammosomatotroph cell tumors, or discreet mammotroph and somatotroph tumors, reflect the common stem cell origin of the somatotroph cell lineage.[2, 24-26] Although acidophil stem cell adenomas secrete GH, their predominant product is PRL, thus accounting for the high incidence of hyperprolactinemic symptoms (galactorrhea, amenorrhea, infertility) initially seen in these patients.[27] Patients with McCune-Albright syndrome may also have acromegaly, although the presence of a discreet GH cell adenoma has been inconsistently reported in

TABLE 22–1. Causes of Acromegaly

Cause	Prevalence (%)
Excess GH secretion	
Pituitary	98
Densely or sparsely granulated GH cell adenoma	60
Mixed GH cell and PRL cell adenoma	25
Mammosomatotroph cell adenoma	10
Plurihormonal adenoma	
GH cell carcinoma or metastases	
Multiple endocrine neoplasia-1 (GH cell adenoma)	
McCune-Albright syndrome (rarely adenoma)	
Ectopic sphenoid or parapharyngeal sinus pituitary adenoma	
Extrapituitary tumor	
Pancreatic islet cell tumor	<1
Excess GH-releasing hormone secretion	
Central	<1
Hypothalamic hamartoma, choristoma, ganglioneuroma	<1
Peripheral	1
Bronchial carcinoid, pancreatic islet cell tumor, small cell lung cancer, adrenal adenoma, medullary thyroid carcinoma, pheochromocytoma	
Excess growth factor activity	
Acromegaloidism	<1

GH, growth hormone; PRL, prolactin.
Adapted from Melmed S: Acromegaly. N Engl J Med 322:966–977, 1990.

TABLE 22–2. **Clinical and Pathologic Characteristics of GH-Secreting Pituitary Tumors**

Cell Type	Hormonal Products	Clinical Features	Histologic Features
Densely granulated somatotroph	GH	Slow growing	Numerous somatotrophs with large secretory granules
Sparsely granulated somatotroph	GH	Rapidly growing Often invasive	Cellular pleomorphism
Mixed cell (somatotroph/lactotrope)	GH and PRL	Variable	Densely and sparsely granulated somatotrophs and lactotrophs
Mammosomatotroph	GH and PRL	Commonly in children Gigantism Mild hyperprolactinemia	Both GH and PRL in same cell, often same secretory granule
Acidophil stem cell	PRL and GH	Rapidly growing/invasive Hyperprolactinemia dominant	Distinctive ultrastructure Giant mitochondria
Plurihormonal cell	GH (PRL) with α-GSU, FSH/LH, TSH, or ACTH	Often, secondary hormonal products are clinically silent Rarely hyperthyroidism or Cushings disease	Variable: either monomorphous or plurimorphous
Somatotroph carcinoma	GH	Aggressive and invasive	Rigorously documented extracranial metastasis

ACTH, adrenocorticotropic hormone; GH, growth hormone; GSU, α-glycoprotein subunit; LH, lutenizing hormone; PRL, prolactin; TSH, thyroid-stimulating hormone.
Adapted from Melmed S: Pathogenesis of pituitary tumors. Endocrinol Metab Clin North Am 21:553–574, 1992.

these cases.[28] Rarely, acromegaly may occur in patients with a partially empty sella.[29] The rim of pituitary tissue surrounding the empty sella may harbor a small endocrinologically active GH-secreting adenoma not visible on magnetic resonance imaging (MRI) (i.e., <2 mm in diameter). Because embryonic pituitary tissue originates from the nasopharyngeal Rathke's pouch, ectopic pituitary adenomas may arise in remnant nasopharyngeal tissue along the line of primitive adenohypophysial migration. These adenomas may not be detected on normal pituitary MRI fields, and more extensive skull base imaging may be required. Very rarely, ectopic GH production by a pancreatic,[30] lung,[31] or ovarian[32] neoplasm may result in acromegaly.[1]

Excess Growth Hormone–Releasing Hormone Secretion

Excessive circulating levels of GHRH may overstimulate the pituitary and cause somatotroph hyperplasia, GH hypersecretion, and acromegaly.[33] Central overproduction of GHRH may occur in patients harboring hypothalamic hamartomas or gangliocytomas.[33] These rare tumors are usually diagnosed by pathologic examination of a surgically resected sellar mass causing GH hypersecretion and acromegaly.[34] Ectopic GHRH production by carcinoid tumors, although rare, accounts for most cases of acromegaly.[35] Although the clinical association of acromegaly with carcinoid disease had long been recognized, the pathogenesis of ectopic GHRH production has only recently been elucidated. Subclinical GHRH immunoreactivity has been demonstrated in about 40% of lung, abdominal, and bony carcinoid tissue specimens.

Pituitary somatotroph hyperplasia plus acromegaly associated with ectopic GHRH production has now been reported in over 100 patients, and the original isolation of GHRH was in fact accomplished from a pancreatic carcinoid tumor.[36] Because the peripheral features of hypersomatotropism are quite similar in all forms of pituitary and nonpituitary acromegaly, diagnosis of the etiology of the disease may be clinically challenging.[1]

Acromegaloidism is a very rare syndrome characterized by acromegalic features with no discernible pituitary tumor and normal serum GH and IGF-1 concentrations. It has been presumed that this disorder is due to excess secretion of a putative, as yet unidentified growth factor.[37]

Role of the Hypothalamus in the Etiology of Acromegaly

Hypothalamic GHRH and SRIF selectively regulate GH gene expression and secretion.[8] These hypothalamic peptide hormones are expressed both within the anterior pituitary gland itself and within GH-secreting pituitary tumors.[38, 39] GHRH, in addition to its hormonal regulation of GH production, induces somatotroph DNA synthesis.[40] Mice bearing an overexpressing GHRH transgene are subject to somatotroph hyperplasia and ultimately to pituitary adenomas.[41, 42] In patients with carcinoid tumors and ectopic GHRH production, somatotroph hyperplasia and occasionally adenomas may also develop, which suggests that disordered endocrine or paracrine GHRH or SRIF action may be permissive for pituitary tumor growth.[43] GHRH signaling defects have also been identified in acromegaly. Constitutive activation of the GHRH receptor G protein signaling unit facilitates ligand-independent induction of GH gene expression. This *gsp* mutation results in guanosine triphosphatase (GTPase) inactivation with subsequent elevated cyclic adenosine monophosphate (cAMP) levels and GH hypersecretion.[44, 45] Excessive CREB (cAMP response element–binding protein) serine phosphorylation may also account for activation of the CREB–Pit-1 (pituitary-specific transcription factor-1) signaling unit in a subset of GH cell adenomas.[46]

Pituitary tumor–derived paracrine GHRH and/or SRIF may also regulate tumor growth or function, although no consistent activating hormone receptor structural mutations have been identified. A truncated alternatively spliced GHRH receptor transcript has been described, but its functional significance is unclear.[47] In light of compelling evidence favoring intrinsic genetic defects occurring in GH-secreting pituitary tumors as discussed below, it is apparent that hypothalamic influences may be permissive of tumor growth rather than being proximally involved in the initiation of somatotroph tumorigenesis.[43, 48]

Intrinsic Pituitary Lesions

Virtually all GH cell adenomas arise as discreet clonal expansions of a single transformed cell[22] (Table 22–3). This monoclonal origin implies that intrinsic genetic alterations account for tumorigenic initiating events and supports abundant earlier clinical observations that resection of small well-circumscribed adenomas often results in surgical cure of GH-secreting adenomas.[24, 43, 49] Because adenohypophysial tissue surrounding the pituitary adenoma is usually histologically normal, it is unlikely that multiple independent cellular events (e.g., generalized hyperplasia) precede adenoma formation. Increasing evidence points to complex molecular cascades accounting for the cellular progression resulting in pituitary cell transformation and, ultimately, tumor formation. Multistep development of pituitary acromegaly involves a spectrum of genetic alterations associated with disregulation of cell proliferation, differentiation, and GH production.[43] Activation of oncogene function and/or inactivation of tumor suppressor genes may account for these changes[43, 50, 51] (see Table 22–3).

TABLE 22–3. Evidence for an Intrinsic Pituitary Defect in the Pathogenesis of Acromegaly

GH-secreting adenomas are monoclonal

Absence of somatotroph hyperplasia in normal pituitary tissue surrounding pituitary adenomas

Successful surgical cure of well-circumscribed GH cell adenomas is achieved in >75% of patients

Adenoma transformation is rarely associated with generalized somatotroph hyperplasia

Unrestrained GH hypersecretion occurs independently of physiologic hypothalamic feedback control

Normalization of GH pulsatility often occurs after complete adenoma resection

GH, growth hormone.

Adapted from Drange MR, Melmed S: IGFs in the evaluation of acromegaly. *In* Rosenfeld RG, Roberts CT (eds): Contemporary Endocrinology. The IGF System: Molecular Biology, Physiology, and Clinical Applications. Totowa, NJ, Humana, 1999, pp 699–720.

Candidate Genes in the Etiology of Acromegaly

Inactivating Mutations

Several transgenic animal models have shown that disruption of tumor suppressor genes (including RB [retinoblastoma] and p27) results in a high incidence of pituitary tumor formation in afflicted mice.[52–54] Because a variety of chromosomal loss of heterozygosity (LOH) patterns are observed in human adenomas, loss of tumor suppressor gene activity was similarly postulated for human tumors (Table 22–4).

Several chromosomal lesions occur in pituitary tumor tissue derived from patients with sporadic nonfamilial acromegaly. LOH involving chromosomes 11q13, 13, and 9 occurs in up to 20% of sporadic[50, 55, 56] pituitary tumors. Despite the multiple endocrine neoplasia type 1 (MEN-1) gene location on chromosome 11, non–MEN-1 patients with sporadic pituitary tumors and 11q LOH harbor intact coding and intronic sequences, with appropriately expressed MEN-1 mRNA.[56] Lesions in chromosomes 13 and 9 are also more prevalent in invasive or larger adenomas.[51] Chromosome 13q LOH occurs in proximity to the RB locus and was found in 13 aggressive pituitary tumors, whereas small circumscribed tumors exhibit intact RB alleles.[57] These results suggest the presence of putative tumor suppressor genes located on chromosomes 11 and 13 that may be involved in controlling the propensity for pituitary tumor proliferation. Despite these heterogeneous chromosomal LOH patterns, no consistent loss of tumor suppressor gene activity has been identified for acromegaly. Although tumor invasiveness or size correlates with an increased propensity for chromosomal LOH,[51] identification of a specific molecular lesion leading to loss of antiproliferative activity in GH-secreting tumors remains elusive[43] (see Table 22–3).

Activating Mutations

GTPase acts to inactivate stimulatory G (Gs) proteins that induce adenyl cyclase and intracellular cAMP accumulation.[58] Missense muta- tions replacing residue 201 (Arg → Cys or His) or 227 (Gln → Arg or Leu), termed *gsp*, result in persistently elevated ligand-independent Gs activity and constitutively elevated cAMP and GH hypersecretion.[44] *Gsp* mutations occur in a subset of GH adenomas, with a prevalence ranging from 30% to 40% in whites[58–63] to only 10% in Japanese[64] patients with acromegaly. No clinically or biochemically significant correlations have been associated with *gsp* mutations.[44, 65] Thus although these mutational events suggest a compelling mechanism for explaining GH cell hypersecretion, their clinical significance has not been apparent (see Table 22–4).

Rarely, *ras* mutations have been observed in highly invasive pituitary tumors or their extrapituitary metastases.[66–68] Development of true GH cell carcinoma with documented extracranial metastases, however, is exceedingly rare[67] (see Table 22–4).

Recently, a novel pituitary tumor–transforming gene (PTTG) was isolated from rat GH-secreting pituitary tumor cells.[69] PTTG overexpression results in cell transformation in vitro and experimental tumor formation in vivo. The PTTG gene is located on chromosome 5q33, a region with a known propensity for development of several malignancies.[43] Increased PTTG mRNA abundance was detected in all GH-producing tumors, with more than 10-fold increases evident in larger tumors.[70] Thus the strong transforming potential of PTTG, as well as its widespread and abundant expression in pituitary tumors, probably indicates a key role in early induction of GH cell transformation, possibly by regulating the expression and action of pituitary growth factors[71] (see Table 22–4).

Familial Syndromes

Acromegaly may occur as a component of MEN syndromes, including the Carney complex or MEN-1. The Carney complex consists of myxomas, spotty skin pigmentation, and testicular, adrenal, and pituitary tumors.[72–75] About 20% of patients with this autosomal dominant syndrome associated with chromosome 2p16 harbor GH-secreting pituitary tumors.[50, 72]

The MEN-1 gene is located on chromosome 11q13, and LOH of chromosome 11q13 occurs in pancreatic, parathyroid, and pituitary tumors of patients with MEN-1.[56, 76] Inactivation of the MEN-1 tumor suppressor gene probably accounts for the syndrome, in accordance with Knudson's "two hit" theory whereby both inherited allelic germ-line mutations and a somatic deletion are required for inactivation of both specific alleles and subsequent tumor formation.[77] MEN-1, an autosomal dominant syndrome, consists of hyperplastic or adenomatous parathyroid glands, endocrine pancreas, and anterior pituitary.[76] Pituitary adenomas develop in almost half these patients, with GH cell adenomas reported in about 10% of afflicted subjects.

Isolated familial acromegaly or gigantism not associated with MEN has rarely been reported.[50, 78, 79] Chromosome 11q13 LOH with no discernible MEN-1 mutation was detected in the pituitary adenomas of two brothers with gigantism.[80]

Epidemiology of Acromegaly

Acromegaly is a rare disease, and accurate assessment of its prevalence in the community has been difficult to ascertain. In Newcastle,

TABLE 22–4. Tumor Suppressor Genes and Oncogenes Associated with GH Cell Adenomas

Gsα	Protein	Defect	Function
Tumor suppressor genes			
Men1	Menin	Mutation or deletion	Nuclear; function unknown
P16INK4a	p16	Methylation	CDK4 inhibitor; loss of cell cycle regulation
Oncogenes			
gsp (GNAS1)	Gsα subunit of G protein	Missense mutation at codon 201 or 227	Inactivates intrinsic GTPase; constitutive activation of adenyl cyclase
H-*ras*	Ras	Missense mutation at codon 12, 13, or 61	Constitutive activation; associated with metastases
Pttg	PTTG	Overexpression	Promotes transformation

GH, growth hormone; GTPase, guanosine triphosphatase; PTTG, pituitary tumor–transforming gene.

Adapted from Drange M, Melmed S: Etiopatogenia de la acromegalia. *In* Webb S (ed): Libro De La Acromegalia. Accion Medica, Barcelona, Spain, 1998.

England, an annual incidence of 2.8 new patients per million adult population was reported, with an approximate point prevalence of 38 cases per million adult population.[81] A higher incidence was reported in Sweden, where the average prevalence of the disease was reported to be 69 cases per million.[2, 82] If these data are projected to the population of the United States, 750 to 900 new cases would be expected annually, and GH-secreting pituitary adenomas would be present, but undiagnosed, in another 10,000 to 20,000 persons. The mean age at diagnosis is 40 to 45 years, and its insidious onset may cause the disease to not be diagnosed until 10 to 12 years after symptom onset.[82–84] This long delay in diagnosis is often due to the subtle and slow onset of common symptoms, including headache, joint pains, jaw malocclusion, or mild type 2 diabetes. Furthermore, this relatively long time delay allows prolonged exposure of peripheral tissues to unacceptably elevated GH and IGF-1 levels.

DIAGNOSIS

Persistent GH hypersecretion is the hallmark of acromegaly. Excess GH stimulates hepatic production of IGF-1, which is responsible for most of the clinical manifestations of acromegaly.[85–87] The diagnosis is often delayed for up to 12 years because of slow clinical progression over many years. Although serum GH and IGF-1 concentrations are both increased in virtually all patients with acromegaly, increases in serum IGF-1 are often disproportional to increases in GH. When a patient is suspected to have acromegaly, biochemical testing is required to confirm the clinical diagnosis, and imaging techniques are used to localize the cause of excess GH secretion (Table 22–5).

Documenting Growth Hormone Hypersecretion

The diagnosis of acromegaly is confirmed by measurement of serum GH after a glucose load and by assessing levels of GH-dependent circulating molecules such as IGF-1 and IGF-binding protein-3 (IGFBP-3).[29] IGF-1 levels reflect the integrated bioeffects of GH hypersecretion, and age- and sex-matched elevated IGF-1 levels are pathognomonic of acromegaly.[88]

Measurement of the serum IGF-1 concentration is the most precise single screening test for acromegaly. Unlike GH, serum IGF-1 concentrations do not fluctuate hourly according to food intake, exercise, or sleep, but instead reflect integrated GH secretion during the preceding day or longer. Serum IGF-1 concentrations, which are gender and age dependent, are elevated in virtually all patients with acromegaly, thus providing excellent discrimination from normal subjects.[2, 85] In normal subjects, serum IGF-1 concentrations are highest during puberty and decline gradually thereafter; values are significantly lower in adults older than 60 years than in younger subjects. Females have higher levels than males do, and pregnancy may also be associated with elevated IGF-1 levels. Thus an inappropriately controlled "normal" IGF-1 value in an elderly male patient may in fact be truly elevated and indicative of acromegaly. Serum GH should be measured in patients with equivocal or elevated age- and sex-adjusted serum IGF-1 values.

Although all patients with acromegaly have increased GH secretion, it may be difficult to distinguish elevated random GH levels from normal. GH levels fluctuate widely throughout the day and night, and measuring random GH levels rarely provides useful information for

TABLE 22–5. Diagnosis of Acromegaly

Biochemical testing
  GH nadir >1 ng/mL during oral glucose load
  Elevated age- and gender-matched IGF-1 level
MRI
  Visualization of pituitary adenoma

GH, growth hormone; IGF-1, insulin-like growth factor-1; MRI, magnetic resonance imaging.

diagnosis of the disorder.[2] Short-term fasting, exercise, stress, and sleep are all associated with elevated GH, and the availability of ultrasensitive GH assays has indicated that this pulsatile GH rhythm may in fact occur at levels below the detectable sensitivity of previously available assays. Serum GH concentrations fluctuate widely, from less than 0.5 to 1 ng/mL (less than 0.1 ng/mL with ultrasensitive assays) during most of the day, to 2 to 5 ng/mL after exercise, to as high as 20 or 30 ng/mL at night or after vigorous exercise. Random serum GH concentrations also may be elevated in patients with uncontrolled diabetes mellitus, liver disease, and malnutrition. Thus several dynamic tests have been proposed to confirm GH hypersecretion. The mean GH concentration obtained from 6-hourly samplings will generally provide an integrated summation of net GH secretion, and averaged pooled levels greater than 5 ng/mL are usually encountered in acromegaly.[2]

The diagnostic hallmark of excess GH hypersecretion is failure to suppress GH levels to less than 2 ng/mL (standard radioimmunoassay) or less than 1 ng/mL (chemiluminescent; immunoradiometric assay) during a 2-hour period after a 75-g oral glucose load.[29] Invariably, these patients will exhibit elevated total IGF-1 levels with a strong log-linear association between the 24-hour mean GH output and IGF-1 levels.[2, 89] About 10% or less of patients may have apparently "normal" GH and/or IGF-1 levels at the time of diagnosis. Repeating the assays in a reputable laboratory may often resolve an apparent clinical-biochemical discordance. Alternatively, reinterpretation of a glucose suppression test or using a rigorous GH assay may confirm the diagnosis.

About 60% of patients with acromegaly also exhibit an evoked GH response (>50%) to thyrotropin-releasing hormone (TRH) (500 μg given intravenously) or, less commonly, to gonadotropin-releasing hormone administration. These discordant responses are seen only in patients with tumorous GH hypersecretion and not in normal subjects. Conversely, levodopa (500 mg orally) reduces serum GH concentrations by 50% or more in about half of patients with acromegaly, whereas it increases GH concentrations in normal subjects.[2]

Because IGFBP-3 secretion is GH dependent, concentrations may be elevated in patients with acromegaly, thus suggesting that IGFBP-3 measurement may prove useful in diagnosis.[90] However, in contrast to the tight correlation of integrated mean 24-hour serum GH with total and free IGF-1 levels, IGFBP-3 levels do not appear to correlate with disease activity.[91, 92] Thirty-two percent of subjects with active acromegaly had normal IGFBP-3 levels, and in patients who failed to suppress GH, no consistent elevation of IGFBP-3 was observed.[91] Thus the utility of IGFBP-3 measurements for diagnosis or follow-up of acromegaly is limited.

Localizing the Source of Excess Growth Hormone

Once a biochemical diagnosis of excess GH hypersecretion is confirmed, MRI of the pituitary to localize the source of hormone excess is indicated. MRI effectively delineates soft tissue pituitary masses, and gadolinium-enhanced MRI may detect adenomas 2 mm in diameter. In about 75% of patients the tumor is a macroadenoma (tumor diameter of 10 mm or more) and may extend to parasellar or suprasellar regions or invade the cavernous sinus. Over 90% of patients will exhibit a discrete pituitary adenoma on MRI, whereas about 10% of patients may in fact harbor a partial or even apparently total empty sella. Functional GH-secreting adenomas may arise in the remnant rim of pituitary tissue surrounding the empty sella and may not be visible on MRI. Rarely, other nonpituitary causes of acromegaly (see above) will require abdominal or chest imaging to localize the source of ectopic GHRH or GH production. Lateral skull radiographs with sellar coned-down tomography or pituitary computed tomographic scans are not usually indicated because they expose patients to unnecessary ionizing radiation and, when compared with MRI techniques, are insensitive, especially in delineating soft tissue changes.

NONPITUITARY ACROMEGALY. Rare nonpituitary causes of acromegaly include a hypothalamic tumor secreting GHRH,[33, 93] a nonendocrine tumor secreting GHRH,[36, 94] or ectopic GH secretion by a nonendocrine tumor.[1, 31, 32] MRI of the head and pituitary should identify some of these tumors. If pituitary MRI findings are normal, abdominal and chest imaging should be performed, followed by catheterization studies in an attempt to demonstrate an arteriovenous GHRH gradient over the suspected tumor bed. In patients with ectopic GHRH secretion, serum GHRH and GH concentrations are both elevated and pituitary MRI reveals a normal-sized or enlarged hyperplastic gland.[95]

An algorithm for the diagnostic evaluation of patients suspected of having acromegaly is shown in Figure 22–1. A normal age- and gender-controlled serum IGF-1 concentration is strong evidence excluding the diagnosis of acromegaly. If the serum IGF-1 concentration is high (or equivocal), serum GH should be measured within 2 hours after oral glucose administration. If pituitary MRI fails to reveal the presence of a discreet adenoma in the presence of clear-cut biochemical evidence of hypersomatotropism, studies to identify the rarely encountered GHRH- or GH-secreting tumors should be undertaken.

Clinical Manifestations

The somatotroph adenoma itself, especially if a macroadenoma, may cause local symptoms such as headache, visual field defects (classically bitemporal hemianopia), and cranial nerve palsies. These compressive features are not unique to acromegaly and may occur with any enlarging sellar mass. Nevertheless, the headache associated with acromegaly is uniquely debilitating and may not be exclusively caused by pressure effects.

The systemic clinical features of acromegaly occur as a consequence of the deleterious impact of elevated serum concentrations of both GH and IFG-1 on peripheral tissues (Table 22–6). The somatic impact of elevated GH includes growth stimulation of a variety of tissues, such as skin, connective tissue, cartilage, bone, and many epithelial tissues, including mucosal surfaces. The metabolic effects of excess GH include nitrogen retention, insulin antagonism, and enhanced lipogenesis.

The onset of acromegaly is insidious and disease progression usually slow. At diagnosis, about 75% of patients are shown to harbor macroadenomas (tumor diameter of 10 mm or greater), and some tumors extend to the parasellar or suprasellar regions.[15] Headaches are the initial symptoms in approximately 60% of patients, and 10% have visual symptoms.

ACRAL OVERGROWTH. Acral and soft tissue overgrowth is invariably a feature of acromegaly. Characteristic findings include an enlarged protruding jaw (macrognathia) with associated mandibular overbite and enlarged, swollen hands and feet resulting in increasing shoe and glove size and the need to enlarge rings. Facial features are coarse, with enlargement of the nose and frontal bones, as well as the jaw; the upper incisors are consequently spread apart. Despite the prominence of these findings, the rate of change is so slow that few

TABLE 22–6. Risks of Long-Term Exposure to Elevated Growth Hormone Levels

Arthropathy
  Unrelated to age of onset or to GH levels
  Usually occurs with acromegaly of long duration
  Reversibility
    Rapid symptomatic improvement with treatment
    Irreversibility of bone and cartilage lesions
Neuropathy
  Peripheral nerves affected
    Intermittent anesthesias, paresthesias
    Sensorimotor polyneuropathy
    Impaired sensation
  Reversibility
    Onion bulbs (whorls) do not regress with lowered GH levels
Cardiovascular disease
  Cardiomyopathy
    Left ventricular diastolic function decreased
    Left ventricular mass increased; arrhythmias
    Fibrous hyperplasia of connective tissue
  Hypertension
    Exacerbates cardiomyopathic changes
  Reversibility
    May progress even with normalized GH levels
Respiratory disease
  Upper airway obstruction
    Caused by soft tissue overgrowth and decreased pharyngeal
      muscle tone
  Reversibility
    Improved with reduction of GH levels
Malignancy
  Increased risk of malignancy
  Increased soft tissue polyps
  Reversibility
    Effect of therapy on risk of malignancy unknown
Carbohydrate intolerance
  Occurs in one-fourth of acromegalics, more often with family
    history of diabetes mellitus
  Reversibility
    Improves with reduced GH levels

GH, growth hormone.
From Melmed S, Dowling RH, Frohman L, et al: Acromegaly: Consensus for cure. Am J Med 97:468, 1994. Copyright 1994, with permission from Excerpta Medica, Inc.

patients seek care because their appearance has changed (e.g., only 13% of 256 patients in one series[5]).

RHEUMATOLOGIC FEATURES. Musculoskeletal symptoms are leading causes of morbidity and serious functional disability in patients with acromegaly.[96, 97] In several studies encompassing large series, at least half of all patients exhibited minor arthralgias, and severe, debili-

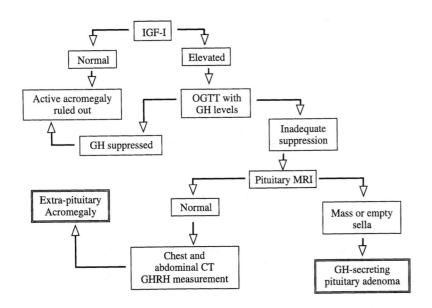

FIGURE 22–1. Diagnosis of acromegaly. CT, computed tomography; GH, growth hormone; GHRH, GH-releasing hormone; IGF-1, insulin-like growth factor-1; MRI, magnetic resonance imaging; OGTT, oral glucose tolerance test. (Adapted from Melmed S: Anterior pituitary. In Korenman S (ed): Current Practice of Medicine. New York, Churchill Livingstone, 1996.)

tating arthritic features ultimately developed in over one-third of patients.[97, 98] The pathogenesis of joint disease in acromegaly generally begins with a noninflammatory osteoarthritic disorder and culminates in severe secondary joint and cartilage degeneration.[97] Excess GH and IGF-1 exposure leads to uneven cartilage proliferation that results in a mechanically unstable joint surface. Joint spaces then narrow as weight-bearing surfaces erode cartilage and cause excess intra-articular new fibrocartilage deposits. Subchondral cysts and osteophytes then develop in an irreversible self-perpetuating process. Severe physical deformity and functional disability result from these inexorable pathologic and mechanical stresses. Although symptomatic and functional relief of arthritic disorders is observed in most patients after lowering GH levels, structural changes are unfortunately not reversible.[98, 99]

Joint arthralgias are a common initial feature of the disease, and back pain and kyphosis are common.[5] Synovial tissue and cartilage enlarge and cause hypertrophic arthropathy of the knees, ankles, hips, spine, and other joints.[97] Back pain may also occur because of osteoporosis caused either by GH excess itself or concurrent gonadal insufficiency from the enlarging pituitary tumor. Spine and hip bone density may be increased in women with acromegaly, but not if estrogen deficiency is present.[100] When excess GH secretion begins before epiphyseal fusion, linear growth increases and causes pituitary gigantism.

SKIN AND SOFT TISSUES. The skin thickens, and multiple recurrent skin tags may appear.[3, 101] Hyperhidrosis at rest is common (present in 50% of patients)[2, 3, 5] and often malodorous. Hair growth increases, and some women have hirsutism.[2, 5, 102] Other manifestations of soft tissue overgrowth include macroglossia, deepening of the voice, and paresthesias of the hands (carpal tunnel syndrome) from nerve entrapment.[2, 5–7, 15, 98] Other patients have a symmetric sensorimotor peripheral (rarely hypertrophic) neuropathy unrelated to entrapment.[96]

THYROID. Thyroid enlargement may be diffuse or multinodular. In a study of 37 patients with acromegaly, 92% had an enlarged thyroid gland when assessed by ultrasound; mean thyroid size was increased more than five times normal.[103] Thyroid function is, however, usually normal.

CARDIOVASCULAR. Impaired cardiovascular function in acromegaly is an important determinant of morbidity and mortality.[3, 104] The deleterious direct impact of excess GH and IGF-1, as well as the effect of hypertension, which is present in 30% of patients, contributes to the disorder.[5, 105, 106] Cardiac enlargement is disproportionate to the increased size of internal body organs,[107–109] and the severity of cardiomyopathy correlates significantly with the duration of exposure to hypersomatotropism.[104, 108, 110] Mean left ventricular mass may be significantly increased to over 200 g, as opposed to a normal mean weight of 140 g, and end-systolic and diastolic volumes are attenuated. Concentric ventricular hypertrophy is associated with interstitial fibrosis, lymphocytic infiltration, and necrosis.[108] Resting diastolic blood pressure and left and right ventricular peak filling rates are elevated. Postexercise systolic and diastolic blood pressure may also be elevated, and the left ventricular ejection fraction is attenuated.[111] Because physiologic doses of replacement GH may also actually improve cardiac function in patients with adult GH deficiency, there appears to be a fine equilibrium for the respective impacts of GH excess and GH deficiency on maintaining healthy myocardial function.[108]

SLEEP APNEA. Peripheral airway obstruction caused by macroglossia, mandible deformation, mucosal hypertrophy, and inspirational laryngeal collapse has long been recognized as causing airway obstruction,[5] snoring, and sleep apnea in up to two-thirds of patients.[3] Macroglossia and enlargement of the soft tissues of the pharynx and larynx lead to obstructive sleep apnea in about 50% of patients; others have central sleep apnea, possibly resulting from altered central respiratory control.[112] Sleep apnea may be an important cause of mortality in these patients. Recently, a central form of sleep apnea has been recognized in acromegaly.[112–114] This disorder appears to correlate more closely with elevated GH and IGF-1 levels and may reflect central respiratory suppression caused by the disregulated hypothalamic-GH axis. Clearly, the strong association of sleep apnea with hypertension, coronary artery disease, and cardiac arrest also reflects the clinical phenotype of patients with acromegaly. Attenuation of GH levels, especially with octreotide, improves or abrogates sleep apnea.[112, 115] After 6 months'

treatment of 14 apneic acromegalic patients with octreotide, a 40% decrease in the number of apneic events per hour was seen, as well as a decrease in total apneic time from 28% to 15%. Maximum O_2 saturation rose from 76% to 84%, accompanied by a decline in daytime sleepiness, as well as improvement in central and obstructive apneic parameters.[112]

DIABETES. GH is a potent antagonist of insulin action, and glucose intolerance is encountered in up to 60% of patients. About 25% of patients may require insulin, and thus diabetes is an important systemic complication of hypersomatotropism. Diabetes is a major determinant of mortality, and only 30% of patients with diabetes at the time that acromegaly is diagnosed appear to survive 20 years.[83, 116]

GONADAL FUNCTION. Women with acromegaly may have amenorrhea, with or without galactorrhea,[3, 15, 117] and some have hot flashes and vaginal atrophy. Men may have impotence, loss of libido, decreased facial hair growth, and testicular atrophy.[3, 7, 117] Hypogonadism is caused either by hyperprolactinemia (present in about 30% of patients)[102, 117] or by impairment of gonadotropin secretion as the expanding pituitary tumor compresses normal pituitary gonadotroph cells. Asymptomatic reversible prostatic enlargement is also common, even in men with hypogonadism.[118, 119]

NEOPLASMS. Acromegaly is associated with a significantly enhanced risk for the development of colonic polyps and gastrointestinal cancer.[101, 120–122] Retrospective studies have reported premalignant adenomatous colonic polyps in up to 30% of patients.[101, 122–124] Patients with acromegaly are more likely to have multiple adenomatous polyps, as well as polyps proximal to the splenic flexure, which are less likely to be diagnosed during sigmoidoscopy.[121, 125] No difference in the duration or degree of acromegaly is evident in patients with or without adenomatous polyps. In a retrospective review, malignant tumors, including adenocarcinomas of the colon, stomach, and esophagus and melanoma, developed in approximately 10% of patients with acromegaly.[126] The increase in colon cancer (odds ratio of 3.1–13.5) reflects the high rate of adenoma formation in these patients. However, a multicenter retrospective study of 1362 patients with acromegaly found a lower cancer rate than in the general population (standardized incidence ratio of 0.76) but an increased colon cancer mortality rate.[127] The enhanced mortality correlated with persistently elevated serum GH concentrations but was not observed in patients with posttreatment serum GH levels below 2.5 ng/mL.[128, 129] Colonoscopy is therefore recommended at diagnosis for all patients and periodically thereafter.

Laboratory Findings

Patients with acromegaly exhibit increased serum GH and IGF-1 concentrations and may have hyperglycemia, with frank diabetes occurring in 25% of patients. Some patients have hypertriglyceridemia. Hypercalciuria and hyperphosphatemia (not >5.5 mg/dL) occur in approximately 70% of patients as a result of direct stimulation of renal tubular phosphate reabsorption by IGF-1.[102]

Hyperprolactinemia occurs in about 30% of patients and is due to co-secretion of PRL and GH by the tumor or to stalk interference with hypothalamic-pituitary portal delivery of dopamine. Secretion of other pituitary hormones, especially gonadotropins, may also be decreased. Elevated plasma fibrinogen concentrations revert to normal with therapy, which suggests that effective treatment of acromegaly may prevent cardiovascular morbidity.[130]

Mortality

The overall mortality rate in acromegaly is about two to four times that of the general population.[129, 131, 132] Up to 50% of patients die before 50 years of age, and up to 89% die before the age of 60 years.[2, 133] In a series of 151 patients, survival was reduced an average of 10 years in comparison to age-matched controls.[83]

Although mortality and morbidity in acromegaly are significantly correlated with cardiovascular, pulmonary, and neoplastic disorders, the single most significant determinant of survival is the level of

TABLE 22–7. Outcome Determinants of Acromegaly

Causes of Death	%	Survival Determinants	P Value
Cardiovascular	38–62	Last known GH	.0001
Respiratory	0–25	Hypertension	.02
Malignancy	9–25	Cardiac disease	.03
		Diabetes	.03
		Symptom duration	.04

Elevated mortality is reversed by suppressing growth hormone (GH).
Data from Wright, 1969; Alexander et al., 1980; Nabarro, 1987; Bengtsson et al., 1988; Rajasoorya, 1994; Bates, 1994; Swearingen et al., 1998; Abosch et al., 1998; and Freda et al., 1998.

posttreatment GH[83] (Table 22–7). Several retrospective studies now indicate that survival in acromegaly may be normalized to a control age-matched rate by controlling GH levels[128, 129, 131]; in particular, life-table analysis showed that GH levels less than 2.5 ng/mL were associated with survival rates equal to those of the general population.[131, 134] Thus tight control of GH through aggressive multimodal therapy appears to reduce mortality risk to that expected for nonacromegalic subjects.[84, 128, 129]

MANAGEMENT

Treatment Goals for Acromegaly

Treatment goals for acromegaly embody principles that apply to treating hormonal hypersecretory tumors. Treatment should be both safe and efficacious. GH and IGF-1 levels should be normalized, especially because elevated GH levels have been associated with mortality in these patients. Thus tight GH control is an important therapeutic endpoint.[84] Tumor mass effects, especially central compression of visual tracts, should be alleviated. Pituitary function should also be preserved, and if hypopituitarism develops, patients require lifelong pituitary replacement. Importantly, clinical features of the disease that lead to the characteristic morbidity and ultimately to mortality should be ameliorated. Several treatment options are available for acromegaly. Transsphenoidal surgical resection of the adenoma, pharmacologic therapy with somatostatin analogues and dopamine agonists, and various modes of radiation therapy are used to treat GH-secreting adenomas. The challenge of tight GH control in acromegaly can now be met with greater stringency by using single or multimodal forms of therapy. Effective disease control should thus include sustained hormone suppression, a contained adenoma mass, improved systemic morbidity, and ultimately, normalized mortality (Table 22–8).

Surgery

Surgery for the treatment of GH-secreting pituitary tumors was pioneered in the early part of the century by Dr. Harvey Cushing, who demonstrated successful resection of such tumors by a transsphenoidal approach. This technique is standard, and only very rarely do large masses that extend far beyond the sella turcica require a transfrontal approach. The most important determinant of a successful surgical outcome is the experience of the surgeon. Recently, endoscopic approaches to pituitary adenoma resection have proved to be efficacious.[135, 136]

Surgery rapidly alleviates acromegaly symptoms, removes the tumor mass, relieves optic tract pressure effects, and relieves headache. Tumor debulking, even if partial, may also be helpful in enhancing the effectiveness of subsequent therapy. Surgical control is also inversely correlated with initial tumor size and GH levels.[137, 138] Not all patients are appropriate surgical candidates, usually because of coexisting cardiovascular and pulmonary disease, which may be a contraindication to anesthesia. If the tumor is sufficiently large or invasive and portends intraoperative damage to vital structures, the benefits of the procedure should be weighed against surgical risks.

Results of surgical resection of GH-secreting adenomas have only recently included more stringent biochemical criteria. Short-term remission (GH, 5 μg/L) was achieved in 76% of 254 patients, with most of 129 patients remaining in long-term remission.[129] Although the biochemical parameter of "basal" GH less than 5 μg/L used in this study does not reflect normalization of GH hypersecretion, even with this less stringent criterion the postsurgical mortality outcome was equivalent to that of age- and sex-matched controls, in contrast to the 2.4- to 4.8-fold enhanced mortality observed in patients with persistent disease (GH, >5 ug/L). In another study that used more stringent criteria (normalized IGF-1 levels or GH suppression to 2 μg/L after glucose loading), over 90% of patients harboring microadenomas successfully achieved these criteria.[128] However, less than 50% of patients harboring macroadenomas are biochemically controlled.[128, 138, 139] Unfortunately, most tumors encountered at diagnosis are large macroadenomas. In these invasive tumors, surgical resection is invariably followed by persistent GH and or IGF-1 hypersecretion. Visible residual tumor mass is often contiguous with or involves the cavernous sinus, internal carotid arteries, or suprasellar regions. Mortality risk in patients cured at surgery does not differ from that of controls, whereas in patients with persistent disease, even after adjuvant irradiation or medical therapy, mortality remains significantly increased (almost 2-fold). Thus the level of GH attained postsurgically is the most important determinant of mortality outcome.[83] However, regardless of the treatment mode, normalization of GH restores mortality risk to that of age-matched population controls and postoperative disease persistence is associated with a 3.5-fold relative mortality risk.[128]

TABLE 22–8. Treatment Options for Acromegaly

Surgery	Somatostatin Analogue	Radiotherapy	Dopamine Agonists (High Dose)
Efficacy			
Microsurgery GH controlled in 80%	GH controlled in ~65% of patients within weeks	GH <5 ng/mL in 905 of patients in 18 yr	GH <5 ng/mL in 15%
Macrosurgery GH controlled in <50%			
Normal IGF-1 in ~50%	Normal IGF-1 in ~70%	Normal IGF-1 in <5%	Normal IGF-1 in <10%
Advantages			
Rapid onset	No hypopituitarism	Permanent	Oral administration
One-time cost	Rapid onset	One-time cost	Low cost
May be permanent	Continued efficacy	Good patient compliance	No hypopituitarism
Disadvantages			
New hypopituitarism (10%)	Cost of drug and monitoring	Ineffective and slow onset	Relatively ineffective
Diabetes insipidus (2–3%)	Asymptomatic gallstones (25%)	Hypopituitarism (50%)	Adverse events (~30%)
Local complications (~6%)	Injections required	Visual/CNS dysfunction (~2%)	High dose required
Cranial nerve/CNS damage (~1%)		Cost of interim medical therapy	
Tumor persistence			

CNs, central nervous system; GH, growth hormone; IGF-1, insulin-like growth factor.
Adapted from Melmed S, Jackson I, Kleinberg D, et al: Current treatment guidelines for acromegaly. J Clin Endocrinol Metab 83:2646–2652, 1998. © The Endocrine Society.

SIDE EFFECTS. The most important adverse surgical event is failure to totally resect invasive tumor and, consequently, persistent hormonal hypersecretion. Postoperative complications occur in approximately 10% of patients, and their incidence is largely dependent on the experience of the operating surgeon.[140] Complications include permanent diabetes insipidus, cerebrospinal fluid leaks requiring repair, meningitis, severe sinusitis, and hypopituitarism.[82, 133, 139–141] Perioperative morbidity and residual pituitary failure remain of concern in patients with invasive tumors, especially when operated on by less experienced surgeons.

In summary, surgical success is based largely on skill and experience and on tumor size or invasiveness. Surgery is useful for prompt lowering of GH levels, and tumor debulking may enhance the effectiveness of medical therapy. After apparent successful resection, however, up to 8% of tumors recur within 10 years. GH levels should be measured in the immediate postoperative period, and evidence of GH hypersecretion at this time portends either disease persistence or long-term recurrence. By immunoradiometric GH assay, postglucose GH values less than 1.0 µg/L are found in 50% of patients after surgery, and in 39% of patients with normalized IGF-1 levels, GH levels still fail to be suppressed.[142]

Pituitary Irradiation

Techniques for pituitary radiotherapy include external radiation using either a cyclotron or a cobalt-60 source, and the radiotherapy is administered as a total dose of 4500 to 5000 rad. Higher doses are associated with a high incidence of side effects, whereas lower doses, although safer, appear to be less clinically effective. The total dose is given as 25 daily 180- to 200-rad fractions administered over a 6-week period.[143] Maximal tumor irradiation with minimal damage to nontumorous surrounding tissue has been achieved by advances in stereotactic MRI-directed tumor localization, focused beam direction, field size simulation, head immobilization, and isocentral rotational techniques.[144]

Proton-beam therapy also decreases GH secretion but is not widely available. Stereotactic ablation of GH-secreting adenomas by gamma knife radiosurgery is a promising new technique for which long-term results are not yet available. In 16 postsurgical patients monitored for up to 2.6 years, GH levels of less than 5 ng/mL and normalized IGF-1 concentrations were observed within 16 months of stereotactic radiosurgery.[145] However, the short follow-up precludes an assessment of complication outcome.

Tumor growth is invariably arrested after fractionated radiotherapy, but GH decline is slow, dropping by approximately 20% per year. Within 18 years, 90% of patients have random serum GH concentrations lower than 5 ng/mL.[143] The degree and rapidity of GH attenuation are highly dependent on pretreatment GH levels.[143] However, few patients achieve the currently accepted rigorous goal of therapy, that is, a glucose-suppressed serum GH concentration less than 1 ng/mL. In one series, only 5 of 30 patients monitored for 10 or more years achieved this goal. After radiotherapy in 38 patients, 20 of whom had preradiotherapy IGF-1 data available, GH levels fell by about 60% 3.5 years after irradiation and by about 80% 7 years after radiotherapy. However, plasma levels of IGF-1 remained almost unchanged and did not decrease below 80% of the initial value, even 7 years after radiotherapy. Only 2 patients ultimately exhibited normalized IGF levels.[146] The failure of irradiation to effectively normalize IGF-1 levels in the long term implies persistent, albeit low levels of GH hypersecretion in these patients.[146]

SIDE EFFECTS. Pituitary failure will develop in 50% of patients undergoing deep x-ray therapy by 10 years and require thyroid, gonadal, and/or adrenal steroid replacement.[1, 29] Rarely, optic tract damage results in visual deficits. Ten years after radiotherapy, patients have a small, but significant risk of a secondary brain malignancy, including glioma, in up to 1.7% of patients (relative risk of 16 vs. expected).[147–149] Radiation may also rarely induce brain parenchymal changes[149–151] and brain dysfunction manifested as depression, decreased memory, decreased general quality of life, loss of vision, and

cranial nerve palsies.[141, 152] Long-term controlled results and side effect profiles for gamma knife radiosurgery are not yet available.

Thus radiotherapy is effective in acromegaly, although its benefits are dose and time dependent and GH reduction is delayed by 10 to 15 years. Even with the best techniques, GH levels below 2.0 ng/mL and normalization of IGF-1 levels are infrequently achieved.[146, 153] Therefore, radiation therapy may be useful for patients with growing pituitary tumors whose condition is not controlled by surgery or who are resistant to medical therapy.

Medical Management

Octreotide

Octreotide is a synthetic octapeptide analogue of native naturally occurring somatostatin. This eight–amino acid analogue (molecular weight of 1019) binds selectively to the SSTR2 somatostatin receptor subtype.[154] After subcutaneous injection, octreotide is rapidly absorbed, and peak drug concentrations (5.5 ng/mL) are achieved within 24 minutes of a 100-µg injection. The plasma distribution is about 12 minutes, and the elimination half-life is 1.5 hours, as compared with 2 minutes for natural SRIF.[154, 155]

Octreotide inhibits GH, glucagon, and insulin release, but the analogue exhibits greater selectivity in suppressing GH and glucagon than does somatostatin.[154] In normal subjects, octreotide attenuates GH stimulation evoked by arginine,[156] exercise, and insulin-induced hypoglycemia.[157, 158] The drug may also abrogate the postprandial release of gastrointestinal and pancreatic peptides.[158] Because native somatostatin suppresses thyroid-stimulating hormone (TSH) secretion, it is not surprising that octreotide also blocks the TRH-induced release of TSH.[156, 158, 159] In acromegaly, octreotide lowers GH levels (by >50%) in over 95% of all patients.

In the long term, about 70% of patients will have integrated GH levels suppressed to below 5 ng/mL, and about 55% of patients have GH levels suppressed to less than 2 ng/mL. Seventy percent or more of patients will have their IGF-1 levels normalized after long-term treatment with octreotide (Fig. 22–2). Hypopituitarism will not develop while taking octreotide because octreotide binds selectively to the somatostatin receptor subtype that regulates GH secretion.[160] In addition to its effects on suppressing GH and IGF-1 levels, headache, fatigue, perspiration, joint pains, carpal tunnel syndrome, and paresthesias improve in most patients treated long term.

The starting dose of octreotide is 50 µg given subcutaneously in 8-hourly doses, and after 2 weeks, the dose can be increased to 100 µg three times daily. Thereafter, dose titrations to a maximum of 1500 µg/day may be made depending on the nadir 2-hour postinjection GH level. The efficacy of octreotide can also be improved by increasing the dose frequency, although not necessarily increasing the total daily drug dose, or by administering the drug in a continuous-infusion minipump. Interestingly, long-term (>3 years) use of the drug is associated with enhanced sensitivity and improved biochemical control. Tachyphylaxis does not occur, and downregulation of receptor responses does not appear to be manifested clinically.[159] About half of all patients will exhibit tumor shrinkage (30% average tumor volume change).

GROWTH HORMONE RESPONSE TO LONG-TERM DEPOT PREPARATIONS. Several long-term depot somatostatin preparations are now available. The best-studied drugs are octreotide LAR (long-acting release) and lanreotide.[155, 159, 161, 162] Octreotide LAR incorporates octreotide into microspheres of a biodegradable poly-D,L-lactide-co-glycolide glucose polymer. After three monthly injections of the depot preparation, sustained octreotide concentrations are maintained.

Figure 22–3 depicts the pharmacokinetic response to octreotide LAR in acromegaly. After a single injection of octreotide LAR, drug levels peak at about 28 days after injection and fall slowly thereafter. GH levels decline after the injection and, by day 14, are suppressed to less than 2 µg/L. GH suppression (as determined by measurement of integrated secretion over a 4-hour period) is sustained through day 49 and starts rising thereafter. From the pharmacokinetic curve it is

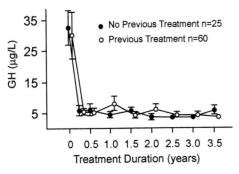

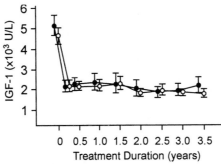

FIGURE 22–2. Growth hormone (GH) and insulin-like growth factor-1 (IGF-1) concentrations with long-term octreotide treatment. (From Newman C, Melmed S, George A, et al: Octreotide as primary therapy for acromegaly. J Clin Endocrinol Metab 83:3034, 1998. © The Endocrine Society.)

apparent that a single injection administered every 30 days will allow GH levels to be persistently suppressed throughout the month. Figure 22–4 depicts the effects of a single, monthly injection of octreotide LAR in a group of patients with acromegaly whose average GH levels were suppressed for the duration of the study (up to 31 months). GH suppression appears to be sustained as long as patients receive monthly injections of octreotide LAR.

Long-term treatment with octreotide LAR reduces mean 4-hour serum GH values to less than 5 µg/L in 90% of subjects and to less than 2.5 µg/L in 70% of subjects. IGF-1 values are normalized in over 65%. Clinical improvement is sustained, with little systemic or local intolerance. Thus administration of octreotide LAR results in persistent therapeutic serum drug concentrations and sustained suppression of both GH and IGF-1 values. The incidence of gallstones, microlithiasis, biliary sediment, or biliary sludge does not differ from that after subcutaneous octreotide (see below).

SIDE EFFECTS. Although octreotide is relatively safe in the long term, several important adverse events are reported. Asymptomatic echogenic gallbladder lesions develop in about 25% of patients.[29] These lesions include both sludge and gallstones, which are usually diagnosed within the first 2 years of treatment, with few, if any new echogenic events encountered thereafter. The prevalence of gallstones during octreotide therapy appears to vary geographically. In China, gallstones will ultimately develop in most patients taking octreotide[163]; on the other hand, patients in southern Europe exhibit a far lower incidence. Clearly, dietary and/or other environmental factors play a role in their pathogenesis. Transient gastrointestinal symptoms, including anorexia, nausea, vomiting, flatulence, and loose stools, may occur, especially during the first 2 weeks of therapy; these symptoms may be ameliorated by injecting the medication between meals or at night. Rarely, fat malabsorption and bradycardia have been reported.

In summary, long-acting somatostatin analogues[84] are effective and safe in managing GH hypersecretion in patients in whom surgical resection has failed to achieve a stringent biochemical remission. Somatostatin analogues may also be offered as primary therapy for patients who refuse surgery, have medical risk factors that contraindicate surgery, or have undergone irradiation, in whom GH levels may yet remain unacceptably elevated for up to 15 years or more.[29, 84, 164] Most patients harboring macroadenomas have persistent postsurgical GH hypersecretion, and the use of SRIF analogues should be weighed against radiotherapy for these patients. Long-acting injectable depot analogues administered once every 14 to 30 days provide enhanced patient convenience and compliance while retaining drug sensitivity.[84, 165, 166] Prior surgery appears to not alter the long-term efficacy of somatostatin analogues in attaining biochemical control. However, drug cost and patient compliance need to be factored in when deciding on therapeutic options.

Dopamine Agonists

High doses of dopamine agonists have been used for several years in the management of these patients, and bromocriptine is associated with GH normalization in less than 15% of patients. A large meta-analysis revealed that only 20% of patients will achieve GH levels less than 5 ng/mL, which is not a maximal criterion for control. Only 10% or less of all patients will actually have IGF-1 levels normalized. However, bromocriptine does not carry with it a risk for hypopituitarism, and because it is an orally available medication, it is extremely convenient and cost-effective for the patient.[168] Cabergoline, a long-acting dopamine agonist, has recently been used in acromegaly, but the long-term results are not yet compelling.[168–170]

ADVERSE EVENTS. Because high doses (>20 mg/day) are required to achieve even moderate efficacy, the incidence of adverse events is far higher than usually seen when treating patients with prolactinomas. Patients receiving high doses of dopamine agonists complain of gastrointestinal symptoms, including nausea, vomiting, and abdominal cramps. Rarely, arrhythmias have been reported. Nasal stuffiness and sleep disturbances are common complaints.[167, 171, 172]

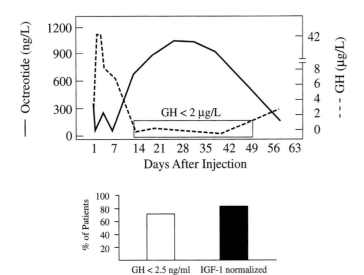

FIGURE 22–3. Pharmacokinetics of octreotide, long-acting release (LAR). GH, growth hormone; IGF-1, insulin-like growth factor.

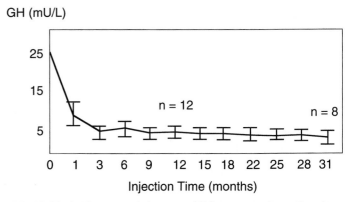

FIGURE 22–4. Mean growth hormone (GH) concentration with octreotide (long-acting release) long-term treatment. (From Davies PH, Stewart SE, Lancranjan I, et al: Long-term therapy with long-acting octreotide (Sandostatin-LAR) for the management of acromegaly. Clin Endocrinol 48:311, 1998.)

Integrated Approach to the Management of Acromegaly

Treatment Approach for Acromegaly: Patients with Likelihood of Good Surgical Outcome

Once acromegaly is diagnosed, the likelihood of surgical cure is assessed (Fig. 22–5). For small well-circumscribed tumors, surgical excision by an experienced pituitary surgeon is the treatment of choice. Surgical cure rates are maximal for noninvasive, well-encapsulated smaller tumors. If a good surgical outcome is predicted, that is, a 60% chance or better that the disease will be controlled by tumor excision, surgery is indicated. After surgery, patients are monitored to ensure that GH responses to a glucose load are less than 1 ng/mL and that IGF-1 levels are normalized. If, however, after surgery hormone levels are not controlled, indicative of disease persistence or recurrence, either short- or long-acting somatostatin analogues are indicated.[29]

After drug initiation, GH responses to glucose and IGF-1 levels are monitored for assessment of disease control. If the patient is still not biochemically controlled by these criteria, a dopamine agonist is added or reoperation or irradiation is considered.

Patients with a Poor Likelihood of Successful Surgical Outcome

Patients with large adenomas are likely to have a poor surgical outcome, and less than half of them will be biochemically controlled. Most patients in whom acromegaly is newly diagnosed harbor large macroadenomas, which portend a poor surgical outcome. These patients can be offered primary treatment with somatostatin analogues, as would patients in whom surgery is contraindicated or who decline surgery. Because the drug may reduce tumor bulk, subsequent surgery may in fact be rendered easier, although no prospective data yet support this principle. If biochemical control is not achieved, drug efficacy may be improved by dose increases and the addition of a dopamine agonist, and ultimately these patients are candidates for surgery, irradiation, or investigational treatment with a GH receptor antagonist.[29]

Follow-up

Laboratory follow-up of patients includes performance of an oral glucose load and measurement of GH levels during the subsequent 2 hours. Stringent responses include GH less than 1 ng/mL, accompanied by a normalized IGF-1 level. If these goals are not achieved, medical treatment should be initiated, and if already being administered, efficacy may be improved by increasing medication dose frequency or adding a dopamine agonist. Reoperation and radiation therapy are further adjuvant options. Pituitary MRI should be repeated after 6 to 12 months in patients with macroadenomas, depending on the degree of local pressure signs. In patients with tumors that have been effectively excised, serial MRI is warranted only once every 2 years after surgery. Invasive residual tumors require more frequent MRI evaluation. Although tumor mass may not invariably shrink with somatostatin analogue therapy, further progressive tumor growth rarely occurs while patients are taking the medication.

General

Patients with acromegaly require management of multiple associated medical disorders. Colonoscopy should be performed at the time of diagnosis. The presence of risk factors for colon cancer, including more than three skin tags, a family history, age older than 50 years, or the presence of previous polyps, requires more aggressive colonoscopic monitoring. Because cardiovascular morbidity is so high in patients with acromegaly, aggressive management of hypertension, left ventricular hypertrophy, cardiac failure, and arrhythmias should be pursued. Pulmonary function and sleep evaluation should be undertaken in all patients early in the course of the disorder, and debilitating arthritis requires aggressive rheumatologic management. Screening and therapy for insulin resistance and diabetes are important, and somatostatin analogues usually improve diabetes control dramatically. Insulin requirements may immediately drop to 90% of pretreatment needs as GH is effectively suppressed. Headache is an extremely common symptom and usually improves with somatostatin analogues; if not, potent analgesics may be indicated. Maxillofacial disorders may require dental, maxillary, and facial cosmetic surgery. Fertility is commonly of concern to patients, and several recent reports of successful pregnancies in women treated with octreotide provide optimistic guidelines for pregnancy management.[111, 173] Nevertheless, octreotide is not approved by the Food and Drug Administration for use during pregnancy. Patients with acromegaly may be depressed and suffer from low self-esteem and other psychosocial sensitivity.[174] Thus careful individual or group counseling may be indicated to assist patients with these issues. Finally, because all the available treatment modes for

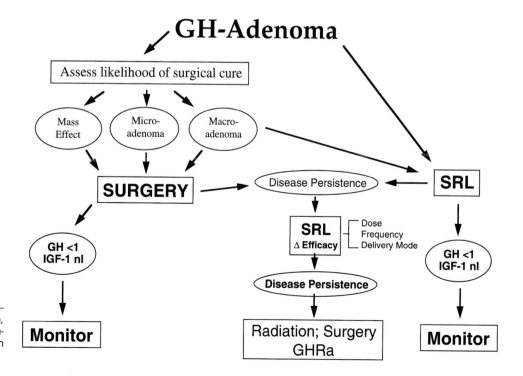

FIGURE 22–5. Management of acromegaly. GH, growth hormone; GHRa, GH receptor antagonist; IGF-1, insulin-like growth factor-1; SRL, somatostatin receptor ligand.

acromegaly are associated with therapy-specific complications, they should be carefully watched for and, if they occur, promptly treated.

The availability of long-acting depot preparations of somatostatin analogues has changed the approach to management inasmuch as patient compliance and medication acceptance are expected to improve markedly. These slow-release formulations requiring single injections once every 2 to 4 weeks are at least as effective as subcutaneous octreotide in normalizing IGF-1 in 75% of patients; their side effect profile appears quite similar. In the future, the potential availability of injectable GH receptor antagonists[175] and oral formulations of selective somatostatin receptor ligands[160] will provide promising new therapeutic avenues for patients manifesting GH hypersecretory syndromes.

REFERENCES

1. Melmed S: Acromegaly. N Engl J Med 322:966–977, 1990.
2. Barkan AL: Acromegaly: Diagnosis and therapy. Endocrinol Metab Clin North Am 18:277–310, 1989.
3. Molitch ME: Clinical manifestations of acromegaly. Endocrinol Metab Clin North Am 21:597–614, 1992.
4. Marie P: Sur deux cas d'acromegalie: Hypertrophie singuliere non congenitale des extremites superieures et cephalique. Rev Med 6:297–333, 1886.
5. Nabarro JDN: Acromegaly. Clin Endocrinol (Oxf) 26:481–512, 1987.
6. Reichlin S: Acromegaly. Med Grnd Rnds 1:9–24, 1982.
7. Jadresic A, Banks LM, Child DF, et al: The acromegaly syndrome: Relation between clinical features, growth hormone values and radiological characteristics of the pituitary tumours. Q J Med 51:189–204, 1982.
8. Frohman LA, Jansson JO: Growth hormone–releasing hormone. Endocr Rev 7:223–253, 1986.
9. Thorner MO, Vance ML: Growth hormone, 1988. J Clin Invest 82:745–747, 1988.
10. Yamashita S, Melmed S: Insulin-like growth factor I regulation of growth hormone gene transcription in primary rat pituitary cells. J Clin Invest 79:449–452, 1987.
11. Berelowitz M, Szabo M, Frohman LA, et al: Somatomedin-C mediates growth hormone negative feedback by effects on both the hypothalamus and the pituitary. Science 212:1279–1281, 1981.
12. Melmed S, Yamashita S, Yamasaki H, et al: IGF-1 receptor signaling: Lessons from the somatotroph. Recent Prog Horm Res 51:189–215, 1996.
13. Veldhuis JD, Liem AY, South S, et al: Differential impact of age, sex steroid hormones, and obesity on basal versus pulsatile growth hormone secretion in men as assessed in an ultrasensitive chemiluminescence assay. J Clin Endocrinol Metab 80:3209–3222, 1995.
14. Carter-Su C, Schwartz J, Smit LS: Molecular mechanism of growth hormone action. Annu Rev Physiol 58:187–207, 1996.
15. Daniels GH, Martin JB: Neuroendocrine regulation and diseases of the anterior pituitary and hypothalamus. In Wilson JD, Braunwald E, Isselbacher KJ, et al (eds): Harrison's Principles of Internal Medicine, ed 12. New York, McGraw-Hill, 1991, pp 1655–1679.
16. D'Ercole AJ, Stiles AD, Underwood LE: Tissue concentrations of somatomedin C: Further evidence for multiple sites of synthesis and paracrine or autocrine mechanisms of action. Proc Natl Acad Sci U S A 81:935–939, 1984.
17. Drange MR, Melmed S: IGFs in the evaluation of acromegaly. In Rosenfeld RG, Roberts CT (eds): Contemporary Endocrinology. The IGF System: Molecular Biology, Physiology, and Clinical Applications. Clifton, NJ, Humana, 1999, pp 699–720.
18. Jones JI, Clemmons DR: Insulin-like growth factors and their binding proteins: Biological actions. Endocr Rev 16:3–34, 1995.
19. Van Wyk JJ: The somatomedins: Biological and physiologic control mechanisms. In Growth Factors. Orlando, FL, Academic, 1984, pp 81–125.
20. Isaksson OG, Lindahl A, Nilsson A, et al: Mechanism of the stimulatory effect of growth hormone on longitudinal bone growth. Endocr Rev 8:426–438, 1987.
21. Spencer GS, Hodgkinson SC, Bass JJ: Passive immunization against insulin-like growth factor-I does not inhibit growth hormone–stimulated growth of dwarf rats. Endocrinology 128:2103–2109, 1991.
22. Herman V, Fagin J, Gonsky R, et al: Clonal origin of pituitary adenomas. J Clin Endocrinol Metab 71:1427–1433, 1990.
23. Melmed S, Braunstein GD, Horvath E, et al: Pathophysiology of acromegaly. Endocr Rev 4:271–290, 1983.
24. Drange MR, Melmed S: Molecular pathogenesis of acromegaly. Pituitary 2:43–50, 1999.
25. Frawley LS, Boockfor FR: Mammosomatotropes: Presence and functions in normal and neoplastic pituitary tissue. Endocr Rev 12:337–355, 1991.
26. Asa SL, Kovacs K, Horvath E, et al: Human fetal adenohypophysis: Electron microscopic and ultrastructural immunocytochemical analysis. Neuroendocrinology 48:423–431, 1988.
27. Horvath E, Kovacs K, Singer W, et al: Acidophil stem cell adenoma of the human pituitary: Clinicopathologic analysis of 15 cases. Cancer 47:761–771, 1981.
28. Weinstein LS, Shenker A, Gejman PV, et al: Activating mutations of the stimulatory G protein in the McCune-Albright syndrome. N Engl J Med 325:1688–1695, 1991.
29. Melmed S, Jackson I, Kleinberg D, et al: Current treatment guidelines for acromegaly. J Clin Endocrinol Metab 83:2646–2652, 1998.
30. Melmed S, Ezrin C, Kovacs K, et al: Acromegaly due to secretion of growth hormone by an ectopic pancreatic islet-cell tumor. N Engl J Med 312:9–17, 1985.
31. Sparagana M, Phillips G, Hoffman C, et al: Ectopic growth hormone syndrome associated with lung cancer. Metabolism 20:730–736, 1971.
32. Kaganowicz A, Farkouh NH, Frantz AG, et al: Ectopic human growth hormone in ovaries and breast cancer. J Clin Endocrinol Metab 48:5–8, 1979.
33. Sano T, Asa SL, Kovacs K: Growth hormone–releasing hormone–producing tumors: Clinical, biochemical, and morphological manifestations. Endocr Rev 9:357–373, 1988.
34. Asa SL, Scheithauer BW, Bilbao JM, et al: A case for hypothalamic acromegaly: A clinicopathological study of six patients with hypothalamic gangliocytomas producing growth hormone–releasing factor. J Clin Endocrinol Metab 58:796–803, 1984.
35. Oberg K, Norheim I, Wide L: Serum growth hormone in patients with carcinoid tumours: Basal levels and response to glucose and thyrotrophin releasing hormone. Acta Endocrinol (Copenh) 109:13–18, 1985.
36. Thorner MO, Perryman RL, Cronin MJ, et al: Somatotroph hyperplasia: Successful treatment of acromegaly by removal of a pancreatic islet tumor secreting a growth hormone–releasing factor. J Clin Invest 70:965–977, 1982.
37. Ashcraft MW, Hartzband PI, Van Herle AJ, et al: A unique growth factor in patients with acromegaloidism. J Clin Endocrinol Metab 57:272–276, 1983.
38. Levy A, Lightman SL: Growth hormone–releasing hormone transcripts in human pituitary adenomas. J Clin Endocrinol Metab 74:1474–1476, 1992.
39. Levy L, Bourdais J, Mouhieddine B, et al: Presence and characterization of the somatostatin precursor in normal human pituitaries and in growth hormone secreting adenomas. J Clin Endocrinol Metab 76:85–90, 1993.
40. Billestrup N, Swanson LW, Vale W: Growth hormone–releasing factor stimulates proliferation of somatotrophs in vitro. Proc Natl Acad Sci U S A 83:6854–6857, 1986.
41. Mayo KE, Hammer RE, Swanson LW, et al: Dramatic pituitary hyperplasia in transgenic mice expressing a human growth hormone–releasing factor gene. Mol Endocrinol 2:606–612, 1988.
42. Kovacs M, Kineman RD, Schally AV, et al: Effects of antagonists of growth hormone–releasing hormone (GHRH) on GH and insulin-like growth factor I levels in transgenic mice overexpressing the human GHRH gene, an animal model of acromegaly. Endocrinology 138:4536–4542, 1997.
43. Shimon I, Melmed S: Genetic basis of endocrine disease: Pituitary tumor pathogenesis. J Clin Endocrinol Metab 82:1675–1681, 1997.
44. Spada A, Arosio M, Bochicchio D, et al: Clinical, biochemical, and morphological correlates in patients bearing growth hormone–secreting pituitary tumors with or without constitutively active adenylyl cyclase. J Clin Endocrinol Metab 71:1421–1426, 1990.
45. Vallar L, Spada A, Giannattasio G: Altered Gs and adenylate cyclase activity in human GH-secreting pituitary adenomas. Nature 330:566–568, 1987.
46. Bertherat J, Chanson P, Montminy M: The cyclic adenosine 3′,5′-monophosphate-responsive factor CREB is constitutively activated in human somatotroph adenomas. Mol Endocrinol 9:777–783, 1995.
47. Hashimoto K, Koga M, Motomura T, et al: Identification of alternatively spliced messenger ribonucleic acid encoding truncated growth hormone–releasing hormone receptor in human pituitary adenomas. J Clin Endocrinol Metab 80:2933–2939, 1995.
48. Molitch ME: Prolactinoma. In Melmed S (ed): The Pituitary. Cambridge, Blackwell, 1995, pp 443–477.
49. Melmed S, Ho K, Klibanski A, et al: Clinical review 75: Recent advances in pathogenesis, diagnosis, and management of acromegaly. J Clin Endocrinol Metab 80:3395–3402, 1995.
50. Gadelha MR, Prezant TR, Une KN, et al: Loss of heterozygosity on chromosome 11q13 in two families with acromegaly/gigantism is independent of mutations of the multiple endocrine neoplasia type I gene. J Clin Endocrinol Metab 84:249–256, 1999.
51. Bates AS, Farrell WE, Bicknell EJ, et al: Allelic deletion in pituitary adenomas reflects aggressive biological activity and has potential value as a prognostic marker. J Clin Endocrinol Metab 82:818–824, 1997.
52. Fero ML, Rivkin M, Tasch M, et al: A syndrome of multiorgan hyperplasia with features of gigantism, tumorigenesis, and female sterility in p27(Kip1)-deficient mice. Cell 85:733–744, 1996.
53. Jacks T, Fazeli A, Schmitt EM, et al: Effects of an Rb mutation in the mouse. Nature 359:295–300, 1992.
54. Nakayama K, Ishida N, Shirane M, et al: Mice lacking p27(Kip1) display increased body size, multiple organ hyperplasia, retinal dysplasia, and pituitary tumors. Cell 85:707–720, 1996.
55. Herman V, Drazin NZ, Gonsky R, et al: Molecular screening of pituitary adenomas for gene mutations and rearrangements. J Clin Endocrinol Metab 77:50–55, 1993.
56. Prezant TR, Levine J, Melmed S: Molecular characterization of the MEN-1 tumor suppressor gene in sporadic pituitary tumors. J Clin Endocrinol Metab 83:1388–1391, 1998.
57. Pei L, Melmed S, Scheithauer B, et al: Frequent loss of heterozygosity at the retinoblastoma susceptibility gene (RB) locus in aggressive pituitary tumors: Evidence for a chromosome 13 tumor suppressor gene other than RB. Cancer Res 55:1613–1616, 1995.
58. Spada A, Lania A, Ballare E: G protein abnormalities in pituitary adenomas. Mol Cell Endocrinol 142:1–14, 1998.
59. Barlier A, Gunz G, Zamora AJ, et al: Prognostic and therapeutic consequences of Gs alpha mutations in somatotroph adenomas. J Clin Endocrinol Metab 83:1604–1610, 1998.
60. Landis CA, Masters SB, Spada A, et al: GTPase inhibiting mutations activate the alpha chain of Gs and stimulate adenylyl cyclase in human pituitary tumours. Nature 340:692–696, 1989.
61. Clementi E, Malgaretti N, Meldolesi J, et al: A new constitutively activating mutation of the Gs protein alpha subunit–gsp oncogene is found in human pituitary tumours. Oncogene 5:1059–1061, 1990.
62. Lyons J, Landis CA, Harsh G, et al: Two G protein oncogenes in human endocrine tumors. Science 249:655–659, 1990.
63. Boggild MD, Jenkinson S, Pistorello M, et al: Molecular genetic studies of sporadic pituitary tumors. J Clin Endocrinol Metab 78:387–392, 1994.
64. Hosoi E, Yokogoshi Y, Horie H, et al: Analysis of the Gs alpha gene in growth hormone–secreting pituitary adenomas by the polymerase chain reaction—direct

sequencing method using paraffin-embedded tissues. Acta Endocrinol (Copenh) 129:301–306, 1993.

65. Adams EF, Brockmeier S, Friedmann E, et al: Clinical and biochemical characteristics of acromegalic patients harboring gsp-positive and gsp-negative pituitary tumors. Neurosurgery 33:198–203, 1993.

66. Cai WY, Alexander JM, Hedley-Whyte ET, et al: Ras mutations in human prolactinomas and pituitary carcinomas. J Clin Endocrinol Metab 78:89–93, 1994.

67. Pei L, Melmed S, Scheithauer B, et al: H-ras mutations in human pituitary carcinoma metastases. J Clin Endocrinol Metab 78:842–846, 1994.

68. Karga HJ, Alexander JM, Hedley-Whyte ET, et al: Ras mutations in human pituitary tumors. J Clin Endocrinol Metab 74:914–919, 1992.

69. Pei L, Melmed S: Isolation and characterization of a pituitary tumor-transforming gene (PTTG). Mol Endocrinol 11:433–441, 1997.

70. Zhang X, Horwitz GA, Heaney AP, et al: Pituitary tumor transforming gene (PTTG) expression in pituitary adenomas. J Clin Endocrinol Metab 84:761–767, 1999.

71. Zhang X, Horwitz GA, Prezant TR, et al: Structure, expression, and function of human pituitary tumor–transforming gene (PTTG). Mol Endocrinol 13:156–166, 1999.

72. Stratakis CA, Carney JA, Lin JP, et al: Carney complex, a familial multiple neoplasia and lentiginosis syndrome: Analysis of 11 kindreds and linkage to the short arm of chromosome 2. J Clin Invest 97:699–705, 1996.

73. Stratakis CA, Jenkins RB, Pras E, et al: Cytogenetic and microsatellite alterations in tumors from patients with the syndrome of myxomas, spotty skin pigmentation, and endocrine overactivity (Carney complex). J Clin Endocrinol Metab 81:3607–3614, 1996.

74. Carney JA, Hruska LS, Beauchamp GD, et al: Dominant inheritance of the complex of myxomas, spotty pigmentation, and endocrine overactivity. Mayo Clin Proc 61:165–172, 1986.

75. Carney JA, Gordon H, Carpenter PC, et al: The complex of myxomas, spotty pigmentation, and endocrine overactivity. Medicine (Baltimore) 64:270–283, 1985.

76. Teh BT, Kytola S, Farnebo F, et al: Mutation analysis of the MEN1 gene in multiple endocrine neoplasia type 1, familial acromegaly and familial isolated hyperparathyroidism. J Clin Endocrinol Metab 83:2621–2626, 1998.

77. Knudson AGJ: Mutation and cancer: Statistical study of retinoblastoma. Proc Natl Acad Sci U S A 68:820–823, 1971.

78. Benlian P, Giraud S, Lahlou N, et al: Familial acromegaly: A specific clinical entity—further evidence from the genetic study of a three-generation family. Eur J Endocrinol 133:451–456, 1995.

79. Ackermann F, Krohn K, Windgassen M, et al: Acromegaly in a family without a mutation in the menin gene. Exp Clin Endocrinol Diabetes 107:93–96, 1999.

80. Yamada S, Yoshimoto K, Sano T, et al: Inactivation of the tumor suppressor gene on 11q13 in brothers with familial acrogigantism without multiple endocrine neoplasia type 1. J Clin Endocrinol Metab 82:239–242, 1997.

81. Alexander L, Appleton D, Hall R, et al: Epidemiology of acromegaly in the Newcastle region. Clin Endocrinol (Oxf) 12:71–79, 1980.

82. Bengtsson BA, Edén S, Ernest I, et al: Epidemiology and long-term survival in acromegaly. Acta Med Scand 223:327–335, 1988.

83. Rajasoorya C, Holdaway IM, Wrightson P, et al: Determinants of clinical outcome and survival in acromegaly. Clin Endocrinol 41:95–102, 1994.

84. Melmed S: Tight control of growth hormone: An attainable outcome for acromegaly treatment. J Clin Endocrinol Metab 83:3409–3410, 1998.

85. Clemmons DR, Van Wyk JJ, Ridgway EC, et al: Evaluation of acromegaly by radioimmunoassay of somatomedin-C. N Engl J Med 301:1138–1142, 1979.

86. Rieu M, Kuhn JM, Bricaire H, et al: Evaluation of treated acromegalic patients with normal growth hormone levels during oral glucose load. Acta Endocrinol 107:1–8, 1984.

87. Lee PD, Durham SK, Martinez V, et al: Kinetics of insulin-like growth factor (IGF) and IGF-binding protein responses to a single dose of growth hormone. J Clin Endocrinol Metab 82:2266–2274, 1997.

88. Melmed S: Confusion in clinical laboratory GH and IGF-1 reports. Pituitary 2:171–172, 1999.

89. Barkan AL, Beitins IZ, Kelch RP: Plasma insulin-like growth factor-I/somatomedin-C in acromegaly: Correlation with the degree of growth hormone hypersecretion. J Clin Endocrinol Metab 67:69–73, 1988.

90. Grinspoon S, Clemmons D, Swearingen B, et al: Serum insulin-like growth factor–binding protein-3 levels in the diagnosis of acromegaly. J Clin Endocrinol Metab 80:927–932, 1995.

91. de Herder WW, van der Lely AJ, Janssen JA, et al: IGFBP-3 is a poor parameter for assessment of clinical activity in acromegaly. Clin Endocrinol (Oxf) 43:501–505, 1995.

92. van der Lely AJ, de Herder WW, Janssen JA, et al: Acromegaly: The significance of serum total and free IGF-I and IGF-binding protein-3 in diagnosis. J Endocrinol 155(suppl):9–16, 1997.

93. Shibasaki T, Kiyosawa Y, Masuda A, et al: Distribution of growth hormone–releasing hormone–like immunoreactivity in human tissue extracts. J Clin Endocrinol Metab 59:263–268, 1984.

94. Guillemin R, Brazeau P, Bohlen P, et al: Growth hormone–releasing factor from a human pancreatic tumor that caused acromegaly. Science 218:585–587, 1982.

95. Melmed S, Ziel FH, Braunstein GD, et al: Medical management of acromegaly due to ectopic production of growth hormone–releasing hormone by a carcinoid tumor. J Clin Endocrinol Metab 67:395–399, 1988.

96. Lieberman SA, Bjorkengren AG, Hoffman AR: Rheumatologic and skeletal changes in acromegaly. Endocrinol Metab Clin North Am 21:615–631, 1992.

97. Colao A, Marzullo P, Vallone G, et al: Reversibility of joint thickening in acromegalic patients: An ultrasonography study. J Clin Endocrinol Metab 83:2121–2125, 1998.

98. Bluestone R, Bywaters EG, Hartog M, et al: Acromegalic arthropathy. Ann Rheum Dis 30:243–258, 1971.

99. Dons RF, Rosselet P, Pastakia B, et al: Arthropathy in acromegalic patients before

100. Lesse GP, Fraser WD, Farquharson R, et al: Gonadal status is an important determinant of bone density in acromegaly. Clin Endocrinol (Oxf) 48:59–65, 1998.

101. Klein I, Parveen G, Gavaler JS, et al: Colonic polyps in patients with acromegaly. Ann Intern Med 97:27–30, 1982.

102. Thorner MO, Vance ML, Horvath E, et al: The anterior pituitary. *In* Wilson JD, Foster DW (eds): Williams Textbook of Endocrinology, ed 8. Philadelphia, WB Saunders, 1992, pp 221–310.

103. Cheung NW, Boyages SC: The thyroid gland in acromegaly: An ultrasonographic study. Clin Endocrinol (Oxf) 46:545–549, 1997.

104. Lombardi G, Colao A, Ferone D, et al: Effect of growth hormone on cardiac function. Horm Res 48:38–42, 1997.

105. Chanson P, Megnien JL, del Pino M, et al: Decreased regional blood flow in patients with acromegaly. Clin Endocrinol (Oxf) 49:725–731, 1998.

106. Lieberman SA, Hoffman AR: Sequelae to acromegaly: Reversibility with treatment of the primary disease. Horm Metab Res 22:313–318, 1990.

107. Colao A, Cuocolo A, Marzullo P, et al: Effects of 1-year treatment with octreotide on cardiac performance in patients with acromegaly. J Clin Endocrinol Metab 84:17–23, 1999.

108. Lombardi G, Colao A, Marzullo P, et al: Is growth hormone bad for your heart? Cardiovascular impact of GH deficiency and of acromegaly. J Endocrinol 155(suppl):33–39, 1997.

109. Sacca L, Cittadini A, Fazio S: Growth hormone and the heart. Endocr Rev 15:555–573, 1994.

110. Colao A, Cuocolo A, Marzullo P, et al: Impact of patient's age and disease duration on cardiac performance in acromegaly: A radionuclide angiography study. J Clin Endocrinol Metab 84:1518–1523, 1999.

111. Colao A, Merola B, Ferone D, et al: Acromegaly. J Clin Endocrinol Metab 82:2777–2781, 1997.

112. Grunstein RR, Ho KK, Sullivan CE: Effect of octreotide, a somatostatin analog, on sleep apnea in patients with acromegaly. Ann Intern Med 121:478–483, 1994.

113. Grunstein RR, Ho KY, Sullivan CE: Sleep apnea in acromegaly. Ann Intern Med 115:527–532, 1991.

114. Grunstein RR, Ho KY, Berthon-Jones M, et al: Central sleep apnea is associated with increased ventilatory response to carbon dioxide and hypersecretion of growth hormone in patients with acromegaly. Am J Respir Crit Care Med 150:496–502, 1994.

115. Chanson P, Timsit J, Benoit O, et al: Rapid improvement in sleep apnoea of acromegaly after short-term treatment with somatostatin analogue SMS 201-995 (letter). Lancet 1:1270–1271, 1986.

116. Melmed S: Unwanted effects of growth hormone excess in the adult. J Pediatr Endocrinol Metab 9:369–374, 1996.

117. Duncan E, Wass JAH: Investigation protocol: Acromegaly and its investigation. Clin Endocrinol (Oxf) 50:285–293, 1999.

118. Colao A, Marzullo P, Spiezia S, et al: Effect of growth hormone (GH) and insulin-like growth factor I on prostate diseases: An ultrasonographic and endocrine study in acromegaly, GH deficiency, and healthy subjects. J Clin Endocrinol Metab 84:1986–1991, 1999.

119. Colao A, Marzullo P, Ferone D, et al: Prostatic hyperplasia: An unknown feature of acromegaly. J Clin Endocrinol Metab 83:775–779, 1998.

120. Ituarte EA, Petrini J, Hershman JM: Acromegaly and colon cancer. Ann Intern Med 101:627–628, 1984.

121. Jenkins P: Cancer in acromegaly. Trends Endocrinol Metab 9:360–366, 1998.

122. Ezzat S, Melmed S: Clinical review 18: Are patients with acromegaly at increased risk for neoplasia? J Clin Endocrinol Metab 72:245–249, 1991.

123. Ezzat S, Strom C, Melmed S: Colon polyps in acromegaly. Ann Intern Med 114:754–755, 1991.

124. Pines A, Rozen P, Ron E, et al: Gastrointestinal tumors in acromegalic patients. Am J Gastroenterol 80:266–269, 1985.

125. Jenkins PJ, Fairclough PD, Richards T, et al: Acromegaly, colonic polyps and carcinoma. Clin Endocrinol (Oxf) 47:17–22, 1997.

126. Ron E, Gridley G, Hrubec Z, et al: Acromegaly and gastrointestinal cancer [published erratum appears in Cancer 69:549, 1992]. Cancer 68:1673–1677, 1991.

127. Orme SM, McNally RJ, Cartwright RA, et al: Mortality and cancer incidence in acromegaly: A retrospective cohort study. United Kingdom Acromegaly Study Group. J Clin Endocrinol Metab 83:2730–2734, 1998.

128. Swearingen B, Barker FG, Katznelson L, et al: Long-term mortality after transsphenoidal surgery and adjunctive therapy for acromegaly. J Clin Endocrinol Metab 83:3419–3426, 1998.

129. Abosch A, Tyrrell JB, Lamborn KR, et al: Transsphenoidal microsurgery for growth hormone–secreting pituitary adenomas: Initial outcome and long-term results. J Clin Endocrinol Metab 83:3411–3418, 1998.

130. Landin-Wilhelmsen K, Tengborn L, Wilhelmsen L, et al: Elevated fibrinogen levels decrease following treatment of acromegaly. Clin Endocrinol (Oxf) 46:69–74, 1997.

131. Bates AS, Van't Hoff W, Jones JM, et al: An audit of outcome of treatment in acromegaly. Q J Med 86:293–299, 1993.

132. Wright AD, Hill DM, Lowy C, et al: Mortality in acromegaly. Q J Med 39:1–16, 1970.

133. Ross DA, Wilson CB: Results of transsphenoidal microsurgery for growth hormone–secreting pituitary adenoma in a series of 214 patients. J Neurosurg 68:854–867, 1988.

134. Bates AS, Van't Hoff W, Jones JM, et al: Does treatment of acromegaly affect life expectancy? Metabolism 44(suppl 1):1–5, 1995.

135. Jho HD, Carrau RL: Endoscopic endonasal transsphenoidal surgery: Experience with 50 patients. J Neurosurg 87:44–51, 1997.

136. Jho HD, Carrau RL, Ko Y, et al: Endoscopic pituitary surgery: An early experience. Surg Neurol 47:213–222, 1997.

137. Davis DH, Laws ER Jr, Ilstrup DM, et al: Results of surgical treatment for growth hormone–secreting pituitary adenomas. J Neurosurg 79:70–75, 1993.

138. Ahmed S, Elsheikh M, Stratton IM, et al: Outcome of transsphenoidal surgery for acromegaly and its relationship to surgical experience. Clin Endocrinol (Oxf) 50:561–567, 1999.
139. Fahlbusch R, Honegger J, Buchfelder M: Surgical management of acromegaly. Endocrinol Metab Clin North Am 21:669–692, 1992.
140. Ciric I, Ragin A, Baumgartner C, et al: Complications of transsphenoidal surgery: Results of a national survey, review of the literature, and personal experience. Neurosurgery 40:225–236, 1997.
141. Long H, Beauregard H, Somma M, et al: Surgical outcome after repeated transsphenoidal surgery in acromegaly. J Neurosurg 85:239–247, 1996.
142. Freda PU, Post KD, Powell JS, et al: Evaluation of disease status with sensitive measures of growth hormone secretion in 60 postoperative patients with acromegaly. J Clin Endocrinol Metab 83:3808–3816, 1998.
143. Eastman RC, Gorden P, Glatstein E, et al: Radiation therapy of acromegaly. Endocrinol Metab Clin North Am 21:693–712, 1992.
144. Laws JE, Vance ML: Radiosurgery for pituitary tumors and craniopharyngiomas. Neurosurg Clin North Am 10:327–336, 1999.
145. Landolt AM, Haller D, Lomax N, et al: Stereotactic radiosurgery for recurrent surgically treated acromegaly: Comparison with fractionated radiotherapy. J Neurosurg 88:1002–1008, 1998.
146. Barkan AL, Halasz I, Dornfeld KJ, et al: Pituitary irradiation is ineffective in normalizing plasma insulin-like growth factor I in patients with acromegaly. J Clin Endocrinol Metab 82:3187–3191, 1997.
147. Tsang RW, Laperriere NJ, Simpson WJ, et al: Glioma arising after radiation therapy for pituitary adenoma. A report of four patients and estimation of risk [published erratum appears in Cancer 73:492, 1994]. Cancer 72:2227–2233, 1993.
148. Ahmed M, Kanaan I, Rifai A, et al: An unusual treatment-related complication in a patient with growth hormone–secreting pituitary tumor. J Clin Endocrinol Metab 82:2816–2820, 1997.
149. Brada M, Ford D, Ashley S, et al: Risk of second brain tumour after conservative surgery and radiotherapy for pituitary adenoma. BMJ 304:1343–1346, 1992.
150. Al-Mefty O, Kersh JE, Routh A, et al: The long-term side effects of radiation therapy for benign brain tumors in adults. J Neurosurg 73:502–512, 1990.
151. Alexander MJ, DeSalles AA, Tomiyasu U: Multiple radiation-induced intracranial lesions after treatment for pituitary adenoma: Case report. J Neurosurg 88:111–115, 1998.
152. Crossen JR, Garwood D, Glatstein E, et al: Neurobehavioral sequelae of cranial irradiation in adults: A review of radiation-induced encephalopathy. J Clin Oncol 12:627–642, 1994.
153. Thalassinos NC, Tsagarakis S, Ioannides G, et al: Megavoltage pituitary irradiation lowers but seldom leads to safe GH levels in acromegaly: A long-term follow-up study. Eur J Endocrinol 138:160–163, 1998.
154. Lamberts SWJ, van der Lely AJ, de Herder WW, et al: Octreotide. N Engl J Med 334:246–254, 1996.
155. Flogstad AK, Halse J, Haldorsen T, et al: Sandostatin LAR in acromegalic patients: A dose-range study. J Clin Endocrinol Metab 80:3601–3607, 1995.
156. Del Pozo E, Neufeld M, Schluter K, et al: Endocrine profile of a long-acting somatostatin derivative SMS 201-995. Study in normal volunteers following subcutaneous administration. Acta Endocrinol (Copenh) 111:433–439, 1986.
157. Lightman SL, Fox P, Dunne MJ: The effect of SMS 201-995, a long-acting somato-

statin analogue, on anterior pituitary function in healthy male volunteers. Scand J Gastroenterol Suppl 119:84–95, 1986.
158. Battershill PE, Clissold SP: Octreotide: A review of its pharmacodynamic and pharmacokinetic properties, and therapeutic potential in conditions associated with excessive peptide secretion. Drugs 38:658–702, 1989.
159. Gillis JC, Noble S, Goa KL: Octreotide long-acting release (LAR): A review of its pharmacological properties and therapeutic use in the management of acromegaly. Drugs 53:618–699, 1997.
160. Shimon I, Yan X, Taylor JE, et al: Somatostatin receptor (SSTR) subtype–selective analogues differentially suppress in vitro growth hormone and prolactin in human pituitary adenomas: Novel potential therapy for functional pituitary tumors. J Clin Invest 100:2386–2392, 1997.
161. Flogstad AK, Halse J, Bakke S, et al: Sandostatin LAR in acromegalic patients: Long term treatment. J Clin Endocrinol Metab 82:23–28, 1997.
162. Giusti M, Gussoni G, Cuttica CM, et al: Effectiveness and tolerability of slow release lanreotide treatment in active acromegaly: Six-month report on an Italian Multicenter Study. Italian Multicenter Slow Release Lanreotide Study Group. J Clin Endocrinol Metab 81:2089–2097, 1996.
163. Shi YF, Zhu XF, Harris AG, et al: Prospective study of the long-term effects of somatostatin analog (octreotide) on gallbladder function and gallstone formation in Chinese acromegalic patients. J Clin Endocrinol Metab 76:32–37, 1993.
164. Stewart PM, Kane KF, Stewart SE, et al: Depot long-acting somatostatin analog (Sandostatin-LAR) is an effective treatment for acromegaly. J Clin Endocrinol Metab 80:3267–3272, 1995.
165. Newman CB, Melmed S, Snyder PJ, et al: Safety and efficacy of long-term octreotide therapy of acromegaly: Results of a multicenter trial in 103 patients—a clinical research center study. J Clin Endocrinol Metab 80:2768–2775, 1995.
166. Caron P, Cogne M, Gusthiot-Joudet B, et al: Intramuscular injections of slow-release lanreotide (BIM 23014) in acromegalic patients previously treated with continuous subcutaneous infusion of octreotide (SMS 201-995). Eur J Endocrinol 132:320–325, 1995.
167. Jaffe CA, Barkan AL: Treatment of acromegaly with dopamine agonists. Endocrinol Metab Clin North Am 21:713–735, 1992.
168. Jackson SN, Fowler J, Howlett TA: Cabergoline treatment of acromegaly: A preliminary dose finding study. Clin Endocrinol (Oxf) 46:745–749, 1997.
169. Abs R, Verhelst J, Maiter D, et al: Cabergoline in the treatment of acromegaly: A study in 64 patients. J Clin Endocrinol Metab 83:374–378, 1998.
170. Muratori M, Arosio M, Gambino G, et al: Use of cabergoline in the long-term treatment of hyperprolactinemic and acromegalic patients. J Endocrinol Invest 20:537–546, 1997.
171. Colao A, Ferone D, Marzullo P, et al: Effect of different dopaminergic agents in the treatment of acromegaly. J Clin Endocrinol Metab 82:518–523, 1997.
172. Vance ML, Evans WS, Thorner MO: Drugs five years later: Bromocriptine. Ann Intern Med 100:78–91, 1984.
173. Herman-Bonert V, Seliverstov M, Melmed S: Pregnancy in acromegaly: Successful therapeutic outcome. J Clin Endocrinol Metab 83:727–731, 1998.
174. Furman K, Ezzat S: Psychological features of acromegaly. Psychother Psychosom 67:147–153, 1998.
175. Chen WY, Chen NY, Yun J, et al: In vitro and in vivo studies of antagonistic effects of human growth hormone analogs. J Biol Chem 269:15892–15897, 1994.

Chapter 23

Gonadotroph Adenomas

Peter J. Snyder

DEFINITION AND BACKGROUND

Gonadotroph adenomas are pituitary adenomas that arise from gonadotroph cells of the pituitary gland. They are among the most common of pituitary adenomas, constituting 40% to 50% of all macroadenomas. For many years they were not recognized as being of gonadotroph cell origin, probably for two reasons. First, they secrete inefficiently. Second, what they do secrete—intact gonadotropins and their subunits—usually do not produce a recognizable clinical syndrome. Consequently, these adenomas are usually not recognized until they become so large that they cause neurologic symptoms. They make up a large percentage of clinically nonfunctioning adenomas.

ETIOLOGY

Gonadotroph adenomas appear to be true neoplasms, arising from a somatic mutation of a single progenitor cell that divides repetitively. The evidence for this view comes from studies that show that virtually all pituitary adenomas, including gonadotroph adenomas, are monoclonal, that is, they arise from a somatic mutation of a single cell. These studies utilized the technique of restriction fragment length polymorphism to determine if pituitary adenomas in women whose other somatic cells are heterozygous for the enzymes hypoxanthine phosphoribosyltransferase (HPRT) and phosphoglycerate kinase (PGK) are homozygous or heterozygous. This technique relies on the fact that early in embryogenesis in females, one X chromosome, either of maternal or paternal origin, is inactivated. Because the inactivation is random, normal somatic tissues from women who are heterozygous for a gene express approximately equal amounts of both alleles of that gene. In contrast, a neoplasm that occurs after embryogenesis in a heterozygous woman arises from a single progenitor cell and therefore expresses only one of the alleles. In one study of five women whose pituitary macroadenomas expressed some combination of follicle-stimulating hormone β (FSH-β), luteinizing hormone β (LH-β), and α subunit, and whose peripheral leukocytes were heterozygous for HPRT, the adenomas had predominantly one allele or the other[1] (Fig. 23–1). This study suggests that gonadotroph adenomas arise from a somatic mutation of a single progenitor cell which then proliferates, but what mutation and what causes the transformation remain unknown.

Specific mutations are known that appear to cause development of about 40% of somatotroph adenomas[2] and pituitary adenomas associated with multiple endocrine neoplasia type 1 (MEN-1),[3] but the mutations that cause other pituitary adenomas, including gonadotroph adenomas, are not known. Investigators have searched, directly or indirectly, for many other mutations that might be causally related to the development of other pituitary adenomas, including genes that express the *c-myc, c-fos, c-myb,*[4] and *ras* genes,[5, 6] retinoblastoma

suppressor,[7–9] interleukin-6 (IL-6),[10] pituitary adenylate cyclase activating peptides,[11] protein kinase C,[12] basic fibroblast growth factor,[13] epidermal growth factor (EGF),[14] transforming growth factor β (TGF-β),[15] gonadotropin-releasing hormone (GnRH),[16] GnRH receptor,[17] steroidogenic factor-1,[18] activin,[19, 20] and follistatin,[20, 21] but none has been clearly associated with the pathogenesis of any pituitary adenomas.

External hormonal stimulation from the hypothalamus now seems unlikely to be a primary cause of gonadotroph adenomas, but it might have a secondary effect on adenoma growth and it probably has an effect on adenoma secretion. The possibility that gonadotroph adenomas could arise from stimulation of the gonadotroph cells as a consequence of testosterone deficiency in long-standing primary hypogonadism was raised because of the observation that patients who have long-standing primary hypogonadism do develop some degree of pituitary enlargement.[22] Even before the recent demonstration that gonadotroph adenomas are monoclonal, however, a principal etiologic role of primary hypogonadism in the development of gonadotroph adenomas seemed unlikely, because the historical, clinical, and hormonal characteristics of patients with gonadotroph adenomas are quite distinct from those of patients with primary hypogonadism, as discussed later under Differential Diagnosis. And yet, hormonal secretion by gonadotroph adenomas does seem to be dependent on endogenous GnRH, since administration of the GnRH antagonist Nal-Glu GnRH to patients with gonadotroph adenomas and supranormal serum FSH concentrations lowers the FSH values to normal.[23] Histologic evidence also supports the view that gonadotroph adenomas are true neoplasms. Gonadotroph adenomas are composed of sheets of similar pituitary cells, rather than a mixture of various kinds of pituitary cells arranged in a sinusoidal pattern, as occurs in the normal pituitary. Hyperplasia of one kind of pituitary cell, in contrast, is manifest by an increase in that type of cell but not by an effacement of the normal pituitary sinusoidal architecture or the absence of other pituitary cell types.

PATHOPHYSIOLOGY

Secretion by gonadotroph adenomas can be characterized as inefficient, incomplete, and inconsistent. Secretion is inefficient compared to other pituitary adenomas; whereas a lactotroph adenoma 2 cm in diameter usually produces a serum prolactin concentration 100 to 1000 times normal, a gonadotroph adenoma of that size produces a serum FSH concentration no more than 10 times normal and sometimes not supranormal at all.[24] Secretion is incomplete, in that secretion of both intact FSH and LH—and only of them—is unusual; instead, secretion is usually of some combination of intact FSH and α, FSH-β, and LH-β subunits.[24–26] Secretion is inconsistent among adenomas in the relative amounts of intact FSH and LH and their subunits that each secretes.

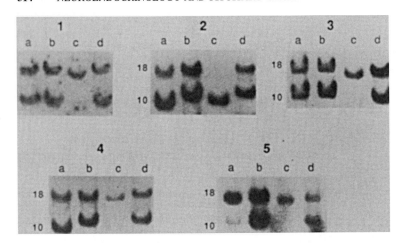

FIGURE 23-1. Demonstration of the apparent monoclonality of five pituitary adenomas. The bands represent DNA fragments of the hypoxanthine phosphoribosyltransferase gene from the peripheral leukocytes (lanes *a* and *b*) and pituitary adenoma cells (lanes *c* and *d*) of five women. The leukocytes of each patient show both alleles (lane *a*), but the adenoma cells show only one allele (lane *c*), supporting the hypothesis that these adenomas arose from clonal expansion of a single cell. (From Alexander JM, Biller BMK, Bikkal H, et al: Clinically nonfunctioning pituitary tumors are monoclonal in origin. J Clin Invest 86:336–340, 1990.)

These characteristics can be recognized both in vivo and in vitro, and both basally and in response to stimulation. In spite of these subtleties of secretion, one or more of these secretory abnormalities can be recognized in vivo in approximately 50% to 75% of patients with gonadotroph adenomas.

Basal Secretion

Intact Follicle-Stimulating Hormone and Luteinizing Hormone

Gonadotroph adenomas more often produce supranormal serum concentrations of intact FSH than of intact LH.[24] This conclusion is drawn from data obtained in men, because of the difficulty in interpreting basal values of gonadotropins and their subunits in women with pituitary macroadenomas. In a series of 38 men who had clinically nonfunctioning pituitary adenomas, most of which had in vitro evidence of gonadotroph origin, 10 had supranormal serum FSH concentrations[26] (Fig. 23–2). The degree of FSH elevation may range from minimal to 10 times the upper limit of normal. The intact FSH secreted by gonadotroph adenomas appears to be normal, or nearly normal, qualitatively. The size of the FSH is similar to that of intact FSH, and not to FSH-β or α subunits, by gel filtration.[27] The charge on the FSH molecules secreted by gonadotroph adenomas also appears to be normal, as judged by chromatofocusing patterns.[28] Biologic activity of the FSH when tested in vitro is even greater than that from normal men,[29] but biologic activity has not been tested in vivo.

Gonadotroph adenomas uncommonly produce supranormal serum concentrations of intact LH, and rarely of sufficient degree to cause a supranormal serum testosterone concentration.[30–32] More common than an actual elevation of intact LH is an artifactual elevation resulting from a supranormal serum α subunit concentration cross-reacting in a polyclonal assay for LH; this artifact can be circumvented by using an immunoradiometric or immunofluorimetric assay, which has much greater specificity for the intact molecule.

Gonadotropin Subunits: α, FSH-β, and LH-β

About 15% of men who have gonadotroph adenomas have supranormal basal serum concentrations of α, or FSH-β, or LH-β subunits, often in combination with supranormal concentrations of another subunit or intact FSH or LH.[26] Occasionally, a single subunit will be supranormal. When α subunit alone is supranormal,[33, 34] the source can be either a gonadotroph or a thyrotroph adenoma, and in vitro studies are needed to make the distinction.

Stimulated Secretion

Administration of thyrotropin-releasing hormone (TRH) to patients who have gonadotroph adenomas often produces an increase in the serum concentrations of intact gonadotropins and their subunits, especially of the LH-β subunit.[26, 35, 36] These responses are interpretable as being characteristic of gonadotroph adenomas, because normal men and women show no response of intact gonadotropins and their subunits to TRH, or, in the case of intact LH and LH-β, no more than a

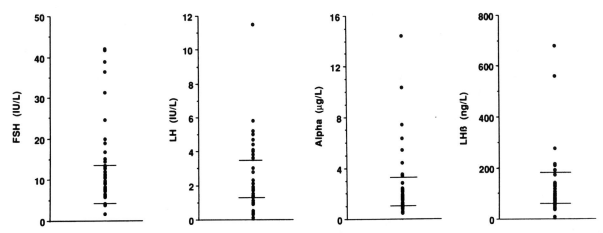

FIGURE 23-2. Basal serum concentrations of intact follicle-stimulating hormone (FSH) and luteinizing hormone (LH) and α and LH-β subunits in 38 men with pituitary macroadenomas that were considered "clinically nonfunctioning." Eleven had elevations of FSH, 10 of LH, 8 of α subunit, and 6 of LH-β subunit. Of the 38 adenomas, 36 were studied in cell culture and 29 could be identified as gonadotroph adenomas by their secretion in culture. (From Daneshdoost L, Gennarelli TA, Bashey HM, et al: Identification of gonadotroph adenomas in men with clinically nonfunctioning adenomas by the LH-β subunit response to TRH. J Clin Endocrinol Metab 77:1352–1355.)

33% increase. In a study of 16 women with pituitary macroadenomas that were clinically nonfunctioning, 11 could be identified as being of gonadotroph origin by their LH-β subunit responses to TRH; 4 had responses of LH and 3 of FSH[36] (Fig. 23–3). Of 38 men who had pituitary macroadenomas that were clinically nonfunctioning, 14 had responses of LH-β, 5 of intact LH, and 4 of intact FSH.[26]

Administration of GnRH to patients who have gonadotroph adenomas results in greatly variable FSH and LH responses, ranging from subnormal to normal,[37] but the responses cannot be interpreted, because either normal or adenomatous gonadotroph cells could be the source of the FSH or LH.

Secretion In Vitro

Gonadotroph adenomas that are recognized in vivo by supranormal basal or stimulated serum concentrations of intact gonadotropins or subunits usually secrete in culture relatively large amounts of the same intact hormones and subunits they secreted in vivo. Of 11 women whose clinically nonfunctioning adenomas could be recognized as being of gonadotroph origin by their LH-β responses to TRH, 9 were established in dispersed cell culture, and all 9 secreted readily detectable amounts of LH-β.[36] In addition, gonadotroph adenomas often secrete relatively large amounts of other gonadotroph cell products in culture as well.[36] For example, some adenomas, associated in vivo only with a supranormal serum basal concentration of intact FSH, also secrete large amounts of LH in culture. Other adenomas, associated in vivo only with a supranormal concentration of α subunit, secrete intact FSH in culture, which identifies them as gonadotroph adenomas. Yet other adenomas, associated with normal basal serum concentrations of intact gonadotropins and their subunits but with a large LH-β response to TRH, secrete large amounts of intact FSH as well as LH-β in culture. Gonadotroph adenomas in culture respond to both TRH and GnRH by secreting both FSH and LH.[38, 39] They respond to somatostatin[40] and bromocriptine[41] by decreased secretion of gonadotropins and their subunits.

DIAGNOSIS

Clinical Presentation

Gonadotroph adenomas usually come to clinical attention when they become so large that they cause neurologic symptoms (Table 23–1).

TABLE 23–1. Clinical Presentations of Gonadotroph Adenomas

Neurologic symptoms (most common)
   Visual impairment
   Headache
   Other (diplopia, seizures, cerebrospinal fluid rhinorrhea, etc.)
Incidental finding
   When an imaging procedure is performed because of an unrelated symptom
Hormonal symptoms (least common)
   Oligomenorrhea or amenorrhea in a premenopausal woman
   Premature puberty when intact luteinizing hormone is secreted in a prepubertal boy
   Symptoms of hormonal deficiencies (common but uncommonly the presenting symptoms)

The large size is illustrated by a series of 100 patients whose gonadotroph adenomas, documented immunocytochemically, averaged 2.5 ± 0.7 cm in diameter and ranged from 1.1 to 4.5 cm.[42] They may also be an incidental finding when an imaging procedure of the head is performed for an unrelated reason. Least commonly, they may come to medical attention because of hormonal hypersecretion. The large size of gonadotroph adenomas commonly causes hormonal hyposecretion from the nonadenomatous pituitary, but these deficiencies usually do not impel the patient to seek medical attention. Gonadotroph adenomas are probably not recognized when they are microadenomas, because they are so inefficient that when they are of that size they probably do not result in supranormal serum concentrations of intact gonadotropins or their subunits.

Impaired vision is the neurologic symptom that most commonly leads a patient with a gonadotroph adenoma to seek medical attention, because suprasellar extension of the adenoma elevates and compresses the optic chiasm. Although a bitemporal visual field defect is considered the most typical abnormality, asymmetrical defects are also common. When compression becomes more severe, central visual acuity may also be impaired. The onset of the deficit is usually so gradual that patients often do not seek ophthalmologic consultation for months or even years.

Other neurologic symptoms that may cause a patient with a gonadotroph adenoma to seek medical attention are headaches, caused presumably by expansion of the sella; diplopia, caused by oculomotor

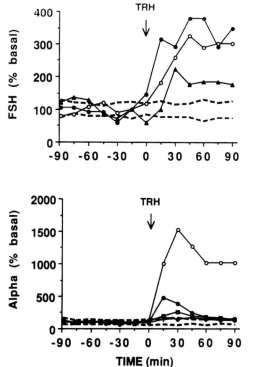
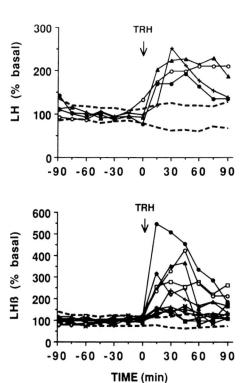

FIGURE 23–3. Increases in the serum concentrations of intact follicle-stimulating hormone (FSH), luteinizing hormone (LH), α subunit, and, mostly, LH-β subunit to thyrotropin-releasing hormone (TRH) in 16 women with adenomas that had been thought to be "nonsecreting" on the basis of basal hormone concentrations. The *dashed lines* show the ranges of serum concentrations in 16 age-matched healthy women. Eleven women with "nonsecreting" adenomas exhibited significant responses to TRH of LH-β subunit, four of intact LH and α subunit, and three of FSH. (From Daneshdoost L, Gennarell TA, Bashey HM, et al: Recognition of gonadotroph adenomas in women. N Engl J Med 324:589–594, 1991.)

nerve compression due to lateral extension of the adenoma; cerebrospinal fluid (CSF) rhinorrhea, caused by inferior extension of the adenoma; and the excruciating headache and diplopia caused by pituitary apoplexy.

Detection of a gonadotroph adenoma as an incidental finding when an imaging procedure of the head is performed for an unrelated reason, such as a motor vehicle accident, is the next most common presentation. The least common presentation is consequent to hormonal hypersecretion by the adenoma. This includes oligo-or amenorrhea in a premenopausal woman due to excessive FSH secretion, ovarian hyperstimulation syndrome in a premenopausal woman due to excessive FSH secretion,[43, 44] and premature puberty in a prepubertal boy due to an adenoma secreting intact LH.[45, 46]

At the time of initial presentation with a neurologic symptom, many patients with gonadotroph adenomas, when questioned, admit to symptoms of hormonal deficiencies. Ironically, the most common pituitary hormonal deficiency is of LH, the result of compression of the normal gonadotroph cells by the adenoma and lack of secretion of a substantial amount of intact LH by the adenomatous gonadotroph cells. The result in men is a subnormal serum testosterone concentration, which produces decreased energy and libido. The result in premenopausal women is amenorrhea. Thyroid-stimulating hormone (TSH) and adrenocorticotropic hormone (ACTH) deficiencies, leading to thyroxine and cortisol deficiencies, may also occur.

Diagnostic Tests

The process of making the diagnosis of a gonadotroph adenoma usually proceeds from recognizing that a patient's visual abnormality or other neurologic symptom could represent an intrasellar lesion, to confirming the presence of a sellar lesion by an imaging procedure, to finding the secretory abnormalities characteristic of a gonadotroph adenoma (Table 23–2).

Tests of Vision and Imaging of the Pituitary

Neuro-ophthalmologic evaluation should include a computerized test of visual fields and assessment of visual acuity. The pituitary should be imaged by magnetic resonance (MR) (Fig. 23–4). Magnetic resonance imaging (MRI) will not, however, show calcification in a craniopharyngioma as well as a computed tomography (CT) scan, will often not distinguish a pituitary adenoma from other intrasellar lesions, and will not distinguish a pituitary adenoma from the nonadenomatous pituitary or one kind of pituitary adenoma from another.

Hormonal Tests

Intrasellar mass lesions detected by MRI should be evaluated further by measurement of serum concentrations of pituitary hormones to determine if the lesion is of pituitary or nonpituitary origin, and if

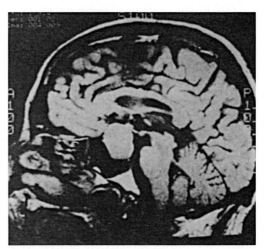

FIGURE 23–4. Magnetic resonance imaging showing in a sagittal view of the head a large gonadotroph adenoma extending superiorly to elevate the optic chiasm. Gonadotroph adenomas are often not recognized until they become this large.

pituitary, the cell of origin. An adenoma of gonadotroph or thyrotroph origin should be suspected if the serum prolactin concentration is less than 100 ng/mL, the patient does not appear acromegalic and the serum insulin-like growth factor I (IGF-I) concentration is not supranormal, and the patient does not have Cushing's syndrome or supranormal urine cortisol excretion. Preoperative recognition that an intrasellar mass lesion is of gonadotroph origin depends on finding specific combinations of basal gonadotropins and stimulated concentrations of intact gonadotropins and their subunits. The combinations differ somewhat in men and women.

In a man who has a pituitary macroadenoma, elevated basal serum concentrations of intact gonadotropins or their subunits alone or in combination with responses of any of these to TRH are strong evidence that the adenoma is of gonadotroph origin. An elevated basal FSH concentration is common, as are elevated concentrations of basal α, FSH-β, and LH-β subunits. Patients who have elevated basal intact hormone and subunit secretion often exhibit responses of any one of them to TRH.

In a woman who has a pituitary macroadenoma, basal serum concentrations of intact FSH or its subunits are usually of little diagnostic value, because of the difficulty in interpreting elevated values in a woman over 50 years old, the age at which these adenomas usually present. In that situation, differentiation between the adenoma and nonadenomatous postmenopausal gonadotroph cells as the source of the elevated gonadotropins and their subunits is usually not possible. In a few situations, however, the distinction can be made, such as when intact FSH is markedly elevated but LH is not elevated at all, or when one of the gonadotropin subunits is distinctly elevated but intact FSH and LH are not elevated.[36] In a woman, therefore, the in vivo diagnosis depends on finding a response to TRH of intact FSH or LH or, most commonly, of LH-β subunit.

Differential Diagnosis

Gonadotroph adenomas need to be distinguished from other kinds of pituitary adenomas, nonpituitary lesions arising within and around the sella, and long-standing primary hypogonadism. Although adenomas arising from other pituitary cells usually are recognized readily by the clinical syndromes they produce and by their secretory products, some somatotroph,[47, 48] corticotroph,[49] and even lactotroph adenomas are clinically silent. These appear to be nonsecreting in vivo and are recognized only when studied in vitro, such as by immunospecific staining. Intra- and parasellar lesions of nonpituitary origin can sometimes be distinguished from pituitary adenomas on the basis of their imaging characteristics, but not always, and sometimes are not recognized for what they are until examined histologically. Neither other

---

TABLE 23–2. Hormonal Criteria for the Diagnosis of Gonadotroph Adenomas*

Men	Women
Supranormal Basal Serum Concentrations of	
FSH†	FSH but not LH
α, LH-β, or FSH-β subunits	Any subunit relative to intact FSH and LH
LH and testosterone	
Supranormal Response to TRH of	
FSH	FSH
LH	LH
LH-β (most common)	LH-β (most common)

*Assuming the patient has a pituitary macroadenoma. Approximately 50% to 75% of patients with gonadotroph adenomas will have one or more of these abnormalities.
†Assuming the patient does not have a history of primary hypogonadism.
FSH, follicle-stimulating hormone; LH, luteinizing hormone; TRH, thyrotropin-releasing hormone.

pituitary adenomas nor nonpituitary lesions exhibit the hormonal abnormalities characteristic of gonadotroph adenomas. Long-standing primary hypogonadism can lead to gonadotroph cell hypertrophy and thus to pituitary enlargement as well as to elevated serum gonadotropin concentrations, and in this way is similar to gonadotroph adenomas. The pituitary enlargement seen with primary hypogonadism, however, is not nearly so great as that with gonadotroph adenomas at the time of presentation. In primary hypogonadism, LH as well as FSH is elevated, and neither intact gonadotropins nor their subunits respond to TRH.[35]

Clinical Utility of Diagnosis

Making the diagnosis of a gonadotroph adenoma in vivo is of value in distinguishing a lesion as being of pituitary rather than nonpituitary origin and in providing a marker by which to monitor the response to treatment. Distinguishing an intrasellar lesion as pituitary rather than nonpituitary in origin is of value because it can influence treatment. If surgery is needed, for example, a pituitary lesion is almost always approached transsphenoidally, no matter how large, because it is infradural, but a meningioma should be approached transcranially if it arises above the dura. Finding tumor markers characteristic of gonadotroph adenomas, such as elevated basal FSH or α or LH-β subunit concentrations, not only identifies the lesion as being of gonadotroph origin but provides a means by which to follow the response to treatment. When the basal serum FSH concentration is elevated prior to surgery, for example, the decrease after surgery correlates with reduction in adenoma mass seen by imaging.[50]

TREATMENT

Because gonadotroph adenomas are usually not detected until they become so large that they cause significant visual impairment, treatment usually must be directed at reducing adenoma mass and restoring vision as soon as possible. Surgery, usually transsphenoidal, is the only treatment that meets these criteria (Table 23–3). Gonadotroph adenomas are usually sensitive to radiation, which may be used to prevent regrowth if substantial adenoma tissue remains after surgery, or as primary treatment if an adenoma is detected before it becomes large enough to cause neurologic symptoms. Several pharmacologic treatments have been tried, but none reduce adenoma size much.

Surgery

Surgical Approaches

Transsphenoidal surgery via an operating microscope is usually the preferred treatment for gonadotroph adenomas that impair vision significantly. Transsphenoidal surgery may also be performed because of severe headaches, diplopia, or other neurologic abnormalities, or

elevation of the optic chiasm in the absence of visual impairment. The transsphenoidal approach is usually preferred over the transcranial as the initial procedure no matter how great the suprasellar extension, because pituitary adenomas are infradural and the risk of serious side effects is less. An endoscopic approach to sellar masses has been reported by some surgeons.[51–53] This approach, which appears to be evolving, employs an endoscope in a similar fashion to endoscopic surgery of the sinuses. Some patients with hormonally active pituitary adenomas appear to have been cured by this procedure while others have not. Some of the same complications that occur with the microsurgical technique have been reported. Transcranial surgery may be performed when suprasellar adenoma tissue that remains after transsphenoidal surgery continues to cause clinically significant neurologic impairment. Neurologic side effects are somewhat more likely with this approach than with transsphenoidal surgery.

Efficacy

Seventy percent to 80% of patients in one series who had abnormal visual fields due to a gonadotroph adenoma experienced improvement following transsphenoidal surgery.[50] This improvement is similar to that of all macroadenomas. In one series of 230 patients whose visual fields were abnormal before transsphenoidal surgery, the fields improved in 73%, remained the same in 23%, and worsened in 4%.[54] In another series of 113 pituitary adenomas that extended beyond the sella, 81% of those with visual field defects before surgery experienced improvement in fields after surgery, 19% remained the same, and none worsened.[55] The improvement in vision was paralleled by a decrease in hormonal hypersecretion.[50]

Complications

Serious complications of transsphenoidal surgery are uncommon, but appear to be greater when the adenoma is very large and the surgeon has had relatively little experience with transsphenoidal procedures. In a survey in which neurosurgeons were asked to report their own experience, serious complications reported by the 958 respondents included carotid artery injury (1.1%), central nervous system injury (1.3%), loss of vision (1.8%), ophthalmoplegia (1.4%), hemorrhage or swelling of the residual tumor (2.9%), CSF leak (3.9%), meningitis (1.5%), and death (0.9%).[56] The chances of anterior pituitary insufficiency (19.4%) and diabetes insipidus (17.8%) were higher. The incidence of each complication was higher among less experienced surgeons. Among neurosurgeons who reported performing fewer than 200 transsphenoidal procedures, 1.2% of procedures resulted in death, but among neurosurgeons who reported performing more than 500 procedures, only 0.2% resulted in death. Although these results are based on retrospective self-reporting via questionnaire, they provide a broader assessment of complications of transsphenoidal surgery than that provided by the most experienced pituitary surgeons,[57–59] whose complication rates are closer to those of the most experienced group above.[56]

TABLE 23–3. Comparison of Treatments for Gonadotroph Adenomas

Treatment	Indications	Complications
Transsphenoidal surgery	Intrasellar mass with suprasellar extension and severe visual impairment	Worsening of vision, oculomotor palsy, hematoma, cerebrospinal fluid rhinorrhea, meningitis, seizures, diabetes insipidus, hypopituitarism
Transcranial surgery	Large, residual symptomatic extrasellar tissue following transsphenoidal surgery	Same as above, but more likely
Supervoltage radiation	Primary treatment: intrasellar mass with only mild suprasellar extension	Transient: fatigue, nausea, hair loss, loss of taste and smell
	Adjuvant treatment: substantial residual adenoma tissue after surgery	Permanent: hypopituitarism
Observation	Adenoma confined to sella; patient elderly or infirm	Visual impairment
Medications (dopamine agonists, gonadotropin-releasing hormone antagonists)	Experimental protocol; generally ineffective	

Complication rates are also greater in patients who have had prior pituitary surgery than in those who have not, and even greater in those whose prior surgery was via craniotomy than in those whose prior surgery was transsphenoidal.[60]

Evaluation of the Results

The results of surgery should initially be evaluated 4 to 6 weeks afterward. Residual adenoma tissue should be evaluated by MRI and by measurement of whatever hormones or subunits had been elevated before surgery. The functions of the nonadenomatous anterior pituitary should also be reevaluated postoperatively, as should vasopressin secretion. Neuro-ophthalmologic function should likewise be reevaluated.

Radiation

Techniques

Radiation therapy has been used for decades to treat pituitary adenomas. The standard technique has employed a supervoltage source to deliver a total of 45 to 50 Gy in daily 2-Gy doses via three external portals. Other techniques have recently been utilized which employ various radiation sources delivered stereotactically, to attempt to minimize the amount of radiation to which the brain is exposed. One group of techniques, collectively called stereotactic radiosurgery, involves administration of a large single dose of radiation from one of several possible sources, including protons from a cyclotron, high-energy x-rays from a linear accelerator, or gamma radiation from a ^{60}Co source (gamma knife). Another technique, called "conformal radiation," involves administration of supervoltage radiation in fractionated doses, as in conventional radiotherapy, but from multiple portals and guided by a computer-generated model so that the radiation conforms to the boundaries of the lesion.

Efficacy

When conventional radiation is administered following surgery for a pituitary macroadenoma, it is usually effective in preventing regrowth of the adenoma.[61–63] In one study of men who had conventional radiation therapy following surgery for clinically nonfunctioning pituitary macroadenomas, only 4 (6%) of the 63 patients who received radiation following surgery developed new visual impairment requiring additional treatment during the subsequent 15 years, but 42 (66%) of the 63 who did not receive radiation developed new visual impairment.[63] The efficacy of stereotactic methods of radiation delivery in preventing recurrence of pituitary adenomas and other sellar tumors remains to be determined.

Complications and Side Effects

There are both short-term and long-term side effects of conventional radiation. The short-term side effects include nausea, lethargy, loss of taste and smell, and loss of hair at the radiation portals. The first two remit within 2 months, and the latter two usually remit within 6 months but may be permanent. The long-term adverse effects include hypopituitarism and neurologic complications. Hypopituitarism may begin as soon as 1 month after completion of radiation, but usually not until a year or more. By 10 years, about 50% of patients have a deficiency of ACTH, TSH, or LH.[64–66] Neurologic side effects occur less commonly. Blindness due to optic neuritis,[67, 68] brain tumors, and cerebrovascular accidents attributed to accelerated local atherosclerosis have been reported,[69, 70] but other series that have evaluated possible neurologic sequelae have found no neurologic side effects.[71] Because the various stereotactic techniques for administering radiation to the sella area are designed to expose the structures surrounding the sella and the brain to less radiation than does the conventional technique, it is possible that some of these may not be as likely to cause neurologic sequelae, but it is too soon to know if this hope will be realized. The larger amount of radiation given per dose during stereotactic radiosurgery, however, poses a potentially greater risk of optic neuritis than does conventional radiation. In fact, radiation-induced optic neuritis has been reported following this procedure.[72]

Management of Patients after Radiation

Hormonal evaluation, both for excessive secretion of whichever intact gonadotropins and their subunits were secreted excessively by the adenoma prior to treatment and for deficient secretion by the nonadenomatous pituitary, should be performed 6 and 12 months after radiation and once a year thereafter. Evaluation of size by MRI should be performed 1 year after radiation and, if the mass is smaller, less frequently thereafter. Neuro-ophthalmologic evaluation should be repeated after radiation if it was abnormal before.

Pharmacologic Treatment

Several drugs have been administered in attempts to treat gonadotroph adenomas, but so far none have been found that reduce their size consistently and substantially.

Although dopamine does not decrease gonadotropin secretion to an appreciable degree in normal subjects, bromocriptine has been reported to decrease the secretion of intact gonadotropins and α subunit in a few patients and even to improve vision in one, but not to reduce adenoma size.[73, 74] CV 205-504 has also been reported to reduce secretion and adenoma size in occasional patients.[75]

The somatostatin analogue, octreotide, has been used to treat gonadotroph adenomas because of the demonstration that somatostatin itself may decrease secretion by gonadotroph adenomas in vitro. Although there have been occasional reports of dramatic decreases in size of gonadotroph adenomas associated with octreotide administration[76, 77] and some improvement in vision, the majority of patients have shown little if any improvement in adenoma size or vision.[76–78]

Several agonist analogues of GnRH have been administered to patients with gonadotroph adenomas, based on the rationale that chronic administration of these agonists causes downregulation of GnRH receptors on, and decreased secretion of FSH and LH from, normal gonadotroph cells. Administration of GnRH agonist analogues to patients with gonadotroph adenomas, however, generally produces either an agonist effect or no effect on secretion and no effect on adenoma size.[79, 80]

Potent antagonist analogues of GnRH have recently been developed. Administration for 1 week of the GnRH antagonist Nal-Glu GnRH, to men with gonadotroph adenomas reduced their elevated FSH concentrations to normal.[23] However, when Nal-Glu administration was continued for 6 months, although FSH remained suppressed, adenoma size did not decrease.[81]

REFERENCES

1. Alexander JM, Biller BMK, Bikkal H, et al: Clinically nonfunctioning pituitary tumors are monoclonal in origin. J Clin Invest 86:336–340, 1990.
2. Landis CA, Masters SB, Spada A, et al: GTPase inhibiting mutations activate the α chain of G$_s$ and stimulate adenylate cyclase in human pituitary tumors. Nature 340:692–696, 1989.
3. Chandrasekhapappa SC, Guru SC, Manickam P, et al: Positional cloning of the gene for multiple endocrine neoplasia-type 1. Science 276:404–407, 1997.
4. Woloschak M, Roberts JL, Post K: c-myc, c-fos, and c-myb gene expression in human pituitary adenomas. J Clin Endocrinol Metab 79:253–257, 1994.
5. Cai WY, Alexander JM, Hedley-Whyte ET, et al: ras mutations in human prolactinomas and pituitary carcinomas. J Clin Endocrinol Metab 78:89–93, 1994.
6. Pei L, Melmed S, Scheithauer B, et al: H-ras mutations in human pituitary carcinoma metastases. J Clin Endocrinol Metab 78:842–846, 1994.
7. Cryns VL, Alexander JM, Klibanski A, Arnold A: The retinoblastoma gene in human pituitary tumors. J Clin Endocrinol Metab 77:644–646, 1993.
8. Zhu J, Leon SP, Beggs AH, et al: Human pituitary adenomas show no loss of heterozygosity at the retinoblastoma gene locus. J Clin Endocrinol Metab 78:922–927, 1994.
9. Ikeda H, Beauchamp RL, Yoshimoto T, Yandell DW: Detection of heterozygous mutation in the retinoblastoma gene in a human pituitary adenoma using pcr-sscp analysis and direct sequencing. Endocr Pathol 6:189–196, 1995.
10. Jones TH, Daniels M, James RA, et al: Production of bioactive and immunoreactive interleukin-6 (IL-6) and expression of IL-6 messenger ribonucleic acid by human pituitary adenomas. J Clin Endocrinol Metab 78:180–187, 1994.

11. Robberecht P, Vertongen P, Velkeniers B, et al: Receptors for pituitary adenylate cyclase activating peptides in human pituitary adenomas. J Clin Endocrinol Metab 77:1235–1239, 1993.
12. Alvaro V, Levy L, Dubray C, et al: Invasive human pituitary tumors express a point-mutated alpha-protein kinase-C. J Clin Endocrinol Metab 77:1125–1129, 1993.
13. Ezzat S, Smyth HS, Ramyar L, Asa SL: Heterogeneous in vivo and in vitro expression of basic fibroblast growth factor by human pituitary adenomas. J Clin Endocrinol Metab 80:878–884, 1995.
14. LeRiche V, Asa SL, Ezzat S: Epidermal growth factor and its receptor (EGF-R) in human pituitary adenomas: EGF-R correlates with tumor aggressiveness. J Clin Endocrinol Metab 81:656–662, 1996.
15. Ezzat S, Walpola IA, Ramyar L, et al: Membrane-anchored expression of transforming growth factor alpha in human pituitary adenoma cells. J Clin Endocrinol Metab 80:534–539, 1995.
16. Miller GM, Alexander JM, Klibanski A: Gonadotropin-releasing hormone messenger RNA expression in gonadotroph tumors and normal human pituitary. J Clin Endocrinol Metab 81:80–83, 1996.
17. Alexander JM, Klibanski A: Gonadotropin-releasing hormone receptor mRNA expression by human pituitary tumors in vitro. J Clin Invest 93:2332–2339, 1994.
18. Asa SL, Bamberger A-M, Cao B, et al: The transcription activator steroidogenic factor-1 is preferentially expressed in the human pituitary gonadotroph. J Clin Endocrinol Metab 81:2165–2170, 1996.
19. Haddad G, Penabad JL, Bashey HM, et al: Expression of activin/inhibin subunit messenger ribonucleic acids by gonadotroph adenomas. J Clin Endocrinol Metab 79:1399–1403, 1994.
20. Alexander JM, Swearingen B, Tindall GT, Klibanski A: Human pituitary adenomas express endogenous inhibin subunit and follistatin messenger ribonucleic acids. J Clin Endocrinol Metab 80:147–152, 1995.
21. Penabad JL, Bashey HM, Asa SL, et al: Decreased follistatin gene expression in gonadotroph adenomas. J Clin Endocrinol Metab 81:3397–3403, 1996.
22. Samaan NA, Stephans AV, Danziger J, Trujillo J: Reactive pituitary abnormalities in patients with Klinefelter's and Turner's syndromes. Arch Intern Med 139:198–201, 1979.
23. Daneshdoost L, Pavlou S, Molitch ME: Inhibition of follicle-stimulating hormone secretion from gonadotroph adenomas by repetitive administration of a gonadotropin-releasing hormone antagonist. J Clin Endocrinol Metab 71:92–97, 1990.
24. Snyder PJ: Gonadotroph cell adenomas of the pituitary. Endocr Rev 6:552–563, 1985.
25. Lanzi R, Montorsi F, Losa M, et al: Laparoscopic bilateral adrenalectomy for persistent Cushing's disease after transsphenoidal surgery. Surgery 123:144–150, 1998.
26. Daneshdoost L, Gennarelli TA, Bashey HM, et al: Identification of gonadotroph adenomas in men with clinically nonfunctioning adenomas by the LHβ subunit response to TRH. J Clin Endocrinol Metab 77:1352–1355, 1993.
27. Snyder PJ, Bashey HM, Kim SU, Chappel SC: Secretion of uncombined subunits of luteinizing hormone by gonadotroph cell adenomas. J Clin Endocrinol Metab 59:1169–1175, 1984.
28. Chappel SC, Bashey HM, Snyder PJ: Similar isoelectric profiles of FSH from gonadotroph cell adenomas and non-adenomatous pituitaries. Acta Endocrinol 113:311–316, 1986.
29. Galway AB, Hsueh JW, Daneshdoost L, et al: Gonadotroph adenomas in men produce biologically active follicle-stimulating hormone. J Clin Endocrinol Metab 71:907–912, 1990.
30. Snyder PJ, Sterling FH: Hypersecretion of LH and FSH by a pituitary adenoma. J Clin Endocrinol Metab 42:544–550, 1976.
31. Peterson RD, Kourides IA, Horwith M, et al: Luteinizing hormone and α-subunit-secreting pituitary tumor: Positive feedback of estrogen. J Clin Endocrinol Metab 51:692–698, 1981.
32. Klibanski A, Deutsch PJ, Jameson JL, et al: Luteinizing hormone–secreting pituitary tumor: Biosynthetic characterization and clinical studies. J Clin Endocrinol Metab 64:536–542, 1987.
33. Ridgway EC, Klibanski A, Ladenson PW, et al: Pure alpha-secreting pituitary adenomas. N Engl J Med 304:1254–1259, 1981.
34. Klibanski A, Ridgway EC, Zervas NT: Pure alpha subunit-secreting pituitary tumors. J Neurosurg 59:585–589, 1983.
35. Snyder PJ, Muzyka R, Johnson J, Utiger RD: Thyrotropin-releasing hormone provokes abnormal follicle-stimulating hormone (FSH) and luteinizing hormone responses in men who have pituitary adenomas and FSH hypersecretion. J Clin Endocrinol Metab 51:744–748, 1980.
36. Daneshdoost L, Gennarelli TA, Bashey HM, et al: Recognition of gonadotroph adenomas in women. N Engl J Med 324:589–594, 1991.
37. Snyder PJ, Bigdeli H, Gardner DF, et al: Gonadal function in 50 men with untreated pituitary adenomas. J Clin Endocrinol Metab 48:309–314, 1979.
38. Mashiter K, Adams E, Van Noorden S: Secretion of LH, FSH and PRL shown by cell culture and immunocytochemistry of human functionless pituitary adenomas. Clin Endocrinol 15:103–112, 1981.
39. Kwekkeboom DJ, Dejong FH, Lamberts SWJ: Gonadotropin release by clinically nonfunctioning and gonadotroph pituitary adenomas in vivo and in vitro relation to sex and effects of thyrotropin-releasing hormone, gonadotropin-releasing hormone and bromocriptine. J Clin Endocrinol Metab 68:1128–1135, 1989.
40. Klibanski A, Alexander JM, Bikkal HA, et al: Somatostatin regulation of glycoprotein hormone and free subunit secretion in clinically nonfunctioning and somatotroph adenomas in vitro. J Clin Endocrinol Metab 1248:1255, 1991.
41. Lamberts SWJ, Verleun T, Oosterom R: The effects of bromocriptine, thyrotropin-releasing hormone, and gonadotropin-releasing hormone on hormone secretion by gonadotropin-secreting pituitary adenomas in vivo and in vitro. J Clin Endocrinol Metab 64:524–530, 1987.
42. Young WF Jr, Scheithauer BW, Kovacs KT, et al: Gonadotroph adenoma of the pituitary gland: A clinicopathologic analysis of 100 cases. Mayo Clin Proc 71:649–656, 1996.
43. Djerassi A, Coutifaris C, West VA, et al: Gonadotroph adenoma in premenopausal woman secreting follicle-stimulating hormone and causing ovarian hyperstimulation. J Clin Endocrinol Metab 80:591–594, 1995.
44. Christin-Maitre S, Rongieres-Bertrand C, Kottler et al: A spontaneous and severe hyperstimulation of the ovaries revealing a gonadotroph adenoma. J Clin Endocrinol Metab 83:3450–3453, 1998.
45. Faggiano M, Criscuolo T, Perrone I, et al: Sexual procecity in a boy due to hypersecretion of LH and prolactin by a pituitary adenoma. Acta Endocrinol 102:167–172, 1983.
46. Ambrosi B, Basstti M, Ferrario R, et al: Precocious puberty in a boy with a PRL, LH- and FSH-secreting pituitary tumour: Hormonal and immunocytochemical studies. Acta Endocrinol 122:569–576, 1990.
47. Klibanski A, Zervas NT, Kovacs K, Ridgway EC: Clinically silent hypersecretion of growth hormone in patients with pituitary tumors. J Neurosurg 66:806–811, 1987.
48. Yamada S, Sano T, Stefaneanu L, et al: Endocrine and morphological study of a clinically silent somatotroph adenoma of the human pituitary. J Clin Endocrinol Metab 76:352–356, 1993.
49. Asa SL, Ezzat S: The cytogenesis and pathogenesis of pituitary adenomas. Endocr Rev 19:798–827, 1998.
50. Harris RI, Schatz NJ, Gennarelli TA, et al: Follicle-stimulating hormone–secreting pituitary adenomas: Correlation of reduction of adenoma size with reduction of hormonal hypersecretion after transsphenoidal surgery. J Clin Endocrinol Metab 56:1288, 1983.
51. Sethi DS, Pillay PK: Endoscopic management of lesions of the sella turcica. J Laryngol Otol 109:956–962, 1995.
52. Jho H-D, Carrau RL: Endoscopic endonasal transsphenoidal surgery: Experience with 50 patients. J Neurosurg 87:44–51, 1997.
53. Yaniv E, Rappaport H: Endoscopic transseptal transsphenoidal surgery for pituitary tumors. Neurosurg 40:944–946, 1997.
54. Trautmann JC, Laws ER Jr: Visual status after transsphenoidal surgery at the Mayo Clinic. Am J Ophthalmol 96:200, 1983.
55. Black PM, Zervas NT, Candia G: Management of large pituitary adenomas by transsphenoidal surgery. Surg Neurol 29:4434, 1988.
56. Ciric I, Ragin A, Baumgartner C, Pierce D: Complications of transsphenoidal surgery: Results of a national survey, review of the literature, and personal experience. Neurosurgery 40:225–237, 1997.
57. Wilson CB: A decade of pituitary microsurgery. J Neurosurg 61:814–833, 1984.
58. Black PM, Zervas NT, Candia GL: Incidence and management of complications of transsphenoidal operations for pituitary adenomas. Neurosurgery 20:920–924, 1987.
59. Barrow DL, Tindall GT: Loss of vision after transsphenoidal surgery. Neurosurgery 27:60–68, 1990.
60. Laws ER Jr, Fode NC, Redmond MJ: Transsphenoidal surgery following unsuccessful prior therapy. J Neurosurg 63:823–829, 1985.
61. Zaugg M, Adamman O, Pescia R, Landolt AM: External irradiation of macroinvasive pituitary adenomas with telecobalt: A retrospective study with long-term follow-up in patients irradiated with doses mostly of between 4045 Gy. Int J Radiat Oncol Biol Phys 32:671–680, 1995.
62. McCord MW, Buatti JM, Fennel EM, et al: Radiotherapy for pituitary adenoma: Long-term outcome and sequellae. Int J Radiat Oncol Biol Phys 39:437–444, 1987.
63. Gittoes NJL, Bates AS, Tse W, et al: Radiotherapy for non-functioning pituitary adenomas. Clin Endocrinol 48:331–337, 1998.
64. Snyder PJ, Fowble B, Schatz et al: Hypopituitarism following radiation therapy of pituitary adenomas. Am J Med 81:457–462, 1986.
65. Littley MD, Shalet SM, Beardwell CG, Lillehei KO: Hypopituitarism following external radiotherapy for pituitary tumours in adults. Q J Med 145:160, 1970.
66. Nelson P, Goodman M, Flickenger J, et al: Endocrine function in patients with large pituitary tumors treated with operative decompression and radiation therapy. Neurosurgery 24:398–400, 1989.
67. Schatz NJ, Lichenstein S, Corbett JJ: In Glaser MS, Smith JL (eds): Neuro-Ophthalmopathy Symposium of the University of Miami and the Bascom Palmer Eye Institute. St Louis, Mosby–Year Book, 1978, pp 131–139.
68. Millar JL, Spry NA, Lamb DS, Delahunt J: Blindness in patients after external beam irradiation for pituitary adenoma: Two cases occuring after small daily fractional doses. Clin Oncol 3:291–294, 1991.
69. Brada M, Ford D, Ashley S, et al: Risk of second brain tumour after conservative surgery and radiotherapy for pituitary adenoma. BMJ 304:1343–1346, 1993.
70. Fisher BJ, Gaspar LE, Noone B: Radiation therapy of pituitary adenoma: Delayed sequelae. Radiology 187:843–846, 1993.
71. Dowsett RJ, Fowble B, Sergott RC, et al: Results of radiotherapy in the treatment of acromegaly: Lack of ophthalmologic complications. Int J Radiat Oncol Biol Phys 19:453–459, 1990.
72. Girkin CA, Comey CH, Lunsford LD, et al: Radiation optic neuropathy after stereotactic radiosurgery. Ophthalmology 104:1634–1643, 1997.
73. Berezin M, Olchovsky D, Pines A, et al: Reduction of follicle-stimulating hormone (FSH) secretion in FSH-producing pituitary adenoma by bromocriptine. J Clin Endocrinol Metab 59:1220–1222, 1984.
74. Vance ML, Ridgway EC, Thorner MO: Follicle-stimulating hormone and alpha subunit-secreting pituitary tumor treated with bromocriptine. J Clin Endocrinol Metab 61:580–584, 1985.
75. Kwekkeboom DJ, Lamberts SJ: Long-term treatment with the dopamine agonist CV 205-502 of patients with a clinically non-functioning, gonadotroph, or α-subunit secreting pituitary adenoma. Clin Endocrinol 36:171–176, 1992.
76. Sy RAG, Bernstein R, Chynn KY, Kourides IA: Reduction in size of a thyrotropin- and gonadotropin-secreting pituitary adenoma treated with octreotide acetate (somatostatin analog). J Clin Endocrinol Metab 74:690–694, 1992.
77. Warnet A, Harris AG, Renard E, et al: A prospective multicenter trial of octreotide in 24 patients with visual defects caused by nonfunctioning and gonadotropin-secreting adenomas. Neurosurgery 41:786–797, 1997.
78. Katznelson L, Oppenheim DS, Coughlin F, et al: Chronic somatostatin analog adminis-

tration in patients with alpha subunit–secreting pituitary adenomas. J Clin Endocrinol Metab 75:1318–1325, 1992.

79. Roman SH, Goldstein M, Kourides IA, et al: The luteinizing hormone–releasing hormone (LHRH) agonist [D-Trp6-Pro9-NEt] LHRH increased rather than lowered LH and alpha subunit levels in a patient with an LH-secreting pituitary tumor. J Clin Endocrinol Metab 58:313–319, 1984.

80. Klibanski A, Jameson JL, Biller BMK, et al: Gonadotropin and alpha subunit re-

sponses to chronic gonadotropin-releasing hormone analog administration in patients with glycoprotein hormone-secreting pituitary tumors. J Clin Endocrinol Metab 68:81–86, 1989.

81. McGrath GA, Goncalves RJ, Udupa JK, et al: New technique for quantitation of pituitary adenoma size: Use in evaluating treatment of gonadotroph adenomas with gonadotropin-releasing hormone antagonist. J Clin Endocrinol Metab 76:1363–1368, 1993.

Chapter 24

TSH-Producing Adenomas

Paolo Beck-Peccoz ▪ Luca Persani

Pituitary thyrotropin-producing adenomas (TSH-omas) are rare tumors that cause hyperthyroidism by chronically stimulating an intrinsically normal thyroid gland.[1-4] The first case of hyperthyroidism secondary to TSH-oma (central hyperthyroidism) was reported in 1960 by measuring serum TSH levels with a bioassay.[5] In 1970, Hamilton and coworkers[6] documented the first case of TSH-oma that was indisputably proved by modern radioimmunoassay techniques. Since then, about 300 patients have been reported in the literature. Although early reports describe these tumors as invasive macroadenomas that cause high morbidity and, in general, are difficult to be remove surgically, some cases are now more easily cured owing to earlier diagnosis. In fact, with the advent of ultrasensitive immunometric assays for TSH measurement, which are routinely performed in association with direct measurement of circulating free thyroid hormones (free thyroxine [FT$_4$] and free triiodothyronine [FT$_3$]), it is expected that patients with TSH-oma at the stage of microadenoma will be recognized with increasing frequency, thus permitting an improved clinical outcome.

Classically, TSH-omas, together with resistance to thyroid hormone,[7-9] were defined as syndromes of "inappropriate secretion of TSH," based on the common hormonal profile characterized by high levels of FT$_4$ and FT$_3$ in the presence of measurable TSH concentrations, a finding that contrasted with that observed in primary hyperthyroidism in which TSH is always undetectable. Nonetheless, the term *central hyperthyroidism* seems to be more pertinent for these disorders. However, clinically and biochemically euthyroid patients with pituitary adenomas that secrete TSH molecules, possibly with reduced bioactivity, have been described but not clearly documented.[10, 11] Moreover, pituitary hyperplasia and, in rare instances, true adenoma[12, 13] secondary to long-standing primary hypothyroidism are well-known clinical conditions, recently reviewed by us and others.[4] In the majority of these so-called feedback tumors, resolution of the pituitary lesion and normalization of TSH levels occur after levothyroxine replacement therapy, thus bringing into question the actual functional autonomy of such tumors (see Chapter 105).

The clinical importance of these rare entities is based on the diagnostic and therapeutic challenges they present. Failure to recognize these different diseases may result in dramatic consequences, such as improper thyroid ablation in patients with central hyperthyroidism or unnecessary pituitary surgery in patients with resistance to thyroid hormone. In contrast, early diagnosis and correct treatment of pituitary tumors prevent the occurrence of complications (visual defects by compression of the optic chiasm, hypopituitarism) and should improve the rate of cure.

OCCURRENCE

TSH-producing adenoma is a rare disorder accounting for about 0.5% to 1% of all pituitary adenomas in both clinical and surgical or pathologic series.[14, 15] The prevalence in the general population is 1 to 2 cases per million. However, it is worth considering that these data were calculated many years ago, when probably only a minority of these tumors was diagnosed. Indeed, the number of reported cases of

TSH-omas has tripled since the late 1980s (Fig. 24–1). A recent report confirms this trend in a large surgical series, indicating that the occurrence of TSH-omas increased from less than 1% to 2.8% from 1989 to 1991.[16] This increased number of recorded cases results from the introduction of ultrasensitive immunoradiometric assays for TSH as a first-line test for the evaluation of thyroid function. Based on the finding of measurable serum TSH levels in the presence of elevated thyroid hormone concentrations, many patients previously thought to have Graves' disease can be correctly diagnosed as having a TSH-secreting pituitary adenoma or, alternatively, resistance to thyroid hormone. Moreover, an increased awareness by the endocrinologist and general practitioner regarding the existence of central hyperthyroidism has greatly contributed to the disclosure of a higher number of patients with such a rare disorder.

PATHOLOGY AND ETIOPATHOGENESIS

The thyrotroph is the cell type of origin in TSH-omas. These tumors are nearly always benign; at present, transformation of a TSH-oma into a carcinoma with multiple metastases has been reported in only one patient.[17] The majority of them (72%) secrete TSH alone, although this is often accompanied by unbalanced hypersecretion of the α subunit. About one fourth of TSH-omas are mixed adenomas, characterized by concomitant hypersecretion of other anterior pituitary hormones, mainly growth hormone (GH) or prolactin (PRL), or both, which are known to share with TSH the common transcription factor Pit-1. Indeed, hypersecretion of TSH and GH is the most frequent association (16%), followed by hypersecretion of TSH and PRL (10.4%) and occasionally TSH and gonadotropins (1.4%) (Fig. 24–2).

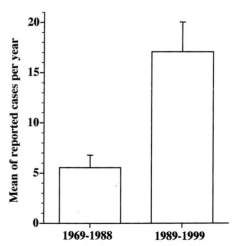

FIGURE 24–1. *The significant increase of reported cases of TSH-producing adenoma in the last decade, when ultrasensitive TSH assay and direct methods for free thyroid hormone measurement became available as first-line tests of thyroid function.*

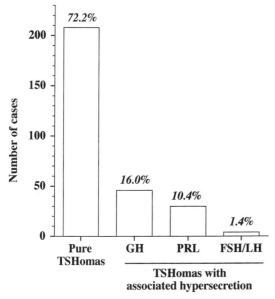

FIGURE 24–2. Classification of TSH-producing adenomas based on hormone secretion into circulation.

No association with adrenocorticotropic hormone (ACTH) hypersecretion has been documented to date. An ectopic TSH-producing adenoma has been documented in the pharyngeal hypophysis.[18]

At morphologic and histopathologic analysis, most TSH-omas are macroadenomas (87%), frequently with fibrous consistency, even in the absence of prior surgery or radiotherapy, and high local invasiveness.[19] However, previous thyroid ablation by surgery or radioiodine has deleterious effects on the size and invasiveness of the tumor (Fig. 24–3).[4, 20] In fact, invasive macroadenomas were found in 49% of patients who had undergone thyroid ablation versus 27% in those who were untreated, whereas the figure was reversed in patients with microadenomas (diameter <1 cm) or intrasellar macroadenomas. Therefore, previous thyroid ablation may induce an aggressive transformation of the tumor, as observed in Nelson's syndrome after adrenalectomy for Cushing's disease.

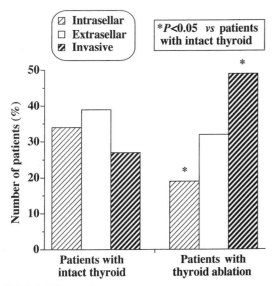

FIGURE 24–3. Effects of previous thyroid ablation on the size of TSH-producing adenomas. *Intrasellar* refers to both microadenomas and intrasellar macroadenomas, *extrasellar* to macroadenomas with suprasellar extension, and *invasive* to invasive macroadenomas. Data have been calculated from 253 reported patients (163 with intact thyroid and 90 with thyroid ablation). Statistical analysis has been carried out by Fisher's exact test.

Light microscopy shows that adenoma cells are chromophobic, although they occasionally stain with either basic or acid dyes. Ultrastructurally, adenomatous cells frequently appear monomorphous, even if they hypersecrete TSH, α subunit, and other pituitary tropins.[21, 22] Cells with abnormal morphologic features or mitoses,[23] which may be misinterpreted as pituitary malignancy or metastases from distant carcinomas, are present in poorly differentiated adenomas that are characterized by the presence of fusiform cells with sparse and small secretory granules (80 to 200 nm). Indeed, there are no clear criteria of malignancy for TSH-omas except for the presence of metastases. It is worth noting that the only carcinoma reported so far exhibited a progressive malignant transformation accompanied by a decline of TSH and α subunit secretion.[17]

Immunostaining studies show the presence of TSH-β, either free or combined with the α subunit. By using double immunostaining, the existence of mixed TSH-α subunit adenomas composed of one cell type secreting α subunit alone and another cosecreting α subunit and TSH has been documented.[24] In addition to α subunit, TSH frequently colocalizes with other pituitary hormones in the same tumoral cell[25] or even in the same secretory granule.[21, 24, 26, 27] Nonetheless, positive immunohistochemistry panels for one or more pituitary hormones does not necessarily correlate with hypersecretion in vivo.[28] Indeed, positive immunostaining for ACTH and gonadotropins without evidence of in vivo hypersecretion has been reported.[29–33]

TSH-omas have been shown to be monoclonal in origin,[34] and several studies have screened a substantial number of adenomas for proto-oncogene activation[28, 29, 35–37] or loss of antioncogenes,[36, 38] yielding negative results.[4] A highly variable expression of thyrotropin-releasing hormone (TRH) and dopamine receptors was documented in several adenomas,[39–41] whereas functional somatostatin receptors were constantly detected in TSH-omas,[42–45] thus providing the rationale for their medical treatment with somatostatin analogues.

CLINICAL FEATURES

Patients with TSH-oma present with the signs and symptoms of either hyperthyroidism or the mass effect of an expanding intracranial tumor (Table 24–1). TSH-omas may occur at any age (range, 11 to 84 years), although most patients are in the third to sixth decade of life. Unlike the female predominance seen in the other common thyroid disorders, TSH-omas occur with equal frequency in males and females. Goiter and clinical thyrotoxicosis are the most common presenting symptoms. Most patients presented with a long history of thyroid dysfunction, often mistakenly diagnosed as Graves' disease, and one third had inappropriate thyroidectomy or radioiodine thyroid ablation, or both. Thus, patients with TSH-omas may present to the specialist with hyperthyroidism that has been refractory to prior therapeutic attempts. In general, clinical features of hyperthyroidism are sometimes milder than expected on the basis of serum thyroid hormone

TABLE 24–1. Clinical Characteristics of Patients with TSH-oma*

	Patients with TSH-oma % (n/Total)†
Age, yr	40.8 ± 14.1 (191)‡
Female sex	55 (148/268)
Previous thyroid ablation	33 (95/290)
Severe thyrotoxicosis	24 (44/181)
Goiter	93 (173/185)
Thyroid nodules	72 (46/64)
Macroadenomas	87 (221/253)
Visual field defect	41 (56/137)
Headache	20 (22/113)
Menstrual disorders§	32 (24/74)

*Data from reports published until January 1999.
†n/Total refers to the number of patients for whom the information was available.
‡Mean ± SD (n).
§Data include women with or without associated prolactin hypersecretion.

levels. Moreover, individual patients with untreated TSH-oma were reported to be clinically euthyroid.[10, 46, 47] This emphasizes the importance of systematic measurement of TSH and FT$_4$ in all patients with pituitary tumor to disclose those with central hyper- or hypothyroidism. In some acromegalic patients, signs or symptoms of hyperthyroidism are missed, as they are overshadowed by those of acromegaly.[21, 48] Severe thyrotoxic features clinically, such as atrial fibrillation, cardiac failure, and episodes of periodic paralysis,[49, 50] are observed in one fourth of cases.

The presence of a goiter is the rule (93%), even in patients who have undergone previous partial thyroidectomy. As the thyroid is intrinsically normal in this disorder, it may regrow even after near total resection as a consequence of TSH hyperstimulation. Occurrence of multinodular goiter has been reported in several patients,[51] and differentiated thyroid carcinoma has been reported in two patients.[52, 53] Progression towards functional autonomy seems to be infrequent.[54, 55] In contrast to Graves' disease, the occurrence of circulating antithyroid autoantibodies is similar to that found in the general population. Unilateral exophthalmos due to orbital invasion by pituitary tumor was reported in only three patients with TSH-omas, whereas Graves-associated bilateral ophthalmopathy was reported in five patients.[4]

Most patients bearing a TSH-producing macroadenoma seek medical attention with signs and symptoms of an expanding intracranial tumor. Indeed, as a consequence of tumor suprasellar extension or invasiveness, signs and symptoms of tumor mass prevail over those of thyroid hyperfunction in many patients. Visual field defects are present in about two thirds and headache in one fifth of patients. Moreover, partial hypopituitarism is common and loss of gonadal function is present in about one third of patients.[19, 56] Galactorrhea was recorded in almost all patients with mixed TSH- and PRL-secreting tumors.[57, 58]

Finally, TSH-omas may occur in families with multiple endocrine neoplasia type 1[59–61] and in McCune-Albright syndrome.[62]

BIOCHEMICAL FINDINGS

TSH and Thyroid Hormone Levels

High concentrations of thyroid hormones in the presence of detectable TSH levels are typically present in patients with hyperthyroidism due to a TSH-oma or with resistance to thyroid hormone. In the case of replacement therapy for prior thyroidectomy or thyroid ablation, it is crucial to assess patients in steady-state, as TSH levels need 4 to 6 weeks to adjust to a change in levothyroxine dose. Thus, the diagnosis of TSH-producing adenoma may be difficult to establish in any patient who has had a dramatic change in thyroid hormone replacement therapy resulting from either physician instruction or poor compliance. Conversely, the finding of elevated TSH levels in patients who have undergone thyroid ablation and have been overtreated with levothyroxine, should be regarded as a possible sign of previously undiagnosed TSH-oma.[63]

Various abnormalities in the pituitary-thyroid axis, as well as laboratory artifacts, may cause a biochemical profile similar to that characterizing central hyperthyroidism. These different conditions are more common than are TSH-omas and resistance to thyroid hormone and should be excluded before performing the extensive clinical assessment of the possible presence of central hyperthyroidism. Either familial or drug- or estrogen-induced increases of circulating thyroxine binding globulin (TBG) or variants of albumin or transthyretin lead to increases in the levels of total serum thyroid hormone, particularly T$_4$, thus producing a biochemical profile that may be confused with TSH-omas. Therefore, the measurement of free thyroid hormones is mandatory in these conditions and should be performed by means of direct "two-step" methods, that is, methods that are able to avoid contact between serum proteins and tracer at the time of assay.[64, 65] Indeed, normal levels of total T$_4$ were recorded in several patients with TSH-oma, and only the measurement of FT$_4$ allowed the right diagnosis of central hyperthyroidism. Furthermore, inhibition of T$_4$ to T$_3$ conversion induced by iodine-containing drugs or nonthyroidal illness may cause hyperthyroxinemia and nonsuppressed TSH that are, however, associated with normal or low-normal T$_3$. In clinically ambiguous situations, the differential diagnosis rests on the recognition of the underlying disorder as well as documenting normalization of thyroid function test results at a later stage or after recovery of drug withdrawal.

Several laboratory artifacts may cause falsely high serum levels of either TSH or thyroid hormones (Table 24–2). The more common factors interfering in TSH measurement are heterophilic antibodies directed against mouse gamma globulins[66] or anti-TSH antibodies. However, preventing the formation of the "sandwich", anti-TSH antibodies usually leads to an underestimation of the actual levels of TSH and rarely to an overestimation. The presence of anti-T$_4$ or anti-T$_3$ autoantibodies, or both, may cause FT$_4$ or FT$_3$, or both, to be overestimated, particularly when "one-step" analogue methods are employed.[65] Finally, because patients with a TSH-oma may have T$_3$ toxicosis as in other forms of hyperthyroidism, there is a need to measure T$_3$ and, in particular, free T$_3$ when T$_4$ levels are normal.

In TSH-omas, extremely variable levels of serum TSH and thyroid hormones have been reported (Table 24–3). Interestingly, in patients previously treated with thyroid ablation, TSH levels are dramatically higher than in untreated patients, although free thyroid hormone levels were still in the hyperthyroid range and the reduction of total thyroid hormone levels was minimal. The conserved sensitivity of tumoral thyrotroph cells to even small reductions of circulating free thyroid hormone levels is confirmed by the rapidly increased rate of TSH secretion during antithyroid drug administration.[48]

Although patients with TSH-oma have a TSH-dependent hyperstimulation of the thyroid gland, any significant correlation between immunoreactive TSH and free thyroid hormone levels is lacking, even though only untreated patients are taken into account. Moreover, in one third of these patients, high levels of free thyroid hormones are associated with immunoreactive TSH levels within the normal range. Variations of the biologic activity of secreted TSH molecules most likely account for these findings.[67] The first demonstration that circulating TSH in patients with TSH-oma may possess an enhanced bioactivity was made in one patient with a mixed GH-TSH–secreting pituitary adenoma in whom a ratio between biologic and immunologic activities of TSH significantly higher than that of controls was documented.[21] Other studies indicate that the circulating TSH biologic/immunologic activity ratio may be normal, reduced, or increased in patients with TSH-oma,[19, 67, 68] probably because of altered glycosylation of circulating TSH molecules. In fact, both intrapituitary and circulating TSH exist as multiple isoforms characterized by heterogeneity of oligosaccharide chains, which has a great impact on hormone biologic properties, such as biologic activity and metabolic clearance rate. Tumoral transformation may be accompanied by variable alterations of the post-translational processing within thyrotrophs, leading to the secretion of TSH molecules with peculiar glycosylation and biologic properties.[67, 69, 70]

Glycoprotein Hormone α Subunit

TSH-omas commonly secrete excessive quantities of the free α subunit, resulting in high levels of circulating free α subunit in two

TABLE 24–2. Circulating Factors That May Interfere with Measurement Hormone, Thus Simulating the Presence of a TSH-Producing Adenoma

Heterophilic antibodies directed against mouse γ-globulins leading to interference with monoclonal antibodies used in the immunometric assay*
Anti-TSH autoantibodies or antibodies cross-reacting with TSH†
Anti-iodothyronine autoantibodies (anti-T$_4$ or anti-T$_3$ or both)‡
Abnormal forms of albumin or transthyretin (e.g., familial dysalbuminemic hyperthyroxinemia)‡

*This interference is commonly prevented by the addition of a few microliters of mouse serum to the assay buffer.
†Overestimation of thyroid-stimulating hormone (TSH) is rare in the presence of such antibodies. The interference cannot be prevented, but it can be documented by performing dilution and recovery tests in the immunoassay.
‡To prevent misdiagnosis, measure free T$_4$ and free T$_3$ by direct "two-step" methods.[64, 65]

TABLE 24–3. Biochemical Data of Patients with TSH-oma

Parameter	Patients with Intact Thyroid	Patients with Thyroid Ablation	P
TSH, mU/L*	9.4 ± 1.1 (116)	55.8 ± 10.2 (79)	<0.0002
α Subunit, μg/L*	17.6 ± 5.6 (66)	14.54 ± 2.7 (46)	NS
α Subunit/TSH, molar ratio*,†	43.8 ± 15.2 (66)	3.7 ± 0.7 (46)	<0.03
TT₄, nmol/L*	243.5 ± 19.9 (30)	177.1 ± 9.8 (45)	<0.002
FT₄, pmol/L*	43.2 ± 2.5 (64)	28.6 ± 2.4 (29)	<0.0006
TT₃, nmol/L*	5.2 ± 0.3 (27)	4.1 ± 0.3 (42)	NS
FT₃, pmol/L*	16.6 ± 0.9 (52)	10.5 ± 0.9 (20)	<0.0005
Normal TSH levels‡	33% (52/159)	11% (9/78)	<0.0005
High α subunit levels‡	65% (63/97)	73% (35/48)	NS
High α subunit/TSH, molar ratio‡	88% (83/94)	77% (37/48)	NS
High SHBG levels‡	90% (19/21)	67% (6/9)	NS
Abnormal TSH response to TRH test†,§	83% (109/132)	83% (58/70)	NS
Abnormal TSH response to T₃ suppression test‡,‖	100% (46/46)	100% (33/33)	NS

Data from reports published until January 1999.
*Mean ± SE (n).
†To calculate α subunit//TSH molar ratio divide α subunit (μg/L) by TSH (mU/L) and multiply by 10 provided that TSH International Reference Preparation 80/558 is used in the immunometric assay.
‡% (n/total).
§Net TSH increment <4.0 mU/L.
‖Lack of complete TSH inhibition after 8 to 10 days of L-T₃ administration (80–100 μg/day).
TSH, thyroid-stimulating hormone; TT₄, total thyroxine; FT₄, free thyroxine; TT₃, total triiodothyronine; FT₃, free triiodothyronine; SHBG, sex hormone-binding globulin; TRH, thyrotropin-releasing hormone.

thirds of patients (see Table 24–3). This is another expression of the altered synthetic process within tumoral thyrotrophs and represents a helpful diagnostic clue to the presence of a TSH-oma. Secretion of the α subunit in these tumors is in excess not only of the TSH-β subunit but also of the intact TSH molecule. This results in a molar ratio of α subunit to TSH, which is generally higher than 1. Although previous studies have suggested that a ratio greater than 1.0 is indicative of the presence of TSH-producing adenoma,[1, 71] similar values have been observed in normal controls, particularly in postmenopausal women, indicating the need for appropriate control groups matched for TSH and gonadotropin levels.[4, 51, 72] Interestingly, microadenomas that frequently have α subunit levels within the normal range may show a high α subunit/TSH molar ratio. Furthermore, it has been suggested that extremely high levels of free α subunit might portend future malignant behavior and that a spontaneous and marked decrease of both TSH and α subunit might indicate that the tumor is becoming less differentiated and correlate with invasive and metastatic behavior.[17]

Parameters Evaluating Peripheral Thyroid Hormone Action

The measurements of several parameters of peripheral thyroid hormone action both in vivo (basal metabolic rate, cardiac systolic time intervals, Achilles' reflex time) and in vitro (sex hormone–binding globulin [SHBG], cholesterol, angiotensin-converting enzyme, osteocalcin, blood red cell sodium content, carboxyterminal cross-linked telopeptide of type I collagen [ICTP], and so on)[73] may help in quantifying the degree of peripheral hyperthyroidism, particularly in patients with mild clinical signs and symptoms[30, 48, 51, 74–77] (see Table 24–3). In particular, evaluations of SHBG and ICTP may help differentiate hyperthyroid patients with TSH-oma, in whom these parameters are elevated, from those with resistance to thyroid hormone, in whom they are in the range of those of euthyroid subjects.

DYNAMIC TESTING

Several stimulatory and inhibitory tests have been employed to evaluate TSH secretory dynamics in patients with TSH-oma. None of these tests is of clear-cut diagnostic value, and the combination of some of them may increase their accuracy in disclosing the pituitary adenoma. Among the stimulatory tests, TRH-induced TSH secretion is absent or blunted in 83% of patients (see Table 24–3). Although the

α subunit response to the preceding stimulatory agents usually paralleled that of TSH, in some cases discrepancy between α subunit and TSH response to TRH has been recorded. Such a discrepancy may be due to the presence of mixed adenomas, composed of distinct cell types that possess different receptor expression.[21, 24] Most TSH-omas are unable to increase TSH secretion after administration of dopamine antagonists such as domperidone or sulpiride. Chronic treatment with antithyroid drugs induces an increase in serum TSH levels in most patients because of both the high sensitivity of adenomatous cells to the reduction of circulating levels of FT₄ and FT₃[48] and the recovered TSH secretion by normal thyrotrophs surrounding the adenoma in response to the activated feedback mechanism.[4, 78] In keeping with this are the observations of significantly higher TSH levels in patients who have undergone thyroid ablation, as well as the more active proliferation of tumoral cells in treated patients.

Among inhibitory tests, a complete inhibition of both basal and TRH-stimulated TSH secretion after a T₃ suppression test (Werner test: 80 to 100 μg/day of levothyronine for 8 to 10 days) has never been recorded in a patient with a TSH-oma (see Table 24–3), although a slight TSH reduction may occur in a minority of patients. In patients who have undergone previous thyroid ablation, this test is the most sensitive and specific in documenting the possible presence of a TSH-oma. However, high doses of T₃ are contraindicated in elderly patients or in those with coronary heart disease. Dopamine (1 to 4 μg/kg body weight/min intravenously) or dopamine agonists, such as bromocriptine (2.5 mg orally), are generally ineffective in inhibiting TSH secretion, whereas native somatostatin or its analogues reduce TSH levels in the majority of cases and may be predictive of the efficacy of long-term treatment in the majority of patients.[51, 79, 80]

IMAGING STUDIES AND LOCALIZATION

When considering the diagnosis of a TSH-oma, full imaging studies, particularly high-resolution computed tomography (CT) or nuclear magnetic resonance imaging (MRI), are necessary. However, since most TSH-omas are macroadenomas, alterations of the sella profile on plain radiographs are present in many cases. Curiously, in two patients, pituitary stones have been described.[81] Various degrees of suprasellar extension or sphenoidal sinus invasion are present in two thirds of cases.

Microadenomas are now reported with increasing frequency, accounting for about 13% of all recorded cases. In contrast to other secreting pituitary tumors,[82] no correlation between serum TSH levels and tumor size was found in untreated patients with TSH-oma. Pituitary scintigraphy with radiolabeled Tyr³-substituted octreotide has been shown to successfully image TSH-omas.[83] Moreover, in vivo evidence for both somatostatin and dopamine D_2-receptors was obtained by using single-photon emission tomography with ¹¹¹In-pentetreotide and ¹²³I-iodobenzamide.[80, 84] The presence of these receptors correlates with the sensitivity of the tumor to chronic medical treatment. ¹¹¹In-pentetreotide scintigraphy may also be useful in localizing possible ectopic TSH-producing adenomas. Finally, bilateral petrosal sinus sampling has been used in difficult cases, allowing the identification and lateralization of a microadenoma not seen on radiographic scans.[85] However, one should expect a certain number of false lateralizations, as already observed for ACTH-secreting pituitary tumors.

DIFFERENTIAL DIAGNOSIS

The presence of detectable TSH levels in a hyperthyroid patient rules out primary hyperthyroidism, whereas in patients receiving levothyroxine replacement for primary hypothyroidism, poor compliance is by far the most common cause of apparent inappropriate secretion of TSH, with TSH still too high for the levels of the thyroid hormones. This underscores the importance of studying patients in steady-state. The first step in the case of hyperthyroxinemia and detectable TSH is to measure free thyroid hormone levels and repeat TSH measurement by ultrasensitive assays. The finding of normal TSH, FT_4 and FT_3 levels suggests euthyroid hyperthyroxinemia, whereas high FT_4 and FT_3 concentrations and suppressed TSH definitively indicate the presence of primary hyperthyroidism due to Graves' disease and other forms of thyrotoxicosis. If FT_4 and FT_3 concentrations are elevated in the presence of measurable TSH levels, it is important to exclude methodologic interference. When the existence of central hyperthyroidism is eventually confirmed, several diagnostic steps have to be carried out to differentiate a TSH-oma from resistance to thyroid hormone. This is particularly true for the variant of resistance to thyroid hormone with predominant pituitary resistance where there are clear clinical signs of hyperthyroidism.[7–9] Indeed, alterations of pituitary content on CT or MRI, as well as the possible presence of neurologic signs and symptoms (visual defects, headache) or clinical features of concomitant hypersecretion of other pituitary hormones (acromegaly, galactorrhea, amenorrhea) definitely point to the presence of a TSH-oma. Nevertheless, the differential diagnosis may be difficult when the pituitary adenoma is undetectable by CT or MRI or in the case of confusing (empty sella) or incidental pituitary lesions.[86, 87] No significant differences in age, sex, previous thyroid ablation, TSH levels, or free thyroid hormone concentrations occur between patients with TSH-oma and those with resistance to thyroid hormone (Table 24–4). However, in contrast with resistance to thyroid hormone pa-

tients, familial cases of TSH-oma have never been documented. The finding of measurable TSH levels and high concentrations of FT_4 and FT_3 in one relative definitely points to the diagnosis of resistance to thyroid hormone. Serum TSH levels within the normal range are more frequently found in resistance to thyroid hormone, whereas elevated α subunit concentrations or high α subunit/TSH molar ratio is typically present in patients with TSH-omas. Moreover, absent or impaired TSH responses to TRH administration and to the T_3 suppression test favor the presence of a TSH-oma. Circulating SHBG levels are in the hyperthyroid range in patients with TSH-oma, the only patients with low SHBG being those with concomitant hypersecretion of GH, which potently inhibits SHBG secretion. The few patients with thyroid hormone resistance and high SHBG levels were those treated with estrogens or those showing profound hypogonadism.[76] Other parameters that may be useful in the differential diagnosis are the markers of bone turnover, such as ICTP (altered in TSH-omas, normal in resistance to thyroid hormone), or total cholesterol (rarely high in TSH-omas).[9, 77] In difficult cases, particularly after thyroidectomy, genetic investigations on the thyroid hormone receptor–β_1 mutations may be the only diagnostic test. Finally, an apparent association between TSH-oma and resistance to thyroid hormone has been reported in a young Japanese woman.[74] Although genetic studies and familial investigations were not carried out in this case, the occurrence of TSH-omas in patients with resistance to thyroid hormone is theoretically possible and, therefore, should be carefully considered.

TREATMENT AND OUTCOME

Pituitary Surgery and Radiation Therapy

The primary goal in the treatment of TSH-omas is to remove the pituitary tumor and restore euthyroidism. Therefore, the first therapeutic approach to TSH-producing adenomas should be to surgically remove or debulk the tumor by transsphenoidal or subfrontal adenomectomy, the choice of route depending on the tumor volume and its suprasellar extension.[88, 89] This may be particularly difficult because of the marked fibrosis of these tumors and the local invasion involving the cavernous sinus, internal carotid artery, or optic chiasm. In order to restore euthyroidism before surgery, antithyroid drugs or octreotide along with propranolol can be administered. If surgery is contraindicated or declined, pituitary radiotherapy (no less than 45 Gy fractionated at 2 Gy/day or 10 to 25 Gy in a single dose if a stereotactic gamma unit is available) and subsequent somatostatin analogue administration should be considered.

Surgery alone or combined with radiotherapy induces normalization of thyroid hormone levels and apparent complete removal of tumor

TABLE 24–4. Differential Diagnosis Between TSH-Producing Adenomas (TSH-omas) and Resistance to Thyroid Hormones

Parameter	TSH-omas	Resistance to Thyroid Hormones	P
Age, yr	11–84	0.1–80	NS
Sex, F/M ratio	1.28	1.17	NS
TSH, mU/L*	2.7 ± 0.6	2.2 ± 0.3	NS
FT_4, pmol/L*	40.0 ± 4.2	29.5 ± 2.5	NS
FT_3, pmol/L*	14.5 ± 1.4	11.7 ± 1.0	NS
SHBG, nmol/L*	113.0 ± 17.2	62.0 ± 4.0	<0.0001
Familial cases	0%	81%	<0.0001
Lesions at CT or MRI	98%	2%	<0.0001
High α subunit levels	65%	2%	<0.0001
High α subunit/TSH, molar ratio	81%	2%	<0.0001
Abnormal TSH response to TRH test†	83%	4%	<0.0001
Abnormal TSH response to T_3 suppression test‡	100%	100%§	NS

*Only patients with an intact thyroid were taken into account. Data are obtained from patients followed at the Institute of Endocrine Sciences, University of Milan, Milan, Italy (13 cases of TSH-omas and 59 cases of resistance to thryoid hormones) and are expressed as mean ± SE.

†Net TSH increment <4.0 mU/L.

‡Werner's test (80–100 μg T_3 for 8–10 days). Quantitatively normal responses to T_3, that is, complete inhibition of both basal and thyrotropin-releasing hormone (TRH)-stimulated thyroid-stimulating hormone (TSH) levels, have never been recorded in either group of patients.

§Although abnormal in quantitative terms, TSH response to T_3 suppression test is qualitatively normal in the majority of patients with resistance to thyroid hormones.[7–9]

mass in about one third of patients, whereas the normalization of thyroid hormones without a complete removal of the adenoma occurs in an another third of patients (Table 24–5). Collectively, about two thirds of TSH-omas are under control with surgery or irradiation, or both. In the remaining patients, the large size and the invasiveness of the tumor prevent successful removal of the tumor. Elevation of α subunit or cosecretion of other pituitary hormones does not seem to be an unfavorable prognostic factor. Postsurgical deaths were reported in five cases. Partial or complete hypopituitarism may be the result of surgery. Evaluation of other pituitary functions, particularly ACTH secretion, should be carefully undertaken soon after surgery and checked again every year, especially in patients treated by radiotherapy. In addition, in the case of surgical cure, postoperative TSH is undetectable and may remain low for many weeks or months, causing central hypothyroidism. The time necessary for the recovery of normal thyrotrophs is variable, and occasionally permanent central hypothyroidism may occur because of damage to the normal thyrotroph by the tumor or during surgery. Thus, temporary or permanent levothyroxine replacement therapy may be necessary. In a few cases, total thyroidectomy was performed after pituitary surgery failed because the patients were at risk of thyroid storm.

Medical Treatment

In terms of pharmacologic therapy of TSH-omas, antithyroid drugs must not be used as medical treatment of TSH-omas because they may cause more rapid growth and invasiveness of the tumors, and their use is recommended only as preparation of the patient for neurosurgery. For alleviating the symptoms of hyperthyroidism, β-blockers such as propranolol may be used. Glucocorticoids are effective in reducing TSH secretion but they induce deleterious side effects in long-term treatment. Dopamine agonists, particularly bromocriptine, have been employed in some TSH-omas with variable results, the positive effects observed in some patients with mixed TSH- and PRL-secreting adenoma diminishing with time.[90] Currently, the medical treatment of TSH-omas rests on somatostatin analogues such as octreotide[44, 79, 80, 91] or the new slow-release formulation of lanreotide.[92] Octreotide leads to a reduction of TSH and α subunit secretion in almost all cases, with restoration of the euthyroid state in the majority of them (see Table 24–5). Moreover, modifications of the TSH glycoisomer distribution pattern during octreotide treatment have been documented in one patient,[93] suggesting that restoration of euthyroidism in some patients showing no reduction in immunoreactive levels of TSH during octreotide therapy may be due to a reduction of the bioactivity of secreted molecules.[79, 94] During octreotide therapy, tumor shrinkage occurs in about half of patients (see Table 24–5) and vision improvement is seen in 75%.

Tachyphylaxis occurred in 22% of patients and responded to increasing octreotide doses, whereas long-term studies demonstrated true escape from the inhibitory effects in few cases. In only 5% of cases was a true resistance to octreotide treatment documented. Octreotide treatment was effective in restoring euthyroidism in one pregnant woman with central hyperthyroidism and had no side effects on fetal development and thyroid function.[95] Patients taking octreotide have

to be carefully monitored because untoward side effects, such as cholelithiasis and carbohydrate intolerance, may become manifested. The dose administered should be tailored for each patient, depending on therapeutic response and tolerance (including gastrointestinal side effects). The marked octreotide-induced suppression of TSH secretion and consequent biochemical hypothyroidism seen in some patients may require levothyroxine substitution. Whether somatostatin analogue treatment may be an alternative to surgery and irradiation in patients with TSH-oma remains to be established. However, the slow-release preparation of somatostatin, lanreotide-SR, and octreotide-LAR, may represent a useful tool for long-term treatment of such a rare pituitary adenoma.[92]

CRITERIA OF CURE AND FOLLOW-UP

Evidence has accumulated about the criteria of cure and follow-up of patients undergoing operation or irradiation for TSH-omas.[4, 48, 51] In untreated hyperthyroid patients, it is reasonable to assume that cured patients have clinical and biochemical reversal of thyroid hyperfunction. However, normal free thyroid hormone concentrations or indices of peripheral thyroid hormone action in the euthyroid range may be associated with a partial removal or destruction of tumoral cells, since transient clinical remission and euthyroidism are frequently observed.[48, 51] As it occurs for other pituitary tumors, disappearance of neurologic signs and symptoms only partially reflects the radicality of tumor removal, since it may occur even in the presence of an incomplete debulking of the tumor. Pituitary imaging performed after surgery has a low predictivity because of the high frequency of false-negative imaging results. The criteria of normalization of circulating TSH are not applicable to previously thyroidectomized patients or to those with normal basal values of TSH. In our experience, undetectable TSH levels 1 week after surgery are likely to indicate complete adenomectomy provided that the patient was hyperthyroid and presurgical treatments were stopped at least 10 days before surgery.[48] Similarly, although normalization of α subunit or α subunit/TSH molar ratio is in general a good index for the evaluation of therapy efficacy; both parameters are normal in a remarkable number of patients with TSH-oma. The most sensitive and specific test to document the complete removal of the adenoma remains the T_3 suppression test (in the absence of clinical contraindication). In fact, regardless of the restoration of euthyroidism, only patients in whom T_3 administration completely inhibits basal and TRH-stimulated TSH secretion appear to be truly cured (Fig. 24–4).

Data on the recurrence rate of TSH-oma in patients judged cured after surgery or radiotherapy are still lacking. However, the recurrence of the adenoma does not appear to be frequent, at least in the first years after successful surgery. In general, the patient should be evaluated clinically and biochemically two or three times the first year postoperatively and then every year. Pituitary imaging should be performed every 2 or 3 years but should be performed promptly whenever an increase in TSH and thyroid hormone levels or clinical symptoms occur. In the case of persistent macroadenoma, a close visual field follow-up is required, as the visual function is threatened.

CONCLUSIONS

Central hyperthyroidism due to TSH-secreting pituitary adenomas is a rare cause of thyrotoxicosis. The diagnosis is now facilitated by the recent introduction of ultrasensitive TSH immunoassays as well as direct free thyroid hormone measurement, which are not obscured by abnormal serum transport proteins. Increased awareness and early recognition of these tumors will prevent inappropriate treatment, such as thyroid ablation or long-term antithyroid drug administration, which undoubtedly increases TSH secretion, tumor size, and invasiveness. Although no single diagnostic test is pathognomonic in establishing the diagnosis, the elevation of α subunit levels and serum SHBG concentrations, as well as the frequently absent or impaired TSH responses to TRH and T_3 suppression tests, are the most useful markers to distinguish patients with TSH-omas from those with thyroid hor-

TABLE 24–5. Results of Various Treatments in Patients with TSH-Producing Adenoma

	Surgery (n = 123)	Surgery + Radiation (n = 56)	Somatostatin Analogues (n = 75)
Reduction of tumor mass			
Complete	33%	29%	0%
Partial	33%	41%	53%
Absent	34%	30%	48%
Resolution of clinical symptoms			
Yes	56%	61%	95%
No	44%	39%	5%

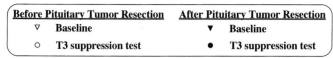

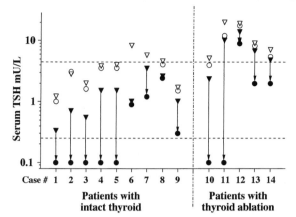

FIGURE 24–4. Results of T$_3$ suppression test carried out before and after pituitary surgery in patients with TSH-producing adenoma. *Horizontal dashed lines* indicate the normal range of serum TSH. Note the lack of TSH suppression in all patients before neurosurgery. Complete suppression of serum TSH levels (i.e., complete removal of the adenoma) was seen in about half of patients after neurosurgery, independent of previous thyroid ablation.

mone resistance. Furthermore, high resolution CT and MRI may help in detecting tumors as small as 3 mm. Surgery still remains the first therapeutic approach to the disease, followed by radiotherapy in the case of failure. The finding of measurable TSH levels after a simple T$_3$ suppression test definitely indicates that the removal of the tumor cells was incomplete, thus requiring a closer follow-up of the patient or additional therapies, or both. If needed, treatment with somatostatin analogues is worthwhile, allowing restoration of euthyroidism and even tumor shrinkage in many cases.

Acknowledgment

The authors thank Dr. Anna Spada for the critical reading of the manuscript.

REFERENCES

1. Smallridge RC: Thyrotropin-secreting tumors. *In* Mazzaferri EL, Samaan NA (eds): Endocrine Tumors. Boston, Blackwell, 1993, p 136.
2. Samuels MH, Ridgway EC: Glycoprotein-secreting pituitary adenomas. Baillieres Clin Endocrinol 9:337, 1995.
3. Greenman Y, Melmed S: Thyrotropin-secreting pituitary tumors. *In* Melmed S (ed): The Pituitary. Boston, Blackwell Science, 1995, p 546.
4. Beck-Peccoz P, Brucker-Davis F, Persani L, et al: Thyrotropin-secreting pituitary tumors. Endocr Rev 17:610, 1996.
5. Jailer JW, Holub DA: Remission of Graves' disease following radiotherapy of a pituitary neoplasm. Am J Med 28:497, 1960.
6. Hamilton C, Adams LC, Maloof F: Hyperthyroidism due to thyrotropin-producing pituitary chromophobe adenoma. N Engl J Med 283:1077, 1970.
7. Refetoff S, Weiss RE, Usala SJ: The syndromes of resistance to thyroid hormone. Endocr Rev 14:348, 1993.
8. Beck-Peccoz P, Asteria C, Mannavola D: Resistance to thyroid hormone. *In* Braverman LE (ed): Contemporary Endocrinology: Diseases of the Thyroid. Totowa, NJ, Humana Press, 1997, p 199.
9. Chatterjee VKK, Clifton-Bright RJ, Gurnell M: Thyroid hormone resistance. *In* Jameson JL (ed): Contemporary Endocrinology: Hormone Resistance Syndromes. Totowa, NJ, Humana Press, 1999, p 145.
10. Felix I, Asa SL, Kovacs K, et al: Recurrent plurihormonal bimorphous pituitary adenoma producing growth hormone, thyrotropin, and prolactin. Arch Pathol Lab Med 118:66, 1994.
11. Bertholon-Grégoire M, Trouillas J, Guigard MP, et al: Mono and plurihormonal thyrotropic pituitary adenomas: Pathological, hormonal and clinical studies in twelve patients. Eur J Endocrinol 140:519, 1999.
12. Katz MS, Gregerman RI, Horvath E, et al: Thyrotroph cell adenoma of the human pituitary gland associated with primary hypothyroidism: Clinical and morphological features. Acta Endocrinol 95:41, 1980.
13. Pioro EP, Scheithauer BW, Laws ER Jr, et al: Combined thyrotroph and lactotroph

14. Saeger W, Lüdecke DK: Pituitary adenomas with hyperfunction of TSH. Virchows Arch Am Pathol Anat Histol 394:255, 1982.
15. Wilson CB: A decade of pituitary microsurgery. The Herbert Olivecrona lecture. J Neurosurg 61:814, 1984.
16. Mindermann T, Wilson CB: Thyrotropin-producing pituitary adenomas. J Neurosurg 79:521, 1993.
17. Mixson AJ, Friedman TC, David AK, et al: Thyrotropin-secreting pituitary carcinoma. J Clin Endocrinol Metab 76:529, 1993.
18. Cooper DS, Wenig BM: Hyperthyroidism caused by an ectopic TSH-secreting pituitary tumor. Thyroid 6:337, 1996.
19. Gesundheit N, Petrick P, Nissim M, et al: Thyrotropin-secreting pituitary adenomas: Clinical and biochemical heterogeneity. Ann Intern Med 111:827, 1989.
20. Weintraub BD, Petrick PA, Gesundheit N, et al: TSH-secreting pituitary tumors. *In* Medeiros-Neto G, Gaitan S (eds): Frontiers in Thyroidology. New York, Plenum, 1986, p 71.
21. Beck-Peccoz P, Piscitelli G, Amr S, et al: Endocrine, biochemical, and morphological studies of a pituitary adenoma secreting growth hormone, thyrotropin (TSH), and α-subunit: Evidence for secretion of TSH with increased bioactivity. J Clin Endocrinol Metab 62:704, 1986.
22. Ozawa Y, Kameya T, Kasuga A, et al: A functional thyrotropin- and growth hormone-secreting pituitary adenoma with ultrastructurally monomorphic feature: A case study. Endocr J 45:211, 1998.
23. Trouillas J, Girod C, Loras B, et al: The TSH secretion in the human pituitary adenomas. Pathol Res Pract 183:596, 1988.
24. Terzolo M, Orlandi F, Bassetti M, et al: Hyperthyroidism due to a pituitary adenoma composed of two different cell types, one secreting alpha-subunit alone and another cosecreting alpha-subunit and thyrotropin. J Clin Endocrinol Metab 72:415, 1991.
25. Jaquet P, Hassoun J, Delori P, et al: A human pituitary adenoma secreting thyrotropin and prolactin: Immunohistochemical, biochemical and cell culture study. J Clin Endocrinol Metab 59:817, 1984.
26. Kuzuya N, Inoue K, Ishibashi M, et al: Endocrine and immunohistochemical studies on thyrotropin (TSH)-secreting pituitary adenomas: Responses of TSH, alpha-subunit and growth hormone to hypothalamic releasing hormones and their distribution in adenoma cells. J Clin Endocrinol Metab 71:1103, 1990.
27. Malarkey WB, Kovacs K, O'Dorisio T: Response of GH- and TSH-secreting pituitary adenoma to a somatostatin analogue (SMS 201–995): Evidence that GH and TSH coexist in the same cell and secretory granules. Neuroendocrinology 49:267, 1989.
28. Sanno N, Teramoto A, Matsuno A, et al: Clinical and immunohistochemical studies on TSH-secreting pituitary adenoma: Its multihormonality and expression of Pit-1. Modern Pathol 7:893, 1994.
29. Dong Q, Brucker-Davis F, Weintraub BD, et al: Screening of candidate oncogenes in human thyrotroph tumors: Absence of activating mutations of the Gα$_q$, Gα$_{11}$, Gα$_s$, or thyrotropin-releasing hormone receptor genes. J Clin Endocrinol Metab 81:1134, 1996.
30. Lind P, Langsteger W, Költringer P, et al: Transient prealbumin-associated hyperthyroxinemia in a TSH-producing pituitary adenoma. Nuklearmedizin 29:40, 1990.
31. Waldhäusl W, Brautsch-Marrain P, Nowotony P, et al: Secondary hyperthyroidism due to thyrotropin hypersecretion: Study of pituitary tumor morphology and thyrotropin chemistry and release. J Clin Endocrinol Metab 49:879, 1979.
32. Stanley JM, Najjar SS: Hyperthyroidism secondary to a TSH-secreting pituitary adenoma in a 15-year-old-male. Clin Pediatr 30:109, 1991.
33. Patrick AW, Atkin SL, MacKenzie J, et al: Hyperthyroidism secondary to a pituitary adenoma secreting TSH, FSH, alpha-subunit and GH. Clin Endocrinol (Oxf) 40:275, 1994.
34. Mantovani S, Beck-Peccoz P, Saccomanno K, et al: TSH-secreting pituitary adenomas are monoclonal in origin. Proceedings of the 77th Annual Meeting of the Endocrine Society, (P2–485 Abstract), 1995, p 412.
35. Pellegrini I, Barlier A, Gunz G, et al: Pit-1 gene expression in the human pituitary and pituitary adenomas. J Clin Endocrinol Metab 79:189, 1994.
36. Boggild MD, Jenkinson S, Pistorello M, et al: Molecular genetics studies of sporadic pituitary tumors. J Clin Endocrinol Metab 78:387, 1994.
37. Friedman E, Adams EF, Höög A, et al: Normal structural dopamine type 2 receptor gene in prolactin-secreting and other pituitary tumors. J Clin Endocrinol Metab 78:568, 1994.
38. Sumi T, Stefaneanu L, Kovacs K, et al: Immunohistochemical study of p53 protein in human and animal pituitary tumors. Endocr Pathol 4:95, 1993.
39. Chanson P, Orgiazzi J, Derome PJ, et al: Paradoxical response of thyrotropin to L-dopa and presence of dopaminergic receptor in a thyrotropin-secreting pituitary adenoma. J Clin Endocrinol Metab 59:542, 1984.
40. Chanson P, Li JY, LeDafniet M, et al: Absence of receptors for thyrotropin (TSH)-releasing hormone in human TSH-secreting pituitary adenomas associated with hyperthyroidism. J Clin Endocrinol Metab 66:447, 1988.
41. LeDafniet M, Brandi A-M, Kujas M, et al: Thyrotropin-releasing hormone (TRH) binding sites and thyrotropin response to TRH are regulated by thyroid hormones in human thyrotropic adenomas. Eur J Endocrinol 130:559, 1994.
42. Polak M, Bertherat J, Li JY, et al: A human TSH-secreting adenoma: Endocrine, biochemical and morphological studies. Evidence of somatostatin receptors by using quantitative autoradiography. Clinical and biological improvement by SMS 201–995 treatment. Acta Endocrinol 124:479, 1991.
43. Takano K, Ajima M, Teramoto A, et al: Mechanism of action of somatostatin on human TSH-secreting adenoma cells. Am J Physiol 268:E558, 1995.
44. Bertherat J, Brue T, Enjalbert A, et al: Somatostatin receptors on thyrotropin-secreting pituitary adenomas: Comparison with the inhibitory effects of octreotide upon in vivo and in vitro hormonal secretions. J Clin Endocrinol Metab 75:540, 1992.
45. Levy A, Eckland DJA, Gurney AM, et al: Somatostatin and thyrotropin-releasing hormone response and receptor status of a thyrotropin-secreting pituitary adenoma: Clinical and "in vitro" studies. J Neuroendocrinol 1:321, 1989.

46. Koide Y, Kugai N, Kimura S, et al: A case of pituitary adenoma with possible simultaneous secretion of thyrotropin and follicle-stimulating hormone. J Clin Endocrinol Metab 54:397, 1982.

47. Scanlon MF, Howells S, Peters JR, et al: Hyperprolactinaemia, amenorrhoea and galactorrhoea due a pituitary thyrotroph adenoma. Clin Endocrinol 23:35, 1985.

48. Losa M, Giovanelli M, Persani L, et al: Criteria of cure and follow-up of central hyperthyroidism due to thyrotropin-secreting pituitary adenomas. J Clin Endocrinol Metab 81:3084, 1996.

49. Kiso Y, Yoshida K, Kaise K, et al: A case of thyrotropin (TSH)-secreting tumor complicated by periodic paralysis. Jpn J Med 29:399, 1990.

50. Alings AM, Fliers E, de Herder WW, et al: A thyrotropin-secreting pituitary adenoma as a cause of thyrotoxic periodic paralysis. J Endocrinol Invest 21:703, 1998.

51. Brucker-Davis F, Oldfield EH, Skarulis MC, et al: Thyrotropin-secreting pituitary tumors: Diagnostic criteria, thyroid hormone sensitivity, and treatment outcome in 25 patients followed at the National Institutes of Health. J Clin Endocrinol Metab 84:476, 1999.

52. Calle-Pascual AL, Yuste E, Martin P, et al: Association of a thyrotropin-secreting pituitary adenoma and a thyroid follicular carcinoma. J Endocrinol Invest 14:499, 1991.

53. Gasparoni P, Rubello D, Persani L, et al: Unusual association between a thyrotropin-secreting pituitary adenoma and a papillary thyroid carcinoma. Thyroid 8:181, 1998.

54. Beckers A, Abs R, Mahler C, et al: Thyrotropin-secreting pituitary adenomas: Report of seven cases. J Clin Endocrinol Metab 72:477, 1991.

55. Abs R, Stevenaert A, Beckers A: Autonomously functioning thyroid nodules in a patient with a thyrotropin-secreting pituitary adenoma: Possible cause-effect relationship. Eur J Endocrinol 131:355, 1994.

56. Sy ARG, Bernstein R, Chynn KI, et al: Reduction in size of a thyrotropin- and gonadotropin-secreting pituitary adenoma treated with octreotide acetate (somatostatin analogue). J Clin Endocrinol Metab 74:690, 1992.

57. Horn K, Erhardt F, Fahlbusch R, et al: Recurrent goiter, hyperthyroidism, galactorrhoea and amenorrhoea due to a thyrotropin and prolactin-producing pituitary tumor. J Clin Endocrinol Metab 43:137, 1976.

58. Adriaanse R, Brabant G, Endert E, et al: Pulsatile thyrotropin and prolactin secretion in a patient with a mixed thyrotropin- and prolactin-secreting pituitary adenoma. Eur J Endocrinol 130:113, 1994.

59. Lamberg BA, Ripatti J, Gordin A, et al: Chromophobe pituitary adenoma with acromegaly and TSH-induced hyperthyroidism associated with parathyroid adenoma. Acta Endocrinol 69:157–172, 1969.

60. Burgess JR, Greenaway TM: Thyrotropinomas in multiple endocrine neoplasia type 1 (MEN-1). Aust NZ J Med 24:740, 1994.

61. Wynne AG, Gharib H, Scheithauer BW, et al: Hyperthyroidism due to inappropriate secretion of thyrotropin in 10 patients. Am J Med 92:15–24, 1992.

62. Gessl A, Freissmuth M, Czech T, et al: Growth hormone-prolactin-thyrotropin-secreting pituitary adenoma in atypical McCune-Albright syndrome with functionally normal Gsα protein. J Clin Endocrinol Metab 79:1128, 1994.

63. Langlois M-F, Lamarche JB, Bellabarba D: Long-standing goiter and hypothyroidism: An unusual presentation of a TSH-secreting adenoma. Thyroid 6:329, 1996.

64. Ekins R: Measurement of free hormones in blood. Endocr Rev 11:5, 1990.

65. Beck-Peccoz P, Piscitelli G, Cattaneo MG, et al: Evaluation of free thyroxine methods in the presence of iodothyronine binding autoantibodies. J Clin Endocrinol Metab 58:736, 1984.

66. Zweig MH, Csako G, Spero M: Escape from blockade of interfering heterophile antibodies in a two-site immunoradiometric assay for thyrotropin. Clin Chem 34:2589, 1988.

67. Beck-Peccoz P, Persani L: Variable biological activity of thyroid-stimulating hormone. Eur J Endocrinol 131:331, 1994.

68. Bevan JS, Burke CW, Esiri MM, et al: Studies of two thyrotropin-secreting pituitary adenomas: Evidence for dopamine receptor deficiency. Clin Endocrinol 31:59, 1989.

69. Magner JA, Kane J: Binding of thyrotropin to lentil lectin is unchanged by thyrotropin-releasing hormone administration in three patients with thyrotropin-producing pituitary adenomas. Endocr Res 8:163, 1992.

70. Magner JA, Klibanski A, Fein H, et al: Ricin and lentil lectin affinity chromatography reveals oligosaccharide heterogeneity of thyrotropin secreted by 12 human pituitary tumors. Metabolism 41:1009, 1992.

71. Kourides IA, Ridgway EC, Weintraub BD, et al: Thyrotropin-induced hyperthyroidism: Use of alpha and beta subunit levels to identify patients with primary tumors. J Clin Endocrinol Metab 45:534, 1977.

72. Beck-Peccoz P, Persani L, Faglia G: Glycoprotein hormone α-subunit in pituitary adenomas. Trends Endocrinol Metab 3:41, 1992.

73. Smallridge RC: Metabolic, physiologic, and clinical indexes of thyroid function. In Braverman LE, Utiger RD (eds): Werner and Ingbar's The Thyroid, ed 7. Philadelphia, JB Lippincott, Philadelphia, 1996, p 397.

74. Watanabe K, Kameya T, Yamauchi A, et al: Thyrotropin-producing adenoma associated with pituitary resistance to thyroid hormone. J Clin Endocrinol Metab 76:1025, 1993.

75. Azarnivar A, Chopra IJ: Tension pneumoencephalus after transsphenoidal resection of a thyrotropin (TSH)-secreting pituitary adenoma. Endocrinologist 5:308–311, 1995.

76. Beck-Peccoz P, Roncoroni R, Mariotti S, et al: Sex hormone-binding globulin measurement in patients with inappropriate secretion of thyrotropin (IST): Evidence against selective pituitary thyroid hormone resistance in nonneoplastic IST. J Clin Endocrinol Metab 71:19, 1990.

77. Persani L, Preziati D, Matthews CH, et al: Serum levels of carboxyterminal cross-linked telopeptide of type I collagen (ICTP) in the differential diagnosis of the syndromes of inappropriate secretion of TSH. Clin Endocrinol 47:207, 1997.

78. Rubello D, Busnardo B, Girelli ME, et al: Severe hyperthyroidism due to neoplastic TSH hypersecretion in an old man. J Endocrinol Invest 12:571, 1989.

79. Chanson P, Weintraub BD, Harris AG: Octreotide therapy for thyroid stimulating hormone–secreting pituitary adenomas. A follow-up of 52 patients. Ann Intern Med 119:236, 1993.

80. Losa M, Magnani P, Mortini P, et al: Indium-111 pentetreotide single-photon emission tomography in patients with TSH-secreting pituitary adenomas: Correlation with the effect of a single administration of octreotide on serum TSH levels. Eur J Nucl Med 24:728, 1997.

81. Webster J, Peters JR, John R, et al: Pituitary stone: Two cases of densely calcified thyrotropin-secreting pituitary adenomas. Clin Endocrinol 40:137, 1994.

82. Nabarro JDN: Acromegaly. Clin Endocrinol (Oxf) 26:481–512, 1987.

83. Lamberts SWJ, Krenning EP, Reubi J-C: The role of somatostatin and its analogs in the diagnosis and treatment of tumors. Endocr Rev 12:450, 1991.

84. Verhoeff NPLG, Bemelman FJ, Wiersinga WM, et al: Imaging of dopamine D2 and somatostatin receptors in vivo using single-photon emission tomography in a patient with a TSH/PRL-producing pituitary macroadenoma. Eur J Nucl Med 20:555, 1993.

85. Frank SJ, Gesundheit N, Doppman JL, et al: Preoperative lateralization of pituitary microadenomas by petrosal sinus sampling: Utility in two patients with non–ACTH-secreting tumors. Am J Med 87:679, 1989.

86. Mariotti S, Anelli S, Bartalena L, et al: Familial hyperthyroidism due to nonneoplastic inappropriate TSH secretion associated with sellar abnormalities. (Abstract) J Endocrinol Invest 10(suppl 1):20, 1987.

87. Hall WA, Luciano MG, Doppman JL, et al: Pituitary magnetic resonance imaging in normal human volunteers: Occult adenomas in the general population. Ann Intern Med 120:817, 1994.

88. McCutcheon IE, Weintraub BD, Oldfield EH: Surgical treatment of thyrotropin-secreting pituitary adenomas. J Neurosurg 73:674, 1990.

89. Barbarino A, DeMarinis L, Anile C, et al: Normal pituitary function and reserve after selective transsphenoidal removal of a thyrotropin-producing pituitary adenoma. Metabolism 29:739, 1980.

90. Carlson H, Linfoot J, Braunstein G, et al: Hyperthyroidism and acromegaly due to a thyrotropin- and growth hormone–secreting pituitary tumor. Lack of hormonal response to bromocriptine. Am J Med 74:915, 1983.

91. Comi R, Gesundheit N, Murray L, et al: Response of thyrotropin-secreting pituitary adenomas to a long-acting somatostatin analogue. N Engl J Med 317:12, 1987.

92. Gancel A, Vuillermet P, Legrand A, et al: Effects of a slow-release formulation of the new somatostatin analogue lanreotide in TSH-secreting pituitary adenomas. Clin Endocrinol 40:421, 1994.

93. Francis TB, Smallridge RC, Kane J, et al: Octreotide changes serum thyrotropin (TSH) glycoisomer distribution as assessed by lectin chromatography in a TSH macroadenoma patient. J Clin Endocrinol Metab 77:183, 1993.

94. Hill S, Falko J, Wilson C, et al: Thyrotropin-producing pituitary adenomas. J Neurosurg 57:515, 1982.

95. Caron P, Gerbaud C, Pradayrol L, et al: Successful pregnancy in an infertile woman with a thyrotropin-secreting macroadenoma treated with somatostatin analog (octreotide). J Clin Endocrinol Metab 81:1164, 1996.

Chapter 25

Prolactinomas and Hyperprolactinemic Syndrome

Giovanni Faglia

Pathologic hyperprolactinemia, defined as persistently elevated serum prolactin (PRL) levels in the absence of pregnancy or physiologic postpartum lactation, is a common finding in clinical endocrinology practice and indicates the existence of a hypothalamic-pituitary disorder. The corresponding clinical picture, the hyperprolactinemic syndrome, is characterized by menstrual disturbances, infertility, and galactorrhea in women and loss of sexual desire and potency in men. The association of menstrual disorders, infertility, and galactorrhea has been known since the thirties.[1, 2] Three different clinical pictures were described: one characterized by postpartum amenorrhea, galactorrhea, low urinary gonadotropin levels, and no sellar enlargement (Chiari-Frommel syndrome)[3]; one consisting of nonpuerperal amenorrhea, galactorrhea, low urinary gonadotropin levels, and no sellar enlargement (Ahumada-Argonzdel Castillo syndrome)[4]; and one in which amenorrhea and galactorrhea were associated with a chromophobe pituitary tumor (Forbes-Henneman-Griswold-Albright syndrome).[5] It took several decades before PRL was identified in humans as a hormone distinct from somatotropin,[6] and radioimmunoassay enabled measurement of PRL circulating levels, which proved that all the above-mentioned syndromes were characterized by elevated levels of circulating PRL. A proportion of patients showed an enlarged sella, whereas others, without any detectable sella alteration on plain skull radiographs, were surgically demonstrated to bear very tiny pituitary tumors (microadenomas),[7] a finding confirmed years later by the introduction of high-resolution imaging techniques such as dynamic computed tomography (CT) and then magnetic resonance imaging (MRI).[8] Positive PRL immunostaining of the excised tumors,[9] cure of the syndrome after radical adenomectomy,[7] and demonstration of PRL release by tumor fragments in vitro[10] led to introduction of the term "prolactinoma" into current use and obsolescence of the previous eponymic classification. However, prolactinoma is not the sole cause of hyperprolactinemia. Because PRL secretion is mainly under the inhibitory control of dopamine,[11] every process interfering with dopamine synthesis and release by dopaminergic neurons, transport from the median eminence to the pituitary, or action at the lactotroph level has been recognized as capable of sustaining PRL hypersecretion. Knowledge of the PRL-inhibiting role of dopamine has allowed the introduction of treatment with dopamine agonists,[12] which have proved effective not only in reducing PRL secretion but also in causing the pituitary tumor to shrink in patients with prolactinoma,[13] thus becoming the first-choice therapy for hyperprolactinemic syndrome.

In this chapter, the causes, epidemiology, clinical findings, and diagnostic and therapeutic approaches to hyperprolactinemia will be briefly reviewed, with particular emphasis on prolactinomas.

CAUSES OF HYPERPROLACTINEMIA

The multitude of events that cause chronic PRL elevation above normal limits (<20 ng/mL in women and <15 ng/mL in men) are listed in Table 25–1.

Physiologic Hyperprolactinemia

PRL secretion is increased in several physiologic conditions that should be taken into account when patients are being investigated for hyperprolactinemia. Prolactin is secreted in a pulsatile manner, and spontaneous episodic PRL peaks occur 8 to 12 times in 24 hours. Moreover, a sleep-associated elevation in serum PRL levels occurs a couple of hours after the onset of sleep and lasts for about 1 hour after awakening.[14] PRL secretion is part of the physiologic response to stress, and both physically and psychologically stressful events can cause serum PRL to rise, possibly through mechanisms mediated by endogenous opioid stimulation.[15] During pregnancy, serum PRL levels increase steadily until term in response to high estrogen levels, when values about 10-fold over baseline are reached. Breast-feeding is accompanied by episodic PRL peaks, 5- to 8-fold times basal levels, that promptly follow suckling and presumably aimed to prepare the breast for the next nursing episode. Independent of nursing, nipple stimulation causes serum PRL to increase. Sexual orgasm may also induce hyperprolactinemia.[16]

Drug-Induced Hyperprolactinemia

Chronic use of neuroactive drugs is one of the major causes of hyperprolactinemia. Because PRL secretion is under the inhibitory control of dopamine,[11] every drug affecting dopamine synthesis and release or action at the lactotroph receptor or postreceptor levels may cause hyperprolactinemia. Thus antipsychotic drugs such as chlorpromazine, perphenazine, and haloperidol, compounds of the tiapride family, including those mainly used as antiemetic or gastric motility regulators such as metoclopramide and domperidone, are able to increase serum PRL levels by acting as dopamine receptor blockers. Elevated serum PRL levels are also caused by antihypertensive drugs acting as inhibitors of catecholamine synthesis, such as α-methyldopa, or as catecholamine depletors, such as reserpine. Opioids are direct stimulators of PRL secretion. The H_2 antagonists cimetidine and ranitidine cause serum PRL to rise when administered intravenously. Antidepressants such as the imipramines and fluoxetine increase serum PRL levels by acting through serotonin-mediated pathways. Estrogens,

TABLE 25–1. Causes of Hyperprolactinemia

Physiologic
 Sleep
 Stress (physical, psychologic)
 Pregnancy
 Nursing
 Orgasm
Pharmacologic
 Dopamine receptor blockers
  Phenothiazines: chlorpromazine, perphenazine, etc.
  Butyrophenones: haloperidol
  Thioxanthenes
  Tiaprides: sulpiride, metoclopramide, domperidone, cisapride,
   raclopride, etc.
 Dopamine synthesis inhibitors
  α-Methyldopa
 Catecholamine depletors
  Reserpine
 Opioids
 H₂ antagonists
  Cimetidine, ranitidine
 Imipramines
  Amitriptyline, amoxapine
 Serotonin reuptake inhibitors
  Fluoxetine (Prozac)
 Calcium antagonists
  Verapamil
 Estrogens
Pathologic
 Lesions of the hypothalamus or pituitary stalk
  Hypothalamic tumors
  Inflammatory or granulomatous diseases
  Other expanding lesions
  Cranial irradiation
 Pituitary lesions
  Prolactinomas
  Plurihormonal adenomas
  Lesions deconnecting the pituitary from the hypothalamus
  Infiltrative diseases
  Empty sella
 Primary hypothyroidism
 Polycystic ovary syndrome
 Neurogenic
  Nipple stimulation
  Lesions of the mammary region
  Spinal cord lesions
 Chronic renal failure
 Liver cirrhosis
 Idiopathic (?)

which stimulate PRL secretion and induce lactotroph hyperplasia, induce marked elevations in serum PRL levels when administered at high doses (e.g., male-to-female transsexual individuals[17]), whereas at low doses, such as in oral contraceptives or hormone replacement therapy for menopause, estrogens have much less effect or no effect on PRL levels.[18]

Pathologic Hyperprolactinemia

Lesions of the Hypothalamus or Pituitary Stalk

Lesions of the hypothalamus or pituitary stalk may impair dopamine transport from the median eminence to the pituitary and cause hyperprolactinemia. Such lesions include hypothalamic tumors (e.g., craniopharyngioma, Rathke's cyst, hamartoma, germinoma, glioma, deposits from other tumors), inflammatory or granulomatous diseases (such as sarcoidosis, histiocytosis X, tuberculosis), and other expanding lesions involving the hypothalamic-pituitary region (such as pituitary nonfunctioning macroadenoma [pseudoprolactinoma], meningioma, pseudotumor cerebri, ventricular cyst, empty sella, aneurysm of the carotid artery).[19] Cranial irradiation for craniofacial tumors or for bone marrow transplantation frequently results in hyperprolactinemia.

Prolactin-Secreting Pituitary Tumors

PRL-secreting pituitary adenomas are the most frequent cause of pathologic hyperprolactinemia. They may consist of lactotrophs only (prolactinomas) or be mixed tumors secreting growth hormone (GH)/PRL, adrenocorticotropic hormone (ACTH)/PRL, and thyroid-stimulating hormone (TSH)/PRL, in descending order of frequency. In the latter, hyperprolactinemia is associated with acromegaly, Cushing's disease, and TSH-dependent hyperthyroidism, respectively. Mixed follicle-stimulating hormone (FSH) and/or luteinizing hormone (LH)/PRL-secreting tumors are rare and may be clinically indistinguishable from prolactinomas except in children, in whom they may cause precocious puberty.[20] PRL-secreting pituitary carcinomas are exceedingly rare.[21]

Prolactinomas account for 40% to 50% of pituitary adenomas.[22–24] According to their dimensions, they are conventionally distinguished into microprolactinomas (<10 mm in diameter) and macroprolactinomas (>10 mm in diameter). A positive correlation between tumor size and serum PRL levels has been reported.[25] Although macroprolactinomas represent the final stage of progressive enlargement of initially small tumors, the risk that microprolactinomas may evolve and expand to a macroadenoma is relatively low, not exceeding 3% to 7%, as deduced from longitudinal studies in patients monitored for several years by pituitary imaging.[26–30] If serum PRL levels are taken as an index of the disease, most patients with moderate hyperprolactinemia (<200 ng/mL) do not change the order of magnitude of their PRL levels throughout years, about one-third have decreased or even normalized levels, and less than one-fifth show significant increases.[27] Progression during estrogen therapy has been reported only anecdotally.[31]

As far as prolactinoma formation is concerned, the pathogenetic role of a primary hypothalamic dysfunction causing reduced central dopaminergic tone has been debated for a long time.[32, 33] The observation of prompt PRL suppressibility by dopamine agonists initially favored this hypothesis, which was subsequently abandoned as evidence was accumulating of augmented central dopaminergic tone in response to PRL excess. In fact, it was observed that in patients with prolactinomas, dopaminergic disinhibition by the dopamine receptor blocker domperidone was followed by an exaggerated TSH increase with respect to normal controls.[33] Because TSH is also under dopaminergic inhibitory control, this evidence was in favor of increased neuronal production of dopamine that was normally transported to the pituitary. Subsequently, other causes of diminished dopamine activity at the lactotroph level were considered, such as abnormalities in pituitary vasculature or intrinsic abnormalities of dopamine receptors or intracellular effectors. In fact, evidence was presented that the blood supply of prolactinomas was coming mainly from pituitary arteries rather than from portal capillaries (the number of which is actually reduced in prolactinomas), that patients with prolactinomas were less sensitive to the PRL-suppressive effects of dopamine,[29, 34, 35] and that dopaminergic receptors were less expressed in the subset of dopamine-resistant prolactinomas.[36] Thus quantitative and/or qualitative alterations of D₂ receptors were hypothesized to occur in prolactinomas.[37] Recent cloning of the D₂ receptor and its localization in the long arm of chromosome 11,[38] a region that may have allelic losses in pituitary tumors,[39] have stimulated screening for mutations in the D₂ receptor–coding gene in prolactinomas. However, no inactivating mutation was found.[40] Moreover, the concentration and affinity constant of the D₂ receptors present in prolactinomas were found to be similar to those in normal pituitary, although extremely variable.

Because studies of pituitary adenoma clonality by X chromosome inactivation analysis have demonstrated that even prolactinomas are monoclonal in origin,[41] the hypothesis of an initiating oncogenic mutation associated with hypothalamic malfunction or stimulatory action by other promoting factors was put forward.[42] However, no specific mutation has been discovered until recently, except for an H-ras mutation in one single malignant prolactinoma.[43, 44] Loss of heterozygosity in 11q13 has been reported in some familial cases or in association with multiple endocrine neoplasia type 1 (MEN-1), but not in the common type of prolactinomas.[45, 46] In summary, the ultimate cause of prolactinomas still remains obscure, although a multifactorial, multistep origin is highly probable.[42]

Other Pituitary Lesions

Nonfunctioning pituitary adenomas constitute about one-quarter of all pituitary tumors. They are frequently associated with hyperprolactinemia because the tumor mass may cause deconnection from the hypothalamus, which is why they are commonly called "nonprolactinomas" or "pseudoprolactinomas." Although serum PRL levels are generally moderately elevated with respect to tumor volume, differentiation from prolactinomas may be a real diagnostic problem.

Infiltrative lesions of the pituitary and empty sella may also cause hyperprolactinemia.[47, 48]

Other Causes

Moderate hyperprolactinemia may be present in primary hypothyroidism[49, 50] and probably results either from increased thyroid-releasing hormone (TRH) production in response to low thyroid hormone levels or, in more severe and long-lasting cases, from hypothalamic disconnection secondary to pituitary enlargement caused by thyrotroph hyperplasia or feedback tumor.

Polycystic ovary syndrome may be associated (15%–40% of cases)[51, 52] with mild hyperprolactinemia resulting from acyclic hyperestrogenism and diminished central dopaminergic and GABA-ergic tone.

Peripheral neurogenic stimulation is the cause of the hyperprolactinemia observed in patients with irritative lesions of the thoracic wall (particularly those involving the mammary region) or the thoracic portion of the spinal cord.

Other diseases that may alter central regulation of PRL secretion, such as chronic renal failure and liver cirrhosis, may be associated with moderate hyperprolactinemia.

It is still debated whether so-called idiopathic hyperprolactinemia is a distinct disease sustained by neurosecretory dysfunction of the tubero-infundibular dopaminergic system or is instead due to microadenomas so tiny that they go undetected radiologically.

PATHOLOGY

This section covers the pathology of PRL-secreting tumors. As far as other lesions of the pituitary and hypothalamus leading to hyperprolactinemia are concerned, the reader is addressed to other contributions.[53]

Lactotroph Hyperplasia

Human pathology involving PRL cell hyperplasia as the sole cause of PRL hypersecretion is not well known because of the rare availability of such specimens. Also very rare is the finding of hyperplastic nontumorous lactotrophs adjacent to prolactinomas that have been described as well-defined nodular areas.[54–56] In contrast, in the vast majority of cases, the extratumoral lactotrophs show ultrastructural features of involution. Lactotroph hyperplasia has also been described in patients with long-standing primary hypothyroidism[57] and in peritumoral tissue of patients with Cushing's disease.[58]

Prolactin-Secreting Pituitary Adenomas

Because of the expanding use of medical treatment with dopamine agonists as first-choice therapy, the percentage of prolactinomas is progressively decreasing in surgical series and in pathologic reports,[53] even though they account for 50% to 60% of all pituitary tumors in clinical and autopsy series.[22–24, 59] PRL-secreting tumors usually originate in the lateral wings of the anterior pituitary. Microprolactinomas are generally well-delimited lesions that may induce swelling of the corresponding hemipituitary, which causes the superior profile of the gland to become convex and dislocate the pituitary stalk toward the contralateral lobe. They may impress the ipsilateral cavernous sinus and cause thinning and bulging of the sella floor. Light microscopy

reveals that although small in size, about 30% to 40% of microadenomas infiltrate the surrounding pituitary tissue and eventually the dura, the adjacent bony structures, and the cavernous sinus. Macroprolactinomas show wide variability in size, from larger than 10 mm to several centimeters in diameter (giant prolactinomas). Depending on their dimensions, they may remain intrasellar; expand downward in the sphenoidal sinus or upward to occupy the suprasellar spaces and impinge on the optic chiasm and the hypothalamus, sometimes reaching and occluding Monro's foramina and causing enlargement of cerebral ventricles; or expand laterally, invade the cavernous sinuses, and englobe the internal carotid artery.

Most prolactinomas are composed of sparsely granulated lactotrophs that are chromophobic or tenuously acidophilic by classic histology, uniformly distributed within the tumor, or more rarely, arranged in papillary structures.[53, 60] Calcifications are common.[61] By electron microscopy the adenomatous lactotrophs appear irregular, with large nuclei and wide nucleoli. Rough endoplasmic reticulum (RER) is abundant, and the Golgi complex is prominent. Secretory granules are small (150–300 nm), spherical, sparse, and frequently extruded into the extracellular space. They are usually poorly immunoreactive; however, greater positivity to anti-PRL antisera is found in the immature granules within the sacculi of the Golgi complex.[53, 60]

A small proportion of prolactinomas are densely granulated.[53, 60] These tumors are intensely acidophilic and show strong positivity for immunoreactive PRL. On electron microscopy, the RER is less developed than in sparsely granulated adenomas, whereas the Golgi complex is similarly prominent. The secretory granules are abundant, strongly electron dense, highly variable in size (200–700 nm) within the Golgi apparatus and cytoplasm, and frequently extruded into the extracellular space. A higher frequency of densely granulated lactotrophs has been reported to occur in adenomas from patients previously treated with dopamine agonists.[56] Some prolactinomas are characterized by the deposition of abundant spherical amyloid,[62] the origin of which has recently been reported to be from a 4-kDa amyloidogenic peptide. Because amino acid sequencing revealed that this peptide was identical to the first 34 amino acids of intact PRL, it has been suggested that spherical amyloid originates from abnormally processed PRL.[63]

Mixed Pituitary Adenomas

The most frequent mixed pituitary tumors are GH/PRL-secreting adenomas. These tumors characteristically co-secrete PRL and GH. They include mixed somatotroph-lactotroph adenomas, mammosomatotroph adenomas, and acidophilic stem cell adenomas. Mixed somatotroph-lactotroph adenomas are composed of two different cell populations (generally, densely granulated somatotrophs and sparsely granulated lactotrophs) or composed of bihormonal cells co-secreting both hormones.[64] Mammosomatotroph adenomas predominantly produce GH and are clinically associated with acromegaly and mild hyperprolactinemia. They are characterized by very large secretory granules (up to 2000 nm). Acidophilic stem cell adenomas, which predominantly produce PRL, may show oncocytic changes consisting of the presence of ballooned giant mitochondria, the abundance of which may obscure morphologic assessment of RER and Golgi features.

Other PRL-secreting mixed pituitary adenomas are represented by the rare mixed ACTH/PRL-, TSH/PRL-, and FSH/LH/PRL-secreting adenomas, which are easily identified by immunocytochemistry.[53, 65]

Pituitary Prolactin-Secreting Carcinomas

Pituitary PRL-secreting carcinomas are extremely rare, but aggressive neoplasms that not only expand toward adjacent structures but also infiltrate the sella floor and walls, invade the sphenoidal sinus, the cavernous sinuses, and the suprasellar region, and most importantly, give rise to distant metastases usually localized in other intracranial or extracranial areas of the nervous system; more rarely, visceral deposits have been described.[21, 66–68] Morphologic findings do not differ too much from those of sparsely granulated prolactinoma and do not help in diagnosing PRL-secreting carcinoma, provided that no distant deposit(s) are present and the number of mitoses observed does not exceed that observed in benign prolactinomas, which is usually very low.

EPIDEMIOLOGY

The hyperprolactinemic syndrome is common in women, but less frequently observed in men. It has been reported to cause alterations in the menstrual cycle in 25% to 30% of women, whereas only 1% to 3% of men report loss of libido and sexual potency.[69, 70] Because the clinical manifestations are essentially those of hypogonadism, this difference has been ascribed to the more prominent manifestation of symptoms in women (menstrual disorders eventually associated with galactorrhea), which leads to early medical observation and endocrinologic evaluation. In contrast, in men, who are generally reluctant to seek medical attention in relation to gradual loss of libido and sexual potency, the underlying hyperprolactinemia may go undetected. Such reasoning has led to suggestions that the frequency of hyperprolactinemia is substantially similar in both sexes. This hypothesis seems to be supported by the finding that the female-to-male ratio of about 20 reported in most series of patients with microprolactinomas falls to about 1 in unselected autopsy series,[59, 71] and no sex-related differences are found in the distribution of macroprolactinomas[22] when the initial symptoms (headache, visual field defects, etc.) are equally severe in both sexes. However, hyperprolactinemia is reported to occur in about one-third of women with menstrual disturbances,[69] but supranormal PRL levels are observed in only a minute proportion of men with sexual impotence and/or sterility,[70] which is in favor of a much higher frequency of hyperprolactinemia in women, probably as a consequence of their higher exposure to estrogen.[72] As already mentioned, prolactinomas are the most frequent cause of organic hyperprolactinemia. They represent 40% to 50% of all pituitary adenomas. Their prevalence is estimated to be about 0.008% to 0.012% and their incidence is about 2.7 per 100,000 per year. Microprolactinomas account for about 65% to 70% of PRL-secreting adenomas and are more frequently diagnosed in women than in men (20:1), whereas the frequency of macroprolactinomas is on the same order of magnitude in the two sexes (F/M, 1.04:1).[22, 73, 74] The median age at the time of diagnosis is 21 to 30 years for microprolactinomas and 41 to 50 for macroprolactinomas. Hyperprolactinemia in postmenopausal women is more frequently due to macroprolactinomas than microprolactinomas.[75] Prolactinoma is the pituitary tumor most frequently encountered in children and during adolescence,[76-79] and in a recent study it represented 70% of 48 pituitary adenomas occurring in teenagers.[80] In contrast, of 44 patients in whom pituitary tumors were diagnosed at the age of 65 to 83 years, only 2 had prolactinoma.[81] Prolactinoma is the most frequent pituitary tumor occurring in MEN-1 syndrome.[45] Consistent with this finding, the frequency of MEN-1 syndrome in patients with prolactinomas appears to be higher than in those with other pituitary tumors: 14.3% in 42 prolactinomas vs. 1.6% in a recently described series of 124 other pituitary tumors.[82] Rarely, prolactinomas may occur in a familial setting as recently reported in four families.[83]

CLINICAL PICTURE

In women of reproductive age, the earliest and most frequent manifestations of hyperprolactinemia are amenorrhea, galactorrhea, and infertility. In most cases, alterations in the menstrual cycle span from hypo-oligomenorrhea to secondary amenorrhea; in rare instances, hypermenorrhea/polymenorrhea may occur as a result of the shortened luteal phase[84] and, very rarely, no menstrual dysfunction will be seen at all. Amenorrhea is usually secondary and may appear after pregnancy or oral contraceptive use. More rarely, when PRL hypersecretion occurs before menarche, amenorrhea may appear primary in origin. Almost invariably, menstrual disorders are associated with anovulation and infertility, and in rare cases these last disturbances may be the only manifestations of hyperprolactinemia. Galactorrhea, either sponta-

neous or provoked by gentle breast expression, occurs in about 30% to 80% of hyperprolactinemic women in association with menstrual disorders, depending on the series.[29] As already mentioned, on rare occasion galactorrhea may occur even in the absence of any menstrual alterations.

Hyperprolactinemia is the only recognizable alteration in most cases of infertility caused by anovulatory menses and in about 15% of spontaneous recurrent miscarriages. It has recently been reported that of 352 women with recurrent spontaneous abortion, about 18% were hyperprolactinemic and that the percentage of subsequent successful pregnancies was significantly higher after normalization of serum PRL levels.[85]

Dyspareunia resulting from reduced vaginal secretion caused by hypoestrogenism is a frequent accompanying symptom and may be, at least in part, responsible for the loss of libido that is also frequently present in women.

Long-lasting exposure to low estrogen levels may cause osteopenia, and hyperprolactinemic women might be at risk for the development of osteoporosis.[86, 87] In fact, a spinal bone mineral content 20% to 25% lower in hyperprolactinemic women than in age-matched controls and an increased annual rate of spinal bone loss (3.8%) that tended to improve after the restoration of normoprolactinemia and regular menses have been reported.[88, 89]

Seborrhea and moderate hirsutism may be present, typically accompanied by elevated levels of the two weak androgens androstenedione and dehydroepiandrosterone sulfate (DHEAS). The association of DHEAS with hyperprolactinemia has suggested a stimulatory effect of PRL on adrenocortical androgen secretion.[90]

In men, the most common clinical manifestation of hyperprolactinemia is the progressive loss of libido and sexual potency. These symptoms are present in about 90% of men with PRL-secreting pituitary adenoma and almost invariably improve after normalization of serum PRL levels.[91, 92] Diminution of ejaculate volume, which may be associated with oligospermia, is also frequently reported. Galactorrhea and/or gynecomastia is present in about 15% to 30% of patients[91] (Fig. 25–1). Physical signs of hypogonadism such as decreased secondary and primary androgen-dependent hair growth, muscular hypotrophy, and increased abdominal fat may also be present. In contrast, testicular hypotrophy is less frequently described,[93] and some patients may paradoxically have testicular enlargement.[94]

Increased body weight or a recent history of weight gain is fre-

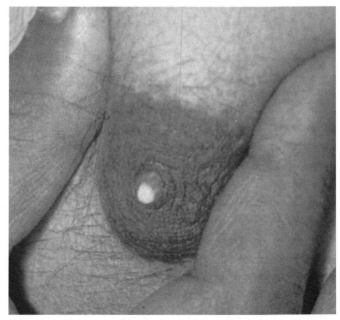

FIGURE 25–1. Galactorrhea is not a rare symptom in hyperprolactinemic men. Gentle breast expression provoked galactorrhea in this 42-year-old male patient with a macroprolactinoma. His serum prolactin concentration was 600 ng/mL.

quently observed and may be an initial symptom in both women and men.[95] In women the weight gain is often associated with fluid retention that may cause swelling of the hands and feet.

Hyperprolactinemic patients of both sexes may suffer from anxiety, depression, fatigue, emotional instability, irritability, and hostility,[15, 96] all psychologic or behavioral symptoms that in women may resemble those observed in menopause.

In patients with prolactinoma, the clinical picture of hyperprolactinemic syndrome may be associated with signs and symptoms of an expanding pituitary lesion. Headache, which is common in patients with macroadenoma, is also frequently present in those with microprolactinoma and even in patients with idiopathic hyperprolactinemia. The size of the adenoma does not appear to strictly correlate with the frequency of headache, which is similar in patients with microadenomas and macroadenomas (50%–60% vs. 60%–70%). However, more severe, persistent, and heavy headache is reported in patients with macroadenomas and significantly ameliorates after tumor shrinkage.[97] In addition, no strict correlation has been found between the frequency of headache episodes and serum PRL levels. Nevertheless, headache is generally reported to regress after PRL normalization.

In macroadenomas, diminished visual acuity and/or visual field defects are frequent and even today are common initial symptoms. Ophthalmoplegia may occur when tumors expand laterally and invade the cavernous sinus. A rare symptom is rhinorrhea, which may occur spontaneously in tumors invading the sphenoidal and/or ethmoidal sinuses or, more frequently, as a consequence of rapid drug-induced tumor shrinkage.[98] Moreover, macroadenomas may cause hypopituitarism either by primary pituitary impairment or by hypothalamic disconnection.[99] The frequency of deficiencies of other anterior pituitary hormones, both in macroadenomas and in microadenomas, is outlined in Table 25–2.

In mixed tumors, the clinical picture related to the co-secreted hormone may prevail, and hyperprolactinemia might emerge only at hormonal investigation. Conversely, particularly as far as GH and TSH are concerned, sometimes the hyperprolactinemic syndrome may obscure the initially vague clinical manifestations of acromegaly and TSH-induced hyperthyroidism, respectively.

PATHOPHYSIOLOGY

Hyperprolactinemic hypogonadism is a functional disorder that promptly regresses after PRL levels are normalized. PRL excess impairs reproductive function by acting at both the hypothalamic and gonadal level. It has been reported that hyperprolactinemia causes central dopaminergic as well as opioidergic tone to increase,[16, 33, 100] which results in suppression of the pulsatile gonadotropin-releasing hormone. The importance of the role exerted by opioids is corroborated by the finding that administration of the opioid antagonist naloxone may restore ovulatory menses in hyperprolactinemic women. In addition, hyperprolactinemia blocks the estrogen-positive feedback of LH secretion and causes abolition of the LH ovulatory surge.[101] Therefore, in hyperprolactinemic women, gonadotropin secretion is not pulsatile, estrogen-positive feedback on LH is abolished, and the ovulatory LH peak does not usually occur. Moreover, at the gonadal level, hyperprolactinemia inhibits the synthesis of 17β-estradiol and progesterone, thereby impairing follicle development.

In men, LH pulsatile secretion is also altered, and evidence indicates that testicular steroidogenesis, as well as the peripheral conversion of testosterone to 5α-dihydrotestosterone, is negatively affected by PRL excess. Altered gonadotropin and androgen secretion leads to defective semen maturation.[29, 91–93]

Milk production requires the concurrent action of several hormones, including PRL, estrogens, progesterone, and insulin, which is why galactorrhea is not present in most hyperprolactinemic patients, particularly those with the highest circulating PRL levels leading to the most severe sex hormone deficiency.

HORMONAL EVALUATION

Hormonal evaluation of patients with suspected hyperprolactinemic syndrome should be mainly based on the measurement of basal circulating PRL levels. Reliable results are obtained only if PRL assay methods are well standardized and validated and blood samples taken in an appropriate manner from carefully prepared patients. Although commercially available immunometric assays using specific monoclonal anti-PRL antibodies generally give reliable results, falsely low serum PRL levels may be observed in patients with a very high PRL concentration because of the so-called high-dose hook effect,[102–104] which can be eliminated by diluting serum samples 1:10 or 1:20. In contrast, the presence of endogenous anti-PRL autoantibodies can cause false hyperprolactinemia, as well as the presence of poorly biologically active "large" (50–60 kDa) and "very large" (150 kDa) molecular forms of PRL (macroprolactinemia).[105–107] These conditions should be taken into account, particularly in patients with pituitary macroadenomas, because the "hook effect" may lead to misdiagnosis of nonfunctioning pituitary tumors for prolactinoma, with negative consequences on the therapeutic strategy.

Because the serum PRL profile varies according to the sleep-awake rhythm, on which are superimposed episodic peaks,[14] and because PRL secretion is sensitive to stressful events and physical exercise, serum PRL levels may be elevated when measured on a single blood sample. Therefore, serum PRL levels should be measured on multiple samples (at least three in 1 hour) taken in the morning, a couple hours after awakening, during slow saline infusion to avoid multiple venipuncture, in the absence of any stress, in a comfortable room, and in fasting and resting patients not taking any drug known to affect PRL secretion. Normal reference limits may vary from laboratory to laboratory; in general, however, normal women have levels less than 20 ng/mL and normal men, less than 15 ng/mL.

In the past, several dynamic tests intended to discriminate patients with idiopathic hyperprolactinemia or pseudoprolactinoma from those with prolactinoma were proposed. However, soon after their introduction it became clear that inhibitory tests with high or low doses of dopamine infused over a 120-minute period (4 μg/kg/min or 0.04/μg/kg/min) or with the administration of direct dopaminergic agents such as L-dopa and bromocriptine were unable to achieve this goal, although they might give some information concerning the sensitivity of lactotrophs to dopamine. In addition, tests designed to selectively enhance central dopaminergic tone, such as the administration of L-dopa in association with carbidopa (because it does not cross the blood-brain barrier, carbidopa prevents L-dopa conversion into dopamine in the peripheral circulation, but not at the central level) or nomifensine (which stimulates endogenous dopamine production by blocking dopamine reuptake by dopaminergic neurons), failed in discriminating idiopathic from tumoral hyperprolactinemia.[108]

TRH, antidopaminergic drugs, vasoactive intestinal polypeptide, insulin-induced hypoglycemia, and opioidergic compounds were proposed as stimulatory tests with the same purpose because it was promptly documented that most prolactinomas are unable to enhance serum PRL levels in response to these agents. The agents still used today are TRH (200 μg intravenously) and D_2 receptor blockers (domperidone, 10 mg intravenously, metoclopramide, 10 mg intravenously, or sulpiride, 50 mg intramuscularly). In normal subjects these agents cause serum PRL levels to increase by at least 100% over

TABLE 25–2. Anterior Pituitary Hormone Deficiencies* in Patients with Prolactinomas

Hormone (Testing)	Macroprolactinomas	Microprolactinomas
ACTH (ITT, CRH)	37/153 (24.2%)	6/168 (3.6%)
GH (ITT, arginine)	34/53 (64.1%)	2/86 (2.3%)
TSH (TRH)	45/142 (31.7%)	5/207 (2.4%)
LH/FSH (GnRH)	32/108 (29.6%)	7/175 (4.0%)

*As evaluated by currently accepted anterior pituitary function testing. Unpublished data from the author's file.

ACTH, adrenocorticotropic hormone; CRH, corticotropin-releasing hormone; FSH, follicle-stimulating hormone; GH, growth hormone; GnRH, gonadotropin-releasing hormone; ITT, insulin-induced hypoglycemia; LH, luteinizing hormone; TRH, thyrotropin-releasing hormone; TSH, thyroid-stimulating hormone.

TABLE 25–3. Efficiency and Predictive Value of TRH (200 μg IV) and a Dopamine Receptor Blocker (Sulpiride, 50 mg IM) in Diagnosing Prolactinomas in 452 Hyperprolactinemic Women*

Finding	No. of Patients	Predictive Value (%)		Efficiency (%)	
		TRH	*DARB*	*TRH*	*DARB*
Pituitary tumor					
Macroadenoma	142	66	61	69	69
Microadenoma	207	74	74	67	70
No evidence of	103	65	68	62	64
Total	452	83	82	77	76
Prolactin levels (ng/mL)					
>20–50	104	48	39	64	54
50–200	168	75	81	73	77
>200	180	93	93	65	89

*All patients had MRI with contrast-enhanced imaging of the sella region. Data were subgrouped according to the presence of pituitary adenoma and its size and basal serum prolactin levels. Efficiency and predicted value were calculated according to the following formulas:

$$\text{Predictive value} = \text{TP}/(\text{TP} + \text{FP}) \times 100$$
$$\text{Efficiency} = (\text{TP} + \text{TN})/(\text{TP} + \text{FP} + \text{TN} + \text{FN}) \times 100$$

where TP = true positive, FP = false positive, TN = true negative, and FN = false negative.
DARB, dopamine receptor blocker; TRH, thyrotropin-releasing hormone.
Unpublished data from the author's file.

baseline. Theoretically, patients with idiopathic hyperprolactinemia are expected to increase serum PRL after both provocative stimuli, whereas those with prolactinomas are expected to not increase serum PRL in response to both TRH and dopamine receptor blockers. Patients with pseudoprolactinomas, whose hyperprolactinemia is the result of hypothalamic deconnection, are expected to respond to TRH but not to dopamine receptor blockers. In this light, these tests have been claimed to facilitate the differential diagnosis between radiologically undetectable microprolactinomas and idiopathic hyperprolactinemia and between prolactinomas and pseudoprolactinomas. However, the specificity and sensitivity of these tests, as well as their predictive value and efficiency, have not been ideal (Table 25–3). In particular, these tests are poorly effective in patients with serum PRL levels less than 50 ng/mL, which represents the most problematic group, and in discriminating patients with macroprolactinoma from those with pseudoprolactinoma or suprasellar nonpituitary lesions.[109–112]

Because primary hypothyroidism may cause hyperprolactinemia, thyroid function should be investigated. Pituitary hormone secretion should also be carefully evaluated, particularly in patients with macroprolactinomas, in order to detect hypothalamic-pituitary insufficiency (see Table 25–2).

IMAGING

Since the introduction of high-resolution techniques, imaging of the pituitary gland and hypothalamus has attained fundamental importance in the diagnosis of hyperprolactinemic states, particularly in patients who do not have any alteration of the sella turcica on plain radiographs of the skull.[8, 113–116] High-resolution CT scanning of coronal and sagittal sections with contiguous images, 1.5 mm collimation, contrast enhancement, and dynamic conditions enables precise study of the pituitary gland and the surrounding structures, including the sella bones. Microprolactinomas usually appear as unique, round, hypodense lesions in a thickened pituitary. The superior profile of the pituitary is convex, and the sella floor may be lowered, thinned, and sometimes eroded or discontinuous, depending on the lesion. The pituitary stalk is displaced toward the side opposite the lesion. The quality of the images is even better with the use of MRI (Fig. 25–2); even without good visualization of osseous structures, MRI has the advantage of avoidance of radiation exposure and the use of paramagnetic contrast medium (gadolinium), which is better tolerated than the iodinated contrast media used for CT.

As far as sensitivity is concerned, both CT and MRI are 81% to 94% sensitive, whereas specificity is still matter of discussion. In one recent study of 74 women with serum prolactin levels above 52 ng/mL investigated by MRI, microadenomas were found in 38 patients (51.3%), macroadenomas in 6 (8.1%), an infundibular glioma in 1,

and normal pituitary glands in 29 patients (39.2%).[114] In another study, the presence of microprolactinoma was investigated by CT in 51 hyperprolactinemic women who underwent pituitary surgery: 85% had abnormal CT results, but in only 34% of them was an adenoma found at surgery.[115] In addition, it should be noted that the presence of minute focal signal alterations has been reported in variable, but not negligible percentages of normal subjects (16%–36%) with both techniques. From the available data it may be concluded that (1) MRI is preferable to CT and (2) this sensitive tool for the detection of pituitary microadenomas cannot be used as a screening investigation—unless in the presence of clinical and biochemical evidence consistent with suspicion of prolactinoma.[8, 114]

In macroadenomas, MRI helps in the evaluation of tumor extension but is unable to determine its nature, which largely rests on hormonal and clinical assessment or histopathology. MRI is also extremely sensitive in detecting other sellar, parasellar, stalk, or hypothalamic lesions causing hyperprolactinemia, in detecting intracranial or intrasphenoidal ectopic prolactinomas, or in differentiating intracranial or intrathecal deposits from malignant prolactinomas.[117]

Recently, in vivo imaging of prolactinomas with the use of radiolabeled dopamine D_2 receptor radioligands such as ^{123}I-epidepride (^{123}I-IBZM [iodobenzamide]–single-photon emission CT) has been proposed for the acquisition of functional information.[118–120] This technique, although potentially providing a means of identifying pituitary tumors possessing dopamine receptors, is of limited practical value in view of its high cost.

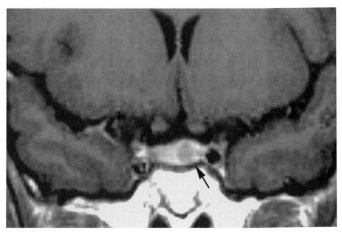

FIGURE 25–2. Typical magnetic resonance image of a pituitary microprolactinoma (coronal view). The lesion *(arrow)* is hypodense and makes the superior profile of the pituitary convex.

DIAGNOSIS

Taking a careful history of drug ingestion is recommended in every patient suspected of having hyperprolactinemia because the history may obviate the need for further investigation. Routine blood tests should be carried out to exclude hypothyroidism, chronic renal failure, and liver cirrhosis.

Because some patients have marginally elevated serum PRL levels, often measured on a single sample taken in stressful conditions or after drug ingestion, the first question to be addressed is whether they have pathologic hyperprolactinemia. About 43% of patients referred to the author's center for further investigation of hyperprolactinemia previously diagnosed elsewhere (in general, young women with menstrual disturbances and serum PRL levels ranging from >20 to <100 ng/mL) have normal serum PRL concentrations after appropriate multiple sampling carried out as previously described in Hormonal Evaluation. Serum PRL levels lower than 100 ng/mL that progressively drop to within normal limits during multiple sampling exclude the diagnosis of hyperprolactinemia. In contrast, serum PRL levels greater than 200 ng/mL are distinctive of prolactinoma. Patients with serum PRL levels persistently above the normal reference limits but lower than 200 ng/mL constitute the "intriguing" group. First of all it is necessary to establish whether they are harboring a pituitary tumor. For this purpose, they need to undergo MRI, which may help in distinguishing pituitary adenoma from other conditions associated with elevations in PRL. If an image consistent with microadenoma is found, the diagnosis of microprolactinoma is acceptable. If a pituitary macroadenoma is found, it is mandatory to establish whether it is a real prolactinoma. In fact, in the presence of serum PRL levels lower than 200 ng/mL, the diagnosis of pseudoprolactinoma is the most likely. Unfortunately, the diagnosis of pseudoprolactinoma or a nonpituitary lesion is not always feasible with certainty on a biochemical or radiologic basis and often requires histopathologic confirmation. Although TRH and/or dopamine receptor blocker tests are of limited value for discriminating between prolactinomas and pseudoprolactinomas, the finding of a positive response to TRH favors the diagnosis of pseudoprolactinoma. The absence of any tumor shrinkage during chronic dopamine agonist therapy in spite of serum PRL normalization also points to pseudoprolactinoma.

The diagnosis of idiopathic hyperprolactinemia is based only on "exclusion criteria." Although high-resolution imaging techniques able to detect even lesions 2 to 3 mm in diameter have reduced the number of patients in whom idiopathic hyperprolactinemia is diagnosed, it is still possible that some of them are harboring microadenomas below the present limits of detectability. TRH and dopamine receptor blocker testing do not help in making this distinction,[112] which nowadays is of minor practical importance because of the effectiveness of treatment with dopamine agonists and the documented modest trend toward progression of the disease in both conditions.[27–30]

THERAPY

Treatment of hyperprolactinemic syndromes is aimed not only at normalizing circulating PRL levels, thereby causing the associated symptoms to regress, but in prolactinomas, also at decreasing or stabilizing the size of the tumor, thereby alleviating symptoms of mass effect, preserving or restoring anterior pituitary function, and preventing progression of the disease.

Immediate effects of lowering PRL levels are restoration of menstrual function and fertility in women and libido and potency in men. Also, lowering PRL levels helps prevent the functional sequelae of exposure to chronic PRL excess, including estrogen deficiency–associated osteopenia.[50, 88, 121–123]

In patients with prolactinoma, the ideal treatment would be radical ablation of the tumor and restoration of normal hypothalamic-pituitary function without a need for additional treatment. However, these results are achieved in only a limited number of patients by surgery.[124, 125] In contrast, the efficacy of dopaminergic drugs in lowering PRL secretion and in shrinking the tumor mass in patients with prolactinoma is far better and has made these agents first-choice

therapy.[126] Unfortunately, this quality has also led to the widespread malpractice of immediate institution of treatment with dopamine agonists as soon as hyperprolactinemia is documented, but before the cause of the hyperprolactinemia is diagnosed. A precise diagnosis is in fact mandatory to plan an appropriate therapeutic strategy because treatment of hyperprolactinemia varies according to its nature.

Treatment Planning

Antidopaminergic drug withdrawal in patients treated with agents known to enhance serum PRL levels is generally followed by normalization of circulating PRL levels and regression of the hyperprolactinemic syndrome. However, particularly in psychiatric patients,[127] simply stopping antidopaminergic medication is not always feasible, so an alternative plan of treatment should be designed with collaboration between the endocrinologist and psychiatrist. Similarly, removal of stressful conditions or habits may normalize PRL secretion.

Adequate L-thyroxine replacement therapy usually causes PRL secretion to normalize in hypothyroid patients.[49] Kidney transplantation, but not hemodialysis reduces serum PRL levels to normal in patients with chronic renal failure. Irritative lesions of the spine, thoracic wall, or mammary region causing PRL to rise via neurogenic pathways should be treated as appropriate.

In hyperprolactinemic patients with polycystic ovary syndrome, treatment with dopamine agonists may be used as adjuvant therapy to facilitate the resumption of ovulatory menses.

In the presence of nonneoplastic hypothalamic lesions or idiopathic hyperprolactinemia or even in patients with microprolactinoma, particularly when the symptoms are modest and pregnancy is not desired, the "no treatment" option should be considered. In fact, it has been reported that in a group of 70 hyperprolactinemic patients (not including macroprolactinomas) monitored for up to 15 years, a spontaneous significant fall in the median PRL concentration occurred in 31 women not receiving therapy, with stable normalization in 11 of them.[30] Serum PRL also fell to normal in 3 of 10 women who had no treatment at all. These data confirm that hyperprolactinemia is, in a not negligible proportion of cases, a self-limiting process.

In hyperprolactinemic patients with a space-occupying mass of the hypothalamic-pituitary region other than prolactinoma, the ideal therapy is treatment of the primary lesion.[19, 47] Sarcoidotic granulomas may be reduced by corticosteroid administration.[128] Transcranial neurosurgery is indicated for removal of hypothalamic tumors such as gliomas, meningiomas, craniopharyngiomas, and cysts. Radiotherapy, eventually associated with appropriate chemotherapy, may be effective in reducing other surgically unapproachable neoplastic masses and hypothalamic-pituitary deposits from malignant tumors.

As far as prolactinomas are concerned, three therapeutic options are available: pituitary surgery, radiotherapy, and medical treatment with dopaminergic agonists.[122–126, 129–131] In some patients, individualized therapeutic strategies must be designed and more than one treatment used. Several factors should be taken into account when designing therapeutic plans, such as the specific clinical problem of individual patients, the different natural history of microadenomas and macroadenomas, the risks and benefits of each treatment, the desire for pregnancy, and the patient's preference for treatment.

Pituitary Surgery

The choice of pituitary surgery should take into account the volume of the adenoma, the age of the patient, the desire for restoration of fertility, the efficacy and tolerability of the dopamine agonists, and the type of surgical approach indicated. In general, the extent of the neurosurgical approach is inversely related to adenoma volume and serum PRL levels.[124–125] Also, the presence of local microinvasion of the dura and adjacent bony structures or fibrosis resulting from previous radiation or medical treatment may affect the surgical outcome. In macroprolactinomas approached by either transcranial or transnasosphenoidal surgery, the success rate is poor (<40%), the frequency of postoperative hypopituitarism is relatively high, and adjunctive therapy is needed in the vast majority of cases. These considerations and the availability of effective and generally well tolerated dopamine agonist therapy have limited the indications for pituitary surgical treatment of macroprolactinomas to debulking of huge tumors before allowing pregnancy, restoration of visual function, or alleviation of neurologic symptoms in giant tumor type adenomas that do not adequately shrink with medical therapy.

In microprolactinomas, which are always approached through the transnasosphenoidal route, the immediate success rate is as high as 80% to 90% and postoperative hypopituitarism is rare, but the recurrence rate is relatively high (17%–50%).[132–137] Thus pituitary surgery has been relegated to patients who are intolerant or resistant to dopamine agonists or want to be free of long-term medication.

Because dopamine agonist treatment reduces the tumor mass of most prolactinomas,[13, 138–140] the effects of dopaminergic pretreatment on surgical outcome have been investigated. The morphologic changes observed in tumors removed from treated patients reflect the effects of dopamine agonists on PRL synthesis and release.[141] Tumor shrinkage results from the reduction in volume of each individual lactotroph. At light and electron microscopy, the adenoma appears to be composed of small lactotrophs with reduced cytoplasm and involution of the Golgi complex and RER. Nuclei are irregular and heterochromatic. Secretory granules do not show peculiar alterations. The changes observed are promptly reversed after withdrawal of short-term treatment. In contrast, prolonged treatment with dopamine agonists may result in permanent regressive changes and proliferation of fibrous tissue.[142] Thus a worse outcome has been reported for microadenomas treated long-term and has been attributed to the marked interstitial and perivascular fibrosis of the adenoma.[143, 144] This finding has been confirmed by several studies,[125, 142] but not by others.[145] On the other hand, in macroprolactinomas, short-term pretreatment with dopamine agonists has been reported to improve the surgical outcome,[145–149] whereas more prolonged treatment reduces the success rate.

Radiotherapy

Radiotherapy is generally limited to a minority of patients with macroprolactinoma unsuccessfully treated by neurosurgery, with macroprolactinoma refractory to medical treatment, or in conjunction with medical treatment. Serum PRL levels decrease only gradually over a period of years, and the frequency of delayed loss of hypothalamic-pituitary function is high. More rarely, radiotherapy, particularly by gamma knife, is used as primary treatment.[150–154]

Medical Treatment

Dopamine agonists are the ideal treatment for prolactinomas because after binding D_2 receptors on the lactotroph membrane, they inhibit PRL synthesis and release and are able to reduce tumor volume in the vast majority of patients (Fig. 25–3); moreover, they are generally well tolerated and do not have any negative effects on anterior pituitary hormone secretion other than PRL. Their mechanism of action is the same as that of native dopamine. D_2 receptor is a seven-membrane–spanning protein, the occupancy of which by dopamine (agonists) produces multiple intracellular responses. These responses lead to the inhibition of adenylyl cyclase activity and consequently cyclic adenosine monophosphate formation, to activation of K^+ channels, and to a reduction in intracellular Ca^{2+} concentration, ultimately resulting in diminished PRL gene transcription and lactotroph mitotic activity. The morphologic changes, previously described, initially lead to a reduction in cytoplasmic volume, then to regressive changes, and finally to fibrosis. After short-term treatment, drug withdrawal is followed by tumor re-expansion, serum PRL increment to pretreatment levels, and reappearance of clinical symptoms, whereas after long-term treatment, PRL levels may remain below pretreatment levels and responsiveness to TRH and dopamine receptor blockers may reappear.[155] Several dopamine agonists have been developed.[12, 126, 156, 157] Those most extensively used today are the ergot derivatives bromocriptine and cabergoline and the nonergot D_2 agonist quinagolide (CV 205-502). They differ in doses and the time required to achieve clinical results, in the duration of action, and in the frequency and severity of untoward effects.[29, 74, 123, 130, 131, 140, 156, 158–170]

In general, treatment should be initiated at very low doses, taken after meals, and increased stepwise up to the optimal dose. Diminution of serum PRL levels is rapid, and clinical effects are usually seen in a few days or weeks, although in some patients normalization of serum PRL levels and disappearance of clinical symptoms are achieved only after several months. Treatment should be continuous because the therapeutic effects usually disappear after drug withdrawal in a variable period of time. However, after a couple of years of treatment, persistent normoprolactinemia or a significant reduction with respect to pretreatment levels, accompanied by normal ovulatory menses, has been reported to occur in about 10% to 15% of patients with microprolactinoma,[155] a percentage not dissimilar, however, from that recorded in observational studies of untreated patients.[27] Although rare cases of progressively acquired resistance to dopamine agonists have been reported, particularly in giant or malignant prolactinomas,[171–172] long-term administration of dopamine agonists does not usually induce tachyphylaxis, and the therapeutic dose may even be tapered to minimal in a good percentage of patients.[173] The question of whether dopaminergic treatment of prolactinomas should be lifelong is still open.[174] As a general rule, in medically treated patients with macroprolactinoma, treatment is necessarily lifelong, at the minimal dose required to maintain normoprolactinemia and reduced tumor volume, whereas in patients with microprolactinoma, treatment may be safely stopped after menopause, provided that no tumor expansion occurs.

Although the adverse effects of dopamine agonists are similar in nature because they are intrinsic to dopaminergic stimulation, they differ in frequency and severity from drug to drug, depending on the selectivity of D_2 receptor occupancy, the ability to cross the blood-brain barrier, and the individual sensitivity of patients. The dopamine receptors on lactotrophs are of the D_2 type, and the pituitary lies outside the blood-brain barrier, whereas the side effects are produced mainly by the occupancy of other dopamine receptor subtypes inside the blood-brain barrier. The most common side effects are abdominal discomfort, nausea, vomiting, constipation, orthostatic hypotension, vertigo, and nasal congestion. They are generally mild and tend to attenuate or disappear over time. Rarely, they may be severe enough to require discontinuation of treatment, particularly in patients who also complain of paresthesias, drowsiness, hallucinations, and psychosis. Alcohol ingestion may aggravate the side effects of dopamine agonists.

The widest experience has been accumulated with bromocriptine, which is considered the reference standard in clinical pharmacology investigations with other dopamine agonists. Bromocriptine, administered orally once or twice a day at doses of 2.5 to 20 mg/day causes a prompt reduction in serum PRL levels to within the normal range in 60% to 100% of cases, followed by clinical remission of the hyperprolactinemic syndrome. Women resume regular ovulatory menses and galactorrhea disappears after 1 to 3 months of treatment in 57% to 100% and 64% to 100% of cases, respectively. Pituitary tumors shrink in about 70% to 90% of cases. However, sporadic patients in whom tumor expanded during bromocriptine therapy have been reported,[175] thus emphasizing the need for careful surveillance of dopamine agonist therapy.

In men, libido, potency, and normal sperm counts are promptly restored in most cases.

Tumor shrinkage, which in some cases has been reported to occur in a few days, is usually fully evident after 2 to 3 months of therapy and may be impressive in macroprolactinomas (see Fig. 25–3). The extrasellar portion of the adenoma seems to be most sensitive to the shrinking effect, which facilitates rapid improvement of visual field defects and regression of mass symptoms. In invasive tumors expanding in the sphenoidal and/or ethmoidal sinuses, rapid and massive tumor shrinkage may cause rhinorrhea requiring surgical treatment.

The effects of dopamine agonist therapy on osteopenia are well documented in women.[88, 121, 122, 176] They are attributed to the restoration of normal estrogen secretion rather than PRL lowering per se. In fact, it has recently been reported that in hyperprolactinemic males after 18 months of therapy, bone mineral density values at both the lumbar spine and femoral neck did not significantly change, regardless of the dopamine agonist used (bromocriptine, cabergoline, or CV 205-502),

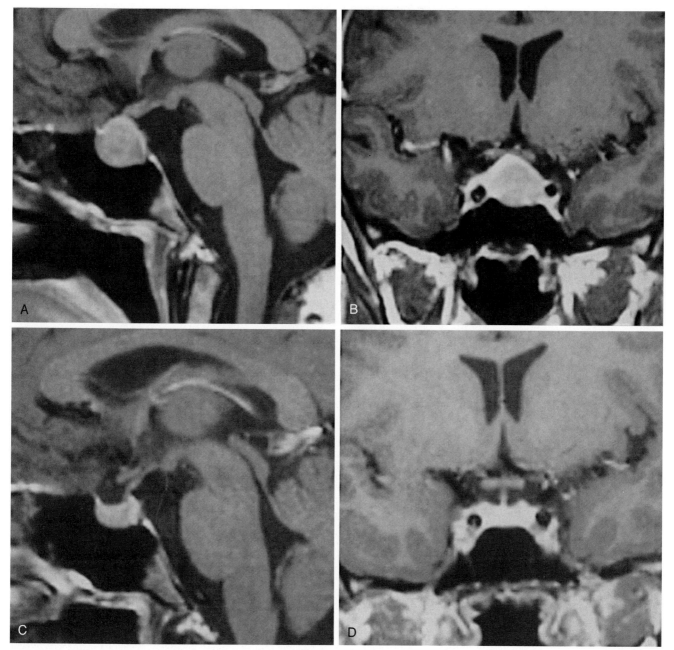

FIGURE 25–3. Effect of dopamine agonist on tumor volume. Magnetic resonance imaging shows the prolactinoma size in sagittal (*A* and *C*) and coronal (*B* and *D*) views, in basal conditions (*A* and *B*), and after 3 months of cabergoline, 1.5 mg/week (*C* and *D*).

although serum PRL levels, testosterone, and dihydrotestosterone were normalized.[177]

A not negligible minority (10% to 25%) of patients are partially or totally resistant to bromocriptine. It is clinically difficult to clearly distinguish refractoriness from intolerance to doses of bromocriptine (up to 40–60 mg/day) high enough to produce clinical effects. The reasons for resistance to dopamine agonists are not fully understood yet. The concentration and affinity constant of dopamine receptors in prolactinomas, although highly variable from tumor to tumor, were reported to not be substantially dissimilar from those in normal pituitary.[178] However, in studies carried out in dopamine agonist–resistant prolactinomas, a marked reduction in spiroperidol-binding sites was observed in responsive tumors,[179] a finding that was even more marked in tumors that had grown during dopamine agonist treatment. Other studies have demonstrated that resistant prolactinomas have decreased expression of the two isoforms of D_2 receptor. In particular, it has been shown that the mRNA corresponding to the short D_2 receptor isoform is poorly expressed.[36, 180] This finding has suggested that

resistance to dopamine might involve defects in posttranscriptional splicing,[180] perhaps in association with diminished $G_{i\alpha}$ expression.[180, 181]

Recent studies have emphasized the role of nerve growth factor in pituitary development, particularly in the control of proliferation and differentiation of lactotrophs and the expression of functional D_2 receptors.[182] These researchers have claimed that exposure of bromocriptine-resistant prolactinoma cells to nerve growth factor suppresses the tumoral phenotype and restores dopamine sensitivity.[183]

With the aim of improving tolerability and overcoming resistance to treatment, a number of other dopamine agonists have been developed, including lisuride, lergotrile, metergoline, mesulergine, dihydroergo-cristine, dihydroergocryptine, pergolide, terguride, cabergoline, and quinagolide.[131] Among them, cabergoline[157] and quinagolide[156] seem to meet these goals (Tables 25–4 and 25–5). Cabergoline ia a naturally long-acting ergot derivative; prolonged suppression of serum PRL concentrations lasting 7 to 14 days was obtained after the administration of single oral doses ranging between 0.3 and 1.0 mg. The prolonged action seems to be due to the generation of active metabolites.

TABLE 25–4. Effects of Bromocriptine, Quinagolide, and Cabergoline in Patients with Microprolactinoma or Idiopathic Hyperprolactinemia

Drug	Patients (No.)	PRL Normalized (% of Pts)	Regular Menses Resumption (% of Pts)	Pregnancies (No.)	Intolerance (Drug Stopped) (% of Pts)	Authors
BRC	236	59	68	16	12	Webster et al.,[161] 1994
CV	40	77	77	NR	15	Merola et al.,[184] 1994
Cab	223	83	82	25	3	Webster et al.,[161] 1994

Brc, bromocriptine; Cab, cabergoline; CV, quinagolide (CV 205-502); NR, not reported; PRL, prolactin; Pts, patients.

Cabergoline is usually administered at a dose of 0.25 to 1.0 mg twice a week, although once-a-week administration (0.5–3.0 mg) has been reported to be equally effective in patients with macroadenoma.[166] The success rate is superior to that of bromocriptine, and the side effects are remarkably much less frequent and severe.[161, 167, 168, 170, 185, 186] This favorable profile allows doses to be increased up to 6 mg/week, which normalizes serum PRL levels in about 85% of patients with microadenomas, in 75% with macroprolactinomas, and notably, in a proportion of bromocriptine- or quinagolide-resistant patients[164-166, 168, 169] (Table 25–6).

Quinagolide, a nonergot compound, is usually effective at a dose of 0.15 to 0.75 mg/day. The success rate in controlling hyperprolactinemic syndrome is comparable to that of bromocriptine, but side effects are significantly less frequent and intense.[162] Normalization of serum PRL has been reported in some bromocriptine-resistant patients[153, 156, 159, 160] (Table 25–7).

Malignant Prolactinomas

Treatment of malignant prolactinomas remains to be identified. Surgery and radiotherapy are only temporarily effective, as are dopamine agonists, to which patients become progressively resistant. Octreotide and chemotherapy are usually ineffective.[187]

Prolactinoma and Pregnancy

The restored fertility requires precise patient counseling. If the patient does not desire children, oral contraceptives are allowed because it has been proved that the small amount of estrogen in the pill does not promote tumor expansion.[18] In patients who desire children, pregnancies are easily obtained; pregnancy rates of 37% to 81% have been reported in patients with prolactinoma. The risk of tumor expansion is less than 5% with microprolactinomas, whereas it is as high as 15% to 25% with macroprolactinomas.[188, 189] In these last patients, depending on the size of the tumor, pregnancy is not advisable without previous tumor debulking. In addition, intra-adenomatous hemorrhage may occur and lead to brisk enlargement of the tumoral mass and consequently headache, blindness, cranial nerve palsies, or even fatal intracranial blood diffusion.[190]

In women with microprolactinoma, pregnancies are generally uneventful and deliveries occur normally; the frequency of miscarriage, premature birth, or congenital malformations is not different from that in healthy women. As a rule, dopamine agonist administration should be stopped as soon as pregnancy is diagnosed and eventually reinstituted if tumor expansion occurs.[29, 74, 188, 191, 192] Although no adverse effects of cabergoline on pregnancy and the fetus have been reported,[193] they have not been extensively investigated yet. Therefore, the long-lasting presence in the circulation of cabergoline active metabolites suggests that treatment should be shifted to bromocriptine or CV 205-502 at least 1 to 2 months before conception.

Serum PRL levels and visual field perimetry should be carefully monitored throughout the entire period of pregnancy, particularly in patients with macroprolactinoma, because no preferred time for complications has been identified. If complications occur, appropriate treatment should be promptly instituted according to the severity of the complication, from the reinstitution of dopamine agonist therapy to transsphenoidal surgery in the case of brisk tumor expansion or pituitary apoplexy. The prophylactic use of low doses of bromocriptine has been suggested as a means of preventing complications without any detrimental effect on pregnancy and the newborn. After pregnancy, PRL secretion and pituitary imaging should be re-evaluated. It is noteworthy that spontaneous normalization of PRL secretion and disappearance of the pituitary microadenoma on imaging have been reported to occur after pregnancy.[194] The most likely explanation is that changes in the pituitary microcirculation occurring during pregnancy may cause a silent infarction of the lactotroph adenoma. In a retrospective study over a 15-year period of follow-up, the final PRL concentration was normal in 35% of women who had at least one pregnancy. These data confirm that pregnancy may be one factor favoring PRL normalization.[30]

Surgical vs. Medical Treatment

The general criteria about the therapeutic choices have already been enunciated. However, further comments on surgical vs. medical treatment are advisable inasmuch as the role of pituitary surgery in the management of prolactinomas has recently been reconsidered.[173] In both microprolactinomas and macroprolactinomas, pituitary surgery is still recommended for patients who are refractory or intolerant to dopamine agonists, those in whom medical treatment is unable to shrink the adenoma, or patients with cystic or rapidly expanding tumors. As already mentioned, pituitary surgery to debulk the tumor mass and prevent tumor expansion is indicated for women with macroprolactinoma who wish to become pregnant. Also, the surgical option should be considered in patients who do not want to be medically treated for life, particularly those with microprolactinoma. In fact, these patients have at least a 70% probability of being definitely cured by transsphenoidal selective adenomectomy, and medical treatment may hamper the results of subsequent pituitary surgery. In contrast, at variance with previous reports,[145-149] a recent retrospective study of patients with macroprolactinomas that examined the results of surgery

TABLE 25–5. Effects of Bromocriptine, Quinagolide, and Cabergoline in Patients with Macroprolactinoma

Drug	Patients (No.)	PRL Normalized (% of Pts)	Tumor Shrinkage (% of Pts)	Visual Field Improvement (% of Pts)	Regular Menses (% of Pts)	Intolerance (Drug Stopped) (% of Pts)	Author
Brc	27	66.6	66.6	90	86	14.8	Molitch et al.,[129] 1985
CV	26	58.0	38.4	66.6	73	3.7	Vance et al.,[158] 1990
Cab	85	61.2	66.1	66.6	79	4.7	Ferrari et al.,[168] 1997

Brc, bromocriptine; Cab, cabergoline; CV, quinagolide (CV 205-502); PRL, prolactin; Pts, patients.

TABLE 25–6. Effects of Cabergoline on Serum Prolactin Levels in Patients Resistant to Bromocriptine and/or Quinagolide*

No. of Patients	Max Dose of Cabergoline (mg/wk)	Pts with Prolactin Normalized (Normal/Total)	Author
3 (1μ + 2M)	3.0	2/3	Delgrange et al.,[164] 1996
5 (5M)	3.0	3/5	Biller et al.,[166] 1996
27 (8μ + 19M)	3.0	23/27	Colao et al.,[169] 1997
16 (16M)	10.5	8/16	Ferrari et al.,[168] 1997
51 (9μ + 42M)		36/51 (70.6%)	Total

*Resistance to bromocriptine or quinagolide is defined by the lack of prolactin suppression below 50% of basal levels with daily doses of 15 mg or 600 μg, respectively.
μ, microprolactinomas; M, macroprolactinomas.

combined with dopamine agonists vs. dopamine agonists alone in long-term treatment did not show any difference in the two groups in anterior pituitary function, imaging changes, stability, or progression of the disease.[195] Thus initial surgical reduction of the tumor mass followed by medical therapy does not seem to result in a better long-term outcome than dopamine agonist therapy does alone. These data argue in favor of medical treatment as first-line therapy for macroprolactinomas, provided that patients are responsive, tolerant, and compliant with dopamine agonist therapy. A short course (6–8 weeks) of dopamine agonist therapy is still advisable before surgery in patients with giant prolactinomas and neurologic complications because tumor shrinkage may either render surgery unnecessary or facilitate more radical excision of the tumor.

Monitoring Hyperprolactinemic Patients

The way to monitor hyperprolactinemic patients varies from patient to patient, depending on the therapeutic strategy adopted, and should be carefully planned. Thus no precise and rigid schedules can be proposed, only flexible general guidelines. Patients for whom the "no treatment" option has been chosen should be re-evaluated for serum PRL levels every 6 months and should have visual field evaluation and imaging of the hypothalamic pituitary region at 1 and 2 years and then every 3 to 5 years. Pituitary imaging should be anticipated in the event of a significant increase in serum PRL levels.

In the days after pituitary surgery, serum PRL levels and plasma and urine osmolality should be evaluated. Thyroid hormones and urinary free cortisol should also be determined a short distance from the point of surgical intervention, and complete reassessment of pituitary function should be carried out after 3 months to evaluate the need for adjunctive therapy and hormone replacement therapy. Imaging and visual field evaluation should be done 3 months after surgery and then every 1 to 3 years.

Pituitary function should be reassessed annually in patients who undergo radiotherapy while taking into account the fact that endocrine defects may appear several years after irradiation. Imaging should be also periodically performed to evaluate not only adenoma size but also the possible, although rare onset of radiation-induced intracranial tumors.[29, 131]

Monitoring patients treated with dopamine agonists includes monthly medical consultation with evaluation of serum PRL levels until the optimal dose is achieved (i.e., the minimal dose able to

maintain normoprolactinemia, or in partially resistant patients, the dose able to maintain the lowest levels of serum PRL with the minimal side effects) and then every 6 to 12 months. Visual fields should be evaluated after 3 and 6 months and then annually in patients with pretreatment visual defects. MRI should be carried out after 6 months and then every 1 to 2 years.

SUMMARY

The hyperprolactinemic syndrome is characterized by menstrual disturbances, infertility, and galactorrhea in women and loss of libido and potency in men. It is the most common hypothalamic-pituitary disorder in clinical endocrinology practice. It may be due to either disrupted PRL inhibitory control by dopamine or the presence of an autonomous PRL-secreting pituitary tumor. The most frequent causes among the former group include the use of drugs that interfere with endogenous dopamine synthesis, release, or binding to D_2 receptors on the lactotroph and lesions of the hypothalamic-pituitary region (of tumoral, granulomatous, inflammatory, or traumatic origin) that are able to prevent hypothalamic dopamine from reaching the lactotroph through the portal vessels. The latter group of causes includes pure PRL-secreting adenomas (microadenomas or macroprolactinomas, depending on adenoma size less than or greater than 10 mm) and mixed tumors. The diagnosis is based on a careful clinical and pharmacologic history, an accurate and reliable estimation of basal serum PRL levels, and MRI of the hypothalamic-pituitary region. Inhibitory and stimulatory dynamic tests are of limited or no value in discriminating the origin of hyperprolactinemia. Correct diagnosis is the necessary premise for an appropriate therapeutic approach, the indiscriminate use of dopamine agonists in any undiagnosed hyperprolactinemia being clinical malpractice. Withdrawal of antidopaminergic agents in patients being treated with these drugs, relief from stressful situations, adequate thyroid hormone therapy in hypothyroid patients, corticosteroid treatment of hypothalamic sarcoidosis, and removal of masses impinging on the hypothalamus are appropriate therapeutic strategies in some patients, depending on the origin of the hyperprolactinemia. Dopamine agonist treatment, which has proved effective not only in reducing PRL secretion but also in causing the pituitary tumor to shrink, is the first-choice therapy in patients with prolactinoma. The new dopamine agonists cabergoline and quinagolide, which are much better tolerated and able to overcome, at least in some cases, dopamine resistance, have enlarged the number of successfully medically treated patients.

TABLE 25–7. Effects of Quinagolide on Serum Prolactin Levels in Patients Resistant to Bromocriptine*

No. of Patients	Max Dose of Quinagolide (μg/day)	Pts with Prolactin Normalized (Normal/Total)	Author
7 (1μ + 6M)	600	2/7	Duranteau et al.,[159] 1991
21 (6μ + 15M)	500	11/21	Brue et al.,[160] 1992
8 (6μ + 2M)	450	4/8	Vilar et al.,[156] 1994
28 (7μ + 21M)	300	12/28	Morange et al.,[163] 1996
64 (20μ + 44)		29/64 (45.3%)	Total

*Resistance to bromocriptine is defined by the lack of prolactin suppression below 50% of basal levels with daily doses of 15 mg.
μ, microprolactinomas; M, macroprolactinomas.

Pituitary surgery still has a role in debulking huge tumors, particularly in women who want to become pregnant, and in patients resistant or intolerant to or not compliant with medical treatment. Radiotherapy is rarely indicated as first-choice therapy.

REFERENCES

1. Ahumada R, del Castillo EB: Amenorrea y galactorrea. Biol Soc Obstet Ginecol 11:64–67, 1932.
2. Krestin D: Spontaneous lactation associated with enlargement of the pituitary. Lancet 1:928–930, 1932.
3. Mendel EB: Chiari-Frommel syndrome. Am J Obstet Gynecol 51:889–892, 1946.
4. Argonz J, del Castillo EB: A syndrome characterized by estrogenic insufficiency, galactorrhea and decreased urinary gonadotropin. J Clin Endocrinol Metab 13:79–87, 1953.
5. Forbes AP, Henneman PH, Griswold GC, Albright F: Syndrome characterized by galactorrhea, amenorrhea, and low urinary FSH: Comparison with acromegaly and normal lactation. J Clin Endocrinol Metab 14:264–271, 1954.
6. Friesen HG: The discovery of human prolactin: A very personal account. Clin Invest Med 18:66–72, 1995.
7. Hardy J: Transsphenoidal surgery of hypersecreting pituitary tumors. In Kolhler G, Ross GT (eds): Diagnosis and Treatment of Pituitary Tumors. New York, Elsevier, 1973, pp 179–194.
8. Elster AD: Modern imaging of the pituitary. Radiology 187:1–14, 1993.
9. Kovacs K, Horvat E: Pituitary adenomas associated with hyperprolactinemia: Morphological and immunological aspects. In Faglia G, Giovanelli M, MacLeod RM (eds): Pituitary Microadenomas. London, Academic, 1980, p 123.
10. Anniko M, Eneroth P, Werner S, Wersall J: Human pituitary microadenomas in organ culture. In Faglia G, Giovanelli M, MacLeod RM (eds): Pituitary Microadenomas. London, Academic, 1980, pp 143–149.
11. Cooke NE: Prolactin: Basic physiology. In DeGroot LJ, Jamieson JL (eds): Endocrinology, ed 3. Philadelphia, WB Saunders, 1994, pp 368–393.
12. Flückiger E, Doepfner W, Marko M, et al: Effects of ergot alkaloids on the hypothalamic-pituitary axis. Postgrad Med 52:57–61, 1976.
13. Bevan JS, Webster J, Burke CW, Scanlon MF: Dopamine agonists and pituitary tumour shrinkage. Endocr Rev 13:220–240, 1992.
14. Sassin JF, Frantz AG, Kapen S, Weitzman ED: The nocturnal rise of human prolactin is dependent on sleep. J Clin Endocrinol Metab 37:436, 1975.
15. Reavley S, Fisher AD, Owen D, et al: Psychological distress in patients with hyperprolactinaemia. Clin Endocrinol 47:343–348, 1997.
16. Neill JD: Prolactin secretion and its control. In Knobil Z, Neill JD (eds): The Physiology of Reproduction. New York, Raven, 1988, pp 1379–1390.
17. Serri O, Noiseux D, Robert F, Hardy J: Lactotroph hyperplasia in an estrogen treated male-to-female transsexual patient. J Clin Endocrinol Metab 81:3177–3179, 1996.
18. Testa G, Vegetti W, Motta T, et al: Two-year treatment with oral contraceptives in hyperprolactinemic patients. Contraception 58:69–73, 1998.
19. Rohmer V, Chanson P, Dupas B, Beckers A: Non pituitary tumours of the sellar region. Ann Endocrinol 58:11–19, 1997.
20. Ambrosi B, Bassetti IM, Ferrario R, et al: Precocious puberty in a boy with a PRL-, LH- and FSH-secreting pituitary tumour: Hormonal and immunocytochemical studies. Acta Endocrinol 122:569–576, 1990.
21. Pernicone PJ, Scheithauer BW, Sebo TJ, et al: Pituitary carcinoma: A clinicopathologic study of 15 cases. Cancer 79:804–812, 1997.
22. Ambrosi B, Faglia G, Multicenter Pituitary Tumor Study Group Lombardy Region: Epidemiology of pituitary tumors. In Faglia G, Beck-Peccoe P, Ambrosi B, et al (eds): Pituitary Adenomas. New Trends in Basic and Clinical Research. Int Congr Series, vol 961. Amsterdam, Excerpta Medica, 1991, pp 159–168.
23. Stoffel Wagner B, Stoger P, Klingmuller D: Prediagnostic natural history and initial symptoms in 517 patients with hypophyseal adenoma. Dtsche Med Wochenschr 122:213–219, 1997.
24. Terada T, Kovacs K, Stefaneanu L, Horvath E: Incidence, pathology, and recurrence of pituitary adenomas: Study of 647 unselected surgical cases. Endocr Pathol 6:301–310, 1995.
25. von Werder K, Eversmann T, Fahlbusch R, Rjosk HK: Treatment of hyperprolactinemia. In Ganong WF, Martini L (eds): Frontiers in Neuroendocrinology. New York, Raven, 1982, pp 123–159.
26. March CM, Kletsky OA, Davajan V, et al: Longitudinal evaluation of patients with untreated prolactin-secreting pituitary adenomas. Am J Obstet Gynecol 139:835–844, 1981.
27. Martin TL, Kim M, Malarkey WB: The natural history of idiopathic hyperprolactinemia. J Clin Endocrinol Metab 60:855–858, 1985.
28. Sisam DA, Sheehan JP, Sheedar LR: The natural history of untreated microprolactinomas. Fertil Steril 48:67–71, 1987.
29. von Werder: Prolactinomas: Clinical finding and endocrinology. In Landolt AM, Vance ML, Reilly PL (eds): Pituitary Adenomas. New York, Churchill Livingstone, 1996, pp 111–126.
30. Jeffcoate WJ, Pound N, Sturrock NDC, Lambourne J: Long-term follow-up of patients with hyperprolactinaemia. Clin Endocrinol 45:299–303, 1996.
31. Garcia MM, Kapcala LP: Growth of a microprolactinoma to a macroprolactinoma during estrogen therapy. J Endocrinol Invest 18:450–455, 1995.
32. Fine SA, Frohman LA: Loss of central nervous system component of dopaminergic inhibition of prolactin secretion in patients with prolactin-secreting pituitary tumors. J Clin Invest 61:973–980, 1978.
33. Scanlon MF, Rodriguez-Arnao MD, Gregor AM, et al: Altered dopaminergic regulation of thyrotropin release in patients with prolactinomas. Comparison with other tests of hypothalamic-pituitary function. Clin Endocrinol 12:133–139, 1984.
34. Bansal S, Lee LA, Wolff PD: Abnormal prolactin responsivity to dopaminergic suppression in hyperprolactinemic patients. Am J Med 71:961–966, 1981.
35. Connel JMC, Padfield PL, Bunting EA, et al: Inhibition of prolactin secretion by low-dose dopamine infusion in patients with hyperprolactinemia. Clin Endocrinol 16:527–532, 1983.
36. Melmed S: The structure and function of pituitary dopamine receptors. Endocrinologist 7:385–389, 1997.
37. Wood DF, Johnston JM, Johnston DG: Dopamine, the dopamine D2 receptor and pituitary tumours. Clin Endocrinol 35:455–466, 1991.
38. Civelli O, Bunzow JR, Grandy DK: Molecular diversity of dopamine receptors. Annu Rev Pharmacol Toxicol 32:281, 1993.
39. Thakker RV, Pook MA, Wooding C, et al: Association of somatotropinomas with loss of alleles on chromosome 11 and with gsp mutations. J Clin Invest 91:2815–2821, 1993.
40. Friedman E, Adams E, Hoog A, et al: Normal structural dopamine type 2 receptor gene in prolactin-secreting and other pituitary tumors. J Clin Endocrinol Metab 78:568–574, 1994.
41. Herman V, Fagin J, Gonski R, et al: Clonal origin of pituitary adenomas. J Clin Endocrinol Metab 71:1427–1433, 1990.
42. Faglia G: Genesis of pituitary adenomas. In Landolt AM, Vance ML, Reilly PL (eds): Pituitary Adenomas. New York, Churchill Livingstone, 1996, pp 3–13.
43. Karga HJ, Alexander JM, Hedley-Whyte ET, et al: Ras mutations in human pituitary tumors. J Clin Endocrinol Metab 74:914–919, 1992.
44. Yi Cai W, Alexander JM, Hedley-Whyte ET, et al: Ras mutations in human prolactinomas and pituitary carcinomas. J Clin Endocrinol Metab 78:89–93, 1994.
45. Burgess JR, Shepherd JJ, Parameswaran V, et al: Prolactinomas in a large kindred with multiple endocrine neoplasia type 1: Clinical features and inheritance pattern. J Clin Endocrinol Metab 81:1841–1845, 1996.
46. Olufemi SE, Green JS, Manickam P, et al: Common ancestral mutation in the MEN1 gene is likely responsible for the prolactinoma variant of MEN1 (MEN1(Burin)) in four kindreds from Newfoundland. Hum Mutat 11:264–269, 1998.
47. Folkerth RD, Price DL, Schwartz M, et al: Xanthomatous hypophysitis. Am J Surg Pathol 22:736–741, 1998.
48. Valensi P, Combes ME, Perret G, Attali JR: TSH and prolactin responses to thyrotropin releasing hormone (TRH) and domperidone in patients with empty sella syndrome. J Endocrinol Invest 19:293–297, 1996.
49. Notsu K, Ito Y, Furuya H, et al: Incidence of hyperprolactinemia in patients with Hashimoto's thyroiditis. Endocr J 44:89–94, 1997.
50. Vanderpump MPJ, French JM, Appleton D, et al: The prevalence of hyperprolactinaemia and association with markers of autoimmune thyroid disease in survivors of the Whickham Survey cohort. Clin Endocrinol 48:39–44, 1998.
51. Luciano AA, Chapler FK, Sherman BM: Hyperprolactinemia in polycystic ovary syndrome. Fertil Steril 41:719–725, 1984.
52. Isik AZ, Gulekli B, Zorlu CG, et al: Endocrinological and clinical analysis of hyperprolactinemic patients with and without ultrasonically diagnosed polycystic ovarian changes. Gynecol Obstet Invest 43:183–185, 1997.
53. Horvath E, Kovacs K: The adenohypophysis. In Kovacs K, Asa SL (eds): Functional Endocrine Pathology, vol 1. Cambridge, Blackwell, 1991, pp 245–281.
54. Saeger W, Lüdecke D: Pituitary hyperplasia. Definition, light and electron microscopy structures and significance in surgical specimens. Virchows Arch Pathol Anat 399:277–287, 1983.
55. Landoldt AM, Minder H: Immunohistochemical examination of the paradenomatous "normal" pituitary. An evaluation of prolactin cell hyperplasia. Virchows Arch Pathol Anat 403:181–193, 1984.
56. Horvath E, Kovacs K: Tumors of the pituitary glands. In Hartmann WH (ed): Atlas of Tumor Pathology, vol 21. Washington, DC, Armate Forces Institute of Pathology, 1986, pp 1–264.
57. Pioro EP, Scheithauer RW, Laws ER Jr, et al: Combined thyrotroph and lactotroph cell hyperplasia simulating prolactin-secreting pituitary adenoma in longstanding primary hypothyroidism. Surg Neurol 29:218, 1988.
58. Saad MF, Adams F, Mackay H, et al: Occult Cushing's disease presenting with acute psychosis. Am J Med 76:759–766, 1984.
59. Burrow GN, Wortzman G, Rewcastle NB, et al: Microadenomas of the pituitary and abnormal sellar tomograms in an unselected autopsy series. N Engl J 304:156–158, 1981.
60. Saeger W, Mohr K, Caselitz J, Lüdeche DK: Light and electron microscopical morphometry of pituitary adenomas in hyperprolactinemia. Pathol Res Pract 181:544–550, 1986.
61. Rilliet B, Mohr G, Robert F: Calcifications in pituitary adenomas. Surg Neurol 15:249–255, 1981.
62. Landoldt AM, Kleihues P, Heitz PU: Amyloid deposits in pituitary adenomas. Arch Pathol Lab Med 111:453–458, 1987.
63. Hinton DR, Polk RK, Linse KD, et al: Characterization of spherical amyloid protein from a prolactin-producing pituitary adenoma. Acta Neuropathol 93:43–49, 1997.
64. Bassetti M, Spada A, Arosio M, et al: Morphological studies on mixed growth hormone-(GH) and prolactin-(PRL) secreting human pituitary adenomas. Coexistence of GH and PRL in the same secretory granule. J Clin Endocrinol Metab 62:1093–1100, 1986.
65. Scheithauer BW, Horvath E, Kovacs K, et al: Plurihormonal pituitary adenomas. Semin Diagn Pathol 3:69–82, 1987.
66. Gollard R, Kosty M, Cheney C, et al: Prolactin-secreting pituitary carcinoma with implants in the cheek pouch and metastases to the ovaries: A case report and literature review. Cancer 76:1814–1820, 1995.
67. Saeger W, Bosse U, Pfingst E, et al: Prolactin-secreting pituitary carcinoma. Case report of a very rare metastasizing tumor. Pathologe 16:354–358, 1995.
68. Rockwell BH, Pica R, Raji MR, et al: Case report—intrathecal metastatic pituitary prolactinoma. AJR 167:1295–1296, 1996.
69. Franks S, Murray MAF, Jequier AM, et al: Incidence and significance of hyperprolactinaemia in women with amenorrhoea. Clin Endocrinol 4:597–607, 1975.

70. Buvat J, Lemaire A: Endocrine screening in 1,022 men with erectile dysfunction: Clinical significance and cost-effective strategy. J Urol 158:1764–1767, 1997.

71. Molitch ME, Russel EJ: The pituitary "incidentaloma." Ann Intern Med 112:925–931, 1990.

72. Allen DL, Mitchner NA, Uveges TE, et al: Cell-specific induction of c-fos expression in the pituitary gland by estrogen. Endocrinology 138:2128–2135, 1997.

73. Mindermann T, Wilson CB: Age-related and gender-related occurrence of pituitary adenomas. Clin Endocrinol 41:359–364, 1994.

74. von Werder K, Müller OA, Fink U, Gräf K: Diagnosis and treatment of hyperprolactinemia. *In* Imura H (ed): The Pituitary. New York, Raven, 1994, pp 453–489.

75. Maor Y, Berezin M: Hyperprolactinemia in postmenopausal women. Fertil Steril 67:693–698, 1997.

76. Lüdecke DK, Herrmann HD, Schulte FJ: Special problems with neurosurgical treatment of hormone-secreting pituitary adenomas in children. Prog Exp Tumor Res 40:362–370, 1987.

77. Kane LA, Leinung MC, Scheithauer BW, et al: Pituitary adenomas in childhood and adolescence. J Clin Endocrinol Metab 79:1135–1140, 1994.

78. Mindermann T, Wilson CB: Pediatric pituitary adenomas. Neurosurgery 36:259–268, 1995.

79. Dissaneevate P, Warne GL: Hyperprolactinaemia and pituitary adenomas in adolescence. J Pediatr Endocrinol Metab 11:531–541, 1998.

80. Artese R, D'Osvaldo DH, Molocznik I, et al: Pituitary tumors in adolescent patients. Neurol Res 20:415–417, 1998.

81. Benbow SJ, Foy P, Jones B, et al: Pituitary tumours presenting in the elderly: Management and outcome. Clin Endocrinol 46:657–660, 1997.

82. Corbetta S, Pizzocaro A, Peracchi M, et al: Multiple endocrine neoplasia type 1 in patients with recognized pituitary tumours of different types. Clin Endocrinol 47:507–512, 1997.

83. Berezin M, Karasik A: Familial prolactinoma. Clin Endocrinol 42:483–486, 1995.

84. Del Pozo E, Wyss H, Tolis G, et al: Prolactin and deficient luteal function. Obstet Gynecol 53:282, 1979.

85. Hirahara F, Andoh N, Sawai K, et al: Hyperprolactinemic recurrent miscarriage and results of randomized bromocriptine treatment trials. Fertil Steril 70:246–252, 1998.

86. Koppelman MCS, Kurtz DW, Morrish KA, et al: Vetebral body mineral content in hyperprolactinemic women. J Clin Endocrinol Metab 39:1050–1043, 1984.

87. Wardlaw SL, Bilezikian JP: Hyperprolactinemia and osteopenia. J Clin Endocrinol Metab 75:690–691, 1992.

88. Schlechte J, El-Khouri G, Kathol M, Walkner L: Forearm and vertebral bone mineral in treated and untreated hyperprolactinemic amenorrhea. J Clin Endocrinol Metab 64:1021–1026, 1987.

89. Biller BMK, Baum HBA, Rosenthal DI, et al: Progressive trabecular osteopenia in women with hyperprolactinemic amenorrhea. J Clin Endocrinol Metab 75:692–697, 1992.

90. Vermeulen A, Andò S: Prolactin and adrenal androgen secretion. Clin Endocrinol 8:295–301, 1978.

91. Carter JN, Tyson JE, Tolis G, et al: Prolactin-secreting tumors and hypogonadism in 22 men. N Engl J Med 299:847, 1978.

92. Berezin M, Shimon I, Hadani M: Prolactinoma in 53 men: Clinical characteristics and of treatment (male prolactinoma). J Endocrinol Invest 18:436–441, 1995.

93. Walsh JP, Pullan PT: Hyperprolactinaemia in males: A heterogeneous disorder. Aust N Z J Med 27:385–390, 1997.

94. Ruvalcaba RHA, Castro Magana M, Angulo M: Macrotestes associated with hyperprolactinemia. J Pediatr Endocrinol Metab 9:617–622, 1996.

95. Greenman Y, Tordjman K, Stern N: Increased body weight associated with prolactin secreting pituitary adenomas: Weight loss with normalization of prolactin levels. Clin Endocrinol 48:547–553, 1998.

96. Sobrinho LG: The psychogenic effects of prolactin. Acta Endocrinol 129:39–40, 1993.

97. Kemmann E, Jones JB: Hyperprolactinemia and headaches. Am J Obstet Gynecol 145:668–671, 1983.

98. Siegel RD, Lee SL: Pneumocephalus and cerebrospinal fluid rhinorrhea after bromocriptine therapy of an invasive prolactinoma: A case report and review of the literature. Endocrinologist 6:148–152, 1996.

99. Faglia G, Travaglini P, Beck-Peccoz P, et al: Anterior pituitary hormones other than those hypersecreted in patients with functioning microadenomas. *In* Faglia G, Giovanelli M, MacLeod RM (eds): Pituitary Microadenomas. London, Academic, 1980, pp 277–294.

100. Weiner RI, Findell PR, Kordon C: Role of classic and peptide neuromediators in the regulation of LH and prolactin. *In* Knobil Z, Neill JD (eds): The Physiology of Reproduction. New York, Raven, 1988, pp 1235–1281.

101. Evans WS, Cronin MJ, Thorner MO: Hypogonadism in hyperprolactinemia. Proposed mechanisms. *In* Ganong WF, Martini L (eds): Frontiers in Neuroendocrinology. New York, Raven, 1982, pp 77–122.

102. Stjean E, Blain F, Comtois R: High prolactin levels may be missed by immunoradiometric assay in patients with macroprolactinomas. Clin Endocrinol 44:305–309, 1996.

103. Barkan AL, Chandler WF: Giant pituitary prolactinoma with falsely low serum prolactin: The pitfall of the "high-dose hook effect": Case report. Neurosurgery 42:913–915, 1998.

104. Petakov MS, Damjanovic SS, Nikolic Durovic MM, et al: Pituitary adenomas secreting large amounts of prolactin may give false low values in immunoradiometric assays. The hook effect. J Endocrinol Invest 21:184–188, 1998.

105. Hattori N, Inagaki C: Anti-prolactin (PRL) autoantibodies cause asymptomatic hyperprolactinemia: Bioassay and clearance studies of PRL–immunoglobulin G complex. J Clin Endocrinol Metab 82:3107–3110, 1997.

106. Sulimani RA: Idiopathic hyperprolactinemia: What should we do about it? Endocrinologist 8:31–33, 1998.

107. Tritos NA, Guay AT, Malarkey WB: Asymptomatic "big" hyperprolactinemia in two men with pituitary adenomas. Eur J Endocrinol 138:82–85, 1998.

108. Moriondo P, Travaglini P, Nissim M, Faglia G: Evaluation of two inhibitory tests (nomifensine and L-dopa + carbidopa) for the diagnosis of hyperprolactinemic states. Clin Endocrinol 13:525–533, 1980.

109. Klijn JCM, Lamberts SWJ, DeJong FH, Birkenhager JC: The value of the thyrotropin-releasing hormone test in patients with prolactin-secreting pituitary tumors and suprasellar non-pituitary tumors. Fertil Steril 35:155–161, 1981.

110. Ferrari C, Rampini F, Benco R, et al: Functional characterization of hypothalamic hyperprolactinemia. J Clin Endocrinol Metab 55:987–991, 1982.

111. Arafah BM, Nekl KE, Gold RS, Selman WR: Dynamics of prolactin secretion in patients with hypopituitarism and pituitary macroadenomas. J Clin Endocrinol Metab 80:3507–3512, 1995.

112. Sawers HA, Robb OJ, Walmsley D, et al: An audit of the diagnostic usefulness of PRL and TSH responses to domperidone and high resolution magnetic resonance imaging of the pituitary in the evaluation of hyperprolactinaemia. Clin Endocrinol 46:321–326, 1997.

113. Stadnik F, Spruyt D: Pituitary microadenomas: Diagnosis with dynamic serial CT, conventional CT and T1 weighted MR imaging before and after the injection of gadolinium. Eur J Radiol 15:675–679, 1994.

114. Rand T, Kink E, Sator M, et al: MRI of microadenomas in patients with hyperprolactinaemia. Neuroradiology 38:744–746, 1996.

115. Davis PC, Hoffman JC, Tindall JT, Braun JF: Prolactin-secreting pituitary microadenomas: Inaccuracy of high resolution CT imaging. Am J Neuroradiol 5:721–726, 1984.

116. Farabola M, Bettinelli A, Resta F, et al: Clinical value of dynamic MRI in the diagnosis of pituitary microadenoma. Riv Neuroradiol 10:17–28, 1997.

117. Hattori N, Ishihara T, Saiwai S, et al: Ectopic prolactinoma on MRI. J Comput Assist Tomogr 18:936–938, 1994.

118. de Herder WW, Reijs AEM, Kwekkeboom DJ, et al: In vivo imaging of pituitary tumours using a radiolabelled dopamine D2 receptor radio-ligand. Clin Endocrinol 45:755–767, 1996.

119. Pirker W, Riedl M, Luger A, et al: Dopamine D2 receptor imaging in pituitary adenomas using iodine-123-epipride and SPECT. J Nucl Med 37:1931–1937, 1996.

120. Ferone D, Lastoria S, Colao A, et al: Correlation of scintigraphic results using I-123-methoxybenzamide with hormone levels and tumor size response to quinagolide in patients with pituitary adenomas. J Clin Endocrinol Metab 83:248–252, 1998.

121. Klibanski A, Greenspan SL: Increase in bone mass after treatment of hyperprolactinemic amenorrhea. N Engl J Med 315:542–546, 1986.

122. Klibanski A: Indications for treatment of hyperprolactinemia: An overview. Endocrinologist 7:376–378, 1997.

123. Vance ML: New directions in the treatment of hyperprolactinemia. Endocrinologist 7:153–159, 1997.

124. Giovanelli M, Losa M, Mortini P: Surgical therapy of pituitary adenomas. Metabolism 45(suppl 1):115–116, 1996.

125. Reilly PL: Prolactinomas: Surgical results and prognosis. *In* Landolt AM, Vance ML, Reilly PL (eds): Pituitary Adenomas. New York, Churchill Livingstone, 1996, pp 363–374.

126. Kleinberg DL: Pharmacological therapies and surgical options in the treatment of hyperprolactinemia. Endocrinologist 7:379–384, 1997.

127. Nordstrom AL, Farde L: Plasma prolactin and central D-2 receptor occupancy in antipsychotic drug–treated patients. J Clin Psychopharmacol 18:305–310, 1998.

128. Cannavò S, Romano C, Buffa R, Faglia G: Granulomatous sarcoidotic lesion of hypothalamic pituitary region associated with Rathke's cleft cyst. J Endocrinol Invest 20:77–81, 1997.

129. Molitch ME, Elton RL, Blackwell LE, et al: Bromocriptine as primary therapy for prolactin-secreting macroadenomas: Results of a perspective multicentric study. J Clin Endocrinol Metab 60:690–705, 1985.

130. Lamberts SWJ, MacLeod RM: Prolactinomas: Medical treatment. *In* Landolt AM, Vance ML, Reilly PL (eds): Pituitary Adenomas. New York, Churchill Livingstone, 1996, pp 431–442.

131. Molitch ME: Prolactinoma. *In* Melmed S (ed): The Pituitary. Cambridge, Blackwell, 1995, pp 443–477.

132. Serri O, Rasio E, Beauregard H: Recurrence of hyperprolactinemia after selective transsphenoidal adenomectomy in women with prolactinomas. N Engl J Med 309:280–283, 1983.

133. Rodman EF, Molitch ME, Post KD, et al: Long term follow-up of transsphenoidal selective adenomectomy for prolactinomas. JAMA 252:921–924, 1984.

134. Schlechte JA, Sherman BM, Chapler FK, Van Gilder J: Long term follow-up of women with surgically treated prolactin-secreting pituitary tumors. J Clin Endocrinol Metab 62:1296–1301, 1986.

135. Webster J, Page MD, Bevan JS: Low recurrence rate after partial hypophysectomy for prolactinomas: The predictive value of prolactin dynamic function tests. Clin Endocrinol 36:35–44, 1992.

136. Ciccarelli E, Ghigo E, Miola C, et al: Prolonged follow-up of "cured" prolactinoma patients after successful adenomectomy. Clin Endocrinol 32:583–592, 1992.

137. Feigenbaum SL, Downey DE, Wilson CB, Jaffe RB: Transsphenoidal pituitary resection for preoperative diagnosis of prolactin-secreting adenoma in women: Long term follow-up. J Clin Endocrinol Metab 81:1711–1719, 1996.

138. Thorner MO, Schran HF, Evans WS, et al: A broad spectrum of prolactin suppression by bromocriptine in hyperprolactinemic women: A study of serum prolactin and bromocriptine levels after acute and chronic administration of bromocriptine. J Clin Endocrinol Metab 50:1026–1033, 1980.

139. Thorner MO, Perryman RL, Rogol AD, et al: Rapid changes of prolactinoma after withdrawal and reinstitution of bromocriptine. J Clin Endocrinol Metab 53:480–483, 1981.

140. Molitch M: Macroprolactinoma size reduction with dopamine agonists. Endocrinologist 7:390–398, 1997.

141. Bassetti M, Spada A, Pezzo G, Giannattasio G: Bromocriptine treatment reduces the cell size in human macroprolactinomas. J Clin Endocrinol Metab 58:268–273, 1984.

142. Esiri MM, Bevan JS, Burke CW, Adams CBI: Effect of bromocriptine treatment on the fibrous tissue component of prolactin-secreting and nonfunctioning macroadenomas of the pituitary gland. J Clin Endocrinol Metab 63:383–388, 1986.

143. Landoldt AM: Prolactinomas: Preoperative bromocriptine treatment. Perspect Neurol Surg 1:105–119, 1990.

144. Soule SG, Farhi J, Conway GS, et al: The outcome of hypophysectomy for prolactinomas in the era of dopamine agonist therapy. Clin Endocrinol 44:711–716, 1996.

145. Perrin G, Tretuyer C, Trouillas J, et al: Surgical outcome and pathological effects of bromocriptine preoperative treatment in prolactinomas. Pathol Res Pract 187:587–592, 1991.

146. Barrow DL, Tindall GT, Kovacs K, et al: Clinical and pathological effects of bromocriptine on prolactin-secreting and other pituitary tumors. J Neurosurg 60:1–7, 1984.

147. Weiss MH, Wycoff RR, Yadley, et al: Bromocriptine treatment of prolactin-secreting tumors: Surgical implications. Neurosurgery 12:640–642, 1984.

148. Fahlbusch R, Buchfelder M, Schrell U: Short-term preoperative treatment of macroprolactinomas with dopamine agonists. J Neurosurg 67:807–815, 1987.

149. Saeki N, Nakamura M, Sunami K, Yamaura A: Surgical indication after bromocriptine therapy on giant prolactinomas: Effects and limitations of the medical treatment. Endocr J 45:529–537, 1998.

150. Plowman PN: Radiotherapy for pituitary tumours. Baillieres Clin Endocrinol Metab 9:407–420, 1995.

151. Zierhut D, Flentje M, Adolph J, et al: External radiotherapy of pituitary adenomas. Int J Radiat Oncol Biol Phys 33:307–314, 1995.

152. Motti EDF, Losa M, Pieralli S, et al: Stereotactic radiosurgery of pituitary adenomas. Metabolism 45:111–114, 1996.

153. Tsang RW, Brierley JD, Panzarella T, et al: Role of radiation therapy in clinical hormonally-active pituitary adenomas. Radiother Oncol 41:45–53, 1996.

154. Yoon SC, Suh TS, Jang HS, et al: Clinical results of 24 pituitary macroadenomas with linac-based stereotactic radiosurgery. Int J Radiat Oncol Biol Phys 41:849–853, 1998.

155. Moriondo P, Travaglini P, Nissim M, et al: Bromocriptine treatment of microprolactinomas: Evidence of stable prolactin decrease after drug withdrawal. J Clin Endocrinol Metab 60:764–772, 1985.

156. Vilar L, Burke CW: Quinagolide efficacy and tolerability in hyperprolactinaemic patients who are resistant to or intolerant of bromocriptine. Clin Endocrinol 41:821–826, 1994.

157. Rains CP, Bryson HM, Fitton A: Cabergoline: A review of the pharmacological properties and therapeutic potential in the treatment of hyperprolactinemia and inhibition of lactation. Drugs 49:255–279, 1995.

158. Vance ML, Lipper M, Kibanski A, et al: Treatment of prolactin-secreting macroadenomas with the long-acting non ergot agonist CV 105-502. Ann Intern Med 112:668–673, 1990.

159. Duranteau L, Chanson P, Horlait S, et al: Effect of the new dopaminergic agonist CV 205-502 on plasma prolactin levels and tumor size in bromocriptine-resistant prolactinomas. Clin Endocrinol 34:25–29, 1991.

160. Brue T, Pellegrini I, Gunz G, et al: Effects of the new dopamine agonist CV 205-502 in human prolactinomas resistant to bromocriptine. J Clin Endocrinol Metab 74:577–584, 1992.

161. Webster J, Piscitelli G, Polli A, et al: A comparison of cabergoline and bromocriptine in the treatment of hyperprolactinemic amenorrhea. N Engl J Med 331:905–909, 1994.

162. Colao A, Merola B, Sarnacchiaro F, et al: Comparison among different dopamine-agonists of new formulation in the clinical management of macroprolactinomas. Horm Res 44:222–228, 1995.

163. Morange I, Barlier A, Pellegrini I, et al: Prolactinomas resistant to bromocriptine: Long-term efficacy of quinagolide and outcome of pregnancy. Eur J Endocrinol 135:413–420, 1996.

164. Delgrange E, Maiter D, Donckier J: Effects of the dopamine agonist cabergoline in patients with prolactinoma intolerant or resistant to bromocriptine. Eur J Endocrinol 134:454–456, 1996.

165. Delgrange E, Donckier J: Prolactinomas apparently resistant to quinagolide respond to cabergoline therapy. J Clin Endocrinol Metab 82:2755–2756, 1997.

166. Biller BMK, Molitch ME, Vance ML, et al: Treatment of prolactin-secreting macroadenomas with the once-weekly dopamine agonist cabergoline. J Clin Endocrinol Metab 81:2338–2343, 1996.

167. Muratori M, Arosio M, Gambino G, et al: Use of cabergoline in the long-term treatment of hyperprolactinemic and acromegalic patients. J Endocrinol Invest 20:537–546, 1997.

168. Ferrari CI, Abs R, Bevan JS, et al: Treatment of macroprolactinoma with cabergoline: A study of 85 patients. Clin Endocrinol 46:409–413, 1997.

169. Colao A, Di Sarno A, Sarnacchiaro F, et al: Prolactinomas resistant to standard dopamine agonists respond to chronic cabergoline treatment. J Clin Endocrinol Metab 82:876–883, 1997.

170. Webster J: A comparative review of the tolerability profiles of dopamine agonists in the treatment of hyperprolactinemia and inhibition of lactation. Drug Saf 14:118–238, 1998.

171. Kovacs K, Stefaneanu L, Horvath E, et al: Prolactin-producing pituitary tumor: Resistance to dopamine agonist therapy. J Neurosurg 82:886–890, 1995.

172. Loh KC, Shlossberg AH, Rittmaster RS, Holness RO: Giant prolactinomas: A retrospective review. Endocrinologist 6:257–263, 1996.

173. Liuzzi A, Oppizzi G: Microprolactinomas: Why requiem for surgery? J Endocrinol Invest 19:196–198, 1996.

174. Faglia G: Should dopamine agonist treatment for prolactinomas be life-long? Clin Endocrinol 34:173–174, 1991.

175. Crosignani PG, Mattei A, Ferrari CI, Giovanelli M: Enlargement of a prolactin-secreting pituitary macroadenoma during bromocriptine. Br J Obstet Gynaecol 89:199–170, 1982.

176. Schlechte JA: Clinical impact of hyperprolactinaemia. Baillieres Clin Endocrinol Metab 9:359, 1995.

177. Di Somma C, Colao A, Di Sarno A, et al: Bone marker and bone density responses to dopamine agonist therapy in hyperprolactinemic males. J Clin Endocrinol Metab 83:807–813, 1998.

178. Bression D, Brandi AM, Martes MP, et al: Dopaminergic receptors in human prolactin-secreting adenomas: A quantitative study. J Clin Endocrinol Metab 51:1037–1042, 1980.

179. Pellegrini I, Rasolonjanahary R, Gunz G, et al: Resistance to bromocriptine in prolactinomas. J Clin Endocrinol Metab 69:500–509, 1989.

180. Caccavelli L, Feron F, Morange I, et al: Decreased expression of the two D-2 dopamine receptor isoforms in bromocriptine-resistant prolactinomas. Neuroendocrinology 60:314–322, 1994.

181. Caccavelli L, Morange Ramos I, Kordon C, et al: Alteration of g alpha subunits mRNA levels in bromocriptine resistant prolactinomas. J Neuroendocrinol 8:737–746, 1996.

182. Missale C, Spano P: Nerve growth factor in pituitary development and pituitary tumors. Front Neuroendocrinol 19:128–150, 1998.

183. Missale C, Sigala S, Fiorentini C, et al: Nerve growth factor suppresses the tumoral phenotype of human prolactinomas. Horm Res 47:240–244, 1997.

184. Merola B, Sarnacchiaro F, Colao A: CV 205-502 in the treatment of tumoral and non-tumoral hyperprolactinemic states. Biomed Pharmacother 48:167–174, 1994.

185. Bevan JS, Davis JRE: Cabergoline: An advance in dopaminergic therapy. Clin Endocrinol 41:709–712, 1994.

186. Ciccarelli E, Grottoli S, Razzore P, et al: Long-term treatment with cabergoline, a new long-lasting ergoline derivative, in idiopathic or tumorous hyperprolactinaemia and outcome of drug-induced pregnancy. J Endocrinol Invest 20:547, 1997.

187. Hurel SJ, Harris PE, McNicol AM, et al: Metastatic prolactinoma: Effect of octreotide, cabergoline, carboplatin and etoposide: Immunocytochemical analysis of proto-oncogene expression. J Clin Endocrinol Metab 82:2962–2965, 1997.

188. Gemzell C, Wang CF: Outcome of pregnancy in women with pituitary adenoma. Fertil Steril 121:363–372, 1979.

189. Kupersmith MJ, Rosenberg C, Kleinberg D: Visual loss in pregnant women with pituitary adenomas. Ann Intern Med 121:473–477, 1994.

190. Bergh T, Nillius SJ, Wide L: Clinical course and outcome of pregnancies in amenorrheic women with hyperprolactinemia and pituitary tumors. BMJ 2:875–880, 1977.

191. Turkalj I, Braun P, Krupp P: Surveillance of bromocriptine during pregnancy. JAMA 247:1589–1591, 1982.

192. Rau H, Badenhoop K, Usadel KH: Treatment of prolactinoma during pregnancy and lactation. Dtsche Med Wochenschr 121:28–32, 1996.

193. Robert E, Musatti L, Piscitelli G, Ferrari CI: Pregnancy outcome after treatment with the ergoline derivative cabergoline. Reprod Toxicol 10:333–337, 1996.

194. Mornex R, Hugues B: Remission of hyperprolactinemia after pregnancy. N Engl J Med 324:60, 1991.

195. Hofle G, Gasser R, Mohsenipour I, Finkenstedt G: Surgery combined with dopamine agonists versus dopamine agonists alone in long-term treatment of macroprolactinoma: A retrospective study. Exp Clin Endocrinol Diabetes 106:211–216, 1998.

Chapter 26

Surgical Management of Pituitary Tumors

Reza Jarrahy ▪ Hrayr K. Shahinian

HISTORICAL BACKGROUND

The development of pituitary surgery over the past century is largely credited to the pioneering work of Harvey Cushing in the early 1900s.[47, 106] Cushing's early experience with transsphenoidal approaches to the sella built on the work of his mentor Halstead and his contemporaries, including Giordano, Schloffer, Kanavel, and Hirsch.[21, 52, 53, 99] Similarly, Cushing's interpretation of the transcranial approach draws from the prior experiences of, among others, Caton, Paul, Horsley, Krause, and Kiliani.[18, 21, 52, 55, 85] Cushing would ultimately focus his practice on the transcranial technique and cited its direct and wide exposure of the gland from a suprasellar perspective as paramount to the effective surgical management of pituitary disease.[22, 23, 51, 106] Reports of Cushing's success with this procedure helped establish widespread acceptance of the transcranial method throughout Europe.[79] Hirsch's continued practice of the transsphenoidal technique, however, contributed to a polarization of opinions on treatment options in pituitary surgery. Claiming that transsphenoidal exposure of the gland was adequate for thorough resection of tumor, he argued that the less invasive nature of this procedure made it the technique of choice in pituitary surgery. His opinions were shared by other prominent surgeons, as were those of Cushing. Practice of both methods continued, as did lively discussions within the medical community regarding the indications, merits, and pitfalls of each.

Cushing's assistant Norman Dott sustained this debate. Dott acquired experience in both procedures under Cushing's tutelage. In his own practice at the University of Edinburgh he wrote and lectured in favor of the transsphenoidal technique.[30] He also began developing instruments designed specifically for use in the procedure. Among those who studied and applied Dott's experience to their own practice was Gerard Guiot, who credited his revival of transsphenoidal hypophysectomy in France during the 1950s to Dott's influence.[47] Guiot's adaptation of the procedure is especially noteworthy in its correlation with the introduction of intraoperative radiofluoroscopic imaging.[106] Jules Hardy followed the work of Dott and Guiot and incorporated newly developed medical technology into his technique.[44–46] His work is distinguished for his description of the use of the operating microscope, pictures of which he first presented in 1965.[48]

The introduction of fluoroscopy and microscopy to pituitary surgery in effect ended the debate on how to maximally expose the gland with the least morbidity. With these instruments available, adequate exposure and thorough exploration of intrasellar and suprasellar extensions of the gland became possible without the need for a large frontal craniotomy or prolonged brain retraction. With these advances, the transseptal transsphenoidal approach came to be accepted as the procedure of choice for the surgical management of most pituitary lesions. Transcranial techniques were reserved for use in the resection of tumors with extensive invasion into the anterior and middle cranial cavities. With specific roles for these two procedures thus identified, the indications for microscopic transseptal transsphenoidal and transcranial pituitary surgery have remained relatively well defined for several decades.

Recently, however, discussion regarding the most effective and least invasive way to perform pituitary surgery has been renewed as the above-described standards have been challenged. Developments in the field of sinus endoscopy[66, 80, 86, 95, 118] originally prompted surgeons to attempt endoscope-assisted surgery of the pituitary gland via the traditional transseptal approach.[40, 50, 57, 84, 95, 105, 109, 130, 131] Experimental and clinical models of fully endoscopic pituitary surgery via a transnasal transsphenoidal approach have since been described.[16, 49, 58–61] This procedure is proving to be equally, if not more effective than microscopy as the primary imaging modality in pituitary surgery. Additional experience with this procedure and its outcomes will determine its ultimate role in pituitary surgery.

SURGICAL ANATOMY

Because of its position at the interface of the anterior and middle cranial fossae, frontal and lateral transcranial approaches to the pituitary gland require familiarity with the anatomic relationships between the critical structures that reside within these spaces, as well as the surgical anatomy of the sella turcica. Moreover, the inferior microscopic and endoscopic approaches call for specific knowledge of intranasal and infranasal anatomy and architecture.

The Anterior and Middle Cranial Cavities

The embryologic development of the anterior and middle cranial fossae is predicted upon the formation of ossification centers within the chondral template of the developing skull base. This sheet of cartilage provides the framework for the base of the cranium, as well as parts of the midface and nose. Deposition of bone within this cartilage gives rise to most of the occipital, temporal, sphenoid, and ethmoid bones and determines their ultimate shape.[38, 69, 70, 75, 103]

The frontal bone defines the rostral limit of the anterior cranial cavity. The mature bone represents the fusion of separate ossification centers within the embryonic membranous neurocranium that articulate in the midline at the metopic suture.[38, 111] An osseous projection called the frontal crest extends posteriorly from the inner surface of the frontal bone along the floor of the cavity. The frontal crest points to the cribriform plate and is separated from it by the foramen cecum.[14] This foramen passes an emissary vein. The cribriform plate is a punctate bony surface that forms the roof of the nasal cavities bilaterally. Its perforate nature is derived from its formation around the differentiated nerves of the upper nasal passages, which pass into the anterior fossa to synapse on the olfactory bulbs.[71, 73, 119, 126] These are the distal limits of the olfactory tracts, the purely sensory nerves that lie on the surface of the cribriform plate to provide the sense of smell. The cribriform plate is bisected by the falx cerebri and crista galli, which represents the intracranial extension of the perpendicular plate of the ethmoid bone.[14, 24, 73, 87]

The remainder of the floor of the anterior fossa is made up of the thin orbital plates of the frontal bone.[7] These irregularly surfaced platforms form the roofs of the orbits and support the frontal lobes. They articulate medially with the cribriform plate. At this interface the anterior and posterior ethmoidal arteries—distal branches of the ophthalmic artery—pass through foramina in the plate to supply the nasal septum and lateral nasal walls.[15] Posterior to the cribriform plate, the body and lesser wings of the sphenoid mark the caudal limits of the anterior cavity and the anterior margin of the middle cranial fossa.

The middle fossa houses the temporal lobes laterally and the pituitary gland anteriorly. Most of the floor of the cavity is made up of the sphenoid bone.[103] Various foramina in the floor of the middle fossa allow for passage of neurovascular structures into and out of the cranium. These structures include the carotid artery, the middle meningeal artery and vein, and the branches of the trigeminal nerve.[65, 107] A gap at the medial junction of the greater and lesser sphenoid wings—the superior orbital fissure—is occupied by the first branch of the trigeminal nerve, by the oculomotor, trochlear, and abducens nerves, and by the ophthalmic veins. The bony optic canal provides a route for passage of the optic nerve into the apex of the orbit.[91, 103, 114]

The Sella Turcica and Pituitary Gland

The sella turcica, also commonly referred to as the hypophysial fossa, contains the pituitary gland. Structurally, it represents a rounded excavation of the sphenoid bone that is flanked by numerous critical structures. The dorsum sellae is the uppermost extension of the clivus and forms the posterior wall of the sella. It has lateral protuberances that are referred to as the posterior clinoid processes. The anterior boundary of the sella is set by the tuberculum sellae, a raised prominence on the superior surface of the sphenoid bone immediately in front of the hypophysial fossa.[37, 103] The curving projections of the lesser wings of the sphenoid terminate medially in the anterior clinoid processes, which rest above and posterolateral to the tuberculum.[94] Anterior to the tuberculum sellae is a depression in the sphenoid called the prechiasmic groove, to either side of which lie the intracranial openings of the optic canals.[119]

The development and ultrastructure of the pituitary gland itself are thoroughly discussed elsewhere in this text. However, knowledge of its anatomic relationships is of paramount importance in the surgical management of hypophysial disease. The hypophysis sits in the cavity of the sella turcica at the distal end of the hypophysial stalk. The stalk serves as a direct conveyance of hormones to the posterior pituitary and as a conduit for hormone-releasing signals to the anterior pituitary via its portal vessels.[32] It descends from the median eminence of the hypothalamus and passes through a central hiatus in the diaphragma sellae, a dural reflection between the anterior and posterior clinoid processes that covers the hypophysial fossa.[36, 37, 101, 102] Above the diaphragma, the hypophysial stalk is anteriorly related to the optic chiasm. Most commonly, the chiasm directly overlies the sella and pituitary. (This anatomic arrangement is the basis of the incidence of visual symptoms—most notably bitemporal hemianopia—seen in

patients with pituitary tumors that have suprasellar extension.) Alternatively, the chiasm may lie over the tuberculum ("prefixed" position) or over the dorsum sellae ("postfixed" position).[101] The optic nerves emerge from the optic canals anteromedial to the tips of the anterior clinoid processes to run posteromedially toward the chiasm. Knowledge of these normal and variant anatomic patterns is especially important when performing transcranial operations in which the approach to the sella is conducted along the floor of the anterior fossa directly toward the optic nerves and chiasm.

The parasellar vascular anatomy must also be fully appreciated to minimize the chance of intraoperative vascular injury. Subfrontal approaches to the sella expose the carotid arteries and the anterior arc of the circle of Willis, as well as perforating branches from these major vessels. Vascular structures in the suprasellar area may be displaced by superior extensions of tumors that distort normal anatomic relationships and make manipulation of these vessels extremely dangerous.[12, 72, 90, 100]

The carotid artery emerges from the roof of the cavernous sinus beneath the optic nerve and immediately gives off its ophthalmic branch, which turns into the optic canal on the underside of the nerve.[62] The carotid turns back toward the posterior clinoid process, where it meets the posterior communicating artery and gives off the anterior cerebral artery.[25, 94, 101, 102] This artery courses over the superior surface of the optic chiasm and gives off an anterior communicating branch to its contralateral counterpart. The length of this segment determines how tightly it is draped over the chiasm and any underlying tumor. Longer communicating arteries are generally related to the optic nerves rather than the chiasm.[119] This anatomy must be fully identified in both midline and oblique transcranial subfrontal approaches. Surgeons using these methods must carefully work around the optic nerves and chiasm and associated neurovascular structures while removing tumor from the sella and sphenoid.[27, 28]

The carotid arteries are also at risk during transsphenoidal approaches to the sella. Their tortuous intracranial course carries them alongside the lateral margins of the sphenoid sinus.[101] Here they are at risk when the anterior wall and mucosa of the sinus are dissected. The intracavernous segments of the arteries are susceptible to overly aggressive curettage of tumor from within the sphenoid or sella. This risk also applies to cavernous sinus injury without carotid artery involvement. The barriers between the lateral walls of the sella turcica and the medial boundaries of the cavernous sinuses are often negligible and therefore quite vulnerable to damage from dissecting instruments.[26–28, 79, 101, 102]

The Nasal Cavities

Pituitary surgeons must navigate the neurovascular anatomy of the anterior and middle cranial fossae in transcranial pituitary surgery, as well as the length of the nasal septum in the transseptal transsphenoidal approach. The introduction of transnasal endoscopic pituitary surgery has further underscored the necessity for surgeons to become familiar with the relationships of the sella and pituitary gland to the bony, cartilaginous, and mucosal architecture of the nasal cavities and the paranasal sinuses.

During embryonic development, bilateral invaginations of ectoderm located superior to the opening of the mouth pass posteriorly through the mesoderm of the head to form the left and right nasal pits. These meet and fuse with the endoderm of the most cranial extension of the primitive foregut and create a passageway from the external environment to the gut lumen. Thus connected, the nasal pits are referred to as the right and left nasal cavities and the part of involved foregut is called the nasopharynx.[119] The common medial wall of each nasal cavity is the embryonic nasal septum, and the floors of these cavities form the primary palate.[9, 76, 103, 119]

Cartilage forms in the mesoderm of the roof of each nasal cavity and extends into the adjacent upper regions of the lateral walls and the septum. Connective tissue develops in the inferior lateral walls, inferior septum, and cavity floors. Bony deposition begins in ossification centers found throughout the cartilaginous and membranous portions of the nasal capsule.[6, 69] The posterior and inferior parts of the nasal septum become ossified to form the perpendicular plate of the ethmoid and the vomer, respectively.[43] The crista galli—the superior extension of the perpendicular plate of the ethmoid—is also formed in this process.[24] The anterior extent of the septum remains cartilaginous. The roof of the nasal cavities ossifies around nerve fibers that communicate superiorly with the olfactory bulbs. The cribriform plate of the ethmoid is thereby formed, as previously discussed.

A "gap" in the deposition of cartilage in the lateral nasal cavity wall results in the hiatus semilunaris.[6, 24, 87] In its mature form, it is identified as a depression in the lateral nasal wall at the level of the middle meatus. Cartilage formation resumes at the inferior aspect of this hiatus in the uncinate process, which invaginates to create the inferior turbinate. This structure in turn ossifies and runs nearly the entire anteroposterior distance of the nasal cavity. The remainder of the cartilage of the lateral wall ossifies to generate the ethmoid labyrinth.[6, 24, 76, 87] As the paranasal air sinuses develop, the labyrinth is polarized into lateral and medial walls. The former makes up the medial wall of the orbit. The latter generates two additional invaginating bony processes, the precursors of the middle and inferior turbinates. Like the inferior turbinate, the middle spans nearly the entire length of the nasal cavity. The superior turbinate, however, is more limited in length and sits near the roof of the nasal cavity. The recesses created by the curvatures of the turbinates are referred to as meati and are the sites of origin of the paranasal sinuses.[24, 76, 87]

The mucous membranes lining the lateral nasal walls evaginate into the skeleton of the midface to create air pockets surrounded by bone.[76, 87, 113] Posteriorly, the mucous membrane covering the anterior surface of the sphenoid bone pushes back to create the sphenoid sinus.[76] Formation of a thin bony septum divides the sinus into left and right cavities. Although normally a midline structure, the nature of the septation may vary widely.[101] The sphenoid sinus communicates with the nasal cavities via ostia that are anteriorly related to the sphenoethmoid recesses behind the superior turbinates.[104] The mucous membranes of the superior meatus generate the posterior ethmoidal air cells, whereas those of middle meatus contribute to the anterior ethmoidal air cells.[6, 76, 87] The anterior ethmoidal air cells, frontal sinus, and maxillary sinus all communicate with the nasal cavity via the hiatus semilunaris.[13]

Not all the cartilage of the external nose is ossified. The atrium is the intranasal space that lies anterior to the turbinates; it remains enclosed by cartilaginous walls after development is complete. That part of the anterior nasal cavity bounded by the alae of the nose is specifically referred to as the vestibule.

During endoscopic transnasal pituitary surgery, endoscopes are advanced into the vestibule to first identify the inferior turbinate and the anterior portion of the septum. As discussed above, the inferior and middle turbinates span almost the entire depth of the nasal cavity. Therefore, with slight superior and posterior advancement of the endoscope, the anterior limit of the middle turbinate comes into view. With further caudal progress, the remainder of the middle turbinate and the superior turbinate are appreciated. The goal of the intranasal portion of this procedure is to create a wide passage from the exterior to the sphenoid rostrum. The space of the middle meatus is therefore obliterated as the middle turbinate is outfractured. The sphenoid ostia may or may not be readily apparent until mucosa is dissected from the anterior surface of the body of the sphenoid. The superior and middle turbinates serve as valuable landmarks for identifying the approximate locations of the ostia until they are directly visualized.

Mucosal bleeding encountered intraoperatively may come from distal branches of either the internal or external carotid arteries.[15] The maxillary branch of the external carotid artery feeds the sphenopalatine artery, which branches into posterior lateral nasal and posterior septal arteries. These arteries ramify within the mucosa of the deep nasal cavities. As noted above, the anterior lateral nasal and anterior septal branches of the anterior ethmoidal artery provide rostral circulation. The posterior ethmoidal artery, although less constant in its anatomic course, also contributes to the posterior nasal vascular supply.[15, 62]

TRANSCRANIAL SURGERY OF THE PITUITARY GLAND

Indications

Most pituitary tumors, including those with parasellar and suprasellar extensions, can be successfully treated by microscopic transseptal or endoscopic transnasal approaches to the sella.[28, 120, 121] These techniques are less invasive and less timely and are associated with fewer complications, as will be discussed below. They provide adequate exposure of the gland, even when tumor extends beyond the boundaries of the hypophysial fossa. If tumor invasion of the middle or anterior cranial cavities is significant, however, transcranial approaches offer a greater chance of complete or near-complete tumor removal. Often a transcranial method will be reserved for the second stage of a two-stage operation.[28, 121] The primary procedure is performed via microscopic or endoscopic exposure of the sella turcica in which the bulk of the tumor is removed transsphenoidally. Residual tumor is then targeted in a subsequent transcranial exploration.

The transcranial approach is well suited to the management of other lesions affecting the parasellar areas that tend to spread regionally, including chordomas, craniopharyngiomas, meningiomas, and vascular lesions.[34, 41, 82, 121]

Patient Positioning

After the induction of general anesthesia and rotation of the patient so that the head is away from the anesthesiologist, the procedure begins. The patient is placed supine on the operating room table and the head of the bed is raised approximately 15 degrees. The position of the patient's head is determined by using the floor of the anterior cranial fossa as a guide to the surgical landmarks of the suprasellar area. In the midline subfrontal approach, the head is extended 30 degrees in a vertical plane toward the surgeon. At this angle the frontal lobes will fall back and the surgeon will have a direct path to the pituitary along the orbital plates of the frontal bone.[27, 121] When adequate head position is achieved, the head is fixed in place with a three-pin horseshoe clamp.

The head is shaved from the hairline to the apex of the cranial vault, and both the head and an area of the lower right quadrant of the abdominal wall are washed with aqueous iodine-based aseptic solution. The latter area is prepared in anticipation of intraoperative harvesting of an abdominal fat graft to fill the space of the sphenoid sinus once the tumor is removed.

Surgical Technique

Four variations of the transcranial technique (Fig. 26–1) remain in popular use: the midline subfrontal approach, the oblique subfrontal approach, the pterional approach, and the subtemporal approach. Whereas the first two approaches are still regularly used to reach pituitary tumors with extensive extrasellar involvement, the pterional and subtemporal methods are of greater benefit in the management of nonpituitary lesions that occur in the posterior parasellar areas.

Midline Subfrontal Approach

The midline subfrontal approach remains the most common method for transcranial pituitary surgery because it affords direct exposure of the optic nerves and carotid arteries while providing ready access to the hypophysial stalk.[121] A hemicoronal flap is developed on the ipsilateral side of the tumor in a subperiosteal plane superiorly and to the depth of the deep temporalis fascia laterally where the muscle overlies bone. The incision is carried from the level of the lateral canthus of the eye to just beyond the midline. The temporalis muscle is disinserted to reveal the juncture of the zygoma and the lateral orbital rim. Bur holes placed at this site and in the midline at the level of the orbital roof are used to direct the craniotomy.

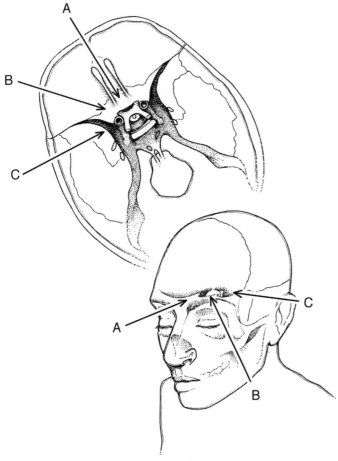

FIGURE 26–1. Transcranial approach. Arrows denote vectors of approach to the pituitary gland. *A,* Midline subfrontal approach. *B,* Oblique subfrontal approach. *C,* Pterional/subtemporal approach.

With the bone flap removed, the dura is incised and the brain lifted from the floor of the fossa. Throughout the procedure, retraction must be kept to a minimum because postoperative swelling of the frontal lobe can be problematic.[78, 121, 123] Avulsion of the olfactory nerve is also a significant operative risk that results in postoperative anosmia.[35, 39, 116] Dissection is carried out along the midline, with the crista galli and invested falx cerebri serving as initial landmarks. By proceeding posteriorly along the cribriform plate, the optic nerve is seen emerging from the optic canal. Once the ipsilateral optic nerve is revealed, it should be fully exposed and used as a guide to expose the contralateral optic nerve and the optic chiasm. The anatomy of the anterior circle of Willis is further defined in this dissection. Once the neurovascular anatomy is fully detailed, the surgeon can work around the relevant structures to remove tumor from the sella.[98, 99, 112, 121] An assortment of dissecting curettes are used for this purpose.

In the case of a prefixed chiasm or large tuberculum sellae, direct access to the sella is impeded. If so, the tuberculum may be removed or drilled to gain entry into the sphenoid sinus below.[99] The anterior wall of the sella is then removed and resection of tumor progresses. A fat graft may be placed within the space of the sinus after tumor resection is complete.

After resection, the dura is reapproximated to achieve a water-tight seal. If it is compromised during the initial craniotomy, the frontal sinus is cranialized by removal of its posterior wall and obliteration of the frontonasal duct. The craniotomy bone flap is replaced and affixed with microplates and screws, and the soft tissues of the scalp are tightly reapproximated. The patient is extubated at the end of the procedure and transferred to the intensive care unit. In addition to monitoring for potential sequelae specific to pituitary surgery (diabetes insipidus, visual field deficits, etc.), particular attention is paid to the development of signs indicative of frontal lobe edema in the postoperative period.

Oblique Subfrontal Approach

The oblique subfrontal approach is identical to the midline subfrontal approach in the development of scalp and bone flaps. It also proceeds along the floor of the anterior fossa to reach the suprasellar area. However, this approach is undertaken at an angle to the midline to allow less aggressive retraction of the frontal lobe and minimize the risk of postoperative anosmia.[99] Unfortunately, this lateral approach yields incomplete access to the sella turcica, thus making thorough removal of contralateral tumor more difficult. In addition, the surgeon is forced to work over the optic nerves, which increases the likelihood of a major complication. The beneficial decrease in frontal lobe retraction that this procedure offers must be carefully weighed against the added risks to the regional neurovascular structures that it entails.

Pterional Approach

The pterional approach is most often used in the management of lesions such as chordomas or meningiomas that, in addition to pituitary lesions, may also occupy the extrasellar space. Exposure in this approach may be widened through wide retraction of the sylvian fissure.[11, 34, 82, 121] Excellent exposure of most of the clivus is achieved. However, retraction of the frontal lobe in this technique may also place the olfactory nerve at risk for avulsion.[10]

Subtemporal Approach

Finally, the subtemporal approach is conducted along the floor of the middle fossa via a temporal craniotomy and middle fossa craniectomy. The retrosellar area is exposed in this procedure, but only with heavy and potentially deleterious retraction of the temporal lobe. At risk as well are the neurovascular structures that traverse the floor of the middle fossa.[41, 54, 112, 121] Its usefulness in light of other less morbid options is therefore limited.

TRANSSEPTAL TRANSSPHENOIDAL MICROSCOPIC PITUITARY SURGERY

In current practice, transseptal transsphenoidal surgery closely resembles Cushing's originally described method.[47] The development of intraoperative fluoroscopy and microscopy approximately one-half century after his initial contributions enabled surgeons to more precisely localize and visualize critical structures during surgery.[66, 129] Today, the success of this operation is vitally dependent on these imaging modalities.

Indications

This procedure is indicated for the surgical management of pituitary lesions causing endocrinopathies characterized by hypofunction or hyperfunction of the gland that have not adequately responded to medical treatment, for lesions interfering with the optical apparatus and causing visual disturbances, or for lesions invading the cavernous sinus and causing cranial nerve palsies. Microadenomas and macroadenomas are amenable to resection by this method, including those with mild suprasellar and parasellar extension.[5, 47, 74, 93, 128, 129]

In tumor-induced hypopituitarism, compression of the normal pituitary gland and hypophysial stalk interferes with the synthesis and release of pituitary hormones.[1, 5, 47, 97] The resultant clinical syndromes require hormonal replacement therapy, which is costly, wrought with deleterious side effects, and usually of lifelong duration. Surgical intervention may completely eliminate the need for exogenous administration of hormone and restore the pituitary axis.

If the tumor is productive of one or more pituitary hormones, the histologic diagnosis can usually be made before surgery with the use of serum hormonal assays.[4, 5, 19, 64, 83] The patient's signs and symptoms guide physicians in choosing which laboratory tests to perform. Excessive secretion from lactotrophs, somatotrophs, or corticotrophs results in galactorrhea/amenorrhea (females) and decreased sexual function and libido (males), gigantism, and Cushing's disease, respectively. Correlation between clinical and hormonal profiles is similarly used to diagnose tumors of thyrotroph and gonadotroph origin. When medical treatment of these conditions fails, surgical intervention is called for to remove the source of the problem.

Regardless of the functional status of the tumor, ophthalmoplegia and visual field deficits signal its extension beyond the confines of the sella turcica to involve the optic nerves or the cavernous sinuses.[20, 128, 129] Evidence of an optical or visual defect is cause for concern and calls for urgent tumor resection to decompress the involved structures. Compression of the optic chiasm may cause a mild deficit or complete bitemporal hemianopia. Tumor invasion into the cavernous sinus may generate a clinical picture that suggests involvement of one or more of the associated cranial nerves. Tumor anatomy, as documented by computed tomography or magnetic resonance imaging (MRI), usually correlates with the patient's condition.[5, 63, 83, 127]

Suprasellar extensions of macroadenomas will naturally descend into the sella turcica as the tumors are removed through the sphenoid sinus.[45, 47, 128] Tumor removal may be facilitated by Valsalva maneuvers conducted by the anesthesiologist, which transiently raise intracranial pressure and cause inferior displacement of the mass. Parasellar extensions of pituitary tumors, however, are more difficult to manage in as much as the lateral perspectives offered by the microscope are greatly limited. Given the proximity of the optic nerves, optic chiasm, carotid arteries, and cavernous sinuses to the sella, blind curettage of any tumor remnants extending beyond the limits of the sella is potentially catastrophic. Patients with extrasellar extension of tumor into the anterior and middle cranial fossae must be considered for two-stage procedures. In these cases a primary transsphenoidal procedure serves to debulk as much of the tumor as possible from below, whereas a secondary operation via one of the aforementioned transcranial approaches allows resection of tumor remnants.[2, 27, 28, 96] Such improvisation allows complete surgical removal of extensive lesions with minimal morbidity.

Patient Positioning and Operating Room Setup

The patient is placed supine on the operating room table. After induction of general anesthesia and endotracheal intubation, the bed is rotated such that the head is opposite the anesthesiologist, who uses tubing of extended length to maintain the respiratory circuit. The anesthesiologist secures the endotracheal tube in place at the corner of the mouth to leave the opening of the oral cavity free of obstruction. An absorbent sponge is passed through the mouth into the posterior of the oropharynx to collect blood and mucous secretions that collect intraoperatively. This maneuver must be done attentively to not disturb the position of the endotracheal tube.

The head of the bed is raised to make a 20-degree angle with the floor. The patient's head is placed in a carbon horseshoe three-pin clamp. The neck is extended while the head is tilted slightly to the left and rotated approximately 15 degrees to the right, toward the surgeon. The head clamp is then securely fastened to the bed. In this position and with the microscope in place, the surgeon will be operating along a direct anteroposterior axis toward the pituitary gland.[45] The fluoroscopic image intensifier is positioned so that the beam is perpendicular to a sagittal plane through the sella turcica. The contours of the sphenoid sinus and sella turcica must occupy the center of the monitor, which is placed over the patient's right shoulder. The surgeon need therefore only make a slight adjustment in position to view the fluoroscopic image while working under the microscope. Although fluoroscopy is only selectively necessary throughout the procedure, it must be readily and unobtrusively available.

With the patient thus positioned, attention is turned to preparing the surgical site. An aqueous antibacterial solution is applied to the nose, face, and upper gingival mucosa. Cotton-tipped applicators that have been soaked in the solution are placed in the nares. The upper gums are infiltrated with a solution of 1% lidocaine containing epinephrine (1:100,000). This maneuver both lifts the buccal mucosa off the premaxilla and limits the amount of intraoperative bleeding from the oral incision site. A site on the lower right quadrant of the abdomen is also prepared with antibiotic scrub solution and draped with sterile towels. A fat graft is harvested from this site during the procedure. It is used to pack the sella and sphenoid sinus after extirpation of the tumor. An alternative site for fat harvesting is the periumbilicus, where the resultant scar is more discrete. The lateral aspect of the thigh may also be used by surgeons who prefer muscle and fascia as graft substrates.[132] The face is draped so that only the nose and upper lip remain uncovered. After administration of antibiotics, the procedure begins.

Surgical Technique

While the upper lip is retracted by an assistant, an upper buccal sulcus incision is extended between the molar roots. The incision is carried down to the periosteum of the premaxilla. Appropriate placement of the incision is extremely important because enough soft tissue must be left above the teeth to allow for adequate closure. However, if the incision is made too far above the cleft of the sulcus, scar contracture may lead to complaints of lip tightness, as well as aesthetic changes in the appearance of the teeth and gums during smiling. The soft tissues are elevated from the bone to reveal the anterior nasal spine centrally and the piriform apertures bilaterally. The former may be removed with a rongeur, and the apertures may be enlarged to facilitate visualization.

The anterior nasal spine is followed superiorly to the anteroinferior border of the septal cartilage. Once this structure is identified, attention is turned to the development of mucoperichondrial and mucoperiosteal flaps. An elevator is used to free the septal mucosa bilaterally from the level of the nasal spine to a point above the attachment of the cartilaginous septum to the maxillary crest. This dissection is continued caudally along the entire face of the septum on one side until the articulation of the septum with the perpendicular plate of the ethmoid bone is reached. Elevators are also used to lift the mucosa from the floor of both nasal cavities. On the side of the septum from which the surgeon will approach the sella, the inferior mucoperiosteal flap is joined to the septal flap to create a large submucosal tunnel. The choice of side depends on the observed septal architecture. The preferred nasal cavity through which a right-handed surgeon should operate is the left. Alterations in this plan may be required in the event of significant septal deviation.[34, 124] The integrity of the mucosa is maintained during this dissection, and the nares are not violated. Bleeding from distal septal branches of the sphenopalatine artery may be controlled by packing the submucosal spaces with strips of dense cotton sponges.

Once the interface between septal cartilage and ethmoid bone is identified, the base of the septum is gently liberated from the maxillary crest and retracted to the side opposite the developed rhinoseptal submucosal tunnel. The posterior edge of the septum is cut with a swivel knife to facilitate this maneuver. However, the superior attachments of the septum to the ethmoid bone and lateral nasal cartilage are left intact. Separation of these attachments leads to a loss of projection of the nasal tip and must be avoided.[56, 67, 89, 110] The inferior part of the perpendicular plate of the ethmoid bone is then removed and preserved in saline for later use in reconstruction of the floor of the sella. Submucosal dissection is again continued until the vomer comes into view.

Until this point, dissection is performed under direct vision with the aid of magnifying loupes and a headlamp. After removal of the perpendicular plate of the ethmoid and identification of the vomer, however, microscopic dissection begins. First, an adjustable bivalve retractor is placed into the nasal cavity (Fig. 26–2). Its blades are advanced to the rostrum of the sphenoid bone and positioned so that they retract the mucosal flaps off this surface. Excessive retraction of the blades should be avoided because fractures of the bony nasal walls, the piriform apertures, the pterygoid plates, or the palate may

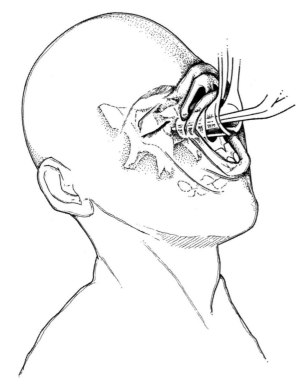

FIGURE 26–2. Microscopic transseptal transsphenoidal approach. Intraoral dissection allows for placement of a bivalve retractor, through which the operation is conducted.

otherwise result. All subsequent operative maneuvers are conducted through the space between the blades of this retractor.

The vomer is removed with the use of a rongeur and the rostral surface of the sphenoid bone is exposed. With the sphenoid ostia used as reference points, the anterior wall of the sphenoid sinus is resected with a combination of rongeurs and graspers. Subsequent examination of the sella is entirely dependent on this exposure. Caution must be used at the lateral boundaries of the sphenoid where the carotid arteries ascend. Additionally, superior dissection must be guarded because injury to the cribriform plate introduces the likelihood of a subsequent cerebrospinal fluid leak.[87, 126]

The anatomy of the sphenoid sinus will depend on the age of the patient, as well as the pituitary pathology.[45] The sphenoid sinus may be nonaerated in pediatric patients, multiseptated, or completely filled with tumor that has invaded through the floor of the sella. Imaging studies provide useful clues to its anatomy before surgery. Once the sphenoid is completely exposed, its mucosal lining is stripped to minimize the risk of postoperative mucocele.[34] The posterior wall of the sinus, which makes up the floor of the sella turcica, is immediately recognizable. Usually, with benign adenomas the floor of the sella is intact. However, the bony border between the pituitary gland and the sphenoid may be thinned, fractured, or even completely obliterated by expanding tumor.[34, 128] In the most common instance of an intact sella, however, the bone must be resected to provide access to the gland.

The first step in resection of the sella turcica is to carefully fracture the floor of the sella with an osteotome. Once a bone flap is removed, rongeurs can be inserted in the space between bone and dura to remove the remainder of the floor in a piecemeal manner. Maximal exposure of the gland is achieved only with thorough removal of bone. Again, as in dissection of the wall of the sphenoid, serious consideration must be given to the surrounding structures, including the carotid arteries and cavernous sinuses laterally and the optic nerves and chiasm superiorly.[34]

Deep to the floor of the sella is the dura, identifiable by its azure hue. The dura must be incised to gain access to the pituitary gland and tumor. A sharp hook or blade is used to make a cruciate incision. Through this incision, ring curettes of different diameters and spatial orientation are introduced to resect the tumor.

The appearance and consistency of tumor tissue are determined by several variables. Histologic type, preoperative therapies (e.g., radiation), tumor age, and other variables (e.g., hemorrhage) can all potentially affect tumor phenotype.[88] A high-quality contrast-enhanced MRI scan of the pituitary gland helps the surgeon differentiate between normal and abnormal tissue. The MRI should allow the surgeon to identify the hypophysial stalk and normal pituitary gland, as well as the mass effect of the tumor on the gland's position.[3, 63, 83, 117, 127] Knowledge of the quadrant in the sella where the normal gland is located must be incorporated into the surgical plan. The histology of tissue of questionable appearance near surgical margins can be confirmed via intraoperative frozen section pathologic analysis.

Resection of tumor is carried out until all grossly identifiable parts of the lesion are removed. As the sella is emptied of tumor, the boundaries of normal pituitary gland are identified, as are the diaphragma sellae, arachnoid, and optic chiasm. Suprasellar and parasellar extensions of tumor must be approached cautiously. The locations of dissecting curettes placed into the suprasellar and parasellar spaces can be confirmed fluoroscopically by using the bony parasellar structures as radiographic landmarks.[47] Extreme care must be taken to avoid the cavernous sinuses, carotid arteries, and optic chiasm because dire complications may ensue if these structures are damaged. Similarly, trauma to the arachnoid membrane increases the risk of damage to neural structures and the risk of postoperative cerebrospinal fluid leak.[128] Preoperative radiologic studies should be available for intraoperative review; as surgical "roadmaps," they help the surgeon define relevant anatomic relationships at the time of surgery.

While the surgeon is conducting a final survey of the operative site for any remaining fragments of tumor, an assistant harvests a fat graft from the abdomen or a graft of muscle and fascia from the lateral portion of the thigh. Several graft design models may be used,[20, 33, 67, 68, 88, 129] and each has as a common goal prevention of subsequent leakage of cerebrospinal fluid. A fragment of the perpendicular plate of the ethmoid bone or a piece of septal cartilage may be used as supportive struts during reconstruction of the floor of the sella in conjunction with either fat, muscle, fascia, or synthetic material.[20, 128, 129] In most cases, however, a simple fat graft that plugs the hole in the floor of the sella and obliterates the space of the sphenoid sinus will suffice.[128] The graft is held in place by a fibrin-based sealant liberally applied around the graft in liquid form. Within seconds it congeals into a firm gelatinous matrix.

With the graft in place, the retractor is removed, the septum and mucosal flaps are repositioned, and the gingival incision is reapproximated with absorbable sutures. Both nares are packed with petroleum jelly–impregnated gauze strips. This packing remains in place for up to 48 hours postoperatively to absorb any draining fluid and provide structural support to the nose as it heals internally.

Postoperative Monitoring

After the operation, the patient is extubated and taken to the intensive care unit for overnight monitoring. Medical staff specifically look for evidence of developing neurologic impairment, visual field deficits, cerebrospinal fluid leak, or diabetes insipidus. Barring any such complications, the patient is transferred to the ward on the day after surgery and is generally transfered home within 72 hours.

Follow-up is dependent on the nature of the tumor and extent of resection and should always be planned in concert with the referring endocrinologist.

Outcomes

Outcomes of microscopic transsphenoidal pituitary surgery are measured along several lines, first and foremost of which are complications related to surgery. Mortality rates are low, generally occurring at a rate of less than 1%.[20, 33, 74] Morbidity arises from damage to neurovascular structures in or proximal to the surgical field. These structures include both the anterior and posterior lobes of the normal pituitary gland, optic chiasm, cavernous sinuses, and carotid arteries. Damage to these structures can in general be entirely avoided with scrupulous and meticulous surgical technique.

The most common complication of this procedure is cerebrospinal fluid leak, which occurs in approximately 1% to 3% of patients.[20, 33, 122, 129] When tumor involves the diaphragma sellae, it should be included in the margins of resection. Doing so unfortunately increases the likelihood of a cerebrospinal fluid leak; intraoperative manifestations of a leak may become apparent immediately after the diaphragma is removed. In such cases, thorough packing of the sella and sphenoid sinus is paramount. Persistent leaks may be treated by placement of a lumbar drain[33, 128, 129] or, when more aggressive intervention is required, by re-exploration and packing of the sphenoid and sella.[20, 95, 132]

The next most common type of complication is related to glandular injury. Damage to the posterior lobe results in diabetes insipidus of either a transient or permanent nature.[33, 88, 129] Administration of desmopressin acetate is the indicated treatment. Treatment of anterior pituitary failure depends on the postoperative pituitary deficiencies that are observed but, in most cases, requires exogenous steroid delivery perioperatively.[33, 88] Again, a well-devised surgical plan and careful surgical technique, including the use of intraoperative frozen section pathology to aid in the demarcation of surgical margins, should enable surgeons to resect tumor while leaving normal gland behind.

Outcome measures used to evaluate surgical efficacy most commonly include clinical parameters such as improvement in preoperative visual deficits and improvement in endocrine function. A review of clinical series indicates that on average, visual disturbances are improved in approximately 80% of cases.[20, 74, 129] Reported rates of normalization of endocrine function vary widely and range from 50% to 90%,[5, 20, 74, 122, 129] depending on tumor size and histology, the hormonal parameters studied, and the criteria used in analysis.

FULLY ENDOSCOPIC PITUITARY SURGERY

The design of endoscopes has been revolutionized over the past several decades, and we now have endoscopes of varying lengths, diameters, and directions of view. In turn, sophisticated light sources, video cameras, digital processors, and lens cleansing and irrigation systems have been developed.[81] The availability of this equipment, without which this procedure cannot be performed safely or effectively, has made the next step in the evolution of pituitary surgery possible.

Indications

Indications for fully endoscopic pituitary surgery are identical to those for the traditional transseptal transsphenoidal microscopic approach, including the surgical management of productive and nonproductive pituitary microadenomas and macroadenomas that either fail medical management or cause visual or cranial nerve deficits.[58–61] Additional indications for this procedure stem from its minimally invasive nature. Because the fully endoscopic approach to the sella and pituitary is less invasive than transseptal microscopic surgery, in some instances it should be considered the first line of surgical therapy. A minimally invasive technique provides a distinct benefit over traditional methods in terms of operating time and perioperative morbidity in the biopsy of intrasellar lesions, and it is useful for pediatric patients and for patients with pituitary tumors whose medical histories put them at greater risk for complications of general anesthesia.

Instruments

Endoscopes

The rod lens design of endoscopes, first introduced in the 1960s by the English physicist H.H. Hopkins,[31, 77] provided the basis for the future manufacture of endoscopes and continues to set the standard for the industry. By integrating a series of lens systems within the rod,

the endoscope could be lengthened and yield an image of unparalleled depth and resolution.[31, 77] The development of endoscopes of varying directions of view has provided for visualization of structures previously hidden from the direct anteroposterior imaging capability of the microscope. Zero-, 30-, 70-, and 120-degree endoscopes offer panoramic perspectives of structures once completely obscured by anatomic "corners." Scopes of different diameters (4.0 and 2.7 mm) also provide valuable options to a surgeon faced with variations in surgical anatomy.[81]

Light Sources

Illumination of tungsten halogen, metal halide, or xenon arc origin is generated by a light source and transmitted to the endoscope via a fiberoptic cable. Light then travels along the length of the endoscope—also fiberoptically—to illuminate the surgical field.[31, 77, 81] The different types of devices offer light of varying brightness and whiteness and also offer hardware in a range of prices and sizes.

Cameras

Hopkins rod endoscopes are manufactured with standard eyepieces through which the endoscopic image can be directly viewed or to which video cameras can be attached. The image can then be projected onto one or several monitors or electronically processed and recorded. Three-chip cameras contain individual chips for each of the primary colors. These cameras produce the highest-quality images and feature automatic control over color, exposure, white balance, and digital contrast enhancement. Single-chip cameras, although less expensive and offering fewer options, also produce high-quality images that are more than adequate for the operating room.[31, 81]

Other devices geared toward improving the quality and flexibility of the images derived from the endoscope are regularly appearing on the market. Devices that digitally process the video image allow detail enhancement and image manipulation. Video processing systems have also made "picture-in-picture" viewing—simultaneous viewing of endoscopic and microscopic images on one monitor—possible.[92, 125] All these options contribute to the great versatility of endoscopy as a surgical tool and make it easily adaptable to highly specialized and intricate procedures.

Holding Arms

Bimanual operating is a necessity in endoscopic pituitary surgery. Multiple instruments are needed during the intranasal approach to the gland and during resection of the tumor. The development of different models of holding arms has obviated the need for surgeons to dedicate one hand to wield the camera and has therefore freed both hands for operating.

In general, holding arms must be sturdy, stable, and adjustable. They must be able to hold the endoscopes securely in place but must allow the surgeon to manipulate them at will and with ease. Originally derived from existing surgical instruments adapted to new applications, early designs combined long metallic rods at movable joints and placed clamps on each end: one to grip the operating table and the other to hold the endoscope. The latest generation of holding arms is designed to work via ball bearing joints that are pneumatically powered. These devices are remarkably flexible and extremely reliable.

Irrigation Sheaths

Invariably, blood, debris, mucus, and mist will cover the lens of the endoscope during surgery and obscure the image. Without a device to clean the surface of the lens *in situ*, the entire endoscope must be removed from the nasal cavity, wiped clean, and replaced. This maneuver must be repeated as many times as necessary to maintain a clear image.

Irrigation sheaths are available in different diameters to accommodate different-sized endoscopes. They are connected to a reservoir of sterile saline via tubing that threads through a motorized pedal-activated gear system. Upon demand, the sheath delivers a cleansing stream of saline over the tip of the endoscope, which is immediately followed by a brief period of suction whereby any remaining drops of saline that would otherwise blur the resolution of the image are removed from the lens. With this system in place, continuity of the procedure is guaranteed.

Positioning and Operating Room Setup

Patient positioning in the fully endoscopic procedure is similar to that used in the traditional transseptal transsphenoidal microscopic technique. However, addition of the endoscopic tower must be considered when organizing the operating room. (The viewing monitor sits atop a movable "tower." The tower combines the camera, light source, and video recording and processing equipment in a single unit.)

The patient is placed supine with the head of the bed raised, the neck extended, and the head rotated and fixed in position with a carbon horseshoe three-pin clamp. Thus situated, the operating instruments and imaging hardware are positioned appropriately. The C-arm fluoroscopy image intensifier is brought to the head of the table and rotated so that the trajectory of the beam yields centrally positioned sphenoid and pituitary contours on the fluoroscopy monitor. Next, the endoscopic tower is placed over the patient's left shoulder, directly in the line of vision of the surgeon, while the fluoroscopy monitor is placed over the patient's right shoulder. This setup provides the surgeon with an unobstructed view of the visual information provided by the endoscope and ready access to real-time and still fluoroscopic imaging. Because the surgeon is not looking down into the eyepieces of a microscope and instead directly forward at the video screen, proper alignment of these components is essential to keep the surgeon oriented to a surgical plane that is perpendicular to the sphenoid rostrum.

Finally, an endoscope holding arm is affixed to the bed on the side opposite the surgeon and wrapped in a sterile drape. The arm reaches over the upper half of the patient's body and the grasping end rests above the patient's nose. Its orientation can be adjusted to alter the position of the endoscope as necessary.

This standard of positioning is appropriate for all cases in which the operation is conducted through the patient's right nostril. As the surgeon stands to the patient's right, use of the right nostril creates a natural axis along which the long, slender endoscopes and surgical instruments can be used comfortably and effectively. The extension and rotation of the patient's neck provide for easy intranasal access to the sphenoid sinus, as well as the bilateral cavernous sinuses and suprasellar areas. A left-sided approach, by comparison, should be considered in patients with significantly deviated nasal septa that effectively obliterate the working space of the right naris or in those with histories of right-sided sinus surgeries or structural abnormalities.[16, 59]

The face, nares, and abdomen or thigh are prepared with antibacterial surgical scrub, as in the transseptal transsphenoidal technique. Some authors[17, 49, 58, 105, 108] support the use of intranasal epinephrine- or cocaine-soaked sponges to obtain mucosal vasospasm. Sterile towels are used to cover the face, with only the nose left exposed during surgery. After the intravenous administration of a third-generation cephalosporin for surgical prophylaxis, the operation is begun.

Surgical Technique

The first step in the endoscopic procedure is to choose the appropriate endoscope. The initial dissection is invariably performed with a zero-degree lens, but the diameter of the scope may vary. The advantages of the 4.0-mm over the 2.7-mm endoscope include higher resolution of the image and better illumination of the surgical field. The 4.0-mm endoscope, however, occupies a significantly greater amount of space in a region that is already confined. Preoperative physical examination of the nasal passages provides the surgeon with an idea of which will be more appropriate. Nevertheless, nasal passages that may initially appear sufficiently large may front a deeper surgical anatomy that precludes the advancement of multiple surgical instruments alongside a 4-mm endoscope. The surgeon must have scopes of both diameters available and must be able to improvise intraoperatively, depending on the intranasal and skull base anatomy of the patient.

Furthermore, every endoscope must be fitted with an irrigation sheath before use. As described above, these sheaths bathe the endoscope lenses with streams of saline when they become clouded with blood or debris. Surgery without a properly functioning lens irrigation system is extremely difficult in that the redundant removal and replacement of endoscopes for cleaning is both tedious to the surgeon and hazardous to the patient.

When the appropriate endoscope is chosen, it is attached to the grasping end of the holder, advanced into the right naris, and used to conduct a brief survey of the anterior nasal vestibule. The middle turbinate and the architecture of the nasal septum are identified. Because the ultimate target of the endoscope is the sphenoid ostium, the goal of the intranasal portion of the procedure is to create a passage to the ostium that is wide enough to accommodate the endoscope and accompanying instruments. This goal can be achieved rapidly but should be meticulously and atraumatically performed because bleeding from traumatized mucosa anteriorly can obscure visualization throughout the procedure posteriorly.

The endoscope is advanced to the anteroinferior border of the middle turbinate. An elevator is passed under the shaft of the endoscope until it is visualized on the monitor. A long straight suction device may also be introduced to clear the naris of any blood or mucoid secretions that accumulate during the subsequent steps. The elevator is placed flatly against the surface of the septum, and firm, sustained pressure is applied in a medial direction. The spongy septal mucosa is flattened and the underlying cartilage is moved. The elastic nature of the cartilage gives it a tendency to recoil to its native position after each thrust. The maneuver is therefore repeated along the entire face of the septum until it yields and is definitively displaced. The elevator is then carefully rotated intranasally and a similar force is applied to the middle turbinate in a lateral direction. The fragile skeleton of the middle nasal turbinate will often crack as it yields, but fracturing the bone is not explicitly necessary. As the nasal passage is widened, the holding arm is released and the endoscope advanced further posteriorly, where medial and lateral displacement of the septum and turbinate continues. Ultimately, the posterior nasopharyngeal wall and the right sphenoid ostium are revealed and mark the caudal extent of the intranasal dissection (Fig. 26–3). Correct localization is confirmed radiographically by passage of a long suction tip through the nostril into the nasopharynx. Placement of the metallic tip against the bony contour of the anterior wall of the sphenoid sinus is confirmed fluoroscopically.

The sphenoid ostium is often difficult to detect, possibly because of diminutive size or mucosal inflammation. However, fluoroscopic identification of surgical instruments against the anterior wall of the sphenoid sinus serves as an adequate test of localization. Some authors have described alternative localization techniques, including the use of various imaging modalities and frame-based stereotactically guided methods.[8, 29, 42]

The mucosal lining of the anterior wall of the sphenoid sinus must be dissected before the sinus can be entered. The mucosa is cauterized with a combination suction-cautery device and then lifted from the surface of the bone with an elevator. This dissection is carried out bilaterally to expose both sphenoid ostia and to the superior and inferior limits of the anterior sphenoid, as defined by the cribriform plate and vomer, respectively. Again, fluoroscopic examination of the bony contours of these structures confirms these limits. The vomer may be removed with a rongeur to more completely expose the surface of the sphenoid bone.

Endoscopic resection of the rostral surface of the sphenoid, the mucosal lining of the sinus, and the floor of the sella proceeds as described above for the microscopic transseptal procedure. The holding arm is released and the endoscope is advanced further toward the pituitary with each subsequent step. The same rongeurs, graspers, and osteotomes are passed through the nostril, below the shaft of the endoscope, and into the surgical field to gain access to the sphenoid sinus and sella turcica. Similarly, the same principles of awareness for

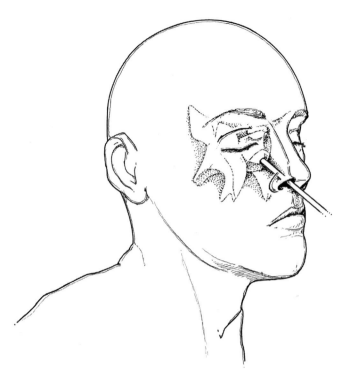

FIGURE 26–3. *Endoscopic transnasal approach. A long, thin rod endoscope provides direct access to the gland without the need for oral or nasal dissection.*

the limits of dissection apply.[57] Under endoscopic imaging, the distal recesses of the sphenoid sinus are better visualized. However, injuries to the cavernous sinuses, carotid arteries, optic nerves and chiasm, and cribriform plate are still possible if caution is not exercised while working within the sinus or sella.

When the sphenoid sinus is completely exposed, the endoscope is advanced into the cavity. There it remains until most of the tumor resection is completed. The floor of the sella, if intact, is fractured and removed to reveal the dural covering of the pituitary gland. Incision of the dura and removal of tumor are conducted as previously described with suction and ring curettes of varying diameter and orientation. Consideration must be given to displacement of the normal gland by tumor as observed on MRI scans. Valsalva maneuvers are implemented in an attempt to deliver suprasellar extensions of tumor into the sella.[59]

Until this point all procedures are carried out under the zero-degree endoscope. Its lens provides near-complete exposure of the sella turcica and a partial view of the suprasellar structures, including the optic chiasm and the arachnoid membrane investing the median eminence. This panorama is remarkably more comprehensive than the microscopic view of the same region.[84, 115] However, the extent of visualization under this scope is limited by its optical capabilities. Therefore, once tumor resection under the zero-degree endoscope is deemed complete, it is replaced with a 30-degree endoscope. By advancing the 30-degree scope into the sella turcica and then rotating it in clockwise and counterclockwise directions about the anteroposterior axis, the parasellar and suprasellar areas are thoroughly visualized.[59, 61] This maneuver reveals the strength of the endoscope in pituitary surgery: areas that are not revealed during microscopic examination are directly exposed. Tumor remnants in these areas are removed and sources of potential tumor recurrence are thereby eliminated. All of this is accomplished with superb visual appreciation of the critical surrounding structures.

A 70-degree endoscope may also be implemented in this examination. However, the information obtained under a 30-degree lens is in most cases sufficient to identify any remaining tumor fragments. (Although available to the surgeon, the 120-degree endoscope adds little to this application. Because of its viewing angle, its progress

cannot be directly viewed as it is passed through the nostril. This blind insertion and advancement pose a significant threat to the patient and therefore severely limit the usefulness of this particular endoscope in this procedure.)

Tumor resection is considered to be complete only after examination with the angled endoscopes is performed and all residual tumor removed. A fat graft from the abdomen or a graft of muscle and fascia lata from the lateral aspect of the thigh is harvested and used to reconstruct the floor of the sella and fill the sphenoid sinus.[16, 49, 58–61, 108] Fibrin sealant is also used to secure its position.

With no mucoperichondrial or mucoperiosteal dissection to speak of, the need for postoperative nasal packings is eliminated.[16, 58, 105] A thin sheet of absorbent sponge material is placed loosely in the nasal vestibule to collect residual secretions from the naris. A small gauze sponge fastened beneath the nose (a "mustache" dressing) serves a similar purpose. Both are extremely well tolerated by patients and are removed the morning after surgery.

Postoperative Monitoring

The patient is extubated in the operating room and observed in the intensive care unit overnight. Again, particular attention is paid to the development of any neurologic sequelae, alterations in vision, evidence of rhinorrhea, or signs of diabetes insipidus. In the absence of any such problems, patients are moved out of the intensive care unit the day after surgery and may be discharged home on the same or following day.

Outcomes

Because this procedure is relatively new, the amount of data generated by centers using this technique to perform pituitary tumor resection must increase before meaningful comparisons to the microscopic technique can be drawn. However, some general statements and preliminary conclusions can be made. As in the microscopic technique, complications with the fully endoscopic procedure can be almost completely avoided with careful technique. The incidence of morbidity is related to injuries to the normal gland or to surrounding neurovascular structures.

Preliminary evidence suggests that complication rates and surgical outcomes compare favorably with those that have been reported in large series of transseptal transsphenoidal microscopic pituitary surgeries.[16, 49, 58, 59] More extensive data over longer follow-up are required to substantiate these early trends. However, it is currently clear that transnasal endoscopic pituitary surgery does offer a minimally invasive and effective means of addressing pituitary lesions requiring surgical intervention.

REFERENCES

1. Abboud CF: Anterior pituitary failure. *In* Melmed S (ed): The Pituitary, ed 1. Cambridge, Blackwell, 1995, pp 341–410.
2. Abe T, Iwata T, Kawamura N, et al: Staged transsphenoidal surgery for fibrous nonfunctioning pituitary adenomas with suprasellar extension. Neurol Med Chir (Tokyo) 37:830–835, 1997.
3. Ahmadi H, Larsson EM, Jinkins JR: Normal pituitary gland: Coronal MR imaging of infundibular tilt. Radiology 177:389–392, 1990.
4. Annergers JF, Coulam CB, Abboud CF, et al: Pituitary adenoma in Olmsted County, Minnesota, 1935–1977. A report of an increasing incidence of diagnosis in women of childbearing age. Mayo Clin Proc 53:641–643, 1978.
5. Aron DC, Tyrrell JB, Wilson CB: Pituitary tumors. Current concepts in diagnosis and management. West J Med 162:340–352, 1995.
6. Arredondo de Arreola G, Lopez Serna N, de Hoyos Parra R, et al: Morphogenesis of the lateral nasal wall from 6 to 36 weeks. Otolaryngol Head Neck Surg 114:54–60, 1996.
7. Asano T, Ohno K, Takada Y, et al: Fractures of the floor of the anterior cranial fossa. J Trauma 39:702–706, 1995.
8. Auer LM: Ultrasound stereotaxic endoscopy in neurosurgery. Acta Neurochir Suppl (Wien) 54:34–41, 1992.
9. Avery JA (ed): Oral Development and Histology, ed 1. Los Angeles, Williams & Wilkins, 1987.
10. Aydin IH, Kadioglu HH, Tuzun Y, et al: Postoperative anosmia after anterior communicating artery aneurysms surgery by the pterional approach. Min Invas Neurosurg 39(3):71–73, 1996.

11. Aydin IH, Tuzun Y, Takci E, et al: The anatomical variations of sylvian veins and cisterns. Min Invas Neurosurg 40(2):68–73, 1997.
12. Batjer HH, Kopitnik TA, Giller CA, et al: Surgery for paraclinoidal carotid artery aneurysms. J Neurosurg 80:650–658, 1994.
13. Becker SP: Anatomy for endoscopic sinus surgery. Otolaryngol Clin North Am 22:677–682, 1989.
14. Belden CJ, Mancuso AA, Kotzur IM: The developing anterior skull base: CT appearance from birth to 2 years of age. AJNR Am J Neuroradiol 18:811–818, 1997.
15. Caliot P, Plessis JL, Midy D, et al: The intraorbital arrangement of the anterior and posterior ethmoidal foramina. Surg Radiol Anat 17:29–33, 1995.
16. Cappabianca P, Alfieri A, de Divitiis E: Endoscopic endonasal transsphenoidal approach to the sella: Towards functional endoscopic pituitary surgery (FEPS). Min Invas Neurosurg 41(2):66–73, 1998.
17. Carrau RL, Jho HD, Ko Y: Transnasal-transsphenoidal endoscopic surgery of the pituitary gland. Laryngoscope 106:914–918, 1996.
18. Caton R, Paul FT: A case of acromegaly treated by operation. BMJ 2:1421–1423, 1893.
19. Chang-DeMoranville BM, Jackson IM: Diagnosis and endocrine testing in acromegaly. Endocrinol Metab Clin North Am 21:649–668, 1992.
20. Ciric I, Mikhael M, Stafford T, et al: Transsphenoidal microsurgery of pituitary macroadenomas with long-term follow-up results. J Neurosurg 59:395–401, 1983.
21. Cope VZ: The pituitary fossa, and the methods of surgical approach thereto. Br J Surg 4:107–144, 1916.
22. Cushing H: Surgical experiences with pituitary disorders. JAMA 63:1515–1525, 1914.
23. Cushing H: Disorders of the pituitary gland. Retrospective and prophetic. JAMA 76:1721–1726, 1921.
24. Davis WE, Templer J, Parsons DS: Anatomy of the paranasal sinuses. Otolaryngol Clin North Am 29:57–74, 1996.
25. De Jesus O: The clinoidal space: Anatomical review and surgical implications. Acta Neurochir (Wien) 139:361–365, 1997.
26. Dietemann JL, Kehrli P, Maillot C, et al: Is there a dural wall between the cavernous sinus and the pituitary fossa? Anatomical and MRI findings. Neuroradiology 40:627–630, 1998.
27. Dolenc VV: Surgery of tumors originating in or invading the cavernous sinus. In Long DM (ed): Surgery for Skull-Base Tumors, ed 1. Boston, Blackwell, 1992, pp 211–221.
28. Dolenc VV: Transcranial epidural approach to pituitary tumors extending beyond the sella. Neurosurgery 41:542–550, 1997.
29. Dorward NL, Alberti O, Zhao J, et al: Interactive image-guided neuroendoscopy: Development and early clinical experience. Min Invas Neurosurg 41(1):31–34, 1998.
30. Dott NM, Bailey P, Cushing H: A consideration of the hypophyseal adenomata. Br J Surg 13:314–365, 1925.
31. Eaves FF 3rd, Bostwick J 3rd, Nahai F: Instrumentation and setup for endoscopic plastic surgery. Clin Plast Surg 22:591–603, 1995.
32. Elster AD: Modern imaging of the pituitary. Radiology 187:1–14, 1993.
33. Fahlbusch R, Buchfelder M: The transsphenoidal approach to invasive sellar and clival lesions. In Sekhar LN, Janecka IP (eds): Surgery of Cranial Base Tumors, ed 1. New York, Raven, 1993, pp 337–349.
34. Fahlbusch R, Honegger J, Paulus W, et al: Surgical treatment of craniopharyngiomas: Experience with 168 patients. J Neurosurg 90:237–250, 1999.
35. Favre JJ, Chaffanjon P, Passagia JG, et al: Blood supply of the olfactory nerve. Meningeal relationships and surgical relevance. Surg Radiol Anat 17:133–138, 1995.
36. Ferreri AJ, Garrido SA, Markarian MG, et al: Relationship between the development of diaphragma sellae and the morphology of the sella turcica and its content. Surg Radiol Anat 14:233–239, 1992.
37. FitzPatrick M, Tartaglino LM, Hollander MD, et al: Imaging of sellar and parasellar pathology. Radiol Clin North Am 37:101–121, 1999.
38. Friede H: Normal development and growth of the human neurocranium and cranial base. Scand J Plast Reconstr Surg 15:163–169, 1981.
39. Fukuta K, Saito K, Takahashi M, et al: Surgical approach to midline skull base tumors with olfactory preservation. Plast Reconstr Surg 100:318–325, 1997.
40. Gamea A, Fathi M, el-Guindy A: The use of the rigid endoscope in trans-sphenoidal pituitary surgery. J Laryngol Otol 108:19–22, 1994.
41. Goel A: Middle fossa sub-Gasserian ganglion approach to clivus chordomas. Acta Neurochir (Wien) 136:212–216, 1995.
42. Goodman RR: Magnetic resonance imaging–directed stereotactic endoscopic third ventriculostomy. Neurosurgery 32:1043–1047, 1993.
43. Gruber R, Lesavoy M: Closed septal osteotomy. Ann Plast Surg 40:283–286, 1998.
44. Hardy J: La chirurgie de l'hypophyse par voie transsphénoïdale. Union Med Can 96:702–712, 1967.
45. Hardy J: Transsphenoidal microsurgery of the normal and pathological pituitary. Clin Neurosurg 16:185–217, 1969.
46. Hardy J: Transsphenoidal hypophysectomy. J Neurosurg 34:582–594, 1971.
47. Hardy J: Trans-sphenoidal approach to the pituitary gland. In Wilkins RH, Rengachary SS (eds): Neurosurgery, vol ed 2. New York, McGraw-Hill, 1996, pp 1375–1384.
48. Hardy J, Wisger SM: Transsphenoidal surgery of pituitary fossa tumors with televised radiofluoroscopic control. J Neurosurg 23:612–620, 1965.
49. Heilman CB, Shucart WA, Rebeiz EE: Endoscopic sphenoidotomy approach to the sella. Neurosurgery 41:602–607, 1997.
50. Helal MZ: Combined micro-endoscopic trans-sphenoid excisions of pituitary microadenomas. Eur Arch Otorhinolaryngol 252:186–189, 1995.
51. Henderson WR: The pituitary adenomata. Br J Surg 26:811–921, 1939.
52. Heuer GJ: The surgical approach and treatment of tumors and other lesions about the optic chiasm. Surg Gynecol Obstet 53:489–518, 1931.
53. Hirsch O: Pituitary tumors. A borderland between cranial and trans-sphenoidal surgery. N Engl J Med 254:937–939, 1956.
54. Holliday MJ: Lateral subtemporal approach to the management of sphenoid and temporal-infratemporal fossa lesions. In Long DM (ed): Surgery for Skull-Base Tumors, ed 1. Boston, Blackwell, 1992, pp 191–203.
55. Horsley V: On the techniques of operations on the central nervous system. BMJ 2:411–423, 1906.
56. Ikeda K, Watanabe K, Suzuki H, et al: Nasal airway resistance and olfactory acuity following transsphenoidal pituitary surgery. Am J Rhinol 13:45–48, 1999.
57. Jankowski R, Auque J, Simon C, et al: Endoscopic pituitary tumor surgery. Laryngoscope 102:198–202, 1992.
58. Jarrahy R, Young J, Berci G, et al: Endoscopic skull base surgery I: A new animal model for pituitary surgery. J Invest Surg 12:1–6, 1999.
59. Jho HD, Carrau RL: Endoscopy assisted transsphenoidal surgery for pituitary adenoma. Technical note. Acta Neurochir (Wien) 138:1416–1425, 1996.
60. Jho HD, Carrau RL: Endoscopic endonasal transsphenoidal surgery: Experience with 50 patients. J Neurosurg 87:44–51, 1997.
61. Jho HD, Carrau RL, Ko Y: Endoscopic pituitary surgery. In Rengachary SS, Wilkins RH (eds): Neurosurgical Operative Atlas, vol 5. Baltimore, Williams & Wilkins, 1996, pp 1–12.
62. Jimenez-Castellanos J, Carmona A, Castellanos L, Catalina-Herrera CJ: Microsurgical anatomy of the human ophthalmic artery: A mesoscopic study of its origin, course and collateral branches. Surg Radiol Anat 17:139–143, 1995.
63. Johnson MR, Hoare RD, Cox T, et al: The evaluation of patients with a suspected pituitary microadenoma: Computer tomography compared to magnetic resonance imaging. Clin Endocrinol (Oxf) 36:335–338, 1992.
64. Kaye TB, Crapo L: The Cushing syndrome: An update on diagnostic tests. Ann Intern Med 112:434–444, 1990.
65. Kehrli P, Ali M, Reis M Jr, et al: Anatomy and embryology of the lateral sellar compartment (cavernous sinus) medial wall. Neurol Res 20:585–592, 1998.
66. Kennedy DW, Zinreich SJ, Rosenbaum AE, Johns ME: Functional endoscopic sinus surgery: Theory and diagnostic evaluation. Arch Otolaryngol 111:576–582, 1985.
67. Kern EB: Grand rounds: Transnasal pituitary surgery. Arch Otolaryngol 107:183–190, 1981.
68. Kern EB, Laws ER Jr: The rationale and technique of selective transsphenoidal microsurgery for the removal of pituitary tumors. In Laws ER, Randall RV, Kern EB, Abboud CF (eds): Management of Pituitary Adenomas and Related Lesions with Emphasis on Transsphenoidal Microsurgery. New York, Appleton-Century-Crofts, 1982, pp 219–233.
69. Kjaer I: Ossification of the human fetal basicranium. J Craniofac Genet Dev Biol 10:29–38, 1990.
70. Kjaer I: Human prenatal craniofacial development related to brain development under normal and pathologic conditions. Acta Odontol Scand 53:135–143, 1995.
71. Kral T, Zentner J, Vieweg U, et al: Diagnosis and treatment of frontobasal skull fractures. Neurosurg Rev 20:19–23, 1997.
72. Krisht AF, Barrow DL, Barnett DW, et al: The microsurgical anatomy of the superior hypophyseal artery. Neurosurgery 35:899–903, 1994.
73. Krmpotic-Nemanic J, Padovan I, Vinter I, et al: Development of the cribriform plate and of the lamina mediana. Anat Anz 180:555–559, 1998.
74. Laws ER Jr: Pituitary surgery. Endocrinol Metab Clin North Am 16:647–665, 1987.
75. Lee SK, Kim YS, Jo YA, et al: Prenatal development of cranial base in normal Korean fetuses. Anat Rec 246:524–534, 1996.
76. Libersa C, Laude M, Libersa JC: The pneumatization of the accessory cavities of the nasal fossae during growth. Anat Clin 2:265–273, 1981.
77. Linder TE, Simmen D, Stool SE: Revolutionary inventions in the 20th century. The history of endoscopy. Arch Otalaryngol Head Neck Surg 123:1161–1163, 1997.
78. Long DM: Subfrontal approach to the frontal meningioma. In Long DM (ed): Surgery for Skull-Base Tumors, ed 1. Boston, Blackwell, 1992, pp 93–103.
79. Luft R, Olivecrona H: Experiences with hypophysectomy in man. J Neurosurg 10:301–316, 1953.
80. Lund VJ: Extended applications of endoscopic sinus surgery—the territorial imperative. J Laryngol Otol 111:313–315, 1997.
81. Magnan J, Sanna M (eds): Endoscopy in Neuro-Otology, ed 1. New York, Thieme, 1999.
82. Maira G, Anile C, Rossi GF, et al: Surgical treatment of craniopharyngiomas: An evaluation of the transsphenoidal and pterional approaches. Neurosurgery 36:715–724, 1995.
83. Maroldo TV, Dillon WP, Wilson CB: Advances in diagnostic techniques of pituitary tumors and prolactinomas. Curr Opin Oncol 4:105–115, 1992.
84. Matula C, Tschabitscher M, Day JD, et al: Endoscopically assisted microneurosurgery. Acta Neurochir 134:190–195, 1995.
85. McArthur LL: An aseptic surgical access to the pituitary body and its neighborhood. JAMA 58:2009–2011, 1912.
86. Metson R, Gliklich RE: Endoscopic treatment of sphenoid sinusitis. Otolaryngol Head Neck Surg 114:736–744, 1996.
87. Miller AJ, Amedee RG: Functional anatomy of the paranasal sinuses. J La State Med Soc 149(3):85–90, 1997.
88. Mohr G, Hardy J, Comtois R, et al: Surgical management of giant pituitary adenomas. Can J Neurol Sci 17:62–66, 1990.
89. Nabe-Nielsen J: Nasal complications after transsphenoidal surgery for pituitary pathologies. Acta Neurochir (Wien) 96:122–125, 1989.
90. Nagai H, Moritake K, Nagao S, Yamasaki T: Ultrasonic bruits in the circle of Willis due to a large nonfunctioning pituitary adenoma. J Neuroimaging 7:251–254, 1997.
91. Natori Y, Rhoton AL Jr: Microsurgical anatomy of the superior orbital fissure. Neurosurgery 36:762–775, 1995.
92. Nishioka NS, Mycek MA: Initial experience with a real-time video processor for enhancing endoscopic image contrast. Gastrointest Endosc 48:62–66, 1998.
93. Nishizawa S, Yokoyama T, Ohta S, et al: Surgical indications for and limitations of staged transsphenoidal surgery for large pituitary tumors. Neurol Med Chir (Tokyo) 38:213–219, 1998.

94. Oikawa S, Kyoshima K, Kobayashi S: Surgical anatomy of the juxta-dural ring area. J Neurosurg 89:250–254, 1998.
95. Papay FA, Benninger MS, Levine HL, et al: Transnasal transseptal endoscopic repair of sphenoidal cerebral spinal fluid fistula. Otolaryngol Head Neck Surg 101:595–597, 1989.
96. Patterson RH: The role of transcranial surgery in the management of pituitary adenoma. Acta Neurochir Suppl (Wien) 65:16–17, 1996.
97. Randall RV: Clinical presentation of pituitary adenomas. *In* Laws ER, Randall RV, Kern EB, Abboud CF (eds): Management of Pituitary Adenomas and Related Lesions with Emphasis on Transsphenoidal Microsurgery. New York, Appleton-Century-Crofts, 1982, pp 15–30.
98. Ray BS: Intracranial hypophysectomy. J Neurosurg 28:180–186, 1968.
99. Ray BS, Patterson RH Jr: Surgical treatment of pituitary adenomas. J Neurosurg 19:1–8, 1962.
100. Reisch R, Vutskits L, Patonay L, et al: The meningohypophyseal trunk and its blood supply to different intracranial structures. An anatomical study. Min Invas Neurosurg 39(3):78–81, 1996.
101. Rhoton AL Jr: Microsurgical anatomy of the sellar region. *In* Wilkins RH, Rengachary SS (eds): Neurosurgery, vol 1, ed 2. New York, McGraw-Hill, 1996, pp 1243–1253.
102. Rhoton AL Jr, Hardy DG, Chambers SM: Microsurgical anatomy and dissection of the sphenoid bone, cavernous sinus and sellar region. Surg Neurol 12:63–104, 1979.
103. Ricciardelli EJ: Embryology and anatomy of the cranial base. Clin Plast Surg 22:361–372, 1995.
104. Rice DH, Schaefer SD (eds): Endoscopic Paranasal Sinus Surgery, ed 2. New York, Raven, 1993.
105. Rodziewicz GS, Kelley RT, Kellman RM, et al: Transnasal endoscopic surgery of the pituitary gland: Technical note. Neurosurgery 39:189–192, 1996.
106. Rosegay H: Cushing's legacy to transsphenoidal surgery. J Neurosurg 54:448–454, 1981.
107. Sejrsen B, Jakobsen J, Skovgaard LT, et al: Growth in the external cranial base evaluated on human dry skulls, using nerve canal openings as references. Acta Odontol Scand 55:356–364, 1997.
108. Sethi DS, Pillay PK: Endoscopic management of lesions of the sella turcica. J Laryngol Otol 109:956–962, 1995.
109. Sethi DS, Stanley RE, Pillay PK: Endoscopic anatomy of the sphenoid sinus and sella turcica. J Laryngol Otol 109:951–955, 1995.
110. Sharma K, Tyagi I, Banerjee D, et al: Rhinological complications of sublabial transseptal transsphenoidal surgery for sellar and suprasellar lesions: Prevention and management. Neurosurg Rev 19:163–167, 1996.
111. Silau AM, Hansen BF, Kjaer I: Normal prenatal development of the human parietal bone and interparietal suture. J Craniofac Genet Dev Biol 15(2):81–86, 1995.
112. Sloan AE, Black KB, Becker DP: Lesions of the sella turcica. *In* Donald PJ (ed): Surgery of the Skull Base, ed 1. Philadelphia, Lippincott-Raven, 1998, pp 555–582.
113. Smith TD, Siegel MI, Mooney MP, et al: Formation and enlargement of the paranasal sinuses in normal and cleft lip and palate human fetuses. Cleft Palate Craniofac J 34:483–489, 1997.
114. Spektor S, Piontek E, Umansky F: Orbital venous drainage into the anterior cavernous sinus space: Microanatomic relationships. Neurosurgery 40:532–539, 1997.
115. Spencer WR, Das K, Nwagu C, et al: Approaches to the sellar and parasellar region: Anatomic comparison of the microscope versus endoscope. Laryngoscope 109:791–794, 1999.
116. Spetzler RF, Herman JM, Beals S, et al: Preservation of olfaction in anterior craniofacial approaches. J Neurosurg 79:48–52, 1993.
117. Stadnik T, Stevenaert A, Beckers A, et al: Pituitary microadenomas: Diagnosis with two- and three-dimensional MR imaging at 1.5 T before and after injection of gadolinium. Radiology 176:419–428, 1990.
118. Stankiewicz JA: The endoscopic approach to the sphenoid sinus. Laryngoscope 99:218–221, 1989.
119. Stern JT (ed): Essentials of Gross Anatomy, ed 1. Philadelphia, FA Davis, 1988.
120. Sullivan LJ, O'Day J, McNeill P: Visual outcomes of pituitary adenoma surgery. St. Vincent's Hospital 1968–1987. J Clin Neuroophthalmol 11:262–267, 1991.
121. Taub E, Patterson RH: Transcranial approaches to the pituitary gland and sellar region. *In* Wilkins RH, Rengachary SS (eds): Neurosurgery, vol 1, ed 2. New York, McGraw-Hill, 1996, pp 1385–1388.
122. Tyrrell JB, Lamborn KR, Hannegan LT: Transsphenoidal microsurgical therapy of prolactinomas: Initial outcomes and long-term results. Neurosurgery 44:254–261, 1999.
123. Tzortzidis F, Bejjani G, Papadas T, et al: Craniofacial osteotomies to facilitate resection of large tumours of the anterior skull base. J Craniomaxillofac Surg 24:224–229, 1996.
124. Urquhart AC, Bersalona FB, Ejercito VS, et al: Nasal septum after sublabial transseptal transsphenoidal pituitary surgery. Otolaryngol Head Neck Surg 115:64–69, 1996.
125. Vakil N, Bourgeois K: A prospective, controlled trial of eight-bit, 16-bit, and 24-bit digital color images in electronic endoscopy. Endoscopy 27:589–592, 1995.
126. Vinter I, Krmpotic-Nemanic J, Hat J, et al: The frontal sinus and the ethmoidal labyrinth. Surg Radiol Anat 19:295–298, 1997.
127. Webb SM, Ruscalleda J, Schwarzstein D, et al: Computerized tomography versus magnetic resonance imaging: A comparative study in hypothalamic-pituitary and parasellar pathology. Clin Endocrinol (Oxf) 36:459–465, 1992.
128. Wilson CB: Neurosurgical management of large and invasive pituitary tumors. *In* Tindall GT, Collins WF (eds): Clinical Management of Pituitary Disorders. New York, Raven, 1979, pp 335–342.
129. Wilson CB, Dempsey LC: Transsphenoidal microsurgical removal of 250 pituitary adenomas. J Neurosurg 48:13–22, 1978.
130. Wurster CF, Smith DE: The endoscopic approach to the pituitary gland. Arch Otolaryngol Head Neck Surg 120:674, 1994.
131. Yaniv E, Rappaport H: Endoscopic transseptal transsphenoidal surgery for pituitary tumors. Neurosurgery 40:944–946, 1997.
132. Yoon JH, Lee JG, Kim SH, et al: Microscopical surgical management of cerebrospinal fluid rhinorrhoea with free grafts. Rhinology 33:208–211, 1995.

▲▲▲

Chapter 27

Sellar and Parasellar Tumors in Children

Sandeep Kunwar ▪ Charles B. Wilson

CLINICAL PRESENTATION
RADIOGRAPHIC STUDIES
TUMORS
  Craniopharyngiomas

Pituitary Adenomas
  Surgical Treatment
Optic Pathway and Hypothalamic
Gliomas

Germ Cell Tumors
Rare Lesions

Parasellar and sellar tumors account for approximately one fourth of pediatric brain tumors and slightly more than one half of supratentorial tumors in children.[1, 2] A variety of lesions are encountered in the parasellar region that vary in aggressiveness from malignant teratomas to arachnoid cysts and in size from a pituitary microadenoma to a large cystic craniopharyngioma. Lesions in this region have characteristic clinical presentations, and clinicians treating pediatric patients should be aware of them.

The most common pediatric parasellar tumor is the craniopharyngioma, accounting for 5% to 13% of all intracranial tumors in children and approximately 55% of parasellar lesions.[1, 3] Parasellar gliomas, including those involving the optic nerve and hypothalamus, account for 19% of pediatric parasellar tumors, followed by pituitary adenomas, which account for 1% to 10%, and germ cell tumors, which make up 4% to 6%.[1, 4] The clinical presentation, preoperative assessment, differential diagnosis, and management of children with parasellar and sellar tumors is presented.

CLINICAL PRESENTATION

Richmond and Wilson[5] reviewed the clinical findings in 74 children with parasellar masses treated at the University of California, San Francisco. Presenting symptoms are listed in Table 27–1. The most common presenting symptom was headache (39%) which occurred more often in patients with craniopharyngiomas and diencephalic gliomas. In most patients with headache, increased intracranial pressure secondary to obstruction of cerebrospinal fluid flow was present from distortion of the third ventricle or compression of the aqueduct. Visual failure occurred in 22% of all patients, more frequently with craniopharyngiomas and optic nerve or hypothalamic lesions. Endocrinologic abnormalities occurred in 12% to 19% of patients. Although pituitary hypersecretion was primarily seen in pituitary adenomas, nonspecific hyperprolactinemia may be present in any lesion that compresses or distorts the pituitary stalk and, as a consequence, impairs the flow of

dopamine from hypothalamic neurons through the portal circulation into the anterior pituitary. Menstrual irregularity was the most frequent manifestation of pituitary adenomas of all types and was not dependent on hyperprolactinemia. Growth arrest and short stature occurred with all types of pituitary adenomas except for growth hormone (GH)–releasing adenomas, and was particularly striking in patients with Cushing's disease who had adrenocorticotropic hormone (ACTH)–secreting tumors. One third of patients with craniopharyngiomas also presented with growth failure.

Diabetes insipidus (DI) is rarely seen in patients with pituitary adenomas, and occurs in only 6% to 12% of patients with craniopharyngiomas.[1, 6] However, DI is a common presentation in patients with parasellar germinomas and intrasellar teratomas. These patients present with the triad of DI, pituitary insufficiency, and visual failure. Pituitary insufficiency exists in the majority of patients with craniopharyngiomas (57%) and occurs less often with pituitary adenomas (25%) because most adenomas are small at the time of presentation.[5, 7–11] Precocious puberty is a feature of patients with diencephalic gliomas and hypothalamic hamartomas, but can also be seen in patients with a GH-producing pituitary adenoma.

Patients undergoing evaluation of parasellar lesions require visual assessment by formal neuro-ophthalmologic evaluation. Although the textbook descriptions of the visual field defects that accompany parasellar lesions emphasize bitemporal hemianopsia characteristic of chiasmal compression, monocular and homonymous defects also occur frequently and are associated with involvement of the optic nerve or tract, respectively. Furthermore, pediatric patients are less likely to complain of visual disturbances than are adults and instead acquire adaptive measures. The frequency and severity of abnormal vision is greatest in patients with tumors that directly involve the optic nerve, such as optic gliomas, hypothalamic gliomas, and germinomas. Preoperative visual field deficits were present in 57% of pediatric patients with craniopharyngiomas and in 20% of those with pituitary adenomas.[5]

Abnormalities of the hypothalamic-pituitary axis are a major source of morbidity and possible mortality in children with parasellar tumors. Endocrinologic evaluation of children with pituitary lesions has shown decreased gonadotropin function in 78% of patients of pubertal age.[5] An elevated serum prolactin level is very common in pediatric patients with sellar lesions as a result of either primary hypersecretion (prolactinoma), stalk effect (impairment of the hypothalamic feedback mechanism), or coproduction of prolactin and GH in patients with acromegaly.[12, 13] GH deficiency was most common in ACTH-secreting tumors. High levels of glucocorticoids are associated both clinically and experimentally with hypothalamic suppression of GH release and subsequent growth arrest.[14–19] Growth arrest is also a prominent feature in 57% of patients with craniopharyngiomas, relating either to direct pituitary compression or to hypothalamic dysfunction. Pituitary insufficiency is uncommon with pituitary adenomas, as would be expected by the infrequency of macroadenomas in the pediatric population, and is more likely to be caused by craniopharyngiomas (30% to 55%) and germinomas (79%), emphasizing the importance of preoperative

TABLE 27–1. **Presenting Symptoms of Parasellar Tumors in Children**

Presenting Symptoms	All Patients (%)	Craniopha-ryngioma (%)	Pituitary Adenoma (%)
Headache	39	62	8
Failure of sexual maturation	24	10	52
Visual failure	22	43	8
Pituitary hypersecretion	19	0	80
Growth failure	16	33	0
Diabetes insipidus	12	10	0
Precocious puberty	1	0	0

Adapted from Mindermann T, Wilson CB: Pediatric pituitary adenomas. Neurosurgery 36:259–269, 1995.

TABLE 27–2. Common Findings Among Parasellar and Sellar Tumors

Signs and Symptoms	Craniopharyngioma	Pituitary Adenoma	Germinoma	Parasellar Glioma
Pituitary hypersecretion	−	+ + +	−	−
Preoperative panhypopituitarism	+ +	+	+ +	+
Preoperative diabetes insipidus	+	−	+ + +	+
Visual defect	+ +	+	+ + +	+ + +
Papilledema	+	−	+	+ +
Hydrocephalus/headache	+	−	+	+ +
Parasellar calcification	+ + +	−	−	+
Abnormal sella	+ +	+ + +	−	−
Precocious puberty	−	+ *	−	+
Growth delay	+ +	+ +	+	−

*Among growth hormone–releasing adenomas.

endocrine studies as part of the workup of all sellar and parasellar masses.[4, 5, 20] Characteristic clinical presentations for sellar and parasellar tumors are presented in Table 27–2.

RADIOGRAPHIC STUDIES

Plain skull films, although rarely used today except in head injuries, reveal abnormalities in 87% of children with parasellar lesions, showing evidence of an expanded or asymmetrical sella in 96% of pituitary adenomas, calcification typical of craniopharyngiomas in 70% to 93% of cases, or changes due to hydrocephalus.[5] Axial computed tomography (CT) scans reveal similar bony changes, including abnormalities of the optic canal or tuberculum sella and hyperostosis associated with meningiomas. However, magnetic resonance (MR) imaging, with and without contrast, should be the initial radiographic procedure when a sellar or parasellar mass is suspected because it provides the greatest information about the parasellar anatomy and pathology of the lesion. Kollias et al.[21] reviewed the MR images in 53 pediatric patients with suprasellar tumors and found characteristic features that, in conjunction with clinical data, enable the clinician to differentiate between most suprasellar tumors, although significant overlap does exist. Craniopharyngiomas are predominantly cystic masses with macrocystic components. The solid portion is irregular, heterogeneous, and often contains areas of signal void representing calcification. These tumors also have a smooth ring of cyst wall enhancement after contrast administration (Fig. 27–1). Most pituitary adenomas are less than 1 cm in diameter and are intrasellar, although they can have suprasellar extension and cystic components (Fig. 27–2). Chiasmatic and hypothalamic astrocytomas are predominantly solid and frequently contain microcysts. The solid portion is enhanced intensely after contrast administration (Fig. 27–3). Focal enhancement of a mass in the hypothalamus or pituitary stalk with the clinical presentation of DI is strongly suggestive of a suprasellar germinoma (Fig. 27–4). Teratomas can be distinguished on the basis of their heterogeneity, with the presence of fat, calcification, and various soft tissue densities. In addition to visualizing the parasellar region, MR imaging may be used to assess additional lesions elsewhere in the brain, particularly in the region of the pineal gland. In patients with intrasellar lesions, a supplemental MR image of the sella provides greater detail and can define the exact location of a pituitary microadenoma, or involvement of adjacent structures (carotid arteries; optic nerve, chiasm, or tract; cavernous sinus; or hypothalamus).

TUMORS

Craniopharyngioma

Craniopharyngiomas are the most common tumor of the sellar and parasellar region in children. In the 19th century, these tumors were postulated to arise from the hypophysial duct or Rathke's pouch[22] although current opinion favors their origin from embryonic squamous cell rests of an incompletely involuted hypophysial-pharyngeal duct, and thus a result of disordered embryogenesis.[23, 24] Microscopically,

these tumors have an external layer of high columnar epithelium and a central network of epithelial cells supported by a mesodermal connective tissue stroma. A collagenous basement membrane often forms the boundary between the tumor and the surrounding meninges or brain, and may explain the tight adherence to these structures. Craniopharyngiomas often cause an intense glial reaction in surrounding brain tissue and vascular structures, contributing to tissue adherence and a primary reason for incomplete resections.[24] There are two primary histologic variants, squamous papillary and adamantinomatous; nearly all pediatric craniopharyngiomas are of the latter type.[10, 25, 26]

Craniopharyngiomas are slow-growing, extra-axial tumors that often become quite large before they cause symptoms, including visual loss, headaches, and endocrine dysfunction[1, 5, 10, 25] (Table 27–3). Hyperphagia and obesity, reported in 12% to 32% of patients with craniopharyngiomas, can be quite profound and may be related to insensitization of the hypothalamus to leptin.[27, 28]

The diagnostic workup for craniopharyngiomas has been simplified by the availability of CT and MR imaging. Calcification of the cyst wall is seen in 70% to 93% of childhood craniopharyngiomas.[21] Cyst fluid is usually of low density on CT scans and can have variable signal characteristics on MR images. Invariably, there is a solid component of tumor within the cyst and, rarely, these tumors are entirely

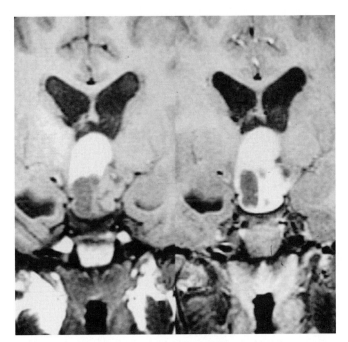

FIGURE 27–1. Coronal T1-weighted precontrast *(left)* and postcontrast *(right)* magnetic resonance image of a craniopharyngioma. The bright signal at the superior aspect of the tumor on the precontrast study represents proteinaceous fluid or acute blood. Note the cyst wall enhancement and the nodular soft tissue component of the tumor.

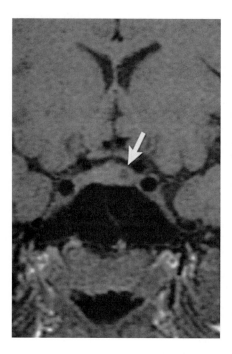
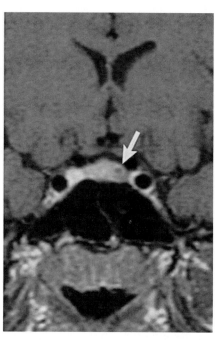

FIGURE 27-2. Coronal T1-weighted precontrast *(left)* and postcontrast *(right)* magnetic resonance image of a microadenoma (prolactinoma) involving the left side of the gland *(arrows)*. The tumor is hyperintense in relationship to the normal gland on precontrast imaging and hypointense compared with the gland on the postcontrast image.

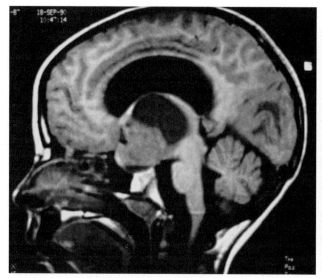
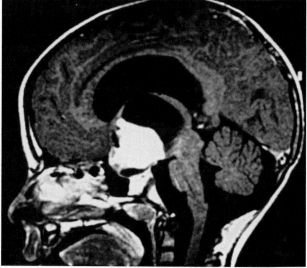

FIGURE 27-3. Sagittal precontrast *(left)* and postcontrast *(right)* magnetic resonance images of a hypothalamic juvenile pilocytic astrocytoma. The solid mass has homogeneous enhancement and the cyst wall does not show enhancement. The sella is expanded by the mass.

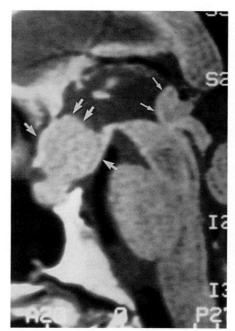
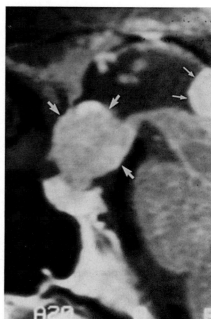

FIGURE 27–4. Sagittal precontrast *(left)* and postcontrast *(right)* magnetic resonance images of a pituitary stalk and pineal gland germinoma. The stalk *(large arrows)* and the pineal region *(small arrows)* masses have strong enhancement and lack cystic components.

solid. Pituitary function and visual field testing should be performed preoperatively, although postoperative endocrine status is more important for patient management because the endocrine profile frequently changes after surgical intervention.[10, 25, 26]

The optimal treatment of craniopharyngiomas remains controversial. Most neurosurgeons agree that gross total resection of a craniopharyngioma is the most desirable operative outcome and offers the best chance of cure.[7, 29, 30] The surgeon's judgment at the time of surgery determines whether an attempt at total removal is justifiable based on the potential for operative mortality and functional impairment. Excellent results with gross total resection have been reported, but in general, mortality rates of 2% to 10% are reported in larger series in which attempts at total removal were made.[10, 25, 26] Recurrence after gross total resection has been reported to be less than 20%.[10, 25, 31, 32] In some reports, partial resection followed by radiotherapy has been as effective as aggressive resection after long-term follow-up.[33–35] Subtotal resection followed by radiotherapy increases survival, prolongs the interval before tumor recurrence, and results in recurrence rates of less than 30%.[20, 29, 36–38] Radiation therapy, particularly in children, carries the risk of radiation necrosis, panhypopituitarism, optic neuropathy, and later, the development of radiation-induced tumors.

Tumor recurrence poses a difficult problem, because attempted complete resection is associated with greater morbidity and mortality,[10] and for this reason most surgeons advocate limited surgery, focusing on debulking or treating cyst recurrence. Treatment of recurrent cysts has included catheter placement and attachment to a reservoir for repeated aspiration, fenestration into sphenoid sinus via a transsphenoidal approach, radiosurgery in selected cases, and intracystic treatment of the cyst wall with instillation of radioisotopes or sclerosing agents (bleomycin).[39–43]

Pituitary Adenomas

Childhood pituitary adenomas constitute 1% to 10% of pediatric brain tumors and 3.6% to 6.0% of all pituitary adenomas treated surgically.[2, 44, 45] The estimated annual incidence of childhood pituitary adenomas ranges from 0.04 to 0.5 per 100,000 depending on the method of survey.[2, 46] Most pituitary adenomas in children present as microadenomas with symptoms associated with pituitary hormone hypersecretion. Unlike in adults, in whom endocrine-inactive tumors constitute more than one third of pituitary adenomas, nonsecreting adenomas are rare in children (3% to 6%) and present clinically as macroadenomas with symptoms of mass effect on adjacent structures (primarily visual defects).[8, 9, 47, 48] Table 27–4 gives the distribution of adenomas encountered in the pediatric population. Among children, occurrences of various adenoma types are age-related. As a generalization, prepubertal children most likely have ACTH-releasing adenomas, whereas older children are more likely to have prolactinomas.[49]

Review of 136 pediatric patients with pituitary adenomas treated by one of us (C.B.W.) indicated that the onset of symptoms, tumor size, and frequency with respect to age varied with the type of adenoma

TABLE 27–3. Presenting Signs and Symptoms in Children with Craniopharyngiomas

	Tomita & McLone[11] (n = 27)	Hoffman et al.[30] (n = 50)	Yasargil et al.[10] (n = 70)*
Median age (range)	8 yr (1–15)	9 yr (1.5–17.5)	NR (1.5–15)
Male to female ratio	13:14	28:22	39:31
Headache (%)	56	68	NR
Visual disturbance (%)	37	48	38
Growth retardation (%)	26	40	46
Obesity (%)	12	18	32
Diabetes insipidus (%)	15	24	35
Hydrocephalus (%)	49	48	36
Delayed puberty (%)	4	14	3
Precocious puberty (%)	8	2	NR

NR, not recorded.
*Series includes primary and recurrent tumors.

TABLE 27–4. Occurrence of Pediatric Adenoma by Secretory Product

	Partington et al.[9] (n = 36)	Dyer et al.[48] (n = 66)	Mindermann & Wilson[8] (n = 136)	Total (n = 238)
Prolactinoma (%)	15 (42)	18 (28)	72 (53)	105 (44)
ACTH-releasing				
Cushing's disease (%)	14 (39)	33 (50)	42 (31)	89 (37)
Nelson's disease (%)	2 (6)	3 (5)	6 (5)	11 (5)
GH-releasing (%)	3 (8)	8 (13)	12 (9)	23 (10)
Endocrine-inactive (%)	2 (5)	4 (6)	4 (3)	10 (4)

ACTH, adrenocorticotropic hormone; GH, growth hormone.

(Fig. 27–5). A summary of the clinical signs and symptoms is presented in Table 27–5. All types of adenomas except for GH-releasing adenomas can cause growth arrest and short stature. Menstrual irregularities are also common symptoms in all adenomas except for those causing Nelson's syndrome.[8] The most common type of pituitary adenoma was a prolactinoma, which occurred in 53% of patients in this series and typically presented in children older than 12 years and in girls.[8] These tumors presented with primary amenorrhea in girls and with gynecomastia and hypogonadism in boys. The size of the tumor correlated directly with the prolactin level. The second most common adenoma in this series was the ACTH-releasing adenoma causing Cushing's disease (31%). These tumors were the most common adenomas in prepubertal children and decreased in frequency with age (see Fig. 27–5). They are the adenoma most often associated with growth arrest and short stature (64%). The adenomas causing Cushing's disease are significantly smaller than all other adenoma types and, rarely, may be associated with multiple coexisting adenomas (4.7%).[44, 47, 50] The least common of the endocrine-active adenomas are GH-releasing, which have a fairly even distribution among the various age groups. These tumors account for only 10% of pituitary adenomas among children. Not surprisingly, rapid growth and acromegalic features are common. Among patients with GH-releasing adenomas, 50% of the girls have menstrual irregularity and 10% of the boys have hypogonadism. Weight gain and precocious puberty may be caused by GH-releasing adenomas.

Endocrine-inactive adenomas account for only 3% of pediatric pituitary adenomas and can cause growth arrest as well as menstrual irregularities secondary to mild elevations of prolactin as a result of stalk compression. These tumors are the largest of all adenomas at presentation and consequently focal neurologic deficits are common.

Surgical Treatment of Pituitary Adenomas

Transsphenoidal resection of pituitary adenomas is safe and has a high potential for cure. Patients with macroadenomas or symptomatic microadenomas should be referred for surgery. Asymptomatic (incidental) and minimally symptomatic microadenomas may also be an indication for surgery because these tumors have the potential to impair pituitary function and invade adjacent tissue as they increase in size. Once a tumor has invaded the cavernous sinus, surgical cure is precluded. With surgical management of pituitary adenomas, outcome varies depending on tumor type.

ACTH-releasing tumors, slightly more common in girls, are the most likely tumors to recur (15% to 25%).[8, 9, 48, 51–53] These tumors are sometimes difficult to identify intraoperatively because of their small size, and preoperative inferior petrosal or cavernous sinus sampling has been performed in some centers on patients with no radiographically lateralizing tumor. For unexplained reasons, negative transsphenoidal exploration of the sella resulted in long-term remissions in 4 of 11 children with Cushing's disease.[8] Hemihypophysectomy, radiation therapy, or adrenalectomy can be used to manage recurrent disease. After pituitary radiotherapy for recurrent Cushing's disease, low-normal adult height may be achievable with GH replacement therapy and additional replacement therapy if needed to restore thyroid and gonadal function.[54] However, the risk of producing or aggravating pituitary insufficiency remains a major drawback to parasellar radiotherapy.

Occurring more frequently in girls and during adolescence,[8, 9, 48] prolactinomas have good surgical outcome, resulting in a cure in 86% to 94% of patients.[8, 48, 55] Medical management of prolactinomas involves treatment with dopamine agonists that can normalize prolactin levels and result in tumor shrinkage.[56] Pharmacologic treatment with bromocriptine in 26 pediatric patients with prolactinomas resulted in normalization of prolactin levels in 5 patients (19%), whereas 21 patients (81%) were intolerant of, or had tumors resistant to, bromocriptine. Quinagolide or cabergoline resulted in prolactin normalization in 15 patients (65%) and 4 patients (15%) remained hyperprolactinemic.[55] Despite dramatic reduction in tumor size in the majority of the patients treated with dopamine agonists, elimination of the tumor has not been reported, and subsequently these patients require lifelong pharmacologic treatment. Although pregnancy has been reported in patients whose prolactinomas were medically managed, we believe that in the pediatric age group definitive treatment with surgery provides an excellent alternative means for allowing conception and delivery.

Among pediatric GH-releasing tumors treated surgically, 83% were cured.[8] A greater degree of invasiveness correlated with a higher recurrence rate for these tumors. For patients for whom surgical management fails, somatostatin analogues provide biochemical normalization of GH levels and insulin-like growth factor-1 (IGF-1)

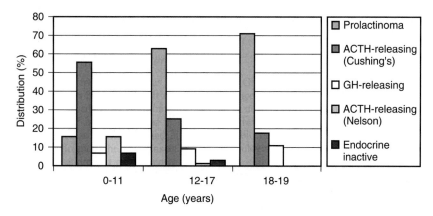

FIGURE 27–5. Age distribution for pediatric pituitary adenomas. ACTH, adrenocorticotropic hormone; GH, growth hormone. (Adapted from Mindermann T, Wilson CB: Pediatric pituitary adenomas. Neurosurgery 36:259–269, 1995.)

TABLE 27–5. Clinical Findings and Tumor Characteristics in Pediatric Adenomas

	Prolactinoma (n = 72)	ACTH-Releasing (Cushing's Disease) (n = 42)	GH-Releasing (n = 12)	ACTH-Releasing (Nelson's Syndrome) (n = 6)	Endocrine-Inactive n = 4 (22)*
Age at onset of symptoms	14.5 ± 2.6	11.9 ± 3.4	13.4 ± 4.8	8.2 ± 3.2	12.5 ± 2.4
Female-male ratio	4.5:1	2:1	1:2	5:1	1:1.5
Median tumor size (mm)	13.8 ± 8.7	5.5 ± 5.8	21.2 ± 9.9	10.6 ± 5.6	35 ± 7
Focal neurologic deficit (%)	18	2	8	0	77
Increased growth (%)	—	—	58	—	—
Short stature (%)	11	64	—	50	18
Cushingoid features (%)	—	91	—	83	—
Primary amenorrhea (%)†	25	—	25	—	10
Secondary amenorrhea (%)†	58	36	—	—	—
Irregular menses (%)†	5	10	25	—	—
Oligomenorrhea (%)†	3	7	—	—	—
Galactorrhea (%)†	36	—	—	—	—
Hypogonadism (%)‡	23	—	13	—	—
Gynecomastia (%)‡	23	7	—	—	—
Delayed puberty (%)	10	7	—	—	23
Precocious puberty (%)	—	5	13	17	—
Weight gain (%)	4	64	13	50	—
Hypertension (%)	—	10	—	17	—
Hyperpigmentation (%)	—	7	—	83	—

ACTH, adrenocorticotropic hormone; GH, growth hormone.
*Combined series with Abe T, Ludecke DK, Saeger W: Clinically nonsecreting pituitary adenomas in childhood and adolescence. Neurosurgery 42:744–751, 1998.
†Among female patients.
‡Among male patients.
Adapted from Mindermann T, Wilson CB: Pediatric pituitary adenomas. Neurosurgery 36:259–269, 1995.

levels in adults,[57, 58] although significant experience in the pediatric population has not been reported.

Finally, in the surgical treatment of clinically endocrine-inactive adenomas, it is critical to adequately decompress neural structures, specifically the optic chiasm. Under appropriate circumstances, curative resection of these tumors can be performed with preservation of remaining pituitary function. Determination of the cell line of origin may be important in the future because medical therapy may be available for certain subgroups.

Optic Pathway and Hypothalamic Gliomas

Optic pathway and hypothalamic gliomas are common in children and constitute 3.6% to over 6.0% of pediatric brain tumors.[3, 59] Tumors can be restricted to the optic nerve (primarily in patients with neurofibromatosis type 1 (NF-1), or involve the chiasm or hypothalamus, or both. Visual symptoms relate to the location of the tumor and range from unilateral visual loss to homonymous visual defects. Frequently, headaches, vomiting, and papilledema accompany tumors involving the hypothalamus associated with raised intracranial pressure secondary to hydrocephalus. When the hypothalamus is involved, children may present with precocious puberty or hypersomnia. Other endocrine abnormalities, such as hyperphagia and diabetes insipidus, are relatively uncommon but may follow radiation therapy. The majority of these tumors are low-grade astrocytomas, and rarely gangliogliomas. About 40% of optic pathway astrocytomas are fibrillary and 60% are pilocytic. Rarely, a malignant optic glioma occurs in a child.[60, 61] Management of optic gliomas of childhood is individualized because the course may vary widely between an indolent hamartoma and a rapidly progressive astrocytoma.[61–63] NF-1 patients with optic nerve gliomas have a better prognosis than patients with gliomas unassociated with neurofibromatosis.[61, 64] Tumors restricted to one orbit that are causing proptosis and significant visual loss can be surgically resected. For more posterior lesions in patients with NF-1 that are not affecting vision, the tumor is followed radiographically, and symptoms are treated with shunting for hydrocephalus and medical therapy for endocrinologic dysfunction. Posteriorly placed tumors in patients without NF-1 or in those who show progression should be treated with resection followed by chemotherapy. In children, radiation therapy is reserved for those tumors in which chemotherapy proves ineffective in arresting progressive clinical deterioration. Treatment of these tumors with surgery, radiation, or chemotherapy results in further endocrine dysfunction in 42% of children.[65] Radiotherapy is significantly associated with GH deficiency, whereas DI, hypoadrenalism, and hypothyroidism are more likely among the complications of aggressive surgery.

Germ Cell Tumors

Primary intracranial germ cell tumors have an incidence of 0.3% to 3.4% of pediatric brain tumors in Western countries and 5% to 15% of pediatric brain tumors in Japan.[66] Intracranial germ cell tumors are separated into germinomas and nongerminomatous germ cell tumors. For germinomas, boys are affected twice as often as girls, whereas in nongerminomatous germ cell tumors, the male-to-female ratio is higher (3.2:1).[67] Most intracranial germ cell tumors are diagnosed in the first and second decades of life, with the peak age of incidence being 11 years. They are most likely to occur in the suprasellar or pineal region. Overall, germinomas and teratomas are the most frequent of the suprasellar germ cell tumors and present with the triad of hypopituitarism, diabetes insipidus, and visual disturbances. Hydrocephalus and precocious puberty may also be present when the hypothalamus is involved. The radiologic appearance of these tumors is not sufficiently distinctive to allow subtyping, and surgical biopsy is often necessary for histologic diagnosis. Serum and cerebrospinal fluid markers may be helpful (the β subunit of human chorionic gonadotropin for embryonal and choriocarcinoma; α-fetoprotein for endodermal sinus tumor) in diagnosis. Germinomas are extremely radiosensitive and long-term survival can be achieved with radiotherapy. However, in young children, chemotherapy should be used as the primary treatment in an effort to limit the intellectual decline associated with radiotherapy in children. Germ cell tumors have a predilection for disseminating within the subarachnoid space, and thus neuraxis staging is essential. Large series have shown survival for patients with intracranial germinoma can be as high as 90% at 10 years.[68, 69] Nongerminomatous germ cell tumors are frequently radioresistant, and patients fare far worse, with a 5-year survival rate that is less than 25%.[38]

Rare Lesions

Other reported parasellar and sellar pediatric lesions include Langerhans' cell histiocytosis (histiocytosis X), involving the pituitary stalk, the hypothalamus, or both, in which patients present with DI and possibly hyperprolactinemia.[5, 70] Meningiomas arising from the sphenoid wing or tuberculum sella may extend into the sella and radiographically mimic a macroadenoma.[71–73] These patients may present with pituitary dysfunction or visual disturbance. Symptomatic Rathke's cleft cysts have also been reported among adolescents and can present with hypopituitarism and growth retardation.[74]

REFERENCES

1. Koos WT, Miller MH: Intracranial Tumors of Infants and Children. Stuttgart, Thieme, 1971.
2. Odom GL, Davis CH, Woodhal B: Brain tumors in children: Clinical analysis of 164 cases. Pediatrics 18:856–869, 1956.
3. Matson DD: Neurosurgery of Infancy and Childhood, ed 2. Springfield IL, Thomas, 1969, p 523.
4. Rueda-Pedraza ME, Heifetz SA, Sesterhenn IA, Clark GB: Primary intracranial germ cell tumors in the first two decades of life. A clinical, light-microscopic, and immunohistochemical analysis of 54 cases. Perspect Pediatr Pathol 10:160–207, 1987.
5. Richmond IL, Wilson CB: Parasellar tumors in children. I. Clinical presentation, preoperative assessment, and differential diagnosis. Childs Brain 7:73–84, 1980.
6. Banna M, Hoare RD, Stanley P, Till K: Craniopharyngioma in children. J Pediatr 83:781–785, 1973.
7. Carmel PW: Craniopharyngiomas. In Wilkins RR, Rengachary SA (eds): Neurosurgery. New York, McGraw-Hill, 1985, pp 905–916.
8. Mindermann T, Wilson CB: Pediatric pituitary adenomas. Neurosurgery 36:259–268, 1995.
9. Partington MD, Davis DH, Laws ER, Scheithauer BW: Pituitary adenomas in childhood and adolescence—Results of transsphenoidal surgery. J Neurosurg 80:209–216, 1994.
10. Yasargil MG, Curcic M, Kis M, et al: Total removal of craniopharyngiomas—Approaches and long-term results in 144 patients. J Neurosurg 73:3–11, 1990.
11. Tomita T, McLone DG: Radical resections of childhood craniopharyngiomas. Pediatr Neurosurg 19:6–14, 1993.
12. Ross DA, Wilson CB: Results of transsphenoidal microsurgery for growth hormone–secreting pituitary adenoma in a series of 214 patients. J Neurosurg 68:854–867, 1988.
13. Li J, Stefaneanu L, Kovacs K, Horvath E, Smyth HS: Growth hormone (GH) and prolactin (PRL) gene expression and immunoreactivity in GH- and PRL-producing human pituitary adenomas. Virchows Arch 422:193–201, 1993.
14. Blodgett FM: Effects of prolonged cortisone therapy on the statural growth, skeletal maturation and metabolic status of children. N Engl J Med 254:636–641, 1956.
15. Karnofsky DA, Ridgway LP: Patterson PA: Growth-inhibiting effect of cortisone acetate on the chick embryo. Endocrinology 48:596–616, 1951.
16. Talbot NB: Endocrine and other factors determining the growth of children. Adv Pediatr 2:238–297, 1947.
17. Van Metre TE, Pinkerton HL: Growth suppression in asthmatic children receiving prolonged therapy with prednisone and methylprednisolone. J Allergy 30:103–113, 1959.
18. Van Metre TE, Niermann WA: Rosen LJ: A comparison of the growth suppressive effect of cortisone, prednisone, and other adrenal cortical hormones. J Allergy 31:531–542, 1960.
19. Wehrenberg WB, et al: Glucocorticoids: Potent inhibitors and stimulators of growth hormone secretion. Endocrinology 126:3200–3203, 1990.
20. Tomita T: Management of craniopharyngiomas in children. Pediatr Neurosci 14:204–211, 1988.
21. Kollias SS, Barkovich AJ, Edwards MS: Magnetic resonance analysis of suprasellar tumors of childhood. Pediatr Neurosurg 17:284–303, 1991.
22. Mott FW, Barrett JOW: Three cases of tumor of the third ventricle. Arch Neurol 1:417–440, 1999.
23. Carmel PW: Brain Tumors of Disordered Embryogenesis. In Youmans J (ed): Neurological Surgery. Philadelphia, WB Saunders, 1996, pp 2761–2781.
24. Carmel PW, Antunes JL, Chang CH: Craniopharyngiomas in children. Neurosurgery 11:382–389, 1982.
25. Adamson TE, Weistler OD, Kleihues P, Yasargil MG: Correlation of clinical and pathological features in surgically treated craniopharyngiomas. J Neurosurg 73:12–17, 1990.
26. Weiner HL, Wisoff JH, Rosenberg ME, et al: Craniopharyngiomas—a clinicopathological analysis of factors predictive of recurrence and functional outcome. Neurosurgery 35:1001–1010, 1994.
27. Roth C, Wilken B, Hanefeld F, et al: Hyperphagia in children with craniopharyngioma is associated with hyperleptinaemia and a failure in the downregulation of appetite. Eur Endocrinol 138:89–91, 1998.
28. Brabant G, Horn R, Mayr B, et al: Serum leptin levels following hypothalamic surgery. Horm Metab Res 28:728–731, 1996.
29. Amacher AL: Craniopharyngioma: The controversy regarding radiotherapy. Childs Brain 6:57–64, 1980.
30. Hoffman HJ, De Silva M, Humphreys RP, et al: Aggressive surgical management of craniopharyngiomas in children. J Neurosurg 76:47–52, 1992.

31. Hoffman HJ: Craniopharyngiomas. Can J Neurol Sci 12:348–352, 1985.
32. Hoffman HJ: Craniopharyngiomas. Prog Exp Tumor Res 30:325–334, 1987.
33. Baskin DS, Wilson CB: Surgical management of craniopharyngiomas. A review of 74 cases. J Neurosurg 65:22–27, 1986.
34. Wen BC, Hussey DH, Staples J, et al: A comparison of the roles of surgery and radiation therapy in the management of craniopharyngiomas. Int J Radiat Oncol Biol Phys 16:17–24, 1989.
35. Weiss M, Sutton L, Marcial V, et al: The role of radiation therapy in the management of childhood craniopharyngioma. Int J Radiat Oncol Biol Phys 17:1313–1321, 1989.
36. Hoff JT, Patterson RH Jr: Craniopharyngiomas in children and adults. J Neurosurg 36:299–302, 1972.
37. Kramer D: Craniopharyngioma: The best treatment is conservative surgery and postoperative radiation therapy. In Morley TP (ed): Current Controversies in Neurosurgery. Philadelphia, WB Saunders, 1976, pp 336–343.
38. Richmond IL, Wilson CB: Parasellar tumors in children. II. Surgical management, radiation therapy, and follow-up. Childs Brain 7:85–94, 1980.
39. Backlund EO, Axelsson B, Bergstrand CG, et al: Treatment of craniopharyngiomas—the stereotactic approach in a ten to twenty-three years' perspective. I. Surgical, radiological and ophthalmological aspects. Acta Neurochir (Wien) 99:11–19, 1989.
40. Julow J, Lányi F, Hajda M, et al: The radiotherapy of cystic craniopharyngioma with intracystic instillation of ⁹⁰Y silicate colloid. Acta Neurochir (Wien) 74:94–99, 1985.
41. Julow J, Lányi F, Hajda M, et al: Further experiences in the treatment of cystic craniopharyngiomas with yttrium 90 silicate colloid. Acta Neurochir Suppl (Wien) 42:113–119, 1988.
42. Kobayashi T, Kageyama N, Ohara K: Internal irradiation for cystic craniopharyngioma. J Neurosurg 55:896–903, 1981.
43. Kodama T, Matsukado Y, Uemura S: Intracapsular irradiation therapy of craniopharyngiomas with radioactive gold: Indication and follow-up results. Neurol Med Chir (Tokyo) 21:49–58, 1981.
44. Laws ER, Scheithauer BW, Groover RV: Pituitary adenomas in childhood and adolescence. Prog Exp Tumor Res 30:359–361, 1987.
45. Lüdecke DK, Herrmann HD, Schulte FJ: Special problems with neurosurgical treatments of hormone-secreting pituitary adenomas in children. Prog Exp Tumor Res 30:362–370, 1987.
46. Annegers JF, Coulam CB, Abboud CF, et al: Pituitary adenoma in Olstead County, Minnesota, 1935–1977. A report of an increasing incidence of diagnosis in women of childbearing age. Mayo Clin Proc 53:641–643, 1978.
47. Mindermann T, Wilson CB: Pituitary adenomas in childhood and adolescence. J Pediatr Endocrinol Metab 8:79–83, 1995.
48. Dyer EH, Civit T, Visot A, et al: Transsphenoidal surgery for pituitary adenomas in children. Neurosurgery 34:207–212, 1994.
49. Mindermann T, Wilson CB: Age-related and gender-related occurrence of pituitary adenomas. Clin Endocrinol 41:359–364, 1994.
50. Kane LA, Leinung MC, Scheithauer BW, et al: Pituitary adenomas in childhood and adolescence. J Clin Endocrinol Metab 79:1135–1140, 1994.
51. Knappe UJ, Ludecke DK: Transnasal microsurgery in children and adolescents with Cushing's disease. Neurosurgery 39:484–492, 1996.
52. Magiakou MA, Mastorakos G, Oldfield EH, et al: Cushing's syndrome in children and adolescents—Presentation, diagnosis, and therapy. N Engl J Med 331:629–636, 1994.
53. Devoe DJ, Miller WL, Conte FA, et al: Long-term outcome in children and adolescents after transsphenoidal surgery for Cushing's disease. J Clin Endocrinol Metab 82:3196–3202, 1997.
54. Johnston LB, Grossmann AB, Plowman PN, et al: Normal final height and apparent cure after pituitary irradiation for Cushing's disease in childhood: Long-term follow-up of anterior pituitary function. Clin Endocrinol 48:663–667, 1998.
55. Colao A, Loche S, Cappa M, et al: Prolactinomas in children and adolescents. Clinical presentation and long-term follow-up. J Clin Endocrinol Metab 83:2777–2780, 1998.
56. Molitch ME, Thorner MO, Wilson C: Management of prolactinomas. J Clin Endocrinol Metab 82:996–1000, 1997.
57. Newman CB, Melmed S, George A, et al: Octreotide as primary therapy for acromegaly [see comments]. J Clin Endocrinol Metab 83:3034–3040, 1998.
58. Davies PH, Stewart SE, Lancranjan L, et al: Long-term therapy with long-acting octreotide (Sandostatin-LAR) for the management of acromegaly [erratum appears in Clin Endocrinol (Oxf) 48:673, 1998]. Clin Endocrinol 48:311–316, 1998.
59. Hoffman HJ: Optic pathway gliomas. In Amador LU (ed): Brain Tumors in the Young. Springfield IL, Thomas, 1983, pp 622–643.
60. McCullough DC, Johnson DL: Optic nerve gliomas and other tumors involving the optic nerve and chiasm. In McLaurin RL (ed): Pediatric Neurosurgery. Philadelphia, WB Saunders, 1989, pp 391–397.
61. Hoffman HJ, Humphreys RP, Drake JM, et al: Optic pathway hypothalamic gliomas—a dilemma in management. Pediatr Neurosurg 19:186–195, 1993.
62. Imes RK, Hoyt WF: Childhood chiasmal gliomas. Update on the fate of patients in the 1969 San Francisco Study. Prog Exp Tumor Res 30:108–112, 1987.
63. Hoyt WF, Baghdassarian SA: Optic glioma of childhood. Natural history and rationale for conservative management. Br J Ophthalmol 53:793–798, 1969.
64. Stern J, DiGiacinto GV, Housepian EM: Neurofibromatosis and optic glioma: Clinical and morphological correlations. Neurosurgery 4:524–528, 1979.
65. Collett-Solberg PF, Sernyak H, SatinSmith M, et al: Endocrine outcome in long-term survivors of low-grade hypothalamic/chiasmatic glioma. Clin Endocrinol 47:79–85, 1997.
66. Hoffman HJ, Otsubo H, Hendrick EB, et al: Intracranial germ-cell tumors in children. J Neurosurg 74:545–551, 1991.
67. Jennings MT, Gelman R, Hochberg F: Intracranial germ-cell tumors: Natural history and pathogenesis. J Neurosurg 63:155–167, 1985.
68. Neuwelt EA, Frenkel EP, Smith RG: Suprasellar germinomas (ectopic pinealomas):

Aspects of immunological characterization and successful chemotherapeutic responses in recurrent disease. Neurosurgery 7:352–358, 1980.

69. Uematsu Y, Tsuura Y, Miyamoto K, et al: The recurrence of primary intracranial germinomas. Special reference to germinoma with STGC (syncytiotrophoblastic giant cell). J Neurooncol 13:247–256, 1992.

70. Nishio S, Mizuno J, Barrow DL, et al: Isolated histiocytosis X of the pituitary gland: Case report. Neurosurgery 21:718–721, 1987.

71. Taylor SL, Barakos JA, Harsh GRt, Wilson CB: Magnetic resonance imaging of tuberculum sellae meningiomas: Preventing preoperative misdiagnosis as pituitary macroadenoma. Neurosurgery 31:621–627, 1992.

72. Germano IM, Edwards MS, Davis RL, Schiffer D: Intracranial meningiomas of the first two decades of life. J Neurosurg 80:447–453, 1994.

73. Drake JM, Hoffman HJ: Meningiomas in childhood, *In* Al-Mefty O (ed): Meningiomas. New York, Raven Press, 1991, pp 145–152.

74. Voelker JL, Campbell RL, Muller J: Clinical, radiographic, and pathological features of symptomatic Rathke's cleft cysts. J Neurosurg 74:535–544, 1991.

Chapter 28

Vasopressin, Diabetes Insipidus, and Syndrome of Inappropriate Antidiuresis

Peter H. Baylis

SYNTHESIS AND METABOLISM OF VASOPRESSIN

Vasopressin, the antidiuretic hormone of most vertebrates, is the major determinant of renal solute-free water excretion and therefore plays a central role in the maintenance of water balance.

History and Background

In 1895, Oliver and Schäfer[1] reported potent hypertensive effects of fresh pituitary gland extracts injected intravenously into mammals; the pressor activity was subsequently shown to reside solely in the neurohypophysis.[2] The renal effects of posterior pituitary extracts were described later by Schäfer.[3] Profound polyuria caused by mechanical injury to dog pituitaries was reversed by injection of pituitary extracts. The discovery of pituitary extract efficacy in the treatment of patients with diabetes insipidus is attributed to two independent workers.[4, 5]

The chemical structure of arginine vasopressin (AVP), found in most mammals (Table 28–1), was elucidated in du Vigneaud's laboratory and synthesized within a few months of its discovery.[6] It is a nonapeptide, molecular weight 1084 Da, and a strongly basic molecule (isoelectric point pH 10.9).[7] Lysine vasopressin is the antidiuretic hormone of the pig family. Biologic activity is readily destroyed by oxidation or reduction of the disulfide bond.[8] Nonmammalian species

have a variety of nonapeptides related closely to vasopressin and oxytocin (see Table 28–1). Single nucleotide changes account for most of the amino acid substitutions, which tend to occur at positions 3, 4, and 8. Thus, considerable structural uniformity is conserved, which has led to the hypothesis that a single ancestral gene evolved along two evolutionary lines, one being vasotocin-vasopressin and the other isotocin-mesotocin-oxytocin.[9] Some recent evidence, however, indicates that multiple genes may encode numerous vasopressin-like hormones.[10]

Molecular Biology

AVP is derived from a large 145–amino acid precursor molecule comprising a signal peptide, AVP, AVP-specific neurophysin, and a glycosylated moiety[11] (Fig. 28–1). Sequence analysis of the genes encoding the bovine AVP precursor molecule and recombinant DNA techniques have confirmed the structure of the AVP-neurophysin complex.[11] The gene for this complex is located on chromosome 20 and is linked closely to the oxytocin gene separated by only 11 kilobases.[12] The gene has three exons encoding the AVP-neurophysin complex, which are separated by two introns (see Fig. 28–1). In all species analyzed at the DNA level thus far, the part of neurophysin moiety is highly conserved.

Studies on the regulation of mammalian AVP gene suggest a close

TABLE 28–1. Amino Acid Sequences of Arginine Vasopressin and Related Neurohypophysial Nonapeptides

	1	2	3	4	5	6	7	8	9	Distribution
Arginine vasopressin	Cys-Tyr-Phe-Glu(NH₂)-Asp(NH₂)-Cys-Pro-Arg-Gly(NH₂)									Most mammals
Lysine vasopressin			Phe	Glu(NH₂)				Lys		Pig family
Arginine vasotocin			Ile	Glu(NH₂)				Arg		Nonmammalian vertebrates
Oxytocin			Ile	Glu(NH₂)				Leu		Mammals, birds
Mesotocin			Ile	Glu(NH₂)				Ile		Reptiles
Isotocin			Ile	Ser				Ile		Fish
Glumitocin			Ile	Ser				Glu(NH₂)		Fish
Valitocin			Ile	Glu(NH₂)				Val		Fish
Aspartocin			Ile	Asp(NH₂)				Leu		Fish

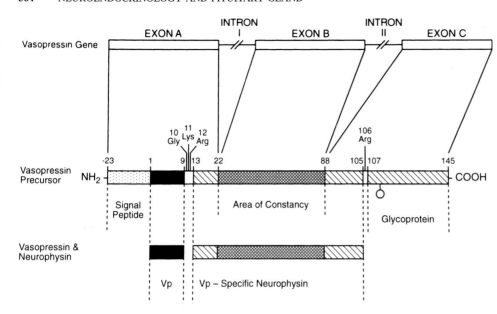

FIGURE 28–1. Bovine vasopressin gene, vasopressin precursor molecule, and AVP with its specific neurophysin. Three exons code for the precursor molecule, which comprises a signal protein, AVP hormone, AVP-specific neurophysin, and a glycoprotein moiety, coupled by amino acids. (Adapted from Land H, Schütz G, Schmale H, Richter D: Nucleotide sequence of cloned cDNA encoding for bovine arginine vasopressin-neurophysin II precursor. Nature 295:299–303, 1982.)

correlation with the expression of oxytocin in some animals. Osmotic salt loading not only causes dramatic accumulation of AVP mRNA in the neurohypophysis[13] and upregulation of the AVP gene but also concomitantly increases oxytocin gene transcription.[14] Conversely, lactation triggers transcription of both oxytocin and vasopressin genes.[15] In rats, AVP and oxytocin genes are expressed in separate groups of hypothalamic neurons, each specific for either vasopressin or oxytocin. Expression of the AVP gene has been observed in extrahypothalamic tissues, such as adrenal gland, gonads, cerebellum, and probably the pituicytes of the posterior pituitary gland.[16]

Studies in lower vertebrates (e.g., teleost fish) suggest that at least two genes encode the vasotocin precursor, the counterpart of the mammalian AVP precursor.[16] A second AVP gene would be convenient to explain the observation that the Brattleboro rat (genetically deficient in hypothalamic AVP) has normal concentrations of AVP in peripheral tissues.[17] It is well recognized that the Brattleboro rat has a single nucleotide deletion in the portion of the hypothalamic gene encoding the AVP-specific neurophysin, which causes a frame shift in the translation product, leading to intracellular degradation of the mutant AVP precursor.[18]

Biosynthesis and Metabolism

Synthesis of the AVP precursor occurs principally in the hypothalamic neurons of the supraoptic and paraventricular nuclei. As the precursor complex migrates along the neuronal axons at a rate of about 2 mm/hour, it undergoes specific cleavage, and the products that include AVP are stored as neurosecretory granules in the posterior pituitary.[19] Release of AVP from the neural lobe is associated with an increase in the rate of phasic firing of electrical impulses.[20] Exocytosis of AVP is calcium dependent. Only a percentage of the peptides are ever released, as some AVP-containing neurosecretory granules migrate from the nerve endings as a result of an aging process and their contents become unavailable for release.[21]

AVP and its specific neurophysin are co-secreted into the systemic circulation in equimolar quantities.[22] Apart from acting as a transport protein for AVP in the neuronal axons, neurophysin appears to serve no other biologic function. The half-life of AVP in the blood volume is about 5 to 15 minutes.[23] After release from the neurohypophysis, AVP circulates unbound to proteins in the blood[23] but does bind to platelet receptors, causing platelet-rich AVP plasma concentrations to be about fivefold higher than those of platelet-depleted plasma.[24]

At least four main sites of enzymatic cleavage have been identified on the AVP molecule.[23] During pregnancy and the immediate postpartum period, an extremely active cysteine aminopeptidase or vasopres-

sinase (E.C.3.4.11.3) of placental syncytiotrophoblastic origin degrades AVP rapidly.[23]

NEUROANATOMY

The posterior lobe of the pituitary gland is an extension of the forebrain. Vasopressor activities from the neurohypophysis have been detected as early as the 10th week of gestation[25] in humans. At birth, the weight of the whole pituitary gland is approximately 100 mg, and it attains an adult human weight of about 600 mg, 20% of which is contributed by the posterior lobe.[26]

Figure 28–2 shows the neuroanatomic relationships of the posterior pituitary in humans. The major site of AVP synthesis is in the magnocellular neurons of the supraoptic and paraventricular nuclei; additional magnocellular neurons containing AVP are found in and near the hypothalamus. Smaller neurons (parvocellular) synthesizing AVP are present in the suprachiasmatic and paraventricular nuclei.[27] Three major vasopressinergic neuronal projections arise from the supraoptic and paraventricular nuclei. The principal pathway originates mainly from the supraoptic nucleus and travels to the posterior lobe; another important pathway terminates in the zona externa of the median eminence, these fibers arising from the medial parvocellular paraventricular nucleus.[27] Extrahypothalamic vasopressinergic neurons project to the forebrain, brain stem, and spinal cord, most of which originate from the paraventricular nucleus.[28, 29] Complex neuronal interconnections exist among paraventricular and supraoptic nuclei and the brain stem nuclei, the nucleus of tractus solitarius, and the locus caeruleus, via dorsal and ventral ascending noradrenergic bundles.

Release of AVP is controlled and modulated by a series of sensory influences. Osmotic regulation is mediated by putative osmoreceptors, anatomically distinct from the supraoptic and paraventricular nuclei. They are located in the anterior circumventricular structures, probably in the organum vasculosum of the lamina terminalis, the subfornical organ, or the anteroventral third ventricle (AV3V) region.[30, 31] The appreciation of thirst, although a cortical function, depends on osmotically sensitive nuclei situated in the anterior or lateral hypothalamus and the integrity of neuronal pathways projecting to the ventromedial nucleus.[30, 31] It is probable that osmoreceptors for thirst are distinct from AVP osmoreceptors. Baroregulatory influences on vasopressin-synthesizing neurons arise from peripheral high- and low-pressure receptors located in the arch of the aorta, the carotid vessels, the atria of the heart, and the great veins within the thorax.[32] Afferent fibers in the vagus and glossopharyngeal nerves terminate in the brain stem nuclei, sensory information then being passed to the AVP neurons in the hypothalamus.

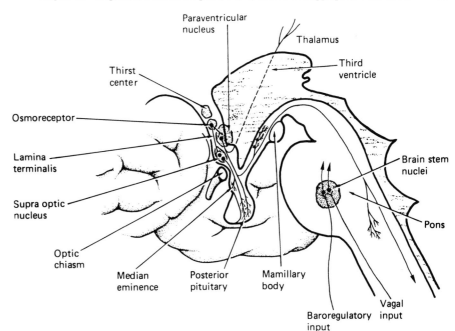

FIGURE 28–2. Schematic representation of hypothalamus, posterior pituitary, and surrounding structures. Major neuronal tracts arise from the supraoptic and paraventricular nuclei, which pass to the posterior lobe of the pituitary, the median eminence, the brain stem and spinal cord, and the forebrain. Afferent fibers to these nuclei originate from the osmoreceptors and baroreceptors, the latter passing via brain stem nuclei.

CONTROL OF SECRETION

Neurotransmitters

Two major classes of substances, the biogenic amines and peptides, act as neurotransmitters that regulate the secretion of AVP.[33] Catecholamines certainly influence AVP secretion. Dopamine is the most abundant amine to be found in the neurohypophysis, together with both D_1 and D_2 receptors. Although evidence indicates that dopamine may act as an inhibitory neurotransmitter in the posterior pituitary, it is a potent stimulant of AVP from rat hypothalami.[34] Dopamine appears to be involved in the release of AVP after nausea and/or emesis,[33] but data conflict on whether cerebral dopamine stimulates or inhibits osmoregulated AVP secretion.[34, 35] Norepinephrine has been found in the supraoptic and paraventricular nuclei by histochemical and immunocytochemical techniques.[36] Central norepinephrine fibers stimulate AVP release via α_1 receptors.[37] Comprehensive studies by Schrier and colleagues[38] provide clear evidence for hemodynamic roles for α- and β-adrenergic agonists, causing inhibition and stimulation of neurohypophysial AVP, respectively.

Acetylcholine is also present in both supraoptic and paraventricular nuclei. Although data that acetylcholine stimulates basal and enhances osmoregulated AVP secretion are unequivocal, controversy remains about whether its action is mediated by the muscarinic or nicotinic receptors.[33]

Excitatory amino acids, glutamate, and aspartate play an important role as mediators of excitatory transmission in the central nervous system and influence osmoregulated vasopressin release and mRNA content of the neurohypophysis.[39] Recent evidence suggests that *N*-methyl-D-aspartic acid receptors play a role in osmotic control of vasopressin secretion and may mediate the inhibitory effect of estrogen on vasopressin release in the rat.[40]

The peptide angiotensin II enhances osmotically stimulated AVP secretion from the posterior pituitary when administered by peripheral infusion or intracerebroventricular injection. Its site of action is either the organum vasculosum of the lamina terminalis[41] or the subfornical organ,[42] which are both putative sites for the osmoreceptor.

Interleukin-1β (IL-1β), a cytokine, has numerous physiologic and pathophysiologic effects, which include the stimulation of vasopressin and oxytocin in the rat.[43] It has been realized that a complex interrelationship exists among IL-1β, prostaglandin, and α-adrenergic mechanisms, which influence rat vasopressin secretion.[44, 45]

Rat studies suggest that atrial natriuretic peptide inhibits AVP secretion[46] by acting on the subfornical organ, but there is little evidence in

humans that circulating physiologic concentrations have an influence on osmoregulated AVP release.[47] Recent work indicates that brain natriuretic peptide inhibits the activity of the supraoptic neurons and those in the AV3V region of the anterior hypothalamus.[48]

Opioid peptides also influence AVP secretion. Leu-enkephalin is present in the supraoptic and paraventricular nuclei and in the nerve terminals containing AVP in the neurohypophysis.[49] The consensus is that the enkephalins and β-endorphin inhibit AVP secretion, probably via a κ opioid receptor.[50, 51]

Many other substances have been implicated in the neurotransmitter control of AVP (steroids, prostaglandins, serotonin, γ-aminobutyric acid [GABA]), but their physiologic significance remains to be determined.[33]

Osmoregulation

After a series of elegant studies on dogs, Verney[52] in 1947 first proposed the concept that secretion of AVP is regulated by the osmolality of body water. He concluded that intracranial osmoreceptors very sensitive to changes in blood sodium concentration and other solutes control AVP release. Initial confirmation of Verney's proposals came from bioassay techniques.[53] Recent studies[54–56] from a variety of laboratories have clearly demonstrated the exquisitely sensitive relationship between plasma osmolality and AVP concentrations. In healthy adults, the infusion of concentrated saline (855 mmol/L) to steadily increase plasma osmolality results in a progressive rise in peripheral plasma AVP concentrations. Although pulsatile release of AVP can be detected in the internal jugular vein, no evidence exists of minute-to-minute fluctuation in AVP concentration in peripheral veins.[57] A direct correlation exists between the two variables (Fig. 28–3), which is defined by the following function:

$$pAVP = 0.43 (pOs - 284), r = +0.96, P < 0.001$$

where pAVP indicates plasma AVP concentration, and pOs indicates plasma osmolality. The abscissal intercept, 284 mOsm/kg, indicates the plasma osmolality at which plasma AVP starts to increase, thus providing a measure of the set of the osmoreceptor mechanism or the osmotic threshold for AVP release. Whether AVP secretion can be completely suppressed remains unclear,[58] but using an exquisitely sensitive cytochemical method to measure plasma AVP levels, the secretion of AVP could not be switched off by hypotonicity.[59] Nevertheless, the concept of a threshold of AVP release remains a pragmatic

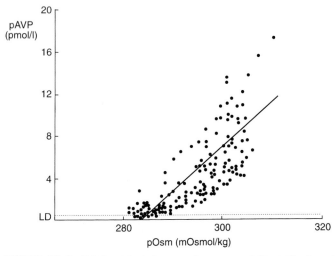

FIGURE 28–3. *Relationship between plasma osmolality (pOsm) and plasma AVP (pAVP) levels. Increases in plasma AVP levels in response to hypertonicity induced by infusion of 855 mmol/L of saline in a group of healthy adults. The mean regression line (dashed line) is defined by pAVP = 0.43 (pOs − 284); r = +0.96; P < 0.001. LD represents the limit of detection of the assay, 0.3 pmol/L. (Adapted from Thompson CJ: Polyuric states in man. In Baylis PH (ed): Water and Salt Homeostasis in Health and Disease. London, Bailliére Tindall, 1989, pp 473–497.)*

means to characterize osmoregulatory function and analyze disorders of osmoregulation.[56] The slope of the regression line reflects the sensitivity or gain of the osmoreceptor–AVP releasing unit. Estimates of osmoreceptor gain and threshold for AVP release obtained by indirect methods of assessing AVP concentrations by measuring urine osmolality correspond well to the above values.[60] Fast rates of hypertonic saline infusion result in exaggerated AVP responses,[54] thereby creating a curvilinear relationship between plasma AVP and plasma osmolality. Complete disconnection of AVP-secreting neurons from their osmoreceptors appears to cause persistent low-grade AVP release, resulting in plasma AVP values about 1.0 pmol/L.[61] Thus, AVP secretion is increased from this "basal" rate by stimulation of facilitatory osmoreceptor cells but is decreased to minimal values by activation of inhibitory cells.

Despite considerable variations in osmoreceptor sensitivity and threshold for AVP release between individuals, these constants remain unchanged within an individual tested over a short period of time.[62] Recent studies have shown that the constants for slope and threshold are similar in monozygotic twins, suggesting a genetic determinant for the set of the osmoregulatory system.[63] Pregnancy causes a lowering of the threshold for AVP secretion without alteration of the gain of the osmoreceptor in both rats[64] and humans,[65] which accounts for the hypo-osmolality of pregnancy. In the luteal phase of the normal human ovulatory menstrual cycle, a small but significant fall in plasma osmolality occurs as a result of lowering of thresholds for thirst and vasopressin release.[66]

The response of the osmoreceptor to solutes other than sodium chloride is variable. In the presence of insulin, moderate hyperglycemia fails to stimulate AVP secretion,[67] but insulinopenic rats do release AVP following severe hyperglycemia.[68] Furthermore, urea has about one third the stimulatory effect on AVP release than that of sodium chloride,[67] and alcohol suppresses AVP secretion.[69] As plasma AVP level rises, antidiuresis and urinary concentration increase. At plasma concentrations of immunoreactive AVP of 0.5 pmol/L or less, maximum diuresis occurs (Fig. 28–4). In response to rising plasma osmolality from 284 mOsm/kg (osmotic threshold for AVP release), plasma AVP concentration rises progressively to achieve increases in urinary concentration. When plasma osmolality exceeds, on average, 295 mOsm/kg of plasma AVP attains about 3 to 4 pmol/L, producing maximum antidiuresis. Greater hyperosmolality, although releasing more AVP, fails to conserve any more renal water, which exposes the body to potentially severe dehydration if fluid is not ingested. This is

avoided in healthy individuals by the stimulation of thirst to promote drinking.[54, 70] The intake of fluid results in lowering of plasma osmolality to levels at which renal water excretion can again be regulated by changes in AVP secretion (i.e., <295 mOsm/kg). In a healthy individual who has elevated plasma AVP concentration due to osmotic stimulation, the act of drinking causes a precipitous fall in plasma AVP shortly after drinking copious amounts of fluid, resulting in lowered plasma AVP but still elevated plasma osmolality[71] (Fig. 28–3). An oropharyngeal reflex is probably responsible for this observation. If fluid volumes greater than those demanded by thirst are consumed, then AVP secretion is suppressed to very low levels (<0.3 pmol/L), at which stage the kidney is capable of excreting 15 to 20 L of urine in 24 hours. Only ingestion of fluid volumes in excess of this results in further lowering of plasma osmolality in healthy adults. It can therefore be appreciated that the osmoregulatory system for thirst and AVP secretion maintains plasma osmolality within the narrow limits of about 284 to 295 mOsm/kg.

The aging process has a considerable effect on osmoregulation and fluid and electrolyte homeostasis.[72] In contrast to many other hormonal systems, basal circulating vasopressin concentrations increase with age[73]; furthermore, an enhanced response of vasopressin release to osmotic stimulation seems to occur.[74] Thirst appreciation, however, is blunted, and fluid intake is reduced.[75] The renal response to fluid overload is decreased, and maximum renal concentrating ability is depressed with aging, exposing the elderly to enhanced risks of both hyponatremia and hypernatremia.[76, 77]

Baroregulation

Blood volume and pressure are widely recognized as having an influence on AVP secretion. Early work in sheep suggested that reductions of at least 10% were necessary to increase antidiuretic activity.[78] In humans, falls in arterial blood pressure on the order of 5% to 10% are necessary to significantly increase circulating immunoreactive AVP concentrations (Fig. 28–5).[79] In contrast to the simple linear correlation between plasma osmolality and plasma AVP, the pressure-AVP relationship is exponential. Changes in blood volume are mediated by low-pressure receptors in the left atrium and great veins within the

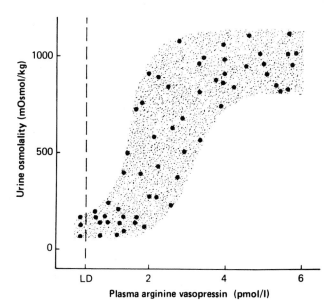

FIGURE 28–4. *Relationship between plasma AVP and urine osmolality during water load and fluid restriction in a group of healthy adults. Maximum urine concentration is achieved by plasma AVP values greater than 3 to 4 pmol/L. LD represents the limit of detection of the assay, 0.3 pmol/L. (From Baylis PH, Robertson GL: Physiological control of vasopressin secretion. In Baylis PH, Padfield PL (eds): The Posterior Pituitary: Hormone Secretion in Health and Disease. New York, Marcel Dekker, 1985, pp 119–139.)*

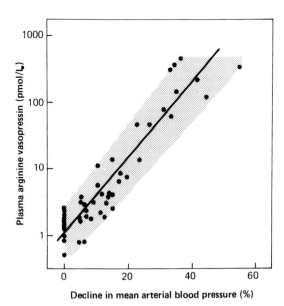

FIGURE 28–5. Relationship of plasma AVP to the percentage decline in mean arterial blood pressure (MABP) induced by infusion of increasing doses of trimethaphan in healthy man. The regression line is defined by log (pAVP) = 0.06 (MABP + 0.67), r = +0.98, P < 0.001, n = 48. (From Baylis PH: Posterior pituitary function in health and disease. Clin Endocrinol Metab 12:747–770, 1983.)

chest, whereas arterial blood pressure regulation is mediated by baroreceptors situated in the arch of the aorta and the carotid walls.[80] Recent evidence suggests that ventricular receptors may also be involved in baroregulation.[81]

Baroregulation of AVP does not operate in isolation; responses are modified by neurohumoral influences. Atrial natriuretic peptides appear to inhibit baroregulated AVP responses, whereas norepinephrine augments responses.[82] Similarly, an interrelationship exists between osmoregulatory and baroregulatory AVP secretion such that the AVP osmoregulatory line is shifted to the left of normal as hypovolemia develops.[83, 84] Thus, under conditions of moderate hypovolemia, osmoregulation is preserved around a lower set-point of plasma osmolality (Fig. 28–6).[83] As hypovolemia becomes more severe, very high plasma AVP values are attained that override the osmoregulatory system.

Other Regulatory Mechanisms

Nausea and emesis are potent stimuli to AVP secretion. In primates, circulating AVP values in excess of 500 pmol/L have been recorded[85, 86]

that are independent of osmotic and hemodynamic input. Traction on the intestines during surgery, for example, is a similar powerful nonosmotic stimulus to AVP release.[87] Both phenomena probably contribute to the high plasma AVP values observed after gastrointestinal surgery and cause hyponatremia if excess fluid is administered in the postoperative period.

Neuroglycopenia is another independent stimulus to AVP secretion, but plasma values attained are only moderate, up to about 6 pmol/L.[88] Whether AVP is a true stress hormone remains controversial.

THIRST

For many decades a "thirst center" has been postulated,[52] but only in the last few years has it been located to the anterior hypothalamic structures, the organum vasculosum of the lamina terminalis, the AV3V region, or the subfornical organ.[89] Whether they are sodium sensors or respond to total osmotic change is not clear.[90] Little doubt exists, however, that thirst is an extremely powerful sensation that drives the seeking and ingestion of water.

A major experimental obstacle has been quantitation of thirst sensation, but recent work in humans using visual analogue scales has overcome the problem to an extent. In contrast to previous concepts, it is now apparent that a simple linear correlation exists between thirst and plasma osmolality, and small changes in blood tonicity are readily appreciated by thirst.[70] A function defining the relationship between thirst and plasma osmolality can be derived as follows:

$$\text{Th} = 0.39 \, (\text{pOsm} - 285), r = +0.95, P < 0.001$$

where Th indicates thirst, and pOsm indicates plasma osmolality. The abscissal intercept, 285 mOsm/kg, represents the osmotic threshold for thirst perception (Fig. 28–7), which is statistically no different from the threshold for AVP release. Despite wide individual variations in the value of the thirst osmotic threshold, it remains remarkably consistent within individuals.[62] Indeed, the functional characteristics of the osmoregulatory lines for AVP release and thirst are very similar. Drinking causes a dramatic fall in osmotically stimulated thirst analogue scores identical to the rapid decline in circulating AVP concentrations.[71]

In addition, thirst can be stimulated by extracellular volume depletion. Underfill of the low-pressure thoracic circulation leads to drinking in animals,[91] an effect probably mediated by the left atrium via the vagus nerve. Angiotensin II is a powerful dipsogen that is present in

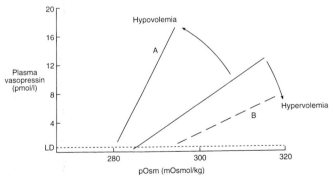

FIGURE 28–6. The effect of hypovolemia and hypervolemia on the slope and osmotic threshold of the osmoregulatory line for vasopressin, expressed diagrammatically. Osmoregulatory lines based on rat data are represented by solid lines. The position of the *dashed line* is the estimated osmoregulatory response with hypervolemia. (Adapted from data of Dunn FL, Brennan TJ, Nelson AE, Robertson GL: The role of blood osmolality and volume in regulating vasopressin secretion in the rat. J Clin Invest 52:3212–3219, 1973.)

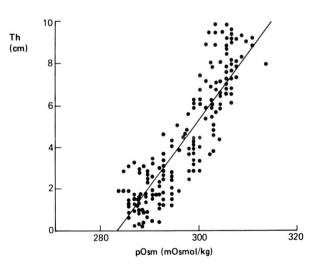

FIGURE 28–7. Relationship between thirst (Th) and plasma osmolality (pOsm) during a hypertonic saline (855 mmol/L) infusion in a group of healthy adults. The mean regression line is defined by Th = 0.39 (pOsm − 285), r = +0.95, P < 0.001. (Adapted from Thompson CJ: Polyuric states in man. *In* Baylis PH (ed): Water and Salt Homeostasis in Health and Disease. London, Bailliére Tindall, 1989, pp 473–497.)

the anterior circumventricular organs but may also act as a peripheral agent, having been generated in the circulation from angiotensinogen by the action of renin released by an underperfused kidney.[92, 93] The effect of aging on thirst and fluid intake has been discussed above.

ACTIONS OF VASOPRESSIN

The effects of AVP are mediated by two major classes of receptor (Table 28–2).[94] The V_1 receptor is coupled to phospholipase C and thus increases the turnover of the inositol phosphates and diacylglycerol and allows the influx of Ca^{2+} to raise intracellular Ca^{2+} concentrations. This receptor is subdivided into V_{1a} and V_{1b} because the binding properties of the pituitary corticotrope (V_{1b}) to a variety of vasopressin agonists and antagonists differ from those of other V_1 receptor tissues. The rat V_{1a} AVP receptor has recently been cloned in hepatocytes and has seven transmembrane domains.[95] The V_2 receptor is coupled via the regulatory G proteins to adenylate cyclase and is found principally in the kidney.[96] Both the human and the rat V_2 receptor have been cloned.[97, 98] The gene, located on the long arm of the X chromosome, encodes a 370–amino acid protein with transmembrane topography characteristic of G protein–coupled receptors.

Renal Effects

Two well-recognized sites of action of AVP have been located in the mammalian kidney: (1) the collecting tubule and (2) the medullary thick ascending limb of Henle's loop. AVP may also act on other parts of the nephron, including the glomerulus. It also decreases medullary blood flow and activates a distinct urea transporter in the inner medullary nephron.[99]

Its effect on the collecting tubule to concentrate urine depends on a solute gradient across the tubular cells, which arises from a hypertonic renal interstitium and hypotonic luminal fluid in the tubule.[100, 101] The hypertonic interstitium results from the active transport of solute from the loops of Henle, which act as a countercurrent multiplier. The vasa recta following the course of the loops function as the countercurrent exchanger. Consequently, a small solute gradient is created between ascending and descending limbs of Henle's loop, which allows the formation of a progressively more concentrated interstitium from the corticomedullary junction to the papilla. In the presence of AVP, the water permeability of the collecting tubules that pass through the hypertonic interstitium is increased. This allows water to move along the gradient from lumen to renal medulla, resulting in urinary concentration.[101]

The increase in water permeability is mediated by a complicated

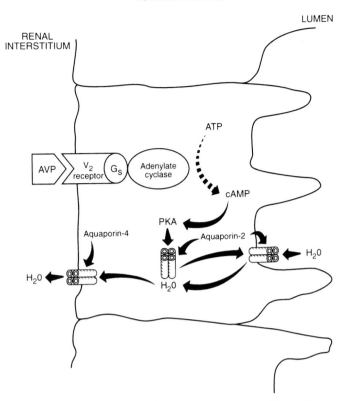

FIGURE 28–8. *Schematic representation of an AVP-sensitive collecting tubule showing the binding of AVP to the basolateral membrane, activating adenylate cyclase via the stimulatory G protein to generate cAMP, which stimulates protein kinase A. The latter inserts aquaporin-2, the water channel protein, as a tetramer into the luminal membrane. Aquaporin-4 on the basolateral membrane is not AVP-sensitive.*

cascade of intracellular events, starting with activation of adenylate cyclase, which increases intracellular cAMP concentration. Stimulation of a cAMP-dependent protein kinase A rearranges intracellular proteins, the water channels known as *aquaporins*. Aquaporin-2 is the vasopressin-responsive water channel protein specific to renal collecting ducts. Tetramers of aquaporin-2 are inserted into the luminal membrane, whereas aquaporin-3 and aquaporin-4 are constitutively expressed on the basolateral membrane to allow water to follow across the tubular cell.[102] The human aquaporin-2 gene is located on chromosome 12 (Fig. 28–8).[103]

In addition to AVP-sensitive water channels in the terminal collecting duct, a distinct AVP-regulated urea transporter is present in the distal collecting tubule of the mammalian kidney.[99, 104] By cycling urea into the renal interstitium, urea is conserved to contribute to the osmotic gradient essential for the water channels.

The other major renal site of AVP action is the medullary thick ascending limb of Henle's loop, which possesses, in some species, an AVP-sensitive adenylate cyclase.[105, 106] Clear evidence exists that sodium can be actively transported into the renal interstitium following AVP stimulation of the thick ascending limb.[107] The effect of AVP on this part of the nephron assists the generation of a hypertonic interstitial renal medulla and increases the osmotic gradient across the collecting tubules, resulting in augmentation of its antidiuretic action.

Cardiovascular Effects

Although AVP is a potent pressor agent, plasma concentrations required to increase arterial blood pressure in healthy individuals are many times higher than those observed under normal basal conditions.[108] Nevertheless, AVP can produce considerable constriction of numerous regional arteries and arterioles (e.g., splanchnic, renal, he-

TABLE 28–2. Classification of Arginine Vasopressin (AVP) Receptors

V_{1a} receptor	Phospholipase C coupled to G protein
	Production of intracellular inositol phosphates increasing ionized calcium and calmodulin phosphorylation
	Production of intracellular diacylglycerol enhancing protein kinase C activity
Sites	Vascular smooth muscle
	Liver
	Platelets
	Cerebrum
V_{1b} receptor	Intracellular actions similar to V_{1a} receptor
	AVP analogue-binding characteristics different than V_{1a} receptor
Site	Pituitary corticotroph
V_2 receptor	Adenylate cyclase coupled to stimulatory G protein
	Production of intracellular cAMP activating protein kinase A
	Mobilization and insertion of aquaporin-2 water channels into luminal cellular membrane
Sites	Renal collecting tubule
	Renal medullary thick ascending limb of Henle's loop

patic) at nearly physiologic plasma concentrations (10 pmol/L).[109] Using specific V_{1a} antagonists, the importance of endogenous AVP in maintaining blood pressure in mild volume depletion has emerged.[110, 111] The pressor effect of AVP varies according to the vascular bed, and differential pressor effects on intrarenal vessels account for the shunting of blood from the medulla to the cortex under the influence of AVP.[112] Cardiac output and oxygen consumption are reduced by AVP through a variety of mechanisms.[113]

However, little evidence indicates that AVP plays a substantial role in the development of essential hypertension in humans, although it may be important in the cause and maintenance of hypertension in some animal models (e.g., deoxycorticosterone-salt hypertension in the rat).[114]

Effect on the Pituitary

Corticotropin-releasing factor (CRF) and AVP are the main secretagogues for corticotropin release from the anterior pituitary. They act synergistically. AVP, synthesized in the parvocellular part of the paraventricular nucleus, is released from the median eminence into the portal blood to supply the anterior pituitary gland. The corticotroph expresses a large number of V_{1b} receptors.[115]

Adrenalectomy in the rat results in elevated CRF and AVP levels in the paraventricular neurons, where the two peptides co-localize in the same cell.[116] Administration of corticosterone reverses the effect of adrenalectomy. Recent studies indicate that these steroid manipulations regulate AVP mRNA.[117] Regulation of corticotropin secretion by AVP is physiologically important. AVP does not influence the secretion of other anterior pituitary hormones. Miscellaneous effects of AVP are given in Table 28–3.[118–129]

DIABETES INSIPIDUS

Classification

Diabetes insipidus or polyuria can be defined by the excretion of copious urine, in excess of 3 L per 24 hours (>40 mL/kg per 24 hours in adults, >100 mL/kg per 24 hours in infants). One of three pathogenetic mechanisms may be responsible for polyuria.[128–130] The first mechanism is a deficiency, usually not absolute, of AVP and is called *hypothalamic diabetes insipidus* (HDI). The second mechanism is partial or total renal resistance to the antidiuretic action of AVP, termed *nephrogenic diabetes insipidus* (NDI). NDI has many causes, from the severe congenital forms to the acquired types that may be reversible if they are due to metabolic disturbances (diabetes mellitus, hypercalcemia). Excessive inappropriate drinking, termed *dipsogenic*

TABLE 28–3. Miscellaneous Effects of Arginine Vasopressin (AVP)

Action	Receptor	Reference
Clotting Factors		
Factor VII release from hepatocytes	V_2	Mannucci et al[118]
von Willebrand factor release from vascular endothelium	V_2	Hashemi et al[119]; Mannucci & Federici[120]
Bone		
Maintenance of bone mineral density	V_2	Pivonello et al[121]
Liver		
Glycogen phosphorylase A activation	V_{1a}	Hems et al[122]; Spruce et al[123]
Brain		
Central blood pressure control	V_{1a}	Pittman & Landgraf[124]
Central temperature control	V_{1a}	Pittman & Landgraf[124]
Animal behavior stimulated		Ferris et al[125]
Retrieval of information (possibly)	V_{1a}	Sangal et al[126]
Function of CSF AVP (possibly)		Schwartz et al[127]

TABLE 28–4. Classification of Diabetes Insipidus

Hypothalamic diabetes insipidus
  Primary
    Genetic (autosomal dominant)
    DIDMOAD (Wolfram) syndrome
    Idiopathic
  Secondary
    Head injury
    After cranial surgery
    Tumors (craniopharyngioma, pinealoma, germinoma, pituitary macroadenoma, hypothalamic metastases)
    Granulomata (sarcoidosis, histyocytosis)
    Infections (meningitis, encephalitis)
    Infundibuloneurohypophysitis
    Vascular (infarction, aneurysms, sickle cell anemia)
    Pregnancy (associated with vasopressinase)
    Autoimmune
Nephrogenic diabetes insipidus
  Primary
    Genetic (X-linked recessive, V_2 receptor gene)
    Genetic (autosomal recessive, aquaporin-2 gene)
    Idiopathic
  Secondary
    Chronic renal disease (polycystic kidneys, obstructive uropathy)
    Metabolic disease (hypercalcemia, hypokalemia)
    Drug induced (lithium, demeclocycline)
    Osmotic diuresis (glucose, mannitol)
    Systemic disorders (amyloidosis, myelomatosis)
    Pregnancy
Dipsogenic diabetes insipidus
  Primary hyperdipsia
  Idiopathic
  Associated with psychosis
  Hypothalamic disease (sarcoidosis)
  Drug induced (anticholinergic, tricyclic antidepressants, lithium)
  Autoimmune (multiple sclerosis)

diabetes insipidus (DDI) or *primary polydipsia* (PP) is the third cause of polyuria. Table 28–4 gives a classification of conditions leading to polyuria.[129, 130]

Hypothalamic Diabetes Insipidus

HDI is a disorder of urinary concentration resulting from impaired osmoregulated AVP secretion. It is also known as neurogenic, central, or cranial diabetes insipidus. Most patients have detectable plasma AVP concentrations that are inappropriately low with respect to the concomitant plasma osmolalities. Persistent polyuria leads to hypertonic dehydration, and patients maintain water balance through an intact thirst mechanism.

It is an uncommon disorder, with an estimated prevalence of 1:25,000 and an equal gender distribution. Destruction of at least 80% of hypothalamic neurons synthesizing AVP is necessary before symptoms of polyuria and polydipsia are manifest.

Etiology

The majority of causes of HDI are secondary to disease acquired during life (see Table 28–4). Blotner's review[131] in 1958 suggested that the most common form of HDI, accounting for 45% of cases, was idiopathic, but recent surveys indicate that the current figure is lower (30%).[132] Some patients have circulating antibodies to hypothalamic AVP-secreting neurons, a possible manifestation of an autoimmune process.[133] The presence of plasma AVP antibodies in untreated patients is exceedingly rare.[134] Occasionally, a "triple-phase response" to trauma of the pituitary stalk has been observed.[135] Immediately after the insult, transient polyuria occurs for a few days, followed by a period of continual antidiuresis lasting up to 1 week, after which permanent HDI ensues. Pituitary tumors that compress or invade the posterior lobe rarely cause HDI, although metastatic deposits in the hypothalamus, often from carcinoma of the breast or bronchus, result in HDI. Lymphocytic infiltration of the neurohypophysis, recognized by a thickened pituitary stalk and inflammatory infiltrates of T-lymphocytes and plasma cells with eosinophils, is an unusual but well-described cause of diabetes insipidus.[136] In childhood, tumors affecting the hypothalamus (e.g., craniopharyngioma, germinoma) and cerebral malformations account for up to 50% of all cases of HDI.[130] Sheehan's syndrome remains an uncommon cause of HDI, but maximal urine-concentrating ability appears to be impaired in some patients, implying a minimal defect in osmoregulated AVP release.[137] Very rarely, diabetes insipidus occurs in pregnancy, which, in some instances, is due to increased activity of circulating vasopressinase,[138] the aminopeptidase of placental origin. The hypothalamic form of pregnancy-associated diabetes insipidus must be differentiated from the transient nephrogenic type that is very occasionally seen in pregnancy.[139]

A number of familial varieties of HDI have been described, inherited usually as a dominant trait. Numerous studies of families with a dominant inheritance show single nucleotide substitutions, deletions or frameshifts causing abnormal processing of the precursor vasopressin molecule.[140–142] Another type of familial HDI can be associated with diabetes mellitus, optic atrophy, nerve deafness, and abnormalities of the renal tract (the DIDMOAD [*d*iabetes *i*nsipidus, *d*iabetes *m*ellitus, *o*ptic *a*trophy, *d*eafness] syndrome).[143, 144]

Investigation

Because no specific clinical features definitely identify the cause of polyuria in a particular patient, diagnosis must rest on the results of investigations. Direct measurement of plasma AVP during osmotic stimulation establishes the diagnosis of HDI, but reliable methods to measure AVP are not always readily available. Consequently, indirect methods of assessing antidiuretic activity during a period of fluid deprivation are commonly used.

Having established that the adult patient is polyuric (24-hour urine volume >3 L), a fluid deprivation test can be performed, with subsequent assessment of renal concentrating ability in response to exogenous AVP. Although a variety of tests have been described,[79, 145, 146] a common protocol is given in Table 28–5. Patients with severe HDI can be distinguished by their low urine osmolality (<300 mOsm/kg), high plasma osmolality (>295 mOsm/kg) after dehydration, and urine concentration to greater than 750 mOsm/kg following administration of desmopressin. Severe NDI can be identified by failure to increase urine osmolality above 300 mOsm/kg after dehydration and administration of desmopressin. Unfortunately, many patients have partial defects, and mild forms of HDI, NDI, and DDI cannot always be differentiated by this type of test.[147] Prolonged periods of fluid deprivation have been advocated to improve diagnosis,[146] as have the infusions of hypertonic saline to raise plasma osmolality quickly,[148] but with little advantage over standard protocols.

Difficulties in establishing a diagnosis arise with fluid deprivation tests because prolonged polyuria from any cause leads to partial resistance to the antidiuretic action of AVP, probably owing to reduction in tonicity of the renal medullary interstitium.[149] Accurate diagnosis of HDI can be made, however, by direct measurement of plasma AVP concentration during infusion of hypertonic saline[147, 150] (Fig. 28–9A). Patients with HDI are identified by subnormal or undetectable plasma AVP concentrations with respect to plasma osmolalities that fall to the right of the normal distribution. Patients with DDI and NDI have plasma AVP responses that fall into the normal range, but these two diagnoses can be distinguished by relating plasma AVP concentration to urine osmolality after a short period of dehydration. NDI is characterized by inappropriately high plasma AVP values for the concomitant urine osmolality, whereas DDI patients show an appropriate relationship (see Fig. 28–9B).

As accurate AVP assays may not be readily available, an alternative approach to diagnosis can be made by instituting a careful therapeutic trial of desmopressin, preferably with the patient in the hospital. Administration of 10 μg of desmopressin intranasally once daily for 2 to 4 weeks causes progressive dilutional hyponatremia in DDI. Patients with NDI remain unaffected, whereas those with HDI experience an improvement in thirst and polyuria but remain normonatremic.

Imaging of the pituitary gland and the surrounding structures, including the pineal gland, is mandatory in all patients with HDI. Magnetic resonance images are preferable to CT scans. The majority of patients with HDI lose the normal hyperintense signal seen in the healthy posterior pituitary with T1-weighted MRI.[151]

Treatment

With severe HDI, profound polyuria is a great inconvenience and may lead to bladder distention, hydroureter, hydronephrosis, and secondary NDI. The treatment of choice for these patients is desmopressin, a synthetic, long-acting vasopressin analogue that possesses minimal pressor activity and has twice the antidiuretic potency of AVP.[152] It can be administered as an intranasal spray (5 to 100 μg daily) or parenterally (0.5 to 2.0 μg daily), but the individual variation in the dose required to control symptoms is considerable.[152] Desmopressin may also be administered orally in the dose range 100 to 1200 μg/day in divided doses. To avoid the potential complication of dilutional hyponatremia, desmopressin should be withdrawn at regular intervals, perhaps once weekly, to allow patients to become polyuric and avoid hyponatremia. If desmopressin is too potent, then lysine vasopressin can be prescribed, which acts for up to 4 hours but has the disadvantage of possessing considerable pressor activity. Pitressin tannate in oil for intramuscular administration or pitressin snuff is poorly tolerated and has been replaced by desmopressin.

Patients with mild forms of HDI (urine volume, <4 L per 24 hours) can be managed with adequate fluids to quench thirst. Others with mild HDI may be treated with a variety of oral agents. Chlorpropamide (250 to 500 mg daily) has been the most frequently used agent and appears to potentiate the antidiuretic action of circulating AVP,[153] reducing urine output by 50%, but troublesome side effects of hypoglycemia and hyponatremia do occur. Thiazides, carbamazepine, clofibrate, and tolbutamide increase antidiuresis in some patients with HDI but are generally less effective than chlorpropamide.

Nephrogenic Diabetes Insipidus

The causes of NDI, renal resistance to the antidiuretic action of AVP, are given in Table 28–4. The rare yet severe X-linked form usually presents in the first year of life.[154] The abnormal gene has been localized to the Xq28 region of the long arm of the X chromosome,[155] which accounts for the numerous abnormalities of the V_2 receptor.[156, 157] A few children with congenital nephrogenic diabetes insipidus have been described who are homozygous for a mutation in the aquaporin-2 gene, which encodes for the renal water channels.[157] Recent studies

---

TABLE 28–5. Protocol for Water Deprivation/ Desmopressin Test

Preparation
    Fluid given overnight prior to test
    Avoid caffeine and smoking
    Weigh patient
Dehydration phase
    Draw blood and collect urine for osmolality and urine volume measurements at 8 A.M.
    Restrict fluids up to 8 hr
    Weigh patient at 2-hr intervals
    Collect blood and urine for osmolality and volume measurements at 2-hr intervals
    Stop test if weight loss exceeds 5% of starting weight or thirst is intolerable
    Supervise patient closely to avoid surreptitious drinking
Desmopressin phase
    Inject 1 μg of desmopressin intramuscularly
    Allow patient to eat and drink up to 1.5–2.0 times the volume of urine passed during dehydration phase
    Collect urine for osmolality and volume at 8 P.M.
    Draw blood and collect urine for osmolality and volume measurements at 9 A.M. the next day

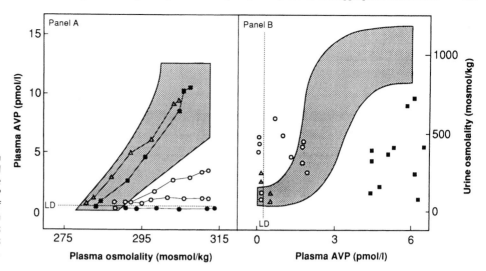

FIGURE 28-9. Results of dynamic tests in patients with polyuria. Plasma osmolality and plasma AVP responses to hypertonic saline (855 mmol/L) infusion *(panel A)*. Plasma AVP and urine osmolality responses to a period of fluid restriction *(panel B)*. The *stippled* area defines the normal response; *circles*, patients with HDI; *squares*, NDI; *triangles*, DDI. LD is the limit of detection of the assay, 0.3 pmol/L.

have identified three independent families with autosomal dominant and recessive phenotypes due to novel mutations in the aquaporin-2 gene.[158] Various metabolic disorders, including hypokalemia, hypercalcemia, and prolonged polyuria, can produce acquired NDI, which is often reversible with correction of the underlying cause. Lithium administration is a common cause of NDI that may not always be reversible.[159] Diagnosis is confirmed by recording inappropriately low urine osmolality with respect to the circulating plasma AVP concentration after a period of controlled fluid restriction (see Fig. 28–9B).

Other than removal of the underlying cause and maintenance of adequate hydration, specific therapy for diabetes insipidus is difficult. For patients with congenital NDI, thiazide diuretics in conjunction with salt restriction, prostaglandin synthetase inhibitors (e.g., indomethacin), and very high dose desmopressin, singly or in combination, are useful but rarely reduce urine volumes by more than 50%.[154, 160]

Dipsogenic Diabetes Insipidus (Primary Polydipsia)

DDI is a syndrome characterized by excessive fluid intake and polyuria. It is often observed in psychotic patients, who may be motivated by irrational beliefs rather than genuine thirst (see Table 28–4). Rarely, structural abnormalities such as hypothalamic sarcoidosis may cause DDI. Recent work using visual analogue scales to assess thirst has identified a group of patients with lowered osmotic thirst thresholds (see Fig. 28–7) but normal osmoregulated AVP secretion and renal function.[161] Confirmation of the diagnosis of primary polydipsia is obtained by observing normal osmoregulated AVP secretion and renal function (see Fig. 28–9). Reduction of fluid intake is the only rational treatment.

SYNDROME OF INAPPROPRIATE ANTIDIURESIS

Hypotonic Hyponatremia

Hyponatremia, defined as a serum sodium level less than 130 mmol/L, is a common electrolyte disorder, occurring in about 15% of hospitalized patients.[162] A pragmatic classification is given in Table 28–6. Clinical assessment identifies the extracellular volume status of most patients, although problems can arise in distinguishing mild forms of hypervolemia and hypovolemia from euvolemia. Pseudohyponatremia due to excessive concentrations of blood glucose, proteins, or lipids is readily excluded because plasma is not hypotonic. Clinical features of hyponatremia (Table 28–7) develop as serum sodium falls slowly below 115 mmol/L or if a very rapid decrease occurs in serum sodium.[163–165] Otherwise patients can remain asymptomatic. Values of serum sodium around 100 mmol/L are life-threatening. Most hyponatremic patients have detectable or elevated plasma AVP concentrations, and their urine osmolality tends to be higher than plasma osmolality,[166, 167] so that neither is diagnostic of the syndrome of inappropriate antidiuresis (SIAD). Measurement of urinary sodium concentration aids classification (see Table 28–6).

Background

Inappropriate antidiuretic hormone secretion was proposed many years ago to account for serum hypochloremia observed in tuberculosis,[168] but it reemerged as a syndrome associated with a variety of conditions described and defined by Bartter and Schwartz [169] (Table 28–8). Support for the hypothesis of inappropriate antidiuretic hormone secretion came from early studies on healthy adults given exoge-

TABLE 28–6. Classification of Hypotonic Hyponatremia

	Hypovolemia		Euvolemia		Hypervolemia	
Extracellular sodium	↓ ↓		→		↑	
Total body water	↓		↑		↑ ↑	
Common causes	Renal loss	Extrarenal loss	SIAD		Cardiac failure	Renal failure
	Diuretics	Vomiting	Hypothyroidism		Cirrhosis	
	Mineralocorticoid deficiency	Diarrhea	Glucocorticoid deficiency		Nephrotic syndrome	
	Salt-losing nephritis	Burns	"Sick cell" syndrome			
	Cerebral salt wasting					
Urinary sodium concentration, mmol/L	>20	<10	>20		<10	>20

Adapted from Berl T, Anderson RJ, McDonald KM, Schrier RW: Clinical disorders of water metabolism. Kidney Int 10:117–132, 1976.

TABLE 28–7. Progressive Clinical Features of Hypotonic Hyponatremia

Anorexia	Muscle cramps	Headache
Nausea	Myoclonus	Confusion
Vomiting	Abdominal ileus	Convulsions
Fatigue	Ataxia	Coma

nous vasopressin and oral fluids to produce dilutional hyponatremia.[170] Studies have now confirmed a variety of abnormalities of AVP secretion in the syndrome.[171]

Etiology

Many conditions associated with dilutional hyponatremia have been reported in which the cause has been attributed to SIAD (Table 28–9).

Small cell carcinoma of the bronchus is probably the most common neoplastic cause of SIAD. AVP has been demonstrated in tumor extracts, suggesting that the tumor was the source of AVP, and evidence that tumorous tissue can synthesize AVP has come from studies on in vitro biosynthesis of AVP.[172] However, not all patients with SIAD associated with neoplastic disease have ectopic AVP production, because abnormal excessive AVP secretion from the posterior pituitary has been demonstrated.[173] Studies have suggested that abnormal forms of AVP are secreted by some tumors and that others synthesize AVP ectopically, but SIAD does not result.

Pathophysiology

The basic abnormality in most cases of SIAD is a failure to maximally suppress AVP secretion as plasma osmolality falls below the theoretical osmotic threshold for AVP release. Thus, AVP continues to circulate at concentrations that are inappropriately high in relation to the hypo-osmolality of body fluids, although the absolute AVP values may not be particularly elevated. For reasons not well understood, patients continue to drink, and this, combined with a degree of persistent antidiuresis due to circulating AVP, leads to dilutional hyponatremia.[174] Investigation of osmoregulated AVP secretion in a large group of patients, all of whom fulfilled the criteria laid down by Bartter and Schwartz and who had a variety of underlying disorders, revealed four distinct patterns of AVP release[173] (Fig. 28–10).

The first pattern (type A; see Fig. 28–10) is characterized by wide fluctuations in plasma AVP concentration that occur at random and bear no relationship to changes in plasma osmolality. Such erratic release could be accounted for by ectopic secretion from neoplastic tissue, but similar patterns occur in non-neoplastic disease, suggesting a lesion in the posterior pituitary or any of its regulatory afferent neurons. Type A accounts for about 35% of cases of SIAD.

A second group, accounting for a third of cases, demonstrates resetting of the osmostat to the left of normal (type B). In these patients, plasma AVP is responsive to changes in plasma osmolality, but the threshold for AVP release is subnormal. Such patients retain the ability to osmoregulate water excretion and to dilute and concentrate urine, but this occurs at a plasma osmolality level that is lower than normal. In this situation, urine osmolality can be lower than plasma osmolality. Again, this pattern of AVP release is observed in both neoplastic and non-neoplastic disease. Because similar shifts to the left of normal are observed in hypovolemia and hypotension, one suspected cause is a lesion in the afferent baroregulatory pathways. Sick-cell syndrome results in a similar pattern of osmoregulated vasopressin release.

TABLE 28–8. Cardinal Features of the Syndrome of Inappropriate Antidiuretic Hormone Secretion

Hyponatremia with appropriately low plasma osmolality
Urine osmolality greater than plasma osmolality
Excessive renal sodium excretion
Absence of hypotension, hypovolemia, and edema-forming states
Normal renal and adrenal function

TABLE 28–9. Some Causes of the Syndrome of Inappropriate Antidiuretic Hormone Secretion

Neoplastic disease	Chest disorders
Carcinoma (bronchus, duodenum, pancreas, bladder, ureter, prostate)	Pneumonia
	Tuberculosis
	Empyema
Thymoma	Cystic fibrosis
Mesothelioma	Pneumothorax
Lymphoma, leukemia	Asthma
Ewing's sarcoma	Aspergillosis
Carcinoid	Drugs
Bronchial adenoma	Vasopressin and analogues
Central nervous system disorders	Oxytocin
Head injury, neurosurgery	Chlorpropamide
Brain abscess or tumour	Clofibrate
Meningitis, encephalitis	Vincristine, vinblastine, cisplatin
Guillain-Barré syndrome	Thiazides
Cerebral hemorrhage	Phenothiazines
Cavernous sinus thrombosis	Monoamine oxidase inhibitors
Hydrocephalus	Selective serotonin reuptake inhibitors
Cerebellar and cerebral atrophy	
Shy-Drager syndrome	"Ecstasy"
Porphyria	Miscellaneous
Peripheral neuropathy	Idiopathic
Epilepsy	Psychosis
Subdural hematoma	AIDS
Delirium tremens	Abdominal surgery

In some cases, AVP secretion cannot be entirely suppressed and the hormone "leaks out" at low plasma osmolality (type C). However, increasing plasma osmolality results in a normal plasma AVP response. The last group (type D), accounting for less than 10% of cases, has entirely normal osmoregulated AVP secretion. Nevertheless, the patients fulfill the criteria of Bartter and Schwartz: they fail to excrete a water load and cannot maximally dilute urine. It is not known whether this abnormality is due to increase in renal sensitivity to extremely low concentrations of AVP or to another antidiuretic factor.

Treatment

Patients with chronic SIAD who have plasma sodium concentrations greater than 125 mmol/L rarely have significant symptoms from hypo-

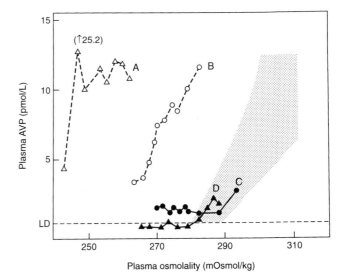

FIGURE 28–10. Four patterns of AVP response to infusion of hypertonic saline in a group of hyponatremic patients with the syndrome of inappropriate antidiuretic hormone secretion. *A,* Erratic release. *B,* Reset osmostat. *C,* AVP leak. *D,* Normal osmoregulated AVP release. (Adapted from Zerbe R, Stropes L, Robertson GL: Vasopressin function in the syndrome of inappropriate antidiuresis. Ann Rev Med 31:315–327, 1980.)

natremia itself and may not require specific treatment to raise plasma sodium levels. With more severe degrees of hyponatremia, some form of therapy may be required.

Adequate treatment directed toward the underlying cause of SIAD is most appropriate, but if this fails, and the patient requires therapy for life-threatening or symptomatic chronic hyponatremia, total fluid intake should be restricted to 500 mL per 24 hours, with the intention of raising serum sodium levels slowly to no higher than 125 to 130 mmol/L.[165, 175–177] Because fluid restriction can be distressing, particularly when it is prolonged, additional drug therapy is advocated to manage chronic hyponatremia. The antidiuretic action of AVP can be blocked by demeclocycline (600 to 1200 mg daily) or the less reliable and more toxic lithium carbonate (600 to 1800 mg daily).[178] The NDI induced by these drugs may take up to 6 weeks to develop fully. Specific antagonists to the V_2 receptor have been synthesized. Although their efficacy has been confirmed in animals, peptide antagonists have failed to fulfill their potential in humans.[179] The long search for a V_2-receptor antagonist has resulted in the identification of a very promising synthetic linear nonpeptide compound, OPC-31260, which increases renal solute-free water excretion.[180] This aquaretic drug has no effect on renal salt excretion. Recent studies in patients with SIAD treated with OPC-31260 have shown substantial improvement in their degree of hyponatremia.[181] Drugs to suppress neurohypophysial AVP secretion (e.g., phenytoin) have met with limited success.[182] An alternative therapeutic approach is the administration of oral furosemide (40 to 80 mg daily) together with salt supplementation (3 g daily).[183] If the serum sodium level is chronically very low (100 to 110 mmol/L), hypertonic saline can be infused slowly to raise serum sodium levels no more rapidly than 0.5 mmol/L/hour to attain a final concentration of about 125 mmol/L, with an increment of no more than 10 mmol/L in 24 hours. Acute symptomatic hyponatremia (for <3 days) may be corrected more quickly but no faster than 2.0 mmol/L/hour, with a limit on the incremental rise in sodium to 25 mmol/L during the initial 24 to 48 hours.[176]

Severe hyponatremia and its treatment are associated with high mortality and morbidity. Rapid correction of chronic low serum sodium levels (<115 mmol/L) by any method can cause central pontine and extrapontine myelinolysis or osmotic demyelination syndrome,[184, 185] in which the patient develops brain edema, seizures, and coma and risks death. This often occurs 2 to 4 days after correction of the hyponatremia. Recent studies have confirmed that both the rate and magnitude of the increase in serum sodium during correction are risk factors for the development of demyelinating lesions in chronically hyponatremic rats.[186]

HYPODIPSIA

Isolated defects in osmoregulated thirst are uncommon. They lead to chronic inadequate intake of fluid, which, in the majority of cases, causes profound hypernatremia.[165, 187, 188] These disorders are referred to as *hypodipsic* or *adipsic hypernatremia*. Not infrequently, an associated disturbance of osmoregulated AVP release is present.

Etiology

Thirst deficiency syndromes develop as a result of a variety of pathologic processes involving the putative thirst osmoreceptor cells in the anterior circumventricular organs of the hypothalamus or their neuronal connections. Table 28–10 lists the specific diseases recognized to cause hypodipsic or adipsic hypernatremia.[165, 187] Tumors due to either neoplastic conditions or granulomatous diseases account for the majority of cases.

Pathophysiology

With the development of visual analogue scales to estimate thirst and precise AVP assays, it is now possible to classify these syndromes into different pathogenetic entities.

TABLE 28–10. Causes of Thrist Deficiency Syndromes

Neoplastic (50%)	Granulomatous (20%)
Primary	Histiocytosis
Craniopharyngioma	Sarcoidosis
Pinealoma	Miscellaneous (15%)
Meningioma	Hydrocephalus
Pituitary tumor	Ventricular cyst
Secondary	Trauma
Bronchial carcinoma	Idiopathic
Breast carcinoma	
Vascular (15%)	
Internal carotid ligation	
Anterior communicating artery aneurysm	
Intrahypothalamic hemorrhage	

Adapted from Robertson GL, Aycinena P, Zerbe RL: Neurogenic disorders of osmoregulation. Am J Med 72:339–353, 1982.

Resetting of the osmotic thresholds for thirst and AVP release to the right of normal (see Figs. 28–3 and 28–7) accounts for patients with "essential" hypernatremia.[189] These patients have persistent hypernatremia but are still able to dilute and concentrate urine and appreciate thirst, but they do so at a higher plasma osmolality set-point.[56, 188]

Complete destruction of the osmoreceptors leads to total adipsia and, interestingly, to a persistently low level of AVP secretion that fails to respond to osmotic stimuli. There are, however, normal AVP responses to nonosmotic stimuli. Severe hypernatremia ensues, as these patients never experience thirst and, if left to themselves, do not drink. Because of persistent minimal nonosmoregulated AVP secretion, hyponatremia can develop if patients are given large fluid loads, as hypo-osmolality does not suppress AVP release.[188]

A third type of defect has been described in which there is normal osmoregulated AVP secretion, but osmoregulated thirst is totally absent.[190] This clinical observation supports the concept of two populations of osmoreceptor cells, one serving AVP pathways and the other thirst appreciation.

Treatment

The cornerstone of management of patients with thirst deficiency syndromes, if the underlying cause cannot be treated, is adequate fluid intake. Hypodipsic patients rarely develop life-threatening hypernatremia because thirst develops when plasma osmolality levels rise sufficiently. Fluid intake then returns serum sodium levels toward normal.

Adipsia with absent osmoregulated AVP secretion presents a major management problem, and these patients run the risk of profound hypernatremia. One therapeutic approach is the oral administration of fluid, the volume of which is based on the previous day's body weight change. Frequent intermittent checks of serum sodium are essential to avoid extreme fluctuations in serum sodium levels.[191] Nevertheless, wide swings from hypernatremia to hyponatremia can still occur.[56] This form of adipsia is indeed life-threatening.

REFERENCES

1. Oliver G, Schäfer EA: On the physiological actions of the pituitary body and certain other glands. J Physiol 18:277–279, 1895.
2. Howell TH: The physiological effects of extracts of the hypophysis cerebri and infundibular body. J Exp Med 3:245–248, 1898.
3. Schäfer EA: The functions of the pituitary body. Proc R Soc 81(series B):442–468, 1909.
4. Farini F: Diabete insipido ed opoterapia ipofisaria. Gazz Osp Clin 34:1135–1139, 1913.
5. von den Velden RL: Die Nierenwirkung von Hypophysenextrakten beim Menschen. Berl Klin Wochenschr 50:2083–2086, 1913.
6. du Vigneaud V, Gish DT, Katsoyannis PG: A synthetic preparation possessing biological properties associated with arginine-vasopressin. J Am Chem Soc 76:4751–4752, 1954.
7. Schally AV: Hormones of the neurohypophysis. *In* Lock W, Schally AV (eds): The Hypothalamus and Pituitary in Health and Disease. Springfield, IL, Charles C Thomas, 1972, pp 154–171.

8. Schally AV, Bowers CY, Kuroshima A, et al: Effect of lysine vasopressin dimers on blood pressure and some endocrine functions. Am J Physiol 207:378–384, 1964.
9. Acher R: Chemistry of the neurohypophysial hormones: An example of molecular evolution. *In* Knobil E, Sawyer WH (eds): Handbook of Physiology, section 7: Endocrinology, vol 4, pt 1. Washington, DC, American Physiological Society, 1974, pp 119–130.
10. Acher R, Chauvet J: Structure, processing and evolution of the neurohypophyseal, hormone-neurophysin precursors. Biochemie 70:1197–1207, 1988.
11. Land H, Schütz G, Schmale H, Richter D: Nucleotide sequence of cloned cDNA encoding for bovine arginine vasopressin-neurophysin II precursor. Nature 295:299–303, 1982.
12. Mohr E, Schmitz E, Richter D: A single rat genomic cDNA fragment encodes both the oxytocin and vasopressin genes separated by 11 kilobases and orientated in opposite transcriptional directions. Biochemie 70:649–654, 1988.
13. Murphy D, Levy A, Lightman S, Carter D: Vasopressin RNA in the neural lobe of the pituitary: Dramatic accumulation in response to salt loading. Proc Natl Acad Sci USA 86:9002–9005, 1989.
14. van Tol HHM, Voorhuis DTAM, Burbach JPH: Oxytocin gene expression in discrete hypothalamic magnocellular cell groups is stimulated by prolonged salt loading. Endocrinology 120:71–76, 1987.
15. Zingg HH, Lefebvre DL: Oxytocin and vasopressin gene expression during gestation and lactation. Mol Brain Res 4:1–6, 1988.
16. Richter D, Mohr E, Schmale H: Molecular aspects of the vasopressin gene family: Evolution, expression and regulation. *In* Jard S, Jamison R (eds): Vasopressin. Montrouge, France, John Libbey, 1991, pp 3–10.
17. Ivell R, Burback JPH: The molecular biology of vasopressin and oxytocin genes. J Neuroendocrinol 3:583–585, 1991.
18. Schmale H, Richter D: Single base deletion in the vasopressin gene is the cause of diabetes insipidus in the Brattleboro rat. Nature 308:705–709, 1984.
19. Russell JT, Brownstein MJ, Gainer H: Biosynthesis of vasopressin, oxytocin and neurophysins: Isolation and characterization of two common precursors (propressophysin and prooxyphysin). Endocrinology 107:1880–1891, 1980.
20. Dutton A, Dyball REJ: Phasic firing enhances vasopressin release from the rat neurohypophysis. J Physiol 290:433–440, 1979.
21. Nordmann JJ, Labouesse J: Neurosecretory granules: Evidence for an aging process within the neurohypophysis. Science 211:595–597, 1981.
22. Sinding C, Robinson AG: A review of neurophysins. Metabolism 26:1355–1370, 1977.
23. Lauson HD: Metabolism of neurohypophysial hormones. *In* Knobil E, Sawyer WH (eds): Handbook of Physiology, section 7: Endocrinology, vol 4, pt 1. Washington, DC, American Physiological Society, 1974, pp 287–393.
24. Bichet DG, Arthus M-F, Barjon JN, et al: Human platelet fraction arginine-vasopressin: Potential physiological role. J Clin Invest 79:881–887, 1987.
25. Dicker SE, Tyler C: Vasopressor and oxytocic activities of pituitary glands of rats, guinea pigs and cats and of human foetuses. J Physiol 121:206–214, 1953.
26. Rasmussen AT: The weight of the principal components of the normal male adult human hypophysis cerebri. Am J Anat 42:1–27, 1928.
27. Zimmerman EA, Nilaver G, Hou-yu A, Silverman AJ: Vasopressinergic and oxytocinergic pathways in the central nervous system. Fed Proc 43:91–96, 1984.
28. Sofroniew MV: Projections from vasopressin, oxytocin and neurophysin neurons to neural targets in the rat and human. J Histochem Cytochem 28:475–478, 1980.
29. Buijs RM, Hermes MLHJ, Kalsbeek A, et al: Vasopressin distribution, origin and functions in the central nervous system. *In* Jard S, Jamison R (eds): Vasopressin. Montrouge, France, John Libbey, 1991, pp 149–158.
30. Carithers JR, Johnson AK: Fine structural studies on the effects of AV3V lesions on the hypothalamoneurohypophyseal neurosecretory system. *In* Cowley AW, Liard J-F, Ausiello DA (eds): Vasopressin: Cellular and Integrative Functions. New York, Raven Press, 1988, pp 301–319.
31. Thrasher TN, Ramsay DJ: Anatomy of osmoreception. *In* Jard S, Jamison R (eds): Vasopressin. Montrouge, France, John Libbey, 1991, pp 267–278.
32. Gauer OH, Henry JP: Circulatory basis of fluid volume control. Physiol Rev 43:423–481, 1963.
33. Carter DA, Lightman SL: Neuroendocrine control of vasopressin secretion. *In* Baylis PH, Padfield PL (eds): The Posterior Pituitary: Hormone Secretion in Health and Disease. New York, Marcel Dekker, 1985, pp 53–118.
34. Bridges TE, Hillhouse EW, Jones MT: The effect of dopamine on neurohypophysial hormones release in vivo and from the rat neural lobe and hypothalamus in vitro. J Physiol 260:647–666, 1976.
35. Lightman SL, Forsling M: Evidence for dopamine as an inhibitor of vasopressin release in man. Clin Endocrinol 12:39–46, 1980.
36. Sladek JR, McNeill TH: Simultaneous monoamine histofluorescence and neuropeptide immunocytochemistry: IV. Verification of catecholamine-neurophysin interactions through single section analysis. Cell Tissue Res 210:181–190, 1980.
37. Willoughby JO, Jervois PM, Menadue MF: Noradrenaline, by activation of alpha-1-adreno-receptors in the region of the supraoptic nucleus, causes secretion of vasopressin in the unanesthetized rat. Neuroendocrinology 45:219–226, 1987.
38. Schrier RW, Berl T, Anderson RJ: Osmotic and nonosmotic control of vasopressin release. Am J Physiol 236:F321–F332, 1979.
39. Sladek CD, Fisher KY, Sidorowicz HE, Mathiasen JR: Osmotic stimulation of vasopressin mRNA content in the supraoptic nucleus requires synaptic activation. Am J Physiol 268:R1034–R1039, 1995.
40. Swenson KL, Badre SE, Morsette DJ, Sladek CD: N-Methyl-D-aspartic acid stimulation of vasopressin release: Role in osmotic regulation and modulation by gonadal steroids. J Neuroendocrinol 10:679–685, 1998.
41. Iovino M, Steardo L: Vasopressin response to central and peripheral angiotensin II in rats with lesion of the subfornical organ. Brain Res 322:365–368, 1984.
42. Iovino M, Steardo L: Vasopressin release to central and peripheral angiotensin II in rats with lesion of the subfornical organ. Brain Res 422:365–368, 1984.

43. Naita Y, Fukata J, Shindo K: Effects of interleukins on plasma arginine vasopressin and oxytocin levels in conscious, freely moving rats. Biochem Biophys Res Commun 174:1189–1195, 1991.
44. Landgraf R: Mortyn Jones Memorial Lecture: Intracerebrally released vasopressin and oxytocin: Measurement, mechanisms and behavioural consequences. J Neuroendocrinol 7:243–253, 1995.
45. Wilson BC, Fulop K, Summerlee AJS: Changing effect of i.c.v. 1L-1β on vasopressin release in anaesthetized female rats at different stages of lactation: Role of prostaglandins and noradrenaline. J Neuroendocrinol 8:915–920, 1996.
46. Samson WK: Atrial natriuretic factor inhibits dehydration and hemorrhage-induced vasopressin release. Neuroendocrinology 40:277–279, 1985.
47. Burrell LM, Lambert HJ, Baylis PH: Effect of atrial natriuretic peptide on thirst and vasopressin release in man. Am J Physiol 60:R475–R479, 1991.
48. Yamamoto S, Inenaga K, Yamashita H: Inhibition by brain natriuretic peptide of vasopressin neurons in the supraoptic nucleus and neurons in the region of the anteroventral third ventricle in rat hypothalamic slice preparations. J Neuroendocrinol 3:45–49, 1991.
49. Martin R, Voigt KH: Enkephalins coexist with oxytocin and vasopressin in nerve terminals of rat neurohypophysis. Nature 289:502–504, 1981.
50. Carter DA, Lightman SL: Inhibition of vasopressin secretion by a kappa-opiate receptor agonist. Neuroendocrinol Lett 6:95–100, 1984.
51. Rossi NF, Kim JK, Summers SN, Schrier RW: Kappa opiate agonist RU 51599 inhibits vasopressin gene expression and osmotically induced vasopressin secretion in vitro. Life Sci 61:2271–2282, 1997.
52. Verney EB: The antidiuretic hormone and the factors which determine its release. Proc R Soc London 135(series B):25–105, 1947.
53. Baratz RA, Ingraham RC: Sensitive bioassay method for measuring antidiuretic hormone in mammalian plasma. Proc Soc Exp Biol Med 100:296–299, 1959.
54. Robertson GL, Shelton RL, Athar S: The osmoregulation of vasopressin. Kidney Int 10:25–37, 1976.
55. Hammer M, Ladefoged J, Olgaard K: Relationship between plasma osmolality and plasma vasopressin in human subjects. Am J Physiol 238:E313–E317, 1980.
56. Baylis PH, Thompson CJ: Osmoregulation of vasopressin secretion and thirst in health and disease. Clin Endocrinol 29:549–576, 1988.
57. Baylis PH, Gill GV: Investigation of polyuria. Clin Endocrinol Metab 13:295–310, 1984.
58. Bie P: Osmoreceptors, vasopressin and control of renal water excretion. Physiol Rev 60:962–1048, 1980.
59. Baylis PH, Pippard C, Gill GV, Burd J: Development of a cytochemical assay for plasma vasopressin: Application to studies on water loading normal man. Clin Endocrinol 24:383–392, 1986.
60. Moses AM, Miller M: Osmotic threshold for vasopressin release as determined by hypertonic saline infusion and dehydration. Neuroendocrinology 7:219–226, 1971.
61. Robertson GL: Physiology of ADH secretion. Kidney Int 32(suppl 21):S20–S26, 1987.
62. Thompson CJ, Selby P, Baylis PH: Reproducibility of osmotic and non-osmotic tests of vasopressin secretion in man. Am J Physiol 60:R533–R539, 1991.
63. Zerbe RL: Genetic factors in normal and abnormal regulation of vasopressin secretion. *In* Schrier RW (ed): Vasopressin. New York, Raven Press, 1985, pp 213–220.
64. Dürr JA, Stamoutsos BA, Lindheimer MD: Osmoregulation during pregnancy in the rat. Evidence for resetting of the threshold for vasopressin secretion during gestation. J Clin Invest 68:337–346, 1981.
65. Davison JM, Gilmore EA, Dürr J, et al: Altered threshold for vasopressin secretion and thirst in human pregnancy. Am J Physiol 246:F105–F109, 1984.
66. Spruce BA, Baylis PH, Burd J, Watson MJ: Variation in osmoregulation of arginine vasopressin during the human menstrual cycle. Clin Endocrinol 22:37–42, 1985.
67. Zerbe RL, Robertson GL: Osmoregulation of thirst and vasopressin secretion in human subjects: Effect of various solutes. Am J Physiol 244:E607–E614, 1983.
68. Vokes TP, Aycinena PR, Robertson GL: Effect of insulin on osmoregulation of vasopressin. Am J Physiol 252:E538–E548, 1987.
69. Eisenhofer G, Johnson RH: Effect of ethanol ingestion on plasma vasopressin and water balance in humans. Am J Physiol 242:R522–R527, 1982.
70. Thompson CJ, Bland J, Burd J, Baylis PH: The osmotic thresholds for thirst and vasopressin release are similar in healthy man. Clin Sci 71:651–656, 1986.
71. Thompson CJ, Burd JM, Baylis PH: Acute suppression of plasma vasopressin and thirst after drinking in hypernatremic humans. Am J Physiol 252:R1138–R1142, 1987.
72. Miller M: Fluid and electrolyte homeostasis in the elderly: Physiological changes of ageing and clinical consequences. Baillieres Clin Endocrinol Metab 11:367–387, 1997.
73. Johnson AG, Crawford GA, Kelly D: Arginine vasopressin and osmolality in the elderly. J Am Geriatr Soc 42:399–404, 1994.
74. Helderman JH, Vestal RE, Rowe JW, et al: The response of arginine vasopressin to intravenous alcohol and hypertonic saline in man: The impact of ageing. J Gerontol 33:39–47, 1978.
75. Phillips PA, Rolls BJ, Ledingham JGG: Reduced thirst after water deprivation in healthy elderly men. N Engl J Med 311:753–759, 1984.
76. Crowe MJ, Forsling ML, Rolls BJ: Altered water excretion in healthy elderly men. Age Ageing 16:285–293, 1987.
77. Lewis WH, Alving AS: Changes with age in the renal function in adult men. Am J Physiol 123:500–515, 1938.
78. Johnson JA, Zehr JE, Moore WW: Effects of separate and concurrent osmotic and volume stimuli on plasma ADH in sheep. Am J Physiol 218:1273–1280, 1970.
79. Baylis PH: Posterior pituitary function in health and disease. Clin Endocrinol Metab 12:747–770, 1983.
80. Goetz K, Bond GC, Bloxham DD: Atrial receptors and renal function. Physiol Rev 55:157–205, 1975.
81. Wang BC, Flora-Ginter G, Leadley RJ, Goetz KL: Ventricular receptors stimulate vasopressin release during hemorrhage. Am J Physiol 254:R204–R211, 1988.

82. Goetz KL, Zhu JL, Leadley RJ, et al: Hemodynamic and hormonal influences on the secretion of vasopressin. *In* Jard S, Jamison R (eds): Vasopressin. Montrouge, France, John Libbey, 1991, pp 279–286.

83. Dunn FL, Brennan TJ, Nelson AE, Robertson GL: The role of blood osmolality and volume in regulating vasopressin secretion in the rat. J Clin Invest 52:3212–3219, 1973.

84. Goldsmith SR, Dodge D, Cowley AW: Nonosmotic influences on osmotic stimulation of vasopressin in humans. Am J Physiol 252:H85–H88, 1987.

85. Rowe JW, Shelton RL, Helderman JH, et al: Influence of the emetic reflex on vasopressin release in man. Kidney Int 16:729–735, 1979.

86. Verbalis JG, Richardson DW, Stricker EM: Vasopressin release in response to nausea-producing agents and cholecystokinin in monkeys. Am J Physiol 252:R749–R753, 1987.

87. Ukei M, Moran WH, Zimmerman B: The role of visceral afferent pathways on vasopressin secretion and urinary excretory patterns during surgical stress. Ann Surg 168:16–28, 1968.

88. Baylis PH, Robertson GL: Arginine vasopressin response to insulin-induced hypoglycemia in man. J Clin Endocrinol Metab 53:935–940, 1981.

89. Thrasher TN, Keil LC, Ramsay DJ: Lesions of the organum vasculosum of the lamina terminalis (OVLT) attenuate osmotically-induced drinking and vasopressin secretion in the dog. Endocrinology 110:1837–1839, 1982.

90. McKinley MJ, Denton DA, Weisinger RW: Sensors for antidiuresis and thirst osmoreceptors or CSF sodium detectors? Brain Res 141:89–103, 1978.

91. Andersson B, Rundgroen M: Thirst and its disorders. Ann Rev Med 33:231–239, 1982.

92. Fitzsimons JT: The physiological basis of thirst. Kidney Int 10:3–11, 1976.

93. McKinley MJ, Denton DA, Park RG, Weisinger RS: Ablation of subfornical organ does not prevent angiotensin-induced water drinking in sheep. Am J Physiol 250:R1052–R1059, 1986.

94. Carmichael MC, Kumar R: Molecular biology of vasopressin receptors. Semin Nephrol 14:341–348, 1994.

95. Morel A, O'Carroll A-M, Brownstein MJ, Lolait SJ: Molecular cloning and expression of a rat V_{1a} arginine vasopressin receptor. Nature 356:523–529, 1992.

96. Kokko JP, Rector FC Jr: Countercurrent multiplication system without active transport in inner medulla. Kidney Int 2:214–223, 1972.

97. Birnbaumer M, Seibold A, Gilbert S, et al: Molecular cloning of the receptor for human antidiuretic hormone. Nature 357:333–335, 1992.

98. Lolait SJ, O'Carroll A-M, McBride OW, et al: Cloning and characterization of a vasopressin V_2 receptor and possible link to nephrogenic diabetes insipidus. Nature 357:336–339, 1992.

99. Nielson S, Knepper MA: Vasopressin activates collecting duct urea transporters and water channels by distinct physical processes. Am J Physiol 265:F204–F213, 1993.

100. Ausiello D: G-protein function in vasopressin-sensitive epithelia. *In* Jard S, Jamison R (eds): Vasopressin. Montrouge, France, John Libbey, 1991, pp 135–145.

101. Bankir L: Vasopressin and the urinary concentrating mechanism. *In* Jard S, Jamison R (eds): Vasopressin. Montrouge, France, John Libbey, 1991, pp 437–447.

102. Cheng A, van Hoek AN, Yeager M, et al: Three-dimensional organisation of a human water channel. Nature 387:627–630, 1997.

103. Deen PMT, Verdijk MAJ, Knoers NVAM: Requirement of human renal water channel aquaporin-2 for vasopressin-dependent concentration of urine. Science 264:92–95, 1994.

104. Knepper MA, Sands JM, Chou CL: Independence of water and urea transport in the rat inner medullary collecting duct. Am J Physiol 256:F610–F621, 1989.

105. Imbert-Teboul M, Chabardès D, Montégut M, et al: Vasopressin-dependent adenylate cyclase activities in the rat kidney medulla: Evidence for two separate sites of action. Endocrinology 102:1254–1261, 1978.

106. Wittner M, Di Stefano A, Wangemann P, et al: Differential effects of ADH on sodium, chloride, potassium, calcium and magnesium transport in cortical and medullary thick ascending limbs of mouse nephron. Pflugers Arch 412:516–523, 1988.

107. Hebert SC, Culpepper RM, Andreoli TE: NaCl transport in mouse medullary thick ascending limbs: I. Functional nephron heterogeneity and ADH-stimulated NaCl cotransport. Am J Physiol 241:412–431, 1981.

108. Montani JP, Liard JF, Schoun J, Möhring J: Hemodynamic effects of exogenous and endogenous vasopressin at low plasma concentrations in conscious dogs. Circ Res 47:346–355, 1980.

109. Altura BM, Altura BT: Actions of vasopressin, oxytocin, and synthetic analogs on vascular smooth muscle. Fed Proc 43:80–86, 1984.

110. Aisenbrey GA, Handelman WA, Arnold P, et al: Vascular effects of arginine vasopressin during fluid deprivation. J Clin Invest 67:961–968, 1981.

111. Liard J-F: Acute hemodynamic effects of antidiuretic agents. *In* Cowley AW, Liard J-F, Ausiello DA (eds): Vasopressin: Cellular and Integrative Functions. New York, Raven Press, 1988, pp 461–466.

112. Johnson MD, Park CS, Malvin RL: Antidiuretic hormone and the distribution of renal cortical blood flow. Am J Physiol 232:F111–F116, 1977.

113. Liard J-F: Vasopressin reduces oxygen uptake in intact dogs but not in sinoaortic denervated dogs. Am J Physiol 257:R1–R9, 1989.

114. Share L, Crofton JT: The role of vasopressin in hypertension. Fed Proc 43:103–106, 1984.

115. Du Pasquier D, Loup F, Dubois-Dauphin M, et al: Binding sites for vasopressin in the human pituitary are associated with corticotrophs and may differ from other known vasopressin receptors. J Neuroendocrinol 3:237–247, 1991.

116. Sawchenko PE, Swanson LW, Vale WW: Co-expression of corticotrophin-releasing factor and vasopressin immunoreactivity in parvocellular neurosecretory neurons of the adrenalectomized rat. Proc Natl Acad Sci USA 81:1877–1883, 1984.

117. Baldino F, Davis LG: Glucocorticoid regulation of vasopressin messenger RNA. *In* Uhl GR (ed): In Situ Hybridization in the Brain. New York, Plenum Press, 1986, p 97.

118. Mannucci PM, Ruggeri ZM, Pareti FI, Capitanio A: DDAVP: A new pharmacological approach to the management of hemophilia and von Willebrand disease. Lancet 1:869–872, 1977.

119. Hashemi S, Tackaberry ES, Palmer DS, et al: DDAVP induced release of von Willebrand factor from endothelial cells in vitro: The effect of plasma and red cells. Biochim Biophys Acta 1052:63–70, 1990.

120. Mannucci PM, Federici AB: Release of factor VIII and von Willebrand factor by vasopressin and derivatives. *In* Jard S, Jamison R (eds): Vasopressin. Montrouge, France, John Libbey, 1991, pp 331–337.

121. Pivonello R, Colao A, di Somma C, et al: Impairment of bone status in patients with central diabetes insipidus. J Clin Endocrinol 83:2275–2280, 1998.

122. Hems DA, Rodrigues LM, Whitton PD: Rapid stimulation by vasopressin, oxytocin and angiotensin II of glycogen degradation in hepatocyte suspensions. Biochem J 172:311–312, 1978.

123. Spruce BA, McCulloch AJ, Burd J, et al: The effect of vasopressin infusion on glucose metabolism in man. Clin Endocrinol 22:463–468, 1985.

124. Pittman QJ, Landgraf R: Vasopressin in thermoregulation and blood pressure control. *In* Jard S, Jamison R (eds): Vasopressin. Montrouge, France, John Libbey, 1991, pp 177–184.

125. Ferris CF, Singer EA, Meenan DM, Albers HE: Inhibition of vasopressin-stimulated flank marking behaviour by V_1-receptor antagonists. Eur J Pharmacol 154:153–159, 1988.

126. Sangal A, Keith AB, Wright C, Edwardson JA: Failure of vasopressin to enhance memory in a passive avoidance task in rats. Neurosci Lett 28:87–92, 1982.

127. Schwartz WJ, Coleman RJ, Reppert SM: A daily vasopressin rhythm in rat cerebrospinal fluid. Brain Res 263:105–112, 1983.

128. Thompson CJ: Polyuric states in man. *In* Baylis PH (ed): Water and Salt Homeostasis in Health and Disease. London, Baillière Tindall, 1989, pp 473–497.

129. Robertson GL: Diabetes insipidus. Endocrinol Metab Clin North Am 24:549–572, 1995.

130. Baylis PH, Cheetham T: Diabetes insipidus. Arch Dis Child 79:84–89, 1998.

131. Blotner H: Primary or idiopathic diabetes insipidus: A system disease. Metabolism 7:191–206, 1958.

132. Moses AM, Notman DD: Diabetes insipidus and syndrome of inappropriate antidiuretic hormone secretion (SIADH). Adv Intern Med 27:73–110, 1982.

133. Scherbaum WA, Bottazzo GF: Autoantibodies to vasopressin cells in idiopathic diabetes insipidus: Evidence for an autoimmune variant. Lancet 1:897–901, 1983.

134. Vokes TJ, Gaskill MB, Robertson GL: Antibodies to vasopressin in patients with diabetes insipidus. Ann Intern Med 108:190–195, 1988.

135. Hollinshead WH: The interphase of diabetes insipidus. Proc Mayo Clin 39:95–100, 1964.

136. Imura H, Nakao K, Shimatsu A, et al: Lymphocytic infundibuloneurohypophysitis as a cause of central diabetes insipidus. N Engl J Med 329:683–689, 1993.

137. Jialal I, Desai K, Rajput MC: An assessment of posterior pituitary function in patients with Sheehan's syndrome. Clin Endocrinol 27:91–95, 1987.

138. Baylis PH, Thompson CJ, Burd JM, et al: Recurrent pregnancy-induced polyuria and thirst due to hypothalamic diabetes insipidus: An investigation into possible mechanisms responsible for polyuria. Clin Endocrinol 24:459–466, 1986.

139. Barron WM, Cohen LH, Ulland LA, et al: Transient vasopressin-resistant diabetes insipidus of pregnancy. N Engl J Med 310:442–444, 1984.

140. Ito M, Mori Y, Oiso Y, Saito H: A single base substitution in the coding region for neurophysin II associated with familial central diabetes insipidus. J Clin Invest 87:725–728, 1991.

141. Miller WL: Molecular genetics of familial central diabetes insipidus. J Clin Endocrinol Metab 77:592–595, 1993.

142. Heppner C, Kotzka J, Bullmann C, et al: Identification of mutations of the arginine vasopressin-neurophysin II gene in two kindreds with familial central diabetes insipidus. J Clin Endocrinol 83:693–696, 1998.

143. Cremers CWRJ, Wijdeveld PGAB, Pinckers AJLG: Juvenile diabetes mellitus, optic atrophy, hearing loss, diabetes insipidus, atonia of the urinary tract and bladder, and other abnormalities (Wolfram syndrome). Acta Paediatr Scand Suppl 264:1–16, 1977.

144. Barrett TG, Bundey SE: Wolfram (DIDMOAD) syndrome. J Med Genet 34:838–841, 1997.

145. Dashe AM, Cramm RE, Crist CA, et al: A water deprivation test for the differential diagnosis of polyuria. JAMA 185:699–703, 1963.

146. Miller M, Dalakos T, Moses AM, et al: Recognition of partial defects in antidiuretic hormone secretion. Ann Intern Med 73:721–729, 1970.

147. Zerbe RL, Robertson GL: A comparison of plasma vasopressin measurements with a standard indirect test in the differential diagnosis of polyuria. N Engl J Med 305:1539–1546, 1981.

148. Moses AM, Streeten DHP: Differentiation of polyuric states by measurement of responses to changes in plasma osmolality induced by hypertonic saline infusion. Am J Med 42:368–377, 1967.

149. Robertson GL: Diagnosis of diabetes insipidus. *In* Czernichow P, Robinson AG (eds): Diabetes Insipidus in Man: Frontiers of Hormone Research, vol 13. Basel, S. Karger, 1985, pp 176–189.

150. Baylis PH, Robertson GL: Vasopressin response to hypertonic saline infusion to assess posterior pituitary function. J R Soc Med 73:255–260, 1980.

151. Sato N, Ishizaka H, Yagi H, et al: Posterior lobe of the pituitary in diabetes insipidus: Dynamic MR imaging. Radiology 186:357–360, 1993.

152. Cobb WE, Spare S, Reichlin S: Neurogenic diabetes insipidus: Management with DDAVP (1-desamino-8-D arginine vasopressin). Ann Intern Med 88:183–188, 1978.

153. Miller M, Moses AM: Potentiation of vasopressin action by chlorpropamide in vivo. Endocrinology 86:1024–1027, 1970.

154. Niaudet P, Dechaux M, Trivinc C, et al: Nephrogenic diabetes insipidus: Clinical and pathophysiological aspects. Adv Nephrol 13:247–260, 1984.

155. Kambouris M, Dlouhy SR, Trofatter JA, et al: Localization of the gene for X-linked nephrogenic diabetes insipidus to Xq28. Am J Med Genet 29:239–246, 1988.

156. Moses AM, Miller JL, Levine MA: Two distinct pathophysiological mechanisms in

congenital nephrogenic diabetes insipidus. J Clin Endocrinol Metab 66:1259–1264, 1988.

157. Mulders SM, Knoers NV, van Lieburg AF, et al: New mutations in the AQP2 gene in nephrogenic diabetes insipidus resulting in functional but misrouted water channels. J Am Soc Nephrol 8:242–248, 1997.

158. Deen PMT, Croes H, van Aubel RAMH, et al: Water channels encoded by mutant aquaporin-2 genes in nephrogenic diabetes insipidus are impaired in their routing. J Clin Invest 95:2291–2296, 1995.

159. Simon NM, Garber E, Arieff AL: Persistent nephrogenic diabetes insipidus after lithium carbonate. Ann Intern Med 86:446–447, 1977.

160. Niaudet P, Dechaux M, Leroy D, Boyer M: Nephrogenic diabetes insipidus in children. In Czernichow P, Robinson AG (eds): Diabetes Insipidus in Man: Frontiers of Hormone Research, vol 13. Basel, Karger, 1985, pp 224–231.

161. Robertson G, Aycinena P, Vokes T, Weiss N: Dipsogenic diabetes insipidus: A variant of primary polydipsia caused by abnormal osmoregulation of thirst. In Yoshida S, Share L (eds): Recent Progress in Posterior Pituitary Hormones 1988. Amsterdam, Elsevier, 1988, pp 411–418.

162. Flear CTG, Gill GV, Burn J: Hyponatremia: Mechanisms and management. Lancet 2:26–31, 1981.

163. Berl T, Anderson RJ, McDonald KM, Schrier RW: Clinical disorders of water metabolism. Kidney Int 10:117–132, 1976.

164. Arieff AL, Flach F, Massry SG: Neurological manifestations and morbidity of hyponatremia, correlation with brain, water and electrolytes. Medicine 55:121–129, 1976.

165. Fried LF, Palevsky PM: Hyponatremia and hypernatremia. Med Clin North Am 81:585–609, 1997.

166. Anderson RJ, Chung H-M, Kluge R, Schrier RW: Hyponatremia: A prospective analysis of its epidemiology and the pathogenetic role of vasopressin. Ann Intern Med 102:164–168, 1985.

167. Gross PA, Pehrisch H, Rascher W, et al: Pathogenesis of clinical hyponatremia: Observations of vasopressin and fluid intake in 100 hyponatremic medical patients. Eur J Clin Invest 17:123–129, 1987.

168. Winkler AW, Crankshaw OF: Chloride depletion in conditions other than Addison's disease. J Clin Invest 17:1–6, 1938.

169. Bartter FC, Schwartz WB: The syndrome of inappropriate secretion of antidiuretic hormone. Am J Med 42:790–806, 1967.

170. Leaf A, Bartter FC, Sautos RF, Wrong O: Evidence in man that urinary electrolyte loss induced by pitressin is a function of water retention. J Clin Invest 32:868–878, 1952.

171. Verbalis JG: Hyponatremia. In Baylis PH (ed): Water and Salt Homeostasis in Health and Disease. London, Baillière Tindall, 1989, pp 499–530.

172. Carney DN, Gazdar AF, Oie HK, et al: The in vitro growth and characterization of small cell lung cancer. In Greco FA (ed): Biology and Management of Lung Cancer. Boston, Martinus Nijhoff, 1983, pp 1–24.

173. Zerbe R, Stropes L, Robertson GL: Vasopressin function in the syndrome of inappropriate antidiuresis. Ann Rev Med 31:315–327, 1980.

174. Rolls B: Thirst in human hypo- and hypernatremic states. In Jard S, Jamison R (eds): Vasopressin. Montrouge, France, John Libbey, 1991, pp 549–556.

175. Kovacs L, Robertson GL: Disorders of water balance hyponatremia and hypernatremia. Clin Endocrinol Metab 6:107–127, 1992.

176. Arieff AI: Management of hyponatremia. Br Med J 307:305–308, 1993.

177. Ellis SJ: Severe hyponatremia: Complications and treatment. Q J Med 88:905–909, 1995.

178. Forrest JN Jr, Cox M, Hong C, et al: Superiority of demeclocycline over lithium in the treatment of chronic syndrome of inappropriate secretion of antidiuretic hormone. N Engl J Med 298:173–177, 1978.

179. Kinter LB, Ilson BE, Caltabianol S, et al: Antidiuretic hormone antagonism in humans: Are there predictors? In Jard S, Jamison R (eds): Vasopressin. Montrouge, France, John Libbey, 1991, pp 321–329.

180. Ohnishi A, Orita Y, Okahara R, et al: Potent aquaretic agent: A novel non-peptide selective vasopressin 2 antagonist (OPC-31260) in men. J Clin Invest 92:2653–2659, 1993.

181. Saito T, Ishikawa S, Abe K, et al: Acute aquaresis by the non-peptide arginine vasopressin (AVP) antagonist OPC-31260 improves hyponatremia in patients with syndrome of inappropriate secretion of antidiuretic hormone. J Clin Endocrinol Metab 82:1054–1057, 1997.

182. Tanay A, Yust I, Peresecenschi G, et al: Long-term treatment of the syndrome of inappropriate antidiuretic hormone secretion with phenytoin. Ann Intern Med 90:50–52, 1979.

183. Decaux G, Waterlot Y, Gennette F, et al: Inappropriate secretion of antidiuretic hormone treated with furosemide. Br Med J 285:89–90, 1982.

184. Sterns RH, Riggs J, Schochet SS: Osmotic demyelination syndrome following correction of hyponatremia. N Engl J Med 314:1535–1542, 1986.

185. Verbalis JG: Adaptation to acute and chronic hyponatremia: Implications for symptomatology, diagnosis and treatment. Semin Nephrol 18:3–19, 1998.

186. Verbalis JG, Martinez AJ: Determinants of brain myelinolysis following correction of chronic hyponatremia. In Jard S, Jamison R (eds): Vasopressin. Montrouge, France, John Libbey, 1991, pp 539–547.

187. Robertson GL, Aycinena P, Zerbe RL: Neurogenic disorders of osmoregulation. Am J Med 72:339–353, 1982.

188. Robertson GL: Abnormalities of thirst regulation. Kidney Int 25:460–469, 1984.

189. de Rubertis FR, Michelis MF, Beck N, et al: "Essential hypernatremia" due to ineffective osmotic and intact volume regulation of vasopressin secretion. J Clin Invest 50:97–111, 1971.

190. Hammond DN, Moll GW, Robertson GL, Chelmicka-Schorr E: Hypodipsic hypernatremia with normal osmoregulation of vasopressin. N Engl J Med 315:433–436, 1986.

191. Ball SG, Vaidja B, Baylis PH: Hypothalamic adipsic syndrome: Diagnosis and management. Clin Endocrinol 47:405–409, 1997.

192. Baylis PH, Robertson GL: Physiological control of vasopressin secretion. In Baylis PH, Padfield PL (eds): The Posterior Pituitary: Hormone Secretion in Health and Disease. New York, Marcel Dekker, 1985, pp 119–139.

Chapter 29

The Pineal Gland: Basic Physiology and Clinical Implications

Josephine Arendt

STRUCTURE AND BIOCHEMISTRY OF THE PINEAL GLAND

Structure

The pineal gland (epiphysis cerebri) is a small, unpaired central structure, essentially an appendage of the brain. Great variation in size and position is seen even within species.[1] In humans the pineal weighs around 100 to 150 mg. It assumes a shape resembling a pine cone (hence pineal) and, again owing to its shape, has been referred to as the "penis of the brain."

The mammalian pineal gland is a secretory organ, whereas in fish and amphibians it is directly photoreceptive and in reptiles and birds it has a mixed photoreceptor and secretory function.[2] The extracranial parietal (parapineal, frontal) organ found in some lower vertebrates has been referred to as the "third eye."[1, 2] The principal cellular component is the pinealocyte, and elements of its photoreceptive evolutionary history remain in both structure and function.[1–3] In some species, including humans, calcified lumps are frequently present in pineal tissue after puberty, although this calcification does not appear to be associated with a decline in metabolic activity except in the sense that activity declines in general with aging.[4–6] The gland is richly vascularized. Its principal innervation is sympathetic and arises from the superior cervical ganglion.[7] In addition, good evidence has been presented for parasympathetic, commissural, and peptidergic innervation.[8] Its primary function in all species studied to date is to transduce information concerning light-dark cycles to body physiology, particularly for the organization of body rhythms.[9] This information is encoded in the secretion patterns of the major pineal hormone melatonin (5-methoxy-*N*-acetyltryptamine).[10]

Synthesis and Metabolism of Melatonin

Melatonin is synthesized within pinealocytes—cell types derived from photoreceptors—from tryptophan via the pathway shown in Figure 29–1.[11, 12] Most synthetic activity occurs during the dark phase, with a major increase (7- to 150-fold) in the activity of serotonin-*N*-

acetyltransferase (arylalkylamine N-acetyltransferase [AA-NAT]). The rhythm of production is endogenous in that it is generated in the suprachiasmatic nucleus (SCN), the major central rhythm-generating system or "clock" in mammals[12] (the pineal itself is a self-sustaining "clock" in some, if not all, lower vertebrates[13]). The rhythm is synchronized to 24 hours primarily by the light-dark cycle acting via the retina and the retinohypothalamic projection to the SCN. The cDNAs encoding both AA-NAT and the *O*-methylating enzyme hydroxyindole-*O*-methyltransferase (see Fig. 29–1) have been cloned, and studies of molecular regulation of melatonin production show some species differences.[14] It is likely that the human enzyme is regulated primarily at a posttranscriptional level, whereas in rodents the key event appears

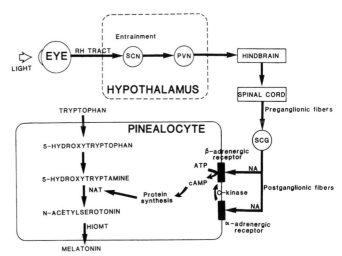

FIGURE 29–1. Control of melatonin synthesis in the pineal gland. The rhythm of secretion is generated in the suprachiasmatic nucleus (SCN) and entrained by the light-dark cycle. HIOMT, hydroxyindole-*O*-methyltransferase; NA, norepinephrine; NAT, 5-hydroxytryptamine (serotonin)-*N*-acetyltransferase; PVN, paraventricular nucleus; RH, retinohypothalamic; SCG, superior cervical ganglion.

to be cyclic adenosine monophosphate (cAMP)-dependent phosphorylation of a transcription factor that binds to the AA-NAT promoter. Rapid decline in activity with light treatment at night appears to depend on proteasomal proteolysis.[15] Phosphorylation of the transcription factor CREB (cAMP-responsive element–binding protein) appears to be an important step in the signal transduction cascade that activates melatonin biosynthesis in the mammalian pineal organ.[16] According to distribution studies of AA-NAT mRNA, this enzyme is expressed in the pineal gland, retina, and to a much lesser extent, some other brain areas, the pituitary, and the testis,[14] but apart from the pineal, these structures contribute little to circulating concentrations in mammals.[9] Within the rodent retina a self-sustaining "clock" maintains rhythmic production of melatonin in vitro as it does in many lower vertebrates.[17] Whether this pattern is true in humans remains to be seen.

Melatonin is metabolized primarily within the liver by 6-hydroxylation, followed by sulfate and/or glucuronide conjugation. A number of minor metabolites are also formed through ring splitting, cyclization of the side chain, or demethylation (see Arendt[9] for a bibliography). In humans and rodents, exogenous oral or intravenous melatonin has a short metabolic half-life (20–60 minutes, depending on the author and species), with a large hepatic first-pass effect and a biphasic elimination pattern. In ruminants, longer half-lives are seen after oral administration.[9, 18–20]

Other Pineal Factors

Although the pineal contains and synthesizes a multitude of other indoles together with biologically active peptides (for review, see Pevet[21, 22]), they have not yet been attributed important physiologic functions. Most effects of pinealectomy can be reversed by melatonin in physiologic concentrations; hence it is difficult to consider other compounds major pineal hormones.

Neural Control of Melatonin Synthesis

In mammals, pineal denervation, or ganglionectomy, abolishes the rhythmic synthesis of melatonin and the light-dark control of its production. Norepinephrine is clearly the major transmitter and acts via β_1-adrenoceptors with potentiation by α_1-stimulation, but the role of neural serotonin is probably not negligible. A day-night variation is seen in pineal norepinephrine, with highest values at night, approximately 180 degrees out of phase with the pineal serotonin rhythm. cAMP acts as a second messenger and stimulates AA-NAT activity. β-Adrenergic receptor–binding sites in the rat pineal vary over a 24-hour period, the lowest number being found toward the end of the dark phase and increasing shortly after lights on.[11, 12, 23, 24]

Other Control Mechanisms

The pineal contains very large numbers of other neuroreceptors and hormone receptors, but evaluation of their physiologic importance is in its infancy.[25–27]

PHYSIOLOGY OF THE PINEAL

Light-Dark Control of Melatonin Synthesis

A Darkness Hormone

In virtually all species studied to date, whether nocturnal or diurnal, melatonin is synthesized and secreted during the dark phase of the day.[9] Remarkably, even the unicellular alga *Gonyaulax* appears to produce melatonin during the dark phase, and it appears to be present in higher plants.[28, 29] Melatonin production is clearly a highly evolutionarily conserved phenomenon. In most vertebrates the rhythm is endogenous, that is, internally generated. It persists in the absence of

time cues, in general assuming a period deviating slightly from 24 hours, and is thus a true circadian rhythm.[30, 31] Lesions of the SCN lead to loss of the vast majority of circadian rhythms such as locomotor activity, sleep, behavior,[32] hormones including melatonin, and urinary constituents. Circadian rhythms are entrained (synchronized) to the 24-hour day primarily by light-dark cycles. Factors (zeitgebers) other than light-dark cycles that are involved in entrainment include behavioral imposition such as forced activity and rest, social and nutritional (rhythmic feeding) cues, temperature variations, knowledge of clock time, certain drugs, possibly electromagnetic fields, and melatonin itself.[31–33]

Melatonin Secretion in Relation to Day Length

In most species, melatonin secretion is related to the length of the night: the longer the night, the longer the duration of secretion.[9] This phenomenon has been particularly well demonstrated in sheep, in which melatonin levels rise within a few minutes of lights off and, in photoperiods of more than around 14 hours of light, do not decline until lights on. In such photoperiods, light serves to entrain the rhythm and suppress secretion at the beginning and/or the end of the dark phase (Fig. 29–2).

The most consistent observation in humans is that melatonin profiles show a phase change from winter to summer, with earlier secretion in summer than in winter (see Arendt[9] for references). However, if humans are kept strictly in darkness for 14 hours per day for a period of 2 months, the melatonin secretion pattern expands to cover almost

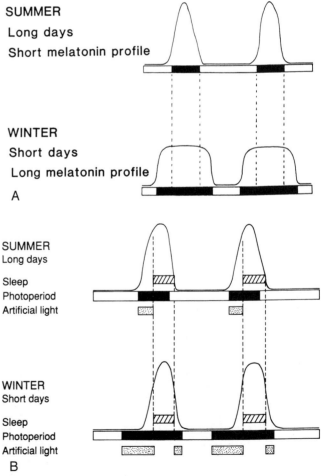

FIGURE 29–2. Diagrammatic representation of melatonin secretion in relation to day length. *A,* The change in duration with length of the natural dark phase acts as a seasonal time cue in photoperiodic species. *B,* Social behavior and artificial lighting in humans lead to minimal change in duration but phase advances in summer. If a long or short dark phase is imposed, the pattern reverts to that shown in *A.*

the entire dark period, and concomitantly, in extended periods of 16 hours of light, the rhythm contracts to less than 9 hours, with accompanying changes in body temperature and sleep.[34]

Light Suppression of Melatonin Secretion

Even brief exposure to light of sufficient intensity at night rapidly suppresses melatonin production.[35] In general, the most effective light appears to be in the green band (540 nm); however, a precise definition is lacking to date.[36] The amount of light required to suppress melatonin secretion during the night varies from species to species, with the time of night, and with previous light exposure.[36] In humans, Lewy et al. observed that 2500 lux (domestic light is around 300–500 lux) is required to completely suppress melatonin at night.[37] However, lower intensities will partially suppress and shift the rhythm in humans.[38, 39]

This observation has been of very considerable importance for a general appreciation of the role of light in human physiology, in particular, its importance in the control of human rhythms and in the treatment of winter depression (seasonal affective disorder[40]).

Entrainment of the Melatonin Rhythm

A single daily light pulse of suitable intensity and duration in otherwise constant darkness is sufficient to phase-shift and synchronize the melatonin rhythm to 24 hours in animals.[41] Phase shifting and entrainment have been demonstrated in humans with suitable intensity and duration of light treatment.[9, 42, 43] However, the relative contribution of light to the entrainment of melatonin in a normal environment remains to be fully determined. Studies in Antarctica suggest that a structured social routine in a dim light environment suffices to synchronize melatonin to 24 hours.[9] However, many blind people with no conscious or unconscious light perception living in a normal social environment show desynchronized melatonin and other circadian rhythms.[44–46]

Role in Photoperiodic Seasonal Functions

Photoperiodism

Most species show seasonal variations in their physiology and behavior, even humans. The reproductive cycle is timed so that environmental conditions are propitious for growth of the young, and variations in behavior, pelage (coat growth and color), appetite, body weight, and fat are such that survival in ambient temperature conditions is optimized and camouflage protects against predators. When seasonal functions are primarily timed by day length, species are referred to as photoperiodic.[47] Photoperiod is often critical for the timing of pubertal development.[48] In general, puberty is reached only during the adult mating season. It is now clear that in photoperiodic mammals and marsupials, an intact innervated pineal gland is essential for the perception of photoperiodic change.[30, 49, 50] Most information is derived from studies on reproductive function in hamsters and sheep.

Role of Melatonin

Pinealectomy removes the vast majority of circulating melatonin in rodents, primates, and ungulates.[49] It was therefore the first pineal hormone to be investigated as a pineal photoneuroendocrine transducer. It is possible to administer melatonin by daily infusion or feeding to generate at will circulating profiles with a duration characteristic of particular photoperiods in an intact or pinealectomized animal.[30, 40–51] In this way it has become clear that a particular melatonin duration is a necessary and sufficient condition for induction of a given seasonal response and is equipotent with a particular photoperiod. Long-duration melatonin is equivalent to short days, and short-duration melatonin is equivalent to long days (see Fig. 29–2). Interpretation of the signal, as with day length, depends on the physiology (for example, long- or short-day breeder) of the species in question. In sheep the evidence is good that long days or short-duration melatonin can time the whole seasonal cycle, at least of reproduction, and act as a seasonal zeitgeber for a presumed endogenous annual rhythm.[51] Animals become refractory to a specific duration of melatonin as they do to a particular photoperiod. For example, a period of long days (or a long-day melatonin signal) is required before a short-day melatonin signal advances the reproductive cycle in sheep.[49–51]

Puberty

The photoperiod via melatonin secretion determines the timing of puberty in some species, provided that a sufficient degree of physical maturity has been reached.[48] Interestingly, photoperiod perception by the fetus is present before birth in rodents and ungulates and ensures a rate of development appropriate to environmental conditions.[52] Melatonin crosses the placenta in a number of species, and melatonin injection in the mother can dictate the timing of postnatal reproductive development.

The laboratory rat is only marginally photoperiodic. Nevertheless, injections of melatonin during the late light phase, during a small window in the late dark phase, or even via continuous release implants, specifically during the period of pubertal development, delay reproductive maturity in both males and females.[53] Full sexual maturity is eventually achieved; thus the system is not permanently compromised. Moreover, in vitro melatonin inhibits gonadotropin-releasing hormone (GnRH)-induced luteinizing hormone (LH) release by cultured rat pituitary glands from prepubertal animals.[54] These observations constitute the main evidence for a possible causal role of melatonin in the pubertal development of humans.

Nonreproductive Seasonal Functions

The pineal gland via melatonin secretion probably plays a role in all photoperiod-dependent functions in mammals. Evidence exists to substantiate this statement with respect to behavior, body weight, coat constitution and color (for example, the white winter coat of some polar species), prolactin variations, antler growth, thyroid activity, appetite, thermoregulation, delayed implantation, embryonic diapause, and hibernation.[30, 49–51, 55, 55a] Partly because the ability to control reproduction is of applied interest in commercially important domestic species such as sheep, this aspect has received more attention than others. The winter coat of animals such as mink, arctic foxes, and cashmere goats also has commercial significance and can be manipulated by photoperiod and melatonin administration. Implanted melatonin induces short-day effects, and a number of commercial preparations of melatonin have been developed to this end.

Role of the Pineal Gland and Melatonin in Circadian Rhythms

Nonmammalian Vertebrates

An extensive literature has described the importance of the pineal (and also the retina) in the control of circadian rhythms in lower vertebrates. Melatonin is produced rhythmically by both the pineal and the retina in many lower vertebrates and probably serves as the common humoral signal for circadian organization.[9, 33]

Role of the Pineal in Mammalian Circadian Rhythms

Until quite recently, opinion was that the pineal did not have a role in the mammalian circadian system. However, in rats, pinealectomy increases the rate of re-entrainment to forced phase shifts of the light-dark cycle, and pinealectomy of hamsters in constant light leads to major disruption of the circadian system.[56, 57] In parallel, a substantial body of work implicates melatonin in circadian thermoregulation (see Badia et al.[55] for a review). Many such effects may involve the thyroid gland.[58]

Effects of Timed Administration of Melatonin

BEHAVIOR, HORMONES, AND TEMPERATURE. In rats, daily melatonin injections synchronize free-running activity and temperature rhythms in constant darkness and are reported to partially or completely synchronize disrupted activity rhythms in constant light, although the latter observation is somewhat controversial.[57, 59, 60] A phase-response curve to single injections of melatonin can be demonstrated with small phase advances of at most 1 hour during the late subjective day.[59] Timed administration hastens adaptation of activity and melatonin production to forced phase shift and can change the direction of re-entrainment.[59, 60, 61] Some but not all strains of adult hamster can be synchronized by melatonin administration,[62] and fetal hamsters can be entrained by maternal injections of melatonin at 24-hour intervals in specific circadian phases.[63]

GESTATION. In the rat, gestation length depends on the ambient light-dark cycle. Small advances or delays in parturition can be induced by day lengths shorter or longer than 24 hours, and the effect can partially be mimicked by timed melatonin administration.[64]

ESTROUS CYCLE. Because the pineal is involved in circadian timing, the presumption must be that it is concerned with timing of the LH surge and, indeed, with general estrous timing. In rats, timed melatonin administration has been demonstrated to mimic the effects of extending the light-dark cycle on timing of the LH surge. Observations of the melatonin rhythm itself show a decreased amplitude during proestrus in rodents but with conflicting reports in other species (see elsewhere[9, 65] for reviews).

AGING. A fairly consistent observation in pineal research is the decline in amplitude of the melatonin rhythm in old age (see Arendt[9] for references). Pinealectomy accelerates the aging process, and the possible antiaging effects of melatonin has generated considerable publicity. Several hypotheses have been put forward to explain these often flawed,[67, 68] insubstantial, but interesting observations. One proposes that melatonin enhances immune responses via an opiatergic mechanism. Another considers that appropriately timed daily melatonin administration optimizes circadian relationships, especially of phase, and increases circadian amplitude (see Armstrong and Redman[69] for references). The most widely published explanation is that melatonin acts as a free radical scavenger and antioxidant.[70–72] Being an easily oxidized molecule, melatonin does indeed have some antioxidant activity. Whether this property is physiologically relevant in mammals remains an open question. It has been suggested that this activity was its primary evolutionary function in primitive species.[71] Certainly, much publicity has attended this property of the molecule; however, the quantities of exogenous melatonin required to generate significant antioxidant activity in vivo remain to be specified.

IN VITRO PHASE SHIFTS. The metabolic activity of the rodent SCN in vivo and the electrical activity of various in vitro SCN preparations can be modified by melatonin; it inhibits 2-deoxyglucose uptake into the nuclei in the late subjective day with no effect at other times and inhibits electrical activity, also during the late subjective day.[60] By far the most convincing evidence is the phase-advancing effect of melatonin on the circadian rhythm of electrical activity in cultured SCN.[73] The effect was large, acute, and time dependent, with shifts of up to several hours being observed. Thus melatonin acts directly on a central biologic clock to change its phase.

RETINAL RHYTHMS. Melatonin appears to function as a paracrine signal within the retina. It enhances retinal function in low-intensity light by inducing photomechanical changes and regulating turnover rates of the photoreceptive apparatuses of rods, cones, and the surrounding pigment epithelium.[73, 74]

SUMMARY. The pineal, the retina, and the SCN together form the basic structures perceiving and transducing the nonvisual effects of light. Melatonin provides a closed loop to this system (Fig. 29–3). It is reasonable to conclude that in adult mammals, melatonin serves to modulate circadian phase and strengthen coupling. In fetal and neonatal mammals, it helps program the circadian system and determine the timing of developmental stages, especially puberty.

THE PINEAL IN HUMAN PHYSIOLOGY AND PATHOLOGY

Clearly, the importance of the pineal in humans depends on the importance of light in human physiology. It is reasonable to assume

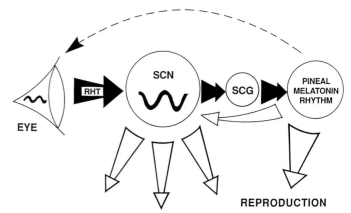

FIGURE 29–3. A model for closed-loop feedback of melatonin within the circadian system. Functional melatonin receptors are found in both the suprachiasmatic nucleus (SCN) and the retina. Rhythm generation in the SCN can be modulated in phase and amplitude by melatonin. The mammalian retina generates rhythmic melatonin production in vitro, which together with pineal-derived melatonin may serve to influence retinal processes.

that the pineal conveys information concerning light-dark cycles for the organization of seasonal and circadian rhythms in humans as in animals. Pinealectomy in humans removes virtually all plasma melatonin.[75] Other consequences of the operation consist of diffuse neurologic problems that do not add up to a consistent functional effect as yet and may be more related to nonspecific effects of the operation.

Human Melatonin Production

Basic Characteristics

MECHANISMS. Early work demonstrated the presence of hydroxyindole-*O*-methyltransferase activity in tissue from postmortem pineal glands. The melatonin content of human pineals is related to the time of death, with higher values at night, as expected. Pathologic or traumatic denervation of the pineal abolishes the plasma melatonin rhythm. β-Adrenergic antagonists suppress melatonin production, and increased availability of norepinephrine and serotonin is stimulatory (see reviews elsewhere[9, 76, 77]). Good evidence has thus been presented that the neural and biochemical pathways known to control pineal function in rats are similar in humans.

MELATONIN AND 6-SULFATOXYMELATONIN PRODUCTION. In a "normal" environment, melatonin is secreted during the night in healthy humans as in all other species. The average maximum levels attained in plasma in adults are on the order of 60 to 70 pg/mL when measured with high-specificity assays. Mean maximum concentrations of 6-sulfatoxymelatonin attain 80 to 100 pg/mL (different mammalian species have a relatively narrow range of circulating concentrations, although birds have more). Minimum concentrations of both compounds are usually below 10 pg/mL. Peak concentrations of melatonin in plasma normally occur between 2 and 4 AM. The onset of secretion is usually around 9 to 10 PM and the offset at 7 to 9 AM in adults in temperate zones. The appearance and peak levels of 6-sulfatoxymelatonin in plasma are delayed by 1 to 2 hours and the morning decline by 3 to 4 hours[9] (Fig. 29–4). In urine, 50% to 80% of 6-sulfatoxymelatonin appears in the overnight sample (midnight to 8 AM), and it is low but rarely undetectable in the afternoon and early evening.

The rhythm is endogenous, with a period usually greater than 24 hours.[30, 43, 78] Possibly the most striking characteristic of the normal human melatonin rhythm is its reproducibility from day to day and from week to week in normal individuals, rather like a hormonal fingerprint.[79] In spite of intraindividual stability, very large variability

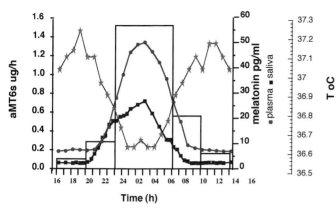

FIGURE 29–4. *Plasma melatonin (circles), saliva melatonin (squares), and urinary 6-sulfatoxymelatonin (aMT6s, histogram) in relation to core body temperature (stars). Mean normal values from the author's laboratory are represented diagrammatically. Note the close correspondence of the temperature nadir with the melatonin peak.*

in amplitude of the rhythm is noted between subjects. A small number of apparently normal individuals have no detectable melatonin in plasma at all times of day.[80]

ASSOCIATION WITH TEMPERATURE. Many associations of melatonin with temperature exist in humans. The most striking is the reciprocal relationship in circadian profiles, where the temperature nadir correlates closely with the peak of melatonin. The ovulatory rise in temperature during the menstrual cycle is associated with a reported decline in the amplitude of melatonin, but the decline in melatonin is not a consistent observation. A causal relationship is probably in effect inasmuch as exogenous melatonin can acutely depress body temperature in humans.[81, 82]

ASSOCIATION WITH SLEEP. Obvious correlations are noted between melatonin production at night and sleep, and again, some specific causal relationships may exist. However, sleep deprivation does not abolish the melatonin rhythm and, in dim light, does not affect secretion.[81] During sleep deprivation, self-rated fatigue exhibits a circadian rhythm that is closely correlated with plasma melatonin levels.[81] Many studies have attempted to relate sleep stages to detailed melatonin profiles, but few associations have emerged, with the exception of a relationship between the timing of sleep spindles and certain other electroencephalographic (EEG) characteristics and the circadian phase of melatonin.[83] Possibly the most striking association concerns the appearance of daytime naps in free-running blind subjects (usually with no light perception), when the peak of melatonin (and of course the temperature nadir) occurs during the daytime.[84] It has been proposed that the initial rise in melatonin opens a "sleep gate," that is, increases sleep propensity.[85]

OTHER ASSOCIATIONS. Obviously, any variable with a marked circadian rhythm shows correlations with melatonin, if necessary, displaced in time. Examples include cortisol, prolactin, thyroid-stimulating hormone, aspects of the immune system, and many others.[9] The relationships of stress, exercise,[86] and some other nonpharmacologic interventions in modification of melatonin production are somewhat unclear and do not appear to play a major role in humans. Insufficient data are available to make further judgments.

Development, Puberty, and Aging

Shortly after birth, very little melatonin or 6-sulfatoxymelatonin is detectable in body fluids. A robust melatonin rhythm appears around 6 to 8 weeks of life.[86] Whether in specific individuals this rhythm corresponds to the organization and synchronization of other circadian variables such as sleep remains a question of very considerable interest. If melatonin serves to set the circadian phase in humans, as it does in rodents, it is quite possible that circadian organization develops in breast-fed babies absorbing maternal melatonin before it does in bottle-fed babies.

The plasma concentration of melatonin increases rapidly thereafter

and reaches a lifetime peak on average at 3 to 5 years of age.[87] The increment is much greater at night. Subsequently, a steady decrease is seen, with mean adult concentrations attained in the mid to late teens and the major decline occurring before puberty[88] (Fig. 29–5). Values remain relatively unchanged until 35 to 40 years of age, and a final decline in amplitude then takes place until (on average) low levels are seen in old age (see Arendt[9] for references). Reports of association of differences in secretion in adults with gender, height, or body weight are not consistent. However, the measured plasma concentrations of melatonin in children are probably related to body weight.[6]

The decline in plasma melatonin in early life in no way proves that it is involved in human pubertal development. Although a lower melatonin concentration has been reported in children with precocious puberty and higher concentrations in those with delayed puberty and hypothalamic amenorrhea than in age-matched controls,[89–91] these associations remain correlative and not causal. Ovarian suppression with a GnRH analogue in precocious girls is not accompanied by changes in melatonin secretion.[92] However, in one case report, induction of sexual development with estrogen was associated with a very rapid decline in melatonin metabolite excretion.[93]

Menstrual Cycle

Some of the very earliest reports on human melatonin described low preovulatory concentrations the morning before ovulation and suggested that low melatonin was facilitatory to the preovulatory LH peak.[9] This observation is inconsistent, however, and more recent work indicates that neither the amplitude nor the phase of melatonin is altered in the course of the normal cycle.[9, 65] The effects of melatonin on core body temperature are reported to vary in the course of the cycle, and herein may lie a physiologic function.[94] LH pulses are amplified in the early follicular phase by oral melatonin at 8 AM.[95] Attempts to develop melatonin as a contraceptive pill in combination with a synthetic progestin minipill have not been successful.[96]

Very large doses (100 mg daily) potentiate testosterone-induced LH suppression.[97] A series of studies in males with and without hypogonadism has reinforced the perception that melatonin is essentially inhibitory to human reproductive function (e.g., Luboshitzky et al.[98, 99]). Because humans appear to conceive more readily in long photoperiods, an explanation may reside in residual human photoperiodism.[100] The results of these studies partially support the contention that melatonin, suitably administered, can inhibit human reproductive activity.

In the author's opinion, low, timed doses of melatonin used to reinforce circadian organization are likely to improve fertility in humans.

Pathology

Pineal Hyperplasia and Hypoplasia

A number of reports of variations in postmortem pineal weight as a function of the cause of death have been summarized by Tapp.[5] Of the most interesting, hypoplasia of the pineal in association with retinal disease may be causally interrelated. Tapp has reported that pineal glands in patients dying of carcinoma of the breast or melanoma are heavier than those from patients with other cancers. Very large pineals (1 g) have been described in a rare genetic syndrome with insulin resistance.[101] Sudden infant death syndrome is associated with small pineals and decreased melatonin production.[102, 103] Such deaths usually occur at night and may be associated with abnormalities of sleep. If melatonin helps coordinate circadian organization in the developing infant, its underproduction may contribute to the disorder.

Pineal Tumors

Tumors of the pineal region in children are frequently associated with abnormal pubertal development.[104] The original hypothesis to explain precocious puberty in boys with pineal tumors was that the tumors destroyed the capacity of the pineal to inhibit sexual develop-

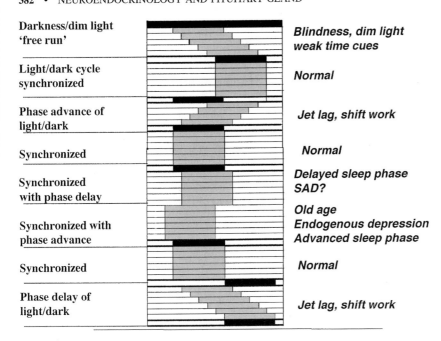

Darkness/dim light 'free run'

Blindness, dim light weak time cues

Light/dark cycle synchronized

Normal

Phase advance of light/dark

Jet lag, shift work

Synchronized

Normal

Synchronized with phase delay

Delayed sleep phase SAD?

Synchronized with phase advance

Old age
Endogenous depression
Advanced sleep phase

Synchronized

Normal

Phase delay of light/dark

Jet lag, shift work

FIGURE 29–5. Circadian rhythm disorders. *White and black filled bars* represent the light-dark cycle. *Grey filled bars* represent the timing of an endogenous circadian rhythm. In constant darkness or dim light with weak time cues, circadian rhythms free run, usually by delay, and show endogenous periodicity *(top panel)*. In a normal environment, rhythms are synchronized to 24 hours *(second panel)*. After an abrupt advance shift (eastward) of time cues, endogenous rhythms adapt via "transients"; during this time of desynchrony, sleep, alertness, performance, gastrointestinal function, metabolism, and other systems are disturbed *(third panel)*. In the *fourth panel*, rhythms are synchronized to the new time cues. The *fifth panel* shows synchronized rhythms but with a phase delay relative to the environment. In the *sixth panel*, rhythms are synchronized but with a phase advance relative to the environment. The *seventh panel* shows normally synchronized rhythms. In the *eighth panel* is an abrupt phase delay (westward) of the light–dark cycle and adaptation by transients. Westward adaptation is usually faster than eastward. All these conditions are susceptible to timed treatment by substances (such as melatonin) that shift rhythms or by manipulating rhythms with light of suitable intensity and duration. (Adapted from Arendt J: Melatonin and the Mammalian Pineal Gland. London, Chapman Hall, 1995, p 71. With kind permission of Kluwer Academic Publishers.)

ment. In fact, much evidence suggests that precocity is due to production of the β subunit of human chorionic gonadotropin (β-hCG) by germ cell tumors of the pineal.[105, 106] This relationship has nevertheless stimulated much work on the possible role of the pineal through the secretion of melatonin as a means of timing human puberty.

Pineal tumors are heterogeneous and may arise from germ cells (teratomas, germinomas, choriocarcinomas, endodermal sinus tumors, mixed germ cell tumors), pineal parenchymal cells (pineoblastoma and pineocytoma), and the supporting stroma (gliomas).[107] All are rare (less than 1% of intracranial space-occupying lesions) and tend to occur in individuals younger than 20 years, with the exception of parenchymal cell tumors, which occur equally in adults and children. Germinomas respond well to radiation therapy, whereas primary surgery is more frequently the treatment of choice in other types. Tumor markers in cerebrospinal fluid, such as α-fetoprotein and β-hCG, together with cerebrospinal fluid cytology and imaging (computed tomography or magnetic resonance imaging) aid in the differential diagnosis. The most common symptoms are secondary to hydrocephalus (headache, vomiting, and drowsiness), together with the triad of visual problems, diabetes insipidus, and reproductive abnormalities.[107] Germinomas and teratomas occur predominantly in males. Both precocious puberty and delayed puberty have been associated with pineal tumors. Precocious puberty is more commonly associated with teratoma. Cohen and coworkers[106] have reviewed the occurrence of precocious puberty in parallel with β-hCG–secreting pineal tumors. Because β-hCG is identical to β-LH, they conclude that pubertal development can be directly attributed to ectopic β-hCG production in many cases. Moreover, the predominance in boys may be explained on the basis that LH alone can stimulate testosterone production, whereas in girls, both LH and follicle-stimulating hormone (FSH) are required for ovarian follicular development and estrogen production.

No information is consistent on overproduction or underproduction of melatonin with specific types of tumor. However, pinealectomy removes circulating melatonin,[9, 75] and radiation therapy appears to greatly suppress melatonin. At present, long-term evaluation of patients after surgery is under way in a number of centers.

Other Solid Tumors

The relationship of the pineal and melatonin to cancer is a subject that has aroused much interest after early work suggesting that the pineal contains oncostatic activity. Cohen and coworkers proposed in 1978 that human breast cancer is a melatonin-deficient disease.[108]

Since that time, many clinical studies have been performed to assess melatonin secretion in cancer patients. Low levels may be associated at least with (stage-dependent) breast and prostatic cancer[109, 110]; however, not all studies are consistent. A number of broad studies that have included various oncologic conditions report significant differences, both increases and decreases, in plasma melatonin between types of cancer and control populations. At present, these studies are uninterpretable. Recent data suggest that the growth of human benign prostate epithelial cells depends on both steroids and melatonin.[111]

General Pathology

Many clinical attempts have been made to relate circulating melatonin to endocrine and other pathology. The results on the whole are difficult to interpret and are inconsistent (see elsewhere[9, 76, 112] for reviews). Liver disease such as cirrhosis, which impairs metabolic function, leads to higher than normal plasma concentrations of melatonin.[76] Drugs that stimulate or suppress hydroxylation and conjugation mechanisms or that compete for metabolic pathways can be expected to affect circulating melatonin. Surprisingly, little evidence exists for a disturbance in melatonin secretion in major sleep disorders such as narcolepsy and Kleine-Levin syndrome, and in delayed–sleep phase insomnia, only a small delay in the rhythm is found.[113, 114]

Psychiatry

Abnormalities in circadian function have been postulated in depression and mania. Melatonin is arguably the best index of biologic clock function; only bright light and, to a smaller extent, posture "mask" expression of the endogenous rhythm,[31, 115] and it has been extensively used in psychiatry and other fields to assess biologic clock status. Studies have shown a decline in amplitude of the melatonin rhythm in patients with depression, together with an increase in cortisol and possibly an increase in mania, although not all studies are consistent.[77]

Little evidence for abnormal timing of melatonin has been found, although Lewy et al. have reported exceptionally delayed melatonin rhythms in winter in patients with seasonal affective disorder as compared with the small delay seen in normal individuals,[116] and Parry and coworkers have observed abnormal melatonin patterns and response to light in patients with premenstrual dysphoric disorder.[117] At present, no consensus has been reached regarding what causes seasonal affective disorder. The treatment originally proposed for patients with this disorder was the creation of an artificial summer day length by using 3 hours of bright full-spectrum light (Vitalite, 2500 lux) in the morning and evening.[40] The "melatonin hypothesis" predicted that such light treatment would shorten the duration of melatonin secretion, thus generating a summer day length signal by analogy with animal work. The light treatment appears to be efficient (albeit with a large placebo effect), but it does not appear to work through suppression of melatonin.

Many pharmacologic antidepressant treatments stimulate melatonin secretion by acting through increased availability of the precursors tryptophan and serotonin and the major pineal neurotransmitter norepinephrine, or by direct action on serotonin and catecholamine receptors.[77] A link between an increase in melatonin production and the efficacy of treatment may be possible, and this prospect merits exploration.

EFFECTS OF MELATONIN IN HUMANS

Therapeutic Potential and Significance to Health

A very large number of people would benefit from the ability to manipulate rhythms at will. Circadian rhythm disturbance is associated with shift work, jet lag, blindness, insomnia, and old age (among other things). A search for a general chronobiotic—a compound able to rapidly shift the biologic clock in all its manifestations—occupies much scientific time and effort. To date, bright light is the only treatment that in suitable intensity and duration is able to shift the biologic clock. A number of pharmaceutical products and steroid hormones have been shown to shift aspects of the circadian system in animals, usually the activity-rest cycle. The possible use of melatonin and its analogues in this area has become evident.

Early Work

Enormous doses of up to 6.6 g (the daily production of about 200,000 people!) in the daytime had no beneficial effects on parkinsonism, Huntington's chorea, depression (which was worsened), and schizophrenia. Skin pigmentation was not affected; human pigment cells do not resemble amphibian melanophores in pigment migration phenomena. Small decreases in plasma LH and FSH were observed (see Arendt[9] for references). Large amounts of melatonin such as these may produce headache, abdominal cramps, and somnolence.

Much lower (2 mg intranasally, 0.3 to 240 mg orally or intravenously) doses of melatonin can induce transient sleepiness or sleep in suitably controlled circumstances (posture is important).[118, 119] Once again, much publicity has surrounded the reported beneficial effects on sleep. However, without a doubt, melatonin does affect sleep. The first evidence dates from 40 years ago when Aaron Lerner, who first isolated the substance, took 100 mg and described sleepiness after the dose.[120] Early investigations used EEG characteristics to delimit an acute mild sedative and "hypnotic" effect in both animals (cats, rats, chickens) and humans.[118, 119] Subsequently, a substantial body of literature, generally using much lower doses, has described advance shifts in the timing of sleep after early evening administration, transient sleepiness at several different times of day within 2 to 4 hours of the dose, time-dependent increases in sleep propensity, effects on the waking EEG comparable to but not identical with benzodiazepines, a lengthening of the first rapid eye movement episode after early evening administration, increases in the fast EEG frequencies after evening naps or nighttime sleep, and "beneficial effects" when taken at bedtime. The latter are usually a reduction in awakening after sleep onset and an increase in total sleep time evaluated subjectively, by actigraphy, and rarely, by EEG. When melatonin was used to hasten adaptation to a 9-hour phase advance, total sleep time, sleep efficiency, and stage 2 sleep were increased, whereas slow wave sleep was decreased. The subject has been extensively reviewed recently.[118, 119, 121] The findings are still inconsistent, however, and some studies have found no effects of any importance on sleep. Differences between study conditions, subjects, dose, and timing are likely to be the reason for apparently contradictory effects, and much more information is needed for solid conclusions to be drawn.

A brief decline in visual reaction time, accompanied by an increase in fatigue ratings but with no effect on memory, has been reported after melatonin administration.[122] Acute oral doses of melatonin stimulate prolactin secretion.[123] This enhanced prolactin secretion may relate to the ability of melatonin in pharmacologic amounts to inhibit some dopaminergic functions. Acute effects on other pituitary hormones are somewhat inconsistent, although recently a relationship between melatonin and vasopressin secretion has been established.[124] The acute pharmacologic properties of melatonin in animals include sedation, hypothermia, anxiolysis, muscle hypotonia, decrease in locomotor activity with a rebound increase on increasing the dose, slight analgesia, slight protection against electroconvulsive shock, constriction of cerebral arteries, potentiation of noradrenalin-induced vasoconstriction, and very low toxicity.[125–127]

Timed Administration

In early work, daily feeding of low-dose (2 to 5 mg) melatonin in the late afternoon advanced the timing of evening self-rated fatigue, the endogenous melatonin rhythm, and the morning decline in prolactin when compared with placebo. No significant effects were seen on self-rated mood or on LH, FSH, testosterone, cortisol, growth hormone, or thyroxine. No deleterious effects were reported by the subjects.[9] Thus in low doses, melatonin has some chronobiotic effects in humans. Melatonin has rapid, transient, mild sleep-inducing effects and lowers alertness and body temperature during the 3 to 4 hours after low doses (0.5–5 mg) during the daytime, these effects being opposite to the acute effects of bright light given at night.[82, 128] In the same dose range it is able to shift timing of the internal clock to both later and earlier times when administration is appropriately timed.[128–130] As for light, the appropriate timing can be predicted from a phase-response curve in subjects whose body clock phase is known. The phase-response curve to melatonin is essentially the reverse of that to light.[131] Melatonin given approximately 8 to 13 hours before core temperature minimum will produce phase advances and, when given around 1 to 4 hours after core temperature minimum, will produce phase delays. However, its effects on the circadian system appear to be both more complicated and much weaker than those of light. For example, it is unable to consistently entrain free running circadian rhythms of core temperature.[130]

Jet Lag and Shift Work

Melatonin treatment timed to induce phase advances and delays has been used in the alleviation of jet lag in at least 12 real-life and simulation conditions, 10 of which reported beneficial effects. Field studies show that self-rated jet lag both westward and eastward can be reduced on average by 50% with appropriately timed treatment.[132, 133] The improvement appears to be greater with larger numbers of time zones. The subjective impressions are reinforced by improved latency and quality of sleep, greater daytime alertness, and slightly more rapid resynchronization of melatonin and cortisol rhythms. Comparable simulation studies have shown a significant increase in the rate of re-entrainment of both hormonal and electrolyte rhythms and an immediate effect of lowering body temperature that persists as more rapid re-entrainment.[134] Neither the dose nor the timing of melatonin administration has been fully optimized, although the most recent and largest successful study reported, with respect to alleviating sleep problems, that 5 mg was more effective than 0.5 mg and a slow-release preparation taken at bedtime after flight.[135] Two studies have shown no effect—a common factor was that the subjects were not adapted to local time before departure (see Arendt et al.[136] for references). In these cases, the individual circadian status is probably a major determinant of response in that undesirable changes in the direction of entrainment may occur with inappropriate timing of treatment. Moreover, unpredictable exposure to bright light can theoretically act in opposition to the desired result.

Very little work has been published on the use of melatonin in shift work, although exposure to bright light sufficient to suppress melatonin secretion during the night is clearly beneficial to night shift workers. Preliminary work suggests improved sleep and increased daytime alertness in night shift workers receiving melatonin at the desired bedtime during a night shift week as compared with placebo and baseline conditions.[137] One other study showed greater circadian adaptation to the night shift, but a third study reported improvement only in sleep.[138,139]

Blindness

Only a small number of studies have been reported, but the consensus suggests that most blind/visually impaired subjects reporting sleep problems derive benefit from melatonin ingestion at the desired bedtime or specifically timed according to the circadian phase.[133, 140, 141] Whether circadian variables other than sleep are entrained in these circumstances remains controversial. Melatonin was strikingly effective at improving sleep and behavior in multiply handicapped children with or without visual impairment.[142]

Sleep Problems of Old Age

Initially encouraging results using melatonin to alleviate sleep disorders in the elderly have proved inconsistent; however, some subjects will undoubtedly derive benefit. Dose timing and formulation remain to be optimized.[143]

Delayed–Sleep Phase Insomnia

Patients with delayed–sleep phase insomnia cannot sleep at the socially acceptable time of night; they delay sleep onset until the early hours of the morning and sleep through much of the day. This condition has been successfully treated with bright light in the early morning to induce phase advances of the clock. In others, evening melatonin (5 mg at 10 PM[114] or 5 hours ahead of endogenous melatonin onset[144]) also advances sleep time significantly. Judicious, timed application of both melatonin and bright light as time cues may well be the treatment of choice for rhythm disturbances.

Cancer

Animal studies have provided good evidence for photoperiod dependency and/or melatonin responsiveness of the initiation and evolution of certain cancers, particularly hormone-dependent cancers. Oncostatic effects are reported in some human cell lines, and in general, the pineal gland and melatonin appear to have antitumor activity.[9, 145–147] In dimethylbenzanthracene-induced mammary tumors in rats, pinealectomy greatly increased the incidence of induced tumor growth, and daily melatonin administration in the late light phase greatly decreased its incidence.[145] Not all reports show positive results, however. A few early reports of positive effects of combination therapy—melatonin and tamoxifen, melatonin and interleukin—require confirmation.[146, 147] Melatonin, when appropriately administered, has generally stimulatory effects on aspects of the immune system, and positive effects on cancer may be a consequence.[147] The evidence that melatonin may also act as a free radical scavenger has been discussed previously.

SITES AND MECHANISM OF ACTION OF MELATONIN

Target Sites

The actions of melatonin are multiple, and many must derive essentially from modification of events in the central nervous system. However, peripheral actions are not excluded. Obvious potential target sites in mammals, from the foregoing discussion, are the retina, the SCN and other central neuroendocrine control systems, and the pituitary gland. Lesions of the SCN and the anterior hypothalamic area can block the photoperiodic and/or circadian effects of melatonin in some rodents, but with a degree of disparity between laboratories.[148] Implants or infusion of melatonin in the hypothalamus mimics or blocks photoperiodic responses in several species.[148–151] In prepubertal rats, melatonin inhibits GnRH-induced LH release in pituitary cultures at concentrations comparable to those circulating in the blood.[54] There is evidence that melatonin influences GnRH secretion from the hypothalamus in cocultures of the median eminence and pars tuberalis.[152]

Uptake and Binding Studies

The development of 2-^{125}I-iodomelatonin as a high–specific activity ligand has permitted the identification of high-affinity (K_d of 25 to 175 pM), saturable, specific, and reversible melatonin binding to cell membranes in the central nervous system, initially in the SCN[153] and the pars tuberalis of the pituitary[154] and subsequently in many brain and other areas, including cells of the immune system, a number of cancer cell lines, the gonads, the kidney, and importantly, the cardiovascular system. The SCN shows clear binding in human postmortem tissue.[155–157] Species variation of melatonin-binding sites in the brain is of course apparent. The most consistent (but not universal) binding site between mammalian species is the pars tuberalis. Studies have shown that the pars tuberalis transduces the effects of photoperiod, via melatonin, on seasonal variations in prolactin secretion in ruminants.[158] Morgan and colleagues have proposed that pars tuberalis cells secrete an entirely new hormone that subsequently mediates the physiologic effects of melatonin—an exciting prospect.[159] When compared with mammals, much more extensive binding can be seen in the brains of birds and lower vertebrates, especially in retinorecipient areas.[155]

Changes in detectable binding are seen with age; for example, in fetal rats the first appearance of binding is in the pituitary: pars distalis and pars tuberalis, with SCN labeling appearing in later gestation. Pars distalis binding is absent in adult rats but persists after birth in the neonate.[160] This finding suggests that binding may indeed underlie function inasmuch as melatonin inhibits GnRH-induced pituitary LH release in prepuberty but not in adulthood. Moreover, binding is detectable in the brain of neonatal Syrian hamsters whose circadian system responds to melatonin,[53] whereas it is lost in adults that do not respond. Changes are also seen with the time of day, with season, and as a function of exposure to melatonin.[161–164]

Krause and Dubocovich have demonstrated a functional melatonin receptor initially in rabbit and chicken retina (inhibition of calcium-dependent dopamine release) that is localized in rabbit dopamine-containing amacrine cells in the inner plexiform, in the outer and inner segments in mice, and possibly in the pigmented layer in some mammals.[164]

Melatonin Receptor Pharmacology

White and coworkers initially demonstrated that melatonin-induced pigment aggregation in amphibian melanophores is a pertussis toxin–sensitive system and that melatonin inhibits forskolin-activated cAMP formation.[165] Inhibition of cAMP production may be a general feature of melatonin receptors. Intensive investigation of the properties of the pars tuberalis–binding site has revealed that physiologic doses of melatonin inhibit forskolin-activated cAMP production in vitro in a time- and dose-related manner.[154] Other studies have provided good evidence that most binding sites are coupled to G proteins. Guanosine triphosphate analogues, which interfere with the regeneration of G_i-coupled receptors, decrease the affinity and sometimes the capacity of ^{125}I-melatonin binding in reptiles, birds, and mammals.[154, 155]

Melatonin receptors have now been cloned, and three subtypes have thus far been identified—Mel-1a, Mel-1b, and Mel-1c.[166] They are G protein coupled, have high affinity (K_d of 20–160 pM), and inhibit cAMP. The Mel-1a receptor gene has been mapped to human chromosome 4q35.1. Tissue expression is restricted to the SCN and the pars tuberalis, which suggests that the circadian and reproductive effects are mediated through this receptor. However, results to date using gene knockout technology are confusing.[167, 168] Mel-1b has been mapped to chromosome 11q21-22, and its expression is in the retina and the brain. It is thought to be concerned with dopaminergic functions in both the retina and the brain. Mel-1c is not found in mammals. A new nomenclature has very recently been devised and accepted by the International Union of Pharmacology.[169]

Melatonin Antagonists and Agonists

Large numbers of putative and actual melatonin agonists together with some antagonists have now been described.[170–172] Most available data concern a series of agonists developed from naphthalene derivatives. They show a range of affinity for the pars tuberalis melatonin receptor, some being of much higher affinity than melatonin.[172] The most interesting have similar effects to melatonin on rhythm physiology in both rodents and humans.[173, 174] It is anticipated that much new information in this area will be available shortly.

SUMMARY

To date, evidence indicates that ^{125}I-melatonin–binding sites are genuine receptors, although by no means have all binding sites been investigated. It is likely that SCN receptors mediate the circadian effects of melatonin, those in the mediobasal hypothalamus and pars tuberalis influence photoperiodic seasonal reproduction with regard to gonadotropin secretion and prolactin, respectively, and those in the retina mediate the retinal processes influenced by melatonin. Which subtypes carry out specific functions remains to be clarified.

REFERENCES

1. Vollrath L: The Pineal Organ. Heidelberg, Germany, Springer-Verlag, 1981.
2. Collin JP: Differentiation and regression of the cells of the sensory line in the epiphysis cerebri. *In* Wolstenholme GEW, Knight J (eds): The Pineal Gland. Edinburgh, Churchill Livingstone, 1972, pp 79–125.
3. Korf H-W, Moller M, Gery I, et al: Immunocytochemical demonstration of retinal S antigen in the pineal organ of four mammalian species. Cell Tissue Res 239:81–85, 1985.
4. Welsh MG: Pineal calcification: Structural and functional aspects. Pineal Res Rev 3:41–68, 1985.
5. Tapp E: The histology and pathology of the human pineal gland. Prog Brain Res 52:481–500, 1979.
6. Bojkowski C, Arendt J: Factors influencing urinary 6-sulphatoxymelatonin, a major melatonin metabolite, in normal human subjects. Clin Endocrinol 33:435–444, 1990.
7. Kappers JA: Innervation of the epiphysis cerebri in the albino rat. Anat Rec 136:220–221, 1960.
8. Moller M, Korf H-W: The innervation of the mammalian pineal gland with special reference to central pinealopetal projections. Pineal Res Rev 2:41–86, 1984.
9. Arendt J: Melatonin and the Mammalian Pineal Gland. London, Chapman & Hall, 1995.
10. Lerner AB, Case JD, Takahashi Y, et al: Isolation of melatonin, pineal factor that lightens melanocytes. J Am Chem Soc 80:2587, 1958.
11. Axelrod J: The pineal gland: A neurochemical transducer. Science 184:1341–1348, 1974.
12. Klein DC: Photoneural regulation of the mammalian pineal gland. *In* Evered D, Clark S (eds): Photoperiodism, Melatonin and the Pineal. Ciba Foundation Symposium 117. London, Pitman, 1985, pp 38–56.
13. Cassone VM, Natesan AK: Time and time again: The phylogeny of melatonin as a transducer of biological time. J Biol Rhythms 12:489–497, 1997.
14. Klein DC, Coon SL, Roseboom PH, et al: The melatonin rhythm generating enzyme: Molecular regulation of serotonin-*N*-acetyl transferase in the pineal gland. Rec Prog Horm Res 52:307–358, 1997.
15. Gastel J, Roseboom PH, Rinaldi PA, et al: Melatonin production: Proteasomal proteolysis in serotonin N-acetyltransferase regulation. Science 279:1358–1360, 1998.
16. Maronde E, Schomerus C, Stehle JH, Korf HW: Control of CREB phosphorylation and its role for induction of melatonin synthesis in rat pinealocytes. Biol Cell 89:505–511, 1998.
17. Tosini G, Menaker M: Circadian rhythms in cultured mammalian retina. Science 272:419–421, 1996.
18. Vakkuri O, Leppaluoto J, Kauppila A: Oral administration and distribution of melatonin in human serum, saliva and urine. Life Sci 37:489–495, 1985.
19. Cavallo A, Ritschel WA: Pharmacokinetics of melatonin in human sexual maturation. J Clin Endocrinol Metab 81:1882–1886, 1996.
20. Lane EA, Moss HB: Pharmacokinetics of melatonin in man: First pass hepatic metabolism. J Clin Endocrinol Metab 61:1214–1216, 1985.
21. Pevet P: The 5-methoxyindoles different from melatonin: Their effects on the sexual axis. *In* Axelrod J, Fraschini F, Velo GP (eds): The Pineal Gland and Its Endocrine Role. New York, Plenum, 1983, pp 331–348.
22. Pevet P: Physiological role of neuropeptides in the mammalian pineal gland. Adv Pineal Res 6:275–282, 1991.
23. Sugden D, Weller JL, Klein DC, et al: α-Adrenergic potentiation of β-adrenergic stimulation of rat pineal *N*-acetyltransferase: Studies using citazoline and fluorine analogs of norepinephrine. Biochem Pharmacol 33:3947–3950, 1984.
24. Pangerl B, Pangerl A, Reiter RJ: Circadian variations of adrenergic receptors in the mammalian pineal gland: A review. J Neural Transm 81:17–29, 1990.
25. Ebadi M, Govitrapong P: Orphan transmitters and their receptor sites in the pineal gland. Pineal Res Rev 4:1–54, 1986.
26. Cardinali DP, Vacas MI: Feedback control of pineal function by reproductive hormones—a neuroendocrine paradigm. J Neural Transm Suppl 13:175–201, 1978.
27. Cardinali DP, Ritta MN: Role of prostaglandins in neuroendocrine junctions: Studies in the pineal gland and the hypothalamus. Neuroendocrinology 36:152–160, 1983.
28. Poggeler B, Balzer I, Hardeland R, Lerchl A: Pineal hormone melatonin oscillates also in the dinoflagellate *Gonyaulax polyedra*. Naturwissenschaften 78:268–269, 1991.
29. Murch SJ, Simmons CB, Saxena PK: Melatonin in feverfew and other medicinal plants. Lancet 350:1598–1599, 1997.
30. Evered D, Clark S (eds): Photoperiodism, Melatonin and the Pineal. Ciba Foundation Symposium 117. London, Pitman, 1985.
31. Wever RA: Light effects on human circadian rhythms: A review of recent Andechs experiments. J Biol Rhythms 4:161–185, 1989.
32. Rusak B, Zucker I: Neural regulation of circadian rhythms. Physiol Rev 59:449–526, 1979.
33. Cassone VM: Effects of melatonin on vertebrate circadian systems. Trends Neurosci 13:457–463, 1990.
34. Wehr TA: The durations of human melatonin secretion and sleep respond to changes in daylength (photoperiod). J Clin Endocrinol Metab 73:1276–1280, 1991.
35. Illnerova H: Entrainment of mammalian circadian rhythms in melatonin production by light. Pineal Res Rev 6:173–217, 1988.
36. Reiter RJ: Action spectra, dose-response relationships and temporal aspects of light's effects on the pineal gland. Ann N Y Acad Sci 453:215–230, 1985.
37. Lewy AJ, Wehr TA, Goodwin FK, et al: Light suppresses melatonin secretion in humans. Science 210:1267–1269, 1980.
38. Bojkowski CJ, Aldhous M, English J, et al: Suppression of nocturnal plasma melatonin and 6-sulphatoxymelatonin by bright and dim light in man. Horm Metab Res 19:437–440, 1987.
39. Boivin DB, Czeisler CA: Resetting of circadian melatonin and cortisol rhythms in humans by ordinary room light. Neuroreport 9:779–782, 1998.
40. Rosenthal NE, Sack DA, Gillin JC, et al: Seasonal affective disorder. A description of the syndrome and preliminary findings with light therapy. Arch Gen Psychiatry 41:72–79, 1984.
41. Lincoln GA, Ebling FJP, Almeida OFX: Generation of melatonin rhythms. *In* Evered D, Clark S (eds): Photoperiodism, Melatonin and the Pineal. Ciba Foundation Symposium 117. London, Pitman, 1985, pp 129–141.
42. Shanahan TL, Czeisler CA: Light exposure induces equivalent phase shifts of the endogenous circadian rhythms of circulating plasma melatonin and core body temperature in man. J Clin Endocrinol Metab 73:227–235, 1991.
43. Wever RA: Characteristics of circadian rhythms in human functions. J Neural Transm Suppl 21:323–374, 1986.
44. Lewy AJ, Newsome DA: Different types of melatonin circadian secretory rhythms in some blind subjects. J Clin Endocrinol Metab 56:1103–1107, 1983.
45. Lockley SW, Skene DJ, Arendt J, et al: Relationship between melatonin rhythms and visual loss in the blind. J Clin Endocrinol Metab 82:3763–3770, 1997.
46. Czeisler CA, Shanahan TL, Klerman EB, et al: Suppression of melatonin secretion in some blind patients by exposure to bright light. N Engl J Med 332:6–11, 1995.
47. Hoffman K: Photoperiodism in vertebrates. *In* Aschoff J (ed): Handbook of Behavioural Neurobiology, suppl 4. 1981, pp 449–473.
48. Ebling FJP, Foster DL: Pineal melatonin rhythms and the timing of puberty in mammals. Experientia 45:946–955, 1989.
49. Arendt J: Role of the pineal gland and melatonin in seasonal reproductive function in mammals. Oxf Rev Reprod Biol 8:266–320, 1986.
50. Bartness TJ, Goldman BD: Mammalian pineal melatonin: A clock for all seasons. Experientia 45:939–945, 1989.
51. Woodfill CJI, Robinson JE, Malpaux BM, Karsch FJ: Synchronisation of the circannual reproductive rhythm of the ewe by discrete photoperiodic signals. Biol Reprod 45:110–121, 1991.
52. Weaver DR, Reppert SM: Maternal melatonin communicates daylength to the fetus in Djungarian hamsters. Endocrinology 119:2861–2863, 1986.
53. Davis F: Melatonin: Role in development. J Biol Rhythms 12:498–508, 1997.
54. Martin JE, Klein DC: Melatonin inhibition of neonatal pituitary response to luteinising hormone–releasing factor. Science 191:301–302, 1975.
55. Reiter RJ: The pineal and its hormones in the control of reproduction in mammals. Endocr Rev 1:109–131, 1980.
55a. Badia P, Myers B, Murphy P: Melatonin and thermoregulation. *In* Reiter RJ, Yu HS (eds): Melatonin: Biosynthesis, Physiological Effects, and Clinical Applications. Boca Raton, FL, CRC Press, 1992.
56. Quay WB: Precocious entrainment and associated characteristics of activity patterns following pinealectomy and reversal of photoperiod. Physiol Behav 5:1281–1290, 1970.
57. Cassone V: The pineal gland influences rat circadian activity rhythms in constant light. J Biol Rhythms 7:27–40, 1992.
58. Vriend J: Evidence for pineal gland modulation of the neuroendocrine-thyroid axis. Neuroendocrinology 36:68–78, 1983.
59. Armstrong SM: Melatonin and circadian control in mammals. Experientia 45:932–939, 1989.
60. Chesworth MJ, Cassone VM, Armstrong SM. Effects of daily melatonin injections on activity rhythms of rats in constant light. Am J Physiol 253:R101–R107, 1987.
61. Illnerova H: *In* Klein DC, Moore RY, Reppert SM (eds): Suprachiasmatic Nucleus, The Minds Clock. Oxford, Oxford University Press, 1991, pp 197–219.
62. Hastings MH, Duffield GE, Ebling FJ, et al: Non-photic signalling in the suprachiasmatic nucleus. Biol Cell 89:495–503, 1998.
63. Davis FC, Mannion J: Entrainment of hamster pup circadian rhythms by prenatal melatonin injections. Am J Physiol 255:R439–R448, 1988.

64. Bosc MJ: Time of parturition in rats after melatonin administration or change of photoperiod. J Reprod Fertil 80:563–568, 1987.

65. Reiter RJ: Melatonin and human reproduction. Ann Med 1:103–108, 1998.

66. Pierpaoli W, Regelson W: The Melatonin Miracle. New York, Simon & Schuster, 1995.

67. Reppert SM, Weaver DR: Melatonin madness. Cell 83:1059–1062, 1995.

68. Arendt J: Melatonin. BMJ 312:1242–1243, 1996.

69. Armstrong SM, Redman J: Melatonin: A chronobiotic with anti-aging properties. Med Hypotheses 34:300–309, 1991.

70. Reiter R, Tang L, Garcia JJ, Munoz-Hoyos A: Pharmacological actions of melatonin in oxygen radical pathophysiology. Life Sci 60:2255–2271, 1997.

71. Hardeland R, Behrmann G, Fuhrberg B, et al: Evolutionary aspects of indoleamines as radical scavengers. Presence and photocatalytic turnover of indoleamines in a unicell, Gonyaulax polyedra. Adv Exp Med Biol 398:279–284, 1996.

72. Marshall KA, Reiter RJ, Poeggeler B, et al: Evaluation of the antioxidant activity of melatonin in vitro. Free Radic Biol Med 21:307–315, 1996.

73. Gillette MU, McArthur AJ: Circadian actions of melatonin at the suprachiasmatic nucleus. Behav Brain Res 73:135–139, 1996.

74. Iuvone M: In Djamgoz MBA, Archer S, Vallerga S (eds): Neurobiology and Clinical Aspects of the Outer Retina. London, Chapman & Hall, 1995, pp 25–55.

75. Neuwelt EA, Mickey B, Lewy AJ: The importance of melatonin and tumour markers in pineal tumours. J Neural Transm Suppl 21:397–413, 1986.

76. Vaughan GM: Melatonin in humans. Pineal Res Rev 2:141–201, 1984.

77. Arendt J: Melatonin: A new probe in psychiatric investigation? Br J Psychiatry 155:585–590, 1989.

78. Middleton B, Arendt J, Stone B: Human circadian rhythms in constant dim light (< 8 lux) with knowledge of clock time. J Sleep Res 5:69–76, 1996.

79. Arendt J: Melatonin. Clin Endocrinol 29:205–229, 1988.

80. Arendt J: Mammalian pineal rhythms. Pineal Res Rev 3:161–213, 1985.

81. Akerstedt T, Froberg JE, Friberg W, Wetterberg L: Melatonin excretion, body temperature and subjective arousal during 64 hours of sleep deprivation. Psychoneuroendocrinology 4:219, 1979.

82. Cagnacci A, Elliot JA, Yen SS: Melatonin: A major regulator of the circadian rhythm of core body temperature in humans. J Clin Endocrinol Metab 75:447–452, 1992.

83. Dijk DJ, Shanahan TL, Duffy JF, et al: Variation of electroencephalographic activity during non–rapid eye movement and rapid eye movement sleep with phase of circadian melatonin rhythm in humans. J Physiol (Lond) 505:851–858, 1997.

84. Lockley SW, Skene DJ, Tabandeh H, et al: Relationship between napping and melatonin in the blind. J Biol Rhythms 12:16–25, 1997.

85. Shochat T, Haimov I, Lavie P: Melatonin—the key to the gate of sleep. Ann Med 30:109–114, 1998.

86. Strassman RJ, Appenzeller O, Lewy AJ, et al: Increase in plasma melatonin, beta-endorphin, and cortisol after a 28.5-mile mountain race: Relationship to performance and lack of effect of naltrexone. J Clin Endocrinol Metab 69:540–545, 1989.

87. Kennaway D, Stamp G, Goble F: Development of melatonin production in infants and the impact of prematurity. J Clin Endocrinol Metab 75:367–369, 1992.

88. Waldhauser F, Frisch H, Waldhauser M, et al: Fall in nocturnal serum melatonin during prepuberty and pubescence. Lancet 1:362–365, 1984.

89. Attanasio A, Borrelli P, Marini R, et al: Serum melatonin in children with early and delayed puberty. Neuroendocrinol Lett 5:387, 1984.

90. Waldhauser F, Boepple P, Schemper M, Crowley WF: Serum melatonin in central precocious puberty is lower than in age matched pre-pubertal children. J Clin Endocrinol Metab 73:793–796, 1991.

91. Berga SL, Mortola JF, Yen SSC: Amplification of nocturnal melatonin secretion in women with functional hypothalamic amenorrhea. J Clin Endocrinol Metab 66:242–244, 1988.

92. Berga SL, Jones KL, Kaufmann S, Yen SSC: Nocturnal melatonin levels are unaltered by ovarian suppression in girls with central precocious puberty. Fertil Steril 52:937–941, 1989.

93. Arendt J, Labib MH, Bojkowski C, et al: Rapid decrease in melatonin production during treatment of delayed puberty with oestradiol in a case of craniopharyngioma. Lancet 1:1326, 1989.

94. Cagnacci A, Krauchi K, Wirz-Justice, Volpe A: Homeostatic versus circadian effects of melatonin on core body temperature in humans. J Biol Rhythms 12:509–517, 1997.

95. Cagnacci A, Elliot JA, Yen SSC: Amplification of pulsatile LH secretion by exogenous melatonin in women. J Clin Endocrinol Metab 73:210–212, 1991.

96. Voordow BCG, Euser R, Verdonk RER, et al: Melatonin and melatonin-progestin combinations alter pituitary-ovarian function in women and can inhibit ovulation. J Clin Endocrinol Metab 74:108–117, 1992.

97. Anderson RA, Lincoln GA, Wu FCW: Melatonin potentiates testosterone-induced suppression of luteinising hormone secretion in normal men. Hum Reprod 8:1819–1822, 1993.

98. Luboshitzky R, Wagner O, Lavi S: Abnormal melatonin secretion in male patients with hypogonadism. J Mol Neurosci 7:91–98, 1996.

99. Luboshitzky R, Wagner O, Lavi S, et al: Abnormal melatonin secretion in hypogonadal men: The effect of testosterone treatment. Clin Endocrinol 47:463–469, 1997.

100. Roenneberg T, Aschoff J: Annual rhythms in human reproduction: I. Biology, sociology or both? J Biol Rhythms 5:195–216, 1990.

101. West RJ, Leonard JV: Familial insulin resistance with pineal hyperplasia: Metabolic studies and effect of hypophysectomy. Arch Dis Child 55:619–621, 1980.

102. Sparks DL, Hunsaker JC III: The pineal gland in sudden infant death syndrome: Preliminary observations. J Pineal Res 5:111–118, 1988.

103. Sturner WQ, Lynch HJ, Deng MH, Wurtman RJ: Melatonin levels in the sudden infant death syndrome. Forensic Sci Int 45:171–180, 1990.

104. Axelrod L: Endocrine dysfunction in patients with tumours of the pineal region. In Schmidek HH (ed): Pineal Tumours. New York, Masson, 1977, pp 61–77.

105. Wass JAL, Jones AE, Rees LH, Besser GM: hCGb producing pineal choriocarcinoma. Clin Endocrinol 17:423–431, 1982.

106. Cohen AR, Wilson JA, Sadeghi-Nejad A: Gonadotrophin-secreting pineal teratoma causing precocious puberty. Neurosurgery 28:597–602, 1991.

107. Horowitz MB: Central nervous system germinomas, a review. Arch Neurol 48:652–657, 1991.

108. Cohen M, Lippman M, Chabner B: Role of pineal gland in aetiology and treatment of breast cancer. Lancet 2:814–816, 1978.

109. Tamarkin L, Danforth D, Lichter A, et al: Decreased nocturnal plasma melatonin peak in patients with estrogen receptor positive breast cancer. Science 216:1003–1005, 1982.

110. Bartsch C, Bartsch H: Modulation of melatonin secretion in cancer patients. Possible mechanisms and significance for prognosis, diagnosis and treatment. In Grossman AB (ed): Frontiers of Hormone Research, vol 23. Maestroni GJM, Conti A, Reiter RJ (eds): Therapeutic Potential of Melatonin. Basel, Karger, 1997, pp 115–124.

111. Gilad E, Matzkin H, Zisapel N: Interplay between sex steroids and melatonin in regulation of human benign prostate epithelial cell growth. J Clin Endocrinol Metab 82:2535–2541, 1997.

112. Gupta D, Attanasio A: Pathophysiology of pineal function in health and disease in children. Pineal Res Rev 6:261–300, 1988.

113. Thompson C, Obrecht R, Franey C, et al: Neuroendocrine rhythms in a patient with the Kleine-Levin syndrome. Br J Psychiatry 147:440–443, 1985.

114. Dahlitz M, Alvarez B, Vignau J, et al: Delayed sleep phase syndrome response to melatonin. Lancet 1:1121–1124, 1991.

115. Deacon S, Arendt J: Posture influences melatonin concentrations in plasma and saliva in humans. Neurosci Lett 167:191–194, 1994.

116. Lewy AJ, Sack RL, Miller LS, Hoban TM: Anti-depressant and circadian phase-shifting effects of light. Science 235:352–354, 1987.

117. Parry BL, Berga SL, Mostofi N, et al: Plasma melatonin circadian rhythms during the menstrual cycle and after light therapy in premenstrual dysphoric disorder and normal control subjects. J Biol Rhythms 12:47–64, 1997.

118. Zhadnova IV, Wurtman RJ: Efficacy of melatonin as a sleep promoting agent. J Biol Rhythms 12:644–650, 1997.

119. Arendt J: Sleep Science: Integrating basic research and clinical practice. In Schwartz W (ed): Melatonin. Karger Monographs in Clinical Neuroscience. Basel, Karger, 1997, pp 196–228.

120. Lerner AB, Nordlund JJ: Melatonin: Clinical pharmacology. J Neural Transm Suppl 13:339–347, 1978.

121. Wirz-Justice A, Armstrong SM: Melatonin: Nature's soporific? J Sleep Res 5:137–141, 1996.

122. Lieberman HR, Waldhauser F, Garfield G, et al: Effects of melatonin on human mood and performance. Brain Res 323:201–207, 1984.

123. Waldhauser F, Steger H, Vorkapic P: Melatonin secretion in man and the influence of exogenous melatonin on some physiological and behavioural variables. Adv Pineal Res 2:207–223, 1987.

124. Kostoglou-Athanassiou I, Treacher DF, Wheeler MJ, Forsling ML: Melatonin administration and pituitary hormone secretion. Clin Endocrinol 48:31–37, 1998.

125. Sugden D: Psychopharmacological effects of melatonin in mouse and rat. J Pharmacol Exp Ther 227:587–591, 1983.

126. Guardiola-Lemaitre B: Toxicology of melatonin. J Biol Rhythms 12:697–706, 1997.

127. Mahle CD, Coggins GD, Agarwal P, et al: Melatonin modulates vascular smooth muscle tone. J Biol Rhythms 12:690–696, 1997.

128. Deacon S, Arendt J: Melatonin-induced temperature suppression and its acute phase-shifting effects correlate in a dose-dependent manner in humans. Brain Res 688:77–85, 1995.

129. Lewy AJ, Ahmed S, Jackson JML, Sack RL: Melatonin shifts human circadian rhythms according to a phase-response curve. Chronobiol 9:380–392, 1993.

130. Middleton B, Arendt J, Stone B: Complex effects of melatonin on human circadian rhythms in constant dim light. J Biol Rhythms 12:467–475, 1997.

131. Lewy AJ, Bauer VK, Ahmed S, et al: The human phase response curve (PRC) to melatonin is about 12 hours out of phase with the PRC to light. Chronobiol Int 15:71–83, 1998.

132. Arendt J, Deacon S: Treatment of circadian rhythm disorders: Melatonin. Chronobiol Int 14:185–204, 1997.

133. Arendt J, Skene DJ, Middleton B, et al: Efficacy of melatonin treatment in jet lag, shift work, and blindness. J Biol Rhythms 12:604–617, 1997.

134. Samel A, Wegman HM, Vejvoda M, Maas H: Influence of melatonin treatment on human circadian rhythmicity before and after a simulated 9 hour time shift. J Biol Rhythms 6:235–248, 1991.

135. Suhner A, Schlagenhauf P, Johnson R, et al: Comparative study to determine the optimal melatonin dosage form for the alleviation of jet lag. Chronobiol Int 15:655–666, 1998.

136. Arendt J, Stone B, Skene DJ: Jet lag and sleep disruption. In Turek F (ed): Principles and Practice of Sleep Medicine, 3rd ed (in press).

137. Folkard S, Arendt J, Clarke M: Can melatonin improve shiftworkers' tolerance of the night shift? Some preliminary findings. Chronobiol Int 10:315–320, 1993.

138. Sack RL, Lewy AJ: Melatonin as a chronobiotic: Treatment of circadian desynchrony in night workers and the blind. J Biol Rhythms 12:595–603, 1997.

139. Dawson D, Encel N, Lushington K: Improving adaptation to simulated night shift: Timed exposure to bright light versus daytime melatonin administration. Sleep 18:11–21, 1995.

140. Arendt J: Safety of melatonin in long term use. J Biol Rhythms 12:673–681, 1997.

141. Palm L, Blennow G, Wetterberg L: Long-term melatonin treatment in blind children and young adults with circadian sleep-wake disturbances. Dev Med Child Neurol 39:319–325, 1997.

142. Jan JE, Espezel H, Appleton RE: The treatment of sleep disorders with melatonin. Dev Med Child Neurol 96:97–107, 1994.

143. Hughes RJ, Sack RL, Lewy AJ: The role of melatonin and circadian phase in age-related sleep-maintenance insomnia: Assessment in a clinical trial of melatonin replacement. Sleep 21:52–68, 1998.

144. Nagtegaal JE, Kerkhof GA, Smits MG, et al: Delayed sleep phase syndrome: A placebo-controlled cross-over study on the effects of melatonin administered five hours before the individual dim light melatonin onset. J Sleep Res 7:135–143, 1998.

145. Tamarkin L, Cohen M, Roselle D, et al: Melatonin inhibition and pinealectomy enhancement of 7,12-dimethylbenz(a)anthracene–induced mammary tumours in the rat. Cancer Res 41:4432–4436, 1981.

146. Lissoni P, Paolorossi F, Meregalli S, et al: Melatonin as a modulator of cancer endocrine therapy. *In* Grossman AB (ed): Frontiers of Hormone Research, vol 23. Maestroni GJM, Conti A, Reiter RJ (eds): Therapeutic Potential of Melatonin. Basel, Karger, 1997, pp 132–136.

147. Conti A, Maestroni GJM: The clinical neuroimmunotherapeutic role of melatonin in oncology. J Pineal Res 19:103–110, 1995.

148. Hastings MH, Maywood ES, Ebling FJP, et al: Sites and mechanism of action of melatonin in the photoperiodic control of reproduction. Adv Pineal Res 5:147–157, 1991.

149. Maywood ES, Hastings MH: Lesions of the iodomelatonin-binding sites of the mediobasal hypothalamus spare the lactotropic, but block the gonadotropic response of male Syrian hamsters to short photoperiod and to melatonin. Endocrinology 136:144–149, 1995.

150. Lincoln GA: Administration of melatonin into the mediobasal hypothalamus as a continuous or intermittent signal affects the secretion of follicle-stimulating hormone and prolactin in the ram. J Pineal Res 12:135–144, 1992.

151. Lincoln G, Maeda K: Effects of placing micro-implants of melatonin in the mediobasal hypothalamus and preoptic area on the secretion of prolactin and β-endorphin in rams. J Endocrinol 134:437–448, 1992.

152. Nakazawa K, Marubayashi U, McCann SM: Mediation of the short-loop feedback of luteinising hormone (LH) on LH-releasing hormone release by melatonin-induced inhibition of LH release from the pars tuberalis. Proc Natl Acad Sci U S A 88:7576–7579, 1991.

153. Vanecek J, Pavlik A, Illnerova H: Hypothalamic melatonin receptor sites revealed by autoradiography. Brain Res 453:359–362, 1987.

154. Morgan PJ, Williams LM: Central melatonin receptors; implications for a mode of action. Experientia 45:955–965, 1989.

155. Weaver DR, Rivkees SA, Carlson LL, Reppert SM: Localisation of melatonin receptors in mammalian brain. *In* Klein DC, Moore RY, Reppert SM (eds): Suprachiasmatic Nucleus: The Mind's Clock. New York, Oxford University Press, 1991, pp 289–308.

156. Dubocovich ML. Melatonin receptors: Are there multiple subtypes? Trends Pharmacol Sci 16:50–56, 1995.

157. Reppert SM, Weaver DR, Godson C: Melatonin receptors step into the light: Cloning and classification of subtypes. Trends Pharmacol Sci 17:100–102, 1996.

158. Lincoln GA, Clarke IJ: Photoperiodically induced cycles in the secretion of prolactin in hypothalamo-pituitary disconnected rams: Evidence for translation of the melatonin signal in the pituitary gland. J Neuroendocrinol 6:251–260, 1994.

159. Morgan PJ, King TP, Lawson W, et al: Ultrastructure of melatonin responsive cells in the ovine pars tuberalis. Cell Tissue Res 263:529–534, 1991.

160. Williams LM, Martinoli MG, Titchener LT, Pelletier G: The ontogeny of central melatonin binding sites in the rat. Endocrinology 128:2083–2090, 1991.

161. Skene DJ, Masson-Pevet M, Pevet P: Seasonal changes in melatonin binding sites in the pars tuberalis of male European hamsters and the effect of testosterone manipulation. Endocrinology 132:1682–1686, 1993.

162. Recio J, Pévet P, Masson-Pévet M: Regulation of melatonin receptors in the pars tuberalis of Syrian hamsters transferred from long to short photoperiod: Implication of melatonin and testosterone. J Neuroendocrinol 10:303–308, 1998.

163. Hazlerigg DG, Gonzalez-Brito A, Lawson W, et al: Prolonged exposure to melatonin leads to time dependent sensitization of adenylate cyclase and down regulates melatonin receptors in pars tuberalis cells from ovine pituitary. Endocrinology 132:285–292, 1993.

164. Krause DN, Dubocovich ML: Regulatory sites in the melatonin system of mammals. Trends Neurosci 13:464–470, 1990.

165. White BH, Sekura RD, Rollag MD: Pertussis toxin blocks melatonin-induced aggregation in *Xenopus* dermal melanophores. J Comp Physiol [B] 157:153–159, 1987.

166. Reppert SM: Melatonin receptors: Molecular biology of a new family of G-protein–coupled receptors. J Biol Rhythms 12:528–531, 1997.

167. Reppert SM: Nature's knockout: The Mel1b receptor is not necessary for reproductive and circadian responses to melatonin in Siberian hamsters. Mol Endocrinol 10:1478–1487, 1996.

168. Dubocovich ML, Yun K, Al-Ghoul WM, et al: Selective MT2 melatonin receptor antagonists block melatonin-mediated phase advances of circadian rhythms. FASEB J 12:1211–1220, 1998.

169. Dubocovich ML, Cardinali DP, Guardiola-Lemaitre B, et al: Melatonin receptors. *In* The IUPHAR Compendium of Receptor Characterization and Classification. London, IUPHAR Media, 1998, pp 187–193.

170. Spadoni G, Balsamini C, Diamantini G, et al: Conformationally restrained melatonin analogues: Synthesis, binding affinity for the melatonin receptor, evaluation of the biological activity, and molecular modeling study. J Med Chem 40:1990–2002, 1997.

171. Dubocovich ML, Masana MI, Iacob S, Sauri DM: Melatonin receptor antagonists that differentiate between the human Mel1a and Mel1b recombinant subtypes are used to assess the pharmacological profile of the rabbit retina ML1 presynaptic heteroreceptor. Naunyn Schmiedebergs Arch Pharmacol 355:365–375, 1997.

172. Yous S, Antrieux J, Howell HE, et al: Novel naphthalenic ligands with a high affinity for the melatonin receptor. J Med Chem 35:1484–1486, 1992.

173. Redman JR, Francis AJ: Entrainment of rat circadian rhythms by the melatonin agonist S-20098 requires intact suprachiasmatic nuclei but not the pineal. J Biol Rhythms 13:39–51, 1998.

174. Krauchi K, Cajochen C, Moeri D, et al: Early evening melatonin and S-20098 advance circadian phase and nocturnal regulation of core body temperature. Am J Physiol 272:R1178–R1188, 1997.

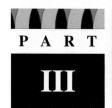

PART III

Growth and Maturation

Editor: Shlomo Melmed

BASIC PHYSIOLOGY

Chapter 30

Growth Hormone

John J. Kopchick

GROWTH HORMONE

A growth-promoting principle of the pituitary gland was discovered in 1921.[1] In 1944, bovine growth hormone (bGH) was isolated,[2] and in the early 1960s, human GH (hGH) was first used in GH-deficient children. In 1979 the cDNA encoding hGH was cloned,[3] and in 1985 recombinant hGH was approved for clinical use. During this time a major scientific goal was the correlation of GH structure with its biologic activities. Toward this end a combination of in vitro and in vivo assays for GH activity have been used. Throughout this chapter the predominant theme will be directed at the structure of the GH molecule as it relates to function. The molecular events at the cellular level that lead to GH-induced biologic activity will then be summarized.

General Background

GH, chorionic somatomammotropin (CS, placental lactogen [PL]), and prolactin (PRL) belong to a family of hormones thought to have evolved from a common precursor.[4, 5] Members of the GH family are encoded by genes that span approximately 2.0 kilobases (kb) and contain five exons and four intervening sequences. The translation start and stop codons are located in exons 1 and 5 of the genes, respectively.[4]

Members of the GH family of proteins contain approximately 200 amino acids with two (GH) or three (PRL) disulfide bonds.[6] The proteins' molecular masses are approximately 22,000 with similar sedimentation and diffusion coefficients.[6, 7] The amino acid composition and sequence of molecules are comparable and approximately 60% to 90% identical. The molecules are synthesized as precursor proteins; that is, they contain N-terminal secretory signal peptides.[4] A comprehensive list of the amino acid sequences of GH molecules from various species has been presented,[8] and a pictorial representation of the percent identity between amino acid sequences has been compiled.[9]

The hGH gene family consists of the 191–amino acid hGH molecule, a GH variant termed hGH-V, hCS, and hPRL. Unlike hGH, which is expressed primarily in the pituitary and is not glycosylated, hGH-V is glycosylated, is expressed in the placenta, and is found in the serum during pregnancy.[10–12] It differs from pituitary hGH in 13 of 191 amino acid residues,[4] and like hGH, it promotes growth.[13] Also, another variant of hGH, termed 20-kDa (20K), has been found in the pituitary. It is produced by alternative splicing of the hGH precursor mRNA and lacks amino acids 32 to 46.[14] Two forms of hCS have been found, hCS-A and hCS-B, that differ by only one amino acid residue located in the secretory signal peptide. hCS is expressed by the placenta and, despite possessing 161 amino acid residues in common with hGH, retains minimal growth-promoting activity.[15] hPRL is expressed by the pituitary gland and contains 199 amino acids, although only 30 are identical to hGH in amino acid alignment.[4] hPRL has been reported to be phosphorylated and glycosylated and is the subject of Chapter 15.

The hGH gene family members are located on the long arm of chromosome 17. The 5′ to 3′ order of these genes are GH, a CS pseudogene, CS-A, GH-V, and CS-B.[16]

GH Action

During the late 1950s and early 1960s a great deal of work was performed on GH and GH isoforms. Several heterogeneous types of GH have been reported.[6, 17–22] The heterogeneity of GH genes, isohormones, and variants has been reviewed and will not be described here.[23]

As the name implies, GH's major function is growth promotion. In vertebrates, hyposecretion of GH during development leads to dwarfism, whereas hypersecretion of GH before puberty leads to gigantism. In adults, hypersecretion of GH from pituitary adenomas results in a clinical condition known as acromegaly, which is characterized by enlarged bones of the face, hands, and feet; enlarged heart, liver, and kidney tissue; fatigue; and weight gain. In approximately 25% of individuals with acromegaly, type 2 diabetes develops in response to chronically elevated circulating insulin levels and subsequent insulin resistance.[24] The subject of acromegaly has been nicely reviewed[25–30] and is the subject of Chapter 22. In healthy adults, GH exerts several metabolic effects, including effects on protein, fat, and carbohydrate.

Among the many metabolic activities of GH, two contradictory actions have been described: acute or early insulin-like activities and chronic or late anti-insulin effects, also called diabetogenic activities. Acute insulin-like activities include hypoglycemia,[31, 32] increased glucose and amino acid transport and metabolism,[33–36] augmented protein synthesis,[34] increased glycogenesis,[37, 38] and heightened lipogenesis.[39, 40] These insulin-like activities are seen primarily in vitro or under special circumstances such as after hypophysectomy. GH's anti-insulin activities include hyperglycemia,[41] hyperinsulinemia,[42] increased lipolysis,[43, 44] decreased glucose transport,[45] increased serum levels of nonesterified fatty acids,[46] decreased glucose metabolism,[47] and insulin resistance.[48–50] These anti-insulin activities have been found after relatively long periods of GH treatment, such as after chronic exposure both in cultured cells and in vivo, and are thought to represent a major physiologic effect of GH.

To explain these two related, but opposite activities, as well as other multiple GH activities, three hypotheses have been presented: (1) the existence of multiple GH receptors (GHRs),[51, 52] (2) the presence of multiple "active centers" in the GH molecule,[53] and (3) the presence of small active GH fragments that result in the multiple activities of GH.[54–58] Work continues to test these three hypotheses.

In addition to the insulin-like and anti-insulin–like activities of the molecule, other in vivo effects of GH activity include an influence on rat tibia size,[59] metabolic and growth effects in hypophysectomized animals,[60] and enhancement of growth rates in transgenic mice.[61–68] Additionally, in vitro or cultured cell–based assays include those in which the GHR gene is either endogenously expressed or expressed via transfection of cells. Assays using these types of cells demonstrate GH-stimulated transcription of cotransfected reporter genes or GH's ability to stimulate cell division.

Many of the functional effects of GH actually result from the action of insulin-like growth factor type 1 (IGF-1), which is produced in the liver, bone, and other tissues in response to GH.[69] In 1985 Green and colleagues put forth the dual-effector theory of GH action.[70] This theory postulates that GH acts directly on cells to promote differentiation whereas IGF-1 promotes cell multiplication. At present an important experimental task is to determine which of the GH-associated effects are directly due to GH and which are an indirect result of the activity of IGF-1. The results of these important experiments will either support or reject the dual-effector theory of GH action.[70]

A great deal of work describing the structure of the GH molecule as it relates to GH's biologic activities has been performed, and several excellent reviews concerning this subject have been presented.[4, 6, 8, 9, 23, 40, 71–75]

GH Fragments

Considerable work to determine the biologic activity of GH and various GH fragments has proceeded. For example, Li and Graf showed that cleavage of hGH by plasmin results in two fragments, residues 1–134 and 141–191, each of which possesses reduced biologic activity.[76] These two fragments were shown to react noncovalently and result in an hGH molecule that possessed full biologic activity[77] when evaluated with the pigeon crop-sac assay[78] and the rat tibia assay.[59] Additionally, Li and Bewley in 1976 presented the first structural representation of GH that included 191 amino acids and two disulfide bonds.[77]

Sonenberg and colleagues found that a tryptic peptide of bGH (fragment A-2) that included amino acid residues 96 to 133 possessed low but significant levels of GH activity in the rat tibia width and weight gain assays[79, 80] and stimulated hGH-like effects in humans.[81] However, the remaining fragment, termed A-1 (bGH 1–95, 134–191), possessed little activity.[81] Upon analysis of the fragments by far ultraviolet circular dichroism and intrinsic fluorescence emission spectroscopy and with the use of Chou-Fasman protein structure predictions,[82, 83] a two-dimensional representation of the three-dimensional structure of GH was presented[84] (Fig. 30–1). Three α helical regions were predicted in this model. Note that the fragment containing residues 96 to 133 included an α helix. Thus the first predicted secondary structure of GH was presented in 1978, complete with α helical regions, β sheets, and disulfide bonds (see Fig. 30–1).

Several lines of research suggested that endogenous GH fragments do in fact exist. Although most of these GH fragments were found to be artifacts of experimental manipulation,[23] several studies were performed on such GH fragments. For example, hGH (1–15) was found to possess insulin-like activity[54–57] whereas hGH (177–191) had anti-insulin activity.[58, 85] Also, an hGH variant (20K) generated by alternative GH precursor mRNA splicing and lacking amino acid residues 32 to 46 also lacked insulin-like activity but possessed growth-promoting, lactogenic, and diabetogenic activity.[19, 51, 86, 87] Salem in 1988 showed that an hGH N-terminal peptide (1–43) was an insulin potentiator that increased insulin-stimulated glucose clearance and glucose metabolism without affecting insulin secretion.[88] Also, Towns et al. found that the N terminus of hGH is involved in the growth-promoting, diabetogenic, and insulin-like activities of the molecule.[89]

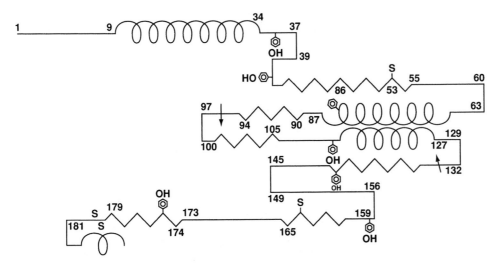

FIGURE 30–1. Schematic representation of bovine growth hormone. *Arrows* indicate the trypsin cleavage sites located between amino acids 96 and 97 and between 132 and 133. Also shown are three α helical regions. (Adapted from Hara K, Hsu Chen CJ, Sonenberg M: Recombination of the biologically active peptides from a tryptic digest of bovine growth hormone. Biochemistry 17:550–556, 1978. Reprinted with permission from the American Chemical Society.)

Additionally, the ability of the 22-kDa, the 20K, and the 5-kDa N-terminal peptide forms of hGH to promote growth in transgenic mice has been evaluated.[90] Both the 22-kDa and 20K forms of hGH stimulated linear mouse growth whereas the 5-kDa form did not.

A wide variety of experiments have been performed on other GH fragments. The reader is referred to a list of approximately 90 GH fragments with their corresponding biologic activities.[91]

Crystal Structure of GH

The crystal structure of the GH molecule, in particular, porcine GH, was solved by Abdel-Meguid and coworkers in 1987[92] (Fig. 30–2). This momentous disclosure came 11 years after the first graphic representation of the GH molecule[77] and 66 years after discovery of the growth-promoting principle of the pituitary gland.[1] GH was found to be an elongated molecule with approximate dimensions of 55 × 35 × 35 Å. The molecule contains four α helixes that are tightly packed as antiparallel bundles aligned in a *up-up-down-down* orientation. Fifty-four percent of GH's 191 amino acids are contained in these four helixes. The molecule also contains a "large loop" between residues 33 and 75, a "smaller loop" between residues 129 and 154, and a "small loop" located at the C terminus.[92] This model has been used by many investigators in the field and represents the prototypic model for GH family members.

Disulfide Bonds in GH

Members of the GH family possess either two (GH) or three (PRL) disulfide bonds. bGH has four Cys residues located at positions 53, 164, 181, and 189. When aligned to optimize amino acid similarity, the four Cys residues were found to be conserved among all GH, PRL, and PL molecules.[6, 73] This conservation may indicate that these residues are important for the structural integrity and biologic activity of the molecules. The four Cys residues form two disulfide bridges: one located between Cys53 and Cys164, which results in a large loop, and the other between Cys181 and Cys189, which forms a small C-terminal loop. The integrity of the small loop has been found to be nonessential for the biologic activity of GH[68, 93] or ovine PRL.[94]

When both disulfide bonds of hGH were split and the sulfur atoms carbamidomethylated, total hGH potency was retained when analyzed in the rat tibia and pigeon crop-sac GH-dependent bioassays.[95] In a similar manner, Campbell et al. found that the two disulfide bridges

pGH

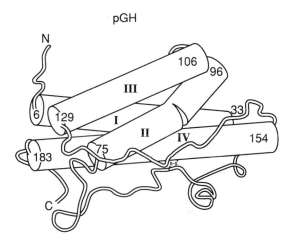

FIGURE 30–2. Crystal representation of porcine growth hormone (pGH) at the 2.8-Å resolution level. Four α helixes are depicted (cylindric rods). The nonhelical region is shown as a thin tube. Also, one of the two disulfide bonds is shown, with the other hidden behind helix IV. The N and C termini are located in the upper left and lower left corners, respectively. (From Abdel-Meguid SS, Shieh HS, Smith WW, et al: Three-dimensional structure of a genetically engineered variant of porcine growth hormone. Proc Natl Acad Sci U S A 84:6434–6437, 1987.)

of hGH are not required for lipolytic or antilipolytic activity in chicken adipose tissue.[96] However, when hGH was reduced and alkylated, substantial loss of biologic activity was noted.[97] Loss of biologic activity was also found when both of the disulfide bonds of porcine GH were reduced and aminoethylated.[98] These contrasting results suggest that the biologic significance of the disulfide bonds' integrity may be species specific.

Site-directed mutagenesis techniques have been used to perform Cys residue conversion experiments. When Cys165 of hGH (equivalent to Cys164 of bGH) was changed to Ala, this hGH analogue retained full biologic activity with respect to native hGH.[99] However, when the disulfide bonds in bGH were disrupted by amino acid substitution of Cys for Ser residues and assayed for their ability to enhance growth in transgenic mice, only animals that expressed bGH analogues with the large loop intact demonstrated a growth-enhanced phenotype. These results suggested that integrity of the large loop, but not the small loop, is essential for GH's growth-enhancing activity.[68]

Homologue and Alanine Scanning of GH

Information about the functional domains of GH obtained through fragment experiments is limited because the overall conformation of the protein has been altered. In the early 1990s, understanding of the structure of GH was advanced by using a novel approach entailing recombinant DNA techniques. Cloned DNA sequences encoding hPRL, which possesses minimal GHR-binding affinity, were substituted for the corresponding regions of hGH. Because PRL and GH are somewhat homologous, the term "homologue scanning" was used to describe these experiments. The PRL/GH chimeric molecules were assayed for their ability to bind PRL or GHR. This approach was very effective in defining the receptor-binding domains of hGH,[100] which were found to be located mainly in the N-terminal portion of α helix I, a loop region between amino acid residues 54 to 74, and the C-terminal portion of α helix IV.[100]

Systematic replacement of fragments of hGH with sequences derived from nonbinding GH homologues has generated information regarding GH/GHR-binding parameters. However, these experiments could not identify the specific residues involved in the ligand-receptor interaction.

After the GH homologue-scanning studies, a more refined approach was applied to the structure/binding relationships of GH and GHR. In this approach, alanine codons were systematically substituted for numerous codons in the GH gene encoding residues found in α helix I, the loop, and α helix IV. This "alanine scanning" approach was used to define specific amino acid residues important for GHR binding.[101] It was reported that amino acid residues 10, 54, 56, 58, 64, and 68 (loop region) and 171, 172, 175, 178, 182, and 185 (C terminus) were involved in GHR binding.[100–102] The scanning mutagenesis studies largely ignored the third α helix of GH because amino acid substitutions in this area resulted in little change in receptor-binding affinity.

The Third α Helix of GH

As stated above, search for a growth-related domain in GH was pioneered by Sonenberg's group in late 1960s and early 1970s.[79, 84, 103, 104] Their main finding was that a short sequence produced by tryptic digestion of bGH to generate residues 96 to 133 (see Fig. 30–1) retained low, but significant rat tibia bone growth–stimulating activity whereas segments 1 to 95 and 134 to 191 had much less activity. The tryptic peptide, consisting of residues 96 to 133, contains the third α helix of GH. Subsequently, it was reported that an hGH fragment (1–134) was fully active in the IM-9 human lymphocyte assay[105] and had lower but significant bioactivity in the rat tibia test.[76] Recently, recombinant hormones possessing different portions of GH, PRL, or PL have been generated and analyzed. hGH (1–134) was linked to hPL (141–191), and hPL (1–134) was linked to hGH (141–191) through a Cys53-Cys165 disulfide bond.[22] These recombinant hormones were then tested for immunoreactivity, as well as their receptor-binding properties. It was found that the recombinant hGH (1–134)-hPL (141–191) retains hGH immunoreactivity and full somatogenic receptor–binding ability but had little hPL activity. On the other hand, the recombinant hPL (1–134)-hGH (141–191) possessed mostly hPL immunoreactivity and lactogenic receptor–binding characteristics, with negligible hGH activity. These results suggested that the immunoreactivity and biologic activity of the hormones are determined primarily by the N-terminal fragment (residues 1–134). The C terminus appears to have little effect in determining the specificity of biologic activity. Together, these results suggested that GH activity could be ascribed to different regions of the GH molecule and that the 96–133 segment might be an "active core" required for growth promotion. These two lines of evidence laid the foundation for the structure-function studies of the third α helix of GH.

Mutagenesis of the GH Gene Encoding α Helix III

By combining site-specific mutagenesis of the GH gene with the ability of bGH analogues to enhance the growth of transgenic mice, we found that a growth-promoting region of GH is localized in the third α helix.[62–67] This α helix possesses amphiphilic characteristics; that is, the hydrophobic residues are geographically separated from the hydrophilic residues (Fig. 30–3). The third α helix is imperfect in that Glu117 (a hydrophilic residue) is found in the lower hydrophobic half of the α helix whereas Ala122 (a hydrophobic residue) and Gly119 are positioned in the hydrophilic portion of the α helix.

Importance of Amphiphilic α Helixes

Amphiphilic secondary structures have been proposed to be important functional domains for many peptide hormones.[106–114] It has been demonstrated that a GH-releasing hormone (GHRH) analogue with an optimized amphiphilic α helix possessed enhanced biologic activity in comparison to native GHRH.[113] In addition, a calcitonin analogue was designed such that it had no amino acid sequence similarity to native calcitonin but maintained identical length and amphiphilic properties. This analogue was nearly as potent as native calcitonin in mobilizing calcium.[110, 111] Also, a yeast transcriptional activator, GCN4, contains an activation domain composed of 19 amino acids that is located outside its DNA-binding region. This short stretch of amino acids forms an amphiphilic α helix that is sufficient for transcriptional activation.[112] It was suggested that this 19–amino acid region in GCN4 might serve as a recognition signal for one or more components of the transcriptional apparatus.[112]

Designing a GH Analogue with a Perfect Amphiphilic α Helix

To convert GH's imperfect third amphiphilic α helix to a "perfect" α helix, we modified Glu117, Gly119, and Ala122 with Leu, Arg, and Asp, respectively[62] (see Fig. 30–3). When these amino acid substitutions were performed and the resulting GH analogue purified and assayed, we found that it bound to GHRs with the same affinity as native GH. However, when the Glu117Leu, Gly119Arg, Ala122Asp GH analogue (termed M8) was assayed for its ability to enhance growth in transgenic mice, this GH analogue did not enhance growth, as does expression of wild-type GH transgenes,[61] but actually suppressed growth. These animals possessed a dwarf phenotype[62] (Fig. 30–4).

Thus three amino acid substitutions (Glu117Leu, Gly119Arg, Ala122Asp) in the third α helix of bGH altered the activities of GH from that of a growth enhancer to a growth suppressor or antagonist.[62] In a subsequent study, we extended this observation by individually modifying Glu117, Gly119, and Ala122 with Leu, Arg, and Asp, respectively. When assayed for their ability to bind to GHRs and to enhance growth in transgenic mice, the substitution of Leu117 for Glu117 resulted in a GH analogue that behaved identically to native GH[63] (Fig. 30–5). Glu117 is conserved in GHs from mammals to chickens.[6] Because the substitution mutation at this position (bGH Glu117Leu) showed no effect on bGH growth-promoting activity, we concluded that residue 117 of bGH is not likely to be involved in growth-promoting activity. Again, this analogue retains the same activities as native bGH.

However, the bGH analogue Gly119Arg was found to bind to GHRs with the same affinity as native GH, but surprisingly, transgenic mice that expressed this analogue were about half the size of their nontransgenic littermates[63] (see Fig. 30–5). We further confirmed this observation by generating hGH Gly120Arg dwarf transgenic mice.[66] Additionally, several other amino acids were substituted for bGH Gly119. All substitutions at amino acid position 119 (bGH Gly119X; X = Arg, Lys, Leu, Pro, Trp) resulted in GH analogues in which the ability to bind to GHRs was uncoupled from the ability to enhance growth in transgenic mice. When these analogues were present at relatively high levels in the serum of transgenic mice, a dwarf phenotype resulted.[63]

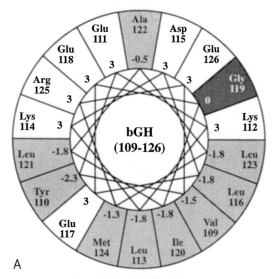
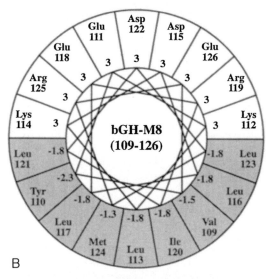

FIGURE 30–3. Axial projection of the third α helix (109–126) of native bovine growth hormone (bGH) *(A)* and amino acid–substituted bGH *(B)*. Amino acid residues and corresponding hydrophilicity values are given. Amino acids in the *open boxes* are hydrophilic (top half of the wheel), and those in the *shaded boxes* are hydrophobic (bottom half). The Gly residue (119) is depicted with *dots*. (From Chen WY, Wight DC, Wagner TE, et al: Expression of a mutated bovine growth hormone gene suppresses growth of transgenic mice. Proc Natl Acad Sci U S A 87:5061–5065, 1990.)

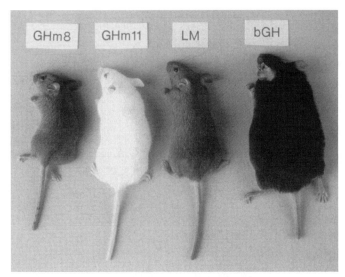

FIGURE 30–4. Growth phenotypes of mice that express different growth hormone (GH) analogues. The animals shown are 6-month-old males. A nontransgenic control animal is indicated as the littermate (LM). A mouse that expresses wild-type bovine GH (bGH) is shown on the right and labeled bGH. A mouse that expresses the bGH antagonist bGH-Gly119Arg is shown on the left and is labeled GHm8. A mouse that expresses a bGH analogue in which the third α helix is destabilized by substitution of proline residues at selected sites[123] is shown and is labeled GHm11. Note that the LM and GHm11 mice are approximately the same size whereas the bGH animal is approximately twice the size of LM and GHm8 is approximately half the size of LM. The LM and GHm8 mice live to approximately 3 years of age whereas the bGH animal dies at 9 to 12 months of age and GHm11 dies at 12 to 15 months of age. (From Yang CW, Striker LJ, Pesce C, et al: Glomerulosclerosis and body growth are mediated by different portions of bovine growth hormone. Studies in transgenic mice. Lab Invest 68:62–70, 1993.)

Finally, substitution of Asp for Ala at residue 122 results in a bGH analogue that binds to GHR but does not enhance (or suppress) growth in transgenic mice. However, unlike bGH Gly119X analogues, the ability to retard mouse growth at relatively high serum levels was diminished. Thus it appears that amino acid substitutions at position 119 (bGH) or 120 (hGH) are more effective than substitutions at position 122 in growth suppression when the analogues are expressed at similar levels in transgenic mice. bGH Ala122Asp may be acting as a partial agonist. Regardless, the salient feature of bGH Ala122Asp and bGH Gly119X is the apparent uncoupling of the ability to bind GHR from the ability to enhance growth in transgenic mice.[62, 63, 66] These studies were the first to document the discovery of GH antagonists (GHAs).

GH Antagonists

Gly119 is conserved among all members of the GH family, including PRL and PL.[6] Gly is unique among amino acids in that it possesses a single hydrogen atom as a side chain. This small side chain has been suggested to increase molecule flexibility.[82] Consequently, it is the least favored residue for the formation of a stable α helical structure.[82] The absolute conservation of this α helix–destabilizing amino acid within a strong α helical–forming region of GH's helix III implies a crucial role for this residue. When bGH Gly119 or hGH Gly120 was replaced with a variety of amino acids and the mutated genes were expressed in transgenic mice, dwarf animals resulted[62, 63, 66] (see Fig. 30–5). We also tested for the ability of the GH-substituted molecules to inhibit GH-dependent conversion of mouse preadipocytes to adipocytes. The bGH Gly119Arg or hGH Gly120Arg analogues were found to inhibit this reaction by 50% at equal molar concentrations of GH and analogue.[115, 116] Thus these GH molecules, in which α helix III

Gly amino acids were replaced by a variety of amino acids, acted as GHAs both in vitro and in vivo.[62–67, 115–117]

Another hGH gene mutation has resulted in a "natural" GHA.[118, 119] In this case the codon for Arg77 was found to be mutated to encode Cys. The child in which this mutation was discovered possessed a dwarf phenotype. The molecule was shown to inhibit GH-stimulated Janus kinase 2 (JAK2) phosphorylation in vitro.[119] However, the molecular mechanism by which this molecule acts as a GHA is not known.

GH Antagonists as Therapeutic Agents

In vitro and in vivo studies of hGHAs have demonstrated that they possess great potential to counteract the pathologic conditions of excess hGH in clinical settings.[62–67, 115, 117, 120, 121] These pathologic situations include acromegaly, diabetic nephropathy,[117, 122, 123] diabetic retinopathy,[124, 125] and certain cancers. For example, GH-induced glomerulosclerosis does not develop in transgenic mice that express GHAs[122] (Fig. 30–6). Also, these animals are resistant to diabetes-induced kidney end-organ damage.[117, 127] Similarly, GHA mice have reduced levels of ischemia-induced retinal neovascularization when compared with nontransgenic mice.[125] Additionally, when GH (giant) and GHA (dwarf) mice are crossed, the resulting offspring are intermediate in size, which suggests that GHAs may overcome the growth-enhancing properties of GH.[128] Thus the use of transgenic animals that express GHAs have yielded data supporting the concept that this type of molecule may be used as a new class of therapeutic agent.

However, to elicit a sufficient pharmacologic effect, GHA should be present in the plasma long enough to antagonize the endogenous effects of GH. Preliminary studies on a GHA (hGH Gly120Lys) have

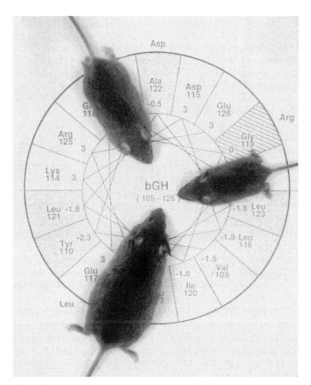

FIGURE 30–5. Representative transgenic mice that express different bovine growth hormone (bGH) analogues superimposed on the Edmonson wheel projection of the third α helix of bGH. The mouse at the lower left expresses bGH-Glu117Leu and possesses an enhanced growth phenotype similar to animals that express wild-type bGH. The animal at the top expresses bGH-Ala122Asp and, despite having elevated serum levels of this GH analogue, possesses a normal growth phenotype. The mouse on the right expresses bGH-Gly119Arg (the first reported GH antagonist) and possesses a dwarf phenotype. (From Chen WY, Wight DC, Mehta BV, et al: Glycine 119 of bovine growth hormone is critical for growth-promoting activity. Mol Endocrinol 5:1845–1852, 1991.)

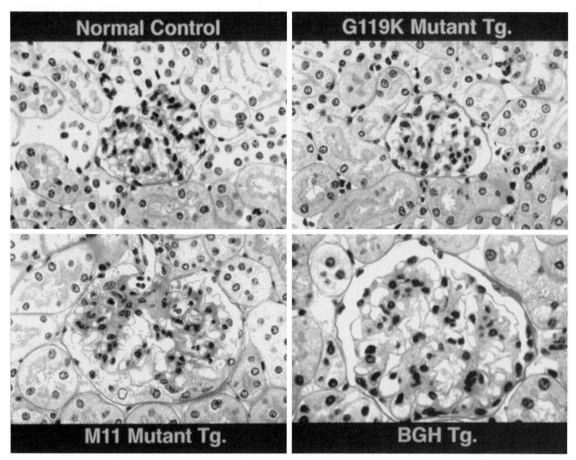

FIGURE 30–6. Kidney histopathology of 9-month-old transgenic and control mice. A glomerulus of a control (Normal Control) and that of a growth hormone (GH) antagonist (G119K) mouse are shown in the upper right and left portions of the figure, respectively. Glomeruli of bGH M11 (M11 Mutant Tg) and that of a bGH (BGH TG) transgenic mouse are shown in the lower left and right sectors, respectively. Kidneys from normal control and antagonists animals show no abnormal pathology. However, severe glomerulosclerosis is seen in kidneys from M11 and bGH transgenic mice.[122, 123, 126] (Modified from Yang CW, Striker LJ, Pesce C, et al: Glomerulosclerosis and body growth are mediated by different portions of bovine growth hormone. Studies in transgenic mice. Lab Invest 68:62–70, 1993.)

shown that this molecule has a serum half-life of less than 1 hour when injected intraperitoneally in mice.[129] This short half-life may render an hGHA impractical for routine clinical use. The half-life of a therapeutic reagent may be improved in several ways. One is to conjugate the therapeutic molecules with polyethylene glycol (PEG), which prolongs the half-life of the molecules.[130–134]

hGHAs have been pegylated[135] and used in vivo. We have found that hGH Gly120Lys, when pegylated with four to six PEGs, has a half-life of approximately 18 hours after a single intravenous, intraperitoneal, or subcutaneous injection.[129] When mice received a daily subcutaneous single injection of various doses (0.25–4 mg/kg) of Gly120-Lys-PEG or vehicle for 5 days, significant, dose-dependent suppression of IGF-1 became obvious starting at day 3. Maximum suppression (up to 70%) of IGF-1 production was achieved by 1-mg/kg dosing at day 6 after the first injection. Also, hepatic GHRs were significantly increased on day 8, also in a dose-dependent manner (Chen et al., unpublished data). These results suggest that exogenous administration of Gly120Lys-PEG can dramatically decrease serum IGF-1 levels and may lead to the use of GHAs as therapeutic agents. In this regard it has recently been shown that injection of a pegylated GHA (hGH Gly120Lys) into mice results in inhibition of diabetes-induced kidney damage.[136]

Other Amino Acid Substitutions in the Hydrophilic Region of GH's Third α Helix

We further generated a series of bGH analogues with single– or double–amino acid substitutions in the hydrophilic region of the α

helix.[67] Corresponding transgenic mice lines were generated and analyzed. Based on the growth rates of these transgenic mice, the analogues were categorized as full growth-promoting analogues (Glu111Ala, Lys112Leu-Lys114Trp, Leu116Ala, Glu117Leu, Glu111Ala-Glu118Ala, Arg125Leu, Glu126Gly), partial growth-promoting analogues or partial agonists (Asp115Ala, Leu123Ile), growth inhibitory analogues (Gly119Xs), or non–growth-promoting analogues (deletion of residue 119, Δ119).

It is important to note that analogues with amino acid substitutions that result in changes in growth-promoting activity are located within a region of nine amino acids, that is, between Asp115 and Leu123. These amino acids form two turns of the α helix. By viewing the side chains of these potentially important amino acids, it appeared that Gly119 and Ala122, two amino acids with relatively small side chains, form a "hingelike" or "cleft" structure that we had predicted[63] (Fig. 30–7) and has been shown to exist in the crystal structure of hGH.[137] The "cleft" is located near the center of this α helix, primarily because of Gly119. Ala122 is at the same phase of the α helix that extends the cleft because of its relatively small side chain. We postulated that this cleft is important for the growth-promoting activity of the GH molecule.[63] If this cleft is important for growth-related biologic activity of the molecule, Gly may be the only residue tolerable at this position. Extension of this model would yield the prediction that any other amino acid substitution at this position would decrease the flexibility of the molecule and/or "fill" the cleft, which would ultimately result in decreased biologic activity.

The amino acid residues chosen to substitute for Gly119 in our study were representative of various amino acid groups and included Leu (hydrophobic, 2.8), Lys (hydrophilic and positive charged, 2.8), Trp (bulky hydrophobic, 3.8), and Pro (helix breaker with a bulky side

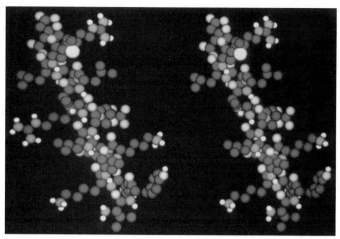

FIGURE 30–7. A space-filling model of the third α helix of growth hormone (GH) *(right)* and a GH antagonist *(left)*. The N terminus of the helixes is located at the *bottom* and the COOH end at the *top*. Note the cleft that is located in the middle of the wild-type helix *(right)* and the occupancy of this cleft with the side chain of Arg *(left)*. (From Chen WY, Wight DC, Mehta BV, et al: Glycine 119 of bovine growth hormone is critical for growth-promoting activity. Mol Endocrinol 5:1845–1852, 1991.)

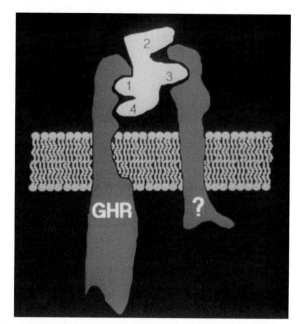

FIGURE 30–8. The growth hormone (GH)-mediated second-target hypothesis regarding GH action. The membrane-spanning GH receptor (GHR) is indicated. GH α helixes are labeled 1, 2, 3, and 4. The unknown "second target" that interacts with Gly119 of bovine GH or Gly120 of human GH is labeled (?) and in this representation is shown as a membrane-spanning protein.

chain, 2.2). The numbers in parentheses indicate the relative volume increase in the amino acid side chain in comparison to Gly after the substitution mutation at position 119.

Finally, Asp115 and Leu123, amino acids with negatively charged (Asp) and long (Leu) side chains, respectively, flank the cleft and may be involved in the interaction with GH targets such as GHR or cellular targets.

To further substantiate the importance of the cleft in the third α helix, we designed a bGH analogue with a deletion at Gly119 (Δ119). Transgenic mice that expressed this analogue had a phenotype similar to their litter mates.[67] These data provide supportive evidence for the importance of the cleft structure in the third α helix. It is interesting to point out that all bGH analogues tested in this study, including Δ119 (deletion mutation, inactive analogue), SAP (scrambled helix, weak antagonist), and Gly119Arg (potent antagonist), were able to bind to the GHR with an affinity similar to that of bGH.

To accommodate all the data concerning the amino acid substitutions in GH, including those derived from the alanine-scanning studies[101] and those directed at the third α helix of GH,[62] we proposed the second-target hypothesis for GH action (Fig. 30–8). In this model, residues in α helices I and IV and the large loop region interact with the GHR as reported by Cunningham and Wells.[101] Additionally, we postulated that the cleft region in α helix III interacts with an unidentified target and that the tripartite complex is the functional unit responsible for induction of GH action.[62]

Co-crystallization of GH with GH Receptor

The second-target hypothesis of GH action predicted that the cleft region in the third α helix of GH would interact with an unidentified target to form a GH/GHR/second-target complex. In 1992, the crystal structure of hGH and the GH-binding protein (GHBP) was solved[137] (Fig. 30–9). Again, four GH α helixes were detected: α helix I (residues 9–34), α helix II (residues 72–92), α helix III (residues 106–128), and α helix IV (residues 155–184). Two small minihelixes, residues 38 to 47 and 64 to 79, were also found in the large loop between α helixes I and II. Importantly, in the crystal two identical GHBP molecules were identified with one GH molecule. Amino acids predicted from the alanine-scanning data[101] were found to form the first contact site with GHBP (site 1), whereas the cleft region in the third α helix, in particular, Gly120, and several amino acids at the N terminus were found to make contact with a second GHBP (site 2).

This observation was a substantial finding in the general field of molecular endocrinology and in the area of growth factor and cytokine molecular and cellular biology. Significantly, it is one of the most fundamental findings in the GH field. Details concerning the interaction are described below. Thus the co-crystallization of one GH molecule with two GHRs[137] supported the GH second-target hypothesis of GH action[62, 63]; the "second target" was a second GHR.

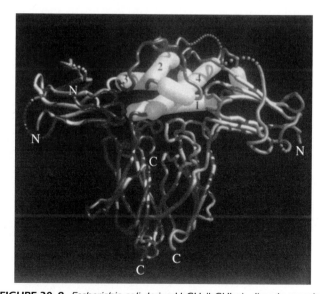

FIGURE 30–9. *Escherichia coli*–derived hGHs(hGHbp)₂ dimeric complex: representation of the growth hormone (GH)/GH receptor cocrystal structure. The GH α helixes are indicated as cylinders and labeled 1, 2, 3, and 4. α Helixes 1 and 4 (site 1) are shown interacting with one GH-binding protein (GHBP), whereas α helix 3 (site 2) is shown interacting with a second GHBP. (Reprinted with permission from de Vos AM, Ultsch M, Kossiakoff AA: Human growth hormone and extracellular domain of its receptor: Crystal structure of the complex. Science 255:306–312, 1992. Copyright 1992 American Association for the Advancement of Science.)

GROWTH HORMONE RECEPTOR

Background

Somatotropic cells of the anterior pituitary are the major site of GH synthesis and secretion. Production is regulated by the opposing actions of two hypothalamic neuropeptides: GHRH, which stimulates the synthesis and secretion of GH, and somatostatin, which inhibits the secretion of GH[69, 138] (see Chapters 31 and 32). GH's essential role in growth promotion was once thought to be accomplished indirectly by the GH-induced synthesis of IGF-1 (see Chapter 33). However, this point is still controversial because the growth phenotype may be a combination of GH's direct tissue effects and the indirect effect of inducing synthesis of IGF-1. In contrast, GH's effect on energy metabolism in nongrowing adults probably results from direct interaction with GHRs on target tissues.[139]

GHRs have been found on the cell surface of many tissues throughout the body, including liver, muscle, adipose, and kidney[140] and in early embryo and fetal tissue,[141–146] where it has an effect on embryonic tooth development.[147] Evidence linking the importance of the GHR to the "growth" phenotype has come from studies on dwarf individuals who are GH resistant. In these individuals, expression of different mutations located throughout the GHR gene results in the dwarf phenotype called the Laron syndrome.[148–151] GHR gene mutations have also been found in certain strains of sex-linked dwarf chickens.[152, 153] Ultimate proof of the importance of the GHR has come recently from disruption of the GHR and GHBP genes.[154] "Knockout" of these genes results in dwarf mice (Fig. 30–10). These mice are approximately half the size of wild-type mice.

GHR and GH-Binding Protein

The GHR is a member of the class 1 hematopoietic cytokine family.[155] The human GHR gene encompasses 10 exons and approximately 90 kb and encodes an extracellular domain, a small transmembrane domain, and an intracellular domain. The protein-coding region of the receptor gene is encoded by exons 2 to 10.[156] Exon 2 of the GHR gene encodes the secretory signal peptide and first six amino acids of the mature form of the protein; exons 3 to 7 encode the extracellular domain; exon 8, the transmembrane domain; and exons 9 and 10, the intracellular domain.

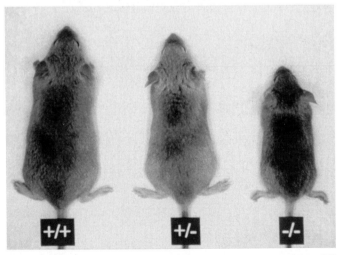

FIGURE 30–10. Growth hormone receptor (GHR)/binding protein (BP) gene–disrupted mice. A wild-type mouse is shown on the *left* (+/+), a heterozygous mouse in the *center* (+/−), and the GHR/BP "knockout" mouse on the *right* (−/−). The GHR/BP −/− mouse is approximately half the size of the normal wild-type (+/+) and heterozygous (+/−) animals. (From Zhou Y, Xu BC, Maheshwari HG, et al: A mammalian model for Laron syndrome produced by targeted disruption of the mouse growth hormone receptor/binding protein gene (the Laron mouse). Proc Natl Acad Sci U S A 94:13215–13220, 1997. Copyright 1997 National Academy of Sciences, U.S.A.)

The structure of the extracellular portion of the GHR consists of two domains, each containing seven β strands arranged to form a sandwich of two antiparallel β sheets.[137] This arrangement is also found in immunoglobulins, CD4, and fibronectin. Stabilizing the GHR structure is a salt bridge between Arg39 and Asp132 and hydrogen bonds between Arg43 and Glu169.[137] Also, three disulfide bonds exist between Cys38–48, Cys83–94, and Cys108–122[137, 157] and are thought to be important in the overall structural integrity of the GHR. The reader is referred to excellent reviews on the GHR and PRL receptor.[158, 159]

A soluble portion of the GHR extracellular domain is termed the GHBP. In mice and rats it is encoded by an additional exon, exon 8A,[160–162] and is produced by alternative splicing of the GHR precursor mRNA.[163, 164] In other vertebrates it is believed to be generated by proteolytic cleavage of the extracellular domain of the GHR. The function of GHBP is unknown, but it may increase the activity of GH by enhancing its half-life or reduce the activity of GH by sequestering the molecule from the GHR. Until the GHBP gene alone is disrupted, the ultimate function of the molecule will remain unknown. The reader is referred to several reviews and papers on GHBP.[23, 71, 163–169]

GH/GHR Dimerization

Examination of the 2.8-ÅA crystal structure of the complex between the hormone and the extracellular domain of the GHR produced by *Escherichia coli* (hGHBP) demonstrated that the complex consisted of one molecule of GH and two molecules of receptor.[137] Furthermore, the crystal structure reveals how a nonsymmetric molecule (i.e., GH) binds to two copies of the receptor via identical epitopes (see Fig. 30–9).

Amino acid residues in the hGHR (actually, hGHBP) involved in contact with hGH have been determined from cocrystallization analysis of the GH/GHR complex.[137, 170, 171] The major binding determinants in the GH molecule (site 1) are located in the two minihelixes between α helixes I and II and between the center and C terminus of helix IV. GHR site 1 residues are amino acids 40 to 45 and 101 to 106, which interact with GH amino acids 168 to 176 in α helix IV, and residues 60 to 63 in the second minihelix. GHR Trp169 interacts with hGH residues 171 to 179 in α helix IV. The site 2 binding determinants in the GHR are the same residues (except for Asn218) as for GHR site 1, especially Trp104 and Trp109. In terms of GH site 2 residues important for contact and dimerization, only Phe1, Ile4, and Asp116 in the third α helix are significant.[172] Of particular interest is the close encounter with GH Gly120 and GHR Trp104 in this site 2 interaction. An exhaustive review of the contact points between GH and the GHR has been presented.[159]

Attempts to generate more potent GH agonist by altering site 1 have been successful. For example, monovalent phage display techniques have yielded GH analogues with increased binding affinity to GHR.[173] Also, GH analogues in which residues have been altered in the C terminus of helix I have resulted in GH agonists with increase GHR-binding affinity.[174, 175]

In the GHR, a GH-induced dimerization domain exists. A Cys residue, Cys241, has been reported to undergo GH-induced intermolecular disulfide bonding, thus bridging together two GHR.[176] Also, eight hGHR amino acid residues are involved in salt bridge and hydrogen bond interaction across the extracellular dimerization domain.[137] For hGHR1 the residues are Ser145, Leu146, Thr147, His150, Asp152, and Ser201 and for hGHR2 they are Asp152, Ser201, Asn143, and Tyr200. Of these eight residues, five are important for GH/GHR-mediated signal transduction: Ser145, His150, Asp152, Try200, and Ser201 but not Leu146 or Thr147.[177] This study, as well as those using monoclonal antibodies to induce a GH response,[178] suggests that a GH-induced conformational change in the GHR is required for a full biologic response. Additionally, the subtle but significant differences between the one hGH/two GHR[137] and the one hGH/one GHR[179] cocrystal structures suggest that a conformational change does occur in the one ligand–two receptor complex.

Members of the cytokine receptor family possess disulfide bonds and a WSXWS "box" in their extracellular domain. The GHR, unlike the other members of the cytokine receptor family, does not possess a WSXWS box, but an equivalent YGEFS sequence has been noted.[180] A similar sequence has been found in the extracellular domain of the PRL receptor.[181] This sequence has been reported to be important for binding GHR accessory molecules,[182] or it provides a stabilizing effect on the receptor's structure.[180, 183]

I have only touched on a few of the structural characteristics of the GHR. For a more exhaustive review of this subject the reader is referred to an excellent review by Waters.[159]

GH/GHR Interaction—A Model

The cocrystallization of GH with GHBP[137] was and is a remarkable scientific finding. However, one must remember that in this crystal structure, GHBP and not the full-length GHR was used. Also, because GHBP was produced by *E. coli*, it was not glycosylated as is native GHBP and GHR. Nonetheless, the interaction of one GH with two GHBPs has been extrapolated to the in vivo interaction of GH with GHR. This finding has led to the theory of a sequential binding mechanism in which hGH binds to two GHRs[172] (Fig. 30–11). In this model, hGH must first bind to one GHR at a high-affinity receptor-binding site that subsequently allows binding of the second receptor. Binding site 1 of hGH is located at residues identified by alanine-scanning mutagenesis studies,[101] that is, α helix I, the loop between amino acids 54 to 74, and α helix IV. Binding site 2 is located at the N terminus (Ile4) and the third α helix, namely, Gly120. The model predicts that a Typ104 residue of the receptor "fits" into the "cleft" of the third α helix of GH. The authors also proposed that hGH Gly120Arg acted as a GHA because the substitution of Arg for Gly at position 120 blocked binding site 2 on the ligand. These data nicely supported the "cleft" theory pertaining to the interaction of GH Gly120 with a second target.[62–67, 115–117]

The importance of GH-induced GHR dimerization has recently been shown in humans. An adenine-to-guanine mutation was found in the hGH gene that results in conversion of Asp112 to Gly112. In the heterozygous state the mutation is believed to be the cause of dwarfism in girls.[184] This hGH analogue binds to hGHR in vitro but does not induce GHR dimerization and does not activate JAK2 and STAT5 (signal transducer and activator of transcription-5).[184]

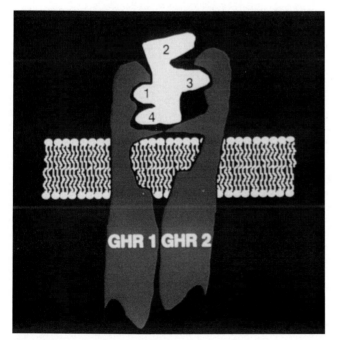

FIGURE 30–11. The one growth hormone (GH)/two GH receptor (GHR) model. The GH α helixes are represented by the numbers 1, 2, 3, and 4 and are shown outside the cell membrane. The two identical single-membrane–spanning GHRs are labeled GHR1 and GHR2. Not shown are the several N-linked glycosylation sites on the GHR.

Together, the results cited above raise the possibility that the one ligand/two receptor model of GH action is not universal and that other GHRs may mediate a subset of GH effects.

GROWTH HORMONE–INDUCED SIGNAL TRANSDUCTION

The molecular mechanisms by which GH transmits its signals via its receptor have been largely elucidated by experiments in cultured cells or hypophysectomized rats.[185] GH-induced in vivo signal transduction systems are still largely unknown and the subject of continued research in our own laboratory,[186] as well as others.[187, 188] Below is summarized several GH-mediated intracellular signal transduction pathways (Fig. 30–12). Some of these pathways may overlap with signal transduction intermediates induced by insulin and other hormones, thus providing opportunities of "biologic crosstalk" between these molecules. Several excellent reviews on the subject have recently been published.[158, 185, 189–191]

JAK Activation

In the early 1990s, GH treatment of responsive cells was found to induce association of a tyrosine kinase with the GHR.[192–194] This kinase was later identified as a 121-kDA protein[195] and found to be a member of the JAK family of proteins, in particular, JAK2.[196, 197] Activation of JAKs appears to be an initial step in one of the GH-induced signal transduction systems (see Fig. 30–12). Although three JAK molecules are involved in GH/GHR signal transduction, JAK2 exhibits the greatest degree of activation.[196, 198–200] GH-dependent JAK2 activation requires interaction between JAK2 and the membrane-proximal, proline-rich motif (termed box 1) located in the intracellular region of the GHR.[201–204] Because GHR itself has no intrinsic kinase activity, it is thought that the colocalization of two JAK2 molecules by the dimerized GHR leads to transphosphorylation of one JAK2 by the other, thereby resulting in JAK2 activation.[185, 190] Activated JAK2, in turn, is thought to phosphorylate GHR on multiple tyrosine residues, possibly providing docking sites for STAT5.[205, 206]

STAT Signaling Pathway

Many of the physiologic effects of GH result from transcriptional regulation of a variety of genes. Several different signaling pathways contribute to this regulation (see Fig. 30–12), but the pathway that was discovered in the mid-1990s and perhaps the most universal pathway implicated in GH action involves STAT proteins. Upon phosphorylation, cytoplasmic STAT proteins form either homodimers or heterodimers, translocate into the nucleus, bind DNA, and activate transcription.[190, 207]

GH-dependent tyrosyl phosphorylation requiring JAK2 activation has been demonstrated for STAT1, STAT3, and STAT5.[198, 204, 208–213] In addition, STAT5 activation requires regions of GHR not involved in JAK2 activation, which suggests that STAT5 also interacts directly with GHR.[198, 204, 205, 214] Docking of STAT5 with GHR requires phosphorylated tyrosine residues presumably mediated by JAK2. The tyrosine residues found to be phosphorylated and important in STAT5 docking and subsequent activation have been reported.[205, 213] Whereas STAT5 has been found to directly associate with GHR,[212] STAT1 and STAT3 probably do not but interact with JAK2 instead.[198, 204, 214] A model of this interaction has been presented.[205]

STAT1, STAT3, STAT5, and possibly STAT4 have also been identified in the GH-induced DNA-binding complexes of several genes. For example, STAT1, STAT3, and in some cells STAT4 have been shown to bind to the *sis*-inducible element of the c-*fos* promoter/enhancer.[209–211, 215] Similarly, STAT5 has been shown to bind to the interferon-γ–activated sequence (GAS)-like response element (GLE) in the serine protease inhibitor (*spi*) 2.1 gene.[216] Their presence is required for maximum transcriptional gene activation.[217, 218]

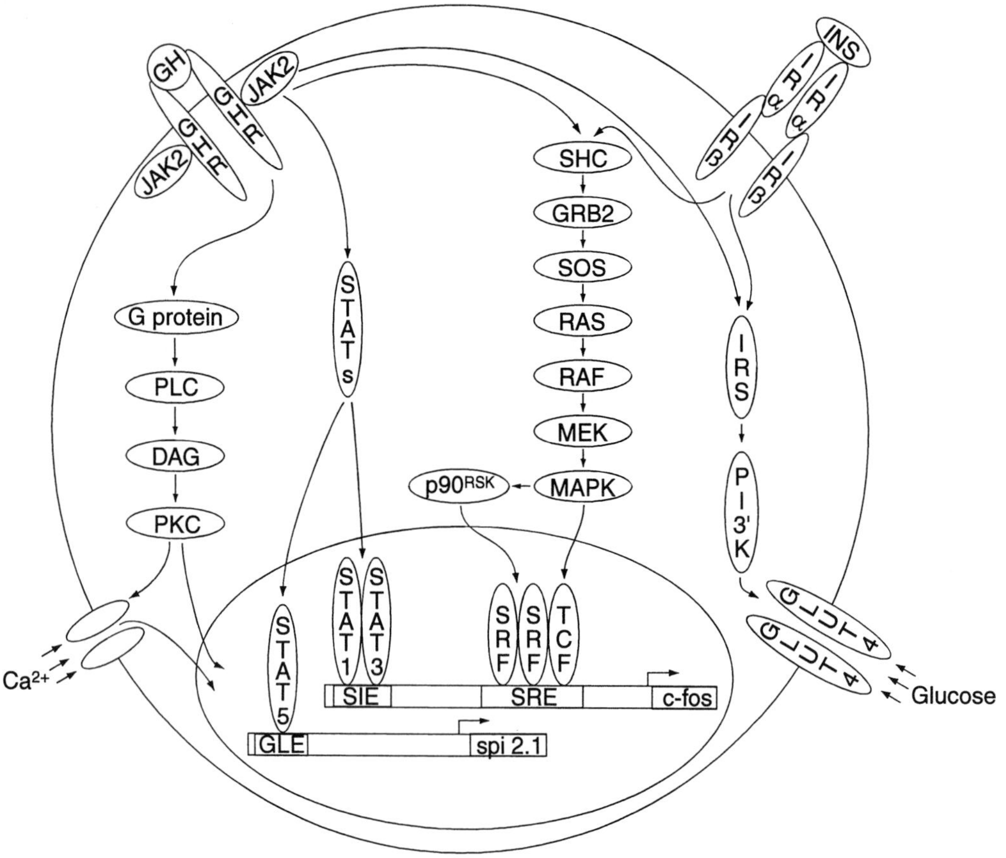

FIGURE 30–12. A model depicting intracellular signaling intermediates induced by binding of growth hormone (GH) with the GH receptor (GHR). DAG, diacylglycerol; ERK, extracellular signal–regulated kinase; GLE, interferon-γ–activated sequence (GAS)-like response element; GLUT, glucose transporter; GRB, growth factor receptor–binding protein; JAK, Janus kinase; INS, insulin; IRα, insulin receptor alpha subunit; MAPK, mitogen-activated protein kinase; MEK, MAPK-ERK kinase; PKC, protein kinase C; PLC, phospholipase C; SIE, sis-inducible element; SOS, son of sevenless; SRE, serum response element; SRF, serum response factor; STAT, signal transducer and activator of transcription; TCF, ternary complex factor. (From Kopchick JJ, Bellush LL, Coschigano KT: Transgenic models of growth hormone action. Annu Rev Nutr 19:437–461, 1999. With permission from the Annual Review of Nutrition, Volume 19, © 1999, by Annual Reviews http://www.AnnualReviews.org.)

MAPK Signaling Pathway

Another GH-inducible pathway that ultimately culminates in transcriptional regulation of a number of genes involves the activation of two mitogen-activated protein kinases (MAPKs): extracellular signal–regulated kinase-1 (ERK1) and ERK2[219–222] (see Fig. 30–12). This pathway was first described for insulin-mediated signal transduction. The pathway most likely begins with GH-stimulated binding of SHC family members to phosphorylated residues in both GHR and JAK2, followed by phosphorylation of the SHCs by JAK2.[223] Subsequently, the tyrosyl-phosphorylated SHC proteins interact with growth factor receptor binding protein-2 (Grb2), which in turn interacts with *son of sevenless* (SOS).[223, 224] Finally, GH activates Ras, Raf and mitogen-activated protein kinase/extracellular regulated kinase (MAPK/ERK) kinase (MEK).[224] These studies, as well as studies by Winston and Hunter,[225] implicate GH as the inducer of the SHC-Grb2-SOS-Ras-Raf-MEK pathway for activation of MAPK. GH has also been shown to activate insulin receptor substrate-1 (IRS-1)[226, 227] and IRS-2,[228] which can also lead to activation of the RAS-MEK signaling pathway (see below).

GH has been shown to activate the S6 kinase p90[RSK], most likely via MAPK.[219] p90[RSK], in turn, can phosphorylate a transcription factor termed serum response factor (SRF) that binds to the GH-responsive serum response element (SRE) of the c-*fos* promoter/enhancer.[215, 229] GH may activate another protein, the ternary complex factor p62[TCF]/ELK1, that interacts with SRF to bind SRE but is directly activated by ERK1 and ERK2.[230, 231] Further evidence that MAPKs are involved in the GH-dependent transcriptional regulation of c-*fos* comes from the observation that the same regions of GHR required for activation of MAPK are also required for c-*fos* gene induction.[232] As mentioned above, STAT proteins are also involved in c-*fos* gene regulation, thus demonstrating a convergence of at least two divergent GH signaling pathways in the regulation of a single gene. MAPK activation, which can be induced by a number of growth factors, may represent a common signal transduction system, whereas activation of STAT proteins (in particular, STAT5) may be more specific to GH.[233]

The MAPK signaling pathway may also contribute to the insulin-like activity of GH, specifically, stimulation of glucose uptake.[232] An inhibitor that blocks GH-induced tyrosyl phosphorylation of ERK1 and ERK2 but not JAK2 also partially inhibits GH-stimulated glucose uptake, thus implicating involvement of inhibitor-sensitive kinases downstream of JAK2 but upstream of ERK1 and ERK2 in this activity.[232]

IRS Signaling Pathway

In addition to the MAPK pathway intermediates, GH also activates members of an additional insulin signaling pathway, IRS-1 and IRS-2[226, 228] (see Fig. 30–12). Although the nature of the interaction between the IRS molecules and the GHR/JAK2 complex is not clear, it does appear that JAK2 activation results in tyrosyl phosphorylation of IRS-1 and IRS-2, which is involved in the insulin-like effects of GH.[227, 228, 234, 235] Phosphatidylinositol (PI) 3′-kinase also appears to be involved in the insulin-like effects of GH inasmuch as a GH-induced interaction between the regulatory subunit of PI 3′-kinase and tyrosyl-phosphorylated IRS-1 and IRS-2 has been demonstrated.[228, 229, 236, 237] PI 3′-kinase, in turn, has been implicated in translocation of the insulin-dependent glucose transporter GLUT4 from low-density microsomes to the plasma membrane, nuclear translocation of ERK1, and regulation of protein kinase C (PKC). Whether these activities are directly GH inducible remains speculative.[228, 237–239] Also, it has not been determined whether the IRS signaling pathway is involved in the more physiologically relevant anti-insulin effects of GH.

PKC Signaling Pathway

Experiments designed to inhibit or deplete PKC activity have suggested the involvement of this family of enzymes in a number of physiologic responses to GH. These responses include the insulin-like stimulation of lipogenesis,[240] induction of c-*fos* gene expression,[241, 242] and stimulation of Ca^{2+} uptake.[243] GH-induced Ca^{2+} oscillations have in turn been implicated in GH-dependent *spi* 2.1 gene transcription[244] and the refractoriness of certain cells to GH's insulin-like effects.[245]

One pathway for PKC activation involves GH-induced 1,2-diacyl-glycerol production by phospholipase C that is possibly coupled to GHR via a G protein.[246, 247] Another proposed pathway for PKC activation involves the IRS/PI 3'-kinase pathway, but its inability to act independently on GH is unclear.[185, 239] We have shown that GH promotes activation and translocation of a protein kinase isoform, PKC-ε, from the cytosol to the plasma membrane, thus suggesting that GH-dependent activation of PKC may involve the IRS/PI 3'-kinase pathway.[248]

As mentioned earlier, the GH-responsive pathways described above have been elucidated primarily by experiments performed in cell culture or under special in vivo circumstances. An important challenge that is just beginning to be addressed is the verification of these pathways in normal animals.[187, 188] The ultimate challenge, however, will be the correlation of physiologic GH functions with a particular signal transduction pathway.

MECHANISM OF GROWTH HORMONE ACTION—PROBLEMS AND OPPORTUNITIES

Problems with the One GH/Two GHR Dimerization Model

Dimerization of the GHR appears to be essential for GH action and has become the model when describing the molecular interaction of GH with the GHR.[121, 137] However, several results, listed below, should lead to more exhaustive testing of the model.

One must remember that in this crystal structure, GHBP and not the full-length GHR was used. Also, because the GHBP was produced by *E. coli*, it was not glycosylated as are the native GHBP and GHR.

GH-induced GHR dimerization and subsequent internalization of the GH/GHR complex are not sufficient for GH-induced intracellular signaling because GHAs do form dimers with the GHR and are internalized.[249] In addition, experiments with monoclonal antibodies indicate that binding of GH but not GHAs appears to lead to a conformational change in the extracellular domain of GHR and gives rise to an active dimer configuration necessary for signal transduction.[250] These data fit nicely with the subtle differences in the cocrystal structures of the GH/GHR 2:1 complex vs. the 1:1 GHA/GHR complex.[179] Thus although GHA can bind to and promote GHR dimer formation, "proper" dimer formation is apparently not induced. Proper GHR dimerization evidently leads to a conformational change in the GHR that is required for subsequent GH-specific intracellular signal transduction.

Data presented in studies using transgenic mice as an in vivo assay for various GH analogues have resulted in mouse phenotypes that cannot be explained simply by using the one GH/two GHR model for GH action.[67, 251] Different mouse growth phenotypes ranging from dwarf to giant were found. These results cannot be explained simply by the altered interaction at binding site 2 of GH with its receptor. In these studies,[67] amino acid substitutions in bGH at positions Asp115 (Asp116 of hGH), Ala122 (Thr123 of hGH), or Leu123 (Leu124 of hGH) have been shown to have less than a sixfold decrease in the ability to induce GHR dimerization in vitro[121] and yet have a significant and different effect on growth-promoting activities.[66] Thus GH-induced GHR dimerization cannot simply explain the different mouse growth phenotypes.

One alternative explanation for these results is that the third α helical region of GH interacts with an unknown second target(s) that participates in the regulation of growth. The second-target postulation is substantiated by the finding that hGH (108–129), a sequence encompassing the third α helix of hGH, binds to a site other than the GHR and evokes a mitogenic responses.[252]

hGH Ile4 has been shown to be an important residue in the site 2 interaction between GH and the GHR. Replacement of Ile4 with alanine greatly diminishes the ability of GH-induced GHR dimerization.[172] Yet expression of this GH analogue (hGH Ile4Ala) in transgenic mice results in large animals or full GH activity.[66] Thus if the hGH analogue (Ile4Ala) is decreasing GHR dimerization, it is not affecting the ability of GH to promote growth in transgenic mice.

In the cocrystal structure of hGH with hGHBP, Trp104 of the GHR closely aligns with hGH Gly120.[137] Transgenic mice that express hGH Gly120Lys possess a dwarf phenotype.[66] However, if hGH Gly120 is replace by Ala, one would predict that GHR Trp104 would be somewhat displaced from the hGH molecule because it cannot "fit" into the cleft of the third α helix. This molecule would be predicted to inhibit or destabilize GHR dimerization. However, this molecule acts as a full agonist in its ability to promote growth in transgenic mice.[66]

Thus, is GH-induced GHR dimerization the universal mechanism by which GH elicits its many activities?

Are There Other GHRs?

As stated above, although the cocrystal structure of GH and the GH/GHBP complex has been solved,[137] one should not become dogmatic in terms of the one ligand/two receptor hypothesis when attempting to explain all of GH's in vivo activities.

In the spirit of an additional GHR, it has been reported that hGH fragment 44–191 binds with low affinity to the GHR and at high, nonphysiologic levels stimulates proliferation of a myeloid cell transfected with the hGHR. Also, the 44–191 fragment can antagonize GH action presumably by blocking GHR dimerization. In contrast, hGH fragment 44–191 has been shown to have an order of magnitude higher diabetogenic activity than hGH.[253] Could another GHR be responsible for these activities?

In addition, when one compares the ability of GH to induce differentiation with its ability to stimulate glucose uptake (GH's insulin-like activity) in 3T3-L1 cells (preadipocytes), one finds a difference in the median effective dose (ED_{50}) for these two activities.[254, 255] The ED_{50} for GH promotion of differentiation is approximately 0.1 nM,[254] whereas that of its insulin-like activity is 1.0 nM.[255] If GH were acting via the same GHR and intracellular signaling system, the same ED_{50} values may be predicted for each activity. However, such is clearly not the case.

Waters and coworkers have reported that hGH analogues with amino acid substitutions at site 1 result in GH analogues with affinities for the GHR similar to or greater that wild-type GH; however, they have markedly decreased bioactivity.[175]

Staten et al. have shown that bovine PL forms a 1:1 complex with bGHR but that bGH will induce a 1:2 complex under similar conditions.[256] Surprisingly, both are able to induce an increase in circulating IGF-1 and nitrogen retention in cattle.

Additionally, the first described GHA (bGH Gly119Arg) represses growth in transgenic mice[62] and inhibits GH-induced preadipocyte differentiation.[115, 116] Surprisingly, this molecule antagonizes the lipolytic effect but retains full insulin-like activity of GH in chicken adipose tissue.[256]

Thus GH may be interacting with another GHR.

GH Assays

One of the most important issues concerning discoveries in the GH area, or perhaps the most important issue, is the types of assays used. One cannot screen for the ability of GH analogues to bind to GHRs in vitro and expect to predict the activity of the molecule in vivo. If such were the only assay used, GHAs would not have been discovered by our group.[62] Additional assays involving the in vivo action of GH are needed.

At times, somewhat unexpected, yet important results are derived from in vivo studies. For example, in a structure-function approach to the activities of GH in which mutated GH genes are expressed in transgenic mice and the growth of the animals is monitored, our group has shown that one can uncouple the ability of GH to enhance IGF-1 production and promote growth from a deleterious effect, such as GH-induced glomerulosclerosis (see Figs. 30–4 and 30–6). Expression of the wild-type GH gene in transgenic mice results in animals with elevated serum IGF-1 levels and a corresponding enhanced growth phenotype.[61, 62] These "giant" GH transgenic mice have been found to die prematurely with glomerulosclerosis as one of the primary causes of death[258] (see Fig. 30–6). Importantly, glomerulosclerosis does not develop in transgenic IGF-1 mice.[257, 258] Thus GH appears to be acting directly on the kidney independent of IGF-1. Support for this concept of GH direct action on peripheral tissue comes from studies on another strain of transgenic mice. When the third α helix of GH was destabilized by the substitution of proline residues at selected sites and these mutated GH genes (termed M11) were subsequently expressed in transgenic mice, animals with normal growth phenotypes and normal serum IGF-1 levels resulted (see Fig. 30–4). However, severe glomerulosclerosis was observed in these animals[122, 123] (see Fig. 30–6). Thus the ability of GH to promote growth and enhance IGF-1 production was uncoupled from the ability to induce glomerulosclerosis. Therefore, it appears that GH is acting directly on the kidney independent of IGF-1. This observation is important because it is the first report that GH may indeed act independent of IGF-1.

Data from in vitro binding studies, cell-based assays, or in vivo assays must be carefully interpreted to precisely define the function of novel GH analogues. For example, the ability of GH analogues to act as mitogenic agents may not be the proper cell-based assay to uncover GH's mechanism of action inasmuch as some believe that GH is not a mitogenic agent.[54] Although a variety of cell-based and several in vivo assays abound, none sufficiently depict the action of the molecule because it acts in "normal" conditions. Thus an important future challenge is to develop assays that reflect the action of GH. Because the in vivo molecular actions of GH are not known, the opportunity exists for the discovery and development of these assays.

CONCLUSIONS

Study of the mechanism by which GH elicits its many and varied responses has proceeded vigorously for nearly five decades. Recent advances in determining the crystal structure of GH[92] (see Fig. 30–2), the discovery of GHAs[62] (see Fig. 30–5), cocrystallization of GH with GHBP[137] (see Fig. 30–9), and gene disruption of the mouse GHR/GHBP[153] (see Fig. 30–10) have resulted in new ideas and research directions in the GH area. With this new information and technologies, the future for testing hypotheses based on the action of GH remains fertile. Important areas for new discovery include elucidation of in vivo GH/GHR-induced signal transduction pathways, the possibility of other novel GHRs, and breakthroughs concerning therapeutic molecules that may influence the activity of GH.

Finally, several important questions arise in regard to the above discussion: (1) do all of GH's biologic activities arise via GH-induced dimerization of the GHR? (2) Do other GHRs exist? (3) Does GH act directly on tissue independent of the action of IGF-1? The answers to these questions will be solved in the future; however, inspection of the preliminary data would suggest the following respective answers: no, yes, yes.

Acknowledgment

My work on GH is currently supported by grants from Ohio University, Sensus Corp, Ohio University College of Medicine, and the Ohio Eminent Scholar's Program, which includes a grant from Milton and Lawrence Goll. Previously, the GH work was supported by the above with additional funding derived from the U.S. Department of Agriculture, National Institutes of Health, Merck & Co., the Juvenile Diabetes International Foundation, and the Central Ohio Diabetes Association.

I would like to thank all my current and former graduate students, postdoctoral fellows, technicians, undergraduate students, and visiting scientists who participated in many of the studies reported in this review. I would also like to thank Markus Riders and Karen Coschigano, Ph.D., for help in preparing this review.

REFERENCES

1. Evans HM, Long JA: The effect of the anterior lobe administered intraperitoneally upon growth, maturity and oestrus cycles of the rat. Anat Rec 21:62–63, 1921.
2. Li CH, Evans HM: The isolation of pituitary growth hormone. Science 99:183–184, 1944.
3. Martial JA, Hallewell RA, Baxter JD, et al: Human growth hormone: Complementary DNA cloning and expression in bacteria. Science 205:602–607, 1979.
4. Miller WL, Eberhardt NL: Structure and evolution of the growth hormone gene family. Endocr Rev 4:97–130, 1983.
5. Niall HD, Hogan ML, Sauer R, et al: Sequences of pituitary and placental lactogenic and growth hormones: Evolution from a primordial peptide by gene reduplication. Proc Natl Acad Sci U S A 68:866–870, 1971.
6. Watahiki M, Yamamoto M, Yamakawa M, et al: Conserved and unique amino acid residues in the domains of the growth hormones. Flounder growth hormone deduced from the cDNA sequence has the minimal size in the growth hormone prolactin gene family. J Biol Chem 264:312–316, 1989.
7. Li CH: The chemistry of human pituitary growth hormone: 1967–1973. *In* Li CH (ed): Hormonal Proteins and Peptides, vol 3. New York, Academic, 1975, pp 1–33.
8. Scanes CG, Campbell RM: Growth hormone: Chemistry. *In* Harvey S, Scanes CG, Daughaday WH (eds): Growth Hormone. Boca Raton, FL, CRC Press, 1995, pp 1–24.
9. Kopchick JJ, Chen WY: Structure function relationships of growth hormone (GH) and other members of the GH gene family. *In* Kostyo JL, Goodman HM (eds): Handbook of Physiology. New York, Oxford, 1999, pp 145–162.
10. Hennen G, Frankenne F, Closset J, et al: A human placental GH: Increasing levels during second half of pregnancy with pituitary GH suppression as revealed by monoclonal antibody radioimmunoassays. Int J Fertil 30:27–33, 1985.
11. Daughaday WH, Trivedi B, Winn HN, et al: Hypersomatotropism in pregnant women, as measured by a human liver radioreceptor assay. J Clin Endocrinol Metab 70:215–221, 1990.
12. Frankenne F, Rentier-Delrue F, Scippo ML, et al: Expression of the growth hormone variant gene in human placenta. J Clin Endocrinol Metab 64:635–637, 1987.
13. Selden RF, Wagner TE, Blethen S, et al: Expression of the human growth hormone variant gene in cultured fibroblasts and transgenic mice. Proc Natl Acad Sci U S A 85:8241–8245, 1988.
14. Lewis UJ: Variants of growth hormone and prolactin and their posttranslational modifications. Annu Rev Physiol 46:33–42, 1984.
15. Wallis M: The molecular evolution of pituitary growth hormone prolactin and placental lactogen: A protein family showing variable rates of evolution. J Mol Evol 17:10, 1981.
16. Chen EY, Liao YC, Smith DH, et al: The human growth hormone locus: Nucleotide sequence, biology, and evolution. Genomics 4:479–497, 1989.
17. Kaplan SL, Grumbach MM: Electrophoretic and immunological characteristics of native and purified human growth hormone. Nature 196:336–338, 1962.
18. Lewis UJ, Brink NC: Crystalline human growth hormone. J Am Chem Soc 80:4429–4430, 1958.
19. Lewis UJ, Dunn JT, Bonewald LF, et al: A naturally occurring structural variant of human growth hormone. J Biol Chem 253:2679–2687, 1978.
20. Li CH, Liu WK, Dixon JS: Human pituitary growth hormone. VI. Modified procedure of isolation and NH2-terminal amino acid sequence. Arch Biochem Biophys 99(suppl 1):327–332, 1962.
21. Roos P, Fevold HR, Gemzell CA: Preparation of human growth hormone by gel filtration. Biochim Biophys Acta 74:525–531, 1965.
22. Russell J, Sherwood LM, Kowalski K, et al: Recombinant hormones from fragments of human growth hormone and human placental lactogen. J Biol Chem 256:296–300, 1981.
23. Baumann G: Growth hormone heterogeneity: Genes, isohormones, variants, and binding proteins. Endocr Rev 12:424–449, 1991.
24. Sonksen PH, Salomon F, Cuneo R: Metabolic effects of hypopituitarism and acromegaly. Horm Res 36:27–31, 1991.
25. Daughaday WH: Growth hormone, insulin-like growth factors, and acromegaly. *In* DeGrout LJ (ed): Endocrinology, vol 3. Philadelphia, WB Saunders, 1995, pp 303–329.
26. Melmed S, Braunstein GD, Horvath E, et al: Pathophysiology of acromegaly. Endocr Rev 4:271–290, 1983.
27. Melmed S, Ho K, Klibanski A, et al: Clinical review 75: Recent advances in pathogenesis, diagnosis, and management of acromegaly. J Clin Endocrinol Metab 80:3395–3402, 1995.
28. Melmed S: Acromegaly. Metabolism 45:51–52, 1996.
29. Melmed S: Unwanted effects of growth hormone excess in the adult. J Pediatr Endocrinol Metab 9(suppl 3):369–374, 1996.
30. Melmed S: Medical management of acromegaly—what and when? Acta Endocrinol (Copenh) 129(suppl 1):13–17, 1993.
31. Milman AE, Russell JA: Some aspects of purified pituitary growth hormone on carbohydrate metabolism in the rat. Endocrinology 47:114–119, 1950.
32. Swislocki NL: Effects of nutritional status and the pituitary on the acute plasma free fatty acid and glucose responses of rats to growth hormone administration. Metabolism 17:174–180, 1968.
33. Hjalmarson A, Ahren K: Sensitivity of the rat diaphragm to growth hormone. II. Early and late effects of growth hormone on amino acid and pentose uptake. Acta Endocrinol (Copenh) 56:347–358, 1967.
34. Kostyo JL, Nutting DF: Acute in vivo effects of growth hormone on protein synthesis in various tissues of hypophysectomized rats and their relationship to the levels of thymidine factor and insulin in the plasma. Horm Metab Res 5:167–172, 1973.
35. Batchelor BR, Mahler RJ: Growth hormone–induced enhancement of insulin sensitivity in adipose tissue. Horm Metab Res 4:87–92, 1972.

36. Goodman HM: The effects of growth hormone on the utilization of L-leucine in adipose tissue. Endocrinology 102:210–217, 1978.

37. Newman JD, Armstrong JM, Bornstein J: Effects of part sequences of human growth hormone on in vivo hepatic glycogen metabolism in the rat. Biochim Biophys Acta 544:234–244, 1978.

38. Porterfield SP: The effects of growth hormone, thyroxine and insulin on the activities of reduced nicotinamide adenine dinucleotide phosphate dehydrogenase, glucose-6-phosphatase and glycogen phosphorylase in fetal rat liver. Horm Metab Res 11:444–448, 1979.

39. Goodman HM, Schwartz J: Growth hormone and lipid metabolism. *In* Knobil E, Sawyer WH (eds): Handbook of Physiology, vol 4. Washington, DC, American Physiological Society, 1974, pp 211–232.

40. Pandian MR, Gupta SL, Talwar GP: Studies on the early interactions of growth hormone: Effect in vitro on lipogenesis in adipose tissue. Endocrinology 88:928–936, 1971.

41. de Bodo R, Altszuler N: The metabolic effects of growth hormone and their physiological significance. Vitam Horm 15:206–211, 1957.

42. Altszuler N, Steele R, Rathgeb I, et al: Influence of growth hormone on glucose metabolism and plasma insulin levels in the dog. *In* Pecile A, Muller EE (eds): Growth Hormone, Proceedings of the First International Symposium. Amsterdam, Excerpta Medica Int Congress Ser 158, 1968, pp 309–315.

43. Fain JN, Kovacev VP, Scow RO: Effect of growth hormone and dexamethasone on lipolysis and metabolism in isolated fat cells of the rat. J Biol Chem 240:3522–3529, 1965.

44. Goodman HM, Grichting G: Growth hormone and lipolysis: A reevaluation. Endocrinology 113:1697–1702, 1983.

45. Goodman HM, Grichting G: Growth hormone action on adipocytes. *In* Raiti S, Tolman RH (eds): Human Growth Hormone. New York, Plenum, 1986, pp 499–512.

46. Hollobaugh SL, Tzagournis M, Folk RL, et al: The diabetogenic action of human growth hormone: Glucose–fatty acid interrelationships. Metabolism 17:485–491, 1968.

47. Altszuler N, Steele R, Rathgeb I, et al: Glucose metabolism and plasma insulin level during epinephrine infusion in the dog. Am J Physiol 212:677–682, 1967.

48. Fraser R, Joplin JF, Opie M, et al: The augmented insulin tolerance test for detecting insulin resistance. J Endocrinol 25:299–303, 1962.

49. MacGorman LR, Rizza RA, Gerich JE: Physiological concentrations of growth hormone exert insulin-like and insulin antagonistic effects on both hepatic and extrahepatic tissues in man. J Clin Endocrinol Metab 53:556–559, 1981.

50. Maloff BL, Levine JH, Lockwood DH: Direct effects of growth hormone on insulin action in rat adipose tissue maintained in vitro. Endocrinology 107:538–544, 1980.

51. Smal J, Closset J, Hennen G, et al: The receptor binding properties of the 20K variant of human growth hormone explain its discrepant insulin-like and growth promoting activities. Biochem Biophys Res Commun 134:159–165, 1986.

52. Sigel MB, Thorpe NA, Kobrin MS, et al: Binding characteristics of a biologically active variant of human growth hormone (20K) to growth hormone and lactogen receptors. Endocrinology 108:1600–1603, 1981.

53. Kostyo JL: The multivalent nature of growth hormone. *In* Raiti S, Tolman RH (eds): Human Growth Hormone. New York, Plenum, 1986, pp 449–454.

54. Armstrong JM, Bornstein J, Bromley JO, et al: Parallel insulin-like actions of human growth hormone and its part sequence hGH 7–13. Acta Endocrinol (Copenh) 102:492–498, 1983.

55. Ng FM, Bornstein J, Welker C, et al: Insulin potentiating action of synthetic peptides relating to the amino terminal sequence of human growth hormone. Diabetes 23:943–949, 1974.

56. Ng FM, Bornstein J: Insulin-potentiating action of a synthetic amino-terminal fragment of human growth hormone (hGH 1–15) in streptozotocin-diabetic rats. Diabetes 28:1126–1130, 1979.

57. Ng FM, Harcourt JA: Stimulation of 2-deoxyglucose uptake in rat adipocytes by a human growth hormone fragment (hGH 4–15). Diabetologia 29:882–887, 1986.

58. Wade JD, Ng FM, Bornstein J, et al: Effect of C-terminal chain shortening on the insulin-antagonistic activity of human growth hormone 177–191. Acta Endocrinol (Copenh) 101:10–14, 1982.

59. Greenspan FS, Li CH, Simpson ME, et al: Bioassay of hypophyseal growth hormone: The tibia test. Endocrinology 45:455–463, 1949.

60. Davidson MB: Effect of growth hormone on carbohydrate and lipid metabolism. Endocr Rev 8:115–131, 1987.

61. Palmiter RD, Brinster RL, Hammer RE, et al: Dramatic growth of mice that develop from eggs microinjected with metallothionein-growth hormone fusion genes. Nature 300:611–615, 1982.

62. Chen WY, Wight DC, Wagner TE, et al: Expression of a mutated bovine growth hormone gene suppresses growth of transgenic mice. Proc Natl Acad Sci U S A 87:5061–5065, 1990.

63. Chen WY, Wight DC, Mehta BV, et al: Glycine 119 of bovine growth hormone is critical for growth-promoting activity. Mol Endocrinol 5:1845–1852, 1991.

64. Chen WY, White ME, Wagner TE, et al: Functional antagonism between endogenous mouse growth hormone (GH) and a GH analog results in dwarf transgenic mice. Endocrinology 129:1402–1408, 1991.

65. Chen WY, Wight DC, Chen NY, et al: Mutations in the third alpha-helix of bovine growth hormone dramatically affect its intracellular distribution in vitro and growth enhancement in transgenic mice. J Biol Chem 266:2252–2258, 1991.

66. Chen WY, Chen N, Yun J, et al: In vitro and in vivo studies of the antagonistic effects of human growth hormone analogs. J Biol Chem 269:20806, 1994.

67. Chen WY, Chen NY, Yun J, et al: Amino acid residues in the third alpha-helix of growth hormone involved in growth promoting activity. Mol Endocrinol 9:292–302, 1995.

68. Chen XZ, Shafer AW, Yun JS, et al: Conversion of bovine growth hormone cysteine residues to serine affects secretion by cultured cells and growth rates in transgenic mice. Mol Endocrinol 6:598–606, 1992.

69. Strobl JS, Thomas MJ: Human growth hormone. Pharmacol Rev 46:1–34, 1994.

70. Green H, Morikawa M, Nixon T: A dual effector theory of growth-hormone action. Differentiation 29:195–198, 1985.

71. Baumann G: Growth hormone binding proteins and various forms of growth hormone: Implications for measurements. Acta Paediatr Scand Suppl 370:72–80, 1990.

72. Kostyo JL: The search for the active core of pituitary growth hormone. Metabolism 23:885–899, 1974.

73. Nicoll CS, Mayer GL, Russell SM: Structural features of prolactins and growth hormones that can be related to their biological properties [published erratum appears in Endocr Rev 1987 Feb;8(1):43]. Endocr Rev 7:169–203, 1986.

74. Goffin V, Martial JA, Summers NL: Use of a model to understand prolactin and growth hormone specificities. Protein Eng 8:1215–1231, 1995.

75. Goffin V, Shiverick KT, Kelly PA, et al: Sequence-function relationships within the expanding family of prolactin, growth hormone, placental lactogen, and related proteins in mammals. Endocr Rev 17:385–410, 1996.

76. Li CH, Graf L: Human pituitary growth hormone: Isolation and properties of two biologically active fragments from plasmin digests. Proc Natl Acad Sci U S A 71:1197–1201, 1974.

77. Li CH, Bewley TA: Human pituitary growth hormone: Restoration of full biological activity by noncovalent interaction of two fragments of the hormone. Proc Natl Acad Sci U S A 73:1476–1479, 1976.

78. Nicoll CS: Bio-assay of prolactin. Analysis of the pigeon crop-sac response to local prolactin injection by an objective and quantitative method. Endocrinology 80:641–655, 1967.

79. Sonenberg M, Kikutani M, Free CA, et al: Chemical and biological characterization of clinically active tryptic digests of bovine growth hormone. Ann N Y Acad Sci 148:532–558, 1968.

80. Yamasaki N, Shimanaka J, Sonenberg M: Studies on the common active site of growth hormone. Revision of the amino acid sequence of an active fragment of bovine growth hormone. J Biol Chem 250:2510–2514, 1975.

81. Levine LS, Sonenberg M, New MI: Metabolic effects in children of a 37 amino acid fragment of bovine growth hormone. J Clin Endocrinol Metab 37:607–615, 1973.

82. Chou PY, Fasman GD: Prediction of protein conformation. Biochemistry 13:222–245, 1974.

83. Garnier J, Osguthorpe DJ, Robson B: Analysis of the accuracy and implications of simple methods for predicting the secondary structure of globular proteins. J Mol Biol 120:97–120, 1978.

84. Hara K, Hsu Chen CJ, Sonenberg M: Recombination of the biologically active peptides from a tryptic digest of bovine growth hormone. Biochemistry 17:550–556, 1978.

85. Wade JD, Pullin CO, Ng FM, et al: The synthesis and hyperglycaemic activity of the amino acid sequence 172–191 of human growth hormone. Biochem Biophys Res Commun 78:827–832, 1977.

86. Frigeri LG, Peterson SM, Lewis UJ: The 20,000-dalton structural variant of human growth hormone: Lack of some early insulin-like effects. Biochem Biophys Res Commun 91:778–782, 1979.

87. Shaar CJ, Grinnan EL, Short WG, et al: Hyperglycemic activity in dogs of recombinant DNA–derived 20,000 dalton variant of methionyl human growth hormone. Endocr Res 12:21–35, 1986.

88. Salem MA: Effects of the amino-terminal portion of human growth hormone on glucose clearance and metabolism in normal, diabetic, hypophysectomized, and diabetic-hypophysectomized rats. Endocrinology 123:1565–1576, 1988.

89. Towns R, Kostyo JL, Vogel T, et al: Evidence that the N-terminus of human growth hormone is involved in expression of its growth promoting, diabetogenic, and insulin-like activities. Endocrinology 130:1225–1230, 1992.

90. Stewart TA, Clift S, Pitts-Meek S, et al: An evaluation of the functions of the 22-kilodalton (kDa), the 20-kDa, and the N-terminal polypeptide forms of human growth hormone using transgenic mice. Endocrinology 130:405–414, 1992.

91. Paladini AC, Pena C, Parks E: Molecular biology of growth hormone. CRC Crit Rev Biochem 15:25–56, 1984.

92. Abdel-Meguid SS, Shieh HS, Smith WW, et al: Three-dimensional structure of a genetically engineered variant of porcine growth hormone. Proc Natl Acad Sci U S A 84:6434–6437, 1987.

93. Graf L, Li CH, Bewley TA: Selective reduction and alkylation of the COOH-terminal disulfide bridge in bovine growth hormone. Int J Pept Protein Res 7:467–473, 1975.

94. Doneen BA, Bewley TA, Li CH: Studies on prolactin. Selective reduction of the disulfide bonds of the ovine hormone. Biochemistry 18:4851–4860, 1979.

95. Dixon JS, Li CH: Retention of the biological potency of human pituitary growth hormone after reduction and carbamidomethylation. Science 154:785–786, 1966.

96. Campbell RM, Kostyo JL, Scanes CG: Lipolytic and antilipolytic effects of human growth hormone, its 20-kilodalton variant, a reduced and carboxymethylated derivative, and human placental lactogen on chicken adipose tissue in vitro. Proc Soc Exp Biol Med 193:269–273, 1990.

97. Necessary PC, Andersen TT, Ebner KE: Activity of alkylated prolactin and human growth hormone in receptor and cell assays. Mol Cell Endocrinol 39:247–254, 1985.

98. Nutting DF, Kostyo JL, Mills JB, et al: A cyanogen bromide fragment of reduced and S-aminoethylated porcine growth hormone with anabolic activity. Biochim Biophys Acta 200:601–604, 1970.

99. Tokunaga T, Tanaka T, Ikehara M, et al: Synthesis and expression of a human growth hormone (somatotropin) gene mutated to change cysteine-165 to alanine. Eur J Biochem 153:445–449, 1985.

100. Cunningham BC, Jhurani P, Ng P, et al: Receptor and antibody epitopes in human growth hormone identified by homolog-scanning mutagenesis. Science 243:1330–1336, 1989.

101. Cunningham BC, Wells JA: High-resolution epitope mapping of hGH-receptor interactions by alanine-scanning mutagenesis. Science 244:1081–1085, 1989.

102. Cunningham BC, Bass S, Fuh G, et al: Zinc mediation of the binding of human growth hormone to the human prolactin receptor. Science 250:1709–1712, 1990.

103. Hara K, Sonenberg M: Polyalanylation of bovine somatotropin peptide 96–133. Biochim Biophys Acta 492:95–101, 1977.
104. Yamasaki N, Kangawa K, Kobayashi S, et al: Amino acid sequence of a biologically active fragment of bovine growth hormone. J Biol Chem 247:3874–3880, 1972.
105. Aston R, Ivanyi J: Antigenic, receptor-binding and mitogenic activity of proteolytic fragments of human growth hormone. EMBO J 2:493–497, 1983.
106. Blanc JP, Taylor JW, Miller RJ, et al: Examination of the requirement for an amphiphilic helical structure in beta-endorphin through the design, synthesis, and study of model peptides. J Biol Chem 258:8277–8284, 1983.
107. Blanc JP, Kaiser ET: Biological and physical properties of a beta-endorphin analog containing only D-amino acids in the amphiphilic helical segment 13–31. J Biol Chem 259:9549–9556, 1984.
108. Edmundson AB: Amino-acid sequence of sperm whale myoglobin. Nature 205:883–887, 1965.
109. Kaiser ET, Kezdy FJ: Amphiphilic secondary structure: Design of peptide hormones. Science 223:249–255, 1984.
110. Moe GR, Kaiser ET: Design, synthesis, and characterization of a model peptide having potent calcitonin-like biological activity: Implications for calcitonin structure/activity. Biochemistry 24:1971–1976, 1985.
111. Moe GR, Miller RJ, Kaiser ET: Design of a peptide hormone: Synthesis and characterization of a model peptide with calcitonin-like activity. J Am Chem Soc 105:4100–4102, 1983.
112. Stanojevic D, Verdine GL: Deconstruction of GCN4/GCRE into a monomeric peptide-DNA complex. Nat Struct Biol 2:450–457, 1995.
113. Tou JS, Kaempfe LA, Vineyard BD, et al: Amphiphilic growth hormone releasing factor (GRF) analogs: Peptide design and biological activity in vivo. Biochem Biophys Res Commun 139:763–770, 1986.
114. Xing H, Shapiro DJ: An estrogen receptor mutant exhibiting hormone-independent transactivation and enhanced affinity for the estrogen response element. J Biol Chem 268:23227–23233, 1993.
115. Okada S, Chen WY, Wiehl P, et al: A growth hormone (GH) analog can antagonize the ability of native GH to promote differentiation of 3T3-F442A preadipocytes and stimulate insulin-like and lipolytic activities in primary rat adipocytes. Endocrinology 130:2284–2290, 1992.
116. Okada S, Kopchick JJ: Effects of growth hormone antagonist (hGH-G120R) on 3T3-F442A adipocytes, vol 55. The American Diabetes Association, 1995, pp 135A.
117. Chen NY, Chen WY, Bellush L, et al: Effects of streptozotocin treatment in growth hormone (GH) and GH antagonist transgenic mice. Endocrinology 136:660–667, 1995.
118. Takahashi Y, Kaji H, Okimura Y, et al: Brief report: Short stature caused by a mutant growth hormone [published erratum appears in N Engl J Med 1996 May 2;334(18):1207]. N Engl J Med 334:432–436, 1996.
119. Chihara K, Takahashi Y, Kaji H, et al: Short stature caused by a natural growth hormone antagonist. Horm Res 49:41–45, 1998.
120. Dattani MT, Hindmarsh PC, Brook CG, et al: G120R, a human growth hormone antagonist, shows zinc-dependent agonist and antagonist activity on Nb2 cells. J Biol Chem 270:9222–9226, 1995.
121. Fuh G, Cunningham BC, Fukunaga R, et al: Rational design of potent antagonists to the human growth hormone receptor. Science 256:1677–1680, 1992.
122. Yang CW, Striker LJ, Kopchick JJ, et al: Glomerulosclerosis in mice transgenic for native or mutated bovine growth hormone gene. Kidney Int Suppl 39:90–94, 1993.
123. Yang CW, Striker LJ, Pesce C, et al: Glomerulosclerosis and body growth are mediated by different portions of bovine growth hormone. Studies in transgenic mice. Lab Invest 68:62–70, 1993.
124. Foley ED, Aiello LP, Pierce EA, et al: The effect of growth hormone on a mouse model of proliferative retinopathy (abstract). Invest Ophthalmol Vis Sci 36(suppl):1047, 1995.
125. Smith LE, Kopchick JJ, Chen W, et al: Essential role of growth hormone in ischemia-induced retinal neovascularization. Science 276:1706–1709, 1997.
126. Yang CW, Striker GE, Chen WY, et al: Differential expression of glomerular extracellular matrix and growth factor mRNA in rapid and slowly progressive glomerulosclerosis: Studies in mice transgenic for native or mutated growth hormone. Lab Invest 76:467–476, 1997.
127. Chen NY, Chen WY, Kopchick JJ: Liver and kidney growth hormone (GH) receptors are regulated differently in diabetic GH and GH antagonist transgenic mice. Endocrinology 138:1988–1994, 1997.
128. Chen NY, Chen WY, Striker LJ, et al: Co-expression of bovine growth hormone (GH) and human GH antagonist genes in transgenic mice. Endocrinology 138:851–854, 1997.
129. Chen WY, Zhao GH, Gu Y, et al: Pharmacokinetic & pharmacodynamic studies of human growth hormone antagonist G120K-PEG in mice, vol 10. San Francisco, International Congress of Endocrinology, 1996, pp 275.
130. Allen TM, Hansen C, Martin F, et al: Liposomes containing synthetic lipid derivatives of poly(ethylene glycol) show prolonged circulation half-lives in vivo. Biochim Biophys Acta 1066:29–36, 1991.
131. Inoue H, Kadoya T, Kabaya K, et al: A highly enhanced thrombopoietic activity by monomethoxy polyethylene glycol–modified recombinant human interleukin-6. J Lab Clin Med 124:529–536, 1994.
132. Klibanov AL, Maruyama K, Beckerleg AM, et al: Activity of amphipathic poly(ethylene glycol) 5000 to prolong the circulation time of liposomes depends on the liposome size and is unfavorable for immunoliposome binding to target. Biochim Biophys Acta 1062:142–148, 1991.
133. Tsutsumi Y, Kihira T, Tsunoda S, et al: Intravenous administration of polyethylene glycol–modified tumor necrosis factor-alpha completely regressed solid tumor in Meth-A murine sarcoma model. Jpn J Cancer Res 85:1185–1188, 1994.
134. Yamaoka T, Tabata Y, Ikada Y: Distribution and tissue uptake of poly(ethylene glycol) with different molecular weights after intravenous administration to mice. J Pharm Sci 83:601–606, 1994.
135. Olson K, Gehant R, Mukku V, et al: Preparation and characterization of poly(ethylene glycol)ylated human growth hormone antagonist. In Harris JM, Zalipsky S (eds): Poly(ethylene Glycol) Chemistry and Biological Applications. Washington, DC, American Chemical Society, 1997, pp 170–181.
136. Flyvbjerg A, Bennet WF, Rasch R, et al: Inhibitory effect of a growth hormone receptor antagonist (G120K-PEG) on renal enlargement, glomerular hypertrophy and urinary albumin excretion in experimental diabetes in mice. Diabetes 48:377–382, 1999.
137. de Vos AM, Ultsch M, Kossiakoff AA: Human growth hormone and extracellular domain of its receptor: Crystal structure of the complex. Science 255:306–312, 1992.
138. Kopchick JJ, Woodley FW: Regulation of growth hormone gene expression. In LeRoith D (ed): Advances in Molecular and Cellular Endocrinology, vol 1. Stamford, CT, JAI Press, 1997, pp 51–82.
139. Goodman HM: Growth hormone and metabolism. In Schreibman MP, Scanes CG, Pang PKT (eds): The Endocrinology of Growth, Development, and Metabolism in Vertebrates. San Diego, CA, Academic, 1993, pp 93–115.
140. Roupas P, Herington AC: Cellular mechanisms in the processing of growth hormone and its receptor. Mol Cell Endocrinol 61:1–12, 1989.
141. Garcia-Aragon J, Lobie PE, Muscat GE, et al: Prenatal expression of the growth hormone (GH) receptor/binding protein in the rat: A role for GH in embryonic and fetal development? Development 114:869–876, 1992.
142. Klempt M, Bingham B, Breier BH, et al: Tissue distribution and ontogeny of growth hormone receptor messenger ribonucleic acid and ligand binding to hepatic tissue in the midgestation sheep fetus. Endocrinology 132:1071–1077, 1993.
143. Barnard R, Thordarson G, Lopez MF, et al: Expression of growth hormone–binding protein with a hydrophilic carboxyl terminus by the mouse placenta: Studies in vivo and in vitro. J Endocrinol 140:125–135, 1994.
144. Hill DJ, Riley SC, Bassett NS, et al: Localization of the growth hormone receptor, identified by immunocytochemistry, in second trimester human fetal tissues and in placenta throughout gestation. J Clin Endocrinol Metab 75:646–650, 1992.
145. Werther GA, Haynes K, Waters MJ: Growth hormone (GH) receptors are expressed on human fetal mesenchymal tissues—identification of messenger ribonucleic acid and GH-binding protein. J Clin Endocrinol Metab 76:1638–1646, 1993.
146. Ohlsson C, Lovstedt K, Holmes PV, et al: Embryonic stem cells express growth hormone receptors: Regulation by retinoic acid. Endocrinology 133:2897–2903, 1993.
147. Zhang CZ, Li H, Young WG, et al: Evidence for a local action of growth hormone in embryonic tooth development in the rat. Growth Factors 14:131–143, 1997.
148. Laron Z, Pertzelan A, Mannheimer S: Genetic pituitary dwarfism with high serum concentration of growth hormone—a new inborn error of metabolism? Isr J Med Sci 2:152–155, 1966.
149. Laron Z, Klinger B, Erster B, et al: Serum GH binding protein activities identifies the heterozygous carriers for Laron type dwarfism. Acta Endocrinol (Copenh) 121:603–608, 1989.
150. Laron Z, Lilos P, Klinger B: Growth curves for Laron syndrome. Arch Dis Child 68:768–770, 1993.
151. Laron Z: Laron syndrome—from description to therapy. Endocrinologist 3:21–28, 1993.
152. Duriez B, Sobrier ML, Duquesnoy P, et al: A naturally occurring growth hormone receptor mutation: In vivo and in vitro evidence for the functional importance of the WS motif common to all members of the cytokine receptor superfamily. Mol Endocrinol 7:806–814, 1993.
153. Huang N, Cogburn LA, Agarwal SK, et al: Overexpression of a truncated growth hormone receptor in the sex-linked dwarf chicken: Evidence for a splice mutation. Mol Endocrinol 7:1391–1398, 1993.
154. Zhou Y, Xu BC, Maheshwari HG, et al: A mammalian model for Laron syndrome produced by targeted disruption of the mouse growth hormone receptor/binding protein gene (the Laron mouse). Proc Natl Acad Sci U S A 94:13215–13220, 1997.
155. Bazan JF: Haemopoietic receptors and helical cytokines. Immunol Today 11:350–354, 1990.
156. Godowski PJ, Leung DW, Meacham LR, et al: Characterization of the human growth hormone receptor gene and demonstration of a partial gene deletion in two patients with Laron-type dwarfism. Proc Natl Acad Sci U S A 86:8083–8087, 1989.
157. Fuh G, Mulkerrin MG, Bass S, et al: The human growth hormone receptor. Secretion from Escherichia coli and disulfide bonding pattern of the extracellular binding domain. J Biol Chem 265:3111–3115, 1990.
158. Kelly PA, Ali S, Rozakis M, et al: The growth hormone/prolactin receptor family. Recent Prog Horm Res 48:123–164, 1993.
159. Waters MJ: The growth hormone receptor. In Kostyo JL, Goodman HM (eds): Handbook of Physiology. New York, Oxford, 1999, pp 397–444.
160. Zhou Y, He L, Kopchick JJ: An exon encoding the mouse growth hormone binding protein (mGHBP) carboxy terminus is located between exon 7 and 8 of the mouse growth hormone receptor gene. Receptor 4:223–227, 1994.
161. Zhou Y, He L, Kopchick JJ: Structural comparison of a portion of the rat and mouse growth hormone receptor/binding protein genes. Gene 177:257–259, 1996.
162. Edens A, Southard JN, Talamantes F: Mouse growth hormone–binding protein and growth hormone receptor transcripts are produced from a single gene by alternative splicing. Endocrinology 135:2802–2805, 1994.
163. Sadeghi H, Wang BS, Lumanglas AL, et al: Identification of the origin of the growth hormone–binding protein in rat serum. Mol Endocrinol 4:1799–1805, 1990.
164. Baumbach WR, Horner DL, Logan JS: The growth hormone–binding protein in rat serum is an alternatively spliced form of the rat growth hormone receptor. Genes Dev 3:1199–1205, 1989.
165. Talamantes F: The structure and regulation of expression of the mouse growth hormone receptor and binding protein. Proc Soc Exp Biol Med 206:254–256, 1994.
166. Frick GP, Tai LR, Baumbach WR, et al: Tissue distribution, turnover, and glycosylation of the long and short growth hormone receptor isoforms in rat tissues. Endocrinology 139:2824–2830, 1998.

167. Bingham B, Oldham ER, Baumbach WR: Regulation of growth hormone receptor and binding protein expression in domestic species. Proc Soc Exp Biol Med 206:195–199, 1994.

168. Oldham ER, Bingham B, Baumbach WR: A functional polyadenylation signal is embedded in the coding region of chicken growth hormone receptor RNA. Mol Endocrinol 7:1379–1390, 1993.

169. Baumann G: Growth hormone binding proteins. *In* Melmed ES (ed): Endocrine Update Book Series. Norwell, MA, Kluwer, 1999.

170. Clackson T, Wells JA: A hot spot of binding energy in a hormone-receptor interface. Science 267:383–386, 1995.

171. Clackson T, Ultsch MH, Wells JA, et al: Structural and functional analysis of the 1:1 growth hormone:receptor complex reveals the molecular basis for receptor affinity. J Mol Biol 277:1111–1128, 1998.

172. Cunningham BC, Ultsch M, De Vos AM, et al: Dimerization of the extracellular domain of the human growth hormone receptor by a single hormone molecule. Science 254:821–825, 1991.

173. Lowman HB, Wells JA: Affinity maturation of human growth hormone by monovalent phage display. J Mol Biol 234:564–578, 1993.

174. Rowlinson SW, Barnard R, Bastiras S, et al: Evidence for involvement of the carboxy terminus of helix 1 of growth hormone in receptor binding: Use of charge reversal mutagenesis to account for calcium dependence of binding and for design of higher affinity analogues. Biochemistry 33:11724–11733, 1994.

175. Rowlinson SW, Barnard R, Bastiras S, et al: A growth hormone agonist produced by targeted mutagenesis at binding site 1. Evidence that site 1 regulates bioactivity. J Biol Chem 270:16833–16839, 1995.

176. Frank SJ, Gilliland G, Van Epps C: Treatment of IM-9 cells with human growth hormone (GH) promotes rapid disulfide linkage of the GH receptor. Endocrinology 135:148–156, 1994.

177. Chen C, Brinkworth R, Waters MJ: The role of receptor dimerization domain residues in growth hormone signaling. J Biol Chem 272:5133–5140, 1997.

178. Rowlinson SW, Behncken SN, Rowland JE, et al: Activation of chimeric and full-length growth hormone receptors by growth hormone receptor monoclonal antibodies. A specific conformational change may be required for full-length receptor signaling. J Biol Chem 273:5307–5314, 1998.

179. Ultsch MH, Somers W, Kossiakoff AA, et al: The crystal structure of affinity-matured human growth hormone at 2 Å resolution. J Mol Biol 236:286–299, 1994.

180. Baumgartner JW, Wells CA, Chen CM, et al: The role of the WSXWS equivalent motif in growth hormone receptor function. J Biol Chem 269:29094–29101, 1994.

181. Somers W, Ultsch M, De Vos AM, et al: The x-ray structure of a growth hormone–prolactin receptor complex. Nature 372:478–481, 1994.

182. Kossiakoff AA, Somers W, Ultsch M, et al: Comparison of the intermediate complexes of human growth hormone bound to the human growth hormone and prolactin receptors. Protein Sci 3:1697–1705, 1994.

183. Rozakis-Adcock M, Kelly PA: Identification of ligand binding determinants of the prolactin receptor. J Biol Chem 267:7428–7433, 1992.

184. Takahashi Y, Shirono H, Arisaka O, et al: Biologically inactive growth hormone caused by an amino acid substitution. J Clin Invest 100:1159–1165, 1997.

185. Argetsinger LS, Carter-Su C: Mechanism of signaling by growth hormone receptor. Physiol Rev 76:1089–1107, 1996.

186. Cataldo LA, Kopchick JJ: Characterization of growth hormone mediated signal transduction in mouse liver, vol 80. New Orleans, The Endocrine Society, 1998, pp 143.

187. Chow JC, Ling PR, Qu Z, et al: Growth hormone stimulates tyrosine phosphorylation of JAK2 and STAT5, but not insulin receptor substrate-1 or SHC proteins in liver and skeletal muscle of normal rats in vivo. Endocrinology 137:2880–2886, 1996.

188. Thirone ACP, Carvalho CRO, Saad MJA: Growth hormone stimulates the tyrosine kinase activity of JAK2 and induces tyrosine phosphorylation of insulin receptor substrates and shc in rat tissues. Endocrinology 140:55–62, 1999.

189. Carter-Su C, Schwartz J, Smit LS: Molecular mechanism of growth hormone action. Annu Rev Physiol 58:187–207, 1996.

190. Ihle JN, Witthuhn BA, Quelle FW, et al: Signaling by the cytokine receptor superfamily: JAKs and STATs. Trends Biochem Sci 19:222–227, 1994.

191. Kopchick JJ, Bellush LL, Coschigano KT: Transgenic models of growth hormone action. Annu Rev Nutr 19:437–461, 1999.

192. Carter-Su C, Stubbart JR, Wang XY, et al: Phosphorylation of highly purified growth hormone receptors by a growth hormone receptor–associated tyrosine kinase. J Biol Chem 264:18654–18661, 1989.

193. Campbell GS, Christian LJ, Carter-Su C: Evidence for involvement of the growth hormone receptor–associated tyrosine kinase in actions of growth hormone. J Biol Chem 268:7427–7434, 1993.

194. Wang X, Uhler MD, Billestrup N, et al: Evidence for association of the cloned liver growth hormone receptor with a tyrosine kinase. J Biol Chem 267:17390–17396, 1992.

195. Wang X, Moller C, Norstedt G, et al: Growth hormone–promoted tyrosyl phosphorylation of a 121-kDa growth hormone receptor–associated protein. J Biol Chem 268:3573–3579, 1993.

196. Argetsinger LS, Campbell GS, Yang X, et al: Identification of JAK2 as a growth hormone receptor–associated tyrosine kinase. Cell 74:237–244, 1993.

197. Carter-Su C, Argetsinger LS, Campbell GS, et al: The identification of JAK2 tyrosine kinase as a signaling molecule for growth hormone. Proc Soc Exp Biol Med 206:210–215, 1994.

198. Smit LS, Meyer DJ, Billestrup N, et al: The role of the growth hormone (GH) receptor and JAK1 and JAK2 kinases in the activation of Stats 1, 3, and 5 by GH. Mol Endocrinol 10:519–533, 1996.

199. Johnston JA, Kawamura M, Kirken RA, et al: Phosphorylation and activation of the Jak-3 Janus kinase in response to interleukin-2. Nature 370:151–153, 1994.

200. Argetsinger LS, Carter-Su C: Growth hormone signalling mechanisms: Involvement of the tyrosine kinase JAK2. Horm Res 45:22–24, 1996.

201. VanderKuur JA, Wang X, Zhang L, et al: Domains of the growth hormone receptor required for association and activation of JAK2 tyrosine kinase. J Biol Chem 269:21709–21717, 1994.

202. Frank SJ, Gilliland G, Kraft AS, et al: Interaction of the growth hormone receptor cytoplasmic domain with the JAK2 tyrosine kinase. Endocrinology 135:2228–2239, 1994.

203. Dinerstein H, Lago F, Goujon L, et al: The proline-rich region of the GH receptor is essential for JAK2 phosphorylation, activation of cell proliferation, and gene transcription. Mol Endocrinol 9:1701–1707, 1995.

204. Wang YD, Wood WI: Amino acids of the human growth hormone receptor that are required for proliferation and Jak-STAT signaling. Mol Endocrinol 9:303–311, 1995.

205. Wang X, Darus CJ, Xu BC, et al: Identification of growth hormone receptor (GHR) tyrosine residues required for GHR phosphorylation and JAK2 and STAT5 activation. Mol Endocrinol 10:1249–1260, 1996.

206. VanderKuur JA, Wang X, Zhang L, et al: Growth hormone–dependent phosphorylation of tyrosine 333 and/or 338 of the growth hormone receptor. J Biol Chem 270:21738–21744, 1995.

207. Schindler C, Darnell JE Jr: Transcriptional responses to polypeptide ligands: The JAK-STAT pathway. Annu Rev Biochem 64:621–651, 1995.

208. Gronowski AM, Rotwein P: Rapid changes in nuclear protein tyrosine phosphorylation after growth hormone treatment in vivo. Identification of phosphorylated mitogen-activated protein kinase and STAT91. J Biol Chem 269:7874–7878, 1994.

209. Meyer DJ, Campbell GS, Cochran BH, et al: Growth hormone induces a DNA binding factor related to the interferon-stimulated 91-kDa transcription factor. J Biol Chem 269:4701–4704, 1994.

210. Campbell GS, Meyer DJ, Raz R, et al: Activation of acute phase response factor (APRF)/Stat3 transcription factor by growth hormone. J Biol Chem 270:3974–3979, 1995.

211. Gronowski AM, Zhong Z, Wen Z, et al: In vivo growth hormone treatment rapidly stimulates the tyrosine phosphorylation and activation of Stat3. Mol Endocrinol 9:171–177, 1995.

212. Gouilleux F, Pallard C, Dusanter-Fourt I, et al: Prolactin, growth hormone, erythropoietin and granulocyte-macrophage colony stimulating factor induce MGF-Stat5 DNA binding activity. EMBO J 14:2005–2013, 1995.

213. Xu BC, Wang X, Darus CJ, et al: Growth hormone promotes the association of transcription factor STAT5 with the growth hormone receptor. J Biol Chem 271:19768–19773, 1996.

214. Sotiropoulos A, Moutoussamy S, Renaudie F, et al: Differential activation of Stat3 and Stat5 by distinct regions of the growth hormone receptor. Mol Endocrinol 10:998–1009, 1996.

215. Meyer DJ, Stephenson EW, Johnson L, et al: The serum response element can mediate induction of c-fos by growth hormone. Proc Natl Acad Sci U S A 90:6721–6725, 1993.

216. Wood TJ, Sliva D, Lobie PE, et al: Mediation of growth hormone–dependent transcriptional activation by mammary gland factor/Stat 5. J Biol Chem 270:9448–9453, 1995.

217. Chen C, Clarkson RW, Xie Y, et al: Growth hormone and colony-stimulating factor 1 share multiple response elements in the c-fos promoter. Endocrinology 136:4505–4516, 1995.

218. Bergad PL, Shih HM, Towle HC, et al: Growth hormone induction of hepatic serine protease inhibitor 2.1 transcription is mediated by a Stat5-related factor binding synergistically to two gamma-activated sites. J Biol Chem 270:24903–24910, 1995.

219. Anderson NG: Growth hormone activates mitogen-activated protein kinase and S6 kinase and promotes intracellular tyrosine phosphorylation in 3T3-F442A preadipocytes. Biochem J 284:649–652, 1992.

220. Campbell GS, Pang L, Miyasaka T, et al: Stimulation by growth hormone of MAP kinase activity in 3T3-F442A fibroblasts. J Biol Chem 267:6074–6080, 1992.

221. Winston LA, Bertics PJ: Growth hormone stimulates the tyrosine phosphorylation of 42- and 45-kDa ERK-related proteins. J Biol Chem 267:4747–4751, 1992.

222. Moller C, Hansson A, Enberg B, et al: Growth hormone (GH) induction of tyrosine phosphorylation and activation of mitogen-activated protein kinases in cells transfected with rat GH receptor cDNA. J Biol Chem 267:23403–23408, 1992.

223. VanderKuur J, Allevato G, Billestrup N, et al: Growth hormone–promoted tyrosyl phosphorylation of SHC proteins and SHC association with Grb2. J Biol Chem 270:7587–7593, 1995.

224. Vanderkuur JA, Butch ER, Waters SB, et al: Signaling molecules involved in coupling growth hormone receptor to mitogen-activated protein kinase activation. Endocrinology 138:4301–4307, 1997.

225. Winston LA, Hunter T: JAK2, Ras, and Raf are required for activation of extracellular signal–regulated kinase/mitogen-activated protein kinase by growth hormone. J Biol Chem 270:30837–30840, 1995.

226. Souza SC, Frick GP, Yip R, et al: Growth hormone stimulates tyrosine phosphorylation of insulin receptor substrate-1. J Biol Chem 269:30085–30088, 1994.

227. Argetsinger LS, Hsu GW, Myers MG Jr, et al: Growth hormone, interferon-gamma, and leukemia inhibitory factor promoted tyrosyl phosphorylation of insulin receptor substrate-1. J Biol Chem 270:14685–14692, 1995.

228. Argetsinger LS, Norstedt G, Billestrup N, et al: Growth hormone, interferon-gamma, and leukemia inhibitory factor utilize insulin receptor substrate-2 in intracellular signaling. J Biol Chem 271:29415–29421, 1996.

229. Rivera VM, Miranti CK, Misra RP, et al: A growth factor–induced kinase phosphorylates the serum response factor at a site that regulates its DNA-binding activity. Mol Cell Biol 13:6260–6273, 1993.

230. Gille H, Kortenjann M, Thomae O, et al: ERK phosphorylation potentiates Elk-1–mediated ternary complex formation and transactivation. EMBO J 14:951–962, 1995.

231. Hill CS, Treisman R: Transcriptional regulation by extracellular signals: Mechanisms and specificity. Cell 80:199–211, 1995.

232. Gong TW, Meyer DJ, Liao J, et al: Regulation of glucose transport and c-fos and

egr-1 expression in cells with mutated or endogenous growth hormone receptors. Endocrinology 139:1863–1871, 1998.

233. Harding PA, Wang XZ, Kopchick JJ: Growth hormone (GH)-induced tyrosine-phosphorylated proteins in cells that express GH receptors. Receptor 5:81–92, 1995.

234. Eriksson H, Ridderstrale M, Tornqvist H: Tyrosine phosphorylation of the growth hormone (GH) receptor and Janus tyrosine kinase-2 is involved in the insulin-like actions of GH in primary rat adipocytes. Endocrinology 136:5093–5101, 1995.

235. Ridderstrale M, Tornqvist H: PI-3-kinase inhibitor Wortmannin blocks the insulin-like effects of growth hormone in isolated rat adipocytes. Biochem Biophys Res Commun 203:306–310, 1994.

236. Ridderstrale M, Degerman E, Tornqvist H: Growth hormone stimulates the tyrosine phosphorylation of the insulin receptor substrate-1 and its association with phosphatidylinositol 3-kinase in primary adipocytes. J Biol Chem 270:3471–3474, 1995.

237. Cheatham B, Vlahos CJ, Cheatham L, et al: Phosphatidylinositol 3-kinase activation is required for insulin stimulation of pp70 S6 kinase, DNA synthesis, and glucose transporter translocation. Mol Cell Biol 14:4902–4911, 1994.

238. Urich M, el Shemerly MY, Besser D, et al: Activation and nuclear translocation of mitogen-activated protein kinases by polyomavirus middle-T or serum depend on phosphatidylinositol 3-kinase. J Biol Chem 270:29286–29292, 1995.

239. Toker A, Meyer M, Reddy KK, et al: Activation of protein kinase C family members by the novel polyphosphoinositides PtdIns-3,4-P2 and PtdIns-3,4,5-P3. J Biol Chem 269:32358–32367, 1994.

240. Smal J, De Meyts P: Role of kinase C in the insulin-like effects of human growth hormone in rat adipocytes. Biochem Biophys Res Commun 147:1232–1240, 1987.

241. Gurland G, Ashcom G, Cochran BH, et al: Rapid events in growth hormone action. Induction of c-fos and c-jun transcription in 3T3-F442A preadipocytes. Endocrinology 127:3187–3195, 1990.

242. Slootweg MC, de Groot RP, Herrmann-Erlee MP, et al: Growth hormone induces expression of c-jun and jun B oncogenes and employs a protein kinase C signal transduction pathway for the induction of c-fos oncogene expression. J Mol Endocrinol 6:179–188, 1991.

243. Gaur S, Yamaguchi H, Goodman HM: Growth hormone increases calcium uptake in rat fat cells by a mechanism dependent on protein kinase C. Am J Physiol 270:C1485–C1492, 1996.

244. Billestrup N, Bouchelouche P, Allevato G, et al: Growth hormone receptor C-terminal domains required for growth hormone–induced intracellular free Ca^{2+} oscillations and gene transcription. Proc Natl Acad Sci U S A 92:2725–2729, 1995.

245. Schwartz Y, Yamaguchi H, Goodman HM: Growth hormone increases intracellular free calcium in rat adipocytes: Correlation with actions on carbohydrate metabolism. Endocrinology 131:772–778, 1992.

246. Rogers SA, Hammerman MR: Growth hormone activates phospholipase C in proximal tubular basolateral membranes from canine kidney. Proc Natl Acad Sci U S A 86:6363–6366, 1989.

247. Catalioto RM, Ailhaud G, Negrel R: Diacylglycerol production induced by growth hormone in Ob1771 preadipocytes arises from phosphatidylcholine breakdown. Biochem Biophys Res Commun 173:840–848, 1990.

248. Okada S, Kopchick JJ: Growth hormone inhibits translocation of protein kinase C-α and -γ stimulated by insulin in 3T3-F422A cells, vol 78. San Francisco, The Endocrine Society, 1996.

249. Harding PA, Wang X, Okada S, et al: Growth hormone (GH) and a GH antagonist promote GH receptor dimerization and internalization. J Biol Chem 271:6708–6712, 1996.

250. Mellado M, Rodriguez-Frade JM, Kremer L, et al: Conformational changes required in the human growth hormone receptor for growth hormone signaling. J Biol Chem 272:9189–9196, 1997.

251. Kopchick J, Chen XZ, Li Y, et al: Differential in vivo activities of bovine growth hormone analogues. Transgenic Res 7:61–71, 1998.

252. Jeoung DI, Allen DL, Guller S, et al: Mitogenic and receptor activities of human growth hormone 108–129 [published erratum appears in J Biol Chem 1995 Nov 3;270(44):26721]. J Biol Chem 268:22520–22524, 1993.

253. Lewis UJ, Lewis LJ, Salem MA, et al: A recombinant-DNA–derived modification of human growth hormone (hGH44-191) with enhanced diabetogenic activity. Mol Cell Endocrinol 78:45–54, 1991.

254. Nixon T, Green H: Contribution of growth hormone to the adipogenic activity of serum. Endocrinology 114:527–532, 1984.

255. Silverman MS, Mynarcik DC, Corin RE, et al: Antagonism by growth hormone of insulin-sensitive hexose transport in 3T3-F442A adipocytes. Endocrinology 125:2600–2604, 1989.

256. Staten NR, Byatt JC, Krivi GG: Ligand-specific dimerization of the extracellular domain of the bovine growth hormone receptor. J Biol Chem 268:18467–18473, 1993.

257. Campbell RM, Chen WY, Wiehl P, et al: A growth hormone (GH) analog that antagonizes the lipolytic effect but retains full insulin-like (antilipolytic) activity of GH. Proc Soc Exp Biol Med 203:311–316, 1993.

258. Doi T, Striker LJ, Quaife C, et al: Progressive glomerulosclerosis develops in transgenic mice chronically expressing growth hormone and growth hormone releasing factor but not in those expressing insulinlike growth factor-1. Am J Pathol 131:398–403, 1988.

▲▲▲

Growth Hormone–Releasing Hormone and Growth Hormone Secretagogues: Basic Physiology and Clinical Implications

Bruce D. Gaylinn ▪ Ralf Nass ▪ Andrew A. Toogood
Michael O. Thorner

BASIC PHYSIOLOGY

Growth Hormone–Releasing Hormone

History

Growth hormone–releasing hormone (GHRH), the last of the originally proposed hypophysiotropic factors, was identified structurally in 1982. A generation earlier Reichlin[1, 2] proposed the existence of a GHRH because selective hypothalamic lesions yielded a growth hormone (GH) deficiency state and growth failure. Although many groups attempted to isolate GHRH, success was achieved first by isolation of GHRH from GHRH-producing abdominal tumors rather than from the traditional physiologic source, the hypothalamus. In 1973 it was first reported that extracts of various human tumors enhance GH release.[3] Eight cases of presumed ectopic GHRH-secreting tumors were described,[4–13] and a partial purification of GHRH from an extrapituitary tumor was reported in 1980.[14] In October 1980 we studied in Charlottesville, Virginia, a patient with acromegaly and Turner's syndrome. Her acromegaly was due to somatotroph hyperplasia rather than a pituitary adenoma,[15] a diagnosis that became evident after her acromegaly persisted despite transsphenoidal surgery. Therefore, we sought a source for ectopic GHRH secretion and found a 5-cm tumor in the tail of the pancreas. It was from this tumor that two different teams isolated a 40–amino acid peptide, GHRH(1–40)-OH, then designated growth hormone–releasing factor (GH-RF).[16–18] Simultaneously, the Guillemin laboratory sequenced three GHRH peptides from a tumor obtained in Lyon, France: GHRH(1–44)-NH$_2$, GHRH(1–40)-OH, and GHRH(1–37)-OH.[19, 20] The amino acid sequences were identical for all three factors, with varying C-terminal extensions indicating the possibility of processing prior to release. The full biologic activity resided in residues 1 to 29,[21] and the sequence demonstrated that this was a member of the glucagon-secretin family of peptides. There were no disulfide bonds and no evidence of glycosylation of this peptide factor. These GHRHs eventually fulfilled the requirements of a hypophysiotropic GHRH. This chapter provides a limited summary of basic and clinical GHRH research.

Molecular and Cellular Biology

GHRH is a peptide hormone produced predominantly by neurons in the arcuate nucleus of the hypothalamus. These neurons send processes to the median eminence where GHRH is released into the pituitary portal circulation. GHRH then acts to stimulate the pulsatile release of GH from somatotrophs of the anterior pituitary.[22] Both GHRH(1–44)-NH$_2$ and GHRH(1–40)-OH can be found in the human hypothalamus[23–25] and in pituitary tumors of acromegalic patients.[26] GHRH is also produced in other tissues where it may serve autocrine or paracrine roles. GHRH can be made synthetically[17, 27] and recombinantly in *Escherichia coli*.[28] Human GHRH has also been introduced into transgenic mice.[29]

GHRH PEPTIDE. GHRH is a member of a family of homologous peptides that includes secretin, glucagon, glucagon-like peptides (GLP-1, GLP-2), vasoactive intestinal peptide (VIP), pituitary adenylate cyclase–activating peptide (PACAP), PACAP-related peptide (PRP), peptide histidine-methionine (PHM, known as PHI in other species where the C-terminal residue is isoleucine), and glucose-dependent insulinotrophic polypeptide (GIP, also called gastric inhibitory peptide).[30–32] These peptides are thought to have arisen from a common ancestor through a series of gene duplications.[32] They retain sequence and structural similarities and can, to varying extents, interact at each other's receptors.[30]

The GHRH peptide sequence is known for several mammals, and GHRH-like sequences have been found in birds, fish, and even protochordate invertebrates.[33–35] GHRH sequences shown in Table 31–1 demonstrate that the N-terminal (1–29) residues that are required for receptor binding in the human[21] are 62% identical in the mouse (the most divergent known mammal) and less conserved in more distant species. This is in contrast to related peptides like PACAP, VIP, and glucagon, which are 100% identical in many mammals and better than 90% identical in more distant species.[32, 35]

It has been proposed that the active tertiary structure of the GHRH peptide is an amphiphilic α helix that runs from residue 4 onward.[36, 37] This helical structure, with polar and hydrophobic faces, is presumably stabilized when the peptide is bound to its receptor but is not stable in aqueous solution.[38] Circulating GHRH is rapidly inactivated in vivo by dipeptidylaminopeptidase IV (DPP-IV) acting at alanine 2[39] and is also partially inactivated by oxidation at methionine 27.[21]

Medicinal chemists have used the GHRH scaffold to develop peptidic GHRH analogues with increased stability and potency. These efforts have utilized combinations of strategies that include increasing the stability of the α helix with helix-forming residues or ring structures; introducing unnatural amino acids or polyethylene glycol resi-

TABLE 31–1.   Growth Hormone–Releasing Hormone (GHRH) Sequences*

	1	29	44	Identity (%)†
Human	YADAIFTNSYRKVLGQLSARKLLQDIMSR	QQGESNQERGARARL		100
Porcine	YADAIFTNSYRKVLGQLSARKLLQDIMSR	QQGERNQEQGARVRL		100
Bovine‡	YADAIFTNSYRKVLGQLSARKLLQDIM**N**R	QQGERNQEQGAKVRL		97
Ovine	YADAIFTNSYRK**I**LGQLSARKLLQDIM**N**R	QQGERNQEQGAKVRL		93
Hamster	YADAIFT**S**SYRKVLGQLSARKLLQDIMSR	QQGERNQEQGPRVRL		97
Rat	**H**ADAIFT**S**SYR**RI**LGQL**Y**ARKLL**HE**IM**N**R	QQGERNQEQRSRFN		72
Murine	**H**VDAIFT**TNY**RK**LL**SQL**Y**ARK**VI**QDIMNK	Q.GERIQEQRARLS		62
Chicken	**H**ADGIF**SKA**YRK**LL**GQLSARN**YLH**SLMAK	RVGGASSGLGDEAEPLS		55
Carp	**H**ADG**MFNKA**YRK**AL**GQLSARK**YLH**TLMAK	RVGGG.SMIEDDNEPLS		55
Catfish	**H**ADG**LLDRALRDILV**QLSARK**YLH**SLTAV	RVGEE.EEDEEDSEPLS		38
Tunicate	**H**SDGIFTK**DY**RK**Y**LGQL**RAQKFLQ**W**L**MKR			59
Related human peptides				
VIP	**H**SDA**V**FT**DNY**T**RLRKQ**M**AVKKY**LN**S**ILN			31
PACAP	**H**SDGIFTD**SY**S**RYRKQ**M**AVKKY**LAAVLG**K	RYKQRVKNK		31
PHM	**H**AD**GVF**T**SDFS**KLLGQLSA**KKY**LE**S**LM			48
GHRH-RP	**QVDSMWAE**.....**QKQMELESILVALL**..	.QKHSRNSQG		10

*Ellipsis points indicate gap in alignment.
†Identity calculated for residues 1–29 that are required for activity at the GHRH receptor. Residues that differ from the human in the 1–29 region are shown in **boldface.**
‡Bovine and caprine sequences are identical.
VIP, vasoactive intestinal peptide; PACAP, pituitary adenylate cyclase–activating peptide; PHM, peptide-histidine-methionine; GHRH-RP, GHRH-related peptide.

dues to decrease DPP, tryptic, and chymotryptic protease susceptibility and thereby prolong the half-life of the peptide in the circulation and subcutaneous tissues; and replacing the oxidizable methionine.[21, 40–44] Substituting the alanine at position 2 with D-arginine was found to produce GHRH antagonists.[45, 46] More stable, higher-affinity versions of this type of antagonist have recently been developed[47, 48] and may prove useful to block the mitogenic affects of GHRH.[49] While GHRH acts as a low-affinity agonist at the VIP receptor, GHRH analogues such as N-Ac-Tyr[1], D-Phe[2]GHRH(1–29)-NH$_2$ have been developed as VIP antagonists.[50]

GENE AND mRNA. Messenger RNA extracted from human tumors allowed complementary DNA (cDNA) probes to be constructed and the single-copy GHRH gene to be identified on human chromosome 20.[51] The human,[52] rat,[53] and mouse[54] genes span about 10 kb of DNA and include five exons. The third exon encodes the 1–31 sequence which is sufficient for the known biologic activities of GHRH. The human mRNA encodes a 108–amino acid precursor protein, the middle region of which is processed to form the mature GHRH peptide. Brain-, placental-, and gonadal-specific forms of GHRH mRNA are known.[53, 55, 56] These tissue-specific messages initiate at different gene promotors and result in mRNAs of different sizes, but the encoded precursor protein remains identical. Immunologic evidence shows that the C-terminal fragment of the precursor protein is processed into an additional peptide known as GHRH-related peptide (GHRH-RP; see Table 31–1). GHRH-RP is expressed in the human hypothalamus[57] where its role is not known and in rat testis where it is reported to regulate Sertoli cell function.[58] An additional alternatively spliced mRNA found in rat placenta but not hypothalamus encodes the normal GHRH but includes an altered GHRH-RP.[59]

TISSUE DISTRIBUTION. In the human and a number of species GHRH immunoreactivity is present in the basal hypothalamus, appropriate anatomically for release into the pituitary portal vessels.[25, 60–64] GHRH cell bodies directing processes to the median eminence originate from both the perifornical nucleus[63] and the arcuate (rat) or infundibular (human) nucleus.[25, 60, 61, 63] GHRH perikarya are also found in the ventromedial nucleus,[62, 63, 65] a region that can induce increased GH release upon electrical stimulation.[9] There is a reciprocal innervation between GHRH and somatostatin neurons in the rat hypothalamus,[66] providing the potential for direct communication between the major stimulatory and inhibitory neurons governing GH release. This relationship may participate in the ultradian oscillation of hypothalamic GHRH and somatostatin mRNAs.[67] GHRH neurons also directly express somatostatin receptors.[68] A number of other brain regions outside of the hypothalamus contain immunoreactive GHRH.[61–63] The ontogeny of GHRH neurons suggests that they appear in the human fetus between 18 and 29 weeks of gestation[60, 69] and in the rat on embryonic day 18, reaching adult levels by postnatal day 30.[70]

There is much evidence for GHRH outside the central nervous system (CNS) in a number of cell types and tissues in humans and in rodents, but its function outside the GH axis remains to be established. mRNA for GHRH, immunoactive GHRH, or bioactive GHRH content is reported in anterior pituitary,[71] ovary,[72] testis,[56, 73] placenta,[55, 56, 74–76] leukocytes,[77–79] adrenal medulla,[80] pancreas,[81, 82] gastrointestinal tract,[82, 83] and in tumors associated with the GH axis,[26, 71, 84, 85] as well as many other tumor types, including tumors of the human breast, endometrium, and ovary.[86] Ultrasensitive reverse transcriptase–polymerase chain reaction (RT-PCR) techniques can detect trace amounts of GHRH mRNA in most rat tissues examined.[87] Studies in the somatotroph found immunoreactive GHRH in secretory granules and the cell nuclei.[88] Additional data demonstrate somatotroph uptake of labeled GHRH into secretory granules, lysosomes, and the nuclear membrane.[89, 90]

GHRH Signaling

GHRH RECEPTOR. GHRH acts through a high-affinity G protein–coupled receptor (GHRH-R) found in anterior pituitary and coupled to cyclic adenosine monophophate (cAMP) signaling.[91] Upon the molecular cloning of the receptor from human pituitary tumor and rat and mouse pituitary,[92–94] it was found to be a member of the G protein–coupled receptor family B, also called the secretin family. The GHRH-R protein has 47%, 42%, 35%, and 28% sequence identity with receptors for VIP, secretin, calcitonin, and parathyroid hormone, respectively.[92, 93] The isolated cDNAs encoded a 423–amino acid protein that has seven putative transmembrane domains, and a 108-residue N-terminal extracellular domain (after signal peptide cleavage) containing one glycosylation site (Fig. 31–1). The rat and human protein sequences are 82% identical.[92] The GHRH-R sequence predicts 10 extracellular cysteine residues that are also found in secretin, VIP, and PACAP receptors. Eight of these 10 are conserved in nearly all reported members of this receptor family. These cysteine residues are proposed to form sulfhydral cross-links that stabilize an extracellular domain involved in hormone binding.[95]

The cloned pituitary GHRH-R expressed in cell lines demonstrated saturable, high-affinity, GHRH-specific binding and also stimulated the accumulation of intracellular cAMP in response to physiologic concentrations of GHRH.[92–94] Unlike some related receptors that could signal through both cAMP–protein kinase A (PKA) and phospholipase C–inositol triphosphate–protein kinase C (PKC) pathways, only cAMP activation could be detected. Though GHRH was not seen to activate the phospholipase C pathway in somatotroph cells, it does stimulate phospholipid turnover. A specific GHRH antagonist blocked both binding and second messenger responses.

Data from the cloned receptor were consistent with photoaffinity cross-linking studies of GHRH-R in sheep pituitary membranes that revealed high-affinity binding sites with an apparent molecular weight of 55 kDa and one glycosylation site. After deglycosylation and taking into account the mass of the coupled GHRH analogue, the molecular weight of the native ovine receptor protein was estimated at 42 kDa,[96] in agreement with the prediction from the human cDNA sequence of 45 kDa, assuming cleavage of a signal peptide.[93] Further, the binding characteristics of the natural sheep receptor and the cloned human receptor are largely in agreement with a single high-affinity site with a dissociation constant (K_d) of approximately 0.2 nM.

Various radiolabeled forms of GHRH bind to membranes of the pituitary, thymus, and spleen. The dissociation constants estimated in these studies vary wildly from 41 pM[97] to 590 nM.[98] No binding was measurable in three nonfunctional pituitary adenomas, while there was consistent GHRH binding to five acromegalic adenomas, with dissociation constants averaging 0.3 nM.[99]

Studies attempting to delineate the receptor's GHRH binding domains using chimeric receptor constructs[95] or GHRH cross-linking[100] suggest that while the large N-terminal extracellular domain plays a major role in GHRH binding, other domains are also essential for ligand selectivity and binding.

GHRH RECEPTOR mRNA AND GENE. Two GHRH-R mRNA transcripts of approximately 2.5 and 4.0 kb were identified in rat pituitary, 2.0 and 2.1 kb in mouse, and 3.5 kb in ovine pituitary.[92–94] Further, in mouse it has been shown that the receptor is expressed in a spatial and temporal pattern corresponding to GH gene expression.[94] In the mouse, the first evidence of Pit-1 (a pituitary-specific transcription factor) expression occurred at embryonic day 14.5, while transcripts encoding the cloned receptor first appeared on embryonic day 16.5.[94] Mutations that cause a loss of Pit-1 expression, such as in dw/dw mice, lead to a lack of GHRH-R gene expression and somatotroph hypoplasia.[94]

The human GHRH-R gene is divided into 13 exons separated by variably sized introns that spread its length to over 15 kb, the complete sequence of which is known.[101] Fluorescent in situ hybridization localized the gene to human chromosome 7p14–15.[96, 102] Studies of the receptor gene's promoter region found no traditional initiator motifs such as a TATA box.[103, 104] Putative binding sites for several transcription factors including Pit-1, Oct-1, Brn-2, NF-1, cAMP response element (CRE), and estrogen receptor response elements (EREs) were identified. An in vitro reporter system demonstrated that expression was enhanced by Pit-1 and glucocorticoids and inhibited by estrogen.[103] Pit-1 stimulation is consistent with previous studies in Snell and Jackson dwarf mice showing Pit-1 dependence of receptor expression.[94] The glucocorticoid effect on the promoter may be the mechanism for glucocorticoid upregulation of GHRH binding sites[105] and receptor mRNA[106, 107] in rats. The estrogen inhibition of promoter transcription is consistent with the observed sexual dimorphism in receptor mRNA expression.[108] Studies have suggested that GHRH-R expression is upregulated by GHRH itself.[109–111] While a putative CRE that could explain this effect was found in the receptor gene promoter, in vitro regulation of the promoter by forskolin could not be demonstrated.

The structure of the rat GHRH-R gene[112] closely matches that of the human, but includes an additional exon that would predict an alternatively spliced receptor message. This alternative long form encodes 41 additional amino acids in the third intracellular loop. Rat and mouse GHRH-R cDNA clones demonstrate this alternative long form.[92, 94] However, analysis of rat pituitary mRNA by PCR revealed only evidence of the shorter form.[92] Alternative splicing at the homologous site in the PACAP receptor results in functional receptors that differ in their relative signaling through cAMP and phospholipase C second messenger pathways.[113] When the long form of the rat GHRH-R is stably expressed in cell lines, it binds GHRH but no intracellular signaling through any pathway, cAMP or phospholipase C, could be detected.[112]

In mouse there is evidence of alternative splicing encoding a receptor devoid of the first transmembrane domain.[94] Alternatively spliced GHRH mRNA encoding a receptor lacking the last two transmembrane domains has been reported in human pituitary tumors and in normal pituitary.[114] In the rat an alternative splice replacing the last five amino acid residues at the C-terminus with a new 17-residue sequence has been found by PCR.[115] This receptor variant appears to signal cAMP normally. No functional role for any of these alternatively spliced GHRH-R messages has been established, though it is proposed that a truncated receptor variant expressed in tumors can act as a dominant negative in inhibiting GHRH signaling.[116]

GHRH-R mutations resulting in dwarfism have recently been identified in mouse and humans. The first such mutation was found in the *little* mouse. This dwarf strain has an inherited autosomal defect resulting in low levels of GH and pituitary hypoplasia, but is still responsive to exogenous GH. The mutation was mapped by linkage analysis to mouse chromosome 6.[117] Pituitary cells from these mice would not respond to GHRH but could release GH in response to other activators of cAMP, suggesting a receptor defect.[118] After the cloning of the GHRH-R cDNA, two groups localized the mouse gene to the midregion of chromosome 6 and went on to sequence the receptor from the *little* mouse.[119, 120] They found an Asp-to-Gly point mutation at residue 60 of the receptor's extracellular domain. This residue is highly conserved in related receptors and its mutation resulted in a complete loss of cAMP signaling. Further studies demonstrated that the mutant *little* mouse receptor was properly expressed and localized in the cell membrane, but was unable to bind GHRH.[121]

In studies of human dwarfs, a GHRH-R mutation has been identified in three distantly related kindreds from India,[122] Pakistan,[123] and Sri Lanka.[124] These patients all share a recessive mutation mapping to

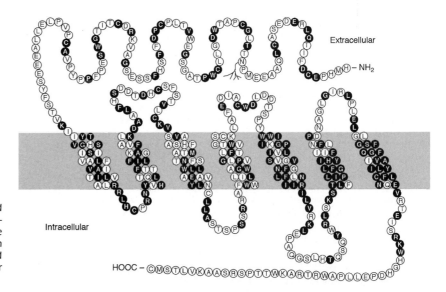

FIGURE 31–1. *Cartoon representation of the deduced sequence of the human pituitary growth hormone–releasing hormone receptor. Shaded amino acids are conserved in closely related receptors. (From Gaylinn BD, Harrison JK, Zysk JR, et al: Molecular cloning and expression of a human anterior pituitary receptor for GHRH. Mol Endocrinol 7:77–84, 1993.)*

chromosome 7p14. A single base pair change encodes a premature stop codon at residue 72 resulting in a severe receptor truncation and loss of all function. Another receptor mutation has been identified in a large Brazilian kindred.[125] In this case the mutation interferes with a splice donor site resulting in the retention of intron 1. The translational reading frame is disrupted at residue 20 within the signal peptide and no part of the mature receptor protein can be made. It is likely that other receptor mutations will be identified in GH-deficient patients and it is possible that activating mutations may be associated with some cases of acromegaly.

INTRACELLULAR SIGNALING. At the somatotroph, GHRH activates many of the classic signaling systems, including cAMP, calmodulin, calcium mobilization, and phospholipid pathways, indicating a significant commitment of the somatotroph to respond to GHRH. As with many secretory cells, GHRH-accelerated GH release requires both calcium[126-130] and calmodulin.[127, 131] Intracellular calcium is elevated within seconds of a GHRH stimulus, both in pituitary cells[132-134] and thymocytes.[135] This calcium response is dependent on influx of extracellular calcium and is not due to the release of intracellular stores.[136] cAMP also signals to the cell nucleus regulating multiple transcription factors to affect gene expression.[137]

cAMP METABOLISM. cAMP analogues and calcium stimulate GHRH release from cultured hypothalamus, while PKC modulates these effectors.[138]

At the somatotroph GHRH stimulates cAMP accumulation and GH release and these responses are blocked by somatostatin.[126-128, 139-149] Glucocorticoid pretreatment enhances both the potency and efficacy of GHRH in driving cAMP accumulation and GH release[150]; this steroid is necessary for GHRH-induced cAMP accumulation after several days in culture. Adenylate cyclase activity in membranes of normal rat pituitary or human acromegalic tumors[151] is enhanced by GHRH in a guanine nucleotide-[131, 152] and calmodulin-sensitive[131] manner. Pertussis toxin enhances GHRH-initiated cAMP accumulation and GH release.[139, 142, 146] The spontaneous reduction in GHRH-stimulated cAMP levels that occurs over time can be blocked by cycloheximide,[139] while the stimulatory ability of GHRH is potentiated by PKC activation.[145, 146, 149, 153] This indicates that another receptor system which stimulates PKC may directly enhance the productivity of the GHRH-R-coupling protein–adenylate cyclase complex,[154, 155] a candidate for which is growth hormone secretagogue (GHS) receptor.[153]

PHOSPHOLIPIDS. GHRH increases phosphatidylinositol labeling[156] as well as free arachidonate levels[157] in the pituitary. Although in most systems no effect of GHRH on polyphosphoinositide hydrolysis is detectable,[158] a report shows that in a specific subclass of porcine somatotrophs (low-density somatotrophs) GHRH stimulates both cAMP and inositol phosphate–dependent second messenger pathways.[159] Other metabolic pathways involving phospholipid metabolism may be activated by or modulate GHRH activity.[133, 144] cAMP metabolism can be dissociated from GH release after GHRH with some phospholipid metabolic enzyme inhibitors, indicating they can act distal to the cAMP system to evoke exocytosis.[144]

MITOGENIC SIGNALING. In vivo, insufficient GHRH signaling during development through a GHRH-R defect[120] or as a result of GHRH antisera administration[160] results in somatotroph hypoplasia. Excess GHRH signaling through tumor expression,[15] Gs mutation,[161] or transgenic overexpression[162] stimulates somatotroph hyperplasia. In vitro, GHRH is a mitogenic signal for somatotroph proliferation.[163] The mitogen-activated protein kinase (MAPK) pathway is a potential mechanism for this action. Recent preliminary evidence demonstrates a dose-dependent GHRH stimulation of the tyrosine phosphorylation of MAPK.[164, 165] The pathways through which GHRH activates MAPK are not established.

GH mRNA AND RELEASE DYNAMICS IN CULTURE. GHRH stimulates the level or transcription rate of GH mRNA,[166, 167] the release of newly synthesized GH[168] and total GH (stored plus released),[169] as well as the proliferation of somatotrophs in vitro.[163] The GHRH effect on the somatotroph varies according to the anatomic location of the somatotroph within the pituitary[170] and the GH-releasing effect is further enhanced by acute administration of glucocorticoids,[27, 150, 171] possibly through increased GHRH binding.[97] Like glucocorticoids, triiodothyronine[171] and GH-releasing peptide (GHRP)[153] can

amplify GHRH-stimulated GH secretion. In contrast, insulin-like growth factor-1 (IGF-I)[27] and somatostatin[147, 171] are noncompetitive inhibitors of GHRH-accelerated GH release in vitro.

Accelerated GH release occurs immediately after exposure to GHRH[139, 141, 172-175] and remains elevated for the duration of the GHRH pulse,[139, 141, 172, 174, 175] albeit at declining rates of release after about 10 minutes.[141, 169, 172, 175-178] This spontaneous decline could occur without GH content depletion[176] and could be blocked by cycloheximide, suggesting the participation of a rapidly turning-over inhibitory protein.[139] The reciprocal interaction of GHRH and somatostatin, suggested neuroanatomically,[66] and in pituitary portal blood measurements,[179, 180] results in a greater mass of GH release per GHRH pulse. This has been demonstrated in perifusion culture.[181]

Picomolar to nanomolar concentrations of GHRH that likely are present in pituitary portal blood[179, 180] regulate a graded GH response from the somatotroph.[17, 20, 27, 140] GHRH also stimulates modest prolactin (PRL) release at low GHRH concentrations in vitro[182, 183] and the secretion of a protein known as peptide 23 (identical to pancreatitis-associated protein and a member of the C-type lectin supergene family).[184, 185] As GHRH can interact with VIP receptors (VIP is a PRL secretagogue) in intestinal epithelium[186] and GH3 cells,[187] it is possible that pharmacologic or pathologic levels of GHRH can activate these and other receptor types.

Animal Studies

GHRH RELEASE. The pulsatile release of GH is influenced by numerous factors, including nutrition, body composition, metabolism, age, sex steroids, adrenal corticoids, thyroid hormones, and renal and hepatic functions.[188] A major common pathway for these factors is through their effects on GHRH release from the hypothalamus through direct actions on GHRH neurons and also through interplay with somatostatin neurons. These effects may be mediated through other factors such as GHSs,[189] catacholamines,[190] interleukin-1,[191] somatostatin,[191] opioids,[190] leptin,[192-194] inhibin,[195] and neuropeptide Y (NPY).[196]

GHRH EFFECTS ON THE GH AXIS. GHRH was first demonstrated to stimulate GH release in vivo using anesthetized rats.[197, 198] These GH responses to GHRH could be enhanced by passive immunization against somatostatin[199-201] or blocked by passive immunization against rat GHRH.[199, 200] It was soon found that GHRH could enhance GH secretion in every vertebrate species tested, including monkey,[202] bovine,[203-206] swine,[207] chicken,[208] and carp.[34]

GHRH is necessary for endogenous pulsatile GH secretion as anti-GHRH antisera treatment eliminated these pulses in rats and sheep.[209, 210] Antisera to GHRH also decreased statural growth[211] and GHRH-R mRNA expression[110] in the rat. Conversely, GHRH administered over several days to weeks enhances body or organ growth and function in experimental animals.[206, 212-214] The effect is particularly striking in mice transgenic for GHRH.[215, 216] Pulses of GHRH are measured in pituitary portal plasma of unanesthetized sheep with peak values of 25 to 40 pg/mL, and a period of 71 minutes.[180] Temporal analysis of GH pulses in these sheep suggested a complex regulation that can only be partially explained by GHRH and somatostatin pulses and suggest the involvement of other factors such as an endogenous ligand corresponding to the synthetic GH secretagogues.[153]

During development basal GH responses to exogenous GHRH decrease from postnatal day 1 to day 28 in the rhesus monkey.[217] Passive immunization against GHRH shows that endogenous GHRH is an active secretagogue up to day 9.[218] In the rat, GHRH injections do not increase GH levels at postnatal day 2,[219] whereas stimulatory responses of similar magnitude to those seen in the rhesus monkey are measured at postnatal days 10, 30, and 75 as well as at 14 months.[220] Likewise, 5 days of GHRH injections elevate GH biosynthesis in rat pituitaries at postnatal day 10.[221] Rat pituitary GHRH-R mRNA expression was highest in early gestation, declined to a nadir at 12 days of age, increased at the onset of sexual maturation, and then declined with aging.[222]

There are significant changes in GHRH status during aging. In the hypothalamus there is a reduction in GHRH gene expression and content,[223] as well as a decrease in GHRH binding to pituitary in 18-

month-old rats.[224] GHRH-R mRNA is correspondingly decreased in 18-month-old rats, but can be brought back toward levels observed in younger animals by treatment with GHRH.[225] Decreased GHRH-R expression may contribute to the diminished pituitary response to GHRH in aged male rats[226–228] and humans.[83, 229]

The GHRH system is also strongly influenced by sex (or gonadal steroids). Hypothalamic GHRH mRNA levels are greater in male than female rats,[230, 231] are reduced by orchiectomy, and increased by testosterone treatment in intact[232] or castrated[233] male rats. Estradiol has no effect on hypothalamic GHRH mRNA.[232, 234] The ability of GHRH to elicit a GH response in vivo varies during the rat estrous cycle,[235] is of greater magnitude in the male than female,[220, 236] and is strongly sex steroid–dependent.[236] Somatotrophs from male rats likewise have a greater cAMP and GH response to GHRH than those from female rats when studied in static[143] or perfusion[236] cultures. Furthermore, the intact and castrate male rat treated with testosterone yields the most GHRH-responsive somatotrophs,[236] as does direct testosterone treatment of cultured somatotrophs.[237] Sex differences can be measured at the level of the single somatotroph using the hemolytic plaque assay[238]; testosterone (administered in vivo) increases secretory capacity and recruits a subpopulation of somatotrophs, while estradiol has the opposite effects.[239] GHRH receptor message levels are dramatically lower in female than in male rats[108] and estrogen acts as the receptor gene to inhibit GHRH-R mRNA expression.[103]

In addition to sex steroid effects, free fatty acids[240] and GH itself[241] reduce the in vivo release of GH in response to GHRH. GH treatment decreases hypothalamic GHRH content in intact rats[231] and after hypophysectomy GHRH levels in the hypothalamus rise,[242] suggesting feedback regulation of GHRH by GH. Thyroxine replacement can restore hypothalamic immunoreactive GHRH levels reduced by thyroidectomy in rats,[243] and both triiodothyronine and cortisol can protect against the reduction in GHRH-stimulated GH release in hypothyroid,[244] or adrenalectomized rats,[245, 246] respectively. Indeed, chronic glucocorticoids in vivo decrease GHRH expression in GHRH neurons of the arcuate nucleus.[247, 248]

Months of excess GHRH exposure in transgenic mice is associated with increased pituitary mass and mammosomatotroph hyperplasia[215, 216] that eventually results in adenoma formation after 12 months.[249, 250] This is reminiscent of the clinical findings in patients with ectopic GHRH secretion. What was surprising was the rapidity of this effect; GHRH infusions were capable of inducing enlargement of the anterior pituitary within days in intact, normal rats.[251] The dose range of this acute effect has yet to be defined, and this observation does not address the potential risks of replacement of GHRH in deficiency states. In pituitary allograph studies in orchiectomized hamsters, exogenous GHRH maintains somatotroph size without affecting the percentage of GH cells.[252]

GHRH EFFECTS ON FUNCTIONS OUTSIDE OF THE GH AXIS. GHRH stimulates gastrin release and epithelial cell proliferation in the digestive tract.[253] It also stimulates insulin, glucagon, and somatostatin secretion from the pancreas.[254–256] In the brain, GHRH coexists with tyrosine hydroxylase[257] and can enhance its activity,[258] as well as that of choline acetyltransferase,[259] while inhibiting thyrotropin-releasing hormone (TRH) secretion from the rat hypothalamus.[260] GHRH influences eating behavior[261–264] and circulating GHRH is increased by feeding in humans.[265] The latter effect is due to release of GHRH from extra-CNS sites. GHRH enhances non–rapid eye movement sleep in rats.[266] GHRH antisera[267] or GHRH antagonist[268] inhibits sleep, and sleep deprivation enhances hypothalamic GHRH mRNA levels.[269, 270] Most of these activities, including the control of GH status, suggest that GHRH predominantly acts as a nutrient-partitioning hormone, to regulate body composition.

Growth Hormone Secretagogues

History

Opiates have been recognized to stimulate GH secretion. The GHS story evolved from the seminal observation by Bowers and colleagues[271] that met-enkephalin analogues, which lacked analgesic ac-

tivity, preserved their GH-releasing activity. Bowers and colleagues developed these GHRPs and the most promising of the initial compounds they developed was GHRP-6, a hexapeptide with two D-amino acids.[272] This compound did not interact with the GHRH-R and in vivo synergized with GHRH.[273, 274] A characteristic of GHSs is that they have rather weak effects on GH stimulation from the pituitary in vitro while they are very efficacious when administered in vivo. This observation, together with the simple structure of the GHRPs, made them attractive molecules to be developed to enhance GH secretion. Thus the pharmaceutical industry became interested and expended major resources to developing peptide and nonpeptide compounds. A remarkable achievement by the Merck group was that they took one of their synthetic compounds, MK-677, as a tool, and succeeded in the expression cloning of the GHS receptor (GHS-R).[275] Thus we now have the structure of the GHS-R prior to the isolation and characterization of the natural ligand for the receptor.[276] In a sense this is a repeat of the opiate peptide story. Opiates have been used since antiquity; our knowledge about the natural compounds that they mimic has only been available for about two decades and the receptors were only cloned more recently (see footnote on p. 411).

Physiology and Molecular Biology

PROPERTIES OF SYNTHETIC PEPTIDE AND PEPTIDOMIMETIC GHS COMPOUNDS. The first GHS developed by Bowers and colleagues was GHRP (Table 31–2), a synthetic peptide derived from met-enkephalin that retained the ability to release GH from somatotrophs in vitro, but had little opioid activity.[271, 277] This compound showed no in vivo activity. Refinement of GHRP resulted in GHRP-6, which has significantly improved stability and potency.[272] GHRP-6 is active both in vitro and in vivo, and has served as the model GHS from which many new compounds have been developed. GHRP-2 (KP 102)[278] is an improved structure with sixfold greater potency in rats. In an effort to extend the in vivo half-life of GHRP-6, the first tryptophan was stabilized by the addition of a methyl group.[279] The resulting compound, known as hexarelin, appears equivalent to GHRP-2 in human studies.[280] GHRP-6, GHRP-2, and hexarelin are generally administered intravenously (IV) or subcutaneously (SC). These peptides can stimulate GH following administration intranasally[281] or orally (PO), although much higher doses are required.

In a pioneering effort to develop an orally active GHS that would be better absorbed, a group at Merck Research Laboratories engineered a nonpeptide benzolactam compound that closely mimicked the structure of GHRP-6.[282] This compound, referred to as MK-751 (L-692,429), was active and well tolerated in humans,[283, 284] but had low bioavailability PO. An alternative spiroindane structure was developed and modified to produce MK-677 (L-163,191) which had significantly improved potency PO and duration of action (>60% bioavailability PO in dogs with 5- to 6-hour half-life).[285] These nonpeptide GHSs were shown to act specifically and through the same mechanism as GHRP-6, being synergistic with GHRH, not blocked by GHRH antagonists, ineffective after saturating GHRP-6, and competing at the cloned GHS-R.[286]

A large number of pharmaceutical companies and research groups

TABLE 31–2. Synthetic Peptide and Peptidomimetic Growth Hormone Secretagogue (GHS) Compounds

Name	Structure	K_i (nM)*	ED_{50} (nM)†
GHRP	Tyr-D-Trp-Gly-Phe-Met-NH$_2$		
GHRP-6	His-D-Trp-Ala-Trp-D-Phe-Lys-NH$_2$	1.9	10
Hexarelin	His-D-Mrp-Ala-Trp-D-Phe-Lys-NH$_2$		
GHRP-2	D-Ala-D-βNal-Ala-Trp-D-Phe-Lys-NH$_2$	0.21	
MK-751	L-692,429 Benzolactam peptidomimetic		60
MK-677	L-163,191 Spiroindoline peptidomimetic	0.1	1.3

*K_i for competing (^{35}S)MK-677 at the cloned GHS receptor.[275]
†ED_{50} in rat pituitary cell growth hormone release assay.[285]
ED_{50}, median effective dose; GHRP, growth hormone–releasing peptide; D-Mrp, 2-methyl-D-tryptophan; D-βNal, β-(2-naphthyl)D-alanine.

are actively developing GHSs, and many new peptide and nonpeptide compounds have been identified. The GHSs discussed here are difficult to compare as they differ in their pharmacokinetics and pharmacodynamics, potency in different assays, and species specificity. Though some compounds are reported to elevate PRL, adrenocorticotropic hormone (ACTH), and cortisol,[280] others may have greater specificity.[287, 288] GHSs are also reported to have specific effects on appetite,[289, 290] sleep,[291] and cardiac function.[292, 293] Different GHSs seem to differ in their relative potencies for these effects, suggesting differing cross-reactivities at unknown receptor subtypes and raising hopes for new compounds tailored specifically for these sites.

GHSs: SITES OF ACTION. Considerable evidence suggests that GHSs act at the level of the hypothalamus as well as at the pituitary.[294–298] The major site of GHS action, however, seems to be at the hypothalamus.[273, 298–300] This hypothalamic action is thought to explain why GHSs are much more effective in vivo than in vitro, and also, the marked synergy that is seen when GHSs and GHRH are given together in vivo. The dominant role of this hypothalamic action is demonstrated by the fact that GHSs are unable to release GH in children and adults with pituitary stalk transection.[301, 302] An alternative explanation is that GHRH is required for GH synthesis and in its absence GHSs are largely ineffective. This is supported by studies in pigs where exogenous GHRH overcomes the effect of stalk transection and allows GHS responses.[303]

GHS RECEPTOR. While no corresponding endogenous factor has yet been identified (see footnote on p. 411), evidence suggests that GHSs act on somatotrophs through a phospholipase C–inositol triphosphate-PKC signaling pathway distinct from the cAMP-PKA pathway activated by GHRH.[304, 305] Studies demonstrated a high-affinity, low-abundance (^{35}S)MK-677 binding site in anterior pituitary and hypothalamus that has the Mg^{2+} and guanosine triphosphate (GTP) dependence characteristic of a G protein–coupled receptor.[306] This allowed MK-677-induced calcium-activated chloride currents in *Xenopus* oocytes to be used as a method for the expression cloning of a GHS-R from swine pituitary mRNA.[275] When this cDNA was used as a probe, two types (Ia and Ib) of receptor cDNA were identified in both swine and human pituitary libraries. The human type Ia cDNA encodes a 366–amino acid seven-transmembrane receptor of the rhodopsin family. This cDNA conferred high affinity (K_d = 0.4 nM), saturable, and specific binding of MK-677 that was competed by both peptide and nonpeptide GHSs. The type Ib GHS-R cDNA represented an alternatively spliced message from the same gene, but encoded only five transmembrane domains and appeared to be nonfunctional.[275]

At the time it was cloned, the GHS-R represented a new branch in the rhodopsin family of the G protein–coupled receptors, with only 35% and 29% identity with the closest known sequences, which were for neurotensin and TRH receptors. More recently, several orphan receptors more closely related to the GHS-R have been cloned,[307, 308] and the one most similar to GHS-R (52% identity) has been identified as a receptor for the gut peptide motilin.[309] This suggests that the endogenous ligand for the GHS-R is a peptide with homology to motilin.

Ribonuclease (RNase) protection assays demonstrated that GHS-R mRNA was a rare message present in low abundance in human pituitary and hippocampus.[275] In the rat brain, in situ hybridization showed GHS-R in the arcuate and ventromedial nuclei of the hypothalamus,[275] two sites thought to be involved in the regulation of GH secretion. Other brain regions not traditionally associated with GH secretion express GHS-R, including the choroid plexus and the hippocampus.[295, 310, 311] This finding suggests a wider role for GHS in the brain, for example, in the control of feeding behavior.[289, 290, 312] In peripheral tissues, very low but detectable levels of GHS-R mRNA are reported in pancreas and renal pelvis.[311, 313]

GHS-R mRNA has also been demonstrated in human pituitary adenomas.[314–316] The highest abundance has been demonstrated in GH-secreting pituitary adenomas of which 100% expressed the receptor message, some at 200-fold the levels of normal pituitary.[314, 315, 317] GHS-R message was also present in some thyroid-stimulating hormone (TSH)–secreting, ACTH-secreting, and gonadotroph adenomas, as well as in prolactinomas.

REGULATION OF GHS RECEPTOR. Because the natural ligand of the GHS-R has not yet been identified, investigation of the regulation of this system has focused on changes in the expression of GHS-R. The few existing studies, using the dw/dw rat model or normal rats[300, 318] to investigate the effects of GH on hypothalamic and pituitary GHS-R expression, suggested that GHS-Rs are involved in feedback regulation of GH. Whether these effects occur directly at the pituitary level or are mediated indirectly through the hypothalamus has yet to be determined. In addition, the expression of the pituitary GHS-R mRNA seems to be sex-dependent, whereas the hypothalamic expression of this receptor showed no significant sex difference.[319] GHRH appears to positively regulate the pituitary GHS-R in rats.[320]

EVIDENCE FOR GHS RECEPTOR SUBTYPES. GHSs are synthetic compounds that appear to be quite specific for stimulating GH release, but do have other actions. To date only one type of GHS-R is well characterized. In examining GHS effects, it is difficult to distinguish possible coincidental effects at unrelated receptors from specific actions at related receptor subtypes. Data suggesting GHS-R subtypes are beginning to accumulate. Binding studies at pituitary and hypothalamic membranes have shown GHS binding sites with different relative affinity for peptidyl and nonpeptidyl GHS. Whereas the non-peptidyl GHS MK-677 binds specifically to the high-affinity site, GHRP-6 binds preferentially to medium- and low-affinity sites.[306, 321, 322] Characterization of high-affinity hexarelin binding and cross-linking sites in pituitary and brain has suggested the existence of different GHS-R subtypes. In these studies, the relative affinities for different GHSs and the molecular size of the cross-linked binding site do not seem to match the properties of the cloned GHS-R.[310, 323] While hexarelin stimulates both GH release and feeding behavior, new hexarelin analogues appear specific for one effect or the other, suggesting that they act at different brain receptors.[290] Hexarelin is also reported to have GH-independent beneficial cardiac effects that persist after hypophysectomy and have been attributed to specific hexarelin binding sites in the heart.[292, 293, 324]

REGULATION OF GH RELEASE. At the pituitary GHSs can directly stimulate the release of GH.[153, 282, 297, 304, 325–327] GHSs cause somatotroph depolarization and raise intracellular Ca^{2+} but use a different receptor and signaling mechanism from GHRH.[328–332] At the level of individual pituitary cells examined with the reverse hemolytic plaque assay, GHSs increased the number of GH-secreting cells without altering the amount of GH released per cell. In contrast, GHRH increased both the amount of GH secreted per cell and the number of GH-secreting cells, while somatostatin predominantly acted to decrease the number of secreting cells; this is the opposite of the effect of GHSs and supports the view that GHSs act as functional antagonists of somatostatin.[328]

It is widely accepted that the synthesis of GH in the pituitary is under the control of GHRH.[167] In the absence of GHRH, GHSs can also stimulate GH synthesis. In rat pups treated with GHRH antiserum from birth, 5-day treatment with hexarelin results in a restoration of pituitary GH mRNA levels to that of controls.[299, 333] Similar findings were made in GHRH-deficient young adult male rats.[333]

At the level of the hypothalamus, the mechanisms underlying GHS stimulation of pituitary GH release are not yet defined. Many data explain GHS actions through indirect effects on the hypothalamus and the involvement of GHRH[334–337] and somatostatin,[330] though other evidence suggests that GHSs increase GH secretion independently of GHRH or somatostatin.[299, 336, 338]

In the hypothalamus a subset of GHRH neurons express GHS-R[339] and GHSs have been shown to enhance the expression of c-*fos* in some GHRH and NPY neurons.[340] But GHSs do not appear to stimulate GHRH release from hypothalamic explants.[341] GHS treatment does decrease hypothalamic somatostatin mRNA levels in the aged rat to levels seen in young controls.[342]

The direct actions of GHSs, together with interactions with GHRH and somatostatin, are proposed by some to be insufficient to explain the observed synergism with GHRH and GHS responses when GHRH action is blocked.[189, 273] This suggests the alternative hypothesis that in addition to the known mechanisms, GHSs can also act to release an unknown hypothalamic factor (U factor) which acts as a potent stimulator of GH release from the pituitary.[273] Such a U factor could explain why the major actions of GHS require an intact hypophysial stalk, but also points out that there is much we do not know about the actions of GHRH.*

CLINICAL IMPLICATIONS

Growth Hormone–Releasing Hormone

Measurement of GHRH Levels

Following the synthesis of GHRH, radioimmunoassays (RIAs) to measure the peptide were developed rapidly and have been utilized to document concentrations of the releasing hormone in tissues and body fluids. Initially it was hoped that GHRH in the peripheral circulation would be principally of hypothalamic origin and its measurement would thus serve as an index of hypothalamic secretion. However, it is clear that most circulating GHRH is not of hypothalamic origin, but instead comes from the gut.[343-346] Further, an RIA would ideally measure intact biologically active hormone. However, GHRH(1–44)-NH_2 has a very short half-life in the circulation of 6.8 minutes and the metabolite GHRH(3–44)-NH_2 appears within 1 minute of an IV injection of GHRH(1–44)-NH_2.[347] GHRH is cleaved by a DPP-IV in the circulation. The biologic activity of GHRH(3–44)-NH_2 is less than 10^{-3} that of GHRH(1–44)-NH_2.[39] Unfortunately, most RIAs measure GHRH(1–44)-NH_2 and GHRH(3–44)-NH_2 with equal efficiency and therefore do not reflect biologic activity in the circulation. Most assays are directed to the midportion of the GHRH molecule and therefore do not distinguish between different circulating forms. Besides the RIA, more sensitive enzyme immunoassays for GHRH measurement have been developed.[348] One of the few indications for measuring serum GHRH is GHRH-producing tumors.

GHRH LEVELS IN ACROMEGALY. There has been intense interest in the frequency of ectopic GHRH as a cause of acromegaly. Two extensive studies have addressed this issue. In a study of 80 patients with acromegaly, 76 had GHRH levels in the normal range.[344] Of the 4 with elevated levels, one was known to harbor a GHRH-secreting tumor. Extensive evaluation of the other 3 failed to determine a source for the GHRH. In a second study, 3 of 177 patients with acromegaly exhibited elevated serum levels of GHRH.[349] In all cases, the GHRH levels were markedly elevated (i.e., in the nanogram per milliliter range), and the patients were previously known to have GHRH-secreting tumors. Thus, although apparently rare, ectopic secretion of GHRH must be considered as a possible cause of acromegaly and measurement of peripheral GHRH seems prudent as a part of the evaluation. Since it is known that the release of ectopic hormones may be intermittent, and since only 300 pg/mL of GHRH is necessary to stimulate GH release in normal subjects, a single normal or modestly elevated GHRH determination may not exclude ectopic GHRH-associated acromegaly.

The subject of GHRH-producing tumors has been previously reviewed.[350, 351] GHRH-producing tumors associated with acromegaly are rare. Unique features of patients with acromegaly harboring tumors secreting GHRH were young age, female preponderance, foregut derivation of the tumors, benign biologic behavior, small secretory granules in the tumor, and frequent association with multiple endocrine neoplasia, type 1 (MEN-1) syndrome. The pancreas and lung are common primary sites. GHRH-containing tumors unassociated with acromegaly include those of gut and thymus, small cell carcinoma of lung, and medullary carcinoma of thyroid. Several tumors are plurihormonal. In contrast to somatotroph adenoma seen in patients with classic acromegaly, the hypophysial lesion represents somatotroph hyperplasia in acromegalic patients with GHRH-producing tumor. This finding indicates that GHRH not only increases somatotroph secretory activity but causes somatotroph proliferation. Studies of GHRH-pro-

ducing tumors are of fundamental importance to obtain insight into endocrine activity of pituitary somatotrophs and the pathogenesis of GH-secreting pituitary adenomas associated with acromegaly; the importance of GHRH in the etiology of acromegaly is still unresolved. Preliminary evidence suggests that the amount of GHRH mRNA expression in somatotroph adenomas is associated with the progression and aggressiveness of these tumors.[85] The GHRH receptor mRNA is specifically expressed in GH-producing adenomas and somatotrophs.[84] To address whether GHRH can produce tumors, transgenic mice expressing the human GHRH gene have been developed. These animals, exposed to excessive quantities of GHRH throughout development and life, developed mammosomatotroph or somatotroph adenomas.[247, 250] The significance of these observations to the human disease is unclear and further studies are needed. Early studies have investigated the beneficial effects of GHRH antagonists in animal and human studies. Treatment of transgenic mice overexpressing the human GHRH gene with GHRH antagonists resulted in suppression of GH and IGF-I secretion.[352] The relationship between GHRH-secreting tumors and MEN-1 syndrome is controversial; further studies are required to elucidate whether they represent two distinct entities or whether GHRH-producing tumors accompanied by acromegaly are only *forme fruste* manifestations of MEN-1 syndrome. Several cases of acromegaly due to ectopic GHRH secretion associated with MEN-1 syndrome have been described.[353-357]

EUTOPIC GHRH SECRETION. Occasionally hypothalamic gangliocytomas may be associated with acromegaly. Immunocytochemical staining of such tumors for GHRH has been described. It has been suggested that these tumors should be considered as an unusual cause of acromegaly.[358] On occasion these tumors are intrasellar; in such cases, the observation that somatotrophs are in close anatomic association with neurons suggests that GHRH not only stimulates GH secretion but may also cause adenoma formation. An intrasellar gangliocytoma with somatotroph adenoma has been described. The gangliocytoma was strongly positive for gastrin and weakly positive for GHRH. Since gastrin administered intracerebroventricularly increases GH secretion, it has been suggested that gastrin release may act in a paracrine fashion on gangliocytoma to enhance GHRH secretion and thus cause somatotroph adenoma.[359-361]

GHRH LEVELS IN GH-DEFICIENT CHILDREN. Many reports concerning serum and cerebrospinal fluid (CSF) concentrations of GHRH in children with various forms of growth deficiency have appeared. Of 22 children with the diagnosis of constitutional short stature (defined as 2 to 3 SD below the predicted mean height for age, peak levels of GH in excess of 10 μg/L during at least one provocation test, and bone age approximating chronologic age), basal GHRH levels (8 to 148 pg/mL) were no different from those noted in normal children.[362] In addition, in 5 of 9 children, GHRH levels rose twofold 15 minutes after administration of levodopa (500 mg PO). In another study of 16 children with idiopathic delayed puberty the peak serum GHRH concentration following levodopa was 41 ± 10 pg/mL and this compared with 96 ± 25 pg/mL in children with constitutional short stature.[363] Similarly, in patients with hypothalamic hypopituitarism there was no increase in circulating GHRH levels after levodopa, which contrasts with responses in normal subjects.[364, 365] These patients with hypothalamic hypopituitarism do respond to exogenous GHRH administration. Insulin-induced hypoglycemia increased circulating GHRH levels in normal subjects, but not in 6 patients with isolated GH deficiency.[366] In 10 children with short stature, GHRH levels increased at 15 minutes after hypoglycemia, from 10 ± 0.5 to 17.1 ± 3.1 pg/mL.[367] There was no increase in GHRH after arginine, even though hypoglycemia alone or arginine alone increased GH concentrations.

However, in contrast to children with constitutional short stature, five children with GH deficiency associated with hypothalamic germinomas were reported to have undetectable concentrations of GHRH in the CSF.[368] In addition, children with idiopathic GH deficiency have GHRH present in the CSF but at concentrations lower than those in normal children (15.1 ± 1.0 vs. 29.3 ± 2.0 pg/mL; mean ± SEM).

GHRH as a Diagnostic Agent

Until 1985 the use of cadaveric GH was strictly controlled and limited to use in children with short stature due to severe GH defi-

---

*Since this chapter was written, ghrelin, an endogenous ligand specific for the GHS receptor, has been identified. See the following article and NCBI GenBank submission for more information about this important discovery: Kojima M, Hosoda H, Date Y, et al: Ghrelin is a growth-hormone–releasing acylated peptide from stomach. Nature 402:656–660, 1999; and Tomasetto CL, Karam SM, Rio MC: GenBank, direct submission, accession number AJZ43503. Washington, DC, National Center for Biotechnology Information (NCBI), 1999.

ciency. Dynamic tests of GH reserve were, therefore, of clinical significance in pediatric endocrinology and were performed primarily for academic interest in adults with hypothalamic-pituitary disease. With the advent of recombinant human GH, now available in unrestricted quantities, and its approval for use in adults with GH deficiency resulting from hypothalamic pituitary disease in the United States, Europe, and Australia, the need to diagnose GH deficiency safely and effectively has become an important issue in adult endocrinology.[369]

Many of the tests used to determine GH status are either hazardous under certain circumstances (the insulin tolerance test [ITT] is contraindicated in the elderly, and in patients with ischemic heart disease or a history of seizures) or associated with unpleasant side effects, (glucagon causes nausea and delayed hypoglycemia, clonidine is associated with drowsiness and hypotension, and arginine causes dizziness and phlebitis). Tests that are effective in children, such as those using arginine or clonidine as the stimulus, are less effective at releasing GH in adults.[370] The ITT is frequently quoted as the gold standard investigation for diagnosing GH deficiency in children and adults, but many endocrinologists shy away from this procedure because of concerns about the effects of hypoglycemia in their patients and because the test has to be supervised for its duration by a physician.

GHRH and the GH-releasing substances (e.g., GHRP-6, GHRP-1, GHRP-2, hexarelin, MK-677) are powerful GHSs that are safe and well tolerated in both adults and children. These agents have attracted increasing attention as stimuli used to determine GH status in both adults and children.

Typically, tests of GH reserve in both children and adults have utilized procedures that depend on effects mediated by the hypothalamus. For example, agents such as arginine, glucagon, clonidine, or levodopa and insulin-induced hypoglycemia are assumed to elicit a hypothalamic signal that acts upon the somatotrophs to stimulate the release of GH. A lesion of the hypothalamus or the pituitary may produce an abnormal GH response to these stimuli. The use of GHRH to stimulate GH release directly from the somatotrophs allows a theoretical distinction to be made between patients with a pituitary abnormality, who will have an abnormal response to GHRH, and those with hypothalamic lesions who may respond normally to GHRH. This may be important when determining the therapeutic strategy for an individual patient.

ADMINISTRATION OF GHRH TO NORMAL SUBJECTS. The effects of GHRH and its analogues given as a bolus have been studied in healthy men, women, and children.[371–381] Following an IV injection of GHRH, GH levels begin to rise within 5 minutes and reach a peak between 30 and 60 minutes. The ability of GHRH to release GH is dose-dependent,[380] the maximal response being observed following a dose of 1 μg/kg or higher.[375] In adults the GH response to GHRH is similar in men and women, although women are more sensitive to GHRH than men; the dose of GHRH required for half-maximal GH secretion is 0.4 μg/kg in men and 0.2 μg/kg in women. The GH response to GHRH in women is not altered by the changes in sex steroid hormones that occur during the menstrual cycle.[379]

The effect of pubertal development on the GH response to GHRH is slight.[382, 383] When 68 prepubertal children were compared with 66 children at various stages of puberty, no overall difference in GH response to GHRH was observed.[382] In a more detailed study that examined children at each stage of puberty, a slight decrease in GH response to GHRH was seen in boys during midpuberty. Although a similar decrease was not observed in girls, the GH response to GHRH did not differ significantly between the sexes during puberty.[383] In prepubertal children being evaluated for poor growth, priming the hypothalamic-pituitary-GH axis with sex steroids can normalize a suboptimal GH response to some stimuli. The GH response to GHRH is not affected by priming with estrogen,[384] suggesting that sex steroids assert their effects at the hypothalamus, either reducing somatostatin tone or increasing GHRH release, not at the pituitary.

The ability of GHRH to release GH is similar in prepubertal and pubertal children and in young adults. Over the course of the adult life span, however, the magnitude of the GH peak following GHRH declines with increasing age.[228, 371, 385, 386] The likely mechanism for the age-related decline of the response to GHRH is an increase in somatostatin tone.[387] Support for this is found in studies that utilize GHRH

in combination with pyridostigmine or arginine.[388, 389] These agents have both been used alone as diagnostic tests for GH deficiency, producing a GH pulse by reducing somatostatin tone.[390, 391] Arginine and pyridostigmine act synergistically with GHRH, producing large GH pulses similar to those seen in younger adults.

THE GHRH TEST. Which Analogue to Use? The potency of the two naturally occurring analogues of GHRH, GHRH(1–40) and GHRH(1–44), has been compared and found to be equal. These two compounds have also been compared with the synthetic analogue GHRH(1–29)-NH₂ and have been found to be equipotent in terms of stimulating GH release.[392] At the present time GHRH(1–29)-NH₂ is the analogue commercially available in the United States and Europe for use in clinical practice as a diagnostic agent and in the United States for the treatment of children with GH deficiency.

Test Procedure. The GHRH test is typically performed in the morning, after an overnight fast. GHRH is administered as an IV bolus through a cannula inserted into a forearm vein. The dose of GHRH is determined by the weight of the patient; 1 μg/kg is used in both adults and children. Blood is drawn for estimation of GH levels 15 minutes and immediately before the injection of GHRH is given, then at 15, 30, 45, and 60 minutes following the administration of GHRH.

Side Effects. Overall, side effects are uncommon following the administration of GHRH, and when they occur they are usually mild. The most frequently reported side effect is transient warmth and flushing of the face that passes within 5 minutes of administration. Other side effects reported are pain and redness at the injection site, nausea, vomiting, headache, a strange taste in the mouth, and tightness in the chest. These symptoms are transient and resolve rapidly.

What Constitutes a Normal GH Response to GHRH? With any test used in clinical practice, it is important to determine what constitutes a normal response. Accordingly, several studies have addressed this question for the GHRH test. Ranke et al.[393] defined the normal range of GH responses to GHRH in 86 children with a normal GH axis as 11.8 to 172.4 μg/L, by determining the mean response ±2 SD. This study also concluded that a GH response of less than 10 μg/L should be used as the diagnostic threshold for GH deficiency in children.

The diagnostic threshold of 10 μg/L has been used in other studies utilizing the GHRH test[394–396] and is now generally accepted in pediatric practice. This peak is similar to that used to define GH deficiency when using the majority of stimuli in children despite it being recognized that the different stimuli are not equal in their ability to release GH.[382] Such thresholds are defined arbitrarily, despite attempts to rationalize them.[397] This may reflect the fact that the diagnosis of GH deficiency in a child depends primarily on the clinical finding of poor growth, and that the stimulation test is used to confirm the presence of GH deficiency.

In adults, the diagnostic threshold used to identify patients with GH deficiency is lower than that used in pediatric practice. For example a GH peak of less than 3 μg/L during an ITT is considered to be indicative of severe GH deficiency that warrants therapy with exogenous GH. If arginine were to be used as the stimulus the diagnostic cutoff would be even lower than this.[397, 398] In adults the GHRH test is generally a more potent stimulus of GH secretion, resulting in higher pulses than those seen following the ITT, arginine, or glucagon.[399] This would suggest that the diagnostic cutoff for severe GH deficiency might be higher than 3 μg/L using the GHRH test in adults, but this has not been determined.

THE GHRH TEST IN CHILDREN WITH SHORT STATURE. Normal Hypothalamic-Pituitary-GH Axis. The GH response elicited by GHRH in children with short stature due to a variety of causes has been well characterized.[393–395, 400–409] Children who have constitutional short stature, with no underlying pathologic condition, have a normal GH peak following GHRH administration,[393, 402, 404, 405, 407, 409] but the timing of that peak may be delayed.[400, 403] Children that are short as a result of intrauterine growth retardation also have a normal GH response to GHRH.

GH Deficiency. GHRH is a powerful secretagogue and generally elicits a greater GH response than many of the traditional tests of GH status. Children with GH deficiency defined using conventional tests frequently have a greater response to GHRH than to other tests of GH status.[400] In a study of prepubertal children undergoing investigation of abnormal growth, subjects were divided into groups according to their response to conventional tests. GH status was considered normal if the peak GH response to a conventional test was greater than 10 μg/L; partial and severe GH deficiency were defined as a peak GH response between 5 and 10 μg/L and less than 5 μg/L, respectively.

Assuming a diagnostic cutoff of 10 μg/L for the GHRH test, 76% of the children with partial and 39% with severe GH deficiency had a GH peak greater than 10 μg/L during the GHRH test. Conversely, 10% of the children considered to have a normal GH axis had a peak GH response less than 10 μg/L, a figure consistent with the findings of other studies. This study demonstrated a considerable discordance between conventional tests of GH status and the GHRH test. It also indicated that, in a significant proportion of children with GH deficiency diagnosed clinically and confirmed using conventional tests, somatotroph function may be preserved, the cause of their impaired GH status being hypothalamic rather than pituitary dysfunction.

Patients who develop GH deficiency following cranial irradiation also exhibit discordance between the GHRH test and conventional tests of GH status. Typically, such patients have received radiotherapy for a tumor distant from the hypothalamic-pituitary axis, but this region was included in the radiation field, or cranial irradiation was given prophylactically during the treatment of acute lymphoblastic leukemia. The GH response to GHRH in such patients was greater than the response to the ITT and the arginine test in 80% of patients in one study.[410] This suggests that radiation primarily affects the hypothalamic mechanisms that regulate GH secretion from the anterior pituitary. The magnitude of the GH peak during the GHRH test decreases as the time from radiation increases, suggesting that the effects of radiation do, ultimately, impinge upon somatotroph function. This may be a direct effect of radiation on the somatotrophs or the indirect effect of long-standing GHRH deficiency depleting the available GH pool within the somatotroph. The latter is supported by the observation that priming with GHRH for several days prior to the GHRH test can increase the GH response to GHRH significantly.[411]

GHRH AND THE DIAGNOSIS OF GH DEFICIENCY IN ADULTS. There are surprisingly few data on the use of GHRH alone as a diagnostic test in adults. Much of the work was carried out before the advent of recombinant human GH when the diagnosis of GH deficiency in adults was not an issue. The few studies in the literature were performed on small numbers of patients, the majority of whom had childhood-onset GH deficiency. More recently, studies that have investigated GHRH as a diagnostic agent in adults have utilized it in combination with other agents, the aim being to normalize the GH response across the adult life span (see below).

LIMITATIONS OF THE GHRH TEST. The use of GHRH alone as a diagnostic test for GH deficiency is limited by several factors. The discordance observed between the results of the GHRH test and the results of other stimulation tests such as the ITT can lead to difficulties interpreting the results of the GHRH test. There is considerable inter- and intraindividual variation in the results of the GHRH test. The coefficient of variation for the GHRH test has been reported as 60% for children[412] and 45% for adults,[399] although the variability diminishes with increasing age in adults.[413] The sensitivity of the GHRH test is relatively poor in children with short stature and varies with the severity of the GH deficiency as determined by other tests of GH status. In one study the sensitivity of the GHRH test was 24% in patients with GH insufficiency (GH peak 5.0 to 10.0 μg/L to conventional tests) and 61% in patients with severe GH deficiency (GH peak <5.0 μg/L).[400] The specificity of the GHRH test has been reported to be 85% to 90%.[382, 400]

The ability to interpret the GHRH test is confounded further by the inhibition of the GH response in obese subjects.[414–416] This may be particularly important when assessing patients with GH deficiency who have abnormal body composition with a propensity to abdominal obesity. The GH response to GHRH in obese patients with pituitary tumors is reduced, making it difficult to define their GH status accurately, particularly if the GH deficiency is isolated.[417]

The GHRH test is safe, associated with few side effects, and requires minimal medical supervision, making it an attractive test for use in the outpatient setting. However, the problems outlined above make it difficult to interpret the results of the GHRH test in clinical practice and it must, therefore, be used with caution. A GH peak greater than 10 μg/L does not exclude GH deficiency in a child with poor growth, and further evaluation of the hypothalamic-pituitary axis should be undertaken. A positive result (i.e., a GH peak <10 μg/L) will be indicative of GH deficiency, but, because 10% to 15% of normal children fall into this group, further evaluation to confirm the diagnosis of GH deficiency will be necessary. The relatively good specificity of the GHRH test suggests that a positive result is significant and the child should be evaluated further with additional investigations and monitoring. At the present time, the primary role of the GHRH test is to determine which children are candidates for GHRH therapy.

TESTS UTILIZING GHRH IN COMBINATION WITH OTHER AGENTS. The observation that GHRH acts synergistically with agents that reduce somatostatin tone has led to the development of tests which combine GHRH with arginine, pyridostigmine, and clonidine. GHRH acts synergistically with these agents producing large GH pulses, the magnitude of which frequently exceeds 50 μg/L in healthy subjects.[382, 388, 399, 418–420] The addition of these agents to GHRH increases the reproducibility of the test and improves diagnostic accuracy.

GHRH in combination with pyridostigmine or arginine causes profound release of GH. In one study of normal children and adolescents the normal range for GHRH plus pyridostigmine was 22.6 to 90.0 μg/L (n = 94), and that of GHRH plus arginine, 22.4 to 108 μg/L (n = 81).[382] The results of these tests were not influenced by pubertal stage in either girls or boys.[382, 421] In children with GH deficiency the GHRH-pyridostigmine test, used with the diagnostic threshold of 20 μg/L, the diagnosis was confirmed in 100% of patients with organic GH deficiency (caused by craniopharyngioma) and 80% of patients with idiopathic GH deficiency.[419]

GHRH in combination with arginine has been extensively evaluated in adults with pituitary disease in the hope that it will provide a safer alternative to the ITT, which is currently considered to be the gold standard investigation of GH status in adults. The combination of GHRH with arginine was chosen over pyridostigmine because the side effects with pyridostigmine were unpleasant and the GH response to GHRH plus arginine is not affected by age.[422]

In adults the GH response to GHRH and arginine is not affected by sex or age; similar results are achieved in male and female subjects and young and old adults.[420, 422, 423] Across the adult life span the 3rd percentile limit of GH response to GHRH plus arginine is 16.5 μg/L and the 1st percentile limit is 9 μg/L.

Adults with GH deficiency all had a peak GH response to GHRH plus arginine that fell below 16.5 μg/L, and 92% of patients had a peak below 9 μg/L. The GH peaks achieved during the GHRH-arginine test correlate well with those during the ITT, although the absolute GH response to GHRH plus arginine is considerably greater than that to the ITT. Of the seven patients that had achieved a peak GH greater than 9 μg/L during the GHRH-arginine test, six had achieved a GH peak higher than the diagnostic threshold for the ITT (3 μg/L). It was suggested by the authors that the diagnostic cutoff for the GHRH-arginine test should be 9 μg/L for severe GH deficiency in adults and 16.5 μg/L for GH insufficiency.

GHRH Therapy in GH-Deficient Children

The potential of GHRH as a therapeutic agent for GH-deficient children has been examined in several studies. The majority of GH-deficient children with short stature and growth failure have a disorder of hypothalamic regulation of the pituitary rather than a defect of the somatotroph. In these children injections of GHRH, as well as other GHSs, might be a useful treatment option. One of the first studies published in 1985 reported the use of GHRH (1–40)-OH administered SC with a peristaltic pump every 3 hours to two children with organic hypopituitarism (post-traumatic, hydrocephalus).[424] The children received 3-hourly doses of 1 or 3 μg/kg GHRH for 6 months. Both children increased their growth rate by about 1.5- to 6.0-fold compared to the growth rate before administration of GHRH(1–40)-OH. The rationale for using this dose regimen was based on the observation

TABLE 31–3. Children Treated with Subcutaneous Growth Hormone–Releasing Hormone (GHRH) by Pump

References	n	Diagnosis* (Peak GH μg/L)	GHRH	Dose (μg/kg)	Total Dose (μg/day)†	Growth Velocity (cm/yr) (Mean ±SEM) Pre	Growth Velocity (cm/yr) (Mean ±SEM) During	Responders	Comments
Thorner et al.[425]	10	GHD (<10)	1–40	1–3 q 3 hr	200–600	3.5 ±1.4 (±SD)	10.0 ±2.2 (6 mo)	100%	Ab 11/20
	10	GHD (<10)	1–40	1–2 q 3 hr overnight only	100–200	3.4 ±1.0	6.2 ±2.1 (6 mo)	80%	
Low[426]	7	GHD (<2)	1–44	1–2 q 3 hr	200–400	2.7 ±0.2	8.4 ±2.5 (2 mo) 5.4 ±0.7 (12 mo)	71%	Ab—none
Brain et al.[427]	5 (12 mo) 3 (3–6 mo)	Partial GHD (<10)	1–29	Continuous	2150	4.6 ±0.3 (±SD)	7.0 ±1.4 (12 mo) (similar GV in 3 at 3–6 mo)	100%	Ab—all

*Peak GH response to standard pharmacologic tests.
†Assumes 25-kg child.
GH, growth hormone; GHD, growth hormone deficiency; Ab, antibodies; GV, growth velocity.

that in growing children, five to nine pulses of GH are detected every 24 hours.

Since then, several studies have been performed to evaluate the benefits of GHRH therapy in GH-deficient children with different GHRH injection regimens and different doses. However the groups of children who were treated were not homogeneous; their diagnoses varied from GH deficiency and short stature to normal variant short stature without GH deficiency. The GHRH preparations used included GHRH(1–40)-OH, GHRH(1–44)-NH$_2$, and GHRH(1–29)-NH$_2$.

GHRH GIVEN BY PUMP. Table 31–3 shows the results of GHRH treatment by pump.[425–427] The response with this kind of treatment varied from 71% to 100%. The growth rate on GHRH therapy varied from 6.2 to 10 cm/year over the first 6 months and was maintained in patients for up to 5 years. The growth velocity appears to be related to the total daily dosage, which ranged from 10 to 2150 μg/day. So far no studies have evaluated whether it is the frequency of administration or the total daily dose which has the greatest impact on the

therapeutic outcome. The first study which looked at administration by pump or single injections of GHRH was published in 1988.[425] It described the effects of different routes of GHRH administration in 24 GH-deficient children. GHRH(1–40) was given either by pump every 3 hours SC or every 3 hours SC overnight only. Alternatively, GHRH was given twice daily in a dose of 1 to 4 μg/kg per dose for 6 months. In all three circumstances the growth velocity increased between 1.8- and 2.9-fold, with the greatest effects seen during the pump therapy with injections every 3 hours.

Unfortunately there are no long-term comparative studies examining the growth-promoting effects of GHRH with GH. Two short-term studies (6 months' treatment) provided conflicting results: one suggested a comparable growth response with GHRH similar to GH treatment,[428] whereas the other suggested that GHRH was less effective.[429]

GHRH GIVEN SC TWICE A DAY (Table 31–4).[425, 430–437] The most impressive results with GHRH injections given twice daily were

TABLE 31–4. Children Treated with Subcutaneous Growth Hormone–Releasing Hormone (GHRH) by Twice-Daily Injections

References	n	Diagnosis* (μg/L)	GHRH	Dose (μg/kg)	Total Dose (μg/day)†	Growth Velocity (cm/yr) (Mean ±SD) Pre	Growth Velocity (cm/yr) (Mean ±SD) During	Responders	Comments
Ross et al.[430]	18	GHD (<3.5) (including 10 IGHD, 4 MPHD, 3 cranial irradiation, 1 septo-optic dysplasia)	1–29	≤25‡	500–1000	1.7 ±1.2 (after 3 mo 3.4 ±1.6)	7.2 ±2.5 (6 mo) 3.0 ±1.2 (6 mo)	44%	Ab 14/17
Takano et al.[431]	4	2 IGHD (<7), 2 germinoma	1–44	50–100 μg/dose	100–200	#1 3.5 #2 3.1 #3 2.0 #4 1.0	8.2 (6 mo) 3.8 (# 1 & 3) 9.8 0.8	50%	Ab 2/4
Thorner et al.[425]	4	GHD (<10)	1–40	4	200	3.2 ±1.8	7.9 ±2.4 (6 mo)	100%	Ab 1/4
Smith & Brook[432]	8	GHD (8.5), some MPHD	1–29	4–8	200–400		5.1 ±0.3 (4 μg) 5.9 ±0.4 (8 μg) (mean—9 mo)	63%	Ab not done
Butenandt & Staudt[433]	7	GHD (<3)	1–29	4–6	200–300	3.0 (1.9–3.8)	4.0 (0.5–8.2) (6–15 mo)	29%	7/7 respond to subsequent GH; Ab not done
Duck et al.[434]	20	GHD (<10)	1–44	10–20§	500–1000	3.6 ±1.1	8.6 ±2.5 (6 mo) 8.1 ±1.5 (12 mo)	100%	Ab—none
Kirk et al.[435]	18	Height <3rd percentile	1–29	20	1000	4.8	7.2		
Pasqualini et al.[436]	9	Growth retardation because of CRF: 3 treated conservatively, 3 on dialysis, 3 after renal transplantation	1–29	26	1300	3.8	8.0		
Ogilvy-Stuart et al.[437]	9	GHD, radiation-induced (<20 mU/L)	1–29	15	750	3.3	6.0		

*Peak GH to standard pharmacologic tests.
†Assumes 25-kg child.
‡Dose 250 μg if weight <20 kg (n = 8) or 500 μg dose if weight >20 kg (n = 10).
§Sixteen subjects, 10-μg dose for 1 year; 4 subjects, 10 μg for 6 months and 20 μg for second 6 months.
GHD, growth hormone deficiency; IGHD, isolated GHD; MPHD, multiple pituitary hormone deficiency; Ab, antibodies; CRF, chronic renal failure.

TABLE 31–5. Children Treated with Subcutaneous Growth Hormone–Releasing Hormone (GHRH) by Once-Daily Injection

References	n	Diagnosis (μg/L)*	GHRH	Dose (μg/kg)	Total Dose (μg/day)†	Growth Velocity (cm/yr) (Mean ±SEM)		Responders	Comments
						Pre	During		
Rochiccioli et al.[438]	6	Partial GHD (<11)	1–44	10	250	4.2 ±1.1 (±SD)	10 ±3.3 (6 mo) 8.6 ±1.8 (12 mo)	83% (at 12 mo)	Reduced GV at 9–12 mo; Ab 1/6
Bozzola et al.[439]	25	10 GHD (<5)	1–44	1.6–18	40–450	3.5 ±0.2	7.3 ±0.4 (6 mo)‡	40% (at 6 mo)	Responders
		15 partial GHD (<10)				3.7 ±0.2	4.1 ±0.3	32% (at 12 mo)	Nonresponders Ab 6/25
Romer et al.[411]	11	GHD (<5)	1–44	10	250		2.6 (6 mo)	0%	Older children 19/21 pretreated with GH; 2/20 > 2 cm/yr
	9	GHD (<3)	1–44	10 (3 ×/wk)		3.3 (n = 20)	3.0 (for all 20)		
Lievre et al.[440]	111	GHD (<10)	1–44	1.3–23.1	30–300	≤ − 2 SD 3.8 ±0.1	> 2 cm/yr (6 mo) 6 ±0.2	50% increased GV	Ab 13.5%; 42% had catch-up growth
Wit et al.§[441]	5	GHD (<10)	1–44	7.5	190	2.5	4.6 (3 mo)	40% >2 cm/yr	"Insufficient response"; 10 pretreated with GH; Ab–none
	6			15	380	2.7	7.0 (3 mo)	50%	
Lanes et al.[442]	16	GHD (<10)	1–29	30	750	3.4 ±0.7	6.8 ±0.1 (6 mo) 6.2 ±0.9 (12 mo) 6.6 ±1.0 (18 mo) 6.5 ±0.7 (24 mo)	68% > 2 cm/yr over baseline	GHRH Ab were detected in 4/11 and 6/11 responders at 6 and 12 mo and in 2/5 nonresponders at 6 mo
Thorner et al.[443]	110	GHD (<10)	1–29	30	750	4.1 ±0.9	8.0 ±1.5 (6 mo) 7.2 ±1.3 (12 mo)	74% > 2 cm/yr	Overall 62% had at least 1 positive Ab result at some point during treatment

*Peak GH to standard pharmacologic tests.
†Assumes 25 kg child.
‡After withdrawal of GHRH, responders' growth velocity decreased from 7.3 ± 0.4 to 5.1 ± 1.7; treated with GH (0.6 IU/kg for 6 mo).
§Three-month study of 10/12 pretreated with GH.
See Table 31–3 for abbreviations.
Subsequent methionyl-GH treatment (8 IU/wk): at 3-months average growth velocity similar for those on higher dose of GHRH; 3 had better response on GHRH.

achieved in a multicenter study using GHRH(1–44)-NH$_2$ in 20 GH-deficient children.[434] All of the children responded with accelerated growth velocity. The growth velocity increased from 3.6 cm/year before treatment to 8.6 after 6 months, and 8.1 after 12 months. Ogilvy-Stuart et al.[437] reported a significant beneficial effect of GHRH(1–29) given in a dose of 30 μg/kg/day over 1 year, which resulted in a 1.8-fold increase of growth velocity per year in 9 children with radiation-induced GH deficiency.

The effects of GHRH(1–29) therapy in growth retardation caused by chronic renal failure were examined in nine children by Pasqualini and coworkers.[436] They either were treated conservatively or with dialysis or had renal transplantation. GHRH(1–29) 52 μg/kg/day was administered for 3 to 6 months. The growth velocity increased from 3.8 to 8 cm/year.

GHRH GIVEN SC ONCE A DAY. Several groups have investigated the effects of GHRH given SC by once-daily injections and the results are summarized in Table 31–5.[411, 438–443] A study investigating 110 GH-deficient children treated with a dose of 30 μg/kg/day of GHRH(1–29)[443] showed a significant increase in linear growth velocity with 4.1 cm/year before treatment and 7.2 cm/year after 1 year of treatment (Fig. 31–2). The largest number of children was investigated in the GHRH European Multicenter Study,[440] which reported the treatment of 111 GH-deficient children.

Height velocity increased from 3.8 cm/year before to 6 cm/year

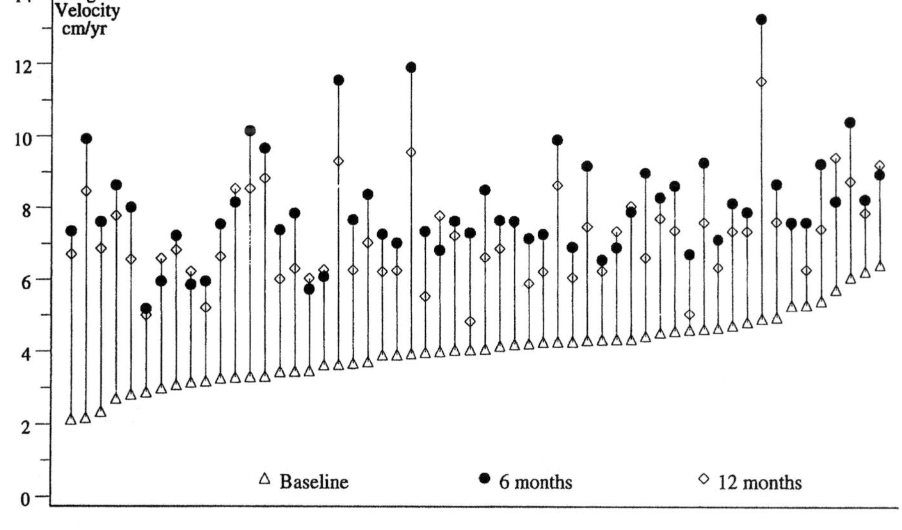

FIGURE 31–2. The effect of 6 and 12 months' growth hormone–releasing hormone (1–29) treatment in growth hormone–deficient children. The height velocities at baseline *(triangle)* and after 6 months *(circle)* and 12 months *(diamond)* of treatment are plotted by increasing baseline values. (From Thorner MO, Rochiccioli P, Colle M, et al: Once daily subcutaneous growth hormone–releasing hormone therapy accelerates growth in growth hormone–deficient children during the first year of therapy. J Clin Endocrinol Metab 81:1189–1196, 1996.)

during 6 months of treatment. The group of Bozzola[439] reported an increase of growth velocity from 3.5 cm/year to 7.3 cm/year after 6 months of treatment in 10 GH-deficient children with GHRH(1–44). The optimal growth velocity was observed in the first 9 months of therapy in most of the studies.[438] Lanes and Carrillo[442] reported that therapy with GHRH(1–29) in 16 prepubertal GH-deficient children given once daily SC over 12 to 24 months resulted in a significant increase in growth velocity.

WHICH CHILDREN SHOULD BE CONSIDERED FOR GHRH THERAPY? The use of GHRH(1–29)-NH$_2$ treatment of idiopathic GH deficiency in children with growth failure has now been approved by the Food and Drug Administration (FDA). The recommended daily dose is 30 μg/kg/day given SC at bedtime. The patients should be selected according to the following criteria: All children should be prepubertal, with a bone age of less than 7.5 years for females and less than 8.0 years for males. Children who do not adequately respond (i.e., peak GH level of ≤2 μg/L) to a GH stimulation test with GHRH prior to the study should not be treated with GHRH.

ADVERSE EFFECTS. Development of antibodies during GHRH treatment has been described.[425, 427, 430, 431, 438–440, 442, 443] Treatment-related adverse events have been reported, including local injection reactions characterized by pain, swelling, or redness, as well as headache, flushing, dysphagia, dizziness, hyperactivity, and urticaria. There are few reported data on thyroid function in children with GH deficiency. One study reported an increase in thyroid replacement requirements in one of seven patients[444]; another study reported a 5% incidence of hypothyroidism.[425] The mechanism underlying the change in thyroid function is unclear, but it has been hypothesized that an increase in GH levels results in an increase in somatostatin tone with subsequent inhibition of TSH secretion.[445]

GHRH Treatment in Adults

Optimal GHRH therapy requires the functional integrity of somatotroph cells.[446] While in GH-deficient adults this is no longer the case, older adults in whom the somatotroph hyposecretion is thought to be caused by the decreased activity of GHRH-secreting neurons still have an intact hypothalamic-pituitary axis. In addition, the pituitary GH-releasable pool in the elderly is comparable to that in young adults.

In fact, the few available studies dealing with the administration of GHRH in adults have been performed in the elderly to investigate whether GHRH treatment could counteract the age-dependent decline of GH. Twice-daily injections of GHRH(1–29) for 2 weeks,[447] as well as continuous GHRH(1–44) infusions for 2 weeks in healthy older men,[448] partially reversed the age-related decrease of GH as well as IGF-I levels. Another study, performed over 6 weeks,[449] suggested that GHRH administration to the elderly might attenuate some effects of aging on muscle strength. The results of further long-term studies on the effects of GHRH treatment in the elderly are awaited.

Growth Hormone Secretagogues

Since the first studies reporting the GH-releasing capabilities of GHSs in humans there has been interest in their potential as diagnostic agents. Peptide and nonpeptide GHSs are powerful stimulators of GH release, effective when administered IV, SC, intranasally,[450] or PO.[284] These agents typically cause GH release in excess of that observed following GHRH or during the ITT.

GHS Action in Healthy Subjects

The GHSs cause the release of GH in a dose-dependent fashion.[451] They are more potent than GHRH: 1 μg/kg of GHRP-6 peptide results in significantly greater GH release than the same dose of GHRH. The effect of GHS on GH release is more reproducible than the effect of GHRH. The peptide GHSs (e.g., GHRP-6, GHRP-1, GHRP-2, and hexarelin) and the nonpeptide GHSs (e.g., MK-677) differ in terms of their pharmacokinetics. MK-677 has been developed specifically as an orally active agent. The peptidyl GHSs are active PO, but only at doses several hundred times higher than that required when administered IV.

An intact hypothalamic-pituitary axis is vital to facilitate the maximal effect of GHS on GH release. GHRH and somatostatin both influence the action of GHS, augmenting and diminishing the magnitude of the GH pulse, respectively. When GHRH is administered in combination with GHS the effect is synergistic, the magnitude of the GH pulse being greater than that obtained from the sum of the two agents administered separately.[274, 452–457] The presence of GHRH is required for GHSs to exert their effects on GH secretion. In a family from the remote Valley of Sind in Pakistan, a missense mutation in the GHRH receptor that changes the glycine at residue 72 in the extracellular domain to a stop results in a phenotype analogous to the little mouse.[458] When members of the family that were homozygous for the mutation were challenged with hexarelin there was no detectable GH response. In addition, studies performed in children who are GH-deficient as a result of pituitary stalk transection are unresponsive to GHSs.[459] Thus, somatotroph exposure to GHRH is necessary for GHSs to exert their action.

Manipulation of somatostatin tone also affects the GH response to GHSs. When hexarelin was given to subjects in combination with somatostatin the amount of GH released was significantly reduced.[460] When arginine was administered to the elderly, a group proposed to have increased somatostatin tone, GH levels following the administration of GHRP-6 increased significantly, to levels seen in younger subjects.[461]

GHSs demonstrate GH-releasing activity during the neonatal period at a level which persists during prepubertal life.[462] During puberty there is an increased GH response to GHS which persists into adult life.[463–465] Subsequently, over the course of the adult life span, the GH response to GHS declines, in line with the reduction in spontaneous GH secretion.[453, 461, 466]

The response to GHS does not vary with sex apart from during puberty, when girls exhibit a greater response to GHS than do boys.[464] The response in adult women is similar to that observed in men. Over the course of the adult life span, as with other stimuli, the magnitude of the GH response to GHS diminishes in line with the fall in spontaneous GH secretion observed with aging.[446] Women who received GHSs at various times during the menstrual cycle achieved similar peaks whether studied during the early follicular, late follicular, or luteal phase.[467]

GHSs and the Diagnosis of GH Deficiency

Although the effects of acute administration of GHSs have been extensively studied in healthy adults and children, few studies have evaluated their potential as diagnostic agents in patients with GH deficiency. The primary reason for this is the age-dependent decline in secretagogue-stimulated GH release, making it necessary to determine age-specific normative data. Instead of undertaking this considerable task, efforts have concentrated on finding ways of overcoming the effects of age by administering a GHS in combination with arginine or GHRH.

The combination of GHRH and GHS is the most potent stimulus of GH release known to endocrinologists and provides a promising alternative to the ITT. In normal subjects the lower limit of the normal range (3rd percentile) of responses to GHRH and hexarelin was 55.5 μg/L, which was considerably higher than the lower limit of normal following GHRH and arginine (3rd percentile = 17.5 μg/L). The response to GHS plus GHRH is reproducible within an individual; the GH levels attained are similar among individuals and do not appear to decline with age.[455, 468] Perhaps the most important feature of the GHS-GHRH test is its ability to discriminate GH-deficient patients from normal subjects. In two studies the combination of GHS and GHRH had a specificity and sensitivity of 100%.[469, 470] The combination of GHS and GHRH is safe and well tolerated; side effects are similar to those seen when the two agents are administered separately.

The GHRH and GHS Test in Difficult Diagnostic Situations

The power of the combined stimulus of GHRH and GHS has resulted in its application to difficult diagnostic situations in which

GH release, both spontaneous and stimulated, is reduced by a coexisting process. The problem of aging has already been discussed, but other situations, particularly obesity and syndromes of glucocorticoid excess, may confound the diagnosis of GH deficiency.

OBESITY. Spontaneous and stimulated GH secretion is reduced in obese subjects.[415] The exact cause of the hyposomatotropism is uncertain, but a variety of mechanisms have been suggested. Among the hypotheses put forward are increased somatostatin tone, a reduction in the secretion of GHRH or of the natural ligand for the GHS receptor, or any combination of these.[471] What is known for certain is that the GH response to a number of stimuli, including GHRH,[414] GHRP-6,[454] and hexarelin,[472] is inversely correlated with body fat mass, specifically abdominal fat mass. The diminished GH response can make it difficult to accurately define the GH status of an obese patient with hypothalamic-pituitary disease, particularly those in whom GH deficiency may be the only hormone abnormality.

The combination of GHRH with either arginine[416] or GHS[454] administered to an obese subject causes a GH response far greater than any other stimulus, although the GH level does not quite reach that seen in normal controls. These tests are useful tools in the differentiation of true GH deficiency from hyposomatotropism caused by obesity.

SYNDROMES OF GLUCOCORTICOID EXCESS. In rats glucocorticoids potentiate GHRH action and enhance spontaneous GH secretion. In normal humans there is a biphasic effect of pharmacologic doses of glucocorticoids. When normal men were treated with a single IV bolus of dexamethasone 4 mg and 3 hours later were challenged with a bolus injection of GHRH, the peak GH response to GHRH increased from 9.9 ± 2.0 µg/L to 29.2 ± 5.7 µg/L. When the dexamethasone dose was increased to 8 mg IV 12 hours prior to a GHRH bolus, the peak GH response to GHRH was attenuated to 3 ± 1.1 µg/L. These results suggest an acute stimulatory response followed by a later inhibitory effect.[473] The pretreatment with pyridostigmine before administering GHRH partially reversed the effects of 48 hours of dexamethasone therapy, suggesting that somatostatin tone may be increased by glucocorticoids.[474]

Patients with glucocorticoid excess caused by Cushing's syndrome or by exogenous steroids have markedly impaired GH secretion.[475] This may result from the combined effects of chronic exposure to glucocorticoids and the changes in body composition associated with Cushing's syndrome, particularly the central adiposity. The suppression of GH in these patients may persist for up to 1 year after resolution of the glucocorticoid excess[476] which may give rise to misinterpretation of a patient's GH status. GHRH and GHRP-6 have been administered to patients with Cushing's syndrome separately and in combination. The effect of GHRH in these patients was almost abolished and the response to GHRP-6 was considerably reduced compared to controls. The combination of GHRH and GHRP-6 was considerably more potent than either GHRH or GHRP-6 used alone, but the GH peaks were only 20% of those seen in normal subjects.[477] An earlier study had shown that the response to GHRH and pyridostigmine increased threefold following 7 days' priming with GHRH.[478] These data suggest that the effects of chronic glucocorticoid excess are primarily caused by reduced GHRH secretion. Whether the combination of GHRH and GHS will be able to predict which patients with Cushing's disease will recover normal GH secretion is a matter for further study.

The combination of GHS and GHRH provides a promising alternative to the ITT as the gold standard investigation to determine GH deficiency in adults and possibly children. Once GHSs are freely available, this test can be evaluated in everyday clinical practice by endocrinologists and may replace the ITT as the first-line investigation when diagnosing GH deficiency. Until then, the use of GHSs in the diagnosis of GH deficiency will be limited to a handful of academic centers around the world.

Therapeutic Potential of GHSs

Since the discovery of GHRPs in 1976, 5 years before the discovery of GHRH,[479] several different types of GHSs have been developed, including a series of nonpeptidyl GHSs.[285, 297, 330, 480] The concept that these agents amplify the pulsatile GH secretory pathway, instead of overriding normal physiology, has made this group of drugs the target

of intensive research. The initial enthusiasm which accompanied the concept of orally available peptidergic and nonpeptidergic GHSs, however, has been mitigated by the controversial results of several studies suggesting that there are no benefits in terms of changes in body composition, as well as a report of tolerance.[481] Others could not find development of tolerance and described beneficial effects on body composition.[482]

Therefore, the area of GHSs as therapeutic agents remains controversial. Some areas are discussed below where GHS might be a useful agent, especially under the assumption that new compounds with higher efficacy and better oral availability will be developed. It is essential for the reader to recognize that each GHS is unique in terms of its bioavailability profile, its metabolism, and its specificity of action. Thus no two GHSs may be compared except on a superficial level. It is not sound to extrapolate from one GHS to another.

THERAPEUTIC POTENTIAL OF GHSs IN CHILDREN. The use of GHSs in children with growth retardation has been thought to have therapeutic potential. Several studies have proved the GH-releasing effects of these compounds, peptidergic as well as non-peptidergic, in short-term infusion studies in children. As a GH stimulus, they are as potent or even more potent than GHRH. Loche and coworkers[483] demonstrated that IV bolus infusions of hexarelin, 2 µg/kg of body weight, can increase GH release in short-statured children (familial short stature and constitutional delay of growth).

In a trial performed by Mericq et al.,[484] GHRP-2 was administered subcutaneously to six prepubertal children of short stature with GH deficiency, defined as a GH response of less than 7 µg/L to at least two standard provocative tests and a growth velocity of 4 cm/year or less. The agents were administered for 6 months at increasing doses (0.3, to 1.0, to 3.0 µg/kg/day). At months 7 and 8 the children received GHRP-2 3 µg/kg/day together with GHRH 3 µg/kg/day. The maximal overnight GH and GH peak amplitude showed a progressive increase at the higher doses. Growth velocities were increased when compared to baseline (5.3 ± 0.8 vs. 3.0 ± 0.5 cm/year, $P < .05$). During the long treatment period the GHRP-2 injections were well tolerated. However, the study was not placebo-controlled.

The only data available to date about the effects of a nonpeptidergic GHS have been reported by Yu et al.[485] In this double-blind placebo-controlled study with the GHS MK-677 with 94 previously untreated, prepubertal GH-deficient children (height < 5th percentile, growth velocity < 25th percentile, peak GH < 10 ng/mL on two tests), the GHS was well tolerated. The children were treated for 6 months with either 0.4 mg/kg/day or 0.8 mg/kg/day. Mean growth velocity increased by more than 3 cm/year at 6 months.[485]

Similar results have been reported[486] in a group of prepubertal non–GH-deficient children. In this study eight prepubertal children with constitutional short stature were treated with hexarelin administered three times daily intranasally. After treatment for up to 8 months the growth velocity increased significantly (mean $\pm$SD) from 5.3 ± 0.8 to 8.3 ± 1.7 cm/year in this group. Whether these changes would translate into increased adult height in these children after a longer therapy period is unclear to date.

Altogether, in preliminary studies the growth response to GHS in GH-deficient children has been lower than that seen with GH treatment. Whether this is explained by the type of GH-deficient children selected for the trials or a suboptimal dosing regimen has yet to be determined. The development of new compounds with improved pharmacodynamic properties might bring improved results.

The use of GHSs in children with non–GH-deficient short stature has to be evaluated very carefully in the future.

THERAPEUTIC POTENTIAL OF GHS IN ADULTS. GH therapy has been approved in adults with organic GH deficiency[369] caused by hypothalamic-pituitary disease and for the AIDS-related wasting syndrome[487] in the United States. As adults with GH deficiency very often do not have an intact hypothalamic-pituitary axis, only some of these patients would probably benefit from the use of GHSs.[488] Currently no data exist to date investigating the potential positive effects of GHS treatment in the AIDS-related wasting syndrome. Another potential field of research is the catabolic state of severe illness.

It seems that in the prolonged catabolic state of critical severe illness, a relative hyposomatotropism occurs, which seems to be partly of hypothalamic origin.[489] Infusion studies with GHRP-2 showed that given alone or together with GHRH, the somatotrophs can respond in this condition. In addition, there seems to occur a significant responsiveness to GH under GHRP infusion to these patients.[490–492] A 5-day infusion of GHRP-2 and TRH in protracted critical illness not only reactivated the blunted GH and TSH secretion but also showed metabolic effectiveness in this condition.[493] A double-blind placebo-controlled study[494] showed in a small number of healthy volunteers that diet-induced nitrogen wasting can be reduced after 7 days of treatment with an oral GH secretagogue (MK-677). These findings support the concept of GHS use in the catabolic state. Further evaluation of the merits of the use of GHSs in adult patients on maintenance hemodialysis is warranted.[495]

The use of GHSs for treatment of critically ill patients has to be evaluated carefully. A recent study[496] showed that treatment with high doses of GH (0.07 to 0.13 mg/kg/day) leads to an increase in morbidity and mortality in these patients.

Another potential field of application for GHS is in the normal older population, as there is an age-dependent decrease in GH secretion.[387] Some of the changes in body composition seen in the elderly resemble the changes seen in the GH-deficient adults.[387] Studies investigating the effects of GH treatment in the elderly have shown that GH treatment in the elderly might have beneficial effects on lean body mass, adipose tissue, and bone mineral density.[497] In addition, the releasable GH pool of the pituitary is preserved in the elderly.

The few existing studies investigating the effects of GHSs in the elderly have shown conflicting results. One study, using the peptidergic GHS hexarelin, could not show a beneficial effect on body composition after 16 weeks of SC treatment. The same investigators reported a partial and reversible attenuation of the GH response to hexarelin, measured 4 weeks after cessation of hexarelin therapy. IGF-I did not change significantly.[481]

Studies performed with an oral nonpeptidergic GHS (MK-677) resulted in a significant increase in IGF-I concentration compared to that of young adults after 4 weeks of treatment with 25 mg given once a day. This increase was accompanied by an increase in the mean 24-hour GH concentration, GH pulse height, and interpulse nadir concentrations of these volunteers. There were no significant changes in the pulse number observed. No desensitization of the hypothalamic-pituitary GH axis occurred. Despite the fact that GHSs have been shown to have adrenocorticotropic hormone (ACTH) and PRL-releasing activity,[462] no change in cortisol secretion was found in this study.[498] The PRL levels rose slightly but remained within the normal range. Fasting insulin levels, as well as glucose levels, have been reported to increase under MK-677 treatment.[499]

These divergent results underline once again that each GHS is unique in terms of its bioavailability and specificity profiles. Long-term studies are needed to further investigate the potential benefits of GHSs in the older population, that is, an increase in muscle mass and strength, as well as positive changes in body composition such as reduction in visceral fat.

Whether the use of GHSs in obesity will be of any benefit is questionable and requires further careful evaluation. The GH-releasing effects in obesity are decreased when compared with a normal population.[414, 500] Eight weeks of treatment with the GHS MK-677 at a dose of 25 mg/day in 24 obese men showed no change in total or visceral fat.[482] Of interest, the fat-free mass increased significantly and IGF-I levels increased approximately 40% in this study. Another potential therapeutic use for GHSs might be their use to improve cardiac function in certain stages of heart failure.[293] This is most likely caused by a direct effect of the GHS at the heart, where cardiac-specific GHS binding sites have been identified.[501]

REFERENCES

1. Reichlin S: Growth and the hypothalamus. Endocrinology 67:760–773, 1960.
2. Reichlin S: Growth hormone content of pituitaries from rats with hypothalamic lesions. Endocrinology 69:225–230, 1961.
3. Beck C, Larkins RG, Martin TJ, et al: Stimulation of growth hormone release from superfused rat pituitary by extracts of hypothalamus and of human lung tumours. J Endocrinol 59:325–333, 1973.
4. Dabek FT: Bronchial carcinoid tumour with acromegaly in two patients. J Clin Endocrinol Metab 38:329–333, 1974.
5. Sonksen PH, Ayres AB, Braimbridge M, et al: Acromegaly caused by pulmonary carcinoid tumours. Clin Endocrinol (Oxf) 5:503–513, 1976.
6. Caplan RH, Koob L, Abellera RM, et al: Cure of acromegaly by operative removal of an islet cell tumor of the pancreas. Am J Med 64:874–882, 1978.
7. Shalet SM, Beardwell CG, MacFarlane IA, et al: Acromegaly due to production of a growth hormone releasing factor by a bronchial carcinoid tumor. Clin Endocrinol (Oxf) 10:61–67, 1979.
8. Saeed uz Zafar M, Mellinger RC, Fine G, et al: Acromegaly associated with a bronchial carcinoid tumor: Evidence for ectopic production of growth hormone–releasing activity. J Clin Endocrinol Metab 48:66–71, 1979.
9. Leveston SA, McKeel DW Jr, Buckley PJ, et al: Acromegaly and Cushing's syndrome associated with a foregut carcinoid tumor. J Clin Endocrinol Metab 53:682–689, 1981.
10. Southern AL: Functioning metastatic bronchial carcinoid with elevated levels of serum and cerebrospinal fluid serotonin and pituitary adenoma. J Clin Endocrinol Metab 20:298–305, 1960.
11. Weiss L, Ingram M: Adenomatoid bronchial tumors: A consideration of the carcinoid tumors and the salivary tumors of the bronchial tree. Cancer 14:161–178, 1961.
12. Buse J, Buse MG, Roberts WJ: Eosinophilic adenoma of the pituitary and carcinoid tumors of the rectosigmoid area. J Clin Endocrinol Metab 21:735–738, 1961.
13. Ballard HS, Frame B, Hartsock RJ: Familial multiple endocrine adenoma-peptic ulcer complex. Medicine (Baltimore) 43:481–516, 1964.
14. Frohman LA, Szabo M, Berelowitz M, et al: Partial purification and characterization of a peptide with growth hormone–releasing activity from extrapituitary tumors in patients with acromegaly. J Clin Invest 65:43–54, 1980.
15. Thorner MO, Perryman RL, Cronin MJ, et al: Somatotroph hyperplasia: Successful treatment of acromegaly by removal of a pancreatic islet tumor secreting a growth hormone–releasing factor. Trans Assoc Am Physicians 95:177–187, 1982.
16. Spiess J, Rivier J, Thorner M, et al: Sequence analysis of a growth hormone releasing factor from a human pancreatic islet tumor. Biochemistry 21:6037–6040, 1982.
17. Rivier J, Spiess J, Thorner M, et al: Characterization of a growth hormone–releasing factor from a human pancreatic islet tumour. Nature 300:276–278, 1982.
18. Esch FS, Bohlen P, Ling NC, et al: Characterization of a 40 residue peptide from a human pancreatic tumor with growth hormone releasing activity. Biochem Biophys Res Commun 109:152–158, 1982.
19. Sassolas G, Chayvialle JA, Partensky C, et al: Acromegaly, clinical expression of the production of growth hormone releasing factor in pancreatic tumors. Ann Endocrinol (Paris) 44:347–354, 1983.
20. Guillemin R, Brazeau P, Bohlen P, et al: Growth hormone-releasing factor from a human pancreatic tumor that caused acromegaly. Science 218:585–587, 1982.
21. Campbell RM, Lee Y, Rivier J, et al: GRF analogs and fragments: Correlation between receptor binding, activity and structure. Peptides 12:569–574, 1991.
22. Frohman LA, Jansson JO: Growth hormone–releasing hormone. Endocr Rev 7:223–253, 1986.
23. Bohlen P, Brazeau P, Bloch B, et al: Human hypothalamic growth hormone releasing factor (GRF): Evidence for two forms identical to tumor derived GRF-44-NH2 and GRF-40. Biochem Biophys Res Commun 114:930–936, 1983.
24. Ling N, Esch F, Bohlen P, et al: Isolation, primary structure, and synthesis of human hypothalamic somatocrinin: Growth hormone–releasing factor. Proc Natl Acad Sci U S A 81:4302–4306, 1984.
25. Lin HD, Bollinger J, Ling N, et al: Immunoreactive growth hormone–releasing factor in human stalk median eminence. J Clin Endocrinol Metab 58:1197–1199, 1984.
26. Asa SL, Kovacs K, Thorner MO, et al: Immunohistological localization of growth hormone–releasing hormone in human tumors. J Clin Endocrinol Metab 60:423–427, 1985.
27. Brazeau P, Ling N, Bohlen P, et al: Growth hormone releasing factor, somatocrinin, releases pituitary growth hormone in vitro. Proc Natl Acad Sci U S A 79:7909–7913, 1982.
28. Engels JW, Glauder J, Mullner H, et al: Enzymatic amidation of recombinant (Leu27) growth hormone releasing hormone-Gly45. Protein Eng 1:195–199, 1987.
29. Brar AK, Downs TR, Heimer EP, et al: Biosynthesis of human growth hormone–releasing hormone (hGRH) in the pituitary of hGRH transgenic mice. Endocrinology 129:3274–3280, 1991.
30. Christophe J, Svoboda M, Dehaye J-P, et al: The VIP/PHI/secretin/helodermin/helospectin/GRF family: Structure-function relationships of the natural peptides, their precursors and synthetic analogues as tested in vitro on receptors and adenylate cyclase in a panel of tissue membranes. In Martinez J (ed): Peptide Hormones as Prohormones: Processing, Biological Activity, Pharmacology. Chichester, UK, Ellis Horwood, 1989.
31. Bell GI: The glucagon superfamily: Precursor structure and gene organization. Peptides 7:27–36, 1986.
32. Campbell RM, Scanes CG: Evolution of the growth hormone–releasing factor (GRF) family of peptides. Growth Regul 2:175–191, 1992.
33. McRory JE, Parker RL, Sherwood NM: Expression and alternative processing of a chicken gene encoding both growth hormone–releasing hormone and pituitary adenylate cyclase–activating polypeptide. DNA Cell Biol 16:95–102, 1997.
34. Vaughan JM, Rivier J, Spiess J, et al: Isolation and characterization of hypothalamic growth-hormone releasing factor from common carp, Cyprinus carpio. Neuroendocrinology 56:539–549, 1992.
35. McRory J, Sherwood NM: Two protochordate genes encode pituitary adenylate cyclase–activating polypeptide and related family members. Endocrinology 138:2380–2390, 1997.
36. Kaiser ET, Kezdy FJ: Amphiphilic secondary structure: Design of peptide hormones. Science 223:249–255, 1984.
37. Campbell RM, Bongers J, Felix AM: Rational design, synthesis, and biological evaluation of novel growth hormone releasing factor analogues. Biopolymers 37:67–88, 1995.
38. Clore GM, Martin SR, Gronenborn AM: Solution structure of human growth hor-

mone releasing factor. Combined use of circular dichroism and nuclear magnetic resonance spectroscopy. J Mol Biol 191:553–561, 1986.

39. Frohman LA, Downs TR, Heimer EP, et al: Dipeptidylpeptidase IV and trypsin-like enzymatic degradation of human growth hormone–releasing hormone in plasma. J Clin Invest 83:1533–1540, 1989.

40. Kovacs M, Gulyas J, Bajusz S, et al: An evaluation of intravenous, subcutaneous, and in vitro activity of new agmatine analogs of growth hormone–releasing hormone hGH-RH (1–29)NH2. Life Sci 42:27–35, 1988.

41. Coy DH, Hocart SJ, Murphy WA: Human growth hormone–releasing hormone analogues with much improved in vitro growth hormone–releasing potencies in rat pituitary cells. Eur J Pharmacol 204:179–185, 1991.

42. Zarandi M, Serfozo P, Zsigo J, et al: Potent agonists of growth hormone–releasing hormone. Part I. Int J Pept Protein Res 39:211–217, 1992.

43. Campbell RM, Heimer EP, Ahmad M, et al: Pegylated peptides. V. Carboxy-terminal PEGylated analogs of growth hormone–releasing factor (GRF) display enhanced duration of biological activity in vivo. J Pept Res 49:527–537, 1997.

44. Cervini LA, Donaldson CJ, Koerber SC, et al: Human growth hormone–releasing hormone hGHRH(1–29)-NH2: Systematic structure-activity relationship studies. J Med Chem 41:717–727, 1998.

45. Coy DH, Murphy WA, Sueiras-Diaz J, et al: Structure-activity studies on the N-terminal region of growth hormone releasing factor. J Med Chem 28:181–185, 1985.

46. Robberecht P, Coy DH, Waelbroeck M, et al: Structural requirements for the activation of rat anterior pituitary adenylate cyclase by growth hormone–releasing factor (GRF): Discovery of (N-Ac-Tyr1, D-Arg2)-GRF(1–29)-NH2 as a GRF antagonist on membranes. Endocrinology 117:1759–1764, 1985.

47. Zarandi M, Horvath JE, Halmos G, et al: Synthesis and biological activities of highly potent antagonists of growth hormone–releasing hormone. Proc Natl Acad Sci U S A 91:12298–12302, 1994.

48. Toth K, Kovacs M, Zarandi M, et al: New analogs of human growth hormone–releasing hormone (1–29) with high and prolonged antagonistic activity. J Pept Res 51:134–141, 1998.

49. Jungwirth A, Schally AV, Pinski J, et al: Growth hormone–releasing hormone antagonist MZ-4–71 inhibits in vivo proliferation of Caki-I renal adenocarcinoma. Proc Natl Acad Sci U S A 94:5810–5813, 1997.

50. Waelbroeck M, Robberecht P, Coy DH, et al: Interaction of growth hormone–releasing factor (GRF) and 14 GRF analogs with vasoactive intestinal peptide (VIP) receptors of rat pancreas. Discovery of (N-Ac-Tyr1,D-Phe2)-GRF(1–29)-NH2 as a VIP antagonist. Endocrinology 116:2643–2649, 1985.

51. Gubler U, Monahan JJ, Lomedico PT, et al: Cloning and sequence analysis of cDNA for the precursor of human growth hormone–releasing factor, somatocrinin. Proc Natl Acad Sci U S A 80:4311–4314, 1983.

52. Mayo KE, Cerelli GM, Lebo RV, et al: Gene encoding human growth hormone–releasing factor precursor: Structure, sequence, and chromosomal assignment. Proc Natl Acad Sci U S A 82:63–67, 1985.

53. Mayo KE, Cerelli GM, Rosenfeld MG, et al: Characterization of cDNA and genomic clones encoding the precursor to rat hypothalamic growth hormone–releasing factor. Nature 314:464–467, 1985.

54. Frohman MA, Downs TR, Chomczynski P, et al: Cloning and characterization of mouse growth hormone–releasing hormone (GRH) complementary DNA: Increased GRH messenger RNA levels in the growth hormone–deficient lit/lit mouse. Mol Endocrinol 3:1529–1536, 1989.

55. Gonzalez-Crespo S, Boronat A: Expression of the rat growth hormone–releasing hormone gene in placenta is directed by an alternative promoter. Proc Natl Acad Sci U S A 88:8749–8753, 1991.

56. Berry SA, Srivastava CH, Rubin LR, et al: Growth hormone–releasing hormone-like messenger ribonucleic acid and immunoreactive peptide are present in human testis and placenta. J Clin Endocrinol Metab 75:281–284, 1992.

57. Bloch B, Baird A, Ling N, et al: Immunohistochemical evidence that growth hormone–releasing factor (GRF) neurons contain an amidated peptide derived from cleavage of the carboxyl-terminal end of the GRF precursor. Endocrinology 118:156–162, 1986.

58. Breyer PR, Rothrock JK, Beaudry N, et al: A novel peptide from the growth hormone releasing hormone gene stimulates Sertoli cell activity. Endocrinology 137:2159–2162, 1996.

59. Perez-Riba M, Gonzalez-Crespo S, Boronat A: Differential splicing of the growth hormone–releasing hormone gene in rat placenta generates a novel pre-proGHRH mRNA that encodes a different C-terminal flanking peptide. FEBS Lett 402:273–276, 1997.

60. Bloch B, Gaillard RC, Brazeau P, et al: Topographical and ontogenetic study of the neurons producing growth hormone–releasing factor in human hypothalamus. Regul Pept 8:21–31, 1984.

61. Bugnon C, Gouget A, Fellmann D, et al: Immunocytochemical demonstration of a novel peptidergic neurone system in the cat brain with an anti-growth hormone–releasing factor serum. Neurosci Lett 38:131–137, 1983.

62. Jacobowitz DM, Schulte H, Chrousos GP, et al: Localization of GRF-like immunoreactive neurons in the rat brain. Peptides 4:521–524, 1983.

63. Merchenthaler I, Vigh S, Schally AV, et al: Immunocytochemical localization of growth hormone–releasing factor in the rat hypothalamus. Endocrinology 114:1082–1085, 1984.

64. Sawchenko PE, Swanson LW, Rivier J, et al: The distribution of growth-hormone–releasing factor (GRF) immunoreactivity in the central nervous system of the rat: An immunohistochemical study using antisera directed against rat hypothalamic GRF. J Comp Neurol 237:100–115, 1985.

65. Bloch B, Brazeau P, Bloom F, et al: Topographical study of the neurons containing hpGRF immunoreactivity in monkey hypothalamus. Neurosci Lett 37:23–28, 1983.

66. Horvath S, Palkovits M, Gorcs T, et al: Electron microscopic immunocytochemical evidence for the existence of bidirectional synaptic connections between growth hormone–releasing hormone– and somatostatin-containing neurons in the hypothalamus of the rat. Brain Res 481:8–15, 1989.

67. Zeitler P, Tannenbaum GS, Clifton DK, et al: Ultradian oscillations in somatostatin and growth hormone–releasing hormone mRNAs in the brains of adult male rats. Proc Natl Acad Sci U S A 88:8920–8924, 1991.

68. Tannenbaum GS, Zhang WH, Lapointe M, et al: Growth hormone–releasing hormone neurons in the arcuate nucleus express both Sst1 and Sst2 somatostatin receptor genes. Endocrinology 139:1450–1453, 1998.

69. Bresson JL, Clavequin MC, Fellmann D, et al: Ontogeny of the neuroglandular system revealed with HPGRF 44 antibodies in human hypothalamus. Neuroendocrinology 39:68–73, 1984.

70. Ishikawa K, Katakami H, Jansson JO, et al: Ontogenesis of growth hormone–releasing hormone neurons in the rat hypothalamus. Neuroendocrinology 43:537–542, 1986.

71. Joubert D, Benlot C, Lagoguey A, et al: Normal and growth hormone (GH)–secreting adenomatous human pituitaries release somatostatin and GH-releasing hormone. J Clin Endocrinol Metab 68:572–577, 1989.

72. Bagnato A, Moretti C, Ohnishi J, et al: Expression of the growth hormone–releasing hormone gene and its peptide product in the rat ovary. Endocrinology 130:1097–1102, 1992.

73. Tsagarakis S, Ge F, Besser GM, et al: Similar high molecular weight forms of growth hormone–releasing hormone are found in rat brain and testis. Life Sci 49:1627–1634, 1991.

74. Suhr ST, Rahal JO, Mayo KE: Mouse growth-hormone–releasing hormone: Precursor structure and expression in brain and placenta. Mol Endocrinol 3:1693–1700, 1989.

75. Margioris AN, Brockmann G, Bohler HC Jr, et al: Expression and localization of growth hormone–releasing hormone messenger ribonucleic acid in rat placenta: In vitro secretion and regulation of its peptide product. Endocrinology 126:151–158, 1990.

76. Meigan G, Sasaki A, Yoshinaga K: Immunoreactive growth hormone–releasing hormone in rat placenta. Endocrinology 123:1098–1102, 1988.

77. Weigent DA, Blalock JE: Immunoreactive growth hormone–releasing hormone in rat leukocytes. J Neuroimmunol 29:1–13, 1990.

78. Stephanou A, Knight RA, Lightman SL: Production of a growth hormone–releasing hormone-like peptide and its mRNA by human lymphocytes. Neuroendocrinology 53:628–633, 1991.

79. Weigent DA, Riley JE, Galin FS, et al: Detection of growth hormone and growth hormone–releasing hormone–related messenger RNA in rat leukocytes by the polymerase chain reaction. Proc Soc Exp Biol Med 198:643–648, 1991.

80. Nicholson WE, DeCherney GS, Jackson RV, et al: Pituitary and hypothalamic hormones in normal and neoplastic adrenal medullae: Biologically active corticotropin-releasing hormone and corticotropin. Regul Pept 18:173–188, 1987.

81. Shibasaki T, Kiyosawa Y, Masuda A, et al: Distribution of growth hormone–releasing hormone-like immunoreactivity in human tissue extracts. J Clin Endocrinol Metab 59:263–268, 1984.

82. Bosman FT, Van Assche C, Nieuwenhuyzen Kruseman AC, et al: Growth hormone releasing factor (GRF) immunoreactivity in human and rat gastrointestinal tract and pancreas. J Histochem Cytochem 32:1139–1144, 1984.

83. Christofides ND, Stephanou A, Suzuki H, et al: Distribution of immunoreactive growth hormone–releasing hormone in the human brain and intestine and its production by tumors. J Clin Endocrinol Metab 59:747–751, 1984.

84. Lopes MB, Gaylinn BD, Thorner MO, et al: Growth hormone–releasing hormone receptor mRNA in acromegalic pituitary tumors. Am J Pathol 150:1885–1891, 1997.

85. Thapar K, Kovacs K, Stefaneanu L, et al: Overexpression of the growth-hormone–releasing hormone gene in acromegaly-associated pituitary tumors. An event associated with neoplastic progression and aggressive behavior. Am J Pathol 151:769–784, 1997.

86. Kahan Z, Arencibia JM, Csernus VJ, et al: Expression of growth hormone–releasing hormone (GHRH) messenger ribonucleic acid and the presence of biologically active GHRH in human breast, endometrial, and ovarian cancers. J Clin Endocrinol Metab 84:582–589, 1999.

87. Matsubara S, Sato M, Mizobuchi M, et al: Differential gene expression of growth hormone (GH)–releasing hormone (GRH) and GRH receptor in various rat tissues. Endocrinology 136:4147–4150, 1995.

88. Morel G, Mesguich P, Dubois MP, et al: Ultrastructural evidence for endogenous growth hormone–releasing factor-like immunoreactivity in the monkey pituitary gland. Neuroendocrinology 38:123–133, 1984.

89. Mentlein R, Buchholz C, Krisch B: Binding and internalization of gold-conjugated somatostatin and growth hormone–releasing hormone in cultured rat somatotropes. Cell Tissue Res 258:309–317, 1989.

90. Morel G: Uptake and ultrastructural localization of a [125I] growth hormone releasing factor agonist in male rat pituitary gland: Evidence for internalization. Endocrinology 129:1497–1504, 1991.

91. Mayo KE, Miller TL, DeAlmeida V, et al: The growth-hormone–releasing hormone receptor: Signal transduction, gene expression, and physiological function in growth regulation. Ann N Y Acad Sci 805:184–203, 1996.

92. Mayo KE: Molecular cloning and expression of a pituitary-specific receptor for growth hormone–releasing hormone. Mol Endocrinol 6:1734–1744, 1992.

93. Gaylinn BD, Harrison JK, Zysk JR, et al: Molecular cloning and expression of a human anterior pituitary receptor for growth hormone-releasing hormone. Mol Endocrinol 7:77–84, 1993.

94. Lin C, Lin SC, Chang CP, et al: Pit-1-dependent expression of the receptor for growth hormone releasing factor mediates pituitary cell growth. Nature 360:765–768, 1992.

95. DeAlmeida VI, Mayo KE: Identification of binding domains of the growth hormone–releasing hormone receptor by analysis of mutant and chimeric receptor proteins. Mol Endocrinol 12:750–765, 1998.

96. Gaylinn BD, Lyons CE, Zysk JR, et al: Photoaffinity cross-linking to the pituitary receptor for growth hormone–releasing factor. Endocrinology 135:950–955, 1994.

97. Seifert H, Perrin M, Rivier J, et al: Binding sites for growth hormone releasing factor on rat anterior pituitary cells. Nature 313:487–489, 1985.

98. Abribat T, Boulanger L, Gaudreau P: Characterization of [125I-Tyr10]human growth hormone–releasing factor (1–44) amide binding to rat pituitary: Evidence for high and low affinity classes of sites. Brain Res 528:291–299, 1990.
99. Ikuyama S, Natori S, Nawata H, et al: Characterization of growth hormone–releasing hormone receptors in pituitary adenomas from patients with acromegaly. J Clin Endocrinol Metab 66:1265–1271, 1988.
100. Gaylinn BD, Lyons CE, Thorner MO: Mapping of the GHRH receptor binding site by photoaffinity crosslinking from different residues of GHRH. Presented at 79th Annual Meeting of the Endocrine Society, Minneapolis, June 11–14, 1997, p 156.
101. Andrews S, Dubbelde C, Ryan E: The sequence of *Homo sapiens* PAC clone DJ0877J02. 1998, US National Center for Biotechnology Information, National Library of Medicine: GenBank Accession AC005155. Available at: http://www.ncbi.nlm.gov/.
102. Wajnrajch MP, Chua SC, Green ED, et al: Human growth hormone–releasing hormone receptor (GHRHR) maps to a YAC at chromosome 7p15. Mamm Genome 5:595, 1994.
103. Petersenn S, Rasch AC, Heyens M, et al: Structure and regulation of the human growth hormone–releasing hormone receptor gene. Mol Endocrinol 12:233–247, 1988.
104. Iguchi G, Okimura Y, Takahashi T, et al: Cloning and characterization of the 5-flanking region of the human growth hormone–releasing hormone receptor gene. J Biol Chem 274:12108–12114, 1999.
105. Seifert H, Perrin M, Rivier J, et al: Growth hormone–releasing factor binding sites in rat anterior pituitary membrane homogenates: Modulation by glucocorticoids. Endocrinology 117:424–426, 1985.
106. Tamaki M, Sato M, Matsubara S, et al: Dexamethasone increases growth hormone (GH)–releasing hormone (GRH) receptor mRNA levels in cultured rat anterior pituitary cells. J Neuroendocrinol 8:475–480, 1996.
107. Miller TL, Mayo KE: Glucocorticoids regulate pituitary growth hormone–releasing hormone receptor messenger ribonucleic acid expression. Endocrinology 138:2458–2465, 1997.
108. Ono M, Miki N, Murata Y, et al: Sexually dimorphic expression of pituitary growth hormone–releasing factor receptor in the rat. Biochem Biophys Res Commun 216:1060–1066, 1995.
109. Bilezikjian LM, Seifert H, Vale W: Desensitization to growth hormone–releasing factor (GRF) is associated with down-regulation of GRF-binding sites. Endocrinology 118:2045–2052, 1986.
110. Horikawa R, Hellmann P, Cella SG, et al: Growth hormone–releasing factor (GRF) regulates expression of its own receptor. Endocrinology 137:2642–2645, 1996.
111. Aleppo G, Moskal SF II, De Grandis PA, et al: Homologous down-regulation of growth hormone–releasing hormone receptor messenger ribonucleic acid levels. Endocrinology 138:1058–1065, 1997.
112. Miller TL, Godfrey PA, DeAlmeida VI, et al: The rat growth hormone–releasing hormone receptor gene: Structure, regulation, and generation of receptor isoforms with different signaling properties. Endocrinology 140:4152–4165, 1999.
113. Journot L, Waeber C, Pantaloni C, et al: Differential signal transduction by six splice variants of the pituitary adenylate cyclase–activating peptide (PACAP) receptor. Biochem Soc Trans 23:133–137, 1995.
114. Tang J, Lagace G, Castagne J, et al: Identification of human growth hormone–releasing hormone receptor splicing variants. J Clin Endocrinol Metab 80:2381–2387, 1995.
115. Zeitler P, Stevens P, Siriwardana G: Functional GHRH receptor carboxyl terminal isoforms in normal and dwarf (dw) rats. J Mol Endocrinol 21:363–371, 1998.
116. Motomura T, Hashimoto K, Koga M, et al: Inhibition of signal transduction by a splice variant of the growth hormone–releasing hormone receptor expressed in human pituitary adenomas. Metabolism 47:804–808, 1998.
117. Eicher EM, Beamer WG: Inherited ateliotic dwarfism in mice. Characteristics of the mutation, little, on chromosome 6. J Hered 67:87–91, 1976.
118. Jansson JO, Downs TR, Beamer WG, et al: Receptor-associated resistance to growth hormone–releasing factor in dwarf "little" mice. Science 232:511–512, 1986.
119. Godfrey P, Rahal JO, Beamer WG, et al: GHRH receptor of little mice contains a missense mutation in the extracellular domain that disrupts receptor function. Nat Genet 4:227–232, 1993.
120. Lin SC, Lin CR, Gukovsky I, et al: Molecular basis of the little mouse phenotype and implications for cell type-specific growth. Nature 364:208–213, 1993.
121. Gaylinn BD, DeAlmeida VI, Lyons CE, et al: The mutant growth hormone–releasing hormone (GHRH) receptor of the little mouse does not bind GHRH. Endocrinology 140:5066–5074, 1999.
122. Wajnrajch MP, Gertner JM, Harbison MD, et al: Nonsense mutation in the human growth hormone–releasing hormone receptor causes growth failure analogous to the little (lit) mouse. Nat Genet 12:88–90, 1996.
123. Baumann G, Maheshwari H: The Dwarfs of Sindh: Severe growth hormone (GH) deficiency caused by a mutation in the GH-releasing hormone receptor gene. Acta Paediatr Suppl 423:33–38, 1997.
124. Netchine I, Talon P, Dastot F, et al: Extensive phenotypic analysis of a family with growth hormone (GH) deficiency caused by a mutation in the GH-releasing hormone receptor gene. J Clin Endocrinol Metab 83:432–436, 1998.
125. Salvatori R, Hayashida CY, Aguiar-Oliveira MH, et al: Familial dwarfism due to a novel mutation of the growth hormone–releasing hormone receptor gene. J Clin Endocrinol Metab 84:917–923, 1999.
126. Bilezikjian LM, Vale WW: Stimulation of adenosine 3′,5′-monophosphate production by growth hormone–releasing factor and its inhibition by somatostatin in anterior pituitary cells in vitro. Endocrinology 113:1726–1731, 1983.
127. Mougin C, Brazeau P, Ling N, et al: Roles of cyclic AMP and calcium in the mechanism of the release of growth hormone by somatocrinin. C R Acad Sci III 299:83–88, 1984.
128. Brazeau P, Ling N, Esch F, et al: Somatocrinin (growth hormone releasing factor) in vitro bioactivity: Ca^{++} involvement, cAMP mediated action and additivity of effect with PGE2. Biochem Biophys Res Commun 109:588–594, 1982.
129. Beck-Peccoz P, Volpi A, Maggioni AP, et al: Evidence for an inhibition of thyroid hormone effects during chronic treatment with amiodarone. Horm Metab Res 18:411–414, 1986.
130. Hart GR, Ray KP, Wallis M: Mechanisms involved in the effects of TRH on GHRH-stimulated growth hormone release from ovine and bovine pituitary cells. Mol Cell Endocrinol 56:53–61, 1988.
131. Schettini G, Cronin MJ, Hewlett EL, et al: Human pancreatic tumor growth hormone–releasing factor stimulates anterior pituitary adenylate cyclase activity, adenosine 3′,5′-monophosphate accumulation, and growth hormone release in a calmodulin-dependent manner. Endocrinology 115:1308–1314, 1984.
132. Holl RW, Thorner MO, Leong DA: Intracellular calcium concentration and growth hormone secretion in individual somatotropes: Effects of growth hormone–releasing factor and somatostatin. Endocrinology 122:2927–2932, 1988.
133. Snyder GD, Yadagiri P, Falck JR: Effect of epoxyeicosatrienoic acids on growth hormone release from somatotrophs. Am J Physiol 256:E221–E226, 1989.
134. Rawlings SR, Hoyland J, Mason WT: Calcium homeostasis in bovine somatotrophs: Calcium oscillations and calcium regulation by growth hormone–releasing hormone and somatostatin. Cell Calcium 12:403–414, 1991.
135. Guarcello V, Weigent DA, Blalock JE: Growth hormone releasing hormone receptors on thymocytes and splenocytes from rats. Cell Immunol 136:291–302, 1991.
136. Thorner MO, Holl RW, Leong DA: The somatotrope: An endocrine cell with functional calcium transients. J Exp Biol 139:169–179, 1988.
137. Bertherat J: Nuclear effects of the cAMP pathway activation in somatotrophs. Horm Res 47:245–250, 1997.
138. Cugini CD, Millard WJ, Leidy JW: Signal transduction systems in growth hormone–releasing hormone and somatostatin release from perfused rat hypothalamic fragments. Endocrinology 129:1355–1362, 1991.
139. Cronin MJ, Hewlett EL, Evans WS, et al: Human pancreatic tumor growth hormone (GH)–releasing factor and cyclic adenosine 3′,5′-monophosphate evoke GH release from anterior pituitary cells: The effects of pertussis toxin, cholera toxin, forskolin, and cycloheximide. Endocrinology 114:904–913, 1984.
140. Cronin MJ, Rogol AD, Dabney LG, et al: Selective growth hormone and cyclic AMP stimulating activity is present in human pancreatic islet cell tumor. J Clin Endocrinol Metab 55:381–383, 1982.
141. Cronin MJ, Rogol AD, MacLeod RM, et al: Biological activity of a growth hormone–releasing factor secreted by a human tumor. Am J Physiol 244:E346–353, 1983.
142. Cronin MJ, Rogol AD: Sex differences in the cyclic adenosine 3′:5′-monophosphate and growth hormone response to growth hormone–releasing factor in vitro. Biol Reprod 31:984–988, 1984.
143. Cronin MJ, Rogol AD, Myers GA, et al: Pertussis toxin blocks the somatostatin-induced inhibition of growth hormone release and adenosine 3′,5′-monophosphate accumulation. Endocrinology 113:209–215, 1983.
144. Cronin MJ, MacLeod RM, Canonico PL: Modification of basal and GRF-stimulated cyclic AMP levels and growth hormone release by phospholipid metabolic enzyme inhibitors. Neuroendocrinology 40:332–338, 1985.
145. Cronin MJ, Canonico PL: Tumor promoters enhance basal and growth hormone releasing factor stimulated cyclic AMP levels in anterior pituitary cells. Biochem Biophys Res Commun 129:404–410, 1985.
146. Cronin MJ, Summers ST, Sortino MA, et al: Protein kinase C enhances growth hormone releasing factor (1–40)–stimulated cyclic AMP levels in anterior pituitary. Actions of somatostatin and pertussis toxin. J Biol Chem 261:13932–13935, 1986.
147. Arimura A, Culler MD, Turkelson CM, et al: In vitro pituitary hormone releasing activity of 40 residue human pancreatic tumor growth hormone releasing factor. Peptides 4:107–110, 1983.
148. Culler MD, Kenjo T, Obara N, et al: Stimulation of pituitary cAMP accumulation by human pancreatic GH-releasing factor-(1–44). Am J Physiol 247:E609–615, 1984.
149. Ray KP, Wallis M: Regulation of growth hormone secretion and cyclic AMP metabolism in ovine pituitary cells: Interactions involved in activation induced by growth hormone–releasing hormone and phorbol esters. Mol Cell Endocrinol 58:243–252, 1988.
150. Michel D, Lefevre G, Labrie F: Dexamethasone is a potent stimulator of growth hormone–releasing factor–induced cyclic AMP accumulation in the adenohypophysis. Life Sci 35:597–602, 1984.
151. Spada A, Vallar L, Giannattasio G: Presence of an adenylate cyclase dually regulated by somatostatin and human pancreatic growth hormone (GH)–releasing factor in GH-secreting cells. Endocrinology 115:1203–1209, 1984.
152. Labrie F, Gagne B, Lefevre G: Growth hormone–releasing factor stimulates adenylate cyclase activity in the anterior pituitary gland. Life Sci 33:2229–2233, 1983.
153. Cheng K, Chan WW, Barreto A Jr, et al: The synergistic effects of His-D-Trp-Ala-Trp-D-Phe-Lys-NH_2 on growth hormone (GH)–releasing factor–stimulated GH release and intracellular adenosine 3′,5′-monophosphate accumulation in rat primary pituitary cell culture. Endocrinology 124:2791–2798, 1989.
154. Summers ST, Cronin MJ: Phorbol esters induce two distinct changes in GH3 pituitary cell adenylate cyclase activity. Arch Biochem Biophys 262:12–18, 1988.
155. Summers ST, Cronin MJ: Phorbol esters enhance basal and stimulated adenylate cyclase activity in a pituitary cell line. Biochem Biophys Res Commun 135:276–281, 1986.
156. Canonico PL, Cronin MJ, Thorner MO, et al: Human pancreatic GRF stimulates phosphatidylinositol labeling in cultured anterior pituitary cells. Am J Physiol 245:E587–590, 1983.
157. Canonico PL, Speciale C, Sortino MA, et al: Growth hormone releasing factor (GRF) increases free arachidonate levels in the pituitary: A role for lipoxygenase products. Life Sci 38:267–272, 1986.
158. Dobson PRM, Merritt JE, Baird JG, et al: The effect of growth hormone releasing factor on cyclic AMP accumulation and phosphatidylinositol breakdown. Presented at International Conference on Cyclic Nucleotides Protein Phosphorylation, Milan, June 27–July 1, 1983.
159. Ramirez JL, Torronteras R, Malagon MM, et al: Growth hormone–releasing factor

mobilizes cytosolic free calcium through different mechanisms in two somatotrope subpopulations from porcine pituitary. Cell Calcium 23:207–217, 1998.

160. Cella SG, Locatelli V, Broccia ML, et al: Long-term changes of somatotrophic function induced by deprivation of growth hormone–releasing hormone during the fetal life of the rat. J Endocrinol 140:111–117, 1994.

161. Landis CA, Masters SB, Spada A, et al: GTPase inhibiting mutations activate the alpha chain of Gs and stimulate adenylyl cyclase in human pituitary tumours. Nature 340:692–696, 1989.

162. Lloyd RV, Jin L, Chang A, et al: Morphologic effects of hGRH gene expression on the pituitary, liver, and pancreas of MT-hGRH transgenic mice. An in situ hybridization analysis. Am J Pathol 141:895–906, 1992.

163. Billestrup N, Swanson LW, Vale W: Growth hormone–releasing factor stimulates proliferation of somatotrophs in vitro. Proc Natl Acad Sci U S A 83:6854–6857, 1986.

164. Zeitler PS, Siriwardana G: Ligand binding to the growth hormone–releasing hormone (GHRH) receptor (GHRHr) activates the MAP kinase pathway in rat somatotrophs. Presented at 80th Annual Meeting of the Endocrine Society, New Orleans, June 24–27, 1998, p 219.

165. Mayo KE, Miller T, DeAlmeida V, et al: GHRH receptor signal transduction and gene regulation. Presented at 81st Annual Meeting of the Endocrine Society, San Diego, June 12–15, 1999, p 44.

166. Barinaga M, Yamonoto G, Rivier C, et al: Transcriptional regulation of growth hormone gene expression by growth hormone–releasing factor. Nature 306:84–85, 1983.

167. Barinaga M, Bilezikjian LM, Vale WW, et al: Independent effects of growth hormone releasing factor on growth hormone release and gene transcription. Nature 314:279–281, 1985.

168. Stachura ME, Tyler JM, Farmer PK: Fractional reduction of somatostatin concentration interacted with rat growth hormone releasing hormone to titrate the magnitude of pulsatile growth hormone and prolactin release in perfusion. Neuroendocrinology 48:500–506, 1988.

169. Dieguez C, Foord SM, Shewring G, et al: The effects of long term growth hormone releasing factor (GRF 1–40) administration on growth hormone secretion and synthesis in vitro. Biochem Biophys Res Commun 121:111–117, 1984.

170. Perez FM, Hymer WC: A new tissue-slicing method for the study of function and position of somatotrophs contained within the male rat pituitary gland. Endocrinology 127:1877–1886, 1990.

171. Vale W, Vaughan J, Yamamoto G, et al: Effects of synthetic human pancreatic (tumor) GH releasing factor and somatostatin, triiodothyronine and dexamethasone on GH secretion in vitro. Endocrinology 112:1553–1555, 1983.

172. Borges JL, Uskavitch DR, Kaiser DL, et al: Human pancreatic growth hormone–releasing factor-40 (hpGRF-40) allows stimulation of GH release by TRH. Endocrinology 113:1519–1521, 1983.

173. Almeida OF, Schulte HM, Rittmaster RS, et al: Potency and specificity of a growth hormone–releasing factor in a primate and in vitro. J Clin Endocrinol Metab 58:309–312, 1984.

174. Vigh S, Schally AV: Interaction between hypothalamic peptides in a superfused pituitary cell system. Peptides 5:241–247, 1984.

175. Badger TM, Millard WJ, McCormick GF, et al: The effects of growth hormone (GH)–releasing peptides on GH secretion in perfused pituitary cells of adult male rats. Endocrinology 115:1432–1438, 1984.

176. Zafar MS, Mellinger RC, Fine G, et al: Acromegaly associated with a bronchial carcinoid tumor: Evidence for ectopic production of growth hormone–releasing activity. J Clin Endocrinol Metab 48:66–71, 1979.

177. Ceda GP, Hoffman AR: Growth hormone–releasing factor desensitization in rat anterior pituitary cells in vitro. Endocrinology 116:1334–1340, 1985.

178. Gelato MC, Rittmaster RS, Pescovitz OH, et al: Growth hormone responses to continuous infusions of growth hormone–releasing hormone. J Clin Endocrinol Metab 61:223–228, 1985.

179. Plotsky PM, Vale W: Patterns of growth hormone–releasing factor and somatostatin secretion into the hypophysial-portal circulation of the rat. Science 230:461–463, 1985.

180. Frohman LA, Downs TR, Clarke IJ, et al: Measurement of growth hormone–releasing hormone and somatostatin in hypothalamic-portal plasma of unanesthetized sheep. Spontaneous secretion and response to insulin-induced hypoglycemia. J Clin Invest 86:17–24, 1990.

181. Weiss J, Cronin MJ, Thorner MO: Periodic interactions of GH-releasing factor and somatostatin can augment GH release in vitro. Am J Physiol 253:E508–514, 1987.

182. Law GJ, Ray KP, Wallis M: Effects of growth hormone–releasing factor, somatostatin and dopamine on growth hormone and prolactin secretion from cultured ovine pituitary cells. FEBS Lett 166:189–193, 1984.

183. Stachura ME, Tyler JM, Farmer PK: Human pancreatic growth hormone–releasing factor-44 differentially stimulates release of stored and newly synthesized rat growth hormone in vitro. Endocrinology 116:698–706, 1985.

184. Tachibana K, Marquardt H, Yokoya S, et al: Growth hormone–releasing hormone stimulates and somatostatin inhibits the release of a novel protein by cultured rat pituitary cells. Mol Endocrinol 2:973–978, 1988.

185. Katsumata N, Chakraborty C, Myal Y, et al: Molecular cloning and expression of peptide 23, a growth hormone–releasing hormone–inducible pituitary protein. Endocrinology 136:1332–1339, 1995.

186. Bergstrom RW, Hansen KL, Clare CN, et al: Hypogonadotropic hypogonadism and anosmia (Kallmann's syndrome) associated with a marker chromosome. J Androl 8:55–60, 1987.

187. Zeytin F, Brazeau P: GRF (somatocrinin) stimulates release of neurotensin, calcitonin and cAMP by a rat C cell line. Biochem Biophys Res Commun 123:497–506, 1984.

188. Muller EE, Locatelli V, Cocchi D: Neuroendocrine control of growth hormone secretion. Physiol Rev 79:511–607, 1999.

189. Casanueva FF, Dieguez C: Growth hormone secretagogues: Physiological role and clinical utility. Trends Endocrinol Metab 10:30–38, 1999.

190. Miki N, Ono M, Shizume K: Evidence that opiatergic and alpha-adrenergic mechanisms stimulate rat growth hormone release via growth hormone–releasing factor (GRF). Endocrinology 114:1950–1952, 1984.

191. Honegger J, Spagnoli A, Honegger J, et al: Interleukin-1 beta modulates the acute release of growth hormone–releasing hormone and somatostatin from rat hypothalamus in vitro, whereas tumor necrosis factor and interleukin-6 have no effect. Endocrinology 129:1275–1282, 1991.

192. Tannenbaum GS, Gurd W, Lapointe M: Leptin is a potent stimulator of spontaneous pulsatile growth hormone (GH) secretion and the GH response to GH-releasing hormone. Endocrinology 139:3871–3875, 1998.

193. Cocchi D, De Gennaro Colonna V, Bagnasco M, et al: Leptin regulates GH secretion in the rat by acting on GHRH and somatostatinergic functions. J Endocrinol 162:95–99, 1999.

194. Carro E, Senaris RM, Seoane LM, et al: Role of growth hormone (GH)–releasing hormone and somatostatin on leptin-induced GH secretion. Neuroendocrinology 69:3–10, 1999.

195. Carro E, Senaris RM, Mallo F, et al: Regulation of hypothalamic somatostatin and growth hormone releasing hormone mRNA levels by inhibin. Brain Res Mol Brain Res 66:191–194, 1999.

196. Carro E, Seoane LM, Senaris R, et al: Interaction between leptin and neuropeptide Y on in vivo growth hormone secretion. Neuroendocrinology 68:187–191, 1998.

197. Wehrenberg WB, Ling N, Bohlen P, et al: Physiological roles of somatocrinin and somatostatin in the regulation of growth hormone secretion. Biochem Biophys Res Commun 109:562–567, 1982.

198. Wehrenberg WB, Ling N, Brazeau P, et al: Somatocrinin, growth hormone releasing factor, stimulates secretion of growth hormone in anesthetized rats. Biochem Biophys Res Commun 109:382–387, 1982.

199. Wehrenberg WB, Bloch B, Phillips BJ: Antibodies to growth hormone–releasing factor inhibit somatic growth. Endocrinology 115:1218–1220, 1984.

200. Wehrenberg WB, Brazeau P, Luben R, et al: Inhibition of the pulsatile secretion of growth hormone by monoclonal antibodies to the hypothalamic growth hormone releasing factor (GRF). Endocrinology 111:2147–2148, 1982.

201. Tannenbaum GS, Ling N: The interrelationship of growth hormone (GH)–releasing factor and somatostatin in generation of the ultradian rhythm of GH secretion. Endocrinology 115:1952–1957, 1984.

202. Koritnik DR, Cronin MJ, Orth DN, et al: Pituitary response to intravenous hypothalamic releasing peptides in cynomolgus monkeys treated with contraceptive steroids. J Clin Endocrinol Metab 65:37–45, 1987.

203. Johke T, Hodate K, Ohashi S, et al: Growth hormone response to human pancreatic growth hormone releasing factor in cattle. Endocr J 31:55–61, 1984.

204. Moseley WM, Krabill LF, Friedman AR, et al: Administration of synthetic human pancreatic growth hormone–releasing factor for five days sustains raised serum concentrations of growth hormone in steers. J Endocrinol 104:433–439, 1985.

205. Moseley WM, Krabill LF, Friedman AR, et al: Growth hormone response of steers injected with synthetic human pancreatic growth hormone–releasing factors. J Anim Sci 58:430–435, 1984.

206. Enright WJ, Chapin LT, Moseley WM, et al: Growth hormone–releasing factor stimulates milk production and sustains growth hormone release in Holstein cows. J Dairy Sci 69:344–351, 1986.

207. Peticlerc D, Pelletier G, Lapierre H, et al: Dose response of two synthetic human growth hormone–releasing factors on growth hormone release in heifers and pigs. J Anim Sci 65:996–1005, 1987.

208. Leung FC, Taylor JE: In vivo and in vitro stimulation of growth hormone release in chickens by synthetic human pancreatic growth hormone releasing factor (hpGRFs). Endocrinology 113:1913–1915, 1983.

209. Ono M, Miki N, Demura H: Effect of antiserum to rat growth hormone (GH)–releasing factor on physiological GH secretion in the female rat. Endocrinology 129:1791–1796, 1991.

210. Magnan E, Mazzocchi L, Cataldi M, et al: Effect of actively immunizing sheep against growth hormone–releasing hormone or somatostatin on spontaneous pulsatile and neostigmine-induced growth hormone secretion. J Endocrinol 144:83–90, 1995.

211. Cella SG, Locatelli V, Mennini T, et al: Deprivation of growth hormone–releasing hormone early in the rat's neonatal life permanently affects somatotropic function. Endocrinology 127:1625–1634, 1990.

212. Thorner MO, Cronin MJ, Growth hormone–releasing factor: Clinical and basic studies. *In* Mueller EE, MacLeod RM, Frohman LA (eds): Neuroendocrine Perspectives. Amsterdam, Elsevier, 1985.

213. Ling N, Zeytin F, Bohlen P, et al: Growth hormone releasing factors. Annu Rev Biochem 54:403–423, 1985.

214. Clark RG, Robinson IC: Growth induced by pulsatile infusion of an amidated fragment of human growth hormone releasing factor in normal and GHRF-deficient rats. Nature 314:281–283, 1985.

215. Mayo KE, Hammer RE, Swanson LW, et al: Dramatic pituitary hyperplasia in transgenic mice expressing a human growth hormone–releasing factor gene. Mol Endocrinol 2:606–612, 1988.

216. Stefaneanu L, Kovacs K, Horvath E, et al: Adenohypophysial changes in mice transgenic for human growth hormone–releasing factor: A histological, immunocytochemical, and electron microscopic investigation. Endocrinology 125:2710–2718, 1989.

217. Wheeler MD, Wehrenberg WW, Styne DM: Growth hormone regulation by growth hormone–releasing hormone in infant rhesus monkeys. Biol Neonate 60:19–28, 1991.

218. Wheeler MD, Styne DM: Longitudinal changes in growth hormone response to growth hormone–releasing hormone in neonatal rhesus monkeys. Pediatr Res 28:15–18, 1990.

219. Acs Z, Lonart G, Makara GB: Role of hypothalamic factors (growth-hormone–releasing hormone and gamma-aminobutyric acid) in the regulation of growth hormone secretion in the neonatal and adult rat. Neuroendocrinology 52:156–160, 1990.

220. Ge F, Tsagarakis S, Rees LH, et al: Relationship between growth hormone–releasing

hormone and somatostatin in the rat: Effects of age and sex on content and in-vitro release from hypothalamic explants. J Endocrinol 123:53–58, 1989.

221. Cozzi MG, Zanini A, Locatelli V, et al: Growth hormone–releasing hormone and clonidine stimulate biosynthesis of growth hormone in neonatal pituitaries. Biochem Biophys Res Commun 138:1223–1230, 1986.

222. Korytko AI, Zeitler P, Cuttler L: Developmental regulation of pituitary growth hormone–releasing hormone receptor gene expression in the rat. Endocrinology 137:1326–1331, 1996.

223. Colonna VD, Zoli M, Cocci D, et al: Reduced growth hormone releasing factor (GHRF)-like immunoreactivity and GHRF gene expression in the hypothalamus of aged rats. Peptides 10:705–708, 1989.

224. Abribat T, Deslauriers N, Brazeau P, et al: Alterations of pituitary growth hormone–releasing factor binding sites in aging rats. Endocrinology 128:633–635, 1991.

225. Girard N, Boulanger L, Denis S, et al: Differential in vivo regulation of the pituitary growth hormone–releasing hormone (GHRH) receptor by GHRH in young and aged rats. Endocrinology 140:2836–2842, 1999.

226. Sonntag WE, Gough MA: Growth hormone releasing hormone induced release of growth hormone in aging male rats: Dependence on pharmacological manipulation and endogenous somatostatin release. Neuroendocrinology 47:482–488, 1988.

227. Ceda GP, Valenti G, Butturini U, et al: Diminished pituitary responsiveness to growth hormone–releasing factor in aging male rats. Endocrinology 118:2109–2114, 1986.

228. Lang I, Kurz R, Geyer G, et al: The influence of age on human pancreatic growth hormone releasing hormone stimulated growth hormone secretion. Horm Metab Res 20:574–578, 1988.

229. Pavlov EP, Harman SM, Merriam GR, et al: Responses of growth hormone (GH) and somatomedin-C to GH-releasing hormone in healthy aging men. J Clin Endocrinol Metab 62:595–600, 1986.

230. Argente J, Chowen JA, Zeitler P, et al: Sexual dimorphism of growth hormone–releasing hormone and somatostatin gene expression in the hypothalamus of the rat during development. Endocrinology 128:2369–2375, 1991.

231. Maiter DM, Gabriel SM, Koenig JI, et al: Sexual differentiation of growth hormone feedback effects on hypothalamic growth hormone–releasing hormone and somatostatin. Neuroendocrinology 51:174–180, 1990.

232. Zeitler P, Argente J, Chowen-Breed JA, et al: Growth hormone–releasing hormone messenger ribonucleic acid in the hypothalamus of the adult male rat is increased by testosterone. Endocrinology 127:1362–1368, 1990.

233. Zeitler P, Vician L, Chowen Breed JA, et al: Regulation of somatostatin and growth hormone–releasing hormone gene expression in the rat brain. Metabolism 39:46–49, 1990.

234. Maiter D, Koenig JI, Kaplan LM: Sexually dimorphic expression of the growth hormone–releasing hormone gene is not mediated by circulating gonadal hormones in the adult rat. Endocrinology 128:1709–1716, 1991.

235. Aguilar E, Pinilla L: Ovarian role in the modulation of pituitary responsiveness to growth hormone–releasing hormone in rats. Neuroendocrinology 54:286–290, 1991.

236. Evans WS, Krieg RJ, Limber ER, et al: Effects of in vivo gonadal hormone environment on in vitro hGRF-40-stimulated GH release. Am J Physiol 249:E276–280, 1985.

237. Hertz P, Silbermann M, Even L, et al: Effects of sex steroids on the response of cultured rat pituitary cells to growth hormone–releasing hormone and somatostatin. Endocrinology 125:581–585, 1989.

238. Leong DA, Lau SK, Sinha YN, et al: Enumeration of lactotropes and somatotropes among male and female pituitary cells in culture: Evidence in favor of a mammosomatotrope subpopulation in the rat. Endocrinology 116:1371–1378, 1985.

239. Ho KY, Thorner MO, Krieg RJ Jr, et al: Effects of gonadal steroids on somatotroph function in the rat: Analysis by the reverse hemolytic plaque assay. Endocrinology 123:1405–1411, 1988.

240. Alvarez CV, Mallo F, Burguera B, et al: Evidence for a direct pituitary inhibition by free fatty acids of in vivo growth hormone responses to growth hormone–releasing hormone in the rat. Neuroendocrinology 53:185–189, 1991.

241. Grings EE, Scarborough R, Schally AV, et al: Response to a growth hormone-releasing hormone analog in heifers treated with recombinant growth hormone. Domest Anim Endocrinol 5:47–53, 1988.

242. Levy A, Matovelle MC, Lightman SL, et al: The effects of pituitary stalk transection, hypophysectomy and thyroid hormone status on insulin-like growth factor 2–, growth hormone releasing hormone–, and somatostatin–mRNA prevalence in rat brain. Brain Res 579:1–7, 1992.

243. Katakami H, Downs TR, Frohman LA: Decreased hypothalamic growth hormone–releasing hormone content and pituitary responsiveness in hypothyroidism. J Clin Invest 77:1704–1711, 1986.

244. Edwards CA, Dieguez C, Scanlon MF: Effects of hypothyroidism, triiodothyronine and glucocorticoids on growth hormone responses to growth hormone–releasing hormone and His-D-Trp-Ala-Trp-D-Phe-Lys-NH₂. J Endocrinol 121:31–36, 1989.

245. Wehrenberg WB, Baird A, Ling N: Potent interaction between glucocorticoids and growth hormone–releasing factor in vivo. Science 221:556–558, 1983.

246. Wehrenberg WB, Baird A, Klepper R, et al: Interactions between growth hormone–releasing hormone and glucocorticoids in male rats. Regul Pept 25:147–155, 1989.

247. Miell J, Corder R, Miell PJ, et al: Effects of glucocorticoid treatment and acute passive immunization with growth hormone–releasing hormone and somatostatin antibodies on endogenous and stimulated growth hormone secretion in the male rat. J Endocrinol 131:75–86, 1991.

248. Senaris RM, Lago F, Coya R, et al: Regulation of hypothalamic somatostatin, growth hormone–releasing hormone, and growth hormone receptor messenger ribonucleic acid by glucocorticoids. Endocrinology 137:5236–5241, 1996.

249. Asa SL, Kovacs K, Stefaneanu L, et al: Pituitary mammosomatotroph adenomas develop in old mice transgenic for growth hormone–releasing hormone. Proc Soc Exp Biol Med 193:232–235, 1990.

250. Asa SL: The role of hypothalamic hormones in the pathogenesis of pituitary adenomas. Pathol Res Pract 187:581–583, 1991.

251. Cronin MJ, Burnier J, Clarke RG: Growth hormone releasing hormone infusion in normal rats enlarges the pituitary within days. J Endocrinol Invest 14:34, 1991.

252. Horacek MJ, Campbell GT, Blake CA: Effects of growth hormone–releasing hormone on somatotrophs in anterior pituitary gland allografts in hypophysectomized, orchidectomized hamsters. Cell Tissue Res 253:287–290, 1988.

253. Lehy T, Accary JP, Dubrasquet M, et al: Growth hormone–releasing factor (somatocrinin) stimulates epithelial cell proliferation in the rat digestive tract. Gastroenterology 90:646–653, 1986.

254. Hermansen K, Kappelgaard AM: Characterization of growth hormone–releasing hormone stimulation of the endocrine pancreas: Studies with alpha- and beta-adrenergic and cholinergic antagonists. Acta Endocrinol 114:589–594, 1987.

255. Bailey CJ, Wilkes LC, Flatt PR, et al: Effects of growth hormone–releasing hormone on the secretion of islet hormones and on glucose homeostasis in lean and genetically obese-diabetic (ob/ob) mice and normal rats. J Endocrinol 123:19–24, 1989.

256. Green IC, Southern C, Ray K: Mechanism of action of growth hormone–releasing hormone in stimulating insulin secretion in vitro from isolated rat islets and dispersed islet cells. Horm Res 33:199–204, 1990.

257. Horvath S, Mezey E, Palkovits M: Partial coexistence of growth hormone–releasing hormone and tyrosine hydroxylase in paraventricular neurons in rats. Peptides 10:791–795, 1989.

258. Kentroti S, Vernadakis A: Growth hormone–releasing hormone influences neuronal expression in the developing chick brain. I. Catecholaminergic neurons. Brain Res 49:275–280, 1989.

259. Kentroti S, Vernadakis A: Growth hormone–releasing hormone and somatostatin influence neuronal expression in developing chick brain. II. Cholinergic neurons. Brain Res 512:297–303, 1990.

260. Mitsuma T, Nogimori T, Hirooka Y: Effects of growth hormone–releasing hormone and corticotropin-releasing hormone on the release of thyrotropin-releasing hormone from the rat hypothalamus in vitro. Exp Clin Endocrinol 90:365–368, 1987.

261. Imaki T, Shibasaki T, Hotta M, et al: The satiety effect of growth hormone–releasing factor in rats. Brain Res 340:186–188, 1985.

262. Dickson PR, Vaccarino FJ: Characterization of feeding behavior induced by central injection of GRF. Am J Physiol 259:R651–657, 1990.

263. Vaccarino FJ, Bloom FE, Rivier J, et al: Stimulation of food intake in rats by centrally administered hypothalamic growth hormone–releasing factor. Nature 314:167–168, 1985.

264. Ruckebusch Y, Malbert CH: Stimulation and inhibition of food intake in sheep by centrally-administered hypothalamic releasing factors. Life Sci 38:929–934, 1986.

265. Penny ES, Sopwith AM, Patience RL, et al: Characterization by high-performance liquid chromatography of circulating growth hormone–releasing factors in normal subjects. J Endocrinol 111:507–511, 1986.

266. Wehrenberg WB, Ehlers CL: Effects of growth hormone–releasing factor in the brain. Science 232:1271–1273, 1986.

267. Obal F Jr, Payne L, Opp M, et al: Growth hormone–releasing hormone antibodies suppress sleep and prevent enhancement of sleep after sleep deprivation. Am J Physiol 263:R1078–1085, 1992.

268. Zhang J, Obal F Jr, Zheng T, et al: Intrapreoptic microinjection of GHRH or its antagonist alters sleep in rats. J Neurosci 19:2187–2194, 1999.

269. Toppila J, Alanko L, Asikainen M, et al: Sleep deprivation increases somatostatin and growth hormone–releasing hormone messenger RNA in the rat hypothalamus. J Sleep Res 6:171–178, 1997.

270. Zhang J, Chen Z, Taishi P, et al: Sleep deprivation increases rat hypothalamic growth hormone–releasing hormone mRNA. Am J Physiol 275:R1755–1761, 1998.

271. Bowers CY, Momany F, Reynolds GA, et al: Structure-activity relationships of a synthetic pentapeptide that specifically releases growth hormone in vitro. Endocrinology 106:663–667, 1980.

272. Bowers CY, Momany FA, Reynolds GA, et al: On the in vitro and in vivo activity of a new synthetic hexapeptide that acts on the pituitary to specifically release growth hormone. Endocrinology 114:1537–1545, 1984.

273. Bowers CY, Sartor AO, Reynolds GA, et al: On the actions of the growth hormone-releasing hexapeptide, GHRP. Endocrinology 128:2027–2035, 1991.

274. Bowers CY, Reynolds GA, Durham D, et al: Growth hormone (GH)–releasing peptide stimulates GH release in normal men and acts synergistically with GH-releasing hormone. J Clin Endocrinol Metab 70:975–982, 1990.

275. Howard AD, Feighner SD, Cully DF, et al: A receptor in pituitary and hypothalamus that functions in growth hormone release. Science 273:974–977, 1996.

276. Conn PM, Bowers CY: A new receptor for growth hormone–release peptide. Science 273:923, 1996.

277. Momany FA, Bowers CY, Reynolds GA, et al: Design, synthesis, and biological activity of peptides which release growth hormone in vitro. Endocrinology 108:31–39, 1981.

278. Bowers CY, Reynolds GA, Bowers CV, et al: Dimensions of GH releasing peptides (GHRPs). Presented at 75th Annual Meeting of the Endocrine Society, Las Vegas, June 9–12, 1993, 413 (abstract).

279. Deghenghi R, Cananzi MM, Torsello A, et al: GH-releasing activity of hexarelin, a new growth hormone releasing peptide, in infant and adult rats. Life Sci 54:1321–1328, 1994.

280. Arvat E, di Vito L, Maccagno B, et al: Effects of GHRP-2 and hexarelin, two synthetic GH-releasing peptides, on GH, prolactin, ACTH and cortisol levels in man. Comparison with the effects of GHRH, TRH and hCRH. Peptides 18:885–891, 1997.

281. Ghigo E, Arvat E, Camanni F: Orally active growth hormone secretagogues: State of the art and clinical perspectives. Ann Med 30:159–168, 1998.

282. Cheng K, Chan WW, Butler B, et al: Stimulation of growth hormone release from rat primary pituitary cells by L-692,429, a novel non-peptidyl GH secretagogue. Endocrinology 132:2729–2731, 1993.

283. Gertz BJ, Barrett JS, Eisenhandler R, et al: Growth hormone response in man to L-692,429, a novel nonpeptide mimic of growth hormone–releasing peptide-6. J Clin Endocrinol Metab 77:1393–1397, 1993.

284. Aloi JA, Gertz BJ, Hartman ML, et al: Neuroendocrine responses to a novel growth hormone secretagogue, L-692,429, in healthy older subjects. J Clin Endocrinol Metab 79:943–949, 1994.
285. Patchett AA, Nargund RP, Tata JR, et al: Design and biological activities of L-163,191 (MK-0677): A potent, orally active growth hormone secretagogue. Proc Natl Acad Sci U S A 92:7001–7005, 1995.
286. Smith RG, Van der Ploeg LH, Howard AD, et al: Peptidomimetic regulation of growth hormone secretion. Endocr Rev 18:621–645, 1997.
287. Chapman IM, Hartman ML, Pezzoli SS, et al: Enhancement of pulsatile growth hormone secretion by continuous infusion of a growth hormone–releasing peptide mimetic, L-692,429, in older adults—a clinical research center study. J Clin Endocrinol Metab 81:2874–2880, 1996.
288. Raun K, Hansen BS, Johansen NL, et al: Ipamorelin, the first selective growth hormone secretagogue. Eur J Endocrinol 139:552–561, 1998.
289. Locke W, Kirgis HD, Bowers CY, et al: Intracerebroventricular growth-hormone–releasing peptide-6 stimulates eating without affecting plasma growth hormone responses in rats. Life Sci 56:1347–1352, 1995.
290. Torsello A, Luoni M, Schweiger F, et al: Novel hexarelin analogs stimulate feeding in the rat through a mechanism not involving growth hormone release. Eur J Pharmacol 360:123–129, 1998.
291. Frieboes RM, Murck H, Maier P, et al: Growth hormone–releasing peptide-6 stimulates sleep, growth hormone, ACTH and cortisol release in normal man. Neuroendocrinology 61:584–589, 1995.
292. Bisi G, Podio V, Valetto MR, et al: Acute cardiovascular and hormonal effects of GH and hexarelin, a synthetic GH-releasing peptide, in humans. J Endocrinol Invest 22:266–272, 1999.
293. Broglio F, Valetto MR, Podio V, et al: The acute administration of hexarelin, a synthetic GHRP, but not of growth hormone increases left ventricular ejection fraction in normal man. Presented at 80th Endocrine Society Meeting, New Orleans, June 24–27, 1998, abstract 15–3.
294. Locatelli V, Torsello A: Growth hormone secretagogues: Focus on the growth hormone–releasing peptides. Pharmacol Res 36:415–423, 1997.
295. Dickson SL, Leng G, Dyball RE, et al: Central actions of peptide and non-peptide growth hormone secretagogues in the rat. Neuroendocrinology 61:36–43, 1995.
296. Sirinathsinghji DJ, Chen HY, Hopkins R, et al: Induction of c-*fos* mRNA in the arcuate nucleus of normal and mutant growth hormone–deficient mice by a synthetic non-peptidyl growth hormone secretagogue. Neuroreport 6:1989–1992, 1995.
297. Elias KA, Ingle GS, Burnier JP, et al: In vitro characterization of four novel classes of growth hormone–releasing peptide. Endocrinology 136:5694–5699, 1995.
298. Torsello A, Grilli R, Luoni M, et al: Mechanism of action of hexarelin. I. Growth hormone–releasing activity in the rat. Eur J Endocrinol 135:481–488, 1996.
299. Locatelli V, Grilli R, Torsello A, et al: Growth hormone–releasing hexapeptide is a potent stimulator of growth hormone gene expression and release in the growth hormone–releasing hormone–deprived infant rat. Pediatr Res 36:169–174, 1994.
300. Bennett PA, Thomas GB, Howard AD, et al: Hypothalamic growth hormone secretagogue-receptor (GHS-R) expression is regulated by growth hormone in the rat. Endocrinology 138:4552–4557, 1997.
301. Loche S, Cambiaso P, Merola B, et al: The effect of hexarelin on growth hormone (GH) secretion in patients with GH deficiency. J Clin Endocrinol Metab 80:2692–2696, 1995.
302. Popovic V, Damjanovic S, Micic D, et al: Blocked growth hormone–releasing peptide (GHRP-6)–induced GH secretion and absence of the synergic action of GHRP-6 plus GH-releasing hormone in patients with hypothalamopituitary disconnection: Evidence that GHRP-6 main action is exerted at the hypothalamic level. J Clin Endocrinol Metab 80:942–947, 1995.
303. Hickey GJ, Drisko J, Faidley T, et al: Mediation by the central nervous system is critical to the in vivo activity of the GH secretagogue L-692,585. J Endocrinol 148:371–380, 1996.
304. Cheng K, Chan WW, Butler B, et al: Evidence for a role of protein kinase-C in His-D-Trp-Ala-Trp-D-Phe-Lys-NH_2-induced growth hormone release from rat primary pituitary cells. Endocrinology 129:3337–3342, 1991.
305. Akman MS, Girard M, O'Brien LF, et al: Mechanisms of action of a second generation growth hormone–releasing peptide (Ala-His-D-beta Nal-Ala-Trp-D-Phe-Lys-NH_2) in rat anterior pituitary cells. Endocrinology 132:1286–1291, 1993.
306. Pong SS, Chaung LY, Dean DC, et al: Identification of a new G-protein–linked receptor for growth hormone secretagogues. Mol Endocrinol 10:57–61, 1996.
307. McKee KK, Tan CP, Palyha OC, et al: Cloning and characterization of two human G protein–coupled receptor genes (GPR38 and GPR39) related to the growth hormone secretagogue and neurotensin receptors. Genomics 46:426–434, 1997.
308. Tan CP, McKee KK, Liu Q, et al: Cloning and characterization of a human and murine T-cell orphan G-protein–coupled receptor similar to the growth hormone secretagogue and neurotensin receptors. Genomics 52:223–229, 1998.
309. Feighner SD, Tan CP, McKee KK, et al: Receptor for motilin identified in the human gastrointestinal system. Science 284:2184–2188, 1999.
310. Muccioli G, Ghe C, Ghigo MC, et al: Specific receptors for synthetic GH secretagogues in the human brain and pituitary gland. J Endocrinol 157:99–106, 1998.
311. Guan XM, Yu H, Palyha OC, et al: Distribution of mRNA encoding the growth hormone secretagogue receptor in brain and peripheral tissues. Brain Res Mol Brain Res 48:23–29, 1997.
312. Okada K, Ishii S, Minami S, et al: Intracerebroventricular administration of the growth hormone–releasing peptide KP-102 increases food intake in free-feeding rats. Endocrinology 137:5155–5158, 1996.
313. Yokote R, Sato M, Matsubara S, et al: Molecular cloning and gene expression of growth hormone–releasing peptide receptor in rat tissues. Peptides 19:15–20, 1998.
314. Adams EF, Huang B, Buchfelder M, et al: Presence of growth hormone secretagogue receptor messenger ribonucleic acid in human pituitary tumors and rat GH3 cells. J Clin Endocrinol Metab 83:638–642, 1998.
315. Skinner MM, Nass R, Lopes B, et al: Growth hormone secretagogue receptor expression in human pituitary tumors. J Clin Endocrinol Metab 83:4314–4320, 1998.
316. Korbonits M, Jacobs RA, Aylwin SJ, et al: Expression of the growth hormone secretagogue receptor in pituitary adenomas and other neuroendocrine tumors. J Clin Endocrinol Metab 83:3624–3630, 1998.
317. Renner U, Brockmeier S, Strasburger CJ, et al: Growth hormone (GH)–releasing peptide stimulation of GH release from human somatotroph adenoma cells: Interaction with GH-releasing hormone, thyrotropin-releasing hormone, and octreotide. J Clin Endocrinol Metab 78:1090–1096, 1994.
318. Kamegai J, Wakabayashi I, Miyamoto K, et al: Growth hormone–dependent regulation of pituitary GH secretagogue receptor (GHS-R) mRNA levels in the spontaneous dwarf rat. Neuroendocrinology 68:312–318, 1998.
319. Kamegai J, Wakabayashi I, Kineman RD, et al: Growth hormone–releasing hormone receptor (GHRH-R) and growth hormone secretagogue receptor (GHS-R) mRNA levels during postnatal development in male and female rats. J Neuroendocrinol 11:299–306, 1999.
320. Kineman RD, Kamegai J, Frohman LA: Growth hormone (GH)–releasing hormone (GHRH) and the GH secretagogue (GHS), L692,585, differentially modulate rat pituitary GHS receptor and GHRH receptor messenger ribonucleic acid levels. Endocrinology 140:3581–3586, 1999.
321. Sethumadhavan K, Veeraragavan K, Bowers CY: Demonstration and characterization of the specific binding of growth hormone–releasing peptide to rat anterior pituitary and hypothalamic membranes. Biochem Biophys Res Commun 178:31–37, 1991.
322. Codd EE, Shu AY, Walker RF: Binding of a growth hormone releasing hexapeptide to specific hypothalamic and pituitary binding sites. Neuropharmacology 28:1139–1144, 1989.
323. Ong H, McNicoll N, Escher E, et al: Identification of a pituitary growth hormone–releasing peptide (GHRP) receptor subtype by photoaffinity labeling. Endocrinology 139:432–435, 1998.
324. De Gennaro Colonna V, Rossoni G, Bernareggi M, et al: Cardiac ischemia and impairment of vascular endothelium function in hearts from growth hormone–deficient rats: Protection by hexarelin. Eur J Pharmacol 334:201–207, 1997.
325. Cheng J, Wu TJ, Butler B, et al: Growth hormone releasing peptides: A comparison of the growth hormone releasing activities of GHRP-2 and GHRP-6 in rat primary pituitary cells. Life Sci 60:1385–1392, 1997.
326. Lei T, Buchfelder M, Fahlbusch R, et al: Growth hormone releasing peptide (GHRP-6) stimulates phosphatidylinositol (PI) turnover in human pituitary somatotroph cells. J Mol Endocrinol 14:135–138, 1995.
327. Mitani M, Kaji H, Abe H, et al: Growth hormone (GH)–releasing peptide and GH releasing hormone stimulate GH release from subpopulations of somatotrophs in rats. J Neuroendocrinol 8:825–830, 1996.
328. Goth MI, Lyons CE, Canny BJ, et al: Pituitary adenylate cyclase activating polypeptide, growth hormone (GH)–releasing peptide and GH-releasing hormone stimulate GH release through distinct pituitary receptors. Endocrinology 130:939–944, 1992.
329. Soliman EB, Hashizume T, Kanematsu S: Effect of growth hormone (GH)–releasing peptide (GHRP) on the release of GH from cultured anterior pituitary cells in cattle. Endocr J 41:585–591, 1994.
330. Smith RG, Pong SS, Hickey G, et al: Modulation of pulsatile GH release through a novel receptor in hypothalamus and pituitary gland. Recent Prog Horm Res 51:261–285[discussion 285–266], 1996.
331. Chen C, Wu D, Clarke IJ: Signal transduction systems employed by synthetic GH-releasing peptides in somatotrophs. J Endocrinol 148:381–386, 1996.
332. Giustina A, Bonfanti C, Licini M, et al: Hexarelin, a novel GHRP-6 analog, stimulates growth hormone (GH) release in a GH-secreting rat cell line (GH1) insensitive to GH-releasing hormone. Regul Pept 70:49–54, 1997.
333. Torsello A, Luoni M, Grilli R, et al: Hexarelin stimulation of growth hormone release and mRNA levels in an infant and adult rat model of impaired GHRH function. Neuroendocrinology 65:91–97, 1997.
334. Guillaume V, Magnan E, Cataldi M, et al: Growth hormone (GH)–releasing hormone secretion is stimulated by a new GH-releasing hexapeptide in sheep. Endocrinology 135:1073–1076, 1994.
335. Bercu BB, Yang SW, Masuda R, et al: Role of selected endogenous peptides in growth hormone–releasing hexapeptide activity: Analysis of growth hormone–releasing hormone, thyroid hormone–releasing hormone, and gonadotropin-releasing hormone. Endocrinology 130:2579–2586, 1992.
336. Conley LK, Teik JA, Deghenghi R, et al: Mechanism of action of hexarelin and GHRP-6: Analysis of the involvement of GHRH and somatostatin in the rat. Neuroendocrinology 61:44–50, 1995.
337. Jansson J-O, Downs TR, Beamer WG, et al: The dwarf "little" (lit/lit) mouse is resistant to growth hormone (GH)–releasing peptide (GH-RP-6) as well as to GH-releasing hormone (GRH). Presented at the 68th Annual Meeting of the Endocrine Society, Anaheim, CA, 1986, abstract 397.
338. Fletcher TP, Thomas GB, Willoughby JO, et al: Constitutive growth hormone secretion in sheep after hypothalamopituitary disconnection and the direct in vivo pituitary effect of growth hormone releasing peptide 6. Neuroendocrinology 60:76–86, 1994.
339. Tannenbaum GS, Lapointe M, Beaudet A, et al: Expression of growth hormone secretagogue-receptors by growth hormone–releasing hormone neurons in the mediobasal hypothalamus. Endocrinology 139:4420–4423, 1998.
340. Dickson SL, Luckman SM: Induction of c-*fos* messenger ribonucleic acid in neuropeptide Y and growth hormone (GH)–releasing factor neurons in the rat arcuate nucleus following systemic injection of the GH secretagogue, GH-releasing peptide-6. Endocrinology 138:771–777, 1997.
341. Korbonits M, Little JA, Forsling ML, et al: The effect of growth hormone secretagogues and neuropeptide Y on hypothalamic hormone release from acute rat hypothalamic explants. J Neuroendocrinol 11:521–528, 1999.
342. Cattaneo L, Luoni M, Settembrini B, et al: Effect of long-term administration of hexarelin on the somatotrophic axis in aged rats. Pharmacol Res 36:49–54, 1997.
343. Rosskamp R, Becker M, Haverkamp F, et al: Plasma levels of growth hormone–releasing hormone and somatostatin in response to a mixed meal and during sleep in children. Acta Endocrinol 116:549–554, 1987.

344. Penny ES, Penman E, Price J, et al: Circulating growth hormone releasing factor concentrations in normal subjects and patients with acromegaly. BMJ 289:453–455, 1984.
345. Inoue S, Katakami H, Hidaka H, et al: Peripheral plasma levels of human growth hormone releasing hormone (GHRH) during the sleep test in short children. Endocr J 45:S71–75, 1998.
346. Sopwith AM, Penny ES, Lytras N, et al: Dissociation between circulating concentrations of immunoreactive growth hormone releasing factor and growth hormone in normal human subjects. Clin Sci 72:181–185, 1987.
347. Frohman LA, Downs TR, Williams TC, et al: Rapid enzymatic degradation of growth hormone–releasing hormone by plasma in vitro and in vivo to a biologically inactive product cleaved at the NH_2 terminus. J Clin Invest 78:906–913, 1986.
348. Katakami H, Hashida S, Hidaka H, et al: Development and clinical application of a highly sensitive enzyme immunoassay (EIA) for human growth hormone–releasing hormone (hGHRH) in plasma. Endocr J 45:S67–70, 1998.
349. Thorner MO, Frohman LA, Leong DA, et al: Extrahypothalamic growth-hormone–releasing factor (GRF) secretion is a rare cause of acromegaly: Plasma GRF levels in 177 acromegalic patients. J Clin Endocrinol Metab 59:846–849, 1984.
350. Sano T, Asa SL, Kovacs K: Growth hormone–releasing hormone–producing tumors: Clinical, biochemical, and morphological manifestations. Endocr Rev 9:357–373, 1988.
351. Faglia G, Arosio M, Bazzoni N: Ectopic acromegaly. Endocrinol Metab Clin North Am 21:575–595, 1992.
352. Kovacs M, Kineman RD, Schally AV, et al: Effects of antagonists of growth hormone–releasing hormone (GHRH) on GH and insulin-like growth factor I levels in transgenic mice overexpressing the human GHRH gene, an animal model of acromegaly. Endocrinology 138:4536–4542, 1997.
353. Sano T, Yamasaki R, Saito H, et al: Growth hormone–releasing hormone (GHRH)–secreting pancreatic tumor in a patient with multiple endocrine neoplasia type I. Am J Surg Pathol 11:810–819, 1987.
354. Asa SL, Singer W, Kovacs K, et al: Pancreatic endocrine tumour producing growth hormone–releasing hormone associated with multiple endocrine neoplasia type I syndrome. Acta Endocrinol 115:331–337, 1987.
355. Ramsay JA, Kovacs K, Asa SL, et al: Reversible sellar enlargement due to growth hormone–releasing hormone production by pancreatic endocrine tumors in an acromegalic patient with multiple endocrine neoplasia type I syndrome. Cancer 62:445–450, 1988.
356. Yamasaki R, Saito H, Sano T, et al: Ectopic growth hormone–releasing hormone (GHRH) syndrome in a case with multiple endocrine neoplasia type I. Endocr J 35:97–109, 1988.
357. Liu SW, van de Velde CJ, Heslinga JM, et al: Acromegaly caused by growth hormone–relating hormone in a patient with multiple endocrine neoplasia type I. Jpn J Clin Oncol 26:49–52, 1996.
358. Asa SL, Scheithauer BW, Bilbao JM, et al: A case for hypothalamic acromegaly: A clinicopathological study of six patients with hypothalamic gangliocytomas producing growth hormone–releasing factor. J Clin Endocrinol Metab 58:796–803, 1984.
359. Bevan JS, Asa SL, Rossi ML, et al: Intrasellar gangliocytoma containing gastrin and growth hormone–releasing hormone associated with a growth hormone–secreting pituitary adenoma. Clin Endocrinol (Oxf) 30:213–224, 1989.
360. Kojima K, Miyake M, Nakagawa H, et al: Multiple gastric carcinoids and pituitary adenoma in type A gastritis. Intern Med 36:787–789, 1997.
361. Garcia-Rojas JF, Mangas A, Barba A, et al: Role of growth hormone–releasing hormone on pentagastrin-induced growth hormone release in normal subjects. J Endocrinol Invest 14:241–244, 1991.
362. Donnadieu M, Evain-Brion D, Tonon MC, et al: Variations of plasma growth hormone (GH)–releasing factor levels during GH stimulation tests in children. J Clin Endocrinol Metab 60:1132–1134, 1985.
363. Argente J, Evain Brion D, Donnadieu M, et al: Impaired response of growth hormone–releasing hormone (GHRH) measured in plasma after L-dopa stimulation in patients with idiopathic delayed puberty. Acta Paediatr Scand 76:266–270, 1987.
364. Mitsuhashi S, Yamasaki R, Miyazaki S, et al: Effect of oral administration of L-dopa on the plasma levels of growth hormone–releasing hormone (GHRH) in normal subjects and patients with various endocrine and metabolic diseases. Nippon Naibunpi Gakkai Zasshi 63:934–946, 1987.
365. Chihara K, Kashio Y, Kita T, et al: L-dopa stimulates release of hypothalamic growth hormone–releasing hormone in humans. J Clin Endocrinol Metab 62:466–473, 1986.
366. Kashio Y, Chihara K, Kita T, et al: Effect of oral glucose administration on plasma growth hormone–releasing hormone (GHRH)-like immunoreactivity levels in normal subjects and patients with idiopathic GH deficiency: Evidence that GHRH is released not only from the hypothalamus but also from extrahypothalamic tissue. J Clin Endocrinol Metab 64:92–97, 1987.
367. Rosskamp R, Becker M, Tegeler A, et al: Effect of insulin-induced hypoglycemia on circulating levels of plasma growth hormone–releasing hormone and somatostatin in children. Horm Res 27:121–125, 1987.
368. Kashio Y, Chihara K, Kaji H, et al: Presence of growth hormone–releasing factor-like immunoreactivity in human cerebrospinal fluid. J Clin Endocrinol Metab 60:396–398, 1985.
369. Growth Hormone Research Society: Consensus guidelines for the diagnosis and treatment of adults with growth hormone deficiency: Summary statement of the Growth Hormone Research Society workshop on adult growth hormone deficiency. J Clin Endocrinol Metab 83:379–381, 1998.
370. Rahim A, Toogood AA, Shalet SM: The assessment of growth hormone status in normal young adult males using a variety of provocative tests. Clin Endocrinol (Oxf) 45:557–562, 1996.
371. Shibasaki T, Shizume K, Nakahara M, et al: Age-related changes in plasma growth hormone response to growth hormone–releasing factor in man. J Clin Endocrinol Metab 58:212–214, 1984.
372. Thorner MO, Rivier J, Spiess J, et al: Human pancreatic growth-hormone–releasing factor selectively stimulates growth-hormone secretion in man. Lancet 1:24–28, 1983.
373. Wood SM, Ch'ng JL, Adams EF, et al: Abnormalities of growth hormone release in response to human pancreatic growth hormone releasing factor (GRF (1–44)) in acromegaly and hypopituitarism. BMJ 286:1687–1691, 1983.
374. Rosenthal SM, Schriock EA, Kaplan SL, et al: Synthetic human pancreas growth hormone–releasing factor (hpGRF1–44-NH_2) stimulates growth hormone secretion in normal men. J Clin Endocrinol Metab 57:677–679, 1983.
375. Gelato MC, Pescovitz OH, Cassorla F, et al: Dose-response relationships for the effects of growth hormone–releasing factor-(1–44)-NH_2 in young adult men and women. J Clin Endocrinol Metab 59:197–201, 1984.
376. Sassolas G, Chatelain P, Cohen R, et al: Effects of human pancreatic tumor growth hormone–releasing hormone (hpGRH1–44-NH_2) on immunoreactive and bioactive plasma growth hormone in normal young men. J Clin Endocrinol Metab 59:705–709, 1984.
377. Lang I, Schernthaner G, Pietschmann P, et al: Effects of sex and age on growth hormone response to growth hormone–releasing hormone in healthy individuals. J Clin Endocrinol Metab 65:535–540, 1987.
378. Chihara K, Kashio Y, Abe H, et al: Idiopathic growth hormone (GH) deficiency, and GH deficiency secondary to hypothalamic germinoma: Effect of single and repeated administration of human GH-releasing factor (hGRF) on plasma GH level and endogenous hGRF-like immunoreactivity level in cerebrospinal fluid. J Clin Endocrinol Metab 60:269–278, 1985.
379. Evans WS, Borges JL, Vance ML, et al: Effects of human pancreatic growth hormone-releasing factor-40 on serum growth hormone, prolactin, luteinizing hormone, follicle-stimulating hormone, and somatomedin-C concentrations in normal women throughout the menstrual cycle. J Clin Endocrinol Metab 59:1006–1010, 1984.
380. Vance ML, Borges JL, Kaiser DL, et al: Human pancreatic tumor growth hormone–releasing factor: Dose-response relationships in normal man. J Clin Endocrinol Metab 58:838–844, 1984.
381. Gelato M, Malozowski S, Nicoletti M: Responses to growth hormone releasing hormone during development and puberty in normal boys and girls. *In* Symposium on Recent Developments in the Study of Growth Factors: GRF and Somatomedin. Basel, S Karger, 1985.
382. Ghigo E, Bellone J, Aimaretti G, et al: Reliability of provocative tests to assess growth hormone secretory status. Study in 472 normally growing children. J Clin Endocrinol Metab 81:3323–3327, 1996.
383. Gelato MC, Malozowski S, Caruso-Nicoletti M, et al: Growth hormone (GH) responses to GH-releasing hormone during pubertal development in normal boys and girls: Comparison to idiopathic short stature and GH deficiency. J Clin Endocrinol Metab 63:174–179, 1986.
384. Ross RJ, Grossman A, Davies PS, et al: Stilboestrol pretreatment of children with short stature does not affect the growth hormone response to growth hormone–releasing hormone. Clin Endocrinol (Oxf) 27:155–161, 1987.
385. Iovino M, Monteleone P, Steardo L: Repetitive growth hormone–releasing hormone administration restores the attenuated growth hormone (GH) response to GH-releasing hormone testing in normal aging. J Clin Endocrinol Metab 69:910–913, 1989.
386. Coiro V, Volpi R, Cavazzini U, et al: Restoration of normal growth hormone responsiveness to GHRH in normal aged men by infusion of low amounts of theophylline. J Gerontol 46:M155–M158, 1991.
387. Corpas E, Harman SM, Blackman MR: Human growth hormone and human aging. Endocr Rev 14:20–39, 1993.
388. Ghigo E, Goffi S, Nicolosi M, et al: Growth hormone (GH) responsiveness to combined administration of arginine and GH-releasing hormone does not vary with age in man. J Clin Endocrinol Metab 71:1481–1485, 1990.
389. Ghigo E, Goffi S, Arvat E, et al: Pyridostigmine partially restores the GH responsiveness to GHRH in normal aging. Acta Endocrinol 123:169–173, 1990.
390. Alba-Roth J, Muller OA, Schopohl J, et al: Arginine stimulates growth hormone secretion by suppressing endogenous somatostatin secretion. J Clin Endocrinol Metab 67:1186–1189, 1988.
391. Ross RJ, Tsagarakis S, Grossman A, et al: GH feedback occurs through modulation of hypothalamic somatostatin under cholinergic control: Studies with pyridostigmine and GHRH. Clin Endocrinol (Oxf) 27:727–733, 1987.
392. Grossman A, Savage MO, Besser GM: Growth hormone releasing hormone. Clin Endocrinol Metab 15:607–627, 1986.
393. Ranke MB, Gruhler M, Rosskamp R, et al: Testing with growth hormone–releasing factor (GRF(1–29)NH_2) and somatomedin C measurements for the evaluation of growth hormone deficiency. Eur J Pediatr 145:485–492, 1986.
394. Bozzola M, Tato L, Cisternino M, et al: Synthetic growth hormone–releasing hormone (GHRH 1–44) in the differential diagnosis between hypothalamic and pituitary GH deficiency. J Endocrinol Invest 9:503–506, 1986.
395. Takano K, Hizuka N, Shizume K, et al: Plasma growth hormone (GH) response to GH-releasing factor in normal children with short stature and patients with pituitary dwarfism. J Clin Endocrinol Metab 58:236–241, 1984.
396. Schonberg D: Diagnosis of growth hormone deficiency. Baillieres Clin Endocrinol Metab 6:527–546, 1992.
397. Shalet S, Toogood A, Rahim A, et al: The diagnosis of growth hormone deficiency in children and adults. Endocr Rev 19:203–223, 1998.
398. Toogood A, Jones J, O'Neill P, et al: The diagnosis of severe growth hormone deficiency in elderly patients with hypothalamic-pituitary disease. Clin Endocrinol (Oxf) 48:569–576, 1998.
399. Hoeck HC, Jakobsen PE, Vestergaard P, et al: Differences in reproducibility and peak growth hormone responses to repeated testing with various stimulators in healthy adults. Growth Horm IGF Res 9:18–24, 1999.
400. Chatelain P, Alamercery Y, Blanchard J, et al: Growth hormone (GH) response to a single intravenous injection of synthetic GH-releasing hormone in prepubertal children with growth failure. J Clin Endocrinol Metab 65:387–394, 1987.
401. Schriock EA, Lustig RH, Rosenthal SM, et al: Effect of growth hormone (GH)–releasing hormone (GRH) on plasma GH in relation to magnitude and duration of

GH deficiency in 26 children and adults with isolated GH deficiency or multiple pituitary hormone deficiencies: Evidence for hypothalamic GRH deficiency. J Clin Endocrinol Metab 58:1043–1049, 1984.

402. Laron Z, Keret R, Bauman B, et al: Differential diagnosis between hypothalamic and pituitary hGH deficiency with the aid of synthetic GH-RH 1–44. Clin Endocrinol (Oxf) 21:9–12, 1984.

403. Pintor C, Puggioni R, Fanni V, et al: Growth-hormone releasing factor and clonidine in children with constitutional growth delay. Evidence for defective pituitary growth hormone reserve. J Endocrinol Invest 7:253–256, 1984.

404. Reiter JC, Craen M, van Vliet G: Decreased growth hormone response to growth hormone–releasing hormone in Turner's syndrome: Relation to body weight and adiposity. Acta Endocrinol 125:38–42, 1991.

405. Sartorio A, Spada A, Conti A, et al: Effect of two consecutive administrations of GHRH in children with constitutional growth delay. Eur J Pediatr 149:678–679, 1990.

406. Lannering B, Albertsson-Wikland K: Growth hormone release in children after cranial irradiation. Horm Res 27:13–22, 1987.

407. Takano K, Shizume K, Imura H, et al: Plasma growth hormone (GH) response to GH-releasing factor (SM-8144) in children of short stature and patients with GH deficiency. Endocr J 34:117–128, 1987.

408. Cappa M, Loche S, Borrelli P, et al: Growth hormone response to growth hormone releasing hormone 1–40 in Turner's syndrome. Horm Res 27:1–6, 1987.

409. Rogol AD, Blizzard RM, Johanson AJ, et al: Growth hormone release in response to human pancreatic tumor growth hormone–releasing hormone 1–40 in children with short stature. J Clin Endocrinol Metab 59:580–586, 1984.

410. Ahmed SR, Shalet SM: Hypothalamic growth hormone releasing factor deficiency following cranial irradiation. Clin Endocrinol (Oxf) 21:483–488, 1984.

411. Romer TE, Rymkiewicz-Kluczynska B, Olivier M, et al: Growth hormone–releasing hormone reverses secondary somatotroph unresponsiveness. J Clin Endocrinol Metab 72:503–506, 1991.

412. Hindmarsh PC, Swift PG: An assessment of growth hormone provocation tests. Arch Dis Child 72:362–367[discussion 367–368], 1995.

413. Dysken MW, Skare SS, Burke MS, et al: Intrasubject reproducibility of growth hormone–releasing hormone–stimulated growth hormone in older women, older men, and younger men. Biol Psychiatry 33:610–617, 1993.

414. Williams T, Berelowitz M, Joffe SN, et al: Impaired growth hormone responses to growth hormone–releasing factor in obesity. A pituitary defect reversed with weight reduction. N Engl J Med 311:1403–1407, 1984.

415. Scacchi M, Pincelli AI, Cavagnini F: Growth hormone in obesity. Int J Obes Relat Metab Disord 23:260–271, 1999.

416. Ghigo E, Procopio M, Boffano GM, et al: Arginine potentiates but does not restore the blunted growth hormone response to growth hormone–releasing hormone in obesity. Metabolism 41:560–563, 1992.

417. Bing-You RG, Bigos ST, Oppenheim DS: Serum growth hormone response to growth hormone–releasing hormone in non-obese and obese adults with hypopituitarism. Metabolism 42:790–794, 1993.

418. Cordido F, Casanueva FF, Dieguez C: Cholinergic receptor activation by pyridostigmine restores growth hormone (GH) responsiveness to GH-releasing hormone administration in obese subjects: Evidence for hypothalamic somatostatinergic participation in the blunted GH release of obesity. J Clin Endocrinol Metab 68:290–293, 1989.

419. Ghigo E, Imperiale E, Boffano GM, et al: A new test for the diagnosis of growth hormone deficiency due to primary pituitary impairment: Combined administration of pyridostigmine and growth hormone–releasing hormone. J Endocrinol Invest 13:307–316, 1990.

420. Valetto MR, Bellone J, Baffoni C, et al: Reproducibility of the growth hormone response to stimulation with growth hormone–releasing hormone plus arginine during lifespan. Eur J Endocrinol 135:568–572, 1996.

421. Cappa M, Loche S, Salvatori R, et al: The growth hormone response to pyridostigmine plus growth hormone releasing hormone is not influenced by pubertal maturation. J Endocrinol Invest 14:41–45, 1991.

422. Ghigo E, Aimaretti G, Gianotti L, et al: New approach to the diagnosis of growth hormone deficiency in adults. Eur J Endocrinol 134:352–356, 1996.

423. Aimaretti G, Corneli G, Razzore P, et al: Comparison between insulin-induced hypoglycemia and growth hormone (GH)–releasing hormone + arginine as provocative tests for the diagnosis of GH deficiency in adults. J Clin Endocrinol Metab 83:1615–1618, 1998.

424. Thorner MO, Reschke J, Chitwood J, et al: Acceleration of growth in two children treated with human growth hormone–releasing factor. N Engl J Med 312:4–9, 1985.

425. Thorner MO, Rogol AD, Blizzard RM, et al: Acceleration of growth rate in growth hormone–deficient children treated with human growth hormone–releasing hormone. Pediatr Res 24:145–151, 1988.

426. Low LC: The therapeutic use of growth-hormone–releasing hormone. J Pediatr Endocrinol 6:15–20, 1993.

427. Brain CE, Hindmarsh PC, Brook CG: Continuous subcutaneous GHRH(1–29)NH2 promotes growth over 1 year in short, slowly growing children. Clin Endocrinol (Oxf) 32:153–163, 1990.

428. Neyzi O, Yordam N, Ocal G, et al: Growth response to growth hormone–releasing hormone(1–29)-NH$_2$ compared with growth hormone. Acta Paediatr Suppl 388:16–21[discussion 22], 1993.

429. Chen RG, Shen YN, Yei J, et al: A comparative study of growth hormone (GH) and GH-releasing hormone(1–29)-NH$_2$ for stimulation of growth in children with GH deficiency. Acta Paediatr Suppl 388:32–35[discussion 36], 1993.

430. Ross RJ, Rodda C, Tsagarakis S, et al: Treatment of growth-hormone deficiency with growth-hormone–releasing hormone. Lancet 1:5–8, 1987.

431. Takano K, Hizuka N, Asakawa K, et al: Human growth hormone–releasing hormone (hGH-RH; hGRF) treatment of four patients with GH deficiency. Endocr J 35:775–781, 1988.

432. Smith PJ, Brook CG: Growth hormone releasing hormone or growth hormone treatment in growth hormone insufficiency? Arch Dis Child 63:629–634, 1988.

433. Butenandt O, Staudt B: Comparison of growth hormone releasing hormone therapy and growth hormone therapy in growth hormone deficiency. Eur J Pediatr 148:393–395, 1989.

434. Duck SC, Schwarz HP, Costin G, et al: Subcutaneous growth hormone–releasing hormone therapy in growth hormone–deficient children: First year of therapy. J Clin Endocrinol Metab 75:1115–1120, 1992.

435. Kirk JM, Trainer PJ, Majrowski WH, et al: Treatment with GHRH(1–29)NH$_2$ in children with idiopathic short stature induces a sustained increase in growth velocity. Clin Endocrinol (Oxf) 41:487–493, 1994.

436. Pasqualini T, Ferraris J, Fainstein-Day P, et al: Growth acceleration in children with chronic renal failure treated with growth-hormone–releasing hormone (GHRH). Medicina (B Aires) 56:241–246, 1996.

437. Ogilvy-Stuart AL, Stirling HF, Kelnar CJ, et al: Treatment of radiation-induced growth hormone deficiency with growth hormone–releasing hormone. Clin Endocrinol (Oxf) 46:571–578, 1997.

438. Rochiccioli PE, Tauber MT, Coude FX, et al: Results of 1-year growth hormone (GH)–releasing hormone-(1–44) treatment on growth, somatomedin-C, and 24-hour GH secretion in six children with partial GH deficiency. J Clin Endocrinol Metab 65:268–274, 1987.

439. Bozzola M, Biscaldi I, Cisternino M, et al: Long term growth hormone (GH)–releasing hormone and biosynthetic GH therapy in GH-deficient children: Comparison of therapeutic effectiveness. J Endocrinol Invest 13:235–239, 1990.

440. Lievre M, Chatelain P, Van Vliet G, et al: Treatment with growth hormone–releasing hormone (GHRH) 1–44 in children with idiopathic growth hormone deficiency: A randomized double-blind dose-effect study. The GHRH European Multicenter Study (GEMS) Group. Fundam Clin Pharmacol 6:359–366, 1992.

441. Wit JM, Otten BJ, Waelkens JJ, et al: Short-term effect on growth of two doses of GRF 1–44 in children with growth hormone deficiency: Comparison with growth induced by methionyl-GH administration. Horm Res 27:181–189, 1987.

442. Lanes R, Carrillo E: Long-term therapy with a single daily subcutaneous dose of growth hormone releasing hormone (1–29) in prepubertal growth hormone deficient children. Venezuelan Collaborative Study Group. J Pediatr Endocrinol 7:303–308, 1994.

443. Thorner M, Rochiccioli P, Colle M, et al: Once daily subcutaneous growth hormone–releasing hormone therapy accelerates growth in growth hormone–deficient children during the first year of therapy. Geref International Study Group. J Clin Endocrinol Metab 81:1189–1196, 1996.

444. Low LC, Wang C, Cheung PT, et al: Long term pulsatile growth hormone (GH)–releasing hormone therapy in children with GH deficiency. J Clin Endocrinol Metab 66:611–617, 1988.

445. Lippe BM, Van Herle AJ, LaFranchi SH, et al: Reversible hypothyroidism in growth hormone–deficient children treated with human growth hormone. J Clin Endocrinol Metab 40:612–618, 1975.

446. Ghigo E, Arvat E, Aimaretti G, et al: Diagnostic and therapeutic uses of growth hormone–releasing substances in adult and elderly subjects. Baillieres Clin Endocrinol Metab 12:341–358, 1998.

447. Corpas E, Harman SM, Pineyro MA, et al: Growth hormone (GH)–releasing hormone-(1–29) twice daily reverses the decreased GH and insulin-like growth factor-I levels in old men. J Clin Endocrinol Metab 75:530–535, 1992.

448. Corpas E, Harman SM, Pineyro MA, et al: Continuous subcutaneous infusions of growth hormone (GH) releasing hormone 1–44 for 14 days increase GH and insulin-like growth factor-I levels in old men. J Clin Endocrinol Metab 76:134–138, 1993.

449. Vittone J, Blackman MR, Busby-Whitehead J, et al: Effects of single nightly injections of growth hormone–releasing hormone (GHRH 1–29) in healthy elderly men. Metabolism 46:89–96, 1997.

450. Laron Z, Frenkel J, Gil-Ad I, et al: Growth hormone releasing activity by intranasal administration of a synthetic hexapeptide (hexarelin). Clin Endocrinol (Oxf) 41:539–541, 1994.

451. Imbimbo BP, Mant T, Edwards M, et al: Growth hormone–releasing activity of hexarelin in humans. A dose-response study. Eur J Clin Pharmacol 46:421–425, 1994.

452. Casanueva FF, Micic D, Pombo M, et al: Role of the new growth hormone–releasing secretagogues in the diagnosis of some hypothalamopituitary pathologies. Metabolism 45:123–126, 1996.

453. Arvat E, Gianotti L, Grottoli S, et al: Arginine and growth hormone–releasing hormone restore the blunted growth hormone–releasing activity of hexarelin in elderly subjects. J Clin Endocrinol Metab 79:1440–1443, 1994.

454. Cordido F, Penalva A, Dieguez C, et al: Massive growth hormone (GH) discharge in obese subjects after the combined administration of GH-releasing hormone and GHRP-6: Evidence for a marked somatotroph secretory capability in obesity. J Clin Endocrinol Metab 76:819–823, 1993.

455. Micic D, Popovic V, Doknic M, et al: Preserved growth hormone (GH) secretion in aged and very old subjects after testing with the combined stimulus GH-releasing hormone plus GH-releasing hexapeptide-6. J Clin Endocrinol Metab 83:2569–2572, 1998.

456. Penalva A, Carballo A, Pombo M, et al: Effect of growth hormone (GH)–releasing hormone (GHRH), atropine, pyridostigmine, or hypoglycemia on GHRP-6-induced GH secretion in man. J Clin Endocrinol Metab 76:168–171, 1993.

457. Micic D, Mallo F, Peino R, et al: Regulation of growth hormone secretion by the growth hormone releasing hexapeptide (GHRP-6). J Pediatr Endocrinol 6:283–289, 1993.

458. Maheshwari HG, Rahim A, Shalet SM, et al: Selective lack of growth hormone (GH) response to the GH-releasing peptide hexarelin in patients with GH-releasing hormone receptor deficiency. J Clin Endocrinol Metab 84:956–959, 1999.

459. Maghnie M, Spica-Russotto V, Cappa M, et al: The growth hormone response to hexarelin in patients with different hypothalamic-pituitary abnormalities. J Clin Endocrinol Metab 83:3886–3889, 1998.

460. Arvat E, Gianotti L, Di Vito L, et al: Modulation of growth hormone–releasing activity of hexarelin in man. Neuroendocrinology 61:51–56, 1995.

461. Ghigo E, Arvat E, Rizzi G, et al: Arginine enhances the growth hormone–releasing activity of a synthetic hexapeptide (GHRP-6) in elderly but not in young subjects after oral administration. J Endocrinol Invest 17:157–162, 1994.

462. Ghigo E, Arvat E, Muccioli G, et al: Growth hormone–releasing peptides. Eur J Endocrinol 136:445–460, 1997.

463. Laron Z, Bowers CY, Hirsch D, et al: Growth hormone–releasing activity of growth hormone–releasing peptide-1 (a synthetic heptapeptide) in children and adolescents. Acta Endocrinol 129:424–426, 1993.

464. Bellone J, Aimaretti G, Bartolotta E, et al: Growth hormone–releasing activity of hexarelin, a new synthetic hexapeptide, before and during puberty. J Clin Endocrinol Metab 80:1090–1094, 1995.

465. Loche S, Cambiaso P, Carta D, et al: The growth hormone–releasing activity of hexarelin, a new synthetic hexapeptide, in short normal and obese children and in hypopituitary subjects. J Clin Endocrinol Metab 80:674–678, 1995.

466. Ghigo E, Arvat E, Rizzi G, et al: Growth hormone–releasing activity of growth hormone–releasing peptide-6 is maintained after short-term oral pretreatment with the hexapeptide in normal aging. Eur J Endocrinol 131:499–503, 1994.

467. Penalva A, Pombo M, Carballo A, et al: Influence of sex, age and adrenergic pathways on the growth hormone response to GHRP-6. Clin Endocrinol (Oxf) 38:87–91, 1993.

468. Micic D, Popovic V, Kendereski A, et al: The sequential administration of growth hormone–releasing hormone followed 120 minutes later by hexarelin, as an effective test to assess the pituitary GH reserve in man. Clin Endocrinol (Oxf) 45:543–551, 1996.

469. Gasperi M, Aimaretti G, Scarcello G, et al: Low dose hexarelin and growth hormone (GH)–releasing hormone as a diagnostic tool for the diagnosis of GH deficiency in adults: Comparison with insulin-induced hypoglycemia test. J Clin Endocrinol Metab 84:2633–2637, 1999.

470. Peino R, Leal A, Garcia-Mayor RV, et al: The use of growth hormone (GH) secretagogues in the diagnosis of GH deficiency in humans. Growth Horm IGF Res 9:101–105, 1999.

471. Casanueva FF, Dieguez C: Interaction between body composition, leptin and growth hormone status. Baillieres Clin Endocrinol Metab 12:297–314, 1998.

472. Rahim A, O'Neill PA, Shalet SM: The effect of body composition on hexarelin-induced growth hormone release in normal elderly subjects. Clin Endocrinol (Oxf) 49:659–664, 1998.

473. Casanueva FF, Burguera B, Tome MA, et al: Depending on the time of administration, dexamethasone potentiates or blocks growth hormone–releasing hormone–induced growth hormone release in man. Neuroendocrinology 47:46–49, 1988.

474. Trainer PJ, Kirk JM, Savage MO, et al: Pyridostigmine partially reverses dexamethasone-induced inhibition of the growth hormone response to growth hormone–releasing hormone. J Endocrinol 134:513–517, 1992.

475. Frantz AG, Rabkin MT: Human growth hormone: Clinical measurement, response to hypoglycaemia and suppression by corticosteroids. N Engl J Med 271:1375–1381, 1964.

476. Magiakou MA, Mastorakos G, Gomez MT, et al: Suppressed spontaneous and stimulated growth hormone secretion in patients with Cushing's disease before and after surgical cure. J Clin Endocrinol Metab 78:131–137, 1994.

477. Leal-Cerro A, Pumar A, Garcia-Garcia E, et al: Inhibition of growth hormone release after the combined administration of GHRH and GHRP-6 in patients with Cushing's syndrome. Clin Endocrinol (Oxf) 41:649–654, 1994.

478. Leal-Cerro A, Pumar A, Villamil F, et al: Growth hormone releasing hormone priming increases growth hormone secretion in patients with Cushing's syndrome. Clin Endocrinol (Oxf) 38:399–403, 1993.

479. Momany FA, Bowers CY, Reynolds GA, et al: Conformational energy studies and in vitro and in vivo activity data on growth hormone–releasing peptides. Endocrinology 114:1531–1536, 1984.

480. McDowell RS, Elias KA, Stanley MS, et al: Growth hormone secretagogues: Characterization, efficacy, and minimal bioactive conformation. Proc Natl Acad Sci U S A 92:11165–11169, 1995.

481. Rahim A, O'Neill PA, Shalet SM: Growth hormone status during long-term hexarelin therapy. J Clin Endocrinol Metab 83:1644–1649, 1998.

482. Svensson J, Lonn L, Jansson JO, et al: Two-month treatment of obese subjects with the oral growth hormone (GH) secretagogue MK-677 increases GH secretion, fat-free mass, and energy expenditure. J Clin Endocrinol Metab 83:362–369, 1998.

483. Loche S, Colao A, Cappa M, et al: The growth hormone response to hexarelin in children: Reproducibility and effect of sex steroids. J Clin Endocrinol Metab 82:861–864, 1997.

484. Mericq V, Cassorla F, Salazar T, et al: Effects of eight months treatment with graded doses of a growth hormone (GH)–releasing peptide in GH-deficient children. J Clin Endocrinol Metab 83:2355–2360, 1998.

485. Yu H, Cassorla F, Tiulpakov A, et al: A double blind placebo-controlled efficacy trial of an oral growth hormone (GH) secretagogue (MK-0677) in GH deficient (GHD) children. Presented at 80th Annual Meeting of the Endocrine Society, New Orleans, June 24–27, 1998.

486. Laron Z, Frenkel J, Deghenghi R, et al: Intranasal administration of the GHRP hexarelin accelerates growth in short children. Clin Endocrinol (Oxf) 43:631–635, 1995.

487. Schambelan M, Mulligan K, Grunfeld C, et al: Recombinant human growth hormone in patients with HIV-associated wasting. A randomized, placebo-controlled trial. Serostim Study Group. Ann Intern Med 125:873–882, 1996.

488. Chapman IM, Pescovitz OH, Murphy G, et al: Oral administration of growth hormone (GH) releasing peptide-mimetic MK-677 stimulates the GH/insulin-like growth factor-I axis in selected GH-deficient adults. J Clin Endocrinol Metab 82:3455–3463, 1997.

489. Van den Berghe G, DeZegher F, Bouillon R: The somatotrophic axis in critical illness: Effects of growth hormone secretagogues. Growth Horm IGF Res 8:153–155, 1998.

490. Van den Berghe G, de Zegher F, Bowers CY, et al: Pituitary responsiveness to GH-releasing hormone, GH-releasing peptide-2 and thyrotrophin-releasing hormone in critical illness. Clin Endocrinol (Oxf) 45:341–351, 1996.

491. Van den Berghe G, de Zegher F, Veldhuis JD, et al: The somatotropic axis in critical illness: Effect of continuous growth hormone (GH)–releasing hormone and GH-releasing peptide-2 infusion. J Clin Endocrinol Metab 82:590–599, 1997.

492. Van den Berghe G, de Zegher F, Baxter RC, et al: Neuroendocrinology of prolonged critical illness: Effects of exogenous thyrotropin-releasing hormone and its combination with growth hormone secretagogues. J Clin Endocrinol Metab 83:309–319, 1998.

493. Van den Berghe G, Wouters P, Weekers F, et al: Reactivation of pituitary hormone release and metabolic improvement by infusion of growth hormone–releasing peptide and thyrotropin-releasing hormone in patients with protracted critical illness. J Clin Endocrinol Metab 84:1311–1323, 1999.

494. Murphy MG, Plunkett LM, Gertz BJ, et al: MK-677, an orally active growth hormone secretagogue, reverses diet-induced catabolism. J Clin Endocrinol Metab 83:320–325, 1998.

495. Jenkins RC, Meguid El Nahas A, Wilkie ME, et al: The effect of dose, nutrition, and age on hexarelin-induced anterior pituitary hormone secretion in adult patients on maintenance hemodialysis. J Clin Endocrinol Metab 84:1220–1225, 1999.

496. Takala J, Ruokonen E, Webster NR, et al: Increased mortality associated with growth hormone treatment in critically ill adults. N Engl J Med 341:785–792, 1999.

497. Rudman D, Feller AG, Nagraj HS, et al: Effects of human growth hormone in men over 60 years old. N Engl J Med 323:1–6, 1990.

498. Chapman IM, Bach MA, Van Cauter E, et al: Stimulation of the growth hormone (GH)–insulin-like growth factor I axis by daily oral administration of a GH secretagogue (MK-677) in healthy elderly subjects. J Clin Endocrinol Metab 81:4249–4257, 1996.

499. Copinschi G, Van Onderbergen A, L'Hermite-Baleriaux M, et al: Effects of a 7-day treatment with a novel, orally active, growth hormone (GH) secretagogue, MK-677, on 24-hour GH profiles, insulin-like growth factor I, and adrenocortical function in normal young men. J Clin Endocrinol Metab 81:2776–2782, 1996.

500. Kirk SE, Gertz BJ, Schneider SH, et al: Effect of obesity and feeding on the growth hormone (GH) response to the GH secretagogue L-692,429 in young men. J Clin Endocrinol Metab 82:1154–1159, 1997.

501. Locatelli V, Rossoni G, Schweiger F, et al: Growth hormone–independent cardioprotective effects of hexarelin in the rat. Endocrinology 140:4024–4031, 1999.

Somatostatin

Agnes Schonbrunn

Somatostatin was identified in 1973 as a 14–amino acid cyclic peptide present in hypothalamic extracts that was capable of inhibiting growth hormone secretion by dispersed rat pituitary cells and thus named somatotropin release–inhibiting factor (SRIF).[1] Since this landmark discovery, our understanding of somatostatin's actions and importance has exploded. The gene for somatostatin has been cloned, and the biosynthesis of two biologically active peptides, somatostatin-14 (SS14) and somatostatin-28 (SS28), both encoded by this single gene, has been elucidated. These peptides have been found in virtually all mammalian neuroendocrine tissues, as well as in the central and peripheral nervous systems, and their wide and tissue-specific distribution has been characterized in detail. In addition, the genes for two new peptides with a great deal of structural similarity to somatostatin, namely, cortistatin and urotensin II, have been discovered. Numerous physiologic and pathologic functions of somatostatin-like peptides have been demonstrated, showing that they act not only as hormones by transport via the blood stream but also as neurotransmitters or neuromodulators and as paracrine regulators of neighboring cells. We now know that somatostatins modulate secretion, neurotransmission, smooth muscle contractility, and cell proliferation and affect physiologic processes ranging from learning and growth to digestion. In addition, they inhibit a variety of neuroendocrine, neural, and hormone-responsive tumors. Five different somatostatin receptor genes have been cloned, and exploration of their unique expression patterns and functional properties is well under way. Most exciting, as our understanding of the physiologic roles played by this peptide family and its receptors has increased, the number and variety of diagnostic and therapeutic uses for somatostatin analogues and nonpeptidic, somatostatin receptor–specific ligands have also proliferated.

MOLECULAR DIVERSITY OF SOMATOSTATIN-RELATED PEPTIDES

Somatostatins are a phylogenically ancient, multigene family; somatostatin-like immunoreactivity has been identified in all vertebrates, as well as in many invertebrates, including ciliated protozoa.[2–4] New insight into evolution of the somatostatin gene was recently provided by the discovery of cortistatin and urotensin II, two mammalian peptides structurally similar to somatostatin (Fig. 32–1). Like other protein hormones, somatostatin-like peptides are synthesized as high-molecular-weight precursors (prepropeptides) that are cleaved at specific residues by processing enzymes to generate the mature secreted products (see below). Further increasing the complexity within the somatostatin peptide family, somatostatin prepropeptides can be cleaved at different sites in different species and in different tissues, thereby generating products of varying length.[3, 4]

To date, three genes encoding somatostatin-like peptides have been identified in mammals. The human preprosomatostatin-I (PSS-I) gene encodes a 116–amino acid biosynthetic precursor that is processed in a tissue-specific manner to two different mature peptides, SS14 and SS28 (see Fig. 32–1). This gene has been highly conserved during evolution: the primary structure of SS14 has been maintained in all vertebrate species examined with only three exceptions: (1) the lam-

prey, which contains the substitution Thr12→Ser; (2) the Pacific ratfish, which contains an Asn5→Ser substitution, and (3) the sturgeon *Acipenser gueldenstaedti*, which contains a Gly2→Pro substitution. Whereas PSS-I is the only gene that encodes somatostatin in most vertebrates, including humans, teleost fish have two different preprosomatostatin genes, PSS-I and PSS-II. The latter codes for a precursor that contains [Tyr7,Gly10]SS14 at its C terminus. No evidence of PSS-II gene expression has been seen in species other than teleosts. However, two distinct somatostatin-like genes have also been isolated from frogs. One shows strong sequence similarity with PSS-I from mammals, and the other, termed PSS-2, encodes [Pro2,Met13]SS14 at its C terminus but otherwise shows little structural similarity with either PSS-I or PSS-II.[3]

The second mammalian gene encoding a somatostatin-like peptide is preprocortistatin (PCS), so named because it is expressed mainly in the cortex and hippocampus of rats.[5] The human gene would be expected to produce a primary product of 105 amino acid residues.[6] Although the posttranslation processing of PCS has not been elucidated, it is likely that this precursor is processed to cortistatin-29 in addition to (or perhaps instead of) cortistatin-17 (or cortistatin-14 in the rat)[5, 7] (see Fig. 32–1). Interestingly, cortistatin contains the Gly2→Pro substitution found in the sturgeon and the Thr12→Ser substitution present in the lamprey. Thus the unexpected discovery of cortistatin more than 20 years after the identification of somatostatin has led to the suggestion that duplication of a preprosomatostatin gene occurred early in evolution and gave rise to the highly conserved PSS-I gene, as well as the mammalian PCS gene and the amphibian PSS-2 gene[3] (see Fig. 32–1). However, the possibility that a homologue of the amphibian PSS-2 gene is expressed in mammals in addition to PSS-I and PCS cannot be excluded and may imply that other somatostatin-like genes remain to be discovered.

The third mammalian somatostatin-like gene encodes preprourotensin II, a 124–amino acid peptide in humans that contains the 11–amino acid urotensin II at its C terminus.[8] However, even though urotensin II is structurally similar to SS14, especially in the functionally important central region of the molecule containing the Phe-Trp-Lys sequence (see Fig. 32–1), urotensin II appears to be derived from an ancestral precursor different from that giving rise to somatostatin and cortistatin.[3]

The recent discovery of peptides with a great deal of structural similarity to somatostatin raises several important questions that are only now beginning to be answered. (1) Is some of the immunoreactivity previously attributed to somatostatin due to cortistatin or urotensin II? (2) Do these peptides act at overlapping or distinct receptors? (3) Do somatostatin analogues such as octreotide, a stable peptide agonist used for the treatment of various endocrine and malignant disorders (see Fig. 32–1), also activate cortistatin or urotensin II receptors?

BIOSYNTHESIS OF SOMATOSTATIN PEPTIDES

The gene encoding human somatostatin is located on chromosome 3 in the region 3q28 and contains a single intron that interrupts

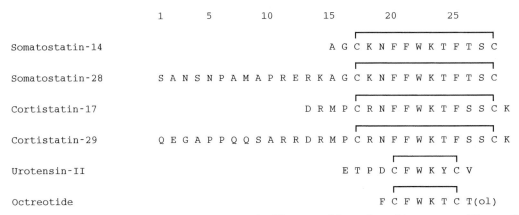

FIGURE 32–1. Structure of bioactive peptides homologous to somatostatin. Alignment of the amino acid sequences of five peptides homologous to somatostatin is shown: mammalian SS14 and SS28, the rat and human cortistatins, and human urotensin II. The position of the intramolecular disulfide bond between the two cysteine residues is indicated in each peptide and results in the formation of a cyclic structure. The amino acid residues critical for high-affinity binding to somatostatin receptors comprise the central FWKT sequence. The structure of the synthetic, stable somatostatin analogue octreotide is shown for comparison, with D-amino acids substituted at the 1(F) and 4(W) positions.

the coding sequence in the propeptide portion of the somatostatin precursor.[9–11] Splicing of the primary transcript generates an mRNA that codes for a 116–amino acid preprosomatostatin peptide containing SS14 and SS28 at its C terminus. As for other secreted molecules, the N terminus of preprosomatostatin contains a signal or leader sequence that targets the nascent peptide together with the associated mRNA and ribosomal translational machinery to the rough endoplasmic reticulum (RER). Specific proteins in the RER recognize and bind the leader sequence and facilitate transfer of the nascent peptide into the lumen of the ER cisternae, thereby ensuring that the peptide enters the secretory pathway. After this transfer, but before translation is completed, the 24–amino acid signal sequence is cleaved. The final translation product is a 92-residue propeptide that is subsequently transported from the RER to the trans-Golgi network (Fig. 32–2). Prosomatostatin (ProSS) is further hydrolyzed at specific prohormone cleavage sites as it traverses the secretory pathway from the Golgi to secretory granules.[12–14] Tissues vary in the relative amount of the two biologically active end-products that they produce, SS14 and SS28, presumably as a result of the nature and the level of the different processing enzymes expressed in each cell type.[14] However, because the affinities of most sst receptor subtypes for these two somatostatin peptides are the same or very similar (see below), the physiologic importance of such differential processing is still unclear.

Several endopeptidases have been implicated in the cleavage of ProSS, most of them related to the subtilisin/kexin-like serine proteinases of the proprotein convertase (PC) family.[14–17] Members of this enzyme family exhibit characteristic specificities for the type of site cleaved, patterns of tissue expression, and subcellular localization. For a particular endopeptidase to catalyze a processing step physiologically requires that the enzyme both be able to recognize the appropriate sequence in the substrate and colocalize with the propeptide in the same cell and subcellular compartment.

The sites in ProSS that are cleaved to generate SS14 and SS28 fall into different classes[14, 16] (see Fig. 32–2). The sequence hydrolyzed to produce SS14 (RERK ↓, where ↓ denotes the position of cleavage) is a typical type II processing site of the general form (K/R)X(K/R)(K/R) ↓.[16] Thus hydrolysis occurs C-terminal to a pair of basic residues forming SS14 and an 8-kDa peptide, ProSS(1–76). The sequence that is cleaved to produce SS28 (RLELQR ↓) is a typical type III site that is cleaved C-terminal to a monobasic Arg residue with the subsequent release of SS28 and a 7-kDa peptide, ProSS(1–63).[16] Cleavage of type III precursor proteins requires the presence of a basic amino acid 4, 6, or 8 residues N-terminal to the cleavage site, as seen in ProSS.[16] Although further cleavage of SS28 could theoretically generate SS14, this pathway does not appear to be used to a significant extent. Rather, SS14 is produced independently of SS28 by direct

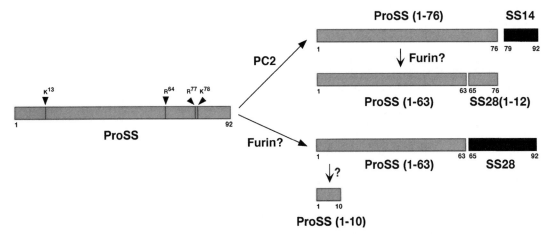

FIGURE 32–2. Biosynthesis of somatostatin peptides. The primary transcript of the mammalian somatostatin gene is preprosomatostatin (116 amino acids). Prosomatostatin (ProSS) (92 amino acids) is derived from preprosomatostatin by cleavage of the 24-residue N-terminal signal sequence by a signal peptidase during translation of the mRNA in the rough endoplasmic reticulum. Further posttranslational cleavage of ProSS occurs in the Golgi complex and in the vesicular compartments of the secretory pathway. The figure shows the peptide products that have been isolated from somatostatin-producing tissues. Cleavage at the C-terminal end of the molecule occurs either at a monobasic Arg site to yield SS28 or at a dibasic Arg-Lys site to produce SS14. ProSS can also be processed by hydrolysis at a monobasic Lys site near the N terminus to generate ProSS(1–10). Carboxypeptidases are thought to remove the basic residues on the C terminus of the primary peptide products formed by endoprotease cleavage.

hydrolysis of ProSS, and the two other products, SS28(1–12) and ProSS(1–63), are subsequently formed by further hydrolysis of ProSS(1–76).[18, 19] A third cleavage occurs at an atypical site that is C-terminal to a monobasic Lys and contains an Arg that is six residues N-terminal to the cleavage site.[20] The direct precursor for this reaction is probably ProSS(1–63),[20] and after carboxypeptidase action, the final product is ProSS(1–10). Although this peptide is released from many somatostatin-producing cells, it has no known biologic activity. After endopeptidase cleavage, carboxypeptidases usually remove the basic amino acids from the C terminus of the products produced by endopeptidase hydrolysis.

Several enzymes have been implicated in the processing of ProSS. PC1 and PC2 are neural/neuroendocrine-specific enzymes that are mainly localized in secretory granules and can efficiently cleave ProSS at the type II site to form SS14.[14, 16] The observation that processing of ProSS to SS14 was completely blocked in the pancreas of mice lacking active PC2 as a result of targeted gene disruption provides strong evidence for the physiologic importance of PC2 in SS14 biosynthesis.[21] Interestingly, SS28 was the major end-product of ProSS processing in these mice, which suggests that it may be formed in a default pathway. Furin, which is expressed in all tissues and cell lines examined to date, has been proposed as the endoprotease that cleaves ProSS to generate SS28 inasmuch as it can increase the formation of this product when exogenously expressed together with ProSS.[14] This suggestion is consistent with the predominant localization of furin in the trans-Golgi network, a site where significant ProSS processing occurs.[12–14] However, the type III site in ProSS that is cleaved to produce SS28 is not an optimal substrate for furin.[16] In fact, this enzyme has been implicated primarily in the processing of constitutively secreted proteins rather than peptide hormones and neuropeptides.[16, 22] Hence other PCs may be involved in the physiologic formation of SS28 either instead of or in addition to furin.[23] Little is known about the enzyme that cleaves ProSS to generate ProSS(1–10) or about the carboxypeptidases that hydrolyze the basic residues from the endopeptidase cleavage products.

The human cortistatin gene has been localized to chromosome 1p36,[6] but the human urotensin II gene has not yet been mapped. Human preprocortistatin contains dibasic sites whose cleavage could yield either CS29 (REVARR ↓) or CS17 (SARR ↓). Similarly, an 11-residue human urotensin II could be formed from preprourotensin II by cleavage at the highly basic KPYYKKR ↓ sequence. However, although both these genes code for the synthesis of prohormones, neither the mechanisms involved in the processing of these precursors to mature peptides nor the nature of the peptide products formed in different tissues has been elucidated.

THE SOMATOSTATIN RECEPTOR FAMILY

High-affinity binding sites for somatostatin were first identified in pituitary tumor cell lines by using the radioiodinated SS14 analogue [^{125}I-Tyr^1]SS14.[24, 25] The presence of these binding sites was correlated with the ability of somatostatin to inhibit hormone secretion, which indicates that they represent functional receptors.[24, 25] Because [^{125}I-Tyr^1]SS14 binding was regulated by guanine nucleotides, somatostatin receptors were recognized to be members of the G protein–coupled

receptor family long before any information about their structure was available.[26]

The receptors in the GH$_4$C$_1$ pituitary cell line appeared homogeneous and bound both SS14 and SS28 with nanomolar affinity.[24, 27] However, subsequent studies with small synthetic somatostatin analogues such as octreotide (see Fig. 32–1) revealed the existence of two different somatostatin receptor subtypes in rat cortical membranes.[28, 29] One of these subtypes, initially called SS$_A$ and subsequently labeled SRIF1, bound octreotide with nanomolar affinity, whereas the SS$_B$/SRIF2 receptor subtype bound this analogue at least 1000 times more poorly. Both these somatostatin receptor types had high affinity for the two natural ligands SS14 and SS28. Interestingly, pancreatic and pituitary membranes appeared to express only the SS$_A$/SRIF1 receptor.[28, 29] These observations provided the first evidence for multiple somatostatin receptor subtypes, as well as tissue-specific expression of different somatostatin receptors.

Molecular cloning of five somatostatin receptor genes in 1992 demonstrated that this receptor family was far more complex than suspected from earlier pharmacologic studies.[30–34] The five genes have been named *sst1* to *sst5* in the order of their discovery,[35] although initially there was some confusion in nomenclature such that the sst4 and sst5 receptors were sometimes reversed. The somatostatin receptor genes are all located on different chromosomes (Table 32–1). In four of the genes—*sst1*, *sst3*, *sst4*, and *sst5*—the coding region is present in a single exon. However, *sst2* has been shown to undergo alternative splicing in mice and rats at the 3′ end of the mRNA and give rise to two protein products.[36, 37] The *sst2A* variant corresponds to the product of the unspliced mRNA, whereas the *sst2B* variant contains an alternative exon at the 3′ end that codes for a slightly shorter C terminus with a different sequence than coded for by *sst2A*.[36] Splicing may affect the specificity of sst2 receptor signaling or its regulation.[38] Recent cloning of the first nonmammalian sst receptors has provided evidence for the existence of multiple sst receptor subtypes in lower vertebrates as well.[39, 40]

Analysis of their amino acid sequences demonstrated that the five *sst* genes were homologous to those for the G protein–coupled receptor family.[41, 42] This family is the largest known receptor family, and its members share a common secondary structure consisting of seven transmembrane domains (7TMDs) connected by three intracellular and three extracellular loops. Signal transduction by 7TMD receptors involves activation of specific guanosine triphosphate–binding, heterotrimeric transducing proteins, called G proteins, by direct interaction between the G proteins and the cytoplasmic loops of the agonist-occupied receptor.[43, 44] Activated G proteins then regulate effector enzymes or ion channels, thereby altering the levels of second messengers such as cyclic adenosine monophosphate, inositol triphosphate, and calcium. Consistent with their sequence similarity to the 7TMD receptor family, all sst receptors have been shown to signal via G proteins.[45–47]

Each sst receptor subtype is highly conserved between species. For example, in the case of the sst1 receptor, which is the most highly conserved subtype, the rat, mouse, and human sequences diverge less than 3%.[47] Even with the least conserved somatostatin receptor subtype, namely, sst5, the rat and human receptor sequences diverge less than 20%.[47] Sequence comparisons among the five sst receptor subtypes demonstrated that they are all also similar to each other, exhibiting 40% to 55% amino acid identity (Fig. 32–3).

TABLE 32–1. Properties of Human Somatostatin Receptor Subtypes

Property	sst1	sst2A	sst3	sst4	sst5
Chromosomal localization	14q13	17q24	22q13.1	20p11.2	16p13.3
Amino acids	391	369	418	388	363
Asn glycosylation sites	4, 44, 48	9, 22, 29, 32	17, 30	24	13, 26, 187
Cys palmitoylation site	339	328	None	327	320
Receptor phosphorylation	+	+	+	−	?
Receptor internalization	Low	High	High	Low	High
SS-binding affinity	SS14 = SS28	SS14 = SS28	SS14 = SS28	SS14 = SS28	SS28 > SS14
Octreotide affinity	Low	High	Moderate	Low	High

SS, somatostatin.

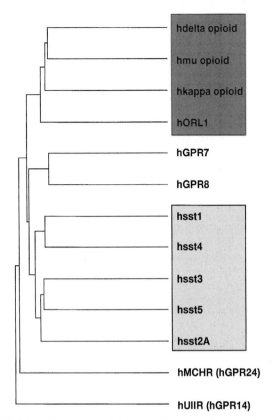

FIGURE 32–3. Sequence relationships between the receptors for somatostatin, opioid peptides, urotensin II, and homologous orphan receptors. The dendrogram was generated by aligning the polypeptide sequences of the human somatostatin receptors (hsst1, P30872; hsst2A, P30874; hsst3, P32745; hsst4, P31391; hsst5, P35346), the human opioid receptors (κ, P41145; μ, P42866; δ, P41143; ORL1, P41146), the human urotensin II receptor (GPR14, AAD55578), the human melanin-concentrating hormone receptor (hGPR24, Q997005), and the orphan receptors hGPR7 (P48145) and hGPR8 (P48146). Sequences obtained from either the Swiss Prot or the GenPept database were aligned by using the default settings of the PILEUP program (Genetics Computer Group, GCG, Madison, WI). The length of the lines is proportional to percent sequence identity. The plot shows that hsst1 and hsst4 form one subgroup and hsst2, hsst5, and hsst3 form a second subgroup within the somatostatin receptor family.

Somatostatin receptors fall into two groups based on sequence comparisons: sst1 and sst4 show greater sequence overlap with each other than with the other sst receptor subtypes, and the same is true for sst2, sst3, and sst5 (see Fig. 32–3). Structural features shared by members within each of these groups are likely to be responsible for common pharmacologic specificities and functional properties, and indeed, sequence comparisons have helped identify critical residues involved in ligand binding.[48] The next closest G protein–coupled receptor family consists of the four known opioid receptors, which exhibit about 30% amino acid identity with sst receptors (see Fig. 32–3). Although SS14 does not itself bind significantly to opioid receptors and the opioid peptides are not ligands for sst receptors, octreotide is a moderately potent antagonist at the μ opioid receptor.[49]

An extensive search for new G protein–coupled receptors has led to the isolation of several new mammalian receptor clones with sequence similarity to sst receptors[50] (see Fig. 32–3). The ligands for many of these receptors remain to be identified. However, peptides with high affinity for two such "orphan" receptors have been characterized recently. Urotensin II (see Fig. 32–1) appears to be the endogenous ligand for GPR14,[51] and melanin-concentrating hormone is the native ligand for SLC-1 (also called GPR24).[52–54] Neither SLC-1 nor GPR14 binds SS14,[51, 52, 55] and hence these receptors would not be expected to mediate any of the biologic actions of native somatostatin. A cortistatin-specific receptor has not been described, although the existence

of such a receptor is suggested by the distinct effects of cortistatin on sleep physiology, locomotor behavior, and hippocampal function.[56] Thus it is quite likely that additional sst-like receptors remain to be discovered in mammals.[57] The extent to which the numerous available somatostatin analogues activate any of the sst-like receptors remains to be investigated.

Somatostatin receptors are integral membrane proteins whose amino acid sequences have seven hydrophobic segments.[30] A model of the human sst2A receptor is shown in Figure 32–4, and Table 32–1 summarizes some of the structural features that the sst receptors share with other 7TMD receptors.[41, 42] The seven α helical transmembrane domains, which are thought to be clustered around a common core,[58] are connected via three intracellular (IL) and three extracellular (EL) loops (ILs and ELs, respectively). The greatest sequence similarity between sst receptor subtypes occurs within these transmembrane domains, and hence these domains have been proposed to be involved in ligand binding, a hypothesis corroborated by site-directed mutagenesis.[48, 59, 60] The sequence differences between the sst receptor subtypes, which reside primarily in the intracellular and extracellular domains, are presumably responsible for their distinct properties.

By analogy with other 7TMD receptors, ILs are likely to be involved in signaling and receptor regulation, whereas ELs are thought to provide important structural and targeting information.[42, 43] The sst2A receptor contains two highly conserved cysteine residues, one in EL1 and one in EL2, which probably form a disulfide bond (see Fig. 32–4, Table 32–1). Although the existence of this disulfide bond has not been demonstrated in any of the sst receptors, it is believed to be important for stabilizing the conformation of other 7TMD receptors. The extracellular N-terminal tail of sst2A contains four potential sites for N-glycosylation, a posttranslational modification catalyzed in the RER and Golgi that is believed to help target receptors to the plasma membrane. Although the actual sites of glycosylation on the sst2A receptor have not been identified, this receptor is known to be glycosylated from two observations. First, N-glycosidase treatment dramatically alters the migration pattern of the sst2A receptor on sodium dodecyl sulfate (SDS) gels. The molecular mass of the sst2A receptor is predicted to be 41 kDa from its amino acid sequence. In fact, this receptor migrates as a broad band of approximately 85 kDa on SDS polyacrylamide gels and is converted to a sharp 40-kDa band by N-glycosidase treatment.[61, 62] Second, the sst2A receptor binds tightly to lectins.[63] Based on similar observations, sst1, sst3, and sst5 are also glycosylated, whereas sst4, whose mobility is not affected by N-glycosidase, may not be.[62, 64] Interestingly, variation in the degree and/or the nature of receptor glycosylation between tissues and cell types produces slight differences in receptor migration (see Gu et al.[61, 65] and Reubi et al.,[66] for example). The functional significance of such differences in receptor glycosylation is unknown.

The ILs of 7TMD receptors are also targets for covalent modification. The highly conserved Cys in the C-terminal tail of sst2A is probably palmitoylated, although this modification has not been demonstrated.[41, 42] However, the sst2A receptor is known to be phosphorylated on both the third IL and the C-terminal tail.[63, 67] Sst2A receptor phosphorylation appears to be catalyzed by at least two different classes of enzymes: G protein receptor kinases and protein kinase C.[63, 67] The sst1 and sst3 receptors are also phosphorylated,[68, 69] whereas phosphorylation of sst4 could not be detected.[70] As for other 7TMD receptors, phosphorylation is likely to be important in desensitization and internalization of somatostatin receptors, although the molecular mechanisms involved remain to be elucidated.

Expression of individual sst receptor subtypes has permitted each of their pharmacologic specificities to be investigated, and these studies have been extensively reviewed.[46, 47, 71, 72] Somatostatin receptor subtypes sst1 through sst4 do not distinguish between SS14 and SS28. In contrast, sst5 binds SS28 approximately five times more avidly than it does SS14, although the physiologic importance of this preference is still unknown. The structural features of SS14 known to be essential for biologic activity include a cyclic structure, which is formed by the disulfide bond between Cys3 and Cys14, and amino acid side chain functional groups at four central residues: Phe at position 7, Trp at position 8, Lys at position 9, and Thr at position 10 (see Fig. 32–1).[27, 73] These features are present in cortistatin (see Fig. 32–1) and, as would

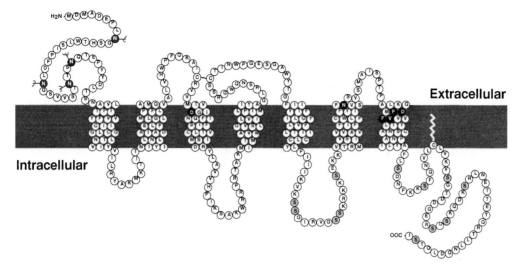

FIGURE 32–4. *Proposed structure of the human sst2A receptor. The four potential glycosylation sites within the N-terminal extracellular region are indicated with little trees. The Cys in the C-terminal tail, which is in a position to act as a potential palmitoylation site, is shown with an attached lipid moiety. Potential serine phosphorylation sites in the third IL and C terminal tail of the receptor are shown in gray. Residues implicated in ligand binding by site-directed mutagenesis are indicated in black in the third, fifth, and sixth transmembrane domains.*

be predicted, cortistatin binds to all five sst receptor subtypes with high affinity ($K_d \approx 0.1$ nmol/L).[74] These features are also present in the metabolically stable somatostatin analogue octreotide (see Fig. 32–1). However, octreotide only binds with high affinity ($K_d \approx 0.1$ nmol/L) to sst2 and sst5.[75] Even though it also binds with moderate affinity to sst3, it does not bind to either sst1 or sst4.[46, 47, 71, 72, 76] Thus although the cyclic structure and central Phe-Trp-Lys-Thr sequence are essential for the biologic activity of somatostatins, they are not sufficient. In fact, the binding selectivity of different sst receptor subtypes for octreotide and other short somatostatin analogues has resulted in the pharmacologic classification of sst2, sst3, and sst5 as SRIF1 receptors and sst1 and sst4 as SRIF2 receptors, in parallel with their grouping based on sequence identity.[35]

Until recently, no somatostatin receptor agonists were available that had sufficient specificity for individual sst receptor subtypes to allow biologic activities to be unambiguously assigned to particular sst receptors. However, this situation changed with the identification of several nonpeptide agonists that exhibited high selectivity for each of the five sst receptor subtypes.[77] The first somatostatin receptor antagonists were also reported recently, although these compounds are not as specific for individual sst receptors as the most selective agonists.[78–80] The availability of high-affinity, subtype-specific agonists and antagonists is clearly essential for defining the physiologic functions of individual sst receptors, and such compounds have already provided insight into their respective biologic activities.

WHY SO MANY SOMATOSTATIN RECEPTORS?

To understand the physiologic role of somatostatin fully, one must appreciate the distinct functional properties of the individual somatostatin receptor subtypes. Because sst1, sst2, sst3, and sst4 do not distinguish between SS14 and SS28, ligand selectivity between the endogenous SS peptides cannot be an important aspect of their biology, although such selectivity may be significant for the sst5 receptor. Rather, the distinct functions of sst receptor subtypes are likely to involve differences in the intracellular signaling cascades that are activated upon hormone binding, differences in the regulation of receptor action, or differences in the control of receptor expression, either by tissue-specific transcription factors or by endocrine or paracrine regulators.

Because many tissues express multiple sst receptor subtypes and since receptor specific agonists have only recently become available, studies of the signal transduction mechanisms activated by individual sst receptors have mostly involved heterologous expression of one sst

subtype at a time in receptor-negative hosts such as COS, CHO, HEK, or fibroblastic cells. Although this approach has helped to define how the sst receptor subtypes differ in function, it has two significant disadvantages. First, the cellular environment provided by the transfected host may be quite different from the secretory or excitatory cells in which sst receptors normally reside. For example, in nontransformed endocrine cells, somatostatin leads to a reduction in intracellular calcium due to a decrease in calcium influx through voltage-dependent calcium channels. However, a reduction in calcium has not been observed in most sst-transfected hosts, presumably because the cell lines utilized do not express the necessary channels. In fact, somatostatin has been shown to increase intracellular calcium in these cells.[81, 82] Second, the receptor level produced by transfection is often 10 to 100 times higher than that found in cells expressing sst receptors endogenously. It is well recognized that at such high receptor concentrations, low-affinity receptor-effector interactions may become significant, leading to activation of signaling cascades that are not affected at endogenous receptor levels.[83] However, despite these limitations, heterologous expression systems can provide useful information about the unique capabilities of each sst receptor subtype, and studies using such model systems have been intensively investigated in the last few years (reviewed in references 45–47 and 84).

All sst receptors inhibit adenylyl cyclase via pertussis toxin–sensitive G proteins.[45–47, 84] This class of G proteins, which includes the five Gα subunits (G$_{\alpha i\text{-}1}$, G$_{\alpha i\text{-}2}$, G$_{\alpha i\text{-}3}$, G$_{\alpha o\text{-}1}$, and G$_{\alpha o\text{-}2}$), also links sst receptors to effectors other than adenylyl cyclase, including voltage-sensitive calcium channels,[85–88] potassium channels,[89–91] ser/thr phosphatases,[89] and tyrosine phosphatases.[92–95] Comprehensive summaries listing the effectors known to be regulated by each sst receptor subtype have been compiled in several recent reviews.[45–47, 84] Although the data are incomplete, it is clear that different sst subtypes vary in their ability to regulate many effectors. For example, sst2, sst3, sst4, and sst5, but not sst1, can activate the G protein–gated inwardly rectifying K channel, GIRK1, when co-expressed in *Xenopus* oocytes.[91] Similarly, somatostatin inhibits high voltage–activated (HVA) Ca^{2+} currents in the rat insulinoma cell line RINm5F expressing sst2 but not sst1.[96] However, in a different rat insulinoma cell line (1046–38 cells), the sst1-selective ligand CH-275 caused a marked inhibition of voltage-operated Ca^{2+} channels, while the sst2-specific analogue octreotide elicited a less pronounced effect, suggesting that in this rat insulinoma cell line, inhibition of Ca^{2+} channels is preferentially mediated by sst1.[97] Hence, effector coupling is both receptor subtype– and cell type–specific. The numerous reports of differences in signaling among sst receptor subtypes expressed in the same cellular host indicate that receptor-specific activation of different signal transduction pathways is likely to be physiologically important.[45–47, 84]

Although most sst receptor signaling is blocked by pertussis toxin, some biochemical and biologic effects of sst receptors are partially or completely toxin-*insensitive,* indicating that they are mediated either by pertussis toxin–resistant G proteins or possibly by other protein-protein interactions. Examples of pertussis toxin–insensitive effects include inhibition of Na/H exchange by sst1 in fibroblastic Ltk-cells,[98] stimulation of adenylyl cyclase by sst5 in CHO cells,[99] and inhibition of cell proliferation in Ar4–2J cells, probably mediated by sst2.[100] Inhibition of the Na/H transporter by sst1 may involve $\alpha 12$,[101] and stimulation of adenylyl cyclase is likely to occur via Gs.[99] However, the identity of the pertussis toxin–insensitive G protein(s), which might mediate somatostatin inhibition of cell proliferation in Ar4–2J cells, is unknown.

A variety of different strategies have been used to identify the specificity of sst receptor–G protein interactions. These approaches have included isolation and biochemical characterization of sst-receptor G protein complexes,[61, 64, 102, 103] examination of specific sst signaling pathways following reduction or elimination of individual G protein subunits by antisense nucleotides,[104, 105] use of pertussis–toxin insensitive G_i/G_o mutants to reconstitute somatostatin signaling after inactivation of endogenous G_i/G_o proteins,[106] and covalent labeling of specific G protein subunits with radioactively labeled GTP analogues on sst receptor stimulation.[88] Unfortunately, results from the different experimental systems are not always in total agreement. Further, many of the studies did not identify the sst subtype being investigated and, indeed, may have been studying several receptor subtypes simultaneously. Hence, a complete picture of the specificity of sst receptor–G protein interactions is not yet available. Nevertheless, several conclusions can be drawn at this stage. Individual sst receptor subtypes can couple to multiple G proteins, sometimes with clearly different affinities.[61] Several of the pertussis toxin–sensitive G proteins can link sst receptors to adenylyl cyclase. One G protein subunit may couple sst receptors to multiple effectors. Both the α and the β-γ G protein subunits are involved in signaling, and these subunits usually couple receptors to different effectors. For example, in intestinal smooth muscle cells, which express only the sst3 receptor subtype, α subunits of both G_{i1} and G_o mediate inhibition of adenylyl cyclase, whereas the β-γ subunits mediate activation of phospholipase $C_{\beta 3}$.[107] Similarly, in transfected CHO cells, sst1 and sst4 both inhibit adenylyl cyclase via the α subunits of pertussis toxin–sensitive G proteins, but stimulate mitogen-activated protein (MAP) kinase via the β-γ subunits.[94, 95] Future studies are likely to identify the spectrum of G protein subunits activated by each sst receptor subtype in normal tissues, and thereby define the events at this critical junction, which determines the specificity of sst receptor signaling.

How the different second messenger systems regulated by somatostatin are linked to biologic responses is better understood for some of somatostatin's actions than others. For example, in pituitary cells, somatostatin reduces intracellular calcium and cyclic adenosine monophosphate (cAMP) by independent mechanisms.[26, 108] The reduction in cAMP is due to direct inhibition of adenylyl cyclase. The reduction in cytosolic calcium is due both to a stimulation of potassium channel activity, which hyperpolarizes the cell membrane and consequently decreases influx through voltage-dependent calcium channels indirectly, and to direct inhibition of calcium channel activity.[109] The ensuing reduction in both intracellular cAMP and calcium concentrations contributes to somatostatin inhibition of secretion, and when either signaling pathway is blocked, the magnitude of the inhibitory effect of somatostatin is reduced.[110, 111] In contrast, the mechanisms by which sst receptors regulate cell growth are rather poorly understood. Because MAP kinase (also called extracellular signal–regulated kinase, or ERK) is recognized as a critical component in the signal transduction cascade regulating cell proliferation, the mechanisms by which sst receptors modulate its activity have been investigated in detail.[94, 95, 112–114] The sst1, sst2, and sst5 receptors, when recombinantly expressed in CHO cells, can all inhibit cell growth,[95, 115] whereas the sst4 receptor stimulates CHO cell proliferation.[94] Yet despite their opposite growth effects, both the sst1 receptor[95] and the sst4 receptor[94] activate MAP kinase by a pertussis toxin–sensitive mechanism. In contrast, although sst1 and sst5 both inhibit CHO cell proliferation, the former stimulates MAP kinase, whereas the latter decreases it.[95, 112] Detailed

molecular studies have indicated that multiple pathways can lead to MAP kinase regulation by sst receptors and have suggested that differences in the duration of the sst effect, as well as in its direction, may determine whether stimulation or inhibition of cell proliferation is produced by somatostatin treatment.[94, 95, 112–114] Alternatively, other signaling pathways, such as tyrosine phosphatase activation, may provide the critical signal. Many questions remain, however, and the mechanisms by which somatostatin regulates cell growth and apoptosis are under intense investigation.

In addition to specificity in signaling, differences in the regulation of sst receptor subtypes are also likely to be important determinants of somatostatin action. Alterations in sst receptor responsiveness during somatostatin exposure vary dramatically between tissues, depending both on the response being measured and on the nature of the target cell. In some instances, desensitization occurs within minutes after initiation of somatostatin treatment; in others, no desensitization is detected even after years of somatostatin analogue exposure. Perhaps the most compelling evidence for somatostatin desensitization comes from studies with neurons, a target cell that must be able to rapidly modulate its responsiveness to stimulation. In chick sympathetic neurons, somatostatin inhibits an N-type Ca^{2+} current, and this inhibition desensitizes with a half-time of 3 minutes.[116, 117] In guinea pig submucosal neurons, somatostatin-induced hyperpolarization also desensitizes within minutes.[118] Exposure to somatostatin or to selective somatostatin agonists, such as octreotide, leads to a slower desensitization in pituitary cells, occurring over the course of hours, days, or weeks, depending on the system examined.[119–122] However, desensitization, at least to pharmacologic doses of octreotide, does not occur during long-term octreotide treatment of many human pituitary tumors.[123] In fact, the suppressive effect of octreotide on growth hormone secretion in patients with acromegaly is usually maintained after 10 years of uninterrupted therapy.[124] Some, but probably not all, of these differences are probably due to sst receptor–specific regulation, because receptor subtype differences exist among sst receptors in their ability to undergo acute desensitization. For example, sst2 inhibition of adenylyl cyclase is rapidly desensitized, whereas sst4 inhibition is not.[63, 70] However, not all of the observed differences in the regulation of somatostatin responsiveness in different tissues can be attributed to receptor-specific behavior. For example, the sst2 receptor desensitizes after 15 minutes of somatostatin treatment in a growth hormone–secreting pituitary tumor cell line,[63] and yet growth hormone–secreting tumors that express this receptor remain sensitive to octreotide therapy for years.[124] These observations suggest that susceptibility to somatostatin desensitization depends not only on the sst receptor subtype expressed, but also on its cellular environment and they imply that differential regulation of sst receptors may occur in normal tissues and tumors. To understand how and why such differences occur, attention has been focused on elucidating the manner in which somatostatin responsiveness is regulated in different tissues and on understanding the molecular basis for sst receptor subtype-specific regulation.

Multiple molecular mechanisms are likely to be responsible for changes in responsiveness to somatostatin. Regulation of cellular reactivity can occur at the level of the receptor, at the level of the G protein signal transducers, or at the level of effectors, and is, in fact, known to be modulated at all these molecular targets for other GPCRs. By analogy to studies with rhodopsin and the β-adrenergic receptor (α_2AR), the GPCRs that have been examined in greatest detail,[125–128] acute regulation of somatostatin receptor responsiveness, occurring over minutes, is likely to involve uncoupling of receptors from G proteins and/or a translocation of the receptor from the cell surface to intracellular compartments, where it is no longer accessible to stimulation. The molecular events involved in the regulation of *individual* sst receptor subtypes have also been examined by expression of specific sst receptors in heterologous cell expression systems and have focused to a large extent on receptor internalization (for reviews see references 45–47 and 84). These studies have shown that different receptor subtypes are internalized at substantially different rates following agonist binding. In general, sst1 and sst4 are internalized to a lesser extent than that noted for sst2, sst3, and sst5. However, there are substantial differences among the various studies, possibly attributable to the different host cell lines used for sst receptor expression or to species-specific differences in receptor behavior. For example, the human sst4 was rapidly internalized in CHO cells,[129] whereas the rat sst4 was poorly internalized in HEK cells.[130] Such rationalizations cannot, however, explain the observation that in CHO cells the human sst2A receptor may be either decreased[131] or increased[129] by somatostatin pretreatment. However, the recent recognition that protein kinase C stimulates sst2A internalization[132] suggests that heterologous regulation by serum factors may be responsible for some of the discrepant results reported.

Little is known about the cellular and tissue-specific mechanisms that might be involved in sst receptor regulation, as only fragmentary information is available regarding the molecular events involved in the modulation of sst receptor signaling. Somatostatin binding leads to an increase in the phosphorylation of the sst1[68], the sst2A[63], and the sst3[6a] receptor.[69] In contrast, no phosphorylation of the sst4 receptor was detected,[70] and data are not available regarding the phosphorylation of the other sst receptor subtypes. Although the enzyme(s) catalyzing the phosphorylation of the sst2A and sst3 receptors have not been identified, the G protein receptor kinase, GRK2, has been implicated in the phosphorylation of sst2A by the observation that somatostatin treatment of S49 cells, which express primarily the sst2A receptor,[114] leads to translocation of the GRK2 to the plasma membrane.[133] In addition, protein kinase C activation also stimulates sst2A receptor phosphorylation concomitantly with increased receptor internalization.[132] Thus, by analogy with other GPCRs, receptor phosphorylation is likely to be an early step leading to sst receptor internalization and/or desensitization. Pharmacologic studies have suggested that sst receptors internalize primarily, but not uniformly, via a clathrin-coated vesicular pathway.[46, 47, 84] However, the trafficking and recycling of various sst receptor subtypes in different intracellular compartments are only now being investigated in detail.

The mechanisms of sst receptor desensitization and internalization not only are important for understanding somatostatin physiology, but are of clinical relevance as well. Desensitization to drug treatment is of central importance in pharmacology. Although desensitization does not appear to be a problem during tumor therapy with somatostatin analogues, it may be important in other therapeutic applications. SS receptor scintigraphy, which is used for the preoperative localization of sst receptor–expressing tumors, is performed 24 to 48 hours following injection of radiolabeled SS analogues and hence is thought to detect not only receptor-ligand binding interactions but also, and probably largely, internalized ligands that accumulate in endosomes or lysosomes because of their resistance to degradation.[134] Thus, the ability of different sst receptor subtypes to internalize bound radiolabeled peptides is likely to be important in their sensitivity to imaging.

Chronic regulation of somatostatin receptor signaling also occurs and can be observed after many hours or days of continuous analogue exposure. Such long-term regulation, which is likely to be of greater clinical than physiologic relevance, may involve changes in the rates of receptor degradation[135] or synthesis.[136] Indeed, regulation of receptor mRNA levels by both somatostatin and other hormones, such as glucocorticoids and estrogens, has been observed (for reviews, see references 45–47 and 84). Because the promoter regions of several sst receptor subtypes have recently been sequenced (reviewed in Kreienkamp[84]), the mechanisms by which sst receptor transcription is regulated by hormonal as well as tissue-specific factors is likely to be elucidated in the near future. It is noteworthy in this regard that the sequence similarity observed in the coding region of sst receptor subtypes is absent in the 5′ and 3′ flanking regions of the receptor genes, consistent with distinct patterns of gene expression and regulation. Even slower changes in responsiveness to octreotide treatment, occurring in tumors after months or years of therapy, are likely to involve changes in tumor differentiation and selection of resistant cell populations, and little is known about the mechanisms involved.

Tissue-specific expression of sst receptor subtypes has been extensively documented in studies examining the distribution of receptor mRNAs as well as, more recently, the distribution of receptor subtype proteins (for reviews, see references 45–47 and 84). These studies are discussed in detail later in the context of the physiologic functions of individual sst subtypes. The role of tissue-specific transcription factors

in the expression of individual sst receptor genes is currently under investigation.[137]

Although we do not yet fully understand the biologic functions of individual somatostatin receptors, a large body of work indicates that each of the six known receptor subtypes plays a unique role. This role is determined by where and when the receptor is expressed, how it signals in each cellular context, and how it is regulated.

PHYSIOLOGIC ROLES OF SOMATOSTATIN

The numerous functions of somatostatin in vivo have been elucidated using a combination of different approaches. In early studies to determine whether somatostatin was capable of eliciting particular effects, somatostatin itself was administered, whereas more recently, the biologic responses to stable somatostatin analogues or receptor-specific nonpeptide agonists have been examined. Evidence for the physiologic significance of any biologic effects produced by exogenously administered analogues is obtained by demonstrating that endogenous SS14 or SS28 could reach the target site, by showing that the responsive cells express somatostatin receptors with the appropriate pharmacologic specificity, and, in the absence of receptor-specific antagonists, by demonstrating that neutralizing antibodies to somatostatin block the effects under investigation. Recently, mice deficient either in somatostatin[138, 139] or in individual somatostatin receptor subtypes[140, 141] have been developed. Because these mice are viable, they are being used as model organisms to illuminate the importance of individual sst receptors in some of the major targets of somatostatin action: the pituitary, the central and peripheral nervous systems, the pancreas, and the gastrointestinal tract.

The Pituitary

The best-established physiologic action of somatostatin is in the inhibitory control of GH secretion: somatostatin interacts with growth hormone–releasing hormone (GHRH) to produce the pulsatile secretion of GH essential for normal growth in mammals (for reviews, see references 142–145). Exogenous somatostatin inhibits GH responses to all known physiologic and pharmacologic stimuli, including exercise, insulin-induced hypoglycemia, and GHRH. Moreover, active immunization of rats against somatostatin increases basal GH levels and diminishes episodic bursts of GH secretion.[142] Finally, GH levels are elevated in null mutant mice lacking somatostatin expression as a result of targeted mutagenesis.[138, 139]

Somatostatin is synthesized in both hypothalamic periventricular and arcuate neurons. Axons of somatostatin-containing cell bodies in the hypothalamic periventricular area project to the median eminence and terminate near portal capillaries. These nerve terminals secrete somatostatin into the hypophyseal portal system, which transports it to the anterior pituitary gland, where it interacts with an abundance of high-affinity somatostatin receptors. Consistent with the observation that sst2A and sst5 receptor immunoreactivity is present on rat somatotrophs,[146, 147] nonpeptidyl somatostatin agonists with either sst2 or sst5 selectivity each inhibit GHRH-stimulated GH release from rat pituitary cells.[148] In addition, an sst2 receptor antagonist induced release of GH when given to anesthetized rats.[149] Thus, both sst2 and sst5 receptor subtypes appear to inhibit GH release in the rat.

Somatostatin also regulates thyroid-stimulating hormone (TSH) secretion and inhibits prolactin release in female or estrogen-primed male animals.[143, 150–152] However, somatostatin does not affect basal or stress-induced ACTH secretion in normal human subjects and rodents and does not affect basal or GnRH-stimulated gonadotropin secretion.[143] The receptor subtypes involved in somatostatin regulation of pituitary hormones other than GH remain to be determined.

The Nervous System

Somatostatin fulfills the requirements for a neurotransmitter: it is present in nerve terminals in synaptic vesicles, it is released by a calcium-dependent mechanism on depolarization of cultured neurons or brain slices, it acts on specific neuronal receptors to cause hyperpolarization and a reduction in calcium influx, and it can modulate the release of other neurotransmitters.[153, 154] Injection of exogenous somatostatin in the brain increases arousal, decreases sleep, stimulates grooming, and causes analgesia and motor impairments.[153, 154] Behavioral studies suggest that somatostatin may be involved in the control of appetite as well as in learning and memory.

The distribution of somatostatin, as well as that of several sst receptor subtypes, has been characterized in detail both in the brain and in the peripheral nervous system and has been recently summarized.[47, 154] Although there is some overlap in the expression of different sst receptor subtypes in certain brain regions, each receptor exhibits a unique pattern consistent with distinct functions.[47, 153–157] Mice lacking sst2 receptor expression do not show any gross defects in either development or behavior,[140] although this receptor is widely distributed in brain. However, somatostatin null mice showed a significant impairment in motor learning.[138] Nonetheless, the precise neurologic role of either sst2 or other sst receptor subtypes is not yet known.

The Pancreas

Exogenous somatostatin regulates both endocrine and exocrine pancreatic secretion.[158, 159] In the rat, it inhibits the release of insulin, glucagon, pancreatic polypeptide, and somatostatin itself. It also inhibits pancreatic exocrine secretion, particularly the pancreatic enzyme responses to cholecystokinin and the pancreatic bicarbonate responses to secretin.[158, 159]

Somatostatin is produced by D cells within the endocrine pancreas. Infusion of a somatostatin antibody significantly increased insulin secretion in human pancreas and also reversed the inhibitory effect of exogenous SS14 on insulin, indicating that intraislet somatostatin has an inhibitory role in the regulation of β-cell secretion in the human islet.[160] Similarly, somatostatin inhibits glucagon secretion by a paracrine action.

Immunohistochemical staining showed that in the rat, all acinar cells and the glucagon and pancreatic polypeptide cells were intensely labeled for sst2A.[161] No signal was detected in somatostatin-producing D cells, and most insulin-containing cells were negative. In addition, the sst2A receptor is abundantly expressed in acinar cells. In contrast, the sst5 receptor is present primarily in the insulin-secreting cells of the rat pancreas.[162] These results are consistent with the effects of nonpeptidyl sst ligands in wild-type mice (WT) and sst2 knockout mice (sst2KO).[163] There was no difference in basal glucagon and insulin secretion between islets isolated from sst2KO and WT mice; however, potassium/arginine-stimulated glucagon secretion was approximately twofold higher in islets isolated from sst2KO mice. SS14 potently inhibited stimulated glucagon secretion in islets from WT mice but was much less effective in islets from sst2KO mice. An sst2-selective analogue inhibited glucagon secretion in islets from WT but was inactive in islets from sstKO mice, whereas an sst5-selective analogue slightly reduced glucagon release in both animal groups. In contrast sst1-, sst3-, and sst4-selective analogues were inactive. Somatostatin and the sst5-selective analogue inhibited glucose-stimulated insulin release in islets from WT and sst2KO mice, whereas the sst2 analogue was less effective. Overall, the results indicate that somatostatin inhibition of glucagon release in mouse and rat islets is primarily mediated via sst2, whereas insulin secretion is regulated primarily via sst5.

When the localization of the sst2A receptor was examined in the normal human pancreas, striking species differences in receptor distribution were observed.[164] The sst2A receptor was present in insulin- as well as glucagon-producing cells, but not in acinar tissue. Thus, in humans, unlike in rats, the action of somatostatin on pancreatic exocrine secretion must be mediated either indirectly or through a different somatostatin receptor subtype on acinar cells. Moreover, in human pancreatic islets, the sst2A receptor appears not to be differentially expressed by the A and B cells, as it is in the rat and mouse. In fact, studies with somatostatin analogues have shown that insulin secretion

in the human islet is primarily inhibited via sst2.[165] These observations emphasize that caution is needed when extrapolating conclusions regarding specific somatostatin functions from one species to another.

The Gastrointestinal Tract

Intravenous somatostatin inhibits the secretion of a wide variety of gastrointestinal hormones, including gastrin, cholecystokinin, secretin vasoactive intestinal polypeptide, gastric inhibitory polypeptide (GIP), motilin, and enteroglucagon.[166–169] In addition, secretory volume and gastric acid and pepsin production are decreased by somatostatin, and gastrointestinal motility, gallbladder contraction, and blood flow are also reduced. Thus, somatostatin controls, by a variety of means, the rate at which nutrients enter the circulation.

Somatostatin is produced both in specific endocrine cells (D cells) in the gastrointestinal tract as well as in neurons of the visceral autonomic nervous system. Most of the somatostatin in the stomach and duodenum is found in D cells, and only a small fraction is found in nerve terminals. Somatostatin is also found in the myenteric plexus of the intestinal tract, in submucosal neurons, and in the lumen of the stomach and duodenum. Thus, somatostatin can act as a neuromodulator, a paracrine regulator, or a luminal hormone to modulate gastrointestinal function.

Nutrient intake, particularly fat, causes a rise in circulating somatostatin levels, and most of the measured circulating somatostatin is thought to arise from the gastrointestinal tract. After meals, the plasma level of somatostatin increases, primarily owing to secretion by D cells of the pancreas and the stomach.

The distribution of sst receptor subtypes in the gastrointestinal tract is only beginning to be elucidated. The sst2A receptor protein was shown by immunohistochemical studies to be present in the human gastrointestinal lymphatic and nervous components, but not in gastrointestinal circular and longitudinal smooth muscle.[170] In the rat enteric nervous system, sst2A immunoreactivity was found primarily in neurons of the myenteric and submucosal plexuses, and abundant fibers distributed to the muscle, mucosa, and vasculature.[171] Immunoreactive staining was also observed in non-neuronal cells, including presumed interstitial cells of Cajal of the intestine and enterochromaffin-like cells of the stomach.[171] Fibers expressing sst2A receptor immunoreactivity were often in close proximity to D cells of the gastric and intestinal mucosa. Co-localization of somatostatin and sst2A receptor immunoreactivities was not observed in endocrine cells nor in enteric neurons. The multiple types of cells expressing the sst2A receptor, including enteric neurons and non-neuronal structures, in addition to the relationship between somatostatin and sst2A receptor elements provide evidence that the sst2A receptor mediates somatostatin effects in the gastrointestinal tract via neuronal and paracrine pathways.[171] Studies with sst2 knockout mice have shown that this somatostatin receptor subtype is mainly responsible for somatostatin suppression of gastric acid secretion.[141] However, the role of this and other sst receptor subtypes in the many gastrointestinal effects of somatostatin remain to be determined.

SUMMARY

Enormous progress has been made in our understanding of somatostatin action in the almost 30 years since its isolation. Nonetheless, we continue to be surprised by unexpected discoveries, such as identification of the cortistatin family of somatostatin-like peptides. Thus the future holds the promise of a more complete understanding of the specific physiologic roles of the different somatostatins and their receptors, as well as the expectation for exciting new discoveries that we cannot yet even foresee.

Acknowledgments

I am grateful to David Steffen, Biomedical Computing, Inc., for sequence analysis and the past and present members of my laboratory for their contributions to our understanding of somatostatin action.

REFERENCES

1. Brazeau P, Vale W, Burgus R, et al: Hypothalamic polypeptide that inhibits the secretion of immunoreactive pituitary growth hormone. Science 179:77–79, 1973.
2. Berelowitz M, LeRoith D, von Schenk H, et al: Somatostatin-like immunoactivity and biological activity is present in *Tetrahymena pyriformis*, a ciliated protozoan. Endocrinology 110:1939–1344, 1982.
3. Conlon JM, Tostivint H, Vaudry H: Somatostatin- and urotensin II–related peptides: Molecular diversity and evolutionary perspectives. Regul Pept 69:95–103, 1997.
4. Lin XW, Otto CJ, Peter RE: Evolution of neuroendocrine peptide systems: Gonadotropin-releasing hormone and somatostatin. Comp Biochem Physiol C Pharmacol Toxicol Endocrinol 119:375–388, 1998.
5. de Lecea L, Criado JR, Prospero-Garcia O, et al: A cortical neuropeptide with neuronal depressant and sleep-modulating properties. Nature 381:242–245, 1996.
6. de Lecea L, Ruiz-Lozano P, Danielson PE, et al: Cloning, mRNA expression, and chromosomal mapping of mouse and human preprocortistatin. Genomics 42:499–506, 1997.
7. Fukusumi S, Kitada C, Takekawa S, et al: Identification and characterization of a novel human cortistatin-like peptide. Biochem Biophys Res Commun 232:157–163, 1997.
8. Coulouarn Y, Lihrmann I, Jegou S, et al: Cloning of the cDNA encoding the urotensin II precursor in frog and human reveals intense expression of the urotensin II gene in motoneurons of the spinal cord. Proc Natl Acad Sci U S A 95:15803–15808, 1998.
9. Shen LP, Rutter WJ: Sequence of the human somatostatin I gene. Science 224:168–171, 1984.
10. Zabel BU, Naylor SL, Sakaguchi AY, et al: High-resolution chromosomal localization of human genes for amylase, proopiomelanocortin, somatostatin, and a DNA fragment (D3S1) by in situ hybridization. Proc Natl Acad Sci U S A 80:6932–6936, 1983.
11. Montminy MR, Goodman RH, Horovitch SJ, Habener JF: Primary structure of the gene encoding rat preprosomatostatin. Proc Natl Acad Sci U S A 81:3337–3340, 1984.
12. Lepage-Lezin A, Joseph-Bravo P, Devilliers G, et al: Prosomatostatin is processed in the Golgi apparatus of rat neural cells. J Biol Chem 266:1679–1688, 1991.
13. Xu H, Shields D: Prohormone processing in permeabilized cells: Endoproteolytic cleavage of prosomatostatin in the trans-Golgi network. Biochimie 76:257–264, 1994.
14. Patel YC, Galanopoulou A: Processing and intracellular targeting of prosomatostatin-derived peptides: The role of mammalian endoproteases. Ciba Found Symp 190:26–40, 1995.
15. Cohen P, Rholam M, Boussetta H: Methods for the identification of neuropeptide processing pathways. *In* Smith IA (ed): Peptidases and Neuropeptide Processing. New York, Academic, 1995.
16. Seidah NG, Day R, Marcinkiewicz M, Chretien M: Precursor convertases: An evolutionary ancient, cell-specific, combinatorial mechanism yielding diverse bioactive peptides and proteins. Ann N Y Acad Sci 839:9–24, 1998.
17. Steiner DF: The proprotein convertases. Curr Opin Chem Biol 2:31–39, 1998.
18. Brakch N, Rholam M, Nault C, et al: Differential processing of hormone precursor. Independent production of somatostatins 14 and 28 in transfected neuroblastoma 2A cells. FEBS Lett 282:363–367, 1991.
19. Brakch N, Cohen P, Boileau G: Processing of human prosomatostatin in AtT-20 cells: S-28 and S-14 are generated in different secretory pathways. Biochem Biophys Res Commun 205:221–229, 1994.
20. Benoit R, Esch F, Bennett HP, et al: Processing of prosomatostatin. Metabolism 39(suppl 2):22–25, 1990.
21. Furuta M, Yano H, Zhou A, et al: Defective prohormone processing and altered pancreatic islet morphology in mice lacking active SPC2. Proc Natl Acad Sci U S A 94:6646–6651, 1997.
22. Nakayama K: Furin: A mammalian subtilisin/Kex2p-like endoprotease involved in processing of a wide variety of precursor proteins. Biochem J 327:625–635, 1997.
23. Bourdais J, Pierotti AR, Boussetta H, et al: Isolation and functional properties of an arginine-selective endoprotease from rat intestinal mucosa. A putative prosomatostatin convertase. J Biol Chem 266:23386–23391, 1991.
24. Schonbrunn A, Tashjian AHJ: Characterization of functional receptors for somatostatin in rat pituitary cells in culture. J Biol Chem 253:6473–6783, 1978.
25. Richardson UI, Schonbrunn A: Inhibition of adrenocorticotropin secretion by somatostatin in pituitary cells in culture. Endocrinology 108:281–290, 1981.
26. Koch BD, Schonbrunn A: The somatostatin receptor is directly coupled to adenylate cyclase in GH4C1 pituitary cell membranes. Endocrinology 114:1784–1790, 1984.
27. Schonbrunn A, Rorstad OP, Westendorf JM, Martin JB: Somatostatin analogs: Correlation between receptor binding affinity and biological potency in GH pituitary cells. Endocrinology 113:1559–1567, 1983.
28. Reubi J-C: Evidence for two somatostatin-14 receptor types in rat brain cortex. Neurosci Lett 49:259–263, 1984.
29. Tran VT, Beal MF, Martin JB: Two types of somatostatin receptors differentiated by cyclic somatostatin analogs. Science 228:492–495, 1985.
30. Yamada Y, Post SR, Wang K, et al: Cloning and functional characterization of a family of human and mouse somatostatin receptors expressed in brain, gastrointestinal tract, and kidney. Proc Natl Acad Sci U S A 89:251–255, 1992.
31. Kluxen F-W, Bruns C, Lubbert H: Expression cloning of a rat brain somatostatin receptor cDNA: Proc Natl Acad Sci U S A 89:4618–4622, 1992.
32. Yamada Y, Reisine T, Law SF, et al: Somatostatin receptors, an expanding gene family: Cloning and functional characterization of human SSTR3, a protein coupled to adenylyl cyclase. Mol Endocrinol 6:2136–2142, 1992.
33. Bruno JF, Xu Y, Song J, Berelowitz M: Molecular cloning and functional expression of a brain-specific somatostatin receptor. Proc Natl Acad Sci U S A 89:11151–11155, 1992.
34. O'Carroll A-M, Lolait SJ, König M, Mahan LC: Molecular cloning and expression

35. of a pituitary somatostatin receptor with preferential affinity for somatostatin-28. Mol Pharmacol 42:939–946, 1992.
35. Hoyer D, Bell GI, Berelowitz M, et al: Classification and nomenclature of somatostatin receptors. Trends Pharmacol Sci 16:86–88, 1995.
36. Vanetti M, Kouba M, Wang X, et al: Cloning and expression of a novel mouse somatostatin receptor (SSTR2B). FEBS Lett 311:290–294, 1992.
37. Schindler M, Kidd EJ, Carruthers AM, et al: Molecular cloning and functional characterization of a rat somatostatin sst2(b) receptor splice variant. Br J Pharmacol 125:209–217, 1998.
38. Lin X, Vogt G, Höllt V: The two isoforms of the mouse somatostatin receptor (mSSTR2A and mSSTR2B) differ in coupling efficiency to adenylate cyclase and in agonist-induced receptor desensitization. FEBS Lett 331:260–266, 1993.
39. Lin X, Janovick JA, Brothers S, et al: Molecular cloning and expression of two type one somatostatin receptors in goldfish brain. Endocrinology 140:5211–5219, 1999.
40. Zupanc GK, Siehler S, Jones EM, et al: Molecular cloning and pharmacological characterization of a somatostatin receptor subtype in the gymnotiform fish *Apteronotus albifrons*. Gen Comp Endocrinol 115:333–345, 1999.
41. Kolakowski LF Jr: GCRDb: A G-protein–coupled receptor database. Receptors Channels 2:1–7, 1994.
42. Bockaert J, Pin JP: Molecular tinkering of G protein–coupled receptors: An evolutionary success. EMBO J 18:1723–1729, 1999.
43. Bourne HR: How receptors talk to trimeric G proteins. Curr Opin Cell Biol 9:134–142, 1997.
44. Hamm HE: The many faces of G protein signaling. J Biol Chem 273:669–672, 1998.
45. Schonbrunn A: Somatostatin receptors present knowledge and future directions. Ann Oncol 10(suppl 2):17–21, 1999.
46. Patel YC: Somatostatin and its receptor family. Front Neuroendocrinol 20:157–198, 1999.
47. Meyerhof W: The elucidation of somatostatin receptor functions: A current view. Rev Physiol Biochem Pharmacol 133:55–108, 1998.
48. Kaupmann K, Bruns C, Raulf F, et al: Two amino acids, located in transmembrane domains VI and VII, determine the selectivity of the peptide agonist SMS 201–995 for the SSTR2 somatostatin receptor. EMBO J 14:727–735, 1995.
49. Maurer R, Gaehwiler BH, Buescher HH, et al: Opiate antagonistic properties of an octapeptide somatostatin analog. Proc Natl Acad Sci U S A 79:4815–4817, 1982.
50. Marchese A, George SR, Kolakowski LF Jr, et al: Novel GPCRs and their endogenous ligands: Expanding the boundaries of physiology and pharmacology. Trends Pharmacol Sci 20:370–375, 1999.
51. Ames RS, Sarau HM, Chambers JK, et al: Human urotensin-II is a potent vasoconstrictor and agonist for the orphan receptor GPR14. Nature 401:282–286, 1999.
52. Chambers J, Ames RS, Bergsma D, et al: Melanin-concentrating hormone is the cognate ligand for the orphan G-protein–coupled receptor SLC-1. Nature 400:261–265, 1999.
53. Saito Y, Nothacker HP, Wang Z, et al: Molecular characterization of the melanin-concentrating-hormone receptor. Nature 400:265–269, 1999.
54. Bachner D, Kreienkamp H, Weise C, et al: Identification of melanin concentrating hormone (MCH) as the natural ligand for the orphan somatostatin-like receptor 1 (SLC-1). FEBS Lett 457:522–524, 1999.
55. Kolakowski LF Jr, Jung BP, Nguyen T, et al: Characterization of a human gene related to genes encoding somatostatin receptors. FEBS Lett 398:253–258, 1996.
56. Criado JR, Li H, Jiang X, et al: Structural and compositional determinants of cortistatin activity. J Neurosci Res 56:611–619, 1999.
57. Darlison MG, Richter D: Multiple genes for neuropeptides and their receptors: Coevolution and physiology. Trends Neurosci 22:81–88, 1999.
58. Baldwin JM: The probable arrangement of the helices in G protein–coupled receptors. EMBO J 12:1693–1703, 1993.
59. Strnad J, Hadcock JR: Identification of a critical aspartate residue in transmembrane domain three necessary for the binding of somatostatin to the somatostatin receptor SSTR2. Biochem Biophys Res Commun 216:913–921, 1995.
60. Ozenberger BA, Hadcock JR: A single amino acid substitution in somatostatin receptor subtype 5 increases affinity for somatostatin-14. Mol Pharmacol 47:82–87, 1995.
61. Gu YZ, Schonbrunn A: Coupling specificity between somatostatin receptor sst2a and G proteins—isolation of the receptor G protein complex with a receptor antibody. Mol Endocrinol 11:527–537, 1997.
62. Helboe L, Moller M, Norregaard L, et al: Development of selective antibodies against the human somatostatin receptor subtypes sst1–sst5. Brain Res Mol Brain Res 49:82–88, 1997.
63. Hipkin RW, Friedman J, Clark RB, et al: Agonist-induced desensitization, internalization, and phosphorylation of the sst2a somatostatin receptor. J Biol Chem 272:13869–13876, 1997.
64. Gu YZ, Brown PJ, Loose-Mitchell DS, et al: Development and use of a receptor antibody to characterize the interaction between somatostatin receptor subtype 1 and G proteins. Mol Pharmacol 48:1004–1014, 1995.
65. Reubi JC, Kappeler A, Waser B, et al: Immunohistochemical localization of somatostatin receptors sst2A in human tumors. Am J Pathol 153:233–245, 1998.
66. Hofland LJ, Liu Q, van Koetsveld PM, et al: 1999 Immunohistochemical detection of somatostatin receptor subtypes sst1 and sst2A in human somatostatin receptor positive tumors. J Clin Endocrinol Metab 84:775–780, 1999.
67. Hipkin RW, Schonbrunn A: Protein kinase C activation stimulates somatostatin receptor 2A (sst2A) internalization. *In* Proceedings of the 80th Meeting of the Endocrine Society. New Orleans, 1998, p 74.
68. Liu Q, Prejusa A, Schonbrunn A: Agonist induced phosphorylation of the sst1 somatostatin receptor: Relationship to desensitization and internalization. *In* Proceedings of the 82nd Meeting of the Endocrine Society. Toronto, 2000.
69. Roth A, Kreienkamp HJ, Meyerhof W, Richter D: Phosphorylation of four amino acid residues in the carboxyl terminus of the rat somatostatin receptor subtype 3 is crucial for its desensitization and internalization. J Biol Chem 272:23769–23774, 1997.

70. Kreienkamp HJ, Roth A, Richter D: Rat somatostatin receptor subtype 4 can be made sensitive to agonist-induced internalization by mutation of a single threonine (residue 331). DNA Cell Biol 17:869–878, 1998.
71. Coy DH, Taylor JE: Receptor-specific somatostatin analogs—correlations with biological activity. Metab Clin Exp 45:21–23, 1996.
72. Bruns C, Raulf F, Hoyer D, et al: Binding properties of somatostatin receptor subtypes. Metab Clin Exp 45(suppl 1):17–20, 1996.
73. Rivier J, Brazeau P, Vale W, Guillemin R: Somatostatin analogs. Relative importance of the disulfide bridge and of the Ala-Gly side chain for biological activity. J Med Chem 18:123–126, 1975.
74. Siehler S, Seuwen K, Hoyer D: [^{125}I]Tyr10-cortistatin14 labels all five somatostatin receptors. Naunyn Schmiedebergs Arch Pharmacol 357:483–489, 1998.
75. Siehler S, Seuwen K, Hoyer D: [^{125}I][Tyr3]octreotide labels human somatostatin sst2 and sst5 receptors. Eur J Pharmacol 348:311–320, 1998.
76. Siehler S, Seuwen K, Hoyer D: Characterisation of human recombinant somatostatin receptors. 1. Radioligand binding studies. Naunyn Schmiedebergs Arch Pharmacol 360:488–499, 1999.
77. Rohrer SP, Birzin ET, Mosley RT, et al: Rapid identification of subtype-selective agonists of the somatostatin receptor through combinatorial chemistry. Science 282:737–740, 1998.
78. Bass RT, Buckwalter BL, Patel BP, et al: Identification and characterization of novel somatostatin antagonists. Mol Pharmacol 50:709–715, 1996.
79. Hocart SJ, Jain R, Murphy WA, et al: Highly potent cyclic disulfide antagonists of somatostatin. J Med Chem 42:1863–1871, 1999.
80. Hocart SJ, Jain R, Murphy WA, et al: Potent antagonists of somatostatin: Synthesis and biology. J Med Chem 41:1146–1154, 1998.
81. Tomura H, Okajima F, Akbar M, et al: Transfected human somatostatin receptor type 2, SSTR2, not only inhibits adenylate cyclase but also stimulates phospholipase C and Ca^{2+} mobilization. Biochem Biophys Res Commun 200:986–992, 1994.
82. Akbar M, Okajima F, Tomura H, et al: Phospholipase C activation and Ca^{2+} mobilization by cloned human somatostatin receptor subtypes 1–5, in transfected COS-7 cells. FEBS Lett 348:192–196, 1994.
83. Milligan G: Mechanisms of multifunctional signalling by G protein-linked receptors. Trends Pharmacol Sci 14:239–244, 1993.
84. Kreienkamp HJ: Molecular biology of the receptors for somatostatin and cortistatin. Results Probl Cell Differ 26:215–237, 1999.
85. Schmidt A, Hescheler J, Offermanns S, et al: Involvement of pertussis toxin–sensitive G-proteins in the hormonal inhibition of dihydropyridine-sensitive Ca^{2+} currents in an insulin-secreting cell line (RINm5F). J Biol Chem 266(27):18025–18033, 1991.
86. Shapiro MS, Hille B: Substance P and somatostatin inhibit calcium channels in rat sympathetic neurons via different G protein pathways. Neuron 10:11–20, 1993.
87. Viana F, Hille B: Modulation of high voltage-activated calcium channels by somatostatin in acutely isolated rat amygdaloid neurons. J Neurosci 16(19):6000–6011, 1996.
88. Degtiar VE, Harhammer R, Nurnberg B: Receptors couple to L-type calcium channels via distinct Go proteins in rat neuroendocrine cell lines. J Physiol (Lond) 502(pt 2):321–333, 1997.
89. White RE, Schonbrunn A, Armstrong DL: Somatostatin stimulates Ca^{2+}-activated K^+ channels through protein dephosphorylation. Nature 351:570–573, 1991.
90. Armstrong DL, White RE: An enzymatic mechanism for potassium channel stimulation through pertussis-toxin–sensitive G proteins. Trends Neurosci 15:403–408, 1992.
91. Kreienkamp HJ, Honck HH, Richter D: Coupling of rat somatostatin receptor subtypes to a G-protein gated inwardly rectifying potassium channel (GIRK1). FEBS Lett 419(1):92–94, 1997.
92. Lopez F, Esteve JP, Buscail L, et al: The tyrosine phosphatase SHP-1 associates with the sst2 somatostatin receptor and is an essential component of sst2-mediated inhibitory growth signaling. J Biol Chem 272(39):24448–24454, 1997.
93. Reardon DB, Dent P, Wood SL, et al: Activation in vitro of somatostatin receptor subtypes 2, 3, or 4 stimulates protein tyrosine phosphatase activity in membranes from transfected Ras-transformed NIH 3T3 cells: Coexpression with catalytically inactive SHP-2 blocks responsiveness. Mol Endocrinol 11(8):1062–1069, 1997.
94. Sellers LA: Prolonged activation of extracellular signal-regulated kinase by a protein kinase C-dependent and N17Ras-insensitive mechanism mediates the proliferative response of G(i/o)-coupled somatostatin sst(4) receptors. J Biol Chem 274(34): 24280–24288, 1999.
95. Florio T, Yao H, Carey KD, et al: Somatostatin activation of mitogen-activated protein kinase via somatostatin receptor 1 (SSTR1). Mol Endocrinol 13(1):24–37, 1999.
96. Fujii Y, Gonoi T, Yamada Y, et al: Somatostatin receptor subtype SSTR2 mediates the inhibition of high-voltage-activated calcium channels by somatostatin and its analogue SMS 201–995. FEBS Lett 355:117–120, 1994.
97. Roosterman D, Glassmeier G, Baumeister H, et al: A somatostatin receptor 1 selective ligand inhibits Ca^{2+} currents in rat insulinoma 1046–38 cells. FEBS Lett 425(1):137–140, 1998.
98. Barber DL, McGuire ME, Ganz MB: Beta-adrenergic and somatostatin receptors regulate Na-H exchange independent of cAMP. J Biol Chem 264:21038–21042, 1989.
99. Carruthers AM, Warner AJ, Michel AD, et al: Activation of adenylate cyclase by human recombinant sst5 receptors expressed in CHO-K1 cells and involvement of $G\alpha s$ proteins. Br J Pharmacol 126(5):1221–1229, 1999.
100. Viguerie N, Tahiri-Jouti N, Ayral AM, et al: Direct inhibitory effects of a somatostatin analog, SMS201–995, on AR4–2J cell proliferation via pertussis toxin-sensitive guanosine triphosphate–binding protein–independent mechanisms. Endocrinology 124:1017–1025, 1989.
101. Lin X, Voynoyasenetskaya TA, Hooley R, et al: $G\alpha_{12}$ differentially regulates Na^+-H^+ exchanger isoforms. J Biol Chem 271:22604–22610, 1996.
102. Brown PJ, Schonbrunn A: Affinity purification of a somatostatin receptor-G-protein complex demonstrates specificity in receptor-G-protein coupling. J Biol Chem 268(9):6668–6676, 1993.
103. Luthin DR, Eppler CM, Linden J: Identification and quantification of G_i-type GTP-binding proteins that copurify with a pituitary somatostatin receptor. J Biol Chem 268(8):5990–5996, 1993.
104. Liu YF, Jakobs KH, Rasenick MM, Albert PR: G protein specificity in receptor-effector coupling: Analysis of the roles of G_o and G_{i2} in GH4C1 pituitary cells. J Biol Chem 269:13880–13886, 1994.
105. Kalkbrenner F, Dippel E, Wittig B, Schultz G: Specificity of interaction between receptor and G protein: Use of antisense techniques to relate G-protein subunits to function (review). Biochem Biophys Acta 1314:125–139, 1996.
106. Senogles SE: The D_2 dopamine receptor isoforms signal through distinct $G_{i\alpha}$ proteins to inhibit adenylyl cyclase: A study with site-directed mutant $G_{i\alpha}$ proteins. J Biol Chem 269(37):23120–127, 1994.
107. Murthy KS, Coy DH, Makhlouf GM: Somatostatin receptor-mediated signaling in smooth muscle: Activation of phospholipase $C_{\beta 3}$ by $G_{\alpha\text{-}\gamma}$ and inhibition of adenylyl cyclase by $G_{\alpha i1}$ and $G_{\alpha ao}$. J Biol Chem 271:23458–23463, 1996.
108. Koch BD, Blalock JB, Schonbrunn A: Characterization of the cyclic AMP-independent actions of somatostatin in GH cells: I. An increase in potassium conductance is responsible for both the hyperpolarization and the decrease in intracellular free calcium produced by somatostatin. J Biol Chem 263:216–225, 1988.
109. Schonbrunn A, Gu YZ, Dournard P, et al: Somatostatin receptor subtypes: Specific expression and signaling properties. Metab Clin Exp 45:8–11, 1996.
110. Koch BD, Schonbrunn A: Characterization of the cyclic AMP-independent actions of somatostatin in GH cells: II. An increase in potassium conductance initiates somatostatin-induced inhibition of prolactin secretion. J Biol Chem 263:226–234, 1988.
111. Hsu WH, Xiang HD, Rajan AS, et al: Somatostatin inhibits insulin secretion by a G-protein-mediated decrease in Ca^{2+} entry through voltage-dependent Ca^{2+} channels in the beta cell. J Biol Chem 266(2):837–843, 1991.
112. Cordelier P, Esteve JP, Bousquet C, et al: Characterization of the antiproliferative signal mediated by the somatostatin receptor subtype sst5. Proc Natl Acad Sci U S A 94(17):9343–9348, 1997.
113. Reardon DB, Wood SL, Brautigan DL, et al: Activation of a protein tyrosine phosphatase and inactivation of Raf-1 by somatostatin. Biochem J 314(pt 2):401–404, 1996.
114. Dent P, Wang Y, Gu YZ, et al: S49 cells endogenously express subtype 2 somatostatin receptors which couple to increase protein tyrosine phosphatase activity in membranes and down-regulate Raf-1 activity in situ. Cell Signal 9(7):539–549, 1997.
115. Buscail L, Esteve J-P, Saint-Laurent N, et al: Inhibition of cell proliferation by the somatostatin analogue RC-160 is mediated by somatostatin receptor subtypes SSTR2 and SSTR5 through different mechanisms. Proc Natl Acad Sci U S A 92:1580–1584, 1995.
116. Golard A, Role LW, Siegelbaum SA: Protein kinase C blocks somatostatin-induced modulation of calcium current in chick sympathetic neurons. J Neurophysiol 70:1639–1643, 1993.
117. Golard A, Siegelbaum SA: Kinetic basis for the voltage-dependent inhibition of N-type calcium current by somatostatin and norepinephrine in chick sympathetic neurons. J Neurosci 13:3884–3894, 1993.
118. Shen KZ, Surprenant A: Somatostatin-mediated inhibitory postsynaptic potential in sympathetically denervated guinea-pig submucosal neurones. J Physiol (Lond) 470:619–635, 1993.
119. Smith MA, Yamamoto G, Vale WW: Somatostatin desensitization in rat anterior pituitary cells. Mole Cell Endocrinol 37:311–318, 1984.
120. Welsh JB, Szabo M: Impaired suppression of growth hormone release by somatostatin in cultured adenohypophyseal cells of spontaneously diabetic BB/W rats. Endocrinology 123:2230–2234, 1988.
121. Kelijman M, Frohman LA: Impaired inhibitory effects of somatostatin on growth hormone (GH)-releasing hormone stimulation of GH secretion after short term infusion. J Clin Endocrinol Metab 71:157–163, 1990.
122. Koper JW, Hofland LJ, Van Koetsveld PM, et al: Desensitization and resensitization of rat pituitary tumor cells in long-term culture to the effects of the somatostatin analogue SMS201–995 on cell growth and prolactin secretion. Cancer Res 50:6238–6242, 1990.
123. Ducasse MC, Tauber JP, Tourre A, et al: Shrinking of a growth hormone-producing pituitary tumor by continuous subcutaneous infusion of the somatostatin analog SMS 201–995. J Clin Endocrinol Metab 65:1042–1046, 1987.
124. Lamberts SW, van der Lely AJ, de Herder WW, Hofland LJ: Octreotide. N Engl J Med 334(4):246–254, 1996.
125. Bunemann M, Hosey MM: G-protein coupled receptor kinases as modulators of G-protein signalling. J Physiol (Lond) 517(pt 1):5–23, 1999.
126. Krupnick JG, Benovic JL: The role of receptor kinases and arrestins in G protein-coupled receptor regulation. Annu Rev Pharmacol Toxicol 38:289–319, 1998.
127. Ferguson SS, Caron MG: G protein-coupled receptor adaptation mechanisms. Semin Cell Dev Biol 9:119–127, 1998.
128. Pitcher JA, Freedman NJ, Lefkowitz RJ: G protein-coupled receptor kinases. Annu Rev Biochem 67:653–692, 1998.
129. Hukovic N, Panetta R, Kumar U, Patel YC: Agonist-dependent regulation of cloned human somatostatin receptor types 1–5 (hsstr1–5)-subtype selective internalization or upregulation. Endocrinology 137:4046–4049, 1996.
130. Roth A, Kreienkamp HJ, Nehring RB, et al: Endocytosis of the rat somatostatin receptors: Subtype discrimination, ligand specificity, and delineation of carboxy-terminal positive and negative sequence motifs. DNA Cell Biol 16:111–119, 1997.
131. Rens-Domiano S, Law SF, Yamada Y, et al: Pharmacological properties of two cloned somatostatin receptors. Mol Pharmacol 42:28–34, 1992.
132. Hipkin RW, Wang Y, Schonbrunn A: Protein kinase C activation stimulates the phosphorylation and internalization of the sst2A somatostatin receptor. J Biol Chem 275:5591–5599, 2000.
133. Mayor FJ, Benovic JL, Caron MG, Lefkowitz RJ: Somatostatin induces translocation of the beta-adrenergic receptor kinase and desensitizes somatostatin receptors in S49 lymphoma cells. J Biol Chem 262:6468–6471, 1987.

134. Hofland LJ, van Koetsveld PM, Waaijers M, Lamberts SW: Internalisation of isotope-coupled somatostatin analogues. Digestion 57(suppl 1):2–6, 1996.

135. Presky DH, Schonbrunn A: Somatostatin pretreatment increases the number of somatostatin receptors in GH4C1 pituitary cells and does not reduce cellular responsiveness to somatostatin. J Biol Chem 263:714–721, 1988.

136. Bruno JF, Xu Y, Berelowitz M: Somatostatin regulates somatostatin receptor subtype mRNA expression in GH3 cells. Biochem Biophys Res Commun 202:1738–1743, 1994.

137. Baumeister H, Wegner M, Richter D, Meyerhof W: Dual regulation of somatostatin receptor subtype 1 gene expression by pit-1 in anterior pituitary GH3 cells. Mol Endocrinol 14:255–271, 2000.

138. Zeyda T, Diehl N, Paylor R, et al: Phenotype screening of somatostatin null mutant mice reveals impairment in motor learning. (Submitted for publication.)

139. Juarez RA, Rubinstein M, Chan EC, Low MJ: Increased growth following normal development in middle-aged somatostatin-deficient mice. Soc Neurosci

140. Zheng H, Bailey A, Jiang MH, et al: Somatostatin receptor subtype 2 knockout mice are refractory to growth hormone-negative feedback on arcuate neurons. Mol Endocrinol 11(11):1709–1717, 1997.

141. Martinez V, Curi AP, Torkian B, et al: High basal gastric acid secretion in somatostatin receptor subtype 2 knockout mice. Gastroenterology 114(6):1125–1132, 1998.

142. Tannenbaum GS: Somatostatin as a physiological regulator of pulsatile growth hormone secretion. Horm Res 29(2–3):70–74, 1988.

143. Gillies G: Somatostatin: The neuroendocrine story. Trends Pharmacol Sci 18(3):87–95, 1997.

144. Bluet-Pajot MT, Epelbaum J, Gourdji D, et al: Hypothalamic and hypophyseal regulation of growth hormone secretion. Cell Mol Neurobiol 18(1):101–123, 1998.

145. Muller EE, Locatelli V, Cocchi D: Neuroendocrine control of growth hormone secretion. Physiol Rev 79(2):511–607, 1999.

146. Mezey E, Hunyady B, Mitra S, et al: Cell specific expression of the sst2A and sst5 somatostatin receptors in the rat anterior pituitary. Endocrinology 139:414–419, 1998.

147. Kumar U, Laird D, Srikant CB, et al: Expression of the five somatostatin receptor (SSTR1–5) subtypes in rat pituitary somatotrophes: Quantitative analysis by double-layer immunofluorescence confocal microscopy. Endocrinology 138:4473–4476, 1997.

148. Parmar RM, Chan WW, Dashkevicz M, et al: Nonpeptidyl somatostatin agonists demonstrate that sst2 and sst5 inhibit stimulated growth hormone secretion from rat anterior pituitary cells. Biochem Biophys Res Commun 263:276–280, 1999.

149. Baumbach WR, Carrick TA, Pausch MH, et al: A linear hexapeptide somatostatin antagonist blocks somatostatin activity in vitro and influences growth hormone release in rats. Mol Pharmacol 54(5):864–873, 1998.

150. Kimura N, Hayafuji C, Konagaya H, Takahashi K: 17-β-Estradiol induces somatostatin inhibition of prolactin release and regulates somatostatin receptors in rat anterior pituitary cells. Endocrinology 119:1028–1036, 1986.

151. Gooren LJG, Harmsen-Louman W, van Kessel H: Somatostatin inhibits prolactin release from the lactotroph primed with oestrogen and cyproterone acetate in man. J Endocrinol 103:333–335, 1984.

152. Djordjijevic D, Zhang J, Priam M, et al: Effect of 17beta-estradiol on somatostatin receptor expression and inhibitory effects on growth hormone and prolactin release in rat pituitary cell cultures. Endocrinology 139:2272–2277, 1998.

153. Epelbaum J, Dournaud P, Fodor M, Viollet C: The neurobiology of somatostatin. Crit Rev Neurobiol 8(1–2):25–44, 1994.

154. Schindler M, Humphrey PP, Emson PC: Somatostatin receptors in the central nervous system. Prog Neurobiol 50(1):9–47, 1996.

155. Dournaud P, Gu YZ, Schonbrunn A, et al: Localization of the somatostatin receptor sst2a in rat brain using a specific anti-peptide antibody. J Neurosci 16:4468–4478, 1996.

156. Dournaud P, Boudin H, Schonbrunn A, et al: Interrelationships between somatostatin sst2A receptors and somatostatin-containing axons in rat brain: evidence for regulation of cell surface receptors by endogenous somatostatin. J Neurosci 18:1056–1071, 1998.

157. Stroh T, Kreienkamp HJ, Beaudet A: Immunohistochemical distribution of the somatostatin receptor subtype 5 in the adult rat brain: predominant expression in the basal forebrain. J Comp Neurol 412:69–82, 1999.

158. Reichlin S: Somatostatin: I. N Engl J Med 309:1495–1501, 1983.

159. Reichlin S: Somatostatin: II. N Engl J Med 309:1556–1563, 1983.

160. Kleinman R, Gingerich R, Wong H, et al: Use of the Fab fragment for immunoneutralization of somatostatin in the isolated perfused human pancreas. Am J Surg 167:114–119, 1994.

161. Hunyady B, Hipkin RW, Schonbrunn A, Mezey E: Immunohistochemical localization of somatostatin receptor Sst2a in the rat pancreas. Endocrinology 138(6):2632–2635, 1997.

162. Mitra SW, Mezey E, Hunyady B, et al: Colocalization of somatostatin receptor sst5 and insulin in rat pancreatic beta-cells. Endocrinology 140(8):3790–3796, 1999.

163. Strowski MZ, Parmar RM, Blake AD, Schaeffer JM: Somatostatin inhibits insulin and glucagon secretion via two receptors subtypes: an in vitro study of pancreatic islets from somatostatin receptor 2 knockout mice. Endocrinology 141(1):111–117, 2000.

164. Reubi JC, Kappeler A, Waser B, et al: Immunohistochemical localization of somatostatin receptor sst2A in human pancreatic islets. J Clin Endocrinol Metab 83:3746–3749, 2000.

165. Atiya AW, Moldovan S, Adrian TE, et al: Intraislet somatostatin inhibits insulin (via a subtype-2 somatostatin receptor) but not islet amyloid polypeptide secretion in the isolated perfused human pancreas. J Gastrointest Surg 1(3):251–256, 1997.

166. Tulassay Z: Somatostatin and the gastrointestinal tract. Scand J Gastroenterol Suppl 228:115–121, 1998.

167. Reubi JC, Laissue J, Waser B, et al: Expression of somatostatin receptors in normal, inflamed, and neoplastic human gastrointestinal tissues. Ann N Y Acad Sci 733:122–137, 1994.

168. Lucey MR, Yamada T: Biochemistry and physiology of gastrointestinal somatostatin. Dig Dis Sci 34(suppl):5S–13S, 1989.

169. Schusdziarra V: Physiological significance of gastrointestinal somatostatin. Horm Res 29(2–3):75–78, 1988.

170. Reubi JC, Laissue JA, Waser B, et al: Immunohistochemical detection of somatostatin sst2a receptors in the lymphatic, smooth muscular, and peripheral nervous systems of the human gastrointestinal tract: Facts and artifacts. J Clin Endocrinol Metab 84(8):2942–2950, 1999.

171. Sternini C, Wong H, Wu SV, et al: Somatostatin 2A receptor is expressed by enteric neurons, and by interstitial cells of Cajal and enterochromaffin-like cells of the gastrointestinal tract. J Comp Neurol 386(3):396–408, 1997.

Insulin-Like Growth Factor-1 and Its Binding Proteins

David R. Clemmons

The family of insulin-like growth factors (IGFs) and related substances is unusual when considered in the context of traditional hormones. Although these substances are secreted into extracellular fluids and act on cells in distal target organs, much like traditional hormones, they also act on cells that are adjacent to the cells of origin and on the cells of origin themselves, such as fibroblasts, resulting in autocrine or paracrine growth stimulation. Therefore, these substances can be viewed as either traditional hormones or as locally produced growth factors. The ability to genetically manipulate animals has resulted in a greater understanding of the role of locally produced IGF-1 in regulating growth in vivo. Although knowledge is still evolving in this area, it is clear that the full understanding of the mechanism of action of polypeptide growth factors, such as IGF-1, cannot be elucidated without an appreciation of both their systemic endocrine effects, which can be demonstrated in classic in vivo infusion experiments, and their local tissue effects, which can be analyzed indirectly by using gene knockout experiments. Clearly, both of these sources of peptide, that is, autocrine-produced and endocrine-transported, are important for regulation of growth in vivo. Likewise, attempts in clinical medicine to manipulate growth factor activities, as in treating cancers that are growth factor–dependent, may rely both on ablation of systemically produced circulating hormonal concentrations and ablation of local tissue production. Thus, a true understanding of the physiologic mechanisms that regulate both types of production is necessary.

The IGFs belong to a family of polypeptides that evolved from a common ancestral precursor into IGF-1 and IGF-2 and, later, into IGF-1, IGF-2, and proinsulin. All three members of the family probably evolved before the emergence of a pituitary gland, although growth hormone (GH) control of IGF-1 evolved at the time IGF-1 and insulin diverged. Unlike insulin, both IGF-1 and IGF-2 circulate bound to high-affinity binding proteins. This results in a markedly different type of regulation of their actions as compared to insulin. Similarly, the IGFs have distinct receptors that bind them with much higher affinity than insulin, and the insulin receptor has similar selectivity. Because they are ubiquitously secreted in all tissues, the IGFs represent important systemic regulators of growth, and no doubt this production in multiple target tissues is a major determinant of balanced organ and tissue growth.

IGF-1 was originally discovered based on its property of stimulating sulfation of proteoglycans that are present in cartilage.[1] It was later determined that it was an important stimulant of cartilage DNA synthesis.[2] This property was discovered while trying to develop in vitro assays for GH activity. When GH was added to cartilage in vitro, it was a poor stimulant of cartilage sulfation. However, the administration of GH to hypophysectomized animals resulted in induction of a substance in serum that was a potent stimulant of cartilage sulfation. This suggested that a separate growth factor was induced in the serum of these animals. Purification of this substance led to determination of its primary amino acid sequence and to studies that showed that it could stimulate the growth of whole animals.[3, 4]

Molecular technology has made it possible to determine the structure of the receptors for the IGFs and for GH. These studies have also led to the identification of signal transduction pathways that are linked to each receptor. All three substances can induce activation of similar signaling molecules, although in several cases activation of the receptors clearly induces distinct substances. A more complete description of the relative roles of IGF-1, insulin, and GH in growth and metabolic regulation ultimately awaits the elucidation of all of the genes that are induced by activation of each receptor. This should lead to a better definition of their respective target cell roles, as well as their relative hierarchical importance in growth regulation.

COMPONENTS OF THE INSULIN-LIKE GROWTH FACTOR SYSTEM

IGF-1 Gene and Protein Structures

The IGF-1 gene is a complex, multicomponent gene, with six exons.[5] The gene structure is shown in Figure 33–1. The first and second exons encode the 5′ untranslated and prepropeptide regions of IGF-1. Exon 3 encodes the distal propeptide sequence and the regions of the mature peptide that are homologous to the B chain of insulin, the region homologous to the C peptide, and to the A chain region. Exon 4 encodes a D extension peptide. The fifth and sixth exons are shuffled and can encode one of two sequences termed IGF-1A and IGF-1B.[6] This alternative splicing occurs in multiple tissues, and both IGF-1A and IGF-1B have been found as gene products of specific cell types in culture.[7, 8]

Several forms of IGF-1 messenger RNA (mRNA) are transcribed, and at least four specific transcripts are often detected in tissues.[9] The most abundant transcript that is detected is the 6-kb IGF-1 transcript, which includes multiple polyadenylation sites and a long 3′ untranslated sequence. The abundance of this transcript is regulated by GH.[10] Several different fetal and tissue-specific promoters of IGF-1 have been identified, and they account for distinct transcript patterns in various tissues and the appearance of various forms at specific periods in development.[11] Other abundant transcripts include a 3.2-kb transcript, a 2.7-kb transcript, and a 0.9-kb transcript. Stimuli other than GH have been shown to influence the abundance of these transcripts in various tissues.[12, 13] The small 0.9-kb transcript is one source of the mature 70–amino acid IGF-1 peptide. This transcript is present in the liver and is believed to be an important source of the peptide that is present in the systemic circulation. Alternative processing of the mRNA following its transcription has been described for multiple tissues and may be physiologically relevant in specific situations. Variable polyadenylation sites and regulation of processing of the 3′ untranslated RNA extensions have been shown to occur and can result in transcripts of different length.[14]

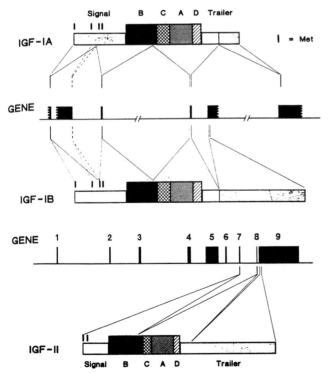

FIGURE 33–1. Structure of the human IGF-1 gene and the precursor proteins it encodes. The black boxes that are shown represent exons. The portions of each exon that encode parts of the precursor protein are shown by lines. The IGF-1 A and -1 B precursor forms are represented by boxes. The B, C, A, and D domains of the mature peptides are noted.

TABLE 33–1. Specific Amino Acids in Insulin-Like Growth Factor-1 (IGF-1) That Mediate Binding Protein and Receptor Association

Region of IGF-1	Ligand Interaction
B chain	
Glu3, Thr4, Gln15, Phe16	Required for binding to IGF binding proteins (IGFBPs) 1–6
A chain	
Phe49, Arg50, Ser51	Required for optimal binding to IGFBP-1, -2, -4, -5
Tyr24, Tyr31, Tyr60	IGF-1 receptor
Tyr24-Arg37	Contains the primary binding site
Tyr60	Necessary for a stable conformation

The polypeptide structures of three members of the IGF gene family are shown in Figure 33–2. Mature IGF-1 and IGF-2 contain 70 and 67 amino acids, respectively.[15] Proinsulin has a longer C peptide region compared to the C peptide region in IGF-1 or IGF-2. The sequence in this region is not conserved. The A chain and B chain peptide regions are of similar length. The sequences in this region are 41% and 43% homologous to proinsulin. IGF-1 and -2 contain D domain extensions of 8 and 6 amino acids, respectively. Unlike proinsulin, IGF-1 and -2 are not cleaved into two-chain polypeptides during intracellular processing, but rather they are secreted as intact single-chain proteins. Forms of IGF-1 have been isolated from serum and from cell culture supernatants that contain the E peptide extensions (e.g., both A and B), but the relative abundance of these forms in most tissues is not well defined.[7, 8] The frequency of processing of the E peptide domains is unclear, since longer forms of IGF-1A or IGF-1B have been shown to be secreted by cells in culture. However, some cells do not secrete IGF-1 with the E peptide extension.

Specific amino acids within the IGF-1 molecule have been shown by site-directed mutagenesis to account for receptor or binding protein association, or both (Table 33–1). Specifically Tyr24, Tyr60, and, to some extent, Tyr31 are critical for IGF-1 receptor recognition.[16, 17] The tyrosines at positions 24 and 60 are conserved within IGF-2, but Tyr31 is not present. The residue that is homologous to Tyr24 in proinsulin, for example, Phe25, is important for insulin binding to its receptor. Tyr60 appears to be necessary to maintain IGF-1 in its stable conformation. Studies using mutant forms of IGF-1 with large deletions indicate that the region between residues 24 and 37 contains the primary receptor binding site.[18] Mutations in this region have very little effect on binding protein affinity.

IGF-1 and -2 contain four amino acids that account for most of the binding protein activity. These include the amino acids at positions 3, 4, 15, and 16 of the B chain region of IGF-1 and the homologous residues 6, 7, 18, and 19 in IGF-2.[19] These residues are critical for recognition by all six forms of IGF binding proteins (IGFBPs). Mutant forms of IGF-1 with substitution of proinsulin residues in these four positions have a nearly total loss of binding protein activity.[20] In addition, residues at amino acids 49, 50, and 51 in the A chain are critical for recognition by four of the six high-affinity binding proteins.[21] The major exception is IGFBP-3, wherein only the B chain residues appear to be important. Studies of the tertiary structures of IGF-1 and IGF-2 have predicted that these residues are surface-exposed and therefore should be available for protein binding. The C peptide regions in each of the three proteins are divergent and this accounts for most of the heterogeneity of sequence between IGF-1 and IGF-2. The disulfide linkages are conserved in all three peptides.

The structure of IGF-1 is highly conserved across species. Bovine IGF-1 is identical to human, and rat differs by only three amino acids.[22] IGF-1-like molecules have been detected in all vertebrates that have been analyzed, and even species as low on the phylogenetic tree as *Caenorhabditis elegans* contain IGF-1-like molecules. Computer modeling studies have indicated that the three-dimensional structure of IGF-1 is probably similar to that of insulin, which has been analyzed by x-ray crystallography.[23] Different forms of IGF-1 have been found to be present in human serum and tissues. The most extensively

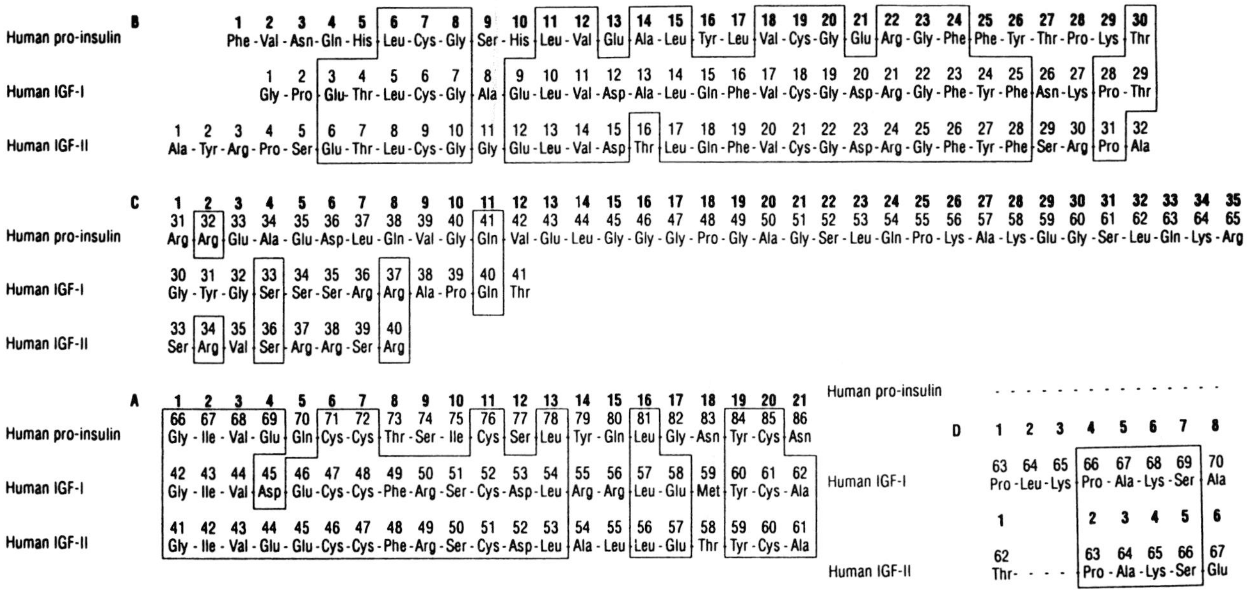

B

Human pro-insulin (1–30): Phe-Val-Asn-Gln-His-[Leu-Cys-Gly]-Ser-His-[Leu-Val]-Glu-Ala-Leu-Tyr-Leu-[Val-Cys-Gly]-Glu-Arg-Gly-Phe-[Phe-Tyr-Thr-Pro-Lys]-[Thr]

Human IGF-I (1–29): Gly-Pro-[Glu-Thr-Leu-Cys-Gly]-Ala-Glu-Leu-Val-Asp-Ala-Leu-Gln-Phe-Val-Cys-Gly-Asp-Arg-Gly-Phe-Tyr-Phe-[Asn-Lys]-[Pro-Thr]

Human IGF-II (1–32): Ala-Tyr-Arg-Pro-Ser-[Glu-Thr-Leu-Cys-Gly]-Gly-[Glu-Leu-Val-Asp]-[Thr]-Leu-Gln-Phe-Val-Cys-Gly-Asp-Arg-Gly-Phe-Tyr-Phe-[Ser-Arg]-[Pro]-[Ala]

C

Human pro-insulin (residues 31–65): Arg-[Arg]-Glu-Ala-Glu-Asp-Leu-Gln-Val-Gly-[Gln]-Val-Glu-Leu-Gly-Gly-Gly-Pro-Gly-Ala-Gly-Ser-Leu-Gln-Pro-Lys-Ala-Lys-Glu-Gly-Ser-Leu-Gln-Lys-Arg

Human IGF-I (residues 30–41): Gly-Tyr-Gly-[Ser]-Ser-Ser-Arg-[Arg]-Ala-Pro-[Gln]-Thr

Human IGF-II (residues 33–40): Ser-[Arg]-Val-[Ser]-Arg-Arg-Ser-[Arg]

A

Human pro-insulin (residues 66–86): [Gly-Ile-Val-Glu]-Gln-[Cys-Cys]-Thr-Ser-Ile-[Cys]-Ser-[Leu]-Tyr-Gln-[Leu]-Gly-Asn-[Tyr-Cys]-Asn

Human IGF-I (residues 42–62): [Gly-Ile-Val]-[Asp]-Glu-[Cys-Cys]-Phe-Arg-Ser-Cys-Asp-Leu-Arg-Arg-Leu-Glu-[Met]-Tyr-Cys-Ala

Human IGF-II (residues 41–61): [Gly-Ile-Val-Glu]-Glu-[Cys-Cys]-Phe-Arg-Ser-Cys-Asp-Leu-Ala-Leu-Leu-Glu-Thr-Tyr-Cys-Ala

D

Human pro-insulin: - - - - - -

Human IGF-I (residues 63–70): Pro-Leu-Lys-[Pro-Ala-Lys-Ser]-Ala

Human IGF-II (residues 62–67): Thr- - - -[Pro-Ala-Lys-Ser]-Glu

FIGURE 33–2. *The sequences of proinsulin, IGF-1, and IGF-2. The sequences are divided into the B, C, A, and D domains.*

studied form is des-(1–3)-IGF-1, which occurs in brain and in serum.[24, 25] This molecule is believed to be important because it has much lower affinity for binding proteins and therefore, if generated in vivo, can provide a more biologically active form of IGF-1.

IGF-1 Receptor

The IGF-1 receptor is omnipresent and has been shown to be present in cell types derived from all three embryonic lineages. When animal tissues have been analyzed, this receptor can be detected uniformly. This probably accounts for the ability of IGF-1 to stimulate growth of all tissues. The receptor number appears to be very tightly controlled since receptor number per cell varies within the range of 20,000 to 35,000. This may be an important, protective regulatory function, since cellular transformation in response to IGF-1 usually requires more than 1 million receptors per cell.[26] This hypothesis is supported by the fact that, when cells are genetically engineered to contain more than a million IGF-1 receptors per cell, they become tumorigenic, whereas cells that have less than 100,000 receptors per cell do not induce tumors. Thus, the variables that regulate IGF-1 receptor number could be important in terms of the genesis of neoplasia.

The hormonal regulation of receptor number has been analyzed in great detail. Hormones such as GH, FSH (follicle-stimulating hormone), LH (luteinizing hormone), progesterone, estradiol, and thyroxine (T_4), have been shown to increase receptor expression.[27, 28] Similarly, platelet-derived growth factor (PDGF), epidermal growth factor (EGF), fibroblast growth factor (FGF), and angiotensin II upregulate expression in specific cell types.[29, 30] Following hormone binding, there is classic downregulation of receptor number with internalization of receptors. However, possibly owing to IGFBPs, the rate of internalization of IGF-1 receptors is substantially less than that of other growth factors, such as EGF or insulin.

The biochemical structure of the receptor is similar to other polypeptide growth factor receptors (Fig. 33–3). The receptor is a heterotetrameric glycoprotein composed of two ligand-binding subunits termed α subunits, which contain 706 amino acids, and two β subunits, which contain 627 amino acids. Only the β subunits have a transmembrane domain (see Fig. 33–3). In humans, the protein is translated from a single mRNA transcript derived from a 21-exon gene located on chromosome 15, Q25–Q26.[31] The prepropeptide contains 1367 amino acids. It is cleaved between Lys708 and Arg709 to generate the α and β subunits, which are linked together by disulfide bonds to form the α2β2 heterotetrameric receptor. Amino acid sequence comparison with the insulin receptor reveals 46% amino acid identity.[31]

The α subunit contains a cysteine-rich domain between residues 148 and 302. This region contains the ligand-binding region of the receptor. Antibodies directed against this region have been shown to block binding. The ligand-binding domain of the α subunit binds IGF-1 with an association constant of approximately 10^{-9}M. IGF-2 binds with sixfold lower affinity, and insulin with a 200- to 300-fold lower affinity.[5, 32]

The β subunit of the receptor is composed of a transmembrane domain between positions 906 and 929 that is followed by a long, intracytoplasmic domain. This region contains intrinsic tyrosine kinase (TK) activity and critical sites of tyrosine and serine phosphorylation. The TK domain is 84% homologous to the insulin receptor TK domain.[33] The catalytic domain contains an adenosine triphosphate (ATP) binding motif and a catalytic lysine at position 1003. Substitution for this lysine abolishes IGF-1-stimulated biologic actions.[34] Ligand binding to the α subunit triggers a conformational change and dimerization that leads to autoactivation.[35, 36] This, in turn, leads to transreceptor phosphorylation, wherein specific tyrosines located on one β subunit are transphosphorylated by the TK activity located on the paired β subunit. This mode of TK activation that results in tyrosine autophosphorylation is similar to that which occurs in the insulin receptor.[36–38]

There are at least six important tyrosines contained within the cytoplasmic domain that are phosphorylated by the intrinsic TK. The most important is a triple tyrosine motif at positions 1149, 1150, and 1151. Substitutions for these tyrosines abolish IGF-1 signaling.[34, 39] Following phosphorylation of these residues in response to activation of intrinsic TK activity by hormone binding to the receptor, the TK is further activated to phosphorylate intracellular substrates, such as insulin receptor substrate-1 and -2 (IRS-1 and -2) (see below). Following its phosphorylation, IRS-1 binds tightly to the receptor at Tyr950. Substitution for this residue does not alter autophosphorylation but attenuates IRS-1 phosphorylation and biologic signaling.[40] Following adherence of IRS-1 to the receptor, the intrinsic TK activity is further activated, and it phosphorylates additional sites on IRS-1. This leads to the binding adapter proteins, such as Grb-2, or other kinases, such as phosphotidylinositol-3′-OH kinase (PI-3-kinase). Substitutions for Tyr1131, Tyr1135, and Tyr1136 also results in major loss of autophosphorylation and no phosphorylation of exogenous substrates, such as IRS-1.[39] Mutation of Tyr1316 abrogates the ability to activate PI-3-kinase, and alteration of Tyr1250 and Tyr1251, which are not found in the insulin receptor, induces a major reduction in the cellular proliferation response.[41] The C-terminal tyrosines 1150 and 1151 are also phosphorylated. The receptor can also directly phosphorylate other substrates, including Shc, Crk, and Grb-10.[42, 43] Phosphorylation

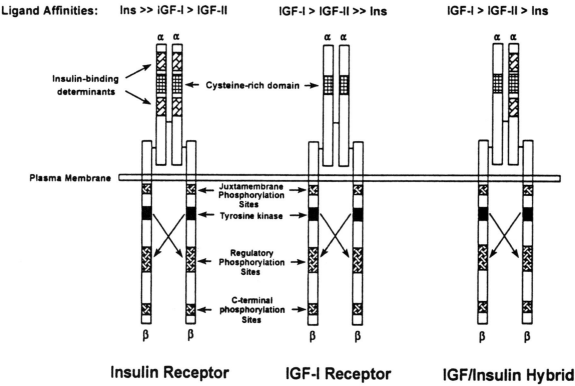

FIGURE 33–3. Structural characteristics of the insulin, IGF-1, and hybrid receptors.

of residues 1280 and 1283 is necessary for binding to 14–3–3, an additional signaling intermediate. The NPXY motif on the receptor C-terminal domain is required for internalization.[44, 45]

Chimeric receptors that contain αβ dimers of the IGF-1 receptor and insulin receptor have been described.[46] These αβ dimers are disulfide-bonded. Receptor hybrids have been detected in several tissue and cell types. It is possible that they exist in all cells in which both IGF-1 and insulin receptors are expressed. The ligand specificity and affinity properties of hybrid receptors are much closer to those of the IGF-1 receptor as compared to the insulin receptor. The biologic significance of hybrid receptor formation has not been determined.

The receptor has been overexpressed in several types of cells in culture. Overexpression can lead to the ability of cells to grow in soft agar and form tumors in nude mice.[26] This suggests that tight regulation of receptor number is responsible for controlling the ability of IGF-1 to transform cells. Importantly, deletion of specific tyrosines, mainly substitution for Tyr1251, results in a marked diminution in the transforming property of the IGF-1 receptor, although mitogenesis in vitro is still preserved.[47, 48] In addition to its ability to transform, the receptor appears to be extremely important for IGF-1 to modulate the effects of other growth factors. Mouse fibroblasts containing deficient numbers of IGF-1 receptors do not increase DNA synthesis in response to EGF. Similarly, overexpression of the EGF and PDGF receptors does not lead to proliferation of fibroblasts in soft agar in the absence of IGF-1 receptors.[49, 50] Cellular transformation by simian virus 40 (SV40) requires expression of the IGF-1 receptor, and wild-type Ras activation has less of an effect on cellular transformation if the IGF-1 receptor is absent.[51] Likewise, *Src* oncogene expression results in transforming activity only in the presence of an IGF-1 receptor. Blocking phosphorylation of Tyr1250 and Tyr1251, Tyr1316, His1293, or Lys1294 results in loss of the ability of the receptor to be transforming, although mitogenesis and IRS-1 phosphorylation responses are intact.[52]

The IGF-1 receptor has an important role in normal development and normal fetal growth. Animals that have had the IGF-1 receptor deleted by homologous recombination are born approximately 40% of normal size.[53] These animals were not viable at birth, due to hypoplasia of diphragmatic muscle. Defects in the development of the nervous system, skin, and bones are present. These developmental abnormali-ties occur relatively late in gestation. Fibroblasts obtained from these embryos have a markedly attenuated growth response to serum compared to fibroblasts from normal embryos.[54]

The receptor is also important for prevention of apoptosis. IGF-1 and its receptor support the viability of nonproliferating cells in culture, such as neurons. The extent of apoptosis that can be induced in neurons by osmotic hyperglycemia, ischemia, or potassium shock is dependent upon normal IGF-1 receptor expression, suggesting that it is neuroprotective.[55] Hematopoietic cells that are dependent on interleukin-3 (IL-3) for proliferation, and undergo apoptosis if IL-3 is withdrawn, are protected by IGF-1 exposure if IGF-1 receptors are present. Plating tumor cells on a surface that does not involve ligand binding to integrins results in susceptibility to apoptosis, and this susceptibility can be reversed by incubation with IGF-1.[56] Mutation of Tyr1251, Lys1294, or His1293 eliminates the capacity of the receptor to protect against apoptosis, whereas mutations of Tyr1250, Tyr1316, or Tyr950 have no effect.[57]

In contrast to the IGF-1 receptor, overexpression of the insulin receptor is nontransforming. Likewise, overexpression of a chimeric receptor bearing the β subunit of the insulin receptor is nontransforming, but if the IGF-1 receptor β subunit is expressed with the insulin receptor α subunit, then mitogenic activity of insulin is detected at much lower ligand concentrations and this receptor construct allows transformation to occur.[58]

Receptor-Mediated Signal Transduction Systems

Following activation of the intrinsic TK activity and phosphorylation of the triple tyrosine domain of the receptor, the docking protein, IRS-1, binds directly to the receptor (Fig. 33–4). A functionally similar protein termed IRS-2 has been shown to bind by a similar mechanism.[59] Following binding, IRS-1 is then tyrosine-phosphorylated by the receptor at multiple sites, creating docking motifs that are critical for binding of intracellular proteins that contain Src homology-2 (SH-2) domains. These domains contain approximately 100 amino acids that share similarity with a segment first identified in the cellular oncogene, *Src*. Six of the tyrosines in IRS-1 occur within YMXM sequences, a kinase recognition motif within SH-2 domains.[60] Other proteins that bind directly to the phosphorylated tyrosines on IRS-1 include the adapter proteins Nck and Grb-2.[61] Grb-2 forms a complex with the Ras activating protein (son of sevenless, SOS), and this complex leads to subsequent P-21 Ras activation, which activates Raf and downstream components of the mitogen-activated protein kinase (MAPK) pathway. Activation of this pathway is important for the mitogenic function of IGF-1.[42, 62] The IGF-1 receptor can directly phosphorylate Src homology–containing protein (SHC), and this can lead to activation of Grb-2 independently of IRS-1. An additional signaling molecule that is activated by the receptor is Crk, a Grb-2-like protein, with SH-2 and SH-3 domains. Crk then activates Grb-2 and SOS after it is phosphorylated by the IGF-1 receptor.[43] Other signaling pathways that have been shown to be activated include protein kinase C, phospholipase C, and direct stimulation of calcium-permeable ion channels.[63–65]

IRS-1 also induces the two subunits of PI-3-kinase to associate. This results in catalytic activation, the generation of inositol triphosphate and activation of protein tyrosine kinase B.[66, 67] This kinase activates P70 S6 kinase and GSK-3, a kinase that is involved in glucose transport. This pathway is also important for IGF-1-induced increases in cell motility and for inhibition of apoptosis.[68]

Since there is great specificity between insulin and IGF-1 in terms of molecular mechanisms of action, it was presumed that major differences would be detected in the signal transduction pathways that each hormone utilized. However, IGF-1 and insulin receptor kinase domains are 84% identical, and similar residues are autophosphorylated. Presumably, either distinct domains are activated in the IRS-1 and -2 or separate combinations of signaling pathways are activated. Although activation of IRS-1, IRS-2, and SHC appears to be nondistinguishable between insulin and IGF-1 receptors, activation of Crk-2 is specific for the IGF-1 receptor.[43] Since Crk-2 has transforming activity, its activation may partially account for the ability of overexpression of IGF-1 receptors to be transforming. Likewise, insulin receptor activation results in dephosphorylation of tyrosine residues on focal adhesion kinase, whereas IGF-1 receptor does not have this effect.[69] A more detailed molecular explanation has been provided by the observation that activation of IRS-1 by the respective receptors results in binding to phosphorylated tyrosines in different domains.[70] The insulin receptor binds preferentially to Tyr987 and Tyr727, whereas the IGF-1 receptor binds preferentially to Tyr895. Finally, it should be noted that activation of Src kinase results in phosphorylation of the IGF-1 receptor, but not the insulin receptor.[71] Gene targeting experiments have shown that the IGF-1 receptor clearly has effects that are different from those

of the insulin receptor, but how these effects are mediated in vivo beyond receptor ligand-binding selectivity remains undetermined.

Blocking specific functions of intracellular signaling pathways has been shown to attenuate specific IGF-1 actions. The PI-3-kinase pathway appears important for glucose transport and for cell migration.[66, 67] Specific inhibitors of PI-3-kinase result in attenuation of these IGF-1-stimulated actions. Similarly, the MAPK pathway appears to be the predominant pathway for mitogenesis and rescue from apoptosis, and specific blockade of these phosphorylation reactions results in a preferential effect on these IGF-1-stimulated effects.[57] However, the requirement for either pathway is not absolute, since high concentrations of specific inhibitors of these pathways result in inhibition of overlapping functions. For example, 1.0 μM PD98059 inhibits MAPK effectively, and it is a potent inhibitor of IGF-1-stimulated DNA synthesis, but it has no effect on cell migration. However, a 50-μM concentration of this compound will inhibit cell migration significantly, even though it has a weak effect on PI-3-kinase activity. This suggests that there may be overlapping contributions of these pathways to multiple cellular functions. Protein kinase C also appears to be essential to IGF-1-stimulated migration and stimulation of gene transcription of specific genes.

IGF-2–Mannose 6-Phosphate Receptor

The IGF-2 cation-independent mannose 6-phosphate receptor is a single-chain membrane spanning a glycoprotein that contains 2451 amino acids. It binds mannose 6-phosphate residues on lysosomal enzymes, as well as IGF-2. There is a large extracellular domain, a 23–amino acid transmembrane domain, and a 164-residue C-terminal intracytoplasmic domain. The extracellular domain is composed of 15 repeating motifs.[72] Motifs 7 to 9 bind mannose 6-phosphate, and motif 11 contains the IGF-2 binding region.[73] Intracellularly, this receptor functions to translocate newly synthesized lysosomal enzymes into endosomes. On the cell surface, it binds to mannose 6-phosphate–containing extracellular glycoproteins, which are endocytosed into endosomes. The receptors are then recycled back to the cell surface. Proteins other than lysosomal enzymes that have been described as binding to this receptor include proliferin, thyroglobulin, and latent transforming growth factor-β (TGF-β). Binding of latent TGF-β has been shown to result in cleavage of the inactive form into active TGF-β.[74] In adipocytes, it has been shown that insulin is a potent stimulant of redistribution of mannose 6-phosphate receptors from intracellular

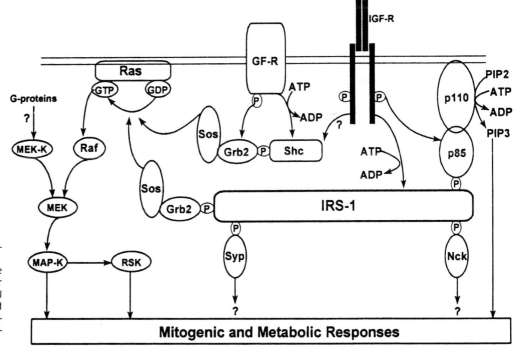

FIGURE 33–4. Major signaling pathways that are utilized by the IGF-1 receptor. Shown for comparison are the pathways utilized by other growth factors, such as epidermal growth factor and platelet-derived growth factor. P-110 and P-85 represent the major subunits of phosphatidylinositol-3'-kinase.

locations to the plasma membrane.[75] The receptor binds IGF-2 with an affinity in the range of K_d 1 to 3 nM. The affinity for IGF-1 is 80-fold lower, and the receptor does not bind insulin.[76] The mannose 6-phosphate–containing proteins are binding at a site that is distinct from IGF-1, and the receptor can bind both ligands simultaneously. Once IGF-2 is bound, it is internalized and degraded. The extracellular portion of the receptor can be proteolytically cleaved in certain cell types, and the cleavage product is released. This soluble form has been detected in plasma; however, the physiologic significance of its release into plasma has not been determined.[77]

The role of this receptor in IGF physiology is incompletely understood. Deletion of the receptor or mutations that result in loss of IGF-2 binding result in death of fetal mice at approximately 15 days of gestation.[78] The receptor is subject to parental imprinting, such that only the maternal allele of the IGF-2 receptor and the paternal allele of IGF-2 are expressed. Therefore, mice that inherit a receptor allele containing a mutation from the mother lack functional IGF-2 receptors. These mice develop severe edema in utero prior to death.[79] They are also larger than fetuses of comparable developmental age. If IGF-2 is concomitantly deleted, approximately 50% of the fetuses survive birth; however, postnatal survival is poor. These mice presumably lack the scavenging function of the IGF-2 receptor and accumulate toxic levels of IGF-2. While the scavenging function of the receptor is well accepted, it is less clear whether this receptor mediates important actions mediated by the IGF-1 receptor, such as growth stimulation. The receptor does not contain a TK domain. Whether it has a signaling mechanism is unknown. In certain cell types in culture, mutant forms of IGF-2 that bind poorly to the IGF-1 receptor stimulate some cellular events, such as cell migration. Increases in calcium flux have been shown to occur following stimulation of 3T3 cells by IGF-2 binding to this receptor. Additionally, the receptor has been shown to activate guanosine triphosphate (GTP) binding proteins, but the exact functional significance of this is undetermined. The cytoplasmic portion of the receptor encodes regions that are necessary for specific subcellular localization and endocytosis, as well as binding to GTP binding proteins.[80] In addition, it contains residues that are phosphorylated by intracellular kinases, but the role of this phosphorylation is unknown. Partitioning of the receptor following internalization can be hormonally regulated. Treatment with insulin results in translocation of a large number of receptors to the cell surface. Mannose 6-phosphate stimulates a similar increase, and this can be blocked by pretreatment with pertussis toxin, implying both stimulatory and inhibitory GTP binding protein regulation.[80] A specific antibody that blocks IGF-1 receptor action can completely inhibit IGF-2-mediated cellular growth responses in several cell types. This suggests that many of the growth-promoting effects of IGF-2 are mediated through the IGF-1 receptor.

IGF Binding Proteins

A characteristic of IGF-1 and IGF-2 that distinguishes them from proinsulin is the ability to bind to high-affinity IGFBPs. The IGFBPs are a family of six proteins that each have high affinity for IGF-1 and -2.[81] In each case, this affinity is greater than the affinity of the type 1 IGF receptor for IGF-1. One or more members of this family are present in all extracellular fluids. Therefore, they control the ability of IGF-1 and -2 to bind to receptors. In addition to this property, the major functions of the IGFBPs include (1) transporting the IGFs in the vasculature, (2) controlling their access to the extravascular space, (3) controlling tissue localization and distribution, and (4) controlling access to receptors and thereby modulating the biologic responses of cells to IGF-1.

The gene structure of the IGFBPs has been presented in several reviews. All of the six forms of IGFBPs contain four exons.[82] The mRNA species range in size from 1.4 kb (IGFBP-2) to 6.0 kb (IGFBP-5). When their protein structures are examined, there is a great deal of similarity among the IGFBPs. Of the 18 cysteines, all are conserved in four of the six binding proteins. IGFBP-4 has two additional cysteines, and IGFBP-6 has only 16 cysteines. If the cysteine structure is disrupted, IGF-1 binding is markedly attenuated. All are secreted proteins and contain a hydrophobic leader sequence. The affinity of

TABLE 33–2. Affinities of Insulin-Like Binding Proteins (IGFBPs) for Insulin-Like Growth Factor (IGF) 1 and 2

IGFBPs	Affinity ($K_a \times 10^9$) L/M	
	IGF-1	*IGF-2*
IGFBP-1	1.1	1.2
IGFBP-2	3.4	10.9
IGFBP-3	8.9	22.1
IGFBP-4	2.6	6.0
IGFBP-5	38	41
IGFBP-6	0.1	4.4

each protein for IGF-1 and -2 is shown in Table 33–2. As can be seen from the table, the greatest discrepancy is in IGFBP-6, which has a 40-fold higher affinity for IGF-2.

An important general property of the IGFBPs is their conservation of sequence in the N-terminal and C-terminal thirds of each protein. There is a high degree of sequence homology in these two modules among each protein.[82] Similarly, the sequences in these regions are highly conserved across species. In contrast, the middle third sequence diverges completely. This may be important functionally, since this is the major site of proteolytic cleavage for IGFBPs and suggests that distinct proteases cleave specific forms.

IGFBP-1 has an estimated mass of approximately 25,271 Da. It is not glycosylated, but it contains an Arg-Gly-Asp near its C-terminus.[83] This sequence has been shown to bind to the $\alpha5\beta1$ integrin.[84] IGFBP-1 is relatively unique in that it appears intact in multiple types of extracellular fluids and is, of the six, the most resistant to proteolytic cleavage. The affinity of IGFBP-1 for IGF-1 and -2 are nearly equal.

IGFBP-2 contains 289 amino acids and has a mass estimate of 32,444 Da. Its sequence is highly conserved across species, especially in the C-terminus.[85] IGFBP-2 is not glycosylated. It also has an Arg-Gly-Asp sequence near its C-terminus, but no one has been able to demonstrate that this protein binds to $\alpha5\beta1$ integrin. The protein is cleaved in many types of physiologic fluids, and the fragments have remarkably reduced affinity for IGF-1 and -2.[86]

IGFBP-3 contains 266 amino acids and is variably N-glycosylated.[87] This accounts for varying molecular weight estimates between 43 and 56 kDa. There are three potential N-linked glycosylation sites, all of which are used. Digestion within N-glycanase reduces the estimated molecular mass to 34 kDa. Glycosylation does not alter the affinity of this protein. There is no Arg-Gly-Asp sequence. IGFBP-3 contains a highly basic region between residues 216 and 244, in which 10 of 18 amino acids are basic. This region accounts for its heparin-binding activity and its ability to adhere to glycosaminoglycans.[88, 89]

IGFBP-4 is a 24,532 Da protein containing 237 amino acids. It is N-glycosylated and therefore migrates with molecular masses of 28 kDa in the glycosylated form and 24 kDa in the nonglycosylated form.[90] Glycosylation does not affect the affinity for IGF-1 or -2. There are two extra cysteines in the central core region of IGFBP-4, but their functional significance is undefined. IGFBP-4 is cleaved in most physiologic fluids to 16- and 14-kDa fragments that have very low affinity for IGF-1 and -2.[91]

IGFBP-5 has a molecular mass of 31,393 Da, and human IGFBP-5 contains 252 amino acids. IGFBP-5 is the most highly conserved form of IGFBP, with 97% homology in sequence between mouse and human.[92] It is most closely related in sequence to IGFBP-3, with approximately 50% homology in the N- and C-terminal ends. There is no Arg-Gly-Asp sequence present. IGFBP-5 contains the same heparin-binding domain as IGFBP-3, located between amino acids 201 and 218.[89] Mutagenesis of these residues results in loss of heparin binding.[93] This sequence also mediates binding to extracellular matrix (ECM).[94, 95] IGFBP-5 is O-glycosylated and has size estimates between 31 and 34 kDa. This protein has a high affinity for IGF-1 and -2. It is proteolytically cleaved into a 22-kDa fragment in physiologic fluids that has a much lower affinity for these ligands.[96]

IGFBP-6 has a molecular weight estimated at 31,413 Da. Its cysteine content differs among species, with 14 cysteines in the rat and 16 cysteines in the human.[97] There is no Arg-Gly-Asp sequence. The protein is O-glycosylated, but not N-glycosylated.[98] It has a high affinity for IGF-2 compared to IGF-1, but the physiologic significance of this difference has not been ascertained.[99] IGFBP-6 is proteolytically cleaved in physiologic fluids.

REGULATION OF INSULIN-LIKE GROWTH FACTOR-1 AND ITS BINDING PROTEINS

Control of IGF-1 Concentrations in Serum

Prior to the advent of molecular biologic techniques that made it possible to obtain sufficient, highly purified IGF-1 to administer to humans, the primary means of assessing its effects on anabolism was to make inferences from changes in plasma or tissue IGF-1 concentrations.[100] Correlations between IGF-1 levels and indices of anabolism, such as growth rate, rates of total body protein synthesis, and nitrogen balance, were undertaken and inferences were drawn based on changes in IGF-1 serum levels in response to variables such as GH administration.[100, 101] These studies formed the basis of several principles of IGF-1 physiology that have been confirmed directly by manipulation of IGF-1 expression in transgenic animals and by infusion of IGF-1 into animals and humans, and indirectly by measurements of changes in IGF-1 concentrations in states of GH deficiency (GHD) or excess.

Age is an important determinant of normal serum IGF-1 concentration. Plasma concentrations rise from very low levels, 20 to 60 ng/mL at birth, to peak values between 600 and 1100 ng/mL at puberty.[102] The concentrations fall rapidly in the second decade, reaching mean values of 350 ng/mL by age 20, and then decline more slowly over each decade. They are 50% of the 20-year-old values by age 60 years.[103] A portion of this change is due to age-dependent changes in GH secretion. Although this may account for much of the decline that occurs during adulthood, it clearly does not account for all of the major increase that occurs during childhood.

There are important genetic determinants of plasma IGF-1 concentrations. Studies in twins have shown that approximately 40% of each individual's IGF-1 variability can be accounted for on the basis of undefined genetic factors, which are linked to height.[104] There is a very close correlation between IGF-1 concentrations and height in many different types of populations that have been studied, and these appear to be due, at least partly, to this genetic factor. This genetic determinant is independent of intrinsic GH secretion.

The major hormonal determinant of plasma IGF-1 concentrations is GH. Children with definitive evidence of GHD usually have IGF-1 values that are below the 95% confidence interval.[105, 106] Because values vary so much throughout childhood, however, age-adjusted normative data are required to interpret low plasma IGF-1 values (Fig. 33–5). Consideration of developmental stage (skeletal age) is also important for interpreting low values.[107] A normal IGF-1 value is strong evidence that GHD is not present. Conversely, a low value does not definitively prove that GHD is present.[101, 108] Other causes of growth retardation can be associated with a low IGF-1, although causes such as constitutional growth delay are usually associated with normal levels. However, values less than the 95% confidence interval can occur in such children, usually when nutritional intake is suboptimal. Administration of GH to patients with GHD results in a substantial rise in IGF-1, and this occurs in the first 4 to 6 hours following an injection.[109] The values peak at 24 hours and then begin to attenuate. Because GH also increases the plasma concentrations of IGFBP-3 and a third protein, termed acid labile subunit (ALS), the duration of this change is due to altered IGF-1 clearance. The IGF-1 response of a short child to GH administration has not proved to be a useful diagnostic test.[110, 111] In spite of these problems in interpreting low values, basal IGF-1 measurements have proved very useful as a screening test for selecting individuals who should undergo stimulation testing to assess their GH secretory response.[101, 105, 106, 108]

In states of GH excess, IGF-1 values are invariably increased. The

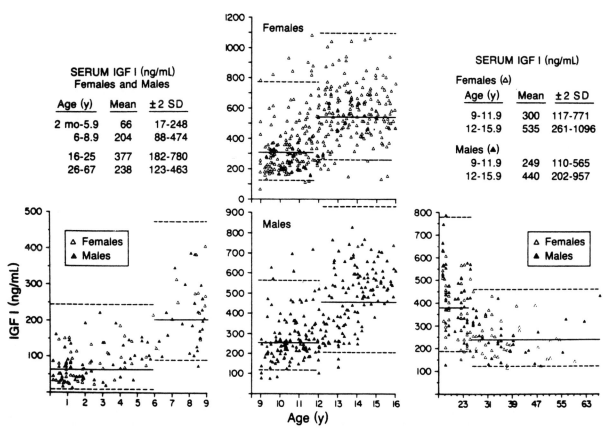

SERUM IGF I (ng/mL) Females and Males		
Age (y)	Mean	± 2 SD
2 mo-5.9	66	17-248
6-8.9	204	88-474
16-25	377	182-780
26-67	238	123-463

SERUM IGF I (ng/mL)		
Females (△)		
Age (y)	Mean	± 2 SD
9-11.9	300	117-771
12-15.9	535	261-1096
Males (▲)		
9-11.9	249	110-565
12-15.9	440	202-957

FIGURE 33–5. *Serum concentrations of IGF-1 in healthy subjects, ages 2 months to 68 years. The 95% confidence intervals are shown as dashed lines.*

mean IGF-1 for patients with acromegaly is approximately seven times the normal age-adjusted control value.[112] The sensitivity and specificity of a single IGF-1 measurement for diagnosing acromegaly in patients above 20 years are greater than 97%.[113] The severity of the IGF-1 abnormality appears to correlate with disease activity, and values correlate with measurement of soft tissue growth, such as heel pad thickness.[112] IGF-1 measurements are useful in monitoring the response to therapy and correlate well with residual GH secretion in these patients.[114] Generally, if 24-hour mean GH values are less than 1.6 ng/mL, then IGF-1 will be within the age-adjusted 95% confidence interval. IGF-1 values are also elevated during the last trimester of pregnancy, presumably due to increases in placental GH secretion.[115]

Another hormonal variable that controls IGF-1 concentrations is T_4. Plasma IGF-1 concentrations are low in severe T_4 deficiency and rise with thyroid hormone replacement.[116] Values are not suppressed in Turner's syndrome, and estrogen replacement results in little change. Prolactin has a weak, stimulatory effect on plasma IGF-1. In subjects with severe GHD, prolactin concentrations of 200 ng/mL or greater can maintain IGF-1 in the normal range.

Nutritional status is an important determinant of plasma IGF-1 concentrations. An adequate caloric and protein intake has to be maintained to maintain an adequate serum IGF-1, both in children and adults.[117, 118] Fasting for 3 days results in substantial reduction in total serum IGF-1 and a blunted response to the administration of GH.[119] Ten days of fasting results in a 70% decrease in plasma IGF-1. Following a 5-day fast, values decline by 53%, and subjects must be refed for at least 8 days for values to return to normal. During fasting and refeeding, the change in IGF-1 correlates with the change in nitrogen balance.[120] The change is due to both energy and protein deficiency. An energy intake of 20 kcal/kg and an intake of 0.6 g/kg of protein are required to maintain a normal IGF-1. Children with severe protein-calorie malnutrition have low IGF-1 values that respond to treatment.[117] Other catabolic conditions, such as hepatic failure, inflammatory bowel diseases, or renal failure, are associated with low serum IGF-1 concentrations.[121, 122] Insulin is an important determinant of IGF-1 concentrations. Although it is difficult to differentiate between nutritional regulation and insulin action, insulin perfusion of the liver in diabetic animals results in a substantial increase in plasma IGF-1.[123] Patients with poorly controlled type 1 diabetes mellitus have low-normal IGF-1 values that rise to the normal range with adequate insulin treatment.[124] Furthermore, in poorly controlled type 1 diabetes, there is a correlation between hemoglobin A_{1c} values and IGF-1.[125] Similarly, patients with severe insulin resistance have low IGF-1 values.[126]

Control of IGFBP Concentrations in Blood and Extracellular Fluids

Four forms of IGFBPs are easily detected in plasma: IGFBP-1, -2, -3, and -4. IGFBP-3 is not only the most abundant but has the highest affinity for IGF-1 and -2.[127] The IGFBPs in serum perform three functions. The first is to act as transport proteins for the IGFs, the second is to regulate their half-lives, and the third is to provide a specific means for transcapillary transport into extravascular fluid compartments.

The plasma concentrations of IGFBP-3 are regulated by GH. IGFBP-3 concentrations are low in patients with GHD and increase following GH treatment.[128] This increase is partially due to a direct effect of GH on IGFBP-3 synthesis; however, it is also due to the fact that the half-life of IGFBP-3 is prolonged by binding to the two other proteins to form a ternary complex (consisting of IGF-1 or -2, IGFBP-3, and ALS). ALS is an 88-kDa glycoprotein containing several leucine-rich domains that are known to facilitate protein-protein interaction, and it is this domain structure that accounts for its binding to IGFBP-3.[129] Since IGF-1 and ALS synthesis are also increased by GH, all three components are increased, and this acts to prolong the half-life of each component. The binding of IGF-1 to this complex in plasma functions to prolong its half-life from 6 minutes in the free form, which is similar to that of insulin, to 16 hours.[130] The prolongation of the half-life of ALS-associated IGF-1-IGFBP-3 complexes is also due to the fact that this macromolecular complex (150 kDa)

cannot freely cross capillary barriers, and therefore is not excreted by the kidney. If sufficient IGF-1 and IGFBP-3 are infused to exceed the binding capacity of ALS, then their half-lives are shortened substantially, indicating that it is the ternary complex that maintains the stability and prolongs their half-lives. The molar concentration of IGFBP-3 in serum is generally equal to the sum of IGF-1 and -2, and therefore it is usually saturated or nearly saturated. The affinity of IGFBP-3 for IGF-1 and -2 is not lowered by binding to ALS, and therefore its high affinity is maintained. This high affinity and its long half-life account for the fact that approximately 75% of the IGF-1 and -2 in plasma is carried in this complex.[131] The exact function of this large storage pool of IGF-1 and -2 in serum is unknown. However, it is clear that changes in the IGF-1 concentrations within this large complex correlate with the anabolic response to GH administration. Plasma IGFBP-3 levels are elevated in patients with acromegaly, low in patients with GHD, as are ALS levels.[132, 133] Age is an important determinant of IGFBP-3 concentration, and it varies with age in a manner that is similar to IGF-1.[107]

Hormones other than GH can influence the synthesis of IGFBP-3, and therefore its plasma concentration. This protein is low in prepubertal males and increases following testosterone administration. It decreases 40% following menopause and can be increased in postmenopausal females with physiologic estrogen replacement.[134] IGFBP-3 concentrations are low in patients with hypothyroidism and increase 55% following administration of T_4.[135]

Insulin improves the IGFBP-3 synthesis response to GH, but it does not appear to have a direct effect. Insulin also stimulates ALS, and severe diabetes results in reduced ALS levels and reduced complex formation. Although GH directly stimulates IGFBP-3 and ALS synthesis, infusion of IGF-1, while increasing serum IGFBP-3 transiently, acts to suppress its concentrations over time by suppressing GH release from the pituitary and thereby lowering ALS synthesis.[136] Since the ALS concentration is rate-limiting for complex formation, the total complex levels decrease after infusion of high doses of IGF-1 for several days.

IGFBP-3 abundance in serum is also regulated by protease activity.[137, 138] Several proteases that degrade IGFBP-3 have been described, including prostate-specific antigen (PSA) and plasmin, but the exact identity of the serum protease has not been determined.[139] Protease concentrations are abundant in human pregnancy serum[137, 138] and are also present in GH-deficient states.[140] Proteolytic cleavage reduces the affinity of IGFBP-3 greatly, and therefore the IGF-1 that is reduced binds to unsaturated IGFBP-1, -2, and -4 wherein it can equilibrate much more readily with the extracellular compartments.[141] An important function of proteases that cleave IGFBP-3 may be to liberate IGF-1 from the IGFBP-3-ALS complex and allow greater extravascular equilibration by binding to the lower-molecular-weight forms of IGFBPs that are in better equilibrium with those in the extravascular space.

The next most abundant IGFBP in plasma is IGFBP-2.[142] The affinity of IGFBP-2 for IGF-1 is less than that of IGFBP-3, and its plasma concentrations are substantially lower. IGFBP-2 concentrations are inversely regulated by GH; that is, they are high in GHD, suppressed by administration of GH, and low in acromegaly.[143] Unlike IGFBP-3, IGFBP-2 does not bind to ALS, and there is no ternary complex in plasma; therefore, its half-life when bound to IGF-1 is approximately 90 minutes. It is also not saturated, and excess binding capacity exists. Intact IGFBP-2 crosses the capillary barriers.[144] IGFBP-2 is also degraded by a protease, and fragments with reduced affinity have been detected in plasma. Hepatocytes appear to be the major source of serum IGFBP-2, and the abundance of its mRNA in liver is regulated in parallel with its plasma concentrations.[145] Hypophysectomy in experimental animals results in a major increase in IGFBP-2 mRNA expression in liver. GH administration to GH-deficient humans results in substantial lowering of plasma IGFBP-2. One of the major stimuli of IGFBP-2 concentrations in serum is IGF-1. Following IGF-1 administration to GH-deficient humans or patients with diabetes, there is a three- to fourfold increase in IGFBP-2.[146] Plasma IGFBP-2 concentrations are also increased by IGF-2, and they are elevated in patients with retroperitoneal tumors that produce IGF-2.[147] Hepatic IGFBP-2 mRNA expression is significantly increased in diabetic rats and suppressed with insulin administration.[148] Severely limiting nutrient intake in humans results in increases in plasma IGFBP-2, as does poorly controlled type 1 diabetes.[143] Prolonged nutrient deprivation results in approximately a twofold increase in plasma IGFBP-2 concentrations. This appears to be dependent upon protein intake, since this can be mimicked with low protein diets that are relatively normal in caloric content, and IGFBP-2 expression in animals is increased during protein restriction.[149, 150] Since the half-life of the IGF-1 bound to IGFBP-2 is considerably less than IGF-1 bound to IGFBP-3, it has been assumed that this IGF-1 is in more rapid equilibrium with that in the extravascular space. Whether this shift in the proportion of IGF-1 bound to IGFBP-2 as opposed to IGFBP-3 accounts for some of the biologic effects that occur when IGF-1 is administered in the absence of increased IGFBP-3 is a topic of current investigation.

A third abundant protein in serum is IGFBP-1. IGFBP-1 also circulates in binary complexes with IGF-1 and -2. Its affinity for the two growth factors is coequal (Table 33–2). IGFBP-1 is acutely regulated by insulin.[151, 152] Insulin-deficient states, such as fasting or type 1 diabetes, are associated with very high concentrations of IGFBP-1, whereas administration of insulin or ingestion of a meal results in marked suppression (five- to sixfold) of serum IGFBP-1 concentrations.[152, 153] Major sites of synthesis of IGFBP-1 are highly restricted, and the liver is the principle site of synthesis, although kidney, maternal placenta, and uterus are other sources of this peptide. Plasma concentrations are controlled primarily by hepatic synthesis and release. Hepatic synthesis is primarily under the control of insulin,[151] although other hormones, such as GH and cortisol, also have effects.[154] IGFBP-1 in blood is unsaturated, and therefore IGFBP-1 is proposed to be a major modulator of free IGF-1 levels, particularly in response to food intake. Postprandially, changes in serum insulin result in a four- to fivefold decrease in IGFBP-1. This change is due to direct suppression of synthesis in the liver. IGFBP-1 mRNA expression also decreases in experimental animals after insulin administration to diabetic animals.[151] This is due to a direct effect of insulin on IGFBP-1 gene transcription, and there is an insulin response element in the 5′ flanking region of the IGFBP-1 gene.[155] IGFBP-1 crosses intact capillary beds, and the amount that crosses in a fixed time period is dependent upon ambient insulin concentrations.[156]

Because IGFBP-1 can bind free IGF-1, it has been proposed to have a glucoregulatory function. That is, since IGF-1 enhances insulin sensitivity, factors that lead to excessive IGFBP-1 may lead to reduced insulin sensitivity. In states of significant insulin resistance, there is enhanced phosphorylation of IGFBP-1, which increases its affinity for IGF-1 and therefore results in further attenuation of its ability to enhance insulin sensitivity.[157] Both fasting and diabetes have been shown to be causes of disproportionate increases in serum IGFBP-1 concentrations.[152, 153] In addition, administration of glucocorticoid increases IGFBP-1, presumably by a direct effect on IGFBP-1 gene transcription.[154] Unlike the other IGFBPs in serum, no protease for IGFBP-1 serum has been described, and the intact molecule is frequently the only form that is detected, although it is probably proteolytically degraded by the kidney, since fragments of IGFBP-1 can be detected in urine. Administration of large concentrations of IGFBP-1 to hypophysectomized rats has resulted in slight increases in glucose concentrations, suggesting that IGFBP-1 may have some role in regulating the insulin-like actions of IGF-1.[158] Since IGF-1 increases insulin sensitivity, the high concentrations of IGFBP-1 that occur in diabetes may contribute to insulin resistance.[159]

The exact roles of IGFBP-1 and IGFBP-2 in controlling the distribution of the IGFs has not been determined. In catabolic states, such as nutritional deprivation, GHD, or renal failure, IGFBP-1 and IGFBP-2 levels are increased and they may become the major binding component.[160–162] Similarly, in these conditions, the amount of IGF-1 that is bound to IGFBP-3 is decreased.

IGFBP-4 concentrations in serum have been shown to correlate with changes in bone physiology. Specifically, in states of low bone turnover and low parathyroid hormone (PTH) concentrations, serum IGFBP-4 concentrations are increased. There is a correlation between sunlight exposure and IGFBP-4, suggesting that vitamin D, or one of its active metabolites, regulates IGFBP-4.[163]

IGFBP-5 exists in serum almost solely as proteolytic fragments, and intact IGFBP-5 is present at very low concentrations. The fragments that are present have very low affinity for IGF-1 and -2, and therefore their plasma concentrations are unlikely to be major regulators of IGF-1 action. IGFBP-5 concentrations in serum are regulated by GH and both intact IGFBP-5 and its major fragment increase substantially when GH is administered to GH-deficient patients.[164]

IGFBPs have been detected in several extracellular fluids. Table 33–3 lists the various forms of IGFBPs in these fluid compartments and the major variables that have been shown to regulate their concentrations.

Control of IGF-1 Synthesis in Tissues

While it is beyond the scope of this chapter to discuss the expression of IGF-1 in all tissues that have been studied, some general principles are important for a fundamental understanding of the autocrine- and paracrine-mediated actions of this growth factor. Connective tissue cells within a given tissue or organ are often the origin of IGF-1 transcripts.[165] In situ hybridization studies have shown that fibroblasts and other cells of mesenchymal origin are the primary extrahepatic sources of IGF-1 in vivo.[166] Importantly, the abundance of this transcript in connective tissue cells is increased in response to GH.[167] Fibroblast synthesis is also regulated by growth factors such as PDGF.[168]

In cartilage, both GH and FGF have been shown to be potent stimuli of IGF-1 synthesis by prechondrocytes.[169] Its synthesis is greatest in cells that are actively differentiating. When chondrocytes reach the hypertrophic state, IGF-1 synthesis is diminished.

Similar to cartilage, bone osteoblasts are a source of IGF-1 peptide, and it is synthesized in fetal calvarial tissue.[170] GH also increases IGF-1 synthesis by osteoblasts. IGF-1 synthesis rates correlate with changes in osteoblast DNA synthesis, type I collagen synthesis, and synthesis of other components of bone ECM.[171] Several bone trophic factors, such as bone morphogenic proteins, stimulate the synthesis of IGF-1 mRNA by these cells. In bone, IGF-1 mRNA expression is downregulated by glucocorticoids. In contrast, estrogen stimulates the expression of IGF-1.[172] Prostaglandins are also potent inducers of IGF-1 gene transcription by osteoblasts, and PTH is a potent stimulator of IGF-1 gene transcription.[165, 173] In contrast, the bone growth factors, FGF, PDGF, and TGF-β, downregulate IGF-1 expression. IGF-1 appears to be an important factor in erythropoiesis. Rates of red blood cell mass synthesis are decreased in GH-deficient animals and are restored with IGF-1 administration.[174] Erythroid precursor cells have been shown to synthesize IGF-1, and its synthesis can be stimulated in these cells both by GH and erythropoietin. Similarly, granulocyte precursor cells synthesize IGF-1 mRNA, and this is stimulated by granulocyte-macrophage colony-stimulating factor.[175]

Reproductive Tract

IGF-1 expression is decreased in the ovary of the hypophysectomized rat, and ovarian expression increases in response to GH. Estrogen can increase ovarian IGF-1 expression, and this has been localized primarily to the thecal cells of the early follicle.[176] IGF-1 receptors are also present in these follicles, indicating the possibility of an autocrine loop. Follicular fluid contains IGF-1 and -2, and their concentrations are increased following FSH administration.[177] Several studies suggest that IGF-2 effects are more dominant in the ovary, and much more IGF-2 is produced in that organ. In the oviduct, IGF-1 and -2 have been shown to be present in oviductal fluid, and oviductal cells express mRNA encoding both IGF-1 and -2, as well as IGF-1 receptors. Endometrium normally expresses IGF-1 mRNA, and, in rats, a 20-fold increase can be induced with estradiol administration.[9] Estrogen induces IGF-1 expression primarily in the epithelium, whereas progesterone induces it in the endometrial stroma. In the late proliferative phase, IGF-1 mRNA is present almost exclusively in the stroma. Similarly, IGF-1 receptor mRNA is upregulated during the secretory phase of the menstrual cycle. The testes express IGF-1 mRNA, and

TABLE 33–3. *The Various Forms of Insulin-Like Growth Factor Binding Proteins (IGFBPs)*

Tissue	Primary Cell Type of Origin or Area	Form of IGFBP Secreted	Variables That Control Synthesis or Secretion
Uterus, decidua	Stroma and epithelium	IGFBP-1	Estrogen, progesterone
	Stroma	IGFBP-2, -4, -5, -6	
	Endothelium	IGFBP-3	
	Myometrium	IGFBP-2, -3, -5	
Placenta	Epithelium	IGFBP-1	Hypoxia, dexamethasone
		IGFBP-2, -3, -4	Fetal development
Brain	Choroid plexus, meninges	IGFBP-2	
	Capillaries	IGFBP-3	
	Olfactory bulb, Schwann cells	IGFBP-2, -6	
	White matter, nerves	IGFBP-5	
	Glial cells	IGFBP-2, -3	Hypoxic injury
	Focal neuronal concentrations	IGFBP-4	
Kidney	Collecting ducts	IGFBP-1	
	Distal tubules	IGFBP-2	Work induction by furosemide
	Mesangial cells	IGFBP-5	
Lung	Mesenchymal cells (fetus)	IGFBP-2	
	Epithelium (fetus)	IGFBP-2	
	Pneumatocytes	IGFBP-4	
	Interstitial cells	IGFBP-5	
Breast	Epithelium	IGFBP-2, -3	Increased IGFBP-5 during lactation
	Stroma	IGFBP-3, -4, -5	Increased IGFBP-5 during lactation withdrawal
Cartilage	Prechondrocytes	IGFBP-3, -4, -5	
	Hypertrophic chondrocytes	IGFBP-3, -5	
Bone	Osteoblasts	IGFBP-5	Age-related decrease
		IGFBP-4	Vitamin D
	Capillaries	IGFBP-3	
Gut	Epithelium	IGFBP-2, -4	
		IGFBP-3	Nutrient deprivation
	Lamina propria	IGFBP-3, -5	Increase in response to injury
Bladder	Smooth muscle	IGFBP-2, -4, -5	Hypertrophy increases IGFBP-2
Prostate	Stroma	IGFBP-2, -3	
Liver	Hepatocytes	IGFBP-1, -2, -4, -6	Fasting increases IGFBP-1, -2; insulin deprivation increases IGFBP-1, -2
	Sinusoids, stroma	IGFBP-3, -5	GH increases IGFBP-3
Ovary	Theca	IGFBP-2, -4	LH increases IGFBP-2; involution increases IGFBP-4
	Stroma	IGFBP-5	
	Stroma, capillaries	IGFBP-3	
	Corpus luteum	IGFBP-3	
Connective tissue	Fibroblasts	IGFBP-3, -4, -5	IGF-1, IGF-2, RA increase IGFBP-3; TNF-α, IL-1 increase IGFBP-4; dexamethasone increases IGFBP-4 and decreases IGFBP-5; IGF-1 increases IGFBP-5
Skeletal muscle	Myoblasts, myocytes	IGFBP-2, -4, -5	Differentiation increases IGFBP-2 and -5
Blood vessels	Endothelium	IGFBP-2, -3, -4, -6	
	Smooth muscle	IGFBP-2, -4, -5	Injury increases IGFBP-5

GH, growth hormone; LH, luteinizing hormone; RA, rheumatoid arthritis; TNF-α, tumor necrosis factor-α; IL-1, interleukin-1.

the source of origin is the Leydig cell.[178] IGF-1 expression by Leydig cells is downregulated by interleukin-1 (IL-1) and upregulated by LH.

Neural Tissue

Circulating plasma IGF-1 crosses the blood-brain barrier. However, much of the IGF-1 that is present in cerebrospinal fluid (CSF) is believed to arise from IGF-1 synthesis within the central nervous system (CNS). The major sites of IGF-1 mRNA are the Purkinje cells of the cerebellum, the olfactory bulb, and hippocampus.[179] The retina is also a site of postnatal expression. Astroglial cells in the cerebellum are also an important site of IGF-1 expression. Immunohistochemical staining has shown that IGF-1 is transported along axons and dendrites, and that IGF-1 is present in the choroid plexus.

Muscle

IGF-1 mRNA is expressed in the satellite cells and myoblasts of skeletal muscle.[180, 181] Following an ischemic or toxic injury there is a major increase in IGF-1 mRNA expression.[180] The wave of increase of expression after skeletal muscle injury coincides with the appearance of regenerating tissue and rapid cell division. Work-induced hypertrophy in muscle of hypophysectomized rats can also lead to an increase in expression of IGF-1 and -2, indicating that this change is GH-independent. Cardiac muscle is also a site of IGF-1 synthesis, and it is increased in models of cardiac hypertrophy that have been induced either by pressure or volume overload.[182, 183] Blood vessels are also an important site of IGF-1 synthesis. Both endothelial and smooth muscle cells contain IGF-1 mRNA. Pressure overload results in increased IGF-1 expression.[184] Following blood vessel injury, there is an increase in IGF-1 expression by smooth muscle cells.[185]

Liver

IGF-1 expression in liver correlates extremely well with changes in plasma GH concentrations. Expression in hepatic tissue is low in hypophysectomized animals and increases after administration of

GH.[186] Likewise, nutritional deprivation results in a major decrease in IGF-1 mRNA, and this can be restored with refeeding.[187] Some of these changes are due to changes in transcription, and some are due to changes in mRNA stability. Following partial hepatectomy, there is no increase in IGF-1 synthesis at 36 hours in the remaining hepatic lobes; however, IGF-1 receptors increase.

Development

IGF-1 transcripts are easily detected in developing rats, in intestine, liver, lung, and brain. Expression is present as early as 11-day embryos, and IGF-1 mRNA increases 8.6-fold by day 13.[188] In early embryos, IGF-1 is detected in yolk sac, hepatic bud, in dermal myotomes and sclerotomes, and in brachial arch mesoderm. In late fetal development, labeling is more intense in muscle, precartilagenous mesenchymal condensations, perichondrium, and the immature chondrocyte periosteum, as well as in ossification centers.[189] In human fetal embryos, IGF-1 mRNA levels are relatively low at 16 weeks, and the highest levels are found in placenta and stomach. At 20 weeks, fetal kidney, placental lung, brain, cartilage, and liver have detectable transcripts. The perisinusoidal cells of the liver and perichondrium appear to be foci of intense expression in 20-week fetuses, and the cells of origin appear to be fibroblast-like. Postnatally, expression increases markedly in skin, nerve, and muscle.

Kidney

IGF-1 is expressed at low levels in the fetal kidney; however, in the adult kidney in rats, IGF-1 mRNA is abundant.[190] Immunohistochemical staining shows moderate amounts of IGF-1 in both the proximal and distal tubules of human fetuses. In adult rats, IGF-1 is localized primarily over the collecting ducts. Overexpression of IGF-1 in transgenic animal kidneys has been shown to result in renal growth, and GH administration to GH-deficient rats results in increased expression of IGF-1 in the kidney. In rats, unilateral nephrectomy with compensatory growth of the contralateral kidney results in increased mRNA expression 24 hours after nephrectomy in the remaining kidney.[191] This increase in compensatory synthesis is partly dependent on GH, since it is less intense in hypophysectomized animals. After ischemic injury, there is increased IGF-1 immunoreactivity in the regenerating cells of the proximal tubules.

Control of IGFBP Concentrations in Tissues

Since IGF-1 and -2 function not only as endocrine hormones but also as paracrine regulators of growth and differentiation in tissues, the primary role of the IGFBPs in tissues may be to control the amount of locally produced IGF that is accessible to receptors. The exact regulation of each of the six binding proteins in each tissue in which they are expressed is beyond the scope of this chapter. As shown in Table 33–3, each tissue appears to express different combinations of binding proteins differentially.

BIOLOGIC ACTIONS OF INSULIN-LIKE GROWTH FACTOR-1

IGF-1 Stimulation of DNA Synthesis in Vitro

IGF-1 receptors are present in almost all cell types and mediate most of the effects of IGF-1 and -2 in vitro, as well as the growth-promoting effects of insulin, when it is present in sufficiently high concentrations to activate this receptor (e.g., concentrations $>10^{-7}$ M). Several biologic actions of IGF-1 have been studied using cells in culture, including anabolic effects such as increases in protein synthesis and cell size; effects on carbohydrate metabolism, such as glucose transport, glucose oxidation, and lipid synthesis; and effects

on cell growth, including stimulation of DNA synthesis, mitogenesis, and inhibition of cell death. Other generalized processes that have been analyzed include cell cycle progression, cell differentiation, and cellular migration. Specific events, such as synthesis of individual proteins, have been analyzed, as well as the ability of IGF-1 to augment specific functions of differentiated cells that are stimulated by other hormones or growth factors.

One of the most commonly studied effects of IGF-1 in vitro is its ability to stimulate DNA synthesis. IGF-1 appears to act principally by stimulating entry into DNA synthesis from the latter part of the G_1 phase of the cell cycle.[192] In some systems, its presence is required for progression through all 12 hours of G_1. IGF-1 is not as potent in stimulating quiescent cells to enter G_1 compared to other growth factors, such as PDGF or FGF, but once cells have entered the cycle, it is often sufficient to stimulate progression through to the S phase.[193] In some cell types, it is possible to alter this requirement by overexpressing EGF, the c-*myb* proto-oncogene, or SV40 T antigen.[194] Generally, these manipulations cause cells to secrete more autocrine-produced IGF-1 and thereby stimulate the IGF-1 receptor. Support for the hypothesis that constitutively synthesized IGF-1 is required in such systems derives from studies in which antibodies that inhibit IGF-1 binding to its receptor block DNA synthesis, and cells that have had the IGF-1 receptor deleted do not grow in response to stimulation by other growth factors.[195] Similarly, in some systems, overexpression of the IGF-1 receptor will abrogate the need for PDGF or FGF.[196]

Other growth factors have been shown to work cooperatively with IGF system components. PDGF and FGF increase the number of IGF-1 binding sites, and FGF increases constitutive tyrosine phosphorylation of the IGF-1 receptor kinase.[197] IGF-1 is a mitogen for essentially every type of cell that possesses IGF-1 receptors. These include all mesenchymal cell types and many types of epithelial cells, including neuronal epithelial, and multiple endodermally derived cell types. Cell lines in culture that have been shown to have an increased number of IGF-1 receptors are more sensitive to the growth-promoting actions of IGF-1. A factor complicating the interpretation of all experiments in which IGF-1 is added in vitro is the autocrine secretion of IGF-1. This autocrine-synthesized IGF-1 is capable of binding to receptors and stimulating anabolic effects.[198] Therefore, analysis of the effects of IGF-1 added to cells in culture often must take into account this confounding variable. In many of the studies in which synergism between IGF-1 and other growth factors has been observed, their effects are partially due to autocrine-secreted IGF-1. Hormones such as TSH and FSH and growth factors such as PDGF and EGF may exert part of their proliferative effects by stimulating autocrine secretion of IGF-1.[199]

Cell Type and Tissue Responses

Cartilage

Many of the growth-promoting actions of GH on skeletal growth are believed to be due to the local production of IGF-1 by prechondrocytes or early differentiating chondrocytes within the epiphysial growth plate.[200] In vitro, IGF-1 stimulates cartilage cell division and size, as well as proteoglycan synthesis, which contributes to enhanced ECM synthesis.[201] In addition, IGF-1 may mediate some of the growth-promoting effects of triiodothyronine (T_3) on cartilage, since exposure of cartilage in vitro to an anti-IGF-1 antibody results in attenuated responses to T_3 administration.

Bone

IGF-1 stimulates several anabolic effects on bone cells in culture. Exposure of preosteoblast cells to IGF-1 results in stimulation of type I collagen synthesis, DNA and RNA synthesis, and total protein synthesis.[202] In addition, skeletal tissue is a rich source of stored IGF-1. Osteoblasts themselves can synthesize IGF-1, and several of the IGFBPs that bind to bone ECM can act as a storage reservoir.[90] IGF-1 expression has been shown to be stimulated by a number of hormones and cytokines that are potent trophic growth factors for bone, implying that many of their effects may be mediated locally through IGF-1 production.

Skin

Proliferation of primary human keratinocytes in culture has been shown to be stimulated by IGF-1, and IGF-1 is produced by dermal fibroblasts, but not by skin epithelial cells, which suggests that paracrine stimulation of skin epithelium by IGF-1 derived from dermal fibroblasts may be the primary mechanism by which this growth factor contributes to epithelial proliferation.[203]

Skeletal Muscle

Several types of myoblasts in culture have been shown to respond to the addition of IGF-1. Both IGF-1 and -2 stimulate muscle cell protein synthesis, as well as DNA synthesis.[204] Their effects are complex, because they are linked to the differentiation program of these cells (see below). IGF-1 is synthesized by the satellite cells which are premyoblast precursors and synthesis in satellite cells is controlled by the need to maximize the proliferative pool. Following stimulation of myoblast proliferation, prolonged exposure to higher concentrations of IGF-1 results in terminal differentiation.[205] This effect is linked to the ability of IGF-1 to enhance the expression of the myogenic differentiation protein, myogenin.

Nervous System

The major cell types that grow in response to IGF-1 are astrocytes and glial cell precursors. In end-terminally differentiated neurons IGF-1 has been shown to stimulate neurite outgrowth and myelin synthesis.[206] Cells derived from the sympathetic nervous system, such as adrenal chromaffin cells, are stimulated to divide by IGF-1.[207] IGF-1 is a stimulant of neurite outgrowth in axons damaged by denervation.[208, 209]

Other Cell Types

Other cell types that have been shown to be IGF-1-responsive include mammary epithelial cells, vascular smooth muscle cells, endothelial cells, mesangial cells, erythroid progenitor cells, oocytes, adrenal fasciculata cells, granulosa cells, promyelocytic cells, glanulocyte colony-forming cells, fetal hepatocytes, pancreatic islet cells, oligodendrocytes, Sertoli cells, and spermatogonia.[199]

Other Biologic Actions of IGF-1

Effect on Cell Death

In many systems, IGF-1 has been shown to be a potent inhibitor of programmed cell death. The systems that have been best characterized are hematopoietic and neuronal cell precursors. In hematopoietic cells, erythroid progenitor cells can be induced to undergo apoptosis with serum or erythropoietin deprivation, and this effect is suppressed by IGF-1.[210] IGF-1 inhibits apoptosis in myeloid precursors that occurs following the withdrawal of stimulatory cytokines, such as interleukin-3 (IL-3).[211] In many tumor cell types transfection with a dominant negative form of the IGF-1 receptor (a form of IGF receptor that has a TK defective subunit) results in enhancement of the apoptotic effect that is induced by cytotoxic agents.[212] During ovarian follicle development, IGF-1 stimulation by gonadotrophins may prevent apoptosis of the developing follicular cells.[213] IGF-1 has been shown to inhibit the apoptosis that occurs during development in myoblasts, neurons, and oligodendrocytes.[73]

Effect on Differentiation

In cultured myoblasts, IGF-1 induces the expression of myogenin, a specific myoblast differentiation factor, and myogenin induction can be blocked with antisense oligonucleotides that inhibit the synthesis

of autocrine-stimulated IGF-1.[214] Autocrine-produced IGF-2 may have similar effects. The programmed events that occur during differentiation in response to IGF-1 are time-specific since, in L-6 myoblasts, cellular exposure to high concentrations of IGF-1 early in the differentiation program acts to inhibit differentiation, but at later time points it is accelerated.[214] IGF-2 may also inhibit apoptosis that occurs during transition from proliferation to differentiation in myoblastic cell lines. Differentiation markers have also been shown to be preferentially stimulated in response to IGF-1 or -2 in osteoclasts, chondrocytes, and neural cells.[215–217] The addition of IGF-1 to different types of cultured neurons has been shown to enhance neuronal differentiation. Maintenance of neuroepithelial cultures in several model systems has been shown to be enhanced by IGF-1, probably by inhibiting apoptosis.

Effect on Specialized Functions

Production of steroids by ovarian granulosa cells and thecal cells has been shown to be stimulated by IGF-1 and -2, and the effects are synergistic with FSH.[177] IGF-1 also stimulates steroid hormone secretion by adrenocorticotropic hormone (ACTH)–responsive adrenocortical cells.[218] IGF-1 stimulates testosterone secretion from Leydig cells and acts synergistically with LH to increase the response.[219] Similarly, thyroglobulin production by thyroid follicular cells is synergistically enhanced with TSH plus IGF-1.[220] Thymulin is a specific secretory product of thymic epithelium that is stimulated by IGF-1. GH secretion by pituitary cells is inhibited by IGF-1.[221] Histamine release from β cells in response to immunoglobulin E is potentiated by IGF-1. IGF-1 inhibits glutamate-stimulated release of γ-aminobutyric acid (GABA) from Purkinje cells. IGF-1 is a specific stimulant of IGFBP-5 synthesis by muscle cells and fibroblasts.[222] Other specific proteins whose synthesis is stimulated by IGF-1 include elastin by smooth muscle cells,[223] crystallin by lens epithelial cells,[224] and cholesterol side cleavage enzyme by adrenal cortical cells.[225]

Several generalized metabolic processes that are stimulated by IGF-1 in a variety of cell types have been analyzed. These include glucose uptake, glycolysis, glycogen synthesis, and glucose oxidation in fat cells and skeletal muscle cells.[226] These metabolic effects can be mediated by the insulin receptor if sufficient IGF-1 is added in vitro (e.g., concentrations $>10^{-8}$ M); however, antibody blocking studies have indicated that IGF-1 can have direct effects on this process through its own receptor in some cell types. Similarly, the hybrid IGF-1–insulin receptor may play a role in mediating these effects in some cell types. Total protein synthesis, ECM protein synthesis, cell migration, and the synthesis of proteoglycans and collagen, in particular, have been analyzed extensively in connective tissue cells. IGF-1 often acts in concert with other growth factors to stimulate connective tissue cell protein synthesis. IGF-1 is a potent stimulant of cell migration and stimulates this process by both chemotaxis and chemokinesis.[227] IGF-1 is not directly angiogenic, but it can stimulate the synthesis of angiogenic peptides, such as vascular endothelial cell growth factor.

Role in Malignant Tumors

Because IGF-1 is a potent inhibitor of apoptosis, it has been proposed that it may function to enhance tumor formation in several experimental animal models. The presence of an intact IGF-1 receptor is required for tumor propagation.[19, 228] In the absence of IGF-1 receptor, C6 glioma cells do not form tumors and undergo apoptosis.[212] Often, the presence of a normal IGF-1 receptor number is inadequate for tumor formation, and the IGF-1 receptors need to be overexpressed.[26] However, several processes that are necessary for tumor formation can be facilitated by IGF-1, even in the absence of enhanced receptor number, such as prevention of cell death. Deletion of the receptor results in inability of cells that would normally be tumorigenic in nude mice to form tumors, and mutation of specific tyrosine residues on the receptor and expression of these mutated receptors results in lack of tumor formation.[47, 229] In human tumors a direct causal role for the receptor in pathogenesis has been difficult to prove. All of the data that exist are correlative. In Wilms' tumor, small cell lung carcinoma, and uterine cancer, IGF-1 receptor number is increased.[230] No mutations of the receptor have been identified in human tumors.

Several cell types that form tumors in animals have been shown to overproduce IGF-1 or IGF-2. However, in these systems, antisense IGF-1 often does not inhibit tumor formation or induce apoptosis, in contrast to the effects that are induced by blocking receptor synthesis. Transgenic mice that overexpress IGF-2 have a higher rate of hepatic tumor formation.[231] Precancerous liver nodules that occur in virally induced models of hepatic cancers overexpress IGF-2. Pancreatic tumor cells that have been transformed with SV40 T antigen require IGF-2 for continued growth.[232] Certain fetal tumors, such as Wilms' tumor and neuroblastoma, are accompanied by loss of imprinting of the IGF-2 gene, and overproduction of IGF-2 accompanies tumor formation.[233] The IGF-2 receptor has also been implicated in a role as a tumor suppressor in hepatocellular carcinomas, possibly through its role in the clearance and degradation of IGF-2.[234] The only paraneoplastic syndrome that is known to be definitively linked to IGF-2 overproduction occurs with retroperitoneal sarcomas. Overproduction of IGF-2 by the tumor results in hypoglycemia.[235] The mechanism that has been proposed is that IGF-2 binds to lower-molecular-weight forms of IGFBPs in plasma (such as IGFBP-2) and this allows accelerated equilibration of IGF-1 and -2 with IGFBPs in extravascular fluids, thus leading to hypoglycemia.

CONTROL OF INSULIN-LIKE GROWTH FACTOR-1 ACTION IN CELLS AND TISSUES BY INSULIN-LIKE GROWTH FACTOR BINDING PROTEINS

Since the IGFBPs are omnipresent in all tissues and have high affinity for IGF-1, they function to regulate IGF-1 actions by controlling access to receptors. The most important determinant of this capacity to modulate IGF-1 action is their affinity for IGF-1, although other variables, such as binding to their own receptors, which leads to IGF-1-independent actions, may play a role.

Regulation of IGFBP Affinity

The affinity of each binding protein is shown in Table 33–2. The estimates vary, but they range between 2- and 50-fold greater than the affinity of the type 1 IGF receptor for IGF-1. The biologic implication of this high affinity is obvious, since, in the soluble form, high-affinity binding proteins will prevent receptor association. Variables that lower the affinity to levels that are much less than the IGF-1 receptor, such as proteolysis, function to allow a sudden increase in the amount of IGF-1 receptor–associated IGF-1. In contrast, variables that lower IGFBP affinity to a range where it approximates that of the receptor but leaves the form of IGFBP intact may result in prolonged, enhanced diffusion of IGF-1 and -2 onto receptors. Either process may result in enhancement of IGF-1 actions, but the type of effect that is enhanced may differ. Additionally, IGFBPs may function to alter the clearance rate of IGF-1 and -2 in tissues and thereby provide a more stable reservoir of peptides. At present, three variables have been identified that significantly alter the affinity of one or more of the IGFBPs. These include proteolysis, phosphorylation, and adherence to cell surfaces or ECM.

Proteolysis

Proteolysis of IGFBP-3 by serum proteases has been shown to result in marked loss of affinity for IGF-1 and a significant, but less intense change in affinity for IGF-2. The principle fragment that is retained, the 32-kDa fragment, has at least a 20-fold reduction in affinity for IGF-1.[141] This protease is present in high concentrations in serum in pregnancy and following nutritional deprivation.[236] It is also detectable in states of GHD. The nature of the protease is unknown, although a significant amount of data support the hypothesis that it is a cation-dependent serine protease. Matrix metalloproteases (MMPs), such as

MMP-1, MMP-2, and MMP-9, degrade several forms of IGFBPs, including IGFBP-3, and constitute part of the IGFBP-3 serum protease activity that is noted during pregnancy.[237] Several well-defined proteases have been shown to degrade IGFBP-3, including plasmin, cathepsin-D, and PSA.[238, 239] IGFBP-3 proteolytic activity has been noted in lymph, follicular fluid, peritoneal fluid, and amniotic fluid. The IGFBP-2 protease is also a cation-dependent serine protease and cleaves IGFBP-2 into fragments that have very low affinity for IGF-1 and -2. To cleave IGFBP-2 optimally, this protease requires that IGF-1 or -2 be bound to IGFBP-2.[240] IGFBP-5 has been shown to be cleaved by proteases in a variety of physiologic fluids, including serum, and by a cation-dependent 95-kDa serine protease that is present in cell culture supernatants from fibroblasts, osteoblasts, and smooth muscle cells.[241] IGFBP-5, like IGFBP-3, is also cleaved by MMP-2 and -9.[242] The fragments of IGFBP-5 that are generated have very low affinity. Blocking proteolytic cleavage by incubating IGF-1 with a mutated, protease-resistant form of IGFBP-5 was shown to inhibit IGF-1-stimulated cell growth. IGFBP-4 proteases are also present in several physiologic fluids. Like IGFBP-2, IGFBP-4 proteolytic activity is enhanced by IGF binding to IGFBP-4.[243] There are correlative data suggesting that degradation of IGFBP-4 results in relief of inhibition of IGF-1 actions.[244]

Phosphorylation

Three of the six forms of IGFBP have been shown to be phosphorylated: IGFBP-1, -3, and -5. IGFBP-1 is phosphorylated on serine residues at positions 101, 119, and 169. Caseine kinase-2 is one of two kinases that can phosphorylate IGFBP-1.[245] Phosphorylation increases the affinity of IGFBP-1 for IGF-1 by sixfold. Different degrees of phosphorylated IGFBP-1 have been found in different physiologic fluids, and during poorly controlled diabetes there is a very highly phosphorylated form of IGFBP-1 that predominates.[152] IGFBP-3 is phosphorylated at positions 111 and 113.[246] The identity of the kinase responsible for IGFBP-3 phosphorylation has not been determined.

Adherence to Cell Surface, Extracellular Matrix, and Glycosaminoglycans

Both IGFBP-3 and IGFBP-5 have been shown to adhere to cell surfaces. Proteoglycan-containing cell surface proteins may be an important cell surface binding component for both proteins. Specific receptors have been postulated to exist for IGFBP-3. The type V TGF-β receptor is an important cell surface moiety that binds IGFBP-3.[247] IGF-1 that is bound to ECM or cell-associated IGFBP-3 is in more favorable equilibrium with receptors, since IGFBP-3 binding to cells lowers its affinity by approximately 10-fold.[248] IGFBP-5 binding to ECM or to proteoglycans causes an eightfold reduction in affinity.[94] However, proteoglycans are not the only type of ECM protein that can bind to IGFBP-5. Plasminogen activator inhibitor-1 has been shown to bind to IGFBP-5 with high affinity. Localization of IGFBP-5 within the ECM may provide an important means for focally concentrating IGF-1 or -2 in the pericellular environment.

Effects of Specific Forms of IGFBPs on IGF-1 Actions

IGFBP-1

Detailed analysis of IGFBP-1 actions in vitro has shown that this protein, when added in excess over IGF-1, is generally inhibitory. That is, if highly phosphorylated, high-affinity forms of IGFBP-1 are added in a 4:1 molar excess over IGF-1, they inhibit DNA synthesis, as well as glucose incorporation and glucose transport.[249, 250] IGFBP-1 has been shown to block IGF-1 binding to receptors on human endometrial membranes, and it inhibits differentiated functions such as the steroidogenic response of human granulosa cells to IGF-1. IGFBP-1 can also enhance the cellular response to IGF-1. If the dephosphorylated form of IGFBP-1 is utilized and added in an equimolar ratio or less with IGF-1, IGFBP-1 can potentiate the in vitro response of smooth muscle cells, keratinocytes, and fibroblasts to IGF-1.[251, 252] IGFBP-1 has been shown to directly stimulate migration of Chinese hamster ovary cells, fibroblasts, and smooth muscle cells by binding to the $\alpha5\beta1$ integrin receptor through its Arg-Gly-Asp sequence.[84] This effect does not require IGF-1 binding to IGFBP-1.

IGFBP-2

IGFBP-2 has also been shown to be inhibitory in most in vitro experiments. Using purified IGFBP-2, it was shown to inhibit IGF-1-stimulated thymidine incorporation to chick embryo fibroblasts and rat astroglial cells, as well as a human lung carcinoma cell line.[253] IGFBP-2 inhibited IGF-1- and -2-stimulated protein synthesis in Madin-Darby bovine kidney (MDBK) cells, and des-(1–3)-IGF-1, which did not bind to IGFBP-2, was fully stimulatory.[254] IGFBP-2 has been shown to stimulate IGF-1-stimulated glucose incorporation and aminoisobutyric acid (AIB) transport in microvascular endothelial cells and DNA synthesis in smooth muscle cells.[255, 256]

IGFBP-3

IGFBP-3, if added in molar excess, inhibits glucose incorporation into fat cells, as well as IGF-1-stimulated DNA synthesis in human fibroblasts. Maximum inhibition was noted at a 5:1 molar ratio. IGFBP-3 inhibits IGF-1-stimulated glucose incorporation.[257] If IGFBP-3 is preincubated with muscle cells and then removed from the medium, it can potentiate their AIB transport response to IGF-1.[258] Using this experimental paradigm, IGFBP-3 was also shown to stimulate the IGF-1-stimulated DNA synthesis response of human fibroblasts, but coincubation with IGFBP-3 was inhibitory.[259] IGFBP-3 inhibited IGF-1-stimulated cyclic adenosine monophosphate (cAMP) generation by rat granulosa cells and inhibited IGF-1-stimulated collagen synthesis by osteoblasts.[260]

IGFBP-3 has been shown to bind to the type V TGF-β receptor. Direct addition of IGFBP-3 has been shown to attenuate the effects of several growth factors, including FGF, on cell growth.[261] TGF-β is believed to cause part of its growth inhibitory effect in breast carcinoma cells through induction of IGFBP-3.[262] Antibodies to IGFBP-3 block the stimulation of apoptosis by TGF-β in prostate carcinoma cells. IGFBP-3 can inhibit growth of fibroblasts that do not possess IGF-1 receptors. These findings indicate that IGFBP-3 clearly has some growth-suppressive effects, at least in vitro, that are independent of IGF-1. IGFBP-3 has also been shown to stimulate apoptosis in certain cell lines, including cells that do not possess IGF-1 receptors.

IGFBP-4

IGFBP-4 has been consistently shown in in vitro experiments to inhibit the actions of IGF-1 on cartilage and bone growth.[263] IGFBP-4 that is synthesized constitutively by intestinal carcinoma cells inhibits this growth.[264] Several differentiated functions of IGF-1 have been shown to be inhibited by IGFBP-4, including the generation of cAMP by osteoblasts, protein synthesis by prostatic cells, and glycogen synthesis by osteosarcoma cells, as well as the steroidogenic response of granulosa cells to FSH. IGFBP-4 potently inhibits smooth muscle cell replication, as well as AIB transport.[265]

IGFBP-5

IGFBP-5 has been shown to potentiate the effects of IGF-1 in stimulating protein synthesis and DNA synthesis in skeletal tissue, including myoblasts, smooth muscle cells, fibroblasts, osteoblasts, and chondrocytes.[241] The potentiation of fibroblasts and smooth muscle cell growth is believed to occur by association of IGFBP-5 with ECM.[94] ECM binding requires a specific region of basic amino acids that are located between positions 201 and 218, and mutation of specific basic residues within this motif results in the loss of ECM association and an inability to potentiate the effects of IGF.[266] IGFBP-5 can also potentiate the effect of IGF-2 on mouse osteoblast, DNA, and protein synthesis. A fragment of IGFBP-5 has also been shown to potentiate the effect of IGF-1 on osteoblast DNA synthesis.[267] Schwann cell differentiation that is stimulated by IGF-1 has been shown to be potentiated by IGFBP-5.[268]

IGFBP-6

Studies with IGFBP-6 are quite limited. IGFBP-6 appears to preferentially inhibit the effects of IGF-2 in bone, and the response of neuroblastoma cells in culture to IGF-1 is inhibited by IGFBP-6.[269, 270]

In summary, IGFBPs are important modulators of IGF action. They function to control the half-life of IGF in blood and its distribution among tissues and extracellular fluids. In extracellular fluids, they clearly control the ability of IGF-1 and -2 to associate with receptors. Factors that alter the affinity of IGFBPs for IGF-1 and -2 can result in enhancement of IGF action. The exact role of each of these binding proteins in particular tissues in vivo is currently a major focus of research.

ACTIONS OF INSULIN-LIKE GROWTH FACTOR-1 IN VIVO

IGF-1 was termed "somatomedin" initially because it mediated the growth-promoting actions of GH, and it was presumed to be a growth stimulant for all tissues. Several correlative types of experiments were conducted to support this hypothesis. These included hypophysectomy of animals, resulting in low serum GH and IGF-1 concentrations and a balanced reduction in growth.[271] Likewise, states of GH excess induced by implanting GH-producing tumors into animals resulted in generalized tissue overgrowth and high circulating IGF-1 concentrations. Serum IGF-1 concentrations were shown to correlate well with changes in GH secretion and growth rates that occurred during postnatal life.[128] Based on these observations, it was presumed that GH acted primarily by stimulating IGF-1 synthesis in the liver with concomitant rises in plasma IGF-1, and that IGF-1 was transported to skeletal tissues where it acted to stimulate growth. The development of complementary DNA (cDNA) probes for IGF-1 allowed new types of experiments that led to refinement of this hypothesis. Hepatic IGF-1 expression was shown to be decreased after hypophysectomy, and it was increased following GH administration.[187] Subsequently, it was shown that IGF-1 was synthesized in multiple extrahepatic tissues and that paracrine-synthesized IGF-1 could stimulate growth.[199, 273] This raised the question as to what percentage of the generalized growth-promoting actions of IGF-1 were mediated by autocrine or paracrine secretion and what percentage were mediated by endocrine effects?

Administration of IGF-1

Administration of IGF-1 to whole animals results in balanced growth.[4] If the animal has been hypophysectomized, the effect is enhanced. A rate-limiting factor is the amount of IGF-1 that can be infused, since very high concentrations will induce hypoglycemia.[274] IGF-1 also feeds back on the pituitary and suppresses GH. This results in a reduction in total serum IGF-1 concentrations due to suppression of ALS and IGFBP-3. If animals are made catabolic, either by nutritional deprivation[275] or administration of glucocorticoids,[276] administration of IGF-1 results in a partial reversal of this catabolic effect. Likewise, systemic administration of IGF-1 has been shown to improve wound healing, recovery of renal function after kidney injury,[277] and whole-body protein accretion.[276] In nutritionally compromised models, the increase in organ weight, as in spleen and kidneys, appears to be enhanced preferentially compared to changes in skeletal growth.[278] In contrast, in well-nourished, hypophysectomized rats and mice, there is proportionate body growth, with skeletal tissue being stimulated in a manner nearly identical to nonskeletal tissue.[278] IGF-1 stimulates an increase in glomerular filtration rate and has a direct, trophic effect on gut epithelial proliferation.[279] Infusion of IGF-1 tends to lower IGFBP-3 and raise IGFBP-2, changes that are similar to those that occur in GHD. Infusion of IGF-1 to insulin-deficient, diabetic rats results in improved growth and more utilization of glucose.[280] Similarly, peripheral glucose uptake and glycerol synthesis are stimulated. Infusion of IGF-1 into the insulin-deficient BB/W rat results in suppression of hepatic glucose output, possibly due to a suppressive effect on glucagon and GH, and these actions lead to enhanced sensitivity to insulin.[281]

Modulation of IGF-1 Actions by IGFBPs in Vivo

IGFBP-1

In vivo studies have been performed wherein specific forms of IGFBP have been administered with IGF-1. Administration of an equimolar amount of IGFBP-1 with IGF-1 to animals reduces the growth response of hypophysectomized rats compared to IGF-1 alone.[282] Administration of a large single dose of IGFBP-1 without IGF-1 resulted in a modest increase (6%) in plasma glucose concentration.[158] In contrast, administration of IGFBP-1 with IGF-1 (1:4 molar ratio) to wounds resulted in enhanced wound healing, including increases in reepithelialization and formation of granulation tissue.[283, 284] These findings indicate that in some specialized circumstances, tissue expression of IGFBP-1 may enhance IGF-1 actions as compared to global inhibition when IGFBP-1 is infused into blood with an equimolar amount of IGF-1.

IGFBP-3

Because of its role in carrying IGFs in serum, animal studies in which IGF-1 and IGFBP-3 are infused together have been important for determining the endocrine actions of IGF-1. In vivo administration of a combination of IGF-1 and IGFBP-3 has consistently shown enhancement of the trophic effects of IGF-1.[285] Administration of an equimolar concentration of IGF-1 plus IGFBP-3 to hypophysectomized rats showed increased bone mineralization and increased growth rates compared with IGF-1 alone. Administration of equimolar concentrations of IGF-1 plus IGFBP-3 to estrogen-deficient rats resulted in approximately 30% improvement in bone mineral density.[285] Muscle mass was also increased in these animals. A polyclonal anti-IGF-1 antibody that functions like an IGFBP also enhances the effects of IGF-1 when administered concomitantly with IGF-1 to experimental animals.[286]

Transgenic Animal Studies

Initially, transgenic animal models of IGF-1 action were utilized in which IGF-1 was overexpressed. One particularly interesting model was utilized in which GH secretion was attenuated by cytotoxic destruction of somatotrophs, and then IGF-1 replacement therapy was performed by expressing IGF-1 mRNA in several tissues.[287] These animals grew normally, although there was some disproportionate growth of the kidneys, liver, pancreas, and spleen.[287] Likewise, brain size appeared to be particularly sensitive to IGF-1 transgene overexpression. If IGF-1 is overexpressed on a background of no GHD, then more modest increases in somatic growth compared to control animals are noted; however, total body size can be increased by 30%.[288] Brain size is increased disproportionately by approximately 50%. Whether suppression of GH results in inability to attain greater growth rates is unknown. Interestingly, the GH-deficient mice have a somewhat hypoplastic liver, and this effect is not totally reversed by IGF-1 transgene overexpression.[287] The major conclusion from these studies was that the majority of the growth-promoting effects of GH were mediated by IGF-1 using both autocrine and paracrine as well as endocrine mechanisms and that local expression of IGF-1 in tissues such as brain results in disporportionate increases in growth.

Attempts to determine the effects of IGFBPs have also utilized transgenic animals. IGFBP-1 transgenic animals show variable phenotypes, depending upon which organs express the transgene. Mice who had expression predominantly in pancreas, kidney, and brain had normal organ sizes, except brain, which was decreased in size.[289] Since

IGFBP-1 is not constitutively expressed there, it presumably bound to IGF-1 or IGF-2, and the animals had a reduction in brain growth. In contrast, in mice with abundant liver expression, there was a slight growth retardation at birth and a 10% to 15% reduction in postnatal growth.[290] Similarly, there was moderate glucose intolerance. Abundant expression of IGFBP-1 in the liver has been shown to result in very modest fetal growth retardation. In IGFBP-3 transgenic animals, there is an increase in liver, spleen, and kidney size, although total body weight and length were not significantly greater than controls.[291]

A great deal of information regarding the skeletal and postnatal growth-promoting effects of IGF-1 has been obtained by homologous recombination experiments. In experiments in which the IGF-1 gene was deleted, the fetuses were born alive and were 60% of normal birth length and weight.[292] Homozygous animals had extremely high juvenile mortality rates, and only approximately 10% to 20% of these animals survived to adulthood. This appears to be due somewhat to the gene dosage effects, since animals that were created by one group that had a leaky promoter and resulted in partial IGF-1 deletion, but not total attenuation, were larger at birth, but more important, had nearly 100% survival into adulthood.[293] This suggests that there is some threshold lower limit of IGF-1 concentration that accounts for the excessive mortality. The animals that do survive to adulthood are disporportionately short and have an abnormal growth rate during the normal juvenile period.[292, 293] They reach 30% of normal adult size. They also have poor Leydig cell development and a small brain size. Skeletal abnormalities were also noted. The cause for the increase in premature death is unknown. No apparent abnormalities of differentiation have been noted. Fetal growth retardation begins at day 13.5 in utero and body size is reduced progressively at each stage up to birth.

Deletion of the IGF-1 receptor results in a much more severe phenotype. The animals are 45% of normal size at birth.[52] None survive birth. All have a hypoplastic diaphragm and fail to take a normal first breath. Likewise, there are multiple skeletal and skin defects, indicating that the receptor is necessary for normal muscle, skin, and bone development in utero.

IGF-2 gene deletion gives a very different phenotype. The animals are approximately 60% of normal size at birth, but unlike the IGF-1 mice, they grow normally postnatally and do not die in excessive numbers.[294] No differentiation defects or structural tissue defects are noted. Deletion of both IGF-1 and -2 results in extremely small mice that are approximately 30% of normal size. This manipulation is lethal, since the mice cannot generate a normal inspiration. They are phenotypically similar to the mice lacking the IGF-1 receptor.

Deletion of the IGFBP-2 gene results in animals with large spleens, but no other change in organ growth is noted.[295] Body size is unchanged at birth and remains normal through juvenile development. This implicates a role for IGFBP-2 in fetal splenic development.

Although IGFBP-4 has consistently been shown to inhibit IGF action in vitro, deletion of this gene in vivo resulted in a slight enhancement of fetal growth, for example, a 15% increase in size at birth.[296] These differences persisted postnatally, but there was no further acceleration in growth rate. This suggests that the in vitro actions may not always mimic the in vivo activity.

Autocrine and Paracrine Regulation of IGF-1-Mediated Growth

Experimental animal models have been useful in readdressing the question of the autocrine and paracrine effects of IGF-1. Since multiple animal studies had shown that IGF-1 mRNA transcripts were expressed in connective tissue cells, principally fibroblasts, and in the equivalent cell types in some organs, such as the intestine, wherein the cells in the lamina propria express abundant IGF-1 transcripts, a major question was whether this material was regulated in a similar way to IGF-1 that was expressed in the liver and secreted into blood. Administration of GH to hypophysectomized rats showed that IGF-1 transcripts were increased in skeletal tissue, such as cartilage, bone, muscle, skin, and other organs, such as the brain, indicating that this autocrine- or paracrine-produced IGF-1, much of which was presumed not to enter the circulation, could be regulated locally. This raised the important question of the extent to which autocrine- or paracrine-produced IGF-1 contributed to growth, as opposed to IGF-1 produced in the liver.

Cell culture experiments reinforced the hypothesis that IGF-1 production was widespread and regulated by many factors. PDGF was shown to stimulate IGF-1 synthesis by fibroblast cells, suggesting that autocrine-paracrine IGF-1 might be regulated by factors other than GH. An example of local control of IGF-1 is the response to injury that occurs following several types of injury models, such as freezing ear cartilage or thermal burns.[297] Fibroblast or chondrocyte precursor cells surrounding the damaged area immediately begin to synthesize IGF-1, and the peak of synthesis usually occurs between 3 and 7 days after injury. Balloon denudation of blood vessels is another example of such injury. The wave of IGF-1 synthesis usually coincides with an increase in the number of precursor cells that are entering the proliferative pool.[298, 299] This continues for several days and then begins to subside. Therefore, it has been assumed that local regulation of growth, particularly in response to injury, but also in response to other stimuli, such as unilateral nephrectomy, wherein the contralateral kidney makes more IGF-1 and enlarges, may be more responsive to local IGF-1 regulation.

Another method of analyzing this problem has been to use hypophysectomized or GH-deleted animal models, in which the IGF-1 gene is expressed in tissues other than liver. In this setting, if IGF-1 expression is ubiquitous and can be maintained at high enough levels, the animals develop reasonably normal IGF-1 plasma concentrations and grow normally. Another model of regulation has been analysis of brain growth. The blood-brain barrier provides some partitioning between blood IGF-1 and locally produced IGF-1. Transgenic animals in which there is intense expression of IGF-1 within the CNS show larger brains than animals that do not have this intense expression, indicating a paracrine regulation of growth that is probably partially independent of blood IGF-1 concentrations.[185, 287, 288] However, the excellent correlation between changes in blood concentrations and IGF-1 after GH administration to hypophysectomized animals and growth rates suggest that there is also an excellent correlation between endocrine-produced IGF-1 and growth.

A recent experimental animal model has helped to further understand the relative components of autocrine- and paracrine-produced IGF-1 as compared to blood-transported IGF-1. Yakar and coworkers,[300] using the Cre-Lox expression system, were able to selectively target IGF-1 expression in the liver. There was no IGF-1 expression in the liver, and plasma IGF-1 concentrations were only 20% of normal. In contrast to IGF-1 knockout animals, in which the expression of IGF-1 in peripheral tissues, as well as liver, is destroyed, all other tissues in these animals synthesized IGF-1 normally. Deletion of IGF-1 expression from the liver was not associated with growth inhibition. These animals were of normal size at birth and grew normally postnatally. This indicates that deletion of IGF-1 expression in the liver results in a major reduction in endocrine-produced IGF-1 and that autocrine or paracrine IGF-1 in these experimental mice is adequate to allow normal statural growth. Since peripheral tissue IGF-1 expression is also under the control of GH, this type of experiment does not distinguish between how much of the locally produced IGF-1 is regulated by factors other than GH and how much is under GH control. It does eliminate the possibility that, in order to grow normally, one has to have a completely normal blood IGF-1 concentration, and proves definitively that the major source of blood IGF-1 is the liver. Although it might not be surprising that fetal growth was normal in these animals, since IGF-2 is an important fetal growth factor, it is striking that there was no juvenile growth retardation, in spite of these low plasma IGF-1 concentrations.

EFFECTS OF INSULIN-LIKE GROWTH FACTOR-1 IN HUMANS

Anabolism

The data regarding IGF-1 infusion into humans as compared to administration of GH need to be evaluated in light of recent findings regarding the autocrine and paracrine actions of IGF-1. As noted previously, when GH is administered, IGF-1 mRNA is clearly induced in multiple tissues in experimental animals that have been made GH-deficient, and there is a rise in serum IGF-1. This indicates that both autocrine and paracrine mechanisms, as well as endocrine ones, are activated by GH. In contrast, administration of IGF-1 alone intravenously to GH-deficient animals or humans does not result in autocrine or paracrine activation of IGF-1 gene expression. Similarly, other undefined but important growth-regulatory molecules that are synthesized in response to GH may not be increased by IGF-1; therefore IGF-1 administration may not always induce the same anabolic changes as GH.

Administration of IGF-1 to normal humans results in changes that are comparable to those noted previously in animal studies. A large bolus of rapidly administered IGF-1 (e.g., 100 μg/kg) results in hypoglycemia.[301] When analyzed on a molar basis, IGF-1 is one-twelfth as potent as insulin in reducing glucose and free fatty acid levels. A continuous infusion of 24 μg/kg/hour of IGF-1 to normal humans results in a 50% reduction in C peptide but maintenance of euglycemia. Peripheral glucose uptake is increased at these infusion rates of IGF-1, and hepatic glucose production and free fatty acid levels are suppressed. Protein breakdown is also decreased.[302] However, using lower infusion rates (5 μg/kg/hour), which do not necessitate supplemental glucose to avoid hypoglycemia, there is no effect on protein breakdown.[303] Insulin sensitivity is also enhanced, as assessed by insulin-to-glucose ratios measured during the IGF-1 infusion. IGF-1 has consistently suppressed insulin levels and resulted in more efficient glucose responsiveness to insulin.[304] Since GH is also suppressed, inhibition of several of the known insulin antagonist actions of GH may contribute to this change. IGF-1 also suppresses glucagon, and such suppression probably contributes to the enhanced insulin sensitivity that is observed during IGF-1 infusion.[302, 304]

Administration of exogenous IGF-1 to catabolic subjects results in improvement in nitrogen balance at an infusion rate of 12 μg/kg/hour and the degree of improvement is comparable to that achieved with GH administration.[305] A second study that used the same design (i.e., 6 days of a 50% caloric restriction) showed that concomitant administration of GH with 12 μg/kg/hour infusion of IGF-1 resulted in further enhancement of nitrogen retention compared to either treatment alone. GH inhibited the development of symptomatic hypoglycemia. Infusion of IGF-1 alone resulted in suppression of IGFBP-3 concentrations and suppression of ALS, but administration of concomitant GH resulted in maintenance of normal levels of this complex in plasma.[136] This high level of the IGF-1-IGFBP-3 complex may have contributed to improved nitrogen balance. Several other studies have suggested that maintenance of complex activity results in a better anabolic response.

IGF-1 alone also caused a threefold increase in IGFBP-2 concentrations, suggesting that a larger fraction of the IGF-1 would be bound to IGFBP-2 under these conditions, and thus have a shorter half-life. A reduced anabolic response to IGF-1 alone may occur as a consequence of these changes in IGFBP profiles. Cholesterol is also lowered in response to IGF-1 infusion, as is potassium. Renal function improves, with an approximately 25% increase in glomerular filtration rate and renal blood flow.[306] The fractional excretion of phosphate is decreased, which probably contributes to the antiphosphaturic effect noted in acromegaly.

Although GH selectively stimulates whole-body protein synthesis without a lesser effect on proteolysis acutely, IGF-1 infusions at relatively high concentrations inhibit proteolysis but have no effect on protein synthesis. With prolonged administration of IGF-1 (e.g., 5 to 7 days given as a subcutaneous injection), there is no effect on proteolysis, but a marked increase in protein synthesis, and the effects are indistinguishable from those of GH.[307] Therefore, the mode of administration and the actual dose of IGF-1 that is given are important determinants of whether IGF-1 has an acute insulin-like effect on protein synthesis (e.g., inhibiting proteolysis) or a chronic GH-like effect in preferentially stimulating protein synthesis. The combination of GH plus IGF-1 has a greater effect on decreasing protein oxidation in GH-deficient subjects compared to either substance given alone.[308] Others were not able to demonstrate a greater protein anabolic effect in normal, healthy, fed subjects when the GH and IGF-1 were given simultaneously compared to GH alone.[309] When catabolism is induced by administering high doses of glucocorticoids, IGF-1 has a significant effect on attenuating proteolysis and a small effect on increasing protein synthesis.[310] These effects are less dramatic than those with GH. The effect of IGF-1 in enhancing insulin sensitivity appears to be preserved even in dexamethasone-treated patients.

Bone Metabolism

Shorter IGF-1 administration to normal subjects results in increased bone turnover, with a preferential effect on bone formation.[311] Young women with anorexia nervosa and severe osteopenia also respond by increasing bone turnover, and there is a short-term anabolic effect.[312] IGF-1 is also an effective stimulant of bone formation in men with osteoporosis.[313] Patients with GHD also respond to IGF-1 with increased bone turnover.[314] The peptide has been given to elderly subjects with osteoporosis and results in improved markers of bone formation, such as pyridiniline cross-links in the urine. However, there are also increases in markers of bone resorption, indicating that bone turnover is stimulated.[315] The net effect of long-term administration of IGF-1 alone on bone mineral content is unknown. Studies in rats have shown that administration of IGF-1, in combination with IGFBP-3, may be a potent stimulant of cortical bone formation, and a preliminary report of a 3-month treatment in humans with osteoporosis also supports this conclusion. These enhanced effects of IGF-1 plus IGFBP-3 compared to IGF-1 alone may be due to the inability of IGF-1 administration to sustain high plasma IGF-1 concentrations over prolonged time periods.

Diabetes

When insulin sensitivity is assessed formally with a euglycemic hyperinsulinemic clamp method, IGF-1 administration results in a substantial improvement in sensitivity to insulin.[126] This occurs in normal subjects, in insulin-deficient diabetic patients, and in patients with extreme insulin resistance syndromes, including those involving mutations of the insulin receptor.[316, 317] Administration of IGF-1 to patients with severe insulin resistance results in long-term lowering of glucose and improved insulin sensitivity.[318] Adolescents with type 1 diabetes who were treated for 4 weeks with subcutaneously administered IGF-1, had reduced insulin requirements and improved their metabolic control.[319] Administration of IGF-1 to patients with type A extreme insulin resistance has resulted in improved metabolic control. Some studies, however, have not seen the same degree of improvement in patients with type A insulin resistance. Administration of IGF-1 to subjects with type 2 diabetes shows that it results in a 2.4-fold improvement in insulin resistance as assessed by direct measurement.[320] More important, IGF-1 lowers hemoglobin A_{1c} by approximately 1.7% and results in improved glucose tolerance. Insulin concentrations are lowered in these patients, suggesting that a change in insulin sensitivity is the primary mechanism accounting for this improvement. Similarly, the requirement for exogenous insulin can be lowered in type 1 diabetes by IGF-1 while maintaining good glycemic control.[321] In a large (N = 208) group of type 2 diabetic patients who were treated with four different doses of IGF-1 for 3 months, the groups that received the two highest doses had a 1.6% reduction in hemoglobin A_{1c}, indicating that long-term improvement in diabetic control is achievable with IGF-1.

Side effects have been noted both in normal subjects and in diabetic patients who have received high concentrations of IGF-1 for several weeks. These include parotid gland tenderness, subcutaneous edema, and increase in heart rate of approximately 10%. In rare subjects, there is edema of the retina and, occasionally, pseudotumor cerebri has been noted. Other unusual side effects include Bell's palsy and severe myalgias. All of these side effects have been noted to reverse within several weeks of stopping the IGF-1.[320, 321]

Other Effects of IGF-1

In addition to its effects in suppressing free fatty acids, ketone bodies, and triglycerides acutely, IGF-1 suppresses apolipoprotein B-100 levels. IGF-1 administration also suppresses plasminogen activator inhibitor-1 levels, and this has the potential to lower the risk of thrombosis in patients with atherosclerosis. IGF-1 has been shown to be neurotrophic in humans, and trials in amyotrophic lateral sclerosis have shown some improvement in nerve regeneration and a slight prolongation of survival, indicating improved muscle function.

Growth Hormone Insensitivity Syndrome

Short-term administration of IGF-1 to patients with GH insensitivity syndrome in which there are mutations of the GH receptor results in improvement in nitrogen retention, phosphate retention, and decreases in glucose and insulin.[322] Analysis of growth rates in nine such subjects who were treated for 1 year showed that they grew approximately 7.5 cm in the first year, as compared to pretreatment growth rates of approximately 4 cm/year. Longer-term follow-up, administering IGF-1 at 50 μg/kg twice a day subcutaneously to patients with GH insensitivity syndrome has shown that the first-year growth velocity cannot be maintained in the second year, and the growth rates are reduced to 6 cm/year.[323–326] This growth rate has been maintained for periods as long as 4 years in subjects who received IGF-1, and therefore there appears to be a growth benefit, which, if projected to adulthood, would result in significant improvement in final adult stature. However, the growth rates during the second through fifth years are not as robust as those in GH-deficient subjects who received GH during a similar interval. Hypoglycemia occurs occasionally in these patients but is usually avoidable by a dosage adjustment. Other side effects that have been noted with acute, high-dose administration of IGF-1 to adults have not been observed in these children. One child with a GH insensitivity syndrome did develop pseudotumor cerebri, which resolved while treatment was continued. Another troublesome feature, however, that has been noted is a coarsening of the facial features, particularly in those subjects who are receiving the treatment during initiation of adolescence. This effect appears to be more significant than that noted with GH administration during puberty, but its ultimate significance is undetermined at present. Whether the suboptimal growth rates and coarsening of facial features are due to stimulation by IGF-1 in the absence of the direct actions of GH that are mediated through the GH receptor is unknown.

REFERENCES

1. Salmon WD Jr, Daughaday WH: A hormonally controlled serum factor which stimulates sulfate incorporation by cartilage in vitro. J Lab Clin Med 49:825, 1957.
2. Daughaday WH, Reeder C: Synchronous activation of DNA synthesis in hypophysectomized rat cartilage by growth hormone. J Lab Clin Med 68:357, 1966.
3. Rinderknecht E, Humbel RE: The amino acid sequence of human insulin-like growth factor I and its structural homology with proinsulin. J Biol Chem 253:2769, 1978.
4. Schoenle E, Zapf J, Humbel RE, et al: Insulin-like growth factor I stimulates growth in hypophysectomized rats. Nature 296:252, 1982.
5. Ullrich A, Gray A, Tam AW, et al: Insulin-like growth factor-I receptor primary structure: Comparison with insulin receptor suggests structural determinants that define functional specificity. EMBO J 5:2503, 1986.
6. Rotwein P, Pollack KM, Didier DK, et al: Organization and sequence of the human insulin-like growth factor I gene. J Biol Chem 261:4828, 1986.
7. Conover CA, Baker BK, Hintz RL: Cultured fibroblasts secrete insulin-like growth factor-I A. J Clin Endocrinol Metab 69:25, 1989.
8. Clemmons DR, Shaw DS: Purification and biologic properties of fibroblast somatomedin. J Biol Chem 263:2841, 1986.
9. Murphy LJ, Friesen HG: Differential effects of estrogen and growth hormone on uterine and hepatic insulin-like growth factor-I gene expression in ovariectomized and hypophysectomized rat. Endocrinology 122:325, 1988.
10. Murphy LJ, Bell GI, Duckworth ML, et al: Identification, characterization, and regulation of complementary deoxyribonucleic acid which evokes insulin-like growth factor I. Endocrinology 121:684, 1987.
11. Holt EC, Van Wyk JJ, Lund PK: Tissue and development specific regulation of a complex family of insulin-like growth factor I messenger ribonucleic acids. Mol Endocrinol 2:1077, 1988.
12. Carlsson B, Carlsson L, Billig H: Estrus cycle dependent covariation of the insulin-

like growth factor I (IGF-I) messenger ribonucleic acid and protein in rat ovary. Mol Cell Endocrinol 64:271, 1989.

13. McCarthy TL, Centrella M, Canalis E: Cortisol inhibits the synthesis of insulin-like growth factor-I in skeletal cells. Endocrinology 126:1569, 1990.

14. Hepler JE, VanWyk JJ, Lund PK: Different half lives of insulin-like growth factor-I mRNA that differ in length of 3′ untranslated sequence. Endocrinology 127:155, 1990.

15. Rinderknecht E, Humbel RE: Primary structure of human insulin-like growth factor II. FEBS Lett 89:283, 1978.

16. Cascieri MA, Chicchi GC, Applebaum J, et al: Mutants of human insulin-like growth factor I with reduced affinity for the type I insulin-like growth factor receptor. Biochemistry 27:3229, 1988.

17. Bayne ML, Applebaum J, Chicchi GG, et al: The roles of tyrosines 24, 31, and 60 in the high affinity binding of insulin-like growth factor-I to the type 1 insulin-like growth factor receptor. J Biol Chem 265:15648, 1990.

18. Bayne ML, Applebaum J, Underwood D, et al: The C region of human insulin-like growth factor (IGF) I is required for high affinity binding to the type I IGF receptor. J Biol Chem 264:11004, 1989.

19. Clemmons DR, Dehoff MH, Busby WH, et al: Competition for binding to insulin-like growth factor (IGF) binding protein-2, 3, 4, and 5 by the IGFs and IGF analogs. Endocrinology 131:890, 1992.

20. Bayne ML, Applebaum J, Chicchi GG, et al: Structural analogues of human insulin-like growth factor-I with reduced affinity for serum binding protein and the type II insulin-like growth factor receptor. J Biol Chem 263:6233, 1988.

21. Clemmons DR, Cascieri MA, Camacho-Hubner C, et al: Discrete alterations of the IGF-I molecule that alter its affinity for IGF binding proteins result in changes in bioactivity. J Biol Chem 265:12210, 1990.

22. Tamura K, Kobayashi M, Ishii Y, et al: Primary structure of rat insulin-like growth factor I. Endocrinology 112:2215, 1983.

23. Blundell TL, Bedarkar S, Rinderknecht E, et al: Insulin-like growth factor: A model for tertiary structure accounting for immunoreactivity and receptor binding. Proc Natl Acad Sci U S A 75:180, 1978.

24. Sara V, Carlsson-Skwirut C, Anderson C, et al: Characterization of somatomedin from fetal brain: Identification of a variant form of insulin-like growth factor-I. Proc Natl Acad Sci U S A 83:4904, 1986.

25. Yamamoto H, Murphy LJ: Generation of des 1–3 insulin-like growth factor-I in serum by acid protease. Endocrinology 135:2432, 1994.

26. Kaleko M, Rutter WJ, Miller D: Overexpression of the human insulin-like growth factor-I receptor promotes ligand dependent neoplastic transformation. Mol Cell Biol 10:464, 1990.

27. Hernandez ER: Regulation of the genes for insulin-like growth factor (IGF) I and II and their receptors by steroids and gonadotrophins in the ovary. J Steroid Biochem Mol Biol 53:219, 1995.

28. Moreno B, Rodriguez MJ, Perez CA, et al: Thyroid hormone controls expression of insulin-like growth factor-I receptor gene at different levels in lung and heart in developing and adult rats. Endocrinology 138:1194, 1997.

29. Hernandez-Sanchez C, Werner H, Roberts CT, et al: Differential regulation of insulin-like growth factor-I receptor gene expression by IGF-I and basic fibroblast growth factor. J Biol Chem 272:4663, 1997.

30. Du J, Meng XP, Delafontaine P: Transcriptional regulation of the insulin-like growth factor-I receptor gene: Evidence for protein kinase C dependent and independent pathways. Endocrinology 138:1378, 1996.

31. Abbott AM, Bueno R, Pedrin MT, et al: Insulin-like growth factor-I receptor gene structure. J Biol Chem 267:10759, 1992.

32. LeRoith D, Werner H, Beitner-Johnson D, et al: Molecular and cellular aspects of the insulin-like growth factor-I receptor. Endocr Rev 16:143, 1995.

33. Sepp-Lorczino L: Structure and function of the insulin-like growth factor-I receptor. Breast Cancer Res Treat 47:235, 1998.

34. Kato H, Faria TN, Stannard B, et al: Role of tyrosine kinase activity in signal transduction by the insulin-like growth factor receptor. J Biol Chem 268:2655, 1992.

35. Gual P, Baron U, Adengian F, et al: A conformational change in the beta subunit of the insulin-like growth factor-I receptor identified by anti-peptide antibodies. Endocrinology 136:5298, 1995.

36. Iterie N, Yoshino H, Moses AC, et al: Evidence that receptor aggregation may play a role in transmembrane signaling through the insulin-like growth factor-I receptor. Mol Endocrinol 2:831, 1998.

37. Treadway JL, Frattali AL, Pessin JE: Intramolecular subunit interactions between insulin and insulin-like growth factor-I alpha beta half receptors induced by ligand and Mn/Mg ATP binding. Biochemistry 31:11801, 1992.

38. Longolis WJ, Sasaroka T, Yip CL, et al: Functional characterization of hybrid receptors composed of a truncated insulin receptor and wild type insulin-like growth factor-I or insulin receptors. Endocrinology 136:1978, 1995.

39. Gronberg M, Wulff BS, Rasmussen JS, et al: Structure-function relationship of the insulin-like growth factor receptor tyrosine kinase. J Biol Chem 268:23435, 1990.

40. Yamasaki H, Pager D, Gebremedhin S, et al: Human insulin-like growth factor-I receptor 950 tyrosine is required for somatotroph growth factor signal transduction. J Biol Chem 267:20953, 1992.

41. Blakesley VA, Scrimgeour A, Esposito D, et al: Signaling via the insulin-like growth factor-I receptor: Does it differ from insulin receptor signaling? Cytokine Growth Factor Rev 7:153, 1996.

42. Giorgetti S, Pelicci PG, Pelicci G, et al: Involvement of Src-homology/collagen SHC proteins in signaling through the insulin and IGF-I receptors. Eur J Biochem 233:195, 1994.

43. Beitner-Johnson D, LeRoith D: Insulin-like growth factor-I stimulates tyrosine phosphorylation of endogenous c-crk. J Biol Chem 270:5187, 1995.

44. Prager D, Li HL, Yamasaki H, et al: Human insulin-like growth factor-I receptor internalization. Role for juxtamembrane domain. J Biol Chem 269:11934, 1994.

45. Hsu D, Knudson PE, Zapf J, et al: NPXY motif in the insulin-like growth factor-I receptor is required for efficient ligand mediated receptor internalization and biologic signaling. Endocrinology 134:744, 1994.

46. Soos MA, Field CE, Siddle K: Purified hybrid insulin/insulin-like growth factor-I receptors bind insulin-like growth factor-I but not insulin with high affinity. Biochem J 290:419, 1993.

47. Esposito D, Blakesley VA, Koval AP, et al: Tyrosine residues in the C-terminal domain of the insulin-like growth factor I (IGF-I) receptors mediate mitogenic and tumorigenic signals. Endocrinology 138:2979, 1997.

48. Li S, Resnicoff M, Boneya R: Effect of mutations at serines 1280–1281 on the mitogenic and transforming activities of the IGF-I receptor. J Biol Chem 271:12254, 1996.

49. Coppola D, Ferber A, Miura M, et al: A functional IGF-I receptor is a requirement for mitogenic and transforming activities of the epidermal growth factor receptor. Mol Cell Biol 14:4588, 1994.

50. DeAngelis T, Ferber A, Baserga R: The insulin-like growth factor I receptor is a requirement for the mitogenic and transforming activities of the platelet derived growth factor receptor. J Cell Physiol 164:214, 1995.

51. Sell C, Rubini R, Rubin R, et al: Simian virus 40 large tumor antigen is unable to transform mouse embryo fibroblasts lacking type I insulin-like growth factor receptor. Proc Natl Acad Sci U S A 90:11217, 1993.

52. Surmacz E, Sell C, Swantek J, et al: Dissociation of mitogenesis and transforming activity by C-terminal truncation of the insulin-like growth factor-I receptor. Exp Cell Res 218:370, 1995.

53. Liu JP, Baker J, Perkins AS, et al: Mice carrying null mutations of the genes encoding insulin-like growth factor I (IGF-I) and type 1 IGF receptor (IGF/r). Cell 75:73, 1993.

54. Sell C, Dumenil G, Deneaud C, et al: Effect of a null mutation of the insulin-like growth factor I receptor gene on growth and transformation of mouse embryo fibroblasts. Mol Cell Biol 14:3604, 1994.

55. D'Mello SR, Galli C, Ciott T, et al: Induction of apoptosis in cerebellar granule neurons by low potassium: Inhibition of death by insulin-like growth factor-I and cAMP. Proc Natl Acad Sci U S A 90:10989, 1993.

56. Rubin R, Baserga R: Biology of disease: Insulin-like growth factor-I receptor: Its role in cell proliferation, apoptosis, and tumorigenicity. Lab Invest 13:311, 1995.

57. O'Connor R, Kauffman ZA, Liu Y, et al: Identification of domains of the insulin-like growth factor-I receptor that are required for protection from apoptosis. Mol Cell Biol 17:427, 1997.

58. Faria TN, Blakesley VA, Kato H, et al: Role of the carboxy-terminal domain of the insulin and insulin-like growth factor-I receptors in receptor function. J Biol Chem 269:13922, 1994.

59. Sun XJ, Wang LM, Zhang Y, et al: Role of IRS-2 in insulin and cytokine signaling. Nature 377:173, 1995.

60. Sun XJ, Rothenberg P, Kahn CR, et al: Structure of the insulin receptor substrate IRS-1 defines a unique signal transduction protein. Nature 351:73, 1991.

61. Myers MJ, White MF: The IRS-1 signaling system. Trends Biol Sci 19:289, 1994.

62. Skolnik EY, Batzer A, Li N, et al: The function of Grb-2 in linking the insulin receptor to ras signaling pathways. Science 260:1953, 1993.

63. Takasu W, Takasu M, Komiya I, et al: Insulin-like growth factor-I stimulates inositol phosphate accumulation, a rise in cytosol free calcium, and proliferation in cultured thyroid cells. J Biol Chem 264:18485, 1989.

64. Kojima I, Mogami H, Ogata E: Oscillation of cytoplasmic free calcium concentration induced by insulin-like growth factor-I. Am J Physiol 262:E307, 1992.

65. Neri LM, Billi AM, Monzoli L, et al: Selective nuclear translocation of protein kinase C alpha in Swiss 3T3 cells treated with IGF-I. FEBS Lett 347:63, 1991.

66. Myers MJ, White MF: Insulin signal transduction and the IRS proteins. Annu Rev Pharmacol 36:615, 1996.

67. Myers MG, Sun XJ, Cheatham B, et al: IRS-I is a common element in insulin and insulin-like growth factor I signaling to the phosphatidylinositol 5′-kinase. Endocrinology 132:1421, 1993.

68. Baserga R: The insulin-like growth factor receptor a key to tumor growth? Cancer Res 55:249, 1995.

69. Pillay TS, Sasoka T, Olefsky JM: Insulin stimulates tyrosine dephosphorylation of pp125 focal adhesion kinase. J Biol Chem 270:991, 1995.

70. Xu B, Bird VG, Miller WT: Substrate specificity of the insulin and insulin-like growth factor I receptor tyrosine kinase catalytic domains. J Biol Chem 270:29825, 1995.

71. Peterson JE, Jelinik T, Kaleko M, et al: C phosphorylation and activation of the IGF-I receptor in Src-transformed cells. J Biol Chem 269:27315, 1994.

72. Kornfeld S: Structure and function of the mannose 6 phosphate insulin-like growth factor II receptors. Annu Rev Biochem 61:307, 1992.

73. Stewart CS, Rotwein P: Growth, differentiation, and survival: Multiple physiologic functions for insulin-like growth factors. Physiol Rev 76:1005, 1966.

74. Flaument RS, Kojima S, Abe M, et al: Activation of latent transforming growth factor beta. Adv Pharmacol 24:51, 1993.

75. Appell KC, Simpson IA, Cushman SW: Characterization of the stimulatory action of insulin and insulin-like growth factor II binding in rat adipose cells. Differences in the mechanism of insulin action on insulin like growth factor II receptors and glucose transporters. J Biol Chem 263:10824, 1998.

76. Nielsen FC: The molecular and cellular biology of insulin-like growth factor II. Prog Growth Factor Res 4:257, 1992.

77. Keiss W, Greenstein LA, White RM, et al: Type II insulin-like growth factor receptor is present in rat serum. Proc Natl Acad Sci U S A 84:7720, 1987.

78. Lau MM, Stewart CHE, Liu Z, et al: Loss of imprinted IGF-II cation independent mannose 6 phosphate receptor results in fetal overgrowth and perinatal lethality. Genes Dev 8:2953, 1994.

79. Filson AJ, Louvi A, Efstratiadis A, et al: Rescue of T-associated maternal effect in mice carrying null mutations in IGF-II and IGF-IIr, two reciprocally imprinted genes. Development 118:731, 1993.

80. Okomoto T, Katada T, Murayama Y, et al: A simple structure encodes G protein activity function of the IGF-I/mannose 6 phosphate receptor. Cell 62:709, 1990.

81. Jones JI, Clemmons DR: Insulin-like growth factor and their binding proteins: Biologic actions. Endocr Rev 16:3, 1995.

82. Clemmons DR: Insulin like growth factor binding proteins. *In* Kostyo JL (ed): Handbook of Physiology: Hormonal Control of Growth, vol 5. New York, Oxford University Press, 1999, p 1901.

83. Brewer MT, Stetler GL, Squires CH, et al: Cloning, characterization and expression of a human insulin-like growth factor binding protein. Biochem Biophys Res Commun 152:1289, 1988.

84. Jones JI, Gockerman A, Busby WH Jr, et al: Insulin-like growth factor binding protein 1 stimulates cell migration and binds to the α5β1 integrin by means of its Arg-Gly-Asp sequence. Proc Natl Acad Sci U S A 90:10553, 1993.

85. Rechler MM: Insulin-like growth factor binding proteins. Vitam Horm 47:1, 1993.

86. Pucilowska JB, Davenport ML, Kabir I, et al: The effect of dietary protein supplementation on insulin-like growth factors (IGF's) and IGF binding proteins in children with shigellosis. J Clin Endocrinol Metab 77:1516, 1993.

87. Hossenlopp P, Seurin D, Segovia-Quinson B, et al: Analysis of serum insulin-like growth factor binding proteins using Western blotting: Use of the method for titration of the binding proteins and competitive binding studies. Anal Biochem 154:138, 1986.

88. Booth BA, Boes M, Dake BL, et al: Structure function relationships in the heparin binding C-terminal region of insulin-like growth factor binding protein-3. Growth Regul 6:206, 1996.

89. Baxter RC: Glycosaminoglycans inhibit formation of the 140 kDa insulin-like growth factor binding protein complex. Biochem J 271:773, 1990.

90. Bautista CM, Baylink DJ, Mohan S: Isolation of a novel insulin-like growth factor (IGF) binding protein from human bone: A potential candidate for fixing IGF-II in human bone. Biochem Biophys Res Commun 176:756, 1991.

91. Durham SK, Keifer MR, Riggs BL, et al: Regulation of insulin-like growth factor binding protein-4 by a specific insulin-like growth factor binding protein-4 protease in normal human osteoblast-like cells. Implications for human cell physiology. J Bone Miner Res 9:111, 1994.

92. James PL, Jones SB, Busby WH, et al: IGF binding protein-5 is expressed in myoblast differentiation and is highly conserved. J Biol Chem 268:22305, 1993.

93. Arai T, Clarke JB, Parker A, et al: Substitution of specific amino acids in insulin-like growth factor–binding protein-5 alters heparin binding and its change in affinity for IGF-I in response to heparin. J Biol Chem 271:6099, 1996.

94. Jones JI, Gockerman A, Busby WH, et al: Extracellular matrix contains insulin-like growth factor binding protein-5: Potentiation of the effects of IGF-I. J Cell Biol 121:679, 1993.

95. Nam TJ, Busby WH, Clemmons DR: Insulin-like growth factor binding protein-5 binds to plasminogen activator inhibitor-I. Endocrinology 138:2972, 1997.

96. Camacho-Hubner C, Busby WH, McCusker RH, et al: Identification of the forms of insulin-like growth factor binding proteins produced by human fibroblasts and the mechanisms that regulate their secretion. J Biol Chem 267:11949, 1992.

97. Keifer MD, Masiarz FR, Bauer D, et al: Identification and molecular cloning of two new 30 kDa insulin-like growth factor binding proteins isolated from adult human serum. J Biol Chem 266:9043, 1991.

98. Bach LA, Thotakura NR, Rechler MM: Human IGFBP-6 is O-glycosylated. Biochem Biophys Res Commun 186:301, 1992.

99. Martin JL, Willetts KE, Baxter RC: Purification and properties of a novel insulin-like growth factor-II binding protein from transformed human fibroblasts. J Biol Chem 265:4124, 1990.

100. Clemmons DR, Van Wyk JJ: Factors controlling blood concentrations in somatomedin-C. J Clin Endocrinol Metab 13:113, 1984.

101. Underwood LE, D'Ercole AJ, Van Wyk JJ: Somatomedin-C and the assessment of growth. J Pediatr Clin North Am 27:771, 1980.

102. Underwood LE, VanWyk JJ: Normal and aberrant growth. *In* Wilson JD, Foster DW (eds): Williams Textbook of Endocrinology, ed 8. Philadelphia, WB Saunders, 1991, pp 1079–1104.

103. Rudman DG, Kutner MH, Rogers CM: Impaired growth hormone secretion in the adult population: Relation to age and adiposity. J Clin Invest 67:1361, 1981.

104. Hong Y, Pedesen NL, Brismar K, et al: Quantitative genetic analyses of insulin-like growth factor I (IGF-I), IGF binding protein-1 and insulin levels in middle-aged and elderly twins. J Clin Endocrinol Metab 81:1791, 1996.

105. Zapf J, Walter H, Froesch ER: Radioimmunological determinations of IGF-I and IGF-II in normal subjects and in patients with growth disorders and extrapancreatic tumor hypoglycemia. J Clin Invest 68:1321, 1981.

106. Nunez SB, Municchi G, Barnes KM, et al: Insulin-like growth factor I (IGF-I) and IGF binding protein-3 concentrations compared to stimulated and night growth hormone in the evaluation of short children—A clinical research center study. J Clin Endocrinol Metab 81:1927, 1996.

107. Juul A, Dalgaard P, Blum WF, et al: Serum levels of insulin-like growth factor (IGF) binding protein-3 (IGFBP-3) in healthy infants, children, and adolescents: The relation to IGF-I, IGF-II, IGFBP-1, IGFBP-2, age, sex, body mass index, and pubertal maturation. J Clin Endocrinol Metab 80:2534, 1995.

108. Hasegawa Y, Hasegawa T, Aso T, et al: Comparison between insulin-like growth factor-I (IGF-I) and IGF binding protein-3 (IGFBP-3) measurement in the diagnosis of growth hormone deficiency. Endocr J 40:185, 1996.

109. Copeland KC, Johnson DM, Kuehl RJ, et al: Estrogen stimulates growth hormone and somatomedin-C in castrate and intact female baboons. J Clin Endocrinol Metab 58:698, 1984.

110. Dean HJ, Kellet JG, Bala RM: The effect of growth hormone treatment on somatomedin levels in growth hormone deficient children. J Clin Endocrinol Metab 55:1167, 1982.

111. Moore DC, Rogelio HA, Smith EK, et al: Plasma somatomedin-C as a screening test for growth hormone deficiency in children and adolescents. Horm Res 16:49, 1982.

112. Clemmons DR, Underwood LE, Ridgway EC: Evaluation of acromegaly by radioimmunoassay of somatomedin-C. N Engl J Med 301:1138, 1979.

113. Melmed S: Acromegaly. N Engl J Med 322:966, 1990.

114. Juul A, Main K, Blum WF, et al: The ratio between serum levels of insulin-like growth factor-I (IGF-I) and the IGF binding proteins (IGFBP-1, 2 and 3) decreases with age in healthy adults and is increased in acromegalic patients. Clin Endocrinol (Oxf) 41:85, 1994.

115. Furlanetto RW, Underwood LE, Van Wyk JJ, et al: Serum immunoreactive somatomedin-C is elevated in late pregnancy. J Clin Endocrinol Metab 47:695, 1979.

116. Chernausek SD, Underwood LE, Utiger RD, et al: Growth hormone secretion and plasma somatomedin-C in primary hypothyroidism. Clin Endocrinol (Oxf) 19:337, 1983.

117. Phillips LS, Unterman TG: Somatomedin activity in disorders of nutrition and metabolism. J Clin Endocrinol Metab 13:145, 1984.

118. Clemmons DR, Klibanski A, Underwood LE, et al: Reduction of plasma immunoreactive somatomedin-C during fasting in humans. J Clin Endocrinol Metab 53:1247, 1981.

119. Merimee TJ, Zapf J, Froesch ER: Insulin-like growth factors in fed and fasted states. J Clin Endocrinol Metab 55:999, 1982.

120. Isley WL, Underwood LE, Clemmons DR: Dietary components that regulate serum somatomedin-C in humans. J Clin Invest 71:175, 1983.

121. Tonshoff B, Blum WF, Wingen A, et al: Serum insulin-like growth factors (IGFs) and IGF binding proteins 1, 2, and 3 in children with chronic renal failure: Relationship to height and glomerular filtration rate. J Clin Endocrinol Metab 80:2684, 1995.

122. Mock DM: Growth retardation in chronic inflammatory bowel disease. Gastroenterology 11:1019, 1986.

123. Goldstein S, Sertich GJ, Levan KR, et al: Nutrition and somatomedin XIX molecular regulation of insulin-like growth factor I in streptozotocin-diabetic rats. Mol Endocrinol 2:1093, 1988.

124. Bereket A, Lang CH, Blethen SL, et al: Insulin-like growth factor binding protein-2 and insulin: Studies in children with type I diabetes mellitus and maturity-onset diabetes of the young. J Clin Endocrinol Metab 80:3647, 1995.

125. Dills DG, Allen C, Palta M, et al: Insulin-like growth factor-I is related to glycemic control in children and adolescents with newly diagnosed insulin-dependent diabetes. J Clin Endocrinol Metab 80:2139, 1995.

126. Morrow LA, O'Brien MB, Moller DE, et al: Recombinant human insulin-like growth factor-I therapy improves glycemic control and insulin action in the type A syndrome of severe insulin resistance. J Clin Endocrinol Metab 79:205, 1994.

127. Baxter RC, Martin JL: Radioimmunoassay of growth hormone dependent insulin-like growth factor binding protein in human plasma. J Clin Invest 78:1504, 1986.

128. Blum WF, Albertsson-Wikland K, Rosberg S, et al: Serum levels of insulin-like growth factor I (IGF-I) and IGF binding protein 3 reflect spontaneous growth hormone secretion. J Clin Endocrinol Metab 76:1610, 1993.

129. Leogney SR, Baxter RC, Carrerato T, et al: Structure and functional expression of acid labile subunit of the insulin-like growth factor binding protein complex. Mol Endocrinol 6:870, 1992.

130. Guler H-P, Zapf J, Schmid C, et al: Insulin-like growth factors I and II in healthy man. Estimations of half-lives and production rates. Acta Endocrinol 121:753, 1989.

131. Baxter RC, Martin JL: Structure of the Mr 140,000 growth hormone–dependent insulin-like growth factor binding protein complex: Determination by reconstitution and affinity labeling. Proc Natl Acad Sci U S A 86:6898, 1989.

132. De Boer H, Blok GJ, Popp-Snijders C, et al: Monitoring of growth hormone replacement therapy in adults, based on measurements of serum markers. J Clin Endocrinol Metab 81:1371, 1996.

133. Grinspoon S, Clemmons DR, Swearingen B, et al: Serum insulin-like growth factor–binding protein-3 levels in the diagnosis of acromegaly. J Clin Endocrinol Metab 80:927, 1995.

134. Pfeilschifter J, Scheidt-Nave C, Leidig-Bruckner G, et al: Relationship between circulating insulin-like growth factor components and sex hormones in a population based sample of 50- to 80-year-old men and women. J Clin Endocrinol Metab 81:2534, 1996.

135. Miell JP, Taylor AM, Zini M, et al: Effects of hypothyroidism and hyperthyroidism on insulin-like growth factors (IGFs) and growth hormone– and IGF-binding proteins. J Clin Endocrinol Metab 76:950, 1993.

136. Kupfer SR, Underwood LE, Baxter RC, et al: Enhancement of the anabolic effects of growth hormone and insulin-like growth factor-I by the use of both agents simultaneously. J Clin Invest 91:391, 1993.

137. Guidice LC, Farrell EM, Pham H, et al: Insulin-like growth factor binding proteins in maternal serum throughout gestation and in the puerperium. J Clin Endocrinol Metab 71:806, 1990.

138. Hossenlopp P, Segovia B, Lassare C, et al: Enzymatic evidence of degradation of insulin-like growth factor binding protein in 150 k complex during pregnancy. J Clin Endocrinol Metab 71:797, 1990.

139. Bang P: Serum proteolysis of IGFBP-3. Prog Growth Factor Res 6:285, 1995.

140. Walker JL, Baxter RC, Young S, et al: Effects of recombinant insulin-like growth factor I on IGF binding proteins and the acid-labile subunit in growth hormone insensitivity syndrome. Growth Regul 3:109, 1993.

141. Lassare C, Binoux M: Insulin-like growth factor binding protein-3 is functionally altered in pregnancy plasma. Endocrinology 134:1254, 1994.

142. Blum WF, Brier BH: Radioimmunoassays for IGFs and IGFBPs. Growth Regul 4:11, 1994.

143. Clemmons DR, Busby WH, Snyder DK: Variables controlling the secretion of insulin-like growth factor binding protein-2 in normal human subjects. J Clin Endocrinol Metab 73:727, 1991.

144. Bar RS, Clemmons DR, Boes M, et al: Transcapillary permeability and subendothelial distribution of endothelial and amniotic fluid IGF-binding proteins in rat heart. Endocrinology 127:1078, 1990.

145. Ooi GT, Orlowski CC, Brown AL, et al: Different tissue distribution and hormonal

regulation of messenger RNAs encoding rat insulin-like growth factor binding proteins-1 and 2. Mol Endocrinol 4:321, 1990.

146. Young SCJ, Smith-Banks A, Underwood LE, et al: Effects of recombinant IGF-I and GH treatment upon serum IGF binding proteins in calorically restricted adults. J Clin Endocrinol Metab 75:603, 1992.

147. Daughaday WH, Trivedi B, Baxter RC: Serum "big" insulin-like growth factor-II from patients with tumor hypoglycemia lacks normal E-domain O-linked glycosylation, a possible determinant of normal propeptide processing. Proc Natl Acad Sci U S A 90:5283, 1993.

148. Schmid C, Schlapfer I, Waldvogel M, et al: Differential regulation of insulin-like growth factor binding protein (IGFBP)-2 mRNA in liver and bone cells by insulin and retinoic acid in vitro. FEBS Lett 303:205, 1992.

149. Smith WJ, Underwood LE, Clemmons DR: Effects of caloric or protein restriction on insulin-like growth factor-I (IGF-I) and IGF-binding proteins in children and adults. J Clin Endocrinol Metab 80:443, 1995.

150. Straus DS, Takemoto CD: Effect of dietary protein deprivation insulin-like growth factor IGF-I and II, IGF binding protein-2 and serum albumin gene expression in the rat. Endocrinology 127:1849, 1990.

151. Ooi GT, Tseng LY, Tran MQ, et al: Insulin rapidly decreases insulin-like growth factor-binding protein-1 gene transcription in streptozotocin-diabetic rats. Mol Endocrinol 6:2219, 1992.

152. Suikkari A-M, Koivisto VA, Koistinen R, et al: Dose-response characteristics for suppression of low molecular weight plasma insulin-like growth factor binding protein by insulin. J Clin Endocrinol Metab 68:135, 1989.

153. Busby WH, Snyder DK, Clemmons DR: Radioimmunoassay of a 26,000 dalton plasma insulin-like growth factor binding protein: Control by nutritional variables. J Clin Endocrinol Metab 67:1225, 1988.

154. Powell DR, Lee PDK, DePaolis LA, et al: Dexamethasone stimulates expression of insulin-like growth factor-binding protein-1 gene expression in human hepatoma cells. Growth Regul 3:11, 1993.

155. Unterman T, Oehler DT, Ngyuen H, et al: A novel DNA/protein complex interacts with the insulin-like growth factor binding protein-1 (IGFBP-1) insulin response sequence and is required for maximal effects of insulin and glucocorticoids on promoter function. Prog Growth Factor Res 6:119, 1995.

156. Bar RS, Boes M, Clemmons DR, et al: Insulin differentially alters transcapillary movement of intravascular IGFBP-1, IGFBP-2 and endothelial cell IGF binding proteins in rat heart. Endocrinology 127:497, 1990.

157. Westwood M, Gibson JM, Williams AC, et al: Hormonal regulation of circulating insulin-like growth factor–binding protein-1 phosphorylation status. J Clin Endocrinol Metab 80:3520, 1995.

158. Lewitt MS, Denyer GS, Cooney GJ, et al: Insulin-like growth factor binding protein-1 modulates blood glucose levels. Endocrinology 129:2254, 1991.

159. Bereket A, Lang CH, Blethen SL, et al: Effect of insulin on the insulin-like growth factor system in children with new onset insulin-dependent diabetes mellitus. J Clin Endocrinol Metab 80:1312, 1995.

160. Davies SC, Wass JAH, Ross RJM, et al: Induction of a specific protease for insulin-like growth factor binding protein-3 in the circulation during severe illness. J Endocrinol 130:469, 1991.

161. Davenport ML, Isley WL, Pucilowska J, et al: Insulin-like growth factor binding protein-3 proteolysis is induced following elective surgery. J Clin Endocrinol Metab 130:2505, 1992.

162. Holt RI, Jones JS, Stone NM, et al: Sequential changes in insulin-like growth factor I and IGF-binding proteins in children with end-stage liver disease before and after orthotopic liver transplantation. J Clin Endocrinol Metab 81:160, 1996.

163. Scharla SH, Strong DD, Mohan S, et al: 1,25-Dihydroxyvitamin D₃ differentially regulates the production of insulin-like growth factor I (IGF-I) and IGF-binding protein-4 in mouse osteoblasts. Endocrinology 129:3139, 1991.

164. Ono T, Kanzaki S, Seino Y, et al: Growth hormone (GH) treatment of GH-deficient children increases serum levels of insulin-like growth factors (IGFs), IGF-binding protein-3 and -5, and bone alkaline phosphatase isoenzyme. J Clin Endocrinol Metab 81:2111, 1996.

165. Roberts CT, Lasky SR, Lowe WL, et al: Molecular coding of rat insulin-like growth factor-I complementary DNA: Differential messenger RNA processing of regulation by growth hormone in extrahepatic tissue. Mol Endocrinol 1:243, 1987.

166. Han VKM, D'Ercole AJ, Lund PK: Cellular location of somatomedin (insulin-like growth factor) messenger RNA in the human fetus. Science 236:193, 1987.

167. Hynes MA, Van Wyk JJ, Brooks PJ, et al: Growth hormone dependence of somatomedin-C/insulin-like growth factor I and insulin-like growth factor II messenger ribonucleic acids. Mol Endocrinol 1:233, 1987.

168. Clemmons DR, Underwood LE, Van Wyk JJ: Hormonal control of immunoreactive somatomedin production by cultured human fibroblasts. J Clin Invest 67:10, 1981.

169. Isgaard J, Nilsson A, Vikma A, et al: Growth hormone regulates the level of IGF-I mRNA in rat growth plate. Endocrinology 122:1515, 1988.

170. McCarthy TL, Centrella M, Canalis E: Parathyroid hormone enhances transcript and polypeptide levels of insulin-like growth factor-I in osteoblast enriched cultures from fetal rat bone. Endocrinology 124:1247, 1989.

171. Silver DM, Fudo H, Halperin D, et al: Differential expression of insulin-like growth factor I (IGF-I) and IGF-II messenger ribonucleic acid in growing rat bone. Endocrinology 132:1158, 1993.

172. Earnst M, Heath JK, Rodan GA: Estradiol effects on proliferation of messenger ribonucleic acid for collagen and insulin-like growth factor I and parathyroid hormone stimulation of adenylate cyclase activity in osteoblast cells from calvaric and long bones. Endocrinology 125:825, 1989.

173. Bichell DP, Rotwein P, McCarthy TL: Prostaglandin E2 avidly stimulates insulin-like growth factor I gene expression in primary osteoblast cultures: Evidence for transcriptional control. Endocrinology 133:1020, 1993.

174. Phillips AF, Persson B, Hall K, et al: The effects of biosynthetic insulin-like growth factor I supplementation on somatic growth, nutrition and erythropoiesis on the neonatal rat. Pediatr Res 23:298, 1988.

175. Adamo ML: Regulation of insulin-like growth factor I gene expression. Diabetes Rev 3:2, 1995.

176. Hernandez ER, Horowitz A, Vera A, et al: Expression of genes encoding the insulin-like growth factors and their receptors in the human ovary. J Clin Endocrinol Metab 74:419, 1992.

177. Guidice LC: Insulin-like growth factors and ovarian follicular development. Endocr Rev 13:641, 1992.

178. Smith EP, Dickson BA, Chernausek SD: Insulin-like growth factor binding protein-3 secretion from cultured rat Sertoli cells: Dual regulation by follicle stimulating hormone and IGF-I. Endocrinology 127:27441, 1990.

179. Bondy CA, Lee WH: Patterns of insulin-like growth factor gene expression in brain: Functional implications. Ann N Y Acad Sci 692:33, 1993.

180. Edwall D, Schalling M, Jennische E, et al: Induction of insulin-like growth factor I messenger ribonucleic acid during regeneration of rat skeletal muscle. Endocrinology 124:820, 1989.

181. Tollefsen SE, Lajara R, McCusker RH, et al: Insulin-like growth factors (IGF) in muscle development. J Biol Chem 264:13810, 1989.

182. Donohue TJ, Lance DD, Largo MN, et al: Induction of myocardial insulin-like growth factor I gene expression in left ventricular hypertrophy. Circulation 89:799, 1994.

183. Hanson MC, Kenneth AF, Alexander RW, et al: Induction of cardiac insulin-like growth factor-I gene expression in pressure overload hypertrophy. Am J Med Sci 306:69, 1993.

184. Fath KA, Alexander RW, Delafontaine P: Abdominal coarctation increases insulin-like growth factor I mRNA levels in rat aorta. Circ Res 72:271, 1993.

185. Cercek B, Fishbein MC, Forrester JS, et al: Induction of insulin-like growth factor I messenger RNA in rat aorta after balloon denudation. Circ Res 66:1755, 1990.

186. Adamo ML, Bach MA, Roberts CT, LeRoith D: Regulation of insulin, IGF-I, and IGF-II gene expression. In LeRoith D (ed): Insulin-Like Growth Factors: Molecular and Cellular Aspects. Boca Raton, FL, CRC Press, 1990, p 271.

187. Lowe WL, Adam OM, Werner H, et al: Regulation by fasting of insulin-like growth factor I and its receptor: Effects on gene expression and binding. J Clin Invest 84:619, 1989.

188. Rotwein P, Pollack KM, Watson M, et al: Insulin-like growth factor gene expression during rat embryonic development. Endocrinology 121:2141, 1987.

189. DePaulo F, Scott LA, Roth J: Insulin and insulin-like growth factor I in early development: Peptides, receptors, and biological events. Endocr Rev 4:558, 1990.

190. Hirschberg R: The physiology and pathophysiology of IGF-I in the kidney. Adv Exp Med Biol 343:345, 1993.

191. Fagin JA, Melmed S: Relative increase in insulin-like growth factor-I messenger ribonucleic acid levels in compensatory renal hypertrophy. Endocrinology 120:718, 1987.

192. Stiles CD, Capone GT, Scher CD, et al: Dual control of cell growth by somatomedin and platelet-derived growth factor. Proc Natl Acad Sci U S A 76:1279, 1979.

193. Leof EB, Wharton W, Van Wyk JJ, et al: Epidermal growth factor and somatomedin-C regulate G₁ progression in competent BALB/c 3T3 cell. Exp Cell Res 141:107, 1982.

194. Travali S, Reiss K, Ferber A, et al: Constituitively expressed c-myb abrogates the requirement for insulin-like growth factor-I in 3T3 fibroblasts. Mol Cell Biol 11:731, 1991.

195. Sell C, Dumenil G, Deveaud C, et al: Effect of null mutation of the type I IGF receptor gene on growth and transformation of mouse embryo fibroblasts. Mol Cell Biol 14:3604, 1994.

196. Pietrzkowski Z, Lammers R, Carpenter G, et al: Constitutive expression of insulin-like growth factor-I and insulin-like growth factor I receptor abrogates all requirements for exogenous growth factors. Cell Growth Differ 3:199, 1992.

197. Pfeifle B, Boeder H, Ditschuneit H: Interaction of receptors for insulin-like growth factor I, platelet-derived growth factor, and fibroblast growth factor in rat aortic cells. Endocrinology 120:2251, 1987.

198. Clemmons DR, Van Wyk JJ: Evidence for a functional role of endogenously produced somatomedin-like peptides in the regulation of DNA synthesis in cultured human fibroblasts and porcine smooth muscle cells. J Clin Invest 75:1914, 1985.

199. Lowe WL: Biologic actions of the insulin-like growth factors. In LeRoith D (ed): Insulin-Like Growth Factors: Molecular and Cellular Aspects. Boca Raton, FL, CRC Press, 1991, p 49.

200. Vetter U, Zapf J, Heit W, et al: Human fetal and adult chondrocytes. Effect of insulin-like growth factors I and II, insulin, and growth hormone on clonal growth. J Clin Invest 77:1903, 1986.

201. Kemp SF, Kearns GL, Smith WG, et al: Effects of IGF-I on the synthesis and processing of glycosaminoglycans in cultured chick chondrocytes. Acta Endocrinol 119:245, 1988.

202. Hock JM, Centrella M, Canalis E: Insulin-like growth factor-I has independent effects on bone matrix formation and cell replication. Endocrinology 122:254, 1988.

203. Barreca A, Delena P, Del Monte S, et al: In vitro paracrine regulation of human growth by fibroblast derived growth factors. J Cell Physiol 151:262, 1992.

204. Dodson MV, Allen RE, Hossner KL: Ovine somatomedin, muliplication stimulating activity, and insulin promote skeletal muscle satellite cell proliferation in vitro. Endocrinology 117:2357, 1985.

205. Florini JR, Ewton DZ, Root SL: IGF-I stimulates terminal myogenic differentiation by induction of myogenin gene expression. Mol Endocrinol 5:718, 1991.

206. Caroni P, Grandes P: Nerve sprouting in innervated adult skeletal muscle induced by exposure to high levels of insulin-like growth factor-I. J Cell Biol 110:1307, 1990.

207. Frondin M, Gammeltoft S: Insulin-like growth factors act synergistically with fibroblast growth factor and nerve growth factor to promote chromaffin cell proliferation. Proc Natl Acad Sci U S A 91:1771, 1994.

208. Caroni P, Schneider C: Signalling by insulin-like growth factors in paralyzed skeletal muscle: Rapid induction of IGF-I expression in muscle fiber and prevention of interstial cell proliferation by IGFBP-5 and IGFBP-4. J Neurosci 14:3378, 1994.

209. Hansson HA, Dahlin LB, Danielsen N, et al: Evidence indicating trophic importance of IGF-I in regenerating peripheral nerves. Acta Physiol Scand 126:609, 1986.
210. Muta K, Krontes B: Apoptosis of human erythroid colony forming cells is decreased by stem cell factor and insulin-like growth factor-I as well as erythropoietin. J Cell Physiol 156:264, 1993.
211. Rodriguez-Tarduchy G, Collins MKL, Garcia I, et al: Insulin-like growth factor I inhibits apoptosis in IL-3 dependent hematopoetic cells. J Immunol 149:535, 1992.
212. Resnicoff MD, Abraham W, Yutaboonchai HL, et al: The insulin-like growth factor-I receptor protects tumor cells from apoptosis *in vitro*. Cancer Res 55:2463, 1995.
213. Claun SY, Billig H, Tilly JL, et al: Gonadotrophin suppression of apoptosis in cultured preovulatory follicles: Mediatory role of endogenous insulin-like growth factor-I. Endocrinology 135:1845, 1994.
214. Florini JR, Ewton DZ, Root SL: Insulin-like growth factors, muscle growth and myogenesis. Diabetes Rev 3:73, 1995.
215. Mochizuki H, Hakeda Y, Watatsuki N, et al: Insulin-like growth factor I supports formation and activation of osteoblasts. Endocrinology 131:1075, 1992.
216. Geduspen JS, Solursh M: Effects of the mesonephros and insulin-like growth factor-I on chondrogenesis. Dev Biol 156:500, 1993.
217. Palmer S, Myerson G, Lindgren E, et al: Insulin-like growth factor-I shifts from promoting cell division to potentiating maturation during normal differentiation. Proc Natl Acad Sci U S A 88:9994, 1991.
218. Penhoat A, Naville D, Jaillard L, et al: Hormonal regulation of insulin-like growth factor-I secretion by bovine adrenal cells. J Biol Chem 264:6858, 1989.
219. Kasson BC, Hseuh AJ: Insulin-like growth factor-I augments androgen biosynthesis by rat testicular cells. Mol Cell Endocrinol 52:27, 1987.
220. Satisteban P, Kohn DL, DiLauro R: Thyroglobulin gene expression is regulated by insulin and insulin-like growth factor I as well as thyrotropin in FRTL 5 cells. J Biol Chem 262:4068, 1987.
221. Yamasaki H, Prager D, Gebremedhin S, et al: Insulin-like growth factor-I (IGF-I) attenuation of growth hormone is enhanced by overexpression of pituitary IGF-I receptors. Mol Endocrinol 5:890, 1991.
222. Duan C, Hawes S, Prevette T, et al: Insulin like growth factor-I (IGF-I) stimulates IGF binding protein-5 synthesis through transcriptional activation of the gene in aortic smooth muscle cells. J Biol Chem 271:4280, 1996.
223. Wolfe BL, Rich CB, Goud HD, et al: Insulin-like growth factor-I regulates transcription of the elastin gene. J Biol Chem 268:124418, 1993.
224. Alemany J, Borras T, dePablo F: Transcriptional stimulation of the delta 1-crystallin gene by insulin-like growth factor I and insulin requires DNA cis elements in chicken. Proc Natl Acad Sci U S A 87:3353, 1990.
225. Urban RJ, Shupnik MA, Bodenburg YH: Insulin-like growth factor-I increases expression of the porcine P-450 cholesterol side chain cleavage gene through a GC-rich domain. J Biol Chem 269:25761, 1994.
226. Dimitridas G, Billings M, Bevan S, et al: Effects of insulin-like growth factor-I on the rates of glucose transport and utilization in rat skeletal muscle *in vitro*. Biochem J 285:269, 1992.
227. Zheng B, Clemmons DR: Blocking ligand occupancy of the αVβ3 integrin inhibits IGF-I signaling in vascular smooth muscle cells. Proc Natl Acad Sci U S A 95:11217, 1998.
228. Morrione A, DeAngelis T, Baserga R: Evidence of the bovine papilloma virus to transform mouse embryo fibroblasts with targeted gene disruption of the insulin-like growth factor-I receptor gene. J Virol 169:5260, 1995.
229. Li S, Resnicoff MD, Baserga R: Effect of substituting tyrosines 1280–1283 on the mitogenic and transforming actions of the insulin like growth factor-I receptor. J Biol Chem 271:12254, 1996.
230. LeRoith D, Werner H, Beitner-Johnson D, et al: Molecular and cellular aspects of the insulin like growth factor I receptor. Endocr Rev 16:143, 1995.
231. Schiramacher P, Held WA, Yang D, et al: Reactivation of insulin-like growth factor II during hepatocarcinogenesis in transgenic mice suggests a role in malignant growth. Cancer Res 5:2549, 1992.
232. Christofori G, Naiki P, Hanahan D: A second signal supplied by insulin like growth factor II in oncogene induced tumorigenesis. Nature 369:414, 1994.
233. Ogawa O, Eccles MA, Szeto J, et al: Relation of insulin like growth factor II gene imprinting implicated in Wilms tumor. Nature 362:749, 1993.
234. De Sousa AT, Hinbrirs GR, Washington MK, et al: Frequent loss of heterozygosity on 6q at the mannose 6 phosphate/insulin like growth factor II receptor locus in human hepatocellular tumors. Oncogene 10:1725, 1995.
235. Baxter RC, Daughaday WH: Impaired function of the ternary insulin-like growth factor binding complex in patients with hypoglycemia due to non–islet cell tumors. J Clin Endocrinol Metab 73:696, 1991.
236. Davenport ML, D'Ercole AJ, Underwood LE: Effects of maternal fasting on fetal growth serum insulin-like growth factors (IGF's) and tissue IGF messenger ribonucleic acids. Endocrinology 126:2062, 1990.
237. Fowlkes J, Enghild JJ, Suzukik N, et al: Matrix metalloproteases degrade insulin like growth factor binding protein-3 in dermal fibroblast cultures. J Biol Chem 269:25742, 1994.
238. Cohen P, Graves HC, Peehl D, et al: Prostate specific antigen PSA is an insulin-like growth factor binding protein-3 protease found in seminal plasma 2. J Clin Endocrinol Metab 75:1046, 1992.
239. Nunn SE, Peehl DM, Cohen P: Acid-activated insulin-like growth factor binding protein protease activity of cathepsin D in normal and malignant prostatic epithelial cells and seminal plasma. J Cell Physiol 171:196, 1997.
240. Gockerman A, Clemmons DR: Porcine aortic smooth muscle cells secrete a serine protease for insulin-like growth factor binding protein-2. Circ Res 76:514, 1995.
241. Clemmons DR: Insulin-like growth factor binding proteins and their role in controlling IGF actions. Cytokine Growth Factor Rev 8:45, 1997.
242. Thrailkill KM, Quarles P, Nagase H, et al: Characterization of insulin-like growth factor binding protein 5 degrading proteases produced throughout murine osteoblast differentiation. Endocrinology 136:3527, 1995.
243. Conover CA: A unique receptor independent mechanism by which insulin-like growth factor I regulates the availability of insulin-like growth factor binding protein in normal and transformed fibroblasts. J Clin Invest 88:1354, 1991.
244. Rees C, Clemmons DR, Horvitz GD, et al: A protease-resistant form of insulin-like growth factor binding protein-4 (IGFBP-4) inhibits IGF-I actions. Endocrinology 139:4182, 1998.
245. Ankrapp DP, Jones JI, Clemmons DR: Characterization of insulin like growth factor binding protein-1 kinases from human hepatoma cells. J Cell Biochem 60:387, 1996.
246. Coverley JA, Baxter RC: Regulation of insulin-like growth factor (IGF) binding protein-3 phosphorylation by IGF-I. Endocrinology 136:5778, 1995.
247. Leal SM, Liu Q, Huang GS, et al: The type V transforming growth factor beta receptor is a putative insulin-like growth factor binding protein 3 receptor. J Biol Chem 272:20572, 1997.
248. McCusker RH, Camacho-Hubner C, Bayne ML, et al: Insulin-like growth factor (IGF) binding to human fibroblast and glioblastoma cells: The modulating effect of cell released IGF binding proteins (IGFBPs). J Cell Physiol 144:244, 1990.
249. Burch WW, Correa J, Shaveley JE, et al: The 25 kDa insulin-like growth factor (IGF) binding protein inhibits both basal and IGF mediated growth in chick embryonic pelvic cartilage in vitro. J Clin Endocrinol Metab 70:173, 1990.
250. Okajimina T, Iwashita M, Takeda Y, et al: Inhibitory effects insulin-like growth factor binding proteins 1 and 3 on IGF activated glucose consumption in mouse Balb/c3T3 fibroblasts. J Endocrinol 133:457, 1993.
251. Elgin RG, Busby WH, Clemmons DR: An insulin-like growth factor binding protein enhances the biologic response to IGF-I. Proc Natl Acad Sci U S A 84:3254, 1987.
252. Kratz G, Lake M, Ljungstrom K, et al: Effect of recombinant IGF binding protein-1 on primary cultures of human keratinocytes and fibroblasts: Selective enhancement of IGF-I but not IGF-II induced cell proliferation. Exp Cell Res 202:381, 1992.
253. Knauer DJ, Smith GL: Inhibition of biologic activity of multiplication stimulating activity by binding to its carrier protein. Proc Natl Acad Sci U S A 77:7252, 1980.
254. Ross M, Francis GL, Szabo L, et al: Insulin-like growth factor (IGF)–binding proteins inhibit the biological activities of IGF-I and IGF-2 but not des-(1–3)-IGF-I. Biochem J 258:267, 1989.
255. Bar RS, Booth BA, Bowes M, et al: Insulin-like growth factor binding proteins from cultured endothelial cells: Purification, characterization, and intrinsic biologic activities. Endocrinology 125:1910, 1989.
256. Bourner MJ, Busby WH, Siegel NR, et al: Cloning and sequence determination of bovine insulin-like growth factor binding protein-2 (IGFBP-2): Comparison of its structural and functional properties with IGFBP-1. J Cell Biochem 48:215, 1992.
257. Zapf J, Schoenle E, Jagars G, et al: Inhibition of the action of nonsuppressible insulin-like activity on isolated fat cells by binding to its carrier protein. J Clin Invest 63:1077, 1979.
258. Conover CA: Potentiation of insulin-like growth factor (IGF) action by IGF-binding protein-3: Studies of underlying mechanism. Endocrinology 130:3191, 1992.
259. DeMellow JSM, Baxter RC: Growth hormone dependent insulin-like growth factor binding protein both inhibits and potentiates IGF-I stimulated DNA synthesis in skin fibroblasts. Biochem Biophys Res Commun 156:199, 1988.
260. Schmid C, Rutishauser J, Schlapfer I, et al: Intact but not truncated insulin-like growth factor binding protein-3 blocks IGF-I induced stimulation of osteoblasts: Control of IGF signalling to bone cells by IGFBP-3 specific proteolysis. Biochem Biophys Res Commun 179:579, 1991.
261. Blat C, Delbe J, Villaudy J, et al: Inhibitory diffusible factor-45 bifunctional activity as a cell growth inhibitor and as an insulin-like growth factor I-binding protein. J Biol Chem 264:12449, 1989.
262. Oh Y, Muller HL, Ng L, et al: Transforming growth factor-beta–induced cell growth inhibition in human breast cancer cells is mediated through insulin-like growth factor–binding protein-3 action. J Biol Chem 270:13589, 1995.
263. Mohan S, Bautista CM, Wergedal J, et al: Isolation of inhibitory insulin-like growth factor (IGF) binding protein from bone cell conditioned medium: A potential local regulator of IGF action. Proc Natl Acad Sci U S A 86:8338, 1989.
264. Coulouscou JM, Shoyab M: Purification of a colon cancer cell growth inhibitor and its identification as insulin-like growth factor binding protein-4. Cancer Res 51:2813, 1991.
265. Conover CA, Durham SK, Zapf J, et al: Cleavage analysis of insulin-like growth factor (IGF)–dependent IGF-binding protein-4 proteolysis and expression of protease-resistant IGF-binding protein-4 mutants. J Biol Chem 270:4395, 1995.
266. Parker A, Rees C, Clarke JB, et al: Binding of insulin-like growth factor binding protein-5 to smooth muscle cell extracellular matrix is a major determinant of the cellular response to IGF-I. Mol Biol Cell 9:2383, 1998.
267. Andress DL, Birnbaum RS: A novel human insulin-like growth factor binding protein secreted by osteoblast cells. Biochem Biophys Res Commun 176:213, 1991.
268. Cheng HL, Feldman EL: Insulin-like growth factor-I (IGF-I) and IGF binding protein-5 in Schwann cell differentiation. J Cell Physiol 171:161, 1997.
269. Gabbitas B, Canalis E: Cortisol enhances the transcription of insulin-like growth factor-binding protein-6 in cultured osteoblasts. Endocrinology 137:1687, 1996.
270. Babajko S, Leneuve P, Loret C, et al: IGF-binding protein-6 is involved in growth inhibition in SH-SY5Y human neuroblastoma cells: Its production is both IGF- and cell density–dependent. J Endocrinol 152:221, 1997.
271. Van Wyk JJ, Underwood LE, Hintz RL, et al: The somatomedins: A family of insulin-like hormones under growth hormone control. Recent Prog Horm Res 30:259, 1974.
272. Juul A, Dalgaard P, Blum WF, et al: Serum levels of insulin-like growth factor (IGF) binding protein-3 (IGFBP-3) in healthy infants, children, and adolescents: The relation to IGF-I, IGF-II, IGFBP-1, IGFBP-2, age, sex, body mass index, and pubertal maturation. J Clin Endocrinol Metab 80:2534, 1995.
273. D'Ercole AJ, Stiles AD, Underwood LE: Tissue concentrations of somatomedin-C: Further evidence for multiple sites of synthesis and paracrine or autocrine mechanisms of action. Proc Natl Acad Sci U S A 81:935, 1984.
274. Jacob RJ, Barrett E, Plewe G, et al: Acute effects of insulin-like growth factor-I on glucose and amino acid metabolism in the awake fasted rat. J Clin Invest 83:1717, 1989.

275. Douglas RG, Gluckman PD, Ball B, et al: The effects of infusion of insulin-like growth factor I (IGF-I), IGF-II and insulin on glucose and protein metabolism in fasted lambs. J Clin Invest 88:614, 1991.

276. Tomas FM, Knowles SE, Owens PC, et al: Insulin-like growth factor-I (IGF-I) and especially IGF-I variants are anabolic in dexamethasone-treated rats. Biochem J 282:91, 1992.

277. Miller SB, Martin DR, Kissone J, et al: Insulin-like growth factor I accelerates recovery from ischemic acute tubular necrosis in the rat. Proc Natl Acad Sci U S A 89:11876, 1992.

278. Thissen JP, Underwood LE, Maiter DM, et al: Failure of IGF-I infusion to promote growth in protein-restricted rats despite normalization of serum IGF-I concentrations. Endocrinology 128:885, 1991.

279. Olanrewaju H, Patel L, Seidel ER: Trophic action of local intraileal infusion of insulin-like growth factor I: Polyamine dependence. Amer J Physiol 263:E282, 1992.

280. Schweiller E, Guler H-P, Merryweather J: Growth restoration of insulin deficit diabetic rats by recombinant human insulin-like growth factor I. Nature 323:169, 1986.

281. Jacob RJ, Sherwin RS, Bowen L, et al: Metabolic effects of IGF-I and insulin in spontaneously diabetic BB/w rats. Am J Physiol 260:E262, 1991.

282. Cox GN, McDermott MJ, Merkel E, et al: Recombinant human insulin-like growth factor binding protein-1 inhibits growth stimulated by IGF-I and growth hormone in hypophysectomized rats. Endocrinology 35:1913, 1994.

283. Jyung RW, Mustoe T, Busby WH, et al: Increased wound breaking strength induced by insulin-like growth factor-1 in combination with IGF binding protein-1. Surgery 115:223, 1994.

284. Galiano RD, Zhao L, Clemmons DR, et al: Interaction between the insulin-like growth factor family and the integrin receptor family in tissue repair processes. J Clin Invest 98:2462, 1996.

285. Bagi CM, Brommage R, Adams SO, et al: Benefit of systemically administered rh IGF-I and rh IGF-I/IGBP-3 on cancellous bone in oophorectomized rats. J Bone Miner Res 9:1301, 1994.

286. Stewart CH, Bates DC, Calder TA, et al: Potentiation of insulin-like growth factor (IGF-I) activity by an antibody: Supportive evidence for enhancement of IGF-I bioavailability in vivo by IGF binding proteins. Endocrinology 133:1462, 1993.

287. Behringer RR, Lewin TM, Quaife CJ, et al: Expression of insulin-like growth factor I stimulates normal somatic growth in growth hormone deficient transgenic mice. Endocrinology 127:1033, 1990.

288. Matthews LS, Hammer RE, Beheringer R, et al: Growth enhancement of transgenic mice expressing human insulin-like growth factor-I. Endocrinology 123:2827, 1988.

289. Dai A, Xing Y, Boney CM, et al: Human insulin-like growth factor binding protein-1 (hIGFBP-1) transgenic mice: Characterization and insights into the regulation of IGFBP-1 expression. Endocrinology 135:1316, 1994.

290. Rajkumar K, Barron D, Lewitt M, et al: Growth retardation and hyperglycemia in insulin-like growth factor binding protein-1 transgenic mice. Endocrinology 136:4029, 1995.

291. Murphy LJ, Molnar P, Lu X, et al: Expression of human insulin-like growth factor-binding protein-3 in transgenic mice. J Mol Endocrinol 15:293, 1995.

292. Baker J, Liu JP, Robertson EJ, et al: Role of insulin like growth factors in embryonic and postnatal growth. Cell 75:83, 1993.

293. Powell-Braxton L, Hollingshead P, Warburton C, et al: IGF-I is required for normal embryonic development in mice. Genes Dev 7:2609, 1993.

294. DeChiara RM, Efstratiadis A, Robertson EJ: A growth deficiency phenotype in heterozygous mice carrying an insulin-like growth factor II gene disruption. Nature 345:78, 1990.

295. Pintar JE, Schuller A, Cerro JA, et al: Genetic ablation of IGFBP-2 suggests functional redundancy in the IGFBP family. Prog Growth Factor Res 6:437, 1995.

296. Shuller AGP, Pintar JE. Embryonic growth deficit in IGFBP-4 deficient mice. Presented at the 80th Endocrine Society Meeting, New Orleans, June 14–18. 1998,OR6-1.

297. Jennische E, Skottner A, Hansson HA: Dynamic changes in insulin-like growth factor I immunoreactivity correlate with repair events in rat ear after freeze-thaw injury. Exp Mol Pathol 47:193, 1987.

298. Hansson HA, Jennische E, Skottner A: Regenerating endothelial cells express insulin-like growth factor-I immunoreactivity after arterial injury. Cell Tissue Res 250:499, 1987.

299. Khorsondi MJ, Fagin JA, Ginnella-Neto A, et al: Regulation of insulin-like growth factor I and its receptor in rat aorta after balloon degradation: Evidence for local bioactivity. J Clin Invest 90:1926, 1992.

300. Yakar S, Liu JU, Stannard B, et al: Normal growth and development in the absence of insulin-like growth factor-I. Proc Natl Acad Sci U S A 96:734, 1999.

301. Guler H-P, Zapf J, Froesch ER: Short-term metabolic effects of recombinant human insulin-like growth factor-I in healthy adults. N Engl J Med 317:137, 1987.

302. Boulware S, Tamborlane W, Sherwin R: Diverse effects of insulin like growth factor I on glucose lipid-I amino acid metabolism. Am J Physiol 262:130, 1992.

303. Mauras N, Horber FF, Haymond MW: Low dose recombinant human insulin-like growth factor-I fails to affect protein anabolism but alters islet cell secretion in humans. J Clin Endocrinol Metab 75:1192, 1992.

304. Kerr D, Tamborlane V, Rife F, et al: Effect of insulin-like growth factor-I on the responses to and recognition of hypoglycemia in humans. A comparison with insulin. J Clin Invest 91:141, 1993.

305. Clemmons DR, Smith-Banks A, Celniker AC, et al: Reversal of diet-induced catabolism by infusion of recombinant insulin-like growth factor-I (IGF-I) in humans. J Clin Endocrinol Metab 75:234, 1992.

306. Guler H-P, Schmid C, Zapf J, et al: Effects of recombinant insulin-like growth factor-I on insulin secretion and renal function in normal human subjects. Proc Natl Acad Sci U S A 86:2868, 1989.

307. Mauras N: Combined recombinant human growth hormone and recombinant human insulin-like growth factor I: Lack of synergy on whole body protein anabolism in normally fed subjects. J Clin Endocrinol Metab 80:2633, 1995.

308. Hussain MA, Schmitz O, Mengel A, et al: Insulin-like growth factor I stimulates lipid oxidation, reduces protein oxidation, and enhances insulin sensitivity in humans. J Clin Invest 92:2249, 1993.

309. Berneis K, Nianis R, Girard J, et al: Effects of insulin-like growth factor I combined with growth hormone on glucocorticoid induced whole body protein catabolism. J Clin Endocrinol Metab 82:2528, 1997.

310. Mauras N, Beaufree B: Recombinant human insulin like growth factor I enhances whole body protein anabolism and significantly diminishes the protein catabolic effects of prednisone in humans without a diabetogenic effect. J Clin Endocrinol Metab 80:869, 1995.

311. Ebling PR, Jones JD, O'Fallon WM, et al: Short term effects of recombinant human insulin like growth factor I on bone turnover in normal women. J Clin Endocrinol Metab 77:1384, 1993.

312. Grinspoon S, Baum HBA, Lee K, et al: Effects of short term rhIGF-I on bone turnover in osteopenic women with anorexia nervosa. J Clin Endocrinol Metab 81:3364, 1996.

313. Johansson AG, Lindh E, Blum WF, et al: Effects of growth hormone and insulin-like growth factor-I in men with osteoporosis. J Clin Endocrinol Metab 81:44, 1996.

314. Biandi T, Glatz Y, Bouillon R, et al: Effects of short term insulin-like growth factor-I (IGF-I) or growth hormone treatment on bone metabolism and on production of 1,25-dihyroxycholecalciferol in GH deficient adults. J Clin Endocrinol Metab 83:81, 1998.

315. Ghiron L, Thompson JL, Holloway L: Effects of recombinant insulin-like growth factor I and growth hormone on bone turnover in elderly women. J Bone Miner Res 10:1844, 1995.

316. Russell-Jones D, Bates AT, Umpleby AM: A comparison of the effects of IGF-I and insulin on glucose metabolism, fat metabolism and the cardiovascular system in normal human volunteers. Eur J Clin Invest 25:403, 1995.

317. Donath MY, Sutsch G, Yan YW, et al: Acute cardiovascular effects of insulin like growth factor I in patients with chronic heart failure. J Clin Endocrinol Metab 183:3177, 1998.

318. Kuzuya H, Matsuura N, Sakamoto M, et al: Trial of insulin-like growth factor-I therapy for patients with extreme insulin resistance syndromes. Diabetes 42:696, 1993.

319. Cheetham TD, Jones J, Taylor AM, et al: The effects of recombinant insulin-like growth factor I administration or growth hormone levels and insulin requirements in adolescents with type 1 insulin-dependent diabetes mellitus. Diabetologia 36:678, 1993.

320. Moses AC, Young SCJ, Morrow LA, et al: Recombinant human insulin-like growth factor I increases insulin sensitivity and improves glycemic control in type II diabetes. Diabetes 45:95, 1996.

321. Quattrin T, Thrailkill K, Baler L, et al: Dual hormonal replacement with insulin and recombinant insulin like growth factor I in insulin dependent diabetes mellitus: Effects on glycemic control, IGF-I levels, and safety profiles. Diabetes Care 20:374, 1997.

322. Walker JL, Ginalska-Malinowska M, Romer TC, et al: Effects of infusion of insulin-like growth factor-I in a child with growth hormone insensitivity syndrome. N Engl J Med 324:1483, 1991.

323. Walker JL, VanWyk JJ, Underwood LE: Stimulation of statural growth by recombinant insulin-like growth factor I in a child with growth hormone insensitivity syndrome (Laron-type). J Pediatr 121:641, 1992.

324. Rosenfeld RG, Rosenbloom AL, Guevara-Aguirre J: Growth hormone (GH) insensitivity due to primary GH receptor deficiency. Endocr Rev 15:369, 1994.

325. Guevara-Aguirre J, Vasconez O, Martinez V, et al: A randomized double blind placebo controlled trial of safety and efficacy of recombinant human insulin-like growth factor I in children with growth hormone receptor deficiency. J Clin Endocrinol Metab 80:1393, 1995.

326. Backeljaw PF, Underwood LE: Prolonged treatment with recombinant insulin-like growth factor I in children with growth hormone insensitivity syndrome—a clinical research center study. J Clin Endocrinol Metab 81:3312, 1996.

Chapter 34

Peptide Growth Factors Other Than Insulin-like Growth Factors or Cytokines

Peter S. Rotwein

GENERAL PRINCIPLES OF GROWTH FACTOR BIOLOGY

Growth factors are secreted proteins that exert diverse effects on cell growth, metabolism, differentiation, and on the growth and development of organisms as distinct as fish, worms, flies, frogs, and humans.[1] Although the term *growth factor* was used initially to describe secreted substances that enhanced cell division, the term now includes proteins that stimulate or inhibit progression through the cell cycle, that control cell death, or that act principally to regulate cellular differentiation.[1, 2] To accomplish these and other biologic actions, growth factors activate specific cellular receptors. Receptors are modular transmembrane proteins that can bind growth factors at their extracellular domains with high affinity and specificity, and can transmit the information generated by binding into changes in cellular economy.[3] Growth factors also may interact with other cell-associated or secreted binding proteins. In general binding proteins do not mediate biologic effects directly, but modulate growth factor availability or stability.

The last few decades have seen an explosive increase in knowledge about growth factors and their actions. This has included the characterization of many growth factors, their receptors, and binding proteins. The structural information derived from the determination of the amino acid sequences of these proteins, and results of studies of biologic function, have led to the classification of growth factors into several discrete families. The information explosion has been enhanced by the advent of molecular cloning in the early 1980s, and by the ability to produce pure recombinant growth factors through molecular biologic techniques. Table 34–1 lists the major growth factor families.

Distinguishing among Hormones, Growth Factors, and Cytokines

As discussed throughout this book, hormones also regulate the growth and development of cells and tissues, and thus could be classified as growth factors. In general, hormones are substances that are produced in endocrine glands, are secreted into the blood stream,

and act at locations distant from their sites of synthesis. Although this *endocrine* mode of action is shared by some growth factors (e.g., see Chapter 31 on the insulin-like growth factor [IGF] family), fundamental differences exist between these two classes of molecules. Unlike hormones, growth factors are produced by many tissues in the body, and thus are not exclusively synthesized by specific glands. Growth factors are proteins, while hormones may be proteins, small peptides, or lipid derivatives. Growth factors also employ modes of action that distinguish them from hormones, termed *paracrine*, *autocrine*, and *juxtacrine* modes. A paracrine mode of action occurs when a growth factor that is secreted by one cell has an effect on adjacent cells. A juxtacrine mode is similar, although the growth factor is bound to the cell membrane or extracellular matrix. Autocrine actions are mediated by a growth factor on its cell of origin after its secretion into the extracellular environment. A variation on this theme has been termed *intracrine* and was first described for an oncogenic variant of platelet-derived growth factor (PDGF) termed *v-sis*.[4, 5] Intracrine actions occur inside the cell of origin and are thus independent of growth factor secretion. These modes of action are outlined in Figure 34–1.

Cytokines are secreted proteins produced principally by lymphocytes, macrophages, and precursors of blood cells. These proteins act to regulate the function of the immune and hematopoietic systems. Cytokines are thus similar to traditional growth factors in their modes of action. They are described in detail in other chapters.

Growth Factor Receptors and Signaling Pathways

As noted above, the effects of growth factors are mediated by activation of specific receptors. Growth factor receptors are transmembrane proteins that consist of at least three domains: an extracellular region that binds the growth factor with high affinity and specificity, a membrane-spanning segment, and one or more intracellular domains that interact with signaling molecules inside the cell.[6–8] Despite the diversity of growth factors and receptors characterized to date, all receptors share these structural features. All growth factor receptors also function as ligand-activated intracellular enzymes. With the exception of receptors for the transforming growth factor-β (TGF-β)

TABLE 34–1. Major Growth Factor Families

Name	Abbreviation	No. of Members
Epidermal growth factor	EGF	8
Fibroblast growth factor	FGF	>15
Insulin-like growth factor	IGF	2
Nerve growth factor	NGF	4
Platelet-derived growth factor	PDGF	2
Transforming growth factor-β	TGF-β	>24

family, all growth factor receptors studied to date show tyrosine kinase activity. Receptors for TGF-β and related molecules phosphorylate substrates on serine and threonine residues rather than tyrosine.[9, 10]

Several general principles govern the steps by which growth factors activate their receptors, although the specific details differ for each growth factor–receptor combination. Binding of a growth factor to the extracellular domain of its receptor first leads to receptor dimerization or oligomerization. Dimerization of the receptor occurs either because the growth factor exists as a dimer and binds to two receptors (e.g., PDGF, TGF-β, nerve growth factor [NGF][7, 8]), because a growth factor monomer has two binding sites for its receptor (e.g., epidermal growth factor [EGF][7, 8]), or because the receptor is a preformed dimer (e.g. IGF-1 [7, 8]). The conformational changes induced by ligand binding then activate the intracellular kinase domain of the receptor, leading sequentially to phosphorylation of the receptor itself (usually on multiple amino acids) by a transphosphorylation mechanism, and then to the phosphorylation of other substrates.[6–8] Autophosphorylation, particularly on tyrosine residues, creates a series of docking sites for other intracellular proteins that contain modules termed SH2 domains, for their similarity with a region of approximately 100 amino acids first identified in the cellular oncogene, *c-src*.[3, 11–13] Different proteins containing SH2 domains bind to distinct docking sites on the receptor, based on the context of each phosphorylated tyrosine, which is defined by the sequence of amino acids adjacent to this modified residue.[6] Recently, another class of phosphotyrosine binding sites, termed the *PTB domain*, has been identified.[14] Although structurally distinct from the SH2 domain, it appears to be functionally equivalent in mediating interactions between a phosphorylated tyrosine residue and a signaling protein. Thus, activated growth factor receptors with multiple phosphorylated tyrosines in different amino acid contexts become the focal point for the transient intracellular aggregation of many SH2- or PTB-containing proteins (Fig. 34–2). These proteins include a variety of intermediates in signal transduction pathways, with the ultimate effects being amplification and diversification of the initial signal induced upon growth factor binding to its receptor. As an example, the activated PDGF receptor binds a series of adapter molecules (Shc, Nck, Grb2), enzymes (PI3 kinase regulatory subunit, phospholipase C γ [PLCγ], protein tyrosine phosphatase 1D [PTP1D], *c-src*), and other proteins, which together participate in the pleiotropic biologic effects of PDGF.[15] Analogous pathways are stimulated by other growth factor receptors. See other chapters for more detailed discussions of signal transduction pathways.

Nuclear Actions of Growth Factors

The long-term changes within cells induced by growth factors are secondary to alterations in gene expression. These changes are but several outcomes of the multiple signaling pathways induced after the assembly of proteins on the activated growth factor receptor. For example, the binding of the adapter molecule Grb2 to a phosphorylated tyrosine of an activated receptor brings this protein and its partner, termed *Son-of-Sevenless (SOS)*, a guanine nucleotide exchange protein, to the cell membrane. SOS can then physically associate with the membrane-bound signaling intermediate, *c-ras*, leading to ras activation through stimulation of its guanosine triphosphate (GTP)–bound form.[16, 17] This sets into motion a series of enzymatic reactions which lead to the phosphorylation and activation of a pair of serine-threonine protein kinases, the mitogen-activated protein (MAPK) or extracellular signal–regulated (ERK) kinases-1 and -2.[16–18] MAPK in turn phosphorylate and activate several cytoplasmic and nuclear proteins, including the transcriptional activator, ternary complex factor, which stimulates expression of the gene encoding *c-fos*.[19–21] This pathway reflects a primary response to growth factors, since it is dependent upon a series of protein-protein interactions and enzymatic steps that do not require new synthesis of cellular proteins. The protein *c-fos* combines with *c-jun* as components of the transcription factor activator protein-1 (AP-1), which in turn regulates the activity of a variety of genes.[19, 21, 22] Thus, gene expression and protein biosynthesis are altered after growth factor signaling is stimulated.

A related pathway mediated by activated growth factor receptors leads to the stimulation of another member of the MAPK family termed c-Jun N-terminal kinase (JNK, also known as stress-activated protein kinase, or SAPK). JNK or SAPK phosphorylates *c-jun* on two serine residues that are critical for its activation as a transcription factor.[21, 23, 24] Thus, both *c-jun* and *c-fos* may be induced through growth factor–stimulated signaling pathways. Other MAPK cascades with different nuclear effects also are activated by growth factor receptors.[18, 22]

Summary

Peptide growth factors are multifunctional proteins that regulate diverse biologic processes through interactions with cellular receptors that function as ligand-activated intracellular enzymes. The enzymatic pathways that are initiated by the binding of a growth factor to its receptor lead to long-term changes in gene expression and protein synthesis that alter the phenotype of individual cells and tissues, and have profound effects on growth and development in the whole animal. Table 34–2 summarizes some of the salient features of growth factor biology. Specific details pertinent to individual growth factor families are described in the following sections.

EPIDERMAL GROWTH FACTOR AND RELATED MOLECULES

EGF was one of the first peptide growth factors to be identified.[25] The EGF family now consists of six structurally similar proteins that

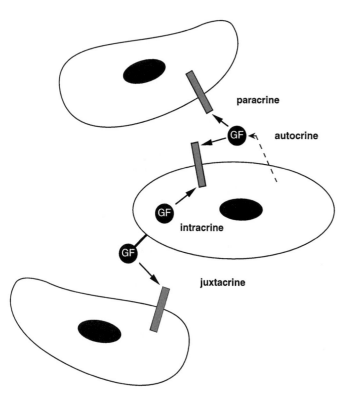

FIGURE 34–1. Modes of growth factor action: autocrine, paracrine, intracrine, and juxtacrine.

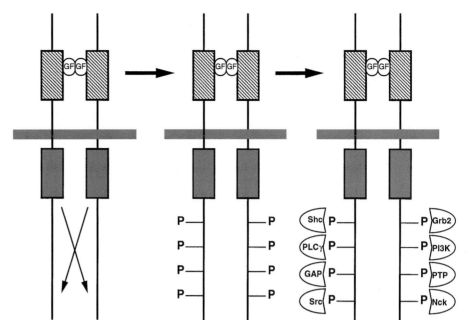

FIGURE 34–2. *An overview of signal transduction by tyrosine kinase receptors. The left panel shows that binding of a growth factor (GF) to the extracellular part of its receptor leads to receptor dimerization and activates the receptor kinase. The center panel demonstrates that tyrosine phosphorylation of the receptor occurs by transphosphorylation. The right panel shows that intracellular substrates with SH2 (see homology-2) domains bind to phosphorylated tyrosine residues of the activated receptor. The ligand-binding domain of the receptor and the tyrosine kinase domain are indicated by boxes. The GF is shown as a dimer. Shc, Nck, Grb2, adapter molecules; PLC, phospholipase C; GTPase-activating protein (GAP), P13K, P13 kinase regulatory subunit; PTP, protein tyrosine phosphatase.*

are capable of binding to and activating the EGF receptor (also known as ErbB1), and two groups of neuregulins, related proteins that bind to and activate other receptors of the ErbB family.[26–29] The four ErbB proteins are receptor tyrosine kinases that function as homo- and heterodimers to activate a variety of intracellular signaling processes.[26, 27] Both the EGF ligands and their ErbB receptors are widely expressed, and are active in embryonic development and adult life.

Structure

The eight members of the EGF and neuregulin families, and three related proteins are listed in Table 34–3. A common feature of this family is that the proteins are synthesized as large transmembrane precursors that are proteolytically cleaved to release the soluble form of the mature growth factor. The larger, membrane-anchored protein precursors also appear to be biologically active and exert their actions through a juxtacrine mechanism.[27, 30] All members of the EGF family share a region of amino acid similarity of 45 to 55 residues known as the EGF-like domain[27] which is necessary and sufficient for binding to ErbB receptors. This protein segment contains six characteristically spaced cysteine residues that form three intramolecular disulfide bonds and define a characteristic three-loop secondary structure that is required for binding to ErbB receptors.[27]

EGF is a conserved 53–amino acid single-chain protein that is synthesized from a 1217–amino acid membrane-bound precursor.[31] The precursor contains eight additional segments with structural homology to EGF, as well as a transmembrane domain, and a short

intracellular C-terminal tail. TGF-α, the second member of the EGF family to be characterized, is a 50-residue peptide derived from a 160–amino acid precursor.[32] The EGF-like domain is 44% identical to EGF. Amphiregulin consists of either a 78- or 84-residue mature protein, and is derived from a 252–amino acid precursor.[33] It was isolated initially from the MCF7 breast cancer cell line.[33] Heparin-binding EGF-like growth factor (HB-EGF) was first identified in the conditioned culture medium derived from the U937 macrophage cell line.[34] The 184–amino acid transmembrane precursor is processed into a series of biologically active mature proteins of 72 to 87 residues that differ at their N-termini.[29, 34] HB-EGF is distinguished from other members of the EGF family by being heavily O-glycosylated and by containing amino acid motifs that allow the protein to interact strongly with heparan sulfate proteoglycans.[29, 35] The membrane-based precursor of HB-EGF also has been identified as the cell surface receptor for diphtheria toxin, and has been shown to be required for toxin entry into susceptible cells.[36] Betacellulin, an 80-residue protein derived from a larger precursor, was characterized from pancreatic β-cell tumors derived from transgenic mice expressing SV40 T antigen in their insulin-producing cells.[37] Epiregulin, a 46–amino acid peptide, was purified from a subclone of the mouse NIH3T3 cell line.[38]

The neuregulins constitute a discrete subclass of the EGF family that do not bind to the EGF receptor, ErbB1, but interact with other ErbBs. The neuregulins, including glial growth factor, acetylcholine receptor–inducing activity, sensory and motor neuron–derived factor, and others,[39–42] are protein products of a single gene that is alternatively

TABLE 34–2. Principles of Growth Factor Biology

1. Growth factors are secreted peptides that exert major effects on cell growth, differentiation, and metabolism, and on the growth and development of the whole organism.
2. Growth factors may be grouped into families that share structural and functional properties.
3. Growth factor action is mediated by interactions with cellular receptors and with cell-associated or secreted binding proteins.
4. Growth factor receptors are transmembrane proteins that function as ligand-activated protein kinases. Changes in phosphorylation of intracellular substrates regulate signaling pathways that ultimately transmit the biologic effects of growth factors, resulting in changes in cell motility, survival, proliferation, differentiation, or metabolism.
5. Abnormalities in growth factors or their receptors may contribute to disorders of growth, development, and differentiation.

TABLE 34–3. Epidermal Growth Factor Family

Epidermal growth factor
Transforming growth factor-α
Amphiregulin
Heparin-binding epidermal growth factor
Betacellulin
Epiregulin
Neuregulin-1 subfamily
    Heregulin/neu-differentiation factor
    Glial growth factor
    Acetylcholine receptor inducing activity
    Sensory and motor neuron–derived factor
Neuregulin-2 subfamily
Distantly related proteins
    Cripto
    Cryptic-1
    Vaccinia virus growth factor

processed into multiple messenger RNA (mRNA) species.[28] Neuregulins contain a shared EGF-like domain of either 77 amino acids (α) or 62 residues (β) in addition to other isoform-specific protein sequences. In general, β neuregulins have been shown to exert more potent biologic effects than α-containing proteins.[28] Related molecules termed *neuregulin-2* have been characterized recently, and have a motif structure similar to neuregulins, including the existence of both α and β versions.[43, 44]

Three additional proteins share structural similarity with EGF family members. Cripto, a gene cloned serendipitously from a human embryonal cancer cell line,[45, 46] and cryptic-1, a gene characterized in differentiating mouse embryonic stem cells,[47] each contain an EGF-like motif with six cysteine residues. Because the spacing of the cysteines differs from other members of the EGF family, with the first disulfide loop being absent, these proteins appear not to bind to ErbB receptors.[48] Receptors mediating their biologic actions have not been identified. Poxviruses, such as vaccinia virus, encode a gene product termed *vaccinia virus growth factor* that is 37% identical to EGF.[49] This 77–amino acid protein, secreted when cells are infected with vaccinia, can bind to and activate the EGF receptor.[49] The role of this factor, as well as activation of the EGF receptor in viral infection or replication, is not clear.

ErbB Receptors and Signaling Mechanisms

The four ErbB receptors are structurally related transmembrane proteins consisting of an extracellular domain with two cysteine-rich segments, a single membrane-spanning region, and a large intracellular segment composed of a tyrosine kinase domain and several tyrosines that become phosphorylated upon receptor activation (Fig. 34–3). The human receptors are also known as HER1 through HER4; ErbB2, or HER2, is also called Neu.[26, 27] As described earlier for receptor tyrosine kinases, binding of EGF family members to ErbB molecules induces receptor dimerization, which triggers kinase activation and autophosphorylation of tyrosine residues in the intracytoplasmic region of the receptors, leading to creation of docking sites for intracellular signaling intermediates and effector proteins.[26, 27]

Despite overall sequence and structural similarities, the four ErbB receptors mediate signal diversification and discrimination through at least three different mechanisms.[27] First, individual receptors are able to bind distinct subsets of EGF family members. EGF, TGF-α, amphiregulin, HB-EGF, betacellulin, and epiregulin can bind to the EGF receptor, ErbB1. Neuregulin, neuregulin-2, HB-EGF, betacellulin, and epiregulin are able to bind to ErbB4. Neuregulin or neuregulin-2 can bind to ErbB3. ErbB2 has no known ligand and thus appears to be an orphan receptor.[26, 27, 50] Second, ligand binding may lead to either receptor homodimerization or to heterodimerization, with the dimerization pattern being defined through both ligand specificity and receptor availability. For example, EGF binding to ErbB1 may lead to the formation of ErbB1 homodimers or to heterodimers of ErbB1 with ErbB2, ErbB3, or ErbB4.[26, 27, 50] Since each ErbB family member has a distinct but overlapping profile of preferred interactions with intracellular signaling intermediates, each combination of receptor dimers has the potential to induce a unique pattern of biologic effects depending upon the signaling molecules activated. Third, ErbB3 does not contain any functional kinase, but rather is a substrate for other ErbB kinases.[26, 27, 50] This effectively limits the range of signaling intermediates activated by receptor heterodimers containing ErbB3.

In addition to the mechanisms described above, several other types of molecular interactions have the potential to extend or modify the range of biologic actions of ErbB receptors. Decorin is a proteoglycan that plays a structural role in modulating assembly of the extracellular matrix.[51] It also may bind to and inhibit some of the actions of TGF-β.[51] Decorin is able to activate the EGF receptor, ErbB1, by directly binding to its extracellular domain, leading to stimulation of receptor kinase activity and to sustained activation of the MAPK signal transduction pathway.[51] The growth hormone receptor (GHR) also uses ErbB1 as a signaling component, but in a mechanistically different way than decorin. The GHR is a member of the cytokine receptor family. Members of this family lack intrinsic protein kinase activity but associate with and activate nonreceptor tyrosine kinases of the Janus kinase (JAK) family (see other chapters for details). In liver cells, stimulation of the GHR by its ligand GH leads to induction of MAPKs through tyrosine phosphorylation of ErbB1 by JAK2.[52] The tyrosine kinase activity of ErbB1 appears to be dispensable for this effect, implying that ErbB1 acts as a substrate for JAK2, and as an intermediate in the signal transduction pathway leading to activation of MAPKs by the GHR. An analogous pattern of receptor crosstalk has been observed between another member of the cytokine receptor family, the gp130 subunit of the interleukin-6 receptor, and ErbB2, which also leads to activation of MAPKs.[53] The physiologic significance of these signaling interactions between cytokine receptors and ErbB receptors and between decorin and ErbB1 remain to be determined.

Crosstalk also occurs between ErbB receptors and G protein–coupled receptors.[54–56] Several ligands that activate different G protein–coupled receptors, including thrombin, lysophosphatidic acid, and endothelin-1, also stimulate tyrosine phosphorylation of ErbB1 and ErbB2 in cultured fibroblasts, leading to induction of MAPKs.[54, 55] In other cultured cells, ErbB1 appears able to activate G proteins through phosphorylation of $G_s\alpha$, leading to stimulation of adenylate cyclase activity.[55, 56] As with cytokine receptors, the biologic significance of such crosstalk remains to be defined.

Biologic Effects

As revealed by targeted gene disruption experiments in mice, EGF family members play key roles in the differentiation of tissues composed principally of epithelial cells, in mesenchymal-epithelial interactions, and in development of components of the central and peripheral nervous systems. Targeted deficiency of ErbB1 caused defective or delayed epithelial development.[57–59] These abnormalities were manifested by reduced placental size, by immature and poorly inflated lungs, by progressive cystic dilation of renal collecting ducts, by diminished thickness of epidermis of the skin, by decreased hair growth secondary to abnormalities of hair follicles, and by diminished development of the eyelids and cornea.[57–59] Depending on strain-specific modifiers, these defects and others led to a host of phenotypic alterations ranging from death at the peri-implantation period to the birth of live mice with multiorgan abnormalities.[57–59] Since lack of one

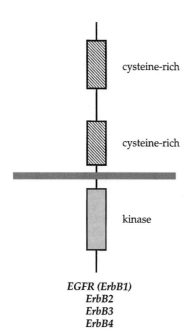

cysteine-rich

cysteine-rich

kinase

EGFR (ErbB1)
ErbB2
ErbB3
ErbB4

FIGURE 34–3. *Epidermal growth factor receptor (EGFR) and related receptors. The two cysteine-rich segments in the extracellular region and the intracellular tyrosine kinase domain are depicted by boxes.*

of the ligands for ErbB1, TGF-α, caused only a subset of defects seen in the ErbB1 knockout mice,[60] these results indicate that the multiple ligands for ErbB1 are required to appropriately regulate receptor actions during development.

Targeted disruption of the genes encoding ErbB2, ErbB4, and neuregulin-1 also showed an overlapping spectrum of developmental abnormalities.[61–64] These mice all died before embryonic day 11 secondary to cardiac malfunction caused by defects in the trabecular extensions of the ventricular myocardium.[61–63] Since ErbB2 and ErbB4 are expressed in myocardial cells, and neuregulin-1 is produced by the adjacent endocardium, these results define a paracrine signaling network in which activation of ErbB2 and ErbB4 by neuregulin-1 is required for proper myocardial differentiation and function. As these mice had distinct but overlapping defects in their nervous systems, it seems likely that other ligands that activate the two receptors in different combinations play important roles in differentiation and maturation in regions of the brain, spinal cord, and peripheral nervous system.[61–63]

A mutation in cripto, one of the divergent members of the EGF family, also was a lethal abnormality.[65] Mice engineered to lack this protein died before embryonic day 11, and had major defects in mesoderm and endoderm formation, and in organization of the anteroposterior body axis.[65]

ErbB signaling pathways are also involved in postnatal development. Treatment of developing mammary glands with EGF, TGF-α, or neuregulin-1 enhanced terminal alveolar differentiation.[66–68] At least three ErbB receptors—ErbB1, -3, and -4—are expressed during mammary development and mediate these biologic effects.[26, 69]

ErbB receptors also play roles in epithelial carcinogenesis. Amplification and overexpression of ErbB2 in breast cancer correlates with both cancer recurrence and poor survival.[70] Other ErbB receptors are also overexpressed or mutated in breast, lung, and other cancers, and have been implicated in disease progression.[71, 72]

Therapeutic Uses

EGF treatment induces the shedding of wool and is used as an alternative to shearing sheep. Antibodies to ErbB2 provide diagnostic information for clinical staging of breast cancer.[71, 72]

FIBROBLAST GROWTH FACTOR FAMILY

Fibroblast growth factors (FGFs) comprise a family of heparin-binding growth factors with diverse effects on wound healing, development, angiogenesis, and other biologic processes. The term *fibroblast growth factor* was initially applied to two proteins, acidic FGF (now FGF-1) and basic FGF (FGF-2), that were isolated from brain and pituitary gland extracts based on their ability to stimulate DNA synthesis in fibroblasts.[73, 74] The FGF family now contains at least 15 members.[74] FGF action is mediated by interactions with transmembrane FGF receptors (FGFRs) and with heparin sulfate proteoglycans (HSPGs). FGFRs also comprise a family that consists of four related genes termed *FGFR1* through *FGFR4*.[75–77] Several different receptor isoforms are the products of alternative RNA splicing.[76, 77]

Structure

The 15 known FGFs show structural similarities in a core region that is required for binding to FGFRs. FGF-1 and -2 are both highly conserved 155–amino acid proteins that are 55% identical to each other.[73, 74] Both proteins lack classic N-terminal signal sequences for directing protein secretion. Despite considerable investigation, how these proteins reach the extracellular environment remains an unsolved problem. FGF-2 mRNA also can be translated beginning with upstream CUG codons, leading to variants with extended N-termini. The FGF-3 precursor also exhibits alternative translation initiation, although this protein contains a signal peptide, as do FGF-4 through 8, and FGF-10. Like FGF-1 and -2, FGF-9, and FGF-11 through FGF-14 lack a signal peptide, and their mechanisms of secretion are unknown.[73, 74]

FGF Receptors and Binding Proteins

FGFRs are the protein products of four highly related genes and share between 60% and 95% amino acid similarity.[75, 77] They function as ligand-activated tyrosine protein kinases with different specificities for the 15 FGF ligands.[75, 77] FGFRs are composed of an extracellular, ligand-binding domain, a single transmembrane segment, and an intracellular region consisting of a tyrosine kinase domain that is split into two parts by a kinase insert region and a C-terminal tail of 55 to 66 residues (Fig. 34–4A). This last segment is divergent in sequence among FGFRs, and may be responsible for interactions with cellular substrates that are distinct for each receptor.[73, 75, 77]

The extracellular domains of FGFRs are composed of two or three immunoglobulin (Ig)-like motifs (Fig. 34–4B) that result from different combinations of alternative RNA splicing of each primary gene transcript.[75, 77] A short unique segment, known as the acidic box domain (because of the high concentration of glutamic and aspartic acid residues), is found between Ig1 and Ig2.[75]

FGFRs exist in both transmembrane and secreted forms (see Fig.

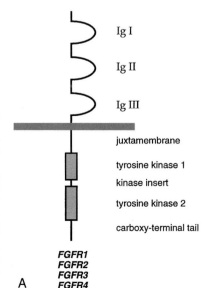

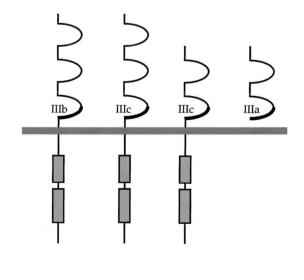

FIGURE 34–4. *A*, Diagram of fibroblast growth factor (FGF) receptors (FGFRs). The different domains are labeled. Ig indicates immunoglobulin-like domains. *B*, Alternative RNA splicing of the *FGFR1* gene regulates synthesis of multiple receptor isoforms. Receptors with two or three Ig domains and with different exons encoding the C-terminal part of Ig domain III are illustrated. Additional receptor subtypes with minor variations on these patterns have been described.

Ig I

Ig II

Ig III

juxtamembrane

tyrosine kinase 1

kinase insert

tyrosine kinase 2

carboxy-terminal tail

FGFR1
FGFR2
FGFR3
FGFR4

A

IIIb   IIIc   IIIc   IIIa

B

34–4B). Transmembrane versions of FGFR1 contain three Ig domains or lack domain 1. The absence of the first Ig region does not alter binding to FGF-1 or -2.[75, 77] Binding affinity may be modified depending upon which of three alternatively spliced exons is used to code for the C-terminal half of the third Ig domain. Receptors using segment IIIb bind FGF-1 with higher affinity than FGF-2, while receptors containing region IIIc bind both growth factors equally, and also bind FGF-4 equivalently.[78] Binding of FGF-3, and FGF-5 through FGF-9 is more variable.[78] Receptors containing segment IIIa are secreted and potentially function as FGF-binding proteins (see Fig. 34–4B). Additional minor receptor variants have been characterized that do not affect ligand binding.

Expression of different FGFRs and splicing variants is controlled in both tissue-specific and developmental-specific ways.[74, 75] In addition, it has been shown that several receptor isoforms are co-expressed in the same tissues.[74, 75] This receptor diversity provides one mechanism for regulating FGF action in different tissues and at different developmental stages.

In addition to the FGFRs, FGFs also bind with lower affinity to several heparin sulfate proteoglycans (HSPGs), including syndecans 1 to 4, glypican, and perlecan.[79] Interactions with HSPGs are essential to high-affinity binding to FGFRs.[80, 81] HSPGs in the extracellular matrix also serve as storage pools for FGFs, providing mechanisms for modulating biologic effects by enhancing local concentrations, limiting degradation, and regulating access to receptors.[82, 83]

Other ligands besides FGFs also bind to FGFRs. Human FGFR1 functions as a coreceptor with HSPGs for adeno-associated virus 2.[79] Cells that express only one of these components fail to bind virus, and are thus resistant to infection. In addition, FGF-1 antagonizes viral infection by competing for binding to FGFR1.[79] Since adeno-associated virus 2–based vectors are being tested for application to human gene therapy, these observations have potential clinical implications.

Binding of FGFs to FGFRs leads to rapid receptor dimerization and to autophosphorylation by a transphosphorylation mechanism. Since FGFs do not form dimers and are not bivalent ligands, the mechanism of receptor dimerization has been unclear. One potential role for cell surface HSPGs is to provide the equivalent of a dimerization interface for FGFs by binding several growth factor molecules simultaneously.[84] This would allow the FGF-HSPG complex to interact with several receptor molecules at the same time and thus stimulate receptor oligomerization. Experimental evidence for this idea has been demonstrated for the interaction of FGF-1 with FGFR2.[81]

Biologic and Clinical Effects

A variety of studies have underscored the critical roles of different members of the FGF family in growth, development, and morphogenesis in many different species. Experiments employing dominant negative FGFRs and other approaches have demonstrated a requirement for FGF signaling in the induction and patterning of mesoderm that occurs early in the development of the frog, *Xenopus laevis*.[85] FGF action is needed for induction of a subset of mesodermal cell types, particularly skeletal muscle. FGFs also may collaborate with activins (members of the TGF-β family) in induction of the notochord.[85] Similar collaborative interactions may be required for induction of other tissue types.[74]

Several FGFs and their receptors have been shown to play critical roles in mouse development, as assessed by targeted gene disruptions and overexpression strategies. A knockout of the *FGFR1* gene in mice led to early embryonic death. Nullizygous embryos died before midgestation, soon after the onset of gastrulation, and had multiple defects in mesodermal derivatives.[86, 87] Heterozygotes developed normally. FGF-3 deficiency caused abnormalities in formation of the tail and inner ear.[88] The absence of FGF-5 led to mice with abnormally long hair, implying a key role for this growth factor in regulation of the hair growth cycle.[89] A homozygous knockout of the FGF-4 gene was a lethal abnormality[90]; embryos developed minimally after implantation into the uterus. FGF-10–deficient embryos failed to form lung buds.[91] Mice with diminished expression of FGF-8 developed abnormalities in the left–right axis during early gestation, with failure to establish normal patterning on the left side.[92] This contrasts with the situation in the chick embryo, where FGF-8 appears to function as a determinant of right-sided identity.[92]

A key role for FGF action in limb development has been defined in the chicken, mouse, and human. Implantation of beads soaked in FGF-1, FGF-2, FGF-4, FGF-6, or FGF-10 into the flank of an early chick embryo caused the appearance of an extra limb bud, and led to the formation of supernumerary limbs.[74] It is likely that this concentrated source of FGF mimics the normal situation by enhancing local cell proliferation, and also by modulating the expression of several other factors that control limb patterning and morphogenesis.[74]

Regulated FGF action also is required for normal bone growth during embryonic development. In mice, targeted deficiency of FGFR3 caused larger than normal bone length, and enhanced expression of proliferating and hypertrophic chondrocytes within the growth plate.[93] In humans, a variety of heterozygous gain-of-function mutations of FGFRs cause craniosynostosis syndromes and chondrodysplasias (Table 34–4).

Craniosynostosis is the premature fusion of skull bone sutures. Different syndromes have been defined based on the association of craniosynostosis with other malformations.[94] Pfeiffer's syndrome consists of craniosynostosis plus flattening of the midface, abnormalities in the great toes and thumbs, and occasionally syndactyly (cutaneous and bony fusion of the digits) affecting other fingers and toes. Crouzon's syndrome includes craniosynostosis with ptosis. In Apert's syndrome craniosynostosis is associated with severe syndactyly of the hands and feet. In the Jackson-Weiss syndrome craniosynostosis is accompanied by variable other malformations, and in Barre-Stevenson syndrome craniosynostosis occurs with furrowed skin and acanthosis nigricans (thickening and darkening of the skin). Achondroplasia is the most common form of dwarfism associated with shortened limbs. Thanatophoric dysplasia is a severe form of achondroplasia, in which the ribs also are shortened. Hypochondroplasia is a milder form of achondroplasia.

TABLE 34–4. Human Fibroblast Growth Factor (FGF) Receptor Mutations

Syndrome	Phenotype	Receptor	Mutation
Pfeiffer's	Craniosynostosis; flattening of midface; abnormal great toes and thumbs; syndactyly	FGFR1	Pro252Arg
		FGFR2	Multiple residues
Crouzon's	Craniosynostosis; ptosis	FGFR2	Multiple residues
		FGFR3	Ala391Glu
Apert's	Craniosynostosis; severe syndactyly	FGFR2	Ser252Trp
			Pro253Arg
Jackson-Weiss	Craniosynostosis; syndactyly; other abnormalities	FGFR2	Cys342Arg
			Ala344Gly
Beare-Stevenson	Craniosynostosis; furrowed skin; acanthosis nigricans	FGFR2	Ser372Cys
			Tyr375Cys
Achondroplasia	Shortening of limbs	FGFR3	Transmembrane domain
Hypochondroplasia	Shortening of limbs	FGFR3	Asn540Lys
Thanatophoric dysplasia	Severe shortening of limbs; abnormalities in vertebrae, ribs, skull	FGFR3	Linker between Ig II and III; C-terminal tail (type I); Lys650Glu (type II)

Known causes for each of these syndromes are heterozygous activating mutations of FGFR1, FGFR2, or FGFR3 (see Table 34–4). One general class of lesions leads to an unpaired cysteine residue within the extracellular region of the affected FGFR. It has been hypothesized that these mutations alter patterns of disulfide bonding within a given receptor, leading to an activating conformational change.[94] Other classes of mutations represent substitutions of highly conserved amino acids in conserved segments of the receptors. These mutations also may lead to activating conformational alterations.[94] The amino acid substitutions that cause the different craniosynostosis syndromes tend to be located in the extracellular domains of FGFR1 through FGFR3, while the mutations responsible for achondroplasias and related abnormalities mostly have been found in the transmembrane and intracellular regions of FGFR3 (see Table 34–4). Surprisingly, to date, mutations in FGFR4 have not been identified in these disorders.

Potential Diagnostic and Therapeutic Uses

DNA-based diagnostic tests are potentially available for craniosynostosis and achondroplasia syndromes, although not all cases of these disorders have been linked to FGFR genes. If gene therapy with vectors based on adeno-associated viruses becomes a clinical reality, then manipulation of expression of FGFR1 will have important implications.

NERVE GROWTH FACTOR FAMILY AND OTHER NEUROTROPHIC FACTORS

NGF was the first growth factor characterized,[95] and was the first trophic agent shown to be critical for survival of sympathetic neurons.[96] There are currently four members of the NGF or neurotrophin family (Table 34–5). These proteins exert diverse effects on the survival and differentiation of different components of the nervous system by activating three related neurotrophic receptors, TrkA, TrkB, and TrkC, and by binding to a low-affinity NGF receptor (NGFR).

Structure of Neurotrophins

Human NGF is a 120–amino acid protein with three intrachain disulfide bonds. It is synthesized as a precursor with an N-terminal extension.[97, 98] Brain-derived neurotrophic factor (BDNF), and neurotrophins 3 and 4 (NT3, NT4) are secreted proteins of 118 to 130 residues with three intrachain disulfide bonds.[97, 98] The four neurotrophic factors are approximately 50 to 60% identical in amino acid sequence and their structures are similar. All four proteins bind to their receptors as homodimers.[97]

Neurotrophin Receptors and Signaling

The high-affinity neurotrophin receptors or Trk family of tyrosine protein kinases was identified initially through studies of an oncogene found in colon cancer. A gene rearrangement resulted in the fusion of a then novel tyrosine kinase with tropomyosin.[99] Analysis of the cellular proto-oncogene led to the characterization of a receptor-like molecule, TrkA, whose tissue distribution corresponded with that of NGF-responsive neurons.[100] Later studies identified two additional members of this family, TrkB and TrkC. The Trks are conserved

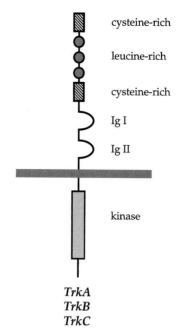

FIGURE 34–5. *Trk A, B,* and *C* encode high-affinity receptors for neurotrophins. Different domains are labeled. Ig indicates an immunoglobulin-like domain.

structurally (Fig. 34–5). They share approximately 80% amino acid identity in their intracellular tyrosine kinase domains but diverge in the extracellular ligand-binding regions.[98] Like other growth factor receptors, Trks are activated by ligand binding to their extracellular domain, which leads to receptor dimerization, kinase activation, and transphosphorylation of sites within the intracytoplasmic region. The phosphorylated tyrosines then serve as docking sites for intracellular proteins with SH2 domains. There are distinct specificities for ligand binding. TrkA binds NGF, TrkB binds BDNF, NT3, and NT4, and TrkC binds NT3.[101]

In addition to the Trks, a structurally distinct lower-affinity NGFR termed p75 also has been described.[102] It is related to Fas/ApoA1, and to the receptors for tumor necrosis factor and lymphotoxin B.[103] These proteins have typical cysteine-rich motifs in their extracellular domains, a single transmembrane segment, and a characteristic short region, termed the "death domain," in their intracellular portions.[102] Binding of NGF to p75 triggers activation of at least two signaling pathways, one leading to stimulation of the transcription factor, nuclear factor-κβ (NF-κβ), and the other enhancing conversion of sphingomyelin to ceramide.[102, 103] Although other neurotrophins also bind to p75, they are not able to trigger sustained signaling responses.[103, 104]

Biologic Effects

The key role of NGF was first shown when injected neutralizing antibodies led to the disappearance of the peripheral sympathetic nervous system in newborn rats.[96] Subsequent studies indicated that target tissues synthesized neurotrophic peptides that maintained neuronal survival and promoted innervation. These observations led to the concept of "target-derived neurotrophic factors."[98, 104] Gene disruption studies in mice have validated this hypothesis, and have defined specific and essential functions for neurotrophins and their receptors. Homozygous mutation of TrkA resulted in loss of peripheral sympathetic neurons and disappearance of distinct populations of pain- and temperature-sensitive neurons.[105] This lethal mutation caused alterations that were similar to those seen after treatment of newborn rodents with NGF antibodies. TrkB-deficient mice exhibited defects in cranial and spinal sensory neurons, and loss of some cranial and spinal motor neurons.[106] The sensory deficits were more severe than those seen with homozygous deficiency of either BDNF or NT4, a result consistent with the observation that both neurotrophins are ligands of

TABLE 34–5. Nerve Growth Factor Family

Nerve growth factor
Brain-derived neurotrophic factor
Neurotrophin 3
Neurotrophin 4

TrkB.[107, 108] TrkB deficiency also was lethal, as was TrkC deficiency. In these latter mice, loss of proprioceptive neurons in the spinal chord and the muscle spindle was seen.[109] Proprioceptive neurons mediate awareness of limb position. Spinal proprioceptive neurons also were diminished in NT3-deficient mice.[110]

Ablation of p75 led to defects in a portion of the peripheral sensory nervous system responsible for sensing changes in skin temperature.[111] The mice were otherwise viable and the sympathetic nervous system was normal.[111]

Although marked abnormalities were observed throughout the spinal chord and peripheral nervous system in Trk-deficient and neurotrophin-deficient mice, minimal changes were seen in the central nervous system (CNS), despite the widespread distribution of TrkB and TrkC in the CNS. This may reflect functional redundancy of neurotrophin signaling in the CNS, or the collaborative effects of other neurotrophic molecules. It has been reported that NGF induces cell death of retinal neurons during early development in the chick.[112] These results and other observations have implicated p75 as a NGF-activated death receptor under certain circumstances.[102]

Other Neurotrophic Factors

Glial-derived neurotrophic factor (GDNF) is a 134–amino acid protein first characterized by its ability to promote survival of midbrain dopaminergic neurons.[101, 113] It is the founding member of a new family of putative neurotrophic agents that includes neurturin (NTN) and persephin.[101, 114, 115] These three proteins are approximately 40% identical in primary amino acid sequence.[101] Members of the GDNF family are unrelated in structure or sequence to the NGF family, but show distant kinship with the TGF-β superfamily.[9] GDNF signaling is initiated by its binding to a heterodimeric receptor composed of α and β subunits that are products of separate genes.[101] The α subunit, termed GDNF-family receptor α (GFRα), is a glycoprotein that is linked to the extracellular face of the cell membrane by a glycophosphatidylinositol anchor.[101] To date, three GFRα proteins have been characterized.[116–120] GFRα1 preferentially binds GDNF, and GFRα2 binds NTN.[115, 117–119] Persephin does not bind to GFRα1, -2, or -3.[115] The β subunit is the proto-oncogene, *ret*, a transmembrane, ligand-activated tyrosine protein kinase.[101] Activating mutants in *ret* cause multiple endocrine neoplasia, type 2, and familial medullary thyroid carcinoma,[121] while inactivating mutations are found in Hirschsprung's disease, a congenital disorder characterized by absence of parasympathetic ganglia from the enteric nervous system.[121]

Gene disruption experiments have revealed identical phenotypes for mice lacking *ret* or GDNF. In both cases there was renal agenesis, neuronal loss in peripheral ganglia, and profound defects in the enteric nervous system, with nearly all neurons distal to the stomach being absent.[122–124] Similar abnormalities in development of the kidney and the enteric nervous system were seen in mice engineered to lack GFRα1.[125] Although NTN and persephin appear to be capable of maintaining survival of cultured ventral midbrain dopaminergic neurons, as well as other neuronal types,[114, 115] their primary physiologic functions have not been elucidated.

Therapeutic Uses

There is presently little information linking abnormalities in neurotrophic factors or their receptors with any disorders, except for the connection between mutations in *ret* and both Hirschsprung's disease and multiple endocrine neoplasia, type 2, as noted above. Nevertheless pharmacologic treatment with these agents, either alone or in concert with other growth factors, may prove beneficial in treating neurodegenerative disorders.

PLATELET-DERIVED GROWTH FACTOR FAMILY

PDGF was discovered as a protein released from the α granules of platelets that was responsible for much of the effect of serum on the proliferation of cells in culture. It was purified from platelets as a highly basic 30-kDa dimeric protein.[126, 127] Purified PDGF was found to consist of two related chains, PDGF-A and PDGF-B, that are products of separate genes.[127] PDGF binds to two cell surface receptors, PDGFR-α and PDGFR-β, which are also related in structure and sequence, but are distinct gene products.[128] Both growth factors and their receptors are expressed in a wide variety of cell and tissue types.[127, 129]

Structure

Mature PDGF-A and -B chains are 109 amino acids in length and are 60% identical.[127, 128] Eight cysteine residues are completely conserved between the two proteins. Both PDGF chains are synthesized as precursor proteins that undergo processing to yield mature glycoproteins.[106] The B chain is homologous to *v-cis*, the transforming protein of simian sarcoma virus.[129] All three combinations of growth factor dimers have been isolated from tissues: AA, AB, BB. In addition to platelet α granules, PDGF has been isolated from several cell types, including macrophages, and from aortic smooth muscle cells.[127]

PDGF Receptors and Signaling

The two PDGFRs are ligand-activated tyrosine protein kinases.[128] The receptors are composed of an extracellular region that contains five Ig-like domains, a transmembrane segment, and an intracellular region with a tyrosine kinase domain that is split by a kinase insert of approximately 100 amino acids (Fig. 34–6). The binding of PDGF to the extracellular region of the receptor induces receptor dimerization. Both homo- and heterodimers can form, depending upon the ligand and the relative receptor abundance. PDGFR-β homodimers bind only PDGF-BB; PDGFR-α homodimers bind all three ligand isoforms, and PDGFR-αβ heterodimers bind PDGF-BB and PDGF-AB.[127] As indicated for other growth factor receptors, ligand binding triggers the receptor kinase, leading to autophosphorylation by a transphosphoryla-

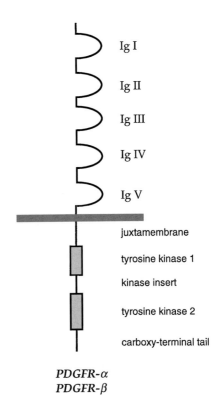

Ig I

Ig II

Ig III

Ig IV

Ig V

juxtamembrane

tyrosine kinase 1

kinase insert

tyrosine kinase 2

carboxy-terminal tail

PDGFR-α
PDGFR-β

FIGURE 34–6. Structure of the two platelet-derived growth factor receptors: PDGFR-α and PDGFR-β. Different regions are labeled. Ig indicates an immunoglobulin-like domain.

tion mechanism. Tyrosine phosphorylation creates docking sites for signal transduction molecules that contain SH2 domains. At least 10 different SH2-containing proteins have been shown to bind to different sites on the two PDGFRs,[130, 131] including adapters (Grb2, Grb7, Nck, Crk); enzymes (PI3 kinase; Src kinases; PLCγ; the tyrosine phosphatase, SHP-2/PTP-1D; and GTPase-activating protein for Ras); and transcription factors (Stats 1, 3, and 5).

Biologic Effects

PDGF action is essential to normal development. A mutation in each component of the PDGF system is associated with lethal developmental anomalies in mice. Absence of the PDGFR-α gene caused death by midgestation, with major defects in formation of bones of the skull and face, spina bifida, and fusions of cervical vertebrae and ribs.[132] A targeted homozygous mutation in the PDGFR-β gene also was lethal,[133] with death during late gestation secondary to hemorrhage. PDGFR-β–deficient mice also showed maldevelopment of the kidneys, with absence of mesangial cells.[133] A similar phenotype is seen in mice with a homozygous null mutation in the PDGF-B chain gene, as predicted, since it is the sole ligand for the β receptor.[134] The cause of hemorrhage in these mice appears to be secondary to absence of microvascular pericytes, which normally contribute to the mechanical stability of the capillary wall.[134] A defect in PDGF-A chain expression also led to a lethal phenotype.[135] In some populations of mice death occurred before midgestation by unknown mechanisms.[135] Other mice lived for up to several weeks after birth but died secondary to emphysema because of loss of alveolar myofibroblasts in the lung. These latter cells are responsible for production of elastin during the phase of lung maturation that occurs normally during the first 2 postnatal weeks.[135]

One of the major actions of PDGF in the adult is in wound healing.[127, 136] Tissue injury leads to the rapid release of abundant PDGF-AB by degranulating platelets. Other acute sources of growth factor include activated macrophages and endothelial cells. Later in the history of a wound, keratinocytes also are induced to produce PDGF. PDGF has several actions during wound healing. It is chemotactic for smooth muscle cells, fibroblasts, neutrophils, and monocytes, and stimulates macrophage activation. It acts as a vasoconstrictor to assist in closure of damaged blood vessels. It is a potent mitogen for fibroblasts and smooth muscle cells, and stimulates their proliferation in collaboration with other growth factors.[136] PDGF induces expression of fibronectin, of collagenase, and of some types of collagen,[136] and these proteins participate in the tissue remodeling that occurs during wound healing.

The actions of PDGF that follow injury to the intima of blood vessels are similar to those occurring after a wound, and contribute to the pathophysiology of atherosclerosis.[128] Release of PDGF by aggregating platelets will trigger the same effects seen in a peripheral wound, leading to the proliferative changes that are associated with atherosclerotic plaques.[128, 136]

Therapeutic Uses

Exogenous PDGF accelerates the healing of incisional wounds in experimental animals,[136] and has been shown to enhance closure of chronic pressure ulcers in human studies.[137] In several models of wound healing, PDGF is most active when used in combination with other growth factors.

TRANSFORMING GROWTH FACTOR-β FAMILY

TGF-β is a dimer of 25 kDa composed of two identical disulfide-linked 12.5-kDa proteins. In mammals three isoforms have been described, TGF-β1, TGF-β2, and TGF-β3.[138] These proteins are prototypic members of a large family of growth factors with diverse biologic

effects in many different species.[9, 138] TGF-β and related proteins control aspects of development, differentiation, and determination; regulate immune function and the response to inflammation; and play pivotal roles in reproduction.[9, 139–141] TGF-β action is controlled by interactions with several classes of receptors, and with cell-associated and extracellular binding proteins. Two classes of high-affinity TGF-β receptors have been defined. Type I and type II receptors are each ligand-activated serine-threonine protein kinases.[9] A type III receptor modulates binding of TGF-β to type I and type II receptors, but lacks its own signaling capability.[9]

TGF-β and Related Proteins

The TGF-β superfamily contains over two dozen members in vertebrates (Table 34–6); multiple homologues exist in invertebrates as well.[138] These proteins are all synthesized as larger precursors with N-terminal extensions. Amino acid sequence similarity among family members is confined to the mature 110- to 140-residue growth factor.[138] Proteolytic cleavage releases the mature protein, which in biologically active form is a dimer.[142] Members of the TGF-β family share seven cysteine residues that are nearly invariant. Six cysteines are involved in the formation of intrachain disulfide bonds which link the protein into a rigid structure termed a "cysteine knot," as initially defined in the crystal structure of TGF-β2.[138] The seventh cysteine forms the interchain disulfide bridge which joins two monomers into a TGF-β dimer.

TGF-β. Three structurally related TGF-β molecules have been characterized in mammals, TGF-β1, TGF-β2, and TGF-β3, and two others have been identified in nonmammalian vertebrates, TGF-β4 from the chicken, and TGF-β5 from *X. laevis*.[138] The mature proteins are 64% to 82% identical. Mammalian TGF-β monomers are 112

TABLE 34–6. Transforming Growth Factor-β (TGF-β) Family

TGF-β subfamily
TGF-β1
TGF-β2
TGF-β3
Activin subfamily
Activin AA
Activin AB
Activin BB
Bone morphogenetic protein 2 (BMP2) subfamily
BMP2
BMP4
BMP3 subfamily
BMP3
GDF10
BMP5 subfamily
BMP5
BMP6/Vgr1
BMP7
BMP8
Vegetal 1 (Vg1) subfamily
Growth differentiation factor 1 (GDF1)/Vg1
GDF3/Vgr2
GDF5 subfamily
GDF5
GDF6
GDF7
Intermediate members
Nodal
Dorsalin
GDF8
GDF9
Distantly related members
Müllerian inhibitory substance
Inhibins
Glial-derived neurotrophic growth factor
Neurturin
Persephin

amino acids in length and contain nine cysteines. They are synthesized as precursors of approximately 350 to 400 residues and are secreted as latent complexes of approximately 100 kDa.[138, 142] Latent complexes consist of the mature TGF-β dimer noncovalently associated with a dimer of the remainder of the precursor protein, which is termed latency-associated peptide (LAP). This small latent complex is unable to bind to TGF-β receptors. A larger latent complex also exists. It consists additionally of a 125- to 160-kDa cysteine-rich glycoprotein known as latent TGF-β binding protein (LTBP). Activation of latent complexes provides one mechanism for regulating growth factor availability.[142] Although the precise pathway of activation has not been elucidated, it appears to involve proteolysis at the cell surface. LAP is a glycoprotein and several of its sugar side chains contain mannose 6-phosphate residues. The IGF-2–/cation-independent mannose 6-phosphate receptor can bind the latent TGF-β complex through these sugar residues and this binding appears essential to activation in tissue culture cells.[142] Activation also requires proteases such as plasmin.[142]

INHIBINS AND ACTIVINS. Inhibins were identified as proteins found in ovarian follicular fluid that inhibited pituitary secretion of follicle-stimulating hormone (FSH). The two inhibins are heterodimers between a distinct α subunit and one of two β subunits, βA and βB. Activins were characterized as stimulators of FSH secretion, and are composed of dimers of inhibin β chains. Three isoforms have been isolated: AA, AB, and BB. Inhibins and activins are functional antagonists.[143] The biologic properties of these proteins are described in detail in other chapters.

BONE MORPHOGENETIC PROTEINS (BMPs). Seven BMPs have been characterized, BMP2 through BMP8.[9, 138] These proteins are composed of dimers of molecular weight 26 to 31 kDa. BMPs were identified initially by their ability to induce cartilage and bone.[144–146] BMP2 and BMP4 are closely related in sequence to each other and to the *Drosophila* protein decapentaplegic (dpp). Dpp plays essential roles in morphogenesis and in bodily patterning in the fly.[138] BMP5 through BMP8 are 74% to 91% identical to one another.[147] BMP6 is also known as vegetal-related 1 (Vgr1).[9] Additional proteins that are closely related to the BMPs include vegetal 1 (Vg1), also termed growth-differentiation factor 1 (GDF1), and GDF3, also known as Vgr2.[9] Other, more distant relatives include nodal, dorsalin, and GDF5 through GDF10.[9, 138] The biologic actions of some of the BMPs and related proteins are described below. A more comprehensive review of BMPs may be found elsewhere.[146, 148]

MÜLLERIAN INHIBITORY SUBSTANCE (MIS). MIS was characterized as a factor secreted by male mammalian embryos that caused regression of the müllerian duct, which otherwise would develop into the oviducts, uterus, and upper one third of the vagina.[149] It is a disulfide-linked dimer that is secreted as a dimeric precursor of approximately 140 kDa. MIS is distantly related in sequence to TGF-β (~30% amino acid similarity). Its biologic actions are described elsewhere in this book.

GLIAL-DERIVED NEUROTROPHIC GROWTH FACTOR. GDNF was isolated through its ability to promote survival and differentiation of dopaminergic neurons.[101] It is less than 25% identical to other members of the TGF-β family. The biologic actions of GDNF and related proteins were described earlier in this chapter.

TGF-β Receptors

TYPE I AND TYPE II RECEPTORS. TGF-β binds to three major cell surface proteins that were initially termed type I, type II, and type III, based on approximate molecular weights of 53, 70, and greater than 200 kDa.[9] Several complementary DNAs (cDNAs) encoding each class of receptor were subsequently cloned. Type I and Type II receptors are structurally related glycoproteins (Fig. 34–7). Both are composed of extracellular ligand-binding domains of 102 to 196 amino acids containing a short cysteine-rich box, a single transmembrane region, and an intracytoplasmic portion of approximately 400 to 500 residues. The intracytoplasmic portion contains a kinase domain that will phosphorylate itself and exogenous substrates on serine and threonine residues.[9, 10, 150] Related receptors have been identified by their ability to bind activins or BMPs. Evidence has accumu-

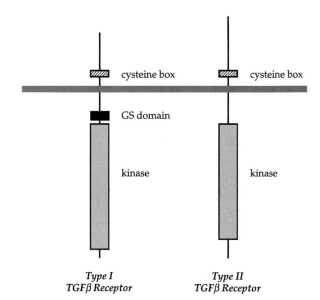

FIGURE 34–7. Structure of type I and type II transforming growth factor-β (TGF-β) receptors. Different regions are labeled. The glycine-serine rich (GS) domain is unique to type I receptors.

lated demonstrating that type I and type II proteins interact to create functional signaling receptors. The type I receptor will bind TGF-β or activin only when associated with the appropriate type II receptor.[9] BMP type I and II receptors each individually have low affinity for BMPs, but cooperatively bind ligand with high affinity.[9]

TYPE III RECEPTORS AND TGF-β BINDING PROTEINS. The type III receptor acts as an accessory molecule in TGF-β action. Type III receptors do not have an intrinsic signaling function but regulate access to signaling receptors.[9] Two related molecules make up the type III TGF-β receptors.[151] Betaglycan is a transmembrane proteoglycan with a protein core molecular weight of 130 kDa. It can bind TGF-β1, -β2, or -β3 with high affinity.[152, 153] Betaglycan is structurally related to endoglin, the other type III receptor protein, a transmembrane glycoprotein composed of two disulfide-linked 95-kDa subunits.[154] Endoglin has been shown to bind TGF-β1 and TGF-β3.[154] Betaglycan and endoglin both consist of large extracellular domains, a single transmembrane segment, and a short intracytoplasmic region. In addition to presenting TGF-β to signaling receptors, type III receptors also may function in the storage and clearance of TGF-β.[9] No comparable type III receptors have been identified yet for activins, BMPs, or other members of the TGF-β superfamily.

Other TGF-β binding proteins include LTBP, described earlier, and follistatin, a widely distributed, secreted glycoprotein that binds activin and inhibits its actions.[143] In addition, α₂-macroglobulin, a serum protein, binds both mature TGF-β and activin, and may play a role in growth factor clearance from the circulation.[9]

Receptor Activation and Signal Transduction Pathways

Ligand binding induces formation of a heteromeric complex of type I and type II receptors (see Chapter 5).[9, 10, 150] Current evidence indicates that this complex contains two or more type I receptor molecules and two or more type II molecules per TGF-β dimer[9, 150] (Fig. 34–8). Complex formation leads to phosphorylation of type I receptors on serine and threonine residues by the type II receptor kinase.[9, 150] Type I receptors then phosphorylate and activate their major substrates, Smad proteins, which are then transduced to the nucleus[9, 10, 150] (see Fig. 34–8). Smads are intracellular proteins composed of two conserved regions, an N-terminal MH1 domain of approximately 130 residues, and a Cl-terminal MH2 domain of approximately 200 amino acids, separated by a central linker segment of variable length.[10, 150] There are three classes of Smads, based on both functional and structural considerations. Receptor-regulated Smads are direct substrates of

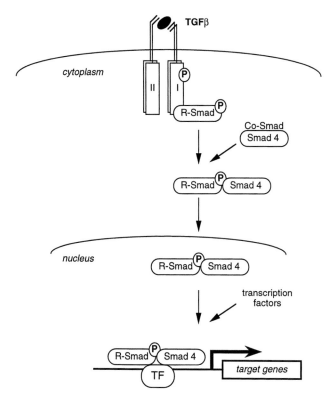

FIGURE 34–8. *The transforming growth factor-β (TGFβ) receptor–Smad pathway. Receptor-regulated Smads (R-Smads) are phosphorylated by the activated receptor complex, leading to binding of the Co-Smad, Smad4. The Smad complex is then transduced to the nucleus, where in association with distinct transcription factors (TF) it binds to sites on target genes to regulate their transcription.*

type I receptors.[10] Smads 2 and 3 are phosphorylated by the type I TGF-β receptor, and Smads 1, 5, and 8, by type I BMP receptors.[10] A second class of Smads participates in signaling through association with receptor-activated Smads. Smad 4 is the only such co-Smad identified to date.[10, 150] Smad 4 binds to a receptor-activated Smad when the latter becomes phosphorylated by the type I receptor kinase.[10, 150] The dimer is then translocated to the nucleus (see Fig. 34–8). Antagonistic Smads, including Smads 6 and 7, block the signaling functions of receptor-activated Smads.[10, 150] Smad 7 inhibits signaling induced by TGF-β and BMPs while Smad 6 preferentially blocks BMP signaling.[10, 150]

Once in the nucleus the Smad complex functions to stimulate gene transcription. The first transcriptional target to be characterized was part of the promoter of an activin-induced gene from *X. laevis*, termed *Mix.2.* The "activin response element" of *Mix.2* binds Smads 2 and 4 complexed with the DNA-binding protein, Fast-1, a member of the forkhead family of transcription factors.[155] It is likely that in other genes regulated by TGF-β, Smads will be shown to interact with additional coregulatory molecules to control transcriptional responses.[156, 157] The Smad pathway is diagrammed in Figure 34–8.

Other signaling pathways also may modulate the actions of TGF-β. A novel MEK kinase termed TAK1 (for TGF-β–activated kinase) was characterized based on its complementation of a MAPK pathway in yeast.[158] TAK1 potentially regulates TGF-β–stimulated expression of reporter genes containing AP-1 sites,[158] but does not appear to be involved in other biologic effects of TGF-β.[9] A TAK1 interacting protein, TAB1, appears able to enhance this transcriptional response.[147] The MAP kinase, JNK/SAPK, also may play a role in the same TAK1-regulated transcriptional pathway.[159]

Biologic Effects

As noted earlier, members of the TGF-β family exert diverse biologic effects. The actions of activins, inhibins, and MIS are described in other chapters. This section outlines some of the functions of other members of this growth factor family.

DEVELOPMENT. Genetic studies indicate major roles for several TGF-β–related proteins in early development. The *Drosophila* protein dpp is essential to normal dorsoventral patterning, to development of the gastrointestinal tract, and to other aspects of cell lineage determination.[138, 144] In the nematode *Caenorhabditis elegans*, homologs of type I and type II receptors (daf-1 and daf-4, respectively) control a signal transduction pathway that is required for formation of a special larval stage (dauer larva) when population density exceeds food supply.[138] During the early development of *X. laevis*, Vg1, activins, and BMPs exert striking effects on the formation and patterning of mesoderm. Similarly, in mice, mutations in *nodal* disrupt normal mesoderm formation.[138] GDF8, also termed *myostatin*, is an inhibitor of skeletal muscle growth.[160]

Mutations in the BMP genes also cause marked developmental abnormalities. Deletion of BMP2 or BMP5 genes in mice causes embryonic lethality.[148] A null mutation in BMP5 leads to alterations in the size, shape, and number of skeletal components and a diminution in the size of the external ear.[148] Mutation of BMP7 causes death in the perinatal period secondary to malformations of kidneys and eyes.[148]

TGF-β1 also is important in mouse development. A targeted disruption of the TGF-β1 gene leads to neonatal death secondary to cardiac abnormalities.[161] This phenotype is seen only in progeny of TGF-β1–deficient mothers, because transplacental passage of TGF-β1 and absorption of TGF-β1 in mother's milk normally compensate for the lack of growth factor production by the nullizygous fetus and infant.[161]

CONTROL OF INFLAMMATION AND THE RESPONSE TO TISSUE INJURY. Mice born from heterozygous mothers with a homozygous null mutation for TGF-β1 have no morphologic abnormalities at birth but die soon after weaning of multiple organ failure secondary to massive infiltration of inflammatory cells.[162, 163] This result potentially reflects the bivalent actions of TGF-β in inflammation and repair of tissue injury. Normally after an injury, TGF-β1 is released by platelets and functions as a strong chemotactic agent for neutrophils, monocytes, lymphocytes, and fibroblasts.[139] Monocytes and lymphocytes are then induced to produce other growth factors and cytokines, while fibroblasts are stimulated to synthesize extracellular matrix proteins. More TGF-β also is synthesized by these cells, which then downregulates the inflammatory process by inhibiting the functions of activated inflammatory cells. The normal result is cessation of inflammation as the wound heals. This last step does not occur in TGF-β1–deficient mice once the source of maternal TGF-β has dissipated, and massive inflammation persists.[161]

Excessive production of TGF-β may enhance tissue fibrosis and contribute to the pathogenesis of fibrotic disorders, including glomerulopathies, liver cirrhosis, rheumatoid arthritis, and others.[140] In experimental glomerulonephritis, neutralizing antibodies to TGF-β1 are able to prevent accumulation of extracellular matrix proteins, and minimize fibrosis.[140]

Mutations and Disease

One of the major actions of TGF-β is to inhibit cell proliferation.[9] It was thus postulated that mutations in TGF-β signaling pathways might be found in cancer, since enhanced proliferation contributes to tumorigenesis. This prediction was demonstrated in analysis of human colon cancers with microsatellite instability, in which inactivating mutations of the type II TGF-β receptor were identified.[164] Microsatellite instability is a common feature of hereditary nonpolyposis colorectal cancer and also has been found in nonhereditary gastrointestinal cancers.[164] Other mutations in the type II receptor have been detected in squamous carcinomas of the head and neck, gastric cancers, and others.[9]

Smad mutations also have been found in human cancers. Smad 4 was initially characterized as a candidate tumor suppressor gene that was mutated or deleted in nearly half of human pancreatic carcinomas.[165] Inactivating mutations were subsequently found in colorectal tumors, and in a small population of other cancers.[9] Smad 2 mutations also have been identified in colon cancer.[166]

Mutations in other components of TGF-β signaling pathways are found in several inherited disorders of humans. The type III receptor, endoglin, and the type I receptor, Alkl, are expressed at high levels in the vascular endothelium. Inactivating mutations in each of these genes have been linked to hereditary hemorrhagic telangiectasia, a disorder characterized by a tendency toward bleeding in the gastrointestinal tract and nasal mucosa secondary to vascular epithelial dysplasia at these sites.[167–169] A potentially inactivating mutation in the *GDF5* gene has been found in Hunter-Thompson acromesomelic chondrodysplasia, a recessive disorder with skeletal abnormalities limited to the distal bones.[170] A phenotypically similar disorder has been observed in mice with mutations in the same gene.[171]

Therapeutic Uses

One use of TGF-β is in wound healing. A single local treatment accelerates wound repair in experimental animals.[139, 140] Topical TGF-β2 has clinical application in repair of retinal tears. Antagonists of TGF-β action also have potential as antifibrotic agents.[140] BMPs may have potential use in repair of bone and joint defects.[146]

OTHER GROWTH FACTOR FAMILIES

Many growth factors have been identified that do not fit into the framework of the families described earlier. Several of these proteins have not been characterized completely, or their biologic effects have not been examined fully. They are not reviewed here. For several others, specific actions have been defined. Two examples, whose properties are summarized below, are hepatocyte growth factor (HGF), and vascular endothelial growth factor (VEGF).

Hepatocyte Growth Factor

HGF is a disulfide-linked heterodimer consisting of a 69-kDa α chain and a 34-kDa β chain that was identified as a potent serum-derived stimulator of liver cell growth in tissue culture[172] and as an effector of enhanced cell motility ("scatter factor"[173]). HGF binds to and activates a heterodimeric tyrosine kinase receptor that is the cellular homologue of the *v-met* oncogene (c-met).[174] This receptor has a wide tissue distribution, and HGF has been shown to exert diverse effects on multiple cell types.[175]

HGF is synthesized as a 728–amino acid single-chain protein.[176, 177] The secreted inactive precursor is cleaved between arginine 494 and valine 495 to generate the biologically active two-chain molecule.[177, 178] The HGF precursor is a substrate for several proteases found in serum, including urokinase-type and tissue-type plasminogen, blood coagulation factor XII, and another serine protease structurally similar to factor XII.[178]

HGF is related in amino acid sequence and overall structure to macrophage-stimulating protein (MSP), which was originally characterized as an activator of peritoneal macrophages,[179] and to plasminogen.[178] All three proteins contain a series of N-terminal "kringle" domains in the α chain,[175, 178] followed by a serine protease domain in the C-terminal segment of the β chain (Fig. 34–9). Kringles are segments of approximately 80 amino acids in length that form a double-looped structure that resembles a pretzel.[175, 178] Alterations of critical amino acids at the putative catalytic site in the β chain have rendered HGF and MSP devoid of protease activity.[175, 176]

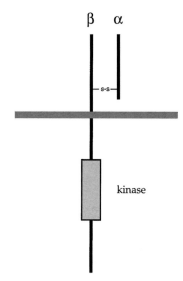

FIGURE 34–10. *Structure of the hepatocyte growth factor receptor. The two chains are indicated, as is the disulfide bond that joins them. The kinase domain in the intracellular portion of the β chain is depicted as a box.*

As noted above, the receptor for HGF is a ligand-activated tyrosine kinase encoded by the cellular homolog of the *c-met* oncogene. The receptor is synthesized as a glycosylated single-chain precursor that undergoes post-translational cleavage to generate the mature disulfide-linked αβ heterodimer (Fig. 34–10). The 50-kDa α chain is extracellular; the transmembrane 145-kDa β chain contains an extracellular ligand-binding region, a single membrane-spanning segment, and an intracellular region with a tyrosine kinase domain and two tyrosine residues near the C-terminus that bind signal transduction molecules when phosphorylated.[177] Ligand binding activates the receptor kinase, leading to autophosphorylation, and recruitment and activation of signaling intermediates, including MAPK and PI3-kinase pathways, src kinases, and others.[175, 177]

The HGF receptor is closely related to two other tyrosine kinases, termed Ron and Sea (an acronym for *s*arcoma, *e*rythroblastosis, and *a*nemia).[180, 181] Both glycoproteins are proto-oncogenes. Ron is the receptor for MSP.[180] The natural ligand for Sea has not been identified.

Activation of Met by HGF initiates a diverse series of biologic actions. Mice with a targeted disruption of the HGF gene die in midgestation secondary to abnormal development of the placenta and liver.[182, 183] Inactivation of Met is also a lethal mutation.[184] These mice also die during midgestation with placental and hepatic abnormalities, and additionally show severe defects in limb musculature,[184] indicating the importance of Met in promoting the normal migration of skeletal myoblasts.

HGF expression is potently induced in the kidney in rats during experimentally stimulated compensatory renal hypertrophy.[178] Because of its strong mitogenic and morphogenic effects on renal tubular cells, HGF is considered to be a potentially therapeutically important renotropic factor.[178] It is also a potent locally produced mitogen and motility factor for gastric epithelial cells,[185] and thus may be of therapeutic benefit in peptic ulcer disease.[185] A similar role for HGF has been postulated in response to liver injury,[175] and protective effects of HGF gene therapy have been demonstrated in experimental liver cirrhosis in rats.[186]

Vascular Endothelial Growth Factor

Development of the vasculature and delivery of blood to tissues are essential to organogenesis during embryonic development, and to normal wound healing and tissue maintenance in the adult. Conversely, abnormal angiogenesis plays a central role in the pathogenesis of a diverse array of diseases, including the growth and metastasis of malignant neoplasms, development of proliferative retinopathies, and

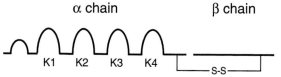

FIGURE 34–9. *Structure of hepatocyte growth factor. The four kringle domains in the α chain, K1 to K4, are indicated, as is the disulfide bond joining the α and β chains.*

other disorders.[187] Although several different growth factors and cytokines have been implicated as potential regulators of normal and pathologic angiogenesis, recent studies have established a critical role for VEGF and its receptors in development of the vasculature and in mediating abnormal vasculogenesis in disease.[187, 188]

VEGF is a disulfide-linked dimeric glycoprotein of approximately 36 to 56 kDa that is distantly related to PDGF. Human VEGF consists of four isoforms of 121, 165, 186, and 206 amino acids that are the protein products of alternatively spliced transcripts of the VEGF gene.[187] VEGF$_{165}$, the major isoform, is a 45-kDa heparin-binding glycoprotein.[187]

VEGF was the first member characterized of a gene family that currently contains at least four distinct proteins. Placental growth factor (PlGF) is a dimeric glycoprotein whose amino acid sequence is approximately 40% identical to VEGF.[189, 190] VEGF-B is a 188-residue protein with approximately 43% identity to VEGF.[191–193] Several isoforms of both proteins have been characterized. VEGF-C is a 399-residue protein that is 32% identical to VEGF in its N-terminal domain.[193, 194]

VEGF binds with high affinity to two related transmembrane tyrosine kinase receptors, VEGFR-1 (also called flt-1 for fms-like tyrosine kinase), and VEGFR-2 (also known as flk-1/KDR for fetal liver kinase-1/kinase domain region).[187, 188] PlGF also binds to VEGFR-1, but with an affinity approximately 10- to 20-fold lower than VEGF.[195] Both receptors have seven Ig-like segments in their extracellular region, a single membrane-spanning domain, and a tyrosine kinase region that is interrupted by a kinase-insert domain (Fig. 34–11). The second Ig-like domain contains the binding site for VEGF.[187] A related protein, flt-4, may be the receptor for VEGF-C.[196] All three receptors are structurally related to the two PDGFRs.[187] VEGFR-1 and VEGFR-2 are expressed predominantly in vascular endothelium,[197, 198] thus accounting for the specific actions of VEGF in the vasculature. The signal transduction pathways responsible for mediating the different biologic actions of VEGF have not been characterized completely. Upon ligand binding, both receptors are able to activate signaling molecules containing SH2 domains, which appear to interact with phosphorylated tyrosine residues located within the intracellular segment of each receptor.[187, 188]

As demonstrated by results of targeted gene disruption experiments, both VEGFRs are essential to vasculogenesis in the embryo.[199, 200] Mice lacking VEGFR-1/flt-1 died in utero before embryonic day 10, and failed to organize normal vascular channels.[199] Mice homozygous for disruption of the VEGFR-2/flk-1 gene also died before embryonic day 10. These mice lacked blood vessels, and additionally had marked deficits in precursors of blood cells.[200] Mice heterozygous for a targeted mutation in VEGF died before embryonic day 12, and had severe abnormalities in the developing forebrain, heart, and aorta, major defects in the vasculature of many organs and tissues, and showed deficient blood cell formation.[201, 202]

VEGF and its receptors also play key roles in the vascular repair that accompanies wound healing.[187] VEGF has been shown to be a potent mitogen for endothelial cells,[203] and has been found to stimulate angiogenesis in both in vitro and in vivo model systems.[204, 205] VEGF also stimulates microvascular leakage, and was identified during its initial characterization as a vascular permeability factor.[206, 207] Enhanced microvascular permeability has been hypothesized to be a key step in angiogenesis, by giving rise to a extravascular fibrin gel that can serve as a substrate for endothelial cell growth.[208]

VEGF is a central component of the pathologic angiogenesis that accompanies tumor growth and metastasis, and other disorders.[209] VEGF gene expression is enhanced in the majority of human cancers.[187] Inhibition of VEGF function with neutralizing antibodies or by blocking receptor function has been shown to abrogate growth of human tumor cell lines in mice.[210–212] The neovascularization that characterizes advanced diabetic retinopathy is a consequence of retinal ischemia, which leads to increased local production of VEGF and subsequent pathologic angiogenesis.[213, 214] Neovascularization is also a major cause of visual loss in age-related macular degeneration,[215] and is thought to be secondary to local production of VEGF in the eye.

Because of the broad roles that VEGF and its receptors play in normal and pathogenic vasculogenesis, several therapeutic interventions are under development to modulate expression and function of this growth factor system. Inhibition of VEGF receptors may effectively block angiogenesis in malignant neoplasms, or may interfere with neovascularization in diabetic retinopathy. Alternatively, therapy with VEGF or bioactive derivatives may be of benefit in vascular deficiency disorders, including chronic limb ischemia and ischemic heart disease.[187, 216, 217]

SUMMARY AND PERSPECTIVE

Growth factors are multifunctional proteins that exert their diverse biologic effects by activating specific transmembrane receptors, which are ligand-regulated protein kinases. The actions of growth factors lead to short-term alterations in cellular function and to long-term changes in the whole organism. As described in this chapter, growth factors play critical roles in many aspects of development, regulate somatic growth of a variety of tissues and organs, and modulate tissue maturation and repair. Although as emphasized in this chapter, each growth factor is able to mediate a unique spectrum of biologic effects, in the whole organism different growth factors collaboratively regulate different functions. Only recently has the potential of growth factors for therapeutic use been recognized. Studies in the coming decade should lead to further understanding of the roles of growth factors in many areas of biology and medicine.

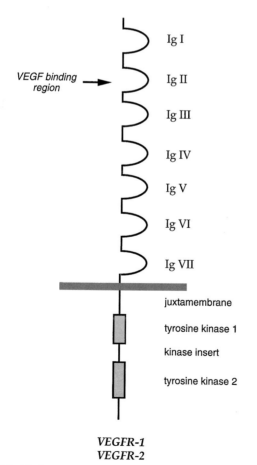

VEGF binding region →

Ig I

Ig II

Ig III

Ig IV

Ig V

Ig VI

Ig VII

juxtamembrane

tyrosine kinase 1

kinase insert

tyrosine kinase 2

VEGFR-1
VEGFR-2

FIGURE 34–11. *Structure of the two vascular endothelial growth factor (VEGF) receptors: VEGFR-1 and VEGFR-2. Different regions are depicted. Ig indicates an immunoglobulin-like domain. The region binding VEGF in Ig II is labeled.*

REFERENCES

1. Sporn MB, Roberts AB: Peptide growth factors are multifunctional. Nature 332:217–218, 1988.
2. Raff MC: Size control: The regulation of cell numbers in animal development. Cell 86:173–175, 1996.

3. Pazin MJ, Williams LT: Triggering signaling cascades by receptor tyrosine kinases. Trends Biochem Sci 17:374–378, 1992.

4. Keating MT, Williams LT: Autocrine stimulation of intracellular PDGF receptors in v-sis-transformed cells. Science 239:914–916, 1988.

5. Bejcek BE, Li DY, Deue TF: Transformation by v-sis occurs by an internal autoactivation mechanism. Science 245:1496–1499, 1989.

6. Fantl WJ, Johnson DE, Williams LT: Signalling by receptor tyrosine kinases. Annu Rev Biochem 62:453–481, 1993.

7. Lemmon MA, Schlessinger J: Regulation of signal transduction and signal diversity by receptor oligomerization. Trends Biochem Sci 19:459–463, 1994.

8. Heldin C-H: Dimerization of cell surface receptors in signal transduction. Cell 80:213–223, 1995.

9. Massague J: TGF-β signal transduction. Annu Rev Biochem 67:853–891, 1998.

10. Attisano L, Wrana JL: Mads and smads in TGFβ signalling. Curr Opin Cell Biol 10:188–194, 1998.

11. Koch CA, Anderson D, Moran MF, et al: SH2 and SH3 domains: Elements that control interactions of cytoplasmic signaling proteins. Science 252:668–674, 1991.

12. Anderson D, Koch CA, Grey L, et al: Binding of SH2 domains of phospholipase C gamma 1, GAP, and Src to activated growth factor receptors. Science 250:979–982, 1990.

13. Matsuda M, Mayer BJ, Fukui Y, Hanafusa H: Binding of transforming protein, P47gag-crk, to a broad range of phosphotyrosine-containing proteins. Science 248:1537–1539, 1990.

14. Kavanaugh WM, Williams LT: An alternative to SH2 domains for binding tyrosine-phosphorylated proteins. Science 266:1862–1865, 1994.

15. Claesson-Welsh L: Platelet-derived growth factor receptor signals. J Biol Chem 269:32023–32026, 1994.

16. Egan SE, Weinberg RA: The pathway to signal achievement. Nature 365:781–783, 1993.

17. Roberts TM: A signal chain of events. Nature 360:534–565, 1992.

18. Davis RJ: MAPKs: New JNK expands the group. Trends Biochem Sci 19:470–473, 1994.

19. Karin M: Signal transduction from the cell surface to the nucleus through the phosphorylation of transcription factors. Curr Opin Cell Biol 6:415–424, 1994.

20. Whitmarsh AJ, Shore P, Sharrocks AD, Davis RJ: Integration of MAP kinase signal transduction pathways at the serum response element. Science 269:403–407, 1995.

21. Karin M: The regulation of AP-1 activity by mitogen-activated protein kinases. J Biol Chem 270:16483–16486, 1995.

22. Hill CS, Treisman R: Transcriptional regulation by extracellular signals: Mechanisms and specificity. Cell 80:199–211, 1995.

23. Derijard B, Hibi M, Wu I-H, et al: JNK1: A protein kinase stimulated by UV light and Ha-Ras that binds and phosphorylates the c-Jun activation domain. Cell 76:1025–1037, 1994.

24. Sanchez I, Hughes RT, Mayer BJ, et al: Role of SAPK/ERK kinase-1 in the stress-activated pathway regulating transcription factor c-Jun. Nature 372:794–798, 1994.

25. Cohen S: Isolation of a mouse submaxillary gland protein accelerating incisor eruption and eyelid opening in the new-born animal. J Biol Chem 237:1555–1562, 1962.

26. Alroy I, Yarden Y: The ErbB signaling network in embryogenesis and oncogenesis: Signal diversification through combination ligand-receptor interactions. FEBS Lett 410:83–86, 1997.

27. Riese DJ II, Stern DF: Specificity within the EGF family/ErbB receptor family signaling network. Bioessays 20:41–48, 1998.

28. Fischbach GD, Rosen KM: ARIA: A neuromuscular junction neuregulin. Annu Rev Neurosci 20:429–458, 1997.

29. Raab G, Klagsbrun M: Heparin-binding EGF-like growth factor. Biochim Biophys Acta 1333:F179–199, 1997.

30. Massague J, Pandiella A: Membrane-anchored growth factors. Annu Rev Biochem 62:515–541, 1993.

31. Bell G, Fong NM, Stempien MM, et al: Human epidermal growth factor precursor: cDNA sequence, expression in vitro and gene organization. Nucleic Acids Res 14:8427–8433, 1986.

32. Derynck R, Roberts AB, Winkler ME, et al: Human transforming growth factor-alpha; Precursor structure and expression in E. coli. Cell 38:287–297, 1984.

33. Shoyab M, Plowman GD, McDonald VL, et al. Structure and function of human amphiregulin: A member of the epidermal growth factor family. Science 243:1074–1076, 1989.

34. Higashiyama S, Abraham JA, Miller J, et al: A heparin-binding growth factor secreted by macrophage-like cells that is related to EGF. Science 251:936–939, 1991.

35. Thompson SA, Higashiyama S, Wood K, et al: Characterization of sequences within heparin-binding EGF-like growth factor that mediate interaction with heparin. J Biol Chem 229:2541–2549, 1994.

36. Naglieh JG, Metherall JE, Russell DW, Eidels L: Expression cloning of a Diphtheria toxin receptor: Identity with a heparin-binding EGF-like growth factor precursor. Cell 69:1051–1061, 1992.

37. Shing Y, Christofori G, Hanahan D, et al: Betacellulin: A mitogen from pancreatic β cell tumors. Science 259:1604–1607, 1993.

38. Toyoda H, Komurasaki T, Uchida D, et al: Epiregulin: A novel epidermal growth factor with mitogenic activity for rat primary hepatocytes. J Biol Chem 270:7495–7500, 1995.

39. Wen D, Peles E, Cupples R, et al: Neu differentiation factor: A transmembrane glycoprotein containing an EGF domain and an immunoglobulin homology unit. Cell 69:559–572, 1992.

40. Holmes WE, Sliwkowski MX, Akita RW, et al: Identification of heregulin, a specific activator of p185erbB2. Science 256: 1205–1210, 1992.

41. Marchionni MA, Goodearl AD, Chen MS, et al: Glial growth factors are alternatively spliced erbB2 ligands expressed in the nervous system. Nature 362:312–318, 1993.

42. Falls DL, Rosen KM, Corfas G, et al: ARIA, a protein that stimulates acetylcholine receptor synthesis, is a member of the neu ligand family. Cell 72:801–815, 1993.

43. Carraway KL III, Weber JL, Unger MJ, et al: Neuregulin-2, a new ligand of ErbB3/ErbB4-receptor tyrpsine kinases. Nature 387:512–516, 1997.

44. Chang H, Riese DJ II, Gilbert W, et al: Ligands for ErbB-family receptors encoded by a neuregulin-like gene. Nature 387:509–512, 1997.

45. Ciccodicola A, Dono R, Obici S, et al: Molecular characterization of a gene of the "EGF family" expressed in undifferentiated human NTERA2 teratocarcinoma cells. EMBO J 8:1987–1997, 1989.

46. Brandt R, Normanno N, Gullick WJ, et al: Identification and biological characterization of an epidermal growth factor–related protein: Cripto-1. J Biol Chem 269:17320–17328, 1994.

47. Shen MM, Wang H, Leder P: A differential display strategy identifies Cryptic, a novel EGF-related gene expressed in the axial and lateral mesoderm during mouse gastrulation. Development 124:429–442, 1997.

48. Kannan S, DeSantis M, Lohmeyer M, et al: Cripto enhances the tyrosine phosphorylation of Shc and activates mitogen-activated protein kinase (MAPK) in mammary epithelial cells. J Biol Chem 272:3330–3335, 1997.

49. Stroobant P, Rice AP, Gullick WJ, et al: Purification and characterization of vaccinia virus growth factor. Cell 42:383–393, 1985.

50. Carraway III KL, Cantley LC: A Neu acquaintance for ErbB3 and ErbB4: A role for receptor heterodimerization in growth signaling. Cell 78:5–8, 1994.

51. Iozzo RV, Moscatello DK, McQuillan DJ, Eichstetter I: Decorin is a biological ligand for the epidermal growth factor receptor. J Biol Chem 274:4489–4492, 1999.

52. Yamauchi T, Ueki K, Tobe K, et al: Tyrosine phosphorylation of the EGF receptor by the kinase Jak2 is induced by growth hormone. Nature 390:91–96, 1997.

53. Qiu Y, Ravi L, Kung HJ: Requirement of ErbB2 for signaling by interleukin-6 in prostate carcinoma cells. Nature 393:83–85, 1998.

54. Daub H, Weiss FU, Wallasch C, Ullrich A: Role of transactivation of the EGF receptor in signalling by G-protein–coupled receptors. Nature 379:557–560, 1996.

55. Nair BG, Parikh B, Miligan G, Patel TB: Gsα mediates epidermal growth factor–elicited stimulation of rat cardiac adenylate cyclase. J Biol Chem 265:23117–23122, 1990.

56. Poppleton H, Sun H, Fulgham D, et al: Activation of Gsα by the epidermal growth factor receptor involves phosphorylation. J Biol Chem 271:6947–6951, 1996.

57. Miettinen PJ, Berger JE, Meneses J, et al: Epithelial immaturity and multiorgan failure in mice lacking epidermal growth factor receptor. Nature 376:337–341, 1995.

58. Threadgill DW, Dlugosz AA, Hansen LA, et al: Targeted disruption of mouse EGF receptor effect of genetic background on mutant phenotype. Science 269:230–233, 1995.

59. Sibilia M, Wagner EF: Strain-dependent epithelial defects in mice lacking the EGF receptor. Science 269:234–237, 1995.

60. Luetteke NC, Qiu TH, Peiffer RL, et al: TGFα deficiency results in hair follicle and eye abnormalities in targeted and waved-1 mice. Cell 73:263–278, 1993.

61. Meyer D, Birchmeier C: Multiple essential functions of neuregulin in development. Nature 378:386–398, 1995.

62. Gasman M, Casagranda F, Orioli D, et al: Aberrant neural and cardiac development in mice lacking the ErbB4 neuregulin receptor. Nature 378:390–394, 1995.

63. Lee K-F, Simon H, Chen H, et al: Requirement for neuregulin receptor erbB2 in neural and cardiac development. Nature 378:394–398, 1995.

64. Kramer R, Bucay N, Kane DJ, et al: Neuregulins with an Ig-like domain are essential for mouse myocardial and neuronal development. Proc Natl Acad Sci U S A 93:4833–4838, 1996.

65. Ding J, Yang L, Yan Y-T, et al: Cripto is required for correct orientation of the anterior-posterior axis in the mouse-embryo. Nature 395:702–707, 1998.

66. Halter SA, Dempsey P, Matsui Y, et al: Distinctive patterns of hyperplasia in transgenic mice with mammary tumor virus transforming growth factor-alpha. Characterization of mammary gland and skin proliferations. Am J Pathol 140:1131–1146, 1992.

67. Spitzer E, Zschiesche W, Binas B, et al: EGF and TGF alpha modulate structural and functional differentiation of the mammary gland from pregnant mice in vitro: Possible role of the arachidonic acid pathway. J Cell Biochem 57:495–508, 1995.

68. Yang Y, Spitzer E, Meyer D, et al: Sequential requirement of hepatocyte growth factor and neuregulin in the morphogenesis and differentiation of the mammary gland. Cell Biol 131:215–226, 1995.

69. Jones FE, Jerry DJ, Guarino BC, Andrews GC: Heregulin induces in vivo proliferation and differentiation of mammary epithelium into secretory lobuloalveoli. Cell Growth Differ 7:1031–1038, 1996.

70. Slamon DJ, Godolphin W, Jones LA, et al: Studies of the HER-2/neu proto-oncogene in human breast andovarian cancer. Science 244:707–712, 1989.

71. Bacus SS, Zelnick CR, Plowman G, Yarden Y: Expression of the erbB-2 family of growth factor receptors and their ligands in breast cancers. Implications for tumor biology and clinical behavior. Am J Clin Pathol 102:S13–S24, 1994.

72. Plowman GD, Culousco JM, Whitney GS, et al: Ligand-specific activation of HER4/p180erbB4, a fourth member of the epidermal growth factor receptor family. Proc Natl Acad Sci U S A 90:1746–1750, 1993.

73. Galzie Z, Kinsella AR, Smith JA: Fibroblast growth factors and their receptors. Biochem Cell Biol 75:669–685, 1997.

74. Szebenyi G, Fallon JF: Fibroblast growth factors as multifunctional signaling factors. Int Rev Cytol 185:45–106, 1999.

75. McKeehan WL, Wang F, Kan M: The heparan sulfate–fibroblast growth factor family: Diversity of structure and function. Prog Nucleic Acid Res Mol Biol 59:135–176, 1998.

76. Gorlin RJ: Fibroblast growth factors, their receptors and receptor disorders. J Craniomaxillofac Surg 25:69–79, 1997.

77. Johnson DE, Williams LT: Structural and functional diversity in the FGF receptor multigene family. Adv Cancer Res 60:1–41, 1993.

78. Ornitz DM, Xu J, Colvin JS, et al: Receptor specifity of the fibroblast growth factor family. J Biol Chem 271:15292–15297, 1996.

79. Qing K, Mah C, Hansen J, et al: Human fibroblast growth factor receptor 1 is a co-receptor for infection by adeno-associated virus 2. Nat Med 5:71–75, 1999.

80. Ornitz DM, Yayon A, Flanagan JG, et al: Heparin is required for cell free binding of basic fibroblast growth factor to a soluble receptor and for mitogenesis. Mol Cell Biol 12:240–247, 1992.
81. Yayor A, Klagsbrun M, Esko JD, et al: Cell surface, heparin like molecules are required for binding of basic fibroblast growth factor to its high affinity receptor. Cell 64:841–848, 1991.
82. Baird N, Ling N: Fibroblast growth factors are present in the extracellular matrix produced by endothelial cells in vitro: Implication for a role of heparinase-like enzymes in the neovascular response. Biochem Biophys Res Commun 142:428–435, 1987.
83. Vlodavsky I, Bar-Shavit R, Ishai-Michaeli R, et al: Extracellular sequestration and release of fibroblast growth factor. A regulatory mechanism? Trends Biochem Sci 16:268–271, 1991.
84. Spivak-Kroizman T, Lemmon MA, Dikic I, et al: Heparin-induced oligomerization of FGF molecules is responsible for FGF receptor dimerization, activation and cell proliferation. Cell 79:1015–1024, 1994.
85. Isaacs HV: New perspectives on the role of the fibroblast growth factor family in amphibian development. Cell Mol Life Sci 53:350–361, 1997.
86. Deng C-X, Wynshaw-Boris A, Shen MM, et al: P. Murine FGFR-1 is required for early postimplantation growth and axial organization. Genes Dev 8:3045–3057, 1994.
87. Yamaguchi TP, Harpal K, Henkemeyer M, Rossant J: fgfr-1 is required for embryonic growth and mesodermal paterning during mouse gastrulation. Genes Dev 8:3032–3044, 1994.
88. Mansour SL: Targeted disruption of int-2 (fgf-3) causes developmental defects in the tail and inner ear. Mol Reprod Dev 39:62–68, 1994.
89. Hebert JM, Rosenquist T, Gotz J, Martin GR: FGF5 as a regulator of the hair growth cycle: Evidence from targeted and spontaneous mutations. Cell 78:1017–1025, 1994.
90. Feldman B, Poueymirou W, Papaioannou VE, et al: Requirement of FGF-4 for postimplantation mouse development. Science 267:246–249, 1995.
91. Min H, Danilenko DM, Scully SA, et al: Fgf-10 is required for both limb and lung development and exhibits striking functional similarity to *Drosophilia* branchless. Genes Dev 12:3156–3161, 1998.
92. Meyers EN, Martin GR: Differences in left-right axis pathways in mouse and chick: Functions of FGF8 and SHH. Science 285:403–406, 1999.
93. Deng C, Wynshaw-Boris A, Zhou F, et al: P. Fibroblast growth factor receptor 3 is a negative regulator of bone growth. Cell 84:911–921, 1996.
94. Webster MK, Donoghue DJ: FGFR activation in skeletal disorders: Too much of a good thing. Trends Genet 13:178–182, 1997.
95. Cohen S: Purification of a nerve-growth promoting protein from the mouse salivary gland and its neuro-cytotoxic antiserum. Proc Natl Acad Sci U S A 46:302–311, 1960.
96. Levi-Montalcini R, Booker B: Destruction of the sympathetic ganglia in mammals by an antiserum to a nerve growth protein. Proc Natl Acad Sci U S A 46:384–391, 1960.
97. Lindsay RM: Neutrophins and receptors. Prog Brain Res 103:3–14, 1994.
98. Barde Y-A: Neutrophins: A family of proteins supporting the survival of neurons. Prog Clin Biol Res 390:45–46, 1994.
99. Pulciani S, Santos E, Lauver AV, et al: Oncogenes in solid human tumors. Nature 300:539–542, 1982.
100. Martin-Zanca D, Barbacid M, Parada LF: Expression of the trk proto-oncogene is restricted to the sensory cranial and spinal ganglia of neural crest origin in mouse development. Genes Dev 4:683–694, 1990.
101. Ibanez CF: Emerging themes in structural biology of neurotropic factors. Trends Neurosci 21:438–444, 1998.
102. Chao M, Casaccia-Bonnefil P, Carter B, et al: Neurotrophin receptors: Mediators of life and death. Brain Res Rev 26:295–301, 1998.
103. Bothwell M: p75^{ntr}: A receptor after all. Science 272:506–507, 1996.
104. Frade JM, Barde Y: Nerve growth factor: Two receptors, multiple functions. Bioessays 20:137–145, 1998.
105. Smeyne RJ, Klein R, Schnapp A, et al: Severe sensory and sympathetic neuropathies in mice carrying a disrupted trk/NGF receptor gene. Nature 368:246–249, 1994.
106. Klein R, Smeyne RJ, Wurst W, et al: Targeted disruption of the trkB neurotrophin receptor gene results in nervous system lesions and neonatal death. Cell 75:113–122, 1993.
107. Ernfors P, Lee KF, Jaenisch R: Mice lacking brain-derived neurotrophic factor develop sensory deficits. Nature 368:147–150, 1994.
108. Conover JC, Erickson JT, Katz DM, et al: Neuronal deficits, not involving motor neurons, in mice lacking BDNF and/or NT4. Nature 375:235–238, 1995.
109. Klein R, Silos-Santiago I, Smeyne RJ, et al: Disruption of the neutrophin 3 receptor gene trkC eliminates Ia muscle afferents and results in abnormal movements. Nature 368:249–251, 1994.
110. Ernfors P, Lee KF, Kucera J, Jaenisch R: Lack of neurotrophin 3 leads to deficiencies in the peripheral nervous system and loss of limb proprioceptive afferents. Cell 77:503–512, 1994.
111. Lee K-F, Davies AM, Jaenisch R: p75-deficient embryonic dorsal root sensory and neonatal sympathetic neurons display a decreased sensitivity to NGF. Development 120:1027–1033, 1994.
112. Frade J-M, Rodriguez-Tebar A, Barde Y-A: Induction of cell death by endogenous nerve growth factor through its p75 receptor. Nature 383:166–168, 1996.
113. Lin L-FH, Doherty DH, Lile JD, et al. GDNF: A glial cell line-derived neurotrophic factor for midbrain dopaminergic neurons. Science 260:1130–1132, 1993.
114. Kotzbauer PT, Lampe PA, Heuckeroth RO, et al: Neurturin, a relative of glial-cell-line-derived neurotropic factor. Nature 384:467–470, 1996.
115. Milbrandt J, deSauvage FJ, Fahrner TJ, et al: Persephin, a novel neurotrophic factor related to GDNF and neurturin. Neuron 20:245–253, 1998.
116. Baloh RH, Gorodinsky A, Golden JP, et al: GFRα3 is an orphan member of the GDNF/neurturin/perephin receptor family. Proc Natl Acad Sci U S A 95:5801–5806, 1998.
117. Jing S, Wen D, Yu Y, et al: GDNF-induced activation of the ret protein tyrosine kinase is mediated by GDNFR-alpha, a novel receptor for GDNF. Cell 85:1113–1124, 1996.
118. Treanor JJ, Goodman L, de Sauvage F, et al: Characterization of a multicomponent receptor for GDNF. Nature 382:80–83, 1996.
119. Baloh RH, Tansey MG, Golden JP, et al: TrnR2, a novel receptor that mediates neurturin and GDNF signaling through Ret. Neuron 18:793–802, 1997.
120. Sanicola M, Hession C, Worley D, et al: Glial cell line–derived neurotrophic factor–independent RET activation can be mediated by two different cell-surface accessory proteins. Proc Natl Acad Sci U S A 94:6238–6243, 1997.
121. Ip N: The neurotrophins and neuropoietic cytokines: Two families of growth factors acting on neural and hematopoietic cells. Ann N Y Acad Sci 840:97–106, 1998.
122. Pichel JG, Shen. L., Hui SZ, et al: Defects in enteric innervation and kidney development in mice lacking GDNF. Nature 382:73–76, 1996.
123. Sanchez MP, Silos-Santiago I, Frisen J, et al. Renal agenesis and the absence of enteric neurons in mice lacking GDNF. Nature 382:70–73, 1996.
124. Schuchardt A, D'Agati V, Larsson-Blomberg L, et al: Defects in the kidney and enteric nervous system of mice lacking the tyrosine kinase receptor Ret. Nature 367:380–383, 1994.
125. Enomoto H, Araki T, Jackman A, et al: GFRα1-deficient mice have deficits in the enteric nervous system and kidneys. Neuron 21:317–324, 1998.
126. Ross R, Glomset J, Kariya B, Harker I: A platelet-dependent serum factor that stimulates the proliferation of arterial smooth muscle cells in vitro. Proc Natl Acad Sci U S A 71:1207–1210, 1974.
127. Heldin C-H, Westermark B: Platelet-derived growth factor: Mechanism of action and possible in vivo function. Cell Regul 1:555–566, 1990.
128. Heldin CH, Ostman A, Ronnstrand L: Signal transduction via platelet-derived growth factor receptors. Biochim Biophys Acta 1378:F79–113, 1998.
129. Westermark B, Heldin C-H: Platelet-derived growth factor: Structure, function and implications in normal and malignant cell growth. Acta Oncol 32:101–105, 1993.
130. Heldin CH: Simultaneous induction of stimulatory and inhibitory signals by PDGF. FEBS Lett 410:17–21, 1997.
131. Eriksson A, Siegbahn B, Westermark B, et al: PDGF α- and β-receptors activate unique and common signal transduction pathways. EMBO J 11:543–550, 1992.
132. Soriano P: The PDGFα receptor is required for neural crest cell development and for normal patterning of the somites. Development 124:2691–2700, 1997.
133. Soriano P: Abnormal kidney development and hematological disorders in PDGF β-receptor mutant mice. Genes Dev 8:1888–1896, 1994.
134. Lindahl P, Johansson BR, Leveen P, Betsholtz C: Pericyte loss and microaneurysm formation in PDGF-B–deficient mice. Science 277:242–244, 1997.
135. Bostrom H, Willetts K, Pekny M, et al: PDGF-A signaling is a critical event in lung alveolar myofibroblast development and alveogenesis. Cell 85:863–873, 1996.
136. Betsholtz C, Raines EW: Platelet-derived growth factor: A key regulator of connective tissue cells in embryogenesis and pathogenesis. Kidney Int 51:1361–1369, 1997.
137. Robson MC, Phillips LG, Thomason A, et al: Platelet-derived growth factor BB for the treatment of chronic pressure ulcers. Lancet 339:23–25, 1992.
138. Kingsley DM: The TGF-β superfamily: New members, new receptors, and new genetic tests of function in different organisms. Genes Dev 8:133–146, 1994.
139. Letterio JJ, Roberts AB: Regulation of immune responses by TGF-β. Annu Rev Immunol 16:137–161, 1998.
140. Border WA, Nobel NA: Transforming growth factor β in tissue fibrosis. N Engl J Med 331:1286–1292, 1994.
141. Roberts AB, Sporn MB: Physiological actions and clinical applications of transforming growth factor-β (TGF-β). Growth Factors 8:1–9, 1993.
142. Flaumenhaft R, Kojima S, Abe M, Rifkin DB: Activation of latent transforming growth factor β. Adv Pharmacol 24:51–76, 1993.
143. Ying SY: Inhibins, activins and follistatins. J Steroid Biochem 33:705–713, 1989.
144. Wozney JM: The bone morphogenetic protein family and osteogenesis. Mol Reprod Dev 32:160–167, 1992.
145. Wozney JM, Rosen V, Celeste AJ, et al: Novel regulators of bone formation: Molecular clones and activities. Science 242:1528–1534, 1988.
146. Sakou T: Bone morphogenetic proteins: From basic studies to clinical approaches. Bone 22:591–603, 1998.
147. Shibuya H, Yamagichi K, Shirakabe K, et al: TAB1: An activator of the TAK1 MAPKKK in TGF-β signal transduction. Science 272:1179–1182, 1996.
148. Wozney JM: The bone morphogenetic protein family: Multifunctional cellular regulators in the embryo and adult. Eur J Oral Sci 106:160–166, 1998.
149. Josso N, Cate RL, Picard JY, et al: Anti-müllerian hormone: The Jost factor. Recent Prog Horm Res 48:1–59, 1993.
150. Padgett RW, Das P, Krishna S: TGF-β signaling, Smads, and tumor suppressors. Bioessays 20:382–391, 1998.
151. Cheifetz S, Weatherbee JA, Tsang ML, et al: The transforming growth factor-beta system, a complex pattern of cross-reactive ligands and receptors. Cell 48:409–415, 1987.
152. Segarini PR, Rosen DM, Seyedin SM: Binding of transforming growth factor-beta to cell surface proteins varies with cell type. Mol Endocrinol 3:261–272, 1989.
153. Gougos A, Letarte M: Primary structure of endoglin, an RGD-containing glycoprotein of human enthothelial cells. J Biol Chem 265: 8361–8364, 1990.
154. Cheifetz S, Bellon T, Cales C, et al: Endoglin is a component of the transforming growth factor-beta receptor system in human endothelial cells. J Biol Chem 267:19027–19030, 1992.
155. Chen X, Weisberg E, Fridmacher V, et al: Smad4 and FAST-1 in the assembly of activin-responsive factor. Nature 389:85–89, 1997.
156. Zhou S, Zawel L, Lengauer C, et al: Characterization of human FAST-1, a TGFβ and activin signal transductor. Mol Cell 2:121–127, 1998.
157. Labbe E, Silvestri C, Hoodless PA, et al: Smad2 and Smad3 positively and negatively regulate TGF-β-dependent transcription through the forkhead DNA-binding protein FAST2. Mol Cell 2:109–120, 1998.
158. Yamaguchi K, Shirakabe K, Shibuya H, et al: Identification of a member of the

MAPKKK family as a potential mediator of TGF-beta signal transduction. Science 270:2008–2011, 1995.

159. Atfi A, Djelloul S, Chastre E, et al: Evidence for a role of Pho-like GTPases and stress-activated protein kinase/c-Jun N-terminal kinase (SAPK/JNK) in transforming growth factor beta-mediated signaling. J Biol Chem 272:1429–1932, 1997.

160. McPherron AC, Lawler AM, Lee SJ: Regulation of skeletal muscle mass in mice by a new TGF-β superfamily member. Nature 387:83–90, 1997.

161. Letterio JJ, Geiser AG, Kulkarni AB, et al: Maternal rescue of transforming growth factor-β1 null mice. Science 264:1936–1938, 1994.

162. Shull MM, Ormsby I, Kier AB, et al: Targeted disruption of the mouse transforming growth factor-beta 1 gene results in multifocal inflammatory disease. Nature 359:639, 1992.

163. Kulkarni AB, Huh CG, Becker D, et al: Transforming growth factor beta 1 null mutation in mice causes excessive inflammatory response and early death. Proc Natl Acad Sci U S A 90:770, 1993.

164. Markowitz S, Wang J, Myeroff L, et al: Inactivation of the type II TGF-β receptor in colon cancer cells with microsatellite instability. Science 268:1336–1338, 1995.

165. Hahn SA, Schutte M, Hoque AT, et al: DPC4, candidate tumor suppressor gene at human chromosome 18q21.1. Science 271:350–353, 1996.

166. Eppert K, Scherer SW, Ozcelik H, et al: MADR2 maps to 18q21 and encodes a TGFbeta-regulated MAD-related protein that is functionally mutated in colorectal carcinoma. Cell 86:543–552, 1996.

167. McAllister KA, Grogg KM, Johnson DW, et al: Endoglin, a TGF-beta binding protein of endothelial cells, is the gene for hereditary haemorrhagic telangiectasia type 1. Nat Genet 8:345–351, 1994.

168. McAllister KA, Baldwin MA, Thukkani AK, et al: Six novel mutations in the endoglin gene in hereditary hemorrhagic telangiectasia type 1 suggest a dominant-negative effect of receptor function. Hum Mol Genet; 4:1983–1985, 1995.

169. Johnson DW, Berg JN, Baldwin MA, et al: Mutations in the activin receptor-like kinase 1 gene in hereditary haemorrhagic telangiectasia type 2. Nat Genet 13:189–195, 1996.

170. Polinkovsky A, Robin NH, Thomas JT, et al: Mutations in CDMP1 cause autosomal dominant brachdactyly type C. Nat Genet 17:18–19, 1997.

171. Storm EE, Huynh TV, Copeland NG, et al: Limb alterations in brachypodism mice due to mutations in a new member of the TGF beta superfamily. Nature 368:639–643, 1994.

172. Nakamura T, Teramoto H, Ichihara A: Purification and characterization of a growth factor from rat platelets for mature parenchymal hepatocytes in primary cultures. Proc Natl Acad Sci U S A 83:6489–6493, 1986.

173. Stoker M, Gherardi E, Perryman M, Gray J: Scatter factor is a fibroblast-derived modulator of epithelial cell motility. Nature 327:239–242, 1987.

174. Bottaro DP, Rubin JS, Faletto DL, et al: Identification of the hepatocyte growth factor receptor as the c-met proto-oncogene product. Science 251:802–804, 1991.

175. Trusolino L, Pugliese L, Comoglio PM: Interactions between scatter factors and the receptors: Hints for therapeutic applications. FASEB J 12:1267–1280, 1998.

176. Chirgadze DY, Hepple J, Byrd RA, et al: Insights into the structure of hepatocyte growth factor/scatter factor (HGF/SF) and implications for receptor activation. FEBS Lett 430:126–129, 1998.

177. Maggiora P, Gambarotta G, Olivero M, et al: Control of invasive growth by the HGF receptor family. J Cell Physiol 173:183–186, 1997.

178. Balkovetz DF, Lipschutz JH: Hepatocyte growth factor and the kidney: It is not just for the liver. Int Rev Cytol 186:225–260, 1999.

179. Skeel A, Yoshimura T, Showalter SD, et al: Macrophage stimulating protein: Purification, partial amino acid sequence, and cellular activity. J Exp Med 173:1227–1234, 1991.

180. Gaudino G, Follenzi A, Naldini L, et al: RON is a heterodimeric tyrosine kinase receptor activated by the HGF homologue MSP. EMBO J 13:3524–3532, 1994.

181. Hayman MJ, Kitchener G, Vogt PK, Beug H: The putative transforming protein of S13 avian erythroblastosis virus is a transmembrane glycoprotein with an associated protein kinase activity. Proc Natl Acad Sci U S A 82:8237–8241, 1985.

182. Schmidt C, Bladt F, Goedecke E, et al: Scatter factor/hepatocyte growth factor is essential for liver development. Nature 373:699–702, 1995.

183. Uehara Y, Minowa O, Mori C, et al: Placental defect and embryonal lethality in mice lacking hepatocyte growth factor/scatter factor. Nature 373:702–705, 1995.

184. Bladt F, Riethmacher D, Isenmann S, et al: Essential role for the c-met receptor in the migration of myogenic precursor cells into the limb bud. Nature 376:768–771, 1995.

185. Takahashi M, Ota S, Shimda T, et al: Hepatocyte growth factor is the most potent endogenous stimulant of rabbit gastric epithelial cell proliferation and migration in primary culture. J Clin Invest 95:1994–2003, 1995.

186. Ueki T, Kaneda Y, Tsutsui H, et al: Hepatocyte growth factor gene therapy of liver cirrhosis in rats. Nat Med 5:226–230, 1999.

187. Ferrara N, Davis-Smyth T: The biology of vascular endothelial growth factor. Endocr Rev 18:4–25, 1997.

188. Plate KH, Warnke PC: Vascular endothelial growth factor. J Neurooncol; 35:365–372, 1997.

189. Maglione D, Guerrerio V, Viglietto G, et al: Isolation of a human placenta cDNA coding for a protein related to the vascular permeability factor. Proc Natl Acad Sci U S A 88:9267–9271, 1991.

190. Hauser S, Weich HA: A heparin-binding form of placenta growth factor (PIGF-2) is expressed in human umbilical vein endothelial cells and in placenta. Growth Factors 9:259–268, 1993.

191. Olofsson B, Pajusola K, Kaipainen A, et al: Vascular endothelial growth factor B, a novel growth factor for endothelial cells. Proc Natl Acad Sci U S A 93:2576–2581, 1996.

192. Grimmond S, Lagercrantz J, Drinkwater C, et al: Cloning and characterization of a human gene related to vascular endothelial growth factor. Genome Res 6:124–131, 1996.

193. Joukov V, Kaipainen A, Jeltsch M, et al: Vascular endothelial growth factors VEGF-B and VEGF-C. J Cell Physiol 173:211–215, 1997.

194. Joukov V, Pajusola K, Kaipainen A, et al: A novel vascular endothelial growth factor, VEGF-C, is a ligand for the FLT (VEGFR-3) and KDR (VEGFR-2) receptor tyrosine kinases. EMBO J 15:290–298, 1996.

195. Park JE, Chen H, Winer J, et al: Placenta growth factor. Potentiation of vascular endothelial growth factor bioactivity, in vitro and in vivo, and high affinity binding to Flt-1 but not to Flk-1/KDR. J Biol Chem 269:25646–25654, 1994.

196. Pajusola K, Aprelikova O, Pelicci G, et al: Signalling properties of FLT4, a proteolytically processed receptor tyrosine kinase related to two VEGF receptors. Oncogene 9:3545–3555, 1994.

197. Jakeman LB, Winer J, Bennett GL, et al: Binding sites for vascular endothelial growth factor are localized on endothelial cells in adult rat tissues. J Clin Invest 89:244–253, 1992.

198. Jakeman LB, Armanini M, Phillips HS, Ferrara N: Developmental expression of binding sites and mRNA for vascular endothelial growth factor suggests a role for this protein in vasculogenesis and angiogenesis. Endocrinology 133:848–859, 1993.

199. Fong G-H, Rossant J, Gertenstein M, et al: Role of Flt-1 receptor tyrosine kinase in regulation of assembly of vascular endothelium. Nature 376:66–67, 1995.

200. Shalabi F, Rossant J, Yamaguchi TP: Failure of blood island formation and vasculogenesis in Flk-1 deficient mice. Nature 376:62–66, 1995.

201. Carmeliat P, Ferreira V, Breier G, et al: Abnormal blood vessel development and lethality in embryos lacking a single VEGF allele. Nature 380:435–439, 1996.

202. Ferrara N, Carvermoore K, Chen H, et al: Heterozygous embryonic lethality induced by targeted inactivation of the VEGF gene. Nature 380:439–442, 1996.

203. Leung DW, Cachianes G, Kuang W-J, et al: Vascular endothelial growth factor is secreted angiogenic mitogen. Science 246:1306–1309, 1989.

204. Wilting J, Christ B, Weich HA: The effects of growth factors on the day 13 chorioallantoic membrane (CAM): A study of VEGF$_{165}$ and PDGF-BB. Anat Embryol 186:251–257, 1992.

205. Takeshita S, Zheng LP, Brogi E, et al: Therapeutic angiogenesis. J Clin Invest 59:662–670, 1994.

206. Senger DR, Galli SJ, Dvorak AM, et al: Tumor cells secrete a vascular permeability factor that promotes accumulation of ascites fluid. Science 219:983–985, 1983.

207. Connolly DT, Olander JV, Heuvelman D, et al: Human vascular permeability factor. Isolation from U937 cells. J Biol Chem 254:20017–20024, 1989.

208. Dvorak HF, Harvey VS, Estrella P, et al: Fibrin containing gels induce angiogenesis: Implications for tumor stroma generation and wound healing. Lab Invest 57:673–686, 1987.

209. Zetter BR: Angiogenesis and tumor metastasis. Annu Rev Med 49:407–424, 1998.

210. Kim KJ, Li B, Winer J, et al: Inhibition of vascular endothelial growth factor–induced angiogenesis suppresses tumor growth in vivo. Nature 362:841–844, 1993.

211. Millauer B, Shawver LK, Plate KH, et al: Glioblastoma growth is inhibited in vivo by a negative dominant Flk-1 mutant. Nature 367:576–579, 1994.

212. Millauer B, Longhi MP, Plate KH, et al: Dominant-negative inhibition of Flk-1 suppresses the growth of many tumor types in vivo. Cancer Res; 56:1615–1620, 1996.

213. Aiello LP, Avery R, Arrigg R, et al: Vascular endothelial growth factor in ocular fluid of patients with diabetic retinopathy and other retinal disorders. N Engl J Med 331:1480–1487, 1994.

214. Adamis AP, Miller JW, Bernal M-T, et al: Increased vascular endothelial growth factor in the vitreous of eyes with proliferative diabetic retinopathy. Am J Ophthalmol 118:445–450, 1994.

215. Kvanta A, Algvere PV, Berglin L, Seregard S: Subfoveal fibrovascular membranes in age-related macular degeneration express vascular endothelial growth factor. Invest Ophthalmol Vis Sci 37:1929–1934, 1996.

216. Banai S, Jaklitsch MT, Shou M, et al: Angiogenic-induced enhancement of collateral blood flow to ischemic myocardium by vascular endothelial growth factor in dogs. Circulation 89:2183–2189, 1994.

217. Isner JM, Pieczak A, Schainfeld R, et al: Clinical evidence of angiogenesis following arterial gene transfer of phVEGF$_{165}$ in patient with ischemic limbs. Lancet 348:370–374, 1996.

CLINICAL DISORDERS

Chapter 35

Somatic Growth and Maturation

Robert L. Rosenfield ▪ Leona Cuttler

Growth is an inherent property of life. Normal somatic growth requires the integrated function of many of the hormonal, metabolic, and other growth factors discussed in preceding chapters. This chapter will first briefly review the determinants of growth. Then it will deal in detail with the overall result of these processes—normal linear growth patterns. Finally, the differential diagnosis and management of disorders of growth will be discussed.

DETERMINANTS OF NORMAL GROWTH: BIOLOGIC, BIOCHEMICAL, AND ENDOCRINOLOGIC

Cellular Growth

Normal growth requires an intrinsically normal cell that is nourished by an optimal milieu (with respect to pH, trace minerals, and substrates for structural and energy purposes) and that is exposed to the necessary growth factors. It is regulated by the same molecular mechanisms that determine physiologic responses in the mature cell.

The body grows primarily through proliferation of cells by mitosis.[1, 2] An increase in cell size generally plays more of a role in organ growth as development approaches completion. Growth factors and other environmental signals affect cell division by modulating passage through the first phase of the mitotic cell cycle (G_1).[3, 4] The first subphase of G_1 requires "competence factors," such as fibroblast growth factor, that induce cells to become competent to synthesize DNA. Cells then require essential amino acids to progress to a critical point in the cycle at which "progression factors" can induce completion of G_1. Progression factors are exemplified by insulin-like growth factors (IGFs), insulin, thyroxine, and hydrocortisone. Growth factors modulate the internal regulatory pathways governed by cyclins and cyclin-dependent kinases (CDKs), which are *proto-oncogenes*, and CDK inhibitors (CDKIs), which are *tumor suppressors*. The balance between cyclin-CDK and CDKI activity determines the start of DNA synthesis (S phase of the cell cycle). From this point onward, cell cycle processes depend entirely on intracellularly triggered controls involving cyclins. After completing DNA synthesis, the cell finishes doubling its entire contents (G_2 phase) and then undergoes the M phase of the cycle, during which cell division is completed.

Somatic Growth

Postnatal Growth

Genetic determinants exist for both prenatal and postnatal growth.[5] Some of the determinants for bone growth reside on the sex chromo-somes: genes on the Y chromosome seem to enhance stature commencing in antenatal life,[5] whereas the X chromosome clearly carries genetic determinants that promote linear growth and regulate body proportions.[5, 6] Recently, several clusters of autosomal genes were found to be involved in growth because they behave differently when they come from the mother than when they come from the father. This difference is due to the epigenetic process of genomic imprinting, which like X inactivation, is due to genes being methylated to silence them.[7] Although the exact nature of most imprinted genes is unknown, the IGF-2 and IGF-2 receptor genes on chromosome 15 are known to be imprinted. The IGF-2 gene is silenced in eggs and thus in the maternal contribution to the embryo's genome ("maternal imprinting"). The IGF-2 receptor is imprinted the opposite way: it is paternally imprinted, that is, only the gene derived from the mother's egg is expressed.

Skeletal linear growth commences with chondrocytes of the epiphyses laying down an orderly cartilage template and proceeds mainly by endochondral bone formation.[8] The cycle of bone cell remodeling for structural purposes is closely linked to the overall metabolic needs for calcium and phosphorus homeostasis, primarily by the actions of parathormone and calciferol. Fibroblast growth factors negatively regulate growth plate chondrogenesis.

Nutrition and metabolism must be adequate for normal growth. Adult height has been used as a marker for the nutritional status of populations during childhood and has been shown to relate to cognitive function.[9, 10] Calories seem particularly critical for cell multiplication. Two percent to 13% of normal energy consumption goes into promoting growth.[1, 11] Protein intake is particularly important for normal growth in cellular size. It must be adequate with respect to both the amount and provision of essential amino acids or their ketoanalogues.[12–14] Essential fatty acids are necessary for normal growth in lower animals, but this requirement may not hold true for primates.[15] Vitamins A and D are important for normal growth.[1, 16] Trace metals such as zinc and copper are probably essential for normal growth and sexual maturation[17–20] because of their role as cofactors for enzyme function. The pH must be maintained at optimal levels to conserve mineral homeostasis.[21]

The general level of *activity* seems to promote overall body growth, just as normal muscular activity is necessary for limb growth. The mechanism is unclear; it may be related to neural trophic factors or blood flow. The efficiency of nitrogen accretion and growth are decreased in inactive rats.[22]

Hormones are essential "catalysts" of growth, and growth hormone (GH) is especially important for cell multiplication.[1] GH secretion is normally mainly controlled by the balance between hypothalamic

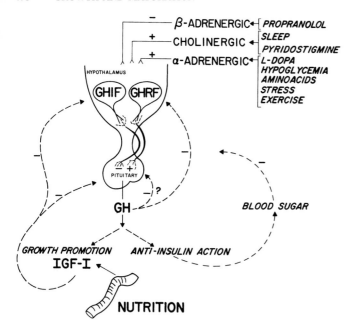

FIGURE 35–1. Major factors in regulation of growth hormone (GH) secretion (+, stimulators of GH release; −, inhibitors of GH release). GH secretion is stimulated primarily by hypothalamic GH-releasing factor (GHRF) and inhibited by neuronal secretion of the hypothalamic GH-inhibiting factor (GHIF) somatostatin. GH is secreted after integration of diverse hypothalamic stimuli. Secretion of GH is facilitated by α-adrenergic, dopaminergic, and cholinergic neurons to the hypothalamus. It is inhibited by β-adrenergic tracts. GH directly exerts negative feedback at the level of the hypothalamus and possibly at the pituitary gland. GH secretion is also inhibited by insulin-like growth factor-1 (IGF-I), which appears to inhibit GH secretion directly at the pituitary gland and indirectly through stimulation of somatostatin release. (Modified from Schaff-Blass E, Burstein S, Rosenfield RL: Advances in diagnosis and treatment of short stature, with special reference to the role of growth hormone. J Pediatr 104:801, 1984.)

secretion of GH-releasing factor and somatostatin, which are in turn subject to complex, intermittent regulation by higher cerebral centers[23–25] (Fig. 35–1). Serum GH is approximately 50% bound to GH-binding protein, levels of which rise through childhood.[26] The GH-binding protein is an alternatively spliced form of the extracellular domain of the GH receptor, although the two may be differentially regulated.[27] GH appears to stimulate growth through dual effects.[28, 28a] It stimulates the production of endocrine IGF-1 (somatomedin-C) and

its major binding protein (IGFBP-3) by the liver. It also directly induces the clonal expansion and differentiation of target stem cells (such as prechondrocytes), and these differentiating cells (chondrocytes) then respond to GH by forming IGF-1 and IGF-1 receptors, which makes them responsive to the growth-promoting effect of both endocrine IGF-1 and IGFs secreted locally (autocrine and paracrine IGFs).

Endocrine IGF-1 production is primarily regulated by GH when nutrition is normal. The pubertal increase in IGF-1 is mediated by sex hormone stimulation of GH secretion.[29–31] IGF-2 is produced by cells independently of GH[32] and seems to be normally important only for local growth regulation.[33] IGF-2 levels seem to be modulated locally by the activity of a metabolizing receptor complex consisting of the IGF-2 receptor and glypican-3.[34]

Regulation of plasma IGF-1 concentrations and bioactivity involves more than just GH. Endocrine IGF-1 is fundamentally under broad regulation by nutrition. Undernutrition decreases plasma IGF-1 levels despite normal or elevated GH concentrations. Overnutrition (i.e., obesity) has the opposite effect.[25] Studies in rats suggest that insulin plays a role in mediating nutritional effects on hepatic IGF-1 formation through its stimulation of amino acid uptake.[35, 36] Thyroid hormone and cortisol are necessary for hepatic IGF-1 production, and prolactin has a slight effect on it.[37] The increased plasma free IGF-1 concentration of obese patients has been attributed to the suppressive effect of their insulin excess on IGFBP-1.[38]

Factors other than GH and nutrition regulate IGF production, but the details are poorly understood. Plasma IGF-1, IGFBP-3 levels,[39] and somatomedin activity[40] rise slowly during the prepubertal years without any change in GH production[41] (Fig. 35–2). When GH production increases during puberty, IGF-1 levels rise more strikingly than those of IGFBP-3; therefore, free plasma IGF-1 rises even more markedly.[39]

The relationship of plasma IGF-1 levels to normal growth is not a simple one. Plasma IGF-1 levels do not correlate with the growth rate in childhood except during the pubertal growth spurt.[23] Peripheral responsiveness to IGF-1 seems to decrease with age.[42] IGFBPs in plasma determine the unbound concentration of IGF-1, and a tissue IGFBP-protease system modulates IGF-1 bioavailability to target cells.[28, 43] IGF bioactivity is also influenced by circulating somatomedin inhibitory activity, which is attributable to both glucocorticoids and incompletely characterized peptides.[44, 45]

Growth may be normal with subnormal GH production in the "growth without growth hormone syndrome."[46] Most often this syndrome has been identified after treatment of pituitary tumors, but the syndrome has occasionally been recognized in benign forms of hypopituitarism. IGF-1 levels may be low, but with normal bioactivity. Most such patients are obese, so insulin excess has been suspected to

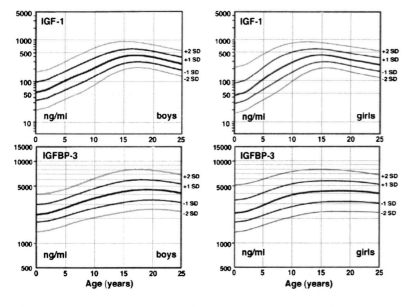

FIGURE 35–2. Plasma insulin-like growth factor-1 (IGF-1) and IGF-binding protein-3 (IGFBP-3) normal ranges from infancy to adulthood. The increases after 10 years of age are related to pubertal stage rather than age. IGF-1 values are given in terms of the World Health Organization reference preparation 87/518, which is of low (44%) purity with respect to authentic recombinant human IGF-1, so the values shown are in excess of the true IGF-1 concentration.[41] (Data from Diagnostic Systems Laboratories, 1997.)

be the growth factor. Hyperprolactinemia is seldom found. The syndrome may prove to be due to a GH variant or an unidentified growth factor.

Thyroid hormone is necessary for bone growth because of both indirect effects on the GH-IGF axis and direct effects on bone growth.[47] Thyroid hormone is required for normal GH secretion in response to GH-releasing hormone (GHRH) and for normal GH action as indexed by GH-binding protein, IGF, and IGFBP levels. Mutation of the thyroid β-receptor produces short stature and delays bone maturation, but not to the same extent as deficiency of thyroid hormone.

Glucocorticoids in above-normal amounts are inhibitors of linear growth.[45, 48] The mechanism is both indirect and direct. Corticoid excess inhibits spontaneous GH secretion by stimulating somatostatin tone. The bioactivity of plasma IGF-1 falls during corticoid therapy, but the nature of the inhibitory change is poorly characterized. Glucocorticoids themselves directly hinder mitogenesis in chondrocytes by inhibiting GH and IGF-1 induction of their respective receptors.[49]

Increased secretion of sex hormones clearly initiates the pubertal growth spurt. About half the contribution of sex hormones to the pubertal growth spurt is due to their stimulation of the GH-IGF axis, which appears to be primarily mediated by estrogen.[29, 30, 32] The remainder of the effects of sex steroids on growth is direct.[50–52] Both estrogens and androgens stimulate epiphyseal growth, but only estrogens bring about epiphyseal closure.[50] Early pubertal amounts of estradiol (about 0.25 mg/month) stimulate growth in girls, in contrast to inhibition of growth with high doses of estrogen.[53] The peak growth velocity of boys occurs at a testosterone production rate of about 50 to 100 mg/month.[54] Whether other sex steroids play an independent role in growth is unknown. It has been reported that dehydroepiandrosterone sulfate promotes calcification of cartilage and that subandrogenic doses of androstenedione promote growth.[55]

Prenatal Growth

Prenatal and postnatal requirements for growth differ in several respects. Embryonic growth is primarily determined by genetic programming of local sequential inductions.[56] Fetal growth is a special case because it depends heavily on the delivery of nutrients, metabolic substrates, and oxygen by the mother and placenta and because the hormonal milieu is regulated in part by the placenta.[57, 58] Familial and environmental variables that correlate with birth size independently of gestational age include maternal weight, sibling birth weight, parity, and inversely, the number of fetuses carried and altitude.[59–64] Monozygous twins are more discordant in size (and anomalies) than are dizygotic ones,[65] which has been attributed to a higher frequency of placental arteriovenous anastomoses causing unequal distribution of blood flow. Placental growth is itself influenced by genomic factors,[7] maternal nutrition, and uterine blood flow. The placenta also influences fetal growth through its elaboration of hormones. For example, human placental lactogen seems to play a modest role in regulating fetal IGF-1 and placental GH influences maternal IGF-1.

Some of the hormonal requirements for fetal growth also differ. Prenatal growth is less dependent than postnatal growth on GH and thyroxine: birth length is usually normal in congenital GH deficiency or resistance, although on average it is reduced by 1 SD,[58, 66] and bone maturation of congenitally hypothyroid fetuses lags only during the last trimester.[67]

Although the serum IGF level is even lower prenatally than in infancy, it rises during gestation and correlates with size at birth.[58] Plasma IGF-1 seems to be virtually independent of GH and is primarily determined by nutritional status, particularly glucose availability and the consequent fetal insulin secretion.[56, 58, 66] IGF-2 blood levels are higher than those of IGF-1 in the fetus, and it is as important as IGF-1 for fetal growth.[33, 68] Fetal rat cartilage has been reported to be resistant to IGF action.[42]

Sex hormones may also play a subtle role in normal fetal and prepubertal growth. After midgestation, plasma testosterone, estradiol, and dehydroepiandrosterone levels of the fetus are equal to or greater than those of the pubertal male, and estrogen promotes fetal bone

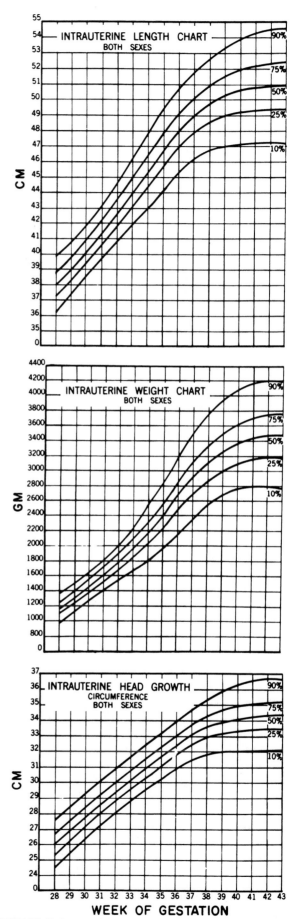

FIGURE 35–3. Intrauterine growth chart. (From Naeye RL, Dixon JB: Distortions in fetal growth standards. Pediatr Res 12:987, 1978, © 1978, The Williams & Wilkins Company, Baltimore.)

development.[55] Androgen action seems to account for the greater birth weight of boys than girls.[56, 66]

PATTERNS OF NORMAL SOMATIC GROWTH

Intrauterine Growth

Standards for intrauterine growth of the general American population are shown in Figure 35–3.[69] Fetal growth is more rapid than postnatal growth. The first fetal epiphyseal center to ossify is the calcaneus (at an average gestational age of 24 weeks), followed by the talus (28 weeks), distal femoral epiphysis (36 weeks), proximal tibial epiphysis (38 weeks), and cuboid (42 weeks).[70] Weight increases out of proportion to length during the third trimester because of the accumulation of fat and muscle.

Healthy infants born prematurely have weights appropriate for gestational age and continue to grow at the same rate that they would have grown in utero.[71] When corrected for postconceptional age, length and weight follow postnatal standards. Consequently, the lengths of children born prematurely remain slightly less through infancy than those of children born at term, but the differences become negligible with time.

Postnatal Growth

Linear growth standards derived from cross-sectional data are shown in Figure 35–4.[72] A "secular trend" toward increasing height of the population with time has been noted.

Growth occurs in three phases—infantile, childhood, and pubertal—each of which has distinct characteristics.[73] Linear growth velocity is most rapid in infancy. Two-thirds of infants cross percentile channels on linear growth curves.[74] The growth of infants seems to result from an initial steep vector, which is generated by the GH- and thyroxine-independent cell proliferation that uniquely drives intrauterine growth, superimposed on a shallow vector, which is dependent on the endocrine factors that determine subsequent growth during childhood.

In childhood, after infancy until puberty begins, growth normally proceeds along a channel that closely corresponds to a given height-attained percentile on cross-sectional growth standards. A child normally establishes this channel by 2 to 3 years of age,[74] although on rare occasions a gradual drift by as many as 40 percentile positions in height attained may occur over a period of several years in normal children.[75] These channels have a slightly decelerating velocity averaging about 6 cm/year[76] (Fig. 35–5). However, normal children cross height velocity percentiles to maintain their height-attained channel[77–79] (Fig. 35–6). Growth consistently along the 3rd percentile for height velocity will lead to subnormal height.

The growth channel seems to be genetically determined. Children grow as though to reach a predetermined target height. This target height can be approximated by calculating the midparent height (the average of the parents' heights) and adding 6.5 cm for boys or subtracting 6.5 cm for girls (to adjust for the average differences between men and women). Alternative functions have been proposed for children with short parents. However, all such predictions are only accurate within a range of 7 to 10 cm.[80]

Deflections from this channel are firmly resisted, as though growth is being developmentally canalized.[81] The mechanisms by which the growth channel is maintained are unknown. They may involve recognition of cell density, which is a determinant of the cell population in culture systems.[82] In the course of a year, healthy children maintain their percentile position with respect to height attained by means of short-term fluctuations in growth velocity termed stasis and saltation.[83] These oscillations may be marked, growth sometimes seeming nil over 3-month periods, and are a potential source of error in growth diagnosis. The variations tend to be seasonal, a "blooming" trend most often occurring in the spring.

During puberty, children again cross height-attained percentiles because the pubertal growth spurts of individuals occur out of phase. The magnitude of this pubertal growth spurt is only apparent from growth velocity standards based on age of menarche or longitudinal data. Peak growth velocity occurs in midpuberty, approximately 1 year before menarche[84] and at a bone age (BA) of approximately 12 years in girls and 13 years in boys.[85] Girls on average achieve only 7 cm further growth after menarche.[86] During the course of sexual maturation, the epiphyseal cartilage plates become progressively obliterated, and growth ceases when the process is complete. Only about 1 cm of growth occurs after fusion is complete in the femur and tibia.

Some of the greater ultimate height of boys than girls results from their later puberty and consequently longer period of prepubertal growth[79]; additionally, boys have a slightly greater peak linear growth velocity than girls do.[78] Early maturers have more brisk pubertal growth than late maturers do.[78] This tendency occurs at comparable levels of bone maturation[87] (Table 35–1). The growth patterns of nonwhite American children differ from those of whites in some particulars.[88, 89] Immigrant children go into a phase of catch-up growth in an optimum nutritional environment.[88]

Body proportions change in concert with growth. The limbs are relatively short in infancy. By about 11 years of age, adult proportions are reached[90, 91] (Figs. 35–7 and 35–8). Occasional marked changes in segmental proportions appear during puberty.[92] Facial physiognomy matures as well. The change in nasal root configuration can be documented by measuring the intercanthic and interorbital distances.[93]

Head circumference increases most rapidly during early infancy[94] (Fig. 35–9). It is related to both skeletal and brain growth, and about half the variation is familial.[95–97]

Weight is a labile parameter relative to height in that it is sensitive to acute illnesses and short-term changes in feeding and activity patterns, as well as muscle mass. Whether nutrition is appropriate can be quickly estimated by comparing a child's percentile position for weight with respect to height age (HA). Percentile standards of weight for height are now available for infants and children,[72] at menarche and maturity in women,[98] and in terms of body mass index for children.[99] During puberty, fat stores tend to increase slightly in girls and decrease in boys. The waist-hip ratio decreases during adolescence in girls because of a relatively great increase in hip circumference.[100]

The postnatal growth of most organs follows the general somatic model.[9] Consequently, blood volume closely approximates 7% of body weight throughout life. However, the brain, lymphoid organs, and reproductive organs follow different growth patterns. Fifty percent of adult brain weight is achieved at 1 year, and lymphoid mass is maximal at 12 years of age. Because the readily exchangeable extracellular compartment is relatively larger in children than adults, water and electrolyte requirements are more closely related to surface area than to weight. Water requirements approximate 1500 mL/m² throughout life, with electrolyte, calorie, and drug dosage requirements generally changing in proportion.[101, 102]

Primary teeth begin to calcify before birth. Calcification and eruption of the permanent teeth are dependent on many of the nutritional and hormonal factors that determine somatic growth.[103] Nevertheless, the correlation between dental and bone maturation is not a good one.

Catch-up Growth and Compensatory Growth

Catch-up growth occurs after relief from any disorder that has caused deviation from a child's genetic growth channel and restores the child to the original channel.[81] In classic ("type 1") catch-up growth, the rate of growth is supranormal and exceeds that expected for the age at which growth had been arrested. During adolescence, it may resemble the pubertal growth spurt. A different kind of catch-up growth ("type 2") occurs after adequate therapy for sexual precocity.[104] In this situation, restoration of height potential occurs because restitutional linear growth proceeds without bone maturation advancement, that is, HA catches up to BA (Table 35–2). Complete compensation for growth failure can occur upon correction of the disorder. However, catch-up may be incomplete if the growth disorder is of many years' duration and extends into the age at which puberty

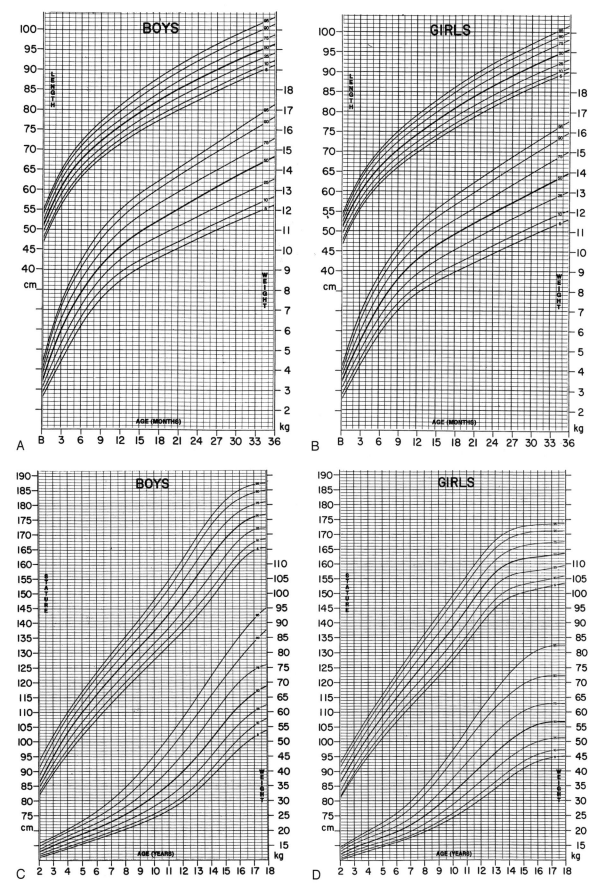

FIGURE 35–4. Current standards for height and weight of normal children in the United States. Smoothed percentiles from the 5th to the 95th are shown; the data are not normally distributed. *A* and *B*, Infant growth charts for length and weight from the Fels Research Institute. *C* and *D*, Older children's growth charts for standing height and weight from the National Health Examination Survey, 1963–1975.

HEIGHT VELOCITY (cm/yr)

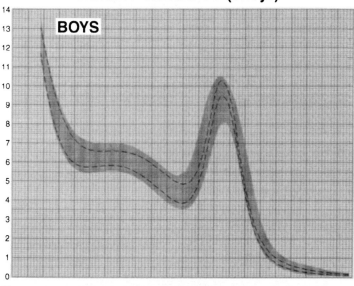

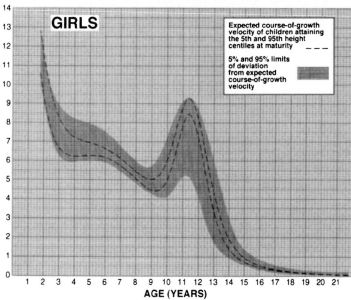

FIGURE 35–5. Longitudinal height velocity standards derived from the Fels, Berkely, and Denver growth studies.[76] (Courtesy of R.D. Bock.)

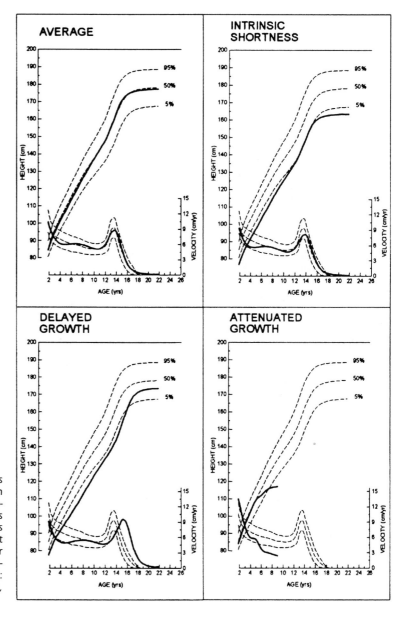

FIGURE 35–6. Linear growth curves in children with various types of growth patterns. Note that three prepubertal children of similar short stature at 9 years of age have different prognoses for growth. The growth curve of an average-size child is shown for comparison. On each chart, the upper scale shows the height attained, and the lower scale shows the height velocity. Normal percentiles are from the National Center for Health Statistics.[72] Growth curves were generated by the TRI-FOUR program of Bock et al. (Bock RD, du Toit SHC, Thissen D: A.U.X.A.L.: Auxological Analysis of Longitudinal Data. Chicago, Scientific Software, 1993. Courtesy of R.D. Bock.)

TABLE 35–1. Percentage of Adult Height Achieved at Successive Bone Ages, Variation in Height Prediction from Bone Age, and Variation in Bone Age in Relation to Chronologic Age

	Bone Age (yr)												
	6.0	7.0	8.0	9.0	10.0	11.0	12.0	13.0	14.0	15.0	16.0	17.0	18.0
Percentage of mature height													
Boys													
Average*		69.5	72.3	75.2	78.4	80.4	83.4	87.6	92.7	96.8	98.2	99.1	99.6
Accelerated*		67.0	69.6	72.0	74.7	76.7	80.9	85.0	90.5	95.8	98.0	99.0	
Retarded*	68.0	71.8	75.6	78.6	81.2	82.3	84.5	88.0					
Girls													
Average	72.0	75.7	79.0	82.7	86.2	90.6	92.2	95.8	98.0	99.0	99.6	99.9	100
Accelerated		71.2	75.0	79.0	82.8	88.3	90.1	94.5	97.2	98.6	99.3	99.8	
Retarded	73.3	77.0	80.4	84.1	87.4	91.8	93.2	96.4	98.3	99.4	99.8	100.0	
	Chronologic Age (yr)												
	6.0	7.0	8.0	9.0	10.0	11.0	12.0	13.0	14.0	15.0	16.0	17.0	18.0
Height prediction standard deviation (inches)													
Boys		1.47	1.27	1.33	1.14	1.09	1.21	1.21	0.88	0.49	0.41		
Girls		1.73	1.46	1.37	1.15	1.06	0.6	0.42	0.38	0.26	0.20		
Bone age standard deviation (mo)													
Boys	9.3	10.1	10.8	11.0	11.4	10.5	10.4	11.1	12.0	14.2	15.1	15.4	
Girls	9.0	8.3	8.8	9.3	10.8	12.3	14.0	14.6	12.6	11.2			

*With respect to whether bone age is within 1 year of chronologic age.
From Gruelich WW, Pyle SI: Radiographic Atlas of Skeletal Development of the Hand and Wrist. Palo Alto, CA, Stanford University Press, 1959.

normally occurs. The mechanism of catch-up growth is unclear; GH is permissive, but the intrinsic epiphyseal factors determining developmental canalization of growth seem to be key.

Compensatory growth is the term used for the local organ regeneration that occurs after the mass of an *organ* has been reduced, as by removal or destruction of a portion of that organ.[81] Examples include the compensatory growth that occurs after partial hepatectomy or loss of a kidney. Local IGF-1 and IGF-2 are involved in this type of growth.[33]

Bone Age in Prediction of Adult Height and Pubertal Milestones

Bone growth is accompanied by a predictable pattern of bone maturation. After epiphyseal ossification centers first appear, they undergo modeling in shape and then fuse with the shaft. Bone maturation is assessed as BA (i.e., skeletal age) (see Table 35–2). Figures 35–10 and 35–11 schematically show the Gruelich and Pyle BA standards.[105, 106] The normal range for BA is indicated in Table 35–1. The evaluation is most reliable if the maturation of each center is assessed to calculate an average[107] in order to circumvent normal variations in the epiphyseal ossification pattern.[108] Other atlas methods are available for assessing bone maturation.[109] Skeletal development of young black children is about 0.67 SD advanced over whites of comparable economic status.[110] Other ethnic differences exist and are to an unknown extent nutritional.[109]

BA is a better predictor of pubertal milestones than chronologic age is. It is as though bone and neuroendocrine maturation have common determinants. A BA of 11 to 12 years corresponds better to the onset of puberty in girls and boys, respectively, than do these chronologic ages. Peak height velocity phase differences are 25% less when plotted against BA instead of chronologic age.[77] In girls, menarche has been demonstrated to occur at a mean skeletal age of approximately 13 years.[105, 111]

The degree of bone maturation is inversely proportional to the amount of epiphyseal cartilage growth remaining. It follows that if a child's BA and HA (see Table 35–2) are equal, the child has the potential to reach an average adult height. The fraction of final height achieved at each BA is known (see Table 35–1). Therefore, adult

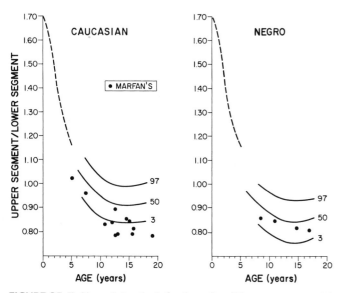

FIGURE 35–7. Normal standards for the ratio of the upper segment to the lower segment of the body. The lower segment is the measurement from the top of the symphysis pubis to the heel; the upper segment is computed by subtracting the lower segment from height. The *dotted line* shows the average for young children in 1932. (Percentile and Marfan data from McKusick VA: Heritable Disorders of Connective Tissue, ed 4. St Louis, Mosby, 1972.)

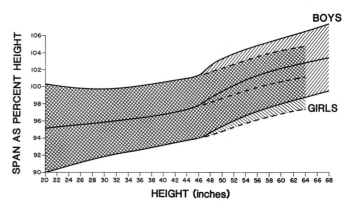

FIGURE 35–8. Standards for arm span as a percentage of height. The *shaded area* represents the normal range, smoothed. (Data from Engelbach W: Endocrine Medicine, vol 1. Springfield, IL, Charles C Thomas, 1932, p 261.)

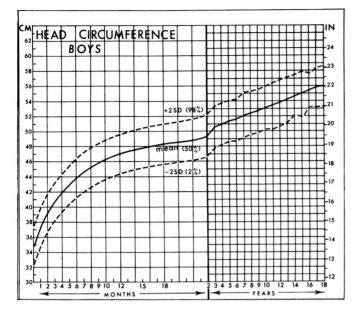

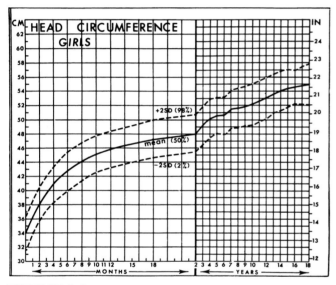

FIGURE 35-9. *Interracial standards for maximal fronto-occipital head circumference. Boys' measurements are about 1 cm greater than those of girls at all ages. (From Nellhaus G: Head circumference from birth to eighteen years. Pediatrics 41:106, 1968. Copyright American Academy of Pediatrics 1968.)*

height can be predicted by dividing a child's current height by this fraction (method of Bayley and Pinneau).[87] The error inherent in this method is less than 1.5 inches in normal children (see Table 35-1). However, spontaneous shifts by as much as 5 inches in predicted height may occur in 3% of the population for reasons that are unclear.[112] The error is not reduced by serial readings[107] and is greater in children who are very short[113] or have bone dysplasias.

To reduce the error in height prediction, elaborate tables have been devised that take into consideration not only a child's BA and height

TABLE 35-2.   Definitions of Growth Parameters

Parameter	Definition
Bone age	Age for which bone maturation is average
Chronologic age	Calendar age
Height age	Age for which height is average
Weight age	Age for which weight is average

but also the genetic target height and weight.[114] Genetic influences on height predicted from BA can be roughly accounted for by adding one-third the amount that the midparent height differs from the average.[86] Weight is inversely related to the age of attainment of pubertal milestones because metabolic signals related to nutrition, one of which is leptin generated by body fat, are necessary for sexual maturation.[98, 115]

GROWTH DISORDERS

Children assessed for inadequate or excessive linear growth generally have either a genetically based, normal-variant growth pattern or a disorder of the congenital, nutritional, metabolic, or endocrine factors discussed above. The following section first categorizes the disorders that cause short stature according to the factors that influence growth. Endocrinopathies are discussed here only insofar as they affect growth; detailed discussion of these disorders can be found in other chapters. Then we present an approach to the differential diagnosis of these disorders according to clinical assessment of the patient's growth pattern: patients are either intrinsically short, that is, literally small boned, or have delayed or attenuated growth patterns in which height potential is normal if properly managed. Treatment of short stature is then discussed. Tall stature is discussed later in a parallel manner in the final section.

Short Stature

Causes of Short Stature

Genetic normal variants dominate as the most frequent causes of this problem. Two nonpathologic familial patterns of growth cause the great majority of cases of short stature (Table 35-3). One pattern is *familial intrinsic short stature* (sometimes termed *familial* or *genetic short stature*), in which a normal child's growth approximates that of the child's short parents. The other pattern is *constitutional delay in growth and pubertal development,* in which healthy children who are short (delayed puberty may be the most prominent symptom) spontaneously achieve their normal growth potential at a later than average age. Characteristically, a parent or close relative has a similar growth pattern. In both these normal-variant growth patterns, the typical patient is of normal birth size, and length progressively crosses growth channels to fall below the 5th percentile by 2 to 3 years of age. HA and BA then characteristically advance at a normal rate so that height is below, but closely parallel to the 5th percentile through the prepubertal years. However, these two normal variants differ in that in the former, BA is normal and puberty occurs at a normal age, whereas in the latter, BA is delayed and puberty is correspondingly delayed until the child reaches a pubertal BA, at which time a normal growth spurt results in a generally normal adult height.

Genetic disorders of bone growth—namely, chromosomal aneuploidy, bone dysplasias, and various dysmorphic and intrauterine growth-retarding syndromes—cause inherent limitations of height that cannot be corrected easily if at all (intrinsic short stature). Stunting of growth and cerebral dysfunction are virtually uniform features of autosomal aneuploidy. Down syndrome (trisomy 21 and variants thereof) is the most common multiple malformation syndrome in humans. Adult height averages 155 cm in affected males, 145 cm in females.[116]

Turner's syndrome (gonadal dysgenesis), caused by deletion of X chromosomal material, is the most common pathologic cause of short stature in girls. The incidence of Turner's syndrome is 1 in 2500 newborn girls. The average birth size of these children is at the lower end of the normal range. Height typically drops below the 3rd percentile by 3 years of age and then nearly parallels this percentile during childhood.[117] Growth becomes further attenuated in the teenage years, in part because of hypogonadism.[118] The most characteristic features of Turner's syndrome are short stature and gonadal dysgenesis. Short-

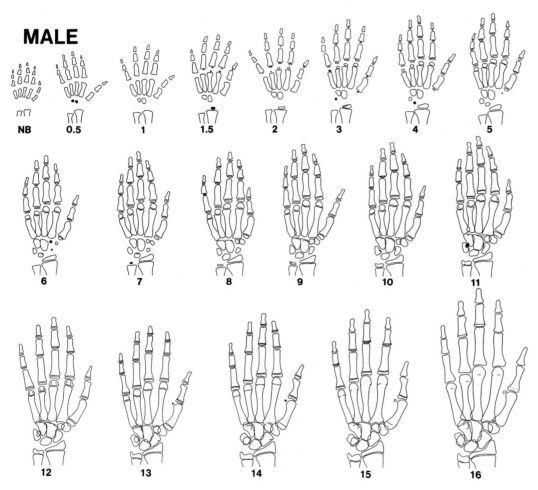

MALE

NB 0.5 1 1.5 2 3 4 5

6 7 8 9 10 11

12 13 14 15 16

FIGURE 35–10. Progression of ossification of the hand and wrist in boys. Tracings are modified from the standards of Gruelich and Pyle[105] according to the manner of Wilkins.[106] Newly apparent ossification centers are shown in *black.* Late prefusion is depicted as a *single line* at the junction of the epiphysis and shaft. Bony projections, which appear as a *double contour* within the outlines of a center, are not illustrated after their appearance has matured.

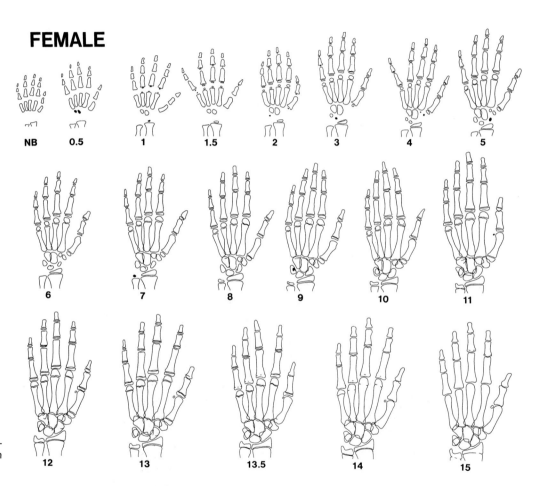

FEMALE

NB 0.5 1 1.5 2 3 4 5

6 7 8 9 10 11

12 13 13.5 14 15

FIGURE 35–11. Progression of ossification of the hand and wrist in girls. See legend for Figure 35–10.

ness is a more consistent finding in patients who partially lack genetic material on the distal end of the short arm of the X chromosome[6] than is gonadal failure. The presence of pubertal development should not deter consideration of the diagnosis because about 10% of patients have some residual ovarian tissue rather than streak gonads. Thus these patients may have spontaneous menarche, although few sustain regular menses.[119] Additional manifestations of Turner's syndrome include lymphedema, particularly in the newborn period, and the dysmorphic features and congenital anomalies listed in Table 35–4. Variations in the physical manifestations of Turner's syndrome are illustrated in Figure 35–12.[93] Aortic root dilatation and renal anomalies are infrequent, but important.[125] The frequency of autoimmune thyroiditis and diabetes mellitus is increased. Karyotype analysis is essential in the investigation of any girl with unexplained short stature. Without growth-promoting therapy, adult height averages 56.5 inches.[117]

Current treatment of Turner's syndrome includes GH therapy. Although Turner's syndrome does not involve GH deficiency as a cause of the growth impairment, GH treatment (particularly in doses higher than those used for GH deficiency) appears to improve growth, and results to date suggest that long-term treatment increases adult height

in many recipients.[117] GH treatment is recommended when the height of a girl with Turner's syndrome drops below the 5th percentile on the normal female growth curve. Studies also suggest that oxandrolone, together with GH, may stimulate growth. The side effects of GH are discussed below under GH deficiency. To induce pubertal development in girls with ovarian failure resulting from Turner's syndrome, very low-dose exogenous estrogen therapy (and eventually cycling with progesterone) is needed in adolescence and beyond.[53]

Bone dysplasias (chondrodysplasias) are often associated with short stature. Abnormal body proportions (e.g., upper body segment abnormally longer than the lower body segment[90]; see Fig. 35–7) or arm span disproportionate to height[91] (see Fig. 35–8) indicate that one is dealing with such a disorder. The most common is achondroplasia, an autosomal dominant condition that has a frequency of about 1 in 10,000, with about 90% of cases representing fresh mutations.[93] It causes short stature (often apparent at birth and with deceleration of the growth rate in infancy), short limbs, macrocephaly, a low nasal bridge, caudal narrowing of the spinal canal, and occasionally hydrocephalus[93] (Fig. 35–13). The average adult height is about 125 cm in females and 131 cm in males.[93] Achondroplasia is generally caused

TABLE 35–3. Factors Causing Short Stature, with Representative Clinical Conditions

Factors Affecting Height	Representative Conditions	Clinical and Laboratory Features
Genetic		
Normal variants	Familial intrinsic shortness	Family history of shortness, normal bone age; no clinical or laboratory abnormalities
	Constitutional delay in growth	Family history of delayed growth, delayed bone age; no other clinical or laboratory abnormalities
Genetic disorders		
Chromosomal aneuploidy	Turner's syndrome	Short, gonadal dysgenesis, otherwise variable phenotype; karyotype necessary to exclude
Bone dysplasias	Achondroplasia	Abnormal body proportions, macrocephaly, short limbs, low nasal bridge, occasional hydrocephalus, abnormal skeletal survey
	Hypochondroplasia	Short stature, short limbs, relative lack of craniofacial abnormalities in contrast to achondroplasia, abnormal skeletal survey
Dysmorphic syndromes	Noonan's syndrome	Similar to Turner's syndrome (see Table 35–4), normal karyotype, and present in both sexes
	Russell-Silver syndrome	IUGR, relative macrocephaly, small triangular face, asymmetry
	Prader-Willi syndrome	Obesity, hypogonadism, hypotonia, intellectual and behavioral deficits, chromosome 15 abnormalities
	Pseudohypoparathyroidism (type IA)	Hypocalcemia, moon face, brachydactyly, mental retardation, abnormal $G_{s\alpha}$
Intrauterine		
Growth retardation	Small for gestational age	Ongoing growth failure in a minority of nonsyndromic cases; diverse maternal, placental, and fetal disorders
Nutritional		
Inadequate intake	Starvation Psychosocial feeding problems Anorexia from chronic disease	Weight generally depressed more than height
Vitamin/mineral deficiency	Rickets	Nutritional deficiency in vitamin D is the most common cause, but diverse other acquired and genetic causes are possible; alkaline phosphatase elevated in most types
Nutrient loss	Zinc deficiency Malabsorption	Symptoms of gastrointestinal, liver, or pancreatic disease; respiratory problems (cystic fibrosis)
	Chronic vomiting	Obstruction to gastrointestinal tract, achalasia of the esophagus, electrolyte disturbances, increased intracranial pressure
Metabolic wastage	Uncontrolled diabetes mellitus	High glycohemoglobin, hepatomegaly (Mauriac syndrome); exclude other causes of poor growth; fetal diabetes causes IUGR
Hormonal		
GH/IGF-1 deficiency	Congenital	May have neonatal hypoglycemia, midline defects; may have only short stature
	Acquired	May have history of trauma, CNA insult, or abnormal CNS examination
	Psychosocial deprivation	May show abnormal behavior, hyperphagia; may mimic panhypopituitarism; growth improves with better environment
	GH/IGF-1 resistance	
Hypothyroidism		Growth failure may be only symptom
Glucocorticoid	Excess	Supraphysiologic levels attenuate growth; often associated with obesity
Sex steroids	Deficiency	Deficiency after 10–11 yr of age impairs growth
Chronic illness		May have history or symptoms of chronic condition or short stature may be the initial feature; weight often impaired more than height

CNS, central nervous system; GH, growth hormone; IGF-1, insulin-like growth factor-1; IUGR, intrauterine growth retardation.

TABLE 35–4. Approximate Incidence of Somatic Abnormalities in Turner's and Noonan's Syndromes*

Abnormality	Turner's Syndrome[93, 118, 119] (%)	Noonan's Syndrome[93, 120–124] (%)
Short stature (<10%)	100/80†	90/90
Gonadal failure	99/85?	≤10/≤10‡
Cryptorchidism	NA/33	NA/75
Hypertelorism	<25	100
High palate	80	75
Neck webbed	50	10
Neck short	68	100
Cubitus valgus	68	30
Chest deformity§	50	50
Coarctation of aorta	20	<1
Pulmonic stenosis	10	50¶
Mental retardation	10**	25
Pigmented moles, multiple	50	<10

*Defined on the basis of the presence (Turner) or absence (Noonan) of a sex chromosome abnormality. Turner's syndrome in females results from deletion of genetic material on the X chromosome. Various sex chromosomal abnormalities have been reported in Turner's syndrome in males—for example, XO, XXY, XO/XY, XO/XY/XYY, XX/XXY.
†Female/male.
‡The distinction between delayed puberty and hypogonadism has seldom been made.
§Pectus or an apparent increase in internipple distance.
¶The high incidence of congenital heart disease in Noonan's syndrome may be due to ascertainment bias, Dr. Noonan being a cardiologist. A variety of other congenital heart defects have been reported in both syndromes.
**Males seem to have a greater incidence of mental retardation, although finding this may be a matter of ascertainment.
NA, not applicable.

by a gain-of-function mutation in the fibroblast growth factor receptor 3 (*FGFR3*) gene.[126, 127] Hypochondroplasia is an allelic variant of achondroplasia.[126, 127] It is manifested as short stature and dysmorphic features that are often more mild than seen in achondroplasia. Newborns may be slightly small, but short stature generally becomes evident by 3 years of age. Few craniofacial abnormalities are associated with hypochondroplasia. These children are minimally short limbed. The hands and feet are usually stubby, and genu varum may occur. The most objective radiologic finding is narrowing of the lower lumbosacral interpedicular distances.

Chondrodysplasias may cause specific patterns of disproportion. In spondyloepiphyseal dysplasia, the spine is disproportionately affected and slowing of growth in midchildhood causes an attenuated growth pattern. On the other hand, some bone dysplasias cause proportionate dwarfism. Tubular stenosis is a proportionate form of bone dysplasia associated with congenital hypoparathyroidism.[128] An activating muta-

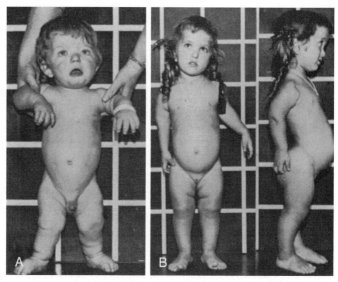

FIGURE 35–13. Achondroplasia. *A,* One-year-old boy with a height age of 4 months. *B,* Four-year-old girl with a height age of 20 months. (From Jones KL (ed): *Smith's Recognizable Patterns of Human Malformation,* 4th ed. Philadelphia, WB Saunders, 1988.)

tion of the parathyroid hormone–related receptor has recently been discovered to cause Jansen's metaphyseal dysplasia, which is associated with asymptomatic hypercalcemia.[129] Various atlases are available to distinguish among the known types of bone dysplasia.[81, 93, 130, 131] In recent years it has become possible to make a specific genetic diagnosis in many cases.[126]

Dysmorphic syndromes caused by a variety of cellular and molecular abnormalities may be associated with intrinsic short stature.[93] Some prominent examples are Noonan's syndrome, Russell-Silver syndrome, Prader-Willi syndrome, and pseudohypoparathyroidism. The parent of origin of the genetic defect influences gene expression to a successively greater extent in the latter three of these disorders through the mechanism of genomic imprinting.[7, 132] Congenital anomalies can be a clue to these and other intrinsic growth disorders because they may be manifested as short stature at birth or in postnatal life[93, 133–139] (Table 35–5).

Noonan's syndrome, originally called "male Turner's syndrome," is now diagnosed in patients of either sex with normal external genitalia who have a Turner-like phenotype but normal sex chromosomes.[120–124] It may be transmitted as an autosomal dominant disorder and has been linked to chromosome 12.[140] Although the anomalies in an individual

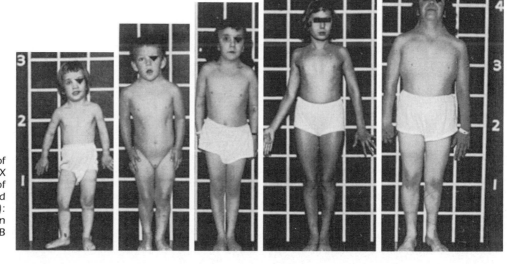

FIGURE 35–12. Variable phenotypes of Turner's syndrome: five girls with 45,X syndrome illustrating the variability of features such as webbed neck and broad chest. (From Jones KL (ed): *Smith's Recognizable Patterns of Human Malformation,* 4th ed. Philadelphia, WB Saunders, 1988.)

TABLE 35–5. Representative Congenital Syndromes Causing Proportionate Short Stature

Syndrome	Common Features
Intrauterine onset of short stature	
Autosomal trisomy	
D (13–15)	Mental retardation, congenital heart disease, bilateral cleft palate and lip, microphthalmos, colobomas, holoprosencephaly
E (16–18)	Mental retardation, congenital heart disease, foot and hand deformities
Genetic	
Russell-Silver	Pseudohydrocephalus
Seckel's	Bird-headed (microcephaly, micrognathia, "beaked" nose), mental retardation
Cornelia de Lange's	Synophrys, small hands and feet
Williams	"Elfin" facies, supravalvular aortic stenosis, ± infantile hypercalcemia[139]
Leprechaunism	Congenital lipodystrophy, "puckish" facies, insulin resistance
Bloom	Photosensitive dermatitis with telangiectatic erythema, malar hypoplasia, small nose[138]
Congenital infection	
Rubella	Hepatosplenomegaly, pancytopenia, patent ductus arteriosus, cataract, deafness
Drugs	
Ethanol	Characteristic facies (short palpebral fissure length, thin upper lip, indistinct philtrum), microcephaly, mental retardation
Hydantoin	Hypertelorism, terminal digit hypoplasia, mental retardation, seizures
Postnatal onset of short stature	
Autosomal trisomy	
Down (21)	Mongoloid facies, hypotonia, mental retardation
Calcium disturbance	
Pseudohypoparathyroidism	Hypocalcemia, brachydactyly, "moon" facies, mental retardation
Genital abnormalities	
Smith-Lemli-Opitz	Male pseudohermaphroditism, microcephaly, syndactyly, characteristic facies
Aarskog	Scrotal anomalies, cryptorchidism, hand webbing, characteristic facies
Robinow's	Mesomelia, hemivertebrae
Bone anomalies	
Fanconi's	Radial aplasia, growth hormone deficiency[134]
Rubinstein-Taybi	Broad thumbs, antimongoloid eyes, hypoplastic maxilla, mental retardation[137]
Mucopolysaccharidoses	Bony deformities, corneal clouding, mental deterioration, ± hepatosplenomegaly
Contractures	
Freeman-Sheldon	"Whistling face," finger contractures, clubfeet
Moore-Federman	Joint limitation, short limbs
Premature senility	
Progeria (Hutchinson-Gilford)	Onset in infancy, characteristic facies, arteriosclerosis, lipodystrophy, mental retardation[133]
Cockayne's	Onset in early childhood, lipodystrophy, retinitis pigmentosa, photosensitivity, mental retardation, microcephaly[135]
Werner's	Onset in late childhood, characteristic facies, atherosclerosis, cataract
Skin and hair defects	
Poikiloderma congenita	"Marbled" pigmentation ± photosensitivity, cataract, ± ectodermal dysplasia
Sjogren-Larsson	Ichthyosis, spasticity

From Jones K: Smith's Recognizable Patterns of Human Malformation. Philadelphia, WB Saunders, 1988.

may resemble those in Turner's syndrome, the overall incidence of malformations is different, with predominantly right-sided cardiac lesions in Noonan's and left-sided lesions in Turner's syndrome (see Table 35–4). Patients with Noonan's syndrome have a better prognosis for gonadal function (delayed puberty rather than gonadal failure) and become somewhat taller than patients with Turner's syndrome, with adult heights averaging 162.5 cm in males and 152.7 cm in females.[141]

In Prader-Willi syndrome, short stature is associated with neonatal failure to thrive and hypotonicity, onset of obesity at about 2 years of age because of the development of a voracious appetite, intellectual impairment, and hypogonadism. It is associated with deletion of a critical region of the proximal part of the long arm of chromosome 15 in 70% of cases and unimaternal disomy of this region in the others[142, 143] (Fig. 35–14). Some may have GH deficiency. GH therapy may improve growth and weight, although the response to GH therapy is inconsistent.[144–146]

Russell-Silver syndrome is a term applied to some children with intrauterine growth retardation in association with dysmorphic features such as pseudohydrocephalus (a relatively large head with a small face), clinodactyly, and subtle body asymmetry. It is a heterogeneous condition. About half of patients with Russell-Silver syndrome simply have delayed puberty and reach a normal adult height,[147] but the remainder may be quite short.[148] Approximately 10% have uniparental disomy of maternal chromosome 7.[149]

Intrauterine growth retardation (IUGR) eventuates in postnatal short stature in approximately 10% to 15% of babies born small for gesta-tional age.[57, 66] Sometimes IUGR occurs as part of a distinct growth-retarding syndrome, such as Russell-Silver syndrome, or as part of a genetic disorder, such as congenital IGF-1 deficiency[150] or uniparental disomy of chromosomes 2, 6, 7, 9, 14, or 16.[149, 151] Congenital diabetes mellitus and insulin receptor mutations are uniformly associated with IUGR.[36, 58] Other cases of IUGR with ongoing growth failure postnatally are nonsyndromic and occur as the seemingly nonspecific result of such dissimilar disorders as maternal heroin addiction,[152] intrauterine infection,[153] placental insufficiency,[154] fetal malnutrition,[155, 156] or hypoxia-related congenital anomalies.[157] The common thread in these causes may be a decreased endowment in total body cell number.[158] However, unexplained IUGR may have genomic roots in view of the fact that uniparental disomy has occasionally only become apparent as the cause of IUGR when it unmasks an autosomal recessive trait.[151] Although some reports suggest that GH therapy increases growth in children with postnatal growth failure after IUGR, the overall benefit remains undetermined and responses are highly variable.[66, 159]

Undernutrition sufficient to reduce calorie intake below 82% to 91% of the recommended level will arrest growth.[160] This degree of undernutrition is suggested by weight below the 90th percentile for height and is associated with a body fat content of less than 10%.[98, 161] Undernutrition may result from inadequate nutrient intake (because of psychosocial feeding or eating disorders, poor appetite from chronic disease), excessive nutrient output (chronic vomiting or malabsorption as in inflammatory bowel disease, celiac disease, cystic fibrosis, or hepatic disease), or metabolic wastage (e.g., as in poorly controlled

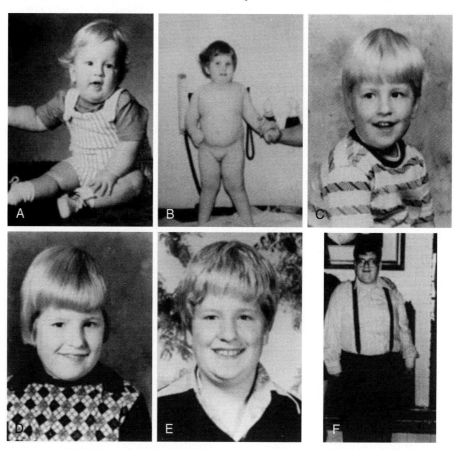

FIGURE 35–14. Evolution of the phenotype in Prader-Willi syndrome in a patient with a 15q deletion. *A,* 11 months; *B,* 2.5 years; *C,* 3.5 years; *D,* 7 years; *E,* 13 years; *F,* 27 years. (From Cassidy SB: Prader-Willi syndrome. J Med Genet 34:917–923, 1997.)

diabetes mellitus).[162, 163] A unique cause of malnutrition in infants is the diencephalic syndrome, which is characterized by a paucity of body fat resembling lipodystrophy in a hyperalert, otherwise healthy child. Radiosensitive brain tumors in the anterior hypothalamic area are the usual cause. Disturbance of the regulation of appetite, secretion of pituitary lipolytic hormones such as GH, or increased energy expenditure has been postulated as the mechanism.[164, 165] Deficiency of trace metals such as zinc and copper causes growth failure.[19, 20]

Metabolic disorders may affect growth. Either chronic acidosis[21] or chronic alkalosis[166] causes growth failure. Chronic anemia[167] and rickets cause a delayed growth pattern.[168, 169] A defect in zinc action has resulted in growth failure.[170]

Hormonal causes of growth failure are the final consideration. GH deficiency is the most difficult to diagnose because it may cause no phenotypic abnormalities other than slow linear growth. If untreated, GH deficiency can result in adults with proportionate extreme short stature (formerly termed "midgets"). Recent advances in our understanding of molecular loci influencing GH synthesis and secretion have elucidated specific etiologies of previously unexplained GH-related growth failure.

GH deficiency can be congenital or acquired and may be isolated or coexist with other pituitary hormone deficiencies (panhypopituitarism). Congenital forms of GH deficiency may be due to primary hypothalamic disorders (reflecting inadequate GHRH) or to primary pituitary defects. Hypothalamic disorders may be associated with midline defects such as septo-optic dysplasia (involving varying degrees of hypoplasia of the optic nerves, chiasm, and infundibular region of the hypothalamus), cleft palate, or a single central incisor.[171–174] Primary pituitary disorders include defects in the GH gene,[175] bioinactive GH,[176] mutations in the GHRH receptor gene,[177] and inactivating mutations of transcription factors essential for pituitary development, such as Pit-1,[178] Prop-1, and HESX-1.[178, 179] Most cases of isolated GH deficiency are currently considered idiopathic and occur in 1 in 3500 children.[180] Half of the cases of sporadic congenital GH deficiency are associated with hypoplasia or maldescent of the pituitary gland identified on magnetic resonance imaging as an ectopic posterior pituitary lobe.[181, 182]

Congenital GH deficiency may lead to neonatal hypoglycemia. The combination of neonatal hypoglycemia, prolonged neonatal jaundice, and in males, micropenis suggests panhypopituitarism.[183] Congenital GH deficiency may be manifested as short stature in early infancy or childhood. In addition to shortness, GH deficiency typically causes relative adiposity, reduced musculature, a cherubic appearance, and a high-pitched voice. However, these manifestations are not present in all children with the disorder. The diagnosis of GH deficiency should be considered in all children with subnormal growth velocity.

Acquired GH deficiency may result from head trauma, tumors such as craniopharyngioma, histiocytosis X, cranial irradiation, or chemotherapy.[184–188] These children show attenuation of growth after an initial period of normal growth.

Functional hypopituitarism is another form of acquired GH deficiency. The prototypic cause of this condition is the psychosocial deprivation syndrome. This "deprivation dwarfism" may be seen in children who are not malnourished or overtly disturbed but who show abnormal behavior patterns, including hyperphagia, hoarding food, drinking from toilets, or sleepwalking.[189–191] GH deficiency in this condition rapidly resolves in a nurturing environment. Anorexia nervosa may also occasionally cause functional GH deficiency.[192]

The diagnosis of GH deficiency classically rests on demonstration of a subnormal GH response to two or more provocative pharmacologic tests of GH reserve (i.e., a GH peak under 10 ng/dL using a polyclonal GH assay; monoclonal antibodies yield GH values that are about half the values of assays using polyclonal antisera[193]) in a child with slow growth velocity, delayed BA, and no other disorder to account for the slow growth. Provocative tests include arginine, L-dopa, clonidine, and insulin-induced hypoglycemia.[194, 195] Two pharmacologic tests are used because approximately 15% to 20% of apparently normal children have a poor response to a single given test of GH reserve. Untreated hypothyroidism, obesity, and glucocorticoid treatment may falsely lower GH levels. Sex steroid priming with estrogen or androgen for 1 to 7 days before the GH provocative test is sometimes used to distinguish GH deficiency from constitutional delay in growth and development.[196–198] Although this classic definition continues to have widespread support, concern has recently been raised because of potential false-positive and false-negative diagnoses when this approach is used and because of inconsistencies in GH assays.[196, 199-201] Alternative approaches have been proposed to diagnose forms of GH deficiency, such as neurosecretory defects and bioinactive GH. These approaches include 12- to 24-hour measurement of spontaneous GH secretion, measurement of IGF-1 and/or IGFBP-3, and therapeutic trials of GH. However, no single method has yet emerged as a gold standard alternative to the classic definition.[202] IGF-1 and IGFBP-3 levels are affected by undernutrition, chronic systemic diseases, and delayed puberty, and they must be interpreted in terms of age and pubertal stage[203, 204] (see Fig. 35-2). After the diagnosis of GH deficiency, magnetic resonance imaging is indicated to determine whether the hypopituitarism is due to structural lesions or tumors.

Recombinant GH therapy (0.18–0.3 mg/kg/week subcutaneously, divided daily or 6 days/week) is the standard treatment for GH deficiency and is remarkably successful in this condition (Fig. 35-15). In GH-deficient children treated with GH daily, the growth rate during the first year of treatment is on average 11.5 cm[205]; although it declines somewhat thereafter, it remains markedly above pretreatment growth velocity. Recombinant GH therapy is effective in bringing adult height into the normal range when it is begun early.[206] GH treatment also increases bone mass and lean tissue mass in children with GH deficiency.[207]

Potential adverse effects of recombinant GH include fluid retention (sometimes with cerebral edema), pancreatitis, glucose intolerance, transient gynecomastia, slipped capital femoral epiphysis, and growth of nevi.[208, 209] Concerns about leukemia and second tumors have not been confirmed among children who do not have other predisposing factors, although ongoing surveillance continues.[210-214] Growth deceleration associated with high-affinity, high-capacity antibodies to GH has been reported but appears to be very rare. Retinopathy has recently been described in patients with renal failure receiving GH to improve growth.[215] In addition to GH treatment, children with GH deficiency associated with other pituitary hormone deficiencies (i.e., panhypopituitarism) require adequate replacement of these hormones. A recent review of the Canadian experience suggests that adrenal insufficiency represents a potentially avoidable cause of death in children with panhypopituitarism.[216]

Traditionally, GH therapy for GH-deficient children has been stopped after adult height is reached and the epiphyses have fused. It is important to not discontinue GH therapy before secondary sex characteristics are advanced because GH potentiates sex hormone effects.[52, 217, 218] A major emerging issue is that of GH treatment beyond the end of linear growth; some studies indicate that low doses of GH improve metabolic status, body composition, and well-being in adults with GH deficiency.[196] Alternatives to standard GH therapy—including depot GH injections, GH-releasing factor, and oral secretagogues—are also available or under development.[219-222]

Although GH deficiency is the most common disorder of the GH-IGF axis that causes short stature, resistance to GH has also been described. GH insensitivity may be due to hereditary defects in the GH receptor (Laron syndrome and its variants).[223-225] Children with a mutant GH receptor have the same clinical manifestations as children with congenital GH deficiency, but they have elevated GH levels, low IGF-1 levels, and failure of GH to stimulate IGF generation. GH-binding protein is usually low because it is an alternatively spliced version of the GH receptor.[224] Inactivating mutation of IGF-1 differs from GH receptor defects in causing IUGR, deafness, and mental retardation.[150] Treatment with recombinant IGF-1 seems to be effective in these conditions.[223, 225, 226] IGF-1 receptor defects appear to account for the short stature of pygmies.[227, 228]

GH resistance may also be secondary to a variety of illnesses. This GH resistance may be due to malnutrition or inhibitors of GH action, among which are glucocorticoids. Antibodies to exogenous GH on rare occasion impair the response to GH therapy.[229]

Hypothyroidism in childhood invariably slows linear growth velocity and, if chronic, causes short stature and retards BA. Congenital hypothyroidism additionally causes profound mental retardation if not treated within the first 3 months of life. Fortunately, neonatal screening programs in many countries enable early detection and treatment of most cases. It is claimed that mild central hypothyroidism causes 10% of cases of idiopathic short stature.[230] The replacement dose of thyroid hormone in children averages 100 μg/m²/day.[231] Catch-up growth is expected after treatment of juvenile hypothyroidism if the diagnosis is made early.[81]

Glucocorticoid excess profoundly slows growth. Doses of cortisol above about 12 to 15 mg/m²/day (prednisone, 3–5 mg/m²/day) impair growth in normal prepubertal children.[45] Growth failure may be the only clear clinical sign of glucocorticoid excess in children.[232, 233] Cushing's syndrome is usually iatrogenic and results from supraphysiologic doses of glucocorticoid by any route, including topical. Endogenous glucocorticoid excess may be due to adrenal tumors (particularly in infants), primary pigmented nodular adrenocortical disease, bilateral adrenal hyperplasia secondary to adrenocorticotropic hormone (ACTH)-producing pituitary adenoma (Cushing's disease), or ectopic ACTH production. The growth attenuation with Cushing's syndrome of any cause contrasts with exogenous obesity, in which children tend to be tall. Significant virilization also occurs with adrenal tumors that secrete androgen as well as glucocorticoids, and growth inhibition may be counteracted by androgen.[234] The diagnosis of endogenous glucocorticoid excess is based on clinical evidence, assessment of suppressibility of endogenous glucocorticoids by exogenous glucocorticoid (dexamethasone suppression test), and radiologic studies to attempt localization of the lesion. Treatment of endogenous glucocorticoid excess focuses on removal or ablation of the underlying lesion (transsphenoidal removal of pituitary microadenoma in the case of Cushing's disease).[235-237] Early and effective treatment of glucocorticoid excess enables catch-up growth.[81] In cases in which growth inhibition is attributable to glucocorticoid treatment of nonendocrine disease, four alternative therapies may be tried: (1) use another form of therapy, (2) lower the daily steroid dose if the underlying disease can be controlled in this manner, (3) switch the patient to alternate-morning prednisone therapy,[238] or (4) switch the patient to topical (e.g., inhaled) steroid therapy.[239] Alternate-day "pulses" of prednisone or topical administration often results in preservation of the desired therapeutic effect while avoiding the unwanted cushingoid changes, but neither are certain solutions to the dilemma. GH therapy may partially counterbalance growth suppression caused by modest doses of glucocorticoid, with considerable variability in response.[48]

Chronic disorders of virtually any organ system may attenuate growth. Such attenuation results from inadequate nutritional intake,

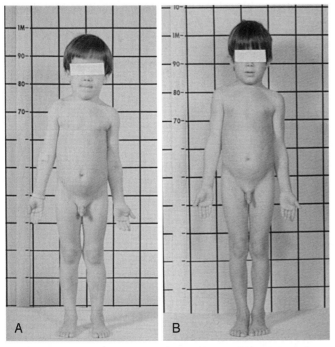

FIGURE 35–15. Growth hormone (GH)-deficient patient before *(A)* and after *(B)* treatment with GH for 1 year. Note that the growth spurt is accompanied by normal maturation of body proportions.

medication that stunts growth (such as supraphysiologic doses of glucocorticoids), secondary endocrine disorders, and organ dysfunction that disrupts growth processes. For example, chronic renal failure is associated with anorexia, anemia, acidosis, hypovitaminosis D, IGFBP retention, GH receptor deficiency, and inadequate (although elevated) compensatory GH secretion.[240-242] Primary gastrointestinal disturbances such as inflammatory bowel disease and celiac disease may cause short stature. The growth disturbance of congenital heart disease usually resolves with surgical correction,[243] but persistence of short stature in some cases suggests an intrinsic component to the short stature.[1, 158] Although the primary disorder is evident in many cases of short stature caused by chronic illness, short stature is sometimes the primary initial feature, notably in inflammatory bowel disease, celiac disease, and renal dysfunction.

The term *idiopathic short stature* (short stature of unknown cause) is sometimes used to include children who appear to have none of the above conditions. It typically includes children with familial intrinsic short stature, constitutional delay, or IUGR. Because the natural histories of these conditions differ, it is important to carefully examine entry criteria when assessing studies of treatment effectiveness for this "diagnosis."

Differential Diagnosis of Short Stature by Growth Pattern

To individualize the work-up of short stature, it is useful to classify patients according to the relationships among chronologic age, weight age, BA, and growth rate. These terms are defined in Table 35–2.

Diagnostic decisions can be simplified by first categorizing the disorder of growth with regard to whether it is a primary disturbance of weight (undernutrition) or height by the relationship between HA and weight age. If the child's weight age is depressed out of proportion to HA (e.g., weight below the 10th percentile for height), primary nutritional disorders or chronic disease should be the principal diagnostic considerations. If the height and weight are proportionately depressed (or height is depressed out of proportion to weight) genetic, endocrinologic, or metabolic disorders are more likely to be responsible.

Primary linear growth disturbances result from inherent aberrations in bone growth or systemic factors extrinsic to bone that affect its rate of growth. Disturbances in linear growth can be understood on the basis of three general principles: (1) normal linear growth during childhood proceeds toward a genetically determined target height by following a predictable channel that is achieved by the end of infancy, (2) normal bone growth is accompanied by a predictable rate of advance of BA, and (3) children normally enter puberty at a pubertal BA. Based on these principles, linear growth disturbances can be categorized into three growth patterns: *intrinsic* shortness, *delayed* growth, or *attenuated* growth[244] (Fig. 35–6 and Table 35–6).

Intrinsic shortness is characterized by an inherent limitation of bone growth that destines affected children to be short adults. By 3 years of age, the growth curves of these children are below but closely parallel to the normal percentiles, with growth rates within or close to the normal range. BA typically approximates chronologic age. Puberty occurs at a normal age (barring associated hypogonadism, as in Turner's syndrome). For example, a 9-year-old child with an HA of 6.5 and a BA of 9 years will be small as an adult. Examples of this growth pattern include normal-variant familial intrinsic short stature, Turner's syndrome, bone dysplasias, primary dysmorphic syndromes (such as Prader-Willi syndrome, Russell-Silver syndrome), severe IUGR-related short stature, and impaired spinal growth secondary to irradiation.

Children with a *delayed* growth pattern have delayed puberty and continue to grow longer than their peers do, thus typically reaching normal adult height. By 3 years of age, the growth curves of these children closely parallel the normal growth channels, with growth rates within or close to the normal range. In contrast to children with intrinsic shortness, BA is significantly delayed, typically to approximately the same extent as HA. For example, a 9-year-old child with an HA of 6.5 and a BA of 6.5 years ordinarily has normal growth potential.

Constitutional delay in growth and pubertal development is by far the most common cause of a delayed growth pattern. Other examples of conditions that may be associated with a delayed growth pattern are mild undernutrition and mild chronic disease, such as anemia and chronic asthma. Because familial intrinsic short stature and constitutional delay are each so common, they occur together about as often as they occur alone. When they coexist, the growth rate is likely to be slightly subnormal and resemble the attenuated pattern.

Children with an *attenuated* growth pattern have low growth rates that result in progressive deviation from their normal growth channels. BA is approximately equal to HA (or even less in hypothyroidism). The delayed BA indicates that adult height potential is normal—*if* the underlying disorder is treated effectively. Beyond 3 years of age this pattern virtually always indicates underlying pathology. However, these underlying disorders, unless optimally treated, preclude normal achievement of height potential. Thus a 9-year-old child with an HA and BA of 6.5 years who has subnormal growth velocity has an attenuated growth pattern; this child has an endocrine, metabolic, or systemic disease until proved otherwise. Examples of conditions causing this growth pattern are GH deficiency, hypothyroidism, glucocorticoid excess, severe chronic illness, and malnutrition. When this growth pattern develops after 10 to 12 years of age, hypogonadism and delayed puberty are major diagnostic considerations.

TABLE 35–6. Differential Diagnosis of Short Stature by Growth Pattern

Type of Growth Pattern	Bone Age Approximations	Growth Rate	Differential Diagnostic Categories

Intrinsic shortness	Chronologic age (BA ≃ CA > HA)	Approximates normal	Familial normal variant
			Genetic syndromes
			    Chromosomal anomalies
			    Bone dysplasia
			    Dysmorphic syndromes
			    Intrauterine growth retardation, nonspecific
			Spinal irradiation

Delayed growth	Height age (BA ≃ CA < HA)	Approximates normal	"Constitutional" normal variant Chronic disease Undernutrition

Attenuated growth	Height age (BA ≃ CA < HA)	Subnormal	Endocrinopathies
			    Growth hormone deficiency related
			    Hypothyroidism
			    Cushing's syndrome
			    Hypogonadism after 10–12 yr of age
			Acid-base disturbances
			Chronic disease, severe (e.g., Crohn's disease)
			Malnutrition

BA, bone age; CA, chronologic age; HA, height age.

Diagnostic Evaluation

Given the many potential causes of short stature, establishing a diagnosis depends on eliciting several features on the history, physical examination, and laboratory studies. Documentation of the growth rate and BA are key, as discussed in the previous section on growth patterns. If the child has a normal BA, indicating an intrinsically short growth pattern, it is important to seek a history of IUGR, the presence or absence of neonatal lymphedema (suggestive of Turner's syndrome), a history of tetany or seizures (compatible with pseudohypoparathyroidism), and a family history of short stature. Physical examination in this group of patients should be directed toward a search for body disproportion and dysmorphisms, as well as pubertal status. When the clinical assessment strongly suggests a particular diagnosis, appropriate and specific diagnostic tests, such as karyotype, gonadotropin and calcium levels, and a skeletal survey, can proceed.

In a child with significantly delayed BA indicating a delayed or attenuated growth pattern, review of systems should be comprehensive; it should focus on weight changes, appetite, food intolerance, vomiting, abdominal cramping, and stool characteristics; genitourinary symptoms, particularly polyuria and enuresis; as well as headache and visual disturbances (suggestive of a central nervous system lesion), lethargy or cold intolerance (suggestive but not necessarily present in hypothyroidism), and pubertal development. The past medical history and history of the use of medications, particularly glucocorticoids in any form, may be important. The classic triad for congenital hypopituitarism is perinatal hypoglycemia, prolonged jaundice, and in boys, micropenis. A family history of delay of puberty or extreme short stature should be sought. A careful general physical examination should be performed. Specific features on physical examination include the weight-height ratio, a search for finger clubbing or perianal sores (inflammatory bowel disease), funduscopy and examination of visual fields (to assess perichiasmatic central nervous system lesions such as craniopharyngiomas), assessment for goiter, and pubertal staging.

Constitutional delay in growth and development is principally a diagnosis of exclusion and, in extreme cases, is difficult to distinguish from isolated defects of gonadotropin or GH production. While puberty is delayed, the growth rate may fall to subnormal levels. Testing shows a delayed BA, and the IGF-1 level remains at a prepubertal level, compatible with the BA. Gonadotropin secretion may remain in the prepubertal range until BA has reached 11 to 12 years. The distinction between hypogonadism and delayed puberty can often be made by determination of gonadotropin levels during sleep or in response to a gonadotropin-releasing hormone (GnRH) agonist test by 14 years of age.[245] GH tests may be compatible with GH deficiency unless performed after sex steroid priming.[196–198] Indeed, transient GH deficiency is sometimes associated with delayed puberty.

When the clinical assessment strongly suggests a particular diagnosis, appropriate and specific diagnostic tests can proceed. If the weight is below the 10th percentile for height, it may be difficult to distinguish undernutrition from constitutional underweight. Calorie counting, the sweat test, and screening tests for occult chronic disease may be helpful. These tests include a complete blood count, chemistry profile, erythrocyte sedimentation rate, and antiendomysial antibodies. The great majority of patients with inflammatory bowel disease and short stature will have anemia, an elevated sedimentation rate, or hypoalbuminemia; an upper gastrointestinal series may be necessary for diagnosis.

If the cause of poor growth is still not clear but the child's growth rate is subnormal (i.e., leading to an attenuated growth pattern) or the child's height is markedly below age-appropriate standards or the family target height, additional tests to assess possible hypothyroidism (free thyroxine, thyrotropin), GH deficiency (IGF-1, IGFBP-3, provocative tests of GH reserve such as clonidine, L-dopa, arginine, insulin), and in girls, karyotype for assessment of Turner's syndrome are indicated. Controversies in interpretation of diagnostic tests for GH deficiency are described at the beginning of this section. Less common tests are generally based on clinical suspicion of the underlying condition (e.g., methylation analysis to diagnose Prader-Willi syndrome).

Not uncommonly, previous measurements are unavailable and the child's pattern of growth is not clear, although the child seems healthy overall. In this situation, it would be reasonable to monitor the child's height at regular intervals to establish a pattern of growth that dictates whether further tests are indicated.

Management

When at all possible, treatment should be directed at the primary cause of pathologic short stature. Examples include nutritional counseling for undernutrition, a gluten-free diet for celiac disease, psychotherapy for eating disorders, thyroid hormone for hypothyroidism, and GH for GH deficiency. Many disorders are hereditary; genetic counseling should not be overlooked. Surgical lengthening of congenitally short legs is a controversial option.[245a]

For conditions considered normal variants (familial short stature, constitutional delay), reassurance and explanation of the wide range of normal are often very helpful. In discussing therapeutic options, the child and family must be advised about the unknown factors (for example, errors are inherent in height predictions). Many parents and children often choose to forgo medical intervention at this point.

Low-dose sex steroid therapy is indicated for the treatment of hypogonadism if puberty is delayed beyond 13 (girls) or 14 (boys) years of age.[246, 247] In extreme cases of constitutional delay, this modality is useful for a limited period to boost self-image by advancing secondary sex characteristics gently with a mild corresponding growth spurt. To minimize the possibility of loss of growth potential, we recommend that the initial course of therapy for the induction of sexual development consist of six monthly injections of 50 mg/m^2 of repository testosterone in boys and 0.2 mg depot estradiol in girls.[53, 247] Such a course of therapy has no deleterious effect on height potential and has positive effects on self-image. The patient's growth, development, and predicted height should be carefully re-evaluated immediately on completion of the therapeutic regimen and again 6 months later before undertaking a second course of therapy. Depot testosterone, 100 mg/m^2/month, and depot estradiol, 1.0 mg/month, closely approximate midpubertal sex hormone production in boys and girls, respectively. We prefer administering injections of repository forms of sex hormones to avoid the occasional side effects of 17-alkylated steroid analogues. However, the anabolic steroid oxandrolone, 0.1 mg/kg/day for 3 to 6 months, has been used without compromising final height.[248] Premature use of adult replacement doses of androgen or estrogen (about twofold greater than the midpubertal doses) will cause a disproportionate advance of BA relative to linear growth and compromise height potential. Children with delayed puberty should be monitored closely from 10 years of age onward because particularly in the most severely delayed cases with the most immature body proportions, puberty inexplicably occurs at an earlier than expected BA, which leads to children falling well short of predicted height.[113, 246]

GH therapy is currently approved by the Food and Drug Administration for the treatment of short stature caused by GH deficiency (0.18–0.3 mg/kg/week, divided into daily subcutaneous doses), Turner's syndrome (up to 0.375 mg/kg/week), and chronic renal failure before kidney transplantation (up to 0.35 mg/kg/week).[144] Varying lines of data suggest that long-term GH therapy may promote growth in a variety of other conditions (including IUGR, Noonan's syndrome, Prader-Willi syndrome, bone dysplasias, spina bifida, idiopathic short stature), although findings in these conditions have been inconsistent.[113, 145, 188, 249–258] Together, these issues have raised the suggestion of therapeutic trials of GH for children with short stature caused by conditions not traditionally treated with GH. However, difficulties remain regarding criteria for assessing trial outcomes and regarding the translation of short-term data on growth velocity into longer-term height gains for individual children. Medical, ethical, and policy issues concerning GH therapy for nontraditional indications are reviewed elsewhere.[144, 160, 259–267a]

Because long-term GnRH agonist therapy is successful in improving the adult height of children with idiopathic sexual precocity by delaying epiphyseal fusion, as discussed at the end of this chapter, attempts have been made to use this therapy as a nonstandard method to promote growth in children with idiopathic short stature. The final height prognosis after 2 years of treatment was improved by 1.0 ±

2.3 (SD) cm, which is statistically significant but of limited efficacy.[268] The height prognosis in isolated GH deficiency seems to be improved by adding GnRH agonist to GH therapy.[269, 270] Although significant improvement in the predicted height of normal short children was achieved by 2 years of combined GH and GnRH agonist therapy, final height was not significantly increased.[271] A report suggests that prolonged therapy modestly improves the outcome.[272]

Tall Stature

Causes of Tall Stature

Genetic normal variants cause most cases of tall stature (Table 35–7). Two distinct familial variants can be identified that lead to different outcomes in tall children. One variant is *familial intrinsic tall stature* (sometimes called genetic tallness): children are typically normal size at birth and a high-normal growth rate is established by 3 years of age. Thus the child typically crosses the height percentile during the first 3 years of life and thereafter maintains a height-attained channel above and closely parallel to the 95th percentile. Children with *constitutionally advanced growth and pubertal development* grow similarly during childhood, but they have an advanced BA and go into puberty early, so they stop growing at a normal height. Both these groups of children have a family history of a similar growth pattern, and the child does not show clinical or biochemical features of the disorders described below.

Genetic and chromosomal disorders are known causes of tall stature. Hyperploidy of sex chromosomes predisposes to tall stature.[5] The most common of these disorders is Klinefelter's syndrome (47,XXY), which is characterized by long-legged proportions dating from the prepubertal years, as well as hypogonadism. The prototypic genetic syndrome associated with tall stature is Marfan syndrome, which usually segregates with mutations in the fibrillin gene.[5, 273] It is classically characterized by musculoskeletal signs (such as arachnodactyly and hyperextensibility), cardiovascular findings (such as aortic aneurysm), ocular signs (such as lens subluxation), and autosomal dominant heredity. Arachnodactyly can be quantitated from either the body proportions or the metacarpal index (ratio of the length to the midshaft breadth of metacarpals II to V; normal: male <8.0:1, female <8.7:1) on a BA radiograph. Congenital contractural arachnodactyly is a genetically closely related syndrome. Homocystinuria is associated with marfanoid features but may also involve mental retardation, joint contractures, and a tendency to thromboembolism. Sipple's syndrome (type 2 poly-

endocrine syndrome) may also have marfanoid features; the presence of mucosal neuromas may be a specific clue to its presence.

Cerebral gigantism (Sotos' syndrome) is characterized by the presence of acromegaloid facial features usually associated with developmental retardation; GH dynamics are normal.[274] Most affected persons are long and slender at birth; all grow rapidly in early childhood with a slightly advanced BA, and they reach an above average, occasionally excessive adult height. It can be mimicked by fragile X syndrome. Macrocephaly is characteristic of other congenital overgrowth disorders such as Weaver's syndrome.[275]

The prototypic congenital macrosomia syndrome is Beckwith-Weidemann syndrome. The most consistent features are overgrowth, macroglossia, umbilical defects ranging from hernia to omphalocele, and earlobe pits. Hyperplasia of various visceral (especially the kidney) and endocrine organs (especially pancreatic β cells) is the rule. Birth size is above average, growth velocity is high until midchildhood, and adult height is 2.5 SD above normal. These children are predisposed to embryonal intra-abdominal tumors in early childhood, most commonly Wilms' tumor and adrenocortical carcinoma. The disorder is associated with loss of heterozygosity at chromosomal locus 11p15.5 as a result of duplications, translocation/inversion, uniparental disomy, or mutation of the CDKI p57[KIP2], which causes an imbalance between the function of growth-promoting genes such as IGF-2 and tumor suppressor genes on this imprinted region.[276] The Simpson-Golabi-Behmel syndrome is similar in having macrosomia, macroglossia, omphalocele, and Wilms' tumor, but it has a different pattern of associated features, such as "bulldog" facies, polydactyly, fingernail hypoplasia, even greater adult height.[34] It is caused by an X-linked mutation of glypican-3, a receptor that modulates IGF-2 action.

Lipodystrophy, particularly the total forms, whether congenital or acquired, are associated with tall stature.[277] Insulin resistance is frequently so severe that it causes pseudoacromegaly, and hyperlipidemia is prominent.

Overnutrition (exogenous obesity) during childhood typically accelerates growth slightly and advances BA comparably to HA. IGF-1 levels are normal in the presence of low GH levels.[25]

Hormonal disorders of GH, sex steroids, and thyroid hormone can cause tall stature. *GH excess i*s a rare, but important cause of accelerated growth. This condition, termed gigantism during childhood, may be associated with acromegaloid features in older children[278, 279] (Fig. 35–16). It is usually due to a pituitary somatotroph adenoma or to somatotroph hyperplasia. Activating mutations of $G_{s\alpha}$ have been described in isolated pituitary adenomas and in patients with McCune-

TABLE 35–7. Factors Causing Tall Stature, with Representative Clinical Conditions

Factors Affecting Height	Representative Conditions	Clinical and Laboratory Features
Genetic		
Normal variants	Familial intrinsic tallness	Growth parallels 95th percentile; family history of tall stature; normal physical examination, puberty, and BA
	Constitutionally advanced	Growth parallels 95th percentile; puberty and BA slightly advanced
Chromosomal abnormalities	Klinefelter's syndrome	Hypogenitalism and hypogonadism, eunuchoid; 47,XXY
	Fragile X syndrome	Mental retardation; macro-orchidism in males
Dysmorphic syndromes	Marfan syndrome	Arachnodactyly, hyperextensibility, lens subluxation, aortic dilation
	Beckwith-Wiedemann syndrome	Infant gigantism, macroglossia, umbilical defects, neonatal hypoglycemia from pancreatic β cell hyperplasia, embryonal tumors may develop
	Cerebral gigantism	Sotos' syndrome: dolichocephalic large head, coarse facies, cerebral dysfunction
Nutrition		
Primary obesity		IGF-1 blood level nutrition driven, "growth without GH"
Hormones		
GH excess		Accelerated growth, acromegaloid signs with advancing age, occasional hyperprolactinemia; may be associated with McCune-Albright syndrome
Hyperthyroidism		Hypermetabolic features, goiter, eye abnormalities
Sex steroid	Excess	Precocious puberty: premature secondary sexual characteristics and epiphyseal fusion leading to compromise in adult height
	Deficiency	Deficiency beyond teenage years permits prolonged growth and eunuchoid habitus

BA, bone age; GH, growth hormone; IGF-1, insulin-like growth factor-1.

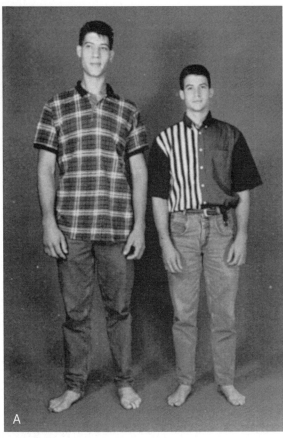
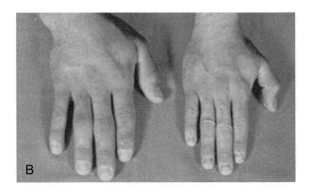
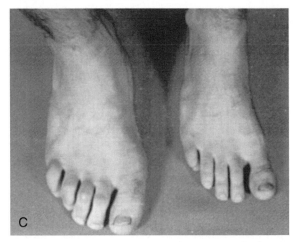

FIGURE 35–16. Pituitary gigantism. A 22-year-old-man with gigantism caused by excess growth hormone is shown to the left of his identical twin. The increased height *(A)* and enlarged hand *(B)* and foot *(C)* of the affected twin are apparent. Their height and features began to diverge at approximately 13 years of age. (From Gagel RF, McCutcheon IE: Images in clinical medicine. Pituitary gigantism. N Engl J Med 340:524, 1999. Copyright © 1999 Massachusetts Medical Society. All rights reserved.)

Albright syndrome associated with hypersecretion of hormones such as GH.[261, 280] Hyperprolactinemia may coexist.

Hyperthyroidism accelerates bone growth and maturation.[277] Affected infants may have premature cranial synostosis.[281]

Sexual precocity accelerates height. Classically, BA is stimulated disproportionately, which leads to premature epiphyseal fusion. Thus these children become tall but stop growing prematurely, so their adult height is stunted. However, slowly progressive forms of precocious puberty do not necessarily deleteriously affect adult height.[282]

Sex hormone deficiency, conversely, prolongs the growing period because the epiphyses do not close. This condition leads to increased height and eunuchoid proportions in hypogonadal individuals.[283] Through the discovery of patients deficient in aromatase or with an inactivating mutation of the estrogen receptor, estradiol has been found to be the critical hormone that brings about epiphyseal fusion.[50]

Differential Diagnosis of Tall Stature by Growth Pattern

Because supranormal height occurs as a result of either inherent endowment or excessive stimulation of the rate of bone growth, the diagnostic approach based on the relationships of chronologic age, HA, BA, and growth velocity is analogous to that described for short stature. Four patterns of growth causing tall stature can be distinguished: intrinsic tallness, advanced growth, accelerated growth, and prolonged growth[244, 284] (Table 35–8, Fig. 35–17).

Intrinsic tallness is the term applied to literally long-boned individuals. They come to grow above, but approximately parallel to the 95th percentile on height-attained curves. Their BA and age of puberty are normal. This condition is usually a normal variant (familial intrinsic tallness), but it is rarely due to genetic disorders such as Marfan syndrome or homocystinuria.

Advanced growth is a pattern with similar growth in childhood; the growth velocity of such children maintains them approximately parallel to the 95th percentile on height-attained curves, but they go into puberty early and thus stop growing at a normal size. This pattern is indicated by a BA advanced in proportion to HA. Examples include normal variant (constitutionally advanced), obesity, and hyperthyroidism. Mild forms of sexual precocity also cause this growth pattern.

Accelerated growth refers to a pattern in which the growth rate is excessive. Adult height is abnormal unless the underlying disorder is corrected; it is subnormal in rapidly progressive sexual precocity, excessive in GH excess.

Prolonged growth results from a deficiency of sex hormones, particularly estrogen.[50] Such patients continue growing into adulthood.

Diagnostic Evaluation

A tall child whose height parallels the 95th percentile and has tall parents, no dysmorphic features, a normal pace of puberty, and normal BA is likely to have *intrinsic tallness* on a familial basis without a pathologic cause. Further investigations are often not needed. However, chromosomal disorders, Marfan syndrome, homocystinuria, and occasionally, excessive GH can simulate the clinical picture. The presence of dysmorphic features, macro-orchidism, or intellectual impairment in a tall child suggests the need for chromosome analysis, plasma amino acid assay, or genetics consultation to evaluate these possibilities.

A tall child with an *advanced growth pattern* (i.e., BA advanced in proportion to HA) is likely to have "constitutional" normal-variant tallness—particularly if the height parallels the 95th percentile, a compatible family history is present, and the clinical examination is otherwise normal. Because hyperthyroidism may mimic these findings, the clinical examination includes evaluation for goiter, ophthalmologic

TABLE 35–8. **Differential Diagnosis of Tall Stature by Growth Pattern**

Type of Growth Pattern	Bone Age Relationships	Growth Rate	Differential Diagnostic Categories

Intrinsic tallness	BA ≃ CA < HA	Approximates normal	Familial tallness
			Chromosomal disorders
			  XXY, fragile X, XXX
			  XYY
			  8p trisomy
			Genetic disorders
			  Marfanoid syndromes
			  Cerebral gigantism syndromes
			  Congenital macrosomia syndromes

Advanced growth	BA ≃ HA > CA	Approximates normal	"Constitutional" normal variant Obesity Lipodystrophy Hyperthyroidism
Accelerated growth	BA > HA > CA	Supranormal	Sexual precocity
	BA ≤ HA > CA	Supranormal	GH or IGF excess
Prolonged growth	BA < HA > CA	Normal	Hypogonadism Estrogen deficiency

BA, bone age; CA, chronologic age; GH, growth hormone; HA, height age; IGF, insulin-like growth factor.

abnormalities, and hypermetabolism; thyroid function studies will provide confirmation. Exogenous obesity, in the absence of dysmorphic features or intellectual impairment, may cause this pattern of tall stature. In the absence of puberty or symptoms or signs suggestive of a hypothalamic disturbance or hypoglycemia, the tall stature virtually excludes an endocrine basis.

An *accelerated growth pattern* (involving progressive deviation of height above the 95th percentile and an advanced BA) requires assessment for sexual precocity, including clinical assessment of primary and secondary sexual characteristics, as well as evaluation for the possibility of central nervous system disorders or abdominal masses and a search for nevi and bone deformities. If the BA is significantly advanced, screening should commence with determination of blood levels of estradiol, testosterone, dehydroepiandrosterone sulfate, gonadotropins (preferably in a third-generation assay), and possibly serum human chorionic gonadotropin. Screening for excessive GH secretion should be initiated with random GH, IGF-1, and IGFBP-3 blood levels. The definitive test for the diagnosis of GH excess is failure of serum GH to become suppressed below 2 ng/mL after an oral glucose load (1.75 g/kg, maximum of 100 g), although some false-positive tests have been reported.[278] Hyperprolactinemia often exists together with GH excess. The most reliable confirmatory test is one of suppressibility of serum GH after a glucose load. If evidence of GH excess is noted, serum GHRH may be measured (to assess the rare possibility of ectopic GHRH production) and appropriate imaging studies performed. The possibilities of McCune-Albright syndrome, multiple endocrine adenomatosis type I, and carcinoid syndrome should also be considered in children and adolescents with GH excess.

A *prolonged growth pattern* suggests sex hormone deficiency or resistance. Evaluation of pubertal development, sense of smell (to evaluate for Kallmann's syndrome), and body proportions (an eunuchoid habitus with long legs and a low upper-lower body segment ratio is characteristic of sex hormone deficiency) is needed. Laboratory studies include ascertainment of circulating sex hormone and gonadotropin levels, chromosome analysis, and—when indicated—imaging studies.

Management

Because familial intrinsic tall stature represents a variant of normal, reassurance and support are needed. In certain cases (particularly predicted adult height in excess of 183 cm for girls), familial tall stature may be particularly distressing, and treatment to curtail growth by accelerating epiphyseal fusion can be undertaken. Estrogen in large

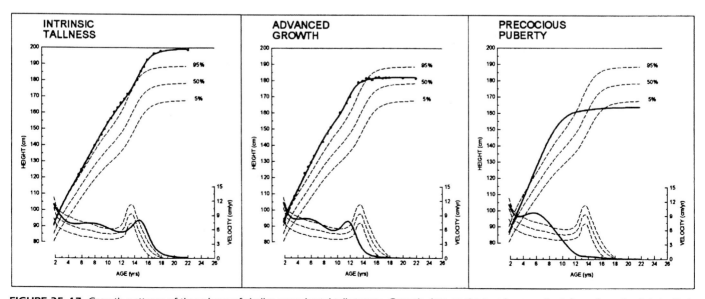

FIGURE 35–17. Growth patterns of three boys of similar prepubertal tall stature. Growth data on the two boys on the left are from the Fels Institute files. One became a tall adult (intrinsic tall stature); the other grew to be of normal adult height after undergoing an early pubertal growth spurt (advanced height). Growth data on the boy with precocious puberty are derived from the data of Thamdrup.[284] (Courtesy of R.D. Bock.)

amounts (e.g., 0.3 mg/day of ethinyl estradiol) can be begun just before or early in puberty, be given daily without interruption, and be continued until epiphyseal fusion has occurred. A progesterone-like compound (e.g., medroxyprogesterone acetate, 10 mg) daily for the first 10 days of each month is also given to yield regular menses. Potential risks of estrogen therapy include thrombosis, hyperlipidemia, glucose intolerance, nausea, mild hypertension, and weight gain. Although evidence indicates that estrogen therapy can reduce adult height as much as 3.5 to 7.3 cm below that predicted, the results cannot be ensured.[285, 286] The use of high-dose estrogen in otherwise normal children must be weighed against the potential adverse effects, including the risk of venous thromboembolism, especially when risk factors for thrombosis are present.[286, 286a] Somatostatin analogue may be an alternative treatment to reduce adult height in selected cases; some authors have reported comparable treatment with estrogen for girls with Marfan syndrome, androgen insensitivity, and other overgrowth problems.[285] Depot testosterone in highly virilizing doses (about 400 mg every 2 weeks) has been used to reduce predicted adult height in selected tall boys, but experience is limited.[285]

Hypersecretion of GH from pituitary adenomas is generally treated by surgery and/or a somatostatin analogue. Pituitary radiation has also been used. Pituitary hyperplasia causing GH excess (as in McCune-Albright syndrome) can be treated with somatostatin analogues. In ectopic GHRH-producing tumors, surgical removal is the first treatment of choice.

The compromised height potential resulting from gonadotropin-dependent sexual precocity is treated by suppressing gonadotropins with long-acting GnRH agonists. The most widely used agents in the United States are leuprolide (ordinarily given as a monthly depot intramuscular injection) and nafarelin (a twice-daily nasal spray). Treatment is effective when started at an early age, with an average height gain above pretreatment height prediction of about 1.4 cm for each year of therapy.[287] Coincident GH deficiency must be treated for optimal growth.[270] Furthermore, GH-sufficient patients with central precocity who start treatment relatively late and whose height velocity falls below the prepubertal normal range after 2 to 3 years gain an average of 2 cm/year when GH therapy is added.[288] Otherwise, premature puberty is treated by specific therapy where possible, for example, cortisol replacement for congenital adrenal hyperplasia or inhibitors of steroidogenesis for McCune-Albright syndrome. Conversely, sex hormones can be replaced in sex hormone deficiency.

REFERENCES

1. Cheek DB: Human Growth. Philadelphia, Lea & Febiger, 1968.
2. Winick M, Noble A: Quantitative changes in DNA, RNA, and protein during prenatal and postnatal growth in the rat. Dev Biol 12:451–466, 1965.
3. Orlowski CC, Furlanetto RW: The mammalian cell cycle in normal and abnormal growth. Endocrinol Metab Clin North Am 25:491–502, 1996.
4. Meredith JE Jr, Winitz S, Lewis JM, et al: The regulation of growth and intracellular signaling by integrins. Endocr Rev 17:207–220, 1996.
5. Sotos JF: Overgrowth. Section IV. Genetic disorders associated with overgrowth. Clin Pediatr (Phila) 36:39–49, 1997.
6. Kosho T, Muroya K, Nagai T, et al: Skeletal features and growth patterns in 14 patients with haploinsufficiency of SHOX: Implications for the development of Turner syndrome. J Clin Endocrinol Metab 84:4613–4621, 1999.
7. Lindgren V: Genomic imprinting in disorders of growth. Endocrinol Metab Clin North Am 25:503–521, 1996.
8. De Luca F, Baron J: Control of bone growth by fibroblast growth factors. Endocrinologist 10:61–65, 1999.
9. Tanner JM: Growth at Adolescence. London, Blackwell, 1962, p 130.
10. Abbott RD, White LR, Ross GW, et al: Height as a marker of childhood development and late-life cognitive function: The Honolulu-Asia aging study. Pediatrics 102:602–609, 1998.
11. Hommes FA, Drost YM, Geraets WXM, Reijenga MAA: The energy requirement for growth: An application of Atkinson's metabolic price system. Pediatr Res 9:51, 1975.
12. Holt LE Jr: Some problems in dietary amino acid requirements. Am J Clin Nutr 21:367, 1968.
13. Fisch RO, Gravem HJ, Feinberg SB: Growth and bone characteristics of phenylketonurics. Comparative analysis of treated and untreated phenylketonuric children. Am J Dis Child 112:3–10, 1966.
14. Cahill CF Jr: Nitrogen versatility in bats, bears, and man. N Engl J Med 290:686, 1974.
15. Holman RT: Essential fatty acid deficiency. Prog Chem Fats Lipids 9:275, 1968.
16. Chesney RW: Requirements and upper limits of vitamin D intake in the term neonate, infant, and older child. J Pediatr 116:159–166, 1990.
17. Clement DH, Fomon SJ, Forbes GB, et al: Trace elements in infant nutrition. Pediatrics 26:715, 1960.
18. Ulmer DD: Trace elements. N Engl J Med 297:318–321, 1977.
19. Nakamura T, Nishiyama S, Futagoishi-Suginohara Y, et al: Mild to moderate zinc deficiency in short children: Effect of zinc supplementation on linear growth velocity. J Pediatr 123:65–69, 1993.
20. Danks DM, Campbell PE, Walker-Smith J, et al: Menkes kinky-hair syndrome. Lancet 1:1100, 1972.
21. Cooke RE, Boyden DG, Haller E: The relationship of acidosis and growth retardation. J Pediatr 57:326, 1960.
22. Viteri FE: The effect of inactivity on the growth of rats fed diets adequate or restricted with respect to normal caloric intake. In New Concepts about Old Aspects of Malnutrition. Academia Mexicana de Pediatria, 1973.
23. Schaff-Blass E, Burstein S, Rosenfield RL: Advances in diagnosis and treatment of short stature, with special reference to the role of growth hormone. J Pediatr 104:801–813, 1984.
24. Cuttler L: The regulation of growth hormone secretion. Endocrinol Metab Clin North Am 25:541–572, 1996.
25. Giustina A, Veldhuis JD: Pathophysiology of the neuroregulation of growth hormone secretion in experimental animals and the human. Endocr Rev 6:717–797, 1998.
26. Wallis M: Growth hormone–binding proteins. Clin Endocrinol 35:291–293, 1991.
27. Walker JL, Moats-Staaats BM, Stiles AD, Underwood LE: Tissue-specific developmental regulation of the messenger ribonucleic acids encoding the growth hormone receptor and the growth hormone binding protein in rat fetal and postnatal tissues. Pediatr Res 31:335–339, 1992.
28. Spagnoli A, Rosenfeld RG: The mechanisms by which growth hormone brings about growth: The relative contributions of growth hormone and insulin-like growth factors. Endocrinol Metab Clin North Am 25:615–631, 1996.
28a. Le Roith D, Butler AA: Insulin-like growth factors in pediatric health and disease. J Clin Endocrinol Metab 84:4355–4361, 1999.
29. Clark PA, Rogol AD: Growth hormones and sex steroid interactions at puberty. Endocrinol Metab Clin North Am 25:665–682, 1996.
30. Roemmich JN, Clark PA, Mai V, et al: Alterations in growth and body composition during puberty: III Influence of maturation, gender, body composition, fat distribution, aerobic fitness, and energy expenditure on nocturnal growth hormone release. J Clin Endocrinol Metab 83:1440–1447, 1998.
31. Rosenfield RL, Furlanetto R: Physiologic testosterone or estradiol induction of puberty increases plasma somatomedin-C. J Pediatr 107:415, 1985.
32. Daughaday WH, Rotwein P: Insulin-like growth factors I and II peptide, messenger ribonucleic acid and gene structures, serum, and tissue concentrations. Endocr Rev 10:68–91, 1989.
33. D'Ercole AJ: Insulin-like growth factors and their receptors in growth. Endocrinol Metab Clin North Am 25:573–590, 1996.
34. Weksberg R, Squire JA, Templeton DM: Glypicans: A growing trend. Nat Genet 12:225–227, 1996.
35. Pao C-I, Farmer PK, Begovic S, et al: Regulation of insulin-like growth factor-I (IGF-I) and IGF-binding protein 1 gene transcription by hormones and provision of amino acids in rat hepatocytes. Mol Endocrinol 7:1561–1568, 1993.
36. Menon RK, Sperling MA: Insulin as a growth factor. Endocrinol Metab Clin North Am 25:633–648, 1996.
37. Schalch DS, Heinrich UE, Draznin B, et al: Role of the liver in regulating somatomedin activity: Hormonal effects on the synthesis and release of insulin-like growth factor and its carrier protein by the isolated perfused rat liver. Endocrinology 104:1044, 1979.
38. Argente J, Caballo N, Barrios V, et al: Multiple endocrine abnormalities of the growth hormone and insulin-like growth factor axis in prepubertal children with exogenous obesity: Effect of short-and long-term weight reduction. J Clin Endocrinol Metab 82:2076–2083, 1997.
39. Juul A, Holm K, Kastrup KW, et al: Free insulin-like growth factor I serum levels in 1430 healthy children and adults, and its diagnostic value in patients suspected of growth hormone deficiency. J Clin Endocrinol Metab 82:2497–2502, 1997.
40. Van Den Brande JL, DeCaju MVL: Plasma somatomedin activity in children with growth disturbances. In Raiti S (ed): Advances in Human Growth Hormone Research. Washington, DC, US Government Printing Office, 1974, p 98.
41. Quarmby V, Quan C, Ling V, et al: How much insulin-like growth factor I (IGF-I) circulates? Impact of standardization on IGF-I assay accuracy. J Clin Endocrinol Metab 83:1211–1216, 1998.
42. Heins JN, Carland JI, Daughaday WH: Incorporation of ^{35}S-sulfate into rat cartilage explants in vitro: Effects of aging on responsiveness to stimulation by sulfation factor. Endocrinology 87:688, 1970.
43. Collett-Solberg PF, Cohen P: The role of the insulin-like growth factor binding proteins and the IGFBP proteases in modulating IGF action. Endocrinol Metab Clin North Am 25:591–614, 1996.
44. Phillips LS, Fusco AC, Unterman TC, del Creco F: Somatomedin inhibitor in uremia. J Clin Endocrinol Metab 59:764, 1984.
45. Allen DB: Growth suppression by glucocorticoid therapy. Endocrinol Metab Clin North Am 25:699–717, 1996.
46. Geffner ME: The growth without growth hormone syndrome. Endocrinol Metab Clin North Am 25:649–664, 1996.
47. Weiss RE, Refetoff S: Effect of thyroid hormone on growth: Lessons from the syndrome of resistance to thyroid hormone. Endocrinol Metab Clin North Am 25:719–730, 1996.
48. Allen DB, Julius JR, Breen TJ, Attie KM: Treatment of glucocorticoid-induced growth suppression with growth hormone. J Clin Endocrinol Metab 83:2824–2829, 1998.
49. Canalis E: Inhibitory actions of glucocorticoids on skeletal growth. Is local insulin-like growth factor I to blame (editorial)? Endocrinology 139:3041–3042, 1998.
50. Bachrach BE, Smith EP: The role of sex steroids in bone growth and development: Evolving new concepts. Endocrinologist 6:362–368, 1996.
51. Abu AO, Horner A, Kusec V, et al: The localization of androgen receptors in human bone. J Clin Endocrinol Metab 82:3493–3497, 1997.

52. Zachmann M, Prader A, Sobel E, et al: Pubertal growth in patients with androgen insensitivity: Indirect evidence for the importance of estrogens in pubertal growth of girls. J Pediatr 108:694–697, 1986.

53. Rosenfeld RL, Perovic N, Devine N, et al: Optimizing estrogen replacement treatment in Turner syndrome. Pediatr 102:486–488, 1998.

54. Rosenfeld R: Low-dose testosterone effect on somatic growth. Pediatrics 77:853–857, 1986.

55. Rosenfeld RL: Role of androgens in growth and development of the fetus, child, and adolescent. Adv Pediatr 19:171, 1972.

56. Styne DM: Fetal growth. Clin Perinatol 25:917–938, 1998.

57. Hay WW Jr, Catz CS, Grave GD, Yaffe SJ: Workshop summary: Fetal growth: Its regulation and disorders. Pediatrics 99:585–591, 1997.

58. Gluckman PD: The endocrine regulation of fetal growth in late gestation: The role of insulin-like growth factors. J Clin Endocrinol Metab 80:1047–1050, 1994.

59. Lubchenco LO, Hansman C, Dressler M, Boyd E: Intrauterine growth as estimated from liveborn birth-weight data at 24 to 42 weeks gestation. Pediatrics 32:793, 1963.

60. Thomson AM, Billewicz WZ, Hytten FE: The assessment of fetal growth. J Obstet Gynaecol Br Commonw 75:90, 1968.

61. Wingerd V, Schoen EJ: Factors influencing length at birth and height at five years. Pediatrics 53:737, 1974.

62. Beck GJ, van der Berg BJ: The relationship of the rate of intrauterine growth of low-birth-weight infants to later growth. J Pediatr 86:504, 1975.

63. Gardoni J, Chang A, Kalyan B, et al: Customized antenatal growth charts. Lancet 339:283–287, 1991.

64. Yip R, Binkin NJ, Trowbridge FL: Altitude and childhood growth. J Pediatr 113:486–489, 1988.

65. Schinzel AGI, Smith DW, Miller JR: Monozygotic twinning and structural defects. J Pediatr 95:921, 1979.

66. de Zegher F, Francois I, van Helvoirt M, Van den Berghe G: Small as fetus and short as child: From endogenous to exogenous growth hormone. J Clin Endocrinol Metab 82:2021–2026, 1997.

67. Smith DW, Popick C: Large fontanels in congenital hypothyroidism. A potential clue toward earlier recognition. J Pediatr 80:753, 1972.

68. Lassarre C, Hardouin S, Daffos F, et al: Serum insulin like growth factors and insulin-like growth factor binding proteins in the human fetus. Relationships with growth in normal subjects and in subjects with intrauterine growth retardation. Pediatr Res 29:219, 1991.

69. Naeye RL, Dixon JB: Distortions in fetal growth standards. Pediatr Res 12:987, 1978.

70. Pryse-Davies J, Smithan JH, Napier KA: Factors influencing development of secondary ossification centres in the fetus and newborn. Arch Dis Child 59:425, 1974.

71. Shaffer SG, Quimiro CL, Anderson JV, Hall RT: Postnatal weight changes in low birth weight babies. Pediatrics 79:702, 1983.

72. Hamill PVV, Drizd TA, Johnson CL, et al: Physical growth: National Center for Health Statistics Percentiles. Am J Clin Nutr 32:607, 1979.

73. Karlberg J: On the construction of the infancy-childhood-puberty growth standard. Acta Paediatr Scand Suppl 356:26–37, 1989.

74. Smith DW, Truog W, Rogers JE, et al: Shifting linear growth during infancy: Illustration of genetic factors in growth from fetal life through infancy. J Pediatr 89:225–230, 1976.

75. Reed RB, Stuart HC: Patterns of growth in height and weight from birth to eighteen years of age. Pediatrics 29:904, 1959.

76. Bock RD, Rosenfield RL: Course-of-growth norms for longitudinal height velocity. Hummanbiol Budapest 25:575–586, 1994.

77. Tanner JM, Whitehouse RH, Takaishi M: Standards from birth to maturity for height, weight, height velocity, and weight velocity: British children, 1960. Arch Dis Child 41:454, 1966.

78. Tanner JW, Davies PWS: Clinical longitudinal standards for height and height velocity for North American children. J Pediatr 107:317–329, 1985.

79. Bock RD, Thissen D: Statistical problems of fitting individual growth curves. *In* Johnson F, Roche A (eds): Human Physical Growth and Maturation. New York, Plenum, 1980, p 265.

80. Tanner J, Goldstein H, Whitehouse R: Standards for children's height at ages 2–9 years allowing for height of parents. Arch Dis Child 45:755, 1970.

81. Boersma B, Wit JM: Catch-up growth. Endocr Rev 18:646–661, 1997.

82. Glinos AD: Density dependent regulation of growth and differentiated function in suspension cultures of mouse fibroblasts. *In* Kulonen E, Pikkarainen J (eds): Biology of Fibroblast. New York, Academic, 1973, p 155.

83. Tillmann V, Thalange NK, Foster PJ, et al: The relationship between stature, growth, and short-term changes in height and weight in normal prepubertal children. Pediatr Res 44:882–886, 1998.

84. Shuttleworth FK: Sexual maturation and physical growth of girls age six to nineteen. Monogr Soc Res Child Dev 2:5, 1937.

85. Cara JF, Rosenfield RL, Furlanetto RW: A longitudinal study of the relationship of plasma somatomedin-C concentration to the pubertal growth spurt. Am J Dis Child 41:562–564, 1987.

86. Tanner JM, Whitehouse RH, Marshall WA, Carter BS: Prediction of adult height, bone age, and occurrence of menarche, at ages 4 to 16 with allowance for midparent height. Arch Dis Child 50:14, 1975.

87. Bayley N, Pinneau S: Tables for predicting adult height from skeletal age: Revised for use with the Gruelich-Pyle hand standards. J Pediatr 40:432–441, 1952.

88. Barr GD, Allen CM, Shinefield HR: Height and weight of 7500 children of three skin colors. Am J Dis Child 124:866, 1972.

89. Schumacher LB, Pawson IG, Kretchmer N: Growth of immigrant children in newcomer schools of San Francisco. Pediatrics 80:861, 1987.

90. McKusick VA: Heritable Disorders of Connective Tissue. St Louis, Mosby, 1972.

91. Engelbach W: Endocrine Medicine. Springfield, IL, Charles C Thomas, 1932, p 261.

92. Maresh MM: Linear growth of long bones of extremities from infancy through adolescence. Am J Dis Child 89:725, 1955.

93. Jones K: Smith's Recognizable Patterns of Human Malformation. Philadelphia, WB Saunders, 1988.

94. Nellhaus G: Head circumference from birth to eighteen years. Pediatrics 41:106, 1968.

95. Weaver DD, Christian JC: Familial variation of head size and adjustment for parental head circumference. J Pediatr 96:990–994, 1980.

96. Krieger I: Head circumference, mental retardation and growth failure. Pediatrics 37:384, 1966.

97. Cloutier MD, Stickler GB: Head circumference in children with idiopathic hypopituitarism. Pediatrics 42:209–210, 1968.

98. Frisch RE, McArthur JW: Menstrual cycles: Fatness as a determinant of minimum weight for height necessary for their maintenance or onset. Science 185:949–951, 1974.

99. Rolland-Cachera M, Sempe M, Guilloud-Bataille M, et al: Adiposity indices in children. Am J Clin Nutr 36:178–184, 1982.

100. Hammer LD, Wilson DM, Litt IF, et al: Impact of pubertal development on body fat distribution among white, Hispanic, and Asian female adolescents. J Pediatr 118:975–980, 1991.

101. Holliday MA: Fluid and electrolyte disturbances in pediatrics. *In* Maxwell MH, Kleeman CR (eds): Clinical Disorders of Fluid and Electrolyte Metabolism. New York, McGraw-Hill, 1962.

102. Butler AM, Richie RH: Simplification and improvement in estimating drug dosage and fluid and dietary allowances for patients of varying sizes. N Engl J Med 262:903, 1960.

103. Rosenstein SN: The teeth. *In* Barnett H (ed): Pediatrics. New York, Appleton-Century-Crofts, 1977, p 931.

104. Bongiovanni AM, Moshang T Jr, Parks JS: Maturtional deceleration after treatment of congenital adrenal hyperplasia. Helv Paediatr Acta 28:127, 1973.

105. Gruelich WW, Pyle SI: Radiographic Atlas of Skeletal Development of the Hand and Wrist. Palo Alto, CA, Stanford University Press, 1959.

106. Wilkins L: The Diagnosis and Treatment of Endocrine Disorders in Childhood and Adolescence. Springfield, IL, Charles C Thomas, 1965.

107. Roche AF, Eyman SL, Davila GH: Skeletal age prediction. J Pediatr 78:997, 1971.

108. Baer MJ, Durkatz J: Bilateral asymmetry in skeletal maturation of the hand and wrist. Am J Phys Anthopol 15:180, 1957.

109. Tanner J, Oshman D, Bahhage F, Healy M: Tanner-Whitehouse bone age reference values for North American children. J Pediatr 131:34–40, 1997.

110. Garn SM, Sanduskjy ST, Nagy JM, McCann MB: Advanced skeletal development in low-income Negro children. J Pediatr 80:965, 1972.

111. Frisancho AR, Garn SM, Rohmann CG: Age at menarche: A new method of prediction and retrospective assessment based on hand x-rays. Hum Biol 41:42, 1969.

112. Bayer LM, Bayley N: Growth pattern shifts in healthy children spontaneous and induced. J Pediatr 62:631, 1963.

113. Hintz RL, Attie KM, Baptista J, Roche A: Effect of growth hormone treatment on adult height of children with idiopathic short stature. N Engl J Med 340:502–507, 1999.

114. Roche A, Wainer H, Thissen D: The RWT method for the prediction of adult stature. Pediatrics 62:631, 1975.

115. Ahima RS, Dushay J, Flier SN, et al: Leptin accelerates the onset of puberty in normal female mice. J Clin Invest 99:391–395, 1997.

116. Cronk C, Crocker AC, Pueschel SM, et al: Growth charts for children with Down syndrome: 1 month to 18 years of age. Pediatrics 81:102–110, 1988.

117. Rosenfeld RG, Attie KM, Frane J, et al: Growth hormone therapy of Turner's syndrome: Beneficial effect on adult height. J Pediatr 132:319–324, 1998.

118. Saenger P: Turner syndrome. Curr Ther Endocrinol Metab 6:239–243, 1997.

119. Pasquino AM, Passeri F, Pucarelli I, et al: Spontaneous pubertal development in Turner syndrome. J Clin Endocrinol Metab 82:1810–1813, 1997.

120. Summitt RL: Turner syndrome and Noonan's syndrome. J Pediatr 75:730–731, 1969.

121. Carballo EC: Turner syndrome and Noonan's syndrome. J Pediatr 75:729–730, 1969.

122. Curts FL, Pucci E, Scappaaticci S, et al: XO and male phenotype. Am J Dis Child 128:90, 1974.

123. Heller RH: The Turner phenotype in the male. J Pediatr 66:48, 1965.

124. Noonan's syndrome. Lancet 340:22–23, 1992.

125. Health supervision for children with Turner syndrome. American Academy of Pediatrics. Committee on Genetics. Pediatrics 96:1166–1173, 1995.

126. Horton WA: Molecular genetic basis of the human chondrodysplasias. Endocrinol Metab Clin North Am 25:683–696, 1996.

127. Vajo Z, Francomano CA, Wilkin DJ: The molecular and genetic basis of fibroblast growth factor 3 disorders: The achondroplasia family of skeletal dysplasias, Muenke craniosynostosis, and Crouzon syndrome with acanthosis nigricans. Endocrin Rev 21:23–39, 2000.

128. Fanconi S, Fischer JA, Wieland P, et al: Kenny syndrome: Evidence for idiopathic hypoparathyroidism in two patients and for abnormal parathyroid hormone in one. J Pediatr 109:469, 1986.

129. Schipani E, Langman CB, Parfitt AM, et al: Constitutively activated receptors for parathyroid hormone and parathyroid hormone–related peptide in Jansen's metaphyseal chondrodysplasia. N Engl J Med 335:708–714, 1996.

130. Silverman RN: Caffey's Pediatric X-Ray Diagnosis. Chicago, Year Book, 1985.

131. Shapiro F: Epiphyseal disorders. N Engl J Med 317:1702–1710, 1987.

132. Weinstein LS, Yu S: The role of genomic imprinting of Gsa in the pathogenesis of Albright hereditary osteodystrophy. Trends Endocrinol Metab 10:81–85, 1999.

133. Allsop RC, Vaziri H, Patterson C, et al: Telomere length predicts replicative capacity of human fibroblasts. Proc Natl Acad Sci U S A 89:10114–10118, 1992.

134. Zachman M, Illig R, Prader A: Fanconi's anemia with isolated growth hormone deficiency. J Pediatr 80:159, 1972.

135. Sugita K, Arima M, Iai M, et al: UV or X-ray sensitivity of cells from Cockayne syndrome. No To Hattatsu 18:286–291, 1986.

136. Epstein CJ, Martin GM, Schultz SL, Motulsky AG: Werner's syndrome. Medicine (Baltimore) 45:177, 1966.

137. Petrij F, Giles RH, Dauwerse HG, et al: Rubinstein-Taybi syndrome caused by mutations in the transcriptional co-activator CBP. Nature 376:348–351, 1995.

138. Keller C, Keller KR, Shew SB, Plon SE: Growth deficiency and malnutrition in Bloom syndrome. J Pediatr 134:472–479, 1999.

139. Partsch C-J, Dreyer G, Gosch A, et al: Longitudinal evaluation of growth, puberty, and bone maturation in children with Williams syndrome. J Pediatr 134:82–89, 1999.

140. Tonoki H, Saitoh S, Kobayashi K: Patient with del(12)(q12q13.12) manifesting abnormalities compatible with Noonan syndrome. Am J Med Genet 75:416–418, 1998.

141. Ranke MB, Heidemann P, Knupfer C, et al: Noonan syndrome: Growth and clinical manifestations in 144 cases. Eur J Pediatr 148:220–227, 1988.

142. Holm VA, Cassidy SB, Butler MG, et al: Prader-Willi syndrome: Consensus diagnostic criteria. Pediatrics 91:398–402, 1993.

143. Cassidy SB: Prader-Willi syndrome. J Med Genet 34:917–923, 1997.

144. Furlanetto RW, Allen DB, Gertner JM, et al: Guidelines for the use of growth hormone in children with short stature: A report by the Drug and Therapeutics Committee of the Lawson Wilkins Pediatric Endocrine Society. J Pediatr 127:857–867, 1995.

145. Carrel AL, Myers SE, Whitman BY, Allen DB: Growth hormone improves body composition, fat utilization, physical strength and agility, and growth in Prader-Willi syndrome: A controlled study. J Pediatr 134:215–221, 1999.

146. Lindgren AC, Hagenaas L, Muller J, et al: Growth hormone treatment of children with Prader-Willi syndrome affects linear growth and body composition favorably. Acta Paediatr 87:28–31, 1998.

147. Saal HM, Pagon RA, Pepin MG: Reevaluation of Russell-Silver syndrome. J Pediatr 107:733–737, 1985.

148. Davies PS, Valley R, Preece MA: Adolescent growth and pubertal progression in the Silver-Russell syndrome. Arch Dis Child 63:130–135, 1988.

149. Eggermann T, Wollmann HA, Kuner R, et al: Molecular studies in 37 Silver-Russell syndrome patients: Frequency and etiology of uniparental disomy. Hum Genet 100:415–419, 1997.

150. Woods KA, Camacho-Hubner C, Savage MO, Clark AJL: Intrauterine growth retardation and postnatal growth failure associated with deletion of the insulin-like growth factor I gene. N Engl J Med 335:1363–1367, 1996.

151. Spiro RP, Christian SL, Ledbetter D, et al: Intrauterine growth retardation associated with maternal uniparental disomy for chromosome 6 unmasked by congenital adrenal hyperplasia. Pediatr Res 46:510–513, 1999.

152. Kandall SR, Albin S, Lowinson J, et al: Differential effects of maternal heroin and methadone use on birthweight. Pediatrics 58:681–685, 1976.

153. Chiriboga-Klein S, Oberfield SE, Casullo AM, et al: Growth in congenital rubella syndrome and correlation with clinical manifestations. J Pediatr 115:251–255, 1989.

154. Soothill P, Nicolaides KH, Bilardo CM, Campbell S: Relation of fetal hypoxia in growth retardation to mean blood velocity in the fetal aorta. Lancet 2:1118, 1986.

155. Bergner L, Susser MW: Low birth weight and prenatal nutrition: An interpretative review. Pediatrics 46:946–966, 1970.

156. Naeye RL, Blanc W, Paul C: Effects of maternal nutrition on the human fetus. Pediatrics 52:494–503, 1973.

157. Naeye R: Organ abnormalities in a human parabiotic syndrome. Am J Pathol 46:299, 1965.

158. Medovy H: New parameters in neonatal growth-cell number and cell size. J Pediatr 711:951, 1967.

159. Chernausek SD: The growth hormone/insulin-like growth factor axis in intrauterine growth retardation: Pathophysiological and therapeutic implications. Endocrinologist 6:294–300, 1996.

160. Sandberg DE, Smith MM, Fornari V, et al: Nutritional dwarfing: Is it a consequence of disturbed psychosocial functioning? Pediatrics 88:926–933, 1991.

161. Pugliese MT, Lifshitz F, Grad G, et al: Fear of obesity. A cause of short stature and delayed puberty. N Engl J Med 309:513–518, 1983.

162. Winter RJ, Phillips LS, Green OC, Traisman HS: Somatomedin activity in the Mauriac syndrome. J Pediatr 97:598–600, 1980.

163. Taylor AM, Sharma AK, Avasthy N, et al: Inhibition of somatomedin-like activity by serum from streptozotocin-diabetic rats: Prevention by insulin treatment and correlation with skeletal growth. Endocrinology 121:1360–1365, 1987.

164. Addy DP, Hudson FP: Diencephalic syndrome of infantile emaciation. Analysis of literature and report of further 3 cases. Arch Dis Child 47:338–343, 1972.

165. Vlachopapadopoulou E, Tracey KJ, Capella M, et al: Increased energy expenditure in a patient with diencephalic syndrome. J Pediatr 122:922, 1993.

166. Simopoulos AP, Bartter FC: Growth characteristics and factors influencing growth in Bartter's syndrome. J Pediatr 81:56, 1972.

167. Platt OS, Rosenstock W, Espeland MA: Influence of sickle hemoglobinopathies on growth and development. N Engl J Med 311:7, 1984.

168. Glorieux FH: Rickets, the continuing challenge (editorial). N Engl J Med 325:1875–1877, 1991.

169. Alon U, Donaldson DL, Hellerstein S, et al: Metabolic and histologic investigation of the nature of nephrocalcinosis in children with hypophosphatemic rickets and in the Hyp mouse. J Pediatr 120:899–905, 1991.

170. Sampson B, Kovar IZ, Rauscher A, et al: A case of hyperzincemia with functional zinc depletion: A new disorder? Pediatr Res 42:219–225, 1997.

171. Ellenberger C, Runyan TE: Holoprosencephaly with hypoplasia of the optic nerve, dwarfism and agenesis of the septum pellucidum. Am J Ophthalmol 70:960, 1970.

172. Rudman D, Davis T, Priest JH, et al: Prevalence of growth hormone deficiency in children with cleft lip or palate. J Pediatr 93:378–382, 1978.

173. Roessler E, Belloni E, Gaudenz L, et al: Mutations in the human sonic hedgehog gene cause holoprosencephaly. Nat Genet 14:357–360, 1996.

174. Berry SA, Pierpont ME, Gorlin RJ: Solitary maxillary central incisor and short stature. J Pediatr 104:877, 1984.

175. Wagner JK, Eble A, Hindmarsh PC, Mullis PE: Prevalence of human GH-1 gene alterations in patients with isolated growth hormone deficiency. Pediatr Res 43:105–110, 1998.

176. Takahashi Y, Kaji H, Okimura Y, et al: Brief report: Short stature caused by a mutant growth hormone [published erratum appears in N Engl J Med 1996 May 2;334(18):1207]. N Engl J Med 334:432–436, 1996.

177. Gertner JM, Wajnrajch MP, Leibel RL: Genetic defects in the control of growth hormone secretion. Horm Res 49(suppl):9–14, 1998.

178. Cohen LE, Wondisford FE, Radovick S: Role of Pit-1 in the gene expression of growth hormone, prolactin, and thyrotropin. Endocrinol Metab Clin North Am 25:523–540, 1996.

179. Parks JS, Brown MR, Hurley DL, et al: Heritable disorders of pituitary development. J Clin Endocrinol Metab 84:4362–4370, 1999.

180. Lindsay R, Feldkamp M, Harris D, et al: Utah growth study: Growth standards and the prevalence of growth hormone deficiency. J Pediatr 125:29–35, 1994.

181. Triulzi F, Scotti G, di Natale B, et al: Evidence of a congenital midline brain anomaly in pituitary dwarfs: A magnetic resonance imaging study in 101 patients. Pediatrics 93:409–416, 1994.

182. Bozzola M, Adamsbaum C, Biscaldi I, et al: Role of magnetic resonance imaging in the diagnosis and prognosis of growth hormone deficiency. Clin Endocrinol 45:21–26, 1996.

183. Choo-Kang LR, Sun CC, Counts DR: Cholestasis and hypoglycemia: Manifestations of congenital anterior hypopituitarism. J Clin Endocrinol Metab 81:2786–2789, 1996.

184. Newman CB, Levine LS, New MI: Endocrine function in children with intrasellar and suprasellar neoplasms. Am J Dis Child 135:259, 1981.

185. Thomsett MJ, Conte FA, Kaplan SL, Grumbach MM: Endocrine and neurologic outcome in childhood craniopharyngioma: Review of effect of treatment in 42 patients. J Pediatr 97:728, 1980.

186. Sklar CA, Grumbach MM, Kaplan SL, Conte FA: Hormonal and metabolic abnormalities associated with central nervous system germinoma in children and adolescents and the effect of therapy: Report of 10 patients. J Clin Endocrinol Metab 52:9–16, 1981.

187. Shalet SM: Radiation and pituitary dysfunction (editorial). N Engl J Med 328:131–133, 1993.

188. Román J, Villaizdán CJ, Garcia-Foncillas J, et al: Growth and growth hormone secretion in children with cancer treated with chemotherapy. J Pediatr 131:105–112, 1997.

189. Silver HK, Finkelstein M: Deprivation dwarfism. J Pediatr 70:317, 1967.

190. Powell GF, Brasel JA, Blizzard RM: Emotional deprivation and growth retardation simulating idiopathic hypopituitarism. I Clinical evaluation of the syndrome. N Engl J Med 276:1271–1278, 1967.

191. Skuse D, Albanese A, Stanhope R, et al: A new stress-related syndrome of growth failure and hyperphagia in children, associated with reversibility of growth-hormone insufficiency. Lancet 348:353–358, 1996.

192. Huseman C, Johanson A: Growth hormone deficiency in anorexia nervosa. J Pediatr 87:946–948, 1975.

193. Blethen SL, Chasalow FI: Use of a two-site immunoradiometric assay for growth hormone (GH) in identifying children with GH-dependent growth failure. J Clin Endocrinol Metab 57:1031, 1983.

194. Frasier SD: A review of growth hormone stimulation tests in children. Pediatrics 53:979, 1974.

195. Cara JF, Johanson AJ: Growth hormone for short stature not due to classic growth hormone deficiency. Pediatr Clin North Am 37:1229–1254, 1990.

196. Shalet SM, Toogood A, Rahim A, Brennan BMDI: The diagnosis of growth hormone deficiency in children and adults. Endocr Rev 19:203–223, 1998.

197. Moll GW Jr, Rosenfield RL, Fang VS: Administration of low-dose estrogen rapidly and directly stimulates growth hormone production. Am J Dis Child 140:124–127, 1986.

198. Marin G, Domene HM, Barnes KM, et al: The effects of estrogen priming and puberty on the growth hormone response to standardized treadmill exercise and arginine-insulin in normal girls and boys. J Clin Endocrinol Metab 79:537–541, 1994.

199. Rosenfeld RG, Albertsson-Wikland K, Cassorla F, et al: Diagnostic controversy: The diagnosis of childhood growth hormone deficiency revisited. J Clin Endocrinol Metab 80:1532–1540, 1995.

200. Ghigo E, Bellone J, Aimaretti G, et al: Reliability of provocative tests to assess growth hormone secretory status. Study in 472 normally growing children. Endocrinol Metab 81:3323–3327, 1996.

201. Carel JC, Tresca J-P, Letrait M, et al: Growth hormone testing for the diagnosis of growth hormone deficiency in childhood: A population register–based study. J Clin Endocrinol Metab 82:2117–2121, 1997.

202. Rose SR, Ross JL, Uriarte M, et al: The advantage of measuring stimulated as compared with spontaneous growth hormone levels in the diagnosis of growth hormone deficiency. N Engl J Med 319:201–207, 1988.

203. Juul A, Dalgaard P, Blum WF, et al: Serum levels of insulin-like growth factor (IGF)-binding protein-3 (IGFBP-3) in healthy infants, children, and adolescents: The relation to IGF-I, IGF-II, IGFBP-1, IGFBP-2, age, sex, body mass index, and pubertal maturation. J Clin Endocrinol Metab 80:2534–2542, 1995.

204. Oliv ié MAA, Garcia-Mayor R, Leston DG, et al: Serum insulin-like growth factor (IGF) binding protein-3 and IGF-I levels during childhood and adolescence. A cross-sectional study. Pediatr Res 38:149–155, 1995.

205. MacGillivray MH, Baptista J, Johanson A: Outcome of a four-year randomized study of daily versus three times weekly somatotropin treatment in prepubertal naive growth hormone–deficient children. Genetech Study Group. J Clin Endocrinol Metab 81:1806–1809, 1996.

206. Blethen SL, Baptista J, Kuntze J, et al: Adult height in growth hormone (GH) deficient children treated with biosynthetic GH. The Genentech Growth Study Group. J Clin Endocrinol Metab 82:418–420, 1997.

207. Boot AM, Engels MA, Boerma GJ, et al: Changes in bone mineral density, body composition, and lipid metabolism during growth hormone (GH) treatment in children with GH deficiency. J Clin Endocrinol Metab 82:2423–2428, 1997.

208. Blethen SL, Allen DB, Graves D, et al: Safety of recombinant deoxyribonucleic

acid–derived growth hormone: The National Cooperative Growth Study experience. J Clin Endocrinol Metab 80:1704–1710, 1996.

209. Malozowski S, Tanner LA, Wysowski D, Fleming GA: Growth hormone, insulin-like growth factor I, and benign intracranial hypertension (letter). N Engl J Med 329:665–666, 1993.

210. Fradkin J, Mills J, Schonberger L, et al: Risk of leukemia after treatment with pituitary growth hormone. JAMA 270:2829–2832, 1993.

211. Nishi Y, Tanaka T, Takano K, et al: Recent status in the occurrence of leukemia in growth hormone-treated patients in Japan. J Clin Endocrinol Metab 84:1961–1965, 1999.

212. Shalet SM, Brennan BM, Reddingius RE: Growth hormone therapy and malignancy. Horm Res 48(suppl):29–32, 1997.

213. Moshang T Jr, Rundle AC, Graves DA, et al: Brain tumor recurrence in children treated with growth hormone: The National Cooperative Growth Study experience. J Pediatr 128(suppl):4–7, 1996.

214. Moshang T Jr, Grimberg A: The effects of irradiation and chemotherapy on growth. Endocrinol Metab Clin North Am 25:731–742, 1996.

215. Koller DA, Green L, Gertner JM, et al: Retinal changes mimicking diabetic retinopathy in two nondiabetic, growth hormone–treated patients. J Clin Endocrinol Metab 83:2380–2383, 1998.

216. Taback SP, Dean HJ: Mortality in Canadian children with growth hormone (GH) deficiency receiving GH therapy 1967–1992. J Clin Endocrinol Metab 81:1693–1696, 1996.

217. Zachman MM, Prader A: Anabolic and androgenic effect of testosterone on sexually immature boys and its dependency on growth hormone. J Clin Endocrinol Metab 40:85, 1970.

218. Rilemma JA: Development of the mammary gland and lactation. Trends Endocrinol Metab 5:149, 1994.

219. Johnson OL, Cleland JL, Lee HJ, et al: A month-long effect from a single injection of microencapsulated human growth hormone. Nat Med 2:795–799, 1996.

220. Smith RG, Van der Ploeg LH, Howard AD, et al: Peptidomimetic regulation of growth hormone secretion. Endocr Rev 18:621–645, 1997.

221. Pihoker C, Badger TM, Reynolds GA, et al: Treatment effects of intranasal growth hormone releasing peptide-1 in children with short stature. J Endocrinol 155:79–86, 1997.

222. Thorner M, Rochiccoli P, Collee M, et al: Once daily subcutaneous growth hormone–releasing hormone therapy accelerates growth in growth hormone deficient children during the first year of therapy. J Clin Endocrinol Metab 81:1189–1196, 1996.

223. Rosenbloom AL, Rosenfeld RG, Guevara-Aguirre J: Growth hormone insensitivity. Pediatr Clin North Am 44:423–442, 1997.

224. Attie KM, Carlsson LM, Rundle AC, Sherman BM: Evidence for partial growth hormone insensitivity among patients with idiopathic short stature. The National Cooperative Growth Study. J Pediatr 127:244–250, 1995.

225. Guevara-Aguirre J, Rosenbloom AL, Vasconez O,et al: Two-year treatment of growth hormone (GH) receptor deficiency with recombinant insulin-like growth factor I in 22 children: Comparison of two dosage levels and to GH-treated GH deficiency. J Clin Endocrinol Metab 82:629–633, 1997.

226. Backeljauw PF, Underwood LE: Prolonged treatment with recombinant insulin-like growth factor I in children with growth hormone insensitivity syndrome—a clinical research center study. J Clin Endocrinol Metab 81:3312–3317, 1996.

227. Van Wyk JJ, Smith EP: Insulin-like growth factors and skeletal growth: Possibilities for therapeutic interventions. J Clin Endocrinol Metab 84:4349–4354, 1999.

228. Heath-Monnig E, Wohltmann HJ, Mills-Dunlap B, Daughaday WH: Measurement of insulin-like growth factor I (IGF-I) responsiveness of fibroblasts of children with short stature: Identification of a patient with IGF-I resistance. J Clin Endocrinol Metab 64:501–507, 1987.

229. Kaplan SL, Savage DCL, Suter S, et al: Antibodies to human growth hormone arising in patients treated with human growth hormone: Incidence, characteristics, and effects on growth. *In* Raiti S (ed): Advances in Human Growth Hormone Research. Washington, DC, US Government Printing Office, 1974, 725.

230. Pitukcheewanont P, Rose SR: Nocturnal TSH surge: A sensitive diagnostic test for central hypothyroidism in children. Endocrinologist 7:226–232, 1997.

231. Rezvani I, DiGeorge AM: Reassessment of the daily dose of oral thyroxine for replacement therapy in hypothyroid children. J Pediatr 90:291–297, 1977.

232. Lee PA, Weldon W, Migeon CV: Short stature as the only clinical sign of Cushing's syndrome. J Pediatr 86:89, 1975.

233. McArthur RG, Hayles AB, Salassa RM: Growth retardation in Cushing disease. J Pediatr 96:783–784, 1979.

234. Shahidi NT, Crigler JF Jr: Evaluation of growth and/or endocrine systems in testosterone-corticosteroid–treated patients with aplastic anemia. J Pediatr 70:233, 1967.

235. Leinung MC, Zimmerman D: Cushing's disease in children. Endocrinol Clin North Am 23:629–639, 1994.

236. Leinung MC, Kane LA, Scheithauer BW, et al: Long-term follow-up for transsphenoidal surgery for the treatment of Cushing's disease in childhood. J Clin Endocrinol Metab 80:2475–2479, 1995.

237. Styne DM, Grumbach MM, Kaplan SL: Treatment of Cushing's disease in childhood and adolescence by transsphenoidal microadenomectomy. N Engl J Med 310:889, 1984.

238. Soyka LF: Alternate-day corticosteroid therapy. Adv Pediatr 19:47, 1972.

239. Hollman GA, Allen DB: Overt glucocorticoid excess due to inhaled corticosteroid therapy. Pediatrics 81:452–455, 1988.

240. Schaefer F, Veldhuis JD, Stanhope R, et al: Alterations in growth hormone secretion and clearance in peripubertal boys with chronic renal failure and after renal transplantation. J Clin Endocrinol Metab 78:1298–1306, 1994.

241. Potter DE, Greifer I: Statural growth of children with renal disease. Kidney Int 14:334–339, 1978.

242. Tonshoff B, Cronin MJ, Reichert M, et al: Reduced concentration of serum growth hormone (GH)-binding protein in children with chronic renal failure: Correlation

with GH insensitivity. The European Study Group for Nutritional Treatment of Chronic Renal Failure in Childhood. The German Study Group for Growth Hormone Treatment in Chronic Renal Failure. J Clin Endocrinol Metab 82:1007–1013, 1997.

243. Schuurmans FM, Pulles-Heintzberger CFM, Gerver WJM, et al: Long-term growth of children with congenital heart disease: A retrospective study. Acta Paediatr 87:1250–1255, 1998.

244. Rosenfield RL: Essentials of growth diagnosis. Endocrinol Metab Clin North Am 25:743–758, 1996.

245. Ghai K, Cara JF, Rosenfield RL: Gonadotropin releasing hormone agonist (nafarelin) test to differentiate gonadotropin deficiency from constitutionally delayed puberty in teen-age boys—a clinical research center study. J Clin Endocrinol Metab 80:2980–2986, 1995.

245a. Gross R: Leg lengthening. Lancet 354:1574–1575, 1999.

246. Albanese A, Stanhope R: Predictive factors in the determination of final height in boys with constitutional delay of growth and puberty. J Pediatr 126:545–550, 1995.

247. Rosenfield RL: Diagnosis and management of delayed puberty. J Clin Endocrinol Metab 70:559–562, 1990.

248. Tse W-Y, Buyukgebiz A, Hindmarsh PC, et al: Long-term outcome of oxandrolone treatment in boys with constitutional delay of growth and puberty. J Pediatr 117:588, 1990.

249. Oberfield S: Growth hormone use in normal, short children—a plea for reason. N Engl J Med 340:55–59, 1999.

250. Wit JM, Kamp GA, Rikken B: Spontaneous growth and response to growth hormone treatment in children with growth hormone deficiency and idiopathic short stature. Pediatr Res 39:295–302, 1996.

251. Hindmarsh PC, Brook CGD: Final height of short normal children treated with growth hormone. Lancet 348:13–16, 1996.

252. Ramaswami U, Rumsby G, Spoudeas HA, et al: Treatment of achondroplasia with growth hormone: Six years of experience. Pediatr Res 46:435–439, 1999.

253. Buchlis JG, Irizarry L, Crotzer BC, et al: Comparison of final heights of growth hormone–treated vs untreated children with idiopathic growth failure. J Clin Endocrinol Metab 83:1075–1079, 1998.

254. Rotenstin D, Reigel DH: Growth hormone treatment of children with neural tube defects: Results from 6 months to 6 years. J Pediatr 128:184–189, 1996.

255. Rivkees SA, Bode HH, Crawford JD: Long-term growth in juvenile acquired hypothyroidism: The failure to achieve normal adult stature. N Engl J Med 318:599–602, 1988.

256. Petryk A, Richton S, Sy JP, Blethen SL: The effect of growth hormone treatment on stature in Aarskog syndrome. J Pediatr Endocrinol Metab 12:161–165, 1999.

257. Bridges NA, Hindmarsh PC: Growth of children with hypochondroplasia treated with growth hormone for up to three years. Horm Res 36(suppl):56–60, 1991.

258. Romano AA, Blethen SL, Dana K, Noto RA: Growth hormone treatment in Noonan syndrome: The National Cooperative Growth Study experience. J Pediatr 128 (suppl): 18–21, 1996.

259. Lantos J, Siegler M, Cuttler L: Ethical issues in growth hormone therapy. JAMA 261:1024, 1989.

260. Underwood LE: Growth hormone therapy for short stature: Yes or no? Hosp Pract 27:192–198, 1992.

261. Cuttler L, Silvers JB, Singh J, et al: Short stature and growth hormone therapy: A national study of physician recommendation patterns. JAMA 276:531–537, 1996.

262. Finkelstein BS, Silvers JB, Marrero U, et al: Insurance coverage, physician recommendations, and access to emerging treatments: Growth hormone therapy for childhood short stature. JAMA 279:663–668, 1998.

263. Zimet G, Oweens RP, Dahms WT, et al: Psychosocial outcome of children evaluated for short stature. Arch Pediatr Adolesc Med 151:1017–1023, 1997.

264. Zimet GD, Cutler M, Litvene M, et al: Psychological adjustment of children with non–growth hormone deficient short stature. J Pediatr Adolesc Psychol 16:264–170, 1995.

265. Kodish E, Cuttler L: Ethical issues in emerging new treatments such as growth hormone therapy for children with Down syndrome and Prader-Willi syndrome. Curr Opin Pediatr 8:401–405, 1996.

266. Downie AB, Mulligan J, McCaughey ES, et al: Psychological response to growth hormone treatment in short normal children. Arch Dis Child 75:32–35, 1996.

267. Lippe BM, Nakamoto JM: Conventional and nonconventional uses of growth hormone. Recent Prog Horm Res 48:179–235, 1993.

267a. Jeffcoate W: Can growth hormone therapy cause diabetes? Lancet 355:589–590, 2000.

268. Carel JC, Hay F, Coutant R, et al: Gonadotropin-releasing hormone agonist treatment of girls with constitutional short stature and normal pubertal development. J Clin Endocrinol Metab 81:3318–3322, 1996.

269. Mericq V, Eggers M, Avila A, et al: Near final height in pubertal growth-hormone (GH)-deficient patients treated with GH alone or in combination with luteinizing hormone-releasing hormone analogue: Results of a prospective, randomized trial. J Clin Endocrinol Metab 85:569–573, 2000.

270. Adan L, Souberbielle JC, Zucker JM: Adult height in 24 patients treated for growth hormone deficiency and early puberty. J Clin Endocrinol Metab 82:229–233, 1997.

271. Lanes R, Gunczier P: Final height after combined growth hormone and gonadotropin-releasing hormone analogue therapy in short healthy children entering into normally timed puberty. Clin Endocrinol 49:197–202, 1998.

272. Pasquino AM, Pucarelli I, Roggini M, Segni M: Adult height in short normal girls treated with gonadotropin-releasing hormone analogs and growth hormone. J Clin Endocrinol Metab 85:619–622, 2000.

273. Pereira L, Levran O, Ramirez F, et al: A molecular approach to the stratification of cardiovascular risk in families with Marfan's syndrome. N Engl J Med 331:148–153, 1994.

274. Sotos JF: Overgrowth. Section V. Syndromes and other disorders associated with overgrowth. Clin Pediatr (Phila) 36:89–103, 1997.

275. Sotos JF: Overgrowth. Section VI. Genetic syndromes and other disorders associated with overgrowth. Clin Pediatr (Phila) 36:157–170, 1997.

276. Li M, Squire JA, Weksberg R: Molecular genetics of Wiedemann-Beckwith syndrome. Am J Med Genet 79:253–259, 1998.
277. Sotos JF: Overgrowth. Section III. Other hormonal causes. Clin Pediatr (Phila) 35:637–648, 1996.
278. Sotos JF: Overgrowth. Section II. Hormonal causes. Clin Pediatr (Phila) 35:579–590, 1996.
279. Gagel RF, McCutcheon IF: Images in Clinical Medicine. Pituitary gigantism. N Engl J Med 340:524, 1999.
280. Dotsch J, Kiess W, Hanze J, et al: Gs alpha mutation at codon 201 in pituitary adenoma causing gigantism in a 6-year-old boy with McCune-Albright syndrome. J Clin Endocrinol Metab 81:3839–3842, 1996.
281. Wilroy RS Jr, Etteldorf JN: Familial hyperthyroidism including two siblings with neonatal Graves disease. J Pediatr 78:625, 1971.
282. Brauner R, Adan L, Malandry A, Zantleifer D: Adult height in girls with idiopathic true precocious puberty. J Clin Endocrinol Metab 79:415–420, 1994.
283. Uriarte MM, Baron J, Garcia HB, et al: The effect of pubertal delay on adult height in men with isolated hypogonadotropic hypogonadism [published erratum appears in J Clin Endocrinol Metab 1992 Oct;75(4):1009]. J Clin Endocrinol Metab 74:436–440, 1992.
284. Thamdrup E: Precocious Sexual Development. Springfield, IL, Charles C Thomas, 1961.
285. Sotos JF: Overgrowth. Section I. Overgrowth disorders. Clin Pediatr (Phila) 35:517–529, 1996.
286. Drop SLS, de Waal WJ, Keizer-Schrama SM: Sex steroid treatment of constitutionally tall stature. Endocr Rev 19:540–558, 1998.
286a. van Ommen CH, Fijnvandraat K, Vulsma T, et al: Acquired protein S deficiency caused by estrogen treatment of tall stature. J Pediatr 135:477–481, 1999.
287. Paul D, Conte FA, Grumbach MM, Kaplan SL: Long-term effect of gonadotropin-releasing hormone agonist therapy on final and near-final height in 26 children with true precocious puberty treated at a median age of less than 5 years. J Clin Endocrinol Metab 80:546–551, 1995.
288. Pasquino AM, Pucarelli I, Segni M, et al: Adult height in girls with central precocious puberty treated with gonadotropin-releasing hormone analogues and growth hormone. J Clin Endocrinol Metab 84:449–452, 1999.

Chapter 36

Growth Hormone Deficiency in Children

Ron G. Rosenfeld

Statural growth along predictable growth curves is one of the hallmarks of the healthy child. Deviation from normal growth standards is a cardinal manifestation of underlying illness, and can reflect a wide variety of genetic, constitutional, and pathologic conditions, of which growth hormone deficiency (GHD) represents a small subset. Nevertheless, because GHD (1) may be symptomatic of serious underlying abnormalities of the central nervous system (CNS), (2) may represent a genetically transmitted condition, (3) may indicate multiple pituitary deficiencies, and (4) is a treatable condition, it is critical that this diagnosis be considered in any child who is growing abnormally.

For the most part, GHD in childhood can be considered a form of insulin-like growth factor (IGF) deficiency.[1, 2] There are some limitations to this identity, as in some older children with acquired GHD (see below), but the classifications of etiologies of GHD and IGF deficiency are largely overlapping (Tables 36–1 and 36–2). Because IGF-1 is the major mediator of skeletal growth in children, the phenotypes of the various forms of IGF deficiency share many common features, necessitating sophisticated and comprehensive clinical, biochemical, radiologic, and genetic analysis to fully tease apart the various causes. Nevertheless, such analysis is often warranted in light of the important prognostic, therapeutic, and genetic implications of the various diagnoses.

The reported incidence of GHD is, to a large extent, a product of the criteria employed to establish the diagnosis, and clearly reflects wide variation in the stringency of diagnostic tests. An incidence of 1 in 60,000 live births has been reported from the United Kingdom.[3] A survey of Scottish schoolchildren, on the other hand, led to a calculated prevalence of 1 per 4000 live births.[4] The Utah Growth Study provided an estimated prevalence of 1 in 3480 live births.[5]

TABLE 36–1. Categorization of Insulin-like Growth Factor Deficiency

I. Hypothalamic dysfunction
II. Pituitary growth hormone (GH) deficiency
III. GH insensitivity
   A. Primary
   B. Secondary

ETIOLOGY OF GROWTH HORMONE DEFICIENCY AND INSULIN-LIKE GROWTH FACTOR DEFICIENCY

Several large surveys have indicated that approximately one-fourth of children diagnosed currently with GHD have an "organic" cause for their condition, such as trauma, CNS tumors, inflammation, irradiation, or anatomic abnormalities of the hypothalamus or pituitary[6, 7] (see Table 36–2). This leaves approximately 75% of diagnosed patients with having "idiopathic" GHD. It is highly likely, however, that such surveys greatly overestimate the number of true cases of idiopathic GHD. Many such cases undoubtedly reflect overdiagnosis, based on nonstringent criteria for a diagnosis of GHD; this is evidenced by the poor reproducibility of the many diagnostic tests for idiopathic GHD (see below). Furthermore, as we have learned more about the multiple genes involved in the development of a functional hypothalamic-pituitary axis, it has become apparent that many patients previously labeled as idiopathic GHD have genetic abnormalities or subtle anatomic abnormalities affecting the hypothalamus or pituitary, or both. It appears likely that true idiopathic GHD is, in actuality, a rare, if not nonexistent, condition.

Destructive Lesions of the Hypothalamus and Pituitary

A wide range of destructive lesions involving the hypothalamus or pituitary may present with isolated GHD or with multiple pituitary hormonal deficiencies. Birth trauma, associated, for example, with abrupt delivery, prolonged labor, or extensive use of forceps, has been associated frequently with subsequent hypothalamic or pituitary dysfunction.[8, 9] An increased incidence of GHD has been reported in breech deliveries, although it is still unclear whether such deliveries lead to acquisition of pituitary dysfunction, or, on the other hand, whether pre-existing CNS abnormalities result in higher rates of abnormal birth presentations.

Tumors

CNS tumors are an important cause of GHD and combined pituitary hormone deficiency (CPHD), and must be excluded in every child

TABLE 36–2. Etiologic Classification of Growth Hormone Deficiency (GHD) and Insulin-like Growth Factor (IGF) Deficiency

I. Destructive lesions of the hypothalamus or pituitary
   A. Trauma
   B. Tumors
   C. Infiltrative diseases (tuberculosis, sarcoidosis, hemochromatosis)
   D. Vascular lesions
   E. Surgery
   F. Irradiation
   G. Autoimmune hypophysitis
II. Developmental abnormalities of the hypothalamus or pituitary
   A. Anencephaly
   B. Holoprosencephaly
   C. Septo-optic dysplasia
   D. Posterior pituitary ectopia
   E. Empty sella
III. Genetic abnormalities of hypothalamic or pituitary hormone synthesis or secretion
   A. Autosomal recessive GHD (type 1), due to mutations or deletions of the *GH1* gene
   B. Autosomal dominant GHD (type 2), due to mutations or deletions of the *GH1* gene
   C. X-linked GHD (type 3)
   D. Defects in the receptor for growth hormone–releasing hormone (GHRH)
   E. Combined pituitary hormone deficiencies
      1. Abnormalities of pituitary transcription factors
IV. Psychosocial dwarfism
V. Growth hormone insensitivity
   A. Primary
   B. Secondary
VI. Primary IGF deficiency
VII. IGF insensitivity
   A. Abnormalities of IGF binding proteins (IGFBPs)
   B. Abnormalities of IGF receptors

with GHD who does not have an obvious alternative explanation for growth failure.[10] Midline brain tumors include germinomas, meningiomas, gliomas, colloid cysts of the third ventricle, ependymomas, and optic nerve gliomas. GHD or CPHD may also occur from local extension of tumors affecting the head or neck, such as craniopharyngeal carcinomas and lymphomas. The major pediatric tumor involving the pituitary is craniopharyngioma, which is probably an evolving congenital malformation which develops from remnants of Rathke's pouch.[11, 12] Arising from rests of squamous cells at the embryonic junction of the adenohypophysis and neurohypophysis, it forms an enlarging cyst filled with degenerating cells, leading to "machinery oil" cyst fluid or calcifications, but never to malignant degeneration. These calcifications may be seen, at times, on skull films, and constitute an important diagnostic sign. Although craniopharyngiomas represent the consequences of a congenital malformation, they may present clinically at any age. While significant growth failure may be observed at the time of diagnosis, patients most commonly present with complaints of increased intracranial pressure, such as headaches, vomiting, and oculomotor disturbances; visual field defects are frequently noted at the time of diagnosis.[13–16] Fifty percent to 80% of patients have deficiency of at least one pituitary hormone, most commonly growth hormone (GH) or gonadotropins; diabetes insipidus is reported in 25% to 50% of patients at diagnosis. Pituitary adenomas are much less common in children than in adults, and account for less than 5% of patients with organic GHD.[17, 18] The majority of pediatric pituitary adenomas stain positive for prolactin (PRL), and GH-secreting adenomas are extremely rare in childhood.

Langerhans' cell histiocytosis, previously known as histiocytosis X and characterized by a localized or generalized proliferation of histiocytes, may also present at any age.[19] The term encompasses at least three clinical forms: (1) eosinophilic granuloma, usually presenting as solitary bone disease; (2) Hand-Schüller-Christian disease, which is a chronic form of the disease, typically manifesting with diabetes insipidus, exophthalmos, and multiple calvarial lesions; and (3) Letterer-

Siwe disease, a disseminated form, typically affecting infants. Depending upon the sites and extent of histiocytic infiltration, these disorders may involve isolated GHD or multiple pituitary deficiencies, with or without diabetes insipidus.[20–22]

Infiltrative and Inflammatory Disorders

Infiltrative diseases are uncommon causes of GHD in the pediatric population, but pituitary insufficiency may be observed in CNS involvement in tuberculosis,[23] sarcoidosis,[24] or toxoplasmosis. Inflammation associated with bacterial, viral, fungal, or parasitic disease may also result in hypothalamic-pituitary dysfunction. Lymphadenoid hypophysitis has been reported to present as a pituitary tumor.[25]

Vascular Lesions

Aneurysms may behave as space-occupying lesions and cause hypothalamic or pituitary destruction. Such lesions are usually evident on radiographic evaluation.

Irradiation of the Central Nervous System

The pituitary gland and, in particular, the hypothalamus are sensitive to radiation; often, both regions of the CNS are involved.[26–40] Such damage is, typically, difficult to assess precisely, since the hypothalamus and pituitary may differ in the extent of involvement, and the loss of function may evolve with time. Sensitivity to CNS radiation may differ among patients, although the majority of children will experience some degree of hypothalamic or pituitary dysfunction within 5 years of receiving 3000 Gy.[31, 32] Spontaneous GHD is frequently decreased by doses as low as 1800 to 2400 Gy,[34] and subtle dysfunction may be observed at even lower doses. GH secretion, generally, appears to be the most sensitive to irradiation, followed by thyroid-stimulating hormone (TSH) and gonadotropins, and, finally, adrenocorticotropic hormone (ACTH).

Because pituitary dysfunction evolves over several years following irradiation, it is important that all children subjected to cranial irradiation be monitored for growth deceleration. While provocative GH testing may be within normal limits, measures of spontaneous GH secretion frequently demonstrate abnormalities.[29] Serum concentrations of IGF-1 or insulin-like growth factor binding protein-3 (IGFBP-3) are not invariably reduced in the early years following cranial irradiation.[41, 42] Given these complexities, it is recommended that, in patients receiving cranial irradiation, a diagnosis of GHD be considered in any child with growth deceleration plus any biochemical evidence of GHD, including provocative GH levels, spontaneous GH secretion, or IGF-1 or IGFBP-3 concentrations. Delay of therapy until biochemical tests are "totally conclusive" may result in unfavorable adult height.[30, 40] This is further complicated by the fact that spinal irradiation may lead to compromised spinal growth, even in the face of GH replacement. Furthermore, cranial irradiation may also result in precocious puberty, with early and unfavorable epiphyseal fusion.[38, 43–45] Low-dose irradiation is frequently associated with such precocious onset of puberty; higher doses may result in gonadotropin deficiency and pubertal delay.[43–46] In the irradiated child with early puberty, therapy with gonadotropin-releasing hormone (GnRH) analogues should be considered, with or without GH treatment, to delay epiphyseal fusion.[47] As in all patients with GHD, it is critical that nutrition be optimized and that euthyroidism be maintained.

GHD may also be observed in patients who have received cranial irradiation as part of the regimen for bone marrow transplantation (BMT).[48–56] Total body irradiation may also result in abnormal vertebral growth, as well as gonadal failure and pubertal delay. Recent studies have shown that final heights in 28 long-term survivors of BMT were, generally, in the lower part of the normal range.[56] Although subtle foms of partial GHD may occur in this population, if the dosage of irradiation has been modest, a conservative approach, accompanied by careful monitoring of the growth rate, may be warranted.

Developmental Abnormalities of the Hypothalamus and Pituitary

Both severe and subtle malformations of the brain, hypothalamus, or pituitary may result in isolated GHD or CPHD. The possibility of pituitary dysfunction should be considered in any child with a congenital midbrain or midfacial abnormality. Anencephaly results in hypothalamic and pituitary insufficiency, frequently with a small, abnormally formed, or ectopic pituitary gland[57, 58]; detailed endocrine evaluations of affected patients are not readily available, however. Holoprosencephaly, which results from abnormal midline development of the embryonic forebrain, is also associated with hypothalamic insufficiency.[59, 60] Milder manifestations of midline developmental defects include cyclopia, hypertelorism, absence of the midline nasal septum, midline clefts of the palate or lip, and a single central incisor. Controversy continues around the issue of whether simple clefts of the palate or lip are also associated with pituitary dysfunction.[61] In the absence of a definitive answer to this question, growth rates in such children should be monitored carefully.

Septo-optic dysplasia may be considered another example of midbrain structural abnormality potentially associated with hypothalamic insufficiency.[62–64] In its complete form, this condition combines hypothalamic insufficiency with hypoplasia or absence of the optic chiasm or optic nerves, and agenesis or hypoplasia of the corpus callosum and septum pellucidum. Wide variability in this syndrome has been described, and the clinical phenotype may, similarly, cover a wide range. Accordingly, all patients with congenital GHD should have magnetic resonance imaging (MRI) or computed tomography (CT) scan of the brain, with careful attention paid to the hypothalamus, pituitary, and optic chiasm. Pituitary insufficiency has been described in patients with optic nerve hypoplasia evident only on radiographic studies.[63] Similarly, the possibility of septo-optic dysplasia must be considered in any child with growth failure associated with pendular or rotary nystagmus, or with significant impairment of vision associated with a small optic disk.

As methods of radiologic evaluation of the CNS have improved, an increasing percentage of patients with idiopathic GHD have been found to have structural abnormalities.[65–73] In a recent MRI study of 101 consecutive patients with a diagnosis of congenital idiopathic GHD, ectopia of the posterior pituitary (PPE) was found in 59[73]; extremely small pituitary volume was seen in patients with PPE, as well as normal-appearing posterior pituitaries combined with severely narrowed pituitary stalks. Patients with PPE differed from those with normal posterior pituitaries in higher male-female ratios (3:1 vs. 1:1), greater frequency of CPHD (49% vs. 12%), breech delivery (32% vs. 7%), and associated congenital brain anomalies (12% vs. 7%). In a number of studies involving 341 children with isolated GHD or CPHD, 54% had the characteristic MRI findings of PPE (often identified as a posterior pituitary "bright" spot), pituitary stalk dysgenesis, or hypoplasia or aplasia of the anterior pituitary, either singly or severally.[68–73] MRI abnormalities were more readily identified in patients with CPHD (93%) than in isolated GHD (32%).

These findings appear to be best explained by a defect in induction of the mediobasal structure of the brain in the early embryo, rather than the product of birth trauma, as previously suggested.[67, 69] Whether pituitary insufficiency is the result of hypothalamic or pituitary dysgenesis, or the product of hypoplasia or sectioning of the pituitary stalk, is not always clear. Perinatal problems, however, including breech presentation, may prove to be the consequence, rather than the cause, of underlying CNS abnormality. The concept that PPE, stalk section

or hypoplasia, and pituitary hypoplasia may represent abnormal embryonic development, rather than the consequences of birth trauma, is supported by the finding of similar anatomic abnormalities[72, 74, 75] in patients with septo-optic dysplasia, type I Arnold-Chiari syndrome, and holoprosencephaly. Furthermore, the occasional presence of genital hypoplasia in affected infants strongly supports the belief that hypothalamic-pituitary insufficiency began in utero.[74–76]

In the empty sella syndrome, abnormalities of the sellar diaphragm allow herniation of the suprasellar subarachnoid space into the region of the sella turcica.[77] This may result in damage to the sella, including the pituitary. Empty sella syndrome may be the consequence of surgery or irradiation, or may be idiopathic.

Genetic Abnormalities of Hypothalamic and Pituitary Hormone Synthesis and Secretion

It has been estimated that as many as 5% to 30% of patients with GHD have an affected first-degree relative.[78, 79] These numbers may, in fact, underestimate the incidence of genetic abnormalities in patients with GHD or CPHD, and recent years have seen a broadening of our understanding of genetic abnormalities in hypothalamic and pituitary development and function.[80, 81]

Isolated Human Growth Hormone Deficiency

Four forms of genetically transmitted isolated GHD have been described, although the distinctions between these forms occasionally blur[78–83] (Table 36–3). Isolated GHD IA results from mutations or deletions of the *GH1* gene, located as part of a cluster of five structurally related genes (*GH1*, *CSHP* [chorionic somatomammotropin pseudogene], *CSH* [chorionic somatomammotropin], *GH2*, and *CSH2*) on chromosome 17. This disorder is transmitted as an autosomal recessive trait and, typically, presents with severe congenital GHD.[84] In GHD IA, complete loss of pituitary GH secretion occurs, secondary to deletions resulting from nonhomologous crossing over at different sites in the GH and chorionic somatomammotropin (CS) gene cluster. The most common deletion is 6.7 kb, but deletions of 7.0, 7.6, and greater than 45 kb have also been observed. Wagner et al.[81] have also described the GHD IA phenotype in a patient with a point mutation in codon 23 of the GH signal peptide, converting GAG to TAG (stop codon; E23X), resulting in premature termination of translation. These deletions have been reported in a wide variety of ethnic groups, including northern European, Mediterranean, and Asian. Patients experience severe GHD and, typically, have an excellent initial response to GH therapy. Because of the absence of a normal GH molecule in fetal life, an attenuation of the growth response to exogenous GH may result from the development of anti-GH antibodies,[84] although this event has been described less frequently with newer GH preparations.

GHD lB displays a more heterogeneous phenotype, reflecting the degree of GHD or the bioactivity of the GH molecule produced.[81] Some such children have 1- or 2-bp deletions in the *GH1* gene, leading to frameshifts and, potentially, early translational stop signals. Other mutations have been reported within the fourth intron of the the *GH1* gene, resulting in abnormal pre–messenger RNA (mRNA) splicing at the exon 3 to exon 4 splice boundary. Other genetic causes of GHD IB may include abnormalities of the promoter region. GHD may range from severe to partial, and, typically, responds well to GH treatment, without development of clinically significant anti-GH antibodies.

TABLE 36–3. McKusick Classification of Familial Isolated Human Growth Hormone (GH) Deficiency

Form	Genetics	Endogenous GH	Response to GH	Associated Deficiencies	Molecular Basis
IA	AR	Absent	May be transient	−	*GH1* deletion/mutation
IB	AR	Decreased	+	−	?*GH1* mutation
II	AD	Decreased	+	−	?Dominant negative
III	X-linked	Decreased	+	−	?

AR, autosomal recessive; AD, autosomal dominant.

Unlike GHD IA and IB, GHD II is transmitted as an autosomal dominant trait. It has been reported to result, at least in some cases, from mutations in intron 3, leading to a loss of exon 3. The resulting 17 kDa protein is lacking amino acids 32–71, including one of the cysteines involved in formation of intramolecular disulfide bonds. A dominant negative effect is speculated to arise from the formation of abnormal intermolecular bonds between abnormal and normal GH molecules, resulting in defective secretion. GHD III, an X-linked form of isolated growth hormone deficiency (IGHD), has been reported in patients with hypogammaglobulinemia. To date, no alteration in the *GH1* gene has been identified in this condition.

IGHD has also been reported recently in cousins with a mutation of the growth hormone–releasing hormone (GHRH) receptor.[85] The mutation resulted in formation of a truncated receptor molecule, lacking the transmembrane region and the G protein binding site. A group of 18 interrelated patients were identified subsequently in Pakistan, with a Glu72Stop mutation.[86] Over 120 patients in a single province of northeastern Brazil were found to share a donor splice mutation in position 1 of intron 1.[87] All patients reported to date have been homozygous for mutations of the GHRH receptor gene. Serum GH concentrations fail to rise following standard provocative testing, as well as after GHRH administration. The patients thus resemble the *little* mouse (lit/lit), which has a mutation of the GHRH receptor gene affecting the ligand-binding domain.[88] At the time of this writing, no mutations of the human GHRH gene have been identified.

Combined Pituitary Hormone Deficiency

Recent studies have elucidated the critical roles of a variety of transcription factors that are involved in pituitary organogenesis cell commitment and proliferation, and differentiation of specific hormone synthesis and secretion[80] (Table 36–4). The embryonic anterior pituitary gland develops from a midline structure that is contiguous with the primordium of the ventral diencephalon. The various cell types of the anterior pituitary, such as somatotrophs corticotrophs, lactotrophs, thyrotrophs, and gonadotrophs, must undergo highly selective differentiation that requires specific temporal sequences and spatial localization. This process is regulated, at least in part, by a group of DNA-binding homeodomain transcription factors. Abnormalities of these transcription factors can result in familial CPHDs. Not all of these proteins have been associated with human pituitary dysplasia to date, but they appear, nevertheless, to play critical roles in normal pituitary development, and may prove to be involved in various forms of pituitary agenesis, hypoplasia, and dysgenesis. Since some of these transcription factors are expressed outside of the embryonic pituitary as well, developmental defects may be complex.

Rpx is an acronym for the murine *Rathke's pouch homeobox*[89, 90] It is a paired-like homeodomain protein which appears in the mouse at embryonic day 8.5 and is gone by embryonic day 14.5. It is intially expressed throughout the prosencephalic plate, but is later restricted to Rathke's pouch, in the regions that contain precursors of all five anterior pituitary cell types. Abnormalities of the *Rpx* gene would be expected to result in anterior pituitary agenesis, although no spontaneous mutations in the mouse or human have been identified to date.

The pituitary OTX (P-OTX) protein binds to the transcriptional activation domain of Pit-1, an important pituitary-specific transcription factor itself (see below).[91] In the mouse, it appears at the same time as Rpx (embryonic day 8.5); the protein persists in the anterior and intermediate lobes of the pituitary and can be identified in all anterior pituitary cell types. As with Rpx, abnormalities of P-OTX would be expected to cause pituitary agenesis or hypoplasia. Given the wide embryonic distribution of P-OTX, pituitary dysplasia might be associated with developmental abnormalities of the oral epithelium, tongue, mandible, salivary gland, duodenum, and hindlimb.

P-Lim, also known as mouse LIM-3 (mLIM-3) and LIM homeobox 3 (Lhx3), is present in Rathke's pouch by embryonic day 9.5, and persists in the anterior pituitary.[92] Animals homozygous for targeted disruption of P-Lim developed Rathke's pouch, but failed to progress to formation of discrete anterior and intermediate lobes of the anterior pituitary.[93] Although P-Lim interacts with β-TSH, PRL, and Pit-1, no effect on the GH promoter has been identified to date.

Abnormalities of the gene for Prop-1 (Prophet of Pit-1) have been shown to be responsible for Ames dwarfism in mice.[94] The phenotype appears to be the result of failure of initial determination of the Pit-1 lineage required for production of GH, PRL, and TSH, leading to dyshormonogenesis and failure to activate Pit-1 gene expression. The Ames mouse pituitary gland contains less than 1% of the normal complement of somatotrophs, and decreased numbers of lactotrophs and thyrotrophs. Wu et al.[95] identified four CPHD families with homozygosity or compound heterozygosity for inactivating mutations of Prop-1. In addition to the anticipated deficiencies of GH, PRL, and TSH, patients were found to be also gonadotropin-deficient. Delayed puberty was common, but patients appeared capable of entering puberty spontaneously. To date, at least 11 families with CPHD resulting from Prop-1 gene defects have been identified, with wide variability among the different gene mutations, and even among siblings sharing the same mutation.[96, 97]

Pit-1 was the first of the pituitary transcription factors to be identified and is still the best characterized.[98, 99] It is a member of the POU family, and contains a highly conserved bipartite DNA-binding domain, consisting of the POU homeodomain, required for low-affinity DNA binding, and the POU-specific domain, responsible for the specificity of DNA binding and potential interactions with other proteins. Presumably, Pit-1 binds in a highly specific manner to target DNA regions; then, possibly in concert with other transcription factors, it forms a transactivation complex on the DNA, through an N-terminal transcriptional activation domain. Thus, the Pit-1 protein binds to and activates transcription from the GH, PRL, β-TSH, and Pit-1 genes.

Expression of Pit-1 begins on embryonic day 14.5, and continues to be expressed in mature somatotrophs, lactotrophs, and thyrotrophs. The Snell mouse, characterized by pituitary hypoplasia, and GH, PRL, and TSH deficiencies, has been shown to have a point mutation of the Pit-1 gene, affecting the third α helix of the POU homeodomain, and thereby abrogating binding of Pit-1 to promoter sequences. Multiple mutations and deletions of the Pit-1 gene have now been identified in humans with CPHD, characterized by the combination of GH, PRL, and TSH deficiency.[100–102] Mutations have been described which separately affect the DNA-binding capacity of Pit-1 or its transactivation properties. Autosomal dominant transmission, resulting from a dominant negative effect, has been observed in mutations affecting Pit-1 dimerization, the transactivation domain (P24L), or in the relatively common R271W mutation, which results in increased binding to promoter elements and disruption of transcriptional activatioin.[103] Autosomal recessive transmission is found in most other mutations, such

TABLE 36–4. Sites and Timing of Expression of Pituitary Transcription Factors

Factor	Cells	Start of Expression (Embryonic Day)	End of Expression (Embryonic Day)	Independent Activation	Interaction with Pit-1
Rpx	All	8.5	14.5	?	None
P-OTX	All	8.5	Persists	All but β-TSH	GH, PRL
P-Lim	All	9.5	Persists	All	β-TSH, PRL, Pit-1
Prop-1*	S, P, T	10.5	14.5	Inhibits Rpx	None
Pit-1*	S, P, T	14.5	Persists	GH, PRL, β-TSH	Not applicable

S, somatotrophs; P, lactotrophs; T, thyrotrophs; β-TSH, β-thyroid-stimulating hormone; GH, growth hormone; PRL, prolactin.

*Known human clinical syndromes have been identified to date. Pit-1 deficiency is characterized by GH, PRL, and variable TSH deficiency. Prop-1 deficiency is characterized by GH, PRL, TSH, variable gonadotropin, and, in some cases, partial ACTH deficiency.

as A172stop, E250stop, R143G, A158P, and P239S.[104] Variability in phenotype has been reported, although most patients exhibit growth retardation during the first year of life. Typically, GH and PRL deficiency is complete; TSH secretion may be observed during infancy, but declines progressively during the early months of life. After appropriate GH and thyroid replacement, patients appear to enter puberty normally and have normal fertility. Lactation, however, may be impaired.

Psychosocial Dwarfism

Psychosocial dwarfism, also known as "emotional deprivation dwarfism," was first described by Powell et al. in 1967.[105, 106] In this extreme form of failure to thrive, children display bizarre eating and drinking behavior, social withdrawal, delayed speech, and, on occasion, other evidence of developmental delay. Periodic hyperphagia is associated with decreased GH responsiveness to standard provocative stimuli, but also with subnormal responses to exogenous GH therapy.[107] Removal from the stressful environment, which usually involves removal from the home, is accompanied by a restoration of normal GH secretion, typically within weeks, and a period of catch-up growth.[108, 109] The mechanisms for this reversible form of GHD are unclear, but it is of note that a variety of psychiatric conditions in adults may be associated with decreased spontaneous and provocative GH secretion. Establishment of the diagnosis of psychosocial dwarfism requires documentation of catch-up growth and restoration of normal GH secretion following correction of the environmental situation.

Growth Hormone Insensitivity

The spectrum of growth hormone insensitivity (GHI) has greatly expanded since the original description of this syndrome by Laron and Pertzelan in 1966.[110] A classification of GHI was published in 1990[111] and recently modified by Savage and Rosenfeld.[112] Primary GHI results from hereditary defects in the GH receptor, GH signal transduction, or GH activity. In its expanded form, primary GHI includes not only various forms of GH resistance but also specific defects in IGF synthesis, transport, or receptors (Table 36–5). Secondary GHI results from acquired resistance to GH action, as occurs with antibodies to GH or the GH receptor, malnutrition, liver disease, and other chronic catabolic states.[113, 114]

Growth Hormone Receptor Defects

To date, more than 200 cases of GH receptor defects around the world have been identified and confirmed by biochemical or molecular

TABLE 36–5. Classification of Growth Hormone (GH) Insensitivity

I. Primary GH insensitivity (hereditary defects)
  A. GH receptor defect (may be positive or negative for GH-binding protein)
    1. Extracellular mutation/deletion
    2. Cytoplasmic mutation/deletion
    3. Intracellular mutation/deletion
  B. GH signal transduction defect (distal to cytoplasmic domain of GH receptor)
  C. IGF-1 synthetic defect
  D. IGF-1 transport defect
  E. IGF-1 receptor defect
  F. Bioactive GH molecule
II. Secondary GH insensitivity (acquired defects)
  A. Circulating antibodies to GH that inhibit GH action
  B. Antibodies to the GH receptor
  C. GH insensitivity caused by malnutrition, liver disease, catabolic states, etc.
  D. Other conditions that cause GH insensitivity

IGF-1, insulin-like growth factor-1.

studies.[113, 114] Originally described in Israel and the Mediterranean region, patients with GH receptor defects have been identified now in a wide variety of ethnic and racial groups. Most patients have been shown to have deletions or point mutations in the portion of the GH receptor gene that encodes the extracellular domain of the transmembrane GH receptor molecule. This portion of the GH receptor is the GH-binding domain and, as a result of proteolytic cleavage, circulates in serum as a GH-binding protein (GHBP). Thus, the overwhelming majority of patients demonstrate decreased GH-binding activity in serum. At least one mutation of the extracellular domain of the GH receptor gene, however, results in defective dimerization of GH receptor molecules at the cell membrane; as a result, serum GHBP activity may be normal in such patients, even with mutations affecting the extracellular domain.[115] Woods et al.[116] have identified two cousins with severe GH resistance resulting from homozygosity for a mutation at the splice site of exon 8. The resulting GH receptor molecule lacks a functional transmembrane and intracellular domain, but actually has increased serum GHBP levels due to release of the truncated GH receptor molecule from the cell.

In its classic form, GHI resulting from abnormalities of the GH receptor is transmitted in an autosomal recessive manner. Given the requirement for GH receptor dimerization to elicit action, however, it was predicted that certain mutations might behave in a dominant negative manner, and demonstrate the clinical phenotype in a heterozygous state.[117, 118] This appears to be the case for at least one mutation of the intracellular domain, in which dominant inheritance results from a heterozygous 876-1 G to C transversion of the 3' splice acceptor site preceding exon 9.[119] The severely truncated cytoplasmic domain is incapable of transmitting a normal GH signal, even when it forms a heterodimer with the wild-type GH receptor. Such heterozygous transmission, perhaps in a milder form, has been hypothesized to be a cause of some cases of "idiopathic short stature."[117, 118] To accept this diagnosis, however, growth failure and low serum concentrations of IGF-1 and IGFBP-3 must be shown to be unresponsive to GH therapy.

Growth Hormone Signal Transduction Defects

To date, no cases of GHI resulting from specific defects of the GH receptor signaling cascade distal to the intracellular domain of the GH receptor (and proximal to IGF-1 synthesis) have been documented. It is to be anticipated, however, that short stature might result from such a defect. Since neither GH nor IGF-1 is required for fetal survival, a patient with this kind of defect would be expected to be viable, unless the distal GH signal cascade (or portions of it) proves necessary for survival when stimulated by some ligand other than GH.

IGF-1 Synthetic Defects

Studies involving targeted disruption of the genes for IGF-1, IGF-2, and the IGF-1 receptor in mice have demonstrated the pivotal role of the IGF axis in growth.[120–122] Unlike GH, which seems essential for postnatal growth only (GH may be necessary for totally normal fetal growth during the final weeks of gestation), IGF-1 is critically involved in both prenatal and postnatal skeletal growth. Woods et al.[123] described a 15-year-old boy with a partial deletion of the IGF-1 gene, resulting in both intrauterine growth retardation and severe postnatal growth failure (height −6.7 SD). As expected, growth was not responsive to exogenous GH treatment. Additional features of this patient included sensorineural deafness, microcephaly, and mental retardation; the role of IGF-1 deficiency in these features is unclear.

IGF-1 Transport Defects

On a theoretic basis, growth failure may result from abnormalities of IGFBPs by two distinct mechanisms: (1) severe deficiencies of IGFBPs may result in abnormal half-lives and increased clearance of IGF molecules[124]; (2) increased concentrations of IGFBPs may inhibit IGF action by competing with receptors for binding of IGF. Patients with classic GHI resulting from defects of the GH receptor typically have decreased serum concentrations of IGFBP-3 and IGFBP-5, as well as the acid labile subunit (ALS) required for formation of the ternary complex.[113, 114, 125–127] These patients have been demonstrated to have a greatly decreased half-life of IGF-1 in serum, although the contribution of the shortened IGF half-life to growth failure is unclear. Barreca et al.[128] have reported a case of short stature apparently due to high circulating concentrations of IGFBP-1. This patient had both intrauterine and postnatal growth failure, associated with 10- to 20-fold increases in fasting serum IGFBP-1. The authors speculated that increased IGFBP-1 concentrations inhibited IGF-1 action, interfered with formation of the ternary complex and led to accelerated clearance of IGF peptides, and inhibited IGF feedback on GH secretion.

IGF-1 Receptor Defects

Targeted disruption of the IGF-1 receptor gene also has been reported to cause severe intrauterine growth retardation and postnatal growth failure in mice.[122] In fact, growth failure is more severe in such mice than in mice with IGF-1 gene knockouts, presumably reflecting the inability of IGF-1, IGF-2, and insulin to elicit biologic action through the IGF-1 receptor. Such mice typically die within the first few hours or days of life. IGF-1 receptor defects have been hypothesized to play a factor in the short stature characteristic of African pygmies.[129]

Bioinactive Growth Hormone Molecule

Since the GH molecule exists in multiple molecular forms, resulting from alternative splicing or post-translational processing,[130, 131] some cases of short stature have been hypothesized to be the consequence of abnormal ratios of the various normal GH forms.[132, 133] To date, no totally convincing cases of growth failure resulting from this mechanism have been reported. Kowarski et al.[133] described several cases of growth failure which they ascribed to GH molecules with normal immunoreactivity but decreased bioactivity. The first convincing case, however, was not reported until 1996, when Takahashi et al.[134, 135] described two individuals heterozygous for point mutations in the GH gene. The mutant GH molecules (R77C and D112G) were capable of binding to the GH receptor, perhaps even with increased affinity, but were unable to stimulate tyrosine phosphorylation of GH-activated intracellular signaling intermediates in a normal manner. The ability of the R77C mutant to behave in a dominant negative manner was demonstrated by its ability to inhibit the in vitro actions of wild-type GH.

Secondary Growth Hormone Insensitivity

GH resistance, in the presence of structurally normal GH receptors, has been reported in patients with GHD IA treated with exogenous GH.[84] It has been speculated that since such patients have GH gene deletions, and have never synthesized normal pituitary GH, exogenous GH is capable of acting as a foreign antigen, thereby stimulating production of GH-inhibitory antibodies. Not all patients with GHD IA, however, develop such antibodies. GH receptor antibodies theoretically could similarly inhibit GH action, although such cases have not been demonstrated to date. Relative GHI has also been observed in chronic liver disease, malnutrition, and a variety of chronic catabolic disease states. GH resistance in such cases is, typically, relative, rather than absolute.

CLINICAL FEATURES OF GROWTH HORMONE DEFICIENCY AND INSULIN-LIKE GROWTH FACTOR DEFICIENCY

Recent studies in humans and in animal models have demonstrated marked similarities, but also critical differences, between the clinical features of GHD and various forms of IGF deficiency. The clinical features of classic GHI, resulting from mutations or deletions of the gene for the GH receptor, and presenting with severe IGF-1 deficiency despite elevated serum GH concentrations, are virtually indistinguishable from congenital absence of GH, as in GHD IA.[113, 114, 136] Prenatal

growth is near normal in both conditions. Although mild reductions in birth length and weight have been observed in both conditions (newborns are, generally, within 10% of normal size for gestation), neither GHI resulting from GH receptor defects nor congenital GHD is a cause of severe intrauterine growth retardation.[74, 137, 138] On the other hand, mice with targeted disruption of the gene for IGF-1, IGF-2, or, especially, the IGF-1 receptor, have marked intrauterine growth failure.[120–122] The same was observed for the single reported case of IGF-1 deficiency resulting from homozygosity for a deletion of the IGF-1 gene.[123] These findings appear to indicate that while IGF-1 and the IGF-1 receptor are critically involved in intrauterine growth, IGF-1 synthesis and secretion in utero are not regulated primarily by pituitary GH.

IGF-1 production comes under GH regulation either in the last few months of fetal life or shortly after birth, as GHI and congenital GHD are both characterized by severe postnatal growth failure, which may be evident in the early months of life.[113, 114, 139] Growth failure is greater for skeletal growth than for body weight, so infants and young children have an appearance of relative adiposity. Neonatal problems that suggest the possibility of pituitary deficiencies, especially CPHD, include neonatal hypoglycemia[140]; this may be severe, although it is readily correctable by administration of glucose. Measurement of serum concentrations of IGFBP-1 may be of value in the neonate with hypoglycemia, as low levels would be consistent with hyperinsulinemia, while normal concentrations are consistent with GHD.[141] The presence of concomitant gonadotropin deficiency is suggested by the presence of microphallus, cryptorchidism, and scrotal hypoplasia, but genital ambiguity would not be expected.[76] Prolonged jaundice with direct hyperbilirubinemia and cholestasis may also be observed, typically in patients with CPHD.[142, 143] The relative contributions of GH, ACTH, and TSH deficiency to this presentation are unclear. It is imperative that the diagnosis of pituitary insufficiency be considered in any infant (especially term) with hypoglycemia, cryptorchidisim, and microphallus, or direct hyperbilirubinemia. In such infants, it may be expedient and even cost-effective to immediately perform MRI of the brain, looking for evidence of septo-optic dysplasia, pituitary hypoplasia, stalk hypoplasia or disruption, and PPE (see Diagnosis).

After the perinatal period, the defining feature of IGF deficiency, resulting from either GHD or GHI, is growth failure.[113, 114, 144] Careful documentation of growth may demonstrate defective skeletal growth during the first 6 months of life in congenital GHD or GHI; by 6 to 12 months of age, growth failure is inevitable in these conditions. Height velocity is, typically, at −2 to −5 SD for chronologic age, leading to a progressive deviation from the normal growth curves. In severe, long-standing GHD or GHI, heights may be as much as −10 SD.[113, 114] In patients with acquired GHD, the critical feature is documentation of a change in the growth rate. Thus, a child who has been growing at the 75th percentile, but falls off to the 25th percentile, warrants an evaluation, even though his or her height may still be within the normal range. A good rule of thumb is that between the age of 2 years and the onset of puberty, children normally maintain their height percentile with remarkable integrity. Deviation from this percentile (either acceleration or deceleration) should lead to further investigation.

Skeletal proportions are maintained normally in GHD and GHI, but tend to correlate better with bone age than with chronologic age. Bone age is delayed, typically, often to less than 60% of chronologic age. In acquired GHD, bone age delay may not be present; when acquired GHD is accompanied by accelerated puberty, as occasionally seen in patients with intracranial tumors, bone age may be accelerated.[45, 47] Weight-to-height ratios tend to be high, resulting in the appearance of relative adiposity and immaturity. This is supported by the infantile facial appearance of many patients, reflecting relative hypoplasia of facial bones, with a hypoplastic nasal bridge, frontal bossing, and delayed closure of sutures.[113, 114, 145] Head circumference is, generally, near the lower limits of normal, indicating relatively normal brain growth. As a result, the head-to-trunk and cephalofacial ratios may appear abnormally high, and patients may be believed, mistakingly, to be hydrocephalic. Where musculature is poorly developed and gross motor milestones delayed, an erroneous impression of mental retardation may be given.[146, 147] Hypoplasia of the larynx may lead to a high-pitched, infantile voice. Hair growth in early years may be sparse. Blue sclerae are observed occasionally, and are thought to result from decreased growth of scleral connective tissue.[113, 114, 136] Delayed dentition may be observed, but in the absence of midline craniofacial abnormalities, it is otherwise normal. Genital growth, prior to the onset of puberty, is usually proportional to body size. Puberty may be delayed, but in the absence of other endocrine deficiencies is otherwise normal.

Limited data are available on the adult heights of untreated patients with GHD. These results are often difficult to interpret because of (1) heterogeneity in the timing of GHD; (2) heterogeneity in the severity of GHD; (3) the presence or absence of other pituitary deficiencies; and (4) delay in puberty, resulting in late epiphyseal fusion. Wit et al.[148] summarized the results from studies of 22 untreated men and 14 untreated women with severe isolated GHD, and reported a mean adult height of -4.7 SD.[149–151] In patients with untreated autosomal recessive GHD, Rimoin and colleagues[149] reported mean adult heights of -7.4 SD. In GHI, adult heights as short as -11.9 SD have been reported.[113, 114] It is of note that in patients with GHI, a striking correlation has been observed between height and measures of serum IGF-1 or IGFBP-3, indicating that even in the absence of GH action, non–GH-dependent production of IGF-1 is still a major regulator of skeletal growth.[113, 114, 152, 153] In patients with CPHD, adult height is often not as severely affected as in IGHD, presumably reflecting pubertal delay and late epiphyseal fusion.[151]

DIAGNOSIS OF INSULIN-LIKE GROWTH FACTOR DEFICIENCY AND GROWTH HORMONE DEFICIENCY IN CHILDHOOD

The diagnostic evaluation of children with growth failure is complex.[1, 2, 154] The underlying principle must be that any evaluation should be based upon careful auxologic considerations, always placed in the context of the family history of growth. Because the biochemical diagnosis of GH and IGF deficiency remains imperfect, it is all the more critical that careful consideration be given to the issue of which children should be evaluated. The following categories of growth failure, warranting diagnostic evaluation, should be taken as flexible guidelines and not arbitrary and rigid rules:

1. Short stature (severe: height >3 SD below mean) in the absence of an alternative explanation (such as Turner's syndrome, renal disease, severe intrauterine growth retardation [IUGR], etc.)
2. Short stature (moderate: height -2 to -3 SD) and growth deceleration (height velocity <25%)
3. Severe growth deceleration
4. Predisposing condition (tumor, radiation, etc.) and growth deceleration (height velocity <25%)
5. Neonatal signs consistent with pituitary deficiencies (hypoglycemia, microphallus, direct hyberbilirubinemia) in the absence of an alternative explanation

These guidelines must be interpreted, however, in light of the known errors in measurement of height and calculation of height velocities. Voss et al.[155] have reported that serial height velocity calculations in short normal children vary considerably from year to year, with no significant correlations from one year to another. As a result, auxology, by itself, may not allow discrimination between a short normal child and a child with partial GHD.

Diagnosis in the Neonate

As stated above, IGF deficiency resulting from classic GHD or GHI is not associated with severe intrauterine growth failure, although birth length may be only 90% of normal term dimensions.[137, 138] In the single reported case of IGF-1 deficiency resulting from an IGF-1 gene deletion,[123] severe IUGR was noted, as predicted from the targeted gene disruption model in mice.[120–122] Accordingly, GHD and GHI need not be part of the differential diagnosis of severe IUGR, especially

when other explanations are available, such as placental insufficiency, dysmorphic syndromes, and so on. However, GHD should be considered in the infant with unexplained hypoglycemia, cryptorchidism or microphallus, direct hyperbilirubinemia, or midline craniofacial abnormalities. The diagnosis may be facilitated by allowing the infant to fast and, when the glucose has fallen below 30 mg/dL, obtaining blood samples for measurement of GH and cortisol. On an arbitrary basis, a serum GH of less than 10 ng/mL is considered consistent with a diagnosis of GHD under these considerations.[154] MRI of the brain should be obtained to look for PPE, hypoplasia of the anterior pituitary, hypoplasia or absence of the pituitary stalk, hypoplasia of the optic chiasm, and absence or hypoplasia of the corpus callosum and septum pellucidum.[65–73] If the clinical features of a neonate are believed to be consistent with pituitary insufficiency, it may be reasonable to perform MRI of the brain immediately, as the diagnosis may be readily established if a hypothalamic or pituitary abnormality is identified.

Diagnosis in the Child

Diagnostic evaluation in children must be based upon auxology, as described above. In children, broad overlap exists between GHD or GHI and IGF deficiency. Given the diagnostic controversies surrounding GHD, it may make more sense to establish a diagnosis of IGF deficiency, and then search for the cause (see Tables 36–1 and 36–2).

Diagnosis of IGF Deficiency

With the development of sensitive and specific assays for the various components of the IGF system, assessment of the IGF axis has become relatively straightforward.[2, 156] Radioimmunoassays and other derivative assays are readily available and allow direct measurement of the three components of the IGF axis known to be GH-dependent: IGF-1,[127, 156–158] IGFBP-3,[127, 156, 159, 160] and the ALS.[127, 161, 162] Supportive data may come from assessment of serum concentrations of IGF-2[157] or IGFBP-2,[163] but these proteins are not directly GH regulated. Serum levels of IGF-1, IGFBP-3, and ALS are relatively constant throughout the day and are not greatly affected by feeding, sleep, or exercise level[158, 160, 162]; accordingly, multiple sampling is not necessary, and a single blood specimen is usually sufficient.

There are a number of issues concerning IGF-related assays that are worth noting:

1. IGFBPs potentially interfere with radioimmunoassays for IGF-1 and IGF-2, as well as with radioreceptor assays and bioassays.[156, 164, 165] Ideally, IGFBPs should be removed from serum samples prior to assay for IGF peptides. This is best done by acid gel chromatography,[166] a laborious procedure which many laboratories have replaced with an acid-ethanol extraction method.[167] The latter strategy, however, is not ideal, and assays employing such methodologies should be validated carefully. An alternative approach is to block the IGFBPs by addition of an excess of either IGF-1 or IGF-2, but this mandates the use of a highly specific antibody for the other IGF ligand.[168] A third approach has been the use of radiolabeled IGF analogues with decreased affinity for interfering IGFBPs.[167]
2. Serum concentrations of IGF-1 are markedly age-dependent[169–172]; the same is true for IGF-2,[169–171] IGFBP-3,[160] and ALS,[162] although to a considerably lesser extent. Serum concentrations of IGF-1 are lowest during early childhood,[158, 169, 170] the time when one would wish to establish a biochemical diagnosis. Because discrimination between abnormal IGF-1 levels and low-normal levels may be particularly problematic in this age group, it is all the more important that the IGF-1 assay be sensitive and rigorous. Serum concentrations of IGF-1 should always be interpreted in light of the patient's chronologic age and pubertal status.[156, 169–172] There is, however, no particular advantage to relating IGF-1 or IGFBP-3 concentrations to bone age rather than chronologic age.
3. Serum IGF-1 concentrations may be affected by malnutrition and chronic disease.
4. Decreased serum concentrations of IGF-1, IGFBP-3, and ALS

will be seen in GHI, as well as GHD.[113, 114, 127, 152, 153] Discrimination between GHI and GHD requires measurement of serum GH concentrations, as well as assessment of a number of other biochemical indices (see below).

5. There are a number of theoretic and practical advantages to IGFBP-3 assays, compared to IGF-1 assays: they are technically simpler because they do not require removal of interfering IGFBPs; IGFBP-3 is less affected than IGF-1 by chronic disease and malnutrition; serum concentrations of IGFBP-3 are typically in the range of 1000 to 5000 ng/mL, so assay sensitivity is not an issue; IGFBP-3 concentrations, while age-dependent, do not vary as greatly as IGF-1 levels.

Despite these caveats, much can be said to support the use of IGF-related assays in the diagnosis of IGF deficiency, GHD, and GHI. Concurrent measurement of IGF-1, IGFBP-3 and ALS is an effective way of assessing the integrated GH-IGF axis.[2]

Diagnosis of Growth Hormone Deficiency

Assessment of GH secretion is problematic, in part because of the pulsatile nature of GH secretion.[173] The most consistent GH surges accompany slow-wave electroencephalographic rhythms during phases 3 and 4 of sleep. Although this rhythmicity is characteristic of GH secretion at all ages, the size of the amplitudes and the total integrated GH secretion varies with sex, age, pubertal status, and nutrition.[174, 175] Between pulses, serum GH concentrations are extremely low, often less than 0.1 ng/mL. Consequently, measurement of random serum GH concentrations is unlikely to be of value in the diagnosis of GHD, as a low GH level cannot discriminate between GHD and the normal interpulse nadir. Measurement of spontaneous GH secretion requires multiple sampling, typically every 5 to 30 minutes over a 12 to 24-hour period.[173–177] Such methodologies are inconvenient and expensive, and while they allow identification of the patient with severe GHD, it is not clear that they can discriminate between partial GHD and normal secretory variation.[178] Continual blood withdrawal over 12 to 24 hours permits measurement of mean serum GH concentrations, but is inconvenient and provides less information than multiple sampling.[179–181] However, even the reproducibility of GH secretory patterns in children from day to day is uncertain. Rose and colleagues[178] reported that measurement of spontaneous GH secretion identified only 57% of children diagnosed as GHD by provocative testing. Lanes[182] reported that approximately 25% of normally growing children have low overnight GH concentrations. A longitudinal study of GH secretion in normal boys during puberty indicated wide intersubject variation,[174, 175] and day-to-day variation has been noted among normal subjects.[183]

The label of "neurosecretory dysfunction" has been applied to slowly growing children with normal provocative GH levels, but with abnormally low spontaneous GH secretory patterns.[176, 177] There is little doubt that this combination may be observed in children who have been cranially irradiated,[29] but its applicability and utility in the evaluation of short children in general remains unproven. An alternative approach has been the measurement of urinary GH concentrations.[184–188] This methodology requires a timed urinary collection and a GH assay of high sensitivity, as urinary GH concentrations are, typically, low. The theoretic advantages of this approach include its relative ease of performance and noninvasive nature, as well as the requirement for only a single GH measurement. This must be balanced, however, by the need to assess the effects of renal function, the wide interindividual variation, and the lack of adequate age- and sex- related standards.

For over 25 years, the standard for the diagnosis of GHD has been provocative testing of GH "secretory reserve"[154, 189] (Table 36–6). Physiologic stimuli for such tests have included sleep[190] and exercise,[191, 192] and pharmacologic stimuli have included a wide variety of agents.[189, 193–203] None of these tests truly mimics normal GH secretory physiology and none has been evaluated adequately in normal children and normal short children. The limitations of these tests have led to the widely practiced approaches of obtaining multiple sequential blood samples during stimulation, and of combining two or more tests, in an effort to adequately screen out normal children; "passing" any one test is commonly accepted as indicating normal GH secretory capability.[199–202] In general, these tests are capable of identifying the child with complete or severe GHD; such children however, rarely pose a diagnostic problem, and can be identified readily by a variety of simpler methodologies, such as measurement of IGF-1 and IGFBP-3. Some of the limitations of provocative GH testing in the diagnosis of milder forms of GHD are described below:

1. Provocative testing, by its nature, is nonphysiologic. None of the commonly used stimuli truly mimics normal regulation of GH secretion.

2. The definition of a "normal" response to stimulation is totally arbitrary, and reflects, at least in part, the availability of GH as a therapeutic agent. Thus, when only pituitary-derived GH was available, the commonly accepted threshold for a "normal" GH response was 5 ng/mL. This was gradually increased to 7 and, later, to 10 ng/mL. The package inserts employed by pharmacologic producers of GH reflect this vagueness, with statements such as "lack of *adequate* endogenous GH secretion,"[204] and "*inadequate* secretion of *normal* endogenous GH"[205] (my italics reflect terms lacking sufficient definition).

3. The age- and sex-dependence of GH secretion in children has not been given adequate consideration. GH secretion rises during puberty, generally reflecting an increase in pulse amplitude.[174, 175, 206, 207] Despite this, the same criteria have been employed for defining GH deficiency throughout the pediatric and adolescent age groups. There has been numerous documentation of children who "failed" provocative GH testing at a preadolescent age, only to "pass" when retested

TABLE 36–6. Growth Hormone Stimulation Tests*

Stimulus	Dosage	Timing of Samples (min)	Comments
Exercise	Steep climbing or exercise cycle for 10–15 min	0, 10–15, 20–30	
Levodopa	<15 kg, 125 mg; 15–30 kg, 250 mg; >30 kg, 500 mg	0, 60, 90	Nausea
Clonidine	0.15 mg/m²	0, 30, 60, 90	Tiredness; postural hypotension
Arginine HCl	0.5 g/kg (max, 30 g) IV, given as 10% arginine HCl in 0.9% NaCl over 30 min	0, 15, 30, 45, 60	
Insulin	0.05–0.1 U/kg IV	0, 15, 30, 60, 75, 90, 120	Hypoglycemia; requires supervision
Glucagon	0.03 mg/kg IM (max, 1 mg)	0, 30, 60, 90, 120, 150, 180	Nausea
GHRH	1 μg/kg IV	0, 15, 30, 45, 60, 90, 120	Flushing; metallic taste

*Tests should be performed after an overnight fast.
Patients should be documented to be euthyroid.
Prepubertal children should be primed with gonadal steroids. Recommended regimens include (1) conjugated estrogens 2.5–5.0 mg by mouth the night before and the morning of the test (males/females); (2) ethinyl estradiol 50–100 μg/day for 3 consecutive days before testing (males/females); (3) depot testosterone 100 mg (males)
Insulin stimulation is designed to induce hypoglycemia, with a lowering of blood sugar to <50% of baseline levels. Such testing should only be performed under appropriate medical supervision. In young children with a high suspicion of pituitary deficiencies, the lower dosage of insulin may be employed.
IV, intravenous; IM, intramuscular; GHRH, GH-releasing hormone.
Adapted from Reiter EO, Rosenfeld RG: Normal and abnormal growth. *In* Wilson JD, Foster DW, Kronenberg HM, Larsen PR (eds): Williams Textbook of Endocrinology, ed 9. Philadelphia, WB Saunders, 1998, pp 1427–1507.

after administration of exogenous sex steroids[208] or after spontaneous puberty.[209, 210] Although such cases have sometimes been labeled as "transient" GHD, it is far more likely that they represent the inadequacies of provocative testing.[211] Marin and colleagues[212] demonstrated that when exercise and arginine stimulation tests were performed on normal-stature children without sex steroid priming, the lower-limits-of-normal (−2 SD) peak serum GH concentration for prepubertal children was as low as 1.9 ng/mL. For children who were in Tanner stage 5 of puberty, this value was 9.3 ng/mL. When estrogen was administered as a "priming" agent to prepubertal children before provocative GH testing, the lower 95% confidence limit for peak serum GH concentration rose to 7.2 ng/mL. When estrogen was not administered, the peak serum GH failed to exceed 7 ng/mL during three provocative tests in 61% of normal prepubertal children. Such children would have been diagnosed erroneously as having GHD on the basis of their non–estrogen-primed provocative GH test. While it has been argued that priming prepubertal children with gonadal steroids is not physiologic, it is clear that the false-positive rate in nonprimed GH tests is unacceptably high. We conclude that sex steroid priming must be performed in GH provocative tests of prepubertal children if these tests are to have any discriminatory capability.

4. GH assays are frequently nonspecific, and measure a variety of immunoreactive molecular forms of GH.[130, 131] These GH variants do not necessarily possess equivalent growth-promoting actions. Furthermore, considerable interassay variability exists in the measurement of these GH molecular variants.[213–216] This limitation is not necessarily overcome by the use of monoclonal antibodies, since the specificity of the antibody is a key issue; other issues include GH standards, diluents, and labeling methodologies. It is not likely that these problems will be resolved by immunofunctional GH assays, which may face many of the same issues.[217] Such difficulties are further complicated by the fact that most physicians ordering GH measurements have little knowledge of the specifics and limitations of the assays performed.[218]

5. The effect of obesity on responsiveness to provocative GH testing has not been assessed adequately.[219]

6. The effect of depression, anxiety, and a variety of psychosocial factors on GH responsiveness has not been studied adequately in children.[220] These factors are well known to affect GH secretory dynamics in adults.[221–223]

7. In addition to evaluating the pubertal status of patients prior to GH testing, it is essential that patients be documented to be euthyroid.

8. Provocative testing fails to give any consideration to the effect of negative feedback by serum IGF-1.[224–230] It probably makes more sense to interpret GH levels in light of serum IGF concentrations, much as TSH concentrations are best assessed with a knowledge of circulating thyroxine levels.

9. Provocative GH testing is expensive, uncomfortable, and potentially risky. Insulin-induced hypoglycemia should only be performed in a supervised setting. Deaths have been documented in patients rendered hypoglycemic and corrected in an overly vigorous manner.[231]

Of the provocative tests listed in Table 36–6, it should be noted that stimulation with GHRH is not designed to document if a patient has GHD, but rather whether GHD, established by other methodologies, is the result of pituitary or hypothalamic dysfunction.[232, 233] Failure to respond to GHRH suggests that the abnormality is at the pituitary level. This test may be enhanced by the addition of arginine or pyridostigmine,[234] which act to inhibit endogenous somatostatin, but, again, will fail to identify the child with GHD on a hypothalamic basis.

Correlations Between IGF and Growth Hormone Measurements

Multiple studies have investigated the correlations between assays of the IGF axis and GH provocative tests, in an effort to ascertain the reliability of each diagnostic test.[1, 2, 154, 156, 157, 159, 162, 163, 235–240] All such studies are inherently flawed, as they frequently are comprised of subjects in whom the underlying diagnosis is uncertain; discrepancies between measures of GH and components of the IGF system are therefore difficult to resolve. In pediatric patients with complete or severe GHD, stimulated GH concentrations and serum IGF-1 and IGFBP-3 are invariably low. It is in the group of patients with partial or evolving GHD that the correlations between serum GH and IGF concentrations begin to falter (see below).

In one study, which assessed serum concentrations of both IGF-1 and IGF-2, 18% of patients with low provocative GH levels had IGF-1 concentrations in the normal range, but only 4% of children with GHD (defined by provocative GH testing) had normal serum concentrations of both IGF-1 and IGF-2.[157] Blum and colleagues[159] reported that serum IGFBP-3 concenrations were below the 5th percentile for chronologic age in 97% of children diagnosed with GHD by both provocative GH levels and auxologic criteria. In the same study, 95% of non–GH-deficient short children had normal serum IGFBP-3. Juul and Skakkebaek[236] have reported sensitivity and specificity of the IGFBP-3 assay in the diagnosis of GHD as 60% and 98%, respectively, in children less than 10 years of age, and 57% and 79%, respectively, in patients aged 10 to 20 years. The addition of IGFBP-2 assays has been reported to enhance the value of IGF-1 and IGFBP-3 assays in the diagnosis of GHD.[163] In studies involving measurement of spontaneous GH secretion, correlations with serum IGF-1 and IGFBP-3 have been imperfect.[186]

The failure to see perfect correlations between measurements of the IGF axis and either provocative or spontaneous GH concentrations can be ascribed to several factors:

1. By far the most important is likely to be erroneous identification of GHD patients. As stated above, multiple problems in GH testing have led to a diagnosis of GHD in many children who are endocrinologically normal.[154, 210, 240] It should not be surprising if some of these children prove to have normal IGF-1 or IGFBP-3 concentrations. In studies that have been limited to severe childhood GHD the correlation between IGF and GH measurements is excellent.

2. Flaws exist in IGF-related assays, just as they do in GH assays.[156] There exist important assay issues concerning removal of interfering IGFBPs and specificity of antibodies that need to be addressed.[164–168] It is also critical that IGF, IGFBP-3, and ALS concentrations be compared with accurate age-related normative values.[158, 160, 162]

3. The value of IGF-related assays breaks down when dealing with evolving GHD, especially in pubertal or postpubertal patients. The best example of this is in irradiation-induced growth failure, where evolving GHD, characterized by growth failure and biochemical evidence of impaired GH secretion, is frequently accompanied by normal IGF-1 and IGFBP-3 concentrations.[41, 42, 240, 241] This is particularly true in the pubertal patient. It is clear from patients with severe GHI that a pubertal rise in serum IGF-1 and IGFBP-3 occurs, even in the absence of any GH action[113, 114]; this pubertal increase means that in the adolescent and adult, serum IGF-1 and IGFBP-3 concentrations are only partially GH dependent.

Diagnosis of Growth Hormone Insensitivity

GHI is another form of IGF deficiency.[113, 114] Originally reported by Laron and Pertzelan,[110] in its classic form GHI is an autosomal recessive disorder characterized by an abnormality of the GH receptor (GH receptor deficiency; see Table 36–5).[111, 112] The criteria used for establishing the diagnosis in this classic form are summarized in Table 36–7.[136, 153] These criteria are best-suited to the patient who is homozygous for a mutation or deletion involving the extracellular, GH-binding domain of the GH receptor. Such patients, typically, have decreased serum GH-binding activity, accompanied by decreased serum concentrations of IGF-1 and IGFBP-3, increased serum levels of GH, and defective IGF-1 and IGFBP-3 responsiveness to exogenous GH (IGF generation test).[113, 114, 136, 153] Ideally, the biochemical diagnosis should be corroborated by molecular studies, designed to identify abnormalities of the GH receptor gene.[113, 114, 136, 242–244]

A number of recent studies have broadened the concept of GHI.[117, 118, 243–246] Mutations affecting the GH receptor dimerization domain and regions involved in intracellular trafficking (in the extracellular portion of the receptor),[115, 247] as well as the transmembrane or intracellular domains,[116, 119, 248] have been shown to cause GHI, despite normal or even increased serum GH-binding activity. Milder forms of GHI have

TABLE 36–7. Scoring System for the Diagnosis of Growth Hormone (GH) Insensitivity Syndrome*

Test	Parameter	Criterion	Score
Auxology	Height	< -3 SD	1
Basal GH	Random GH	>2.5 ng/mL	1
Basal IGFs	IGF-1	<50 ng/mL	1
	IGFBP-3	< -2 SD	1
IGF-1 generation	IGF-1 increase	<15 ng/mL	1
	IGFBP-3 increase	<400 ng/mL	1
GH binding	Percentage GH bound	$<10\%$	1

*A score of 5 points or greater is considered consistent with classic GHI.[251]
IGF, insulin-like growth factor; IGFBP, insulin-like growth factor binding protein.

been ascribed to heterozygosity for certain mutations which may have a dominant negative effect.[117, 118, 245, 246] A diagnosis of an atypical or partial form of GHI should be supported by molecular studies and demonstration of an impaired IGF generation response to exogenous GH.[112, 249–253] Unfortunately, normative data for IGF generation are not available currently, so the definition of "impaired response" is empiric and arbitrary.

A Practical Approach to Diagnostic Evaluation

A practical approach to the diagnosis of a child with GHD or GHI is grounded on auxology, and necessitates careful selection of which children require biochemical evaluation. The best way to avoid false positives in the diagnosis of GHD is to not test children who fail to meet the auxologic or predisposing criteria described above.

In the prepubertal child with abnormal growth, serum concentrations of IGF-1, IGFBP-3, and perhaps ALS, IGF-2, and IGFBP-2, provide a means for establishing a diagnosis of IGF deficiency. In the child with low levels of these components of the IGF system, a systematic evaluation will allow determination of whether hypothalamic or pituitary dysfunction exists, or whether GHI is causative. Provocative GH testing with two or more agents and with appropriate sex steroid priming will provide some information on GH secretory capability; GHRH stimulation, with or without arginine or pyridostigmine, will allow determination of whether the defect is at the hypothalamic or pituitary level.

It is our recommendation that GH therapy is justified in the patient with abnormal auxology supported by biochemical data demonstrating *either* abnormally low provocative GH concentrations or IGF deficiency. This recommendation acknowledges the failure of either GH testing or IGF testing to identify partial GH deficiency with 100% certainty. It is clear that most prepubertal children with true GHD will demonstrate abnormalities of both GH and IGF secretion, and that some children will have unequivocally low IGF-1 and IGFBP-3 concentrations but a seemingly normal GH response, whereas others will unequivocally fail GH stimulation testing but have borderline or normal IGF concentrations. Ultimately, the diagnosis of GHD requires that the clinician integrate clinical data, serial height measurements, family history, and a variety of biochemical values, all of which may not always be completely concordant.

In the pubertal patient, especially when GHD has been acquired, it should not be surprising to see discrepancies between GH testing and IGF measurement. This will be true, particularly, in the presence of an evolving GHD, as is seen in patients receiving cranial irradiation. Documentation of growth failure in such patients may be sufficient to warrant initiation of GH therapy if either GH testing or the IGF concentration is abnormal. Indeed, an argument can be made for starting GH treatment in patients who are experiencing unequivocal growth failure, even before their GH and IGF levels fall. This recommendation requires careful clinical judgment and an assessment of the likelihood that the patient will have sufficient time before epiphyseal closure to achieve normal growth.

Documentation of GHD also requires that other pituitary functions be assessed periodically, including TSH, ACTH, and gonadotropin status. Other pituitary deficiencies may not be evident upon initial assessment, but may develop over time. MRI of the hypothalamus and pituitary should be performed initially, to determine if there is evidence of intracranial tumors, pituitary hypoplasia, midline defects, and so on. Even if the baseline MRI is normal, in the absence of an alternative explanation for GHD or CPHD, the possibility of tumors or structural defects should not be dismissed permanently.

The recent recommendations that GH replacement be administered to adults with GHD have made it all the more critical that the diagnosis of GHD be established firmly. A number of studies have indicated that as many as 20% to 87% of children diagnosed with GHD test normally as adults.[207, 208, 254–257] This is particularly true for patients with IGHD or who carry a diagnosis of idiopathic GHD. It is therefore recommended that all pediatric patients diagnosed as having GHD be retested as young adults.[240, 258, 259] In the patient with known organic disease or a molecular defect, measurement of serum concentrations of IGF-1 and IGFBP-3 might be sufficient. In the patient whose GHD has no known cause, it is imperative that retesting include measurements of both the IGF axis and GH secretion.

TREATMENT

Growth Hormone

Initial efforts to treat hypopituitarism with bovine or ovine GH failed, because of the specific requirement for primate-derived GH preparations.[260–262] The first successful treatment of human GHD with human pituitary–derived GH (hGH) was in the 1950s.[263, 264] This use of human cadaver pituitary–derived hGH represented a remarkable therapeutic breakthrough for children with GHD, but necessitated national cooperative efforts to collect pituitaries and extract and purify hGH.[264–267] Although it has been estimated that over 27,000 children were treated with pituitary-derived hGH over a 30-year period, limited supplies mandated the use of suboptimal dosages, interrupted treatment periods, and frequent cessation of therapy before maximal height had been attained. The distribution of hGH was halted in the United States in early 1985, following the discovery of several cases of Creutzfeldt-Jakob disease associated with its use.[268–271] To date, more than 60 cases of this fatal spongiform encephalopathy have been traced to the use of hGH. Fortunately, clinical trials of recombinant DNA–derived hGH (rhGH) had begun in the early 1980s and the safety and efficacy of such preparations were soon verified.[272–274] By November 1985, the U.S. Food and Drug Administration approved the use of rhGH in children with GHD, and other countries soon followed. The initial rhGH preparations included an N-terminal methionine; met-rhGH proved to be fully active biologically, but was ultimately replaced by the mature 191–amino acid protein. The biopotency of current preparations of rhGH, expressed as international units per milligram of the new World Health Organization (WHO) rhGH reference reagent for somatropin (88/624), is 3 IU/mg.[275]

Investigations of optimal dosing of rhGH have been complicated by the use of heterogeneous study populations, so that studies frequently include patients with unequivocal and complete GHD, together with patients with partial (or perhaps nonexistent) GHD. Several studies have demonstrated a dose-response relationship for hGH, but the slope of the response is relatively shallow.[264, 276] MacGillivray and colleagues[277] compared the growth responses of 99 children treated with pituitary hGH at a mean dosage of 0.1 mg/kg/week, with those of 77 children treated with rhGH at a dosage of 0.3 mg/kg/week. The mean time required to reach normal height (> -2.0 SD) was 48 months for the low-dose group and 27 months for the high-dose group. Fifty-one percent of the low-dose group never attained normal height (> -2.0 SD), compared to 23% in the high-dose group. Cohen and Rosenfeld[278] compared the growth responses of prepubertal, naive patients randomized to rhGH at a dosage of 0.175, 0.35, or 0.7 mg/kg/week for the first 2 years of treatment. Significantly greater height velocities and gains in height SD resulted from the 0.35 mg/kg/week vs. 0.175 mg/kg/week, but no further significant improvement was observed with the 0.7 mg/kg/week dosage. Ultimately, the issues that should determine dosage in the child with GHD are (1) how best to return the growth-retarded child to the normal growth curve; (2) how best to ensure that the child attains his or her genetic height potential;

(3) risks; and (4) cost. For the child with severe GHD, weekly dosages of 0.175 mg/kg, administered in seven daily doses, either by a subcutaneous or intramuscular route, are usually sufficient to increase growth rates from 3 to 4 cm/year to more than 10 cm/year. Indeed, Ranke and colleagues[279] have reported that in children with GHD, auxologic parameters, such as chronologic age (the younger the patient, the better the response), and the difference between target height and actual height (the smaller the patient, the better the response) are better predictors of growth response than the cumulative weekly GH dosage. Although this lower dosage appears to be more than sufficient for initial therapy of most children with true GHD, there has been a gradual movement toward higher dosages, with many patients now being started on 0.35 mg/kg/week. Prolonged treatment almost invariably results in a waning response to hGH, with growth rates typically falling to 7 to 9 cm/year in the second and third year. MacGillivray and colleagues[277, 280] have compared daily rhGH with thrice-weekly rhGH at the same cumulative dosage of 0.30 mg/kg/week. The mean total height gain over a 4-year period was 9.7 cm greater in the daily treated patients (38.4 vs. 28.7 cm, $P<.0002$). Studies are currently underway to assess the efficacy of sustained-release rhGH preparations, which may be administered as infrequently as every 2 to 4 weeks.[281]

The physician is, thus, frequently faced with the quandary of choosing between a high dosage of rhGH, designed to correct growth deficiency as rapidly as possible, vs. a more economical use of an expensive medication. This, in part, can be addressed by early and proper diagnosis of the child with GHD, so that therapy can be initiated at as young an age as possible, before the growth deficit becomes difficult to surmount. In the young child with a modest growth deficiency, it would seem reasonable to initiate therapy with the lower dosage (0.175 mg/kg/week, given daily) and monitor the growth response. If the growth rate in the first year is less than 10 cm/year, or if the growth response wanes excessively, the dosage of rhGH can be increased. In the older child, or where the growth deficit is great, initiation of therapy with a higher dosage (0.35 mg/kg/week) may be indicated. Daily administration appears to be preferable to thrice-weekly, and it is critical that compliance be maintained and that dosages be adjusted periodically for weight gain. In the patient with multiple pituitary deficiencies, it is important that a euthyroid status be maintained and that glucocorticoid replacement not be excessive.

Early initiation of therapy, combined with careful attention to dosage adjustments and compliance, is the best predictor of cumulative growth response in patients with GHD. Final height correlates with height at the initiation of puberty, so it is important to maximize growth during the prepubertal period, within the limits of safety and economy.[281–294] Analysis of data on final heights of rhGH-treated GHD is complicated by the heterogeneity of patient groups and dosage, but the most common observation is a general failure of children to reach their full genetic height potential, especially in the case of IGHD.[282–294] Price and Ranke[295] have reported final heights of −1.26 SD and −1.45 SD in males and females, respectively, with IGHD, and −0.22 SD and −0.52 SD in males and females, respectively, with CPHD. MacGillivray and colleagues[296] reported mean adult heights of −1.5 SD in both IGHD and CPHD. In patients with longer durations of treatment and higher dosages of rhGH, adult heights tended to be greater, although still failing to achieve full genetic height potential. In 121 children treated for 8 years with 0.3 mg/kg/week, the mean adult height was −0.7 SD. De Luca and colleagues[297] reported that in 13 GHD children, in whom treatment was initiated prior to 5 years of age and continued for at least 9 years, 8 children exceeded their respective target heights, and only 3 failed to attain an adult height within the target range.

It is clear that the timing of puberty has a significant impact on adult height of rhGH-treated GHD.[293, 294, 298, 299] The duration of rhGH treatment and the height gained prepubertally are, typically, greater when puberty is induced rather than spontaneous. In a study by Ranke and colleagues[298] final height was attained at 17.8 and 19.2 years in boys and at 16.0 and 17.0 years in girls following spontaneous and induced puberty, respectively. Final heights were greater after induced puberty compared with spontaneous puberty in boys (171.3 vs. 166.0 cm) and in girls (157.0 vs. 155.0 cm). Therapy designed at delaying the onset of puberty (both normal and precocious) may augment the cumulative growth response to rhGH (see below).

Adverse Effects of Human Growth Hormone

rhGH has had an excellent track record of safety.[300–303] Reports of anti-GH antibodies in patients employing rhGH have been few, and these antibodies have only proved rarely to attenuate the growth response.[274, 304, 305] Fluid retention, carpal tunnel syndrome, and insulin resistance are observed in adults, but are seldom significant in children. Idiopathic intracranial hypertension (pseudotumor cerebri) has been observed occasionally, but resolves with cessation of treatment, or even if treatment is continued.[300, 306, 307] Slipped capital femoral epiphysis has been reported, but it is not clear that its incidence is greater than that observed in normal children during rapid periods of growth, or in hypothyroid children treated with thyroxine.[308–310] Other possible rare and still unproven complications include acute pancreatitis,[311] increased growth of pigmented nevi,[312] and prepubertal gynecomastia.[313]

The most important theoretic risk that has been raised with rhGH therapy has been that of malignancy.[300, 301, 314–323] Epidemiologic assessment has been complicated by the fact that many rhGH recipients are at increased risk of malignancy because of chromosomal abnormalities, prior malignancies, or prior histories of chemotherapy or irradiation. Additionally, it has been suggested that, in some cases, GH deficiency itself may predispose to development of malignancy.[301, 302] Although a number of early reports suggested a link between hGH treatment and leukemia, Blethen and colleagues[300] reported that an analysis of 47,000 patient-years of treatment in greater than 19,000 children indicated that in children without known risk factors, rhGH therapy was not associated with an increased occurrence of tumors or recurrence rate of leukemia or CNS tumors. Despite these assurances, it is customary to delay rhGH treatment in children with treated brain tumors until they have been shown to be tumor-free for at least 1 to 2 years.

Growth Hormone–Releasing Hormone

In children whose GHD is due to a hypothalamic abnormality, treatment with GHRH would appear to be an appropriate therapeutic option.[324–326] Both GHRH (1–4) and (1–29) have been shown to be biologically active in humans. Unfortunately, although it can be absorbed nasally, this route of administration has not proved to be effective[327] and treatment must be via subcutaneous or intramuscular injection, as is the case with rhGH. Direct comparisons of rhGH and GHRH have not been performed, but a number of studies indicate that GHRH, administered once or twice daily, can increase the growth rates of children with GHD on a hypothalamic basis, although the response in most reports appears to be less than that expected with rhGH therapy.[324–326] No specific therapeutic advantage of GHRH over rhGH has been demonstrated to date, although further studies are warranted to investigate optimization of dosage and frequency of administration. Short-term growth responses have been noted with intranasal administration of GHRH, but waning appears to occur rapidly and local side effects, such as rhinorrhea, were observed. It is of note that Lifschitz et al.[328] reported that six of nine children showed sustained increases in height velocity and spontaneous overnight GH secretion for 4 to 24 months after a brief period of treatment with GHRH (2 to 13 months). These findings must be confirmed, but suggest that GHRH may "reprogram" pituitary GH secretion.

Patients should be demonstrated to respond to GHRH by increasing their serum GH concentrations before GHRH is administered therapeutically. It is noteworthy, however, that a number of studies have indicated little correlation between the growth response to GHRH and the initial GH response to intravenous therapy.[233, 324, 325, 329] Whether this is due to inadequate GHRH dosing, decreased pituitary content of releasable GH, or downregulation of GHRH receptors on somatotropic cells is unclear.[325, 326] Prolonged administration of GHRH may prove to be necessary to adequately define potential pituitary responsiveness.

TABLE 36–8. Growth Response to Insulin-like Growth Factor-1 (IGF-1) Treatment of Growth Hormone Insensitivity

Study Group	n	IGF-1 Dose (μg/kg)	Growth Velocity (cm/yr)(SD)		
			Pretreatment	Year 1	Year 2
Israel[340]	9	150–200/day	4.6 (1.3)	8.2 (0.8)	—
	6*	150–200/day	5.0 (1.2)	8.3 (1.0)	6.0 (1.3)
Multicenter study group[339]	26	40–120 b.i.d.	NA	8.5 (2.1)	—
	18*	40–120 b.i.d.	NA	8.6 (1.7)	6.4 (0.2)
North Carolina[341]	5	80–120 b.i.d.	4.2 (0.9)	9.3	6.2
Ecuador[337,338]	15	120 b.i.d.	3.4 (1.4)	8.8 (1.1)	6.4 (1.1)
	7	80 b.i.d.	3.0 (1.8)	9.1 (2.2)	5.6 (2.1)

NA, not available.

*Subjects included in prior cohort for year 1 data.

Adapted from Rosenfeld RG: IGF-I treatment of growth hormone insensitivity. *In* Takano T, Hizuka N, Takahashi S-I (eds): Molecular Mechanisms to Regulate the Activities of Insulin-like Growth Factors. Amsterdam, Elsevier, 1998, pp 359–364.

Growth Hormone–Releasing Peptides and Nonpeptidyl Growth Hormone Secretagogues

Since the discovery of growth hormone–releasing peptides (GHRPs) by Bowers et al. in the 1980s,[330] a variety of small GHRPs and nonpeptidyl small-molecule GH secretagogues have been manufactured.[326, 331] These small molecules are potent stimulators of GH release, especially when administered together with GHRH, and may be active when administered by intravenous, intramuscular, subcutaneous, nasal, and oral routes.[326, 331] These potential advantages must be balanced by the likelihood that normal GHRH production is required to see maximal benefit from such agents.[332, 333] Trials are currently in progress to assess the utility of these agents in the treatment of children and adults with GHD.

Insulin-like Growth Factor-1

Complete or severe GHI cannot be treated with conventional dosages of rhGH, although it is conceivable that partial GHI may respond to superphysiologic dosages. The development of recombinant IGF-1, however, has provided the potential for bypassing defects in the GH

TABLE 36–9. Comparison of Insulin-like Growth Factor-1 Treatment of Growth Hormone Insensitivity (GHI) and Growth Hormone Treatment of Growth Hormone Deficiency (GHD)

	GHI	GHD	*P*-Value
Growth velotcity (cm/yr) (SD)			
Year 1	8.9 (1.5)	10.9 (1.6)	<.0001
Year 2	6.1 (1.5)	8.1 (2.2)	<.02
Year 3	5.7 (1.4)	8.3 (1.9)	<.001
Increment of growth velocity above baseline (cm/yr) (SD)			
Year 1	5.5 (1.4)	8.8 (2.5)	<.0001
Year 2	2.9 (1.6)	6.1 (3.1)	<.01
Year 3	2.9 (1.2)	6.5 (2.4)	<.005
Change in height SD score (SD)*	1.4 (0.6)	2.2 (1.0)	<.01
Change in height age (SD)*	1.7 (0.8)	2.5 (0.7)	<.01
Change in bone age (SD)*	2.0 (1.1)	2.6 (1.3)	NS

*Over 2 years of treatment.

NS, not significant.

Adapted from Rosenfeld RG: IGF-I treatment of growth hormone insensitivity. *In* Takano T, Hizuka N, Takahashi S-I (eds): Molecular Mechanisms to Regulate the Activities of Insulin-like Growth Factors. Amsterdam, Elsevier, 1998, pp 359–364; and Guevara-Aguirre J, Rosenbloom AL, Vasconez O: Two-year treatment of growth hormone (GH) receptor deficiency with recombinant insulin-like growth factor I in 22 children. Comparison of two-dosage levels and to GH-treated GH deficiency. J Clin Endocrinol Metab 82:629–633, 1997.

receptor, GH signaling cascade, or IGF-1 biosynthesis.[334] Laron and colleagues[335] reported growth acceleration to rates of 8.8 to 13.6 cm/year in five children with GHI treated with a single daily dose of 150 μg/kg for 3 to 10 months. Subsequent studies, however, have indicated a more modest response to IGF-1 treatment[334, 336–343] (Table 36–8). In a randomized, double-blind, placebo-controlled trial of IGF-1 therapy, growth rates in subjects receiving IGF-1 increased from 2.9 to 8.6 cm/year during the first year of treatment, and 6.4 cm/year in the second year.[339] As with rhGH treatment of GHD, growth is best during the first year of treatment, with a subsequent waning effect. In general, the growth response to IGF-1 does not match that observed with rhGH treatment of naive GHD[334, 340] (Table 36–9). This may be due to a number of factors: (1) inadequate dosage of IGF-1; (2) failure of IGF-1 treatment to correct deficiencies of IGFBP-3 and ALS, with a resulting short half-life for IGF-1 in serum; and (3) growth-promoting actions of rhGH that are independent of its ability to stimulate IGF-1 production.

REFERENCES

1. Rosenfeld RG: Disorders of growth hormone/IGF secretion and action. *In* Sperling M (ed): Pediatric Endocrinology. Philadelphia, WB Saunders, 1996, pp 117–169.
2. Rosenfeld RG: Is growth hormone deficiency a viable diagnosis? J Clin Endocrinol Metab 82:349–351, 1997.
3. Parkin JM: Incidence of growth hormone deficiency. Arch Dis Child 49:904–905, 1974.
4. Vimpani GV, Vimpani AF, Lidgard GP, et al: Prevalence of severe growth hormone deficiency. BMJ 2:427–430, 1977.
5. Lindsay R, Feldkamp M, Harris D, et al: Utah Growth Study: Growth standards and the prevalence of growth hormone deficiency. J Pediatr 125:29–35, 1994.
6. Wilton P: Progress in Growth Hormone Therapy—5 Years of KIGS. Mannheim, Germany, JJ Verlag, 1994, pp 62–66.
7. Genentech National Cooperative Growth Study Summary Report 18. San Francisco, Genentech, 1994, pp 6–13.
8. Albertsson-Wikland K, Niklasson A, Karlberg P: Birth data for patients who later develop growth hormone deficiency: Preliminary analysis of a national register. Acta Paediatr Suppl 370:115–120, 1990.
9. Craft WH, Underwood LE, Van Wyk JJ: High incidence of perinatal insult in children with idiopathic hypopituitarism. J Pediatr 96:397–402, 1980.
10. Costin G: Endocrine disorders associated with tumors of the pituitary and hypothalamus. Pediatr Clin North Am 26:15–31, 1979.
11. Jenkins JS, Gilberg CJ, Ang V: Hypothalamic-pituitary function in patients with craniopharyngiomas. J Clin Endocrinol Metab 43:394–399, 1976.
12. Thomsett MJ, Conte FA, Kaplan SL, et al: Endocrine and neurologic outcome in childhood craniopharyngioma. J Pediatr 97:728–735, 1980.
13. Laws ER, Thapar K: The diagnosis and management of craniopharyngioma. Growth Genet Horm 10:6–10, 1994.
14. Paja M, Lucas T, Garcia-Uria J, et al: Hypothalamic-pituitary dysfunction in patients with craniopharyngioma. Clin Endocrinol (Oxf) 42:467–473, 1995.
15. Rivarola M, Mendilaharzu H, Warman M, et al: Endocrine disorders in 66 suprasellar and pineal tumors of patients with prepubertal and pubertal ages. Horm Res 37:1–6, 1992.
16. Devile CJ, Grant DB, Hayward RD, et al: Growth and endocrine sequelae of craniopharyngioma. Arch Dis Child 75:108–114, 1996.
17. Kane LA, Leinung MC, Scheithauer BW, et al: Pituitary adenomas in childhood and adolescence. J Clin Endocrinol Metab 79:1135–1140, 1994.
18. Frailioli B, Ferrante L, Celli P: Pituitary adenomas with onset during puberty: Features and treatments. J Neurosurg 59:590–595, 1983.
19. Egeler RM, D'Angio GJ: Langerhans' cell histiocytosis. J Pediatr 127:1–11, 1996.
20. Braunstein GD, Kohler PO: Pituitary function in Hand-Schüller-Christian disease. Evidence for deficient growth hormone release in patients with short stature. N Engl J Med 286:1225–1229, 1972.
21. Broadbent V, Dunger DN, Yeomans E, et al: Anterior pituitary function and computed tomography/magnetic resonance imaging in patients with Langerhans cell histiocytosis and diabetes insipidus. Med Pediatr Oncol 21:649–654, 1993.
22. Dean HJ, Bishop A, Winter JSD: Growth hormone deficiency in patients with histiocytosis X. J Pediatr 109:615–618, 1996.
23. Bartsocas CS, Pantelakis SN: Human growth hormone therapy in hypopituitarism due to tuberculous meningitis. Acta Paediatr Scand 62:304–306, 1973.
24. Stuart CA, Neelon FA, Lebovitz HE: Hypothalamic insufficiency: The cause of hypopituitarism in sarcoidosis. Ann Intern Med 88:589–594, 1978.
25. Mayfield RK, Levine JH, Gordon L, et al: Lymphadenoid hypophysitis presenting as a pituitary tumor. Am J Med 69:619–623, 1980.
26. Albertsson-Wikland K, Lannering B, Marky I, et al: A longitudinal study on growth and spontaneous growth hormone (GH) secretion in children with irradiated brain tumors. Acta Paediatr Scand 76:966–973, 1987.
27. Brauner R, Rappaport R, Prevot C, et al: A prospective study of the development of growth hormone deficiency in children given cranial irradiation, and its relation to statural growth. J Clin Endocrinol Metab 68:346–351, 1989.
28. Shalet SM: Irradiation-induced growth. Pediatr Clin North Am 15:591–606, 1986.
29. Blatt J, Bercu BB, Gillin JC, et al: Reduced pulsatile growth hormone secretion in children after therapy for acute lymphoblastic leukemia. J Pediatr 104:182–186, 1984.

30. Sklar CA, Constine LS: Chronic neuroendocrinological sequelae of radiation therapy. Int J Radiat Oncol Biol Phys 31:1113–1121, 1995.
31. Clayton PE, Shalet SM: Dose dependency of time of onset of radiation-induced growth hormone deficiency. J Pediatr 118:226–228, 1991.
32. Rappaport R, Brauner R: Growth and endocrine disorders secondary to cranial irradiation. Pediatr Res 25:561–567, 1989.
33. Littley MD, Shalet SM, Beardwell CG, et al: Radiation-induced hypopituitarism is dose-dependent. Clin Endocrinol (Oxf) 31:361–373, 1989.
34. Sklar C, Mertens A, Walter A, et al: Final height after treatment for childhood acute lymphoblastic leukemia: Comparison of no cranial irradiation with 1800 and 2400 centigrays of cranial irradiation. J Pediatr 123:56–64, 1993.
35. Stubberfield TG, Byrne GC, Jones TW: Growth and growth hormone secretion after treatment for acute lymphoblastic leukemia in childhood. J Pediatr Hematol Oncol 17:167–171, 1995.
36. Katz JA, Pollack BH, Jacaruso D, et al: Finally attained height in patients successfully treated for childhood acute lymphoblastic leukemia. J Pediatr 123:546–552, 1993.
37. Donaldson SS, Kaplan H: Complications of treatment of Hodgkin's disease in children. Cancer Treat Rep 66:977–989, 1982.
38. Davies HA, Didcock E, Didi A, et al: Growth, puberty, obesity after treatment for leukemia. Acta Paediatr Scand 411:45–50, 1995.
39. Constine LS, Woolf PD, Cann D, et al: Hypothalamic-pituitary dysfunction after radiation for brain tumors. N Engl J Med 328:87–94, 1993.
40. Sklar CA: Growth following therapy for childhood cancer. Cancer Invest 13:511–516, 1995.
41. Sklar CA, Sarafoglou K, Whittam E: Effects of insulin-like growth factor binding protein 3 in predicting the growth hormone response to provacative testing in children treated with cranial irradiation. Acta Endocrinol 129:511–515, 1993.
42. Nivot S, Benelli C, Clot JP, et al: Nonparallel changes of growth hormone (GH) and insulin-like growth factor binding protein-3, and GH-binding protein, after craniospinal irradiation and chemotherapy. J Clin Endocrinol Metab 78:597–601, 1995.
43. Leiper AD, Stanhope R, Kitching P, et al: Precocious and premature puberty associated with treatment of acute lymphoblastic leukemia. Arch Dis Child 62:1107–1112, 1962.
44. Ogilvy-Stuart AL, Shalet SM: Growth and puberty after growth hormone treatment after irradiation for brain tumors. Arch Dis Child 73:141–146, 1973.
45. Quigley C, Cowell C, Jimenez M, et al: Normal or early development of puberty despite gonadal damage in children treated for acute lymphoblastic leukemia. N Engl J Med 321:143–151, 1989.
46. Oberfield SE, Soranno D, Nirenbert A, et al: Age at onset of puberty following high dose central nervous system radiation. Arch Pediatr Adolesc Med 150:589–592, 1996.
47. Cara JF, Kreiter ML, Rosenfield RL: Height prognosis of children with true precocious puberty and growth hormone deficiency: Effect of combination therapy with gonadotropin releasing hormone agonist and growth hormone. J Pediatr 120:709–715, 1992.
48. Sklar C: Growth and endocrine disturbances after bone marrow transplantation in childhood. Acta Paediatr Suppl 411:57–61, 1995.
49. Bushhouse S, Ramsay NKC, Pescovitz OH, et al: Growth in children following irradiation for bone marrow transplantation. Am J Pediatr Hematol Oncol 11:134–140, 1989.
50. Clement-De Boers A, Oostdijk W, Van Weel-Sipman MH: Final height and hormonal function after bone marrow transplantation in children. J Pediatr 129:544–550, 1996.
51. Giri N, Davis EAC, Vowels MR: Long-term complications following BMT in children. J Pediatr Child Health 29:201–205, 1993.
52. Bozzola M, Giorgiani G, Locatelli F, et al: Growth in children after bone marrow transplantation. Horm Res 39:122–126, 1993.
53. Brauner R, Fontoura M, Zucker JM, et al: Growth and growth hormone secretion after bone marrow transplantation. Arch Dis Child 68:458–463, 1993.
54. Thomas BC, Stanhope R, Plowman PN, et al: Endocrine function following single fraction and fractionated total body irradiation for bone marrow transplantation in childhood. Acta Endocrinol 128:508–512, 1993.
55. Ogilvy-Stuart AL, Clark DJ, Wallace WHB, et al: Endocrine deficit after fractionated total body irradiation. Arch Dis Child 67:1107–1110, 1992.
56. Cohen A, Rovelli A, Van-Lint MT, et al: Final height of patients who underwent bone marrow transplantation during childhood. Arch Dis Child 74:437–440, 1996.
57. Chin KY: The endocrine glands of anencephalic foetuses. Chin Med J (Engl) 2(suppl):63–90, 1938.
58. Lemire RI, Beckwith JB, Warkany J: Anencephaly. New York, Raven Press, 1978.
59. Hintz RL, Menking M, Sotos JF: Familial holoprosencephaly with endocrine dysgenesis. J Pediatr 72:81–87, 1968.
60. Lieblich JM, Rosen SW, Guyda H, et al: The syndrome of basal encephalocele and hypothalamic pituitary dysfunction. Ann Intern Med 89:910–916, 1978.
61. Rudman D, Davis GT, Priest JH, et al: Prevalence of growth hormone deficiency in children with cleft lip or palate. J Pediatr 93:378–381, 1978.
62. Izenberg N, Rosenblum M, Parks JS: The endocrine spectrum of septo-optic dysplasia. Clin Pediatr 23:632–636, 1984.
63. Wilson DM, Enzmann DR, Hintz RL, et al: Cranial computed tomography in septo-optic dysplasia: Discordance of clinical and radiological features. Neuroradiology 26:279–283, 1984.
64. Willnow S, Kiess W, Butenandt O, et al: Endocrine disorders in septo-optic dysplasia (De Morsier syndrome)—evaluation and follow-up of 18 patients. Eur J Pediatr 155:179–184, 1996.
65. Fujisawa I, Kikuchi K, Nishimura K, et al: Transection of the pituitary stalk: Development of an ectopic posterior lobe assessed with MR imaging. Radiology 165:487–489, 1987.
66. Abrahams JJ, Trefelner E, Boulware SD: Idiopathic growth hormone deficiency MR findings in 35 patients. Am J Neuroradiol 12:155–160 1991.
67. Kuroiwa T, Okabe Y, Hasuo K, et al: MR imaging of pituitary dwarfism. Am J Neuroradiol 12:161–164 1991.
68. Cacciari E, Zucchini S, Carla G, et al: Endocrine function and morphological findings in patients with disorders of the hypothalamo-pitutitary area: A study with magnetic resonance. Arch Dis Child 65:1199–1202, 1990.
69. Maghnie M, Larizza D, Triulzi F, et al: Hypopituitarism and stalk agenesis: A congenital syndrome worsened by breech delivery? Horm Res 35:104–108, 1991.
70. Brown RS, Bhatia V, Hayes E: An apparent cluster of congenital hypopituitarism in central Massachusetts: Magnetic resonance imaging and hormonal studies. J Clin Endocrinol Metab 72:12–18, 1991.
71. Root AW, Martinez CR: Magnetic resonance imaging in patients with hypopituitarism. Trends Endocrinol Metab 3:283–287, 1992.
72. Argyopoulou M, Perignon F, Brauner R, et al: Magnetic resonance imaging in the diagnosis of growth hormone deficiency. J Pediatr 120:886–891, 1992.
73. Triulzi F, Scotti G, diNatale B, et al: Evidence of a congenital midline brain anomaly in pituitary dwarfs: A magnetic resonance imaging study in 101 patients. Pediatrics 93:409–416, 1994.
74. DeLuca F, Bernasconi S, Blandino A, et al: Auxological, clinical, and neuroradiological findings in infants with early onset growth hormone deficiency. Acta Paediatr Scand 84:561–565, 1995.
75. Grumbach MM, Gluckman PD: The human fetal hypothalamic and pituitary gland: The maturation of neuroendocrine mechanisms controlling secretion of fetal pituitary growth hormone, prolactin, gonadotropin, adrenocorticotropin-related peptides and thyrotropin. *In* Tulchinsky D, Little AB (eds): Maternal and Fetal Endocrinology. Philadelphia, WB Saunders, 1994, pp 193–261.
76. Lovinger RD, Kaplan SL, Grumbach MM: Congenital hypopituitarism associated with neonatal hypoglycemia and microphallus: Four cases secondary to hypothalamic hormone deficiences. J Pediatr 87:1171–1181, 1975.
77. Wilkinson IA, Duck SC, Gager WE, et al: Empty sella syndrome. Occurrence in childhood. Am J Dis Child 136:245–248, 1982.
78. Parks JS, Pfaffle RW, Brown MR: Growth hormone deficiency. *In* Weintraub BD (ed): Molecular Endocrinology: Basic Concepts and Clinical Correlations. New York, Raven Press, 1995, pp 473–490.
79. Phillips JA, Cogan JD: Molecular basis of familial human growth hormone deficiency. J Clin Endocrinol Metab 76:11–16, 1994.
80. Parks JS, Adess ME, Brown MR: Genes regulating hypothalamic and pituitary development. Acta Paediatr Suppl 423:28–32, 1997.
81. Wagner JK, Eble A, Hindmarsh PC, et al: Prevalence of human GH-1 gene alterations in patients with isolated growth hormone deficiency. Pediatr Res 43:105–110, 1998.
82. Perez Juarado LA, Argente J: Molecular basis of familial growth hormone deficiency. Horm Res 42:189–197, 1994.
83. Phillips JA, Hjell BL, Seeburg PH, et al: Molecular basis for familial isolated growth hormone deficiency. Proc Natl Acad Sci U S A 78:63–72, 1981.
84. Illig R, Prader A, Ferrandez A, et al: Hereditary prenatal growth hormone deficiency with increased tendency to growth hormone antibody formation ("A-type" of isolated growth hormone deficiency). Acta Paediatr Scand 60:607, 1971.
85. Wajnrajch MP, Gertner JM, Harbison MD, et al: Nonsense mutations of the human growth hormone releasing hormone receptor (GHRHR) causes growth failure analogous to that of the little (lit) mouse. Nat Genet 12:88–90, 1996.
86. Baumann G, Maheshwari H: Severe growth hormone (GH) deficiency caused by a mutation in the GH-releasing hormone receptor gene. Acta Paediatr Suppl 423:33–38, 1997.
87. Salvatori R, Hagashida CY, Aguiar-Olivera MH, et al: Familial dwarfism due to a novel mutation of the growth hormone–releasing hormone receptor gene. J Clin Endocrinol Metab 84:917–923, 1999.
88. Godfrey P, Rahal JO, Beamer WG, et al: GHRH receptor of little mouse contains missense mutation in the extracellular domain that disrupts receptor function. Nat Genet 4:227–232, 1993.
89. Hermesz E, Mackem S, Mahox KA: *Rpx:* A novel anterior-restricted homeobox gene progressively activated in the prechordal plate, anterior neural plate and Rathke's pouch of the mouse embryo. Development 122:41–52, 1996.
90. Gage PJ, Brinkmeier ML, Scarlett LM: The Ames dwarf gene, df, is required early in pituitary ontogeny for the extinction of *Rpx* transcription and initiation of lineage-specific cell proliferation. Mol Endocrinol 10:1570–1581, 1996.
91. Szeto DP, Ryan AK, O'Connell SM, et al: P-OTX, a Pit-1-interacting homeodomain factor expressed during anterior pituitary gland development. Proc Natl Acad Sci U S A 93:7706–7710, 1996.
92. Seidah NG, Barale JC, Marcinkiewicz M, et al: The mouse homeoprotein mLIM-3 is expressed early in cells derived from the neuroepithelium and persists in adult pituitary. DNA Cell Biol 13:1163–1180, 1994.
93. Sheng HZ, Zhadanov AB, Mosinger B Jr, et al: Specification of pituitary cell lineages by the LIM homeobox gene *L-hx.* Science 272:1004–1007, 1996.
94. Sornson MW, Wu W, Daser JS, et al: Pituitary lineage determination by the Prophet of Pit-1 homeodomain factor defective in Ames dwarfism. Nature 384:327–333, 1996.
95. Wu W, Cogan JD, Pfäffle RW, et al: Mutations in PROP1 cause familial combined pituitary hormone deficiency. Nat Genet 18:147–149, 1998.
96. Fofanova O, Takamura N, Kinoshita E, et al: Compound heterozygous deletion of the PROP-1 gene in children with combined pituitary hormone deficiency. J Clin Endocrinol Metab 83:2601–2604, 1998.
97. Flück C, Deladoey J, Rutishauser K, et al: Phenotype variability in familial combined pituitary hormone deficiency caused by a PROP-1 gene mutation resulting in the substitution Arg → Cys at codon 120 (R120C). J Clin Endocrinol Metab 83:3727–3734, 1998.
98. Bodner M, Castrillo J-L, Theill LE, et al: The pituitary-specific transcription factor GHF-1 is a homeobox-containing protein. Cell 55:505–518, 1988.
99. Mangalam HJ, Albert VR, Ingraham HA, et al: A pituitary POU domain protein, pit-1, activates both growth hormone and prolactin promoters transcriptionally. Genes Dev 3:946–958, 1989.
100. Li S, Crenshaw EB, Rawson EJ, et al: Dwarf locus mutants lacking three pituitary cell types result from mutations in the POU-domain gene. Nature 347:528–533, 1990.

101. Tatsumi K, Miyai K, Notomi T, et al: Cretinism with combined hormone deficiency caused by a mutation in the *PIT1* gene. Nat Genet 1:56–58, 1992.

102. Radovick S, Nations M, Du Y, et al: A mutation in the POV-homeodomain of Pit-1 responsible for combined pituitary hormone deficiency. Science 257:1115–1118, 1992.

103. Pfäffle R, Kim C, Otten B, et al: Pit-1:Clinical aspects. Horm Res 45(suppl 1):25–28, 1996.

104. Pernasetti F, Milner RDG, Al Ashwal AAL, et al: Pro239Ser: A novel recessive mutation of the *Pit-1* gene in seven Middle Eastern children with growth hormone, prolactin, and thyrotropin deficiency. J Clin Endocrinol Metab 83:2079–2083, 1998.

105. Powell GF, Brasel JA, Blizzard RM: Emotional deprivation and growth retardation simulating idiopathic hypopituitarism. N Engl J Med 276:1271–1278, 1967.

106. Blizzard RM, Bulatovic A: Psychosocial short stature: A syndrome with many variables. Clin Endocrinol Metab 6:687–712, 1992.

107. Stanhope R, Adlard P, Hamill G, et al: Physiological growth hormone (GH) secretion during the recovery from psychosocial dwarfism: A case report. Clin Endocrinol (Oxf) 28:335–339, 1988.

108. Skuse D, Albanese A, Stanhope R: A new stress-related syndrome of growth failure and hyperphagia in children, associated with reversibility of growth-hormone insufficiency. Lancet 348:353–358, 1996.

109. Albanese A, Hamill G, Jones J, et al: Reversibility of physiological growth hormone secretion in children with psychosocial dwarfism. Clin Endocrinol 40:687–692, 1994.

110. Laron Z, Pertzelan AMS: Genetic pituitary dwarfism with high serum concentration of growth hormone—a new inborn error of metabolism? Isr J Med Sci 2:152–155, 1966.

111. Rosenbloom AL, Guevara-Aguirre J, Rosenfeld RG, et al: The little women of Loja: Growth hormone receptor deficiency in an inbred population of southern Ecuador. N Engl J Med 323:1367–1374, 1990.

112. Savage MO, Rosenfeld RG: Growth hormone insensitivity: A proposed revised classification. Acta Paediatr Suppl 428:147, 1999.

113. Rosenfeld RG, Rosenbloom AL, Guevara-Aguirre J: Growth hormone (GH) insensitivity due to primary GH receptor deficiency. Endocr Rev 15:369–390, 1994.

114. Rosenfeld RG, Rosenbloom AL, Guevara-Aguirre J: Abnormalities of growth hormone action. *In* Kelnar CJH, Savage MO, Stirling HF, Saenger P (eds): Growth Disorders. Pathophysiology and Treatment. London, Chapman & Hall, 1998, pp 549–564.

115. Douquesnoy P, Sobrier ML, Duriez B: A single amino acid substitution in the exoplasmic domain of the human growth hormone (GH) receptor confers familial GH resistance (Laron syndrome) with positive GH-binding activity by abolishing receptor homodimerization. EMBO J 13:1386–1395, 1994.

116. Woods KA, Fraser NC, Postel-Vinay MC, et al: A homozygous splice site mutation affecting the intracellular domain of the growth hormone (GH) receptor resulting in Laron syndrome with elevated GH-binding protein. J Clin Endocrinol Metab 81:1686–1690, 1996.

117. Goddard AD, Covello R, Luoh S-M, et al: Mutations of the growth hormone receptor in children with idiopathic short stature. N Engl J Med 333:1093–1098, 1995.

118. Rosenfeld RG: Broadening the growth hormone insensitivity syndrome. N Engl J Med 333:1145–1146, 1995.

119. Ayling RM, Ross R, Towner P, et al: A dominant-negative mutation of the growth hormone receptor gene causes familial short stature (abstract). Nat Genet 16:13–14, 1997.

120. DeChiara TM, Efstratiadis A, Robertson EJ: A growth-deficiency phenotype in heterozygous mice carrying an insulin-like growth factor II gene disrupted by targeting. Nature 345:78–80, 1990.

121. Baker J, Lizarralde G, Robertson EJ, et al: Role of insulin-like growth factors in embryonic and postnatal growth. Cell 75:73–82, 1993.

122. Liu JP, Baker J, Perkins AS, et al: Mice carrying null mutations of the genes encoding insulin-like growth factor I (Igf-1) and type 1 IGF receptor (Igf1r). Cell 75:73–82, 1993.

123. Woods KA, Camacho-Hubner C, Savage MO, et al: Intrauterine growth retardation and postnatal growth failure associated with deletion of the insulin-like growth factor I gene. N Engl J Med 335:1342–1349, 1996.

124. Vaccarello MA, Diamond FB Jr, Guevara-Aguirre J, et al: Hormonal and metabolic effects and pharmacokinetics of recombinant insulin-like growth factor-I in growth hormone receptor deficiency (GH receptor deficiency) Laron syndrome. J Clin Endocrinol Metab 77:273–280, 1993.

125. Gargosky SE, Wilson KF, Fielder PJ, et al: The composition and distribution of insulin-like growth factors (IGFs) and IGF-binding proteins (IGFBPs) in the serum of growth hormone receptor–deficient patients: Effects of IGF-1 therapy on IGFBP-3. J Clin Endocrinol Metab 77:1683–1689, 1993.

126. Gargosky SE, Wilson KF, Fielder PJ, et al: Effects of insulin-like growth factor I treatment on the molecular distribution of insulin-like growth factors among different proteins. Acta Paediatr Suppl 399:159–162, 1994.

127. Burren CP, Wanek D, Mohan S, et al: Serum insulin-like growth factor binding protein levels in growth hormone insensitivity: Studies in Ecuadorian children with short stature and GH-receptor mutation. Acta Paediatr Suppl 88:185–191, 1999.

128. Barreca A, Bozzola M, Cesarone A, et al: Short stature associated with high circulating insulin-like growth factor (IGF)–binding protein-1 and low circulating IGF-II: Effect of growth hormone therapy. J Clin Endocrinol Metab 83:3534–3541, 1998.

129. Jain S, Golde DW, Bailey R, et al: Insulin-like growth factor-I resistance. Endocr Rev 19:625–646, 1998.

130. Lewis UJ, Singh RNP, Tutwiler GH, et al: Human growth homone: A complex of proteins. Recent Prog Horm Res 36:477–508, 1980.

131. Baumann G: Heterogeneity of growth hormone. *In* Bercu B (ed): Basic and Clinical Aspects of Growth Hormone. New York, Plenum Press, 1988, pp 13–31.

132. Valenta LJ, Sigtel MB, Lesniak MA, et al: Pituitary dwarfism in a patient with circulating abnormal growth hormone polymers. N Engl J Med 312:214–217, 1985.

133. Kowarski AA, Schneider J, Ben-Galim E, et al: Growth failure with normal serum RIA-GH and low somatomedin activity: Somatomedin restoration and growth acceleration after exogenous GH. J Clin Endocrinol Metab 47:461–464, 1978.

134. Takahashi Y, Kaji H, Okimura Y, et al: Short stature caused by a mutant growth hormone. N Engl J Med 334:432–436, 1996.

135. Takahashi Y, Shirono H, Arisaka O, et al: Biologically inactive growth hormone caused by an amino acid substitution. J Clin Invest 100:1159–1165, 1997.

136. Woods KA, Dastot F, Preece MA, et al: Phenotype:genotype relationships in growth hormone insensitivity syndrome. J Clin Endocrinol Metab 82:3529–3535, 1997.

137. Wit JM, van Unen H: Growth of infants with neonatal growth hormone deficiency. Arch Dis Child 67:920–924, 1992.

138. Gluckman PD, Gunn AJ, Wray A, et al: Congenital idiopathic growth hormone deficiency associated with prenatal and early postnatal growth failure. J Pediatr 121:920–923, 1992.

139. Goodman HG, Grumbach MM, Kaplan SL: Growth and growth hormone II. A comparison of isolated growth hormone deficiency and multiple pituitary hormone deficiency, in 35 patients with idiopathic hypopituitary disease. N Engl J Med 278:57–68, 1968.

140. Herber SM, Milner RDG: Growth hormone deficiency presenting under age 2 years. Arch Dis Child 59:557–560, 1984.

141. Katz LEL, Satin-Smith MS, Collett-Solberg P, et al: Insulin-like growth factor binding protein-I levels in the diagnosis of hypoglycemia caused by hyperinsulinism. J Pediatr 131:193–199, 1997.

142. Copeland KC, Franks RC, Ramamurthy R: Neonatal hyperbilirubinemia and hypoglycemia in congenital hypopituitarism. Clin Pediatr 20:523–526, 1981.

143. Choo-Kang LR, Sun C-CJ, Counts DR: Cholestasis and hypoglycemia: Manifestations of congenital anterior hypopituitarism. J Clin Endocrinol Metab 81:2786–2789, 1996.

144. Laron Z, Lilos P, Klinger B: Growth curves for Laron syndrome. Arch Dis Child 68:768–770, 1993.

145. Schaefer GB, Rosenbloom AL, Guevara-Aguirre J, et al: Facial morphometry of Ecuadorian patients with growth hormone receptor deficiency. J Med Genet 31:635–640, 1994.

146. Kranzler JH, Rosenbloom AL, Martinez V, et al: Normal intelligence with severe insulin-like growth factor I deficiency due to growth hormone receptor deficiency. A controlled study in a genetically homogeneous population. J Clin Endocrinol Metab 83:1953–1958, 1998.

147. Laron Z, Galafzer A: A comment on normal intelligence in growth hormone receptor deficiency. J Clin Endocrinol Metab 83:4528, 1998.

148. Wit JM, Kamp G, Rikken B: Spontaneous growth and response to growth hormone treatment in chidren with growth hormone deficiency and idiopathic short stature. Pediatr Res 39:295–302, 1996.

149. Rimoin DL, Merimee TJ, Rabinowitz D, et al: Genetic aspects of clinical endocrinology. Recent Prog Horm Res 24:365–437, 1968.

150. Ranke MB: A note on adults with growth hormone deficiency. Acta Paediatr Suppl 331:80–82, 1987.

151. van der Werff ten Bosch JJ, Bot A: Growth of males with idiopathic hypopituitarism without growth hormone treatment. Clin Endocrinol (Oxf) 32:707–717, 1990.

152. Guevara-Aguirre J, Rosenbloom AL, Fielder PJ, et al: Growth hormone receptor deficiency in Ecuador: Clinical and biochemical phenotype in two populations. J Clin Endocrinol Metab 76:417–423, 1993.

153. Savage MO, Blum WF, Ranke MB, et al: Clinical features and endocrine status in patients with growth hormone insensitivity (Laron syndrome). J Clin Endocrinol Metab 77:1465–1471, 1993.

154. Rosenfeld RG, Albertsson-Wikland K, Cassorla F, et al: The diagnosis of childhood growth hormone deficiency revisited. J Clin Endocrinol Metab 80:1532–1540, 1995.

155. Voss LD, Wilkin TJ, Bailey BJR, et al: The reliability of height and height velocity in the assessment of growth (the Wessex Growth Study). Arch Dis Child 66:833–837, 1991.

156. Rosenfeld RG, Gargosky SE: Assays for insulin-like growth factors and their binding proteins: Practicalities and pitfalls. J Pediatr 128 (suppl):S52–S57, 1996.

157. Rosenfeld RG, Wilson DM, Lee PDK: Insulin-like growth factors I and II in the evaluation of growth retardation. J Pediatr 109:428–433, 1986.

158. Juul A, Bang P, Hertel NT, et al: Serum insulin-like growth factor-I in 1,030 healthy children, adolescents and adults: Relation to age, sex, stage of puberty, testicular size, and body mass index. J Clin Endocrinol Metab 78:744–752, 1994.

159. Blum WF, Ranke MB, Kietzmann K, et al: A specific radioimmunoassay for the growth hormone–dependent somatomedin-binding protein: Its use for diagnosis of GH deficiency. J Clin Endocrinol Metab 70:1292–1298, 1990.

160. Juul A, Dalgaard P, Blum WF, et al: Serum levels of insulin-like growth factor (IGF) binding protein-3 in healthy infants, children and adolescents: The relation of IGF-I, IGF-II, IGFBP-1, IGFBP-2, age, sex, body mass index, and pubertal maturation. J Clin Endocrinol Metab 80:2534–2542, 1995.

161. Labarta JI, Gargosky SE, Simpson DM, et al: Immunoblot studies of the acid-labile subunit (ALS) in biological fluids, normal human serum and in children with GH deficiency and GH receptor deficiency before and after long-term therapy with GH or IGF-I respectively. Clin Endocrinol (Oxf) 47:657–666, 1997.

162. Juul A, Moller S, Mosfeldt-Laursen E, et al: The acid-labile subunit of human ternary insulin-like growth factor binding protein complex in serum: Hepatosplanchnic release, diurnal variation, circulating concentrations in healthy subjects, and diagnostic use in patients with growth hormone deficiency. J Clin Endocrinol Metab 83:4408–4415, 1998.

163. Smith WJ, Nam TJ, Underwood LE, et al: Use of insulin-like growth factor binding protein-2 (IGFBP-2), IGFBP-3, and IGF-1 for assessing growth hormone status in short children. J Clin Endocrinol Metab 77:1294–1299, 1993.

164. Daughaday WH, Kapadia M, Mariz I: Serum somatomedin binding proteins: Physiologic significance and interference in radioligand assay. J Lab Clin Med 109:355–363, 1986.

165. Powell DR, Rosenfeld RG, Baker BK, et al: Serum somatomedin levels in adults with chronic renal failure: The importance of measuring insulin-like growth factor (IGF)-1 and -2 in acid chromatographed uremic serum. J Clin Endocrinol Metab 63:1186–1192, 1986.

166. Horner JM, Liu F, Hintz RL: Comparison of [125I] somatomedin-A and [125I] somatomedin C radioreceptor assays for somatomedin peptide content in whole and acid-chromatographed plasma. J Clin Endocrinol Metab 47:1287–1295, 1978.

167. Bang P, Ericksson U, Sara V, et al: Comparison of acid ethanol extraction and acid gel filtration prior to IGF-I and IGF-II radioimmunoassays: Improvement of determinations in acid ethanol extracts by the use of a truncated IGF-I as radioligand. Acta Endocrinol (Copenh) 124:620–629, 1991.

168. Blum WF, Ranke MB, Bierich JR: A specific radioimmunoassay for IGF-II: The interference of IGF binding proteins can be blocked by excess IGF-I. Acta Endocrinol 118:374–380, 1988.

169. Bennett A, Wilson DM, Liu F, et al: Levels of insulin-like growth factor-I and -II in human cord blood. J Clin Endocrinol Metab 57:609–612, 1983.

170. Gluckman PD, Barrett-Johnson JJ, Butler JH, et al: Studies of insulin-like growth factor I and II by specific radioligand assays in umbilical cord blood. Clin Endocrinol 19:405–413, 1983.

171. Luna AM, Wilson DM, Wibbelsman CJ, et al: Somatomedins in adolescence: A cross-sectional study of the effect of puberty on plasma insulin-like growth factor I and II levels. J Clin Endocrinol Metab 57:258–271, 1983.

172. Cara JF, Rosenfield RL, Furlanetto RW: A longitudinal study of the relationship of plasma somatomedin-C concentration to the pubertal growth spurt. Am J Dis Child 147:562–564, 1987.

173. Thomas GB, Robinson ICAF: Central regulation of growth hormone secretion. *In* Kelnar CJH, Savage MO, Stirling HF, Saenger P (eds): Growth Disorders. Pathophysiology and Treatment. London, Chapman & Hall, 1998, pp 99–125.

174. Martha PM Jr, Rogol AD, Veldhuis JD, et al: Alterations in the pulsatile properties of circulating growth hormone concentrations during puberty in boys. J Clin Endocrinol Metab 69:563–570, 1989.

175. Martha PM, Gorman KM, Blizzard RM, et al: Endogenous growth hormone secretion and clearance rates in normal boys as determined by deconvolution analysis: Relationship to age, pubertal status and body mass. J Clin Endocrinol Metab 74:336–344, 1992.

176. Spiliotis BE, August GP, Hung W, et al: Growth hormone neurosecretory dysfunction: A treatable cause of short stature. JAMA 252:2223–2230, 1984.

177. Bercu BB, Shulman D, Root AW, et al: Growth hormone (GH) provocative testing frequently does not reflect endogenous GH secretion. J Clin Endocrinol Metab 86:709–716, 1986.

178. Rose SR, Ross JL, Uriarte M, et al: The advantage of measuring stimulated as compared with spontaneous growth hormone levels in the diagnosis of growth hormone deficiency. N Engl J Med 319:201–207, 1988.

179. Thompson RG, Rodriguez A, Kowarski AA, et al: Growth hormone: Metabolic clearance rates, integrated concentrations and production rates in normal adults and the effects of prednisone. J Clin Invest 51:3193–3199, 1972.

180. Zadik Z, Chalew SA, McCarter RJ, et al: The influence of age on the 24-hour integrated concentrations of growth hormone in normal individuals. J Clin Endocrinol Metab 60:153, 1985.

181. Zadik Z, Chalew SA, Gilula Z, et al: Reproducibility of growth hormone testing procedures: A comparison between 24-hour integrated concentration and pharmacological stimulation. J Clin Endocrinol Metab 71:1127–1130, 1990.

182. Lanes R: Diagnostic limitations of spontaneous growth hormone measurements in normally growing prepubertal children. Am J Dis Child 143:1284–1286, 1989.

183. Donaldson DL, Hollowell JG, Pan F, et al: Growth hormone secretory profiles: Variation on consecutive nights. J Pediatr 115:51–56, 1989.

184. Hourd P, Edwards R: Current methods for the measurement of growth hormone in urine. Clin Endocrinol (Oxf) 40:155–170, 1994.

185. Albini CH, Quattrin T, Vandlen RL, et al: Quantitation of urinary growth hormone in children with normal and subnormal growth. Pediatr Res 23:89–92, 1988.

186. Granada ML, Sanmarti ALA, et al: Clinical usefulness of urinary growth hormone measurements in normal and short children according to different expressions of urinary growth hormone data. Pediatr Res 32:73–76, 1992.

187. Phillip M, Chalew SA, Stene MA, et al: The value of urinary growth hormone determination for assessment of growth hormone deficiency and compliance with growth hormone therapy. Am J Dis Child 147:553–557, 1993.

188. Skinner AM, Clayton PE, Price DA, et al: Urinary growth hormone excretion in the assessment of children with disorders of growth. Clin Endocrinol (Oxf) 39:201–206, 1993.

189. Frasier SD: A review of growth hormone stimulation tests in children. Pediatrics 53:929–937, 1974.

190. Underwood LE, Azumi K, Voina SJ, et al: Growth hormone levels during sleep in normal and growth hormone deficient children. Pediatrics 48:946–954, 1971.

191. Buckler JMH: Plasma growth hormone response to exercise as a diagnostic aid. Arch Dis Child 48:565–567, 1973.

192. Lacey KA, Hewison A, Parkin JM: Exercise as a screening test for growth hormone deficiency in children. Arch Dis Child 48:508–512, 1973.

193. Coller R, Leboeuf G, Letarte J: Stimulation of growth hormone secretion by levodopa propranolol in children and adolescents. Pediatrics 56:262–266, 1975.

194. Lanes R, Hurtado E: Oral clonidine—an effective growth hormone–releasing agent in prepubertal subjects. J Pediatr 100:710–714, 1982.

195. Mitchell ML, Bryne MJ, Sanchez Y, et al: Detection of growth deficiency. The glucagon simulation test. N Engl J Med 282:539–541, 1970.

196. Merimee TJ, Rabinowitz D, Fineberg SE: Arginine-inititated release of human growth hormone. N Engl J Med 280:1434–1438, 1969.

197. Kaplan SL, Abrams CAL, Bell JJ: Growth and growth hormone. I: Changes in serum levels of growth hormone following hypoglycemia in 134 children with growth retardation. Pediatr Res 2:43–63, 1968.

198. Root AW, Rosenfeld RL, Bongiovanni AM, et al: The plasma growth hormone response to insulin-induced hypoglycemia in children with retardation of growth. Pediatrics 39:844–852, 1967.

199. Penny R, Blizzard RM, Davis WT: Sequential arginine and insulin tolerance tests on the same day. J Clin Endocrinol Metab 29:1499–1501, 1969.

200. Fass B, Lippe BM, Kaplan SA: Relative usefulness of three growth hormone stimulation screening tests. Am J Dis Child 133:931–933, 1979.

201. Weldon VV, Gupta SK, Klingensmith G: Evaluation of growth hormone release in children using arginine and L-dopa in combination. J Pediatr 87:540–544, 1975.

202. Reiter EO, Martha PM Jr: Pharmacological testing of growth hormone secretion. Horm Res 33:121–127, 1990.

203. Raiti S, Davis WT, Blizzard RM: A comparison of the effects of insulin hypoglycemia and arginine infusion on release of human growth hormone. Lancet 2:1182–1183, 1967.

204. Physicians' Desk Reference: Montvale, NJ, Medical Economics Data Production, 1994, p 1004.

205. Physicians' Desk Reference: Montvale, NJ, Medical Economics Data Production, 1994, p 1228.

206. Iranmanesh A, Lizarralde G, Veldhuis ID: Age and relative adiposity are specific negative determinants of the frequency and amplitude of growth hormone (GH) secretory bursts and the half-life of endogenous GH in healthy men. J Clin Endocrinol Metab 73:1081–1088, 1991.

207. Finkelstein JW, Roftwarg HP, Boyar RM, et al: Age-related change in twenty-four-hour spontaneous secretion of growth hormone. J Clin Endocrinol Metab 35:665–670, 1972.

208. Lippe BM, Wong S, Kaplan SA: Simultaneous assessment of growth hormone and ACTH reserve in children pretreated with diethylstilbestrol. J Clin Endocrinol 33:949–956, 1971.

209. Cacciari E, Tassoni P, Parisi G, et al: Pitfalls in diagnosing impaired growth hormone (GH) secretion: Retesting after replacement therapy of 63 children defined as GH deficient. J Clin Endocrinol Metab 74:1284–1289, 1974.

210. Tauber M, Moulin P, Pienkowski C, et al: Growth hormone (GH) retesting and auxological data in 131 GH-deficient patients after completion of treatment. J Clin Endocrinol Metab 82:352–356, 1982.

211. Trygstad O: Transitory growth hormone deficiency successfully treated with human growth hormone. Acta Endocrinol 84:11–22, 1977.

212. Marin G, Domene HM, Barnes KM, et al: The effects of estrogen priming and puberty on the growth hormone response to standardized treadmill exercise and arginine-insulin in normal girls and boys. J Clin Endocrinol Metab 79:537–541, 1994.

213. Blethen SL, Chaslow FI: Use of a two-site radioimmunometric assay for growth hormone (GH). J Endocrinol Metab 57:1031–1035, 1983.

214. Reiter EO, Morris AH, MacGillivray MH, et al: Variable estimates of serum growth hormone concentrations by difference radioassay systems. J Clin Endocrinol Metab 66:68–71, 1988.

215. Celniker AC, Chem AB, Wert RM Jr, et al: Variability in the quantitation of circulating growth hormone using commercial immunoassays. J Clin Endocrinol Metab 68:469–476, 1989.

216. Barth JH, Smith JH, Clarkson P: Wide diversity in measurements of growth hormone after stimulation tests in short children are due to assay variability. Ann Clin Biochem 32:369–372, 1995.

217. Strasburger CJ, Wu Z, Pflaum C-D, et al: Immunofunctional assay of human growth hormone (hGH) in serum: A possible concensus for quantitative hGH measurement. J Clin Endocrinol Metab 81:2613–2620, 1996.

218. Wyatt DT, Mark D, Slyper A: Survey of growth hormone treatment practices by 251 pediatric endocrinologists. J Clin Endocrinol Metab 80:3292–3297, 1995.

219. Veldhuis JD, Iranmanesh A, Ho KKY, et al: Dual defects in pulsatile growth hormone secretion and clearance subserve the hyposomatotropism of obesity in man. J Clin Endocrinol Metab 72:519–526, 1991.

220. Jensen JB, Garfinkel BD: Growth hormone dysregulation in children with major depressive disorder. J Am Child Adolesc Psychiatry 29:295–301, 1990.

221. Brambilla F, Perna G, Garberi A, et al: Alpha-2 adrenergic receptor sensitivity in panic disorder. I: GH response to GHRH and clonidine stimulation in panic disorder. Psychoneuroendocrinology 20:1–9, 1995.

222. Charney DS, Heninger GR, Sternberg DE, et al: Adrenergic receptor sensitivity in depression. Effects of clonidine in depressed patients and healthy subjects. Arch Gen Psychiatry 39:290–294, 1982.

223. Pine DS, Cohen P, Brook J: Emotional problems during youth as predictors of stature during early adulthood: Results from a prospective epidemiologic study. Pediatrics 97:856–863, 1996.

224. Berelowitz M, Szabo M, Frohman LA, et al: Somatomedin-C mediates growth hormone negative feedback by effects on both the hypothalamus and pituitary. Science 212:1279–1281, 1981.

225. Yamashita S, Melmed S: Insulin-like growth factor I action on rat anterior pituitary cells: Suppression of growth hormone secretion and messenger ribonucleic acid levels. Endocrinology 118:176–182, 1986.

226. Abe H, Molitch M, Van Wyk JJ, et al: Human growth hormone and somatomedin-C suppress the spontaneous release of growth hormone in unanesthetized rats. Endocrinology 113:1319–1324, 1983.

227. Ceda GP, Hoffman AR, Silverberg GD, et al: Regulation of growth hormone release from cultured human pituitary adenomas by somatomedins and insulin. J Clin Endocrinol Metab 60:1204–1209, 1985.

228. Ceda GP, Davis WT, Rosenfeld RG, et al: The growth hormone (GH) releasing hormone (GHRH)-GH-somatomedin axis: Evidence for rapid inhibition of GHRH-elicited GH release by insulin-like growth factors I and II. Endocrinology 120:1658–1662, 1987.

229. Guler HP, Zapf J, Froesch ER: Short-term metabolic effects and half-lives of intravenously administered insulin-like growth factor I in healthy adults. N Engl J Med 317:137–140, 1987.

230. Vaccarello MA, Diamond FB Jr, Guevara-Aguirre J, et al: Hormonal and metabolic effects and pharmacokinetics of recombinant insulin-like growth factor-I in growth hormone receptor deficiency (GH receptor deficiency) Laron syndrome. J Clin Endocrinol Metab 77:273–280, 1993.
231. Shah A, Stanhope R, Matthews D: Hazards of pharmacological tests of growth hormone secretion in childhood. BMJ 304:173–174, 1992.
232. Shriock EA, Hulse JA, Harris DA, et al: Evaluation of hypothalamic dysfunction in growth hormone (GH)–deficient patients using single versus multiple doses of growth hormone–releasing hormone (GHRH-44) and evidence for diurnal variation in somatotroph responsiveness to GHRH in GH deficient patients. J Clin Endocrinol Metab 65:1177–1182, 1987.
233. Rochiccioli PE, Tauber MT, Coude F-X, et al: Results of 1 year growth hormone–releasing hormone (1-44) treatment on growth, somatomedin-C, and 24-hour GH secretion in 6 children with partial GH deficiency. J Clin Endocrinol Metab 65:268–274, 1987.
234. Ghigo E, Bellone J, Aimasetti G, et al: Reliability of provocative tests to assess growth hormone secretory status. Study in 472 normally growing children. J Clin Endocrinol Metab 81:3323–3327, 1996.
235. Tillmann V, Bickler JMH, Kibirige MS, et al: Biochemical tests in the diagnosis of childhood growth hormone deficiency. J Clin Endocrinol Metab 82:531–535, 1997.
236. Juul A, Skakkeback NE: Prediction of the outcome of growth hormone provocative testing in short children by measurement of serum levels of insulin-like growth factor I and insulin-like growth factor binding protein-3. J Pediatr 130:197–204, 1997.
237. Hasegawa Y, Hasegawa T, Aso T, et al: Clinical utility of insulin-like growth factor binding protein-3 in the evaluation and treatment of short children with suspected growth hormone deficiency. Eur J Endocrinol 131:27–32, 1994.
238. Clanfarani S, Boemi S, Spagnoli A, et al: Is IGF binding protein-3 assessment helpful for the diagnosis of GH deficiency? Clin Endocrinol (Oxf) 43:43–47, 1995.
239. Nunez SB, Municchi G, Barnes KM, et al: Insulin-like growth factor-I and IGF-binding protein-3 concentrations compared to stimulated and night growth hormone in the evaluation of short children—a clinical research center study. J Clin Endocrinol Metab 81:1927–1932, 1996.
240. Shalet SM, Toogood A, Rahim A, et al: The diagnosis of growth hormone deficiency in children and adults. Endocr Rev 19:203–223, 1998.
241. Souberbielle JC, Zucker JM, Rappaport R, et al: Nonparallel changes of growth hormone (GH) and insulin-like growth factor-I, insulin-like growth factor binding protein-3 and GH-binding protein, after craniospinal irradiation and chemotherapy. J Clin Endocrinol Metab 78:597–601, 1994.
242. Rosenfeld RG: The molecular basis of the growth hormone insensitivity syndrome. Clin Pediatr Endocrinol 6(suppl 10):13–17 1997.
243. Rosenfeld RG: Growth hormone insensitivity: Perspectives on genotypic and phenotypic heterogeneity. Clin Pediatr Endocrinol 7(suppl 11): 1–7, 1998.
244. Johnston LB, Woods KA, Rose SJ, et al: The broad spectrum of inherited growth hormone insensitivity syndrome. Trends Endocrinol Metab 9:228–232, 1998.
245. Attie KM, Carlsson LMS, Russell-Fraser T, et al: Evidence for partial growth hormone insensitivity among patients with idiopathic short stature. J Pediatr 127:244–250, 1995.
246. Saenger P: Partial growth hormone insensitivity—idiopathic short stature is not always idiopathic. Acta Paediatr Suppl 428:194–198, 1999.
247. Wocjik J, Berg MA, Exposito N, et al: Four contiguous amino acid substitutions, identified in patients with Laron syndrome, differently affect the binding affinity and intracellular trafficking of the growth hormone receptor. J Clin Endocrinol Metab 83:4481–4489, 1998.
248. Ida K, Takahashi Y, Kaji H, et al: Growth hormone (GH) insensitivity syndrome with high serum GH-binding protein levels caused by a heterozygous splice site mutation of the GH receptor gene producing a lack of intracellular domain. J Clin Endocrinol Metab 83:531–537, 1998.
249. Rosenfeld RG, Kemp SF, Hintz RL: Constancy of somatomedin response to growth hormone treatment of hypopituitary dwarfism, and lack of correlation with growth rate. J Clin Endocrinol Metab 53:611–617, 1981.
250. Thalange NKS, Price DA, Gill MS, et al: Insulin-like growth factor binding protein-3 generation: An index of growth hormone insensitivity. Pediatr Res 39:849–855, 1996.
251. Blum WF, Ranke MB, Savage MO, et al: Insulin-like growth factors and their binding proteins in patients with growth hormone receptor deficiency: Suggestions for new diagnostic criteria. Acta Paediatr Suppl 383:125–126, 1992.
252. Cotterill AM, Camacho-Hübner C, Woods K, et al: The insulin-like growth factor I generation test in the investigation of short stature. Acta Paediatr Suppl 399:128–130, 1994.
253. Schwarze CP, Wollmann HA, Binder G, et al: Short-term increments of insulin-like growth factor I (IGF-I) and IGF-binding protein-3 predict the growth response to growth hormone (GH) therapy in GH-sensitive children. Acta Paediatr Suppl 428:200–208, 1999.
254. Clayton PE, Price DA, Shalet SM: Growth hormone state after completion of treatment with growth hormone. Arch Dis Child 62:222–226, 1987.
255. Wacharasindhu S, Cotterill AM, Camacho-Hübner C, et al: Normal growth hormone secretion in growth hormone insufficient children after completion of linear growth. Clin Endocrinol (Oxf) 45:553–556, 1996.
256. Longobardi S, Merola B, Pivonello R, et al: Re-evaluation of growth hormone (GH) secretion in 69 adults diagnosed as GH deficient patients during childhood. J Clin Endocrinol Metab 81:1244–1247, 1996.
257. Nicolson A, Toogood AA, Rahim A, et al: The prevalence of severe growth hormone deficiency in adults who received growth hormone replacement in childhood. Clin Endocrinol (Oxf) 44:311–316, 1996.
258. De Boer H, van der Veen E: Why retest young adults with childhood-onset growth hormone deficiency? J Clin Endocrinol Metab 82:2032–2036, 1997.
259. Shalet SM, Rosenfeld RG: Growth hormone replacement therapy during transition of patients with childhood-onset growth hormone deficiency into adulthood: What are the issues? Growth Horm IGF Res 8: 177–184, 1998.
260. Bennett LL, Weinberger H, Escamilla R, et al: Failure of hypophyseal growth hormone to produce nitrogen storage in a girl with hypophyseal dwarfism. J Clin Endocrinol Metab 10:492–495, 1950.
261. Knobil E, Greep RO: Physiological effects of growth hormone of primate origin in the hypophysectomized monkey. Fed Proc 15:111–112, 1956.
262. Knobil E, Wolf RC, Greep RO: Some physiologic effects of primate pituitary growth-hormone preparations in the hypophysectomized rhesus monkey. J Clin Endocrinol 16:916, 1956.
263. Raben MS: Treatment of a pituitary dwarf with human growth hormone. J Clin Endocrinol Metab 18:901–903, 1958.
264. Frasier SD: Human pituitary growth hormone (hGH) therapy in growth hormone deficiency. Endocr Rev 4:155–170, 1983.
265. Milner RCG, Russell-Fraser T, Brook CGD, et al: Experience with human growth hormone in Great Britain: The report of the MRC Working Party. Clin Endocrinol (Oxf) 11:15–18, 1979.
266. Job JC, Joab N, Toublane TE, et al: Résultats à terme des traitements par l'hormone de croissance humaine. Arch Franc Pediatr 41:477–482, 1984.
267. Raiti S: The national hormone and pituitary program: Achievements and current goals. *In* Raiti S, Tolman R (eds): Human Growth Hormone. New York, Plenum Press, 1986, pp 1–12.
268. Fradkin JE: Creutzfeldt-Jakob disease in pituitary growth hormone recipients. Endocrinologist 3:108–114, 1993.
269. Buchanan CR, Preece MA, Milner RDG: Mortality, neoplasia, and Creutzfeldt-Jakob disease in patients treated with human pituitary growth hormone in the United States. BMJ 302:824–828, 1991.
270. Tintner R, Brown P, Hedley-Whyte ET, et al: Neuropathologic verification of Creutzfeldt-Jakob disease in the exhumed American recipient of human growth hormone: Epidemiologic and pathogenetic implications. Neurology 36:932–936, 1986.
271. Hintz RL: The prismatic case of Creutzfeldt-Jakob disease associated with pituitary growth hormone treatment. J Clin Endocrinol Metab 80:2298–2301, 1995.
272. Rosenfeld RG, Aggarwal BB, Hintz RL, et al: Recombinant DNA-derived methionyl growth hormone is similar in membrane binding properties to human pituitary growth hormone. Biochem Biophys Res Commun 106:202–209, 1982.
273. Hintz RL, Rosenfeld RG, Wilson DM, et al: Biosynthetic methionyl–human growth hormone is biologically active in adult humans. Lancet 1:1276–1279, 1982.
274. Kaplan SL, Underwood LE, August GP, et al: Clinical studies with recombinant DNA-derived methionyl-hGH in GH deficient children. Lancet 1:697–700, 1986.
275. MacGillivray MH, Blizzard RM: Rationale for dosing recombinant human growth hormone by weight rather than units. Growth Genet Horm 10:7–9, 1994.
276. Frasier SD, Costin G, Lippe BM, et al: A dose-response curve for human growth hormone. J Clin Endocrinol Metab 53:1213–1217, 1981.
277. MacGillivray MH, Baptista J, Johanson A, et al: Outcome of a four year randomized study of daily versus three times weekly somatropin treatment in prepubertal naive growth hormone deficient children. J Clin Endocrinol Metab 81:1806–1809, 1996.
278. Cohen P, Rosenfeld RG: Dose response effects of growth hormone on auxological and biochemical parameters in GH deficient children. Pediatrics 1999, in press.
279. Ranke MB, Lindberg A, Guilbaud O: Prediction of growth in response to treatment with growth hormone. *In* Ranke MB, Gunnarsson R (eds): Progress in Growth Hormone Therapy— 5 Years of KIGS. Mannheim, Germany, JJ Verlag, 1994, pp 97–111.
280. MacGillivray MH, Blethen SL, Buchlis JG, et al: Current dosing of growth hormone in children with growth hormone deficiency: How physiologic? Pediatrics 102:527–530, 1998.
281. Johnson OL, Cleleand TL, Lee HJ, et al: A month-long effect from a single injection of microencapsulated human growth hormone. Nat Med 2:795–799, 1996.
282. Bundak R, Hindmarsh PC, Brook CGD: Long-term auxologic effects of human growth hormone. J Pediatr 112:875–879, 1988.
283. Libber SM, Plotnick LP, Johanson AJ, et al: Long-term follow-up of hypopituitary patients treated with human growth hormone. Medicine (Baltimore) 69:46–55, 1990.
284. Bierich JR: Final height in hypopituitary patients after treatment with hGH. *In* Bierich JR, Cacciari E, Raiti S (eds): Growth Abnormalities. New York, Raven Press, 1989, pp 161–174.
285. Bramswig JH, Schlosser H, Kiese K: Final height in children with growth hormone deficiency. Horm Res 43:126–128, 1995.
286. Blethen SL, Foley T, LaFranchi S, et al: Adult height (AH) in growth hormone deficiency (abstract). Pediatr Res 27:85A, 1995.
287. Chipman JJ, Hicks JR, Holcombe JH, et al: Approaching final height in children treated for growth hormone deficiency. Horm Res 43:129–131, 1995.
288. Frisch H, Birnbacher R: Final height and pubertal development in children with growth hormone deficiency after long-term treatment. Horm Res 43:132–134, 1995.
289. Severi F: Final height in children with growth hormone deficiency. Horm Res 43:138–140, 1995.
290. Josefsberg Z, Bauman B, Pertzelan A, et al: Greater efficiency of human growth hormone therapy in children below five years of age with growth hormone deficiency: A 5-year follow-up study. Horm Res 27:126–133, 1987.
291. Blethen SL, Compton P, Lippe BM, et al: Factors predicting the response to growth hormone (GH) therapy in prepubertal children with GH deficiency. J Clin Endocrinol Metab 74:574–579, 1993.
292. Arrigo T, DeLuca F., Bernasconi S, et al: Catch-up growth and height prognosis in early treated children with congenital hypopituitarism. Horm Res 44(suppl):26–31, 1996.
293. Burns EC, Tanner JM, Preece MA, et al: Final height and pubertal development in 55 children with idiopathic growth hormone deficiency, treated for between 2 and 15 years with human growth hormone. Eur J Pediatr 137:155–164, 1981.
294. Bourguignon JP, Vandeweghe M, Vanderschuren-Lodeweyckx M, et al: Pubertal growth and final height in hypopituitary boys: A minor role of bone age at onset of puberty. J Clin Endocrinol Metab 63:376–382, 1986.
295. Price DA, Ranke MB: Final height following growth hormone treatment. *In* Ranke

MB, Gunnarsson R (eds): Progress in Growth Hormone Therapy—5 Years of KIGS. Mannheim, Germany, JJ Verlag, 1994, pp 574–579.
296. MacGillivray MH, Clopper RR, Sandberg DE, et al: Growth responses of hypopituitary children to growth hormone (GH) treatment during the pituitary (pGH) and recombinant (rGH) eras. Horm Res 48(suppl 2):85, 1997.
297. De Luca F, Maghnie M, Arrigo T, et al: Final height outcome of growth hormone–deficient patients treated since less than five years of age. Acta Paediatr 85:1167–1171, 1996.
298. Ranke MB, Price DA, Albertsson-Wikland K, et al: Factors determining pubertal growth and final height in growth hormone treatment of idiopathic growth hormone deficiency. Horm Res 48:62–71, 1997.
299. Blethen SL, Baptista J, Kuntze J, et al: Adult height in growth hormone (GH)–deficient children treated with biosynthetic GH. J Clin Endocrinol Metab 82:418–420, 1997.
300. Blethen SL, Alster DK, Graves D, et al: Safety of recombinant DNA–derived growth hormone (rhGH): The National Cooperative Growth Study experience. J Clin Endocrinol Metab 81:1704–1710, 1996.
301. Wilton P: Adverse events during growth hormone treatment: 5 years' experience. *In* Ranke B, Gunnarsson R (eds): Progress in Growth Hormone Therapy—5 Years of KIGS. Mannheim, Germany, JJ Verlag, 1994, pp 291–307.
302. Blethen SL: Complications of growth hormone therapy in children. Curr Opin Pediatr 7:466–471, 1995.
303. Cowell CT, Dietsch S: Adverse events during growth hormone therapy. J Pediatr Endocrinol Metab 8:243–252, 1995.
304. Massa G, Vanderschuren-Lodeweyckx M, Bouillon R: Five-year follow-up of growth hormone antibodies in growth hormone deficient children treated with recombinant human growth hormone. Clin Endocrinol 38:137–142, 1993.
305. Pirazzoli P, Cacciari E, Mandini M, et al: Follow-up of antibodies to growth hormone in 210 growth hormone–deficient children treated with different commercial preparations. Acta Paediatr 84:1233–1236, 1995.
306. Malozowski S, Tanner LA, Wysoluski D, et al: Growth hormone, insulin-like growth factor-I, and benign intracranial hypertension. N Engl J Med 329:665–666, 1993.
307. Ranke MB: Effects of growth hormone on the metabolism of lipids and water and their potential causing adverse events during growth hormone treatment. Horm Res 39:104–106, 1993.
308. Harris WR: The endocrine basis for slipping of the upper femoral epiphysis: An experimental study. J Bone Joint Surg Br 32:5–11, 1950.
309. Kelsey JL: Epidemiology of slipped capital femoral epiphysis: A review of the literature. Pediatrics 51:1042–1050, 1973.
310. Rappaport EB, Fife D: Slipped capital femoral epiphysis in growth hormone–deficient patients. Am J Dis Child 139:396–399, 1985.
311. Malozowski S, Hung W, Scott DC: Acute pancreatitis associated with growth hormone therapy for short stature. N Engl J Med 332:401–402, 1995.
312. Bourguignon JP, Pierard GE, Ernould C, et al: Effects of human growth hormone therapy on melanocytic naevi. Lancet 341:1505–1506, 1993.
313. Malozowski S, Stadel BV: Prepubertal gynecomastia during growth hormone therapy. J Pediatr 126:659–661, 1995.
314. Watanabe S, Yamagucki N, Tsunematsu Y, et al: Risk factors for leukemia occurrence among growth hormone users. Jpn J Cancer 80:822–825, 1989.
315. Fisher DA, Job J, Preece M, et al: Leukemia in patients treated with growth hormone. Lancet 1:1159–1160, 1988.
316. Fradkin JE, Mills JL, Schonberger LB, et al: Risk of leukemia after treatment with pituitary growth hormone. JAMA 270:2829–2832, 1993.
317. Oglivy-Stuart AL, Ryder WD, Gattamaneni HR, et al: Growth hormone and tumor recurrence. BMJ 304:1601–1605, 1992.
318. Tuffli GA, Johanson A, Rundle AC, et al: Lack of increased risk for extracranial, nonleukemic neoplasms in recipients of recombinant deoxyribonucleic acid growth hormone. J Clin Endocrinol Metab 80:1416–1422, 1995.
319. Arslanian SA, Becker DJ, Lee PA, et al: Growth hormone therapy and tumor recurrence: Findings in children with brain neoplasms and hypopituitarism. Am J Dis Child 139:347–350, 1985.
320. Clayton PE, Shalet SM, Gattamaneni HR, et al: Does growth hormone cause relapse of brain tumors? Lancet 1:711–713, 1987.
321. Rodens KP, Kaplan SL, Grumbach MM, et al: Does growth hormone therapy increase the frequency of tumor recurrence in children with brain tumors? Acta Endocrinol 28(suppl):188–189, 1987.

322. Moshang T Jr: Is brain tumor recurrence increased following growth hormone treatment? Trends Endocrinol Metab 6:205–209, 1995.
323. Moshang T, Rundle AC, Graves DA, et al: Brain tumor recurrence in children treated with growth hormone: The National Cooperative Growth Study experience. J Pediatr 128:S4–S7, 1996.
324. Thorner MO, Rogol AD, Blizzard RM, et al: Acceleration of growth rate in growth hormone–deficient children treated with human growth hormone–releasing hormone. Pediatr Res 24:145–151, 1988.
325. Thorner MO, Rochiccioli P, Colle M, et al: Once daily subcutaneous growth hormone–releasing hormone therapy accelerates growth in growth hormone–deficient children during the first year of therapy. Geraf International Study Group. J Clin Endocrinol Metab 81:1189–1196, 1996.
326. Huerta MG, Rogol AD: Growth hormone–releasing hormone and other growth hormone secretagogues. *In* Kelnar CJH, Savage MO, Stirling HF, Saenger P (eds): Growth Disorders. Pathophysiology and Treatment. London, Chapman & Hall, 1998, pp 701–720.
327. Hummelink R, Sippell WG, Benoit KG: Intranasal administration of growth hormone–releasing hormone (1–29)-NH₂ in children with growth hormone deficiency: Effects on growth hormone secretion and growth. Acta Paediatr Suppl 388:23–26, 1993.
328. Lifschitz F, Lanes R, Puliese M, et al: Sustained improvement in growth velocity and recovery from suboptimal growth hormone (GH) secretion after treatment with human pituitary GH-releasing hormone (1–44)-NH₂. J Clin Endocrinol Metab 75:1255–1260, 1992.
329. Duck SC, Schwartz HP, Costin G, et al: Subcutaneous growth hormone–releasing hormone therapy in growth hormone deficient children: First year of therapy. J Clin Endocrinol Metab 75:1115–1120, 1992.
330. Bowers CY, Momany F, Reynolds GA, et al: Structure-activity relationships of a synthetic pentapeptide that specifically releases growth hormone in vitro. Endocrinology 106:663–667, 1980.
331. Bowers CY, Alster DK, Frentz JM: The growth hormone–releasing activity of a synthetic hexapeptide in normal men and short stature children after oral administration. J Clin Endocrinol Metab 74:292–298, 1992.
332. Bowers CY: On a peptidomimetic growth hormone–releasing peptide. J Clin Endocrinol Metab 79:940–942, 1994.
333. Smith RG, van der Ploey LHT, Howard AD, et al: Peptidomimetic regulation of growth hormone secretion. Endocr Rev 18:621–645, 1997.
334. Rosenfeld RG: IGF-I treatment of growth hormone insensitivity. *In* Takano T, Hizuka N, Takahashi S-I (eds): Molecular Mechanisms to Regulate the Activities of Insulin-like Growth Factors. Amsterdam, Elsevier, 1998, pp 359–364.
335. Laron Z, Anin S, Klipper-Auerback Y, et al: Effects of insulin-like growth factor-I on linear growth, head circumference and body fat in patients with Laron-type dwarfism. Lancet 339:1258–1261, 1992.
336. Walker J, Van Wyk JJ, Underwood LE: Stimulation of statural growth by recombinant insulin-like growth factor-I in a child with growth hormone insensitivity syndrome (Laron type). J Pediatr 121:641–646, 1992.
337. Wilton P: Treatment with recombinant insulin-like growth factor-I of children with growth hormone receptor deficiency (Laron syndrome). Acta Paediatr Suppl 282:137–141, 1992.
338. Savage MO, Wilton P, Ranke MB, et al: Therapeutic response to recombinant IGF-I in thirty-two patients with growth hormone insensitivity (abstract). Pediatr Res 33:S5, 1993.
339. Guevara-Aguirre J, Vasconez O, Martinez V, et al: A randomized, double-blind, placebo-controlled trial on safety and efficacy of recombinant human insulin-like growth factor-I in children with growth hormone receptor deficiency. J Clin Endocrinol Metab 80:1393–1398, 1995.
340. Guevara-Aguirre J, Rosenbloom AL, Vasconez O: Two-year treatment of growth hormone (GH) receptor deficiency with recombinant insulin-like growth factor I in 22 children: Comparison of two-dosage levels and to GH-treated GH deficiency. J Clin Endocrinol Metab 82:629–633, 1997.
341. Ranke MB, Savage MO, Chatelain PG, et al: Insulin-like growth factor I improves height in growth hormone insensitivity: Two years' results. Horm Res 44:264, 1995.
342. Klinger B, Laron Z: Three year IGF-I treatment of children with Laron syndrome. J Clin Endocrinol Metab 82:149–158, 1995.
343. Backeljauw PF, Underwood LE, The GHIS Collaborative Group: Prolonged treatment with recombinant insulin-like growth factor-I in children with growth hormone insensitivity syndrome—a clinical research center study. J Clin Endocrinol Metab 81:3312–3317, 1996.

Chapter 37

Growth Hormone Deficiency in Adults

Ken K.Y. Ho

Adult patients with organic hypopituitarism receive substitutive hormone treatment for secondary glucocorticoid, sex steroid, and thyroid hormone deficiency. Until recently, growth hormone (GH) deficiency in these patients was not regarded as a clinical problem, as it was assumed that GH had no physiologic relevance after cessation of childhood growth.

The critical role of GH in stimulating childhood growth is well recognized and its use in treating dwarfism due to GH deficiency is an unchallenged indication worldwide. Body growth represents the result of the stimulation by GH of a complex and integrated series of metabolic processes which are readily demonstrable in adults even after cessation of body growth. Growth stops at the end of childhood as a result of fusion of the growth plates in long bones. However, GH continues to be produced throughout adult life and is the most abundant hormone in the adult pituitary gland. Hormones exert their actions by binding to specific receptors on tissues. All body tissues examined to date contain receptors for GH. This observation suggests that the effects of GH are widespread and that the hormone plays a general role in maintaining the metabolic process and the integrity of many tissues.

Raben[1] first reported, nearly four decades ago, improved vigor and well-being in an adult woman with hypopituitarism treated with GH. A major reason for past neglect of treating adult patients with hypopituitarism with GH was the very limited availability of pituitary-derived GH outside the pediatric setting. The advent of genetic engineering resulting in abundant supplies of recombinant GH has been accompanied by a major reappraisal of its physiologic role in adult life.

EPIDEMIOLOGY

There is limited information on the epidemiology of hypopituitarism. A Swedish survey estimates the prevalence of hypopituitarism to be approximately 175 cases per million.[2] Pituitary and parasellar tumors are the commonest causes of hypopituitarism in adults. Data from two studies with a combined total of 505 patients with adult hypopituitarism revealed that approximately 70% arise from pituitary tumors, 12% from craniopharyngiomas, 5% are idiopathic, and 10% from unknown causes.[3, 4]

The etiology of adult GH deficiency from a recent survey of 258 patients is shown in Table 37–1. As the majority of these patients had multiple anterior hormone deficiencies, the disorders that result in hypopituitarism are similar to those that cause GH deficiency. The treatment of pituitary tumors is a significant cause of GH deficiency. In 165 patients with pituitary tumors evaluated before surgery, about 50% of patients already had evidence of GH deficiency.[5] After surgery, about 80% had evidence of GH deficiency. In patients who received

postoperative radiotherapy, endocrine evaluation after 5 years revealed that all patients were GH-deficient.[5]

CONSEQUENCES OF GROWTH HORMONE DEFICIENCY

One of the first indications of possible deleterious effects of GH deficiency in adults came from an epidemiologic study in 1990[3] which reported a two-fold increase in cardiovascular mortality in patients with hypopituitarism on conventional hormone replacement (Fig. 37–1). Two more recent reports provide further evidence that adults with hypopituitarism have reduced life expectancy from cardiovascular and cerebrovascular mortality.[4, 6]

In addition to the epidemiologic findings, adults with GH deficiency, whether dating from childhood or acquired in later adult life, suffer from a range of metabolic, body compositional, and functional abnormalities. These patients have a recognizable clinical syndrome, associated with characteristic history, symptoms, signs, and investigative findings (Table 37–2).

Metabolism

Hypopituitarism patients unreplaced with GH display biochemical abnormalities which are strongly linked to the development of vascular

TABLE 37–1. Etiology of Adult Growth Hormone (GH) Deficiency in 258 Patients

	Frequency (%)
Pituitary tumors	58
Functioning	29
Nonfunctioning	29
Parasellar tumors	23
Craniopharyngioma	13
Brain (glioma, pinealoma, dysgerminoma, histiocytosis X)	5
Meningioma	4
Metastatic malignancy	1
Idiopathic	6
Vascular (Sheehan's syndrome, apoplexy)	5
Others (developmental, trauma)	7
Lymphocytic hypophysitis	1
Total	100

Adapted from Christ ER, Carroll PV, Sonksen PH: The etiology of growth hormone deficiency in human adult. In Bengtsson B-A (ed): Growth Hormone. Boston, Kluwer Academic, 1999, pp 97–108.

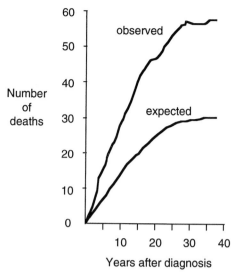

FIGURE 37–1. Mortality rate in adult patients with hypopituitarism on conventional hormone replacement therapy. (From Rosen T, Bengtsson BA: Premature mortality due to cardiovascular disease in hypopituitarism. Lancet 336:285–288, 1990. © by The Lancet Ltd., 1990.)

disease. These patients have higher concentrations of total and low-density lipoprotein (LDL) cholesterol, as well as apolipoprotein B.[7–9] Evidence has been obtained from ultrasonographic studies of premature atherosclerosis.[10] These patients also have a higher level of plasminogen activator inhibitory activity and higher concentration of fibrinogen,[11] both markers of increased atherothrombotic propensity, with fibrinogen being a known risk factor for stroke and myocardial infarction.

Body Composition

There is marked abnormality of body composition characterized by increased proportion of body fat and reduced lean mass.[12, 13] These

TABLE 37–2. Syndrome of Adult Growth Hormone (GH) Deficiency

Symptoms

Increased body fat
Reduced muscle bulk
Reduced strength and physical fitness
Reduced sweating
Impaired psychological well-being
   Depressed mood
   Anxiety
   Reduced physical stamina
   Reduced vitality and energy
   Increased social isolation

Signs

Overweight
Increased adiposity, especially abdominal
Poor muscular development
Reduced exercise performance
Thin, dry skin
Depressed affect

Investigations

Peak GH response to hypoglycemia <3 μg/L (all patients)
Low IGF-1 (60% of patients)
Hyperlipidemia: high LDL cholesterol, low HDL cholesterol
Elevated fasting insulin
Reduced bone mineral density

IGF-1, insulin-like growth factor; LDL, low-density lipoprotein; HDL, high-density lipoprotein.

changes are a consequence of the loss of the lipolytic and anabolic actions of GH. The effects of GH on body fat and muscle can be seen in Figure 37–2 which shows the striking changes in body physique in an adult male before and 5 years after acquiring GH deficiency following surgery for a pituitary tumor.

These patients are not only more obese but also display a disproportionate increase in central abdominal fat.[13] The tendency for central fat deposition is important since visceral obesity is linked to the development of insulin resistance, diabetes, and cardiovascular disease.[14] Indeed, adults with GH deficiency have evidence of insulin resistance[15] and a higher prevalence of impaired glucose tolerance.[16]

The reduction of lean body mass in adult GH deficiency arises from combined reduction of bone, muscle, and visceral mass and extracellular fluid volume. Bone mass at different skeletal sites is reduced in patients with childhood-onset and adult-onset GH deficiency.[17, 18] There is preliminary evidence that risk of fractures is increased.[9]

Physical Performance

The abnormalities of body composition are accompanied by a significant impairment of physical performance and muscle strength.[19, 20] Physical fitness, as determined by cycle ergometry, has been consistently shown to be reduced in adult GH deficiency with rates of maximal oxygen uptake reduced on average by about 30%.[21] Exercise performance is a complex parameter dependent on a number of factors, including cardiorespiratory function, as well as skeletal muscle function. These patients have impaired cardiac function with reduced ventricular muscle mass, reduced ejection fraction, impaired ventricular filling,[22–24] and reduced lung size, all of which contribute to reduced exercise capacity. As the skin is a target tissue of GH action, another likely contributing factor to reduced exercise endurance is impairment of sweating, which arises from hypoplasia of the eccrine sweat glands. Indeed, the skin of GH-deficient subjects is atrophic and dry.[9] Reduced sweating increases susceptibility to hyperthermia during exercise and may limit exercise performance.[25]

Quality of Life

The metabolic, body compositional, and functional abnormalities in adult GH deficiency are accompanied by significant impairment of

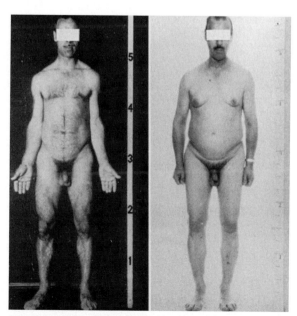

FIGURE 37–2. Body physique in a normal adult male before and 5 years after acquiring growth hormone deficiency as a result of pituitary surgery for a macroadenoma. Note the striking change in body composition with an accumulation of body fat, particularly in the abdomen, and marked loss of musculature. (Courtesy of Professor Peter Sonksen.)

psychological well-being and reduced quality of life. Fatigue, easy exhaustion, and lack of vitality are common symptoms. A number of studies have investigated self-perception of affective and emotional state, health problems, and the extent to which these affect daily activities using validated questionnaires. GH-deficient adults had lower energy scores, lacked physical stamina, and tended to have dysfunctional emotional reactions.[26, 27] There was lower self-perception of quality of life with patients regarding themselves as having reduced health, self-control, vitality, and experiencing more anxiety. A Dutch survey of social integration reported that GH-deficient adults had impaired social status.[28] These patients were on a lower professional scale, had lower income, were generally without partners, and living at home with their parents.

Thus the collective evidence indicates that adults who lack GH are not normal but suffer from metabolic abnormalities, disordered body composition, reduced physical fitness, impaired psychological well-being, and reduced quality of life.

DIAGNOSIS OF ADULT GROWTH HORMONE DEFICIENCY

Although the features of GH deficiency are recognizable, they are not particularly distinct, and mimic body compositional and biochemical changes of the aging process.[29] GH secretion itself falls progressively with aging, which is associated with a progressive increase in adiposity, which itself reduces GH secretion.[30, 31] Thus, clinical suspicion must be confirmed by accurate biochemical diagnosis to ensure that GH-deficient patients are accurately identified and treated.

Whom to Test

GH deficiency should be defined biochemically within an appropriate clinical context. The Growth Hormone Research Society has recommended that biochemical testing for GH deficiency be considered in patients with a high probability of hypothalamus-pituitary disease and manifesting clinical features of the syndrome.[32] This includes patients with a past history of organic hypothalamic-pituitary dysfunction, cranial irradiation, or known childhood-onset GH deficiency. In patients with organic hypothalamic-pituitary disease, the prevalence of GH deficiency is strongly linked to the number of pituitary hormone deficits, ranging from approximately 45% with no deficit, to virtually 100% if three or four pituitary hormone deficiencies are present.[33]

Patients with childhood-onset GH deficiency should be retested as adults before committing them to long-term GH replacement. About one-fourth of patients demonstrate normal GH responses when retested in adulthood using the same stimulation test.[34] Patients with a childhood diagnosis of isolated GH deficiency are the least likely to have demonstrable GH deficiency in adult life. Whether this is due to an error in initial diagnosis or recovery of GH secretion is not known.

Biochemical Diagnosis

There are three widely accepted approaches to assessing GH secretory status. These are measuring (1) the peak GH response to a provocative test, (2) spontaneous GH secretion, and (3) serum concentrations of GH-regulated proteins such as insulin-like growth factor-1 (IGF-1) and IGF binding protein-3 (IGFBP3). The merits of each have been carefully investigated.

Provocative Tests

The diagnosis of adult GH deficiency is established by provocative testing of GH secretion. Patients should be on adequate and stable hormone replacement for other hormonal deficits prior to testing. A number of provocative tests are available and include the insulin tolerance test (ITT), and arginine, glucagon, clonidine, or growth

hormone–releasing hormone (GHRH) testing alone or in combination with arginine or pyridostigmine. However, GH-releasing potency differs among these agents, with the ITT being a better stimulator of GH release than arginine or clonidine.

The Growth Hormone Research Society has recommended the ITT as the diagnostic test of choice.[32] It is superior to measuring integrated 24-hour GH concentration or IGF-1[35] (Fig. 37–3). Provided adequate hypoglycemia (<2.2 mmol/L or 40 mg/dL) is achieved, the ITT distinguishes GH deficiency from the reduced GH secretion that accompanies normal aging and obesity. The ITT should be performed in experienced endocrine units under supervision. The test is contraindicated in patients with electrocardiographic evidence or history of ischemic heart disease, or in patients with seizure disorders. Given these precautions, the ITT is safe with a risk of an adverse event of less than 1 in 450.[36] Normal subjects respond to insulin-induced hypoglycemia with a peak GH concentration of greater than 5 μg/L.[36] Severe GH deficiency is defined by a peak GH response to hypoglycemia of less than 3 μg/L. These cutoff values were defined in GH

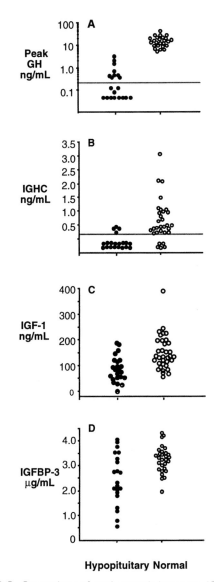

FIGURE 37–3. Comparison of peak growth hormone (GH) concentration obtained during an insulin tolerance test (A), integrated GH concentration (IGHC) obtained from blood withdrawal every 20 minutes for 24 hours (B), insulin-like growth factor-1 (IGF-1) (C) and IGF binding protein-3 (IGFBP-3) concentrations (D) in patients with organic hypopituitarism and age- and sex-matched normal subjects. The *dotted line* denotes the limit of reading. (From Hoffman DM, O'Sullivan AJ, Baxter RC, Ho KKY: Diagnosis of growth hormone deficiency in adults. Lancet 343:1064–1068, 1994. © by The Lancet Ltd., 1994.)

assays employing polyclonal competitive radioimmunoassays. However, GH immunoassay results vary among different methods and therefore the cutoff value may need to be adjusted appropriately.

In patients in whom the ITT is contraindicated, alternative provocative tests of GH secretion must be used with appropriate cutoffs because of their varying ability to stimulate GH release. At present, the combined administration of arginine and GHRH is the most promising alternative.[37] Other alternatives include arginine alone or glucagon. These tests have less well-established diagnostic value compared to the ITT. Other stimulatory tests, including the use of GH secretagogues, may prove to be useful but require further validation.

Spontaneous Secretion

Spontaneous secretion is most commonly estimated by measuring GH from frequent samples obtained over a 24-hour period. Integrated GH measurements obtained in this way do not readily discriminate GH-deficient patients from normal subjects even with the use of highly sensitive assays.[38] Together with the labor-intensive nature of the procedure, this procedure is more suitable as a research tool and cannot be recommended as a practical or reliable diagnostic test for GH deficiency (see Fig. 37–3).[35]

Biochemical Markers of Growth Hormone Action

Biochemical markers of GH action include IGF-1, IGFBP3, and the acid-labile subunit of the IGF-1–IGFBP complex. Of the three biochemical markers, the merit of IGF-1 has been the most intensively studied. Serum IGF-1 concentrations are only useful when age-adjusted normal ranges are used. While IGF-1 levels are reduced in adult GH deficiency, a normal concentration does not exclude the diagnosis (see Fig. 37–3). A subnormal IGF-1 level in an adult patient with coexisting pituitary hormone deficits is strongly suggestive of GH deficiency, particularly in the absence of conditions known to reduce IGF-1 levels, such as malnutrition, liver disease, poorly controlled diabetes mellitus, and hypothyroidism. The separation of IGF-1 values between GH-deficient and normal subjects is greatest in the young. As IGF-1 levels decline in normal subjects with aging, IGF-1 becomes less reliable as a biochemical marker of GH deficiency in patients over 50 years old when the values merge with those of normal subjects.[37] Measurement of IGFBP3 or the acid labile subunit does not offer any advantage over IGF-1.

Thus, the biochemical diagnosis of adult GH deficiency is normally established by the ITT in patients with a history of pituitary disease. A low IGF-1 level in such patients signifies hyposomatotropism, although a normal level dose not exclude the diagnosis.

GROWTH HORMONE REPLACEMENT THERAPY

The beneficial effects of GH replacement in hypopituitary adults were first reported in 1989.[13, 39] Since then, numerous studies have confirmed the initial observations[9] and are summarized in Table 37–3.

Metabolism

GH treatment induces profound effects on protein and fat metabolism which result in significant changes in body composition. The anabolic effects arise from direct stimulation of protein synthesis and reduction of protein oxidation. GH stimulates lipolysis and fat oxidation, enhancing the utilization of fat for energy metabolism. The marked effects of GH on substrate metabolism are accompanied by a significant stimulation of resting energy expenditure.[13]

In addition to exerting effects on the oxidative metabolism of fat, GH also induces significant effects on lipoprotein metabolism. Most studies report a decrease in total cholesterol.[9] Less consistently reported are effects on increasing high-density lipoprotein (HDL) cholesterol and reducing levels of LDL cholesterol and apolipoprotein B.[40–42] The favorable effects of improving the lipoprotein profile are more evident after treatment for longer than a year. Most studies report little effect on triglyceride levels. Mechanisms accounting for a less atherogenic profile include GH induction of hepatic LDL receptors and reduction in central adiposity accompanied by an improvement in insulin sensitivity.

Body Composition

GH replacement induces striking changes in body composition.[9, 13, 39, 41, 43] One of the first studies of adult replacement reported a significant reduction of 18% of body fat and a corresponding increase of lean body mass of 10% over 6 months of treatment (Fig. 37–4). These changes in body composition occurred without a significant change in body weight. Regional studies of body composition show that the greatest reduction of body fat occurs in abdominal and visceral fat.[44] Longer-term studies demonstrate that restoration of body composition is largely completed by the first 12 months of treatment. GH replacement also causes progressive thickening of skin and restoration of eccrine function leading to correction of skin dryness.

The increase in lean body mass arises from combined increase in skeletal muscle mass, visceral mass, and bone mass, as well as in extracellular fluid volume. Studies using computed tomography (CT) scanning show that cross-sectional area of thigh muscle increases by 5% to 8% after 6 months of treatment, with values becoming normal after 3 years of continuous treatment.[20, 45] A significant increase in extracellular water also occurs. These changes occur as a consequence of the antinatriuretic properties of GH, which are dose-dependent and involve activation of the renin-angiotensin system, as well as a direct renal tubular effect.[46]

Bone remodeling is activated by GH. Markers of bone formation such as osteocalcin, alkaline phosphatase, and bone Gla protein along with markers of resorption, such as urinary hydroxyproline, are increased by GH treatment.[9] Initial studies reporting changes in bone mineral density (BMD) over 6 to 12 months of treatment gave conflicting results. However, more recent studies reporting long-term data show progressive increase in BMD beyond 12 to 18 months of treatment[47–49] (Fig. 37–5). The gain is more marked in those with low densities before starting GH treatment.[47] The collective findings suggest that GH induces a biphasic effect, an initial predominance of bone resorption followed by a net gain in bone mass after 12 months of treatment. Whether these changes translate in the longer term to reduced fracture rates requires future study.

TABLE 37–3. Summary of the Clinical Consequences of Growth Hormone (GH) Deficiency in Adults and the Impact of GH Replacement Treatment

	GH Deficiency	GH Replacement
Metabolism		
Lipolysis	Decreased	Restored
Protein anabolism	Decreased	Restored
Glucose tolerance	Impaired	Restored
Total cholesterol	Increased	Decreased
LDL	Increased	Decreased
HDL	Decreased	Increased
Body composition		
Body fat	Increased	Restored
Abdominal fat	Increased	Restored
Lean body mass	Decreased	Restored
Muscle bulk	Decreased	Restored
Function		
Muscle strength	Decreased	Restored
Exercise capacity	Decreased	Restored
Quality of life	Impaired	Improved

LDL, low-density lipoprotein; HDL, high-density lipoprotein.

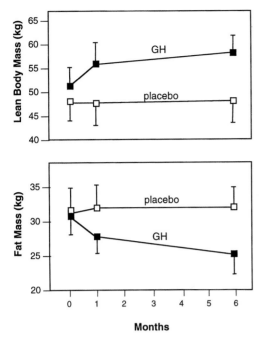

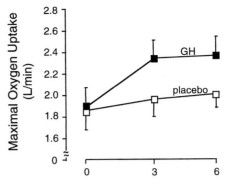

FIGURE 37–6. Maximal exercise capacity in growth hormone (GH)–deficient adults during treatment with either GH or placebo for 6 months. Exercise capacity was measured as maximal oxygen uptake during incremental cycle ergometry. (From Cuneo RC, Salomon F, Wiles CM, et al: Growth hormone treatment of growth hormone deficient adults: II. Effects on exercise performance. J Appl Physiol 70:695–700, 1991.)

FIGURE 37–4. Body composition in growth hormone (GH)–deficient adults during treatment with either GH or placebo for 6 months. (From Salomon F, Cuneo RC, Hesp R, Sonksen PH: The effects of treatment with recombinant human growth hormone on body composition and metabolism in adults with growth hormone deficiency. N Engl J Med 321:1797–1803, 1989. Copyright © 1989 Massachusetts Medical Society. All rights reserved.)

Physical Performance

Several studies have reported that the increase in lean body and muscle mass during GH treatment is accompanied by an improvement in muscle strength. Quadriceps or hip muscle strength improves significantly after 6 months of treatment.[20, 45] The strongest data have recently been provided by Johannsson et al.[50] who reported normalization of isometric quadriceps force and torque after 2 years of treatment. Many studies have also reported improvement in exercise capacity and performance in parallel with an increase in maximal oxygen uptake[21, 51] (Fig. 37–6). Submaximal exercise performance, estimated as anaerobic threshold, also increases significantly during GH treatment, suggesting that physical activities of daily living may be accomplished by less metabolic stress and less subjective perception of effort. In addition to increases in muscle strength, many other factors may contribute to an

improvement in exercise performance. These include enhanced cardiac function and improved heat dissipation through increased sweating. The data of a positive effect of GH on cardiac function are strong. Stroke volume, cardiac output, and diastolic function improve during GH treatment, which also increases ventricular mass.[21, 52, 53]

Quality of Life

The psychological well-being and quality of life of GH-deficient patients on replacement have been assessed using self-administered questionnaires which address general health and well-being. Although these tools are not disease-specific, several double-blind, placebo-controlled studies have reported improvement in mood, energy, sleep, and vitality scores with GH treatment,[26, 41, 42, 44] with continued improvement in these domains during the open phase. In general, GH replacement improved perceived health status and subjective well-being in the domains of health-related quality of life within 6 months. These findings were confirmed in a large randomized placebo-controlled blinded trial based on partner evaluation by questionnaire. According to the partner, the patients were more alert, active, and industrious, and had greater vitality and endurance during GH treatment.[54]

A 1997 study reported significant differences in clinical and biochemical presentation and responses to GH therapy between patients with childhood-onset and those with adult-onset GH deficiency.[43] Height, body weight, and lean body mass were lower in those with childhood-onset GH deficiency. They demonstrated greater change in body composition but lesser improvements in lipid profiles and quality-of-life measures than the group with adult-acquired GH-deficiency. The interesting differences at baseline and in responses to GH are likely to reflect the biologic roles of GH at difference phases of life, as well as the psychological impact of GH injections in the developing child. A patient with adult-onset disease is likely to recognize the restoration of a quality of life to a level experienced before acquiring GH deficiency. In contrast, adults who received GH as a developing child have grown up with and adapted to the condition and are likely to harbor negative recollections of enforced daily injections. As GH therapy is terminated on epiphysial closure, which occurs before somatic maturation, conventionally GH-treated children may not reach their physical and developmental potential on termination of GH treatment for short stature.[55] The data suggest the existence of two clinical entities, developmental and metabolic, reflecting the function of GH at different stages of life.[43]

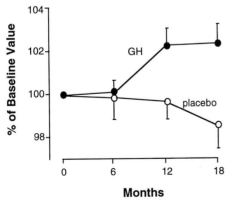

FIGURE 37–5. Bone mineral density of the lumbar spine in growth hormone (GH)–deficient adults during treatment with either GH or placebo for 18 months. (From Baum HB, Biller BM, Finkelstein JS, Klibanski A: Effect of physiologic growth hormone therapy on bone density and body composition in patients with adult onset growth hormone deficiency. A randomized, placebo-controlled trial. Ann Intern Med 125:883–890, 1996.)

TREATMENT

The key issues concerning treating and monitoring GH treatment in adults with GH deficiency are summarized in Table 37–4.

TABLE 37–4. Treatment Guidelines for Growth Hormone (GH) Replacement in Adult GH Deficiency

Pretherapy	Adequate replacement of other hormone deficiencies
	Pituitary imaging
	Body composition
	IGF-1, BSL, lipids
Starting dose	0.15–0.3 mg/day (0.5–1.0 IU)
Adjustments	Small monthly increment 0.01–0.15 mg/day
Monitor	IGF-1 (dose titration)
	BSL, lipids
	Weight, body composition, quality-of-life measures
Side effects	Edema, arthralgia, myalgia, parasthesia
Dosage considerations	Avoid weight-based regimens
	Women require more GH than men
	Elderly require less GH than the young
	Requirements greater with oral than transdermal estrogen therapy in women
Contraindications	Malignancy, intracranial hypertension, proliferative retinopathy

IGF-1, insulin-like growth factor-1; BSL, blood sugar level.

Dosage

A difficulty in integrating information from GH replacement trials stems from the lack of uniformity in the expression of units of GH dosage between centers. Treatment regimens are variably expressed in terms of body weight or surface area, milligrams or international units, as daily or weekly dosage regimens. To facilitate the comparison of various replacement regimens, Table 37–5 shows the conversion for a reference dose of 0.25 IU/kg/week, a dosage regimen employed in a number of multicenter trials. The conversion is normalized for an adult weighing 70 kg having a body surface area of 1.8 m^2 to provide an approximation for a daily dose expressed in either milligrams or international units. For most commercial preparations of GH, 1 mg is equivalent to 3 IU of GH. Most studies to date have employed a fixed-dose regimen based on body weight. This may not be appropriate since it commits obese patients to a larger dose, which is not compatible with the known physiologic reduction in GH secretion with adiposity, nor does it allow for reduced GH requirements with aging.[30]

The Growth Hormone Research Society has recommended that the replacement dosage not be weight-based. Patients are to be commenced on a low dose (0.15 to 0.3 mg/day, or 0.45 to 0.9 IU/day) with the dose gradually increased in accordance with clinical and biochemical responses.[32] The maintenance dosage may vary considerably, is influenced by sex and age, but rarely exceeds 1 mg/day (3 IU/day). Women appear to require higher doses than men,[56] while the elderly require lower doses. A recent study of dose optimization designed to achieve normal IGF-1 levels reported the average daily maintenance dose to be 1.2 IU in women and 0.8 IU in men.[57] GH should be administered subcutaneously each day in the evening.

What clinical endpoints should be monitored? A physical examination and careful history with particular attention to quality-of-life questions are of great value in monitoring treatment and where possible the partner's input should be sought. Serum IGF-1 is the most useful biochemical marker of GH response, the level of which should be maintained within an age-adjusted normal range. Clinical monitoring should include assessment of body composition (e.g., waist circumference, skin folds, or dual x-ray absorptiometry) and lipid measurements.

Interactions

GH may influence the metabolism of many substances, including hormones and medications. GH stimulates the activity of the hepatic cytochrome P450 system, which is a major pathway of the oxidative metabolism of several drugs, including anticonvulsants and theophylline. It is likely that dosage adjustments may be necessary in patients commencing GH treatment. Cortisol is also metabolized by the hepatic cytochrome P450 system. There is biochemical evidence that GH increases the metabolic disposal of cortisol and may increase the risk of adrenal insufficiency,[58] which has been reported in some studies.[41] While a causal relationship remains unproven, GH-deficient patients on GH therapy should be strongly advised to increase the dosage of glucocorticoids when unwell, as is generally recommended.

GH stimulates the peripheral conversion of thyroxine (T_4) to triiodothyronine (T_3). This effect may be frequently seen as a fall in circulating T_4 levels, particularly in patients on thyroid hormone replacement for hypopituitarism.[59] If T_3 is not monitored during GH replacement, a fall in T_4 may be misinterpreted as inadequate substitution and may lead to an unnecessary increase in the dosage of thyroid hormone replacement.

Estrogen has significant effects on the metabolic and endocrine functions of the liver which are dependent on the route of administration. When compared to the transdermal route, oral estrogen reduces IGF-1 and fat oxidation, effects that are opposite to those of GH.[60] The possibility that oral estrogens may antagonize GH action is supported by the observation that women are less responsive than men to GH.[56] GH-deficient women who are also hypogonadal should receive estrogen by a nonoral route during GH replacement.

Safety

The principle of hormone replacement therapy predicates that hormone replacement restore the untreated, morbid hormone-deficient state to normal. Side effects may be encountered as a consequence of inappropriate dosage or the failure of the mode of hormone replacement to induce a pharmacokinetic profile that mimics normal physiology. The same issues apply to GH replacement therapy. The experience from several large multicenter clinical trials indicates that GH treatment is safe and well tolerated.[41, 61, 62]

The most common side effects arise from the antinatriuretic action of GH which causes fluid retention (see Table 37–4). These manifest as dependent edema, paresthesia, and carpal tunnel syndrome, and occur with greater frequency in older patients. However, these symptoms are mild, dose-related, and resolve in the majority of patients, either spontaneously or with dosage reduction.[63] The early trials employed somewhat supraphysiologic doses of GH and encountered these side effects in up to 50% of patients. More recent trials employing a dosage regimen designed to maintain IGF-1 levels in the normal range have encountered virtually no untoward effects.[48] GH replacement dosage needs to be individualized, as is the case for other types of hormone replacement therapies.

Although GH antagonizes insulin action, the risk of developing hyperglycemia is very low. Only two cases of reversible diabetes were reported from two European multicenter trials with a combined total

TABLE 37–5. Conversion of Dosage Regimen of Growth Hormone (GH) Expressed in Body Weight or Body Surface, International Units (IU), or Milligrams (mg) to an Approximate Daily Dose (1 mg = 3 IU)

GH Units	Dosage			Daily Dose*
	kg/wk	kg/day	m^2/day	
IU	0.25	0.035	1.4	2.5
mg	0.08	0.01	0.46	0.83

*70-kg man with a body surface area of 1.8 m^2.

of 400 patients,[61, 62] while none of 166 patients developed diabetes in an Australian study.[41] Insulin sensitivity improves and may normalize after some months of treatment.[64] This paradoxical effect arises from the reduction in central abdominal fat which ameliorates insulin resistance.

As GH promotes the growth of tissues, concern has been expressed that GH therapy may increase the risk of pituitary tumor recurrence or the development of neoplasia. Analysis of the extensive pediatric experience shows no convincing evidence for a causal link between GH treatment and tumor recurrence or the development of neoplasia, including leukemia.[65] It has recently been reported that mean IGF-1 levels are higher in patients with prostate and breast cancers than in controls.[66, 67] One interpretation of these observations is that elevating IGF-1, which occurs with GH treatment, may increase the risk of developing prostate and breast cancers. If this is true, patients with acromegaly who have sustained elevated IGF-1 levels should have a higher incidence of these malignancies. There are conflicting reports about whether cancer incidence is increased in this disease and many studies have lacked statistical power. The biggest study to date, involving over one thousand acromegalic patients, found overall cancer incidence rates to be lower than in the general population. There was no significant increase in site-specific cancer rates, including breast cancer.[68] These data in acromegaly provide the strongest evidence against a causal association between IGF-1 and malignancy. Current recommendations for cancer prevention and early detection should be practiced in the adult with hypopituitarism treated with GH. It should be emphasized that the issues should be viewed in the context of restoring a GH-deficient state to normal. Nevertheless, it is important for future studies to establish whether the incidence of cancer or tumor recurrence in GH-replaced patients is different from that in untreated patients.

Contraindications

Contraindications to GH replacement include active malignancy, benign intracranial hypertension, and proliferative retinopathy. Pregnancy is not a contraindication, although treatment should be discontinued in the second trimester as GH is produced by the placenta.[32]

CONCLUSION

Adult patients with GH deficiency have impaired health characterized by abnormalities of fuel metabolism, body composition, physical performance, and psychological function which adversely affect quality of life. Most, if not all, of these abnormalities improve or normalize with GH replacement. Side effects are minor, mostly relate to fluid retention, and can be minimized by individualizing dosage requirements. Because GH remains expensive, it is important that its use in adults be restricted to patients with proven GH deficiency. Based on the global evidence of efficacy and safety, adults with GH deficiency should receive replacement with GH, a principle consistent with the tenet of hormone replacement for hormone deficiency in the practice of endocrinology.

REFERENCES

1. Raben MS: Growth hormone: 2. Clinical uses of human growth hormone. N Engl J Med 266:82–86, 1962.
2. Rosen T, Bengtsson BA: Epidemiology of adult onset hypopituitarism in Göteborg, Sweden during 1956–1987 (abstract). In International Symposium on Growth Hormone and Growth Factors, Göteborg, Sweden 1994, p 60.
3. Rosen T, Bengtsson B-A: Premature mortality due to cardiovascular disease in hypopituitarism. Lancet 336:285–288, 1990.
4. Bates AS, Van't Hoff W, Jones JP, Clayton RN: The effect of hypopituitarism on life expectancy. J Clin Endocrinol Metab 81:1169–1172, 1996.
5. Littley MD, Shalet SM, Beardwell CG, et al: Hypopituitarism following external radiotherapy for pituitary tumours in adults. QJM 70:145–160, 1989.
6. Bulow B, Hagmart L, Mikoczy Z, et al: Increased cerebrovascular mortality in patients with hypopituitarism. Clin Endocrinol 46:75–81, 1997.
7. Libber SM, Plotnick LP, Johanson AJ, et al: Long-term follow up of hypopituitary patients treated with human growth hormone. Medicine (Baltimore) 69:46–55, 1990.

8. De Boer H, Blok GJ, Voerman HJ, et al: Serum lipid levels in growth hormone deficient men. Metabolism 43:199–203, 1994.
9. Carroll PV, Christ ER, Bengtsson BA, et al: Growth hormone deficiency in adulthood and the effects of growth hormone replacement: A review. J Clin Endocrinol Metab 83:382–395, 1998.
10. Markussis V, Beyshah SA, Fisher C, et al: Detection of premature atherosclerosis by high resolution ultrasonography in symptom-free hypopituitary adults. Lancet 340:1188–1192, 1992.
11. Johansson JO, Landin K, Tengborn L, et al: High fibrinogen and plasminogen activator inhibitory activity in growth hormone-deficiency adults. Arteriosclerosis Thromb 14:434–437, 1994.
12. Hoffman DM, O'Sullivan AJ, Freund J, Ho KKY: Adults with growth hormone deficiency have abnormal body composition but normal energy metabolism. J Clin Endocrinol Metab 80:72–77, 1995.
13. Salomon F, Cuneo RC, Hesp R, Sonksen PH: The effects of treatment with recombinant human growth hormone on body composition and metabolism in adults with growth hormone deficiency. N Engl J Med 321:1797–1803, 1989.
14. Reaven G: Banting Lecture, 1988: Role of insulin resistance in human disease. Diabetes 37:1595–1607, 1988.
15. Hew FL, Koschmann M, Christopher M, Alford K: Insulin resistance in growth hormone deficient adults: Defects in glucose utilisation and glycogen synthetase activity. J Clin Endocrinol Metab 81:555–564, 1996.
16. Beyshah SA, Henderseon A, Nithayanathan R, et al: Metabolic abnormalities in growth hormone deficient adults: Carbohydrate tolerance and lipid metabolism. Endocrinol Metab 1:173–180, 1994.
17. Kaufman J, Taelman P, Vermelen A, Vandeweghe M: Bone mineral status in growth hormone deficient males with isolated and multiple pituitary deficiencies. J Clin Endocrinol Metab 74:118–123, 1992.
18. Holmes SJ, Economou G, Whitehouse RW, et al: Reduced bone mineral densities in in patients with adult onset growth hormone deficiency. J Clin Endocrinol Metab 78:669–674, 1994.
19. Rutherford OM, Beshyah SA, Johnston DG: Quadriceps strength before and after growth hormone replacement in growth hormone deficient adults. Endocrinol Metab 1:44–47, 1994.
20. Cuneo RC, Salomon F, Wiles CM, et al: Growth hormone treatment of growth hormone deficient adults. I. Effects on muscle mass and strength. J Appl Physiol 70:688–694, 1991.
21. Cuneo RC, Salomon F, Wiles CM, et al: Growth hormone treatment of growth hormone deficient adults. II. Effects on exercise performance. J Appl Physiol 70:695–700, 1991.
22. Amato G, Carella C, Fazio S, et al: Body composition, bone metabolism, and heart structure and function in growth hormone (GH) deficient adults before and after GH replacement therapy. J Clin Endocrinol Metab 77:1671–1676, 1993.
23. Merola B, Cittadini A, Coloa A, et al: Cardiac structural and functional abnormalities in adult patients with growth hormone deficiency. J Clin Endocrinol Metab 77:1658–1661, 1993.
24. Shahi M, Beshyah SA, Hackett D, et al: Myocardial dysfunction in treated adult hypopituitarism: A possible explanation for increased cardiovascular mortality. Br Heart J 67:92–96, 1992.
25. Juul A, Behrenscheer A, Tims T, et al: Impaired thermoregulation in adults with growth hormone deficiency during heat exposure and exercise. Clin Endocrinol 38:237–244, 1993.
26. McGauley GA, Cuneo RC, Salomon FC, Sonksen PH: Psychological well-being before and after growth hormone treatment in adults with growth hormone deficiency. Horm Res 33(suppl):52–54, 1990.
27. Rosen T, Wiren L, Wilhemsen L, et al: Decreased psychological well-being in adult patients with growth hormone deficiency. Clin Endocrinol 40:111–116, 1994.
28. Rikken B, Van Busschbach J, Le Cessie S, et al: Impaired social status of growth hormone deficient adults as compared to controls with short or normal stature. Clin Endocrinol 43:205–211, 1995.
29. Rudman D: Growth hormone, body composition and aging. J Am Geriatr Soc 33:800–807, 1985.
30. Ho KY, Evans WS, Blizzard RM, et al: Effects of sex and age on the 24 hour secretory profile of GH secretion in man: Importance of endogenous estradiol concentrations. J Clin Endocrinol Metab 64:51–58, 1987.
31. Iranmanesh A, Lizarralde G, Veldhuis JD: Age and relative adiposity are specific negative determinants of the frequency and amplitude of growth hormone (GH) secretory bursts and the half-life of endogenous GH in healthy men. J Clin Endocrinol Metab 73:1081–1088, 1991.
32. Growth Hormone Research Society: Consensus guidelines for the diagnosis and treatment of adults with growth hormone deficiency: Summary statement of the Growth Hormone Research Society Workshop on Adult Growth Hormone Deficiency. J Clin Endocrinol Metab 83:379–381, 1998.
33. Toogood AA, Beardwell C, Shalet SM: The severity of growth hormone deficiency in adults with pituitary disease is related to the degree of hypopituitarism. Clin Endocrinol 41:511–516, 1994.
34. Nicholson A, Toogood AA, Rahim A, Shalet SM: The prevalence of severe GH-deficiency in adults who received GH replacement in childhood. Clin Endocrinol 44:311–316, 1996.
35. Hoffman DM, O'Sullivan AJ, Baxter RC, Ho KKY: Diagnosis of growth hormone deficiency in adults. Lancet 343:1064–1068, 1994.
36. Hoffman DM, Ho KKY: Diagnosis of GH deficiency in adults. In Juul A, Jorgensen JOL (eds): Growth Hormone in Adults. Cambridge, Cambridge University Press, 1996, pp 168–185.
37. Ghigo E, Aimaretti G, Gianotti L, et al: New approach to the diagnosis of growth hormone deficiency in adults. Eur J Endocrinol 134:352–356, 1996.
38. Reutens AT, Hoffman DM, Leung KC, Ho KKY: Evaluation and application of a highly sensitive assay for serum growth hormone (GH) in the study of adult GH deficiency. J Clin Endocrinol Metab 80:480–485, 1995.

39. Jorgensen JOL, Theusen L, Ingemann-Hansen T, et al: Beneficial effects of growth hormone treatment in GH-deficient adults. Lancet 1:1221–1225, 1989.
40. Weaver JU, Monson JP, Noonan K, et al: The effect of low dose recombinant human growth hormone replacement on regional fat distribution, insulin sensitivity and cardiovascular risk factors in hypopituitary patients. J Clin Endocrinol Metab 80:153–159, 1995.
41. Cuneo RC, Judd S, Wallace JD, et al: The Australian multicenter trial of growth hormone treatment in GH-deficient adults. J Clin Endocrinol Metab 83:107–116, 1998.
42. Beyshah SA, Henderson A, Niththyananthan R, et al: The effects of short and long term growth hormone replacement in hypopituitary adults on lipid metabolism and carbohydrate tolerance. J Clin Endocrinol Metab 80:356–363, 1995.
43. Attanasio AF, Lamberts SWJ, Matranga AMC: Adult growth hormone deficient patients demonstrate heterogeneity between childhood-onset and adult-onset before and during human GH treatment. J Clin Endocrinol Metab 82:82–88, 1997.
44. Bengtsson B-A, Eden S, Lonn L, et al: Treatment of adults with growth hormone (GH) deficiency with recombinant human GH. J Clin Endocrinol Metab 76:309–317, 1993.
45. Jorgensen JOL, Theusen L, Muller J, et al: Three years of growth hormone treatment in growth-hormone deficient adults: Near normlisation of body composition and physical performance. Acta Endocrinol 130:224–228, 1994.
46. Hoffman DM, Crampton L, Sernia C, et al: Short term growth hormone (GH) treatment of GH deficient adults increases body sodium and extracellular water but not blood pressure. J Clin Endocrinol Metab 81:1123–1128, 1996.
47. Johannsson G, Rosen T, Bosaues I, et al: Two years of growth hormone treatment increases bone mineral content and density in hypopituitary patients with adult-onset growth hormone deficiency. J Clin Endocrinol Metab 81:2865–2873, 1996.
48. Baum HB, Biller BM, Finkelstein JS, Klibanski A: Effect of physiologic growth hormone therapy on bone density and body composition in patients with adult onset growth hormone deficiency. A randomized, placebo-controlled trial. Ann Intern Med 125:883–890, 1996.
49. Vandeweghe M, Taelman P, Kaufman J-M: Short and long term effects of growth hormone treatment on bone turnover and bone mineral content in adult growth hormone-deficient males. Clin Endocrinol 39:409–415, 1993.
50. Johannsson G, Grimby G, Sunnerhagen KS, Bengtsson BA: Two years of growth hormone treatment increases isometric and isokinetic muscle strength in GH-deficient adults. J Clin Endocrinol Metab 82:2877–2884, 1997.
51. Nass R, Huber RM, Klauss V, et al: Effect of growth hormone (hGH) replacement therapy on physical work capacity and cardiac and pulmonary function in patients with hGH deficiency acquired in adulthood. J Clin Endocrinol Metab 80:552–557, 1995.
52. Caidahl K, Eden S, Bengtsson BA: Cardiovascular and renal effects of growth hormone. Clin Endocrinol 40:393–400, 1994.
53. Valcavi R, Gaddi O, Zini M, et al: Cardiac performance and mass in adults with hypopituitarism: Effect of one year of growth hormone treatment. J Clin Endocrinol Metab 80:659–666, 1995.
54. Burman P, Broman JE, Hetta J, et al: Quality of life in adults with growth hormone (GH) deficiency: Response to treatment with recombinant GH in a placebo-controlled 21 month trial. J Clin Endocrinol Metab 80:3585–3590, 1995.
55. Rutherford OM, Jones DA, Round JM, et al: Changes in skeletal muscle and body composition after discontinuation of growth hormone treatment in growth hormone deficient young adults. Clin Endocrinol 34:469–475, 1991.
56. Burman P, Johansson AG, Siegbahn A, et al: Growth hormone (GH)–deficient men are more responsive to GH replacement therapy than women. J Clin Endocrinol Metab 82:550–555, 1997.
57. Drake WM, Coyte D, Camacho-Hubner C, et al: Optimizing growth hormone replacement therapy by dose titration in hypopituitary adults. J Clin Endocrinol Metab 83:3913–3919, 1998.
58. Weaver JU, Thaventhiran L, Noonan K, et al: The effect of growth hormone replacement on cortisol metabolism and glucocorticoid sensitivity in hypopituitary adults. Clin Endocrinol 41:639–648, 1994.
59. Jorgensen JOL, Pedersen SA, Lauberg P, et al: Effects of growth hormone therapy on thyroid function of growth hormone–deficient adults with and without concomitant thyroxine-substituted central hypothyroidism. J Clin Endocrinol Metab 69:1127–1132, 1989.
60. O'Sullivan AJ, Crampton L, Freund J, Ho KKY: Route of estrogen replacement confers divergent effects on energy metabolism and body composition in postmenopausal women. J Clin Invest 102:1035–1040, 1998.
61. Mardh G, Lundin K, Borg G, et al: Growth hormone replacement therapy in adult hypopituitary patients with growth hormone deficiency: Combined data from 12 European placebo-controlled trials. Endocrinol Metab 1(suppl A):43–49, 1994.
62. Chipman JJ, Attanasio AF, Birkett MA, et al: The safety profile of growth hormone replacement therapy in adults. Clin Endocrinol 46:473–481, 1997.
63. De Boer H, Blok GJ, Popp-Snijders C, et al: Monitoring of growth hormone replacement therapy in adult based on measurement of serum markers. J Clin Endocrinol Metab 80:2069–2076, 1996.
64. Hwu CM, Kwok CF, Lai TY, et al: Growth hormone replacement reduces total body fat and normalizes insulin sensitivity in GH-deficient adults: A report of one-year clinical experience. J Clin Endocrinol Metab 82:3285–3292, 1997.
65. Allen D: National Cooperative Growth Study Safety Symposium: Safety of human growth hormone therapy. J Pediatr 128:S8–13, 1996.
66. Chan JM, Stampfe MJ, Giovannucci E, et al: Plasma insulin-like growth factor 1 and prostate cancer risk: A prospective study. Science 279:563–566, 1998.
67. Hankinson SE, Willett WC, Colditz GA, et al: Circulating concentrations of insulin-like growth factor-I and risk of breast cancer. Lancet 351:1393–1396, 1998.
68. Orme SM, McNally RI, Cartwright RA, Belchez PE: Mortality and cancer incidence in acromegaly: A retrospective cohort study. J Clin Endocrinol Metab 83:2730–2734, 1998.

▲▲▲▲

Chapter 38

Aging, Endocrinology, and the Elderly Patient

Jesse Roth ▪ Christian A. Koch ▪ Kristina I. Rother

Leaders in medicine, through their academic organizations and with support from foundations, and practicing geriatricians have fretted for the last decade over the need to intercalate advances in geriatric medicine into the practice of specialties, including endocrinology. This chapter has been written with their collective wisdom in mind. The opening focuses on the art of medicine exemplified in care of the elderly. The next section surveys aging of populations, individuals, organ systems, cells, and molecules and concludes with theories of aging. Then drugs, depression, dementia, and delirium (as well as sleep) are covered because of their multifaceted interplay with the endocrine system in elderly patients. In the last part of the chapter, major endocrine areas are reviewed with respect to special features in the elderly patient (Table 38–1); the presentations here are intended to complement the more extensive presentations on the same topics elsewhere in this book.

THE ART OF MEDICINE

Contemporary science and medicine have conferred on clinicians a very large array of tests and treatments. With the elderly, especially the frail elderly, a great deal of judgment must be used by the physician in deciding which of the large number of tests and treatments should be used and which should thoughtfully and knowingly be withheld. Two forces from the extremes pull at the middle. One is to systematically undertreat because of agism, a prejudice that blocks access of

the elderly to the full benefits of modern medicine. The other extreme is to manage elderly patients as though they were robust young patients. To achieve the golden mean, the clinician must set lofty goals but approach them gently, with frequent follow-up observations and contact with the patient, best done outside the hospital. (Often the hospital is a very inhospitable place for an elderly patient.[1–3]) Although the growth of science in medicine has progressively subordinated the art of medicine in many disciplines, geriatric medicine with its focus on the elderly patient remains a fountainhead for practice of the art of medicine. For the elderly patient with an endocrine disorder, the clinician must be in charge, not the computer-driven protocol.

The rich skills of excellent physicians are best tested by the typical elderly patient: multiple interacting illnesses and drugs; subtle manifestations of new disorders camouflaged by the pre-existing ones; restricted homeostatic capabilities, both biologically and socially; and the sparse database of direct evidence.[4, 5] In return, modern medicine's modest capabilities often match the patient's constrained expectations, and the complexities are so intricate that each contact between patient, family, and physician provides a fresh opportunity to do some good. In approaching an elderly patient concerning endocrine disturbances, physicians should remember to be alert to four widespread opportunities for good: to seek unappreciated depression (or other neuropsychiatric disturbances), to review drugs for possible mischief, to find ways to avoid hospitalization, and to seek opportunities to bring comfort to the patient and the patient's family, a skill that physicians have practiced for millennia before science was ever introduced to medicine.

TABLE 38–1. Circulating Levels of Hormones in Advanced Age (Relative to Younger Adults)

	Elevated	Same	Reduced
Men and women	Follicle-stimulating hormone	Adrenocorticotropic hormone	Growth hormone
	Luteinizing hormone	Cortisol	Insulin-like growth factor-1
	Vasopressin	Epinephrine	Renin
	Atrial natriuretic hormone	Thyrotropin*	Aldosterone
	Parathyroid hormone	Thyroxine	3,5,3′-Triiodothyronine
	Insulin	Glucagon	Androsterone
	Leptin		DHEA
			DHEA sulfate
			1,25(OH)$_2$ vitamin D
			25-OH vitamin D
Women	Ovarian testosterone		Estrone
			Estradiol
			Progesterone
			Testosterone
Men	Free estrone		Testosterone
	Free estradiol		Free testosterone

*Although overall thyrotropin levels in the elderly are unchanged, thyrotropin in many elderly individuals will be above and below the normal range established for younger patients.
DHEA, Dehydroepiandrosterone.
Adapted from Cobbs EL, Duthie EH, Murphy JB (eds): Geriatrics Review Syllabus: A Core Curriculum in Geriatric Medicine, ed 4. New York, American Geriatrics Society, and Dubuque, IA, Kendall/Hunt, 1999.

AGING OF POPULATIONS, INDIVIDUALS, ORGAN SYSTEMS, CELLS, AND MOLECULES

The Demographics and Their Consequences

The elderly population, predominantly female, is increasing, both absolutely and relatively in the industrialized and developing nations[6] (Fig. 38–1). The frail elderly and the "oldest old," those 85 and older, are showing the most rapid rate of growth[4–7] (see Fig. 38–1). Because of the remarkable shortage of published data on patients older than 65, especially the frail elderly, most normal values, tests, and therapies that have been devised are based on much younger subjects. When evaluating a young adult, often the clinician is interpolating between points from the archival database, whereas with older patients the clinician is extrapolating from the database. The older the patient, the more tenuous the extrapolation. In the absence of age-specific data, more caution needs to be exercised in interpretation of tests and construction of management plans based on published data on younger adults.

The Aging Process vs. Disease

To distinguish normal aging from the disease processes that accumulate in old age,[8, 9] imagine a graph that plots the shortest time to run a marathon as a function of chronologic age. To run a marathon requires excellent health and training, yet with age older than 40 comes an inexorable lengthening of how much time it takes. That is normal aging, but aging also brings with it heightened susceptibility to disease, growing frailty, and an increased likelihood of dying. With regard to the endocrine system, another feature of aging is the loss of homeostatic reserve; the boundaries of control widen, and the subtleties of control systems diminish, spoken of as a "loss of complexity." [10]

Longevity and Genetics

Longevity has very strong genetic influences.[11–13] The maximum life span of any member of a species is nearly absolute. A Methuselah among mice would be equivalent to a young child among humans or elephants. Among monozygotic twins, longevity is more closely correlated than in dizygotic twins, and the details of the aging process may be remarkably similar. A recent twin study of women older than 80 showed that cognition was much more similar in the monozygotic

pairs, thus fortifying the place of inheritance even late in life with complex multifactorial traits.[14]

A series of rare single-gene defects associated with premature aging and mortality in humans have garnered a great deal of attention from researchers.[12, 13, 15] Genomic instability has been noted in some, and in several of these disorders, the molecular defects have been localized to genes for helicases, enzymes vital to DNA repair.[15, 16] (See later about the potential role of DNA damage in aging.) The intensive search for longevity genes in the yeast (*Saccharomyces cerevisiae*), worm (*Caenorhabditis elegans*), and fruit fly (*Drosophila melanogaster*) has been explosively productive.[17] Among the discoveries is a molecule similar to the insulin receptor that is found in the worm.[18, 19]

Environmental Influences on Aging

One maneuver that prolongs life in rodents and in nonhuman primates is systematic severe calorie restriction.[20, 21] The biochemical events responsible for the extended life span are not yet known but are under intense study. The reduction in blood glucose is particularly intriguing in light of suggestions that glycosylated proteins may mediate some effects of aging (see later). In humans, exercise and a normal body mass index each favor longevity. Diabetes and obesity, both syndromes characterized by substrate excess, accelerate aging and reduce the life span (effectively through their phenotypes, not their genotypes). Long-lived individuals who remain healthy commonly exercise a great deal more than the mean for their ages.[22] Cause-and-effect relationships have not been established. Higher socioeconomic status, independent of other variables, promotes better health and longer life, but the biologic correlates of this phenomenon remain obscure.[23–25]

Genetics and Environment in Diseases of Old Age

Most of the common disorders of old age have strong genetic influences that interact with environmental factors over time to produce the disorders[13, 26, 27] (Fig. 38–2). Single-gene defects with mendelian inheritance patterns typically account for a very small minority; ordinarily, heredity is the result of the interaction of several susceptibility genes. As seen in Figure 38–2, obesity susceptibility genes interact over time with patterns of diet and exercise to cause obesity. The obesity in turn becomes an environmental factor that interacts with susceptibility genes for diabetes to produce hyperglycemia. A similar pattern holds for hypertension. The hyperglycemia and hypertension become environmental factors that interact with other genes

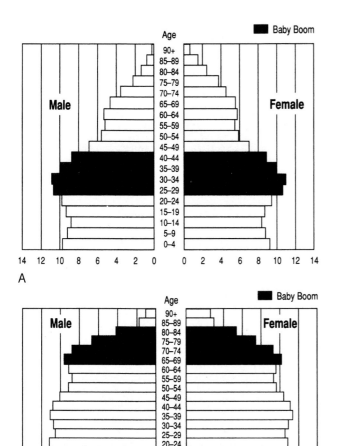

FIGURE 38–1. Expansion of the elderly population by sex and age from 1990 *(A)* to 2030 *(B)*. With increasing age, females are an increasingly larger proportion of the population than males. Between 1990 and 2030, the proportion of the population older than 65 and that older than 80 years will grow in absolute and relative numbers. In effect, the outline of the population figure shifts from triangle-like in 1990 to a rectangle-like polygon in 2030. *(A from US Bureau of the Census: Current Population Reports, Special Studies, P23-178RV, Sixty-Five Plus in America.* US Government Printing Office, Washington, DC, 1992, pp 1–2; *B* based on data from Current Population Report P25-1092, *Populations Projections of the United States by Age, Sex, Race, and Hispanic Origin: 1992–2050.* US Government Printing Office, Washington, DC, 1992, p 48.)

that confer susceptibility to diabetic complications such as nephropathy and retinopathy (Fig. 38–2). In every patient, genetic and environmental elements interact over time to pattern the aging process. In turn, the aging process influences the timetable of the diseases that characteristically afflict the elderly.

Aging of Systems with Endocrinologic Consequences

Reproductive organs age earlier and more dramatically in women than in men. Bone and skeletal muscle diminish by about one-third, whereas fat and connective tissue increase.[8] (Sarcopenia, the loss of muscle mass, has received attention as a key feature in frailty and many of its consequences.[28]) The endocrine system is also affected by aging of the nervous system and the immune system. In the central nervous system (CNS), neurons, glia, and blood vessels are affected. Changes are common in dendrites and cytoskeletal elements. Increases can be seen in cellular infiltrates and protein deposits, both extracellu-

lar and intracellular. These changes correlate clinically with both global and focal effects. For example, the elderly show heightened susceptibility to delirium with even modest metabolic insults. They also have diminished sensitivity to hyperosmolality in the subjective recognition of thirst and vigor of water-seeking behavior. The age-related diminution of immune function[29] has broad general (as well as endocrinologic) implications: diminished efficacy of vaccines (pneumonia/diabetes), as well as heightened susceptibility to infection (diabetes), cancer (ectopic hormone secretion), and autoimmunity (hypothyroidism; β cell autoimmunity). The mechanisms are unclear but the clinical consequences are apparent.

Maintenance of Cell Populations

For endocrine systems to sustain function into old age, ideally the populations of secretory cells and target cells remain constant and fully functioning. Constancy of cell numbers requires that births equal deaths. Cell death can occur by accident (necrosis) or more often by triggering the endogenous program of cell death (apoptosis).[30–32] The cell is continuously receiving signals from intracellular and extracellular sources that both favor and discourage apoptosis.[33] Small changes in this balance will change cell numbers. (Insulin-like growth factor-1 [IGF-1] is among the most potent antiapoptotic factors known; does the age-dependent diminution in circulating IGF-1 contribute? Cytokines and damaged DNA can each trigger apoptosis. Does their increase with age favor apoptosis?)

The production of a fully competent replacement for the dead cell is a complex process.[33] A stem cell or precursor cell must be stimulated to divide, migrate to its proper final position, and mature into a fully functioning differentiated cell. Each of these processes is highly regulated by internal and external signals. With aging, the stem cell population may be depleted. Stem cells may no longer replicate (see later under Telomeres and Replicative Senescence). Signals that direct migration or maturation, often derived from other cells, may be altered with age. These signals may be short lived, such as cytokines and other hormone-like agents, or be long-lived molecules such as those in the intercellular matrix.[33]

Maintenance of Cell Function

As noted, differentiation of a stem cell into a fully functioning mature cell depends on an orderly array of internal and external signals. It is now clear that maintenance of the fully functioning mature state requires a continuous input of similar signals, many of which were among the menu of signals needed for the initial maturation of that cell type.[33] An alteration in any of these maintenance signals with aging may be the cause of changes in cell function. In addition to a full complement of cells and a full menu of maintenance factors, maintenance of full function requires the *absence* of interfering substances that disrupt normal cell function, such as cytokines, amyloids, advanced glycosylation end-products (AGEs, see later), hyperglycemia, and altered matrix molecules. For example, with autoimmune diabetes, cell loss is the dominant force late in the illness; earlier, hyperglycemia may cause β cell dysfunction. Earlier yet, cytokines that are released from infiltrating inflammatory cells may be the dominant mechanism of impaired release of insulin, before measurable loss of β cells.[34, 35]

Telomeres and Replicative Senescence

Most cells undergo "replicative senescence" with age. The original observations were made with fibroblasts in culture, which undergo a finite number of cell divisions before ceasing reproduction.[36–40] The cells function well but remain in reproductive arrest, a state referred to as "replicative senescence." The number of divisions before arrest is inversely related to the age of the donor. Cells from young individuals with Werner's syndrome, an inborn illness that has features of accelerated aging, behave like cells of an aged donor.[38, 39] With cells

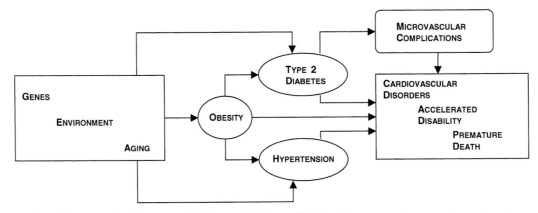

FIGURE 38–2. Interaction of genes and environment with diseases of old age. Obesity, diabetes, and hypertension each has its own group of genes that predispose an individual to that disorder. With each disorder, the genetic factors interact with a group of environmental factors and, over time, produce cardiovascular disorders, accelerated disability, and premature death. Furthermore, these diseases interact with each other. For example, the increased fat mass in obesity becomes an additional environmental factor for both diabetes and hypertension. With the microvascular complications of diabetes, which have their own independent genetic predispositions (not shown), the hypertension (not shown) and hyperglycemia become environmental factors. Finally, the microvascular complications contribute as environmental factors to the macrovascular or cardiovascular disorders and their consequences.

from a range of animal species, the number of divisions before replicative senescence is proportional to the life span of the species; short-lived species exhibit fewer divisions before arrest.[38, 39]

The number of replications is tabulated in the cell's *telomeres*, the noncoding ends of chromosomes.[41–45] Every chromosome terminates at each end with a telomere, which is composed of a long series of identically repeating hexanucleotide units that confer stability to the chromosome. (Broken ends of chromosomes that lack telomeres are unstable.) In only a few cell types is each telomere reproduced to its full length along with the rest of the chromosome when the cell's DNA is reproduced. Reproduction of the distal end of each telomere requires *telomerase*, a unique transferase that synthesizes the repeating units.[46] Most somatic cells lack telomerase activity; when the whole chromosome is being reproduced, the last few units of the telomere are left off. Thus the daughter chromosomes are ever so slightly shorter at both ends than the mother chromosomes; the rest of the chromosome, including the entire coding region, will be reproduced identically. Progressive shortening of the telomeres ultimately leads to a certain critical length of telomere that prevents further cell division. This process is the molecular basis for "replicative senescence." Germ cells, lymphocytes, and cancer cells have telomerase activity and thereby escape replicative senescence. Supporting the evidence for the role of telomeres are studies showing that somatic cells engineered to contain constitutively active telomerase can escape replicative senescence.[47]

Aging of Molecules

Proteins often undergo oxidative damage over time that may alter their function and metabolic fate, typically by heightening their susceptibility to degradation.[48–50] Also, glucose can bind to the amino groups of proteins, first reversibly and then irreversibly.[51, 52] The glucose moiety covalently linked to the protein can transform into ring structures known as AGEs. In addition to their effect on the function and fate of that protein, AGEs linked to any protein can bind to and activate cell surface receptors for the AGEs (known as RAGEs). These complexes activate cells probably by mechanisms similar to those of hormones and other signaling systems, which is how AGEs mediate many complications of diabetes. For example, AGEs can promote cell division or cell death, mimic cytokines, or stimulate their release. Substantial amounts of AGEs are also present in euglycemic individuals, but at levels well below those found with hyperglycemia. The accumulation of AGEs and other covalent modifications with aging is most prominent in long-lived proteins, such as in the lens.[51–53] It has been proposed that agents that reduce the level of AGEs may be useful in blunting some aspects of the aging process.

Amyloid Formation

An intact protein or protein fragment, when present at high concentrations intracellularly, can form organized arrays that may become insoluble fibrils known collectively as amyloid.[54] Among neurodegenerative disorders, Alzheimer's disease, Huntington's disease, and some forms of familial Parkinson's disease have each been associated with time- and age-dependent accumulations of a specific amyloid that is characteristic for that illness and thought to be closely linked to its particular pathophysiology.[55–58] Endocrine cells, such as the C cells of the parathyroid gland or the β cells of the pancreas, which have very high concentrations of protein hormones, are susceptible to amyloid deposits. The accumulation of insoluble deposits of protein may in some circumstances alter cell function and life span. (Small soluble aggregates of proteins may exist for a long time before rapidly coalescing into large insoluble aggregates typical of amyloid. A delay at the molecular level might correspond to the delay in the onset of clinical disease often observed even with congenital disorders. The sickling of hemoglobin is a carefully studied model of this type of process.[59–61])

Lipid Accumulations

Long-lived cells such as neurons and cardiac myocytes accumulate lipofuscin (so-called age pigment). Auto-oxidation products of unsaturated lipids are believed to be the major precursors.[62] Other lipid-derived elements accumulate in a wide range of cells.[63]

Free Radicals

A free radical (e.g., superoxide, $\dot{O}_2$) is a short-lived, highly reactive small molecule with an unpaired electron that can chemically alter DNA, proteins, and lipids by multiple mechanisms to produce a multiplicity of effects (oxidative stress).[64–67] In addition, free radicals can activate and mimic cellular signals (e.g., NFκB or nuclear factor kappa B, a broadly acting cell regulator), thereby modifying gene expression. Consequences include both specific disease processes and generalized changes associated with aging (e.g., cataract formation). In vivo, metabolic processes at multiple intracellular loci (involving O_2 as well as NO) and environmental elements (chemical as well as physical) generate free radicals continuously. Enzymes (e.g., superoxide dismutase and catalase) and small molecules (e.g., glutathione and vitamins E and C) scavenge and inactivate them. Mechanisms are also present to repair oxidative damage. Accumulation of oxidative damage has been proposed as a major mechanism in the aging process and in many disorders of old age, including cancer, atherosclerosis, and Alzheimer's disease.

DNA Repair

The nucleotides in DNA are continuously being damaged.[65–72] What prevents damaged DNA from becoming a mutation is the highly organized DNA repair process. Until the damaged DNA is reproduced, the error is not permanent, but rather very likely to be repaired. With aging, DNA repair mechanisms become less efficient.[72] Mutations accumulate. Surveillance mechanisms inside the cell detect damaged DNA and prevent cells from reproducing until the DNA is repaired; unrepaired DNA may also trigger apoptotic cell death.[30–32] Inborn errors of DNA repair have been associated with reduced longevity.[11–13] In addition, the accumulation of mutations is an important part of carcinogenesis and probably also autoimmunity, both of which are relevant to endocrine disorders in the elderly. (As noted earlier, immune function declines with old age, and diminutions in immunity are associated with both cancer and autoimmunity.)

Mitochondrial DNA

Aging is associated with the progressive accumulation of mitochondria with defective genes.[71–77] In contrast to nuclear DNA, the tiny fraction of total DNA that resides in the genome of the mitochondrion is derived solely from maternal sources; a multiplicity of copies is present per cell, and great heterogeneity of the mitochondrial genome is seen within cells as well as between cells. Several cellular mechanisms (e.g., proximity to sites of free radical production and less efficient DNA repair) favor a time-dependent accumulation of mutations in mitochondrial DNA that can lead to diminution in cellular production of ATP, diminished function, or (apoptotic) cell death. At the level of the organ or tissue this process will be manifested as slowly progressive loss of function. Based on observations of patients who have inborn defects in mitochondrial DNA, cells with very high energy demands, such as brain, muscle, and secretory cells (e.g., pancreas, gonads), may be especially vulnerable.

Theories of Aging

In experimental animals, both genetic and environmental studies support clinical evidence for the existence and operation of a biologic clock that coordinates the aging process.[78] Experimentally, a change in a gene or an environmental element (e.g., ambient temperature or access to sexual partners) that alters the life span is associated with an across-the-board change in essentially all components of the aging process. Current theories of aging tend to select for emphasis one or two of the many biologic concomitants of aging described in this chapter.[79–83] Free radical or oxidative damage is probably the most popular. Time-dependent accumulation of DNA damage or intrinsic mutagenesis is the focus of another leading theory, with recent attention also on mitochondrial DNA. Several forms of stress associated with the release of catecholamines, glucocorticoids, or cytokines, especially interleukin-6, have been key to other theories.[79, 84–86] Progressive accumulation of abnormal proteins is at the center of the error catastrophe theory.[50, 55, 79] More recently, glycated proteins have gained ascendancy.[51, 52] Programmed senescence of organ systems (e.g., immune system or alterations in the neuroendocrine pacemakers that govern the hypothalamic-pituitary-adrenal axis) has also been championed.[29, 55, 79] Theories based on replicative senescence of somatic cells have gained adherents recently.[39, 40, 43, 44] Each of the theories provides fuel for the engines of research but so far explains only a limited portion of the observations.

DRUGS AND THE ELDERLY

Drugs in Diagnostic Evaluation

Drugs often have such a dominating presence in elderly patients that early in the diagnostic work-up it is prudent to consider the possibility that one or more drugs are causing a syndrome that is mimicking an endocrinopathy (or other illness) and that drug withdrawal will result in full recovery.[87–96] Elderly patients on average take seven to eight medications. A complete inventory is essential but requires effort. To ensure completeness, the patient should bring in every medication at every visit, including those applied to the skin and eyes. Nowadays, nonprescription drugs (including herbs and supplements, as well as other alternative therapies) deserve special attention. The fragmentation of medical care aggravates the problem; a new physician pressed for time who has just met the patient may rubber-stamp the old medications while adding new ones to meet the current complaints. All drugs individually have significant side effects, but patients taking multiple drugs are at exponentially greater risk than patients taking only one or two drugs; the multiplicity of interactions defies practical definition. (The poorly cataloged side effects of alternative therapies add further complexities.) *Polypharmacy* has traditionally been a neutral term to indicate the need for a combination of drugs to treat one medical condition. For contemporary geriatricians, polypharmacy is a pejorative intimating that the patient is using too many drugs and that *pharmaceutical debridement* is in order. Often, with supervision, an elderly patient can safely discontinue the use of multiple drugs, feel better, and save money. (We suggest facetiously that a physician should collect a commission for 1 year for each medication whose use is discontinued.) The final item in the drug history is alcohol abuse. Both de novo and recrudescent alcohol abuse is often overlooked in the elderly, especially women, in the wealthy and well educated, and in those who live alone with few links to the outside.[97–99]

Special Considerations when Prescribing Drugs for the Elderly

The response of elderly patients to a drug may be quite different than the response of young people because of age-related changes in body composition and organ function, as well as the accumulation of diseases[87–91, 93–96, 100] (Table 38–2). When prescribing drugs (especially for women), consider age-dependent reductions in lean body mass, muscle mass, and total body water with effects on initial volumes of drug distribution. Also present is an age-related diminution in hepatic metabolism (especially phase 1) and renal function, such as a lower glomerular filtration rate. Pathologic loss of cardiac, hepatic, or renal function may further alter responses to the drug. (It is worth recalling that in the elderly, serum creatinine may be in the normal range, despite a diminution in renal function, because of the fall-off in creatinine production associated with the atrophy of skeletal muscle. Similarly, malnutrition may keep the blood urea nitrogen value in the normal range despite a decline in renal function.) Overall, drugs typically have increased potency with advances in age of the patient; that is, a left shift in the dose-response curve is common. Therefore it is wise to start with small doses and work toward defined endpoints

TABLE 38–2. Physiologic Changes Associated with Aging that May Affect Drug Disposition

Absorption	Distribution
Decreased gastric acidity	Decreased total body water
Decreased gastrointestinal motility	Decreased lean body mass
Decreased absorptive surface	Increased body fat proportion
Decreased splanchnic blood flow	Decreased serum albumin
Metabolism	Increased α_1-acid glycoprotein
Decreased hepatic mass	Elimination
Decreased hepatic blood flow	Decreased renal mass
	Decreased renal blood flow
	Decreased glomerular filtration rate
	Decreased tubular secretion

Modified from Cobbs EL, Duthie EH, Murphy JB (eds): Geriatrics Review Syllabus: A Core Curriculum in Geriatric Medicine, ed 4. New York, American Geriatrics Society, and Dubuque, IA, Kendall/Hunt, 1999; based on Montamat SC, Cusack BJ, Vestal RE: Management of drug therapy in the elderly. N Engl J Med 321:303–309, 1989.

of response. Prolongation of the half-life of drugs dictates a need for (1) longer intervals between dose changes and (2) longer periods to allow dissipation of discontinued drugs. When selecting drugs to prescribe to older patients, consider giving preference to drugs that have been in wide use for long periods. They are less likely to bring surprises than new drugs are. In general, new drugs are much less well tested on older people.

Setting a specific therapeutic goal for every medication that the patient is taking provides discipline to avoid the accumulation of medications and reduces the risk of undesirable side effects.[87, 95, 96, 100] Contingency plans for a drug's discontinuation can be recorded when the drug is started; if the drug fails to achieve its goals, use of the medication can be discontinued expeditiously.

Noncompliance in the elderly is quite common[90, 91, 100, 101] and aggravated by current trends in medical practice. Reductions in the patient's hearing, vision, manual dexterity, and speed of understanding may be partially compensated by written instructions in large print and follow-up calls. A review of the treatment regimen by the clinician at each visit, possibly reinforced by an assistant in the presence of an involved relative, would be very helpful. A great risk for serious error occurs at the transitions from outpatient to inpatient status and vice versa. Thus a phone call at home immediately after discharge to review the discharge instructions would be most valuable.

When drugs are mentioned, the physician immediately thinks of the classic dictum "first do no harm." A second dictum to follow is to "do some good." In young patients this principle may consist of giving an appropriate medication, whereas in the elderly another common possibility is to do good by reducing the dose or eliminating one or more medications.

NEUROPSYCHIATRY AND THE ELDERLY

Interaction of Endocrine and Neuropsychiatric Disorders

In geriatric patients, changes in cognition and behavior often herald physical illnesses. Endocrine and metabolic disorders in the elderly will often have cerebral consequences such as depression, dementia, or delirium. Neuropsychiatric signs and symptoms are often prominent and may dominate the clinical picture. Furthermore, neuropsychiatric disorders (e.g., depression or Alzheimer's disease) may produce significant endocrine changes. Finally, this area is one where an insightful clinician can especially help the patient.

Nomenclature Changes

The *Diagnostic and Statistical Manual of Mental Disorders*, edition 4 (DSM-IV), uses *cognitive disorder* to replace *organic mental disorder*. Other obsolete terms include *functional* and *organic*, as well as *organic brain syndrome* and *senility*.

Depression

Depression, which is more common in the elderly, is frequently serious and affects multiple aspects of the patient's life; depression is complicated by a high rate of suicide, especially among elderly white males.[84, 102–115] In contrast to younger patients, in whom depression is typically idiopathic, depression in the elderly is more often associated with a definable etiology. Prescription and nonprescription drugs are frequent culprits.[87–89, 94–96] Among the endocrine disorders most often cited are diabetes, hypercalcemia, thyroid hormone deficiency and excess, and glucocorticoid deficiency and excess. (The complex link between depression and glucocorticoid excess is expanded on later.) Other conditions include vitamin B_{12} or folate deficiency, inflammatory disorders, cancer, cerebrovascular disorders, and neurodegenerative diseases. Parkinson's disease and Alzheimer's disease may be heralded by depression. Post-stroke patients and caregivers of patients with

Alzheimer's disease are particularly prone to depression. Depression in the elderly is often subtle and referred to as "masked depression" or "depression without sadness."[116–118] Especially in functionally impaired elderly patients, anxiety is often a prominent feature but responds along with improvement in mood. The regular use of a geriatrics depression screen is highly recommended. (Depression is more common in the elderly than anemia is, so a routine screen for it should be performed as often as measurements of hemoglobin.[119–121]) A recently published screen that tested well against longer standard tests, even in patients older than 65, asks the patient to answer two questions[113]: "During the past month, have you often been bothered by feeling down, depressed, or hopeless? During the past month, have you often been bothered by little interest or pleasure in doing things?" A "yes" to either was considered positive and had high sensitivity (>90%) for the diagnosis. A "no" to both made depression quite unlikely.[113] A longer, more detailed screen is included for use as needed to confirm results or help resolve ambiguities[120] (Table 38–3).

Depression brings disturbances in sleep patterns, which in turn may aggravate the depression. Circadian rhythms, typically more erratic among older people, are even more disturbed with depression, thus making interpretations of tests that depend on circadian rhythms more difficult. The elevated plasma adrenocorticotropic hormone (ACTH) and cortisol levels that often occur in patients with depression are so similar to those observed in patients with mild Cushing's syndrome that they are frequently very difficult, if not impossible to distinguish on a biochemical basis.[122–128] Until recently, the medical significance of this biochemical abnormality was not appreciated. One group (but not another) has shown in recent studies that long-standing depression with disturbed pituitary-adrenal relationships results in osteoporosis that is typical of patients with steroid excess, which suggests that the hypercortisolemia of depression is not simply a biochemical abnormality but has pathologic consequences.[109, 129, 130] Although it is not yet standard practice to treat the hypercortisolemia of depression, physicians should be alert in the future for solid data to support this path.[131] The high cortisol is another reason to be more aggressive in the recognition and management of depression; restoration of mood and normalization of cortisol go together. Depression (untreated) appears

TABLE 38–3. Screening Estimate of Depression in the Elderly (Short Form)

Choose the best answer for how you felt over the past *week*		One point each
1. Are you basically satisfied with your life?	Yes/no	No
2. Have you dropped many of your activities and interests?	Yes/no	Yes
3. Do you feel that your life is empty?	Yes/no	Yes
4. Do you often get bored?	Yes/no	Yes
5. Are you in good spirits most of the time?	Yes/no	No
6. Are you afraid that something bad is going to happen to you?	Yes/no	Yes
7. Do you feel happy most of the time?	Yes/no	No
8. Do you often feel helpless?	Yes/no	Yes
9. Do you prefer to stay at home rather than going out and doing new things?	Yes/no	Yes
10. Do you feel you have more problems with memory than most?	Yes/no	Yes
11. Do you think it is wonderful to be alive now?	Yes/no	No
12. Do you feel pretty worthless the way you are now?	Yes/no	Yes
13. Do you feel full of energy?	Yes/no	No
14. Do you feel that your situation is hopeless?	Yes/no	Yes
15. Do you think that most people are better off than you are?	Yes/no	Yes

Score zero or 1 point for each answer. Evaluation: normal, 0 to 5; above 5 suggests depression.

Modified from Cobbs EL, Duthie EH, Murphy JB (eds): Geriatrics Review Syllabus: A Core Curriculum in Geriatric Medicine, ed 4. New York, American Geriatrics Society, and Dubuque, IA, Kendall/Hunt, 1999; based on Sheikh JI, Yesavage JA: Geriatric depression scale: Recent evidence and development of a shorter version. Clin Gerontol 5:165–172, 1986.

to contribute to poorer outcomes of other disorders.[108, 110, 111, 114, 119] In addition, depression can be associated with a dementia (or "pseudodementia") that is quite difficult to distinguish from dementia of the Alzheimer type, except that it is reversible with successful antidepressant therapy.[132] More common are patients with Alzheimer's disease who are also depressed; successful therapy for depression may result in measurable improvement in function.[133, 134] In general, depression is underdiagnosed and undertreated, especially in the elderly. Typically, the benefits of therapy greatly outweigh the side effects.[112, 114, 135] Psychotherapy (especially for hopelessness), drugs (which may take days up to a couple of months to work), and electric shock therapy (in selected cases) all have a useful role.[136, 137]

Dementia

Dementia is a syndrome characterized by a constellation of cognitive defects often associated with behavioral disturbances and has over 100 etiologies, including vascular diseases, space-occupying masses, and infections involving the CNS, as well as vitamin B_{12} deficiency and hypothyroidism.[133-135, 138-141] Medications that are commonly implicated include long-acting benzodiazepines and anticonvulsants.[94-96] Some of the dementias can be fully reversed by reversing the primary process, especially dementias that are drug-induced. Most patients with late-onset, slowly developing progressive dementia have Alzheimer's disease, designated in the DSM-IV as dementia of the Alzheimer type, but the final diagnosis still depends on postmortem histology. When dementias were first sharply redefined 25 years ago, it was proposed that a significant minority of dementias might be fully reversible. The early optimism is not justified by recent studies. Some dementias are reversible, especially drug-induced ones, but they constitute a much smaller fraction of the total than previously thought. Still, reversible causes of cognitive disorders should be searched for zealously, especially depression, subdural hematoma, normal-pressure hydrocephalus, hypothyroidism, vitamin B_{12} deficiency, and drug toxicity. However, optimism that the cognitive disorder will be fully reversed by removing the inciting agent must be guarded. On the other hand, most patients with dementia will show some improvement after successful treatment of other serious illnesses, depression being a particularly good example.[95, 133, 134, 138]

For diagnostic purposes and follow-up, a formal mini–mental examination is highly recommended.[142*] The examiner needs to exclude a confusional state or delirium before testing and to make sure that the patient is attentive. Minimal levels of dementia may be missed, especially in highly educated, sophisticated individuals. Another diagnostic maneuver, as a short screen or to complement the mini–mental status examination when the scores are unexpectedly high, is to ask the patient to draw the face of a clock.[143, 144] The emergence of drugs that enhance cognition (or slow the decline) in patients with Alzheimer's disease has heightened the motivation of clinicians to make the diagnosis early.[139]

Benign senescent forgetfulness and age-associated memory impairment are diagnostic synonyms now applied to elderly patients with isolated memory disorders or other minor defects in cognition. They do not qualify at this point for the diagnosis of Alzheimer's disease (e.g., score okay on a formal mini–mental examination, despite points lost for recall), but up to 50% will qualify as having Alzheimer's disease within 5 years.[138]

Delirium

Delirium (which some authorities also refer to as confusion) is a very common acute manifestation of drug toxicity or medical illness.[145-161] The long list of etiologies includes hypoxia, hypotension, electrolyte abnormalities (Na^+, K^+, Ca^{2+}, Mg^{2+}), hypothyroidism, and glucocorticoid deficiency or excess, as well as hyperglycemia and hypoglycemia. Delirium needs to be recognized and distinguished from dementia and from depression. The official diagnostic criteria

*Also see the Website http://www.minimental.com

TABLE 38–4. Diagnostic Criteria for Delirium (DSM-IV)

Disturbances of consciousness (i.e., reduced clarity of awareness of the environment) with reduced ability to focus, sustain, or shift *attention*
Development of a *change in cognition* (such as memory deficit, disorientation, language disturbance) or *perceptual disturbance* that is not better accounted for by a pre-existing established or evolving dementia
Disturbance that *develops over a short period* (usually hours to days) and *tends to fluctuate* during the course of the day
Evidence from the history, physical examination, or laboratory findings that the disturbance is *caused by* the direct physiologic consequences of one or more *medical conditions* or *medications*

Modified from Cobbs EL, Duthie EH, Murphy JB (eds): Geriatrics Review Syllabus: A Core Curriculum in Geriatric Medicine, ed 4. New York, American Geriatrics Society, and Dubuque, IA, Kendall/Hunt, 1999; adapted from American Psychiatric Association: Diagnostic and Statistical Manual of Mental Disorders, ed 4. Washington, DC, American Psychiatric Association, 1994, p 129.

are listed in Table 38–4. Distinction between dementia and delirium alone or delirium superimposed on dementia is a substantial clinical challenge (as is the distinction of depression-induced pseudodementia from dementia alone or dementia with superimposed depression).

It is extremely important to recognize delirium early because it is frequently the earliest or *only* sign of a potentially catastrophic medical condition. Inouye et al. provide a four-point assessment[150] (Table 38–5). Nurses' notes are often prophetic. Severe illness, advanced age, and impaired physical function all enhance the risk for delirium. An underlying dementia magnifies the other risk factors (Table 38–6). In a patient with delirium, medications should be reviewed in detail to eliminate all except those absolutely essential. In theory, any drug is capable of producing delirium by itself; equally often, drugs contribute collectively. Metabolic status should be evaluated carefully, especially electrolytes, Ca^{2+}, Mg^{2+}, and glucose. The acute onset, the change in level of consciousness, and the cognitive impairment will help clinicians correctly diagnose delirium. In some series, 10% to 15% of older medical patients admitted to a hospital met the criteria for delirium. Of those admitted without delirium, the disorder subsequently developed in 20%, especially among the frail and the ill. Although delirium per se has little impact on mortality, it is associated with a high mortality rate inasmuch as many of the patients are elderly and frail and have serious medical conditions. Delirium was once considered to be a transient reversible disorder with few long-term effects, reversible when the cause of the delirium was removed. Now

TABLE 38–5. Assessment of Delirium

1. Acute onset and fluctuating course
   Is there evidence of an acute change in mental status from the patient's baseline?
   Did this behavior fluctuate during the past day, come and go, increase and decrease in severity?
2. Inattention
   Is the patient having difficulty focusing attention and keeping track of what is being said or easily distractible?
3. Disorganized thinking
   Is the patient's speech disorganized or incoherent, rambling or irrelevant, unclear or illogical with unpredictable switching from subject to subject?
4. Altered level of consciousness
   Overall, how would you rate this patient's level of consciousness?
   Vigilant (hyperalert)
   Alert (normal)
   Lethargic (drowsy, easily aroused)
   Stuporous (difficult to arouse)
   Comatose (unarousable)

The diagnosis of delirium requires the presence or an abnormal rating for criteria 1 and 2 plus either 3 or 4.

Modified from Tune LE: Delirium. *In* Hazzard WR, Blass JP, Ettinger WH Jr, et al (eds): Principles of Geriatric Medicine and Gerontology, ed 4. New York, McGraw-Hill, 1999, pp 1229–1237; based on Inouye SK, van Dyck CH, Alessi CA, et al: Clarifying confusion: The confusion assessment method: A new method for detection of delirium. Ann Intern Med 113:941–948, 1990.

TABLE 38–6. Delirium: Outline of Risk Factors and Common Etiologies (with a View to Prevention and Early Treatment)

Environment: hospitalization, procedures, other disruptions
Drugs: individually and collectively
Endocrine and metabolic dysregulation: salt, water, calcium, magnesium, thyroid hormone, glucose
Infection
Organ dysfunction
    Cardiopulmonary (hypoxia, hypercapnia)
    Renal
    Hepatic
    CNS, especially dementia
Demographics: age older than 80 yr, male, diminished level of physical function, fractures

Data from Cobbs et al.[4] and Hazard et al.[5]

it is recognized that when the inciting cause has been detected and remedied, full recovery may often take many months or be elusive.[159–161] The reason for this poor long-term prognosis is obscure but serves as a caution in the use of drugs and hospitalization, two major precipitants of delirium, and adds motivation for prevention, early recognition, and treatment (Tables 38–6 and 38–7).

Sleep

Sleep disturbances are common among the elderly. Etiologies are multiple.[162–171] Reduced physical activity, depression, dementia, delirium, drugs, sleep apnea, and nocturnal vasopressin deficiency (see later) are among the contributors to a long list. Circadian rhythms in the elderly are often damped.[165, 172–174] Sleep disorders disturb the rhythm and vice versa, which complicates the interpretation of tests that depend on circadian rhythms.[172–175] Obstructive sleep apnea has been described with obesity, hypothyroidism, acromegaly, and with testosterone replacement; each responds to appropriate specific therapy, in addition to general measures applicable to all.[176] Other conditions linked to obstructive sleep apnea in the elderly are post-stroke status, multi-infarct dementia, Alzheimer's disease, depression, and sedative drugs.[170, 171] Less well appreciated is that otherwise normal, thin elderly individuals also show an age-dependent increase in prevalence of the same syndrome; the etiology is unknown and the overall

TABLE 38–7. Delirium—Prevention and Early Recognition

Anticipation
    Inventory the risk factors to identify high-risk patients
    Record results of the history from the family and a brief cognitive test (of orientation, attentiveness, sensorium) as baseline for follow-up
Prevention
    Shorten (or better yet, avoid) hospital stay
    Reduce medications as much as possible
    Stabilize and control the physical environment
        Plan lighting
        Avoid overstimulation and understimulation
    Plan people in the environment
        Caregivers
            Limit (and orient) the cast of characters
            Encourage early alert for infections, dehydration, hypoxia, etc.
        Family—encourage constant presence and continuous involvement
    Hospital routine
        Avoid the mindless fragmentation of sleep typical of hospitals
        Family or trusted caregiver in constant attendance for all procedures
    Cues to the patient
        Clock, calendar, verbal reminders of time and place
        Introduce personnel, procedures, and medications
Early recognition
    Review with staff and peruse nursing notes for disorientation, inappropriate speech or behavior, sensory misperceptions, and hallucinations
    Regularly retest orientation, attentiveness, and sensorium

prognosis less gloomy.[167, 168] Nonpharmacologic therapies can be quite effective and safe and should be given precedence, especially in the elderly.[169–171]

REVIEW OF INDIVIDUAL HORMONES

Melatonin

Synthesis and release of melatonin, the hormone of the pineal gland, are stimulated by darkness and inhibited by light.[177–184] Melatonin secretion progressively declines in old age.[177–179] Insomnia in the elderly is accompanied by serum melatonin levels that are lower and with a delayed nighttime peak in comparison to age-matched controls without insomnia.[178] Orally administered doses in the range of 0.2 to 0.3 mg achieve peak blood levels similar to normal endogenous bedtime levels and are helpful in initiating normal sleep. Higher doses such as 3 mg may be needed for sustained sleep. So far, the drug appears to be quite safe; doses many times that level have been given without serious side effects, but the total organized experience is still very limited.[180–184] The broad-spectrum antiaging effects of melatonin administration are thus far unsupported by systematic studies.

Hypercortisolism

An unresolved diagnostic problem is distinguishing the heightened and dysrhythmic secretion of ACTH and cortisol associated with depression or with Alzheimer's disease, two common disorders, from mild, early, or episodic forms of Cushing's syndrome, much less common afflictions that are often subtle in their clinical features, especially in the elderly.[122–127, 185–187] A recent study containing a catalog of the shortcomings of extant tests and a proposal for a new test showed that the midnight cortisol level was above 7.5 µg/dL in 96% of patients with Cushing's syndrome but in none of 23 patients with a "pseudo-Cushing state"; most patients in the latter group were obese and none were older than 65 years.[185] Thus the distinction in an elderly patient between mild Cushing's syndrome and a "pseudo-Cushing" state is still challenging, especially with midnight plasma cortisol levels 10 µg/dL or lower. In general, Cushing's disease is less common in the elderly than in younger adults, whereas ectopic ACTH production, cortisol-producing adrenal carcinomas, and incidentalomas are more common.[177, 186] Overall, interpretation of the usual tests for adrenal hyperfunction in the elderly needs to be done cautiously.[177, 185–187]

Adrenal Insufficiency

In the elderly, as in other adults, glucocorticoid withdrawal is the major cause of adrenal insufficiency. Among other etiologies, autoimmunity is less common than in younger patients, whereas metastases, hemorrhage (most often in a patient taking anticoagulant drugs), and infections (especially recrudescent tuberculosis) are more common.[177, 186] Symptoms are typically nonspecific: anorexia, weight loss, weakness, confusion, and failure to thrive. The usual signs (hypotension, hyperpigmentation) and laboratory abnormalities (azotemia, hypoglycemia, hyponatremia, and hyperkalemia) may be mild or absent. In the elderly the diagnosis is delayed or missed even more often than in the young, with potentially fatal consequences. Fortunately, provocative testing, such as the ACTH stimulation test, remains valid with aging. Even more than in young people, when the diagnosis is suspected on clinical grounds, the immediate collection of specimens, including an abbreviated ACTH stimulation test, can be followed safely by acute glucocorticoid replacement therapy intravenously and by other routes until laboratory results are available to validate the diagnostic conclusion.

Sexuality and Aging

The medical community is showing increasing interest in the sexual activities of the elderly.[188] Given that the decline in ovarian function in women and testicular function in males is but one of the factors in a very complex array of components that go into normal sexual interest and performance, it is not surprising that replacement of sex steroids alone is effective in only a minority of patients. The suggestion of a stimulatory effect of dehydroepiandrosterone (DHEA) on the sexuality of women with adrenal insufficiency and the success of sildenafil on erectile and intromission capabilities in many normal men raise the possibility that in the future new agents will be developed to treat individual components of the many that disturb sexual function.[189] The reader is referred elsewhere for a detailed and thoughtful discussion of this complex and important issue, including the frequent role of depression and drugs as major contributors to sexual dysfunction.[188]

Sex Hormone Replacement Strategies in the Elderly

Guidelines have been established for estrogen replacement in women because of its benefits on bone and the cardiovascular system. Epidemiologic and other data suggesting a benefit in delaying or improving dementia of the Alzheimer type (along with the well-accepted cardioprotection potential) are promoting more estrogen use in elderly women, but overall the studies are not yet definitive.[138] The newer guidelines for testosterone replacement in men are resting on better data.[190, 191] Studies of effects on cognition are in progress. Again, the reader is referred to Chapter 158 for more complete coverage of the pros and cons of sex hormone replacement in the elderly.

Growth Hormone and IGF-1

With aging comes a progressive diminution in growth hormone secretion, defined as the area under the curve of serum growth hormone measured for 24 hours or just at night.[172–174, 192–196] An increase in the inhibitory influence of somatostatin has been considered at least as important as a diminution in stimulatory inputs through growth hormone–releasing hormone and other secretagogues.[174, 197–200] Some of the broad-spectrum changes associated with aging (e.g., decrease in lean body mass, strength, stamina, and bone density) may be contributed to by this decline in growth hormone, but growth hormone therapy in normal elderly (which stimulates IGF-1 release) has been disappointing; the side effects outweigh the measurable benefits.[192–194, 201–208] (Support is growing for consideration of growth hormone replacement, along with replacement of other pituitary-dependent hormones, in adults of all ages who have a bona fide growth hormone deficiency as part of a pituitary disorder.[209–219]) A progressive age-dependent decline is seen in circulating IGF-1 levels.[200, 218, 220, 221] Clinical studies in this arena are turning to oral agents that stimulate secretion of endogenous growth hormone.[200, 222–225]

Adrenal Androgens

A very substantial age-dependent decrement in secretion of androgens from the adrenal has been noted.[191] Of these substances, DHEA has been studied the most. Overall, DHEA replacement has been disappointing, except possibly for the enhancement of sexuality in women with adrenal insufficiency.[189] It has been suggested that psychologic benefits (antidepressant, anxiolytic, sense of well-being) may require therapy for 4 months.[189] Short-term androgenic side effects may be disturbing.[191] The long-term adverse effects of adrenal androgens have not been sufficiently evaluated, but their androgenic and estrogenic potential is a serious factor to be considered. Potential toxicity caused by non–Food and Drug Administration–sanctioned manufacturing processes is also a consideration.[191]

ENDOCRINE REGULATION OF SALT AND WATER

Depletion and excess of salt or water, the most common serious metabolic disorders in the elderly, are often dominated by CNS symp-

TABLE 38–8. Decreased Fluid Intake in Elderly Patients

Limited access to fluids
  Physical restraints
  Restricted mobility
  Poor vision
Fluid restriction
  Preprocedure
  Prevention (by family) of incontinence, nocturia, or aspiration
  Therapy for edema or hyponatremia
Altered sensorium
  Medications
  Central nervous system insults
  Febrile illness
  Dementia, delirium, depression, psychosis
Gastrointestinal disorders
  Swallowing disorders
  Bowel obstruction—mechanical, metabolic, ischemic
  Anticholinergic medication
Alteration in thirst mechanism
  Age dependent: diminution in sense of thirst and water intake in
    response to hyperosmolality
  Medication related, e.g., cardiac glycosides
  Focal central nervous system pathology

Modified from Davis KM, Minaker KL: Disorders of fluid balance: Dehydration and hyponatremia. *In* Hazzard WR, Blass JP, Ettinger WH Jr, et al (eds): Principles of Geriatric Medicine and Gerontology, ed 4. New York, McGraw-Hill, 1999, pp 1429–1436.

toms and are frequently associated with serious illnesses and poor outcomes. Age-dependent loosening of homeostatic controls, coupled with the effects of cognitive decline, diseases, diet, and drugs, contributes to the high prevalence and seriousness of these disorders[226–233] (Table 38–8).

Body Composition

Changes in body composition with age predispose the elderly to disturbances in fluid and electrolyte balance.[8] Lean body mass diminishes along with a diminution in total body water, 10% or more, from youth to old age; the intracellular fluid compartment is especially affected. (In planning replacement of fluid deficits, goals need to be scaled down with increasing age.)

Fluid Intake

Thirst is a defense mechanism to prevent dehydration. In normal young individuals, thirst becomes evident when plasma osmolality rises to values greater than 292 mOsm/kg.[234] Healthy older persons aged 65 to 85 years demonstrated a diminished awareness of thirst when exposed to plasma osmolality of up to 296 mOsm/kg achieved by water deprivation or saline infusion[235–242] (see Table 38–8). Healthy elderly also show diminished water intake when presented with water. Why healthy elderly have diminished thirst perception remains unclear; a selectively altered sensitivity of osmoreceptors to thirst may play a role. Cognitive and physical disabilities, especially diminution of mobility, further contribute to the reduced ingestion of fluids. Recovering stroke victims and those with Alzheimer's disease (see later) in particular show a relative insensitivity to drinking in the face of water deprivation. (Planned fluid intake may be essential to prevent dehydration in the elderly.)

Aging of the Kidney

With aging, the kidney diminishes in size with a reduction in the number of glomeruli, renal blood flow, and the glomerular filtration rate[231, 243–245] (Table 38–9). The latter is probably the major factor in the kidney's reduced ability to dilute urine and excrete a water load.[246–248] In the elderly the most dilute urine is almost twice as

TABLE 38–9. The Aging Kidney

Anatomic changes
    Decreased size and volume of the kidney
    Decreased number of functioning glomeruli
    Decreased mass of tubules
    Sclerosis of preglomerular and postglomerular arterioles
Changes in function
    Progressive decrease in the glomerular filtration rate
    Progressive decrease in renal blood flow
    Decrease in maximal concentration of urine
    Reduction in maximal dilution of urine
    Sluggish response to sodium deprivation
    Decreased rate of response to an acid load

Modified from Beck LH: Aging changes in renal function. *In* Hazzard WR, Blass JP, Ettinger WH Jr, et al (eds): Principles of Geriatric Medicine and Gerontology, ed 4. New York, McGraw-Hill, 1999, pp 767–776.

concentrated as in the young. The increased tendency to passive reabsorption of fluid enhances the possibility of water overload.

At the other end of the scale is also a progressive decline in the kidney's ability to concentrate urine with increasing age.[249–251] As in chronic renal failure, the reduced number of functioning nephrons may contribute to an obligatory solute diuresis in the remaining intact nephrons. Water conservation in response to acute dehydration, which occurs promptly in young people, is delayed in the elderly. Renal tubular sensitivity to vasopressin is diminished[252, 253]; the mild persistent elevation in plasma vasopressin in the normal elderly may contribute.

As with water, the aged kidney has a reduced capacity to compensate for sodium losses and sodium deprivation. Overall, age-related changes in the kidney favor sodium wasting, including a heightened tendency to excess sodium loss after a water load or after the institution of salt restriction[254–256] (see Table 38–9).

Vasopressin

Multiple groups have studied basal levels of plasma vasopressin (arginine vasopressin, antidiuretic hormone [ADH]) in the elderly, but disagreement reigns.[257–266] The sleep-associated rise in plasma vasopressin is absent in healthy elderly and may contribute to the nocturnal diuresis that is common among the elderly (see later).[267, 268] Vasopressin metabolism is unchanged, which suggests that changes in plasma concentrations reflect changes in secretory rates. With hypertonic saline infusion and with water deprivation, plasma vasopressin levels are higher in the elderly than in the young at comparable levels of osmolality, thus suggesting that the osmoreceptors linked to vasopressin secretion are more sensitive in the elderly.[234, 257] (Other studies disagree.[260, 261, 269]) On the other hand, vasopressin release in response to an upright posture is diminished, probably as a result of impaired baroreceptor function.[270–272] Ethanol-induced inhibition of vasopressin secretion is markedly diminished among the elderly, possibly because of overriding by the enhanced sensitivity to osmolality.[257] Patients with Alzheimer's disease, when fluid deprived, show an impaired vasopressin response.[273] This defect, coupled with their reduction in thirst, heightens the risk of dehydration in these patients.

Atrial Natriuretic Hormone

Atrial natriuretic hormone (ANH), a product of the heart, acts on the kidney to promote sodium excretion and diuresis (and on blood vessels to enhance vasodilatation and diminish blood pressure).[261, 274] It also inhibits the renin-angiotensin-aldosterone system.[275–277] In the elderly, ANH levels are elevated in the basal state and after stimuli of secretion; the kidney's sensitivity to ANH is heightened and aldosterone production is suppressed.[278–282]

Renin-Angiotensin-Aldosterone

Aldosterone levels in healthy elderly are reduced in both the supine and upright positions because of a decline in the conversion of inactive to active renin and the suppressive effect of ANH.[283] The elevated ANH, reduced aldosterone, and age-related changes in the kidney all contribute to sodium wasting.

Hyporeninemic Hypoaldosteronism

Hyporeninemic hypoaldosteronism, the most frequent form of isolated hypoaldosteronism, is common in the elderly. Risk factors include renal disease, angiotensin-converting enzyme inhibitors, and hyperglycemia associated with diabetes mellitus.[284, 285] The hyperkalemia is aggravated by potassium-sparing drugs. It is ameliorated by diuretics or mineralocorticoid replacement, one sodium losing and the other sodium retaining, respectively.

Hyponatremia

Untreated or poorly treated hypothyroidism, hypoadrenalism, and diabetes mellitus may traditionally be associated with hyponatremia. Hyponatremia (<136 mEq/L) typically represents water excess relative to sodium, or dilutional hyponatremia. Total extracellular volume may be elevated (e.g., congestive heart failure), normal (e.g., inappropriate ADH), or diminished (e.g., diuretics or gastrointestinal losses). Hyponatremia is common among healthy elderly, with an even higher prevalence among geriatric outpatients, hospitalized elderly, and residents of long-term care facilities.[227, 228, 286–292] Contributors to hyponatremia include hypotonic fluid intake, low sodium diet, low sodium tube feeding, renal sodium loss, and inappropriate ADH secretion.[227, 228, 286–292]

The syndrome of inappropriate ADH (SIADH) is common in the elderly, particularly those with CNS disorders, malignancies, inflammatory lung diseases, and certain drugs (especially antipsychotics, angiotensin-converting enzyme inhibitors, and diuretics).[293, 294] In addition, a high prevalence of idiopathic SIADH is seen in the elderly.[293–297] Sodium depletion may dominate over water retention in patients treated excessively with diuretics or those maintained on tube feeding for a long time. Primary polydipsia (>10 L/day) is most commonly observed in psychiatric patients with drug-induced dry mouth. In younger patients it rarely causes hyponatremia because of the kidney's capacity to excrete free water, but in elderly patients this rare syndrome can cause hyponatremia as a result of the kidney's reduced capacity for free water excretion.[298]

Mild hyponatremia is usually asymptomatic and may be treated simply by restricting free water intake.[299] When associated with SIADH, fluid restriction often needs to be strict (800–1000 mL/day) to be effective. (When the hyponatremia of SIADH presents serious problems, demeclocycline or lithium, which counters the effects of vasopressin, may be useful adjuncts.[293]) Symptoms of hyponatremia (lethargy, somnolence, coma, seizures) occur with severe (<120 mEq/L) or rapidly progressing reductions in serum sodium.[293, 298] Treatment of symptomatic hyponatremia should be immediate but controlled, with an intermediate goal of serum sodium of 125 mEq/L.[300] At that level, treatment should be slowed to avoid risk of CNS damage, including central pontine myelinolysis. With a normal or expanded extracellular fluid volume, normal saline combined with a loop diuretic such as furosemide is effective and safer than saline alone; furosemide will produce an increased volume of dilute urine.[301] Because symptomatic hyponatremia and overzealous therapy (too fast or too much) can cause CNS damage, therapy needs to be very prompt but controlled.[292, 293, 298–302] Neurologic symptoms of hyponatremia may not resolve for several days after full correction of the salt and water abnormalities.[300, 302]

Hypernatremia and Dehydration

The combination of hypernatremia and dehydration (Na$^+$ >148 mEq/L) occurred in 1% of 16,000 hospitalized patients older than 60, half on admission and half within 1 week[229, 293, 298, 303] (Table 38–10). Mortality in these patients was very high.[303, 304] Excess fluid loss and insufficient fluid replacement are greater in the elderly than the young. The consequences are magnified by the age-related decrease in baseline fluid volume.

TABLE 38–10. Factors Associed with Hypernatremia in Elderly Patients

Factors	Patients (%)
Febrile illness	70
Infirmity	40
Surgery	21
Nutritional supplementation	20
Intravenous solutes	18
Diabetes mellitus	15
Diarrhea	11
Gastrointestional bleeding	9
Diuretics	9
Diabetes insipidus	7

Modified from Davis KM, Minaker KL: Disorders of fluid balance: Dehydration and hypernatremia. *In* Hazzard WR, Blass JP, Ettinger WH Jr, et al (eds): Principles of Geriatric Medicine and Gerontology, ed 4. New York, McGraw-Hill, 1999, pp 1429–1436; based on Snyder NA, Feigal DW, Arieff AI: Hypernatremia in elderly patients: A heterogeneous, morbid, and iatrogenic entity. Ann Intern Med 107:309–319, 1987.

Endocrine-related causes of excess fluid loss include diabetes mellitus, hypercalcemia, drug-induced nephrogenic diabetes insipidus, vasopressin deficiency or suppression, and aldosterone deficiency (Addison's disease or decreased renin).[293, 298] Rehydration planning for the elderly should favor oral replacement. Subcutaneous fluid may also be very useful.[298] Total deficit calculations and replacement plans need to consider the reduced fluid compartments in the elderly, the limited capability of the aged kidney to handle an overload, and the slowness of homeostatic responses in the elderly. Cerebral edema is one of the more dramatic and tragic endpoints of overzealous therapy.[229] Hypernatremia in the setting of normal volume status or fluid overload is uncommon.[305–307] Treatment of these patients consists of restriction of sodium and fluid intake.

Deaths during heat waves occur largely in elderly people and are caused by excessive loss of salt and water combined with impaired homeostatic mechanisms, both physiologic and psychosocial.[304] It is wise to educate the elderly and their families to anticipate the problem, including precise suggestions on fluid replacement.

Alzheimer's Disease

Patients with Alzheimer's disease often have progressive diminution in the thirst perception and water-seeking behavior. Some, but not all investigators have also found inappropriate reductions in vasopressin secretion and vasopressin action, which result in a greatly increased risk of dehydration and hypernatremia.[308–311] They also may have a reversal of the normal day/night urine flow with nocturnal polyuria (see below).[166]

Nocturnal Diabetes Insipidus in the Elderly

In younger people, daytime urine volume is significantly greater than that produced at night, in part due to a burst of vasopressin secretion near bedtime.[166, 268] In some normal elderly and especially patients with Alzheimer's disease, nighttime urine flow exceeds daytime flow, possibly related to the loss of nocturnal vasopressin secretion.[268] The polyuria associated with this nocturnal vasopressin deficiency–like syndrome can be manifested as disturbed sleep patterns and urinary incontinence.[168, 312] While recognizing that the differential diagnosis of disordered sleep, nocturia, and incontinence is complex, it is worth noting that in some patients the administration of 0.1 mg desmopressin orally at bedtime has been reported to produce substantial improvement in sleep, nocturnal polyuria, and incontinence, with considerable lightening of the caregiver's burden and without change in 24-hour urine volume or body weight.[313–315] Although no serious side effects were noted at this dose in these studies, water intoxication can occur with the use of desmopressin.[313–317]

DIABETES MELLITUS

The aim of this section is to highlight problems specific to elderly persons with diabetes.[318–322] Even diabetologists and geriatricians harbor ambivalence and uncertainty when managing elderly patients with diabetes because studies in the elderly are sparse.[323] Recommended therapy consists of a fusion of data from younger patients (65 or younger) with general approaches for management of the elderly. The art of medicine stands side by side with the science.

Half of all people with diabetes are older than 65 years. In this group the disease has probably been diagnosed in only half.[324–326] The number of elderly with diabetes will increase rapidly over the next several decades inasmuch as the incidence of diabetes increases as a function of age and the proportion of elderly in the population is increasing, patients with early-onset diabetes are living longer, and the extraordinary epidemic of obesity in the United States and worldwide is driving up the incidence of diabetes.[327–329] The frequent comorbid conditions along with their medications have an impact on diabetes in the elderly, as do the biologic changes we associate with aging, including progressive diminution in physical activity and loss of lean body mass.[330] A substantial fraction of those older than 65 with diabetes are overweight and would benefit from weight reduction.[328, 331, 332] Fat cells themselves may have important effects on the metabolic alterations in obesity; fat cells are a source of internal secretions, including free fatty acids, tumor necrosis factor-α, leptin, and plasminogen activator inhibitor type 1, that influence insulin resistance, insulin secretion, glucose metabolism, and atherosclerotic risk.[333–335]

In the elderly, diabetes is associated with accelerated functional decline, more chronic disease, more outpatient and inpatient medical care, self-perception of ill health, diminished quality of life, and a doubling of the death rate.[336–338] Cognition and mood may be negatively affected, both of which may be improved by glycemic control.[339–342] Vascular dementia is increased, as is Alzheimer's disease.[342–345] Does this increase reflect the accelerated biologic clock associated with diabetes? Can these global consequences be affected by prudently aggressive therapy?[346–349]* The prudently aggressive approach to diabetes that is favored here and based on the improved outcome demonstrated for microvascular complications may at the same time provide an answer to these other unresolved questions.

Diagnosis

The recognition that hyperglycemia per se causes many of the pathologic alterations in diabetes has led to the repeal of age-dependent standards.[346–349]

The fasting blood glucose level has returned to primacy in the diagnosis and also appears to be predictive of diabetes in older people.[349, 350] The official recommendation of the American Diabetes Association is that fasting blood sugar be screened every 3 years in high-risk individuals. Most elderly are in the high-risk group. Being 65 or older by itself garners 9 points; a first-degree relative with diabetes or modestly overweight is enough to reach the 10 points needed to qualify for the label of *high risk*.[349] (Extrapolations of current data and scientific policy lead us to predict that in the future, officially sanctioned standards for blood glucose levels that trigger therapeutic intervention will continue to go lower.)

Autoimmunity

Traditionally, hyperglycemia that begins late in life has been assumed to be type 2 diabetes, where insulin resistance dominates and insulin deficiency is subordinate. Increasing evidence indicates that the risk of autoimmunity directed at pancreatic β cells is lifelong.[325, 351] In contrast to young people with autoimmunity, who often have dramatic deterioration in glucose metabolism, in the elderly autoimmunity may result in an indolent course that mimics type 2 diabetes in

---

*Also see the list of references to Technical Reviews and Consensus Statements,[349] pp. 113–116.)

its early stages; over time, the insulin deficiency progresses to insulin dependence within several years after onset of the hyperglycemia.[351] Identification of individual patients in this subgroup of older patients may become important in the future when immune-directed therapy for autoimmune diabetes becomes practical; now, its importance is only conceptual and serves to alert physicians to the existence of this subgroup, who have an elevated prevalence of insulin dependence.

Onset

In the elderly, both those with typical type 2 and those with autoimmune diabetes, the onset of hyperglycemia tends to be insidious, often asymptomatic or characterized by nonspecific symptoms.[352] Polyuria, polydipsia, and polyphagia are less common, in part because of the heightened threshold for glycosuria. In elderly patients the onset of incontinence (from polyuria), infection, gangrene, delirium, coma, or a neuropathy or vascular event may be the heralding event. In occasional patients the onset of hyperglycemia may be dramatic, often associated with a major disorder that exaggerates the hyperglycemia, such as stroke, myocardial infarction, or systemic infection. Among older patients, hyperglycemia may be present for some time before coming to medical attention ("hyperglycemia unawareness").[324, 353] The time from recognition of the hyperglycemia medically to onset of the macrovascular (and microvascular) complications of diabetes can be substantially shorter in the elderly than in the typical young patient with type 1 diabetes, possibly because the clock had started so much before medical recognition of the hyperglycemia.[324, 353, 354] As the age of patients with diabetes increases, macrovascular complications will progressively dominate the overall outcome relative to microvascular complications.[354–356]

Other Consequences of Hyperglycemia

In addition to the traditional microvascular and macrovascular complications, other pathophysiologic consequences of hyperglycemia, especially in the elderly, may also be significant, including abnormalities in platelet adhesiveness, vascular reactivity, cellular signaling, osmotic stress, cellular differentiation, and defense against infections.[357–360]

Infections

Hyperglycemia and aging are each associated with reduced defenses, more severe infections, and reduced warning signs and symptoms.[361] Infection control is one more motivating force for prudently aggressive control of hyperglycemia in the elderly, both for prevention and for treatment of infections. Among infections linked to diabetes in the elderly are osteomyelitis, infectious monarticular arthritis, infections of prosthetic joints, and reactivation of tuberculosis, as well as malignant otitis externa with *Pseudomonas aeruginosa* and necrotizing fasciitis.[361, 362]

With regard to lung infections, certain organisms (*Staphylococcus aureus*, gram negatives, and *Mycobacterium tuberculosis*) are more common in patients with diabetes. Diabetes heightens the mortality and morbidity associated with *Streptococcus pneumoniae* and influenza virus; immunizations against both should be current. (Responses to vaccines in diabetic patients are similar to those in euglycemic peers.[361])

With regard to the urinary tract, bacteriuria, upper tract infections, bilateral infections, urinary tract emphysema, fungal infections (especially *Candida*), perinephric abscesses, and papillary necrosis are more common in patients with diabetes. Subtlety of manifestation may delay recognition.[361]

Foot infection with associated cellulitis, osteomyelitis, and amputation, an ever-present sword of Damocles in all patients with diabetes, is an especially serious threat in the elderly. Preventive measures should be emphasized, particularly in the elderly. Infections need an aggressive coordinated team approach.[363]

Necrotizing fasciitis, typically caused by *S. aureus* or of polymicrobial origin, may occur innocently with pain and local signs before gas accumulation and systemic toxicity are recognized. A high level of suspicion, emergency evaluation, and prompt treatment with multiple antibiotics and surgical debridement are necessary to reduce the high mortality rate.[361]

Emphysematous cholecystitis, a virulent infection with gas accumulation, is associated with a high prevalence of gangrene, perforation, and death. Prompt recognition, antibiotics, and surgery are essential.[361]

Invasive (so-called malignant) otitis externa caused by *Pseudomonas* may lead to bone and intracranial involvement; the lack of fever and similarity to typical otitis externa often result in delay in diagnosis. Early involvement of an otolaryngologist is essential. Rhinocerebral mucormycosis is another unusual infection with a large predominance of victims with diabetes.[361]

Hyperosmolar Coma and Other Diabetes-Related Syndromes in the Elderly

Other conditions that are sometimes linked to the elderly with diabetes are accidental hypothermia, taste dysfunction, constipation, intradermal bullae, periarthrosis of the shoulder, diabetic amyotrophy, and diabetic neuropathic cachexia, where a painful neuropathy and severe depression dominate.[364–369]

Hyperosmolar coma is characterized by severe dehydration with volume depletion and severe hyperglycemia. ("Coma" is a traditional part of the name but is not a necessary component for the diagnosis.) It occurs largely in the elderly with a severe illness, such as pneumonia, and results from the highly accelerated outpouring of glucose from the liver that is typical of insulin-deficient diabetes, superimposed upon age-related defects in salt and water metabolism.[320, 370–372] The glycosuria is inadequate to prevent the glucose from rising to extremely high levels. For multiple reasons, fluid intake is insufficient to prevent severe hyperosmolality. Insulin levels are insufficient to prevent hyperglycemia but sufficient to prevent ketoacidosis. "Nonketotic" coma is another name for this syndrome; despite its name, ketonuria from prolonged fasting may sometimes be present, but ketonemia is absent, which clinically distinguishes it from ketoacidosis.[373] Both ketoacidosis and lactic acidosis, two key alternatives in the differential diagnosis, are typically associated with tachypnea and hyperpnea, whereas hyperosmolar coma is not. Often the hyperglycemia/hyperosmolarity syndrome camouflages the acute precipitating illness or vice versa.

Early rapid *partial* replacement of the fluid loss is urgent, with normal saline initially, followed later by hypotonic saline. Glucose levels will drop with fluids alone. Modest doses of intravenous insulin (10 U initially, followed by 5 U/hour) should commence at the same time or after fluid therapy has begun, along with vigilant monitoring of blood glucose.[370–372] A search for infection and other treatable conditions must also be undertaken early. It is not possible to predict the glycemic level that will prevail after recovery. Glucose metabolism may be remarkably restored. Interestingly, when survivors of hyperosmolar coma were deprived of water, they were less thirsty, drank less, and became more hyperosmolar than other patients with type 2 diabetes or normal controls. The authors suggest that their subnormal thirst and drive to ingest fluids may have predisposed them to this unusual condition.[374]

Philosophy Behind Prudent Aggressiveness in Therapy

The Diabetes Control and Complications Trial (DCCT) (in type 1 diabetes) and the U.K. Prospective Diabetes Study Group (UKPDS) (in type 2 diabetes), along with other pioneering but smaller studies, have forged a consensus in the field that the level of plasma glucose is a major determinant of all microvascular outcomes.[346–349] These studies showed that aggressive management improved glycemia but that euglycemia was elusive in most patients because the incidence and severity of hypoglycemia increased as the blood glucose was pushed to euglycemic levels. Although absolute euglycemia is rarely achieved, all decrements in glucose toward normal were beneficial, which should encourage patients and caregivers. In the elderly, the

TABLE 38–11. Factors to Consider in Setting Diabetes Treatment Goals for Elderly Patients

Estimate of patient's life expectancy
Patient's preferences and commitment
Primary care provider beliefs: effect of glycemia on sequelae
Risk factors for hypoglycemia
Availability of support services
Coexisting serious health problems
   Psychiatric
   Cognitive
   Complications of diabetes
   Major limitations of function
Complexity of the medical regimen
Economic issues

Adapted from Halter JB: Diabetes mellitus. *In* Hazzard WR, Blass JP, Ettinger WH Jr, et al (eds): Principles of Geriatric Medicine and Gerontology, ed 4. New York, McGraw-Hill, 1999, pp 991–1012.

benefit-vs.-risk equation is pushed to higher glucose levels: the elderly have fewer years to gain and hypoglycemia may be more damaging (Table 38–11). Although the target level for control (glucose and hemoglobin A_{1c}) must be raised, the zeal for control must be sustained. Today's patients will be living and functioning longer than previous generations; we must treat them for the long term. A prudent, straightforward philosophy to adopt at this time is that in our hearts we set the goal of achieving euglycemia and in our heads we recognize that maintaining euglycemia in most patients is impossible and we must make concessions to the dangers of hypoglycemia. An aggressive but prudent approach is helped by the current generation of elderly patients who are increasingly more willing to actively participate in the management of their illness.

It had been typical for many physicians to target treatment in elderly patients so that the patient is maintained "asymptomatic," that is, free of gross glycosuria. (For the same degree of glycosuria the elderly are likely to have more hyperglycemia because of the elevated renal threshold.) Data indicating that in young and middle-aged patients any improvement in blood glucose can be expected to reduce the incidence of microvascular (and possibly also macrovascular) complications has probably made this standard of therapy obsolete for most patients, including the elderly.[345–349]

Treatment

The approach here is focused on treatment of the hyperglycemia[375, 376] (Table 38–11). These patients often have hypertension and dyslipidemia as well.[377–379] Practitioners are urged to give equal attention to control of hypertension (see later).[377] Most elements of the dyslipidemia will initially respond to improvement in the hyperglycemia. When the glycemia reaches its new plateau is an appropriate time to begin specific therapy for the lipid disorders.[378] Evidence is growing about the benefits of improving the lipid profile in elderly patients with diabetes.[379] Unfortunately, adequate control of glucose, blood pressure, and plasma lipids may require a total of six to eight medications, which is both costly and risky because of drug side effects and interactions. In our opinion, in the elderly with diabetes, considerations of blood pressure should take precedence over considerations of glucose, which should dominate over considerations of lipids.

The standard recommendations apply regarding diet (hypocaloric for weight loss or eucaloric balanced) and exercise (aerobic and muscle strengthening).[332, 349] A benefit of even modest exercise is heightened sensitivity to endogenous insulin, independent of weight loss. Customized approaches are especially advisable in the elderly.[320, 380, 381] In particular, many older patients are underweight, so rotely prescribed restrictive diets can be counterproductive. Of special importance is incorporation of a bedtime snack for every elderly patient who is taking antihyperglycemic medications to reduce the likelihood of hypoglycemia during the night. Postprandial hypotension (20 mm Hg systolic or more) without a compensatory increase in heart rate within an hour or so of a meal is surprisingly common among the elderly.[382–384]

Symptoms of hypotension, which can include syncope, transient ischemic attack, angina, weakness, or dulled sensorium, need to be distinguished from symptoms of hypoglycemia. Suggestions for management of this common form of hypotension include frequent small meals, favoring complex over simple carbohydrates, avoidance of alcohol, avoidance of hypovolemia, addition of caffeine at mealtime, and moderate postprandial walking.[382–385]

When diet and exercise fall short, drugs should be introduced.[386–388] No drug regimen is ideal. Single agents are often effective initially. Later, better control can be achieved with a combination of agents. The UKPDS showed that over time, most patients have progressive deterioration in glucose metabolism and control, so more effort needs to be exerted to achieve a reduced return on the investment.[389] Early awareness of the natural history by patients and caregivers will prevent discouragement later in the course of the illness.

Hypoglycemia

Hypoglycemia, the major barrier to excellent control of diabetes at all ages, is an especially formidable barrier in the elderly[390–399] (Table 38–12). For example, euglycemic elderly men (aged 60–70) subjected to insulin-induced hypoglycemia were more prone to severe cognitive impairment and much less likely to recognize warning signs than were their young (aged 22–26) counterparts, although counterregulatory hormone responses were indistinguishable in these studies.[392] Insulin or oral agents are associated with a potential for serious, even fatal hypoglycemia.[392, 396, 397] (Studies in type 1 diabetes has shown that the targets are not fixed. The ambient glucose levels that trigger counterregulatory events and cerebral dysfunction are reset to correspond to glucose levels in blood in the most recent hours or days—up with hyperglycemia and down with hypoglycemia.)

Multiple factors make the elderly more susceptible to hypoglycemia (Table 38–12). In the elderly, glycemic sensitivity to epinephrine is reduced.[395] In response to hypoglycemia, glucose production and endogenous glucagon release, the major hormonal defense against hypoglycemia, are significantly reduced.[391, 395, 398] Epinephrine release, which is spared in aging, may be diminished by recent bouts of hypoglycemia, by diabetic neuropathy, or by β-blockers. (β-Blockers are not absolutely contraindicated, but added caution is needed.) Recognition of hypoglycemia and corrective action to counter it are reduced in the elderly. Inadequate education, irregularity of food intake, drugs for other conditions, diminution in cognition (basal, hypoglycemia-induced, effects of other drugs), and decrements in the hepatic and especially renal clearance of drugs are other potential contributors.[388, 392, 399]

Other Considerations of Treatment

Undiagnosed depression, often subtle in the elderly, may need to be managed at the same time.[320, 337, 339] The cost and complexity of the regimen need to be considered more carefully than with younger patients. The psychologic (and other) barriers among physicians, other caregivers, and patients to the introduction of insulin therapy for the elderly should be confronted early.[400] ("Insulin resistance" is the term facetiously applied to this phenomenon.) Except for metformin, the hypoglycemic drugs, when effective, typically produce a modest gain in weight that is especially pronounced with insulin.[401] The patient and

TABLE 38–12. Risk Factors for Hypoglycemia in Older Patients with Diabetes

Diminished glucagon response (age related)
Impaired autonomic nervous system function
Cognitive disorder
Nutrition: poor or irregular
Polypharmacy: alcohol or other sedative
Kidney or liver failure

Adapted from Halter JB: Diabetes mellitus. *In* Hazzard WR, Blass JP, Ettinger WH Jr, et al (eds): Principles of Geriatric Medicine and Gerontology, ed 4. New York, McGraw-Hill, 1999, pp 991–1012.

the family should be forewarned and exonerated. Only in exceptional cases is the weight gain so great that a change in therapy is required. Fears of adverse effects of insulin or sulfonylureas on cardiovascular disease have dissipated.[347–349, 402, 403] Treatment of advanced renal disease in the elderly is now much more similar in patients with and without diabetes.[349]

Selection of Medications

SULFONYLUREAS. When nonpharmacologic measures are inadequate, the sulfonylureas and other nonsulfonylureas that act on the same receptor in the pancreatic β cell are effective as initial pharmacologic therapy.[386, 387, 389] Short-acting sulfonylureas are preferred in the elderly; severe hypoglycemia, sometimes quite delayed, is a well-recognized side effect, especially with longer-acting agents such as chlorpropamide and glyburide.[404, 405] SIADH has been recognized with some of the sulfonylureas (e.g., chlorpropamide, glyburide, and tolbutamide).[406, 407] It appears likely that drugs designed to be taken with each meal will give therapeutic results that are adequate with less propensity to severe hypoglycemia than noted with the once-daily drugs. Because these drugs are metabolized in the liver and excreted in urine, they should be used carefully when diminution in liver or kidney function is a factor; short-acting drugs at reduced levels would seem wise.[386–388]

BIGUANIDES. Metformin, widely used in Europe for decades, is an effective agent alone and in combination with other agents in the elderly.[408–412] In addition to lowering glucose effectively, it does not cause hypoglycemia or weight gain, which are common with other agents. It also reduces lipid abnormalities and attenuates the weight gain that accompanies insulin therapy.[411] Although lactic acidosis is much less of a threat with metformin than with other biguanides, the drug should be avoided or withdrawn in conditions that may favor lactic acidosis, such as acute intercurrent illnesses, administration of contrast media, or reduced cardiac, hepatic, or renal function (creatinine >1.5 mg/dL).[413–415] The reduced appetite or anorexia, which contributes to the stable weight, may be a problem in frail or undernourished elderly patients.

ACARBOSE. The α-glucosidase inhibitor acarbose, by preventing full digestion of carbohydrates, reduces postprandial glycemia with negligible effect on fasting levels.[416] Evidence is mounting that postprandial (rather than fasting) glycemia may correlate best with hyperglycemia-induced pathology.[417–419] Another advantage is that it does not cause hypoglycemia. The major side effects are intestinal: flatulence, cramps, and diarrhea, which may subside with continuation of the drug. Although these effects may be less bothersome in many elderly (than in younger patients), this therapy might be unsuitable for some elderly patients. Because the drug blocks the breakdown of disaccharides, oral sucrose is ineffective in combating the hypoglycemia that is induced by concomitant use of insulin or sulfonylurea; the patient needs to be prepared to use glucose or fructose.

THIAZOLIDINEDIONES. These drugs, which may take days to weeks to act initially, lower blood glucose effectively and improve lipid profiles in the elderly when used as monotherapy or in combination with insulin, metformin, or a sulfonylurea-like drug.[420, 421] Alone, thiazolidinediones do not cause hypoglycemia, but because they act to heighten cellular sensitivity to insulin, they can trigger hypoglycemia by insulin or sulfonylurea. Weight gain with therapy is common and is only partly due to fluid retention. Troglitazone, the first to market, has now been withdrawn from the market due to serious liver toxicity.[422–425] The two new (1999) members of this class, rosiglitazone and pioglitazone, appear to be quite a bit less likely to be associated with this complication, but patients need to be observed for it.[426–432] At this time all drugs of this class should be avoided by patients with abnormal liver function test results, and patients taking these drugs should be screened often for liver abnormalities during the first 1 to 2 years.

INSULIN. Insulin is the oldest and best studied drug for diabetes. It can reduce the blood glucose level when other drugs fail and is the obvious choice for emergencies such as hyperosmolar coma or ketoacidosis.[318, 370, 371, 373, 433] Hypoglycemia and weight gain are the chief side effects. Insulin can be used in elderly patients, but rituals and routines need to be established to minimize errors. Premixed preparations are now available and are especially useful in elderly patients.[434] New preparations of insulin that do not dimerize (e.g., lispro insulin) may provide more reproducible patterns of absorption of insulin from subcutaneous sites, along with better glycemic regulation.[435] For many, a bedtime dose of insulin in conjunction with oral medications at other times will be suitable.[412] Later, the patient may require two or, occasionally, more insulin injections per day. Even when insulin is the dominant therapy, some patients gain by the addition of an oral agent.

Therapy for most patients undergoes progression.[389] In most elderly patients, especially the frail, the geriatric dictum start low and go slow is especially relevant when treating hyperglycemia. Most start with diet and exercise. As needed, sulfonylurea therapy is started. Later, many physicians add metformin.[408] After that, one of the two oral agents should be replaced with a thiazolidinedione, or a glucosidase inhibitor should be added.[386] If necessary, 10 U of NPH should be added at bedtime in place of the evening dose of oral antidiabetic medication. At the next stage, if needed, twice-daily insulin can replace all the other drugs. Premixed combinations of insulins with short and medium durations of action may be preferred.[435] If after careful adjustment of the twice-daily doses of insulin hyperglycemia is not adequately regulated, the addition of metformin may be helpful. If a thiazolidinedione is added, the insulin dose should be initially reduced to prevent hypoglycemia.

Notes on Monitoring of Therapy

Self-monitoring can be used in older as in younger patients.[436] Although fasting glucose is becoming a favorite for diagnosis, growing evidence suggests that postprandial levels of glucose may be stronger influences on hemoglobin A_{1c} and therefore a better target to track for treatment.[417–419] The hemoglobin A_{1c} level in some elderly subjects may not reflect glucose levels as well as in younger subjects, which suggests to some that serum fructosamine may be a more reliable and preferred method.[437, 438]

Treatment of Hypertension

As with hyperglycemia, the UKPDS study of middle-aged patients with diabetes showed that aggressive control of hypertension with medication markedly improves outcomes but ideal control is impossible to achieve because of the increase in adverse events as normal levels of blood pressure are approached.[377, 439, 440] Based on these and other data, a prudently aggressive program of blood pressure control is warranted while keeping in mind that in the elderly, safeguards against hypotension are reduced and the consequences (e.g., falls, ischemia) are more threatening.

Thus the elderly may be an ideal group for the use of mainstream nondrug therapies for hypertension, such as exercise, diet, and weight loss alone and in combination with medications.

THYROID FUNCTION

A discussion of thyroid disorders in the elderly, of value in itself, also provides a general approach to the problem of endocrine disorders in this population. Abnormalities of the thyroid are common in individuals older than 60 years, with an increase in both prevalence and incidence.[441–443] About 5% of the population older than 60 takes thyroxine (T_4), the large majority for appropriate reasons.[444]

All thyroid disorders in the elderly are represented in younger age groups, but the emphasis shifts. Subclinical hypothyroidism, postablative hypothyroidism, nonthyroidal diseases that affect thyroid function tests, drug-induced thyroid dysfunction, and the hyperthyroidism of multinodular goiter are more common in the elderly than in a younger cohort.[445] Clinical signs and symptoms are often more muted relative to the severity of the dysfunction, and interpretation of function tests may be more uncertain because the standard ranges are derived from younger and healthier patients.[445–448] Autoimmunity typically increases with increasing age. Likewise, the elderly have more tumors both benign and malignant, some of which are hyperfunctioning. Both the fraction of tumors that are malignant and the aggressiveness of the malignant tumors increase with age.[445, 447, 448]

Changes with Aging

Many changes have been documented in the hypothalamus, pituitary, and thyroid with aging, especially in rats. Comments here are restricted to changes that are most clinically relevant. The thyroid gland itself changes little in size, possibly shrinking somewhat in synchrony with changes in lean body mass.[449, 450] A normal gland may be more difficult to palpate. Tumors detected by palpation, scans, function tests, and autopsy examination are more common.

With aging, the half-life of T_4 is substantially prolonged (offset in the euthyroid by a reduction in endogenous T_4 production).[451] In patients who have been receiving long-standing suppression or replacement therapy, especially those totally dependent on exogenous hormone, doses of hormone that were appropriate years ago may need to be reduced.[452] Similarly, when hormone replacement is initiated in the elderly, starting doses are typically low (12.5–25 μg of thyroxine) when compared with those in younger adults, and the optimal dose is best achieved by small step increases every 4 to 8 weeks monitored by both clinical criteria and laboratory tests, especially thyroid-stimulating hormone (TSH) and T_4. Treatment with liothyronine (triiodothyronine [T_3]) is hardly ever indicated in the elderly. Rare exceptions (see later) include some patients with amiodarone-induced hypothyroidism (to circumvent this drug's inhibition of T_4 deiodination) and most patients with myxedema coma (where a very rapid response is highly desired).

Radioactive iodine uptake by the thyroid is unchanged or diminished. Iodide clearance by the thyroid and by the kidney is diminished. The most serious implication is in patients who are to receive very large doses of radioactive iodine for the treatment of thyroid cancer; dosimetry calculations must be very accurate.[453, 454]

The normal circulating levels of T_4 and thyroxine-binding globulin are unchanged, whereas circulating T_3 may be slightly diminished because of reduced production without a change in clearance.[445, 455] TSH levels remain within the normal range for younger adults but may fall somewhat in centenarian males and possibly in elderly females.[445, 456–458] An increase is seen in the fraction of asymptomatic elderly who have TSH values that exceed or fall short of the normal range. In one study, TSH measurements above or below the normal range were found in 20% of women and 10% of men.[459] It is uncertain what fraction of these patients represent an age effect on the values of the normal range or early stages of ("subclinical") hypothyroidism and hyperthyroidism, respectively.

Routine Testing

Because of the high prevalence of thyroid disorders and their subtlety in the elderly, routine testing or having a very low threshold for testing is warranted.[460–463] The best single test for the measurement of thyroid function in the elderly is a serum TSH done well in a sensitive assay; a free T_4 level is a good alternative.[445] For reasons of cost, plasma T_4 is an acceptable substitute for routine purposes.[445] Measurement of antithyroid antibodies, although predictive of hypothyroidism, is probably not cost-effective as a routine test.

Extrathyroidal Influences and the Euthyroid Sick Syndrome

Extrathyroidal influences on the thyroid and on thyroid function tests are more common among the elderly. Interpretation of thyroid function tests, especially T_3 levels, may be complicated by effects of acute or chronic alterations in diet, especially carbohydrates.[464–468] Drugs, more widely used in the elderly, can alter thyroid test results in euthyroid patients (e.g., sex steroids and glucocorticoids) or affect thyroid function (e.g., lithium and amiodarone).[469–477] Amiodarone has

a multiplicity of sites of interaction, including effects on hormone synthesis, hormone metabolism, and interaction with target cells for hormone action.[478–482] It can precipitate both hypothyroidism (especially in those with thyroid autoimmune disease) and hyperthyroidism (especially in those with multinodularity).[479, 481, 483]

Among disorders in this group, the most vexing conceptually is the *euthyroid sick syndrome* (now also known as the *nonthyroidal illness syndrome*).[445, 473, 474, 484, 485] Because of its tight link with serious illness, it is associated with a high mortality rate and is widespread among the elderly.[445, 484–486] In its mild form, serum T_3 (and free T_3) are reduced whereas serum T_4 and TSH are normal. (The free T_4 in this syndrome is in dispute because of vagaries in methodology.[486]) With more advanced disease, serum T_4 is reduced, as is TSH. The low T_4 levels (e.g., <4 μg/dL) in this syndrome are associated with very high mortality rates, which is not surprising because these patients are severely ill from other causes. The reigning consensus is that this condition represents a normal adaptive response to illness, that the patients are euthyroid, and that no therapy for the thyroid is indicated.[445, 484, 485] A novel speculative interpretation is that in its mild form, conversion of T_4 to T_3 is inhibited. At this stage the response may be adaptive, but more severe illness results in central hypothyroidism (probably hypothalamic in origin) with a reduction in thyrotropin-releasing hormone (possibly mediated by cytokines); this leads to a reduction in TSH, a reduction in T_4, and a reduction in T_3, which results in a hypothyroid state that is detrimental to the individual.[486] This hypothetic interpretation leads to the suggestion of an imaginative research protocol wherein patients with severe forms (T_4 <4 μg/dL) would be treated with low doses of T_3 and T_4 to restore hormone levels to the lower reaches of the normal range.[486, 487] This conceptualization is attractive, although far from ready for the clinic, and reminds us of some of the cytokine-mediated syndromes in which low levels of activation appear to be adaptive whereas higher levels are deleterious. Many challenges to this approach are being raised.[488–490]

Hypothyroidism

In overt hypothyroidism, free T_4 levels are reduced and serum TSH levels are elevated. In subclinical hypothyroidism, TSH levels are elevated but the free T_4 concentration is within the normal range. Elderly patients have an increased prevalence of both forms of hypothyroidism (and of pathologic levels of antithyroid antibodies).[441–443, 445–448] The vast majority have primary hypothyroidism with chronic autoimmune thyroiditis as the major cause, augmented by a series of iatrogenic etiologies, including prior therapy for hyperthyroidism, radiation to the head and neck, thyroid surgery, and drugs (see earlier). Patients with normal TSH levels but high levels of thyroid antibodies have a higher than expected likelihood of an elevated TSH level developing over the ensuing years.[441, 445, 491, 492]

The clinical features of hypothyroidism in the elderly are thought to be less obvious than in younger patients.[462, 445, 492] A systematic study tested this traditional view.[463] In the elderly they found fewer signs or symptoms and a diminished frequency of classic signs, especially less weight gain, cold intolerance, paresthesias, and muscle cramps. One interpretation is that the typical constellation of relatively nonspecific findings may be more difficult to recognize because of the insidious onset and because the elderly have a higher background of other illnesses, medications, and cognitive changes.[445]

In the elderly, psychiatric symptoms may dominate.[493–495] Textbooks of geropsychiatry list hypothyroidism as a cause of depression, delirium, and dementia. However, the overall prevalence of hypothyroidism in each of these diagnostic categories is small, and cure of these conditions with thyroid hormone replacement is far from uniform.[495, 496] In practice, every patient with these three conditions should be tested for hypothyroidism (and hyperthyroidism) while recognizing that the yield will be low diagnostically and the response to therapy, although positive, will be far less than 100%. "Myxedema madness" is the quaint term applied when agitation dominates the delirium, dementia, or other psychosis in a patient with hypothyroidism. To qualify for this diagnostic category, substantial reversibility with hormone replacement is implied.[497–499]

In general, when the causative agent of delirium is removed, the delirium may resolve dramatically, as with drug withdrawal. However, it is being increasingly recognized in the elderly that delirium may take months to resolve after the agent is removed and that full resolution may not always be achieved.[159, 160]

The cardiovascular consequences of hypothyroidism (bradycardia, hypertension, hyperlipidemia, atherosclerosis, and pericardial effusion) are more worrisome in the elderly because of the high prevalence of background cardiovascular disease.[487, 500–502] Hypothyroidism is among the most frequent causes of secondary hypertension; its frequency increases with age and responds well to thyroid hormone therapy.[503, 504] Sleep apnea can be triggered or aggravated by hypothyroidism.[176, 505] Both myopathy and extracellular fluid accumulations induced by hypothyroidism may contribute. The apnea usually responds well to thyroid hormone replacement. The anemia of hypothyroidism, although classically thought of as macrocytic, can also be microcytic or normocytic.[506, 507] Other causes of anemia such as deficiencies of iron, vitamin B_{12}, or folate are also common in the elderly.[507]

Therapy

The optimal dose of thyroid hormone for replacement in the elderly is typically less than that in younger adults but shows wide variation.[445, 447, 448, 452, 508–511] Caution must be exercised because cardiovascular and other disorders can be deleteriously affected by excessive thyroid hormone.[500, 512] A starting dose of thyroxine at 12.5 to 25 μg/day, seems prudent, with dose adjustments at 1- to 2-month intervals until the serum TSH level is within the normal range or close to it. Because some drugs interfere with thyroxine absorption, the thyroxine should probably be given separately from other medications. Some drugs accelerate serum T_4 clearance or inhibit conversion of T_4 to T_3 (e.g., amiodarone), so occasional patients may require higher replacement doses.[511]

Myxedema Coma

Myxedema coma is a true medical emergency.[513–517] It is a rare syndrome that occurs after severe long-standing untreated hypothyroidism, classically in elderly women during the winter. It is associated with a high mortality rate and requires early recognition and prompt treatment with thyroid hormone. (Obviously, this syndrome needs to be distinguished from other disorders that produce obtundation in patients who also have much milder hypothyroidism that is only a modest coincidental complication.) Cold weather, infections, trauma, and drugs (especially those that affect thyroid function, e.g., amiodarone and lithium, or those that depress the CNS) are common precipitating agents; severe depression of CNS, cardiovascular, and pulmonary function may be both causes and effects.[517] Clinical evidence of previous thyroid disease, radioiodine therapy, or thyroidectomy is helpful diagnostically. Hypothermia, hypoventilation, bradycardia, hypotension, anemia, dilutional hyponatremia, and hypoglycemia, as well as elevations in cholesterol, lactate dehydrogenase, and creatine kinase, are findings supportive of the diagnosis.[517] Hypothermia, which is common and can be extraordinary in degree, may be the herald for the diagnosis; hypoglycemia, when present, can contribute further to the depression in temperature.[517] A very low T_4 and a very high TSH are typical, but severe illness alone can diminish TSH.[518] (A very low T_4 with a low TSH would occur with the very rare pituitary etiology for the severe hypothyroidism.[517]) Typically, the diagnosis must first be made on clinical grounds. Blood should be obtained for thyroid tests and for plasma cortisol determination before treatment, but initiation of intravenous hormone replacement should follow immediately, before the test results become available. With current methods and dogged diplomacy, many test results should be available from the laboratory within hours.

Many therapeutic suggestions have appeared in the literature. Because of (1) the uncertainty of diagnosis (before completing thyroid function tests), (2) the urgency of treatment, (3) the unpredictability of conversion of T_4 to T_3 at multiple sites, (4) the retarded access of T_4 to the CNS,[519] (5) respect for the potential lethality of exogenous thyroid hormone in very sick elderly, and (6) the paucity of data,

Wartofsky's regimen is especially appealing to us[517]: prompt commencement of therapy with thyroxine, 4 μg/kg lean body weight (about 200 μg) intravenously followed in 24 hours with an additional 100-μg dose, and 50 μg daily, orally if possible, starting on the third day.[517] At the same time, T_3 at a dose of 20 μg is given, followed by 10 μg every 8 hours. Because T_3 is fully absorbed from the gastrointestinal tract, choice of the oral vs. the intravenous route is determined by the severity of the patient's illness. When thyroid tests have been completed and the patient's improvement permits, it is appropriate to switch to oral thyroxine maintenance. For the first several days, each dose of thyroid hormone should be preceded by clinical evaluation for signs of excess.[517] Many experts recommend co-administration of intravenous hydrocortisone because of the possibility of coexistent adrenal insufficiency, before or precipitated by thyroid hormone therapy.[517]

Hyperthyroid States

Hyperthyroidism is common among the elderly.[447, 520–527] Graves' disease is the most common cause, but both the goiter and the eye disease associated with it are less frequent and less severe. Toxic multinodular goiter (Plummer's disease) becomes almost as common as Graves' disease as a cause of hyperthyroidism in the elderly, especially in regions of relative iodine deficiency and often in patients with a long history of simple or multinodular goiter and euthyroidism.[445]

Iatrogenic Causes

Among the elderly it is common to find thyroxine replacement at doses that were appropriate but are now too high (see earlier).[452, 509, 510] Nodular goiters predispose patients to iodine-induced hyperthyroidism when given large quantities of iodine-containing medications such as amiodarone or diagnostic agents.[478–483, 528] (T_4 levels are elevated, TSH is suppressed, and radioiodine uptake is low, similar to patients with exogenous thyroxine administration.)

T_3 Toxicosis

Common forms of hyperthyroidism are associated with a disproportionate increase in T_3 production. In a minority of patients the hyperthyroidism is due solely to an elevation in T_3; TSH is suppressed whereas measurements of T_4 are in the normal range.[529, 530] (The clinical and laboratory findings with this condition can be re-created by the ingestion of T_3.[531]) T_3 toxicosis is thought to be more common in the elderly, especially (1) in regions of iodine deficiency, (2) in the early stages of hormone overproduction, and (3) in patients with recurrence after subtotal thyroidectomy. Remission with antithyroid therapy may be rapid and long lasting.[445]

Clinical Manifestations in the Elderly

With hyperthyroidism in the elderly, signs and symptoms in one system, for example, the cardiovascular, neuropsychiatric, muscular, or gastrointestinal system, may dominate the clinical picture.[426, 445, 495, 496, 524–526, 532–534] Some symptoms in the elderly are atypical in younger patients: lethargy, apathy, depression, pseudodementia, weakness and atrophy of muscles, anorexia, and constipation.[445, 526] Goiter is absent in half, and hyperactive reflexes, excessive sweating, heat intolerance, and diarrhea are much less common.[520, 521, 529, 530, 533–535]

Diagnosis

Because serum (total) T_4 is a sensitive test but has low specificity, diagnosis of hyperthyroidism requires the demonstration of suppressed TSH with an elevated level of free T_4, total T_3, or both.[445, 521–525, 532–534] Suppression of the serum TSH level may occur without elevation of thyroid hormone levels in a small fraction of euthyroid elderly,[445, 529, 530, 535] in patients treated with glucocorticoids, in patients treated with slightly excessive T_4 replacement, and in patients with hyperthyroidism in flux, that is, just starting or resolving.[445]

Treatment of Hyperthyroidism in the Elderly

One recommended treatment is ^{131}I preceded by several weeks or months of an antithyroid drug.[445, 447, 448, 508, 520–525, 532–545] During this time intrathyroidal stores of hormone are depleted, thereby greatly reducing the likelihood that the radiation will cause an explosive release of active hormone that can aggravate the thyrotoxicosis.[546–549] (Given the subtleties of the clinical and laboratory findings in the elderly and the resultant uncertainty of the diagnosis, the response to antithyroid drugs may also serve to clarify the true diagnosis before ablation with radioactive iodine.) The drugs need to be withdrawn about a week before the administration of radioactive iodine and then started again a week after the treatment. Other experts, respecting the potential adverse effects of the drugs as more serious than the threat of radiation-induced exacerbation of the hyperthyroidism, prescribe antithyroid drugs for only a few days or not at all before radioiodine administration.[550, 551] A standard dose of radioactive iodine is given for Graves' disease, whereas three times that amount is recommended for large multinodular goiters.[445, 541] The age-related diminution in urinary clearance of iodide needs to be considered in calculation of the dose. β-Blockers can also be used, especially for tachycardia, but many elderly patients have contraindications to their use. The incidence of postradiation hypothyroidism is probably greater in the elderly and needs to be monitored and treated.

Antithyroid drugs can be used as definitive therapy for Graves' disease. Those who favor this approach point out that in the elderly discontinuation of the drugs at a later time is typically associated with very low recurrence rates. Except in special circumstances, surgery is not advisable in the elderly. Our overall recommendation is as follows: the greater the age of the patient, typically the greater the number of extrathyroidal concerns; the broad range of acceptable approaches to treat the hyperthyroidism should encourage the practitioner to create an individualized plan for each patient that clearly balances the benefits and risks for that patient.

Thyroid Storm

Severe hyperthyroidism is a true medical emergency; thyroid storm and thyrotoxic crisis are fanciful names for this condition.[445, 514, 515, 548, 549, 551–557] In patients with inadequately treated hyperthyroidism caused by Graves' disease or multinodular goiter, thyrotoxic crisis or thyroid storm can be precipitated by external events, including infection, trauma, surgery, or a therapeutic dose of radioactive iodine. Fever combined with serious cardiovascular and neuropsychiatric complications may dominate the clinical picture. The diagnosis is a clinical one; blood samples are drawn (plasma hormone levels are typically not distinguishable from those of run-of-the-mill hyperthyroidism), but therapy must be undertaken immediately before the results are available because untreated, the condition has a high mortality rate. Because of its added property of blocking conversion of T_4 to T_3 propylthiouracil is the drug of choice, accompanied shortly thereafter by iodide (ipodate or a saturated solution of potassium iodide) and glucocorticoids to diminish conversion of T_4 to T_3.[549] When not contraindicated, a β-blocker is often effective. (Lithium, to inhibit hormone release, or cholestyramine, to deplete the hormone pool, may be useful in very special circumstances.[544, 558]) Response to effective therapy is prompt (within 1 to 2 days). To avoid a further increase in levels of free hormone, salicylates or other drugs that displace bound hormone from the circulating thyroxine-binding proteins should be avoided when possible.

Thyroid Tumors in the Elderly

Age has distinct influences on the incidence, prevalence, and biology of thyroid tumors and therefore has an impact on patient management. The prevalence of solitary and multiple thyroid nodules increases with age and with the efficiency of the diagnostic tools used:

palpation (less satisfactory in the elderly) vs. ultrasonography (incidentalomas are more common) vs. autopsy (clinically silent neoplasms are more common).[559–562] Clinically, women are much more afflicted than men, but the ratio of malignant to benign is clearly greater among men. Papillary carcinomas remain the most common malignancies by far; the incidence declines after age 50, whereas their aggressiveness clearly increases.[563, 564] (Follicular carcinomas are the second most common and follow a similar pattern, but the age profile is pushed up about a decade.)[564, 565] Radiation to the head or neck before age 15 confers heightened susceptibility to papillary carcinoma that appears to be lifelong, although the incidence of cancer does decline in later years. The large cohort of children irradiated in the 1940s is just reaching the age of 65.[565, 566] In monitoring this group of patients for thyroid neoplasms it should be kept in mind that this radiation may also predispose individuals to tumors of the parathyroid (with hypercalcemia) and salivary glands.[567, 568]

The sporadic, nonfamilial form of medullary carcinoma is much more common in the elderly than is the familial form of this neoplasm.[569–571] Medullary carcinomas in this age group have an overall pattern and prognosis that roughly resemble those of follicular carcinomas. (The familial tumors, which often occur with multiple endocrine neoplasia type 2, have several differences, including an earlier age at diagnosis.[570, 571]) In addition to the secretion of thyrocalcitonin, which is asymptomatic (but can have prognostic value), secretion of one or more ectopic hormones from the C cell tumor may affect the clinical course.

Anaplastic carcinomas—malignant, invasive, and metastasizing—account for 5% to 10% of all thyroid cancers.[572–575] They typically occur after age 60 with a painful, rapidly enlarging mass (often in a pre-existing asymptomatic nodule). The mass may be stone hard, tender, and fixed, with restricted movement on swallowing. Hoarseness, stridor, and dysphagia may all be associated complaints. Node involvement and distant metastases may be detected at the initial evaluation. Although the short-term and ultimate prognosis is typically grim, a combination of therapies may yield disease-free intervals of several years in a minority of patients.[572–575]

Thyroid lymphomas, essentially all of B cell origin, account for 1% to 5% of thyroid malignancies.[576, 577] The key point here is that they be distinguished from anaplastic cancers. They share many clinical features (rapidly enlarging neck mass, often with swelling, hoarseness, and dysphagia) but differ widely in treatment and prognosis. Thyroid lymphomas typically afflict females older than 60 years who have a long history of Hashimoto's disease. The diagnosis is established by microscopic examination of tumor tissue, including specific immunologic markers to distinguish lymphoma from the small cell form of anaplastic cancer. External radiation and systemic chemotherapy are very effective, even when the tumor has extended to extrathyroidal sites.

ENDOCRINE CONTROL OF CALCIUM HOMEOSTASIS

Bone is the major storage site for calcium and a major support for the body. With aging, the serum calcium levels are maintained in the normal range via changes in hormonal milieu, but the integrity of the bones as a support system diminishes.[578–581] Cortical bone, which accounts for approximately 75% of the weight of the skeleton, undergoes a reduction in overall thickness and an increase in porosity with aging. Trabecular bone, which accounts for 25% of the skeletal weight, but a majority of bone remodeling surface, shows a loss due to both a thinning and loss of normal trabeculae. Fractures of both types of bone, with their potentially devastating consequences, become a major hazard in women and are increasingly recognized as a problem for elderly men.[582–586] The diminution of bone mineral is labeled as osteopenia, and when more severe as osteoporosis.[587, 588] Traditionally in women, two types of primary osteoporosis have been distinguished: postmenopausal osteoporosis or type I, associated with estrogen deficiency, and over the age of 65, so-called senile osteoporosis or type II, associated with calcium malabsorption, vitamin D deficiency, and secondary hyperparathyroidism.[587–598] In older men, there is the additional effect of a progressive diminution in androgens; the anabolic effects of testosterone on bone are probably mediated via its own receptor as well as via the estrogen receptor after its conversion to estrogen by aromatase.[599, 600] Bone resorption is promoted by IL-6 released from osteoclasts; sex hormones exercise strong negative feedback on the release of IL-6.[578–580, 587, 588, 601, 602] (In both sexes, the demineralization process is accelerated by glucocorticoid excess of exogenous or endogenous origin; even the mild elevations associated with depressive disorders can diminish the bone mineral density.[109]) Severe deficiencies or defects in the vitamin D system cause osteomalacia, a metabolic bone disease characterized by the accumulation of unmineralized matrix, independent of bone mass.[578, 579] We have limited our review here to the contributions of parathyroid hormone and vitamin D derivatives to calcium homeostasis in the elderly and their effects on the aging process in bones. The reader is referred to other chapters for detailed descriptions of the effects of sex hormones, growth factors and cytokines, and other bone disorders, their diagnosis and management.

PARATHYROID HORMONE. Parathyroid hormone (PTH) stimulates the kidney to reabsorb more calcium from the urine and to convert more 25(OH) vitamin D (*calcidiol*, abbreviated 25(OH)D) to 1,25(OH)$_2$ vitamin D (*calcitriol*, abbreviated 1,25(OH)$_2$).[578, 581, 587, 588] Parathyroid hormone, by multiple mechanisms, stimulates osteoclasts to reabsorb bone and mobilize calcium. Parathyroid hormone concentrations in serum increase with age, resulting from an increase in secretion and a decrease in metabolism, possibly owing to an age-dependent diminution in renal function[587, 588, 596]; the latter also contributes to the increase in the concentration of bioinactive forms of the hormone in the circulation. The newer assays, which measure only the bioactive hormone, have confirmed that the level of bioactive PTH is elevated. PTH secretion by the parathyroid gland is exquisitely sensitive to small drops in ionized calcium within the normal range. Multiple elements related to aging have been implicated, but the precise mechanisms have not been definitely established (see later). The striking inverse relationship between PTH and 25(OH)D levels (Fig. 38–3) illustrates the link between the deficiency of vitamin D with aging and secondary hyperparathyroidism.[603] This relationship extends to seasonal variations where the winter nadir of 25(OH)D is associated

with a PTH peak; in summer, these are reversed.[604, 605] In the Baltimore Longitudinal Study of Aging, lower radial bone densities in men were related to higher PTH levels and lower 25-OHD levels.[606] Similarly, in a study of 133 community-based elderly men aged 65 to 76, the higher the PTH level, the lower the bone mineral density of the proximal femur.[599]

VITAMIN D. Vitamin D, the hormone precursor, comes in food and is also synthesized in the skin from 7-dehydrocholesterol, a process that becomes less efficient in the elderly.[603, 607, 608] In addition, the elderly often have less exposure to sunlight, especially among the homebound or residents of regions closer to the poles.[603, 609] Gastrointestinal causes of vitamin D deficiency in the elderly include malabsorption and avoidance of vitamin D containing dairy products.[598, 610, 611] Vitamin D is hydroxylated in the liver to 25(OH) vitamin D in a hormone independent fashion. With age, there is a linear decrease of serum 25(OH)D, which is a good reflection of total vitamin D stores.[612] In addition to reduced production, degradation of 25(OH)D may be accelerated by drugs (e.g., diphenylhydantoin). 25(OH)D is: (1) the principal precursor of 1,25(OH)$_2$D, (2) an inconsequential hormone surrogate, and (3) a strong competitor of 1,25(OH)$_2$ vitamin D for binding sites in plasma. When 25(OH)D drops to very low levels, as happens among the elderly, mechanisms are in place for both a decrease in the free fraction of circulating 1,25(OH)$_2$D and a fall in production of 1,25(OH)$_2$D.[595, 613, 614]

With aging, the converting enzyme, 1α-hydroxylase, in the kidney is reduced in concentration and activity, in addition to the decrement in the concentration of its substrate.[595, 614] Probably the reduction in 25(OH)D and 1,25(OH)$_2$D levels both contribute to the increase in PTH (see Fig. 38–3).

The proposed sequence of events appears to be a diminution in vitamin D (from both skin and gastrointestinal tract) leading to a progressive fall in 25(OH)D, which leads ultimately to a fall in 1,25(OH)$_2$D. The low level of 1,25(OH)$_2$D is due to a decrement in the level of 25(OH)D and a reduced efficiency of its conversion to 1,25(OH)$_2$D. The decrease in 1,25(OH)$_2$D, mainly through its negative effects on calcium metabolism, is followed by a compensatory increase in PTH, which elevates the serum 1,25(OH)$_2$D toward normal, associated with an increase in bone resorption. In the elderly, there is a modest resistance to the action of 1,25(OH)$_2$D on intestinal calcium absorption due to an age-related decrease in vitamin D receptors.[615, 616] With regard to the elderly and secondary hyperparathyroidism, it remains to be determined whether there is also an age-dependent decrement in serum calcium concentration or reduced sensitivity of the parathyroid gland to negative feedback by calcium or reduced sensitivity to the negative feedback effects of 1,25(OH)$_2$D.

Many elderly in Europe and in the US are deficient in vitamin D and its derivatives. The threshold concentration of serum 25(OH)D to define vitamin D deficiency is controversial. The vitamin D assays in the early studies from Europe had lower values than those with the radioimmunoassays typically used in the US.[617, 618] Overt osteomalacia and rickets are usually found when 25-OHD levels fall below 12.5 nmol/L (5 ng/ml). Whereas 25-OHD concentrations below 30 nmol/L (12 ng/ml) generally indicate vitamin D deficiency, adverse skeletal effects may even be seen with 25-OHD concentrations at 77 nmol/L (~30 ng/ml), because among individuals PTH levels may start to increase at that 25-OHD concentration or below.[597, 619] Among homebound elderly in Baltimore, 54% had low 25-OHD levels.[603, 614] Among 290 inpatients, 57% had vitamin D deficiency with serum 25-OHD levels at or below 38 nmol/L.[620] Among postmenopausal women with hip fractures, 50% had 25-OHD levels below 30 nmol/L; 37% of these women had PTH levels greater than 6.8 pmol/L with elevated levels of markers of bone resorption.[592] During the winter in Boston, postmenopausal women had a severe decline in mineral density of the spine that could be prevented by vitamin D supplementation during the winter to maintain 25-OHD at summer levels of 90 nmol/L.[621] As noted earlier, vitamin D levels are diminished in elderly residents of higher latitudes.[607, 622, 623] In Finland, the annual injection in autumn of ergocalciferol (150,000 to 300,000 IU) for 5 years led to a 44% reduction in the fracture rate in women.[624] Vitamin D deficiency in the elderly can also produce pain, weakness, and decrements in function that are reversed with replacement therapy.[614, 625–627]

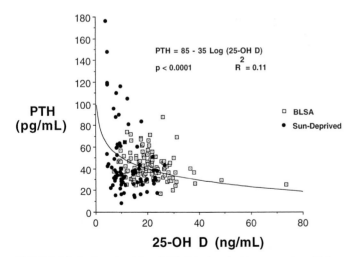

FIGURE 38–3. *Relationship of 25-OH vitamin D to parathyroid hormone. The concentration of circulating parathyroid hormone (PTH, picograms per milliliter) is plotted as a function of the circulating level of 25-OH vitamin D (nanograms per milliliter). Two populations were studied: healthy adults in the Baltimore Longitudinal Study on Aging and a group of sun-deprived homebound elderly. High levels of 25-OH vitamin D are shown to be associated with low levels of parathyroid hormone. When the 25-OH vitamin D level is below 40 ng/mL, the PTH concentration tends to be elevated. With 25-OH vitamin D levels below 10, a significant proportion of the population have clearly elevated levels of PTH. The favorable response to vitamin D therapy suggests that diminution in vitamin D derivatives may trigger the secondary hyperparathyroidism that is common among the elderly, especially in those who are homebound and thereby have little exposure to ultraviolet light.*

CALCIUM. With aging, the extracellular concentration of calcium remains within the normal range, but the mass of calcium in bone is progressively lost. The intake of calcium and the efficiency of calcium absorption from the small intestine diminish.[598, 615, 616, 628–630] The latter is in part due to the age-dependent decrements in serum levels of 1,25(OH)$_2$D, to decreases in 1,25(OH)$_2$D receptors in the gastrointestinal tract, and other changes with age including diminution in gastric acidity (low pH improves absorption of ingested calcium). The small intestine in the aged individual is less effective in compensating for a low calcium diet (i.e., of maximizing efficiency of absorption). In the kidney, the elevated PTH promotes calcium reabsorption.[628–630] Overall, with aging, the kidney is unchanged with respect to its capacity to handle calcium. Compared with young adults in whom bone resorption and bone formation are balanced, in the elderly, calcium balance in bone tends to move into negative territory and stay there.

IMMOBILIZATION AND OTHER INFLUENCES ON BONE. Immobilization in the elderly warrants special mention.[631–635] Immobility results in the mobilization of calcium from bone that suppresses PTH and thus diminishes synthesis of 1,25(OH)$_2$D and also produces a deficiency of 25(OH)D. The absence of an elevated PTH level should not confuse the clinician. In addition to drugs to suppress bone resorption (see elsewhere), replacement therapy with calcitriol should be considered to bypass the 1α-hydroxylase deficiency. Weight bearing and exercise obviously should be promoted.

Among the other important influences on bone density in the elderly are: (1) long standing harmful elements in life style (e.g., low calcium diet; low BMI; nicotine, caffeine, alcohol, sedentary behavior); (2) diminution in hormones and hormone-related messengers including sex hormones (especially estrogen in women and both androgens and estrogens in men) and also possibly GH and IGF-1 (discussed elsewhere in this chapter), and (3) the peak level bone density achieved in early adult life (which has strong genetic and environmental influences). Studies of the genetics of bone mass and bone loss have uncovered a number of allelic variances of genes related to hormone effects on bone, including the vitamin D receptor. The significance of the genetic polymorphisms is under active study.[636–643]

PROPHYLAXIS. The overall goal is to prevent fractures. In this important area, the details are under discussion, but the principles are clear. In addition to sex hormones (see elsewhere), it is likely that vitamin D and calcium, and probably supplements of other nutrients, will become universal. Recommended dietary allowances (RDA) in the elderly are not rigorously established including those for calcium. At present, the RDA for elemental calcium is at 800 mg/day for men and women older than age 50. It is based on estimates of efficiency of calcium absorption (~40%) and obligatory losses (about 250 mg/day) and far below the NIH consensus conference recommendation of 1500 mg/day for those over age 65 (best given as 500 mg t.i.d. with meals; one should recall that gastric acidity promotes calcium absorption, while dietary fiber interferes).[598, 644–648]

One measure to reduce vitamin D deficiency is fortification of foods, because natural dietary sources of vitamin D are limited. Milk is fortified with vitamin D in the US and Canada but is not universally in Europe. The vitamin D content of fortified foods can vary.[649] The emerging consensus now is that the elderly should consume vitamin D 800 IU/day (or 100,000 units every 3 to 6 months), instead of the classic RDA of 200 IU/day.

A prospective, randomized study of 3270 elderly women (age range, 69 to 106) with a mean calcium intake of 500 mg/day and a mean serum 25-OHD level of 15 ng/ml, showed that the incidence of hip and other osteoporotic fractures was reduced after supplementation with cholecalciferol 800 IU/day and calcium 1 g/day.[645–647] Dietary supplementation with 1500 mg elemental calcium and 700 IU cholecalciferol, given daily for 3 years, reduced bone loss and the incidence of nonvertebral fractures in a group aged 65 years and older.[645]

REFERENCES

1. Creditor MC: Hazards of hospitalization of the elderly. Ann Intern Med 118:219–223, 1993.
2. Sager MA, Rudberg MA, Jalaluddin M, et al: Hospital admission risk profile (HARP): Identifying older patients at risk for functional decline following acute medical illness and hospitalization. J Am Geriatr Soc 44:251–257, 1996.
3. Inouye SK, Wagner DR, Acampora D, et al: A predictive index for functional decline in hospitalized elderly medical patients. J Gen Intern Med 8:645–652, 1993.
4. Cobbs EL, Duthie EH, Murphy JB (eds): Geriatrics Review Syllabus: A Core Curriculum in Geriatric Medicine, ed 4. New York, American Geriatrics Society, and Dubuque, IA, Kendall/Hunt, 1999.
5. Hazzard WR, Blass JP, Ettinger WH Jr, et al (eds): Principles of Geriatric Medicine and Gerontology, ed 4. New York, McGraw-Hill, 1999.
6. Martin LG, Preston SH (eds): Demography of Aging. Washington, DC, National Academy Press, 1994.
7. Rosenwaike I: A demographic portrait of the oldest old. Milbank Mem Fund Q Health Soc 63:187–205, 1985.
8. Taffet GE: Age-related physiologic changes. In Cobbs EL, Duthie EH, Murphy JB (eds): Geriatrics Review Syllabus: A Core Curriculum in Geriatric Medicine, ed 4. New York, American Geriatrics Society, and Dubuque, IA, Kendall/Hunt, 1999, pp 10–23.
9. Rowe JW, Kahn RL: Human aging: Usual and successful. Science 237:143–149, 1987.
10. Lipsitz LA, Goldberger AL: Loss of 'complexity' and aging: Potential applications of fractals and chaos theory to senescence. JAMA 267:1806–1809, 1992.
11. Finch CE, Tanzi R: Genetics of aging. Science 278:407–411, 1997.
12. Martin GM: The genetics of aging. Hosp Pract 32:47–50, 55–56, 59–61, 1997.
13. Turker MS, Martin GM: Genetics of human disease, longevity, and aging. In Hazzard WR, Blass JP, Ettinger WH Jr, et al (eds): Principles of Geriatric Medicine and Gerontology, ed 4. New York, McGraw-Hill, 1999, pp 21–44.
14. McClearn GE, Johansson B, Berg S, et al: Substantial genetic influence on cognitive abilities in twins 80 or more years old. Science 276:1560–1563, 1997.
15. Bohr VA, Dianov G, Balajee A, et al: DNA repair and transcription in human premature aging disorders. J Invest Dermatol Symp Proc 3:11–13, 1998.
16. Gray MD, Shen JC, Kamath-Loeb AS, et al: The Werner syndrome protein is a DNA helicase. Nat Genet 17:100–103, 1997.
17. Jazwinski SM: Longevity, genes, and aging. Science 273:54–59, 1996.
18. Thomas JH, Inoue T: Methuselah meets diabetes. Bioessays 20:113–115, 1998.
19. Roush W: Worm longevity gene cloned. Science 277:897–898, 1997.
20. Sohal RS, Weindruch R: Oxidative stress, caloric restriction, and aging. Science 273:59–63, 1996.
21. Masoro EJ: Dietary restriction and aging. J Am Geriatr Soc 41:994–999, 1993.
22. Rowe JW, Kahn RL: Successful aging. Aging (Milano) 10:142–144, 1998.
23. Kennedy BP, Kawachi I, Prothrow-Stith D: Income distribution and mortality: Cross sectional ecological study of the Robin Hood index in the United States. BMJ 312:1004–1007, 1996.
24. House JS, Kessler RC, Herzog AR: Age, socioeconomic status, and health. Milbank Q 68:383–411, 1990.
25. House JS, Lepkowski JM, Kinney AM, et al: The social stratification of aging and health. J Health Soc Behav 35:213–234, 1994.
26. Silver K, Shuldiner AR: Candidate genes for type 2 diabetes mellitus. In LeRoith D, Olefsky JM, Taylor SI (eds): Diabetes Mellitus: A Fundamental and Clinical Text, ed 2. Philadelphia, JB Lippincott, 2000, pp 705–711.
27. Shuldiner AR: Obesity and diabetes: Research points to genetic connection. Geriatrics 52:57–60, 1997.
28. Evans WJ: What is sarcopenia? J Gerontol A Biol Sci Med Sci 50:5–8, 1995.
29. Miller RA: The aging immune system: Primer and prospectus. Science 273:70–74, 1996.
30. Tomei LD, Umansky SR: Aging and apoptosis control. Neurol Clin 16:735–745, 1998.
31. Warner HR: Aging and regulation of apoptosis. Curr Top Cell Regul 35:107–121, 1997.
32. Warner HR, Hodes RJ, Pocinki K: What does cell death have to do with aging? J Am Geriatr Soc 45:1140–1146, 1997.
33. Roth J, Yen C-J: The role of intercellular communication in diseases of old age. In Hazzard WR, Blass JP, Ettinger WH Jr, et al (eds): Principles of Geriatric Medicine and Gerontology, ed 4. New York, McGraw-Hill, 1999, pp 45–59.
34. Atkinson MA, Maclaren NK: The pathogenesis of insulin-dependent diabetes mellitus. N Engl J Med 331:1428–1436, 1994.
35. Eizirik DL, Sandler S, Welsh N, et al: Cytokines suppress human islet function irrespective of their effects on nitric oxide generation. J Clin Invest 93:1968–1974, 1994.
36. Hayflick L: The limited in vitro lifetime of human diploid cell strains. Exp Cell Res 37:614–616, 1965.
37. Hayflick L, Moorehead PF: The serial cultivation of human diploid cell strains. Exp Cell Res 25:585–621, 1961.
38. Hayflick L: The cell biology of human aging. Sci Am 242:58–66, 1980.
39. Hayflick L: Cell aging. In Eisdorfer C (ed): Annual Review of Gerontology and Geriatrics. New York, Springer, 1980, pp 26–67.
40. Smith JR, Pereira-Smith OM: Replicative senescence: Implications for in vivo aging and tumor suppression. Science 273:63–67, 1996.
41. Allsopp RC, Vaziri H, Patterson C, et al: Telomere length predicts replicative capacity of human fibroblasts. Proc Natl Acad Sci U S A 89:10114–10118, 1992.
42. Chiu C, Harley CB: Replicative senescence and cell immortality: The role of telomeres and telomerase. Proc Soc Exp Biol Med 214:99–106, 1997.
43. Greider CW: Telomeres and senescence: The history, the experiment, the future. Curr Biol 8:178–181, 1998.
44. Olovnikov AM: Telomeres, telomerase, and aging: Origin of the theory. Exp Gerontol 31:443–448, 1996.
45. Harley CB, Futcher AB, Greider CW: Telomeres shorten during aging of human fibroblasts. Nature 345:458–460, 1990.
46. Morin GB: The human telomere terminal transferase enzyme is a ribonucleoprotein that synthesizes TTAGGG repeats. Cell 59:521–529, 1989.
47. Bodnar AG, Ouellette M, Frolkis M, et al: Extension of life-span by introduction of telomerase into normal human cells. Science 279:349–352, 1998.

48. Stadtman ER: Protein oxidation and aging. Science 257:1220–1224, 1992.
49. Stadtman ER: Role of oxidized amino acids in protein breakdown and stability. Methods Enzymol 258:379–393, 1995.
50. Levine RL, Stadtman ER: Protein modifications with aging. *In* Schneider EL, Rowe JW (eds): Handbook of the Biology of Aging. San Diego, CA, Academic, 1996, pp 184–197.
51. Vlassara H: Recent progress on the biologic and clinical significance of advanced glycosylation end products. J Lab Clin Med 124:19–30, 1994.
52. Brownlee M: Advanced protein glycosylation in diabetes and aging. Annu Rev Med 46:223–234, 1995.
53. Wells-Knecht MC, Huggins TG, Dyer DG, et al: Oxidized amino acids in lens protein with age: Measurement of *o*-tyrosine and dityrosine in the aging human lens. J Biol Chem 268:12348–12352, 1993.
54. Sipe JD: Amyloidosis. Annu Rev Biochem 61:947–975, 1992.
55. Martin JB: Molecular basis of the neurodegenerative disorders. N Engl J Med 340:1970–1980, 1999.
56. Sisodia SS: Alzheimer's disease: Perspectives for the new millennium. J Clin Invest 104:1169–1170, 1999.
57. Huang CC, Faber PW, Persichetti F, et al: Amyloid formation by mutant huntingtin: Threshold, progressivity and recruitment of normal polyglutamine proteins. Somat Cell Mol Genet 24:217–233, 1998.
58. Clayton DF, George JM: Synucleins in synaptic plasticity and neurodegenerative disorders. J Neurosci Res 58:120–129, 1999.
59. Harper JD, Lansbury PT Jr: Models of amyloid seeding in Alzheimer's disease and scrapie: Mechanistic truths and physiological consequences of the time-dependent solubility of amyloid proteins. Annu Rev Biochem 66:385–407, 1997.
60. Eaton WA, Hofrichter J: Sickle cell hemoglobin polymerization. Adv Protein Chem 40:63–279, 1990.
61. Mozzarelli A, Hofrichter J, Eaton WA: Delay time of hemoglobin S polymerization prevents most cells from sickling in vivo. Science 237:500–506, 1987.
62. Terman A, Brunk UT: Lipofuscin: Mechanisms of formation and increase with age. APMIS 106:265–276, 1998.
63. Yin D: Biochemical basis of lipofuscin, ceroid, and age pigment–like fluorophores. Free Radic Biol Med 21:871–888, 1996.
64. Ames BN, Shigenaga MK, Hagen TM: Oxidants, antioxidants, and the degenerative diseases of aging. Proc Natl Acad Sci U S A 90:7915–7922, 1993.
65. Martin GM, Austad SN, Johnson TE: Genetic analysis of aging: Role of oxidative damage and environmental stresses. Nat Genet 13:25–34, 1996.
66. Fraga CG, Shigenaga MK, Park JW, et al: Oxidative damage to DNA during aging: 8-Hydroxy-2′-deoxyguanosine in rat organ DNA and urine. Proc Natl Acad Sci U S A 87:4533–4537, 1990.
67. Shigenaga MK, Gagen TM, Ames BN: Oxidative damage and mitochondrial decay in aging. Proc Natl Acad Sci U S A 91:10771–10778, 1994.
68. Singh NP, Danner DB, Raymond RT, et al: Basal DNA damage in individual human lymphocytes with age. Mutat Res 256:1–6, 1991.
69. Mann DB, Springer DL, Smerdon MJ: DNA damage can alter the stability of nucleosomes: Effects are dependent on damage type. Proc Natl Acad Sci U S A 94:2215–2220, 1997.
70. Hanawalt PC: Evolution of concepts in DNA repair. Environ Mol Mutagen 23:78–85, 1994.
71. Croteau DL, Bohr VA: Repair of oxidative damage to nuclear and mitochondrial DNA in mammalian cells. J Biol Chem 272:25409–25412, 1997.
72. Gilchrest BA, Bohr VA: Aging processes, DNA damage, and repair. FASEB J 11:322–330, 1997.
73. Shigenaga MK, Gagen TM, Ames BN: Oxidative damage and mitochondrial decay in aging. Proc Natl Acad Sci U S A 91:10771–10778, 1994.
74. Mecocci P, MacGarvey U, Kaufman AE, et al: Oxidative damage to mitochondrial DNA shows marked age-dependent increases in human brain. Ann Neurol 34:609–616, 1993.
75. Melov S, Hinerfeld D, Esposito L, Wallace DC: Multi-organ characterization of mitochondrial genomic rearrangements in ad libitum and caloric restricted mice show striking somatic mitochondrial DNA rearrangements with age. Nucleic Acids Res 25:974–982, 1997.
76. Wallace DC: Mitochondrial DNA in aging and disease. Sci Am 277:40–47, 1997.
77. Croteau DL, Stierum RH, Bohr VA: Mitochondrial DNA repair pathways. Mutat Res 434:137–148, 1999.
78. Rogina B, Benzer S, Helfand SL: *Drosophila* drop-dead mutations accelerate the time course of age-related markers. Proc Natl Acad Sci U S A 94:6303–6306, 1997.
79. Miller RA: The biology of aging and longevity. *In* Hazzard WR, Blass JP, Ettinger WH Jr, et al (eds): Principles of Geriatric Medicine and Gerontology, ed 4. New York, McGraw-Hill, 1999, pp 3–19.
80. Austad SN: Theories of aging: An overview. Aging (Milano) 10:146–147, 1998.
81. Kirkwoood TB: Biological theories of aging: An overview. Aging (Milano) 10:144–146, 1998.
82. Masoro EJ: Theories of aging: A pathophysiological perspective. Aging (Milano) 9:428–429, 1997.
83. Troen BR, Cristofalo VJ: The biology of aging. *In* Cobbs EL, Duthie EH, Murphy JB (eds): Geriatrics Review Syllabus: A Core Curriculum in Geriatric Medicine, ed 4. New York, American Geriatrics Society, and Dubuque, IA, Kendall/Hunt, 1999, pp 5–10.
84. Dentino AN, Pieper CF, Rao MK, et al: Association of interleukin-6 and other biologic variables with depression in older people living in the community. J Am Geriatr Soc 47:6–11, 1999.
85. Harris TB, Ferrucci L, Tracy RP, et al: Associations of elevated interleukin-6 and C-reactive protein levels with mortality in the elderly. Am J Med 106:506–512, 1999.
86. Ershler WB: Interleukin 6: A cytokine for gerontologists. J Am Geriatr Soc 41:176–181, 1993.
87. Leipzig RA: Pharmacology and appropriate prescribing. *In* Cobbs EL, Duthie EH, Murphy JB (eds): Geriatrics Review Syllabus: A Core Curriculum in Geriatric Medicine, ed 4. New York, American Geriatrics Society, and Dubuque, IA, Kendall/Hunt, 1999, pp 30–35.
88. Walker J, Wynne H: The frequency and severity of adverse drug reactions in elderly people. Age Ageing 23:255–259, 1994.
89. Hanlon JT, Schmader KE, Koronkowski MJ, et al: Adverse drug events in high risk older outpatients. J Am Geriatr Soc 45:945–948, 1997.
90. Vestal RE, Montamat SC, Nielson CP: Drugs in special patient groups: The elderly. *In* Melmon KL, Morrelli HF, Hoffman BB, Nierenberg DF (eds): Clinical Pharmacology: Basic Principles in Therapeutics, ed 3. New York, McGraw-Hill, 1992, pp 851–874.
91. Montamat SC, Cusack BJ, Vestal RE: Management of drug therapy in the elderly. N Engl J Med 321:303–309, 1989.
92. Thomas JA: Drug-nutrient interactions. Nutr Rev 53:271–282, 1995.
93. Pharmacokinetics and Drug Interactions in the Elderly and Special Issues in Elderly African-American Populations, Institute of Medicine Report. Washington, DC, National Academy Press, 1997.
94. Seymour RM, Routledge PA: Important drug-drug interactions in the elderly. Drugs Aging 12:485–494, 1998.
95. Moore AR, O'Keeffe ST: Drug-induced cognitive impairment in the elderly. Drugs Aging 15:15–28, 1999.
96. Schwartz JB: Clinical pharmacology. *In* Hazzard WR, Blass JP, Ettinger WH Jr, et al (eds): Principles of Geriatric Medicine and Gerontology, ed 4. New York, McGraw-Hill, 1999, pp 303–331.
97. Adams WL, Barry KL, Fleming MF: Screening for problem drinking in older primary care patients. JAMA 276:1964–1967, 1996.
98. Atkinson RM: Aging and alcohol use disorders: Diagnostic issues in the elderly. Int Psychogeriatr 2:55–72, 1990.
99. Patricia P, Ackerman B, Ackerman K: Chemical dependency in the elderly. *In* Hazzard WR, Blass JP, Ettinger WH Jr, et al (eds): Principles of Geriatric Medicine and Gerontology, ed 4. New York, McGraw-Hill, 1999, pp 1357–1363.
100. Rochon PA, Gurwitz JH: Drug therapy. Lancet 346:32–36, 1995.
101. Corlett AJ: Aids to compliance with medication. BMJ 313:926–929, 1996.
102. Blazer DG, Bachar JR, Manton KG: Suicide in late life: Review and commentary. J Am Geriatr Soc 34:519–525, 1986.
103. Blazer DG: Depression in the elderly: Myths and misconceptions. Psychiatr Clin North Am 20:111–119, 1997.
104. Blazer DG, Landerman LR, Hays JC, et al: Symptoms of depression among community-dwelling elderly African-American and white older adults. Psychol Med 28:1311–1320, 1998.
105. Blazer D, Burchett B, Service C, George LK: The association of age and depression among the elderly: An epidemiologic exploration. J Gerontol 46:M210–M215, 1991.
106. German PS, Shapiro S, Skinner EA: Mental health of the elderly: Use of health and mental health services. J Am Geriatr Soc 33:246–252, 1985.
107. Blazer DG: Depression. *In* Hazzard WR, Blass JP, Ettinger WH Jr, et al (eds): Principles of Geriatric Medicine and Gerontology, ed 4. New York, McGraw-Hill, 1999, pp 1331–1340.
108. Glassman AH, Shapiro PA: Depression and the course of coronary artery disease. Am J Psychiatry 155:4–11, 1998.
109. Michelson D, Stratakis C, Hill L, et al: Bone mineral density in women with depression. N Engl J Med 335:1176–1181, 1996.
110. Koenig HG, George LK, Larson DB, et al: Depressive symptoms and nine-year survival of 1,001 male veterans hospitalized with medical illness. Am J Geriatr Psychiatry 7:124–131, 1999.
111. Rabins PV, Harvis K, Koven S: High fatality rates of late-life depression associated with cardiovascular disease. J Affect Disord 9:165–167, 1985.
112. Lebowitz BD, Pearson JL, Schneider LS, et al: Diagnosis and treatment of depression in late life: Consensus statement update. JAMA 278:1186–1190, 1997.
113. Whooley MA, Avins AL, Miranda J, Browner WS: Case-finding instruments for depression: Two questions are as good as many. J Gen Intern Med 12:439–445, 1997.
114. Glassman AH, Rodriguez AI, Shapiro PA: The use of antidepressant drugs in patients with heart disease. J Clin Psychiatry 59(suppl 10):16–21, 1998.
115. Cole MG: Age, age of onset and course of primary depressive illness in the elderly. Can J Psychiatry 28:102–104, 1983.
116. Gallo JJ, Rabins PV, Lyketsos CG, et al: Depression without sadness: Functional outcomes of nondysphoric depression in later life. J Am Geriatr Soc 45:570–578, 1997.
117. Gallo JJ, Cooper-Patrick L, Lesikar S: Depressive symptoms of whites and African Americans aged 60 years and older. J Gerontol B Psychol Sci Soc Sci 53:P277–P286, 1998.
118. Gallo JJ, Rabins PV: Depression without sadness: Alternative presentations of depression in late life. Am Fam Physician 60:820–826, 1999.
119. Borson S, Barnes RA, Kukull WA, et al: Symptomatic depression in elderly medical outpatients: I. Prevalence, demography, and health service utilization. J Am Geriatr Soc 34:341–347, 1986.
120. Sheikh JI, Yesavage JA: Geriatric depression scale: Recent evidence and development of a shorter version. Clin Gerontol 5:165–172, 1986.
121. Salive ME, Cornoni-Huntley J, Guralnik JM, et al: Anemia and hemoglobin levels in older persons: Relationship with age, gender, and health status. J Am Geriatr Soc 40:489–496, 1992.
122. Pfohl B, Sherman B, Schlechte J, Winokur G: Differences in plasma ACTH and cortisol between depressed patients and normal controls. Biol Psychiatry 20:1055–1072, 1985.
123. Pfohl B, Sherman B, Schlechte J, Stone R: Pituitary-adrenal axis rhythm disturbances in psychiatric depression. Arch Gen Psychiatry 42:897–903, 1985.
124. Schlechte JA, Coffman T: Plasma free cortisol in depressive illness: A review of findings and clinical implications. Psychiatr Med 3:23–31, 1985.
125. Miller TP, Taylor J, Rogerson S, et al: Cognitive and noncognitive symptoms in

dementia patients: Relationship to cortisol and dehydroepiandrosterone. Int Psychogeriatr 10:85–96, 1998.

126. Weiner MF, Vobach S, Olsson K, et al: Cortisol secretion and Alzheimer's disease progression. Biol Psychiatry 42:1030–1038, 1997.

127. Deuschle M, Weber B, Colla M, et al: Effects of major depression, aging and gender upon calculated diurnal free plasma cortisol concentrations: A re-evaluation study. Stress 2:281–287, 1998.

128. Ferrier IN, Pascual J, Charlton BG, et al: Cortisol, ACTH, and dexamethasone concentrations in a psychogeriatric population. Biol Psychiatry 23:252–260, 1988.

129. Michelson D, Gold PW: Pathophysiologic and somatic investigations of hypothalamic-pituitary-adrenal axis activation in patients with depression. Ann N Y Acad Sci 840:717–722, 1998.

130. Amsterdam JD, Hooper MB: Bone density measurement in major depression. Prog Neuropsychopharmacol Biol Psychiatry 22:267–277, 1998.

131. Wolkowitz OM, Reus VI, Chan T, et al: Antiglucocorticoid treatment of depression: Double-blind ketoconazole. Biol Psychiatry 45:1070–1074, 1999.

132. Alexopoulos GS, Meyers BS, Young RC, et al: The course of geriatric depression with "reversible dementia": A controlled study. Am J Psychiatry 150:1693–1699, 1993.

133. Raskind MA: The clinical interface of depression and dementia. J Clin Psychiatry 59(suppl 10):9–12, 1998.

134. Pearson JL, Teri L, Reifler BV, Raskind MA: Functional status and cognitive impairment in Alzheimer's patients with and without depression. J Am Geriatr Soc 37:1117–1121, 1989.

135. Raskind MA: Geriatric psychopharmacology: Management of late-life depression and the noncognitive behavioral disturbances of Alzheimer's disease. Psychiatr Clin North Am 16:815–827, 1993.

136. Benbow SM: The role of electroconvulsive therapy in the treatment of depressive illness in old age. Br J Psychiatry 155:147–152, 1989.

137. Baldwin RC, Jolley DJ: The prognosis of depression in old age. Br J Psychiatry 149:574–583, 1986.

138. Kawas CH: Alzheimer's disease. *In* Hazzard WR, Blass JP, Ettinger WH Jr, et al (eds): Principles of Geriatric Medicine and Gerontology, ed 4. New York, McGraw-Hill, 1999, pp 1257–1270.

139. Small GW, Rabins PV, Barry PP, et al: Diagnosis and treatment of Alzheimer disease and related disorders. Consensus statement of the American Association for Geriatric Psychiatry, the Alzheimer's Association, and the American Geriatrics Society. JAMA 278:1363–1371, 1997.

140. Barrett JJ, Haley WE, Harrell LE, Powers RE: Knowledge about Alzheimer disease among primary care physicians, psychologists, nurses, and social workers. Alzheimer Dis Assoc Disord 1:99–106, 1997.

141. Mega MS, Cummings JL, Fiorello T, Gornbein J: The spectrum of behavioral changes in Alzheimer's disease. Neurology 46:130–135, 1996.

142. Folstein MF, Folstein S, McHugh PR: "Mini-mental state": A practical method of grading the cognitive state of patients for the clinician. J Psychiatr Res 12:189–198, 1975.

143. Wolf-Klein GP, Silverstone FA, Levy AP, Brod MS: Screening for Alzheimer's disease by clock drawing. J Am Geriatr Soc 37:730–734, 1989.

144. Watson YI, Arfken CL, Birge SJ: Clock completion: An objective screening test for dementia. J Am Geriatr Soc 41:1235–1240, 1993.

145. Tune LE: Delirium. *In* Hazzard WR, Blass JP, Ettinger WH Jr, et al (eds): Principles of Geriatric Medicine and Gerontology, ed 4. New York, McGraw-Hill, 1999, pp 1229–1237.

146. Sandberg O, Gustafson Y, Brannstrom B, Bucht G: Clinical profile of delirium in older patients. J Am Geriatr Soc 47:1300–1306, 1999.

147. Rudberg MA, Pompei P, Foreman MD, et al: The natural history of delirium in older hospitalized patients: A syndrome of heterogeneity. Age Ageing 26:169–174, 1997.

148. Chan D, Brennan NJ: Delirium: Making the diagnosis, improving the prognosis. Geriatrics 54:28–30, 36, 39–42, 1999.

149. Inouye SK, Schlesinger MJ, Lydon TJ: Delirium: A symptom of how hospital care is failing older persons and a window to improve quality of hospital care. Am J Med 106:565–573, 1999.

150. Inouye SK, Bogardus ST Jr, Charpentier PA, et al: A multicomponent intervention to prevent delirium in hospitalized older patients. N Engl J Med 340:669–676, 1999.

151. Inouye SK: Predisposing and precipitating factors for delirium in hospitalized older patients. Dement Geriatr Cogn Disord 10:393–400, 1999.

152. Francis J, Kapoor WN: Delirium in hospitalized elderly. J Gen Intern Med 5:65–79, 1990.

153. Francis J, Martin D, Kapoor WN: A prospective study of delirium in hospitalized elderly. JAMA 263:1097–1101, 1990.

154. Foreman MD, Mion LC, Tryostad L, Fletcher K: Standard of practice protocol: Acute confusion/delirium. Geriatr Nurs 20:147–152, 1999.

155. Jacobson SA: Delirium in the elderly. Psychiatr Clin North Am 20:91–110, 1997.

156. Blair, BD: Delirium. *In* Cobbs EL, Duthie EH, Murphy JB (eds): Geriatrics Review Syllabus: A Core Curriculum in Geriatric Medicine, ed 4. New York, American Geriatrics Society, and Dubuque, IA, Kendall/Hunt, 1999, pp 111–115.

157. Inouye SK, van Dyck CH, Alessi CA, et al: Clarifying confusion: The confusion assessment method: A new method for detection of delirium. Ann Intern Med 113:941–948, 1990.

158. Lerner AJ, Hedera P, Koss E, et al: Delirium in Alzheimer disease. Alzheimer Dis Assoc Disord 11:16–20, 1997.

159. Levkoff SE, Evans DA, Liptzin B, et al: Delirium: The occurrence and persistence of symptoms among elderly hospitalized patients. Arch Intern Med 152:334–340, 1992.

160. Rockwood K: The occurrence and duration of symptoms in elderly patients with delirium. J Gerontol 48:M162–M166, 1993.

161. Murray AM, Levkoff SE, Wetle TT, et al: Acute delirium and functional decline in the hospitalized elderly patient. J Gerontol 48:M181–M186, 1993.

162. Prinz PN, Vitiello MV, Raskind MA, Thorpy MJ: Geriatrics: Sleep disorders and aging. N Engl J Med 323:520–526, 1990.

163. Floyd JA: Sleep promotion in adults. Annu Rev Nurs Res 17:27–56, 1999.

164. Ancoli-Israel S: Sleep problems in older adults: Putting myths to bed. Geriatrics 52:20–30, 1997.

165. Dijk DJ, Duffy JF: Circadian regulation of human sleep and age-related changes in its timing, consolidation and EEG characteristics. Ann Med 31:130–140, 1999.

166. Asplund R: The nocturnal polyuria syndrome (NPS). Gen Pharmacol 26:1203–1209, 1995.

167. Schwartz AR, Smith PL: Sleep apnea in the elderly. Clin Geriatr Med 5:315–329, 1989.

168. Levy P, Pepin JL, Malauzat D, et al: Is sleep apnea syndrome in the elderly a specific entity? Sleep 19(suppl):29–38, 1996.

169. Vitiello MV: Effective treatments for age-related sleep disturbances. Geriatrics 54:47–52, 1999.

170. Haponik EF, McCall WV: Sleep problems. *In* Hazzard WR, Blass JP, Ettinger WH Jr, et al (eds): Principles of Geriatric Medicine and Gerontology, ed 4. New York, McGraw-Hill, 1999, pp 1413–1428.

171. Kwentus JA: Sleep problems. *In* Cobbs EL, Duthie EH, Murphy JB (eds): Geriatrics Review Syllabus: A Core Curriculum in Geriatric Medicine, ed 4. New York, American Geriatrics Society, and Dubuque, IA, Kendall/Hunt, 1999, pp 159–164.

172. Kern W, Dodt C, Born J, Fehm HL: Changes in cortisol and growth hormone secretion during nocturnal sleep in the course of aging. J Gerontol A Biol Sci Med Sci 51:M3–M9, 1996.

173. Van Cauter E, Plat L: Physiology of growth hormone secretion during sleep. J Pediatr 128(suppl):32–37, 1996.

174. Van Cauter E, Plat L, Copinschi G: Interrelations between sleep and the somatotropic axis. Sleep 21:553–566, 1998.

175. Magri F, Locatelli M, Balza G, et al: Changes in endocrine circadian rhythms as markers of physiological and pathological brain aging. Chronobiol Int 14:385–396, 1997.

176. Rosenow F, McCarthy V, Caruso AC: Sleep apnoea in endocrine diseases. J Sleep Res 7:3–11, 1998.

177. Gruenewald DA, Matsumoto AM: Aging of the endocrine system. *In* Hazzard WR, Blass JP, Ettinger WH Jr, et al (eds): Principles of Geriatric Medicine and Gerontology, ed 4. New York, McGraw-Hill, 1999, pp 949–965.

178. Brzezinski A: Melatonin in humans. N Engl J Med 336:186–195, 1997.

179. Zeitzer JM, Daniels JE, Duffy JF, et al: Do plasma melatonin concentrations decline with age? Am J Med 107:432–436, 1999.

180. Wetterberg L: Melatonin and clinical application. Reprod Nutr Dev 39:367–382, 1999.

181. Zisapel N: The use of melatonin for the treatment of insomnia. Biol Signals Recept 8:84–89, 1999.

182. Bubenik GA, Blask DE, Brown GM, et al: Prospects of the clinical utilization of melatonin. Biol Signals Recept 7:195–219, 1998.

183. Avery D, Lenz M, Landis C: Guidelines for prescribing melatonin. Ann Med 30:122–130, 1998.

184. Sack RL, Lewy AJ, Hughes RJ: Use of melatonin for sleep and circadian rhythm disorders. Ann Med 30:115–121, 1998.

185. Papanicolaou DA, Yanovski JA, Cutler GB Jr, et al: A single midnight serum cortisol measurement distinguishes Cushing's syndrome from pseudo-Cushing states. J Clin Endocrinol Metab 83:1163–1167, 1998.

186. Berwaerts JJ, Verhelst JA, Verhaert GC, et al: Corticotropin-dependent Cushing's syndrome in older people: Presentation of five cases and therapeutical use of ketoconazole. J Am Geriatr Soc 46:880–884, 1998.

187. Wilkinson CW, Peskind ER, Raskind MA: Decreased hypothalamic-pituitary-adrenal axis sensitivity to cortisol feedback inhibition in human aging. Neuroendocrinology 65:79–90, 1997.

188. Butler RN, Lewis MI: Sexuality and aging. *In* Hazzard WR, Blass JP, Ettinger WH Jr, et al (eds): Principles of Geriatric Medicine and Gerontology, ed 4. New York, McGraw-Hill, 1999, pp 171–178.

189. Arlt W, Callies F, van Vlijmen JC, et al: Dehydroepiandrosterone replacement in women with adrenal insufficiency. N Engl J Med 341:1013–1020, 1999.

190. Basaria S, Dobs AS: Risks versus benefits of testosterone therapy in elderly men. Drugs Aging 15:131–142, 1999.

191. Tenover LJ: Trophic factors and male hormone replacement. *In* Hazzard WR, Blass JP, Ettinger WH Jr, et al (eds): Principles of Geriatric Medicine and Gerontology, ed 4. New York, McGraw-Hill, 1999, pp 1029–1040.

192. Hoffman AR, Lieberman SA, Butterfield G, et al: Functional consequences of the somatopause and its treatment. Endocrine 7:73–76, 1997.

193. Savine R, Sonksen PH: Is the somatopause an indication for growth hormone replacement? J Endocrinol Invest 22(5 suppl):142–149, 1999.

194. von Werder K: The somatopause is no indication for growth hormone therapy. J Endocrinol Invest 22(5 suppl):137–141, 1999.

195. O'Connor KG, Harman SM, Stevens TE, et al: Interrelationships of spontaneous growth hormone axis activity, body fat, and serum lipids in healthy elderly women and men. Metabolism 48:1424–1431, 1999.

196. Toogood AA, Shalet SM: Ageing and growth hormone status. Baillieres Clin Endocrinol Metab 12:281–296, 1998.

197. Russell-Aulet M, Jaffe CA, Demott-Friberg R, Barkan AL: In vivo semiquantification of hypothalamic growth hormone–releasing hormone (GHRH) output in humans: Evidence for relative GHRH deficiency in aging. J Clin Endocrinol Metab 84:3490–3497, 1999.

198. degli Uberti EC, Ambrosio MR, Cella SG, et al: Defective hypothalamic growth hormone (GH)-releasing hormone activity may contribute to declining GH secretion with age in man. J Clin Endocrinol Metab 82:2885–2888, 1997.

199. Mulligan T, Jaen-Vinuales A, Godschalk M, et al: Synthetic somatostatin analog (octreotide) suppresses daytime growth hormone secretion equivalently in young and older men: Preserved pituitary responsiveness to somatostatin's inhibition in aging. J Am Geriatr Soc 47:1422–1424, 1999.

200. Smith RE, Feighner S, Prendergast K, et al: A new orphan receptor involved in pulsatile growth hormone release. Trends Endocrinol Metab 10:128–135, 1999.

201. Boonen S, Lesaffre E, Aerssens J, et al: Deficiency of the growth hormone–insulin-like growth factor-I axis potentially involved in age-related alterations in body composition. Gerontology 42:330–338, 1996.

202. Boonen S, Aerssens J, Dequeker J: Age-related endocrine deficiencies and fractures of the proximal femur: I. Implications of growth hormone deficiency in the elderly. J Endocrinol 149:7–12, 1996.

203. Thorner MO: Theodore R. Woodward Award. Age-related decline in growth hormone secretion: Clinical significance and potential reversibility. Trans Am Clin Climatol Assoc 108:99–108, 1996.

204. Welle S: Growth hormone and insulin-like growth factor-I as anabolic agents. Curr Opin Clin Nutr Metab Care 1:257–262, 1998.

205. Morley JE: Growth hormone: Fountain of youth or death hormone? J Am Geriatr Soc 47:1475–1476, 1999.

206. Papadakis MA, Grady D, Black D, et al: Growth hormone replacement in healthy older men improves body composition but not functional ability. Ann Intern Med 124:708–716, 1996.

207. Bouillanne O, Rainfray M, Tissandier O, et al: Growth hormone therapy in elderly people: An age-delaying drug? Fund Clin Pharmacol 10:416–430, 1996.

208. Cuttica CM, Castoldi L, Gorrini GP, et al: Effects of six-month administration of recombinant human growth hormone to healthy elderly subjects. Aging (Milano) 9:193–197, 1997.

209. Toogood AA, Jones J, O'Neill PA, et al: The diagnosis of severe growth hormone deficiency in elderly patients with hypothalamic-pituitary disease. Clin Endocrinol (Oxf) 48:569–576, 1998.

210. Toogood AA, Shalet SM: Growth hormone replacement therapy in the elderly with hypothalamic-pituitary disease: A dose-finding study. J Clin Endocrinol Metab 84:131–136, 1999.

211. Toogood AA, O'Neill PA, Shalet SM: Beyond the somatopause: Growth hormone deficiency in adults over the age of 60 years. J Clin Endocrinol Metab 81:460–465, 1996.

212. Toogood AA, Adams JE, O'Neill PA, Shalet SM: Body composition in growth hormone deficient adults over the age of 60 years. Clin Endocrinol (Oxf) 45:399–405, 1996.

213. Toogood AA, Shalet SM: Growth hormone deficiency in the elderly. Curr Ther Endocrinol Metab 6:645–649, 1997.

214. Toogood AA, Adams JE, O'Neill PA, Shalet SM: Elderly patients with adult-onset growth hormone deficiency are not osteopenic. J Clin Endocrinol Metab 82:1462–1466, 1997.

215. Gill MS, Toogood AA, O'Neill PA, et al: Urinary growth hormone (GH), insulin-like growth factor I (IGF-I), and IGF-binding protein-3 measurements in the diagnosis of adult GH deficiency. J Clin Endocrinol Metab 83:2562–2565, 1998.

216. Nicolson A, Toogood AA, Rahim A, Shalet SM: The prevalence of severe growth hormone deficiency in adults who received growth hormone replacement in childhood. Clin Endocrinol (Oxf) 44:311–316, 1996.

217. Colao A, Cuocolo A, Di Somma C, et al: Impaired cardiac performance in elderly patients with growth hormone deficiency. J Clin Endocrinol Metab 84:3950–3955, 1999.

218. Span JP, Pieters GF, Sweep CG, et al: Plasma IGF-I is a useful marker of growth hormone deficiency in adults. J Endocrinol Invest 22:446–450, 1999.

219. Hilding A, Hall K, Wivall-Helleryd IL, et al: Serum levels of insulin-like growth factor I in 152 patients with growth hormone deficiency, aged 19–82 years, in relation to those in healthy subjects. J Clin Endocrinol Metab 84:2013–2019, 1999.

220. Hall K, Hilding A, Thoren M: Determinants of circulating insulin-like growth factor-I. J Endocrinol Invest 22(5 suppl):48–57, 1999.

221. O'Connor KG, Tobin JD, Harman SM, et al: Serum levels of insulin-like growth factor-I are related to age and not to body composition in healthy women and men. J Gerontol A Biol Sci Med Sci 53:M176–M182, 1998.

222. Chapman IM, Bach MA, Van Cauter E, et al: Stimulation of the growth hormone (GH)–insulin-like growth factor I axis by daily oral administration of a GH secretogogue (MK-677) in healthy elderly subjects. J Clin Endocrinol Metab 81:4249–4257, 1996.

223. Merriam GR, Buchner DM, Prinz PN, et al: Potential applications of GH secretagogs in the evaluation and treatment of the age-related decline in growth hormone secretion. Endocrine 7:49–52, 1997.

224. Arvat E, Camanni F, Ghigo E: Age-related growth hormone–releasing activity of growth hormone secretagogues in humans. Acta Paediatr Suppl 423:92–96, 1997.

225. Vittone J, Blackman MR, Busby-Whitehead J, et al: Effects of single nightly injections of growth hormone–releasing hormone (GHRH 1–29) in healthy elderly men. Metabolism 46:89–96, 1997.

226. Lavizzo-Mourey R, Johnson J, Stolley P: Risk factors for dehydration among elderly nursing home residents. J Am Geriatr Soc 36:213–218, 1988.

227. Kennedy PG, Mitchell DM, Hoffbrand BI: Severe hyponatremia in hospital inpatients. BMJ 2:1251–1253, 1978.

228. Tierney WM, Martin DK, Greenlee MC, et al: The prognosis of hyponatremia at hospital admission. J Gen Intern Med 1:380–385, 1986.

229. Snyder NA, Feigal DW, Arieff AI: Hypernatremia in elderly patients: A heterogeneous, morbid, and iatrogenic entity. Ann Intern Med 107:309–319, 1987.

230. Palevsky PM, Bhagrath R, Greenberg A: Hypernatremia in hospitalized patients. Ann Intern Med 124:197–203, 1996.

231. Kaysen GA, Myers BD: The aging kidney. Clin Geriatr Med 1:207–222, 1985.

232. Hoffman NB: Dehydration in the elderly: Insidious and manageable. Geriatrics 46:35–38, 1991.

233. Rolls BJ, Phillips PA: Aging and disturbances of thirst and fluid balance. Nutr Rev 48:137–144, 1990.

234. Robertson GL: Thirst and vasopressin function in normal and disordered states of water balance. J Lab Clin Med 101:351–371, 1983.

235. Phillips PA, Rolls BJ, Ledingham JG, et al: Reduced thirst after water deprivation in healthy elderly men. N Engl J Med 311:753–759, 1984.

236. Phillips PA, Bretherton M, Johnston CI, Gray L: Reduced osmotic thirst in healthy elderly men. Am J Physiol 261:R166–R171, 1991.

237. Phillips PA, Bretherton M, Risvanis J, et al: Effects of drinking on thirst and vasopressin in dehydrated elderly men. Am J Physiol 264:R877–R881, 1993.

238. Mack GW, Weseman CA, Langhans GW, et al: Body fluid balance in dehydrated healthy older men: Thirst and renal osmoregulation. J Appl Physiol 76:1615–1623, 1994.

239. Davies I, O'Neill PA, McLean KA, et al: Age-associated alterations in thirst and arginine vasopressin in response to a water or sodium load. Age Ageing 24:151–159, 1995.

240. Mukherjee AP, Coni NK, Davison W: Osmoreceptor function among the elderly. Gerontol Clin (Basel) 15:227–233, 1973.

241. McAloon Dyke M, Davis KM, Clark BA, et al: Effects of hypertonicity on water intake in the elderly: An age-related failure. Geriatr Nephrol Urol 7:11–16, 1997.

242. de Castro JM: Age-related changes in natural spontaneous fluid ingestion and thirst in humans. J Gerontol 47:321–330, 1992.

243. Rowe JW, Andres RA, Tobin JD, et al: The effect of age on creatinine clearance in men: A cross-sectional and longitudinal study. J Gerontol 31:155–163, 1976.

244. Davies DF, Shock NW: Age changes in glomerular filtration, effective renal plasma flow and tubular excretory capacity in adult males. J Clin Invest 29:496–506, 1950.

245. Hollenberg NK, Adams DF, Solomon HS, et al: Senescence and the renal vasculature in normal man. Circ Res 34:309–316, 1974.

246. Crowe MJ, Forsling ML, Rolls BJ, et al: Altered water excretion in healthy elderly men. Age Ageing 16:285–293, 1987.

247. Dontas AS, Karkenos S, Papanayioutou P: Mechanisms of renal tubular defects in old age. Postgrad Med J 48:295–303, 1972.

248. Lye M: Electrolyte disorders in the elderly. Clin Endocrinol Metab 13:377–398, 1984.

249. Lindeman RD, Van Buren C, Raisz LG: Osmolar renal concentrating ability in healthy young men and hospitalized patients without renal disease. N Engl J Med 262:1306–1309, 1960.

250. Rowe JW, Shock NW, DeFronzo RA: The influence of age on the renal response to water deprivation in man. Nephron 17:270–278, 1976.

251. Lewis WH, Alving AS: Changes with age in the renal function in adult men. Am J Physiol 123:500–515, 1938.

252. Miller JH, Shock NW: Age differences in the renal tubular response to antidiuretic hormone. J Gerontol 8:446–450, 1953.

253. Miller M: Influence of aging on vasopressin secretion and water regulation. In Schrier RW (ed): Vasopressin. New York, Raven, 1985, pp 249–258.

254. Epstein M, Hollenberg NK: Renal salt wasting despite apparently normal renal, adrenal and central nervous system function. Nephron 24:121–126, 1979.

255. Macias Nunez JF, Bondia Roman AB, Rodriguez Commes JL: Physiology and disorders of water balance and electrolytes in the elderly. In Macias Nunez JF, Cameron JS (eds): Renal Function and Disease in the Elderly. London, Butterworth, 1987, pp 67–93.

256. Macias Nunez JF, Iglesias GC, Bondia RA, et al: Renal handling of sodium in old people: A functional study. Age Ageing 7:178–181, 1978.

257. Helderman JH, Vestal RE, Rowe JW, et al: The response of arginine vasopressin to intravenous ethanol and hypertonic saline in man: The impact of aging. J Gerontol 33:39–47, 1978.

258. Chiodera P, Capretti L, Marchesi M, et al: Abnormal arginine vasopressin response to cigarette smoking and metoclopramide (but not to insulin-induced hypoglycemia) in elderly subjects. J Gerontol 46:M6–M10, 1991.

259. Duggan J, Kilfeather S, Lightman SL, O'Malley K: The association of age with plasma arginine vasopressin and plasma osmolality. Age Ageing 22:332–336, 1993.

260. Faull CM, Holmes C, Baylis PH: Water balance in elderly people: Is there a deficiency of vasopressin? Age Ageing 22:114–120, 1993.

261. Clark BA, Elahi D, Fish L, et al: Atrial natriuretic peptide suppresses osmostimulated vasopressin release in young and elderly humans. Am J Physiol 261:E252–E256, 1991.

262. Frolkis VV, Golovchenko SF, Medved VI, Frolkis RA: Vasopressin and cardiovascular system in aging. Gerontology 28:290–302, 1982.

263. Crawford GA, Johnson AG, Gyory AZ, Kelly D: Change in arginine vasopressin concentrations with age. Clin Chem 39:2023, 1993.

264. Kirkland J, Lye M, Goddard C, et al: Plasma arginine vasopressin in dehydrated elderly patients. Clin Endocrinol (Oxf) 20:451–456, 1984.

265. Rondeau L, de Lima J, Caillens H, et al: High plasma antidiuretic hormone in patients with cardiac failure: Influence of age. Miner Electrolyte Metab 8:267–274, 1982.

266. Johnson AG, Crawford GA, Kelly D, et al: Arginine vasopressin and osmolality in the elderly. J Am Geritar Soc 42:399–404, 1994.

267. Kirkland JL, Lye M, Levy DW, Banerjee AK: Patterns of urine flow and electrolyte excretion in healthy elderly people. BMJ 287:1665–1667, 1983.

268. George CP, Messerli FH, Genest J, et al: Diurnal variation of plasma vasopressin in man. J Clin Endocrinol Metab 41:332–338, 1975.

269. Li CH, Hsieh SM, Nagai I: The response of plasma arginine vasopressin to 14 h water deprivation in the elderly. Acta Endocrinol (Copenh) 105:314–317, 1984.

270. Rowe JW, Minaker KL, Sparrow D, Robertson GL: Age-related failure of volume-pressure mediated vasopressin release. J Clin Endocrinol Metab 54:661–664, 1982.

271. Vargas E, Lye M, Faragher EB, et al: Cardiovascular haemodynamics and the response of vasopressin, aldosterone, plasma renin activity and plasma catecholamines to head-up tilt in young and old healthy subjects. Age Ageing 15:17–28, 1986.

272. Robertson GL, Rowe JW: The effect of aging on neurohypophysial function. Peptides 1(suppl):159–162, 1980.

273. Albert SG, Nakra BR, Grossberg GT, Caminal ER: Drinking behavior and vasopressin responses to hyperosmolality in Alzheimer's disease. Int Psychogeriatr 6:79–86, 1994.

274. Espiner EA, Richards AM, Yandle TG, Nicholls MG: Natriuretic hormones. Endocrinol Metab Clin North Am 24:481–509, 1995.

275. Genest J, Larochelle P, Cusson JR, et al: The atrial natriuretic factor in hypertension. State of the art lecture. Hypertension 11(suppl):13–17, 1988.

276. Cuneo RC, Espiner EA, Nicholls MG, et al: Effect of physiological levels of atrial natriuretic peptide on hormone secretion: Inhibition of angiotensin-induced aldosterone secretion and renin release in normal man. J Clin Endocrinol Metab 65:765–772, 1987.

277. Clinkingbeard C, Sessions C, Shenker Y: The physiological role of atrial natriuretic hormone in the regulation of aldosterone and salt and water metabolism. J Clin Endocrinol Metab 70:582–589, 1990.

278. McKnight JA, Roberts G, Sheridan B, Atkinson AB: Relationship between basal and sodium stimulated plasma atrial natriuretic factor, age, sex, and blood pressure in normal man. J Hum Hypertens 3:157–163, 1989.

279. Tajima F, Sagawa S, Iwamoto J, et al: Renal and endocrine responses in the elderly during head-out water immersion. Am J Physiol 254:R977–R983, 1988.

280. Kario K, Nishikimi T, Yoshihara F, et al: Plasma levels of natriuretic peptides and adrenomedullin in elderly hypertensive patients: Relationships to 24 h blood pressure. J Hypertens 16:1253–1259, 1998.

281. Ohashi M, Fujio N, Nawata H, et al: Pharmacokinetics of synthetic alpha-human atrial natriuretic polypeptide in normal men: Effect of aging. Regul Pept 19:265–271, 1987.

282. Heim JM, Gottmann K, Weil J, et al: Effects of a bolus dose of atrial natriuretic factor in young and elderly volunteers. Eur J Clin Invest 19:265–271, 1989.

283. Weidmann P, DeMyttenaere-Bursztein S, Maxwell MH, de Lima J: Effect of aging on plasma renin and aldosterone in normal man. Kidney Int 8:325–333, 1975.

284. Perez GO, Lespier L, Jacobi J, et al: Hyporeninemia and hypoaldosteronism in diabetes mellitus. Arch Intern Med 137:852–855, 1977.

285. Phelps KR, Lieberman RL, Oh MS, Carroll HJ: Pathophysiology of the syndrome of hyporeninemic hypoaldosteronism. Metabolism 29:186–199, 1980.

286. Miller M, Hecker MS, Friedlander DA, Carter JM: Apparent idiopathic hyponatremia in an ambulatory geriatric population. J Am Geriatr Soc 44:404–408, 1996.

287. Miller M, Morley JE, Rubenstein LZ: Hyponatremia in a nursing home population. J Am Geriatr Soc 43:1410–1413, 1995.

288. Baglin A, Prinseau J, Aegerter P, et al: Electrolytic abnormalities in elderly people: Prevalence and relations with medical treatment. Multicentric study of 631 subjects aged 70 years and over. Presse Med 21:1459–1463, 1992.

289. Kleinfeld M, Casimir M, Borra S: Hyponatremia as observed in a chronic disease facility. J Am Geriatr Soc 27:156–161, 1979.

290. Rudman D, Racette D, Rudman IW, et al: Hyponatremia in tube-fed elderly men. J Chronic Dis 39:73–80, 1986.

291. Sunderam SG, Mankikar GD: Hyponatremia in the elderly. Age Ageing 12:77–80, 1983.

292. Beck LH: Aging changes in renal function. In Hazzard WR, Blass JP, Ettinger WH Jr, et al (eds): Principles of Geriatric Medicine and Gerontology, ed 4. New York, McGraw-Hill, 1999, pp 767–776.

293. Miller M: Water balance in older persons. In Morley JE, van den Berg L (eds): Endocrinology of Aging. Totowa, NJ, Humana, 2000, pp 73–92.

294. Castrillon JL, Mediavilla A, Mendez MA, et al: Syndrome of inappropriate antidiuretic hormone secretion (SIADH) and enalapril. J Intern Med 233:89–91, 1993.

295. Crowe M: Hyponatremia due to syndrome of inappropriate antidiuretic hormone secretion in the elderly. Ir Med J 73:482–483, 1980.

296. Goldstein CS, Braunstein S, Goldfarb S: Idiopathic syndrome of inappropriate antidiuretic hormone secretion possibly related to advanced age. Ann Intern Med 99:185–188, 1983.

297. Hirshberg B, Ben-Yehuda A: The syndrome of inappropriate antidiuretic hormone secretion in the elderly. Am J Med 103:270–273, 1997.

298. Davis KM, Minaker KL: Disorders of fluid balance: Dehydration and hyponatremia. In Hazzard WR, Blass JP, Ettinger WH Jr, et al (eds): Principles of Geriatric Medicine and Gerontology, ed 4. New York, McGraw-Hill, 1999, pp 1429–1436.

299. Zarinetchi F, Berl T: Evaluation and management of severe hyponatremia. Adv Intern Med 41:251–283, 1996.

300. Spital A: Hyponatremic encephalopathy. Am J Med 103:251–252, 1997.

301. Hantman D, Rossier B, Zohlman R, Schrier R: Rapid correction of hyponatremia in the syndrome of inappropriate secretion of antidiuretic hormone: An alternative treatment to hypertonic saline. Ann Intern Med 78:870–875, 1973.

302. Sterns RH, Cappuccio JD, Silver SM, Cohen EP: Neurologic sequelae after treatment of severe hyponatremia: A multicenter perspective. J Am Soc Nephrol 4:1522–1530, 1994.

303. Palevsky PM, Bhagrath R, Greenberg A: Hypernatremia in hospitalized patients. Ann Intern Med 124:197–203, 1996.

304. Borra SI, Beredo R, Kleinfeld M: Hypernatremia in the aging: Causes, manifestations, and outcome. J Natl Med Assoc 87:220–224, 1995.

305. Baylis PH, Thompson CJ: Osmoregulation of vasopressin secretion and thirst in health and disease. Clin Endocrinol 29:549–576, 1988.

306. Moore FD: Common patterns of water and electrolyte change in injury, surgery and disease. N Engl J Med 238:377–384, 1958.

307. Kahn T: Hypernatremia with edema. Arch Intern Med 159:93–98, 1999.

308. Albert SG, Nakra BR, Grossberg GT, Caminal ER: Vasopressin response to dehydration in Alzheimer's disease. J Am Geriatr Soc 37:843–847, 1989.

309. Reding MJ, DiPonte P: Vasopressin in Alzheimer's disease. Neurology 33:1634–1635, 1983.

310. Peskind ER, Pascualy M, Edland SD, et al: Plasma arginine vasopressin response to hypertonic saline infusion in Alzheimer disease. Alzheimer Dis Assoc Disord 9:238–242, 1995.

311. Norbiato G, Bevilacqua M, Carella F, et al: Alterations in vasopressin regulation in Alzheimer's disease. J Neurol Neurosurg Psychiatry 51:903–908, 1988.

312. Ouslander JG, Johnson TM II: Incontinence. In Hazzard WR, Blass JP, Ettinger WH Jr, et al (eds): Principles of Geriatric Medicine and Gerontology, ed 4. New York, McGraw-Hill, 1999, pp 1595–1614.

313. Seiler WO, Stahelin HB, Hefti U: Desmopressin reduces night urine volume in geriatric patients: Implications for treatment of the nocturnal incontinence. Clin Invest 70:619, 1992.

314. Asplund R, Sundberg B, Bengtsson P: Desmopressin for the treatment of nocturnal polyuria in the elderly: A dose titration study. Br J Urol 82:642–646, 1998.

315. Asplund R, Sundberg B, Bengtsson P: Oral desmopressin for nocturnal polyuria in elderly subjects: A double-blind, placebo-controlled randomized exploratory study. Br J Urol 83:591–595, 1999.

316. Hourihane J, Salisbury AJ: Use caution in prescribing desmopressin for nocturnal enuresis. BMJ 306:1545, 1993.

317. Bernstein SA, Williford SL: Intranasal desmopressin–associated hyponatremia: A case report and literature review. J Fam Pract 44:203–208, 1997.

318. Singh I, Marshall MC: Diabetes mellitus in the elderly. Endocrinol Metab Clin North Am 24:255–272, 1995.

319. Samos LF, Roos BA: Diabetes mellitus in older persons. Med Clin North Am 82:791–803, 1998.

320. Morley JE: An overview of diabetes mellitus in older persons. Clin Geriatr Med 15:211–224, 1999.

321. Sinclair AJ: Diabetes in the elderly: A perspective from the United Kingdom. Clin Geriatr Med 15:225–237, 1999.

322. Halter JB: Diabetes mellitus. In Hazzard WR, Blass JP, Ettinger WH Jr, et al (eds): Principles of Geriatric Medicine and Gerontology, ed 4. New York, McGraw-Hill, 1999, pp 991–1012.

323. Glynn RJ, Monane M, Gurwitz JH, et al: Aging, comorbidity, and reduced rates of drug treatment for diabetes mellitus. J Clin Epidemiol 52:781–790, 1999.

324. Harris MI: Undiagnosed NIDDM: Clinical and public health issues. Diabetes Care 16:642–652, 1993.

325. Harris MI, Robbins DC: Prevalence of adult-onset IDDM in the U.S. population. Diabetes Care 17:1337–1340, 1994.

326. Stolk RP, Pols HA, Lamberts SW, et al: Diabetes mellitus, impaired glucose tolerance, and hyperinsulinemia in an elderly population. The Rotterdam Study. Am J Epidemiol 145:24–32, 1997.

327. Burke JP, Williams K, Gaskill SP, et al: Rapid rise in the incidence of type 2 diabetes from 1987 to 1996: Results from the San Antonio Heart Study. Arch Intern Med 159:1450–1456, 1999.

328. Cassano PA, Rosner B, Vokonas PS, Weiss ST: Obesity and body fat distribution in relation to the incidence of non–insulin-dependent diabetes mellitus. A prospective cohort study of men in the normative aging study. Am J Epidemiol 136:1474–1486, 1992.

329. Mokdad AH, Serdula MK, Dietz WH, et al: The spread of the obesity epidemic in the United States, 1991–1998. JAMA 282:1519–1522, 1999.

330. Meneilly GS: Pathophysiology of type 2 diabetes in the elderly. Clin Geriatr Med 15:239–253, 1999.

331. Mott JW, Wang J, Thornton JC, et al: Relation between body fat and age in 4 ethnic groups. Am J Clin Nutr 69:1007–1103, 1999.

332. Reaven GM: Beneficial effect of moderate weight loss in older patients with non–insulin-dependent diabetes mellitus poorly controlled with insulin. J Am Geriatr Soc 33:93–95, 1985.

333. Spiegelman B, Peraldi P: TNF-alpha and insulin resistance: Summary and future prospects. Mol Cell Biochem 182:169–175, 1998.

334. Sethi JK, Hotamisligil GS: The role of TNF alpha in adipocyte metabolism. Semin Cell Dev Biol 10:19–29, 1999.

335. Alessi MC, Peiretti F, Morange P, et al: Production of plasminogen activator inhibitor 1 by human adipose tissue: Possible link between visceral fat accumulation and vascular disease. Diabetes 46:860–867, 1997.

336. Rosenthal MJ, Fajardo M, Gilmore S, et al: Hospitalization and mortality of diabetes in older adults: A 3-year prospective study. Diabetes Care 21:231–235, 1998.

337. Petterson T, Lee P, Hollis S, et al: Well-being and treatment satisfaction in older people with diabetes. Diabetes Care 21:930–935, 1998.

338. Sinclair AJ, Robert IE, Croxson SC: Mortality in older people with diabetes mellitus. Diabet Med 14:639–647, 1997.

339. Viinamaki H, Niskanen L, Uusitupa M: Mental well-being in people with non–insulin-dependent diabetes mellitus. Acta Psychiatr Scand 92:392–397, 1995.

340. Meneilly GS, Cheung E, Tessier D, et al: The effect of improved glycemic control on cognitive functions in the elderly patient with diabetes. J Gerontol 48:M117–M121, 1993.

341. Gradman TJ, Laws A, Thompson LW, Reaven GM: Verbal learning and/or memory improves with glycemic control in older subjects with non–insulin-dependent diabetes mellitus. J Am Geriatr Soc 41:1305–1312, 1993.

342. Ott A, Stolk RP, van Harskamp F, et al: Diabetes mellitus and the risk of dementia. The Rotterdam Study. Neurology 53:1937–1942, 1999.

343. Stewart R, Liolitsa D: Type 2 diabetes mellitus, cognitive impairment and dementia. Diabet Med 16:93–112, 1999.

344. Boston PF, Dennis MS, Jagger C: Factors associated with vascular dementia in an elderly community population. Int J Geriatr Psychiatry 14:761–766, 1999.

345. Lovestone S: Diabetes and dementia: Is the brain another site of end-organ damage? Neurology 53:1907–1909, 1999.

346. Diabetes Control and Complications Trial Research Group: The effect of intensive treatment of diabetes on the development and progression of long-term complications in insulin-dependent diabetes mellitus. N Engl J Med 329:977–986, 1993.

347. UK Prospective Diabetes Study Group (UKPDS 33): Intensive blood-glucose control with sulphonylureas or insulin compared with conventional treatment and risk of complications in patients with type 2 diabetes. Lancet 352:837–853, 1998.

348. UK Prospective Diabetes Study Group (UKPDS 34): Effect of intensive blood-glucose control with metformin on complications in overweight patients with type 2 diabetes. Lancet 352:854–865, 1998.

349. American Diabetes Association: Clinical practice recommendations 2000. Diabetes Care 23(suppl 1):1–116, 2000.

350. Edelstein SL, Knowler WC, Bain RP, et al: Predictor of progression from impaired glucose tolerance to NIDDM: An analysis of six prospective studies. Diabetes 46:701–710, 1997.

351. Leslie RD, Pozzilli P: Type I diabetes masquerading as type II diabetes: Possible implications for prevention and treatment. Diabetes Care 17:1214–1219, 1994.

352. Gambert SR: Atypical presentation of diabetes mellitus in the elderly. Clin Geriatr Med 6:721–729, 1990.

353. Muggeo M: Accelerated complications in type 2 diabetes mellitus: The need for greater awareness and earlier detection. Diabet Med 15(suppl 4):60–62, 1998.

354. Cohen DL, Neil HA, Thorogood M, Mann JI: A population-based study of the incidence of complications associated with type 2 diabetes in the elderly. Diabet Med 8:928–933, 1991.

355. Naliboff BD, Rosenthal M: Effects of age on complications in adult onset diabetes. J Am Geriatr Soc 37:838–842, 1989.

356. Greene DA: Acute and chronic complications of diabetes mellitus in older patients. Am J Med 80:39–53, 1986.

357. Yki-Jarvinen H: Toxicity of hyperglycaemia in type 2 diabetes. Diabetes Metab Rev 14(suppl 1):45–50, 1998.

358. Vehkavaara S, Seppala-Lindroos A, Westerbacka J, et al: In vivo endothelial dysfunction characterizes patients with impaired fasting glucose. Diabetes Care 22:2055–2060, 1999.

359. Jonas JC, Sharma A, Hasenkamp W, et al: Chronic hyperglycemia triggers loss of pancreatic beta cell differentiation in an animal model of diabetes. J Biol Chem 274:14112–14121, 1999.

360. Virkamaki A, Yki-Jarvinen H: Allosteric regulation of glycogen synthase and hexokinase by glucosamine-6-phosphate during glucosamine-induced insulin resistance in skeletal muscle and heart. Diabetes 48:1101–1107, 1999.

361. Joshi N, Caputo GM, Weitekamp MR, Karchmer AW: Infections in patients with diabetes mellitus. N Engl J Med 341:1906–1912, 1999.

362. Bradley SF: Infectious diseases. In Reuben DR, Yoshikawa TT, Besdine RW (eds): Geriatrics Review Syllabus: A Core Curriculum in Geriatric Medicine, ed 3. New York, American Geriatrics Society, and Dubuque, IA, Kendall/Hunt, 1996, pp 264–273.

363. Levin ME: Preventing amputation in the patient with diabetes. Diabetes Care 18:1383–1394, 1995.

364. Morley JE, Kaiser FE: Unique aspects of diabetes mellitus in the elderly. Clin Geriatr Med 6:721–729, 1990.

365. Neil HA, Dawson JA, Baker JE: Risk of hypothermia in elderly patients with diabetes. BMJ 293:416–418, 1986.

366. Hofbauer MH, Puleo D: Idiopathic diabetic bullosum. J Am Podiatr Med Assoc 81:613–617, 1991.

367. Friedman NA, LaBan MM: Periarthrosis of the shoulder associated with diabetes mellitus. Am J Phys Med Rehabil 68:12–14, 1989.

368. Sander HW, Chokroverty S: Diabetic amyotrophy: Current concepts. Semin Neurol 16:173–178, 1996.

369. Ellenberg M: Diabetic neuropathic cachexia. Diabetes 23:418–423, 1974.

370. Lorber D: Nonketotic hypertonicity in diabetes mellitus. Med Clin North Am 79:39–52, 1995.

371. Matz R: Management of the hyperosmolar hyperglycemic syndrome. Am Fam Physician 60:1468–1476, 1999.

372. Arieff AI: Cerebral edema complicating nonketotic hyperosmolar coma. Miner Electrolyte Metab 12:383–389, 1986.

373. Malone ML, Gennis V, Goodwin JS: Characteristics of diabetic ketoacidosis in older versus younger adults. J Am Geriatr Soc 40:1100–1104, 1992.

374. McKenna K, Morris AD, Azam H, et al: Exaggerated vasopressin secretion and attenuated osmoregulated thirst in human survivors of hyperosmolar coma. Diabetologia 42:534–538, 1999.

375. American Diabetes Association: Implications of the Diabetes Control and Complications Trial (position statement). Diabetes Care 23(suppl 1):24–26, 2000.

376. American Diabetes Association: Implications of the United Kingdom Prospective Diabetes Study (position statement). Diabetes Care 23(suppl l):27–31, 2000.

377. UK Prospective Diabetes Study Group: Tight blood pressure control and risk of macrovascular and microvascular complications in type 2 diabetes (UKPDS 38). BMJ 317:703–713, 1998.

378. American Diabetes Association: Management of dyslipidemia in adults with diabetes (position statement). Diabetes Care 23(suppl 1):57–60, 2000.

379. Heller FR: Prevention of cardiovascular events by hypolipidemic therapy: Evidence-based medicine criteria. Acta Clin Belg 54:299–301, 1999.

380. Evans WJ: Exercise and nutritional needs of elderly people: Effects on muscle and bone. Gerontology 15:15–24, 1998.

381. Evans WJ, Cyr-Campbell D: Nutrition, exercise, and healthy aging. J Am Diet Assoc 97:632–638, 1997.

382. Aronow WS: Dizziness and syncope. In Hazzard WR, Blass JP, Ettinger WH Jr, et al (eds): Principles of Geriatric Medicine and Gerontology, ed 4. New York, McGraw-Hill, 1999, pp 1519–1534.

383. Jansen RW, Lipsitz LA: Postprandial hypotension: Epidemiology, pathophysiology, and clinical management. Ann Intern Med 122:286–295, 1995.

384. Vaitkevicius PV, Esserwein DM, Maynard AK, et al: Frequency and importance of postprandial blood pressure reduction in elderly nursing-home patients. Ann Intern Med 115:865–870, 1991.

385. Oberman AS, Harada RK, Gagnon MM, et al: Effects of postprandial walking exercise on meal-related hypotension in frail elderly patients. Am J Cardiol 84:1130–1132, 1999.

386. Jennings PE: Oral antihyperglycaemics. Considerations in older patients with non–insulin-dependent diabetes mellitus. Drugs Aging 10:323–331, 1997.

387. Scheen AJ, Lefebvre PJ: Oral antidiabetic agents: A guide to selection. Drugs 55:225–236, 1998.

388. Harrower AD: Pharmacokinetics of oral antihyperglycaemic agents in patients with renal insufficiency. Clin Pharmacokinet 31:111–119, 1996.

389. Turner RC, Cull CA, Frighi V, Holman RR: Glycemic control with diet, sulfonylurea, metformin, or insulin in patients with type 2 diabetes mellitus: Progressive requirement for multiple therapies (UKPDS 49). UK Prospective Diabetes Study (UKPDS) Group. JAMA 281:2005–2012, 1999.

390. Cryer PE: Symptoms of hypoglycemia, thresholds for their occurrence, and hypoglycemia unawareness. Endocrinol Metab Clin North Am 28:495–500, 1999.

391. Marker JC, Cryer PE, Clutter WE: Attenuated glucose recovery from hypoglycemia in the elderly. Diabetes 41:671–678, 1992.

392. Matyka K, Evans M, Lomas J, et al: Altered hierarchy of protective responses against severe hypoglycemia in normal aging in healthy men. Diabetes Care 20:135–141, 1997.

393. Cryer PE: Symptoms of hypoglycemia, thresholds for their occurrence, and hypoglycemia unawareness. Endocrinol Metab Clin North Am 28:495–500, 1999.

394. Cryer PE: Hypoglycemia is the limiting factor in the management of diabetes. Diabetes Metab Res Rev 15:42–46, 1999.

395. Marker JC, Clutter WE: Cryer PE: Reduced epinephrine clearance and glycemic sensitivity to epinephrine in older individuals. Am J Physiol 275:E770–E776, 1998.

396. Stepka M, Rogala H, Czyzyk A: Hypoglycemia: A major problem in the management of diabetes in the elderly. Aging (Milano) 5:117–121, 1993.

397. Thomson FJ, Masson EA, Leeming JT, Boulton AJ: Lack of knowledge of symptoms of hypoglycaemia by elderly diabetic patients. Age Ageing 20:404–406, 1991.

398. Ortiz-Alonso FJ, Galecki A, Herman WH, et al: Hypoglycemia counterregulation in elderly humans: Relationship to glucose levels. Am J Physiol 267:E497–E506, 1994.

399. Shorr RI, Ray WA, Daugherty JR, Griffin MR: Incidence and risk factors for serious hypoglycemia in older persons using insulin or sulfonylureas. Arch Intern Med 157:1681–1686, 1997.

400. Smith NL, Heckbert SR, Bittner VA, et al: Antidiabetic treatment trends in a cohort of elderly people with diabetes: The Cardiovascular Health Study, 1989–1997. Diabetes Care 22:736–742, 1999.

401. Hauner H: The impact of pharmacotherapy on weight management in type 2 diabetes. Int J Obes Relat Metab Disord 23(suppl 7):12–17, 1999.

402. Boyne MS, Saudek CD: Effect of insulin therapy on macrovascular risk factors in type 2 diabetes. Diabetes Care 22(suppl 3):45–53, 1999.

403. Lebovitz HE: Effects of oral antihyperglycemic agents in modifying macrovascular risk factors in type 2 diabetes. Diabetes Care 22(suppl 3):C41–C44, 1999.

404. Stahl M, Berger W: Higher incidence of severe hypoglycaemia leading to hospital admission in type 2 diabetic patients treated with long-acting versus short-acting sulphonylureas. Diabet Med 16:586–590, 1999.

405. Robertson DA, Home PD: Problems and pitfalls of sulphonylurea therapy in older patients. Drugs Aging 3:510–524, 1993.

406. Kadowaki T, Hagura R, Kajinuma H, et al: Chlorpropamide-induced hyponatremia: Incidence and risk factors. Diabetes Care 6:468–471, 1983.

407. Miller M: Water balance in older persons. In Morley JE, van den Berg L (eds): Endocrinology of Aging. Totowa NJ, Humana, 2000, pp 73–92.

408. Brown JB, Pedula KL: Metformin as secondary therapy in a defined population with type 2 diabetes. Clin Ther 21:1678–1687, 1999.

409. Inzucchi SE, Maggs DG, Spollett GR, et al: Efficacy and metabolic effects of metformin and troglitazone in type II diabetes mellitus. N Engl J Med 338:867–872, 1998.

410. Lalau JD, Vermersch A, Hary L, et al: Type 2 diabetes in the elderly: An assessment of metformin (metformin in the elderly). Int J Clin Pharmacol Ther Toxicol 28:329–332, 1990.

411. Makimattila S, Nikkila K, Yki-Jarvinen H: Causes of weight gain during insulin therapy with and without metformin in patients with type II diabetes mellitus. Diabetologia 42:406–412, 1999.

412. Yki-Jarvinen H, Ryysy L, Nikkila K, et al: Comparison of bedtime insulin regimens in patients with type 2 diabetes mellitus. A randomized, controlled trial. Ann Intern Med 130:389–396, 1999.

413. Chan NN, Brain HP, Feher MD: Metformin-associated lactic acidosis: A rare or very rare clinical entity? Diabet Med 16:273–281, 1999.

414. Thomsen HS, Morcos SK: Contrast media and metformin: Guidelines to diminish the risk of lactic acidosis in non–insulin-dependent diabetics after administration of contrast media. ESUR Contrast Media Safety Committee. Eur Radiol 9:738–740, 1999.

415. McCartney MM, Gilbert FJ, Murchison LE, et al: Metformin and contrast media—a dangerous combination? Clin Radiol 54:29–33, 1999.

416. Johnston PS, Lebovitz HE, Coniff RF, et al: Advantages of alpha-glucosidase inhibition as monotherapy in elderly type 2 diabetic patients. J Clin Endocrinol Metab 83:1515–1522, 1998.

417. Gerstein HC: Glucose: A continuous risk factor for cardiovascular disease. Diabet Med 14(suppl 3):25–31, 1997.

418. Haller H: Postprandial glucose and vascular disease. Diabet Med 14(suppl 3):50–56, 1997.

419. Jovanovic L: Rationale for prevention and treatment of postprandial glucose-mediated toxicity. Endocrinologist 9:87–92, 1999.

420. Schwartz S, Raskin P, Fonseca V, Graveline JF: Effect of troglitazone in insulin-treated patients with type II diabetes mellitus: Troglitazone and Exogenous Insulin Study Group. N Engl J Med 338:861–866, 1998.

421. Plosker GL, Faulds D: Troglitazone: A review of its use in the management of type 2 diabetes mellitus. Drugs 57:409–438, 1999.

422. Wagenaar LJ, Kuck EM, Hoekstra JB: Troglitazone: Is it all over? Neth J Med 55:4–12, 1999.

423. Misbin RI: Troglitazone-associated hepatic failure. Ann Intern Med 130:330, 1999.

424. Herrine SK, Choudhary C: Severe hepatotoxicity associated with troglitazone. Ann Intern Med 130:163–164, 1999.

425. Imura H: A novel antidiabetic drug, troglitazone—reason for hope and concern. N Engl J Med 338:908–909, 1998.

426. Riddle MC: Oral pharmacologic management of type 2 diabetes. Am Fam Physician 60:2613–2620, 1999.

427. Anonymous: Rosiglitazone for type 2 diabetes mellitus. Med Lett Drugs Ther 41:71–73, 1999.

428. Balfour JA, Plosker GL: Rosiglitazone. Drugs 57:921–930, 1999.

429. Yamasaki Y, Kawamori R, Wasada T, et al: Pioglitazone (AD-4833) ameliorates insulin resistance in patients with NIDDM. AD-4833 Glucose Clamp Study Group, Japan. Tohoku J Exp Med 183:173–183, 1997.

430. Forman LM, Simmons DA, Diamond RH: Hepatic failure in a patient taking rosiglitazone. Ann Intern Med 132:118–121, 2000.

431. Al-Salman J, Arjomand H, Kemp DG, Mittal M: Hepatocellular injury in a patient receiving rosiglitazone: A case report. Ann Intern Med 132:121–124, 2000.

432. Freid J, Everitt D, Boscia J: Rosiglitazone and hepatic failure. Ann Intern Med 132:164, 2000.

433. Wolffenbuttel BH, Sels JP, Rondas-Colbers GJ, et al: Comparison of different insulin regimens in elderly patients with NIDDM. Diabetes Care 19:1326–1332, 1996.

434. Coscelli C, Calabrese G, Fedele D, et al: Use of premixed insulin in the elderly: Reduction of errors in patient preparation of mixtures. Diabetes Care 15:1628–1630, 1992.

435. Heise T, Weyer C, Serwas A, et al: Time-action profiles of novel premixed preparations of insulin lispro and NPL insulin. Diabetes Care 21:800–803, 1998.

436. Gilden JL, Casia C, Hendryx M, Singh SP: Effects of self-monitoring of blood glucose on quality of life in elderly diabetic patients. J Am Geriatr Soc 38:511–515, 1990.

437. Hom FG, Ettinger B, Lin MJ: Comparison of serum fructosamine vs glycohemoglobin as measures of glycemic control in a large diabetic population. Acta Diabetol 35:48–51, 1998.

438. Cefalu WT, Prather KL, Murphy WA, Parker TB: Clinical evaluation of serum fructosamine in monitoring elderly outpatient diabetics. J Am Geriatr Soc 37:833–837, 1989.

439. UK Prospective Diabetes Study Group (UKPDS 39): Efficacy of atenolol and captopril in reducing risk of macrovascular and microvascular complications in type 2 diabetes. BMJ 317:713–720, 1998.

440. UK Prospective Diabetes Study Group (UKPDS 40): Cost effectiveness analysis of improved blood pressure control in hypertensive patients with type 2 diabetes. BMJ 317:720–726, 1998.

441. Vanderpump MP, Tunbridge WM, French JM, et al: The incidence of thyroid disorders in the community: A twenty-year follow-up of the Whickham Survey. Clin Endocrinol (Oxf) 43:55–68, 1995.

442. Tunbridge WM, Evered DC, Hall R, et al: The spectrum of thyroid disease in a community: The Whickham Survey. Clin Endocrinol (Oxf) 7:481–493, 1977.

443. Sawin CT, Castelli WP, Hershman JM, et al: The aging thyroid: Thyroid deficiency in the Framingham Study. Arch Intern Med 145:1386–1388, 1985.

444. Sawin CT, Geller A, Hershman JM, et al: The aging thyroid: The use of thyroid hormone in older persons. JAMA 261:2653–2655, 1989.

445. Hassani S, Hershman JM: Thyroid diseases. In Hazzard WR, Blass JP, Ettinger WH Jr, et al (eds): Principles of Geriatric Medicine and Gerontology, ed 4. New York, McGraw-Hill, 1999, pp 973–989.

446. Feit H: Thyroid function in the elderly. Clin Geriatr Med 4:151–161, 1988.

447. Levy EG: Thyroid disease in the elderly. Med Clin North Am 75:151–167, 1991.

448. Chiovato L, Mariotti S, Pinchera A: Thyroid diseases in the elderly. Baillieres Clin Endocrinol Metab 11:251–270, 1997.

449. Wesche MF, Wiersinga WM, Smits NJ: Lean body mass as a determinant of thyroid size. Clin Endocrinol (Oxf) 48:701–706, 1998.

450. Hegedus L, Perrild H, Poulsen LR, et al: The determination of thyroid volume by ultrasound and its relationship to body weight, age, and sex in normal subjects. J Clin Endocrinol Metab 56:260–263, 1983.

451. Gregerman RI: Mechanisms of age-related alterations of hormones secretion and action: An overview of 30 years of progress. Exp Gerontol 21:345–365, 1991.

452. Sawin CT, Herman T, Molitch ME, et al: Aging and the thyroid: Decreased requirement for thyroid hormone in older hypothyroid patients. Am J Med 75:206–209, 1983.

453. Gaffney GW, Gregerman RI, Shock NW: Relationship of age to the thyroidal accumulation, renal excretion and distribution of radioiodide in euthyroid man. J Clin Endocrinol Metab 22:784–794, 1962.

454. Oddie TH, Myhill J, Pirnique FG, Fisher DA: Effect of age and sex on the radioiodine uptake in euthyroid subjects. J Clin Endocrinol Metab 28:776–782, 1968.

455. Kabadi UM, Rosman PM: Thyroid hormone indices in adult healthy subjects: No influence of aging. J Am Geriatr Soc 36:312–316, 1988.

456. Sawin CT, Geller A, Kaplan MM, et al: Low serum thyrotropin (thyroid-stimulating hormone) in older persons without hyperthyroidism. Arch Intern Med 151:165–168, 1991.

457. Lewis GF, Alessi CA, Imperial JG, Refetoff S: Low serum free thyroxine index in ambulating elderly is due to a resetting of the threshold of thyrotropin feedback suppression. J Clin Endocrinol Metab 73:843–849, 1991.

458. Monzani F, Del Guerra P, Caraccio N, et al: Age-related modifications in the regulation of the hypothalamic-pituitary-thyroid axis. Horm Res 46:107–112, 1996.

459. Parle JV, Franklyn JA, Cross KW, et al: Prevalence and follow-up of abnormal thyrotrophin (TSH) concentrations in the elderly in the United Kingdom. Clin Endocrinol (Oxf) 34:77–83, 1991.

460. Goldberg TH, Chavin SI: Preventive medicine and screening in older adults. J Am Geriatr Soc 45:344–354, 1997.

461. Danese MD, Powe NR, Sawin CT, Ladenson PW: Screening for mild thyroid failure at the periodic health examination: A decision and cost-effectiveness analysis. JAMA 276:285–292, 1996.

462. Gambert SR: Atypical presentation of thyroid disease in the elderly. Geriatrics 40:63–65, 68–69, 1985.

463. Doucet J, Trivalle C, Chassagne P, et al: Does age play a role in clinical presentation of hypothyroidism? J Am Geriatr Soc 42:984–986, 1994.

464. DeLany JP, Hansen BC, Bodkin NL, et al: Long-term calorie restriction reduces energy expenditure in aging monkeys. J Gerontol A Biol Sci Med Sci 54:B5–B11, 1999.

465. Goichot B, Schlienger JL, Grunenberger F, et al: Thyroid hormone status and nutrient intake in the free-living elderly: Interest of reverse triiodothyronine assessment. Eur J Endocrinol 130:244–252, 1994.

466. Portnay GI, O'Brian JT, Bush J, et al: The effect of starvation on the concentration and binding of thyroxine and triiodothyronine in serum and on the response to TRH. J Clin Endocrinol Metab 39:191–194, 1974.

467. Spaulding SW, Chopra IJ, Sherwin RS, Lyall SS: Effect of caloric restriction and dietary composition of serum T3 and reverse T3 in man. J Clin Endocrinol Metab 42:197–200, 1976.

468. Hugues JN, Burger AG, Pekary AE, Hershman JM: Rapid adaptations of serum thyrotrophin, triiodothyronine and reverse triiodothyronine levels to short-term starvation and refeeding. Acta Endocrinol (Copenh) 105:194–199, 1984.

469. Gittoes NJ, Franklyn JA: Drug-induced thyroid disorders. Drug Saf 13:46–55, 1995.

470. O'Connor P, Feely J: Clinical pharmacokinetics and endocrine disorders: Therapeutic implications. Clin Pharmacokinet 13:345–364, 1987.

471. Miller LG: Herbal medicinals: Selected clinical considerations focusing on known or potential drug-herb interactions. Arch Intern Med 158:2200–2211, 1998.

472. Sauvage MF, Marquet P, Rousseau A, et al: Relationship between psychotropic drugs and thyroid function: A review. Toxicol Appl Pharmacol 149:127–135, 1998.

473. Cavalieri RR: The effects of nonthyroid disease and drugs on thyroid function tests. Med Clin North Am 75:27–39, 1991.

474. Hennemann G, Krenning EP: Pitfalls in the interpretation of thyroid function tests in old age and non-thyroidal illness. Horm Res 26:100–104, 1987.

475. Wenzel KW: Disturbances of thyroid function tests by drugs. Acta Med Austriaca 23:57–60, 1996.

476. Davies PH, Franklyn JA: The effects of drugs on tests of thyroid function. Eur J Clin Pharmacol 40:439–451, 1991.

477. Ramsay I: Drug and non-thyroid induced changes in thyroid function tests. Postgrad Med J 61:375–377, 1985.

478. Nademanee K, Singh BN, Callahan B, et al: Amiodarone, thyroid hormone indexes, and altered thyroid function: Long-term serial effects in patients with cardiac arrhythmias. Am J Cardiol 58:981–986, 1986.

479. Sato K, Miyakawa M, Eto M, et al: Clinical characteristics of amiodarone-induced thyrotoxicosis and hypothyroidism in Japan. Endocr J 46:443–461, 1999.

480. Nademanee K, Piwonka RW, Singh BN, Hershman JM: Amiodarone and thyroid function. Prog Cardiovasc Dis 31:427–437, 1989.

481. Trip MD, Wiersinga W, Plomp TA: Incidence, predictability, and pathogenesis of amiodarone-induced thyrotoxicosis and hypothyroidism. Am J Med 91:507–511, 1991.

482. Harjai KJ, Licata AA: Effects of amiodarone on thyroid function. Ann Intern Med 126:63–73, 1997.

483. Martino E, Aghini-Lombardi F, Bartalena L, et al: Enhanced susceptibility to amiodarone-induced hypothyroidism in patients with thyroid autoimmune disease. Arch Intern Med 154:2722–2726, 1994.

484. Docter R, Krenning EP, de Jong M, Hennemann G: The sick euthyroid syndrome: Changes in thyroid hormone serum parameters and hormone metabolism. Clin Endocrinol (Oxf) 39:499–518, 1993.

485. Wartofsky L: The low T3 or "sick euthyroid syndrome": Update 1994. Endocr Rev 3:248–251, 1994.

486. DeGroot LJ: Dangerous dogmas in medicine: The nonthyroidal illness syndrome. J Clin Endocrinol Metab 84:151–164, 1999.

487. Klemperer JD, Ojamaa K, Klein I: Thyroid hormone therapy in cardiovascular disease. Prog Cardiovasc Dis 38:329–336, 1996.

488. Wartofsky L, Burman KD, Ringel MD: Trading one "dangerous dogma" for another? Thyroid hormone treatment of the "euthyroid sick syndrome." J Clin Endocrinol Metab 84:1759–1760, 1999.

489. Glinoer D: Comment on dangerous dogmas in medicine—the nonthyroidal illness syndrome. J Clin Endocrinol Metab 84:2262–2263, 1999.

490. Caplan RH: Comment on dangerous dogmas in medicine: The nonthyroidal illness syndrome. J Clin Endocrinol Metab 84:2261–2263, 1999.

491. Geul KW, van Sluisveld IL, Grobbee DE, et al: The importance of thyroid microsomal antibodies in the development of elevated serum TSH in middle-aged women: Associations with serum lipids. Clin Endocrinol (Oxf) 39:275–280, 1993.

492. Griffin JE: Hypothyroidism in the elderly. Am J Med Sci 299:334–345, 1990.

493. McGaffee J, Barnes MA, Lippmann S: Psychiatric presentations of hypothyroidism. Am Fam Physician 23:129–133, 1981.

494. Moss R, D'Amico S, Maletta G: Mental dysfunction as a sign of organic illness in the elderly. Geriatrics 42:35–42, 1987.

495. Fava M, Labbate LA, Abraham ME, Rosenbaum JF: Hypothyroidism and hyperthyroidism in major depression revisited. J Clin Psychiatry 56:186–192, 1995.

496. Ordas DM, Labbate LA: Routine screening of thyroid function in patients hospitalized for major depression or dysthymia? Ann Clin Psychiatry 7:161–165, 1995.

497. Reed K, Bland RC: Masked "myxedema madness." Acta Psychiatr Scand 56:421–426, 1977.

498. Cook DM, Boyle PJ: Rapid reversal of myxedema madness with triiodothyronine. Ann Intern Med 104:893–894, 1986.

499. Davidoff F, Gill J: Myxedema madness: Psychosis as an early manifestation of hypothyroidism. Conn Med 41:618–621, 1977.

500. Aronow WS: The heart and thyroid disease. Clin Geriatr Med 11:219–229, 1995.

501. Gomberg-Maitland M, Frishman WH: Thyroid hormone and cardiovascular disease. Am Heart J 135:187–196, 1998.

502. Polikar R, Burger AG, Scherrer U, Nicod P: The thyroid and the heart. Circulation 87:1435–1441, 1993.

503. Streeten DH, Anderson GH Jr, Howland T, et al: Effects of thyroid function on blood pressure: Recognition of hypothyroid hypertension. Hypertension 11:78–83, 1988.

504. Anderson GH Jr, Blakeman N, Streeten DH: The effect of age on prevalence of

secondary forms of hypertension in 4429 consecutively referred patients. J Hypertens 12:609–615, 1994.

505. VanDyck P, Chadband R, Chaudhary B, Stachura ME: Sleep apnea, sleep disorders, and hypothyroidism. Am J Med Sci 298:119–122, 1989.

506. Fein HG, Rivlin RS: Anemia in thyroid diseases. Med Clin North Am 59:1133–1145, 1975.

507. Quaglino D, Ginaldi L, Furia N, De Martinis M: The effect of age on hemopoiesis. Aging (Milano) 8:1–12, 1996.

508. Vanderpump MP, Ahlquist JA, Franklyn JA, Clayton RN: Consensus statement for good practice and audit measures in the management of hypothyroidism and hyperthyroidism. The Research Unit of the Royal College of Physicians of London, the Endocrinology and Diabetes Committee of the Royal College of Physicians of London, and the Society for Endocrinology. BMJ 313:539–544, 1996.

509. Toft AD: Thyroxine therapy. N Engl J Med 331:174–180, 1994.

510. Kabadi UM: Influence of age on optimal daily levothyroxine dosage in patients with primary hypothyroidism grouped according to etiology. South Med J 90:920–924, 1997.

511. Mandel SJ, Brent GA, Larsen PR: Levothyroxine therapy in patients with thyroid disease. Ann Intern Med 119:492–502, 1993.

512. Gammage M, Franklyn J: Hypothyroidism, thyroxine treatment, and the heart. Heart 77:189–190, 1997.

513. Blum M: Myxedema coma. Am J Med Sci 264:432–443, 1972.

514. Menendez CE, Rivlin RS: Thyrotoxic crisis and myxedema coma. Med Clin North Am 57:1463–1470, 1973.

515. Urbanic RC, Mazzaferri EL: Thyrotoxic crisis and myxedema coma. Heart Lung 7:435–447, 1978.

516. Nicoloff JT, LoPresti JS: Myxedema coma. A form of decompensated hypothyroidism. Endocrinol Metab Clin North Am 22:279–290, 1993.

517. Wartofsky L: Myxedema coma. In Braverman LE, Utiger RD (eds): Werner and Ingbar's The Thyroid, ed 7. Philadelphia, JB Lippincott, 1996, pp 871–877.

518. Hooper MJ: Diminished T.S.H. secretion during acute non-thyroidal illness in untreated primary hypothyroidism. Lancet 1:48–49, 1976.

519. Chernow B, Burman KD, Johnson DL, et al: T$_3$ may be a better agent than T$_4$ in the critically ill hypothyroid patient: Evaluation of transport across the blood-brain barrier in a primate model. Crit Care Med 11:99–104, 1983.

520. Ronnov-Jessen V, Kirkegaard C: Hyperthyroidism—a disease of old age? BMJ 1:41–43, 1973.

521. Kawabe T, Komiya I, Endo T, et al: Hyperthyroidism in the elderly. J Am Geriatr Soc 27:152–155, 1979.

522. Gambert SR: Hyperthyroidism in the elderly. Clin Geriatr Med 11:181–188, 1995.

523. Dumitriu L, Ursu H: Hyperthyroidism in the elderly. I. Clinical manifestations. Endocrinologie 23:83–90, 1985.

524. Dumitriu L, Ursu H: Diagnosis and treatment of hyperthyroidism in elderly patients. Endocrinologie 22:167–176, 1984.

525. Bailes BK: Hyperthyroidism in elderly patients. AORN J 69:254–258, 1999.

526. Trivalle C, Doucet J, Chassagne P, et al: Differences in the signs and symptoms of hyperthyroidism in older and younger patients. J Am Geriatr Soc 44:50–53, 1996.

527. Bagchi N, Brown TR, Parish RF: Thyroid dysfunction in adults over age 55 years. A study in an urban US community. Arch Intern Med 150:785–787, 1990.

528. Newman CM, Price A, Davies DW, et al: Amiodarone and the thyroid: A practical guide to the management of thyroid dysfunction induced by amiodarone therapy. Heart 79:121–127, 1998.

529. Figge J, Leinung M, Goodman AD, et al: The clinical evaluation of patients with subclinical hyperthyroidism and free triiodothyronine (free T$_3$) toxicosis. Am J Med 96:229–234, 1994.

530. Hennemann G, Krenning EP: Pitfalls in the interpretation of thyroid function tests in old age and non-thyroidal illness. Horm Res 26:100–104, 1987.

531. Sylvia Vela B, Dorin RI: Factitious triiodothyronine toxicosis. Am J Med 90:132–134, 1991.

532. Griffin MA, Solomon DH: Hyperthyroidism in the elderly. J Am Geriatr Soc 34:887–892, 1986.

533. Martin FI, Deam DR: Hyperthyroidism in elderly hospitalised patients. Clinical features and treatment outcomes. Med J Aust 164:200–203, 1996.

534. Francis T, Wartofsky L: Common thyroid disorders in the elderly. Postgrad Med 92:225–230, 233–236, 1992.

535. Wallace K, Hofmann MT: Thyroid dysfunction: How to manage overt and subclinical disease in older patients. Geriatrics 53:32–38, 41, 1998.

536. Farrar JJ, Toft AD: Iodine-131 treatment of hyperthyroidism: Current issues. Clin Endocrinol (Oxf) 35:207–212, 1991.

537. Cooper DS: Which anti-thyroid drug? Am J Med 80:1165–1168, 1986.

538. Yamada T, Aizawa T, Koizumi Y, et al: Age-related therapeutic response to antithyroid drug in patients with hyperthyroid Graves' disease. J Am Geriatr Soc 42:513–516, 1994.

539. Wartofsky L: Radioiodine therapy for Graves' disease: Case selection and restrictions recommended to patients in North America. Thyroid 7:213–216, 1997.

540. Wartofsky L: Treatment options for hyperthyroidism. Hosp Pract 31:69–73, 76–78, 81–84, 1996.

541. Hamburger JI, Hamburger SW: Diagnosis and management of large toxic multinodular goiters. J Nucl Med 26:888–892, 1985.

542. Gittoes NJ, Franklyn JA: Hyperthyroidism. Current treatment guidelines. Drugs 55:543–553, 1998.

543. Wartofsky L, Glinoer D, Solomon B, Lagasse R: Differences and similarities in the treatment of diffuse goiter in Europe and the United States. Exp Clin Endocrinol 97:243–251, 1991.

544. Solomon BL, Wartofsky L, Burman KD: Adjunctive cholestyramine therapy for thyrotoxicosis. Clin Endocrinol (Oxf) 38:39–43, 1993.

545. Kennedy JW, Caro JF: The ABCs of managing hyperthyroidism in the older patient. Geriatrics 51:22–24, 27, 31–32, 1996.

546. Tamagna EI, Levine GA, Hershman JM: Thyroid-hormone concentrations after radio-iodine therapy for hyperthyroidism. J Nucl Med 20:387–391, 1979.

547. Shafer RB, Nuttall FQ: Acute changes in thyroid function in patients treated with radioactive iodine. Lancet 2:635–637, 1975.

548. Shafer RB, Nuttall FQ: Thyroid crisis induced by radioactive iodine. J Nucl Med 12:262–264, 1971.

549. Kidess AI, Caplan RH, Reynertson RH, Wickus G: Recurrence of ^{131}I-induced thyroid storm after discontinuing glucocorticoid therapy. Wisc Med J 90:463–465, 1991.

550. Werner MC, Romaldini JH, Bromberg N, et al: Adverse effects related to thionamide drugs and their dose regimen. Am J Med Sci 297:216–219, 1989.

551. Cooper DS, Goldminz D, Levin AA, et al: Agranulocytosis associated with antithyroid drugs. Effects of patient age and drug dose. Ann Intern Med 98:26–29, 1983.

552. Ingbar SH: Management of emergencies. IX. Thyrotoxic storm. N Engl J Med 274:1252–1254, 1966.

553. Carter JN, Eastman CJ, Kilham HA, Lazarus L: Rational therapy for thyroid storm. Aust N Z J Med 5:458–461, 1975.

554. Burch HB, Wartofsky L: Life-threatening thyrotoxicosis. Thyroid storm. Endocrinol Metab Clin North Am 22:263–277, 1993.

555. Wartofsky L: Thyrotoxic storm. In Braverman LE, Utiger RD (eds): Werner and Ingbar's The Thyroid, ed 7. Philadelphia, JB Lippincott, 1996, pp 701–707.

556. Dillmann WH: Thyroid storm. Curr Ther Endocrinol Metab 6:81–85, 1997.

557. Roth RN, McAuliffe MJ: Hyperthyroidism and thyroid storm. Emerg Med Clin North Am 7:873–883, 1989.

558. Solomon B, Glinoer D, Lagasse R, Wartofsky L: Current trends in the management of Graves' disease. J Clin Endocrinol Metab 70:1518–1524, 1990.

559. Wiest PW, Hartshorne MF, Inskip PD, et al: Thyroid palpation versus high-resolution thyroid ultrasonography in the detection of nodules. J Ultrasound Med 17:487–496, 1998.

560. Vander JB, Gaston EA, Dawber TR: The significance of nontoxic thyroid nodules. Final report of a 15-year study of the incidence of thyroid malignancy. Ann Intern Med 69:537–540, 1968.

561. Hintze G, Windeler J, Baumert J, et al: Thyroid volume and goitre prevalence in the elderly as determined by ultrasound and their relationships to laboratory indices. Acta Endocrinol (Copenh) 124:12–18, 1991.

562. Mortensen JD, Woolner LB, Bennett WA: Gross and microscopic findings in clinically normal thyroid glands. J Clin Endocrinol Metab 15:1270–1280, 1955.

563. Mazzaferri EL: Papillary thyroid carcinoma: Factors influencing prognosis and current therapy. Semin Oncol 14:315–332, 1987.

564. Mazzaferri EL: An overview of the management of papillary and follicular thyroid carcinoma. Thyroid 9:421–427, 1999.

565. DeGroot LJ, Kaplan EL, Shukla MS, et al: Morbidity and mortality in follicular thyroid cancer. J Clin Endocrinol Metab 80:2946–2953, 1995.

566. Ron E, Lubin JH, Shore RE, et al: Thyroid cancer after exposure to external radiation: A pooled analysis of seven studies. Radiat Res 141:259–277, 1995.

567. Schneider AB, Gierlowski TC, Shore-Freedman E, et al: Dose-response relationships for radiation-induced hyperparathyroidism. J Clin Endocrinol Metab 80:254–257, 1995.

568. Schneider AB, Lubin J, Ron E, et al: Salivary gland tumors after childhood radiation treatment for benign conditions of the head and neck: Dose-response relationships. Radiat Res 149:625–630, 1998.

569. Dottorini ME, Assi A, Sironi M, et al: Multivariate analysis of patients with medullary thyroid carcinoma. Prognostic significance and impact on treatment of clinical and pathologic variables. Cancer 77:1556–1565, 1996.

570. Modigliani E, Cohen R, Campos JM, et al: Prognostic factors for survival and for biochemical cure in medullary thyroid carcinoma: Results in 899 patients. The GETC Study Group. Groupe d'etude des tumeurs a calcitonine. Clin Endocrinol (Oxf) 48:265–273, 1998.

571. Samaan NA, Schultz PN, Hickey RC: Medullary thyroid carcinoma: Prognosis of familial versus nonfamilial disease and the role of radiotherapy. Horm Metab Res Suppl 21:21–25, 1989.

572. Lo CY, Lam KY, Wan KY: Anaplastic carcinoma of the thyroid. Am J Surg 177:337–339, 1999.

573. Voutilainen PE, Multanen M, Haapiainen RK, et al: Anaplastic thyroid carcinoma survival. World J Surg 23:975–979, 1999.

574. Kanaseki T, Harabuchi Y, Wakashima J, et al: A case of anaplastic thyroid carcinoma surviving disease free for over 2 years. Kanaseki Auris Nasus Larynx 26:217–220, 1999.

575. Udelsman R, Chen H: The current management of thyroid cancer. Adv Surg 33:1–27, 1999.

576. Matsuzuka F, Miyauchi A, Katayama S, et al: Clinical aspects of primary thyroid lymphoma: Diagnosis and treatment based on our experience of 119 cases. Thyroid 3:93–99, 1993.

577. Holm LE, Blomgren H, Lowhagen T: Cancer risks in patients with chronic lymphocytic thyroiditis. N Engl J Med 312:601–604, 1985.

578. Favus MJ (ed): Primer on the Metabolic Bone Diseases and Disorders of Mineral Metabolism, ed 4. Philadelphia, Lippincott Williams & Wilkins, 1999.

579. Ott SM: Osteoporosis and osteomalacia. In Hazzard WR, Blass JP, Ettinger WH Jr, et al (eds): Principles of Geriatric Medicine and Gerontology, ed 4. New York, McGraw-Hill, 1999, pp 1057–1084.

580. Binkley N: Osteoporosis and osteomalacia. In Reuben DR, Yoshikawa TT, Besdine RW (eds): Geriatrics Review Syllabus: A Core Curriculum in Geriatric Medicine, ed 3. New York, American Geriatrics Society, Dubuque, Kendall/Hunt, 1996, pp 152–159.

581. Baylink DJ, Jennings JC, Mohan S: Calcium and bone homeostasis and changes with aging. In Hazzard WR, Blass JP, Ettinger WH Jr, et al (eds): Principles of Geriatric Medicine and Gerontology, ed 4. New York, McGraw-Hill, 1999, pp 1041–1056.

582. Orwoll ES: Osteoporosis in men. Endocrinol Metabl Clin North Am 27:349–367, 1998.

583. Ebeling PR: Osteoporosis in men: New insights into aetiology, pathogenesis, prevention and management. Drugs Aging 13:421–434, 1998.

584. Jackson JA, Kleerekoper M: Osteoporosis in men: Diagnosis, pathophysiology, and prevention. Medicine 69:137–152, 1990.

585. Khosla S, Melton LJ III, Riggs BL: Osteoporosis: Gender differences and similarities. Lupus 8:393–396, 1999.

586. Fatayerji D, Eastell R: Age-related changes in bone turnover in men. J Bone Miner Res 14:1203–1210, 1999.

587. Epstein S, Bryce G, Hinman JW, et al: The influence of age on bone mineral regulating hormones. Bone 7:421–425, 1986.

588. Wemeau JL: Calciotropic hormones and aging. Horm Res 43:76–79, 1995.

589. Baker MR, McDonald H, Peacock M, Nordin BE: Plasma 25-hydroxy vitamin D concentrations in patients with fractures of the femoral neck. BMJ 1:589, 1979.

590. Hordon LD, Peacock M: Osteomalacia and osteoporosis in femoral neck fracture. Bone Miner 11:247–259, 1990.

591. Bettica P, Bevilacqua M, Vago T, Norbiato G: High prevalence of hypovitaminosis D among free-living postmenopausal women referred to an osteoporosis outpatient clinic in northern Italy for initial screening. Osteoporos Int 9:226–229, 1999.

592. LeBoff MS, Kohlmeier L, Hurwitz S, et al: Occult vitamin D deficiency in postmenopausal US women with acute hip fracture. JAMA 281:1505–1511, 1999.

593. Bruce DG, St John A, Nicklason F, Goldswain PR: Secondary hyperparathyroidism in patients from Western Australia with hip fracture: Relationship to type of hip fracture, renal function, and vitamin D deficiency. J Am Geriatr Soc 47:354–359, 1999.

594. Boonen S, Aerssens J, Dequeker J: Age-related endocrine deficiencies and fractures of the proximal femur: II implications of vitamin D deficiency in the elderly. J Endocrinol 149:13–17, 1996.

595. Slovik DM, Adams JS, Neer RM, et al: Deficient production of 1,25-dihydroxyvitamin D in elderly osteoporotic patients. N Engl J Med 305:372–374, 1981.

596. Quesada JM, Coopmans W, Ruiz B, et al: Influence of vitamin D on parathyroid function in the elderly. J Clin Endocrinol Metab 75:494–501, 1992.

597. Haden S, Fuleihan GE, Angell JE, et al: Calcidiol and PTH levels in women attending an osteoporosis program. Calcif Tissue Int 64:275–279, 1999.

598. McKane WR, Khosla S, Egan KS, et al: Role of calcium intake in modulating age-related increases in parathyroid function and bone resorption. J Clin Endocrinol Metab 81:1699–1703, 1996.

599. Murphy S, Khaw KT, Cassidy A, Compston JE: Sex hormones and bone mineral density in elderly men. Bone Miner 20:133–140, 1993.

600. Carani C, Qin K, Simoni M, et al: Effect of testosterone and estradiol in a man with aromatase deficiency. N Engl J Med 337:91–95, 1997.

601. Bellido T, Jilka RL, Boyce BF, et al: Regulation of interleukin-6, osteoclastogenesis, and bone mass by androgens: The role of the androgen receptor. J Clin Invest 95:2886–2895, 1995.

602. Manolagas SC, Jilka RL: Bone marrow, cytokines, and bone remodeling: Emerging insights into the pathophysiology of osteoporosis. N Engl J Med 332:305–311, 1995.

603. Gloth FM III, Gundberg CM, Hollis BW, et al: Vitamin D deficiency in homebound elderly persons. JAMA 274:1683–1686, 1995.

604. Lips P, Hackeng WH, Jongen MJ, et al: Seasonal variation in serum concentrations of parathyroid hormone in elderly people. J Clin Endocrinol Metab 57:204–206, 1983.

605. Hegarty V, Woodhouse P, Khaw KT: Seasonal variation in 25-hydroxyvitamin D and parathyroid hormone concentrations in healthy elderly people. Age Ageing 23:478–482, 1994.

606. Sherman SS, Hollis BW, Tobin JD: Vitamin D status and related parameters in a healthy population: The effects of age, sex, and season. J Clin Endocrinol Metab 71:405–413, 1990.

607. Webb AR, Holick MF: The role of sunlight in the cutaneous production of vitamin D₃. Annu Rev Nutr 8:375–399, 1988.

608. MacLaughlin J, Holick MF: Aging decreases the capacity of human skin to produce vitamin D₃. J Clin Invest 76:1536–1538, 1985.

609. Melin AL, Wilske J, Ringertz H, Saaf M: Vitamin D status, parathyroid function and femoral bone density in an elderly Swedish population living at home. Aging (Milano) 11:200–207, 1999.

610. Avioli LV, McDonald JE, Lee SW: The influence of age on the intestinal absorption of 47-Ca absorption in post-menopausal osteoporosis. J Clin Invest 44:1960–1967, 1965.

611. Barragry JM, France MW, Corless D, et al: Intestinal cholecalciferol absorption in the elderly and in younger adults. Clin Sci Mol Med 55:213–220, 1978.

612. Jacques PF, Felson DT, Tucker KL, et al: Plasma 25-hydroxyvitamin D and its determinants in an elderly population sample. Am J Clin Nutr 66:929–936, 1997.

613. Bouillon RA, Auwerx JH, Lissens WD, Pelemans WK: Vitamin D status in the elderly: Seasonal substrate deficiency causes 1,25-dihydroxycholecalciferol deficiency. Am J Clin Nutr 45:755–763, 1987.

614. Gloth FM III, Tobin JD: Vitamin D deficiency in older people. J Am Geriatr Soc 43:822–828, 1995.

615. Ebeling PR, Sandgren ME, DiMagno EP, et al: Evidence of an age-related decrease in intestinal responsiveness to vitamin D: Relationship between serum 1,25-dihydroxyvitamin D₃ and intestinal vitamin D receptor concentrations in normal women. J Clin Endocrinol Metab 75:176–182, 1992.

616. Ebeling PR, Yergey AL, Vieira NE, et al: Influence of age on effects of endogenous 1,25-dihydroxyvitamin D on calcium absorption in normal women. Calcif Tissue Int 55:330–334, 1994.

617. Lips P, Chapuy MC, Dawson-Hughes B, et al: International comparison of serum 25-hydroxyvitamin D measurements. Osteoporos Int 9:394–397, 1999.

618. Jongen MJ, Van Ginkel FC, van der Vijgh WJ, et al: An international comparison of vitamin D metabolite measurements. Clin Chem 30:399–403, 1984.

619. Chapuy MC, Preziosi P, Maamer M, et al: Prevalence of vitamin D insufficiency in an adult normal population. Osteoporos Int 7:439–443, 1997.

620. Thomas MK, Lloyd-Jones DM, Thadhani RI, et al: Hypovitaminosis D in medical inpatients. N Engl J Med 338:777–783, 1998.

621. Dawson-Hughes B, Dallal GE, Krall EA, et al: Effect of vitamin D supplementation on wintertime and overall bone loss in healthy postmenopausal women. Ann Intern Med 115:505–512, 1991.

622. Dubbelman R, Jonxis JH, Muskiet FA, Saleh AE: Age-dependent vitamin D status and vertebral condition of white women living in Curacao (the Netherlands Antilles) as compared with their counterparts in the Netherlands. Am J Clin Nutr 58:106–109, 1993.

623. McKenna MJ: Differences in vitamin D status between countries in young adults and the elderly. Am J Med 93:69–77, 1992.

624. Heikinheimo RJ, Inkovaara JA, Harju EJ, et al: Annual injections of vitamin D and fractures of aged bones. Calcif Tissue Int 51:105–110, 1992.

625. Gloth FM III, Lindsay JM, Zelesnick LB, Greenough WB III: Can vitamin D deficiency produce an unusual pain syndrome? Arch Intern Med 151:1662–1664, 1991.

626. Gloth FM III, Smith CE, Hollis BW, Tobin JD: Functional improvement with vitamin D replenishment in a cohort of frail, vitamin D-deficient older people. J Am Geriatr Soc 43:1269–1271, 1995.

627. Bischoff HA, Stahelin HB, Urscheler N, et al: Muscle strength in the elderly: Its relation to vitamin D metabolites. Arch Phys Med Rehabil 80:54–58, 1999.

628. Heaney RP, Recker RR, Stegman MR, Moy AJ: Calcium absorption in women: Relationship to calcium intake, estrogen status, and age. J Bone Miner Res 4:469–475, 1989.

629. Nordin BE, Wilkinson R, Marshall DH, et al: Calcium absorption in the elderly. Calcif Tissue Res 215:442–451, 1976.

630. Gallagher JC, Riggs BL, Eisman J, et al: Intestinal calcium absorption and serum vitamin D metabolites in normal subjects and osteoporotic patients. J Clin Invest 64:729–736, 1979.

631. Stewart AF, Adler M, Byers CM, et al: Calcium homeostasis in immobilization: An example of resorptive hypercalciuria. N Engl J Med 306:1136–1140, 1982.

632. Sato Y, Oizumi K, Kuno H, Kaji M: Effect of immobilization upon renal synthesis of 1,25-dihydroxyvitamin D in disabled elderly stroke patients. Bone 24:271–275, 1999.

633. Sato Y, Kuno H, Asoh T, et al: Effect of immobilization on vitamin D status and bone mass in chronically hospitalized disabled stroke patients. Age Ageing 27:265–269, 1999.

634. Bischoff H, Stahelin HB, Vogt P, et al: Immobility as a major cause of bone remodeling in residents of a long-stay geriatric ward. Calcif Tissue Int 64:485–489 1999.

635. Theiler R, Stahelin HB, Tyndall A, et al: Calcidiol, calcitriol and parathyroid hormone serum concentrations in institutionalized and ambulatory elderly in Switzerland. Int J Vitam Nutr Res 69:96–105, 1999.

636. Audi L, Garcia-Ramirez M, Carrascosa A: Genetic determinants of bone mass. Horm Res 51:105–123, 1999.

637. Seeman E, Hopper JL, Bach LA, et al: Reduced bone mass in daughters of women with osteoporosis. N Engl J Med 320:554–558, 1989.

638. Morrison NA, Qi JC, Tokita A, et al: Prediction of bone density from vitamin D receptor alleles. Nature 367:284–287, 1994.

639. Krall EA, Parry P, Lichter JB, Dawson-Hughes B: Vitamin D receptor alleles and rates of bone loss: Influences of years since menopause and calcium intake. J Bone Miner Res 10:978–984, 1995.

640. Ferrari S, Manen D, Bonjour JP, et al: Bone mineral mass and calcium and phosphate metabolism in young men: Relationship with vitamin D receptor allelic polymorphisms. J Clin Endocrinol Metab 84:2043–2048, 1999.

641. Gennari L, Becherini L, Mansani R, et al: Fokl polymorphism at translation initiation site of the vitamin D receptor gene predicts bone mineral density and vertebral fractures in postmenopausal Italian women. J Bone Miner Res 14:1379–1386, 1999.

642. Masi L, Becherini L, Colli E, et al: Polymorphisms of the calcitonin receptor gene are associated with bone mineral density in postmenopausal Italian women. Biochem Biophys Res Commun 248:190–195, 1998.

643. Kurabayashi T, Tomita M, Matsushita H, et al: Association of vitamin D and estrogen receptor gene polymorphism with the effect of hormone replacement therapy on bone mineral density in Japanese women. Am J Obstet Gynecol 180:1115–1120, 1999.

644. Looker AC, Orwoll ES, Johnston CC Jr, et al: Prevalence of low femoral bone density in older U.S. adults from NHANES III. J Bone Miner Res 12:1761–1768, 1997.

645. Dawson-Hughes B, Harris SS, Krall EA, Dallal GE: Effect of calcium and vitamin D supplementation on bone density in men and women 65 years of age or older. N Engl J Med 337:670–676, 1997.

646. Chapuy MC, Arlot ME, Duboeuf F, et al: Vitamin D₃ and calcium to prevent hip fractures in elderly women. N Engl J Med 327:1637–1642, 1992.

647. Chapuy MC, Arlot ME, Delmas PD, Meunier PJ: Effect of calcium and cholecalciferol treatment for three years on hip fractures in elderly women. BMJ 308:1081–1082, 1994.

648. Ooms ME, Roos JC, Bezemer PD, et al: Prevention of bone loss by vitamin D supplementation in elderly women: A randomized double-blind trial. J Clin Endocrinol Metab 80:1052–1058, 1995.

649. Holick MF, Shao Q, Liu WW, Chen TC: The vitamin D content of fortified milk and infant formula. N Engl J Med 326:1178–1181, 1992.

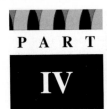

Immunology and Endocrinology

Editor: Leslie J. DeGroot

Chapter *39*

Immunologic Mechanisms Causing Autoimmune Endocrine Disease

Kevan C. Herold ▪ Jeffrey A. Bluestone

Over the past two decades it has become increasingly clear that many endocrine disorders are mediated by autoimmune mechanisms. These autoimmune attacks can target almost any of the endocrine glands and lead to diverse clinical manifestations ranging from destruction of the organ (e.g., Hashimoto's disease or type 1 diabetes mellitus [T1DM]) to overstimulation of the endocrine gland and hypersecretion of hormones (e.g., Graves' disease) (Table 39–1). Recent studies point to common pathways that lead to these diseases, including dysregulation of immune T and B lymphocytes and/or the mechanisms that control their activity. In this chapter we will provide an overview of the basic processes that control the immune response and relate these pathways to the pathogenesis of autoimmune endocrine diseases. Identification and better understanding of these pathways may unveil targets for immune therapy.

TABLE 39–1. Endocrine Diseases Most Likely Caused by Autoimmune Mechanisms

Chronic lymphocytic thyroiditis (Hashimoto's disease)
Graves' disease
Postpartum thyroiditis
Type 1 diabetes mellitus
Type B insulin resistance
Autoimmune hypoglycemia (insulin autoantibodies)
Autoimmune oophoritis
Autoimmune orchitis
Addison's disease
Autoimmune hypophysitis
Autoimmune hypoparathyroidism
Type 1 polyendocrine autoimmunity
  Chronic mucocutaneous candidiasis
  Hypoparathyroidism
  Addison's disease
Adrenal medullary autoantibodies
Primary (adrenal) pigmented and nodular forms of Cushing's syndrome

T LYMPHOCYTES: STRUCTURAL AND FUNCTIONAL BIOLOGY

In most experimental models of autoimmune endocrine disease, T cells play a central role in pathogenesis of the disease. For example, in the OS chicken, an animal model of spontaneous thyroiditis, the disease is mediated by T cells. T cell depletion, within a day of hatching, prevents the later development of thyroiditis.[1] In all animal models of T1DM, T cell depletion prevents disease and diabetes can be adoptively transferred by T cells or splenocytes.[2–4] Roep et al. isolated a T cell clone from a patient with newly diagnosed type 1 diabetes that proliferates specifically in response to insulin secretory granule proteins.[5]

The precise prevalence of cellular responses to endocrine tissue in the general population is not known. It is likely, however, that cell-mediated responses are more frequent than initially suspected. For example, focal thyroiditis can be found at autopsy in as many as 6% of men and 22% of women without known thyroid disease.[6] Thus low levels of cellular autoimmunity are tolerated in many normal individuals without progression to autoimmune disease. Identifying the factors that modulate progression from tolerable levels to autoimmune disease is key to understanding disease pathogenesis and designing interventions to prevent disease.

Structure and Activation Pathways of the T Cell Receptor

T cells express a receptor complex consisting of unique antigen-specific receptors (T cell receptors [TCRs]) associated with a multimolecular complex of molecules, CD3ε, CD3δ, CD3γ, and CD3ζ. These associated monomorphic proteins are responsible for signal transduction[7–10] (Fig. 39–1). The part of the TCR complex that binds to antigen includes a heterodimer consisting of α/β or γ/δ chains. In humans,

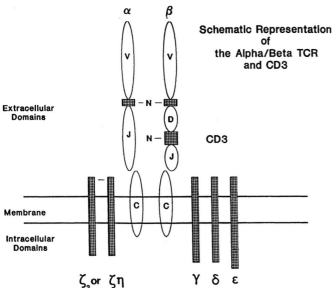

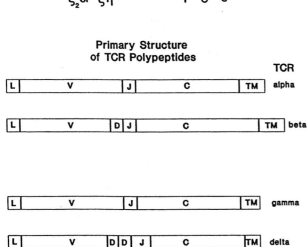

FIGURE 39–1. *A schematic representation of the T cell receptor (TCR) polypeptides. This diagram shows the structural relationships of the αβ TCR and other chains of the CD3 complex. The primary structure of the TCR polypeptides is also illustrated. C, constant gene segments; D, diversity; N, areas of N region addition; TM, transmembrane portions; V, variable. (Reproduced, with permission, from Moss PAH, Rosenberg WMC, Bell JI: The human T cell receptor in health and disease. Annu Rev Immunol 10:71–96, © 1992 by Annual Reviews www.AnnualReviews.org.)*

95% of circulating T cells are α/β and the remainder express γ/δ chains. α/β T cells can be further differentiated by expression of CD4 or CD8 molecules on their cell surfaces. These molecules are members of the immunoglobulin family of cell surface molecules and bind to class II and class I major histocompatibility complex (MHC) molecules on antigen-presenting cells (APCs), respectively, thus playing a critical role in both T cell development and subsequent antigen recognition.[10, 11]

Over the past decade, signaling through the TCR/CD3 complex has been shown to depend on a cascade of biochemical events involving tyrosine phosphorylation and subsequent downstream kinase activation[12] (Fig. 39–2). Ligation of the TCR leads to immediate activation of the associated src kinases (p56lck and p59fyn), which results in phosphorylation of the tyrosines localized within intracellular domains of the TCR/CD3 complex proteins CD3γ, CD3δ, CD3ε, and CD3ζ. These tyrosines are part of a regulatory sequence of amino acids, termed the immune receptor tyrosine activation motif (ITAM), in a 70-kDa kinase designated ZAP-70, which selectively binds to the phosphorylated TCR-ζ chain.[13] Phosphorylation of the ITAMs leads to a cascade of subsequent kinase activation, phosphorylation, and

dephosphorylation of downstream proteins, including another tyrosine kinase ZAP-70 and two adapter proteins, SLF-76 and LAT.[14] These adapters set in motion two major signaling cascades, one involving phospholipase C$_{\gamma 1}$ activation and the other, activation of ras. These events result in additional biochemical signals ultimately leading to the activation of ERK1/ERK2 (extracellular signal–regulated kinases), JNK (c-Jun N-terminal kinase), and the phosphatase calcineurin, which promotes nuclear transcription factor activation (AP-1, NFAT, NF-κB) and thereby leads to cytokine transcription. Thus protein phosphorylation after receptor engagement controls T lymphocyte behavior

Delovitch and colleagues have described an impairment in the ability of T cells from the nonobese diabetic (NOD) mouse, a model of T1DM, to function in TCR activation pathways.[15] They have identified defective TCR-mediated signaling along the protein kinase C/Ras/ mitogen-activated protein kinase pathway of T cell activation. In addition, the non–FcR-binding anti-CD3 monoclonal antibody (mAb) or altered peptide ligands (see below) proposed for the treatment of autoimmune diseases are thought to alter the normal T cell activation cascade.[16, 17]

Phenotypically and Functionally Distinct T Cell Subsets

Initial studies of T lymphocytes demonstrated two distinct subsets based on expression of CD4 or CD8 glycoproteins. These subsets differentially recognize peptides in the context of class II vs. class I MHC molecules, respectively.[11] However, over the last decade it has become increasingly clear that CD4$^+$ and CD8$^+$ T cells can be further subclassified into functionally distinct subsets. Naive T cells activated by antigen/MHC complexes can differentiate into mature effector phenotypes based on the production of different soluble mediators, or cytokines.[15, 16] This paradigm, delineated initially in murine systems, occurs in humans as well.[18, 19] The most distinctive subsets of CD4$^+$, or "helper," T cells are designated T$_H$0, T$_H$1, and T$_H$2 (also abbreviated Th0, Th1, and Th2). T$_H$0 cells, the least differentiated subset, can be driven by stimulation with antigen and costimulatory signals to differentiate into T$_H$1 cells that secrete interleukin-2 (IL-2) and interferon-γ (IFN-γ) or into T$_H$2 cells that secrete IL-4, IL-5, and IL-10.[20] T$_H$1 cells mediate classic delayed hypersensitivity reactions, whereas T$_H$2 cells provide help for B cells as they differentiate into antibody-

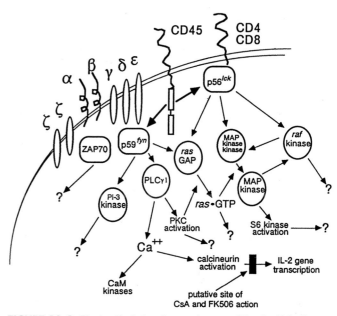

FIGURE 39–2. *Biochemical signaling pathways of T cells. This diagram illustrates the complex signaling pathways that are set in motion after T cell activation. The arrows in each case define potential regulatory influences. (Reproduced, with permission, from Perlmutter RM, Levine SD, Appleby MW, et al: Regulation of lymphocyte function by protein phosphorylation. Annu Rev Immunol 11:451–499, © 1993 by Annual Reviews www.AnnualReviews.org.)*

producing plasma cells. However, even T_H1 cells influence antibody production by altering the isotypes produced during an immune response. For example, in humans, IgG4 isotypes are associated with T_H2 responses (IgG1 in mice), whereas IgG1 isotypes are associated with T_H1 responses (IgG2a in mice).[21] Several families of T cell transcription factors have been identified, including Ikaros, LKLF, GATA3, and cmaf, that control differentiation of T cells at the molecular level.[22]

Studies in murine systems indicate that the affinity of the TCR for its ligand, costimulatory interactions, and the cytokines themselves can alter T cell differentiation into one or another phenotype.[23, 24] This process is most apparent in mouse models, where T cells from TCR transgenic mice can differentiate into either T_H1 or T_H2 cells, depending on the inflammatory milieu in which they differentiate. For example, IFN-γ and IL-12 promote the differentiation of precursor cells into T_H1 cells by preventing the outgrowth of T_H2 cells and by augmentation of T_H1 differentiation. IL-4 has the greatest influence in driving T_H2 differentiation.[24, 25]

Several variables associated with T cell activation affect development of the final phenotype.[21] For example, the antigen dose and the antigen itself may affect differentiation. However, both "low" and "high" doses of antigen have been found to cause differentiation to T_H2 phenotypes. Likewise, ligands that provide an altered signal to the TCR, such as altered peptide ligands and non–FcR-binding anti-CD3 antibody, have also been shown to skew differentiation toward a T_H2 response.[16, 17, 26] In addition to the TCR signal, costimulatory signals (see below) are another important variable in the net effect of the activation signal and the phenotype that results. The involvement of particular costimulatory ligands in turn depends on several other factors such as the tissue involved and other associated cells.

The final phenotype of a cell has important implications for the cell's ability to mediate autoimmune disease. In most instances, the cell-mediated immune responses involved in autoimmune endocrine diseases have been associated with T_H1 cytokines (IFN-γ, and IL-2), and protection from autoimmune endocrine disease has been associated with T_H2 cytokines (IL-4 and IL-5). For example, after treatment of mice with multiple low doses of streptozotocin, the inflamed islets have an increased content of IFN-γ, and treatment with anti–IFN-γ antibody prevents diabetes.[27]

The relationship between T cell phenotype and autoimmune endocrine disease has been extensively studied in the NOD mouse, a model of T1DM. In these mice insulitis initially appears between 2 and 4 weeks of age, and diabetes is first detected after 15 weeks of age. As discussed below, T cells are mediators of the disease, although B lymphocytes are required for the initiation of insulitis. In NOD mice, expression of T_H1 cytokines can be detected as early as 1 to 2 months of age. Increased expression of T_H1 cytokines is seen in females, in whom diabetes develops in 70% to 90% of mice, but decreased expression in males, in whom diabetes occurs only in 10% to 20% of mice.[28] Interestingly, genetic absence of IFN-γ delays, but does not prevent diabetes in the NOD mouse, which suggests that IFN-γ is an enhancer rather than a requirement for disease.[29] Monoclonal T cells expressing a TCR reactive with islet antigen will cause autoimmune diabetes when they differentiate in vitro into cells that produce IFN-γ and are transferred into young NOD mice, but not when they differentiate in vitro into IL-4 producers.[30] In addition, differentiation of cells to a T_H1 phenotype, which is enhanced by the administration of IL-12, can exacerbate NOD diabetes.[31] The defective TCR signaling in NOD mice described by Delovitch et al. has been associated with impaired IL-4 production.[32] Treatment of NOD mice with IL-4 or expression of this cytokine in the islets leads to protection from diabetes.[33] However, the situation is not as simple as progression of disease with T_H1 cytokines and protection with T_H2 cytokines. Although treatment of NOD mice with IL-10 protected against diabetes, Wogensen et al. found that in NOD mice producing IL-10 in the islets as a transgene, accelerated diabetes occurred even though the islet-infiltrating cells were of a T_H2 phenotype.[34, 35] Although TCR transgenic T cells of a T_H2 phenotype will not transfer diabetes into young NOD mice, they will do so into NOD/*scid* animals.[36] Thus this and other observations, discussed below, suggest that interaction between the cytokine milieu at the time of antigen recognition and a diverse population of cells present at that site ultimately determines the pathogenicity of the response.

Requirement for Costimulation for T Cell Activation

Engagement of the TCR alone is insufficient to cause conventional activation of T cells and differentiation into effector cells. In fact, delivery of the TCR signal alone, in the absence of a "costimulatory" signal, may result in T cell unresponsiveness (or anergy) or even apoptosis (programmed cell death).[37, 38] Thus a second "costimulatory" signal is required for the development of fully competent T cells and B cells. Costimulation regulates expansion of antigen-reactive populations of T cells, migration of cells to sites of inflammation, production of soluble mediators of inflammation, and differentiation of T cells into the subsets discussed above. It is therefore expected that these interactions can control autoimmune endocrine disease.

Costimulatory signals are generated through the interaction of receptors on the surfaces of T cells with ligands on the surfaces of APCs. The interactions between these molecules are not antigen specific. The combination of signals delivered through the TCR with costimulatory signals is synergistic for T cell activation. Activation leads to the production of IL-2 and other cytokines and chemokines, rescues cells from apoptosis, and leads to the expansion of mature effector cells capable of mediating a sustained immune response.[39, 40] Most peripheral tissues do not express costimulatory signals, and therefore interaction between T cells reactive with peripheral antigens would not normally be expected to result in competent T cell activation. This control of T cell activation may be important in regulating tolerance to peripheral tissues, including endocrine organs. Several costimulatory receptors have been described, the most notable being CD28 and CD40 ligand (CD40L) (Table 39–2).

CD28 interacts with molecules on the APC termed B7-1 (CD80) and B7-2 (CD86).[51] CD28 is a cell surface glycoprotein that was originally identified by the ability of anti-CD28 molecules to block the anergy induced in T cells after their encounter with antigen plus MHC complexes. B7-1 (CD80) was the first identified ligand for CD28, and B7-1 transfectants can costimulate antigen- and mitogen-driven T cell proliferation and IL-2 production and block induction of anergy in T cell clones.[52–55] Transgenic expression of B7-1 on islet cells in the NOD mouse leads to accelerated diabetes, and its expression on the islets of normal mice leads to susceptibility to autoimmune diabetes induced by multiple low doses of streptozotocin.[56, 57] These studies indicated that provision of a CD28 costimulatory signal subsequent to antigen recognition is sufficient to activate islet antigen–reactive cells.

However, antibodies against B7-1 do not completely block T cell stimulation, and cells from mice deficient in B7-1 can still stimulate antigen-specific T cell responses. In contrast, a soluble high-affinity homologue of CD28, cytotoxic T lymphocyte antigen-4 (CTLA-4), fully blocked CD28-dependent responses.[51] These results suggested that a second CD28 ligand exists. This B7-1 homologue was later identified in both the human and mouse and termed CD86 and B7-2, respectively.[58, 59] A combination of antibodies against B7-1 and B7-2 will completely inhibit antigen-specific T cell responses in vitro.

TABLE 39–2. Costimulatory Receptors and Ligands

Costimulatory Molecule	Ligand(s)	Reference
Activation molecules		
CD28	CD80, CD86	39
?	B7h	41, 42
ICOS	B7-H1	41, 43
CD40L (gp39) (CD154)	CD40	44, 45
OX40	OX40R	46
4-1BB (CD137)	4-1BBL	47, 48
ICAM-1	LFA-1, LFA-3	49
Inhibitory molecules		
CTLA-4 (CD152)	CD80, CD86	39
CD30	CD30L	50

Considerable evidence attesting to the relevance of CD28 costimulatory signals in endocrine disease has accumulated. Lenschow et al. found that a soluble form of human CTLA-4 immunoglobulin (hCTLA4Ig) can prevent diabetes in the NOD mouse.[60] Prevention of disease was shown to be due to the blockade of B7-2/CD28 interactions. Herold et al. made similar observations in diabetes induced with multiple low doses of streptozotocin.[61] In murine autoimmune thyroiditis, blockade of B7-2 inhibited priming and in vitro activation of effector cells.[62] By virtue of their ability to induce cytokine production, costimulatory signals can affect autoimmune responses in positive and negative ways. For example, Arreaza et al. found that treatment of young NOD mice with an agonistic anti-CD28 mAb restored deficient IL-4 production in the mice and prevented autoimmune diabetes.[44]

CD28/B7 interactions may regulate differentiation of T cells into the phenotypes described above. For example, prevention of autoimmune diabetes in the NOD mouse after treatment with hCTLA4Ig is associated with a shift in the isotypes of autoantibodies and thus suggests a shift from a T_H1- to a T_H2-mediated response (D. Lenschow, K. Herold, J. Bluestone, B. Singh, unpublished observations). However, the effects of B7-2 and B7-1 ligands may not be the same at all anatomic sites. In an experimental allergic encephalomyelitis model of multiple sclerosis, blockade of B7-1 reduces IFN-γ production and prevents disease, whereas blockade with anti–B7-2 exacerbates disease.[45] Thus CD28/B7 costimulation can affect the phenotype of the immune response, which may ultimately determine its ability to induce disease.

CD40L (CD154) was first identified as the receptor on T cells for the costimulatory ligand CD40 on B lymphocytes.[63] Humans with a genetic mutation in CD40L are subject to the development of an immunodeficiency, the hyper-IgM syndrome, that is characterized by elevated levels of IgM, low levels of IgA, IgG, and IgE, and an absence of germinal centers. This observation and other murine studies indicate a primary role of CD40/CD154 interactions in the regulation of B cell proliferation, production of immunoglobulin, immunoglobulin class switching, rescue of B cells from apoptotic death, germinal center formation, and generation of B cell memory.[64] Furthermore, CD40/CD154 interactions can regulate the APC function of B and dendritic cells through the induction of other costimulatory ligands, especially B7. Initial studies suggested that CD40/CD40L interaction may be important primarily as an inducer of B7 expression on APCs because full reconstitution of cellular and humoral immunity was achieved in CD40L-deficient mice by administration of an activating antibody to CD40 that increased expression of B7-2.[65] However, more recent observations, in a cardiac allograft model, indicate that CD40/CD40L interactions provide functional effects in addition to B7-1 and B7-2 interactions and that this pathway can independently costimulate T cells.[66] Nonetheless, CD40L/CD40 interactions are thought to be important early in the immune response but less important after initiation. Blockade of CD40/CD40L interactions can prevent diabetes only if implemented early in life but cannot block recurrent insulitis.[46, 67]

Other costimulatory interactions have also been found to be important in autoimmune responses, particularly in the absence of costimulation by CD28, CD40L, and/or the cytokines IL-2 or IL-4. The OX-40 receptor (OX-40R) is a transmembrane protein found on the surface of activated CD4$^+$ T cells. When engaged by an agonist such as anti–OX-40 antibody or the OX-40 ligand during antigen presentation to T cell lines, OX-40R generates a costimulatory signal that is as potent as CD28 costimulation.[47] Engagement of OX-40R enhances effector and memory-effector T cell function by upregulating IL-2 production and increasing the life span of effector T cells. Blocking OX-40/OX-40R interactions has been found to decrease experimental allergic encephalomyelitis, a model of multiple sclerosis.[48]

4-1BB is a member of the tumor necrosis factor (TNF) receptor superfamily expressed on activated CD4$^+$ and CD8$^+$ T cells.[68] 4-1BB can costimulate IL-2 production by resting primary T cells independent of CD28 ligation. 4-1BB (CD137) appears to play a role in T cell–dependent humoral immune responses and in CD8-dependent responses. This molecule may also be important in promoting T_H2 responses though production of IL-10.[69] Finally, certain T cell surface molecules such as CD30 and CTLA-4 are *negative* regulators of immune responses as discussed below.

FUNCTIONAL BIOLOGY OF B LYMPHOCYTES

The hallmark of autoimmune endocrine disease is the presence of autoantibodies directed against organ-specific antigens. Autoantibodies to endocrine antigens are not uncommon in the general population. In one cross-sectional study, 10.3% of women and 2.7% of men without thyroid dysfunction were found to have thyroid autoantibodies.[70] Likewise, 3.1% of first-degree relatives of patients with type 1 diabetes have islet cell antibodies. However, only 1% of relatives progress to diabetes over a 7-year period.[71] These clinical observations suggest that autoreactive B cells do not always result in clinical disease and are tolerated by the host. Moreover, these observations also indicate that autoantibodies alone are not sufficient to cause autoimmune endocrine disease.

The antigen-specific binding receptor on B cells is membrane immunoglobulin (mIg), which is a tetrameric complex of immunoglobulin heavy and light chains.[72] Similar to T cells, B cell function is also dependent on signal transduction pathways.[73] The signal transduction component of mIg consists of a disulfide-bonded heterodimer of the Ig-α and Ig-β molecules. Within the Ig-α and Ig-β subunits of mIg is an ITAM that induces protein tyrosine kinase activation and calcium mobilization. The signaling function of the ITAM is dependent on two conserved tyrosine residues that are sites of phosphorylation after B cell receptor (BCR) engagement. Two distinct signals are delivered through the BCR: an activation signal that leads to cell entry into the cell cycle and upregulation of costimulatory molecules, as well as a persistence signal, which is needed for normal B cell development. mIg is associated with a protein complex that is homologous to the CD3 complex associated with the TCR. The components of this disulfide-linked heterodimeric complex bind to cytoplasmic effectors, including src family tyrosine kinases. The receptor-associated src family kinases associate with downstream effectors, including phospholipase C$_\gamma$, P21^{ras}, guanosine triphosphatase–activating protein, phosphatidylinositol 3-kinase, and microtubule-associated protein kinase.[72] A unique feature of B cells is their ability to respond to antigen in different structural contexts with different biologic responses.[72, 74] For example, the encounter of a B cell with antigen may lead to clonal deletion or receptor editing (see below), which represent inhibited responses, whereas if the antigen is encountered in multimeric form complexed with carbohydrate, the B cell is induced to proliferate. In the latter situation, anergy can result if T cell help is not provided.

In contrast to T cells, B lymphocytes cannot be unequivocally grouped into subsets on the basis of unique surface markers alone. All B cells make and secrete antibodies, although two major subpopulations of B cells display sufficient functional diversity to justify their classification as distinct subsets.[75] CD5$^+$ B cells (B1) differentiate in the omentum and constitute the predominant B cell type during fetal life.[76, 77] They tend to produce IgM antibodies with broad specificity for bacterial and self-antigens. Although rheumatoid factor activity and anti-DNA antibodies are most frequently produced by B1 cells, they are not responsible for autoantibodies against endocrine cells. The responses of B1 cells are thymus independent and provide a first line of defense against common bacterial antigens. B1 responses do not lead to immunologic memory.

B2 cells represent the conventional B cells that secrete all immunoglobulin classes, and these cells are the subset most relevant to autoimmune endocrine diseases.[78] B2 cells are thymus dependent and require physical interaction with T cells specific for the same antigen (cognate help). These cells are the probable source of autoantibodies such as antithyroglobulin, antimicrosomal, anti–glutamic acid decarboxylase (GAD), and anti–IA-2/ICA512 antibodies.

The B2 cell relies on its surface immunoglobulin clonal receptors to bind and internalize antigen, which is then processed and presented on class II MHC molecules to helper T cells.[79] After engagement of the TCR with the MHC plus peptide complex, many pairs of cell adhesion molecules actively participate in the T-B cell interaction.

Several of these pairs deliver costimulatory signals to the B cell to promote its clonal expansion and differentiation. In addition, activated T cells secrete cytokines such as IL-4, IL-5, and others that in turn stimulate B cell differentiation. The process of T cell–dependent B cell differentiation is complex and highly regulated, and several possible outcomes may result, including the generation of memory cells and highly differentiated effector cells that secrete immunoglobulin.[80]

ANTIGEN PRESENTATION TO LYMPHOCYTES

The immune responses that cause autoimmune endocrine diseases are antigen specific. That is, they are focused toward certain target peptides rather than involving generalized immune dysregulation. The specificity of this response is conferred by the ability of immune cells to respond exclusively to organ-specific antigens. However, antigen recognition by T and B lymphocytes differs: the antigen receptors on T cells recognize protein sequences of 8 to 20 amino acids in length trapped in an MHC basket, whereas immunoglobulins, which are the antigen receptors on B cells, recognize three-dimensional structures present on unprocessed antigens.[81–87] Processing of proteins and presentation of their peptide components to T cells require a complex series of interrelated events that take place in specialized APCs, including cells such as macrophages, dendritic cells, and in certain situations, B cells. APCs perform two essential functions required for the initiation of immune responses: first, they display antigenic fragments associated with specialized antigen-presenting molecules, and second, they deliver costimulatory signals required for lymphocyte activation and differentiation.

The specialized antigen-presenting molecules are the cell surface glycoproteins encoded in the highly polymorphic MHC genes called class I and class II. MHC molecules are peptide-binding molecules that present intracellular peptides for recognition by T cells. Conventional (CD4$^+$ and CD8$^+$) T cells recognize only the complex of MHC plus peptide, and therefore T cell recognition is said to be MHC restricted. In this manner, only peptides that can bind to MHC molecules can be "seen" by T cells.

MHC molecules sample the contents of the intracellular compartments and bring representative peptides to the cell surface for T cell scrutiny. MHC class I molecules specialize in the binding of endogenous peptides in the endoplasmic reticulum and in their subsequent transport to the cell surface for recognition by T cells expressing the MHC class I–binding molecule CD8 (CD8$^+$ T cells). Class I MHC molecules are found on all cells, although the relative level of expression may differ considerably between organs, cell types, and even individual cells.[83] In contrast, MHC class II molecules (also referred to as Ia) bind exogenous peptides generated by proteolysis of extracellular material in the endosomal compartment and present them on the surface for recognition by T cells expressing the MHC class II–binding molecule CD4 (CD4$^+$ T cells).[84, 86] Expression of class II MHC molecules is more restricted than that of class I. They are found on APCs such as macrophages and dendritic cells, B lymphocytes, thymic epithelial cells, and in humans, activated T lymphocytes.

The structures of MHC class I and II molecules reflect their specialized functions. Class I and II molecules both contain N-terminal peptide-binding baskets sitting on a structural platform made up of two immunoglobulin domains. MHC class I consists of an α chain with three extracellular domains associated noncovalently with the non-MHC peptide β$_2$-microglobulin. The MHC class I basket is made up of the α$_1$ and β$_2$ domains supported by the immunoglobulin α$_3$- and β$_2$-microglobulin domains.[81] MHC class II is a heterodimer of α and β chains, both of which are integral membrane proteins with two extracellular domains. The α$_1$ and β$_1$ domains create the MHC class II basket that sits on top of the immunoglobulin α$_2$ and β$_2$ domains.[84] For both classes of MHC molecules, the peptide-binding basket is made up of two domains, each contributing four β pleated sheets and one α helix. The β sheets form the bottom of the basket and the α helix forms the sides. Most of the polymorphic residues in MHC molecules reside in the sites involved in peptide binding.

More recently, the human CD1 family of cell surface molecules has been characterized as non-MHC antigen-presenting molecules.[86] Unlike class I and II MHC molecules, the antigen-binding groove of CD1 is made up of hydrophobic residues, which suggests that CD1 binds hydrophobic ligands such as lipids. Thus antigens presented by CD1 are lipid and glycoprotein in nature instead of peptides. CD1 molecules are recognized by natural killer (NK)-like T cells.[88] These cells are thought to be a source of IL-4 in the early stages of an immune response. As discussed above, the local cytokine environment at the time of T cell activation affects the differentiation of T cells. It was therefore of note that in humans, NK-like cells that express the Vα24-JαQ TCR had reduced production of IL-4 in relatives of patients who progress to diabetes when compared with relatives of patients who do not progress to diabetes.[89] These investigators suggest that the reduced IL-4 production by this subset of cells leads to immune responses skewed toward production of IFN-γ, which is involved in the development of autoimmune diabetes.

It follows from the previous discussion that the ability of a T cell to respond to any given antigen is dependent not only on the binding characteristics of antigenic peptides but also on the physical properties of the MHC molecules. Thus it is not surprising that genes of the MHC have been most strongly associated with autoimmune endocrine diseases. For example, multiple associations with Graves' and class I and class II HLA alleles have been reported—HLA-B8 was among the first associations with the disease.[90, 91] The strongest association in whites is found with DR3.[91, 92] HLA-DQA1*0501 has been found to be independently associated in some studies,[93, 94] whereas in others this apparent linkage has been found to be the result of linkage disequilibrium with DR3.[91] HLA-DR3 has been specifically associated with clinically isolated autoimmune adrenal disease.[95] Specific antigens associated with autoimmune adrenal disease include DPB1*0101, DQA*0501, DQB*0201, and DRB1*0301.[91] A specific arginine substitution in DQA1*0501 has also been linked with autoimmune adrenal disease.[94]

The association of T1DM with genes in the MHC region is very strong—in several studies,[96] mean lod (logarithm of odds) scores are greater than 10. Among whites, HLA-DR3 and HLA-DR4 alleles confer increased susceptibility to T1DM, and as many as 94% of white T1DM patients carry these alleles.[97–99] The strength of the association with the MHC is reflected by comparing the risk in HLA-nonidentical siblings (1.2%) with the age-corrected empiric risk of T1DM in HLA-identical siblings (15.5%). Studies of North American white patients with these alleles showed that the association is closer to the DQ region of the MHC. In fact, Todd et al. found that absence of an aspartic acid at position 57 of the DQ-β chain best explained susceptibility to T1DM.[100] Interestingly, an analogous finding exists in the unique I-A^{g7} class II allele of the NOD mouse.[101] Thus DQ haplotypes lacking aspartic acid, such as DQ*0201 (DQw2) and DQ*0302 (DQw8), are associated with increased risk whereas alleles with aspartic acid, such as DQ*0602 (Dqw1.2) and DQ*0102, are protective. The phenotype of protective alleles is dominant.[99]

The fact that specific sequences of the DQ-β chain conferred susceptibility suggested that by virtue of the antigen-binding properties conferred by the protein sequence of DQ, T cell activation, T cell tolerance, and/or other functional immune responses regulating islet antigen–reactive T cells might be affected. Transgenic expression of another amino acid residue at position 57 inhibited diabetes development in the NOD mouse.[102–104] The unique diabetes-susceptible class II MHC molecules have unique peptide-binding properties. Peptides eluted from I-A^{g7} have sequences that implicate an acidic residue in the C terminus of the peptide as important for binding. Reich et al. have shown the role of this residue in binding by direct peptide-binding analysis.[105] This C-terminal acidic amino acid may interact with an arginine residue in the MHC class II α chain that is exposed when β chain residue 57 is mutated to serine or to the unique β chain residue histidine 56. However, other than the C-terminal amino acid, the I-A^{g7} class II–binding peptides lack other identifiable binding motifs but rather interact via general hydrophobic amino acid residues.

More recently, another molecular basis of MHC linkage that is based on the unusual physical properties of the DQ and I-A^{g7} molecules is beginning to be elucidated. First, these class II molecules fail to form stable αβ dimers in association with binding peptides. In contrast to murine alleles such as I-A^d, I-A^b, and I-A^k, very few stable αβ dimers are located on the surfaces of NOD APCs, the dimers are short lived, and they present antigenic peptides to T cells poorly.[106, 107] These features may preclude negative selection of autoreactive T cells in the thymus (see below) and/or affect activation of diabetogenic T cells in the periphery.

MECHANISMS OF TOLERANCE

The development of endocrine disease by immunologic mechanisms represents a failure to develop or maintain tolerance to self-antigens. In this setting tolerance refers to the absence of immunologic destruction of a tissue and does not necessarily imply the absence of autoreactive cells or antibodies. In most instances the initiators of the immune response that results in disease have not been identified. Among those antigens that have been described as targets of autoimmunity, most are constitutively expressed cellular components (e.g., thyroid peroxidase, GAD, insulin). Thus recent interest has focused on understanding how tolerance toward self-proteins is established and maintained by the immune system and comprehending how failures of this system result in endocrine diseases.

The random rearrangement of individual variable components of the TCR and BCR genes is designed to maximize diversity in anticipation of all possible MHC/antigenic structures.[108] An important implication of the random nature of TCR and BCR gene arrangement is that every individual, even monozygotic twins, will have a unique immune cell repertoire. This fact has been invoked to explain the discordance of autoimmune endocrine diseases, such as T1DM, among identical twins.

The chance rearrangement of TCR and BCR genes that leads to such diverse reactivity implies that self-reactive receptors will be present in the repertoire. Mechanisms to eliminate/control/restrict responses to self are therefore paramount to avoid autoimmune disease.

Clonal Deletion

The most important and efficacious mechanism for tolerance is clonal deletion. Clonal deletion occurs predominantly in the thymus (T cells) and bone marrow (B cells) as a consequence of the elimination of immature lymphocytes.[109] In the thymus, several developmental steps occur that ultimately lead to the export of T cells reactive with antigens in the context of self-MHC molecules (Fig. 39–3). First, to ensure that only cells that are capable of responding to antigens presented by self-MHC molecules constitute the final repertoire, cells that respond to antigen in the context of self-MHC undergo a process termed "positive selection," whereas those not restricted by self-MHC molecules do not mature further and die by apoptosis. Clonal deletion occurs predominantly in immature lymphocytes. Apoptosis is developmentally regulated in lymphocytes to ensure their timely death after encounters with self-antigens. The success of clonal deletion is dependent on the availability of self-antigens at tolerogenic concentrations and correct functioning of the lymphocyte's apoptotic machinery. In general, self-reactive clones with high-affinity receptors are more likely to be clonally deleted than those expressing low affinity for self. For example, studies in transgenic mice expressing TCR specific for the male antigen (H-Y), selective class II or class I MHC molecules, or specific peptides, as well as intrathymically transplanted islet cells, have been used to show that clonal deletion occurs between migration from the thymic cortex to the medulla and is responsible for the elimination of potentially autoreactive T cells from the repertoire of mature peripheral T cells.[50, 110–113]

It follows that the ability of clonal deletion to eliminate autoreactive T cells is dependent on the following: (1) the ability of the MHC molecules to bind and present autoantigens, (2) expression of the antigen in the thymus at the time of development, and (3) function of the activation pathways needed for negative selection. In animal models, inhibiting clonal deletion by treatment of neonatal mice with cyclosporine causes autoimmune disease manifested by lesions in the testes, pancreas, and islets of Langerhans.[114, 115] As discussed above, the

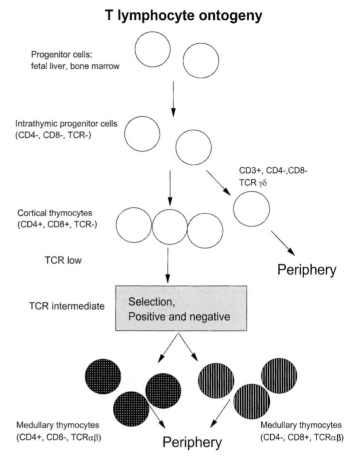

FIGURE 39–3. T cell ontogeny. Bone marrow precursors that lack the phenotype of mature T cells migrate to the thymus during fetal life. Most T cells do not mature further. Through events termed positive and negative selection, cells that are able to react with foreign peptide plus major histocompatibility complex but are not reactive with self-peptides expressed in the thymus at the time of ontogeny are selected for maturation. As the cells mature through these stages, they first express T cell receptor with both CD4 and CD8 and then lose expression of either CD4 or CD8 and acquire the phenotype of mature T cells.

failure to delete autoreactive lymphocytes from the repertoire may be tightly linked to the MHC genes by virtue of the unique set of self-peptides that they bind and/or their binding characteristics, which may be poor in the case of DQ or I-A^{g7} molecules associated with type 1 diabetes. Expression of known islet antigens in the thymus at the time of T cell development has been shown to result in loss of the susceptibility to autoimmune diabetes induced with multiple low doses of streptozotocin or in the biobreeding/Worcester (BB/W) rat and NOD mouse.[6, 112, 113, 116] Therefore, transplantation of islets into the thymus of younger patients has been suggested as one approach to induction of tolerance to islets for prevention of T1DM or rejection of transplanted islet allografts.

Clonal deletion affects only antigens that are expressed or that traffic into the thymus, and therefore cells reactive with antigens expressed outside the thymus will not be deleted from the repertoire. Interestingly, many antigens previously considered to be expressed exclusively in the periphery are actually expressed in the thymus. For example, both insulin and GAD, thought to be important autoantigens in human type 1 diabetes, are expressed in the thymus.[117] It has been postulated that the association between polymorphisms of the insulin gene and T1DM may be accounted for by the effects of these polymorphisms on expression of insulin in the thymus and the effects of the relative expression of this antigen on negative selection of autoreactive T cells.[118] Finally, recent data have suggested that the costimulatory molecule CTLA-4 may be associated with clonal deletion in the thymus of potentially autoreactive T cells. Intrathymic CTLA-4 blockade dramatically inhibits anti-CD3–mediated depletion of CD4$^+$, CD8$^+$ double-positive immature thymocytes.[119]

Clonal deletion is also a mechanism for removal of self-reactive B cells from the peripheral lymphoid compartment. Immature B cells that encounter self-antigen are eliminated from the immune repertoire by negative selection.[120, 121] For example, lysozyme-binding B cells in the spleen and lymph nodes are deleted in double-transgenic mice expressing antilysozyme immunoglobulin and a membrane-bound form of lysozyme. Negative selection has been proposed to take place by two distinct mechanisms: (1) deletion by apoptosis and (2) alteration of antigen receptor specificity by receptor editing. Receptor editing refers to a process by which selection occurs at the level of the BCR, and self-reactive receptors that encounter autoantigen in the bone marrow are altered through secondary rearrangement.[122] Whether receptor editing is effective in preventing autoreactivity to organ-specific B cells has not been shown.

Studies of B cell tolerance to endocrine organs suggest that clonal deletion does not occur in cells reactive with organ-specific antigens. For example, systemic expression of membrane-bound hen-egg lysozyme (mHEL) results in elimination or inactivation of circulating HEL-reactive B cells. However, when mHEL is expressed exclusively on thyroid cells, elimination or inactivation of circulating HEL-reactive B cells does not occur.[123] Other mechanisms must therefore be operational to avoid autoreactivity. One possibility is that antigens are sequestered from circulating preimmune B cells, similar to clonal ignorance discussed below.

Peripheral Tolerance via Cell Death

After activation of T cells in the periphery, T lymphocyte death occurs through two mechanisms: activation-induced cell death (AICD) and growth factor withdrawal.[124] In AICD, death of activated cells is mediated by TNF and Fas/Fas ligand (FasL) interactions, which deliver death signals to activated T cells that result in apoptosis.[125, 126] Thus elimination of activated cells by death signals is one means of preventing autoreactivity. One of the unique characteristics of "immune-privileged" sites is expression of FasL, which causes death of activated T cells that express Fas and thereby prevents T cell responses against the FasL-expressing organ. IL-2 is also a key regulator of this process.[127] Recent data support a primary role for AICD and growth factor withdrawal in allotransplantation. Turka, Strom, and others have demonstrated that apoptosis of activated, alloreactive T cells is essential for the induction of tolerance. In sharp contrast, global immunosuppression with drugs such as FK-506 and cyclosporine blocks T cell activation and apoptosis and precludes the induction of tolerance.[128]

Clonal Ignorance

In general, naive T cells do not circulate into peripheral tissues. Clonal ignorance refers to a situation in which self-reactive lymphocytes with the functional capacity to respond to their target antigens coexist with that antigen.[129–132] In one example, expression of the alloantigen I-A^d on the β cells of H-2^b mice failed to induce an inflammatory response and subsequent development of diabetes even though cells reactive with the alloantigen were present in the animal and responded to the alloantigen in vitro.[133] This state is precarious because self-reactive lymphocyte clones operationally ignore self-antigens only as long as local conditions permit. The condition may be reversed by the presence of inflammatory mediators, antigen mimicry, or other mechanisms that can induce T cell migration to sites of antigen and expression of activation molecules.[134] For example, mice expressing a transgene encoding a glycoprotein from the lymphocytic choriomeningitis virus (LCMV) in the pancreatic β cells, as well as a TCR that recognizes the glycoprotein plus MHC, are functionally tolerant of the glycoprotein.[135] The tolerance is broken if the mouse is infected with live LCMV. Interestingly, if in addition a third gene is present, termed adenovirus E3, that among other things inhibits expression of class I molecules on β cells, tolerance is not broken by infection with LCMV even though LCMV-reactive cells are found in

the spleen.[136] This example illustrates that functional tolerance may be local.

Control of T cell migration may also be related to induction of tolerance to peripheral antigens induced in neonates. In mouse bone marrow chimeras generated at different ages, recent thymic emigrants were tolerized to a skin-expressed MHC class I antigen only during the neonatal period but not during adulthood.[137] Blockade of T cell migration neonatally prevented tolerance induction. Thus T cell trafficking through nonlymphoid tissues in the neonate is crucial for the establishment of self-tolerance to sessile, skin-expressed antigens.

Clonal Anergy

Clonal anergy refers to a state of functional nonresponsiveness of lymphocytes. Over 30 years ago Bretcher and Cohn suggested that B cells required two signals for effective activation, the first provided by the antigen-specific receptor and the second by another noncognate "costimulatory" receptor.[138] The notion was that the autoreactive response could be controlled, at least in part, by alterations in activation involving the TCR/BCR or costimulatory signals. Lafferty and Gill hypothesized that these types of intervention would lead to the development of anergy.[139] There is now ample evidence that this form of peripheral regulation occurs in vivo.[39, 51] Under certain circumstances of signal 1 or signal 2 blockade, the T cells not only fail to respond to antigen but also do not respond when rechallenged with the antigen even when appropriate activating signals are delivered.

Clonal anergy can be induced in T cells by providing an altered "signal 1" or by providing signal 1 in the absence of "signal 2." Allen et al. found that "altered peptide ligands" that bind TCR can induce nonresponsiveness in antigen-reactive T cells, and Smith et al. reported that non–FcR–binding anti-CD3 mAb can induce anergy of T$_H$1 cells by delivering an altered signal to activated T cells.[16, 17, 28] The molecular mechanisms that are thought to underlie this induced nonresponsiveness involve qualitative changes in the phosphorylation of TCR components. The basis for the selective effects on phenotypic subsets is not clear inasmuch as similar changes in TCR signaling have been observed in T$_H$1 and T$_H$2 cells. Nonetheless, the selective effects make this approach very attractive for immune therapies. These observations are also consistent with the notion of tolerance induction as an active process that involves delivery of "altered" activation signals.[128]

Tolerance of B cells involves changes in antigen receptor signaling.[140] B cells in transgenic mice expressing a BCR for HEL and circulating HEL populate the peripheral lymphoid organs but do not respond to HEL.[140] These same cells will proliferate in response to lipopolysaccharide and retain responsiveness to stimulation via CD40 and IL-4. The anergic cells are characterized by downregulation of IgM but not IgD and by the accumulation of B cells in the splenic follicular mantle zone. BCR ligation in these mice fails to activate signaling pathways and the nuclear transcription factor NF-κB. This clonal anergy is analogous to the effects of TCR activation in the absence of costimulatory signals. Silencing of autoreactive B cells involves changes in antigen receptor function and changes in the cells' potential to differentiate.

Inhibitory T Cell Ligands

As discussed above, the absence of costimulatory molecules on resting cells may serve to inhibit activation of T cells reactive with the self-antigens expressed by those same cells and even induce anergy of the antigen-reactive cells because "signal 1" (via the TCR) will be delivered in the absence of "signal 2" (costimulatory signal). In addition, other "costimulatory signals" can inhibit immune responsiveness. This concept is illustrated by the fact that mAbs against B7-1 actually exacerbate autoimmune diabetes in the NOD mouse.[60] This surprising observation suggested that B7-1 may be the ligand for an inhibitory signal to the T cell that regulates development of autoimmune diabetes. At least two surface molecules have been identified that may deliver "inhibitory" signals to T cells (see Table 39–2).

CTLA-4 was originally identified in 1987 as a homologue of CD28 and was thought to be a costimulatory molecule.[141] Like CD28, CTLA-4 binds both B7-1 and B7-2 but does so with much higher affinity. However, in contrast to CD28, which activates T cells when ligation of CTLA-4 inhibits T cell responses and IL-2 production.[142–145] Whereas CD28 is expressed on resting T cells, there is little evidence for expression of CTLA-4. After activation, CTLA-4 can be detected on the cell surface, although an even greater pool of the molecule is present intracellularly.[146] Significant expression of CTLA-4 occurs approximately 48 hours after T cell activation and is enhanced by inflammatory mediators.

Mice deficient in CTLA-4 die at a young age of autoimmune disease involving the heart, pancreas, and other organs.[147] Treatment of TCR transgenic NOD mice with anti–CTLA-4 mAb will precipitate diabetes.[148] Thus these functional and experimental observations suggest that CTLA-4 is an important negative regulator of activated T cells and indicate that perturbation of the "balance" of inhibitory and regulatory signals that control T cell behavior may be implicated in the pathogenesis of autoimmune endocrine disease.

It is therefore of interest that Yanagawa et al. found an association between polymorphisms in the CTLA-4 gene and Graves' disease.[149] Similarly, in the NOD mouse, a diabetes susceptibility locus has been found on chromosome 1 within a region that encompasses CTLA-4 and CD28 (Iddm5), but Iddm5 has not been precisely identified. Colucci et al. found defective expression of CD28 and CTLA-4 in these mice.[150] Studies in patients with T1DM have also suggested an association of the CTLA-4 gene and disease, although this finding has not been reproducible in all populations studied.[151, 152] The role of CTLA-4 in controlling T cell responsiveness makes this locus an interesting candidate gene for disease susceptibility. It has been suggested that failure to deliver T cell inhibitory signals in the periphery or even during thymic development because of functional differences in CTLA-4 alleles may result in unchecked T cell responses or failure to delete autoreactive cells during T cell ontogeny.

In addition, depending on the cells that are activated by costimulatory signals (see below), the net effect of costimulatory signals may be inhibition of disease. For example, although CTLA4Ig prevented diabetes in the NOD mouse, accelerated diabetes develops in mice deficient in CD28, and they express high levels of IFN-γ in their islets.[153] It has been postulated that CD28 costimulatory signals may be necessary for the development and/or activation of a regulatory population of cells.

CD30 is another T cell ligand that may deliver inhibitory signals, particularly for cells that have not been deleted through the Fas pathway of AICD. In a transplantation model, Kurts et al. found that CD8+, CD30− cells were 6000 times more aggressive for pancreatic islets than were wild-type CD8+ T cells.[154]

Thus both stimulatory and inhibitory mechanisms are controlled by costimulatory signals. It is clear from this discussion that manipulation of costimulatory signals would be an attractive target for immune therapy because it would specifically target autoantigen-reactive T cells and spare naive cells. However, because both inhibition and activation signals are delivered to T cells through "costimulatory" ligands, a clearer understanding of the role of these ligands is needed before considering clinical studies.

Immune Regulatory Cells

More recent data have provided evidence for populations of cells that can inhibit the activity of effector T cells. Control or inhibition of autoreactive T cells may represent as important a control mechanism as activation and may also be attributed to thymus-derived cells. Seddon and Mason have identified a population of CD4+ peripheral T cells or CD4+ thymocytes that can prevent the induction of autoimmune thyroiditis.[155] Development of these cells is antigen specific, and their activity depends on endogenously produced IL-4 and transforming growth factor-β (TGF-β) (see below). Generation of "regulatory" T cells from thymic emigrant precursors is driven by peripheral autoantigen. BB/W rats are lymphopenic and subject to spontaneous development of autoimmune diabetes.[156] T cells expressing RT6, which

have been shown to inhibit diabetes, fail to develop in these rats. Depletion of RT6+ T cells in diabetes-resistant BB rats precipitates disease. In the NOD mouse, Herbelin et al. have identified a population of thymocyte-derived cells that are positive for CD4 and L-selectin and are able to inhibit transfer of diabetes by T cells from diabetic mice.[157] These observations in experimental systems suggest that in addition to autoimmune effector cells, cells with a regulatory role also develop in the thymus and may play an important role in controlling activation of the disease-causing cells. Several groups have described CD8+ cells that are reactive with activated CD4+ T cells and restricted by the minor histocompatibility antigen Qa-1 and that inhibit the CD4+ T cell responses potentially involved in autoimmunity.[158]

Although not a physiologic mechanism for maintaining tolerance, tolerance induced with anti-CD4 and anti-CD8 mAbs has shed light on cellular mechanisms that may be normally operative. A combination of anti-CD4 and anti-CD8 mAbs could induce long-lasting tolerance to skin grafts in mice.[159] This tolerance developed over a 4-week period, but once established, the tolerance could affect naive cells transferred into the mice (dominant tolerance). Tolerance depended on the presence of host CD4+ T cells focused to the site of antigen. Further studies with a third-party graft indicated that regulation operated in a local microenvironment where antigen acts to focus naive antigen-specific T cells into the vicinity of regulatory CD4+ T cells. However, even naive T cells would acquire tolerance by cohabitation with the tolerant cells. This phenomenon was termed "infectious tolerance."[160]

Cytokines as Regulators of Peripheral Tolerance

As discussed above, many autoimmune endocrine diseases have been found to involve a T_H1-type cytokine response whereas T_H2 cytokines are protective. Moreover, by modifying the cytokine milieu, cytokines can prevent or exacerbate autoimmune disease. Therefore the cytokine environment at the time of T cell activation, as well as the cells' ability to produce cytokines, is likely to be an important determinant of progression of disease.

In addition, just as cytokines can affect differentiation of endocrine-reactive T cells, the other T cells that are present also play a role in mediating the protective effects of cytokines. For example, expression of IL-4 as a transgene in the islets of wild-type NOD mice will prevent diabetes but fail to do so when the TCR repertoire is limited to a single TCR.[161] These findings suggest that the effects of cytokines are on the heterogeneous population of cells involved in the autoimmune response rather than a single cell population.

Finally, in addition to the effects of IL-4 and IL-10 in favoring differentiation of T_H2 cells, the cytokine TGF-β, produced by a third subset of T cells designated T_H3 that also produce IL-4 and IL-10, has been postulated to regulate peripheral tolerance. TGF-β is thought to be involved in tolerance induced to ingested antigens (oral tolerance).[162] It has been postulated that this mechanism may be invoked to prevent autoimmune disease. Indeed, in the NOD mouse it has been possible to prevent diabetes by feeding insulin to the animals.[163] This observation forms the basis for the "oral tolerization" arm of the Diabetes Prevention Trial-1.

CHARACTERIZATION OF THE AUTOIMMUNE RESPONSE

Antigenic Targets of the Endocrine Autoimmune Response

Work over the past several years has identified antigenic targets of the immune response in autoimmune endocrine diseases.[164–174] Some of these targets of T1DM and autoimmune thyroid disease are listed in Tables 39–3 and 39–4. In general, the antigens represent intracellular proteins without structural anomalies. The fact that these proteins have a vital role in normal human physiology and that they are expressed at high levels in the organism highlights the importance of the various control mechanisms discussed previously in regulating responses to them.

TABLE 39–3. Autoantigens Identified in Type 1 Diabetes Mellitus

Antigen	Reference
Insulin B chain*	164
IA-2/ICA512*	165
IA-2β/phogrin	166
GAD65*	167
ICA69	168
Imogen	169

*Autoantibodies against these antigens are most predictive of type 1 diabetes mellitus.

Alternatively, several lines of evidence support the notion that mimicry between foreign peptides and autoantigens may result in autoreactivity. For example, GAD, which has been shown to be the target of autoantibodies in human type 1 diabetes and pathogenic T cells in the NOD mouse, has molecular homology with the coxsackievirus protein P2-C.[175] The similarities between these two epitopes may lead to autoreactivity in genetically predisposed persons. A similar mechanism may also account for the high rate of development of type 1 diabetes in the offspring of women who have had congenital rubella. Karjalainen et al. reported that patients with type 1 diabetes have antibodies that react with a discrete segment of bovine serum albumin (ABBOS), which suggests the possibility that mimicry between the bovine serum albumin antigen and an islet antigen may trigger an anti-islet immune response.[176] However, although these mechanisms of molecular mimicry are suggested by epidemiologic data, little direct evidence supports their role in human disease at this time. Furthermore, from the discussion of clonal ignorance above, it is clear that other factors are needed for activation of antigen-reactive T cells.

In animal models of autoimmune endocrine disease, heat shock proteins (hsp60) have been implicated as targets of the autoimmune response.[177] Furthermore, tolerization to these normal stress products has been found to prevent autoimmune diabetes.[178] This induction of tolerance is believed to occur by deviation of pathogenic T_H1 cells to a T_H2 phenotype.

An important recent development elucidated primarily from studies of autoreactive T cells from animal models is the concept of spreading and diversification of the antigenic targets of autoimmune responses, or epitope spreading.[179] Although the initial immune response may be to a particular peptide sequence of an antigen, with time, other peptides of the same antigen become targets of the autoimmune response (intramolecular spreading), and even additional antigens are involved (intermolecular spreading). Such spreading has been shown in the NOD mouse for T cell responses to GAD as well as insulin.[180, 181] The extent to which the response to the primary antigen or to the spread antigens accounts for tissue destruction is not clearly understood. An implication of this understanding is that it may be difficult to identify inciting antigens by studying the autoimmune response in its late course. Furthermore, immune interventions with specific antigens must take place early in the evolving response because with time, the proportion of T cells reactive with the inciting antigen diminishes.

Role of Cytokines in the Autoimmune Response

Activated T cells produce soluble products that also affect the differentiation of an immune response and may directly affect its

TABLE 39–4. Autoantigens Identified in Human Autoimmune Thyroid Diseases

Antigen	Reference
Heat shock protein	170
Flavoprotein subunit of mitochondrial succinate dehydrogenase (formerly unidentified 64-kDa protein)	171
Na/I transporter	172
TG	173
TPO (formerly microsomal antigen)	174
TSH receptor	174

TG, thyroglobulin; TPO, thyroperoxidase; TSH, thyroid-stimulating hormone.

pathogenicity. One of the important early mediators of differentiation of autoimmune cells is IFN-α; its presence has been detected in the pancreas in early lesions of autoimmune diabetes, and transgenic expression of IFN-α in islet cells causes diabetes.[182]

As discussed above, in most instances cell-mediated immune responses associated with autoimmune endocrine disease have been associated with T_H1 cytokines (IFN-γ and IL-2), and protection from autoimmune endocrine disease has been associated with T_H2 cytokines (IL-4 and IL-5). However, rather than a clear distinction between progression of disease with T_H1 cytokines and prevention with T_H2 cytokines, most studies have suggested an evolving process that can exhibit a varying phenotype. In NOD mice, expression of T_H1 cytokines can initially be detected by 1 to 2 months of age, and increased expression of T_H1 cytokines is seen in female mice, in whom diabetes develops in 70% to 90%, but a decrease is seen in male mice, in whom diabetes occurs only in 10% to 20%.[28] Fathman et al. reported that expression of IFN-γ in islets from NOD mice occurs as a relatively late process, soon before the clinical appearance of hyperglycemia.[183] More recently, Andre-Schmutz et al. found in TCR transgenic NOD mice that treatment with cyclophosphamide precipitates diabetes, which required coordinate expression of IL-18, IL-12, and TNF-α. In fact, no cellular or molecular evidence of cell contact–mediated mechanisms of cell death could be found in their studies.[184] In autoimmune thyroid disease, the response may vary with the phenotype and stage of the disease. Both T_H1 and T_H2 phenotypes can be found in glands from patients with Graves' and Hashimoto's diseases. The difference between diseases may be the effect of a functionally dominant population at a given time.[185]

The precise mechanism whereby cytokines affect the autoimmune response is not clear and may involve maintenance/loss of tolerance and direct toxic effects on target tissues, as well as their effects on differentiation of effector T cells. Sarvetnick et al. showed that insulitis, loss of tolerance to islet antigens, and diabetes occurred with transgenic expression of class II MHC molecules and IFN-γ in β cells.[186] Other studies using IFN-γ receptor mutant mice suggest that the important effect of this cytokine is on APCs.[187]

Cytokines produced by T_H1 cells, including IFN-γ together with IFN-α, have direct toxic effects on islet cells.[188] In vitro, these soluble mediators can inhibit glucose-stimulated insulin release from islets. It is postulated that these cytokines can induce the production of free radicals that may directly injure or destroy β cells. This hypothesis underlies the ongoing European nicotinamide diabetes intervention trial.[189]

Role of Immunoglobulins in Autoimmune Endocrine Diseases

In a few examples, including Graves' disease (antibodies against the thyroid-stimulating hormone receptor), autoimmune hypoglycemia (antibodies against insulin), and type B insulin resistance (antibodies against the insulin receptor), autoantibodies are direct mediators of disease. However, in most other autoimmune endocrine diseases, autoantibodies are markers of the autoimmune process and have helped elucidate the pathogenesis of the disease, but they are not the direct mediators of disease.[190–193] For example, autoantibodies have identified islet antigens such as ICA512 (IA-2), GAD65, and insulin in T1DM that may be the target of pathogenic T cells. Because T cell help is needed for B2 cells, it should therefore not be unexpected that immunoglobulin-producing B cells are required for disease pathogenesis. In the NOD mouse, diabetes does not occur in the absence of B cells.[194, 195] However, this result does not prove that autoantibodies are important effectors in this disease. The B cells may serve as APCs and may also provide the necessary costimulatory signals for early T cell activation. This notion is supported by the observation that later in the disease process, B lymphocytes appear to be dispensable inasmuch as diabetes can be adoptively transferred by B cell–depleted spleen cells from diabetic mice.[196]

Regardless of the pathogenic role of autoantibodies in disease progression, autoantibodies have facilitated study of the natural history of autoimmune endocrine diseases and identified autoantigens. In type 1 diabetes, studies of discordant twins and triplets in whom diabetes later developed have shown that autoimmunity may be present for years before disease is clinically apparent and at a time when only subtle abnormalities in insulin secretion can be detected.

The antigens recognized by the autoantibodies have more recently identified the natural progression of disease. The three most predictive antibodies—anti-insulin, anti-GAD65, and anti-ICA512—appear sequentially, thus suggesting an evolution of the disease process[193] (G. Eisenbarth, personnel communication). Studies of autoantibodies in T1DM support the notion that the disease develops over a period of about 3 years.

In addition, autoantibodies have led to the identification of antigens involved in the pathogenesis of disease (see Table 39–3) and the targets of autoreactive T cells. The antigen GAD65 was originally found through a search for the antigen recognized by antibodies reactive with a 64-kDa islet cell membrane protein that was identified in the serum of patients and BB/W rats, a rat model of T1DM.[167, 197–199] Autoantibodies to GAD65 are found in 70% of children with newly diagnosed diabetes and in 4.1% of control children.[198] In the NOD mouse, loss of tolerance to GAD65 has been found to correlate with the development of disease.[181, 200] Restoration of tolerance to GAD65 through a number of different immune manipulations such as intrathymic injection of GAD, intravenous injection of GAD, oral feeding of GAD, or intraislet GAD antisense expression can prevent T1DM and recurrence in islets transplanted into diabetic animals.[200–203] The insulin B chain is also the target of autoantibodies, particularly in young patients.[193, 204, 205] Insulin autoantibodies have been found in 56% of patients with newly diagnosed diabetes and in 2.8% of control children. This antigen is also recognized by pathogenic T cells in animal models of the disease. Importantly, pathogenic CD4+ and CD8+ T cell clones from NOD mice that are reactive with insulin have been isolated.[180, 205]

Other Factors Involved in Activation of Autoimmune Endocrine Responses

The discussion above has highlighted the fact that the microenvironment of activation of T cells may affect the activation of cells and their differentiation into mature phenotypes. The fact that soluble products of activated T and other immune cells can activate the T cell response should not come as a surprise inasmuch as the first identified "costimulatory" factor was IL-2. Consistent with this role of soluble factors is the observation that subclinical thyroiditis may become exacerbated by treatment of patients with IL-2 (see below).[206] Likewise, IFN-γ has been found early in islet inflammatory lesions of the BB/W rat and in diabetes induced with multiple low doses of streptozotocin.[207] Hypothyroidism may evolve from subclinical thyroiditis after treatment of patients with IFN-α. Importantly, soluble factors produced by T and other cells may affect the access of T cells to sites of antigen, as well as affect sites of antigen presentation.[208, 209] For example, Picarella et al. found that transgenic expression of TNF-α leads to invasive insulitis and TNF-β peri-insulitis.[210] Chemokines are produced by activated T cells and may induce recruitment of other activated cells into the organ.[211]

Mechanisms of Cell Death

Recent studies of sequential involvement of T cell subsets in the NOD mouse have begun to shed light on mechanisms of cell death in this model of type 1 diabetes. Insulitis and diabetes fail to develop in mice deficient in the expression of class I MHC molecules (β_2-microglobulin negative).[212, 213] Further studies involving adoptive transfer of splenocytes from NOD mice into immune-deficient NOD/scid mice have suggested that CD8+ cells are needed early in the disease and CD4+ cells are involved in later stages of islet destruction.[214] Consistent with this notion is the observation that insulitis or diabetes does not develop in NOD mice deficient in perforin, an enzyme from cytotoxic granules in CD8+ T cells.[215] Thus these studies suggest that tissue destruction, mediated by CD8+ T cells, is a required early event

in the pathogenesis of autoimmune disease in this model. However, the final mechanisms of islet destruction are still under investigation, including whether cell contact is necessary.[184] In this regard, immunohistochemical analysis suggests that apoptotic mechanisms are involved in β cell death.[216] The molecular and possibly chemical mediators of this final event are unresolved. The cytokine milieu created by activated T_H/T_C1 T cells in which the β cell finds itself is toxic to insulin-producing cells. TNF-α and IFN-γ are perhaps the most important cytokines.[205] Using transgenic and knockout NOD mice, Pakala et al. have recently shown the role of these molecules in tissue destruction.[217] Islets deficient in Fas, IFN-γ receptor, or inducible nitric oxide synthase had normal diabetes development. However, the specific lack of TNF-α receptor 1 caused protection from diabetes by altering the ability of islet-reactive CD4+ T cells to establish insulitis and destroy β cells.

Fas/FasL interactions leading to apoptosis of target cells have been incriminated in autoimmune endocrine diseases. Chervonsky et al. found that the ability to upregulate Fas is acquired by β cells during the natural course of diabetes in NOD mice.[218] Their studies using Fas-deficient, NOD$^{lpr/lpr}$ mice, which are resistant to spontaneous diabetes, support a critical role for this pathway in causing β cell destruction. However, the importance of Fas/FasL interactions has also taken an interesting turn in studies of FasL-expressing islets and in studies of thyroid glands from patients with Hashimoto's thyroiditis.[219] These studies suggest that fratricide rather than homicide may account for cell death. Giordano et al. found that thyrocytes from glands with Hashimoto's thyroiditis, but not normal thyroids, express Fas. FasL was shown to be constitutively expressed in both normal and diseased glands. They postulated that expression of Fas, induced in glands with Hashimoto's disease, FasL expressed by the same or a neighboring cell and led to cell death. This theory was consistent with their finding that exposure to IL-1β induced thyrocyte apoptosis, which was prevented by antibodies that block Fas. Therefore, induction of Fas expression by IL-1β (or another inflammatory cytokine) could lead to death by suicide or fratricide.

TREATMENT OF AUTOIMMUNE ENDOCRINE DISEASES BY IMMUNE MODULATION

As understanding of the mechanisms of autoimmune endocrine disease has developed, novel immunotherapies have evolved to prevent or treat these diseases. Most of the trials have involved treatment of new-onset T1DM. Initial trials used conventional, broad-spectrum immunosuppressive agents including cyclosporine and azathioprine with prednisone.[220–225] Treatment with these agents was able to alter the natural history of the disease over the first year from diagnosis. In an analysis of responders to cyclosporine, investigators found that the most important predictor of response to drug treatment was the metabolic status (plasma C peptide level) at entry into the trial. Unfortunately, treatment with these drugs was unable to induce a lasting clinical remission of the disease, and by 3 years after treatment with cyclosporine,[223] none of the patients remained in a non–insulin-requiring remission. Importantly, the toxicity of these broad-spectrum immunosuppressive agents has led most investigators to abandon their use in this setting.

The identification of insulin as an important antigen in the disease has led to more specific approaches to immunotherapy. Keller et al. reported that the onset of diabetes could be prevented in nondiabetic relatives at high risk for development of the disease by treatment with insulin at a time when their tolerance to oral glucose was normal.[226] This initial clinical observation has led to a large multicenter trial to test the ability of treatment with insulin to prevent or modify the onset of diabetes in relatives of patients who are at high risk for the disease. This trial is now in progress and should be completed in the year 2003. Furthermore, the observation that oral administration of insulin was able to prevent disease in the NOD mouse has led to the inclusion of a treatment arm in this trial involving oral administration of insulin. It should be noted that the mechanism of this effect of insulin in animal models of the disease and in patients is not certain. In addition

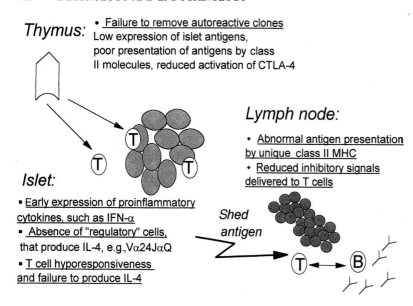

Thymus:
• Failure to remove autoreactive clones
Low expression of islet antigens,
poor presentation of antigens by class
II molecules, reduced activation of CTLA-4

Lymph node:
• Abnormal antigen presentation
by unique class II MHC
• Reduced inhibitory signals
delivered to T cells

Islet:
■ Early expression of proinflammatory
cytokines, such as IFN-α
■ Absence of "regulatory" cells,
that produce IL-4, e.g.,Vα24JαQ
■ T cell hyporesponsiveness
and failure to produce IL-4

Shed antigen

FIGURE 39–4. Immune dysregulation and autoimmune diabetes. This figure illustrates points in control of autoreactivity that have been postulated to be affected during the development of type 1 diabetes. The sites of immune regulation include the thymus, peripheral tissue (islet), and the lymph node.

to a mechanism involving induction of tolerance to a diabetes-specific antigen, it is possible that as a result of metabolic rest of the cell, pathogenically important antigens are no longer presented to the immune system. However, Muir et al. reported that metabolically inactive insulin B chain was also able to prevent diabetes in NOD mice.[227]

A clinical trial with a non–FcR-binding anti-CD3 mAb is in progress in T1DM. As discussed, this agent has been shown to selectively anergize activated T_H1 cells, possibly by delivering an altered TCR signal similar to "altered peptide ligands." Preclinical studies by Chatenoud et al. in the NOD mouse suggested that the agent could reverse diabetes at the appearance of hyperglycemia and that it was most effective when administered at that time. Activated T_H1 cells are found in the islets at the time of diagnosis of diabetes in the NOD mouse, which may explain the effectiveness of the agent at this late stage of disease pathogenesis.

The experience with clinical trials to treat autoimmune thyroiditis is more limited. Investigators have examined the effects of immune suppression on the exacerbation of ophthalmopathy that occurs after radioiodine therapy for hyperthyroidism.[228] This manifestation is thought to be related to an increase in levels of circulating thyroid autoantibodies associated with leakage of antigens after radioactive iodine therapy. Bartalena et al. reported that exacerbation of this manifestation was prevented by corticosteroid treatment at the time of radioiodine therapy.[229]

One of the more interesting clinical observations has been the *appearance* of autoimmune thyroiditis after the administration of cytokines for other conditions. Both hypothyroidism and hyperthyroidism have been reported after treatment with IFN-α. The mean incidence of IFN-α–induced thyroid dysfunction has been reported to be 6%, but at least one antithyroid antibody has been found in 17% of these patients. Spontaneous resolution occurs in more than half of affected individuals after discontinuation of IFN-α treatment. The presence of thyroid autoantibodies before therapy was a predictor for thyroid dysfunction. Hypothyroidism is also a frequent occurrence after lymphokine-activated killer cell therapy. The hypothyroidism appears to be due to activation of intrathyroidal lymphocytes by IL-2 and induction of IFN-γ, a potent inhibitory cytokine for thyroid cells. These studies suggest a mechanism of thyroid dysfunction in which primed cells are activated by the administration of high doses of cytokines and support the models of pathogenesis suggested above.

CONCLUSION

Experimental data, primarily based on animal models of human diseases, would suggest that autoimmune endocrine diseases result from dysregulated immune responses directed against normal constituents of the endocrine glands. The fact that these diseases often follow

a progressive course resulting in complete cellular destruction may reflect activation of the response by the continued presence of the antigen, the impact of local inflammation, epitope spreading, and genetically predetermined sensitivity to the target tissue. Ongoing studies of genetic predisposition to these diseases have suggested new testable hypotheses about pathologic mechanisms, including failure to remove autoreactive cells from the repertoire because of the unusual binding properties of certain class II MHC molecules, low, nontolerogenic levels of autoantigen expression in the thymus, and/or defective costimulatory and negative regulatory signals (Fig. 39–4).

However, in the periphery, other events are needed for activation of the autoimmune response, such as costimulatory signals and chemokine and cytokine activity, which may also be awry in the autoimmune setting. Little is known about how these events are initiated and regulated in human disease—the possibility of an infectious event resulting in cross-reactivity between antigens of that agent and the islet cells remains. Under these circumstances, normal mechanisms of immune tolerance, such as clonal anergy, deletion, or immunoregulation via cytokines, may fail and lead to unwanted pathogenic autoreactivity.

New developments in understanding the mechanisms of autoimmune endocrine disease have suggested novel approaches to immunotherapy, in particular, targeting lymphocyte activation pathways and induction of lymphocyte anergy. The new developments have also indicated that previous attempts to induce sustained reversal of disease by broad immune suppression are not likely to be successful and, in fact, may counteract the new tolerogenic protocols. These newer strategies will attempt to target "antigen-specific" immune pathways, both pathogenic and regulatory, so that lasting tolerance can be achieved.

REFERENCES

1. Pointes de Carvallio LP, Templeman J, Wick G, Roitt IM: The role of self-antigen in the development of autoimmunity in obese strain chickens with spontaneous autoallergic thyroiditis. J Exp Med 155:1255–1266, 1982.
2. Miller BH, Appel MC, O'Neil JJ, Wicker LS: Both the Lyt2+ and L3T4+ T cell subsets are required for the transfer of diabetes in non-obese diabetic (NOD) mice. J Immunol 140:52–62, 1988.
3. Koevary S, Rossini AA, Stoller W, et al: Passive transfer of diabetes in the BB/W rat. Science 220:727–729, 1983.
4. Herold KC, Montag AG, Fitch FW: Treatment with anti–T lymphocyte antibodies prevents induction of insulitis in mice given multiple low doses of streptozotocin. Diabetes 36:796–801, 1987.
5. Roep BO, Arden SD, deVries RRP, Hutton JC: T cell clones from a type 1 diabetes patient respond to insulin secretory granule proteins. Nature 345:632–634, 1990.
6. Williams ED, Donaich I: The post-mortem incidence of focal thyroiditis. J Pathol 83:255–264, 1962.
7. Davis M: T cell receptor gene diversity and selection. Annu Rev Biochem 59:475–496, 1990.
8. Jorgensen JL, Reay PA, Ehrich EW, Davis M: Molecular components of T cell recognition. Annu Rev Immunol 10:835–873, 1992.

9. Alberola-Ila J, Takaki S, Kerner JD, Perlmutter R: Differential signaling by lymphocyte antigen receptors. Annu Rev Immunol 15:125–154, 1997.
10. Janeway CA Jr: The T cell receptor as a multicomponent signaling machine: CD4/CD8 coreceptors and CD45 in T cell activation. Annu Rev Immunol 10:645–674, 1992.
11. Fleury SG, Crouteau G, Sekaly R-P: CD4 and CD8 recognition of class II and class I molecules of the major histocompatibility complex. Semin Immunol 3:177–186, 1991.
12. Qian D, Griswold-Prenner I, Rosner RM, Fitch FW: Multiple components of the T cell antigen receptor complex become tyrosine-phosphorylated upon activation. J Biol Chem 268:4488–4494, 1993.
13. Weiss A, Littman DR: Signal transduction by lymphocyte antigen receptors. Cell 76:263–278, 1994.
14. Perlmutter RM, Levine SD, Appleby MW, et al: Regulation of lymphocyte function by protein phosphorylation. Annu Rev Immunol 11:451–499, 1993.
15. Rapoport MJ, Lazarus AH, Jaramillo A, et al: Thymic T cell anergy in autoimmune nonobese diabetic mice is mediated by defective T cell receptor regulation of the pathway of p21ras activation. J Exp Med 177:1221–1232, 1993.
16. Smith JA, Tang Q, Bluestone JA: Partial TCR signals delivered by FcR-nonbinding anti-CD3 monoclonal antibodies differentially regulate individual Th subsets. J Immunol 160:4841–4849, 1998.
17. Pfeiffer C, Stein K, Southwood SHK, et al: Altered peptide ligands can control CD4 T lymphocyte differentiation in vivo. J Exp Med 181:1569–1574, 1995.
18. Kelso A, Troutt AB, Maraskovsky E, et al: Heterogeneity in lymphokine profiles of CD4+ and CD8+ T cells and clones activated in vivo and in vitro. Immunol Rev 123:85–114, 1991.
19. Rogmani S: Lymphokine production by human T cells in disease states. Annu Rev Immunol 12:227–258, 1994.
20. Constant SL, Bottomly K: Induction of the Th1 and Th2 CD4+ T cell responses: Alternative approaches. Annu Rev Immunol 15:297–322, 1997.
21. Coffman RL, Seymour BWP, Lebman DA, et al: The role of helper T cell products in mouse B cell differentiation and isotype regulation. Immunol Rev 102:5–28, 1988.
22. Nakamura T, Kamogawa Y, Bottomly K, Flavell RA: Polarization of IL-4– and IFN-gamma–producing CD4+ T cells following activation of naive CD4+ T cells. J Immunol 158:1085–1094, 1997.
23. Kuo CT, Leiden JM: Transcriptional regulation of T lymphocyte development and function. Annu Rev Immunol 17:149–188, 1999.
24. Swain SL, Weinberg AD, English M, Huston G: IL-4 and IFN direct the development of distinct subsets of helper T cells. J Immunol 145:3796, 1990.
25. Seder RA, Gazzinelli R, Sher A, Paul WE: IL-12 acts directly on CD4+ T cells to enhance priming for IFN production and diminishes IL-4 inhibition of such priming. Proc Natl Acad Sci U S A 90:10188–10192, 1993.
26. Smith JA, Tso JY, Clark MR, et al: Nonmitogenic anti-CD3 monoclonal antibodies deliver a partial T cell receptor signal and induce clonal anergy. J Exp Med 185:1413–1422, 1997.
27. Herold KC, Vezys V, Sun Q, et al: Regulation of cytokine production during development of autoimmune diabetes induced with multiple low-doses of streptozotocin. J Immunol 156:3521–3527, 1996.
28. Fox CJ, Danska JS: IL-4 expression at the onset of islet inflammation predicts nondestructive insulitis in nonobese diabetic mice. J Immunol 158:2414–2424, 1997.
29. Hultgren B, Huang X, Dybdal N, Stewart TA: Genetic absence of gamma-interferon delays but does not prevent diabetes in NOD mice. Diabetes 45:812–817, 1996.
30. Katz JD, Benoist C, Mathis D: T helper cell subsets in insulin dependent diabetes. Science 268:1185–1188, 1995.
31. Trembleau S, Penna G, Bosi E, et al: Interleukin 12 administration induces T helper type 1 cells and accelerates autoimmune diabetes in NOD mice. J Exp Med 181:817–821, 1995.
32. Rapoport M, Jaramillo A, Zipris D, et al: Interleukin 4 reverses T cell proliferative unresponsiveness and prevents the onset of diabetes in nonobese diabetic mice. J Exp Med 178:87–98, 1993.
33. Gallichan WS, Balasa B, Davies JD, Sarvetnick N: Pancreatic IL-4 expression results in islet-reactive Th2 cells that inhibit diabetogenic lymphocytes in the nonobese diabetic mouse. J Immunol 163:1696–1703, 1999.
34. Pennline KH, Roque-Gaffrey E, Monahan M: Recombinant human IL-10 prevents the onset of diabetes in the nonobese diabetic mouse. Clin Immunol Immunopathol 71:169–175, 1994.
35. Wogensen L, Lee MS, Sarvetnick N: Production of interleukin 10 by islet cells accelerates immune-mediated destruction of beta cells in nonobese diabetic mice. J Exp Med 179:1379–1384, 1994.
36. Pakala SV, Kurrer MO, Katz JD: T helper 2 (Th2) T cells induce acute pancreatitis and diabetes in immune-compromised nonobese diabetic (NOD) mice. J Exp Med 186:299–306, 1997.
37. Jenkins MK: The ups and downs of T cell costimulation. Immunity 1:442–446, 1994.
38. Jenkins MK, Schwartz RH: Antigen presentation by chemically modified splenocytes induces antigen-specific T cell unresponsiveness in vitro and in vivo. J Exp Med 165:302–319, 1987.
39. Mueller DL, Jenkins MK, Schwartz RH: Clonal expansion versus functional clonal inactivation: A costimulatory signalling pathway determines the outcome of T cell receptor occupancy. Annu Rev Immunol 7:4545–4580, 1989.
40. Herold KC, Lu J, Rulifson I, et al: Regulation of chemokine production by CD28/B7 costimulation. J Immunol 159:4150–4153, 1997.
41. Abbas AK, Sharpe AH: T cell stimulation: An abundance of B7s. Nat Med 5:1345–1346, 1999.
42. Swallow MM, Wallin JJ, Sha WC: B7h, a novel costimulatory homolog of B7.1 and B7.2 is induced by TNF-alpha. Immunity 11:423–432, 1999.
43. Dong H, Zhy G, Tamada K, Chen L: B7-H1, a third member of the B7 family, co-stimulates T cell proliferation and interleukin-10 secretion. Nat Med 5:1365–1369, 1999.
44. Arreaza GA, Cameron MJ, Jaramillo A, et al: Neonatal activation of CD28 signaling overcomes T cell anergy and prevents autoimmune diabetes by an IL-4–dependent mechanism. J Clin Invest 100:2243–2255, 1997.
45. Kuchroo VK, Das MP, Brown JA, et al: B7-1 and B7-2 costimulatory molecules activate differentially the Th1/Th2 developmental pathways: Application to autoimmune disease therapy. Cell 80:707–718, 1995.
46. Balasa B, Krahl T, Patstone G, et al: CD40 ligand–CD40 interactions are necessary for the initiation of insulitis and diabetes in nonobese diabetic mice. J Immunol 159:4620–4627, 1997.
47. Akiba H, Miyahira Y, Atsuta M, et al: Critical contribution of OX40 ligand to T helper cell type 2 differentiation in experimental leishmaniasis. J Exp Med 191:275–380, 2000.
48. Weinberg AD, Wegmann KW, Funatake C, Whitham RH: Blocking OX-40/OX-40 ligand interaction in vitro and in vivo leads to decreased T cell function and amelioration of experimental allergic encephalomyelitis. J Immunol 162:1818–1826, 1999.
49. Kim JJ, Tsai A, Nottingham LK, et al: Intracellular adhesion molecule-1 modulates beta-chemokines and directly costimulates T cells in vivo. J Clin Invest 103:869–877, 1999.
50. Posselt AM, Barker CF, Friedman AI, Naji A: Prevention of autoimmune diabetes in the BB rat by intrathymic islet transplantation at birth. Science 256:1321–1324, 1992.
51. Lenschow DJ, Walunas TL, Bluestone JA: CD28/B7 system of T cell costimulation. Annu Rev Immunol 14:233–258, 1996.
52. Linsley PS, Ledbetter JA: The role of the CD28 coreceptor during T cell responses to antigen. Annu Rev Immunol 11:191–212, 1993.
53. June CH, Ledbetter JA, Linsley PS, Thompson CB: Role of the CD28 receptor in T cell activation. Immunol Today 11:211–216, 1990.
54. Harding RA, McArthur JG, Gross JA, et al: CD28-mediated signalling costimulates murine T cells and prevents induction of anergy in T cell clones. Nature 356:607–609, 1992.
55. Linsley PS, Brady W, Grosmaire L, et al: Binding of the B cell activation antigen B7 to CD28 costimulates T cell proliferation and interleukin 2 mRNA accumulation. J Exp Med 173:721–730, 1991.
56. Wong S, Guerder S, Visintin I, et al: Expression of the costimulatory molecule B7-1 in pancreatic beta cells accelerates diabetes in the NOD mouse. Diabetes 44:326–329, 1995.
57. Harlan DM, Barnett MA, Abe R, et al: Very-low dose streptozotocin induces diabetes in insulin promoter mB7-1 transgenic mice. Diabetes 44:816–823, 1995.
58. Freeman GH, Gribben JG, Boussiotis VA, et al: Cloning of B7-2: A CTLA-4 counter-receptor that costimulates human T cell proliferation. Science 262:909–911, 1993.
59. Lenschow DJ, Su GH, Zuckerman LA, et al: Expression and functional significance of an additional ligand for CTLA-4. Proc Natl Acad Sci U S A 90:11054–11063, 1993.
60. Lenschow DJ, Ho SC, Sattar H, et al: Differential effects of B7-1 and B7-2 mAb treatment on the development of diabetes in the NOD mouse. J Exp Med 181:1145–1155, 1995.
61. Herold KC, Vezys V, Koons A, et al: CD28/B7 co-stimulation regulates autoimmune diabetes induced with multiple low doses of streptozotocin. J Immunol 158:984–991, 1997.
62. Peterson KE, Sharp GC, Tang H, Braley-Mullen H: B7.2 has opposing roles during the activation versus effector stages of experimental autoimmune thyroiditis. J Immunol 162:1859–1867, 1999.
63. Noelle RJ, Ledbetter JA, Aruffo A: CD40 and its ligand, an essential ligand-receptor pair for thymus-dependent B-cell activation. Immunol Today 13:431–433, 1992.
64. Foy TM, Aruffo A, Bajorath J, et al: Immune regulation by CD40 and its ligand GP39. Annu Rev Immunol 14:591–617, 1996.
65. Yang Y, Wilson JM: CD40 ligand–dependent T cell activation: Requirement of B7-CD28 signaling through CD40. Science 273:1862–1864, 1996.
66. Judge TA, Wu Z, Zheng XG, et al: The role of CD80, CD86, and CTLA4 in alloimmune responses and the induction of long-term allograft survival. J Immunol 162:1947–1951, 1999.
67. Markees TG, Serreze DV, Phillips NE, et al: NOD mice have a generalized defect in their response to transplantation tolerance induction. Diabetes 48:967–974, 1999.
68. Kienzle G, von Kempis J: CD137 (ILA/4-1BB), expressed by primary human monocytes, induces monocyte activation and apoptosis of B lymphocytes. Int Immunol 12:73–82, 2000.
69. Mittler RS, Bailey TS, Klussman K, et al: Anti-4-1BB monoclonal antibodies abrogate T cell–dependent humoral immune responses in vivo through the induction of helper T cell anergy. J Exp Med 190:1535–1540, 1999.
70. Turnbridge WMG, Evered DC, Hall R, et al: The spectrum of thyroid disease in the community: The Whickham survey. Clin Endocrinol 7:481–492, 1977.
71. Riley WJ, Maclaren NK, Krisher J, et al: A prospective study of the development of diabetes in relatives of patients with insulin-dependent diabetes. N Engl J Med 323:1167–1172, 1990.
72. Cambier JC, Pleiman CM, Clark MR: Signal transduction by the B cell antigen receptor and its coreceptors. Annu Rev Immunol 12:457–486, 1994.
73. Kurosaki T: Genetic analysis of B cell antigen receptor signaling. Annu Rev Immunol 17:555–592, 1999.
74. Reth M, Hombach J, Weinands J, et al: The B-cell antigen receptor complex. Immunol Today 12:196–201, 1991.
75. Casali P, Notkins AL: CD5+ B lymphocytes, polyreactive antibodies and the human B cell repertoire. Immunol Today 10:364–369, 1989.
76. Solvason N, Kearney JF: THe human fetal omentum: A site of B cell generation. J Exp Med 175:397–404, 1992.
77. Hardy RR: Variable gene usage, physiology and development of Ly-1+ (CD5+) B cells. Curr Opin Immunol 4:181–185, 1992.
78. Tarlinton DM, McLean M, Nossal GJ: B1 and B2 cells differ in their potential to switch immunoglobulin isotype. Eur J Immunol 25:3388–3393, 1995.

79. Finkelman FD, Lees A, Morris SC: Antigen presentation by B lymphocytes to CD4+ T lymphocytes in vivo: Importance for B lymphocytes and T lymphocyte activation. Semin Immunol 4:247–256, 1992.
80. Williams AF, Barclay AN: The immunoglobulin superfamily—domains for cell surface recognition. Annu Rev Immunol 6:381–405, 1988.
81. Bjorkman PH, Saper MA, Samraoui B, et al: The foreign antigen binding site and T cell recognition regions of class I histocompatibility antigens. Nature 329:512–518, 1987.
82. Brown JH, Jardetzky T, Saper MA, et al: A hypothetical model of the foreign antigen binding site of class II histocompatibility molecules. Nature 332:845–850, 1988.
83. van Bleek GM, Nathenson SG: Presentation of antigenic peptides by MHC class I molecules. Trends Cell Biol 2:202–207, 1992.
84. Germain RN, Hendrix LR: MHC class II structure, occupancy and surface expression determined by post–endoplasmic reticulum antigen binding. Nature 353:134–139, 1991.
85. Rothbard JB, Gefter MC: Interactions between immunogenic peptides and MHC proteins. Annu Rev Immunol 9:527–565, 1991.
86. Watts C: Capture and processing of exogenous antigens for presentation on MHC molecules. Annu Rev Immunol 15:821–850, 1997.
87. Porcelli SA, Modlin RL: The CD1 system: Antigen-presenting molecules for T cell recognition and glycolipids. Annu Rev Immunol 17:297–330, 1999.
88. Exley M, Garcia J, Balk SP, Porcelli S: Requirements for CD1d recognition by human invariant V2+CD4−CD8− T cells. J Exp Med 186:109–120, 1997.
89. Wilson SB, Kent SC, Patton KT, et al: Extreme Th1 bias of invariant Vα24JαQ T cells in type 1 diabetes. Nature 391:177–181, 1998.
90. Farid NR, Bear J: The human major histocompatibility complex and endocrine disease. Endocr Rev 2:50, 1981.
91. Baker Jr: Autoimmune endocrine disease. JAMA 278:1931, 1997.
92. Brix TH, Kyvik KO, Hegedus L: What is the evidence of genetic factors in the etiology of Graves' disease? A brief review. Thyroid 8:627, 1998.
93. Badenhoop K, Walfish PG, Rau H, et al: Susceptibility and resistance alleles of human leukocyte antigen (HLA) DQA1 and HLA DQB1 are shared in endocrine autoimmune disease. J Clin Endocrinol Metab 80:2112, 1995.
94. Lavard L, Madsen HO, Perrild H, et al: HLA class II associations in juvenile Graves' disease: Indication of a strong protective role of the DRB1*0701,DQA1*0201 haplotype. Tissue Antigens 50:639, 1997.
95. Maclaren N, Riley W: Inherited susceptibility to autoimmune Addison's disease is linked to human leukocyte antigens-DR3 and/or DR4, except when associated with type I autoimmune polyglandular syndrome. J Clin Endocrinol Metab 62:455, 1986.
96. Todd JA: Genetics of type 1 diabetes. Pathol Biol 45:219–227, 1997.
97. Nepom G: Immunogenetics of HLA-associated diseases. Concepts Immunopathol 5:80, 1988.
98. Bach FH, Rich SS, Barbosa R, et al: Insulin-dependent diabetes–associated HLA-D region encoded determinants. Hum Immunol 12:59, 1985.
99. Baisch JM, Weeks T, Giles R, et al: Analysis of HLA-DQ genotypes and susceptibility in insulin-dependent diabetes mellitus. N Engl J Med 322:1836, 1990.
100. Todd JA, Bell JI, McDevitt H: HLA-DQB gene contributes to susceptibility and resistance to insulin-dependent diabetes mellitus. Nature 329:599, 1987.
101. Davies J, Kawaguchi Y, Bennett S, et al: A genome-wide search for human type 1 diabetes susceptibility genes. Nature 371:130, 1994.
102. Lund T, O'Reilly L, Hutchings P, et al: Prevention of insulin-dependent diabetes mellitus in non-obese diabetic mice by transgenes encoding modified I-A beta-chain or normal I-E alpha-chain. Nature 345:727–729, 1990.
103. Miyazaki T, Uno M, Uehira M, et al: Direct evidence for the contribution of the unique I-ANOD to the development of insulitis in non-obese diabetic mice. Nature 345:722–724, 1990.
104. Slattery RM, Kjer-Nielsen L, Allison J, et al: Prevention of diabetes in non-obese diabetic I-A^k transgenic mice. Nature 345:724–726, 1990.
105. Reich EP, von Grafenstein H, Barlow A, et al: Self peptides isolated from MHC glycoproteins of non-obese diabetic mice. J Immunol 152:2279–2288, 1994.
106. Kanagawa O, Shimizu J, Unanue ER: The role of I-Ag7 beta chain in peptide binding and antigen recognition by T cells. Int Immunol 9:1523–1526, 1997.
107. Carrasco-Marin E, Shimizu J, Kanagawa O, Unanue ER: The class II MHC I-Ag7 molecules from non-obese diabetic mice are poor peptide binders. J Immunol 156:450–458, 1996.
108. Schatz DG, Oettinger MA, Schlissel: V(D)J recombination: Molecular biology and regulation. Annu Rev Immunol 10:359–384, 1992.
109. Von Boehmer H: The developmental biology of T lymphocytes. Annu Rev Immunol 6:309–326, 1988.
110. MacDonald HR, Hengartner H, Pedrazzini T: Intrathymic deletion of self reactive cells prevented by neonatal anti-CD4 antibody treatment. Nature 335:730–733, 1988.
111. Blackman M, Kappler J, Marrack P: The role of the T cell receptor in positive and negative selection of developing T cells. Science 248:1335–1337, 1990.
112. Koevary SB, Blomberg M: Prevention of diabetes in BB/Wor rats by intrathymic islet injection. J Clin Invest 89:512–520, 1992.
113. Herold KC, Montag AG, Buckingham F: Induction of tolerance to autoimmune diabetes with islet antigens. J Exp Med 176:1107–1114, 1992.
114. Jankins MK, Schwartz, RH, Pardoll DH: Effects of cyclosporin A on T cell development and clonal deletion. Science 241:1655–1658, 1988.
115. Gao E-K, Lo D, Cheney R, et al: Abnormal differentiation of thymocytes in mice treated with cyclosporin A. Nature 336:176–179, 1988.
116. Gerling IC, Atkinson MA, Leiter EH: The thymus as a site for evaluating the potency of candidate beta cell autoantigens in NOD mice. J Autoimmun 7:851–858, 1994.
117. Jolicoeur C, Hanahan D, Smith KM: T-cell tolerance toward a transgenic beta-cell antigen and transcription of endogenous pancreatic genes in thymus. Proc Natl Acad Sci U S A 91:6707–6711, 1994.
118. Pugliese A, Zeller M, Fernandez A Jr: The insulin gene is transcribed in the human thymus and transcription levels correlated with allelic variation at the INS VNTR-IDDM2 susceptibility locus for type 1 diabetes. Nat Genet 15:293–297, 1997.
119. Cilio CM, Daws MR, Malashicheva A, et al: Cytotoxic T lymphocyte antigen 4 is induced in the thymus upon in vivo activation and its blockade prevents anti-CD3–mediated depletion of thymocytes. J Exp Med 188:1239–1246, 1998.
120. Goodnow CC: Transgenic mice and analysis of B cell tolerance. Annu Rev Immunol 10:489–518, 1992.
121. Nemazee D, Russell D, Arnold B, et al: Clonal deletion of autospecific B lymphocytes. Immunol Rev 122:117–132, 1991.
122. Retter MW, Nemazee D: Receptor editing: Genetic reprogramming of autoreactive lymphocytes. Cell Biochem Biophys 31:81–88, 1999.
123. Akkaraju S, Canaan K, Goodnow C: Self-reactive B cells are not eliminated or inactivated by autoantigen expressed on thyroid epithelial cells. J Exp Med 186:2005–2012, 1997.
124. Rudin CM, Thompson CB: Apoptosis and disease: Regulation and clinical relevance of programmed cell death. Annu Rev Med 48:267–281, 1997.
125. Webb S, Morris C, Sprent J: Extrathymic tolerance of mature T cells: Clonal elimination as a consequence of immunity. Cell 63:1249–1256, 1990.
126. Ashkenazi A, Dixit VM: Death receptors: Signaling and modulation. Science 281:1305–1308, 1998.
127. Lenardo M, Chan KM, Hornung F, et al: Mature T lymphocyte apoptosis—immune regulation in a dynamic and unpredictable antigenic environment. Annu Rev Immunol 17:221–253, 1999.
128. Li Y, Li XC, Zheng XX, et al: Blocking both signal 1 and signal 2 of T-cell activation prevents apoptosis of alloreactive T cells and induction of peripheral allograft tolerance. Nat Med 11:1298–302, 1999.
129. Miller JFAP, Morahan G: Peripheral T cell tolerance. Annu Rev Immunol 10:51–70, 1992.
130. Miller J, Daitch L, Rath P, Selsing E: Tissue specific expression of allogeneic class II molecules induces neither islet rejection nor clonal inactivation of alloreactive T cell. J Immunol 144:334–341, 1990.
131. Hammerling G, Schonrich G, Momburg R, et al: Non-deletional mechanisms of peripheral and central tolerance: Studies with transgenic mice with tissue specific expression of a foreign MHC class I antigen. Immunol Rev 122:47–67, 1991.
132. Ransdell F, Fowlkes BJ: Maintenance of in vivo tolerance of persistence of antigen. Science 257:1130–1133, 1992.
133. Lo D, Burkly LC, Widera G, et al: Diabetes and tolerance in transgenic mice expressing class II MHC molecules in pancreatic beta cells. Cell 53:159–168, 1988.
134. Ohashi PS, Oehen S, Buerki K, et al: Ablation of "tolerance" and induction of diabetes by virus infection in viral antigen transgenic mice. Cell 65:305–317, 1991.
135. Oldstone MBA, Nerenberg M, Southern P, et al: Virus infection triggers insulin dependent diabetes mellitus in a transgenic model. Cell 65:319–331, 1991.
136. Von Herrath MG, Efrat S, Oldstone MB, Horwitz MS: Expression of adenoviral E3 transgenes in β cells prevents autoimmune diabetes. Proc Natl Acad Sci U S A 94:9808–9813, 1997.
137. Alferink J, Aigner S, Reibke R, et al: Peripheral T-cell tolerance: The contribution of permissive T-cell migration into parenchymal tissues of the neonate. Immunol Rev 169:255–261, 1999.
138. Bretcher P, Cohn M: A theory of self-nonself discrimination. Science 169:1042–1046, 1970.
139. Lafferty K, Gill RG: The maintenance of self-tolerance. Immunol Cell Biol 71:209–214, 1993.
140. Nossal GJV, Pike BL: Clonal anergy: Persistence in tolerant mice of antigen-binding B lymphocytes incapable of responding to antigens or mitogen. Proc Natl Acad Sci U S A 77:1602–1606, 1980.
141. Brunet JF, Denizot F, Luciani MF, et al: A new member of the immunoglobulin superfamily CTLA-4. Nature 328:267–270, 1987.
142. Walunas TL, Lenschow DJ, Bakker CY, et al: CTLA-4 can function as a negative regulator of T cell activation. Immunity 1:405–413, 1994.
143. Krummel MF, Allison JP: CTLA-4 engagement inhibits IL-2 accumulation and cell cycle progression upon activation of resting T cells. J Exp Med 183:2533–2540, 1996.
144. Walunas TL, Bakker CY, Bluestone JA: CTLA-4 ligation blocks CD28-dependent T cell activation. J Exp Med 183:2541–2550, 1996.
145. Karandiker NJ, Vanderglut CL, Walunas TL, et al: CTLA-4: A negative regulator of autoimmune disease. J Exp Med 184:783–788, 1996.
146. Alegre ML, Noel PJ, Eisfelder BJ, et al: Regulation of surface and intracellular expression of CTLA4 on mouse T cells. J Immunol 157:4762–4770, 1996.
147. Tivol EA, Borriello F, Schweitzer AN, et al: Loss of CTLA-4 leads to massive lymphoproliferation and fatal multiorgan tissue destruction, revealing a critical negative regulatory role of CTLA-4. Immunity 5:541–547, 1995.
148. Luhder F, Hoglund P, Allison JP, et al: Cytotoxic T lymphocyte–associated antigen 4 (CTLA-4) regulates the unfolding of autoimmune diabetes. J Exp Med 187:427–432, 1998.
149. Yanagawa T, Hidaka Y, Guimaraes V, et al: CTLA-4 gene polymorphism associated with Graves' disease in a Caucasian population. J Clin Endocrinol Metab 80:41–45, 1995.
150. Colucci F, Bergman ML, Penha-Goncalves C, et al: Apoptosis resistance of nonobese diabetic peripheral lymphocytes linked to the Idd5 diabetes susceptibility region. Proc Natl Acad Sci U S A 94:8670–8674, 1997.
151. Nistico L, Buzzetti F, Pritchard LE, et al: The CTLA-4 gene region of chromosome 2q33 is linked to and associated with, type 1 diabetes. Belgian Diabetes Registry. Hum Mol Genet 5:1075–1080, 1996.
152. Djilali-Saiah I, Larger E, Harfouch-Hammoud E, et al: No major role for the CTLA-4 gene in the association of autoimmune thyroid disease with IDDM. Diabetes 47:125–127, 1998.
153. Lenschow DJ, Herold KC, Rhee L, et al: CD28/B7 regulation of Th1 and Th2 subsets in the development of autoimmune diabetes. Immunity 5:285–293, 1996.
154. Kurts S, Carbone FR, Krummel MF, et al: Signalling through CD30 protects against autoimmune diabetes mediated by CD8 T cells. Nature 398:341–344, 1999.

155. Seddon B, Mason D: Regulatory T cells in the control of autoimmunity: The essential role of transforming growth factor beta and interleukin 4 in the prevention of autoimmune thyroiditis in rats by peripheral CD4(+)CD45FC− cells and CD4+CD8− thymocytes. J Exp Med 189:279–288, 1999.
156. Greiner DL, Mordes JP, Handler ES, et al: Depletion of RT6.1+ T lymphocytes induces diabetes in resistant biobreeding/Worcester (BB/W) rats. J Exp Med 166:461–475, 1987.
157. Herbelin A, Gombert J-M, Lepault F, et al: Mature mainstream TCRαβ+CD4+ thymocytes expressing L-selectin mediate "active tolerance" in the nonobese diabetic mouse. J Immunol 161:2620–2628, 1998.
158. Jiang H, Kashleva H, Xu LX, et al: T cell vaccination induces T cell receptor Vβ-specific Qa-1–restricted regulatory CD8(+) T cells. Proc Natl Acad Sci U S A 95:4533–4537, 1998.
159. Waldmann H, Cobbold S: How do monoclonal antibodies induce tolerance? A role for infectious tolerance? Annu Rev Immunol 16:619–644, 1998.
160. Cobbold S, Waldmann H: Infectious tolerance. Curr Opin Immunol 10:518–524, 1998.
161. Mueller R, Bradley LM, Krahl T, Sarvetnick N: Mechanism underlying counterregulation of autoimmune diabetes by IL-4. Immunity 7:411–418, 1997.
162. Weiner HL, Freidman A, Miller A, et al: Oral tolerance: Immunologic mechanisms and treatment of animal and human organ specific autoimmune diseases by oral administration of autoantigens. Annu Rev Immunol 12:809–838, 1994.
163. Zhang ZJ, Davidson L, Eisenbarth G, et al: Suppression of diabetes in nonobese diabetic mice by oral administration of porcine insulin. Proc Natl Acad Sci U S A 88:10252–10261, 1991.
164. Palmer JP, Asplin C, Clemons P, et al: Insulin antibodies in insulin-dependent diabetics before insulin treatment. Science 222:1337, 1983.
165. Rabin D, Pleasic S, Shapiro H, et al: Islet cell antigen 512 is a diabetes-specific islet autoantigen related to protein tyrosine phosphatases. J Immunol 152:3183, 1994.
166. Hawkes K, Wasmeier C, Christie MR, et al: Identification of the 37k-antigen in insulin-dependent diabetes as a tyrosine phosphatase–like protein (phogrin) related to IA-2. Diabetes 45:1187, 1996.
167. Baekkeskov S, Aanstoot H-J, Christgau S: Identification of the 64K autoantigen in insulin-dependent diabetes as the GABA-synthesizing enzyme glutamic acid decarboxylase. Nature 347:151, 1990.
168. Pietropaolo M, Castãno L, Babu S, et al: Islet cell autoantigen 69 kD (ICA69): Molecular cloning and characterization of a novel diabetes-associated autoantigen. J Clin Invest 92:359, 1993.
169. Arden SD, Roep BO, Neophytou PI, et al: Imogen 38: A novel 38-kD islet mitochondrial autoantigen recognized by T cells from a newly diagnosed type 1 diabetic patient. J Clin Invest 97:551, 1996.
170. Appetecchia M, Castelli M, Delpino A: Anti–heat shock protein autoantibodies in autoimmune thyroiditis. Preliminary study. J Exp Clin Cancer Res 16:395, 1997.
171. Kubota S, Gunji K, Ackrell BAC, et al: The 64-kilodalton eye muscle protein is the flavoprotein subunit of mitochondrial succinate dehydrogenase: The corresponding serum antibodies are good markers of an immune-mediated damage to the eye muscle in patients with Graves' hyperthyroidism. J Clin Endocrinol Metab 83:443, 1998.
172. Morris JC, Bergert ER, Bryant WP: Binding of immunoglobulin G from patients with autoimmune thyroid disease to rat sodium-iodide symporter peptides: Evidence for the iodide transporter as an autoantigen. Thyroid 7:527, 1997.
173. Tomer Y: Anti-thyroglobulin autoantibodies in autoimmune thyroid diseases: Cross-reactive or pathogenic? Clin Immunol Immunopathol 82:3, 1997.
174. McKenzie JM, Zakarija M: Antibodies in autoimmune thyroid disease. *In* Braverman L, Utiger R (eds): The Thyroid: A Fundamental and Clinical Text, ed 7. Philadelphia, JB Lippincott, 1996, p 416.
175. Endl J, Otto H, Jung G, et al: Identification of naturally processed T cell epitopes from glutamic acid decarboxylase presented in the context of HLA-DR alleles by T lymphocytes of recent onset IDDM patients. J Clin Invest 99:2405–2415, 1997.
176. Karjalainen J, Martin JM, Knip M, et al: A bovine albumin peptide as a possible trigger of insulin-dependent diabetes. N Engl J Med 327:302–307, 1992.
177. Elias D, Cohen IR: Treatment of autoimmune diabetes and insulitis in NOD mice with heat shock protein 60 peptide p277. Diabetes 44:1132–1138, 1995.
178. Elias D, Meilin A, Ablamunits V, et al: Hsp60 peptide therapy of NOD mouse diabetes induces a Th2 cytokine burst and downregulates autoimmunity to various β-cell antigens. Diabetes 46:758–764, 1997.
179. Lehmann PV, Sercarz EE, Forsthuber T, et al: Determinant spreading and the dynamics of the autoimmune T-cell repertoire. Immunol Today 14:203–208, 1993.
180. Wong FS, Karttunen J, Dumont C, et al: Identification of an MHC class I–restricted autoantigen in type 1 diabetes by screening an organ-specific cDNA library. Nat Med 5:1026–1031, 1999.
181. Kaufman DL, Clare-Salzler M, Tian J, et al: Spontaneous loss of T-cell tolerance to glutamic acid decarboxylase in murine insulin-dependent diabetes. Nature 366:69, 1993.
182. Stewart TA, Hultgren B, Huang X, et al: Induction of type I diabetes by interferon-alpha in transgenic mice. Science 260:1942–1946, 1993.
183. Shimada A, Charlton B, Taylor-Edwards C, Fathman CG: Beta-cell destruction may be a late consequence of the autoimmune process in nonobese diabetic mice. Diabetes 45:1063–1067, 1996.
184. Andre-Schmutz I, Hindelang C, Benoist C, Mathis D: Cellular and molecular changes accompanying the progression from insulitis to diabetes. Eur J Immunol 29:245–255, 1999.
185. Roura-Mir C, Catalfamo M, Sospedra M, et al: Single-cell analysis of intrathyroidal lymphocytes shows differential cytokine expression in Hashimoto's and Graves' disease. Eur J Immunol 27:3290–3302, 1997.
186. Sarvetnick N, Shizuru J, Liggitt D, et al: Loss of pancreatic islet tolerance induced by β cell expression of interferon γ. Nature 346:844–847, 1990.
187. Thomas HE, Parker JL, Schreiber RD, Kay TW: IFN-gamma action on pancreatic beta cells causes class I MHC upregulation but not diabetes. J Clin Invest 102:1249–1257, 1998.
188. Rabinovitch A, Sumoski W, Rajotte RV, Warnock GL: Cytotoxic effects of cytokines on human pancreatic islet cells in monolayer culture. J Clin Endocrinol Metab 71:152–156, 1990.
189. Reimers JI, Andersen HU, Pociot F: Nikotinamid og forebyggelse af insulinkraevende diabetes mellitus. Rationale, virkningsmekanisme, toksikologi og kliniske erfaringer. ENDIT Gruppe. [Nicotinamide and prevention of insulin-dependent diabetes mellitus. Rationale, effects, toxicology, and clinical experience. ENDIT Group.] Ugeskr Laeger 156:461–465, 1994.
190. Kriss JP, Pleshakow V, Chien JR: Isolation and identification of the long-acting thyroid stimulator and its relation to hyperthyroidism and circumscribed pretibial myxedema. J Clin Endocrinol Metab 24:1005–1028, 1964.
191. Goldman J, Baldwin D, Rubenstein AH, et al: Characterization of circulating insulin and proinsulin binding antibodies in autoimmune hypoglycemia. J Clin Invest 63:1050–1059, 1979.
192. Moller DE, Flier JS: Insulin resistance: Mechanisms, syndromes, and implications. N Engl J Med 325:938–948, 1991.
193. Eisenbarth G: Type 1 diabetes mellitus. A chronic autoimmune disease. N Engl J Med 314:1360, 1986.
194. Noorchashm H, Noorchashm N, Kern J, et al: B-cells are required for the initiation of insulitis and sialitis in nonobese diabetic mice. Diabetes 46:941, 1997.
195. Serreze DV, Chapman HD, Varnum DS, et al: B lymphocytes are essential for the initiation of T cell–mediated autoimmune diabetes: Analysis of a new "speed congenic" stock of NOD.Ig^{null} mice. J Exp Med 184:2049, 1996.
196. Miller BJ, Appel MC, O'Neil JJ, et al: Both the Lyt-2+ and L3T4+ T cell subsets are required for the transfer of diabetes in nonobese diabetic mice. J Immunol 140:52, 1988.
197. Kaufman DL, Erlander MG, Clare-Salzler M, et al: Autoimmunity to two forms of glutamate decarboxylase in insulin-dependent diabetes mellitus. J Clin Invest 89:283, 1992.
198. Hagopian W, Michelsen B, Karlsen AE: Autoantibodies in IDDM primarily recognize the 65,000-Mr rather than the 67,000-Mr isoform of glutamic acid decarboxylase. Diabetes 42:631, 1993.
199. Hagopian W, Sanjeevi C, Kockum I, et al: Glutamate decarboxylase-, insulin-, and islet cell-autoantibodies and HLA typing to detect diabetes in a general population-based study of Swedish children. J Clin Invest 95:1505, 1995.
200. Tisch R, Yang X, Singer SM, et al: Immune response to glutamic acid decarboxylase correlates with insulitis in non-obese diabetic mice. Nature 366:72, 1993.
201. Ma S-W, Zhao D-L, Yin Z-Q, et al: Transgenic plants expressing autoantigens fed to mice to induce oral immune tolerance. Nat Med 3:793–801, 1997.
202. Tian J, Clare-Salzler M, Herschenfeld A, et al: Modulating autoimmune responses to GAD inhibits disease progression and prolongs islet graft survival in diabetes-prone mice. Nat Med 2:1348–1354, 1996.
203. Zhang ZJ, Davidson L, Eisenbarth G, et al: Suppression of diabetes in nonobese diabetic mice by oral administration of porcine insulin. Proc Natl Acad Sci U S A 88:10252, 1991.
204. Atkinson MA, Maclaren NK, Luchetta R: Insulitis and diabetes in NOD mice reduced by prophylactic insulin therapy. Diabetes 39:933, 1990.
205. Haskins K, Wegmann D: Diabetogenic T-cell clones. Diabetes 45:1299–1305, 1996.
206. Atkins MH, Mier JW, Parkinson DR, et al: Hypothyroidism after treatment with interleukin-2 and lymphokine-activated killer cells. N Engl J Med 318:1557–1563, 1988.
207. Huang X, Hultgren B, Dybdal N, Stewart TA: Islet expression of interferon-alpha precedes diabetes in both the BB rat and streptozotocin-treated mice. Immunity 1:469–478, 1994.
208. Vial T, Descotes J: Immune-mediated side-effects of cytokines in humans. Toxicology 105:31–57, 1995.
209. Conlon KC, Urba WJ, Smith JW 2d: Exacerbation of symptoms of autoimmune disease in patients receiving alpha-interferon therapy. Cancer 65:2237–2242, 1990.
210. Picarella DE, Kratz A, Li CB, et al: Transgenic tumor necrosis factor (TNF)-alpha production in pancreatic islets leads to insulitis, not diabetes. Distinct patterns of inflammation in TNF-alpha and TNF-beta transgenic mice. J Immunol 150:4136–4150, 1993.
211. Baggiolini M, Dewald B, Moser B: Human chemokines: An update. Annu Rev Immunol 15:675–705, 1997.
212. Serreze DV, Chapman HD, Varnum DS, et al: Initiation of autoimmune diabetes in NOD/Lt mice is MHC class I–dependent. J Immunol 158:3978–3986, 1997.
213. Wicker LS, Leiter EH, Todd JA, et al: Beta 2-microglobulin–deficient NOD mice do not develop insulitis or diabetes. Diabetes 43:500–504, 1994.
214. Christianson SW, Shultz LD, Leiter EH: Adoptive transfer of diabetes into immunodeficient NOD-scid/scid mice. Relative contributions of CD4+ and CD8+ T-cells from diabetic versus prediabetic NOD.NON-Thy-1a donors. Diabetes 42:44–55, 1993.
215. Kagi D, Odermatt B, Seiler P, et al: Reduced incidence and delayed onset of diabetes in perforin-deficient nonobese diabetic mice. J Exp Med 7:989–997, 1997.
216. Kurrer MO, Pakala SV, Hanson HL, Katz JD: β Cell apoptosis in T cell–mediated autoimmune diabetes. Proc Natl Acad Sci U S A 94:213–218, 1997.
217. Pakala SV, Chivetta M, Kelly CB, Katz JD: In autoimmune diabetes the transition from benign to pernicious insulitis requires an islet cell response to tumor necrosis factor alpha. J Exp Med 189:1053–1062, 1999.
218. Chervonsky AV, Wang Y, Wong FS, et al: The role of Fas in autoimmune diabetes. Cell 89:17–24, 1997.
219. Giordano C, Stassi G, De Maria R, et al: Potential involvement of Fas and its ligand in the pathogenesis of Hashimoto's. Science 275:960–963, 1997.
220. The Canadian-European randomized control trial group: Cyclosporin-induced remission of IDDM after early intervention. Association of 1 yr of cyclosporin treatment with enhanced insulin secretion. Diabetes 37:1574–1582, 1988.

221. Stiller CF, Dupre J, Gent M: Effects of cyclosporine immunosuppression in insulin-dependent diabetes mellitus of recent onset. Science 223:1362–1367, 1984.

222. Bougneres FP, Carel JC, Castano L, et al: Factors associated with early remission of type 1 diabetes in children treated with cyclosporine. N Engl J Med 318:663–670, 1988.

223. Bougneres PF, Landais P, Boisson C: Limited duration of remission of insulin dependency in children with recent overt type I diabetes treated with low-dose cyclosporin. Diabetes 39:1264–1272, 1990.

224. Cook JJ, Hudson I, Harrison LC, et al: Double-blind controlled trial of azathioprine in children with newly diagnosed type I diabetes. Diabetes 38:779–783, 1989.

225. Silverstein J, MacLaren N, Riley W, et al: Immunosuppression with azathioprine and prednisone in recent-onset insulin-dependent diabetes mellitus. N Engl J Med 319:599–604, 1988.

226. Keller RJ, Eisenbarth GS, Jackson RA: Insulin prophylaxis in individuals at high risk of type I diabetes. Lancet 341:927–928, 1993.

227. Muir A, Peck A, Clare-Salzler M, et al: Insulin immunization of nonobese diabetic mice induces a protective insulitis characterized by diminished intraislet interferon-gamma transcription. J Clin Invest 95:628–634, 1995.

228. Tallstedt L, Lundell G, Torring O, et al: Occurrence of ophthalmopathy after treatment for Graves' hyperthyroidism. The Thyroid Study Group. N Engl J Med 326:1733–1738, 1992.

229. Bartalena L, Marcocci C, Bogazzi F, et al: Relation between therapy for hyperthyroidism and the course of Graves' ophthalmopathy. N Engl J Med 338:73–78, 1998.

Chapter 40

Interactions of the Endocrine and Immune Systems*

George P. Chrousos ▪ Ilia J. Elenkov

The neuroendocrine and immune systems play major roles in adaptation. Any "stressor" or threat to the stability of the steady state or homeostasis of the organism is counteracted by responses of the organism—*the adaptive responses.* The effectors of these responses are the corticotropin-releasing hormone (CRH)/arginine-vasopressin (AVP) and locus ceruleus–noradrenaline (LC-NA)/autonomic (sympathetic) neurons of the hypothalamus and brain stem, which respectively regulate the peripheral activities of the hypothalamic-pituitary-adrenal (HPA) axis and the systemic/adrenomedullary sympathetic nervous systems (SNS). Activation of the HPA axis and LC-NA/autonomic system results in systemic elevations of glucocorticoids and catecholamines (CAs), respectively, that act in concert to maintain homeostasis.[1]

Since Selye's time, in the late 1930s, stress hormones, and especially glucocorticoids, have been progressively known to shrink the thymus and lymph nodes; to inhibit lymphocyte proliferation, migration, and cytotoxicity; and to suppress the secretion of certain cytokines, such as interleukin-2 (IL-2) and interferon-γ (IFN-γ). These early observations and the broad use of glucocorticoids as potent anti-inflammatory/immunosuppressant agents led to the initial conclusion that stress was, in general, immunosuppressive. Recently, however, there has been convincing evidence that glucocorticoids and CAs, at levels that can be achieved during stress, influence the immune response in a less monochromatic way. This new understanding helps explain some well-known, but often contradictory, effects of stress on the immune system and on the onset and course of certain infectious, autoimmune/inflammatory, allergic, and neoplastic diseases. This chapter provides a brief up-to-date review of this understanding.

HISTORIC MILESTONES

Neuroendocrinology and immunology developed independently of each other for many years. Celsus defined four of the five cardinal signs of inflammation almost 2000 years ago, while Eustachius described the adrenal glands in 1563. The question, however, as to how the brain communicates with the immune system remained unknown or enigmatic until recently. Evidence that lymphoid organs are innervated date back to the end of the 19th century when nerves, independently of blood vessels, were found to enter lymph nodes.[2] In 1898, von Fürth described a bioactive principle in extracts from animal

adrenal glands, which he called "suprarenin." Three years later, Takamine and Aldrich independently isolated suprarenin in crystalline form (cf. ref. 3) and named it adrenaline; their investigation determined the correct formula ($C_9H_{13}NO_3$) of this substance, which represents the first hormone to be isolated from animal tissues. During later experiments, in 1907, a "by-product" of the synthesis of adrenaline or epinephrine was identified; this substance became commercially available as "arterenol" in 1908. It was in fact, noradrenaline or norepinephrine, formally discovered and isolated from tissues 40 years later.

At the end of the 19th century and at the beginning of the 20th century, Metchnicoff and Ehrlich, respectively, developed the concepts of cellular and humoral immunity (see ref. 4). In 1904, Loeper and Crouzon[5] were the first to describe a pronounced leukocytosis after subcutaneous injection of epinephrine in humans. In the 1920s Metal'nikov and Chorine[6] showed that immune reactions could be conditioned by classic pavlovian means. In the 1930s, Selye described involution of the thymus in animals exposed to stressors and expanded upon the concept of the stress response initially introduced by Cannon.[7] Cannon had called this response the "fight or flight" reaction and had linked it to stress and to CA secretion. Cannon had also emphasized the "generalized" sympathetic response or the "wisdom of the body" that occurs during stress, contrasting it with the more "discrete" functions of parasympathetic pathways (see refs. 8, 9).

In the 1940s, von Euler[10] isolated from a lymphoid organ, the spleen, norepinephrine (NE) and later provided evidence that NE was the major neurotransmitter released from sympathetic nerves. Cortisone, the precursor of the active principle of the adrenal glands, was isolated by Kendal and Reichstein in the late 1940s and shown to suppress immune functions. These scientists, along with Hench, received the Nobel Prize in Medicine or Physiology, after Hench showed that cortisone produced a spectacular amelioration of rheumatoid arthritis.[11, 12] Interestingly, in the 1950s Dougherty and Frank[13] noticed a 400% increase of what they called "stress-lymphocytes" within 10 minutes after subcutaneous injection of epinephrine. These cells had the morphology of large granular lymphocytes or natural killer (NK) cells, whose function and characteristics were described in the late 1970s (see Benschop et al.[3]).

It was in the 1970s and 1980s that Besedovsky and co-workers demonstrated that classic hormones and newly described cytokines were involved in a functionally relevant *cross-talk* between the brain and the immune system.[14–16] They showed that an immune response induced an increase of plasma glucocorticoid concentrations,[14, 16, 17] altered the activity of hypothalamic noradrenergic neurons,[18] and decreased the content of NE in the spleen.[15, 19] At about the same time, the first comprehensive morphologic studies provided evidence that both primary and secondary lymphoid organs were innervated by sympathetic/noradrenergic nerve fibers. Furthermore, it was shown that classic behavioral conditioning,[20] stressful stimuli,[1, 21, 22] or lesions in specific regions of the brain[23] reproducibly altered immune function. Finally, evidence was obtained in experimental animals that the susceptibility to autoimmune diseases was determined to a great extent by the activity of the stress system[24–26] or that stress mediators exert both pro- and anti-inflammatory effects.[1, 27] Subsequently, we witnessed an explosive growth of a new interdisciplinary research area that studies the neuroimmune communication, and our understanding of the interactions between the neuroendocrine system and the immune and inflammatory reaction has expanded enormously.

ORGANIZATION OF THE STRESS SYSTEM

The HPA axis and the systemic sympathetic and adrenomedullary (sympathetic) system are the peripheral limbs of the stress system, whose main function is to maintain basal and stress-related homeostasis.[8, 28] The central components of this system are located in the hypothalamus and the brain stem (Fig. 40–1). They include the parvocellular neurons of the paraventricular nuclei of the hypothalamus that CRH and AVP; the CRH neurons of the paragigantocellular and parabrachial nuclei of the medulla; and the A1, A2, A3 and A6 (locus ceruleus), mostly noradrenergic cell groups of the medulla and pons.

Each of the paraventricular nuclei has three parvocellular divisions: a medial group, producing mostly CRH and projecting and secreting into the hypophysial portal system; an intermediate group, producing mostly AVP and also projecting and secreting into the hypophysial portal system, and a lateral group, producing primarily CRH and projecting to and innervating noradrenergic and other neurons of the stress system in the brain stem (Fig. 40–2).[8, 28, 29] Some parvocellular neurons contain and secrete both CRH and AVP, and this neural population increases with stress.[30, 31] Other paraventricular CRH neurons project to and innervate proopiomelanocortin-containing neurons of the central stress system in the arcuate nucleus of the hypothalamus, as well as neurons of pain control areas of the hind brain and spinal cord (see Figs. 40–1 and 40–2). Activation of the stress system leads to CRH-induced secretion of proopiomelanocortin-derived and other opioid peptides,[32, 33] which enhance analgesia.[8, 28] These peptides also simultaneously inhibit the activity of the stress system by suppressing CRH and norepinephrine secretion.[8, 28]

CRH stimulates the secretion of adrenocorticotropic hormone (ACTH) by the corticotrophs of the anterior pituitary.[34, 35] Its effect on the pituitary is also permissive, since when CRH is absent, very little ACTH secretion takes place. AVP alone has very little ACTH secretagogue activity but is a potent synergistic factor with CRH. CRH and AVP may act synergistically on other target tissues with CRH and AVP receptors in the CNS and perhaps the periphery.[36]

Every hour, the parvocellular neurons secrete two or three mostly synchronous pulses of CRH and AVP into the hypophysial portal system.[37–41] In early morning, the amplitudes of these pulses are highest, increasing the amplitude and apparent frequency of ACTH and cortisol secretory episodes. The frequency appears to increase, because previously undetectable pulses of ACTH and cortisol become measurable by standard assays. During acute stress, the amplitude of CRH and AVP pulses also increases, resulting in increases in the amplitude and apparent frequency of ACTH and cortisol pulses; in this case, the stress system recruits additional secretagogues of CRH, AVP, or ACTH, such as magnocellular AVP, and angiotensin II.[8, 28, 42, 43]

Circulating ACTH of pituitary origin is the key regulator of glucocorticoid secretion by the adrenal gland's *zona fasciculata*. Other hormones, including CAs, neuropeptide Y (NPY), from the adrenal medulla, and additional autonomic neural input to the adrenal cortex also take part in the regulation of glucocorticoid secretion.[41, 44–47] ACTH participates in the control of aldosterone secretion by the *zona glomerulosa* and of adrenal androgen secretion by the *zona reticularis*.

The sympathetic system originates in nuclei within the brain stem and gives rise to preganglionic efferent fibers that leave the CNS through the thoracic and lumbar spinal nerves ("thoracolumbar sys-

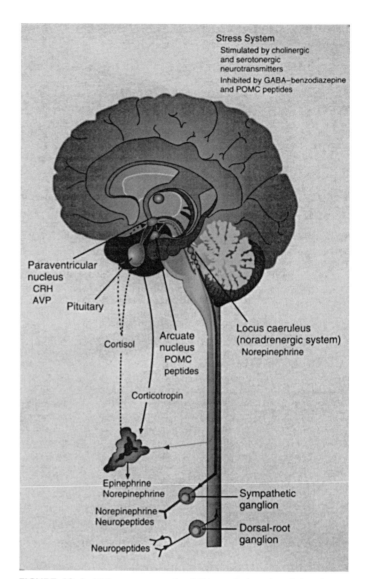

FIGURE 40–1. Major components of the central and peripheral stress system. The paraventricular nucleus and the locus ceruleus/noradrenergic system are shown along with their peripheral limbs, the pituitary-adrenal axis, and the adrenomedullary and systemic sympathetic systems. The hypothalamic corticotropin-releasing hormone (CRH) and central noradrenergic neurons mutually innervate and activate each other, while they exert presynaptic autoinhibition through collateral fibers. Arginine vasopressin (AVP) from the paraventricular nucleus synergizes with CRH on stimulating corticotropin (ACTH) secretion. The cholinergic and serotonergic neurotransmitter systems stimulate both components of the central stress system, while the γ-aminobutyric acid/benzodiazepine (GABA/BZD) and arcuate nucleus proopiomelanocortin (POMC) peptide systems inhibit it. The latter is directly activated by the stress system and is important in the enhancement of analgesia that takes place during stress. (From Chrousos G: The hypothalamic-pituitary-adrenal axis and immune-mediated inflammation. N Engl J Med 332:1351–1362, 1995. Copyright © 1995 Massachusetts Medical Society. All rights reserved.)

tem"). Most of the sympathetic preganglionic fibers terminate in ganglia located in the paravertebral chains that lie on either side of the spinal column. The remaining sympathetic ganglia are located in prevertebral ganglia, which lie in front of the vertebrae. From these ganglia, postganglionic sympathetic fibers run to the tissues innervated. Most postganglionic sympathetic fibers release NE; they are noradrenergic fibers, i.e., they act by releasing NE. Adrenal medulla contains chromaffin cells, embryologically and anatomically homologous to the sympathetic ganglia also derived from the neural crest. The adrenal medulla, unlike the postganglionic sympathetic nerve terminals, releases mainly epinephrine, and to a lesser extent NE (the approximate

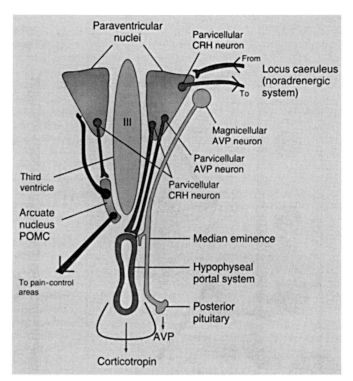

FIGURE 40–2. A close-up view of the paraventricular nuclei of the hypothalamus. Parvocellular CRH- and arginine vasopressin (AVP)–secreting neurons project to and secrete into the hypophysial portal system. Parvocellular CRH neurons also project to the brain stem to innervate neurons of the locus ceruleus/noradrenergic system. Magnocellular AVP-secreting neurons terminate at the posterior pituitary and secrete into the systemic circulation; however, they also have collateral terminals in the portal system. CRH is permissive for and stimulates pituitary corticotropin (ACTH) secretion, while AVP has a major synergistic role with CRH in the secretion of ACTH. The arcuate proopiomelanocortin (POMC) nucleus is shown, along with the mutual innervation between CRH and POMC-peptide–secreting neurons. (From Chrousos G: The hypothalamic-pituitary-adrenal axis and immune-mediated inflammation. N Engl J Med 332:1351–1362, 1995. Copyright © 1995 Massachusetts Medical Society. All rights reserved.)

ratio is 4:1); typical preganglionic sympathetic nerve terminals, whose main neurotransmitter is acetylcholine, innervate the chromaffin cells of the adrenal medulla.

CAs are synthesized from tyrosine that is transported into the noradrenergic endings or varicosities by a sodium-dependent carrier. Tyrosine is converted to dopamine (the rate-limiting step in the NE synthesis) by the enzyme tyrosine hydroxylase (TH) and a carrier that can be blocked by reserpine transports dopamine into the secretory vesicles. Dopamine (DA) is converted to NE within these vesicles by dopamine-hydroxylase (DBH). In the adrenal medulla, NE is further converted to epinephrine.

Role of Stress System in Maintaining Basal and Stress-Related Homeostasis

Living organisms survive by maintaining an immensely complex dynamic steady state of the internal milieu. When homeostasis is disturbed or threatened, by internal or external challenges, both the HPA axis and the SNS become activated, resulting in increased peripheral levels of glucocorticoids and CAs that act in concert to maintain homeostasis. Selye defined this reaction in the 1930s as the "general adaptation or stress syndrome."[8]

The stress system has a baseline, circadian activity, but also responds on demand to physical and emotional stressors. At rest, via glucocorticoids and CAs it maintains basal homeostasis, as a major regulator of fuel metabolism, heart rate, blood vessel tone, and thermogenesis, while during stress it adjusts these functions accordingly. This

system integrates and responds to a great diversity of distinct circadian, neurosensory, blood-borne, and limbic signals. This also includes humoral signals from the immune system and inflammatory reaction. Indeed, any immune challenge that threatens the stability of the internal milieu can be regarded as a stressor, i.e., a stimulus to the organism that activates the stress system to help re-attain homeostasis.

The last 15 years have provided evidence that certain cytokines, and particularly the proinflammatory ones, including tumor necrosis factor (TNF)–α, IL-1, and IL-6, activate both the HPA axis and the SNS.[1, 48] Moreover, these cytokines, alone, or in conjunction with components of the stress system, induce fever, sleepiness, fatigue, loss of appetite, and decreased libido, and activate the hepatic synthesis of acute phase proteins, changes referred to as *sickness behavior* and *acute phase response,* respectively. Stress that is associated with an immune challenge has been called *immune* or *inflammatory stress,*[1] and like other forms of stress, is coordinated by the central stress system and its peripheral arms.

Functionally, the CRH and LC/NE/sympathetic systems seem to participate in a positive, reverberatory feedback loop so that activation of one system tends to activate the other as well.[8, 28, 49, 50] This includes projections of CRH-secreting neurons from the lateral paraventricular nuclei (PVN) to the central sympathetic systems in the hindbrain, and conversely, projections of catecholaminergic fibers from the LC-NE system, via the ascending noradrenergic bundle, to the PVN in the hypothalamus. Thus, CRH stimulates norepinephrine secretion through its specific receptors, while norepinephrine stimulates CRH secretion through primarily α1-noradrenergic receptors.[8, 28, 50] Autoregulatory, ultrashort negative feedback loops are also present in these neurons, with CRH and norepinephrine collateral fibers acting in an inhibitory fashion on presynaptic CRH and β2-noradrenergic receptors, respectively. The CRH, AVP, and noradrenergic neurons receive stimulatory input from the serotonergic, cholinergic, and histaminergic systems and inhibitory input from the γ-aminobutyric acid (GABA)/benzodiazepine and opioid peptide neuronal systems of the brain.[8, 28, 49, 50] Centrally secreted substance P has inhibitory actions on the hypothalamic CRH but not AVP neurons and stimulatory effects on the central noradrenergic system.[50–52]

Activation of the stress system leads to adaptive behavioral and physical changes.[8, 28] Centrally, the behavioral changes include enhanced arousal and accelerated motor reflexes, better attention span and cognitive function, decreased feeding and sexual behavior, and increased ability to withstand pain. Peripherally, the activation of the stress system results in increased sympathetic output, i.e., increase of the release of NE from the sympathetic nerve terminals and epinephrine/NE from the adrenal medulla, and in increased secretion of glucocorticoids by the adrenal cortex. These changes are related to the physical adaptation that includes changes in cardiovascular function, intermediary metabolism, and modulation of the immune and inflammatory reaction.

Innervation of Lymphoid Organs

Sympathetic/noradrenergic and sympathetic/NPY postganglionic nerve fibers innervate both the smooth muscle of the vasculature and the parenchyma of specific compartments of primary and secondary lymphoid organs.[53, 54] These nerve fibers and their varicosites do travel in plexuses that run adjacent to and along the blood vessels in these organs; it is hence possible that both NE and NPY, released from these fibers, play a role in controlling blood flow to these organs and the traffic of leukocytes within their vessels. However, some noradrenergic fibers, that are not associated with blood vessels, are present in the parenchyma of lymphoid organs tissue.[53, 54] NE released from their nerve fibers may exert immunomodulatory roles by altering the activity of local leukocytes. Noradrenergic innervation of lymphoid tissues appears to be regional and specific; generally, zones of T cells, macrophages and plasma cells are richly innervated, whereas nodular and follicular zones of developing or maturing B cells are poorly innervated.[53]

The main target cells of the noradrenergic innervation of lymphoid organs appear to be immature and mature thymocytes, thymic epithelial cells (TEC), T lymphocytes, macrophages, mast cells, plasma cells, and enterochromaffin cells. Noradrenergic nerve fibers in the thymus are closely associated with mast cells within both the perivascular and parenchymal zones, suggesting a possible humoral role for NE and histamine in the maturation of T cells. Noradrenergic innervation is present early in development, and the arrival of the fibers generally precedes the development of the cellular compartment of the immune system, suggesting a role for NE in the development of this system. For example, at the time of development and reorganization of the periarterial lymphatic sheath (PALS) in the spleen (postnatal day 14 in the rat), the noradrenergic plexus around the central arterioles and its branches increase in density, displaying an adult pattern of both vascular and parenchymal innervation.[55]

In addition to the autonomic/sympathetic innervation, all lymphoid organs also receive sensory peptidergic innervation that is confined mostly to the parenchyma.[56] The most abundantly present neuropeptides are the tachykinins, substance P and neurokinin A, calcitonin gene-related peptide (CGRP), and vasoactive intestinal polypeptide/peptide histidine isoleucine (VIP/PHI). Double immunofluorescence reveals coexistence of tachykinins with CGRP and of TH with NPY. This coexistence pattern conforms to the general scheme described for the peripheral innervation of nonimmune organs.

A close spatial relationship between peptidergic nerve fibers and mast cells, T cells, and macrophages is observed in immune organs.[56] Peptidergic nerves, however, are sparse in pure B cell regions. Neuromast cell contacts are present in lymphoid organs, except the spleen.[56] Mast cells bear receptors for and respond to substance P (SP); the latter triggers the release of granules containing histamine, cytokines, and lipid mediators of inflammation, including leukotrienes. NE, on the other hand, through the stimulation of α_2- or β_2-adrenoreceptors, stimulates or inhibits the release of histamine from mast cells. Thus, apart from their direct immunomodulatory effects, SP antidromically released from sensory nerves, or NE released from postganglionic noradrenergic nerve terminals may exert indirect immunomodulatory effects via changes in mast cell degranulation within the parenchyma of lymphoid organs.

Neuromast cell connections and neuromacrophage connections, as well as neuro-T cell contacts, are not restricted to the preformed lymphoid organs and tissues, but are also regularly encountered in most nonimmune tissues.[56] Mast cells, T cells, and macrophages are regularly seen in contact with peripheral nerves and in both sympathetic and sensory ganglia. In the skin, postcapillary venules, macrophages, mast cells, and peptidergic nerves stained for tachykinins/CGRP form a typical quadrad, while in the outer wall of larger blood vessels, the quadrad is joined by TH/NPY fibers. Further, close interrelations but no coincidence of TH/NPY and SP/CGRP immunoreactive fibers are frequently observed in perivascular regions.[56]

THE IMMUNE RESPONSE AND THE INFLAMMATORY REACTION

Any immune response involves, firstly, recognition of a pathogen, and secondly, mounting of a reaction against it. Broadly speaking, the different types of immune response fall into two categories: the *innate* (or nonspecific), and *adaptive* (or specific) immune response.

Phagocytic cells, such as monocytes, macrophages, and polymorphonuclear neutrophils, bind to microorganisms, internalize them, and kill them. Because they use primitive nonspecific recognition systems, which allow them to bind to a variety of microbial products, they mediate innate immune responses, acting as a first line of defense.[57] However, a subgroup of lymphocytes known as large granular lymphocytes (LGLs) also have the capacity to recognize surface changes that occur on a variety of tumor or virally infected cells and to destroy these cells using nonspecific recognition systems; this action is often called "natural killer (NK)" cell activity. Both monocytes/macrophages and LGLs may also recognize and destroy target cells (or pathogens) coated with specific antibody.

Lymphocytes, such as T lymphocytes (or T cells) and B lymphocytes (or B cells), are central components of the adaptive immune response, since they specifically recognize individual pathogens,

whether they are inside host cells or outside in the tissue fluids or blood. B cells combat extracellular pathogens and their products by releasing antibodies, which specifically recognize and bind target molecules, the antigens. Antigens may be molecules on the surface of pathogens, or soluble toxins, produced by them. One group of lymphocytes, the T-helper (Th) cells, exerts regulatory function, i.e., they interact with B cells and help them divide, differentiate, and make antibody; this group also interacts with mononuclear lymphocytes and helps them destroy intracellular pathogens. Another group of T cells, the T-cytotoxic (Tc), is responsible for the destruction of host cells, which have become infected by viruses or other intracellular pathogens. T cells use a specific receptor, the T cell antigen receptor (TCR), to recognize antigens, but only in association with familiar markers on host cells. This receptor is related, both in structure and function, to the surface antibody, which B cells use as their antigen receptors. T cells generate their effects, either by releasing cytokines or by direct cell-cell interactions.[57]

The cells of the immune system are widely distributed throughout the body, but if an infection occurs, it is necessary to mobilize a large number of them at the site of infection. The process by which this occurs manifests itself as inflammation and includes (1) increased blood supply to the infected area by local vasodilation, and (2) increased capillary permeability to permit diapedesis of leukocytes and exudation of plasma containing soluble mediators of immunity. The migration of leukocytes is assisted by a process of chemical attraction known as chemotaxis (Fig. 40–3).

The cells that participate in the inflammatory reaction are monocytes, polymorphonuclear leukocytes, including neutrophils, basophils, and eosinophils, and lymphocytes, all attracted from the blood to the inflammatory site, and local immune accessory cells, such as endothelial cells, mast cells, tissue fibroblasts, and resident macrophages. In the earliest stages of inflammation, neutrophils are particularly prevalent, but in the later stages monocytes and lymphocytes take on a primary role. Local generation of secretory products, including cytokines, lipid mediators of inflammation, and neuropeptides, is crucial for further chemoattraction of cells and for the coordinated activation of the effector cells.[58, 59] Most of the time, these events are clinically undetectable. Occasionally, however, clinical inflammation occurs, generating high concentrations of local and circulating levels of cytokines and other mediators of inflammation associated with activation of the stress system and sickness behavior.

The sensory afferent fibers and postganglionic sympathetic neurons of the peripheral nervous system also influence inflammation (see Fig. 40–3).[60-64] The sensory fibers sense the local threat and not only send signals to the central nervous system, but also secrete pro-inflammatory or anti-inflammatory substances, such as, respectively, the neuropeptides substance P or somatostatin, in the site of inflammation. The neurotransmitter NE that is released from the postganglionic sympathetic nerve fibers exerts mostly anti-inflammatory effects locally (see text below).

Role of Th1 and Th2 Cells and Type 1 and Type 2 Cytokines in the Regulation of Cellular and Humoral Immunity

Immune responses are regulated by antigen-presenting cells (APC), such as monocytes/macrophages, dendritic cells, and other phagocytic cells, that are components of *innate immunity*, and by the recently described lymphocyte subclasses Th1 and Th2 (also abbreviated T_H1 and T_H2), that are components of *adaptive immunity*.[65, 66] Th1 cells primarily secrete IFN-γ, IL-2, and TNF-β, which promote cellular immunity; whereas Th2 cells secrete a different set of cytokines, primarily IL-4, IL-10, and IL-13, which promote humoral immunity (Fig. 40–4).

Naive CD4$^+$ (antigen-inexperienced) Th0 cells are clearly bipotential and serve as precursors of Th1 and Th2 cells. Among the factors currently known to influence the differentiation of these cells toward Th1 or Th2, cytokines produced by cells of the innate immune system are the most important. Thus, IL-12, produced by activated monocytes/macrophages or other APCs, is a major inducer of Th1 differentiation

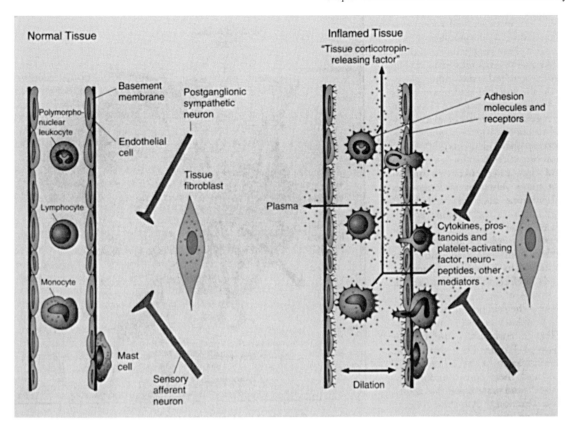

FIGURE 40–3. Major components and events of inflammation. Quiescent circulating leukocytes, local immune accessory cells, and the terminals of peripheral postganglionic sympathetic and sensory afferent neurons are shown *(left-hand panel)*. In inflamed tissue *(right-hand panel)*, there is vasodilation, increased permeability of the vessel, and exudation of plasma. Activated leukocytes and endothelial cells express adhesion molecules and adhesion-molecule receptors. Cells attach to the vessel wall and diapedesis takes place, with chemotaxis toward a chemokine gradient at the focus of inflammation. Activated circulating cells, migrant cells, local immune accessory cells, and peripheral nerves secrete cytokines, prostanoids, platelet activating factor, neuropeptides, and other mediators of inflammation. Some of these substances, such as interleukin-6, leukotrienes, complement component 5α, corticotropin-releasing hormone, and transforming growth factor–β, have chemokinetic activity. Some substances, such as the inflammatory cytokines tumor necrosis factor–α, interleukin-1, and interleukin-6, escape in the systemic circulation, causing systemic symptoms and activating the hypothalamic-pituitary-adrenal axis. Because of such effects, these substances were historically referred to as "tissue corticotropin releasing factor (CRF)" (see text). (From Chrousos G: The hypothalamic-pituitary-adrenal axis and immune-mediated inflammation. N Engl J Med 332:1351–1362, 1995. Copyright © 1995 Massachusetts Medical Society. All rights reserved.)

and hence cellular immunity; this cytokine acts in concert with NK-derived IFN-γ to further promote Th1 responses.[67] APC-derived IL-12 and TNF-α in concert with NK cell- and Th1 cell-derived IFN-γ stimulate the functional activity of T cytotoxic (Tc) cells, NK cells, and activated macrophages, i.e., the major components of cellular immunity. All three cytokines, IL-12, TNF-α, and IFN-γ, also stimulate the synthesis of nitric oxide (NO) and other inflammatory mediators that drive chronic delayed type inflammatory responses. Because of these crucial and synergistic roles in inflammation, IL-12, TNF-α, and IFN-γ are considered the major pro-inflammatory cytokines.[65–67]

Th1 and Th2 responses are mutually inhibitory. Thus, IL-12 and IFN-γ inhibit Th2 and, vice versa, IL-4 and IL-10 inhibit Th1 responses. IL-4 and IL-10 promote humoral immunity by stimulating the growth and activation of mast cells and eosinophils, the differentiation of B cells into antibody-secreting B cells, and B cell immunoglobulin switching to IgE. Importantly, these cytokines inhibit macrophage activation, T cell proliferation, and the production of pro-inflammatory cytokines.[65, 66] Thus, IL-4 and IL-10 are the major anti-inflammatory cytokines[65, 66] (see Fig. 40–4).

EFFECTS OF THE HPA AXIS AND THE SYMPATHETIC NERVOUS SYSTEM ON THE IMMUNE AND INFLAMMATORY REACTION

Adrenocortical Hormones

The anti-inflammatory and immunosuppressive properties of glucocorticoids, exerted via their ubiquitous intracellular receptors, make

them invaluable therapeutic agents in numerous diseases.[68] The glucocorticoid receptor is a 777-amino-acid cytoplasmic protein with three major functional domains and several subdomains. The carboxyterminal region binds glucocorticoid, and the middle portion domain binds to specific sequences of DNA in the regulatory regions of glucocorticoid-responsive genes (glucocorticoid-responsive elements).[68, 69]

Glucocorticoids influence the traffic of circulating leukocytes and inhibit many functions of leukocytes and immune accessory cells.[8, 28, 68, 69] They suppress the immune activation of these cells, inhibit the production of cytokines and other mediators of inflammation, and cause cytokine resistance. Subgroups of T lymphocytes are particularly affected by glucocorticoids. Thus, these hormones suppress Th1 function and stimulate apoptosis of eosinophils and certain groups of T lymphocytes. Glucocorticoids also inhibit the expression of adhesion and adhesion receptor molecules on the surface of immune and other cell[70] and potentiate the acute phase reaction.[71] All of these effects depend on altering the transcription rates of glucocorticoid-responsive genes or changing the stability of messenger RNAs of several proteins involved in inflammation.[72–74] For instance, glucocorticoids suppress production of IL-6 and IL-1 by decreasing both the transcription rate of the genes for these interleukins and the stability of their messenger RNA.

Among the many proteins regulated by glucocorticoids are the phospholipase A2, cyclooxygenase 2, and inducible nitric oxide synthetase 2 genes.[68, 74–78] Suppression of these proteins decreases production of prostanoids, platelet activating factor, and nitric oxide, three key molecules in the inflammatory response. The activated glucocorticoid receptor also inhibits the proinflammatory activity of many growth factors and cytokines by directly interacting with and blocking

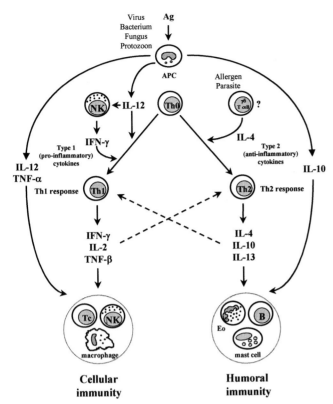

FIGURE 40–4. Role of Th1 and Th2 cells, and type 1 and type 2 cytokines in the regulation of cellular and humoral immunity. Cellular immunity provides protection against intracellular bacteria, protozoa, fungi, and several viruses, whereas humoral immunity provides protection against multicellular parasites, extracellular bacteria, some viruses, soluble toxins, and allergens (see text). Solid lines represent stimulation, while dashed lines inhibition. Ag, antigen; APC, antigen-presenting cell; NK, natural killer cell; T, T cell; B, B cell; Th, T-helper cell; Tc, T-cytotoxic cell; Eo, eosinophil; IL, interleukin; TNF, tumor necrosis factor; IFN, interferon. (From Elenkov I, Chrousos G: Stress hormones, Th1/Th2 patterns, pro/anti-inflammatory cytokines and susceptibility to disease. TEM 10:359–368, 1999.)

the third messenger systems for these hormones.[68, 69] These include the transcription factors c-jun, nuclear factor (NF-κB), and cAMP-responsive element binding (CREB) protein. In a mutual fashion, elevated intracellular concentrations of these factors prevent the activated glucocorticoid receptor from exerting its effects on the genome.

Several circadian immune functions cause disease-associated diurnal changes that correspond to plasma glucocorticoid levels.[79, 80] For example, the delayed hypersensitivity reaction, which is particularly sensitive to glucocorticoids, is greatest in the evening when glucocorticoids are low and least in the morning when they are high.[79]

The secretion of adrenal androgens, which, like cortisol, follow the circadian pattern of ACTH, is associated with a distinct developmental pattern with highest levels in utero, puberty, and early adulthood.[81] Adrenal androgens with the Δ^5 configuration in the A ring have been suggested as modulators of immune function.[82–85] An orphan receptor of the steroid-thyroid receptor superfamily specific for Δ^5-adrenal androgens has been detected in T lymphocytes and presumably mediates the potentiation of Th1 cells by these androgens, enhancing cellular immunity.[85]

Catecholamines

Lymphocyte traffic and circulation are under the influence of SNS and CAs. In the short term, acutely (<30 minutes), CAs mobilize NK cells from depots, whereas in the long term, chronically, CAs decrease the number of lymphocytes, and particularly of NK cells in the peripheral blood.[3] CAs or β-adrenoreceptor (AR) agonists inhibit the T cell proliferation induced by mitogens.[86, 87] This is usually accompanied by

an increase of cAMP in lymphocytes, and the amount of cAMP produced by T cells stimulated with isoproterenol, a β-AR agonist, is proportional to the degree of inhibition of the proliferation.[88, 89] β-ARs agonists exert similar inhibitory effect on the proliferative response of human highly purified T cells stimulated with immobilized anti-CD3 monoclonal antibody through the CD3/TCR complex.[89, 90]

In vitro and in vivo studies reveal that CAs mediate, both acutely and chronically, an inhibition of NK cell activity.[91, 92] Central administration of CRH that is known to increase the sympathetic autonomic outflow is accompanied by decreased NK activity in the periphery, an effect that is independent of adrenocortical activation.[93–95] This effect of central CRH is also rapid: within 20 minutes of the infusion lytic values of splenic NK cells decline by nearly 50%, while the cytotoxicity of peripheral NK cells is reduced within 1 hour.[93, 95]

Moreover, several lines of evidence suggest that stress, which is accompanied by increased levels of peripheral CAs, inhibits several components of cellular immunity and particularly NK cell activity, an effect that is mediated mainly by the CRH-SNS axis.[93] Thus, in animals, the central application of anti-CRH antibodies completely blocks the inhibitory effect of footshock stress on NK activity.[93] It appears that NK cells are the most "sensitive" cells to the suppressive effect of stress, and, not surprisingly, NK cell activity has become a bona fide index of stress-induced suppression of cellular immunity, employed in many studies (see ref. 93). Apart from a direct and acute effect, chronically, during subacute or chronic stress, CAs may suppress NK activity indirectly, though their potent inhibition of the production of IL-12 and IFN-γ,[96] cytokines essential for NK activity (see text below).

CAs appear to mediate both inhibitory and stimulatory effects on macrophage activity. This process is influenced by several factors, such as availability of type 1/pro-inflammatory cytokines; presence or absence of antigen; presence in the microenvironment of pro-inflammatory mediators, such as SP, peripheral (immune) CRH, and histamine, released from the sensory and postganglionic-sympathetic neurons or mast cells, respectively; and the state of activation or differentiation of macrophages, which may determine the β-ARs responsiveness and the expression of α-ARs. CAs also exert enhancing effects on the initiation of Tc responses, in contrast to inhibition of effector Tc cell function. CAs inhibit both neutrophil phagocytosis and the release of lysosomal enzymes from neutrophils.[97] Furthermore, the superoxide generation and formation of oxygen radicals that play an important microbicidal role are suppressed at nanomolar concentrations of epinephrine, an effect mediated by β2-ARs.[98, 99]

When B cells and Th cells are exposed to Th cell–dependent antigen, NE, through stimulation of β2 receptors, exerts an enhancing effect on B cell antibody (Ab) production.[100, 101] One mechanism for this enhancement may involve a β2-AR–induced increase in the frequency of B cells differentiating into Ab-secreting cells. Moreover, Th cells not only activate B cells via cell-to-cell interaction, but they (Th2 cells) also provide the cytokines necessary for B cell growth. Here again, CAs may play important modulatory role through their differential effect on type 1 and type 2 cytokine production (see text below). Thus, the β-AR agonists salbutamol and fenoterol potentiate IL-4–induced IgE production by human peripheral blood mononuclear cells (PBMC), while they inhibit IFN-γ production by the same cells.[102] Furthermore, salbutamol induces an increase of the ex vivo release of IL-4, IL-6, and IL-10 by human PBMC.[103]

Stress Hormones Suppress Cellular and Potentiate Humoral Immunity

Effects of Glucocorticoids

Glucocorticoids suppress the production of TNF-α, IFN-γ, and IL-2 in vitro and in vivo in animals and humans.[1] As recently shown, glucocorticoids also act through their classic cytoplasmic/nuclear receptors on APCs to suppress the production of the main inducer of Th1 responses IL-12 in vitro and ex vivo.[96, 104] Because IL-12 is extremely potent in enhancing IFN-γ and inhibiting IL-4 synthesis by T cells, the inhibition of IL-12 production may represent a major mechanism through which glucocorticoids affect the Th1/Th2 balance. Thus, glucocorticoid-treated monocytes/macrophages produce significantly less IL-12, leading to a decreased capacity of these cells to induce IFN-γ production by antigen-primed CD4⁺ T cells; the same treatment of monocytes/macrophages is also associated with an increased production of IL-4 by T cells, probably resulting from disinhibition from the suppressive effects of IL-12 on Th2 activity[105] (Fig. 40–5).

Furthermore, glucocorticoids potently downregulate the expression of IL-12 receptors on T and NK cells. This explains why human peripheral blood mononuclear cells stimulated with immobilized anti-CD3 lose their ability to produce IFN-γ in the presence of glucocorticoids.[106] Thus, although glucocorticoids may have a direct suppressive effect on Th1 cells, the overall inhibition of IFN-γ production by these cells appears to result mainly from the inhibition of IL-12 production by APCs and from the loss of IL-12 responsiveness of NK and Th1 cells.

It is particularly noteworthy that glucocorticoids have no effect on the production of the potent anti-inflammatory cytokine IL-10 by monocytes; yet, lymphocyte-derived IL-10 production is upregulated by glucocorticoids.[96, 107] Thus, rat CD4⁺ T cells pretreated with dexamethasone exhibit increased levels of mRNA for IL-10.[108] Similarly, during experimental endotoxemia or cardiopulmonary bypass, or in multiple sclerosis patients having an acute relapse, the treatment with glucocorticoids is associated with increased plasma IL-10 secretion.[107, 109, 110] This might have resulted from a direct stimulatory effect of glucocorticoids on T cell IL-10 production and/or from the disinhibi-

tion of the restraining inputs of IL-12 and IFN-γ on monocyte/lymphocyte IL-10 production.

Effects of Catecholamines

CAs drive a Th2 shift, both at the level of APCs and Th1 cells (see Fig. 40–5). We recently demonstrated that NE and epinephrine potently inhibited or enhanced the production of IL-12 and IL-10, respectively, in human whole blood cultures stimulated with lipopolysaccharide (LPS) ex vivo.[96] These effects are mediated by stimulation of β-ARs, since they are completely prevented by propranolol, a β-AR antagonist. Our findings were subsequently extended by other laboratories showing that non-selective β- and selective β₂-AR agonists inhibited the production of IL-12 in vitro and in vivo.[111, 112] In conjunction with their ability to suppress IL-12 production, β₂-AR agonists inhibited the development of Th1-type cells, while promoting Th2 cell differentiation.[111]

β-ARs are expressed on Th1 cells, but not on Th2 cells.[100] This may provide an additional mechanistic basis for a differential effect of CAs on Th1/Th2 functions. In fact, in both murine and human systems, β₂-AR agonists inhibit IFN-γ production by Th1 cells, but do not affect IL-4 production by Th2 cells.[100, 113] Importantly, the differential effect of CAs on Th1/Th2 cytokine production also operates in in vivo conditions. Thus, increasing sympathetic outflow in mice by selective α₂-AR antagonists or application of β-AR agonists results in inhibition of LPS-induced TNF-α and IL-12 production[112, 114, 115]; in humans, the administration of the β₂-AR agonist salbutamol results in inhibition of IL-12 production ex vivo,[111] and acute brain trauma that is followed by massive release of CAs triggers secretion of substantial amounts of systemic IL-10.[116]

CAs exert inhibition on the production of pro-inflammatory cytokines in vivo. Application of propranolol, a β-AR antagonist that blocks their inhibitory effect on cytokine-producing cells, results in substantial increases of LPS-induced secretion of TNF-α and IL-12 in mice.[112, 115] Thus, systemically, both glucocorticoids and CAs, respectively, through inhibition and stimulation of Th1 and Th2 cytokine secretion, cause selective suppression of cellular immunity and a shift toward Th2-mediated humoral immunity. This is further substantiated by studies showing that stress hormones inhibit effector function of cellular immunity components, i.e., the activity of NK, Tc, and activated macrophages.

The preceding general conclusion on the effects of stress hormones on Th1/Th2 balance may not pertain to certain conditions or local responses, at specific compartments of the body. Thus, the synthesis of TGF-β, another type 2 cytokine with potent anti-inflammatory activities, is differentially regulated by glucocorticoids: it is enhanced in human T cells but suppressed in glial cells.[117] In addition, NE, via stimulation of α₂-ARs, can augment LPS-stimulated production of TNF-α from mouse peritoneal macrophages,[118] whereas hemorrhage, a condition associated with elevations of systemic CA concentrations, increases through stimulation of α-AR the expression of TNF-α and IL-1 by lung mononuclear cells.[119]

Since the response to β-AR agonist stimulation wanes during maturation of the human monocyte to macrophage,[120] it is possible that at certain compartments of the body, the α-AR–mediated effect of CAs becomes transiently dominant. Through this mechanism, CAs may actually boost local cellular immune responses in a transitory fashion. This is further substantiated by the finding that CAs potentiate the production of IL-8 from PBMC and epithelial cells of the lung,[121] thus probably promoting recruitment of polymorphonuclear leukocytes to this organ. The "paradoxic" stress-induced potentiation of inflammation in the lung may explain why the "adult respiratory distress" syndrome develops frequently in patients with major infections associated with profound activation of the stress system.[122] Thus, in summary, while stress hormones suppress Th1 responses and pro-inflammatory cytokine secretion and boost Th2 responses systemically, they may affect differently certain local responses. Further studies are needed to address this question.

The CRH–Mast Cell–Histamine Axis

Central, hypothalamic CRH influences the immune system indirectly, through activation of the end-products of the peripheral stress

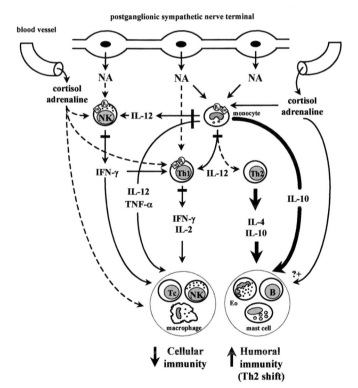

FIGURE 40–5. Effect of glucocorticoids and catecholamines on Th1/Th2 balance, cellular and humoral immunity. Stress influences immunity by stimulating cortisol and adrenaline secretion from the adrenal cortex and medulla, respectively, and the release of noradrenaline from the postganglionic sympathetic nerve terminals in blood vessels and lymphoid organs; systemic effects of glucocorticoids and catecholamines on the production of key regulatory type 1 and type 2 cytokines, Th1 and Th2 functions and, respectively, components of cellular and humoral immunity. NA, noradrenaline; NK, natural killer cell; GR, glucocorticoid receptor; T, T cell; B, B cell; Th, T-helper cell; Tc, T-cytotoxic cell; Eo, eosinophil; IL, interleukin; TNF, tumor necrosis factor; IFN, interferon. (From Elenkov I, Chrousos G: Stress hormones, Th1/Th2 patterns, pro/anti-inflammatory cytokines and susceptibility to disease. TEM 10:359–368, 1999.)

response, i.e., glucocorticoids and CAs. CRH, however, is also secreted peripherally at inflammatory sites (*peripheral* or *immune* CRH) and influences the immune system directly, through local modulatory actions.[1, 27] We first localized immunoreactive CRH in inflamed tissues of animals with experimental carrageenan-induced subcutaneous aseptic inflammation[27] and streptococcal cell wall– and adjuvant-induced arthritis, and retinol-binding protein (RBP)–induced uveitis, and in human tissues from patients with various autoimmune/inflammatory diseases, including rheumatoid arthritis, autoimmune thyroid disease, and ulcerative colitis (cf. ref. 123). The demonstration of CRH-like immunoreactivity in the dorsal horn of the spinal cord, dorsal root ganglia, and sympathetic ganglia support the hypothesis that the majority of immune CRH in early inflammation is of peripheral nerve rather than of immune cell origin (cf. ref. 123).

Peripheral CRH has pro-inflammatory and vascular permeability enhancing and vasodilatory actions. Thus, systemic administration of specific CRH antiserum blocks the inflammatory exudate volume and cell number in carrageenan-induced inflammation and RBP-induced uveitis, and inhibits stress-induced intracranial mast cell degranulation.[27, 124] In addition, CRH administration to humans or nonhuman primates causes major peripheral vasodilation manifested as flushing and increased blood flow and hypotension[125]; an intradermal CRH injection induces a marked increase of vascular permeability and mast cell degranulation.[126] Importantly, this effect is blocked by a CRH type 1 receptor antagonist and is stronger than the effect of an equimolar concentration of C48/80, a potent mast cell secretagogue.[126]

Thus, it appears that the mast cell is a major target of immune CRH. This has an anatomic prerequisite: in blood vessels, periarterial sympathetic plexuses are closely associated with mast cells lining the perivascular regions, and plexuses of nerve fibers (noradrenergic and peptidergic) within lymphoid parenchyma are also closely associated with clusters of mast cells. Histamine, a major product of mast cell degranulation, is a well-recognized mediator of acute inflammation and allergic reactions. These actions are mainly mediated by activation of H1 histamine receptors and include vasodilation, increased permeability of the vessel wall, edema, and, in the lungs, bronchoconstriction. Thus, it is conceivable that CRH activates mast cells via a CRH receptor type 1–dependent mechanism, leading to release of histamine and other contents of the mast cell granules that subsequently cause vasodilation, increased vascular permeability, and other manifestations of inflammation (Fig. 40–6).

The last 10 to 15 years have provided strong evidence that histamine may have important immunoregulatory functions via H2 receptors expressed on immune cells (see ref. 127). We have recently found that histamine, via stimulation of H2 receptors on peripheral monocytes and subsequent elevation of cAMP, inhibits the secretion of human IL-12 and stimulates the production of IL-10.[128] Our data are consistent with previous studies showing that histamine, via H2 receptors, also inhibits TNF-α production from monocytes and IFN-γ production by Th1-like cells, but has no effect on IL-4 production from Th2 clones.[129] Thus, histamine, similarly to CAs, appears to drive a Th2 shift both at the level of APCs and Th1 cells. Thus, the activation of CRH–mast cell–histamine axis through stimulation of H1 receptors may induce acute inflammation and allergic reactions, while through activation of H2 receptors it may induce suppression of Th1 responses and a Th2 shift (see Fig. 40–6).

Stress–immune system interactions are undoubtedly complex. The evidence presented above, accumulated over the last decade, strongly suggests that stress hormones differentially regulate Th1/Th2 patterns and type 1/type 2–cytokine secretion. Although interest in the Th2 response was initially directed at its protective role in helminthic infections and its pathogenic role in allergy, this response may have important regulatory functions in countering the tissue-damaging effects of macrophages and Th1 cells.[65] Thus, an excessive immune response, through activation of the stress system, and hence, through glucocorticoids and CAs, suppresses the Th1 response and causes a Th2 shift. This may protect the organism from "overshooting" by type 1/pro-inflammatory cytokines and other products of activated macrophages with tissue damaging potential.

Locally, as stated above, stress may exert pro- or anti-inflammatory effects. This may be influenced by several factors, such as presence

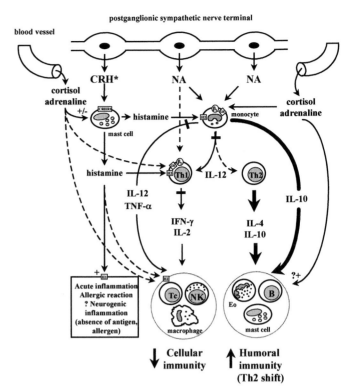

FIGURE 40–6. Effect of corticotropin-releasing hormone–mast cell–histamine axis, glucocorticoid and catecholamines on Th1/Th2 balance, cellular and humoral immunity. Stress and CRH influence immune/inflammatory and allergic responses by stimulating glucocorticoid, catecholamines, and peripheral (immune) CRH secretion and by altering the production of key regulatory cytokines and histamine (see text). *CRH is also released from sensory nerves upon their activation. Solid lines represent stimulation, dashed lines inhibition. CRH, peripheral (immune) corticotropin-releasing hormone; NA, noradrenaline; NK, natural killer cell; GR, glucocorticoid receptor; T, T cell; B, B cell; Th, T-helper cell; Tc, T-cytotoxic cell; Eo, eosinophil; IL, interleukin; TNF, tumor necrosis factor; IFN, interferon. (From Elenkov I, Chrousos G: Stress hormones, Th1/Th2 patterns, pro/anti-inflammatory cytokines and susceptibility to disease. TEM 10:359–368, 1999.)

or absence of antigen, the nature of antigen and/or the presence and relative expression of particular receptor subtypes on the surface of immune cells (e.g., β2- versus α2-adrenergic or H1- versus H2-histaminergic receptors), or the organ involved. In addition, recent evidence indicates that stress is not a uniform, nonspecific reaction[130]; different type of stressors with their own central neurochemical and peripheral neuroendocrine "signatures" might have different effects on the immune response.

EFFECTS OF THE IMMUNE AND INFLAMMATORY REACTION ON THE HPA AXIS AND THE SYMPATHETIC NERVOUS SYSTEM

The last two to three decades provided evidence that during an immune response, certain cytokines can signal the CNS, which through a complex CRH-dependent pathway triggers activation of both the HPA axis and the SNS.[16, 18, 131–136] Most of the HPA axis-stimulating activity in plasma comes from three cytokines, TNF-α, IL-1, and IL-6, which are produced at inflammatory sites and elsewhere in response to inflammation. In most situations, TNF-α appears first, followed by tandem secretion of IL-1 and IL-6.[137–139] All three cytokines stimulate their own secretion from the cells that produce them. In addition, TNF-α and IL-1 stimulate secretion of IL-6, whereas IL-6 inhibits secretion of TNF-α and IL-1. IL-6 acts synergistically with glucocorticoids in stimulating production of acute phase reactants.[68, 71] Secretion of systemic IL-6 is also increased during stress of noninflammatory etiology, presumably stimulated by stress-induced CAs through a β_2-adrenergic receptor mechanism.[140, 141]

All three inflammatory cytokines independently activate the HPA axis; in combination, their effects are synergistic.[132, 134, 142–144] Activation can be blocked with CRH-neutralizing antibodies, glucocorticoids, and prostanoid synthesis inhibitors. All three cytokines also directly stimulate CRH secretion in rat hypothalamic explants, and this effect can also be blocked by glucocorticoids and prostanoid synthesis inhibitors in vitro. The three inflammatory cytokines also mediate the stimulatory effect of bacterial lipopolysaccharide on the HPA axis. Antibodies to IL-6 almost completely inhibit this effect, suggesting a central role for IL-6 in axis stimulation.[145]

The elevations of ACTH and cortisol attained by IL-6 in human beings are well above those observed with maximal stimulating doses of CRH, suggesting that IL-6 in addition to CRH stimulates parvocellular AVP and other ACTH secretagogues.[146, 147] ACTH levels are already maximal at doses of IL-6 that do not increase peripheral AVP levels. At higher doses, however, IL-6 causes peripheral elevations of AVP, indicating that this cytokine can also activate magnocellular AVP-secreting neurons. This suggests that elevations of IL-6 may be a common etiologic factor in the syndrome of inappropriate secretion of antidiuretic hormone observed in diverse states, such as infectious or inflammatory diseases or trauma.[147]

The HPA axis and the SNS are involved in a long feedback loop between the immune system and the CNS. The afferent limb of this loop seems to operate by bloodborne cytokines, which via circulation or through the afferents of the vagus nerve[148] activate the central components of the stress system. How inflammatory cytokines reach the hypothalamic CRH and AVP neurons is unclear, given that the blood-brain barrier protects the cellular bodies of both kinds of neurons.[142, 149, 150] The cytokines may cause the endothelial and glial cells to secrete prostanoids and IL-6, and other mediators of inflammation, which reach the CRH and AVP neurons in a cascade-like fashion.[145, 151] Alternatively, a special transport system may be present for one or more of the inflammatory cytokines. Also, the inflammatory cytokines may directly activate the terminals of the CRH and AVP neurons in the median eminence, which is outside the blood-brain barrier. Because NE released in this region might exert tonic inhibitory control on CRH release through stimulation of α_2-ARs,[152, 153] it was suggested that TNF-α by inhibiting NE release, i.e., by disinhibition of this control, might trigger an increase of CRH release and subsequently an increase of ACTH from the anterior pituitary.[154]

Inflammation may also activate the HPA axis indirectly, by stimulation of the central noradrenergic stress system through cytokines and other mediators, which act first on stress system neurons of the area postrema that lie outside the blood-brain barrier or on neuron bodies inside the barrier through the endothelial-glial-neuronal cascade mentioned above. In addition, nociceptive, visceral, and somatosensory afferent neurons of the peripheral nervous system from inflammatory sites acutely stimulate the noradrenergic and CRH stress systems through an ascending neural spinal or cerebral nerve route.[155, 156] In fact, several lines of evidence indicate that certain cytokines, such as IL-1 and interferon (IFN)-α, stimulate both the central and peripheral components of the SNS. Thus, administration of IL-1 in the periphery increases the turnover of NE in the hypothalamus[133] and increases peripheral NE and epinephrine plasma levels.[157] Intracerebroventricular (i.c.v.) and peripheral injection of IFN-α or IL-1β produces a long-lasting increase of the sympathetic activity of the splenic nerve and an increased turnover of NE in the spleen.[158] As a result, the release of NE in the spleen is enhanced, as indicated by a recent in vivo microdialysis study.[159]

In addition to their acute effects on the hypothalamus, the inflammatory cytokines can apparently directly stimulate pituitary ACTH and adrenal cortisol secretion at high concentrations or given adequate time for interaction with these tissues.[134, 142, 160–164] Normally, the anterior pituitary and adrenal glands produce IL-1 and IL-6, which may influence local hormone production.[142, 165, 166] However, these cytokines may not always stimulate the pituitary gland or the adrenal cortex. IL-6, TNF-α, and IFN-γ inhibit the stimulatory effect of CRH on anterior

pituitary cell cultures,[167, 168] whereas TNF-α is a potent inhibitor of ACTH-induced cortisol production by cultured adrenocortical cells.[169]

Other inflammatory mediators and cytokines, including IFN-α, IL-2, epidermal growth factor, TGF-β, prostanoids, and platelet activating factor (PAF), may also participate in the modulation of the HPA axis activity by inflammation (Table 40–1). The interferons and IL-2 may do so indirectly, by causing secretion of inflammatory cytokines. Prostanoids and platelet activating factor, however, are autacoid amplifiers of hypothalamic CRH and AVP secretion. Receptors for these substances are present in the PVN, and CRH and AVP neurons respond to them.[8, 142, 149]

Certain cytokines or combinations of cytokines have been shown to cause their target tissues to become resistant to glucocorticoids.[170, 171] IL-2 and IL-4 together cause glucocorticoid resistance in T cells by markedly decreasing the affinity of the glucocorticoid receptor for its ligand by an as yet unclear mechanism.[171] In addition, changes in the intracellular metabolism of cortisol into less active or inactive metabolites in cells of the immune system alter the sensitivity of these cells to glucocorticoids.[172]

AMPHIDROMOUS INTERACTIONS BETWEEN THE STRESS AND IMMUNE SYSTEMS

Short- and Long-Term Adaptations

Chronic activation of either the HPA axis or the immune and inflammatory reaction results in reciprocally protective adaptations. Thus, the immune suppression of patients with chronic endogenous Cushing's syndrome is quite mild, suggesting that these patients become somewhat tolerant to glucocorticoids. Indeed, even though neutrophilia and eosinopenia persist, the lymphocyte phenotypes and function in these patients are similar to those of age- and gender-matched controls. Animals with chronic inflammatory disease, on the other hand, have mild rather than severe hypercortisolism, which is surprisingly associated with low CRH and high AVP messenger RNA expression and peptide secretion in the hypothalamus.[173–175]

Peripheral inflammation-induced hypothalamic elevation of substance P, an inhibitor of CRH secretion, has been considered the mechanism by which CRH neuron suppression occurs in certain painful inflammatory states.[50–52] In addition, elevated levels of inflammatory cytokines and interferon may participate in the restraint of the HPA axis by blocking the stimulatory effects of CRH and ACTH on the pituitary gland and adrenal cortex, respectively.[167–169] Human examples of this are certain patients with septic shock or AIDS and most patients with African trypanosomiasis, who have impaired adrenal responses to stress or exogenous stimuli such as CRH and corticotropin.[176–179]

TABLE 40–1. Cytokines and Other Mediators of Inflammation that Influence the Hypothalamic-Pituitary-Adrenal Axis

Inflammatory Cytokines

Tumor necrosis factor–α
Interleukin-1α and interleukin-1β
Interleukin-6

Other Cytokines

Interferon-α
Interferon-γ
Interleukin-2

Growth Factors

Epidermal growth factor
Transforming growth factor–β

Lipid Mediators

Prostanoids
Platelet-activating factor

Chronic activation of the HPA axis is also associated with another adrenocortical adaptation, which leads to a relative decrease in the production of Δ^5-adrenal androgens.[180] This in turn may alter the T-helper phenotype of chronically affected patients toward predominance of Th2.[82–84]

Influences of Reproductive Hormones

In general, autoimmune diseases affect females more than males. In animal models, androgens usually suppress, whereas estrogens stimulate the immune response.[181, 182] The mechanisms of these effects are insufficiently characterized, although estrogens are known to stimulate adhesion molecules and adhesion molecule receptors in immune and immune accessory cells, while the CRH gene and hence immune CRH expression are responsive to estrogen.[70, 183, 184] Prolactin also potentiates the immune and inflammatory reaction in vitro and in animals.[185] Inhibition of pituitary prolactin secretion in humans with autoimmune disease has not been effective therapeutically, perhaps because local, autacoid prolactin production may not respond to dopaminergic inhibition.[25]

DISTURBANCES IN THE INTERACTION BETWEEN THE STRESS AND IMMUNE SYSTEMS

Defects of the HPA Axis

Disturbances of the feedback relationship between the HPA axis and the immune and inflammatory reaction have been observed in animals and human states and can have two kinds of opposing effects (Table 40–2). An excessive HPA response to inflammation can mimic the stress or hypercortisolemic state, and can increase susceptibility to infectious agents and tumors, and cause resistance to autoimmune or inflammatory disease. Conversely, a defective HPA axis response can mimic the glucocorticoid-deficient state and thus cause resistance to infections and neoplasms, but increased susceptibility to autoimmune

TABLE 40–2. States Potentially Associated with Suppression or Activation of the Immune and Inflammatory Reaction through Defects in the Hypothalamic-Pituitary-Adrenal (HPA) Axis or Its Target Tissues

Suppression of Immune and Inflammatory Reaction	Activation of Immune and Inflammatory Reaction
Increased HPA Axis Activity	*Decreased HPA Axis Activity*
Cushing's syndrome	Adrenal insufficiency
Melancholic depression	Rheumatoid arthritis
Chronic active alcoholism	Atypical/seasonal depression
Chronic stress	Chronic fatigue/fibromyalgia
Chronic excessive exercise	Hypothyroidism
Pregnancy (last trimester)	Posttraumatic stress disorder
	Nicotine withdrawal
	Post–Cushing's syndrome cure
	Post glucocorticoid therapy
	Postpartum period
	Post chronic stress
	(Lewis rat)
	(Obese chicken, autoimmune thyroiditis)
Hypersensitivity to Glucocorticoids	*Resistance to Glucocorticoids*
HIV-1 infection (Vpr)	Rheumatoid arthritis
	Steroid-resistant asthma
	AIDS and glucocorticoid resistance
	Degenerative osteoarthritis
	Systemic lupus erythematosus*

*Due to increased catabolism of cortisol in target tissues.[172]
From Chrousos G: The hypothalamic-pituitary-adrenal axis and immune-mediated inflammation. N Engl J Med 332:1351–1362, 1995. Copyright © 1995 Massachusetts Medical Society. All rights reserved.

and inflammatory disease. Indeed, such properties were identified in Fischer and Lewis rats, two highly inbred strains selected for their resistance (Fischer) or susceptibility (Lewis) to inflammatory disease.[24, 186] In the Lewis rat, the responsiveness of the HPA axis to inflammatory stimuli is decreased, whereas in the Fischer rat, HPA axis responsiveness to the same stimuli is increased.

Lewis rats are susceptible to a host of inflammatory diseases such as a rheumatoid arthritis–like syndrome in response to streptococcal cell wall peptidoglycan, uveitis in response to immunization with retinol-binding protein, and encephalomyelitis in response to myelin basic protein. Fischer rats, by contrast, resist these experimentally induced diseases. The defect in the Lewis rat was localized to the hypothalamic CRH neuron, which was globally defective in its response to all stimulatory neurotransmitters.[187] The overall HPA axis response to stress was decreased in the Lewis rat; in addition, these animals exhibited chronic elevations of vasopressin as well as behaviors reminiscent of atypical depression in humans, a state characterized by low hypothalamic CRH secretion.[8, 28, 188, 189]

Do the abnormalities in Lewis rats have parallels in humans? A subgroup of patients with active rheumatoid arthritis might qualify. These patients have low or normal circadian concentrations of ACTH and cortisol despite elevated plasma concentrations of IL-1β and IL-6.[190, 191] Such patients have a poor response to the stress associated with major surgery, such as large joint replacement, despite dramatic postoperative elevations of IL-1β and IL-6.[191] Like Lewis rats, these patients also have consistently elevated levels of circulating AVP. Similar to Lewis rats with streptococcal cell wall peptidoglycan-induced arthritis, the inflamed joints of these patients have markedly elevated concentrations of immunoreactive CRH.[192, 193] None of these abnormalities of the HPA axis were present in "control" patients with osteomyelitis (inflammatory disease) or degenerative osteoarthritis.

A key question about human rheumatoid arthritis is whether the hyporesponsiveness of the HPA axis is genetic constitutional or secondary to a particular type of chronic inflammation or both. To date, the data point to a genetic disturbance that defines increased susceptibility.[194] Prospective studies of families with autoimmune inflammatory disease should test this hypothesis, using a quantifiable benign inflammatory stimulus such as recombinant IL-6.[146, 147]

Other examples suggest that a defective HPA axis increases susceptibility to autoimmune disease or increased immune reactivity[8, 28, 195, 196] (see Table 40–2). Given the many behavioral effects of CRH, it is not surprising that fatigue, dysthymia, irritability, or even frank depression are frequent in many of these low CRH states.[8, 28]

Defects of the Glucocorticoid Target Tissues

Glucocorticoid hypersensitivity of the immune system can mimic the immunosuppression of hypercortisolism, whereas glucocorticoid resistance of the immune system may result in excessive immune and inflammatory activity, which may also arise from glucocorticoid resistance in target tissues[69, 196–201] (see Table 40–2). Four diseases illustrate this mechanism. In rheumatoid arthritis, the concentration of glucocorticoid receptors in circulating leukocytes is reduced by approximately 50%.[196, 197] This phenomenon cannot be attributed to hypercortisolism. Leukocyte resistance to glucocorticoids also occurs in steroid-resistant asthma.[198, 199] Most patients with this disorder have marked but reversible decreases of affinity of glucocorticoid receptors in T lymphocytes, suggesting an acquired problem, probably associated with elevations of transcription factors such as c-*jun*, NF-κB, and CREB, that interact with and neutralize activated glucocorticoid receptors; however, in a small subgroup of patients, glucocorticoid receptor concentrations are irreversibly decreased in all leukocyte subtypes, suggesting a congenital syndrome.[199] In some patients with AIDS, leukocytes also have a marked decrease in the affinity of glucocorticoid receptors for cortisol.[200] In these patients, the glucocorticoid resistance may be generalized, since there are signs of glucocorticoid deficiency, including postural hypotension and hyponatremia, despite elevated levels of corticotropin and cortisol. A fourth disease in which the reduced expression of glucocorticoid receptors and glucocorticoid resistance may have a role is degenerative osteoarthritis.[201] Osteoarthritic chondrocytes contain approximately half of the glucocorticoid receptors of normal chondrocytes and resist dexamethasone-induced suppression of metalloprotease synthesis. Metalloprotease participates in the limited inflammatory destruction of the cartilage in the joints of patients with osteoarthritis. Finally, glucocorticoid resistance has also been observed in patients with Crohn's disease.[202]

Stress-Induced Th2 Shift: Clinical Implications of Excessive or Deficient Responses

Infections

A major factor governing the outcome of infectious diseases is the selection of Th1- versus Th2-predominant adaptive responses during and after the initial invasion of the host. Thus, stress, and hence, a stress-induced Th2 shift, may have a profound effect on the susceptibility of the organism to and/or may influence the course of an infection, the defense against which is primarily through cellular immunity mechanisms (Table 40–3).

Cellular immunity, and particularly IL-12 and IL-12–dependent IFN-γ secretion in humans, seems essential in the control of mycobacterial infections.[203] In the 1950s, Thomas Holmes (cf. ref. 204) reported that individuals who had experienced stressful life events were more likely to develop tuberculosis and less likely to recover from it. Although it is still a matter of some speculation, stress hormone–induced inhibition of IL-12 and IFN-γ production and the consequent suppression of cellular immunity may amply explain the pathophysiologic mechanisms of these observations.

Helicobacter pylori infection is the most common cause of chronic gastritis that in some cases progresses to peptic ulcer disease. The role of stress in promoting peptic ulcers has been recognized for many years. Thus, increased systemic stress hormone levels, in concert with an increased local concentration of histamine, induced by inflammatory or stress-related mediators, may skew the local responses toward Th2 and thus may allow the onset or progression of a *Helicobacter pylori* infection.

HIV+ patients have IL-12 deficiency, while disease progression has been correlated with a Th2 shift. The innervation (primarily sympathetic/noradrenergic) of lymphoid tissue may be particularly relevant to HIV infection, since lymphoid organs represent the primary site of HIV pathogenesis. In fact, as recently shown, NE, the major sympathetic neurotransmitter released locally in lymphoid organs,[54, 205] is able to directly accelerate HIV-1 replication by up to 11-fold in acutely infected human PBMCs.[206] The effect of NE on viral replication is transduced via the β-AR-adenylyl cyclase-cAMP-PKA signaling cascade.[206] The HIV-1 itself may contribute to the induction of intracellular cAMP through an immunosuppressive, retroviral envelope peptide, which causes a shift in the cytokine balance and leads to suppression of cell-mediated immunity.[207]

Progression of HIV infection is also characterized by mildly increased cortisol secretion in both the early and late stages of the disease. Thus, increased glucocorticoid production, triggered by the chronic infection, was recently proposed to contribute to HIV progression.[208] In another recent study, Kino and colleagues found that one of the HIV-1 accessory proteins, Vpr, acts as a potent coactivator of the host glucocorticoid receptor rendering lymphoid cells hyperresponsive to glucocorticoids.[209] Thus, on the one hand, stress hormones suppress cellular immunity and hence HIV replication, whereas, on the other hand, the virus itself may suppress cell-mediated immunity using the same pathways by which stress hormones, including CAs and glucocorticoids, alter the Th1/Th2 balance.

In a recent study, an association was demonstrated between stress and the susceptibility to common cold among 394 persons who had been intentionally exposed to five different upper respiratory viruses. Psychologic stress was associated in a dose-dependent manner with an increased risk of acute infectious respiratory illness, and this risk was attributed to increased rates of infection rather than to an increased frequency of symptoms after infection.[22] Thus, stress hormones through their selective inhibition of cellular immunity may play substantial roles in the increased risk of an individual to acute respiratory infections caused by common cold viruses.

TABLE 40–3. Putative Pathophysiologic Roles of Stress Hormone–Induced Alterations of Th1/Th2 Balance in Certain Infections, Infectious Complications after Major Injury, Autoimmune/Inflammatory, Allergic, or Neoplastic Diseases

Condition	Host Response	Pathogenic Response	Role of Stress
Infections			
Mycobacter tuberculosis *Helicobacter pylori* HIV Common cold viruses	Th1 protects	Suppressed cellular immunity, deficit of IL-12 and IFN-γ, Th2 shift with progression of infection	Stress-induced Th2 shift may contribute to increased susceptibility to or progression of these infections
Major Injury	Th2 protects?	Suppressed cellular immunity and IL-12, and IFN-γ production, overproduction of IL-10, Th2 shift	Increased levels of stress hormones may contribute to suppression of cellular immunity resulting in infectious complications
Autoimmunity			
RA, MS, ATD, type 1 diabetes mellitus	Excessive Th1 response	Th1 shift, overproduction of IL-12, TNF-α, IFN-γ; deficit of IL-10	A hypoactive stress system may facilitate/sustain the Th1 shift and flares of these autoimmune diseases*
SLE	Excessive Th2 response	Th2 shift, deficit of IL-12 and TNF-α, overproduction of IL-10	Stress (Th2 shift) may induce/facilitate flares of SLE
Allergy (Atopy)	Excessive Th2 responses	Th2 shift, deficit of IL-12, overproduction of IL-4, IL-10	Stress hormone- (and histamine)-induced Th2 shift may induce/facilitate/sustain allergic reactions*
Tumors	Th1 protects	Suppressed cellular immunity, deficit of IL-12, TNF-α, overproduction of IL-10	Stress hormone- (and histamine)-induced Th2 shift may contribute to increased susceptibility to or progression of certain tumors

*The role of stress in autoimmunity and atopy is more complex; see text for details.
Th, T-helper; IL, interleukin; TNF, tumor necrosis factor; IFN, interferon; RA, rheumatoid arthritis; MS, multiple sclerosis; ATD, autoimmune thyroid disease; SLE, systemic lupus erythematosus.
From Elenkov I, Chrousos G: Stress hormones, Th1/Th2 patterns, pro/anti-inflammatory cytokines and susceptibility to disease. TEM 10:359–368, 1999.

Major Injury

Major injury (serious traumatic injury and major burns) or major surgical procedures often lead to severe immunosuppression that contributes to delayed wound healing and infectious complications and, in some cases, to sepsis, the most common cause of late death after trauma. A strong stimulation of the SNS and the HPA axis correlates with the severity of both cerebral and extracerebral injury and an unfavorable prognosis (cf. ref. 116). In patients with traumatic major injury, and in animal models of burn injury, the suppressed cellular immunity is associated with diminished production of IFN-γ and IL-12 and increased production of IL-10, i.e., a Th2 shift.[210] A recent study indicated that systemic release of IL-10 triggered by SNS activation might be a key mechanism of immunosuppression after injury. Thus, high levels of systemic IL-10 documented in patients with "sympathetic storm" due to acute accidental or iatrogenic brain trauma were associated with high incidence of infection.[116] In a rat model, the increase of IL-10 was prevented by β-AR blockade,[116] whereas cellular immunity was improved in burned mice after H2 histamine receptor blockade.[127] Therefore, stress hormones and histamine secretion triggered by major injury, via an induction of a Th2 shift, may contribute to the severe immunosuppression observed in these conditions.

Autoimmunity

Several autoimmune diseases are characterized by common alterations of Th1 vs. Th2 and IL-12/TNF-α vs. IL-10 balance (see Table 40–3). In rheumatoid arthritis (RA), multiple sclerosis (MS), type 1 diabetes mellitus, autoimmune thyroid disease (ATD), and Crohn's disease (CD), the balance is skewed toward Th1 and an excess of IL-12 and TNF-α production, while Th2 activity and the production of IL-10 are deficient. This appears to be a critical factor that determines the proliferation and differentiation of Th1-related autoreactive cellular immune responses in these disorders.[211] On the other hand, systemic lupus erythematosus (SLE) is associated with a Th2 shift and an excessive production of IL-10, while IL-12 and TNF-α production appear to be deficient.

The effect of stress on autoimmunity is extremely complex; often stress is related to both induction/exacerbation and amelioration of disease activity.[26, 212] Animal studies and certain clinical observations suggest that a hyperactive or hypoactive stress system may be associated with decreased or increased vulnerability to different types of autoimmune diseases. Thus, Fischer rats, which have a hyperactive stress system, are extremely resistant to experimental induction of Th1-mediated autoimmune states, including arthritis, uveitis, and experimental allergic encephalomyelitis (EAE).[26] Similarly, women in the third trimester of pregnancy, who have increased levels of cortisol, experience remission of Th1 type–mediated autoimmune diseases, such as RA, MS, type 1 diabetes mellitus, and ATD, possibly via suppression of pro-inflammatory (IL-12 and TNF-α) and potentiation of anti-inflammatory (IL-4 and IL-10) cytokine production.[26, 213] Through a reciprocal mechanism, Th2 type–mediated autoimmune disorders mainly driven by IL-10, such as SLE, may flare up in high cortisol and CA output states, i.e., during stress or pregnancy.[26, 213]

Conversely, Lewis rats, which possess a hypoactive HPA axis, are extremely prone to develop experimentally induced Th1-mediated states, such as arthritis, uveitis, or EAE.[26] Similarly, clinical situations associated with decreased stress system activity are associated with increased expression or susceptibility to Th1 type–mediated autoimmune diseases such as RA, MS, and ATD. These are the postpartum period and the period that follows cure of endogenous Cushing's syndrome or discontinuation of glucocorticoid therapy.[1, 26, 96] This might also include the period that follows cessation of chronic stress or a rebound effect upon relief from stressors.

Epidemiologic studies suggest that severe stress, as reported by many patients, often precedes the development of certain Th1-mediated autoimmune states. Viral induction of autoimmunity is thought to occur by either bystander T cell activation or molecular mimicry. Recent studies suggest that tissue-tropic coxsackie B4 virus is associated by bystander damage with the development of type 1 diabetes mellitus, while human parvoviruses may be causative agents for rheu-

matoid arthritis.[214, 215] If future studies confirm these hypotheses, severe stress, and hence, severe suppression of cellular immunity may turn out to be a critical factor that facilitates the establishment of pathogenic and tissue-tropic viral infection followed by "autoimmune" tissue damage. At a later stage, severe stress, by skewing the balance toward Th2, may ameliorate disease activity, whereas acute stress and peripheral release of immune CRH, through its pro-inflammatory effects, may exacerbate, in some cases, disease activity.

Allergy/Atopy

Allergic reactions of type 1 hypersensitivity (atopy), such as asthma, eczema, hay fever, urticaria, and food allergy, are characterized by dominant Th2 responses, overproduction of histamine, and a shift to IgE production. As in the case of autoimmunity, the effects of stress on atopic reactions are complex, at multiple levels, and can be at either direction. Stress hormones acting at the level of APCs and lymphocytes may induce a Th2 shift and, thus, facilitate or sustain atopic reactions; however, this can be antagonized by their effects on the mast cell (see Fig. 40–6). Glucocorticoids and CAs (through β-ARs) suppress the release of histamine by mast cells, thus abolishing its pro-inflammatory, allergic, and bronchoconstrictor effects. Thus, reduced levels of epinephrine and cortisol in the very early morning could contribute to nocturnal wheezing and have been linked to high circulating histamine levels in asthmatics.[216] This may also explain the beneficial effect of glucocorticoids and β2-agonists in asthma. Infusion of high doses of adrenaline, however, causes a rise in circulating histamine levels that may be due to an alpha-adrenergic–mediated increase in mediator release (cf. ref. 216). Thus, severe acute stress associated with high adrenaline concentrations and/or high local secretion of CRH could lead to mast cell degranulation. As a result, a substantial amount of histamine could be released, which consequently would not antagonize, but rather amplify, the Th2 shift through H2 receptors, while in parallel, by acting on H1 receptors, it could initiate a new episode or exacerbate a chronic allergic condition (see Fig. 40–6).

Glucocorticoids alone or in combination with β2-AR agonists are broadly used in the treatment of atopic reactions, and particularly asthma. In vivo, ex vivo, and in vitro exposure to glucocorticoids and β2-agonists result in a reduction of IL-12 production, which persists at least several days.[96, 105, 111] Thus, glucocorticoid and/or β2-AR agonist therapy is likely to reduce the capacity of APC to produce IL-12; to greatly suppress type 2 cytokine synthesis is activated, but not resting T cells; and to abolish eosinophilia.[105] If, however, resting (cytokine-uncommitted) T cells are subsequently activated by APCs preexposed to glucocorticoids and/or β2-AR agonists, enhanced IL-4 production, but limited IFN-γ synthesis, could be induced.[105] Thus, although in the short-term, the effect of glucocorticoids and β2-AR agonists may be beneficial, their long-term effects might be to sustain the increased vulnerability of the patient to the allergic condition. This is further substantiated by the observations that both glucocorticoids and β2-AR agonists potentiate the IgE production in vitro and in vivo.[217, 218]

Tumor Growth

The amount of IL-12 available at the tumor site appears to be critical for tumor regression.[219] Thus, low levels of IL-12 have been associated with tumor growth, as opposed to tumor regression observed with administration of IL-12 delivered in situ or systemically. On the other hand, local overproduction of IL-10 and TGF-β by inhibiting the production of IL-12 and TNF-α, and the cytotoxicity of NK and Tc cells, seems to play an inappropriate immunosuppressive role, allowing increased malignant tumor growth, as seen, for example, in melanoma.[220] These and others studies suggest that Th1 function is locally downregulated during tumor growth.

Several lines of evidence suggest that stress can increase the susceptibility to tumors, tumor growth, and metastases. In animals, β-AR stimulation suppresses NK cell activity and compromises resistance to tumor metastases[221]; stress decreases the potential of spleen cells to turn into antitumor Tc against syngeneic B16 melanoma, and it significantly suppresses the ability of tumor-specific CD4+ cells to produce IFN-γ and IL-2.[222] In humans, the augmentation of the rate of tumor progression and cancer-related death has been associated with stress (cf. ref. 222), whereas treatment with cimetidine, an H2 histamine antagonist, correlated with increased survival in patients with gastric and colorectal cancer.[223] In fact, high concentrations of histamine have been measured within colorectal and breast cancer tissues and large numbers of mast cells have been identified within certain tumor tissues (cf. ref. 128). These data suggest that stress hormone/histamine-induced suppression of cellular immunity may contribute to increased growth of certain tumors.

THERAPEUTIC PERSPECTIVES

Glucocorticoids and agents that potentiate their actions are options for treatment of autoimmune inflammatory diseases.[68] By potentiating the secretion or the effects of hypothalamic CRH with CRH secretagogues, CRH agonists or CRH binding protein antagonists that cross the blood-brain barrier may prevent the development of inflammatory disease in susceptible persons with a hypofunctional HPA axis and at the same time correct central nervous system symptoms of CRH deficiency.[8, 28] Such an action could be envisioned for nonpeptidic substance P antagonists, which would be expected to reverse the CRH suppression that occurs in chronic inflammatory states, and at the same time act as a local anti-inflammatory agent.

Antagonists of pro-inflammatory peptides may control inflammatory diseases or processes in which these peptides have a primary pathogenic role. Depending on their ability to cross the blood-brain barrier and the location of the therapeutic target, these antagonists could be used systemically or in a compartmentalized fashion.

Once the mechanisms of acquired glucocorticoid resistance in rheumatoid arthritis, steroid-resistant asthma, AIDS, and other inflammatory diseases are elucidated, therapy with the appropriate intracellular agents that will sensitize the cascade of glucocorticoid action in immune cells, or treatment with cytokines or their antagonists, or pharmacologic agents that influence their secretion and action may become available for the management of these disorders.

The potential immunopotentiating effects of Δ^5-adrenal androgens on Th1 cells may be useful in the treatment of diseases such as systemic lupus erythematosus and the final stages of AIDS. A preliminary, placebo-controlled study of dehydroepiandrosterone administration to patients with lupus was associated with marked clinical improvement and minimal adverse effects. A similar therapy might be beneficial in other such diseases.

Moreover, blocking the effect of stress by β$_2$-AR and/or H2 antagonists may result in boosting Th1 responses that may be useful in the management of certain infections or tumors, while the combined administration of β$_2$-AR agonists and glucocorticoids may help in the management of certain Th1-mediated autoimmune diseases. Finally, CRH antagonists may help prevent stress-induced Th1-suppression and triggering of stress-induced allergic or vasokinetic phenomena. Such antagonists are at hand and show promise in preclinical studies.

REFERENCES

1. Chrousos GP: The hypothalamic-pituitary-adrenal axis and immune-mediated inflammation. N Engl J Med 332:1351–1362, 1995.
2. Tonkoff W: Zur Kenntnis der Nerven der Lymphdrüsen. Anat Anz 16:456–459, 1899.
3. Benschop RJ, Rodriguez-Feuerhahn M, Schedlowski M: Catecholamine-induced leukocytosis: Early observations, current research, and future directions. Brain Behav Immun 10:77–91, 1996.
4. Paul W (ed): Fundamental Immunology, ed 3. New York, Raven Press, 1993.
5. Loeper M, Crouzon O: L'action de l'adrenaline sur le sang. Arch Med Exp Anat Pathol 16:83–108, 1904.
6. Metal'nikov S, Chorine V: Rôle des réflexes conditionnels dans l'immunité. Ann Inst Pasteur Paris 40:893–900, 1926.
7. Selye H: Thymus and adrenals in the response of the organism to injuries and intoxications. Br J Exp Pathol 17:234–238, 1936.
8. Chrousos GP, Gold PW: The concepts of stress and stress system disorders. Overview of physical and behavioral homeostasis. JAMA 267:1244–1252, 1992.
9. Janig W, McLachlan EM: Characteristics of function-specific pathways in the sympathetic nervous system. Trends Neurosci 15:475–481, 1992.
10. von Euler US: The presence of a substance with sympathin E properties in spleen extracts. Acta Physiol Scand 11:168–173, 1946.
11. Nobelstiftelsen: Les Prix Nobel. In Norstedt and Soner: Imprimerie Royal, Stockholm, 1951.
12. Hench PS, Kendall EC, Slocumb CH, et al: The effect of a hormone of the adrenal cortex (17-hydroxy-11-dehydro-corticosterone: compound E) and of pituitary adrenocorticotropic hormone on rheumatoid arthritis. Mayo Clin Proc 24:181–197, 1949.
13. Dougherty TF, Frank JA: The quantitative and qualitative responses of blood lymphocytes to stress stimuli. J Lab Clin Med 42:530–537, 1953.
14. Besedovsky HO, Sorkin E, Keller M, et al: Changes in blood hormone levels during the immune response. Proc Soc Exp Biol Med 150:466–470, 1975.
15. Besedovsky HO, del Rey A, Sorkin E, et al: Immunoregulation mediated by the sympathetic nervous system. Cell Immunol 48:346–355, 1979.
16. Besedovsky HO, del Rey A, Sorkin E, et al: Immunoregulatory feedback between interleukin-1 and glucocorticoid hormones. Science 233:652–654, 1986.
17. Besedovsky HO, del Rey A, Sorkin E: Lymphokine-containing supernatants from Con A–stimulated cells increase corticosterone blood levels. J Immunology 126:385–389, 1981.
18. Besedovsky HO, del Rey A, Sorkin E, et al: The immune response evokes changes in braion noradrenergic neurons. Science 221:564–566, 1983.
19. del Rey A, Besedovsky HO, Sorkin E, et al: Sympathetic immunoregulation: Difference between high and low-responder animals. Am J Physiol 242:R30–R33, 1982.
20. Ader R, Cohen N: Behaviorally conditioned immunosuppression and murine systemic lupus erythematosus. Science 215:1534–1536, 1982.
21. Keller SE, Weiss JM, Schleifer SJ, et al: Stress-induced suppression of immunity in adrenalectomized rats. Science 221:1301–1304, 1983.
22. Cohen S, Tyrrell DA, Smith AP: Psychological stress and susceptibility to the common cold. N Engl J Med 325:606–612, 1991.
23. Carlson SL, Felten DL: Involvement of hypothalamic and limbic structures in neural-immune communication. In Goetzl EJ, Spector NH: Neuroimmune networks: Physiology and Diseases. New York, Alan R. Liss, 1989.
24. Sternberg EM, Young WS, Bernardini R, et al: A central nervous system defect in biosynthesis of corticotropin-releasing hormone is associated with susceptibility to streptococcal cell wall–induced arthritis in Lewis rats. Proc Natl Acad Sci USA 86:4771–4775, 1989.
25. Sternberg EM, Hill JM, Chrousos GP, et al: Inflammatory mediator–induced hypothalamic-pituitary-adrenal axis activation is defective in streptococcal cell wall arthritis-susceptible Lewis rats. Proc Natl Acad Sci USA 86:2374–2378, 1989.
26. Wilder RL: Neuroendocrine–immune system interactions and autoimmunity. Annu Rev Immunol 13:307–338, 1995.
27. Karalis K, Sano H, Redwine J, et al: Autocrine or paracrine inflammatory actions of corticotropin-releasing hormone in vivo. Science 254:421–423, 1991.
28. Chrousos GP: Regulation and dysregulation of the hypothalamic-pituitary-adrenal axis. The corticotropin-releasing hormone perspective. Endocrinol Metab Clin North Am 21:833–858, 1992.
29. Saper CB, Loewy AD, Swanson LW, et al: Direct hypothalamo-autonomic connections. Brain Res 117:305–312, 1976.
30. Whitnall MH: Stress selectively activates the vasopressin-containing subset of corticotropin-releasing hormone neurons. Neuroendocrinology 50:702–707, 1989.
31. de Goeij DC, Kvetnansky R, Whitnall MH, et al: Repeated stress-induced activation of corticotropin-releasing factor neurons enhances vasopressin stores and colocalization with corticotropin-releasing factor in the median eminence of rats. Neuroendocrinology 53:150–159, 1991.
32. Nikolarakis KE, Almeida OF, Herz A: Stimulation of hypothalamic beta-endorphin and dynorphin release by corticotropin-releasing factor (in vitro). Brain Res 399:152–155, 1986.
33. Burns G, Almeida OF, Passarelli F, et al: A two-step mechanism by which corticotropin-releasing hormone releases hypothalamic beta-endorphin: The role of vasopressin and G-proteins. Endocrinology 125:1365–1372, 1989.
34. Lamberts SW, Verleun T, Oosterom R, et al: Corticotropin-releasing factor (ovine) and vasopressin exert a synergistic effect on adrenocorticotropin release in man. J Clin Endocrinol Metab 58:298–303, 1984.
35. Rittmaster RS, Cutler GBJ, Gold PW, et al: The relationship of saline-induced changes in vasopressin secretion to basal and corticotropin-releasing hormone-stimulated adrenocorticotropin and cortisol secretion in man. J Clin Endocrinol Metab 64:371–376, 1987.
36. Elkabir DR, Wyatt ME, Vellucci SV, et al: The effects of separate or combined infusions of corticotrophin-releasing factor and vasopressin either intraventricularly or into the amygdala on aggressive and investigative behaviour in the rat. Regul Pept 28:199–214, 1990.
37. Redekopp C, Irvine CH, Donald RA, et al: Spontaneous and stimulated adrenocorticotropin and vasopressin pulsatile secretion in the pituitary venous effluent of the horse. Endocrinology 118:1410–1416, 1986.
38. Ixart G, Barbanel G, Conte-Devolx B, et al: Evidence for basal and stress-induced release of corticotropin releasing factor in the push-pull cannulated median eminence of conscious free-moving rats. Neurosci Lett 74:85–89, 1987.
39. Engler D, Pham T, Fullerton MJ, et al: Studies of the secretion of corticotropin-releasing factor and arginine vasopressin into the hypophysial-portal circulation of the conscious sheep. I. Effect of an audiovisual stimulus and insulin-induced hypoglycemia. Neuroendocrinology 49:367–381, 1989.
40. Carnes M, Lent SJ, Goodman B, et al: Effects of immunoneutralization of corticotropin-releasing hormone on ultradian rhythms of plasma adrenocorticotropin. Endocrinology 126:1904–1913, 1990.
41. Calogero AE, Norton JA, Sheppard BC, et al: Pulsatile activation of the hypothalamic-pituitary-adrenal axis during major surgery. Metabolism 41:839–845, 1992.
42. Holmes MC, Antoni FA, Aguilera G, et al: Magnocellular axons in passage through the median eminence release vasopressin. Nature 319:326–329, 1986.
43. Phillips MI: Functions of angiotensin in the central nervous system. Annu Rev Physiol 49:413–435, 1987.

44. Hinson JP: Paracrine control of adrenocortical function: A new role for the medulla? J Endocrinol 124:7–9, 1990.
45. Andreis PG, Neri G, Mazzocchi G, et al: Direct secretagogue effect of corticotropin-releasing factor on the rat adrenal cortex: The involvement of the zona medullaris. Endocrinology 131:69–72, 1992.
46. Vinson GP, Whitehouse BJ, Henvill KL: The actions of alpha-MSh on the adrenal cortex, the melanotrophic peptides. In Hadley ME: Biological Roles. Boca Raton, FL, CRC Press, 1988.
47. Ottenweller JE, Meier AH: Adrenal innervation may be an extrapituitary mechanism able to regulate adrenocortical rhythmicity in rats. Endocrinology 111:1334–1338, 1982.
48. Besedovsky HO, Del Rey A, Sorkin E, et al: Immunoregulatory feedback between interleukin-1 and glucocorticoid hormones. Science 233:652–654, 1986.
49. Sawchenko PE, Imaki T, Potter E, et al: The functional neuroanatomy of corticotrophin-releasing factor. In Chadwick DJ, Marsh J, Ackrill K: Corticotrophin-Releasing Factor. Chichester, John Wiley, 1993.
50. Larsen PJ, Jessop D, Patel H, et al: Substance P inhibits the release of anterior pituitary adrenocorticotrophin via a central mechanism involving corticotrophin-releasing factor–containing neurons in the hypothalamic paraventricular nucleus. J Neuroendocrinol 5:99–105, 1993.
51. Culman J, Tschope C, Jost N, et al: Substance P and neurokinin A induced desensitization to cardiovascular and behavioral effects: Evidence for the involvement of different tachykinin receptors. Brain Res 625:75–83, 1993.
52. Jessop DS, Chowdrey HS, Larsen PJ, et al: Substance P: Multifunctional peptide in the hypothalamo-pituitary system? J Endocrinol 132:331–337, 1992.
53. Felten DL, Felten SY, Carlson SL, et al: Noradrenergic and peptidergic innervation of lymphoid tissue. J Immunol 135:755s–765s, 1985.
54. Vizi ES, Orso E, Osipenko ON, et al: Neurochemical, electrophysiological and immunocytochemical evidence for a noradrenergic link between the sympathetic nervous system and thymocytes. Neuroscience 68:1263–1276, 1995.
55. Ackerman KD, Felten SY, Bellinger DL, et al: Noradrenergic sympathetic innervation of the spleen: III. Development of innervation in the rat spleen. J Neurosci Res 18:49–54, 1987.
56. Weihe E, Nohr D, Michel S, et al: Molecular anatomy of the neuro-immune connection. Int J Neurosci 59:1–23, 1991.
57. Roitt I, Brostoff J, Male D (eds): Immunology, ed 4. London, CV Mosby, 1996.
58. Gallin JI, Goldstein IM, Snyderman R: Overview. In Gallin JI, Goldstein IM, Snyderman R: Inflammation: Basic Principles and Clinical Correlates. New York, Raven Press, 1988.
59. Paul WE, Seder RA: Lymphocyte responses and cytokines. Cell 76:241–251, 1994.
60. Celander DR, Folkow B: The nature and distribution of afferent fibers provided with the axon reflex arrangements. Acta Physiol Scand 359–370, 1953.
61. Payan DG, Goetzl EJ: Modulation of lymphocyte function by sensory neuropeptides. J Immunol 135:783s–786s, 1985.
62. Engel D: The influence of the sympathetic nervous system on capillary permeability. Res Exp Med (Berl) 173:1–8, 1978.
63. Holzer P: Local effector functions of capsaicin-sensitive sensory nerve endings: Involvement of tachykinins, calcitonin gene-related peptide and other neuropeptides. Neuroscience 24:739–768, 1988.
64. Coderre TJ, Basbaum AI, Levine JD: Neural control of vascular permeability: Interactions between primary afferents, mast cells, and sympathetic efferents. J Neurophysiol 62:48–58, 1989.
65. Fearon DT, Locksley RM: The instructive role of innate immunity in the acquired immune response. Science 272:50–53, 1996.
66. Mosmann TR, Sad S: The expanding universe of T-cell subsets: Th1, Th2 and more. Immunol Today 17:138–146, 1996.
67. Trinchieri G: Interleukin-12: A proinflammatory cytokine with immunoregulatory functions that bridge innate resistance and antigen-specific adaptive immunity. Annu Rev Immunol 13:251–276, 1995.
68. Boumpas DT, Chrousos GP, Wilder RL, et al: Glucocorticoid therapy for immune-mediated diseases: Basic and clinical correlates. Ann Intern Med 119:1198–1208, 1993.
69. Chrousos GP, Detera-Wadleigh SD, Karl M: Syndromes of glucocorticoid resistance. Ann Intern Med 119:1113–1124, 1993.
70. Cronstein BN, Kimmel SC, Levin RI, et al: A mechanism for the antiinflammatory effects of corticosteroids: The glucocorticoid receptor regulates leukocyte adhesion to endothelial cells and expression of endothelial-leukocyte adhesion molecule 1 and intercellular adhesion molecule 1. Proc Natl Acad Sci USA 89:9991–9995, 1992.
71. Hirano T, Akira S, Taga T, et al: Biological and clinical aspects of interleukin 6. Immunol Today 11:443–449, 1990.
72. Lee SW, Tsou AP, Chan H, et al: Glucocorticoids selectively inhibit the transcription of the interleukin 1 beta gene and decrease the stability of interleukin 1 beta mRNA. Proc Natl Acad Sci USA 85:1204–1208, 1988.
73. Zanker B, Walz G, Wieder KJ, et al: Evidence that glucocorticosteroids block expression of the human interleukin-6 gene by accessory cells. Transplantation 49:183–185, 1990.
74. Nakano T, Ohara O, Teraoka H, et al: Glucocorticoids suppress group II phospholipase A2 production by blocking mRNA synthesis and post-transcriptional expression. J Biol Chem 265:12745–12748, 1990.
75. Vishwanath BS: Glucocorticoid deficiency increases phospholipase A2 activity in rats. J Clin Invest 92:1974–1980, 1993.
76. O'Banion MK, Winn VD, Young DA: cDNA cloning and functional activity of a glucocorticoid-regulated inflammatory cyclooxygenase. Proc Natl Acad Sci USA 89:4888–4892, 1992.
77. Conrad DJ, Kuhn H, Mulkins M, et al: Specific inflammatory cytokines regulate the expression of human monocyte 15-lipoxygenase. Proc Natl Acad Sci USA 89:217–221, 1992.
78. Moncada S, Higgs A: The L-arginine–nitric oxide pathway. N Engl J Med 329:2002–2012, 1993.
79. Cove-Smith JR, Kabler P, Pownall R, et al: Circadian variation in an immune response in man. Br Med J 2:253–254, 1978.
80. Harkness JA, Richter MB, Panayi GS, et al: Circadian variation in disease activity in rheumatoid arthritis. Br Med J (Clin Res Ed) 284:551–554, 1982.
81. Mastorakos G, Chrousos G: Adrenal hyperandrogenism. In Adashi E, Rock J, Rosenwaks Z: Reproductive Endocrinology, Surgery, and Technology. New York, Raven Press, 1995.
82. Daynes RA, Dudley DJ, Araneo BA: Regulation of murine lymphokine production in vivo. II. Dehydroepiandrosterone is a natural enhancer of interleukin 2 synthesis by helper T cells. Eur J Immunol 20:793–802, 1990.
83. Blauer KL, Poth M, Rogers WM, et al: Dehydroepiandrosterone antagonizes the suppressive effects of dexamethasone on lymphocyte proliferation. Endocrinology 129:3174–3179, 1991.
84. Suzuki T: Dehydroepiandrosterone enhances IL2 production and cytotoxic effector function of human T cells. Clin Immunol Immunopathol 61:202–211, 1991.
85. Meikle AW: The presence of a dehydroepiandrosterone-specific receptor binding complex in murine T cells. J Steroid Biochem Mol Biol 42:293–304, 1992.
86. Hadden JW, Hadden EM, Middleton E Jr: Lymphocyte blast transformation I. Demonstration of adrenergic receptors in human peripheral lymphocytes. Cell Immunol 1:583–595, 1970.
87. Chambers DA, Cohen RL, Perlman RL: Neuroimmune modulation: Signal transduction and catecholamines. Neurochem Int 22:95–110, 1993.
88. Carlson SL, Brooks WH, Roszman TL: Neurotransmitter-lymphocyte interactions: Dual receptor modulation of lymphocyte proliferation and cAMP production. J Neuroimmunol 24:155–162, 1989.
89. Bartik MM, Brooks WH, Roszman TL: Modulation of T cell proliferation by stimulation of the beta-adrenergic receptor: Lack of correlation between inhibition of T cell proliferation and cAMP accumulation. Cell Immunol 148:408–421, 1993.
90. Elliott L, Brooks W, Roszman T: Inhibition of anti-CD3 monoclonal antibody-induced T-cell proliferation by dexamethasone, isoproterenol, or prostaglandin E2 either alone or in combination. Cell Mol Neurobiol 12:411–427, 1992.
91. Whalen MM, Bankhurst AD: Effects of beta-adrenergic receptor activation, cholera toxin and forskolin on human natural killer cell function. Biochem J 272:327–331, 1990.
92. Hellstrand K, Hermodsson S: An immunopharmacological analysis of adrenaline-induced suppression of human natural killer cell cytotoxicity. Int Arch Allergy Appl Immunol 89:334–341, 1989.
93. Irwin M: Stress-induced immune suppression: Role of brain corticotropin releasing hormone and autonomic nervous system mechanisms. Adv Neuroimmunol 4:29–47, 1994.
94. Irwin M, Hauger R, Brown M: Central corticotropin-releasing hormone activates the sympathetic nervous system and reduces immune function: Increased responsivity of the aged rat. Endocrinology 131:1047–1053, 1992.
95. Strausbaugh H, Irwin M: Central corticotropin-releasing hormone reduces cellular immunity. Brain Behav Immun 6:11–17, 1992.
96. Elenkov IJ, Papanicolaou DA, Wilder RL, et al: Modulatory effects of glucocorticoids and catecholamines on human interleukin-12 and interleukin-10 production: Clinical implications. Proc Assoc Am Physicians 108:374–381, 1996.
97. Zurier RB, Weissmann G, Hoffstein S, et al: Mechanisms of lysosomal enzyme release from human leukocytes. II. Effects of cAMP and cGMP, autonomic agonists, and agents which affect microtubule function. J Clin Invest 53:297–309, 1974.
98. Weiss M, Schneider EM, Tarnow J, et al: Is inhibition of oxygen radical production of neutrophils by sympathomimetics mediated via beta-2 adrenoceptors? J Pharmacol Exp Ther 278:1105–1113, 1996.
99. Barnett CCJ, Moore EE, Partrick DA, et al: Beta-adrenergic stimulation down-regulates neutrophil priming for superoxide generation, but not elastase release. J Surg Res 70:166–170, 1997.
100. Sanders VM, Baker RA, Ramer-Quinn DS, et al: Differential expression of the beta2-adrenergic receptor by Th1 and Th2 clones: Implications for cytokine production and B cell help. J Immunol 158:4200–4210, 1997.
101. Sanders VM: The role of adrenoceptor-mediated signals in the modulation of lymphocyte function. Adv Neuroimmunol 5:283–298, 1995.
102. Coqueret O, Dugas B, Mencia-Huerta JM, et al: Regulation of IgE production from human mononuclear cells by beta 2–adrenoceptor agonists. Clin Exp Allergy 25:304–311, 1995.
103. Coqueret O, Lagente V, Frere CP, et al: Regulation of IgE production by beta 2-adrenoceptor agonists. Ann NY Acad Sci 725:44–49, 1994.
104. Blotta MH, DeKruyff RH, Umetsu DT: Corticosteroids inhibit IL-12 production in human monocytes and enhance their capacity to induce IL-4 synthesis in CD4+ lymphocytes. J Immunol 158:5589–5595, 1997.
105. DeKruyff RH, Fang Y, Umetsu DT: Corticosteroids enhance the capacity of macrophages to induce Th2 cytokine synthesis in CD4+ lymphocytes by inhibiting IL-12 production. J Immunol 160:2231–2237, 1998.
106. Wu CY, Wang K, McDyer JF, et al: Prostaglandin E2 and dexamethasone inhibit IL-12 production and IL-12 responsiveness. J Immunol 161:2723–2730, 1998.
107. van der Poll T, Barber AE, Coyle SM, et al: Hypercortisolemia increases plasma interleukin-10 concentrations during human endotoxemia—a clinical research center study. J Clin Endocrinol Metab 81:3604–3606, 1996.
108. Ramierz F, Fowell DJ, Puklavec M, et al: Glucocorticoids promote a TH2 cytokine response by CD4+ T cells in vitro. J Immunol 156:2406–2412, 1996.
109. Tabardel Y, Duchateau J, Schmartz D, et al: Corticosteroids increase blood interleukin-10 levels during cardiopulmonary bypass in men. Surgery 119:76–80, 1996.
110. Gayo A, Mozo L, Suarez A, et al: Glucocorticoids increase IL-10 expression in multiple sclerosis patients with acute relapse. J Neuroimmunol 85:122–130, 1998.
111. Panina-Bordignon P, Mazzeo D, Lucia PD, et al: Beta2-agonists prevent Th1 development by selective inhibition of interleukin 12. J Clin Invest 100:1513–1519, 1997.
112. Hasko G, Szabo C, Nemeth ZH, et al: Stimulation of beta-adrenoceptors inhibits endotoxin-induced IL-12 production in normal and IL-10 deficient mice. J Neuroimmunol 88:57–61, 1998.

113. Borger P, Hoekstra Y, Esselink MT, et al: Beta-adrenoceptor–mediated inhibition of IFN-gamma, IL-3, and GM-CSF mRNA accumulation in activated human T lymphocytes is solely mediated by the beta2-adrenoceptor subtype. Am J Respir Cell Mol Biol 19:400–407, 1998.

114. Hasko G, Elenkov IJ, Kvetan V, et al: Differential effect of selective block of alpha 2-adrenoreceptors on plasma levels of tumour necrosis factor–alpha, interleukin-6 and corticosterone induced by bacterial lipopolysaccharide in mice. J Endocrinol 144:457–462, 1995.

115. Elenkov IJ, Hasko G, Kovacs KJ, et al: Modulation of lipopolysaccharide-induced tumor necrosis factor–alpha production by selective alpha- and beta-adrenergic drugs in mice. J Neuroimmunol 61:123–131, 1995.

116. Woicichowsky C, Asadullah K, Nestler D, et al: Sympathetic activation triggers systemic interleukin-10 release in immunodepression induced by brain injury [in process citation]. Nat Med 4:808–813, 1998.

117. Batuman OA, Ferrero A, Cupp C, et al: Differential regulation of transforming growth factor beta-1 gene expression by glucocorticoids in human T and glial cells. J Immunol 155:4397–4405, 1995.

118. Spengler RN, Allen RM, Remick DG, et al: Stimulation of alpha-adrenergic receptor augments the production of macrophage-derived tumor necrosis factor. J Immunol 145:1430–1434, 1990.

119. Le Tulzo Y, Shenkar R, Kaneko D, et al: Hemorrhage increases cytokine expression in lung mononuclear cells in mice: Involvement of catecholamines in nuclear factor-kappaB regulation and cytokine expression. J Clin Invest 99:1516–1524, 1997.

120. Baker AJ, Fuller RW: Loss of response to beta-adrenoceptor agonists during the maturation of human monocytes to macrophages in vitro. J Leukoc Biol 57:395–400, 1995.

121. Linden A: Increased interleukin-8 release by beta-adrenoceptor activation in human transformed bronchial epithelial cells. Br J Pharmacol 119:402–406, 1996.

122. Meduri GU, Chrousos GP: Duration of glucocorticoid treatment and outcome in sepsis: Is the right drug used the wrong way? Chest 114:355–360, 1998.

123. Webster EL, Torpy DJ, Elenkov IJ, et al: Corticotropin-releasing hormone and inflammation. Ann NY Acad Sci 840:21–32, 1998.

124. Theoharides TC, Spanos C, Pang X, et al: Stress-induced intracranial mast cell degranulation: A corticotropin-releasing hormone–mediated effect. Endocrinology 136:5745–5750, 1995.

125. Udelsman R, Gallucci WT, Bacher J, et al: Hemodynamic effects of corticotropin releasing hormone in the anesthetized cynomolgus monkey. Peptides 7:465–471, 1986.

126. Theoharides TC, Singh LK, Boucher W, et al: Corticotropin-releasing hormone induces skin mast cell degranulation and increased vascular permeability, a possible explanation for its proinflammatory effects. Endocrinology 139:403–413, 1998.

127. Rocklin RE (ed): Histamine and H2 Antagonists in Inflammation and Immunodeficiency. New York and Basel, Marcel Dekker, 1990.

128. Elenkov IJ, Webster E, Papanicolaou DA, et al: Histamine potently suppresses human IL-12 and stimulates IL-10 production via H2 receptors. J Immunol 161:2586–2593, 1998.

129. Lagier B, Lebel B, Bousquet J, et al: Different modulation by histamine of IL-4 and interferon-gamma (IFN-gamma) release according to the phenotype of human Th0, Th1 and Th2 clones. Clin Exp Immunol 108:545–551, 1997.

130. Pacak K, Palkovits M, Yadid G, et al: Heterogeneous neurochemical responses to different stressors: A test of Selye's doctrine of nonspecificity. Am J Physiol 275:R1247–R1255, 1998.

131. Berkenbosch F, van OJ, del RA, et al: Corticotropin-releasing factor–producing neurons in the rat activated by interleukin-1. Science 238:524–526, 1987.

132. Sapolsky R, Rivier C, Yamamoto G, et al: Interleukin-1 stimulates the secretion of hypothalamic corticotropin-releasing factor. Science 238:522–524, 1987.

133. Dunn AJ: Systemic interleukin-1 administration stimulates hypothalamic norepinephrine metabolism paralleling the increased plasma corticosterone. Life Sci 43:429–435, 1988.

134. Bernardini R, Kamilaris TC, Calogero AE, et al: Interactions between tumor necrosis factor–alpha, hypothalamic corticotropin-releasing hormone, and adrenocorticotropin secretion in the rat. Endocrinology 126:2876–2881, 1990.

135. Elenkov IJ, Kovacs K, Kiss J, et al: Lipopolysaccharide is able to bypass corticotrophin-releasing factor in affecting plasma ACTH and corticosterone levels: Evidence from rats with lesions of the paraventricular nucleus. J Endocrinol 133:231–236, 1992.

136. Kovacs KJ, Elenkov IJ: Differential dependence of ACTH secretion induced by various cytokines on the integrity of the paraventricular nucleus. J Neuroendocrinol 7:15–23, 1995.

137. Akira S, Hirano T, Taga T, et al: Biology of multifunctional cytokines: IL 6 and related molecules (IL 1 and TNF). FASEB J 4:2860–2867, 1990.

138. Hesse DG, Tracey KJ, Fong Y, et al: Cytokine appearance in human endotoxemia and primate bacteremia. Surg Gynecol Obstet 166:147–153, 1988.

139. van Deventer SJ, Buller HR, ten Cate JW, et al: Experimental endotoxemia in humans: Analysis of cytokine release and coagulation, fibrinolytic, and complement pathways. Blood 76:2520–2526, 1990.

140. van Gool J, van Vugt H, Helle M, et al: The relation among stress, adrenalin, interleukin 6 and acute phase proteins in the rat. Clin Immunol Immunopathol 57:200–210, 1990.

141. Komaki G, Gottschall PE, Somogyvari-Vigh A, et al: Rapid increase in plasma IL-6 after hemorrhage, and posthemorrhage reduction of the IL-6 response to LPS, in conscious rats: Interrelation with plasma corticosterone levels. Neuroimmunomodulation 1:127–134, 1994.

142. Imura H, Fukata J, Mori T: Cytokines and endocrine function: An interaction between the immune and neuroendocrine systems. Clin Endocrinol (Oxf) 35:107–115, 1991.

143. Naitoh Y, Fukata J, Tominaga T, et al: Interleukin-6 stimulates the secretion of adrenocorticotropic hormone in conscious, freely-moving rats. Biochem Biophys Res Commun 155:1459–1463, 1988.

144. Perlstein RS, Mougey EH, Jackson WE, et al: Interleukin-1 and interleukin-6 act synergistically to stimulate the release of adrenocorticotropic hormone in vivo. Lymphokine Cytokine Res 10:141–146, 1991.

145. Perlstein RS, Whitnall MH, Abrams JS, et al: Synergistic roles of interleukin-6, interleukin-1, and tumor necrosis factor in the adrenocorticotropin response to bacterial lipopolysaccharide in vivo. Endocrinology 132:946–952, 1993.

146. Mastorakos G, Weber JS, Magiakou MA, et al: Hypothalamic-pituitary-adrenal axis activation and stimulation of systemic vasopressin secretion by recombinant interleukin-6 in humans: Potential implications for the syndrome of inappropriate vasopressin secretion. J Clin Endocrinol Metab 79:934–939, 1994.

147. Mastorakos G, Chrousos GP, Weber JS: Recombinant interleukin-6 activates the hypothalamic-pituitary-adrenal axis in humans. J Clin Endocrinol Metab 77:1690–1694, 1993.

148. Maier SF, Goehler LE, Fleshner M, et al: The role of the vagus nerve in cytokine-to-brain communication. Ann NY Acad Sci 840:289–300, 1998.

149. Tilders FJ, DeRijk RH, Van Dam AM, et al: Activation of the hypothalamus-pituitary-adrenal axis by bacterial endotoxins: Routes and intermediate signals. Psychoneuroendocrinology 19:209–232, 1994.

150. Reichlin S: Neuroendocrine-immune interactions. N Engl J Med 329:1246–1253, 1993.

151. De Simoni MG, Sironi M, De Luigi A, et al: Intracerebroventricular injection of interleukin 1 induces high circulating levels of interleukin 6. J Exp Med 171:1773–1778, 1990.

152. Vizi ES, Harsing LGJR, Zimanyi I, et al: Release and turnover of noradrenaline in isolated median eminence: Lack of negative feedback modulation. Neuroscience 16:907–916, 1985.

153. Plotsky PM, Cunningham ET Jr, Widmaier EP: Catecholaminergic modulation of corticotropin-releasing factor and adrenocorticotropin secretion. Endocr Rev 10:437–458, 1989.

154. Elenkov IJ, Kovacs K, Duda E, et al: Presynaptic inhibitory effect of TNF-alpha on the release of noradrenaline in isolated median eminence. J Neuroimmunol 41:117–120, 1992.

155. Gordon ML: An evaluation of afferent nervous impulses in the adrenal cortical response to trauma. Endocrinology 47:347–350, 1950.

156. Chapman LF, Goodell H: The participation of the nervous system in the inflammatory reaction. Ann NY Acad Sci 116:990–1017, 1963.

157. Berkenbosch F, de Goeij DEC, del Rey AE, et al: Neuroendocrine, sympathetic and metabolic responses induced by interleukin-1. Neuroendocrinology 50:570–576, 1989.

158. Katafuchi T, Hori T, Take S: Central administration of interferon-alpha enhances rat sympathetic nerve activity to the spleen. Neurosci Lett 125(1):37–40, 1991.

159. Shimizu N, Hori T, Nakane H: An interleukin-1b–induced noradrenaline release in the spleen is mediated by brain corticotropin-releasing factor: An in vivo microdialysis study in conscious rats. Brain Behavior Immun 7:14–23, 1994.

160. Spangelo BL, Judd AM, Isakson PC, et al: Interleukin-6 stimulates anterior pituitary hormone release in vitro. Endocrinology 125:575–577, 1989.

161. Roh MS: Direct stimulation of the adrenal cortex by interleukin-1. Surgery 102:140–146, 1987.

162. Salas MA, Evans SW, Levell MJ, et al: Interleukin-6 and ACTH act synergistically to stimulate the release of corticosterone from adrenal gland cells. Clin Exp Immunol 79:470–473, 1990.

163. Tominaga T, Fukata J, Naito Y, et al: Prostaglandin-dependent in vitro stimulation of adrenocortical steroidogenesis by interleukins. Endocrinology 128:526–531, 1991.

164. Vankelecom H, Carmeliet P, Van Damme J, et al: Production of interleukin-6 by folliculo-stellate cells of the anterior pituitary gland in a histiotypic cell aggregate culture system. Neuroendocrinology 49:102–106, 1989.

165. Schultzberg M, Andersson C, Unden A, et al: Interleukin-1 in adrenal chromaffin cells. Neuroscience 30:805–810, 1989.

166. Vankelecom H, Carmeliet P, Heremans H, et al: Interferon-gamma inhibits stimulated adrenocorticotropin, prolactin, and growth hormone secretion in normal rat anterior pituitary cell cultures. Endocrinology 126:2919–2926, 1990.

167. Gaillard RC, Turnill D, Sappino P, et al: Tumor necrosis factor alpha inhibits the hormonal response of the pituitary gland to hypothalamic releasing factors. Endocrinology 127:101–106, 1990.

168. Jaattela M, Ilvesmaki V, Voutilainen R, et al: Tumor necrosis factor as a potent inhibitor of adrenocorticotropin-induced cortisol production and steroidogenic P450 enzyme gene expression in cultured human fetal adrenal cells. Endocrinology 128:623–629, 1991.

169. Almawi WY, Lipman ML, Stevens AC, et al: Abrogation of glucocorticoid-mediated inhibition of T cell proliferation by the synergistic action of IL-1, IL-6, and IFN-gamma. J Immunol 146:3523–3527, 1991.

170. Kam JC, Szefler SJ, Surs W, et al: Combination IL-2 and IL-4 reduces glucocorticoid receptor-binding affinity and T cell response to glucocorticoids. J Immunol 151:3460–3466, 1993.

171. Klein A, Buskila D, Gladman D, et al: Cortisol catabolism by lymphocytes of patients with systemic lupus erythematosus and rheumatoid arthritis. J Rheumatol 17:30–33, 1990.

172. Harbuz MS, Lightman SL: Stress and the hypothalamo-pituitary-adrenal axis: Acute, chronic and immunological activation. J Endocrinol 134:327–339, 1992.

173. Dallman MF: Stress update: Adaptation of the hypothalamic-pituitary-adrenal axis to chronic stress. Trends Endocrinol Metabol 62–69, 1993.

174. Swain MG, Patchev V, Vergalla J, et al: Suppression of hypothalamic-pituitary-adrenal axis responsiveness to stress in a rat model of acute cholestasis. J Clin Invest 91:1903–1908, 1993.

175. Rothwell PM, Udwadia ZF, Lawler PG: Cortisol response to corticotropin and survival in septic shock. Lancet 337:582–583, 1991.

176. Kidess AI, Caplan RH, Reynertson RH, et al: Transient corticotropin deficiency in critical illness. Mayo Clin Proc 68:435–441, 1993.

177. Dluhy RG: The growing spectrum of HIV-related endocrine abnormalities. J Clin Endocrinol Metab 70:563–565, 1990.
178. Reincke M, Heppner C, Petzke F, et al: Impairment of adrenocortical function associated with increased plasma tumor necrosis factor–alpha and interleukin-6 concentrations in African trypanosomiasis. Neuroimmunomodulation 1:14–22, 1994.
179. Parker LN, Levin ER, Lifrak ET: Evidence for adrenocortical adaptation to severe illness. J Clin Endocrinol Metab 60:947–952, 1985.
180. Berczi I: Gonadotrophins and sex hormones. In Berczi I: Pituitary Function and Immunity. Boca Raton, FL, CRC Press, 1986.
181. Raveche ES, Steinberg AD: Sex hormones and autoimmunity. In Berczi I: Pituitary Function and Immunity. Boca Raton, FL, CRC Press, 1986.
182. Cid MC, Kleinman HK, Grant DS, et al: Estradiol enhances leukocyte binding to tumor necrosis factor (TNF)–stimulated endothelial cells via an increase in TNF-induced adhesion molecules E-selectin, intercellular adhesion molecule type 1, and vascular cell adhesion molecule type 1. J Clin Invest 93:17–25, 1994.
183. Vamvakopoulos NC, Chrousos GP: Evidence of direct estrogenic regulation of human corticotropin-releasing hormone gene expression. Potential implications for the sexual dimophism of the stress response and immune/inflammatory reaction. J Clin Invest 92:1896–1902, 1993.
184. Berczi I, Nagy E: Prolactin and other iactogenic hormones. In Berczi I: Pituitary Function and Immunity. Boca Raton, FL, CRC Press, 1986.
185. Gellersen B, Kempf R, Telgmann R, et al: Nonpituitary human prolactin gene transcription is independent of Pit-1 and differentially controlled in lymphocytes and in endometrial stroma. Mol Endocrinol 8:356–373, 1994.
186. Calogero AE, Sternberg EM, Bagdy G, et al: Neurotransmitter-induced hypothalamic-pituitary-adrenal axis responsiveness is defective in inflammatory disease-susceptible Lewis rats: In vivo and in vitro studies suggesting globally defective hypothalamic secretion of corticotropin-releasing hormone. Neuroendocrinology 55:600–608, 1992.
187. Patchev VK, Kalogeras KT, Zelazowski P, et al: Increased plasma concentrations, hypothalamic content, and in vitro release of arginine vasopressin in inflammatory disease–prone, hypothalamic corticotropin-releasing hormone–deficient Lewis rats. Endocrinology 131:1453–1457, 1992.
188. Sternberg EM, Glowa JR, Smith MA, et al: Corticotropin releasing hormone related behavioral and neuroendocrine responses to stress in Lewis and Fischer rats. Brain Res 570:54–60, 1992.
189. Neeck G, Federlin K, Graef V, et al: Adrenal secretion of cortisol in patients with rheumatoid arthritis. J Rheumatol 17:24–29, 1990.
190. Chikanza IC, Petrou P, Kingsley G, et al: Defective hypothalamic response to immune and inflammatory stimuli in patients with rheumatoid arthritis. Arthritis Rheum 35:1281–1288, 1992.
191. Masi AT, Josipovic DB, Jefferson WE: Low adrenal androgenic-anabolic steroids in women with rheumatoid arthritis (RA): Gas-liquid chromatographic studies of RA patients and matched normal control women indicating decreased 11-deoxy-17-ketosteroid excretion. Semin Arthritis Rheum 14:1–23, 1984.
192. Crofford LJ, Sano H, Karalis K, et al: Local expression of corticotropin-releasing hormone in inflammatory arthritis. Ann NY Acad Sci 771:459–471, 1995.
193. Crofford LJ, Sano H, Karalis K, et al: Corticotropin-releasing hormone in synovial fluids and tissues of patients with rheumatoid arthritis and osteoarthritis. J Immunol 151:1587–1596, 1993.
194. Sternberg EM: Hyperimmune fatigue syndromes: Diseases of the stress response? [Corrected; published erratum appears in J Rheumatol 1993 May;20(5):925.] J Rheumatol 20:418–421, 1993.
195. Dekaris D, Sabioncello A, Mazuran R, et al: Multiple changes of immunologic parameters in prisoners of war. Assessments after release from a camp in Manjaca, Bosnia. JAMA 270:595–599, 1993.
196. Schlaghecke R, Kornely E, Wollenhaupt J, et al: Glucocorticoid receptors in rheumatoid arthritis. Arthritis Rheum 35:740–744, 1992.
197. Kirkham BW, Corkill MM, Davison SC, et al: Response to glucocorticoid treatment in rheumatoid arthritis: In vitro cell mediated immune assay predicts in vivo responses. J Rheumatol 18:821–825, 1991.
198. Corrigan CJ, Brown PH, Barnes NC, et al: Glucocorticoid resistance in chronic asthma. Peripheral blood T lymphocyte activation and comparison of the T lymphocyte inhibitory effects of glucocorticoids and cyclosporin A. Am Rev Respir Dis 144:1026–1032, 1991.
199. Sher ER, Leung DY, Surs W, et al: Steroid-resistant asthma. Cellular mechanisms contributing to inadequate response to glucocorticoid therapy. J Clin Invest 93:33–39, 1994.
200. Norbiato G, Bevilacqua M, Vago T, et al: Cortisol resistance in acquired immunodeficiency syndrome. J Clin Endocrinol Metab 74:608–613, 1992.
201. DiBattista JA, Martel-Pelletier J, Antakly T, et al: Reduced expression of glucocorticoid receptor levels in human osteoarthritic chondrocytes. Role in the suppression of metalloprotease synthesis. J Clin Endocrinol Metab 76:1128–1134, 1993.
202. Franchimont D, Louis E, Dupont P, et al: Dig Dis Sci (in press).
203. Altare F, Durandy A, Lammas D, et al: Impairment of mycobacterial immunity in human interleukin-12 receptor deficiency. Science 280:1432–1435, 1998.
204. Lerner BH: Can stress cause disease? Revisiting the tuberculosis research of Thomas Holmes, 1949–1961. Ann Intern Med 124:673–680, 1996.
205. Elenkov IJ, Vizi ES: Presynaptic modulation of release of noradrenaline from the sympathetic nerve terminals in the rat spleen. Neuropharmacology 30:1319–1324, 1991.
206. Cole SW, Korin YD, Fahey JL, et al: Norepinephrine accelerates HIV replication via protein kinase A–dependent effects on cytokine production. J Immunol 161:610–616, 1998.
207. Haraguchi S, Good RA, James-Yarish M, et al: Induction of intracellular cAMP by a synthetic retroviral envelope peptide: A possible mechanism of immunopathogenesis in retroviral infections. Proc Natl Acad Sci USA 92:5568–5571, 1995.
208. Clerici M, Bevilacqua M, Vago T, et al: An immunoendocrinological hypothesis of HIV infection. Lancet 343:1552–1553, 1994.
209. Kino T, Gragerov A, Kopp JB, et al: The HIV-1 virion–associated protein vpr is a coactivator of the human glucocorticoid receptor [in process citation]. J Exp Med 189:51–62, 1999.
210. O'Sullivan ST, Lederer JA, Horgan AF, et al: Major injury leads to predominance of the T helper-2 lymphocyte phenotype and diminished interleukin-12 production associated with decreased resistance to infection. Ann Surg 222:482–490, 1995.
211. Segal BM, Dwyer BK, Shevach EM: An interleukin (IL)-10/IL-12 immunoregulatory circuit controls susceptibility to autoimmune disease. J Exp Med 187:537–546, 1998.
212. Rogers MP, Fozdar M: Psychoneuroimmunology of autoimmune disorders. Adv Neuroimmunol 6:169–177, 1996.
213. Elenkov IJ, Hoffman J, Wilder RL: Does differential neuroendocrine control of cytokine production govern the expression of autoimmune diseases in pregnancy and the postpartum period? Mol Med Today 3:379–383, 1997.
214. Horwitz MS, Bradley LM, Harbertson J, et al: Diabetes induced by Coxsackie virus: Initiation by bystander damage and not molecular mimicry [in process citation]. Nat Med 4:781–785, 1998.
215. Takahashi Y, Murai C, Shibata S, et al: Human parvovirus B19 as a causative agent for rheumatoid arthritis. Proc Natl Acad Sci USA 95:8227–8232, 1998.
216. Barnes P, FitzGerald G, Brown M, et al: Nocturnal asthma and changes in circulating epinephrine, histamine, and cortisol. N Engl J Med 303:263–267, 1980.
217. Zieg G, Lack G, Harbeck RJ, et al: In vivo effects of glucocorticoids on IgE production. J Allergy Clin Immunol 94:222–230, 1994.
218. Coqueret O, Lagente V, Frere CP, et al: Regulation of IgE production by beta 2-adrenoceptor agonists. Ann NY Acad Sci 725:44–49, 1994.
219. Colombo MP, Vagliani M, Spreafico F, et al: Amount of interleukin 12 available at the tumor site is critical for tumor regression. Cancer Res 56:2531–2534, 1996.
220. Chouaib S, Asselin-Paturel C, Mami-Chouaib F, et al: The host-tumor immune conflict: From immunosuppression to resistance and destruction. Immunol Today 18:493–497, 1997.
221. Shakhar G, Ben-Eliyahu S: In vivo beta-adrenergic stimulation suppresses natural killer activity and compromises resistance to tumor metastasis in rats. J Immunol 160:3251–3258, 1998.
222. Li T, Harada M, Tamada K, et al: Repeated restraint stress impairs the antitumor T cell response through its suppressive effect on Th1-type CD4+ T cells. Anticancer Res 17:4259–4268, 1997.
223. Matsumoto S: Cimetidine and survival with colorectal cancer. Lancet 346:115, 1995.

Chapter 41

The Autoimmune Polyglandular Syndromes

Qiao-Yi Chen ▪ Anjli Kukreja ▪ Noel K. Maclaren

Constellations of multiple endocrine gland insufficiencies often associated with diseases of nonendocrine organs afflict individual patients and their families. Recognition of those "polyglandular" syndromes has evolved over the last century, as summarized in Table 41–1. In 1849, Thomas Addison first described the clinical and pathologic features of adrenocortical failure in patients who also appeared to have pernicious anemia.[1] In this autopsy series, several patients were also cited with vitiligo in addition to adrenalitis. In their 1908 review of polyglandular insufficiencies (islet, thyroid, gonad, adrenal, anterior hypophysis), Claude and Gourgerot suggested a common pathogenesis for these conditions.[2] Mononuclear leukocyte infiltrates of goitrous thyroid glands were first noted by Hashimoto in 1912,[3] and a similar lesion of pancreatic islets, termed *insulitis,* was described by von Meyenburg in 1940.[6] It was Schmidt in 1926 who documented the association between adrenocortical failure and thyroiditis,[4] whereas Carpenter et al. in 1964 expanded Schmidt's syndrome to include type

1 diabetes.[11] A second association between mucocutaneous candidiasis and hypoparathyroidism was first suggested in 1929 by Thorpe and Handley.[5] Whitaker et al. expanded this latter association to a triad including adrenocortical insufficiency in 1956.[7] The autoimmune pathogenesis of these disorders began to emerge that same year when Roitt et al. discovered circulating precipitating autoantibodies to thyroglobulin in patients with Hashimoto's thyroiditis,[8] and in 1963 Blizzard and Kyle observed antibodies to the adrenal gland in a proportion of patients with Addison's disease.[17] In 1980, Neufeld et al. from our own group distinguished two major autoimmune polyglandular syndromes (APSs) that contain Addison's disease (APS-I and -II) and one APS without the involvement of Addison's disease that was classified as type III APS.[12] Further work is needed to further characterize these latter groups (Table 41–2).

Type I APS is diagnosed when a patient manifests at least two of the following three key features: hypoparathyroidism, hypoadrenocorticism, and recurrent mucocutaneous candidiasis. This rare syndrome usually begins with persistent candidiasis during the first decade of life, often during infancy. It has been reported to affect males and females almost equally in a large American series,[13] but a modest female bias was observed in another collection of smaller reports.[18] The more common type II APS is characterized by adrenocortical insufficiency in conjunction with thyroiditis and/or type 1 diabetes. Its prevalence has not been formally established, but it has been estimated to affect 14 to 20 persons per million population.[19] The diagnosis of type II APS is frequently made during early adulthood through midlife, and it is three to four times more common in females than males. Type III APS revolves around thyrogastric autoimmunities, in association with vitiligo and type 1 diabetes. Should Addison's disease also develop in such patients, their condition would be reclassified as type II APS.

Immunogenetic studies suggest that HLA class II genes are associated with type II and type III APS, whereas a recessive gene that has been mapped to the long arm of chromosome 21 (q22.3) is responsible for type I APS. The recessive gene responsible for APS-I has recently been identified. Multiple mutations were found in this gene, autoimmune regulator (*AIRE*), in patients with APS-I (but not APS-II), thus supporting the clinical classification of APS-I and APS-II. The test for *AIRE* gene mutations can now help distinguish type I from type II APS, which can occasionally become blurred in individual patients, especially if their problems develop when they are adults. Furthermore, the findings of homozygous *AIRE* gene mutations in siblings of patients with APS-I could be used to predict development of the component diseases. Functional studies of the *AIRE* gene product are now needed to promote an understanding of the pathogenic process of type I APS and perhaps give insight into normal immune tolerance mechanisms. Moreover, many autoantigens for the component diseases of APS have been identified in the 1990s. Autoantibodies to these autoantigens can be used as disease markers to either facilitate diagnosis of the involved component diseases or predict them. In addition,

TABLE 41–1. Emergence of the Polyglandular Syndromes

Event	Year	Reference
Description of adrenocortical atrophy in patients with pernicious anemia	1849	1
Hypothesis that polyglandular disease arises from a single process	1908	2
Description of mononuclear leukocyte infiltrate in goitrous thyroid glands	1912	3
Schmidt's syndrome described (thyroiditis and adrenalitis)	1926	4
Description of association between hypoparathyroidism and candidiasis	1929	5
Description of mononuclear leukocyte infiltrate in islets of Langerhans of diabetic patients	1940	6
Triad of hypoadrenocorticism, hypoparathyroidism, and candidiasis described	1956	7
Thyroid autoantibodies observed	1956	8
Thyroiditis induced in rabbits by immunizing with gland extract	1956	9
Indirect immunofluorescence labeling technique described	1959	10
Carpenter et al. expand Schmidt's syndrome to include insulin-dependent diabetes mellitus	1964	11
Clinical classification of distinct polyglandular autoimmune syndromes	1980	12, 13
AIRE gene responsible for APS-I mapped to chromosome 21q22.3	1994	14
AIRE gene identified, thus confirming the clinical classification of APS	1997	15, 16

APS, autoimmune polyglandular syndrome.

587

TABLE 41–2. *The Autoimmune Polyglandular Syndromes*

Type I APS	Type II APS	Type III APS	Frequency (%)
Hypoparathyroidism	Adrenocortical insufficiency	Thyroiditis, type 1 diabetes (IMD), pernicious anemia, vitiligo	>40
Mucocutaneous candidiasis	Thyroiditis		
Adrenocortical insufficiency	Insulin-dependent diabetes mellitus		
Ungual dystrophy, enamel hypoplasia, hypogonadism			
Malabsorption			10–40
Alopecia (totalis or universalis)			
Pernicious anemia (juvenile onset)			
Thyroiditis			
Chronic active hepatitis			
Vitiligo	Hypogonadism	Hypogonadism	<10
Sjögren's syndrome	Vitiligo	Alopecia (adult onset)	
Anterior hypophysitis	Alopecia	Myasthenia gravis	
Type 1 diabetes (IMD)	Pernicious anemia (adult onset)	Celiac disease	
	Myasthenia gravis	Rheumatoid arthritis	
	Celiac disease	Sjögren's syndrome	
	Rheumatoid arthritis		
	Sjögren's syndrome		

APS, autoimmune polyglandular syndrome; IMD, immune-mediated diabetes.

understanding of the cell-mediated immune responses involved in the pathophysiologic mechanism of APS is needed. This chapter is designed to review the pathogenesis of the APSs and current knowledge of their molecular immunogenetics.

PATHOPHYSIOLOGY

Evidence supporting the autoimmune nature of the component diseases of APS is compelling: (1) affected organs demonstrate a chronic inflammatory infiltrate composed mainly of lymphocytes, sometimes aggregating into follicle formation; (2) some of the component diseases are associated with immune response genes encoded by class II loci of the HLA complex; and (3) the syndromes are replete with autoantibodies reacting to target tissue–specific antigens, which are often targeted organ–specific enzymes. The initiating events and autoimmune pathogenic processes of APS remain largely undiscovered, but it is probable that both genetic and environmental factors are involved. In patients with APS-I and the same *AIRE* gene mutations, different disease components develop in different orders with various ages of onset, which suggests the involvement of environmental factors and/or other background genetic factors.

Autoantibodies may arise spontaneously through a breakdown in normal immunologic tolerogenesis or by immunization with an environmental agent that is a molecular mimic of a self-antigen (see below for discussion). They could arise as part of a bystander immune response to self after direct viral infection or damage to the target organ by a chemical agent. Other autoantibodies appear to arise during a secondary immune response and are stimulated by the release of intracellular antigens from damaged glands, which are normally sequestered from the immune system. The three main classes of organ-specific self-antigens to which autoantibodies are directed in APS (Table 41–3) are surface receptor molecules; intracellular enzymes, which have a central role in a vital and unique cellular function of the target cell; and secreted proteins such as hormones produced by the affected organs. Examples of surface receptor molecules affected by autoimmunity include the thyrotropin receptor, which is involved in Graves' disease (stimulatory type), as well as in atrophic thyroiditis (blocking type), and a component of the glucose transport system of the pancreatic β cell, which has been implicated as a target in immune-mediated (type 1) diabetes (IMD). Important enzymes that act as autoantigens include thyroid peroxidase (previously called thyroid "microsomal" antigen) in Hashimoto's thyroiditis and the P450 steroidogenic enzyme 21-hydroxylase (21-OH), essential to steroid hormone biosynthesis, in autoimmune Addison's disease. Thyroglobulin, as targeted in Hashimoto's thyroiditis, or insulin and proinsulin, as

involved in IMD, are examples of autoantigenic endocrine cell products important to their respective autoimmune diseases.

It is perplexing why the component diseases of APS coexist. One possibility is that sharing of target antigenic epitopes between affected glands may be responsible. Experimental evidence for this possibility is most often lacking, but 17-OH and side chain cleavage (scc) enzymes are present in the "steroidal cells" of the testes, ovary, placenta, and adrenal cortex. In addition, partial autoantibody cross-reactivity between the P450 21-OH and 17-OH enzymes has been proposed in view of the amino acid sequence homology of the epitope region of these two molecules.[20] This theory is supported by evidence that absorption by recombinant 17-OH could partially remove the reactivity of sera from patients with APS-I against recombinant 21-OH, and vice versa, thus suggesting both the presence of cross-reactive antibodies to 17-OH and 21-OH and a separate population of antibodies to 21-OH and 17-OH in the sera of patients with APS-I.[21] However, for the remaining component autoimmune diseases, no evidence of antigen cross-reactivity has been found.

Humoral Autoimmunity

One of the prominent features of APS is the presence of circulating autoantibodies to autoantigens normally present in the endocrine organs involved in the disease. Such autoantibodies can occur long before appearance of the respective clinical diseases. Patients with any of the three types of APS may have autoantibodies against the same autoantigen, and many of the targeted autoantigens are enzymes (see Table 41–3). Identification of circulating organ-specific autoantibodies provided the earliest and strongest evidence for an autoimmune pathogenesis of the APSs. Whereas patients with collagen-vascular diseases synthesize immunoglobulins that recognize non–organ-specific cellular targets such as nucleic acids or nucleoproteins, endocrine autoimmunities are associated with autoantibodies that react to organ-specific antigens. Although the pathogenic relevance of organ-specific autoantibodies remains unclear, their importance as diagnostic indicators and predictive markers of future disease is well established.[22–26] Indirect immunofluorescent assay continues to be a useful and convenient method to screen for autoantibodies to the autoantigens present in target organs. Procedures for procurement and processing of fresh frozen human substrate tissues for such testing must be meticulously followed to obtain consistent and reliable results.[27] Biochemical assays, such as immunoprecipitation assays using autoantigens labeled with radioisotopes, are commonly used for measuring specific autoantibodies and have shown high sensitivity and good reproducibility and quantitative capacity.

TABLE 41–3. Types of Autoantigens in Autoimmune Polyglandular Syndromes

Target Organ	Enzymes	Receptors	Secreted Cell Products
Islet	Glutamic acid decarboxylase$_{65}$	Insulin receptor	Insulin
	Tyrosine phosphatase IA2/IA-2β	Glucose transporter (GLUT2)	Proinsulin
Thyroid	Thyroid peroxidase	Thyrotropin	Thyroglobulin
		Parathyroid	
Parathyroid		Calcium-sensing receptor	
Adrenal	21α-Hydroxylase	ACTH	
	17α-Hydroxylase		
Gonad	17α-Hydroxylase, side chain	Gonadotropin	
	cleavage enzyme		
Gastric intestine	H$^+$, K$^+$-ATPase, tryptophan		Intrinsic factor
	hydroxylase, tissue		
	transglutaminase		
Liver	P450IID6, 2C9, 1A2, AADC		
Melanocytes	Tyrosinase		

AADC, amino acid decarboxylase; ACTH, adrenocorticotropic hormone.

ADRENOCORTICAL AUTOANTIBODIES. Adrenocortical autoantibodies (AAs) detected by indirect immunofluorescent labeling have been reported in most patients with nontuberculous Addison's disease when tested at the time of their diagnoses.[28] All layers of the adrenal cortex bind AAs, with striking sparing of the adrenal medulla. Fluorescence of the zona glomerulosa in particular gives a distinctive pattern when viewed by ultraviolet microscopy. Some 15% of AA-positive patients with Addison's disease also have an autoantibody that cross-reacts with other steroid-producing cells such as placental syncytiotrophoblasts, ovarian luteal cells, and/or testicular Leydig cells, and most of these patients have type I APS. These "steroidal cell" autoantibodies (SCAs) are distinguished from AAs by their ability to be adsorbed from serum by preincubation with adrenal, gonadal (ovarian or testicular), or placental homogenates, whereas AAs are exclusively removed from positive sera by prior exposure to adrenal homogenates. When detected, SCAs indicate a high risk for future gonadal failure, especially in females with high titers.[23, 29] Patients with premature ovarian failure and a positive test for AAs have a higher risk for the development of Addison's disease than do those who do not test positive.[30]

The major steroid cell autoantigens involved in the reaction of AAs have been identified, as mentioned above, and include 21-OH, 17α–OH, and P450scc (see Table 41–3). The major antigen for SCA is 17-OH, a 55-kDa gonadal and adrenal steroid biosynthetic P450 microsomal enzyme.[31] Most patients with nontuberculous Addison's disease have antibodies to 21-OH, although the reported frequencies may vary depending on the techniques used.[32–37] Antibodies to 21-OH are generally found at higher frequency and titer in patients with Addison's disease in association with APS than in patients with isolated Addison's disease. The frequency of antibodies to 17-OH and P450scc is also considerably higher in patients with APS than in patients with isolated Addison's disease.[36, 38, 39] Thus the presence of antibodies to 17-OH or P450scc in patients with isolated Addison's disease may indicate progression toward APS. The dominant epitopes on 21-OH commonly recognized by autoantibodies from patients with Addison's disease as an isolated disease or in association with APS are located in the C-terminal end and in a central region of 21-OH.[40, 41] The epitopes on 21-OH can be either conformational[42] or linear in nature.[43]

Autoantibodies to 21-OH or AAs are useful markers indicating a risk for the development of Addison's disease. Occasionally, AA-positive individuals who do not have overt adrenocortical failure can be identified by screening patients with autoimmune diseases, especially autoimmune endocrine diseases, and their family members. About 20% of asymptomatic AA-positive relatives were reported to have elevated basal serum levels of adrenocorticotropic hormone (ACTH) and/or renin or blunted adrenocortical responses to an intravenous infusion of ACTH, features that are indicative of subclinical glandular dysfunction (Fig. 41–1). In two separate studies, autoantibodies to 21-OH were found at frequencies of 2.3% (7/304)[21] and 1.7% (11/629)[44] in patients with IMD. These results are similar to the frequencies of AA found a decade previously.[45] Furthermore, many of

these patients had raised ACTH/renin levels indicative of impending Addison's disease.[24] It is reported that 25% of patients without clinical symptoms of hypoadrenalism but with a positive test for AAs were actually at a stage of subclinical hypoadrenalism.[46] In addition, Addison's disease may subsequently develop in up to 40% of such individuals over a follow-up period of 6 months to 10 years.[24, 46] This risk was observed to be especially high if the autoantibodies fixed complement in vitro or were present at high titer. Thus close attention should be paid to patients with positive tests for autoantibodies to 21-OH and those with risk HLA alleles such as DRB1*03/DQB1*0201, which is associated with both IMD and Addison's disease.[47, 48] In addition, all patients with features suggestive of APS-I but without overt Addison's disease should be tested for AAs because at least 20% of APS-I patients without symptoms of Addison's disease are positive for antibodies to 21-OH.[49] Symptoms of adrenal deficiency may not be manifested unless most of the adrenal cortex has been destroyed.[24] However, 21-OH autoantibody–positive patients with subclinical Addison's disease can be identified by increased levels of resting plasma renin activity and/or raised afternoon serum ACTH levels tested after patients have been recumbent for 1 hour. As the disease progresses, depressed ACTH-stimulated cortisol responses and electrolyte disturbances can eventually be noted.[24]

Whereas cellular immune mechanisms are thought to cause the glandular destruction seen in autoimmune endocrinopathies, a pathogenic role for humoral autoreactivity in autoimmune oophoritis has been suggested by studies showing complement-mediated cytotoxicity of cultured granulosa cells in the presence of sera from affected patients but not in the presence of sera from control patients.[50] Binding of SCAs to granulosa cells by indirect immunofluorescence, however, can be demonstrated only when autoantibodies are present in high titer. Antibodies of patients with Addison's disease had been shown to have inhibitory effects on recombinant 21-OH enzyme activity in vitro,[51] but such enzyme inhibitory effects are not so evident in vivo[52] and are conceptually unlikely to account for the resultant disease because such antibodies cannot penetrate adrenocortical cells to inhibit steroidogenesis.

PARATHYROID GLAND–SPECIFIC AUTOANTIBODIES. Autoantibodies to the parathyroid gland were detected in 38% of 74 patients with idiopathic hypoparathyroidism by indirect immunofluorescent assay.[53] However, subsequent investigations have found that antiparathyroid serologic immunoreactivity is rare in patients with failed glands[54] and is not usually parathyroid specific.[55] Indeed, antibodies considered to be against parathyroid antigens in previous reports have, we believe, been confused with mitochondrial autoantibodies, and humoral sensitivity to parathyroid tissue may have delineated a tissue-specific response to antigens within the endothelial component of the gland.[56] In a recent study from our laboratory involving Western blotting, the calcium-sensing receptor was recognized in 32% (8/25) of patients with hypoparathyroidism associated with either APS-I or hypothyroidism, with the major epitope located on the external domain of the receptor.[57] This finding suggests that such autoantibodies could

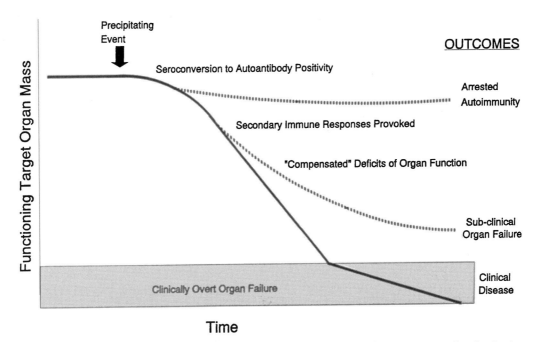

FIGURE 41-1. The proposed natural history of endocrine autoimmunity. Autoimmune attack of target organs often begins in people who have a genetic predisposition after an unknown precipitating event *(arrow)*. The early process manifests itself by provoking autoantibody production, and it may arrest at that stage *(top broken line)*. Progressive disease, associated with secondary responses against antigens released by damaged tissue, is initially detectable by minimal biochemical abnormalities, such as elevations of trophic hormones. Organ function loss may plateau before the critical organ mass threshold is reached *(lower broken line)*, or it may progress to clinically overt disease *(solid line)*. Hormone replacement therapy may decelerate the destruction of surviving tissue, but at this late stage, complete organ atrophy is inevitable.

have a pathogenic role involving downregulation of parathyroid hormone secretion through signal transduction events in parathyroid cells.

PANCREATIC β CELL AUTOANTIBODIES. The intensive studies of humoral autoimmunities against antigens expressed by the pancreatic β cell (e.g., islet gangliosides, insulin, proinsulin, glutamic acid decarboxylase [GAD_{65}], and tyrosine phosphatases [IA-2 and IA2-β]) highlight the complexity of disease-autoantibody relationships. The presence of islet cell autoantibodies detected by immunofluorescence, together with insulin autoantibody and/or anti-GAD or IA-2, has a high predictive value for the development of IMD. However, islet cell autoantibodies, as well as GAD autoantibodies, also occur in many patients with APS-I,[58, 59] a syndrome with only a low likelihood of progression to clinically overt diabetes,[13, 58] at least in U.S. patients. Recent studies indicate that autoantibodies to islet cell autoantigens in patients with APS-I have different reactive characteristics from those of patients with IMD as in APS-II/III. For example, GAD_{65} autoantibodies are readily detectable by Western blotting in the sera of patients with APS-I,[58] similar to the GAD autoantibodies present in the sera of patients with stiff-man syndrome, an autoimmune neurologic disorder,[60] thus indicating that these autoantibodies recognize linear epitopes on denatured GAD_{65}. However, the GAD_{65} autoantibodies present in patients with IMD usually react with conformational epitopes of native or undenatured proteins,[61] which suggests that different immunoregulation mechanisms could have been involved in driving the production of these two sets of GAD_{65} autoantibodies. It also suggests that the presence of islet cell autoimmunity in APS-I is not necessarily an indicator of the destruction of islet cells, at least in APS-I and stiff-man syndrome. It presumably lacks other components of the pathogenic process (e.g., antigen-specific cytotoxic T lymphocytes) that are necessary to produce β cell damage and thus overt hyperglycemia. Alternatively, the islet cell nondestructive autoimmune response in patients with APS-I may result from an impaired cellular immunoregulatory mechanism different from that in APS-II; however, these speculations need to be systematically proved through specific studies.

THYROID GLAND AUTOANTIBODIES. Autoantibodies in patients with APS react with thyroid gland proteins, including thyroid peroxidase, thyroglobulin, and thyrotropin receptors. Although immunoglobulins against the thyrotropin receptor may stimulate or inhibit both thyroid gland activity and the growth of thyrocytes, no consis-

tently discernible effect on thyroid function has yet been attributed to autoantibodies that recognize thyroid peroxidase or thyroglobulin (see Table 41–3). Nevertheless, immunization of susceptible strains of mice with thyroglobulin in complete Freund's adjuvant induces a thyroid-specific immune infiltrate in experimental allergic thyroiditis.[62] Autoimmunity against the thyroid gland is unusual in APS-I.

AUTOANTIBODIES IN OTHER AUTOIMMUNE DISEASES ASSOCIATED WITH APS. Hypogonadism, hypopituitarism, pernicious anemia, malabsorption, alopecia, and/or vitiligo may develop in patients with APS. Screening for marker autoantibodies for these associated diseases facilitates early diagnosis and treatment of the corresponding diseases. Weight loss and malabsorption are most often seen in patients with Addison's disease, especially those with APS-I,[63] which may indicate the underlying celiac disease, intestinal bacterial overgrowth, or loss of intestinal endocrine cells. Thus patients with APS should also be screened for associated endocrine and nonendocrine diseases by testing for the corresponding autoantibodies.

Interestingly, autoantibodies to tryptophan hydroxylase have recently been associated with malabsorption in patients with APS-I.[64] Also, celiac disease, which can occur in patients with APS-I or APS-II, is characterized by damage to absorptive villi and flattening and hypoplasia of the crypts of the small intestine. Autoantibodies have been detected to a newly identified autoantigen, tissue transglutaminase, in patients with celiac disease,[65] in line with the known evidence for its autoimmune nature.[66, 67] Here, ingestion of gliadin in wheat appears to provoke a reversible autoimmunity to transglutaminase-associated symptoms. Thus detection of autoantibodies to tissue transglutaminase in patients with Addison's disease regardless of its association with APS would help identify the existence of celiac disease in the patients tested.

Achlorhydria and pernicious anemia occurring as part of the APSs are associated with the presence of circulating autoantibodies against gastric parietal cells (PCAs) and, less frequently, intrinsic factor. Approximately 10% of patients with IMD have coexisting circulating PCAs, and achlorhydria develops in many of these patients.[68] The pathogenic importance of these immunoglobulins is suggested by their toxic effects on the gastric mucosa of frogs and guinea pigs.[69, 70] The parietal cell proton pump (H^+,K^+-ATPase) represents at least one target of PCA.[71] Thus PCAs appear to be primarily associated with achlorhydria, whereas intrinsic factor may arise secondarily as a consequence of gastric cell damage and is associated with an increased likelihood of clinical pernicious anemia.

Vitiligo is often seen in patients with APS-I, and antimelanocyte autoantibodies have been demonstrated in a small number of individuals with type I APS and vitiligo.[72] We commonly find chronic lymphocyte infiltrations in active vitiligo lesions. Furthermore, tyrosinase, the rate-limiting enzyme for melanin formation, is one target for autoantibodies in patients with vitiligo associated with endocrine diseases.[73] However, controversy on the frequency of autoantibodies to tyrosinase in patients with vitiligo has been reported.[74, 75] It appears that patients with vitiligo in association with APS tend to have higher frequencies of antibodies to tyrosinase than do patients with only vitiligo. Tyrosinase-reactive T cells are present in the normal immune system and are responsible for the stimulation of peptides derived from tyrosinase.[76] Immunization by tyrosinase-related protein-1 has recently been shown to induce destruction of melanocytes in mice,[77] whereas the Smyth chicken model of vitiligo is characterized by autoantibodies to tyrosine-related protein-1.[78]

Antibodies detected by indirect immunofluorescent labeling of hypothalamic vasopressin-producing cells have also been reported in a small number of patients with central diabetes insipidus who had other autoimmune endocrinopathies.[27] In a report of 19 patients with a variety of endocrine autoimmunities, autoantibodies against anterior pituitary lactotrophs were detected,[79] and scattered reports of humoral responses against somatotrophs and perhaps even gonadotrophs have also been published but not independently confirmed. Rarely, if ever have these patients had symptomatic disease of their hypothalamic-pituitary axis, however. In contrast, among 30 reported patients with proven or presumed symptomatic lymphocytic hypophysitis, autoantibodies directed against the pituitary gland have been described.[80] With the use of transformed rodent pituitary cell lines as a substrate in an indirect immunofluorescence assay, immunoglobulins that specifically bound the hypophysial cells in culture were observed in the serum of patients with the empty-sella syndrome.[81] The authors believe that pituitary autoimmunity is an area of potential research that needs more attention.

The antibodies described above that react with cellular enzymes or hormones generally have unknown pathogenic significance. The functional role of autoantibodies that alter organ function by binding to their hormone receptors is, however, readily understandable. Whereas autoantibodies that bind thyrotropin and acetylcholine receptors have long been recognized to have pathogenic importance in Graves' disease and myasthenia gravis, respectively, a similar mechanism has only recently emerged as a potential pathogenic process in other endocrine autoimmunities. Thus immunoglobulins that recognize receptors for gonadotropins, insulin, calcium-sensing receptors, or ACTH receptors may inhibit the action of their respective hormone ligands[82] (see Table 41–3).

In type I APS patients with chronic active hepatitis, autoantibodies against mitochondrial, nuclear, or smooth muscle antigens are frequently found, although their clinical significance is unclear. Cytochrome P450 proteins are often the common targets of autoantibodies from patients with APS and patients with autoimmune liver diseases.[83] Abnormal B lymphocyte function has been variably described in patients with APS. Deficiency of IgA is the most common feature, and high levels of IgG and IgE have also been observed in some patients.[84, 85] Deficient secretion of IgA immunoglobulins by the intestine may result in small intestinal bacterial overgrowth and subsequent diarrhea.

Cellular Autoimmunity

Pathologic observations and experimental investigations of cellular immunity in multiorgan autoimmunity have yielded results similar to those found in the more intensive studies of isolated autoimmune thyroid and pancreatic islet diseases. In this section, therefore, information derived from research into APS and other autoimmune disorders will be combined to review the principles of autoimmunity that are important in APS pathogenesis.

The gross and microscopic pathologic changes in types I and II/III APS are similar to those of component-isolated endocrinopathy. Histologic examination of affected adrenal, thyroid, and parathyroid glands, ovaries, pancreatic islets, and gastric mucosa has yielded similar results.[28, 86–94] A mononuclear leukocyte infiltrate that is composed mainly of lymphocytes with some macrophages, natural killer (NK) cells, and plasma cells is typically seen. Neutrophils are characteristically absent. The infiltrating lymphocytes are of both B and T cell lineage, and the T cell population includes both CD4+ and CD8+ subsets, often displaying activation markers.[86, 90] Sparing of adjacent nontarget tissue is striking in all organs. As the disease approaches its final stages, scarring and atrophy predominate within the gland, mediated in part through target cell–induced apoptosis. Fibrosis eventually becomes a prominent finding in most affected glands and may highlight islands of surviving endocrine tissue that are both hyperplastic and hypertrophied, as illustrated by "regenerative nodules" in the adrenalitis lesions of Addison's disease. Such attempts at regeneration are invariably accompanied by continued inflammation.

Effector Functions

The presence of circulating tissue-specific autoreactive leukocytes in patients with APS was first demonstrated by the elaboration of migration inhibitory factors after the incubation of target organ homogenates with peripheral blood mononuclear cells (PBMCs) from affected individuals. Subsequently, increased levels of PBMCs expressing activation markers such as HLA class II antigens have been observed in patients with early but not end-stage IMD, Graves' disease, thyroiditis, Addison's disease, and oophoritis.[86, 95] Because surface antigen phenotyping does not reliably distinguish lymphocytes with different functions, cytokine production profiles of PBMCs are coming under scrutiny. Decreased production of interleukin-4 and increased production of interferon-γ in response to mitogen has been observed in patients with new-onset IMD.[96, 97] In contrast, autologous thyroid cells elicited interferon-γ production by PBMCs harvested from patients with autoimmune thyroid disease but not from those with nontoxic goiters or thyroid cancer.[98] Examination of affected end organs obtained early in the disease process will ultimately be more informative than examination of circulating lymphocytes. Unfortunately, tissue specimens obtained at or after the time that disease becomes clinically apparent contain infiltrates that represent a complex response against a multitude of antigens. Animal models of disease are now being used to observe the kinetics of leukocyte infiltration of autoimmune targets. In nonobese diabetic (NOD) mice, reports of early insulitis have described initial infiltration by macrophages and CD8+ T lymphocytes, followed by CD4+ T lymphocytes and B lymphocytes.[99]

It appears unlikely that the action of a single T lymphocyte clone can result in clinically important organ failure inasmuch as adoptive transfer of either IMD or thyroiditis requires the transfusion of both CD4+ and CD8+ lymphocytes. Nonetheless, it is likely that autoimmunity against one of several, discrete antigens can initiate disease. One recent report, however, in which insulin gene promotor–linked GAD antisense DNA was used to reduce islet cell expression of the antigen suggested that islet cell autoimmune diabetes was promptly abrogated.[100] Target organ invasion by restricted T cell families, identified by their expression of T cell receptor genes that contain uniquely rearranged variable (V) or complementarity-determining regions (e.g., CDR3) or by monoclonal expansion of B lymphocytes, has not been demonstrated convincingly in APS. Preferential use of certain T cell receptor families may occur, however, in an antigen-specific fashion during the inductive events.[101]

Despite the multitude of investigations, the sequence of effector events leading to eventual cell destruction has not been resolved with any certainty. It has been difficult to determine how the local effects of cytokines (released from either leukocytes, damaged endothelium, or possibly endocrine epithelium)[28, 102] and the aberrant expression of major histocompatibility complex (MHC) antigens (class I and/or class II)[86, 91, 103] and adhesion molecules (intercellular adhesion molecule-1)[104, 105] on the endocrine epithelium surface contribute to the pathologic process. In diabetic rodents, β cell expression of class I MHC is observed early in the pathogenic sequence, perhaps enhancing the ability of CD8+ T cells to lyse these cellular targets. Later, enhanced class II reactivity may occur as a result of the invasion of macrophages and perhaps some patchy aberrant expression of these antigens on pancreatic β cells.

Recurrent mucocutaneous candidal infections in type I APS, which are often resistant to treatment, most certainly reflect an abnormality in T lymphocyte function. No specific T cell defect to account for these findings has been consistently identified, although one must exist.[92] The possible role of the elusive transfer factor remains unclear.[106] Again, this area needs further investigation, especially regarding function of the newly identified *AIRE* gene.

Immunoregulatory Functions

The classic concept of autoimmune disease arising from a "forbidden" lymphocyte clone that has escaped intrathymic deletion is incomplete inasmuch as some potentially autoreactive T lymphocytes are regularly found circulating in healthy individuals. Normal tolerance to self is achieved by the active induction of clonal deletion by the thymus, clone-specific anergy, or cytokine deviation by a peripheral regulatory process that remains poorly defined. Deficiencies in such immunoregulation may allow potentially autoreactive lymphocyte clones to become activated and thus pathogenic. The NOD mouse has low levels of cytokine-rich NK T cells, and transfer of such cells to NOD mice prevents the development of diabetes.[107] Wilson et al. found that NK T cell clones derived from patients with IMD often lacked interleukin-4 and had increased interferon-γ.[108] We find that NK T cells detectable in peripheral blood by antibodies to their restricted $V_{\alpha24}/V_{\beta11}$ T cell receptor are invariably reduced in IMD, as well as in certain otherwise normal persons (unpublished data). Recently, antigen-presenting cells have been shown to play an important role in autoimmune disease, particularly IMD. Antigen-presenting cells, which include dendritic cells, macrophages, and B lymphocytes, are the first cell type to appear in the pancreatic inflammatory process in NOD mice.[109] Furthermore, dendritic cells are abundantly present in progressive human insulitis.[110] It has been indicated in one study that dendritic cells are both phenotypically and functionally impaired in humans at risk for IMD.[111] It has been hypothesized that a defect in dendritic cell function in the thymus in IMD-prone humans reduces the editing of self-reactive T cells or, in the periphery, impairs induction of regulatory T cells to prevent IMD.[111]

Environmental Factors

If environmental precipitators of autoimmunity exist, and they probably do, their identification continues to be elusive. As an environmental factor, virus has long been suspected of being an agent that induces autoimmune disease. The pathogenic effects of virus on autoimmunity could result in a bystander attack on a particular target organ or in molecular mimicry, in which a viral peptide and a peptide of a host protein have immunologic cross-reactivity. Viral infection may also result in an immune response that accelerates an ongoing autoimmune response and eventually precipitates the clinical disease. An infectious trigger of polyglandular autoimmunity has not been reported in human epidemiologic studies. Reovirus type I infection in susceptible mice can cause IMD and growth failure associated with antibodies to the anterior pituitary and pancreatic islets. However, a recent report on the expression of a human endogenous retrovirus (HERVK-10) as a cause of IMD[112] is probably incorrect.[113–115]

Genetics

APS-I is not associated with any class II HLA alleles,[116] but it has been linked to a newly identified gene (*AIRE*) located on chromosome 21. APS-II and APS-III are associated with HLA class II genes with apparently distinctive HLA alleles for each of them. These two latter

syndromes remain to be further defined genetically, especially with respect to their underlying non-HLA genes.

GENETIC STUDIES IN APS-I. APS-I is an autosomal recessive disease with a pattern of inheritance initially derived from analysis of patients with idiopathic Addison's disease and hypoparathyroidism[117] and later reported by others in different racial groups.[12, 63, 118, 119] By allelic association and linkage analysis, a candidate gene was initially mapped to the long arm of chromosome 21 (21q22.3) in 14 Finnish families of patients with APS-I.[14] This gene was later narrowed down to a range of less than 500 kb, around the gene encoding phosphofructokinase of the liver type (PFKL), by linkage analysis and physical mapping in relative homogeneous Finnish and European patients with APS-I,[120, 121] and later in a heterogeneous group of U.S. patients with APS-I.[122] Ultimately, two individual groups identified the responsible gene, *AIRE* (autoimmune regulator), located proximal to the gene for PFKL on the long arm of chromosome 21.[15, 16] The *AIRE* gene consists of 14 exons and encodes a protein with an estimated 545 amino acids that contains two plant homeodomain (PHD) zinc finger motifs, three LXXLL motifs, and a proline-rich region, suggestive of its putative role as a nuclear transcriptional regulator (Fig. 41–2). Multiple mutations have been detected in patients with APS-I and different racial backgrounds, thus indicating that this gene is the disease gene responsible for APS-I.

CHARACTERISTICS OF THE APS-I DISEASE GENE IN PATIENTS WITH APS-I. Nineteen separate mutations in the *AIRE* gene have been detected, either as homozygous or heterozygous forms with different frequencies in APS-I patients of various ethnic backgrounds (see Fig. 41–2). The predicted outcomes for most of the *AIRE* mutations are truncated AIRE proteins in which one or two of its zinc finger motifs are disrupted. This effect is due to the introduction of either a stop codon or a frameshift in the coding gene. However, 4 missense mutations, R15L, L28P, Y90C, and K83E, result in the substitution of a single amino acid in exon 1 or 2. It remains to be confirmed how such missense mutations have a disrupting impact on the function of AIRE protein.

Of 19 separate mutations, 2 are most frequently detected in various racial groups. One is called R257X and is located at exon 6, and the other one is 1094del13 and is located at exon 8 of the *AIRE* gene. The remaining mutations are much less frequent, and some of them have been detected only in a single allele. R257X is a substitution of C for T at amino acid position 257. This substitution results in change of an Arg codon (CCA) to a stop codon (TGA) and would produce a truncated protein with about 256 amino acids.[15] R257X is a dominant mutation in Finnish patients with APS-I and is also frequently present in patients with other ethnic backgrounds, such as in northern Italians, Swiss, British, Germans, New Zealanders, and American whites.[123, 124] 1094del13, a 13-bp deletion at nucleotide positions 1094 to 1106, results in a frameshift to produce a truncated 372–amino acid residue. 1094del13 has been detected in APS-I patients of various ethnic backgrounds.[16, 123–126] We find this form of the *AIRE* gene mutation to be the most common in U.S. patients. In addition, 1094del13 is a dominant *AIRE* gene lesion in British patients with APS-I inasmuch as 74% (17/23) of mutated *AIRE* gene alleles from British patients with APS-I contain this deletion.[126]

Founder effects exist for some genetically isolated populations, as determined by analysis of mutations and haplotypes in patients with polymorphic markers closely associated with the *AIRE* gene locus. Recombination events are less common when two genomic markers are closer, and linkage disequilibrium is thus stronger with polymorphic markers of closely located genes. Therefore, individuals are likely to have common ancestors if they share the same haplotype for polymorphic markers that are in linkage disequilibrium, especially when they arise from genetically isolated populations. Haplotype analysis of polymorphic markers located close to the *AIRE* gene in Finnish patients has suggested that more than 85% of cases of APS-I in Finnish patients are due to one major mutation that is commonly present in the ancestors of the Finnish population.[120] This result is in concordance with the finding that the mutation R257X is present in up to 82% of Finnish patients with APS-I and is accompanied by one predominant haplotype of closely linked polymorphic markers, such as *D21S1912* and *PFKL*.[15, 16] *D21S1912* is located approximately 130

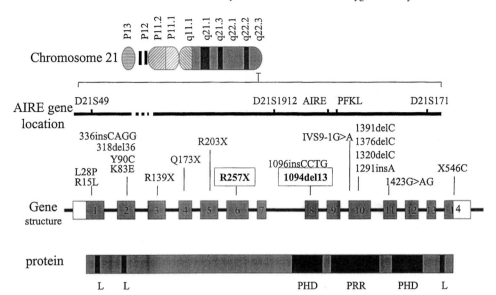

FIGURE 41–2. AIRE gene location, mutations, and characteristics of AIRE protein. The AIRE gene is located on chromosome 21q22.3, close to the gene encoding phosphofructokinase of the liver type (PFKL). R257X and 1094del13 are commonly present in patients with type I autoimmune polyglandular syndrome among the total 19 detected mutations. Two plant homeodomain (PHD) zinc finger motifs, three LXXLL motifs (L), and a proline-rich region (PRR) are present in the AIRE protein. The nomenclature of the mutations was based on the AIRE cDNA sequence (GenBank Accession # AB006682).

kb upstream of the *AIRE* gene, and *PFKL* is located 1.5 kb downstream of the *AIRE* gene.[15, 16] This evidence suggests that R257X occurred as a single mutation event in the relatively homologous Finnish population. Studies of 12 British families with APS-I for *AIRE* gene mutations found that 17 of the 24 possible mutant *AIRE* alleles tested had 1094del13 with a common haplotype spanning the *AIRE* gene locus, which suggests the presence of a founder effect also for the British patients.[126] Similarly, a founder effect may be present in the Sardinian population, which has until recently been a genetically isolated population.[127] Mutation R139X has been found in 90% (18/20) of independent alleles with identical haplotypes for *D21S1912-PFKL* in that ethnic group.[125]

That patients with the same *AIRE* gene mutations often had different closely linked haplotypes suggests that either ancient mutational events or multiple independent events occurred to account for the *AIRE* mutations and haplotypes observed. For example, R257X is also a major mutation present in patients from European countries other than Finland. However, non-Finnish patients with R257X have more diversified haplotypes of *D21S1912-PFKL*.[123] Such is also the case for the other major mutation, 1094del13, inasmuch as different haplotypes are present in patients with different ethnic origins. For example, 9 of 15 alleles of 1094del13 detected in 13 patients from a group of American white patients with APS-I had different *D21S1912-PFKL* haplotypes,[124] thus suggesting that multiple independent events led to the 1094del13 mutation. This result should be expected because the patients were of heterogeneous origins, typical of the North American population. Thus the genetic data are now in hand for diagnosis and genetic counseling in families affected by APS-I.

ROLE OF THE *AIRE* GENE IN THE PATHOGENESIS OF APS-I. An understanding of the biologic role of the AIRE protein should provide needed insight into the mechanism of tolerance and autoimmunity, particularly to APS-I, which displays T cell abnormalities as well as multiple autoimmune endocrinopathies. The *AIRE* gene is well expressed as mRNA in the thymus, as well as in other tissues such as lymph nodes, pancreas, adrenal cortex, and PBMCs.[15, 16] Attention has already been drawn to its nuclear localization and its probable role in transcriptional regulation of the encoded protein based on analysis of the predicted amino acid sequence.[15, 16] The pattern of the two zinc finger motifs in AIRE-1 is similar to the pattern seen in the Mi-2 and TIF1 autoantigens.[128] Mi-2 autoantigen is a 240-kDa human nuclear protein recognized by sera from patients with autoimmune dermatomyositis.[129] The Mi-2 autoantigen is actually a recently identified partial fragment of a chromohelicase DNA (CHD)-binding protein, CHD3.[130] The family of CHD proteins is known to play roles in gene expression and regulation.[130] Also, TIF1 is actively involved in transcriptional control of the estrogen receptor.[126, 129] Accordingly, the *AIRE* gene most likely participates in transcriptional regulation of the expression of another gene(s).

No obvious correlations have been found between mutant genotypes of the *AIRE* gene and clinical phenotypes of APS-I, which suggests that the outcome of the syndrome may be influenced by environmental factors. As mentioned above, the core phenotype of APS-I includes the three diseases mucocutaneous candidiasis, hypoparathyroidism, and Addison's disease. Patients with APS-I also frequently have one or more other autoimmune diseases, such as chronic active hepatitis, alopecia, vitiligo, or evidence of an immunodeficiency state, including chronic diarrhea/malabsorption, chronic mucocutaneous candidiasis, and oropharyngeal carcinomas. Not all patients with APS-I express all three core component diseases or the frequently accompanied diseases. Even patients of the same ethnic origin with the same *AIRE* mutation may have different component diseases of APS-I or a different order of appearance of the component diseases.[123, 125, 126] Different phenotype expressions are also present in affected siblings.

However, specific component diseases may develop in some ethnic groups of patients with APS-I, thus suggesting that the outcome of the syndrome is influenced by background genes within a population. For example, candidiasis is relatively rare in Iranian Jewish patients with APS-I.[119] Also, IMD is rarely seen in patients with APS-I in the United States; however, it does occur in some 15% of Finnish patients with APS-I, especially with increasing age. Finns, however, suffer the world's highest rates of IMD and must have a high gene pool for IMD. Finnish patients with APS-I often have ectodermal and enamel hypoplasia.[63] Calcium deficiency secondary to hypoparathyroidism should not be the primary cause for enamel dystrophy because in Finnish patients, ectodermal and enamel hypoplasia occurs in APS-I patients with or without hypoparathyroidism.[63, 132] In addition, those non-Finnish patients with APS-I who had hypoparathyroidism are seldom seen with enamel hypoplasia.[119, 122] Background genes or genes with epistatic effects may be responsible for variations in the expressed phenotype.[120] Alternatively, more than one gene may be responsible for the development of APS-I, although this possibility is becoming increasingly unlikely. Thus studies on the function of the *AIRE* gene could shed more light on the pathogenic mechanism of APS-I.

GENETIC STUDIES IN APS-II, APS-III. APS-II/III often affects individuals in many generations of the same family, which suggests that APS-II/III is inherited as an autosomal dominant trait with incomplete penetrance.[85, 116, 133] Addison's disease, either as a component disease of APS-II or as an individual disease, is associated with HLA-DR3 and HLA-DR4,[134, 135] but we believe that the HLA-DR4 haplotype, when seen in APS-II, relates to coexisting β cell autoimmunity.[47] However, thyroid autoimmunity in pedigrees with IMD may segregate independently from the HLA complex.[68] DR3-DQB1*0201/DQB1*0302 is associated with APS-II when IMD is present.[136] Such HLA associations suggest that particular molecules of HLA are required for the development of component autoimmune diseases and that the expression of a particular autoimmune phenotype depends on the involvement of these plus other gene products, especially in a multicomponent autoimmune syndrome such as APS-II. Unlike APS-I, the order of appearance of the component diseases of APS-II varies greatly. Individual patients can initially have Addison's disease and, subsequently, IMD and/or autoimmune thyroid disease or any other sequence. This variation could indicate the presence of different pathogenic pathways during the development of APS-II. Thus it might be expected that non-HLA genes plus particular alleles of HLA genes could influence the susceptibility of individual patients to a constellation of diseases. For example, the association of DQB1*0302 with APS-II was abolished in our study when patients with APS-II and overt clinical IMD or positive autoantibodies to islet antigens were excluded from analysis.[47] Also, development of the same disease with different susceptible HLA alleles has been observed in interracial studies of HLA susceptibility.[137] In addition, multigenetic involvement in development of the individual component diseases of APS-II/III has been proved, such as linkage of IMD to more than a dozen loci in non-HLA genomic regions,[138] and autoimmune thyroid disease appears to be polygenic as well.[139–141]

Patients with APS-III lack Addison's disease and definitive genetic features except for their associations with its component diseases and their associated HLA alleles. For example, DQB1*0301 is increased when Hashimoto's thyroiditis is present, DRB1*03 and DRB3 are increased when Graves' disease and/or IMD is present, and DRB1*13 is associated with vitiligo. Non-HLA genes are, however, expected to also be involved in the development of APS-III, and attempts have been made to map for non-HLA genes responsible for the component disease of APS-III. For example, Tomer et al. linked a susceptible locus for Graves' disease to within a 6 centimorgans at the chromosome 20q11.2.[142] Although this susceptible locus is waiting to be confirmed, the finding of a gene for the component disease of APS-III would help in understanding the pathogenesis of the syndrome. The susceptible locus at chromosome 20q11.2 was linked to Graves' disease but not to Hashimoto's thyroiditis. This finding again suggests that the cause of pathogenic autoimmunity may involve different pathogenic processes and that alternative pathways exist for the breakdown in immune system self-tolerance. Thus genetic studies of autoimmune endocrine syndromes should facilitate understanding of the pathogenic process of these diseases, which may be applicable to the component autoimmunities.

CLINICAL SPECTRUM OF AUTOIMMUNE POLYGLANDULAR SYNDROMES

An important responsibility for clinicians managing patients with endocrine gland deficiencies is to consider whether an individual with a single endocrine autoimmunity is at risk for the occurrence of a polyglandular disorder. Clues uncovered by a thorough history and physical examination plus laboratory findings of organ-specific autoantibodies may reveal the true multifocal nature of a patient's condition. Subclinical or "compensated" deficiencies, identified by elevations in tropic hormone levels (e.g., normal thyroxine but elevated thyrotropin in Hashimoto's disease), reflect early gland destruction with initial compensation before overt gland failure with decreases in thyroxine are seen. Once recognized, each individual hormone deficiency should be monitored and treated with the same therapeutic replacement regimens as those used for patients who have isolated gland dysfunction. The authors urge the use of full diagnostic autoantibody panels, followed by monitoring of the function of any targeted organ in all probands with Addison's disease and their immediate relatives. We suggest screening for adrenal autoimmunity in patients with IMD complicated by the presence of circulating thyroid gland autoantibodies. Perhaps all patients with IMD should be screened for 21-OH or adrenocortical autoantibody markers because a missed diagnosis may be unnecessarily fatal.

Type I APS

APS-I is diagnosed when two of the three defining diseases are present (i.e., mucocutaneous candidiasis, hypoparathyroidism, adreno-

cortical insufficiency). The first sign is invariably mucocutaneous candidiasis. Any young person afflicted by troublesome moniliasis should be assessed for a possible T lymphocyte deficiency state and for type I APS as well. In one study, nearly 45% of pediatric patients with refractory monilial infections but no overt underlying T cell defect had an autoimmune endocrinopathy.[143] Of patients with type I APS in whom recurrent monilial infections develop, most have lesions that are restricted to the skin, nails, and oral and perianal mucosa. Although remissions of varying length occur, progressive or relapsing courses are common, and gastrointestinal involvement can become severe, especially when complicated by bacterial overgrowth, chronic diarrhea, or gastrointestinal hemorrhage. Hypoparathyroidism develops in more than 75% of patients with type I APS, usually before 10 years of age. Severe hypocalcemia manifested by carpopedal spasms, seizures, or laryngospasm can be the initial feature of type I APS, especially in young children. Adrenocortical failure typically develops after hypoparathyroidism between the ages of 3 and 30 years. Deficiencies of mineralocorticoids and glucocorticoids usually arise simultaneously, but their onset can be separated by 5 or more years.[63]

Females suffer from gonadal insufficiency more often than males do and usually have maturational arrest after the onset of pubarche or menarche. Autoimmune oophoritis may also be manifested as failed pubertal development or as menstrual irregularities and polycystic ovaries.[144]

Fat malabsorption, which may be episodic, has been linked by some to hypoparathyroidism. More likely causes include IgA deficiency, gluten sensitivity, and bacterial overgrowth of the upper portion of the small bowel. Recently, malabsorption has been found to be linked to autoantibodies to tryptophan hydroxylase and lack of secretion of intestinal endocrine cells.[64] Deficiencies of iron or vitamin B_{12} result from parietal cell autoimmunity, with the subsequent early appearance of achlorhydria followed by intrinsic factor deficiency and pernicious anemia. Typical atrophic gastritis arises in 15% of type I APS cases, with a mean age at onset of 16 years.[63] Studies of Finnish patients have particularly emphasized manifestations of type I APS in the teeth and integument. In decreasing order of frequency, enamel hypoplasia, ungual dystrophy (pitting), keratopathy, and tympanic membrane sclerosis have all been reported at rates from 33% to 77%.[63] Vitiligo may be missed if not specifically sought by ultraviolet light (Wood's lamp examination). Alopecia totalis or universalis is frequent, but all types of alopecia occur. It has been suggested that hair loss may diminish after treatment of hypoparathyroidism is started,[18] but such amelioration does not reflect the authors' experience. The appearance of hepatomegaly or jaundice with dark urine and clay-colored stool often heralds the onset of chronic active hepatitis. It occurs in up to 10% of patients and is not associated with persistent immunologic hypersensitivity to hepatitis viruses. Sjögren's syndrome (parotitis, arthritis, and sicca syndrome) is not infrequent, whereas IMD, chronic thyroiditis, and hypophysitis are distinctly uncommon. We have now seen several patients in whom oropharyngeal carcinomas have developed, a situation sometimes seen in others with chronic defects in T cell immunity or prolonged immunosuppressive therapy.

Type II/III APS

Type II APS is far more common than type I and is diagnosed when a patient has adrenocortical deficiency with combinations of IMD, chronic lymphocytic thyroiditis, and/or pernicious anemia and Graves' disease. Unlike type I APS, this syndrome can be more difficult to recognize before the onset of clinically significant multigland disease. The disease is commonly manifested in the third or fourth decade, but it is not uncommon before or after these ages. It is heralded by adrenocortical failure in almost half the cases, although this estimate may be skewed by a selection bias in the literature. As many as 20 years can elapse before the full extent of the polyglandular involvement becomes evident. Furthermore, isolated thyroiditis and IMD are common enough in these age groups that routine adrenal or 21-OH autoantibody screening of such affected patients is difficult to justify unless adrenocortical insufficiency is clinically suspected. The authors recommend routine thyroid autoantibody screening of all patients with

IMD and adrenal autoantibody testing in those found to be positive. Physicians who wish to test all patients with IMD, however, cannot be faulted. Nevertheless, physicians should routinely elicit historical and physical features relevant to the diagnostic triad in all patients with IMD and/or autoimmune thyroiditis. A family history of polyglandular failure is often present in past generations and can serve as a flag for patients who need extra monitoring. The presence of extra-endocrinologic manifestations such as alopecia or vitiligo is less common than in type I APS, but when such manifestations are present, they are important clinical indicators of widespread autoimmunity, especially if they are profound. The risk of mortality from untreated adrenocortical failure in the 2% of patients with myasthenia gravis in whom associated endocrinopathies develop requires that all such patients younger than 40 years be assessed closely for endocrinologic disorders during their initial investigation.

Type III APS remains to be further characterized. APS-III is notably seen in middle-aged women but can occur at any age. It was defined according to the accompanying autoimmune endocrinopathies, which include autoimmune thyroid diseases and/or IMD, plus one of other autoimmune diseases such as pernicious anemia and vitiligo, but not Addison's disease. It is type II APS without adrenocortical involvement. Once Addison's disease has appeared, such patients are reclassified as having APS-II.

Other Associations with APS

Rare diagnoses have on occasion been reported in association with an APS. The authors and others have monitored patients with type I APS in whom severe, idiopathic, noninflammatory myopathy with eventual respiratory failure developed. Hyposplenism may not be uncommon. Separate reports suggested that pure red cell hypoplasia and male infertility in patients with type I APS responded well to glucocorticoid therapy.[144, 145] In rare cases, neo-osseous porosis and sarcoidosis have been linked to type I and type II APS, respectively.[146, 147] Nephrocalcinosis develops in many patients with APS-I and may be related to vitamin D therapy for hypoparathyroidism. It could be related to antibodies to calcium-sensing receptors on the proximal renal tubules, although this association is speculative.

Differential Diagnosis

The differential diagnosis of APS during the initial assessment varies according to the disease manifested. When evidence of a second autoimmunity is present, consideration should be given to whether the patient has type I or type II/III APS because future monitoring and the prognosis are different for these syndromes. Other diagnostic considerations are summarized in Table 41–4. Chromosomal disorders such as trisomy 21 and Turner's syndrome (45,XO and its genetic variants) are associated with an increased risk of endocrine autoimmunities, especially Hashimoto's thyroiditis (up to 30%) and IMD (approximately 5%).[148, 149] The primary hypogonadism of Turner's syndrome, however, is not of autoimmune origin, and the apparent growth hormone deficiencies in some of these females may resolve after estrogen priming. DiGeorge syndrome is a developmental disorder of the branchial arches that results in facial deformities, aortic arch anomalies, and thymic and parathyroid gland agenesis. Hypoparathyroidism and mucocutaneous candidiasis develop in these patients, with the diagnosis usually made in infancy, and they have few to no circulating T lymphocytes but produce no autoantibodies and Addison's disease never develops. Kearns-Sayre syndrome is a myopathic disease associated with hypoparathyroidism, primary hypogonadism, IMD, and hypopituitarism. Cardiac conduction defects are common, and muscle biopsies are usually diagnostic. Wolfram's syndrome or DIDMOAD (diabetes insipidus, diabetes mellitus, optic atrophy, nerve deafness) is an uncommon congenital condition that occurs in young children. Congenital hypoparathyroidism has been reported to be caused by the biosynthetic effects of parathyroid hormone. Congenital rubella is associated with later onset of IMD and hypothyroidism. The POEMS syndrome (plasma cell dyscrasia with polyneuropathy, organomegaly, endocrinopathy, M protein, and skin changes) occurs mainly in Japanese patients. It is associated with IMD and primary hypogonadism. Thymomas (malignant more so than benign) are associated with myasthenia gravis in up to 50% of cases. They arise most commonly after 40 years of age in myasthenic patients and may be seen in association with Cushing's syndrome, Graves' disease, or Addison's disease.[150] Hemochromatosis is usually manifested as lethargy, malaise, abdominal pain, and hypermelanotic skin lesions. The similarity to Addison's disease can become confusing in patients with either IMD or secondary hypogonadism induced by pancreatic or hypophysial iron deposition. Rarely, thyroid, parathyroid, or adrenocortical insufficiencies have been reported in hemochromatosis. Myotonic dystrophy is associated with primary testicular atrophy, alopecia, and less frequently, diabetes mellitus (usually related to insulin resistance).

Diagnostic Protocols

Three major laboratory approaches are used to diagnose an APS, including serologic test for autoantibodies, function tests for the secretion of organ-specific hormones, and genetic tests for *AIRE* mutations and mutations in HLA-D genes. First, serum screening for autoantibodies is used to (1) verify the autoimmune nature of the disease in patients with polyglandular insufficiency, (2) identify patients affected by an isolated endocrinopathy in whom multiorgan autoimmunity is likely to develop, and (3) screen family members of patients with APS, even if those relatives are currently asymptomatic. A complete screening panel includes assessment of adrenal (21-hydroxylase), steroidal cell (17-OH and P450ssc enzymes), thyroid (peroxidase and thyroglobulin), islet cell (GAD_{65} and IA-2/IA2-β), and parietal cell (H^+,K^+-ATPase) autoantibodies (see Table 41–3). Thyroid-stimulating immunoglobulins may be useful in selected patients. A single negative examination does not rule out the possibility of future disease, and annual to biannual follow-up tests are prudent. The predictive value of a positive result has been presented above.

Second, in autoantibody-positive individuals, assessment of end-organ function is required. Serum levels of thyrotropin, calcium, phosphorus, and fasting glucose determined annually can effectively assess thyroid, parathyroid, and pancreatic islet function of asymptomatic patients. Suspicion of subclinical gland dysfunction should prompt a complete functional evaluation of the suspect gland before determining a final diagnosis. Gonadal dysfunction is diagnosed when random serum gonadotropin levels are elevated in the face of low sex steroid levels.

Although depression of early morning serum cortisol levels and electrolyte disturbances represent changes that occur at or just before the clinical onset of adrenocortical failure, it is best to monitor individuals at high risk for hypoadrenocorticism (those with AAs or SCAs) annually by seeking inappropriate elevations of basal serum ACTH levels (midafternoon or later) and supine (>1 hour) plasma renin

TABLE 41–4. Differential Diagnosis of Autoimmune Polyglandular Syndromes

Type I APS
Type II APS
Type III APS
Thyrogastric autoimmunity
Chromosomal disorder (45X,O; trisomy 21)
Kearns-Sayre syndrome
Congenital rubella
DiGeorge syndrome
Wolfram's syndrome (DIDMOAD)
POEMS
Thymoma
Hemochromatosis
Myotonic dystrophy

APS, autoimmune polyglandular syndrome; DIDMOAD, diabetes insipidus, diabetes mellitus, optic atrophy, and neural deafness; POEMS, polyneuropathy, organomegaly, endocrinopathy, M protein, and skin changes.

activity. To date, the authors have determined no clinically relevant advantage to screening for adrenal gland dysfunction by formal ACTH stimulation testing or plasma renin activity assessment after salt deprivation. In our studies, raised serum ACTH levels beyond early morning indicated that the anterior hypophysis was responding to impending adrenocortical insufficiency and thus warranted follow-up with complete assessment of adrenocortical function.[24]

Annual hemoglobin or hematocrit determinations are essential, with accompanying examination of the blood film for erythrocyte and polymorphonuclear neutrophil morphology. When nutritional deficiencies are suspected, serum levels of ferritin and/or vitamin B_{12} and red cell folate determinations are indicated.

Fat malabsorption in APS may occur for many reasons, some of which are reversed with proper treatment. It is therefore mandatory that fat malabsorption be completely investigated. Stool examination for ova and parasites is helpful for diagnosing *Giardia lamblia* infection, but it may be necessary to obtain duodenal fluid or a jejunal biopsy for direct examination and culture. Bacterial overgrowth can be diagnosed by duodenal aspirates, and a small bowel biopsy is required to diagnose villous atrophy morphologically. Serum IgA levels should also be assessed. Malabsorption/chronic diarrhea is unfortunately refractory to therapy. Antibodies to tryptophan hydroxylase, when present, may indicate absence of intestinal serotonin-containing cells.

Third, *AIRE* gene mutational analyses should be performed in patients with suspected APS-I and in siblings of patients with APS-I, especially those in whom symptoms of component diseases of APS-I have developed. For example, children or adolescents with suspected recurrent mucocutaneous candidal infection that has been refractory to topical medication should have the diagnosis confirmed at least initially by culturing scrapings from the periphery of an affected area. Such patients should be tested for *AIRE* gene mutation to confirm the diagnosis of APS-I. The presence of homozygous *AIRE* gene mutations would indicate the diagnosis of APS-I and may predict development of the component diseases of APS-I. However, failure to detect *AIRE* gene mutations should not exclude a diagnosis of APS-I inasmuch as the known *AIRE* gene mutations are not detected in 10% to 30% of patients with an established diagnosis of APS-I, depending on their racial origin. This observation suggests that defects other than in the *AIRE* gene coding region may have similar effects as *AIRE* gene mutation on the development of APS-I, perhaps through defects in *AIRE* gene regulation.

Therapy

It has already been suggested that the key to successfully managing patients with an APS is to identify and treat their autoimmunities before they cause significant morbidity and mortality. Treatment of organ insufficiency is identical whether it occurs in isolation or as part of an APS. Replacement therapy remains the cornerstone. Patient education about the nature of the disease is often critical to early recognition of new autoimmunities, and as with any chronic disease, individualized needs for psychosocial support must be assessed. Genetic counseling is also warranted, and additional affected family members should be sought by specific tests. Emergency identification should be worn at all times by APS patients, and the use of increased corticosteroid doses at times of acute stress usually averts adrenal crisis in those with Addison's disease. The authors believe that exogenous glucocorticoid supplements given at times of acute stress are well advised in asymptomatic individuals who have biochemical evidence of asymptomatic adrenocortical disease.

Of all the endocrine components of an APS, only IMD does not carry a satisfactory prognosis when managed with well-monitored hormone replacement therapy. The long-term vascular complications have thus made IMD a candidate for aggressive experimental approaches. Results of controlled trials using cyclosporine and azathioprine for treating newly diagnosed IMD have indicated that some metabolic benefits are provided, although they are not often long lived, even with continued immunotherapy.[151, 152] Anecdotal reports of improved orchitis,[153] oophoritis,[154] and hypophysitis[155] after immuno-

suppressive corticosteroid treatment are provocative but require systematic evaluation. For now, all immunomodulating therapies must be considered experimental and should be prescribed only in the setting of a controlled clinical trial. As more autoantigens are identified and the disease pathogenesis becomes better understood, selective antigen-based therapies that do not cause generalized immunosuppression may be developed. The National Institutes of Health is conducting a U.S. IMD prevention trial (DPT-I) using the antigen insulin given orally or as a daily subcutaneous injection. Still further in the future lies the prospect of curative organ transplantation. Pancreatic and, to a lesser extent, islet transplants are currently used in kidney graft recipients with IMD.[156] Adrenal gland transplants have been experimentally successful in rodents[157] and humans.[158]

The introduction of ketoconazole has greatly helped in the treatment of chronic mucocutaneous candidiasis, which is commonly resistant to topical antimicrobials.[159] The drug frequently causes gastrointestinal upset and can interfere with glucocorticoid and sex steroid biosynthesis. Elevations of hepatic transaminases are usually transient, but fatal hepatic necrosis can rarely be caused by ketoconazole.

Management of fat malabsorption should first be aimed at diagnosing and treating reversible causes. Bacterial overgrowth often responds to broad-spectrum oral antibiotics. *G. lamblia* is best treated with quinacrine hydrochloride or metronidazole, and villous atrophy, seen especially in type II APS, typically responds to dietary gluten withdrawal. If no specific cause of fat malabsorption is found, nutritional support with fat-soluble vitamin and medium-chain fatty acid supplements may be required. Such management is best done in consultation with a nutrition or gastroenterology specialist. Unfortunately, in our experience some patients remain refractory to all approaches.

Improved survival for patients with chronic active hepatitis has been achieved with new regimens of immunomodulating agents such as prednisone, cyclosporine, and azathioprine.[156] Tertiary hepatic care is indicated for patients in whom chronic active hepatitis develops.

Prognosis

The impact of an APS on a given patient's life-style varies considerably because of differences in a host of disease-dependent, patient-dependent, family-dependent, and physician-dependent factors. All patients with either type I or type II/III APS are committed to a regimen of lifelong hormone, mineral, and/or vitamin replacement. Although it is usually best to counsel patients to continue participating in all their regular activities, health care providers must be mindful that an APS disease can dramatically alter a patient's life (e.g., an airline pilot in whom IMD develops).

Systematic studies of the long-term prognosis in APS patients are lacking, but clinical impressions are that patients with type II APS have rates of morbidity and mortality that are identical to those of the component diseases when they occur in isolation. Adrenal crises are still a significant cause of preventable mortality, and uncontrolled thyroid hormone imbalances can on rare occasion be emergencies, especially in the elderly. The complications of IMD, both acute and chronic, are as important in the APS setting as in isolated pancreatic disease.

Although many patients in whom type I APS is diagnosed lead a full and vigorous life,[63] poorer outcomes are common. In some, a course of recurrent illness initially develops in their second decade of life. Problems include asthenia, which is often of uncertain etiology; recurrent opportunistic infections, which presumably arise because of a T lymphocyte deficiency; chronic active hepatitis, which continues to be one of the most common causes of mortality in type I APS; and oropharyngeal carcinoma, which can be fatal unless diagnosed early. Mortality near the end of the second or during the third decade is not uncommon.

CONCLUSION

Syndromes of multiorgan failure induced by autoimmunity occur in well-recognized patterns and can be detected at an asymptomatic stage by screening high-risk individuals for circulating autoantibodies. Such autoantibodies are also of diagnostic importance in symptomatic patients. Detection of *AIRE* gene mutations has become a useful indication for the diagnosis of APS-I. Optimal management includes close anticipatory monitoring so that early treatment of organ failure can be instituted, thereby preventing irreversible morbidity or even death, especially for untreated Addison's disease. Currently, treatment is limited to pharmacologic replacement and psychosocial support; however, increases in our understanding of the pathogenesis of these conditions should lead to treatments that will prevent progression to complete end-organ destruction. Over recent years, dramatic progress has been made in the identification of target antigens and epitopes involved in the autoimmune organ-specific diseases that are components of the APSs. Studies of the function of the *AIRE* gene product would promote understanding of the pathogenesis of APS-I and immune tolerance in general. Gene therapies based on the disease gene(s) identified are needed for the eventual cure and prevention of APS.

REFERENCES

1. Addison T: Anaemia: Disease of the suprarenal capsules. Lond Med Gaz 8:517–518, 1849.
2. Claude H, Gourgerot H: Insuffisance pluriglandulaire endocrinienne. J Physiol Pathol Gen 10:469–480, 1908.
3. Hashimoto H: Zur kenntnis der lymphomatosen veranderung der schilddruse (struma lymphatosa). Acta Klin Chir 97:219–248, 1912.
4. Schmidt MB: Eine biglandulare Erkrankung (Nebennieren und Schilddrusse) bei Morbus Addisonii. Verh Dtsch Ges Pathol 21:212–221, 1926.
5. Thorpe ES, Handley HE: Chronic tetany and chronic mycelial stomatitis in a child aged four-and-one-half years. Am J Dis Child 38:328–338, 1929.
6. von Meyenburg H: Uber "Insulitis" bei diabetes. Schweitz Med Wochenschr 71:554–557, 1940.
7. Whitaker J, Landing BH, Esselborn VM, Williams RR: The syndrome of familial juvenile hypoadrenocorticism, hypoparathyroidism and superficial moniliasis. J Clin Endocrinol 16:1374–1387, 1956.
8. Roitt IM, Doniach D, Campbell PN, Hudson RV: Autoantibodies in Hashimoto's disease (lymphadenoid goitre). Lancet 2:820–821, 1956.
9. Rose NR, Witebsky E: Studies on organ specificity: V. Changes in the thyroid gland of rabbits following active immunization with rabbit thyroid extracts. J Immunol 76:417–427, 1956.
10. Holborow EJ, Brown PC, Roitt IM, Doniach D: Cytoplasmic location of "complement-fixing" auto-antigen in human thyroid epithelium. Br J Pathol 40:583–588, 1959.
11. Carpenter CCJ, Solomon N, Silverberg SG, et al: Schmidt's syndrome (thyroid and adrenal insufficiency): A review of the literature and a report of fifteen new cases including ten instances of coexistent diabetes mellitus. Medicine (Baltimore) 43:153–180, 1964.
12. Neufeld M, Maclaren N, Blizzard R: Autoimmune polyglandular syndromes. Pediatr Ann 9:154–162, 1980.
13. Neufeld M, Maclaren NK, Blizzard RM: Two types of autoimmune Addison's disease associated with different polyglandular autoimmune (PGA) syndromes. Medicine (Baltimore) 60:355–362, 1981.
14. Aaltonen J, Bjorses P, Sandkuijl L, et al: An autosomal locus causing autoimmune disease: Autoimmune polyglandular disease type I assigned to chromosome 21. Nat Genet 8:83–87, 1994.
15. Nagamine K, Peterson P, Scott HS, et al: Positional cloning of the APECED gene. Nat Genet 17:393–398, 1997.
16. The Finnish-German APECED Consortium: An autoimmune disease, APECED, caused by mutations in a novel gene featuring two PHD-type zinc-finger domains. Nat Genet 17:399–403, 1997.
17. Blizzard RM, Kyle MA: Studies of the adrenal antigens and antibodies in Addison's disease. J Clin Invest 42:1653–1660, 1963.
18. Brun JM: Juvenile autoimmune polyendocrinopathy. Horm Res 16:308–316, 1982.
19. Maclaren NK, Riley WJ: Autoimmune endocrinopathies. In Samter M, Talmage DW, Frank MM, et al (eds): Immunological Diseases of the Endocrine System. Boston, Little, Brown, 1988, pp 1737–1764.
20. Peterson P, Krohn KJ: Mapping of B cell epitopes on steroid 17 alpha-hydroxylase, an autoantigen in autoimmune polyglandular syndrome type I. Clin Exp Immunol 98:104–109, 1994.
21. Peterson P, Uibo R, Peranen J, Krohn K: Immunoprecipitation of steroidogenic enzyme autoantigens with autoimmune polyglandular syndrome type I (APS-1) sera; further evidence for independent humoral immunity to P450c17 and p450c21. Clin Exp Immunol 107:335–340, 1997.
22. Riley WJ, Maclaren NK, Krischer J, et al: A prospective study of the development of diabetes in relatives of patients with insulin-dependent diabetes. N Engl J Med 323:1167–1172, 1990.
23. Elder M, Maclaren N, Riley W: Gonadal autoantibodies in patients with hypogonadism and/or Addison's disease. J Clin Endocrinol Metab 52:1137–1142, 1981.
24. Ketchum CH, Riley WJ, Maclaren NK: Adrenal dysfunction in asymptomatic patients with adrenocortical autoantibodies. J Clin Endocrinol Metab 58:1166–1170, 1984.
25. Betterle C, Scalici C, Presotto F, et al: The natural history of adrenal function in autoimmune patients with adrenal autoantibodies. J Endocrinol 117:467–475, 1988.
26. Leisti S, Ahonen P, Perheentupa J: The diagnosis and staging of hypocortisolism in progressing autoimmune adrenalitis. Pediatr Res 17:861–867, 1983.
27. Scherbaum WA: Autoimmune hypothalamic diabetes insipidus. Prog Brain Res 93:283–292, 1992.
28. Bigazzi PE: Autoimmunity of the adrenals. In Volpe R (ed): Autoimmunity and Endocrine Disease. New York, Marcel Dekker, 1985, pp 345–373.
29. Ahonen P, Miettinen A, Perheentupa J: Adrenal and steroidal cell antibodies in patients with autoimmune polyglandular disease type I and risk of adrenocortical and ovarian failure. J Clin Endocrinol Metab 64:494–500, 1987.
30. Betterle C, Volpato M, Rees Smith B, et al: Adrenal cortex and steroid 21-hydroxylase autoantibodies in adult patients with organ-specific autoimmune diseases: Markers of low progression to clinical Addison's disease. J Clin Endocrinol Metab 82:932–938, 1997.
31. Krohn K, Uibo R, Aavik E, et al: Identification by molecular cloning of an autoantigen associated with Addison's disease as steroid 17α-hydroxylase. Lancet 339:770–773, 1992.
32. Winqvist O, Karlsson F, Kampe O: 21-Hydroxylase, a major autoantigen in idiopathic Addison's disease. Lancet 339:1559–1562, 1992.
33. Baumann-Antczak A, Wedlock N, Bednarek J, et al: Autoimmune Addison's disease and 21-hydroxylase. Lancet 340:429–430, 1992.
34. Bednarek J, Furmaniak J, Wedlock N, et al: Steroid 21-hydroxylase is a major autoantigen involved in adult onset autoimmune Addison's disease. FEBS Lett 309:51–55, 1992.
35. Falorni A, Nikoshkov A, Laureti S, et al: High diagnostic accuracy for idiopathic Addison's disease with a sensitive radiobinding assay for autoantibodies against recombinant human 21-hydroxylase. J Clin Endocrinol Metab 80:2752–2755, 1995.
36. Chen S, Sawicka J, Betterle C, et al: Autoantibodies to steroidogenic enzymes in autoimmune polyglandular syndrome, Addison's disease, and premature ovarian failure. J Clin Endocrinol Metab 81:1871–1876, 1996.
37. Tanaka H, Perez MS, Powell M, et al: Steroid 21-hydroxylase autoantibodies: Measurements with a new immunoprecipitation assay. J Clin Endocrinol Metab 82:1440–1446, 1997.
38. Winqvist O, Gustafsson J, Rorsman F, et al: Two different cytochrome P450 enzymes are the adrenal antigens in autoimmune polyendocrine syndrome type I and Addison's disease. J Clin Invest 92:2377–2385, 1993.
39. Seissler J, Schott M, Steinbrenner H, et al: Autoantibodies to adrenal cytochrome P450 antigens in isolated Addison's disease and autoimmune polyendocrine syndrome type II. Exp Clin Endocrinol Diabetes 107:208–213, 1999.
40. Wedlock N, Asawa T, Baumann-Antczak A, et al: Autoimmune Addison's disease. Analysis of autoantibody binding sites on human steroid 21-hydroxylase. FEBS Lett 332:123–126, 1993.
41. Volpato M, Prentice L, Chen S, et al: A study of the epitopes on steroid 21-hydroxylase recognized by autoantibodies in patients with or without Addison's disease. Clin Exp Immunol 111:422–428, 1998.
42. Asawa T, Wedlock N, Baumann-Antczak A, et al: Naturally occurring mutations in human steroid 21-hydroxylase influence adrenal autoantibody binding. J Clin Endocrinol Metab 79:372–376, 1994.
43. Song YH, Connor E, Li Y, et al: The role of tyrosinase in autoimmune vitiligo. Lancet 344:1049–1052, 1994.
44. Brewer KW, Parziale VS, Eisenbarth GS: Screening patients with insulin-dependent diabetes mellitus for adrenal insufficiency. N Engl J Med 337:202, 1997.
45. Riley WJ, Maclaren NK, Neufeld M: Adrenal autoantibodies and Addison disease in insulin-dependent diabetes mellitus. J Pediatr 97:191–195, 1980.
46. Betterle C, Volpato M, Rees Smith B, et al: Adrenal cortex and steroid 21-hydroxylase autoantibodies in adult patients with organ-specific autoimmune diseases: Markers of low progression to clinical Addison's disease. J Clin Endocrinol Metab 82:932–938, 1997.
47. Huang W, Connor E, Rosa TD, et al: Although DR3-DQB1*0201 may be associated with multiple component diseases of the autoimmune polyglandular syndromes, the human leukocyte antigen DR4-DQB1*0302 haplotype is implicated only in beta-cell autoimmunity. J Clin Endocrinol Metab 81:2559–2563, 1996.
48. Peterson P, Salmi H, Hyoty H, et al: Steroid 21-hydroxylase autoantibodies in insulin-dependent diabetes mellitus. Childhood Diabetes in Finland (DiMe) Study Group. Clin Immunol Immunopathol 82:37–42, 1997.
49. Uibo R, Aavik E, Peterson P, et al: Autoantibodies to cytochrome P450scc, P450c17, and P450c21 in autoimmune polyglandular disease types I and II and in isolated Addison's disease. J Clin Endocrinol Metab 78:323–328, 1994.
50. McNatty KP, Short RV, Barnes EW, Irvine WJ: The cytotoxic effect of serum from patients with Addison's disease and autoimmune ovarian failure on human granulosa cells in culture. Clin Exp Immunol 22:378–384, 1975.
51. Furmaniak J, Talbot D, Reinwein D, et al: Immunoprecipitation of human adrenal microsomal antigen. FEBS Lett 231:25–28, 1988.
52. Boscaro M, Betterle C, Volpato M, et al: Hormonal responses during various phases of autoimmune adrenal failure: No evidence for 21-hydroxylase enzyme activity inhibition in vivo. J Clin Endocrinol Metab 81:2801–2804, 1996.
53. Blizzard RM, Chee D, Davis W: The incidence of parathyroid and other antibodies in the sera of patients with idiopathic hypoparathyroidism. Clin Exp Immunol 1:119–128, 1966.
54. Chapman CK, Bradwell AR, Dykks PW: Do parathyroid and adrenal autoantibodies coexist? J Clin Pathol 39:813–814, 1986.
55. Betterle C, Caretto A, Zeviani M, et al: Demonstration and characterization of anti-human mitochondria autoantibodies in idiopathic hypoparathyroidism and in other conditions. Clin Exp Immunol 62:353–360, 1985.
56. Fattorossi A, Aurbach GD, Sakaguchi K, et al: Anti-endothelial cell antibodies: Detection and characterization in sera from patients with autoimmune hypoparathyroidism. Proc Natl Acad Sci U S A 85:4015–4019, 1988.
57. Li Y, Song YH, Rais N, et al: Autoantibodies to the extracellular domain of the calcium sensing receptor in patients with acquired hypoparathyroidism. J Clin Invest 97:910–914, 1996.
58. Velloso LA, Winqvist O, Gustafsson J, et al: Autoantibodies against a novel 51 kDa

islet antigen and glutamate decarboxylase isoforms in autoimmune polyendocrine syndrome type I. Diabetologia 37:61–69, 1994.

59. Tuomi T, Bjorses P, Falorni A, et al: Antibodies to glutamic acid decarboxylase in autoimmune polyendocrine syndrome type 1. J Clin Endocrinol Metab 82:147–150, 1997.

60. Solimena M, Folli F, Aparisi R, et al: Autoantibodies to GABA-ergic neurons and pancreatic beta cells in stiff-man syndrome. N Engl J Med 322:1555–1560, 1990.

61. Tuomi T, Rowley MJ, Knowles WJ, et al: Autoantigenic properties of native and denatured glutamic acid decarboxylase: Evidence for a conformational epitope. Clin Immunol Immunopathol 71:53–59, 1994.

62. Elrehewy M, Kong YM, Giraldo AA, Rose NR: Syngeneic thyroglobulin is immunogenic in good responder mice. Eur J Immunol 11:146–151, 1981.

63. Ahonen P, Myllärniemi S, Sipilä I, et al: Clinical variation of autoimmune polyendocrinopathy–candidiasis–ectodermal dystrophy (APECED) in a series of 68 patients. N Engl J Med 322:1829–1836, 1990.

64. Ekwall O, Hedstrand H, Grimelius L, et al: Identification of tryptophan hydroxylase as an intestinal autoantigen. Lancet 352:279–283, 1998.

65. Dieterich W, Ehnis T, Bauer M, et al: Identification of tissue transglutaminase as the autoantigen of celiac disease. Nat Med 3:797–801, 1997.

66. Picarelli A, Maiuri L, Frate A, et al: Production of antiendomysial antibodies after in-vitro gliadin challenge of small intestine biopsy samples from patients with coeliac disease. Lancet 348:1065–1067, 1996.

67. Maki M: Coeliac disease and autoimmunity due to unmasking of cryptic epitopes? Lancet 348:1046–1047, 1996.

68. Maclaren NK, Riley WJ: Thyroid, gastric, and adrenal autoimmunities associated with insulin-dependent diabetes mellitus. Diabetes Care 8(suppl 1):34–38, 1985.

69. Loveridge N, Bitensky L, Chayen J, et al: Inhibition of parietal cell function by human gammaglobulin containing gastric parietal cell antibodies. Clin Exp Immunol 41:264–270, 1980.

70. Tanaka N, Glass GBJ: Effect of prolonged administration of parietal cell antibodies from patients with atrophic gastritis and pernicious anemia on the parietal cell mass and hydrochloric acid output in rats. Gastroenterology 58:482–494, 1970.

71. Burman P, Mardh S, Norberg L, Karlsson FA: Parietal cell antibodies in pernicious anemia inhibit H^+, K^+-adenosine triphosphatase, the proton pump of the stomach. Gastroenterology 96:1434–1438, 1989.

72. Betterle C, Mirakian R, Doniach D, et al: Antibodies to melanocytes in vitiligo. Lancet 1:159, 1984.

73. Song YH, Connor E, Li Y, et al: The role of tyrosinase in autoimmune vitiligo. Lancet 344:1049–1052, 1994.

74. Baharav E, Merimski O, Shoenfeld Y, et al: Tyrosinase as an autoantigen in patients with vitiligo. Clin Exp Immunol 105:84–88, 1996.

75. Xie Z, Chen D, Jiao D, Bystryn JC: Vitiligo antibodies are not directed to tyrosinase. Arch Dermatol 135:417–422, 1999.

76. Visseren MJ, van Elsas A, van der Voort EI, et al: CTL specific for the tyrosinase autoantigen can be induced from healthy donor blood to lyse melanoma cells. J Immunol 154:3991–3998, 1995.

77. Overwijk WW, Lee DS, Surman DR, et al: Vaccination with a recombinant vaccinia virus encoding a "self" antigen induces autoimmune vitiligo and tumor cell destruction in mice: Requirement for CD4(+) T lymphocytes. Proc Natl Acad Sci U S A 96:2982–2987, 1999.

78. Austin LM, Boissy RE: Mammalian tyrosinase-related protein-1 is recognized by autoantibodies from vitiliginous Smyth chickens. An avian model for human vitiligo. Am J Pathol 146:1529–1541, 1995.

79. Bottazzo GF, Pouplard A, Florin-Christensen A, Doniach D: Autoantibodies to prolactin-secreting cells of human pituitary. Lancet 2:97–101, 1975.

80. Cosman F, Kalmon DP, Holub DA, Wardlaw SL: Lymphocytic hypophysitis: Report of 3 new cases and review of the literature. Medicine (Baltimore) 68:240–256, 1989.

81. Komatsu M, Kondo T, Yamauchi K, et al: Antipituitary antibodies in patients with the primary empty sella syndrome. J Clin Endocrinol Metab 67:633–638, 1988.

82. Wilkin TJ: Receptor autoimmunity in endocrine disorders. N Engl J Med 323:1318–1324, 1990.

83. Manns MP: Recent developments in autoimmune liver diseases. J Gastroenterol Hepatol 12(suppl):256–271, 1997.

84. Arulanantham K, Dwyer JM, Genel M: Evidence for defective immunoregulation in the syndrome of familial candidiasis endocrinopathy. N Engl J Med 300:164–168, 1979.

85. Eisenbarth GS, Wilson PN, Ward F, et al: The polyglandular failure syndrome: Disease inheritance, HLA-type, and immune function studies in patients and families. Ann Intern Med 91:528–533, 1979.

86. Volpe R: Immunology of human thyroid disease. In Volpe R (ed): Autoimmune Diseases of the Endocrine System. Boca Raton, FL, CRC Press, 1990, pp 73–239.

87. Brenner O: Addison's disease with atrophy of the cortex of the suprarenals. Q J Med 22:121–144, 1928.

88. Gloor E, Hurlimann J: Autoimmune oophoritis. Am J Clin Pathol 81:105–109, 1984.

89. Sedmak DD, Hart WR, Tubbs RR: Autoimmune oophoritis: A histopathologic study of involved ovaries with immunologic characterization of the mononuclear cell infiltrate. Int J Gynecol Pathol 6:73–81, 1987.

90. Bottazzo GF, Dean BM, McNally JM, et al: In situ characterization of autoimmune phenomena and expression of HLA molecules in the pancreas in diabetic insulitis. N Engl J Med 313:353–360, 1985.

91. Foulis AK, Liddle CN, Farquharson MA, et al: The histopathology of the pancreas in type I (insulin-dependent) diabetes mellitus: A 25-year review of deaths in patients under 20 years of age in the United Kingdom. Diabetologia 29:267–274, 1986.

92. Muir A, Schatz DA, Maclaren NK: Autoimmune Addison's disease. In Bach JF (ed): Immunoendocrinology: Seminars in Immunopathology, vol 14. New York, Springer-Verlag, 1993, pp 275–284.

93. Craig JM, Schiff LH, Boone JE: Chronic moniliasis associated with Addison's disease. Am J Dis Child 89:669–684, 1955.

94. Roitt IM, Doniach D: Gastric autoimmunity. In Miescher PA, Müller-Eberhard HJ (eds): Textbook of Immunopathology. New York, Grune & Stratton, 1976, pp 737–749.

95. Muir A, Maclaren NK: Autoimmune diseases of the adrenal glands, parathyroid glands, gonads, and hypothalamic-pituitary axis. Endocrinol Metab Clin North Am 20:619–644, 1991.

96. Berman MA, Sandborg CI, Wang Z, et al: Decreased IL-4 production in new onset type I insulin-dependent diabetes mellitus. J Immunol 157:4690–4696, 1996.

97. Kallmann BA, Huther M, Tubes M, et al: Systemic bias of cytokine production toward cell-mediated immune regulation in IDDM and toward humoral immunity in Graves' disease. Diabetes 46:237–243, 1997.

98. Aguayo J, Sakatsume Y, Jamieson C, et al: Nontoxic nodular goiter and papillary carcinoma of the thyroid gland are not associated with peripheral blood lymphocyte sensitization to thyroid cells. J Clin Endocrinol Metab 68:145–149, 1989.

99. Jarpe AJ, Hickman MR, Anderson JT, et al: Flow cytometric enumeration of mononuclear cell populations infiltrating the islets of Langerhans in prediabetic NOD mice: Development of a model of autoimmune insulitis for type I diabetes. Reg Immunol 3:305–307, 1991.

100. Yoon JW, Yoon CS, Lim HW, et al: Control of autoimmune diabetes in NOD mice by GAD expression or suppression in beta cells. Science 284:1183–1187, 1999.

101. Davies TF, Martin A, Concepcion ES, et al: Evidence of limited variability of antigen receptors on intrathyroidal T cells in autoimmune thyroid disease. N Engl J Med 325:238–244, 1991.

102. Campbell IL, Harrison LC: Molecular pathology of type I diabetes. Mol Biol Med 7:299–309, 1990.

103. Bottazzo GF, Todd I, Rirakian R, et al: Organ-specific autoimmunity: A 1986 overview. Immunol Rev 94:137–169, 1986.

104. Bagnasco M, Caretto A, Olive D, et al: Expression of intercellular adhesion molecule-1 (ICAM-1) on thyroid epithelial cells in Hashimoto's thyroiditis but not in Graves' disease or papillary thyroid cancer. Clin Exp Immunol 83:309–313, 1991.

105. Campbell IL, Cutri A, Wilkinson D, et al: Intercellular adhesion molecule-1 is induced on endocrine islet cells by cytokines but not by reovirus infection. Proc Natl Acad Sci U S A 86:4282–4286, 1989.

106. Kirkpatrick CH: Transfer factor. CRC Crit Rev Clin Lab Sci 12:87–122, 1980.

107. Baxter AG, Kinder SJ, Hammond KJ, et al: Association between $\alpha\beta TCR^+CD4^-CD8^-$ T-cell deficiency and IDDM in NOD/Lt mice. Diabetes 46:572–582, 1997.

108. Wilson SB, Kent SC, Patton KT, et al: Extreme Th1 bias of invariant $V\alpha24J\alpha Q$ T cells in type 1 diabetes. Nature 391:177–181, 1998.

109. Rosmalen JG, Leenen PJ, Katz JD, et al: Dendritic cells in the autoimmune insulitis in NOD mouse models of diabetes. Adv Exp Med Biol 417:291–294, 1997.

110. Jansen A, Voorbij HA, Jeucken PH, et al: An immunohistochemical study on organized lymphoid cell infiltrates in fetal and neonatal pancreases. A comparison with similar infiltrates found in the pancreas of a diabetic infant. Autoimmunity 15:31–38, 1993.

111. Takahashi K, Honeyman MC, Harrison LC: Impaired yield, phenotype, and function of monocyte-derived dendritic cells in humans at risk for insulin-dependent diabetes. J Immunol 161:2629–2635, 1998.

112. Conrad B, Weissmahr RN, Boni J, et al: A human endogenous retroviral superantigen as candidate autoimmune gene in type I diabetes. Cell 90:303–313, 1997.

113. Lan M, Mason A, Coutant R, et al: HERV-K10s and immune-mediated (type 1) diabetes. Cell 95:14–16, 1998.

114. Lower R, Tonjes RR, Boller K, et al: Development of insulin-dependent diabetes mellitus does not depend on specific expression of the human endogenous retrovirus HERV-K. Cell 95:11–14, 1998.

115. Murphy VJ, Harrison LC, Rudert WA, et al: Retroviral superantigens and type 1 diabetes mellitus. Cell 95:9–11, 1998.

116. Maclaren NK, Riley WJ: Inherited susceptibility to autoimmune Addison's disease is linked to human leukocyte antigens-DR3 and/or DR4, except when associated with type I autoimmune polyglandular syndrome. J Clin Endocrinol Metab 62:455–459, 1986.

117. Spinner MW, Blizzard RM, Childs B: Clinical and genetic heterogeneity in idiopathic Addison's disease and hypoparathyroidism. J Clin Endocrinol Metab 28:795–804, 1968.

118. Ahonen P: Autoimmune polyendocrinopathy–candidosis–ectodermal dystrophy (APECED): Autosomal recessive inheritance. Clin Genet 27:535–542, 1985.

119. Zlotogora J, Shapiro MS: Polyglandular autoimmune syndrome type I among Iranian Jews. J Med Genet 29:824–826, 1992.

120. Bjorses P, Aaltonen J, Vikman A, et al: Genetic homogeneity of autoimmune polyglandular disease type I. Am J Hum Genet 59:879–886, 1996.

121. Aaltonen J, Horelli-Kuitunen N, Fan JB, et al: High-resolution physical and transcriptional mapping of the autoimmune polyendocrinopathy–candidiasis–ectodermal dystrophy locus on chromosome 21q22.3 by FISH. Genome Res 7:820–829, 1997.

122. Chen QY, Lan MS, She JX, Maclaren NK: The gene responsible for autoimmune polyglandular syndrome type 1 maps to chromosome 21q22.3 in US patients. J Autoimmun 11:177–183, 1998.

123. Scott HS, Heino M, Peterson P, et al: Common mutations in autoimmune polyendocrinopathy–candidiasis–ectodermal dystrophy patients of different origins. Mol Endocrinol 12:1112–1119, 1998.

124. Heino M, Scott HS, Chen Q, et al: Mutation analyses of North American APS-1 patients. Hum Mutat 13:69–74, 1999.

125. Rosatelli MC, Meloni A, Meloni A, et al: A common mutation in Sardinian autoimmune polyendocrinopathy–candidiasis–ectodermal dystrophy patients. Hum Genet 103:428–434, 1998.

126. Pearce SH, Cheetham T, Imrie H, et al: A common and recurrent 13-bp deletion in the autoimmune regulator gene in British kindreds with autoimmune polyendocrinopathy type 1. Am J Hum Genet 63:1675–1684, 1998.

127. Cavalli-Sforza LL, Menozzi P, Piazza A: The History and Geography of Human Genes. Princeton, NJ, Princeton University Press, 1994.

128. Thenot S, Henriquet C, Rochefort H, Cavailles V: Differential interaction of nuclear receptors with the putative human transcriptional coactivator hTIF1. J Biol Chem 272:12062–12068, 1997.

129. Ge Q, Nilasena DS, O'Brien CA, et al: Molecular analysis of a major antigenic region of the 240-kD protein of Mi-2 autoantigen. J Clin Invest 96:1730–1737, 1995.

130. Woodage T, Basrai MA, Baxevanis AD, et al: Characterization of the CHD family of proteins. Proc Natl Acad Sci U S A 94:11472–11477, 1997.

131. Le Douarin B, Zechel C, Garnier JM, et al: The N-terminal part of TIF1, a putative mediator of the ligand-dependent activation function (AF-2) of nuclear receptors, is fused to B-raf in the oncogenic protein T18. EMBO J 14:2020–2033, 1995.

132. Lukinmaa PL, Waltimo J, Pirinen S: Polyendocrinopathy–candidiasis–ectodermal dystrophy (APECED): Report of three cases. J Craniofac Genet Dev Biol 16:174–181, 1996.

133. Butler MG, Hodes ME, Conneally PM, et al: Linkage analysis in a large kindred with autosomal dominant transmission of polyglandular autoimmune disease type II (Schmidt syndrome). Am J Med Genet 18:61–65, 1984.

134. Santamaria P, Barbosa JJ, Lindstrom AL, et al: HLA-DQB1–associated susceptibility that distinguishes Hashimoto's thyroiditis from Graves' disease in type I diabetic patients. J Clin Endocrinol Metab 78:878–883, 1994.

135. Tamai H, Kimura A, Dong RP, et al: Resistance to autoimmune thyroid disease is associated with HLA-DQ. J Clin Endocrinol Metab 78:94–97, 1994.

136. Boehm BO, Manfras B, Seidl S, et al: The HLA-DQ beta non–Asp-57 allele: A predictor of future insulin-dependent diabetes mellitus in patients with autoimmune Addison's disease. Tissue Antigens 37:130–132, 1991.

137. She JX: Susceptibility to type I diabetes: HLA-DQ and DR revisited. Immunol Today 17:323–329, 1996.

138. Todd JA: Genetics of type 1 diabetes. Pathol Biol (Paris) 45:219–227, 1997.

139. Yanagawa T, Hidaka Y, Guimaraes V, et al: CTLA-4 gene polymorphism associated with Graves' disease in a Caucasian population. J Clin Endocrinol Metab 80:41–45, 1995.

140. Donner H, Rau H, Walfish PG, et al: CTLA4 alanine-17 confers genetic susceptibility to Graves' disease and to type 1 diabetes mellitus. J Clin Endocrinol Metab 82:143–146, 1997.

141. Sale MM, Akamizu T, Howard TD, et al: Association of autoimmune thyroid disease with a microsatellite marker for the thyrotropin receptor gene and CTLA-4 in a Japanese population. Proc Assoc Am Physicians 109:453–461, 1997.

142. Tomer Y, Barbesino G, Greenberg DA, et al: Linkage analysis of candidate genes in autoimmune thyroid disease. III. Detailed analysis of chromosome 14 localizes Graves' disease-1 (GD-1) close to multinodular goiter-1 (MNG-1). International Consortium for the Genetics of Autoimmune Thyroid Disease. J Clin Endocrinol Metab 83:4321–4327, 1998.

143. Herrod HG: Chronic mucocutaneous candidiasis in childhood and complications of non-*Candida* infection: A report of the pediatric immunodeficiency collaborative study group. Pediatrics 116:377–382, 1990.

144. Mandel M, Etzioni A, Theodor R, Passwell JH: Pure red cell hypoplasia associated with polyglandular autoimmune syndrome type I. Isr J Med Sci 25:138–141, 1989.

145. Tsatsoulis A, Shalet SM: Antisperm autoantibodies in the polyglandular autoimmunity (PGA) syndrome type I: Response to cyclical steroid therapy. Clin Endocrinol 35:299–303, 1991.

146. Vela BS, Dorin RI, Hartshorne MF: Case report 631: Neo-osseous porosis (metaphyseal osteopenia) in polyglandular autoimmune (Schmidt) syndrome. Skeletal Radiol 19:468–471, 1990.

147. Walz B, From GL: Addison's disease and sarcoidosis: Unusual frequency of coexisting hypothyroidism (Schmidt's syndrome). Am J Med 89:692–693, 1990.

148. Jones KL: Smith's Recognizable Patterns of Human Malformation, ed 4. Philadelphia, WB Saunders, 1988, pp 74–79.

149. Hall JG, Gilchrist DM: Turner syndrome and its variants. Pediatr Clin North Am 37:1421–1440, 1990.

150. Engel EG: Myasthenia gravis and other disorders of neuromuscular transmission. *In* Braunwald E, Isselbacher KJ, Petersdorf RG, et al (eds): Harrison's Principles of Internal Medicine. New York, McGraw-Hill, 1987, pp 2079–2082.

151. Silverstein J, Maclaren N, Riley W, et al: Immunosuppression with azathioprine and prednisone in recent onset insulin dependent diabetes mellitus. N Engl J Med 319:599–604, 1988.

152. Martin S, Schernthaner G, Nerup J, et al: Follow up of cyclosporin A treatment in type I (insulin dependent) diabetes mellitus: Lack of long-term effects. Diabetalogia 34:429–434, 1991.

153. Tsatsoulis A, Shalet SM: Antisperm autoantibodies in the polyglandular autoimmunity (PGA) syndrome type I: Response to cyclical steroid therapy. Clin Endocrinol 35:299–303, 1991.

154. Rabinowe SL, Berger M, Welch WR, Dluhy RG: Lymphocyte dysfunction in autoimmune oophoritis. Resumption of menses with corticosteroids. Am J Med 81:347–350, 1986.

155. Mayfield RK, Levine JH, Gordon C, et al: Lymphoid adenohypophysitis presenting as a pituitary tumour. Am J Med 69:619–623, 1980.

156. Sutherland DER: Current status of pancreas transplantation. J Clin Endocrinol Metab 73:461–463, 1991.

157. Ricordi C, Lacy PE, Santiago JV, et al: Transplantation of parathyroid, adrenal cortex and adrenal medulla using procedures which successfully prolonged islet allograft survival. Horm Metab Res Suppl 25:132–135, 1990.

158. Yu XC, Yu TL, Zhang SZ, et al: Homotransplantation of adrenal gland. Chin Med J (Engl) 104:487–490, 1991.

159. Stravinoha MW, Soloway RD: Current therapy of chronic liver disease. Drugs 39:814–840, 1990.

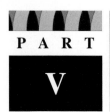

PART V

Obesity, Anorexia Nervosa, and Nutrition in Endocrinology

Editor: John C. Marshall

Chapter 42

Appetite Regulation

Stephen L. Lin ▪ John F. Wilber

PEPTIDES INVOLVED IN TASTE
 PERCEPTION
GASTROINTESTINAL FACTORS INVOLVED
 IN POSTPRANDIAL SATIETY

HYPOTHALAMIC PEPTIDES INVOLVED IN
 STIMULATING THE EXPRESSION OF
 APPETITE

HYPOTHALAMIC PEPTIDES INVOLVED IN
 INHIBITING FEEDING BEHAVIOR
LONG-TERM REGULATION OF ADIPOSE
 TISSUE MASS

Obesity is the oldest and most common metabolic disease in humans. Approximately 30% of Americans suffer from obesity, and the problem is increasing rapidly. Moreover, the cost of dietary programs, special foods, and drugs added together reaches a staggering $100 billion annually in the United States alone. To understand the pathophysiology of obesity, a thorough understanding of appetite regulation is required because obesity ultimately results from an excess of energy intake over energy expenditure.

Assimilation of nutrients in humans involves a homeostatic system with both acute and chronic components. The size, frequency, and composition of meals are regulated day to day by a neuroendocrine peptidergic system integrated in the hypothalamus, primarily in the paraventricular nucleus (PVN). Additional features of the acute system of appetite control include peripheral elements involving taste and temperature perception and gastric and intestinal hormonal satiety factors. The central nervous system integrates these hormonal, thermal, and metabolic signals (Fig. 42–1). Embracing a longer time frame, humoral forces, most importantly leptin, modulate long-term total body adiposity through feedback interactions with the hypothalamic hormonal system of anorexigenic and orexigenic peptides. In humans, hereditary, social, psychological, and cultural factors are particularly important in the regulation of food consumption, and the ultimate pleasures of culinary activities may decompensate these physiologic systems designed to achieve satietal restraint.

PEPTIDES INVOLVED IN TASTE PERCEPTION

Located in the oral cavity are receptors that recognize the taste, texture, and temperature of ingested foods, and taste plays an important role in the selection of foods. Three peptides are particularly important in taste perception. Substance P has been found in fibers innervating taste buds in the tongue. When released from this area by capsaicin, substance P reduces the intake of either water or saline when compared with solutions containing saccharin, sucrose, or quinine.[1] Cholecystokinin (CCK) modulates taste preferences through the gastrointestinal tract in addition to its satietal actions. In rats and monkeys, the suppressive effects of CCK on food intake are positively correlated with the amount of sham feeding through open gastric fistulas, which implies a pregastric effect of CCK on food intake. This particular effect of CCK, in contrast to its satiety properties, involves changes in the taste qualities of substances ingested.[2, 3] Finally, opioid peptides appear to participate in taste perception. This function of opioids has been corroborated by showing that naltrexone, an opioid receptor

antagonist, lowers the intake of highly palatable diets in rodents, whereas naloxone, another opioid receptor antagonist, lowers the ingestion of saccharin-flavored fluids.[1]

GASTROINTESTINAL FACTORS INVOLVED IN POSTPRANDIAL SATIETY

Because animals with open gastric fistulas feed longer than normally and exhibit a marked reduction in feeding behavior when small quantities of nutrients are introduced into the duodenum, a search for humoral factors originating from the gastrointestinal tract yielded the hormone CCK in the pioneering work of Gibbs and colleagues.[4] A large body of literature has now documented the peripheral satiety effects of CCK. Secretin, gastrin, and gastric inhibitory peptide, in contrast, exhibit no appetite-lowering actions. Moreover, suppression of eating by CCK is not accompanied by signs of toxicity or nausea, but rather by behavioral patterns characteristic of satiety. CCK has subsequently been administered in a number of feeding paradigms to many experimental models, including mice, monkeys, and humans. The universal finding has been that subsequent meal sizes are reduced. That these actions of CCK depend on the integrity of vagal afferent projections indicates that initiation of CCK action is peripheral to the central nervous system. Moreover, the role of endogenous CCK in appetite control has been reinforced by the demonstration that administration of foodstuffs that can stimulate the release of CCK, such as the amino acid phenylalanine, results in diminution of food intake in rats and monkeys. Finally, administration of the C-terminal octapeptide of CCK to normal and obese humans decreases food intake.

The possibility that CCK also causes satiety by acting in the central nervous system has been suggested by the demonstration that CCK type B receptors predominate in the brain in the tractus solitarius and the area postrema. However, because vagotomy preempts CCK effects, it is clear that the gastrointestinal tract is the key locus for CCK actions. Moreover, CCK does not cross the blood-brain barrier,[5] which constitutes strong evidence against an important central action of gut-derived CCK.[3, 6]

Other factors of gastrointestinal origin that have some satiety properties include somatostatin, glucagon, calcitonin, bombesin, its mammalian counterpart gastrin-releasing peptide, and neuromedin C. Peptides that cause appetite inhibition through vagal mechanisms, like CCK, include somatostatin and glucagon. The role of these peptides in human obesity, in contrast to that of CCK, is currently speculative.

Finally, several metabolites, including glucose, glycerol, free fatty

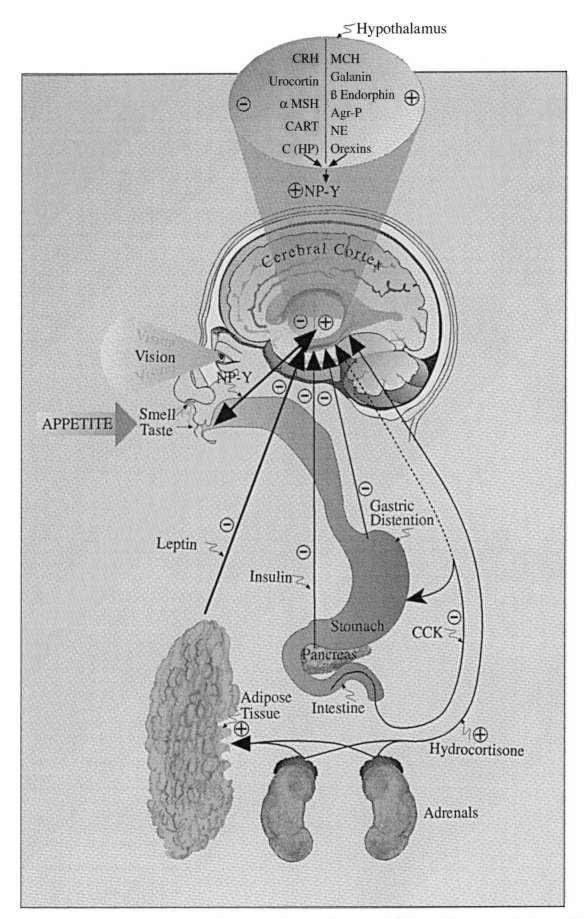

FIGURE 42–1. A model of appetite regulation. Meal size, frequency, and composition are controlled acutely by a neuroendocrine peptidergic system in the hypothalamus, as projected in the cone above. Inhibitory peptides are designated by a *minus sign*, and stimulatory peptides are designated by a *plus sign*. Over a longer time frame, leptin from adipocytes modulates total-body adiposity by negative feedback at hypothalamic nuclei. Additional negative signals from the periphery include insulin, cholecystokinin, and gastric distention. Hydrocortisone stimulates appetite centrally. Sensory inputs such as vision, smell, and taste play a large role in determining the quality and quantity of food intake.

TABLE 42–1. Appetite Stimulatory Factors

Neuropeptide Y
Galanin
Melanin-concentrating hormone
Agouti-related protein
Glucocorticoids
Norepinephrine
Orexins/hypocretins

acids, ketones, and certain amino acids, can modulate feeding behavior as well.

HYPOTHALAMIC PEPTIDES INVOLVED IN STIMULATING THE EXPRESSION OF APPETITE

Regulation of appetite through hypothalamic mechanisms contributes importantly to the maintenance of energy homeostasis and body weight around a set-point. Hypothalamic peptides involved in modifying feeding behavior can be divided into stimulatory and inhibitory groups (Table 42–1). The most important peptide in promoting food intake and energy storage is neuropeptide Y (NPY), which is synthesized and released from neurons in the arcuate (ARC) nucleus. Secretion of NPY, moreover, is negatively regulated by prevailing levels of insulin and leptin, very important in the feedback regulation of energy homeostasis, discussed below. Direct administration of NPY into the hypothalamus stimulates food intake and concomitantly lowers energy expenditure. Chronic NPY administration is a highly effective mechanism for causing obesity in experimental models. The intrinsic NPY pathway in the hypothalamus is stimulated when animals have been subjected to food deprivation, intensive exercise, or lactation or have diabetes mellitus.[7] This intrinsic activation of NPY appears to be a consequence of low levels of insulin and leptin and elevated levels of glucocorticoids.[8]

Four other peptides and a catecholamine appear to play roles as anabolic forces in food intake, including galanin (GAL), melanin-concentrating hormone (MCH), and norepinephrine (NE), which act in concert with NPY to stimulate feeding behavior to reverse reductions in body mass.

GAL, a 29–amino acid peptide, has been shown to stimulate feeding in satiated rodents when injected into the cerebral ventricles or hypothalamus. GAL may exert its effects through mediation of NPY-induced feeding[9] or by stimulating endorphin release, which also stimulates feeding.[10] These effects of GAL are short lived, however, when compared with those of NPY. Other evidence suggests that NE may mediate some of its effects or act in concert with GAL. Injections of GAL into the PVN cause a substantial rise in NE levels while stimulating appetite, and GAL coexists in neurons that innervate the PVN from the medulla and the dorsal pons. NE injections themselves stimulate appetite, and when α-adrenergic antagonists are injected into the PVN, feeding is no longer stimulated by GAL. Also, inhibition of catecholamine synthesis blunts the effects of GAL on appetite stimulation.[11] The question arises that if NE and GAL have the same effect, why would they be co-expressed in the same neuron? One possibility is that NE preferentially stimulates carbohydrate ingestion, whereas GAL preferentially stimulates fat intake. GAL may act through suppression of dopamine release to preferentially stimulate fat ingestion.[12] GAL has also been shown to suppress release of cortisol and insulin, two hormones implicated in the stimulation of carbohydrate intake.[13, 14] Therefore, the overall role of GAL may be to shift feeding behavior from carbohydrates to fat ingestion.

The 19–amino acid peptide MCH also exhibits a stimulatory effect on feeding. Its mechanism of action parallels the NPY pathway in several respects in that MCH augments ongoing feeding, fasting stimulates MCH gene expression, and MCH mRNA transcripts are increased in genetically obese ob/ob mice.[15]

AgrP is an MC4 receptor antagonist, and it causes the obesity syndrome in lethal agouti mice by interrupting anorexigenic signaling by α-MSH through MC4 receptors.[20] AgrP is localized in cells in the ARC, like NPY. Because some of these cells project to the PVN, the simultaneous release of NPY and AgrP stimulates appetite directly, as well as indirectly by decreasing the inhibitory influences of α-MSH.

Recently, a new class of orexigenic peptides, the hypocretins, has been demonstrated by two laboratories.[16, 17] Hypocretin I and II are located in the dorsal and lateral hypothalamic areas. These peptides, however, are much less potent than NPY in stimulating food intake, and much higher amounts of orexins are required than these other feeding signals, including GAL, MCH, and NPY, to elicit significant stimulation of feeding. The potential role of hypocretins in feeding behavior in humans is not presently known.

HYPOTHALAMIC PEPTIDES INVOLVED IN INHIBITING FEEDING BEHAVIOR

A number of peptides, in contrast to NPY, inhibit feeding behavior (Table 42–2). These peptides include corticotropin-releasing hormone (CRH) and α-melanocyte–stimulating hormone (α-MSH), derived from the larger prohormone proopiomelanocortin.

Central injection of CRH in rodents induces anorexia and simultaneously stimulates energy expenditure. These effects can occur at low amounts of administered peptide, on the order of 10^{-10} M. Microinjection studies indicate that the site of anorexic action of CRH lies within the PVN, probably mediated by two receptors, CRH-R1 and CRH-R2. The CRH antagonist α-helical CRH can attenuate the anorexic effects of CRH injected into the PVN. Moreover, food deprivation associated with weight loss is accompanied by reduced hypothalamic CRH gene expression in laboratory rodents. Conversely, when weight gain is induced by nutrient administration to rats in quantities exceeding energy requirements, CRH gene expression is increased, a response identical to that after the administration of leptin into the hypothalamus (see below). These observations indicate that in rodents, overfeeding and weight gain lead to negative feedback by leptin secretion from adipocytes, which stimulates the CRH pathway, causes a reduction in food intake and enhanced energy expenditure, and activates the loss of excess body weight.[7] Urocortin, a recently described member of the CRH family that shares 45% homology with CRH, is even more potent than CRH in suppressing feeding behavior.[18, 19]

α-MSH may be more important than CRH in negatively regulating appetite. α-MSH is synthesized from hypothalamic neurons adjacent to those that synthesize NPY, and its action is initiated by binding to the MC4 receptor. Importantly, animals deficient in the MC4 receptor become severely obese, thus indicating that α-MSH signaling is a critical moiety in body weight homeostasis.[20]

Additional peptides that have the ability to inhibit appetite include glucagon-like peptide-1 (GLP-1), the agouti-related protein (AgrP), the histidyl proline diketopiperazine cyclo-(His-Pro) (C[HP]), and the cocaine- and amphetamine-related transcript (CART).

GLP-1 is present in the central nervous system, like many gastrointestinal peptides, and the hypothalamus is extensively innervated by tracts originating from neurons in the caudal portion of the nucleus of the solitarius tract.[21, 22] Moreover, feeding in fasted animals can be inhibited by the administration of GLP-1 centrally, and this blockage can be reversed by administration of the GLP-1 receptor antagonist exendin.[23-25] Further support for a physiologic role of GLP-1 as an anorexic mediator is strengthened by observations that exendin can

TABLE 42–2. Appetite Inhibitory Factors

Corticotropin-releasing hormone
Urocortin
Cyclo-(His-Pro)
Glucagon-like peptide-1
α-Melanocyte–stimulating hormone
Leptin
Cholecystokinin
Cocaine- and amphetamine-related transcript

activate feeding in fed rats and daily administration of exendin leads to augmentation of food intake and body weight.[24] Kalra and colleagues moreover report that one of the sites of GLP-1 action is the PVN, where GLP immunoreactive fibers terminate and where exendin can block GLP-1–induced activation of cFos.[7]

Our laboratory has been studying the potential role of the novel dipeptide C(HP) derived from thyrotropin-releasing hormone by partial proteolysis. This small molecule exhibits long-lasting appetite suppression when administered intracerebroventricularly and undergoes hypothalamic concentration fluctuations with feeding and fasting. C(HP) can induce sustained inhibition of weight gain in rodents when administered centrally by an Alzet osmotic pump over a 2-week period. The highest concentrations of C(HP) are localized to the PVN, and the elevated levels of C(HP) while fasting, which are rapidly restored to normal after refeeding, are compatible with the concept that during fasting C(HP) secretion is inhibited and C(HP) release is then activated during refeeding to participate in generating satiety. This peptide has been shown by our group to be ubiquitously present in the human brain, and the highest concentrations are in the hypothalamic PVN. Of particular note, C(HP) is completely resistant to enzymatic proteolysis, and administration of this peptide even orally to laboratory rodents can inhibit appetite via the central nervous system and cause weight loss over a 2-week interval.[26]

Finally, CART is a neuropeptide that inhibits feeding in rodents. CART mRNA has been found in the lateral zone of the hypothalamus (LH) and dorsomedial nucleus, as well as in the PVN and ARC, the two most important sites implicated in appetite regulation. CART is believed to play roles in leptin and NPY signaling. Leptin-deficient ob/ob mice have decreased CART levels in the LH and ARC, and when these mice are administered leptin, CART levels are normalized in the ARC and increase in the LH. Moreover, after 24 to 48 hours of fasting, rats also show a decrease in ARC CART mRNA levels. Given the locations of CART mRNA in the brain, it has been proposed that CART affects NPY signaling. Central administration of CART suppressed feeding in both normal rats and rats whose appetite had been stimulated by NPY. The physiologic importance of CART in normal feeding is underscored by the increased feeding of rodents after the administration of specific anti-CART sera.[7, 27]

LONG-TERM REGULATION OF ADIPOSE TISSUE MASS

Several hormones participate over a longer temporal frame in a feedback system to ensure equilibrium between energy intake and energy expenditure. The most important of these hormones is leptin, a 167–amino acid protein synthesized exclusively in white fat adipocytes (Table 42–3). Cloning of this protein, encoded by the obesity (*ob*) gene in adipocytes, has lent considerable strength to the idea that adipose tissue provides an appetite-lowering signal(s) to the hypothalamus in a negative-feedback system for adipose tissue homeostasis. Administration of leptin to the ob/ob, leptin-deficient mouse results in complete reversal of all the abnormal phenotypic features, including

obesity, hyperphagia, hyperlipidemia, diabetes mellitus, insulin resistance, and hypothermia. Receptor mRNA for the leptin receptor (ob-RbmRNA) is strongly expressed in the ARC, PVN, ventromedial nucleus, and LH. Microinjection of leptin into the ARC, the most sensitive site, inhibits food intake in rodents and simultaneously stimulates energy expenditure in brown fat. It is of interest that the db/db mouse, which has a mutation in the leptin receptor that renders it leptin resistant, exhibits a phenotype identical to that of the ob/ob mouse. Expression of the leptin gene is strongly enhanced by insulin, glucocorticoids, and estrogens and is reduced by adrenergic agonists and probably androgens as well.[2, 8, 28]

Levels of circulating leptin in humans are proportional to total body fat mass, are pulsatile, and are characterized by a circadian rhythm with a nocturnal peak. Levels are higher in women than in men. Basal levels occur during the late AM hours, and leptin levels then rise progressively until the early morning, followed by a gradual decline to baseline.[29] This diurnal rhythm is preserved in obese subjects, but at a higher concentration of circulating leptin. During periods of weight loss, plasma leptin concentrations decline and mRNA expression of the leptin gene is lowered in adipose tissue. The reductions in plasma leptin levels are of sufficient magnitude to activate hyperphagia and decreased energy expenditure and are often associated with infertility in rodents. This connection between total body fat and fertility has suggested the concept that leptin functions to optimize total body fat for full reproductive capability. In rodents at least, leptin resistance may be due to structural abnormalities in the leptin receptor or defective transport of leptin across the blood-brain barrier. Another possibility is a defect in signal transduction, as evidenced by the lethal yellow mouse mutant. These mice show elevated mRNA levels of suppressor of cytokine signaling protein-3 (SOC-3), a cytokine-inducible inhibitor that can block leptin signal transduction in a mammalian cell line.[30]

The most important link between adipose tissue–derived peripheral leptin and the hypothalamic appetite integrating centers is NPY. NPY is synthesized in the ARC and projected to the PVN. Importantly, NPY expression is activated by reductions in circulating leptin in states of food deprivation and weight loss. Concomitantly, CRH and MSH release is inhibited. This configuration decreases satiety and brown fat energy expenditure, stimulates food intake, and may also modulate responses to gastric expansion and CCK from the peripheral gut satiety system. The net result is augmented caloric intake to reestablish normal adipose tissue mass. Whether other anorexigenic peptides are also suppressed is under study.[31]

The exact role of leptin in the pathophysiology of human obesity is not yet understood fully. Although a few human subjects have been documented to have single mutations in the *LEP* gene leading to the ob/ob phenotype in humans, most obese humans have elevated plasma leptin concentrations and appear to be leptin resistant.

Deficiency of leptin has been identified in two children from a highly consanguineous lineage; these children have very low circulating leptin levels because of a congenital mutation in the leptin gene. When born, the children were phenotypically normal, including normal body weight, but thereafter they exhibited hyperphagia, impaired satiety, and the development of obesity by 3 to 4 months of age. Both children were homozygous for a single guanine nucleotide mutation in codon 133 of the leptin reacting frame, which resulted in 14 aberrant amino acids after glycine 132 in leptin, followed by a premature stop codon, which renders the leptin protein biologically inactive. The course of these children paralleled that of ob/ob mice in most respects. However, these children have not yet exhibited the stunting of linear growth characteristic of ob/ob mice.[31] Other salient features of affected humans include a normal serum cortisol level (ob/ob mice, in contrast, have elevated corticosterone concentrations), slightly elevated thyroid-stimulating hormone levels (ob/ob mice do not consistently have thyroid abnormalities), and an elevated fasting insulin level in the older child (similar to ob/ob mice). These phenotypic discrepancies may reflect interspecies differences in the physiologic role of leptin, the small number of patients available for study, or the lack of maturity of these prepubertal children.

Finally, these new insights into appetite and fat mass regulation have implications for the pharmacotherapy of obesity. It is probable that the appetite-controlling center(s) in the central nervous system,

TABLE 42–3. Cardinal Features of Leptin

167–amino acid protein product of the *ob* gene in rats (*LEP* gene in humans)

Serum half-life ≈ 90 min

Circadian rhythm of secretion, with basal level in late AM and peak level in early AM

Produced exclusively in adipocytes; levels proportional to fat mass

Leptin deficiency leads to hyperphagia and obesity in both rodents and humans

Leptin resistance: characteristic of human obesity and may contribute to obesity

Leptin-specific receptor is present in many tissues, including adipose tissue, lungs, kidneys, muscle, and brain

Interacts with other appetite regulatory factors, e.g., glucocorticoids, insulin, neuropeptide Y, corticotropin-releasing hormone, androgens, estrogens, and norepinephrine

regulated dynamically by many and redundant mediators around an "adipostat set-point," will ultimately respond best to rectifying abnormal central regulatory mechanisms rather than to intervention at a single point with an anorexigenic peptide or an antagonist of an orexigenic agent. Pharmacotherapy for either prevention or treatment of obesity in the near term will probably improve greatly but remain adjunctive to the classic and keystone roles of caloric restriction and augmented exercise.

REFERENCES

1. Wilber JF: Regulation of appetite by peptides and monoamines. *In* DeGroot LJ (ed): Endocrinology, vol 3, ed 2. Philadelphia, WB Saunders, 1990.
2. Rosenbaum M, Leibel RL, Hirsch J: Obesity. N Engl J Med 337:396–407, 1997.
3. Lee MC, Schiffman SS, Pappas TN: Role of neuropeptides in the regulation of feeding behavior: A review of cholecystokinin, bombesin, neuropeptide Y, and galanin. Neurosci Biobehav Rev 18:313–323, 1994.
4. Gibbs J, Young RC, Smith GP: Cholecystokinin decreases food intake in rats. J Comp Physiol Psychol 84:488–495, 1973.
5. Oldendorf WH: Blood-brain barrier permeability to peptides: Pitfalls in measurement. Peptides 2(suppl 2):109–111, 1981.
6. Morley JE: Neuropeptide regulation of appetite and weight. Endocr Rev 8:256–287, 1987.
7. Kalra SP, Dube MG, Pu S, et al: Interacting appetite-regulating pathways in the hypothalamic regulation of body weight. Endocr Rev 20:68–100, 1999.
8. Schwartz MW: Regulation of appetite and body weight. Hosp Pract 32:109–119, 1997.
9. Kalra SP: Appetite and body weight regulation: Is it all in the brain? Neuron 19:227–230, 1997.
10. Horvath TL, Kalra SP, Naftolin F, Leranth C: Morphological evidence for a galanin-opiate interaction in the rat mediobasal hypothalamus. J Neuroendocrinol 7:579–588, 1995.
11. Kyrkouli SE, Stanley BG, Hutchinson R, et al: Peptide-amine interactions in the hypothalamic paraventricular nucleus: Analysis of galanin and neuropeptide Y in relation to feeding. Brain Res 521:185–191, 1990.
12. Tempel DL, Leibowitz KJ, Leibowitz SF: Effects of PVN galanin on macronutrient selection. Peptides 9:309–314, 1988.
13. Tempel DL, Leibowitz SF: Diurnal variations in the feeding responses to norepinephrine, neuropeptide Y and galanin in the PVN. Brain Res Bull 25:821–825, 1990.
14. Tempel DL, Leibowitz SF: Galanin inhibits insulin and corticosterone release after injection into the PVN. Brain Res 536:353–357, 1990.
15. Qu D, Ludwig DS, Gammeltoft S, et al: A role for melanin-concentrating hormone in the central regulation of feeding behavior. Nature 380:243–247, 1996.
16. de Lecea L, Kilduff TS, Peyron C, et al: The hypocretins: Hypothalamic-specific peptide with neuroexcitatory activity. Proc Natl Acad Sci U S A 95:322–327, 1998.
17. Sakurai T, Amemiya A, Ishii M, et al: Orexins and orexin receptors: A family of hypothalamic neuropeptides and G protein–coupled receptors that regulate feeding behavior. Cell 92:573–585, 1998.
18. Vaughan J, Donaldson C, Bittencourt J, et al: Urocortin, a mammalian neuropeptide related to fish urotensin I and to corticotropin-releasing factor. Nature 378:287–292, 1995.
19. Spina M, Merlo-Pich E, Chan RK, et al: Appetite-suppressing effects of urocortin, a CRF-related neuropeptide. Science 273:1561–1564, 1996.
20. Huszar D, Lynch CA, Fairchild-Huntress V, et al: Targeted disruption of the melanocortin-4 receptor results in obesity in mice. Cell 88:131–141, 1997.
21. Shimizu I, Hirota C, Obhboshi C, Shima K: Identification and characterization of glucagon-like peptide 17–36 amide binding site in the rat brain and lung. FEBS Lett 241:209–212, 1987.
22. Fehmann HC, Goke R, Goke B: Cell and molecular biology of the incretin hormones glucagon-like peptide-I and glucose-dependent insulin releasing polypeptide. Endocr Rev 16:390–410, 1995.
23. Lambert PD, Wilding JPH, Ghatei MA, Bloom SR: A role for GLP-1 (7–36) NH$_2$ in the central control of feeding behavior. Digestion 54:360–361, 1993.
24. Turton MD, O'Shea D, Gunn IN, et al: A role for glucagon-like peptide-1 in the central regulation of feeding. Nature 379:69–72, 1996.
25. Tang-Christensen M, Larsen PJ, Goke R, et al: Central administration of GLP-1-(7–36) amide inhibits food and water intake in rats. Am J Physiol 271:R848–R856, 1996.
26. Wilber JF: Unpublished observation.
27. Kristensen P, Judge ME, Thim L, et al: Hypothalamic CART is a new anorectic peptide regulated by leptin. Nature 393:72–76, 1998.
28. Bray GA, York DA: Leptin and clinical medicine: A new piece in the puzzle of obesity. J Clin Endocrinol Metab 82:2771–2776, 1997.
29. Saladin R, De Vos P, Guerre-Millo M, et al: Transient increase in obese gene expression after food intake or insulin administration. Nature 377:527–529, 1995.
30. Bjorback C, Elmquist JK, Frantz JD, et al: Identification of SOCS-3 as a potential mediator of central leptin resistance. Mol Cell 1:619–625, 1998.
31. Montague CT, Farooqi IS, Whitehead JP, et al: Congenital leptin deficiency is associated with severe early-onset obesity in humans. Nature 387:903–908, 1997.

Chapter 43

▲▲▲▲
Leptin

Rexford S. Ahima ▪ Jeffrey S. Flier

HISTORICAL BACKGROUND

Leptin is an adipocyte-derived hormone discovered through positional cloning of the *ob* gene by Friedman and colleagues in 1994.[1] The discovery of leptin has revolutionized our understanding of nutritional physiology inasmuch as leptin appears to serve a critical link between energy stores and neural networks in the brain involved in the regulation of appetite and energy expenditure.[2–4] In addition, leptin has been recognized to have other roles through effects on regulation of the neuroendocrine axis, immune function, hematopoiesis, endothelial proliferation, and brain development.[2–9] In this chapter we will highlight the major advances leading to our current understanding of the role of leptin as an integrative hormone in these diverse systems.

Two areas of particular historic relevance to leptin are (1) the discovery of *ob/ob* and *db/db* mice and (2) investigations into the physiologic regulation of body weight. More than two decades ago researchers at the Jackson Laboratories discovered recessive mutations in mice, *obese (ob/ob)* and *diabetes (db/db)*, both of which caused syndromes of hyperphagia, decreased energy expenditure, morbid obesity, insulin resistance, and neuroendocrine abnormalities, including hypercorticism and infertility.[10, 11] Subsequently, cross-circulation (parabiosis) experiments carried out by Coleman suggested that the *ob* gene encoded or was necessary for the production of a humoral factor that decreased appetite and increased metabolism whereas the *db* gene encoded a receptor for this factor or was in some other way necessary for reception of this signal.[12] Although Coleman's idea of a circulating satiety factor eventually proved to be correct, it is noteworthy that the studies were viewed with skepticism over the ensuing decades until recent cloning of the *ob* and *db* genes. This skepticism may be partly due to the fact that parabiosis experiments are inherently difficult to perform and interpret. Furthermore, the source of the putative circulating satiety factor was not evident, although adipose tissue was considered likely.

Research carried out about three decades ago by Kennedy, Cahill, Sims, Horton, and other investigators laid the foundation for our current understanding of the physiology of energy balance.[13–16] A detailed discussion of this subject is beyond the scope of this chapter, but it is important to note that studies in humans, rodents, and other mammals over the years have produced compelling evidence in support of a homeostatic mechanism designed to resist pertubations in energy balance.[16, 17] Changes in energy stores, such as from starvation or forced overfeeding, have been shown to result in compensatory changes in voluntary feeding and energy expenditure.[16] The net effect of these adaptations is to restore body weight to a presumed "set point." What was missing until the discovery of leptin was the demonstration of a mechanism for sensing changes in nutritional status and a determination of how such a regulatory mechanism might interact with effector organs such as the brain to maintain energy balance. Expression of the adipose-derived hormone leptin serves both as a sensor of energy and as a signal to hypothalamic targets involved in the regulation of appetite and metabolism.

THE *ob* AND *db* GENES

The *ob* gene was isolated by positional cloning and shown to be expressed as a 4.5-kb mRNA transcript in adipose tissue.[1] Recent studies have also demonstrated *ob* gene expression in placenta, murine fetal tissue, gastric fundic mucosa, and skeletal muscle.[1, 18–21] The *ob* gene encodes a 167–amino acid secreted protein that is unique in the database.[1] At the time of its discovery, ob protein was predicted to act as an afferent hormone signal in a negative feedback loop to regulate adipose mass. In agreement with this hypothesis, injection of recombinant ob protein was shown to decrease body weight and adiposity in *ob/ob* and wild-type mice, but not in *db/db* mice lacking functional receptors for the hormone.[22–24] Based on its ability to cause marked weight reduction, the product of the *ob* gene was named "leptin" (from the Greek root "leptos," meaning thin).[22] The two available strains of *ob/ob* mice each have mutations in the *ob* gene. The more widely studied strain C57Bl/6J*ob/ob* has a C-to-T substitution resulting in a stop codon instead of arginine at position 105, which leads to a truncated protein lacking biologic activity that is subject to intracellular degradation.[1, 25] The truncated protein is not secreted, and *ob* mRNA expression is increased in adipose tissue in this mutant, consistent with the view that expression of the *ob* gene is under negative feedback regulation. The other mutant, *ob²ʲ/ob²ʲ*, has a transposon insertion in the first intron of the *ob* gene that prevents the synthesis of mature ob mRNA.[1] Both *ob/ob* mutants are leptin deficient, hyperphagic, and morbidly obese and manifest similar metabolic and neuroendocrine abnormalities.[4]

Although the *ob* gene has been linked to severe obesity in some family studies, mutations in the coding sequence of the *ob* gene are extremely rare in humans.[26, 27] The first cases of morbid childhood obesity resulting from a frameshift mutation in the *ob* gene were described in two cousins from a highly consanguineous Pakistani family in 1997.[28] In these patients, a single guanine nucleotide deletion in codon 133 resulted in a frameshift mutation, encoding of 14 aberrant amino acids, and a premature stop codon. This alteration results in the synthesis of a truncated leptin protein (14 kDa) incapable of being secreted that undergoes intracellular degradation.[25] A missense mutation (C to T) of codon 105 of the *ob* gene causing morbid obesity was reported in three members of a Turkish family.[29] Leptin deficiency leads to hyperphagia, morbid obesity, and central hypogonadism in humans, as it does in rodents. However, unlike *ob/ob* mice, hypercorticism, severe hyperinsulinemia, diabetes, and hypothermia have as yet not been described in leptin-deficient humans.[28–30]

The leptin receptor (Ob-R) was first isolated by expression cloning from mouse choroid plexus by Tartaglia et al. in 1995.[31] It belongs to the family of class 1 cytokine receptors and includes receptors for interleukin-6, leukemia inhibitory factor, granulocyte-colony stimulating factor, and gp130 and has high affinity (nanomolar range) for leptin.[31, 32] Multiple splice variants of Ob-R mRNA encoding at least six different leptin receptor isoforms have been identified[33, 34] (Fig. 43–1). All Ob-R isoforms share an identical extracellular ligand-binding domain at the N terminus but differ at the C terminus. Five isoforms, Ob-Ra, Ob-Rb, Ob-Rc, Ob-Rd, and Ob-Rf, have transmembrane domains; however, only Ob-Rb (the long receptor isoform) contains all the intracellular motifs required for activation of the JAK/STAT (Janus kinase/signal transducers and activators of transcription) signal transduction pathway.[32, 35–37] Ob-Re, which lacks a transmembrane domain, is secreted and circulates as a soluble receptor.

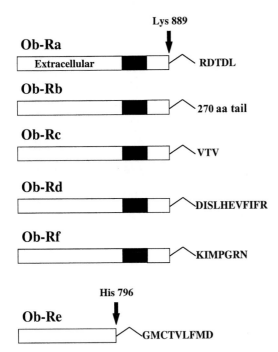

FIGURE 43–1. Domain structure of alternatively sliced leptin receptor (Ob-R) isoforms. Five isoforms, Ob-Ra, Ob-Rb, Ob-Rc, Ob-Rd, and Ob-Re, have been identified in mice and Ob-Rf in rats. Truncation sites are denoted by *arrows*. Ob-R isoforms share a common extracellular (leptin) binding domain but differ at the C terminus (intracellular domain). Terminal amino acid (aa) residues for various Ob-R isoforms are denoted by the alphabet code. Only Ob-Rb, the long isoform, has all intracellular protein motifs necessary for signaling via the JAK/STAT (Janus Kinase/signal transducer and activator of transcription) signal transduction pathway. Ob-Re lacks a transmembrane domain (TM) and circulates as a soluble receptor. (Data from Tartaglia,[32] Lee et al.,[33] Wang et al.,[34] and Chua et al.[35])

As predicted by parabiosis experiments two decades ago, Ob-R mutations lead to obesity in rodents and humans.[12, 33, 35–40] In C57Bl/Ks*db/db* mice, a mutation that results in the insertion of a premature stop codon in the 3′ end of the Ob-Rb mRNA transcript leads to a receptor lacking the intracytoplasmic domain required for signaling through the JAK/STAT pathway.[35] The *db/db* mutation causes hyperphagia, metabolic derangement, and morbid obesity, as in *ob/ob* mice; however, unlike the latter, *db/db* mice do not respond to leptin treatment.[22–24] Other strains of *db/db* mice, such as *db^Pas^/db^Pas^* and *db^3J^/db^3J^*, lack the transmembrane and intracytoplasmic motifs and are phenotypically similar to C57Bl/Ks*db/db* mice.[38] Ob-R defects are also responsible for obesity in *fa/fa* and Koletsky rats. A single amino acid substitution (Gln to Pro) at position 269 of the extracellular domain decreases cell surface expression of Ob-R in obese *fa/fa* rats and also decreases binding affinity and the capacity for signal transduction.[35, 41, 42] *fa/fa* rats are reported to have the capacity to respond to inhibition of food intake by high doses of leptin administered intracerebroventricularly.[43] Obese Koletsky rats have a point mutation at amino acid position 763 that results in a stop codon in the extracellular domain of Ob-R.[39, 44] As would be expected, this mutation leads to a lack of all surface leptin receptors, obesity, and insensitivity to leptin action.[35, 44] Taken together, the above studies in rodents have established that the intracytoplasmic domain of Ob-Rb is critical to regulation of appetite and body weight by leptin. As with mutations of the *ob/ob* gene, Ob-R mutations are extremely rare in humans. Clement et al. described the first cases of human obesity with a mutation resulting in deletions of the intracellular and transmembrane domains of Ob-R in a French family of Kabilian origin in 1998.[40] Three sisters who were homozygous for the mutation had early-onset obesity, impaired linear growth, and hypothalamic amenorrhea. The results of provocative hormone testing were consistent with impairment of growth hormone and thyrotropin secretion.

PHYSIOLOGIC REGULATION OF LEPTIN EXPRESSION AND PLASMA LEVELS

Leptin is synthesized mainly by adipose tissue and is regulated by a variety of factors, including nutrition and hormones.[2–4] A strong positive correlation is found between adipose mass and triglyceride content and between leptin mRNA and plasma leptin levels[45–48] (Fig. 43–2). Accordingly, leptin mRNA and protein levels are higher in obese than lean individuals.[45–47] Leptin levels increase within hours after a meal in rats.[49] In contrast, no acute rise in leptin is seen with meals in humans.[50] Food restriction results in a reduction in leptin over a period of several hours, out of proportion to the changes in fat stores and the fall in body weight in both humans and rodents.[51–54] These findings suggest that leptin is capable of serving as an indicator of short-term energy balance, as well as energy stores.

Several lines of evidence suggest that the effect of feeding on leptin expression is influenced importantly by insulin. Leptin levels do not vary with individual meals as do insulin levels, but rise during the course of the day and peak at night in humans (or at the end of the nighttime feeding cycle in rodents).[49, 54, 55] Peak leptin expression in adipose tissue coincides with a rise in insulin during maximum feeding and is blunted by food deprivation and a fall in insulin.[49] Insulin directly stimulates leptin mRNA and protein expression over a course of several hours.[56] As determined by the euglycemic clamp technique, the decline in insulin levels with fasting precedes the fall in leptin levels in humans and is likely to mediate the latter.[52] Although a direct causal role is not implied, a strong positive correlation has been noted between leptin and insulin levels in obesity, which may reflect the fact that insulin resistance increases with obesity along with a rise in fat mass and leptin.[57, 58]

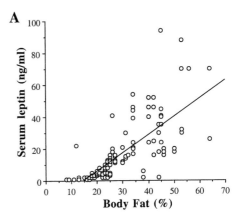

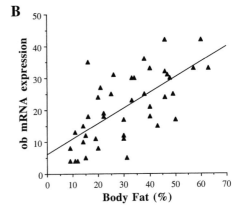

FIGURE 43–2. Relationship between percent body fat (bioelectrical impedance), serum leptin, and subcutaneous *ob* mRNA expression in a group of lean and obese subjects. *A,* A strong positive correlation is seen between percent body fat and serum leptin ($r = 0.86$; $P < .001$; $n = 275$) and *(B)* between percent body fat and *ob* mRNA levels ($r = 0.6$; $P < .001$; $n = 54$). (Data from Considine RV, Sinha MK, Heiman ML, et al: Serum immunoreactive leptin concentrations in normal weight and obese humans. N Engl J Med 334:292–295, 1996.)

Glucocorticoids stimulate leptin expression and may synergize with insulin.[59] Although leptin expression is stimulated directly in isolated adipocytes by glucocorticoids, these studies often involved the administration of pharmacologic doses of glucocorticoids.[60] However, studies in humans have shown that leptin levels are regulated by alterations in glucocorticoids within the physiologic range.[61] Leptin levels are increased by chronic, but not acute elevation of glucocorticoids in patients with Cushing's disease.[62] A circadian leptin rhythm has been described in rodents and humans. In the fed state, an inverse relationship is seen between leptin and glucocorticoids such that peak leptin levels coincide with the nadir of glucocorticoids during the dark cycle in humans (light cycle in rodents).[54, 63–65] Conversely, the nadir of leptin coincides with the rise in glucocorticoids at the beginning of the light cycle in humans (dark cycle in rodents). Circadian rhythms of leptin and glucocorticoids are entrained by feeding such that an alteration in meal timing results in a parallel shift in peak levels of both hormones.[64, 65] An ultradian leptin rhythm is also seen in humans.[63] Frequent blood sampling (every 7 minutes) has revealed a pulsatile pattern of leptin, with a pulse amplitude of 130% and a mean of 30 pulses per day. The mechanism underlying these leptin pulses is unknown but could represent a net effect of pulsatile effectors of leptin release, such as norepinephrine from autonomic nerves and insulin.

Leptin levels are sexually dimorphic, with females having higher levels than males at any given age and body fat content.[66–68] This divergence may partly reflect differences in the expression of leptin in various fat depots inasmuch as higher levels of leptin are expressed in subcutaneous than intra-abdominal adipose tissue and the former is more abundant in women. Leptin synthesis is inhibited by testosterone, so it is possible that low leptin levels in postpubertal males are partly attributable to suppression of leptin synthesis by testosterone.[69] In contrast, because leptin levels are higher in prepubertal girls and postmenopausal women, it is unlikely that female sex steroids play a significant role in the regulation of leptin.[67, 69] This view is consistent with the observation that estrogen and progestins do not alter leptin levels in premenopausal and postmenopausal women.[70] Ultradian and circadian leptin rhythms may modulate reproductive function in females, as suggested by the strong positive correlation between pulsatile leptin secretion, luteinizing hormone, and estradiol levels in women with regular menstrual cycles.[71] Interestingly, the circadian leptin rhythm is blunted in a subset of female athletes with exercise-induced menstrual irregularity.[72]

Leptin expression is influenced by other factors (see Table 43–1). For example, growth hormone deficiency leads to increased adiposity and a rise in leptin levels in adult humans.[73] Although treatment with growth hormone for up to a year decreased adipose mass in these patients, plasma leptin levels were not altered significantly.[73] Administration of thyroxine and triiodothyronine is reported to decrease leptin levels in rats, but short-term hyperthyroxinemia does not appear to alter leptin levels in humans.[74, 75] Leptin expression is increased in response to acute infection and sepsis.[76–78] Based on studies in rodents, it has been suggested that the rise in leptin levels is mediated by endotoxin and cytokines, such as tumor necrosis factor, leukemia inhibitory factor, and interleukin-1.[77, 79, 80] However, different responses have been observed in humans. For example, interleukin-1 causes a transient increase in leptin expression in humans, whereas acute treatment with endotoxin does not alter leptin expression.[81, 82] Cytokines and leptin both potently inhibit appetite, increase energy expenditure, and decrease body weight.[17, 83] Therefore, it is possible that increased leptin expression from cytokine stimulation may worsen anorexia and promote cachexia in acute infection by synergizing with the primary actions of cytokines on appetite and energy homeostasis.

Leptin expression is influenced by factors apart from adipose mass or triglyceride content during the prepubertal period. Thus leptin mRNA in subcutaneous adipose tissue and serum leptin levels are severalfold higher in neonatal mice and are not reduced by food deprivation for up to 12 hours.[64, 84] The prepubertal rise in leptin precedes maturation of the neuroendocrine axis in mice.[64] A similar increase in leptin expression has been reported in a longitudinal study in prepubertal boys. As in mice, the surge in leptin in these boys is independent of adipose mass and precedes gonadal maturation.[85] There appears to be sexual dimorphism in leptin expression. Leptin concentrations are higher in girls than boys before the onset of puberty, do not show a characteristic surge as in boys, and continue to increase after puberty.[85–87] In contrast to the temporal association between leptin levels and puberty in rodents and humans, studies in nonhuman primates have failed to detect a prepubertal rise in leptin.[88]

Leptin is expressed in other cells besides adipocytes. High levels of leptin mRNA and protein have been localized to rodent and human placenta.[18, 19] Leptin levels are higher in the cord blood of full-term than preterm neonates and correlate strongly with birth weight.[89, 90] Leptin expression in placenta appears to be stimulated by insulin and glucocorticoids, as evidenced by higher placental and cord blood leptin in newborns of mothers with untreated gestational diabetes and in response to antenatal glucocorticoid treatment.[90] Placental leptin expression is also increased by hypoxia and may be involved in the pathogenesis of preeclampsia.[91] Leptin is synthesized by mammary epithelial cells, secreted into milk and absorbed into the circulation in infants, and is proposed to regulate feeding and energy balance in infants.[92] De novo expression of leptin mRNA and protein has also been demonstrated in rat gastric fundic mucosa.[20] In addition to the 16-kDa leptin protein, a higher-molecular-weight protein (19 kDa) was detected on immunoblots of gastric fundic mucosal extracts. The functional significance of the higher-molecular-weight protein is not known. Feeding and administration of CCK-8 (the active C-terminal peptide of cholecystokinin) decreased gastric leptin immunoreactivity and protein content and increased plasma leptin concentrations. Thus gastric-derived leptin may act locally in the gastrointestinal tract and the brain to influence satiety.[20]

A potential link between leptin and nutrient flux into adipose tissue and skeletal muscle mediated by the hexosamine biosynthetic pathway has been suggested.[21] Infusion of glucosamine, the end product of the hexosamine pathway, caused rapid increases in leptin mRNA and protein levels in the adipose tissue of rats. The rise in glucosamine levels also stimulated de novo leptin mRNA and protein synthesis in skeletal muscle, albeit at lower concentrations. Hyperglycemia and hyperlipidemia produced similar increases in leptin mRNA and protein levels in adipose tissue and skeletal muscle. It has been proposed that the induction of leptin in skeletal muscle by glucosamine may regulate cellular metabolism by increasing the expression of uncoupling protein.[21]

LEPTIN TRANSPORT AND CLEARANCE

Leptin is secreted by adipose tissue, does not appear to undergo posttranslational modification, and circulates as a protein with a relative molecular weight of 16 kDa.[93] Sedimentation analysis has revealed that leptin binds to plasma proteins and also forms complexes with soluble leptin receptors in the circulation.[40, 94] It is estimated that 5% to 20% of circulating leptin is bound to plasma proteins in lean and

TABLE 43–1. Regulation of Leptin Levels by Nutrition, Hormones, and Other Factors

Increase leptin
    Overfeeding
    Obesity (except *ob/ob* mutation)
    Insulin
    Glucocorticoids
    Acute infection/sepsis
        Endotoxin (lipopolysaccharide)
        Cytokines (IL-1, TNF, LIF)
    Glucosamine
Decrease leptin
    Fasting
    Testosterone
    β-Adrenergic agonists
    Thiazolidinediones (rodents)
    ? Thyroid hormone (in rats)
    Smoking
    Cold exposure (brown adipose tissue)

IL-1, interleukin-1; LIF, leukocyte inhibitory factor; TNF, tumor necrosis factor.

obese individuals. Abundant leptin-binding sites are distributed widely in several tissues and create an additional pool of leptin that contributes to prolongation of the half-life of leptin along with carrier proteins in plasma.[95] Immunoassays appear to detect both free and bound leptin, but it is likely that bound leptin is not biologically active.

Although leptin receptors are distributed widely in various tissues, several lines of evidence suggest that leptin exerts its effects on energy balance mainly by acting in the brain (Fig. 43–3). First, intracerebroventricular leptin injection has manyfold more potent effects on food intake, energy expenditure, and body weight than does peripheral leptin administration.[22, 23, 24] Second, a saturable transport system for leptin has been demonstrated in the rodent brain.[96] Third, peripheral leptin administration activates the hypothalamic and brain stem neuronal circuits involved in the regulation of feeding behavior and autonomic and neuroendocrine function.[97, 98] Given that leptin is a large protein, the mechanism by which it is transported into the brain has attracted considerable attention. Neuronal targets of leptin are located in the arcuate, dorsomedial, ventromedial, and ventral premamillary nuclei, within close proximity to the median eminence.[98–101] As with other circumventricular organs, the median eminence has fenestrated capillaries, so these neurons are potentially accessible to proteins and other large molecules through diffusion.

Leptin may also reach neuronal targets in the brain via cerebrospinal fluid (CSF), presumably by receptor-mediated transport. The expression of high levels of short-form leptin receptors in the choroid plexus (the site of CSF production) is consistent with this view.[101, 102] It is possible that these receptors are involved in blood-to-CSF leptin transport. Alternatively, leptin receptors may mediate the efflux of leptin from the CSF to the venous circulation. Leptin is present in the CSF of obese Koletsky rats despite the lack of all forms of membrane leptin receptors, thus indicating that it is capable of entering CSF by other mechanisms such as diffusion.[44] Furthermore, the CSF leptin concentration is 100 times lower than plasma leptin and 50-fold below the K_d of the leptin receptor (i.e., 0.7 nM).[31, 102, 103] It is therefore unlikely that CSF is a major source of leptin for neuronal targets in the brain.

Another potential route of leptin transport into the central nervous system is across the blood-brain barrier. Although circumventricular regions such as the median eminence have fenestrated capillaries, the endothelial cells in most brain regions have tight junctions that constitute part of the barrier designed to exclude large molecules from the brain parenchyma. Some polypeptides such as insulin are transported into the brain parenchyma by receptor-mediated transcytosis across the blood-brain barrier.[104, 105] Leptin may reach neuronal targets in the brain by a similar transport mechanism. Brain microvessels (i.e., capillaries) express high levels of short-form leptin receptors and are capable of binding and internalizing leptin.[102, 106] Thus leptin receptors in brain capillary endothelial cells may be involved in leptin transport

into the brain parenchyma and/or uptake and degradation of leptin. Expression of short-form leptin receptors is increased in brain microvessels in rats fed a high fat diet, which implies that receptor-mediated leptin transport may be modified by changes in nutrient composition or circulating leptin levels.[107]

Leptin is distributed to several organs and cleared mainly by the kidney.[108–110] The importance of the kidney as a major organ for leptin clearance is suggested by higher plasma leptin concentrations being observed in patients with renal impairment and end-stage renal disease when matched by sex, age, or adiposity.[108, 111] High leptin levels might contribute to cachexia in patients with end-stage renal disease. Studies suggest that leptin is filtered by the glomeruli and degraded by renal epithelial cells.[110] Short-form leptin receptors are highly expressed in the kidney and may mediate renal leptin clearance by internalization and degradation, as has been shown in Chinese hamster ovary (CHO) cells expressing the short-form leptin receptor Ob-Ra.[112] Although short-form leptin receptors are widely distributed in other highly vascular organs, such as the liver and lungs, it is unlikely that these organs are major sites for leptin clearance because no net uptake of leptin occurs in the liver and lung.[109]

CELLULAR MECHANISMS OF LEPTIN ACTION

Leptin regulates cellular function predominantly by binding to the long-form receptor (Ob-Rb), which then leads to activation of the JAK/STAT pathway and transcriptional regulation.[32, 36, 37] The initial role of this leptin receptor is revealed by genetic evidence in that absence of this receptor in *db/db* mice results in severe obesity that is resistant to endogenous and exogenous leptin.[22–24] Brain regions involved in the regulation of energy balance such as the arcuate, ventromedial, and dorsomedial hypothalamic nuclei express high levels of Ob-Rb.[99–101] Although in vitro studies have shown that leptin activates STAT1, STAT3, and STAT5, in vivo leptin injection activates only STAT3 in the hypothalamus.[36, 37] STAT3 protein colocalizes with neuropeptide Y (NPY) and proopiomelanocortin (POMC) in arcuate hypothalamic neurons.[113] These neuropeptides are among the most critical mediators of leptin action in the brain and are directly regulated by leptin. The coexpression of STAT3 protein is consistent with transcriptional regulation of NPY and POMC gene expression by leptin. Leptin regulates the expression of other STAT3-dependent target genes in the hypothalamus, including the immediate-early genes c-*fos*, c-*jun*, and *tis*-11 and SOCS-3, a member of the suppressors of cytokine signaling family.[32, 37, 114] In vivo leptin-mediated regulation of the JAK/STAT pathway has also been demonstrated in the jejunum.[115] The long-form leptin receptor (Ob-Rb) is expressed in jejunal epithelium and mediates the cellular response to intravenous leptin administration by inducing

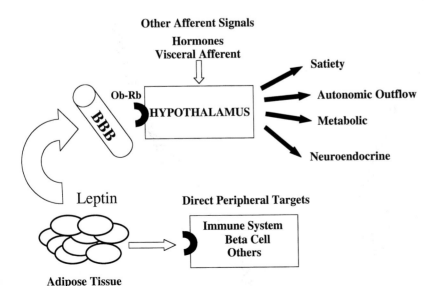

FIGURE 43–3. Sites of leptin action. Leptin is transported to neuronal targets in the hypothalamus and regulates appetite, autonomic outflow, metabolism, and neuroendocrine function. Leptin also exerts direct effects on the immune system and pancreatic β cells. BBB, blood-brain barrier; Ob-Rb, long leptin receptor isoform.

STAT3 and STAT5. As with the hypothalamus, leptin injection induces the expression of immediate-early genes in the jejunum. It is possible that the regulation of cellular function in discrete segments of the gastrointestinal tract by leptin alters nutrient absorption and gut motility.

Leptin is also capable of exerting rapid effects on synaptic transmission in the brain and insulin secretion. For example, leptin hyperpolarizes glucose-responsive neurons in the hypothalamus through activation of ATP-sensitive potassium channels and inhibits insulin secretion by affecting similar channels in pancreatic β cells.[116, 117] Activation of channel activity in both systems is inhibited by tolbutamide.[116, 117] Leptin also directly depolarizes neurons in the paraventricular hypothalamic nucleus, inhibits NPY release from the hypothalamus by modifying calcium channel activity, and modulates vagal discharge in the stomach.[118–120] The signal transduction pathways by which leptin exerts these rapid actions on synaptic transmission and insulin secretion from pancreatic islets are not known. Although Ob-Rb is expressed in the hypothalamus and pancreatic islets, these electrophysiologic actions of leptin are not likely to involve transcriptional regulation via the JAK/STAT pathway.

Low levels of Ob-Rb have been detected in adipose tissue, the pituitary and adrenal glands, T lymphocytes, vascular endothelium, and ovarian follicular cells.[5–7, 121–124] Leptin is reported to stimulate the proliferation of CD4+ lymphocytes, cytokine production, and phagocytosis; promote angiogenesis; and directly modulate the secretion of glucocorticoids, estradiol, and anterior pituitary hormones.[5–7, 121–124] These effects of leptin are probably mediated in part by extrahypothalamic Ob-Rb. Several short leptin receptor isoforms are expressed via alternative splicing of the leptin receptor gene.[4, 33] These isoforms bind leptin through identical extracellular domains, but their expression does not prevent obesity in *db/db* mice and their physiologic role is as yet undefined.[4] A role in leptin transport and/or degradation is likely. Leptin can phosphorylate JAK2, IRS-1 (insulin receptor substrate-1), and ERK2 (extracellular signal–regulated kinase-2) and induce the mRNA of immediate-early genes in CHO cells by binding to Ob-Ra.[125] Although these effects are seen in artificial in vitro systems, it is possible that some of leptin's actions in certain tissues are mediated by short-form leptin receptors.

ROLE OF LEPTIN IN ENERGY HOMEOSTASIS

Leptin as an Anti-obesity Hormone

Discovery of the *ob* gene set the stage for consideration of leptin as the long sought after "adipostatic" hormone. The concept of an adipostatic mechanism for body weight regulation is based on the observation that body weight is relatively stable over long periods in mammals.[13, 16, 17] Most mammals have the capacity to adapt to overfeeding and food deprivation by adjusting food consumption and energy expenditure to restore body weight and adiposity to previous levels. A major feature of this adaptation is the capacity to store excess energy as triglycerides in adipose tissue. In addition to generating more calories per unit weight than carbohydrates and protein, fat can be stored in an almost anhydrous form in subcutaneous, abdominal, and visceral depots, which increases the capacity for storage of excess calories for later use in times of food deprivation. The important role of adipose tissue in energy homeostasis is further exemplified by the observation that surgical resection of subcutaneous adipose tissue in weanling rats results in regeneration and precise restoration of adipose mass over several months.[126]

After discovery of the *ob* gene, several studies showed that peripheral leptin injection and, more potently, intracerebroventricular leptin injection caused marked inhibition of food intake, increased energy expenditure, and weight loss in *ob/ob* mice.[22–24] The rise in energy expenditure in response to leptin treatment is probably the net result of stimulation of sympathetic nervous activity in brown adipose tissue, increased thermogenesis in other tissues in part from increased expression of uncoupling protein, and increased locomotor activity.[2, 23, 127] Although initial studies also suggested that wild-type rodents were

less sensitive to leptin action, recent experiments have clearly demonstrated that minimal elevation of leptin levels by constant peripheral infusion has potent effects on feeding, energy expenditure, and body weight in normal ad lib fed rodents.[22–24, 128] Remarkably, as in *ob/ob* mice, leptin-mediated weight loss in wild-type rodents is limited to adipose tissue and does not affect lean body mass.[128]

These observations on the ability of leptin to decrease body weight formed the basis for the prevailing concept of leptin as an "anti-obesity hormone." However, with the availability of immunoassays for leptin, it was soon clear that circulating leptin levels were elevated in human and rodent obesity (except the *ob* mutation).[45, 47] Similarly, *ob* mRNA expression is increased in adipose tissue in obese individuals.[45–47] The inability of rising endogenous leptin levels to prevent obesity must be reconciled with the concept that leptin's primary role is to act in a negative feedback loop to limit weight gain. Hyperleptinemia is thought to be indicative of "leptin resistance" in obese individuals (akin to hyperinsulinemia in type 2 diabetes); however, the mechanisms underlying this resistance are yet to be defined.[3, 4] Rodent obese models have provided some insight into potential mechanisms for leptin resistance. For example, diet-induced obesity causes resistance to peripheral leptin administration in mice, but these mice are reported to respond to intracerebroventricular leptin injection.[129] A similar response to leptin is observed in New Zealand obese (NZO) mice with a polygenic mutation leading to late-onset obesity.[128] In contrast, obese agouti (*Ay*) mice are resistant to both peripheral and central leptin injection.[128] Because leptin is thought to influence feeding behavior and energy balance by acting primarily in the brain, these results suggest that leptin resistance may be caused by defects in leptin transport into the brain, by abnormalities of leptin signaling in target neurons, or by defects in the downstream neural circuits engaged by leptin. Leptin resistance in NZO mice most likely results from impaired brain leptin transport, whereas central leptin resistance in agouti (*Ay/a*) mice is most probably caused by leptin insensitivity at a downstream step in the brain.[128] Recent studies have confirmed that signaling through the melanocortin-4 receptor is involved in leptin action to inhibit appetite and that this pathway is impaired in *Ay/a* mice because of ectopic expression of the melanocortin antagonist agouti.[130, 131]

Access of leptin to CSF appears to be limited in obese individuals, as evidenced by lower CSF–peripheral leptin ratios.[132] Because the CSF–plasma leptin ratio is also decreased in obese *fa/fa* and Koletsky rats with defects in leptin receptor expression and/or function, it has been suggested that leptin transport into CSF may be mediated by a receptor-mediated process and that this process may be involved in the pathogenesis of leptin resistance.[39, 44, 133] Although leptin levels in plasma are low in patients with anorexia nervosa, the CSF–plasma leptin ratio is elevated during refeeding in such patients and could mediate the abnormal perception of "fatness," as well as resistance to weight gain during refeeding in these patients.[103, 134] Recently, SOCS-3 has been suggested to act as a potential mediator of central leptin resistance.[114] SOCS-3 expression is induced in hypothalamic target neurons by acute leptin administration and thus blocks leptin signaling in cells expressing Ob-Rb.[114] Leptin resistance may also be mediated by the Src homology-2 (SH2)-containing tyrosine phosphatase SHP-2 inasmuch as leptin signaling is reported to be enhanced when the binding site on Ob-Rb for SHP-2 is mutated.[135]

Leptin as a Hormone Mediating Adaptation to Starvation

An alternative view of leptin's role in energy homeostasis is that the fall in leptin with fasting is a signal to the brain that energy stores are declining[3, 54] (Figs. 43–4 and 43–5). Because starvation is a preeminent threat to survival, complex neural, metabolic, hormonal, and behavioral mechanisms have developed in mammals to defend against it (reviewed elsewhere[3, 17]). In the classic response to starvation, a switch from carbohydrate- to fat-based metabolism is seen as glycogen stores in the liver are depleted. This adaptation is mediated by the fall in insulin and a rise in counterregulatory hormones such as glucagon, epinephrine, and glucocorticoids. The growth hormone axis is also involved. Growth hormone increases with fasting in humans,

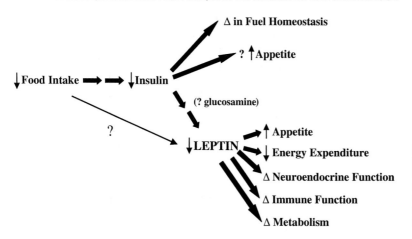

FIGURE 43–4. Insulin and leptin as mediators of the adaptation to fasting. The fall in insulin levels mediates the switch from carbohydrate to fat-based metabolism. Insulin may also stimulate appetite by direct action in the brain. Leptin decreases as a result of the decline in insulin and mediates various metabolic, neuroendocrine, and immune responses to fasting.

whereas insulin-like growth factor-1 (IGF-1) decreases. In contrast, both growth hormone and IGF-1 levels are reduced by fasting in rodents. Other adaptations to starvation include suppression of the thyroid and gonadal axes, a fall in body temperature, and increased appetite. The metabolic effect of these adaptive responses is to stimulate gluconeogenesis to provide glucose for brain metabolism, to supply fatty acids from triglyceride breakdown for energy use in other tissues, and to limit protein catabolism. Energy utilization is reduced during fasting, in part through suppression of thyroid thermogenesis and limitation of procreation and growth.

Inspection of the phenotype of leptin deficiency in *ob/ob* mice and leptin insensitivity in *db/db* mice reveals striking similarities to the adaptation to fasting.[3, 4, 30] In addition to the metabolic and neuroendocrine alterations described above, total leptin deficiency in *ob/ob* mice

and partial leptin deficiency with fasting also lead to immune dysfunction.[5] Proliferation of CD4[+] cells and cytokine production by T_H1 cells are decreased in *ob/ob* mice and normalized by leptin. The hypothesis that the fall in leptin mediates the metabolic and neuroendocrine adaptation to fasting has been directly tested. By preventing the characteristic fall in leptin with a leptin repletion paradigm, activation of the hypothalamic-pituitary-adrenal axis and suppression of thyroid and reproductive hormones were blunted during fasting in mice.[54] A similar role for leptin as a mediator of changes in the growth hormone, reproductive, and thyroid axes in response to fasting has been shown in rats and nonhuman primates.[136–138] Low leptin levels mediate the hormonal response to fasting primarily by acting on neuronal targets in the hypothalamus and possibly through regulation of pituitary function.[3, 54, 122, 136, 137] Metabolic actions of leptin on peripheral tissues have

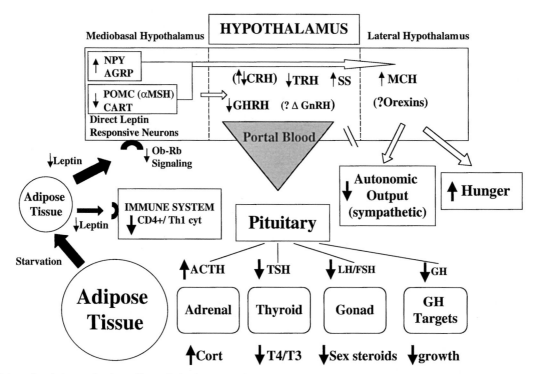

FIGURE 43–5. Interaction between leptin and hypothalamic neuronal targets during starvation. The fall in leptin results in an increase in neuropeptide Y (NPY) and agouti-related peptide (AGRP) levels and a decrease in proopiomelanocortin (POMC) and cocaine- and amphetamine-regulated transcript (CART) levels in the arcuate hypothalamic nucleus. NPY and AGRP stimulate feeding (orexigenic), whereas α-melanocyte–stimulating hormone (α MSH, a product of POMC) and CART inhibit feeding (anorexigenic). Arcuate hypothalamic neurons expressing NPY, POMC, AGRP, and CART are directly responsive to leptin. These neurons project to the lateral hypothalamus and regulate the expression of melanin-concentrating hormone (MCH), a major stimulator of feeding. In addition, leptin targets in the arcuate hypothalamic nucleus regulate the neuroendocrine axis and autonomic output. The fall in leptin also leads to suppression of immune function. ACTH, adrenocorticotropic hormone; CRH, corticotropin-releasing hormone; FSH, follicle-stimulating hormone; GH, growth hormone; GHRH, GH-releasing hormone; GnRH, gonadotropin-releasing hormone; LH, luteinizing hormone; SS, somatostatin; T₃, triiodothyronine; T₄, thyroxine; TRH, thyrotropin-releasing hormone; TSH, thyroid-stimulating hormone.

also been described. Leptin directly regulates CD4[+] proliferation and T$_H$1 cytokine production during fasting, thus indicating that it is an important link between nutritional status and immune function.[5]

Leptin's role as a "starvation hormone" may have important implications for the pathogenesis of human obesity. One study has shown that a subpopulation of Pima Indians with a more rapid than normal weight gain and obesity have relatively low plasma leptin levels.[139] If the leptin concentration is inappropriately low for a given mass of adipose tissue in a subset of patients, the development of obesity could be promoted.[4, 139] Whether such a situation is true in the general population has not yet been established.

PATHWAYS FOR LEPTIN ACTION IN THE CENTRAL NERVOUS SYSTEM

Classic lesion studies carried out more than four decades ago established the hypothalamus as an important site for the regulation of feeding and metabolism (reviewed elsewhere[140, 141]). Lesions of the ventromedial hypothalamus led to a syndrome of overfeeding and obesity, whereas lesions of the lateral hypothalamic area resulted in failure to eat or drink. These findings formed the basis of the "dual-center" model of feeding and body weight regulation in which satiety and feeding centers were proposed to be located in the ventromedial and lateral hypothalamic nuclei, respectively. However, the validity of this model was challenged by subsequent experiments in which the reported abnormalities of feeding behavior and energy balance could not be reproduced by discrete hypothalamic lesions or appropriate chemical stimulation.

The discovery of leptin has rekindled enormous interest in the role of the hypothalamus in feeding behavior and energy balance. Many of the abnormalities of energy balance induced by lesions of the ventromedial hypothalamus are also present in *ob/ob* mice, as well as in obese leptin-insensitive *db/db* mice and *fa/fa* rats.[30, 140, 141] The long-form leptin receptor is highly expressed in neurons in the arcuate, dorsomedial, and ventromedial hypothalamic nuclei,[100–102] and leptin-sensitive neurons in these nuclei project to key sites in the hypothalamus, such as the paraventricular and lateral hypothalamic nuclei, as well as extrahypothalamic sites in the brain stem and cortex to regulate feeding behavior and autonomic and neuroendocrine function.[99, 140, 141] Furthermore, lesions of the ventromedial and adjacent arcuate hypothalamic nuclei prevent the inhibitory effects of leptin on appetite and body weight, consistent with the view that the ventrobasal hypothalamus is an important site for leptin action in the brain.[142]

Neuronal targets of leptin express neurotransmitters/neuropeptides implicated in appetite, energy expenditure, and body weight regulation. A detailed description of the anatomic distribution of neurons expressing these peptides and their projections is presented in excellent reviews.[140, 141, 143] Briefly, populations of neurons in the arcuate hypothalamic nucleus that express high levels of the long-form leptin receptor (Ob-Rb) also express NPY, agouti-related peptide (AGRP), POMC, a precursor of α-melanocortin–stimulating hormone (α-MSH), and cocaine- and amphetamine-regulated transcript (CART) (see Fig. 43–5). Most NPY neurons in the arcuate hypothalamic neurons express AGRP. Similarly, most POMC neurons express CART. Leptin-sensitive neurons in the arcuate hypothalamus that express NPY, AGRP, POMC, and CART project to the medial and ventral parvicellular subdivisions of the paraventricular hypothalamus, where they are likely to regulate neuroendocrine and autonomic function (see Fig. 43–5). Arcuate hypothalamic neurons also project to the lateral hypothalamus and perifornical area, and these circuits are likely to regulate food intake. Neurons in the lateral hypothalamus express high levels of melanin-concentrating hormone (MCH) and orexin/hypocretin, and these neurons project extensively to the neocortex, limbic regions, and sites in the brain stem. Because lateral hypothalamic neurons do not express detectable levels of Ob-Rb, it is likely that regulation of MCH and orexin/hypocretin expression by leptin is mediated indirectly by leptin-sensitive neurons in the arcuate hypothalamus.

Neurotransmitters/peptides involved in the regulation of feeding and energy balance in the brain have been classified as "orexigenic" or "anorexigenic" based on their ability to stimulate or inhibit feeding, respectively (reviewed elsewhere[3, 4, 141, 143]). For example, NPY, MCH, AGRP, galanin, norepinephrine, and orexin/hypocretin each increase food intake in response to intracerebroventricular injection. In contrast, α-MSH, corticotropin-releasing hormone (CRH), CART, CCK, glucagon-like peptide-1 (GLP-1), urocortin, bombesin, and serotonin each decrease food intake (i.e., are anorexigenic). Orexigenic and anorexigenic neuropeptides/neurotransmitters are proposed to function in a homeostatic mechanism to mediate leptin action. The orexigenic peptides NPY, AGRP, and MCH are increased in states of leptin deficiency, such as in *ob/ob* mice and fasting, and decreased by leptin. NPY is the most potent orexigenic peptide known and is also involved in the regulation of autonomic and neuroendocrine function. POMC is a precursor of α-MSH in the brain, and this anorexic peptide is directly regulated by leptin in the arcuate nucleus. POMC expression is decreased in the hypothalamus of *ob/ob* mice and during fasting and is increased by leptin. α-MSH inhibits food intake and also modulates neuroendocrine and autonomic function.[144, 145]

It is likely that the anorexic actions of leptin are mediated by the coordinate fall in levels of orexigenic peptides, such as NPY, AGRP, and MCH, and rise in anorexigenic peptides, such as POMC (α-MSH) and CART. In contrast, hyperphagia from leptin deficiency, such as by fasting, is likely to result from a rise in NPY and AGRP and a fall in α-MSH and CART levels (see Fig. 43–5). Leptin may also influence feeding behavior and metabolism by regulating the expression of CCK and other central mediators listed earlier. Our understanding of the roles of putative central mediators of leptin action is complicated by the fact that induced mutations of these neuropeptides or their receptors sometimes do not produce the expected phenotype. For example, NPY-deficient mice feed normally, do not show any growth or neuroendocrine deficits, and exhibit a normal or exaggerated response to leptin.[146] Similarly, targeted deletion of NPY receptors (Y1 and Y5), which are thought to mediate feeding behavior, do not decrease food intake or prevent weight gain.[147, 148] However, NPY appears to be partially responsible for hyperphagia, obesity, and neuroendocrine abnormalities in totally leptin-deficient *ob/ob* mice, as evidenced by the ability of NPY deficiency to ameliorate these abnormalities.[149] The role of MCH as an orexigenic peptide was confirmed by a recent study showing that MCH deficiency causes hypophagia and decreased weight gain in mice.[150] However, as with NPY-deficient mice, MCH-deficient mice respond normally to leptin.[150] These findings suggest that the central nervous system may have redundant pathways for leptin action and that regulation of appetite and metabolism by leptin is likely to involve complex interactions among various neurotransmitters/peptides and their receptors.

Other neuropeptide targets for leptin include thyrotropin-releasing hormone (TRH), CRH, and gonadotropin-releasing hormone (GnRH). TRH is the probable mediator of suppression of the thyroid axis seen in response to falling leptin levels during fasting.[137] Although some evidence suggests that the fall in TRH mRNA expression with fasting is mediated by leptin-responsive neurons in the arcuate hypothalamus (i.e., NPY and possibly POMC neurons),[151] TRH expression may also be regulated directly by leptin because neurons in the parvicellular hypothalamic nucleus known to express TRH and other hypophysiotropic peptides are activated by leptin.[97] CRH is a potent inhibitor of appetite when administered into the brain and also increases sympathetic activity in brown adipose tissue.[17] However, reports of leptin's effect on CRH neurons are discordant. Leptin inhibits hypoglycemia-induced CRH release from hypothalamic explants, but it has also been shown to increase CRH secretion from the hypothalamus.[152, 153] CRH mRNA expression has been reported to be unchanged or decreased with fasting and stimulated or unaffected by leptin treatment.[3, 17] Thus the role of CRH neurons in leptin action remains unsettled. The actions of leptin to regulate the hypothalamic-pituitary-gonadal axis are well established,[29, 40, 54, 154–157] but the precise site of action is as yet unclear. Leptin stimulates GnRH secretion from hypothalamic explants, but because GnRH neurons appear to not express leptin receptors, it is likely that leptin's actions are mediated indirectly by other neurons.[122, 138] Apart from the hypothalamus, leptin receptors have also been localized to the cerebellum, neocortex, thalamus, and brain stem.[101, 102] The functional role of leptin in these brain regions is unknown. It is possible that these sites are involved in the integration of complex behavior associated with feeding or mediate the diverse sensory, motor, and visceral actions of leptin.

The nature of the interaction between hypothalamic neurotransmitter/peptide expression and physiologic alterations in leptin levels, that is, from low levels during fasting to elevated levels with overfeeding and obesity, is unknown. A recent study has suggested different thresholds for leptin at neuronal targets in the brain involved in the regulation of appetite, metabolism, and neuroendocrine function.[4, 158] By expressing leptin during the prenatal period in ob/ob mice, it was demonstrated that neuroendocrine abnormalities, including pubertal maturation and fertility, are corrected by lower doses of leptin that only partially blunt hyperphagia and obesity. In contrast, thermoregulatory defects are not reversed by expression of normal leptin levels. These findings suggest that responses to low leptin levels with fasting and high leptin levels with overfeeding may be mediated by different subsets of neurons.

OTHER SYSTEMIC EFFECTS OF LEPTIN

Leptin's effects on physiology extend beyond regulation of appetite and body weight. Leptin appears to be a critical signal for maturation of the reproductive axis, as evidenced by its ability to restore puberty and fertility in ob/ob mice, accelerate puberty in wild-type mice, and facilitate normal maturation of the reproductive system in rodents.[154–157] Leptin deficiency or insensitivity from ob and db mutations causes hypothalamic hypogonadism in humans as well.[29, 40] Low leptin or lack of a diurnal leptin rhythm has been associated with amenorrhea in female athletes, although causation has not been established.[71, 72] Leptin regulates the hypothalamic-pituitary-adrenal axis independent of its role in starvation. For example, leptin can blunt adrenocorticotropic hormone and glucocorticoid secretion during restraint stress and has been described to directly regulate hormone secretion by the pituitary and adrenal glands.[122, 123, 152, 159]

Leptin has the capacity to regulate lipid and glucose metabolism by actions independent of its effects on appetite and body weight. For example, leptin acutely stimulates lipolysis, gluconeogenesis, and glucose metabolism.[23, 160, 161] The extent to which these effects are mediated through the central nervous system as opposed to direct actions in peripheral cells is unclear. In addition to increasing energy expenditure through stimulation of sympathetic nerve activity in brown adipose tissue, leptin enhances sympathetic nerve activity in the adrenal gland, kidney, and hind limb skeletal muscle and may thereby be involved in the regulation of cardiovascular and renal function.[2, 162] The latter effects of leptin on autonomic and cardiorenal function may have important implications for cardiovascular complications of obesity. A potential developmental role for leptin is suggested by its expression in placenta, widespread distribution of leptin and leptin receptors in fetal tissue, and the ability of leptin to regulate hematopoiesis.[6, 18, 19] Leptin is also likely to play a role in brain development, as evidenced by structural and synthetic abnormalities in the brains of ob/ob and db/db mice.[8, 9, 163, 164] Leptin deficiency in ob/ob and db/db mice leads to decreased brain weight, structural neuronal defects, impaired myelination, and immature expression of several neuronal and glial proteins in the neocortex, hippocampus, striatum, and brain stem.[8, 9] Chronic leptin treatment initiated after weaning increases brain weight and DNA content and restores whole brain protein content and expression of some neuronal proteins, such as GAP-43 (growth-associated protein-43), syntaxin-1, and SNAP-25 (soluble N-ethylmaleimide-sensitive factor [NSF] attachment protein-25) to normal levels.[8, 9] Leptin may influence neuronal and glial function indirectly by regulating levels of thyroxine, growth hormone, sex hormones, and glucocorticoids.[54, 64, 136, 137] Alternatively, leptin may regulate neuronal and glial function directly inasmuch as leptin receptors have been localized in both cell types in several brain regions.

FUTURE PERSPECTIVES

The discovery of leptin has greatly expanded our understanding of metabolic physiology. As often happens when a new hormone or protein is discovered, the initial concept of leptin as an anti-obesity hormone whose primary role is to limit weight gain by decreasing food intake and increasing energy expenditure has been replaced by a more complex view. Leptin is an important mediator of the adaptation to starvation and also has diverse modulatory effects on the neuroendocrine axis, hematopoiesis, growth, and development. Most of the current knowledge of the effects of leptin is based on studies in rodents. The literature on the role of leptin in humans is filled with studies on associations between leptin and various parameters in patients and healthy subjects. Although these studies have contributed to the understanding of leptin physiology and its relationship to diseases, experiments to directly address the complex role of this adipose-derived hormone in humans are greatly needed. Trials are currently under way to assess the efficacy of human recombinant leptin in the treatment of obesity. It is hoped that future studies will clarify the physiologic role of leptin as an integrator of energy balance and neuroendocrine function in humans and identify the molecular basis for defective leptin action in obesity.

REFERENCES

1. Zhang Y, Proenca R, Maffei M, et al: Positional cloning of the mouse obese gene and its human homologue. Nature 372:425–432, 1994.
2. Spiegelman BM, Flier JS: Adipogenesis and obesity: Rounding out the big picture. Cell 87:377–389, 1996.
3. Flier JS: Clinical review 94: What's in a name? In search of leptin's physiologic role. J Clin Endocrinol Metab 83:1407–1413, 1998.
4. Friedman JM, Halaas JL: Leptin and the regulation of body weight in mammals. Nature 395:763–770, 1998.
5. Lord GM, Matarese G, Howard JK, et al: Leptin modulates the T-cell immune response and reverses starvation-induced immunosuppression. Nature 294:897–891, 1998.
6. Gainsford T, Wilson TA, Metcalf D, et al: Leptin can induce proliferation, differentiation and functional activation of hemopoietic cells. Proc Natl Acad Sci U S A 93:14564–14568, 1996.
7. Sierra-Honigmann MR, Nath AK, Murakami C, et al: Biologic action of leptin as an angiogenic factor. Science 281:1683–1685, 1998.
8. Steppan CM, Swick AG: A role for leptin in brain development. Biochem Biophys Res Commun 256:600–602, 1999.
9. Ahima RS, Bjorbaek C, Osei SY, Flier JS: Regulation of neuronal and glial proteins by leptin: Implications for brain development. Endocrinology 140:2755–2762, 1999.
10. Ingalls AM, Dickie MM, Snell GD: Obesity, a new mutation in the house mouse. J Hered 41:317–318, 1950.
11. Coleman DL: Obese and diabetes: Two mutant genes causing diabetes-obesity syndromes in mice. Diabetologia 14:141–148, 1978.
12. Coleman DL: Effects of parabiosis of obese with diabetes and normal mice. Diabetologia 9:294–298, 1973.
13. Kennedy GC: The role of depot fat in the hypothalamic control of food intake in the rat. Proc R Soc Lond Biol 140:578–596, 1953.
14. Cahill JG, Herrera MG, Morgan AP, et al: Hormone-fuel interrelationships during fasting. J Clin Invest 45:1751–1769, 1966.
15. Sims EA, Horton ES: Endocrine and metabolic adaptation to obesity and starvation. Am J Clin Nutr 21:1455–1470, 1968.
16. Harris RBS, Kasser TR, Martin RJ: Dynamics of recovery of body composition after overfeeding, food restriction or starvation of mature female rats. J Nutr 116:2536–2546, 1986.
17. Schwartz MW, Seeley R: Neuroendocrine responses to starvation and weight loss. N Engl J Med 336:1802–1811, 1997.
18. Masuzaki H, Ogawa Y, Sagawa N, et al: Nonadipose production of leptin: Leptin as a novel placenta-derived hormone in humans. Nat Med 3:1029–1033, 1997.
19. Hoggard N, Hunter L, Duncan JS, et al: Leptin and leptin receptor mRNA and protein expression in the murine fetus and placenta. Proc Natl Acad Sci U S A 94:11073–11078, 1997.
20. Bado A, Levasseur S, Attoub S, et al: The stomach is a source of leptin. Nature 394:790–793, 1998.
21. Wang J, Liu R, Hawkins M, et al: A nutrient-sensing pathway regulates leptin gene expression in muscle and fat. Nature 393:684–688, 1998.
22. Halaas J, Gajiwala K, Maffei M, et al: Weight-reducing effects of the plasma protein encoded by the obese gene. Science 269:543–546, 1995.
23. Pelleymounter M, Cullen M, Baker M, et al: Effects of the obese gene product on body weight regulation in ob/ob mice. Science 269:540–543, 1995.
24. Campfield LA, Smith FJ, Guisez J, et al: Recombinant mouse OB protein: Evidence for a peripheral signal linking adiposity and central neural networks. Science 269:546–549, 1995.
25. Rau H, Reaves BJ, O'Rahilly S, Whitehead JP: Truncated human leptin (Δ133) associated with extreme obesity undergoes proteosomal degradation after defective intracellular transport. Endocrinology 140:1718–1723, 1999.
26. Clement K, Garner C, Hager J, et al: Indication for linkage of human OB gene region with extreme obesity. Diabetes 45:687–690, 1996.
27. Maffei M, Stoffel M, Barone M, et al: Absence of mutations in the human OB gene in obese/diabetic subjects. Diabetes 45:679–682, 1996.
28. Montague CT, Farooqi S, Whitehead JP, et al: Congenital leptin deficiency is associated with severe early onset obesity in humans. Nature 387:903–908, 1997.

29. Strobel A, Issad T, Camoin L, et al: A leptin missense mutation associated with hypogonadism and morbid obesity. Nat Genet 18:213–215, 1998.
30. Bray GA, York DA: Hypothalamic and genetic obesity in experimental animals: An autonomic and endocrine hypothesis. Physiol Rev 59:719–790, 1979.
31. Tartaglia L, Dembski M, Weng X, et al: Identification and expression cloning of a leptin receptor. Cell 83:1263–1271, 1995.
32. Tartaglia LA: The leptin receptor. J Biol Chem 272:6093–6096, 1997.
33. Lee GH, Proenca R, Montez JM, et al: Abnormal splicing of the leptin receptor in diabetic mice. Nature 379:632–635, 1996.
34. Wang M-Y, Zhou YT, Newgard CB, Unger RH: A novel leptin receptor isoform in rat. FEBS Lett 392:87–90, 1998.
35. Chua SC, Chung WK, Wu-Peng XS: Phenotypes of mouse *diabetes* and rat *fatty* due to mutations in the OB (leptin) receptor. Science 271:994–996, 1996.
36. Vaisse C, Halaas JL, Horvarth CM, et al: Leptin activation of Stat3 in the hypothalamus of wild type and ob/ob mice but not db/db mice. Nat Genet 14:95–97, 1996.
37. Ghilardi N, Ziegler S, Wiestner A, et al: Defective STAT signaling by the leptin receptor in diabetic mice. Proc Natl Acad Sci U S A 93:6231–6235, 1996.
38. Li C, Ioffe E, Fidahusein N, et al: Absence of soluble leptin receptor in plasma from db^{Pas}/db^{Pas} and other db/db mice. J Biol Chem 273:10078–10082, 1998.
39. Takaya K, Ogawa Y, Hiraoka J, et al: Nonsense mutation of leptin receptor in the obese spontaneously hypertensive Koletsky rat. Nat Genet 14:130–131, 1996.
40. Clement K, Vaisse C, Lahlous N, et al: A mutation in the human leptin receptor gene causes obesity and pituitary dysfunction. Nature 392:398–401, 1998.
41. White DW, Wang Y, Chua SC, et al: Constitutive and impaired signaling of leptin receptors containing the Gln-Pro extracellular domain mutation. Proc Natl Acad Sci U S A 94:10657–10662, 1997.
42. da Silva BA, Bjorbaek C, Uotani S, Flier JS: Functional properties of leptin receptor isoforms containing the Gln-Pro extracellular domain mutation of the fatty rat. Endocrinology 139:3681–3690, 1998.
43. Cusin I, Rohner-Jeanrenaud F, Stricker-Krongard A, Jeanrenaud B: The weight reducing effect of an intracerebroventricular bolus injection of leptin in genetically obese fa/fa rats. Reduced sensitivity compared with lean animals. Diabetes 45:1446–1450, 1996.
44. Wu-Peng XS, Chua SCJ, Okada N, et al: Phenotype of the obese Koletsky (f) rat due to Tyr763Stop mutation in the extracellular domain of the leptin receptor (Lepr): Evidence for deficient plasma-to-CSF transport of leptin in both the Zucker and Kolestsky obese rat. Diabetes 46:513–518, 1997.
45. Considine RV, Sinha MK, Heiman ML, et al: Serum immunoreactive leptin concentrations in normal weight and obese humans. N Engl J Med 334:292–295, 1996.
46. Lonnqvist F, Arner P, Nordfors, Schalling W: Overexpression of the obese (ob) gene in adipose tissue of human obese subjects. Nat Med 1:950–953, 1995.
47. Maffei MJ, Halaas J, Ravussin E, et al: Leptin levels in human and rodent: Measurement of plasma leptin and ob mRNA in obese and weight-reduced subjects. Nat Med 1:1155–1161, 1995.
48. Frederich RC, Hamann A, Anderson S, et al: Leptin levels reflect body lipid content in mice: Evidence for diet-induced resistance to leptin action. Nat Med 1:1311–1314, 1995.
49. Saladin R, Devos P, Guerre-Millo M, et al: Transient increase in obese gene expression after food intake or insulin administration. Nature 377:527–529, 1995.
50. Korbonits M, Trainer PJ, Little JA, et al: Leptin levels do not change acutely with food administration in normal or obese subjects, but are negatively correlated with pituitary-adrenal activity. Clin Endocrinol 46:751–757, 1997.
51. Kolaczynski JW, Considine RV, Ohannesian J, et al: Responses of leptin to short-term fasting and refeeding in humans. Diabetes 45:1511–1515, 1996.
52. Boden G, Chen X, Mozzoli M, Ryan I: Effect of fasting on serum leptin in normal human subjects. J Clin Endocrinol Metab 81:3419–3423, 1996.
53. Frederich RC, Lollman B, Hamann A, et al: Expression of ob mRNA and its encoded protein in rodents. J Clin Invest 96:1658–1663, 1995.
54. Ahima RS, Prabakaran D, Mantzoros C, et al: Role of leptin in the neuroendocrine response to fasting. Nature 382:250–252, 1996.
55. Sinha MK, Ohannesian JP, Heiman ML, et al: Nocturnal rise of leptin in lean, obese and non–insulin dependent diabetes mellitus subjects. J Clin Invest 97:1344–1347, 1996.
56. Kolaczynski JW, Nyce MR, Considine RV, et al: Acute and chronic effects of insulin on leptin production in humans: Studies in vivo and in vitro. Diabetes 45:699–701, 1996.
57. Boden G, Chen X, Kolacynski JPM: Effects of prolonged hyperinsulinemia on serum leptin in normal human subjects. J Clin Invest 100:1107–1113, 1997.
58. Segal KR, Landt M, Klein S: Relationship between insulin sensitivity and plasma leptin concentration in lean and obese men. Diabetes 45:988–991, 1996.
59. Zakrzewska KE, Cusin I, Sainsbury A, et al: Glucocorticoids as conterregulatory hormones of leptin: Toward understanding of leptin resistance. Diabetes 46:717–719, 1997.
60. De Vos P, Saladin R, Auwerx J, Staels B: Induction of ob gene expression by corticosteroids is accompanied by body weight loss and reduced food intake. J Biol Chem 270:15958–15961, 1995.
61. Elimam A, Knutsson U, Bronnegard M, et al: Variations in glucocorticoid levels within the physiologic range affect plasma leptin levels. Eur J Endocrinol 139:615–620, 1998.
62. Cizza G, Lotsikas AJ, Licinio J, et al: Plasma leptin levels do not change in patients with Cushing's disease shortly after correction of hypercortisolism. J Clin Endocrinol Metab 82:2747–2750, 1997.
63. Licinio J, Mantzoros C, Negrao AB, et al: Human leptin levels are pulsatile and inversely related to pituitary-adrenal function. Nat Med 3:575–579, 1997.
64. Ahima RS, Prabakaran D, Flier JS: Postnatal leptin surge and regulation of circadian rhythm of leptin by feeding: Implications for energy homeostasis and neuroendocrine function. J Clin Invest 101:1020–1027, 1998.
65. Schoeller DA, Cella LK, Sinha MK, Caro JF: Entrainment of the diurnal rhythm of plasma leptin to meal timing. J Clin Invest 100:1882–1887, 1997.
66. Saad ME, Damani S, Gingerich RL, et al: Sexual dimorphism in plasma leptin concentration. J Clin Endocrinol Metab 82:579–584, 1997.
67. Rosenbaum M, Nicolson M, Hirsch J, et al: Effects of gender, body composition and menopause on plasma concentration of leptin. J Clin Endocrinol Metab 81:3424–3427, 1996.
68. Kennedy A, Gettys TW, Watson P, et al: The metabolic significance of leptin in humans: Gender-based differences in relationship to adiposity, insulin sensitivity, and energy expenditure. J Clin Endocrinol Metab 82:1293–1300, 1997.
69. Blum WF, Englaro P, Hanitsch S, et al: Plasma leptin levels in healthy children and adolescents: Dependence on body mass index, fat mass, gender, pubertal stage, and testosterone. J Clin Endocrinol Metab 82:2904–2910, 1997.
70. Castracane VD, Kraemer RR, Franken MA, et al: Serum leptin concentration in women: Effect of age, obesity, and estrogen administration. Fertil Steril 70:472–477, 1998.
71. Licinio J, Negrao AB, Mantzoros C, et al: Synchronicity of frequently sampled 24h concentrations of circulating leptin, luteinizing hormone and estradiol in healthy women. Proc Natl Acad Sci U S A 95:2541–2546, 1998.
72. Laughlin GA, Yen SS: Hypoleptinemia in women athletes: Absence of a diurnal rhythm with amenorrhea. J Clin Endocrinol Metab 82:318–321, 1997.
73. Fisker S, Vahl N, Hansen TB, et al: Serum leptin is increased in growth hormone–deficient adults: Relationship to body composition and effects of placebo-controlled growth hormone therapy for 1 year. Metabolism 46:812–817, 1997.
74. Escobar-Morreale HF, Escobar del Rey F, Morreale de Escobar G: Thyroid hormones influence serum leptin concentrations in the rat. Endocrinology 138:4485–4488, 1997.
75. Mantzoros CS, Rosen HN, Greenspan SL, et al: Short-term hyperthyroidism has no effect on leptin levels in man. J Clin Endocrinol Metab 82:497–499, 1997.
76. Bornstein SR, Licinio J, Tauchnitz R, et al: Plasma leptin levels are increased in survivors of acute sepsis: Associated loss of diurnal rhythm in cortisol and leptin secretion. J Clin Endocrinol Metab 83:280–283, 1998.
77. Grunfeld C, Zhao C, Fuller J, et al: Endotoxin and cytokines induce expression of leptin, the ob gene product, in hamsters. J Clin Invest 97:2152–2157, 1996.
78. Roberts HC, Hardie LJ, Chappell LH, Mercer JG: Parasite-induced anorexia: Leptin, insulin and corticosterone responses to infection with the nematode, *Nippostrogylus brasiliensis*. Parasitology 118:117–123, 1999.
79. Sarraf P, Frederich RC, Turner EM, et al: Multiple cytokines and acute inflammation raise mouse leptin levels: Potential role in inflammatory anorexia. J Exp Med 185:171–175, 1997.
80. Faggioni R, Fantuzzi G, Fuller J, et al: IL-1 beta mediates leptin induction during inflammation. Am J Physiol 274:R204–R208, 1998.
81. Janik JE, Curtis ED, Considine RV, et al: Interleukin 1 alpha increases serum leptin concentrations in humans. J Clin Endocrinol Metab 82:3084–3086, 1997.
82. Bornstein SR, Preas HL, Chrousos GP, et al: Circulating leptin levels during acute experimental endotoxemia and antiinflammatory therapy in humans. J Infect Dis 178:887–890, 1998.
83. Schwartz MW, Dallman MF, Woods SC: Hypothalamic response to starvation: Implications for the study of wasting disorders. Am J Physiol 269:R949–R957, 1995.
84. Devaskar SU, Ollesch C, Rajakumar RA, Rajakumar PA: Developmental changes in obese gene expression and circulating leptin peptide concentrations. Biochem Biophys Res Comm 238:44–47, 1997.
85. Mantzoros C, Flier JS, Rogol AD: A longitudinal assessment of hormonal and physical alterations during normal puberty in boys. V. Rising leptin levels may signal the onset of puberty. J Clin Endocrinol Metab 82:1066–1070, 1997.
86. Hassink SG, Sheslow DV, de Lancey E, et al: Serum leptin in children with obesity: Relationship to gender and development. Pediatrics 98:201–203, 1996.
87. Garcia-Mayor RV, Andrade MA, Rios M, et al: Serum leptin in normal children: Relationship to age, gender, body mass index, pituitary-gonadal hormones, and pubertal stages. J Clin Endocrinol Metab 82:2849–2855, 1997.
88. Plant TM, Durrant AR: Circulating leptin does not appear to provide a signal for triggering the initiation of puberty in the male rhesus monkey (*Macaca mulatta*). Endocrinology 138:4505–4508, 1997.
89. Sivan E, Lin WM, Homko CJ, et al: Leptin is present in human cord blood. Diabetes 46:917–919, 1997.
90. Shekhawat PS, Garland JS, Shivpuri C, et al: Neonatal cord blood leptin: Its relationship to birth weight, body mass index, maternal diabetes, and steroids. Pediatr Res 43:338–343, 1998.
91. Mise H, Sagawa N, Matsumoto T, et al: Augumented placental production of leptin in preeclampsia: Possible involvement of placental hypoxia. J Clin Endocrinol Metab 83:3225–3229, 1998.
92. Casabiell X, Pineiro V, Tome MA, et al: Presence of leptin in colostrum and/or breast milk from lactating mothers: A potential role in the regulation of neonatal food intake. J Clin Endocrinol Metab 82:4270–4273, 1997.
93. Cohen S, Halaas JL, Freidman JM, et al: Human leptin characterization. Nature 382:589, 1996.
94. Houseknecht KL, Mantzoros CS, Kuliawat R, et al: Evidence for leptin binding to proteins in serum of rodents and humans: Modulation with obesity. Diabetes 45:1638–1643, 1996.
95. Hill RA, Margetic S, Pegg GG, Gazzola C: Leptin: Its pharmacokinetics and tissue distribution. Int J Obes Relat Metab Disord 22:765–770, 1998.
96. Banks WA, Kastin AJ, Huang W, et al: Leptin enters the brain by a saturable system independent of insulin. Peptides 17:305–311, 1996.
97. Elmquist JK, Ahima RS, Maratos-Flier E, et al: Leptin activates neurons in ventrobasal hypothalamus and brainstem. Endocrinology 138:839–842, 1997.
98. Elmquist JK, Ahima RS, Elias CS, et al: Leptin activates distinct projections from the dorsomedial and ventromedial hypothalamic nuclei. Proc Natl Acad Sci U S A 741–748, 1998.
99. Schwartz M, Seeley RJ, Campfield LA, et al: Identification of targets of leptin action in rat hypothalamus. J Clin Invest 98:1101–1106, 1996.
100. Mercer JG, Hoggard N, Williams LM, et al: Localization of leptin mRNA and the

long form splice variant (Ob-Rb) in mouse hypothalamus and adjacent brain regions by in situ hybridization. FEBS Lett 387:113–116, 1996.

101. Elmquist JK, Bjorbaek C, Ahima RS, et al: Distributions of leptin receptor isoforms in the rat brain. J Comp Neurol 395:535–547, 1998.
102. Bjorbaek C, Elmquist JK, Michl P, et al: Expression of leptin receptor isoforms in brain microvessels. Endocrinology 139:3485–3491, 1998.
103. Schwartz MW, Peskind E, Raskind M, et al: Cerebrospinal fluid leptin concentrations: Relationship to plasma levels and to adiposity in humans. Nat Med 2:589–593, 1996.
104. Pardridge WM: Receptor-mediated peptide transport through the blood-brain barrier. Endocr Rev 7:314–330, 1986.
105. Schwartz MW, Figlewicz DP, Baskin DG, et al: Insulin in the brain: A hormonal regulator of energy balance. Endocr Rev 13:387–414, 1992.
106. Golden PL, Maccagnan TJ, Padridge WM: Human blood-brain barrier leptin receptor: Binding and endocytosis in isolated human brain microvessels. J Clin Invest 99:14–18, 1997.
107. Boado RJ, Golden PL, Levin N, Padridge WM: Upregulation of blood-brain barrier shortform leptin receptor gene products in rats fed a high fat diet. J Neurochem 71:1761–1764, 1998.
108. Sharma K, Considine RV, Michael B, et al: Plasma leptin is partly cleared by the kidney and elevated in hemodialysis patients. Kidney Int 51:1980–1985, 1997.
109. Jensen MD, Moller N, Nair KS, et al: Regional leptin kinetics in humans. Am J Clin Nutr 69:18–21, 1999.
110. Meyer C, Robson D, Rackovsky N, et al: Role of the kidney in human leptin metabolism. Am J Physiol 273:E903–E907, 1997.
111. Merabet E, Dagogo-Jack S, Coyne DW, et al: Increased plasma leptin concentration in end-stage renal disease. J Clin Endocrinol Metab 82:847–850, 1997.
112. Uotani S, Bjorbaek C, Tornoe J, Flier JS: Functional properties of leptin receptor isoforms. Internalization and degradation of leptin and ligand-induced receptor down-regulation. Diabetes 48:279–286, 1999.
113. Hakanssson ML, Meister B: Transcription factor STAT3 in leptin target neurons of the rat hypothalamus. Neuroendocrinology 68:420–427, 1998.
114. Bjorbaek C, Elmquist JK, Franz JD, et al: Identification of SOCS-3 as a potential mediator of central leptin resistance. Mol Cell 1:619–625, 1998.
115. Morton NM, Emilsson V, Liu YL, Cawthorne MA: Leptin action in intestinal cells. J Biol Chem 273:26194–26201, 1998.
116. Spanswick D, Smith MA, Groppi VE, et al: Leptin inhibits hypothalamic neurons by activation of ATP-sensitive potassium channels. Nature 390:521–525, 1997.
117. Kieffer TJ, Heller S, Leech CA, et al: Leptin suppression of insulin secretion by the activation of ATP-sensitive K$^+$ channels in pancreatic β-cells. Diabetes 46:1087–1093, 1997.
118. Powis JE, Bains JS, Ferguson AV: Leptin depolarizes rat hypothalamic paraventricular nucleus neurons. Am J Physiol 274:R1468–R1472, 1998.
119. Glaum SR, Hara M, Binkodas VP, et al: Leptin, the obese gene product, rapidly modulates synaptic transmission in the hypothalamus. Mol Pharmacol 50:230–235, 1996.
120. Wang YH, Tache Y, Sheibel AB, et al: Two types of leptin-responsive gastric vagal afferent terminals: An in vitro single-unit study in rats. Am J Physiol 273:R833–R837, 1997.
121. Siegrist-Kaiser C, Pauli V, Juge-Aubry C, et al: Direct effect of leptin on brown and white adipose tissue. J Clin Invest 100:2858–2864, 1997.
122. Yu WH, Kimura M, Walczewska A, et al: Role of leptin in hypothalamic-pituitary function. Proc Natl Acad Sci U S A 94:1023–1028, 1997.
123. Bornstein SR, Uhlmann K, Haidan A, et al: Evidence for a novel peripheral action of leptin as a metabolic signal to the adrenal gland: Leptin inhibits cortisol release directly. Diabetes 46:1235–1238, 1997.
124. Zachow RJ, Magoffin DA: Direct intraovarian effects of leptin: Impairment of the synergistic action on insulin-like growth factor I on follicle stimulating hormone dependent estradiol 17 beta production by rat ovarian granulosa cells. Endocrinology 138:847–850, 1997.
125. Bjorbaek C, Uotani S, da Silva B, Flier JS: Divergent signaling capacities of the long and short isoforms of the leptin receptor. J Biol Chem 272:32686–32695, 1997.
126. Faust IM, Johnson PR, Hirsch J: Adipose tissue regeneration following lipectomy. Science 197:391–393, 1977.
127. Scarpace PJ, Matheny M, Pollock BH, et al: Leptin increases uncoupling protein expression and energy expenditure. Am J Physiol 273:E226–E230, 1997.
128. Halaas JL, Boozer C, Blair-West J, et al: Physiological response to long-term peripheral and central leptin infusion in lean and obese mice. Proc Natl Acad Sci U S A 94:8878–8883, 1998.
129. Van Heek M, Compton DS, France CF, et al: Diet-induced obese mice develop peripheral, but not central, resistance to leptin. J Clin Invest 99:385–390, 1997.
130. Seeley RJ, Thiele TE, van Dijk G, et al: Melanocortin receptors in leptin effects. Nature 390:349, 1997.
131. Fan W, Boston BA, Kesterson RA, et al: Role of melanocortinergic neurons in feeding and the agouti obesity syndrome. Nature 385:165–168, 1997.
132. Caro JF, Kolaczynski JW, Nyce MR, et al: Decreased cerebrospinal fluid/serum leptin ratio in obesity: A possible mechanism for leptin resistance. Lancet 348:159–161, 1996.

133. Ishizuka T, Ernsberger P, Liu S, et al: Phenotypic consequences of a nonsense mutation in the leptin receptor gene (fak) in obese spontaneously hypertensive Koletsky rats (SHROB). J Nutr 128:2299–2306, 1998.
134. Mantzoros C, Flier JS, Lesen MD, et al: Cerebrospinal fluid leptin in anorexia nervosa: Correlation with nutritional status and potential role in resistance to weight gain. J Clin Endocrinol Metab 82:1845–1851, 1997.
135. Carpenter LR, Farruggela TJ, Symes A, et al: Enhancing leptin response by preventing SH2-containing phosphatase 2 interaction with ob receptor. Proc Natl Acad Sci U S A 95:6061–6066, 1998.
136. Vuagnat BAM, Pierroz DD, Lalaoui M, et al: Evidence for a leptin–neuropeptide Y axis for the regulation of growth hormone secretion in the rat. Neuroendocrinology 67:291–300, 1998.
137. Legradi G, Emerson CH, Ahima RS, et al: Leptin prevents fasting-induced suppression of prothyrotropin-releasing hormone messenger ribonucleic acid in neurons of the hypothalamic paraventricular nucleus. Endocrinology 138:2569–2576, 1997.
138. Finn PD, Cunningham MJ, Pau KY, et al: The stimulatory effect of leptin on the neuroendocrine reproductive axis of the monkey. Endocrinology 139:4652–4662, 1998.
139. Ravussin E, Pratley RE, Maffei M, et al: Relatively low plasma leptin concentrations precede weight gain in Pima Indians. Nat Med 3:238–240, 1997.
140. Sawchenko PE: Toward a new neurobiology of energy balance, appetite and obesity: The anatomists weigh in. J Comp Neurol 402:435–441, 1998.
141. Elmquist JK, Elias CF, Saper CB: From lesions to leptin: Hypothalamic control of food intake and body weight. Neuron 22:221–232, 1999.
142. Dube MG, Xu B, Kalra PS, et al: Disruption in neuropeptide Y and leptin signaling in obese ventromedial hypothalamic–lesioned rats. Brain Res 816:38–46, 1999.
143. Flier JS, Maratos-Flier E: Obesity and the hypothalamus: Novel peptides for new pathways. Cell 92:437–440, 1998.
144. Hagan MM, Rushing PA, Schwartz MW, et al: Role of the CNS melanocortin system in the response to overfeeding. J Neurosci 19:2362–2367, 1999.
145. Shalts E, Feng YJ, Ferin M, Wardlaw SL: Alpha-melanocyte–stimulating hormone antagonizes the neuroendocrine effects of corticotropin-releasing factor and interleukin-1 alpha in the primate. Endocrinology 131:132–138, 1992.
146. Erickson JC, Clegg KE, Palmiter RD: Sensitivity to leptin and susceptibility to seizures of mice lacking neuropeptide Y. Nature 381:415–418, 1996.
147. Pedrazzini T, Seydoux J, Kunster P, et al: Cardiovascular response, feeding behavior and locomotor activity in mice lacking the NPY Y1 receptor. Nat Med 4:722–726, 1998.
148. Marsh DJ, Hollopeter G, Kafer KE, Palmiter RD: Role of Y5 neuropeptide Y receptor in feeding and obesity. Nat Med 4:718–721, 1998.
149. Erickson JC, Hollopeter G, Palmiter RD: Attenuation of the obesity syndrome of ob/ob mice by the loss of neuropeptide Y. Science 274:1704–1707, 1996.
150. Shimada M, Tritos N, Lowell BB, et al: Mice lacking melanin-concentrating hormone are hypophagic and lean. Nature 396:670–674, 1999.
151. Legradi G, Emerson CH, Ahima RS, et al: Arcuate nucleus ablation prevents fasting-induced suppression of ProTRH mRNA in the hypothalamic paraventricular nucleus. Neuroendocrinology 68:89–97, 1998.
152. Heiman ML, Ahima RS, Craft LS, et al: Leptin inhibition of the hypothalamic-pituitary-adrenal axis in response to stress. Endocrinology 138:3859–3863, 1997.
153. Costa A, Poma A, Martignoni E, et al: Stimulation of corticotropin-releasing hormone release by obese (ob) gene product, leptin, from hypothalamic explants. Neuroreport 8:1131–1134, 1997.
154. Chehab F, Lim M, Lu R: Correction of the sterility defect in homozygous obese female mice by treatment with the human recombinant leptin. Nat Genet 12:318–320, 1996.
155. Barash IA, Cheung CC, Weigle DS, et al: Leptin is a metabolic signal to the reproductive system. Endocrinology 137:3144–3147, 1997.
156. Ahima RS, Dushay J, Flier SN, et al: Leptin accelerates the onset of puberty in normal female mice. J Clin Invest 99:391–395, 1997.
157. Chehab FF, Mounzih K, Lu R, Lim ME: Early onset of reproductive function in normal female mice treated with leptin. Science 275:88–90, 1997.
158. Ioffe E, Moon B, Connolly E, Friedman JM: Abnormal regulation of the leptin gene in the pathogenesis of obesity. Proc Natl Acad Sci U S A 95:11852–11855, 1998.
159. Pralong FP, Roduit R, Waeber G, et al: Leptin inhibits directly glucocorticoid secretion by normal human and rat adrenal gland. Endocrinology 139:4264–4268, 1998.
160. Rossetti L, Massillon D, Barzilai N, et al: Short term effects of leptin on hepatic gluconeogenesis and in vivo insulin action. J Biol Chem 272:27758–27763, 1997.
161. Kamohara S, Burcelin R, Halaas JL, et al: Acute stimulation of glucose metabolism in mice by leptin treatment. Nature 389:374–377, 1997.
162. Haynes WG, Sivitz WJ, Morgan DA, et al: Sympathetic and cardiorenal actions of leptin. Hypertension 30:619–623, 1997.
163. Bereiter DA, Jeanrenaud B: Altered neuroanatomical organization in the central nervous system of genetically obese (ob/ob) mice. Brain Res 165:249–260, 1979.
164. Sena A, Sarlieve LL, Rebel G: Brain myelin of genetically obese mice. J Neurol Sci 68:233–244, 1985.

Chapter 44

Obesity

Jamie Dananberg ▪ Jose F. Caro

Changes in body weight follow the laws of physics and dictate that if caloric intake is greater than caloric output, weight gain will occur. However, *regulation* of body weight homeostasis is a complex integration of genetic, social, behavioral, and physiologic factors, many of which have yet to be fully understood.

The systems that regulate body weight and energy homeostasis developed over an evolutionary time scale. The biologic factors responsible for the increasing prevalence of obesity were set down early in mankind and were probably meant to defend against significant loss of lean mass during times of food scarcity. Presently, we are only beginning to characterize the dietary milieu of our prehistoric ancestors. Answers to basic questions such as whether animal meat was part of the early hominid diet[1] will aid our efforts at understanding the conditions that drove the evolution of weight regulatory systems. Wherever the evidence leads, one thing is certain: the genetic and social adaptations that have been passed down through the millennia have resulted in populations with ever-increasing waistlines and risks for serious morbidity and mortality.

EPIDEMIOLOGY OF OVERWEIGHT AND OBESITY

The diseases of overweight and obesity are global in scope. For every developed country in the world in which data are available, the incidence and prevalence of excessive weight have increased over time.[2] Epidemiologic analysis of obesity is complicated in that the criteria by which overweight and obesity are defined have shifted over time. Currently, it is recommended that body mass index (BMI, weight divided by height squared [kg/m²]) be used for establishing diagnoses of overweight (BMI of 25.0–29.9 kg/m²) and obesity (BMI ≥30.0 kg/m²).[3] These cutoffs were chosen as predictors of morbidity and mortality. Based on these criteria, it is currently estimated that 64 million Americans are overweight and another 44 million are obese,[4] and these figures reflect an increase in the prevalence of obesity over time (Fig. 44–1). The prevalence of both overweight and obesity has increased dramatically in both men and women in the United States between 1960 and 1994. The overall prevalence of overweight has increased from 43.3% of individuals aged 20 to 74 during the period 1960 to 1962[5] to 54.9% of all individuals 20 years and older during the period 1988 to 1994.[6] In parallel, costs for weight-related health

care have skyrocketed. In the United States during 1995, the total cost of health care attributable to obesity approached $100 billion, roughly half of which was spent on direct medical costs to treat obesity-associated disease.[7]

DISEASES ASSOCIATED WITH OBESITY

Mortality

Obesity and overweight themselves independently confer an increased risk of mortality. Although the link between obesity and increased rates of morbidity and mortality has been questioned in older populations,[8] many other studies have established such a direct linkage. The increase in risk begins to rise at a BMI greater than 25 kg/m².[9] The risk rises slowly at levels over 25 kg/m² and then rises

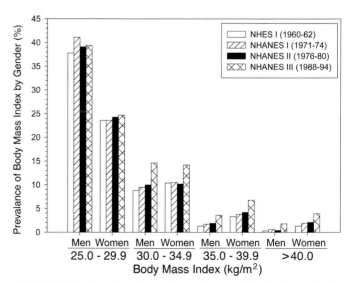

FIGURE 44–1. Age-adjusted prevalence of overweight (body mass index [BMI], 25–29.9) and obesity (BMI, ≥30) as measured in the National Health Assessment Surveys.[6]

steeply at levels greater than 30 kg/m². Individuals with a BMI of 30 kg/m² or greater have a 1.5- to 2-fold excess independent risk of mortality than do individuals with a BMI less than 25 kg/m².[9] Paradoxically, a BMI lower than 20 kg/m² is associated with a modest increase in mortality, even after adjusting for confounding variables.[9] The data relating obesity to mortality risk were drawn from epidemiologic studies of primarily white populations. In other groups, the inflection point at which mortality risk increases with increased BMI may be shifted. For example, in black American populations, mortality risk appears to rise at BMI levels of 27 kg/m² and greater.[10]

Cardiovascular and Cerebrovascular Disease

Overweight, obesity, and abdominal fat increase the risk of both cardiovascular[11, 12] and cerebrovascular[13] disease. The reasons for the increased risk for cardiovascular and cerebrovascular diseases may include elevations of blood pressure, low-density lipoprotein cholesterol (LDL-C), triglycerides, small dense LDL-C, total cholesterol, fibrinogen, plasminogen activator inhibitor-1, and insulin and decreases in high-density lipoprotein cholesterol.

In 1983, the Framingham Study published a 26-year follow-up of participants showing a 26% to 46% increase in the relative risk for cardiovascular disease in individuals who were 30% over ideal body weight vs. individuals at ideal body weight[11] (Fig. 44–2). In the Nurses' Health Study of more than 100,000 women monitored for 14 years, the risk of coronary heart disease (CHD) was nearly two times greater in subjects with a BMI between 25 and 28.9 kg/m² and nearly three times greater in subjects with a BMI of 29 kg/m² or greater than in subjects with a BMI of 21 kg/m² or lower.[14] In a cohort study of middle-aged British men, the incidence of coronary events increased 10% for each 1-kg/m² rise in the BMI over 22.[15] Although in some studies an association between CHD and excess weight was not found, this association has been well established in all studies that controlled for other risk factors such as smoking, age, family history, upper body adiposity, and menopausal and hormone replacement status.

Hypertension

The INTERSALT study involving more then 10,000 men and women reported that a 10-kg increase in weight was associated with a 3.0–mm Hg rise in systolic blood pressure and a 2.3–mm Hg rise in diastolic blood pressure.[16] This degree of blood pressure elevation has been associated with a 12% increase in CHD and a 24% increase in stroke.[17] The precise mechanism by which changes in weight alter blood pressure has not been established.

Dyslipidemia

Increases in BMI are associated with increases in total cholesterol, triglycerides, total LDL,[18] and small dense LDL[19] and with decreases in high-density lipoproteins.[20] The risk of CHD is primarily due to increases in LDL. Increases in the BMI of 10 U from a starting level between 20 and 30 kg/m² will raise LDL-C levels between 10 and 20 mg/dL.[18] Changes of this magnitude can be expected to increase the risk of CHD by 10% over a 5- to 10-year period.[21] The risk may be particularly great for individuals with more prominent upper body obesity, in whom triglyceride, small dense LDL, and apolipoprotein B levels are high.[22]

Congestive Heart Failure

Both overweight and obesity have been shown to be independent risk factors for the development of congestive heart failure.[11] Furthermore, because both hypertension and diabetes are also associated with congestive heart failure, the overall risk when these dependent factors are taken into account is proportionally increased.[23]

Stroke

Fewer studies have carefully examined the association of cerebrovascular disease and weight vs. cardiovascular disease and weight. An association has been established in the evaluation of both fatal and nonfatal strokes, particularly when a subset of patients with ischemic stroke is evaluated.[11, 13] The risk of stroke is nearly twofold higher in women with a BMI greater than 32 kg/m² than in women with a BMI less than 21 kg/m².[13]

Diabetes Mellitus

Numerous studies have shown an association between increases in weight and the development of type 2 diabetes mellitus.[24, 25] In fact, the risk for diabetes increases at BMI levels below that established for the diagnosis of overweight. In the Nurses' Health Study, BMI values above 22 kg/m² were associated with an increased risk of diabetes.[24] It has been estimated that the relative risk for diabetes increases by 25% for each unit of BMI above 22 kg/m².[26] It has also been estimated that more than a quarter of all newly diagnosed cases of diabetes in the United States were due to weight gain of more than 5 kg.[27]

Cancer

Cancer of the colon, particularly the distal end of the colon, has been shown in a number of studies to be strongly associated with obesity in

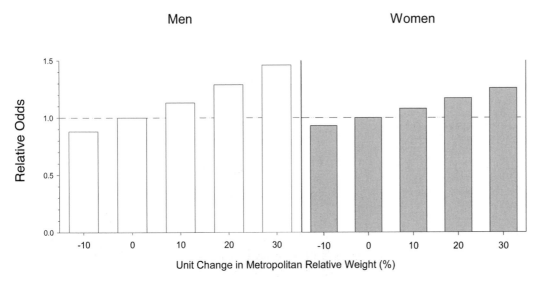

FIGURE 44–2. The relative odds of developing cardiovascular disease corresponding to degrees of change in Metropolitan Relative Weight (weight/ideal weight × 100) between age 25 years and entry into the Framingham Study. The odds ratios reflect adjustments for the effects of relative weight at age 25 years and age and risk factor levels. (From Hubert HB, Feinleib M, McNamara PM, et al: Obesity as an independent rich factor for cardiovascular disease: A 26-year follow-up of participants in the Framingham Heart Study. Circulation 67:968–977, 1983. By permission of The American Heart Association, Inc.)

men, as well as obesity in women, but to a lesser extent.[28, 29] In some cases, the incidence of colon cancer is nearly twofold greater in individuals with a BMI greater than 29 kg/m² than in those with a BMI less than 21 kg/m².

Although obesity has been shown to be inversely associated with the incidence of breast cancer in premenopausal women,[30, 31] that "protection" diminishes approximately 10 years after menopause.[32] Increases of 8 kg over adulthood can lead to a twofold increase in the risk of breast cancer, an association that is particularly evident for women who have not received postmenopausal estrogen replacement therapy.[33]

The risk of endometrial cancer is increased significantly with increases in body weight.[34, 35] Previously, some of this risk has been attributable to the coassociation of diabetes mellitus with obesity. However, in a study of obese and lean women with or without diabetes, obesity conferred a significant proportion of the excess risk of endometrial cancer in women with diabetes.[36]

Female Reproductive Health

Polycystic ovarian syndrome, a disorder that includes hirsutism, obesity, ovulatory and menstrual dysfunction, and insulin resistance, is among the most common causes of altered reproductive function in women who are overweight.[37] Even modest increases in weight in young women can adversely affect fertility,[38] and women with polycystic ovarian syndrome and obesity have an increased risk of infertility.

Obesity during pregnancy is also associated with excessive morbidity. Pregnant women with obesity have a nearly a 10-fold excess risk of hypertension and a significant increase in the risk of gestational diabetes.[39] Furthermore, the risk of congenital malformations, primarily neural tube defects, is increased in the pregnancy of obese women.[40] Finally, increased weight before pregnancy has been shown to result in an increased risk of adverse fetal outcomes.[41]

Other

For women with a BMI greater than 40 kg/m², the risk of gallstones is nearly seven times higher than for women with a BMI less than 24 kg/m².[42] A twin study estimated that for every 1-kg rise in body weight, the risk of osteoarthritis increases by approximately 10%.[43] Conversely, weight loss is associated with an increase in pain-free range of motion and a decrease in analgesic use.[44] Sleep apnea is another morbidity associated directly with weight gain.[45] Diagnosis and treatment of sleep apnea in obese patients are particularly important because of the sequelae of hypoxia, hypertension, myocardial infarction, and cardiac arrythmias.[46]

Relationship to Body Fat Distribution

Diseases associated with obesity are more highly correlated with the presence of intra-abdominal (visceral) fat than with peripheral (subcutaneous) fat. When compared with equal-weight patients with peripheral obesity, patients with abdominal obesity have a greater risk for type 2 diabetes mellitus, CHD, stroke, and hormone-dependent cancers of the breast and endometrium.[47–52] Furthermore, patients with abdominal obesity have higher glucose and insulin levels during an oral glucose tolerance test and higher rates of lipolysis than do patients with peripheral obesity.[53]

INTEGRATED REGULATION OF ENERGY BALANCE

Energy expenditure can be divided into several components. The resting metabolic rate (RMR) is the energy expended during inactivity to fuel the normal, resting, physiologic processes and to maintain normal body temperature. The RMR, or basal metabolic rate, can be thought of as the average metabolic rate during sleep plus the energy cost of arousal. The RMR accounts for approximately 60% to 70% of daily energy expenditure.[54] In contrast, thermogenic processes are processes that increase energy expenditure over the RMR in response to food consumption, changes in ambient temperature, exposure to drugs or changing hormonal concentrations, or psychologic stresses. Of these processes, the thermic effect of food is quantitatively the largest and accounts for approximately 10% of daily energy expenditure.[55] The final, most variable component of energy expenditure is physical activity. For most adults in developed nations, physical activity accounts for approximately 20% to 30% of daily energy expenditure.

Because living organisms exist in a dynamic environment, energy balance should be considered in the context of the time- and weight-dependent rate of energy utilization. For example, an increase in energy intake results in positive energy balance and weight gain. Over time, weight gain slows because of a compensatory increase in energy expenditure and restoration of energy balance. Therefore, conditions at the new steady state include increased energy intake, increased energy expenditure, and an increase in body mass. Consequently, for an individual, change in weight is not just a function of food intake, but also changes in the homeostatic mechanisms that define energy balance.

The positive energy balance responsible for obesity is caused by excessive energy intake, reduced energy expenditure, or a combination of these two factors. In several studies, a reduction in energy expenditure was found in infants in whom obesity developed by 1 year of age,[56] in 5-year-old children in whom obesity was found to develop by adolescence,[57] and in adult Pima Indians, in whom obesity develops with aging.[58] In contrast, several investigators have not found a decrease in energy expenditure in infants[59] or children[60] who become overweight later in life. These differences may be explained, in part, by the imprecision of the technology used to measure energy intake and energy expenditure. Overweight may occur in young children with changes in either food intake or energy expenditure at the limit of detection. Additionally, although the measurements are static, changes in energy balance are temporally dynamic such that assessments occur before or after adaptations. Finally, regulation of energy homeostasis is subject to multiple genetic and environmental influences. A primary abnormality may differ between any two populations given a single environmental perturbation. Conversely, a primary abnormality may differ for any single population exposed to two different milieux.

Signaling Systems

The homeostatic mechanisms of weight that respond to changes in diet or the external environment include signaling, integration, and effector components (Fig. 44–3). The signaling component involves sensory, somatic, and environmental messages that relay information regarding body composition, energy balance, thermogenesis, and food availability and leads to a coordinated response that restores or maintains homeostasis. The signals that are recognized to regulate body weight can be divided into lipostatic, glucostatic, and satiety signals.

Lipostatic Signals

Regulation of body weight requires an integrated system of communication between the storage compartment and the regulatory compartment. White adipose tissue (WAT) is the major site for long-term energy storage in the form of triglycerides. Transmission of information regarding the relative amount of WAT was shown to be dependent on the recently discovered hormone leptin.[61] Leptin is the protein product of the *ob* gene, a deficiency of which was shown to be the etiology for obesity in the *ob/ob* mouse.[61] This protein and its regulation and receptor are discussed in great detail in Chapter 43. The most important support for the role of leptin in regulating weight in humans is the occurrence of genetic defects within the leptin signaling pathway in two families (see Mutations of Leptin or the Leptin Receptor, below).

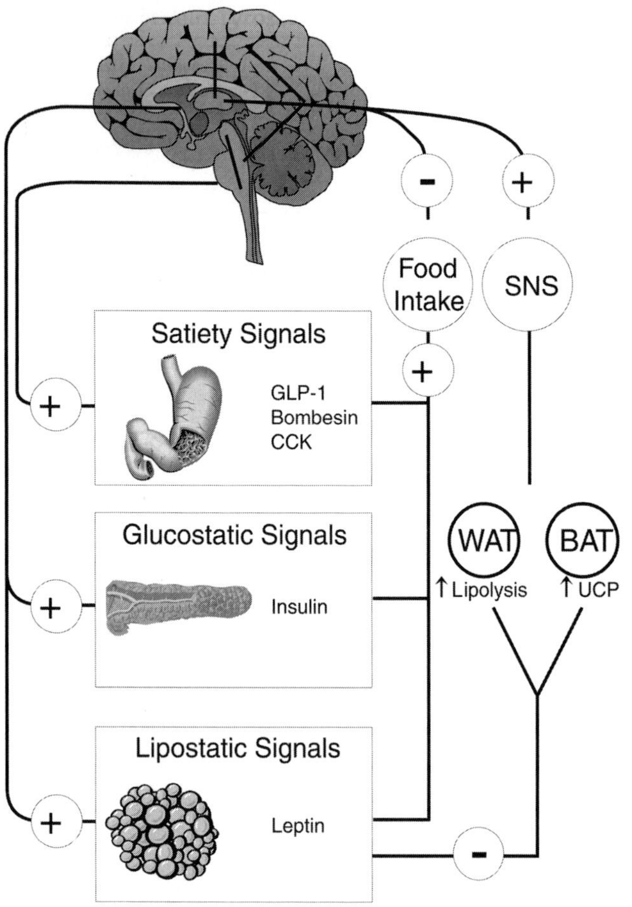

FIGURE 44–3. Integration between feeding-related signals to the brain and food intake and energy expenditure. Food intake initiates a series of signals that reach the hypothalamus via the blood-brain barrier (lipostatic and glucostatic signals) or via the brain stem (satiety signals). The hypothalamus integrates these signals with other sensory, cognitive, and environmental signals from the cerebral cortex. This integrated information, when sent back to the periphery, results in a decrease in food intake and activation of the sympathetic nervous system (SNS). The SNS via the β_3-adrenergic receptor stimulates lipolysis in white adipose tissue (WAT) and thermogenesis in brown adipose tissue (BAT) via activation of uncoupling proteins (UCPs). CCK, cholecystokinin; GLP-1, glucagon-like peptide-1.

Glucostatic Signals

Although insulin clearly plays a role in systemic fuel utilization, data also support its activity within the central nervous system to regulate energy homeostasis. Some evidence indicates that insulin-regulated glucose metabolism within ventromedial hypothalamus neurons may regulate autonomic outflow and, subsequently, the metabolic rate. In humans, insulin infusion during euglycemic clamp procedures increases sympathetic nervous system activity.[62] In animal models, direct injection of insulin into the ventromedial hypothalamus alters sympathetic nervous activity to brown adipose tissue (BAT).[63] Finally, destruction of insulin-sensitive neurons in the ventromedial hypothalamus by injection of gold thioglucose blocks diet-induced increases in thermogenesis.[64]

Satiety Signals

Cholecystokinin

Among the earliest satiety factors identified was the gut peptide cholecystokinin (CCK), which regulates meal size in rats in a dose-dependent manner.[65] In baboons, CCK administered directly by the intraventricular route significantly reduced 30-minute meal consumption, whereas intravenous CCK had no such effect.[66] The importance

of CCK in the regulation of appetite and food intake was further established with the use of selective antagonists. Whereas CCK reduced meal intake by nearly half, a selective antagonist completely reversed this suppression. By itself, the CCK antagonist was able to increase food intake by approximately one-third.[67]

Bombesin Family

Several factors have been identified that may play a role in meal size regulation, including the bombesin family of molecules. These molecules include bombesin, gastrin-releasing peptide, neuromedin C, and neuromedin B, all of which are able to suppress food intake. These molecules appear to act through a family of receptors that have been initially grouped as neuromedin C preferring and gastrin-releasing peptide preferring.[68–70]

Incretins

Another family of gastrointestinal signals is the incretin family of peptides. These peptides, secreted by enteroendocrine cells of the large and small intestine, were first identified as being responsible for the incremental release of insulin that occurs after oral administration of glucose relative to that after an equivalent amount of glucose administered intravenously.[71, 72] Glucose-dependent insulinotropic peptide was the first member of this family to be identified.[73] The most studied member of the incretin peptides is glucagon-like peptide-1 (GLP-1). GLP-1 is derived from proglucagon mRNA. It is now known that GLP-1 lowers blood glucose by increasing glucose-mediated insulin release, delaying gastric emptying, and inhibiting glucagon release. Furthermore, intracerebroventricular administration of GLP-1 significantly decreases food and water intake.[73] In this role, GLP-1 may be important in regulating energy intake and its subsequent metabolism. It was shown that many of these peripheral satiety factors signal the brain via afferent nerves or by acting as circulating factors that interact with specific receptors residing in the brain.[66, 74–76] However, chronic administration has not yet been shown to significantly affect body weight.[77]

Glucocorticoids

Excess glucocorticoids have profound effects on fat and muscle mass and on fat and glucose metabolism. However, their role in signaling to the central nervous system has only more recently been elucidated. Central administration of corticosterone increases fat mass in adrenalectomized rodents.[78] In contrast, deficiency of glucocorticoids significantly enhances the ability of centrally administered leptin to cause weight loss, an effect reversed by the administration of glucocorticoid.[79] Furthermore, centrally administered glucocorticoids significantly increase plasma leptin levels, medial basal hypothalamic corticotropin-releasing hormone (CRH) levels, and arcuate nucleus neuropeptide Y (NPY) protein levels. These data suggest parallel actions of leptin and glucocorticoid in signaling in weight homeostasis. A schematic representing the potential mechanisms of glucocorticoid action on energy balance is shown in Figure 44–4.

Integration of Signals: Central Nervous System Regulation of Weight

A number of orexigenic and anorexigenic signals within the most important areas of the brain have been identified. Much of the input to the brain is integrated within the hypothalamus. This concept is underscored by the observation that mRNA for the functional long form of the leptin receptor has been identified in numerous nuclei throughout the hypothalamus, including the arcuate nucleus, dorsomedial hypothalamus, paraventricular nucleus, ventromedial hypothalamus, lateral hypothalamus, ventral premamillary and medial mamillary nuclei, and lateral olfactory nucleus.[80] The crosstalk within and between these nuclei, even within single neurons, is only now being understood and systematically explored.

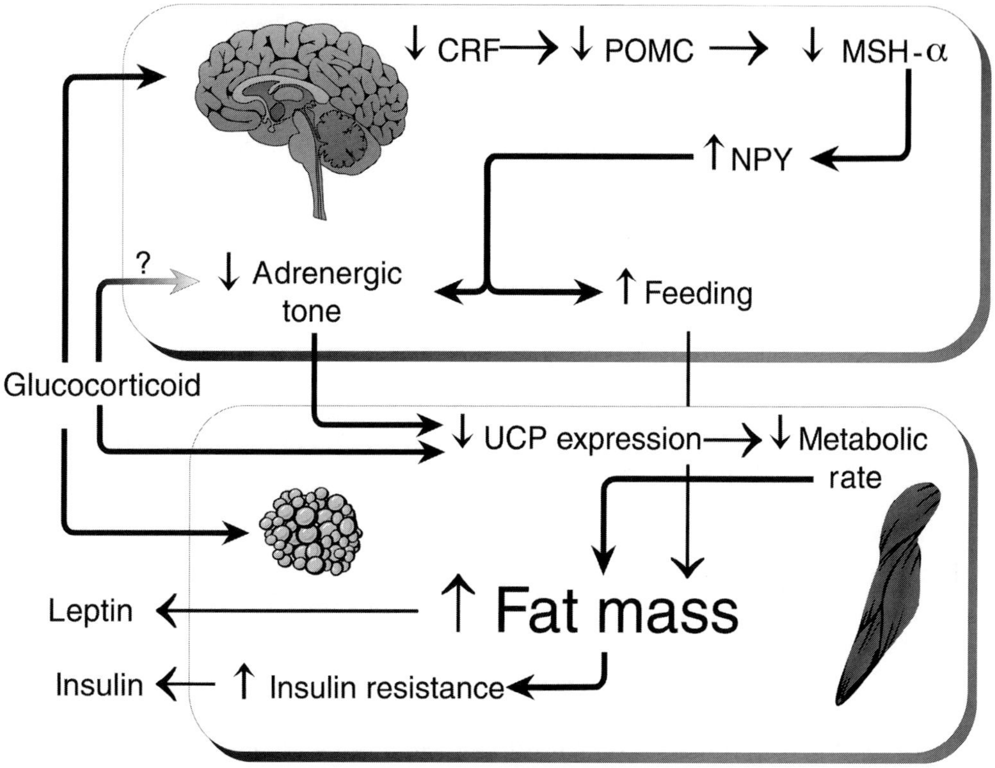

FIGURE 44–4. *Schematic representation of the mechanism(s) by which glucocorticoid may affect energy balance and food intake. CRF, corticotropin-releasing factor; α-MSH, α-melanocyte-stimulating hormone; NPY, neuropeptide Y; POMC, proopiomelanocortin; UCP, uncoupling protein.*

Orexigenic Signals

Neuropeptide Y

Post–leptin receptor signaling, to a great extent, involves the negative inhibition of NPY. NPY is a neurotransmitter widely expressed throughout the brain. However, NPY neurons within the hypothalamus were shown to be an important part of regulating energy consumption and feeding behavior after the discovery of leptin. NPY is highly overexpressed in the leptin-deficient *ob/ob* mouse and in the leptin receptor–deficient *db/db* mouse.[81, 82] Furthermore, NPY overexpression can be reversed by leptin administration in the *ob/ob* mouse, but not the *db/db* mouse.[83] In normal animals, leptin administration to animals that have been fasted prevents the normal increase in hypothalamic NPY with food restriction.[84, 85] NPY is among the most potent orexigenic peptides. When injected directly into the paraventricular nucleus of the hypothalamus, NPY causes a marked increase in food intake, weight, and body fat within 10 days of treatment in female rats.[86] The metabolic changes induced by centrally administered NPY mimic the changes seen in obesity.[79] Furthermore, centrally administered NPY reduces sympathetic nervous system efferent activity to BAT with a subsequent decrease in energy expenditure.[87, 88]

Although NPY and leptin appear to be components of an important feedback loop, experiments in transgenic animals suggest that the role of NPY in weight regulation and feeding behavior is complex. Mice deficient in NPY have normal body weight, feeding behavior, and body composition.[89, 90] At least five NPY receptors have been cloned, including one that appears to be a pseudogene,[91] and at least one additional receptor identified by pharmacologic means has eluded cloning.[91] Although experiments with agonists and antagonists suggest that the NPY-1 and NPY-5 receptors are the most likely candidates for the "feeding" receptor, some degree of uncertainty still surrounds this interpretation.[92] The NPY-5 receptor knockout mouse gains more weight, not less, between 12 and 20 weeks of age than do heterozygous knockout or wild-type mice. This weight gain is associated with increased amounts of food consumption and fat pad weight.[93] In the NPY-1 receptor knockout mouse, weight is increased as well, but it is associated with decreases in energy expenditure during the active period but with no change in food intake when compared with heterozygous knockout or wild-type mice.[94] Therefore, the relative importance of NPY and the various NPY receptor subtypes will require

additional work with more selective antagonists and transgenic animals with combinations of gene disruptions.

Melanin-Concentrating Hormone

Melanin-concentrating hormone (MCH), a circulating peptide first discovered in chub salmon that regulates fish scale color by aggregating melanonosomes,[95] was identified in the hypothalamus of the *ob/ob* mouse by differential-display polymerase chain reaction. Injection of MCH into the lateral ventricles causes an increase in food intake.[96] Recently it has been shown that transgenic mice produced with targeted deletions of the *MCH* gene had lower body weight, hypophagia, and an increased metabolic rate despite lower levels of both leptin and pro-opiomelanocortin (POMC) mRNA within the arcuate nucleus.[97] Interestingly, these mice had a hyperphagic response to starvation,[97] similar to that seen in mice lacking expression of NPY.[90]

Galanin

Galanin, a hypothalamic peptide found in abundance in the paraventricular nucleus, is associated with preference for dietary fat.[98] Galanin expression is significantly upregulated by increases in dietary fat, more so in obese-prone strains than in obese-resistant strains.[99] However, chronic central administration of galanin does not result in hyperphagia or obesity.[100]

Orexins

Two closely related hypothalamic neuropeptides have been identified that may also play a role in weight homeostasis. Orexin-A and orexin-B (hypocretin-1 and hypocretin-2, respectively), derived from the same parent precursor molecule, are upregulated with fasting. Central administration of either protein stimulates food intake.[101]

Opioids

The POMC polypeptide is the parent molecule of several peptides with potential weight-regulating properties (see Chapter 16). Among those with orexigenic properties are the endogenous opioid peptides. Opioids have been known for years to stimulate appetite, but it was

TABLE 44–1. Family of Melanocortin Receptors

Receptor	Tissue	Function	Antagonist
MC-1	Melanocytes	Pigmentation	Agouti
MC-2	Adrenal cortex	Steroid genesis	Agouti
MC-3	Hypothalamus, limbic	Feeding ?	Agouti, AGRP
MC-4	Hypothalamus, brain	Feeding	Agouti, AGRP
MC-5	Peripheral tissues	?	?

AGRP, agouti-related protein.

identification of the endogenous opioid peptides β-endorphin, dynorphin A, and enkephalins that led to increased interest in this system as it relates to energy balance. Long-acting enkephalin analogues (possibly via the δ opioid receptor), β-endorphin (possibly via the μ opioid receptor), and dynorphin A (possibly via the κ opioid receptor) have all been shown to increase feeding behavior.[102, 103]

Anorexigenic Signals

Pro-opiomelanocortin System

In addition to the opioid molecules that stimulate feeding behavior, the POMC polypeptide yields a number of anorexigenic molecules (see Chapter 16). α-Melanocyte–stimulating hormone (α-MSH) elicits effects that are opposed to the effects of NPY and MCH. The action of α-MSH is mediated through the melanocortin family of receptors, five of which have been identified and are summarized in Table 44–1. α-MSH activation of the melanocortin-4 (MC-4) receptor and possibly the MC-3 receptor appears to inhibit eating behavior and increase energy expenditure as deduced from antagonist and gene knockout experiments. Agouti protein, a naturally occurring antagonist to all melanocortin receptors and normally produced only in skin, causes obesity when ectopically overexpressed in the brain of the yellow agouti (A^y) mouse.[104] Furthermore, transgenic mice deficient in MC-4 receptor have a hyperphagic and obese phenotype.[105] Finally, agouti-related protein, another endogenous protein that is an antagonist at the MC-3 and MC-4 receptors, when overexpressed in transgenic mice also produces an obese phenotype.[106] A schematic representation of how these molecules and receptors interact is shown in Figure 44–5.

Corticotropin-Releasing Hormone

CRH[107] and the related urocortin[108] reduce food intake and body weight when administered directly to the brain. Additionally, leptin administration increases the expression of CRH mRNA in the hypothalamus.[84] Finally, the increase in weight seen in glucocorticoid excess states may in part be due to the attendant suppression of CRH.[109, 110]

Cocaine and Amphetamine Regulated Transcript

The neuropeptide cocaine and amphetamine regulated transcript (CART) was discovered by differential display to identify the genes expressed after acute administration of cocaine and amphetamine to rats. The C-terminal 48 amino acids of the prohormone predicted by the sequence of the gene appears to be the biologically active form and is a potent inhibitor of feeding.[111] CART mRNA has been shown to be highly expressed in multiple nuclei of the hypothalamus, many of which are important in feeding behavior and appetite regulation. The potential role of CART in energy balance was suggested by showing that leptin coordinately regulated CART expression and furthermore that CART inhibited the feeding response induced by either fasting or NPY.[112]

Neurotensin

Neurotensin (NT), a 13–amino acid peptide first discovered because of its vasodilatory activity and isolated and purified from bovine hypothalamus, is found throughout the brain and gastrointestinal tract. In the brain, its highest concentrations are in the hypothalamus, with a nuclei pattern consistent with its role as an anorexigenic peptide.[102] NT decreases both spontaneous and norepinephrine-induced feeding. Regulation of NT is inverse to that of NPY in *ob/ob* mice and in Zucker obese (*fa/fa*) rats. However, the role of NT in the daily regulation of feeding behavior, caloric intake, and satiety has not yet been established.

Other Peptides

As discussed above, GLP-1 may be an important signaling peptide from the periphery. However, several lines of evidence also suggest

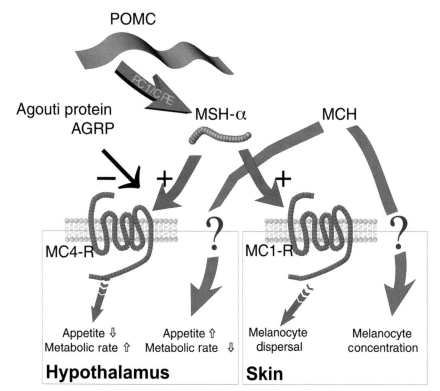

FIGURE 44–5. Schematic representation of the crosstalk and signaling of the proopiomelanocortin (POMC) product α-melanocyte-stimulating hormone (α-MSH), agouti proteins, and melanocyte-concentrating hormone (MCH). POMC cleavage by prohormone convertase-1 and carboxypeptidase E (PC1/CPE) yields α-MSH which inhibits feeding and stimulates the metabolic rate through the melanocortin-4 receptor (MC4-R) in the hypothalamus. Agouti protein and agouti-related protein (AGRP) inhibit this signaling. α-MSH also causes darkening of skin pigments via the MC1 receptor (MC1-R). MCH, acting through unidentified receptor(s), has effects counter to that of α-MSH in the hypothalamus in humans and in pigment cells of fish scales.

that GLP-1 may be a central anorexigenic molecule. It is known that GLP-1 has potent central effects. Furthermore, concentrations of GLP-1 administered centrally have effects that are not reproduced when administered peripherally. Finally, GLP-1 has been found in several hypothalamic nuclei responsible for energy balance.[102]

Other neuropeptides that have been identified and may affect weight homeostasis include somatostatin, thyroid-stimulating hormone (independent of thyroid hormone), calcitonin gene–related peptide, norepinephrine, and growth hormone–releasing hormone.

Effector Components in Energy Homeostasis: Peripheral Systems

The peripheral systems involved in energy balance can be divided into efferent signals from the brain and their respective receptors and the effector molecules that translate the signals into an increase or decrease in energy expenditure. The two most studied efferent signal systems are the adrenergic nervous system and the thyroid hormone axis. Although thyroid hormone clearly plays a role in the basal state of energy utilization, the long half-life of thyroxine, as well as its long-term genomic effects, suggests that this system is most important in affecting energy balance on a long-term basis. The discovery of several isoforms of the thyroid hormone receptor with differential tissue distributions opens the possibility of regulation of energy through specific receptor subtypes.[113] The effect of thyroid hormone on metabolism and the metabolic rate is covered in Chapter 94. The daily variations in energy expenditure are more likely to occur via the adrenergic nervous system. The effector molecules that separate fuel oxidation from ATP synthesis (i.e., potential chemical energy) reside within a subset of the family of mitochondrial transport protein known as uncoupling proteins (UCPs).

Uncoupling Proteins

The first uncoupling protein (now termed UCP-1) was identified in the mid-1970s[114, 115] as a mitochondrial protein that bound to purine nucleotides and fatty acids and was involved in energy dissipation. This protein family belongs to the mitochondrial anion carrier proteins, which also include adenosine diphosphate (ADP)/ATP carrier, phosphate, and oxoglutarate carriers. UCP-1 is primarily expressed in BAT.[116] In mitochondria derived from other cell types, oxidation of fuels is tightly coupled to the generation of ATP. The mitochondrial respiratory chain produces a proton gradient across the inner mitochondrial membrane. ATP synthesis from ADP by the protein ATP synthase is driven by the coupled movement of protons down this electrochemical gradient. If ADP substrate is limited, proton flux through ATP synthase is inhibited and the gradient is maintained. In BAT mitochondria, protons may move down the gradient in a manner that is uncoupled from ATP synthesis.[117] Uncoupling of the potential energy of the gradient from ATP generation provides a mechanism for both the dissipation of excess calories and the production of heat.

The activity of UCPs is highly regulated within BAT. In addition to receptor-mediated changes in cyclic adenosine monophosphate, free fatty acids are important intracellular activators of UCP-1 activity.[118, 119] Cytosolic ATP inhibits UCP-1 activity, perhaps in a negative feedback loop. In addition to allosteric or transport-level regulation, it is likely that transcriptional regulation occurs as well. The UCP-1 protein is acutely upregulated by catecholamines via the β_3-adrenergic receptor,[120] as well as by the other β-receptor subtypes, particularly during development.[121] Adrenergic-mediated upregulation of UCP-1 also accounts for increased expression with cold exposure, as well as explains, to some extent, diet-induced thermogenesis.[122, 123]

Two additional cloned proteins, UCP-2 and UCP-3, have different tissue-specific expression and transcriptional regulation. At least one report has shown that the proton transport activity of UCP-1 is dependent on the presence of an intact histidine pair, which is absent in both UCP-2 and UCP-3.[124] UCP-2 is expressed in BAT but, unlike UCP-1, is also expressed in a broad range of tissues. Figure 44–6 shows the known regulators of expression of the various UCP proteins.

Adrenergic Nervous System

The adrenergic nervous system regulates energy expenditure at the cellular level by regulating the expression of UCPs (see Fig. 44–6) and at the whole animal level by enhancing total and basal oxygen consumption,[125] increasing thermogenic responses, and increasing BAT mass.[126] The α- and β-adrenergic receptors mediate catecholamine responses.

The β-adrenergic receptors were first subtyped by Lands et al. into β_1- and β_2-adrenergic receptors.[127] However, evidence increasingly indicated that the pharmacology of known adrenergic agonists in adipose and gastrointestinal tissue was not explained by the known β-adrenergic receptors.[128] In 1983 it was proposed that the atypical β-adrenergic receptor within adipose tissue be considered a third β-

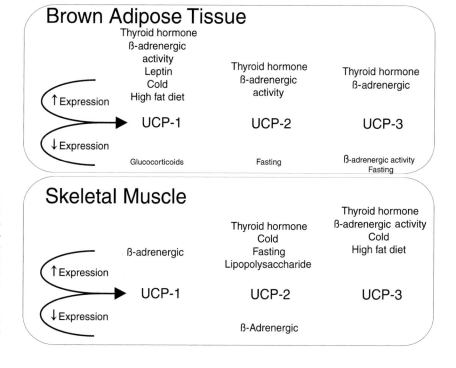

FIGURE 44–6. Known effects of a variety of stimuli on expression of the major uncoupling proteins (UCPs) in brown adipose tissue *(upper panel)* and skeletal muscle *(lower panel)*. Chemicals and physiologic conditions above or below each UCP increase or decrease UCP mRNA expression, respectively. Discrepent results may be explained by data derived from experiments with intact animals that did not control for ambient temperature, age, or obesity propensity of the strain. Data do not represent protein expression or activity, an attribute that is difficult to measure in cell systems and elusive if not impossible to measure in whole animals.

receptor subtype.[129] Although all three receptor subtypes are found within adipocytes, the β_3-adrenergic receptor is most highly expressed in BAT, the tissue most likely responsible for the thermogenic effect of food[130] and acclimation to cold.[131]

The β_3-adrenergic receptor is a member of the seven-transmembrane G protein–coupled receptor family and is 95% homologous to the β_1- and β_2-adrenergic receptors. Despite having sequence information on the β_1- and β_2-adrenergic receptors for a number of years, cloning of the human β_3-adrenergic receptor occurred only in 1989.[132] Additional work led to the discovery that the human isoform of the β_3-receptor was different from the rat receptor in that it had a second exon with an additional six amino acids on the C terminus.[133] This change in protein structure was not expected to cause significant interspecies differences in pharmacology. However, many of the pharmacologic agonists synthesized and optimized for activity at the rat β_3-receptor were actually weak partial agonists at the human receptor. This finding was a possible explanation for failure of β_3-receptor agonists to increase energy expenditure in humans.[134] A unique aspect of the β_3-receptor, in contrast to the β_1- and β_2-adrenergic receptors, was the lack of acute homologous downregulation by serine kinases.[135]

β_3-Receptor pharmacology and/or receptor mRNA has also been identified in the following tissues other than fat, with considerable variation existing between species: skeletal muscle,[120] ileum-colon,[136–138] gastric fundus,[139] neural tissue,[140] bronchial smooth muscle,[141] vasculature,[142] and heart tissue.[143]

A polymorphism in the β_3-adrenergic receptor gene has been identified that leads to a single amino acid substitution within the molecule at position 64, with arginine replacing a tryptophan.[144] Many studies have examined whether the occurrence of this polymorphism is linked to any of a number of abnormalities, including obesity, diabetes, insulin resistance, and glucose intolerance, as well as the relative risk of each of these conditions. Presently, the evidence would suggest that if this polymorphism has any effect on the development of obesity or diabetes, it is relatively minor.

Human adipocytes express α-adrenergic receptors to a high level. The α_2-adrenergic receptors are the predominant subtype. The α-adrenergic receptor, under catecholamine stimulation, acts to suppress lipolysis. Differences in relative expression of the α- and β-adrenergic receptors have been used to explain some of the uniqueness of human forms of obesity. Unlike lower mammals, human adipocytes tend to express relatively fewer β- and more α-adrenergic receptors. Therefore, on balance, human adipose is relatively resistant to the lipolytic effects of catecholamines and hence is more likely to store fat.

SYNDROMES OF OBESITY

Common Obesity

The most common forms of obesity cannot be explained by single, clearly defined defects. In fact, many believe that the obesity epidemic is largely related to a normal physiology built for energy conservation and efficient fuel utilization in the face of environmental and social factors that promote food intake and limit physical activity. In this view, common obesity is a result of the interaction between widely varying environmental influences and polygenically controlled traits. Many genes have been identified that show linkage to obesity, energy balance, feeding behavior, or adipocyte biology. The reader is referred to an excellent review by Comuzzie and Allison.[145] It is unlikely that any single external cause or single gene will explain common obesity and overweight.

Many factors contribute to overeating. Food availability and portion size have increased markedly this century. Rapid and far-reaching deployment of "fast-food" establishments is found in nearly every developed country worldwide. Within the fast-food industry, the use of enticing extra-large portions is commonplace. In addition to size and availability of food, the nutrient composition of typical diets may also contribute to obesity. The importance of fat content as a contributor to the occurrence of human obesity is supported by the observation that the sine qua non of animal models of diet-induced obesity is the administration of a diet containing at least 35% of total calories from fat. Whether this dependence is due to fat per se or that high fat foods have a higher caloric density is unclear.

Reduction in physical activity may also have contributed to the occurrence of obesity. Technologic advances in transportation, telecommunications, and computing have reduced the need for physical exertion as part of the activities of daily living. The electronics revolution, including television and video games, has promoted a more passive form of entertainment. Importantly, many children do not participate in school-associated physical activity because of reductions in funding for physical education, as well as a reduction in the number of specially trained physical education teachers.[146]

Neuroendocrine Obesity

Hypothalamic Obesity

Hypothalamic obesity has been reported after specific injuries to the hypothalamus. Such injuries causing obesity are uncommon, but include trauma, malignancy, and inflammatory disease.[147] Several features of this syndrome are invariably present, including signs and symptoms of increased intracranial pressure, abnormalities in hypothalamic-pituitary function, and hypothalamic neurologic abnormalities (e.g., disorders of thirst and thermal regulation).[147]

Polycystic Ovarian Disease

Polycystic ovarian disease is a constellation of phenotypes that includes, to varying degrees, menstrual dysfunction, hirsutism, hyperandrogenism, cystic ovaries, insulin resistance, and obesity.[37] Obesity is a defined part of the syndrome in as many as half of these patients.[148] The cause of obesity in polycystic ovarian disease is unclear. It is possible that obesity may predate the development of menstrual dysfunction. It has been proposed that obesity may be an etiologic factor in the development of polycystic ovarian disease by an associated increase in adipose conversion of the adrenal androgen Δ^4-androstenedione to the weak estrogen estrone.[149]

Cushing's Syndrome and Cushing's Disease

Central obesity is among the hallmark findings associated with both Cushing's syndrome and Cushing's disease. These two entities are described in detail in Chapter 121.

Hypothyroidism

Obesity may be a feature of primary or secondary hypothyroidism, although most changes in weight associated with thyroid disease are not usually marked. Hypothyroidism is associated with abnormalities in water excretion leading to possible hyponatremia and water retention, which may explain some of the increased weight often seen. The increased subcutaneous thickening noted in skin is not likely to be manifested as significant weight gain.

Genetic Causes of Obesity

Mutations of Leptin or the Leptin Receptor

Two families have been identified that have mutations in either the leptin gene or the leptin receptor gene. In one highly consanguineous family, two cousins were identified as having a homozygous frameshift mutation involving deletion of a single guanine nucleotide in codon 133 of the leptin gene. Both affected individuals had normal weight at birth, but deviation from normal growth curves occurred by 3 months in one and by 4 months in the other. One of the affected patients weighed 86 kg (57% body fat) by 8 years of age. The other patient weighed 29 kg (54% body fat) by 2 years of age. Hyperphagia was present in both patients.[150]

A second family has been described in which three sisters (one deceased at age 19 years) had morbid obesity and significant deviation from normal weight-height growth curves before the age of 1 year. In all three, serum leptin levels were well above (>500 ng/mL) that predicted by weight. The proband was found to have a G → A mutation in the splice donor site of exon 16 of the leptin receptor gene. This mutation was found to encode a protein lacking both the transmembrane and intracellular domains of the leptin receptor.[151]

Other Monogenic Mutations Causing Obesity

In addition to mutations of the leptin and leptin receptor genes, several newly identified mutations involving orexigenic and anorexigenic neuropeptides or an adipocyte-differentiating factor were linked to early-onset, severe obesity. These mutations involved the genes encoding POMC, prohormone convertase-1 (PC1), the MC-4 receptor, and peroxisome proliferator–activated receptor γ2 (PPARγ2).

Linkage of human obesity to chromosome 2 in proximity to the *POMC* locus, as well as the role of α-MSH in the regulation of feeding, led to the hypothesis that POMC or its progeny peptides were associated with obesity. This hypothesis was borne out when two patients were identified with mutations within the *POMC* locus and who displayed the predicted phenotype of obesity, altered pigmentation, and adrenocorticotropic hormone (ACTH) deficiency. One patient was shown to be a compound heterozygote with exon 3, with a single nucleotide substitution at position 7013 leading to a premature stop codon in the paternal allele and a single nucleotide deletion at position 7133 leading to a frameshift and altered ACTH and α-MSH structure, as well as a premature termination, in the maternal allele. This girl was found to have ACTH deficiency as a newborn, which was diagnosed in part because of the presence of adrenal hypoplasia in her first-born brother. She was reported to have hyperphagia and obesity commencing at 4 months of age. A second patient was also identified with a homozygous mutation involving a single nucleotide substitution at position 3804 (exon 2) located 11 bp upstream of the start codon for the wild-type protein. This mutation introduces an additional, out-of-frame start codon within the consensus sequence for translation initiation. Such a mutation could be expected to prevent translation of the wild-type protein. This patient was found to have only trace amounts of circulating POMC-derived peptides.[152]

The processing of POMC into its component neuropeptides is to a great extent accomplished by the action of two endopeptidases, PC1 and carboxypeptidase E. Interest in mutations of these processing enzymes as causes of obesity arose from the knowledge that mutations of carboxypeptidase E lead to an obese phenotype in the *fat/fat* mouse.[153] A patient has been described with compound heterozygous mutations within the *PC1* gene: a single amino acid substitution of arginine for glycine at position 483 prevented processing of pro-PC1 and retention in the endoplasmic reticulum, and a single base pair substitution of the intron-5 donor splice site led to the skipping of exon 5 and loss of 26 amino acids, a frameshift, and occurrence of a premature stop codon within the catalytic domain.[154] With effects attributed to abnormal processing of POMC, the patient was reported to have a complex phenotype including extreme childhood obesity, glucose intolerance, hypogonadotropic hypogonadism, hypocortisolism, hypoinsulinemia, and elevated proinsulin and POMC concentrations.[155]

In mice, targeted disruption of the MC-4 receptor leads to obesity.[105] A description of a frameshift mutation in the MC-4 receptor has now been described in a human patient. This individual was shown to be heterozygous for a 4-bp deletion at codon 211 of the MC-4 receptor that resulted in a frameshift that introduced a five–amino acid substitution; this alteration was followed by a premature stop codon within the region encoding the fifth transmembrane domain that led to a truncated protein. The patient had severe obesity beginning as early as 4 months of age that was associated with hyperphagia and continuous food-seeking behavior.[156]

Although no monogenic mutations of adipocyte differentiation or triglyceride storage genes have been identified in rodents, a missense mutation in the *PPARγ2* gene has been identified in humans that is associated with marked obesity. In screening a population of obese individuals, 4 of 121 were found to have substitution of a glutamine for a proline at position 115 in the PPARγ2 protein. Phenotypically, the patients with the mutation had a significantly higher BMI. Three

of 4 had type 2 diabetes but, interestingly, tended to have lower fasting serum insulin concentrations. Expression of the mutant protein in murine fibroblasts suggested that this mutation decreased serine phosphorylation at position 114, an event that reduces PPARγ2 activity. Transfected fibroblasts were also shown to have an increased rate of adipocyte differentiation and triglyceride accumulation in comparison to cells transfected with wild-type PPARγ2.[157]

Other Genetic Disorders

A number of rare genetic disorders have been identified that are associated with significant changes in body weight and body composition. Several of these syndromes are summarized in Table 44–2.

THERAPY FOR OBESITY

Determination of Treatment Candidates

As in the pharmacologic treatment of all diseases, no risk-free, highly efficacious therapies are available. Therefore, we are left balancing risk and efficacy in a highly heterogeneous group of individuals with a wide range of risk factors for significant disease. Underscoring the risk associated with overweight and obesity, the National Heart, Lung, and Blood Institute of the National Institutes of Health convened an Expert Panel on the Identification, Evaluation, and Treatment of Overweight and Obesity in Adults as part of an overall Obesity Education Initiative. That panel prepublished guidelines for diagnosing and treating patients in June 1998.

Evidence now supports the full range of interventions in patients with a BMI of 30 kg/m² or greater and in patients with BMIs of 27 kg/m² or greater and 29.9 kg/m² or less with at least two associated risk factors (Table 44–3). For patients with a BMI of 25 kg/m² or greater, it is agreed that diet and exercise be instituted. Whether pharmacologic intervention is used at this point depends on the severity and degree of associated risk factors balanced against known risks for a particular treatment. The initial target weight loss should be a minimum of 10% of starting body weight. Efforts should be made, with frequent follow-up and feedback, to establish a rate of weight loss of approximately 1 to 2 lb (0.5–1 kg) per week for a period of up to 6 months. The first step in weight loss is the institution of a diet and exercise program. Depending on the particular risks in any given patient, individuals who are unable to achieve or maintain target weight loss should then begin behavior modification programs, followed as necessary by pharmacotherapy and then, in the most severe cases, weight loss surgery. These options are discussed in greater detail below. In many cases, success will depend on a combination of all strategies. The most successful initial regimens are those that combine diet, exercise, and behavioral therapy.[159]

Diet Therapy

Caloric restriction will lead to weight loss; however, for any single patient, the total calories that will maintain constant weight or initiate weight loss varies significantly. Several formulas have been developed for the calculation of resting or basal metabolic rate.[160–163] These equations are very useful in setting approximate targets for dietary calories in individuals seeking weight loss. However, variability between subjects is high, so regular interval monitoring of weight loss and subsequent adjustments to dietary intake should be undertaken.

A review of the effectiveness of some recent published programs with moderate calorie-restricted diets (approximately 1200 kcal/day for women, 1500 kcal/day for men) indicated that after an average of 21 weeks, weight loss was approximately 8.5 kg from baseline after a 21% attrition rate.[164] After an additional 1 year follow-up period, most of these subjects had regained some, but not all their weight.[164] Regain of weight is among the greatest challenges facing a diet intervention program. It has been shown that over time, weight regain increases and virtually all patients in a moderate calorie-restricted program regained all their pretreatment weight within 5 years.[165]

TABLE 44–2. Characteristics of Genetic Syndromes Causing Obesity

Characteristic	Syndrome				
	Prader-Willi	*AHO*	*Bardet-Biedl*	*Cohen*	*Börjeson-Forssman-Lehmann*
Inheritance	Sporadic	Sex-influenced autosomal dominant*	Autosomal recessive	Autosomal recessive	X-linked
Gene mapping	Loss of expression in 15q11-q13, usually deletion	Loss of *GNAS1*† gene on 20q13 or unknown‡	Unknown	8q22-q23§	Xq26-q27
Stature	Short	Short, stocky build	Usually normal	Usually short	Short
Obesity	Moderate to severe by age 3 Hyperphagia and food-seeking behavior	Moderate by age 4	Moderate to severe, truncal by age 3	Mild to moderate, truncal by midchildhood	Moderate by early childhood
Physical	Neonatal hypotonia Narrow bifrontal diameter Almond-shaped eyes Narrow nasal bridge Down-turned mouth Small, narrow hands and feet Hypopigmentation (50%) Strabismus Scoliosis GH deficiency	Round face Short neck Brachydactyly Ectopic calcifications ± Pseudohypopara- thyroidism and/or multiple hormone resistance Metacarpal (3rd, 4th, and 5th) and metatarsal (3rd and 4th) shortening	Pigmentary retinopathy Postaxial polydactyly Renal abnormalities¶	Infantile hypotonia Narrow hands and feet with long tapering fingers Down-slanting palpebral fissures High nasal bridge Short philtrum High narrow palate Prominent central incisors Occasionally chorioretinal dysplasia	Coarse facies Prominent supraorbital ridges Deep-set eyes with ptosis and narrow palpebral fissures Large ears
Reproductive capacity	Primary hypogonadism		Hypogonadism M: primary F: primary, secondary	Delayed puberty	Genital hypoplasia
Mental retardations	Mild	Mild	Mild	Mild to moderate	Severe: M Normal to severe: F
Other	Thick saliva High pain threshold Sleep disturbances Thermoregulatory disturbances Osteoporosis			Most cases from Finland and Israel Intermittent granulocytopenia	

*Except primary hypoparathyroidism type II and AHO phenocopy types.
†α Subunit of the G protein Gα, gene.
‡Dependent on AHO type.
§In Finnish families.
¶Calyceal distortion, persistent fetal lobulation, tubular concentration defect, renal insufficiency, hypertension, and other heterogeneous parenchymal lesions.
AHO, Albright's hereditary osteodystrophy; GH, growth hormone.
Adapted from Guray-Aygun M, Cassidy SB, Nicholls RD: Prader-Willi and other syndromes associated with obesity and mental retardation. Behav Genet 27:307–324, 1997.

TABLE 44–3. Listing of Risk Factors in Assessing Suitability for Treatment Intervention in Individuals with a Body Mass Index between 25 and 29.9 kg/m²

Risk	Subgroup, Diagnostic Criteria, or Manifestation
Established CHD	History of myocardial infarction
	History of angina pectoris (stable or unstable)
	History of coronary artery surgery
	History of coronary artery procedures (e.g., angioplasty)
Presence of other atherosclerotic diseases	Peripheral arterial disease
	Abdominal aortic aneurysm
	Symptomatic carotid artery disease
Additional cardiovascular risks	Cigarette smoking
	Hypertension (systolic blood pressure $\geq$140 mm Hg *or* diastolic blood pressure $\geq$90 mm Hg)
	High-risk LDL-C ($\geq$160 mg/dL)
	Low-risk HDL-C ($\leq$35 mg/dL)
	Impaired FBG (110–125 mg/dL, inclusive)
	Family history or premature CHD (myocardial infarction or sudden death in father 55 or younger or mother 65 or younger)
	Age (men $\geq$45 yr; women $\geq$55 yr)
Type 2 diabetes	Fasting plasma glucose $\geq$126 mg/dL
	Casual plasma glucose $\geq$200 mg/dL plus symptoms
	2-hr plasma glucose $\geq$200 mg/dL during OGTT[158]
Sleep apnea	Recurrent apnea or hypopnea associated with clinical impairment
Identification of other obesity-associated diseases	Gynecologic abnormalities
	Osteoarthritis
	Gallstones and their complications
	Stress incontinence
Other risk factors	Physical inactivity
	High triglycerides ($\geq$400 mg/dL)

From http://www.nhlbi.nih.gov/nhlbi/cardio/obes/prof/guidelns/ob_gdlns.pdf
CHD, coronary heart disease; FBG, fasting blood glucose; HDL-C, high-density lipoprotein cholesterol; LDL-C, low-density lipoprotein cholesterol; OGTT, oral glucose tolerance test.

Because of the limited efficacy of moderate calorie-restricted weight loss programs, the use of very low calorie diets was investigated. These diets, often providing less than 800 kcal/day, deliver large amounts of high-quality protein sources (>50 g/day) in an effort to spare fat-free mass during the period of weight loss induced by severe caloric restriction. In most cases, under careful medical supervision these diets can safely induce weight loss of 1.5 to 2.5 kg/week.[166] However, a significant increase in the risk of gallstone development has been noted.[167] In the few well-controlled studies evaluating the efficacy of very low calorie diets, mean weight loss over the period of caloric restriction (16–26 weeks) ranged from approximately 10 kg to over 21 kg.[168–171] However, during follow-up intervals, all studies showed partial regain of the lost weight at 1 and 2 years, and in the one study that reported 5-year follow-up data, patients weighed more than their pretreatment weight.[170]

Because very low calorie diets do not seem to offer marked benefit over moderate calorie-restricted diets, it is recommended that a level of caloric restriction could be instituted with less risk and over a longer-term basis. Despite the shortcomings of moderate calorie-restricted diets, it is well agreed that the dietary habits that may be conferred during these programs will be important adjuncts to any additional therapy that may be prescribed. The guidelines recom-

mended for the initial dietary intervention are given in Table 44–4. A 500- to 1000-kcal energy deficit will cause patients to lose 1 to 2 lb/ week. This diet may be maintained for up to 6 months and should lead to the desired 10% weight loss in patients with initial BMI values of 35 kg/m² or greater. For patients with less severe obesity, the caloric deficit should be reduced. For many patients, particularly those with larger BMI values, weight loss beyond 6 months is extremely difficult. Part of this difficulty is explained by a concomitant reduction in metabolic rate and energy expenditure for a given amount of activity, so the caloric deficit is greatly reduced despite similar quantities of food intake. To maintain weight or continue weight loss, adjustments to greater levels of physical exercise must therefore be instituted between 3 and 6 months of a weight loss program. Finally, social factors often make chronic, continuous caloric restriction very difficult.

Exercise

It is not contested that physical activity is a central component of any weight loss program. Given the fact that total caloric intake has not risen dramatically in the United States over the past two decades, many experts believe the rise in obesity rates is more directly attribut-

TABLE 44–4. Initial Dietary Recommendations for Weight Loss

Nutrient	Recommended Intake
Calories	Approximately 500- to 1000-kcal/day reduction from usual intake
Total fat	30% or less of total calories
Saturated fatty acids*	8%–10% of total calories
Monounsaturated fatty acids	Up to 15% of total calories
Polyunsaturated fatty acids	Up to 10% of total calories
Cholesterol*	<300 mg/day
Protein	Approximately 15% of total calories
Carbohydrate	55% or more of total calories
Sodium chloride	No more than 100 mmol/day (approximately 2.4 g of sodium or approximately 6 g of sodium chloride)
Calcium	1000–1500 mg
Fiber	20–30 g

*May require additional modification if coexisting hyperlipidemia is present.

able to a decrease in the amount of physical activity of most Americans. Irrespective of etiology, multiple benefits are derived from any program that incorporates physical activity, including an increase in the likelihood for successful weight loss by both increasing energy expenditure[172] and decreasing appetite, an improvement in cardiovascular fitness and reduction in the risk of CHD,[173, 174] an increase in the success of weight maintenance once targets are achieved, and a reduction in intra-abdominal fat.[175]

As in all forms of physical exertion, it is best to start slowly, gradually building to the target level of activity. Many recommend a starting point of 10 minutes of walking, 3 days weekly, with increased walking to a target of up to 45 minutes 5 or more days per week. This target of exercise will use between 100 and 200 kcal/day. Given time, most patients will have improvements in exercise tolerance and functional capacity, often leading to higher targets and more strenuous sessions. More vigorous sessions may help sustain weight loss over time.

Behavior Modification

Because eating is often undertaken for personal, psychological, or social reasons, associated behaviors are often powerful forces that impede long-term caloric restriction and weight loss. Efforts at weight loss independent of changes in long-term behavior are unlikely to succeed. A range of behavior modification techniques have been devised and tested, each being nearly equally effective at supporting a weight loss program. Irrespective of the specific technique, the goal is generally to alter eating and eating-associated behavior for the long term with common behavior modification techniques.[3]

Pharmacotherapy

Over the past 50 years a large number of pharmacologic agents have been used in the control of weight with varying degrees of success. How health care dollars were spent reflects the relatively low acceptance of pharmacotherapy. In 1995 it was estimated that the amount of money spent in the United States on all weight loss products and services, including diet foods and drinks, exercise programs and equipment, and ancillary products, approached $35 billion, including $12 billion on diet food products alone. Purchase of diet food persists despite the widely held understanding that virtually all these products will do little to promote long-term weight loss and only exercise programs have a potential impact on cardiovascular conditioning. In contrast, the amount of money spent on anti-obesity pharmaceuticals in this same period was less than $500 million. These figures underscore the perception, be it real or imagined, that the agents available are either of relatively limited efficacy or have associated safety issues that make them less desirable alternatives.

However, since 1995, changes have taken place. Several new agents were introduced, several older agents were reinvestigated, and two compounds were withdrawn from the market over safety concerns, as described below. At the present time, several compounds have been studied and used for the treatment of obesity, but these agents, including ephedrine, fluoxetine, and caffeine, have not been approved for use by the U.S. Food and Drug Administration. A number of other compounds, including mazindol, phentermine, benzphetamine, and phendimetrazine, are approved for only short-term use for obesity in a number of countries worldwide. A number of these compounds have limited efficacy.[176]

Despite the advances and changes in pharmacotherapy, few programs have been available that lead to weight loss of more than 10 kg over diet and exercise programs. Nevertheless, although the degree of weight loss induced by pharmacotherapy is modest, such changes could be expected to have an impact on the risk of comorbid conditions and potentially on mortality. However, studies also demonstrate consistent impediments to assessing the durability of efficacy. First, weight loss appears to plateau between 24 and 30 weeks of treatment. Second, both the placebo and active arms appear to have a consistent, albeit modest rise in weight from the plateau point through to the end of the

study. Third, the study effect on weight endpoint is very large. In a study of D-fenfluramine, although weight loss in the active group was substantial (~10% of initial body weight), the placebo effect was also substantial, with a loss of approximately 7% of initial weight.[177] Finally, obesity trials are difficult to conduct in general because of a very large dropout rate. After 12 months, dropout rates approaching 50% in placebo groups are common, and even in active therapy arms, dropout rates may still be as high as 30% to 40%.[176] Given the high rates of dropout, completer analyses are often undertaken in addition to or even in lieu of intention-to-treat analyses. Because the single greatest reason for discontinuation is often dissatisfaction with weight loss, completer analyses will overestimate the a priori effect that any compound would be expected to achieve in a population of obese individuals.

Fenfluramine

D-Fenfluramine (and its racemic relative fenfluramine) is a centrally acting serotoninergic agonist and reuptake inhibitor whose main effect is suppression of appetite. D-Fenfluramine and fenfluramine were studied in several placebo-controlled, randomized, double-blind trials and were shown to cause significant weight loss from baseline.[177–180] The popularity of the use of D-fenfluramine was enhanced by the observation that when used over a 28-week treatment phase in combination with phentermine, a dopaminergic agonist, a significant 15.6% reduction from initial body weight was induced vs. a mean 4.9% decrease in placebo-treated patients.[181] Furthermore, at least partial durability was demonstrated in follow-up open-label studies lasting up to 156 weeks.[182] However, in mid-1997, cardiac valvulopathy was reported in 24 patients treated with D-fenfluramine and phentermine.[183] Follow-up requests from the U.S. Food and Drug Administration led to a total of 113 confirmed cases of D-fenfluramine– or fenfluramine-induced valvulopathy (with or without phentermine).[184] These results ultimately led to the voluntary withdrawal of both D-fenfluramine and fenfluramine from the market.

Orlistat

Orlistat, a synthetic derivative of lipstatin (from *Streptomyces toxytricini*), is an inhibitor of gastric and pancreatic lipases, enzymes critical for the digestion and absorption of fat from the gastrointestinal tract. Inhibition of lipases causes a reduction in the absorption of fat and an increase in the excretion of triglycerides in feces. In a dose-ranging 24-week study of obese subjects (mean BMI ~35 kg/m²), orlistat caused a maximal 9.8% decrease in initial body weight vs. a decrease of 6.5% in the placebo-treated group.[185] In a separate 2-year randomized, crossover study of 688 obese individuals (BMI ~36 kg/m², weight ~100 kg), orlistat, 120 mg three times daily, caused a 10.2% decrease from initial body weight after the first year vs. a 6.1% decrease in the placebo group.[186] Notably, both studies demonstrated a decrease in levels of the fat-soluble vitamins D, E, and β-carotene in a greater number of orlistat-treated patients than in placebo-treated patients. Furthermore, the number of adverse events predominantly related to the gastrointestinal tract and included increased fatty and oily stools, fecal urgency and incontinence, and flatulence. In 1999, orlistat was approved in the United States for the treatment of obesity.

Sibutramine

Sibutramine is a serotonin, dopamine, and norepinephrine reuptake inhibitor. In several published studies it has been shown to cause weight loss by a proposed primary mechanism of appetite suppression. In a dose-ranging 12-week trial of obese patients (BMI ~32 kg/m², weight ~85 kg), sibutramine caused a maximum weight loss of approximately 5 kg (~6% loss from initial weight) vs. a weight loss of approximately 1 kg (~1% loss from initial weight) in the placebo group.[187] In a 1-year placebo-controlled trial, analysis of patients who completed the study showed that 65% of patients taking 15 mg of sibutramine lost 5% of their initial body weight whereas only 29% of placebo-treated patients lost as much.[188] Significant numbers of patients have also been shown to lose greater than 10% of initial body weight. This degree of efficacy should make sibutramine another important tool in an overall weight loss program. Monitoring of blood pressure will be important, however, because sibutramine has been associated with a 3– to 60–beat per minute increase in heart rate and an approximately 4–mm Hg increase in diastolic blood pressure even after weight loss.[189]

Pharmacotherapy—Future

β₃-Adrenergic Receptor Agonists

The β₃-adrenergic receptor is highly expressed in human BAT and to a limited degree in human WAT.[190] Multiple studies in animals have indicated that this receptor is a potential target for anti-obesity therapy. Administration of a β₃-adrenergic receptor agonist has been shown to cause either weight loss, an increase in energy expenditure, or both in multiple species.[191–198] In addition to an anti-obesity effect, β₃-adrenergic receptor agonists have been shown to have antihyperglycemic effects that appear to be, at least in part, independent of their anti-obesity effects.[199, 200]

To date, little or no efficacy of β₃-adrenergic receptor agonists has been demonstrated in humans, although one agent was able to induce a shift in the respiratory quotient, thus indicating an alteration in lipid oxidation.[134] However, all the compounds that have been put into clinical trials were optimized for activity at the rat β₃-adrenergic receptor. As discussed previously, the pharmacology of the rodent receptor is distinct from that of the human and other species. Additionally, it is argued that the small amount of BAT in adult humans limits the maximal effect on energy expenditure. However, this characteristic may not limit efficacy during chronic therapy. Treatment with β₃-adrenergic receptor agonists leads to significant expansion of the BAT compartment.[201, 202] Humans have the potential for induction of BAT as demonstrated in patients with pheochromocytoma, in whom brown fat is markedly increased.[203] Finally, β₃-adrenergic receptors do not appear to undergo acute, agonist-induced downregulation,[135] which suggests that the weight loss effect may require extended activity leading to the induction of energy-regulating proteins such as UCP.

Leptin

The discovery of leptin held great promise for a potential target at which to direct pharmacotherapy. However, the observation that leptin levels rise and fall with weight and reach very high levels in obese patients[204] led many to conclude that most patients with obesity are resistant to the effects of leptin on reducing appetite and increasing energy expenditure. No major leptin receptor defect appears to account for this level of resistance.[205] Therefore, resistance to leptin action appears to be related to either an inability of higher leptin concentrations to penetrate the blood-brain barrier in order to signal to a normally functioning receptor, a postreceptor signaling defect present in patients with obesity, or perhaps a combination of these. A trial of recombinant leptin at approximately 300 mg/day by subcutaneous injection for up to 6 months in humans achieved a significant decrease of approximately 8 kg from the initial weight as opposed to the placebo effect of a decrease of about 2 kg.[206] In a follow-up statement regarding this work, no significant effects on weight were achieved overall; however, a subset of patients did achieve a response that could be the subject of further investigation.[207]

New Targets

Pharmaceuticals are under development for many potential new targets. The receptors for NPY are potentially important sites as drug targets. As noted previously, NPY is among the most potent orexigenic peptides identified, so by selectively blocking NPY at the "feeding" receptor, it is possible that the increased appetite and food-seeking behavior that occur during weight loss can be inhibited. Because the NPY-1 and NPY-5 receptors appear to be the most important subtypes with respect to feeding and weight regulation, several development programs are under way for the identification of selective antagonists.

The melanocortin receptor system has also generated exciting interest. An agonist of the MC-3 or MC-4 receptor may lead to suppression of appetite. Because agouti-related protein increases feeding behavior by inhibiting activity at the MC-4 receptor, agents that prevent this interaction could also have appetite-suppressing properties. The newly discovered neuropeptides MCH and orexins, as well as CRH, galanin, and opioid antagonists, may also be important targets in the race to develop effective anti-obesity agents. In addition to these novel peptides, work is ongoing in the area of selective serotoninergic agents, such as agonists of the 5-HT₂c receptor subtype, that may have a significantly better therapeutic index than any of the predecessor compounds to date.

In the search for agents that work in the periphery, several areas of research may prove promising. The importance of the UCPs is still being understood. It is difficult to target these proteins because the need to deliver compounds to the intracellular and possibly the intramitochondrial compartments represents a true challenge. Furthermore, attempts to upregulate the expression or activity of UCPs in a tissue-specific manner may also be a difficult hurdle. UCP-2, for example, although highly expressed in BAT and skeletal muscle, is also found in immune response tissue, as well as in cardiocytes and brain. Uncoupling oxidated respiration in these tissues may lead to unfavorable toxicology. UCP-1, found only in BAT, may be insufficiently expressed to have an impact on human forms of obesity. Several of the other peripherally circulating peptides have also generated some interest as potential primary or adjunctive therapies for obesity, including CCK,[75] GLP-1,[208] and bombesin.[209] These molecules may be helpful by altering the meal termination signal.

REFERENCES

1. Sponheimer M, Lee-Thorp JA: Isotopic evidence for the diet of an early hominid, *Australopithecus africanus*. Science 283:368–370, 1999.
2. Keil U, Kuulasmaa K: WHO MONICA Project: Risk factors. Int J Epidemiol 18(suppl 1):46–55, 1989.
3. Donato KA, Pi-Suyner FX, Becker DM, et al: Executive summary of the clinical guidelines on the identification, evaluation, and treatment of overweight and obesity in adults. Arch Intern Med 158:1855–1867, 1998.
4. Kuczmarski RJ, Carroll MD, Flegal KM, et al: Varying body mass index cutoff points to describe overweight prevalence among U.S. adults: NHANES III (1988 to 1994). Obes Res 5:542–548, 1997.
5. Stamler R, Stamler J, Riedlinger WF, et al: Weight and blood pressure. Findings in hypertension screening of 1 million Americans. JAMA 240:1607–1610, 1978.
6. Flegal KM, Carroll MD, Kuczmarski RJ, et al: Overweight and obesity in the United States: Prevalence and trends, 1960–1994. Int J Obes Relat Metab Disord 22:39–47, 1998.
7. Seidell JC: The impact of obesity on health status: Some implications for health care costs. Int J Obes Relat Metab Disord 19(suppl 6):13–16, 1995.
8. Stevens J, Cai J, Pamuk ER, et al: The effect of age on the association between body-mass index and mortality. N Engl J Med 338:1–7, 1998.
9. Manson JE, Stampfer MJ, Hennekens CH, et al: Body weight and longevity. A reassessment. JAMA 257:353–358, 1987.
10. Durazo-Arvizu R, Cooper RS, Luke A, et al: Relative weight and mortality in U.S. blacks and whites: Findings from representative national population samples. Ann Epidemiol 7:383–395, 1997.
11. Hubert HB, Feinleib M, McNamara PM, et al: Obesity as an independent risk factor for cardiovascular disease: A 26-year follow-up of participants in the Framingham Heart Study. Circulation 67:968–977, 1983.
12. Anonymous: Health implications of obesity. National Institutes of Health Consensus Development Conference Statement. Ann Intern Med 103:1073–1077, 1985.
13. Rexrode KM, Hennekens CH, Willett WC, et al: A prospective study of body mass index, weight change, and risk of stroke in women. JAMA 277:1539–1545, 1997.
14. Willett WC, Manson JE, Stampfer MJ, et al: Weight, weight change, and coronary heart disease in women. Risk within the 'normal' weight range. JAMA 273:461–465, 1995.
15. Shaper AG, Wannamethee SG, Walker M: Body weight: Implications for the prevention of coronary heart disease, stroke, and diabetes mellitus in a cohort study of middle aged men. BMJ 314:1311–1317, 1997.
16. Dyer AR, Elliott P: The INTERSALT study: Relations of body mass index to blood pressure. INTERSALT Co-operative Research Group. J Hum Hypertens 3:299–308, 1989.
17. Cutler JA, Psaty BM, MacMahon S, et al: Public health issues in hypertension control: What has been learned from clinical trials. *In* Laragh JH, Brenner BM (eds): Hypertension: Pathophysiology, Diagnosis, and Management. New York, Raven, 1995, pp 253–270.
18. Denke MA, Sempos CT, Grundy SM: Excess body weight. An under-recognized contributor to dyslipidemia in white American women. Arch Intern Med 154:401–410, 1994.
19. Reaven GM, Chen YD, Jeppesen J, et al: Insulin resistance and hyperinsulinemia in individuals with small, dense low density lipoprotein particles. J Clin Invest 92:141–146, 1993.

20. Anonymous: National Cholesterol Education Program. Second Report of the Expert Panel on Detection, Evaluation, and Treatment of High Blood Cholesterol in Adults (Adult Treatment Panel II). Circulation 89:1333–1445, 1994.
21. Law MR, Wald NJ, Thompson SG: By how much and how quickly does reduction in serum cholesterol concentration lower risk of ischaemic heart disease? BMJ 308:367–372, 1994.
22. Imbeault P, Lemieux S, Prud'homme D, et al: Relationship of visceral adipose tissue to metabolic risk factors for coronary heart disease: Is there a contribution of subcutaneous fat cell hypertrophy? Metab Clin Exp 48:355–362, 1999.
23. Urbina EM, Gidding SS, Bao W, et al: Effect of body size, ponderosity, and blood pressure on left ventricular growth in children and young adults in the Bogalusa Heart Study. Circulation 91:2400–2406, 1995.
24. Colditz GA, Willett WC, Stampfer MJ, et al: Weight as a risk factor for clinical diabetes in women. Am J Epidemiol 132:501–513, 1990.
25. Chan JM, Rimm EB, Colditz GA, et al: Obesity, fat distribution, and weight gain as risk factors for clinical diabetes in men. Diabetes Care 17:961–969, 1994.
26. Colditz GA, Willett WC, Rotnitzky A, et al: Weight gain as a risk factor for clinical diabetes mellitus in women. Ann Intern Med 122:481–486, 1995.
27. Ford ES, Williamson DF, Liu S: Weight change and diabetes incidence: Findings from a national cohort of US adults. Am J Epidemiol 146:214–222, 1997.
28. Giovannucci E, Ascherio A, Rimm EB, et al: Physical activity, obesity, and risk for colon cancer and adenoma in men. Ann Intern Med 122:327–334, 1995.
29. Martinez ME, Giovannucci E, Spiegelman D, et al: Leisure-time physical activity, body size, and colon cancer in women. Nurses' Health Study Research Group. J Natl Cancer Inst 89:948–955, 1997.
30. Chu SY, Lee NC, Wingo PA, et al: The relationship between body mass and breast cancer among women enrolled in the Cancer and Steroid Hormone Study. J Clin Epidemiol 44:1197–1206, 1991.
31. Willett WC, Browne ML, Bain C, et al: Relative weight and risk of breast cancer among premenopausal women. Am J Epidemiol 122:731–740, 1985.
32. Hunter DJ, Willett WC: Diet, body size, and breast cancer. Epidemiol Rev 15:110–132, 1993.
33. Huang Z, Hankinson SE, Colditz GA, et al: Dual effects of weight and weight gain on breast cancer risk. JAMA 278:1407–1411, 1997.
34. Tornberg SA, Carstensen JM: Relationship between Quetelet's index and cancer of breast and female genital tract in 47,000 women followed for 25 years. Br J Cancer 69:358–361, 1994.
35. Baanders-van Halewyn EA, Blankenstein MA, Thijssen JH, et al: A comparative study of risk factors for hyperplasia and cancer of the endometrium. Eur J Cancer Prev 5:105–112, 1996.
36. Shoff SM, Newcomb PA: Diabetes, body size, and risk of endometrial cancer. Am J Epidemiol 148:234–240, 1998.
37. Ehrmann DA, Barnes RB, Rosenfield RL: Polycystic ovary syndrome as a form of functional ovarian hyperandrogenism due to dysregulation of androgen secretion. Endocr Rev 16:322–353, 1995.
38. Rich-Edwards JW, Goldman MB, Willett WC, et al: Adolescent body mass index and infertility caused by ovulatory disorder. Am J Obstet Gynecol 171:171–177, 1994.
39. Johnson SR, Kolberg BH, Varner MW, et al: Maternal obesity and pregnancy. Surg Gynecol Obstet 164:431–437, 1987.
40. Prentice A, Goldberg G: Maternal obesity increases congenital malformations. Nutr Rev 54:146–150, 1996.
41. Cnattingius S, Bergstrom R, Lipworth L, et al: Prepregnancy weight and the risk of adverse pregnancy outcomes. N Engl J Med 338:147–152, 1998.
42. Stampfer MJ, Maclure KM, Colditz GA, et al: Risk of symptomatic gallstones in women with severe obesity. Am J Clin Nutr 55:652–658, 1992.
43. Cicuttini FM, Baker JR, Spector TD: The association of obesity with osteoarthritis of the hand and knee in women: A twin study. J Rheumatol 23:1221–1226, 1996.
44. Willims RA, Foulsham BM: Weight reduction in osteoarthritis using phentermine. Practitioner 225:231–232, 1981.
45. Young T, Palta M, Dempsey J, et al: The occurrence of sleep-disordered breathing among middle-aged adults. N Engl J Med 328:1230–1235, 1993.
46. Shepard JW Jr: Hypertension, cardiac arrhythmias, myocardial infarction, and stroke in relation to obstructive sleep apnea. Clin Chest Med 13:437–458, 1992.
47. Swanson CA, Potischman N, Wilbanks GD, et al: Relation of endometrial cancer risk to past and contemporary body size and body fat distribution. Cancer Epidemiol Biomarkers Prev 2:321–327, 1993.
48. Ballard-Barbash R, Schatzkin A, Carter CL, et al: Body fat distribution and breast cancer in the Framingham Study. J Natl Cancer Inst 82:286–290, 1990.
49. Ducimetiere P, Richard JL: The relationship between subsets of anthropometric upper versus lower body measurements and coronary heart disease risk in middle-aged men. The Paris Prospective Study. I. Int J Obes 13:111–121, 1989.
50. Lapidus L, Bengtsson C, Larsson B, et al: Distribution of adipose tissue and risk of cardiovascular disease and death: A 12 year follow up of participants in the population study of women in Gothenburg, Sweden. BMJ 289:1257–1261, 1984.
51. Larsson B, Svardsudd K, Welin L, et al: Abdominal adipose tissue distribution, obesity, and risk of cardiovascular disease and death: 13 year follow up of participants in the study of men born in 1913. BMJ 288:1401–1404, 1984.
52. Ohlson LO, Larsson B, Svardsudd K, et al: The influence of body fat distribution on the incidence of diabetes mellitus. 13.5 years of follow-up of the participants in the study of men born in 1913. Diabetes 34:1055–1058, 1985.
53. Kissebah AH, Vydelingum N, Murray R, et al: Relation of body fat distribution to metabolic complications of obesity. J Clin Endocrinol Metab 54:254–260, 1982.
54. Ravussin E, Lillioja S, Anderson TE, et al: Determinants of 24-hour energy expenditure in man. Methods and results using a respiratory chamber. J Clin Invest 78:1568–1578, 1986.
55. Ravussin E, Swindburn BA: Energy metabolism. In Stunkard AJ, Wadden TA (eds): Obesity: Theory and Therapy, ed 2. New York, Raven, 1993, pp 97–123.
56. Roberts SB, Savage J, Coward WA, et al: Energy expenditure and intake in infants born to lean and overweight mothers. N Engl J Med 318:461–466, 1988.
57. Griffiths M, Payne PR, Stunkard AJ, et al: Metabolic rate and physical development in children at risk of obesity. Lancet 336:76–78, 1990.
58. Ravussin E, Lillioja S, Knowler WC, et al: Reduced rate of energy expenditure as a risk factor for body-weight gain. N Engl J Med 318:467–472, 1988.
59. Davies PS, Day JM, Lucas A: Energy expenditure in early infancy and later body fatness. Int J Obes 15:727–731, 1991.
60. Goran MI, Shewchuk R, Gower BA, et al: Longitudinal changes in fatness in white children: No effect of childhood energy expenditure. Am J Clin Nutr 67:309–316, 1998.
61. Zhang Y, Proenca R, Maffei M, et al: Positional cloning of the mouse obese gene and its human homologue [published erratum appears in Nature 1995 Mar 30; 374(6521):479]. Nature 372:425–432, 1994.
62. Rowe JW, Young JB, Minaker KL, et al: Effect of insulin and glucose infusions on sympathetic nervous system activity in normal man. Diabetes 30:219–225, 1981.
63. Sakaguchi T, Bray GA: The effect of intrahypothalamic injections of glucose on sympathetic efferent firing rate. Brain Res Bull 18:591–595, 1987.
64. Young JB, Landsberg L: Impaired suppression of sympathetic activity during fasting in the gold thioglucose–treated mouse. J Clin Invest 65:1086–1094, 1980.
65. Gibbs J, Young RC, Smith GP: Cholecystokinin decreases food intake in rats. J Comp Physiol Psychol 84:488–495, 1973.
66. Figlewicz DP, Sipols A, Porte D Jr, et al: Intraventricular bombesin can decrease single meal size in the baboon. Brain Res Bull 17:535–537, 1986.
67. Reidelberger RD, O'Rourke MF: Potent cholecystokinin antagonist L 364718 stimulates food intake in rats. Am J Physiol 257:R1512–R1518, 1989.
68. Gibbs J, Fauser DJ, Rowe EA, et al: Bombesin suppresses feeding in rats. Nature 282:208–210, 1979.
69. Stein LJ, Woods SC: Gastrin releasing peptide reduces meal size in rats. Peptides 3:833–835, 1982.
70. Ladenheim EE, Wirth KE, Moran TH: Receptor subtype mediation of feeding suppression by bombesin-like peptides. Pharmacol Biochem Behav 54:705–711, 1996.
71. Perley MJ, Kipnis DM: Plasma insulin responses to oral and intravenous glucose: Studies in normal and diabetic subjects. J Clin Invest 46:1954–1962, 1967.
72. Elrick H, Stimmler L, Hald CJ, et al: Plasma insulin response to oral intravenous glucose administration. J Clin Invest 24:1076–1082, 1964.
73. Drucker DJ: Glucagon-like peptides. Diabetes 47:159–169, 1998.
74. Figlewicz DP, Sipols AJ, Porte D Jr, et al: Intraventricular CCK inhibits food intake and gastric emptying in baboons. Am J Physiol 256:R1313–R1317, 1989.
75. Moran TH, Shnayder L, Hostetler AM, et al: Pylorectomy reduces the satiety action of cholecystokinin. Am J Physiol 255:R1059–R1063, 1988.
76. Smith GP, Jerome C, Norgren R: Afferent axons in abdominal vagus mediate satiety effect of cholecystokinin in rats. Am J Physiol 249:R638–R641, 1985.
77. West DB, Fey D, Woods SC: Cholecystokinin persistently suppresses meal size but not food intake in free-feeding rats. Am J Physiol 246:R776–R787, 1984.
78. Green PK, Wilkinson CW, Woods SC: Intraventricular corticosterone increases the rate of body weight gain in underweight adrenalectomized rats. Endocrinology 130:269–275, 1992.
79. Zarjevski N, Cusin I, Vettor R, et al: Chronic intracerebroventricular neuropeptide-Y administration to normal rats mimics hormonal and metabolic changes of obesity. Endocrinology 133:1753–1758, 1993.
80. Elmquist JK, Bjorbaek C, Ahima RS, et al: Distributions of leptin receptor mRNA isoforms in the rat brain. J Comp Neurol 395:535–547, 1998.
81. Chua SC Jr, Brown AW, Kim J, et al: Food deprivation and hypothalamic neuropeptide gene expression: Effects of strain background and the diabetes mutation. Brain Res Mol Brain Res 11:291–299, 1991.
82. Wilding JP, Gilbey SG, Bailey CJ, et al: Increased neuropeptide-Y messenger ribonucleic acid (mRNA) and decreased neurotensin mRNA in the hypothalamus of the obese (ob/ob) mouse. Endocrinology 132:1939–1944, 1993.
83. Stephens TW, Basinski M, Bristow PK, et al: The role of neuropeptide Y in the antiobesity action of the obese gene product. Nature 377:530–532, 1995.
84. Schwartz MW, Seeley RJ, Campfield LA, et al: Identification of targets of leptin action in rat hypothalamus. J Clin Invest 98:1101–1106, 1996.
85. Seeley RJ, van Dijk G, Campfield LA, et al: Intraventricular leptin reduces food intake and body weight of lean rats but not obese Zucker rats. Horm Metab Res 28:664–668, 1996.
86. Stanley BG, Kyrkouli SE, Lampert S, et al: Neuropeptide Y chronically injected into the hypothalamus: A powerful neurochemical inducer of hyperphagia and obesity. Peptides 7:1189–1192, 1986.
87. Billington CJ, Briggs JE, Grace M, et al: Effects of intracerebroventricular injection of neuropeptide Y on energy metabolism. Am J Physiol 260:R321–R327, 1991.
88. Bray GA: Peptides affect the intake of specific nutrients and the sympathetic nervous system. Am J Clin Nutr 55(suppl):265–271, 1992.
89. Erickson JC, Hollopeter G, Palmiter RD: Attenuation of the obesity syndrome of ob/ob mice by the loss of neuropeptide Y. Science 274:1704–1707, 1996.
90. Erickson JC, Clegg KE, Palmiter RD: Sensitivity to leptin and susceptibility to seizures of mice lacking neuropeptide Y. Nature 381:415–421, 1996.
91. Gehlert DR: Subtypes of receptors for neuropeptide Y: Implications for the targeting of therapeutics. Life Sci 55:551–562, 1994.
92. Woldbye DP, Larsen PJ: The how and Y of eating. Nat Med 4:671–672, 1998.
93. Marsh DJ, Hollopeter G, Kafer KE, et al: Role of the Y5 neuropeptide Y receptor in feeding and obesity. Nat Med 4:718–721, 1998.
94. Pedrazzini T, Seydoux J, Kunstner P, et al: Cardiovascular response, feeding behavior and locomotor activity in mice lacking the NPY Y1 receptor. Nat Med 4:722–726, 1998.
95. Nahon JL: The melanin-concentrating hormone: From the peptide to the gene. Crit Rev Neurobiol 8:221–262, 1994.
96. Qu D, Ludwig DS, Gammeltoft S, et al: A role for melanin-concentrating hormone in the central regulation of feeding behaviour. Nature 380:243–247, 1996.

97. Shimada M, Tritos NA, Lowell BB, et al: Mice lacking melanin-concentrating hormone are hypophagic and lean. Nature 396:670–674 1998,.
98. Akabayashi A, Koenig JI, Watanabe Y, et al: Galanin-containing neurons in the paraventricular nucleus: A neurochemical marker for fat ingestion and body weight gain. Proc Natl Acad Sci U S A 91:10375–10379, 1994.
99. Leibowitz SF, Akabayashi A, Wang J: Obesity on a high-fat diet: Role of hypothalamic galanin in neurons of the anterior paraventricular nucleus projecting to the median eminence. J Neurosci 18:2709–2719, 1998.
100. Smith BK, York DA, Bray GA: Chronic cerebroventricular galanin does not induce sustained hyperphagia or obesity. Peptides 15:1267–1272, 1994.
101. Sakurai T, Amemiya A, Ishii M, et al: Orexins and orexin receptors: A family of hypothalamic neuropeptides and G protein–coupled receptors that regulate feeding behavior. Cell 92:573–585, 1998.
102. Kalra SP, Dube MG, Pu SY, et al: Interacting appetite-regulating pathways in the hypothalamic regulation of body weight. Endocr Rev 20:68–100, 1999.
103. Morley JE: Neuropeptide regulation of appetite and weight. Endocr Rev 8:256–287, 1987.
104. Cone RD, Lu D, Koppula S, et al: The melanocortin receptors: Agonists, antagonists, and the hormonal control of pigmentation. Recent Prog Horm Res 51:287–318, 1996.
105. Huszar D, Lynch CA, Fairchild-Huntress V, et al: Targeted disruption of the melanocortin-4 receptor results in obesity in mice. Cell 88:131–141, 1997.
106. Ollmann MM, Wilson BD, Yang YK, et al: Antagonism of central melanocortin receptors in vitro and in vivo by agouti-related protein. Science 278:135–138, 1997.
107. Rothwell NJ: Central effects of CRF on metabolism and energy balance. Neurosci Biobehav Rev 14:263–271, 1990.
108. Spina M, Merlo-Pich E, Chan RK, et al: Appetite-suppressing effects of urocortin, a CRF-related neuropeptide. Science 273:1561–1564, 1996.
109. Schwartz MW, Seeley RJ: Seminars in medicine of the Beth Israel Deaconess Medical Center. Neuroendocrine responses to starvation and weight loss. N Engl J Med 336:1802–1811, 1997.
110. Flier JS, Maratos-Flier E: Obesity and the hypothalamus: Novel peptides for new pathways. Cell 92:437–440, 1998.
111. Kristensen P, Judge ME, Thim L, et al: Hypothalamic CART is a new anorectic peptide regulated by leptin. Nature 393:72–76, 1998.
112. Thim L, Kristensen P, Larsen PJ, et al: CART, a new anorectic peptide. Int J Biochem Cell Biol 30:1281–1284, 1998.
113. Murata Y: Multiple isoforms of thyroid hormone receptor: An analysis of their relative contribution in mediating thyroid hormone action. Nagoya J Med Sci 61:103–115, 1998.
114. Ricquier D, Kader JC: Mitochondrial protein alteration in active brown fat: A sodium dodecyl sulfate–polyacrylamide gel electrophoretic study. Biochem Biophys Res Commun 73:577–583, 1976.
115. Heaton GM, Wagenvoord RJ, Kemp A Jr, et al: Brown-adipose-tissue mitochondria: Photoaffinity labelling of the regulatory site of energy dissipation. Eur J Biochem 82:515–521, 1978.
116. Gura T: Uncoupling proteins provide new clue to obesity's causes. Science 280:1369–1370, 1998.
117. Lowell BB, Flier JS: Brown adipose tissue, beta 3-adrenergic receptors, and obesity. Annu Rev Med 48:307–316, 1997.
118. Strieleman PJ, Schalinske KL, Shrago E: Fatty acid activation of the reconstituted brown adipose tissue mitochondria uncoupling protein. J Biol Chem 260:13402–13405, 1985.
119. Bukowiecki LJ: Regulation of energy expenditure in brown adipose tissue. Int J Obes 9(suppl 2):31–41, 1985.
120. Nagase I, Yoshida T, Kumamoto K, et al: Expression of uncoupling protein in skeletal-muscle and white fat of obese mice treated with thermogenic beta-3-adrenergic agonist. J Clin Invest 97:2898–2904, 1996.
121. Silva JE, Rabelo R: Regulation of the uncoupling protein gene expression. Eur J Endocrinol 136:251–264, 1997.
122. Carmona MC, Valmaseda A, Brun S, et al: Differential regulation of uncoupling protein-2 and uncoupling protein-3 gene expression in brown adipose tissue during development and cold exposure. Biochem Biophys Res Commun 243:224–228, 1998.
123. Florez-Duquet M, Horwitz BA, McDonald RB: Cellular proliferation and UCP content in brown adipose tissue of cold-exposed aging Fischer 344 rats. Am J Physiol 274:R196–R203, 1998.
124. Bienengraeber M, Echtay KS, Klingenberg M: H+ transport by uncoupling protein (UCP-1) is dependent on a histidine pair, absent in UCP-2 and UCP-3. Biochemistry 37:3–8, 1998.
125. Hauge A, Oye I: Effect of adrenaline and adrenergic blocking agents on the basal oxygen consumption of the perfused rat heart. Nature 210:998–1000, 1966.
126. Rothwell NJ, Saville ME, Stock MJ: Sympathetic and thyroid influences on metabolic rate in fed, fasted, and refed rats. Am J Physiol 243:R339–R346, 1982.
127. Lands AM, Arnold A, McAuliff JP, et al: Differentiation of receptor systems activated by sympathomimetic amines. Nature 214:597–598, 1967.
128. Furchgott RF: The classification of adrenoreceptors (adrenergic receptors): An evaluation from the standpoint of receptor theory. In Blaschko H, Muecholl E (eds): Catecholamines. Berlin, Springer, 1972, pp 283–335.
129. Tan S, Curtis-Prior PB: Characterization of the beta-adrenoceptor of the adipose cell of the rat. Int J Obes 7:409–414, 1983.
130. Rothwell NJ, Stock MJ: A role for brown adipose tissue in diet-induced thermogenesis. Obes Res 5:650–656, 1997.
131. Himms-Hagen J: Brown adipose tissue thermogenesis and obesity. Prog Lipid Res 28:67–115, 1989.
132. Emorine LJ, Marullo S, Briend-Sutren MM, et al: Molecular characterization of the human beta 3-adrenergic receptor. Science 245:1118–1121, 1989.
133. Granneman JG, Lahners KN, Rao DD: Rodent and human beta 3-adrenergic receptor genes contain an intron within the protein-coding block. Mol Pharmacol 42:964–970, 1992.
134. Weyer C, Tataranni PA, Snitker S, et al: Increase in insulin action and fat oxidation after treatment with CL 316,243, a highly selective beta3-adrenoceptor agonist in humans. Diabetes 47:1555–1561, 1998.
135. Nantel F, Bonin H, Emorine LJ, et al: The human beta 3-adrenergic receptor is resistant to short term agonist-promoted desensitization. Mol Pharmacol 43:548–555, 1993.
136. McLaughlin DP, MacDonald A: Evidence for the existence of 'atypical' beta-adrenoceptors (beta 3-adrenoceptors) mediating relaxation in the rat distal colon in vitro. Br J Pharmacol 101:569–574, 1990.
137. van der Vliet A, Rademaker B, Bast A: A beta adrenoceptor with atypical characteristics is involved in the relaxation of the rat small intestine. J Pharmacol Exp Ther 255:218–226, 1990.
138. Taneja DT, Clarke DE: Evidence for a noradrenergic innervation to "atypical" beta adrenoceptors (or putative beta-3 adrenoceptors) in the ileum of guinea pig. J Pharmacol Exp Ther 260:192–200, 1992.
139. McLaughlin DP, MacDonald A: Characterization of catecholamine-mediated relaxations in rat isolated gastric fundus: Evidence for an atypical beta-adrenoceptor. Br J Pharmacol 103:1351–1356, 1991.
140. Esbenshade TA, Han C, Theroux TL, et al: Coexisting beta 1- and atypical beta-adrenergic receptors cause redundant increases in cyclic AMP in human neuroblastoma cells. Mol Pharmacol 42:753–759, 1992.
141. Webber SE, Stock MJ: Evidence for an atypical, or beta 3-adrenoceptor in ferret tracheal epithelium. Br J Pharmacol 105:857–862, 1992.
142. Oriowo MA: Different atypical beta-adrenoceptors mediate isoprenaline-induced relaxation in vascular and non-vascular smooth muscles. Life Sci 56:L269–L275, 1995.
143. Kaumann AJ, Molenaar P: Differences between the third cardiac beta-adrenoceptor and the colonic beta 3-adrenoceptor in the rat. Br J Pharmacol 118:2085–2098, 1996.
144. Shuldiner AR, Silver K, Roth J, et al: Beta 3-adrenoceptor gene variant in obesity and insulin resistance. Lancet 348:1584–1585, 1996.
145. Comuzzie AG, Allison DB: The search for human obesity genes. Science 280:1374–1377, 1998.
146. U.S. Department of Health and Human Services: Physical Activity and Health: A Report of the Surgeon General. Atlanta, U.S. Department of Health and Human Services, 1996.
147. Bray GA: Syndromes of hypothalamic obesity in man. Pediatr Ann 13:525–536, 1984.
148. Franks S, Kiddy D, Sharp P, et al: Obesity and polycystic ovary syndrome. Ann N Y Acad Sci 626:201–206, 1991.
149. Longcope C, Pratt JH, Schneider SH, et al: Aromatization of androgens by muscle and adipose tissue in vivo. J Clin Endocrinol Metab 46:146–152, 1978.
150. Montague CT, Farooqi IS, Whitehead JP, et al: Congenital leptin deficiency is associated with severe early-onset obesity in humans. Nature 387:903–908, 1997.
151. Clement K, Vaisse C, Lahlou N, et al: A mutation in the human leptin receptor gene causes obesity and pituitary dysfunction. Nature 392:398–401, 1998.
152. Krude H, Biebermann H, Luck W, et al: Severe early-onset obesity, adrenal insufficiency and red hair pigmentation caused by POMC mutations in humans. Nat Genet 19:155–157, 1998.
153. Naggert JK, Fricker LD, Varlamov O, et al: Hyperproinsulinaemia in obese fat/fat mice associated with a carboxypeptidase E mutation which reduces enzyme activity. Nat Genet 10:135–142, 1995.
154. Jackson RS, Creemers JW, Ohagi S, et al: Obesity and impaired prohormone processing associated with mutations in the human prohormone convertase 1 gene. Nat Genet 16:303–306, 1997.
155. O'Rahilly S, Gray H, Humphreys PJ, et al: Brief report: Impaired processing of prohormones associated with abnormalities of glucose homeostasis and adrenal function. N Engl J Med 333:1386–1390, 1995.
156. Yeo GS, Farooqi IS, Aminian S, et al: A frameshift mutation in MC4R associated with dominantly inherited human obesity (letter). Nat Genet 20:111–112, 1998.
157. Ristow M, Muller-Wieland D, Pfeiffer A, et al: Obesity associated with a mutation in a genetic regulator of adipocyte differentiation. N Engl J Med 339:953–959, 1998.
158. Gavin JR, Alberti KGMM, Davidson MB, et al: Report of the Expert Committee on the Diagnosis and Classification of Diabetes Mellitus. Diabetes Care 20:1183–1197, 1999.
159. Rossner S: Long-term intervention strategies in obesity treatment. Int J Obes Relat Metab Disord 19(suppl 7):29–35, 1995.
160. Owen OE, Kavle E, Owen RS, et al: A reappraisal of caloric requirements in healthy women. Am J Clin Nutr 44:1–19, 1986.
161. Owen OE, Holup JL, D'Alessio DA, et al: A reappraisal of the caloric requirements of men. Am J Clin Nutr 46:875–885, 1987.
162. Schofield WN: Predicting basal metabolic rate, new standards and review of previous work. Human Nutr Clin Nutr 39(suppl 1):5–41, 1985.
163. Hayter JE, Henry CJ: A re-examination of basal metabolic rate predictive equations: The importance of geographic origin of subjects in sample selection. Eur J Clin Nutr 48:702–707, 1994.
164. Wadden TA: Treatment of obesity by moderate and severe caloric restriction. Results of clinical research trials. Ann Intern Med 119:688–693, 1993.
165. Kramer FM, Jeffery RW, Forster JL, et al: Long-term follow-up of behavioral treatment for obesity: Patterns of weight regain among men and women. Int J Obes 13:123–136, 1989.
166. Wadden TA, Stunkard AJ, Brownell KD: Very low calorie diets: Their efficacy, safety, and future. Ann Intern Med 99:675–684, 1983.
167. Everhart JE: Contributions of obesity and weight loss to gallstone disease. Ann Intern Med 119:1029–1035, 1993.
168. Wing RR, Marcus MD, Salata R, et al: Effects of a very-low-calorie diet on long-term glycemic control in obese type 2 diabetic subjects. Arch Intern Med 151:1334–1340, 1991.
169. Miura J, Arai K, Tsukahara S, et al: The long term effectiveness of combined therapy by behavior modification and very low calorie diet: 2 years follow-up. Int J Obes 13(suppl 2):73–77, 1989.

170. Wadden TA, Sternberg JA, Letizia KA, et al: Treatment of obesity by very low calorie diet, behavior therapy, and their combination: A five-year perspective. Int J Obes 13(suppl 2):39–46, 1989.

171. Sikand G, Kondo A, Foreyt JP, et al: Two-year follow-up of patients treated with a very-low-calorie diet and exercise training. J Am Diet Assoc 88:487–488, 1988.

172. Frey-Hewitt B, Vranizan KM, Dreon DM, et al: The effect of weight loss by dieting or exercise on resting metabolic rate in overweight men. Int J Obes 14:327–334, 1990.

173. Verity LS, Ismail AH: Effects of exercise on cardiovascular disease risk in women with NIDDM. Diabetes Res Clin Pract 6:27–35, 1989.

174. Katzel LI, Bleecker ER, Colman EG, et al: Effects of weight loss vs aerobic exercise training on risk factors for coronary disease in healthy, obese, middle-aged and older men. A randomized controlled trial. JAMA 274:1915–1921, 1995.

175. Centers for Disease Control, National Center for Chronic Disease Prevention and Health Promotion: Surgeon General's Report on Physical Activity and Health. Atlanta, Centers for Disease Control and Prevention, 1996.

176. Munro JF: Clinical aspects of the treatment of obesity by drugs: A review. Int J Obes 3:171–180, 1979.

177. Guy-Grand B, Apfelbaum M, Crepaldi G, et al: International trial of long-term dexfenfluramine in obesity. Lancet 2:1142–1145, 1989.

178. Mathus-Vliegen EM, van de Voorde K, Kok AM, et al: Dexfenfluramine in the treatment of severe obesity: A placebo-controlled investigation of the effects on weight loss, cardiovascular risk factors, food intake and eating behaviour. J Intern Med 232:119–127, 1992.

179. Weintraub M, Hasday JD, Mushlin AI, et al: A double-blind clinical trial in weight control. Use of fenfluramine and phentermine alone and in combination. Arch Intern Med 144:1143–1148, 1984.

180. Weintraub M: Long-term weight control: The National Heart, Lung, and Blood Institute funded multimodal intervention study. Clin Pharmacol Ther 51:581–585, 1992.

181. Weintraub M, Sundaresan PR, Madan M, et al: Long-term weight control study. I (weeks 0 to 34). The enhancement of behavior modification, caloric restriction, and exercise by fenfluramine plus phentermine versus placebo. Clin Pharmacol Ther 51:586–594, 1992.

182. Weintraub M, Sundaresan PR, Schuster B, et al: Long-term weight control study. III (weeks 104 to 156). An open-label study of dose adjustment of fenfluramine and phentermine. Clin Pharmacol Ther 51:602–607, 1992.

183. Connolly HM, Crary JL, McGoon MD, et al: Valvular heart disease associated with fenfluramine-phentermine. N Engl J Med 337:581–588, 1997.

184. Centers for Disease Control and Prevention: Cardiac valvulopathy associated with exposure to fenfluramine or dexfenfluramine: U.S. Department of Health and Human Services Interim Public Health Recommendations, November 1997. MMWR 46:1061–1066, 1997.

185. Van Gaal LF, Broom JI, Enzi G, et al: Efficacy and tolerability of orlistat in the treatment of obesity: A 6-month dose-ranging study. Orlistat Dose-Ranging Study Group. Eur J Clin Pharmacol 54:125–132, 1998.

186. Sjostrom L, Rissanen A, Andersen T, et al: Randomised placebo-controlled trial of orlistat for weight loss and prevention of weight regain in obese patients. European Multicentre Orlistat Study Group. Lancet 352:167–172, 1998.

187. Hanotin C, Thomas F, Jones SP, et al: Efficacy and tolerability of sibutramine in obese patients: A dose-ranging study. Int J Obes Relat Metab Disord 22:32–38, 1998.

188. Lean ME: Sibutramine—a review of clinical efficacy. Int J Obes Relat Metab Disord 21(suppl 1):30–39, 1997.

189. Lean ME, Han TS, Morrison CE: Waist circumference as a measure for indicating need for weight management. BMJ 311:158–161, 1995.

190. Krief S, Lonnqvist F, Raimbault S, et al: Tissue distribution of beta 3-adrenergic receptor mRNA in man. J Clin Invest 91:344–349, 1993.

191. Ghorbani M, Himmshagen J: Appearance of brown adipocytes in white adipose tissue during CL316,243-induced reversal of obesity and diabetes in Zucker fa/fa rats. Int J Obes 21:465–475, 1997.

192. Santti E, Huupponen R, Rouru J, et al: Potentiation of the anti-obesity effect of the selective beta 3-adrenoceptor agonist BRL 35135 in obese Zucker rats by exercise. Br J Pharmacol 113:1231–1236, 1994.

193. Umekawa T, Yoshida T, Sakane N, et al: Anti-obesity and anti-diabetic effects of CL316,243, a highly specific beta(3)-adrenoceptor agonist, in Otsuka Long-Evans Tokushima fatty rats: Induction of uncoupling protein and activation of glucose transporter 4 in white fat. Eur J Endocrinol 136:429–437, 1997.

194. Yoshida T, Sakane N, Wakabayashi Y, et al: Anti-obesity effect of CL 316,243, a highly specific beta 3-adrenoceptor agonist, in mice with monosodium-L-glutamate–induced obesity. Eur J Endocrinol 131:97–102, 1994.

195. Yoshida T, Sakane N, Wakabayashi Y, et al: Anti-obesity and anti-diabetic effects of CL 316,243, a highly specific beta 3-adrenoceptor agonist, in yellow KK mice. Life Sci 54:491–498, 1994.

196. Yoshida T, Hiraoka N, Yoshioka K, et al: Anti-obesity and anti-diabetic actions of a beta 3-adrenoceptor agonist, BRL 26830A, in yellow KK mice. Endocrinol Jpn 38:397–403, 1991.

197. Collins S, Daniel KW, Petro AE, et al: Strain-specific response to beta(3)-adrenergic receptor agonist treatment of diet-induced obesity in mice. Endocrinology 138:405–413, 1997.

198. Sasaki N, Uchida E, Niiyama M, et al: Anti-obesity effects of selective agonists to the beta 3-adrenergic receptor in dogs. II. Recruitment of thermogenic brown adipocytes and reduction of adiposity after chronic treatment with a beta 3-adrenergic agonist. J Vet Med Sci 60:465–469, 1998.

199. deSouza CJ, Hirshman MF, Horton ES, et al: CL-316,243, a beta(3)-specific adrenoceptor agonist, enhances insulin-stimulated glucose disposal in nonobese rats. Diabetes 46:1257–1263, 1997.

200. Liu X, Perusse F, Bukowiecki LJ: Mechanisms of the antidiabetic effects of the beta 3-adrenergic agonist CL-316243 in obese Zucker-ZDF rats. Am J Physiol 274:R1212–R1219, 1998.

201. Champigny O, Ricquier D: Evidence from in vitro differentiating cells that adrenoceptor agonists can increase uncoupling protein mRNA level in adipocytes of adult humans: An RT-PCR study. J Lipid Res 37:1907–1914, 1996.

202. Champigny O, Ricquier D, Blondel O, et al: Beta 3-adrenergic receptor stimulation restores message and expression of brown-fat mitochondrial uncoupling protein in adult dogs. Proc Natl Acad Sci U S A 88:10774–10777, 1991.

203. Ricquier D, Nechad M, Mory G: Ultrastructural and biochemical characterization of human brown adipose tissue in pheochromocytoma. J Clin Endocrinol Metab 54:803–807, 1982.

204. Sinha MK, Opentanova I, Ohannesian JP, et al: Evidence of free and bound leptin in human circulation. Studies in lean and obese subjects and during short-term fasting. J Clin Invest 98:1277–1282, 1996.

205. Considine RV, Considine EL, Williams CJ, et al: The hypothalamic leptin receptor in humans: Identification of incidental sequence polymorphisms and absence of the db/db mouse and fa/fa rat mutations. Diabetes 45:992–994, 1996.

206. Greenberg AS, Heymsfield SB, Fujioka K, et al: Preliminary safety and efficacy of recombinant methionyl human leptin administered by SC injection in lean and obese subjects. In Proceedings of the Eighth International Congress on Obesity. Paris, August 1998.

207. Amgen Press Release: Amgen Reports Solid Third-Quarter Results and Announces Additional $1 Billion Stock Repurchase Plan. Thousand Oaks, CA, Amgen, 1998.

208. Wang Z, Wang RM, Owji AA, et al: Glucagon-like peptide-1 is a physiological incretin in rat. J Clin Invest 95:417–421, 1995.

209. Ohki-Hamazaki H, Watase K, Yamamoto K, et al: Mice lacking bombesin receptor subtype-3 develop metabolic defects and obesity. Nature 390:165–169, 1997.

Chapter 45

Anorexia Nervosa and Other Eating Disorders

Robert T. Rubin ▪ Walter H. Kaye

"*A young woman thus afflicted, her clothes scarcely hanging together on her anatomy, her pulse slow and slack, her temperature two degrees below the normal mean, her bowels closed, her hair like that of a corpse—dry and lustreless, her face and limbs ashy and cold, her hollow eyes the only vivid thing about her—this wan creature whose daily food might lie on a crown piece, will be busy with mother's meetings, with little sister's frocks, with university extension and with what you please else of unselfish effort, yet on what funds God only knows.*"[1]

INTRODUCTION

Anorexia nervosa and bulimia nervosa are eating disorders that have been recognized for hundreds of years,[2–5] yet they remain major enigmas of psychiatry.[6–19] These are important illnesses, in that they carry significant morbidity, physical as well as psychologic, and in the case of anorexia nervosa death can occur in severe, untreated cases. Therefore, early recognition and aggressive treatment are particularly important. Because the physical manifestations of these illnesses are so prominent, most patients have their first encounters with medical specialists other than psychiatrists. Not infrequently, lengthy diagnostic work-ups for underlying physical illness are conducted. Often, only when the results of the work-up do not fit a known physical illness is a psychologic disturbance entertained. As described in the first part of this chapter, the psychiatric diagnostic criteria for anorexia and bulimia nervosa, when carefully applied to patients, permit these illnesses to be suspected early in the medical work-up and referral to the psychiatric specialist to be recommended to the patient in a constructive and acceptable way.

HISTORY AND EPIDEMIOLOGY

Anorexia nervosa and bulimia nervosa are diseases primarily of adolescent girls; approximately 95% of anorexia nervosa cases are female. Although there is documentary evidence of anorexia nervosa occurring in the Middle Ages, credit for the first medical account has been given to Richard Morton, an English physician who published *Phthisiologia; or, a Treatise of Consumptions,* in 1689.[3, 20, 21] His first chapter contained a section on "nervous consumption," the etiology of which he attributed to be in "the System of the Nerves proceeding from a Preternatural state of the Animal Spirits, and the destruction of the Tone of the Nerves. . . ." Anorexia nervosa as a modern clinical entity derives from publications by Charles Lasègue, a French physician, and William Gull, an English physician, both in 1873.[22, 23] Both writers referred to the illness as hysterical anorexia. A year later, Gull[24] published a treatise entitled *Anorexia Nervosa,* the current appellation for this illness. Bliss and Branch[3 (p14)] commented that "it is revealing to note the extraordinary differences in the description of

the same condition by the two men. While Gull's comments were as direct and precise as a pathologic report, Lasègue conveyed a sense of the spirit and feeling of these people, the nuances of their disturbed relationships, and the subtleties of their intrapsychic turmoil." Chapters in the early 20th-century history of anorexia nervosa predominantly involve its distinction from physical illnesses such as Simmonds' cachexia.[25]

Although binge eating (bulimia) has long been recognized as part of the symptomatology of anorexia nervosa, bulimia nervosa as a distinct syndrome was first proposed in 1979 by Russell.[26] He elaborated two criteria for bulimia nervosa: an irresistible urge to overeat, followed by self-induced vomiting or purging, and a morbid fear of becoming fat. In common with anorexia nervosa, such patients did keep their body weight somewhat below normal, but not to the same degree as anorexia nervosa patients, and they tended not to develop amenorrhea and were more active sexually. Russell considered bulimia nervosa to be an "ominous variant" of anorexia nervosa, in that comorbid depressive symptoms were often severe and distressing, leading to a high risk of suicide, and the prognosis was less favorable than in uncomplicated anorexia nervosa.

The more recent history of both these diseases parallels the maturation of psychiatry as a medical specialty since World War II. Careful theoretical formulations of the psychodynamics of these eating disorders have been augmented by elucidation of their physiology, especially their neuroendocrinology. Treatment methods, both biologic (e.g., pharmacotherapeutic) and psychotherapeutic have been refined, so that there is now a reasonably effective armamentarium with which to manage these disorders. The focus on them is prominent—for example, a Medline search for January 1996 to December 1999 yielded 804 citations for anorexia nervosa and 677 citations for bulimia.

The incidence of anorexia nervosa reported in epidemiologic studies has varied between approximately 0.5 and 15 cases per 100,000 population per year.[16, 27–29] The large variation is related to the diagnostic criteria used, the methods of case ascertainment, and the population studied (e.g., clinic vs. community). The prevalence of anorexia nervosa is about 1%, although it has been reported in some studies as considerably higher.[30–32] As mentioned, approximately 95% of cases are female.[33] A meta-analysis of 42 mortality studies in anorexia nervosa revealed the crude mortality rate (due to all causes of death) to be 5.9%, which is substantially greater than that for female inpatients and for the general population.[34]

The prevalence of bulimia nervosa varies between 2% and 4%.[31, 32, 35–37] Both anorexia and bulimia nervosa, as well as subsyndromal anorexia and bulimia, are far more common in certain groups of young women, notably athletes and ballet dancers, where occupational demands place a premium on thinness. Primary and secondary amenorrhea in these individuals is extraordinarily common. The occurrence of both anorexia and bulimia nervosa may be on the rise,[28, 38–41] which coincides with the increasing prevalence of obesity throughout the world.[42, 43]

Since the 1980s, emerging evidence from large-scale twin and family studies has suggested that eating disorders are familial.[44, 45] Moreover, there is cross-transmission between anorexia nervosa and bulimia nervosa, and these two disorders appear to share a common vulnerability. The transmissible elements of these disorders remain elusive, however. In addition, twin and family studies suggest that major depressive disorder and substance dependence most likely do not share a common etiology with the eating disorders.

DIAGNOSIS

The fourth edition of the *Diagnostic and Statistical Manual of Mental Disorders* (DSM-IV)[15] provides the current clinical criteria for anorexia nervosa and bulimia nervosa. The DSM has undergone three revisions since it became a criterion-based diagnostic system with DSM-III in 1980, and a number of the major diagnostic categories have undergone considerable change across these revisions. In contrast, the criteria for anorexia nervosa have remained relatively stable, although recent findings suggest future revision should be considered.[46] The criteria for bulimia nervosa have undergone some revision in DSM-IV.[47]

Tables 45–1 and 45–2 show the DSM-IV criteria for anorexia nervosa and bulimia nervosa, respectively. What is striking about these criteria are the many identifiable behavioral and psychologic aspects of these illnesses. If the patient and her family are queried about these aspects, considerable information pointing toward the diagnosis can be gleaned, psychiatric consultation can be considered early in the diagnostic process, and specialized and expensive laboratory testing can often be avoided.

For anorexia nervosa, a particular feature of the weight loss is the patient's refusal to maintain body weight, which often manifests as an active resistance to increasing caloric intake. As illustrated in Figure 45–1, the cachexia can be severe, and, as mentioned, self-starvation can lead to death. If the onset is in childhood or early adolescence, there may be a failure to make the expected weight gain during the active growth phase. This refusal to gain or maintain body weight is rooted psychologically in the second criterion, an intense fear of gaining weight or of becoming fat, even though the patient is underweight. There is a subjective distortion of body image such that the emaciated individual appears to herself to be either at an acceptable weight or even fat. Indeed, initiation of treatment by insisting on the patient's eating can lead to purging behavior that did not occur prior to treatment.

A corollary of this is the third criterion, disturbance of the experience of one's body weight or shape (e.g., undue influence of body

TABLE 45–1. DSM-IV Diagnostic Criteria for Anorexia Nervosa

Refusal to maintain body weight at or above a minimally normal weight for age and height (e.g., weight loss leading to maintenance of body weight less than 85% of that expected; or failure to make expected weight gain during period of growth, leading to body weight less than 85% of that expected).

Intense fear of gaining weight or becoming fat, even though underweight.

Disturbance in the way in which one's body weight or shape is experienced, undue influence of body weight or shape on self-evaluation, or denial of the seriousness of the current low body weight.

In postmenarcheal females, amenorrhea—i.e., the absence of at least three consecutive menstrual cycles. (A woman is considered to have amenorrhea if her periods occur only following hormone—e.g., estrogen—administration.)

Type

Restricting type: During the current episode . . . the person has not regularly engaged in binge-eating or purging behavior (i.e., self-induced vomiting or the misuse of laxatives, diuretics, or enemas).

Binge-eating/purging type: During the current episode . . . the person has regularly engaged in binge-eating or purging behavior (i.e., self-induced vomiting or the misuse of laxatives, diuretics, or enemas).

Reprinted with permission from American Psychiatric Association: Diagnostic and Statistical Manual of Mental Disorders, ed 4. Washington, DC, American Psychiatric Association, 1994.

TABLE 45–2. DSM-IV Diagnostic Criteria for Bulimia Nervosa

Recurrent episodes of binge eating. An episode of binge eating is characterized by both of the following:

Eating, in a discrete period of time (e.g., within any 2-hour period), an amount of food that is definitely larger than most people would eat during a similar period of time and under similar circumstances.

A sense of lack of control over eating during the episode (e.g., a feeling that one cannot stop eating or control what or how much one is eating).

Recurrent inappropriate compensatory behavior in order to prevent weight gain, such as self-induced vomiting; misuse of laxatives, diuretics, enemas, or other medications; fasting; or excessive exercise.

The binge eating and inappropriate compensatory behaviors both occur, on average, at least twice a week for 3 months.

Self-evaluation is unduly influenced by body shape and weight.

The disturbance does not occur exclusively during episodes of anorexia nervosa.

Type

Purging type: During the current episode . . . the person has regularly engaged in self-induced vomiting or the misuse of laxatives, diuretics, or enemas.

Nonpurging type: During the current episode . . . the person has used other inappropriate compensatory behaviors, such as fasting or excessive exercise, but has not regularly engaged in self-induced vomiting or the misuse of laxatives, diuretics, or enemas.

Reprinted with permission from American Psychiatric Association: From Diagnostic and Statistical Manual of Mental Disorders, ed 4. Washington, DC, American Psychiatric Association, 1994.

weight or shape on self-evaluation [e.g., self-esteem] or denial of the seriousness of the weight loss, or both), even though there may be clear adverse physical sequelae in addition to the fourth criterion, secondary amenorrhea. For the endocrinologist, questions that should be asked of the patient and her family to address these psychologic and behavioral aspects of anorexia nervosa include the following (adapted from the Structured Clinical Interview for DSM-IV[48]):

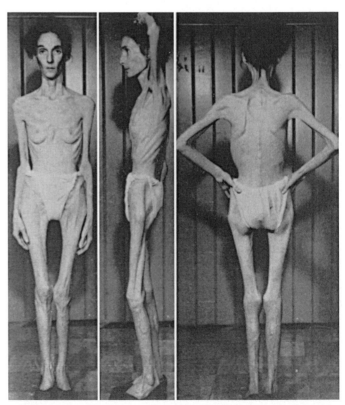

FIGURE 45–1. Extreme cachexia in an anorexia nervosa patient. (From Bliss EL, Branch CHH: Anorexia Nervosa: Its History, Psychology, and Biology. New York, Paul B. Hoeber, 1960.)

How much do you weigh now?

How tall are you?

What foods do you eat?

Why do you limit yourself to those foods?

Do you feel you are fat now?

Are you concerned that you might become fat if you ate more?

Do you weigh less than other people think you should weigh?

Do you need to be very thin in order to feel good about yourself?

Has anyone told you it can be dangerous to be as thin as you are?

What kinds of things do you do to keep from gaining weight?

Have you ever made yourself vomit or take laxatives, enemas, or water pills? How often?

How much do you exercise?

Before now, were you having periods? Were they regular? When did they stop?

For bulimia nervosa, the distinguishing features are uncontrollable binge eating of a definitely larger than normal amount of food (first criterion) that is clearly repetitive (third criterion). Here, too, one's sense of self is unduly influenced by weight and body shape (fourth criterion); compensatory behaviors such as self-induced vomiting, purging, fasting between binges, and exercise are invoked to prevent weight gain (second criterion). The frequency and chronicity of the binging, and especially the compensatory behaviors, help distinguish bulimia nervosa from overeating in general. And, because binge eating and purging can occur as part of anorexia nervosa, a fifth criterion for bulimia nervosa is that it does occur exclusively during episodes of anorexia nervosa. For the endocrinologist, questions that should be asked of the patient and her family to address the criteria for bulimia nervosa include the following (adapted from the Structured Clinical Interview for DSM-IV[48]):

Do you have times when your eating gets out of control? Tell me about these times.

During these times, do you often eat within a 2-hour period what most people would regard as an unusual amount of food?

Can you give me an example of the kinds and amounts of food that you might eat during one of these times?

How often do these times occur?

Do you do anything to counteract the effects of eating that much—like making yourself vomit; taking laxatives, enemas, or water pills; strict fasting between periods of eating a lot of food; or exercising a lot?

How important is your body shape and size in how you feel about yourself?

These questions and those regarding anorexia nervosa should be asked of the patient in a manner comfortable to both the health care professional and the patient, rather than in a fixed manner. Depending on the patient, questions about both bulimic and anorexic behaviors may need to be asked; the patient's history and presenting symptoms should dictate the emphasis of the interview. The sample questions are given to indicate that one can (and should) ask about eating behavior forthrightly. If the topics of the questions are followed, information about all the diagnostic criteria for both anorexia nervosa and bulimia nervosa will be gleaned.

The patient should also be asked if this is the first time these behaviors have occurred or if there have been past episodes; in the case of the latter, a careful history taking about each episode, its severity and duration, and treatments and their success should be done. This information may yield important clues as to how to approach (and how not to approach) the patient therapeutically during the current episode.

The questions listed previously may also help lead to the elucidation of comorbid psychiatric conditions or even primary conditions for which anorexia or bulimia may be just an associated symptom. For example, with regard to the latter, one of the authors was once asked to consult on a young adolescent girl hospitalized on the endocrine service with electrolyte disturbances suggestive of Bartter's syndrome. However, with no confirmatory evidence of somatic causes of the patient's cachexia and with observation by the nurses of bizarre eating habits, a diagnosis of anorexia nervosa was entertained, and psychiatric

interview of the patient by one of the authors during endocrine rounds was requested. After introductions were made by the psychiatrist as to who he was and why he was there, initial questioning began with what the patient ate (lettuce and carrots only) and why she ate only those two items (the computer in the hospital basement was giving her instructions to do so). Additional questioning about symptoms of psychosis led to a presumptive diagnosis of schizophrenia with secondary anorexia, and the patient was referred for psychiatric care.

Symptoms of depression and anxiety often occur in malnourished, cachexic anorexics as well as in persons who are symptomatic with binging and purging.[49–56] These symptoms appear to be exaggerated by malnutrition, as they are reduced by improved nutrition. Mild to moderate negative mood states and obsessive symptoms persist after recovery in both anorexic and bulimic individuals,[56–58] which raises the possibility that these traits contribute to the pathogenesis of eating disorders.

A possible relationship between anorexia nervosa and obsessive-compulsive disorder (OCD) has been hypothesized for more than 50 years. There is a high incidence of comorbid OCD in anorexic and bulimic women and their families, as well as increased rates of anorexia nervosa and bulimia nervosa in persons with primary OCD. It has been questioned whether the core eating disorder symptoms (e.g., fear of fatness, pursuit of thinness) are indeed a specific type of obsession. Symmetry, ordering, and perfectionism are the most common target symptoms in women with anorexia and bulimia nervosa, and these traits persist after recovery. Leckman and others[59] delineated four symptom dimensions of OCD, one of which was symmetry and ordering; these occurred most commonly in men. Whether OCD in men and eating disorders in women are gender-specific expressions of a common psychobiology related to obsessions with symmetry and ordering compulsions remains to be determined. Functional brain neuroimaging of anorexic patients is beginning to delineate activation of limbic and paralimbic areas that may be involved with calorie fear; these areas have also been implicated as a neural substrate of obsessive-compulsive and depressive symptoms.[60]

GENERAL PHYSICAL AND LABORATORY FINDINGS

The general physical and laboratory findings of anorexia nervosa and bulimia nervosa are presented in Tables 45–3 and 45–4, respectively.[61] Medical complications occur secondary to chronic starvation and malnutrition and to bingeing and purging.[14] Neuroimaging studies of anorexics have shown enlargement of cortical sulci and subarachnoid spaces, suggestive of cerebral atrophy, which may or may not be reversible with refeeding.[17, 62] Proton magnetic resonance spectroscopy (P-MRS) indicates higher ratios of choline-containing compounds to creatine and *N*-acetylaspartate, suggesting starvation-associated increased cell membrane turnover.[63] Consistent with these findings, ^{31}P-MRS has shown higher phosphodiester peaks and smaller phosphomonoester peaks in malnourished anorexics, indicating abnormal membrane phospholipid metabolism.[64]

The electrolyte disturbances of anorexia nervosa and bulimia nervosa depend on whether purging is primarily by vomiting or by abuse of laxatives or diuretics (or both). The medical management of these cases can be complex and must be individualized. Comerci[61] presented detailed case histories of an anorexic and a bulimic patient, including critiques of their treatment, which highlighted the intricacies of successful medical management of these disorders.

NEUROENDOCRINOLOGY

Abnormal hormone profiles and responses to challenge are closely related to the "starvation" status of anorexia nervosa and bulimia nervosa patients. Hormone abnormalities may also be present, but to a lesser extent, in normal-weight women with bulimia nervosa. The presence of starvation in anorexia nervosa is evident from the weight loss, but it may not be recognized in normal-weight bulimia: Although bulimic women often maintain a normal weight, they do so by re-

TABLE 45-3. Physical and Laboratory Findings in Anorexia Nervosa

Physical
Cachexia, emaciation, dehydration, shock or impending shock
Covert infectious processes, immunologic problems late in process
Dry skin, desquamation, yellowish palms and soles
Scalp and pubic hair loss, lanugo, increased pigmented body hair
Hypothermia, decreased metabolic rate, bradycardia, hypotension
Bradypnea (respiratory compensation for alkalosis)
Edema of lower extremities, heart murmur (infrequent)
Signs of estrogen deficiency (dry skin, osteoporosis, small uterus and cervix, dry vaginal mucosa) and androgen deficiency (no acne or oily skin)
Chemical
Normal laboratory results early in process
Elevated BUN, secondary to dehydration
Hypercarotenemia
Elevated serum cholesterol early in process; may decrease later
Decreased plasma transferrin, complement, fibrinogen, prealbumin; usually normal protein and albumin:globulin ratio
Elevated serum lactic dehydrogenase and alkaline phosphatase
Depressed serum magnesium, calcium, phosphorus, the last a late and ominous sign
Possibly depressed plasma zinc, urinary zinc, and copper
Hematologic
Panleukopenia with relative lymphocytosis
Thrombocytopenia
Very low erythrocyte sedimentation rate
Anemia late in process, especially with rehydration

Adapted from Comerci GD: Medical complications of anorexia nervosa and bulimia nervosa. Med Clin North Am 74:1293–1310, 1990.

TABLE 45-4. Physical and Laboratory Findings in Bulimia Nervosa

Physical
Usually well groomed with good hygiene
Usually normal weight or mild–moderate obesity
Generalized or localized edema of lower extremities
Swelling of parotid and other salivary glands
Bruises and lacerations of posterior pharynx, lesions of fingers and dorsum of hands, secondary to induced vomiting
Dental enamel discoloration and dysplasia, secondary to vomiting of gastric acid
Pyorrhea and other gum disorders
Diminished reflexes, muscle weakness, paralysis, infrequently peripheral neuropathy
Muscle cramping (with induced hypoxia or positive Trousseau's sign)
Signs of hypokalemia (hypotension, weak pulse, arrythmias, decreased cardiac output, poor-quality heart sounds; shortness of breath; ileus, abdominal distension, acute gastric dilatation; depression, mental clouding)
Additional physical features of anorexia nervosa, if food restriction is part of syndrome
Chemical
Uncomplicated bulimia
No abnormalities reported; possible abnormal glucose metabolism
Bulimia with vomiting
Metabolic alkalosis (hypochloremia, elevated serum bicarbonate)
Hypokalemia (secondary to metabolic alkalosis)
Hypovolemia with secondary hyperaldosteronism (also contributes to hypokalemia), pseudo-Bartter's syndrome
Bulimia with vomiting and purging (laxatives or diuretics)
All the above findings, plus:
Decreased body potassium secondary to diarrhea and renal losses
Metabolic acidosis with spuriously normal serum potassium
Hypokalemic nephropathy (urine concentrating deficit)
Hypokalemic myopathy (including cardiomyopathy)
Hypo- or hypercalcemia, hypomagnesemia, hypophosphatemia

Adapted from Comerci GD: Medical complications of anorexia nervosa and bulimia nervosa. Med Clin North Am 74:1293–1310, 1990.

stricting food intake when not bingeing and purging, and they may have monotonous and poorly balanced meals. Starvation-induced depletion of hepatic glycogen stores results in free fatty acids and ketone bodies replacing glucose as the primary energy source. This shift from glycogenolysis to lipolysis and ketogenesis is associated with an increase in free fatty acids and their metabolites. β-Hydroxybutyric acid levels are elevated in both anorexia and bulimia nervosa,[65] indicating that bulimic patients are nutritionally depleted in spite of their normal body weight.

The relationship of starvation and eating disorders to neuroendocrine function is most clearly seen for the pituitary-gonadal axis. As mentioned, secondary amenorrhea is one of the criteria for anorexia nervosa in postmenarcheal women, and oligomenorrhea occurs in about 50% of bulimics. Table 45–5 lists the major endocrine disturbances that occur in anorexia and bulimia nervosa.[12, 17, 66–73] The secondary amenorrhea is a direct result of altered gonadotropin secretion. Serum sex hormone binding globulin may be increased, and both estrogen and testosterone are decreased.[74] As indicated in Table 45–3, there are physical signs of severe estrogen deficiency. The luteinizing hormone response to luteinizing hormone–releasing hormone stimulation is blunted, but the follicle-stimulating hormone response is usually normal.

TABLE 45-5. Neuroendocrine Disturbances In Anorexia Nervosa and Bulimia Nervosa

	Anorexia Nervosa	Bulimia Nervosa
Pituitary-Gonadal Axis		
Plasma gonadotropins (LH, FSH)	↓	± ↓
Plasma estradiol	↓ ↓	± ↓
Plasma testosterone	↓	?
LHRH stimulation of LH	↓	± ↓
LHRH stimulation of FSH	↔	↔
Pituitary-Adrenocortical Axis		
Plasma and CSF cortisol	↑	± ↑
Plasma ACTH	↔	↔
CSF ACTH	↓	↔ (↓ when abstinent)
CSF CRH	↑	?
CSF vasopressin	↑	↑
CRH stimulation of ACTH	↓	?
ACTH stimulation of cortisol	↑	?
Dexamethasone suppression test	50%–90% nonsuppression	20%–60% nonsuppression
Pituitary-Thyroid Axis		
Plasma total T_4	± ↓	↔ (± ↓ when abstinent)
Plasma T_3	↓ ↓	↓
Plasma reverse T_3	↑	↔ (↓ when abstinent)
Plasma TSH	± ↓	± ↓ (↑ when abstinent)
CSF TRH	↓	?
TRH stimulation of TSH	↓	↓
Other Neuroendocrine Axes		
Growth hormone	↑	↑
Prolactin	↔	± ↓
Prolactin response to serotonergic challenge	↓	↓
Melatonin	± ↑	?

LH, luteinizing hormone; FSH, follicle-stimulating hormone; LHRH, luteinizing hormone–releasing hormone; CSF, cerebrospinal fluid; ACTH, adrenocorticotropic hormone; CRH, corticotropin-releasing hormone; T_4, thyroxine; T_3, triiodothyronine; TSH, thyroid-stimulating hormone; TRH, thyrotropin-releasing hormone, ↑, increased; ↓, decreased; ↔, unchanged; ?, insufficient data.

Figure 45–2 illustrates the circadian serum luteinizing hormone (LH) profiles of girls at different pubertal stages and in a 21-year-old woman with anorexia nervosa of 14 months' duration whose body weight was 60% of ideal weight.[66] This patient's menarche was at age 14, and, during the period of weight loss, her LH profile was that of a prepubertal girl. Bulimia nervosa patients may also have decreased gonadotropin secretion if they have lost 15% or more of their body weight, but they usually have normal circulating gonadotropins and continue their menses.

With reference to the hypothalamic-pituitary-adrenal cortical (HPA) axis (Table 45–5), the abnormalities in anorexia nervosa and in reduced-weight bulimia nervosa[75–78] are strikingly similar to those occurring in 30% to 50% of patients with major depression.[72, 79] Circulating cortisol is increased at all times of the day and night, but its circadian rhythm is preserved in terms of amplitude and timing.[80] Circulating adrenocorticotropic hormone (ACTH) is usually normal, as it is in major depression, when it is determined by radioimmunoassay; the more specific immunoradiometric assay for ACTH$_{1-39}$ has shown decreased ACTH in major depression,[81] which also could be the case for ACTH$_{1-39}$ in these eating disorders. In this regard, cerebrospinal fluid (CSF) ACTH concentrations appear to be decreased, but CSF corticotropin-releasing hormone (CRH) concentrations may be increased,[82, 83] as may be CSF vasopressin,[84, 85] a secretagogue for ACTH in addition to CRH,[86] which appears to play a greater role in stress states than under normal conditions.[87]

Stimulation and suppression tests of the HPA axis have been conducted mainly in anorexia nervosa, and they are in accord with the baseline hormone findings. The ACTH response to CRH administration is reduced, undoubtedly secondary to enhanced negative feedback on the pituitary corticotrophs exerted by elevated circulating cortisol. The cortisol response to ACTH administration is increased, suggesting increased secretory capacity of the adrenal cortex. The low-dose dexamethasone suppression test is abnormal in 50% to 90% of anorexics and in 20% to 60% of bulimics, depending on the weight loss. Because dexamethasone acts primarily at the pituitary,[88] ACTH and cortisol escape from dexamethasone suppression, suggesting increased suprapituitary stimulation of corticotrophs by CRH and vasopressin. Taken together, the pituitary-adrenocortical findings indicate a mild to moderate activation of this hormone axis in anorexia and bulimia nervosa.

With reference to the pituitary-thyroid axis, starvation leads to considerably decreased plasma free triiodothyronine (T$_3$) concentrations, along with somewhat decreased plasma free thyroxine (T$_4$) and increased plasma reverse T$_3$ concentrations. This represents the "euthyroid sick syndrome" hormone profile.[89–91] The decreased circulating T$_3$ helps reduce energy expenditure and minimizes muscle protein catabolism into amino acids for gluconeogenesis.[89] CSF thyrotropin-releasing hormone also appears to be reduced in anorexia nervosa.[92] When bingeing, bulimic patients generally have normal thyroid indices with perhaps reduced T$_3$ and thyroid-stimulating hormone concentrations; however, when they become abstinent, their pituitary-thyroid axis function resembles that of anorexic patients.[93–95]

Insulin-like growth factor, type 1 (IGF-1) concentrations are low in both anorexia nervosa and bulimia nervosa, and circulating growth hormone is increased, perhaps owing to diminished feedback of IGF-1 on growth hormone secretion. Circulating prolactin is usually unchanged in anorexia nervosa and may be reduced in bulimia nervosa. Prolactin responses to serotonergic challenges such as meta-chlorophenylpiperazine, fenfluramine, L-tryptophan, and 5-OH-tryptophan are diminished in both anorexia and bulimia nervosa,[96–100] suggesting decreased central nervous system (CNS) serotonergic neurotransmitter function.[101] (Serotonin uptake–inhibiting antidepressants have shown some promise in the treatment of these eating disorders, as discussed later.) Circulating melatonin has been reported as both unchanged and increased in anorexia nervosa and as unchanged in bulimia nervosa.[102–104]

The effects of reduced caloric intake on these endocrine systems has been studied in healthy individuals.[105, 106] When healthy control women were starved, plasma gonadotropin concentrations declined. The women also experienced increased circulating concentrations of cortisol and growth hormone and decreased plasma T$_3$ concentrations despite normal plasma T$_4$—the "euthyroid sick syndrome" hormone profile.[89] The endocrine abnormalities associated with starvation in the healthy female subjects reversed with the resumption of normal eating patterns.

It is important to emphasize that the endocrine changes in both anorexia nervosa and bulimia nervosa revert to normal with successful treatment of these illnesses, indicating that the endocrine changes are state markers of the metabolic stress of starvation and malnutrition. It should also be emphasized that, in addition to its effects on hormone secretion, starvation can lead to abnormal psychologic states. Semistarvation of male conscientious objectors to military service was associated with increased irritability, labile mood, depression, decreased concentration, decreased libido, and decreased motor activity,[107] and starvation and malnutrition can exaggerate the comorbid psychiatric symptoms of anorexia and bulimia nervosa.[56] These changes reinforce the concept of starvation-related "state" changes, influencing both the behavioral and the endocrine aspects of anorexia and bulimia nervosa.

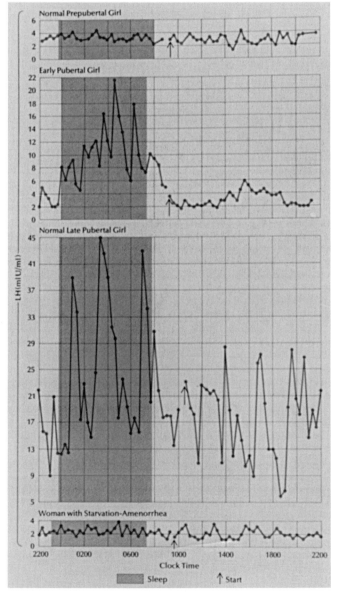

FIGURE 45–2. *Circadian serum luteinizing hormone (LH) profiles in girls at different pubertal stages and in a 21-year-old woman with anorexia nervosa of 14 months' duration whose body weight was 60% of ideal weight. Menarche was at age 14 years, and her LH profile is that of a prepubertal girl. (From Vande Wiele RL: Anorexia nervosa and the hypothalamus. Hosp Pract 12:45–51, 1977. © 1977 The McGraw-Hill Companies, Inc. Illustration by Albert Miller.)*

NEUROPEPTIDES IN THE CENTRAL NERVOUS SYSTEM

Since the 1980s, the realization has evolved that the peripheral hormonal disturbances in anorexia nervosa and bulimia nervosa are a consequence of the malnutrition associated with starvation and bingeing rather than being etiologic. Contemporaneously, an understanding of how CNS neuronal pathways contribute to starvation-induced alterations in peripheral hormonal secretion has been developed. The mechanisms for controlling food intake involve a complex interplay among peripheral (taste, gastrointestinal peptides, vagal afferent nerves) and CNS neurotransmitters and neuromodulators, including monoamines and neuropeptides that influence hunger and satiety.[108] In animals, compounds such as norepinephrine, serotonin, opioids, neuropeptide Y and YY, leptin, CRH, and vasopressin contribute to regulating the rate, duration, and size of meals, as well as the selection of carbohydrates and protein.

Neuropeptides were initially determined to be regulators primarily of hypothalamic functions such as food and water consumption and metabolism, sexuality, sleep, body temperature, pain sensation, and autonomic function. These compounds have also been localized in other areas of the CNS besides the hypothalamus and pituitary, and they appear to regulate complex human mental functions such as mood, obsessionality, attachment formation, and risk-taking and addictive behaviors.[109] Some of the behavioral disturbances occurring during starvation may therefore be related to alterations in function of the following peptides throughout the CNS.

Neuropeptide Y and Peptide YY

These are phylogenetically and structurally related 36 amino acid peptides that share the same receptor superfamily and are potent activators of feeding behavior in animals. Neuropeptide Y (NPY) occurs in high concentrations in limbic structures, including the hypothalamus, and is present throughout the cerebral cortex as well.[110] It is produced in the arcuate nucleus of the hypothalamus and acts on the paraventricular nucleus to help mediate increased eating, especially of carbohydrate-rich sweet foods,[111] and to reduce energy expenditure. In contrast, peptide YY (PYY) occurs in lower concentrations in the CNS, in caudal brain stem and spinal cord. PYY is primarily peripherally located in endocrine cells of the lower gastrointestinal tract, where it helps mediate gastrointestinal motility and function.

Intracerebroventricular (ICV) NPY administration in animals produces many of the physiologic and behavioral changes associated with anorexia nervosa, including gonadal steroid-dependent effects on LH secretion,[112] suppression of sexual activity,[113] increased CRH in the hypothalamus,[114] and hypotension.[115] Significantly elevated concentrations of CSF NPY have been found in underweight anorexics as compared to healthy volunteers, whereas these patients, whether underweight or recovered, had normal CSF PYY concentrations.[116] CSF NPY returned to normal with recovery, although patients with amenorrhea continued to have higher CSF NPY concentrations. Although animal studies indicate that increased NPY activity can stimulate feeding,[117] elevated CSF NPY is not an effective stimulant of feeding in underweight anorexics, as evidenced by their resistance to eating and weight gain. Anorexics typically display an obsessive and paradoxic interest in dietary intake and food preparation, and it may be that increased NPY activity in extrahypothalamic areas of the CNS could contribute to these cognitions and behaviors.

ICV PYY administration in rats causes massive food ingestion, to which tolerance does not develop.[118] This effect on feeding behavior in animals prompted the speculation that increased CNS PYY activity may contribute to bulimia. CSF PYY concentrations of normal-weight bulimic women studied when bingeing and vomiting were similar to those of controls.[116] In contrast, CSF PYY was significantly elevated in bulimic women studied after a month of abstinence from bingeing and vomiting, as compared to healthy volunteer women and anorexia nervosa patients. CSF NPY concentrations were normal in the bulimic women, in contrast to the elevated CSF NPY concentrations in the anorexic women.

It is not known why CSF PYY is normal in bulimics with chronic bingeing and vomiting and becomes elevated after a period of abstinence. Future studies should examine whether abrupt cessation of bingeing or vomiting, or both, results in an overshoot of CNS PYY production. Whatever the cause, this disturbance is of potential importance. Normal-weight bulimia carries a high recidivism rate, despite treatment. Abnormally elevated CNS PYY activity in the abstinent bulimic may contribute to a persistent drive toward bingeing, particularly a desire for sweet, high-caloric foods.

Leptin

Leptin is the recently discovered hormone product of the mouse *ob* gene and human homologue gene *LEP*.[119] Leptin is secreted predominantly by adipose cells and acts as an afferent signal and regulator of body fat stores.[120] It is thought to activate OB receptors, encoded by the *db* gene, primarily in the hypothalamus but also in extraneural tissues including the vascular epithelium, where leptin-induced angiogenesis may aid increased energy expenditure.[121, 122] In rodents, defects in the leptin coding sequence, resulting in leptin deficiency, and defects in leptin receptors[123] are associated with obesity. Treatment with recombinant leptin reduces fat mass in both obese and normal-weight animals in a dose-dependent manner.[124, 125] In humans, serum leptin concentrations are positively correlated with fat mass in individuals in all weight ranges. Women tend to have higher serum leptin than men of the same weight, presumably because of their higher proportion of body fat.[126] Obesity in humans is not thought to be a result of leptin deficiency per se, but obesity may be associated with leptin resistance.[127]

Malnourished and underweight anorexia nervosa patients have significantly reduced plasma and CSF leptin concentrations compared with normal-weight controls,[128–131] implying a normal physiologic response to starvation. Reduced plasma/CSF leptin ratio has been found in anorexics compared with controls, suggesting that the proportional decrease in leptin with weight loss is greater in plasma than in CSF. As in normal control women, serum leptin concentrations in anorexics are correlated with body weight and fat mass. During refeeding in anorexia nervosa patients, CSF leptin concentrations increased to normal values before full weight restoration,[131] possibly as a consequence of the relatively rapid and disproportionate accumulation of fat during refeeding. This suggests that premature normalization of leptin concentrations might contribute to difficulty in achieving and sustaining a normal weight in anorexics.

There have been only a few studies of leptin in bulimia nervosa. In one study, serum leptin concentrations in ill bulimics were similar to those of normal control women and were correlated with body mass.[130] Kaye and colleagues (unpublished data) found normal plasma and CSF leptin concentrations in long-term recovered anorexic and bulimic patients. Taken together, the data suggest that, similar to normal individuals, leptin is correlated with body weight in anorexia and bulimia nervosa, but it is not involved in their etiology.

Leptin also appears to modulate fertility. Its administration to infertile ob/ob and prepubertal mice induces reproductive function.[132, 133] Although feeding of normal meals to lean or obese humans does not affect plasma leptin concentrations or *ob* messenger RNA (mRNA) expression,[134] animal studies have shown that acute fasting and refeeding rapidly decrease and increase, respectively, *ob* mRNA expression[135] and that overfeeding (without weight gain) increases *ob* mRNA expression.[136] Such findings have led to the hypothesis that leptin is the metabolic signal that mediates impaired reproductive ability in extreme overweight and underweight conditions. There appear to have been no studies addressing a potential relationship between leptin and amenorrhea in anorexia nervosa.

In some anorexic patients, amenorrhea may occur before significant weight loss, and leptin may be the mediating hormone. Weight loss generally causes circulating leptin concentrations to fall in proportion to the loss of body fat mass,[71] but acute, fasting-induced weight loss can provoke a fall in leptin disproportionately greater than would be expected from the amount of fat lost.[137] This suggests that, under conditions of intense food deprivation, leptin may instigate metabolic responses before a significant weight or fat loss has occurred. Reduced leptin concentrations appear to be a critical signal that initiates the neuroendocrine response to starvation, including limiting procreation, decreasing thyroid thermogenesis, and increasing secretion of stress steroids.[138] Leptin administration during fasting partially restores LH and testosterone concentrations, blunts falling T_4 concentrations, and attenuates the rise in ACTH and glucocorticoids, without affecting plasma concentrations of insulin, glucose, or ketone bodies.

As mentioned previously, during starvation, circulating concentrations of NPY (a potent appetite stimulator) increase, which inhibits gonadotropin release and activates the HPA axis. Since leptin also inhibits starvation-induced elevations in NPY, leptin may counteract the effects of starvation by regulating the amount of hypothalamic NPY mRNA.[139] Leptin may also reduce food intake and body weight by increasing the metabolic rate through activation of β-adrenergic receptors and possibly through its own anorexigenic properties.[140]

Corticotropin-Releasing Hormone

As mentioned previously, the hypercortisolism in anorexia and bulimia nervosa is most likely due to hypersecretion of CRH, which is most probably a response to weight loss per se. CRH may also have a role beyond the HPA axis, as ICV administration of CRH to animals produces physiologic and behavioral changes associated with anorexia nervosa, including hypothalamic hypogonadism,[141] decreased sexual activity,[142] decreased feeding behavior,[143] and hyperactivity.[144]

Opioid Peptides

CNS opioid agonists increase food intake, and opioid antagonists decrease food intake,[145–147] suggesting that these compounds may mediate some aspects of anorexia nervosa.[31, 148–150] Although assessment of brain opioid activity in vivo in humans is problematic—because of the many CNS neuropeptides with opioid activity and the multiplicity of CNS opioid receptors—the relative activity of a few opioid peptides has been determined in anorexic patients by measurement of their CSF concentrations. Underweight anorexics were found to have significantly reduced CSF β-endorphin concentrations compared with healthy volunteers.[151] CSF β-endorphin concentrations remained significantly below normal after short-term weight restoration but returned to normal after long-term weight restoration. CSF β-endorphin concentrations also have been shown to be reduced in women with bulimia nervosa.[150] CSF dynorphin concentrations have been reported as normal in all stages of anorexia nervosa and in bulimia nervosa.[152, 153]

Open trials of high doses of the opiate antagonist naltrexone have been reported to reduce binge frequency in bulimia nervosa,[154, 155] but double-blind, controlled trials with lower naltrexone doses have shown no effect on binge frequency or macronutrient intake.[156, 157] One double-blind trial indicated that relatively high-dose naltrexone treatment reduced binge and purge frequency and total daily food intake of bulimics, but it did not affect their ability to resist the desire to binge or purge.[158] Whether high-dose opioid antagonist treatment has a role in the treatment of bulimia nervosa is still unclear.

A disturbance in CNS opioid function may also contribute to the neuroendocrine abnormalities in anorexia and bulimia nervosa (e.g., disturbances in HPA and pituitary-gonadal axis function).[159, 160] Brain opioid pathways inhibit ACTH and cortisol release in humans, and they suppress pulsatile gonadotropin secretion in rats and in sexually mature humans. Underweight anorexics frequently have a blunted response of LH secretion to opiate antagonists,[161–164] and weight restoration tends to normalize this response.[165] The failure of opioid antagonists to increase LH secretion in underweight anorexics suggests that another neurotransmitter system (or systems) may be responsible for this neuroendocrine disturbance.

Vasopressin and Oxytocin

In addition to the effects of vasopressin on HPA axis regulation and free-water clearance by the kidney and the effects of oxytocin during the puerperium, these structurally related neuropeptides are distributed throughout the CNS and function as long-acting neuromodulators of complex behaviors. The effects of vasopressin appear to be reciprocal to those of oxytocin: Central administration of vasopressin to rats enhances memory consolidation and retrieval, whereas administration of oxytocin disrupts memory.[166, 167]

In addition to abnormally high CSF vasopressin concentrations[84, 85] and impaired osmoregulation of plasma vasopressin,[168] anorexia nervosa patients have reduced CSF oxytocin concentrations and impaired plasma oxytocin responses to stimulation.[169] Underweight anorexics also have an impaired plasma oxytocin response to challenging stimuli.[170] These abnormalities tend to normalize after weight restoration, suggesting they are secondary to malnutrition or abnormal fluid balance, or both. In underweight anorexics, low CNS oxytocin might interact with high CNS vasopressin to enhance the retention of cognitive distortions of the aversive consequences of eating, thereby reinforcing these patients' perseverative preoccupation with the adverse consequences of food intake.

Patients with normal-weight bulimia were found to have elevated CSF vasopressin concentrations but normal CSF oxytocin both on admission and after 1 month of nutritional stabilization and abstinence from bingeing and purging.[84] In these patients, as well, high CNS vasopressin might contribute to their obsessional preoccupation with the aversive consequences of weight gain.

Long-Term Effects of Multiple Neuropeptide Disturbances

As with the peripheral endocrine changes in pituitary and target gland hormones in anorexia nervosa and bulimia nervosa patients reviewed earlier, multiple neuropeptide disturbances occur when patients engage in pathologic eating behaviors and become malnourished. And, as with the peripheral endocrine markers, these peptide systems tend to become normal with long-term recovery from anorexia nervosa. Fewer studies have been done assessing these systems after recovery from bulimia nervosa, but they also suggest normalization of peptide function. The slow correction of these neuropeptide disturbances with weight restoration in anorexia and bulimia nervosa implies that the disturbances are secondary to malnutrition or weight loss, or both, and are not etiologic. Nevertheless, as indicated previously, an understanding of these neuropeptide disturbances may shed light on why many anorexics cannot easily reverse their illness. Secondary symptoms such as obsessions and dysphoric mood may be exaggerated by CNS neuropeptide alterations and cause the primary illness to be more refractory to treatment.

While these neuropeptide disturbances do not appear to be a permanent feature or cause of anorexia nervosa, they are strongly entrenched and are corrected only slowly with improved nutrition and weight normalization. This may be one explanation for why, even after improved nutrition and weight gain, many anorexics have great difficulty normalizing their behavior. That the neuropeptide disturbances eventually become normal during long-term recovery suggests that treatment of anorexia and bulimia nervosa must be sustained for months after weight normalization, to rectify the many physiologic disturbances.

TREATMENT

Treatment of the eating disorders has been, and continues to be, complex and difficult. In a 20-year follow-up of anorexia nervosa patients, about one third rated their outcomes as good, one third as intermediate, and one third as poor.[171] A range of cognitive-behavior, educational, psychodynamic, and psychopharmacologic treatments have been used,[172–174] none of which has been completely successful over the long term. Consequently, as is often the case in the management of psychiatric patients, a combination of therapies is used; however, for the eating disorders, their rationale may not always be well justified on the basis of scientific studies.

With regard to anorexia nervosa, in contrast to bulimia nervosa, there has been a dearth of large-scale, randomized controlled clinical treatment trials.[175–178] A prominent focus has been on interventions previously tested on comorbid psychiatric disorders, such as depression and substance abuse. However, eating disorders and these comorbid syndromes appear to be independently transmitted familial liabilities,[179, 180] so that treatments also need to be targeted to the eating disorders themselves.

Early controlled treatment studies of anorexia nervosa were narrowly focused on testing the value of behavior modification in increasing the rate of weight gain in hospitalized, emaciated patients and the efficacy of adjunctive pharmacologic treatment with either neuroleptic or antidepressant drugs. Weight gain could be achieved in many patients through a combination of supportive nursing care and behavioral techniques, whereas pharmacotherapy had little incremental advantage in the treatment of severely ill patients.[181]

More recent controlled studies have examined the efficacy of various psychologic therapies in promoting weight gain in acutely ill patients[182–184] and in preventing relapse following restoration of normal body weight.[185] Substantial improvement in body mass and general psychosocial adjustment was achieved in some anorexic subjects through cognitive-behavior, psychoeducational, and family therapy techniques, with or without dietary counseling. Therapeutic gains were not as robust in patients with more chronic disability. Studies also showed that fluoxetine reduced relapse and obsessionality when administered after weight restoration in anorexics.[186, 187] There are, however, several methodologic shortcomings to these studies, including small sample sizes, significant dropout rates, initial use of inpatient treatment for medically compromised patients, and, importantly, absence of follow-up assessment of the durability of these gains in preventing relapse.[178] Improved treatment of anorexia nervosa remains of great clinical and public health importance, in that it is a chronic, relapsing illness[188] with substantial and costly medical morbidity.[189]

Bulimia nervosa has been studied for only two decades, yet a number of controlled clinical trials have shown the efficacy of both antidepressant medications[176, 190] and psychologic therapies, especially cognitive-behavior therapy (CBT), in reducing both the frequency of bingeing and purging and the severity of body dissatisfaction, pursuit of thinness, and perfectionism.[191–193] However, medication alone produces full remission in only a minority of patients; many patients require multiple medication trials before achieving clinically significant improvement; there have been significant dropout rates in controlled clinical trials; and relapse during continuation therapy is high.

CBT alone produces higher rates of full remission in bulimia nervosa than does antidepressant monotherapy.[193, 194] Even so, 40% to 60% of patients receiving CBT remain symptomatic to some degree after acute treatment.[177, 192, 194] The mechanisms by which psychologic treatments are effective are not well understood and appear to be complex. Fairburn and associates,[191] comparing the effects of CBT, interpersonal therapy (IPT), and pure behavior therapy, showed that IPT, which strictly avoided direct reference to abnormal eating attitudes or dietary behaviors, achieved long-term benefits in controlling binge eating and purging equal to those obtained with CBT.

How long to continue treatment once binge eating abates, in order to minimize relapse, remains undetermined. With antidepressant continuation therapy, the risk of relapse in bulimics[195] may be higher than in patients with unipolar depression.[196] Predictors of long-term outcome within and across treatment modalities remain largely unstudied,[178] as is the issue of whether combination therapy with CBT and antidepressants has additive or synergistic effects. Combined treatment may have an advantage over CBT alone in reducing binge eating and purging, but the incremental benefit is modest.[193, 194]

An optimal therapeutic strategy for bulimia nervosa thus remains to be identified. Remaining questions include the duration of continuation of psychosocial and antidepressant therapies needed to sustain the gains achieved during acute treatment, the mechanisms underpinning the possibly synergistic effects of combined treatment, the predictors of differential treatment outcomes, the reasons for a more rapid decay of acute antidepressant treatment effects in bulimia nervosa as compared to in major depression, and the anticipated effects of crossing over to alternative modalities of treatment when initial treatment fails.[178]

The difficulties faced by clinicians in the treatment of anorexia

nervosa and bulimia nervosa will continue, and may even magnify, as trends in health care delivery reduce access to extended care in specialty inpatient and outpatient facilities. These external forces may compromise efforts, certainly for severely ill patients, to suppress the debilitating and sometimes life-threatening behavioral and biologic symptoms and sequelae of these illnesses. The endocrinologist is best advised to seek psychiatric specialist consultation early in the evaluation of patients with these eating disorders, not just to aid in their differential diagnosis but, importantly, to help plan the complex therapeutic approaches currently known to offer the best outcomes in these illnesses.

[Note: Several recent references of interest have been added to the bibliography.[197–200]]

REFERENCES

1. Allbutt TC, Rolleston HD: A System of Medicine. London, Macmillan, 1908, p 398.
2. Berkman JM: Anorexia nervosa, anorexia, inanition, and low basal metabolic rate. Am J Med Sci 180:411–424, 1930.
3. Bliss EL, Branch CHH: Anorexia Nervosa: Its History, Psychology, and Biology. New York, Paul B. Hoeber, 1960.
4. Lucas AR: Toward the understanding of anorexia nervosa as a disease entity. Mayo Clin Proc 56:254–264, 1981.
5. Vandereycken W, Van Deth R: From Fasting Saints to Anorexic Girls: The History of Self-Starvation. London, Althone Press, 1994.
6. Bruch H: Eating Disorders: Obesity, Anorexia Nervosa and the Person Within. New York, Basic Books, 1973.
7. Vigersky RA (ed): Anorexia Nervosa. New York, Raven Press, 1977.
8. Garfinkel PE, Garner DM: Anorexia Nervosa: A Multidimensional Perspective. New York, Brunner/Mazel, 1982.
9. Pirke KM, Ploog D (eds): The Psychobiology of Anorexia Nervosa. Berlin, Springer-Verlag, 1984.
10. Herzog DB, Copeland PM: Eating disorders. N Engl J Med 313:295–303, 1985.
11. Habermas T: The psychiatric history of anorexia nervosa and bulimia nervosa: Weight concerns and bulimic symptoms in early case reports. Int J Eat Disord 8:259–273, 1989.
12. Foster DW: Eating disorders: Obesity, anorexia nervosa, and bulimia nervosa. In Wilson JD, Foster DW (eds): Williams Textbook of Endocrinology, ed 8. Philadelphia, WB Saunders, 1992, pp 1335–1365.
13. Halmi KA (ed): Psychobiology and Treatment of Anorexia Nervosa and Bulimia Nervosa. Washington, DC, American Psychiatric Press, 1992.
14. Kaplan AS, Garfinkel PE: Medical Issues and the Eating Disorders: The Interface. New York, Brunner/Mazel, 1993.
15. American Psychiatric Association: Diagnostic and Statistical Manual of Mental Disorders, ed 4. Washington, DC, American Psychiatric Association, 1994, pp 539–550.
16. Garfinkel PE: Eating disorders. In Kaplan HI, Sadock BJ (eds): Comprehensive Textbook of Psychiatry/VI. Baltimore, Williams & Wilkins, 1995, pp 1361–1371.
17. Warren MP: Anorexia nervosa. In DeGroot LJ, Besser M, Burger HG, et al (eds): Endocrinology, ed 3. Philadelphia, WB Saunders, 1995, pp 2679–2687.
18. Walsh BT: Eating disorders. In Tasman A, Kay J, Lieberman JA (eds): Psychiatry. Philadelphia, WB Saunders, 1997, pp 1202–1216.
19. Walsh BT, Devlin MJ: Eating disorders: Progress and problems. Science 280:1387–1390, 1998.
20. Morton R: Phthisiologia, seu exercitationes de phthisi tribus libris comprehensæ. Totumque opus variis historiis illustratum. London, Smith & Walford, 1689. (Translated as Phthisiologia; or, a Treatise of Consumptions, 1694.)
21. Hunter R, Macalpine I: Three Hundred Years of Psychiatry 1535–1860. London, Oxford University Press, 1963, pp 230–232.
22. Lasègue C: De l'anorexie hystérique. Arch Gén Méd 1:385, 1873.
23. Gull WW: Anorexia hysterica (apepsia hysterica). Brit Med J 2:527, 1873.
24. Gull WW: Anorexia nervosa (apepsia hysterica, anorexia hysterica). Trans Clin Soc Lond 7:22–31, 1874.
25. Simmonds M: Über Hypophysisschwund mit tödlichem Ausgang. Deutsche Med Wochenschr 40:322, 1914.
26. Russell GFM: Bulimia nervosa: An ominous variant of anorexia nervosa. Psychol Med 9:429–448, 1979.
27. Szmukler GI, Tantam D: Anorexia nervosa: Starvation dependence. Br J Med Psychol 57:303–310, 1984.
28. Lucas AR, Beard CM, O'Fallon WM, et al: Anorexia nervosa in Rochester, Minnesota: A 45-year study. Mayo Clin Proc 63:433–442, 1988.
29. Vandereycken W, Hoek HW: Are eating disorders culture-bound syndromes? In Halmi KA (ed): Psychobiology and Treatment of Anorexia Nervosa and Bulimia Nervosa. Washington, DC, American Psychiatric Press, 1992, pp 19–36.
30. Crisp AH, Palmer RL, Kalucy RS: How common is anorexia nervosa? A prevalence study. Br J Psychiatry 128:549–554, 1976.
31. Pope HG, Hudson JI, Yurgulun-Todd D, et al: Prevalence of anorexia nervosa and bulimia in three student populations. Int J Eat Disord 3:45–51, 1984.
32. Szmukler GI: The epidemiology of anorexia nervosa and bulimia. J Psychiatr Res 19:143–153, 1984.
33. Hsu LK: Epidemiology of the eating disorders. Psychiatr Clin North Am 19:681–700, 1996.
34. Sullivan PF: Mortality in anorexia nervosa. Am J Psychiatry 152:1073–1074, 1995.
35. Cooper PJ, Charnock DJ, Taylor MJ: The prevalence of bulimia nervosa: A replication study. Br J Psychiatry 151:684–686, 1987.

36. Ben-Tovim DI, Subbiah N, Scheutz B, et al: Bulimia: Symptoms and syndromes in an urban population. Aust N Z J Psychiatry 23:73–80, 1989.

37. Fairburn CG, Beglin SJ: Studies of the epidemiology of anorexia nervosa. Am J Psychiatry 147:401–408, 1990.

38. Willi J, Grossmann S: Epidemiology of anorexia nervosa in a defined region of Switzerland. Am J Psychiatry 140:564–567, 1983.

39. Pyle RL, Halvorson PA, Neuman PA, et al: The increasing prevalence of bulimia in freshman college students. Int J Eat Disord 5:631–647, 1986.

40. Williams P, King M: The "epidemic" of anorexia nervosa: Another medical myth? Lancet 1:205–207, 1987.

41. Anderson AE: Anorexia nervosa: Who are you? Where are you? Mayo Clin Proc 63:511–512, 1988.

42. Hill JO, Peters JC: Environmental contributions to the obesity epidemic. Science 280:1371–1374, 1998.

43. Taubes G: As obesity rates rise, experts struggle to explain why. Science 280:1367–1368, 1998.

44. Strober M: Family-genetic studies. *In* Halmi KA (ed): Psychobiology and Treatment of Anorexia Nervosa and Bulimia Nervosa. Washington, DC, American Psychiatric Press, 1992, pp 61–76.

45. Lilenfeld LR, Strober M, Kaye WH: Genetics and family studies of anorexia nervosa and bulimia nervosa. *In* Kaye WH, Jimerson DC (eds): Eating Disorders. Ballière's Clinical Psychiatry. London, Ballière Tindall, 1997, pp 177–197.

46. Garfinkel PE, Lin E, Goering P, et al: Should amenorrhea be necessary for the diagnosis of anorexia nervosa? Evidence from a Canadian community sample. Br J Psychiatry 168:500–506, 1996.

47. Garfinkel PE, Kennedy SH, Kaplan AS: Views on classification and diagnosis of eating disorders. Can J Psychiatry 40:445–456, 1995.

48. First MB, Spitzer RL, Gibbon M, et al: Structured Clinical Interview for DSM-IV Axis I Disorders. New York, Biometrics Research Department, New York State Psychiatric Institute, 1996.

49. Strober M: Depression in the eating disorders: A review and analysis of descriptive, family and biological findings. *In* Garner DM, Garfinkel PE (eds): Diagnostic Issues in Anorexia Nervosa and Bulimia Nervosa. New York, Brunner/Mazel, 1980, pp 80–111.

50. Laessle RG, Wittchen HU, Fichter MM, et al: The significance of subgroups of bulimia and anorexia nervosa: Lifetime frequency of psychiatric disorders. Int J Eat Disord 8:569–574, 1989.

51. Herzog DB, Keller MB, Sacks NR, et al: Psychiatric comorbidity in treatment-seeking anorexics and bulimics. J Am Acad Child Adolesc Psychiatry 31:810–818, 1992.

52. Braun DL, Sunday SR, Halmi KA: Psychiatric comorbidity in patients with eating disorders. Psychol Med 24:859–867, 1994.

53. Holderness CC, Brooks-Gunn J, Warren WP: Co-morbidity of eating disorders and substance abuse: Review of the literature. Int J Eat Disord 16:1–34, 1994.

54. Brewerton TD, Lydiard RB, Herzog DB, et al: Comorbidity of Axis I psychiatric diagnosis in bulimia nervosa. J Clin Psychiatry 56:77–80, 1995.

55. Garfinkel PE, Lin E, Goering P, et al: Bulimia nervosa in a Canadian community sample: Prevalence and comparison of subgroups. Am J Psychiatry 152:1052–1058, 1995.

56. Pollice C, Kaye WH, Greeno CG, et al: Relationship of depression, anxiety, and obsessionality to state of illness in anorexia nervosa. Int J Eat Disord 21:367–376, 1997.

57. Srinivasagam NM, Plotnicov KH, Greeno C, et al: Persistent perfectionism, symmetry, and exactness in anorexia nervosa after long-term recovery. Am J Psychiatry 152:1630–1634, 1995.

58. Kaye WH, Greeno CG, Moss H, et al: Alterations in serotonin activity and psychiatric symptomatology after recovery from bulimia nervosa. Arch Gen Psychiatry 55:927–935, 1998.

59. Leckman JF, Grice DE, Boardman J, et al: Symptoms of obsessive-compulsive disorder. Am J Psychiatry 154:911–917, 1997.

60. Ellison Z, Foong J, Howard R, et al: Functional anatomy of calorie fear in anorexia nervosa. Lancet 352:1192, 1998.

61. Comerci GD: Medical complications of anorexia nervosa and bulimia nervosa. Med Clin North Am 74:1293–1310, 1990.

62. Lambe EK, Katzman DK, Mikulis DJ, et al: Cerebral gray matter volume deficits after weight recovery from anorexia nervosa. Arch Gen Psychiatry 54:537–542, 1997.

63. Schlemmer H-P, Möckel R, Marcus A, et al: Proton magnetic resonance spectroscopy in acute, juvenile anorexia nervosa. Psychiatry Res 82:171–179, 1998.

64. Kato T, Shiori T, Murashita J, et al: Phosphorus-31 magnetic resonance spectroscopic observations in 4 cases with anorexia nervosa. Prog Neuropsychopharmacol Biol Psychiatry 21:719–724, 1997.

65. Pirke KM, Pahl J, Schweiger U: Metabolic and endocrine indices of starvation in bulimia: A comparison with anorexia nervosa. Psychiatry Res 15:33–39, 1985.

66. Vande Wiele RI: Anorexia nervosa and the hypothalamus. Hosp Pract 12:45–51, 1977.

67. Vigersky RA, Loriaux DL: Anorexia nervosa as a model of hypothalamic dysfunction. *In* Vigersky RA (ed): Anorexia Nervosa. New York, Raven Press, 1977, pp 109–121.

68. Ferrari E, Brambilla F (eds): Disorders of Eating Behavior: A Psychoneuroendocrine Approach. Oxford, Pergamon Press, 1986.

69. Newman MM, Halmi KA: The endocrinology of anorexia nervosa and bulimia nervosa. Neurol Clin North Am 6:195–212, 1988.

70. Levy AB: Neuroendocrine profile in bulimia nervosa. Biol Psychiatry 25:98–109, 1989.

71. Fichter MM, Pirke KM: Starvation models and eating disorders. *In* Szmukler G, Dare C, Treasure J (eds): Handbook of Eating Disorders: Theory, Treatment and Research. West Sussex, England, Wiley and Sons, 1995, pp 83–107.

72. Licinio J, Wong ML, Gold PW: The hypothalamic-pituitary-adrenal axis in anorexia nervosa. Psychiatry Res 62:75–83, 1996.

73. Kaye WH, Gendall K, Kye C: The role of the central nervous system in the psychoneuroendocrine disturbances of anorexia and bulimia nervosa. Psychiatr Clin North Am 21:381–396, 1998.

74. Tomova A, Kumanov P, Kirilov G: Factors related to sex hormone binding globulin concentrations in women with anorexia nervosa. Horm Metab Res 27:508–510, 1995.

75. Walsh BT, Katz JL, Levin J, et al: Adrenal activity in anorexia nervosa. Psychosom Med 40:499–506, 1978.

76. Casper RC, Chatterton RT, Davis JM: Alterations in serum cortisol and its binding characteristics in anorexia nervosa. J Clin Endocrinol Metab 49:406–411, 1979.

77. Gold PW, Gwirtsman H, Avgerinos PC, et al: Abnormal hypothalamic-pituitary-adrenal function in anorexia nervosa: Pathophysiologic mechanisms in underweight and weight-corrected patients. N Engl J Med 314:1335–1342, 1986.

78. Fichter MM, Pirke KM, Pollinger J, et al: Disturbances in the hypothalamo-pituitary-adrenal and other neuroendocrine axes in bulimia. Biol Psychiatry 27:1021–1037, 1990.

79. Rubin RT, Poland RE, Lesser IM, et al: Neuroendocrine aspects of primary endogenous depression. I. Cortisol secretory dynamics in patients and matched control subjects. Arch Gen Psychiatry 44:329–336, 1987.

80. Boyar RN, Hellman LD, Roffwarg H, et al: Cortisol secretion and metabolism in anorexia nervosa. N Engl J Med 296:190–193, 1977.

81. Rubin RT, Phillips JJ, McCracken JT, et al: Adrenal gland volume in major depression: Relationship to basal and stimulated pituitary-adrenal cortical axis function. Biol Psychiatry 40:89–97, 1996.

82. Hotta M, Shibasaki T, Masuda A, et al: The responses of plasma adrenocorticotropin and cortisol to corticotropin-releasing hormone (CRH) and cerebrospinal fluid immunoreactive CRH in anorexia nervosa patients. J Clin Endocrinol Metab 62:319–324, 1986.

83. Kaye WH, Gwirtsman HE, George DT, et al: Elevated cerebrospinal fluid levels of immunoreactive corticotropin releasing hormone in anorexia nervosa: Relation to state of nutrition, adrenal function and intensity of depression. J Clin Endocrinol Metab 64:203–208, 1987.

84. Gold PW, Kaye WH, Robertson GL, et al: Abnormalities in plasma and cerebrospinal-fluid arginine vasopressin in patients with anorexia nervosa. N Engl J Med 308:1117–1123, 1983.

85. Demitrack MA, Kalogeras KT, Altemus M, et al: Plasma and cerebrospinal fluid measures of arginine vasopressin secretion in patients with bulimia nervosa and in subjects. J Clin Endocrinol Metab 74:1277–1283, 1992.

86. Antoni FA: Vasopressinergic control of pituitary adrenocorticotropin secretion comes of age. Front Neuroendocrinol 14:76–122, 1993.

87. Scott LV, Dinan TG: Vasopressin and the regulation of hypothalamic-pituitary-adrenal axis function: Implications for the pathophysiology of depression. Life Sci 62:1985–1998, 1998.

88. De Kloet ER: Why dexamethasone poorly penetrates in brain. Stress 2:13–20, 1997.

89. Wartofsky L, Burman KD: Alterations in thyroid function in patients with systemic illness: The "euthyroid sick syndrome." Endocr Rev 3:164–217, 1982.

90. Natori Y, Yamaguchi N, Koike S, et al: Thyroid function in patients with anorexia nervosa and depression. Rinsho Byori 42:1268–1272, 1994.

91. Altemus M, Hetherington M, Kennedy B, et al: Thyroid function in bulimia nervosa. Psychoneuroendocrinology 21:249–261, 1996.

92. Lesem MD, Kaye WH, Bissette G, et al: Cerebrospinal fluid TRH immunoreactivity in anorexia nervosa. Biol Psychiatry 35:48–53, 1994.

93. Devlin MJ, Walsh BT, Kral JG, et al: Metabolic abnormalities in bulimia nervosa. Arch Gen Psychiatry 47:144–148, 1990.

94. Altemus M, Hetherington MM, Flood M, et al: Decrease in resting metabolic rate during abstinence from bulimic behavior. Am J Psychiatry 148:1071–1072, 1991.

95. Spalter AR, Gwirtsman HE, Demitrack MA, et al: Thyroid function in bulimia nervosa. Biol Psychiatry 33:408–414, 1993.

96. Hadigan CM, Walsh BT, Buttinger C, et al: Behavioral and neuroendocrine responses to metaCPP in anorexia nervosa. Biol Psychiatry 37:504–511, 1995.

97. Brewerton TD, Jimerson CD: Studies of serotonin function in anorexia nervosa. Psychiatry Res 62:31–42, 1996.

98. Goldbloom DS, Garfinkel PE, Katz R, et al: The hormonal response to intravenous 5-hydroxytryptophan in anorexia nervosa. J Psychosom Res 40:289–297, 1996.

99. Jimerson DC, Wolfe BE, Metzger ED, et al: Decreased serotonin function in bulimia nervosa. Arch Gen Psychiatry 54:529–534, 1997.

100. Levitan RD, Kaplan AS, Joffe RT, et al: Hormonal and subjective responses to intravenous meta-chlorophenylpiperazine in bulimia nervosa. Arch Gen Psychiatry 54:521–527, 1997.

101. Wolfe BE, Metzger ED, Jimerson DC: Research update on serotonin function in bulimia nervosa and anorexia nervosa. Psychopharm Bull 33:345–354, 1997.

102. Mortola JF, Laughlin GA, Yen SS: Melatonin rhythms in women with anorexia nervosa and bulimia nervosa. J Clin Endocrinol Metab 77:1540–1544, 1993.

103. Kennedy SH: Melatonin disturbances in anorexia nervosa and bulimia nervosa. Int J Eat Disord 16:257–265, 1994.

104. Hoffmann G, Pollow K, Nowara D, et al: Circadian blood serotonin and melatonin level in anorexia nervosa patients in comparison with normally menstruating women. Geburtshilfe Frauenheilkd 56:485–490, 1996.

105. Pirke KM, Schweiger U, Lemmel W, et al: The influence of dieting on the menstrual cycle of healthy young women. J Clin Endocrinol Metab 60:1174–1179, 1985.

106. Fichter MM, Pirke KM, Holsboer F: Weight loss causes neuroendocrine disturbances: Experimental studies in healthy starving subjects. Psychiatry Res 17:61–72, 1986.

107. Keys A, Brozek J, Henschel A: The Biology of Human Starvation. Minneapolis, University of Minnesota Press, 1950.

108. Morley JE, Blundell JE: The neurobiological basis of eating disorders: Some formulations. Biol Psychiatry 23:53–78, 1988.

109. Martin JB, Reichlin S: Clinical Endocrinology, ed 2. Philadelphia, FA Davis, 1987, pp 557–605.

110. Allen YS, Adrian TE, Allen JM: Neuropeptide Y distribution in the rat brain. Science 221:877–879, 1983.

111. Stanley BC, Daniel DR, Chin AS, et al: Paraventricular nucleus injections of peptide YY and neuropeptide Y preferentially enhance carbohydrate ingestion. Peptides 6:1205–1211, 1985.
112. Kalra SP, Allen LG, Clark JT, et al: Neuropeptide Y—an integrator of reproductive and appetitive functions. *In* Moody TW (ed): Neural and Endocrine Peptides and Receptors. New York, Plenum Press, 1986, pp 353–366.
113. Clark JT, Kalra PS, Kalra SP: Neuropeptide Y stimulates feeding but inhibits sexual behavior in rats. Endocrinology 117:2435–2442, 1985.
114. Haas DA, George SR: Neuropeptide Y administration acutely increases hypothalamic corticotropin-releasing factor immunoreactivity: Lack of effect in other rat brain regions. Life Sci 41:2725–2731, 1987.
115. Fuxe K, Agnati LF, Harfstrand A: Central administration of neuropeptide Y induces hypotension, bradypnea and EEG synchronization in the rat. Acta Physiol Scand 118:189–192, 1983.
116. Kaye WH, Berrettini W, Gwirtsman H, et al: Altered cerebrospinal fluid neuropeptide Y and peptide YY immunoreactivity in anorexia and bulimia nervosa. Arch Gen Psychiatry 147:548–556, 1990.
117. Sahu A, Kalra PS, Kalra SP: Food deprivation and ingestion induces reciprocal changes in neuropeptide Y concentrations in the paraventricular nucleus. Peptides 9:83–86, 1988.
118. Morley JE, Levine AS, Grace M, et al: Peptide YY (PYY), a potent orexigenic agent. Brain Res 341:200–203, 1985.
119. Zhang Y, Proenca R, Maffei M, et al: Positional cloning of the mouse obese gene and its human homologue. Nature 372:425–432, 1994.
120. Elmquist JK, Maratos-Flier E, Saper CB, et al: Unraveling the central nervous system pathways underlying leptin. Nature Neuroscience 1:445–450, 1998.
121. Tartaglia LA, Dembski M, Weng X, et al: Identification and expression cloning of a leptin receptor, OB-R. Cell 83:1263–1271, 1995.
122. Sierra-Honigman MR, Nath AK, Murakami C, et al: Biological action of leptin as an angiogenic factor. Science 281:1683–1686, 1998.
123. Chen H, Charlat O, Tartaglia LA, et al: Evidence that the diabetes gene encodes the leptin receptor: Identification of a mutation in the leptin receptor gene in db/db mice. Cell 84:491–495, 1996.
124. Pelleymounter MZ, Cullen M, Baker MJ, et al: Effects of the obese gene product on body weight regulation in ob/ob mice. Science 269:540–543, 1995.
125. Collins S, Kuhn CM, Petro AE, et al: Role of leptin in fat regulation. Nature 380:677, 1996.
126. Considine RV, Sinha M, Heiman ML, et al: Serum immunoreactive-leptin concentrations in normal-weight and obese humans. N Engl J Med 334:292–295, 1996.
127. Hamann A, Matthaei S: Regulation of energy balance by leptin. Exp Clin Endocrinol Diabetes 104:293–300, 1996.
128. Hebebrand J, Van der heyden J, Devos R, et al: Plasma concentrations of obese protein in anorexia nervosa. Lancet 346:1624–1625, 1995.
129. Grinspoon S, Gulick T, Askari H, et al: Serum leptin levels in women with anorexia nervosa. J Clin Endocrinol Metab 81:3861–3864, 1996.
130. Ferron F, Considine RV, Peino R, et al: Serum leptin concentrations in patients with anorexia nervosa, bulimia nervosa and non-specific eating disorders correlate with body mass index but are independent of the respective disease. Clin Endocrinol 46:289–293, 1997.
131. Mantzoros C, Flier JS, Lesem MD, et al: Cerebrospinal fluid leptin in anorexia nervosa: Correlation with nutritional status and potential role in resistance to weight gain. J Clin Endocrinol Metab 82:1845–1851, 1997.
132. Chehab FF, Lim ME, Lu R: Correction of the sterility defect in homozygous obese female mice by treatment with the human recombinant leptin. Nature Genet 112:318–320, 1996.
133. Chehab FF, Mounzih K, Lu R, et al: Early onset of reproductive function in normal female mice treated with leptin. Science 265:88–90, 1997.
134. Clapham JC, Smith SA, Moore GBT, et al: Plasma leptin concentrations and OB gene expression in subcutaneous adipose tissue are not regulated by acutely physical hyperinsulinaemia in lean and obese humans. Int J Obes Relat Metab Disord 21:179–183, 1997.
135. Trayhurn P, Thomas MEA, Duncan JS, et al: Effects of fasting and refeeding on ob gene expression in white adipose tissue of lean and obese (ob/ob) mice. FEBS Lett 368:488–490, 1995.
136. Harris RBS, Ramsay TG, Smith SR, et al: Early and late stimulation of ob mRNA expression in meal-fed and overfed rats. J Clin Invest 97:2020–2026, 1996.
137. Boden G, Chen X, Mazzoli M, et al: Effect of fasting on serum leptin in normal subjects. J Clin Endocrinol Metab 81:3419–3423, 1996.
138. Ahima RS, Prabakaran D, Mantzoros C, et al: Role of leptin in the neuroendocrine response to fasting. Nature 382:250–252, 1996.
139. Stephens TW, Basinski M, Bristow PK, et al: The role of neuropeptide Y in the antiobesity action of the obese gene product. Nature 377:530–533, 1995.
140. Erikson JC, Clegg KE, Palmiter RD: Sensitivity to leptin and susceptibility to seizures of mice lacking neuropeptide Y. Nature 381:415–421, 1996.
141. Rivier C, Vale W: Influence of corticotropin-releasing factor on reproductive functions in the rat. Endocrinology 114:914–921, 1984.
142. Sirinathsinghji DJ, Rees LH, Rivier J, et al: Corticotropin-releasing factor is a potent inhibitor of sexual receptivity in the female rat. Nature 305:232–235, 1983.
143. Britton DR, Koob GR, Rivier J, et al: Intraventricular corticotropin-releasing factor enhances behavioral effects of novelty. Life Sci 31:363–367, 1982.
144. Sutton RE, Koob GF, LeMoal M, et al: Corticotropin-releasing factor produces behavioral activation in rats. Nature 297:331–333, 1982.
145. Leibowitz SF, Hor L: Endorphinergic and alpha-noradrenergic systems in the paraventricular nucleus: Effects on eating behavior. Peptides 3:421–428, 1982.
146. Morley JE, Levine AS, Yim GK, et al: Opioid modulation of appetite. Neurosci Biobehav Rev 7:281–305, 1983.
147. Reid LD: Endogenous opioid peptides and the regulation of drinking and feeding. Am J Clin Nutr 42:1099–1132, 1985.
148. Moore R, Mills IH, Forster A: Naloxone in the treatment of anorexia nervosa: Effect on weight. J R Soc Med 74:129–131, 1981.
149. Donohoe TP: Stress-induced anorexia: Implications for anorexia nervosa. Life Sci 34:203–218, 1984.
150. Marrazzi MA, Luby ED: An auto-addiction opioid model of chronic anorexia nervosa. Int J Eat Disord 5:191–208, 1986.
151. Kaye WH, Berrettini WH, Gwirtsman HE, et al: Reduced cerebrospinal fluid levels of immunoreactive pro-opiomelanocortin related peptides (including β-endorphin) in anorexia nervosa. Life Sci 41:2147–2155, 1987.
152. Brewerton TD, Lydiard RB, Laraia MT, et al: CSF beta-endorphin and dynorphin in bulimia nervosa. Am J Psychiatry 149:1086–1090, 1992.
153. Lesem MD, Berrettini WH, Kaye WH, et al: Measurement of CSF dynorphin A 1–8 immunoreactivity in anorexia nervosa and normal-weight bulimia. Biol Psychiatry 29:244–252, 1991.
154. Jonas JM, Gold MS: Treatment of antidepressant resistant bulimia with naltrexone. Int J Psychiatry Med 16:305–309, 1987.
155. Jonas JM, Gold MS: The use of opiate antagonists in treating bulimia: A study of low dose versus high dose naltrexone. Psychiatry Res 24:195–199, 1988.
156. Mitchell JE, Christenson G, Jennings J, et al: A placebo-controlled, double-blind crossover study of naltrexone hydrochloride in outpatients with normal weight bulimia. J Clin Psychopharmacol 9:94–97, 1989.
157. Agger SA, Schwalberg MD, Bigaouette JM, et al: Effect of a tricyclic antidepressant and opiate antagonist on binge eating behavior in normal weight bulimia and obese, binge-eating subjects. Am J Clin Nutr 53:865–871, 1991.
158. Marrazzi MA, Bacon JP, Kinzie J, et al: Naltrexone use in the treatment of anorexia nervosa and bulimia nervosa. Int Clin Psychopharmacol 10:163–172, 1995.
159. Grossman A: Brain opiates and neuroendocrine function. Clin Endocrinol Metab 12:725–746, 1983.
160. Pfeiffer A, Herz A: Endocrine actions of opioids. Horm Metab Res 16:386–397, 1984.
161. Baranowska B, Rozbicka G, Jeske W, et al: The role of endogenous opiates in the mechanism of inhibited luteinizing hormone (LH) secretion in women with anorexia nervosa: The effect of naloxone on LH, follicle-stimulating hormone, prolactin, and beta-endorphine secretion. J Clin Endocrinol Metab 59:412–416, 1984.
162. Baraban JM, Walsh BT, Gladis M, et al: Effect of naloxone on luteinizing hormone secretion in eating disorders: A pilot study. Int J Eat Disord 5:149–155, 1986.
163. Giusti M, Torre R, Traverso L, et al: Endogenous opioid blockade and gonadotropin secretion: Role of pulsatile luteinizing hormone–releasing hormone administration in anorexia nervosa and weight loss amenorrhea. Fertil Steril 49:797–801, 1988.
164. Armeanu M, Berkhout GMJ, Schoemaker J: Pulsatile luteinizing hormone secretion in hypothalamic amenorrhea, anorexia nervosa, and polycystic ovarian disease during naltrexone treatment. Fertil Steril 57:762–770, 1992.
165. Garcia-Rubi E, Vazquez-Aleman D, Mendez J P, et al: The effects of opioid blockade and GnRH administration upon luteinizing hormone secretion in patients with anorexia nervosa during the stages of weight loss and weight recovery. Clin Endocrinol 37:520–528, 1992.
166. De Wied D: The influences of the posterior and intermediate lobe of the pituitary and pituitary peptides on the maintenance of a conditioned avoidance response in rats. Neuropharmacology 4:157–167, 1965.
167. Bohus B, Kovacs GL, De Weid D: Oxytocin, vasopressin and memory: Opposite effects on consolidation and retrial processes. Brain Res 157:414–417, 1978.
168. Nishita JK, Ellinwood EH Jr, Rockwell WJ, et al: Abnormalities in the response of plasma arginine vasopressin during hypertonic saline infusion in patients with eating disorders. Biol Psychiatry 26:73–86, 1989.
169. Demitrack MA, Lesem MD, Listwak S J, et al: CSF oxytocin in anorexia nervosa and bulimia nervosa: Clinical and pathophysiologic considerations. Am J Psychiatry 147:882–886, 1990.
170. Chiodera P, Volpi R, Capretti L, et al: Effect of estrogen or insulin-induced hypoglycemia on plasma oxytocin levels in bulimia and anorexia nervosa. Metabolism 40:1226–1230, 1991.
171. Ratnasuriya RH, Eisler I, Szmuckler GI, et al: Anorexia nervosa: Outcome and prognostic factors after 20 years. Br J Psychiatry 158:495–502, 1991.
172. Garner DM, Garfinkel PE (eds): Handbook of Psychotherapy for Anorexia Nervosa and Bulimia. New York, Guilford Press, 1985.
173. Garner DM, Garfinkel PE (eds): Handbook of Treatment for Eating Disorders, ed 2. New York, Guilford Press, 1997.
174. Walsh BT, Devlin MJ: Psychopharmacology of anorexia nervosa, bulimia nervosa, and binge eating. *In* Bloom FE, Kupfer DJ (eds): Psychopharmacology: The Fourth Generation of Progress. New York, Raven Press, 1995, pp 1581–1589.
175. Agras WS: Nonpharmacologic treatments of bulimia nervosa. J Clin Psychiatry 52(suppl):29–33, 1991.
176. Mitchell JE, Raymond N, Specker S: A review of the controlled trials of pharmacotherapy and psychotherapy in the treatment of bulimia nervosa. Int J Eat Disord 14:229–247, 1993.
177. Wilson GT, Fairburn CG: Cognitive treatments for eating disorders. J Consult Clin Psychol 61:261–269, 1993.
178. Kaye W, Strober M, Stein D, et al: New directions in treatment research of anorexia nervosa and bulimia nervosa. Biol Psychiatry 45:1285–1292, 1999.
179. Strober M, Lampert C, Morrell W, et al: A controlled family study of anorexia nervosa: Evidence of familial aggregation and lack of shared transmission with affective disorders. Int J Eat Disord 9:239–253, 1990.
180. Lilenfeld LR, Kaye WH, Greeno CG, et al: A controlled family study of anorexia nervosa and bulimia nervosa: Psychiatric disorders in first-degree relatives and effects of proband comorbidity. Arch Gen Psychiatry 55:603–610, 1998.
181. Jimerson DC, Wolfe BE, Brothman AW, et al: Medications in the treatment of eating disorders. Psychiatr Clin North Am 19:739–754, 1996.
182. Channon S, de Silva P, Hemsley D, et al: A controlled trial of cognitive-behavioural and behavioural treatment of anorexia nervosa. Behav Res Ther 27:529–535, 1989.

183. Crisp AH, Norton K, Gowers S, et al: A controlled study of the effect of therapies aimed at adolescent and family psychopathology in anorexia nervosa. Br J Psychiatry 159:325–333, 1991.

184. Treasure J, Todd G, Brolly M, et al: A pilot study of a randomized trial of cognitive analytical therapy vs. educational behavioral therapy for adult anorexia nervosa. Behav Res Ther 33:363–367, 1995.

185. Russell GFM, Szmukler GI, Dare C, et al: An evaluation of family therapy in anorexia nervosa and bulimia nervosa. Arch Gen Psychiatry 44:1047–1056, 1987.

186. Kaye WH, Weltzin T, Hsu LKG, et al: An open trial of fluoxetine in patients with anorexia nervosa. J Clin Psychiatry 52:464–471, 1991.

187. Kaye WH: Relapse prevention with fluoxetine in anorexia nervosa: A double-blind placebo-controlled study. *In* New Research Abstracts, 150th Annual Meeting of the American Psychiatric Association, May 1997.

188. Herzog DB, Keller M, Strober M: The current status of treatment for anorexia nervosa and bulimia nervosa. Int J Eat Disord 12:215–220, 1992.

189. McKenzie JM, Joyce PR: Hospitalization for anorexia nervosa. Int J Eat Disord 11:235–241, 1992.

190. Walsh BT: Psychopharmacologic treatment of bulimia nervosa. J Clin Psychiatry 52(suppl 10):34–38, 1991.

191. Fairburn CG, Jones R, Peveler RC, et al: Psychotherapy and bulimia nervosa: The longer-term effects of interpersonal psychotherapy, behavior therapy and cognitive-behavior therapy. Arch Gen Psychiatry 50:419–428, 1993.

192. Garner DM, Rockert W, Davis R, et al: Comparison between cognitive-behavioral and supportive-expressive therapy for bulimia nervosa. Am J Psychiatry 150:37–46, 1993.

193. Walsh BT, Wilson GT, Loeb KL: Medication and psychotherapy in the treatment of bulimia nervosa. Am J Psychiatry 154:523–531, 1997.

194. Agras WS, Rossiter EM, Arnow B, et al: Pharmacologic and cognitive-behavioral treatment for bulimia nervosa: A controlled comparison. Am J Psychiatry 149:82–87, 1992.

195. Walsh BT, Hadigan CM, Devlin MJ, et al: Long-term outcome of antidepressant treatment for bulimia nervosa. Am J Psychiatry 148:1206–1212, 1991.

196. Keller MB, Boland RJ: The implications of failure to achieve successful long-term maintenance treatment of recurrent unipolar depression. Biol Psychiatry 44:348–360, 1998.

197. Becker AE, Grinspoon SK, Klibanski A, et al: Eating disorders. N Engl J Med 340:1092–1098, 1999.

198. Kalra SP, Dube MG, Pu S, et al: Interacting appetite-regulating pathways in the hypothalamic regulation of body weight. Endocr Rev 20:68–100, 1999.

199. Inui A: Feeding and body-weight regulation by hypothalamic neuropeptides—mediation of the actions of leptin. Trends Neurosci 22:62–67, 1999.

200. Sawchenko P: Toward a new neurobiology of energy balance, appetite, and obesity: The anatomists weigh in. J Comp Neurol 402:435–441, 1998.

▲▲▲

Chapter 46

Starvation and Nutritional Therapy

David Heber

Our ability to adapt to starvation is the result of the interplay of the endocrine system and major metabolic pathways and has much in common with the homeostatic processes needed to maintain temperature, salt concentration, or appetite.[1] Different endocrine glands work synergistically in this process, and understanding these interrelationships provides a basis for the recognition and therapy of primary and secondary forms of malnutrition.[2, 3] The discovery and application of well-defined parenteral and enteral nutrition since the 1970s rationalized the metabolic and hormonal treatment of malnutrition.[5] Nutritional therapy has been shown to be essential to survival in the critical care setting and has resulted in metabolic and nutritional insights which have influenced many areas of endocrinology.[4, 5] This chapter attempts to provide an integrated view of the endocrine response to starvation and the treatment of malnutrition using parenteral and enteral nutrition.

ADAPTATION TO UNCOMPLICATED STARVATION

The adaptation to starvation consists of a series of well-coordinated hormonal and metabolic changes. Aspects of these adaptive mechanisms are utilized each day in well-nourished persons between bedtime and breakfast to maintain normal blood sugar levels in the absence of food intake. The changes in hormones and metabolites which occur during this interval are similar to those seen in the earliest stages of the adaptation to starvation. If fasting is continued for up to 6 weeks, a series of adaptations occur to maintain the integrity of body protein stores essential to survival. Ironically, the bulk of the information available on the physiology of the adaptation to uncomplicated starvation has been developed in studies of massively obese subjects fasting voluntarily under metabolic ward conditions.[6–8]

Dietary Sources and Body Stores of Energy

The average distribution of dietary macronutrients consumed in the diet is roughly 20% to 40% as fat, 40% to 60% as carbohydrate, and 10% to 20% as protein. There are variations in the dietary sources of these nutrients throughout the world and some variations in the proportions of these macronutrients. For example, in countries consuming a low fat, high fiber diet, complex carbohydrates are obtained from cereals, grains, fruits, and vegetables, whereas in industrialized countries consuming a high fat, low fiber diet, simple sugars from processed foods will make up a large portion of the carbohydrate consumed. Despite wide variations in the dietary intake of macronutrients among various populations, the body stores these dietary macronutrients in a fairly uniform but different pattern from the ingested proportions. The

distribution of stored calories is ideally adapted to the metabolic needs under conditions of stress and starvation.

In the average 70-kg man, the largest store of calories is in the form of fat in adipose tissue, with approximately 135,000 calories stored in 13.5 kg of adipose tissue. This storage compartment can be greatly expanded with long-term overnutrition in obese individuals. There are approximately 54,000 calories stored as protein both in muscle and viscera. Only half these calories can be mobilized for energy, since depletion below 50% of total protein stores is incompatible with life.[9] In addition to being an energy source, protein plays a functional role in many organs, including the liver, and depletion is associated with impaired immunity to infection.[10] In fact, the most common cause of death in an epidemic of starvation is typically simple bacterial pneumonia. Conservation of protein is an adaptation tightly linked to survival during acute starvation.

There are only 1200 calories stored as carbohydrate in liver and muscle glycogen. There are clear adaptive advantages to storing calories as fat, since fat can provide more energy per gram than carbohydrate or protein. However, since carbohydrate stores are so small, they are depleted in 3 days of uncomplicated starvation or sooner under conditions of increased energy expenditure. This dependence on fat and protein stores in starvation requires metabolic adaptations to minimize the loss of protein stores and a shift to metabolic pathways predominantly utilizing the large fat stores available (Fig. 46–1).

Metabolic Requirements of the Starved Host

The postabsorptive period is defined as 8 to 16 hours after eating and has been defined operationally as the point in time after an overnight fast when a number of hormonal determinations can be made under standard conditions. It can be thought of as a period of very early adaptation to starvation. During this period, the primary metabolic priority is the provision of adequate glucose for essential functions of the brain, red blood cells, peripheral nerves, and renal medulla.

During this postabsorptive phase, insulin levels fall as blood glucose falls from a range of 4 to 5 mmol/L to 3 to 4 mmol/L.[7] Glucose is released from the liver into the circulation via glycogenolysis of stores accumulated after feeding under the influence of insulin. The fall in glucose level is associated with depletion of glycogen stores. Skeletal muscle does not release glucose from stored glycogen directly into the circulation because myocytes lack the enzyme glucose-6-phosphatase. However, muscle releases lactate and amino acids such as alanine which can enter the circulation and are converted to glucose in the liver via gluconeogenesis. Glucagon in the presence of lowered insulin

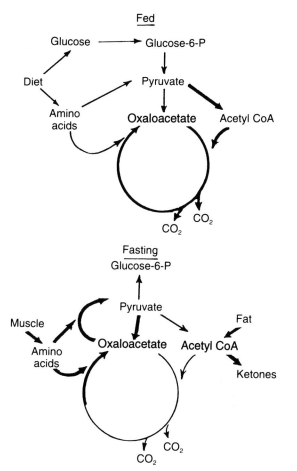

FIGURE 46–1. *The flow of substrate during the fed and fasting states.*

concentrations promotes gluconeogenesis during the postabsorptive period.[11]

In addition, glucagon in the presence of lowered insulin levels promotes lipolysis. As the stored triglyceride in adipocytes is mobilized as free fatty acids, those tissues which do not require glucose as the primary fuel (e.g., skeletal muscle) begin to oxidize free fatty acids. These changes during the early postabsorptive period act to increase free fatty acid oxidation in order to spare protein breakdown. During the first few days of starvation, free fatty acid concentrations increase from a range of 0.5 to 0.8 mmol/L up to 1.2 to 1.6 mmol/L and plateau thereafter as starvation is prolonged.[7] These free fatty acids circulate bound to albumin and are oxidized in the liver to water-soluble ketone bodies, including acetoacetate and β-hydroxybutyrate. In obese subjects with more than adequate triglyceride stores, acetoacetate concentrations rise 25-fold and β-hydroxybutyrate concentrations rise 100-fold from the levels observed in the postabsorptive phase following 4 to 6 weeks of uncomplicated starvation (Fig. 46–2). These are the largest fluctuations seen in any circulating fuel with prolonged starvation.[12]

Protein synthesis and catabolism have been estimated to account for approximately 40% of resting energy expenditure (REE). In addition, the changes in protein metabolism are critical to maintaining the body cell mass during starvation, which directly affects survival.[13] Plasma amino acids measured in venous blood give nonspecific indications of the adaptations taking place in protein metabolism during the course of starvation. In addition, the excretion of protein from the body as urinary urea nitrogen expressed as nitrogen balance provides further insights into overall protein nutriture (see Fig. 46–2).

The total α-amino nitrogen concentration, which reflects total amino acids, increases transiently from 4.6 to 4.8 mmol/L over the first few days of starvation and then decreases to 3.6 mmol/L.[14] These total amino acid changes obscure the changes in several different classes of amino acids. First, the branched-chain amino acids—leucine, isoleucine, and valine—increase transiently approximately twofold in the blood between 3 and 5 days after the onset of starvation. Alanine, which is the primary glucogenic amino acid in the liver during starvation, is released from muscle in amounts larger than the measurable alanine stores of muscle. This is explained by the formation of alanine in muscle through what is known as the *alanine cycle* (Fig. 46–3). Pyruvate from the liver, as well as pyruvate derived by glycolysis of glucose from glycogen stores, enters the muscle, where the branched-chain amino acids donate an amino group, via the action of a specific branched-chain amino acid–targeted enzyme, to produce alanine. This alanine is then released to the liver, where alanine accounts for a significant portion of glucose synthesis. During the period between 3 and 5 days after the onset of starvation, the branched-chain amino acids in the circulation support an increased rate of gluconeogenesis until the full adaptation to a fat-fuel economy has progressed significantly. Second, blood and muscle alanine concentrations decline rapidly over the first 10 days of starvation and then continue to decrease

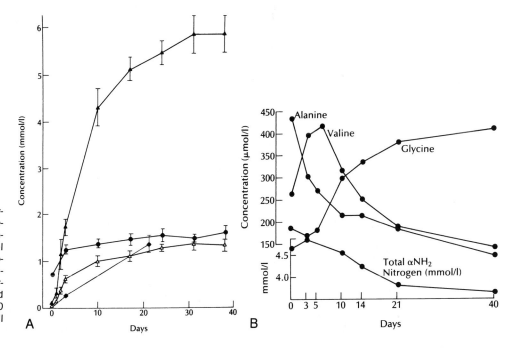

FIGURE 46–2. *A,* Blood 3-hydroxybutyrate (▲), acetoacetate (△), plasma acetone (♦), and free fatty acid (●) concentrations during starvation. *B,* Total α-amino (αNH₂) nitrogen and three representative amino acids during prolonged starvation. (From Cahill GF: Starvation in man. N Engl J Med 282:668–675, 1970. Copyright © 1970 Massachusetts Medical Society. All rights reserved.)

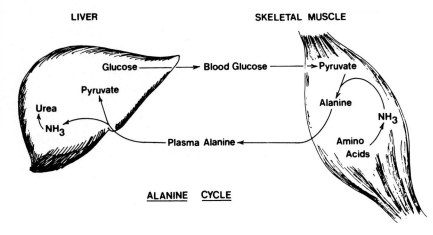

LIVER   SKELETAL MUSCLE

ALANINE   CYCLE

FIGURE 46–3. The alanine cycle allows carbon chains and ammonia to be shuttled from skeletal muscle to the liver, where they are used to synthesize glucose and urea, respectively.

progressively to about 30% of postabsorptive levels several weeks later. Third, blood and muscle glutamine concentrations also decrease progressively during starvation.

In the first few days of starvation, the gut plays an important role in regulating protein and amino acid metabolism. The intestinal synthesis of glutamine increases with a subsequent increase in alanine and ammonia formation. The alanine is used for hepatic gluconeogenesis, while the increased ammonia levels in the portal circulation trigger the liver to produce glutamine, which is utilized by the kidney for gluconeogenesis.[15] After 30 days of fasting, the kidney becomes an important gluconeogenic organ, contributing about half the body's glucose need. Most of this glucose is derived from the *glutamine cycle* (Fig. 46–4). Glutamine from the muscle and liver is converted to glutamate and ammonia in the kidney. Glutamate is then deaminated to α-ketoglutarate, which enters the gluconeogenic pathway.

The basic mechanisms underlying these adaptive changes in protein synthesis and degradation are still not completely understood. Proteolysis occurs in cellular lysosomes via autophagy. This process is stimulated by a shortage of critical regulatory amino acids, including phenylalanine, tryptophan, methionine, leucine, tyrosine, glutamic acid, proline, and histidine.[16] While not conclusively established, it appears that decreased concentrations of specific amino acyl transfer RNAs for these amino acids trigger proteolysis (Fig. 46–5). In terms of protein synthesis, there is a decrease in the amount and activity of RNA subunits involved in initiation, elongation, and termination of protein synthesis. Insulin is the primary hormone known to regulate protein metabolism.[17] Insulin deficiency leads to net protein breakdown, and hyperinsulinemia under euglycemic conditions inhibits proteolysis. There is also evidence that glucagon participates in this regulatory

process by stimulating splanchnic proteolysis.[18] Plasma cortisol levels are increased for several hours and inhibit protein synthesis while increasing protein breakdown. Elevations in epinephrine, previously thought to increase protein breakdown, lead to decreases in the rate of whole-body protein breakdown. Growth hormone (GH) has been shown to increase protein synthesis but to oppose insulin's antiproteolytic effects. The role of the insulin-like growth factors, IGF-I and IGF-II, as both endocrine and paracrine signals is important in the adaptation to starvation. The anabolic effects are mediated via the IGF-I receptor, present in all cells except liver and adipose cells. IGF-I expression is regulated both by nutrition and by other hormones. For example, serum IGF-I concentrations are age-dependent and closely linked to the age-dependent production of GH. IGF levels increase after puberty and decline with age in parallel with anabolic potential in response to nutrition. Recent studies[19] have demonstrated that plasma amino acid levels and amino acid availability also play an important role in modulating the rate of protein breakdown. The magnitude of these amino acid–mediated antiproteolytic effects was equivalent to that of insulin.

The impact of the adaptation to a fat-fuel economy is reflected in the rapid changes in urinary nitrogen excretion, showing net protein sparing through two processes. First, there is less protein breakdown. It has been estimated that protein synthesis decreases in the whole body by 40% between the postprandial and postabsorptive phases,[13] with a further decrease over the first several days of starvation. Second, there is increased reutilization of nitrogen, evidenced by decreased urea formation in the liver through the arginine-citrulline cycle. In obese subjects fasting for 7 days, protein breakdown and urinary urea nitrogen excretion decrease in parallel. Overall nitrogen is conserved

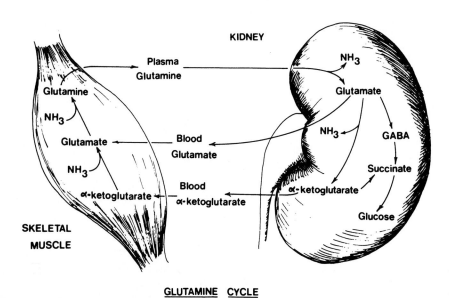

KIDNEY

SKELETAL
MUSCLE

GLUTAMINE   CYCLE

FIGURE 46–4. The glutamine cycle is a shuttle analogous to the alanine cycle which exists between skeletal muscle and the kidney. This cycle increases in importance as a fast extends beyond 30 days.

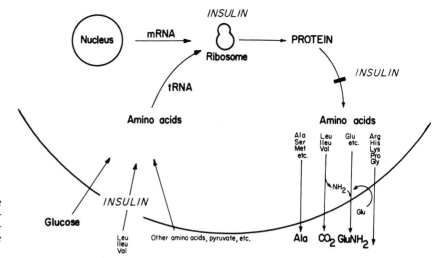

FIGURE 46–5. Effect of insulin in promoting glucose and amino acid uptake into muscle, activation of protein synthesis at the ribosome, and inhibition of proteolysis. Also shown is the predominant release of alanine (Ala) and glutamine ($GluNH_2$).

so that nitrogen excretion decreases from 12 g/day in the postabsorptive state to 5 g/day 7 to 10 days later. This decrease translates into a decrease in muscle protein breakdown from 75 to 20 g/day. Based on theoretical calculations of the time necessary to reach the crucial 50% of body cell mass, survival is extended through these adaptations from approximately 60 days to over 260 days, provided that adequate fluid and electrolytes are administered.[20]

Hormonal Mediators of Metabolic Adaptation

As discussed earlier, insulin is the primary hormone regulating fuel metabolism in the fed and fasted states. However, a number of other hormones participate in the adaptation to uncomplicated starvation. One group of hormones is called *counterregulatory* in recognition of their ability to antagonize the hypoglycemic action of administered insulin. Glucagon, for example, promotes glycogenolysis, gluconeogenesis, ketogenesis, proteolysis, and lipolysis. The levels of circulating catecholamines, norepinephrine, and epinephrine, which rise following insulin-induced hypoglycemia, also increase following acute starvation.[21]

Lipolysis is central to the adaptation to starvation and is regulated by catecholamines, glucagon, and GH. Catecholamines help to inhibit insulin secretion, which permits lipolysis. The lipolytic effects of epinephrine are more pronounced early in starvation,[22] and the rise in catecholamines promotes the metabolic utilization of fat. These hormones act through stimulatory and inhibitory G proteins and the cyclic adenosine monophosphate (cAMP) cascade to modulate hormone-sensitive lipase. β_1-Adrenergic stimulation increases glucagon secretion and inhibits muscle glucose metabolism.[23] β_1-Adrenergic stimulation mediates the effects of glucagon, GH, cortisol, and vasopressin to increase lipolysis.[22] Thyroid hormones and glucocorticoids may act permissively on the processes stimulating lipolysis, while the actions of vasopressin, β-lipotropin, β-endorphin, and α-melanocyte-stimulating hormone have not been established.

The brain plays a critical role in the adaptation to starvation through control of hunger and satiety, influences on the rate of energy expenditure, and regulation of hormones involved in the disposition of energy stores.[24] Neuropeptide Y (NPY), found in the arcuate nucleus of the hypothalamus, is a member of the pancreatic polypeptide family and increases during food restriction, acting to increase food intake. Studies of weight loss following food restriction in rodents support the notion that the brain can sense a signal reflecting total body energy stores. Leptin is produced in adipocytes and is proportional to body fat stores in the fed state, but with food restriction, leptin levels fall rapidly. Therefore, leptin can respond to energy balance acutely during starvation out of proportion to changes in body energy stores while acting as an indicator of energy stores in the fed state. Leptin also acts at the arcuate nucleus via a specific receptor to suppress the increase in NPY

expression seen with food restriction. A complete discussion of the actions and regulation of leptin and NPY is outside the scope of this chapter (see Chapter 43).

IGF-I, or somatomedin-C, stimulates amino acid uptake and protein synthesis while inhibiting lipolysis.[25] IGF peptides in serum are associated with IGF binding proteins (IGFBPs), a family of six polypeptides thought to modulate storage, transport, and action of the IGFs. As noted above, IGF-I secretion parallels GH secretion with age. During starvation, this linkage is broken. In the presence of elevated GH levels, IGF-I levels remain low, and the concentration of IGF-I inhibitors in the circulation is increased.[26]

Within 7 to 10 days of starvation, there is a marked adaptive decrease in energy expenditure. Normally, REE is proportional to lean body mass. However, after 7 to 10 days of starvation, there is a 20% decrease in REE, at a time when lean body mass has decreased by less than 5%.[27] Changes in the peripheral metabolism of thyroid hormones occur which may contribute significantly to the observed decrease in energy expenditure. Among these changes, there is less production of triiodothyronine (T_3), the most metabolically active thyroid hormone, via a decreased activity of 5′-monodeiodinase in the liver and other peripheral tissues.[28] There is a reciprocal rise in reverse T_3, an inactive metabolite, while thyroxine (T_4) levels remain constant.[29] The overall decrease in energy expenditure with starvation is an adaptive change that results in a decreased rate of whole-body lipolysis, proteolysis, and gluconeogenesis (Fig. 46–6). Aerobic exercise in obese dieters does not reverse this adaptive change in energy regulation.[30]

There is a good correlation between the adaptive hormonal changes that occur during starvation (Table 46–1) and the decrease in whole-body protein breakdown that occurs as a result.[31]

ADAPTATION TO PROTEIN-ENERGY MALNUTRITION

Observations of epidemics of starvation in Third World countries led to the classification and definition of two different pathophysiologic syndromes occurring in response to uncomplicated starvation, as well as to the undernutrition associated with illness.[32-35] These concepts, while useful as classifications, are oversimplified, and the entire spectrum of protein and energy malnutrition has been observed in malnourished children throughout the world. Infants and children under 5 years of age have the highest energy requirements per unit body weight of any age group. Since their visceral organs account for a good portion of total body weight, energy expenditures between 50 and 100 kcal/kg/day are commonly measured compared with average energy expenditures of 20 to 30 kcal/kg/day in adults.[36] In fact, in epidemics of starvation, children will die first, men second, and women last, since women have the largest fat stores to allow protein sparing in the face of starvation.

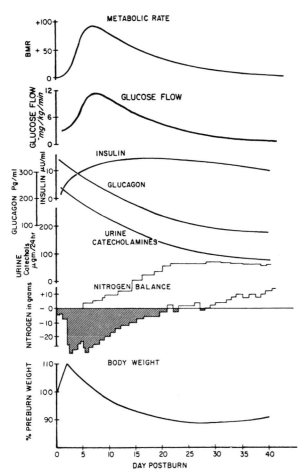

FIGURE 46–6. The hypermetabolism of injury during the flow phase is accompanied by increased glucagon and catecholamines relative to insulin. The hormonal mediators return to normal with recovery.

Clinical Spectrum

Intrauterine undernutrition, prematurity, failure of lactation, and use of dilute formulas can lead to a wasting syndrome called *marasmus* that usually presents in the first 6 months of life.[37] The infant adapts to undernutrition by decreasing its linear growth rate and thereby decreasing energy requirements. If the condition persists, there is loss of muscle and fat tissue. There are no signs of edema or biochemical abnormalities, and immune function is maintained in this condition.

In many parts of Africa, custom dictates that after 1 year of breast-feeding, children are weaned and sent to an adoptive aunt to be fed cassava fruit, a source of carbohydrates but not protein. The Swahili word for "separated from the breast" is *kwashiorkor,* and this name

was given to the syndrome observed in children suffering from protein but not calorie deprivation. The condition occurs most frequently after weaning.[38] The major features distinguishing it from marasmus are edema and hypoalbuminemia. In addition, a fatty liver, mucous membrane sores, and relative preservation of fat stores occur. Since it often occurs in response to acute events, linear growth is not as severely retarded.

Growth retardation without any clinical features is the most common presentation of protein-energy malnutrition in children. The GH–IGF-I axis in children is the most sensitive in demonstrating changes due to malnutrition,[39] just as the reproductive hormonal axis is the most sensitive in adult women who develop amenorrhea in response to undernutrition.

Etiology and Pathophysiology

Marasmus is the childhood equivalent of semistarvation, and the hormonal and metabolic adaptations to acute starvation occur as expected. The changes in insulin, GH, and cortisol observed in obese normal individuals subjected to starvation can be seen in these children even before the development of obvious marasmus.[40]

On the other hand, it is not clear why some children develop kwashiorkor in the same nutritional environment while others develop marasmus. Kwashiorkor is more common in areas where protein intake is lower.[41] However, within a particular population it has not been possible to demonstrate that those children developing kwashiorkor indeed had the lowest protein intake.[42] One of the clearest causes of kwashiorkor due to decreased protein intake comes from North American infants fed coffee creamers containing only 1% protein, 30% carbohydrate, and 69% fat calories in place of milk.[43] Rats fed a low protein-to-energy ratio will consume excess calories.[44] This leads to fatty liver and hypoalbuminemia. Lipolysis is thought to occur secondary to sympathetic stimulation combined with relative insulin resistance, while the fatty liver occurs due to the failure of apoprotein B synthesis to export triglycerides synthesized from the influx of fatty acids. Hepatic ketone production is also impaired. It is not uncommon for up to 40% of the liver mass to be fat compared with the usual 5%.

Higher plasma insulin and lower cortisol levels have been found in children with kwashiorkor than in children with marasmus.[40] It has been proposed that the higher insulin levels will direct amino acids toward muscle protein synthesis at the expense of liver protein synthesis. Overall protein synthesis is reduced in perfused rat liver systems when blood from protein-depleted rats is used.[45] Protein synthesis can be restored by adding branched-chain amino acids. While GH levels are usually elevated in kwashiorkor, these elevated levels are associated with reduced growth. In addition, administration of GH in these children will fail to stimulate growth.[46] These phenomena are accounted for by the decreased levels of IGF-I observed in both kwashiorkor and marasmus.

Since kwashiorkor also tends to occur acutely, there may be processes interfering with the adaptation to starvation, resulting in increased loss of muscle and visceral protein. In this way, kwashiorkor may be a model for the malnutrition seen in the adult with infection or traumatic injuries (see below).

ENDOCRINE RESPONSES TO ILLNESS AND UNDERNUTRITION

Illness and undernutrition are closely related in a number of chronic conditions. In fact, anorexia is one of the earliest symptoms of infectious, inflammatory, and neoplastic diseases. In a number of medical and surgical conditions, the hormonal changes associated with the adaptations to starvation described above do not occur. Nutritional assessment is focused on determining the severity of malnutrition, the underlying metabolic adaptations which pertain, and the form of therapy to be utilized. Following surgical or traumatic injury, there is a well-described series of events in which a specific sequence of hormonal changes occurs and which must be considered in evaluating nutritional therapy. In the patient with critical illness, a hypermetabolic

TABLE 46–1. Changes in Serum Levels of Hormones in Nine Obese Subjects after Fasting (mean ± SEM)

	After 12-Hour Fast	After 7-Day Fast
T₃ (ng/dL)	130 ± 15	59 ± 5.0*
Free T₃ (pg/dL)	322 ± 32	159 ± 1.3*
rT₃ (ng/dL)	35 ± 3	57 ± 5.0*
T₄ (mg/dL)	9.1 ± 0.7	9.3 ± 0.8
Free T₄ (ng/dL)	4.7 ± 0.2	3.0 ± 0.3
Insulin	34 ± 6.0	15 ± 2.0*
Morning cortisol (mg/dL)	19.1 ± 2.1	26.4 ± 3.4*
Urinary free cortisol (mg/24 hr)	27.1 ± 3.2	41.8 ± 6.3*

T_3, triiodothyronine; rT_3, reverse triiodothyronine; T_4, thyroxine.
*P <.05.

state caused by the endocrine and immune responses to illness results in a situation where nutritional therapy is recognized to be essential to survival of the patient. Nutritional therapy can be used to support the malnourished patient, but special modifications are indicated in the metabolic support of patients with renal disease, pulmonary disease, cardiac disease, hepatic insufficiency, critical illness, and multiple organ system failure.

Etiology

Malnutrition in the hospitalized patient can result from decreased intake, increased losses, or increased requirements due to the metabolic effects of injury, sepsis, surgical trauma, or chronic disease. Reduced intake can result from decreased appetite or anorexia. Abnormal tastes, acquired food aversions, and decreased taste may occur in diabetes, renal failure, and cancer, especially following chemotherapy or radiation therapy.[47] Psychosocial disorders, including depression and isolation, can be associated with decreased food intake. When nausea or vomiting is induced as a side effect of any medication, reduced food intake can occur.

Both maldigestion and malabsorption can lead to losses of ingested nutrients.[48] Maldigestion in patients with exocrine pancreatic insufficiency can result from pancreatitis or pancreatic tumors. Malabsorption due to gastrointestinal dysfunction or absence can result from infarction of bowel segments, intestinal pseudo-obstruction due to defects in the neuromuscular functions mediating normal bowel motility, or diseases affecting the absorptive capacity of the gastrointestinal epithelium. Actual loss of nutrients from body stores can occur in so-called protein-losing enteropathies, which can occur in Ménétrier's disease, Crohn's disease, celiac sprue, and Whipple's disease.

Chronic diseases, surgical injury, trauma, and sepsis result in a redistribution of nutrients from reserves in muscle and fat tissue to the liver and bone marrow for host defense, visceral protein synthesis, and thermogenesis.[49–51] These responses interfere with the normal response to undernutrition and thereby make the patient more likely to develop malnutrition in a short period of time. Protein conservation, which is the hallmark of the adaptation to uncomplicated starvation, does not occur. Instead, protein turnover is increased, leading to increased loss of urinary nitrogen and an increase in REE. In fact, rates of hypermetabolism have been found to correlate with increased losses of urinary nitrogen in patients with major burns, sepsis, infection, or surgical trauma. For instance, in patients undergoing elective surgery, urinary nitrogen losses typically are between 7 and 9 g/day, whereas in patients with sepsis or skeletal trauma, nitrogen losses increase to between 11 and 14 g/day.[52]

Organ failure can result from a combination of factors in the critically ill patient, including regional hypoperfusion and hypoxia, toxic medications, immune responses, endocrine dysfunction, and acute starvation. Metabolic support can play a critical role in the survival of such patients.

Pathophysiology

The metabolic response associated with the stress of surgery or infection or the inflammation associated with the active phases of chronic illnesses, including cancer, differs markedly from the metabolic and hormonal adaptations occurring with uncomplicated starvation. This response can be considered to have evolved to help the previously well-nourished individual survive life-threatening injury or hemorrhage. In addition, the immune system is mobilized to counter any infection that might occur. The presence of an illness or chronic disease essentially provides a stimulus to this response system that is not quickly and easily eradicated. The resulting prolonged stress response can cause nutritional status to deteriorate and represents a particularly hazardous response for the previously malnourished individual with an illness.

The injury-stress response can be divided into two phases[53] (see Fig. 46–6). The ebb phase, which lasts for approximately 24 hours after an injury or insult, is dominated by the hemodynamic response

to injury, which includes hypoperfusion, hypometabolism, and cardiac instability. There is a brisk release of hormones during this period, accompanied by a resistance to their action. Following successful resuscitation and restoration of perfusion, the flow phase begins and predominates between 48 and 72 hours after the initial stress. During this phase, metabolic responsiveness to circulating hormones returns, with resulting hypermetabolism, increased glucose production, increased protein breakdown, and lipolysis. In critical illnesses such as sepsis and multiple system organ failure, this phase is prolonged. During this phase, protein loss cannot be reversed despite the administration of apparently adequate nutritional support. During this phase, nutritional support can reduce the net loss of protein, and this is reflected in changes in urinary nitrogen excretion. Only correction of the underlying disease process will halt catabolism in this phase. Nonetheless, the temporizing influence of nutritional support can provide critical maintenance of pulmonary function[54] and gastrointestinal integrity[55] until the therapies directed at the primary disease process can have their intended effects.

The hormones mediating the metabolic changes noted in the ebb and flow phases of the stress response include insulin, glucagon, GH, cortisol, and catecholamines.[56] The secretion of both glucagon and insulin from the pancreas is critically influenced by the balance of α- and β-adrenergic stimulation during the stress response. During the ebb phase, the α-adrenergic inhibition of insulin release predominates even in the face of hyperglycemia. Glucose production rises during this phase, resulting in the characteristic hyperglycemia of injury or sepsis. In the flow phase, β-adrenergic stimulation predominates, with an increase in insulin to normal or higher levels. This phase is characterized by insulin resistance and results in abnormal glucose tolerance. The secretion of glucagon is not affected by α-adrenergic effects immediately after injury, but β-adrenergic stimulation increases glucagon secretion. Therefore, glucagon levels are increased during both phases of the injury response.[57] Inhibition of glucagon but not catecholamines will result in a decrease in endogenous glucose production.[58] The decreased insulin-to-glucagon ratio is consistent with the changes seen in glucose metabolism, but these changes are associated with alterations in the secretion of other hormones as well.

The hypothalamic response to stress results in the release of adrenocorticotropic hormone (ACTH), which stimulates adrenal glucocorticoid secretion. This response is stimulated directly by nerves originating in the area of injury or surgical trauma and does not occur with anesthesia or experimental denervation of the area before injury.[59] Cortisol stimulates hepatic gluconeogenesis and the release of amino acids from muscles via proteolysis. These effects result in a shunting of protein reserves from the periphery to the liver.

While cortisol is permissive of lipolysis, GH stimulates a rise in plasma free fatty acids and lipid oxidation.[60] Following an injury, GH is elevated even in the presence of hyperglycemia. Administration of GH can reverse some of the catabolic effects of glucocorticoids observed in malnourished patients receiving prednisone therapy.[61]

In addition to these hormonal changes, there is an increase in the synthesis of acute phase proteins such as fibrinogen, C-reactive protein, serum amyloid A protein, ceruloplasmin, haptoglobin, α2-macroglobulin, α1-acid glycoprotein, and certain complement components as well as procoagulants.[62] There is also a prominent leukocytosis with neutrophilia and a redistribution of plasma trace minerals evidenced by a decrease in zinc and iron and an increase in copper secondary to increased ceruloplasmin.[63]

The fever, negative nitrogen balance, increased protein metabolism, and other metabolic changes associated with the injury response are mediated in part through the action of cytokines released into the blood stream as part of the immune response described. A complete review of all the actions of the cytokines and their interaction is beyond the scope of this chapter but is available in several excellent reviews.[64–66] The interface of the gastrointestinal tract and the nutritional environment is protected by the gut-associated lymphoid tissue, which is the largest collection of immunocytes in the body.[67] Intraepithelial lymphocytes are found between gut mucosal epithelial cells and are the first population of cells to be exposed to foreign antigens and organisms which reside in the intestinal lumen. Beneath the epithelial basement membrane is the lamina propria, which contains mature plasma cells and lymphocytes as well as dense collections of lympho-cytes called Peyer's patches. These cells work together to process antigens from the intestinal lumen. The intraepithelial lymphocytes interact with the gut mucosal epithelial cells and synthesize a number of cytokines, including interferon-γ, the interleukins (ILs) IL-2, IL-3, IL-4, and IL-6, and tumor necrosis factor-α (TNF-α).[68, 69] Just as malnutrition affects cell-mediated immunity, as evidenced by reduction in skin test reactivity, it is postulated that gut atrophy with malnutrition results in the breakdown of the gut-associated lymphoid tissue, leading to transmigration of bacteria into the blood stream as an important pathogenic event in the injury response in the malnourished patient.

Many components of the injury response have been shown to benefit the host in the presence of infection or inflammation.[70] For instance, fever, reduction of serum iron levels, and acute phase proteins may help to fight certain infections. A prolonged injury response leading to malnutrition can impair the host immune response to pathogens. For instance, protein-malnourished patients fail to become febrile despite obvious sepsis. The ability of malnourished patients to synthesize leukocyte endogenous mediator (a combination of cytokines isolated from white blood cells) is impaired but can be restored following intravenous nutritional support. This improvement in immune respon-siveness also has been associated with improved survival in these patients. As discussed below, there is a close interaction of nutritional therapy with immunity. Overfeeding and the use of certain lipids may impair immune response.[71] It is clear that this is an area where a great deal of additional research must be done to improve the nutritional therapy of the injured, septic, or chronically ill patient.

Clinical Spectrum

Malnutrition in the hospitalized patient and the patient with chronic illness is classified into two major types. First, a kwashiorkor-like malnutrition occurs when sufficient calories are provided but protein is not, or when the acute response to stress interferes with the normal adaptation to starvation. These patients have hypoalbuminemia and edema but do not invariably have decreased body weight or wasting. This process can be relatively acute, accounting for the lack of a wasting response, and the replacement of lean tissue with water ac-counts for the lack of marked weight loss in many patients. Second, a marasmus-like malnutrition or protein-energy malnutrition can occur in which lean tissue and body weight are somewhat decreased, but immune function and albumin secretion are maintained due to the ketoadaptation and energy conservation characteristic of starvation physiology. The imposition of acute stress on preexisting nutrition of either type can lead to a severe form of malnutrition called *combined marasmus-kwashiorkor–type malnutrition.*

While global clinical assessment of nutritional status has been shown to be as effective as formal nutritional assessment in dis-covering malnutrition,[72] the exercise of assessing the patient serves as a device enabling the diet technicians, house officers, and other physi-cians attending malnourished patients with complex problems to focus on the nutritional needs of patients under their care.

DIAGNOSTIC PROTOCOLS

Nutritional Assessment

A nutritionally oriented history should inquire as to the patient's pre-illness weight, height, rate of weight loss prior to presentation, nausea, vomiting, anorexia, and specific ingestive, metabolic, or ab-sorptive problems that could impair nutritional status. Based on these assessments, the percent ideal body weight from standard tables and the percent usual weight at presentation can be calculated. Body weight changes may be misleading in patients with fluid overload, including those with congestive heart failure, liver disease, and renal failure. In uncomplicated starvation, there is an increase in extracellu-lar fluid volume which tends to maintain weight despite loss of metabolically active tissues.

The sensitivity of nutritional evaluation is enhanced by including certain assessments of the functional indices of the body cell mass, including certain proteins synthesized in the liver[73] and the status of host immune function.[74]

Albumin is the major protein synthesized in the liver and carries out significant functions as a carrier protein and to provide oncotic pressure. Its half-life is approximately 20 days, and it does not reflect recent changes in nutritional status. Transferrin has a half-life of only 8.8 days and so can reflect more recent changes in nutritional status. However, transferrin levels are increased in iron deficiency, reducing the specificity of this measurement for nutritional status. Prealbumin has a half-life of 24 hours and can be used to reflect changes in nutritional status over the short term as patients receive nutritional support to assess response to therapy. Biochemical assessment should include, at a minimum, measurement of albumin. An albumin level of greater than 3.5 g/dL is normal. Albumin levels of 3.0 to 3.5 g/dL indicate significant hypoalbuminemia, while levels below 3.0 g/dL indicate severe albumin deficiency.

Immune function is impaired in malnutrition.[70] The quantitation of absolute lymphocyte counts derived from a complete blood cell count and differential and the assessment of delayed hypersensitivity using skin test antigens are techniques used to assess the impact of nutri-tional status on immune function. The routinely utilized skin test antigens include tuberculin (as purified protein derivative, or PPD), mumps, streptokinase-streptodornase (SK-SD), *Candida albicans,* and *Trichophyton.* These tests were chosen on the basis that most normal persons are exposed to them and would be expected to have a positive skin test reaction. In uncomplicated starvation or protein-energy mal-nutrition, skin test reactivity can be restored with renutrition. Anergy is not specific to malnutrition and can be a feature of certain diseases such as Hodgkin's disease, while decreased white blood cell counts can be depressed transiently in the postoperative period and following infection with human immunodeficiency virus. Therefore, these esti-mations of immunocompetence are not simply specific to malnutrition.

Given the variety of nutritional assessment techniques available, most clinicians will have to select a small group of routinely available tests to use on a regular basis. Most clinical centers will have available skin testing, albumin, and transferrin for routine use. These tests should make it possible to assess whether patients are mildly, moder-ately, or severely malnourished and whether marasmic, kwashiorkor-like, or combined severe malnutrition is present (Table 46–2).

The status of the lean body mass can be assessed by measuring urinary creatinine excretion over 24 hours. Creatinine production in most people is directly related to skeletal muscle mass, provided that no rapid catabolism of muscle is in progress, as with severe sepsis or trauma, and that large amounts of dietary creatinine found in animal skeletal muscle are not being ingested. A creatinine-height index is calculated based on the measured 24-hour excretion of creatinine and that expected in a normal adult of the same height as the patient. This index has limited sensitivity, with values between 60% and 80% of ideal representing moderate skeletal muscle depletion and 40% to

TABLE 46–2. Diagnostic Features of Adult Malnutrition

	Marasmus	Kwashiorkor
Clinical setting	Decreased caloric intake	Decreased protein intake plus stress
Time course to develop	Months to years	Weeks to months
Physical examination	Cachectic; fat depletion, muscle wasting	May look well nourished
Anthropometrics		
TSF	Depressed	Relatively preserved
AMC	Depressed	Relatively preserved
Weight for height	Depressed	Relatively preserved
Creatinine-height index	Depressed	Relatively preserved
Skin test responses	Normal or depressed	Relatively preserved
Visceral proteins		
Albumin	Relatively normal	Low
Transferrin	Relatively normal	Low
Lymphocyte cell	Relatively normal	Low

TSF, triceps skinfold; AMC, arm muscle circumference.

50% representing severe skeletal muscle depletion.[75] For purposes of estimation, the ideal creatinine excretion for adults is taken as 23 mg/kg/24 hours for males and 18 mg/kg/24 hours for females.[76]

Assessment of Risk of Nutritional Depletion

Assessment of risk of nutritional depletion can be used to determine which patients require consideration for nutritional therapy, as described below. The presence of any of the following criteria should motivate the physician to conduct a complete nutritional assessment[77] with consideration of appropriate forms of nutritional therapy: (1) recent involuntary weight loss of greater than 5% in 1 month or over 10% in 6 months, especially when associated with anorexia, fatigue, or weakness; (2) history of recent significant physiologic stresses such as organ dysfunction, major surgery, infection, or illness within the last 3 months; (3) absolute lymphocyte count less than 1200/mm³; or (4) serum albumin less than 3.2 g/dL.

Determining Route and Dose of Nutritional Therapy

Nutritional therapy ranges from dietary counseling urging increased voluntary intake of foods and nutritional supplements to forced intake of nutrients via the gastrointestinal tract (enteral nutrition) or via the venous circulation (parenteral nutrition). The therapy of malnutrition is based on meeting the nutritional requirements of the patient for total energy, macronutrients, and micronutrients.

Total energy requirements can be measured using indirect calorimetry or estimated using approximate formulas. For well-nourished normal subjects, the estimated energy expenditure using the Harris-Benedict formula[78] is within 10% of the measured energy expenditure in approximately 90% of all subjects. However, in subjects with a variety of illnesses, hypermetabolism or hypometabolism may occur.[79] For these individuals, measurement of REE using indirect calorimetry is practical and more accurate than estimation methods (Fig. 46–7). In this method, data obtained from the rate of oxygen consumption and carbon dioxide production measured under controlled conditions, together with information on urinary nitrogen excretion, can be used to assess REE. The patient is placed under a ventilated plastic canopy at rest, and measurements are made for approximately 15 minutes. The equipment required for this measurement is available in most hospital pulmonary function laboratories, and newer portable models for bedside use are also available. Many of these newer pieces of equipment perform all necessary calculations internally to provide information on the energy requirements of patients. The ratio of the volume of carbon dioxide produced to oxygen consumed is defined as

the respiratory quotient (RQ). Glucose has an RQ of 1.0, and the oxidation of glucose yields 5.0 kcal/L of oxygen consumed. Fat has an RQ of approximately 0.7, yielding significantly less energy per liter of oxygen consumed. The respiratory quotients and calorie equivalents of different mixtures of carbohydrate and fat per liter of oxygen consumed are shown in Table 46–3. These values are the nonprotein RQ values used to assess energy expenditure once an adjustment has been made for protein oxidation based on an estimate of the amounts of energy liberated (26.51 kcal/g of nitrogen), oxygen consumed (5.91 L/g of nitrogen), and carbon dioxide produced (4.76 L/g of nitrogen) by the metabolism of protein (see Table 46–3). The daily excretion of urinary nitrogen is converted to the rate of nitrogen excretion per hour and is used to calculate REE, as shown in the example adapted from Cantarow and Trumper[80] in Table 46–4.

Once REE has been measured or basal energy expenditure (BEE) estimated using the Harris-Benedict equation, the total caloric requirements of subjects can be estimated. In general, these estimates range from 1.2 to 2.0 times the measured or estimated values based on observations of patients undergoing treatment for a variety of medical and surgical conditions. In moderately catabolic surgical patients, enteral nutrition has been found to lead to positive nitrogen balance at approximately 1.5 times the BEE, while in parenteral nutrition, 1.75 to 2.0 times the BEE is required.[81] Utilization of estimates of 1.75 times the BEE as a standard practice for all patients receiving paren-

TABLE 46–3. Respiratory Quotient (RQ) for Metabolism of Fuel Mixtures

RQ*	Percentage of Total Oxygen Consumed by		Percentage of Heat Produced by		kcal/L O₂
	Carbohydrate	*Fat*	*Carbohydrate*	*Fat*	
0.707	0	100	0	100	4.686
0.75	14.7	85.3	15.6	84.4	4.739
0.80	31.7	68.3	33.4	66.6	4.801
0.82	38.6	61.4	40.3	59.7	4.825
0.85	48.8	51.2	50.7	49.3	4.862
0.90	65.8	34.2	67.5	32.5	4.924
0.95	82.9	17.1	84.0	16.0	4.985
1.00	100	0	100	0	5.047

*Nonprotein RQ.

From Cantarow A, Trumper M: Clinical Biochemistry. Philadelphia, WB Saunders, 1955, p 367.

TABLE 46–4. Energy Expenditure Determination by Indirect Calorimetry and Estimation

Example Calculation

The calculation of energy expenditure using indirect calorimetry is illustrated by the following example adapted from Cantarow and Trumper.[80] These data were obtained from a patient under basal conditions: (1) urinary nitrogen, 0.18 g/hr, (2) oxygen consumption, 12.2 L/hr, and (3) carbon dioxide production, 9.2 L/hr.

0.18 g of urinary N represents:
$0.18 \times 5.91 = 1.06$ L of oxygen
$0.18 \times 4.76 = 0.85$ L of carbon dioxide
$0.18 \times 26.51 = 4.77$ kcal

Nonprotein oxygen consumption = $12.2 - 1.06 = 11.14$ L
Nonprotein carbon dioxide production = $9.2 - 0.85 = 8.35$ L
Nonprotein RQ = 0.75, representing the liberation of 4.739 kcal/L of oxygen
Nonprotein energy expenditure = $4.739 \times 11.14 = 52.79$ kcal/hr
Total energy expenditure = $52.79 + 4.77 = 57.56$ kcal/hr
For men: RME (kcal/day) = $66.4730 + 13.7516(W) + 5.0033(H) - 6.7750(A)$
For women: RME (kcal/day) = $655.095 + 9.563(W) + 1.8496(H) - 4.6756(A)$
where W = present weight in kilograms, H = height in centimeters, and A = age in years.

RQ, respiratory quotient; RME, resting metabolic expenditure.

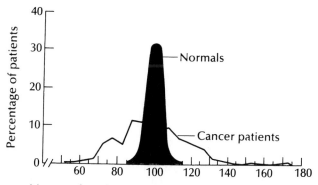

FIGURE 46–7. The distribution of measured resting energy expenditure in "normals" and in cancer patients. (From Knox L, Crosby L, Feurer I, et al: Energy expenditure in malnourished cancer patients. Ann Surg 197:152–162, 1983.)

teral nutritional therapy regardless of metabolic needs has led to overnutrition with resulting complications in certain disease states, as described below.[82]

Evaluation of Response to Nutritional Support

Since the goal of nutritional support is the attainment of an anabolic state or reduction of nitrogen losses, assessment of nitrogen balance is the most useful clinical assessment to determine whether nutritional therapy is effective. *Nitrogen balance* is defined as the difference between nitrogen intake and nitrogen excretion. Nitrogen intake is taken as the protein intake determined from dietary records divided by 6.25 g nitrogen per gram of "average" protein ingested. Nitrogen excretion is taken as the urinary nitrogen excreted per 24 hours plus a fixed estimate of 4.0 g/24 hours for unmeasured nitrogen losses from cellular sloughing into the feces (1 g), losses from the skin (0.2 g), and nonurea nitrogen losses in the urine (2 g).[83] Since nitrogen balance is most usefully applied in a serial fashion in the same patient, the particular constants used to estimate unmeasured excretion are only important for comparison of published results.

At any given level of nitrogen intake, nitrogen balance improves with increased administration of nonprotein calories to a maximum achieved at a ratio of 150:1 of nonprotein calories per gram of nitrogen.[84] Proteins vary in their biologic value based on the mixture of essential and nonessential amino acids they contain. Albumin has the ideal mixture of amino acids for optimal utilization of protein and is assigned a biologic value of 100. Casein is close to albumin in its biologic quality, followed by meat proteins such as those found in steak or tuna, which have a biologic value of 80. Corn and beans, each with biologic values of 40 or less, can be combined in a protein mixture with a biologic value of 80 because the amino acid patterns of the two proteins are complementary. The protein requirement for normal persons is 0.55 g/kg protein for a high-biologic-value protein such as milk or albumin but 0.8 g/kg for the mixture of proteins found in the average American diet.[85]

SPECIAL THERAPEUTIC PROBLEMS

Complications

Complications can occur following either enteral or parenteral nutrition. Complications of enteral nutrition are either mechanical or metabolic, while complications of parenteral nutrition can be mechanical, infectious, or metabolic.[86]

Mechanical problems of enteral feeding include aspiration, especially in semiconscious patients or patients with abnormalities of swallowing. This problem can be minimized by proper feeding tube placement and determination of the residual gastric contents 8 hours after feeding to eliminate the possibility of gastric outlet obstruction or gastric atony. If these latter problems occur, the feeding tube can be placed into the jejunum. Proper placement should be ensured radiologically to avoid misplacement of the feeding tube. Irritation of the oropharynx and the gastric mucosa can occur, especially with the use of larger-bore and less flexible feeding tubes. This problem can be minimized by using inert silicone rubber and polyurethane tubes.

Diarrhea is the most common complication associated with tube feeding.[87] Carefully increasing the rate of administration will help avoid this problem. Most enteral formulations are lactose-free, so lactose intolerance is not likely to cause diarrhea. Nonetheless, prolonged starvation can lead to gastrointestinal epithelial atrophy and maldigestion, which, in turn, could result in diarrhea. Diarrhea also can be due to the effects of other medications, colonic infections (e.g., *Clostridium difficile*), or overly rapid administration of hypertonic enteral formulations. Dehydration with hypernatremia also can be a problem in infants and the elderly, in whom inadequate fluid intake can occur during the administration of a hypertonic enteral formula. Glucosuria can occur in patients without a prior history of diabetes when high carbohydrate enteral formulas are used.

The complications of parenteral nutrition are in many cases more serious than those associated with enteral nutrition.[88] Pneumothorax and subclavian vein thrombosis are the most common catheter-related complications. Pneumothorax should occur in only about 1% to 2% of catheter insertions, but this rate is higher when transthoracic puncture is used rather than open surgical placement of catheters or when less experienced persons insert the catheters.[89] Radiologic confirmation of proper placement and to exclude the presence of pneumothorax is essential. Pneumothorax usually will resolve spontaneously, but a chest tube may be required in some cases. Thrombosis of the catheter in the central veins has been reported in 5% to 10% of patients receiving parenteral nutrition, especially when hypercoagulable states are present, as in sepsis, inflammatory bowel disease, pancreatitis, or cancer.[90] Heparin is given daily in prophylactic doses of 6000 units routinely, but when thrombosis occurs, the catheter must be removed. Peripheral venous nutrition is used while a full course of heparin or other treatment is undertaken to treat thrombosis. Infections most commonly occur from skin contaminants such as gram-positive organisms but can include fungi and unusual bacteria, especially if acquired during hospitalization. Infected catheters must be removed prior to the systemic treatment of catheter-related sepsis. In patients committed to lifelong parenteral nutrition, this decision is made carefully, since only eight external sites are available for central vein catheter placement.

In nutritional support, the goals are simply to provide adequate calories and nutrients to restore nutritional deficiencies and to maintain protein synthesis, positive nitrogen balance, and lean body mass.[91] Metabolic support of the critically ill patient is directed at partial caloric replacement, sustenance of important cellular and organ metabolism, and the avoidance of overfeeding and the metabolic costs of overfeeding, including lipogenesis, gluconeogenesis, and thermogenesis related to inefficient metabolism.

There are a variety of metabolic complications that can occur during parenteral nutrition. The most common is overfeeding, which results in RQs of greater than 1.0. This results in excessive carbon dioxide production, which can complicate the care of patients with chronic lung disease.[92] Hyperglycemia can occur in many patients due to transient insulin resistance or relative insulin deficiency. Both subcutaneous insulin and insulin added to the parenteral solutions can be used to treat this complication.[93] Metabolic acidosis, which occurred commonly when potassium and sodium were administered only as chloride salts, is less frequently a problem since the use of acetate buffers in parenteral solutions. Abnormalities of phosphate, potassium, calcium, and magnesium can occur due to excessive or inadequate administration in the presence of underlying disorders such as renal failure or gastrointestinal fistulas that predispose to electrolyte abnormalities.[94, 95] Deficiencies of trace minerals such as zinc, copper, and chromium rarely occur, since these are now added routinely to parenteral solutions.[96] Azotemia can occur in renal failure patients or with excessive administration of amino acids relative to nonprotein calories given and is treated simply by reducing the amino acid load administered.[97] Essential fatty acid deficiency rarely occurs since the use of intravenous lipid emulsions has become common.[98] In most cases, the metabolic complications associated with parenteral nutrition respond to fluid and electrolyte management with careful monitoring of input and output on a daily basis.[99]

Excessive infusion rates and the choice of the wrong mixture of macronutrients can be harmful in the critically ill patient. One of the most common problems encountered in intravenous nutrition is hepatomegaly resulting from increased hepatic lipogenesis. This occurs when glucose is used as the sole energy source or is given at greater than the endogenous production rate of 3 g/kg/day. Cholestasis also can result from these changes. Replacement of glucose with long-chain triglycerides (LCTs) derived from soybean or safflower oil has been shown to reduce fatty infiltration of the liver. These LCTs are associated with problems related to poor clearance by the reticuloendothelial system, leading to hypertriglyceridemia and possible adult respiratory distress syndrome and increased production of 2- and 4-series prostaglandins and leukotrienes, which can enhance vasoconstriction, platelet aggregation, immunosuppression, inhibition of monokine responses, and free radical formation.[100]

The use of medium-chain triglycerides (MCTs) can avoid some of these problems, at least in experimental systems.[101] MCT oils do not require acylcarnitine transferase action for transport into mitochondria and are metabolized to ketone bodies readily. They contain no essential fatty acids and so should not be used alone. There are research efforts to combine the effects of LCTs and MCTs in structured lipids where the triglyceride contains both types of fatty acids. Additional structured lipids containing *n*-3 fatty acids, so-called fish oils, are also being studied actively.[102]

A breakdown in the physical barrier and immunologic defense function of the gastrointestinal tract can promote multiple organ failure syndrome. The gastrointestinal tract is particularly susceptible to ischemic and reperfusion injury. Glutamine, a preferred fuel in the gut epithelium, may promote gastrointestinal tract epithelial healing after an injury.[103] In animal studies, an enteral formula containing glutamine has been shown to improve gastrointestinal epithelial mucosal integrity and nitrogen balance.[104] Research is underway on the incorporation of these physiologic properties of specific nutrients into therapeutic regimens to prevent multiple organ failure syndrome. However, the crucial difference between the multiple organ failure syndrome and chronic malnutrition is recognized in the need to avoid overfeeding by providing a hypocaloric protein-sparing nutritional regimen.

Nutritional Support as Therapy

Patients with gastrointestinal fistulas often evidence fluid and electrolyte abnormalities, sepsis, and malnutrition. Retrospective analyses suggest that nutritional therapy is beneficial in promoting the closure of these fistulas.[105] It has been noted that 90% of fistulas destined to close did so within 1 month of the control of sepsis. Prior to the advent of total parenteral nutrition (TPN), intensive enteral nutrition resulted in a favorable effect on mortality and a rate of closure comparable with that later observed following parenteral nutrition. While fistula output is more effectively managed with parenteral than enteral nutrition, enteral feedings may be as effective in very proximal or very distal fistulas. Moreover, with chronic low-output fistulas, even oral feeding may be tolerated. In any case, surgery is indicated for those fistulas not closing within 40 days after nutritional support is initiated. Crohn's disease, radiation enteritis, residual tumor, distal intestinal obstruction, epithelialization of a short fistulous tract (<2 cm from bowel to skin), and complete interruption of the gastrointestinal tract make it unlikely that healing will occur. In these instances, early surgical repair should be undertaken.

Short-bowel syndrome results when greater than 75% of the small intestine is absent secondary to extensive disease or massive resection.[106] This syndrome can occur secondary to trauma, infarction, severe Crohn's disease, radiation enteritis, and cancer. Loss of the ileum is more significant than loss of jejunum, since ileal loss leads to decreased enterohepatic circulation of bile salts. This results in entry of bile salts into the colon with resulting diarrhea and decreased absorption of vitamin B_{12}. Compensatory growth occurs in the small intestine following resection, with epithelial hyperplasia.[107] The intensity of epithelial hyperplasia is related directly to the length of intestine resected. The stimuli promoting this response are poorly understood but may include food, enteric secretions, and hormones. Immediately following the initial injury, diarrhea, fluid, and electrolyte disorders are controlled together with provision of parenteral nutrition. After several weeks, fecal output may fall to less than 2 L/day, at which point a trial of enteral feeding may be attempted using a predigested diet that is low in LCTs (elemental diet). As the small bowel adapts, carbohydrates and protein are provided, with fat limited to less than 30 g/day utilizing MCTs. After 6 months to 2 years, complete oral nutrition is possible in many patients. Dietary supplements of calcium and fat-soluble vitamins are prescribed for these patients even after gastrointestinal adaptation, since steatorrhea often persists with malabsorption of fat-soluble vitamins and precipitation of calcium in soaps.

Patients with chronic renal failure can be given nutrition during hemodialysis with improved nitrogen retention. During acute renal failure, electrolyte and fluid abnormalities, as well as azotemia, occur commonly and require appropriate alterations of the parenteral nutrition regimen.[108] Patients with cardiac disease often require fluid and

sodium restriction and may benefit from diuretic administration so that protein and calorie requirements can be met.[109]

Diabetic patients developing hyperglycemia either can be given insulin as described or can be provided with an increased percentage of calories as fat to reduce insulin requirements.[110]

Patients with hepatic insufficiency have abnormal amino acid profiles with increased concentrations of aromatic amino acids and decreased levels of branched-chain amino acids.[111] Decreased plasma levels of branched-chain amino acids are thought to lead to increased central nervous system levels of aromatic amino acids, since these two classes of amino acids compete for uptake at the blood-brain barrier. Increased levels of aromatic amino acids interfere with catecholamine metabolism, resulting in shunting of tyrosine to produce octopamine, a false neurotransmitter. Excess serotonin is thought to develop from increased levels of tryptophan. The combination of decreased catecholamines, false neurotransmitters, and increased serotonin levels is proposed to lead to hepatic coma. Specialized formulas have been used to treat patients with hepatic encephalopathy. Some improvements in neurologic function with administration of specially formulated enteral supplements are noted in patients with chronic hepatic failure. However, in acute hepatic insufficiency, these formulas provided by the parenteral route have not proved beneficial when compared with ordinary parenteral formulations.

THERAPEUTIC PROTOCOLS

Enteral and Parenteral Nutrition

Once malnutrition has been diagnosed and classified as mild, moderate, or severe marasmic, kwashiorkor, or combined protein-energy malnutrition, the choice of route of administration of nutritional therapy depends on the functional status of the gastrointestinal tract, the methods available for provision of nutritional support, and a working understanding of the various nutritional products and types of equipment used for parenteral and enteral nutritional support.

As a general rule, the enteral feeding route should be used whenever the gastrointestinal tract is functional.[88] Enteral feeding results in higher rates of visceral protein synthesis than similar nutrients provided parenterally. Enteral feeding results in a physiologic release of gut peptides, including insulinotropic peptides which enhance anabolism. In addition, provision of nutrients in the gastrointestinal lumen has been shown in animal studies to maintain the barrier function of the gut to translocation of endotoxin and gram-negative bacteria.[112]

Prior to initiation of enteral feeding, every attempt should be made to utilize voluntary feeding techniques. Changes in meal frequency and size, use of flavorings, preparation of favorite foods in the patient's home, consideration of nutrition in the scheduling of diagnostic and therapeutic procedures, and the use of nutritional supplements between meals should be considered.

Consideration should be given as to whether the patient's primary illness is best treated by putting the bowel to rest. For example, patients with gastrointestinal fistulas often require avoidance of enteral feeding.

The gastrointestinal tract must be truly functional. The stomach must be capable of delivering the nutritional mixture to the small intestine, and then digestion and absorption must proceed normally. If there is functional gastric obstruction due to a problem with gastric emptying, diabetic gastropathy, or prior surgery, then a tube can be placed directly into the jejunum.

When the gastrointestinal tract is not functional and there are clear therapeutic goals, parenteral nutrition should be used. There are a number of accepted indications for parenteral nutrition, including short-bowel syndrome, where there is inadequate small bowel surface area for digestion and absorption of nutrients even after adaptation. The ability of this therapy to maintain life under these circumstances is established. The role of parenteral nutrition has been under careful scrutiny in view of the expense and potential side effects of this form of nutritional therapy.[113] While parenteral nutrition is not therapeutic in terms of the conditions themselves, a useful role of parenteral nutrition has been defined in subgroups of patients with pancreatitis, gastrointestinal fistulas, and inflammatory bowel disease.

In some situations, transitional feeding is utilized in which parenteral and enteral nutrition are combined. For example, parenteral nutrition can be used in burn and head trauma patients when the gastrointestinal tract is functional but the total caloric requirement cannot be met by the enteral route.

Prognosis

While it is simple to demonstrate the impact of renutrition on the patient with uncomplicated starvation or an inability to absorb calories due to a loss of intestinal tissue, it is much more difficult to demonstrate the beneficial effects of nutrition in patients with a number of chronic illnesses, including common forms of cancer. Often the course of the underlying illness will mask the beneficial effects of nutritional therapy. The benefits of nutritional support have been well documented in selected reviews.[114]

For a number of indications, the use of TPN is controversial.[115] While many cancer and AIDS patients benefit from renutrition, the routine use of TPN in all cancer patients receiving chemotherapy or in all AIDS patients regardless of nutritional status is not appropriate. In some patients receiving chemotherapy or radiation therapy, mucosal inflammation, nausea, and vomiting impair normal intake. In such patients, TPN may be needed as an adjunct to restore the patient's functional status in order to continue therapy or undertake radiation therapy, chemotherapy, or surgical therapy.

The use of nutritional support in many instances is not supported by clinical trial data. However, a judgment must be made by the physician as to the severity of the effects of malnutrition and whether nutrition can reverse these effects to affect the overall prognosis. There are many instances where nutrition has become a routine part of patient care prior to a careful evaluation of its real benefit. It remains a challenge for nutrition researchers to define the benefits of nutritional support and to determine its best application in clinical practice.

REFERENCES

1. Cahill GF: Starvation in man. N Engl J Med 282:668–675, 1970.
2. Jelliffe DB: The Assessment of the Nutritional Status of the Community (Monograph Series 53). Geneva, World Health Organization, 1966.
3. Bistrian BR, Blackburn GL, Vitale J, et al: Prevalence of malnutrition in general medical patients. JAMA 235:1567–1570, 1976.
4. Wan JM, Han M, Blackburn GL: Nutrition, immune function, and inflammation: An overview. Proc Nutr Soc 48:315–335, 1989.
5. Blackburn GL, Wan JM, Teo TC, et al: Metabolic support of organ failure. In Bihari DJ, Cerra FB (eds): New Horizons: Multiple Organ Failure. Fullerton, CA, Society of Critical Care Medicine, 1989, pp 337–370.
6. Owen OE, Morgan AP, Kemp HG, et al: Brain metabolism during fasting. J Clin Invest 48:574–583, 1969.
7. Owen OE, Felig P, Morgan AP, et al: Liver and kidney metabolism during prolonged starvation. J Clin Invest 48:574–583, 1969.
8. Owen OE, Reichard GA: Human forearm metabolism during progressive starvation. J Clin Invest 50:1536–1545, 1971.
9. Bistrian BR, Blackburn GL, Hallowell E, Heddle R: Protein status of general surgical patients. JAMA 230:858–860, 1974.
10. Chandra RK: Nutrition, immunity, and infection: Present knowledge and future directions. Lancet 1:688–691, 1983.
11. Marliss EB, Aoki TT, Unger RH, et al: Glucagon levels and metabolic effects in fasting man. J Clin Invest 49:2256–2270, 1970.
12. Owen OE, Reichard GA, Kinney JM, et al: Metabolism during catabolic states of starvation, diabetes, and trauma in humans. In Bleicher SJ, Brodoff BN (eds): Diabetes Mellitus and Obesity. Baltimore, Williams & Wilkins, 1982, pp 172–184.
13. Waterlow JC: Protein turnover with special reference to man. Q J Exp Physiol 169:409–438, 1984.
14. Felig P, Owen OE, Wahren J, Cahill GF: Amino acid metabolism during prolonged starvation. J Clin Invest 48:584–594, 1969.
15. Cersosimo E, Williams PE, Radosevich PM, et al: Role of glutamine in adaptations in nitrogen metabolism during fasting. Am J Physiol 250:E622–628, 1986.
16. Mortimore GE, Poso AR: Lysosomal pathways in hepatic protein degradation: Regulatory role of amino acids. Fed Proc 434:1289–1294, 1984.
17. Fukagawa NK, Minaker DL, Rowe JW, et al: Insulin-mediated reduction of whole body protein breakdown: Dose-response effects on leucine metabolism in postabsorptive men. J Clin Invest 76:2306–2311, 1985.
18. Nair KS, Halliday D, Matthews DE, Welle SL: Hyperglucagonemia during insulin deficiency accelerates protein catabolism (abstract). Diabetes 36(suppl 2):74, 1987.
19. Flakoll PJ, Brown LL, Frexes-Steed M, Abumrad NN: Use of amino acid clamps

to investigate the role of insulin in regulating protein breakdown in vivo. JPEN 15:81S–85S, 1991.
20. Young VR: Energy metabolism and requirements in the cancer patient. Cancer Res 37:2336–2347, 1977.
21. Arner P, Engfeldt P, Nowak J: In vivo observations on the lipolytic effect of noradrenaline during therapeutic fasting. J Clin Endocrinol Metab 53:1207–1212, 1981.
22. Jensen MD, Haymond MW, Gerich JE, et al: Lipolysis during fasting. J Clin Invest 79:207–213, 1987.
23. Unger RH: Insulin-glucagon relationship in the defense against hypoglycemia. Diabetes 32:575–583, 1983.
24. Schwartz MW, Dallman MF, Woods SC: Hypothalamic response to starvation: Implications for the study of wasting disorders. Am J Physiol 269:R949–R957, 1995.
25. Froesch ER, Schmid C, Schwander J, Zapf J: Actions of insulin-like growth factor. Annu Rev Physiol 47:443–467, 1985.
26. Phillips LS: Nutrition, somatomedins, and the brain. Metabolism 35:78–87, 1986.
27. Bray GA: The Obese Patient. Philadelphia, WB Saunders, 1976, p 141.
28. Chopra IJ, Huang TS, Beredo A, et al: Evidence for an inhibitor of extrathyroidal conversion of thyroxine to 3,5,3-triiodothyronine in sera of patients with nonthyroidal illnesses. J Clin Endocrinol Metab 60:666–672, 1985.
29. Spencer CA, Lum SM, Wilber JF, et al: Dynamics of serum thyrotropin and thyroid hormone changes in fasting. J Clin Endocrinol Metab 56:883–888, 1983.
30. Henson LC, Poole DC, Donahoe CP, Heber D: Effects of exercise training on resting energy expenditure during caloric restriction. Am J Clin Nutr 46:893–899, 1987.
31. Henson LC, Heber D: Whole body protein breakdown rates and hormonal adaptation during fasting in obese subjects. J Clin Endocrinol Metab 57:316–319, 1984.
32. Torun B, Chew F: Protein-energy malnutrition. In Shils ME, Olson JA, Shike M (eds): Modern Nutrition in Health and Disease, vol 2, ed 8. Baltimore, Williams & Wilkins, 1994, pp 950–976.
33. Latham MC: Protein-energy malnutrition. In Present Knowledge in Nutrition, ed 6. Washington, DC, International Life Sciences Institute, 1990, pp 39–46.
34. Lira PIC, Ashworth A, Morris SS: Low birth weight and morbidity from diarrhea and respiratory infection in northeast Brazil. Pediatrics 128:497–504, 1996.
35. Ruz M, Solomons NW, Mejia LA, Chew F: Alterations of circulating micronutrients with overt and occult infections in anemic Guatemalan preschool children. Int J Food Sci Nutr 46:257–265, 1995.
36. Golden BE, Golden MHN: Protein deficiency, energy deficiency, and the edema of malnutrition. Lancet 1:1261–1265, 1982.
37. Barltrop D, Sandhu BK: Marasmus, 1985. Postgrad Med J 61:915–923, 1985.
38. Frenk S: Protein-energy malnutrition. In Arneil GC, Metcoff J (eds): Pediatric Nutrition. London, Butterworths, 1985, pp 151–193.
39. Hintz RL, Suskind R, Amatayakul K, et al: Plasma somatomedin and growth hormone values in children with protein-energy malnutrition. J Pediatr 92:153–156, 1978.
40. Whitehead RG, Coward WA, Lunn PG, Rutishauser I: A comparison of the pathogenesis of protein-energy malnutrition in Uganda and Gambia. Trans R Soc Trop Med Hyg 71:189–195, 1977.
41. Truswell AS: Protein vs energy in protein energy malnutrition. S Afr Med J 59:753–756, 1981.
42. Gopalan C: Kwashiorkor and marasmus: Evolution and distinguishing features. In McCance RA, Widowson EM (eds): Calorie Deficiencies and Protein Deficiencies. London, Churchill Livingstone, 1968, pp 49–58.
43. Sinatra FR, Merritt RJ: Iatrogenic kwashiorkor in infants. Am J Dis Child 135:21–23, 1981.
44. Kirsch RE, Saunders SJ, Frith L, et al: Plasma amino acid concentration and the regulation of albumin synthesis. Am J Clin Nutr 22:1559–1562, 1969.
45. Lumn PG, Whitehead RG, Baker BA: The relative effects of a low-protein high-carbohydrate diet on free amino acid composition of liver and muscle. Br J Nutr 36:219–230, 1976.
46. Hadden DR, Rutishauser IHE: Effect of human growth hormone in kwashiorkor and marasmus. Arch Dis Child 42:29–33, 1967.
47. Schiffman SS: Taste and smell in disease. N Engl J Med 308:1275–1277, 1983.
48. Baron RB: Malnutrition in hospitalized patients: Diagnosis and treatment. West J Med 144:63–67, 1986.
49. Birkhan RH, Long CL, Fitkin D, et al: Effects of major skeletal trauma on whole body protein turnover in man measured by 14C-leucine. Surgery 88:294–299, 1980.
50. Long CL, Jeevanandam M, Kim BM, Kinney JM: Whole body protein synthesis and catabolism in septic man. Am J Clin Nutr 30:1340–1344, 1977.
51. Bistrian BR, Schwartz J, Istfan NW: Cytokines, muscle proteolysis, and the catabolic response to infection and inflammation. Proc Soc Exp Biol Med 200:220–223, 1992.
52. Blackburn GL, Bistrian BR, Maini BS: Nutritional and metabolic support of the hospitalized patient. JPEN 1:11, 1977.
53. Cuthbertson DP, Tilstone WJ: Metabolism during the post-injury period. Adv Clin Chem 12:1–4, 1969.
54. Bassili HR, Dietel M: Effects of nutritional support on weaning patients off of mechanical ventilators. JPEN 5:161–163, 1981.
55. Alverdy J, Chi HS, Sheldon G: The effect of parenteral nutrition on gastrointestinal immunity: The importance of enteral stimulation. Ann Surg 202:681–684, 1985.
56. Alberti KGMM, Batstone GF, Foster KJ, Johnston DG: Relative roles of various hormones on mediating the metabolic response to injury. JPEN 4:141–145, 1980.
57. Nair KS, Halliday D, Matthews DE, Welle SL: Hyperglucagonemia during insulin deficiency accelerates protein catabolism (abstract). Diabetes 36(suppl 1):74A, 1987.
58. Matthews DE, Pesola G, Campbell RG: Effect of epinephrine on amino acid and energy metabolism in humans. Am J Physiol 258:E948–E956, 1990.
59. Hjortso NC, Christensen NJ, Andersen T, Kehlet H: Effects of the extradural administration of local anesthetic agents and morphine on the urinary excretion of cortisol, catecholamines, and nitrogen following elective surgery. Br J Anaesth 57:400–406, 1985.

60. Ziegler TR, Young LS, Manson JM, Wilmore DW: Metabolic effects of recombinant human growth hormone in patients receiving parenteral nutrition. Ann Surg 208:6–16, 1988.

61. Horber FF, Haymond MW: Human growth hormone prevents the protein catabolic side effects of prednisone in humans. J Clin Invest 86:265–272, 1990.

62. Dinarello CA: Interleukin 1 and the pathogenesis of the acute phase response. N Engl J Med 311:1413–1418, 1984.

63. Kushner I: The phenomenon of the acute phase response. Ann N Y Acad Sci 389:39–48, 1982.

64. Old LJ: Polypeptide mediator network. Nature 326:330–331, 1987.

65. Nathan CF: Secretory products of macrophages. J Clin Invest 79:319–326, 1987.

66. Dinarello CA: Interleukin 1. Rev Infect Dis 6:51–95, 1984.

67. Klein J, Mosley R: Phenotypic and Cytotoxic Characteristics of Intraepithelial Lymphocytes. New York, Raven Press, 1994.

68. Teitelbaum D, Reyas B, Merion R, et al: Intestinal intraepithelial lymphocytes: Identification of an inhibitory sub-population. J Surg Res 63:123–127, 1996.

69. Fujihashi K, McGhee JR, Beagley KW, et al: Cytokine-specific ELISPOT assay. Single cell analysis of IL-2, IL-4, and IL-6 producing cells. J Immunol Methods 160:181–189, 1993.

70. Chandra RK: Nutrition, immunity and infection: Present knowledge and future directions. Lancet 1:688–691, 1983.

71. Hammaway KJ, Moldawer LL, Georgieff M: The effect of lipid emulsions on reticuloendothelial system function in the injured animal. JPEN 9:559–565, 1985.

72. Jeejeebhoy KN: Muscle function and malnutrition. Gut 27(suppl 1):25–39, 1986.

73. Shetty PS, Watrasiewicz KE, Jung RT, James WPT: Rapid-turnover proteins: An index of subclinical protein-energy malnutrition. Lancet 2:230–232, 1979.

74. Kahan BD: Nutrition and host defense mechanisms. Surg Clin North Am 61:557–570, 1981.

75. Bistrian BR, Blackburn GL, Hallowell E, Heddle R: Protein status of general surgical patients. JAMA 230:858–870, 1974.

76. Bistrian BR, Blackburn GL, Shermann M: Therapeutic index of nutritional depletion in hospitalized patients. Surg Gynecol Obstet 141:512–518, 1975.

77. Irving M: ABC of nutrition: Enteral and parenteral nutrition. BMJ 291:1404–1408, 1985.

78. Harris JA, Benedict FG: Biometric Studies of Basal Metabolism in Man. Washington, DC, Carnegie Institute, 1919, publication 279.

79. Knox L, Crosby L, Feurer I, et al: Energy expenditure in malnourished cancer patients. Ann Surg 197:152–162, 1983.

80. Cantarow A, Trumper M: Clinical Biochemistry. Philadelphia, WB Saunders, 1955, p 367.

81. Ang SD, Leskiw MJ, Stein TP: The effect of increasing total parenteral nutrition on protein metabolism. JPEN 7:525–529, 1983.

82. Askanazi J, Rosenbaum SH, Hyman AI: Respiratory changes induced by the large glucose loads of total parenteral nutrition. JAMA 243:1444–1447, 1980.

83. Sirba E: Effect of reduced protein intake on nitrogen loss from the human integument. Am J Clin Nutr 20:1158–1161, 1978.

84. Calloway D, Spector H: Nitrogen balance as related to caloric and protein intake in active young men. Am J Clin Nutr 2:405–412, 1954.

85. Recommended Dietary Allowances, ed 10. Washington, DC, National Academy Press, 1989.

86. Bethel RA, Jansen RD, Heymsfield SB, et al: Nasogastric hyperalimentation through a polyethylene catheter: An alternative to central venous hyperalimentation. Am J Clin Nutr 32:1112–1120, 1979.

87. Voit KAJ, Echave V, Brown RA, Gund FN: Use of elemental diet during the adaptive stage of short gut syndrome. Gastroenterology 65:419–426, 1973.

88. Heymsfield SB, Bethel RA, Ansley JD, et al: Enteral hyperalimentation: An alternative to central venous hyperalimentation. Ann Intern Med 90:63–71, 1979.

89. Feliciano DV, Mattox KL, Graham JM: Major complications of percutaneous subclavian catheters. Am J Surg 138:869–874, 1979.

90. Ryan A, Abel M, Abbot WM: Catheter complications in total parenteral nutrition. N Engl J Med 290:757–761, 1974.

91. Cerra FB: Hypermetabolism, organ failure, and metabolic support. Surgery 101:1–14, 1987.

92. Covelli HD, Black JW, Olsen MS, Beekman JF: Respiratory failure precipitated by high carbohydrate loads. Ann Intern Med 95:579–581, 1981.

93. Ryan JA: Complications of total parenteral nutrition. *In* Fischer JE (ed): Total Parenteral Nutrition. Boston, Little, Brown, 1976, pp 55–100.

94. Ruberg R, Allen T, Goodman M: Hypophosphatemia with hypophosphaturia in hyperalimentation. Surg Forum 22:87–88, 1971.

95. Fleming CR, McGill DB, Hoffman HN, Nelson RA: Total parenteral nutrition. Mayo Clin Proc 51:187–189, 1976.

96. Fleming CR, Hodges RE, Hurley LS: A prospective study of serum copper and zinc levels in patients receiving total parenteral nutrition. Am J Clin Nutr 29:70–77, 1976.

97. Chen WJ, Ohashi E, Kasai M: Amino acid metabolism in parenteral nutrition: With special reference to the calorie/nitrogen ratio and the blood urea nitrogen level. Metabolism 23:1117–1123, 1974.

98. Goodgame JT, Lowry SF, Brennan MF: Essential fatty acid deficiency in total parenteral nutrition: Time course of development and suggestions for therapy. Surgery 84:271–277, 1978.

99. Blackburn GL, Wan JMF, Teo TC, et al: Metabolic support in organ failure. *In* Bihari DJ, Cerra FB (eds): New Horizons—Multiple Organ Failure. Fullerton, CA, Society of Critical Care Medicine, 1989, pp 337–370.

100. Kinsella JE, Lokesh B, Broughton S, Whelan J: Dietary polyunsaturated fatty acids and eicosanoids: Potential effects on modulation of inflammatory and immune cells: An overview. Nutrition 6:24–44, 1990.

101. Holman RT: Nutritional and metabolic interrelationships between fatty acids. Fed Proc 23:1062–1067, 1964.

102. DeMichele SJ, Karlstad MD, Bistrian BR, et al: Enteral nutrition with structured lipid: Effect on protein metabolism in thermal injury. Am J Clin Nutr 50:1295–1302, 1989.

103. Windmueller HG: Glutamine utilization by the small intestine. Adv Enzymol 53:210, 1982.

104. Fox AD, Kripke SA, DePaula JA: Glutamine supplemented diets prolong survival and decrease mortality in experimental enterocolitis. JPEN 12(suppl 1):8S, 1988.

105. Thomas RJS: The response of patients with fistulas of the gastrointestinal tract to parenteral nutrition. Surg Gynecol Obstet 153:77–80, 1981.

106. Weser E, Fletcher JT, Urban E: Short bowel syndrome. Gastroenterology 77:575–532, 1980.

107. Williamson RCN: Intestinal adaptation. N Engl J Med 298:1393–1402, 1444–1450, 1978.

108. Blumenkrantz MJ, Kopple JD, Koffler A: Total parenteral nutrition in the management of acute renal failure. Am J Clin Nutr 31:1830–1840, 1978.

109. Heymsfield SB, Bethel RA, Ansley JD: Cardiac abnormalities in cachectic patients before and during nutritional repletion. Am Heart J 95:584–594, 1978.

110. Fischer JE: Nutritional support in the seriously ill patient. Curr Probl Surg 17:466–532, 1980.

111. Fischer JE, Bower RH: Nutritional support in liver disease. Surg Clin North Am 61:653–660, 1981.

112. Peck MD, Alexander JW, Gonce SJ: Low-protein diets improve survival from peritonitis in guinea pigs. Ann Surg 209:448–454, 1989.

113. Pillar B, Perry S: Evaluating total parenteral nutrition: Final report and statement of the technology assessment and practice guidelines forum. Nutrition 6:313–317, 1990.

114. Meguid MM, Mughal MM, Meguid V, Terry JJ: Risk-benefit analysis of malnutrition and perioperative nutritional support: A review. Nutr Int 3:25–34, 1987.

115. Koretz RL: What supports nutritional support? Dig Dis Sci 29:577–588, 1984.

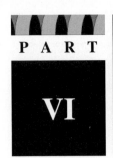

PART VI

Diabetes Mellitus, Carbohydrate Metabolism, and Lipid Disorders

Editor: Arthur H. Rubenstein

BASIC PHYSIOLOGY

Chapter 47

Anatomy, Developmental Biology, and Pathology of the Pancreatic Islets

Brigitte Reusens ▪ Joseph J. Hoet* ▪ Claude Remacle

Fascinating new techniques have resulted in significant advances since the discovery by Paul Langerhans, more than 100 years ago, of "the heaps and clusters of cells" (*Zellhäufchen*), entangled in a very vascularized network rather surprisingly in the "abdominal salivary gland." Laguesse,[1] christening the "little vascular glands" (*véritables petites glandes vasculaires sanguines)* as islets of Langerhans, attributed a functional role to them on the basis of protracted studies of the pancreata of vertebrates and a careful observation of the pancreata of eight men sentenced to death. The role and specific nature of the cells were further confirmed by his observation of the pancreas of a neonate, in whom he characterized voluminous and numerous islets "with astonishment."

Basic β cell structure interrelates with its functional adaptation which starts already during the primary development of the cell in the fetus and extends throughout life. To explore this vital activity of the β cell the research obviously cannot be performed in humans, and therefore one has to resort to the integration of many scattered observations based on phylogenic and comparative morphology and physiology. Shortcomings are obvious, but they stimulate new ventures in research to unravel the mysteries of the β cell. The dominant function of the latter is to foster anabolism from the inception of fetal life throughout the demands and the vicissitudes of existence. The insufficiency of β cells, in either number or function or both, is an etiologic factor in diabetes mellitus. In this respect, the initiation stage of the β cell, its autonomous development, its proliferative capacity during fetal life, the preservation of generative processes during extrauterine life, as well as environmental factors that modulate each of these stages, have to be considered and defined when the etiology of diabetes is being discussed.

The β cell is a specific component of the islets of Langerhans,

whose cellular constituency is contingent on its location within the pancreas. The latter develops from two buds, one dorsal and one ventral, to form the splenic and the duodenal lobes, in which stem cell differentiation will generate a glucagon-rich splenic and pancreatic polypeptide–rich duodenal lobe, respectively. The mode of its vascularization, its innervation, and its contiguity with the gastrointestinal tract are specific to mammals, including humans. It is a significant challenge to explore the dynamics of growth and the life cycle of β cells in connection with such a heterogeneous disease as diabetes.

THE SIGNIFICANCE OF THE PHYLOGENY AND ONTOGENY OF THE β CELL

Phylogeny

In the course of evolution, the neurohormonal regulatory peptides appear to have originated in the nervous system and later also localized in endocrine cells that developed in more highly evolved invertebrate species. The dual localization of regulatory peptides is retained throughout the animal kingdom[2] as exemplified by the "brain-gut axis" of vertebrates.[3]

The neuroendocrine cells regulating carbohydrate metabolism evolve from dispersed cell populations in prevertebrate animals, becoming separate endocrine organs in the most highly developed vertebrates.[4] The scenario envisaged by Falkmer and coworkers[4, 5] involves successive steps. In primitive vertebrates, the insulin cells, followed by somatostatin cells, leave the gut mucosa and form a separate islet organ; the glucagon and PP cells remain scattered in the gut mucosa. Later, glucagon, or glicentin, cells and finally PP cells join their

---

*Deceased.

colleagues in islets within the pancreas. In the most highly evolved vertebrates, a close functional connection persists between the gastrointestinal mucosa with its endocrine cells and the islets via the "enteroinsular" axis,[6] of which gastric inhibitory polypeptide (GIP) is one identified constituent.

Ontogeny

A dorsal pancreatic bud first arises as an evagination of the primitive gut endoderm (Fig. 47–1). Shortly thereafter, a ventral bud appears and rotates around the duodenum. The two buds fuse, grow, and form new folds leading to a highly branched structure. Acini and ducts appear clearly. Three types of epithelial compartments constitute the mammalian pancreas: the ductular system, the exocrine acinar cells, and the islets of Langerhans, which constitute the endocrine tissue. Exocrine acinar cells produce proenzymes, which are drained by the ductal system into the duodenum. Langerhans islets are dispersed throughout the whole pancreas. They are composed of almost one thousand endocrine cells of four different types α, β, δ, and PP cells, whose main function is to secrete, respectively, glucagon, insulin, somatostatin, and pancreatic polypeptide drained by a highly developed blood supply.

After budding of the pancreatic anlagen from the duodenal epithelium, endocrine and exocrine stem cells are believed to derive from common protodifferentiated cells of ductal origin, which under adequate stimuli differentiate into acinar or islet cells. This cell type is not yet identified, but its existence can be suspected from the experiments of pancreatectomy,[7] duct ligation,[8] and wrapping of the pancreas within cellophane,[9] in which a remarkable regeneration of endocrine and exocrine cells from ductal tissue occurs.

The sequential order of appearance during development of the four islet hormones is glucagon, insulin, somatostatin, and pancreatic polypeptide. These peptides tend to be co-expressed with other hormones early in development, but little or no co-expression of the four hormones is observed in adult β cells.

In the human fetus no endocrine cells are present at 7 weeks, but as early as the ninth week, immunostainable glucagon (or glicentin) α cells, insulin β cells, somatostatin δ cells, and PP cells are found in primitive islets or as isolated cells adjacent to duct cells.[10–12] During the sixteenth week, the four hormone-containing cells are abundant and fully recognizable. The splenic lobe contains more α cells and fewer PP cells than the duodenal lobe, but similar densities of β and δ cells. After the tenth week, however, the islets in the posterior part of the duodenal lobe contain a high number of PP cells with fewer α cells.[6, 12] The expression of gastrin in fetal islets is short-lived, and is absent in adult islets.[13]

In human fetal islets, which are small and unevenly distributed in the exocrine parenchyma, β cells are in the center of the islets and grow surrounded by other islet cells, which form a peripheral "mantle."[14]

The ontogeny of mammalian islets seems to follow the phylogenic origin. Based on the observation that during very early embryogenesis endocrine cells may, like neurons, take up amine precursors and decarboxylate them, Pearse formulated the APUD (amine precursor uptake and decarboxylation) theory, which proposed that these endocrine cells derived from the neural crest and migrated to the endoderm during development.[15, 16] This migration was never verified, however, and it is now generally accepted that both the endocrine pancreas and exocrine pancreas are of endodermal origin.[17] Inversion of the polarity of the mitotic axis in certain epithelial cells of growing pancreatic ducts is currently viewed as the mechanical means to separate endocrine islets from the continuous duct epithelium[17, 18] (Fig. 47–2) The pancreas has long been thought to develop from epithelial-mesenchymal interaction wherein undifferentiated epithelium in the duodenal anlage is stimulated by the mesenchyme which overlies it, allowing growth and differentiation into the mature pancreas leading to acinar, endocrine, and ductal structures. Therefore, a mesenchymal factor was suspected,[19] but recent studies demonstrated that the mesenchyme is not required for all aspects of pancreatic development, but rather for the acinar structures only. Ducts will only develop when components of the basement membrane originated from mesenchyme are present.[20] When the mesenchyme is removed from the pancreatic rudiment, the differentiation of the endocrine cells is largely favored. Follistatin is also produced by the embryonic mesenchyme and mimics both the inductive effect of the mesenchyme on the development of the exocrine pancreas and the repressive effect of the mesenchyme on the development of the cells of the endocrine pancreas.[21]

Because the data are rather difficult to gather in humans, the rodent model, especially the rat, provides a useful tool for analyzing the evolution of the β cell mass.

In rodent, the β cell mass develops in three phases, as already proposed.[17] During the first phase, the phase of protodifferentiation (F10–15), a few insulin-containing cells develop. These cells co-express glucagon, but are not associated into islets and do not express the glucose transporter-2 (GLUT2) or molecules associated with secretory granules like IAPP (islet amyloid polypeptide) present in adult β cells. The insulin accumulation within the pancreas parallels the rate of cell proliferation. Around day 15, by way of enhanced transcription and subsequent increased rate of insulin synthesis, the secondary transition takes place. The cytodifferentiation of β cells occurs, characterized by the appearance of secretory granules, and the hormone content per cell increases exponentially. These new insulin-containing cells do not co-express glucagon any more. They are GLUT2-positive, express characteristic molecules associated with adult β cells, and are grouped into islets. It has been shown that the first wave of the insulin-positive cells is under control of the mesenchyme.[21]

To form islets of Langerhans, the differentiated cells migrate into the interstitial matrix and aggregate. This morphogenesis requires extracellular matrix degradation occurring in rodents at F17–19 through activation of a metalloproteinase, which is under the control of transforming growth factor-β (TGF-β).[22] The fully differentiated stage is reached at day 19 to day 20. This sequence of events occurs in the same manner in vivo and in vitro, indicating its autonomy.

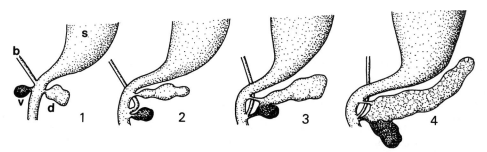

FIGURE 47–1. *Schematic outline of the development of the mammalian pancreas. 1, Two buds arise from the duodenal part of the primitive gut: one dorsal and one ventral (blackened). 2, The ventral bud, following the bile duct, turns and approaches the dorsal bud. 3, The two buds fuse together. 4, The ventral bud becomes part of the head of the pancreas (the PP-rich duodenal lobe), whereas the dorsal bud gives rise to the body and tail (the glucagon-rich splenic lobe); the pancreatic juice is drained off by the main and the accessory pancreatic ducts. s, stomach; b, bile duct; d, dorsal bud; v, ventral bud.*

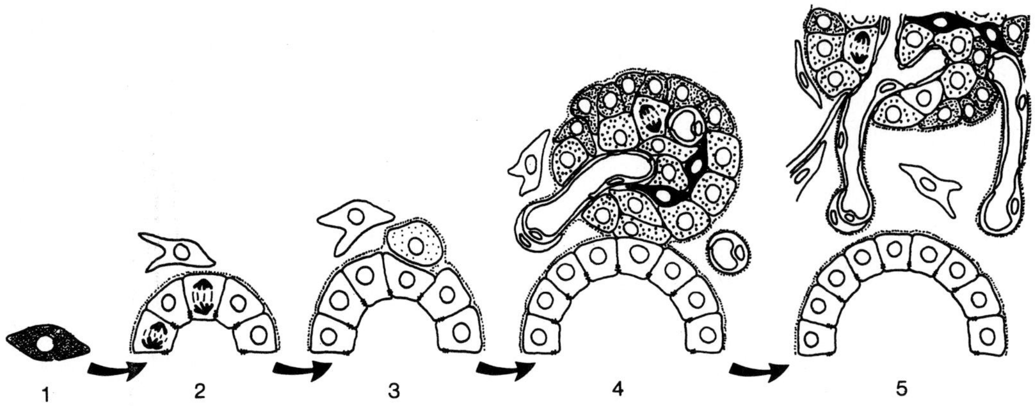

FIGURE 47–2. Schematic view of the differentiation of islet cells. *1,* Postulated primitive precursor cell, characterized by the amine precursor uptake and decarboxylation (APUD) property and the presence of neuron-specific enolase. *2,* Inversion of the polarity of mitotic division in specific epithelial duct cells gives rise to committed endocrine cells. The mesenchyme may intervene in the process. *3,* One daughter cell remains connected with the epithelial layer by junctional complexes; the other is free and penetrates the mesenchymal tissue. *4,* The "ductal" islet is still connected to the duct epithelium. The blood supply invades the islet cell cluster. The various cell types arise either from the same or from different precursors, which may be located within the duct epithelium or within the islet. *5,* In a later stage, the islets separate from the duct. Growth proceeds by mitoses of differentiated cells. Less differentiated precursors within the islet may contribute. A pool of committed cells within the duct epithelium may be present. Islets are innervated.

Cell Lineage

Pancreatic development and differentiation into different pancreatic cells is achieved through the expression or repression of transcription factors at critical moments of pancreatic development. The phenotype differences are presumably determined by the expression of specific sets of transcription factors. They allow cells to react to signals of the surrounding tissue. The interactions between the different transcription factors modulate their activities. A particularly impressive example of this characteristic is the ability of Pdx1 to orchestrate an "exocrine-endocrine switch" in pancreatic cells, depending on the presence or absence of other transcription factors.[23] Phenotypes of the fully differentiated pancreatic cells are also maintained due to the expression of specific transcription factors which, at the same time, may repress genes including transcription factors expressed in other pancreatic cell types.

Comprehensive information on this subject may be found in several reviews.[24–28] This flourishing investigation may be summarized briefly as follows (Fig. 47–3): In mice, the onset of pancreatic development occurs around day F8.5 (10-somite stage) of fetal development in the sonic hedgehog–negative part of the gut wall, with concomitant expression of Pdx1, the master regulator of pancreatic development. At this stage, it confers competence to early epithelial cells to grow, branch, and differentiate. However, other transcription factor(s) must exist upstream of Pdx1, because a few glucagon and insulin cells are still found in Pdx1(-/-) mice characterized by pancreatic agenesis. During the next 2 days several transcription factors appear either in subsets of, or in all precursor cells.

Around day F10.5, Pdx1 expression is downregulated. Future exocrine cells segregate from endocrine cell precursors at this stage, each pancreatic cell type starting its own specific chain of expression and repression of transcription factors. A second burst of Pdx1 expression followed by an increased Nkx6.1 expression is observed around day F13.5 in immature β cells. At birth, exocrine cells and each subpopulation of endocrine cells feature a specific set of transcription factors.

In addition to their roles in pancreatic development, the transcription factors are also involved in pancreatic function.[24–28] The bulk of the data available concerns Pdx1. Through synergistic interactions with other transcription factors it influences hormone expression and repression[24, 25, 27] and is one of the glucose-responsive elements involved in insulin gene transcription.[25–28] Pdx1 also participates in the activation of other genes such as IAPP, glucokinase, and GLUT2 specifically expressed in β cells.[25, 26, 28]

Even if the hypothesis of the neuroectodermal origin of islet cells has become obsolete, the pancreatic endocrine cells maintain close relations with neural elements during development and at the adult stage.

Para- and orthosympathetic innervations, as well as their respective roles in inducing "postprandial hypoglycemic" (acetylcholine) and "stress-induced hyperglycemic" (epinephrine, norepinephrine) effects, have been well evaluated.[29–33] In addition, these innervations contain peptide neurotransmitters with matching activity. For example, orthosympathetic islet nerves contain galanin and neuropeptide Y (NPY), which inhibit insulin secretion,[34–36] while parasympathetic nerves contain vasoactive intestinal polypeptide (VIP) and gastrin-releasing peptide (GRP), which are insulinotropic neurotransmitters.[37] The functional roles of other aminergic or peptidergic pancreatic neurotransmitters such as serotonin,[38–40] dopamine,[41] enkephalin, substance P, and cholecystokinin (CCK)[42–46] remain unclear. Moreover, islet endocrine cells may contain amine or neural peptides beyond their own hormonal products.[42, 46]

During development islet cells also express a variety of neurohormones other than classic islet peptides. Their role is not completely defined, but besides hormonal function, they take part in intraislet homeostasis. IAPP, peptide YY (PYY), and NPY, having inhibitor activity on insulin release, might contribute to the unresponsiveness of the fetal β cell to glucose, thereby protecting the fetus from hypoglycemia during development.[47] These neuropeptides are expressed very early in the endocrine pancreas.[48, 49] In the rat, the first PYY appears at day F12, when the fusion of the ventral and dorsal pancreatic anlage has occurred. PYY is detected in the endocrine cells expressing also insulin and glucagon. At that time NPY is limited to interlobulary nerves around blood vessels and the duct. NPY messenger RNA (mRNA) appears at day F16 and its protein at day F17 in insulin-positive cells, while PYY disappears from the β cell and remains confined to the glucagon-positive cells only. Hence, the two endocrine cell populations can be distinguished. At birth, NPY mRNA disappears from the β cell, and its protein 5 days later. It remains solely in the neural elements as described in adult endocrine pancreas.

γ-Aminobutyric acid (GABA) may also illustrate the complexity of the neural and endocrine relationship within islets. GABAergic nerve cell bodies are present at the periphery of islets with numerous GABA-containing processes extending into the islet mantle.[50] In addition to that intraislet GABAergic innervation, insulin-secreting cells are the only endocrine islet cells that contain, synthesize, and degrade GABA. Its concentration is comparable to that observed in the brain. This amino acid seems to be present in the nuclei, cytosol, and mitochondria and absent from the secretory granules[50, 51] and is not coreleased with insulin.[52] During development, modification of the GABA concentration follows the same evolution as the increase in β cell number. Furthermore, GABA is taken up by somatostatin cells and these, as

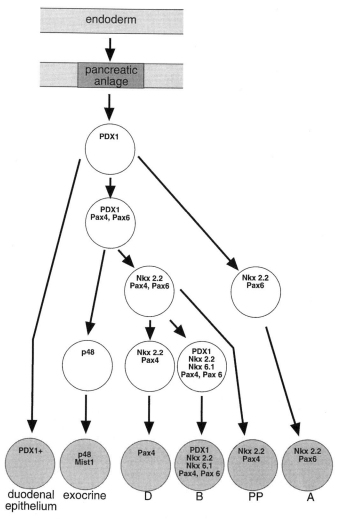

FIGURE 47–3. *Schematic representation of selected markers expressed during the commitment and differentiation of the pancreatic endocrine cells. From the primitive endoderm segregates the pancreatic anlage, which gives rise to the exocrine and endocrine cells (β, α, δ, and PP). This identification is still provisional.*

The IAPP gene is expressed in β cells,[62] and this 37–amino acid peptide is synthesized by the β cell using the same processing enzyme(s) that converts proinsulin to insulin. In many species, IAPP is expressed early during fetal development, possibly before insulin.[63] IAPP is stored in secretory granules of immature pluripotential endocrine cells of the pancreas from 14-week-old human fetuses.[64] IAPP might act as a vasodilator in the islet and also be a growth factor. In rat, IAPP was found in pluripotent islet progenitor cells residing in the primitive ductular epithelium, together with PYY, glucagon, and to a lesser extent with insulin. As development proceeds, the insulin-IAPP phenotype is segregated from that of PYY-glucagon and when islet structures appear, insulin-IAPP–expressing cells primarily occupy their central portions, while PYY-glucagon–expressing cells are found in the periphery.[47]

The functional relation of IAPP and insulin and the timing of gene expression of the two hormones may be different in the human fetus than in adults, indicating that the relation between IAPP and insulin may be less tightly linked in fetal than adult cells. Neonatal somatostatin and glucagon cell lines co-express IAPP together with their respective hormones.[65]

Based on the co-expression of hormones and neuropeptides in immature endocrine cells, an islet cell lineage has been proposed. Other marker proteins may also help to delineate the steps in the lineage. In rodents, GLUt2 is restricted only to β cells. However, during ontogeny a large population of undifferentiated cells from the pancreatic epithelium are GLUt2-positive. Some of these cells maintain this expression, giving rise to β cells, whereas the others lose the ability to express this problem and differentiate into acinar cells.[66]

THE CYTOLOGIC ORGANIZATION OF THE ISLETS

The cytologic organization and cellular ultrastructure of pancreatic islets have been described in detail in a previous edition of this book,[67] and several reviews offer further updated morphologic data.[14, 68–74]

The islets of Langerhans consist of a neuroendocrine complex which comprises islets, neuronal ganglia, and nerve fibers, as well as fenestrated capillaries along which the islet cells are distributed. The fluid mosaic plasma membrane is the site of information input, and the main structurally visible specialization on these endocrine cells is the gap junction, through which transmembrane channels permit transfer of low-molecular-weight substances between adjacent homologous or heterologous endocrine cell types.[75, 76] Changes in the gap junctions may be related to the functional state of the β cells,[77] but how they are involved in pathologic states is not known.

The typical organization of islet cells, which is not random, but organized as a core of β cells surrounded by the three other non–B cell types, depends on cell adhesion molecules (CAMs), which exist on the surface of endocrine cells.[78, 79] They are needed to develop and maintain normal tissue structure and function. They are mediators of cell-cell interactions and regulators of cell fate determination by influencing growth, differentiation, and organization within tissues. The epithelial cell adhesion molecule (Ep-CAM, human pancarcinoma antigen) has a morphoregulatory role in pancreatic islet development[80] where its highest levels are found in islet-like cell clusters budding from the ductal epithelium. The Ca^{2+}-independent neural cell adhesion molecule (NCAM) is required for cell-type segregation during organogenesis and its presence is restricted to the endocrine tissue and nerve endings. In its absence, the islet cell distribution becomes randomized and its initial structure is lost.[81] The initial clustering of β cells is also dependent on cadherins, a Ca^{2+}-dependent family of CAMs. In their absence the clustering of cells disappear except for a specific aggregation of α cells.[82]

Good evidence suggests that the characteristic three-dimensional organization of the islet is of physiologic significance. Experiments involving dissociation of adult rat islets into single cells show a loss of regulated function in vitro, whereas spontaneous reaggregation is associated with restoration of normal basal and glucose-stimulated insulin release.[83–85]

In β cells (Fig. 47–4), besides ancillary cytoplasmic organelles such

well as glucagon cells, seem to possess GABA$_A$ receptors. Although GABA does not appear to affect insulin secretion, it inhibits that of glucagon and somatostatin.[53] The GABA shunt enzymes, glutamate decarboxylase (GAD) and GABA transaminase (GABA-T), have also been localized within the β cells. Lately two isoforms of GAD, the 65-kDa and 67-kDa molecules, have been identified.[54] GAD 65 and 67 are detected in human fetal β, α, and duct epithelial cells.[55] In the bovine and ovine fetal pancreas, GAD 65 is localized predominantly in the β cell, but also is seen in a smaller proportion of α cells, although it is confined to the β cell in adulthood.[56, 57] This suggests a role of GAD 65 in early development of pancreatic islets. In addition, GAD has been recognized as a key immune target during the initial stages of insulin-dependent diabetes mellitus (IDDM).[56, 58, 59]

The functional significance of the intricate nervous system relationships during the development of islets is unknown. Definite innervation seems unnecessary for proper islet formation, as shown by in vitro culture of pancreatic rudiments, but a possible modulating activity of neural interplay may intervene. In late developmental stages, innervation close to endocrine cells and capillaries is apparent, and receptors on islet cells for neuromediators are present.[60]

Special mention should be made of the IAPP. IAPP is closely related to the calcitonin gene–related peptide (CGRP). The presence of CGRP in immunoreactive nerve fibers is a feature common to all vertebrate pancreata, but the localization of CGRP immunoreactivity in the islet endocrine cells is restricted to some mammalian pancreata.[61]

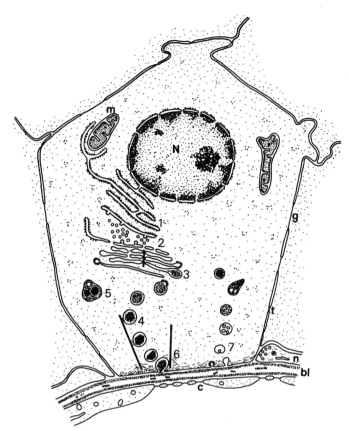

FIGURE 47–4. Schematic summary of the secretory process in the β cell. *1,* Biosynthesis of (pre)proinsulin in the rough endoplasmic reticulum. *2,* Transfer of proinsulin to the Golgi complex, via the microvesicles or the cisternae of the endoplasmic reticulum. *3,* Conversion of proinsulin to insulin and storage in membrane-limited granules. *4,* End of the conversion process and crystallization of hexameric insulin-zinc. *5,* Occasional degradation of the secretory product by crinophagy. *6,* Exocytotic liberation of insulin granules, mediated by the cytoskeleton of microtubules and microfilaments. *7,* Membrane recycling by endocytotic pathway. N, nucleus; m, mitochondria; g, gap junction; t, tight junction; bl, basal lamina; c, fenestrated endothelium; n, nerve.

as mitochondria and lysosomes, the rough endoplasmic reticulum is the site where the hormonal precursor preproinsulin is cleaved to form proinsulin, which is transported to the Golgi complex, where it is packaged in membranous sacs. During this process, the cell takes care of this sequential cleavage of proinsulin into insulin, split 33, 32 proinsulin, and C peptide.

A cytoskeletal structure composed of microtubules interconnected with microfilaments[86–89] is responsible for the transport of the mature insulin granules which are usually released by exocytosis, leaving behind large exocytotic pits. The complex kinetics of insulin secretion may be in part a reflection of multiple insulin compartments within the secretory sac.[90] Ionic movements such as shifts of intracellular calcium[91] are related to the changes of membrane potentials as verified by electrophysiologic studies of β cells.[92–95] They add to the shared specific connections of the islet cells with each other to create a complex and heterogeneous secretory microorgan.[96–97]

Glucose is the major nutrient secretagogue of insulin and mediates insulin secretion mainly by the following process: glucose metabolism and mitochondrial phosphorylation leading to generation of adenosine triphosphate (ATP), depolarization of the plasma membrane due to closure of the ATP-sensitive K^+ channel and an increase in the intracellular free Ca^{2+} through the voltage-dependent channel, is followed by activation of the secretory machinery leading to insulin release.

The development of the normal insulin secretory response in many mammals does not occur before birth which may protect the fetus against hyperglycemia. The β cells of the fetus are able, however, to

synthesize and release insulin in response to agents that increase cyclic adenosine monophosphate (cAMP), activate enzyme protein kinase C,[98] and raise Ca^{2+} levels,[99] although their response to glucose stimulation in vivo or in vitro never displays a biphasic pattern as seen in adult islets. The difference between the fetal and postnatal response could be due to abnormal glucose transport since the synthesis of GLUT2 is reduced by 50% in fetal β cells compared to neonates.[100] Other reasons could be evoked, such as differences in ion channel population of the plasma membrane, or immature glucose metabolism. Fetal β cells are able, however, to secrete insulin when challenged by agents such as leucine, arginine, or sulphonylureas elevating the intracellular Ca^{2+} concentration through glucose-independent pathways. Therefore, the fetal β cells are characterized by being functional, but insensitive to an early stimulation by glucose.

THE LIFE CYCLE OF THE β CELL

Early microscopic studies of pancreatic tissue from diabetic subjects showed a combined picture of disappearing islet cells or their remnants together with evidence of regenerative processes.[101, 102] Under nonpathologic circumstances, β cells were considered for many years to be terminally differentiated and unchanged after birth, but it is clear now that the dynamic balance between β cell growth and degeneration determines the availability of its secretory product and hence the insulin levels present in biologic fluids that reach the target tissues.

In addition, the dynamics of the β cell mass can adapt to various situations to maintain glucose homeostasis. Again, this natural adaptation occurs by a careful balance between β cell birth and death by apoptosis. β cell birth can be achieved by two processes: differentiation from precursor stem cell (neogenesis) and by replication of already differentiated β cells. Diabetes may ensue if the loss is not associated with an appropriate replacement of β cells.

In the fetus, the β cell mass grows exponentially through both β cell replication and recruitment of undifferentiated β cells from pancreatic ducts.[103, 104] The rate of cell death by apoptosis is low. After birth, the growth rate of islet cells, including the β cell, decreases to reach adult values at weaning. However, a considerable turnover of the β cell population occurs within the 3 weeks after birth. A burst of apoptosis occurs in the endocrine pancreas of 10 to 15-day-old rats.[105] Since the total pancreatic β cell mass is not substantially changed, this suggests that a new population of β cells derived from replication or neogenesis compensates for the loss. A similar wave of β cell apoptosis has been recently described in humans.[106] The significance of this peculiar ontogeny may reflect a change in the β cell population which is necessary to evolve from fetal to postnatal life. The fetal β cell population would be suited to intrauterine life in which acute insulin release is not necessary within a stable nutritional environment. After birth the need to rapidly release insulin under the nutritional, endocrine, and neural control characteristics of adult metabolism appears. Insulin-like growth factor (IGF)-2 (IGF-2) is present in 30% of fetal β cells and it declines after birth when IGF-1 begins to increase. The wave of apoptosis after birth has been partially attributed to the decrease of this survival factor, IGF-2.[107]

From the last stage of fetal life, 19 to 20 days in the rat, the β cell mass becomes more sensitive to modulation by various factors. β cell DNA replication occurs in response to various stimuli. The most potent factors are D-glucose and mixtures of amino acids, which are even more potent during fetal life. Amino acids, and in particular branched amino acids, may promote β cell proliferation by stimulating phosphorylation of PHAS-I (phosphorylated heat- and acid-stable protein regulated by insulin), which is a regulator of translation initiation during mitogenesis, and by facilitating the proliferative effects mediated by growth factors.[108] The replication of β cells that express growth hormone (GH) and prolactin receptors can also be stimulated by these two hormones.[109] Although GH stimulates IGF-1 release from both fetal and adult islets, the mediation of the mitogenic activity of GH by IGFs remains elusive.[110, 111] The latter stimulate the expression of insulin and of a preadipocyte factor, a β cell product abundant during the perinatal period and involved in the differentiation and growth of the β cell.[112] IGF-binding proteins (IGFBPs) play a decisive role in the mitogenic stimulation of β cells. Indeed, IGF-BPs do not act solely as carriers of IGFs but also influence the availability and the biologic activity of IGFs at the cellular level.[113, 114] Insulin itself, interacting with IGF-1 receptors,[102] also stimulates islet cell replication.[115] In addition, different polypeptide growth factors may regulate islet cell replication, such as hepatocyte growth factors, epidermal growth factor, TGF-α, and peptides from the gastrointestinal tract.[109, 111] Moreover, β cell replication capacity is a function of the genetic background, as demonstrated in rodent strains.[116] During the last stages of fetal development, nutrients may also reach the fetal gastrointestinal mucosa. By this time, the mucosa has acquired the structural maturation allowing absorption of the glucose- and amino acid–rich amniotic fluid.[117, 118] It is precisely at this period of late fetal life that an enormous growth of β cell mass occurs.

Using in vitro–cultured late fetal islets, the cycle of β cells could similarly be studied.[111, 119] The generation time, which is the time needed for a single parent cell to form two daughter cells, is 14.9 hours for the rat β cell. By comparison, the normal range for an epithelial cell to cycle is 9 to 24 hours. In β cells, the G_1 phase (before DNA synthesis) takes 2.5 hours in vitro; the S phase (DNA synthesis), 6.4 hours; the G_2 phase (premitotic), 5.5 hours; and mitosis, 0.5 hour. Glucose is mitogenic for β cells, and its availability in higher concentration produces an increased number of β cells in vitro and in vivo.[120, 121] Experiments on synchronized islet cells indicate that glucose stimulates the proliferation by regulating the number of β cells passing through the cell cycle rather than altering the duration of the cell cycle. A small pool of β cells has a higher capacity for cell division, but most of the β cells are in an irreversible G_0 phase and are unable to reenter the cell cycle.[111] However, another model emerged from experiments with prolactin stimulation of unsynchronized islet cells. It suggests that a mitogenic response occurs by recruitment of quiescent β cells into the cell cycle and by limiting the exit from the cell cycle by the daughter cells.[119] From the latter study, it was concluded that most of the β cells are not in an irreversible G_0 state and probably retain a rather limited capacity for cell division (Fig. 47–5).

The β cell mass can adapt to physiologic conditions. Indeed, during pregnancy, there is an increase in β cells in the rat as well as in humans,[122] presumably in order to produce more insulin to fulfill the anabolic needs of the fetus. This is ascribable to an increase in cell number, probably due to the direct effect of an increase in prolactin and placental lactogen on the β cell replication pathway, rather than on neogenesis from ductal precursor. During that period, food intake is increased and could also be in part responsible for islet cell proliferation and increased insulin secretion.[123] After pregnancy the hyperplasia of the β cells resolves by apoptosis.[124] Obesity, which leads to insulin resistance, requires an increased insulin secretion which could also be achieved by an augmentation of the β cell mass.[125]

THE VASCULARIZATION OF THE PANCREAS

An adequate islet blood flow is critical for both the oxygen and the nutrient supply to the endocrine cells and the distribution of islet hormones to be supplied to target cells.

The macrovascularization of the pancreas is disparate, since the dorsal lobe is essentially supplied by branches from the celiac trunk (via the gastroduodenal and splenic arteries), while the ventral lobe is vascularized by the superior mesenteric artery (via the inferior pancreaticoduodenal artery).[96] The arterial blood in the rat, as well as in the human pancreas, preferentially flows through the insular-acinar portal route. Neither the insular-venous routes nor the lobular and ductal route interferes with the insular-acinar portal route that conveys high concentrations of insular hormones to the exocrine acini.[126] The specific vascularization of the islet has been calculated to be 10% of the overall pancreatic blood flow, while the total islet mass, at least for rats, is only 1%. When glucose is injected intra-arterially, the islet blood flow increases by 80%, although the total pancreatic blood flow increases by only 10%.[127] Although the whole pancreatic blood flow decreases progressively with age in rats, the islet blood flow increases. Adult and aging animals also showed a marked preferential islet blood flow in response to a glucose stimulus.[127, 128] This was not the case in growing younger animals, in which pancreatic blood flow and islet blood flow increased in concert.[129] In obese animals, islet blood flow increased in the first instance but decreased with age to a level lower than normal, which could be implicated in the impaired islet function in these animals.[130] A decreased islet blood flow is also observed in the Goto-Kakisaki (GK) rat, a model of type 2 diabetes.[112]

The microvascularization of the islets is also heterogeneous and related to islet size. The vascular volume and the numeric density of islet capillaries are lower in the smaller islets. In the classic view,

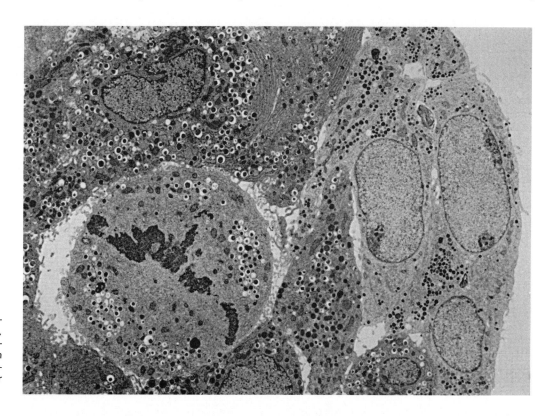

FIGURE 47–5. Electron micrograph of a cultured fetal rat islet, showing mitosis of a differentiated β cell containing insulin granules. The metaphase chromosomes are visible in the center of the cell.

afferent vessels enter the islet through discontinuities of the non–β cell mantle and divide into capillaries, which are surrounded by β cells. The efferent vessels pass through the heterocellular layer of peripheral endocrine cells.[97, 131, 132] It is interesting that after islet transplantation, the capillary glomerulus-like network of the islet graft was found supplied by individual arterioles, which regularly pierced the islet and divided into capillaries within the graft.[133] However, the inverse route, by which blood mainly flows from the α, δ cell mantle to the core, has been suggested after arterial injections of resin causing reduced blood flow to the islets.[126]

The vascular arrangements do not seem to be influenced by age, pregnancy, or lactation, and the structural integrity of the ducts, as well as that of their vascular supply, should help maintain the population of ductal islets. Pathologic damage provoked by congenital, degenerative, or inflammatory disease could be deleterious. If it occurs during prenatal development, the capacity for postnatal β cell multiplication and regeneration might be impaired.

The organization of the capillary network has a prominent functional role that also becomes apparent when considering the precise interrelations between the δ cells.[97, 131] The latter show an alignment with the capillaries of the peripheral area and a preferential mutual connection with each other. Juxtaposition of the δ cells to both β and α cells also exists to a certain extent, as well as privileged heterologous contact with β cells alone. The contiguity of the δ cells with each other, together with their angioarchitectural organization with cytoplasmic extensions, creates a functional unit wherein the secretion is directed toward the vascular poles. The intercellular impulses could preferentially reach a large number of cells through the vascular bed, but could also reach a restricted number of immediately adjacent cells by the perivascular or paracrine route to carry out a coordinated function.

THE PATHOMORPHOLOGY OF THE ENDOCRINE PANCREAS

For the clinician, the onset, evolution, and symptomatology of diabetes are heterogeneous, and the etiology of "idiopathic" diabetes should also be disparate. Since the advent of serum insulin measurements, the metabolic disturbances of diabetes mellitus have been related to absolute or relative insulin deficiency. The clinical evolution of diabetes is characterized by a fascinating heterogeneity.

Technical and methodologic achievements give further support to the clinical distinction that is being made between the different types of diabetes. They also nurture new advances, which may help to untangle the enigma of diabetes by linking the cytology, secretion, and proliferation of β cells to each other.

Variable qualitative and quantitative changes in the morphology of the endocrine and exocrine pancreas should reflect the variety of modulating environmental factors and genetic backgrounds that determine the clinical evolution of the disease. In regard to the life cycle of a β cell, stimulation and insults could induce differential effects depending on their time of occurrence. They may occur during crucial times of fetal life. They may develop in the course of physiologic adaptations, such as in pregnancy, or in stress situations.[134, 135] Later, the development of diabetes depends on the adaptation of β cells to acute or slow destructive processes or to changes in peripheral tissues.[135, 136] In addition, the pathomorphology of the diabetic pancreas can be better interpreted by integrating it into the clinical picture of the individual's diabetic condition.

At least two different types of disease are described. A relatively acute evolution toward major insulinopenia may exist. This is called type 1 diabetes, or insulin-dependent diabetes mellitus, which usually occurs in children or adolescents and is thus growth-related and may be life-threatening. It may also affect adults.[137] IDDM is caused by the progressive autoimmune destruction of insulin-producing pancreatic β cells. The first detailed study of the insulitis was provided by Gepts,[138] who described it in 15 of 22 type 1 diabetic patients who died within 6 months of the clinical onset of their disease. Although the pathogenesis of autoimmune IDDM has been extensively studied since that time, the precise mechanisms involved in the initiation and progression of β cell destruction remain unclear.[139]

Type 1 Diabetes

At the onset of type 1 diabetes, immune disregulation results in the appearance of antibodies against components of the insulin-secreting cells, namely insulin itself, islet cell antigen (ICA), islet cell surface antigen (ICSA), GAD 65 and GAD 67, and heat shock protein 65 (hsp 65).[140, 141] Macrophages or dendritic cells are the first cell types to infiltrate the pancreatic islets. The presentation of β cell–specific autoantigens by these cells to CD4$^+$ T helper cells in association with major histocompatibility complex (MHC) class II molecules is considered the initial step in the development of autoimmune IDDM.[139] The migration of the macrophages, autoreactive lymphocytes, and other leukocytes from the blood stream into the islets is controlled in part by selective expression and functional regulation of CAMs on the surface of the mononuclear cells and vascular endothelial cells or in the extracellular matrix.[142] This is a typical picture of the described "insulitis." A variety of cytokines implicated in the pathogenesis of IDDM have been found to be expressed at the gene or protein level or both in the insulitis lesion of animals with autoimmune diabetes, including the nonobese diabetic (NOD) mouse and the BB rat, as well as in the pancreata of an IDDM patient.[143, 144]

A current hypothesis is that the autoreactive T cells are a T$_H$1 subset identified by its distinct cytokine products interleukin (IL)-2 (IL-2), interferon-γ (IFN-γ), and tumor necrosis factor-β (TNF-β), whereas the protective limb of the immune response may be mediated by T$_H$2 subsets that produce IL-4 and IL-10. According to this concept, T$_H$1 cells and their cytokine products activate macrophages and cytotoxic T cells to destroy β cells, causing IDDM, while T$_H$2 and their cytokine products downregulate T$_H$1 cells and cytokines and thereby prevent IDDM. Activated macrophages produce IL-1 and TNF-α and activated T cells produce TNF-α, TNF-β, and IFN-γ. These cytokines bind to specific receptors on β cells and elicit signals that activate different pathways leading to β cell death.[145, 146]

Besides lesions of insulitis, pseudoatrophic islets, as well as islets with regenerating β cells, are found in individuals with diabetes of recent onset. The destructive process may eventually exceed the regenerative capacity of β cells, resulting in insulinopenia and the characteristic metabolic derangement of type 1 diabetes.

If the process of insulitis is now being deciphered, the cause is still largely unclear. For further information on the pathogenesis of type 1 diabetes, see Chapter 54.

Type 2 Diabetes

Another type of diabetes, type 2 (non–insulin-dependent diabetes mellitus, or NIDDM), features disturbances in the secretory pattern of insulin and may progress to insulinopenia relative to insulin requirements. It occurs predominantly in adults.

The complications of the disease seem comparable in both types of diabetes. Other clinical situations associated with diabetes mellitus are acromegaly, Cushing's disease, pheochromocytoma, glucagonoma, and hemochromatosis; these conditions may be associated with specific changes of structure or function in the endocrine pancreas. In the diabetic syndrome accompanying genetic diseases, characteristic changes in the islets may also be seen. Diabetes in the tropics, in special ethnic groups, in regions with endemic infections, and in cases of undernutrition[147] may also be associated with specific lesions in the pancreas.

The variable clinical course of type 2 diabetes is reflected in morphologic changes in the pancreas, with quantitative changes noted in some type 2 diabetic patients, whereas others do not show obvious pathologic lesions. It should be noted that some individuals with a clinical course characteristic of NIDDM may have circulating ICSAs and develop type 1 diabetes at a later time. These patients should be classified as having late-onset type 1 diabetes, with pancreatic morphologic changes consistent with type 1 diabetes.

Because type 2 diabetes often coexists with obesity, the effect of the latter condition upon the morphology of islets is relevant, although there are few data in humans. Obese but nondiabetic subjects show an increased β cell volume, suggesting that under prediabetic conditions, the β cells still have the capacity to respond to increased functional demand by enhanced proliferation.[148] This finding was also noted in obese rodents.[149] The increased β cell mass results in high circulating insulin levels in obese humans and animals. In manifest diabetes, the β cells have lost their proliferative potential. They are always present, regardless of the duration and severity of the disease, but lack any signs of functional activity.[148]

A significant feature that has been described in the endocrine pancreas of patients with NIDDM is deposits of amyloid, which may occur in 25% to 92% of cases, depending on the particular series.[70, 150, 151] In nondiabetic persons, amyloid deposits are confined to a very few islets in the tail of the pancreas.[150] The extent of the amyloid deposits seems to be related to age and the need for insulin therapy, and therefore to the severity of β cell destruction. Once the lesion has been initiated, a continuous process seems to be set in motion which is not halted by diet or oral hypoglycemic drugs.[152, 153] Islet amyloid is characteristic of type 2 diabetes in every human population examined to date, including whites,[154] Pima Indians,[152] Asian Indians,[155] and Japanese.[156] It seems to be a ubiquitous event, possibly induced by environmental factors and not limited to a specific genetic background. Amyloid deposits do not occur in type 1 diabetes.

Amyloid deposits in the human consist predominantly of IAPP. Occurrence of islet amyloid is paradoxically associated with the loss of IAPP immunoreactivity in the β cell itself.[157] The deposits are situated within the boundaries of the islets between the endocrine cells and the islet capillaries.[158] Fibrils invaginate the margins of the β cell adjacent to the amyloid deposits. The latter also contain other substances, such as apolipoprotein E, heparan sulfate, amyloid P protein, proteoglycan, and perlecan.[159] In addition, cellular debris, such as insulin granules and tubulin, is present. Because amyloid formation precedes the occurrence of hyperglycemia in animals, the impact of a small amount of amyloid on insulin secretion needs to be further assessed. However, amyloid deposits are associated with dead or degenerating β cells, and intracellular IAPP amyloid causes cell death by triggering apoptotic pathways.[160]

The formation of islet amyloid does not seem to depend on an individual's genetic predisposition to form amyloid or on a molecular abnormality of IAPP. It has been hypothesized that an alteration in β cell function resulting in a change in the production, processing, or secretion of IAPP, individually or severally, is critical to the initial formation of islet amyloid fibrils in human diabetes. Local conditions could induce these modifications, but they remain largely unknown. However, one factor that has been involved in such β cell changes resulting in the initiation of amyloid formation is the consumption of increased dietary fat.[159]

In contrast to human IAPP, rodent IAPP does not form amyloid fibrils, but studies in cats and nonhuman primates highlights the significance of amyloid deposits[158, 161, 162] which are detected before the onset of hyperglycemia in the development of spontaneous diabetes in these species. The degree of amyloid formation and the number of islets affected show a progressive increase associated with the severity of the disease.

A limitation in the intrinsic capacity of the β cells to divide might underlie the occurrence of type 2 diabetes in animals. Experimental models indicate the importance of the regenerative capacity of the endocrine pancreas. After pancreatectomy in five strains of rats, the regeneration of β cells was shown to be strain-specific, indicating that cell division could be genetically determined.[163] In other experiments, the regenerative capacity of endocrine pancreatic tissue has been shown to be approximately 42% of its original amount when 90% of the organ has been extirpated.[164] The compensatory growth implicates two pathways: the replication of preexisting exocrine and endocrine cells, and proliferation and differentiation of precursor cells.[165] The islets may appear normal, grossly enlarged, or small, with a markedly reduced number of non–β cells. The experimentally reduced islet mass after partial regeneration shows major functional defects. Insulin output is normal in response to a nonglucose challenge but is reduced after a glucose load. This is reminiscent of the insulin secretory pattern observed in type 2 diabetes.[166, 167] After pancreatectomy, the administration of insulin prevents the reduction of the β cell population and the fibrosis noted in regenerating islets.[136] The lowered blood sugar, the exogenously induced hyperinsulinemia, or both, may be

responsible for the prevention of the aforementioned lesions. It is conjectured that the proliferation of β cells may not be sustained if the amount of insulin secreted by the β cells is not appropriately related to the β cell mass.

In line with what has been observed in experimental models of pancreatectomy, alterations during formation and development of the endocrine pancreas in early life may have consequences for the capacity to face further demands. A pathophysiologic condition, such as diabetic gestation, highlights certain modulating effects upon fetal β cell proliferation. An increased percentage of pancreatic endocrine tissue with β cell hyperplasia and high vascularity is observed in macrosomic human neonates from diabetic mothers. The neonatal β cells from pups born to mildly diabetic rats have an increased proliferative capacity that can be confirmed after 7 days of culture.[168, 169] Cytologic analysis confirmed the higher β cell activity. These pups became glucose-intolerant in adulthood. This is associated with insulin depletion in their islets of Langerhans. The pancreata of pups born to severely diabetic rats show degranulation and degenerative changes, and the β cell replication rate is reduced[168, 169] and remains lower after 7 days of culture.[118] These pups became insulin-resistant and diabetic in adulthood. Thus, pancreatic maturation that has not proceeded through the normal phases during fetal or neonatal periods may have lasting consequences that could impair subsequent replication in response to various stimulating factors.

A major insult, common throughout the world, that may also be responsible for a reduction of the β cell mass is poor nutrition during gestation. Epidemiologic, as well as experimental, data reveal that deficient maternal nutrition during pregnancy, even over a brief period, may lead to irreversible changes in the offspring leading to obesity, diabetes, hypertension, and cardiovascular diseases in adulthood. Poor maternal nutrition during pregnancy results in fetal malnutrition. At the cellular level, the lower β cell mass with reduced vascularization leads to impaired insulin action, and then to decreased fetal growth. Fetal malnutrition may also induce alterations in the development of other organs such as the liver and kidney, and adipose tissue.

Different long-term consequences of fetal malnutrition exist which cannot be reversed by adequate nutrition postnatally. The altered β cell function may precipitate the development of NIDDM when the affected person is exposed to stress situations such as pregnancy or aging. The same is also true when these previously nutritionally deprived offspring become obese, insulin-resistant, or hyperlipidemic. There is also an increased risk of developing hypertension, which results from abnormalities in the kidneys. Ultimately, these phenomena—NIDDM, hypertension, altered organ structure and function—may lead to syndrome X, characterized by hyperlipidemia, hyperinsulinemia, hyperglycemia, insulin resistance, obesity, and hypertension and cardiovascular disease. Animal models of malnutrition show numerous aspects of these events.

Experiments in rats highlight the consequences of inadequate protein ingestion by the mother for the islet cell mass of the offspring. When a low protein isocaloric diet was fed to the mother during gestation, the endocrine pancreas of the fetus showed a reduction in volume density, insulin content, and insulin secretion. In addition, a major reduction in islet vascularization was noted.[171] The fetal and neonatal β cell mass is reduced owing to reduced proliferative capacity of the β cell in which the cell cycle is lengthened and due also to an increased rate of apoptosis in the fetal β cells.[172] Maintaining the animal on a low-protein diet until adult age confirmed these pathologic features, which were associated with a lower insulin secretion after an oral glucose challenge.[173] A normal protein diet after birth did not restore the structure or function of the endocrine pancreas to normal in adulthood.[173] However, in a first step, the progeny are able to adapt to insulinopenia by increasing the number of insulin receptors on peripheral tissues, insulin resistance subsequently develops later with age.[174–176]

Such alterations acquired during development have consequences also for the adaptation of the endocrine pancreas to pregnancy and therefore have deleterious consequences for the next generation.[177] These results indicate the sensitivity of the β cell to the lack of nutrients during development. The latter creates an abnormal metabolic environment in the mother and fetus, with low serum taurine,[178] which seems to be necessary for normal insulin secretion of the fetal β cells.[179]

Development of the endocrine pancreas is also sensitive to the lack of calories in the diet of the mother,[180] since cell mass is decreased at birth due to alteration in islet neogenesis with lasting consequences at adulthood.[181, 182]

Studies in humans are unable to identify the fundamental pathologic defects of NIDDM, which are caused by a combination of genetic and environmental factors. In prediabetic obese populations such as the Pima Indians, β cells can compensate for insulin resistance by sufficiently increasing insulin secretion and enhancing β cell sensitivity to glucose. However, when the β cell response is inadequate, glucose intolerance develops.[183] There is circumstantial evidence suggesting the presence of a primary defect in the endocrine pancreas[184]; however, it is not as convincing as a direct demonstration of specific alterations of the β cell mass. Such investigation is obviously impossible in humans, but different models of spontaneous type 2 diabetic rats have been investigated for these alterations, some of them being present very early in life. The GK rat is a genetic model of NIDDM. Already at 21.5 days, GK fetuses feature hyperglycemia and hyperinsulinemia. Their pancreatic insulin content and total β cell mass are sharply decreased and remain decreased until adulthood.[185] The impaired β cell development does not seem to be related to maternal hyperglycemia.[186] Moreover, the adult GK pancreas exhibits noticeable changes in the architecture of the large islet subpopulation, which displays considerable fibrosis with clusters of β cells widely separated from each other by strands of connective tissue.[185] The Otsuka-Long-Evans-Tokushima fatty (OLETF) rat, another genetic model of spontaneous development of NIDDM, exhibits hyperglycemic obesity with hyperinsulinemia and insulin resistance as observed in humans. Pancreatectomy experiments have demonstrated that these rats have a poor capacity for proliferation of their pancreatic β cells—a defect to which they may be genetically predisposed.[187]

Well-identified genetic defects in humans lead to specific subclasses of type 2 diabetes, such as maturity-onset diabetes of the young (MODY). MODY subtypes 1, 3, 4, and 5 are caused by mutations in four transcription factors: HNF-4α, HNF-1α, Pdx1, and MNF-1β, respectively,[188] whereas MODY 2 results from a mutation in the glucokinase gene.

For further information on the pathogenesis of type 2 diabetes, see Chapter 55.

SUMMARY

Originating from the primitive gut, the β cell differentiates among other endocrine cells with the unique predestination to convert ingested food into energy to be used by the organism by way of anabolic pathways. The number of stem cells and the growth of differentiated β cells are modified by the interaction of genetic factors and environmental events. During fetal development, the emergence of β cells and their differentiation and proliferative potential may be modified by their genetic predisposition, but at each developmental stage they may also be damaged by adverse environmental incidents. The genetic determination of the β cell generative capacity and the hereditary or acquired impairment of β cell survival determine the life course of the β cell mass. Type 1 diabetes in a subject with a characteristic predestined immunologic makeup may evolve to an acute stage by repetitive lysis of the pancreatic β cells. Regenerative processes may at first compensate for these losses, but they eventually fail with the passage of time. The pathomorphologic signs in the pancreas of a patient with type 1 diabetes reflect the degeneration of the β cells as well as their dynamic replacement. Observed first are the macrophages with insulitis (lymphocytic infiltration around the remaining β cells), and second, hyperplasia of the β cells, but the latter may not be long-lasting. The lymphocytic reaction vanishes completely when a state of absolute β cell loss and insulinopenia develops.

Type 2 diabetes appears later in life when growth is completed. This condition is associated with amyloid deposits, which result in reduction in the number of β cells and produce modest insulinopenia. The amyloid deposits occur in nonhuman primates and in humans. The underlying cause is unknown. In addition, the pathomorphologic findings reflect a lack of regenerative activity despite the presence of hyperglycemia, which should be mitogenic for postnatal β cells. Because of genetic

determination or acquired reduction of the proliferative cell pool, the β cell mass fails to regenerate. If the normal proliferation rate of the β cells is reduced, relative or absolute insulinopenia may ensue.

Clinical and experimental observations demonstrate that maternal events affecting the emergence of the β cells in the fetus and damaging their proliferative capacity may lead to diabetes later in life. The health of the mother may therefore be responsible for changes in the structure and function of the β cells of her offspring later in life. The type and degree of the exogenous stimulus, as well as the genetically determined cellular capacity to resist the insult, ultimately regulate the extent of the β cell destruction. The pathomorphologic observations that have been described indicate the basis for conclusions regarding the heterogeneity of the etiology, course, and outcome of diabetes. They provide further grounds for classification of the clinical types of diabetes and should help in understanding and preventing some of the deficiencies that β cells acquire during their life course.

REFERENCES

1. Laguesse E: Le Pancréas. Revue Générale d'Histologie. Lyon, France, A Storck et Cie, 1906.
2. Van Noorden S: The neuroendocrine system in protostomian and deutorostomian invertebrates and lower vertebrates. *In* Falkmer S, Hankanson R, Sundler F (eds): Evolution and Tumor Pathology of the Neuroendocrine System. Fernstrom Foundation Series. Amsterdam, Elsevier, 1984, pp 7–38.
3. Reinecke M, Forssmann WG: Why do we study the phylogeny of neuropeptide hormones? *In* Falkmer S, Hakanson R, Sundler F (eds): Evolution and Tumor Pathology of the Neuroendocrine System. Fernstrom Foundation Series. Amsterdam, Elsevier, 1984, pp 1–6.
4. Falkmer S, El-Salhy M, Titlbach M: Evolution of the neuroendocrine system in vertebrates. A review with particular reference to the phylogeny and postnatal maturation of the islet parenchyma. *In* Falkmer S, Hakanson R, Sundler F (eds): Evolution and Tumor Pathology of the Neuroendocrine System. Fernstrom Foundation Series. Amsterdam, Elsevier, 1984, pp 59–88.
5. Van Noorden S, Falkmer S: Gut islet endocrinology: Some evolutionary aspects. Invest Cell Pathol 3:21–35, 1980.
6. Creutzfeld W: The incretin concept today. Diabetologia 16:75–85, 1979.
7. Bonner-Weir S, Baxter LA, Schuppin GT, et al: A 2nd pathway for regeneration of adult exocrine and endocrine pancreas: A possible recapitulation of embryonic development. Diabetes 42:1715–1720, 1993.
8. Wang RN, Klöppel G, Bouwens L: Duct-to-islet-cell differentiation and islet growth in the pancreas of duct ligated adult rats. Diabetologia 38:1405–1411, 1995.
9. Rosenberg L, Vinik A: Trophic stimulation of the ductular islet cell axis: A new approach to the treatment of diabetes. Adv Expr Med Biol 321:95–104, 1992.
10. Like A, Orci L: Embryogenesis of the human pancreatic islets: A light and electron microscopic study. Diabetes 2(suppl 2): 511–534, 1972.
11. Stefan Y, Grasso S, Perrelet A, et al: The pancreatic polypeptide rich lobe of the human pancreas: Definite identification from the ventral pancreatic primordium. Diabetologia 23:141–142, 1982.
12. Clark A, Grant AM: Quantitative morphology of endocrine cells in human fetal pancreas. Diabetologia 25:31, 1983.
13. El-Salhy M, Wilander E, Grimelius L: Immunocytochemical localization of gastric inhibitory peptide (GIP) in the human fetal pancreas. Ups J Med Sci 87:81–85, 1982.
14. Van Assche FA, Hoet JJ, Jack PMB: Endocrine pancreas of the pregnant mother, fetus and the newhorn. *In* Beard RW, Nathanielsz PW (eds): Fetal Physiology and Medicine, (ed 2). New York, Marcel Dekker, 1984, pp 127–152.
15. Pearse A, Takor-Takor T: Embryology of the diffuse neuro-endocrine system and its relationship to the peptides. Fed Proc 38:2288–2294, 1979.
16. Pearse A: The cytochemistry and ultrastructure of polypeptide hormone producing cells of the APUD series and the embryologic, physiologic and pathologic implications of the concept. J Histochem Cytochem 17:303–313, 1979.
17. Pictet R, Rutter WJ: Development of the embryonic pancreas. *In* Steiner DF, Freinkel N (eds): Handbook of Physiology. Section 7: Endocrinology, vol. 1. Endocrine Pancreas. Washington DC, American Physiological Society, 1972, pp 25–66.
18. Rutter WJ: The development of the endocrine and exocrine pancreas. *In* Fitzgerald PJ, Morrison X (eds): The Pancreas. Baltimore, Williams & Wilkins, 1980, pp 30–38.
19. Rutter WJ, Pictet R, Harding JD, et al: An analysis of pancreatic development: role of mesenchymal factor and other extracellular factors. *In* Papaconstantinou J, Rutter WJ (eds): 35th Symposium of the Society of Developmental Biologists. New York, Academic Press, 1978, pp 205–227.
20. Gittes GK, Galante PE, Hanahan D, et al: Lineage specific morphogenesis in the developing pancreas: Role of mesenchymal factors. Development 122:439–447, 1996.
21. Miralles F, Czernichow P, Scharfmann R: Follistatin regulates the relative proportions of endocrine versus exocrine tissue during pancreatic development. Development 125:1017–1024, 1998.
22. Miralles F, Battelino T, Czernichow P, et al: TGF-beta plays a key role in morphogenesis of the pancreatic islets of Langerhans by controlling the activity of the matrix metalloproteinase MMP-2. J Cell Biol 143:827–836, 1998.
23. Swift GH, Liu Y, Rose SD, et al: An endocrine-exocrine switch in the activity of the pancreatic homeodomain protein PDX1 through formation of a trimeric complex with PBX1b and MRG1 (MEIS2). Mol Cell Biol 18:5109–5120, 1998.
24. Edlund H: Perspectives in diabetes. Transcribing pancreas. Diabetes 47:1817–1823, 1998.
25. Habener JF, Stoffers DA: A newly discovered role of transcription factors involved

in pancreas development and the pathogenesis of diabetes mellitus. Proc Assoc Am Physicians 110:12–21, 1998.

26. Madsen OD, Jensen J, Blume N, et al: Pancreatic development and maturation of the islet B cell. Studies of pluripotent islet cultures. Eur J Biochem 24:435–445, 1996.

27. Sander M, German MS: The β cell transcription factors and development of the pancreas. J Mol Med 75:327–340, 1997.

28. Yamaoka T, Itakura M: Development of pancreatic islets (review). Int J Mol Med 3:247–261, 1999.

29. Bereiter DA, Rohner-Jeanrenaud F, Berthoud HR, et al: CNS modulation of pancreatic endocrine function. Diabetologia 20:417–425, 1981.

30. Rohner-Jeanrenaud F, Jeanrenaud B: L'axe système nerveux central (SNC)-pancréas endocrine. Ann Endocrinol 44:217–227, 1983.

31. Helman A, Marre M, Bobbioni E, et al: The brain-islet axis: The nervous control of the endocrine pancreas. Diabet Metab 8:53–64, 1983.

32. Amenta F, Cavallotti C, De Rossi M, et al: The cholinergic innervation of the human pancreatic islets. Acta Histochem 73:273–278, 1983.

33. Campfield LA, Smith FJ: Neural control of insulin secretion. Interaction of norepinephrine and acetyl-choline. Regul Integrative Comp Physiol 13:629–634, 1983.

34. Dunning BE, Havel PJ, Veith RC, et al: Pancreatic and extrapancreatic galamin release during sympathetic neural activation in dogs. Am J Physiol 258:E436–E440, 1990.

35. Havel P, Parry S, Curry D, et al: Autonomic nervous system conscious rats. Endocrinology 130:2225–2229, 1992.

36. Skoglung G, Gross RA, Bertrand GR, et al: Comparison of effects of neuropeptides Y and norepinephrine on insulin secretion and vascular resistance in perfused rat pancreas. Diabetes 40:660–665, 1991.

37. Ahren B, Ostenson CG, Efendic S: Other islet peptides. In Samols E (ed): The Endocrine Pancreas. New York, Raven Press, 1991, pp 153–173.

38. Bird LJ, Wright EE, Feldman M: Pancreatic islets. A tissue rich in serotonin. Diabetes 29:304–308, 1980.

39. Koevary SB, Azmitia EC, Mc Evoy RC: Rat pancreatic serotoninergic nerves: Morphologic, pharmacologic and physiologic studies. Brain Res 265:328–332, 1983.

40. Koevary SB, Mc Evoy RC, Azmitia EC: Evidence for the presence of serotoninergic perikarya in the fetal rat pancreas as demonstrated by the high affinity uptake of (3H)-5-HT. Brain Res 280:368–372, 1983.

41. Lindstrom P: Modification of mouse islet function by 5-hydroxytryptamine dopamine and their precursors. Acta Biol Med Germ 41:118–1190, 1982.

42. Larsson LI: New aspects on the neural paracrine and endocrine regulation of islet function. Front Horm Res 7:14–29, 1980.

43. Rehfeld JH, Larsson LI, Golterman NR, et al: Neural regulation of pancreatic hormone secretion by the C-terminal tetrapeptide of CCK. Nature 284:33–38, 1980.

44. Smith PM, Madson KL: Interactions between autonomic nerves and endocrine cells of the gastroenteropancreatic system. Diabetologia 20:314–321, 1981.

45. Stach W, Radke R: Zur Innervation der Langerhansschen Inseln. Licht und elektronmikroskopische Untersuchungen am Pankreas von Laboratoriumstieren. Endokrinologie 79:210–220, 1982.

46. Hakanson R, Sundler F: The design of the neuroendocrine system: A unifying concept and its consequences. Trends Pharmacol Sci 4:41–44, 1983.

47. Mulder H, Myrsen-Axcrona U, Gebre-Medhin S, et al: Expression of non-classical islet hormone like peptides during the embryonic development of the pancreas. Microsc Res Tech 15:313–321, 1998.

48. Myrsen-Axcrona U, Ekblad E, Sundler F: Developmental expression of NPY, PYY and PP in the rat pancreas and their coexistence with islet hormones. Regul Pept 26:165–175, 1997.

49. Jackerott M, Oster A, Larsson LI: PYY in developing murine islet cells: comparisons to development of islet hormones, NPY and BrdU incorporation. J Histochem Cytochem 44:809–817, 1996.

50. Sorenson RL, Garry DG, Brelje C: Perspectives in diabetes structural and functional considerations of GABA in islets of Langerhans B cells and nerves. Diabetes 40:1365–1374, 1991.

51. Gilon P, Tappaz M, Remacle C: Localization of GAD-like immunoreactivity in the pancreas and stomach of the rat and mouse. Histochemistry 96:355–365, 1991.

52. Smismans A, Schuit F, Pipeleers D: Nutrient regulation of gamma-aminobutyric acid release from islet beta cells. Diabetologia 43:1411–1415, 1997.

53. Gilon P, Bertrand G, Loubatieres-Mariani MM, et al: The influence of α-aminobutyric acid on hormone release by the mouse and rat endocrine pancreas. Endocrinology 129:2521–2529, 1991.

54. Velloso LA, Kämpe O, Eizirik DL, et al: Human autoantibodies react with glutamic acid decarboxylase antigen in human and rat but not in mouse pancreatic islets. Diabetologia 36:39–46, 1993.

55. Mally MI, Cirulli V, Otonkoski T et al: Ontogeny and tissue distribution of human GAD expression. Diabetes 45:496–501, 1996.

56. Reddy S, Elliott RB, Poole CA, et al: Double-label immunofluorescence study of glutamic acid decarboxylase in the fetal and adult ovine pancreas by light and confocal microscopy: Evidence for predominant beta-cell coexpression. Gen Comp Endocrinol 106:301–309, 1997.

57. Reddy S, Wu D, Poole CA: Glutamic acid decarboxylase 65 and 67 isoforms in fetal, neonatal and adult porcine islets: Predominant beta cell co-localization by light and confocal microscopy. J Autoimmun 9:21–27, 1996.

58. Baekkeskov S, Aanstoot HJ, Christgau S, et al: Identification of the 64K autoantigen in insulin dependent diabetes as the GABA synthesizing enzyme glutamic acid decarboxylase. Nature 347:151–156, 1990.

59. Atkinson MA, Kaufmann D, Campbell L et al: Response of peripheral blood mononuclear cells to glutamate decarboxylase in insulin dependent diabetes. Lancet 399:458–459, 1992.

60. Milner RDG, De Gasparo M: The autonomic nervous system and perinatal metabolism. Ciba Found Symp 83:291–309, 1981.

61. Ding WG, Guo LD, Kitasato H, et al: Phylogenic study of calcitonin gene related

62. Westermark P, Engstrom U, Johnson KH, et al: Islet amyloid polypeptide: Pinpointing amino acid residues linked to amyloid fibril formation. Proc Natl Acad Sci U S A 87:5036–5040, 1990.

63. Rindi G, Terenghi G, Westermark G, et al: Islet amyloid polypeptide in proliferating B cell during development, hyperplasia and neoplasia in humans and mouse. Am J Pathol 138:1321–1325, 1991.

64. Lukinius A, Korsgren O, Grimelius L et al: Expression of islet amyloid polypeptide in fetal and adult porcine and human pancreatic islet cells. Endocrinology 137:5319–5325, 1997.

65. Madsen OD, Nielsen JH, Michelsen B, et al: Islet amyloide polypeptide and insulin expression are controlled differently in primary and transformed islet cells. Mol Endocrinol 5:143–148, 1991.

66. Pang K, Mukonoweshuro C, Wong GG: Beta cells arise from glucose transporter type 2 (GLUT2)-expressing epithelial cells of the developing rat pancreas. Proc Natl Acad Sci U S A 91:9559–9563, 1994.

67. Lacy PE, Greider MH: Anatomy and ultrastructural organization of pancreatic islets. In De Groot LJ, Odell WD, Martini L, et al (eds): Endocrinology, vol 2. New York, Grune & Stratton, 1979, pp 907–919.

68. Gepts W: Pathology of islet tissue in human diabetes. In Freinkel N, Steiner DF (eds): Handbook of Physiology. Section 7: Endocrinology, vol 1. Endocrine Pancreas. Washington, DC, American Physiological Society, 1972, pp 289–304.

69. Volk BW, Wellmann KF: The Diabetic Pancreas. New York, Plenum Press, 1977.

70. Gepts W, Lecompte PM: The pancreatic islets in diabetes. Am J Med 70:105–115, 1981.

71. Munger BL: Morphological characterization of islet cell diversity. In Cooperstein SJ, Watkins D (eds): The Islet of Langerhans. New York, Academic Press, 1981, pp 3–34.

72. Orci L: Patterns of cellular and subcellular organization in the endocrine pancreas. J Endocrinol 102:3–11, 1984.

73. Volk BW, Arquilla E, Allen R: The Diabetic Pancreas, ed 2. New York, Plenum Press, 1985.

74. Federlin KF, Scholtholt J: The Importance of Islets of Langerhans for Modern Endocrinology. New York, Raven Press, 1984.

75. Meda P, Kohen E, Kohen C, et al: Direct communication of homologous and heterologous endocrine islet cells in culture. J Cell Biol 92:221–226, 1982.

76. Meda P, Michaels RL, Halban PA, et al: In vivo modulation of gap junction and dye coupling between B cells of the intact pancreatic islet. Diabetes 32:858–868, 1983.

77. Meda P. Gap junction involvement in secretion: The pancreas experience. Clin Exp Pharmacol Physiol 23:1053–1057, 1996.

78. Rouiller DG, Cirulli V, Halban P: Difference in aggregation properties and levels of the neural cell adhesion molecule (NCAM) between islet cells types. Exp Cell Res 391:305–312, 1990.

79. Rouiller DG, Cirulli V, Halban PA: Uvomorulin mediates calcium-dependent aggregation of islet cells, whereas calcium-independent cell adhesion molecules distinguish between islet cell types. Dev Biol 148:233–242, 1991.

80. Cirulli V, Crisa L, Beattie GM, et al: KSA antigen Ep-CAM mediates cell-cell adhesion of pancreatic epithelial cells: Morphoregulatory roles in pancreatic islet development. J Cell Biol 140:1519–1534, 1998.

81. Esni F, Taljedal IB, Perk AK, et al: Neural cell adhesion molecule (N-CAM) is required for cell type segregation and normal ultrastructure in pancreatic islets. J Cell Biol 144:325–337, 1999.

82. Dahl U, Sjodin A, Semb H: Cadherins regulate aggregation of pancreatic beta cells in vivo. Development 122:2895–2902, 1996.

83. Halban P, Wollheim CB, Blondel B, et al: The possible importance of contact between pancreatic islet cells for the control of insulin release. Endocrinology 111:86–94, 1982.

84. Halban PA, Powers SL, George KL, et al: Spontaneous reassociation of dispersed adult rat pancreatic islet cells into aggregates with three dimensional architecture typical of native islets. Diabetes 36:783–790, 1987.

85. Pipeleers D, In't Veld P, Maes E, et al: Glucose induced insulin release depends on functional cooperation between islet cells. Proc Natl Acad Sci U S A 79:7322–7325, 1982.

86. Malaisse WJ, Malaisse-Lagae F, Van Obberghen E, et al: Role of microtubules in the phasic pattern of insulin release. Ann N Y Acad Sci 253:630–652, 1975.

87. Malaisse WJ, Orci L: The role of the cytoskeleton in pancreatic B cell function. Methods Achiev Exp Pathol 9:112–136, 1979.

88. Mc Daniel ML, Lacy PE: Interaction of cell organelles in insulin secretion. In Cooperstein SJ, Watkins D (eds): The Islet of Langerhans. New York, Academic Press, 1981, pp 97–115.

89. Howell SL, Tyhurst M: The insulin storage granule. In Poisner AM, Trifaro IM (eds): The Secretory Granule. Amsterdam, Elsevier, 1982, pp 155–172.

90. Dudek RW, Boyne AF, Charles TM: Novel secretory granule morphology in physically fixed pancreatic islets. J Histochem Cytochem 32:929–934, 1984.

91. Wollheim CB, Sharp GWG: Regulation of insulin release by calcium. Physiol Rev 61:914–973, 1981.

92. Malaisse WJ, Herchuelz A, Sener A: Inorganic ions and insulin secretion. In Cooperstein SJ, Watkins D (eds): The Islet of Langerhans. New York, Academic Press, 1981, pp 149–171.

93. Henquin JC, Meissner HP: Significance of ionic fluxes and changes in membrane potentials for stimulus secretion coupling in pancreatic B-cells. Experientia 40:1043–1052, 1984.

94. Petersen OH, Findley I: Electrophysiology of the pancreas. Physiol Rev 67:1054–1116, 1987.

95. Henquin JC: The fiftieth anniversary of the hypoglycaemic sulphonamides. How did the mother compound work? Diabetologia 35:907–912, 1992.

96. Orci L: Macro- and micro domains in the endocrine pancreas. Diabetes 31:538–565, 1982.

peptide immunoreactive structures in the pancreas. Histochem Cell Biol 109:103–109, 1998.

97. Grube D, Bohn R: The microanatomy of human islets of Langerhans with special reference to somatostatin (D) cells. Arch Histol Jpn 46:327–353, 1983.
98. Rorsman P, Arkhammaar P, Bokvist K, et al: Failure of glucose to elicit a normal secretory response in fetal pancreatic beta cells results from insensitivity of the ATP-regulated K^+ channels. Proc Natl Acad Sci U S A 86:4505–4509, 1989.
99. Weinhaus AJ, Poronnik P, Cook DL, et al: Insulin secretagogues but not glucose stimulate an increase in Ca^{++} in fetal rat beta cell. Diabetes 44:118–124, 1995.
100. Hughes SJ: The role of reduced glucose transporter content and glucose metabolism in the immature secretory responses of fetal rat pancreatic islets. Diabetologia 37:134–140, 1994.
101. Cecil RL: On hypertrophy and regeneration of the islands of Langerhans. J Exp Med 14:500–518, 1911.
102. King GL, Kahn CR, Rechler MM, et al: Direct demonstration of separate receptors for growth and metabolic activities of insulin and multiplication stimulation activity: Insulin like growth factors using antibodies to the insulin receptor. J Clin Invest 36:130–140, 1980.
103. Hill DJ, Hogg J: Growth factor control of pancreatic β cell hyperplasia. *In* Herington A (ed): Clinical Endocrinology and Metabolism. London, Baillière Tindall, 1991, pp 689–698.
104. Kaung HL: Growth dynamics of pancreatic islet cell populations during fetal and neonatal development of the rat. Dev Dyn 200:163–175, 1994.
105. Scaglia L, Cahill CJ, Finegood DT, et al: Apoptosis participates in the remodeling of the endocrine pancreas in the neonatal rat. Endocrinology 138:1736–1741, 1997.
106. Tornehave D, Larsson LI: Presence of Bcl-X1 during development of the human fetal and rat neonatal endocrine pancreas. Correlation to programmed cell death (abstract). Exp Clin Endocrinol Diabetes 105:A27, 1997.
107. Petrik J, Arany E, McDonald T, et al: Apoptosis in the pancreatic islet cells of the neonatal rat is associated with a reduced expression of insulin like growth factor II that may act as a survival factor. Endocrinology 139:2994–3004, 1998.
108. Xu G, Kwon G, Marshall CA, et al: Branched chain amino acids are essential in the regulation of PHAS-1 and p70 S6 kinase by pancreatic β cells. J Biol Chem 273:28178–28184, 1998.
109. Nielsen JH, Svensson C, Galsgaard ED, et al: Beta cell proliferation and growth factors. J Mol Med 77:62–66, 1999.
110. Billestrup N, Nielsen JH: The stimulatory effect of growth hormone, prolactin, and placental lactogen on beta-cell proliferation is not mediated by insulin like growth factor-I. Endocrinology 129:883–888, 1991.
111. Swenne I. Pancreatic beta cell growth and diabetes mellitus. Diabetologia 35:193–201, 1992.
112. Carlsson PO, Andersson A, Jansson L: Influence of age, hyperglycemia, leptin and NPY on islet blood flow in obese hyperglycemic mice. Am J Physiol 275:E594–E601, 1998.
113. Baxter RC: Insulin like growth factor (IGF) binding proteins: The role of serum IGFBPs in regulating IGF availability. Acta Paediatr Suppl. 272:107–114, 1991.
114. Hogg J, Han VKM, Clemmons DR, et al: Interactions of nutrients, insulin like growth factors (IGFs) and IGF-binding proteins in the regulation of DNA synthesis by isolated fetal rat islets of Langerhans. J Endocrinol 138:401–412, 1993.
115. Romanus JA, Rabinovitch A, Rechler MM: Neonatal rat islet cell cultures synthetize insulin-like growth factor I. Diabetes 34:696–702, 1987.
116. Swenne I, Andersson A: Effect of genetic background on the capacity for islet cell replication in mice. Diabetologia 27:464–467, 1984.
117. De Gasparo M, Desaulles PA: Fetal pancreatic anatomy and late adaptation to the environment. *In* Shafrir E, Renold AE (eds): Lessons from Animal Diabetes. London, John Libbey, 1984, pp 685–694.
118. Reusens-Billen B: Effet du Diabète Maternel sur le Pancréas Endocrine et le Système Digestif chez le Rat Fetal. Ph D thesis, Université Catholique de Louvain, Belgium, 1985.
119. Brelje TC, Parsons JA, Sorenson RL: Regulation of islet β cell proliferation by prolactin in rat islets. Diabetes 43:263–273, 1994.
120. Logothetopoulos J: Islet cell regeneration and neogenesis. *In* Steiner ED, Freinkel N (eds): Handbook of Physiology. Section 7: Endocrinology, vol 1. Endocrine Pancreas. Washington, DC, American Physiological Society, 1972, pp 67–76.
121. Kaung HLC: Effect of glucose on beta cell proliferation and population size in organ culture of fetal and neonatal rat pancreases. J Embryol Exp Morphol 74:303–312, 1983.
122. Sorenson RL, Brelje TC: Adaptations of islets of Langerhans to pregnancy: B-cell growth, enhanced insulin secretion and the role of lactogenic hormones. Horm Metab Res 29:301–307, 1997.
123. Nieuwenhuizen AG, Schuiling GA, Seijsener AF, et al: Effects of food restriction on glucose tolerance, insulin secretion, and islet-cell proliferation in pregnant rats. Physiol Behav 65:671–677, 1999.
124. Scaglia L, Smitth FE, Bonner-Weir S: Apoptosis contributes to the involution of beta cells mass in post partum rat pancreatas. Endocrinology 136:5461–5459, 1995.
125. Vinik A, Rafaeloff R, Pittenger G, et al: Induction of pancreatic islet neogenesis. Horm Metab Res 29:278–293, 1997.
126. Murakami T, Miyake T, Tsubouchi M, et al: Blood flow patterns in the rat pancreas: A simulative demonstration by injection replication and scanning electron microscopy. Microsc Res Tech 37:498–508, 1997.
127. Jansson L, Hellerström C: Stimulation by glucose of the blood flow to the pancreatic islets of the rat. Diabetologia 25:45–50, 1983.
128. Jansson L: The blood flow to the pancreatic and the islets of Langerhans during an intraperitoneal glucose load in rat. Diabetes Res Clin Pract 1:111–114, 1984.
129. Jansson L, Swenne I: Age dependent changes of pancreatic islet blood flow in the rat. Int J Pancreatol 5:157–163, 1989.
130. Carlsson PO, Jansson L, Ostenson CG et al: Islet capillary blood pressure increase mediated by hyperglycemia in NIDDM GK rats. Diabetes 46:947–952, 1997.
131. Grube D, Eckert I, Speck PT, et al: Immunohistochemistry and microanatomy of the islets of Langerhans. Biomed Res 4:25–36, 1983.
132. Bonner-Weier S, Orci L: New perspectives on the microvasculature of the islets of Langerhans in the rat. Diabetes 31:883–889, 1982.
133. Menger MD, Vajkoczy P, Beger C, et al: Orientation of microvascular blood flow in pancreatic islet isografts. J Clin Invest 93:2280–2285, 1994.
134. Cecil RL: A study of the pathological anatomy of the pancreas in ninety cases of diabetes mellitus. J Exp Med 11:266–290, 1909.
135. Hultquist GT, Olding LB: Endocrine pathology of infants of diabetic mothers. Acta Endocrinol 97:1–202, 1981.
136. Ziegler B, Lucke J, Besh W, et al: Pregnancy associated changes in the endocrine pancreas of normoglycaemic streptozotocin-treated Wistar rats. Diabetologia 28:172–175, 1985.
137. Laakso M, Pyorala K: Age of onset and type of diabetes. Diabetes Care 8:114–117, 1985.
138. Gepts W: Pathologic anatomy of the pancreas in juvenile diabetes mellitus. Diabetes 14:619–633, 1965.
139. Yoon JW, Jun HS, Santamaria PP: Cellular and molecular mechanisms for the initiation and progression of beta cell destruction resulting from the collaboration between macrophages and T cells. Autoimmunity 27:109–122, 1998.
140. Wilkin T, Armitage M, Casey C, et al: Value of insulin auto-antibodies as serum markers for insulin dependent diabetes mellitus. Lancet 1:480–482, 1985.
141. Roep BO: T-cell responses to autoantigens in IDDM. The search for the Holy Grail. Diabetes 45:1147–1156, 1996.
142. Yang XD, Michie SA, Mebius RE, et al: The role of cell adhesion molecules in the development of IDDM: Implications for pathogenesis and therapy. Diabetes 45:705–710, 1996.
143. Bach JF: Insulin-dependent diabetes mellitus as an autoimmune disease. Endocr Rev 15:516–542, 1994.
144. Rabinovitch A: An update on cytokines in the pathogenesis of insulin dependent diabetes mellitus. Diabetes Metab Rev 14: 129–151, 1998.
145. Mandrup-Poulsen T, Helqvist S, Wogensen LD, et al: Cytokines and free radicals as effector molecules in the destruction of pancreatic β-cells. Curr Top Microbiol Immunol 164: 169–193, 1990.
146. Corbett JA, McDaniel ML: Intraislet release of interleukin 1 inhibits B cell function by inducing B cell expression of inducible nitric oxide synthase. J Exp Med 181:559–568, 1995.
147. Rao HR: The role of undernutrition in the pathogenesis of diabetes mellitus. Diabetes Care 7:595–601, 1984.
148. Klöppel G, Lohr M, Habich K, et al: Islet pathology and the pathogenesis of type 1 and type 2 diabetes mellitus revisited. Survey Synth Pathol Res 4:110–125, 1985.
149. Coleman DL: Diabetes obesity syndromes in mice. Diabetes 31 (suppl 1):1–6, 1982.
150. Westermark P, Wilanders E: The influence of amyloid deposits on the islet volume in maturity onset diabetes mellitus. Diabetologia 15:417–421, 1978.
151. Westermark P: Islet pathology of non insulin dependent diabetes mellitus (NIDDM). Diabet Med 13:S46–S48, 1996.
152. Clark A, Saad MF, Nezzer T, et al: Islet amyloid polypeptide in diabetic and non-diabetic Pima indians. Diabetologia 33:285–289, 1990.
153. Clark A, Charge SB, Badman MK, et al: Islet amyloid polypeptide: Actions and role in the pathogenesis of diabetes. Biochem Soc Trans 24:594–599, 1996.
154. Guiot Y, Rahier J: Apport de l'anatomo-pathologie à la compréhension des différents types de diabète. Rev Fr Endocrinol Clin Nutr Metab 3:261–272, 1993.
155. Vishwanathan K, Bazaz-Malik G, Dandekar J, et al: A qualitative and quantitative histological study of the islets of Langerhans in diabetes mellitus. Indian J Med Sci 26:807–812, 1972.
156. Saito K, Yaginuma N, Takahashi T: Differential volumetry of A, B and D cells in the pancreatic islets of diabetic and non diabetic subjects. Tohoku J Exp Med 129:273–283, 1979.
157. Westermark GT, Christmanson L, Terenghi G, et al: Islet amyloid polypeptide: Demonstration of mRNA in human pancreatic islets by in situ hybridization in islets with and without amyloid deposits. Diabetologia 36:323–328, 1993.
158. Clark A: Islet amyloid:An enigma of type 2 diabetes. Diabetes Metab Rev 8:117–132, 1992.
159. Kahn SE, Andrikopoulos S, Verchere CB: Islet amyloid: A long recognized but underappreciated pathological feature of type 2 diabetes. Diabetes 48:241–253, 1999.
160. Hiddinga HJ, Eberhardt NL: Intracellular amyloidogenesis by human islet amyloid polypeptide induces apoptosis in COS-1 cells. Am J Pathol 154:1077–1088, 1999.
161. Westermark P, Johnson KH, Engstrom U, et al: Islet amyloid polypeptide: Synthetic peptides for study of the pathogenesis of islet amyloid. *In* Natvig JB, Forre O, Husby G, et al (eds): Amyloid and Amyloidosis. Dordrecht, Netherlands, Kluwer, 1991, pp 449–452.
162. Hellman U, Wernstedt C, Westermark P, et al: Amino-acid sequence from degu islet amyloid derived insulin shows unique sequences characteristics. Biochem Biophys Res Commun 169:571–577, 1990.
163. Kaufmann F, Rodriguez RR: Subtotal pancreatectomy in five different rat strains: Incidence and course of development of diabetes. Diabetologia 27:38–43, 1986.
164. Bonner-Weir S, Trent DF, Weir GC: Partial pancreatectomy in the rat and subsequent defect in glucose induced insulin release. J Clin Invest 71:1544–1553, 1983.
165. Bonner-Weir S: Regulation of pancreatic B cell mass in vivo. Recent Prog Horm Res 49:91–103, 1994.
166. Rubenstein AH: Insulin, proinsulin and C-peptide secretion: Metabolism and regulation in health and disease. *In* De Groot LL, Odell WD, Martini L et al (eds): Endocrinology, vol. 2. New York, Grune & Stratton, 1979, pp 951–957.
167. Kosaka K, Akanuma Y, Hagura R, et al: Plasma insulin response during the 100 gm glucose tolerance test in diabetic patients. *In* Baba S, Kaneko T, Yamaihara N (eds): Proinsulin, Insulin, C-Peptide. Amsterdam, Excerpta Medica, 1979, pp 283–293.
168. Eriksson U, Swenne I: Diabetes in pregnancy: Growth of the fetal pancreatic B cells in the rat. Biol Neonate 42:239–248, 1982.
169. Swenne I, Eriksson U: Diabetes in pregnancy: Islet cell proliferation in the fetal rat pancreas. Diabetologia 23:525–528, 1982.

170. Reusens-Billen B, Remacle C, Daniline J, et al: Cell proliferation in pancreatic islets of rat fetuses and neonates from normal and diabetic mothers. An in vitro and in vivo study. Horm Metab Res 16:565–618, 1984.

171. Snoeck A, Remacle C, Reusens, et al: Effect of a low protein diet during pregnancy on the fetal endocrine pancreas. Biol Neonate 57:107–118, 1990.

172. Petrik J, Reusens B, Arany E, et al: A low protein diet alters the balance of islet cell replication and apoptosis in the fetal and neonatal rat, and is associated with a reduced pancreatic expression of insulin like growth factor-II. Endocrinology 140:4861–4873, 1999.

173. Dahri S, Snoeck A, Reusens-Billen B, et al: Islet function in offspring of mothers on low-protein diet during gestation. Diabetes 40(suppl 2):115–120, 1991.

174. Ozanne SE, Wang CL, Coleman N et al: Altered muscle insulin sensitivity in the male offspring of protein malnourished rats. Am J Physiol 271:E1128–E1134, 1996.

175. Ozanne SE, Nave BT, Wang CL, et al: Poor fetal nutrition causes a long term change in expression of insulin signaling component in adipocytes. Am J Physiol 273:E46–E51, 1997.

176. Ozanne SE, Smith GD, Tikerpae J, et al: Altered regulation of hepatic glucose output in the male offspring of protein malnourished rat dams. Am J Physiol 270:E559–E564, 1996.

177. Reusens B, Remacle C: Effect of maternal malnutrition and metabolism on the developing endocrine pancreas: Experimental findings. *In* Barker DJP (ed): Fetal Origins of Cardiovascular and Lung Diseases. New York, Marcell Dekker (in press).

178. Reusens B, Dahri S, Snoeck A, et al: Long term consequences of diabetes and its complications may have a fetal origin: Experimental and epidemiological evidence. *In* Cowett RM (ed): Diabetes. Nestlé Nutrition Workshop Series, vol. 35. 1995, pp 187–198.

179. Cherif H, Reusens B, Ahn MT, et al: Effects of taurine on the insulin secretion of rat fetal islets from dams fed a low protein diet. J Endocrinol 159:341–348, 1998.

180. Garofano A, Czernichow P, Bréant B: In utero undernutrition impairs rat beta-cell development. Diabetologia 40:1231–1234, 1997.

181. Garofano A, Czernichow P, Bréant B: Effect of ageing on beta-cell mass and function in rats malnourished during the perinatal period. Diabetologia 42:711–718, 1999.

182. Garofano A, Czernichow P, Bréant B: Beta-cell mass and proliferation following late fetal and early postnatal malnutrition in the rat. Diabetologia 41:1114–1120, 1998.

183. Bogardus C, Lillioja S, Howard BV, et al: Relationships between insulin secretion, insulin action and fasting plasma glucose concentration in nondiabetic and non–insulin dependent diabetic subjects. J Clin Invest 74:1238–1245, 1984.

184. McCance DR, Pettitt DJ, Hanson RL, et al: Glucose, insulin concentrations and obesity in childhood and adolescence as predictors of NIDDM. Diabetologia 37:617–623, 1994.

185. Movassat J, Saulnier C, Serradas P, et al: Impaired development of pancreatic beta-cell mass is a primary event during the progression to diabetes in the GK rat. Diabetologia 40:916–925, 1997.

186. Serradas P, Gangnerau MN, Giroix MH, et al: Impaired pancreatic beta cell function in the fetal GK rat. Impact of diabetic inheritance. J Clin Invest 15:899–904, 1998.

187. Zhu M, Noma Y, Mizuno A, et al: Poor capacity for proliferation of pancreatic beta-cells in Otsuka-Long-Evans-Tokushima fatty rat: A model of spontaneous NIDDM. Diabetes 45:941–946, 1996.

188. Froguel P: Nuclear factor and type 2 diabetes. Schweiz Med Wochenschr 128:1936–1939, 1998.

Chemistry and Biosynthesis of the Islet Hormones: Insulin, Islet Amyloid Polypeptide (Amylin), Glucagon, Somatostatin, and Pancreatic Polypeptide*

Donald F. Steiner ▪ Graeme I. Bell ▪ Arthur H. Rubenstein
Shu J. Chan

The classic experiments of Von Mering and Minkowski at the close of the 19th century clearly demonstrated the important role of the pancreas in the prevention of diabetes.[1] Early in the 20th century, a number of investigators undertook to prepare pancreatic extracts to treat diabetes, but it was not until the work of the Canadians—Fred Banting, Charles Best, and John Collip (Fig. 48–1)—working in the laboratory of Prof. J. J. R. Macleod at the University of Toronto in 1921–1922 that potent preparations of insulin were routinely made.[2] The name "insulin" was based on the belief that the hormone was derived from the islets of Langerhans and actually was suggested as early as 1909 by deMayer and later again in 1917 by Sir Edward Sharpey-Schafer. Preparative methods based on the early work of Scott[3] as well as refinements by Banting et al.[4] were rapidly developed for the commercial preparation of the hormone, and within about 1 year insulin began to be administered to patients with diabetes, often with dramatic effects.[2] The chemical nature of insulin was a more elusive problem, although the fact that it was destroyed by proteolytic enzymes suggested that it was indeed a protein.[5] At that time, however, it was not appreciated that proteins might function as hormones as well as enzymes and produce such dramatic biologic effects as the lowering of blood glucose levels and the enhancement of carbohydrate utilization. When J. J. Abel first succeeded in crystallizing insulin in 1926 there was great controversy as to whether the crystals of protein he had obtained were actually the active biologic principle or merely the vehicle for a smaller active moiety.[6] Such controversies seem remarkable in the light of our detailed present-day knowledge of the structure and biologic properties of insulin, but it is important to remember that many of the modern techniques of protein chemistry were developed, in part, through the clinical need for insulin, which made it abundantly available to the biochemist as a model protein for study.

This chapter selectively reviews the chemistry and properties of insulin and the other islet hormones, including islet amyloid polypep-

tide (IAPP or amylin), glucagon, somatostatin, and pancreatic polypeptide (PP) and their precursor forms, the mechanisms of their biosynthesis in the various islet cells in which they are produced, and the structures of the genes that encode them. Studies on the mechanism of biosynthesis of insulin via proinsulin in the pancreatic β cells have long provided a useful model for analysis of the production of the other islet hormones and of many other hormonal and neuroendocrine peptides and growth factors and their receptors, as well as many other proteins that traverse the secretory pathway. Continuing clarification of the enzymic mechanisms underlying the proteolytic cleavage of proproteins now provides a more complete picture of neuroendocrine peptide formation and processing. Most such peptides exist in multiple forms in tissue or in the circulation, and the origin and metabolism of these forms adds additional complexity to the normal physiologic regulation of endocrine and paracrine/neural secretion. This information will be related, wherever possible, to pathologic states in man, particularly diabetes and related metabolic syndromes and benign or malignant endocrine tumors.

ISOLATION, PROPERTIES, AND STRUCTURE OF INSULIN

Isolation and Characterization

Insulin occurs throughout the vertebrate kingdom, and insulin-like substances have been found in the brains and/or digestive systems of a number of invertebrate species.[7] The early recognition that ethanol[3] or acid-ethanol[4] extraction of pancreas inhibited proteolytic destruction of insulin has provided the basis for most modern preparative procedures.[8, 9] Acid-ethanol also efficiently extracts proinsulin, C-peptide, IAPP, glucagon, PP, somatostatin, and their precursor forms from pancreatic tissue in most species. Acid-ethanol extracts can be partially purified by fractional precipitation and isoelectric precipitation in the presence of organic solvents to solubilize fats, which can then be further resolved by gel filtration,[10] ion exchange chromatography,[11, 12]

*Work in our laboratories was supported by National Institutes of Health grants DK13914, DK20595, and by the Howard Hughes Medical Institute.

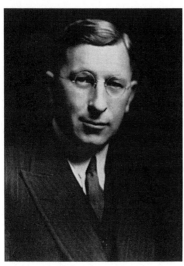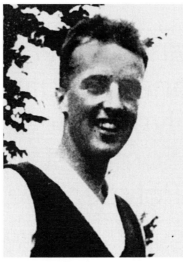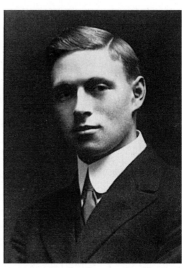

FIGURE 48–1. Photographs of Frederick G. Banting, Charles H. Best, and John B. Collip, the principal developers of successful methods for insulin extraction, taken about the time of insulin's discovery in 1921. (Photographs courtesy of Michael Bliss, Toronto, Canada.)

and high-performance liquid chromatography (HPLC).[13–15] Salting-out from acidic solutions is not effective for recovering small amounts of insulin and may lead to significant losses of C-peptide as well as to loss of the other peptides.[16] Yields of insulin vary according to the source: mammalian pancreas yields 10 to 15 nmol/kg (of wet weight); fetal calf pancreas, 60 to 70 nmol/kg; fish islets, 300 to 500 nmol/kg; and isolated rat islets of Langerhans, 2 to 3 nmol/kg. The biologic activity of most highly purified contemporary mammalian insulin preparations ranges from 26 to 30 IU/mg. The bovine insulin standard of the International Union of Pure and Applied Chemistry is stated to have an activity of 25 IU/mg of dry weight.[8] Although crystallization with zinc was once regarded as a powerful method for purification of insulin, it is now generally recognized that even repeated crystallization does not eliminate all impurities from insulin, and not all species have insulins capable of binding zinc and/or of crystallizing.[12, 17] Most crystalline preparations of animal-derived insulin contain small residual amounts of glucagon, desamido insulin, proinsulin and its intermediate cleavage forms, ethyl esters of insulin, dimers of insulin, and higher aggregates of insulin and proinsulin with unknown components.[12, 18]

The use of modern biosynthetic methods based on recombinant DNA technology[19–21] has eliminated some impurities, such as other hormones, but may introduce new types of trace contaminants derived from the bacterial or yeast host cells.[19] Early gel filtration studies of crystalline bovine insulin preparations separated impurities into essentially three fractions[12]: (1) "a-component"—material of high molecular weight eluting essentially in the void volume and containing insulin cross-linked or aggregated with other proteins; (2) "b-component"—proinsulin, intermediate cleavage products of proinsulin, and insulin dimers; and (3) "c-component"—insulin-like components including desamido forms, arginyl insulins (B_{31} and B_{32} arginine residues), C-peptide, and small amounts of glucagon.[12, 22, 23] The a-component turned out to be highly antigenic in producing insulin antibodies.[18] Further purification of the insulin-containing fractions by ion-exchange chromatography, using urea-containing buffers or 60% ethanol as dispersing agents, yielded preparations that were better than 99% pure, i.e., the "monocomponent" or "single-component" insulins that are now widely available.[11, 18] These preparations are far less antigenic than most of the crystalline insulin preparations of animal origin used formerly, and they have been shown to improve the control of diabetes.[24] The introduction of biosynthetic human insulin for therapy has further reduced the problem of antigenicity, but it has been difficult to eliminate entirely, because even the human hormone can undergo chemical changes during storage that may tend to induce formation of (auto)antibodies.[25, 26]

The assay of insulin, like most other protein hormones, has always presented difficulties with regard to precision and sensitivity. The various in vivo blood glucose-lowering assays that are often used by pharmaceutical houses require too much material to be very useful for most experimental laboratories. The use of polyacrylamide gel electrophoresis and/or HPLC with appropriate standards can provide a wealth of useful information regarding the homogeneity and quality of the preparations.[11–13, 15, 27] These methods also give indications as to the state of amidation of the insulin or proinsulin, which may reflect the harshness of preparative procedures or the extent of autolysis prior to extraction. Other routinely used biochemical methods for assessing the purity of proteins are equally applicable, but it must be born in mind that although all tests indicate that homogeneity has been achieved, the biologic activity of the preparation must be examined directly to ascertain that no chemical damage to the hormone has occurred. This can usually be accomplished by in vitro assays using isolated fat or liver cells, or various cultured cells, and comparing such parameters as glucose oxidation, lipogenesis, glucose transport, or glycogen synthesis with purified standards.[8, 28] The introduction of hormone-binding assays using isolated plasma membrane preparations or purified receptors has provided more sensitive and reliable methods for screening material for biologic potency in vivo; these methods have thus far demonstrated a good correlation between binding and measured biologic potency.[29–31] However, both binding tests and immunoassays can be misleading, as neither necessarily measures the true biologic effectiveness of the hormone. Thus, the thorough characterization of any insulin preparation should include measurements of biologic potency in suitable isolated cell preparations and of binding characteristics, as well as full characterization of the protein in terms of its molecular weight, composition, homogeneity, and, if possible, amino acid composition and sequence. For more detailed information regarding the physicochemical properties of insulin, several reviews are recommended.[8, 17, 25, 32, 33]

Insulin Structure

The determination of the complete primary structure of bovine insulin by Sanger and his associates in 1955[34] provided the first complete structure of a protein and it also proved beyond question that proteins are defined molecular entities. The exploration of species differences in insulin structure led to the recognition of the existence of the genetic code. The primary structures of insulins from about 70 vertebrate species have been determined in the interval since the pioneering studies of Sanger,[34] Smith,[35] and others.[8, 36–48] In addition to these, the structures of several insulin-like peptides from invertebrates have been elucidated. These include a growth-promoting hormone of the light green cells in the snail *Lymnaea*,[49] an unusual insulin-like molecule that regulates carbohydrate metabolism in *Aplysia*,[50] the insulin-like brain peptide from the silkworm *Bombyx mori*,[51] an insulin-like peptide from the locust,[52] and insulin-like peptides from *Caenorhabditis elegans*.[53, 54] Although less closely related to the vertebrate insulins, these are clearly members of the insulin superfamily.[55] In vertebrates, in addition to relaxin, other insulin-like peptides have recently been discovered in reproductive tissues.[56]

The low rate of mutation acceptance of insulin (2%–4% of residues per 100 million years) is comparable to that of many other well-defined globular proteins, such as hemoglobin, cytochrome *c*, or many enzymes.[55, 57] Nonetheless, amino acid substitutions can occur at many positions within either chain without greatly altering the biologic effectiveness of the hormone as measured in various bioassay systems (Fig. 48–2). However, certain structural features are conserved throughout vertebrate evolution, including the positions of the three disulfide bonds, the N-terminal and C-terminal regions of the A chain, and the hydrophobic residues in the C-terminal region of the B chain, as well as others. Chemical modifications in any of these regions tend to markedly reduce or abolish biologic activity, underscoring their roles in maintaining the secondary and tertiary structural features necessary for receptor binding.[8, 17, 58, 59] The C-terminal hydrophobic sequence of the B chain (residues 23–27) also plays an important role in the formation of insulin dimers in solution as described below.

As might be anticipated from the more extensive amino acid replacements (8%–10%) that occur between mammalian and fish insulins,[47] it is not surprising that the immunologic cross-reactivity between these proteins is rather weak. Generally, such low cross-reactivity can easily be detected by conventional immunoassays if the heterologous insulin is used as the labeled tracer. For detailed considerations of insulin antigenicity in relation to its structure, several reviews are recommended.[8, 60]

The elucidation by Blundell and Wood,[17] Blundell and co-workers,[61, 62] and Baker at al.[63] of the three-dimensional structure of porcine insulin, initially at a resolution of 2.8 Å and with more recent refinements at 1.5 Å, was an important breakthrough in the study of peptide hormone structure. The results have proved invaluable in interpreting much of the available chemical data on the properties of insulin.[62, 63] Detailed knowledge of the spatial organization of the molecule has also been helpful in studies on the molecular mechanism of binding and action of insulin. The hexameric unit of crystalline zinc insulin (Fig. 48–3) consists of three dimers arranged around a major threefold axis that passes through two zinc atoms, each of which is coordinated with the imidazole groups of three B10 histidine residues and is located above or below the plane of the hexamer.[61, 62] The insulin dimers are held together in the crystals by hydrogen bonds between the peptide groups of residues 24 and 26 within the C-terminal region of the B chain, forming an antiparallel β-pleated sheet structure. The structure of a porcine insulin monomer is shown in Figure 48–4.

In this high-resolution (1.5 Å) representation, all of the amino acid side chains are shown in their normal orientations, and the putative receptor binding region is outlined. Recent nuclear magnetic resonance

(NMR) studies[64] provide support for the conclusion that the structure of the insulin monomer in solution is closely similar to that in crystals.

X-ray diffraction studies on crystals of insulin from the hagfish, a cyclostome, have defined a very similar arrangement of the molecular backbone of the insulin in this very primitive vertebrate[17, 37, 65] despite replacements at about 40% of sites, which is consistent with its evolutionary divergence of about 500 million years. These results indicate the conservation in this cyclostomian insulin of many primary structural features known to be concerned with the formation of the characteristic folded structure of the hormone. Thus, although increased numbers of amino acid substitutions have occurred in certain New World species, such as the guinea pig, other hystricomorph rodents, and some primates,[17, 35, 40, 41, 66] the native molecular structure of insulin, as well as its tendency to form isologous dimers, has remained remarkably constant throughout vertebrate evolution. This fact is further reflected in the relatively high retention of biologic potency among the known insulins; most fish insulins are only slightly less active than mammalian insulins, and even the much more primitive and highly substituted hagfish insulin has been found to have about 5% of the biologic activity of bovine or porcine insulin in various mammalian test systems.[67, 68]

These findings also imply that the receptors for insulin,[69] as well as their actions, have changed relatively little throughout vertebrate evolution. Similar conservatism is often seen in essential structural proteins and enzymes.[70] The interaction of insulin and its receptor initiates a variety of biochemical functions in the plasma membrane, including catalysis (tyrosine kinase), self-association, and/or interactions with other cellular components leading to various metabolic and anabolic responses, as well as endocytosis of insulin and its degradation or transcellular transport.[71] The insulin receptor and insulin's actions are discussed in greater detail in Chapter 50.

Receptor-Binding Region of Insulin

Recent studies have led to revisions in previously held theories regarding the location of the receptor-binding region in the insulin molecule. Several naturally occurring mutant human insulins (see Defects in the Insulin Gene later in the chapter) have proven to be especially valuable in redefining current views of the location of the receptor-binding surface of the insulin molecule. Earlier views were based on the presumed inflexibility of the C-terminal region of the B chain in the insulin structure, as revealed by x-ray analysis (Fig. 48–5A). Studies of insulin substitutions involving residues B24 or B25 and of despentapeptide insulin, in which the last five residues of the B chain have been deleted, suggest that the C-terminal region of the B chain is reoriented to facilitate receptor binding. The most convincing evidence for this has arisen from studies of a novel miniproinsulin molecule synthesized by Markussen,[72] in which B29 lysine is in direct peptide linkage to A1 glycine. Although this molecule is biologically

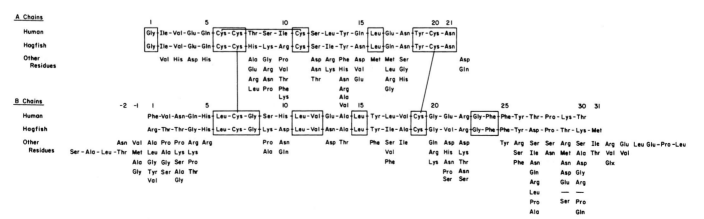

FIGURE 48–2. *Amino acid sequence of human and hagfish insulins, with substitutions occurring at each position in 70 other known vertebrate insulins shown below for comparison. Invariant residues are enclosed in boxes.*

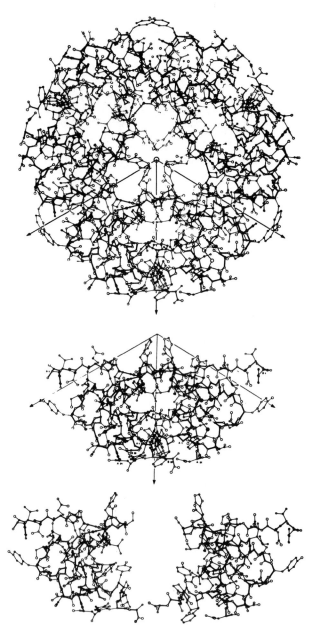

FIGURE 48–3. *View of a hexamer of porcine insulin (2-Zn) along the threefold axis, showing the development of dimers from monomers and their organization into the hexamer. Zinc-binding imidazole side chains of His-B10 residues project toward the central axis above and below the midplane of the hexamers. (From Blundell TL, Dodson GG, Hodgkin DC, et al: Insulin: The structure in the crystals and its reflection in chemistry and biology. Adv Protein Chem 26:279, 1972.)*

by leucine in a mutant human insulin,[15] which would normally be regarded as a biochemically conservative substitution because of their similar aliphatic character, leads to a distortion of the surface exposed to solvent and, upon binding, to the receptor recognition site of the hormone.

Additional studies have helped to further delineate the roles of B24 phenylalanine (Phe), B25 Phe, and A3 valine (Val) in insulin-receptor interactions. The construction of semisynthetic insulin analogues bearing unnatural amino acids at these positions has been particularly helpful in this respect. Three unexpected findings should be noted. First the β-aromatic ring of B25 Phe is required for high-affinity hormone-receptor interactions only in the context of full-length insulin analogues. Because this requirement is lost when residues B26 through B30 are deleted, it appears that B25 Phe somehow directs the conformational changes discussed above without itself contributing direct binding energy.[76, 77] The tolerance for bulk distal to the β-aromatic ring in position B25-substituted analogues further suggests that the B25 Phe side chain defines the edge of intermolecular contact when insulin is bound to its receptor.[78] Second, B24 Phe can be replaced by any of several amino acids in the D-configuration (but not by their corresponding L-enantiomers) or by glycine without major changes in the affinity of the insulin receptor for ligand. Again, the β-aromatic ring of phenylalanine apparently contributes little or no binding energy to insulin-receptor interactions. The role of the phenylalanine side chain in this case (like that in the case of B25 Phe) seems to involve receptor contacts that direct conformational adjustments in the peptide backbone of the insulin molecule.[79] Third, whereas replacement of A3 Val by leucine (a residue with a β-branch) greatly decreases the affinity of the insulin receptor for hormone, replacement of A3 Val by *tertiary* leucine (a residue with a bulky β-branch) does not. Because *tertiary* leucine is one of the most severely α-helix–perturbing residues known, it appears that the somewhat disordered α-helix in the N-terminal domain of the insulin A chain may become even more disordered when the hormone is bound to the insulin receptor.[80]

The findings described above identify in several ways the importance of structural changes and of main-chain conformational adjustments in insulin-receptor interactions. It should be noted, however, that portions of the insulin molecule in addition to the C-terminal B chain domain and the N-terminal A chain domain are also crucial for higher-affinity insulin-receptor interactions. It is important to note that

inactive, when crystals were obtained and analyzed[73] it was evident that its three-dimensional structure was essentially isomorphic to that of normal crystalline insulin. What was different in B29-A1 insulin, however, was the immobility of the C-terminal region of the B chain. Recent NMR data on various insulin derivatives in solution[64, 74, 75] also confirm the importance of significant conformational changes in the C terminus of the B chain for effective receptor binding. When five C-terminal residues of the B chain are deleted from the rest of the molecule, as indicated in Figure 48–5B (yielding despentapeptide insulin), an underlying portion of the hydrophobic core of the molecule is exposed. Although the extent of movement of the B chain C terminus when insulin is bound to the receptor is not known, even small movements would alter insulin's topography and enhance the potential for interactions of valine residue A3 with the receptor (compare A and B parts of Fig. 48–5). Hence, replacement of this valine

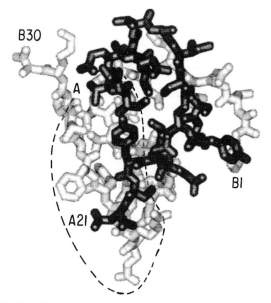

FIGURE 48–4. *View of a porcine insulin monomer (molecule 2) oriented perpendicular to the threefold axis (see Fig. 48–3). The side chains of all the amino acids are shown: the A chain is dark gray and the B chain light gray. Dashes outline the approximate region on the surface of the insulin monomer, which is believed to contact the receptor on binding[500] (this region is shown in greater detail in Fig. 48–5). (Computer graphic representation courtesy of Dr. Bing Xiao, University of York.)*

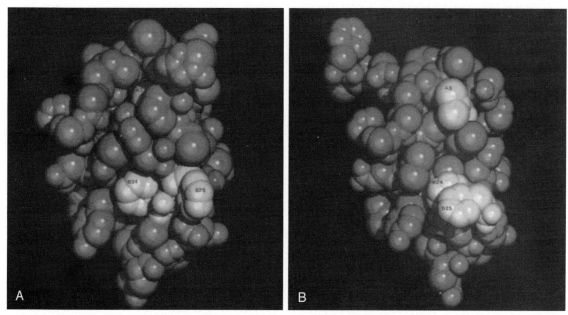

FIGURE 48–5. *A,* The molecule 1 of 2 Zn human insulin with atoms represented with their van der Waals' radii. The residues A3 Val, B24 and B25 Phe, which occur as human mutations, are highlighted by light shading. The view is perpendicular to the dimer-forming surface. The B chain N-terminal residues are extended behind the molecule in this view. *B,* The monomer of beef despentapeptide insulin (DPI). The atoms are represented with their van der Waals' radii. The residues A3 Val, B24 and B25 Phe are highlighted by *light shading,* in the same view as shown in *A.* (The B chain N-terminal residues are extended above B10 histidine in the DPI structure and are therefore visible in this view.) (Courtesy of Drs. Bing Xiao and Guy Dodson, University of York.) (From Steiner DF, Tager HS, Nanjo K, et al: Familial syndromes of hyperproinsulinemia and hyperinsulinemia with mild diabetes. *In* Stanbury JS (ed): The Metabolic Basis of Inherited Disease, ed 7. New York, McGraw-Hill, 1993.)

(1) desoctapeptide insulin (an analogue in which the C-terminal B chain domain has been deleted) retains 0.1% of the receptor-binding potency of insulin, and (2) analogues bearing amino acid replacements in the central B chain α-helix can exhibit either enhanced[81] or diminished[82] receptor-binding potency relative to the native hormone. Although much remains to be learned, studies of naturally occurring mutant human insulins have been very helpful in directing attention and research to crucial regions of the insulin molecule.

BIOSYNTHESIS OF INSULIN

Although earlier studies indicated that insulin was formed via proinsulin, a precursor that includes the B and A chains within a single 9000-Da polypeptide chain,[11, 83, 84] examination by cell-free translation of the initial polypeptide products encoded in insulin messenger ribonucleic acid (mRNA) extracted from islets or islet cell tumors led, in 1975, to the discovery of preproinsulin (see Fig. 48–6). This extended form of proinsulin has a hydrophobic N-terminal 24 residue prepeptide.[85, 86] Such signal peptide extensions have been found at or near the N termini in almost all secretory proteins of animal, plant, or bacterial origin, and they serve to facilitate their segregation from the cytosolic compartment, where protein synthesis is initiated, into the secretory pathway via a complex series of molecular interactions that result in the translocation of the nascent peptide across the membrane of the rough endoplasmic reticulum (RER) into its internal compartments, or cisternae.[87, 88] During, or shortly after, translocation, the signal sequence is cleaved by the signal peptidase, which is located on the inner surface of the RER membrane.[88] Following translocation and cleavage of the signal sequence, the proinsulin molecule folds and undergoes rapid formation of disulfide bonds to achieve its native structure. Evidence suggests that this process is catalyzed by the enzyme protein-thiol reductase, a resident protein of the RER having a C-terminal Lys-Glu-Asp-Leu (KDEL) localization sequence.[89] Proinsulin is then transferred in small coated vesicles from the endoplasmic reticulum (ER) to the *cis* region of the Golgi apparatus.[90, 91] It then passes from the *cis* to the *trans* Golgi, where it is sorted into secretory vesicles. The signal peptide is rapidly degraded in the RER and is thus not a normal secretory product of β cells.[92]

During the intracellular transport of proinsulin from its site of biosynthesis in the rough endoplasmic reticulum of the β cell to the storage granules, it is cleaved to yield insulin and a 26–31 residue peptide fragment, which is designated the *C peptide*; both insulin and C peptide are stored in secretion granules along with small amounts of residual proinsulin and partially cleaved intermediate forms[93] as well as a variety of other more minor β cell secretory products.[94] The

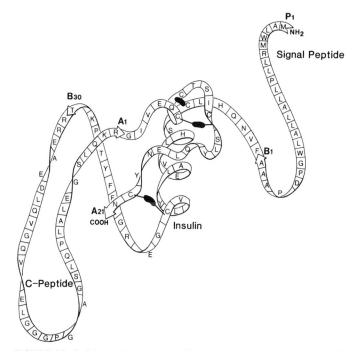

FIGURE 48–6. Schematic structure of human preproinsulin. Removal of the first 24 amino acids (signal peptide) gives rise to proinsulin. Cleavage after B30 (T) and before A1 (G) gives rise to insulin and C peptide. (See text for details and Dayhoff[36] for explanation of single letter amino acid code.)

intracellular processing of precursor proteins (proproteins) is quite distinct from the well-known proteolytic activation of the inactive zymogen forms of many hydrolases, which is a largely extracellular process. Precursor processing is now recognized to be an important feature of almost all endocrine and neural cells, and it also occurs in many other organs (e.g., liver).[95] Certain cellular proteolytic processing enzymes also are coopted in the formation of the envelopes of many viruses.[96–98] Recent progress in the intracellular localization and enzymatic mechanism of these proteolytic events is discussed in greater detail in the section on the conversion of proinsulin to insulin, later in the chapter.

Structure and Properties of Proinsulin

Methods for the isolation of proinsulin and related peptides are discussed in the preceding section. Mammalian proinsulins range in size from 81 (cow) to 86 (human, horse, rat) amino acid residues.[99] The difference is a consequence of the variable size of the connecting polypeptide (C peptide), which links the C terminus of the insulin B chain to the N terminus of the insulin A chain (see Fig. 48–6). All the known mammalian proinsulins have pairs of basic residues at either end of the C peptide that link it to the insulin chains. These residues are excised during the conversion of proinsulin to insulin,[100] and the resulting products are native insulin and the C peptide. The proinsulin-like molecules in invertebrates retain C peptides of roughly similar size that also are excised by cleavage at basic residue pairs.[49, 51] Despite its considerably larger molecular size, proinsulin is remarkably similar to insulin in many properties, including solubility, isoelectric point,[93] self-associative properties,[101] and reactivity with insulin antisera.[83, 102, 103] These observations, and evidence from other studies, strongly suggest that the conformation of the insulin moiety in proinsulin is nearly identical to that of insulin itself.[64, 93] It is of interest that the highly flexible connecting peptide is much larger than would seem to be required to bridge the short 8-Å gap between the ends of the B and A chains in the native insulin molecule (see Fig. 48–6). Although the connecting peptide overlays a portion of the surface of the insulin monomer, it does not completely mask the receptor-binding region, since intact proinsulin exhibits 3% to 5% biologic activity in several systems in vitro.[28, 104] It is unlikely that any significant cleavage or "activation" of proinsulin occurs in the tissues to account for this level of intrinsic activity.[105] The connecting peptide also does not obscure those surfaces of the monomer that interact to form dimers and hexamers.[106, 107] A hypothetical arrangement of the connecting peptide moiety in a proinsulin hexamer is shown in Figure 48–7. As discussed later, this hexameric structure, having the C peptide oriented externally, may play a role in the efficient conversion of proinsulin to insulin in the β cells. The three-dimensional structure of proinsulin has not yet been determined, despite successful crystallization of the hormone in several laboratories.[17, 108]

Precursor Relationship of Proinsulin to Insulin

The precursor-product relationship between proinsulin and insulin has been carefully documented in a variety of studies using isolated islets.*[118–123] The conversion of proinsulin to insulin begins after an initial delay of about 20 minutes and then proceeds as a pseudo–first-

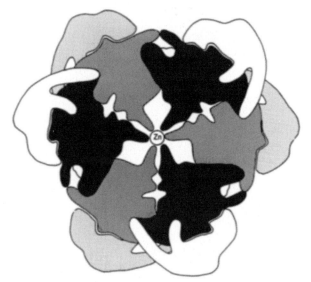

FIGURE 48–7. Hypothetical 2-Zn proinsulin hexamer as viewed along the threefold axis. The connecting peptide is shown in *light gray* and *white* around the periphery of the *darker outline* of an insulin hexamer arranged according to the data of Blundell et al.[62] The central density represents two zinc atoms in coordination linkage to the six (three above and three below hexamer plane) histidine side chains at position 10 in the B chain (compare with Fig. 48–3).

order process over a period of several hours.[118, 119, 124] The intracellular proteolytic conversion of proinsulin to insulin continues even when protein synthesis is inhibited with cycloheximide, indicating that continuous protein synthesis is not necessary for this reaction.[118] The processing of proinsulin normally proceeds to near completion. Hence, the mature secretory granules contain only small amounts (1%–2%) of proinsulin and intermediate materials. Consequently, secreted insulin normally contains only small amounts of these precursor-related peptides.[124] Newly synthesized insulin is selectively released to a slight extent, but the bulk of the secreted material consists of stored preformed hormone and C peptide.[124–126] The major intermediate cleavage forms of mammalian proinsulins have been described by early investigators.[12, 23, 92, 109, 127–129] Comparative studies of insulin biosynthesis in the larger, more readily accessible, single islets (Brockman bodies) of teleost fishes (e.g., the cod[130] and the anglerfish[131, 132]) as well as in the islet parenchyma of such primitive vertebrates as cyclostomes (e.g. the hagfish),[133, 134] have also indicated the formation and intracellular cleavage of proinsulins that are similar in size to the mammalian proteins. Such lower forms exhibit similar requirements for cleavage at paired basic residue sites by the evolutionarily conserved prohormone convertases.

Morphologic Organization of the Insulin Biosynthetic Machinery

The β cells of the islets of Langerhans share many features with other cells that elaborate secretory proteins (Fig. 48–8). The participation of the Golgi apparatus in the formation of secretory vesicles, the so-called β granules, was suggested as early as 1944 by Hard.[135] Later, Munger[136] confirmed, by electron microscopy, that secretory granule formation occurs within the Golgi apparatus. He identified "progranules" with altered morphologic features near the Golgi body. Numerous subsequent studies have confirmed that newly synthesized peptide material passes via the Golgi apparatus into β cell secretory granules. With the exception of the proteolytic processing, the overall process appears to be similar to that occurring in the pancreatic exocrine cells and in many other secretory cells.[137] Immunocytochemical studies using monoclonal antibodies specific for uncleaved proinsulin have demonstrated that newly formed clathrin-clad vesicles derived from the TGN (*trans*-Golgi network) cisternae are rich in proinsulin (Fig.

---

*In rats and mice, two non-allelic insulin genes give rise to two proinsulins, one corresponding to each of the two insulins (I and II).[109, 110] The two insulins differ from each other at only two positions[109] and are identical in both species.[111, 112] These insulins are encoded in nonallelic genes,[55, 112] arising from a duplication event that occurred relatively recently (10–30 million years ago). The gene for insulin I appears to have arisen via a viral retropositional event[113] and lacks the second intervening sequence (see Fig. 48–16). The two rat proinsulins and their corresponding C peptides and intermediate forms have been isolated and their amino acid sequences determined.[109, 114–117] The two rat insulins are synthesized in roughly equal proportions (I/II = 58/42) under basal and stimulated conditions.[84, 109]

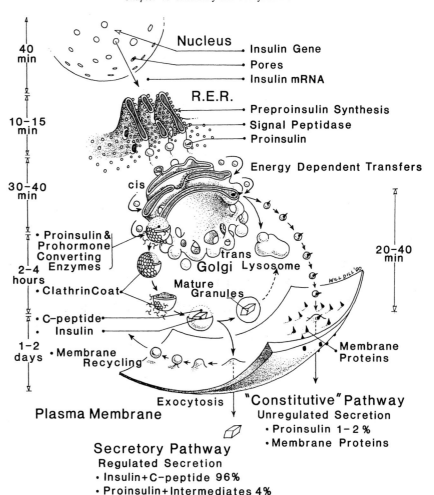

FIGURE 48–8. Schematic model of the subcellular transport of preproinsulin after its synthesis in the rough endoplasmic reticulum (RER) and rapid cleavage to proinsulin (within 1 to 2 minutes). Proinsulin is then released into the intracisternal spaces of the RER, where it folds and forms the native disulfide bonds of insulin. It is then transported to the Golgi apparatus by an energy-dependent process. The clathrin-coated early granules budding from the *trans*-Golgi cisternae are rich in proinsulin and contain the converting proteases, PC2 and PC3. Processing occurs mainly, if not exclusively, in the early secretory granules,[138, 141] giving rise to the more condensed mature granules. Fractionation studies have confirmed that the mature granule-dense cores consist almost entirely of insulin, often in crystalline arrays (see Fig. 48–14), whereas the granule-soluble phase that surrounds the inclusion consists mainly of C peptide and small amounts of proinsulin.[236] The release of newly synthesized proinsulin and insulin begins only about 1 hour after synthesis in the RER; hence, granules must undergo a maturation process that renders them competent for secretion. There is no evidence for significant nongranular routes of secretion of either proinsulin or insulin in normal islets. Exocytosis of granules is regulated by glucose and many other factors, and in humans and dogs it results in the release of insulin and C peptide in approximately equimolar proportions under both basal and stimulated conditions.[246]

48–9), confirming that conversion to insulin occurs principally during the maturation of these secretory "progranules."[138, 139] Proinsulin, in common with many other exportable proteins, is synthesized by ribosomes associated with the RER.[140] Evidence reviewed in the preceding section indicates that proinsulin is in turn derived from a larger precursor, preproinsulin, which is rapidly cleaved to proinsulin in the RER. The proinsulin is then transported from the ER to the Golgi apparatus in small coated vesicles[90] (see Fig. 48–8), in a process that requires about 20 minutes.[93, 138, 139] Addition to pancreatic islets of antimycin or other energy poisons after short labeling periods with tritiated (³H) leucine completely blocks the subsequent transformation of the newly formed proinsulin to insulin.[138, 141, 142] However, if the addition of antimycin is delayed until 30 minutes, there is no inhibition of subsequent conversion, indicating that once newly synthesized proinsulin has reached the *trans* Golgi and/or progranules, its transformation no longer requires energy.[141] The chemical basis of the energy requirement for the intracellular translocation of secretory proteins has been studied by Rothman et al. and is associated with the budding and/or fusion of small vesicles that transport secretory products from the *cis* through the *trans* Golgi cisternae.[143, 144]

The conversion of proinsulin to insulin in intact rat islet cells is a psuedo–first-order reaction having a half-time ranging from about 20 minutes to 1 hour in various studies.[119, 145] Peak labeling of proteins in the Golgi apparatus is observed 30 to 40 minutes after biosynthetic labeling of islets with ³H-amino acids; relatively little radioactivity remains in this region after 1 hour.[146, 147] A similar pattern is observed by means of electron microscopic immunocytochemistry.[138] Thus, it is likely that proinsulin conversion is initiated in the *trans* compartment of the Golgi apparatus or in newly formed secretion granules, or "progranules," as these leave the Golgi region, and that it continues for several hours within these granules as they collect and mature biochemically in the cytosol (see Fig. 48–8).

Conversion of Proinsulin to Insulin

The major proteolytic cleavages required for converting proinsulin to insulin are summarized in Figure 48–10. In early studies it was shown that the conjoint action of trypsin and carboxypeptidase B gave rise to the naturally occurring products—C-peptide and native insulin—essentially quantitatively converting proinsulin to insulin in vitro.[148] This model could also account for the major intermediate forms found in pancreatic extracts[100, 127] and lead to a search for a cellular trypsin-like convertase, assumed to be a serine protease related to trypsin,[93] and for carboxypeptidases related to carboxypeptidase B. Studies in the early 1970s with isolated islet secretion granules already indicated that these were major sites of proinsulin conversion.[149] By labeling proinsulin in intact islets with ³H-arginine, it also could be shown that subsequent conversion of prohormone in an isolated granule fraction in vitro led to the release of free arginine rather than of basic dipeptides,[128] confirming the likely participation of both trypsin-like and carboxypeptidase B–like activities in maturing secretory granules.[150] Carboxypeptidase E, or H—a homologue of pancreatic carboxypeptidase B with a more acidic pH optimum—was first identified in islets[150] and was subsequently identified and characterized in brain and other tissues.[151] Molecular cloning subsequently confirmed its structural and evolutionary relationship to the pancreatic carboxypeptidases.[152] More recently, additional processing carboxypeptidases have been uncovered in brain and other tissues.[153, 154]

Discovery of the Prohormone Convertases. In 1985, a gene encoding an endopeptidase was found in yeast and was shown by genetic manipulations to be necessary for the processing of the α mating factor precursor.[155, 156] This encoded enzyme, which was called Kex2, or kexin, was predicted to be a large (814 residue) integral membrane protein containing a catalytic domain related to the bacterial subtilisins[157, 158] (see Fig. 48–11). Kexin thus arose from a serine protease

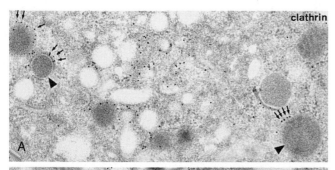

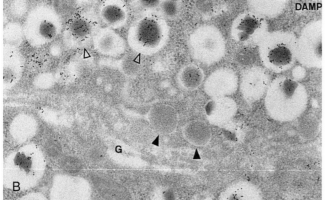

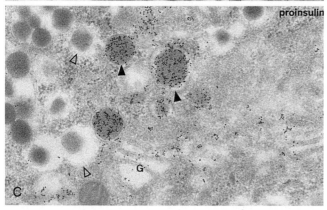

FIGURE 48–9. Clathrin *(A)*, 3-(2,4-dinitroanilino)-3′-amino-*N*-methyldipropylamine (DAMP) *(B)*, and proinsulin *(C)* immunolabeling of Golgi areas (G) of B cells (protein A–gold techniques). These figures show that the population of secretory granules with tightly fitting cores *(black arrowheads)* is clathrin coated *(arrows) (A)*, DAMP poor *(B)*, and proinsulin rich *(C)*. These granules correspond to the maturing coated secretory granules freshly released from the Golgi complex. Conversely, secretory granules with wide clear halos *(white arrowheads)* are deprived of clathrin (not shown here), are DAMP rich *(B)*, and are proinsulin poor *(C)*. These correspond to the noncoated mature (storage) insulin-containing secretory granules. Because DAMP immunoreactivity is assumed to represent an indirect measure of intra-organelle acidity, this may indicate a decreasing pH gradient between proinsulin-rich and insulin-rich granules (i.e., between the converting and the storage compartments). *(A,* ×28,000; *B* and *C,* ×27,000.) (From Orci L: The insulin cell: Its cellular environment and how it processes proinsulin. Diabet Metab Rev 2:71, 1986.)

to process human proinsulin to insulin in vitro through their combined action. The type I activity had a lower calcium requirement (10^{-3} M) and cleaved proinsulin only at the B chain–C peptide junction, whereas the type II activity required a higher calcium concentration for optimal activity (5×10^{-3} M) and cleaved human proinsulin only at the A chain–C peptide junction (see Fig. 48–10). Efforts to further purify these enzymes were partially successful, but quantities available were insufficient for amino acid sequence analysis and/or molecular cloning.

Meanwhile, efforts in many laboratories to find mammalian convertases by screening neuroendocrine cell cDNA libraries with kexin cDNA probes proved unsuccessful. Attempts to express insulinoma, normal islet, or AtT20 cell cDNA libraries in kexin-deficient strains of yeast with appropriate yeast vectors, using the restoration of mating and/or killer factor activity as selective screens, also yielded no positives.[161] However, when the nucleotide and predicted amino acid sequence of kexin in *Saccharomyces cerevisiae* was published by Mizuno et al.[157] in 1988, it became possible to utilize polymerase chain reaction (PCR) methodologies to search for kexin homologues, based on the presumed amino acid sequence conservation surrounding the

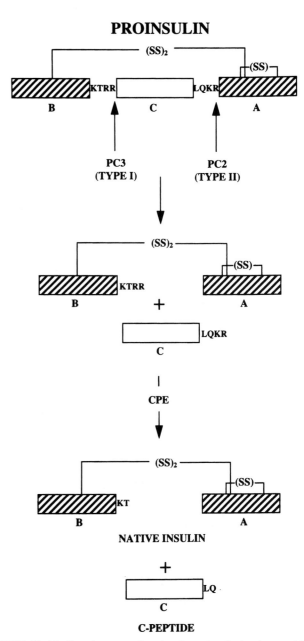

FIGURE 48–10. The cleavage of proinsulin to insulin by the combined action of the subtilisin-like prohormone convertases PC2 and PC1/PC3 and carboxypeptidase H. (See text for details.)

lineage unrelated to that of trypsin, probably via convergent evolution, as it utilizes the same classic charge transfer triad of Asp, His, and Ser as does the trypsin superfamily, but it is embedded in a totally different protein fold. The activity of kexin was shown to be dependent on calcium,[158, 159] and this observation spurred efforts to find mammalian homologues having a similar ionic requirement.

In 1988, Davidson et al.[160] first demonstrated the presence of two calcium-dependent activities (types I and II) in extracts of secretory granules purified from a rat insulinoma, raising the possibility that kexin-like enzymes existed in animal cells. These enzymes were able

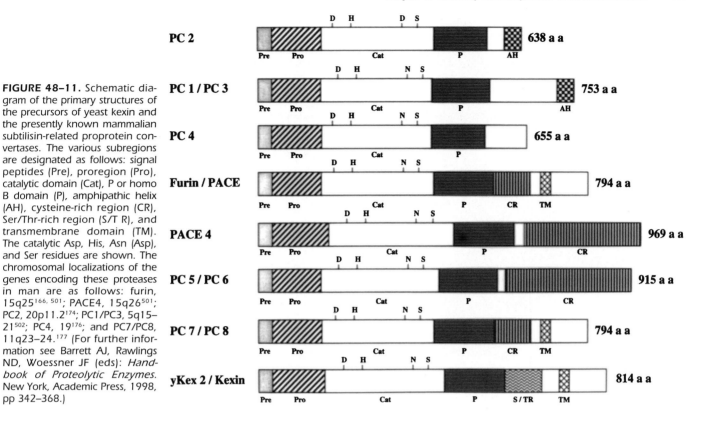

FIGURE 48–11. Schematic diagram of the primary structures of the precursors of yeast kexin and the presently known mammalian subtilisin-related proprotein convertases. The various subregions are designated as follows: signal peptides (Pre), proregion (Pro), catalytic domain (Cat), P or homo B domain (P), amphipathic helix (AH), cysteine-rich region (CR), Ser/Thr-rich region (S/T R), and transmembrane domain (TM). The catalytic Asp, His, Asn (Asp), and Ser residues are shown. The chromosomal localizations of the genes encoding these proteases in man are as follows: furin, 15q25[166, 501]; PACE4, 15q26[501]; PC2, 20p11.2[174]; PC1/PC3, 5q15–21[502]; PC4, 19[176]; and PC7/PC8, 11q23–24.[177] (For further information see Barrett AJ, Rawlings ND, Woessner JF (eds): *Handbook of Proteolytic Enzymes.* New York, Academic Press, 1998, pp 342–368.)

active site Asp, His, or Ser residues. This approach, when used with human insulinoma cDNA, led to the discovery of prohormone convertase 2 (PC2), a 638 residue protein related to kexin in its catalytic domain (49% amino acid identity) but lacking a transmembrane segment, Ser/Thr rich region, and cytosolic domain.[162] Further PCR analysis revealed an additional sequence, related to PC2, at lower abundance in the human insulinoma. A full-length cDNA, designated PC3, was obtained from AtT20 cell cDNA and revealed a 753 residue protein, which, like PC2, also lacked a transmembrane domain.[163] Seidah et al.,[164] in Montreal, using a similar approach based on the conserved Asn and Ser residues of furin,[158] identified PC2 and a second enzyme (that they called PC1/PC3) in mouse pituitary cDNA.[164] The mPC1 proved to be identical to mPC3.[165]

A search of the database with the PC2 sequence revealed *fur*, a related human partial gene sequence, which had been reported by a group in the Netherlands in 1986.[166] Its protein product was designated *furin* because its gene was found in the immediate upstream region of the c-*fes/fps* proto-oncogene. Although furin was believed initially to be a growth factor receptor due to the presence of a downstream cysteine-rich region and putative transmembrane domain, the incomplete N-terminal region was clearly related to the catalytic domains of PC2 and kexin and contained the characteristic catalytic serine residue. Subsequent cloning of full-length furin cDNAs revealed that this protein was structurally analogous to kexin, except that the Ser/Thr-rich domain in kexin was replaced by a cysteine-rich region.[167–170]

Structure and Activation of the Convertases. During the 1990s, a total of seven members of the mammalian prohormone convertase family have been identified.[171, 172] The structures of all these subtilisin-related convertases are compared diagrammatically in Figure 48–11. The genes encoding furin,[166, 173] PC2,[174] PC3,[175] PC4,[176] and PC7/PC8[177] have been cloned and characterized. They show great structural similarity with a high degree of conservation of exon-intron junctions, indicating their probable derivation in evolution from a common ancestral convertase through gene duplication.[174, 178] PC2 differs significantly from other members of this family in having aspartic acid at position 310 (the oxyanion hole residue) instead of a highly conserved asparagine normally present in this position in subtilisin and the other convertases. The δ amide of this asparagine residue in subtilisin is believed to form a hydrogen bond with the carbonyl oxygen of the

scissile peptide bond, which stabilizes the transition state during catalysis.[179] However, if the aspartyl side chain in PC2 is protonated, it should also be able to provide this H bond. Subsequent studies have born out that PC2 is optimally active at pH 5.5, in support of this hypothesis.[180] PC2 also differs from the other enzymes in requiring the coexpression of neuroendocrine protein 7B2 for its activation.[181–183]

PC2 and PC3 are expressed (in varying amounts) only in neuroendocrine tissues, such as the islets of Langerhans, pituitary, and adrenal medulla, and in many regions of the brain.[163, 165] In the islets, both PC2 and PC3 are present in the β cells, whereas only PC2 is present in the α, δ, and γ cells, which produce, respectively, glucagon, somatostatin-14 (SS-14), and pancreatic polypeptide (PP).[184–186] Both PC2 and PC3 have been localized by immunocytochemical staining to the secretory granules in β cells.[185, 187] Immunogold labeling of both proinsulin and PC2 in newly formed secretory vesicles has confirmed the co-localization of the convertases with their putative substrates (Fig. 48–12). PC3 undergoes C-terminal processing to a smaller 66 kDa form in the secretory granules. Western blot tests indicate that mature 66- to 68-kD forms of both PC2 and PC3 are the major forms present in islets of Langerhans, which is indicative of their accumulation in secretory granules.[187] Their tissue and subcellular distribution, along with their more acidic pH optima, contrasting with the more nearly neutral pH optima of kexin, furin, PACE4, PC6, and PC7, support the identification of PC2 and PC3/PC1/PC3 as major convertases of the neuroendocrine system.

In contrast to PC2 and PC3, furin is expressed in almost all tissues, with the highest levels in the kidney and liver,[170, 188] and it may be involved in processing a variety of precursors, including various procoagulant proteins and proalbumin in the liver and some growth factor precursors and/or their receptors in many other tissues.[189, 190] These proteins are not stored in secretory granules but are rapidly secreted via constitutive pathways. In keeping with this role, furin has been localized by immunostaining to the Golgi apparatus within cells.[189] Furin also has a more stringent specificity that allows it to selectively cleave precursors exiting the *trans* Golgi without acting on the dibasic sites of most prohormone precursors, which are cleaved only after they enter the secretory granules. The basis of this greater selectivity is due at least in part to the additional requirement for an arginine residue in the P4 position relative to the cleavage site. This

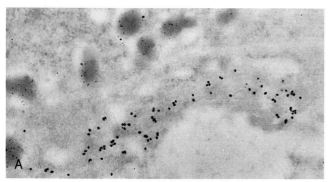

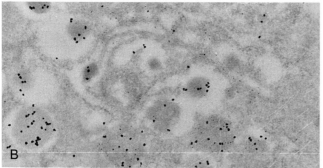

FIGURE 48–12. *A,* Immunogold labeling of proinsulin and PC2 in human islet β cells. Proinsulin-reactive Golgi stack (big colloidal gold particles) lack evident PC2 immunoreactivity (ultra small gold particles), labeling the mature secretory B granules. *B,* Proinsulin-reactive Golgi stack (ultrasmall gold particles) lack evident PC2 immunoreactivity (big gold particles); otherwise, present in the mature haloed and in some immature (proinsulin-reactive) secretory granules. (*A* and *B,* × 50,000). (Electron micrographs courtesy of Dr. Lucio Scopsi, Milan.)

requirement has been demonstrated in a number of studies using a variety of substrates[169, 188–194] and suggests that furin recognizes the general cleavage sequence R-X-K/R-R.[189, 190] Thus, furin substrates often consist of tetrabasic sequences, as in the anthrax toxin protective antigen,[194] the egg laying hormone of *Aplysia,*[195] and the insulin receptor precursor[196]; tribasic sequences, such as R-X-K/R-R[190, 197]; or, less commonly, dibasic sequences in which arginine residues are present only in the essential P1 and P4 positions (R-X-X-R).[194] The polybasic sequences in a number of viral glycoprotein precursors also are likely substrates, and evidence is now mounting that furin and/or related enzymes (e.g., PC6B and PC7) carry out these cleavages, which are essential for full viral virulence.[198–201]

The convertases are synthesized as inactive zymogens due to the presence of an N-terminal 80-residue proregion that follows the signal peptide in the proenzyme (see Fig. 48–11). This sequence usually contains two potential (multibasic residue) processing sites. Kexin is processed autocatalytically at a Lys-Arg (KR) pair at the downstream end of this region during its transport from the ER to the Golgi.[202] The mammalian proteases all have a similar, but more complex (R-X-K/R-R), potential activation cleavage site positioned similarly at the end of their proregions. Studies on furin have indicated that this site is cleaved autocatalytically and intramolecularly in the ER and this cleavage is necessary for the next step—transit to the Golgi. However, the propeptide remains attached after cleavage and serves to inhibit the enzyme until it reaches the TGN, where it dissociates under the more acidic conditions of this compartment; the propeptide is cleaved again at a second, more internal, site, allowing mature furin to gain full activity.[203] Except for PC2, with its unique requirement for 7B2 and relatively late maturation in the secretory granules, the furin model applies to the activation of PC3 and the other convertases.[172]

Role of PC2 and PC3 in Proinsulin Processing. Both PC2 and PC3 are required for proinsulin processing. Earlier studies indicated that PC2 cleaved selectively at the C peptide–A chain junction, whereas PC3 preferentially cleaved at the B chain–C peptide junc-

tion[187, 204] (see Fig. 48–10). However, subsequent results indicate that either convertase is capable of cleaving at both sites when expressed at high enough levels.[205–207] All the available data[204, 208] are consistent with the identification of PC1/PC3 and PC2 as the calcium-dependent type I and type II insulinoma granule-processing activities, respectively, as originally described by Davidson et al.[160] Guest et al.[209] have fully documented the important role of calcium in the transport and proteolytic maturation of proinsulin.

The role and order of action of PC2 and PC3 in proinsulin conversion has also been carefully studied. Rhodes et al.[210] demonstrated that the type II convertase (PC2) prefers the proinsulin intermediate that has already been cleaved at the B chain–C peptide junction (des 31,32 intermediate proinsulin) as a substrate. This observation has led to the scheme for conversion outlined in Figure 48–13, in which PC1/PC3 acts first to generate the des 31,32 intermediate, which is then the preferred substrate for PC2 action. This possible order of action is consistent with observations that PC3 achieves an active form more rapidly than PC2 and has a somewhat higher pH optimum. Thus PC3 may begin cleaving proinsulin in the TGN and very early secretory granules, whereas PC2 acts only in maturing granules. According to this scheme, PC1/PC3 appears to play a more important role in proinsulin processing, and this is born out by observations on islets from mice lacking PC2 due to disruption of its gene.[207, 211]

PC2 null mice are not diabetic, but they exhibit significant hyperproinsulinemia with plasma proinsulin levels in the range of 60%.[211] Pancreatic extracts also show increased proinsulin levels, but only in the homozygous nulls, as indicated in Table 48–1. Pulse-chase studies of insulin biosynthesis in isolated islets, comparing PC2(−/−) mice with wild type (WT) controls, also confirm significantly slower processing of proinsulin to insulin with accumulation of significant levels of des 31,32 intermediate proinsulin.[207] Approximately one-third of the labeled proinsulin remains after a 3- or 4-hour chase, consistent with the levels found by radioimmunoassay in pancreatic extracts. Thus, PC2 converts, at most, about a third of the available proinsulin; therefore, PC3 must be responsible for processing the remaining two-thirds under normal conditions.

Although a PC3 null mouse strain has not yet been generated, it has been possible to examine this issue indirectly in a human subject who is a compound heterozygote with mutations in both copies of the PC3 gene.[212, 213] This 43-year-old woman is obese and had gestational diabetes.[212] Examination of the patient's serum revealed no detectable circulating insulin associated with greatly elevated intact proinsulin and significant amounts of des 64,65 intermediate proinsulin, but little or no des 31,32 proinsulin. This picture is consistent with the conversion scheme outlined in Figure 48–13 and indicates that the pathway shown on the right side of the diagram is the predominant one. It also confirms the likelihood that PC3 is the more important β cell convertase. It is unlikely that no insulin at all is produced in this individual's pancreas; its apparent absence in the circulation is more likely due to the rapid receptor-mediated clearance of the small amounts of mature insulin that probably can be produced in the absence of PC3 in the β cells.

Significance of Proinsulin and Des 31,32 Intermediate in Man. An important clinical issue is the observation that in man, des 31,32 intermediate proinsulin is a major intermediate, making up a very significant proportion of the circulating proinsulin-like material.[214, 215] It has been suggested that the accumulation of des 31,32 proinsulin might be due to a defect in the action of PC2, indicating a defect in the conversion mechanism.[216] At present it is not possible to actually

TABLE 48–1. Percent Proinsulin-like Immunoreactivity in Pancreatic Extracts of Wild Type and PC2 Null Mice

Strain	Male	Female
Wild type	4.5	3.4
PC2 (heterozygous)	4.8	3.7
PC2 (homozygous)	33.0	28.0

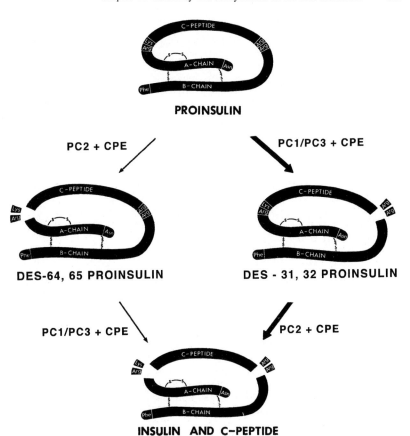

FIGURE 48–13. *Routes of processing of proinsulin in the pancreatic β cell. The pathway on the right is probably more dominant under normal conditions because des-31,32 proinsulin is a preferred substrate for PC2,[210] and the more acidic pH optimum and slower maturation of this enzyme may delay its action during the initial phases of secretory granule maturation. The C-terminal basic residues are removed by CPE (CPH) after endoproteolytic cleavage by the PCs. (Modified from Rouillé Y, Duguay SJ, Lund K, et al: Proteolytic processing mechanisms in the biosynthesis of neuroendocrine peptides. Front Neuroendocrinol 16:322, 1995.)*

measure PC2 activity in human pancreas; however, isolated normal human islets of Langerhans have been reported to convert proinsulin to insulin with significant accumulation of des 31,32 intermediate despite the presence of normal levels of PC2.[217] However, des 31,32 intermediate only reaches levels of 15% to 20% of the total immunoreactive material during biosynthetic pulse-chase studies in the islets of mice lacking PC2 altogether.[207] Thus, even the complete absence of PC2 should not in itself give rise to the very high levels of this intermediate seen in normal human serum samples. This phenomenon can be explained on the basis of the preference of PC2 and PC1/PC3 for a basic residue in the fourth position upstream (P4) from the cleavage site. Such an upstream basic residue is present at the B chain–C peptide junction in human proinsulin but is lacking at the A chain–C peptide junction. This causes an imbalance in the relative susceptibility of these two sites to either of the two convertases and tends to favor the accumulation of des 31,32 intermediate.[207]

Studies on the regulation of the biosynthesis of PC2 and PC3 in β cells suggest that the rates of translation of both of these enzymes are upregulated by glucose, similar to proinsulin on glucose stimulation.[218, 219] However, it is not yet clear whether both PC2 and PC3 mRNA levels are equally elevated along with insulin mRNA during more prolonged stimulation of islets with glucose. Conceivably, under conditions of chronic stimulation, a relative deficiency of PC2 may develop that could exaggerate the abnormalities in circulating proinsulin intermediates seen in diabetics. Thus, the accumulation of des 31,32 proinsulin in man is mainly a reflection of the amino acid sequences at the proteolytic cleavage sites in human proinsulin, whereas increased levels in diabetics may result from a mild deficiency of PC2 when islets are stressed by hyperglycemia. Genetic studies have not indicated a major role for mutations in the PC3,[175, 220] PC2,[221] or CPE[222] genes in susceptibility to any form of diabetes.

Unusual and Rarely Occurring Cleavages. In some species, such as rats, and probably also pigs and humans, additional processive cleavages occur in the C peptide region of proinsulin that appear to be due to a chymotrypsin-like activity.[23, 117, 129, 223] The importance of such additional C peptide cleavages in conversion remains unclear,

however, since they evidently occur only in species in which the C peptide contains sites of high chymotryptic sensitivity. Recently, a novel subtilisin-like convertase was described in several laboratories.[224, 225] This protease is only distantly related to the proprotein convertases and has a cleavage specificity that may be augmented by a P4 arginine residue, like some of the convertases, but it requires a hydrophobic valine or leucine residue at the P1 position of the cleavage site. An activity of this type may be responsible for some of the reported C peptide cleavages at sites with neutral or hydrophobic residues.

In the dog, C peptide cleavage occurs internally at a single arginine residue to produce an N-terminally truncated C peptide having only 23 residues.[226] A number of well-documented instances of such cleavage at single basic residues are known.[227, 228] Some of these may be catalyzed by PC3, especially if a P4 arginine is present and the P1′ residue is not hydrophobic, but others involving Pro-Arg or Arg-Pro sites probably require other enzymes.[229] Taken altogether, these findings suggest that neuroendocrine secretory granules may contain a mixture of processing proteases[223, 230] and that the specific cleavage of precursor forms of insulin or other precursor proteins is dictated, in part, by the high sensitivity to proteolytic digestion of certain regions in these substrate molecules as well as by restrictive specificities in the converting enzymes, which have similar but not identical properties and substrate specificities.

β Granule Formation

One of the mysteries of neuroendocrine and other secretory cells is the mechanism underlying the efficient sorting of proteins destined for regulated secretion into immature secretory vesicles in the TGN. In the β cell, this process is remarkably efficient, resulting in very low levels of unregulated or "constitutive" release of proinsulin (<1%–2%). The early secretory granules have a clathrin coat (see Fig. 48–9), which appears to be involved in some reorganization of the granule contents after and/or during their formation.[231] This granule sorting presumably occurs via small clathrin-clad vesicles that transport some proteins from the granules into cycling endosomal pathways that either recycle to the TGN or to the cell surface. As a consequence of this "constitutive-like" pathway, proteins such as furin, procathepsin B, and possibly others briefly pass through the immature granule compartment where they may play an active, albeit a transient, role (e.g., furin may participate in some away in the processing of prohormones).[231, 232] Also, small amounts of abundant soluble granule components such as proinsulin and/or C peptide may exit the granules within these vesicles.[233] They may also play a role in maintaining synchrony between granule membrane area and granule volume as maturation proceeds.[231]

The newly formed secretory granules in neuroendocrine cells undergo biochemical and morphologic maturation after their formation in the Golgi apparatus. In β cells, the "progranules" characteristically are somewhat larger and less dense than the mature granules and have a uniform appearance.[136, 138] Among the biochemical changes taking place as these progranules mature in the cytoplasm of the cell is the proteolytic conversion of proinsulin to insulin, accompanied by changes in the organization of the products. Electron microscopic studies of maturing insulin-secretory granules indicate that they acquire a dense central core, which often appears to be crystalline (Fig. 48–14). High magnification reveals repeat-unit spacings in the cores that are closely similar to those observed in ordinary zinc insulin crystals.[234–236] Thus, as insulin is liberated from proinsulin, it tends to crystallize with zinc that is concentrated by the β cells. Biochemical fractionation of mature islet secretory granules confirms that the cores contain only insulin, whereas the C peptide liberated in the conversion process remains in solution in the clear fluid space surrounding the dense crystalline core.[236] There is no evidence for co-crystallization of the C peptide with insulin under these conditions or in vitro. However, low levels of proinsulin can co-crystallize with insulin. As a result, the granule cores contain 1% to 2% of intact or partially processed precursor.[236]

The role of zinc in secretory granule formation is not well understood.[237] Most of the zinc in islets is present in the β granules and is liberated proportionately to insulin during secretion, in keeping with its role in crystallization of the hormone.[238, 239] The mechanism for accumulation of zinc within the granules is unclear, but it may be a largely passive process that reflects the ability of both proinsulin and insulin to bind zinc.[106, 240, 241] The insulins of some species, including the guinea pig, coypu, and other hystricomorph rodents[17] and the hagfish,[37, 65] lack the histidine residue at position 10 of the B chain required for zinc binding during the association of insulin dimers into hexamers.[62] As mentioned earlier, most mammalian proinsulins can form soluble hexamers stabilized by two zinc atoms coordinated with the six B10 histidines, as seen in 2-zinc insulin crystals.[63] The proinsulin hexamers can also bind zinc at additional sites without precipitating from solution.[240] This property may allow proinsulin to play a role in zinc accumulation in the islet cells. Another function of the zinc may be to regulate the conversion process by sequestering the newly formed insulin in an osmotically inactive and biochemically stable crystalline form, thus effectively separating the product of this reaction from the enzyme(s) involved.

The pH of the interior of the secretory granule appears to be between pH 5.0 and 6.0 in the mature granules,[128, 139] an optimal pH range for insulin crystallization in vitro. The neutral or slightly alkaline pH in the cisternal spaces of the rough endoplasmic reticulum favors proinsulin folding and sulfhydryl oxidation. The pH remains near neutral throughout the Golgi apparatus but becomes more acidic (pH 6.1) in the TGN as the secretory products are sorted into granules and proteolytic processing begins. Vesicular proton pumps may begin to increase the uptake of protons, which then displace the cationic arginine and lysine residues liberated during conversion. As these move out of the granules and are replaced by hydrogen ions, a downward shift in intragranular pH may occur. Thus, the initially mildly acidic progranules[139] undergo gradual acidification as they mature in the cytosol (see Fig. 48–9), creating appropriate conditions for the crystallization of the newly formed insulin. Clearly, the processes related to the biosynthesis of insulin via preproinsulin and proinsulin and their intracellular transport, sorting, proteolysis, and ultimate storage in

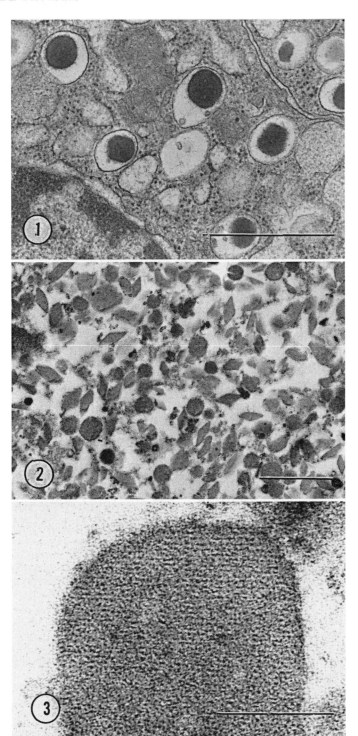

FIGURE 48–14. *1*, Photomicrograph of normal rat β cells (×28,000) showing morphology of mature granules (bar = 1 μm). *2*, Isolated rat β granule cores (×17,000)[236] (bar = 1 μm). *3*, High magnification view (×250,000) showing repeat unit structure of a crystalline core (bar = 0.1 μm). The cores are made up of both rat insulin I and II in approximately equal proportions (Michael J, Steiner DF: unpublished data). Samples were fixed with Karnovsky's solution and stained with osmium tetroxide. (Electron micrographs courtesy of Hewson H. Swift.)

secretory granules are remarkably well integrated, topologically and biochemically. This delicately poised integration of processes leading to the formation and storage of insulin is disturbed in islet cell tumors, which often show unregulated release of insulin together with large amounts of proinsulin; measurements of the latter can provide a useful diagnostic indicator[242, 243] (see Chapter 49).

Biosynthetic Role and Possible Biologic Actions of the C Peptide

Because of its co-secretion with insulin in essentially equimolar amounts,[93, 244–246] the C peptide has been of great value as a marker of insulin secretion in humans under a variety of conditions (see Chapter 49). However, the C peptide radioimmunoassay is limited by the great sequence variability of this region in the proinsulin molecule; cross-reactivity is confined to closely related species, such as mice and rats, in which sequence divergence is minimal. Representative vertebrate C peptide amino acid sequences are compared in Figure 48–15.[99, 247, 248] These peptides exhibit a 15-fold higher rate of mutation acceptance than do the corresponding insulins, a finding that has often been interpreted as indicating that this region in the proinsulin molecule is unlikely to have any specific hormonal function. Among known proteins, only the fibrinopeptides have a higher rate of mutation acceptance than the proinsulin C peptides. Nonetheless, several acidic residues are consistently present at certain positions in the mammalian C peptides (see Fig. 48–15). These offset the added cationic charges due to the pairs of basic residues at the cleavage sites such that the isoelectric pH of proinsulin is nearly the same as that of insulin (i.e. in the range of pH 5.1–5.5) for most of the mammalian prohormones.[88, 249]

Since the early 1990s, a number of reports have appeared describing a number of biologic effects of the C peptide and/or peptides derived from it.[250] These putative effects include enhancement of glucose transport and utilization[250–252]; improvements in microcirculation in muscle,[253] skin, retina, and nerve in diabetics[254–256]; and stimulation of renal tubular Na$^+$,K$^+$-adenosine triphosphatase (ATPase) activity and other parameters of renal function.[250, 252] Stimulation of islet cell proliferation has also been reported.[257] These results suggest that tissue receptors for C peptide might exist and that the circulating C peptide may contribute to improved glycemic control and help to slow the development of the vascular and neural complications of diabetes. What makes these effects even more surprising is that they do not seem to follow the usual rules of ligand-receptor chemistry (i.e., chirality does not matter); a C peptide synthesized entirely of D-amino acids is equally as active as a peptide made with L-amino acids in reversed order.[254] However, a random sequence of the same amino acids leads to loss of activity. These observations suggest that novel interactions with membrane bilayers or other cellular constituents may

underlie the observed effects.[256] These tantalizing data suggest the need for a controlled clinical trial of combined insulin and C peptide therapy in diabetics. However, it should be born in mind that in some of the reported studies, pharmacologic levels of C peptide have been used. It is also difficult to exclude the possibility of chemical impurities in some preparations that might lead to some of the observed effects in the complex biologic systems studied.

In addition to any putative biologic roles, consideration must also be given to the possible biosynthetic role of the C peptide. Thus, the C peptide clearly functions in biosynthesis by converting the insulin A and B chain interaction from an inefficient bimolecular reaction to a highly efficient and concentration-independent unimolecular reaction.[258] Certain regions of the connecting peptide may also facilitate the folding of the proinsulin polypeptide chain and the formation of the correct disulfide bonds, or guide the enzymatic cleavage of proinsulin to insulin by helping to orient the basic residue pairs for efficient binding and cleavage by the convertases.[21, 99] Recent molecular modeling studies indicate that this function of the C peptide may be of particular importance and may require an extended configuration for this region during interaction with the convertases.[259]

It is clear that the length of the C peptide (usually 30 to 35 amino acids) is much greater than that necessary to span the short distance between A1 and B30 in the native insulin molecule (see Figs. 48–4 and 48–6). Not surprisingly, small bifunctional cross-linking reagents inserted between the amino group of A1 glycine and the ε-amino group of B29 lysine of insulin can functionally replace the C peptide in promoting the correct reoxidation of the sulfhydryls in high yield after complete reduction and denaturation.[260, 261] Similarly, mini-proinsulins with greatly shortened or absent connecting peptide segments readily oxidize to form the correct disulfide bridges and can be cleaved to yield insulin.[21, 72] These findings are consistent with the notion that the C peptide region in proinsulin serves other functions in the biosynthetic process in addition to promoting A and B chain combination or has biologic functions as a secreted product.

Another putative function of the relatively long C peptide may be to lengthen the polypeptide chain of proinsulin to facilitate its translocation across the RER membrane. The length of polypeptide chain required to span the large ribosomal subunit and the RER membrane has been estimated to be about 65 residues in extended configuration.[262–264] Moreover, the arrest of translation by the signal recognition

```
              1  2   3   4   5   6   7   8   9  10  11  12  13  14  15  16  17  18  19  20  21  22  23  24  25  26  27  28  29  30  31  32  33  34  35  36  37  38

HUMAN        Glu-Ala-Glu-Asp-Leu-Gln-Val-Gly-Gln-Val-Glu-Leu-Gly-Gly-Gly-Pro-Gly-Ala-Gly-Ser-Leu-Gln-Pro-Leu-Ala-Leu-Glu-Gly-Ser-Leu-Gln

MONKEY       Glu-Ala-Glu-Asp-Pro-Gln-Val-Gly-Gln-Val-Glu-Leu-Gly-Gly-Gly-Pro-Gly-Ala-Gly-Ser-Leu-Gln-Pro-Leu-Ala-Leu-Glu-Gly-Ser-Leu-Gln

HORSE        Glu-Ala-Glu-Asp-Pro-Gln-Val-Gly-Glu-Val-Glu-Leu-Gly-Gly-Gly-Pro-Gly-Leu-Gly-Gly-Leu-Gln-Pro-Leu-Ala-Leu-Ala-Gly-Pro-Gln-Gln

PIG          Glu-Ala-Glu-Asn-Pro-Gln-Ala-Gly-Ala-Val-Glu-Leu-Gly-Gly-Gly-Leu-Gly ——— Gly ——— Leu-Gln-Ala-Leu-Ala-Leu-Glu-Gly-Pro-Pro-Gln

COW, LAMB    Glu-Val-Glu-Gly-Pro-Gln-Val-Gly-Ala-Leu-Glu-Leu-Ala-Gly-Gly-Pro-Gly-Ala-Gly-Gly-Leu — — — — — Glu-Gly-Pro-Pro-Gln

RABBIT       Glu-Val-Glu-Glu-Leu-Gln-Val-Gly-Gln-Ala-Glu-Leu-Gly-Gly-Gly-Pro-Gly-Ala-Gly-Gly-Leu-Gln-Pro-Ser-Ala-Leu-Glu ——— Ala-Leu-Gln

DOG          Glu-Val-Glu-Asp-Leu-Gln-Val-Arg-Asp-Val-Glu-Leu-Ala-Gly-Ala-Pro-Gly-Glu-Gly-Gly-Leu-Gln-Pro-Leu-Ala-Leu-Glu-Gly-Ala-Leu-Gln

RAT I        Glu-Val-Glu-Asp-Pro-Gln-Val-Pro-Gln-Leu-Glu-Leu-Gly-Gly-Gly-Pro-Glu-Ala-Gly-Asp-Leu-Gln-Thr-Leu-Ala-Leu-Glu-Val-Ala-Arg-Gln

RAT II       Glu-Val-Glu-Asp-Pro-Gln-Val-Ala-Gln-Leu-Glu-Leu-Gly-Gly-Gly-Pro-Gly-Ala-Gly-Asp-Leu-Gln-Thr-Leu-Ala-Leu-Glu-Val-Ala-Arg-Gln

GUINEA PIG   Glu-Leu-Glu-Asp-Pro-Gln-Val-Glu-Gln-Thr-Glu-Leu-Gly-Met-Gly-Leu-Gly-Ala-Gly-Gly-Leu-Gln-Pro-Leu-Ala-Leu-Glu-Met-Ala-Leu-Gln

CHINCHILLA   Glu-Leu-Glu-Asp-Pro-Gln-Val-Gly-Gln-Ala-Asp-Pro-Gly-Val-Val-Pro-Glu-Ala-Gly-Arg-Leu-Gln-Pro-Leu-Ala-Leu-Glu-Met-Thr-Leu-Gln

DUCK         Asp-Val-Glu-Gln-Pro-Leu-Val-Asn-Gly-Pro ——— Leu-His-Gly-Glu-Val-Gly-Glu ——— Leu-Pro-Phe-Gln-His-Glu-Glu ——— Tyr-Gln

CHICKEN      Asp-Val-Glu-Gln-Pro-Leu-Val-Ser-Ser-Pro ——— Leu-Arg-Gly-Glu-Ala-Gly-Val ——— Leu-Pro-Phe-Gln-Gln-Glu-Glu-Tyr-Glu-Lys-Val

ANGLERFISH   Asp-Val-Asp-Gln-Leu-Leu-Gly-Phe-Leu-Pro-Pro-Lys-Ser-Gly-Gly-Ala-Ala-Ala-Ala-Gly-Ala-Asp-Asn-Glu-Val-Ala-Glu-Phe-Ala-Phe-Lys-Asp-Gln-Glu-Met-Met-Met-Val

HAGFISH      Asp-Thr-Gly-Ala-Leu-Ala-Ala-Phe-Leu-Pro-Leu-Ala-Tyr-Ala-Gly-Asp-Asn-Glu-Ser-Gln-Asp-Asp-Glu-Ser-Ile-Gly-Ile-Asn-Glu-Val-Leu-Lys-Ser

MOLLUSC      Asn-Ala-Glu-Thr-Asp-Leu-Asp-Asp-Pro-Leu-Arg-Asn-Ile-Lys-Leu-Ser-Ser-Glu-Ser-Ala-Leu-Thr-Tyr-Leu-Thr
```

FIGURE 48–15. Compilation of amino acid sequences of proinsulin C peptides in vertebrates and in a mollusk, *Lymnae stagnalis* (for sources see Steiner[99] and Smit, et al.[503]). The guinea pig C peptide sequence corresponds to that predicted from the nucleotide sequence of the guinea pig insulin gene.[66]

particle (SRP) occurs only after synthesis of a nascent chain of about this length and may play a role in translational control of insulin biosynthesis.[263] Thus, the initial sequestration step in the biosynthesis of secretory peptide precursors may require a minimum peptide chain length that may greatly exceed the size of the final bioactive peptide or peptides, per se.[263, 264] Efficient intracellular transport and correct targeting to secretory granules may impose additional demands on the primary (and tertiary) structure of proinsulin and other precursor proteins.[99, 265, 266] However, mini-proinsulins with deleted C peptides are correctly targeted to the regulated secretory pathway.[265]

The synthesis of several mammalian C peptides has been accomplished by classical fragment-condensation approaches (for refs see Steiner et al.[39]). The synthetic porcine C peptide, containing all four terminal basic residues, was tested for its ability to promote the recombination of insulin A and B chains in vitro, but it failed to influence the yield.[267] Synthetic porcine and bovine C peptides cross-react well with antibodies directed against the corresponding natural proinsulins or C peptides, and fragments of these peptides have been successfully utilized to study the antigenic determinants in this region of the proinsulin molecule.[39, 268] The availability of biosynthetic human proinsulin and insulin, as well as of human C peptide, has opened many new possibilities for studies of the role, metabolism, and antigenicity of these peptides.[25, 269–271]

REGULATION OF INSULIN PRODUCTION

Although the rate of secretion of insulin is subject to elaborate control by glucose and other nutrients, as well as by hormones and neurotransmitters,[272] the renewal and regulation of the granular stores of hormone in the β cells is an important aspect of normal homeostasis. The biosynthesis of insulin is regulated by a variety of mechanisms so as to replenish insulin stores. The amount of insulin and/or proinsulin released via "unregulated," or constitutive, pathways[273] is normally very small, in the range of 1% to 2%.[245] Thus, calcium-dependent exocytosis of preformed storage granules[274] appears to be the major, if not the sole, source of both basal and glucose-stimulated insulin release in vivo.[244] We might ask how this granular compartment is maintained and regulated. The chief positive effectors that have been identified thus far are glucose, augmented by cyclic adenosine monophosphate (cAMP), which may also be generated by a mechanism coupled to glucose metabolism in the β cell.[275] Secretion, however, is not a direct stimulus to insulin biosynthesis, as can be demonstrated by blocking the secretory process via lowering external calcium levels or using inhibitors. These maneuvers do not impair the biosynthetic response to glucose.[93] If inhibition of secretion is prolonged, however, intracellular degradation (autophagy) of secretory granules occurs.[139, 245] Also, in fetal and newborn rat islets, glucose stimulates insulin biosynthesis, although it has little effect on insulin secretion.[276]

It is well known that glucose rapidly stimulates insulin biosynthesis

via stimulation of insulin messenger RNA (mRNA) translation.[93, 277] This response consists of effects of glucose on both the initiation and elongation of proinsulin chains.[277] Glucose stimulation may also reduce the duration of SRP-signal peptide–mediated arrest of nascent preproinsulin chain elongation prior to ribosome docking in the early phases of RER membrane translocation.[266, 277, 278] In addition to this fast-acting translational control mechanism, the rate of transcription of insulin mRNA is also upregulated by glucose and cAMP.[279–282] Increased transcription results in part from phosphorylation of PDX1, a homeodomain protein that binds to regulatory regions of the insulin gene promoter.[283, 284] Insulin mRNA, under normal conditions, turns over very slowly, with a half-life of about 30 hours at normal glucose levels,[280] and its stability is also affected by glucose. Hypoglycemia can lead to rapid declines in insulin mRNA.[285] In contrast, elevated glucose levels increase its half-life dramatically (approximately 2.6-fold), and this action, in combination with increased transcription rates, can effect large increases in insulin mRNA levels over periods of many hours. Prolonged glucose stimulation thus can lead to highly significant increases in insulin production[286] and, eventually, to increased β cell mitosis and hyperplasia as well.[287] Glucose also regulates the turnover of insulin stores within the β cells,[245] but this effect probably plays a less significant regulatory role under normal conditions.

The Insulin Gene Family

The genetic mechanisms controlling the expression of endocrine and neural regulatory peptides in the organism have been explored extensively. The gene for insulin was among the first to be isolated.[288] Its structure in man[289] and several other species[55] is summarized in Figure 48–16. The single copy human gene is located on the short arm of chromosome 11 in band p15.[290, 291] It is flanked on the 5′ side by a unique polymorphic region, composed of tandem repeats, that lies beyond the upstream regulatory region; this polymorphic region does not seem to influence the gene's expression in the pancreas but it provides a useful marker for genetic linkage analysis.[292] Earlier reported correlations of the presence of larger (class III) vs. smaller (class I or class II) repeats in this region with the incidence of type 2 diabetes were confounded by ethnic differences in the distribution of tandem repeats. Further analyses of larger populations failed to support this conclusion but have revealed that class I alleles and genotypes are significantly more frequent in white persons with type 1 diabetes than in those with type 2 diabetes or control subjects.[293] This allele may thus be a marker for a nearby susceptibility gene for type 1 diabetes.

The cDNAs and genes encoding other members of the insulin gene family have been identified and analyzed,[55] and additional members in mammals have been identified more recently.[56, 294] Analysis of the genomic sequences encoding these various peptides substantiates the view that they are all related to insulin and are appropriately consid-

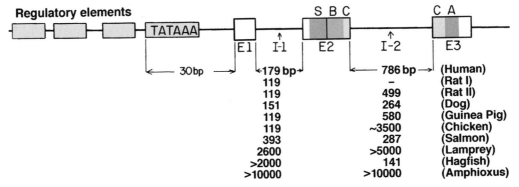

FIGURE 48–16. Diagrammatic representation of the insulin gene in vertebrates. Exons (E) appearing in mature preproinsulin mRNA are shown as bars, and the sizes of the two introns or intervening sequences (I) in various species are tabulated below. U, Untranslated region; P, prepeptide coding region; B, B chain coding region; C, C peptide coding region; and A, A chain coding region. A typical TATA box signaling transcription initiation is shown approximately 30 base pairs upstream from the messenger start site, preceded by a promoter region (unfilled boxes). The human insulin gene, abbreviated INS, is located on the short arm of chromosome 11 in the region p15.[290, 291]

ered members of an insulin superfamily of hormones and/or growth factors. The duplication events that gave rise to genes encoding relaxin and other distantly related insulin-like peptides have not been identified. The genes encoding the insulin-like growth factors (IGFs) appear to have arisen near the time of divergence of the vertebrates. In amphioxus, a primitive protochordate, a single insulin-IGF hybrid molecule has been identified that is equally distant from mammalian insulin and IGF genes.[295] These findings are consistent with the hypothesis that insulin and the IGFs diverged by gene duplication in early vertebrate evolution to better integrate metabolism and growth in these complex organisms. However, in contrast to IGF-1 and -2, which are synthesized by most tissues, at least at some period during development, insulin appears to be produced only in the β cells of the islets of Langerhans in the adult organism.[296]* The selective expression of the insulin gene in the β cells of the islets of Langerhans appears to be brought about by the actions of a number of transactivatng factors that bind to DNA recognition sequences located in the upstream region of the gene between the hypervariable region and the TATA box, i.e., 300 to 400 base pairs upstream (for reviews, see Philippe[297] and Edlund[298]).

Defects in the Insulin Gene: The "Insulinopathies"

Tager and associates were the first to identify a structurally abnormal insulin in the circulation and pancreas of a patient with mild diabetes associated with elevated insulin levels.[299] The development of HPLC systems capable of resolving plasma insulin components then led to the further identification of abnormal insulins differing in hydrophobic character in two additional unrelated lineages.[15] These and similar studies led to the definition of a new clinical syndrome analogous to the hemoglobinopathies—the insulinopathies (i.e., molecular defects involving the insulin molecule). Six families have been identified thus far, all having the syndrome of mild hyperinsulinemic diabetes that is similar, in some respects, to type 2 or non-insulin–dependent diabetes mellitus (NIDDM).[300, 301] Affected individuals have high circulating insulin levels with a distorted C peptide-insulin ratio, resulting most likely from the delayed turnover, in vivo, of circulating insulin variants due to their impaired receptor-binding properties.[302] The disorder is inherited in an autosomal dominant fashion within families, consistent with the mendelian distribution of a defective allele.

The insulin genes (both alleles) have been cloned from affected individuals in these families, and in all six cases a single nucleotide substitution in only one of the two alleles leading to a single amino acid replacement within the insulin molecule was found.[301, 303, 304] The abnormal insulins generated by these missense mutations are all characterized by a very low binding potency, below 5% of normal, as demonstrated by direct assays.[305, 306] However, the replacements occur at different sites within the insulin molecule (at residues B24[Phe → Ser], B25 [Phe → Leu], and A3 [Val → Leu]), and the affected individuals thus far have all been heterozygous for the defective gene. Although not all affected individuals have overt diabetes, it is evident from the high incidence of mild diabetes or glucose intolerance among the affected individuals in these families that the presence of a defective insulin allele can be a significant predisposing factor to the development of diabetes. Hence, such mutations, or still others that might reduce the level of expression of the insulin gene (i.e., leading instead to hypoinsulinemia), could give rise to a picture indistinguishable from the fairly common type 2 diabetes (NIDDM).

Recently a point mutation in one of the two mouse insulin genes (Ins II) has been found to be associated with severe β cell dysfunction in the Mody mouse.[307] This autosomal dominant form of diabetes is not associated with obesity or insulin resistance, but is due instead to impaired insulin production. The mutation of the A7 cysteine to tyrosine evidently causes misfolding, aggregation, and degradation of both mutant and normal proinsulin chains in the endoplasmic reticulum. Molecular chaperones, such as BiP, and enzymes involved in sulfhydryl oxidation, such as protein disulfide isomerase (PDI), are increased in the islets of Mody mice, whereas insulin is greatly decreased. Secretory granules are less abundant and smaller than in controls, whereas ER is enlarged and contains material that is probably composed of proinsulin aggregates. This represents one of the most severe insulinopathies to be found to date, but it clearly indicates the potential for dominant negative structural defects in proinsulin as a cause of diabetes.

In addition to molecular variants involving insulin, others have been identified that give rise to elevated circulating proinsulin levels, with or without clinically significant carbohydrate intolerance.[308, 309] In these families, an autosomal dominant pattern of inheritance is again evident, and in seven cases the defect has been localized to the conversion site in the proinsulin molecule (at the C peptide–A chain junction) at which the arginine of the Lys-Arg pair recognized by the converting enzyme has been replaced by another amino acid, rendering this site uncleavable.[310, 311] In six of these families, molecular cloning has disclosed the substitution of a histidine for Arg 65[312–314]; in another family, leucine replaced Arg 65.[315] An eighth family with hyperproinsulinemia, in which a point mutation changes the histidine at position 10 of the B chain to aspartic acid, has also been identified.[316, 317] This is a particularly interesting mutation because the resultant proinsulin molecule retains the paired basic residues, but it is not processed efficiently due to a defect in its sorting into secretory granules, which leads to its increased secretion as intact proinsulin via constitutive pathways.[318, 319]

The study of molecular variants as exemplified by the cases described above is fascinating and valuable for many reasons. Although rare, these naturally occurring variants shed light on both normal processes and disease mechanisms and thereby assume greater importance and relevance to clinicians. The study of insulin variants have led to significant revisions in theories regarding the location of the receptor-binding region in the insulin molecule (see Receptor Binding Region of Insulin, earlier in the chapter) and has also provided direct evidence that receptor-mediated uptake and degradation of insulin[71, 320, 321] is a major pathway of insulin metabolism in vivo.[300, 301]

Several studies have assessed the frequency of insulin gene mutations in diabetic populations.[322, 323] Variations in both noncoding and coding sequences have been found, but thus far no significant associations with diabetes have been detected. Three promoter variants have also been described.[323, 324] These include a C to G transversion at –56, a C deletion at −90 and an 8-base pair repeat–TGGTCTAA–from positions −322 to −315. This repeat was present in the insulin genes of 5% of subjects with NIDDM and 1% of nondiabetic black American subjects, as well as in 3 of 41 diabetic and 0 of 41 nondiabetic Mauritian Creoles of African ancestry. It was absent in 35 white subjects with NIDDM and 40 Pima Indians. When tested in functional assays, this variant exhibited significantly reduced promoter activity (38%–44% of normal). These results suggest that naturally occurring promoter variants that reduce insulin gene expression may contribute to a small proportion of cases of diabetes in some ethnic groups. Defects in regulatory proteins arising from other loci (e.g., the transcription factor PDX1[325]) also can influence insulin gene expression or its regulation and play an important role in causing diabetes of the MODY type.

IAPP (AMYLIN): A NEW SECRETORY PRODUCT OF THE β CELL

A number of studies during the 1990s have revealed that β cells secrete small amounts of a number of other peptides and proteins in addition to insulin (Table 48–1).[94, 326] Some of these are unique to the islet β cells, whereas others are expressed in other neuroendocrine cells and neoplasms. The chromogranins A, B, and C represent a family of closely related acidic peptides that are expressed in many neuroendocrine cells.[327] Chromogranin A is found in the β, α, and PP cells in the islets, whereas chromogranins B and C are also only present in the islet α cells.[327] The role of these proteins is not under-

---

*Extrapancreatic insulin expression transiently occurs in the yolk sac during embryonic development in the rat[496] and has been detected by in situ hybridization in periventricular cells in rat brain[497]; the latter observation remains to be confirmed.

stood, but it may be related to the formation and organization of the secretory granule or the processing of prohormones. Chromogranin A has been cloned from porcine adrenal medullary tissue[328] as well as from rat pancreatic islet and insulinoma tissue,[329] and some amino acid sequence information on the human peptide from insulinomas is also available.[330] Chromogranin A is processed to release at least two peptides of interest, pancreastatin—a 49–amino acid amidated peptide from the central region of chromogranin A, which was originally isolated from porcine pancreas and which inhibits insulin secretion[331]—and β granin—a 24 kDa peptide derived from the N-terminal region of chromogranin A.[326, 329] Both peptides are stored in insulin granules and are released along with insulin.

Another intriguing co-secreted product is the recently discovered 37–amino acid neuropeptide-like molecule—islet amyloid polypeptide (IAPP), or amylin. IAPP was first described as a major protein constituent of the amyloid deposits that occur in the islets of elderly diabetics (i.e., those with so-called type 2 diabetes, or NIDDM) and in many benign insulinomas of the pancreas as well as in the normal pancreases of the aged.[332–335] Although the presence of amyloid-like material was first noted in specimens of human pancreas as early as 1901 by the pathologist Opie,[336] it was not until 1986 that efforts to solubilize this material were successful.[332] When the soluble material was analyzed, it turned out to be composed mainly of a single peptide, IAPP. Sequence analysis revealed that this peptide (Fig. 48–17) was related to the 37–amino acid neuroendocrine peptides calcitonin gene-related peptide, types 1 and 2 (CGRP-1 and -2).[332–335] CGRP-1 is a second product of the calcitonin type I gene, derived through an alternative splicing event that occurs mainly in neural tissues.[337–339] As a result of this process, a calcitonin encoding exon (exon 4) is replaced by another encoding CGRP (exon 5) in the formation of an mRNA for a preproprotein that gives rise to CGRP via proteolytic processing.[338]

The availability of the amino acid sequence of IAPP led to the identification of both the cDNA and the chromosomal gene encoding this hormone-like polypeptide in humans.[340–343] In addition, cDNAs encoding IAPP precursors from a number of mammalian species have been described.[340, 341, 344] PreproIAPP has a signal peptide followed by a short propeptide ending in Lys-Arg at the N terminus of IAPP (Fig. 48–18). The C-terminal side of the IAPP domain is followed by Gly-Lys-Arg and another short propeptide region. The presence of a glycine residue at the C terminus of the IAPP region preceding the basic dipeptide proteolytic processing signal suggests that IAPP is normally carboxyamidated, as are the CGRPs.[340, 344] Comparison of the sequences of the precursors of IAPP and CGRP also revealed sequence similarities in their signal peptides as well as between the sequences of IAPP and CGRP.

The characterization of the human IAPP gene (see Fig. 48–18) revealed a simpler intron-exon arrangement than described for the genes encoding CGRP-1 and -2,[337] although all are clearly related.[342, 343, 345] The single gene encoding IAPP in humans is located on the short arm of chromosome 12,[342, 343] which is believed to be an evolutionary homologue of chromosome 11, where the CGRP-1 and -2 genes are located.[337] Thus, the available evidence strongly supports the likely divergence of IAPP, CGRP, and calcitonin from a common ancestral gene.

Biosynthesis and Levels of IAPP in Islets

Studies with antibodies specific for IAPP have demonstrated that it is present in islets in significant amounts, as judged by immunocytochemical staining, and is localized to the secretory granules of the β cells.[346–348] Thus, the IAPP precursor is likely transferred along with proinsulin into newly forming secretory vesicles in the TGN of the β cells, where it is then processed into the mature 37-residue carboxy-amidated peptide, stored, and subsequently co-secreted with insulin.[349] The processing of proIAPP appears to require the actions of β cell convertases such as PC2,[350] but the site specificity of PC2 and PC1/PC3 have not yet been determined for this prohormone. The expression of IAPP is stimulated by glucose, comparable to that of insulin under normal conditions, but it may be altered in pathologic states.[351] Very low levels of IAPP mRNA have also been detected in the stomach and other regions of the gastrointestinal tract, in the lung, and also in the dorsal root ganglia of the spinal cord.[352]

The relative levels of IAPP and insulin in the β cell appear to be only a few percent of the level of insulin. HPLC analysis of freshly isolated rat islets shows amounts of IAPP that are in the range of 1% to 2% those of insulin.[94] Biosynthetic labeling experiments in islets have also corroborated these low levels of IAPP expression relative to insulin (Carroll R, Steiner DF: Unpublished data). Although synthetic IAPP has been shown to inhibit insulin secretion from rat islets of Langerhans, the doses (10^{-5} M) required for this affect are extremely high.[353] Most studies[354–356] agree that the levels of IAPP are in the range of 0.2% to 3% of the level of insulin in normal adult rat islets or normal human pancreas. Studies with isolated rat islets have shown that IAPP secretion is stimulated by glucose and that IAPP amounts to about 5% of the amount of insulin released in 1 hour at 16.7 mM of glucose.[356]

Hormonal Effects of IAPP

Leighton and Cooper and others have shown that IAPP inhibits glucose uptake and glycogen synthesis in muscle exposed to IAPP in vitro, an effect it shares with CGRP.[357, 358] In whole animals, efforts to modify glucose tolerance with IAPP infusion have met with mixed success. However, euglycemic glucose clamp studies with dogs have demonstrated that the amidated form of IAPP inhibits insulin-stimulated glucose disposal over short infusion periods of 1 to 2 hours.[359] In these experiments, the rates of IAPP infusion were 3- to 6-fold higher on a molar basis than the rates of insulin infusion. Such high ratios of secretion of IAPP relative to insulin could not be achieved under normal physiologic conditions in vivo. Other studies indicate that the actions of IAPP may be complementary to those of insulin.[360] However, mice lacking IAPP due to a knockout of the gene show increased insulin secretion and more rapid glucose disappearance, suggesting that its normal role is inhibitory with respect to insulin secretion and action.[361, 362]

In view of the distant evolutionary relationship between calcitonin and IAPP, it is of interest that both nonamidated and amidated forms of IAPP have serum calcium–lowering effects in animals in vivo as

FIGURE 48–17. Comparison of IAPP and CGRP amino acid sequences. Note canonical differences between the two peptide families at positions 1, 8, 10, 14, 15, 17, 20 to 28, 35, 36, and 37. The region comprising residues 20 to 29 is believed to nucleate β-pleated sheets in forming amyloid fibrils.[374] (From Nishi M, Sanke T, Nagamatsu S, et al: Islet amyloid polypeptide. A new beta cell secretory product related to islet amyloid deposits. J Biol Chem 265:4173, 1990.)

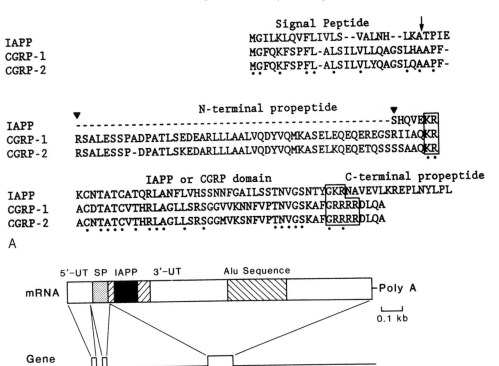

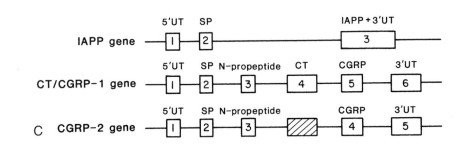

FIGURE 48–18. *A,* Comparison of amino acid sequences of the precursors of human IAPP and CGRPs 1 and 2. The *small arrow* indicates the signal peptide cleavage site; the *arrowheads* show the position of intron exon junctions in the CGRP-1 and 2 genes. *B,* Schematic representation of the mRNA encoding preproIAPP, indicating its relation to the exons of the IAPP gene. This gene in man is located on chromosome 12P12.3.[342, 343] *C,* Comparison of IAPP and CGRP gene structures. The ancestral gene of this superfamily may have been organized similarly to that of the CGRP-2 gene. 5'UT, 5 untranslated region; SP, signal peptide; CT, calcitonin.

well as in cell culture systems.[363, 364] A direct effect on uptake of calcium by bone tissue has been demonstrated, but it is not clear whether this effect is mediated via calcitonin or IAPP receptors.[363] MacIntyre[364] has proposed that IAPP may be secreted along with insulin to promote the utilization of ingested calcium.

Finally, it should be mentioned that because of its extensive homology with CGRP, it seems likely that IAPP may share some actions of CGRP, a family of neuropeptides that are expressed in the nervous system and at nerve endings in many organs throughout the body.[339, 365, 366] Their main functions in peripheral tissues appear to be mediated via cAMP and to involve smooth muscle relaxation leading to bronchial dilation, lowering of blood pressure, and decreases in intestinal motility.[337, 339, 366] It also has been proposed that CGRP may play a role as a growth factor, regulating the development of olfactory bulb neurons during embryogenesis.[367] Recent studies suggest that protein modifiers termed *receptor activity–modifying proteins* (RAMPs) can interact with and modify the specificity of CGRP-like receptors to enhance IAPP binding.[368]

Mechanism of Amyloid Formation

Several studies[369–371] have indicated that islet amyloid formation (Fig. 48–19) occurs more prominently in spontaneously diabetic animals and in certain species more so than others. Among diabetes-prone animals were several different species of nonhuman primates as well as cats, raccoons, and the degu (*Octodon degus*), a New World

rodent related to the guinea pig.[334, 369–373] It is interesting to note that the IAPP sequences in these species differ most significantly in the region that has been defined as amyloidogenic (residues 20–29) in studies by Glenner et al.[374] and Westermark et al.[344, 375] Synthetic peptides from this region had the greatest tendency to form fibrillar stacked β-pleated sheet structures similar to those occurring in amyloid. However, formation of amyloid in the degu occurs via a different mechanism and has been shown to consist mainly of degu insulin, which differs significantly from most other mammalian insulins.[376, 377]

Antibodies raised to various regions of IAPP have verified its presence in islet amyloid by both light and electron microscopic immunocytochemical analysis.[347, 348, 378] Although in normal β cells it is localized within the insulin secretory granules,[347, 348] fibrillar immunoreactive amyloid deposits have also been noted within the cytoplasm of β cells of some patients with type 2 diabetes by Clark and co-workers.[346] Others have also noted the proximity of amyloid deposits to the β cells, suggesting that it has arisen from these cells either by secretion or by some other means of deposition.[375, 379] Clark et al.[380] have found IAPP immunoreactivity in lysosomes and lipofuscin bodies within the β cells of the islets of both normal and diabetic individuals and have suggested that amyloid may begin to form during the intracellular degradation of secretory granules, as occurs in the normal turnover of unused secretory products, a process known as *crinophagy.*

The factors leading to amyloid deposition in diabetes remains unclear,[381, 382] but recent work with transgenic mice hypersecreting human IAPP have demonstrated amyloid deposition under some circum-

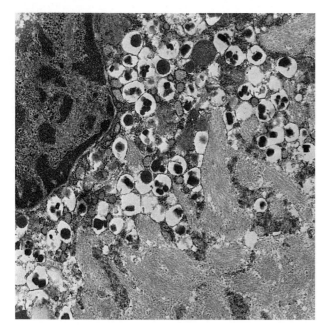

FIGURE 48–19. Photomicrograph showing extensive islet amyloid deposits with adjacent β cells in a human diabetic pancreas (×28,000). (Electron photomicrograph courtesy of Dr. Per Westermark, Linköping, Sweden).

stances, especially with high dietary fat intake.[383] Recent studies have failed to reveal any abnormalities in the predicted sequence of IAPP precursors in 25 subjects with type 2 diabetes,[384] and thus hypotheses involving abnormalities in the structure of either IAPP or its precursor in the formation of islet amyloid are untenable. The amyloid formed in the islets during normal aging appears to be similar to that in diabetic subjects but is usually much less abundant.[385–387]

PROPERTIES AND STRUCTURE OF GLUCAGON

Although the existence of a pancreatic hyperglycemic factor was postulated in the early 1920s,[388] the peptide hormone glucagon was not isolated until 30 years later.[389] Using a crude fraction obtained during the commercial preparation of insulin, Staub et al. succeeded in both purifying and crystallizing the pancreatic stimulator of hyperglycemia.[389] They noted the nearly neutral isoelectric pH of the peptide and its tendency to form fibrils at acidic pH. The availability of the pure hormone thus eliminated any continuing doubt as to the existence of a unique hyperglycemic hormone and made possible a great number of experiments regarding its chemistry and mechanism of action.

In 1957, Bromer et al. reported the amino acid sequence of porcine glucagon and noted the sensitivity of the peptide to digestion by trypsin.[390] Since that time, the glucagons from a number of mammalian, avian, and piscine species have been isolated and their sequences determined (Fig. 48–20).[391–393] Remarkably, the sequence of the glucagons of almost all mammals is identical, except for the guinea pig, in which it differs at five positions.[394–396] The identical glucagons of turkeys and chickens differ from human glucagon at only one position,

and the duck hormone differs at only two.[393, 397, 398] Neither of these changes, however, appears to have a major impact on bioactivity, notwithstanding the reduced reactivity of duck glucagon with antisera directed toward the mammalian hormone.[393] The structure of glucagon in several species of fish has also been reported (see Plisetskaya et al.[399]). These are substituted at from six to ten positions in various species. The high degree of structural conservatism within glucagons, especially among mammals, probably reflects strong evolutionary constraints operating within the glucagon-secretin superfamily of closely related hormones. Guinea pig glucagon is an exception, having five amino acid replacements in its C-terminal region,[394, 395] which reduce its biologic activity to about 10% of that of other species.[396] The amino acid substitutions in the guinea pig protein may represent an adaptation to the markedly altered insulin in this species,[35, 394] which also has greatly reduced biologic potency.[400] An increased rate of mutation acceptance is confined to this region of the guinea pig glucagon gene.[394] Glucagon is structurally related to other neurohormonal peptides, including secretin, vasoactive intestinal polypeptide (VIP), gastric inhibitory peptide (GIP), and growth hormone releasing factor (GHRF), indicating a probable common ancestral origin.[401, 402]

Investigations on the secondary and tertiary structure of glucagon have indicated that the hormone assumes an α-helical conformation, dependent on both peptide concentration and on the characteristics of added solutes (summarized in Steiner et al.[39]). In more concentrated solutions, glucagon monomers associate into trimers and possibly higher oligomers.[17] A major advance in our understanding of glucagon structure came from the work of Sasaki and associates on the complete x-ray analysis of crystalline glucagon at 3 Å resolution.[403] The peptide exists in the crystal as a trimer with a high percentage of helical secondary structure. Residues 10 to 25 occur in α-helix and residues 5 to 9 and 26 to 29 in a less regular, right-handed helical conformation. The N-terminal pentapeptide is apparently more flexible, and its conformation is less well defined. The structure of monomeric glucagon in very dilute solution remains unsolved, but the possibility of the induction of α-helicity by interaction of the peptide with hydrophobic receptor recognition sites has been considered.[17]

The strong evolutionary conservation of glucagon suggests the importance of multiple structural features that contribute to the biologic activity of this gluconeogenic and glycogenolytic hormone. In fact, deletion of either the N-terminal histidyl residue or the C-terminal dipeptide sequence Asn-Thr leads to markedly decreased receptor-binding potency.[404, 405] Glucagon fragments containing fewer than about 25 residues retain no significant ability to bind to glucagon receptors. An exciting advance in the area of glucagon structure-function relationships concerns the chemical synthesis by Unson and co-workers of potent glucagon antagonists[406–408] One such antagonist is a simple glucagon analogue in which the N-terminal histidine has been deleted, Asp9 is replaced by Glu, and the C-terminal threonine exists as its α-carboxamide derivative. Detailed analysis has demonstrated that the loss of His1 and the replacement of Asp9 (actually by any of several amino acids) are critical to the antagonistic properties of the peptide. The antagonist binds to plasma membrane glucagon receptors with high affinity but exhibits no tendency to stimulate adenylyl cyclase or the production of cAMP. Because the analogue competes well for glucagon-receptor interactions, it serves as a glucagon antagonist when the analogue and the natural hormone are present in admixture.[406–408] It is interesting to note that the analogue appears to serve as a partial agonist in stimulating glucose-potentiated insulin secretion from isolated pancreatic islets.[409] Although definitive information is not yet available on differences in secondary structure and general conformation that might apply to the agonist hormone and the antagonist analogue, it is clear that the glucagon receptor is exquisitely sensitive to structural changes in the occupying ligand. Further studies will undoubtedly identify the character of these structural changes and the mechanisms by which both glucagon and antagonist bind to receptor, but glucagon alone exhibits the ability to induce transmembrane signaling events that activate adenylyl cyclase through the intervention of heterotrimeric G proteins. Although the in vivo effects of glucagon antagonists have been studied relatively little,[410] such compounds have the potential for therapeutic use in decreasing the hyperglycemia asso-

```
HUMAN          HSQGTFTSDYSKYLDSRRAQDFVQWLMNT
GUINEA  PIG    ---------------------Q-LK--L-V
CHICKEN        ----------------------------N
DUCK           ---------------T------------N
ANGLERFISH     --E---SN------ED-K--E--R----N
```

FIGURE 48–20. Primary structures of glucagons in several vertebrate species. Residues that differ from the highly conserved sequence of Old World mammals (human, pig, cow, rabbit, rat, hamster) are indicated. (Single letter amino acid code is given in Dayhoff.[36])

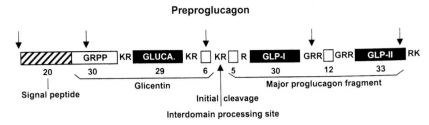

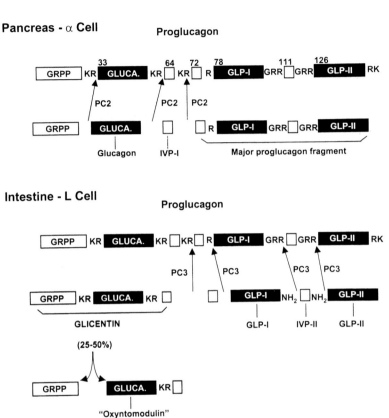

FIGURE 48–21. *Schematic of the human glucagon precursor and its tissue specific processing in α cells vs. intestinal L cells. The processing sites, which must be cleaved to generate glucagon and the glucagon-like peptides, are shown between indicated segments. The C terminus of glucagon-like peptide 1 is amidated; the sequence Gly-Arg-Arg directs cleavage of the precursor and provides a substrate for the polypeptide amidating activity enzyme complex (PAM).[493] The tissue-specific processing of this precursor is indicated. In islet α cells, processing is carried out by PC2 at the more N-terminally located Lys-Arg pairs to produce glucagon. In L cells, residues 1 to 69 are released en bloc as glicentin, or gut glucagon, whereas the C-terminal major proglucagon fragment (residues 72–160) is efficiently processed, most likely by PC1/PC3, to release GLP-1 and -2 peptides (see text for details). Numbers below sequence designate the number of residues; numbers above proglucagon sequence are the residue numbers at the N terminus of each domain. The arrows above the preproglucagon sequence at the top indicate the positions of introns in the human gene; each coding exon of the preproglucagon gene encodes a major domain of preproglucagon. The human glucagon gene, abbreviated GCG, is located on the long arm of chromosome 2 in the region q36 → q37.[504]*

ciated with diabetes.[411] All considered, it is clear that glucagon's biologic activity depends crucially on the necessity to place what may be a great number of its structural features in correct apposition to an equal number of receptor features in a concerted and very precise way. The cloning of the glucagon receptor[412] has opened the way to a more detailed understanding of the mechanism of glucagon binding and action.

Glucagon Biosynthesis

Although the first evidence that glucagon is derived from a higher molecular weight precursor was obtained in 1973, it is only recently that a relatively complete picture of proglucagon and its processing has emerged. Initially, Tager and Steiner isolated from crystalline glucagon an extended form that consisted of the entire sequence of glucagon with a C-terminal octapeptide extension having the sequence Lys-Arg adjacent to the C-terminal threonine of glucagon, suggesting a typical prohormone processing site.[413] Glucagon-like immunoreactivity derived from the intestine (the so-called *gut glucagon* or GLI-1) consisted of a larger component with an apparent molecular mass of 10 kDa and led Moody and co-workers to propose the name *glicentin* for this peptide.[414, 415] On isolation in sufficient quantities for amino acid sequencing, glicentin turned out to consist of only 69 amino acids, and it contained glucagon with the previously described 8-residue C-terminal extension (glucagon 37 or oxyntomodulin), as well as a 32-residue N-terminal extension.[415] Subsequent biosynthetic studies by Patzelt et al. with isolated rat islets led to the definitive

identification of proglucagon as a much larger 18 kDa protein, as estimated by sodium dodecyl sulfate (SDS)-gel electrophoresis under reducing conditions.[416] Pulse-chase experiments revealed that a single proglucagon protein at about 18 kDa appeared very rapidly, but it subsequently split into two similar-sized proteins of 18 to 19 kDa within 10 minutes (shown by Patzelt and Weber[417] to be due to O-glycosylation, i.e., carbohydrate addition to serine or threonine residues), and then resolved back into a single protein of intermediate mobility (about 18.5 kDa), which slowly disappeared over a chase period of 2 hours. An intermediate proteolytic fragment of 13 kDa containing glucagon (by two-dimensional peptide analysis) appeared transiently.[416, 418] By about 1 hour, a major protein of about 10 kDa (termed the *major proglucagon fragment*), which does not contain glucagon, began to accumulate. Normally this component represents a major end product of glucagon processing in rat islets.[416, 419, 420]

The isolation and analysis of cDNA clones for hamster, bovine, and rat proglucagon (for a review see Bell[402]) confirmed the estimated molecular weight of 18 kDa for the mammalian glucagon precursor and revealed several interesting features in addition to a typical prepeptide or signal peptide at its N terminus. The structural organization of a typical mammalian preproglucagon molecule is shown in Figure 48–21. This structure contains the 37-residue extended glucagon first described by Tager and Steiner[413] within the sequence of glicentin,[415] which makes up the N-terminal 69 amino acids of the prohormone. The C-terminal half of the molecule corresponds to the major proglucagon fragment (residues 72–160; Fig. 48–22) observed by Patzelt et al.[416] and subsequently shown to be, along with glucagon, a major co-secretory product of the α cells.[420] The major proglucagon fragment

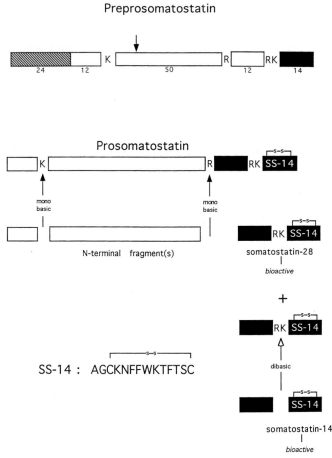

FIGURE 48–22. Sequence of the human somatostatin precursor. The sites which must be cleaved to release somatostatin-28 or somatostatin-14 are shown between indicated segments. The *arrow* above the preprosomatostatin sequence at the top indicates the position of the single intron in the gene encoding this precursor. The human somatostatin gene, abbreviated SST, is located on the long arm of chromosome 3 in the region q28.[505]

contains two glucagon-like sequences, which have been designated GLP-1 and -2. These sequences are bracketed by paired basic amino acids, which are sites of proteolytic processing, and are separated by a short spacer region, as is glucagon from GLP-1. It is interesting to note that islet α cells release predominantly the 29-residue glucagon, whereas GLP-1 and -2 are released mainly[421] or exclusively[422] in the form of the 10 kDa major proglucagon fragment. The reverse occurs in the ileal region of the small intestine, where glicentin, free GLP-1, GLP-1 (residues 7–37), and GLP-2 are the major secretory products (see Fig. 48–21).

Because only a single gene has been found to encode preproglucagon in humans and rats,[402] and the sequence of glicentin derived from porcine intestine is highly homologous to residues 1 to 69 of the predicted prohormonal sequence from humans, hamsters, and cows, the proteolytic processing of proglucagon clearly must differ between the α cells of the islets of Langerhans and the glucagon cells of the intestine.[423] The differential processing of proglucagon in these tissues could be influenced by O-glycosylation, as noted for the pancreatic precursor,[417] but it is more likely to be due to differences in the processing enzymes expressed in these tissues (see Fig. 48–21). The exact site or sites of carbohydrate addition are not known, but they appear to reside in the C-terminal region in either GLP-1 or -2, both of which contain a number of serine and threonine residues that could be glycosylated. It is not known whether a similar modification of proglucagon occurs in intestinal cells. Recent evidence suggests that GLP-1 (residues 7–37) (proglucagon residues 78–107) is a potent stimulator of insulin secretion.[423–425] It appears that this peptide is the most potent "incretin" found to date and may be largely responsible

for the increased insulin response to oral glucose and meal ingestion that has been recognized for many years.[4253] However, no physiologically relevant biologic activity has been ascribed* to the N-terminal extended form of GLP-1 (proglucagon residues 72–107), a polypeptide whose structure was predicted from the position in proglucagon of pairs of basic amino acids, which often represent sites of proteolytic processing.[402] Because processing can also occur at single arginine residues, and residues 78 to 107 of proglucagon are more homologous to the N-terminal sequences of glucagon and GLP-2, perhaps mature GLP-1 should be redefined as proglucagon residues 78–107kDa-amide; the N-terminally extended molecule (proglucagon residues 72–107) could represent an inactive precursor form of GLP-1 (see Fig. 48–21). Recent work by Drucker and colleagues[426] and Litvak et al.[427] has shown that GLP-2 participates in the regulation of intestinal growth. It is interesting to note that some proglucagons in the anglerfish and in other teleosts lack GLP-2 and contain only a glucagon-like sequence and a GLP-1 (residues 7–37)-like sequence.[402]

Recent studies have elucidated the basis for the differential processing of proglucagon in the α cells vs. the intestinal L cells (see Fig. 48–21). The α cell pattern of processing of proglucagon is due to the presence of high levels of PC2 and the absence of significant levels of PC1/PC3 or other convertases.[428] In several studies Rouillé et al. have demonstrated the importance of PC2 for both of the cleavages that release glucagon from proglucagon,[429, 430] and this has been confirmed by studies with isolated islets from PC2 and 7B2 null mice, which show a marked inhibition in glucagon biosynthesis.[211] The phenotype of these mice consists of chronic hypoglycemia, and despite the presence of marked α cell hyperplasia and large amounts of circulating precursor-related glucagon-like immunoreactive material, no active glucagon can be detected. Treatment of these mice with glucagon reverses the hypoglycemia and the α cell hyperplasia (Webb G, Steiner DF: Unpublished results). A similar phenotype is seen in 7B2 null mice, which also lack active PC2.[183]

However, endocrine cells that express high levels of PC1/PC3 can be shown to efficiently process proglucagon to release glicentin and GLP-1, and probably GLP-2 as well.[429, 431] Efforts to conclusively define PC1/PC3 as the major convertase in intestinal L cells of canine origin have not fully supported this notion, though, as both PC2 and PC1/PC3 immunoreactivity are present.[432] The reason for this discrepancy is not clear, but it may represent a species difference between dogs and other mammals. Clearly, cells that express both PC2 and PC1/PC3, such as various β cell lines, process transfected proglucagon completely to glucagon, GLP-1, and GLP-2.[429] PC1/PC3 is also capable of cleaving the single basic residue site in GLP-1 (proglucagon residues 72–107) to release active GLP-1 (residues 7–37).[431] Both PC2 and PC1/PC3 are able to efficiently cleave the interdomain site between glicentin and the major proglucagon fragment (MPGF). These findings suggest that initial cleavage at this site may be required for the further, more specialized processing steps that follow. Proglucagon processing thus provides an excellent example of the regulation of specific hormone production from a multifunctional precursor via differential tissue expression of prohormone convertases PC1/PC3 and PC2. The molecular basis for the sharply defined specificity of the various convertase cleavage sites in proglucagon remains a mystery at this time.

SOMATOSTATIN STRUCTURE AND BIOSYNTHESIS

Somatostatin, a 14-residue peptide (SS-14) containing an internal disulfide bridge (see Fig. 48–22), was first isolated from hypothalamic extracts and shown to inhibit the release of growth hormone.[433] Subsequent studies have shown that somatostatin has a much broader spectrum of inhibitory actions and is much more widely distributed in the body, occurring not only in many regions of the central nervous system but also in many tissues of the digestive tract, including stomach,

---

*Recent studies have confirmed that glucose-dependent insulinotropic peptide (GIP) mediates GLP-1 release from distal intestinal sites in response to feeding.[498, 499]

intestine, and pancreas.[434-436] Somatostatin suppresses the release of many pituitary, pancreatic, and gastrointestinal polypeptide and glycoprotein hormones. In addition, it also inhibits gastric acid and pepsin secretion and intestinal smooth muscle contractility. Moreover, it probably also functions as a neurotransmitter or neuromodulator in the central nervous system.[436] Early studies with isolated islets suggested the existence of a peptide inhibitor of insulin secretion,[437] but the identity of this substance was unknown until the discovery of somatostatin. It soon became apparent that the islet A$_1$ or D cells, first described by Bloom in 1931,[438] were the source of somatostatin in the islets.[434, 439] The mechanism whereby somatostatin inhibits insulin secretion is still unresolved. It is possible that it functions as a paracrine effector, being released from the D cell and only inhibiting insulin and glucagon secretion from adjacent β and α cells within individual islets.[440] The inhibitory effects of somatostatin on secretion of digestive enzymes by surrounding acinar tissue may, however, be mediated by somatostatin secreted from D cells into the blood (i.e., it may be functioning as an endocrine molecule in this situation).[440] In contrast to its effects on insulin secretion, somatostatin does not inhibit insulin biosynthesis in response to glucose in adult rat islets,[441, 442] whereas it reportedly does so in fetal pancreas.[443]

Much study has been devoted to structure activity relationships within the somatostatin molecule in an effort to produce molecules of greater stability and potency, or with altered effectiveness in inhibiting various secretory activities (for reviews, see Reichlin[440] and Gottesman et al.[444]). In the islets, somatostatin and some of its derivatives inhibit glucagon secretion more strongly than insulin. In brittle type 1 diabetes, somatostatin can reduce the magnitude of blood glucose excursions.[440] However, long-term administration poses problems, and it is uncertain whether somatostatin or its derivatives significantly improve glycemic control in diabetic individuals over long periods. The chief utility of somatostatin is in the study of diabetes, in which its infusion can serve to block endogenous islet hormone release, permitting clamp studies and eliminating co-regulatory or counterregulatory influences in studying individual islet hormonal actions or turnover.[444]

Recently, the receptors for somatostatin have been cloned and characterized.[445-449] These studies have identified five structurally related proteins, all members of the G protein–coupled family of receptors having seven transmembrane domains, which bind somatostatin and mediate its diverse cellular actions.

The discovery of larger forms of somatostatin indicated the probable derivation of this peptide from a larger precursor.[436, 450] Much attention has been focused on somatostatin-28 (SS-28), a peptide made up of SS-14 extended through a basic amino acid bridge by a 12 residue N-terminal extension. SS-28 shares many of the actions of the tetradecapeptide form but differs in potency[451] as well as in tissue distribution within and without the central nervous system.[440] The two forms are evidently not interconvertible in the circulation; hence, the relative proportions found in the blood probably reflect differences both in tissue processing of the initial precursor and secretion and in plasma stability, uptake, excretion, and/or degradation.[452] Likewise, the origin of the two circulating forms of somatostatin is unclear and may well reflect the contribution of numerous potential sources throughout the organism.[440, 453]

The biosynthesis of pancreatic somatostatin has been studied both in mammalian islets[454] and in the larger, more readily accessible, single islet of teleostian fishes, known as Brockman bodies.[455, 456] Studies with mammalian islets are complicated by the fact that the somatostatin-producing D cells make up only about 5% of islet cells and usually lie on periphery of the islet,[139] where they are more likely to be damaged by collagenase digestion during islet isolation. Despite these technical difficulties, Patzelt et al.[454] were able to show, using isolated rat islets, that somatostatin is derived from a 12.5 kDa precursor peptide in which the somatostatin moiety occurs at the C terminus. The subsequent cloning of cDNAs for two closely related anglerfish preprosomatostatins,[455, 457] as well as the rat and human precursors,[458-460] confirmed these findings and showed both somatostatin and its precursor structure to be well conserved in vertebrate evolution (see Fig. 48–22). Moreover, the extensive amino acid identity between the rat and human prosomatostatin suggests that the N-terminal 63 residues may have some intrinsic biologic activity as well, although

what these functions might be remains unknown. Somatostatin-like immunoreactivity has been reported in a number of invertebrates and even unicellular organisms, but the identity and relationship of these forms to the SS-14 or -28 products of preprosomatostatin processing in vertebrates remains unclear.

The processing of prosomatostatin has not been studied in sufficient detail in mammalian islets to provide a clear picture of how SS-28 and SS-14 are derived by specific proteolysis of prosomatostatin. In the anglerfish, two prosomatostatins occur, each of which gives rise to only SS-28 or -14.[461] The sequence of prosomatostatin suggests that its cleavage to generate SS-28 requires a trypsin-like enzyme capable of cleaving at a single arginine residue, a feature which occurs in a number of neuropeptide and growth factor precursors, including, among others, the C peptide of dog proinsulin,[226] propancreatic polypeptide,[462] provasopressin/neurophysin[463] and the IGF-1 and -2 precursors,[464, 465] but is relatively rare in comparison with dibasic cleavage sites. Recent studies have identified two distinct proteases involved in the generation of SS-28 or -14 from the anglerfish precursors. The enzyme cleaving at the single arginine site is tentatively identified as an aspartyl protease.[466] It is interesting to note that yeast cells lacking the dibasic processing enzyme kexin retain the ability to cleave rat prosomatostatin to generate SS-28, but not SS-14.[467] In yeast, the aspartyl protease (YAP-2) may be involved in this processing event.[468, 469]

However, generation of SS-14 from SS-28 or larger intermediates of prosomatostatin does occur at a site having paired basic residues. However, the sequence at this site (see Fig. 48–20) is Arg-Lys (R-K), a very rare dibasic combination. Its conservation in all the somatostatin precursors described to date suggests[470] that a special processing enzyme may exist for this site. A 90 kDa endoprotease isolated from rat brain Golgi-neurosecretory granules cleaves SS-28 at this site to yield SS-14.[471, 472] Its high specificity and failure to cleave intact prosomatostatin suggests that it is a highly specialized protease. However, Mackin et al.[473] isolated an enzyme from anglerfish islets that processes prosomatostatin to SS-14, and it provided N-terminal sequence data suggesting that it is related to PC2. Co-expression studies also suggest a role for PC2 in generating SS-14.[474] Studies on PC2 null mice confirm that PC2 is the convertase responsible for generating SS-14.[211] In both islets and brain from PC2 null mice, only SS-28 is found, whereas in the wild type tissues, SS-14 is the major product detected by gel filtration combined with radioimmunoassay (Chiu G, Steiner D: Unpublished data).[211] The D cells are also hyperplastic in the PC2 null mice, but whether this is due to lack of SS-14 or is somehow related to the α cell hyperplasia and/or β cell hypoplasia is unclear. A cAMP-responsive element has been identified in the upstream region of the rat somatostatin gene.[475] However, much remains to be learned regarding the regulation of (pro)somatostatin biosynthesis at both transcriptional and translational levels.

PANCREATIC POLYPEPTIDE

Pancreatic polypeptide (PP) is a 36–amino acid peptide that was originally identified by Kimmel and Chance and their coworkers as a contaminant of some insulin preparations.[476-479] It is the product of a distinct cell type in the islets of Langerhans that is more abundant in the islets in the head of the pancreas—the portion of the pancreas near the duodenum that derives from the ventral anlage during development.[480] Typically the PP-producing cells lie near the periphery of the islets or in clusters among the exocrine tissue,[481] and thus their secretions, like those of the A cells and D cells, are more likely to be born by the blood into the surrounding acinar tissue or directly into the portal circulation. PP secretion is largely under vagal control and it does not appear to regulate carbohydrate metabolism, although levels typically rise promptly following a meal. Instead, its role appears to be to regulate gastrointestinal functions, such as exocrine pancreatic secretion and gallbladder emptying.[479, 482]

PP belongs to a family of structurally related carboxyamidated neuroendocrine peptides that includes PYY and NPY.[483] These peptides occur in many neurons in the peripheral and central nervous system. PP itself is derived from a 9 to 10 kDa precursor, or propancreatic

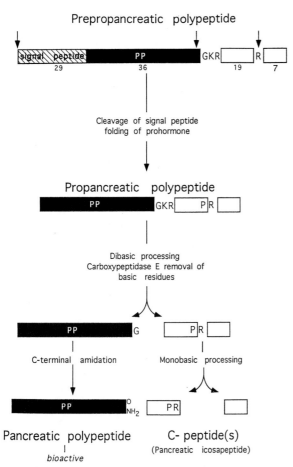

FIGURE 48–23. *Sequence of the human pancreatic polypeptide precursor. The processing sites are shown between indicated segments. The C terminus of pancreatic polypeptide is tyrosine-amide. The peptides generated by processing of this precursor are noted. The* arrows *above the preproPP sequence at the top indicate the positions of introns in the gene encoding the precursor. The human pancreatic polypeptide gene, abbreviated PPY, is located on chromosome 17 in the region p11.1 → qter.*[506]

polypeptide, from which a second peptide co-secretory product is derived, the icosapeptide, in the human, canine, feline, and bovine forms.[463, 484–487] The structure of human prepropancreatic peptide derived from a cDNA clone[488, 489] is shown in Figure 48–23, and the regions corresponding to PP and icosapeptide are indicated. Although the sequence of PP is well conserved in mammals, especially the C-terminal amidated region, the icosapeptide is less well conserved and in fact may not be released as such in the rat[490] or guinea pig,[491] where the single C-terminal arginine processing site (residue 59) is lacking. The icosapeptide has not been found to have any biologic activity. The region following the icosapeptide is even more variable (both in length and sequence), possibly due to differences in splicing of the separate exon(s) that encode this region in the gene.[490, 492]

X-ray crystallographic studies on avian PP indicate an ordered globular structure consisting of an N-terminal polyproline helix (residues 1–8) bent back through a turn to an α-helical region that extends from residues 14 to 32, terminating near a spatially well-defined C-terminal region.[17] It is likely that the structure of the mammalian forms of PP is similar to the avian structure, despite some sequence differences, and that this conformation may exist as well in solution and/or at the receptor-binding site. However, little is known at this time about the PP receptor protein or its tissue distribution.

The biosynthesis of PP appears to follow the general scheme for the other islet hormones as indicated in Figure 48–8. After removal of the prepeptide in the ER, proPP is transferred to the Golgi area, where it is packaged into prosecretory granules and processed by enzymes having specificities for basic residue pairs similar to those responsible

for the processing of proinsulin and proglucagon. Because the N terminus of PP follows immediately after the signal peptide in proPP, only a single site must be processed for its release. The sequence at this site is Gly-Lys-Arg and is most likely processed by at least three enzymes: (1) a paired basic residue endopeptidase recognizing Lys-Arg (i.e., either PC2 or PC3); (2) a carboxypeptidase B-like enzyme (CPase E), which removes the C-terminal arginine and lysine residues successively; and (3) an amidating enzyme system,[493, 494] which oxidatively removes the glycine to yield CO_2 and the carboxyamidated preceding amino acid (tyrosine). Cleavage to produce the icosapeptide then occurs at a single arginine residue in several species, giving rise to the co-secreted icosapeptide. Evidence from studies with cultured dog PP islets indicates that this monobasic processing endopeptidase is distinct from the protease acting on the paired basic residues.[495] However, all these processing activities, as in the case of proinsulin, follow a time course that strongly suggests that they may occur in the maturing progranules, as these collect in the cytosol prior to discharge from the cell in response to cholinergic stimuli. Regulation of the tissue-specific expression of PP as well as modulatory effects of various stimuli on the transcription and translation of its mRNA remain important unexplored areas.

CONCLUSIONS

The general features of the biosynthesis and cell biology of the neuroendocrine hormones and peptides can be summarized as follows:

1. Most neuroendocrine peptides are derived from precursors that are processed within secretory granules prior to their regulated release into the circulation.

2. The processing proteases, as typified by PC2, PC3, and carboxypeptidase E, are usually constituents of the secretory granule and may vary in type or relative quantity, dependent on the particular cell or tissue and the final mixture of peptides that is to be generated.

3. The rate of proteolytic processing is usually kinetically first order, and it is regulated by changes in convertase expression. The half-time for conversion of prohormonal peptides is usually between 30 and 60 minutes.

4. The peptide products of proteolytic cleavage are often retained in the secretory vesicles and co-secreted by exocytosis in a coordinate fashion in response to stimuli (e.g., insulin and C peptide are secreted together in equimolar amounts along with small amounts of proinsulin from the pancreatic islets).

5. Peptide fragments, as exemplified by the proinsulin C peptide, can be utilized as useful markers of secretory activity,[246] although such products may have more prolonged half-lives in the circulation due to the lack of receptor-mediated uptake and degradation.

6. Circulating immunoreactive peptides are usually heterogeneous, consisting of larger or smaller sequence-related or overlapping peptides arising from the incomplete processing of a common precursor, and often have varying potencies, metabolic properties, and immunologic reactivities that can cause discrepancies in the assessment of circulating hormonal bioactivity by radioimmunoassay.

7. The physiology of a secretory cell, whether in the islets, the gastrointestinal tract, or the brain, cannot be fully understood until all the precursor-derived secretory products, in addition to its already known peptide product(s), have been identified and screened for their potential biologic activities. Further studies of the biosynthetic and processing activities of the islet A, B, D, and PP cells have revealed hitherto undiscovered secretory products of potential physiologic significance (e.g. IAPP from the β cells).

Acknowledgments

We thank Rosie Ricks and An Zhou for expert assistance in the preparation of this chapter.

REFERENCES

1. Von Mering J, Minkowski O: Diabetes mellitus nach pankreas extirpation. Arch Exp Pathol Pharmacol Leipzig 26:371, 1890.

2. Bliss M: The Discovery of Insulin. Chicago, University of Chicago Press, 1982.
3. Scott EL: On the influence of intravenous injections of an extract of the pancreas on experimental pancreatic diabetes. Am J Physiol 29:306, 1912.
4. Banting FG, Best CH, Collip JB: Insulin patent. Chem Abstracts 17:3571, 1923.
5. Macleod JJR, Campbell WR: Insulin: Its use in the treatment of diabetes. *In* Medicine Monographs, vol VI, parts I and II. Baltimore, Williams & Wilkins, 1925.
6. Murnaghan JH, Talalay P: John Jacob Abel and the crystallization of insulin. Perspect Biol Med 10:334, 1967.
7. Falkmer S, El-Salhy M, Titlbach M: Evolution of the neuroendocrine system in vertebrates: A review with particular reference to the phylogeny and postnatal maturation of the islet parenchyma. *In* Falkmer S, Håkanson R, Sundler F (eds): Evolution and Tumour Pathology of the Neuroendocrine System. Amsterdam, Elsevier, 1984, p 59.
8. Humbel RE, Bosshard HR, Zahn H: Chemistry of insulin. *In* Steiner DF, Freinkel N (eds): Handbook of Physiology, Endocrinology I. Baltimore, Williams & Wilkins, 1972, p 111.
9. Poulsen JE, Deckert T: Insulin preparations and the clinical use of insulin. *In* Luft R (ed): Insulin: Islet Pathology—Islet Function—Insulin Treatment. Mölndal, Sweden, A. Lindgren & Söner AB, 1976, p 197.
10. Davoren PR: The isolation of insulin from a single cat pancreas. Biochim Biophys Acta 63:150, 1962.
11. Chance RE, Ellis RM, Bromer WW: Porcine proinsulin: Characterization and amino acid sequence. Science 161:165, 1968.
12. Steiner DF, Hallund O, Rubenstein AH, et al: Isolation and properties of proinsulin, intermediate forms and other minor components from crystalline bovine insulin. Diabetes 17:725, 1968.
13. Vigh G, Varga-Puchony Z, Hlavay J, et al: Factors influencing the retention of insulins in reversed-phase high-performance liquid chromatographic systems. J Chromatogr 236:51, 1982.
14. Lloyd LF, Corran PH: Analysis of insulin preparations by reversed-phase high-performance liquid chromatography. J Chromatogr 240:445, 1982.
15. Shoelson S, Haneda M, Blix P, et al: Three mutant insulins in man. Nature 302:540, 1983.
16. Tager H, Rubenstein AH, Steiner DF: Methods for the assessment of peptide precursors: Studies on insulin biosynthesis. *In* O'Malley BW, Hardman JG (eds): Hormones and Cyclic Nucleotides: Methods in Enzymology, vol 37, part B. New York, Academic Press, 1975, p 326.
17. Blundell T, Wood S: The conformation, flexibility, and dynamics of polypeptide hormones. *In* Snell EE, Boyer PD, Meister A, Richardson CC (eds): Annual Review of Biochemistry, vol 51. Palo Alto, Annual Reviews, 1982, p 123.
18. Schlichtkrull J, Heding L: Personal communication, 1970.
19. Gueriguian JL (ed): Insulins, Growth Hormone, and Recombinant DNA Technology. New York, Raven Press, 1981.
20. Chan SJ, Weiss J, Konrad M, et al: Biosynthesis and periplasmic segregation of human proinsulin in E. coli. Proc Natl Acad Sci U S A 78:5401, 1981.
21. Thim L, Hansen MT, Norris K: Secretion and processing of insulin precursors in yeast. Proc Natl Acad Sci U S A 83:6766, 1986.
22. Chance RE: "Discussion." Recent Prog Horm Res 25:272, 1969.
23. Chance RE: Chemical, physical, biological and immunological studies on porcine proinsulin and related polypeptides. *In* Rodriquez RR, Vallance-Owen JJ (eds): Proceedings of the 7th Congress of the International Diabetes Federation. Amsterdam, Excerpta Medica, 1971, p 292.
24. Bruni B, O'Alberto M, Osenda M, et al: Clinical trial with monocomponent lente insulin. Diabetologia 9:492, 1973.
25. Galloway JA, Hooper SA, Spradlin CT, et al: Biosynthetic human proinsulin—review of chemistry, in vitro and in vivo receptor binding, animal and human pharmacology studies, and clinical experience. Diabetes Care 15:666, 1992.
26. Velcovsky HG, Federlin KF: Insulin-specific IgG and IgE antibody response in type I diabetic subjects exclusively treated with human insulin (recombinant DNA). Diabetes Care 5:126, 1982.
27. Mirsky IA, Kawamura K: Heterogeneity of crystalline insulin. Endocrinology 78:1115, 1966.
28. Gliemann J, Sorenson HH: Assay of insulin-like activity by the isolated fat cell method: IV. The biological activity of proinsulin. Diabetologia 6:499, 1970.
29. Freychet P, Roth J, Neville DM: Insulin receptors in the liver: Specific binding of insulin to the plasma membrane and its relation to insulin bioactivity. Proc Natl Acad Sci U S A 68:1833, 1971.
30. Freychet P, Brandenburg D, Wollmer A: Receptor-binding assay of chemically modified insulins: Comparison with in vitro and in vivo bioassays. Diabetologia 10:1, 1974.
31. Glieman J, Gammeltoft S: The biological activity and the binding affinity of modified insulins determined on isolated rat fat cells. Diabetologia 10:105, 1974.
32. Klostermeyer H, Humbel RE: The chemistry and biochemistry of insulin. Angew Chem Int Edit 5:807, 1966.
33. Chance RE, Kroeff EP, Hoffmann JA: Chemical, physical, and biological properties of recombinant human insulin. *In* Guerigian JL (ed): Insulins, Growth Hormone, and Recombinant DNA Technology. New York, Raven Press, 1981, p 71.
34. Sanger F: Chemistry of insulin. Science 129:1340, 1959.
35. Smith LF: Amino acid sequences of insulins. Diabetes 21(suppl 2):457, 1972.
36. Dayhoff MO (ed): Atlas of Protein Sequence and Structure, vol 5(suppl 1). Bethesda, MD, Biochemical Research Foundation, 1973.
37. Peterson JD, Steiner DF, Emdin SO, et al: The amino acid sequence of the insulin from a primitive vertebrate, the Atlantic hagfish (*Myxine glutinosa*). J Biol Chem 250:5183, 1975.
38. Steiner DF: Amino acid sequences of proteins—hormones. *In* Fasman GD (ed): Handbook of Biochemistry and Molecular Biology, Proteins, vol III. Boca Raton, FL, CRC Press, 1976, p 378.
39. Steiner DF, Bell GI, Tager HS: Chemistry and biosynthesis of pancreatic protein hormones. *In* DeGroot L (ed): Endocrinology. Philadelphia, WB Saunders, 1989, pp 1263–1289.
40. Seino S, Steiner DF, Bell GI: Sequence of a new world primate insulin having low biological potency and immunoreactivity. Proc Natl Acad Sci U S A 84:7423, 1987.
41. Yu J-H, Eng J, Yalow RS: Isolation and amino acid sequences of squirrel monkey (*Saimiri sciurea*) insulin and glucagon. Proc Natl Acad Sci U S A 87:9766, 1990.
42. Evans TK, Litthauer D, Oelofsen W: Purification and primary structure of ostrich insulin. Int J Pep Protein Res 31:454, 1988.
43. Conlon JM, Göke R, Andrews PC, Thim L: Multiple molecular forms of insulin and glucagon-like peptide from the Pacific ratfish (*Hydrolagus colliei*). Gen Comp Endocrinol 73:136, 1989.
44. Treacy GB, Shaw DC, Griffiths ME, Jeffrey PD: Purification of a marsupial insulin: Amino-acid sequence of insulin from the eastern grey kangaroo *Macropus giganteus*. Biochim Biophy Acta 990:263, 1989.
45. Berks BC, Marshall CJ, Carne A, et al: Isolation and structural characterization of insulin and glucagon from the holocephalan species *Callorhynchus milii* (elephantfish). Biochem J 263:261, 1989.
46. Conlon JM, Hicks JW: Isolation and structural characterization of insulin glucagon and somatostatin from the turtle, *Pseudemys scripta*. Peptides 11:461, 1990.
47. Conlon JM, Youson JH, Whittaker J: Structure and receptor-binding activity of insulin from a holostean fish, the bowfin (*Amia calva*). Biochem J 276:261, 1991.
48. Conlon JM, Andrews PD, Thim L, Moon TW: The primary structure of glucagon-like peptide but not insulin has been conserved between the American eel, *Anguilla rostrata* and the European eel, *Anguilla anguilla*. Gen Comp Endocrinol 82:23, 1991.
49. Smit AB, Geraerts WPM, Meester I, et al: Characterization of a cDNA clone encoding molluscan insulin-related peptide II of *Lymnaea stagnalis*. Eur J Biochem 199:699, 1991.
50. Lloyd PD, Li L, Rubakhin SS, et al: Insulin prohormone processing, distribution, and relation to metabolism in *Aplysia californica*. J Neurosci 19:7732, 1999.
51. Kawakami A, Iwami M, Nagasawa H, et al: Structure and organization of four clustered genes that encode bombyxin, as insulin-related brain secretory peptide of the silkmoth *Bombyx mori*. Proc Natl Acad Sci U S A 86:6843, 1989.
52. Lagueux M, Lwoff L, Meister M, et al: cDNAs from neurosecretory cells of brains of *Locusta migratoria* (Insecta, Orthoptera) encoding a novel member of the superfamily of insulins. Eur J Biochem 187:249, 1990.
53. Gregoire FM, Chomiki N, Kachinskas D, Warden CH: Cloning and developmental regulation of a novel member of the insulin-like gene family in *Caenorhabditis elegans*. Biochem Biophys Res Comm 249:385, 1998.
54. Duret L, Guex N, Peitsch MC, Bairoch A: New insulin-like proteins with a typical disulfide bond pattern characterized in *Caenorhabditis elegans* by comparative sequence analysis and homology modeling. Genome Res 8:348, 1998.
55. Steiner DF, Chan SJ, Welsh JM, Kwok SDM: Structure and evolution of the insulin gene. Annu Rev Genet 19:463, 1985.
56. Adham IM, Burkhardt E, Benahmed M, Engel W: Cloning of a cDNA for a novel insulin-like peptide of the testicular Leydig cells. J Biol Chem 268:26668, 1993.
57. Dayhoff MO (ed): Atlas of Protein Sequence and Structure, vol 5. Bethesda, MD, Biomedical Research Foundation, 1972.
58. Carpenter FH: Relationship of structure to biological activity of insulin as revealed by degradative studies. Am J Med 40:750, 1966.
59. Brandenburg D, Wollmer A (eds): Insulin: Chemistry, Structure and Function of Insulin and Related Hormones. Proceedings of the Second International Insulin Symposium, Aachen, Germany, September 4–7, 1979. Berlin, Walter de Gruyter, 1980.
60. Arquilla ER, Miles PV, Morris JW: Immunochemistry of insulin. *In* Steiner DF, Freinkel N (eds): Handbook of Physiology, Endocrinology I. Baltimore, Williams & Wilkins 1972, p 159.
61. Blundell TL, Dodson GG, Dodson E, et al: X-ray analysis and the structure of insulin. Recent Prog Horm Res 27:1, 1971.
62. Blundell TL, Dodson GG, Hodgkin DC, et al: Insulin: The structure in the crystals and its reflection in chemistry and biology. Adv Protein Chem 26:279, 1972.
63. Baker EN, Blundell TL, Cutfield JF, et al: The structure of 2Zn pig insulin crystals at 1.5 NA resolution. Philos Trans R Soc Lond 319:369, 1988.
64. Weiss MA, Frank BH, Khait I, et al: NMR and photo-CIDNP studies of human proinsulin and prohormone processing intermediates with application to endopeptidase recognition. Biochemistry 29:8389, 1990.
65. Cutfield JF, Cutfield SM, Dodson EJ, et al: Structure and biological activity of hagfish insulin. J Mol Biol 132:85–100, 1979.
66. Chan SJ, Episkopou V, Zeitlin S, et al: Guinea pig preproinsulin gene: An evolutionary compromise? Proc Natl Acad Sci U S A 81:5046, 1984.
67. Emdin SO, Gammeltoft S, Gliemann J: Degradation, binding affinity and potency of insulin from the Atlantic hagfish (*Myxine glutinosa*) determined in isolated rat fat cells. J Biol Chem 252:602, 1977.
68. Mommsen TP, Plisetskaya EM: Insulin in fishes and agnathans: History, structure, and metabolic regulation. Rev Aquatic Sci 4:225, 1991.
69. Taylor SI, Cama A, Accili D: Mutations in the insulin receptor gene. Endocr Rev 13:566, 1992.
70. Acher R: Recent discoveries in the evolution of proteins. Angew Chem Int Edit 13:186, 1974.
71. Terris S, Hofmann C, Steiner DF: Mode of uptake and degradation of I[125]-labelled insulin by isolated hepatocytes and H4 hepatoma cells. Can J Biochem 57:459, 1979.
72. Markussen J: Proteolytic degradation of proinsulin and of the intermediate forms: Application to synthesis and biosynthesis of insulin. *In* Baba S, Kaneko T, Yanaihara N (eds): Proinsulin, Insulin, C-peptide. Amsterdam, Excerpta Medica, 1979, p 50.
73. Derewnda U, Derewenda Z, Dodson EJ, et al: X-ray analysis of the single chain B29-A1 peptide-linked insulin molecule. J Mol Biol 220:1, 1991.
74. Hua QX, Shoelson SE, Kochoyan NM, Weiss MA: Receptor binding redefined by a structural switch in a mutant human insulin. Nature 354:238, 1991.
75. Kline AD, Justice RM: Complete sequence-specific ^{1}H NMR assignments for human insulin. Biochemistry 29:2906, 1990.

76. Nakagawa SH, Tager HS: Role of the phenylalanine B25 side chain in directing insulin interaction with its receptor. J Biol Chem 261:7332, 1986.

77. Nakagawa SH, Tager HS: Role of the COOH-terminal B-chain domain in insulin-receptor interactions. J Biol Chem 262:12054, 1987.

78. Mirmira RG, Tager HS: Disposition of the phenylalanine B25 side chain during insulin-receptor and insulin-insulin interactions. Biochem 30:8222, 1991.

79. Mirmira RG, Tager HS: Role of phenylalanine B24 side chain in directing insulin interaction with its receptor. J Biol Chem 11:6349, 1989.

80. Nakagawa SH, Tager HS: Importance of aliphatic side-chain structure at positions 2 and 3 of the insulin A chain in insulin-receptor interactions. Biochemistry 31:3204, 1992.

81. Schwartz GP, Burke GT, Katsoyannis PG: A superactive insulin: Insulin (human). Proc Natl Acad Sci 84:6408, 1987.

82. Hu SQ, Burke GT, Schwartz GP, et al: Steric requirements at position B12 for high biological activity in insulin. Biochemistry 32:2631, 1993.

83. Steiner DF, Oyer PE: The biosynthesis of insulin and a probable precursor of insulin by a human islet cell adenoma. Proc Natl Acad Sci U S A 57:473, 1967.

84. Steiner DF, Clark JL, Nolan D, et al: Proinsulin and the biosynthesis of insulin. Recent Prog Horm Res 25:207, 1969.

85. Chan SJ, Keim P, Steiner DF: Cell-free synthesis of rat preproinsulins: Characterization and partial amino acid sequence determination. Proc Natl Acad Sci U S A 73:1964, 1976.

86. Lomedico PT, Chan SJ, Steiner DF, et al: Immunological and chemical characterization of bovine preproinsulin. J Biol Chem 252:7971, 1977.

87. Steiner DF, Quinn PS, Chan SJ, et al: Processing mechanisms in the biosynthesis of proteins. Proc NY Acad Sci 343:1, 1980.

88. Sanders SL, Schekman R: Polypeptide translocation across the endoplasmic reticulum membrane. J Biol Chem 267:13791, 1992.

89. Munro S, Pelham HRB: A C-terminal signal prevents secretion of luminal ER proteins. Cell 48:899, 1987.

90. Orci L, Perrelet A, Ravazzola, et al: Coatomer-rich endoplasmic reticulum. Proc Natl Acad Sci U S A 91:11924, 1994.

91. Pagano A, Letourneur F, Garcia-Estefania D, et al: Sec24 proteins and sorting at the endoplasmic reticulum. J Biol Chem 274:7833, 1999.

92. Patzelt C, Labrecque AD, Duguid JR, et al: Detection and kinetic behavior of preproinsulin in pancreatic islets. Proc Natl Acad Sci U S A 75:1260, 1978.

93. Steiner DF, Kemmler W, Clark JL, et al: The biosynthesis of insulin. In Steiner DF, Freinkel N (eds): Handbook of Physiology, Endocrinology I. Baltimore, Williams & Wilkins, 1972, p 175.

94. Nishi M, Sanke T, Nagamatsu S, et al: Islet amyloid polypeptide: A new β cell secretory product related to islet amyloid deposits. J Biol Chem 265:4173, 1990.

95. Judah JD, Gamble M, Steadman JH: Biosynthesis of serum albumin in rat liver: Evidence for the existence of "proalbumin." Biochem J 134:1083, 1973.

96. Jacobson MR, Baltimore D: Morphogenesis of poliovirus: I. Association of the viral RNA with coat protein. J Mol Biol 33:369, 1968.

97. Kiehn ED, Holland JJ: Synthesis and cleavage of enterovirus polypeptides in mammalian cells. J Virol 5:358, 1970.

98. Arnold E, Luo M, Vriend G, et al: Implications of the picornavirus capsid structure for polyprotein processing. Proc Natl Acad Sci U S A 84:21, 1987.

99. Steiner DF: The biosynthesis of insulin: Genetic, evolutionary and pathophysiologic aspects. In Gotshlich EC (ed): The Harvey Lectures, series 78. New York, Academic Press, 1984, p 191.

100. Steiner DF, Cho S, Oyer PE, et al: Isolation and characterization of proinsulin C-peptide from bovine pancreas. J Biol Chem 246:1365, 1971.

101. Frank BH, Veros AJ: Physical studies on proinsulin: Association behavior and conformation in solution. Biochem Biophys Res Commun 32:155, 1968.

102. Rubenstein AH, Melani F, Pilkis S, et al: Proinsulin: Secretion, metabolism, immunological and biological properties. Postgrad Med J 45(suppl):476, 1969.

103. Rubenstein AH, Mako M, Welbourne WP, et al: Comparative immunology of bovine, porcine, and human proinsulin and C-peptides. Diabetes 19:546, 1970.

104. Narahara HT: Biological activity of proinsulin. In Fritz I (ed): Insulin Action. New York, Academic Press, 1972, p 63.

105. Given BD, Cohen RM, Shoelson SE, et al: Biochemical and clinical implications of proinsulin conversion intermediates. J Clin Invest 76:1398, 1985.

106. Frank BH, Veros AJ: Interaction of zinc with proinsulin. Biochem Biophys Res Commun 38:284, 1970.

107. Steiner DF: Cocrystallization of proinsulin and insulin. Nature 243:528, 1973.

108. Low BW, Fullerton WW, Rosen LS: Insulin/proinsulin, a new crystalline complex. Nature 248:339, 1974.

109. Clark JL, Steiner DF: Insulin biosynthesis in the rat: Demonstration of two proinsulins. Proc Natl Acad Sci U S A 62:278, 1969.

110. Smith LF: Species variation in the amino acid sequence of insulin. Am J Med 40:662, 1966.

111. Markussen J: Mouse insulins—separation and structures. Int J Protein Res 3:149, 1971.

112. Wentworth BM, Schaefer IM, Villa-Komaroff L, et al: Characterization of the two nonallelic genes encoding mouse preproinsulin. J Mol Evol 23:305, 1986.

113. Soares MB, Schon E, Henderson A, et al: RNA-mediated gene duplication: The rat preproinsulin I gene is a functional retroposon. Mol Cell Biol 5:2090, 1985.

114. Sundby F, Markussen J: Rat proinsulins and C-peptides: Isolation and amino acid compositions. Eur J Biochem 25:147, 1972.

115. Markussen J, Sundby F: Rat proinsulin C-peptides: Amino acid sequences. Eur J Biochem 25:153, 1972.

116. Tager HS, Steiner DF: Primary structures of the proinsulin connecting peptides of the rat and horse. J Biol Chem 247:7936, 1972.

117. Verchere CB, Paoletta M, Neerman-Arbez M, et al: Des-(27-31)C-peptide: A novel secretory product of the rat pancreatic beta cell produced by truncation of proinsulin connecting peptide in secretory granules. J Biol Chem 271:27475, 1996.

118. Steiner DF, Cunningham DD, Spigelman L, et al: Insulin biosynthesis: Evidence for a precursor. Science 157:697, 1967.

119. Steiner DF: Evidence for a precursor in the biosynthesis of insulin. Trans NY Acad Sci 30:60, 1967.

120. Tung AK, Yip CC: The biosynthesis of insulin and "proinsulin" in fetal bovine pancreas. Diabetologia 4:68, 1968.

121. Lin BJ, Haist RE: Insulin biosynthesis: Effects of carbohydrates and related compounds. Can J Physiol Pharmacol 47:791, 1969.

122. Morris GE, Korner A: The effect of glucose on insulin biosynthesis by isolated islets of Langerhans in the rat. Biochim Biophys Acta 208:404, 1970.

123. Tanese T, Lazarus NR, Devrim S, et al: Synthesis and release of proinsulin and insulin by isolated rat islets of Langerhans. J Clin Invest 49:1394, 1970.

124. Sando H, Borg J, Steiner DF: Studies on the secretion of newly synthesized proinsulin and insulin from isolated rat islets of Langerhans. J Clin Invest 51:1476, 1972.

125. Sando H, Grodsky GM: Dynamic synthesis and release of insulin and proinsulin from perifused islets. Diabetes 22:354, 1973.

126. Gold G, Gishizky ML, Grodsky GM: Evidence that glucose "marks" β cells resulting in preferential release of newly synthesized insulin. Science 218:56, 1982.

127. Nolan C, Margoliash E, Peterson JD, et al: The structure of bovine proinsulin. J Biol Chem 246:2780, 1971.

128. Kemmler W, Steiner DF, Borg J: Studies on the conversion of proinsulin to insulin: III. Studies in vitro with a crude secretion granule fraction isolated from islets of Langerhans. J Biol Chem 248:4544, 1973.

129. Kuzuya J, Chance RE, Steiner DF, et al: On the preparation and characterization of standard materials for natural human proinsulin and C-peptide. Diabetes 27:161, 1978.

130. Grant PT, Coombs TL: Proinsulin: A biosynthetic precursor of insulin. In Campbell PN, Greville GD (eds): Essays in Biochemistry, vol 6. London, Academic Press, 1971, p 69.

131. Yamaji K, Tada K, Trakatellis AC: On the biosynthesis of insulin in anglerfish islets. J Biol Chem 247:4080, 1972.

132. Hobart PM, Shen L-P, Crawford R, et al: Comparison of the nucleic acid sequence of anglerfish and mammalian insulin mRNA's from cloned cDNA's. Science 210:1360, 1980.

133. Emdin SO, Falkmer S: Phylogeny of insulin: Some evolutionary aspects of insulin production with particular regard to the biosynthesis of insulin in Myxine glutinosa. Acta Paediatr Scand 270(suppl):15, 1977.

134. Chan SJ, Emdin SO, Kwok SCM, et al: Messenger RNA sequence and primary structure of preproinsulin in a primitive vertebrate, the Atlantic hagfish. J Biol Chem 256:7595, 1981.

135. Hard L: The origin and differentiation of the alpha and beta cells in the pancreatic islets of the rat. Am J Anat 75:369, 1944.

136. Munger BL: A light and electron microscopic study of cellular differentiation in the pancreatic islets of the mouse. Am J Anat 103:275, 1958.

137. Farquhar MG, Palade GE: The Golgi apparatus (complex)—(1954–1981)—from artifact to center stage. J Cell Biol 91:77s, 1981.

138. Orci L, Ravazzola M, Amherdt M, et al: Direct identification of prohormone conversion site in insulin-secreting cells. Cell 42:671, 1985.

139. Orci L: The insulin factory: A tour of the plant surroundings and a visit to the assembly line. Diabetolgia 28:528, 1985.

140. Permutt MA, Kipnis DM: Insulin biosynthesis: Studies of islet polyribosomes. Proc Natl Acad Sci U S A 69:505, 1972.

141. Steiner DF, Clark JL, Nolan C, et al: The biosynthesis of insulin and some speculation regarding the pathogenesis of human diabetes. In Cerasi E, Luft R (eds): The Pathogenesis of Diabetes Mellitus. New York, John Wiley & Sons, 1970, p 57.

142. Howell SL: Role of ATP in the intracellular translocation of proinsulin and insulin in the rat pancreatic B cell. Nature (New Biol) 235:85, 1972.

143. Wattenberg BW, Rothman JE: Multiple cytosolic components promote intra-Golgi protein transport: Resolution of a protein acting at a late state, prior to membrane fusion. J Biol Chem 61:2208, 1986.

144. Chappell TG, Welch WF, Schlossman DM, et al: Uncoating ATPase is a member of the 70 kDa family of stress proteins. Cell 45:3, 1986.

145. Nagamatsu S, Bolaffi JL, Grodsky GM: Direct effects of glucose on proinsulin synthesis and processing during desensitization. Endocrinology 120:1225, 1987.

146. Howell SL, Kostianovsky M, Lacy PE: Beta granule formation in isolated islets of Langerhans: A study by electron microscopic radioautography. J Cell Biol 42:695, 1969.

147. Orci L, Lambert AE, Kanazawa Y, et al: Morphological and biochemical studies of B cells in fetal rat endocrine pancreas in organ culture: Evidence for proinsulin biosynthesis. J Cell Biol 50:565, 1971.

148. Kemmler W, Peterson JD, Steiner DF: Studies on the conversion of proinsulin to insulin: I. Conversion in vitro with trypsin and carboxypeptidase B. J Biol Chem 246:6786, 1971.

149. Steiner DF, Kemmler W, Tager HS, et al: Proteolytic mechanisms in the biosynthesis of polypeptide hormones. In Reich E, Rifkin DB, Shaw E (eds): Proteases and Biological Control. Cold Spring Harbor, NY, Cold Spring Harbor Laboratory, 1975, p 531.

150. Zühlke H, Steiner DF, Lernmark NA, et al: Carboxypeptidase B-like and trypsin-like activities in isolated rat pancreatic islets. In CIBA Foundation (ed): Polypeptide Hormones: Molecular and Cellular Aspects. Amsterdam, Excerpta Medica North-Holland, 1976, p 183.

151. Docherty K, Hutton JC: Carboxypeptidase activity in the insulin secretory granule. FEBS Lett 162:137, 1983.

152. Fricker LD, Evans CJ, Esch FS, et al: Cloning and sequence analysis of cDNA for bovine carboxypeptidase E. Nature 323:461, 1986.

153. Song L, Fricker LD: Cloning and expression of human carboxypeptidase Z, a novel metallocarboxypeptidase. J Biol Chem 272:10543, 1997.

154. Song W, Fricker LD, Day R: Carboxypeptidase D is a potential candidate to carry

out redundant processing functions of carboxypeptidase E based on comparative distribution studies in the rat central nervous system. Neuroscience 89:1301, 1999.
155. Julius D, Brake A, Blair L, et al: Isolation of the putative structural gene for the lysine-arginine-cleavage endopeptidase required for processing of yeast prepro-α-factor. Cell 37:1075, 1984.
156. Fuller RS, Sterne RE, Thorner J: Enzymes required for yeast prohormone processing. Annu Rev Physiol 50:345, 1988.
157. Mizuno K, Nakamura T, Ohshima T, et al: Yeast KEX2 gene encodes an endopeptidase homologous to subtilisin-like serine proteases. Biochem Biophys Res Commun 156:246, 1988.
158. Fuller RS, Brake AJ, Thorner J: Intracellular targeting and structural conservation of a prohormone-processing endoprotease. Science 246:482, 1989.
159. Mizuno K, Nakamura T, Ohshima T, et al: Characterization of KEX2-encoded endopeptidase from yeast *Saccharomyces cerevisiae*. Biochem Biophys Res Commun 159:305, 1989.
160. Davidson HW, Rhodes CJ, Hutton JC: Intraorganellar calcium and pH control proinsulin cleavage in the pancreatic β cell via two distinct site-specific endopeptidases. Nature 333:93, 1988.
161. Smeekens SP, Chan SJ, Steiner DF: The biosynthesis and processing of neuroendocrine peptides: Identification of proprotein convertases involved in intravesicular processing. *In* Joosse J, Buijs RM, Tilders FJH (eds): Progress in Brain Res, vol 92. Amsterdam, Elsevier, 1992, p 235.
162. Smeekens SP, Steiner DF: Identification of a human insulinoma cDNA encoding a novel mammalian protein structurally related to the yeast diabasic processing protease Kex2. J Biol Chem 265:2997, 1990.
163. Smeekens SP, Avruch AS, LaMendola J, et al: Identification of a cDNA encoding a second putative prohormone convertase related to PC2 in AtT20 cells and islets of Langerhans. Proc Natl Acad Sci U S A 88:340, 1991.
164. Seidah NG, Gaspar L, Mion P, et al: cDNA sequence of two distinct pituitary proteins homologous to Kex2 and furin gene products: Tissue-specific mRNAs encoding candidates for prohormone processing proteinases. DNA Cell Biol 9:415, 1990.
165. Seidah NG, Marcinkiewicz M, Benjannet S, et al: Cloning and primary sequence of a mouse candidate prohormone convertase PC1 homologous to PC2, furin, and kex2: Distinct chromosomal localization and messenger RNA distribution in brain and pituitary compared to PC2. Mol Endocrinol 5:111, 1990.
166. Roebroek AJM, Schalken JA, Leunissen JAM, et al: Evolutionary conserved close linkage of the c-fes/fps proto-oncogene and genetic sequences encoding a receptor-like protein. EMBO J 5:2197, 1986.
167. Van den Ouweland AMW, van Duijnhoven HLP, Keizer GD, et al: Structural homology between the human fur gene product and the subtilisin-like protease encoded by yeast KEX2. Nucleic Acids Res 18:664, 1990.
168. Van de Ven WJM, Voorberg J, Fontijan R, et al: Furin is a subtilisin-like proprotein processing enzyme in higher eukaryotes. Mol Biol Rep 14:265, 1990.
169. Wise RJ, Baar PJ, Wong PA, et al: Expression of a human proprotein processing enzyme: Correct cleavage of the von Willebrand factor precursor at a paired basic amino acid site. Proc Natl Acad Sci U S A 87:9378, 1990.
170. Barr PJ, Mason OB, Landsberg KE, et al: cDNA and gene structure for a human subtilisin-like protease with cleavage specificity for paired basic amino acid residues. DNA Cell Biol 10:319, 1991.
171. Steiner DF: The proprotein convertases. Curr Opin Chem Biol 2:31, 1998.
172. Zhou A, Webb G, Zhu X, Steiner DF: Proteolytic processing in the secretory pathway. J Biol Chem 274:20745, 1999.
173. Hatsuzawa K, Hosaka M, Nakagawa T, et al: Structure and expression of mouse furin, yeast Kex2-related protease. J Biol Chem 265:22075, 1990.
174. Ohagi S, LaMendola J, LeBeau MM, et al: Identification and analysis of the gene encoding human PC2, a prohormone convertase expressed in neuroendocrine tissues. Proc Natl Acad Sci U S A 89:4977, 1992.
175. Ohagi S, Sakaguchi H, Sanke T, et al: Human prohormone convertase 3 gene: Extron-intron organization and molecular scanning for mutations in Japanese subjects with NIDDM. Diabetes 45:897, 1996.
176. Mbikay M, Raffin-Sanson M-L, Tadros H, et al: Structure of the gene for the testis-specific proprotein convertase 4 and its alternate messenger RNA isoforms. Genomics 20:231, 1994.
177. Goodge KA, Thomas RJ, Martin J, Gillespie MT: Gene organization and alternative splicing of human prohormone convertase PC8. Biochem J 336:353, 1998.
178. Seidah NG, Chrétien M, Day R: The family of subtilisin/kexin like pro-protein and pro-hormone convertases: divergent or shared functions. Biochimie 76:197, 1994.
179. Wells JA, Cunningham BC, Graycar TP, Estell DA: Importance of hydrogen-bond formation in stabilizing the transition state of subtilisin. Philos Trans R Soc Lond 317:415, 1986.
180. Shennan KIJ, Smeekens SP, Steiner DF, Docherty K: Characterization of PC2, a mammalian Kex2 homologue, following expression of the cDNA in microinjected *Xenopus* oocytes. FEBS Lett 284:277, 1991.
181. Muller L, Zhu X, Lindberg I: Mechanism of the facilitation of PC2 maturation by 7B2: involvement in proPC2 transport and activation but not folding. J Cell Biol 139:625, 1997.
182. Muller L, Zhu P, Juliano MA, et al: A 36-residue peptide contains all of the information required for 7B2-mediated activation of prohormone convertase 2. J Biol Chem 274:21471, 1999.
183. Westphal C, Muller L, Zhou A, et al: The neuroendocrine protein 7B2 is required for peptide hormone processing *in vivo* and provides a novel mechanism for pituitary Cushing's disease. Cell 96:689, 1999.
184. Nagamune H, Muramatsu K, Akamatsu T, et al: Distribution of the kexin family proteases in pancreatic islets: PACE4C is specifically expressed in B cells of pancreatic islets. Endocrinology 136:357, 1995.
185. Marcinkiewicz M, Ramla D, Seidah NG, Chrétien M: Developmental expression of the prohormone convertases PC1 and PC2 in mouse pancreatic islets. Endocrinology 135:1651, 1994.
186. Neerman-Arbez M, Cirulli V, Halban PA: Levels of the conversion endoproteases PC1 (PC3) and PC2 distinguish between insulin-producing pancreatic islet β cells and non-β cells. Biochem J 300:57, 1994.
187. Smeekens SP, Albiges-Rizo C, Carroll R, et al: Proinsulin processing by the subtilisin-related proprotein convertases furin, PC2 and PC3. Proc Natl Acad Sci U S A 89:8822, 1992.
188. Rehemtulla A, Kaufman RJ: Preferred sequence requirements for cleavage of pro-von Willebrand factor by propeptide-processing enzymes. Blood 79:2349, 1992.
189. Bresnahan PA, Leduc R, Thomas L, et al: Human fur gene encodes a yeast KEX2-like endoprotease that cleaves pro-β-NGF in vivo. J Cell Biol 111:2851, 1990.
190. Hosaka M, Nagahama M, Kim W-S, et al: Arg-X-Lys/Arg-Arg motif as a signal for precursor cleavage catalyzed by furin within the constitutive secretory pathway. J Biol Chem 266:12127, 1991.
191. Rehemtulla A, Dorner AJ, Kaufman RJ: Regulation of PACE propeptide-processing activity: Requirement for a post-endoplasmic reticulum compartment and autoproteolytic activation. Proc Natl Acad Sci U S A 89:8235, 1992.
192. Korner J, Chun J, O'Bryan L, Axel R: Prohormone processing in *Xenopus* oocytes: Characterization of cleavage signals and cleavage enzymes. Proc Natl Acad Sci U S A 33:11393, 1991.
193. Hatsuzawa K, Nagahama M, Takahashi S, et al: Purification and characterization of furin, Kex2-like processing endoprotease, produced in Chinese hamster ovary cells. J Biol Chem 267:16094, 1992.
194. Molloy SS, Bresnahan PA, Leppla SI, et al: Human furin is a calcium-dependent serine endoprotease that recognizes the sequence Arg-X-X-arg and efficiently cleaves anthrax toxin protective antigen. J Biol Chem 267:16396, 1992.
195. Jung LJ, Scheller RH: Peptide processing and targeting in the neuronal secretory pathway. Science 251:1330, 1991.
196. Yoshimasa Y, Paul JI, Whittaker J, Steiner DF: Effects of amino acid replacements within the tetrabasic cleavage site on the processing of the human insulin receptor precursor expressed in Chinese hamster ovary cells. J Biol Chem 265:17230, 1990.
197. Watanabe T, Nakagawa T, Ikemizu J, et al: Sequence requirements for precursor cleavage within the constitutive secretory pathway. J Biol Chem 267:8270, 1992.
198. Stieneke-Grober A, Vey M, Angliker H, et al: Influenza virus hemagglutinin with multibasic cleavage site is activated by furin, a subtilisin-like endoprotease. EMBO J 11:2407, 1992.
199. Paterson RG, Shaughnessy MA, Lamb RA: Analysis of the relationship between cleavability of a paramyxovirus fusion protein and length of the connecting peptide. J Virol 63:1293, 1989.
200. Spaete RR, Saxena A, Scott PI, et al: Sequence requirements for proteolytic processing of glycoprotein B of human cytomegalovirus strain towne. J Virol 64:2922, 1990.
201. Bosch V, Pawlita M: Mutational analysis of the human immunodeficiency virus type 1 env gene product proteolytic cleavage site. J Virol 64:2337, 1990.
202. Wilcox CA, Fuller RS: Posttranslational processing of the prohormone-cleaving Kex2 protease in the *Saccharomyces cerevisiae* secretory pathway. J Cell Biol 115:297, 1991.
203. Molloy SS, Anderson ED, Jean F, Thomas G: Bi-cycling the furin pathway: From TGN localization to pathogen activation and embryogenesis. Trends Cell Biol 9:28, 1999.
204. Bailyes EM, Shennan KIJ, Seal AJ, et al: A member of the eukaryotic subtilisin family (PC3) has the enzymic properties of the type 1 proinsulin-converting endopeptidase. Biochem J 285:394, 1992.
205. Irminger J-C, Meyer K, Halban P: Proinsulin processing in the rat insulinoma cell line INS after overexpression of the endoproteases PC2 or PC3 by recombinant adenovirus. Biochem J 320:11, 1996.
206. Kaufmann JE, Irminger J-C, Mungall J, Halban PA: Proinsulin conversion in GH3 cells after coexpression of human proinsulin with the endoproteases PC2 and/or PC3. Diabetes 46:978, 1997.
207. Furuta M, Carroll R, Martin S, et al: Incomplete processing of proinsulin to insulin accompanied by elevation of des-31,32 proinsulin intermediates in islets of mice lacking active PC2. J Biol Chem 273:3431, 1998.
208. Bennett DL, Bailyes EM, Nielsen E, et al: Identification of the type 2 proinsulin processing endopeptidase as PC2, a member of the eukaryote substilisin family. J Biol Chem 267:15229, 1992.
209. Guest PC, Bailyes EM, Hutton JC: Endoplasmic reticulum Ca^{2+} is important for the proteolytic processing and intracellular transport of proinsulin in the pancreatic β-cell. Biochem J 323:445, 1997.
210. Rhodes CJ, Lincoln B, Shoelson SE: Preferential cleavage of des-31,32-proinsulin over intact proinsulin by the insulin secretory granule type II endopeptidase: Implications of a favored route for prohormone processing. J Biol Chem 267:22719, 1992.
211. Furuta M, Yano H, Zhou A, et al: Defective prohormone processing and altered pancreatic islet morphology in mice lacking active SPC2. Proc Natl Acad Sci U S A 94:6646, 1997.
212. O'Rahilly S, Gray H, Humphreys PJ, et al: Impaired processing of prohormones associated with abnormalities of glucose homeostasis and adrenal function. N Engl J Med 333:1386, 1995.
213. Jackson RS, Creemers JWM, Ohagi S, et al: Obesity and impaired prohormone processing associated with mutations in the human prohormone convertase 1 gene. Nat Genet 16:303, 1997.
214. Wareham NJ, Byrne CD, Williams R, et al: Fasting proinsulin concentrations predict the development of type 2 diabetes. Diabetes Care 22:262, 1999.
215. Roder ME, Dinesen B, Hartling SG, et al: Intact proinsulin and β-cell function in lean and obese subjects with and without type 2 diabetes. Diabetes Care 22:609, 1999.
216. Rhodes CJ, Alarcón C: What β-cell defect could lead to hyperproinsulinemia in NIDDM? Some clues from recent advances made in understanding the proinsulin-processing mechanism. Diabetes 43:511, 1994.
217. Sizonenko S, Irminger J-C, Buhler L, et al: Kinetics of proinsulin conversion in human islets. Diabetes 42:933, 1993.

218. Martin SK, Carroll R, Benig M, Steiner DF: Regulation by glucose of the biosynthesis of PC2, PC3 and proinsulin in (ob/ob) mouse islets of Langerhans. FEBS Lett 356:279, 1994.
219. Skelly R, Schuppin G, Ishihara H, et al: Glucose-regulated translational control of proinsulin biosynthesis with that of the proinsulin endopeptidases PC2 and PC3 in the insulin-producing MIN6 cell line. Diabetes 45:37, 1996.
220. Kalidas K, Dow E, Saker P, et al: Prohormone convertase 1 in obesity, gestational diabetes mellitus, and NIDDM: no evidence for a major susceptibility role. Diabetes 47:287, 1998.
221. Yoshida H, Ohagi S, Sanke T, et al: Association of the prohormone convertase 2 gene (PCSK2) on chromosome 20 with NIDDM in Japanese subjects. Diabetes 44:389, 1995.
222. Utsunomiya N, Ohagi S, Sanke T, et al: Organization of the human carboxypeptidase E gene and molecular scanning for mutations in Japanese subjects with NIDDM or obesity. Diabetologia 41:701, 1998.
223. Robichon A, Kuks P: Proteolysis in rat hypothalamic neurosecretory granules: Characterization of an α-chymotrypsin–like activity in the pathway of intracellular processing of prohormones. Endocrinology 128:1974, 1991.
224. Sakai J, Rawson RB, Espenshade PJ, et al: Molecular identification of the sterol-regulated luminal protease that cleaves SREBPs and controls lipid composition of animal cells. Molec Cell 2:505, 1998.
225. Seidah NG, Mowla SJ, Hamelin J, et al: Mammalian subtilisin/kexin isozyme SKI-1: A widely expressed proprotein convertase with a unique cleavage specificity and cellular localization. Proc Natl Acad Sci U S A 96:1321, 1999.
226. Kwok SCM, Chan SJ, Steiner DF: Cloning and nucleotide sequence analysis of the dog insulin gene: Coded amino acid sequence of canine preproinsulin predicts an additional C-peptide fragment. J Biol Chem 258:2357, 1983.
227. Benoit R, Ling N, Esch F: A new prosomatostatin-derived peptide reveals a pattern for prohormone cleavage at monobasic sites. Science 238:1126, 1987.
228. Schwartz TW: The processing of precursors. FEBS Lett 200:1, 1986.
229. Nakayama K, Watanabe T, Nakagawa T, et al: Consensus sequence for precursor processing at mono-arginyl sites. J Biol Chem 267:16335, 1992.
230. Docherty K, Steiner DF: Post-translational proteolysis in polypeptide hormone biosynthesis. Annu Rev Physiol 44:625, 1981.
231. Arvan P, Castle D: Protein sorting and secretion granule formation in regulated secretory cells. Trends Cell Biol 2:327, 1992.
232. Kuliawat R, Klumperman J, Ludwig T, Arvan P: Differential sorting of lysosomal enzymes out of the regulated secretory pathway in pancreatic beta-cells. J Cell Biol 137:595, 1997.
233. Arvan P, Kuliawat R, Prabakaran D, et al: Protein discharge from immature secretory granules displays both regulated and constitutive characteristics. J Biol Chem 266:14171, 1991.
234. Greider MH, Howell SL, Lacy PE: Isolation and properties of secretory granules from rat islets of Langerhans: II. Ultrastructure of the beta granule. J Cell Biol 41:162, 1969.
235. Lange RH, Boseck S, Ali SS: Crystallographic interpretation of the ultrastructure of B-granules in the islets of Langerhans of the grass-snake, Natrix n. natrix. Z Zellforsch Mikrosk Anat 131:559, 1972.
236. Michael J, Carroll R, Swift H, Steiner DF: Studies on the molecular organization of rat insulin secretory granules. J Biol Chem 262:16531, 1987.
237. Emdin SO, Dodson GG, Cutfield JM, et al: Role of zinc in insulin biosynthesis. Diabetologia 19:174, 1980.
238. Logothetopoulos J, Maneko M, Wrenshall GA, et al: Zinc, granulation, and extractable insulin of islet cells following hyperglycemia or prolonged treatment with insulin. *In* Brolin SE, Hellman B, Knutson H (eds): The Structure and Metabolism of the Pancreatic Islets Wenner-Gren Center International Symposium Series, vol 3. Oxford, Pergamon Press, 1964, p 333.
239. Falkmer S: Sulfhydryl compounds and heavy metals in islet morphology and metabolism. *In* Rodriquez RR, Vallance-Owne JJ (eds): Proceedings of the 7th Congress of the International Diabetes Federation. Amsterdam, Excerpta Medica, 1971, p 219.
240. Grant PT, Coombs TL, Frank BH: Differences in the nature of the interactions of insulin and proinsulin with zinc. Biochem J 126:433, 1972.
241. Howell SL, Tyhurst M, Duvefelt H, et al: Role of zinc and calcium in the formation and storage of insulin in the pancreatic β-cell. Cell Tissue Res 188:107, 1972.
242. Rubenstein AH, Steiner DF, Horwitz DF: Clinical significance of circulating proinsulin and C-peptide. Recent Prog Horm Res 33:435, 1977.
243. Cohen RM, Given BD, Licinio-Paixao J, et al: Proinsulin radioimmunoassay in the evaluation of insulinomas and familial hyperproinsulinemia. Metabolism 35:1137, 1986.
244. Rubenstein AH, Clark JL, Melani F, et al: Secretion of proinsulin C-peptide by pancreatic B cells and its circulation in blood. Nature 224:697, 1969.
245. Halban PA: Structural domains and molecular lifestyles of insulin and its precursors in the pancreatic beta cell. Diabetologia 34:767, 1991.
246. Polonsky K, Rubenstein AH: Current approaches to measurement of insulin secretion. Diabetes Metab Rev 2:315, 1986.
247. Oyer PE, Cho E, Peterson JD, et al: Studies on human proinsulin: isolation and amino acid sequence of the human pancreatic C-peptide. J Biol Chem 246:1375, 1971.
248. Peterson JD, Nehrlich S, Oyer PE, et al: Determination of the amino acid sequence of the monkey, sheep and dog proinsulin C-peptides by a semi-micro Edman degradation procedure. J Biol Chem 247:4866, 1972.
249. Kohnert KD, Ziegler M, Zühlke H, et al: Isoelectric focusing of proinsulin and intermediates in polyacrylamide gel. FEBS Lett 28:177, 1972.
250. Wahren J, Johansson B-L, Wallberg-Henriksson H: Does C-peptide have a physiological role? Diabetologia 37:S99, 1994.
251. Zierath JR, Galuska D, Johansson B-L, Wallberg-Henriksson, H: Effect of human C-peptide on glucose transport in in vitro incubated human skeletal muscle. Diabetologia 34:899, 1991.
252. Johansson B-L, Sjöberg S, Wahren J: The influence of human C-peptide on renal function and glucose utilization in type 1 (insulin-dependent) diabetic patients. Diabetologia 35:121, 1992.
253. Johansson B-L, Linde B, Wahren J: Effects of C-peptide on blood flow, capillary diffusion capacity and glucose utilization in the exercising forearm of type 1 (insulin-dependent) diabetic patients. Diabetologia 35:1151, 1992.
254. Ido Y, Vindigni A, Chang K, et al: Prevention of vascular and neural dysfunction in diabetic rats by C-peptide. Science 277:563, 1997.
255. Forst T, Kunt T, Pohlmann T, et al: Biological activity of C-peptide on the skin microcirculation in patients with insulin-dependent diabetes mellitus. J Clin Invest 101:2036, 1998.
256. Steiner DF, Rubenstein AH: Proinsulin C-peptide—biological activity? Science 277:531, 1997.
257. Edvell A, Lindström P: Initiation of increased pancreatic islet growth in young normoglycemic mice (Umeå +/?). Endocrinology 140:778, 1999.
258. Steiner DF, Clark JL: The spontaneous reoxidation of reduced beef and rat proinsulins. Proc Natl Acad Sci U S A 60:622, 1968.
259. Lipkind G, Steiner DF: Predicted structural alterations in proinsulin during its interactions with prohormone convertases. Biochemistry 38:890, 1999.
260. Brandenburg D, Wollmer A: The effect of a non-peptide interchain cross-link on the reoxidation of reduced insulin. Hoppe Seylers Z Physiol Chem 354:613, 1973.
261. Busse WD, Hansen SR, Carpenter FH: Carbonylbis (L-methionyl) insulin A proinsulin analog which is convertible to insulin. J Am Chem Soc 96:5949, 1974.
262. Patzelt C, Chan SJ, Duguid J, et al: Biosynthesis of polypeptide hormones in intact and cell-free systems. *In* Magnusson S, Ottesen M, Foltmann B, et al (eds): Regulatory Proteolytic Enzymes and Their Inhibitors. New York, Pergamon Press, 1978, p 69.
263. Okun MM, Shields D: Translocation of preproinsulin across the endoplasmic reticulum membrane. J Biol Chem 267:11476, 1992.
264. Lim SK, Gardella TJ, Baba H, et al: The carboxy-terminus of parathyroid hormone is essential for hormone processing and secretion. Endocrinology 131:2325, 1992.
265. Powell S, Orci L, Craik CS, Moore H-PH: Efficient targeting to storage granules of human proinsulins with altered propeptide domain. J Cell Biol 106:1843, 1988.
266. Steiner DF, Chan SJ, Welsh JM: Models of peptide biosynthesis—the molecular and cellular basis of insulin production. Clin Invest Med 9:318, 1986.
267. Geiger R, Wissman H, Weidenmuller HL, et al: Rekombination der A- und B-ketten von schweine insulin in anwesenheit von synthetischem C-peptid der schweineproinsulins. Z Naturforsch 24b:1489, 1969.
268. Baba S, Kaucko T, Yanaihara N (eds): Proinsulin, Insulin, C-Peptide. Amsterdam, Excerpta Medica, 1979.
269. Glauber HS, Henry RR, Wallace P: The effects of biosynthetic human proinsulin on carbohydrate metabolism in non-insulin-dependent diabetes mellitus. N Engl J Med 316:443, 1987.
270. Madsen OD, Cohen RM, Fitch FW, et al: Production and characterization of monoclonal antibodies specific for human proinsulin using a sensitive micro-dot assay procedure. Endocrinology 113:2135, 1983.
271. Madsen OD, Frank BH, Steiner DF: Human proinsulin specific antigenic determinants identified by monoclonal antibodies. Diabetes 33:1012, 1984.
272. Cook DL, Taborsky GJ Jr: B-cell function and insulin secretion. *In* Porte D Jr, Sherwin RS (eds): Ellenberg and Rifkin's Diabetes Mellitus, ed 5. Stamford, CT, Appleton-Lange, 1997, p 49.
273. Burgess TL, Kelly RB: Constitutive and regulated secretion of proteins. Annu Rev Cell Biol 3:243, 1987.
274. Grodsky GM: Insulin and the pancreas. *In* Harris RS, Munson PL, Diczfalvsy E (eds): Vitamins and Hormones, vol 28. New York, Academic Press, 1970, p 37.
275. Valverde I, Garcia-Morales P, Ghiglione M, et al: The stimulus-secretion coupling of glucose-induced insulin release: LIII. Calcium dependency of the cyclic AMP response to nutrient secretagogues. Horm Metab Res 15:62, 1983.
276. Asplund K: Effects of glucose on insulin biosynthesis in foetal and newborn rats. Horm Metab Res 5:410, 1973.
277. Welsh M, Scherberg N, Gilmore R, et al: Translational control of insulin biosynthesis: Evidence for regulation of elongation, initiation and signal recognition particle-mediated translational arrest by glucose. Biochem J 235:459, 1985.
278. Welsh M, Hammer RE, Brinster RL, et al: Stimulation of growth hormone synthesis by glucose in islets of Langerhans isolated from transgenic mice. J Biol Chem 261:12915, 1986.
279. Nielsen DA, Welsh M, Casadaban MJ, et al: Control of insulin gene expression in pancreatic β-cells and in an insulin-producing cell line, RIN-5F cells: I. Effects on the transcription of insulin mRNA. J Biol Chem 260:13585, 1985.
280. Welsh M, Nielsen DA, MacKrell AJ, et al: Control of insulin gene expression in pancreatic β-cells and in an insulin-producing cell line, RIN-5F cells: II. Regulation of insulin mRNA stability. J Biol Chem 260:13590, 1985.
281. Giddings SJ, Chirgwin JM, Permutt MA: Glucose regulated insulin biosynthesis in isolated rat pancreatic islets is accompanied by changes in proinsulin mRNA. Diabetes Res 2:71, 1985.
282. German MS: Glucose sensing in pancreatic islet beta-cells: The key role of glucokinase and the glycolytic intermediates. Proc Natl Acad Sci U S A 90:1781, 1993.
283. Olson LK, Sharma A, Peshavaria M: Reduction of insulin gene transcription in HIT-T15 β cells chronically exposed to a supraphysiologic glucose concentration is associated with loss of STF-1 transcription factor expression. Proc Natl Acad Sci U S A 92:9127, 1995.
284. Marshak SH, Totary E, Cerasi E, Melloul D: Purification of the β-cell glucose-sensitive factor that transactivates the insulin gene differentially in normal land transformed islet cells. Proc Natl Acad Sci U S A 93:15057, 1996.
285. Shalwitz RA, Herbst T, Carnaghi LR, Giddings SJ: Time course for effects of hypoglycemia on insulin gene transcription in vivo. Diabetes 43:929, 1994.
286. Orland MJ, Chyn R, Permutt MA: Modulation of proinsulin messenger RNA after partial pancreatectomy in rats: Relationships to glucose homeostasis. J Clin Invest 75:2047, 1985.

287. Swenne I: The role of glucose in the in vitro regulation of cell cycle kinetics and proliferation of fetal pancreatic B-cells. Diabetes 31:754, 1982.
288. Ullrich A, Shine J, Chirgwin J, et al: Rat insulin genes: Construction of plasmids containing the coding sequences. Science 196:1313, 1977.
289. Bell GI, Pictet RL, Rutter WJ, et al: Sequence of the human insulin gene. Nature 284:26, 1980.
290. Owerbach D, Bell GI, Rutter WJ, et al: The insulin gene is located on the short arm of chromosome 11 in humans. Diabetes 30:267, 1981.
291. Harper ME, Ullrich A, Saunders GF: Localization of the human insulin gene to the distal end of the short arm of chromosome 11. Proc Natl Acad Sci U S A 78:4458, 1981.
292. Bell GI, Selby MJ, Rutter WJ: The highly polymorphic region near the human insulin gene is composed of simple tandemly repeating sequences. Nature 295:31, 1982.
293. Julier C, Hyer RN, Davies J, et al: Insulin-IGF2 region on chromosome 11p encodes a gene implicated in HLA-DRA-dependent diabetes susceptibility. Nature 354:155, 1991.
294. Koman A, Cazaubon S, Couraud P-O, et al: Molecular characterization and in vitro biological activity of placentin, a new member of the insulin gene family. J Biol Chem 271:20238, 1996.
295. Chan SJ, Cao Q-P, Steiner DF: Evolution of the insulin superfamily: Cloning of a hybrid insulin/insulin-like growth factor cDNA from amphioxus. Proc Natl Acad Sci U S A 87:9319, 1990.
296. Giddings SJ, Chirgwin J, Permutt MA: Evaluation of rat insulin messenger RNA in pancreatic and extrapancreatic tissues. Diabetologia 28:343, 1985.
297. Philippe J: Structure and pancreatic expression of the insulin and glucagon genes. Endocr Rev 12:252, 1991.
298. Edlund H: Transcribing pancreas. Diabetes 47:1817, 1998.
299. Tager H, Given B, Baldwin D, et al: A structurally abnormal insulin causing human diabetes. Nature 281:122, 1979.
300. Haneda M, Polonsky KS, Bergenstal RM, et al: Familial hyper-insulinemia due to a structurally abnormal insulin: Definition of an emerging new clinical syndrome. N Engl J Med 310:1288, 1984.
301. Nanjo K, Sanke T, Miyano M, et al: Diabetes due to secretion of a structurally abnormal insulin (insulin Wakayama): Clinical and functional characteristics of insulin. J Clin Invest 77:514, 1986.
302. Shoelson SE, Polonsky KS, Zeidler A, et al: Human insulin B24 (Phe-Ser): Secretion and metabolic clearance of the abnormal insulin in man and in a dog model. J Clin Invest 73:1351, 1984.
303. Kwok SCM, Steiner DF, Rubenstein AH, et al: Identification of a point mutation in the human insulin gene giving rise to a structurally abnormal insulin (insulin Chicago). Diabetes 32:2, 1983.
304. Haneda M, Chan SJ, Kwok SCM, et al: Studies on mutant human insulin genes: Identification and sequence analysis of a gene encoding SerB24 insulin. Proc Natl Acad Sci U S A 80:6366, 1983.
305. Assoian RK, Thomas NE, Kaiser ET, et al: Insulin and insulin: Altered structures and cellular processing of B24-substituted insulin analogs. Proc Natl Acad Sci U S A 79:5147, 1982.
306. Shoelson S, Fickova M, Haneda M, et al: Identification of a mutant human insulin predicted to contain a serine-for-phenylalanine substitution. Proc Natl Acad Sci U S A 80:7390, 1983.
307. Wang J, Takeuchi T, Tanaka S, et al: A mutation in the insulin 2 gene induces diabetes with severe pancreatic β-cell dysfunction in the Mody mouse. J Clin Invest 103:27, 1999.
308. Gabbay KH, Bergenstal RM, Wolff J, et al: Familial hyperpro-insulinemia: Partial characterization of circulating proinsulin-like material. Proc Natl Acad Sci U S A 76:2881, 1979.
309. Kanazawa Y, Hayashi M, Ikeuchi M, et al: Familial proinsulinemia: A rare disorder of insulin biosynthesis. *In* Baba S, Kaneko T, Yanaihara N (eds): Proinsulin, Insulin, C-Peptide. Amsterdam, Excerpta Medica, 1979, p 262.
310. Robbins DC, Blix PM, Rubenstein AH, et al: A human proinsulin variant at arginine 65. Nature 291:679, 1981.
311. Robbins DC, Shoelson SE, Rubenstein AH, et al: Familial hyper-proinsulinemia: Two cohorts secreting indistinguishable type II intermediates of proinsulin conversion. J Clin Invest 73:714, 1984.
312. Shibasaki Y, Kawakami T, Kanazawa Y, et al: Posttranslational cleavage of proinsulin is blocked by a point mutation in familial hyperproinsulinemia. J Clin Invest 76:378, 1985.
313. Oohashi H, Ohgawara H, Nanjo K, et al: Familial hyperproinsulinemia associated with NIDDM. Diabetes Care 16:1340, 1993.
314. Røder ME, Vissing H, Nauck MA: Hyperproinsulinemia in a three-generation Caucasian family due to mutant proinsulin (arg^{65}6his) not associated with impaired glucose tolerance: The contribution of mutant proinsulin to insulin bioactivity. J Clin Endocrinol Metab 81:1634, 1996.
315. Yano H, Kitano N, Morimoto M, et al: A novel point mutation in the human insulin gene giving rise to hyperproinsulinemia (proinsulin Kyoto). J Clin Invest 89:1902, 1992.
316. Gruppuso PA, Gorden P, Kahn CR, et al: Familial hyperproinsulinemia due to a proposed defect in conversion of proinsulin to insulin. N Engl J Med 311:629, 1984.
317. Chan SJ, Seino S, Gruppuso PA, et al: A mutation in the B chain coding region of the human insulin gene is associated with impaired proinsulin conversion in a family with hyperproinsulinemia. Proc Natl Acad Sci U S A 84:2194, 1987.
318. Gross DJ, Halban PA, Kahn CR, Weir GC: Partial diversion of a mutant proinsulin (B10 aspartic acid) from the regulated to the constitutive secretory pathway in transfected AtT-20 cells. Proc Natl Acad Sci U S A 86:4107, 1989.
319. Carroll RJ, Hammer RE, Chan SJ, et al: A mutant human proinsulin is secreted from islets of Langerhans in increased amounts via an unregulated pathway. Proc Natl Acad Sci U S A 85:8943, 1988.
320. Terris S, Steiner DF: Binding and degradation of ^{125}I-insulin by rat hepatocytes. J Biol Chem 250:8389, 1975.
321. Terris S, Steiner DF: Retention and degradation of ^{125}I-insulin by perfused rat livers. J Clin Invest 57:885, 1976.
322. Sanz N, Karam JH, Horita S, Bell GI: Prevalence of insulin-gene mutations in non–insulin-dependent diabetes mellitus. N Engl J Med 314:1322, 1986.
323. Olansky L, Janssen R, Welling C, Permutt MA: Variability of the insulin gene in American blacks with NIDDM. Diabetes 41:742, 1992.
324. Olansky L, Welling C, Giddings S, et al: A variant insulin promoter in non–insulin-dependent diabetes mellitus. J Clin Invest 89:1596, 1992.
325. Stoffers DA, Stanojevic V, Habener JF: Insulin promoter factor-1 gene mutation linked to early-onset type 2 diabetes mellitus directs expression of a dominant negative isoprotein. J Clin Invest 102:232, 1998.
326. Hutton JC: The insulin secretory granule. Diabetologia 32:271, 1989.
327. Rindi G, Buffa R, Sessa R, et al: Chromogranin A, B and C immunoreactivities of mammalian endocrine cells. Histochemistry 85:19, 1986.
328. Iacangelo AL, Fischer-Colbrie R, Koller KJ, et al: The sequence of porcine chromogranin A messenger RNA demonstrates chromogranin A can serve as the precursor for the biologically active hormone, pancreastatin. Endocrinology 122:2339, 1988.
329. Hutton JC, Nielsen E, Kastern W: The molecular cloning of the chromogranin A-like precursor of β-granin and pancreastatin from the endocrine pancreas. FEBS Lett 236:269, 1988.
330. Schmidt WE, Siegel EG, Kratzin H, Creutzfeldt W: Isolation and primary structure of tumor-derived peptides related to human pancreastatin and chromogranin A. Proc Natl Acad Sci U S A 85:8231, 1988.
331. Tatemoto K, Efendic S, Mutt V, et al: Pancreastatin, a novel pancreatic peptide that inhibits insulin secretion. Nature 324:476, 1986.
332. Westermark P, Wernstedt C, Wilander E, Sletten K: A novel peptide in the calcitonin gene related peptide family as an amyloid fibril protein in the endocrine pancreas. Biochem Biophys Res Commun 140:827–831, 1986.
333. Clark A, Cooper GJS, Lewis CE, et al: Islet amyloid formed from diabetes-associated-peptide may be pathogenic in type 2 diabetes. Lancet 2:231–234, 1987.
334. Westermark P, Wernstedt C, Wilander E, et al: Amyloid fibrils in human insulinoma and islets of Langerhans of the diabetic cat are derived from a neuropeptide-like protein also present in normal islet cells. Proc Natl Acad Sci U S A 84:3881, 1987.
335. Cooper GJS, Willis AC, Clark A, et al: Purification and characterization of a peptide from amyloid-rich pancreases of type 2 diabetic patients. Proc Natl Acad Sci U S A 84:8628, 1987.
336. Opie E: The relation of diabetes mellitus to lesions of the pancreas: Hyaline degeneration of the islands of Langerhans. J Exp Med 5:527, 1901.
337. Breimer LH, MacIntrye I, Zaidi M: Peptides from the calcitonin genes: Molecular genetics, structure and function. Biochem J 255:377, 1988.
338. Amara SG, Jonas V, Rosenfeld MG, et al: Alternative RNA processing in calcitonin gene expression generates mRNAs encoding different polypeptide products. Nature 298:240, 1982.
339. Crenshaw EB III, Russo AF, Swanson LW, Rosenfeld MG: Neuron-specific alternative RNA processing in transgenic mice expressing a metallothionein-calcitonin fusion gene. Cell 49:389, 1987.
340. Sanke T, Bell GI, Sample C, et al: An islet amyloid peptide is derived from an 89-amino acid precursor by proteolytic processing. J Biol Chem 262:17243, 1988.
341. Leffert JD, Newgard CB, Okamoto H, et al: Rat amylin: Cloning and tissue-specific expression in pancreatic islets. Proc Natl Acad Sci U S A 86:3127, 1989.
342. Mosselman S, Höppener JWM, Zandberg J, et al: Islet amyloid polypeptide: Identification and chromosomal localization of the human gene. FEBS Lett 239:227, 1988.
343. Nishi M, Sanke T, Seino S, et al: Human islet amyloid polypeptide gene: Sequence, chromosomal localization and evolutionary history. Mol Endocrinol 3:1775, 1989.
344. Betsholtz C, Svensson R, Rorsman F, et al: Islet amyloid polypeptide (IAPP): cDNA cloning and identification of an amyloidogenic region associated with the species-specific occurrence of age-related diabetes mellitus. Exp Cell Res 183:484, 1989.
345. Mosselman S, Höppener JWM, Lips CJM, Jansz HS: The complete islet amyloid polypeptide precursor is encoded by two exons. FEBS Lett 247:154, 1989.
346. Clark A, Wells CA, Buley ID, et al: Islet amyloid, increased A-cells, reduced B-cells and exocrine fibrosis: Quantitative changes in the pancreas. Diabetes Res 9:1519, 1988.
347. Johnson KH, O'Brien TD, Hayden DW, et al: Immunolocalization of islet amyloid polypeptide (IAPP) in pancreatic beta cells by means of peroxidase-antiperoxidase (PAP) and protein A-gold techniques. Am J Pathol 130:1, 1988.
348. Lukinius A, Wilander E, Westermark GT, et al: Co-localization of islet amyloid polypeptide and insulin in the B cell secretory granules of the human pancreatic islets. Diabetologia 32:240, 1989.
349. Nagamatsu S, Nishi M, Steiner DF: Biosynthesis of islet amyloid polypeptide. J Biol Chem 266:13737, 1991.
350. Badman MK, Shennan KI, Jermany JL, et al: Processing of pro-islet amyloid polypeptide (proIAPP) by the prohormone convertase PC2. FEBS Lett 378:227, 1996.
351. Mulder H, Ahren B, Stridsberg M, Sundler F: Non-parallelism of islet amyloid polypeptide (amylin) and insulin gene expression in rat islets following dexamethasone treatment. Diabetologia 38:395, 1995.
352. Ferrier GJLM, Pierson AM, Jones PM, et al: Expression of the rat amylin (IAPP/DAP) gene. J Mol Endocrinol 3:R1, 1989.
353. Ohsawa H, Kanatsuka A, Yamaguchi T, et al: Islet amyloid polypeptide inhibits glucose-stimulated insulin secretion from isolated rat pancreatic islets. Biochem Biophys Res Commun 160:961, 1989.
354. Nakazato M, Asai J, Kangawa K, et al: Establishment of radioimmunoassay for human islet amyloid polypeptide and its tissue content and plasma concentration. Biochem Biophys Res Commun 164:394, 1989.
355. Asai J, Nakazato M, Kangawa K, et al: Regional distribution and molecular forms of rat islet amyloid polypeptide. Biochem Biophys Res Commun 169:788, 1990.
356. Kanatsuka A, Makino H, Ohsawa H, et al: Secretion of islet amyloid polypeptide in response to glucose. FEBS Lett 259:199, 1989.

357. Leighton B, Cooper GJS: Pancreatic amylin and calcitonin gene-related peptide cause resistance to insulin in skeletal muscle in vitro. Nature 335:632, 1988.

358. Cooper GJS, Leighton B, Dimitriadis GD, et al: Amylin found in amyloid deposits in human type 2 diabetes mellitus may be a hormone that regulates glycogen metabolism in skeletal muscle. Proc Natl Acad Sci U S A 85:7763, 1988.

359. Sowa R, Sanke T, Hirayama J, et al: Islet amyloid polypeptide amide causes peripheral insulin resistance in vivo. Diabetologia 33:118, 1990.

360. Scherbaum WA: The role of amylin in the physiology of glycemic control. Exp Clin Endocrinol Diabetes 106:97, 1998.

361. Gebre-Medhin S, Mulder H, Pekny M, et al: Increased insulin secretion and glucose tolerance in mice lacking islet amyloid polypeptide (amylin). Biochem Biophys Res Commun 250:271, 1998.

362. Ahrén B, Oosterwijk C, Lips CJM, Höppener JWM: Transgenic overexpression of human islet amyloid polypeptide inhibits insulin secretion and glucose elimination after gastric glucose gavage in mice. Diabetologia 41:1374, 1998.

363. Datta HK, Saidi M, Wimalawansa SJ, et al: In vivo and in vitro effects of amylin and amylin-amide on calcium metabolism in the rat and rabbit. Biochem Biophys Res Commun 162:876, 1989.

364. MacIntyre I: Amylinamide, bone conservation, and pancreatic β-cells. Lancet 2:1026, 1989.

365. Mulle C, Benoit P, Pinset C, et al: Calcitonin gene-related peptide enhances the rate of desensitization of the nicotinic acetylcholine receptor in cultured mouse muscle cells. Proc Natl Acad Sci U S A 85:5728, 1988.

366. Lauwerys JM, Van Ranst L: Calcitonin gene-related peptide immunoreactivity in rat lung: A light and electron microscopic study. Thorax 42:183, 1987.

367. Denis-Donini S: Expression of dopaminergic phenotypes in the mouse olfactory bulb induced by the calcitonin gene-related peptide. Nature 339:701, 1989.

368. Christopoulos G, Perry KJ, Morfis M, et al: Multiple amylin receptors arise from receptor activity-modifying protein interaction with the calcitonin receptor gene product. Mol Pharmacol 56:235, 1999.

369. Howard CF: Diabetes in *Macaca nigra*: Metabolic and histologic changes. Diabetologia 10:671, 1974.

370. Westermark P: On the nature of the amyloid in human islets of Langerhans. Histochemistry 38:27, 1974.

371. Yano BL, Hayden DW, Johnson KH: Feline insular amyloid: Association with diabetes mellitus. Vet Pathol 18:621, 1981.

372. Yano BL, Hayden DW, Johnson KH: Feline insular amyloid: Incidence in adult cats with no clinicopathologic evidence of overt diabetes mellitus. Vet Pathol 18:310, 1981.

373. Fox JG, Murphy JC: Cytomegalic virus-associated insulitis in diabetic *Octodon degus*. Vet Pathol 16:625, 1979.

374. Glenner GG, Eanes ED, Wiley CA: Amyloid fibrils formed from a segment of the pancreatic islet amyloid protein. Biochem Biophys Res Commun 155:608, 1988.

375. Westermark P, Johnson KH, O'Brien TD, Betsholtz C: Islet amyloid polypeptide—a novel controversy in diabetes research. Diabetologia 35:297, 1992.

376. Hallman U, Wernstedt C, Westermark P, et al: Amino acid sequence from degu islet amyloid-derived insulin shows unique sequence characteristics. Biochem Biophys Res Commun 169:571, 1980.

377. Nishi M, Steiner DF: Cloning of complementary DNAs encoding islet amyloid polypeptide, insulin, and glucagon precursors from a new world rodent, the degu, *Octodon degus*. Mol Endocrinol 4:1192, 1990.

378. Glenner GG, Ceja F, Mehlhaff P: Antibodies specific for the pancreatic islet amyloid polypeptide associated with type 2 diabetes mellitus. Biochem Biophys Res Commun 159:402, 1989.

379. Westermark P: Fine structure of islets of Langerhans in insular amyloidosis. Virchows Arch 359:1, 1973.

380. Clark A, Edwards CA, Ostle LR, et al: Localisation of islet amyloid peptide in lipofuscin bodies and secretory granules of human β-cells and in islets of type-2 diabetic subjects. Cell Tissue Res 259:179, 1989.

381. Porte D Jr, Kahn SE: Clues to etiology of islet β-cell dysfunction? Diabetes 38:1333, 1989.

382. Westermark G, Westermark P, Eizirik DL, et al: Differences in amyloid deposition in islets of transgenic mice expressing human islet amyloid polypeptide versus human islets implanted into nude mice. Metabolism 48:448, 1999.

383. Kahn SE, Andrikopoulos S, Verchere CB: Islet amyloid: A long-recognized but underappreciated pathological feature of type 2 diabetes. Diabetes 48:241, 1999.

384. Nishi M, Bell GI, Steiner DF: Islet amyloid polypeptide (amylin): No evidence of an abnormal precursor sequence in 25 type 2 (non–insulin-dependent) diabetic patients. Diabetologia 33:628, 1990.

385. Melato M, Antonutto G, Ferronato E: Amyloidosis of the islets of Langerhans in relation to diabetes mellitus and aging. Beitr Pathol 160:73, 1977.

386. Westermark A, Wilander E: The influence of amyloid deposits on the islet volume in maturity onset diabetes mellitus. Diabetologia 15:417, 1978.

387. Maloy AL, Longnecker DS, Greenberg ER: The relation of islet amyloid to the clinical type of diabetes. Hum Pathol 12:917, 1981.

388. Kimball CP, Murlin JR: Aqueous extracts of pancreas: Some precipitation reactions of insulin. J Biol Chem 58:337, 1923.

389. Staub A, Sinn L, Behrens OK: Purification and crystallization of glucagon. J Biol Chem 214:619, 1955.

390. Bromer WW, Sinn LG, Behrens OK: Amino acid sequence of glucagon: V. Location of amide groups, acid-degradation studies, and summary of sequential evidence. J Am Chem Soc 79:2807, 1957.

391. Bromer WW, Boucher ME, Koffenberger JE: Amino acid sequence of bovine glucagon. J Biol Chem 246:2822, 1971.

392. Thomsen J, Kristiansen K, Brunfeldt K, et al: The amino acid sequence of human glucagon. FEBS Lett 21:315, 1972.

393. Sundby F, Frandsen ED, Thomsen J, et al: Crystallization and amino acid sequence of duck glucagon. FEBS Lett 26:289, 1972.

394. Seino S, Welsh M, Bell GI, et al: Mutations in the guinea pig preproglucagon gene are restricted to a specific portion of the prohormone sequence. FEBS Lett 203:25, 1986.

395. Conlon JM, Hansen HF, Schwartz TW: Primary structure of glucagon and a partial sequence of oxyntomodulin (glucagon-37) from the guinea pig. Regul Pept 11:309, 1985.

396. Huang C-G, Eng J, Pan Y-CE, et al: Guinea pig glucagon differs from other mammalian glucagons. Diabetes 35:508, 1986.

397. Markussen J, Frandsen E, Heding LG, et al: Turkey glucagon: Crystallization, amino acid composition and immunology. Horm Metab Res 4:360, 1972.

398. Pollock HG, Kimmel JR: Chicken glucagon, isolation and amino acid sequence studies. J Biol Chem 250:9377, 1975.

399. Plisetskaya E, Pollock HG, Rouse JB, et al: Isolation and structures of coho salmon (*Oncorhynchus kisutch*) glucagon and glucagon-like peptide. Regul Pept 14:57, 1986.

400. Zimmerman AE, Moule ML, Yip CC: Guinea pig insulin: II. Biological activity. J Biol Chem 249:4026, 1974.

401. Falkmer S, Van Noorden S: Ontogeny and phylogeny of the glucagon cell. *In* Lefebvre PJ (ed): Handbook of Experimental Pharmacology, vol 66/I. Berlin, Springer-Verlag, 1983, p 81.

402. Bell GI: The glucagon superfamily: Precursor structure and gene organization. Peptides 7:27, 1986.

403. Sasaki K, Dockerill S, Adamiak DA, et al: X-ray analysis of glucagon and its relationship to receptor binding. Nature 257:751, 1975.

404. Lin MC, Wright DE, Hruby VJ, et al: Structure-function relationships in glucagon: Properties of highly purified des-His'-, monoiodo-, and (homoserine-lactone)-glucagon. Biochemistry 14:1559, 1975.

405. England RD, Jones BN, Flanders KC, et al: Glucagon carboxyl-terminal derivatives: Preparation, purification and characterization. Biochemistry 21:940, 1982.

406. Unson CG, Andreu D, Gurzenda EM, Merrifield RB: Synthetic peptide antagonists of glucagon. Proc Natl Acad Sci U S A 84:4083, 1987.

407. Unson CG, Gurzenda EM, Iwasa K, Merrifield RB: Glucagon antagonists: Contribution to binding and activity of the amino-terminal sequence 1–5, position 12, and the putative α-helical segment 19–27. J Biol Chem 264:789, 1989.

408. Unson CG, MacDonald D, Ray K, et al: Position 9 replacement analogs of glucagon uncouple biological activity and receptor binding. J Biol Chem 266:2763, 1991.

409. Kofod H, Unson CG, Merrifield RB: Potentiation of glucose-induced insulin release in islets by desHis¹ glucagon amide. Int J Pept Protein Res 32:436, 1988.

410. Johnson DG, Goegel CV, Hruby VJ, et al: Hyperglycemia of diabetic rats decreased by a glucagon receptor antagonist. Science 215:1115–1116, 1982.

411. Unger RH: Glucagon and the insulin: Glucagon ratio in diabetes and other catabolic illnesses. Diabetes 20:834, 1971.

412. Jelinek LJ, Lok S, Rosenberg GB, et al: Expression cloning and signaling properties of the rat glucagon receptor. Science 259:1614, 1993.

413. Tager SH, Steiner DF: Isolation of a glucagon-containing peptide: Primary structure of a possible fragment of proglucagon. Proc Natl Acad Sci U S A 70:2321, 1973.

414. Ravazzola M, Siperstein A, Moody AJ, et al: Glicentin immunoreactive cells: Their relationship to glucagon-producing cells. Endocrinology 105:499, 1979.

415. Thim L, Moody A: The primary structure of porcine glicentin (proglucagon). Regul Pept 2:139, 1981.

416. Patzelt C, Tager HS, Carroll RJ, et al: Identification and processing of proglucagon in pancreatic islets. Nature 282:260, 1979.

417. Patzelt C, Weber B: Early O-glycosidic glycosylation of proglucagon in pancreatic islets: An unusual type of prohormonal modification. EMBO J 5:2103, 1986.

418. Patzelt C, Neilsen D, Carroll R, et al: Studies on the biosynthesis of the other peptide hormones of the rat islets of Langerhans. Biochem Soc Trans 8:411, 1980.

419. Patzelt C, Schug G: The major proglucagon fragment: An abundant islet protein and secretory product. FEBS Lett 129:127, 1981.

420. Patzelt C, Schiltz E: Conversion of proglucagon in pancreatic alpha cells: The major endproducts are glucagon and a single peptide, the major proglucagon fragment, that contains two glucagon-like sequences. Proc Natl Acad Sci U S A 81:5007, 1984.

421. Philippe J, Mojsov S, Drucker DJ, et al: Proglucagon processing in a rat islet cell line resembles phenotype of intestine rather than pancreas. Endocrinology 119:2833, 1986.

422. Orskov C, Holst J, Knuhtsen S, et al: Glucagon-like peptides GLP-1 and GLP-2 predicted products of the glucagon gene are secreted separately from pig small intestine but not pancreas. Endocrinology 119:1467, 1986.

423. Mojsov S, Heinrich G, Wilson IB, et al: Preproglucagon gene expression in pancreas and intestine diversifies at the level of post-translational processing. J Biol Chem 261:11880, 1986.

424. Schmidt WE, Siegel EG, Creutzfeldt W: Glucagon-like peptide-1 but not glucagon-like peptide-2 stimulates insulin release from isolated rat pancreatic islets. Diabetologia 28:704, 1985.

425. Orskov C: Glucagon-like peptide-1 a new hormone of the entero-insular axis. Diabetologia 35:701, 1992.

426. Drucker DJ, DeForest L, Brubaker PL: Intestinal response to growth factors administered alone or in combination with human [Gly2]glucagon-like peptide 2. Am J Physiol 273:G1252, 1997.

427. Litvak DA, Hellmich MR, Evers BM, et al: Glucagon-like peptide 2 is a potent growth factor for small intestine and colon. J Gastrointest Surg 2:146, 1998.

428. Rouillé Y, Westermark G, Martin SK, Steiner DF: Proglucagon is processed to glucagon by prohormone convertase PC2 in alpha TC1-6 cells. Proc Natl Acad Sci U S A 91:3242, 1994.

429. Rouillé Y, Martin S, Steiner DF: Differential processing of proglucagon by the subtilisin-like prohormone convertases PC2 and PC3 to generate either glucagon or glucagon-like peptide. J Biol Chem 270:26488, 1995.

430. Rouillé Y, Bianchi M, Irminger J-C, Halban PA: Role of the prohormone convertase PC2 in the processing of proglucagon to glucagon. FEBS Lett 413:119, 1997.

431. Rouillé Y, Kantengwa S, Irminger J-C, Halban PA: Role of the prohormone convertase PC3 in the processing of proglucagon to glucagon-like peptide 1. J Biol Chem 272:32810, 1997.
432. Damholt AB, Buchan AMJ, Holst JJ, Kofod H: Proglucagon processing profile in canine L cells expressing endogenous prohormone convertase 1/3 and prohormone convertase 2. Endocrinol 140:4800, 1999.
433. Guillemin R: Peptides in the brain: The new endocrinology of the neuron. Science 202:390, 1978.
434. Hökfelt T, Efendic S, Hellerström C, et al: Cellular localization of somatostatin in endocrine-like cells and neurons of the rat with special references to the A₁-cells of the pancreatic islets and to the hypothalamus. Acta Endocrinol 80(suppl 200):5, 1975.
435. Arimura A, Sata H, Dupont A, et al: Somatostatin: Abundance of immunoreactive hormone in rat stomach and pancreas. Science 189:1007, 1975.
436. Reichlin S: Somatostatin: I. N Engl J Med 309:1495, 1983.
437. Hellman B, Lernmark NA: A possible role of the pancreatic α₁- and α₂-cells as local regulators of insulin secretion. *In* Falkner S, Hellman B, Täljedal I-B (eds): The Structure and Metabolism of the Pancreatic Islets: A Centennial of Paul Langerhans' Discovery, vol 16. Oxford, Pergamon Press, 1970, p 453.
438. Bloom W: A new type of granular cell in the islets of Langerhans of man. Anat Rec 49:363, 1931.
439. Orci L: General discussion I: Somatostatin—clinical implications. *In* CIBA Foundation (ed): Polypeptide Hormones: Molecular and Cellular Aspects. Amsterdam, Excerpta Medica, 1976, p 313.
440. Reichlin S: Somatostatin: II. N Engl J Med 309:1556, 1983.
441. Olsson S-E, Andersson A, Petersson B, et al: Effects of somatostatin on the biosynthesis and release of insulin from isolated pancreatic islets. Diabete Metab 2:199, 1976.
442. Lernmark NA, Chan SJ, Choy R, et al: Biosynthesis of insulin and glucagon: A view of the current state of the art. *In* CIBA Foundation (ed): Polypeptide Hormones: Molecular and Cellular Aspects. Amsterdam, Excerpta Medica, 1976, p 7.
443. Garcia SD, Jarrousse C, Rosselin G: Biosynthesis of proinsulin and insulin in newborn rat pancreas. J Clin Invest 57:230, 1976.
444. Gottesman IS, Mandarino LJ, Gerich JE: Somatostatin. *In* Cohen M, Foa P (eds): Special Topics in Endocrinology and Metabolism, vol 4. New York, Alan R. Liss, 1982, p 177.
445. Yamada Y, Post Sr, Wang K, et al: Cloning and functional characterization of a family of human and mouse somatostatin receptors expressed in brain, gastrointestinal tract, and kidney. Proc Natl Acad Sci U S A 89:251, 1992.
446. Yasuda K, Res-Domiano S, Breder CD, et al: Cloning of a novel somatostatin receptor, SSTR3, coupled to adenylylcyclase. J Biol Chem 267:20422, 1992.
447. Bell GI, Reisine T: Molecular biology of somatostatin receptors. Trends Neurosci 16:34, 1993.
448. O'Carroll A-M, Lolait SJ, König M, Mahan LC: Molecular cloning and expression of a pituitary somatostatin receptor with preferential affinity for somatostatin-28. Mol Pharmacol 42:939, 1992.
449. Bruno JF, Xu Y, Song J, Berelowitz M: Molecular cloning and functional expression of brain-specific somatostatin receptor. Proc Natl Acad Sci U S A 89:11151, 1992.
450. Schally AV, Huang W-Y, Chang RCC, et al: Isolation and structure of pro-somatostatin: A putative somatostatin precursor from pig hypothalamus. Proc Natl Acad Sci U S A 77:4489, 1980.
451. Brown M, Rivier J, Vale W: Somatostatin-28: Selective action on the pancreatic β-cell and brain. Endocrinology 108:2391, 1981.
452. Shoelson SE, Polonsky KS, Nakabayashi T, et al: Circulating forms of somatostatin-like immunoreactivity in human plasma. Am J Physiol 250:E428, 1986.
453. Patel YC, Srikant CB: Somatostatin mediation of adenohypophysial secretion. *In* Berne RM (ed): Annual Review of Physiology, vol 48. Palo Alto, CA, Annual Reviews, 1986, p 551.
454. Patzelt C, Tager HS, Carroll RJ, et al: Identification of prosomatostatin in pancreatic islets. Proc Natl Acad Sci U S A 77:2410, 1980.
455. Goodman RH, Jacobs JW, Chin WW, et al: Nucleotide sequence of a cloned structural gene coding for a precursor of pancreatic somatostatin. Proc Natl Acad Sci U S A 77:5869, 1980.
456. Noe BD, Spiess J, Rivier JE, Vale W: Isolation and characterization of somatostatin from anglerfish pancreatic islet. Endocrinology 105:1410, 1979.
457. Lund PK, Goodman RH, Montiminy MR, et al: Anglerfish islet pre-proglucagon: II. Nucleotide and corresponding amino acid sequence of the cDNA. J Biol Chem 258:3280, 1983.
458. Goodman RH, Jacobs JW, Dee PC, Habener JF: Somatostatin 28 encoded in a cloned cDNA obtained from a rat medullary thyroid carcinoma. J Biol Chem 257:1756, 1982.
459. Funckes CL, Minth CD, Deschenes R: Cloning and characterization of a mRNA-encoding rat preprosomatostatin. J Biol Chem 258:81, 1983.
460. Shen L-P, Rutter WJ: Sequence of the human somatostatin I gene. Science 224:168, 1984.
461. Danoff A, Shields D: Differential translation of two distinct preprosomatostatin messenger RNAs. J Biol Chem 263:16461, 1988.
462. Nielsen HV, Gether U, Schwartz TW: Cat pancreatic eicosapeptide and its biosynthetic intermediate: Conservation of a monobasic processing site. Biochem J 240:69, 1986.
463. Richter D, Schmale H: A cellular polyprotein from bovine hypothalamus: Structural elucidation of the precursor to the nonapeptide hormone arginine vasopressin. *In* McKerns KW (ed): Regulation of Gene Expression by Hormones. New York, Plenum, 1983, p 235.
464. Jansen M, van Schaik FMA, Ricker AT, et al: Sequence of cDNA encoding human insulin-like growth factor I precursor. Nature 306:609, 1983.
465. Bell GI, Merryweather JP, Sanchez-Pescador R, et al: Sequence of a cDNA clone encoding human preproinsulin-like growth factor II. Nature 310:775, 1984.
466. Mackin RB, Noe BD, Spiess J: The anglerfish somatostatin-28–generating propeptide converting enzyme is an aspartyl protease. Endocrinology 129:1951, 1991.
467. Bourbonnais Y, Danoff A, Thomas DY, Shields D: Heterologous expression of peptide hormone precursors in the yeast *Saccharomyces cerevisiae*. J Biol Chem 266:13203, 1991.
468. Egel-Mitani M, Flygenring HP, Hansen MT: A novel aspartyl protease allowing KEX2-independent MFα propheromone processing in yeast. Yeast 6:127, 1990.
469. Bourbonnais Y, Ash J, Daigle M, Thomas DY: Isolation and characterization of *S. cerevisiae* mutants defective in somatostatin expression: Cloning and functional role of a yeast gene encoding an aspartyl protease in precursor processing at monobasic cleavage sites. EMBO J 12:285, 1993.
470. Argos P, Taylor WL, Minth CD: Nucleotide and amino acid sequence comparisons of preprosomatostatins. J Biol Chem 258:88, 1983.
471. Gluschankof P, Morel A, Gomez S, et al: Enzyme processing somatostatin precursors: An Arg-Lys esteropeptidase from the rat brain cortex converting somatostatin-28 into somatostatin-14. Proc Natl Acad Sci U S A 81:6662, 1984.
472. Lepage-Lezin A, Joseph-Bravo P, Devilliers G, et al: Prosomatostatin is processed in the Golgi apparatus of rat neural cells. J Biol Chem 266:1679, 1991.
473. Mackin RB, Noe BD, Spiess J: Identification of a somatostatin-14-generating propeptide converting enzyme as a member of the kex2/furin/PC family. Endocrinology 129:2263, 1991.
474. Brakch N, Galanopoulou AS, Patel YC, et al: Comparative proteolytic processing of rat prosomatostatin by the convertases PC1, PC2, furin, PACE4 and PC5 in constitutive and regulated secretory pathways. FEBS Lett 362:143, 1995.
475. Montminy MR, Sevarino KA, Wagner JA, et al: Identification of a cyclic-AMP–responsive element within the rat somatostatin gene. Proc Natl Acad Sci U S A 83:6682, 1986.
476. Chance RE, Moon NE, Johnson MG: Human pancreatic polypeptide (HPP) and bovine pancreatic polypeptide (BPP). *In* Jaffe BM, Behrman HR (eds): Methods of Hormone Radioimmunoassay (ed 2). New York, Academic Press, 1979, p 657.
477. Lin T-M: Pancreatic peptide: Isolation, chemistry and biological function. *In* Jerzy Glass GB (ed): Gastrointestinal Hormones. New York, Raven Press, 1980, p 275.
478. Hazelwood RL: Synthesis, storage, secretion and significance of pancreatic polypeptide in vertebrates. *In* Cooperstein SJ, Watkins D (eds): The Islets of Langerhans. New York, Academic Press, 1981, p 275.
479. Kimmel JR, Pollock HG, Chance RE, et al: Pancreatic polypeptide from rat pancreas. Endocrinology 114:1725, 1984.
480. Baetens D, Malaisse-Lagae F, Perrelet A, et al: Endocrine pancreas: Three-dimensional reconstruction shows two types of islets of Langerhans. Science 206:1323, 1979.
481. Orci L: Macro- and micro-domains in the endocrine pancreas: The Banting Memorial Lecture 1981. Diabetes 31:538, 1982.
482. Schwartz TW: Pancreatic polypeptide: A hormone under vagal control. Gastroenterology 85:1411, 1983.
483. Tatemoto K: Neuropeptide Y: Complete amino acid sequence of the brain peptide. Proc Natl Acad Sci U S A 79:5485, 1982.
484. Schwartz TW, Gingerich RL, Tager HS: Biosynthesis of pancreatic polypeptide: Identification of a precursor and a co-synthesized product. J Biol Chem 255:11494, 1980.
485. Schwartz TW, Tager HS: Isolation and biogenesis of a new peptide from pancreatic islets. Nature 294:589, 1981.
486. Schwartz TW, Hansen HF, Håkanson R, et al: Human pancreatic icosapeptide: Isolation, sequence, and immunocytochemical localization of the COOH-terminal fragment of the pancreatic polypeptide precursor. Proc Natl Acad Sci U S A 81:708, 1984.
487. Schwartz TW, Hansen HF: Isolation of ovine pancreatic icosapeptide: A peptide product containing one cysteine residue. FEBS Lett 168:293, 1984.
488. Leiter AB, Keutmann HT, Goodman RH: Structure of a precursor to human pancreatic polypeptide. J Biol Chem 259:14702, 1984.
489. Boel E, Schwartz TW, Norris KE, et al: A cDNA encoding a small common precursor for human pancreatic polypeptide and pancreatic icosapeptide. EMBO J 3:909, 1984.
490. Yamamoto H, Nata K, Okamoto H: Mosaic evolution of prepropancreatic polypeptide. J Biol Chem 261:6156, 1986.
491. Blackstone CD, Seino S, Takeuchi T, et al: Novel organization and processing of the guinea pig pancreatic polypeptide precursor. J Biol Chem 263:2911, 1988.
492. Leiter AB, Montminy MR, Jamieson E: Exons of the human pancreatic polypeptide gene define functional domains of the precursor. J Biol Chem 260:13013, 1985.
493. Eipper BA, Green CB-R, Campbell TA, et al: Alternative splicing and endoproteolytic processing generate tissue-specific forms of pituitary peptidylglycine α-amidating monooxygenase (PAM). J Biol Chem 267:4008, 1992.
494. Takeuchi T, Dickinson CJ, Taylor IL, Yamada T: Expression of human pancreatic polypeptide in heterologous cell lines. J Biol Chem 266:17409, 1991.
495. Schwartz TW: The processing of peptide precursors: "Proline-directed arginyl cleavage" and other monobasic processing mechanisms. FEBS Lett 200:1, 1986.
496. Muglia L, Locker J: Extrapancreatic insulin gene expression in the fetal rat. Proc Natl Acad Sci U S A 81:3635, 1984.
497. Young WS III: Periventricular hypothalamic cells in the rat brain contain insulin mRNA. Neuropeptides 8:93, 1986.
498. Roberge JN, Brubaker PL: Regulation of intestinal proglucagon-derived peptide secretion by glucose-dependent insulinotropic peptide in a novel enteroendocrine loop. Endocrinology 133:233, 1993.
499. Miyawaki K, Yamada Y, Yano H, et al: Glucose intolerance caused by a defect in the entero-insular axis: A study in gastric inhibitory polypeptide receptor knockout mice. Proc Natl Acad Sci U S A 96:14843, 1999.
500. Wood SP, Blundell TL, Wollmer A, et al: The relation of conformation and association of insulin to receptor binding: X-ray and circular-dichroism studies on bovine and hystricomorph insulins. Eur J Biochem 55:531, 1975.

501. Kiefer MC, Tucker JE, Joh R, et al: Identification of a second human subtilisin-like protease gene in the fes/fps region of chromosome 15. DNA Cell Biol 10:757, 1991.
502. Seidah NG, Mattei MG, Gaspar L, et al: Chromosomal assignments of the genes for neuroendocrine convertase PC1 (NEC1) to human 5q15–21, neuroendocrine convertase PC2 (NEC2) to human 20p11.1–11.2, and furin (mouse 7 region). Genomics 11:103, 1991.
503. Smit AB, Vreugdenhil E, Ebberink RHM, et al: Growth-controlling molluscan neurons produce the precursor of an insulin-related peptide. Nature 331:535, 1988.
504. Schroeder WT, Lopez LC, Harper ME, et al: Localization of the human glucagon gene (GCG) to chromosome segment 2q36 6 37. Cytogenet Cell Genet 38:76, 1984.
505. Zabel BU, Naylor SL, Sakaguchi AY, et al: High-resolution chromosomal localization of human genes for amylase, proopiomelanocortin, somatostatin, and a DNA fragment (D3S1) by in situ hybridization. Proc Natl Acad Sci U S A 80:6932, 1983.
506. Takeuchi T, Gumucio DL, Yamada T, et al: Genes encoding pancreatic polypeptide and neuropeptide Y are on human chromosomes 17 and 7. J Clin Invest 77:1038, 1986.

▼▼▼

Chapter 49

Secretion and Metabolism of Insulin, Proinsulin, and C Peptide

Kenneth S. Polonsky ▪ Niall M. O'Meara

Insulin is the most important secretory product of the pancreatic β cell and plays a central role in the regulation of a number of key metabolic processes. Proinsulin is the immediate biosynthetic precursor of insulin and is converted in the β cell secretory granule to form one molecule of C peptide and one molecule of insulin, both of which are secreted into the portal circulation.[1–4] Intact proinsulin is also secreted by the β cell and under normal circumstances constitutes up to 20% of total circulating insulin-like immunoreactivity. The exact physiologic significance of these low concentrations of circulating proinsulin is uncertain, since the in vivo biologic potency of proinsulin is approximately 10% that of insulin.[5, 6]

The weight of current evidence suggests that the role of C peptide relates largely to maintaining the tertiary structure of proinsulin for the insulin biosynthetic process and that it does not possess significant biologic activity after secretion into the circulation.[7, 8] In addition, C peptide has been extremely useful as a peripheral marker of insulin secretion, since it is co-secreted in equimolar concentration with insulin but unlike insulin does not undergo significant hepatic extraction. In this chapter the secretion and metabolism of these three major β cell products—insulin, proinsulin, and C peptide—are reviewed.

THE SECRETION OF INSULIN

Physiologic Regulation of Insulin Secretion

Glucose and Other Carbohydrates

The most important physiologic substance regulating insulin release is glucose.[9–11] The effect of glucose on the β cell is dose-related. Dose-dependent increases in insulin and C peptide concentrations and in insulin secretory rates have been observed following oral and intravenous glucose loads.[12–15] The insulin secretory response is greater following oral as opposed to intravenous glucose administration.[15–18] Otherwise known as the *incretin effect*,[14, 19] this enhanced insulin response to oral glucose is believed to be mediated by a number of gastrointestinal peptide hormones, including glucose-dependent insulinotropic peptide (GIP), cholecystokinin (CKK), and glucagon-like peptide-1 (GLP-1).[19–27] These hormones are released from intestinal endocrine cells postprandially following exposure to glucose and travel in the blood stream to reach the β cells, where they act through second

messengers to increase the sensitivity of these islet cells to glucose. They are not of themselves secretagogues, and their effects are evident only in the presence of hyperglycemia.[20–22] Other intestinal peptide hormones which also may modify the postprandial insulin secretory response in a similar manner include vasoactive intestinal polypeptide (VIP),[28] secretin,[29, 30] and gastrin,[29, 31] but their precise role still remains to be elucidated. In addition to explaining the possible mechanisms underlying the incretin effect, the release of these peptide hormones also may explain how the modest increases in glucose levels seen in nondiabetic subjects postprandially have such a profound effect on the β cell secretory responses, whereas similar glucose concentrations in vitro elicit a much smaller response.[27]

Insulin secretion does not respond as a linear function of the glucose concentration. The relationship of the latter to the rate of insulin release is sigmoidal, with a threshold corresponding to the glucose levels normally seen under fasting conditions and the steep portion of the dose-response curve corresponding to the range of glucose levels normally achieved postprandially.[32–34] This sigmoidal nature of the dose-response curve has been attributed to a gaussian distribution of thresholds for stimulation among the β cells.[34–36]

When glucose is infused intravenously at a constant rate, a biphasic secretory response is observed initially consisting of a rapid early insulin peak followed by a second, more slowly rising peak.[9, 37, 38] The significance of the first-phase insulin release is unclear, but it may reflect a compartment of readily releasable insulin within the β cell or represent the transient rise and fall of a metabolic signal for insulin secretion.[39] Despite earlier suggestions to the contrary,[40, 41] a recent report has demonstrated that the first-phase response to intravenous glucose is highly reproducible[42] in the same subject. Following the acute response, there is a second phase of insulin release which is directly related to the elevation in the glucose level. In the 1980s, in vitro studies using isolated islets and the perfused pancreas suggested a third phase of insulin secretion, which commences 1.5 to 3.0 hours after glucose exposure and is characterized by a spontaneous decline of secretion to 15% to 25% of peak values—a level that is subsequently maintained for more than 48 hours.[43–46]

The effects of a variety of other sugars, sugar derivatives, and sugar alcohols on the β cell also have been studied.[47] In addition to D-glucose, D-mannose, D-glyceraldehyde, dihydroxyacetone, D-glucosamine, N-acetylglucosamine, fructose, and galactose have all been shown to be stimulators or potentiators of insulin secretion in vitro. In vivo studies in dogs and humans suggest that xylitol and sorbitol also enhance β cell function.

The insulin secretory response to glucose exhibits anomeric specificity, the α-anomer being a more potent stimulator of insulin release than the β-anomer.[48] Similar results have been obtained with mannose.[49] Since α-anomers are more readily metabolized by the glycolytic pathway than α-anomers,[50, 51] it has been suggested that the metabolism of glucose and mannose within the β cell is a prerequisite of the production of intracellular signals that trigger insulin release in response to these secretagogues. In support of this observation, iodoacetate, an inhibitor of glyceraldehyde dehydrogenase, and mannoheptulose, an inhibitor of glucokinase, inhibit the insulin-secreting response to glucose in isolated islets.[52] In 1992, a defect in the glucokinase gene was described in a French group of subjects with maturity-onset diabetes of youth (MODY) who also were shown to have impaired β cell responses to glucose.[53, 54]

Amino Acids and Lipids

Amino acids have been shown to stimulate insulin release in the absence of glucose, the most potent secretagogues being the essential amino acids leucine, arginine, and lysine.[55, 56] While leucine was the first amino acid to be studied, experiments with high-protein meals showed that the β cell stimulation observed could not be attributed solely to its leucine content. Indeed, the effects of arginine and lysine on the β cell appear to be more potent. Although the effects of amino acids on insulin secretion are independent of concomitant changes in glucose levels, the effects are potentiated by glucose.[56–58] The response of the islet cells to a series of amino acid metabolites also has been evaluated. Phenylpyruvate, α-ketoisocaproate, α-keto-β-methylvalerate, and α-ketocaproate are potent stimulators of insulin release, and most are effective in the absence of glucose.[47, 59]

In contrast to amino acids, various lipids and their metabolites appear to have only minor effects on insulin release. Although carbohydrate-rich fat meals stimulate insulin secretion, carbohydrate-free fat meals have minimal effects on β cell function.[60] Thus, while ketone bodies as well as short- and long-chain fatty acids have been shown to potentiate the insulin secretory response in islet cells, their exact role under physiologic conditions remains to be elucidated.

Hormones

In addition to the modulating influence of gastrointestinal peptide hormones on the β cell response to glucose, other hormones also influence β cell secretory responses. The pancreatic hormones glucagon and somatostatin have contrasting effects on the β cell. While glucagon has a stimulatory effect,[61] somatostatin suppresses insulin release.[62] It is currently unclear whether these hormones reach the β cell by traveling through the islet cell interstitium (thus exerting a paracrine effect) or through islet cell capillaries. Other hormones exerting a stimulatory role on insulin secretion include growth hormone,[63] glucocorticoids,[64] prolactin,[65–67] placental lactogen,[68] and the sex hormones.[69] Thus, hypophysectomy or adrenalectomy dampens insulin release, while enhanced secretion is a characteristic finding in acromegaly, Cushing's syndrome, and the last trimester of pregnancy. Although all these hormones may stimulate insulin secretion indirectly by inducing a state of insulin resistance, there is evidence that they also act directly on the β cell, possibly enhancing its sensitivity to glucose, since placental lactogen,[70] hydrocortisone,[71] and growth hormone[71, 72] have all been shown to be effective in reversing the reduced insulin response to glucose following hypophysectomy.

Hyperinsulinemia with or without impairment of glucose tolerance has been observed frequently in patients who are hyperthyroid.[73–77] Elevations in serum insulin concentrations have been reported both in the basal state and in response to a glucose load. Despite these observations, the earlier studies quantitating insulin secretory rates in hyperthyroidism yielded conflicting results. Studies in hyperthyroid animals have suggested that insulin secretion rates may be decreased[78, 79] or increased,[80] while in human subjects increased,[75, 76] normal,[81] and reduce[82, 83] C peptide levels had all been reported. Moreover, in many instances, the changes in C peptide levels have not

always been mirrored by similar changes in insulin concentration. The discrepancies between insulin and C peptide in some studies may reflect elevations in proinsulin levels, which are a characteristic finding in hyperthyroidism,[81, 83–85] since most standard insulin radioimmunoassays show cross-reactivity with proinsulin. In 1993 we provided a further explanation for the discrepancies between insulin and C peptide in some of the earlier studies by demonstrating increased C peptide clearance rates in hyperthyroid subjects.[85] Furthermore, in our study, when the individual kinetic parameters derived from the C peptide decay curves of each subject were employed in the calculation of insulin secretion rates from the peripheral C peptide levels using the two-compartment model of Eaton et al.,[86] we demonstrated that insulin secretory responses to meals were increased in subjects who were hyperthyroid.[85] In an additional series of experiments, insulin secretory rates were found to be 50% higher in a group of hyperthyroid subjects during the hyperglycemic clamp technique (Fig. 49–1). These findings taken together suggest that in hyperthyroidism the sensitivity of the β cell to glucose is increased.

The effects of parathyroid hormone (PTH) on β cell function also have been the subject of investigation. Several studies have provided indirect evidence that PTH influences insulin secretion. Experiments using the hyperglycemic clamp technique in dogs and humans with secondary hyperparathyroidism in association with chronic renal failure have demonstrated that insulin secretion is impaired in this clinical setting.[87, 88] In these studies, normalization of the PTH levels through parathyroidectomy in dogs and through the use of medical treatment in the human subjects reversed the abnormalities in insulin secretion. Studies in normocalcemic dogs with normal renal function that previously had a parathyroidectomy have demonstrated that insulin levels during an intravenous glucose tolerance test are significantly higher than in similar dogs with intact parathyroid glands.[87] There are a number of in vitro studies which provide more direct evidence that PTH affects β cell function. Studies using pancreatic islets obtained from normal rats treated with PTH for 6 weeks have demonstrated that the insulin secretory response to glucose is significantly reduced.[89] Indeed, it has been suggested recently that the effect of PTH on the β cell may be dose-related, since the direct incubation of rat islet cells with PTH produces contrasting effects—stimulating insulin secretion at low doses and inhibiting it at higher doses.[90] The stimulatory effect at lower doses was actually inhibited by verapamil, suggesting that calcium may be the crucial second messenger mediating the β cell responses to PTH.

The neurohumoral transmitters of the sympathetic nervous system—norepinephrine and epinephrine—also modify β cell secretory responses. Epinephrine inhibits insulin release by a variety of agents, including glucose.[91, 92] The more potent effect of epinephrine compared with norepinephrine and the fact that α-adrenergic antagonists abolish the inhibitory effect of the former suggest that its action is mediated by stimulation of α-receptors. Similarly, stimulation of sympathetic nerve fibers inhibits insulin secretion, an effect reversed by the α-adrenergic antagonist phentolamine.[93–97] While it is unclear whether the adrenergic limb of the autonomic nervous system has any major influence on normal basal or postprandial secretory responses, it is possible that sympathetic-mediated inhibition of insulin secretion could account for the deteriorating glycemic control reported to occur in diabetic subjects who are under severe stress.

In contrast to the inhibitory effects of the adrenergic neurotransmitters, parasympathomimetic agents stimulate insulin release, and the action is blocked by atropine.[94, 98] The importance of the parasympathetic nervous system in regulating insulin secretion in vivo is unclear, however. Although it is attractive to consider that vagal stimulation of insulin release occurs during meals, its effect may be rather modest. Studies in animals[99, 100] and humans[101, 102] have emphasized the importance of the cephalic phase of insulin release—occurring at the sight, smell, and expectation of food—in regulating the postprandial glucose response. It has been suggested that this reflex, which is under vagal control,[27, 103] may have a key role in minimizing the early rise in glucose levels following meals.[102] Since cholinergic agonists increase the response of the β cell to glucose in vitro,[104] this may be the mechanism by which vagal stimulation achieves its effect. Decreased glucose tolerance has been reported in human subjects following

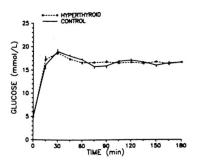

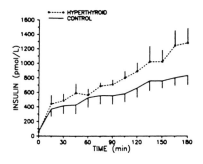

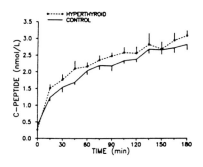

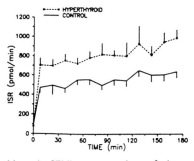

FIGURE 49–1. *Mean (±SEM) concentrations of glucose, insulin, and C peptide and rates of insulin secretion during the hyperglycemic clamp technique in hyperthyroid and control groups. Owing to the impaired clearance rate of C peptide in hyperthyroidism, the C peptide levels in the two graphs were not different. However, when the clearance rates of C peptide in the individual subjects were taken into account in the derivation of insulin secretion rates by deconvolution, significant differences in insulin secretion were observed between the hyperthyroid and control groups.*

vagotomy[105, 106] and in rats in which the islets have been denervated,[107, 108] while the insulin secretory response to meals is delayed in subjects who have undergone pancreas transplantation.[109] However, since many of these patients remain euglycemic off therapy following pancreas transplantation,[109–112] the importance of the vagus in maintaining glucose tolerance is in doubt.

Exercise

The effects of exercise on β cell function also have been evaluated extensively. Individuals who exercise regularly have reduced fasting insulin and C peptide levels,[113–115] and the release of these hormones following a carbohydrate load is also impaired. These latter observations have been made following a 100-g oral glucose load[116, 117] and during a hyperglycemic clamp, in which reduction in both first-phase and second-phase secretory responses has been described.[113–116, 118] Despite these changes, these subjects have normal or even improved glucose tolerance.[113, 118] This suggests that insulin sensitivity is improved in those who exercise regularly, a finding that has been confirmed by the observation of increased glucose disposal rates in athletes during a hyperinsulinemic euglycemic clamp.[113, 118]

Altered β cell responses to glucose are apparent even after short periods of exercise and have been observed in individuals who have been subjected to as little as 1 hour of exercise 24 hours preceding an oral glucose tolerance test.[119] Similarly, even in well-trained athletes, insulin responses to glucose increase dramatically within 2 weeks of cessation of exercise.[114] In this latter study, glucose disposal rates both before and after cessation of exercise were similar, thus supporting the view that those who exercise regularly are more sensitive to the action of insulin. The altered β cell responses to glucose observed in athletic subjects may therefore be a compensatory response to the increased sensitivity to insulin in the periphery.

THE METABOLISM OF INSULIN

Hepatic Metabolism of Insulin

The metabolism of insulin has been studied extensively in vitro as well as in vivo in laboratory animals and humans.[12, 120–134] All studies have come to essentially the same conclusion: the liver is the major site of insulin metabolism. Most workers have demonstrated that approximately 59% of the insulin delivered to the liver is extracted by that organ on the first pass, although some studies have suggested lower values.[135–137] Polonsky et al.,[130, 138] using an in vivo dog model, infused somatostatin in high doses to suppress endogenous β cell secretion. Insulin was infused exogenously via a peripheral vein under steady-state conditions. This experimental design ensured that all measurements were made under steady-state conditions and after complete mixing of insulin in both the portal and hepatic veins had occurred. The hepatic extraction of insulin was between 40% and 60%, and under basal conditions the liver was found to be responsible for 60% of total insulin clearance. The remaining proportion is accounted for predominantly by renal clearance (30%). The fraction of insulin clearance unaccounted for by hepatic and renal uptake mechanisms occurs in other sites, including bowel and muscle.

Hepatic insulin metabolism is thought to be closely related to binding of insulin to the insulin receptor.[139, 140] The first step in degradation of the hormone appears to be binding to receptors in the hepatocyte surface. Insulin is then internalized, and at least some of the internalized insulin serves as the substrate for degradation.

There is considerable controversy surrounding the factors that regulate hepatic insulin metabolism. The only factor that is widely agreed to affect this process is an increase in its plasma concentration beyond the point of saturation. Rubenstein et al.,[123] using an isolated perfused rat liver system, demonstrated that an increase in the insulin concentration in the perfusate above 2000 μU/mL was associated with a fall in the rate at which insulin was cleared. This finding is consistent with saturation of a receptor-mediated removal process. Subsequent studies have confirmed that insulin clearance is saturable, although the level at which saturation occurs is controversial. Most studies have indicated that saturation occurs only at very high insulin levels well above the physiologic range,[123, 134, 141] suggesting that saturation of hepatic insulin metabolism is not an important control mechanism under physiologic conditions. Sonksen et al.,[142] however, infused insulin exogenously to increase peripheral insulin concentrations from basal to approximately 280 μU/mL in normal human volunteers. Over this range there was a progressive reduction in the metabolic clearance rate from 34 to 12 mL/kg/min. Eaton and coworkers[13] also suggested that changes in hepatic insulin uptake may regulate peripheral insulin concentrations under physiologic circumstances. More recent studies have demonstrated that hepatic insulin extraction may fall with intense stimulation of endogenous insulin secretion by either high-dose intravenous glucose infusion or high-dose oral glucose ingestion.[15, 18, 143]

It also has been suggested that glucose is an important factor regulating hepatic insulin metabolism. Studies carried out in dogs by Kaden et al.[124] and by Jaspan and Polonsky[131] demonstrated a significant increase in hepatic insulin extraction following oral glucose ingestion. A number of other authors, including Waddell and Sussman,[144] Kanazawa et al.,[145] and Blackard and Nelson,[146] have reached similar conclusions with different experimental designs and techniques. Honey and Price,[132] however, concluded that glucose administration reduced the fraction of insulin extracted by the liver, and Tranberg and Thorell[147] found that the non–steady-state plasma clearance rate after intraportal infusion of insulin was lower in the face of hyperglycemia than with normoglycemia. Striffler and Curry[133] reported that insulin extraction by an isolated rat pancreas liver system fell to virtually zero in the fed state. Waldhausl et al.,[12] in human studies using C peptide concentrations as an indicator of pancreatic insulin secretion, estimated that hepatic insulin extraction was unchanged after oral glucose. Eaton et al.,[13] using a mathematical model to measure hepatic insulin extraction, concluded that oral glucose per se does not affect hepatic insulin extraction.

It also has been suggested that other factors may affect hepatic insulin metabolism, including glucose, glucagon, somatostatin, and protein ingestion.[126, 128] However, the importance of these factors in the regulation of peripheral insulin concentrations through alterations in hepatic insulin extraction is uncertain.

There is thus considerable evidence that hepatic insulin extraction is a variable process, although the mechanisms by which regulation occurs are controversial, and it is not yet possible to resolve the discrepancies in the different studies. There are two major issues on which there appears to be general agreement: (1) insulin metabolism is closely related to insulin receptor binding, and the substrate for insulin metabolism is bound insulin; and (2) insulin clearance by the liver is a saturable process, but whether hepatic insulin extraction is an important factor that contributes to the regulation of insulin concentrations within the physiologic range is still uncertain.

Renal Metabolism of Insulin

The kidney plays a major role in the degradation of insulin. Arteriovenous differences across the kidney have been measured both in animals and in humans, and renal insulin extraction is approximately 30% to 40%.[128, 148–152] Furthermore, renal uptake mechanisms contribute approximately 30% to the overall clearance of the hormone, Thus the kidney is second only to the liver as an important site of insulin clearance.

The mechanisms involved in the renal degradation of insulin are not agreed on. There appear to be two discrete mechanisms by which the kidney degrades insulin. First, there is glomerular filtration and proximal tubular reabsorption.[153] ^{125}I-insulin has been shown by autoradiographic studies to localize initially to the glomeruli and tubular lumen and subsequently to proximal tubular cells.[153] This pattern of uptake is consistent with endocytosis through endocytotic vesicles and lysosomal metabolism. Only a small proportion of filtered insulin appears intact in the urine, and urinary insulin clearance is less than 1 mL/min.[154–156] In the intact animal, the renal clearance of insulin is greater than the simultaneously measured clearance of insulin, indicating that the hormone is cleared from the kidney by peritubular uptake from postglomerular blood in addition to glomerular filtration. Following ureteral ligation, which eliminates glomerular filtration, the kidney continues to remove and degrade insulin at about 50% of the rate of the filtering kidney.

Other Sites of Insulin Metabolism

Adipose tissue has active insulin-degrading enzyme systems, and isolated fat cells can take up and inactivate insulin.[157, 158] As in the liver, insulin binding and degradation are linked in the adipocytes, although not all the receptor-bound and not even all the internalized insulin are degraded. The reason for this is unclear, and it has even been suggested that some insulin receptors may mediate insulin action and others may mediate degradation.

Several different types of blood cells, including monocytes,[159, 160] red blood cells,[161, 162] and granulocytes, can bind and degrade insulin. The physiologic importance of this is not known.

Placenta is rich in insulin-degrading enzymes, and placental degradation may contribute to the enhanced requirement for insulin in pregnancy.[163, 164] Insulin-degrading activity can be isolated and purified from skeletal muscle, and insulin degradation has been observed in intact muscle preparations. Significant arteriovenous insulin differences across the forearm have been observed in vivo, and it is likely that muscle is quantitatively an important site of insulin degradation following liver and kidney.

THE METABOLISM OF C PEPTIDE

Insulin and C peptide are co-secreted from the β cell on an equimolar basis. Traditionally, it has been believed that C peptide is not biologically active and does not have a physiologic function[8] but is merely a by-product of the insulin biosynthetic process. The major clinical usefulness of the measurement of C peptide is as a peripheral marker of insulin secretion. However, it has been suggested recently that C peptide may increase peripheral glucose utilization and reduce the complications of diabetes when replaced together with insulin in patients with type 1 diabetes.

As discussed earlier, considerable quantities of insulin are extracted by the liver, and the proportion extracted by the liver may vary under different physiologic conditions. Peripheral insulin concentrations therefore reflect the posthepatic delivery rather than the pancreatic secretion of insulin, and insulin secretion rates cannot be derived accurately from peripheral insulin concentrations. In addition, insulin-dependent diabetic patients develop antibodies to the therapeutic exogenous insulin preparations, particularly those containing beef insulin. These antibodies interfere with the insulin radioimmunoassay, making accurate measurement of insulin concentrations in these patients difficult. Furthermore, the insulin radioimmunoassay cannot distinguish between exogenously administered and endogenously secreted insulin and is therefore not useful as a measure of endogenous β cell function. For these reasons, peripheral C peptide concentrations have been used as a more accurate reflection of endogenous β cell secretory activity than peripheral insulin levels, particularly in insulin-treated diabetic patients. The validity of this approach depends on a number of assumptions concerning the metabolism and kinetic distribution of C peptide. The most important assumptions are (1) the hepatic extraction of C peptide is negligible under physiologic conditions, (2) the metabolic clearance rate of C peptide is constant under physiologic conditions and over a wide range of plasma concentrations, and (3) the distribution kinetics of C peptide are such that its plasma concentration accurately reflects its secretion rate even under non–steady-state conditions. The evidence for and against each of these assumptions will now be examined.

The Hepatic Extraction of C Peptide

There is considerable evidence from both animal and human studies that the hepatic extraction of C peptide is negligible. Thus Polonsky et al.[138] measured hepatic fluxes of C peptide under a variety of conditions in conscious fasted dogs with chronic sampling catheters implanted in the portal and hepatic veins and femoral artery. Under basal steady-state conditions following an overnight fast, the hepatic extraction of endogenously secreted as well as exogenously infused C peptide was indistinguishable from zero. Furthermore, hepatic extraction did not increase following stimulation of secretion by either oral or intravenous glucose.[138, 165] Stoll et al.[165] found that the extraction of bovine C peptide by an isolated perfused rat liver system was negligible. Bratusch-Marrain and coworkers[166] infused porcine C peptide into human volunteers with hepatic vein catheters. No concentration gradient of C peptide across the splanchnic bed was detected, indicating that C peptide is not extracted by the liver in humans. On the other hand, Kuhl et al.[167] reported a 30% hepatic extraction of C peptide in experiments conducted in pigs. The authors based their calculations on C peptide concentrations in portal and hepatic veins only, and the contribution of the hepatic artery to hepatic C peptide delivery was not measured. Since under physiologic circumstances the arterial C peptide concentration is lower than in the portal or hepatic vein, their approach would be expected to overestimate hepatic C peptide extraction.

The Metabolic Clearance Rate of C Peptide

If the metabolic clearance rate of C peptide changed significantly under physiologic conditions, or if its clearance kinetics were nonlinear, this would significantly limit its value as a peripheral marker of insulin secretion. The metabolic clearance rate of C peptide has been studied under basal conditions in laboratory animals and humans. Studies performed in rats and dogs have demonstrated that the metabolic clearance rate of C peptide is independent of its plasma concentration over a wide concentration range.[138, 168] Faber et al.[169] injected synthetic human C peptide into normal volunteers and type 1 diabetic patients and found that the metabolic clearance rate was indistinguishable in both groups. The metabolic clearance rate of biosynthetic human C peptide was also measured and found to be similar (4.0 ±0.2 mL/kg/min) at plasma concentrations of 0.8 ±0.23 and 8.93 ±0.5 pmol/mL, indicating linear kinetics within the physiologic concentration range. Furthermore, the metabolic clearance rate of C peptide measured after a bolus injection was similar to that during a constant infusion and was not affected by an increase in the plasma glucose concentration or ingestion of a mixed meal.[170]

Kinetics of Distribution of C Peptide

The availability of biosynthetic human C peptide has allowed the kinetics of human C peptide to be studied in vivo. Following a bolus injection, the decay curve of biosynthetic human C peptide can be described mathematically as the sum of two exponentials with half-disappearance times of approximately 5 and 35 minutes, respectively. Infusion of biosynthetic human C peptide intraportally into dogs or peripherally into humans demonstrated that the peripheral plasma concentration did not change in proportion to the infusion rate. As the infusion rate was increased rapidly, the peripheral concentration increased less than predicted. When the infusion rate was reduced, the peripheral concentration fell more slowly than the infusion rate. These discrepancies were most marked when the infusion rate was increased and decreased rapidly, and least evident when changes were made more slowly. Under steady-state conditions, the infusion rate of C peptide could be derived accurately as the product of plasma concentration and metabolic clearance rate. However, under non–steady-state conditions, more complex mathematical analysis of peripheral C peptide concentrations is necessary to derive the secretion rate of insulin accurately. It has been demonstrated that this can be achieved by use of a two-compartment model initially proposed by Eaton and coworkers.[86] This approach, which has been termed *deconvolution*, involves nonlinear least-squares regression analysis of C peptide decay curves to derive model parameters in individual subjects. Once the fractional rate constants and distribution volume are known, concentrations of peripheral C peptide can be analyzed mathematically and the secretion rate derived. Estimates of the secretion of C peptide and therefore insulin are 98% ± 3% of the actual rate as it is increasing and 100% ± 2% of the rate as it is being reduced. We have demonstrated that the secretion rate of insulin can be derived by deconvolution of peripheral C peptide levels using average mean literature-derived parameters, thus obviating the need for injection of biosynthetic human C peptide in each subject.[171]

Clinical Use and Significance of C Peptide Concentrations

Under steady-state conditions and when insulin secretion changes slowly, the peripheral concentration of C peptide is a good reflection of β cell secretory activity. This is particularly valuable in assessing the extent of endogenous β cell reserve in type 1 diabetes and to study the natural history of this disease. Non–steady-state insulin secretion rates also can be derived from peripheral C peptide concentrations using the two-compartment mathematical model described above with either individual plasma C peptide kinetics derived after intravenous bolus injections of biosynthetic human C peptide or average mean literature-derived parameters.[171] C peptide concentration is also of value as a marker of insulin secretion in non–insulin-dependent diabetic patients with insulin antibodies produced by administration of exogenous insulin.

C peptide is helpful in the diagnosis of surreptitious insulin injection. In these patients, very high insulin concentrations are found in the presence of normal or suppressed C peptide levels. Similarly, C peptide may be helpful in the evaluation of patients with hypoglycemia, as in the diagnosis of insulinoma. During prolonged fasting and in the presence of hypoglycemia, plasma C peptide concentrations are inadequately suppressed in patients with insulinoma in comparison with normal controls. This observation forms the basis for the C peptide suppression test. During this test, insulin is infused intravenously to induce hypoglycemia, and C peptide concentrations are measured. In normal subjects, when the plasma glucose concentration is below 40 mg/dL, plasma C peptide levels fall to 50% of the baseline value or less. In patients with insulinoma, however, incomplete suppression of endogenous β cell secretion is observed.

PROINSULIN KINETICS AND METABOLISM

Circulating Proinsulin-like Components

When samples of human serum and urine are gel-filtered and the fractions measured in the insulin radioimmunoassay, two peaks of immunologically reactive material are identified. The earlier peak corresponds in position to a proinsulin marker and the second to insulin. The high-molecular-weight material in plasma has been characterized in several ways. De Haën and coworkers[172] characterized the nature of proinsulin-like material (PLM) in the circulation using a variety of chemical criteria, including immunoreactivity, electrophoretic mobility, molecular size, and sensitivity to trypsin. They concluded that proinsulin and desdipeptide proinsulin were present in serum in approximately equal amounts accompanied by minor amounts of split proinsulin and monodesamidodesdipeptide proinsulin. Given et al.[173] characterized PLM in human pancreas. Kinetic analysis of proinsulin processing by a mixture of trypsin and carboxypeptidase B (to stimulate in vivo processes catalyzed by as yet unidentified enzymes) revealed (1) a rapid decline in proinsulin concomitant with formation of conversion intermediates, (2) formation of two major conversion intermediates, des-31,32-proinsulin and des-64,65-proinsulin, with predominance of the former intermediate (des-31,32-proinsulin intermediate is formed through removal of the two arginine residues at the junction of the B chain and C peptide [A–C intermediate], while the des-64,65-proinsulin intermediate is formed by removal of the lysine and arginine residues at the A chain–C peptide junction [B–C intermediate]), and (3) complete conversion of the precursor to insulin during extended incubation. Studies on normal human pancreas identified a similar ratio of des-31,32-proinsulin and des-64,65-proinsulin (about 3:1), whereas two insulinomas contained sizable amounts of des-31,32-proinsulin but barely detectable amounts of des-64,65-proinsulin. Small amounts of the split 32,33 and split 65,66 intermediates, in which the corresponding arginine and lysine residues are not removed after formation of the intermediates, may also be present. Typical profiles demonstrating the relative proportions of insulin, des-31,32-proinsulin, and des-64,65-proinsulin in the circulation of a control subject and subjects with impaired glucose tolerance and non–insulin-dependent diabetes mellitus (NIDDM) are shown in Figure 49–5. Studies by Tillil et al.[174] have demonstrated that proinsulin conversion intermediates demonstrate 1% to 20% of the biologic potency of insulin but are considerably more potent than intact proinsulin.

Concentrations of circulating proinsulin-like immunoreactivity (PLI) are elevated in patients with (NIDDM),[175–180] and it has been suggested that the extent of the elevation may be related to the degree of metabolic control.[180] Most published clinical data on proinsulin have been derived using gel-filtration chromatography. The major clinical significance of a raised serum proinsulin concentration is in the diagnosis of pancreatic islet cell tumors. More recent studies with specific radioimmunoassays for proinsulin have confirmed that proinsulin concentrations are elevated above normal in almost all patients with insulinoma.[181] Heding[182] reported similar results in 31 patients with islet cell tumors.

An increase in serum proinsulin may occur as part of a familial autosomal dominant condition (familial hyperproinsulinemia) characterized by the synthesis of a structurally abnormal proinsulin molecule, resulting in impaired intracellular conversion of the precursor to insulin.[183–185]

In addition to diabetes, insulinoma, and familial hyperproinsulinemia, elevated proinsulin concentrations also have been reported in patients with chronic renal failure[186] and thyrotoxicosis.[187, 188]

Metabolism of Proinsulin

Proinsulin constitutes 2% to 4% of the immunoreactive insulin-like material in normal pancreas, a value similar to that found in the portal vein of humans but lower than that found in peripheral serum. This difference is a result of the slower metabolism of proinsulin compared with insulin. A number of studies have shown that proinsulin has a slower metabolic clearance rate than insulin.[5, 142] In contrast to the differences in their metabolic clearance rates, the renal disposition of insulin and proinsulin is similar, being characterized by high extraction and very low urinary clearance.[189] The renal arteriovenous differences of proinsulin and insulin averaged 36% and 40%, respectively, and were linearly related to their arterial concentrations. The fractional urinary clearance never exceeded 0.6%, indicating that more than 90% of the amount filtered was sequestered in the kidney. Thus, elevations in proinsulin concentrations have been reported in patients with chronic renal failure, in whom levels that were five- to sevenfold greater than in healthy fasting subjects have been described.[186] In contrast, insulin concentrations were only two- to fourfold greater in this patient group. These findings are related to the relatively greater proportion of proinsulin that is degraded by the kidneys compared with insulin. On the other hand, studies on the removal of proinsulin and insulin by the isolated perfused rat liver have shown that the hepatic extraction of proinsulin is considerably slower than that of insulin. There is no evidence for conversion of proinsulin to insulin in the circulation.

THE NORMAL INSULIN SECRETORY PROFILE

Postprandial Responses and Circadian Variations in Secretion

In any 24-hour period, it has been estimated that 50% of the total amount of insulin secreted by the pancreas is released under basal conditions and the remainder is secreted in response to meals. Moreover, the β cell response to a particular stimulus appears in part to be dependent on the clock time at which the stimulus was administered. When insulin secretory responses are measured during a 24-hour period, during which time subjects received three standard meals, maximum postprandial responses are observed after breakfast.[190–192] These findings are mirrored by the results of studies in which subjects received oral glucose tolerance tests at different times of the day.[193–195] In these experiments, maximum insulin secretory responses to an oral glucose load were observed in the morning, with lower responses occurring in the afternoon and evening. These diurnal differences are also present following intravenous glucose tolerance tests and during a prolonged 24-hour glucose infusion study, during which the nocturnal rise in glucose concentration was not accompanied by a similar increase in the secretory rate.[196] It has been postulated that these circadian differences may reflect a diminished responsiveness of the β cell to glucose in the afternoon and evening.[195]

Oscillatory Insulin Secretion

In vivo studies of β cell secretory function have demonstrated that insulin is released in a pulsatile manner. This behavior is characterized by rapid oscillations occurring every 8 to 15 minutes[197–205] that are superimposed on slower (ultradian) oscillations occurring at a periodicity of 80 to 150 minutes[191, 196, 206–208] (Fig. 49–2). The rapid oscillations have been observed in a variety of species in addition to humans, including monkeys,[197, 199, 209] baboons,[210] and dogs.[210, 211] Their presence also has been noted in a number of in vitro experiments[212–218] and in subjects who have undergone pancreas transplantation,[219, 220] and, accordingly, neural factors are unlikely to be responsible for their generation. In light of this, it has been suggested that these pulses could be a reflection of the activity of an intrinsic pancreatic pacemaker.[213, 216] However, since these oscillations occur with greater frequency in vitro[214, 217, 218] and following transplantation,[220] it is likely that neural factors may modulate the activity of such a pacemaker.

The rapid oscillations are of small amplitude in the systemic circulation, averaging between 0.4 and 3.2 μU/mL in several published

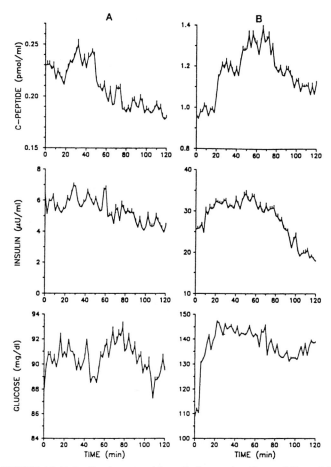

FIGURE 49–2. Profiles in one subject of glucose, insulin, and C peptide during basal conditions (A) and during constant glucose infusion (B). All sample measurements (4 for glucose and 16 for insulin and C peptide) were averaged before profiles were plotted.

human studies.[198, 200, 202, 221] Since these values are very close to the limits of sensitivity of most standard insulin radioimmunoassays, the characterization of these oscillations is subject to considerable pitfalls, not least being the need to differentiate between true oscillations of small amplitude and random assay noise. This latter problem can in part be overcome by increasing the accuracy of laboratory estimations through the use of frequent measurements (six to eight) at each sampling time point in contrast to the standard practice of relying solely on duplicates.[204] Furthermore, we have shown recently that the detection of these pulses in the systemic circulation is greatly facilitated by the use of several different analytic approaches to characterize oscillatory behavior in an individual subject.[204]

The low amplitude of the rapid oscillations in the systemic circulation contrasts sharply with observations in the portal circulation, where pulse amplitudes of 20 to 40 μU/mL have been recorded in dogs.[210, 212] Although the physiologic importance of these low-amplitude rapid pulses in the peripheral circulation is unclear, it is likely that they are of importance in the portal vein, and in this regard it is possible that the liver responds more favorably to insulin delivered in a pulsatile manner than to insulin delivered at a constant rate.[222–224] The discrepancy between the relative amplitudes of the insulin pulses in the portal vs. systemic circulations results in part from the large hepatic extraction of insulin prior to its entry into the systemic circulation. In support of this, we have demonstrated recently that following pancreas transplantation the relative amplitude of the rapid insulin pulses is much greater in a situation where insulin is released from the transplanted β cell directly into the systemic circulation.[220]

In contrast to the rapid oscillations, the slower (ultradian) oscillations are of much larger amplitude in the peripheral circulation. They are present under basal conditions but are amplified postprandially[191, 206] (Fig. 49–3), and they also have been observed in subjects receiving intravenous glucose,[196, 208] suggesting that they are not generated by intermittent absorption of nutrients from the gut. Furthermore, they do not appear to be related to fluctuations in glucagon or cortisol levels[208] and are not regulated by neural factors, since these oscillations are also present in subjects who have undergone pancreas transplantation.[109, 219] Many of these ultradian insulin and C peptide pulses are synchronous with pulses of similar period in glucose,[191, 196, 206] raising the possibility that these oscillations are a product of the insulin-glucose feedback mechanism. In support of this hypothesis, it has been demonstrated that when glucose is administered in an oscillatory pattern, ultradian oscillations in plasma glucose and insulin secretion are generated that are 100% concordant with the oscillatory period of the exogenous glucose infusion.[225] The close relationship between these ultradian oscillations in insulin secretion and similar oscillations in plasma glucose was further exemplified in a recent series of dose-response studies in which the largest-amplitude oscillations in insulin secretion were observed in those subjects exhibiting the largest-amplitude glucose oscillations, which in turn were directly related to the infusion dose of glucose.[226]

ALTERATIONS OF INSULIN SECRETION

Obesity

Subjects who are obese are insulin-resistant and hyperinsulinemic.[227–232] Although decreased insulin clearance has been demon-

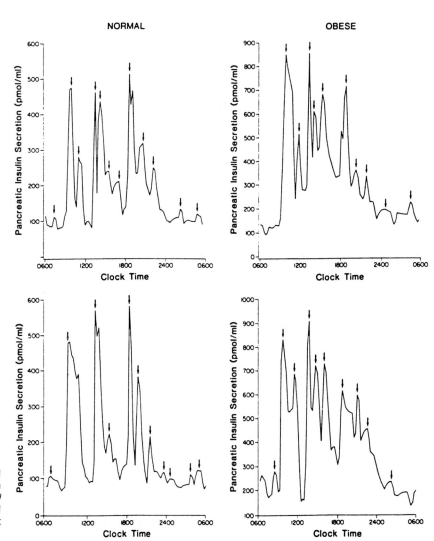

FIGURE 49–3. Patterns of insulin secretion in normal and obese subjects. Four representative 24-hour insulin secretory profiles from two normal-weight subjects *(left)* and two obese subjects *(right)*. Meals were consumed at 0900, 1300, and 1800 hours. Statistically significant pulses of secretion are shown by the *arrows*.

strated in obese subjects,[230, 233] most evidence suggests that the elevated insulin levels in this population subgroup represent a compensatory adaptive response of the β cell to the accompanying insulin resistance.[191] Increased insulin secretory rates both basally and following meals have been demonstrated in obese subjects[143] (Fig. 49–4). The increase in the insulin secretion rate has been shown to be strongly correlated with body mass index. Despite these quantitative changes, qualitative alterations in β cell function have not been demonstrated. As in normal subjects, basal insulin secretion accounts for 50% of the total daily insulin production, and the increased secretion of insulin in obese individuals is not associated with any alteration in the proinsulin-insulin molar ratio.[236] In addition, oscillatory insulin secretion is also preserved in obese subjects. Small-amplitude rapid oscillations in secretion occurring every 10 to 12 minutes[202] and slower oscillations of larger amplitude occurring every 1.5 to 2.0 hours[143, 194] have both been demonstrated, the latter once again being tightly coupled to oscillations of similar period in plasma glucose.[237] It appears, therefore, that the normal regulatory mechanisms controlling insulin secretion in nonobese controls are still operative in hyperinsulinemic obese subjects and that β cell function is intrinsically normal in this setting.

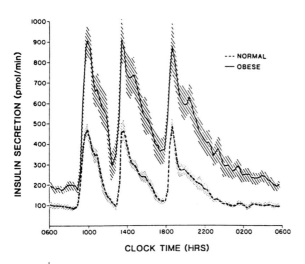

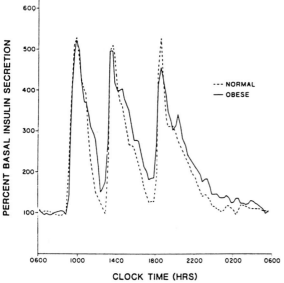

FIGURE 49–4. Mean 24-hour profiles of insulin secretion rates in normal and obese subjects *(top).* The *hatched areas* represent ±1 SEM. The curves in the lower panel were derived by dividing the insulin secretion rate measured in each subject by the basal secretion rate derived in the same subject. Mean data for the normal (– – –) and obese (—) subjects are shown.

Aging

Peripheral insulin resistance, impaired glucose tolerance, and hyperinsulinemia are metabolic changes observed with aging.[234, 238, 239] While the cause of the reduction in insulin sensitivity in the elderly population is not completely understood, lack of exercise appears to be an important factor.[116, 240, 241] Studies in groups of elderly subjects before and after their participation in exercise training programs have demonstrated—using hyperinsulinemic euglycemic clamps—marked improvements in insulin sensitivity following the completion of exercise training programs, which in one study[241] were associated with a corresponding reduction in the β cell secretory responses to glucose.

The initial studies evaluating β cell function in the elderly population yielded conflicting results, with diminished, normal, and increased secretory activity all being reported.[234, 235, 242–246] This discrepancy in the results of the various studies may have resulted in part from the fact that young and elderly subjects were not always studied at comparable levels of insulin sensitivity. This point was emphasized by Gumbiner et al.,[247] who demonstrated that hyperinsulinemia in the elderly was associated with an increased basal secretion of insulin and an increased secretory response to meals. However, when insulin sensitivity was taken into account, the β cell responses during a hyperglycemic clamp—although normal in absolute terms—were deemed to be disproportionately low in elderly subjects. These findings have been confirmed recently in another study in which β cell responses in groups of young and elderly subjects of comparable insulin sensitivity were compared.[248] In this study, insulin secretory responses to glucose and arginine in the elderly group were significantly lower than in the weight-matched younger group. Thus, while elderly subjects have enhanced insulin secretion rates due to insulin resistance, the β cell secretory responses are still inappropriately low for the level of insulin sensitivity. Diminished insulin clearance does not appear to be a contributory factor in the observed hyperinsulinemia in this population subgroup.[246, 247]

Diabetes Mellitus

Insulin-Dependent (Type 1) Diabetes Mellitus

Being insulin-deficient, patients with type 1 diabetes mellitus have practically no β cell response to glucose and nonglucose stimuli.[249] However, the initial period following diagnosis is often associated with an improvement in glucose tolerance to the point where normoglycemia can be maintained for a self-limiting duration in some patients in the absence of any definitive therapy.[250] This so-called honeymoon period is associated with increases in the C peptide and insulin responses to glucose.[251–255] Although β cell secretory capacity is improved during this period, it is still less than that observed in normal subjects, and in addition to this quantitative defect, a qualitative defect is also present, manifested in serum by an increased molar ratio of proinsulin to C peptide.[256–258] Thus, during the honeymoon phase, the pancreas, in addition to secreting less insulin, also releases the contents of immature β cell granules into the circulation. The subsequent and inevitable deterioration in glycemic control heralding the end of the honeymoon period is preceded by a gradual reduction in the secretory capacity of the β cell.[251] However, there are a number of reports suggesting that many patients with type 1 diabetes have some residual insulin production that may be detected many years after the development of overt hyperglycemia.[259, 260]

The β cell secretory responses during the period prior to the onset of type 1 diabetes mellitus are also of interest. Studies in normoglycemic islet cell antibody–positive monozygotic twins whose co-twins were already insulinopenic have demonstrated a progressive diminution in the first-phase insulin response to glucose over a number of years prior to the development of overt diabetes mellitus.[261] During this "early" diabetic phase, the β cell response to other secretagogues, including arginine, tolbutamide, and glucagon, is also impaired.[262] Insulin secretion during this period is still pulsatile. Both rapid and slow (ultradian) oscillations can still be detected. In contrast to those in normal subjects, the rapid pulses do not occur with the same regularity,[221] and the ultradian oscillations are less tightly coupled to corresponding oscillations in plasma glucose.

Non–Insulin-Dependent (Type 2) Diabetes Mellitus

In contrast to those with type 1 diabetes, patients with type 2 diabetes are often hyperinsulinemic, but the degree of hyperinsulinemia is inappropriately low for the prevailing glucose concentrations. Nevertheless, many of these patients have sufficient β cell reserve to maintain a euglycemic state by dietary restriction with or without an oral agent. The β cell defect in patients with NIDDM is characterized by an absent first-phase insulin and C peptide response to an intravenous glucose load and a reduced second-phase response.[57, 249, 263–265] Although in vitro studies using the isolated perfused pancreas have emphasized the importance of hyperglycemia in mediating these changes,[58, 266] the abnormal first-phase response to intravenous glucose persists in patients whose diabetic control has been greatly improved,[249, 263] thus supporting the hypothesis that patients with type 2 diabetes may have an intrinsic defect in the β cell. Furthermore, abnormalities in first-phase insulin secretion also have been observed in first-degree relatives of patients with type 2 diabetes who have only mild glucose intolerance,[267] and an attenuated insulin response to oral glucose has been observed in normoglycemic co-twins of patients with type 2 diabetes[268]—a group at very high risk for NIDDM[269] and who can legitimately be classified as being "prediabetic." This pattern of insulin secretion during the so-called prediabetic phase is also seen in subjects with impaired glucose tolerance who later develop NIDDM[270–273] and in normoglycemic obese subjects with a recent history of gestational diabetes,[274] this latter group also being at high risk for NIDDM.[275] β Cell abnormalities may therefore precede the development of overt type 2 diabetes by many years.

Many studies in recent years have examined the effects of NIDDM on proinsulin levels in serum. These have consistently demonstrated elevated levels of proinsulin in association with increases in the proinsulin-insulin molar ratio.[175, 177, 178, 180, 276, 277] The amount of proinsulin produced in this setting appears to be related to the degree of glycemic control rather than to the duration of the diabetic state, and in one series, proinsulin levels contributed almost 50% of the total insulin immunoreactivity in those NIDDM patients who had marked hyperglycemia.[180] In addition to intact proinsulin, the β cell also secretes one or more of the four major proinsulin conversion products (split 32,33-, split 65,66-, des-31,32-, and des-64,65-proinsulin) into the circulation[172, 173] (Fig. 49–5). These conversion products are produced within the secretory granules of the islet as the result of the activity of specific conversion enzymes at the two cleavage sites in proinsulin linking the C peptide to the A and B chains. The composition of the elevated PLI in patients with NIDDM compared with controls has not been fully characterized. Recently, Hales and colleagues from the University of Cambridge in England have developed immunoradiometric assays for this purpose.[276, 278, 279] Although these assays are clearly more specific than conventional proinsulin assays, they cannot distinguish between des- and split-proinsulin conversion products and have not been validated against high-pressure liquid chromatography (HPLC)–separated immunoreactive insulin and proinsulin, which can make this distinction. In this regard, although Hales et al. reported split 32,33-proinsulin to be the predominant proinsulin conversion product in the circulation, our own preliminary studies using HPLC to separate PLI into its constituent peptides suggest that des-31,32-proinsulin is present in highest concentration. The significance of this distinction is unclear. Utilizing these assays, Hales et al. have measured insulin, proinsulin, and conversion product concentrations 30 minutes after oral glucose in patients with NIDDM.[276] Insulin was reduced in all patients, with no overlap between patients and controls, and concentrations of proinsulin and conversion products were elevated in the patients with NIDDM. These data were interpreted to indicate that NIDDM is primarily a disease of β-cell deficiency and that conventional insulin radioimmunoassays that demonstrate cross-reactivity with proinsulin and the proinsulin conversion products have overestimated the amount of circulating insulin immunoreactivity, thereby minimizing the extent of the β cell defect. Although the elevation in PLI may elevate the circulating immunoreactive insulin level in NIDDM, other published literature has shown considerable overlap between the insulin concentrations in diabetic patients and matched controls, including studies based not only on concentrations of insulin but also on measurements of plasma C peptide.[263, 280–282] Although proinsulin may cross-react to a significant extent in some C peptide assays, in others the cross-reactivity of proinsulin is sufficiently low that the contribution of proinsulin and proinsulin conversion products to total C peptide immunoreactivity is negligible. Nevertheless, these data and the controversy they have generated highlight the importance of the potentially confounding effects of proinsulin and proinsulin conversion products in the interpretation of circulating immunoreactive insulin in patients with NIDDM and emphasize the need to measure the concentrations of the individual peptides.

Abnormalities in the temporal pattern of insulin secretion also have been demonstrated in patients with type 2 diabetes. In contrast to normal subjects in whom equal amounts of insulin are secreted basally and postprandially in a given 24-hour period, patients with NIDDM secrete a greater proportion of their daily insulin under basal conditions[280] (Fig. 49–6). This reduction in the proportion of insulin secreted postprandially appears in part to be related to a reduction in the amplitude of the secretory pulses of insulin occurring after meals rather than to be due to a reduction in the number of pulses. In contrast to normal subjects, in patients with NIDDM the ultradian oscillations in insulin secretion are less tightly coupled with oscillations in plasma glucose[237, 280] (Fig. 49–7). Similar findings were observed in patients with impaired glucose tolerance studied under the same experimental conditions and in a further group of NIDDM patients studied under fasting conditions.[205] The rapid insulin pulses are also abnormal in type 2 diabetes, since the persistent regular rapid

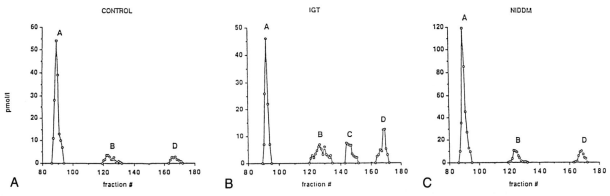

FIGURE 49–5. High-performance liquid chromatography profiles of insulin and proinsulin-like immunoreactivity in three subjects. The column was calibrated with standards of insulin (A), des-31,32-proinsulin (B), des-64,65-proinsulin (C), and intact proinsulin (D).

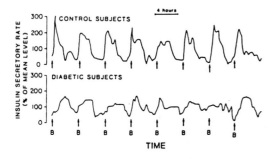

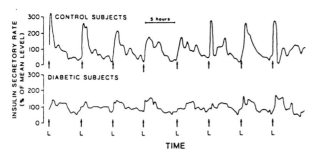

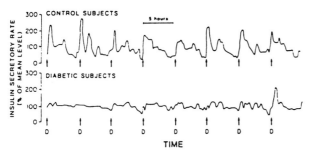

FIGURE 49–6. Temporal variations in postbreakfast, postlunch, and postdinner rates of insulin secretion in control and diabetic subjects. In each subject, the secretion rates during the 30 minutes before the meal and the 4 hours after breakfast or the 5 hours after lunch or dinner were expressed as a percentage of the mean rate of insulin secretion during that interval. The curves were obtain by concatenating the resulting postmeal profiles in eight representative subjects. The times at which the meals were served to successive subjects in the series are indicated by *arrows.*

oscillations present in normal subjects are not observed.[200] Instead, the cycles are of shorter duration and are irregular in nature. Similar findings were observed in a group of first-degree relatives of patients with NIDDM who had only mild glucose intolerance,[283] suggesting that abnormalities in oscillatory activity may be an early manifestation of β cell dysfunction in type 2 diabetes.

The effects of therapy on β cell function in patients with type 2 diabetes also have been investigated. While interpretation of the results in many instances is limited by the fact that β cell function was not always studied at comparable levels before and during therapy,[284] the majority of the studies indicate that improvements in diabetic control are associated with an enhancement of β cell secretory activity.[263, 285–289] This increased endogenous production of insulin appears to be independent of the mode of treatment and is in particular associated with increases in the amount of insulin secreted postprandially.[263, 289] The enhanced β cell secretory activity following meals reflects an increase in the amplitude of existing secretory pulses rather than an increased number of pulses.[289] Despite improvements in glycemic control, β cell function is not normalized following therapy,[263, 286, 289] suggesting that the intrinsic defect in the β cell in type 2 diabetes persists.

Transplantation

Pancreas Transplantation

There are a number of studies which have evaluated β cell function following whole-organ transplantation.[109–112, 290, 291] Since many of those patients who have undergone pancreas transplantation remain euglycemic off therapy in the post-transplant period, it appears that the β cell can function adequately despite being denervated. However, marked alterations in the temporal pattern of insulin secretion have been reported, with basal insulin secretion accounting for up to 75% of the total daily insulin produced in a 24-hour period. Postprandial insulin responses are therefore markedly attenuated.[109] Oscillatory insulin secretion is also preserved following pancreas transplantation. Both rapid and ultradian oscillations in insulin secretion have been demonstrated,[109, 292, 293] but the amplitude of the latter postprandially is significantly reduced.[109] The detection of rapid and slow oscillations in the setting of denervation suggests that the autonomic nervous system is not primarily responsible for their generation. However, since the rapid oscillations occur with greater frequency following transplantation,[293] it is likely that neural factors may modulate the activity of the mechanism responsible for these particular oscillations.

Islet Cell Transplantation

Insulin secretory responses following islet cell transplantation also have been evaluated. Although the procedure of islet cell transplantation should be easier than whole-organ transplantation in humans, there are few reports of transient successful cadaveric transplantation in humans.[294–297] These studies have demonstrated a transient return of the ability to secrete C peptide after the transplantation of 500,000 to 1.3 million islets obtained postmortem from several pancreata. Insulin secretory responses also have been quantitated in a group of five patients who had severe chronic pancreatitis treated by total pancreatectomy followed by isolation and hepatic transplantation of their own islets.[298] Since these patients received their own islets, immunosuppressive agents (which have an adverse effect on β cell function) were not required. In these subjects, the timing of the plasma insulin response to glucose and arginine following transplantation was normal, but the magnitude of the response was diminished. Two of the five subjects were studied before pancreatectomy and following islet cell transplantation. Although both subjects had normal fasting glucose levels and hemoglobin A_{1c} concentrations following transplantation, the insulin and C peptide responses to glucose and arginine were much lower following transplantation. Studies in rats also have demonstrated that the insulin response to a glucose infusion and to a meal is quantitatively reduced but qualitatively intact following islet cell transplantation.[299] The site of transplantation (e.g., liver, spleen, kidney) does not appear to influence these findings.

Insulinoma

In the investigation of hypoglycemia, a detailed knowledge and a correct interpretation of the β cell secretory responses are critical. In distinguishing hypoglycemia due to an islet cell tumor from other causes of hypoglycemia, the measurement of insulin levels may not be sufficient. Under normal physiologic circumstances, β cell secretion is reduced as glucose levels fall. The hypoglycemia seen in patients with an insulinoma, however, is characterized by low glucose levels with inappropriate levels of insulin (which may be normal or elevated).[300, 301] While hypoglycemia induced by the surreptitious administration of insulin also may be associated with hyperinsulinemia, C peptide levels will be elevated in patients with a true insulinoma, while the administration of exogenous insulin may suppress the release of C peptide from the β cell.[302] Moreover, in patients with an insulinoma, a greater proportion of proinsulin is released into the circulation. This latter factor could prove to be important in distinguishing patients with an insulinoma from those rare cases of hypoglycemia resulting from surreptitious ingestion of oral hypoglycemic agents.

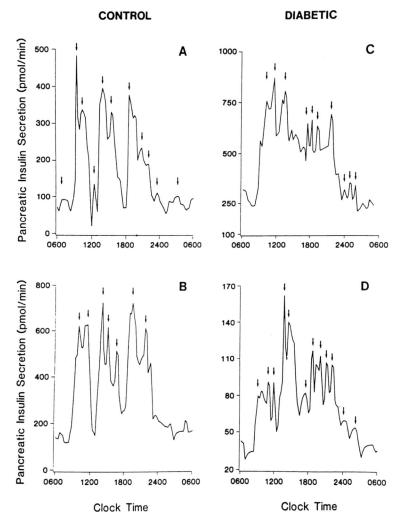

FIGURE 49–7. Patterns of insulin secretion in control and diabetic subjects. Four representative 24-hour insulin secretion profiles from two nondiabetic controls (*A* and *B*) and two diabetic patients (*C* and *D*) are shown. Meals were eaten at 0900, 1300, and 1800 hours. *Arrows* indicate statistically significant pulses of secretion.

REFERENCES

1. Steiner DF, Oyer PE: The biosynthesis of insulin and a probable precursor of insulin by a human islet cell adenoma. Proc Natl Acad Sci U S A 57:473, 1967.
2. Rubenstein AH, Clark JL, Melani F, et al: Secretion of proinsulin, C-peptide by pancreatic β cells and its circulation in blood. Nature 224:697, 1969.
3. Horwitz DL, Starr JI, Mako ME, et al: Proinsulin, insulin, and C-peptide concentrations in human portal and peripheral blood. J Clin Invest 55:1278, 1975.
4. Melani FA, Rubenstein AH, Steiner DF: Human serum proinsulin. J Clin Invest 49:497, 1970.
5. Bergenstal RM, Cohen R, Lever E, et al: The metabolic effects of biosynthetic human proinsulin on carbohydrate metabolism. J Clin Endocrinol Metab 58:973, 1984.
6. Revers RR, et al: The effects of biosynthetic human proinsulin on carbohydrate metabolism in individuals with Type I diabetes. Diabetes 33:762, 1984.
7. Steiner DF: On the role of proinsulin. Diabetes 27(suppl 1):145, 1978.
8. Wojcikowski C, Blackman J, Ostrega D, et al: Lack of effect of high dose biosynthetic human C-peptide on pancreatic hormone release in normal subjects. Metabolism 39:827–832, 1990.
9. Porte D Jr, Puppo AA: Insulin responses to glucose: Evidence for a two-pool system in man. J Clin Invest 48:2309, 1969.
10. Chen M, Porte D Jr: The effect of rate and dose of glucose infusion on the acute insulin response in man. J Clin Endocrinol Metab 42:1168, 1976.
11. Ward WK, Beard JC, Halter JB, et al: Pathophysiology of insulin secretion in non–insulin dependent diabetes mellitus. Diabetes Care 7:491, 1984.
12. Waldhausl W, Bratusch-Marrain P, Gasic S: Insulin production rate following glucose ingestion estimated by splanchnic C-peptide output in normal man. Diabetologia 171:221, 1979.
13. Eaton RP, Allen RC, Schade DS: Hepatic removal of insulin in normal man: Dose response to endogenous insulin secretion. J Clin Endocrinol Metab 56:1294, 1983.
14. Nauck MA, Homberger E, Siegel EG, et al: Incretin effects of increasing glucose loads in man calculated from venous insulin and C-peptide responses. J Clin Endocrinol Metab 63:492, 1986.
15. Tillil H, Shapiro ET, Miller MA, et al: Dose-dependent effects of oral and intravenous glucose on insulin secretion and clearance in normal humans. Am J Physiol 254:E318, 1988.
16. Faber OK, Madsbad S, Kehlet H, et al: Pancreatic beta cell secretion during oral and intravenous glucose administration. Acta Med Scand Suppl 624:61, 1979.
17. Madsbad S, Kehlet H. Hilsted J, et al: Discrepancy between plasma C-peptide and insulin response to oral and intravenous glucose. Diabetes 32:436, 1983.
18. Shapiro ET, Tillil H, Miller AM, et al: Insulin secretion and clearance: Comparison after oral and intravenous glucose. Diabetes 36:1365, 1987.
19. Creutzfeldt W, Ebert R: New developments in the incretin concept. Diabetologia 28:565, 1985.
20. Dupre J, Ross SA, Watson D, et al: Stimulation of insulin secretion by gastric inhibitory polypeptide in man. J Clin Endocrinol Metab 37:826, 1973.
21. Anderson DK, Elahi D, Brown JC, et al: Oral glucose augmentation of insulin secretion: Interaction of gastric inhibitory polypeptide with ambient glucose and insulin levels. J Clin Invest 62:152, 1978.
22. Schmidt WE, Siegel EG, Creutzfeldt W: Glucagon-like peptide-1 but not glucagon-like peptide-2 stimulates insulin release from isolated rat pancreatic islets. Diabetologia 28:704, 1985.
23. Kreymann B, Ghatei MA, Williams G, et al: Glucagon-like peptide-1(7–36), a physiological incretin in man. Lancet 2:1300, 1987.
24. Zawalich WS, Diaz VA: Prior cholecystokinin exposure sensitizes islets of Langerhans to glucose stimulation. Diabetes 36:118, 1987.
25. Zawalich WS: Synergistic impact of cholecystokinin and gastric inhibitory polypeptide on the regulation of insulin secretion. Metabolism 37:778, 1988.
26. Weir GC, Mojsov S, Hendrick GK, et al: Glucagon-like peptide 1(7–37) action on endocrine pancreas. Diabetes 38:338, 1989.
27. Rasmussen H, Zawalich KC, Ganesan S, et al: Physiology and pathophysiology of insulin secretion. Diabetes Care 13:655, 1990.
28. Schebalin M, Said SI, Makhlouf GM: Stimulation of insulin and glucagon secretion by vasoactive intestinal peptide. Am J Physiol 232:E197, 1977.
29. Dupre J, Curtis JD, Unger RH, et al: Effects of secretin, pancreozymin, gastrin on the response of the endocrine pancreas to the administration of glucose or arginine in man. J Clin Invest 48:745, 1969.
30. Halter J, Porte D Jr: Mechanism of impaired acute insulin release in adult onset diabetes: Studies with isoproterenol and secretin. J Clin Endocrinol Metab 46:952, 1978.
31. Rehfield JF, Stadil F: The effect of gastrin on basal and glucose-stimulated insulin secretion in man. J Clin Invest 52:1415, 1973.
32. Pagliara AS, Stillings SN, Hover B, et al: Glucose modulation of amino acid induced glucagon and insulin release in the isolated perfused rat pancreas. J Clin Invest 54:819, 1974.
33. Gerich JE, Charles MA, Grodsky GM: Characterization of the effects of arginine

and glucose on glucagon and insulin release from the perfused rat pancreas. J Clin Invest 54:833, 1974.
34. Grodsky GM: The kinetics of insulin release. *In* Hasselblatt A, Bruchhausen FV (eds): Handbook of Experimental Pharmacology. Vol 32: Insulin II. Berlin, Springer-Verlag, 1975, p 1.
35. Salomon D, Meda P: Heterogeneity and contact dependent regulation of hormone secretion by individual β cells. Exp Cell Res 162:507, 1986.
36. Schuit FC, In't Velo PA, Pipeleers DG: Glucose stimulates proinsulin biosynthesis by a dose dependent recruitment of pancreatic beta cells. Proc Natl Acad Sci U S A 85:3865, 1988.
37. Cerasi E, Luft R: The plasma insulin response to glucose infusion in healthy subjects and in diabetes mellitus. Acta Endocrinol 55:278, 1967.
38. Grodsky GM, Bennett L: Multiphasic aspects of insulin release after glucose and glucagon. *In* Ostman J, Milner RDG (eds): Diabetes. Amsterdam, Excerpta Medica, 1969, p 462.
39. Grodsky GM: Threshold distribution hypothesis for packet storage of insulin and its mathematical modeling. J Clin Invest 51:2047, 1972.
40. Smith CP, Tarn AC, Thomas JM, et al: Between and within subject variation of the first phase insulin response to intravenous glucose. Diabetologia 31:123, 1988.
41. Bardet S, Pasqual C, Mawgendre D, et al: Inter and intra individual variability of acute insulin response during intravenous glucose tolerance tests. Diabetes Metab 15:233, 1989.
42. Rayman G, Clark P, Schneider AE, et al: The first phase insulin response to intravenous glucose is highly reproducible. Diabetologia 33:631, 1990.
43. Bolaffi JL, Heldt A, Lewis LD, et al: The third phase of in vitro insulin secretion: Evidence for glucose insensitivity. Diabetes 35:370, 1986.
44. Curry DL: Insulin content and insulinogenesis by the perfused rat pancreas: Effect of long term glucose stimulation. Endocrinology 118:170, 1986.
45. Hoenig LC, MacGregor LC, Matschinsky FM: In vitro exhaustion of pancreatic β cells. Am J Physiol 250:E502, 1986.
46. Grodsky GM: A new phase of insulin secretion: How will it contribute to our understanding of β-cell function? Diabetes 38:673, 1989.
47. Matschinsky FM, Ellerman J, Stillings S, et al: Hexoses and insulin secretion. *In* Hassellblatt A, Bruchhausen FV (eds): Handbook of Experimental Pharmacology. Vol 32: Insulin II. Berlin, Springer-Verlag, 1975, p 79.
48. Grodsky GM, Fanska R, Lundquist I: Interrelationship between α and β anomers of glucose affecting both insulin and glucagon secretion in the perfused rat pancreas. Endocrinology 97:573, 1975.
49. Niki A, Niki H, Miwa I: Effect of anomers of d-mannose on insulin release from perfused pancreas. Endocrinology 105:1051, 1979.
50. Malaisse WJ, Sener M, Koser M, et al: Stimulus-secretion coupling of glucose-induced insulin release. Metabolism of α and β d-glucose in isolated islets. J Biol Chem 251:5936, 1976.
51. Malaisse WJ, Lagae F, Lebrun P, et al: Metabolic response of pancreatic islets of the rat to the anomers of D-mannose. Diabetologia 23:185, 1982.
52. Zawalich WS, Pagliara AS, Matschinsky FM: Effects of iodoacetate, mannoheptulose and 3-O-methylglucose on the secretory function and metabolism of isolated pancreatic islets. Endocrinology 100:1276, 1977.
53. Froguel P, Vaxillaire M, Sun F, et al: Close linkage of glucokinase locus on chromosome 7p to early-onset non–insulin-dependent diabetes mellitus. Nature 356:162–164, 1992.
54. Velho G, Froguel P, Clement K, et al: Primary pancreatic beta-cell secretory defect caused by mutations in the glucokinase genes in kindreds of maturity onset diabetes of the young. Lancet 340:444, 1992.
55. Levin SR, Karam JH, Kane S, et al: Enhancement of arginine-induced insulin secretion in man by prior administration of glucose. Diabetes 20:171, 1971.
56. Fajans SS, Floyd JC: Stimulation of islet cell secretion by nutrients and by gastrointestinal hormones released during digestion. *In* Steiner DF, Freinkel N (eds): Handbook of Physiology. Washington, DC, American Physiological Society, 1972, p 473.
57. Ward WK, Bolgiano DC, McNight B, et al: Diminished β cell secretory capacity in patients with non–insulin-dependent diabetes mellitus. J Clin Invest 74:1318, 1984.
58. Leahy JL, Bonner-Weir S, Weir GC: Minimal chronic hyperglycemia is a critical determinant of impaired insulin secretion after an incomplete pancreatectomy. J Clin Invest 81:1407, 1988.
59. Matschinsky FM, Fertel R, Kotler-Brajtburg K, et al: Factors governing the action of small calorigenic molecules on the islets of Langerhans. *In* Maussacchia XJ, Breitenbach KP (eds): Proceedings of the 8th Midwest Conference on Endocrinology and Metabolism. Columbia, University of Missouri Press, 1973, p 63.
60. Muller WA, Faloona GR, Unger RH: The influence of the antecedent diet upon glucagon and insulin secretion. N Engl J Med 285:1450, 1971.
61. Samols E, Marri G, Marks V: Promotion of insulin secretion by glucagon. Lancet 2:1299, 1965.
62. Alberti KGMM, Christensen NJ, Christensen SE, et al: Inhibition of insulin secretion by somatostatin. Lancet 2:1299, 1973.
63. Felig P, Marliss EB, Cahill GF Jr: Metabolic response to human growth hormone during prolonged starvation. J Clin Invest 50:411, 1971.
64. Kalhan SC, Adam PAJ: Inhibitory effect of prednisone on insulin secretion in man: Model for duplication of blood glucose concentration. J Clin Endocrinol Metab 41:600, 1975.
65. Landgraf R, Leurs MMC, Weissmann A, et al: Prolactin: A diabetogenic hormone. Diabetologia 13:99, 1977.
66. Gustafson AB, Banasiak MF, Kalkhaff RK, et al: Correlation of hyperprolactinemia with altered plasma insulin and glucagon: Similarity to effects of late human pregnancy. J Clin Endocrinol Metab 51:242, 1980.
67. Brelje Clark T, Sorenson RL: Nutrient and hormonal regulation of the threshold of glucose-stimulated insulin secretion in isolated rat pancreases. Endocrinology 123:1582, 1988.
68. Beck P, Daughaday WH: Human placental lactogen: Studies of its acute metabolic effects and disposition in normal man. J Clin Invest 46:103, 1967.
69. Ensinck JW, Williams RH: Hormonal and non-hormonal factors modifying man's response to insulin. *In* Steiner DF, Freinkel N (eds): Handbook of Physiology. Washington, DC, American Physiological Society, 1972, p 665.
70. Martin JM, Friesen H: Effect of human placental lactogen on the isolated islets of Langerhans in vitro. Endocrinology 84:619, 1969.
71. Curry DL, Bennett LL: Dynamics of insulin release by perfused rat pancreases: Effects of hypophysectomy, growth hormone, adrenocorticotropic hormone and hydrocortisone. Endocrinology 93:602, 1973.
72. Malaisse WJ, Malaisse-Lange F, King S, et al: Effect of growth hormone on insulin secretion. Am J Physiol 215:423, 1968.
73. Doar JWH, Stamp TCB, Wynne V, et al: Effects of oral and intravenous glucose loading in thyrotoxicosis: Studies of plasma glucose, free fatty acid, plasma insulin and blood pyruvate levels. Diabetes 18:633–639, 1969.
74. Ortved AO, Friis T, Ottesen B: Glucose tolerance and insulin secretion in hyperthyroidism. Acta Endocrinol 84:576–587, 1977.
75. Dimitriadis G, Baker B, Marsh H, et al: Effect of thyroid hormone excess on action, secretion and metabolism of insulin in humans. Am J Physiol 248:E593–E601, 1985.
76. Osei K, Falko JM, O'Dorisio TM, et al: Decreased serum C-peptide/insulin molar ratios after oral glucose ingestion in hyperthyroid patients. Diabetes Care 7:471–475, 1984.
77. Cohen P, Barzilai N, Barzilai D, et al: Correlation between insulin clearance and insulin responsiveness: Studies in normal, obese, hyperthyroid and Cushing's syndrome patients. Metabolism 35:744–749, 1986.
78. Malaisse WJ, Malaisse-Lagae F, McCraw EF: Effects of thyroid function on insulin secretion. Diabetes 16:643–646, 1967.
79. Lenzen S: Dose-response studies on the inhibitory effect of thyroid hormones on insulin secretion in the rat. Metabolism 27:81–88, 1977.
80. Wolf E, Eisenstein AB: Portal vein blood insulin and glucagon are increased in experimental hyperthyroidism. Endocrinology 108: 2109–2113, 1981.
81. Taylor R, McCulloch AJ, Zeuzem S, et al: Insulin secretion, adipocyte insulin binding and insulin sensitivity in thyrotoxicosis. Acta Endocrinol 109:96–103, 1985.
82. Roti E, Braverman LE, Robuschi G, et al: Basal and glucose and arginine stimulated serum concentrations of insulin, C-peptide and glucagon in hyperthyroid patients. Metabolism 35:337–342, 1986.
83. Beer SF, Parr JH, Temple RC, et al: The effect of thyroid disease on proinsulin and C-peptide levels. Clin Endocrinol 30:379–383, 1989.
84. Sestoft L, Heding LG: Hypersecretion of proinsulin in thyrotoxicosis. Diabetologia 21:103–107, 1981.
85. O'Meara NM, Blackman JD, Sturis J, et al: Alterations in the kinetics of C-peptide and insulin secretion in hyperthyroidism. J Clin Endocrinol Metab 76:79–84, 1993.
86. Eaton RP, Allen RC, Schade DS, et al: Prehepatic insulin production in man: Kinetic analysis using peripheral connecting peptide behaviour. J Clin Endocrinol Metab 51:520, 1980.
87. Akmal M, Massry SG, Goldstein DA, et al: Role of parathyroid hormone in the glucose intolerance of chronic renal failure. J Clin Invest 75:1037–1044, 1985.
88. Mak RHK, Bettinelli A, Turner C, et al: The influence of hyperparathyroidism on glucose metabolism in uremia. J Clin Endocrinol Metab 60:229–233, 1985.
89. Fadda GZ, Akmal M, Premdas FH, et al: Insulin release from pancreatic islets: Effects of chronic renal failure and excess parathyroid hormone. Kidney Int 33:1066–1072, 1988.
90. Fadda GC, Akmal M, Lipson LG, et al: Direct effect of parathyroid hormone on insulin secretion from pancreatic islets. Am J Physiol 258:E975–E984, 1990.
91. Porte D Jr: A receptor mechanism for the inhibition of insulin release by epinephrine in man. J Clin Invest 46:86–94, 1967.
92. Beard JC, Weinberg C, Pfeifer MA: Interaction of glucose and epinephrine in the regulation of insulin secretion. Diabetes 31:802–807, 1982.
93. Kurose T, Seino Y, Nishi S, et al: Mechanism of sympathetic neural regulation in insulin, somatostatin and glucagon secretion. Am J Physiol 258:E220, 1990.
94. Woods SC, Porte D Jr: Neural control of the endocrine pancreas. Physiol Rev 54:596, 1974.
95. Bloom SR, Edwards AV: The release of pancreatic glucagon and inhibition of insulin in response to stimulation of the sympathetic innervation. J Physiol (Lond) 280:25, 1978.
96. Porte D Jr, Girardier L, Seydoux J, et al: Neural regulation of insulin secretion in the dog. J Clin Invest 52:210, 1973.
97. Roy MW, Lee KC, Jones MS, et al: Neural control of pancreatic insulin and somatostatin secretion. Endocrinology 115:770, 1984.
98. Nishi S, Seino Y, Ishida H, et al: Vagal regulation of insulin, glucagon and somatostatin secretion in vitro in the rat. J Clin Invest 79:1191, 1987.
99. Hommel H, Fischer U, Retzlaff K, et al: The mechanism of insulin secretion after oral glucose administration. II. Reflex insulin secretion in conscious dogs bearing fistulas of the digestive tract by sham-feeding and glucose or tap water. Diabetologia 8:111, 1972.
100. Berthoud HR, Trimble ER, Siegel EG, et al: Cephalic phase insulin secretion in normal and pancreatic islet-transplanted rats. Am J Physiol 238:E336, 1980.
101. Taylor IL, Feldman M: Effect of cephalic-vagal stimulation on insulin, gastric inhibitory polypeptide and pancreatic polypeptide release in humans. J Clin Endocrinol Metab 55:1114, 1982.
102. Bruce DG, Storlein LH, Furler SM, et al: Cephalic phase metabolic responses in normal weight adults. Metabolism 36:721, 1987.
103. Berthoud HR, Bereiter DA, Trimble ER, et al: Cephalic phase, reflex insulin secretion: Neuroanatomical and physicological characterization. Diabetologia 20:393, 1981.
104. Zawalich WS, Zawalich KC, Rasmussen H: Cholinergic agonists prime the β-cell to glucose stimulation. Endocrinology 125:2400, 1989.
105. Hakanson R, Liedberg G, Lundquist I: Effect of vagal denervation on insulin release after oral and intravenous glucose. Experientia 27:460, 1971.
106. Linquette M, Fourlinnie JC, Lagache G: Etude de la glycémie et de l'insulinémie apres vagotomie et pyroplastie chez l'homme. Ann Endocrinol (Paris) 30:96, 1969.

107. Louis-Sylvestre J: Relationship between two stages of prandial insulin release in rats. Am J Physiol 235:E103, 1978.
108. Trimble ER, Siegel EG, Berthoud HR, et al: Intraportal islet transplantation: Functional assessment in conscious unrestrained rats. Endocrinology 106:791, 1980.
109. Blackman JD, Polonsky KS, Jaspan JB, et al: Insulin secretory profiles and C-peptide clearance kinetics at six months and at two years post kidney-pancreas transplantation. Diabetes 41:1346–1354, 1992.
110. Madsbad S, Christiansen E, Andersen HB, et al: β-cell defects after pancreas transplantation in Type I patients. Diabetes 39(suppl 1):15A, 1990.
111. Diem P, Abid M, Redmon J, et al: Systemic venous drainage of pancreas allografts as independent cause of hyperinsulinemia in type I diabetic recipients. Diabetes 39:534, 1990.
112. Pozza G, Bosi E, Secchi A, et al: Metabolic control of type I (insulin dependent) diabetes after pancreas transplantation. BMJ 291:510, 1985.
113. King DS, Dalsky GP, Staten MA, et al: Insulin action and secretion in endurance-trained and untrained humans. J Appl Physiol 63:2247, 1987.
114. King DS, Dalsky GP, Clutter WE, et al: Effects of lack of exercise on insulin secretion and action in trained subjects. Am J Physiol 254:E537, 1988.
115. King DS, Staten MA, Kohrt W, et al: Insulin secretory capacity in endurance-trained and untrained young men. Am J Physiol 259:E155, 1990.
116. Seals DR, Hagberg JM, Allen WK, et al: Glucose tolerance in young and older athletes and sedentary men. J Appl Physiol 56:1521, 1984.
117. Heath GW, Gavin JR III, Hinderliter JM, et al: Effects of exercise and lack of exercise on glucose tolerance and insulin sensitivity. J Appl Physiol 55:512, 1983.
118. King DS, Dalsky GP, Clutter WE, et al: Effects of exercise and lack of exercise on insulin sensitivity and responsiveness. J Appl Physiol 64:1942, 1988.
119. LeBlanc J, Nadeau A, Richard D, et al: Studies on the sparing effect of exercise on insulin requirements in human subjects. Metabolism 30:1119, 1981.
120. Mortimore GE, Tietze F, Stetten D Jr: Metabolism of insulin [131]I: Studies of isolated perfused rat liver and hind limb preparation. Diabetes 8:307, 1959.
121. Solomon SS, Fenster F, Ensinck JW, et al: Clearance studies of insulin and non-suppressible insulin-like activity (NSILA) in the rat liver. Proc Soc Exp Biol Med 126:166, 1967.
122. Mondon CE, Olefsky JM, Dolkas CB, et al: Removal of insulin by perfused rat liver: Effect of concentration. Metabolism 24:153, 1975.
123. Rubenstein AH, Pottenger LA, Mako M, et al: The metabolism of proinsulin and insulin by the liver. J Clin Invest 51:912, 1972.
124. Kaden M, Harding P, Field JB: Effect of intraduodenal glucose administration on hepatic extraction of insulin in the anesthetized dog. J Clin Invest 52:2016, 1973.
125. Harding PE, Bloom G, Field JB: Effect of infusion of insulin into portal vein on hepatic extraction of insulin in anesthetized dogs. Am J Physiol 228:1580, 1975.
126. Rojdmark S, Bloom G, Chou MCY, et al: Hepatic insulin and glucagon extraction after their augmented secretion in dogs. Am J Physiol 235:E88, 1978.
127. Rojdmark S, Bloom G, Chou MCY, et al: Hepatic extraction of exogenous insulin and glucagon in the dog. Endocrinology 102:806, 1978.
128. Ishida T, Rojdmark S, Bloom G, et al: The effect of somatostatin on the hepatic extraction of insulin and glucagon in the anesthetized dog. Endocrinology 106:220, 1978.
129. Jaspan JB, Polonsky KS, Lewis M, et al: Hepatic metabolism of glucagon in the dog: Contribution of the liver to overall metabolic disposal of glucagon. Am J Physiol 3:E233, 1981.
130. Polonsky KS, Jaspan J, Emmanouel D, et al: The hepatic and renal extraction of insulin and glucagon in the dog: Evidence for saturability of insulin metabolism. Acta Endocrinol 102:420, 1983.
131. Jaspan J, Polonsky KS: Glucose ingestion in dogs alters the hepatic extraction of insulin: In vivo evidence for a relationship between biologic action and extraction of insulin. J Clin Invest 69:516, 1982.
132. Honey RN, Price S: The determinants of insulin extraction in the isolated perfused rat liver. Horm Metab Res 11:111, 1979.
133. Striffler JS, Curry DL: Effect of fasting on insulin removal by liver of perfused rat pancreas. Am J Physiol 237:E349, 1979.
134. Ferrannini E, Wahren J, Faber OK, et al: Splanchnic and renal metabolism of insulin in human subjects: A dose response study. Am J Physiol 244:E517, 1983.
135. Misbin RI, Merimere TJ, Lowenstein JM: Insulin removal by isolated perfused rat liver. Am J Physiol 730:171, 1976.
136. Pilo A, Navalesi R, Ferrannini E: Insulin kinetics after portal and peripheral injections of I-insulin. I. Data analysis and modeling. Am J Physiol 230:1626, 1976.
137. Navalesi R, Pilo A, Ferrannini E: Insulin kinetics after portal and peripheral injection of I-insulin. II. Experiments in the intact dog. Am J Physiol 230:1630, 1976.
138. Polonsky KS, Jaspan JB, Pugh W, et al: The metabolism of C-peptide in the dog: In vivo demonstration of the absence of hepatic extraction. J Clin Invest 72:1114, 1983.
139. Kahn RC, Baird K: The fate of insulin bound to adipocytes. J Biol Chem 253:4900, 1978.
140. Terris S, Steiner DF: Binding and degradation of ^{125}I-insulin by rat hepatocytes. J Biol Chem 250:8389, 1981.
141. Polonsky K, Jaspan JB, Emmanouel D, et al: Differences in the hepatic and renal extraction of insulin and glucagon in the dog: Evidence for saturability of insulin metabolism. Acta Endocrinol 102:420, 1983.
142. Sonksen PH, Tompkins CV, Srivastava MC, et al: A comparative study on the metabolism of human insulin and porcine proinsulin in man. Clin Sci Med 45:633, 1973.
143. Polonsky KS, Given BD, Hirsch L, et al: Quantitative study of insulin secretion and clearance in normal and obese subjects. J Clin Invest 81:435, 1988.
144. Waddell WH, Sussman KE: Plasma insulin after diversion of portal and pancreatic blood to the vena cava. Am J Physiol 22:808, 1967.
145. Kanazawa Y, Kuzuya T, Ide T, et al: Plasma insulin responses to glucose in femoral, hepatic and pancreatic veins in dogs. Am J Physiol 211:442, 1966.
146. Blackard WC, Nelson NC: Portal and peripheral vein immunoreactive insulin concentrations before and after glucose infusion. Diabetes 19:302, 1970.
147. Tranberg KG, Thorell J: Variation in the disappearance of unlabelled insulin from plasma: Studies with portal and peripheral infusions. Diabetes 28:846, 1979.
148. Rubenstein AH: Mako ME, Horwitz DL: Insulin and the kidney. Nephron 15:306, 1975.
149. Rabkin R, Simon NM, Steiner S, et al: Effect of renal disease on renal uptake and excretion of insulin in man. N Engl J Med 282:182, 1970.
150. Rabkin R, Colwell JA: The renal uptake and excretion of insulin in the dog. J Lab Clin Med 73:893, 1969.
151. Zaharko DS, Beck LV, Blankenbaker R: Role of the kidney in the disposal of radioiodinated and nonradioiodinated insulin in dogs. Diabetes 15:680, 1966.
152. Chamberlain MJ, Stimmler L: The renal handling of insulin. J Clin Invest 46:911, 1967.
153. Beck LV, Fedynskyj M: Evidence from combined immunoassay and radioautography procedures that intact insulin-I molecules are concentrated by mouse kidney proximal tubule cells. Endocrinology 81:475, 1967.
154. Bourdeau JE, Chen ERY, Carone FA: Insulin uptake in the renal proximal tubule. Am J Physiol 225:1399, 1973.
155. Aun F, Soeldner JS, Mequid MM, et al: Urine insulin levels in health and disease—A concise review. Postgrad Med J 51:622, 1975.
156. Kurokawa K, Lerner RL: Binding and degradation of insulin by isolated renal cortical tubules. Endocrinology 106:655, 1980.
157. Challoner DR: Degradation of porcine insulin and proinsulin by rat adipose tissue. Diabetes 20:276, 1971.
158. Crofford OB, Rogers NJ, Russel WG: The effect of insulin on fat cells: An insulin degrading system extracted from plasma membranes of insulin responsive cells. Diabetes 21 (suppl 2):403, 1972.
159. Beck-Nielsen H, Pederson O: Insulin binding, insulin degradation and glucose metabolism in human monocytes. Diabetologia 17:77, 1979.
160. Powers AC, Solomon SS, Duckworth WC: Insulin degradation by mononuclear cells. Diabetes 29:27, 1980.
161. Kolb HJ, Standl E: An insulin degrading enzyme from human erythrocytes: Isolation and characterization. *In* Brandenburg D, Wollmer A (eds): Insulin, Chemistry, Structure, and Function of Insulin and Related Hormones. Berlin, Walter de Gruyter, 1980, p 509.
162. Gambhir KK, Archer JA, Bradley CJ: Characteristics of human erythrocyte insulin receptors. Diabetes 27:701, 1978.
163. Buse MG, Roberts WJ, Buse J: The role of the human placenta in the transfer and metabolism of insulin. J Clin Invest 41:29, 1962.
164. Freinkel N, Goodner CJ: Carbohydrate metabolism in pregnancy. I. The metabolism of insulin by human placental tissue. J Clin Invest 39:116, 1960.
165. Stoll RW, Touber JL, Menahan LA, et al: Clearance of porcine insulin, proinsulin and connecting peptide by the isolated rat liver. Proc Soc Exp Biol Med 133:894–896, 1970.
166. Bratusch-Marrain PR, Waldhausl WK, Gasic S, et al: Hepatic disposal of biosynthetic human insulin and porcine proinsulin in humans. Metabolism 33:151, 1984.
167. Kuhl C, Faber O, Hornnes P, et al: C-peptide metabolism and the liver. Diabetes 27 (suppl 1):197, 1978.
168. Katz AI, Rubenstein AH: Metabolism of proinsulin, insulin and C-peptide in the rat. J Clin Invest 52:1113, 1973.
169. Faber O, Haben C, Binder C, et al: Kinetics of human connecting peptide in normal and diabetic subjects. J Clin Invest 62:197, 1978.
170. Licinio-Paixao J, Polonsky KS: Ingestion of a mixed meal does not affect the metabolic clearance rate of biosynthetic human C-peptide. J Clin Endocrinol Metab 63:401, 1986.
171. Van Cauter E, Mestrez F, Sturis J, et al: Estimation of insulin secretion rates from C-peptide levels: Comparison of individual and standard kinetic parameters for C-peptide clearance. Diabetes 41:368–377, 1992.
172. De Haën C, Little SA, May JM, et al: Characterization of proinsulin-insulin intermediates in human plasma. J Clin Invest 62:727, 1978.
173. Given BD, Cohen RH, Shoelson SE, et al: Biochemical and clinical implications of proinsulin conversion intermediates. J Clin Invest 76:1398, 1985.
174. Tillil H, Frank BH, Pekar AH, et al: Hypoglycemic potency and metabolic clearance rate of intravenously administered human proinsulin and metabolites. Endocrinology 127:2418, 1990.
175. Ward WK, LaCava EC, Paquette TL, et al: Disproportionate elevation of immunoreactive proinsulin in type 2 (non–insulin-dependent) diabetes mellitus and in experimental insulin resistance. Diabetologia 30:698, 1987.
176. Gorden P, Sherman BM, Simopoulos AP: Glucose intolerance with hypokalemia: An increased proportion of circulating proinsulin-like component. J Clin Endocrinol 34:235, 1972.
177. Duckworth WC, Kitabchi AE, Heinemann M: Direct measurement of plasma proinsulin in normal and diabetic subjects. Am J Med 53:418, 1972.
178. Mako ME, Starr JI, Rubenstein AH: Circulating proinsulin in patients with maturity onset diabetes. Am J Med 63:865, 1977.
179. Heaton DA, Millward BA, Gray IP, et al: Increased proinsulin levels as an early indicator of β-cell dysfunction in non-diabetic twins of type I (insulin-dependent) diabetic patients. Diabetologia 31:182, 1988.
180. Saad M, Kahn SE, Nelson R, et al: Disproportionately elevated proinsulin in Pima Indians with non–insulin dependent diabetes mellitus. J Clin Endocrinol Metab 70:1247, 1990.
181. Cohen RM, Given BD, Licinio-Paixao J, et al: Proinsulin radioimmunoassay in the evaluation of insulinomas and familial hyperproinsulinemia. Metabolism 35:1137, 1986.
182. Heding L: Specific and direct radioimmunoassay for human proinsulin in serum. Diabetologia 13:467, 1973.
183. Gabbay KH, DeLuca K, Fisher JN Jr, et al: Familial hyperproinsulinemia: An autosomal dominant defect. N Engl J Med 294:911, 1976.
184. Robbins DC, Shoelson SE, Rubenstein AH, et al: Familial hyperproinsulinemia: Two

families secreting indistinguishable type II conversion intermediates of proinsulin conversion. J Clin Invest 73:714, 1984.
185. Yano H, Kitano N, Morimoto M, et al: A novel point mutation in the human insulin gene giving rise to hyperproinsulinemia (proinsulin Kyoto). J Clin Invest 89:1902, 1992.
186. Jaspan JB, Mako MD, Kuzuya H, et al: Abnormalities in circulating beta cell peptides in chronic renal failure: Comparison of proinsulin C-peptide and insulin. J Clin Endocrinol Metab 45:441, 1977.
187. Sestoft L, Heding LG: Hypersecretion of proinsulin in thyrotoxicosis. Diabetologia 21:103, 1981.
188. O'Meara NM, Blackman JD, Sturis J, et al: Alterations in the kinetics of C-peptide and insulin secretion in hyperthyroidism. J Clin Endocrinol Metab 76:79–84, 1993.
189. Rubenstein AH, Cho S, Steiner DF: Evidence for proinsulin in human urine and serum. Lancet 1:1353, 1968.
190. Malherbe C, DeGasparo M, DeHertogh R, et al: Circadian variations of blood sugar and plasma insulin levels in man. Diabetologia 5:397, 1969.
191. Polonsky KS, Given BD, VanCauter E: Twenty-four-hour profiles and pulsatile patterns of insulin secretion in normal and obese subjects. J Clin Invest 81:442, 1988.
192. Tasaka Y, Sekine M, Wakatsuki M, et al: Levels of pancreatic glucagon, insulin and glucose during twenty-four hours of the day in normal subjects. Horm Metab Res 7:205, 1975.
193. Jarrett RJ, Baker IA, Keen H, et al: Diurnal variation in oral glucose tolerance: Blood sugar and plasma insulin levels morning, afternoon and evening. BMJ 1:199, 1972.
194. Carroll KF, Nestel PJ: Diurnal variation in glucose tolerance and in insulin secretion in man. Diabetes 22:333, 1973.
195. Alparicio NJ, Puchulu FE, Gadliardino JJ, et al: Circadian variation of the blood glucose, plasma insulin and human growth hormone levels in response to an oral glucose load in normal subjects. Diabetes 23:132, 1974.
196. Van Cauter E, Desir D, Decoster C, et al: Nocturnal decrease in glucose tolerance during constant glucose infusion. J Clin Endocrinol Metab 69:604, 1989.
197. Goodner CJ, Walike BC, Koerker DJ, et al: Insulin, glucagon and glucose exhibit synchronous sustained oscillations in fasting monkeys. Science 195:177, 1977.
198. Lang DA, Matthews DR, Peto J, et al: Cyclic oscillations of basal plasma glucose and insulin concentrations in human beings. N Engl J Med 301:1023, 1979.
199. Hansen BC, Pek S, Koercker DJ, et al: Neural influences on oscillations in basal plasma levels of insulin in monkeys. Am J Physiol 240:E5, 1981.
200. Lang DA, Matthews DR, Burnett M, et al: Brief irregular oscillations of basal plasma insulin and glucose concentrations in diabetic man. Diabetes 30:435, 1981.
201. Lang DA, Matthews DR, Burnett M, et al: Pulsatile, synchronous basal insulin and glucagon secretion in man. Diabetes 31:22, 1982.
202. Hansen BC, Jen KC, Pek SB, et al: Rapid oscillations in plasma insulin, glucagon and glucose in obese and normal weight humans. J Clin Endocrinol Metab 54:785, 1982.
203. Matthews DR, Lang DA, Burnett MA, et al: Control of pulsatile insulin secretion in man. Diabetologia 2:231, 1983.
204. O'Meara NM, Sturis J, Blackman JD, et al: Analytical problems in detecting rapid insulin secretory pulses in normal humans. Am J Physiol 264:E231–238, 1993.
205. Sturis J, Polonsky KS, Shapiro ET, et al: Abnormalities in the ultradian oscillations of insulin secretion and glucose levels in type 2 (non–insulin-dependent) diabetic patients. Diabetologia 35:681–689, 1992.
206. Simon C, Follenius M, Brandenberger G: Postprandial oscillations of plasma glucose, insulin and C-peptide in man. Diabetologia 30:769, 1987.
207. Simon C, Brandenberger G, Follenius M: Ultradian oscillations of plasma glucose, insulin and C-peptide in man during continuous enteral nutrition. J Clin Endocrinol Metab 64:669, 1987.
208. Shapiro ET, Tillil H, Polonsky KS, et al: Oscillations in insulin secretion during constant glucose infusion in normal man: Relationship to changes in plasma glucose. J Clin Endocrinol Metab 67:307, 1988.
209. Koerker DJ, Goodner CJ, Hansen BW, et al: Synchronous sustained oscillations of C-peptide and insulin in the plasma of fasting monkeys. Endocrinology 102:1649–1652, 1978.
210. Jaspan JB, Lever E, Polonsky KS, et al: In vivo pulsatility of pancreatic islet peptides. Am J Physiol 251:E215, 1986.
211. Goodner CJ, Koerker DJ, Weigle DS, et al: Decreased insulin and glucose pulse amplitude accompanying B-cell deficiency induced by streptozotocin in baboons. Diabetes 38:925–931, 1989.
212. Matthews DR, Hermansen K, Connolly AA, et al: Greater in vivo than in vitro pulsatility of insulin secretion with synchronized insulin and somatostatin secretory pulses. Endocrinology 120:2272–2278, 1987.
213. Chou HF, Ipp E: Pulsatile insulin secretion in isolated rat islets. Diabetes 39:112–117, 1990.
214. Goodner CJ, Koerker DJ, Stagner JI, et al: In vitro pancreatic hormonal pulses are less regular and more frequent than in vivo. Am J Physiol 260:E422–E429, 1991.
215. Stagner JI, Samols E, Weir GC: Sustained oscillations of insulin, glucagon and somatostatin from the isolated canine pancreas during exposure to a constant glucose concentration. J Clin Invest 65:939–942, 1980.
216. Bergstrom RW, Fujimoro WY, Teller DC, et al: Oscillatory insulin secretion in perfused isolated rat islets. Am J Physiol 257:E479–E485, 1989.
217. Safarik RH, Joy RM, Curry DL: Episodic release of insulin by rat pancreas: Effects of CNS and state of satiety. Am J Physiol 254:E384–E388, 1988.
218. Stagner J, Samols E: Comparison of insulin and glucagon pulsatile secretion between the rat and dog pancreas in vitro. Life Sci 43:929–934, 1988.
219. Sonnenberg GE, Hoffmann RG, Johnson CP, et al: Low and high frequency insulin secretion pulses in normal subjects and pancreas recipients: Role of extrinsic innervation. J Clin Invest 90:545–553, 1992.
220. O'Meara NM, Sturis J, Blackman JD, et al: Oscillatorv insulin secretion following pancreas transplant. Diabetes 42:855–861, 1993.
221. Bingley PJ, Matthews DR, Williams AJK, et al: Loss of regular oscillatory insulin secretion in islet cell antibody positive non-diabetic subjects. Diabetologia 35:32–38, 1992.
222. Matthews DR, Naylor BA, Jones RG, et al: Pulsatile insulin has greater hypoglycemic effect than continuous delivery. Diabetes 32:617, 1983.
223. Bratusch-Marrain PR, Komjati M, Waldhausl WK: Efficacy of pulsatile versus continuous insulin administration on hepatic glucose production and glucose utilization in type I diabetic humans. Diabetes 35:922, 1986.
224. Ward GM, Walters JM, Aitken PM, et al: Effects of prolonged pulsatile hyperinsulinemia in humans: Enhancement of insulin sensitivity. Diabetes 39:501, 1990.
225. Sturis J, Van Cauter E, Blackman JD, et al: Entrainment of pulsatile insulin secretion by oscillatory glucose infusion. J Clin Invest 87:439, 1991.
226. Sturis J, O'Meara NM, Shapiro ET, et al: Differential effects of glucose stimulation upon rapid pulses and ultradian oscillations of insulin secretion. J Clin Endocrinol Metab 76:895–901, 1993.
227. Olefsky JM, Faquhar JW, Reaven GM: Reappraisal of the role of insulin in hypertriglyceridemia. Am J Med 57:551, 1974.
228. Kissebah AH, Vydelingum N, Murray R, et al: Relation of body fat distribution to metabolic complications of obesity. J Clin Endocrinol Metab 54:254, 1982.
229. Peiris AN, Mueller RA, Smith GA, et al: Splanchnic insulin metabolism in obesity: Influence of body fat distribution. J Clin Invest 78:1648, 1986.
230. Meistas MT, Rendell M, Margolis S, et al: Estimation of the secretion rate of insulin from the urinary excretion rate of C-peptide: Study in obese and diabetic subjects. Diabetes 31:449, 1982.
231. Faber OK, Christensen K, Kehlet H: Decreased insulin removal contributes to hyperinsulinemia in obesity. J Clin Endocrinol Metab 53:618, 1981.
232. Savage PJ, Flock EV, Mako ME, et al: C-peptide and insulin in Pima Indians and Caucasians: Constant fractional hepatic extraction over a wide range of insulin concentrations and in obesity. J Clin Endocrinol Metab 48:594, 1979.
233. Rossell R, Gomis R, Casamitjana R, et al: Reduced hepatic insulin extraction in obesity: Relationship with plasma insulin levels. J Clin Endocrinol Metab 56:608, 1983.
234. DeFronzo RA: Glucose intolerance and aging: Evidence for tissue insensitivity to insulin. Diabetes 28:1095, 1979.
235. Palmer JP, Ensinck JW: Acute-phase insulin secretion and glucose tolerance in young and aged normal men and diabetic patients. J Clin Endocrinol Metab 41:498, 1975.
236. Shiraishi I, Iwamoto Y, Kuzuya T, et al: Hyperinsulinaemia in obesity is not accompanied by an increase in serum proinsulin/insulin molar ratio in groups of human subjects with and without glucose intolerance. Diabetologia 34:737–741, 1991.
237. O'Meara NM, Sturis J, Van Cauter E, et al: Abnormal temporal coupling of glucose and ultradian oscillations of insulin secretion in patients with non-insulin–dependent diabetes mellitus (NIDDM). J Clin Invest 92:262–271, 1993.
238. Davidson MB: The effect of aging on carbohydrate metabolism: A review of the English literature and a practical approach to the diagnosis of diabetes mellitus in the elderly. Metabolism 28:688, 1979.
239. Fink RI, Kolterman OG, Olefsky JM: The physiological significance of glucose intolerance of aging. J Gerontol 39:273, 1984.
240. Tonino RP: Effects of physiological training on the insulin resistance of aging. Am J Physiol 256:E352–E356, 1989.
241. Kahn SE, Larson VG, Beard JC, et al: Effect of exercise on insulin action, glucose intolerance and insulin secretion in aging. Am J Physiol 258:E937–E943, 1990.
242. Dudl RJ, Ensinck JW: Insulin and glucagon relationships during aging in man. Metabolism 26:33, 1977.
243. Schrender HB: Influence of age on insulin secretion and lipid mobilization after glucose stimulation. Isr J Med 8:832, 1972.
244. Crockford PM, Herbeck RJ, Williams RH: Influence of age on intravenous glucose tolerance and serum immunoreactive insulin. Lancet 1:465, 1966.
245. Barbagallo-Sangiori G, Laudicina E, Bompiani GD, et al: The pancreatic beta-cell response to intravenous administration of glucose in elderly subjects. J Geriatr Soc 18:529, 1970.
246. Chen M, Bergman RN, Pacini G, et al: Pathogenesis of age-related glucose intolerance in man: Insulin resistance and decreased β-cell function. J Clin Endocrinol Metab 60:13, 1985.
247. Gumbiner B, Polonsky KS, Beltz WF, et al: Effects of aging on insulin secretion. Diabetes 38:1549, 1989.
248. Kahn SE, Larson VG, Schwartz RS: Exercise training delineates the importance of β-cell dysfunction to the glucose intolerance of human aging. J Clin Endocrinol Metab 74:1336–1342, 1992.
249. Pfeifer MA, Halter JB, Porte D Jr: Insulin secretion in diabetes mellitus. Am J Med 70:579, 1981.
250. Carlstrom S, Ingemanson CA: Juvenile diabetes with long-standing remission. Diabetologia 3:465, 1967.
251. Weber B: Glucose-stimulated insulin secretion during "remission" of juvenile diabetes. Diabetologia 8:189, 1972.
252. Johansen K, Orskov H: Plasma insulin during remission in juvenile diabetes mellitus. BMJ 1:676, 1969.
253. Block MB: Sequential changes in beta-cell function in insulin-treated diabetic patients assessed by C-peptide immunoreactivity. N Engl J Med 288:1144, 1973.
254. Park BN, Soeldner JS, Gleason RE: Diabetes in remission: Insulin secretory dynamics. Diabetes 23:616, 1974.
255. Ludvigsson J, Heding LG: Beta-cell function in children with diabetes. Diabetes 27 (suppl 1):230, 1978.
256. Heding LG, Ludvigsson J, Kasperska-Czyzykowa T: β-Cell secretion in non-insulin and insulin-dependent-diabetics. Acta Med Scand 659:5, 1981.
257. Ludvigsson J, Heding LG: Abnormal proinsulin/C-peptide ration in juvenile diabetes. Acta Diabetol 19:351, 1982.
258. Snorgaard O, Hartling SG, Binder C: Proinsulin and C-peptide at onset and during 12 months of cyclosporin treatment of type I (insulin-dependent) diabetes mellitus. Diabetologia 33:36, 1990.
259. Rogers S, Silink M: Residual insulin secretion in insulin dependent diabetes mellitus. Arch Dis Child 60:200–203, 1985.

260. Sjoberg S, Gunnarsson R, Gjotterberg M, et al: Residual insulin production, glycemic control and prevalence of microvascular lesions and polyneuropathy in long-term Type I (insulin dependent) diabetes mellitus. Diabetologia 30:208–213, 1987.

261. Srikanta S, Ganda OP, Jackson RA, et al: Type I diabetes mellitus in monozygotic twins: Chronic progressive beta cell dysfunction. Ann Intern Med 99:320, 1983.

262. Ganda OP, Srikanta S, Brink SJ, et al: Differential sensitivity to β-cell secretagogues in "early" type I diabetes mellitus. Diabetes 33:516, 1984.

263. Garvey WT, Olefsky JM, Griffin J, et al: The effect of insulin treatment on insulin secretion and insulin action in type II diabetes mellitus. Diabetes 34:222, 1985.

264. Fener RE, Asworth RL, Tronier B, et al: Effects of short-term hyperglycemia on insulin secretion in normal humans. Am J Physiol 250:E655, 1986.

265. Nesher R, Della Casa I, Litvin Y, et al: Insulin deficiency and insulin resistance in type 2 (non–insulin-dependent) diabetes: quantitative contributions of pancreatic and peripheral responses to glucose homeostasis. Eur J Clin Invest 17:266, 1987.

266. Leahy JL, Weir GC: Evolution of abnormal insulin secretory responses during 48-h in vivo hyperglycemia. Diabetes 37:217, 1988.

267. O'Rahilly SP, Nugent Z, Rudenski AS, et al: Beta-cell dysfunction rather than insulin insensitivity is the primary defect in familial type 2 diabetics. Lancet 2:360, 1986.

268. Barnett AH, Spiliopoulos AJ, Pyke DA, et al: Metabolic studies in unaffected co-twins of non-insulin-dependent diabetes. BMJ 282:1656, 1981.

269. Barnett AH, Eff C, Leslie RDG, et al: Diabetes in identical twins: A study of 200 pairs. Diabetologia 20:87, 1981.

270. Kosaka K, Hagura R, Kuzuya T: Insulin responses in equivocal and definite diabetes with special reference to subjects who had mild glucose intolerance but later developed definite diabetes. Diabetes 26:944, 1977.

271. Kadowaki T, Miyake Y, Hagura R, et al: Risk factors for worsening to diabetes in subjects with impaired glucose tolerance. Diabetologia 26:44, 1984.

272. Efendic S, Luft R, Wajngot A: Aspects of the pathogenesis of type 2 diabetes. Endocr Rev 5:395, 1984.

273. Mitrakou A, Kelley D, Mokan M, et al: Role of suppression of glucose production and diminished early insulin release in impaired glucose tolerance. N Engl J Med 326:22–29, 1992.

274. Ward WK, Johnston CLW, Beard JC, et al: Insulin resistance and impaired insulin secretion in subjects with histories of gestational diabetes. Diabetes 34:861, 1985.

275. O'Sullivan JB: Body weight and subsequent diabetes mellitus. JAMA 248:949, 1982.

276. Temple RC, Carrington CA, Luzio SD, et al: Insulin deficiency in non–insulin-dependent diabetes. Lancet 1:293, 1989.

277. Yoshioka N, Kuzuva T, Matsuda A, et al: Serum proinsulin levels at fasting and after oral glucose load in patients with type 2 (non–insulin-dependent) diabetes mellitus. Diabetologia 31:355, 1988.

278. Temple RC, Clark PMS, Nagi DK, et al: Radioimmunoassay may overestimate insulin in non–insulin-dependent diabetics. Clin Endocrinol 32:689, 1990.

279. Nagi DK, Hendra TJ, Ryle AJ, et al: The relationships of concentrations of insulin, intact proinsulin and 32–33 split proinsulin with cardiovascular risk factors in type II (non-insulin-dependent) diabetic subjects. Diabetologia 33:532, 1990.

280. Polonsky KS, Given BD, Hirsch L, et al: Abnormal patterns of insulin secretion in non–insulin dependent diabetes. N Engl J Med 318:1231, 1988.

281. Garvey WT, Olefsky JM, Rubenstein AH, et al: Day-long integrated serum insulin and C-peptide profiles in patients with NIDDM: Correlation with urinary C-peptide excretion. Diabetes 37:590, 1988.

282. Liu G, Coulston A, Chen Y-D, et al: Does day-long absolute hypoinsulinemia characterize the patient with non–insulin-dependent diabetes mellitus? Metabolism 32:754, 1983.

283. O'Rahilly S, Turner RC, Matthews DR: Impaired pulsatile secretion of insulin in relatives of patients with non–insulin-dependent diabetes. N Engl J Med 318:1225, 1988.

284. O'Meara NM, Shapiro ET, Van Cauter E, et al: Effect of glyburide on beta cell responsiveness to glucose in non–insulin-dependent diabetes mellitus. Am J Med 89 (suppl 2A):11, 1990.

285. Turner RC, Holman RR: Beta cell function during insulin or chlorpropamide treatment of maturity-onset diabetes mellitus. Diabetes 27(suppl 1):241, 1978.

286. Kosaka K, Kuzuya T, Akanuma Y, et al: Increase in insulin response after treatment of overt maturity-onset diabetes is independent of the mode of treatment. Diabetologia 18:23, 1980.

287. Hidaka H, Nagulesparan M, Klimes I, et al: Improvement of insulin secretion but not insulin resistance after short-term control of plasma glucose in obese type II diabetics. J Clin Endocrinol Metab 54:217, 1982.

288. Karam JH, Sanz N, Salamon E, et al: Selective unresponsiveness of pancreatic β-cells to acute sulfonylurea stimulation during sulfonylurea therapy in NIDDM. Diabetes 35:1314, 1986.

289. Shapiro ET, Van Cauter E, Tillil H, et al: Glyburide enhances the responsiveness of the β-cell to glucose but does not correct the abnormal patterns of insulin secretion in non–insulin-dependent diabetes mellitus. J Clin Endocrinol Metab 69:571, 1989.

290. Osei K, Henry ML, O'Dorisio TM, et al: Physiological and pharmacological stimulation of pancreatic islet hormone secretion in type I diabetic pancreas allograft recipients. Diabetes 39:1235, 1990.

291. Ostman J, Bolinder J, Gunnarsson R, et al: Metabolic effects of pancreas transplantation: Effects of pancreas transplantation on metabolic and hormonal profiles in IDDM patients. Diabetes 38(suppl 1):88, 1989.

292. Sonnenberg GE, Hoffmann RG, Johnson CP, et al: Low- and high-frequency insulin secretion pulses in normal subjects and pancreas transplant recipients: Role of extrinsic innervation. J Clin Invest 90:545–553, 1992.

293. O'Meara NM, Sturis J, Blackman J, et al: Oscillatory insulin secretion following transplant. Diabetes 42:855–861, 1993.

294. Scharp DW, Lacy PE, Santiago JV, et al: Insulin independence after islet transplantation into type I diabetic patient. Diabetes 39:515–518, 1990.

295. Tzakis AG, Ricordi C, Alejandro R: Pancreatic islet transplantation after upper abdominal exenteration and liver replacement. Lancet 336:402–405, 1990.

296. Scharp DW, Lacy PE, Santiago JV: Results of our first nine intraportal islet allografts in type 1 insulin dependent diabetic patients. Transplantation 51:76–85, 1991.

297. Warnock GL, Kneteman NM, Ryan EA, et al: Long-term follow-up after transplantation of insulin producing pancreatic islets into patients with type 1 (insulin-dependent) diabetes mellitus. Diabetologia 35:85–95, 1992.

298. Pyzdrowski KL, Kendall DM, Halter JB, et al: Preserved insulin secretion and insulin independence in recipients of islet autografts. N Engl J Med 327:220–226, 1992.

299. Van Suylichem PTR, Strubbe JH, Houwing H, et al: Insulin secretion by rat islet isografts of a defined endocrine volume after transplantation to three different sites. Diabetologia 35:917–923, 1992.

300. Grunt JA, Pallotta JA, Soeldner JS: Blood sugar, serum insulin and free fatty acid relationships during intravenous tolbutamide testing in normal young adults and in patients with insulinoma. Diabetes 19:122, 1970.

301. Marks V: Progress report: Diagnosis of insulinoma. Gut 12:835, 1971.

302. Service FJ, Horwitz DL, Rubenstein AH, et al: C-peptide suppression test for insulinoma. J Lab Clin Med 90:180, 1977.

303. Alsever RN, Roberts JP, Gerbe JG, et al: Insulinoma with low circulating insulin levels: The diagnostic value of proinsulin measurements. Ann Intern Med 82:347, 1975.

Chapter 50

The Molecular Basis of Insulin Action

Morris F. White ▪ Martin G. Myers, Jr.

Appropriate storage and release of energy during states of feeding and fasting are essential for survival and are generally controlled by the action of insulin.[1] Insulin is secreted by β cells in the pancreatic islets of Langerhans in response to elevated blood glucose or certain amino acids during and after a meal. Insulin promotes the storage of glucose as glycogen in the liver and muscle, the storage of amino acids in muscle proteins, and the accumulation of triglycerides in adipose tissue (Fig. 50–1). Diabetes mellitus occurs when insulin fails to perform its physiologic function because of either an absolute lack of insulin (type 1) or a relative insulin insufficiency resulting from the inability of pancreatic β cells to overcome peripheral insulin resistance (type 2).[1] Although insulin was discovered over 75 years ago, the molecular mechanisms by which insulin acts are only now being revealed through a multidisciplinary approach including genetics, biochemistry, and cell and molecular biology.[2, 3] Understanding insulin

action and secretion will provide a molecular basis to develop rational treatments for type 1 and type 2 diabetes.

INSULIN AND INSULIN-LIKE GROWTH FACTORS

Members of the Insulin Signaling Family

The mammalian insulin signaling system includes three well-defined ligands, including insulin, insulin-like growth factor-1 (IGF-1), and IGF-2.[4] These factors bind the cell surface insulin receptors and the IGF-1 receptors (IGF1Rs) on target tissues (Fig. 50–2); a related receptor called the insulin receptor–related receptor (IRR) occurs in neuronal tissue, but its physiologic ligand is unknown.[5] Insulin binds

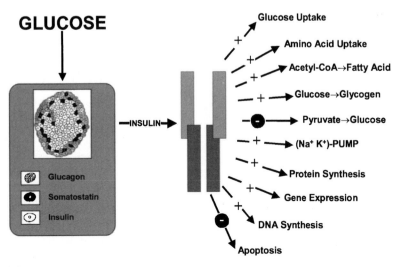

FIGURE 50–1. The role of insulin in physiology. Shown is the architecture of the islets of Langerhans. On the outside are the glucagon-producing α cells next to the somatostatin-producing δ cells. The innermost layer of cells and most of the islet mass consists of the insulin-producing β cells. Glucose (as well as other secretagogues) absorbed from the digestive system stimulates insulin secretion from the β cells. Insulin then circulates via the blood stream to end-organs expressing the insulin receptor (shown in cartoon form). Activation of the insulin receptor regulates a wide variety of processes in target tissues (+ stimulated by insulin; − inhibited by insulin).

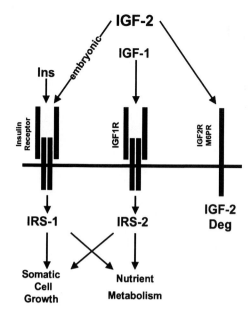

FIGURE 50–2. *The insulin (Ins)/insulin-like growth factor (IGF) family. The insulin/IGF family consists of three hormones: insulin, IGF-1, and IGF-2. These hormones bind three receptors: insulin receptor, IGF-1 receptor (IGF1R), and mannose 6-phosphate receptor (M6PR). The insulin receptor is the primary target for insulin throughout development and life. The IGF-1 receptor is the primary target for IGF-1. IGF-2 binds to the insulin receptor primarily during embryonic development and binds the IGF-1 receptor throughout life. IGF-2 also binds to the mannose 6-phosphate receptor, which targets IGF-2 for degradation instead of signaling. Activation of the insulin receptor or the IGF-1 receptor mediates signals primarily via the cytoplasmic proteins insulin receptor substrate-1 (IRS-1) and IRS-2, which mediate somatic cell growth and metabolism.*

with highest affinity to the insulin receptor (K_d between 0.1 and 1 nmol/L), whereas IGF-1 binds to the IGF1R. Insulin also binds to the IGF1R with low affinity, but this interaction may be irrelevant under ordinary physiologic conditions. Insulin or IGF-1 binding activates the tyrosine kinase on the intracellular portion of these receptors, which initiates a cascade of protein and lipid phosphorylation that regulates cellular responses (see Fig. 50–2). A tyrosine kinase–linked receptor that binds exclusively to IGF-2 has never been identified[6]; however, IGF-2 binds strongly to IGF1R and the type A insulin receptors that predominate during fetal development.[7, 8] IGF-2 also binds to the mannose 6-phosphate receptor, which mediates degradation of IGF-2 and reduces its growth signal.

The Relationship among Metabolism, Growth, and Survival

Members of the insulin receptor family occur throughout evolution and are essential for the development, growth, and survival of *Caenorhabditis elegans* (worms), *Drosophila melanogaster* (fruit flies), and vertebrates.[9, 10] In vertebrates, the insulin receptor has its greatest impact on carbohydrate metabolism and is highly expressed in liver, muscle, and adipose tissue; however, nearly all cells express insulin receptors and display detectable sensitivity to the hormone. IGF1Rs are also expressed in most tissues, where they regulate growth, and they might also regulate carbohydrate metabolism, especially in skeletal muscle.[11, 12] IGF1Rs are also essential for normal β cell development and expansion.[13] Interestingly, the insulin receptor itself also plays a role in insulin secretion.[14] The insulin-related receptor (IRR) is mainly expressed in neuronal tissue, where it might play a specialized role in development or survival.[5, 15] The IRR also occurs in pancreatic β cells, where it might play a role in insulin secretion.[16] Finally, IGF-2 is an important growth factor, especially during devel-

opment.[17] Genetic evidence suggests that the growth-promoting function of IGF-2 during mouse embryogenesis is mediated through the insulin and IGF1Rs.[7, 18]

The distinction between metabolic and growth actions of the receptors for insulin and IGF-1 in mammals is blurry. Although both receptors mediate growth in vitro, mice without insulin receptors are nearly normal size at birth but hyperinsulinemic; they die within 3 to 7 days because of hyperglycemia and ketoacidosis.[19, 20] By contrast, mice without IGF1R are only 45% of normal size at birth and develop slowly.[21] This growth deficit is largely rescued by disruption of the mannose 6-phosphate receptor, which increases the circulating levels of IGF-2 and promotes nearly normal growth through stimulation of the insulin receptor.[7, 18] Like mice, human neonates with diminished IGF-1 signaling are developmentally retarded; however, unlike mice, human infants born without insulin receptors display retarded development in utero together with severe fasting hyperglycemia at birth.[22] This developmental disparity might arise because insulin secretion develops just before birth in mice whereas insulin is involved in the entire last trimester of human pregnancies.[7]

THE INSULIN SIGNALING SYSTEM: AN OVERVIEW

The insulin receptor, like the receptors for other growth factors and cytokines, is composed of an extracellular ligand-binding domain that regulates the activity of an intracellular tyrosine kinase[23, 24] (see Fig. 50–3). During insulin binding, the intracellular tyrosine kinase is partly activated and several regions on the intracellular domain of the insulin receptor become tyrosine-phosphorylated.[25] This process, called autophosphorylation, further activates the tyrosine kinase and promotes the phosphorylation of cellular substrates that coordinate the insulin response.[26]

The principal insulin receptor substrate (IRS) proteins are phosphorylated on multiple tyrosine residues by the activated receptors for insulin and IGF-1.[27] IRS proteins recruit various downstream signaling proteins into a multicomponent complex through interaction between its tyrosine phosphorylation sites and the Src homology-2 (SH2) domains in various signaling proteins (SH2 proteins).[26] Binding of SH2 proteins to IRS proteins initiates cascades of signals that mediate the insulin response (see Fig. 50–2). Signaling proteins regulated by the IRS proteins include phosphatidylinositol 3-kinase (PI-3-kinase), growth factor receptor–binding protein-2 (Grb2), SH2-containing protein tyrosine phosphatase (SHP2), and others.[27]

PI-3-kinase plays a central role downstream of the IRS proteins in activation of a number of signaling cascades.[27] During association with IRS-1 or IRS-2, PI-3-kinase is activated and its phospholipid products promote recruitment to the plasma membrane and activation of various serine kinases. One of these, protein kinase B (PKB), activates additional kinases that regulate multiple biologic responses, including stimulation of glucose transport, protein and glycogen synthesis, and cellular proliferation and survival.[28, 29] In addition to the PI-3-kinase cascade, IRS-1 engages Grb2 to activate the mitogen-activated protein (MAP) kinase cascade.[30, 31] Binding of SHP2 generates a complicated response, including feedback inhibition by dephosphorylation of the IRS protein.[32] Finally, the insulin response is fine-tuned by the action of protein tyrosine phosphatases and various serine kinases on the insulin receptor and the IRS proteins.[33–35] When the relationship between these signaling pathways is disrupted, insulin resistance might result and contribute to the onset of glucose intolerance and ultimately diabetes.

THE INSULIN RECEPTOR

Insulin Receptor Structure

In its native conformation, the insulin receptor is a tetramer composed of two extracellular α subunits linked by disulfide bonds to each other and to the extracellular portion of a β subunit (Fig. 50–3, see also color plate); the β subunit contains a transmembrane domain

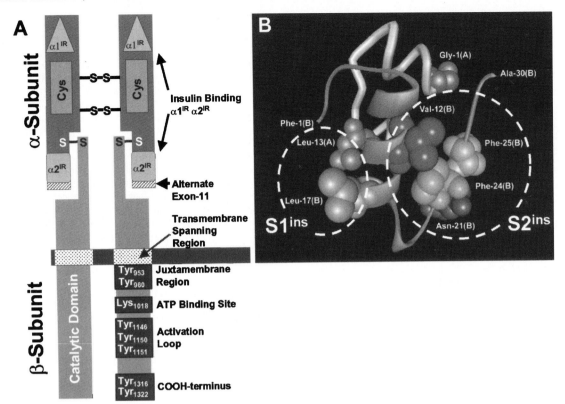

FIGURE 50–3. Structure of insulin and the insulin receptor. *A,* Insulin receptor functional domains. Shown is a cartoon of the insulin receptor with its functional domains. The mature insulin receptor consists of a heterotetramer of two extracellular α subunits linked to two β subunits that contain extracellular, transmembrane, and intracellular components. The holoreceptor is joined by disulfide bonds between cysteine residues in the extracellular α and β subunits, as well as by noncovalent interactions. The α subunit contains the insulin binding regions α1IR and α2IR in addition to a cysteine-rich region and a 12–amino acid alternatively spliced region encoded by exon 11. The β subunit contains a tyrosine kinase catalytic domain with an ATP-binding site and a number of tyrosine phosphorylation sites, including those in the juxtamembrane, activation loop, and COOH-terminal regions. *B,* Structure of insulin. Shown is a ribbon diagram of the mature insulin molecule in which the α chain is light in color and the β chain is dark. Also shown are the side chains of specific amino acids, which form the contact regions for the insulin receptor (S1ins and S2ins).

and an intracellular tail with tyrosine kinase activity.[25] The insulin proreceptor mRNA is the splice product of 22 exons of a 150-kb gene on human chromosome 19.[36, 37] The inclusion of exon 11 is regulated developmentally; the type A isoform of the insulin receptor includes exon 11, whereas the type B isoform lacks exon 11. The type A isoform predominates in most fetal tissues but is limited to the adult central nervous system and hematopoietic cells, whereas the type B isoform predominates in adult liver, muscle, and adipose tissue.[38–41]

Exon 11 encodes 12 amino acids at the end of the β subunit, which slightly reduces insulin-binding affinity and greatly increases IGF-2–binding affinity almost to the level of insulin.[8] The type B insulin receptor has a higher signaling capacity than does the type A receptor based on its greater insulin-stimulated tyrosine kinase activity and ability to phosphorylate IRS proteins in cultured cells.[42] Only the type A receptor mediates IGF-2 signaling. The proportion of type B receptors increases in some patients with type 2 diabetes, but how this increased ratio might contribute to diabetes is not clear.[38, 43]

The α and β subunits are obtained by proteolytic cleavage of the proreceptor chain after proper folding and disulfide bond formation. The holoreceptor ($\alpha_2\beta_2$) is heavily glycosylated on both the α and β subunits and has an apparent molecular weight of approximately 350,000 during sodium dodecyl sulfate–polyacrylamide gel electrophoresis (SDS-PAGE); after reduction of the disulfide bonds, the α and β subunits migrate during SDS-PAGE at 135 and 95 kDa, respectively.[44, 45] The α subunit binds insulin, whereas the intracellular portion of the β subunit contains the tyrosine kinase domain.[25]

Insulin Binds to the Extracellular Region of the Insulin Receptor

Insulin binding has been studied extensively before and after receptor purification from various cell and tissue backgrounds, but a defini-

tive molecular model explaining receptor binding is not yet available. The α subunit is too large to analyze by nuclear magnetic resonance, and crystallization is difficult, in part because of extensive glycosylation. From analysis of naturally occurring and site-directed mutants, structural inferences, and kinetic and isothermal binding data, the insulin molecule has at least two receptor-binding surfaces designated S1ins and S2ins.[46] Each surface interacts preferentially with one of two putative binding sites in each α subunit called α1IR and α2IR (see Fig. 50–3). S1ins binds to α1IR, which might orient S2ins toward the adjacent α subunit to promote binding between S2ins and α2IR. Together, both contacts result in higher-affinity insulin binding than either one achieves alone while altering the conformation of the unoccupied dimer to activate the intracellular tyrosine kinase by releasing it from constitutive inhibition (see Fig. 50–3). Binding of a second insulin molecule to the activated complex occurs at lower affinity resulting in the apparent negative cooperativity, possibly because only one of the contact sites is readily accessible on the α subunit.

The regions of the α subunit that create sites α1IR and α2IR have been identified provisionally by biochemical and genetic approaches. Mutation of 14 amino acid in four discontinuous segments of the N terminus of the insulin receptor α subunit provisionally reveals the location of α1IR. Residues 12 to 15 are critical for insulin binding by making contact points for S1ins; other regions of the N terminus also contribute, including residues 34 to 44, 64 to 67, and 89 to 91.[47] The creation of chimeric molecules between the α subunits of the insulin and IGF1Rs is especially informative.[48] High-affinity insulin binding is transferred to the IGF1R by substituting residues 64 to 137 of the insulin receptor α subunit into the homologous positions of the IGF1R α subunit, thus suggesting that residues 64 to 137 create an insulin-binding domain. Affinity labeling techniques reveal the putative location of α2IR in the C terminus of the α subunit between Thr704 and

Lys718.[49] Only 4 of the residues in this 14–amino acid region can be changed to alanine without reducing insulin binding. Based on the binding and selectivity of IR^A and IR^B, attachment of the 13 amino acids encoded by exon 11 to the end of the IR^B α subunit might destroy contact surfaces for IGF-2 while promoting interaction of S2^ins.

Insulin Binding Activates the Insulin Receptor Tyrosine Kinase

Insulin binding activates the tyrosine kinase located in the intracellular portion of the β subunit.[25] Generally, growth factors and cytokines mediate receptor activation by one of two mechanisms, including dimerization of monomeric receptors and conformational changes in predimerized receptors.[50–52] The dimerization of monomers is well illustrated by the binding of growth hormone to its receptor.[53, 54] For predimerized receptors, such as the receptors for erythropoietin and insulin, constraints placed on the intracellular domains by the unliganded extracellular domains prevent interaction between the intracellular tyrosine kinase domains.[25, 52, 55] Binding of the hormone must relieve this constraint and permit transphosphorylation and signal propagation.

Various experimental findings support the notion that the unliganded α subunit inhibits autophosphorylation of the insulin receptor β subunit.[25] Removal of a portion of the α subunit by incubation of cells with trypsin or by expression of a truncated mutant receptor produces a constitutively active kinase.[56] Thus, like insulin binding, removal of the insulin-binding domains releases the kinase from inhibition and promotes propagation of the insulin signal. Analysis of the trypsinized receptor by nonreducing SDS-PAGE reveals a catalytically active 116-kDa protein composed of an intact β subunit disulfide linked to a 25-kDa C-terminal fragment of the α subunit.[56, 57] The stability of the 25-kDa fragment suggests that it forms a domain of the α subunit. This domain contains four cysteine residues, at least one of which (Cys647) forms a covalent link to the β subunit[58] (see Fig. 50–3A). Substitution of Cys647 with serine disrupts the covalent link, but a noncovalent interaction persists between adjacent α and β subunits.[58] Insulin binds to this mutant receptor, but it fails to activate the kinase, which suggests that the insulin-induced conformational change in the β subunit requires a covalent link between the subunits.

Other point mutations in the α subunit constitutively activate the tyrosine kinase. One of them, Arg86→Pro86, is located in the high-affinity insulin-binding site (α1^IR). Arg82 might promote interactions between the adjacent α subunits, which stabilize the kinase in an inactive conformation, whereas insulin might destabilize this contact to activate the kinase. Certain mutations in the transmembrane spanning region also activate the tyrosine kinase. Substitution of the transmembrane segment in the β subunit with one from the oncogene v-*erb*B-2 that contains a Val664→Glu664 mutation activates the insulin receptor.[59] An analogous point mutation in the transmembrane segment of the insulin receptor (Val938→Asp938) also partially activates the receptor kinase.[60]

Because a strong case exists for activation of the insulin receptor by insulin-induced disruption of α subunit contacts, it seems possible to discover small molecules that could activate the insulin receptor through heterologous interactions residing outside the usual insulin-binding domain. One such recently described natural product opened the way for the rational development of small-molecule insulin mimetics that activate the tyrosine kinase by heterologous mechanisms not involving the usual insulin-binding site.[61]

Function of the Tyrosine Kinase Catalytic Domain

Insulin Receptor Autophosphorylation

The principal mechanism of insulin signaling involves stimulation of β subunit autophosphorylation, which leads to kinase activation and phosphorylation of substrate proteins.[25] Cloning of the insulin receptor and subsequent biochemical studies reveals several important elements, including a specific requirement for ATP, activation by tyrosine autophosphorylation, interactions with specific cellular substrates, and heterologous regulation by serine phosphorylation. The subsequent discovery of naturally occurring mutants without kinase activity and the rational design of in vitro kinase-deficient mutants revealed that insulin-stimulated tyrosine phosphorylation is absolutely essential for biologic activity.[62, 63] This consensus established the importance of tyrosine kinase activity for insulin signaling and anticipated the deleterious consequences of its reduction in humans.[64]

At least seven tyrosine autophosphorylation sites are located in three distinct regions of the insulin receptor β subunit, including two in the intracellular juxtamembrane region, three in the activation loop, and two in the C terminus[25] (see Fig. 50–3). Autophosphorylation of the tyrosine residues in the activation loop increases kinase activity[65–67]; activation may occur by lowering the Michaelis constant (K_m) for ATP.[68] By contrast, the biologic roles of autophosphorylation in the C terminus (Tyr1314 and Tyr1328) remain ambiguous inasmuch as they have been shown to variably regulate tyrosine kinase activity and receptor internalization.[69–73] Under certain conditions, however, the COOH sites might bind SH2 proteins.[74, 75] Autophosphorylation in the juxtamembrane region mediates substrate recognition and is critical for propagation of the insulin signal (see below). In particular, Tyr960 is located in an NPEY motif that binds to the phosphotyrosine-binding (PTB) domain in the IRS proteins and Shc.[76–79] The function of this region reveals the biologic importance of substrate phosphorylation and provided the impetus to purify and clone IRS-1.[80]

The Activation Loop

A central role for the activation loop of the β subunit is well supported by biochemical studies, mutational analysis, and the crystal structure of the β subunit.[66, 67, 81–83] In the purified insulin receptor, the activation loop is the initial region of insulin-stimulated tyrosine phosphorylation; the sequence of autophosphorylation events in intact cells remains difficult to establish but might begin in the juxtambrane region.[66, 84]

Structural studies predict that the unphosphorylated Tyr1162 of the activation loop folds into the catalytic site to prevent substrate binding.[85] A portion of the activation loop also restricts ATP binding in the catalytic site, thereby preventing autophosphorylation of the activation loop before insulin binds; this property may also contribute to the high apparent K_m for ATP before insulin stimulation.[68] The conformational change induced by insulin binding apparently facilitates ATP binding (decreasing the apparent K_m) and promotes autophosphorylation of Tyr1162 (Fig. 50–4, see also color plate). This model, together with early biochemical studies, suggests that the autophosphorylation cascade proceeds rapidly to Tyr1158 and results in a bis-phosphorylated regulatory loop. Although this activity mediates some activation of the kinase toward other substrates, the relatively slow phosphorylation of Tyr1163 to generate the tris-phosphorylated regulatory loop fully activates the kinase toward other substrates.[66] The activation loop undergoes a major conformational change upon tris-autophosphorylation in that it becomes fully removed from the catalytic site to allow unrestricted access by ATP and protein substrates (see Fig. 50–4). Although Tyr1162 and Tyr1158 are the first two sites phosphorylated, phosphorylation of Tyr1163 is critical because it stabilizes the open conformation.[83]

Upon tris-phosphorylation, at least two phosphotyrosine residues in the activation loop are completely exposed by solvent, creating sites for protein interaction (see Fig. 50–4). Several proteins have been found to interact with the regulatory loop. A region of IRS-2 called the kinase regulatory loop binding domain binds to the phosphorylated activation loop.[86, 87] These exposed phosphotyrosine residues may also interact with SH2 proteins that block access to the catalytic domain; a family of small SH2 proteins in the Grb10 family displays such properties.[88]

Substrate Selection

Substrate selectivity by protein kinases, including the insulin receptor, is a two-step process. First, a specific interaction between the

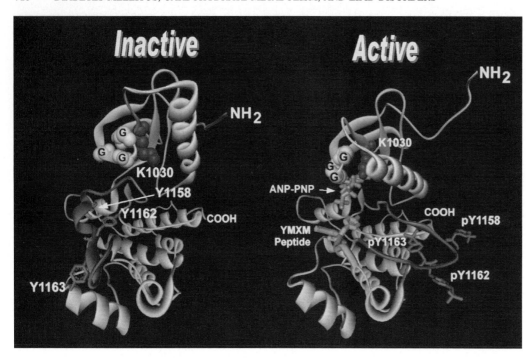

FIGURE 50–4. Structure of the insulin receptor activation loop. Shown are ribbon diagrams of the active site of the insulin receptor tyrosine kinase along with the side chains of important amino acids, including the three glycine residues and K1030 that form the ATP-binding site. The activation loop is shown in *darker gray;* the three activation loop tyrosine residues (Y1158, Y1162, and Y1163) are shown with their side chains. In the inactive, unphosphorylated state *(left panel),* the activation loop blocks access by potential substrates. After phosphorylation, however *(right panel),* the activation loop moves and thus allows substrates such as YMXM peptides (shown in *light gray)* to access the active site. ANP-PNP, nonhydrolyzable ATP analogue.

kinase and the substrate aligns potential substrate phosphorylation sites with the activated catalytic domain. Second, the catalytic domain selects and phosphorylates specific tyrosine residues according to their amino acid contexts. Although phosphorylation of the regulatory loop is important to open up the catalytic domain, phosphorylation of the NPEY motif in the juxtamembrane region is essential for substrate recruitment.[76] Indeed, the juxtamembrane region may compete with the activation loop for access to the catalytic site before insulin stimulation, which suggests that the juxtamembrane region might be phosphorylated before activation loop phosphorylation.[68] In intact cells at physiologic insulin concentrations, the juxtamembrane region appears to contain the first site of autophosphorylation.[84]

After substrate recruitment, the activated insulin receptor kinase phosphorylates tyrosine residues in the context of specific amino acid motifs, including the YMXM, YVNI, and YIDL motifs.[89–91] The structure of the activated β subunit reveals a mechanism by which the catalytic domain selects specific motifs for tyrosine phosphorylation.[83] Substrate peptides bind as short antiparallel β strands to the C-terminal end of the activation loop, thereby allowing hydrophobic residues in the Y + 1 and Y + 3 positions to occupy two small hydrophobic pockets on the C-terminal lobe of the kinase (see Fig. 50–4). Tyrosine residues lying within amino acid motifs that contain charged or bulky side chains at the Y + 1 and Y + 3 positions fit poorly in the kinase active site.[83] These two levels of selectivity ensure the specificity of the insulin and IGF1R.

INSULIN RECEPTOR SUBSTRATES COORDINATE INSULIN SIGNALING

The IRS Proteins

The insulin-stimulated signal transduction cascade depends on an orchestrated set of protein-protein interactions.[92] Although many receptors directly recruit SH2 domain–containing effector and adapter proteins to tyrosine phosphorylation sites in the receptor tail, the predominant signaling mechanism used by the insulin and IGF1Rs involves the recruitment of IRS docking proteins.[26]

The IRS proteins were initially identified as molecules that undergo rapid tyrosine phosphorylation in response to insulin and IGF-1. IRS-1, the prototype member of this family, provided the initial example of a cytoplasmic docking protein coupling an activated receptor tyrosine kinase to various signaling proteins.[80] In addition to IRS-1, the IRS protein family contains at least three other members (Fig. 50–5). IRS-2 was initially identified as a component of the interleukin-4 (IL-4) signaling pathway,[93] IRS-3 is predominantly expressed in adipose tissue,[94] and IRS-4 is expressed predominantly in the pituitary, thymus, and brain.[95] These proteins contain a highly conserved N-terminal pleckstrin homology (PH) domain, followed by a PTB domain, which together are thought to couple these proteins to the activated insulin–IGF-1 receptor.[96] The IRS proteins additionally contain 8 to 18 potential tyrosine phosphorylation sites, depending on the isoform species (see Fig. 50–5). Once tyrosine-phosphorylated, these residues bind and activate SH2-containing effector proteins, including the regulatory subunit of the lipid kinase PI-3-kinase, Grb2, nck, and SHP2. Of these, activation of PI-3-kinase has been implicated in the action of insulin on glucose transport, glycogen synthesis, protein synthesis, antilipolysis, and the control of hepatic gluconeogenesis via regulation of the expression of phosphoenolpyruvate carboxykinase.[97]

The PI-3-Kinase Cascade

PI-3-Kinase Signaling Proteins

The insulin receptor/IRS protein system (like other tyrosine kinase–based systems) recruits and activates type 1A PI-3-kinases.[98, 99] PI-3-kinases phosphorylate PI-4-phosphate and PI-4,5-bisphosphate on the 3′ position of the inositol ring to yield PI-3,4-bisphosphate (PI-3,4-P$_2$) and PI-3,4,5-trisphosphate (PI-3,4,5-P$_3$).[100] PI-3-kinases are heterodimers consisting of one of at least five regulatory subunits (p85α, p55α, p50α, p85β, and p55^{PIK}) and one of three catalytic subunits (p110α, p110β, and p110δ). The regulatory subunits are adapter proteins that contain two SH2 domains surrounding a p110-binding region (Fig. 50–6). Both SH2 domains in the regulatory subunit recognize similar tyrosine-phosphorylated YMXM motifs (Tyr-Met-Xaa-Met). Binding of the SH2 domains to these motifs links the PI-3-kinase holoenzyme directly to activated receptor kinases or to intermediate docking proteins such as IRS-1. Occupancy of both SH2 domains by phosphorylated YMXM motifs activates the PI-3-kinase enzyme and brings it to the membrane, where it has access to phospholipid substrates (PI-4-P, PI-4,5-P$_2$).[101, 102]

The role of the IRS protein/PI-3-kinase pathway in insulin signaling has been studied by a variety of approaches, including the use of inhibitors such as wortmannin and LY294002, as well as by the use of mutant PI-3-kinase or IRS proteins.[103] These approaches generally reveal that PI-3-kinase is critical for cell proliferation and survival

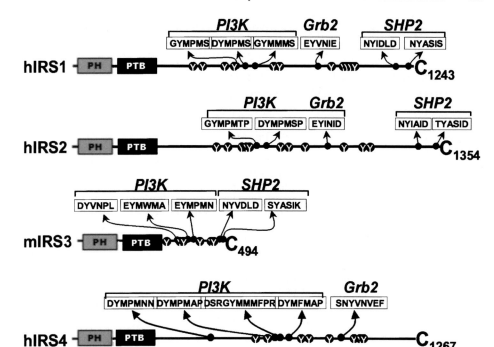

FIGURE 50-5. The insulin receptor substrate (IRS) proteins. Shown are schematic diagrams of the four known IRS proteins (the human sequence is shown for IRS-1, IRS-2, and IRS-4; because human IRS-3 has not been described, mouse IRS-3 is shown). Each of the IRS proteins contains N-teminal pleckstrin homology (PH) and phosphotyrosine-binding (PTB) domains. C-terminal to these domains are extensions of variable length remarkable for a number of conserved tyrosine phosphorylation sites. A number of these sites are shown along with the downstream signaling proteins that they are thought to recruit. Grb2, growth factor receptor–binding protein-2; PI3K, phosphatidylinositol 3-kinase; SHP2, SH2-containing tyrosine phosphatase-2.

during insulin/IGF-1 signaling and for various metabolic signals during insulin stimulation, including antilipolysis, glycogen synthesis, and glucose transport. However, other pathways may synergize with PI-3-kinase to maximally promote these responses.

Genetic Analysis of the PI-3-Kinase Cascade

Recently, *C. elegans* and *Drosophila* genetics revealed novel insight into the molecular mechanisms of insulin/IGF-1 action. These organisms contain an insulin/IGF-1 receptor orthologue that contains a 400–amino acid C terminus possessing some similarity to the C terminus of IRS-1.[9, 104, 105] Interestingly, the *C. elegans* genome does not contain an IRS protein orthologue, whereas *Drosophila* expresses an orthologue called *chico*.[106] The *Drosophila* system might represent an evolutionary hybrid in the transition between worms and vertebrates.[105, 107]

Analysis of the *C. elegans* insulin/IGF-1 receptor orthologue *daf-2* is instructive because many of its downstream elements closely resemble mammalian proteins, including Age-1, a class 1A PI-3-kinase orthologue.[105, 108] Furthermore, the *daf-16* gene, a forkhead transcription factor, lies further downstream in the pathway, which is inactivated by PKB-mediated phosphorylation.[105, 109, 110] These similarities led to the discovery that a number of homologous mammalian forkhead tran-

scription factors might function downstream of the IRS protein in mammalian cells.[29, 111–113] A number of genes controlled by this pathway have already been identified, including those important for the regulation of apoptosis and metabolism.

Regulation of the PI-3-Kinase Pathway by Phosphatidylinositol Phosphatases

The insulin-regulated PI-3-kinase pathway is also regulated by lipid phosphatases, including phosphatase and tensin homologue deleted on chromosome 10 (PTEN) and SH2-containing inositol phosphatase-2 (SHIP2). PTEN, originally identified as a tumor suppressor protein, dephosphorylates the 3′ position of PI polyphosphates, effectively antagonizing the production of PI-3,4-P_2 and PI-3,4,5-P_3 by the type 1 PI-3-kinase and functionally inhibiting insulin signaling.[114, 115] Indeed, the *C. elegans* PTEN homologue *daf-18* antagonizes the insulin receptor–like PI-3-kinase pathway.[116–118]

SHIP2, a 5′ phosphatase, also modifies insulin-stimulated PI phosphate production by catalyzing the conversion of PI-3,4,5-P_3 to PI-3,4-P_2.[119] Whereas the myeloid version of SHIP2 (SHIP) attenuates cytokine signaling, insulin stimulation recruits SHIP2[119–121]; it is thus unclear whether SHIP2 antagonizes insulin signaling by the PI-3-

FIGURE 50-6. Activation of the phosphatidylinositol 3-kinase (PI-3-kinase) signaling system by insulin. Activation of the insulin receptor leads to the recruitment of insulin receptor substrate-1 (IRS-1) and its tyrosine phosphorylation. Some of these tyrosine-phosphorylated sites are recognized by the Src homology-2 (SH2) domains of p85, the regulatory subunit of PI-3-kinase. p85 contains an SH3 domain and two SH2 domains; between the SH2 domains lies a binding site for p110, the PI-3-kinase catalytic subunit. Recruitment of this p85/p110 activates the enzyme and brings it to the membrane, where its substrate phosphatidylinositol-4-phosphate lies. The consequent generation of PI-3,4-P_2 creates binding sites for the pleckstrin homology (PH) domain of protein kinase B (PKB) and phosphoinositide-dependent kinase-1 (PDK1), which are recruited to the cell membrane; PDK1 thus phosphorylates and activates PKB. PKB in turn mediates protein synthesis, glucose transport, and cell survival. PTB, phosphotyrosine-binding domain.

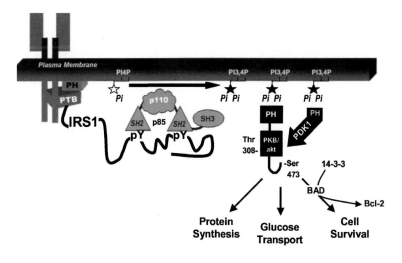

kinase pathway or whether it merely alters the response toward PI-3,4-P$_2$–dependent pathways.[122]

Protein Kinase Cascades Are Regulated by Phospholipid Products of PI-3-Kinase

Products of type 1A PI-3-kinase regulate a number of intracellular serine/threonine kinases, including PKB/Akt, protein kinase C-ζ (PKC-ζ), and p70 S6 kinase (p70^{S6k}).[103] PKB, the cellular homologue of the v-*Akt* oncogene, contains a PH domain that is highly specific for binding PI-3,4-P$_2$.[123, 124] Activation of PI-3-kinases by the insulin receptor/IRS protein pathway generates PI-3,4-P$_2$ (and PI-3,4,5-P$_3$) in the cell membranes (see Fig. 50–6). Binding of the PH domain to PI-3,4-P$_2$ recruits PKB to the plasma membrane, where it encounters the phospholipid-associated protein kinase, phosphoinositide-dependent kinase-1 (PDK1).[55, 108, 125–130] PDK1 contains a PH domain that binds to phospholipid products of PI-3-kinase, which mediates its association with membranes where it catalyzes the phosphorylation of Thr308 of PKB.[127, 128] Phosphorylation of Thr308 partially activates PKB, but full activation occurs after the phosphorylation of Ser473 by a second enzyme tentatively called PDK2.[55, 127] Mutation of the phosphorylation sites in PKB blocks activation and prevents some insulin/IGF-1–stimulated responses.[131]

Activated PKB mediates various metabolic effects of insulin and IGF-1 through the phosphorylation of a growing list of substrates that propagate the insulin/IGF-1 response, including glycogen synthase kinase-3 (GSK3), inducible NO synthase (iNOS), 6-phosphofructo-2-kinase (PFK2), cyclic adenosine monophosphate (cAMP) response element–binding protein (CREB), FKBP (FK506-binding protein)-rapamycin–associated protein (FRAP)/mammalian target of rapamycin (mTOR), forkhead transcription factors, caspase-9, and the proapoptotic Bcl-2 family member, BAD.[131–137] PKB phosphorylates and partially inactivates GSK3, which promotes glycogen synthesis.[138] Inactivation of GSK3 also mediates the effect of many growth factors by inhibiting the phosphorylation of a broad range of substrates, including several transcription factors and the eukaryotic translation initiation factor eIF2B[139] (Fig. 50–7). Phosphorylation of BAD by PKB links extracellular signaling events to the inhibition of apoptosis.[133, 140] During phosphorylation, BAD associates with 14-3-3, which prevents the formation of a pro-apoptotic heterodimer between BAD and Bcl-2/Bcx.[135, 141] Other targets of PKB also promote cell survival, including members of the forkhead family of transcription factors.[111, 142]

The PI-3-kinase cascade includes other serine kinases that mediate the insulin/IGF response, including p70^{s6k} and atypical isoforms of PKC, exemplified by the ζ or λ isoform.[143, 144] Activation of p70^{s6k} is complicated and involves several (PI-3-kinase–regulated) phosphorylation events, including those mediated by mTOR and possibly including PDK1/PDK2 and PKB[145–148] (see Fig. 50–7). p70^{s6k} is important for increasing the rate of translation of certain proteins involved in cell growth, such as myc and fos; however, it does not appear to play a role in carbohydrate metabolism. PKC-ζ and PKC-λ are insensitive to diacylglycerol or Ca^{2+} regulation and appear to be activated during association with PI-3,4-P$_2$ and/or PI-3,4,5-P$_3$; they are also, sensitive to phosphorylation mediated by other phospholipid-dependent proteins kinases, including PDK1.[149] PKC-ζ and PKC-λ might regulate protein synthesis and glucose metabolism in various systems.[150–153]

The p21^{ras} → ERK Cascade

A second critical cascade controlled by insulin is the p21^{ras} → ERK (extracellular signal–regulated kinase; also known as MAP kinase) pathway.[154] Like the PI-3-kinase–mediated pathways, the p21^{ras} → ERK kinase cascade is stimulated by many tyrosine kinases other than the insulin receptor family. One of the earliest recognized oncoproteins, p21^{ras} is a small guanosine triphosphate (GTP)-binding (G) protein. p21^{ras} and other small G proteins transmit signals when bound to GTP; hydrolysis of GTP by the p21^{ras} GTPase function terminates p21^{ras} signaling. The signaling function of p21^{ras} (i.e., the GTP vs. guanosine diphosphate [GDP]-bound state of p21^{ras}) is tightly regulated. GTPase-activating proteins (ras-GAPs) activate p21^{ras} GTPase and thereby result in the hydrolysis of GTP to GDP and deactivation of p21^{ras} signaling. Similarly, p21^{ras} guanine nucleotide exchange factors (ras-GNRFs) facilitate the release of inactivating GDP from p21^{ras} so that GTP binds and activates the signals. In certain cases, these regulatory proteins are coupled to tyrosine kinases through SH2 proteins.

Insulin receptors activate p21^{ras} by recruiting the adapter protein Grb2 (see Fig. 50–7). Grb2 contains two SH3 domains and an SH2 domain, which interacts with tyrosine-phosphorylated IRS proteins and Shc.[30, 31, 155] The second SH3 domain of GRB-2 associates with mammalian son of sevenless (mSOS), a ras-GNRF; thus recruitment of the Grb2/mSOS complex by IRS proteins or Shc results in the activation of p21^{ras} via mSOS-mediated nucleotide exchange.[156, 157] GTP-bound p21^{ras} transmits signals by associating with and activating serine/threonine kinases on the membrane. One such critical kinase is the cellular homologue of the v-*raf* oncogene, c-*raf*.[154] Activated c-raf phosphorylates and activates the MAP/ERK kinases MEK1 and MEK2. Activated MEKs, as their name suggests, phosphorylate and activate the ERK kinases ERK1 and ERK2 (also known as p42 and p44 MAP kinases). A number of alternative MAP kinase pathways are known (e.g., JNK [c-Jun N-terminal kinase] and SAPK [stress-activated protein kinase]), but upstream activation of these kinases does not appear to involve p21^{ras} and raf; a few reports suggest that these kinases may be regulated by insulin.[158]

Downstream of the activated ERK kinases lie a number of transcriptional events. Activated ERK kinases phosphorylate Elk-1, a transcription factor that mediates the expression of a number of immediate early genes, including c-fos.[154] Furthermore, ERK kinases phosphorylate and activate yet another serine kinase, pp90^{rsk}, which translocates to the nucleus and phosphorylates another set of transcription factors, including c-fos. Although the role of these p21^{ras} cascade events in insulin metabolic signaling remains unclear, each of these events is critical to the proliferative effects mediated by the insulin and IGF1Rs.

PROTEIN TRAFFICKING AND INSULIN SIGNALING

Insulin Receptors

Intracellular localization of signaling proteins is critical for the transmission of signals in many systems, so the location and movement of each component is carefully controlled. Before insulin binding, the insulin receptor associates with villous areas of the plasma membrane, possibly in association with microdomains known as caveolae.[159, 160] Whereas unstimulated insulin receptor is taken up into intracellular vesicles at a constant rate, insulin binding to the receptor initiates rapid internalization of the activated receptor.[72, 161, 162] Internalization involves tyrosine kinase–mediated dissociation of the receptor from the villous membrane, followed by association of the receptor with clathrin-coated pits.[163] Association of the insulin receptor with clathrin-coated pits might be mediated by Tyr953 and Tyr960 and by a Leu-Leu motif in the juxtamembrane region of the internal β subunit.[72, 164–166] Involvement of Tyr960 in this mechanism might antagonize signaling inasmuch as the NPEY960 motif binds to the PTB domain in the IRS proteins.

Internalization of the insulin receptor performs at least two distinct functions: first, rapid internalization of the insulin receptor to an internal membrane compartment during insulin stimulation allows rapid association with and tyrosine phosphorylation of the IRS proteins, which are associated with the internal membrane compartment.[159] Second, the internalized insulin receptor enters endosomes, which are acidified to induce dissociation of insulin from the activated insulin receptor to terminate the insulin signal.[167] A small percentage of these receptors might enter lysosomes and be degraded, but most appear to be recycled to the plasma membrane, where they are reactivated by insulin.

IRS Proteins

Unlike the insulin receptor, IRS proteins are soluble proteins. IRS-1 is usually found in the cytosol; however, its distribution between the

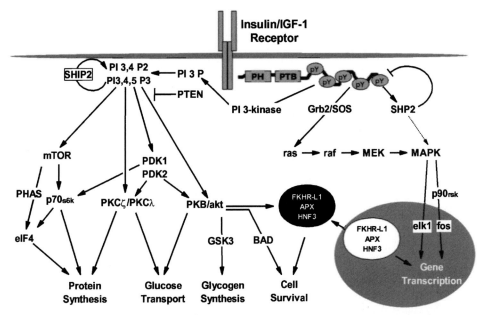

FIGURE 50–7. *The insulin receptor substrate (IRS) protein–dependent insulin/insulin-like growth factor-1 (IGF-1) signaling cascade. Activation of the receptors for insulin and IGF-1 results in tyrosine phosphorylation of the IRS proteins. The IRS proteins thereby bind phosphatidylinositol 3-kinase (PI-3-kinase), growth factor receptor–binding protein-2/son of sevenless (Grb2/SOS), and the SH2-containing tyrosine phosphatase (SHP2). The Grb2/SOS complex mediates the activation of p21^{ras}, thereby activating the ras→raf→mitogen-activated protein (MAP) kinase (MEK)→MAP kinase (MAPK) cascade. SHP2 feeds back to inhibit IRS protein phosphorylation by directly dephosphorylating the IRS protein and may transmit an independent signal to activate MAPK. Activated MAPK phosphorylates p90^{rsk}, which itself phosphorylates c-fos and increases its transcriptional activity. MAPK also phosphorylates the transcription factor, elk1 and increases its transcriptional activity. Activation of PI-3-kinase by IRS protein recruitment results in the generation of PI-3,4-P_2 and PI-3,4,5-P_3 (antagonized by the action of the inositol 3-phosphatase, PTEN). Insulin also activates the inositol 5-phosphatase, SHIP2 which converts PI-3,4,5-P_3 to PI-3,4-P_2. In aggregate, PI-3,4-P_2 and PI-3,4,5-P_3 activate a variety of downstream signaling kinases, including mammalian target of rapamycin (mTOR), which regulates protein synthesis via phosphorylated heat- and acid-stable protein regulated by insulin (PHAS)/p70^{s6k}/eukaryotic initiation factor-4 (eIF4). These lipids also activate alternate protein kinase C (PKC) isoforms and phosphoinositide-dependent kinase (PDK) isoforms. The PDKs activate protein kinase B (PKB), which appears to mediate glucose transport in concert with the atypical PKC isoforms. PKB also regulates glycogen synthase kinase-3 (GSK3), which may regulate glycogen synthesis, and a variety of regulators of cell survival. PKB-mediated of the pro-apoptotic factor, phosphorylation inhibits apoptosis, and phosphorylation of the forkhead proteins results in their sequestration in the cytoplasm, in effect inhibiting their transcriptional activity. HNF3, hepatocyte nuclear factor-3; PH, pleckstrin homology; PTB, phosphotyrosine-binding domain FKHR and APX, forkhead transcription factors.*

cytoplasm and membrane surfaces is readily detected in adipocytes.[159] The reason that IRS proteins are predominantly located in the cytoplasm is not clearly understood. Membrane association of the IRS proteins is critical for interactions with the insulin receptor, as well as for downstream signaling. The association might be mediated through interactions between the PH domain and membrane-associated elements, including phospholipids or acidic membrane proteins.[159, 168–170] Indeed, insulin stimulation rapidly leads to the redistribution of IRS proteins away from the membrane. The ability of IRS proteins to associate reversibly with the membrane is critical to their function: attachment of IRS proteins to the membrane enhances the transmission of certain downstream signals, such as activation of PKB and MAP kinase, but impairs biologic function, including the prevention of apoptosis.[104]

Glucose Transporters

Glucose and other sugars are absorbed into cells from the blood stream through the facilitated glucose transport (GLUT) proteins.[171] GLUT proteins form pores that recognize specific sugars and allow the polar sugar molecules to cross the lipid bilayer and diffuse down their concentration gradient into cells. GLUT1 is expressed in most cells and tissues and regulates so-called housekeeping glucose transport; it is especially highly expressed in liver. GLUT1 resides permanently on the plasma membrane and thus continually transports glucose between the extracellular space and the cell. By contrast, GLUT4 is predominantly expressed in skeletal muscle and adipose tissue. Before insulin stimulation, GLUT4 resides in intracellular vesicles and is unavailable to transport glucose across the plasma membrane.[172] However, insulin does not appreciably alter the activity of either

transporter. Nevertheless, insulin stimulation promotes translocation of GLUT4-containing vesicles to the plasma membrane to increase the rate of glucose influx. Although insulin does not stimulate translocation of GLUT1, chronic insulin treatment increases the levels of cellular GLUT1 via the p21^{ras} → ERK kinase pathway.[173, 174]

Unlike GLUT1, GLUT4 is largely sequestered in intracellular vesicles by sequences unique to its intracellular domains.[175–177] A dileucine motif in the C terminus of GLUT4 is required for its internalization and intracellular localization. Other sequences required for intracellular retention of GLUT4 are complex and poorly characterized. The mechanism coupling insulin signals to the movement of GLUT4 vesicles requires activation of PI-3-kinase by IRS proteins[103, 178]; however, subsequent steps are vague inasmuch as various serine kinases have been implicated, including PKB, PKC-λ, and PKC-ζ.[136, 179] Interestingly, muscle contraction/exercise stimulates GLUT4 translocation in muscle through an entirely independent mechanism that involves activation of the AMP-dependent protein kinase.[180, 181]

THE GENETIC, METABOLIC, AND COUNTERREGULATORY BASIS OF INSULIN RESISTANCE

The balance between peripheral insulin action and islet insulin production maintains normal carbohydrate metabolism throughout life. Mild to moderate insulin resistance is a common occurrence among human populations; given the association of insulin resistance with obesity, age, and physical inactivity, it is especially common in industrialized nations.[182] Increased insulin secretion from the pancreatic β cells usually compensates for this insulin resistance, but when compensation fails, type 2 diabetes occurs. A molecular basis of the imbalance between insulin action and insulin secretion in type 2 diabetes is difficult to establish. The search for molecular causes of type 2 diabetes has followed two directions: identification of gene mutations in family members with diabetes and investigation of mechanisms whereby the insulin signaling system is inhibited. So far, genetic approaches fail to explain the pathophysiology of the common forms of type 2 diabetes; however, they provide important insight into certain early-onset forms of type 2 diabetes (maturity-onset diabetes of youth), including defects in glucokinase and various transcription factors (hepatocyte nuclear factor-1α [HNF-1α], HNF-4α, islet/duodenum homeobox-1 [IDX-1]).[183–186] By contrast, dysfunctional regulation of the insulin signaling system may be a critical step in the progression to type 2 diabetes. Obesity contributes to insulin resistance and β cell dysfunction in type 2 diabetes in humans and in several important animal models of type 2 diabetes, but the mechanism by which these metabolic intermediates interact with and inhibit the insulin signaling pathways is not well understood. In molecular terms, the current search focuses on two mechanisms of inhibiting tyrosine kinase signals—serine phosphorylation of signaling intermediates and dephosphorylation of tyrosine residues on signaling intermediates.

The Insulin Signaling System and the Genetic Basis of Insulin Resistance

A monogenic defect underlying type 2 diabetes would provide the simplest explanation for this disease, and consequently, extensive efforts are under way to identify the "diabetes genes."[187] However, the failure to reveal single mutations responsible for type 2 diabetes suggests that a combination of multiple defects may be involved. Several years ago the insulin receptor was thought to be an ideal locus for linkage to type 2 diabetes. However, after exhaustive analysis, mutations at this locus are rarely observed, and insulin receptor mutations are not associated with type 2 diabetes.[64] A critical role played by the insulin/IGF-1 signaling system during development and fertility might strongly select against these mutations.

Similarly, analysis of gene sequences for the IRS proteins in diabetic populations does not provide a simple genetic basis for insulin resistance. Several polymorphisms in the gene for IRS-1 have been found, some of which are significantly more common in type 2 diabetic patients.[92] The well-characterized Gly972→Arg mutation may moderately decrease insulin-stimulated PI-3-kinase activation in cultured cells.[169, 188] When data from all available studies are pooled, the Gly972→Arg variant might contribute to insulin resistance, although alone it is clearly insufficient to cause diabetes, especially because deletion of the *Irs-1* gene in mice is not diabetogenic.

Two polymorphisms in *Irs-2* were described in a white population, including Gly1057→Asp and Gly879→Ser substitutions; however, neither mutation is associated with diabetes.[189] Similarly, polymorphisms in the human *IRS-4* gene are not associated with diabetes.[190] By contrast, a common polymorphism in p85α is associated with moderately reduced insulin sensitivity during an intravenous glucose tolerance test, but it is not associated with diabetes.[191] Thus genetic defects in the insulin signaling system may partially compromise certain aspects of insulin action in some patients and might contribute to diabetes when β cell compensation fails.

Insulin Resistance in Obesity

The relationship between obesity and insulin resistance and type 2 diabetes is well known, and considerable evidence indicates that insulin signaling is impaired in obese and insulin-resistant humans and rodents.[192, 193] Recent hypotheses explaining obesity-induced diabetes are based on the idea that adipose tissues produce cytokines that might mediate systemic insulin resistance and β cell dysfunction, including leptin and tumor necrosis factor-β (TNF-β).[33, 194–198]

Leptin correlates closely with fasting insulin concentrations and the percentage of body fat, thus making leptin a marker of obesity and insulin resistance.[195] Leptin binding to the long form (LRb) of the leptin receptor activates the Janus kinase-2 (JAK2) tyrosine kinase, which is tightly associated with the cytoplasmic domain of the LRb, the resulting tyrosine phosphorylation of the LRb intracellular tail and JAK2 transmits downstream signals by recruiting SH2 proteins.[199] By this mechanism, LRb activates STAT3 (signal transducer and activator of transcription-3). LRb also promotes activation of the ERK kinases.[200] Leptin might influence β cell physiology by reducing insulin secretion.[201] Thus leptin signaling might provide a rational basis to link obesity to the disruption of β cell function at the molecular level.

TNF-α is an endogenous cytokine produced by macrophages and lymphocytes after inflammatory stimulation. Adipocytes of obese animals and humans overexpress TNF-α in a positive correlation with body mass index and hyperinsulinemia; weight reduction decreases TNF-α expression.[202, 203] Expression of TNF-α by adipose tissue has little effect on systemic TNF-α concentrations, but the concentration of free and membrane-bound TNF-α surrounding adipose tissue is likely to be increased in obesity. TNF-α treatment increases serine phosphorylation of IRS proteins, which inhibits insulin-stimulated tyrosine phosphorylation and impairs insulin signaling.[198, 204, 205] Disruption of both TNF-α receptor isoforms improves insulin sensitivity.[206] Interestingly, troglitazone reduces the ability of TNF-α to cause insulin resistance and thus provides a rational mechanism by which thiazolidinediones might enhance insulin action.[207] Thus localized production of TNF-α might link obesity to insulin resistance (Fig. 50–8).

Heterologous Regulation of the Insulin Signaling System by Serine Phosphorylation

The insulin signaling system is regulated in many ways, including degradation or differential expression of signaling proteins, as well as modification by phosphorylation. Increased serine kinase activity toward the insulin receptor and IRS proteins occurs in type 2 diabetes and insulin resistance.[92] The inhibitory effect of PKC-mediated serine phosphorylation on insulin receptor tyrosine phosphorylation was initially recognized in hepatoma cells.[208] Direct inhibition of insulin receptor function by activated PKC varies considerably between cell background; consequently, the regulatory phosphorylation sites involved are poorly characterized.[209–212] IRS proteins might promote the inhibitory effect of several PKC isoforms on insulin-stimulated tyrosine phosphorylation of the insulin receptor.[213]

IRS-1 and IRS-2 each contain more than 30 serine/threonine residues in consensus sequences for many serine/threonine kinases, including casein kinase II, cAMP-dependent protein kinase, PKC, cdc2 kinase, MAP kinase, and Akt/PKB.[80, 93] Many agents that stimulated serine kinases, including phorbol esters, platelet-derived growth factor, okadaic acid, TNF-α, IL-1α and IL-1β, hyperglycemia, and prolonged insulin stimulation, induce insulin resistance at least partially by decreasing insulin-stimulated tyrosine phosphorylation of the insulin receptor and the IRS proteins (see Fig. 50–8). This serine/threonine phosphorylation in turn impairs insulin-induced tyrosine phosphorylation of IRS proteins, PI-3-kinase activation, and glucose uptake.[198, 205, 214–219] Serine phosphorylation might inhibit IRS protein signaling by impairing its interaction with the activated insulin receptor or by blocking recognition of specific tyrosine phosphorylation sites by the receptor catalytic domain.[216, 218, 220–222]

The Relationship between Insulin Signaling and Metabolism

A relationship between insulin resistance and hyperlipidemia and/or hyperglycemia has been recognized for many years, but the underlying molecular mechanism by which these factors affect the insulin signaling system is not well understood. Insulin receptor tyrosine kinase activity is reduced in rat hepatoma cells incubated in a fatty acid–rich medium when compared with cells grown in normal medium.[223] Moreover, acute elevation in plasma free fatty acid levels induces insulin resistance in rats, which is associated with reduced tyrosine phosphorylation of IRS-1 and insulin-stimulated PI-3-kinase activity.[224]

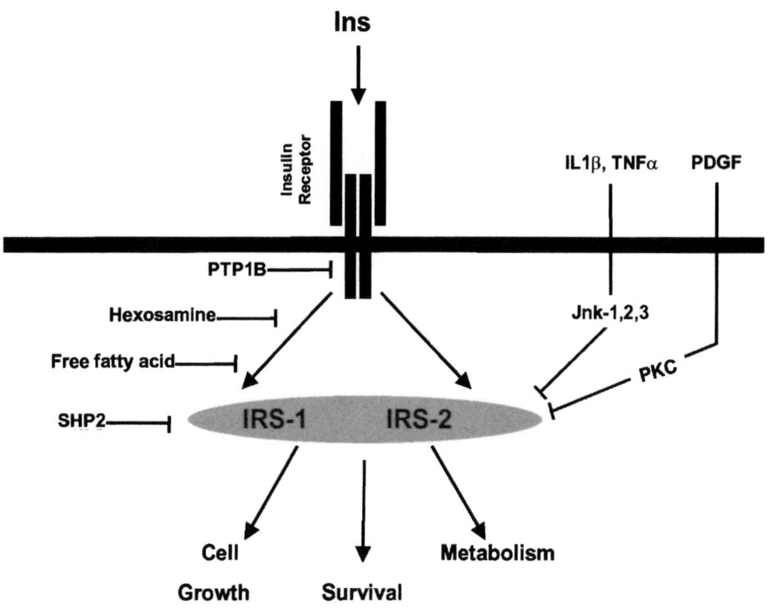

FIGURE 50–8. *Inhibition of the insulin signal. Shown is a cartoon of the early steps in insulin signaling along with negative regulators of these signals. Insulin binding to the receptor activates the insulin receptor tyrosine kinase, which tyrosine-phosphorylates insulin receptor substrate-1 (IRS-1) and IRS-2 and thereby results in the regulation of cell growth, metabolism, and survival. The phosphotyrosine-binding phosphatases PTP1B and SHP2 dephosphorylate the insulin receptor and IRS-1, respectively. The early tyrosine phosphorylation events in insulin signaling are also repressed by metabolites such as hexosamine and free fatty acids, as well as by serine phosphorylation events. Interleukin-1β (IL1β) and tumor necrosis factor-α (TNFα) mediate inhibitory serine phosphorylation events on IRS proteins via the Jnk (c-Jun N-terminal kinase) kinases; protein kinase C (PKC) mediated serine phosphorylation may also inhibit signaling. PDGF, platelet-derived growth factor.*

Infusion of free fatty acids into rats or elevation of muscle triglyceride and long-chain acyl coenzyme A content may activate PKC isoforms, thereby promoting serine phosphorylation of IRS-1 (and potentially IRS-2) and inhibiting activation of the PI-3-kinase cascade during the insulin response.[225, 226]

Chronic hyperglycemia might be related to insulin resistance and β cell failure through the hexosamine pathway. Under ordinary conditions, a portion of intracellular glucose is enzymatically converted to glucosamine, which is used in the posttranslational modification of glycoproteins.[227] Increased flux through this pathway (as in hyperglycemia) increases tissue concentration of uridine diphosphate N-acetylglucosamine (UDP-GlcNAc), which correlates closely with the observed induction of insulin resistance.[227–229] Glucosamine infusion for 2 to 6 hours decreases insulin signaling in a manner that parallels the decrease in insulin-stimulated glucose uptake in skeletal muscle.[230] Elevated levels of UDP-GlcNAc might also cause adventitious *O*-linked glycosylation of serine or threonine phosphorylation sites in certain transcription factors or signaling proteins of the insulin cascade and consequently lead to inhibition of function.[227, 231, 232]

Phosphotyrosine Phosphatases

Soon after it was clear that tyrosine-specific kinases control metabolism and proliferation, the search for phosphotyrosine phosphatases (PTPases) was initiated.[233, 234] Total membrane-bound tyrosine phosphatase activity is increased in the skeletal muscle of type 2 diabetic patients, thus suggesting that PTPase activity might contribute to insulin resistance.[235] Moreover, increased insulin sensitivity associated with weight loss is linked with reduced PTPase activity in adipose tissue.[236] Dozens of such PTPases are known, and overexpression of various PTPases in cells decreases tyrosine phosphorylation and signaling by the insulin receptor and other receptor tyrosine kinases.[237] Phosphatases are rational targets for antidiabetes drugs, but the identification of insulin receptor–specific phosphatases and their specific inhibitors remains difficult.

PTP1B, which was originally cloned from placenta, is the prototype PTPase.[233] PTP1B not only decreases insulin signaling when overexpressed but also associates with the insulin receptor in intact cells, which suggests that it might downregulate the insulin signal in vivo (see Fig. 50–8). Many strategies have been used to design inhibitors for PTP1B, but so far only low-affinity compounds have been reported.[238] Inhibition of PTP1B expressed in adipose cells with phosphotyrosyl-mimetic peptides restores insulin-stimulated glucose uptake.[207] Recently, targeted disruption of PTP1B in mice was shown to increase insulin sensitivity and reduce weight gain because of overeat-

ing without causing undesirable side effects.[35] Thus inhibition of PTP1B is an attractive target for drugs designed to enhance insulin signaling.

SHP2, a cytoplasmic PTPase that contains two SH2 domains, associates with a number of proteins during insulin signaling. The two SH2 domains of SHP2 bind to a pair of tyrosine phosphorylation sites in the tail of IRS-1 during insulin signaling; this interaction activates SHP2 PTPase and results in dephosphorylation of IRS-1, which reduces the ability of IRS-1 to bind PI-3-kinase and mediate certain downstream insulin signals.[239] Mutations in the tail of IRS-1 that eliminate the binding and activation of SHP2 during insulin stimulation increase PI-3-kinase binding and insulin responses promoted by the PI-3-kinase cascade.[32] However, inhibition of SHP2 interferes with the activation of ERK kinases by insulin, which suggests that SHP2 may mediate positive signals or eliminate competitive inhibitory signals.[240] Thus the mechanism linking SHP2 to MAP kinase activation might be complicated and involve the SHP2 family of proteins (known as SHPS or SIRP proteins), which become tyrosine-phosphorylated in response to insulin and bind SHP2.[241]

IRS PROTEINS COORDINATE INSULIN ACTION AND SECRETION

The Role of the Insulin Receptor in Target Tissues

Since the discovery of the insulin receptor and its tyrosine kinase function, we have learned an enormous amount about how insulin functions to transmit intracellular signals and alter cellular metabolism; however, our efforts to integrate molecular knowledge with physiology have been difficult until recently. Valuable data have been derived from humans with natural mutations in signaling molecules such as the insulin receptor. The development of genetically altered mice provides a level of experimental control not previously possible.

Data from human patients with rare mutations in the insulin receptor demonstrated that the insulin receptor mediates critical growth and metabolic signals. These defects impair receptor synthesis, translocation to the plasma membrane surface, insulin binding, transmembrane signaling, and endocytosis.[242] Depending on the allele, severe syndromes of insulin resistance with altered growth, such as leprechaunism or Rabson-Mendenhall syndrome, develop in homozygous or double-heterozygous individuals.[243, 244] Most affected individuals are heterozygous and display severe type A insulin resistance accompanied by polycystic ovarian syndrome and acanthosis nigricans.[242] Interestingly, patients with severe insulin resistance are hyperinsulinemic and possibly glucose intolerant, but not hyperglycemic or diabetic. Thus insulin resistance alone is insufficient to cause diabetes while β cells secrete sufficient insulin to compensate for the resistance, whereas the development of diabetes requires a concomitant defect in insulin secretion. Of course, most of these patients retain some insulin receptor function; complete insulin resistance in the absence of any insulin receptor yields diabetes.

Genetically altered mice reinforce these notions and provide insight into how and where defects in insulin sensitivity and secretion occur. Homozygous disruption of the insulin receptor in mice is lethal (IR$^{-/-}$).[19] Although IR$^{-/-}$ mice undergo relatively normal intrauterine development, they become hyperinsulinemic, hyperglycemic, and ketoacidotic shortly after birth and die during the first few days of life. Thus like humans with homozygous mutations in the insulin receptor, mice that are completely resistant to the effects of insulin exhibit features of diabetes.

In vivo glucose disposal data from humans suggest that muscle is responsible for the vast majority of glucose disposal in the body and that glucose uptake by muscle is critical for glucose homeostasis.[245–247] The partial insulin resistance in type 2 diabetes has long been thought to be predominantly a defect in muscle insulin signaling.[246] By contrast, mice lacking the insulin receptor in skeletal muscle maintain normal glucose homeostasis, and hyperinsulinemia or physiologic insulin resistance never develops.[248] Deletion of the insulin receptor from muscle decreases biochemical insulin signals (e.g., tyrosine phosphorylation of IRS proteins) by greater than 95% and markedly attenuates insulin-stimulated glucose transport in isolated muscle. However, this degree of insulin resistance does not appreciably alter glucose homeostasis in mice and is not sufficient for progression to diabetes.

Perhaps exercise-induced glucose utilization predominates in rodents and masks the insulin-regulated portion. Indeed, genetically altered mice deficient in GLUT4 in skeletal muscle demonstrate insulin resistance and glucose intolerance not observed in mice lacking the insulin receptor in skeletal muscle.[249, 250] Glucose uptake by muscle is impaired in patients with type 2 diabetes, which suggests that muscle glucose transport is clearly important for glucose homeostasis. However, the contraction/exercise-stimulated component of glucose uptake might dominate over the insulin-stimulated component. This hypothesis is consistent with the dramatic improvement in glucose tolerance observed after exercise in animals and humans with type 2 diabetes and fits well with the notion that insulin promotes glucose homeostasis by its action in the liver.

Humans and classic animal models with type 2 diabetes syndromes display relative insulin resistance, unlike the absolute insulin resistance in animals entirely lacking the insulin receptor in certain tissues. Thus in humans and classic animal models, progression to hyperglycemia requires not only the development of insulin resistance but also impairment of the ability of β cells to produce enough insulin to overcome the resistance. Mice with β cell–specific deletion of the insulin receptor display a loss of first-phase insulin secretion in response to glucose, but not arginine.[14] This loss of secretion resembles the defect in insulin secretion observed in humans with type 2 diabetes, which is thought to be one of the earliest abnormalities in glucose homeostasis in these patients.[192] Furthermore, these mice show a progressive loss in glucose tolerance over a 6-month period. Thus although the exact molecular mechanisms and significance of insulin receptor function on insulin release in these animals remain to be elucidated, their impairment may contribute to the onset of type 2 diabetes.

The Role of IRS Proteins in Carbohydrate Metabolism and Diabetes

Deletion of IRS-1 causes a surprisingly mild metabolic phenotype: insulin resistance but essentially normal glucose homeostasis.[251, 252] However, the marked growth retardation found in these animals suggests that IRS-1 is an important mediator of IGF-1 signaling in both prenatal and postnatal somatic growth in mice. This outcome is similar to the finding in *Drosophila*, in which mutation of the IRS protein–like gene (*chico*) produces flies that have small cells, small organs, and small overall size.[253]

Studies have investigated insulin responses in various tissues of the IRS-1$^{-/-}$ mouse to determine the nature of any compensatory signaling. Muscle from IRS-1$^{-/-}$ mice retains only a 20% response to insulin in both metabolic and signaling parameters in vitro (including glucose transport, protein synthesis, PI-3-kinase and MAP kinase activation, among others).[252] Insulin signaling is not as severely reduced in the liver, perhaps because of increased IRS-2 tyrosine phosphorylation.[254, 255] The combined defects in insulin signaling in muscle, adipose tissue, and liver trigger insulin resistance in these mice, but diabetes never develops because of lifelong compensatory hyperinsulinemia. Indeed, IRS-1$^{-/-}$ mice display increased β cell mass. Upon additional insulin resistance achieved by compound heterozygous disruption of the insulin receptor gene, mice display more severe insulin resistance, and diabetes with hyperinsulinemia develops in about one-quarter.[248]

Disruption of IRS-2 in mice results in defects in insulin action and insulin secretion that result in a syndrome similar to human type 2 diabetes.[255] Young IRS-2$^{-/-}$ animals have hyperglycemia and impaired glucose tolerance, as well as peripheral insulin resistance (threefold increase in fasting insulin levels) and a reduced hypoglycemic response during an insulin tolerance test. In hyperinsulinemic euglycemic clamp

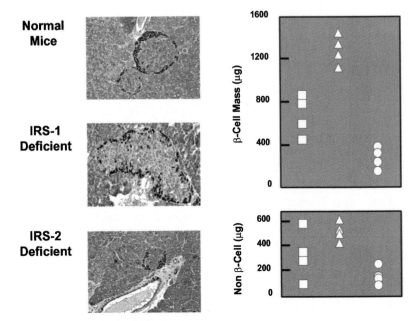

FIGURE 50–9. Impact of insulin receptor substrate (IRS) protein deletion on pancreatic islets. Shown are representative pancreatic islet sections from normal, IRS-1$^{-/-}$, and IRS-2$^{-/-}$ mice, along with quantitation of β cell and non–β cell mass. IRS-1$^{-/-}$ mice, which display insulin resistance and hyperinsulinemia, have greatly increased islet size and β cell mass, whereas IRS-2$^{-/-}$ mice, which have mild insulin resistance and inappropriately low insulin levels, demonstrate decreased islet size and β cell mass.

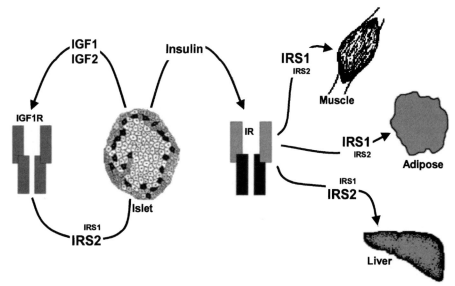

FIGURE 50–10. Model of the relative importance of insulin receptor substrate-1 (IRS-1)/IRS-2 and insulin/insulin-like growth factor (IGF) signaling in mammalian physiology. IGF-1 receptors (IGF1Rs) in the pancreatic islets are critical for islet and β cell growth and survival. IRS-2 is critical for this IGF effect in the islets. Insulin released by the β cells of the islets mediates metabolic signaling in peripheral target tissues such as muscle, adipose, and liver. IRS-1 is relatively more important in mediating the insulin signal in muscle and adipose tissue, whereas IRS-2 signaling dominates in the liver.

studies, these animals have reduced insulin-stimulated whole body glucose disposal and a severe reduction in insulin suppression of hepatic glucose production. Recently we have shown that the defects in insulin-stimulated glucose transport in isolated skeletal muscle and fat are initially mild, thus suggesting that IRS-2 plays a minor role in these tissues or that IRS-1 compensates adequately.[181] However, when diabetes occurs, muscle and fat acquire insulin resistance, but it is unknown whether the resistance is a consequence of hyperglycemia or a long-term result of IRS-2 deficiency.

These data are consistent with the hypothesis that abnormalities in hepatic carbohydrate metabolism constitute the major defect underlying the development of physiologically relevant insulin resistance and suggest that IRS-2–dependent signaling pathways are required for insulin action in hepatocytes.[256] Indeed, recent evidence from insulin receptor–deficient hepatocyte cell lines suggests that IRS-2 mediates most of the metabolic effects of insulin in the liver: the absence of insulin receptors selectively reduces IRS-2 but not IRS-1 phosphorylation and is associated with a failure of insulin to enhance glycogen synthesis and suppress glucose production.

IRS-2 Promotes β Cell Function and Coordinates Nutrient Homeostasis

Although resistance to the action of insulin is important in the early stages of the development of type 2 diabetes, failure of adequate β cell compensation is required for progression to the diabetic state. The hyperglycemia and frank diabetes of IRS-2$^{-/-}$ mice suggest that IRS-2 is critical for proper β cell function. Indeed, young IRS-2$^{-/-}$ mice, before the onset of hyperglycemia, display a 50% reduction in β cell mass when compared with wild-type mice.[255] As these mice age, β cell mass decreases further, almost certainly contributing to the onset of diabetes.[13, 255]

The phenotype of the IRS-2$^{-/-}$ mouse clearly demonstrates that IRS-2 is critical in generating and/or maintaining β cell mass (Fig. 50–9). Thus IRS-2–dependent signals must control either replication of preexisting β cells, the process of neogenesis from islet precursor cells in the pancreatic ductal epithelium, or β cell survival. IRS-2 may play a critical role in mediating insulin secretion as well, although little is currently known about how such mediation may occur. Even though a hierarchy of transcription factors have been implicated in cell development, differentiation, and function, the extracellular factors and intracellular signals underlying these responses are largely unknown.[257] Although both IRS-1 and IRS-2 are expressed in β cells, IRS-2 is the critical signaling element.

The critical role of IRS-2 in the regulation of hepatic carbohydrate metabolism and the appropriate β cell response to insulin resistance

indicates that this molecule and its downstream effector pathways are the central regulatory elements in glucose metabolism. Thus the role of IRS-2 in both peripheral tissues and the β cell provides an elegant model of an integrated mechanism for the regulation of whole body fuel homeostasis (Fig. 50–10). The different physiologic roles of IRS-1 and IRS-2 suggest the existence of critical differences in the signals transmitted by these two proteins that we do not yet understand. They also provide insight into the regulation of glucose homeostasis and the pathogenesis of type 2 diabetes, as well as the role of insulin signaling pathways in β cell function.

REFERENCES

1. Kahn CR: An introduction to type II diabetes. Curr Opin Endocrinol Diabetes 2:283–284, 1995.
2. White MF: The IRS-signalling system: A network of docking proteins that mediate insulin action. Mol Cell Biochem 182:3–11, 1998.
3. Withers DJ, White MF: Insulin action and type 2 diabetes: Lessons from knockout mice. Curr Opin Endocrinol Diabetes 6:141–145, 1999.
4. Roth J, Kahn CR, De Meyts P, et al: Receptors for insulin and other peptide hormones in disease states. *In* Bajaj JS (ed): Insulin and Metabolism. Amsterdam, Excerpta Medica, 1977, pp 73–80.
5. Zhang B, Roth RA: The insulin receptor–related receptor: Tissue expression, ligand binding specificity, and signaling capabilities. J Biol Chem 267:18320–18328, 1992.
6. LeRoith D, Werner H, Beitner-Johnson D, Roberts C: Molecular and cellular aspects of the insulin-like growth factor I receptor. Endocr Rev 16:143–163, 1995.
7. Louvi A, Accili D, Efstratiadis A: Growth-promoting interaction of IGF-II with the insulin receptor during mouse embryonic development. Dev Biol 189:33–48, 1997.
8. Frasca F, Pandini G, Scalia P, et al: Insulin receptor isoform A, a newly recognized, high-affinity insulin-like growth factor II receptor in fetal and cancer cells. Mol Cell Biol 19:3278–3288, 1999.
9. Kimura KD, Tissenbaum HA, Liu Y, Ruvkun G: daf-2, an insulin receptor–like gene that regulates longevity and diapause in *Caenorhabditis elegans*. Science 277:942–946, 1997.
10. Chen C, Jack J, Garofalo RS: The *Drosophila* insulin receptor is required for normal growth. Endocrinology 137:846–856, 1996.
11. Werner H, Beitner-Johnson D, Roberts CT, LeRoith D: Molecular comparisons of the insulin and IGF-1 receptors. *In* Draznin B, LeRoith D (eds): Molecular Biology of Diabetes II. Insulin Action, Effects on Gene Expression and Regulation, and Glucose Transport. Totowa, NJ, Humana, 1994, pp 377–392.
12. Beguinot F, Kahn CR, Moses AC, Smith RJ: Distinct biologically active receptors for insulin, insulin-like growth factor I, and insulin-like growth factor II in cultured skeletal muscle cells. J Biol Chem 260:15892–15898, 1985.
13. Withers DJ, Burks DJ, Towery HH, et al: Irs-2 coordinates Igf-1 receptor–mediated beta-cell development and peripheral insulin signalling. Nat Genet 23:32–40, 1999.
14. Kulkarni RN, Bruning JC, Winnay JN, et al: Tissue-specific knockout of the insulin receptor in pancreatic cells creates an insulin secretory defect similar to that in type 2 diabetes. Cell 96:329–339, 1999.
15. Reinhardt RR, Chin E, Zhang B, et al: Selective coexpression of insulin receptor–related receptor (IRR) and TRK in NGF-sensitive neurons. J Neurosci 14:4674–4683, 1994.
16. Ozaki K: Insulin receptor–related receptor in rat islets of Langerhans. Eur J Endocrinol 139:244–247, 1998.
17. DeChiara TM, Efstratiadis A, Robertson EJ: A growth-deficiency phenotype in heterozygous mice carrying an insulin-like growth factor II gene disrupted by targeting. Nature 345:78–80, 1990.

18. Morrione A, Valentinis B, Xu SQ, et al: Insulin-like growth factor II stimulates cell proliferation through the insulin receptor. Proc Natl Acad Sci U S A 94:3777–3782, 1997.

19. Accili D, Drago J, Lee EJ, et al: Early neonatal death in mice homozygous for a null allele of the insulin receptor gene. Nat Genet 12:106–109, 1996.

20. Joshi RL, Lamothe B, Cordonnier N, et al: Targeted disruption of the insulin receptor gene in the mouse results in neonatal lethality. EMBO J 15:1542–1547, 1996.

21. Baker J, Liu JP, Robertson EJ, Efstratiadis A: Role of insulin-like growth factors in embryonic and postnatal growth. Cell 75:73–82, 1993.

22. Hone J, Accili D, Psiachou H, et al: Homozygosity for a null allele of the insulin receptor gene in a patient with leprechaunism. Hum Mutat 6:17–22, 1995.

23. Ullrich A, Bell JR, Chen EY, et al: Human insulin receptor and its relationship to the tyrosine kinase family of oncogenes. Nature 313:756–761, 1985.

24. Ebina Y, Ellis L, Jarnagin K, et al: The human insulin receptor cDNA: The structural basis for hormone activated transmembrane signalling. Cell 40:747–758, 1985.

25. White MF, Kahn CR: The insulin signaling system. J Biol Chem 269:1–4, 1994.

26. Myers MG Jr, White MF: The new elements in insulin signaling. Insulin receptor substrate-1 and proteins with SH2 domains. Diabetes 42:643–650, 1993.

27. Yenush L, White MF: The IRS-signaling system during insulin and cytokine action. Bioessays 19:491–500, 1997.

28. Alessi DR, Cohen P: Mechanism of activation and function of protein kinase B. Curr Opin Genet Dev 8:55–62, 1998.

29. Brunet A, Bonni A, Zigmond MJ, et al: Akt promotes cell survival by phosphorylating and inhibiting a Forkhead transcription factor. Cell 96:857–868, 1999.

30. Skolnik EY, Lee CH, Batzer AG, et al: The SH2/SH3 domain–containing protein GRB2 interacts with tyrosine-phosphorylated IRS-1 and Shc: Implications for insulin control of ras signalling. EMBO J 12:1929–1936, 1993.

31. Myers MG Jr, Wang LM, Sun XJ, et al: The role of IRS-1/GRB2 complexes in insulin signaling. Mol Cell Biol 14:3577–3587, 1994.

32. Myers MG Jr, Mendez R, Shi P, et al: The COOH-terminal tyrosine phosphorylation sites on IRS-1 bind SHP-2 and negatively regulate insulin signaling. J Biol Chem 273:26908–26914, 1998.

33. Rosen ED, Spiegelman BM: Tumor necrosis factor-alpha as a mediator of the insulin resistance of obesity. Curr Opin Endocrinol Diabetes 6:170–176, 1999.

34. Chen H, Wertheimer SJ, Lin CH, et al: Protein-tyrosine phosphatases PTP1B and syp are modulators of insulin-stimulated translocation of GLUT4 in transfected rat adipose cells. J Biol Chem 272:8026–8031, 1997.

35. Elchebly M, Payette P, Michaliszyn E, et al: Increased insulin sensitivity and obesity resistance in mice lacking the protein tyrosine phosphatase-1b gene. Science 283:1544–1548, 1999.

36. Yang Feng TL, Francke U, Ullrich A: Gene for human insulin receptor: Localization to site on chromosome 19 involved in pre-B-cell leukemia. Science 228:728–731, 1985.

37. Seino S, Seino M, Nishi S, Bell GI: Structure of the human insulin receptor gene and characterization of its promoter. Proc Natl Acad Sci U S A 86:114–118, 1989.

38. Mosthaf L, Grako K, Dull TJ, et al: Functionally distinct insulin receptors generated by tissue-specific alternative splicing. EMBO J 9:2409–2413, 1990.

39. Moller DE, Yokota A, Caro JF, Flier JS: Tissue-specific expression of two alternatively spliced insulin receptor mRNAs in man. Mol Endocrinol 3:1263–1269, 1989.

40. Goldstein BJ, Kahn CR: Analysis of mRNA heterogeneity by ribonuclease H mapping: Application to the insulin receptor. Biochem Biophys Res Commun 159:664–669, 1989.

41. Seino S, Bell GI: Alternative splicing of human insulin receptor messenger RNA. Biochem Biophys Res Commun 159:312–316, 1989.

42. Kosaki A, Pillay TS, Xu L, Webster NJ: The B isoform of the insulin receptor signals more efficiently than the A isoform in HepG2 cells. J Biol Chem 270:20816–20823, 1995.

43. Mosthaf L, Eriksson JW, Haring HU, et al: Insulin receptor isotype expression correlates with risk of non–insulin-dependent diabetes. Proc Natl Acad Sci U S A 90:2633–2635, 1993.

44. Kasuga M, Hedo JA, Yamada KM, Kahn CR: The structure of the insulin receptor and its subunits: Evidence for multiple non-reduced forms and a 210K possible proreceptor. J Biol Chem 257:10392–10399, 1982.

45. Hedo JA, Kahn CR, Hayoshi M, et al: Biosynthesis and glycosylation of the insulin receptor. Evidence for a single polypeptide precursor of the two major subunits. J Biol Chem 258:10020–10026, 1983.

46. De Meyts P: The structural basis of insulin and insulin-like growth factor-1 receptor binding and negative cooperativity, and its relevance to mitogenic versus metabolic signaling. Diabetologia 37(suppl 2):135–148, 1995.

47. Williams PF, Mynarcik DC, Yu GQ, Whittaker J: Mapping of an NH₂-terminal ligand binding site of the insulin receptor by alanine scanning mutagenesis. J Biol Chem 270:3012–3016, 1995.

48. Schumacher R, Soos MA, Schlessinger J, et al: Signaling-competent receptor chimeras allow mapping of major insulin receptor binding domain determinants. J Biol Chem 1993 268:1087–1094.

49. Mynarcik DC, Yu GQ, Whittaker J: Alanine-scanning mutagenesis of a C-terminal ligand binding domain of the insulin receptor alpha subunit. J Biol Chem 271:2439–2442, 1996.

50. Schlessinger J: Signal transduction by allosteric receptor oligomerization. TIBS 13:443–447, 1988.

51. Remy I, Wilson IA, Michnick SW: Erythropoietin receptor activation by a ligand-induced conformation change. Science 283:990–993, 1999.

52. Livnah O, Stura EA, Middleton SA, et al: Crystallographic evidence for preformed dimers of erythropoietin receptor before ligand activation. Science 283:987–990, 1999.

53. Cunningham BC, Ultsch M, de Vos AM, et al: Dimerization of the extracellular domain of the human growth hormone receptor by a single hormone molecule. Science 254:821–825, 1992.

54. Fuh G, Cunningham BC, Fukunaga R, et al: Rational design of potent antagonists to the human growth hormone receptor. Science 256:1677–1680, 1992.

55. Balendran A, Casamayor A, Deak M, et al: PDK1 acquires PDK2 activity in the presence of a synthetic peptide derived from the carboxyl terminus of PRK2. Curr Biol 9:393–404, 1999.

56. Shoelson SE, White MF, Kahn CR: Tryptic activation of the insulin receptor: Proteolytic truncation of the β-subunit releases the β-subunit from inhibitory control. J Biol Chem 263:4852–4860, 1988.

57. Xu QY, Paxton RJ, Fujita-Yamaguchi Y: Substructural analysis of the insulin receptor by microsequence analysis of limited tryptic fragments isolated by sodium dodecyl sulfate–polyacrylamide gel electrophoresis in the absence or presence of dithiothreitol. J Biol Chem 265:18673–18681, 1990.

58. Cheatham B, Kahn CR: Cysteine 647 in the insulin receptor is required for normal covalent interaction between alpha- and beta-subunits and signal transduction. J Biol Chem 267:7108–7115, 1992.

59. Cheatham B, Shoelson SE, Yamada K, et al: Substitution of the erbB-2 oncoprotein transmembrane domain activates the insulin receptor and modulates the action of insulin and insulin-receptor substrate 1. Proc Natl Acad Sci U S A 90:7336–7340, 1993.

60. Longo N, Shuster RC, Griffin LD, et al: Activation of insulin receptor signaling by a single amino acid substitution in the transmembrane domain. J Biol Chem 267:12416–12419, 1992.

61. Zhang B, Salituro G, Szalkowski D, et al: Discovery of a small molecule insulin mimetic with antidiabetic activity in mice. Science 284:974–977, 1999.

62. Chou CK, Dull TJ, Russell DS, et al: Human insulin receptors mutated at the ATP-binding site lack protein tyrosine kinase activity and fail to mediate postreceptor effects of insulin. J Biol Chem 262:1842–1847, 1987.

63. Cama A, de la Luz Sierra M, Ottini L, et al: A mutation in the tyrosine kinase domain of the insulin receptor associated with insulin resistance in an obese woman. J Clin Endocrinol Metab 73:894–901, 1991.

64. Krook A, O'Rahilly S: Mutant insulin receptors in syndromes of insulin resistance. Baillieres Clin Endocrinol Metab 10:97–122, 1996.

65. Rosen OM, Herrera R, Olowe Y, et al: Phosphorylation activates the insulin receptor tyrosine protein kinase. Proc Natl Acad Sci U S A 80:3237–3240, 1983.

66. White MF, Shoelson SE, Keutmann H, Kahn CR: A cascade of tyrosine autophosphorylation in the β-subunit activates the insulin receptor. J Biol Chem 263:2969–2980, 1988.

67. Wilden PA, Siddle K, Haring E, et al: The role of insulin receptor kinase domain autophosphorylation in receptor-mediated activities. J Biol Chem 267:13719–13727, 1992.

68. Cann AD, Kohanski RA: Cis-autophosphorylation of juxtamembrane tyrosines in the insulin receptor kinase domain. Biochemistry 36:7681–7689, 1997.

69. Myers MG Jr, Backer JM, Siddle K, White MF: The insulin receptor functions normally in Chinese hamster ovary cells after truncation of the C-terminus. J Biol Chem 266:10616–10623, 1991.

70. Maegawa H, McClain DA, Freidneberg G, et al: Properties of a human insulin receptor with a COOH-terminal truncation II: Truncated receptors have normal kinase activity but are defective in signaling metabolic effects. J Biol Chem 263:8912–8917, 1988.

71. McClain DA, Maegawa H, Levy J, et al: Properties of a human insulin receptor with a COOH-terminal truncation. I. Insulin binding, autophosphorylation and endocytosis. J Biol Chem 263:8904–8912, 1988.

72. Backer JM, Shoelson SE, Weiss MA, et al: The insulin receptor juxtamembrane region contains two independent tyrosine/beta-turn internalization signals. J Cell Biol 118:831–839, 1992.

73. Baron V, Gautier N, Kaliman P, et al: The carboxyl-terminal domain of the insulin receptor: Its potential role in growth-promoting effects. Biochemistry 30:9365–9370, 1991.

74. Levy-Toledano R, Blaettler DH, Larochelle WJ, Taylor SI: Insulin-induced activation of phosphatidylinositol (PI) 3-kinase. J Biol Chem 270:30018–30022, 1995.

75. Van Horn DJ, Myers MG Jr, Backer JM: Direct activation of the phosphatidylinositol 3'-kinase by the insulin receptor. J Biochem 269:29–32, 1994.

76. White MF, Livingston JN, Backer JM, et al: Mutation of the insulin receptor at tyrosine 960 inhibits signal transmission but does not affect its tyrosine kinase activity. Cell 54:641–649, 1988.

77. Backer JM, Schroeder GG, Cahill DA, et al: The cytoplasmic juxtamembrane region of the insulin receptor: A critical role in ATP binding, endogenous substrate phosphorylation, and insulin-stimulated bioeffects in CHO cells. Biochemistry 30:6366–6372, 1991.

78. Backer JM, Schroeder GG, Kahn CR, et al: Insulin stimulation of phosphatidylinositol 3-kinase activity maps to insulin receptor regions required for endogenous substrate phosphorylation. J Biol Chem 267:1367–1374, 1992.

79. Gustafson TA, He W, Craparo A, et al: Phosphotyrosine-dependent interaction of Shc and IRS-1 with the NPEY motif of the insulin receptor via a novel non-SH2 domain. Mol Cell Biol 15:2500–2508, 1995.

80. Sun XJ, Rothenberg PL, Kahn CR, et al: The structure of the insulin receptor substrate IRS-1 defines a unique signal transduction protein. Nature 352:73–77, 1991.

81. Wilden PA, Backer JM, Kahn CR, et al: The insulin receptor with phenylalanine replacing tyrosine-1146 provides evidence for separate signals regulating cellular metabolism and growth. Proc Natl Acad Sci U S A 87:3358–3362, 1990.

82. Wilden PA, Kahn CR, Siddle K, White MF: Insulin receptor kinase domain autophosphorylation regulates receptor enzymatic function. J Biol Chem 267:16660–16668, 1992.

83. Hubbard SR: Crystal structure of the activated insulin receptor tyrosine kinase in complex with peptide substrate and ATP analog. EMBO J 16:5572–5581, 1997.

84. Feener EP, Backer JM, King GL, et al: Insulin stimulates serine and tyrosine phosphorylation in the juxtamembrane region of the insulin receptor. J Biol Chem 268:11256–11264, 1993.

85. Hubbard SR, Wei L, Ellis L, Hendrickson WA: Crystal structure of the tyrosine kinase domain of the human insulin receptor. Nature 372:746–754, 1994.
86. Sawka-Verhelle D, Tartare-Deckert S, White MF, Van Obberghen E: IRS-2 binds to the insulin receptor through its PTB domain and through a newly identified domain comprising amino acids 591 to 786. J Biol Chem 271:5980–5983, 1996.
87. Sawka-Verhelle D, Baron V, Mothe I, et al: Tyr624 and Tyr628 in insulin receptor substrate-2 mediate its association with the insulin receptor. J Biol Chem 272:16414–16420, 1997.
88. Liu F, Roth RA: Grb-IR: A SH2 domain–containing protein that binds to the insulin receptor and inhibits its function. Proc Natl Acad Sci U S A 92:10287–10291, 1995.
89. Songyang Z, Carraway KL III, Eck MJ, et al: Catalytic specificity of protein-tyrosine kinases is critical for selective signalling. Nature 373:536–539, 1995.
90. Songyang Z, Cantley LC: Recognition and specificity in protein tyrosine kinase–mediated signaling. TIBS 20:470–475, 1995.
91. Shoelson SE, Chatterjee S, Chaudhuri M, White MF: YMXM motifs of IRS-1 define the substrate specificity of the insulin receptor kinase. Proc Natl Acad Sci U S A 89:2027–2031, 1992.
92. Virkamaki A, Ueki K, Kahn CR: Protein-protein interaction in insulin signaling and the molecular mechanisms of insulin resistance. J Clin Invest 103:931–943, 1999.
93. Sun XJ, Wang LM, Zhang Y, et al: Role of IRS-2 in insulin and cytokine signalling. Nature 377:173–177, 1995.
94. Lavan BE, Lane WS, Lienhard GE: The 60-kDa phosphotyrosine protein in insulin-treated adipocytes is a new member of the insulin receptor substrate family. J Biol Chem 272:11439–11443, 1997.
95. Lavan BE, Fantin VR, Chang ET, et al: A novel 160 kDa phosphotyrosine protein in insulin-treated embryonic kidney cells is a new member of the insulin receptor substrate family. J Biol Chem 272:21403–21407, 1997.
96. Yenush L, Makati KJ, Smith-Hall J, et al: The pleckstrin homology domain is the principal link between the insulin receptor and IRS-1. J Biol Chem 271:24300–24306, 1996.
97. Shepherd PR, Withers DJ, Siddle K: Phosphoinositide 3-kinase: The key switch mechanism in insulin signalling. Biochem J 333:471–490, 1998.
98. Leevers SJ, Vanhaesebroeck B, Waterfield MD: Signalling through phosphoinositide 3-kinases: The lipids take centre stage. Curr Opin Cell Biol 11:219–225, 1999.
99. Vanhaesebroeck B, Leevers SJ, Panayotou G, Waterfield MD: Phosphoinositide 3-kinases: A conserved family of signal transducers. Trends Biochem Sci 22:267–272, 1997.
100. Rameh LE, Cantley LC: The role of phosphoinositide 3-kinase lipid products in cell function. J Biol Chem 274:8347–8350, 1999.
101. Backer JM, Myers MG Jr, Shoelson SE, et al: Phosphatidylinositol 3′-kinase is activated by association with IRS-1 during insulin stimulation. EMBO J 11:3469–3479, 1992.
102. Rordorf-Nikolic T, Van Horn DJ, Chen D, et al: Regulation of phosphatidylinositol 3-kinase by tyrosyl phosphoproteins. Full activation requires occupancy of both SH2 domains in the 85 kDa regulatory subunit. J Biol Chem 270:3662–3666, 1995.
103. Myers MG Jr, White MF: Insulin signal transduction and the IRS proteins. Annu Rev Pharmacol Toxicol 36:615–658, 1996.
104. Yenush L, Fernandez R, Myers MG Jr, et al: The *Drosophila* insulin receptor activates multiple signaling pathways but requires IRS-proteins for DNA synthesis. Mol Cell Biol 16:2509–2517, 1996.
105. Gottlieb S, Ruvkun G: daf-2, daf-16 and daf-23: Genetically interacting genes controlling Dauer formation in *Caenorhabditis elegans*. Genetics 137:107–120, 1994.
106. Bohni R, Riesgo-Escovar J, Oldham S, et al: Autonomous control of cell and organ size by CHICO, a *Drosophila* homolog of vertebrate IRS1–4. Cell 97:865–875, 1999.
107. Ruvkun G, Hobert O: The taxonomy of developmental control in *Caenorhabditis elegans*. Science 282:2033–2041, 1998.
108. Paradis S, Ailion M, Toker A, et al: A PDK1 homolog is necessary and sufficient to transduce AGE-1 PI3 kinase signals that regulate diapause in *Caenorhabditis elegans*. Genes Dev 13:1438–1452, 1999.
109. Paradis S, Ruvkun G: *Caenorhabditis elegans* Akt/PKB transduces insulin receptor–like signals from AGE-1 PI3 kinase to the DAF-16 transcription factor. Genes Dev 12:2488–2498, 1998.
110. Ogg S, Paradis S, Gottlieb S, et al: The Forkhead transcription factor DAF-16 transduces insulin-like metabolic and longevity signals in *C. elegans*. Nature 389:994–999, 1997.
111. Kops GJ, de Ruiter ND, de Vries-Smits AM, et al: Direct control of the Forkhead transcription factor AFX by protein kinase B. Nature 398:630–634, 1999.
112. Rena G, Guo S, Cichy SC, et al: Phosphorylation of the transcription factor forkhead family member FKHR by protein kinase B. J Biol Chem 274:17179–17183, 1999.
113. Guo S, Rena G, Cichy S, et al: Phosphorylation of serine 256 by protein kinase B disrupts transactivation by FKHR and mediates effects of insulin on insulin-like growth factor–binding protein-1 promoter activity through a conserved insulin response sequence. J Biol Chem 274:17184–17192, 1999.
114. Sun H, Lesche R, Li DM, et al: PTEN modulates cell cycle progression and cell survival by regulating phosphatidylinositol 3,4,5,-trisphosphate and Akt/protein kinase B signaling pathway. Proc Natl Acad Sci U S A 96:6199–6204, 1999.
115. Maehama T, Dixon JE: PTEN: A tumour suppressor that functions as a phospholipid phosphatase. Trends Cell Biol 9(4):125–128, 1999.
116. Ogg S, Ruvkun G: The *C. elegans* PTEN homolog, DAF-18, acts in the insulin receptor–like metabolic signaling pathway. Mol Cell 2:887–893, 1998.
117. Rouault JP, Kuwabara PE, Sinilnikova OM, et al: Regulation of dauer larva development in *Caenorhabditis elegans* by daf-18, a homologue of the tumour suppressor PTEN. Curr Biol 9:329–332, 1999.
118. Gil EB, Malone LE, Liu LX, et al: Regulation of the insulin-like developmental pathway of *Caenorhabditis elegans* by a homolog of the PTEN tumor suppressor gene. Proc Natl Acad Sci U S A 96:2925–2930, 1999.
119. Lioubin MN, Algate PA, Tsai S, et al: p150^{Ship}, a signal transduction molecule with inositol polyphosphate-5-phosphatase activity. Genes Dev 10:1084–1095, 1996.
120. Liu L, Damen JE, Ware MD, Krystal G: Interleukin-3 induces the association of the inositol 5-phosphatase SHIP with SHP2. J Biol Chem 272:10998–11001, 1997.
121. Habib T, Hejna JA, Moses RE, Decker SJ: Growth factors and insulin stimulate tyrosine phosphorylation of the 51C/SHIP2 protein. J Biol Chem 273:18605–18609, 1998.
122. Deuter-Reinhard M, Apell G, Pot DA, et al: SIP/SHIP inhibits *Xenopus* oocyte maturation induced by insulin and phosphatidylinositol 3-kinase. Mol Cell Biol 17:2559–2565, 1997.
123. Franke TF, Kaplan DR, Cantley LC, Toker A: Direct regulation of the Akt proto-oncogene product by phosphatidylinositol-3,4-bisphosphate. Science 275:665–668, 1997.
124. Klippel A, Kavanaugh WM, Pot D, Williams LT: A specific product of phosphatidylinositol 3-kinase directly activates the protein kinase Akt through its pleckstrin homology domain. Mol Cell Biol 17:338–344, 1997.
125. Cohen P, Alessi DR, Cross DA: PDK1, one of the missing links in insulin signal transduction? Growth Regul 410:3–10, 1997.
126. Kohn AD, Takeuchi F, Roth RA: Akt, a pleckstrin homology domain containing kinase, is activated primarily by phosphorylation. J Biol Chem 271:21920–21926, 1996.
127. Meier R, Hemmings BA: Regulation of protein kinase B. J Recept Signal Transduct Res 19:121–128, 1999.
128. Belham C, Wu S, Avruch J: Intracellular signalling: PDK1—a kinase at the hub of things. Curr Biol 9:R93–R96, 1999.
129. Kapeller R, Chem KS, Yoakim M, et al: Mutations in the juxtamembrane region of the insulin receptor impair activation of phosphatidylinositol 3-kinase by insulin. Mol Endocrinol 5:769–777, 1991.
130. Ruderman N, Kapeller R, White MF, Cantley LC: Activation of phosphatidylinositol-3-kinase by insulin. Proc Natl Acad Sci U S A 87:1411–1415, 1990.
131. Kitamura T, Ogawa W, Sakaue H, et al: Requirement for activation of the serine-threonine kinase Akt (protein kinase B) in insulin stimulation of protein synthesis but not of glucose transport. Mol Cell Biol 18:3708–3717, 1998.
132. Marte BM, Downward J: PKB/Akt: Connecting phosphoinositide 3-kinase to cell survival and beyond. Trends Biochem Sci 22:355–358, 1997.
133. Hemmings BA: Akt signaling linked membrane events to life and death decisions. Science 275:628–630, 1997.
134. Franke TF, Kaplan DR, Cantley LC: PI3K: Downstream AKTion blocks apoptosis. Cell 88:436–437, 1997.
135. Dudek H, Datta SR, Franke TF, et al: Regulation of neuronal survival by the serine-threonine protein kinase Akt. Science 275:661–665, 1997.
136. Kohn AD, Summers SA, Birnbaum MJ, Roth RA: Expression of a constitutively active Akt Ser/Thr kinase in 3T3-L1 adipocytes stimulates glucose uptake and glucose transporter 4 translocation. J Biol Chem 271:31372–31378, 1996.
137. Gingras AC, Kennedy SG, O'Leary MA, et al: 4E-BP1, a repressor of mRNA translation, is phosphorylated and inactivated by the Akt(PKB) signaling pathway. Genes Dev 12:502–513, 1998.
138. Pap M, Cooper GM: Role of glycogen synthase kinase-3 in the phosphatidylinositol 3-kinase/Akt cell survival pathway. J Biol Chem 273:19929–19932, 1998.
139. Hajduch E, Alessi DR, Hemmings BA, Hundal HS: Constitutive activation of protein kinase B alpha by membrane targeting promotes glucose and system A amino acid transport, protein synthesis, and inactivation of glycogen synthase 3 in L6 muscle cells. Diabetes 47:1006–1013, 1998.
140. Datta SR, Dudek H, Tao X, et al: Akt phosphorylation of BAD couples survival signals to the cell-intrinsic death machinery. Cell 91:231–241, 1997.
141. del Peso L, Gonzalez-Garcia M, Page C, et al: Interleukin-3–induced phosphorylation of BAD through the protein kinase Akt. Science 278:687–689, 1997.
142. Hoenack C, Roesen P: Inhibition of angiotensin type 1 receptor prevents decline of glucose transporter (GLUT4) in diabetic rat heart. Diabetes 45(suppl 1):82–87, 1996.
143. Toker A, Cantley LC: Signalling through the lipid products of phosphoinositide-3-OH kinase. Nature 387:673–676, 1997.
144. Avruch J: Insulin signal transduction through protein kinase cascades. Mol Cell Biochem 182:31–48, 1998.
145. Alessi DR, Kozlowski MT, Weng QP, et al: 3-Phosphoinositide–dependent protein kinase 1 (PDK1) phosphorylates and activates the p70 S6 kinase in vivo and in vitro. Curr Biol 8:69–81, 1998.
146. Pullen N, Dennis PB, Andjelkovic M, et al: Phosphorylation and activation of p70s6k by PDK1. Science 279:707–710, 1998.
147. Brown EJ, Beal PA, Keith CT, et al: Control of p70 S6 kinase by kinase activity of FRAP in vivo. Nature 377:441–446, 1995.
148. Weng QP, Andrabi K, Klippel A, et al: Phosphatidylinositol 3-kinase signals activation of p70 S6 kinase in situ through site-specific p70 phosphorylation. Proc Natl Acad Sci U S A 92:5744–5748, 1995.
149. Le Good JA, Ziegler WH, Parekh DB, et al: Protein kinase C isotypes controlled by phosphoinositide 3-kinase through the protein kinase PDK1. Science 281:2042–2045, 1998.
150. Bandyopadhyay G, Standaert ML, Zhao L, et al: Activation of protein kinase C (α, β, and zeta) by insulin in 3T3/L1 cells. Transfection studies suggest a role for PKC-zeta in glucose transport. J Biol Chem 272:2551–2558, 1997.
151. Bandyopadhyay G, Standaert ML, Kikkawa U, et al: Effects of transiently expressed atypical (zeta, lambda), conventional (alpha, beta) and novel (delta, epsilon) protein kinase C isoforms on insulin-stimulated translocation of epitope-tagged GLUT4 glucose transporters in rat adipocytes: Specific interchangeable effects of protein kinases C-zeta and C-lambda. Biochem J 337:461–470, 1999.
152. Kotani K, Ogawa W, Matsumoto M, et al: Requirement of atypical protein kinase lambda for insulin stimulation of glucose uptake but not for akt activation in 3T3-L1 adipocytes. Mol Cell Biol 18:6971–6982, 1998.
153. Mendez R, Kollmorgen G, White MF, Rhoads RE: Requirement of protein kinase C zeta for stimulation of protein synthesis by insulin. Mol Cell Biol 17:5184–5192, 1997.

154. Blenis J: Signal transduction via the MAP kinases: Proceed at your own RSK. Proc Natl Acad Sci U S A 9089:5889–5892, 1993.

155. Skolnik EY, Batzer AG, Li N, et al: The function of GRB2 in linking the insulin receptor to ras signaling pathways. Science 260:1953–1955, 1993.

156. Buday L, Downward J: Epidermal growth factor regulates p21ras through the formulation of a complex of receptor, Grb2 adapter protein, and Sos nucleotide exchange factor. Cell 73:611–620, 1993.

157. Egan SE, Giddings BW, Brooks MW, et al: Association of Sos ras exchange protein with Grb2 is implicated in tyrosine kinase signal transduction and transformation. Nature 363:45–51, 1993.

158. Cobb M, Goldsmith EJ: How MAP kinases are regulated. J Biol Chem 270:14843–14846, 1995.

159. Inoue G, Cheatham B, Emkey R, Kahn CR: Dynamics of insulin signaling in 3T3-L1 adipocytes: Differential compartmentalization and trafficking of insulin receptor substrate (IRS)-1 and IRS-2. J Biol Chem 273:11548–11555, 1998.

160. Yamamoto M, Toya Y, Schwencke C, et al: Caveolin is an activator of insulin receptor signaling. J Biol Chem 273:26962–26968, 1998.

161. Carpentier JL, Paccaud JP, Backer JM, et al: Characterization of the insulin-dependent and -independent steps of insulin receptor internalization. J Cell Biol 122:1243–1252, 1993.

162. Backer JM, Kahn CR, White MF: Tyrosine phosphorylation of the insulin receptor is not required for internalization. Proc Natl Acad Sci U S A 86:3209–3213, 1989.

163. Ceresa BP, Kao AW, Santeler SR, Pessin JE: Inhibition of clathrin-mediated endocytosis selectively attenuates specific insulin receptor signal transduction pathways. Mol Cell Biol 18:3862–3870, 1998.

164. Haft CR, Klausner RD, Taylor SI: Involvement of dileucine motifs in the internalization and degradation of the insulin receptor. J Biol Chem 269:26286–26294, 1994.

165. Backer JM, Shoelson SE, Haring E, White MF: Insulin receptors internalize by a rapid, saturable pathway requiring receptor autophosphorylation and an intact juxtamembrane region. J Cell Biol 115:1535–1545, 1991.

166. Backer JM, Kahn CR, Cahill DA, et al: Receptor-mediated internalization of insulin requires a 12–amino acid sequence in the juxtamembrane region of the insulin receptor β-subunit. J Biol Chem 265:16450–16454, 1990.

167. Backer JM, Kahn CR, White MF: The dissociation and degradation of internalized insulin occur in the endosomes of rat hepatoma cells. J Biol Chem 265:14828–14835, 1990.

168. Burks DJ, Pons S, Towery H, et al: Heterologous PH domains do not mediate coupling of IRS-1 to the insulin receptor. J Biol Chem 272:27716–27721, 1997.

169. Almind K, Inoue G, Pedersen O, Kahn CR: A common amino acid polymorphism in insulin receptor substrate-1 causes impaired insulin signaling. Evidence from transfection studies. J Clin Invest 97:2569–2575, 1996.

170. Yenush L, Zanella C, Uchida T, et al: The pleckstrin homology and phosphotyrosine binding domains of insulin receptor substrate 1 mediate inhibition of apoptosis by insulin. Mol Cell Biol 18:6784–6794, 1998.

171. Mueckler M: Family of glucose-transporter genes. Implications for glucose homeostasis and diabetes. Diabetes 39:6–11, 1990.

172. Gould GW, Derechin V, James DE, et al: Insulin-stimulated translocation of the HepG2/erythrocyte-type glucose transporter expressed in 3T3-L1 adipocytes. J Biol Chem 264:2180–2184, 1989.

173. Hausdorff SF, Frangioni JV, Birnbaum MJ: Role of p21ras in insulin-stimulated glucose transport in 3T3-L1 adipocytes. J Biol Chem 269:21391–21394, 1994.

174. Fingar DC, Birnbaum MJ: A role for raf-1 in the divergent signaling pathways mediating insulin-stimulated glucose transport. J Biol Chem 269:10127–10132, 1994.

175. Haney PM, Levy MA, Strube MS, Mueckler M: Insulin-sensitive targeting of the GLUT4 glucose transporter in L6 myoblasts is conferred by its COOH-terminal cytoplasmic tail. J Cell Biol 129:641–658, 1995.

176. Verhey KJ, Birnbaum MJ: A leu-leu sequence is essential for COOH-terminal targeting signal of GLUT4 glucose transporter in fibroblasts. J Biol Chem 269:2353–2356, 1994.

177. Verhey KJ, Yeh J-I, Birnbaum MJ: Distinct signals in the GLUT4 glucose transporter for internalization and for targeting to an insulin-responsive compartment. J Cell Biol 130:1071–1079, 1995.

178. Cheatham B, Vlahos CJ, Cheatham L, et al: Phosphatidylinositol 3-kinase activation is required for insulin stimulation of pp70 S6 kinase, DNA synthesis, and glucose transporter translocation. Mol Cell Biol 14:4902–4911, 1994.

179. Fingar DC, Hausdorff SF, Blenis J, Birnbaum MJ: Dissociation of pp70 ribosomal protein S6 kinase from insulin-stimulated glucose transport in 3T3-L1 adipocytes. J Biol Chem 268:3005–3008, 1993.

180. Goodyear LJ, Giorgino F, Balon TW, et al: Effects of contractile activity on tyrosine phosphoproteins and phosphatidylinositol 3-kinase activity in rat skeletal muscle. Am J Physiol 268:E987–E995, 1995.

181. Higaki Y, Wojtaszewski JF, Hirshman MF, et al: Insulin receptor substrate-2 is not necessary for insulin- and exercise-stimulated glucose transport in skeletal muscle. J Biol Chem 274:20791–20795, 1999.

182. Roth J: Diabetes and obesity. Diabetes Metab Rev 13:1–2, 1998.

183. Hani EH, Suaud L, Boutin P, et al: A missense mutation in hepatocyte nuclear factor-4 alpha, resulting in a reduced transactivation activity, in human late-onset non–insulin-dependent diabetes mellitus. J Clin Invest 101:521–526, 1998.

184. Carboni JM, Yan N, Cox AD, et al: Farnesyltransferase inhibitors are inhibitors of Ras but not R-Ras2/TC21 transformation. Oncogene 10:1905–1913, 1995.

185. Vaxillaire M, Rouard M, Yamagata K, et al: Identification of nine novel mutations in the hepatocyte nuclear factor 1 alpha gene associated with maturity-onset diabetes of the young (MODY3). Hum Mol Genet 6:583–586, 1997.

186. Comb DG, Roseman S: Glucosamine metabolism. IV. Glucosamine-6-phosphate deaminase. J Biol Chem 232:807–827, 1958.

187. Taylor SI: Deconstructing type 2 diabetes. Cell 97:9–12, 1999.

188. Almind K, Bjorbaek C, Vestergaard H, et al: Amino acid polymorphisms of insulin receptor substrate-1 in non–insulin-dependent diabetes mellitus. Lancet 342:828–832, 1993.

189. Bernal D, Almind K, Yenush L, et al: IRS-2 amino acid polymorphisms are not associated with random type 2 diabetes among Caucasians. Diabetes 47:976–979, 1998.

190. Almind K, Frederiksen SK, Ahlgren MG, et al: Common amino acid substitutions in insulin receptor substrate-4 are not associated with type II diabetes mellitus or insulin resistance. Diabetologia 41:969–974, 1998.

191. Hansen T, Andersen CB, Echwald SM, et al: Identification of a common amino acid polymorphism in the p-85alpha regulatory subunit of phosphatidylinositol 3-kinase: Effects on glucose disappearance constant, glucose effectiveness and the insulin sensitivity index. Diabetes 46:494–501, 1997.

192. DeFronzo RA: Pathogenesis of type 2 diabetes: Metabolic and molecular implications for identifying diabetes genes. Diabetes Rev 5:177–269, 1997.

193. Hansen PA, Han DH, Marshall BA, et al: A high fat diet impairs stimulation of glucose transport in muscle. Functional evaluation of potential mechanisms. J Biol Chem 273:26157–26163, 1998.

194. Flier JS: Leptin expression and action: New experimental paradigms. Proc Natl Acad Sci U S A 94:4242–4245, 1997.

195. Zhang Y, Proenca R, Maffei M, et al: Positional cloning of the mouse obese gene and its human homologue. Nature 372:425–432, 1994.

196. Boden G: Role of fatty acids in the pathogenesis of insulin resistance and NIDDM. Diabetes 46:3–10, 1997.

197. Cohen B, Novick D, Rubinstein M: Modulation of insulin activities by leptin. Science 274:1185–1188, 1996.

198. Hotamisligil GS, Peraldi P, Budvari A, et al: IRS-1 mediated inhibition of insulin receptor tyrosine kinase activity in TNF- and obesity-induced insulin resistance. Science 271:665–668, 1996.

199. Friedman JM, Halaas JL: Leptin and the regulation of body weight in mammals. Nature 395:763–770, 1998.

200. Bjorbaek C, Uotani S, da Silva B, Flier JS: Divergent signaling capacities of the long and short isoforms of the leptin receptor. J Biol Chem 272:32686–32695, 1997.

201. Wang MY, Koyama K, Shimabukuro M, et al: OB-Rb gene transfer to leptin-resistant islets reverses diabetogenic phenotype. Proc Natl Acad Sci U S A 95:714–718, 1998.

202. Hotamisligil GS, Spiegelman BM: Tumor necrosis factor α: A key component of the obesity-diabetes link. Diabetes 43:1271–1278, 1994.

203. Hotamisligil GS, Shargill NS, Spiegelman BM: Adipose expression of tumor necrosis factor-α: Direct role in obesity-linked insulin resistance. Science 259:87–91, 1993.

204. Peraldi P, Hotamisligil GS, Buurman WA, et al: Tumor necrosis factor (TNF)-α inhibits insulin signaling through stimulation of the p55 TNF receptor and activation of sphingomyelinase. J Biol Chem 271:13018–13022, 1996.

205. Kanety H, Feinstein R, Papa MZ, et al: Tumor necrosis factor α–induced phosphorylation of insulin receptor substrate-1 (IRS-1). Possible mechanism for suppression of insulin-stimulated tyrosine phosphorylation of IRS-1. J Biol Chem 270:23780–23784, 1995.

206. Uysal KT, Wiesbrock SM, Hotamisligil GS: Functional analysis of tumor necrosis factor (TNF) receptors in TNF-alpha–mediated insulin resistance in genetic obesity. Endocrinology 139:4832–4838, 1998.

207. Miles PD, Romeo OM, Higo K, et al: TNF-alpha–induced insulin resistance in vivo and its prevention by troglitazone. Diabetes 46:1678–1683, 1997.

208. Takayama S, White MF, Lauris V, Kahn CR: Phorbol esters modulate insulin receptor phosphorylation and insulin action in hepatoma cells. Proc Natl Acad Sci U S A 81:7797–7801, 1984.

209. Tavare JM, Zhang B, Ellis L, Roth RA: Insulin-stimulated serine and threonine phosphorylation of the human insulin receptor. An assessment of the role of serines 1305/1306 and threonine 1348 by their replacement with neutral or negatively charged amino acids. J Biol Chem 266:21804–21809, 1991.

210. Chin JE, Dickens M, Tavare JM, Roth RA: Overexpression of protein kinase C isoenzymes alpha, beta I, gamma, and epsilon in cells overexpressing the insulin receptor. Effects on receptor phosphorylation and signaling. J Biol Chem 268:6338–6347, 1993.

211. Liu F, Roth RA: Identification of serines-967/968 in the juxtamembrane region of the insulin receptor as insulin-stimulated phosphorylation sites. J Biochem 298:1–7, 1994.

212. Liu F, Roth RA: Identification of serines-1035/1037 in the kinase domain of the insulin receptor as protein kinase C-alpha mediated phosphorylation sites. FEBS Lett 352:389–392, 1994.

213. Kellerer M, Mushack J, Seffer E, et al: Protein kinase C isoforms alpha, delta and theta require insulin receptor substrate-1 to inhibit the tyrosine kinase activity of the insulin receptor in human kidney embryonic cells (HEK 293 cells). Diabetologia 41:833–838, 1998.

214. Lawrence JC Jr, Hiken JF, James DE: Stimulation of glucose transport and glucose transporter phosphorylation by okadaic acid in rat adipocytes. J Biol Chem 265:19768–19776, 1990.

215. Haystead TAJ, Weiel JE, Litchfield DW, et al: Okadaic acid mimics the action of insulin in stimulating protein kinase activity in isolated adipocytes. J Biol Chem 265:16571–16580, 1990.

216. Mothe I, Van Obberghen E: Phosphorylation of insulin receptor substrate-1 on multiple serine residues, 612, 662, and 731, modulates insulin action. J Biol Chem 271:11222–11227, 1996.

217. Li J, De Fea K, Roth RA: Modulation of insulin receptor substrate-1 tyrosine phosphorylation by an Akt/phosphatidylinositol 3-kinase pathway. J Biol Chem 274:9351–9356, 1999.

218. De Fea K, Roth RA: Modulation of insulin receptor substrate-1 tyrosine phosphorylation and function by mitogen-activated protein kinase. J Biol Chem 272:31400–31406, 1997.

219. Feinstein R, Kanety H, Papa MZ, et al: Tumor necrosis factor-alpha suppresses insulin-induced tyrosine phosphorylation of insulin receptor and its substrates. J Biol Chem 268:26055–26058, 1993.

220. Paz K, Hemi R, LeRoith D, et al: A molecular basis for insulin resistance. Elevated

serine/threonine phosphorylation of IRS-1 and IRS-2 inhibits their binding to the juxtamembrane region of the insulin receptor and impairs their ability to undergo insulin-induced tyrosine phosphorylation. J Biol Chem 272:29911–29918, 1997.

221. Kennelly PJ, Krebs EG: Consensus sequences as substrate specificity determinants for protein kinases and protein phosphatases. J Biol Chem 266:15555–15558, 1991.

222. De Fea K, Roth RA: Protein kinase C modulation of insulin receptor substrate-1 tyrosine phosphorylation requires serine 612. Biochemistry 36:12939–12947, 1997.

223. Hubert P, Bruneau-Wack C, Cremel G, et al: Lipid-induced insulin resistance in cultured hepatoma cells is associated with a decreased insulin receptor tyrosine kinase activity. Cell Regul 2:65–72, 1991.

224. Dresner A, Laurent D, Marcucci M, et al: Effects of free fatty acids on glucose transport and IRS-1–associated phosphatidylinositol 3-kinase activity. J Clin Invest 103:253–259, 1999.

225. Chalkley SM, Hettiarachchi M, Chisholm DJ, Kraegen EW: Five-hour fatty acid elevation increases muscle lipids and impairs glycogen synthesis in the rat. Metabolism 47:1121–1126, 1998.

226. Griffin ME, Marcucci MJ, Cline GW, et al: Free fatty acid–induced insulin resistance is associated with activation of protein kinase C theta and alterations in the insulin signaling cascade. Diabetes 48:1270–1274, 1999.

227. McClain DA, Crook ED: Hexosamines and insulin resistance. Diabetes 45:1003–1009, 1996.

228. Hebert LF Jr, Daniels MC, Zhou J, et al: Overexpression of glutamine: Fructose-6-phosphate aminotransferase in transgenic mice leads to insulin resistance. J Clin Invest 98:930–936, 1996.

229. Hawkins M, Angelov I, Liu R, et al: The tissue concentration of UDP-N-acetylglucosamine modulates the stimulatory effect of insulin on skeletal muscle glucose uptake. J Biol Chem 272:4889–4895, 1997.

230. Kim YB, Zhu JS, Zierath JR, et al: Glucosamine infusion in rats rapidly impairs insulin stimulation of phosphoinositide 3-kinase but does not alter activation of Akt/protein kinase B in skeletal muscle. Diabetes 48:310–320, 1999.

231. Hart GW, Greis KD, Dong LYD, et al: *O*-linked *N*-acetylglucosamine: The "Yin-Yang" of Ser/Thr phosphorylation? *In* Alavi A, Axford JS (eds): Glycoimmunology. New York, Plenum, 1995, pp 115–123.

232. Snow DM, Hart GW: Nuclear and cytoplasmic glycosylation. Int Rev Cytol 181:43–74, 1998.

233. Tonks NK, Diltz CD, Fischer EH: Characterization of the major protein-tyrosine-phosphatases of human placenta. J Biol Chem 263:6731–6737, 1988.

234. Charbonneau H, Tonks NK, Kumar S, et al: Human placenta protein-tyrosine-phosphatase: Amino acid sequence and relationship to a family of receptor-like proteins. Proc Natl Acad Sci U S A 86:5252–5256, 1989.

235. Ahmad F, Azevedo J, Cortright R, et al: Alterations in skeletal muscle protein-tyrosine phosphatase activity and expression in insulin-resistant human obesity and diabetes. J Clin Invest 100:449–458, 1997.

236. Ahmad F, Considine RV, Bauer TL, et al: Improved sensitivity to insulin in obese subjects following weight loss is accompanied by reduced protein-tyrosine phosphatases in adipose tissue. Metabolism 46:1140–1145, 1997.

237. Goldstein BJ, Ahmad F, Ding W, et al: Regulation of the insulin signalling pathway by cellular protein-tyrosine phosphatases. Mol Cell Biochem 182:91–99, 1998.

238. Taing M, Keng YF, Shen K, et al: Potent and highly selective inhibitors of the protein tyrosine phosphatase 1B. Biochemistry 38:3793–3803, 1999.

239. Kuhne MR, Pawson T, Lienhard GE, Feng GS: The insulin receptor substrate 1 associates with the SH2-containing phosphotyrosine phosphatase Syp. J Biol Chem 268:11479–11481, 1993.

240. Yamauchi K, Milarski KL, Saltiel AR, Pessin JE: Protein-tyrosine-phosphatase SHPTP2 is a required positive effector for insulin downstream signaling. Proc Natl Acad Sci U S A 92:664–668, 1995.

241. Fujioka Y, Matozaki T, Noguchi T, et al: A novel membrane glycoprotein, SHPS-1, that binds the SH2-domain–containing protein tyrosine phosphatase SHP-2 in response to mitogens and cell adhesion. Mol Cell Biol 16:6887–6899, 1996.

242. Taylor SI, Accili D: Mutations in the genes encoding the insulin receptor and insulin receptor substrate-1. *In* LeRoith D, Taylor SI, Olefsky JM (eds): Diabetes Mellitus: A Fundamental and Clinical Text. Philadelphia, Lippincott-Raven, 1996, pp 575–583.

243. Taylor SI, Cama A, Accili D, et al: Mutations in the insulin receptor gene. Endocr Rev 3:566–595, 1992.

244. Taylor SI: Lilly Lecture: Molecular mechanisms of insulin resistance—lessons from patients with mutations in the insulin receptor gene. Diabetes 41:1473–1490, 1992.

245. Yamada K, Goncalves E, Carpentier JL, et al: Transmembrane domain inversion blocks ER release and insulin receptor signaling. J Biol Chem 34:946–954, 1995.

246. Rothman DL, Magnusson I, Cline G, et al: Decreased muscle glucose transport/phosphorylation is an early defect in the pathogenesis of non–insulin-dependent diabetes mellitus. Proc Natl Acad Sci U S A 92:983–987, 1995.

247. Rothenberg PL, White MF, Kahn CR: The insulin receptor tyrosine kinase. *In* Cuatrecasas P, Jacobs S (eds): Handbook of Experimental Pharmacology. Heidelberg, Springer-Verlag, 1990, pp 209–236.

248. Bruning JC, Michael MD, Winnay JN, et al: A muscle specific insulin receptor knockout challenges the current concepts of glucose disposal and NIDDM pathogenesis. Mol Cell 2:559–569, 1998.

249. Galuska D, Ryder J, Kawano Y, et al: Insulin signaling and glucose transport in insulin resistant skeletal muscle. Special reference to GLUT4 transgenic and GLUT4 knockout mice. Adv Exp Med Biol 441:73–85, 1998.

250. Charron MJ, Katz EB: Metabolic and therapeutic lessons from genetic manipulation of GLUT4. Mol Cell Biochem 182:143–152, 1998.

251. Araki E, Lipes MA, Patti ME, et al: Alternative pathway of insulin signalling in mice with targeted disruption of the IRS-1 gene. Nature 372:186–190, 1994.

252. Tamemoto H, Kadowaki T, Tobe K, et al: Insulin resistance and growth retardation in mice lacking insulin receptor substrate-1. Nature 372:182–186, 1994.

253. Bohni R, Riesgo-Escovar J, Oldham S, et al: Autonomous control of cell and organ size by CHICO, a *Drosophila* homolog of vertebrate IRS1-4. Cell 97:865–875, 1999.

254. Yamauchi T, Tobe K, Tamemoto H, et al: Insulin signaling and insulin actions in the muscles and livers of insulin-resistant, insulin receptor substrate 1–deficient mice. Mol Cell Biol 16:3074–3084, 1996.

255. Withers DJ, Gutierrez JS, Towery H, et al: Disruption of IRS-2 causes type 2 diabetes in mice. Nature 391:900–903, 1998.

256. Rother KI, Imai Y, Caruso M, et al: Evidence that IRS-2 phosphorylation is required for insulin action in hepatocytes. J Biol Chem 273:17491–17497, 1998.

257. Sander M, German MS: The β-cell transcription factors and development of the pancreas. J Mol Med 75:327–340, 1997.

Chapter 51

Glucagon Secretion, α Cell Metabolism, and Glucagon Action

Daniel J. Drucker

OVERVIEW

Glucagon and the glucagon-like peptides (GLPs) are derived from a single proglucagon gene in mammals and exhibit an increasing number of biologically important actions. Glucagon, synthesized principally in islet A cells, is a key regulator of glucose homeostasis through its actions on enzymes that regulate glucose production and glycogen synthesis. GLP-1 and GLP-2 are liberated from intestinal endocrine cells, and regulate glucose homeostasis and intestinal epithelial growth, respectively. These three peptides exert their actions via interaction with unique receptors that exhibit distinct patterns of tissue-specific expression. This chapter reviews our current understanding of the biology of glucagon and the proglucagon-derived peptides (PGDPs), emphasizing recent advances in our understanding of glucagon biosynthesis and action and the emerging biologic importance of the GLPs.

BIOSYNTHESIS OF PANCREATIC GLUCAGON

Proglucagon is encoded by a single gene in mammals that gives rise to a proglucagon messenger RNA (mRNA) transcript that is identical in pancreatic islets, brain, and enteroendocrine cells of the small and large intestine. The proglucagon gene contains six exons, several of which encode distinct functional peptide domains (Fig.

51–1). Glucagon, a 29–amino acid peptide, is synthesized in the A cells of the pancreatic islets of Langerhans. Islet A cells are distinguishable from insulin-producing β cells, in part by the morphology of their respective secretory granules and by their anatomic distribution predominantly at the periphery of the islet. The peripheral location of islet A cells, taken together with functional studies demonstrating central (from a core of β cells) to peripheral (A cells) islet blood flow,[1] raises the possibility of a tightly regulated islet microenvironment. Nevertheless, as the distribution of islet α and β cells may vary from species to species, the functional importance of islet cell distribution remains unclear.

Islet Transcription Factors and the A Cell

The pancreas derives from the upper foregut, with dorsal and ventral pancreatic buds giving rise to pancreatic epithelium that eventually forms the exocrine and endocrine pancreas. This process involves signals from mesenchyme, and requires the correct temporal expression of growth factors, transcription factors, and related signaling molecules. Pancreatic islet cells appear to be of endodermal origin and are first detectable by embryonic day 8.5 in the mouse. Intriguingly, the first islet hormone-immunopositive endocrine cells detectable in developing islets contain glucagon immunoreactivity. Insulin-immunopositive cells are detectable by embryonic day 14 in the mouse, followed several days later by the appearance of somatostatin-containing cell types.[2]

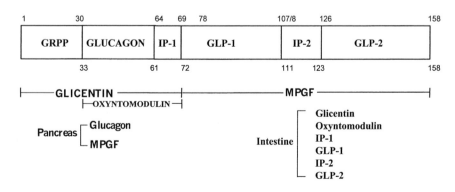

Glucagon   HSQGTFTSDYSKYLDSRRAQDFVQWLMNT
GLP-1   HAEGTFTSDVSSYLEGQAAKEFIAWLVKGRG
GLP-2   HADGSFSDEMNTILDNLAARDFINWLIQTKITD

DPP-IV

FIGURE 51–1. Schematic representation of the proglucagon-derived peptides encoded by the proglucagon gene. The amino acid sequences of human glucagon, glucagon-like peptide-1 (GLP-1), and glucagon-like peptide-2 (GLP-2) are shown. The *arrow* indicates the cleavage site recognized by dipeptidyl-peptidase IV (DPP-IV). IP-1 and IP-2, intervening peptides 1 and 2; MPGF, major proglucagon fragment.

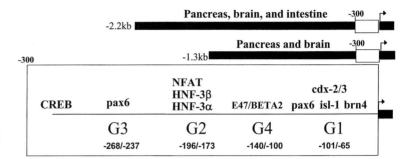

FIGURE 51–2. *Organization of the rat glucagon gene promoter, including the G1–G4 promoter elements, and their cognate transcription factors.*

Although the molecular determinants underlying the anatomic organization of islet cells remain poorly understood, studies of gene disruption in mice have provided new insights into the organization of islet endocrine cells in the pancreas. For example, mice with a null allele in the basic helix-loop-helix (HLH) transcription factor p48 fail to develop exocrine pancreatic tissue; however, hormone-secreting islet cells, including glucagon-producing A cells, are found within the mesentery during embryonic development, and later in the spleen.[3] A key role for cell adhesion molecules in the control of the spatial organization of islet cells is illustrated by analysis of the endocrine pancreas in mice expressing a dominant negative E-cadherin receptor in islet β cells. These mice exhibit abnormal clustering of β cells, yet glucagon-producing α cells are still capable of aggregating into islet-like clusters.[4] In contrast, the normal peripheral distribution of islet α cells is markedly perturbed in neural cell adhesion molecule (NCAM) (−/−)mice; however, the number of α cells and the glucagon content of the pancreas remain unaffected.[5]

Considerable insight into the developmental biology of the endocrine pancreas and islet A cells has been derived from studies of islet transcription factors in mice (Fig. 51–2). Disruption of transcription factor expression via homologous recombination demonstrated that the LIM domain protein *isl*-1 is necessary for the formation of differentiated islet cells, including A cells in the developing pancreas.[6] Remarkably, although mice deficient in the homeobox transcription factor Ipf/Pdx-1 fail to develop a pancreas, a few islet cells, immunopositive for either insulin or glucagon, are observed in Ipf/Pdx-1(−/−) mice at embryonic day 11.[7] These observations suggest that Ipf/Pdx-1 is not essential for the formation of islet A cells.

The homeobox transcription factor *Nkx*2.2 is expressed in adult α, β, and PP islet cells, and mice with targeted disruption of *NKx*2.2 lack β cells, develop diabetes, and exhibit a marked reduction in the numbers of islet α cells.[8] A related phenotype is observed in *NeuroD/BETA2*(−/−) mice, which exhibit marked reductions in the numbers of islet β and α cells and develop diabetes shortly after birth.[9] Similarly, disruption of *pax*6 function in mice results in poorly formed islets with disorganized islet architecture, and markedly reduced but detectable numbers of both β and islet α cells.[10, 11] Intriguingly, mice harboring mutations in islet transcription factors may also exhibit paradoxically increased numbers of islet A cells. For example, mice with a targeted deletion of the *pax*4 gene contain poorly formed islets, with a marked reduction in islet β cells, and comparatively increased numbers of islet A cells.[12] A related phenotype is observed in mice with a homozygous deletion in the glucose transporter-2 (GLUT2) gene, with a marked increase in the ratio of α to β cells observed in GLUT2(−/−) islets.[13] Whether these findings are due to a block in the normal islet differentiation program, or loss of inhibitors that restrain A cell proliferation, is not known. Given the extensive abnormalities that are often evident in transcription factor −/− mice, it is expected that future studies will make more extensive use of tissue- and cell-specific gene targeting, which may permit more detailed analysis of genes important for islet and A cell biology in the embryo and adult mouse.

Proglucagon Gene Transcription Factors

A combination of gene transfection experiments using cell lines in vitro and transgenic studies of promoter function in vivo have yielded considerable insight into the molecular control of glucagon gene transcription. The rat proglucagon gene promoter has been analyzed in considerable detail, and appears to direct transcriptional initiation from a single transcription start site that maps to an identical location in brain, pancreas, and intestine.[14] Cell transfection experiments utilizing islet cell lines have identified four distinct regions, designated G1–G4 (see Fig. 51–2), within the proximal proglucagon promoter that exhibit functional importance for activation of islet cell–specific proglucagon gene transcription.[15, 16] The proximal G1 region is AT-rich, interacts with both widely expressed and islet cell–specific proteins, and is functionally important for specifying expression in islet A cells. G1 interacts with the homeobox transcription factors isl-1, cdx-2/3, brn4, and pax6.[11, 17–20] These transcription factors bind G1 and activate reporter genes containing G$_1$-derived sequences in transfection assays. Reduction of *isl*-1 expression in islet cell lines expressing antisense *isl*-1 RNA leads to reduced G1-dependent proglucagon promoter activity and decreased levels of proglucagon mRNA transcripts.[17] Similarly, increased expression of cdx-3 in islet cells is associated with induction of both transfected G1-dependent reporter genes and endogenous proglucagon gene expression.[18, 21] The G4 element, located just upstream of G1, binds a complex resembling insulin-enhancer factor 1 (IEF1), and recent experiments suggest that IEF1 represents a heterodimer of the HLH proteins E47 and BETA2.[22]

The more distal G3 region functions as an islet enhancer-like element and has been divided into two distinct functional domains. Subdomain A contains a sequence element similar to sequences found within the insulin and somatostatin promoters, leading to the designation of this composite sequence as a *p*ancreatic *is*let cell–specific *e*nhancer *s*equence, or PISCES element.[23, 24] Sequences within domain A of G3 also appear to mediate the inhibition of glucagon gene transcription by insulin.[25–27] The pax6 protein has been identified as a positive activator of proglucagon gene transcription that exerts its function in part through interaction with domain A of the G3 element.[11] pax6 also binds the G1 element, either as a monomer or via heterodimer formation with cdx-2/3.[28] Disruption of *pax*6 expression in gene-targeted mice results in loss of islet A cells.[10, 11] The levels of pancreatic and intestinal proglucagon mRNA transcripts are also markedly reduced in SEY^{NEU} mice that harbor a dominant negative mutation in the *pax*6 gene. Thus pax6, a PISCES binding protein, is functionally important for both islet and enteroendocrine cell development and activation of proglucagon gene transcription via the G3 enhancer and G1 promoter elements.[10, 11, 28, 29]

The G2 element mediates the positive and negative actions of hepatocyte nuclear factor-3 (HNF-3) proteins, with isoforms of HNF-3β and HNF-3α competing for binding to the G2 element and serving as repressors and activators, respectively, of proglucagon gene transcription.[30, 31] HNF-3γ also binds to and transactivates the proglucagon promoter G2 element, but does not appear to be essential to islet cell formation or glucagon gene transcription.[32, 33] Whether HNF-3β plays an essential role in development of islet A cell formation or glucagon gene transcription in vivo remains unknown as targeted inactivation of the HNF-3β gene results in embryonic lethality prior to the formation of the endocrine pancreas.[34, 35] Although the numbers of A cells and the appearance of islets appear histologically normal in HNF3α −/− mice, the development of neonatal hypoglycemia in the face of inappropriately reduced levels of circulating glucagon and proglucagon mRNA transcripts provides importance evidence for the essential role of HNF-3α in pancreatic proglucagon gene transcription.[32]

Activation of the cyclic adenosine monophosphate (cAMP)–dependent pathway leads to transcriptional induction of proglucagon gene expression in both islet and intestinal cells through a cAMP response element (CRE) present, upstream of the G3 element (see Fig. 51–2), in the proximal promoter region of the rat proglucagon gene.[36, 37] The CRE also mediates pharmacologic depolarization-dependent induction of rat proglucagon gene transcription.[38] A second calcium response element has been localized to the G2 element, and calcium responsiveness may be mediated via interaction of NFAT (nuclear factor of activated T cells)-like proteins with members of the HNF-3 family.[39] The sequence of the CRE element is less well conserved in the human proglucagon promoter, and its functional relevance to proglucagon gene expression in human islets has not yet been elucidated.

Transgenic experiments in mice have identified distinct DNA sequences essential for tissue-specific proglucagon gene transcription in vivo. The first 1253 nucleotides of the rat proglucagon promoter direct heterologous transgene expression to the islets and brain but not the intestine in transgenic mice.[40] In contrast, targeting of transgene expression to enteroendocrine cells in vivo requires the presence of additional rat proglucagon gene 5′-flanking sequences between −1253 and −2252.[41] Intriguingly, DNA sequences composing the human proglucagon gene promoter exhibit different functional properties than homologous rat sequences, as the first 1600 bp of the human proglucagon gene 5′-flanking region target transgene expression to appropriate cell types in the brain and intestine, but not the pancreatic islets in transgenic mice.

Islet Proglucagon Biosynthesis

Consistent with the well-described increase in circulating glucagon levels in patients with diabetes, experimental diabetes in rodents is associated with increased levels of pancreatic proglucagon mRNA; correction of the insulin deficiency, but not the hyperglycemia, normalizes the levels of proglucagon mRNA.[42] In contrast to the well-defined role of insulin as a negative regulator of proglucagon biosynthesis, few hormones or metabolites have been identified that clearly increase the synthesis of pancreatic proglucagon in vivo. Although initial experiments using in situ hybridization suggested that 4 days of fasting in the rat leads to a doubling of pancreatic proglucagon mRNA transcript,[43] studies of insulin-induced hypoglycemia failed to demonstrate upregulation of proglucagon mRNA, perhaps due to the confounding inhibitory effects of insulin.[42, 44] Indeed, the majority of studies examining regulators of glucagon secretion fail to demonstrate significant changes in the levels of proglucagon mRNA,[45] suggesting that regulation of secretion, and not biosynthesis, may be a more physiologically relevant locus of control in vivo.

Following transcription of proglucagon mRNA and translation of the proglucagon precursor, 29–amino acid mature glucagon is liberated via posttranslational processing by specific prohormone convertases differentially expressed in the islet α cell. In contrast to processing in the enteroendocrine cell (see Fig. 51–1), the amino acid sequences C-terminal to glucagon remain unprocessed and are secreted as part of a larger polypeptide designated the major proglucagon fragment. Studies using islet cell lines implicate a role for PC2 in processing of proglucagon to glucagon in α cells.[46] The importance of PC2 in the islet A cell was further emphasized by the observation that PC2(−/−) mice exhibit hypoglycemia, α cell hyperplasia, and glucagon deficiency with an accumulation of incompletely processed PGDPs in the pancreas.[47] Whether PC2 directly liberates glucagon from proglucagon, or cleaves proglucagon to glicentin, which is then subsequently processed to glucagon, remains unclear.[47–50] The enzyme PC1 appears to be responsible for cleavage of proglucagon to yield an intestinal profile of PGDPs.[48, 51] The convertases important for proglucagon processing in the brain have not been definitively identified.

GLUCAGON SECRETION

The secretion of glucagon is regulated, both positively and negatively, by neuropeptides, hormones, metabolites, and the autonomic nervous system. The islet A cell plays a central role in the defense of blood glucose, with hypoglycemia stimulating and hyperglycemia suppressing glucagon secretion in vivo. A cells express voltage-dependent Na^+, K^+, and Ca^{2+} channels that interact in the regulation of membrane potential and ultimately, depolarization.[52] Amino acids such as glutamine, alanine, and arginine stimulate both insulin and glucagon secretion, and this observation provides the basis for the use of arginine in the assessment of islet and A cell function in rodent and human physiology.[53] Both α- and β-adrenergic receptors modulate glucagon secretion. Epinephrine stimulates glucagon secretion via a protein kinase A (PKA)–dependent enhancement of Ca^{2+} influx through L-type calcium channels, leading to granule exocytosis.[54] Peptidergic activators of glucagon secretion include cholecystokinin (CCK), pituitary adenylate cyclase–activating polypeptide (PACAP), gastrin, and gastric inhibitory polypeptide (GIP).

In contrast, inhibitors of glucagon secretion include glucose, somatostatin-14, and γ-aminobutyric acid (GABA).[52] Glucose induces GABA release from β cells, providing an indirect mechanism for glucose-mediated suppression of glucagon secretion.[55, 56] Insulin may also directly inhibit glucagon release, possibly via insulin receptors expressed on α cells. The anatomic arrangement of peripheral islet A cell surrounding a core of β cells, taken together with the functional results of immunoneutralization studies, provides additional evidence for intraislet insulin inhibiting downstream A cells.[57]

The effects of glucose on glucagon secretion are integrated with the inhibitory effects of insulin on A cell secretion, as hyperglycemia stimulates insulin secretion, whereas a drop in blood glucose suppresses insulin release from the β cell, thereby relieving the A cell from the tonic inhibitory actions of insulin. These actions are exemplified by meal ingestion, which is associated with increased circulating nutrients, insulin secretion, and reduced levels of circulating glucagon. In contrast, blood glucose is maintained in the fasting state by hepatic glucose production due in part to increased levels of glucagon secretion and suppression of insulin release from the β cell.[58, 59] Consistent with the effect of individual nutrients on A cell function, infusion of arginine stimulates glucagon secretion in both normal subjects and individuals with diabetes mellitus.[59] The response to arginine infusion in normal human subjects, namely stimulation of insulin and glucagon release, is reproducible and as expected, the insulin response is significantly greater, and the glucagon response attenuated, as the glucose concentration increases.[60]

In normal subjects, glucagon secretion rises in the fasting state, and may be further stimulated by exercise, consistent with the physiologic role of glucagon in regulating glucose production. The levels of both glucagon and plasma catecholamines increase with graded exercise in normal human subjects, with the greatest increments in plasma glucagon observed in subjects undergoing prolonged exhaustive exercise.[61] The exercise-induced increment in plasma glucagon appears dependent on the degree and duration of exercise, with some studies demonstrating no significant changes in plasma glucagon during exercise under normoglycemic conditions.[62] Trained healthy male subjects exhibit increased hepatic glucose production following glucagon infusion, implying exercise may be associated with the development of increased glucagon sensitivity.[63] Although prevention of exercise-induced rises in plasma glucagon by concomitant somatostatin infusion may result in mild hypoglycemia,[64] suppression of the rise in plasma glucagon by somatostatin infusion does not always prevent increased hepatic glucose production, likely due to redundant compensatory mechanisms for maintaining normoglycemia.[64, 65]

The control of hepatic glucose production (HGP) is highly sensitive to the glucagon-insulin ratio, and the secretion of these two hormones is generally regulated in a reciprocal manner. The effect of insulin in suppressing HGP may actually be determined in part by the levels of circulating glucagon.[66] Following meal ingestion, nutrient absorption is associated with energy assimilation and suppression of glucagon secretion. Nevertheless, the integrated response of islet A cells is dependent in part on the nutrient composition of the meal, and also reflects positive and negative enteric-derived regulators of glucagon secretion. For example, ingestion of carbohydrate, especially glucose, is associated with a decline in plasma glucagon.[59] Nutrients also promote release of gut-derived peptides such as CCK and GIP that stimulate glucagon release,[67, 68] and GLP-1, which inhibits glucagon release.[69, 70]

Glucagon secretion is increased during times of stress, and "stress-induced hormones" such as cortisol, vasopressin, and β-endorphin, increase glucagon secretion from the A cell. The classic stress hormones epinephrine and norepinephrine also stimulate glucagon secretion, and several distinct mechanisms link the autonomic nervous system to increased secretion from the A cell. Epinephrine secreted from the adrenal medulla increases glucagon secretion in normoglycemic subjects. Furthermore, the pancreas receives innervation from both sympathetic and parasympathetic nerves, and stimulation of these autonomic inputs, all of which are activated by hypoglycemia, increases glucagon secretion.[71] Although specific genetic defects in glucagon secretion have not been described, nondiabetic subjects with mutations in the *MODY1/HNF*-4α gene exhibit decreased arginine-stimulated glucagon secretion and reduced glucose suppression of plasma glucagon,[72] raising the possibility that the HNF-4α transcription factor influences islet α cell function through a direct or indirect mechanism.

Hypoglycemia

Increasing evidence suggests that multiple complementary mechanisms activate A cell secretion during hypoglycemia. Analysis of the glycemic threshold for activation of counterregulatory mechanisms demonstrates that increased epinephrine and glucagon secretion constitute the initial hormonal responses to decreasing blood sugar. Furthermore, the glucose threshold for activation of counterregulatory responses is clearly higher than the threshold for triggering hypoglycemic symptoms in normal subjects.[73] Whether hypoglycemia itself directly stimulates glucagon secretion independent of autonomic input remains unclear. Nevertheless, hypoglycemia suppresses insulin secretion, which removes an important inhibitory influence on glucagon secretion. The finding that A cells express the GLUT1 transporter and glucokinase suggests that glucose transport does not appear to be a critical rate-limiting step for glucose metabolism in A cells, and provides important insight into how A cells directly sense ambient changes in glucose concentrations.[74, 75] Hence, the A cell appears to contain the requisite molecules for sensing and responding to changes in glucose concentrations via glucose metabolism.

The role of circulating epinephrine in the autonomic response to hypoglycemia is well established. Epinephrine also directly stimulates glucagon secretion in normal human subjects, and stimulation of the autonomic sympathetic nervous system innervation to the pancreas elicits an increase in A cell secretion.[76, 77] Furthermore, parasympathetic nerve stimulation, or the neurotransmitter acetylcholine and the neuropeptide VIP (vasoactive intestinal polypeptide), stimulate glucagon secretion. Studies using nerve transection or pharmacologic blockade have illustrated that these pathways exhibit some degree of functional redundancy, providing multiple backup mechanisms to ensure that the A cell responds appropriately to hypoglycemia. Nevertheless, the ganglionic blocker trimethaphan, which impairs autonomic transmission both in ganglia and the adrenal, markedly attenuated the glucagon response to hypoglycemia in normal subjects,[78] emphasizing the important link between autonomic activation and the glucagon counterregulatory response in vivo.

The identity of the specific glucose sensors that trigger the appropriate counterregulatory response to hypoglycemia remains under active investigation. Both the central nervous system (CNS), principally the ventromedial hypothalamus (VMH), and the splanchnic region, specifically the portal system and liver, appear to contain physiologically important glucose-sensing systems. Focal lesions in the VMH, or perfusion of the VMH with 2-deoxyglucose, substantially diminishes or abrogates the peripheral glucagon secretory response to hypoglycemia in rats.[79, 80] Selective perfusion of the portal venous system in rats suggests that the portal vein glucose concentration is a key determinant of the sympathoadrenal response to hypoglycemia, but whether portal glucose sensors are directly or indirectly linked to control of islet glucagon secretion is not clear.[81] Intriguingly, injection of glucose into the portal vein activates glucose-sensitive neurons in the lateral hypothalamus and brain stem, suggesting the possibility of a portal-CNS glucoregulatory axis. The detection of a markedly defective counterregulatory response to hypoglycemia, including absent glucagon and catecholamine secretion, in a patient with hypothalamic sarcoidosis further emphasizes the importance of the hypothalamus in sensing glucose and triggering the release of counterregulatory hormones.[82] Furthermore, human subjects with liver transplants and denervated livers exhibit increased levels of circulating glucagon and defective insulin suppression of glucagon, and human islet transplantation is associated with a defective glucagon response to hypoglycemia.[83, 84] These findings emphasize the importance of the autonomic nervous system and CNS for the regulation of basal and hypoglycemia-stimulated glucagon secretion.

GLUCAGON SECRETION AND DIABETES

Following the development of glucagon radioimmunoassays (RIAs), glucagon levels were noted to be elevated in patients with poorly controlled diabetes, and the lack of the inhibitory action of insulin on the A cell likely contributes to increased glucagon secretion in insulin-deficient diabetic patients. The correction of hyperglucagonemia, using somatostatin pharmacologically or insulin replacement therapeutically, reverses the majority of metabolic derangements associated with insulin-deficient diabetes.[85] These findings have fostered a search for glucagon antagonists that might be employed as adjuncts in the treatment of diabetes, and preliminary evidence obtained using experimental animal models of diabetes suggests the feasibility of this approach in vivo.[86] Despite the central importance of glucagon for control of glucose production, hyperglucagonemia alone, without insulin deficiency, does not significantly increase plasma glucose.[87] In the presence of adequate amounts of insulin, glucose production is suppressible despite glucagon excess, emphasizing the insulin-glucagon ratio, and not just the absolute level of glucagon, as a key determinant of glucose homeostasis.[88] Nevertheless hyperglucagonemia is associated with increased leucine oxidation and resting metabolic rate in subjects with type 1 diabetes, reemphasizing the importance of both insulin and glucagon in the catabolism associated with suboptimally treated diabetes.[89]

The application of intensive insulin therapy to the management of patients with type 1 diabetes has produced an increased incidence of hypoglycemia, and heightened awareness of the importance of counterregulatory mechanisms in maintaining normoglycemia. A number of factors conspire to inhibit glucagon release in insulin-treated patients with type 1 diabetes, including intensive insulin administration, hyperglycemia, and diminished autonomic stimulation of the α cell.[71] Although the glucagon response to hypoglycemia is generally normal in patients with type 1 diabetes of a few years' duration, this response frequently becomes impaired, increasing the susceptibility of patients to hypoglycemia.[90] As intensive insulin treatment regimens become more common, impaired counterregulation and hypoglycemia have been observed in some patients with a very short duration of diabetes, suggesting that frequent episodes of hypoglycemia represent an independent risk for development of an abnormal α cell response. The α cell dysfunction in type 1 diabetes is often selective, as the response to hypoglycemia may be absent, yet glucagon secretion may respond normally to arginine stimulation.[91] Importantly, restoration of normoglycemia for several months may decrease hypoglycemia unawareness in association with improvement in the glucagon response to hypoglycemia in some studies.[92] However, a dissociation between improvement in hypoglycemia unawareness and persistence of defective counterregulatory responses has also been observed.[93]

Multiple defects likely contribute to α cell dysfunction in patients with diabetes. An important issue with therapeutic implications is the understanding of the role of hypoglycemia in the development of α cell dysfunction and deficient glucagon secretion. Patients with some residual β cell function, as assessed by C peptide stimulation, appear to be at decreased risk for hypoglycemia due in part to preserved counterregulatory glucagon responses. Additional contributing factors may include subtle impairment of autonomic stimulation following repeated hypoglycemic episodes. Nevertheless, impaired epinephrine and glucagon responses to insulin-induced hypoglycemia have been observed after a single antecedent hypoglycemic episode in nondiabetic subjects.[94] These observations emphasize the susceptibility of even the normal α cell to episodes of hypoglycemia, with initial reversibility of α cell function superseded, over time, with more sustained defects in the glucagon response to hypoglycemia.

GLUCAGON ACTION

The importance of glucagon in the control of hepatic glucose metabolism provides a useful model for analysis of hormone action in metabolic pathways. Glucagon stimulates glucose production via activation of hepatic glycogenolysis and gluconeogenesis, and by inhibition of glycolysis. Following activation of the glucagon receptor, adenylate cyclase activity is increased, leading to activation of protein kinase A, phosphorylase kinase, and phosphorylase. These actions increase the rate of glycogenolysis via glycogen phosphorylase and inactivate glycogen synthase.[95] Glucagon action serves to modify the activity of enzymes important for glucose production via effects on specific kinases and phosphatases. Glucagon also modulates the expression of genes encoding enzymes of the glycolytic or gluconeogenic pathways[96] and regulates fatty acid metabolism via reduction of malonyl coenzyme A (CoA) and stimulation of fatty acid oxidation.

In adipocytes, glucagon increases cAMP and stimulates lipolysis, thereby providing free fatty acids as substrate for fat-burning tissues. Glucagon also inhibits insulin-stimulated glucose transport in adipocytes through effects on insulin binding and via postreceptor mechanisms.[97] In the peripheral vascular system, glucagon functions as a vasodilator via effects on local vascular tone, and glucagon increases both cardiac output and heart rate, possibly via direct effects on the heart. Pharmacologic doses of glucagon increase renal blood flow, glomerular filtration rate (GFR), and urinary electrolyte excretion, but lower physiologic concentrations of glucagon do not affect renal blood flow, GFR, or solute excretion.[98] The kidney also exhibits significant gluconeogenic capacity and may account for up to 25% of systemic glucose production in humans.[99] Although renal glucose output is markedly increased in subjects with diabetes, and hypoglycemia increases renal glucose output in association with increased release of counterregulatory hormones, the available evidence does not support an important role for glucagon in the control of renal glucose output.[100]

The actions of glucagon are transduced via activation of the glucagon receptor (GR), a seven-transmembrane spanning G protein–coupled receptor. The cloned receptor responds to glucagon with an increase in both intracellular cAMP and intracellular calcium.[101] The human glucagon receptor gene has been localized to chromosome 17q25. Although activating mutations of the GR have been generated by mutagenesis in vitro,[102] no constitutively active GR mutations have been reported in human subjects. Intriguingly, several reports have described an association, initially in populations of French and Sardinian subjects, between a Gly40Ser GR mutation and an increased incidence of type 2 diabetes.[103] Paradoxically, cells expressing a transfected glucagon receptor containing the Gly40Ser mutation exhibit decreased affinity for glucagon in vitro, and subjects with the Gly40Ser mutation exhibit a decreased glycemic response to glucagon infusion in vivo.[104, 105] Furthermore, several population studies have failed to find an association linking the Gly40Ser mutation with an increased prevalence of type 2 diabetes.[104, 106] Hence, whether the Gly40Ser mutation itself contributes to a predisposition, to diabetes, or is associated with other genes that increase diabetes susceptibility in certain populations, remains unclear.

The tissue distribution of GR expression correlates well with results of earlier studies localizing high-affinity glucagon binding sites, with GR mRNA transcripts detected in liver, brain, adipocytes, heart, kidney, and islet β cells. Rat GR mRNA transcripts have also been detected in spleen, thymus, adrenal gland, ovary, and testis, nonclassic target tissues where glucagon action remains poorly defined.[107] Although glucagon action has been extensively studied in the liver and adipocytes, the precise biologic importance of glucagon in the brain remains unclear. The brain stem is the principal site of CNS proglucagon gene expression[108]; however, PGDPs are transported from the brain stem along nerve fibers to multiple brain regions.[109] Consistent with these findings, glucagon binding sites are detected in multiple brain regions[110] and the GR is expressed in cortex, cerebellum, hypothalamus, and brain stem; however, the specific function of glucagon in each of these CNS regions remains unclear. Although intracerebroventricular injection of glucagon in rodents causes hyperglycemia and increases sympathetic nervous system discharge, whether these findings from pharmacologic studies are relevant to physiologic glucose homeostasis requires further analysis.

The β cell expresses receptors for glucagon, GIP, and GLP-1 that are all coupled to cAMP and stimulation of insulin secretion. The threshold for glucagon-stimulated cAMP accumulation in isolated β cells is approximately 1 nM glucagon, higher than the concentrations required for cAMP stimulation by GLP-1 or GIP.[111] The physiologic importance of glucagon for β cell physiology in vivo remains unclear, given the direction of islet blood flow, the peripheral location of islet A cells, and the high concentrations of glucagon required to stimulate the β cell in vitro. Nevertheless, it remains possible that glucagon action on the β cell is also transduced through non–cAMP-dependent pathways, perhaps at a lower-threshold glucagon concentration.

Both the liver and kidney contribute to glucagon clearance from the circulation, but these sites account for less than 50% of glucagon clearance, implicating additional tissues as sites for glucagon clearance or degradation.[112] Glucagon action is terminated via both extracellular and intracellular degradation pathways. Glucagon-degrading activity within hepatic endosomes has been attributed to cathepsins B and D in studies using cathepsin inhibitors,[113] and both glucagon and GLP-1 are substrates for the widely expressed membrane-bound neutral ectopeptidase (NEP) 24.11.[114] An endopeptidase activity has been described that cleaves 29–amino acid glucagon to "miniglucagon," also known as glucagon (19–29) in various tissues. The biologic importance of miniglucagon remains controversial; glucagon (19–29) has positive inotropic actions in ventricular myocyte preparations,[115] and miniglucagon has also been shown to inhibit insulin release via effects on L-type calcium channels in a pertussis toxin–dependent manner.[116, 117] Whether glucagon (19–29) exerts physiologically relevant effects via a separate unique receptor remains unclear.

Pharmaceutic Use of Glucagon in Human Patients

Glucagon is employed as both a diagnostic and therapeutic reagent. Although historically useful for the diagnosis of pheochromocytoma, stimulation of catecholamine secretion in such patients may be dangerous and hence the glucagon stimulation test is not widely used for this purpose. Glucagon may also be employed as part of a diagnostic test in patients with hypoglycemia of unknown origin. Perhaps the most common clinical application of glucagon therapeutically is in the adjunctive management of severe hypoglycemia. Diabetic patients with hypoglycemia generally respond quickly, with a rapid increase in blood glucose, to intranasal, intramuscular, or subcutaneous glucagon administration.[118, 119] Glucagon is also used to inhibit gastrointestinal motility during radiologic investigations, and several studies have reported the efficacy of glucagon administration in small numbers of patients with bronchospasm, or symptomatic bradycardia.[120, 121]

Glucagon Excess and Deficiency

Glucagonomas, presenting as solitary lesions or as part of a multiple endocrine neoplasia syndrome, are most commonly detected in the pancreas, and can be associated with significant elevations in the levels of circulating glucagon and the PGDPs.[122] Rarely, extrapancreatic glucagon-producing tumors have been reported, in sites that include the kidney and ovary. Although many gut carcinoid tumours contain PGDP immunoreactivity, they are not generally associated with the clinical development of a "glucagonoma syndrome." Glucagonoma patients generally present with a pathognomonic skin rash termed *necrolytic migratory erythema*, characterized by a detectable pancreatic mass, weight loss, glossitis, anemia, and some degree of glucose intolerance.[123] The clinical presentation can be variable, likely reflecting adaptation to the metabolic effects of tumor-secreted PGDPS and tumor-specific differences in posttranslational processing of proglucagon. Rarely, patients may present with glucagonomas and associated manifestations of intestinal hyperplasia, presumably due to release of GLP-2.[124] Treatment of benign glucagonomas usually involves surgical resection, whereas chemotherapy, attempted suppression of PGDP secretion and tumor growth with somatostatin analogues, or adjunctive radiotherapy may be indicated in patients with malignant disease. Experimental glucagonomas have also been studied in rodents, and several intriguing phenotypes, including severe anorexia and reduction in islet size, remain poorly understood.[125, 126] Several reports have described isolated cases of glucagon deficiency in infants with hypoglycemia, but these cases are extremely rare. The molecular basis for the putative glucagon deficiency and whether glucagon deficiency is compatible with survival remain unknown.

THE GLUCAGON-LIKE PEPTIDES

The proglucagon gene is expressed in the gastrointestinal tract in the stomach, and both the small and large intestine. The intestinal, brain, and pancreatic proglucagon mRNA transcripts, and by inference, proglucagons, are identical in structure, hence tissue-specific posttranslational processing underlies the liberation of the GLPs in the brain and gastrointestinal tract. In contrast to the pancreas, much less is known about the control of intestinal GLP-1 and GLP-2 biosynthesis. The proglucagon gene islet transcription factors *cdx*-2/3, *pax*6, and members of the HNF-3 family are also expressed in enteroendocrine cells and presumably regulate proglucagon gene transcription in both cell types. Analysis of *SEY^NEU* mice with a dominant negative *pax*6 mutation demonstrated a marked reduction in the levels of proglucagon mRNA transcripts in both small and large intestine. Hence, the *pax*6 gene is essential to both islet and enteroendocrine proglucagon gene transcription. Proglucagon biosynthesis in the gut is regulated by nutrient intake[127] with feeding, and by fiber-enriched diets increasing proglucagon gene expression in the proximal and distal intestine, respectively.

Glucagon-like Peptide I

GLP-1, in both the (7–37) and (7–36^amide) molecular forms, is liberated from proglucagon via posttranslational processing and secreted from intestinal endocrine cells in a nutrient-dependent manner.[128] Although enteroendocrine L cells are distributed along the length of the entire gastrointestinal tract from the stomach to the rectum, the largest numbers of L cells are found in the terminal ileum and proximal colon. The rapid increase in plasma GLP-1 following food ingestion has prompted increasing interest in the existence of a proximal-distal loop, whereby nutrients entering the duodenum and proximal jejunum promote one or more signals that activate GLP-1 secretion from the distal small bowel.[129] Studies in rats have identified GIP as one putative component of such a signaling system. The specific signaling mechanisms utilized by nutrients for stimulation of GLP-1 secretion, perhaps including neural stimuli, are not as completely understood.

The regulation of GLP-1 bioactivity is dependent to a large extent on the rate of GLP-1 degradation in vivo. Both GLP-1 and GLP-2 contain an alanine residue at position 2, rendering these molecules ideal substrates for enzymatic inactivation by dipeptidyl-peptidase IV (DPP-IV). This enzyme, expressed locally in the intestine proximal to sites of GLP-1 synthesis, cleaves circulating GLP-1 to yield the biologically inactive molecule GLP-1 (9–37/9–36^amide).[130, 131] Although GLP-1 (9–37/9–36^amide) displays weak binding affinity for the GLP-1 receptor and is theoretically a circulating antagonist of GLP-1 action, the physiologic importance of circulating GLP-1 (9–37/9–36^amide) has not been established. Nevertheless, a substantial amount of total GLP-1 immunoreactivity circulates as GLP-1 (9–37/9–36^amide), and RIAs that do not distinguish between intact GLP-1 and GLP-1 (9–37/9–36^amide) will overestimate the circulating concentrations of bioactive GLP-1. Due largely to rapid DPP-IV–mediated cleavage of GLP-1,

the half-life of circulating GLP-1 is very short, generally less than 1 minute. These findings, coupled with the proposed pharmaceutic use of GLP-1 for the treatment of diabetes, have encouraged efforts in developing more potent long-acting GLP-1 analogues resistant to DPP-IV–mediated inactivation. Alternatively, inhibitors of the DPP-IV enzyme have also been identified that lower blood sugar and show therapeutic promise in studies of experimental diabetes in rodents.[132]

GLP-1 exerts a number of distinct and complementary actions that serve to control postprandial glycemic excursion (Fig. 51–3). The initial description of GLP-1 bioactivity focused on its actions in the endocrine pancreas, where GLP-1 stimulates glucose-dependent insulin secretion from β cells.[133] GLP-1 also increases proinsulin gene expression and inhibits glucagon secretion, but the mechanism for the effect of GLP-1 on A cells, perhaps indirectly through stimulation of insulin or somatostatin, is not completely delineated.[134] Emerging data raise the possibility that GLP-1 may also play a role in growth and development of pancreatic islets, although the importance of these findings requires further study.

Inhibition of gastric emptying likely accounts for a significant part of the glucose-lowering actions of GLP-1, especially in patients with type 1 diabetes. Indeed, excess GLP-1 administration causes gastric discomfort and cramping in human subjects.[135] Sensations of increased satiety and decreased appetite have also been reported following GLP-1 infusion in human subjects.[136] As GLP-1 administered intracerebroventricularly to rodents inhibits food intake,[137] it remains possible that GLP-1 may decrease appetite via both central effects on the hypothalamic nuclei involved in feeding, and via peripheral effects on gastric emptying. Nevertheless, the end result, namely decreased food intake and a slowing of nutrient transit in the upper gastrointestinal tract, appears to account for a significant portion of the glucose-lowering effect of GLP-1 in vivo. Although administration of GLP-1 and its analogues to rodents also results in decreased water intake, these actions do not appear to be clinically significant in human studies.

GLP-1 exerts its actions through activation of a G protein–coupled receptor structurally related to the glucagon-secretin receptor superfamily.[138] In keeping with studies of glucagon signaling, GLP-1 transduces its signal through both cAMP and calcium-dependent pathways. Although a potential candidate diabetes gene, the GLP-1 receptor (GLP-1R) localized to human 6p21 has not been associated with linkage to families with type 2 diabetes.[139, 140] Similarly, no GLP-1R mutations have been identified in individuals with diabetes, nor have activating mutations of the GLP-1R been described in human subjects. Whether GLP-1 physiologically stimulates cell proliferation in islets remains under investigation; however, GLP-1-dependent activation of the mitogen-activated protein kinase pathway has been described.[141]

Evidence for the physiologic importance of GLP-1 in glucose control derives from studies using GLP-1 antagonists to inhibit GLP-1 action in vivo. Infusion of the GLP-1 antagonist exendin (9–39) into rats or humans increases blood glucose in association with decreased levels of glucose-stimulated insulin.[142, 143] Similarly, immunoneutralization of GLP-1 activity using GLP-1 antiserum increased both fasting and meal-related glycemic excursions in baboons.[144] Furthermore, mice with targeted disruption of the GLP-1 receptor exhibit mild diabetes, with abnormalities in both fasting and postprandial glycemia and subnormal levels of glucose-stimulated insulin.[145] GLP-1R −/− mice do not exhibit changes in insulin sensitivity and basal and glucose-suppressible levels of circulating glucagon are normal. Furthermore, in contrast to the importance of GLP-1 to glucose homeostasis, GLP-1R −/− mice are not obese and do not exhibit abnormalities in food intake, suggesting that long-term disruption of GLP-1 signaling does not produce abnormalities in satiety or body weight.[146]

The multiple actions of GLP-1 in lowering blood glucose in both normal subjects and in patients both with type 1 and type 2 diabetes have raised the possibility that GLP-1 may find a role as a therapeutic agent in diabetes therapy. GLP-1 lowers blood glucose in sulfonylurea-resistant patients, and experimental data from rodents demonstrate that GLP-1 restores glycemic control and increases insulin mRNA in aging rats,[147] providing a rationale for GLP-1 therapy in selected patients with diabetes. Studies in human subjects have demonstrated the safety and efficacy of using GLP-1 to achieve short-term glucose control over several weeks in patients with type 2 diabetes. Nevertheless,

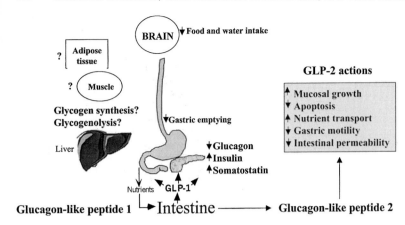

FIGURE 51–3. Biologic actions of the glucagon-like peptides GLP-1 and GLP-2.

GLP-1 is currently administered by injection in the majority of studies, and exhibits a very short half-life in vivo. These limitations emphasize the importance of improving GLP-1 delivery systems, or extending the duration of GLP-1 action through the use of new formulations of GLP-1 analogues to increase the feasibility of developing GLP-1 as a new diabetes therapy.

Glucagon-like Peptide 2

GLP-2 is co-secreted with GLP-1 from intestinal endocrine cells, and is trophic to the mucosal epithelium in both the small and large intestine.[148] The presence of an alanine residue at position 2 (see Fig. 51–1) predicted that GLP-2, like GLP-1, would be a substrate for inactivation by DPP-IV, and significant amounts of biologically inactive GLP-2 (3–33) have been demonstrated in both rodent and human plasma.[149] Similarly, analogues of GLP-2 designed to resist DPP-IV–mediated cleavage are biologically more potent in vivo. Intravenous administration of GLP-2 stimulates intestinal glucose transport within 30 minutes, raising the possibility that GLP-2 exerts both metabolic and growth-promoting actions in the gastrointestinal tract.

The observation that experimental diabetes in rodents is associated with increased mucosal epithelial growth may be explained in part by increased intestinal GLP-2 production, as insulin treatment reverses the changes in mucosal growth and decreases the levels of GLP-2 in rats with diabetes.[150] The importance of GLP-2 for maintenance of the intestinal villous epithelium is further illustrated by studies of rats receiving total parenteral nutrition (TPN), as coinfusion of GLP-2 and TPN prevented mucosal villous hypoplasia in the small intestine.[151] Nevertheless, the physiologic importance of GLP-2 for the physiology or growth of the mucosal epithelium remains unknown, as studies with GLP-2 antagonists or immunoneutralization of GLP-2 have not yet been reported. A G protein–linked GLP-2 receptor, related in sequence to the glucagon and GLP-1 receptors, has recently been isolated, but little is known about the mechanism of GLP-2 action in vivo.[152] Although GLP-2 promotes healing in experimental models of intestinal resection and inflammation,[153, 154] human studies examining the therapeutic potential of GLP-2 administration have not yet been reported.

In summary, the central importance of pancreatic-derived glucagon in the control of glucose homeostasis has focused considerable attention on understanding the physiology of glucagon synthesis, secretion, and action. Furthermore, the delineation of multiple biologic actions of intestinal-derived GLP-1 and GLP-2, and the isolation of distinct receptors for these peptides, has greatly expanded our understanding of the biologic relevance and actions of the PGDPs. It seems reasonable to postulate that additional, as yet undescribed, actions of these and other PGDPs remain to be elucidated. Finally, given the therapeutic potential of both GLP-1 and GLP-2, one or both of these peptides may yet follow glucagon into the clinic as adjunctive therapies for patients with diabetes or intestinal disease, respectively.

REFERENCES

1. Samols E, Stagner JI, Ewart RBL, Marks V: The order of islet microvascular cellular perfusion is B to A to D in the perfused rat pancreas. J Clin Invest 82:350–353, 1988.
2. Edlund H: Transcribing pancreas. Diabetes 47:1817–1823, 1998.
3. Krapp A, Knofler M, Ledermann B, et al: The bHLH protein PTF1-p48 is essential for the formation of the exocrine and the correct spatial organization of the endocrine pancreas. Genes Dev 12:3752–3763, 1998.
4. Dahl U, Sjodin A, Semb H: Cadherins regulate aggregation of pancreatic beta-cells in vivo. Development 122:2895–2902, 1996.
5. Esni F, Taljedal IB, Perl AK, et al: Neural cell adhesion molecule (N-CAM) is required for cell type segregation and normal ultrastructure in pancreatic islets. J Cell Biol 144:325–337, 1999.
6. Ahlgren U, Pfaff SL, Jessell TM, et al: Independent requirement for ISL1 in formation of pancreatic mesenchyme and islet cells. Nature 385:257–260, 1997.
7. Ahlgren U, Jonsson J, Edlund H: The morphogenesis of the pancreatic mesenchyme is uncoupled from that of the pancreatic epithelium in IPF1/IDX1-deficient mice. Development 122:1409–1416, 1996.
8. Sussel L, Kalamaras J, Hartigan-O'Connor DJ, et al: Mice lacking the homeodomain transcription factor Nkx2.2 have diabetes due to arrested differentiation of pancreatic beta cells. Development 125:2213–2221, 1998.
9. Naya FJ, Huang H, Qiu Y, et al: Diabetes, defective pancreatic morphogenesis, and abnormal enteroendocrine differentiation in BETA2/NeuroD-deficient mice. Genes Dev 11:2323–2334, 1997.
10. St-Onge L, Sosa-Pineda B, Chowdhury K, et al: Pax6 is required for differentiation of glucagon-producing α-cells in mouse pancreas. Nature 387:406–409, 1997.
11. Sander M, Neubuser A, Kalamaras J, et al: Genetic analysis reveals that PAX6 is required for normal transcription of pancreatic hormone genes and islet development. Genes Dev 11:1662–1673, 1997.
12. Sosa-Pineda B, Chowdhury K, Torres M, et al: The Pax4 gene is essential for differentiation of insulin-producing β cells in the mammalian pancreas. Nature 386:399–402, 1997.
13. Guillam MT, Hummler E, Schaerer E, et al: Early diabetes and abnormal postnatal pancreatic islet development in mice lacking Glut-2 [see comments] [published errata appear in Nat Genet 17:503, 1997 and 18:88, 1988]. Nat Genet 17:327–330, 1997.
14. Lee YC, Brubaker PL, Drucker DJ: Developmental and tissue-specific regulation of proglucagon gene expression. Endocrinology 127:2217–2222, 1990.
15. Morel C, Cordier-Bussat M, Philippe J: The upstream promoter element of the glucagon gene, G1, confers pancreatic alpha cell–specific expression. J Biol Chem 270:3046–3055, 1995.
16. Philippe J, Drucker DJ, Knepel W, et al: Alpha-cell-specific expression of the glucagon gene is conferred to the glucagon promoter element by the interactions of DNA-binding proteins. Mol Cell Biol 8:4877–4888, 1988.
17. Wang M, Drucker DJ: The LIM domain homeobox gene isl-1 is a positive regulator of islet cell–specific proglucagon gene transcription. J Biol Chem 270:12646–12652, 1995.
18. Jin T, Drucker DJ: Activation of proglucagon gene transcription through a novel promoter element by the caudal-related homeodomain protein cdx-2/3. Mol Cell Biol 16:19–28, 1996.
19. Laser B, Meda P, Constant I, Philippe J: The caudal-related homeodomain protein Cdx-2/3 regulates glucagon gene expression in islet cells. J Biol Chem 271:28984–28994, 1996.
20. Hussain MA, Lee J, Miller CP, Habener JF: POU domain transcription factor brain 4 confers pancreatic α-cell–specific expression of the proglucagon gene through interaction with a novel proximal promoter G1 element. Mol Cell Biol 17:7186–7194, 1997.
21. Jin T, Trinh DKY, Wang F, Drucker DJ: The caudal homeobox protein cdx-2/3 activates endogenous proglucagon gene expression in InR1-G9 islet cells. Mol Endocrinol 11:203–209, 1997.
22. Dumonteil E, Laser B, Constant I, Philippe J: Differential regulation of the glucagon and insulin I gene promoters by the basic helix-loop-helix transcription factors E47 and BETA2. J Biol Chem 273:19945–19954, 1998.
23. Knepel W, Vallejo M, Chafitz JA, Habener JF: The pancreatic islet-specific glucagon G3 transcription factors recognize control elements in the rat somatostatin and insulin-I genes. Mol Endocrinol 5:1457–1466, 1991.

24. Wrege A, Diedrich T, Hochhuth C, Knepel W: Transcriptional activity of domain A of the rat glucagon G3 element conferred by an islet-specific nuclear protein that also binds to similar pancreatic islet cell–specific enhancer sequences (PISCES). Gene Expr 4:205–216, 1995.
25. Philippe J: Glucagon gene transcription is negatively regulated by insulin in a hamster islet cell line. J Clin Invest 84:672–677, 1989.
26. Philippe J, Morel C, Cordier-Bussat M: Islet-specific proteins interact with the insulin-response element of the glucagon gene. J Biol Chem 270:3039–3045, 1995.
27. Philippe J: Insulin regulation of the glucagon gene is mediated by an insulin-responsive DNA element. Proc Natl Acad Sci U S A 88:7224–7227, 1991.
28. Ritz-Laser B, Estreicher A, Klages N, et al: Pax-6 and Cdx-2/3 interact to activate glucagon gene expression on the G1 control element. J Biol Chem 274:4124–4132, 1999.
29. Hill MF, Asa SL, Drucker DJ: Essential requirement for Pax6 in control of enteroendocrine proglucagon gene transcription. Mol Endocrinol 13:1474–1486, 1999.
30. Philippe J, Morel C, Prezioso VR: Glucagon gene expression is negatively regulated by hepatocyte nuclear factor 3b. Mol Cell Biol 14:3514–3523, 1994.
31. Philippe J: Hepatocyte-nuclear factor 3b gene transcripts generate protein isoforms with different transactivation properties on the glucagon gene. Mol Endocrinol 9:368–374, 1995.
32. Kaestner KH, Katz J, Liu Y, et al: Inactivation of the winged helix transcription factor HNF3α affects glucose homeostasis and islet glucagon gene expression in vivo. Genes Dev 13:495–504, 1999.
33. Kaestner KH, Hiemisch H, Schutz G: Targeted disruption of the gene encoding hepatocyte nuclear factor 3γ results in reduced transcription of hepatocyte-specific genes. Mol Cell Biol 18:4245–4251, 1998.
34. Ang SL, Rossant J: HNF-3 beta is essential for node and notochord formation in mouse development. Cell 78:561–574, 1994.
35. Weinstein DC, Ruiz i Altaba A, Chen WS, et al: The winged-helix transcription factor HNF-3 beta is required for notochord development in the mouse embryo. Cell 78:575–588, 1994.
36. Drucker DJ, Jin T, Asa SL, et al: Activation of proglucagon gene transcription by protein kinase A in a novel mouse enteroendocrine cell line. Mol Endocrinol 8:1646–1655, 1994.
37. Knepel W, Chafitz J, Habener JF: Transcriptional activation of the rat glucagon gene by the cyclic AMP-responsive element in pancreatic islet cells. Mol Cell Biol 10:6799–6804, 1990.
38. Schwaninger M, Lux G, Blume R, et al: Membrane depolarization and calcium influx induce glucagon gene transcription in pancreatic islet cells through the cyclic AMP–responsive element. J Biol Chem 268:5168–5177, 1993.
39. Furstenau U, Schwaninger M, Blumes R, et al: Characterization of a novel calcium response element in the glucagon gene. J Biol Chem 274:5851–5860, 1999.
40. Efrat S, Teitelman G, Anwar M, et al: Glucagon gene regulatory region directs oncoprotein expression to neurons and pancreatic alpha cells. Neuron 1:605–613, 1988.
41. Lee YC, Asa SL, Drucker DJ: Glucagon gene 5′-flanking sequences direct expression of SV40 large T antigen to the intestine producing carcinoma of the large bowel in transgenic mice. J Biol Chem 267:10705–10708, 1992.
42. Dumonteil E, Magnan C, Ritz-Laser B, et al: Insulin, but not glucose lowering corrects the hyperglucagonemia and increased proglucagon messenger ribonucleic acid levels observed in insulinopenic diabetes. Endocrinology 139:4540–4546, 1998.
43. Chen L, Komiyo I, Inman L, et al: Effects of hypoglycemia and prolonged fasting on insulin and glucagon gene expression. J Clin Invest 84:711–714, 1989.
44. Shi ZQ, Rastogi KS, Lekas M, et al: Glucagon response to hypoglycemia is improved by insulin-independent restoration of normoglycemia in diabetic rats. Endocrinology 137:3193–3199, 1996.
45. Magnan C, Philippe J, Kassis N, et al: In vivo effects of glucose and insulin on secretion and gene expression of glucagon in rats. Endocrinology 136:5370–5376, 1995.
46. Rouillž Y, Westermark G, Martin SK, Steiner DF: Proglucagon is processed to glucagon by prohormone convertase PC2 in a TC1-6 cells. Proc Natl Acad Sci USA 91:3242–3246, 1994.
47. Furuta M, Yano H, Zhou A, et al: Defective prohormone processing and altered pancreatic islet morphology in mice lacking active SPC2. Proc Natl Acad Sci USA 94:6646–6651, 1999.
48. Dhanvantari S, Seidah NG, Brubaker PL: Role of prohormone convertases in the tissue-specific processing of proglucagon. Mol Endocrinol 10:342–355, 1996.
49. Dhanvantari S, Brubaker PL: Proglucagon processing in an islet cell line: Effects of PC1 overexpression and PC2 depletion. Endocrinology 139:1630–1637, 1998.
50. Rothenberg ME, Eilertson CD, Klein K, et al: Evidence for redundancy in propeptide/prohormone convertase activities in processing proglucagon: An antisense study. Mol Endocrinol 10:331–341, 1996.
51. Rothenberg ME, Eilertson CD, Klein K, et al: Processing of mouse proglucagon by recombinant prohormone convertase 1 and immunopurified prohormone convertase 2 in vitro. J Biol Chem 270:10136–10146, 1995.
52. Rorsman P, Ashcroft FM, Berggren P-O: Regulation of glucagon release from pancreatic A-cells. Biochem Pharmacol 41:1783–1790, 1991.
53. Ward WK, Bolgiano DC, McKnight B, et al: Diminished B cell secretory capacity in patients with noninsulin-dependent diabetes mellitus. J Clin Invest 74:1318–1328, 1984.
54. Gromada J, Bokvist K, Ding W-G, et al: Adrenaline stimulates glucagon secretion in pancreatic A cells by increasing the Ca^{2+} current and the number of granules close to the L-type Ca^{2+} channels. J Gen Physiol 110:217–228, 1997.
55. Smismans A, Schuit F, Pipeleers D: Nutrient regulation of gamma-aminobutyric acid release from islet beta cells. Diabetologia 40:1411–1415, 1997.
56. Gaskins HR, Baldeon ME, Selassie L, Beverly JL: Glucose modulates gamma-aminobutyric acid release from the pancreatic beta TC6 cell line. J Biol Chem 270:30286–30289, 1995.
57. Maruyama H, Hisatomi A, Orci L, et al: Insulin within islets is a physiologic glucagon release inhibitor. J Clin Invest 74:2296–2299, 1984.
58. Marliss EB, Aoki TT, Unger RH, et al: Glucagon levels and metabolic effects in fasting man. J Clin Invest 49:2256–2270, 1970.
59. Unger RH, Aguilar-Parada E, Muller WA, Eisentraut AM: Studies of pancreatic alpha cell function in normal and diabetic subjects. J Clin Invest 49:837–848, 1970.
60. Larsson H, Ahren B: Glucose-dependent arginine stimulation test for characterization of islet function: Studies on reproducibility and priming effect of arginine. Diabetologia 41:772–777, 1998.
61. Galbo H, Holst JJ, Christensen NJ: Glucagon and plasma catecholamine responses to graded and prolonged exercise in man. J Appl Physiol 38:70–76, 1975.
62. Sotsky MJ, Shilo S, Shamoon H: Regulation of counterregulatory hormone secretion in man during exercise and hypoglycemia. J Clin Endocrinol Metab 68:9–16, 1989.
63. Drouin R, Lavoie C, Bourque J, et al: Increased hepatic glucose production response to glucagon in trained subjects. Am J Physiol 274:E23–28, 1998.
64. Hirsch IB, Marker JC, Smith LJ, et al: Insulin and glucagon in prevention of hypoglycemia during exercise in humans. Am J Physiol 260:E695–704, 1991.
65. Coggan AR, Raguso CA, Gastaldelli A, et al: Regulation of glucose production during exercise at 80% of VO_2 peak in untrained humans. Am J Physiol 273:E348–354, 1997.
66. Lewis GF, Vranic M, Giacca A: Glucagon enhances the direct suppressive effect of insulin on hepatic glucose production in humans. Am J Physiol 272:E371–378, 1997.
67. Taminato T, Seino Y, Goto Y, et al: Synthetic gastric inhibitory polypeptide. Stimulatory effect on insulin and glucagon secretion in the rat. Diabetes 26:480–484, 1977.
68. Rossetti L, Shulman GI, Zawalich WS: Physiological role of cholecystokinin in meal-induced insulin secretion in conscious rats. Studies with L 364718, a specific inhibitor of CCK-receptor binding. Diabetes 36:1212–1215, 1987.
69. Wettergren A, Schjoldager B, Mortensen PE, et al: Truncated GLP-1 (proglucagon 78–107-amide) inhibits gastric and pancreatic functions in man. Dig Dis Sci 38:665–673, 1993.
70. Komatsu R, Matsuyama T, Namba M, et al: Glucagonostatic and insulinotropic action of glucagonlike peptide I-(7–36)-amide. Diabetes 38:902–905, 1989.
71. Taborsky Jr GJ, Ahren B, Havel PJ: Autonomic mediation of glucagon secretion during hypoglycemia. Diabetes 47:995–1005, 1998.
72. Herman WH, Fajans SS, Smith MJ, et al: Diminished insulin and glucagon secretory responses to arginine in nondiabetic subjects with a mutation in the hepatocyte nuclear factor-4a/MODY1 gene. Diabetes 46:1749–1754, 1997.
73. Schwartz NS, Clutter WE, Shah SD, Cryer PE: Glycemic thresholds for activation of glucose counterregulatory systems are higher than the threshold for symptoms. J Clin Invest 79:777–781, 1987.
74. Heimberg H, De Vos A, Pipeleers D, et al: Differences in glucose transporter gene expression between rat pancreatic alpha- and beta-cells are correlated to differences in glucose transport but not in glucose utilization. J Biol Chem 270:8971–8975, 1995.
75. Heimberg H, De Vos A, Moens K, et al: The glucose sensor protein glucokinase is expressed in glucagon-producing alpha-cells. Proc Natl Acad Sci USA 93:7036–7041, 1996.
76. Marliss EB, Girardier L, Seydoux J, et al: Glucagon release induced by pancreatic nerve stimulation in the dog. J Clin Invest 52:1246–1259, 1973.
77. Ahren B, Veith RC, Paquette TL, Taborsky GJ Jr: Sympathetic nerve stimulation versus pancreatic norepinephrine infusion in the dog: 2). Effects on basal release of somatostatin and pancreatic polypeptide. Endocrinology 121:332–339, 1987.
78. Havel PJ, Ahren B: Activation of autonomic nerves and the adrenal medulla contributes to increased glucagon secretion during moderate insulin-induced hypoglycemia in women. Diabetes 46:801–807, 1997.
79. Borg WP, During MJ, Sherwin RS, et al: Ventromedial hypothalamic lesions in rats suppress counterregulatory responses to hypoglycemia. J Clin Invest 93:1677–1682, 1994.
80. Borg MA, Sherwin RS, Borg WP, et al: Local ventromedial hypothalamus glucose perfusion blocks counterregulation during systemic hypoglycemia in awake rats. J Clin Invest 99:361–365, 1997.
81. Hevener AL, Bergman RN, Donovan CM: Novel glucosensor for hypoglycemic detection localized to the portal vein. Diabetes 46:1521–1525, 1997.
82. Fery F, Plat L, van de Borne P, et al: Impaired counterregulation of glucose in a patient with hypothalamic sarcoidosis. N Engl J Med 340:852–856, 1999.
83. Perseghin G, Regalia E, Battezzati A, et al: Regulation of glucose homeostasis in humans with denervated livers. J Clin Invest 100:931–941, 1997.
84. Kendall DM, Teuscher AU, Robertson RP: Defective glucagon secretion during sustained hypoglycemia following successful islet allo- and autotransplantation in humans. Diabetes 46:23–27, 1997.
85. Raskin P, Unger RH: Hyperglucagonemia and its suppression. Importance in the metabolic control of diabetes. N Engl J Med 299:433–436, 1978.
86. Van Tine BA, Azizeh BY, Trivedi D, et al: Low level cyclic adenosine 3′,5′-monophosphate accumulation analysis of [des-His1,des-Phe6,Glu9]glucagon-NH_2 identifies glucagon antagonists from weak partial agonists/antagonists. Endocrinology 137:3316–3322, 1996.
87. Sherwin RS, Fisher M, Hendler R, Felig P: Hyperglucagonemia and blood glucose regulation in normal, obese and diabetic subjects. N Engl J Med 294:455–461, 1976.
88. Mittelman SD, Fu YY, Rebrin K, et al: Indirect effect of insulin to suppress endogenous glucose production is dominant, even with hyperglucagonemia. J Clin Invest 100:3121–3130, 1997.
89. Charlton MR, Nair KS: Role of hyperglucagonemia in catabolism associated with type 1 diabetes: Effects on leucine metabolism and the resting metabolic rate. Diabetes 47:1748–1756, 1998.
90. Gerich JE: Lilly lecture 1988. Glucose counterregulation and its impact on diabetes mellitus. Diabetes 37:1608–1617, 1988.
91. Gerich J, Langlois M, Noacco C, et al: Lack of glucagon response to hypoglycemia in diabetes: Evidence for an intrinsic pancreatic alpha cell defect. Science 182:171–173, 1973.

92. Fanelli CG, Epifano L, Rambotti AM, et al: Meticulous prevention of hypoglycemia normalizes the glycemic thresholds and magnitude of most of neuroendocrine responses to, symptoms of, and cognitive function during hypoglycemia in intensively treated patients with short-term IDDM. Diabetes 42:1683–1689, 1993.

93. Dagogo-Jack S, Rattarasarn C, Cryer PE: Reversal of hypoglycemia unawareness, but not defective glucose counterregulation, in IDDM. Diabetes 43:1426–1434, 1994.

94. Heller SR, Cryer PE: Reduced neuroendocrine and symptomatic responses to subsequent hypoglycemia after 1 episode of hypoglycemia in nondiabetic humans. Diabetes 40:223–226, 1991.

95. Bollen M, Keppens S, Stalmans W: Specific features of glycogen metabolism in the liver. Biochem J 336:19–31, 1998.

96. Burcelin R, Katz EB, Charron MJ: Molecular and cellular aspects of the glucagon receptor: Role in diabetes and metabolism. Diabetes Metab 22:373–396, 1996.

97. Sato N, Irie M, Kajinuma H, Suzuki K: Glucagon inhibits insulin activation of glucose transport in rat adipocytes mainly through a postbinding process. Endocrinology 127:1072–1077, 1990.

98. Briffeuil P, Thu TH, Kolanowski J: A lack of direct action of glucagon on kidney metabolism, hemodynamics, and renal sodium handling in the dog. Metabolism 45:383–388, 1996.

99. Stumvoll M, Chintalapudi U, Perriello G, et al: Uptake and release of glucose by the human kidney. Postabsorptive rates and responses to epinephrine. J Clin Invest 96:2528–2533, 1995.

100. Stumvoll M, Meyer C, Kreider M, et al: Effects of glucagon on renal and hepatic glutamine gluconeogenesis in normal postabsorptive humans. Metabolism 47:1227–1232, 1998.

101. Jelinek LJ, Lok S, Rosenberg GB, et al: Expression cloning and signaling properties of the rat glucagon receptor. Science 259:1614–1616, 1993.

102. Hjorth SA, Orskov C, Schwartz TW: Constitutive activity of glucagon receptor mutants. Mol Endocrinol 12:78–86, 1998.

103. Hager J, Hansen L, Vaisse C, et al: A missense mutation in the glucagon receptor gene is associated with non–insulin-dependent diabetes mellitus. Nat Genet 9:299–304, 1995.

104. Tonolo G, Melis MG, Ciccarese M, et al: Physiological and genetic characterization of the Gly40Ser mutation in the glucagon receptor gene in the Sardinian population. The Sardinian Diabetes Genetic Study Group. Diabetologia 40:89–94, 1997.

105. Hansen LH, Abrahamsen N, Hager J, et al: The Gly40Ser mutation in the human glucagon receptor gene associated with NIDDM results in a receptor with reduced sensitivity to glucagon. Diabetes 45:725–730, 1996.

106. Odawara M, Tachi Y, Yamashita K: Absence of association between the Gly40→Ser mutation in the human glucagon receptor and Japanese patients with non–insulin-dependent diabetes mellitus or impaired glucose tolerance. Hum Genet 98:636–639, 1996.

107. Hansen LH, Abrahamsen N, Nishimura E: Glucagon receptor mRNA distribution in rat tissues. Peptides 16:1163–1166, 1995.

108. Drucker DJ, Asa S: Glucagon gene expression in vertebrate brain. J Biol Chem 263:13475–13478, 1988.

109. Larsen PJ, Tang-Christensen M, Holst JJ, et al: Distribution of glucagon-like peptide-1 and other preproglucagon-derived peptides in the rat hypothalamus and brainstem. Neuroscience 77:257–270, 1997.

110. Hoosein NM, Gurd RS: Identification of glucagon receptors in rat brain. Proc Natl Acad Sci USA 81:4368–4372, 1984.

111. Moens K, Heimberg H, Flamez D, et al: Expression and functional activity of glucagon, glucagon-like peptide 1 and glucose-dependent insulinotropic peptide receptors in rat pancreatic islet cells. Diabetes 45:257–261, 1996.

112. Dobbins RL, Davis SN, Neal DW, et al: Compartmental modeling of glucagon kinetics in the conscious dog. Metabolism 44:452–459, 1995.

113. Authier F, Mort JS, Bell AW, et al: Proteolysis of glucagon within hepatic endosomes by membrane-associated cathepsins B and D. J Biol Chem 270:15798–15807, 1995.

114. Hupe-Sodmann K, McGregor GP, Bridenbaugh R, et al: Characterisation of the processing by human neutral endopeptidase 24.11 of GLP-1(7-36) amide and comparison of the substrate specificity of the enzyme for other glucagon-like peptides. Regul Pept 58:149–156, 1995.

115. Sauvadet A, Rohn T, Pecker F, Pavoine C: Synergistic actions of glucagon and miniglucagon on Ca²⁺ mobilization in cardiac cells. Circ Res 78:102–109, 1996.

116. Dalle S, Blache P, Le-Nguyen D, et al: Miniglucagon: A local regulator of islet physiology. Ann NY Acad Sci 865:132–140, 1998.

117. Dalle S, Smith P, Blache P, et al: Miniglucagon (glucagon 19–29), a potent and efficient inhibitor of secretagogue-induced insulin release through a Ca²⁺ pathway. J Biol Chem 274:10869–10876, 1999.

118. Hvidberg A, Djurup R, Hilsted J: Glucose recovery after intranasal glucagon during hypoglycaemia in man. Eur J Clin Pharmacol 46:15–17, 1994.

119. Muhlhauser I, Koch J, Berger M: Pharmacokinetics and bioavailability of injected glucagon: Differences between intramuscular, subcutaneous, and intravenous administration. Diabetes Care 8:39–42, 1985.

120. Melanson SW, Bonfante G, Heller MB: Nebulized glucagon in the treatment of bronchospasm in asthmatic patients. Am J Emerg Med 16:272–275, 1998.

121. Love JN, Sachdeva DK, Bessman ES, et al: A potential role for glucagon in the treatment of drug-induced symptomatic bradycardia. Chest 114:323–326, 1998.

122. Wermers RA, Fatourechi V, Kvols LK: Clinical spectrum of hyperglucagonemia associated with malignant neuroendocrine tumors. Mayo Clin Proc 71:1030–1038, 1996.

123. Mallinson CN, Bloom SR, Warin AP, et al: A glucagonoma syndrome. Lancet 2:1–5, 1974.

124. Drucker DJ: Intestinal growth factors. Am J Physiol 273:G3–G6, 1997.

125. Blume N, Skouv J, Larsson LI, et al: Potent inhibitory effects of transplantable rat glucagonomas and insulinomas on the respective endogenous islet cells are associated with pancreatic apoptosis. J Clin Invest 96:2227–2235, 1995.

126. Ehrlich P, Tucker D, Asa SL, et al: Inhibition of pancreatic proglucagon gene expression in mice bearing subcutaneous endocrine tumors. Am J Physiol Endocrinol Metab 267:E662–E671, 1994.

127. Hoyt EC, Lund PK, Winesett DE, et al: Effects of fasting, refeeding and intraluminal triglyceride on proglucagon expression in jejunum and ileum. Diabetes 45:434–439, 1996.

128. Roberge JN, Brubaker PL: Secretion of proglucagon-derived peptides in response to intestinal luminal nutrients. Endocrinology 128:3169–3174, 1991.

129. Roberge JN, Brubaker PL: Regulation of intestinal proglucagon-derived peptide secretion by glucose-dependent insulinotropic peptide in a novel enteroendocrine loop. Endocrinology 133:233–240, 1993.

130. Deacon CF, Nauck MA, Toft-Nielsen M, et al: Both subcutaneously and intravenously administered glucagon-like peptide 1 are rapidly degraded from the NH₂-terminus in type II diabetic patients and in healthy subjects. Diabetes 44:1126–1131, 1995.

131. Kieffer TJ, McIntosh CHS, Pederson RA: Degradation of glucose-dependent insulinotropic polypeptide and truncated glucagon-like peptide 1 in vitro and in vivo by dipeptidyl peptidase IV. Endocrinology 136:3585–3596, 1995.

132. Holst JJ, Deacon CF: Inhibition of the activity of dipeptidyl-peptidase IV as a treatment for type 2 diabetes. Diabetes 47:1663–1670, 1998.

133. Drucker DJ, Philippe J, Mojsov S, et al: Glucagon-like peptide I stimulates insulin gene expression and increases cyclic AMP levels in a rat islet cell line. Proc Natl Acad Sci USA 84:3434–3438, 1987.

134. Drucker DJ: The glucagon-like peptides. Diabetes 47:159–169, 1998.

135. Willms B, Werner J, Holst JJ, et al: Gastric emptying, glucose responses, and insulin secretion after a liquid test meal: Effects of exogenous glucagon-like peptide-1 (GLP-1)-(7–36) amide in type 2 (non–insulin dependent) diabetic patients. J Clin Endocrinol Metab 81:327–332, 1996.

136. Flint A, Raben A, Astrup A, Holst JJ: Glucagon-like peptide 1 promotes satiety and suppresses energy intake in humans. J Clin Invest 101:515–520, 1998.

137. Turton MD, O'Shea D, Gunn I, et al: A role for glucagon-like peptide-1 in the central regulation of feeding. Nature 379:69–72, 1996.

138. Thorens B, Porret A, Bÿhler L, et al: Cloning and functional expression of the human islet GLP-1 receptor: Demonstration that exendin-4 is an agonist and exendin-(9–39) an antagonist of the receptor. Diabetes 42:1678–1682, 1993.

139. Stoffel M, Espinosa R III, Le Beau MM, Bell GI: Human glucagon-like peptide-1 receptor gene: Localization to chromosome band 6p21 by fluorescence in situ hybridization and linkage of a highly polymorphic simple tandem repeat DNA polymorphism to other markers on chromosome 6. Diabetes 42:1215–1218, 1993.

140. Zhang Y, Cook JTE, Hattersley AT, et al: Non-linkage of the glucagon-like peptide-1 receptor gene with maturity onset diabetes of the young. Diabetologia 37:721–724, 1994.

141. Montrose-Rafizadeh C, Avdonin P, Garant MJ, et al: Pancreatic glucagon-like peptide-1 receptor couples to multiple G proteins and activates mitogen-activated protein kinase pathways in Chinese hamster ovary cells. Endocrinology 140:1132–1140, 1999.

142. Wang Z, Wang RM, Owji AA, et al: Glucagon-like peptide 1 is a physiological incretin in rat. J Clin Invest 95:417–421, 1995.

143. Edwards CM, Todd JF, Mahmoudi M, et al: Glucagon-like peptide 1 has a physiological role in the control of postprandial glucose in humans: Studies with the antagonist exendin 9–39. Diabetes 48:86–93, 1999.

144. D'Alessio DA, Vogel R, Prigeon R, et al: Elimination of the action of glucagon-like peptide 1 causes an impairment of glucose tolerance after nutrient ingestion by healthy baboons. J Clin Invest 97:133–138, 1996.

145. Scrocchi LA, Brown TJ, MacLusky N, et al: Glucose intolerance but normal satiety in mice with a null mutation in the glucagon-like peptide receptor gene. Nat Med 2:1254–1258, 1996.

146. Scrocchi LA, Drucker DJ: Effects of aging and a high fat diet on body weight and glucose control in GLP-1R-/-mice. Endocrinology 139:3127–3132, 1998.

147. Wang Y, Perfetti R, Greig NH, et al: Glucagon-like peptide-1 can reverse the age-related decline in glucose tolerance in rats. J Clin Invest 99:2883–2889, 1997.

148. Drucker DJ, Ehrlich P, Asa SL, Brubaker PL: Induction of intestinal epithelial proliferation by glucagon-like peptide 2. Proc Natl Acad Sci USA 93:7911–7916, 1996.

149. Brubaker PL, Crivici A, Izzo A, et al: Circulating and tissue forms of the intestinal growth factor, glucagon-like peptide 2. Endocrinology 138:4837–4843, 1997.

150. Fischer KD, Dhanvantari S, Drucker DJ, Brubaker PL: Intestinal growth is associated with elevated levels of glucagon-like peptide-2 in diabetic rats. Am J Physiol 273:E815–E820, 1997.

151. Chance WT, Foley-Nelson T, Thomas I, Balasubramaniam A: Prevention of parenteral nutrition–induced gut hypoplasia by coinfusion of glucagon-like peptide-2. Am J Physiol 273:G559–G563, 1997.

152. Munroe DG, Gupta AK, Kooshesh P, et al: Prototypic G protein–coupled receptor for the intestinotrophic factor glucagon-like peptide 2. Proc Natl Acad Sci USA 96:1569–1573, 1999.

153. Scott RB, Kirk D, MacNaughton WK, Meddings JB: GLP-2 augments the adaptive response to massive intestinal resection in rat. Am J Physiol 275:G911–G921, 1998.

154. Drucker DJ, Yusta B, Boushey RP, et al: Human [Gly2]-GLP-2 reduces the severity of colonic injury in a murine model of experimental colitis. Am J Physiol 276:G79–G91, 1999.

Chapter 52

Regulation of Intermediary Metabolism During Fasting and Feeding

Ralph A. DeFronzo ▪ Eleuterio Ferrannini

In the fasting or postabsorptive state, the fasting plasma glucose concentration in a healthy adult is maintained within a very narrow range, 65 to 105 mg/dL (3.6–5.8 mmol/L). Under basal conditions, insulin-independent tissues such as the brain (50%–60%) and splanchnic organs (20%–25%) account for the majority of total body glucose utilization. Muscle, an insulin-dependent tissue, is responsible for most of the remaining 20% to 25% of glucose disposal in the fasting state.[1–3] The basal rate of tissue glucose uptake is precisely equaled by an equivalent rate of glucose output by the liver (80%–85%) and the kidney (15%–20%). After the ingestion or infusion of glucose, this delicate balance between hepatic glucose production (HGP) and tissue glucose utilization is disrupted, and maintenance of normal glucose homeostasis in the fed state depends on three processes that occur simultaneously and in a coordinated, tightly integrated fashion: (1) in response to hyperglycemia, insulin secretion is stimulated; (2) the combination of hyperinsulinemia and hyperglycemia augments glucose uptake by splanchnic (liver and gut) and peripheral (primarily muscle) tissues; and (3) both insulin and glucose suppress HGP. In this chapter we review the whole body and cellular mechanisms by which pancreatic hormones (insulin and glucagon) regulate the normal trafficking of substrates between the splanchnic tissues (liver and gastrointestinal tract) and the glucose-using organs in fed and fasting conditions.

ENERGY METABOLISM

All living organisms require a constant source of energy to maintain their viability. In humans this energy comes in the form of ATP, which is derived from the oxidation of foodstuffs. Because humans feed intermittently, it is necessary to build up a sufficient energy reservoir to supply a constant input of metabolic fuels for oxidation during the interfeeding period. To accomplish this goal the body has developed an intricate metabolic network with multiple checks and balances—hormonal, neural, and substrate—that ensure a steady supply of metabolic fuels to the tissues. This arrangement is particularly crucial for the brain and other neural tissues that use glucose exclusively as their energy source except under unusual conditions of prolonged fasting, when ketone bodies can substitute in part for glucose. Because of the unique dependence of the brain on glucose and because of the intermittent feeding behavior of humans, it is necessary that humans ingest more calories than necessary for immediate energy use and store the excess calories in body depots, which can be mobilized efficiently at a later time for use by the tissues of the body.

From a quantitative standpoint, fat represents the major energy source within the body (Table 52–1). The average 70-kg person who is of ideal body weight possesses approximately 12 kg of triglyceride, which is stored within adipose tissue.[4] If this fat were completely mobilized and oxidized, it would provide approximately 110,000 kcal. Assuming an average metabolic rate of about 2000 kcal/day, this source would be sufficient to sustain the body's energy needs for about 55 days. In addition to its abundance, fat is a more efficient energy source than either glycogen or protein because 9.5 kcal is generated for every gram of fat that is completely oxidized. The comparable energy value for glycogen and protein is 4 kcal/g. Moreover, fat is a less cumbersome storage form of energy because it exists in a nearly anhydrous form in the adipocyte, whereas each gram of glycogen and protein requires about 3 g of water. From these considerations it is obvious that the caloric density of adipose tissue (approximately 8.5 kcal/g of fat) is much greater than the caloric density of either glycogen or protein (approximately 1 kcal/g). Viewed another way, if one were to replace the amount of energy stored in fat with an equivalent amount of energy in the form of glycogen or protein, the body weight of our hypothetic 70-kg man would expand to 196 kg. Such a modification would have major adaptive disadvantages for a species that depends on mobility for survival.

Because the major storage form of energy in the body is fat but the brain and other neural tissues have an obligate need for glucose, the body must have a readily available form of carbohydrate, which is provided by glycogen. In a 70-kg man, approximately 80 g of carbohy-

TABLE 52–1. Tissue and Circulating Energy Content Provided by the Three Major Fuels: Fat, Carbohydrate, and Protein

Tissue	Fuel	Mass (g)	Energy (kcal)
Depots			
Adipose	Triglyceride	12,000	110,000
Muscle	Protein	6000	24,000
Muscle	Glycogen	400	1600
Liver	Glycogen	80	320
Circulation			
Blood	Glucose	20	80
Blood	Fatty acids	0.3	3
Blood	Triglycerides	3	30
Blood	Ketones	0.2	0.8
Blood	Amino acids	6	24

Adapted from Ruderman NB, Tornheim K, Goodman MN: Fuel homeostasis and intermediary metabolism of carbohydrate, fat, and protein. *In* Becker KL (ed): Principles and Practice of Endocrinology and Metabolism. Philadelphia, JB Lippincott, 1992, pp 1054–1064.

drate is stored as liver glycogen and 400 g as muscle glycogen.[4] Because muscle does not contain glucose-6-phosphatase, it cannot generate free glucose for transportation to other tissues. However, glycogenolysis in muscle can provide a readily available source of glucose for local needs in response to acute muscular activity. In addition, muscle-derived lactate, pyruvate, and alanine can be transported via the blood to the liver, where they are used for gluconeogenesis during starvation. In contrast to muscle, the liver contains the necessary enzymatic machinery to produce free glucose from glycogen and to form new glucose from gluconeogenesis precursors. Thus, for short-term metabolic needs, liver glycogen represents the principal carbohydrate reservoir for the energy needs of the brain. As can be seen in Table 52–1, the amount of energy contained in circulating glucose is quite small.

Glycogen metabolism is controlled by a cascade of reversible phosphorylation-dephosphorylation reactions that ultimately converge on the more proximal enzymes that catalyze glycogen synthesis (glycogen synthase) and glycogen degradation (glycogen phosphorylase). Both the synthesis and breakdown of glycogen are regulated by multiple, complex interacting mechanisms involving substrates as well as hormones and neural input. In subsequent sections of this chapter we review certain key aspects of the control of glycogen metabolism.

From a purely theoretic standpoint, protein also represents a large reservoir of energy. A 70-kg man possesses about 6 kg of protein with a potential energy value of 24,000 kcal.[4] However, each protein in the body has a specific function, such as an integral constituent of cell membranes and organelles; an enzyme; a specific transporter of some essential nutrient, element, or vitamin; or a contractile element, specifically, actin or myosin. Excessive breakdown of protein would lead to disruption of normal cell function and eventually to death. Therefore the body has developed a complex metabolic and hormonal response to fasting that minimizes proteolysis and the release of amino acids. Thus when fasting is prolonged beyond 2 to 3 days, a major shift occurs from carbohydrate to fat and ketone body utilization. After 1 to 2 weeks of starvation, the rates of gluconeogenesis and glucose utilization are markedly reduced and ketone bodies become an important substrate for the energy needs of the brain and other neuronal tissues. However, the brain always maintains a need for some glucose. Acetone, which is formed by the nonenzymatic decarboxylation of acetoacetic acid, can serve as a gluconeogenetic precursor by being converted to pyruvoaldehyde in the liver or to 1,2-propanediol in extrahepatic tissues. The rise in circulating blood ketone levels also provides a signal to the muscle to inhibit protein catabolism, thus sparing amino acids for vital cell functions.

GLUCOSE DISTRIBUTION

Carbohydrates, protein, and fat represent the triad of major metabolic fuels. As a metabolic substrate, carbohydrate is present in organisms in its simple monomeric form, α-D-glucopyranose, and as a branched polymer of α-glucose, namely, glycogen. Disaccharides of glucose include lactose, maltose, and sucrose, but these substances are quantitatively less important. In normal healthy subjects, glucose circulates in plasma water at a basal concentration that ranges from 65 to 105 mg/dL (3.6–5.8 mmol/L). After a meal the plasma glucose concentration does not exceed 160 to 180 mg/dL (8.9–10 mmol/L) in normal, healthy individuals. Circulating plasma glucose is in rapid equilibrium with the red blood cell (RBC) glucose concentration.[3] A non–insulin-regulatable transporter effects the facilitated diffusion of glucose from plasma water into the RBC.[5] Because of the abundance of this transporter in erythrocytes, glucose diffuses very rapidly across RBC membranes, with an estimated equilibration time of only 4 seconds. After its transport into the cell, the rate of glucose utilization via glycolysis has been estimated to be about 25 mmol/min or 6 mmol/min/m² of diffusion surface (the total RBC mass is approximately 5 × 10⁹ cells, and each RBC has a mean diameter of 7 mm with a spherical shape that occupies a surface area of approximately 4 m²).[3] Because this rate is about 17,000 times slower than the rate of glucose transport into the erythrocyte, the glucose concentration is, in general, the same in plasma and erythrocyte water. Plasma proteins account for

some 8% of plasma volume, whereas RBC proteins and ghosts occupy about 38% of the packed red cell volume (which in turn averages 40% of the total blood volume). Thus 20% (that is, [0.38 × 0.4] + [0.08 × 0.6] = 0.2) of the total blood volume is inaccessible to glucose. It follows that the glucose concentration should be identical in plasma and RBC water under most circumstances and that a *blood* water glucose concentration of 90 mg/dL (5.0 mmol/L) translates into a *plasma* glucose concentration of 83 mg/dL (4.6 mmol/L) and a *whole blood* glucose concentration of 72 mg/dL (4.0 mmol/L), that is, a 15% systematic difference between plasma and whole blood glucose concentration under typical conditions of hematocrit, proteinemia, and erythrocyte volume.

GLUCOSE METABOLISM: METHODOLOGIC CONSIDERATIONS

Because both RBCs and plasma convey glucose, the total amount of the sugar reaching any given organ is the product of the arterial whole blood glucose concentration times the total blood flow to that organ. Similarly, the total amount of glucose leaving a body region is the product of the whole blood glucose level in the venous effluent times the blood flow rate. Therefore, it follows that the net balance of glucose movement across a body region is the product of blood flow and the arteriovenous whole blood glucose concentration difference; this relation constitutes the Fick principle (Fig. 52–1). It should be emphasized that the use of *plasma* flow rates and plasma glucose concentrations systematically underestimates the net organ balance of glucose (and for that matter, the net organ balance of any substance that is transported in plasma as well as in erythrocytes, such as lactate and some amino acids). Because plasma flow is less than blood flow by an amount equal to the hematocrit (approximately 40%) whereas the plasma glucose concentration is higher than whole blood glucose by only 15% (0.6 × 1.15 = 0.69), the net organ balance is underestimated by 31%.

In muscle, which does not contain glucose-6-phosphatase, the net organ balance is equivalent to the amount of glucose that is taken up and metabolized. The liver, however, can undergo simultaneous uptake and release, that is, from hepatic glycogen stores or from gluconeogenesis. By combining the organ balance technique with radiolabeled glucose, one can calculate the uptake of glucose by an organ bed according to the following equation[6]:

Uptake = (FE) × (blood flow) × (arteriovenous glucose concentration)

where FE equals the fractional extraction of tracer glucose and is calculated as

$$\frac{A^* - V^*}{A^*}$$

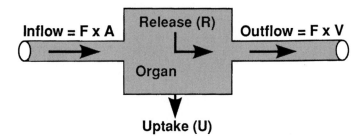

Net Balance = Uptake - Release = (Flow) (A-V)

Inflow = F x A   Release (R)   Outflow = F x V

Organ

Uptake (U)

FIGURE 52–1. *Schematic representation of substrate (glucose) exchange across an organ (the liver) that both irreversibly removes the substrate (glucose) and adds it to the systemic circulation. A, arterial concentration; F, blood flow; V, venous concentration.*

where A* and V* represent the radioactivity of labeled glucose in the artery and vein, respectively. If one knows the net balance of glucose (or any other substrate) across an organ bed and the unidirectional uptake, one can calculate the release of glucose (or any other substrate) according to the following relationship (see Fig. 52–1).

$$\text{Net balance} = \text{uptake} - \text{release}$$

By using the catheter technique to measure the net organ balance of glucose in combination with radiolabeled glucose, much information can be gained about the interorgan exchange of glucose and other substrates, as well as the metabolic pathways involved in the regulation of glucose utilization.

The use of a radioisotope also allows one to measure whole body glucose (or other substrate) turnover.[7] Because of its simplicity, the isotope dilution method has become popular among clinical investigators and has generated large amounts of information. It therefore warrants a brief description here; a more detailed explanation of the tracer technique, as applied to glucose turnover measurement, can be found elsewhere.[7] The choice of a tracer is dictated by cost, ease of measurement, and safety (radiation burden to the patient). The tracer can be administered as a pulse injection or constant intravenous infusion, depending on the type of information desired. For metabolic studies a prime-continuous infusion is generally used. When both the tracer (cold glucose) and tracee (radiolabeled glucose) are in steady state, the glucose turnover rate (milligrams per minute) is calculated simply by dividing the tracer infusion rate (in disintegrations per minute) by the equilibrium specific activity of plasma glucose (in disintegrations per milligram). In normal healthy subjects, equilibrium represents the time (usually about 2 hours after starting the tracer and tracee infusion) when unchanging plasma tracer and tracee concentrations indicate that the specific activity of glucose has become uniform throughout its distribution space. Calculation of the turnover rate as described above (infusion rate divided by the specific activity in plasma) is not based on any assumptions and can be used to quantitate glucose turnover in the postabsorptive state. When non–steady-state conditions prevail, this approach cannot be used. Such is the case after glucose ingestion or infusion. Practical ways to circumvent this problem, however, have been developed. Their common rationale is provided by the theory that the degree and rate of change in the specific activity of glucose are the principal factors that affect non–steady-state analysis of isotope data. The larger the swing in specific activity of glucose, the more uncertain the estimation of actual rates of glucose appearance and disappearance from plasma data. All of the formal models that have been proposed to represent the glucose system become progressively weaker as the specific activity of glucose in plasma is allowed to fluctuate freely. Therefore, one of two strategies can be used: either tracer administration is repeated when the glucose system has reached a new, reasonably steady state, or radioactive and cold glucose infusion rates can be adjusted empirically to "clamp" the specific activity of plasma glucose constant at the basal level. In both cases the aim is to minimize changes in the specific activity of glucose, thereby meeting the conditions under which steady-state equations can be used reliably. Therefore, in reporting results of glucose turnover obtained under non–steady-state conditions, we must make some selection of available data.

GLUCOSE METABOLISM: BASAL (POSTABSORPTIVE) STATE

Glucose Production

By convention, the basal or postabsorptive state is defined as the metabolic condition that prevails in the morning after an overnight (10- to 14-hour) fast. For most individuals this time represents the longest period of fasting in everyday life. For the rest of the day most people are more or less in the fed state. Maintenance of the fasting plasma glucose concentration is primarily the responsibility of the liver,[1, 8] although recent studies have demonstrated that as much as 15% to 20% of basal glucose production is derived from the kidney.[9]

The liver provides glucose for all tissues of the body either by breaking down its own stores of glycogen or by synthesizing glucose from gluconeogenetic precursors, the most important of which are lactate, pyruvate, glycerol, alanine, and other gluconeogenetic amino acids. Glucose production from the kidney is primarily derived from gluconeogenesis. The central role of the liver in providing a constant supply of glucose to the body is related to the presence of glucose-6-phosphatase, which catalyzes the conversion of glucose 6-phosphate (G-6-P) to glucose within the hepatocyte. Although a number of tissues, including muscle and adipocytes, possess the enzymatic machinery necessary to degrade glycogen and to synthesize G-6-P from lactate and amino acids, they either completely lack or possess too little of the key enzyme glucose-6-phosphatase to release significant amounts of free glucose into the circulation. The kidney, like the liver, also possesses the necessary enzymatic apparatus to produce glucose via the gluconeogenetic pathway, although its contribution to the maintenance of basal plasma glucose levels is small in comparison to that of the liver. During prolonged starvation and during metabolic acidosis, renal gluconeogenesis is enhanced and the contribution of the kidney to basal glucose production is increased. Unlike in the liver, the major gluconeogenetic precursor for the kidney is glutamine.

Under postabsorptive conditions, glucose output in healthy adults averages approximately 150 mg/min (approximately 840 mmol/min) or 2.16 mg/min/kg of body weight (12 mmol/min/kg) in a 70-kg individual (Fig. 52–2), and as described above, this glucose is derived primarily from the liver.[1, 8] The variation around this mean is significant (20%–30%), with an unknown contribution of genetic and environmental factors. Little information is available concerning how much the fasting glucose output varies as a consequence of changes in dietary habits, caloric intake, or physical fitness. Intrafamilial covariance of this physiologic variable is also undetermined. Under standard nutritional conditions, the normal liver contains about 80 g of glycogen (see Table 52–1), and during fasting it depletes its liver glycogen stores at a rate of about 110 mg/min (0.6 mmol/min), or 11% per hour.[10] Therefore, it follows that hepatic glycogen depots would become empty after about 12 hours. Because fasting can be prolonged well beyond 12 hours, it is obvious that gluconeogenesis must progressively replace glycogenolysis as the fast continues.[10] In animal species in which the basal rate of glucose turnover is higher than in humans, for example, in dogs (3.6 mg/min/kg) and rats (7.2 mg/min/kg), the limited capacity of the liver to store glycogen confers an increasing role of gluconeogenesis for the maintenance of basal glycemia. This limitation on glycogen accumulation has an anatomic basis in that overcrowding of the cytoplasm with glycogen granules impairs cellular function and results in liver damage, as demonstrated in patients with glycogen storage diseases. In healthy subjects after a 10- to 12-hour overnight fast, gluconeogenesis accounts for approximately 50% of total hepatic glucose release[10] (see Fig. 52–2). The substrates for this

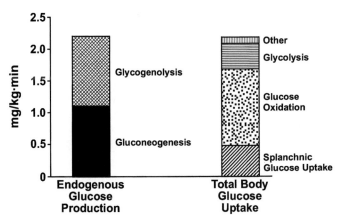

FIGURE 52–2. *Hepatic glucose production and tissue glucose uptake in the postabsorptive state in healthy subjects. See the text for more detailed discussion. (From DeFronzo RA, Bonadonna RC, Ferrannini E: Pathogenesis in NIDDM: A balanced overview. Diabetes Care 15:318–368, 1992. © 1992 by the American Diabetes Association, Inc.)*

de novo glucose synthesis remain somewhat elusive. Circulating lactate, pyruvate, glycerol, alanine, and other gluconeogenetic amino acids are natural candidate precursors and have been shown to transfer their carbons to newly synthesized glucose molecules, as documented by the incorporation of labeled lactate into glucose, that is, the Cori cycle. However, transsplanchnic catheterization in humans and dogs has shown that the net uptake of known circulating gluconeogenetic precursors (lactate, pyruvate, glycerol, amino acids) can account for only about 15% to 20% of the total endogenous glucose production.[11] The discrepancy (180–360 μg/min/kg or 1–2 μmol/min/kg) between radioisotopic estimates of the basal gluconeogenetic rate and accountable circulating precursors suggests that the bloodborne substrates may not be the only source of gluconeogenetic precursors. Within the splanchnic area the intestine returns 10% to 20% of its glucose uptake to the liver as lactate (90 μg/min/kg or 0.5 μmol/min/kg), but this amount fills only part of the gap. It has been suggested that intrahepatic proteolysis and/or lipolysis could provide ample amounts of gluconeogenetic precursors, in addition to those entering from the systemic circulation.[11]

Regulation of basal HGP is controlled by the sum of several neural, hormonal, and metabolic stimuli, some stimulatory and others inhibitory.[8] Figure 52–3 portrays the control system as a simple balance between inhibition and stimulation. Insulin and glucagon provide the primary hormonal signals that regulate production of glucose by the liver under postabsorptive conditions. Of the two, the action of insulin is predominant. HGP is exquisitely sensitive to very small fluctuations in the circulating plasma insulin concentration. Increments in the plasma insulin concentration of as little as 5 to 10 μU/mL cause a marked, rapid suppression of glycogenolysis and decline in hepatic glucose output, whereas inhibition of gluconeogenesis is less sensitive. Regulation of renal glucose production appears to be similar to that of the liver in that it is stimulated by epinephrine and inhibited by insulin.[9]

Moreover, by restraining lipolysis and proteolysis, insulin also reduces the delivery of potential glucose precursors (glycerol and amino acids) from peripheral tissues (adipocytes and muscle) to the liver, which further reduces hepatic glucose output. In its capacity as the inhibitory signal for glucose release, insulin is greatly favored by the anatomic connection between the pancreas and the liver. Because the pancreatic vein is a tributary of the portal vein, insulin that is secreted by β cells reaches the liver in fasting humans at a concentration that is three to four times higher than the peripheral (arterial) concentration. This steep portosystemic gradient is maintained by the high rate of insulin degradation by hepatic tissues (fractional insulin extraction = 50%). Consequently, a small secretory stimulus to β cells disproportionately raises the portal insulin concentration, thereby selectively acting on glucose production rather than enhancing peripheral glucose utilization. In addition to short-circuiting the general circulation, pancreatic insulin release is potentiated by a number of gastrointestinal hormones (such as glucagon-like peptide, cholecystokinin-pancreo-

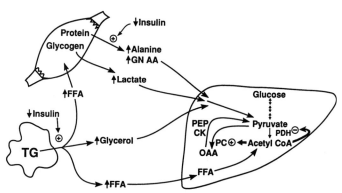

FIGURE 52–4. Metabolic changes during fasting. In the fasting state the decline in basal plasma insulin concentration removes the inhibitory effect of the hormone on lipolysis, and plasma glycerol and free fatty acid (FFA) levels rise. In the hepatocyte, enhanced delivery of FFAs in combination with a decreased insulin-to-glucagon ratio stimulates β oxidation and thereby leads to the accumulation of acetyl coenzyme A (acetyl-CoA). Increased acetyl-CoA, by inhibiting pyruvate dehydrogenase (PDH) and stimulating pyruvate carboxylase in the liver, shuttles pyruvate into the gluconeogenic pathway. Hypoinsulinemia also stimulates proteolysis in muscle, and the enhanced delivery of alanine, other gluconeogenic (GN) amino acids, glycerol, and lactate from peripheral tissues provides the substrates for accelerated hepatic gluconeogenesis.

zymin, gastric inhibitory polypeptide, and secretin) released in response to meal ingestion. Therefore, the anatomic and physiologic connections that constitute the gut-liver-pancreas axis ensure that the primary station for the handling of foodstuff, namely, the liver, is under close control by a nearby, well-informed unit, the β cell.

Conversely, small decrements in the plasma insulin concentration, as little as 1 to 2 μU/mL, lead to a rise in HGP.[12] This highly sensitive interaction between the liver and insulin plays a critical role in the maintenance of fasting glucose levels when fasting is prolonged.[12] As glycogen stores become depleted, the subsequent small decrease in arterial glucose concentration in turn leads to a decline in pancreatic insulin secretion and stimulation of glucagon release. The resultant hypoinsulinemia removes the constraint on lipolysis, and plasma free fatty acid (FFA) levels rise. By mass action FFAs enhance their own uptake by all cells in the body, including liver and muscle. Enhanced FFA oxidation by hepatocytes provides an energy source to drive gluconeogenesis, and the end product of β oxidation, acetyl coenzyme A (acetyl-CoA), stimulates the first committed enzyme, pyruvate carboxylase, in the gluconeogenetic pathway[1, 2] (Fig. 52–4). The combination of hypoinsulinemia, hypoglycemia, and increased FFA as well as amino acid concentration also stimulates hepatic gluconeogenesis.[10] In peripheral tissues, enhanced FFA and ketone oxidation spares glucose utilization (Randle cycle; see the subsequent discussion), thereby minimizing the need for carbohydrate as an energy source.[1, 2]

Another important consequence of the fasting-related decline in plasma insulin concentration is the stimulation of proteolysis.[12] Proteolysis augments the muscle outflow of amino acids, especially alanine, which accounts for approximately 50% of total α-amino nitrogen release. The predominance of alanine in the amino acid efflux from muscle cannot be explained by its presence in cellular proteins, of which alanine accounts for only 7% to 10%. The major source of alanine outflow from muscle during starvation is derived from the transamination of glucose-derived (from muscle glycogen and circulating glucose) pyruvate. The branched-chain amino acids (valine, leucine, isoleucine) provide the amino groups for muscle alanine synthesis. The alanine that is released from muscle is transported via the blood steam to the liver, where it is converted to glucose, thus completing the *glucose-alanine cycle*[9, 13] (see Fig. 52–4).

The *glucose-lactate cycle* (Cori cycle) also provides an important source of three-carbon skeletons for gluconeogenesis during fasting.[12, 13] Insulinopenia enhances the breakdown of glycogen and leads to the accumulation of pyruvate. Because the Krebs cycle has been inhibited by the accelerated rate of FFA oxidation (Randle cycle),

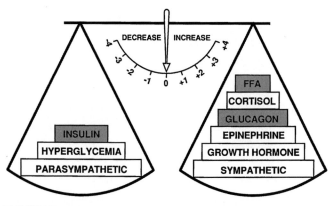

FIGURE 52–3. Balance of factors that regulate hepatic glucose production. Stimulatory factors are shown by the positive numbers to the right; inhibitory factors, of which insulin is dominant, are shown by the negative numbers to the left.

the pyruvate can be either transaminated to alanine (glucose-alanine cycle) or converted to lactate and released into the circulation, where it is carried to the liver and synthesized into glucose (glucose-lactate cycle). From a quantitative standpoint, about twice as many carbon skeletons are recycled to glucose via the Cori cycle as via the alanine cycle.

The counterregulatory hormones (glucagon, epinephrine, growth hormone, cortisol) are all capable of offsetting the action of insulin on the liver and work by stimulating both glycogenolysis and gluconeogenesis.[14] Glucagon has been shown to play a major role in the tonic support of basal hepatic glucose release. In humans and animals, suppression of endogenous glucagon secretion with preservation of basal insulin levels causes a 30% to 40% decline in HGP. This suppression of glucose production involves both the glycogenolytic and gluconeogenetic pathways. The precise quantitative contribution of the other counterregulatory hormones to the maintenance of basal glucose output under normal conditions of fasting has not been assessed. However, it is likely that epinephrine, cortisol, and growth hormone also exert a tonic effect on HGP in the postabsorptive state. These counterregulatory hormones may assume added importance during fasting conditions, when the development of hypoinsulinemia allows their stimulatory effect on glycogenolysis and gluconeogenesis to occur unopposed. The net result of their unopposed action is a rise in hepatic glucose and renal output.

During more pronounced hypoglycemia, as may occur with insulin administration, all of the counterregulatory hormones are released and act synergistically to restore normoglycemia.[14] However, they do so with different dose-response kinetics and time courses. Glucagon and catecholamines act rapidly, whereas cortisol, growth hormone, and thyroid hormones (in that order) are involved in the long-range control of hepatic glucose release. Small increases in plasma glucagon and epinephrine concentrations markedly stimulate both glycogenolysis and gluconeogenesis. Acute elevations in plasma cortisol, growth hormone, and thyroid hormones have no stimulatory effect on total hepatic glucose release. However, both cortisol and growth hormone have been shown to markedly potentiate the effects of epinephrine and glucagon on hepatic glucose release.[14]

In addition to hormonal regulation, the central nervous system has an important role in the maintenance of HGP.[15] Both parasympathetic and sympathetic fibers reach the liver via the splanchnic nerves, thereby supplying autonomic nervous modulation of both glucose production and uptake. In animals, parasympathetic stimulation restrains glycogenolysis and enhances glycogen synthesis, and activation of the sympathetic nerves that innervate the liver stimulates glucose output via potentiation of both glycogenolysis and gluconeogenesis. In humans, the influence of the sympathetic nervous system on hepatic glucose metabolism can be demonstrated under conditions of acute stimulation, but the contribution of the autonomic nervous system to the maintenance of basal HGP remains undetermined.

A number of metabolic signals have been shown to play an important role in the control of HGP in the postabsorptive state.[8, 16, 17] Hyperglycemia per se inhibits liver glucose output. In normal adults, hyperglycemia and hyperinsulinemia occur concurrently, and in combination they provide a potent stimulus to suppress hepatic glucose release. As shown in Figure 52–5, physiologic hyperglycemia (maintained with the hyperglycemic clamp technique), while maintaining basal insulinemia, is as effective as low physiologic levels of insulin in suppressing HGP. More impressive is the observation that hyperglycemia in the presence of hypoinsulinemia (hyperglycemic clamp with somatostatin) causes a greater than 50% suppression of hepatic glucose release (see Fig. 52–5). Conversely, hypoglycemia by itself provides a trigger to increase hepatic glucose release. During insulin-induced hypoglycemia in humans and animals, a rise in plasma glucose occurs even when the counterregulatory hormonal response is inhibited. Recent studies suggest that this effect of hypoglycemia is mediated via glucose sensors in the hypothalamic region of the brain, which then activate hepatic glycogenolysis via sympathetic connections to the liver.[14]

Metabolic signals in the form of altered substrate delivery to the liver can also influence glucose release by the liver.[17] In humans it is very difficult to demonstrate a detectable rise in HGP by infusing

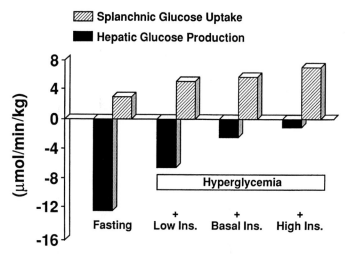

FIGURE 52–5. *Splanchnic glucose uptake (crosshatched bars) and hepatic glucose production (solid bars) in healthy subjects under four experimental conditions: (1) overnight fast, (2) hyperglycemia (+125 mg/dL) with somatostatin blockade of endogenous insulin release (Low Ins), (3) hyperglycemia (+125 mg/dL) with somatostatin plus insulin replacement to maintain the fasting insulin concentration constant (Basal Ins), and (4) hyperglycemia (+125 mg/dL) with endogenous insulin (55 μU/mL) release. Note that hyperglycemia per se inhibits hepatic glucose production and that hyperglycemia acts synergistically with insulin to inhibit liver glucose output. In contrast, hyperglycemia stimulates glucose uptake to approximately the same extent in the presence of low, basal, or high insulin, that is, mostly by mass action. (Drawn from data in DeFronzo RA, Ferrannini E, Hendler R, et al: Regulation of splanchnic and peripheral glucose uptake by insulin and hyperglycemia in man. Diabetes 32:35–45, 1983.)*

large quantities of glycerol, lactate, or a mixture of amino acids as long as physiologic hyperinsulinemia balances out such gluconeogenetic substrate push. However, even though total hepatic glucose output does not increase, the marked stimulation of gluconeogenesis is precisely counterbalanced by inhibition of glycogenolysis. This phenomenon is referred to as hepatic autoregulation. The increased provision of gluconeogenetic precursors leads to a rise in the intrahepatic formation of G-6-P, but the eventual fate of this intermediate is glycogen rather than free glucose because the rate-limiting enzyme for glucose release from the liver, namely, glucose-6-phosphatase, is not simultaneously activated. FFAs play an important role in setting the level of HGP. Only the odd-chain FFAs, such as propionate, can donate their carbon atoms to oxaloacetate in the tricarboxylic acid cycle and thus directly contribute to net gluconeogenesis. The great majority of FFAs in the plasma and within cells are of even-chain configuration, and although they can exchange their carbon moieties with tricarboxylic acid cycle intermediates, they do not contribute to de novo glucose synthesis. Nonetheless, when the perfusion medium of isolated rat liver is enriched with oleate or palmitate, new glucose formation from lactate or pyruvate is enhanced. The biochemical mechanisms involved in this stimulation of gluconeogenesis have been well worked out.[18] The products of FFA oxidation, citrate and acetyl-CoA, activate the key enzymes that control gluconeogenesis (pyruvate carboxylase, phosphoenolpyruvate carboxykinase, and glucose-6-phosphatase) (see Fig. 52–4). In addition, elevated plasma FFA concentrations in vivo are usually accompanied by raised glycerol levels because both glycerol and FFA result from the hydrolysis of triglycerides (see Fig. 52–4). Therefore, accelerated lipolysis supplies both the stimulus (FFA), the substrate (glycerol), and the energy source (ATP from FFA oxidation) to drive gluconeogenesis. In isolated hepatocytes, FFAs in micromolar amounts have also been shown to inhibit glycogen synthase, which suggests that an additional interaction of FFA metabolism with HGP may be at the level of glycogen metabolism. In healthy volunteers, short-term infusion of triglycerides (with heparin to activate lipoprotein lipase) stimulates hepatic glucose output under conditions (such as combined hyperglycemia and insulinopenia induced by somatostatin plus glucose infusion) that mimic the diabetic state. Part of this effect can be reproduced by infusing, under the same experimental circumstances, glycerol alone. On the other hand, when endogenous insulin levels are allowed to rise or when exogenous insulin is administered, the stimulatory effect of triglyceride/heparin infusion on hepatic glucose release is easily overcome. In summary, the long-chain FFAs can regulate HGP both by acting on the key enzymes of gluconeogenesis (that is, through build-up of the products of FFA oxidation) and by virtue of the substrate push of glycerol. This regulatory loop is operative particularly when insulin secretion is not stimulated, such as in the postabsorptive state, when plasma insulin levels are low.

Glucose Disposal

In the basal or postabsorptive state, the rate of whole body glucose disposal equals the rate of hepatic glucose production, and the plasma glucose concentration remains constant.[1, 2] Information about the contribution of individual organs and tissues to total glucose uptake has been obtained by regional catheterization studies performed in combination with radiolabeled isotopes and indirect calorimetry.[19] By collating the available information, the organ-circulation model depicted in Figure 52–6 can be drawn.[3] In this synthesis, calculation of steady-state interorgan exchange of glucose, tissue blood flow, and regional glucose gradients is based on a rate of HGP of 150 mg/min or about 840 mmol/min. For a 70-kg man, the basal glucose flux equals 2.16 mg/min/kg or 12 μmol/min/kg. In the postabsorptive state, approximately 70% of basal glucose disposal takes place in insulin-independent tissues (brain, liver, kidney, intestine, erythrocytes). Of these, the brain predominates and accounts for almost half of total HGP. The liver plus gastrointestinal (splanchnic) tissues account for an additional 20%. It can also be appreciated that the fractional extraction of glucose (as defined earlier) is quite low everywhere in the body (ranging from 1.0%–3.5%) except in the brain (9%) (Table 52–2). Because skeletal muscle represents 40% of total body weight and receives 16% of the cardiac output, one can calculate that it accounts for one-quarter of overall glucose disposal in the basal state, or approximately 440 mg/min (245 μmol/min)[1–3] (see Fig. 52–6). As shown in Table 52–2, muscle glucose clearance averages 1.3 mL/min/kg of tissue. Glucose clearance is a useful metabolic concept and is defined as the amount of plasma that is completely cleared of glucose in a given period; as such, it provides an index of the efficiency of tissue glucose removal. In the rank of efficiency of glucose clearance in the basal state, resting muscle is last, being 10 times less active than the liver and 50 times less active than the brain. It is noteworthy

that tissues (brain, liver, kidneys) that have high glucose clearance in the basal state are insulin independent. Thus, raising the plasma insulin concentration above fasting values has no effect on glucose clearance by these tissues (brain, liver, kidneys), whereas glucose clearance in muscle increases by 10-fold or greater over the physiologic range of insulin concentrations. The intermediate position of heart muscle in the list is accounted for by its constant working state.

These organ-specific glucose clearance characteristics (see Table 52–2) represent the physiologic equivalent of the type and abundance of specific glucose transporters with which the various tissues are endowed[5] (Table 52–3). They also help define the concept of an insulin-independent tissue. Thus, in tissues in which a rise in plasma insulin concentration does not accelerate glucose clearance, the glucose transporter is not responsive to acute changes in the plasma insulin concentration. At present, five glucose transporters have been isolated, each with a unique DNA sequence.[5] A non–insulin-regulatable glucose transporter (GLUT1) effects facilitated glucose transport in the erythrocyte. The abundance of this transporter in the erythrocytes ensures rapid diffusion of glucose across the RBC membrane, and this characteristic confers on the erythrocyte an important role in the interorgan exchange of glucose. The same GLUT1 transporter is present in the brain. Because of its low Michaelis constant, approximately 1 mmol/L, it becomes saturated at low plasma glucose concentrations and is well suited for its function, which is to mediate basal brain glucose uptake. Because the Michaelis constant of the GLUT1 transporter is well below the normal fasting plasma glucose concentration, which is approximately 5 mmol/L, it ensures a constant flux of glucose into brain cells. This important adaptive mechanism provides cerebral tissues with an adequate supply of fuel even in the face of hypoglycemia. Another unique feature of the GLUT1 transporter is its low V_{max}, approximately 3 mmol/L. This characteristic protects the brain against acute fluid shifts and cerebral edema, which would otherwise accompany hyperglycemia. Thus the GLUT1 transporter is well suited for its physiologic function, especially in an insulin-dependent diabetic individual, in whom extreme shifts in plasma glucose concentration (from hypoglycemia to hyperglycemia) are common. Another important corollary of GLUT1 transporter function is that a rise in plasma glucose concentration above fasting levels, that is, greater than 5 mmol/L, necessarily leads to a decline in brain glucose clearance because the transporter becomes saturated at approximately 3 mmol/L. Moreover, because under postabsorptive conditions the brain is responsible for about half of the total body glucose disposal, it also follows that a rise in fasting plasma glucose concentration (with or without a rise in plasma insulin) is associated with a decline in whole body glucose clearance.

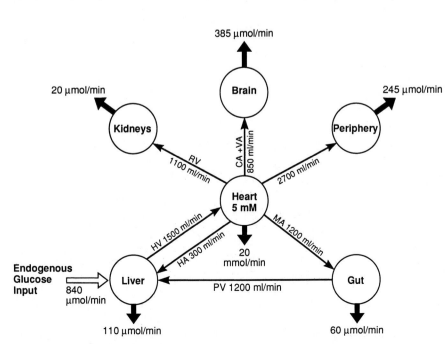

FIGURE 52–6. Schematic representation of organ glucose metabolism and blood flow in the basal or postabsorptive state. Average data compiled for healthy adults from the literature are indicated. "Periphery" encompasses all tissues other than the liver, gut, kidneys, brain, and heart; "gut" includes organs (e.g., intestine, spleen, and pancreas) draining their blood supply into the portal circulation. CA, carotid arteries; HA, hepatic artery; HV, hepatic vein; MA, mesenteric arteries; PV, portal vein; RV, renal veins; VA, vertebral artery. Organ blood flow is shown in milliliters per minute and glucose fluxes in milligrams per minute (micromoles per minute). (Redrawn from Ferrannini E, DeFronzo RA: Insulin actions in vivo: Glucose metabolism. In Alberti KGGM, DeFronzo RA, Keen H, Zimmet P (eds): International Textbook of Diabetes Mellitus. Chichester, England, John Wiley, 1992, pp 409–438.)

TABLE 52–2. Regional Glucose Disposal in the Basal State

Organ	Weight (kg)	Blood Flow (L/min)	Uptake (μmol/min)	Extraction (%)	Clearance* (mL/min/kg)
Brain	1.2	0.85	385	9.1	64
Liver	1.5	1.50	110	2.3	15
Kidneys	0.28	1.10	20	1.9	15
Heart	0.3	0.25	20	1.7	13
Gut	5.0	1.20	60	1.0	2.4
Muscle	28.0	1.05	245	3.5	1.3

*Organ clearance rate divided by organ weight.

A totally distinct (from the physiologic standpoint) glucose transporter, GLUT2, is present in liver and pancreatic β cells.[5] It has a high Michaelis constant, approximately 15 to 20 mmol/L, and as a consequence the free glucose concentration in cells expressing this transporter rises in direct proportion to the increase in plasma glucose concentration. This characteristic allows for these cells to respond as "glucose sensors."[1] Thus as the ambient glucose concentration rises, more glucose enters the β cell, which responds by appropriately augmenting its secretion of insulin, whereas the liver reads the rising plasma glucose level and decreases its output of glucose. As a corollary, a rise in the plasma glucose concentration is associated with a proportional increase in tissue glucose uptake, and liver glucose clearance remains unchanged.[16] Because the GLUT2 transporter does not respond to insulin, hyperinsulinemia is not associated with an increase in hepatic or β cell glucose clearance.[19] Glucose uptake by the pancreas and liver occurs in proportion to the rise in plasma glucose concentration.[16]

It is noteworthy that each glucose transporter is associated with a specific hexokinase with a Michaelis constant that parallels that of its associated glucose transporter.[20] For liver and β cells the phosphorylating enzyme is hexokinase IV or glucokinase. Its high Michaelis constant has led investigators to propose glucokinase as the β cell "sensor." Consistent with this view, studies have demonstrated that maturity-onset diabetes of the young is associated with mutations in the glucokinase gene, and the physiologic result is a defect in insulin secretion.

Insulin-sensitive tissues, such as muscle and adipocytes, contain the GLUT4 transporter[1] and its physiologic coupler hexokinase II. GLUT4 has a Michaelis constant of approximately 5 mmol/L, which is close to that of the plasma glucose concentration. In the basal state, most GLUT4 transporters are not located in the plasma membrane. Rather, they reside in vesicles within the cell. After exposure to insulin, the concentration of GLUT4 in the plasma membrane of adipocytes and muscle increases markedly, with a reciprocal decline in the intracellular GLUT4 pool.[1] Insulin not only enhances their translocation and insertion into the plasma membrane but also augments their intrinsic activity. Thus, muscle glucose clearance rises markedly, 10-fold or greater, in response to increments in plasma insulin concentration within the physiologic range.[1, 21]

The other major glucose transporter, GLUT3, is present in the gut and kidney.[5] It is sodium dependent and does not respond to insulin. In the gut it mediates unidirectional gastrointestinal absorption of glucose in the small intestine, whereas in the kidney it regulates unidirectional glucose absorption in the proximal tubule. Although this transporter is insulin insensitive, it plays a crucial role in glucose homeostasis by regulating its entry into the body and preventing its loss via the kidney.

The intracellular disposition of transported glucose can be studied by using glucose tracers and then localizing the appearance of the label in specific metabolic products such as lactate (in anaerobic glycolysis) or carbon dioxide (in complete oxidation).[7] These techniques, even when correctly applied, provide only estimates of the metabolic fate of plasma glucose, which is in the labeled pool. For example, if glycogen in muscle is oxidized directly, measurement of the specific activity of plasma glucose would miss it completely because plasma glucose does not equilibrate with the intracellular glycogen pool. To circumvent this problem, investigators have used indirect calorimetry, which measures total carbon dioxide production from all carbohydrate sources, both intracellular and extracellular.[22] Although indirect calorimetry depends on a number of assumptions, these assumptions are reasonable under physiologic conditions associated with everyday life and have largely been validated. Moreover, indirect calorimetry is easy to apply, is noninvasive, provides a close estimate of the rate of energy expenditure, and complements information obtained by the tracer method. In the basal state and under ordinary nutritional circumstances, oxygen consumption averages 250 mL/min, and carbon dioxide production is approximately 200 mL/min, for a whole body respiratory quotient (carbon dioxide production divided by oxygen consumption) of about 0.8. From the equations depicted in Table 52–4, whole body carbohydrate oxidation can be estimated to account for about 60% of total glucose uptake under postabsorptive conditions.[19] Because the brain uses 46% of the total glucose turnover (see Table 52–2) and because essentially all of brain glucose uptake is accounted for by oxidation, it follows that about three-quarters (46/60, or 77%) of basal glucose oxidation occurs in the brain. Little is left for other tissues, which preferentially derive their metabolic energy from the oxidation of FFAs and other lipids under postabsorptive conditions. Skeletal muscle, for example, has a respiratory quotient of 0.75 and relies on fat oxidation for the production of 80% of its energy needs in the resting state. Thus, the basal state is characterized by parsimonious use of glucose as a metabolic fuel.[12] Moreover, glucose is selectively channeled to organs that cannot rely on alternative energy sources. In the postabsorptive state, more than half of the total energy production is generated via oxidation of fat, stores of which are plentiful (see Table 52–1). Insulin is the principal regulator that determines the metabolic mix of fuels in the basal state. A small decrement in the circulating hormone level releases the brake on lipolysis and the plasma FFA concentration rises, thereby allowing fat to override glucose in the competition between

TABLE 52–3. Classification of Glucose Transporters and Hexokinases in Various Tissues and Cells

Tissue/Cell	Glucose Transporter	Hexokinase Coupler	Classification
Brain	GLUT1	HK I	Glucose dependent
Erythrocyte	GLUT1	HK I	Glucose dependent
Adipocyte	GLUT4	HK II	Insulin dependent
Muscle	GLUT4	HK II	Insulin dependent
Liver	GLUT2	HK IV$_L$	Glucose sensor
β Cell	GLUT2	HK IV$_B$	Glucose sensor
Gut	GLUT3 symporter		Sodium dependent
Kidney	GLUT3 symporter		Sodium dependent

TABLE 52–4. Indirect Calorimetry: Calculation of Carbohydrate and Lipid Oxidation and Energy Expenditure

Net carbohydrate oxidation (μmol/min)	$25.3\ V_{CO_2} - 17.8\ V_{O_2} - 16.0\ N$
Net lipid oxidation (μmol/min)	$6.5\ (V_{O_2} - V_{CO_2}) - 7.5\ N$
Energy expenditure (kJ/min)	$0.0164\ V_{O_2} + 0.0046\ V_{CO_2} - 0.014\ N$

N, urinary nonprotein nitrogen excretion (mg/min); V_{CO_2}, carbon dioxide production (mL/min); V_{O_2}, oxygen consumption (mL/min).

the two substrates. Although these very small changes in basal plasma insulin concentration are sufficient to promote a shift in fuel metabolism from carbohydrate to fat, the prevailing plasma insulin level is still sufficient to maintain glucose transport and metabolism in target tissues at minimum rates and to restrain protein breakdown, which contributes only about 15% to basal energy metabolism.[12] The role that counterregulatory hormones (glucagon, epinephrine, cortisol, growth hormone, thyroid hormones) play in basal glucose uptake is less well defined but is probably centered on the maintenance of lipolysis because all of the insulin-antagonistic hormones are more or less potent lipolytic stimuli.

Glucose Cycles

After entry of glucose into the cell through a specific glucose transporter, the sugar does not necessarily follow a direct path to its eventual fate, be it glycogen, lactate, carbon dioxide, or pentoses. Rather, it indirectly reaches its destination via a number of circuitous routes that have become known as futile cycles. A metabolic futile cycle is one in which a precursor is converted into a product by a forward reaction and then resynthesized to the precursor. Such a reaction yields no net product accumulation, but energy (ATP) is used. Multiple examples of such futile cycles can be found in the glucose metabolic pathway.[23, 24] The first involves the conversion of glucose to G-6-P by glucokinase and its subsequent reconversion to intracellular free glucose by glucose-6-phosphatase in the liver. Each turn of this cycle uses one molecule of ATP. Another example of a futile cycle is represented by the conversion of G-6-P to fructose 6-phosphate and back through the phosphoglucoisomerase reaction. Perhaps the best-studied futile cycle that is under the control of insulin is the conversion of fructose 6-phosphate to fructose 1,6-bisphosphate in the liver. The reverse reaction is regulated by fructose-1,6-bisphosphatase, whereas the forward reaction is catalyzed by phosphofructokinase (PFK). The latter enzyme is controlled primarily by the energy status of the cell and key intracellular metabolites. High levels of ATP, acidosis, and citrate inhibit whereas adenosine diphosphate and alkalosis stimulate PFK. The most potent activator of PFK is fructose 2,6-bisphosphate, whose synthesis is stimulated by the enzyme fructose 2,6-bisphosphate kinase. This latter enzyme is under the control of insulin, and the PFK step therefore represents an important regulatory control point for insulin action.[25]

In general terms, whenever bidirectional flux through a metabolic pathway is simultaneously operative, there exists a cycle, regardless of the number of intermediate reactions and regardless of whether one or more tissues are involved. In the examples cited above, the cycles occur within individual cells. However, cycles also can exist between organs. In this regard, lipolysis in adipose tissue followed by partial re-esterification of FFA in the liver is a complete cycle. Another important cycle is the breakdown of protein in skeletal muscle with reincorporation of amino acids into proteins in the liver or other tissues. The glucose-alanine and glucose-lactate (Cori) loops[11] also represent important cycles (see previous discussion) that provide conservation of carbon skeletons and transfer of amino groups between muscle and liver.

The derogatory connotation of futility has traditionally been reserved for cycles that go on in the same cell. These cycles are, however, anything but futile. As elegantly discussed by Newsholme and Leech,[23] a metabolic cycle with a reverberating internal loop provides the best kinetic stratagem to maintain the enzymes of a dormant pathway at a minimum of activity while at the same time ensuring a high sensitivity gain for rapid amplification of incoming signals. The ATP cost of these cycles is itself a means of increasing the efficiency of energy dissipation. The fact that the activity of these cycles is under hormonal control (for example, catecholamines, glucagon, and thyroid hormones enhance the cycling rate) establishes a mechanism for rapid modulation. In this way these cycles become components of facultative thermogenesis. Equally important, operation of these futile or substrate cycles allows for the generation of metabolic intermediates that can modulate the activities of key enzymes and allow for allosteric regulation.

GLUCOSE METABOLISM: FED (POSTPRANDIAL) STATE

The fed state refers to the period of active nutrient absorption from the gastrointestinal tract and lasts until the plasma insulin concentration and glucose metabolism have returned to basal values. Normal humans ingest mixed meals that contain carbohydrates along with lipids and protein. In the typical diet carbohydrates represent about 50% of the caloric content, with fat and protein making up approximately 35% and 15%, respectively. However, considerable intraindividual variation is seen in the distribution of the three major dietary constituents. The rate of absorption of dietary carbohydrates is markedly influenced by their chemical form (refined sugars vs. complex carbohydrates) and by the composition of the meal. Protein and fat, in particular, greatly retard gastric emptying and delay carbohydrate absorption. Furthermore, the disposition of dietary carbohydrates is indirectly affected by the dietary fat and protein content to the extent that these latter foodstuffs (1) compete with glucose as substrates in muscle, (2) impair the suppression of HGP by providing gluconeogenetic precursors, and (3) alter the glucoregulatory hormones (FFAs and some amino acids stimulate insulin secretion, whereas most amino acids augment glucagon release).

The rate-limiting factor for the absorption of glucose is gastric emptying. Once glucose enters the small intestine, it is rapidly transported by a specific transport system (GLUT3) that is sodium dependent. This transporter is unique to the intestine and kidney (see Table 52–3), which require glucose to be transported against a steep concentration gradient. The gut (and kidney) epithelial cells use a sodium-glucose cotransport system to overcome the unfavorable glucose concentration gradient.[26] Sodium is transported from the intestinal lumen into the epithelial cell down a favorable sodium gradient. Both sodium and glucose are bound to the transporter, and cellular entry of sodium brings glucose with it. Intracellular glucose exits via the basolateral membrane by means of a different glucose transporter (GLUT1), which is similar to that in the erythrocyte. For glucose transport to continue, sodium must also be pumped out via the basolateral membrane to maintain the favorable sodium gradient for sodium entry from the lumen. This active step is efficiently carried out by an Na^+,K^+-ATPase pump. This coupled system, which effectively and rapidly transports glucose from the intestinal lumen into the interstitial fluid, is independent of insulin. A similar sodium-dependent glucose transport system exists in the proximal tubule of the kidney. In individuals with a normal glomerular filtration rate (180 L/day), the kidney filters approximately 162 g of glucose each day (180 L/day $\times$ 900 mg/L), and this filtered glucose load is completely reabsorbed by the kidney, thereby preserving energy and preventing the loss of fluid and electrolytes, which would otherwise occur with the osmotic diuresis.

Quantitation of Insulin Sensitivity and Insulin Secretion

Because of the difficulties involved in monitoring gastrointestinal absorption of glucose and because of persistently changing plasma glucose and insulin concentrations that preclude the achievement of steady-state conditions, regulation of glucose homeostasis during the fed state has classically been investigated with the use of intravenous glucose, which can be administered in formats that are more suitable for formal analysis. The most detailed information concerning glucose utilization by the whole body, organs, and specific intracellular pathways has come from studies that use the insulin/glucose clamp technique[27] in combination with indirect calorimetry, radioisotope turnover methodology, and limb (forearm and leg) catheterization.[1–3, 16, 19, 21] Because the insulin/glucose clamp technique has become the reference method for the study of glucose metabolism, this procedure is described briefly. The euglycemic insulin version of the clamp technique[27] is shown in Figure 52–7. An exogenous infusion of regular insulin is started at time zero and is given as a priming dose, followed by a constant insulin infusion (usually at a rate of 1 mU/min/kg or 40 mU/min/m²). Such an infusion quickly establishes a hyperinsulinemic

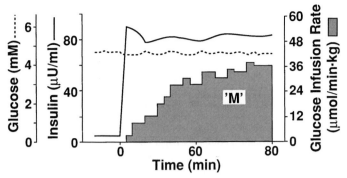

FIGURE 52–7. *Schematic representation of the euglycemic insulin clamp technique. See the text for detailed discussion.*

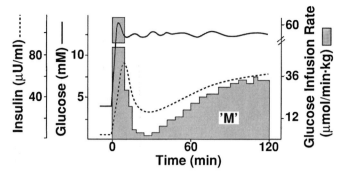

FIGURE 52–8. *Schematic representation of the hyperglycemic clamp technique. See the text for detailed discussion.*

plateau of about 70 mU/mL. A few minutes after starting the insulin, an infusion of 20% glucose is begun. Based on the plasma glucose concentration, which is measured every 5 to 10 minutes, and by using the negative feedback principle, the glucose infusion rate is adjusted periodically to maintain the plasma glucose concentration constant at the basal level. In response to the hyperinsulinemic stimulus, an initial delay in the onset of insulin-stimulated glucose disposal occurs and lasts about 15 to 20 minutes.[21] After this delay comes a rapid rise in glucose utilization from 20 to 80 minutes, which reaches a steady-state plateau value of approximately 5 to 8 mg/min/kg body weight (27–44 μmol/min/kg) during the last 40 minutes of the insulin clamp in healthy young subjects.[21] Because HGP is completely suppressed by insulin in healthy subjects and the plasma glucose concentration is clamped at the basal level, the rate of exogenous glucose infusion must equal the rate of glucose uptake by all tissues of the body and provides a quantitative measure of the amount of glucose metabolized. In some insulin-resistant conditions, such as obesity and type 2 diabetes mellitus,[1–3, 9, 21] HGP (measured independently with radiolabeled glucose) is not completely suppressed and must be added to the rate of exogenous glucose infusion to obtain the true rate of total body glucose utilization. The higher the glucose metabolic rate, the more sensitive the individual to insulin; conversely, the lower the metabolic rate, the more resistant the subject to insulin. The euglycemic insulin clamp technique has the following advantages: (1) any desired combination of plasma glucose and insulin levels can be easily achieved and maintained; (2) the time course of insulin action can be determined with a time resolution of about 10 minutes; (3) other techniques, such as radiolabeled glucose infusion, indirect calorimetry, limb catheterization, and nuclear magnetic resonance spectroscopy, can be readily combined with the clamp protocol; (4) because hypoglycemia is avoided, the release of counterregulatory hormones, which antagonize insulin action, is prevented and one can derive a pure measure of tissue sensitivity to insulin; (5) the effect of other hormones or substrates on insulin action can be quantitated by simultaneously infusing them during a clamp study; and (6) the achievement of constant or nearly constant levels of insulin, glucose, tracer glucose specific activity, and glucose metabolic rate allows one to make quantitative measurements under steady-state conditions and thus avoid interpretive problems encountered when plasma glucose and insulin concentrations and glucose flux rates are constantly changing, such as during oral or intravenous glucose tolerance tests.

The hyperglycemic version of the glucose clamp is depicted in Figure 52–8.[27] In this procedure the plasma glucose concentration is acutely raised by a priming infusion of glucose, which is administered in a logarithmically falling manner over a 15-minute period. Thereafter, the plasma glucose concentration is clamped at the designated plateau by periodically adjusting an exogenous glucose infusion, as described in the euglycemic version of the clamp. The hyperglycemic step-up in plasma glucose concentration evokes an endogenous insulin response that is typically biphasic. Over the initial 10 minutes an early burst of insulin release is followed by a gradual, continuous rise in plasma insulin concentration. The initial peak of insulin (0–10 minutes) represents the release of preformed hormone stored within gran-

ules in the β cell. The late phase (10–120 minutes), which represents the release of newly synthesized insulin within the β cells, lasts until the glucose stimulus is withdrawn. By analogy with the euglycemic insulin clamp counterpart, the hyperglycemic clamp also provides a quantitative measure of the total amount of glucose taken up and metabolized by the body in response to the combined stimuli of endogenous hyperinsulinemia plus hyperglycemia.

Dynamic Interaction Between Insulin Sensitivity and Insulin Secretion

In normal, healthy individuals the euglycemic insulin clamp technique has demonstrated an age-related decline in insulin sensitivity[28] (Fig. 52–9). More important, within the normal population a wide range of insulin sensitivity can be noted. Among 20-year-old subjects, insulin-mediated glucose disposal varies threefold from 4 to 12 mg/min/kg (22–66 μmol/min/kg)[28, 29] (see Fig. 52–9). A number of factors are known to influence insulin sensitivity, including both genetic[30] and acquired[31] factors. Adipose tissue mass, fat distribution, plasma FFA concentration, smoking, and the degree of physical fitness are all powerful determinants of insulin-mediated glucose disposal. Dietary composition has also been shown to influence insulin action, a high fat diet causing insulin resistance. However, even when these factors are taken into account, one cannot explain the wide variation in insulin sensitivity among healthy adult individuals. Studies in whites, Pima Indians, and Mexican Americans[1–3, 30] have demonstrated that genetic factors play an important role in the distribution of insulin sensitivity (as measured by the glucose disposal rate during a euglycemic insulin clamp technique). From these observations it follows that a finely balanced interaction must exist between tissue sensitivity to insulin and insulin secretion by the pancreas to maintain normal glucose

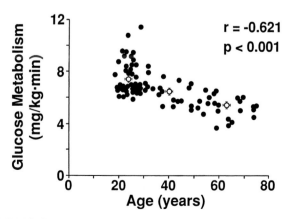

FIGURE 52–9. *Insulin-mediated glucose disposal as a function of age in 84 healthy individuals with normal glucose tolerance. (From DeFronzo RA: Glucose intolerance and aging. Diabetes Care 4:493–501, 1993. © 1993 by the American Diabetes Association, Inc.)*

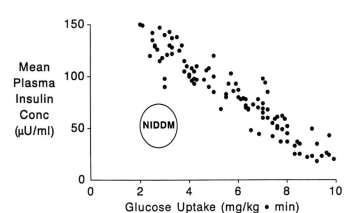

FIGURE 52–10. Relationship between insulin sensitivity (insulin clamp technique) and insulin secretion (hyperglycemic clamp technique) in normal-weight and obese subjects with normal glucose tolerance (solid circles). Non–insulin-dependent diabetic subjects (NIDDM) have a "normal" insulin response, which in the presence of severe insulin resistance results in overt glucose intolerance. (Drawn from data published by DeFronzo[1, 2] and Del Prato et al.[42] and from unpublished observations.)

tolerance. In individuals who fall in the lower quartile of insulin sensitivity, the β cell must be able to sense the defect in insulin action and precisely augment its secretion of insulin to offset the insulin resistance. As can be seen in Figure 52–10, when insulin secretion (measured with the hyperglycemic clamp technique) is plotted against insulin sensitivity (euglycemic insulin clamp technique) in healthy lean and obese subjects with normal oral glucose tolerance, a very strong inverse relationship is noted.[1–3, 29, 32] This relationship between insulin action and insulin secretion has important implications for the development of type 2 diabetes mellitus. As can be seen in Figure 52–10, insulin resistance is uniformly observed in patients with type 2 diabetes mellitus.[1, 2] Their insulin secretory capacity, when viewed in absolute terms, is normal. However, when viewed in context of the severity of insulin resistance, it is clear that they have a major defect in β cell function. In summary, the normal dynamic interaction between insulin secretion and insulin sensitivity represents a key physiologic principle underlying the ability of all individuals to maintain normal glucose homeostasis.

Effect of Insulin on Hepatic and Peripheral Glucose Metabolism

Maintenance of normal glucose homeostasis requires the closely coordinated effects of insulin and hyperglycemia simultaneously to

inhibit HGP and stimulate glucose uptake by peripheral tissues, primarily muscle, and by the liver. Using the euglycemic insulin clamp technique insulin can be shown to exert a potent suppressive action on HGP, such that portal insulin concentrations of less than 100 μU/mL completely abolish glucose entry into the circulation.[16, 33] Figure 52–11 shows the typical time course for suppression of endogenous (primarily hepatic) glucose production after an acute increase in plasma insulin to levels of 60 to 70 μU/mL in healthy subjects.[34] Dose-response curves relating the calculated portal plasma insulin concentration to inhibition of HGP (Fig. 52–12) indicate a half-maximal effect at a level of about 30 μU/mL, which corresponds to an increment in the portal insulin concentration of only 5 to 10 μU/mL.[16, 33] These results indicate the exquisite sensitivity of the liver to very small increments in the circulating plasma insulin concentration. Note that in its capacity as a glucose-producing organ the liver is an insulin-sensitive tissue, whereas it is insulin independent as a glucose consumer. Hyperglycemia, induced by intravenous glucose administration, strongly synergizes this inhibitory action of insulin (see Fig. 52–5). In normal adults, a rise in arterial plasma insulin levels of only 5 to 10 μU/mL is sufficient to rapidly reduce hepatic glucose output by more than 80% (see Fig. 52–12). In addition to insulin's direct suppressive effect on HGP, insulin reduces glucose release from the liver by indirect mechanisms,[17] including inhibition of glucagon secretion and decreased plasma FFA concentrations secondary to inhibition of lipolysis.

Concomitant with suppression of HGP, insulin elicits a dose-response stimulation of whole body glucose disposal[16, 33] (see Fig. 52–12). Under euglycemic conditions the maximum stimulation is approximately 11 to 12 mg/min/kg (61–66 μmol/min/kg) in healthy adult subjects and occurs with plasma insulin concentrations of approximately 250 μU/mL; the half-maximal stimulation of glucose uptake occurs with a plasma insulin concentration of 70 to 110 μU/mL. A dose-response curve of similar shape is derived when progressively higher insulin doses are infused locally into forearm or leg tissue, about 70% of which is composed of skeletal muscle. By extrapolating from forearm or leg to total body muscle mass, it can be estimated that with prevailing peripheral plasma insulin concentrations in the high physiologic range (60–90 μU/mL), approximately 70% of total glucose disposal occurs in muscle tissue.[1–3, 16, 19] Obviously, this percentage increases further with progressively higher insulin levels because the contribution of insulin-independent tissues declines. By combining the insulin clamp technique (plasma insulin concentration approximately 70–80 μU/mL) with leg and hepatic vein catheterization, a composite picture of whole body glucose disposal can be generated (Fig. 52–13). Glucose uptake by the brain (approximately 1.2 mg/min/kg) and splanchnic (liver plus gastrointestinal tissues) region (approximately 0.5 mg/min/kg) is unaffected by insulin infusion.[1–3, 16] Adipose tissue in adult humans is relatively inert and ac-

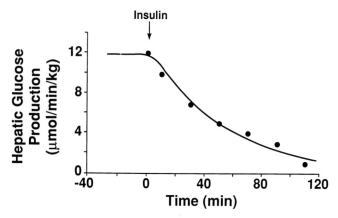

FIGURE 52–11. Time course of suppression of hepatic glucose production in healthy adults during a euglycemic insulin clamp study. (Redrawn from Cobelli C, Mari A, Ferrannini E: The non–steady state problem: Error analysis of Steele's model and developments for glucose kinetics. Am J Physiol 252:E679–E687, 1987.)

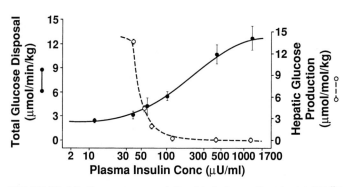

FIGURE 52–12. Dose-response relationship between the plasma insulin concentration (note the log scale) vs. hepatic glucose production and whole body glucose uptake in healthy subjects studied with the euglycemic insulin clamp technique. The insulin concentrations are peripheral levels in the case of total glucose uptake and portal levels in the case of hepatic glucose production. (From DeFronzo DA, Ferrannini E, Hendler R, et al: Regulation of splanchnic and peripheral glucose uptake by insulin and hyperglycemia in man. Diabetes 32:35–45, 1983. © 1983 by the American Diabetes Association, Inc.)

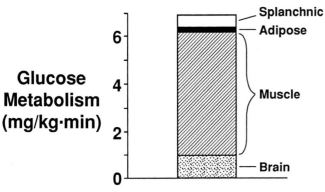

Glucose Metabolism (mg/kg·min)

FIGURE 52–13. Summary of tissue glucose disposal during a euglycemic (90 mg/dL) hyperinsulinemic (+80 μU/mL) clamp technique in healthy subjects. (From DeFronzo RA: Lilly Lecture: The triumvirate: β-Cell, muscle, liver: A collusion responsible for NIDDM. Diabetes 37:667–687, 1988. © 1988 by the American Diabetes Association, Inc.)

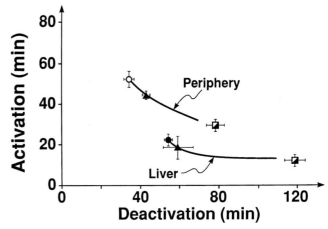

FIGURE 52–15. Relationships between activation and deactivation times for stimulation of peripheral glucose uptake and inhibition of hepatic glucose production during three insulin infusion rates: 15 mU/m²/min *(open circles)*, 40 mU/m²/min *(solid triangles)*, and 120 mU/m²/min *(semisolid squares)*. (Reconstructed from Prager R, Wallace P, Olefsky JM: In vivo kinetics of insulin action on peripheral glucose disposal and hepatic output in normal and obese subjects. J Clin Invest 78:472–481, 1986.)

counts for no more than 2% to 3% of an infused glucose load. However, the role of adipose tissue in insulin-mediated glucose disposal should not be underestimated. Insulin is a potent inhibitor of lipolysis, and the resultant decline in plasma FFA concentrations augments muscle glucose metabolism. From this brief review it is clear that muscle represents the primary tissue responsible for insulin-mediated glucose uptake under euglycemic conditions[1–3, 16, 19] (see Fig. 52–13). When hyperglycemia (plasma glucose raised from 90 to 180 mg/dL) is superimposed on the same level of hyperinsulinemia (70–80 μU/mL), a doubling of total body glucose utilization occurs (Fig. 52–14); consequently, glucose clearance remains unchanged. As can be seen in Figure 52–14, essentially all of the additional increase in glucose disposal above that observed under euglycemic conditions occurs in muscle.

Regulation of glucose production and utilization by insulin depends both on the hormone concentration and on time. At any given insulin concentration there is a finite period before the effect of the hormone is seen and reaches its maximum. Such onset time is the sum of a circulatory delay (delivery of insulin from arterial blood to the cell surface membrane) and a cellular lag (insulin receptor binding and effector activation). Similarly, insulin's effect on glucose metabolism remains for some time (offset) after the circulating concentration has returned to basal levels. Figure 52–15 shows the activation and deactivation times of insulin calculated at euglycemia over a wide range of plasma hormone levels (up to 1000 mU/mL).[35] With the reservations inherent in the analysis of non–steady-state tracer data, the results shown in Figure 52–15 provide evidence that activation

and deactivation are inversely related to one another. Thus at higher plasma insulin concentrations the hormone's effect is more rapid in onset and takes longer to wane. From a physiologic standpoint, it is also noteworthy that the relationship between onset and offset time is different for the liver (suppression of glucose release) and for peripheral tissues (stimulation of glucose uptake). At any insulin dose, the liver is activated more rapidly and the effect persists for a longer duration. The more rapid onset of action in the liver may be related to the shorter diffusion time of bloodborne substances into highly perfused organs (1 mL/min/g of tissue in the liver vs. a corresponding value of 0.04 mL/min/g in resting skeletal muscle, see Table 52–1) and to anatomic differences between liver capillaries (which are fenestrated) and muscle capillaries (which are not fenestrated).

Part of insulin's stimulatory effect on muscle glucose metabolism is related to an increase in limb blood flow[36] and recruitment of newly perfused capillary beds.[37] In response to insulin, a dose-response–related rise in leg blood occurs and correlates closely with the rise in leg muscle glucose uptake (Fig. 52–16). Inhibition of the rise in leg blood flow is associated with a blunted response in insulin-mediated leg glucose uptake, and insulin-resistant conditions such as obesity and diabetes are associated with impairment in insulin-stimulated limb blood flow. The vasodilatory effect of insulin is most prominent with plasma insulin concentrations in the high physiologic to pharmacologic range and after 2 to 4 hours of insulin stimulation.[38] This observation has raised some question about the physiologic significance of the role of increased limb blood in insulin-mediated muscle glucose disposal.[38] Recruitment of previously underperfused muscle beds by insulin is also most prominent at high physiologic to pharmacologic plasma insulin concentrations.[30]

Intracellular Pathways of Glucose Disposal

By combining indirect calorimetry with dose-response studies using the euglycemic insulin clamp technique it has been possible to quantitate the two major components of whole body glucose disposal: glucose oxidation and nonoxidative glucose disposal.[1–3, 19] The latter primarily represents glycogen synthesis, accounting for 90%,[39] whereas the remaining 10% is accounted for by anaerobic metabolism (net lactate production). Figure 52–17 shows that the dose-response curves relating both glucose oxidation and nonoxidative glucose disposal (glycogen synthesis) to the plasma insulin concentration retain the sigmoidal shape of the curve for whole body glucose uptake but with distinctly different dose kinetics. Thus, glucose oxidation is more

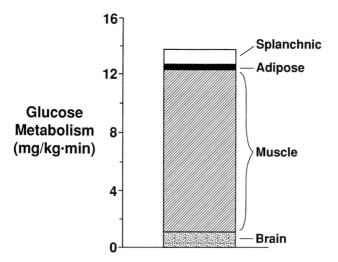

Glucose Metabolism (mg/kg·min)

FIGURE 52–14. Summary of tissue glucose disposal during a hyperglycemic (180 mg/dL) hyperinsulinemic (80 μU/mL) clamp technique.

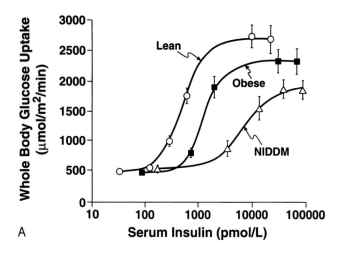

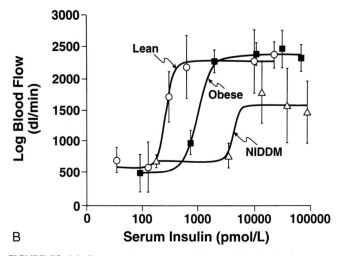

FIGURE 52–16. Dose-response curve relating whole body glucose uptake *(A)* and leg blood flow *(B)* to the plasma insulin concentration during euglycemic insulin clamp studies performed in lean control subjects, normal glucose-tolerant obese subjects, and type 2 diabetic subjects. To convert insulin concentrations from picomoles per liter to microunits per milliliter, divide by 7.175. (From Baron AD: Hemodynamic actions of insulin. Am J Physiol 267:E187–E202, 1994.)

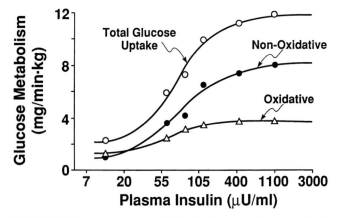

FIGURE 52–17. Dose-response relationship between the plasma insulin concentration and total body glucose uptake, glucose oxidation, and nonoxidative glucose disposal in healthy subjects during a euglycemic insulin clamp study. (Drawn from data in Thiebaud D, Jacot E, DeFronzo RA, et al: The effect of graded doses of insulin on total glucose uptake, glucose oxidation, and glucose storage in man. Diabetes 31:957–963, 1982.)

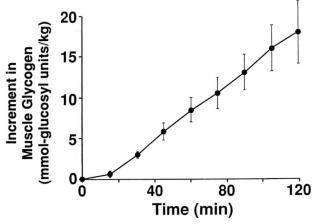

FIGURE 52–18. Time course of stimulation of muscle glycogen formation by combined hyperinsulinemia (100 μU/mL) and hyperglycemia (200 mg/dL) in healthy subjects as determined by nuclear magnetic resonance spectroscopy. (Redrawn from Shulman GI, Rothman DL, Jue T, et al: Quantitation of muscle glycogen synthesis in normal subjects and subjects with non–insulin-dependent diabetes by ^{13}C nuclear magnetic resonance spectroscopy. N Engl J Med 322:223–228, 1990.) Copyright © 1990 Massachusetts Medical Society. All rights reserved.)

sensitive (lower half-maximum) but becomes saturated earlier (lower maximum) than glycogen synthesis does; the latter behaves as a pathway with low sensitivity and high capacity. Skeletal muscle has been identified as the predominant site of insulin-mediated net glycogen synthesis.[39] However, the increment in carbohydrate oxidation that follows systemic insulin administration occurs in muscle as well as other tissues (probably the liver) in an approximate ratio of 1:2. With the use of nuclear magnetic resonance spectroscopy, one can directly quantitate muscle glycogen synthesis. The time course of insulin-stimulated muscle glycogen formation (Fig. 52–18) closely follows the time course of nonoxidative glucose uptake by the whole body.[39] By extrapolation from leg muscle to whole body muscle, one can account for the great majority (80%–90%) of nonoxidative glucose disposal as muscle glycogen formation.

The stimulatory effects of insulin on glucose metabolism in muscle are mediated via the coordinated activation of a number of key cellular regulatory steps. The initial step in insulin action requires binding of the hormone to a specific insulin receptor that is present on the cell surface of all insulin target tissues[1–3, 40] (Fig. 52–19). Trypsinization of cells results in a decrease in insulin action that is directly proportional to the decrease in cell surface insulin receptor number. The insulin receptor is a tetramer consisting of two α subunits and two β subunits.[40] Insulin binds to the α subunit, which communicates its message to the β subunit through sulfhydryl bonds. In healthy subjects insulin binding is associated with the phosphorylation of specific tyrosine

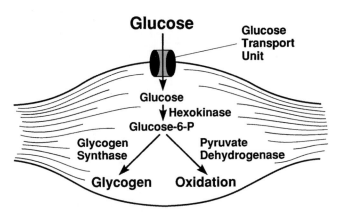

FIGURE 52–19. Schematic representation of glucose transport, glucose phosphorylation, and the intracellular partitioning of glucose into its two major metabolic pathways: glucose oxidation and glycogen synthesis.

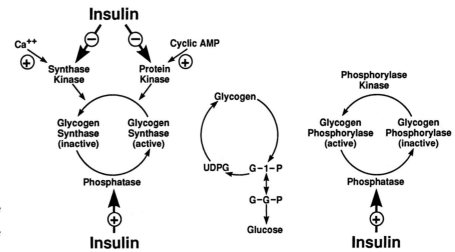

FIGURE 52–20. *Schematic representation of the control of glycogen synthesis and breakdown. Sites of insulin regulation are indicated. See the text for detailed discussion.*

residues in the β subunit. The resultant increase in insulin receptor tyrosine kinase activity initiates a cascade of phosphorylation-dephosphorylation reactions that ultimately lead to the stimulation of glucose transport and metabolism[1, 40] (see Fig. 52–19). The initial step in this complex intracellular signaling cascade involves tyrosine phosphorylation of an intracellular protein called insulin receptor substrate-1 (IRS-1). This system has considerable redundancy, and phosphorylation of IRS-2 and other IRSs is able to substitute for many of the functions of IRS-1. The phosphorylated tyrosine molecules on IRS-1 mediate an association between the SH2 (Src homology-2) domain of IRS-1 and the SH2 domain of the p85-kDa subunit of phosphatidylinositol 3′-kinase (PI-3-kinase), which leads to the activation of PI-3-kinase. PI-3-kinase is an enzyme composed of an 85-kDa binding subunit and a 110-kDa catalytic subunit. The later catalyzes the phosphorylation of phosphatidylinositol, phosphatidylinositol 4-phosphate, and phosphatidylinositol 4,5-diphosphate, which results in the stimulation of glucose transport, increased hexokinase II gene expression, and activation of glycogen synthase.[1, 31] Specific inhibitors of PI-3-kinase impair glucose transport, glucose phosphorylation, and glycogen synthesis. Precisely how products of the PI-3-kinase reaction regulate downstream activity (such as glucose transport and glycogen synthase) remains to be elucidated.

After glucose is transported into the cell, it is rapidly phosphorylated to G-6-P,[20] thus preventing the accumulation of intracellular free glucose, which would otherwise inhibit the transport step. Insulin stimulates glucose transport and phosphorylation by regulating both the amount (transcription and translation) and the activity of the GLUT4 transporter and hexokinase II[1, 5, 20, 41] (see Table 52–3). Insulin also enhances the translocation of glucose transporters from within the cell to the cell membrane.[1, 5] Once glucose has been phosphorylated to G-6-P, it can either be converted to glycogen or enter the glycolytic pathway. Under physiologic conditions of hyperinsulinemia, about two-thirds of G-6-P is converted to glycogen and one-third enters glycolysis[1, 9, 21, 42] (see Fig. 52–17). Of the glucose that enters the glycolytic pathway, most (approximately 80%–90%) is oxidized in the Krebs cycle to carbon dioxide and water, and the remainder is converted to lactate.[42] Insulin regulates flux through the glycogen synthetic and glycolytic pathways by stimulating glycogen synthase and pyruvate dehydrogenase, respectively.[1] Insulin increases the activity of the active form of glycogen synthase, both by stimulating glycogen synthase phosphatase and by inhibiting glycogen synthase kinase/protein kinases[41, 43] (Fig. 52–20). In addition, insulin inhibits glycogen phosphorylase by stimulating glycogen phosphorylase phosphatase, which converts the enzyme to its inactive dephosphorylated form (see Fig. 52–20). Finally, G-6-P, levels of which would be expected to rise as a function of insulin-mediated glucose transport and phosphorylation, both activates the phosphatase reaction and inhibits the kinase reaction.

PFK represents a key functional step in control of glycolysis.[25] However, insulin does not exert any direct effect on this enzyme, which is regulated primarily by the energy (ATP) and fuel (citrate, acyl-CoA) status of the cell. However, insulin indirectly stimulates PFK by increasing fructose 2,6-bisphosphate, a potent activator of PFK. Insulin also regulates flux through glycolysis by increasing the activity of the multienzyme complex pyruvate dehydrogenase.[44] This enzyme is activated by insulin, which stimulates pyruvate dehydrogenase phosphatase, thus converting the enzyme from its inactive phosphorylated form to its active dephosphorylated form (Fig. 52–21). The pyruvate dehydrogenase complex enzyme is also inhibited by its products acetyl-CoA and reduced nicotinamide adenine dehydrogenase (NADH).

Free Fatty Acid–Amino Acid–Glucose Interactions

A major part of insulin's stimulatory action on glucose metabolism is indirect and mediated via changes in substrate metabolism.[1, 17] In contrast to the hormone's stimulatory effect on glucose utilization, insulin is a powerful inhibitor of lipolysis and lipid oxidation.[1, 33, 45] As shown in Figure 52–22, plasma FFA concentrations decline steeply in response to small increments in circulating insulin levels under conditions of euglycemia. This decrease is the result of a marked reduction in the rate of FFA appearance in the circulation. The concomitant decline in plasma glycerol concentration is consistent with in vitro studies and indicates that lipolysis is inhibited. The consequence of the reduced availability of FFA is a parallel reduction in both

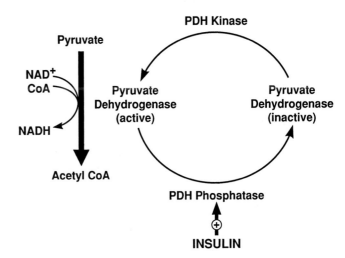

FIGURE 52–21. *Schematic representation of the control of pyruvate dehydrogenase. Sites of insulin regulation are shown. See the text for detailed discussion.*

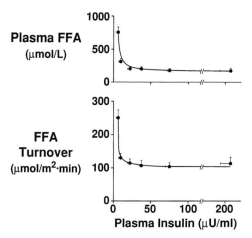

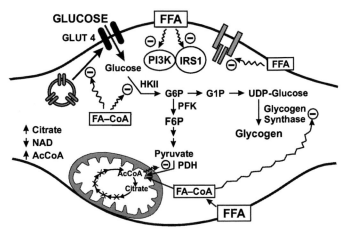

FIGURE 52–22. Dose-response relationship between the plasma insulin concentration and plasma free fatty acid (FFA) concentration *(top)* and rate of plasma FFA turnover *(bottom)* in healthy subjects during euglycemic insulin clamp studies. (Reproduced from Groop LC, Bonadonna RC, Del Prato S, et al: Glucose and free fatty acid metabolism in non–insulin dependent diabetes mellitus: Evidence for multiple sites of insulin resistance. J Clin Invest 84:205–213, 1989 by copyright permission of the American Society for Clinical Investigation.)

FIGURE 52–24. Free fatty acid (FFA)-glucose cycle. Enhanced FFA oxidation depletes nicotinamide adenine dinucleotide (NAD) stores and leads to inhibition of the Krebs cycle and an impairment in glucose oxidation. The increase in intracellular fatty acid acyl-coenzyme A (FA-CoA) concentrations inhibits pyruvate dehydrogenase (PDH), which leads to further impairment in glucose oxidation. Increased FA-CoA levels also inhibit the insulin receptor signal transduction system, glucose transport/phosphorylation, and glycogen synthase, although the precise molecular events involved in inhibition of these insulin-regulated steps have yet to be elucidated. *Dashed lines* represent sites of inhibition of glucose metabolism. See the text for a more detailed description.

FFA oxidation and nonoxidative FFA disposal (re-esterification) (Fig. 52–23). The inverse patterns of change in glucose disposal/oxidation, on the one hand, and lipid utilization, on the other, introduce the important concept of substrate competition. Glucose and long-chain FFAs are the best-known example of substrate competition in insulin-dependent tissues.[1, 45, 46] Physiologically, the rise in plasma glucose (by mass action) and insulin (stimulation of glucose transport) concentrations increases the rate of glucose uptake into fat cells. The resultant increase in intracellular α-glycerol phosphate generated during the stimulation of glycolysis supplies the substrate for augmented re-esterification of tissue FFAs, and at the same time insulin stimulates α-glycerol phosphate acyltransferase, a key enzyme involved in triglyceride synthesis.[47] These combined effects limit the release of FFA into the blood stream. In addition, the glucose-induced rise in plasma insulin concentration quickly inhibits lipolysis by stimulating hormone-sensitive lipase in the adipocyte, which further reduces the

supply of lipid substrates to the oxidative machinery in muscle and liver. A decrease in FFA oxidation by these tissues causes a reciprocal stimulation of glucose oxidation and glycogen synthesis in muscle (see below) and inhibition of gluconeogenesis in the liver.

Glucose-mediated inhibition of FFA metabolism is counterbalanced by FFA-mediated inhibition of glucose metabolism, thus creating an FFA-glucose substrate interaction known as the Randle cycle[45] (Fig. 52–24). When the plasma FFA concentration is elevated, FFAs are transported by mass action into muscle and liver cells by simple diffusion across the membrane. The intracellular FFA concentration is kept low by a specific FFA-binding protein to ensure a favorable transport gradient. Once inside the cell, FFAs are transported into the mitochondria, where they undergo β oxidation (Fig. 52–25). Before

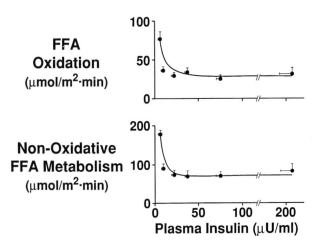

FIGURE 52–23. Dose-response relationship between the plasma insulin concentration vs. the rate of whole body free fatty acid (FFA) oxidation *(top)* and the rate of nonoxidative FFA disposal (re-esterification) *(bottom)* in healthy subjects during euglycemic insulin clamp studies. (Reproduced from Groop LC, Bonadonna RC, Del Prato S, et al: Glucose and free fatty acid metabolism in non–insulin dependent diabetes mellitus: Evidence for multiple sites of insulin resistance. J Clin Invest 84:205–213, 1989 by copyright permission of the American Society for Clinical Investigation.)

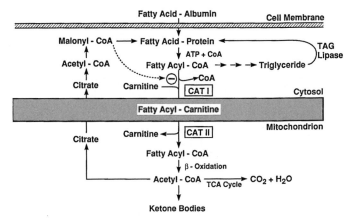

FIGURE 52–25. Free fatty acid (FFA) and ketone body metabolism in the liver. After transport into the hepatocyte, FFAs are activated to their acyl coenzyme A (acyl-CoA) derivative. Depending on the hormonal, metabolic, and energy status of the cell, the fatty acyl-CoA moiety is either transported into the mitochondrion and oxidized or synthesized into triglyceride. Malonyl-CoA, which is a potent inhibitor of carnitine palmitoyltransferase I, plays a pivotal role in the switch from FFA oxidation to lipid synthesis. Insulin enhances the formation of malonyl-CoA by stimulating acetyl-CoA carboxylase. Insulin also favors triglyceride synthesis by inhibiting triacylglycerol lipase, the rate-limiting step for lipolysis.

entering the mitochondria the long-chain fatty acids (oleic, palmitic, stearic, linoleic, and palmitoleic) are first activated to their acyl-CoA derivative by the appropriate acyl-CoA synthetase. Because the inner mitochondrial membrane is not permeable to fatty acid acyl-CoA, a specific transport system is necessary to transport the fatty acyl derivative into the mitochondria[48] (see Fig. 52–25). The enzyme carnitine acyltransferase I in the outer membrane transfers the activated fatty acyl-CoA in the cytosol to carnitine, and the fatty acyl-carnitine derivative is transported through the mitochondrial membrane. At the inner mitochondrial membrane carnitine acyltransferase II, the rate-limiting enzyme for β oxidation, catalyzes transfer of the fatty acyl unit from fatty acyl-carnitine back to CoA, and the fatty acyl-CoA then undergoes β oxidation with the resultant generation of acetyl-CoA.

As β oxidation proceeds, acetyl-CoA accumulates within the cell and becomes a powerful inhibitor of the pyruvate dehydrogenase enzyme complex[46] (see Fig. 52–24). In addition, the accelerated rate of FFA oxidation consumes NAD and generates NADH. This shift in redox potential further inhibits pyruvate dehydrogenase activity and impairs the Krebs cycle. The original Randle cycle proposed that the increased NADH/NAD ratio also leads to the accumulation of citrate, a potent inhibitor of PFK. Inhibition of PFK in turn causes a product feedback inhibition of the early steps involved in glucose phosphorylation and glucose transport. However, this sequence of events has been challenged in humans by the failure to observe an increase in intracellular muscle citrate concentration or inhibition of PFK activity.[49] More recent studies suggest that increased fatty acyl-CoAs have a direct inhibitory effect on the insulin signal transduction system and on glucose transport/phosphorylation[50] (see Fig. 52–24). In the liver there is also evidence that fatty acyl-CoA derivatives directly inhibit glycogen synthase.[51] In healthy humans a physiologic elevation in the plasma FFA concentration (created by lipid/heparin infusion) stimulates FFA oxidation, which in turn inhibits both glucose oxidation and glycogen synthesis,[1, 49, 50, 52] thus providing experimental validation of the Randle cycle,[45] although the biochemical/molecular mechanisms responsible for the FFA-mediated inhibition of muscle glucose metabolism have been altered (from those originally proposed by Randle) by more recent findings (see Fig. 52–24). In nondiabetic subjects a physiologic increment in the plasma insulin level (+50 μU/mL) causes a 50% to 60% decline in plasma FFA concentration and a parallel decline in lipid oxidation (Fig. 52–26). Infusion of Intralipid during the insulin clamp technique to maintain or increase the plasma FFA level (see Fig. 52–26) inhibits insulin-mediated stimulation of both glucose oxidation and

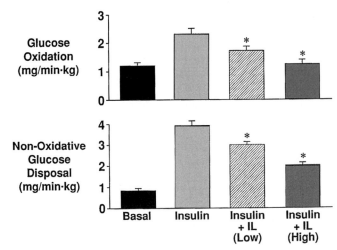

FIGURE 52–27. Inhibitory effect of Intralipid infusion and enhanced lipid oxidation on insulin-mediated rates of glucose oxidation and nonoxidative glucose disposal (see the legend to Fig. 52–25 for a description of the experimental protocol). (From Thiebaud D, DeFronzo RA, Jacot E, et al: Effect of long-chain triglyceride infusion on glucose metabolism in man. Metabolism 31:1128–1136, 1982.)

glucose storage (glycogen synthesis) (Fig. 52–27). These data demonstrate that the Randle cycle operates in vivo in humans in response to physiologic changes in the plasma FFA concentration.

The extent to which insulin action in target tissues is direct rather than mediated by shifts in substrate supply can be appreciated by comparing systemic with local insulin administration. When infused intra-arterially into the human forearm, insulin does not alter the circulating substrate supply in that neither FFA nor glucose concentrations change in the arterial blood that perfuses the forearm tissues. Under these conditions, insulin stimulates forearm glucose uptake and lactate release in a time-dependent manner (Fig. 52–28) but does not induce any detectable change in the local respiratory quotient (0.76) for the blood draining the forearm tissues.[53] This observation indicates that the forearm tissues and the muscle in particular continue to rely mostly on lipid oxidation for energy production and that the vast majority of insulin-stimulated glucose uptake is channeled to glycogen.

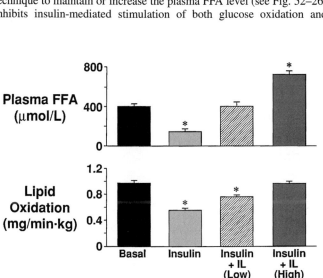

FIGURE 52–26. Plasma free fatty acid (FFA) concentration and total body lipid oxidation (measured by indirect calorimetry) in the basal state and during a 100-μU/mL euglycemic insulin clamp technique performed with and without Intralipid (IL) infusion. Intralipid was infused at two rates to maintain (low IL infusion) or increase (high IL infusion) the basal plasma FFA concentration. The high-dose IL infusion rate maintained the rate of total body lipid oxidation constant at the basal value. (From Thiebaud D, DeFronzo RA, Jacot E, et al: Effect of long-chain triglyceride infusion on glucose metabolism in man. Metabolism 31:1128–1136, 1982.)

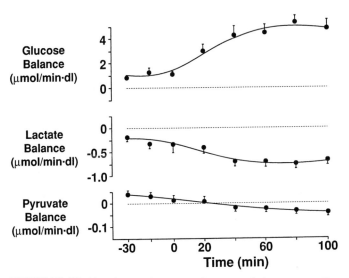

FIGURE 52–28. Net glucose, lactate, and pyruvate balance across the forearm of healthy subjects in the fasting state (−30 to 0 minutes) and during a 100-minute intra-arterial insulin infusion calculated to raise the local insulin concentration by approximately 120 μU/mL. (From Natali A, Buzzigoli G, Taddei S, et al: Effects of insulin on hemodynamics and metabolism in human forearm. Diabetes 39:490–500, 1990. © 1990 by the American Diabetes Association, Inc.)

In contrast, when comparable hyperinsulinemia is created by systemic infusion of insulin, while maintaining euglycemia, the leg respiratory quotient increases from 0.74 to almost 1.00, and glucose oxidation increases whereas lipid oxidation is markedly reduced. In summary, the direct effects of insulin are to promote glucose transport and phosphorylation, glycolysis, and glycogen synthesis; the stimulatory effect of the hormone on glucose oxidation is both direct and indirect, the latter being mediated by a fall in lipid availability.

Increased FFA concentrations also augment HGP. The addition of fatty acids to cultured hepatocytes and to the isolated perfused liver system stimulates gluconeogenesis.[54] In healthy subjects the rate of HGP in the basal state and throughout the range of physiologic plasma insulin concentrations is closely related to the plasma FFA concentration and to the rate of FFA oxidation.[33] Furthermore, FFA infusion in nondiabetic humans under conditions that simulate the diabetic state (hyperglycemia plus hypoinsulinemia) stimulates HGP secondary to stimulation of gluconeogenesis.[55] In nondiabetic subjects with basal levels of insulin and glucose, elevation of the plasma FFA concentration by lipid infusion causes stimulation of gluconeogenesis, but total hepatic glucose output does not increase because of a concomitant decrease in glycogenolysis.[56] This reciprocal interaction between gluconeogenesis and glycogenolysis is referred to as hepatic autoregulation.[57] The relationship between the plasma FFA concentration and HGP can be explained as follows. An increased plasma FFA concentration (by mass action) enhances cellular FFA uptake. The resultant increase in intracellular FFA leads to stimulation of FFA oxidation and the accumulation of acetyl-CoA, which in turn inhibits pyruvate dehydrogenase and stimulates pyruvate carboxylase, the first committed enzyme in the gluconeogenetic pathway (see Fig. 52–4). The net result is an enhanced flux of three-carbon precursors from pyruvate to oxaloacetate and thus into the gluconeogenetic pathway. Finally, the augmented rate of lipid oxidation also provides a continued source of energy (ATP) and substrate to drive gluconeogenesis. In conclusion it should be noted that an increase in plasma FFA concentration need not be associated with an increase in HGP, even though gluconeogenesis is enhanced, as long as hepatic autoregulation is intact.[56, 57] Thus, in dogs and nondiabetic humans, intravenous administration of alanine, lactate, and glycerol augments gluconeogenesis but fails to increase total HGP, because of a reciprocal decline in glycogenolysis. The situation in insulin-resistant states, such as obesity and diabetes, appears to be different. Here, FFA infusion impairs the suppression of HGP by insulin and in some instances may actually elevate the basal rate of HGP.

Amino acids can also enter into a substrate competition cycle with glucose, although somewhat less effectively than FFAs do.[58] Increased amino acid provision enhances glucose production under conditions of insulin deficiency or insulin resistance and limits glucose utilization in the insulinized state. Furthermore, an increase in the plasma FFA concentration exerts a hypoaminoacidemic effect in humans.[59] In summary, each of the three major substrates (glucose, FFAs, and amino acids), if present in excessive amounts (whether by endogenous production or exogenous administration), can lower the level of the other two by stimulating insulin release. Under hyperglycemic conditions in healthy subjects, glucose metabolism is obviously favored because glucose is a much more potent insulin secretagogue than fat or amino acids are. In addition, multiple substrate effects (not mediated by insulin) participate in regulation of the substrates themselves: high FFA or amino acid concentrations raise glucose levels, whereas a high FFA concentration lowers amino acid levels. The net result is the creation of a "glucose–FFA–amino acid" cycle in which each member of the triad influences its fellow members both directly and indirectly through the stimulation of insulin secretion (Fig. 52–29).

Lipid Synthesis

In addition to its potent restraining effect on lipolysis and inhibition of FFA oxidation, the rise in plasma insulin concentration that occurs in the fed state stimulates fatty acid synthesis and storage as triacylglycerol in adipose depots throughout the body.[60] As discussed previously, these fat stores are mobilized during conditions of fasting and

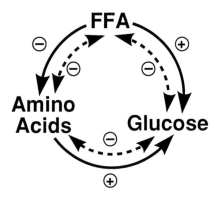

FIGURE 52–29. *The glucose–free fatty acid (FFA)–amino acid cycle. Because glucose, FFA, and amino acids are all insulin secretogogues, isolated increases of each of them lower the circulating levels of the other two via hyperinsulinemia (inner ring). By substrate competition (outer ring), an increased supply of either FFAs or amino acids spares glucose. In addition, FFAs have a hypoaminoacidemic effect of their own. See the text for detailed discussion. (From Ferrannini E, DeFronzo RA: Insulin actions in vivo: Glucose metabolism. In Alberti KGGM, De-Fronzo RA, Keen H, Zimmet P (eds): International Textbook of Diabetes Mellitus. Chichester, England, John Wiley, 1992, pp 409–438.)*

serve as an important metabolic fuel for skeletal muscle, heart, kidney, liver, and other organs. In addition to its important role in lipid synthesis, insulin also enhances cholesterol formation and cholesterol ester storage and promotes phospholipid metabolism.

In humans, adipose tissue and the liver represent the primary sites of fatty acid synthesis. Insulin augments fatty acid synthesis in these tissues primarily by activating acetyl-CoA carboxylase.[36, 46, 47] This enzyme converts acetyl-CoA in the cytosol to malonyl-CoA (see Fig. 52–25). Insulin directly activates acetyl-CoA carboxylase by increasing its phosphorylation state and enhancing its synthesis. Insulin also indirectly activates the enzyme by increasing the supply of citrate, which activates acetyl-CoA carboxylase, and by stimulating the pentose phosphate cycle, thus providing the necessary reducing equivalents (NADH) for fat biosynthesis. Insulin also phosphorylates, thereby activating ATP-citrate lyase, the step immediately preceding that catalyzed by acetyl-CoA carboxylase[46, 47] (see Fig. 52–25). The increase in cytosolic malonyl-CoA concentration simultaneously activates fatty acid synthase and binds to carnitine palmitoyltransferase I, which inactivates the enzyme and inhibits fatty acid oxidation.[48] The net result is enhanced availability of fatty acyl-CoA for triglyceride synthesis. Insulin appears to have little effect on any of the enzymes involved in triacylglycerol synthesis, in marked contrast to insulin's powerful inhibitory action on triacylglycerol lipase, the rate-limiting enzyme in the regulation of lipolysis.[46, 47] In addition to the stimulatory effect of insulin on triglyceride synthesis, the hormone also appears to enhance cholesterol formation through an effect exerted on hydroxymethylglutaryl-CoA reductase.

Ketone Metabolism

Ketones are formed in the liver by the oxidation of FFAs, and their synthesis is tightly regulated by the circulating levels of insulin and glucagon, as well as malonyl-CoA.[47, 48, 61] In the fed state insulin levels rise, lipolysis is inhibited, and intracellular malonyl-CoA levels increase. This latter key intermediate inhibits carnitine acyltransferase I, thus favoring triglyceride synthesis and retarding fatty acid oxidation and ketone body formation (see Fig. 52–25). Conversely, in the starved or diabetic state, plasma insulin levels decline and glucagon rises. The increase in the glucagon-to-insulin ratio is associated with a decrease in malonyl-CoA concentration, and fatty acid oxidation and ketogenesis are favored (see Fig. 52–25). With the exception of the liver, most tissues can oxidize ketone bodies. Their utilization by peripheral tissues, including muscle, is regulated primarily by their plasma concentration. Ketone bodies represent a major fuel for muscle during prolonged fasting once their circulating blood levels increase to 1 to 3 mmol/L. Reversal of the elevated glucagon-to-insulin ratio after feeding rapidly inhibits ketogenesis, and the associated decline in plasma ketone levels abolishes ketone utilization by peripheral tissues.

Oral Glucose

At any given point, the glycemic response to an exogenous glucose load represents the balance between the rate of glucose appearance in the systemic circulation from all sources (ingested glucose entering via the gastrointestinal tract and endogenous glucose production) and the rate at which glucose is disposed of by all tissues in the body. Oral glucose appearance in the systemic circulation depends on (1) the rate at which the gastric contents are passed on to the small intestine, (2) the rate of intestinal glucose absorption, (3) the extent of gut glucose utilization, (4) the amount of glucose taken up by the liver, and (5) the dynamics of glucose transfer through the gut, liver, and posthepatic circulation to the right heart. The contribution of endogenous glucose (which is primarily derived from the liver) production to the glycemic response during feeding depends on the extent and rate of change of hepatic glucose release. Initially, disposition of an ingested glucose load depends on changes in the pattern of hormonal stimuli and substrate availability. Because it represents a summation phenomenon, the response to oral glucose explores the whole of glucose tolerance, not the individual contribution of the various components. As discussed previously in this chapter, the rate-limiting step in the transfer of ingested glucose from the stomach to the liver is the rate of gastric emptying. Gastric emptying depends on the volume, temperature, osmolarity, and sodium content of the glucose solution when glucose alone is ingested. Glucose absorption through the intestinal epithelial cells is rapid, efficient, and well in excess of ordinary needs. Glucose utilization by intestinal tissues is small when glucose is presented from the vascular side, that is, when no oral glucose is supplied (see Table 52–2). The major fuels used by gastrointestinal tissue in the postabsorptive state are FFAs and glutamine. In the presence of glucose at high concentrations on the luminal side, gut glucose metabolism is increased in response to the increased energy needs for absorption. The quantitative aspects of this stimulation of gut glucose utilization remain undetermined in humans. The possibility also exists that systemic hyperglycemia may impede intestinal glucose absorption.

Glucose uptake by the liver is stimulated by portal hyperglycemia (see below),[8, 16] which has a major impact on hepatic glucose release. The traversal of glucose through the hepatic space is relatively quick, and this rapid passage is unlikely to introduce a significant delay in the systemic appearance of oral glucose. In summary, the dynamics of oral glucose appearance are essentially determined by gastric emptying, whereas intestinal transport, transit across the gastrointestinal mucosa into the portal blood, and transhepatic passage together introduce only a small time delay. Stated otherwise, if neither gastrointestinal nor liver tissues used glucose, the time course of oral glucose appearance in the systemic circulation would follow that of gastric emptying, with a time shift of a few minutes. For this reason, the glucose absorption step represents a major component of the shape of the glycemic response to glucose. Figure 52–30 shows the pattern of appearance of ingested glucose in healthy individuals, as reconstructed by a double-isotope tracer technique.[62] Glucose appearance in the systemic circulation peaks within 30 to 45 minutes, declines slowly thereafter, but remains significantly above zero 210 minutes after glucose ingestion. At least 4 to 5 hours is necessary for complete absorption of an oral glucose load, and this time is further prolonged by the presence of fat and protein in the meal. Figure 52–30 also shows the time course of suppression of endogenous glucose release by oral glucose.[62] A sustained nadir is reached between 60 and 120 minutes, followed by a slow return toward the fasting rate. However, hepatic glucose production is still significantly inhibited 210 minutes after the glucose challenge. Overall suppression of HGP during the 3- to 4-hour period after glucose ingestion averages 50%. This proportion is surprisingly less than what would be expected on the basis of the combined portal vein hyperglycemia and hyperinsulinemia (see Fig. 52–5). Because circulating levels of insulin-antagonistic hormones

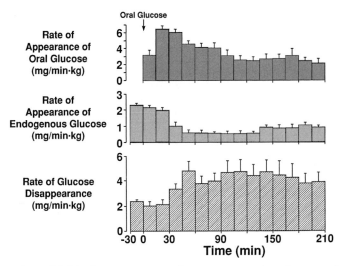

FIGURE 52–30. *Glucose turnover after glucose ingestion. The rate of appearance of the oral glucose load (top), the rate of whole body glucose disappearance (Rd) (bottom), and the rate of endogenous (hepatic) glucose production (middle) are shown after the ingestion of 1 g/kg of glucose in healthy adults. (From Ferrannini E, Bjorkman O, Reichard GA, et al: The disposal of an oral glucose load in healthy subjects: A quantitative study. Diabetes 34:580–588, 1985. © 1985 by the American Diabetes Association, Inc.)*

(except norepinephrine) do not change after oral glucose, it is likely that activation of the sympathetic nervous system, specifically, those nerves innervating the liver, keeps liver glucose outflow open.[15] In Figure 52–31 the observed arterial plasma glucose concentration is broken down into the component contributed by the appearance of oral glucose and that derived from HGP.[62] The resemblance of the oral glucose appearance rate to the plasma glucose curve is readily evident, especially during the first 60 to 90 minutes. Less appreciated is the fact that absorption is still incomplete 3 to 4 hours after ingestion. Figure 52–30 depicts the time course of total body glucose disposal after oral glucose.[62] After a lag of about 30 minutes, tissue glucose uptake is stimulated by 50% to 100% throughout the period of observation. Hyperglycemia (mass action effect of glucose to promote its own uptake) contributes more to whole body glucose disposal during the first half-hour. Thereafter, hyperinsulinemia provides the predominant stimulus. Oral glucose also elicits marked vasodilation of the splanchnic vascular bed, and this regional increase in splanchnic blood flow persists for at least 4 hours. Thus, both the metabolic and the hemodynamic perturbations induced by oral glucose extend beyond the time that it takes for the plasma glucose concentration to return to its preingestion level.

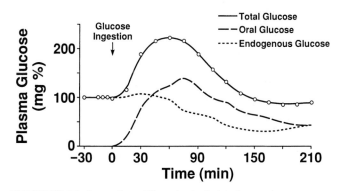

FIGURE 52–31. *Separation of the actual arterial plasma glucose concentration (solid line) into its components based on the amount of glucose that is contributed by endogenous (hepatic) glucose production (dotted line) and oral glucose ingestion (dashed line). (From Ferrannini E, Bjorkman O, Reichard GA, et al: The disposal of an oral glucose load in healthy subjects: A quantitative study. Diabetes 34:580–588, 1985. © 1985 by the American Diabetes Association, Inc.)*

The tissue destination of absorbed glucose has been the subject of intense investigation. Although the liver was classically reputed to be responsible for the eventual disposal of most of an oral glucose load, more recent studies that have used the hepatic vein catheter technique in combination with radioisotope methodology have demonstrated that peripheral tissues dispose of approximately two-thirds of the ingested glucose whereas splanchnic tissues account for the remaining third.[11, 63–65] However, it must be remembered that the splanchnic tissues (liver) also contribute to glucose conservation by reducing the output of glucose. When this amount of glucose is added to what is taken up by splanchnic tissues (liver plus gut), it can be seen that the splanchnic (primarily liver) and peripheral tissues contribute approximately equally to the maintenance of normal glucose homeostasis. Obviously, these approximate proportions vary according to the period over which the study is conducted, as well as with the nature of individual responses to glucose ingestion. A robust insulin secretory response directs more posthepatic glucose to the peripheral tissues, and a large increase in splanchnic blood flow channels the delivery of incoming sugar to the liver. In humans, for example, a glucose drink sipped slowly over a period of 3.5 hours rather than swallowed in one bolus generates the same overall glucose curve but a 50% smaller endogenous insulin response. Finally, in humans and animals the route of glucose administration seems to exert an important influence on the metabolic fate of glucose[11, 65–67] in that the portosystemic glucose concentration gradient per se enhances hepatic glucose uptake independently of portal vein glycemia and total glucose delivery to the liver.[11, 65]

After glucose ingestion, glucose oxidation in the brain continues unabated during the absorptive period. Approximately 50% of the glucose taken up by peripheral tissues (muscle) is oxidized, and the remainder is stored as muscle glycogen or as lactate in the lactate pool. During absorption from the gastrointestinal tract, lactate release by intestinal tissues into the portal vein is markedly increased. It has been estimated that about 5% of the ingested glucose load is converted into three-carbon precursors (lactate, pyruvate, and alanine), which are passed on to the liver and synthesized into glycogen via the indirect pathway of gluconeogenesis. Because the lactate concentration in the hepatic vein also increases after glucose ingestion, it follows that the sum of hepatic lactate production and gut lactate formation must exceed hepatic lactate extraction.[65] Liver glycogen formation during absorption of oral glucose occurs both directly from glucose and indirectly via gluconeogenesis.[68] The relative contributions of the direct (from glucose) and indirect (from gluconeogenetic precursors) pathways to hepatic glycogen synthesis in humans remain uncertain because of methodologic difficulties. However, current data suggest that gluconeogenesis participates in liver glycogen repletion to a much lesser extent in humans than in rats.

Counterregulatory Hormones

A review of the role of the insulin counterregulatory hormones (glucagon, epinephrine, cortisol, growth hormone, and thyroid hormones) and their roles in intermediary metabolism is beyond the scope of this chapter, and the reader is referred to Chapters 51 and 66 and elsewhere.[14] The most important role of the counterregulatory hormones is in defense against hypoglycemia. Glucagon and epinephrine play an important role in the acute recovery from hypoglycemia by stimulating both glycogenolysis and gluconeogenesis. When hypoglycemia is prolonged, cortisol and growth hormone contribute to the restoration of normoglycemia by impairing the tissue's ability to respond to insulin. Epinephrine is also a potent peripheral insulin antagonist. Except for glucagon (whose concentration rises during fasting and stimulates HGP primarily by augmenting gluconeogenesis), it is unclear what role if any these insulin-antagonistic hormones play in glucoregulation during the transition from the fed to the fasted state. More likely, under physiologic conditions these counterregulatory hormones contribute to the mobilization of competitive substrates, especially FFAs, from adipose depots to the liver and muscle, where they serve as an important energy source. Circulating levels of these counterregulatory hormones (except glucagon) do not increase during fasting. Rather, the plasma insulin concentration declines in response to the fall in blood glucose, and the resultant hypoinsulinemia leaves the lipolytic and ketogenic activities of the counterregulatory hormones unopposed, thus facilitating the shift from glucose to FFA metabolism.

REFERENCES

1. DeFronzo RA: Pathogenesis of type 2 diabetes mellitus: Metabolic and molecular implications. Diabet Rev 4:177–269, 1997.
2. DeFronzo RA: Lilly Lecture: The triumvirate: β-Cell, muscle, liver: A collusion responsible for NIDDM. Diabetes 37:667–687, 1988.
3. Ferrannini E, DeFronzo RA: Insulin actions in vivo: Glucose metabolism. In Alberti KGMM, Zimmet P, DeFronzo RA (eds): International Textbook of Diabetes Mellitus. Chichester, England, John Wiley, 1997, pp 505–530.
4. Ruderman NB, Tornheim K, Goodman MN: Fuel homeostasis and intermediary metabolism of carbohydrate, fat, and protein. In Becker KL (ed): Principles and Practice of Endocrinology and Metabolism. Philadelphia, JB Lippincott, 1992, pp 1054–1064.
5. Shepherd P, Kahn BB: Mechanisms of disease: Glucose transporters and insulin action—implications for insulin resistance and diabetes mellitus. N Engl J Med 341:248–257, 1999.
6. Matsuda M, DeFronzo RA: In vivo measurement of insulin sensitivity in humans. In Draznin B, Rizza R (eds): Clinical Research in Diabetes and Obesity, Part I: Methods, Assessments, and Metabolic Regulation. Totawa, NJ, Humana, 1997, pp 23–65.
7. Ferrannini E, Del Prato S, DeFronzo RA: Glucose kinetics: Tracer methods. In Clarke WL, Larner J, Pohl SL (eds): Methods in Diabetes Research, vol 2. Clinical Methods. New York, John Wiley, 1985, pp 107–142.
8. DeFronzo RA, Ferrannini E: Regulation of hepatic glucose metabolism in humans. Diabetes Metab Rev 3:415–459, 1987.
9. Stumvoll M, Meyer C, Mitrakou A, et al: Renal glucose production and utilization: New aspects in humans. Diabetologia 40:749–757, 1997.
10. Chandramouli V, Ekberg K, Schumann WC, et al: Quantifying gluconeogenesis during fasting. Am J Physiol 273:E1209–E1215, 1997.
11. Cherrington AD: Banting Lecture. Control of glucose uptake and release by the liver in vivo. Diabetes 48:1198–1214, 1999.
12. Cahill GF: Starvation in man. N Engl J Med 282:668–675, 1970.
13. DeFronzo RA, Stirewalt WS: Insulin actions in vivo: Protein metabolism. In Alberti GM, Zimmet P, DeFronzo RA (eds): International Textbook of Diabetes Mellitus. Chichester, England, John Wiley, 1997, pp 549–594.
14. Bolli GB, Fanelli CG: Physiology of glucose counterregulation to hypoglycemia. Endocrinol Metab Clin North Am 28:467–493, 1999.
15. Shimazu T: Neuronal regulation of hepatic glucose metabolism in mammals. Diabetes Metab Rev 3:185–206, 1987.
16. DeFronzo RA, Ferrannini E, Hendler R, et al: Regulation of splanchnic and peripheral glucose uptake by insulin and hyperglycemia in man. Diabetes 32:35–45, 1983.
17. Cherrington AD, Edgerton D, Sindeler DK: The direct and indirect effects of insulin on hepatic glucose production in vivo. Diabetologia 41:987–996, 1998.
18. Friedman B, Goodman EH Jr, Weinhouse S: Effects of insulin and fatty acids on gluconeogenesis in the rat. J Biol Chem 242:3620–3627, 1967.
19. DeFronzo RA, Jacot E, Jequier E, et al: The effect of insulin on the disposal of intravenous glucose: Results from indirect calorimetry and hepatic and femoral venous catheterization. Diabetes 30:1000–1007, 1981.
20. Nishi S, Susumu S, Bell GI: Human hexokinase: Sequences of amino- and carboxyl-terminal halves are homologous. Biochem Biophys Res Commun 157:937–943, 1988.
21. DeFronzo RA, Gunnarsson R, Bjorkman O, et al: Effects of insulin on peripheral and splanchnic glucose metabolism in non–insulin dependent diabetes mellitus. J Clin Invest 76:149–155, 1985.
22. Simonson DC, DeFronzo RA: Indirect calorimetry: Methodologic and interpretative problems. Am J Physiol 258:E399–E412, 1990.
23. Newsholme EA, Leech AR: Biochemistry for the Medical Sciences. Chichester, England, John Wiley, 1983, pp 308–310.
24. Vranic M, Wajngot A, Efendic S: New probes to study insulin resistance in men; futile cycles and glucose turnover. Adv Exp Med Biol 189:227–245, 1985.
25. Kurland IJ, Pilkis SJ: Covalent control of 6-phosphofructo-2-kinase/fructose-2,6-bisphosphatase: Insights into autoregulation of a bifunctional enzyme. Protein Sci 4:1023–1037, 1995.
26. Ferrannini E, Barrett E, Bevilacqua S, et al: Sodium elevates the plasma glucose response to glucose ingestion in man. J Clin Endocrinol Metab 54:455–458, 1982.
27. DeFronzo RA, Tobin J, Andres R: Glucose clamp technique: A method for quantifying insulin secretion and insulin resistance. Am J Physiol 237:E214–E223, 1979.
28. DeFronzo RA: Glucose intolerance and aging. Diabetes Care 4:493–501, 1993.
29. Diamond MP, Thornton K, Conally-Diamond MC, et al: Reciprocal variations in insulin-stimulated glucose uptake and pancreatic insulin secretion in women with normal glucose tolerance. J Soc Gynecol Invest 2:708–715, 1995.
30. Lillioja S, Mott DM, Zawadzki JK, et al: In vivo insulin action is familial characteristic in nondiabetic Pima Indians. Diabetes 36:1329–1335, 1987.
31. Groop LC, Tuomi T: Non–insulin-dependent diabetes mellitus: A collision between thrifty genes and affluent society. Ann Med 29:37–53, 1997.
32. Bonadonna RC, Groop L, Kraemer N, et al: Obesity and insulin resistance in man: A dose response study. Metabolism 39:452–459, 1990.
33. Groop LC, Bonadonna RC, Del Prato S, et al: Glucose and free fatty acid metabolism in non–insulin dependent diabetes mellitus: Evidence for multiple sites of insulin resistance. J Clin Invest 84:205–213, 1989.
34. Cobelli C, Mari A, Ferrannini E: The non–steady state problem: Error analysis of Steele's model and developments for glucose kinetics. Am J Physiol 252:E679–E687, 1987.

35. Prager R, Wallace P, Olefsky JM: In vivo kinetics of insulin action on peripheral glucose disposal and hepatic output in normal and obese subjects. J Clin Invest 78:472–481, 1986.

36. Baron AD: Hemodynamic actions of insulin. Am J Physiol 267:E187–E202, 1991.

37. Bonadonna RC, Saccomani MP, Del Prato S, et al: Role of tissue specific blood flow and tissue recruitment in insulin-mediated glucose uptake of human skeletal muscle. Circulation 98:234–241, 1998.

38. Yki-Jarvinen H, Utriainen T: Insulin-induced vasodilatation: Physiology or pharmacology? Diabetologia 41:369–379, 1998.

39. Shulman GI, Rothman DL, Jue T, et al: Quantitation of muscle glycogen synthesis in normal subjects and subjects with non–insulin-dependent diabetes by ^{13}C nuclear magnetic resonance spectroscopy. N Engl J Med 322:223–228, 1990.

40. Virkamaki A, Ueki K, Kahn CR: Protein-protein interaction in insulin signaling and the molecular mechanisms of insulin resistance. J Clin Invest 103:931–943, 1999.

41. Mandarino LJ, Printz RL, Cusi KA, et al: Regulation of hexokinase II and glycogen synthase mRNA, protein, and catalytic activity in human skeletal muscle in vivo. Am J Physiol 32:E701–E708, 1995.

42. Del Prato S, Bonadonna R, Bonora E, et al: Characterization of cellular defects in insulin action in type 2 (non–insulin dependent) diabetes mellitus. J Clin Invest 94:484–494, 1993.

43. Roach PJ, Cheng C, Huang D, et al: Novel aspects of the regulation of glycogen storage. J Basic Clin Physiol Pharmacol 9:139–151, 1998.

44. Mandarino LJ, Wright KS, Verity LS, et al: Effects of insulin infusion on human skeletal muscle pyruvate dehydrogenase, phosphofructokinase, and glycogen synthase: Evidence for their role in oxidative glucose metabolism. J Clin Invest 80:655–663, 1987.

45. Randle PJ, Garland PB, Hales CN, Newsholme EA: The glucose–fatty acid cycle: Its role in insulin sensitivity and metabolic disturbances of diabetes mellitus. Lancet 1:785–789, 1961.

46. Ruderman NB, Saha AK, Vauuas D, Witters LA: Malonyl-CoA, fuel sensing, and insulin resistance. Am J Physiol 276:E1–E18, 1999.

47. Denton RM, Tavare JM: Molecular basis of insulin actions on intracellular metabolism. *In* Alberti KGMM, Zimmet P, DeFronzo RA (eds): International Textbook of Diabetes Mellitus. Chichester, England, John Wiley, 1997, pp 469–488.

48. McGarry JD, Brown NF: The mitochondrial carnitine palmitoyltransferase system. From concept to molecular analysis. Eur J Biochem 144:1–14, 1997.

49. Boden G: Role of free fatty acids in the pathogenesis of insulin resistance in NIDDM. Diabetes 45:3–10, 1996.

50. Dresner A, Laurent D, Marcucci M, et al: Effects of free fatty acids on glucose transport and IRS-1 associated phosphatidylinositol 3-kinase activity. J Clin Invest 103:253–259, 1999.

51. Wititsuwannakul D, Kim K: Mechanism of palmityl coenzyme A inhibition of liver glycogen synthase. J Biol Chem 252:7812–7817, 1977.

52. Bonadonna RC, Zych K, Boni C, et al: Time dependence of the interaction between lipid and glucose metabolism in humans. Am J Physiol 20:E49–E56, 1989.

53. Natali A, Buzzigoli G, Taddei S, et al: Effects of insulin on hemodynamics and metabolism in human forearm. Diabetes 39:490–500, 1990.

54. Blumenthal SA: Stimulation of gluconeogenesis by palmitic acid in rat hepatocytes: Evidence that this effect can be dissociated from provision of reducing equivalents. Metabolism 32:971–976, 1983.

55. Ferrannini E, Barrett EJ, Bevilacqua S, DeFronzo RA: Effect of fatty acids on glucose production and utilization in man. J Clin Invest 72:1737–1747, 1983.

56. Chen X, Iqbal N, Boden G: The effects of free fatty acids on gluconeogenesis and glycogenolysis in normal subjects. J Clin Invest 103:365–372, 1999.

57. Jenssen T, Nurjhan N, Consoli A, Gerich J: Failure of substrate-induced gluconeogenesis to increase overall glucose appearance in normal humans: Demonstration of hepatic autoregulation without a change in plasma glucose concentrations. J Clin Invest 86:489–497, 1990.

58. Ferrannini E, Bevilacqua S, Lanzone L, et al: Metabolic interactions of amino acids and glucose in healthy humans. Diabet Nutr Metab 3:176–186, 1988.

59. Ferrannini E, Barrett EJ, Bevilacqua S, et al: Effect of free fatty acids on blood amino acid levels in humans. Am J Physiol 250:E686–E694, 1986.

60. Hellerstein MK: De novo lipogenesis in humans: Metabolic and regulatory aspects. Eur J Clin Nutr 53(suppl 1):553–565, 1999.

61. Zammit VA: Regulation of ketone body metabolism. Diabet Rev 2:132–155, 1994.

62. Ferrannini E, Bjorkman O, Reichard GA, et al: The disposal of an oral glucose load in healthy subjects: A quantitative study. Diabetes 34:580–588, 1985.

63. DeFronzo RA: Pathogenesis of type 2 (non–insulin dependent) diabetes mellitus. Diabetologia 35:389–397, 1992.

64. Kelley D, Mitrakou A, Marsh H, et al: Skeletal muscle glycolysis, oxidation, and storage of an oral glucose load. J Clin Invest 81:1563–1571, 1988.

65. Cherrington AD, Stevenson RW, Steiner KE, et al: Insulin, glucagon, and glucose as regulators of hepatic glucose uptake and production in vivo. Diabetes Metab Rev 3:307–332, 1987.

66. DeFronzo RA, Ferrannini E, Hendler R, et al: Influence of hyperinsulinemia, hyperglycemia, and the route of glucose administration on splanchnic glucose exchange. Proc Natl Acad Sci U S A 75:5173–5177, 1978.

67. Ferrannini E, Wahren J, Felig P, DeFronzo RA: Role of fractional glucose extraction in the regulation of splanchnic glucose metabolism in normal and diabetic man. Metabolism 29:28–35, 1980.

68. Shulman GI, DeFronzo RA, Rossetti L: Differential effect of hyperglycemia and hyperinsulinemia on the pathway of hepatic glycogen repletion as assessed by ^{13}C-NMR. Am J Physiol 260:E731–E735, 1991.

Chapter 53

Classification and Diagnosis of Diabetes Mellitus

Sean F. Dinneen ▪ Robert A. Rizza

DEFINITION

The term *diabetes mellitus* does not represent a single disease entity but rather a set of disease states sharing certain characteristics. Foremost among these is the presence of elevated plasma glucose levels. As discussed below, the presence of hyperglycemia in a patient is used both to diagnose diabetes and to guide management decisions, which are largely directed at avoiding hyperglycemia. The hyperglycemia itself results from a combination of defects in insulin secretion, insulin action, or both.[1, 2] An important characteristic of the various disease states that are labeled as diabetes is the development of end-organ damage in vital organs of the body, including the retina, the renal glomerulus, and peripheral nerves. The damage results, at least in part, from the chronic effects of hyperglycemia and is mediated through glycation of tissue proteins, increased activity of the polyol pathway, or other, as yet unrecognized, mechanisms.[3] Individual patients vary in their predisposition to develop these so-called microvascular complications. Because of this and because of the length of time they take to develop (frequently decades), the complications of diabetes cannot be used to classify or diagnose the disease. People with diabetes have a considerably greater risk of developing atherosclerotic disease affecting the coronary, cerebrovascular, peripheral arterial, or other parts of the circulation. A cause-and-effect relationship between chronic hyperglycemia and these so-called macrovascular complications of diabetes has not been as clearly established, although evidence is accumulating linking the two.[4] Any definition of diabetes that refers only to carbohydrate metabolism is incomplete. Oskar Minkowski is reputed to have first made the association between the insulin-deficient pancreatectomized state of his laboratory dogs and the sweet taste of their urine. It has been suggested that if Minkowski had lacked a sense of taste but possessed a keen sense of smell, he might have smelled the ketones on the breath of his animals and thereby directed diabetes research toward the study of fat metabolism.[5] Disordered fat and protein metabolism must be included in a complete definition of the disease, although an emphasis on the pathogenesis of hyperglycemia continues to this day. To define a disease purely in biochemical terms is to diminish that component of the disease which leads to much physical, mental, and psychosocial distress for the many millions of people around the world who live with it every day.[6] Chronic rheumatic diseases such as rheumatoid arthritis are not associated with any biochemical hallmark and their definition is based largely on patient-derived symptoms and signs.[7] Therefore, it is important to try to include the patient's perspective in any definition of the chronic disease referred to as diabetes.

CLASSIFICATION

Prior to 1979, a classification system for diabetes was not well established and many different terms were used to describe what was essentially the same clinical entity. Following publication of the report of the National Diabetes Data Group (NDDG)[8] in that year, some order was brought to bear on this area. The recommendations of the NDDG were subsequently endorsed by the World Health Organization (WHO) in a publication in 1980, and minor modifications were later made in a document published in 1985.[9] This classification was in large part based on the pharmacologic therapy of the disease. Insulin-dependent diabetes mellitus (IDDM) and non–insulin-dependent diabetes mellitus (NIDDM) were the two major forms of diabetes identified. The term *insulin-dependent diabetes mellitus* was used to describe patients who were typically lean at presentation, were prone to ketosis, and required insulin for survival. The term *non–insulin-dependent diabetes mellitus* was used to describe patients who were typically obese at presentation, were not prone to ketosis, and did not require insulin for survival. The NDDG also had categories for gestational diabetes, malnutrition-related diabetes mellitus (MRDM), and a category labeled "other types," which included certain forms of diabetes for which a cause had been suggested at that time. As the terms IDDM and NIDDM became widely used during the 1980s and 1990s several problems became apparent. The main problem related to the fact that many patients with NIDDM ended up at some point in the course of their disease being treated with insulin and being either misclassified as IDDM or having the rather confusing term *insulin-requiring NIDDM* applied to them. In addition, as more information became available on the etiology of the various forms of diabetes it became apparent that a classification based on therapy was not always consistent with new insights into the pathogenesis of the various forms of diabetes. For this reason, the American Diabetes Association (ADA) convened an expert panel in 1995 to address the issue of classification. This panel published its recommendations in 1997[10] and these were subsequently endorsed by a WHO consultation group in a 1998 report.[11] The main thrust of this proposal was to move away from a classification based on therapy and toward one based on pathogenesis. Four major categories were proposed: type 1 diabetes, type 2 diabetes, other specific types of diabetes (including categories for which a cause has been established), and gestational diabetes. The details of this system are outlined in Table 53–1 and discussed below.

Type 1 Diabetes

Type 1 diabetes is characterized by the development of a state of complete insulin deficiency. In its fully developed form patients will, if deprived of insulin, develop ketoacidosis, coma, and death. Biochemical testing reveals absence of circulating C peptide (a marker of insulin secretion) despite hyperglycemia. The incidence of type 1 diabetes in the United States is estimated to be approximately 30,000 new cases per year.[12] Although the peak incidence occurs in childhood and early adolescence, this form of diabetes can occur at any age. The incidence of the disease shows marked regional variation, with the highest worldwide incidence reported in Scandinavia.[13] Recent epidemiologic and immunologic research has led to recognition of two major forms of type 1 diabetes based on the presence or absence of certain immunologic markers.

Autoimmune Type 1 Diabetes

Autoimmune type 1 diabetes is a prototypic organ-specific autoimmune disorder. Individuals who develop this form of diabetes are born with a genetic predisposition to autoimmune dysfunction, which may manifest in the development of other autoimmune conditions such as Addison's disease or Hashimoto's thyroiditis. The genetic predisposition is not well understood but is known to be linked to the major histocompatibility locus on chromosome 6.[14] The presence of certain HLA haplotypes appears to predispose the individual to the disease while other HLA haplotypes appear to be protective. In predisposed individuals, a poorly understood environmental trigger sets off a series of immunologic events which culminate in selective cell-mediated

destruction of the β cells of the pancreatic islet. Many antigens have been investigated as potential triggers for the disease. These include certain viral antigens[15] as well as an antigen contained in cow's milk protein.[16] The rate at which β cell destruction occurs varies from individual to individual and may be very brief, as seen when type 1 diabetes presents in the neonatal period, or may be prolonged, as seen in what has been called latent autoimmune diabetes in adults.[17] Antibodies appear in the circulation early in the process of β cell destruction.[18] These autoantibodies are believed to be markers (rather than true instigators) of the immune response. Their presence can help classify a newly diagnosed patient with diabetes. In several studies screening for these autoantibodies has led to recognition of autoimmune type 1 diabetes in individuals who might otherwise have been labeled as having type 2 diabetes[19, 20] (see below). The most frequently encountered autoantibodies are those directed against glutamic acid decarboxylase (GAD), an enzyme involved in γ-aminobutyric acid (GABA) synthesis.[21] Isoforms of GAD are found in the central nervous system as well as in β cells of the pancreatic islet. Other autoantibodies include antibodies directed against a nonspecific islet cell antigen or antibodies directed against insulin itself (anti-insulin antibodies). Anti-GAD antibodies are specific but not very sensitive markers of risk in a population. Testing for these autoantibodies is still restricted to a limited number of laboratories. Greater standardization of assays is required before they can be widely used in clinical practice.

Idiopathic Type 1 Diabetes

The term *idiopathic type 1 diabetes* is used to describe a small subset of individuals with type 1 diabetes who appear not to have an autoimmune basis for their β cell destruction.[22] Other features of this subtype include its occurrence predominantly in individuals of African or Asian ethnicity, its lack of HLA association, and intermittent proneness to ketosis. Recent reports suggest that this form of diabetes may

TABLE 53–1. Classification of Diabetes Mellitus

I. Type 1 diabetes
  A. Immune-mediated
  B. Idiopathic
II. Type 2 diabetes
III. Other specific types
  A. Genetic defects of β cell function
    1. HNF-4α (MODY1)
    2. Glucokinase (MODY2)
    3. HNF-1α (MODY3)
    4. IPF-1 (MODY4)
    5. Mitochondrial DNA
    6. Others
  B. Genetic defects in insulin action
    1. Type A insulin resistance
    2. Leprechaunism
    3. Rabson-Mendenhall syndrome
    4. Lipoatrophic diabetes
    5. Others
  C. Diseases of the exocrine pancreas
    1. Pancreatitis
    2. Trauma/pancreatectomy
    3. Neoplasia
    4. Cystic fibrosis
    5. Hemochromatosis
    6. Fibrocalculous pancreatopathy
    7. Others
  D. Endocrinopathies
    1. Cushing's syndrome
    2. Acromegaly
    3. Glucagonoma
    4. Pheochromocytoma
    5. Somatostatinoma
    6. Aldosteronoma
    7. Hyperthyroidism
    8. Others
	E. Drug- or chemical-induced
	    1. Vacor
	    2. Pentamidine
	    3. Nicotinic acid
	    4. Glucocorticoids
	    5. Thyroid hormone
	    6. Diazoxide
	    7. β-Adrenergic agonists
	    8. Thiazides
	    9. Clozapine
	    10. Protease inhibitors
	    11. Others
	F. Infections
	    1. Congenital rubella
	    2. Cytomegalovirus
	    3. Others
	G. Uncommon forms of immune-mediated diabetes
	    1. Stiff-man syndrome
	    2. Anti-insulin receptor antibodies
	    3. Others
	H. Other genetic syndromes sometimes associated with diabetes
	    1. Downs syndrome
	    2. Klinefelter's syndrome
	    3. Turner's syndrome
	    4. Wolfram's syndrome
	    5. Friedreich's ataxia
	    6. Huntington's chorea
	    7. Lawrence-Moon-Biedl syndrome
	    8. Myotonic dystrophy
	    9. Porphyria
	    10. Prader-Willi syndrome
	    11. Others
	IV. Gestational diabetes mellitus

HNF, hepatocyte nuclear factor; MODY, maturity-onset diabetes of youth; IPF, insulin promoter factor.
Modified from the Report of the Expert Committee on the Diagnosis and Classification of Diabetes Mellitus. Diabetes Care 20:1183–1197, 1997.

be on the increase among African-American youth in the United States.[23]

Type 2 Diabetes

Type 2 diabetes represents the commonest form of diabetes seen in most parts of the developed world. In 1990 to 1992 approximately 625,000 new cases of type 2 diabetes were diagnosed annually in the United States.[24] The condition is characterized by hyperglycemia which results from a combination of defects in insulin secretion and insulin action. In any given individual, the degree to which these defects contribute to the hyperglycemia may vary. The disease usually has its onset after age 40. While progressive β cell failure is believed by many to be an important part of the natural history of this form of diabetes,[25] the β cell destruction is not autoimmune-mediated[26] and does not progress to a point where the patient becomes dependent on insulin for survival. Ketoacidosis is unusual in this form of diabetes, and when it occurs it is usually in the setting of a major intercurrent illness such as myocardial infarction, stroke, or treatment with glucocorticoids. Individuals with type 2 diabetes are not at increased risk for autoimmune diseases but have a higher prevalence of metabolic abnormalities, including obesity, hypertension, and a typical dyslipidemia characterized by hypertriglyceridemia and low levels of high-density lipoprotein (HDL) cholesterol.[27] This combination of metabolic derangements is associated with a marked increase in the risk of atherosclerotic disease. In fact, the prevalence of atherosclerotic disease in people with type 2 diabetes has led to the suggestion that, rather than one leading to the other, the two conditions may share common antecedents.[4] Insulin resistance may be an important predisposing factor for both conditions.[28]

The cause of type 2 diabetes remains to be determined. Any pathogenetic model of the disease must include both genetic and environmental factors. Challenges in establishing the cause of type 2 diabetes include the following: (1) The disease lacks an easy-to-define phenotype but instead is characterized by considerable heterogeneity across different ethnic groups; this heterogeneity is often represented by a spectrum consisting of a predominant defect in insulin secretion on the one hand to a predominant defect in insulin action on the other. (2) The relatively late age of onset makes it difficult to establish large kindreds and therefore limits genetic studies. (3) There are no easy-to-apply methods for screening populations for insulin resistance and defective insulin secretion. (4) The pathways involved in mediating insulin action are complex and not fully understood; most authors believe that a single genetic defect will explain only a subset of the disease; it is much more likely that type 2 diabetes represents a set of disorders. Evidence to support a genetic component of the disease comes from the strong concordance for the disease seen among monozygotic twins.[29] On the other hand, the dramatic increase in incidence and prevalence of type 2 diabetes that accompanies the change to a so-called Westernized life-style strongly supports an environmental component as well.[30]

Other Specific Types of Diabetes

Other specific types of diabetes are included in both the 1979 NDDG and the 1997 ADA classification systems.[8, 10] A number of changes occurred in the subtypes of diabetes listed between the two eras. In particular, the form of diabetes referred to as maturity-onset diabetes of youth (MODY) has been better defined genetically and this is reflected in the 1997 ADA classification system.[10] Another change resulted from removal of MRDM from the classification and the inclusion of fibrocalculous pancreatopathy (which was previously a subtype of MRDM) as a disease of the exocrine pancreas. The decision to remove MRDM as a separate entity resulted from an international conference on this subject.[31, 32] The findings of the conference did not support a direct cause-and-effect relationship between protein-calorie malnutrition and the development of diabetes. Rather, it was felt that the presence of malnutrition could influence the manner in which diabetes might present in an otherwise predisposed individual.

Genetic Defects of β Cell Function

In the past, the term *maturity-onset diabetes of youth* was used to describe a subset of patients with a form of type 2 diabetes characterized by early age of onset of hyperglycemia with an autosomal dominant mode of inheritance. Mutations in certain genes involved in regulating insulin secretion have now been shown to be responsible for the hyperglycemia seen in MODY kindreds.[33] Four major forms of MODY have been described: MODY1 is associated with mutation(s) in the gene encoding hepatocyte nuclear factor (HNF)-4-α[34]; MODY2 is associated with mutation(s) in the gene encoding glucokinase[35]; MODY3 is associated with mutation(s) in the gene encoding HNF-1α[36]; and MODY4 is associated with a mutation in the insulin promoter factor-1 (IPF-1) gene, which regulates pancreatic organogenesis as well as glucose-mediated insulin secretion.[37] All forms of MODY are associated with defective insulin secretion without any significant degree of insulin resistance.[38, 39] In the case of glucokinase, the pathophysiologic mechanism is clear since the enzyme is involved in phosphorylating glucose, one of the first steps in glucose metabolism. A glucokinase mutation therefore decreases the ability of the β cell to sense glucose. MODY2 is associated with relatively mild hyperglycemia that is usually amenable to treatment with diet or oral hypoglycemic agents. MODY1 and MODY3, on the other hand, can be associated with more severe hyperglycemia, a greater likelihood that insulin will be required for management, and a higher propensity to develop complications.[33] The link between diabetes and mutations in the genes for HNF-1α (a hepatocyte transcription factor also expressed in β cells) and HNF-4α (a member of the steroid-thyroid hormone superfamily and an upstream regulator of HNF-1α) remains unknown.[40] To date, only one kindred with MODY4 has been described. It is likely that other variants of MODY will be identified in the future. It has been suggested that MODY may account for between 2% and 5% of cases of type 2 diabetes.[41]

Other genetic disorders associated with impaired β cell function include certain maternally inherited forms of diabetes with a mutation in mitochondrial DNA,[42] disorders which lead to impaired conversion of proinsulin to insulin,[43] and disorders which lead to synthesis of an aberrant form of the insulin molecule.[44] Of the former conditions, diabetes associated with an A to G transition at the nucleotide pair 3243 in mitochondrial transfer RNA (tRNA) has been best characterized and appears to have a wide phenotypic expression from type 2 through to type 1 diabetes. The latter two conditions are inherited in an autosomal dominant manner and are associated with relatively mild glucose intolerance.

Genetic Defects of Insulin Action

For insulin to exert its biologic effect it must first bind to its receptor on the cell surface. Following receptor binding a complex series of postreceptor signaling reactions take place, leading to the hormone's metabolic and mitogenic effects. Disruption of some of these postreceptor mediators (e.g., insulin receptor substrate-1) has been shown to cause diabetes in animals.[45] However, very few human forms of diabetes have been clearly linked to specific genetic defects in the insulin-signaling cascade. Leprechaunism and Rabson-Mendenhall syndrome represent rare congenital disorders of the insulin receptor.[46] Both syndromes are associated with diabetes and hyperinsulinemia and altered growth in utero. As the insulin signaling cascade is further defined, it is likely that additional forms of diabetes will be found to be caused by genetic defects in insulin action.

Diseases of the Exocrine Pancreas

Hyperglycemia can occur during an episode of acute pancreatitis and is associated with a poor prognosis. It is unusual for permanent diabetes to develop following a single episode of acute pancreatitis. Furthermore, removal of up to 90% of the pancreas does not always cause diabetes. On the other hand, diabetes has been reported in association with very small pancreatic adenocarcinomas, leading some investigators to speculate that these tumors produce some diabetogenic factor or factors.[48] Five percent to 15% of patients with cystic fibrosis develop diabetes.[49] Up to half of these patients require insulin either chronically or at times of added stress such as glucocorticoid therapy. Hemochromatosis can cause diabetes.[50] Since glucose tolerance may improve with phlebotomy, this condition represents an important, potentially reversible cause of diabetes. Fibrocalculous pancreatopathy is seen mainly in the Tropics and is associated with abdominal pain and calcification of the pancreas on abdominal imaging.[51]

Endocrinopathies

Cortisol, growth hormone, glucagon, and the catecholamines (epinephrine and norepinephrine) can antagonize insulin action. Tumors that produce these hormones in excess lead to Cushing's syndrome, acromegaly, glucagonoma, and pheochromocytoma, respectively. While all of these conditions are associated with a degree of glucose intolerance, overt diabetes only develops in a subset of patients. The importance of recognizing these secondary forms of diabetes lies in the fact that resection of the underlying tumor can cure the diabetes. The hyperglycemia that is seen in the setting of aldosterone-producing adenomas and somatostatinomas results from alteration of insulin secretion.

Drug- or Chemical-Induced Diabetes

Certain compounds are toxic to β cells.[52, 53] These include the rat poison vacor and the anti-*Pneumocystis* drug pentamidine. The hyperglycemia resulting from these agents is usually not reversible. Thiazide diuretics can inhibit insulin secretion by causing hypokalemia. Glucocorticoids and nicotinic acid cause hyperglycemia by impairing insulin action. Both protease inhibitors used in the treatment of human immunodeficiency virus infection and clozapine, a drug used to treat resistant schizophrenia, can cause hyperglycemia via an as yet undetermined mechanism.

Infections

Certain viral infections, including rubella[54] and coxsackie B virus,[55] have been associated with diabetes. Some studies suggest that a viral infection can trigger autoimmune destruction of β cells in genetically predisposed individuals, leading to autoimmune type 1 diabetes.

Uncommon Forms of Immune-Mediated Diabetes

The stiff-man syndrome is a rare neurologic syndrome characterized by spasticity of the axial muscles. It is associated with very high titers of anti-GAD antibodies and up to one-third of patients develop diabetes.[56] Autoantibodies directed against the insulin receptor represent another rare cause of diabetes.[57] These antibodies have the potential to change from being receptor antagonists (causing insulin resistance) to being receptor agonists (leading to potentially life-threatening hypoglycemia).

Other Genetic Syndromes Sometimes Associated with Diabetes

Many of the genetic syndromes listed under H in Table 53–1 are known to be associated with diabetes. The precise mechanism of the diabetes has not been established for these conditions.

Gestational Diabetes

Gestational diabetes is defined as diabetes with onset or first recognition during pregnancy. The prevalence of gestational diabetes increases in parallel with the prevalence of type 2 diabetes in a population. Approximately 4% of pregnancies in the United States are complicated by gestational diabetes.[58] Risk factors include age (commoner among older women), ethnicity (higher rates are seen among women from ethnic groups with a high incidence of type 2 diabetes), prepregnancy body mass index (risk increases with degree of obesity), parity (risk increases with number of previous pregnancies), and family history of diabetes. A previous pregnancy complicated by gestational diabetes or a history of delivery of a macrosomic infant also represents a strong risk factor for future gestational diabetes. The diagnosis of gestational diabetes is important since, if left untreated, adverse fetal or maternal outcomes can occur. The main adverse fetal outcomes are macrosomia and neonatal hypoglycemia.[59] Maternal complications include a higher rate of dystocia and cesarean section as well as a greater risk of future type 2 diabetes[60] (among women who revert to normal glucose tolerance after completion of the pregnancy).

There are no uniformly agreed upon criteria for the diagnosis of gestational diabetes.[61] The criteria most widely used in North America were developed based on the ability of plasma glucose levels measured during pregnancy to predict future development of type 2 diabetes and not adverse outcomes of that pregnancy. In addition, the 100-g glucose load used in North America is different from the 75-g load used in other parts of the world. Finally, no consensus exists as to who should be screened.[62] In some countries (e.g., the United States) universal screening is routinely undertaken, whereas in other countries (e.g., in Europe) only women believed to be at high risk are screened.

DIAGNOSIS

Diagnostic Criteria

In addition to recommending changes in the classification system for diabetes, the Expert Committee of the ADA also recommended changes in the diagnostic criteria for the disease in their 1997 report.[10] These criteria were subsequently endorsed by WHO[11] and are outlined in Table 53–2. The major differences between the new and the old criteria were a reduction in the fasting plasma glucose cut point used to diagnose the disease and an emphasis on use of fasting plasma glucose as opposed to the oral glucose tolerance test to screen for and diagnose the disease. The fasting plasma glucose level required for a diagnosis of diabetes was reduced from 140 mg/dL to 126 mg/dL. The upper limit of normal for fasting plasma glucose was set at 110 mg/dL. The diagnostic threshold for the 2-hour postglucose challenge plasma glucose level remains at 200 mg/dL. Two other important features of the diagnostic criteria that were retained include the ability to use casual plasma glucose levels in patients with hyperglycemic symptoms and the requirement that a firm diagnosis be based on testing carried out on more than one occasion. The ADA report based its criteria on use of the fasting plasma glucose level, while the WHO report included equivalent cut points for whole-blood venous and capillary glucose (see Table 53–2).

Rationale for the New Diagnostic Criteria

There were three main reasons for the changes recommended in the revised diagnostic criteria. The first reason relates to the lack of equivalence between a fasting plasma glucose value of 140 mg/dL and a 2-hour postglucose challenge value of 200 mg/dL.[63–65] Only approximately 25% of patients with a 2-hour value above 200 mg/dL will have a fasting value above 140 mg/dL. The point at which the two tests approach equivalence (based on receiver operating characteristic curve analysis) is closer to a fasting value of 126 mg/dL. The second reason for changing the criteria comes from epidemiologic studies that have assessed the level of glycemia at which the microvascular complications of diabetes begin to appear.[63, 65] As seen in Figure 53–1 the fasting plasma glucose value at which retinopathy first occurs is closer to 126 mg/dL than 140 mg/dL. This observation was first reported in a population of Pima Indian subjects who have a very high prevalence of diabetes and a bimodal distribution of glucose. It was subsequently confirmed in a population from Egypt and most recently

TABLE 53–2.   Diagnostic Criteria for Diabetes Mellitus and Other Categories of Hyperglycemia

| | Glucose Concentration (mg/dL [mmol/L]) | | |
| | Whole Blood | | |
	Venous	Capillary	Venous Plasma
Diabetes mellitus			
Fasting	≥110 (≥6.1)	≥110 (≥6.1)	≥126 (≥7.0)
or			
2-hr postglucose load	≥180 (≥10.0)	≥200 (≥11.1)	≥200 (≥11.1)
or			
both			
Impaired glucose tolerance			
Fasting concentration (if measured)	<110 (<6.1)	<110 (<6.1)	<126 (<7.0)
and			
2-hr postglucose load	≥120 (≥6.7) and <180 (<10.0)	≥140 (≥7.8) and <200 (<11.1)	≥140 (≥7.8) and <200 (<11.1)
Impaired fasting glucose			
Fasting	≥100 (≥5.6) and <110 (<6.1)	≥100 (≥5.6) and <110 (<6.1)	≥110 (≥6.1) and <126 (<7.0)
2-hr (if measured)	<120 (<6.7)	<140 (<7.8)	<140 (<7.8)

Modified from Alberti KGMM, Zimmet PZ: Definition, diagnosis, and classification of diabetes mellitus and its complications. Part 1: Diagnosis and classification of diabetes mellitus. Provisional report of a WHO consultation. Diabet Med 15:539–553, 1998. Copyright John Wiley & Sons Limited.

in data from the Third National Health and Nutrition Examination Survey in the United States.[10] Because of differences in the design of the studies the retinopathy prevalence data are not comparable across the three populations shown in Figure 53–1. Nevertheless, the cut point at which retinopathy begins to appear is similar in all three studies. The third reason for recommending a change in the diagnostic criteria for diabetes is a pragmatic one and relates to the fact that, outside of pregnancy, the oral glucose tolerance test is seldom used in routine clinical practice. The expert committees of the ADA and WHO acknowledged this fact by emphasizing that the fasting plasma glucose measurement should be considered the preferred method for screening. The ADA also recommended use of the fasting plasma glucose level in epidemiologic studies.

Implications of the New Criteria

A diagnosis of diabetes can have implications for patients not just in terms of their future medical well-being but also in terms of their psychosocial and even economic well-being. Examples of this would include higher life insurance premiums as well as exclusion of patients treated with insulin from certain occupations (e.g., commercial airline pilot). Screening programs should ideally be able to identify individuals who are most likely to benefit from therapy while at the same time minimizing any unnecessary labeling of individuals who do not have the disease. Any change in the diagnostic criteria for diabetes must

take these complex medical, psychosocial, and economic issues into consideration. To date, most of the literature on the impact of the new diagnostic criteria has focused on the medical implications of the change.[66]

New Categories of Hyperglycemia

One impact of the new criteria has been the creation of two new categories of hyperglycemia, namely, normal fasting glucose and impaired fasting glucose. The term *normal fasting glucose* is used to describe individuals with plasma glucose levels less than 110 mg/dL. The choice of 110 mg/dL as the normal cutpoint would appear to be arbitrary. Many laboratories around the country report the upper limit of normal for plasma glucose as 100 mg/dL. Furthermore, plasma glucose represents a continuous variable and there appears to be a continuum of risk for certain events, including future development of diabetes,[67] as well as atherosclerotic coronary or cerebrovascular events.[68] Therefore, while a threshold exists for the risk of microvascular complications (see Fig. 53–1) this may not be the case for the risk of macrovascular complications. Indeed some investigators have proposed the term *dysglycemia* to describe the fact that the higher an individual's plasma glucose level (even if within the "normal" range), the greater their risk of subsequent adverse vascular events.[69]

Impaired fasting glucose represents an intermediate state between normal fasting glucose and overt diabetes. It is the term used to describe individuals with a fasting plasma glucose value between 110

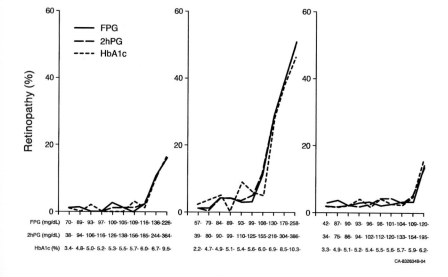

FIGURE 53–1. Prevalence of retinopathy by deciles of the distribution of fasting plasma glucose (FPG), 2-hour postglucose challenge plasma glucose (2hPG), and hemoglobin A1c (HbA1c) level in a population of Pima Indians *(left panel)*, Egyptians *(center panel)*, and a representative sample of the U.S. population aged 40 to 74 years *(right panel)*. (From Report of the Expert Committee on the Diagnosis and Classification of Diabetes Mellitus. Diabetes Care 20:1183–1197, 1997.)

and 125 mg/dL (see Table 53–2). Individuals with impaired fasting glucose are at increased risk of developing diabetes in the future. This state of abnormal glucose homeostasis is analogous but not identical to impaired glucose tolerance. The latter can only be diagnosed by means of an oral glucose tolerance test. A recent report from Mauritius suggests that impaired glucose tolerance may be a better predictor of future diabetes than impaired fasting glucose.[70] Both states represent components of the so-called plurimetabolic syndrome, or syndrome X.[28] This represents a clustering of metabolic abnormalities, including hypertension, dyslipidemia, central obesity, and abnormalities of the fibrinolytic system. Data from the Framingham Offspring Study indicate that these metabolic risk factors worsen across the spectrum of glucose tolerance categories.[71] Together, they greatly increase an individual's risk of atherosclerotic events. It has been suggested that insulin resistance is the factor that provides a link between these metabolic abnormalities. Evidence to support interventions aimed at treating individuals with impaired glucose tolerance or impaired fasting glucose is beginning to accumulate.[72] The main endpoint that has been assessed to date is the development of overt diabetes. Studies assessing the impact of treatment on the rate of atherosclerotic events are anxiously awaited.[73]

Changing the Prevalence and Incidence of Diabetes

Since publication of the initial report recommending new diagnostic criteria for diabetes, many investigators have assessed the impact of the change on the prevalence of the disease in their individual populations.[74–77] The majority of these studies were based on existing data sets in which data on fasting and postchallenge glucose levels were available. The largest of these comparative reports looked at the prevalence of diabetes using the new vs. the old criteria among 16 cohorts comprising 26,190 individuals in eight European countries.[74] As illustrated in Figure 53–2 the new criteria frequently led to a change in the prevalence of the disease, although this was not always in the same direction. The overall change was an increase in prevalence from 7.2% to 7.7%. The risk of disagreement decreased with increasing body mass index and also with increasing age. In contrast, a study which included 4515 elderly people from four centers in North America reported major discrepancies in the prevalence of diabetes using the ADA as opposed to the WHO criteria.[76] The overall prevalence of newly identified diabetes in this study decreased from 14.8% using the WHO criteria to 7.7% using the ADA criteria. An important report from the National Institutes of Health and the National Center for Health Statistics looked at the impact of the new vs. the old criteria on diabetes diagnostic categories in a probability sample of the U.S. population aged 40 to 74 years.[77] The prevalence of undiagnosed

diabetes decreased from 6.4% to 4.4% with use of the new ADA criteria.

More recently, a comparison was made between the new ADA criteria and concomitant glycated hemoglobin levels from two large data sets.[78] The authors reported normal glycated hemoglobin levels in up to 60% of individuals who met the definition of diabetes by fasting plasma glucose criteria. They argue that diabetes should not be diagnosed until evidence of excessive glycosylation is present. Several problems arise with this approach, not least of which is the lack of standardization of assays for glycated hemoglobin. The true test of the appropriateness of the new diagnostic criteria based on fasting plasma glucose levels must await definitive prospective studies looking at the ability of the recommended cut points to predict future diabetic complications.

REFERENCES

1. Gerich J: The genetic basis of type 2 diabetes mellitus: Impaired insulin secretion versus impaired insulin sensitivity. Endoc Rev 19:491–503, 1998.
2. Ferrannini E: Insulin resistance versus insulin deficiency in non–insulin-dependent diabetes mellitus: Problems and prospects. Endoc Rev 19:477–490, 1998.
3. King G, Brownlee M: The cellular and molecular mechanisms of diabetic complications. Endocrinol Metab Clin North Am 25:255–270, 1996.
4. Stern M: Do non–insulin-dependent diabetes mellitus and cardiovascular disease share common antecedents. Ann Intern Med 124:110–116, 1996.
5. McGarry J: What if Minkowski had been ageusic? An alternative angle on diabetes. Science 258:766–770, 1992.
6. Chaufan C: It's my life after all. IDF Bull 42:32–34, 1997.
7. MacGregor A: Classification criteria for rheumatoid arthritis. Baillieres Clin Rheumatol 9:287–304, 1995.
8. National Diabetes Data Group: Classification and diagnosis of diabetes mellitus and other categories of glucose intolerance. Diabetes 28:1039–1057, 1979.
9. Diabetes Mellitus: Report of a WHO study group. Geneva, World Health Organization, 1985.
10. Report of the Expert Committee on the Diagnosis and Classification of Diabetes Mellitus. Diabetes Care 20:1183–1197, 1997.
11. Alberti KGMM, Zimmet PZ: Definition, diagnosis, and classification of diabetes mellitus and its complications. Part 1: Diagnosis and classification of diabetes mellitus. Provisional report of a WHO consultation. Diabet Med 15:539–553, 1998.
12. LaPorte R, Matsushima M, Chang Y: Prevalence and incidence of insulin-dependent diabetes. *In* National Diabetes Data Group (ed): Diabetes in America. Bethesda, MD, National Institutes of Health, 1995, pp 37–46.
13. Karvonen M, Tuomilehto J, Libman I, LaPorte R: A review of the recent epidemiological data on the worldwide incidence of type 1 (insulin-dependent) diabetes mellitus. World Health Organization DIAMOND Project Group. Diabetologia 36:883–892, 1994.
14. Buzzetti R, Quattrocchi C, Nistico L: Dissecting the genetics of type 1 diabetes: Relevance for familial clustering and differences in incidence. Diabetes Metab Rev 14:111–128, 1998.
15. Dahlquist G: The aetiology of type 1 diabetes: An epidemiological perspective. Acta Paediatr 425:5–10, 1998.
16. Scott F, Norris J, Hubert K: Milk and type 1 diabetes: Examining the evidence and broadening the focus. Diabetes Care 19:379–383, 1996.
17. Zimmet P, Tuomi T, Mackay R, et al: Latent autoimmune diabetes mellitus in adults (LADA): The role of antibodies to glutamic acid decarboxylase in diagnosis and prediction of insulin dependency. Diabet Med 11:299–303, 1994.
18. Verge C, Gianani R, Kawasaki E, et al: Predicting type 1 diabetes in first-degree relatives using a combination of insulin, GAD, and ICA512bdc/IA-2 autoantibodies. Diabetes 45:926–933, 1996.
19. Molbak A, Christau B, Marner B, et al: Incidence of insulin-dependent diabetes mellitus in age groups over 30 years in Denmark. Diabet Med 11:650–655, 1994.
20. Humphrey A, McCarty D, Mackay I, et al: Autoantibodies to glutamic acid decarboxylase and phenotypic features associated with early insulin treatment in individuals with adult-onset diabetes mellitus. Diabet Med 15:113–119, 1998.
21. Willis J, Scott R, Brown L, et al: Islet cell antibodies and antibodies against glutamic acid decarboxylase in newly diagnosed adult-onset diabetes mellitus. Diabetes Res Clin Prac 33:89–97, 1996.
22. McLarty D, Athaide I, Bottazzo G, et al: Islet cell antibodies are not specifically associated with insulin-dependent diabetes mellitus in rural Tanzanian Africans. Diabetes Res Clin Pract 9:219–224, 1990.
23. Libman I, LaPorte R, Becker D, et al: Was there an epidemic of diabetes in nonwhite adolescents in Allegheny County, Pennsylvania. Diabetes Care 21:1278–1281, 1998.
24. Kenny S, Aubert R, Geiss L: Prevalence and incidence of non–insulin-dependent diabetes. *In* National Diabetes Data Group (ed): Diabetes in America. Bethesda, MD, National Institutes of Health, 1995, pp 47–67.
25. Rudenski A, Hadden D, Atkinson A, et al: Natural history of pancreatic islet β-cell function in type 2 diabetes mellitus studied over six years by homeostasis model assessment. Diabet Med 5:36–41, 1988.
26. Leahy J: Natural history of beta-cell dysfunction in NIDDM. Diabetes Care 13:992–1010, 1990.
27. Cowie C, Harris M: Physical and metabolic characteristics of persons with diabetes. *In* National Diabetes Data Group (ed): Diabetes in America. Bethesda, MD, National Institutes of Health, 1995, pp 117–164.
28. Reaven G: Role of insulin resistance in human disease. Diabetes 37:1595–1607, 1988.

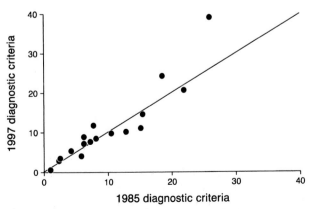

FIGURE 53–2. Prevalence of diabetes in 16 European populations using the 1985 diagnostic criteria of the World Health Organization and the new criteria proposed by the American Diabetes Association in 1997. (From Decode Study Group on Behalf of the European Diabetes Epidemiology Study Group: Will new diagnostic criteria for diabetes mellitus change phenotyped patients with diabetes? Reanalysis of European epidemiological data. BMJ 317:371–375, 1998.)

29. Barnett A, Eff C, Leslie R, Pyke D: Diabetes in identical twins. A study of 200 pairs. Diabetologia 20:87–93, 1981.
30. Knowler W, Saad M, Pettitt D, et al: Determinants of diabetes mellitus in the Pima Indians. Diabetes Care 16:216–227, 1993.
31. Hoet J, Tripathy B, Rao R, Yajnik C: Malnutrition and diabetes in the tropics. Diabetes Care 19:1014–1017, 1996.
32. Tripathy B, Samal K: Overview and consensus statement on diabetes in tropical areas. Diabetes Metab Rev 13:63–76, 1997.
33. Hattersly A: Maturity-onset diabetes of the young: Clinical heterogeneity explained by genetic heterogeneity. Diabet Med 15:15–24, 1998.
34. Yamagata K, Furuta H, Oda N, et al: Mutations in the hepatocyte nuclear factor-4-alpha gene in maturity-onset diabetes of the young (MODY 1). Nature 384:458–460, 1996.
35. Froguel P, Vaxillaire M, Sun F, et al: Close linkage of glucokinase locus on chromosome 7p to early-onset non–insulin-dependent diabetes. Nature 356:162–164, 1992.
36. Yamagata K, Oda N, Kaisaki P, et al: Mutations in the hepatocyte nuclear factor-1-alpha gene in maturity-onset diabetes of the young (MODY 3). Nature 384:455–458, 1996.
37. Stoffers D, Ferrer J, Clarke W, Habener J: Early-onset type-II diabetes mellitus (MODY 4) linked to IPF1. Nat Genet 117:138–139, 1997.
38. Byrne M, Sturis J, Menzel S, et al: Altered insulin secretory response to glucose in diabetic and nondiabetic subjects with mutations in the diabetes susceptibility gene MODY 3 on chromosome 20. Diabetes 45:1503–1510, 1996.
39. Clement K, Pueyo M, Vaxillaire M, et al: Assessment of insulin sensitivity in glucokinase-deficient subjects. Diabetologia 39:82–90, 1996.
40. Habener J, Stoffers D: A newly discovered role of transcription factors involved in pancreas development and the pathogenesis of diabetes mellitus. Proc Assoc Am Physicians 110:12–21, 1998.
41. Velho G, Froguel P: Maturity-onset diabetes of the young (MODY), MODY genes and non–insulin-dependent diabetes mellitus. Diabetes Metab 23:34–37, 1997.
42. Walker M, Turnbull D: Mitochondrial related diabetes: A clinical perspective. Diabet Med 14:1007–1009, 1997.
43. Gruppuso P, Gorden P, Kahn C, et al: Familial hyperproinsulinemia due to a proposed defect in conversion of proinsulin to insulin. N Engl J Med 311:629–634, 1984.
44. Haneda M, Polonsky K, Bergenstal R, et al: Familial hyperinsulinemia due to a structurally abnormal insulin. Definition of an emerging new clinical syndrome. N Engl J Med 310:1288–1294, 1984.
45. Bruning J, Winnay J, Bonner-Weir S, et al: Development of a novel polygenic model of NIDDM in mice heterozygous for IR and IRS-1 null alleles. Cell 88:561–572, 1997.
46. Taylor S: Lilly lecture: Molecular mechanisms of insulin resistance: Lessons from patients with mutations in the insulin-receptor gene. Diabetes 41:1473–1490, 1992.
47. Kahn C, Flier J, Bar R, et al: The syndromes of insulin resistance and acanthosis nigricans. N Engl J Med 294:739–745, 1976.
48. Gullo L, Pezzilli R, Morselli-Labate A, Group IPCS: Diabetes and the risk of pancreatic cancer. N Engl J Med 331:81–84, 1994.
49. Moran A, Doherty L, Wang X, Thomas W: Abnormal glucose metabolism in cystic fibrosis. Pediatr 133:10–17, 1998.
50. Phelps G, Chapman I, Hall P, et al: Prevalence of genetic haemochromatosis among diabetic patients. Lancet 2:233–234, 1989.
51. Yajnik C, Shelgikar K, Naik S, et al: The ketoacidosis-resistance in fibro-calculous-pancreatic-diabetes. Diabetes Res Clin Pract 15:149–156, 1993.
52. Pandit M, Burke J, Gustafson A, et al: Drug-induced disorders of glucose tolerance. Ann Intern Med 118:529–540, 1993.
53. O'Byrne S, Feely J: Effects of drug on glucose tolerance in non–insulin-dependent diabetes (parts I and II). Drugs 40:203–219, 1990.
54. Forrest J, Menser M, Burgess JA: High frequency of diabetes mellitus in young patients with congenital rubella. Lancet 2:332–334, 1971.
55. King M, Bidwell D, Shikh A, et al: Coxsackie-B-virus-specific IgM responses in children with insulin-dependent (juvenile-onset; type 1) diabetes mellitus. Lancet 1:1397–1399, 1983.
56. Solimena M, De Camilli P: Autoimmunity to glutamic acid decarboxylase (GAD) in stiff-man syndrome and insulin-dependent diabetes mellitus. Trends Neurosci 14:452–457, 1991.
57. Flier J: Lilly lecture: Syndromes of insulin resistance: From patient to gene and back again. Diabetes 41:1207–1219, 1992.
58. Engelgau M, Herman W, Smith P, et al: The epidemiology and diabetes and pregnancy in the US, 1988. Diabetes Care 18:1029–1033, 1995.
59. Persson B, Hanson U: Neonatal mobidities in gestational diabetes mellitus. Diabetes Care 21:B79–B84, 1998.
60. Dornhorst A, Rossi M: Risk and prevention of type 2 diabetes in women with gestational diabetes. Diabetes Care 21:B43–B49, 1998.
61. Coustan D, Carpenter M: The diagnosis of gestational diabetes. Diabetes Care 21:B5–B8, 1998.
62. Carr S: Screening for gestational diabetes mellitus. Diabetes Care 21:B14–B18, 1998.
63. McCance D, Hanson R, Charles M, et al: Comparison of tests for glycated haemoglobin and fasting and two hour plasma glucose concentrations as diagnostic methods for diabetes. BMJ 308:1323–1328, 1994.
64. Finch C, Zimmet P, Alberti K: Determining diabetes prevalence: A rational basis for the use of fasting plasma glucose concentrations. Diabet Med 7:603–610, 1990.
65. Engelgau M, Thompson T, Herman W, et al: Comparison of fasting and 2-hour glucose and HbAlc levels for diagnosing diabetes. Diagnostic criteria and performance revisited. Diabetes Care 20:785–791, 1997.
66. McCance D, Hanson R, Pettitt D, et al: Diagnosing diabetes mellitus — do we need new criteria? Diabetologia 40:247–255, 1997.
67. Dinneen S, Maldonado D, Leibson C, et al: Effects of changing diagnostic criteria on the risk of developing diabetes. Diabetes Care 21:1408–1413, 1998.
68. Charles M, Balkau B, Vauzelle-Kervoeden F, et al: Revision of diagnostic criteria for diabetes. Lancet 348:1657–1658, 1996.
69. Gerstein H, Yusuf S: Dysglycaemia and risk of cardiovascular disease. Lancet 347:949–950, 1996.
70. Shaw J, Zimmet P, De Courten M, et al: Impaired fasting glucose or impaired glucose tolerance. What best predicts future diabetes in Mauritius. Diabetes Care 22:399–402, 1999.
71. Meigs J, Nathan D, Wilson P, et al: Metabolic risk factors worsen continuously across the spectrum of nondiabetic glucose tolerance. Ann Intern Med 128:524–533, 1998.
72. Pan X, Li G, Hu Y, et al: Effects of diet and exercise in preventing NIDDM in people with impaired glucose tolerance. The Da Qing IGT and Diabetes Study. Diabetes Care 20:537–544, 1997.
73. The Diabetes Prevention Program Research Group: Design and methods for a clinical trial in the prevention of type 2 diabetes. Diabetes Care 22:623–634, 1999.
74. Decode Study Group on behalf of the European Diabetes Epidemiology Study Group: Will new diagnostic criteria for diabetes mellitus change phenotyped patients with diabetes? Reanalysis of European epidemiological data. BMJ 317:371–375, 1998.
75. De Vegt F, Dekker J, Stehouwer C, et al: American Diabetes Association criteria versus the 1985 World Health Organization criteria for the diagnosis of abnormal glucose tolerance: Poor agreement in the Hoorn Study. Diabetes Care 21:1686–1690, 1998.
76. Wahl P, Savage P, Psaty B, et al: Diabetes in older adults: Comparison of 1997 American Diabetes Association classification of diabetes mellitus with 1985 WHO classification. Lancet 352:1012–1015, 1998.
77. Harris M, Eastman R, Cowie C, et al: Comparison of diabetes diagnostic categories in the US population according to 1997 American Diabetes Association and 1980–1985 World Health Organization diagnostic criteria. Diabetes Care 20:1859–1862, 1997.
78. Davidson M, Schriger D, Peters A, Lorber B: Relationship between fasting plasma glucose and glycosylated hemoglobin. JAMA 281:1203–1210, 1999.

Type 1 (Insulin-Dependent) Diabetes Mellitus: Etiology, Pathogenesis, and Natural History*

Åke Lernmark

HISTORY

Type 1 (insulin-dependent) diabetes mellitus is associated with numerous immune abnormalities. The pancreatic β cells are lost in numbers and volume, and a distinct mode of progression to severe insulin deficiency occurs that requires insulin substitution therapy. In children, type 1 diabetes has a distinct clinical mode of presentation. When age at onset is young, classification of the disease is usually not a problem. In adults, type 1 may masquerade as type 2 diabetes. Although it has been known for decades that diabetes mellitus can occur in various degrees of severity, it was not until approximately 40 years ago that evidence was presented that indicated different modes of inheritance for what were then classified as "maturity-onset" and "juvenile-onset" type diabetes.[1] It is now evident that type 1 diabetes may occur at any age. The fact that type 1 diabetes in adults fulfills clinical criteria for type 2 diabetes demonstrates the limitation of a disease classification, which is based on clinical symptoms rather than on the etiology and pathogenesis of the disease. Current diagnostic criteria for different forms of diabetes mellitus are therefore limited to clinical symptoms,[2] except in rare families with specific mutations (e.g., glucokinase or HNF-1α mutation, which causes specific syndromes of maturity-onset diabetes of the young [MODY]). The basis for the distinction between type 1 and 2 diabetes is the patient's dependence on insulin. Type 1 diabetes in children or nonpregnant adults includes any of the following symptoms or biochemical changes: polyuria, polydipsia, ketonuria, and rapid weight loss together with gross or unequivocal elevation of plasma glucose levels. Stupor and coma may ultimately develop.

The diagnostic criteria to differentiate between type 1 (insulin-dependent) and type 2 (non–insulin-dependent diabetes, or NIDDM) are important to understand the cause and pathogenesis of these two disease entities. The diagnostic criteria are primarily recommendations for classification, the aim of which is to better understand the cause of diabetes and to optimize care of diabetic patients. Using molecular genetics, it has been possible to fully clarify several monogenetic forms of diabetes. The etiology of these diabetes phenotypes, some of them classified as MODY, have been explained by mutations in, for example, the genes for insulin,[3] insulin receptor,[4] glucokinase (MODY-2),[5] HNF-4α (MODY-1), or HNF-1α (MODY-3).[6] The clarification of the etiology of these diabetes phenotypes is a major advancement that has increased the diagnostic precision of diabetes syndromes.[2, 7] The

understanding of the more complex and multifactorial type 1 diabetes syndromes has also undergone significant advances.

Early histologic studies of pancreatic tissue of diabetic patients who died shortly after clinical onset revealed that the pancreatic islets were altered by fibrosis, hyalinosis, atrophy, and infiltration of inflammatory cells.[8] The inflammatory lesion of the islets of Langerhans was later described as insulitis,[9] and quantitative studies of the pancreatic islets showed a specific loss of insulin-producing cells in association with the clinical onset of Type 1 diabetes.[10, 11] The presence of inflammatory cells in and around the islets of Langerhans in about 50% of new-onset patients was also described.[10, 12] The rediscovery of insulitis[10] was of major significance, especially because it was later observed that autoimmune thyroid disease often developed in diabetic patients treated with insulin or, conversely, that patients with diseases of autoimmune character (e.g., Graves' disease, Hashimoto's thyroiditis, pernicious anemia, and Addison's disease) had an increased prevalence of insulin-dependent diabetes.[13, 14] It was therefore suggested that the pathogenesis of insulin-dependent diabetes involved autoimmune reactions directed toward the endocrine pancreas. This notion was supported by delayed hypersensitivity[15] and leukocyte migration inhibition[16, 17] to pancreatic islet antigens. Numerous studies have confirmed the presence of insulitis,[18, 19] whereas blood cell tests indicating presence of β cell–specific autoreactive T cells[20] remain scarce. More recent international workshops confirm that reproducible tests of blood T cell reactivity to islet antigens remain elusive.[21] In contrast, several types of islet cell autoantibodies can now be determined in standardized assays. Long-sought-for islet cell antibodies (ICA) were described in 1974,[22, 23] islet cell surface antibodies (ICSA) in 1978,[24] and complement-dependent antibody-mediated islet cell cytotoxicity in 1980.[25] The first antigen recognized by these antibodies, an islet protein of 64,000 relative molecular mass (Mr), or 64K, was described in 1982.[26] Later, the 64K protein was found to have glutamic acid decarboxylase (GAD) activity,[26] but molecular cloning showed that the enzyme was a novel GAD isoform, GAD65.[27, 28] Autoantibodies to insulin (IAA) were demonstrated in 1983,[29] and a third autoantigen, insulinoma associated antigen-2 (IA-2), a receptor-type protein tyrosine phosphatase, in 1994.[30–32] Since the mid-1980s, numerous studies have used serum from patients with type 1 diabetes in attempts to identify novel β cell target autoantigens by immunoprecipitation or immunoblotting techniques. So far, antibody assays to other autoantigens have failed to show disease sensitivity and specificity superior to that of GAD65, insulin, and IA-2. The presence of autoantibodies against these three autoantigens are shown to replace the more cumbersome ICA indirect immunofluoresence assay.[33] Taken together, ample evidence exists that islet cell autoimmunity is of major importance in the etiopathogenesis of insulin-dependent (type 1) diabetes.

Type 1 diabetes is often thought to be a disorder of acute onset, and

*Studies by the author were supported by the National Institutes of Health (grants DK26190, DK42654, and DK53004), the Diabetes Endocrinology Research Center (NIH grant DK17047), the Juvenile Diabetes Foundation International, the American Diabetes Association, and the Swedish Medical Research Council.

the clinical onset may be dramatic. Over the years, however, numerous reports have noted that symptoms of subclinical diabetes preceded the clinical onset. In addition, in adult diabetes patients classified with type 2 diabetes, a change sometimes occurs from an insulin-independent to an insulin-dependent state. It is now accepted that ICA or autoantibodies against GAD65, insulin, or IA-2 may be present up to several years before the clinical onset of the disease,[34–37] perhaps even at birth.[38]

The possibility that islet autoimmunity might be present long before symptoms of hyperglycemia occur makes it difficult to define a causative factor. The clinical onset is not likely to occur until there is a major loss (80% to 90%) of the islet β cells. An increased frequency of diabetes in conjunction with acute viral illnesses was first described in Norway more than 100 years ago and was subsequently followed by numerous similar case reports. These early reports suggested a relationship between the clinical onset of type 1 diabetes and acute viral illness.[39, 40] Most commonly, type 1 diabetes has been diagnosed in conjunction with infections of mumps, congenital rubella, or Coxsackie virus B4.[39, 40] The true relationship between these viral diseases and later onset of type 1 diabetes remains conjectural. The immunologic responsiveness to viruses among different individuals may be relevant to the disease process. In this respect, type 1 diabetes is both genetically associated with and linked to certain human leukocyte antigen (HLA) genetic factors.[41–43] In fact, using DNA sequence information in the genetic analysis, it is found that more than 95% of all patients in whom type 1 diabetes onset occurred before age 30 years are positive for the chromosome 6 HLA genes DQB1*0302-A1*0301-DRB1*04, DQB1*0201-A1*0501-DRB1*03, or both. Although some 50% to 60% of the background population carry these HLA factors, they represent necessary but insufficient prerequisites for the development of type 1 diabetes. It has been estimated that HLA contributes about 60% of type 1 diabetes risk. Other genetic factors have indeed been identified,[44, 45] but none has shown a level of importance comparable to HLA. In summary, the association with HLA may signify differences in immune responsiveness to certain antigens. The formation of an immune response to an invading antigen (e.g., virus, bacterium) or internal antigen (e.g., a retrovirus) might induce an autoimmune reaction directed against the pancreatic cells.

PREVALENCE

The prevalence of type 1 diabetes is low compared with that of type 2 diabetes. Among individuals 30 years or younger, the prevalence of type 1 diabetes does not usually exceed about 0.3%. The prevalence of type 2 diabetes may be as high as 2% to 3% and increases with advancing age. It has been pointed out[2, 46] that the prevalence figures shown in Table 54–1 should be viewed with caution, because different age groups were studied, and various methods of assessing the cases were used. Both geographic and ethnic differences are seen in the prevalence rates.

TABLE 54–1. The Prevalence of Insulin-Dependent Diabetes in Certain Populations

Location	Age Group Studied (yr)	Method of Ascertainment	Prevalence (per 1000)
China	10–19	Survey	0.09
Cuba	0–15	National registry	0.14
France	0–19	Central registry	0.32
Japan	7–15	School records	0.07
Scandinavian countries	0–14	National registry and hospital records	0.83–2.23
United Kingdom	0–26	National survey of health and development	3.40
United States	5–17	School records	1.93

From Harris MI: Diabetes in America, ed 2. Bethesda, MD, National Institutes of Health, 1995.

TABLE 54–2. Mean Annual Incidence of IDDM (per 100,000) in Children, Adolescents, and Young Adults in Various Locations

Location	Study Population (× 10⁶)	Age (yr)	Incidence Rate (per 10⁵)
North America			
Allegheny County	0.6	0–19	16
Michigan		4–17	20
Canada	0.8	0–16	9
Europe			
Finland	1.0	0–14	34
Sardinia	0.3	0–15	30
Sweden	1.6	0–14	25
Denmark	0.5	0–14	22
Norway	0.9	0–14	21
United Kingdom	14.8	0–15	14
Netherlands	3.2	0–14	11
France	12.5	0–14	7
Oceania			
New Zealand	0.3	0–20	12
Australia	0.5	0–14	12
Asia			
Israel		0–20	4
Jews			4
Arabs			1
Kuwait	3.0	0–20	4
Japan	34.0	0–18	0.8

From Harris MI: Diabetes in America, ed 2. Bethesda, MD, National Institutes of Health, 1995.

INCIDENCE

The incidence rate is the frequency with which new cases of type 1 diabetes are detected during a defined period. The rate is expressed as an annual number of cases per 100,000 age-corrected individuals. A determination of incidence therefore requires a precise knowledge of the total number of individuals in each age group and the number of new patients diagnosed in the particular area during 1 year. Determinations of secular trends constitute an important part of population-based epidemiologic studies. However, such analyses are rare because they require careful follow-up investigations during several subsequent years.

Incidence studies on type 1 diabetes are available[2, 46] from an increasing number of countries and states (Table 54–2). The groups that have been studied are primarily white; only limited information is available for other racial groups. The reliability of data from many countries suffers, however, from the absence of clearly defined degrees of ascertainment and demographics as well as from lack of geographic delineation of the group subjected to investigation. Hence, the average annual incidence rate of type 1 diabetes is increasing and varies between 0.8 and 50 per 100,000 children or young adults.[47–51] Worldwide epidemiologic investigations of type 1 diabetes as a noncommunicable disease indicate 4% to 6% annual increase in incidence rate in Scandinavia,[48, 52] and similar data are being collected in other countries.[51] About 1% of all children born in Scandinavian countries will manifest type 1 diabetes during their lifetime. It is speculated that type 1 diabetes exhibits patterns of epidemic occurrence, suggesting that diabetogenic environmental determinants may exist.[51] Further studies are needed to test this hypothesis, which would require diabetes registries much like those for recognized infectious diseases. Studies from several countries show that the incidence rates vary by geographic region (not only between but also within countries), by age, and by gender.

Geographic Distribution

The annual incidence of type 1 diabetes is higher in northern Europe than in the Mediterranean area, with the exception of Sardinia.[14, 53, 54]

Furthermore, the incidence in Iceland[53] is lower than that in Sweden[55] or Finland.[53] Surprisingly, the type 1 diabetes incidence rate in Estonia is about 25% of the rate in Finland.[54] The incidence rates within countries also show stable differences. The eastern and southern parts of Finland[56] as well as the central and southern parts of Sweden,[55] have higher incidence rates than the northern part of those countries.

The incidence rate in high-level areas is as high as 40 to 50 per 100,000 persons age 0 to 15 years. The cause of geographic variation remains unknown, but it has been speculated that genetic factors, primarily associated with different HLA-DR or DQ genotypes of the major histocompatibility complex (MHC) on chromosome 6, and environmental factors are important. The latter is supported by the observation that monozygotic twins show rates of less than 20% to 30% concordance for IDDM.[57, 58] Also, among HLA-identical siblings of type 1 diabetes-affected patients, about 20% eventually manifest the disease, and the overall lifetime risk for first-degree relatives has been estimated at about 8% for siblings and 5% for children of parents with type 1 diabetes.[59] The mode of inheritance is complex. In addition, the HLA class II molecules from the DQ and DR loci on chromosome 6 that are necessary (but not sufficient) for disease vary greatly between countries and thereby affect disease incidence.[54, 60, 61] In addition, factors in the environment are important in understanding the pathogenesis of type 1 diabetes, and they may also help to explain differences in geographic distribution. Improved epidemiology and better diagnostic criteria to distinguish different forms of diabetes are critical in obtaining reliable incidence rates for various countries and states.

Variation with Age

Until recently, type 1 diabetes was thought to occur almost exclusively in children and adolescents. Epidemiologic studies with rigorous diagnostic criteria[2] suggest, however, that the clinical onset of type 1 diabetes may occur at any age. The incidence rate varies with both age and gender (Fig. 54–1). The peak for both girls and boys, age 11 to 14 years, has been discernible in most studies and seems to be present irrespective of the country or area studied.[47, 51, 53] Little is known about type 1 diabetes in adults. Several studies have revealed difficulties in the classification of diabetes mellitus, whether type 1 or 2, in patients age 25 to 30 years and older.[62]

Patients initially classified and treated as having type 2 diabetes may require insulin after 1 to 5 years of therapy with diet, exercise, or oral hypoglycemic agents.[63, 64] This type of diabetes is referred to as latent autoimmune diabetes in the adult (LADA),[65] slow-onset insulin-dependent diabetes mellitus (SPIDDM),[66] or type 1,5 diabetes. It is speculated that these patients in fact have type 1 diabetes in addition to genetic factors that inhibit rapid progression of β cell killing. Epidemiologic investigation has indicated that the incidence rate of type 1 diabetes in patients older than 20 years remains low, except for a possible peak at around 50 to 65 years.[67]

Although rare, three forms of diabetes mellitus can occur at birth or during the first months of life. One is a transient diabetes mellitus, in which the metabolism and, to a certain extent, normal growth development need to be maintained with insulin for as long as 1 to 2 years. This form of transient diabetes is thought to be caused by delayed islet β cell maturation. The other, more rare, condition is type 1 diabetes resulting from a lack of β cells. This form has autoimmune features and is characterized by a permanent state of insulin dependency. Finally, and very rarely, children can be born without an endocrine pancreas.

In children, minor incidence peaks occur at 4 to 6 years[47] and 7 to 8 years,[68, 69] which have been associated with entrance into preschool or school programs. The major peak, however, is naturally associated with puberty and the maximal velocity of pubertal growth.

Variation with Gender

It has been reported that the peak incidence in girls occurs earlier than in boys.[68] If the clinical onset of type 1 diabetes is linked to

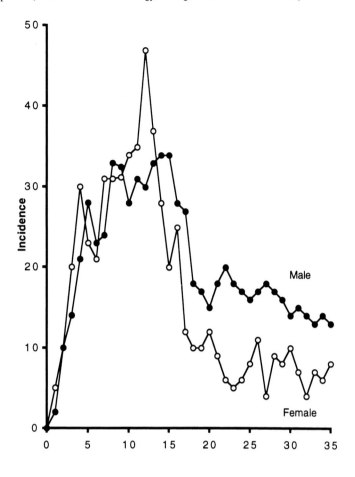

FIGURE 54–1. *Age-adjusted incidence of insulin-dependent diabetes mellitus in relation to age at onset in males and females. (Adapted from data in Nystrom L, Dahlquist G, Ostman J, et al: Risk of developing insulin-dependent diabetes mellitus (IDDM) before 35 years of age: Indications of climatological determinants for age at onset. Int J Epidemiol 21:352–358, 1992.)*

pubertal growth, this difference in incidence rate can be explained by the fact that pubertal growth occurs earlier in girls. Prepubertal boys were found to be taller at the clinical onset of type 1 diabetes.[69] In addition, newly diagnosed children of both genders showed advanced skeletal maturity.[70] Even if boys tend to show an increased height compared with controls, their growth seems to cease about 35 weeks before the clinical onset of type 1 diabetes.[69] It therefore is possible that processes affecting the pancreatic β cell mass and the ability to produce insulin may have profound effects on body growth and function at a young age. Because these processes differ slightly between boys and girls, growth characteristics may offer a simple explanation for the differences seen in incidence rates between the genders.

Surveys based on the registration of all new patients with type 1 diabetes in Sweden[55] and New Zealand[71] have indicated that occurrence of type 1 diabetes before age 15 years is slightly more common among boys. In fact, preliminary evidence[55] suggests that an increased prevalence among boys may be observed only during certain years. A registry of type 1 diabetes among 15- to 34-year-olds (see Fig. 54–1) demonstrates that type 1 diabetes is 1.5 times more common among men than women.[62] Further studies are necessary to document gender-dependent incidence rates and to explain their mechanisms.

ETIOLOGY

The absence of an unambiguous mode of inheritance, the presence of a period of subclinical islet autoimmunity preceding clinical onset of disease, HLA genes that control the immune response, and age and seasonal variation must be taken into account in attempts to explain the cause of type 1 diabetes. A defined etiologic factor, endogenous or exogenous, capable of causing type 1 diabetes remains to be identified (Table 54–3). Because evidence exists of genetic heterogeneity in type 1 diabetes, it is possible that different causative factors are responsible. In experimental animals (see Table 54–3), both viral and chemical agents have been used to reproducibly induce diabetes. In humans, only indirect evidence suggests that such factors are involved in initiating type 1 diabetes. The following is a brief summary of possible genetic or environmental factors that are associated with the appearance of type 1 diabetes.

HLA on chromosome 6 is the major genetic risk factor for type 1 diabetes, regardless of age. The HLA haplotypes DQB1*0302-A1*0301-DRB1*04 and DQB1*0201-A1*0501-DRB1*03 are the two major risk haplotypes.[41, 72] The most important alleles are DQB1*0302 and B1*0201 along with DRB1*03. DRB1*04 is a large family of related molecules, and DRB1*0401 confers an independent risk. DRB1*0403 is negatively associated with diabetes and may protect or decelerate an ongoing disease development.[73] DRB1*03 seems to be more important than DQB1*0201, as it is only DQB1*0201-A1*0501-DRB1*03, not DQB1*0201-A1*0501-DRB1*07, that confers type 1 diabetes risk. The genetic linkage and association between type 1 diabetes and HLA is also remarkable, as certain HLA haplotypes are protective. Most prominently, DQB1*0602-A1*0102 and B1*0603-A1*0102 are protective before age 15 years. The detailed mechanisms by which HLA confer either risk or resistance is not fully understood.[72, 74] The function of these molecules is to display peptide antigens to be recognized by T cell receptors. The disease association may therefore either be related to an inability to induce immunologic tolerance to certain autoantigens or to antigen presentation of an endogenous autoantigen. In the first case, the subject may become vulnerable to infectious agents that mimic autoantigens. Reactivity to the infectious agent sets off an immune response that reacts with self. In the second case, the immune reaction may result in a direct attack on the individual's own cells.

It is estimated that HLA accounts for about 60% of the genetic risk.[75, 76] The genetics of type 1 diabetes mellitus is studied extensively as it represents a paradigm for genetically complex diseases. Genome screens and studies on candidate genes have provided evidence for genetic linkage between polymorphic DNA markers and more than 15 putative type 1 diabetes susceptibility loci.[44, 45, 77] A polymorphism upstream of the insulin gene on chromosome 6 affects type 1 diabetes risk,[78, 79] perhaps by controlling insulin expression in the thymus and thereby the development of immunologic tolerance.[80, 81] The gene for CTLA-4 on chromosome 2 is another candidate.[82, 83] CTLA-4 controls T lymphocyte survival after activation, and it is speculated that regulation of the CTLA-4 gene may affect propensity for autoimmune

TABLE 54–3. Viruses and Other Environmental Factors Implicated in or Able to Induce Type 1 (Insulin-Dependent) Diabetes

Viruses	
Coxsackie	Human, mice
Rubella	Human, hamster
Mumps	Human
Cytomegalovirus	Human
Encephalomyocarditis	Mice
Meningovirus	Mice
Reovirus	Mice
Lymphocytic choriomeningitis	Rats
Rotavirus	Human
Kilham strain (mumps virus)	Rat
Toxins	
Alloxan	
Streptozotocin	
Pyriminyl (Vacor)	
Pentamidine isothiocyanate	
N-3-Pyridylmethyl-*N'*-p'-nitrophenylurea (PNU)	

disease. Taken together, these and other genetic factors have limited effects on the relative risk of type 1 diabetes. The mechanisms by which these factors contribute to appearance of the disease remain to be clarified.

The role of viruses in type 1 diabetes (see Table 54–3) is based on two types of observations. One type is composed of case reports, the first published at the end of the 19th century and followed still by many.[39, 40, 84] Taken together, these reports suggest a relationship between type 1 diabetes and viruses (e.g., rubella, mumps, Coxsackie B virus and rotavirus). Coxsackie B virus has been isolated, propagated in in vitro cultures of endocrine pancreatic cells, and then shown to have diabetic activity in certain mouse strains.[85] Coxsackie virus infection in the mouse seems to be associated with virus replication in the β cells, followed by the formation of GAD65 antibodies.[86, 87] Two important hypotheses follow from these experiments. One hypothesis is that the Coxsackie virus induces β cell neoantigens, which initiate an (auto)immune reaction. This hypothesis can be tested by analyzing the appearance of such neoantigens. The neoantigen may initiate a devastating reaction if its structure mimics a self protein. A sequence in GAD is identical to that in a Coxsackie virus antigen.[88, 89] Another hypothesis is that Coxsackie B virus replication in β cells results in β cell necrosis and the formation of antibodies against β cell constituents or "hidden antigens" not normally surveyed by the immune system. An autoimmune reaction is initiated that may escalate with time.

An epidemic of type 1 diabetes is not expected in humans, although disease epidemiology suggests features of type 1 diabetes as a communicable disease.[51] Many studies in several countries have shown that type 1 diabetes develops in individuals who are positive for HLA-DQ2-DR3, DQ8-DR4, or both (discussed earlier). The DQ6 haplotype confers resistance among children in a dominant manner. Because these specificities are present in about half the population, a diabetogenic virus may not be spread effectively enough to cause disease. Variations in the annual incidence are often taken as evidence of an involvement of virus. In the group of children younger than 6 or 7 years who have type 1 diabetes, however, this annual variation is not always present.[55, 71] An annual variation was also evident in 15- to 34-year-olds, with lower numbers of new patients being identified during the summer months.[52]

The second type of observation is that in epidemics of rubella, pregnant women may acquire a viral infection during the first trimester. Their offspring with congenital rubella have been found to develop type 1 diabetes at a very high frequency,[90, 91] especially HLA-DR3– and/or HLA-DR4–positive children.[91] The clinical onset of type 1 diabetes in many of these patients is preceded by the phenomenon of islet autoimmunity, and most of the patients developing type 1 diabetes have a variety of islet cell autoantibodies. Similarly, these children also have a high prevalence of organ-specific autoantibodies.[92] Congenital rubella therefore offers the most dramatic example of development of type 1 diabetes in association with an environmental factor. Vaccination practices have prevented rubella epidemics but they have not affected the incidence rate of type 1 diabetes. Maternal enteroviral infection during pregnancy is a risk factor for childhood type 1 diabetes.[93, 94] It is therefore possible that gestational infections by many types of viruses affect the maturation of the immune system, causing certain children to be more predisposed to autoimmunity and thereby increasing the risk for type 1 diabetes. Prior exposure to measles, mumps, and rubella, but not vaccination, during adolescence decreased prevalence of pancreatic and thyroid autoantibodies.[95] Maternal virus infections or reduced exposure to natural infections may be associated with an increase in type 1 diabetes.

In experimental animals (see Table 54–3) several viruses, including encephalomyocarditis, rubella, reovirus, and Coxsackie B virus, are capable of inducing diabetes. Some of these virus-induced diabetic syndromes are thought to be caused by β cell destruction alone. Other viruses (e.g., reovirus) were found to primarily affect the immune system of the host to induce a polyclonal autoantibody response. The production of autoantibodies appeared to be closely related to the pathogenesis of disease in mice.[86, 87] The virus-induced disease in mice tends to depend on strain, because some mouse strains are resistant to the pathogenesis of the virus induced in another strain. Similar strain dependency to the β-cytotoxic agent streptozotocin, followed by the inoculation of a diabetogenic virus, rendered otherwise virus-resistant mice diabetic.[96] This observation may be significant to humans because it is possible that repeated injuries to the pancreatic β cells throughout several years of life may eventually induce type 1 diabetes. An additional role of HLA has been suggested because it cannot be excluded that repeated injuries are particularly detrimental if the type 1 diabetes–associated HLA alleles are linked with a poor regenerative capacity of the pancreatic β cells.

Alloxan and streptozotocin are widely used to induce β cell destruction and diabetes in experimental animals. Some species are more resistant to these drugs than others, and the extent to which these agents are able to induce diabetes in humans is uncertain. Streptozotocin is commonly used in treating certain gastroenteric tumors, including glucagonomas; however, insulin-dependent diabetes rarely develops in these patients. The absence of a β-cytotoxic effect could be the result of the dosage used or could reflect the possibility that human β cells are resistant to streptozotocin; in fact, in vitro studies with human islets suggest the absence of cytotoxic effects. A number of compounds structurally related to streptozotocin and alloxan have also been implicated as possible environmental agents. Vacor, an effective rodenticide, is highly diabetogenic in humans.[97] Individuals in whom diabetes developed after ingestion of Vacor were found to be positive for islet cell surface antibodies, which indicates that such autoantibodies may develop after a primary lesion has been inflicted on the β cells.

The nitrosamine moiety that is part of the streptozotocin molecule may be diabetogenic when present on molecules other than D-glucose. Nitrosamines present in cured Icelandic mutton have not only been reported to be diabetogenic in mice, but, in addition, the diabetic activity was transmitted in the germline DNA.[98, 99] Further investigations are needed to substantiate the possibility that environmental chemicals are causative factors in the development of type 1 diabetes.

In summary, viruses and chemical agents have direct effects on the pancreatic β cells and may therefore represent the causative factor that initiates the (auto)immune process against these cells. The alternative hypothesis is that these agents potentiate a β cell–destructive process that is genetically determined or initiated by environmental factors.

PATHOLOGY

Studies of the pancreas in newly diagnosed type 1 diabetes patients have indicated that the gland is diminished in size compared with that in matched controls.[10, 100, 101] An atrophic pancreas with little or negligible residual insulin is typical of a patient with long-standing type 1 diabetes. The atrophy affects primarily the tail of the pancreas. In this part, the composition of the endocrine pancreas is dominated by β and α cells, whereas in the pancreatic head, β and pancreatic polypeptide (PP) cells predominate.

The pancreatic atrophy appears to be reflected in lower serum levels of pancreatic trypsin and isoamylase.[102–104] The levels of these enzymes are decreased at the time of clinical onset and seem to remain lower even after insulin therapy is initiated. It is speculated that the serum trypsin or isoamylase reflects the pancreatic tissue volume and that the atrophy of the gland is a result of an intrapancreatic insulin deficiency affecting the growth of the pancreas.

The insulin deficiency is the result of a specific loss of the β cells, which affects the total mass of the endocrine pancreas in type 1 diabetes (Table 54–4). The islets are small and appear pseudoatrophic.[100, 105] In contrast to the normal pancreas, in which the β cells predominate, the endocrine cells in the diabetic pancreas are primarily α, δ, and PP cells. Lobular variation has been described, and areas with β cell–containing islets without pancreatic atrophy have also been detected, suggesting that parts of the pancreas may be spared.[100] In individuals with newly diagnosed type 1 diabetes, islets with β cells showing signs of hyperactivity have also been found. Sometimes β cells are seen in close proximity to duct cells, suggesting neoformation of cells. The understanding of the developing endocrine pancreas has improved, and a number of transcription factors controlling the process have been identified.[106] However, one of the characteristics of the pancreas in many children with newly diagnosed type 1 diabetes is

TABLE 54–4. Morphometric Analysis of the Endocrine Pancreas in Control Individuals and Patients with Type 1 (Insulin-Dependent) Diabetes Mellitus

Cell Type	Endocrine Pancreas (μg)	
	Controls	*IDDM*
β cells	850	0
α cells	230	150
δ cells	125	97
PP cells	190	166
All cells	1395	413

Adapted from Rahier J, Goebbels RM, Henquin JC: Cellular composition of the human diabetic pancreas. Diabetologia 24:336–371, 1983.

the presence of inflammatory cells adjacent to islets or cords of newly formed β cells.[100]

The presence of inflammatory cells in the diabetic pancreas was first demonstrated at the turn of the 20th century. The term *insulitis* was introduced in 1940.[9] The phenomenon was not established until later quantitative investigations reported insulitis in 16 of 23 individuals with type 1 diabetes who died within 6 months of diagnosis.[10] The total mass of β cells is already markedly reduced at the time of clinical diagnosis,[19, 107, 108] and the presence of inflammatory cells in large numbers is perhaps not to be expected. It is speculated that the antigen attracting the inflammatory cells is a β cell–specific determinant.[108] Immunocytochemical investigation in rare specimens of pancreas from some patients who died shortly after the clinical onset of type 1 diabetes indicates that all cell types considered part of the immune system populate the islets to form the insulitis[12, 19, 109, 110]: T lymphocytes, B lymphocytes, macrophages, and occasional natural killer (NK) cells may be seen. Examination of pancreatic islets in biopsy specimens from newly diagnosed type 1 diabetic patients did not reveal an overwhelming insulitis but rather showed macrophage infiltration and increased expression of HLA class I and II antigens.[111, 112] The sequence of events by which the immunocytes form insulitis may involve an early macrophage or dendritic cell infiltration followed by the recruitment of T and later by B lymphocytes. The initiation of this process is difficult if not impossible to study in humans, because it can be established only during the period preceding the actual clinical onset of the disease. In fact, examination of the pancreas from subjects with high-risk HLA who are positive for islet cell autoantibodies failed to detect insulitis.[113] Conversely, insulitis may not always lead to type 1 diabetes because it has been observed in virus-infected nondiabetic children.[114] However, the role of immune cells in the process leading to the disappearance of β cells is well established in the spontaneously diabetic nonobese diabetic (NOD) mouse and BB rat. It is possible to adoptively transfer diabetes with clonal T lymphocytes. Similarly, transfer of type 1 diabetes between HLA-identical siblings has been achieved by bone marrow transplantation.[115] These observations support the hypothesis that type 1 diabetes is an immune-mediated disease and that immunocytes play a pivotal role in the β cell killing.

The chronic type of inflammatory reaction observed in short-term type 1 diabetes supports the idea that the β cell loss might have been initiated long before the actual clinical onset of insulin dependency. It has not yet been possible to define the sequence of events that triggers the migration or attraction of immune cells to the pancreatic islets. Virus infection, and possibly also chemical modification, may alter antigens that are expressed on the islet β cell surface. Such modified antigens may activate clones of T lymphocytes through accessory (antigen-presenting) cells located either in the islets or in the periphery.

The histopathologic changes of short duration in the endocrine pancreas of type 1 diabetics correspond to a drastic reduction in the ability to produce insulin.[116] Highly sensitive and specific immunoassays for C peptide permit studies of residual β cell function even when the patient is treated with insulin (see Chapter 49). Fasting C peptide levels are reduced, often to the lower level seen in normal subjects. The first months of insulin therapy are associated with an apparent increase in fasting C peptide.[117] After 6 to 9 months' duration, irrespective of whether the residual β cell function was within or below the normal range, the C peptide levels continuously decrease, reaching values below the detection limit of the assay (about 0.05 mmol/mL) after 30 months or longer of type 1 diabetes.[117, 118]

Patients with high titers of islet cell autoantibodies, including ICA and GAD65 autoantibodies, tend to have higher levels of fasting C peptide at clinical onset,[118] whereas IA-2 autoantibody–positive subjects had lower levels.[119] At the same time, however, the presence of ICA, GAD65, or IA-2 autoantibodies may determine a greater rate of loss of endogenous β cells.[119–121] It is therefore possible that the antigen or antigens necessary to maintain levels of islet cell autoantibodies, such as GAD65 or IA-2, are part of the islet β cells. Islet cell autoantibodies may be markers for an immunopathologic process responsible for the continuous eradication of β cells. Further studies are needed to define the extent to which fasting or stimulated levels of C peptide in fact reflect the residual mass of pancreatic β cells. It is not clear, however, whether the residual amount of C peptide and its fluctuation following dietary control or intensified insulin therapy reflect changes either in the number or in the function of residual β cells. Levels of plasma insulin are affected by insulin sensitivity,[122] which may explain why significant loss of endogenous insulin production does not always result in diabetes.[37]

Individuals at risk for development of type 1 diabetes have been found to have hyperproinsulinemia, a condition shown in experimental animals or in vitro experiments to reflect maximally stimulated or perhaps exhausted β cells.[123, 124] When compared with matched controls, HLA-identical siblings of patients with type 1 diabetes have been found to have evidence of both insulin resistance and impaired β cell function.[125] In order to estimate the residual mass of insulin-producing cells in humans, it is important to take into account such factors as the maximal rate of insulin release, extraction of insulin in the liver and peripheral tissues, and resistance to insulin action.[37, 122] Although the total pancreatic insulin content in experimental animals appears to correlate well with the total β cell mass, it cannot be excluded that a diminished β cell mass alters the rate of insulin biosynthesis as well as secretion in the remaining β cells. It has been hypothesized that an increased and sustained demand on remaining β cells exhausts these cells, leading to their death and to a diminished β cell mass. At present, however, no experimental data support this hypothesis. Intensive therapy for type 1 diabetes helps sustain endogenous insulin secretion, which in turn is associated with better metabolic control and lower risk for hypoglycemia and chronic complications.[126–128] Diazoxide treatment at the time of clinical diagnosis also preserves residual insulin secretion.[129] Insulin or diazoxide therapy may allow residual β cells to rest and protect them from further immune-mediated destruction. This possibility is tested in a clinical trial to treat ICA-positive first-degree relatives of type 1 diabetes patients with insulin.[130]

In summary, the pathology of β cell destruction could be the result of (1) cell-mediated cytotoxicity, (2) antibody-mediated cytotoxicity, (3) cytokine-mediated cytotoxicity, or (4) a combination of these. The role of abnormal HLA class II molecule presentation and alterations of the target β cells by chemicals, viruses, or other environmental factors needs to be defined.

PATHOGENESIS

The pathogenesis of type 1 diabetes is strongly associated with several immune abnormalities. These immune abnormalities, in particular autoantibodies directed against specific islet cell autoantigens, such as insulin, GAD65 and IA-2, are dynamic markers of an ongoing disease process. The autoantibodies are studied both before and after the clinical diagnosis as markers of an ongoing pathogenesis. The pathogenetic markers are therefore useful to predict either type 1 diabetes or outcome treatment in patients with new-onset type 1 diabetes. The pathogenetic process is likely to be the same before and after the clinical diagnosis of diabetes. The rate of β cell destruction appears to be influenced by HLA. The HLA DQB1*0302-A1*0301/

DQB1*0201-A1*0501 genotype appears to be associated with accelerated β cell destruction and a more rapid progression to clinical onset of diabetes.[131, 132] The DQB1*0602 or 0603 alleles are dominantly protective, although the negative association is attenuated with increased age at onset.[131] In DQB1*0602/0603-positive patients, the second haplotype is most often DQB1*0302-A1*0201,[133] suggesting that HLA may influence the tempo of the disease process. The HLA DQB1*0302-A1*0301/DQB1*0201-A1*0501 genotype accelerates and DQB1*0602/0603 alleles decelerate type 1 diabetes disease pathogenesis. Because the HLA molecules are important determinants in regulating the immune response in humans, the susceptibility to type 1 diabetes is speculated to be conferred by the functional importance of these molecules in the restriction of the immune response. The role of the class II molecules in the immune response is to convey cell-cell interactions between T-helper (CD4+) lymphocytes and antigen-presenting cells (APC) or B lymphocytes. The CD4+ T cell provides help to cytotoxic T (CD8+) lymphocytes. An antigen taken up, processed, and presented by an APC is recognized only by a T-helper lymphocyte, which has a T cell receptor (TCR) to detect the antigenic epitope in conjunction with the APC HLA class II molecule. A number of "recently identified new genes" (RING) in the HLA region have revealed a final common pathway of antigen presentation by genes controlling proteolysis, peptide transport, and peptide loading onto HLA class I and II molecules.

In summary, the HLA class II molecules which are strongly associated with type 1 diabetes specifically bind short peptides or epitopes. These are recognized by specific TCRs on CD4+ T lymphocytes, which is the signal to initiate the development of cytotoxic T lymphocytes and B lymphocytes, which produce antibodies to the antigen. This entire process is affected by a number of cytokines, which are produced by APCs, T cells, or both. Some of these cytokines, such as interferon gamma (IFN-γ) and interleukin-2 (IL-2) promote an immune response that is predominantly cell mediated and aggressive (often referred to as a Th1 response). Other cytokines, such as IL-4 and IL-10, promote an immune response that is mostly humoral (Th2 response). Dividing an immune reaction into Th1 and Th2 is obviously an oversimplification, but it serves the purpose of better defining immunopathologic mechanisms in type 1 diabetes. The cytokines are local mediators, and changes in plasma levels may not at all reflect the disease pathogenesis.

IMMUNOLOGIC ABNORMALITIES

Cellular Immunopathophysiology

It is possible that the APC activity is altered in patients or in individuals susceptible to type 1 diabetes. Studies with immunoglobulin G (IgG)-sensitized autologous erythrocytes have, for example, shown that normal individuals with a DR3 HLA-haplotype have an abnormally prolonged Fc receptor–mediated mononuclear phagocyte system.[134] Blood monocytes in type 1 diabetes patients may be defective in prostaglandin synthetase.[135] Several observations have been made in which the insulin-deficient diabetic state has markedly influenced cellular function of immunologically competent cells. The importance of studying diabetic patients in good metabolic control cannot be too highly stressed.

Tests for leukocyte migration inhibition or blast formation have indicated that type 1 diabetes patients may be sensitized to pancreatic antigens.[14–16] Migration inhibition was most prominent in patients with type 1 diabetes of short duration. In keeping with the in vitro test, it was noted that these patients often developed a delayed hypersensitivity reaction to subcutaneously injected pancreatic homogenate.[16] These experiments need to be repeated with highly purified specific antigens, such as insulin, GAD65, and IA-2.

Several disorders of autoimmune character have been found to have an imbalance in the peripheral blood between T-helper (CD4+) and suppressor/cytotoxic (CD8+) lymphocytes. Monoclonal antibodies that detect specific cell surface proteins are used to enumerate circulating T lymphocyte subsets, but the results are conflicting, because decreased,

TABLE 54–5. Methods to Detect Islet Cell Autoantibodies

Preparation to Detect Islet Antigen	Method of Detection	Islet Cell (Auto) Antibody	Studies
Recombinant antigens	Immunoassays	GAD antibodies, IA-2 antibodies, insulin antibodies	Greenbaum et al.,[165] Verge et al.,[166] Grubin et al.[167]
Frozen sections of human pancreas	Indirect immunofluorescence	Islet cell cytoplasmic antibodies (ICA, ICCA)	Bottazzo et al.,[23] Atkinson et al.[89]
Dispersed rat islet cells	Indirect immunofluorescence	Islet cell surface antibody (ICSA)	Lernmark et al.[24, 186]
Monolayers of rat islet cells	^{51}Cr release	Islet cell cytotoxic antibody (C′AMC)	Dobersen et al.,[25] Dobersen and Scharff[188]
Purified rat islet β cells	Indirect immunofluorescence	ß cell–specific ICSA	van de Winkel et al.[187]

normal, or slightly elevated suppressor cell numbers have been found.[136, 137] A slight increase in the proportion of class II antigen–positive T lymphocytes was reported, and, as observed in other disorders of autoimmune character, a decrease in suppressor cytotoxic cells was found as well.[138] Patients with type 1 diabetes also have cytotoxic T cells specific for glutamic acid decarboxylase.[139] Several reports indicate an increased frequency of in vitro proliferating T cells in patients with type 1 diabetes, compared to levels in control subjects, in response to autoantigens such as GAD[89, 140, 141] and IA-2.[142] T cell assays in humans are complicated by poor reproducibility and very high interlaboratory variability.[21] Immunodominant epitopes of GAD65[72, 143, 144] and IA-2[142] have been identified and should be useful in improving cellular assays in type 1 diabetes. Mice expressing HLA-DR and -DQ molecules are often used to identify T cell epitopes.[145] Understanding of the recognition of insulin as an autoantigen by human T cells is lacking.[146, 147] When the number of immunoglobulin-secreting cells in peripheral blood was assessed, several patients with type 1 diabetes of short duration had an elevated level of spontaneous secretion of immunoglobulin.[148, 149] It is therefore possible that the clinical onset of type 1 diabetes is associated with a polyclonal B lymphocyte activation. It remains to be determined whether these alterations are acquired, inherited, or related to the pathogenesis of β cell destruction.

In conclusion, antigen-specific tests in HLA-DQ and -DR–matched type 1 diabetic subjects and control individuals should allow a proper test of the hypothesis that a specific immunoregulation abnormality involving β cell antigens is associated with the development of type 1 diabetes.

Humoral Immunopathophysiology

A reaction between antibodies and an autologous tissue preparation is taken as evidence of the presence of autoantibodies, and several assay systems are used to determine the presence of antibodies reactive with pancreatic islet cells (Table 54–5). Immunoprecipitation of human islet proteins has revealed the presence of autoantibodies against a 64K protein,[150, 151] identified as GAD but found to represent an isoenzyme, GAD65, coded for by a gene on human chromosome 10.[27] The previously known GAD67 on chromosome 2 shares 65% of the amino acids, but this isoform is not expressed in human β cells.[28, 152] Trypsin treatment of the 64K immunoprecipitate revealed 40K and 37K fragments of islet antigens,[153, 154] later shown to represent two isoforms of the protein tyrosine phosphatase-like molecules IA-2 (ICA512)[30–32] and IA-2β (phogrin),[155–157] respectively. Finally, insulin antibodies were demonstrated before insulin treatment in about 50% of children with new-onset type 1 diabetes[29, 158] and contribute to type 1 diabetes risk.[159, 160] Other autoantigens have been proposed,[41, 161] but autoantibodies to GAD65, IA-2, and insulin remain the major autoimmune markers for type 1 diabetes. These three autoantibodies appear to replace the indirect immunofluorescence assay for ICA.[33, 36] Because the presence of two or more of these autoantibodies predict type 1 diabetes,[36, 162] it is critical that reliable tests are available to detect these autoantibodies.

ICA standardization was started in 1985[163, 164] and continued with assays for insulin autoantibodies[165] as well as for GAD65 and IA-2 autoantibodies.[166] The insulin autoantibody (IAA) workshops showed

the importance of radiobinding in contrast to enzyme-linked immunosorbent assay (ELISA) or solid-phase assay to detect IAA with high diagnostic sensitivity and specificity.[165] Similarly, the use of coupled in vitro transcription translation to label GAD65[167] and later IA-2[168, 169] in radioligand-binding assays[167, 170] allowed the development of assays with high diagnostic sensitivity and specificity.[166, 171] The following is a summary of the prevalence of autoantibodies to GAD65, IA-2, and insulin using these standardized assay systems.

The frequency of GAD65 antibodies in children with new-onset type 1 diabetes is 70% to 80% (Fig. 54–2), compared with about 8% antibodies against GAD67. Patients with GAD67 antibodies are also GAD65-antibody positive. The GAD65 autoantibody (GAD65Ab) frequency in new-onset patients is little affected by the age at onset; however, in children younger than 10 years, more girls than boys have GAD65Ab. GAD65Ab are evanescent, but less so than ICA (Fig. 54–3). The longer the duration of type 1 diabetes, the lower the frequency of GAD65 antibodies and of ICA. However, almost 50% of patients with a disease duration of 10 years may still be GAD65-antibody positive (see Fig. 54–3). GAD65 autoantibodies are more often detected in DQB1*0201-A1*0501-DRB1*03–positive than in DQB1*0302-A1*0301-DRB1*04–positive patients.[172] All islet cells,

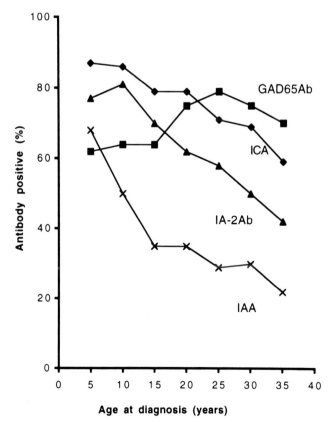

FIGURE 54–2. *Frequency of autoantibodies against GAD65 (GAD65Ab), IA-2 (IA-2Ab), and insulin (IAA) at the time of clinical diagnosis in relation to age at onset.*

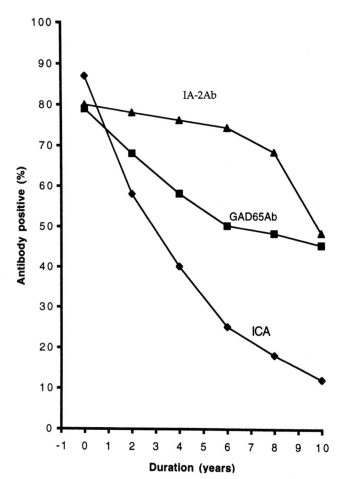

FIGURE 54–3. Frequency of autoantibodies against GAD65 (GAD65Ab) and IA-2 (IA-2Ab) as well as islet cell antibodies (ICA) in relation to the duration of type 1 diabetes. It is noted that patients with type 1 diabetes tend to be positive for one or the other autoantibody despite having had the disease for 10 years.

but β cells in particular, express GAD65. This enzyme produces γ-aminobutyric acid (GABA), which is stored in small neurotransmitter vesicles. It is possible that GABA regulates the secretion of the neighboring glucagon- and somatostatin-producing cells. In an indirect immunofluorescence test with sections of frozen human pancreas, ICA-positive sera give a fluorescence reaction that usually covers all endocrine islet cells. The antigenic determinants GAD65, IA-2, and others are therefore thought to be located in the cytoplasmic compartment of the cells.

Any assessment of an individual's risk of developing diabetes depends on the ability to accurately determine the presence of antibodies in a prospective analysis. This is particularly important because GAD65 antibodies may appear temporarily in healthy individuals.[173] GAD65 antibodies are present in about 1% of the population, but the frequency increases to about 8% among first-degree relatives of patients with type 1 diabetes.[174, 175] The positive predictive value of GAD65 antibodies for type 1 diabetes is about 50% or higher among first-degree relatives. It may be as high as 20% in schoolchildren with high-risk HLA.[158] GAD65 antibodies also predict stiff-man syndrome, although the GAD65 autoantibody epitopes are different from those in type 1 diabetes.[176, 177] Type 1 diabetes is best predicted when the GAD65 antibody assay is combined with IAA and IA-2 antibodies.[36]

IA-2 antibodies are detected in 60% to 70% of patients with new-onset type 1 diabetes.[178] These antibodies are less frequent with increasing age at onset (see Fig. 54–2). The IA-2 antibodies would therefore better predict young age at onset of type 1 diabetes. Longitudinal studies of first-degree relatives suggest that IA-2 autoantibodies tend to appear closer to the clinical onset of type 1 diabetes compared to GAD65 antibodies, which tend to appear earlier in the prodrome.[178]

The IA-2 antibodies are evanescent (see Fig. 54–3), but when present in patients who are young at disease onset, as many as 50% may still be IA-2 antibody–positive after having had diabetes for 10 years (see Fig. 54–3). The IA-2 antibodies are detected for a longer duration than ICA (see Fig. 54–3). IA-2 autoantibodies were associated primarily with DRB1*0401 and not with DQA1*0301-DQB1*0302.[172] IA-2 and IA-2β are both associated with the granule membrane in the cells, but they are also detectable in other endocrine cell types.[155, 179] The mechanisms by which the IA-2 proteins become recognized as autoantigens are not yet understood. The frequency of IA-2 antibodies in the general population is less than 1%.[52] The predictive value of IA-2 antibodies for type 1 diabetes is best estimated in combination with GAD65 and insulin autoantibodies.[36, 162]

It was demonstrated in a radioligand-binding assay that approximately 50% of patients with newly diagnosed but untreated type 1 diabetes have insulin autoantibodies (IAA).[29] These IAA have been standardized, and the measurements carried out in fluid-phase radioimmunoassay were found to have higher diagnostic sensitivity than solid-phase ELISA analyses.[165] IAA are found earlier in childhood and are less frequently found in adults (see Fig. 54–2).[158, 160, 180] IAA were positively associated with DR4, perhaps because they are in linkage disequilibrium with DQB1*0302-DQA1*0301.[172, 181] A first analysis of putative IAA epitope indicates that the amino acids B1–B3 and A8–A13 are important.[182] Further site-directed mutagenesis will be necessary to map IAA in relation to diagnostic sensitivity and specificity because insulin autoantibodies and insulin antibodies that appear after insulin therapy have similar binding characteristics.[183] It has been proposed that IAA predicts type 1 diabetes better in children (see Fig. 54–2) than in adults[159, 184] and that IAA is related to a linear loss of β cell function.[185] Prospective, population-based studies of children, including newborns,[38] are therefore required to determine the possible association between HLA, including the DR4 subtypes, and the production of IAA. In addition, prospective studies would be useful to clarify the predictive value for type 1 diabetes in the general population, considering that many more healthy children will have the IAA marker than will develop diabetes.

Islet cell surface antibodies (ICSA)(see Table 54–5) were demonstrated in dispersed-cell preparations of rat or mouse pancreatic islets in 2% to 4% of control subjects and in about 30% of patients with type 1 diabetes.[24, 186] The ICSA showed a decreased prevalence with increasing duration of disease. Antibodies in type 1 diabetes sera preferentially bind to β cells if the disease is diagnosed before age 30 years.[187] The observation that antibodies are capable of binding to living β cells is important because it allows testing of the possibility that surface-bound antibodies either mediate immune effector mechanisms or directly affect the function of the β cells. The former phenomena may include complement-mediated cytotoxicity or antibody-dependent cellular cytotoxicity. Either mechanism could contribute to killing pancreatic β cells provided that the in vitro phenomenon is also occurring in vivo. The evidence obtained with monolayer cultures of both pancreatic islet cells from newborn rats[25, 188] and cloned rat islet tumor cells[189, 190] is that the cytotoxic islet cell antibodies correlate well with the presence of ICSA but not with ICA. Some patients have both types of antibodies, whereas others have either cytoplasmic or cell surface antibodies.[191]

The concept of a polyclonal activation of the immune system in type 1 diabetes patients is also supported by numerous observations[13, 14, 40, 192–194] of an increased frequency of a variety of autoantibodies (Table 54–6). Because occurrence of these autoantibodies is also increased among first-degree relatives,[195–197] these abnormalities may be a feature of families with type 1 diabetes.

The presence of circulating immune complexes is increased in patients with IDDM of short duration (see Table 54–6). Using the solid-phase C1q or Raji cell tests, the prevalence of immune complexes was 25% to 30%.[198–200] The immune complexes detected by the C1q test were associated with the clinical onset of IDDM rather than with the development of diabetic nephropathy.[200]

In summary, currently available methods for detecting autoantigen-specific autoantibodies (GAD65, IA-2, and insulin) are of value in predicting type 1 diabetes.[36, 162] Standardized assays for these autoantibodies[166] are important when selecting participants in intervention

TABLE 54–6. Autoantibodies and Immune Complexes Found with Increased Frequency among Type 1 Diabetes Patients and Their First-Degree Relatives

Type	Antibody
Organ-specific	
Islets	GAD65, IA-2, or insulin
Thyroid	ICA, ICSA, or C'AMC
	Thyroid peroxidase (TPO)
	Thyroglobulin
Stomach	Gastric-parietal cell or H^+, K^+-ATPase
	Intrinsic factor
Adrenals	Adrenal cell or 21-hydroxylase
Pituitary	Pituitary cell
Non–organ-specific	
Peripheral lymphocytes	Lymphocytotoxic
Nucleic acids	Single-stranded RNA
	Double-stranded RNA
Cell constituents	Tubulin
	Insulin receptor
Plasma proteins	Albumin
Immune complexes	Solid-phase C1q binding
	Raji cell binding

trials.[130] How the uptake, processing, and presentation of these autoantigens by antigen-presenting cells that initiate the formation of islet cell autoantigen reactive T and B lymphocytes are accomplished are important questions that remain to be answered.

SIGNS, SYMPTOMS, AND NATURAL HISTORY

Type 1 diabetes usually produces subjective and objective signs of short duration. The American Diabetes Association[201] and the World Health Organization[202] have recommended several diagnostic criteria for type 1 diabetes (Table 54–7). The onset is primarily among young individuals, but the disease can be manifested at all ages. Most patients have a history of polyuria, polydipsia, and unexplained weight loss. The elevated blood glucose level causes polyuria from the osmotic diuretic effect of glucose. The blood glucose values that lie in the uncertain range require an oral glucose tolerance test to establish a diagnosis (see Table 54–7). An individual who has a fasting blood glucose level greater than 7.0 mmol/L (126 mg/dL) but does not have ketoacidosis or is not in a hyperglycemic hyperosmolar state, is above ideal body weight, and is not pregnant is more likely to have type 2 diabetes. Evidence has been presented that adult-onset type 2 diabetes may progress to type 1 diabetes at a rate of 1% to 2% per year.[1] This

TABLE 54–7. Criteria for the Diagnosis of Diabetes Mellitus*

1. Symptoms of diabetes plus casual plasma glucose concentration ≥200 mg/dL (11.1 mmol/L). *Casual* is defined as any time of day without regard to time since last meal. The classic symptoms of diabetes include polyuria, polydipsia, and unexplained weight loss.

or

2. Fasting plasma glucose (FPG), ≥126 mg/dL (7.0 mmol/L). *Fasting* is defined as no caloric intake for at least 8 hr.

or

3. 2-hr Plasma glucose ≥200 mg/dL (11.1 mmol/L) during an oral glucose tolerance test (OGTT). The test should be performed as described by WHO,[2] using a glucose load containing the equivalent of 75 g of anhydrous glucose dissolved in water.

*In the absence of unequivocal hyperglycemia with acute metabolic decompensation, these criteria should be confirmed by repeat testing on a different day. The third measure (OGTT) is not recommended for routine clinical use.
From Report of the Expert Committee on the Diagnosis and Classification of Diabetes Mellitus, American Diabetes Association: Clinical Practice Recommendations. Diabetes Care 22(suppl 1):S5–S23, 1999.

rate is increased in GAD65 autoantibody–positive patients classified with type 2 diabetes.[63, 64, 203] The symptoms of type 1 diabetes often have an abrupt onset in children and a more insidious onset with increasing age. Girls often have monilial vaginitis. The classic ketoacidosis of diabetes, including air hunger, Kussmaul respiration, acidosis, acetone odor of the breath, dehydration, vomiting, hyperglycemia, glucosuria, ketonemia, and ketonuria, are now uncommon at the initial examination.

The major defect in type 1 diabetes is the deficiency in insulin production. Following an injection of glucose, the β cells in a healthy individual are able to increase the rate of insulin release severalfold. In contrast, a patient with newly diagnosed type 1 diabetes often has a nearly total lack of response to glucose, particularly if signs of diabetic ketoacidosis or metabolic dysregulation are present. Glucose tolerance tests to evaluate the β cell function at the time of clinical onset are not a diagnostic procedure. A variety of glucose tolerance tests, both oral and intravenous (see Chapter 49), are being used to evaluate diabetic states; however, these procedures are more important in disorders of impaired glucose tolerance and type 2 diabetes than they are in providing a distinct diagnosis of type 1 diabetes.

Because type 1 diabetes is detected in the majority of patients following a relatively short period of symptoms, such as increased thirst, polyuria, and unexplained weight loss, the natural history of the disease is unknown. Retrospective analyses of first-degree relatives[204, 205] later found to develop type 1 diabetes have revealed that ICA or autoantibodies to GAD65, IA-2, or insulin, and, later, decreased ability to release insulin in response to glucose, may develop several years before the clinical diagnosis.[36–38, 206] The sequence of events preceding the diagnosis of overt type 1 diabetes would include the following: (1) genetic predisposition, (2) overt immunologic abnormalities with normal glucose levels, (3) development of overt diabetes with C peptide still detectable, and (4) the final stage of insulin dependency, with disappearance of C peptide. The fact that type 1 diabetes develops in persons of all ages should be taken into account when studying the natural history in children and adults. Many first-degree relatives may be positive for immune markers without progressing to type 1 diabetes.[37]

It is important to note that the vast majority of children or young adults developing type 1 diabetes have sporadic, as opposed to familial, disease.[55, 71] Highly effective, precise, and reproducible screening assays for HLA genotypes as well as for GAD65, IA-2, and insulin autoantibodies are therefore required to detect individuals in the background population who are either carriers of islet cell autoimmunity or carriers on their way to developing type 1 diabetes. Specific T lymphocyte proliferation tests against GAD65, IA-2, or insulin, once developed, may also predict type 1 diabetes. Early detection of type 1 diabetes serves several purposes. Among them is the distinct possibility that ketoacidosis associated with a dramatic and traumatic onset of type 1 diabetes would be forestalled. Perhaps early therapy with insulin could prevent accelerated β cell loss. Another possibility is the prevention of β cell destruction by immunosuppression.

Several attempts have been made to treat type 1 diabetic patients with immunosuppressive agents. Plasmapheresis, prednisolone, anti–T cell antibodies, and interferon have had little or no effect, but a controlled trial with cyclosporine suggested that the fall or disappearance of insulin requirement within the first 2 years after the clinical diagnosis was prolonged in about 20% of the patients.[207, 208] The major biologic effect of cyclosporine is to inhibit T cell–mediated immunity. However, the use of the drug was associated with structural renal tubular and glomerular damage.[209] Although immunosuppression successfully prevents autoimmune diabetes in the NOD mouse and the BB rat,[210] it will be necessary to develop novel immunosuppressive drugs to be tested in humans at risk for type 1 diabetes.

SUMMARY

The islet β cells appear to be the specific target in an autoimmune process that leads to the clinical onset of type 1 diabetes. The process of β cell autoimmunity appears to be initiated long before the clinical onset of the disease. The event that initiates this process is not yet understood, and the β cell antigens GAD65, IA-2, or insulin may in fact serve as the recognition structure or structures for the cells in the immune system that eventually produce insulitis. Recent advances in molecular genetics have made it possible to better define the HLA-DQ and -DR molecules that seem to be necessary, but not sufficient, for the development of type 1 diabetes. A screen of the human genome for susceptibility to type 1 diabetes has identified several additional genetic factors that contribute to type 1 diabetes risk. The aim of future studies is to test whether antigen-specific immunosuppression in type 1 diabetes-susceptible individuals will prevent the loss of pancreatic β cells.

REFERENCES

1. Köbberling J, Tattersall B: The Genetics of Diabetes Mellitus. London, Academic Press, 1982.
2. Diabetes Mellitus: Report of a WHO Study Group, technical report series 727. Geneva, World Health Organization, 1985.
3. Steiner DF, Tager HS, Chan SJ, et al: Lessons learned from molecular biology of insulin-gene mutations. Diabetes Care 13:600–609, 1990.
4. Taylor SI, Cama A, Accili D, et al: Mutations in the insulin receptor gene. Endocr Rev 13:566–595, 1992.
5. Bell GI, Pilkis SJ, Weber IT, Polonsky KS: Glucokinase mutations, insulin secretion, and diabetes mellitus. Annu Rev Physiol 58:171–186, 1996.
6. Yamagata K, Oda N, Kaisaki PJ, et al: Mutations in the hepatocyte nuclear factor-1 alpha gene in maturity-onset diabetes of the young (MODY3). Nature 384:455–458, 1996.
7. The Expert Committee on the Diagnosis and Classification of Diabetes Mellitus: Diagnosis and classification of diabetes mellitus. Diabetes Care 22(suppl 1):S5–S23, 1999.
8. Weichselbaum A: Ueber die Veränderungen des Pankreas bei Diabetes Mellitus. Sitzungsber Akad Wissensch Wien 119:189, 1910.
9. von Meyenburg H: Über "Insulitis" bei Diabetes. Schweiz Med Wochenschr 21:554–561, 1940.
10. Gepts W: Pathologic anatomy of the pancreas in juvenile diabetes mellitus. Diabetes 14:619–633, 1965.
11. Gepts W, De Mey J: Islet cell survival determined by morphology. Diabetes 27:251–261, 1978.
12. Foulis AK, McGill M, Farquharson A: Insulitis in type 1 (insulin-dependent) diabetes mellitus in man—macrophages, lymphocytes, and interferon-1 containing cells. J Pathol 165:97–103, 1991.
13. Nerup J, Binder C: Thyroid, gastric and adrenal autoimmunity in diabetes mellitus. Acta Endocrinol 72:279–286, 1973.
14. MacCuish AC, Irvine WJ: Autoimmunological aspects of diabetes mellitus. Clin Endocrinol Metab 4:435–471, 1975.
15. Nerup J, Andersen OO, Bendixen G, et al: Antipancreatic cellular hypersensitivity in diabetes mellitus. Diabetes 20:424–427, 1971.
16. Nerup J, Andersen OO, Bendixen G: Antipancreatic cellular hypersensitivity in diabetes mellitus: Experimental induction of an antipancreatic, cellular hypersensitivity and associated morphological b-cell changes in the rat. Acta Endocrinol (Copenh) 28:231–249, 1973.
17. MacCuish AC, Jordan J, Campbell CJ, et al: Cell-mediated immunity to human pancreas in diabetes mellitus. Diabetes 23:693–697, 1974.
18. Pipeleers D, Ling Z: Pancreatic beta cells in insulin-dependent diabetes. Diabetes Metab Rev 8:209–227, 1992.
19. Lernmark Å, Klöppel G, Stenger D, et al: Heterogeneity of human islet pathology in newly diagnosed childhood insulin-dependent diabetes mellitus: Macrophage infiltrations and expression of HLA-DQ and glutamic acid decarboxylase. Virchows Arch 425:631–640, 1995.
20. Huang S-W, MacLaren NK: Insulin-dependent diabetes: A disease of autoaggression. Science 192:64–66, 1976.
21. Roep BO, Atkinson MA, van Endert PM, et al: Autoreactive T cell responses in insulin-dependent (type 1) diabetes mellitus: Report of the First International Workshop for Standardization of T Cell Assays. J Autoimmun 13:267–282, 1999.
22. MacCuish AC, Irvine JW, Barnes EW, Duncan LJP: Antibodies to pancreatic islet cells in insulin-dependent diabetes with coexistent autoimmune disease. Lancet 2:1529–1531, 1974.
23. Bottazzo GF, Florin-Christensen A, Doniach D: Islet cell antibodies in diabetes mellitus with autoimmune polyendocrine deficiencies. Lancet 2:1279–1283, 1974.
24. Lernmark Å, Freedman ZR, Hofmann C, et al: Islet-cell-surface antibodies in juvenile diabetes mellitus. N Engl J Med 299:375–380, 1978.
25. Dobersen MJ, Scharff JE, Ginsberg-Fellner F, Notkins AL: Cytotoxic autoantibodies to beta-cells in the serum of patients with insulin-dependent diabetes mellitus. N Engl J Med 303:1493–1498, 1980.
26. Baekkeskov S, Aanstoot HJ, Christgau S, et al: Identification of the 64K autoantigen in insulin-dependent diabetes as the GABA-synthesizing enzyme glutamic acid decarboxylase. Nature 347:151–156, 1990.
27. Karlsen AE, Hagopian WA, Grubin CE, et al: Cloning and primary structure of a human islet isoform of glutamic acid decarboxylase from chromosome 10. Proc Natl Acad Sci U S A 88:8337–8341, 1991.
28. Karlsen AE, Hagopian WA, Petersen JS, et al: Recombinant glutamic acid decarboxylase representing a single isoform expressed in human islets detects IDDM associated 64K autoantibodies. Diabetes 41:1355–1359, 1992.
29. Palmer JP, Asplin CM, Clemons P, et al: Insulin antibodies in insulin-dependent diabetics before insulin treatment. Science 222:1337–1339, 1983.
30. Rabin DU, Pleasic SM, Shapiro JA, et al: Islet cell antigen 512 is a diabetes-specific islet autoantigen related to protein tyrosine phosphatases. J Immunol 152:3183–3187, 1994.
31. Lan MS, Lu J, Goto Y, Notkins AL: Molecular cloning and identification of a receptor-type protein tyrosine phosphatase, IA-2, from human insulinoma. DNA Cell Biol 13:505–514, 1994.
32. Payton MA, Hawkes CJ, Christie MR: Relationship of the 37,000- and 40,000-Mr tryptic fragments of islet antigens in insulin-dependent diabetes to the protein tyrosine phosphatase-like molecule IA-2 (ICA512). J Clin Invest 96:1506–1511, 1995.
33. Wiest-Ladenburger U, Hartmann R, Hartmann U, et al: Combined analysis and single-step detection of GAD65 and IA2 autoantibodies in IDDM can replace the histochemical islet cell antibody test. Diabetes 46:565–571, 1997.
34. Gorsuch AN, Spencer KM, Lister J, et al: Evidence for a long prediabetic period in type 1 (insulin-dependent) diabetes mellitus. Lancet 2:1363–1365, 1981.
35. Riley WJ, Maclaren NK, Krischer J, et al: A prospective study of the development of diabetes in relatives of patients with insulin-dependent diabetes. N Engl J Med 323:1167–1172, 1990.
36. Verge CF, Gianani R, Kawasaki E, et al: Prediction of type I diabetes in first-degree relatives using a combination of insulin, GAD, and ICA512bdc/IA-2 autoantibodies. Diabetes 45:926–933, 1996.
37. Greenbaum CJ, Sears KL, Kahn SE, Palmer JP: Relationship of beta-cell function and autoantibodies to progression and nonprogression of subclinical type 1 diabetes: Follow-up of the Seattle Family Study. Diabetes 48:170–175, 1999.
38. Lindberg B, Ivarsson S-A, Landin-Olsson M, et al: Islet autoantibodies in cord blood from children who developed type 1 (insulin-dependent) diabetes mellitus before 15 years of age. Diabetologia 42:181–187, 1999.
39. Yoon JW: A new look at viruses in type 1 diabetes. Diabetes Metab Rev 11:83–107, 1995.
40. Cahill GF, McDevitt HO: Insulin-dependent diabetes mellitus: The initial lesion. N Engl J Med 304:1454–1465, 1981.
41. Schranz D, Lernmark Å: Immunology in diabetes: An update. Diabetes Metab Rev 14:3–29, 1998.
42. Nerup J, Platz P, Anderssen OO: HL-A antigens and diabetes mellitus. Lancet 2:864–866, 1974.
43. Nepom GT: Immunogenetics and IDDM. Diabetes Rev 1:93–103, 1993.
44. Davies JL, Kawaguchi Y, Bennett ST, et al: A genome-wide search for human type 1 diabetes susceptibility genes. Nature 371:130–136, 1994.
45. Concannon P, Gogolin E-KJ, Hinds DA, et al: A second-generation screen of the human genome for susceptibility to insulin-dependent diabetes mellitus. Nature Genet 19:292–296, 1998.
46. Ekoe J-M: Recent trends in prevalence and incidence of diabetes mellitus syndrome in the world. Diabetes Res Clin Pract 1:249–64, 1986.
47. Green A, Gale EA, Patterson CC: Incidence of childhood-onset insulin-dependent diabetes mellitus: The EURODIAB ACE Study. Lancet 339:905–909, 1992.
48. Tuomilehto J, Rewers M, Reunanen A, et al: Increasing trend in type 1 (insulin-dependent) diabetes mellitus in childhood in Finland. Diabetologia 34:282–287, 1991.
49. Dahlquist G, Blom L, Tuvemo T, et al: The Swedish Childhood Diabetes Study: Results from a 9 year case register and 1 year case-referent study indicating that type 1 (insulin-dependent) diabetes mellitus is associated with both type 2 (non-insulin-dependent) diabetes mellitus and autoimmune disorders. Diabetologia 32:2–6, 1989.
50. Bingley PJ, Gale EAM: Rising incidence of IDDM in Europe. Diabetes Care 12:289–295, 1989.
51. Group Study of Diabetes Mellitus: Secular trends in incidence of childhood IDDM in 10 countries. Diabetes 39:858–864, 1990.
52. Nyström L, Dahlquist G, Rewers M, Wall S: The Swedish childhood diabetes study: An analysis of the temporal variation in diabetes incidence 1978–1987. Int J Epidemiol 19:141–146, 1990.
53. Karvonen M, Tuomilehto J, Libman I, et al: A review of the recent epidemiological data on incidence of type 1 (insulin-dependent) diabetes mellitus worldwide. Diabetologia 36:883–892, 1993.
54. Tuomilehto J: Epidemiology of childhood diabetes in the Baltic area. Nord Med 107:244–246, 1992.
55. Dahlquist G, Blom L, Holmgren G, et al: The epidemiology of diabetes in Swedish children 0–14 years old: A 6-year prospective study. Diabetologia 28:802–808, 1985.
56. Reunanen A, Åkerblom HK, Käär ML: Prevalence and 10-year (1970–1979) incidence of insulin-dependent diabetes mellitus in children and adolescents in Finland. Acta Paediatr Scand 71:893–899, 1982.
57. Kaprio J, Tuomilehto J, Koskenvuo M, et al: Concordance for type 1 (insulin-dependent) and type 2 (non-insulin-dependent) diabetes mellitus in a population-based cohort of twins in Finland. Diabetologia 35:1060–1067, 1992.
58. Kyvik KO, Green A, Beck NH: Concordance rates of insulin dependent diabetes mellitus: A population based study of young Danish twins. Br Med J 311:913–917, 1995.
59. Tillil H, Köbberling J: Age-corrected empirical genetic risk estimates for first-degree relatives of IDDM patients. Diabetes 36:93–99, 1987.
60. Todd JA, Farrall M: Genome-wide scanning for linkage in type 1 diabetes. Hum Mol Genet 5:1443–1448, 1996.
61. Awata T, Kuzuya T, Matsuda A, et al: Genetic analysis of HLA class II alleles and susceptibility type 1 (insulin-dependent) diabetes mellitus in Japanese subjects. Diabetologia 35:419–424, 1992.
62. Nyström L, Dahlquist G, Östman J, et al: Risk of developing insulin-dependent diabetes mellitus (IDDM) before 35 years of age: Indications of climatological determinants for age at onset. Int J Epidemiol 21:352–358, 1992.
63. Hagopian WA, Karlsen AE, Gottsater A, et al: Quantitative assay using recombinant human islet glutamic acid decarboxylase (GAD-64) showed 64K autoantibody positivity at onset predicts diabetes type. J Clin Invest 91:368–374, 1993.
64. Tuomi T, Groop LC, Zimmet PZ, et al: Antibodies to glutamic acid decarboxylase

reveal latent autoimmune diabetes mellitus in adults with a non-insulin-dependent onset of disease. Diabetes 42:359–362, 1993.

65. Zimmet PZ, Tuomi T, Mackay IR, et al: Latent autoimmune diabetes mellitus in adults (LADA): The role of antibodies to glutamic acid decarboxylase in diagnosis and prediction of insulin dependency. Diabet Med 11:299–303, 1994.

66. Kobayashi T, Nakanishi K, Murase T, Kosaka K: Small doses of subcutaneous insulin as a strategy for preventing slowly progressive beta-cell failure in islet cell antibody-positive patients with clinical features of NIDDM. Diabetes 45:622–626, 1996.

67. Lorenzen T, Pociot E, Hougaard P, Nerup J: Long-term risk of IDDM in first-degree relatives of patients with IDDM. Diabetologia 37:321–327, 1994.

68. Dahlquist G, Blom L, Lönnberg G: The Swedish Childhood Diabetes Study: A multivariate analysis of risk determinants for diabetes in different age groups. Diabetologia 34:757–762, 1991.

69. Blom L, Persson LA, Dahlquist G: Growth velocity and development of insulin-dependent diabetes mellitus. Diabetologia 35:528–533, 1992.

70. Edelsten AD, Hughes IA, Oakes S: Height and skeletal maturity in children with newly diagnosed juvenile-onset diabetes. Arch Dis Child 56:40–44, 1981.

71. Mason DR, Scott RS, Darlow BA: Epidemiology of insulin-dependent diabetes mellitus in Canterbury, New Zealand. Diabetes Res Clin Pract 3:21–29, 1987.

72. Nepom GT, Kwok WW: Molecular basis for HLA-DQ associations with IDDM. Diabetes 47:1177–1184, 1998.

73. Cucca F, Lampis R, Frau F, et al: The distribution of DR4 haplotypes in Sardinia suggests a primary association of type I diabetes with DRB1 and DQB1 loci. Hum Immunol 43:301–308, 1995.

74. Thorsby E: HLA-associated disease susceptibility: Which genes are primarily involved? Immunologist 3/2:51–58, 1995.

75. Risch N: Genetics of IDDM: Evidence for complex inheritance with HLA. Genet Epidemiol 6:143–148, 1989.

76. Todd JA: Genetic analysis of type 1 diabetes using whole genome approaches. Proc Natl Acad Sci U S A 92:8560–8565, 1995.

77. Owerbach D, Gabbay KH: The search for IDDM susceptibility genes. Diabetes 45:544–550, 1996.

78. Bell GI, Aorita S, Koran JH: A polymorphic locus near the human insulin gene is associated with insulin-dependent diabetes mellitus. Diabetes 33:176–183, 1984.

79. Bennett ST, Wilson AJ, Cucca F, et al: IDDM2-VNTR-encoded susceptibility to type 1 diabetes: Dominant protection and parental transmission of allele of the insulin gene-linked minisatellite locus. J Autoimmun 9:415–421, 1996.

80. Pugliese A, Zeller M, Fernandez J, et al: The insulin gene transcribed in the human thymus and transcription level correlate with allelic variation at the INS VNTR-IDDM2 susceptibility locus for type 1 diabetes. Nature Genet 15:293–297, 1997.

81. Vafiadis P, Bennett ST, Todd JA, et al: Insulin expression in human thymus is modulated by INS VNTR alleles at the IDDM2 locus. Nature Genet 15:289–292, 1997.

82. Nisticó L, Buzzetti R, Pritchard LE, et al: The CTLA-4 gene region on chromosome 2q33 is linked to, and associated with, type 1 diabetes. Belgian-Diabetes Registry. Hum Mol Genet 5:1075–1080, 1996.

83. Van der Auwera BJ, Vandewalle CL, Schuit FC, et al: CTLA-4 gene polymorphism confers susceptibility to insulin-dependent diabetes mellitus (IDDM) independently from age and from other genetic or immune disease markers. The Belgian Diabetes Registry. Clin Exp Immunol 110:98–103, 1997.

84. Yoon JW: Role of viruses in the pathogenesis of IDDM. Ann Med 23:437–445, 1991.

85. Yoon JW, Austin M, Onodera T, Notkins AL: Virus-induced diabetes mellitus: Isolation of a virus from the pancreas of a child with diabetic ketoacidosis. N Engl J Med 300:1173–1179, 1979.

86. Gerling I, Chatterjee NK, Nejman C: Coxsackie virus B4-induced development of antibodies to 64,000 Mr islet autoantigen and hyperglycemia in mice. Autoimmunity 6:49–56, 1991.

87. Hou J, Sheikh S, Martin DL, Chatterjee NK: Coxsackievirus B4 alters pancreatic glutamate decarboxylase expression in mice soon after infection. J Autoimmun 6:529–542, 1993.

88. Kaufman DJ, Erlander MG, Clare-Salzler M, et al: Autoimmunity to two forms of glutamate decarboxylase in insulin-dependent diabetes mellitus. J Clin Invest 89:283–292, 1992.

89. Atkinson MA, Bowman MA, Campbell L, et al: Cellular immunity to a determinant common to glutamate decarboxylase and coxsackie virus in insulin-dependent diabetes. J Clin Invest 94:2125–2129, 1994.

90. Menser MA, Forrest JM, Honeyman MC, Burgess JA: Diabetes, HLA-antigens and congenital rubella. Lancet 2:1508–1509, 1974.

91. Ginsberg-Fellner F, Witt ME, Yagihashi S, et al: Congenital rubella syndrome as a model for type I (insulin-dependent) diabetes mellitus: Increased prevalence of islet cell surface antibodies. Diabetologia 27:87–89, 1984.

92. McIntosh EDG, Menser MA: A 50-year follow-up of congenital rubella. Lancet 340:414–415, 1992.

93. Hyöty H, Hiltunen M, Knip M, et al: A prospective study of the role of coxsackie B and other enterovirus infections in the pathogenesis of IDDM: Childhood Diabetes in Finland (DiMe) Study. Diabetes 44:652–657, 1995.

94. Dahlquist G, Ivarsson S, Lindberg B, Forsgren M: Maternal enteroviral infection during pregnancy as a risk factor for childhood IDDM. Diabetes 44:408–413, 1995.

95. Lindberg B, Ahlfors K, Carlsson A, et al: Previous exposure to measles, mumps and rubella—but not vaccination during adolescence—correlates to the prevalence of pancreatic and thyroid autoantibodies. Pediatrics 104:1–5, 1999.

96. Toniolo A, Onodera T, Yoon J-W, Notkins AL: Introduction of diabetes by cumulative environmental insults from viruses and chemicals. Nature 297:87–89, 1980.

97. Karam JH, Lewitt PA, Young CW, et al: Insulinopenic diabetes after rodenticide (Vacor) ingestion: A unique model of acquired diabetes in man. Diabetes 29:971–978, 1980.

98. Helgason T, Jonasson MR: Evidence for a food additive as a cause of ketosis-prone diabetes. Lancet 2:716–720, 1981.

99. Helgason T, Ewen SWB, Ross IS, Stowers JM: Diabetes produced in mice by smoked/cured mutton. Lancet 2:1017–1022, 1982.

100. Gepts W, LaCompte PM: The pancreatic islets in diabetes. Am J Med 70:105–115, 1981.

101. Klöppel G, Drenck CR, Oberholzer M, Heitz PU: Morphometric evidence for a striking b-cell reduction at the clinical onset of type 1 diabetes. Virchows Arch (Pathol Anat) 403:441–452, 1984.

102. Dandona P, Elias E, Beckett AG: Serum trypsin concentrations in diabetes mellitus. Br Med J 2:1125–1127, 1978.

103. Foo Y, Rosalki SB, Ramdial L: Serum isoamylase activities in diabetes mellitus. J Clin Pathol 33:1102–1105, 1980.

104. Landin-Olsson M, Borgstrom A, Blom L, et al: Immunoreactive trypsin(ogen) in the sera of children with recent-onset insulin-dependent diabetes and matched controls. Pancreas 5:241–247, 1990.

105. Rahier J: The diabetic pancreas: A pathologist's view. *In* Lefebvre P, Pipeleers D (eds): The Pathology of the Endocrine Pancreas. Berlin/Heidelberg, Springer-Verlag, 1988, pp 17–40.

106. Edlund H: Transcribing pancreas. Diabetes 47:1817–1823, 1998.

107. Rahier J, Goebbels RM, Henquin JC: Cellular composition of the human diabetic pancreas. Diabetologia 24:366–371, 1983.

108. Foulis AK, Liddle CN, Farquharson MA, et al: The histopathology of the pancreas in type I (insulin-dependent) diabetes mellitus: A 25-year review of deaths in patients under 20 years of age in the United Kingdom. Diabetologia 29:267–274, 1986.

109. Bottazzo GF, Dean BM, McNally JM, et al: In situ characterization of autoimmune phenomena and expression of HLA molecules in the pancreas in diabetic insulitis. N Engl J Med 313:353–360, 1985.

110. Hänninen A, Jalkanen S, Salmi M, et al: Macrophages, T cell receptor usage, and endothelial cell activation in the pancreas at the onset of insulin-dependent diabetes mellitus. J Clin Invest 90:1901–1910, 1992.

111. Hanafusa T, Miyazaki A, Miyagawa J: Examination of islets in the pancreas biopsy specimens from newly diagnosed type 1 (insulin-dependent) diabetic patients. Diabetologia 33:105–111, 1990.

112. Itoh N, Hanafusa T, Miyazaki A, et al: Mononuclear cell infiltration and its relation to the expression of major histocompatibility complex antigens and adhesion molecules in pancreas biopsy specimens from newly diagnosed insulin-dependent diabetes mellitus patients. J Clin Invest 92:2313–2322, 1993.

113. Lampeter EE, Seifert I, Lohmann D, et al: Inflammatory islet damage in patients bearing HLA-DR3 and/or DR 4 haplotypes does not lead to islet autoimmunity. Diabetologia 37:471–475, 1994.

114. Bennett Jenson A, Rosenberg HS, Notkins AL: Pancreatic islet cell damage in children with fetal viral infections. Lancet 2:354–358, 1980.

115. Lampeter EF, Homberg M, Quabeck K, et al: Transfer of insulin-dependent diabetes between HLA-identical siblings by bone marrow transplantation. Lancet 342:174, 1993.

116. Rubenstein AH, Kuzuya H, Horwitz DL: Clinical significance of circulating C-peptide in diabetes mellitus and hypoglycemic disorders. Arch Intern Med 137:625–632, 1977.

117. Agner T, Damm P, Binder C: Remission in IDDM: Prospective study of basal C-peptide and insulin dose in 268 consecutive patients. Diabetes Care 10:164–169, 1987.

118. Wallensteen M, Dahlquist G, Persson B, et al: Factors influencing the magnitude, duration, and rate of fall of B-cell function in type 1 (insulin-dependent) diabetes children followed for 2 years from their clinical diagnosis. Diabetologia 31:664–669, 1988.

119. Sabbah E, Kulmala P, Veijola R, et al: Glutamic acid decarboxylase antibodies in relation to other autoantibodies and genetic risk markers in children with newly diagnosed insulin-dependent diabetes. Childhood Diabetes in Finland Study Group. J Clin Endocrinol Metab 81:2455–2459, 1996.

120. Marner B, Agner T, Binder C, et al: Increased reduction in fasting C-peptide is associated with islet cell antibodies in type I (insulin-dependent) diabetic patients. Diabetologia 28:875–880, 1985.

121. Nakanishi K, Kobayashi T, Miyashita H, et al: Relationships among islet cell antibodies, residual β-cell function, and metabolic control in patients with insulin-dependent diabetes mellitus of long duration: Use of a sensitive C-peptide radioimmunoassay. Metabolism 39:925–930, 1990.

122. Kahn SE, Prigeon RL, McCulloch DK, et al: Quantification of the relationship between insulin sensitivity and beta-cell function in human subjects: Evidence for a hyperbolic function. Diabetes 42:1663–1672, 1993.

123. Heaton DA, Millward BA, Gray IP: Increased proinsulin levels as an early indicator of b-cell dysfunction in non-diabetic twins of type 1 (insulin-dependent) diabetic patients. Diabetologia 31:182–184, 1988.

124. Roder ME, Knip M, Hartling SG, et al: Disproportionately elevated proinsulin levels precede the onset of insulin-dependent diabetes mellitus in siblings with low first phase insulin responses: The Childhood Diabetes in Finland Study Group. J Clin Endocrinol Metab 79:1570–1575, 1994.

125. Johnston C, Raghu P, McCulloch D, et al: β-cell function and insulin sensitivity in nondiabetic HLA-identical siblings of insulin-dependent diabetics. Diabetes 36:829–837, 1987.

126. Ludvigsson J, Heding LG, Larsson Y, Leander E: C-peptide in juvenile diabetics beyond the postinitial remission period: Relation to clinical manifestations at onset of diabetes, remission and diabetic control. Acta Pædiatr Scand 66:177–184, 1977.

127. The Diabetes Control and Complications Trial Research Group: Effect of intensive therapy on residual beta-cell function in patients with type 1 diabetes in the diabetes control and complications trial. A randomized, controlled trial. Ann Intern Med 128:517–523, 1998.

128. Sochett EB, Daneman D, Clarson C, Ehrlich RM: Factors affecting and patterns of residual insulin secretion during the first year of type 1 (insulin-dependent) diabetes mellitus in children. Diabetologia 30:453–459, 1987.

129. Bjork E, Berne C, Kampe O, et al: Diazoxide treatment at onset preserves residual insulin secretion in adults with autoimmune diabetes. Diabetes 45:1427–1430, 1996.
130. DPT-1 Study Group: The Diabetes Prevention Trial—Type 1 Diabetes (DPT-1): Implementation of screening and staging of relatives. Transplant Proc 27:3377, 1995.
131. Graham J, Kockum I, Sanjeevi CB, et al: Negative association between type 1 diabetes and HLA DQB1*0602-DQA1*0102 is attenuated with age at onset. Eur J Immunogenet 26:117–127, 1999.
132. Knip M, Ilonen J, Mustonen A, Åkerblom HK: Evidence of an accelerated B-cell destruction in HLA-Dw3/Dw4 heterozygous children with type 1 (insulin-dependent) diabetes. Diabetologia 29:347–351, 1986.
133. Sanjeevi CB, Landin-Olsson M, Kockum I, et al: Effects of the second HLA-DQ haplotype on the association with childhood insulin dependent diabetes mellitus. Tissue Antigens 45:148–152, 1994.
134. Lawley TJ, Hall RP, Fauci AS, et al: Defective Fc-receptor functions associated with the HLA-B8/DRw3 haplotype. N Engl J Med 304:185–192, 1981.
135. Litherland SA, Xie XT, Hutson AD, et al: Aberrant prostaglandin synthase 2 expression defines an antigen-presenting cell defect for insulin-dependent diabetes mellitus. J Clin Invest 104:515–523, 1999.
136. Lernmark Å: Cell-mediated immunity in type I (insulin-dependent) diabetes: Update 1984. *In* Andreani D, Di Mario U, Federlin KF, Heding LG (eds): Immunology in Diabetes. London, Kimpton Medical Publications, 1984, pp 121–131.
137. Peakman M, Vergani D: The T lymphocyte in type 1 diabetes. *In* Marshall SM, Home PD (eds): The Diabetes Annual/8. Amsterdam, Elsevier, 1994, pp 53–73.
138. Jackson RA, Morris MA, Haynes BF, Eisenbarth GS: Increased circulation Ia-bearing T cells in type 1 diabetes mellitus. N Engl J Med 306:785–788, 1982.
139. Panina-Bordignon P, Lang R, van Endert PM, et al: Cytotoxic T cells specific for glutamic acid decarboxylase in autoimmune diabetes. J Exp Med 181:1923–1927, 1995.
140. Honeyman MC, Stone N, de Aizpurua H, et al: High T cell responses to the glutamic acid decarboxylase (GAD) isoform 67 reflect a hyperimmune state that precedes the onset of insulin-dependent diabetes. J Autoimmun 10:165–173, 1997.
141. Lohmann T, Leslie RDG, Hawa M, et al: Immunodominant epitopes of glutamic acid decarboxylase 65 and 67 in insulin-dependent diabetes mellitus. Lancet 343:1607–1608, 1994.
142. Lohmann T, Halder T, Engler J, et al: T cell reactivity to DR*0401- and DQ*0302-binding peptides of the putative autoantigen IA-2 in type 1 diabetes. Exp Clin Endocrinol Diabetes 107:166–171, 1999.
143. Endl J, Otto H, Jung G, et al: Identification of naturally processed T cell epitopes from glutamic acid decarboxylase presented in the context of HLA-DR alleles by T lymphocytes of recent onset IDDM patients. J Clin Invest 99:2405–2415, 1997.
144. Wicker LS, Chen SL, Nepom GT, et al: Naturally processed T cell epitopes from human glutamic acid decarboxylase identified using mice transgenic for the type 1 diabetes-associated human MHC class II allele, DRB1*0401. J Clin Invest 98:2597–2603, 1996.
145. Sonderstrup G, McDevitt H: Identification of autoantigen epitopes in MHC class II transgenic mice. Immunol Rev 164:129–138, 1998.
146. Geluk A, vanMeijgaarden KE, Schloot NC, et al: HLA-DR binding analysis of peptides from islet antigens in IDDM. Diabetes 47:1594–1601, 1998.
147. Congia M, Patel S, Cope AP, et al: T cell epitopes of insulin defined in HLA-DR4 transgenic mice are derived from preproinsulin and proinsulin. Proc Natl Acad Sci U S A 95:3833–3838, 1998.
148. Papadopoulos G, Petersen J, Andersen V: Spontaneous in vitro immunoglobulin secretion at the diagnosis of insulin-dependent diabetes. Acta Endocrinol 105:521–527, 1984.
149. Horita M, Suzuki H, Onodera T, et al: Abnormalities of immunoregulatory T cell subsets in patients with insulin-dependent diabetes mellitus. J Immunol 129:1426–1429, 1982.
150. Baekkeskov S, Nielsen JH, Marner B, et al: Autoantibodies in newly diagnosed diabetic children immunoprecipitate human pancreatic islet cell proteins. Nature 298:167–169, 1982.
151. Baekkeskov S, Landin-Olsson M, Kristensen JK, et al: Antibodies to a Mr 64,000 human islet cell antigen precede the clinical onset of insulin-dependent diabetes. J Clin Invest 79:926–934, 1987.
152. Petersen JB, Russel S, Marshall MO, et al: Differential expression of glutamic acid decarboxylase in rat and human islets. Diabetes 42:484–495, 1993.
153. Christie MR, Vohra G, Champagne P, et al: Distinct antibody specificities to a 64-kD islet cell antigen in type 1 diabetes as revealed by trypsin treatment. J Exp Med 172:789–794, 1990.
154. Christie MR, Genovese S, Cassidy D, et al: Antibodies to islet 37k antigen, but not to glutamate decarboxylase, discriminate rapid progression to IDDM in endocrine autoimmunity. Diabetes 43:1254–1259, 1994.
155. Wasmeier C, Hutton JC: Molecular cloning of phogrin, a protein-tyrosine phosphatase homologue localized to insulin secretory granule membranes. J Biol Chem 271:18161–18170, 1996.
156. Cui L, Yu W-P, de Aizpurua HJ, et al: Cloning and characterization of islet cell antigen-related protein-tyrosine phosphatase (PTP), a novel receptor-like PTP and autoantigen in insulin-dependent diabetes. J Biol Chem 271:24817–24813, 1996.
157. LaGasse J, Jelinek L, Sexson S, et al: An islet-cell protein tyrosine phosphatase is a likely precursor to the 37-kDa autoantigen in type 1 diabetes: Human and macaque sequences, tissue distribution, unique and shared epitopes, and predictive autoantibodies. Mol Med 3:163–173, 1997.
158. Hagopian WA, Sanjeevi CB, Kockum I, et al: Glutamate decarboxylase-, insulin- and islet cell-antibodies and HLA typing to detect diabetes in a general population-based study of Swedish children. J Clin Invest 95:1505–1511, 1995.
159. Eisenbarth GS, Jackson GS: Insulin autoimmunity: The rate limiting factor of pre-type 1 diabetes. J Autoimmun 5:214–246, 1992.
160. Ziegler AG, Ziegler R, Vardi P, et al: Life-table analysis of progression to diabetes of anti-insulin autoantibody-positive relatives of individuals with type 1 diabetes. Diabetes 38:1320–1325, 1989.
161. Atkinson MA, Maclaren NK: Islet cell autoantigens in insulin-dependent diabetes. J Clin Invest 92:1608–1616, 1993.
162. Bingley PJ, Bonifacio E, Williams AJK, et al: Prediction of IDDM in the general population: Strategies based on combinations of autoantibody markers. Diabetes 46:1701–1710, 1997.
163. Bottazzo GF, Gleichmann H: Workshop report: Immunology and diabetes workshops: Report of the First International Workshop on the Standardisation of Cytoplasmic Islet Cell Antibodies. Diabetologia 29:125–126, 1986.
164. Greenbaum CJ, Palmer JP, Nagataki S, et al: Improved specificity of ICA assays in Fourth International Immunology of Diabetes Serum Exchange Workshop. Diabetes 41:1570–1574, 1992.
165. Greenbaum CJ, Palmer JP, Kuglin B, Kolb H: Insulin autoantibodies measured by radioimmunoassay methodology are more related to insulin-dependent diabetes mellitus than those measured by enzyme-linked immunosorbent assay: Results of the Fourth International Workshop on the Standardization of Insulin Autoantibody Measurement. J Clin Endcrinol Metab 74:1040–1044, 1992.
166. Verge CF, Stenger D, Bonifacio E, et al: Combined use of autoantibodies (IA-2) autoantibody, GAD autoantibody, insulin autoantibody, cytoplasmic islet cell antibodies) in type 1 diabetes: Combinatorial Islet Autoantibody Workshop. Diabetes 47:1857–1866, 1998.
167. Grubin CE, Daniels T, Toivola B, et al: A novel radioligand binding assay to determine diagnostic accuracy of isoform-specific glutamic acid decarboxylase antibodies in childhood IDDM. Diabetologia 37:344–350, 1994.
168. Kawasaki E, Eisenbarth G, Wasmeier C, Hutton J: Autoantibodies to protein tyrosine phosphatase-like protein in type 1 diabetes: Overlapping specificities to phogrin and ICA512/IA-2. Diabetes 45:1344–1349, 1996.
169. Vandewalle CL, Falorni A, Lernmark Å, et al: Associations of GAD65- and IA-2-autoantibodies with genetic risk markers in new-onset IDDM patients and their siblings. Diabetes Care 20:1547–1552, 1997.
170. Petersen JS, Hejnaes KR, Moody A, et al: Detection of GAD65 antibodies in diabetes and other autoimmune diseases using a simple radioligand assay. Diabetes 43:459–465, 1994.
171. Schmidli RS, Colman PG, Bonifacio E: Disease sensitivity and specificity of 52 assays for glutamic acid decarboxylase antibodies: The Second International GADAB Workshop. Diabetes 44:636–640, 1995.
172. Sanjeevi CB, Hagopian WA, Landin-Olsson M, et al: Association between autoantibody markers and subtypes of DR4 and DR4-DQ in Swedish children with insulin-dependent diabetes reveals closer association of tyrosine pyrophosphatase autoimmunity with DR4 than DQ8. Tissue Antigens 51:281–286, 1998.
173. Rolandsson O, Hägg E, Hampe C, et al: Levels of glutamate decarboxylase (GAD65) and tyrosine phosphatase-like protein (IA-2) autoantibodies in the general population are related to glucose intolerance and body mass index. Diabetologia 42:555–559, 1999.
174. Yu L, Chase HP, Falorni A, et al: Sexual dimorphism in transmission to offspring of expression of islet autoantibodies. Diabetologia 38:1353–1357, 1995.
175. Bonifacio E, Genovese S, Braghi S, et al: Islet autoantibody markers in IDDM: Risk assessment strategies yielding high sensitivity. Diabetologia 38:816–822, 1995.
176. Kim J, Namchuck M, Bugawan T, et al: Higher autoantibody levels and recognition of a linear NH2-terminal epitope in the autoantigen GAD65, distinguish stiff-man syndrome from insulin-dependent diabetes mellitus. J Exp Med 180:595–606, 1994.
177. Li L, Hagopian WA, Brashear HR, et al: Identification of autoantibody epitopes of glutamic acid decarboxylase in stiff-man syndrome patients. J Immunol 152:930–934, 1994.
178. Leslie RD, Atkinson MA, Notkins AL: Autoantigens IA-2 and GAD in type I (insulin-dependent) diabetes. Diabetologia 42:3–14, 1999.
179. Solimena M, Dirkx R Jr, Hermel JM, et al: ICA 512, an autoantigen of type I diabetes, is an intrinsic membrane protein of neurosecretory granules. EMBO J 15:2102–2114, 1996.
180. Landin-Olsson M, Palmer JP, Lernmark Å, et al: Predictive value of islet cell and insulin autoantibodies for type 1 (insulin-dependent) diabetes mellitus in a population-based study of newly-diagnosed diabetic and matched control children. Diabetologia 35:1068–1073, 1992.
181. Ziegler R, Alper CA, Awdeh ZL, et al: Specific association of HLA-DR4 with increased prevalence and level of insulin autoantibodies in first-degree relatives of patients with type 1 diabetes. Diabetes 40:709–714, 1991.
182. Castano L, Ziegler A, Ziegler R, et al: Characterization of insulin autoantibodies in relatives of patients with insulin-dependent diabetes mellitus. Diabetes 42:1202–1209, 1993.
183. Brooks-Worrell BM, Nielson D, Palmer JP: Insulin autoantibodies and insulin antibodies have similar binding characteristics. Proc Assoc Am Phys 111:92–96, 1999.
184. Arslanian SA, Becker DJ, Rabin B, et al: Correlates of insulin antibodies in newly diagnosed children with insulin-dependent diabetes before insulin therapy. Diabetes 34:926–930, 1985.
185. Eisenbarth GS, Gianani R, Yu L, et al: Dual-parameter model for prediction of type I diabetes mellitus. Proc Assoc Am Phys 110:126–135, 1998.
186. Lernmark Å, Hägglöf B, Freedman Z, et al: A prospective analysis of antibodies reacting with pancreatic islet cells in insulin-dependent diabetic children. Diabetologia 20:471–474, 1981.
187. van de Winkel M, Smets G, Gepts W, Pipeleers DG: Islet cell surface antibodies from insulin-dependent diabetics bind specifically to pancreatic β-cells. J Clin Invest 70:41–49, 1982.
188. Dobersen MJ, Scharff JE: Preferential lysis of pancreatic B-cells by islet cell surface antibodies. Diabetes 31:449–462, 1982.
189. Eisenbarth GS, Morris MA, Scearce RM: Cytotoxic antibodies to cloned rat islet cells in serum of patients with diabetes mellitus. J Clin Invest 67:403–408, 1981.
190. Rabinovitch A, MacKay P, Ludvigsson J, Lernmark Å: A prospective analysis of islet cell cytotoxic antibodies in insulin-dependent diabetic children: Transient effects of plasmapheresis. Diabetes 33:224–228, 1984.

191. Freedman ZR, Feed CM, Irvine WJ, et al: Islet-cell cytoplasmic and cell-surface antibodies in diabetes mellitus. Trans Assoc Am Phys 96:64–76, 1979.
192. Scott J, Nerup J, Lernmark Å: Immunologic factors in diabetes mellitus. *In* Rose WF (ed): Clinical Immunology Update. New York, Elsevier, 1985, pp 53–85.
193. Eisenbarth GS: Type 1 diabetes mellitus: A chronic autoimmune disease. N Engl J Med 314:1360–1368, 1986.
194. Maclaren NK, Huang S, Fogh J: Antibody to cultured human insulinoma cells in insulin-dependent diabetics. Lancet 1:997–999, 1975.
195. Huang SW, Hallquist Haedt L, Rich S, Barbosa J: Prevalence of antibodies to nucleic acids in insulin-dependent diabetes and their relatives. Diabetes 30:873–874, 1981.
196. Nordén G, Jensen E, Stilbo I, et al: B-cell function and islet cell and other organ-specific autoantibodies in relatives to insulin-dependent diabetic patients. Acta Med Scand 213:199–203, 1983.
197. Hägglöf B, Rabinovitch A, Mackay P, et al: Islet cell and other organ-specific autoantibodies in healthy first degree relatives to insulin-dependent diabetic patients. Acta Pediatr Scand 75:611–618, 1986.
198. Irvine WJ, Al-Khateeb SF, Di Mario U, et al: Soluble immune complexes in the sera of newly diagnosed insulin-dependent diabetics and in treated diabetics. Clin Exp Immunol 30:16–21, 1977.
199. Abrass CK, Heber D, Lieberman J: Circulating immune complexes in patients with diabetes mellitus. Clin Exp Immunol 52:164–172, 1983.
200. Contreas G, Lernmark Å, Mathiesen EF, Deckert T: Immune complexes in insulin-dependent diabetes. Biomed Biochim Acta 44:129–132, 1985.
201. The Expert Committee on the Diagnosis and Classification of Diabetes Mellitus: Report of the Expert Committee on the Diagnosis and Classification of Diabetes Mellitus. Diabetes 20:1183–1194, 1997.
202. Diabetes mellitus. WHO Tech Rep Ser, 1985, p. 727.
203. Gottsäter A, Landin-Olsson M, Lernmark Å, et al: Glutamate decarboxylase antibody levels predict rate of beta-cell decline in adult onset diabetes. Diabetes Res Clin Pract 27:133–140, 1995.
204. Srikanta S, Ganda OP, Rabizadeh A, et al: First-degree relatives of patients with type 1 diabetes mellitus: Islet-cell antibodies and abnormal insulin secretion. N Engl J Med 313:462–464, 1985.
205. Gorsuch AN, Spencer KM, Lister J: The natural history of type I (insulin-dependent) diabetes mellitus: Evidence for a long prediabetic period. Lancet 2:1363–1365, 1981.
206. Bingley PJ, Christie MR, Bonifacio E, et al: Combined analysis of autoantibodies improves prediction of IDDM in islet cell antibody-positive relatives. Diabetes 43:1304–1310, 1994.
207. Feutren G, Papoz L, Assan R, et al: Cyclosporin increases the rate and length of remission in insulin-dependent diabetes of recent onset: Results of a multicenter double-blind trial. Lancet 2:119–123, 1986.
208. Canadian-European Randomized Control Trial Group: Cyclosporin-induced remission of IDDM after early intervention: Association of 1 year of cyclosporin treatment with enhanced insulin secretion. Diabetes 37:1574, 1988.
209. Feldt R-B, Jensen T, Dieperink H, et al: Nephrotoxicity of cyclosporin A in patients with newly diagnosed type 1 diabetes mellitus. Diabet Med 7:429–433, 1990.
210. Bieg S, Lernmark Å: Animal models for insulin-dependent diabetes mellitus. *In* Volpé R (ed): Autoimmune Endocrinopathies. Totowa, NJ, Humana Press, 1999, pp 113–140.
211. Harris MI: Diabetes in America, ed 2. Bethesda, MD, National Institutes of Health, 1995.

Chapter 55

Type 2 Diabetes Mellitus: Etiology, Pathogenesis, and Natural History

Jerrold M. Olefsky ▪ Yolanta T. Kruszynska

Despite an enormous literature, the pathogenesis of type 2 diabetes mellitus remains unclear. Many reasons for this lack of clarity exist. One important feature that obscures the etiologic picture is that type 2 diabetes mellitus is not a single disease process but, instead, represents a heterogeneous constellation of disease syndromes all leading to a final common pathway—hyperglycemia. It should be clearly recognized that type 2 diabetes is a rather nonspecific diagnosis featuring hyperglycemia as the cardinal clinical finding. Many factors, either alone or in combination, can cause hyperglycemia; thus the complexity of the pathogenesis of type 2 diabetes reflects the heterogeneous genetic, pathologic, environmental, and metabolic abnormalities that can exist in different patients.[1, 2]

Three major metabolic abnormalities coexist in type 2 diabetes,[3–6] each contributing to the hyperglycemic state. These abnormalities are summarized in Figure 55–1. To begin at the hepatic level, the role of the liver in the pathogenesis of type 2 diabetes is overproduction of glucose. Increased basal hepatic glucose production is characteristic of essentially all type 2 diabetic patients with fasting hyperglycemia.[7–9] Skeletal muscle is depicted as the prototypic peripheral insulin target tissue because in the in vivo insulin-stimulated state, 70% to 80% of all glucose is taken up by skeletal muscle. Target tissues are insulin resistant in type 2 diabetes mellitus, and such resistance has been well described in most,[4–7, 10–14] but not all[15] population groups. Finally,

abnormal islet cell function plays a central role in the development of hyperglycemia; decreased β cell function and increased glucagon secretion are frequent concomitants of the diabetic state.[3, 15, 16] Taken together, abnormalities in these three organ systems account for the syndrome of type 2 diabetes mellitus. In subsequent sections of this chapter, each of these abnormalities is considered in further detail. Although the causal mechanisms may be heterogeneous in different type 2 diabetic patient groups, ultimate expression of the hyperglycemic state involves some combination of impaired insulin secretion, insulin resistance, and increased hepatic glucose production, and the relative magnitude and importance of these three common metabolic abnormalities depend on the specific genetic, pathologic, or environmental factors involved in a particular patient. Thus all causes have a final common pathway in these three abnormalities that underlie type 2 diabetes mellitus.

ETIOLOGY OF TYPE 2 DIABETES MELLITUS

Abundant evidence supports the view that a strong genetic component contributes to type 2 diabetes. Thus most patients have a positive family history for this disease, but perhaps the strongest evidence comes from twin studies. For example, in one study 53 twin pairs were examined, 1 of whom was ascertained to have type 2 diabetes. When the other twin was assessed, type 2 diabetes had developed in 91% (48/53) of the co-twins.[17] The five discordant twins had mild glucose intolerance and abnormal insulin responses during oral glucose tolerance tests (GTTs), which suggests that they might ultimately progress to overt disease and push the concordance rate to 100%. Despite the high concordance rate in twins, garden-variety type 2 diabetes is obviously not simply the result of a single gene defect. Thus except in certain families with the unusual condition termed maturity-onset diabetes of the young (MODY; see Chapter 49), the inheritance pattern of type 2 diabetes does not conform to any recognizable mendelian pattern, and the incidence of type 2 diabetes in first-degree relatives is far below what one would expect.

Further evidence for a genetic basis comes from the striking differences in the prevalence of type 2 diabetes in various ethnic groups that are not explained by environmental factors. The prevalence of type 2 diabetes in the United States is 2% to 4% for whites, but it is 4% to 6% for American blacks,[18] 10% to 15% for Mexican-Americans,[19] and 35% for the Pima Indians in Arizona, the group with the highest incidence of type 2 diabetes in the world.[20] In the Pima Indians, 80% of 35- to 44-year-old offspring of two parents with type 2 diabetes mellitus before age 45 have diabetes,[20] and a positive family history of type 2 diabetes is a much better predictor of the incidence

PERIPHERAL TISSUES (MUSCLE)

receptor + post receptor defect

LIVER
INCREASED GLUCOSE PRODUCTION

GLUCOSE

PANCREAS
IMPAIRED INSULIN SECRETION

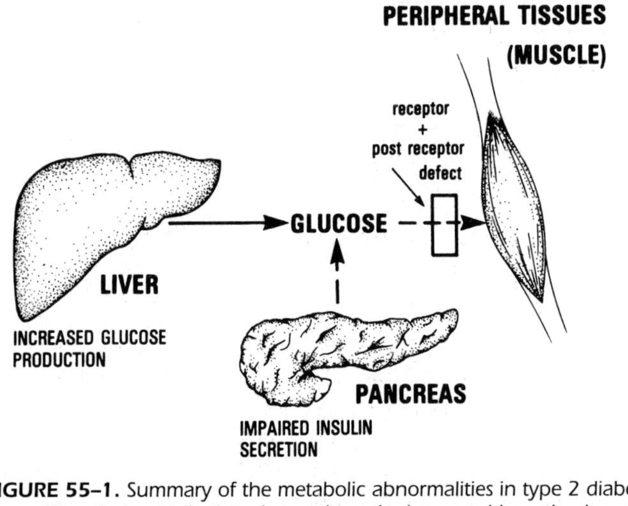

FIGURE 55–1. Summary of the metabolic abnormalities in type 2 diabetes mellitus that contribute to hyperglycemia. Increased hepatic glucose production, impaired insulin secretion, and insulin resistance caused by receptor and postreceptor defects all combine to generate the hyperglycemic state.

of type 2 diabetes than the combined effects of obesity, gender, and physical fitness.[20]

The pathophysiologic findings depicted in Figure 55–1 represent a single point in time after overt type 2 diabetes has developed. However, such an analysis does not reveal the progressive evolution of this disease, a subject that has received considerable attention in recent years. Figure 55–2 presents a schematic description of the natural history or progression to type 2 diabetes. Evidence indicates that in most populations those who evolve to type 2 diabetes begin with insulin resistance. Acquired factors such as obesity, sedentary lifestyle, and aging may be contributory, but insulin resistance is likely to be a primary inherited feature in most type 2 diabetic patients. If β cell function is normal, this condition leads to hyperinsulinemia, which maintains relatively normal glucose tolerance. Impaired glucose tolerance (IGT) eventually develops in a subpopulation of individuals with compensated insulin resistance. Subjects with IGT also typically have fasting and postprandial hyperinsulinemia, but this response is not sufficient to fully compensate for insulin resistance, possibly because of a more profound degree of insulin resistance in some subjects. However, in many it appears to be due to a limited ability to augment their insulin secretion rates.[21] Although a small percentage of subjects with IGT may revert to normal glucose tolerance, many will eventually progress to frank type 2 diabetes mellitus.

The proportion of insulin-resistant subjects who progress to type 2 diabetes depends on the particular ethnic groups studied and the methods of assessment. In most populations the rate of progression of IGT to type 2 diabetes is 2% to 6% per year over 10 years.[22] During the transition from IGT to frank type 2 diabetes, at least three pathophysiologic changes can be observed. First is a marked fall in β cell function and insulin secretion. Whether this decrease is due to preprogrammed genetic abnormalities in β cell function, to acquired defects (such as glucotoxicity), or to both remains to be elucidated. Nevertheless, a marked decrease in β cell function accompanies this transition, and most workers think that this decreased β cell function is the major contributor to type 2 diabetes mellitus. A second metabolic change is at the level of the liver. Subjects with IGT have normal basal rates of hepatic glucose output (HGO), whereas patients with fasting hyperglycemia have increased HGO. Thus the capacity of the liver to overproduce glucose is an important contributory factor (albeit secondary) to the pathogenesis of type 2 diabetes. Finally, many but not all studies have indicated that patients with type 2 diabetes are more insulin resistant than those with IGT. Whether this increase in insulin resistance is secondary to glucotoxicity or to other acquired factors remains to be determined. A number of lines of evidence, largely drawn from population studies, have converged to support the scheme depicted in Figure 55–2.

Using intravenous GTTs, Warram et al. evaluated 155 nondiabetic offspring whose parents both had type 2 diabetes.[23] During a follow-up period averaging 13 years, type 2 diabetes developed in 16% of the offspring. This percentage is eight times the general risk for a corresponding white population of similar age, but it is less than would be expected if type 2 diabetes were the result of a single gene locus. Additionally, this study clearly demonstrated that insulin resistance is present one to two decades before type 2 diabetes is diagnosed. The intravenous GTTs showed impaired glucose clearance accompanied by elevated insulin levels in offspring in whom type 2 diabetes was destined to develop. Thus insulin resistance and hyperinsulinemia (rather than hypoinsulinemia) characterized the prediabetic state, which indicates that the primary defect is peripheral insulin resistance, not an impairment in insulin secretion. The insulin resistance occurred irrespective of obesity and antedated the subsequent development of impaired insulin secretion and overt type 2 diabetes.[23]

Studies in ethnic populations with a high prevalence of type 2 diabetes have also provided data to support the primary role of insulin resistance in its development. Thus in the Pima Indians, hyperinsulinemia and an associated decrease in insulin-mediated glucose disposal are early abnormalities, common in those with normal glucose tolerance, that predict the subsequent development of both IGT and type 2 diabetes.[24–26] Pima Indians with IGT who progress to type 2 diabetes have lower insulin levels 2 hours after a glucose load than do those who continue to have IGT or return to normal glucose tolerance.[24–26] Similar results come from studies of Micronesians in Nauru, a population with a prevalence of type 2 diabetes of approximately 30% in whom family clustering of age-adjusted glucose tolerance levels is seen.[27, 28] Again, in this population, IGT and type 2 diabetes were most likely to develop in those with hyperinsulinemia at baseline, but progression to type 2 diabetes in those with IGT could be predicted by lower baseline insulin responsiveness.

Further evidence that peripheral tissue insulin resistance is a primary inherited defect in those predisposed to type 2 diabetes comes from several studies of insulin sensitivity and insulin secretion in first-degree relatives of type 2 diabetic patients of European ancestry.[29–31] In all these studies, peripheral insulin resistance was found in the normoglycemic relatives and their fasting insulin levels and insulin responses to oral glucose were increased. In two of the studies,[29, 30] some of the first-degree relatives had IGT. Eriksson et al. found that insulin was able to suppress HGO less effectively in the relatives with IGT than in those who were glucose tolerant,[29] thus suggesting a degree of hepatic insulin resistance, although basal HGO rates were normal in both groups. The first-degree relatives with IGT in these studies[29, 30] also had subtle defects in insulin secretion that were not apparent in those with normal glucose tolerance, notably, a delayed early insulin response to oral glucose and decreased first-phase insulin secretion after intravenously administered glucose. Insulin resistance, however, preceded an impairment in insulin secretion in these study populations at high risk for type 2 diabetes mellitus.

In summary, the phenotypic manifestation of type 2 diabetes mellitus involves elevated HGO, impaired insulin secretion, and peripheral insulin resistance. Type 2 diabetes mellitus has a strong genetic component, and studies of prediabetic subjects indicate that in most populations, insulin resistance, accompanied by hyperinsulinemia, exists before any deterioration in glucose homeostasis. After a period of compensatory hyperinsulinemia with normal glucose tolerance or IGT, β cell insulin secretion declines and overt type 2 diabetes mellitus results. In the remainder of this chapter the abnormalities of insulin secretion, insulin action, and hepatic glucose metabolism in type 2

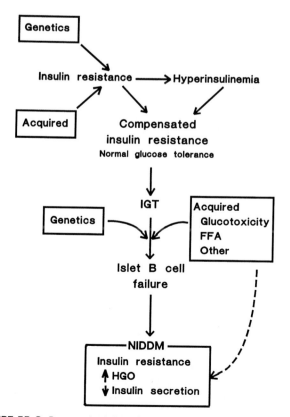

FIGURE 55–2. *Proposed etiology for the development of type 2 diabetes mellitus.*

diabetes are reviewed, with particular attention to basic mechanisms (where known) and their applicability to etiology.

INSULIN SECRETION

Both quantitative and qualitative defects in insulin secretion are found in patients with type 2 diabetes mellitus.[3, 16, 32, 33] The abnormality varies with the severity of diabetes and degree of obesity and may be influenced by the preceding level of diabetic control. As discussed above, evidence indicates that islet β cell function progressively deteriorates during the natural history of type 2 diabetes. This decline in β cell function is evident not only during the progression from compensated insulin resistance to IGT and subsequently to overt type 2 diabetes but also during the course of established type 2 diabetes.[34] The rate of this progression and the relative importance of insulin deficiency vis-à-vis other factors that contribute to the hyperglycemic state vary. Ethnic background and obesity are just two factors that contribute to this variability. For example, in nondiabetic subjects, obesity augments insulin secretion,[3, 16, 35, 36] with a particularly pronounced effect on basal insulin levels, and this effect also occurs in type 2 diabetes.[6, 36, 37] Indeed, higher insulin levels are consistently observed in obese than in lean type 2 diabetic subjects.[36, 37]

In considering the role of insulin deficiency in type 2 diabetes, one must distinguish between impaired β cell secretory function and decreased absolute circulating insulin levels.[3, 16, 36] Thus basal insulin levels are usually normal or increased in type 2 diabetes (see Table 1 in DeFronzo and Ferrannini[38] for review).[16, 36] Indeed, obese type 2 diabetic subjects can have basal insulin levels severalfold higher than normal,[16, 36] but this finding does not mean that basal β cell secretory function is normal because the prevailing plasma glucose level must also be taken into account.[3, 16, 39, 40] Hyperglycemia is the major stimulus for insulin secretion, and when normal individuals are made hyperglycemic by infusion of glucose, circulating insulin levels are higher than those found in type 2 diabetes.[3, 39, 40] Thus type 2 diabetic patients maintain normal or increased basal insulin levels only in the face of the enhanced stimulus of fasting hyperglycemia, which indicates an underlying decrease in the sensitivity of the β cell to glucose. Another factor that bears on our understanding of basal hyperinsulinemia in type 2 diabetes concerns circulating proinsulin levels. Proinsulin is secreted by β cells concomitantly with insulin and cross-reacts with insulin in most insulin immunoassays, thus contributing to the total measured immunoreactive insulin level. In normal subjects, proinsulin represents only a small portion (3%–7%) of the insulin-like material secreted by β cells. However, using proinsulin-specific immunoassays, several groups have shown that in hyperinsulinemic states and in many type 2 diabetic patients, an increased proportion of proinsulin is released and contributes to the measured insulin in standard immuno-

assays, so true insulin levels are overestimated.[16, 32, 36] When corrected for this factor, basal insulin levels are either normal or moderately elevated in type 2 diabetes. The increase in proinsulin secretion relative to insulin in type 2 diabetes parallels the degree of reduced β cell secretory function.[41] The abnormality is unlikely to represent a β cell proinsulin processing defect specific to type 2 diabetes because a similar defect is induced in rats made hyperglycemic by glucose infusion for 48 hours. In these animals, proinsulin is released prematurely in the absence of any specific defect in the proinsulin conversion rate or decreased synthesis of the specific endopeptidases involved.[42]

Stimulated insulin levels can be low, normal, or high in type 2 diabetes,[1, 3, 15, 16, 43] depending on the type of stimulus used and the severity of the diabetes (see Table 1 in DeFronzo and Ferrannini[38] for review). The most profound defects are elicited in response to intravenous glucose. Insulin secretion in response to a sustained intravenous glucose stimulus is normally biphasic; a rapid rise in insulin levels within 1 to 3 minutes of a rise in glucose levels (first phase) is followed by a return to baseline by 6 to 10 minutes and then a gradual increase (second phase). In type 2 diabetes, once fasting plasma glucose levels exceed 126 mg/dL, the first-phase insulin response to intravenous glucose is characteristically completely absent.[3, 16, 44] This relationship is shown in Figure 55–3. Interestingly, acute or first-phase insulin secretion in response to nonglucose stimuli such as arginine[3, 16] or isoproterenol[45] is relatively preserved, even though the response may be lower than in normal individuals when matched for prevailing hyperglycemia. This finding indicates a relatively selective β cell defect in response to glucose stimuli in type 2 diabetes. Because the acute insulin response to intravenously administered arginine or isoproterenol increases along with the prevailing glucose concentration,[3, 40] Porte and colleagues have attempted to quantitate this effect of glucose by plotting the increase in acute insulin response to arginine or isoproterenol pulses as a function of increasing plasma glucose level.[3, 16, 40] The slope of this relationship is termed the glucose potentiation slope, and by this analysis glucose potentiation of β cell function is also reduced in type 2 diabetes.[16, 40]

Second-phase insulin secretion, assessed by using the hyperglycemic clamp or the graded intravenous glucose infusion technique (see Fig. 55–4 for details), is markedly reduced in type 2 diabetes at any given glucose level in comparison with normal or IGT subjects matched for age and body mass index. In general, the more severe the diabetes, the lower the second-phase insulin response.[3, 44]

The loss of first-phase insulin secretion in type 2 diabetes, although a consistent finding, does not appear to be a specific marker for type 2 diabetes. Several findings support this conclusion: (1) in some type 2 diabetic patients, first-phase insulin secretion can be partially or completely restored by salicylates,[46] β-adrenergic blockers,[47] or insulin[48] without ameliorating the basic diabetic state. (2) The defect can be induced by a number of diabetogenic manipulations not related to

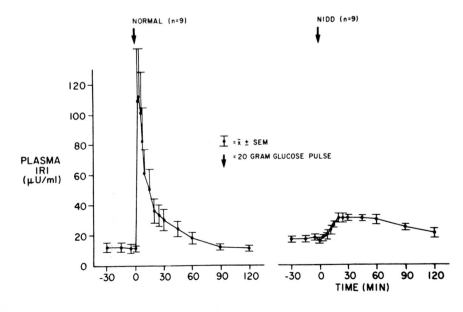

FIGURE 55–3. First-phase insulin release in response to the intravenous administration of glucose in normal and type 2 diabetic (non–insulin-dependent diabetes [NIDD]) subjects. Mean fasting plasma glucose concentrations were 83 ± 3 mg/dL in normal subjects and 160 ± 10 mg/dL in type 2 diabetic subjects. (Reproduced with permission of the American Diabetes Association, Inc., from Ward WWK, Beard JC, Halter JB, et al: Pathophysiology of insulin secretion in non–insulin-dependent diabetes mellitus. Diabetes Care 7:491–502, 1984.)

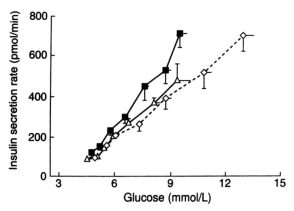

FIGURE 55–4. Relationship between average plasma glucose concentrations and insulin secretion rates during graded glucose infusion studies in a group of lean nondiabetic control subjects *(open triangles)*, nondiabetic obese subjects *(closed squares)*, and matched obese subjects with impaired glucose tolerance *(open diamonds)*. The lowest glucose levels and insulin secretion rates were measured under basal conditions, and subsequent levels were obtained during glucose infusion rates of 1, 2, 3, 4, 6, and 8 mg/kg/min. Values are means ± SEM. (From Polonsky KS: The β-cell in diabetes: From molecular genetics to clinical research. Diabetes 44:705–717, 1995.)

type 2 diabetes, including partial pancreatectomy in rats and hyperglycemic infusions.[49] (3) Islets isolated at laparotomy from type 2 diabetic patients demonstrated substantial glucose-induced insulin secretion, even though in vivo insulin secretion in response to glucose was markedly reduced.[50] This finding suggests that the abnormal in vivo milieu of the type 2 diabetic state may be at least partly responsible for the in vivo defects in insulin secretion. The above findings suggest that the absent first-phase insulin secretion is a nonspecific manifestation of impaired β cell function regardless of the cause of islet damage or dysfunction. Furthermore, hyperglycemia per se may secondarily impair β cell function and lead to a reduced acute insulin response to glucose.

Several points argue that absent first-phase insulin secretion does not play an important role in causing glucose intolerance or hyperglycemia in type 2 diabetes. First, because mildly hyperglycemic and severely hyperglycemic type 2 diabetic patients are equally deficient in first-phase insulin secretion, this deficiency cannot play a role in further deterioration in glucose tolerance from mild to severe fasting hyperglycemia. Second, in selected patients with normal glucose tolerance in whom type 1 diabetes eventually develops, the acute insulin response to intravenous glucose is absent during the normal stage and thus cannot be a cause of the hyperglycemia because it is present months to years before diabetes develops.[51] Finally, salicylates[46] and β-adrenergic blockers[47] can substantially restore the acute insulin response to intravenous glucose with no major improvement in fasting glycemia or glucose tolerance.

After the ingestion of glucose or mixed meals, insulin levels are far more variable in type 2 diabetes than they are in response to intravenous glucose. After oral glucose, insulin levels are usually subnormal in type 2 diabetes,[1, 15, 16, 29] although such may not be the case in patients with mild hyperglycemia.[38, 43] This heterogeneity is depicted in Figure 55–5, which summarizes the results of oral GTTs in a wide spectrum of normal and type 2 diabetic subjects. As can be seen, hyperinsulinemia frequently exists in mild states of glucose intolerance. In individuals with mild diabetes, insulin levels are generally in the normal range, although the rise is delayed and corresponds to the greater and more prolonged rise in plasma glucose levels; with more severe diabetes, insulin levels are low. Even though these studies are cross-sectional, if one thinks of them longitudinally, the concept can be advanced that hyperinsulinemia exists early in the development of type 2 diabetes, whereas in later stages of this disease, β cell function is markedly subnormal.

In type 2 diabetes, the defect in β cell function is relatively (but not completely) specific for glucose stimuli. The relative preservation of insulin responses to nonglucose stimuli, such as certain amino acids and insulinogenic gut peptides released during meal absorption, results in type 2 diabetic patients having a much better insulin response to mixed meals than to oral glucose. Thus in mild type 2 diabetes, insulin responses to mixed meals may be delayed, but the marked postprandial hyperglycemia, coupled with other insulinogenic factors, often leads to exaggerated insulin responses 2 to 4 hours after meal ingestion. This finding is so even when measured insulin levels are corrected for the elevated plasma proinsulin.[36] However, with more severe hyperglycemia (fasting blood sugar greater than 220 mg/dL), decreased insulin levels are more common. Because oral GTTs represent a rather nonphysiologic stress to β cell function, it is important to keep in mind that in the free-living state, although a patient is consuming mixed meals, insulin levels can be relatively preserved in type 2 diabetes.

Because the major abnormality in insulin secretion in type 2 diabetes involves a decreased β cell response to glucose and because this defect is worse with more severe diabetes, two general trends emerge. First, in response to a given stimulus to insulin secretion, the more the stimulus relies on glucose recognition, the more apt insulin levels are to be low in type 2 diabetes. Second, the greater the degree of fasting hyperglycemia, the greater the defect in β cell function.

The cellular mechanisms underlying the decreased β cell responsiveness to glucose are unclear. Whether this decreased responsiveness represents a defect in β cell glucose-sensing mechanisms, a decrease in intracellular glucose metabolism, or some critical stimulatory metabolite requires further studies. Some reports have suggested a decrease in the number of β cells in islets from type 2 diabetic patients,[52, 53] consistent with recent data indicating enhanced β cell apoptosis in

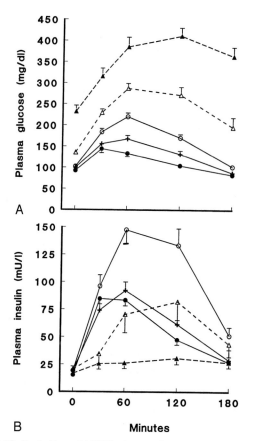

FIGURE 55–5. *A,* Mean (±SEM) plasma glucose response to oral glucose in the five subject groups. *Closed circle,* normal; *cross,* borderline tolerance; *open circle,* impaired glucose tolerance; *open triangle and broken line,* fasting hyperglycemia (110–150 mg/dL); *closed triangle and broken line,* fasting hyperglycemia (>150 mg/dL). *B,* Mean (±SEM) plasma insulin response to oral glucose in the five subject groups. Symbols are the same as in *A.* (From Reaven GM, Olefsky JM: Relationship between heterogeneity of insulin responses and insulin resistance in normal subjects. Diabetologia 13:201–206, 1977.)

diabetic rats.[54, 55] However, the decrease in β cell mass is in the range of 30% to 50%. Because sufficient insulin secretory reserve normally exists to sustain an 80% to 90% loss of β cells without the development of diabetes, it follows that decreased functional capacity of the remaining β cells must exist in type 2 diabetes. Indeed, it has been shown that the maximal insulin secretory capacity may be reduced by as much as 80% in type 2 diabetes.[39] It is possible that the decrease in β cell mass in type 2 diabetes is somehow causally related to the decreased function of the remaining β cells. The constellation of insulin secretory abnormalities that characterizes type 2 diabetes, however, may not be specific. Thus partially pancreatectomized rats and streptozotocin-treated rats display similar insulin secretory defects,[49] which suggests that decreased glucose-stimulated insulin secretion with relative preservation of responsiveness to nonglucose stimuli may be a general type of abnormality in response to a variety of β cell insults.

The strong genetic contribution to the development of type 2 diabetes makes it quite possible that a genetic defect underlies the decline in β cell function. The identification of "diabetes genes" that encode proteins critical for normal β cell function is an area under intensive investigation and is discussed more fully later in this chapter. Acquired factors could also play a role. The insulin secretory abnormalities found in type 2 diabetes may be improved after a period of good blood glucose control irrespective of the treatment used (diet, insulin, or oral hypoglycemic agents).[56–58] This reversibility is consistent with the idea that to some extent at least the abnormalities may be secondary to hyperglycemia or some other factor associated with uncontrolled diabetes. Support for the "glucotoxicity" theory comes from a variety of in vivo and in vitro studies showing that chronic exposure of islets to hyperglycemia can result in a number of different defects in glucose-induced insulin secretion.[49] Importantly, when isolated human islets are incubated under euglycemic and hyperglycemic conditions, islets exposed to previous hyperglycemia demonstrated a marked defect in their ability to secrete insulin in response to subsequent glucose stimuli.[59] Although the precise mechanism is unknown, it seems likely that glucotoxicity plays some role in the impaired β cell function of type 2 diabetes.

Impaired Glucose Tolerance

In subjects with IGT (see Chapter 53), insulin secretory responses are even more variable than in type 2 diabetes.[1, 15, 43, 60] Thus in IGT, insulin levels during oral or intravenous GTTs have been reported as high, normal, or low (see DeFronzo and Ferrannini,[38] Table 1). Part of this variability is explained by the heterogeneity of this category.[22] Thus some subjects have transient IGT and will have normal glucose tolerance when retested. A proportion will progress to frank type 2 diabetes, whereas others will continue to have IGT for many years. In long-term follow-up studies, the proportion of unselected patients with IGT in whom type 2 diabetes developed has ranged from 3% to 60%.[22, 24–26, 60, 61] Thus regardless of the subpopulation studied, it is clear that true diabetes will not eventually develop in all these individuals. Because normoglycemic, insulin-resistant subjects (obese or nonobese) have increased insulin secretion rates,[35, 62, 63] the question arises whether insulin secretion rates in subjects with IGT are appropriately increased for their degree of obesity and/or insulin resistance. It appears that they are not. Polonsky et al. have shown that subjects with IGT secrete less insulin at any given glucose level than do normoglycemic subjects matched for a similar degree of insulin resistance and obesity[21, 33] (see Fig. 55–4). It may be that insulin-resistant IGT subjects who have a progressive impairment in insulin secretion are most prone to development of the full-blown picture of type 2 diabetes.[64]

PERIPHERAL INSULIN RESISTANCE

Insulin resistance is a metabolic state in which a normal concentration of insulin produces a less than normal biologic response. This decreased response to insulin can involve any of the multiple metabolic

effects of insulin, but from the standpoint of relevance to type 2 diabetes, resistance to insulin's effects on glucose metabolism have been the most extensively studied. Because insulin travels from the β cell through the circulation to the target tissue, events at any of these loci can influence the ultimate action of the hormone. Therefore, it is useful to categorize insulin resistance according to known causative mechanisms, and such a classification is presented in Table 55–1. In general, insulin resistance can be due to (1) an abnormal β cell secretory product, (2) circulating insulin antagonists, (3) impaired access of insulin to target cells, or (4) a target tissue defect in insulin action.

Causes of Insulin Resistance

Abnormal β Cell Secretory Product

Several patients have been described who secrete a structurally abnormal, biologically defective insulin molecule resulting from a mutation in the structural gene for insulin.[65] Others have familial hyperproinsulinemia caused by incomplete conversion of proinsulin to insulin within the β cell secretory granule as a result of structural abnormalities at the proteolytic cleavage sites of the proinsulin molecule.[66, 67] These syndromes are dealt with in Chapter 56 and are not discussed further here, except to note that they do not represent insulin-resistant states in the most common usage of this term. Thus in these syndromes the hormone is abnormal and the patients are resistant only to their endogenous insulin and not to exogenous insulin.

Circulating Insulin Antagonists

In general, insulin antagonists may be hormonal or nonhormonal.

HORMONAL ANTAGONISTS. Hormonal antagonists include all the known counterregulatory hormones such as cortisol, growth hormone, glucagon, and catecholamines. Well-known syndromes exist (e.g., Cushing's disease, acromegaly) in which elevated levels of these hormones can induce an insulin-resistant diabetic state. However, in the usual case of obesity or type 2 diabetes, excessive levels of these counterregulatory hormones are not an important contributory factor to insulin resistance. Islet amyloid polypeptide (IAPP), which is co-secreted with insulin from islet β cells, was found to inhibit insulin-stimulated glucose uptake when pharmacologic doses were infused.[68] However, studies to date have shown no anti-insulin actions of IAPP at physiologic levels, nor are circulating concentrations of IAPP elevated in type 2 diabetes.[69] In fact, IAPP may have a beneficial role in glucose homeostasis because it inhibits postprandial glucagon secretion and gastric emptying.[68]

NONHORMONAL ANTAGONISTS. Free Fatty Acids. A number of years ago, Randle et al. hypothesized that the elevated circulating levels of free fatty acids (FFAs) found in obesity and type 2 diabetes impair peripheral glucose utilization.[70] Substantial evidence indicates that FFAs may indeed contribute to insulin resistance, although the intracellular mechanisms may differ from those originally proposed. FFAs also play an important role in the regulation of HGO

TABLE 55–1. Causes of Insulin Resistance

Abnormal β cell secretory product
    Abnormal insulin molecule
    Incomplete conversion of proinsulin to insulin
Circulating insulin antagonists
    Elevated levels of counterregulatory hormones, e.g., growth hormone,
        cortisol, glucagon, or catecholamines
    Cytokines
    Free fatty acids
    Anti-insulin antibodies
    Anti–insulin receptor antibodies
Target tissue defects
    Insulin receptor defects
    Postreceptor defects

and may contribute to hepatic insulin insensitivity in obesity and type 2 diabetes. These issues are discussed later in this chapter.

Anti-Insulin Antibodies. Anti-insulin antibodies develop in essentially all patients treated chronically with insulin.[71] By binding and trapping insulin within the plasma compartment, these antibodies can alter the usual time course of insulin action. However, only in unusual cases do such antibodies actually cause a true insulin-resistant state. A few patients have been described in whom anti-insulin antibodies spontaneously develop in the absence of exogenous insulin therapy.[71] These antibodies can interfere with insulin immunoassays and lead to apparent "hyperinsulinemia," but they do not cause insulin resistance.

Insulin Receptor Antibodies. A fascinating syndrome ("type B insulin resistance") has been described in which patients have antibodies directed against the insulin receptor.[72, 73] This condition is rare. It occurs predominantly in women, and almost all patients have features of other autoimmune disorders such as systemic lupus erythematosus. It is associated with acanthosis nigricans, severe insulin resistance, and diabetes mellitus. Occasional patients have episodes of spontaneous hypoglycemia. The circulating antibodies bind to the insulin receptor in vivo and, by interacting with the insulin-binding domain, block and/or mimic the action of insulin and thereby result in insulin resistance or, occasionally, hypoglycemia.[73]

Cytokines. Increased levels of cytokines such as tumor necrosis factor-α (TNF-α) may contribute to the insulin resistance associated with sepsis, cirrhosis, or other severe illness. In vivo, infusions of TNF-α have major effects on glucose and lipid metabolism.[74, 75] The finding that adipose tissue TNF-α mRNA levels were increased in obese humans[76] and rodents[77] led to the idea that TNF-α may also play a role in the insulin resistance of obesity and type 2 diabetes.[77] Evidence came from in vitro studies showing that incubation of cells with TNF-α impaired insulin receptor signaling.[78] Furthermore, neutralization of TNF-α by infusion of a TNF-α receptor IgG fusion protein reversed insulin resistance in Zucker (fa/fa) rats.[77] However, in subsequent studies in obese type 2 diabetic patients, intravenous infusion of a neutralizing antibody to TNF-α had no effect on insulin resistance,[79] and more recently, TNF-α was found to have no effect in the short term on insulin-stimulated glucose uptake in isolated rat soleus muscle.[80] Clearly, further work is needed to delineate the role of TNF-α in the insulin resistance associated with obesity.

Impaired Access of Insulin to Target Cells

Because insulin must travel from the circulation to target tissues to elicit biologic effects, any defect in this transfer could potentially lead to insulin resistance. The passage of insulin from the plasma compartment to tissue sites of action is marked by substantial delays, and insulin's in vivo effects to stimulate glucose disposal are well correlated with the appearance of insulin in the interstitial fluid.[81] Lymph insulin levels are lower than those in plasma,[81, 82] which indicates that peripheral tissues are more sensitive to insulin than previously recognized. Furthermore, the possibility arises that either the rate or the amount of insulin transferring from the plasma to the interstitial compartment could be abnormal in type 2 diabetes or obesity, thereby contributing to the insulin-resistant state and defects of in vivo insulin action kinetics.[83, 84] Recent studies indicate that transport of insulin across the capillary in vivo is by diffusion[82] and not receptor mediated as has been suggested.[85] Transport by diffusion fits with the finding that transcapillary passage is comparable in normal subjects, insulin-resistant nondiabetic subjects,[86] and patients with type 2 diabetes.[87] Further evidence that the delayed activation of muscle glucose uptake in obesity and type 2 diabetes is not due to impaired transcapillary transport of insulin comes from a study by Nolan et al.[84] This study showed that the kinetic defect in insulin's ability to stimulate leg glucose uptake was not accompanied by any delay in the activation of leg muscle insulin receptors by insulin, thus implying that the kinetic defect is distal to the insulin receptor.

Another physical factor that may relate to insulin resistance is muscle capillary density, which correlates with in vivo insulin sensitivity.[88] Baron et al. have shown that insulin, at least at pharmacologic levels, increases leg blood flow.[89] Because tissue glucose uptake is a product of blood flow and the arteriovenous glucose difference, in-

creased leg blood flow could contribute to overall glucose disposal. Similar studies performed in obese subjects and in subjects with type 2 diabetes revealed a decrease in the insulin-induced increase in leg blood flow, which may explain part of the decrease in total leg glucose uptake.[89] However, others found no effect of insulin on blood flow, nor a decrease in blood flow in either forearm or leg balance studies in type 2 diabetic subjects.[90] More recently, Utriainen and colleagues used [15]O[H2O] and positron emission tomography to confirm an enhancement of leg muscle blood flow by pharmacologic insulin levels, but no difference in the response between type 2 diabetic and normal control subjects.[91]

Taken together, defects in any of the above factors, although possibly contributory, cannot explain the major component of insulin resistance in type 2 diabetes and obesity because numerous studies have demonstrated profound in vitro insulin resistance in tissues and cells from these patients.

Cellular Defects in Insulin Action

Available evidence points to a target tissue defect as the major cause of insulin resistance in type 2 diabetes. Before considering potential causes, it is useful to review some general concepts concerning normal insulin action (Fig. 55–6; also see Chapter 50).

Insulin first binds to its cell surface receptor, a heterotetrameric glycoprotein composed of two α subunits (135 kDa) and two β subunits (95 kDa) linked by disulfide bonds.[92–95] The α subunits, located entirely extracellularly, are responsible for insulin binding. The β subunits are transmembrane proteins containing a small extracellular domain and a larger cytoplasmic domain that contains the insulin-regulated tyrosine kinase activity. Binding of insulin to the receptor rapidly induces a cascade of tyrosine autophosphorylation in the β subunit involving three tyrosine residues in the kinase domain, in addition to tyrosine residues adjacent to the transmembrane domain and in the C terminus of the β subunit.[92–95] Once the receptor is autophosphorylated, its intrinsic tyrosine kinase catalytic activity is markedly enhanced, and it can now phosphorylate tyrosine residues on endogenous protein substrates.[92–95] Activation of the insulin receptor tyrosine kinase is essential both for transduction of the insulin signal and for internalization of the receptor and its bound insulin.[93–95] Patients with naturally occurring mutations in the tyrosine kinase domain of the insulin receptor have syndromes of severe insulin resistance (see Chapter 56).

In recent years, major advances have been made in our understanding of the mechanisms by which the insulin signal is propagated downstream from the activated insulin receptor to the various insulin-regulated enzymes, transporters, and insulin-responsive genes to medi-

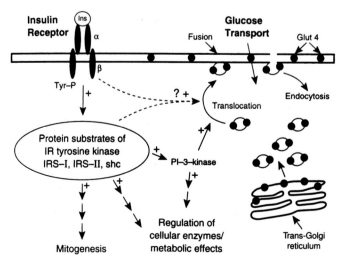

FIGURE 55–6. Model of cellular insulin action. IR, insulin receptor; IRS-I, insulin receptor substrate-1; IRS-II, insulin receptor substrate-2. (From Kruszynska YT, Olefsky JM: Cellular and molecular mechanisms of non–insulin dependent diabetes mellitus. J Invest Med 44:413–428, 1996.)

ate its metabolic and growth effects (see Fig. 55–6). This field is rapidly evolving and complex and is discussed only briefly because it is covered in Chapter 50. A large number of intermediate signaling molecules have been identified, and evidence indicates that after activation of the insulin receptor kinase, more than one signaling pathway may be used (see Fig. 55–6). For example, the pathways leading to the mitogenic effects of insulin consist of elements distinct from those leading to activation of glucose transport. Even a single action of insulin, for example, activation of glucose transport, may involve more than one signaling pathway. Several cytosolic protein substrates of the insulin receptor tyrosine kinase have been identified that are phosphorylated on tyrosine residues within seconds of insulin's binding to its receptor. The first of these substrates to be shown to play a key role in insulin signal transduction was insulin receptor substrate-1 (IRS-1).[95, 96] IRS-1 belongs to a growing family of proteins that includes IRS-2, IRS-3, IRS-4, and a protein termed shc, which are also immediate substrates of the insulin receptor kinase and involved in insulin signaling.[95, 96] These proteins have no enzymatic activity but act as docking proteins. Tyrosine phosphorylation of these substrates enhances their association with proteins that contain src homology-2 (SH2) domains.[95, 96] These domains are sequences of about 100 amino acids that can bind to specific short sequences that encompass a phosphotyrosine moiety. The binding of specific SH2 domain–containing downstream signaling proteins to tyrosine-phosphorylated IRS proteins or shc generates multicomponent signaling complexes, which in turn results in modulation of the activities of several serine and threonine kinases and phosphatases that act on key insulin-regulated enzymes and transcription factors.

One of the most important effects of insulin with respect to type 2 diabetes is to stimulate glucose uptake in skeletal muscle, adipocytes, and heart muscle. Under most physiologic circumstances, glucose transport in these tissues is rate limiting for overall glucose disposal.[97–99] Tissue glucose uptake is mediated by a family of at least five facilitative glucose transporters, each derived from a separate gene. These transporters show a high degree of homology, but each has a tissue-specific distribution.[100, 101] One of them, GLUT4, or the insulin-sensitive glucose transporter, is uniquely expressed in skeletal muscle, adipose tissue, and cardiac muscle.[100, 101] In the unstimulated state, most of the GLUT4 proteins are located in an intracellular vesicular pool. Upon insulin stimulation, recruitment or translocation of these glucose transporter–rich vesicles causes insertion of GLUT4 proteins into the plasma membrane, where they begin to transport glucose into the cell.[102–106] In addition to translocation, insulin may also increase the intrinsic activity of GLUT4. Once the insulin signal dissipates, the GLUT4 proteins return to their intracellular location.

Clearly, insulin action involves a cascade of events, and abnormalities anywhere along this sequence can lead to insulin resistance.

Characteristics of Insulin Resistance in Type 2 Diabetes and Impaired Glucose Tolerance

The frequency of insulin resistance increases as the degree of carbohydrate intolerance worsens.[107] Thus many but not all subjects with IGT are insulin resistant, whereas essentially every type 2 diabetic patient with fasting hyperglycemia displays this abnormality. Some studies indicate that insulin resistance is more marked in type 2 diabetes than in the prediabetic IGT state.[5, 7, 29] However, other reports show only a modest increase in the degree of insulin resistance from IGT to type 2 diabetes. Because most type 2 diabetic patients are overweight, obesity-induced insulin resistance is thought to be an additive factor in the hyperglycemia of these patients. However, obesity can be only a contributory factor because the insulin resistance in obese type 2 diabetic patients exceeds that caused by obesity alone, and nonobese type 2 diabetic patients are also insulin resistant.[5, 7, 38, 107, 108]

In Vivo Studies

All methods of assessing insulin resistance in vivo rely, in one way or another, on measurement of the ability of a fixed dose or concentra-

tion of insulin to promote glucose disposal. Thus a blunted decline in plasma glucose concentration after the administration of intravenous insulin has been demonstrated in type 2 diabetes.[108, 109] Another approach has been to infuse insulin and glucose at fixed rates while endogenous insulin secretion is inhibited either by a combination of epinephrine and propranolol or by somatostatin.[62, 108, 110] With this method, the resulting steady-state plasma glucose level reflects the action of the concomitantly infused insulin; the higher the steady-state plasma glucose, the greater the degree of insulin resistance. Bergman and colleagues' minimal model is yet another method of assessing in vivo insulin resistance.[108] The method entails computer modeling of plasma glucose and insulin levels after an intravenous glucose bolus[108] to generate an index of insulin sensitivity. The test was adapted for type 2 diabetic patients with impaired insulin secretion by giving an injection of insulin 20 minutes after the standard glucose bolus. With all these methods, type 2 diabetic subjects have significantly lower insulin sensitivity than controls do.[5, 108, 110, 111]

Because skeletal muscle is responsible for the great majority of in vivo insulin-stimulated glucose uptake, this tissue must be the major site of the resistance to insulin-stimulated glucose disposal. This conclusion is evidenced by the demonstration of insulin resistance in type 2 diabetic patients during forearm perfusion studies.[112, 113] Leg catheterization studies have shown that skeletal muscle accounts for 80% to 85% of whole body insulin-mediated glucose uptake (IMGU) and that leg skeletal muscle is markedly resistant to insulin's ability to stimulate glucose uptake in type 2 diabetes.[114–116] Thus although other insulin target tissues are insulin resistant in type 2 diabetes, they do not account for a significant proportion of overall glucose uptake, and one can conclude that all measures of in vivo insulin action on glucose disposal have largely assessed the resistance of skeletal muscle in type 2 diabetes to take up glucose under the influence of insulin.

More detailed studies of in vivo insulin resistance have been carried out with the euglycemic glucose clamp method.[108] In this approach, insulin is infused at a constant rate, resulting in a given steady-state plasma insulin level, while plasma glucose is kept constant at a predetermined level by a feedback-controlled variable infusion of glucose. The insulin tends to lower the plasma glucose level, first by suppressing HGO and, second, by stimulating tissue glucose uptake. The amount of glucose that has to be infused to keep plasma glucose constant increases gradually until a steady state is reached. Under these steady-state conditions, the glucose disposal rate provides an excellent quantitative assessment of the biologic effect of a particular steady-state insulin level. If a radioactive or stable isotope of glucose is also infused during the study, HGO during the clamp can also be quantified. In type 2 diabetes, glucose disposal rates are 30% to 60% lower than in matched normal subjects at any given insulin infusion rate, that is, these patients are insulin resistant. If several studies at different insulin levels are performed in a given subject, dose-response curves for insulin-stimulated glucose disposal and suppression of HGO can be constructed. Patients with type 2 diabetes (obese and nonobese) exhibit both a rightward shift in their dose-response curve (diminished sensitivity) and a marked decrease in the maximal rate of glucose disposal[7] (decreased responsiveness) (Fig. 55–7). These changes tend to be more pronounced in obese diabetic patients, particularly at maximal glucose disposal rates (see Fig. 55–7). Obesity per se causes a decrease in insulin sensitivity, and some obese patients show a decrease in insulin responsiveness. However, the insulin resistance of obese type 2 diabetic patients is significantly worse than that of nondiabetic obese subjects. Subjects with IGT tend to have a rightward shift in their dose-response curves with normal maximal glucose disposal rates (see Fig. 55–7).

OXIDATIVE AND NONOXIDATIVE GLUCOSE METABOLISM. By performing indirect calorimetry during glucose clamp studies, one can determine the intracellular fate of glucose by measuring the percentage of glucose that is oxidized in comparison to that which undergoes nonoxidative glucose metabolism (consisting of storage as glycogen plus glycolysis). The insulin concentrations necessary for half-maximal stimulation of glucose oxidation (~50 mU/L in normal subjects) are lower than those required for stimulation of glucose uptake and storage as glycogen (~100 mU/L).[117] Thus at low physiologic insulin levels, oxidative glucose disposal is quantitatively more

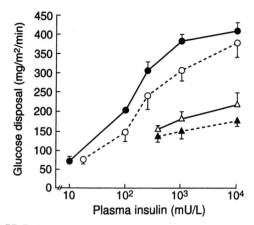

FIGURE 55–7. *Mean insulin dose-response curves for control subjects (closed circles), subjects with impaired glucose tolerance (open circles), and nonobese (open triangles) and obese (closed triangles) type 2 diabetic subjects. The group with impaired glucose tolerance has a rightward shift in the dose-response curve without change in the maximal response (i.e., decreased sensitivity). Lean and obese patients with type 2 diabetes have both a rightward shift and a reduction in the response to a maximally stimulating concentration of insulin (i.e., decreased sensitivity and decreased insulin responsiveness). (From Kolterman OG, Gray RS, Griffin J, et al: Receptor and post-receptor defects contribute to the insulin resistance in non–insulin dependent diabetes mellitus. J Clin Invest 68:957–969, 1981.)*

important, but at higher insulin levels, nonoxidative glucose metabolism predominates.[14, 112] Defects in both oxidative and nonoxidative glucose metabolism exist in type 2 diabetes,[11, 29, 116, 118–122] although the decrease in nonoxidative metabolism is greater. Shulman et al. used nuclear magnetic resonance (NMR) spectroscopy of the gastrocnemius muscle during an infusion of ^{13}C-enriched glucose to show that during a hyperinsulinemic hyperglycemic clamp study, nonoxidative glucose disposal is highly correlated with rates of skeletal muscle glycogen deposition.[11] Moreover, they found a 50% reduction in the rate of muscle glycogen synthesis in type 2 diabetic patients during performance of the glucose clamp technique. The defects in nonoxidative glucose metabolism and muscle glycogen synthesis correlated well with the decrease in whole body glucose uptake.[11]

The reduced muscle glycogen synthesis rate observed in type 2 diabetes could result from a decrease in glucose transport, an impairment in glucose phosphorylation, or an abnormality in the glycogen synthetic pathway. Defects of insulin-stimulated muscle glucose transport in type 2 diabetes are discussed below. Hexokinase II, the predominant isoform in skeletal muscle, phosphorylates incoming glucose to glucose 6-phosphate. Because glucose transport in muscle is by facilitated diffusion, efficient glucose uptake requires that intracellular free glucose be rapidly removed by phosphorylation, thereby maintaining a steep transmembrane glucose gradient. Hexokinase II activity has been found to be decreased in poorly controlled type 2 diabetic patients, and this defect might be expected to contribute to their insulin resistance.[123] Muscle glycogen synthase, which is rate limiting for the synthesis of glycogen from glucose 6-phosphate, is also not activated normally by insulin in type 2 diabetes.[116, 120, 124, 125]

To identify the primary site of the intracellular block in glycogen synthesis, Rothman et al. used ^{31}P-NMR during glucose clamp studies to measure glucose 6-phosphate concentrations in gastrocnemius muscle.[121] They reasoned that a primary block in glycogen synthesis (e.g., resulting from decreased glycogen synthase) would lead to increased glucose 6-phosphate levels, whereas if the decreased flux of glucose to glycogen simply reflected impaired glucose transport and/or phosphorylation, glucose 6-phosphate levels would be low. They found a lower steady-state glucose 6-phosphate concentration in type 2 diabetes, thus indicating that the reduced rate of glycogen synthesis was largely secondary to impaired glucose transport, hexokinase activity, or both. In further muscle NMR studies, these investigators detected a very low intracellular free glucose concentration during hyperinsuli-

nemic hyperglycemic clamp studies in both normal and type 2 diabetic patients.[87] This finding strongly suggests that glucose transport is the rate-controlling step in insulin-stimulated muscle glycogen synthesis in type 2 diabetes. Although these studies do not rule out the possibility that defects in glycogen synthase activation or hexokinase II activity contribute to the impairment in glycogen deposition, they do indicate that decreased insulin-mediated glucose transport is a major contributory defect to the insulin resistance of type 2 diabetes.

FREE FATTY ACIDS, INTRAMYOCELLULAR LIPID, AND INSULIN RESISTANCE. Fasting plasma FFA levels tend to be higher in type 2 diabetic patients than in lean normal subjects, and suppression of FFA levels after meals is impaired.[126, 127] These abnormalities are more pronounced in type 2 diabetic patients with significantly impaired insulin secretion and in obese type 2 diabetic patients.[126–128] Randle et al. showed that glucose and FFAs compete for oxidative metabolism in skeletal muscle and suggested that elevated circulating FFAs may contribute to insulin resistance in type 2 diabetes mellitus and obesity.[70, 129, 130] Studies using the glucose clamp technique have confirmed that elevated FFAs can induce mild insulin resistance.[126, 131–133] Roden et al., using ^{31}P- and ^{13}C-NMR, found that gastrocnemius muscle glucose 6-phosphate levels progressively declined with elevation of plasma FFAs during a hyperinsulinemic euglycemic clamp. This decline preceded the defect in glycogen deposition that developed after about 3 hours.[132] They suggested that increased FFAs produce a progressive inhibition of glucose transport through some mechanism other than that described by Randle, perhaps through the accumulation of long-chain fatty acyl coenzyme A.[134] Recent data support their hypothesis. Thus in rats, Griffin et al. found that FFAs induced a defect at the level of either glucose transport or phosphorylation in association with defects in the insulin signaling pathway, notably, reduced activation of phosphatidylinositol 3-kinase (PI-3-kinase), which is thought to be important for insulin's enhancement of glucose transport.[135] A similar FFA-induced defect in PI-3-kinase activation by FFAs was found in human studies.[133]

Skeletal muscle also uses FFAs from intramuscular triglyceride depots. In nondiabetic subjects, skeletal muscle triglyceride levels vary over a wide range and are inversely related to whole body insulin sensitivity.[136–138] The intramyocyte triglyceride content was found to be a much stronger predictor of insulin sensitivity than was body mass index or percent body fat.[136–138] Muscle triglyceride levels have been found to be markedly increased in type 2 diabetes.[139] Nondiabetic insulin-resistant offspring of type 2 diabetic patients also have a much higher intramyocyte lipid content than do insulin-sensitive offspring matched for age, body mass index, physical activity, and percent body fat.[138, 140]

Cellular Mechanisms of Insulin Resistance

The overall scheme of insulin action represents a multistep sequence in which the binding of insulin to receptors is only the initial event. A defect in any of the effector systems distal to receptor binding can also lead to impaired insulin action and insulin resistance. These defects can involve abnormal coupling between insulin receptor complexes and the glucose transport system, decreased activity of the glucose transport system per se, or a variety of intracellular enzymatic defects located in various pathways of glucose metabolism.

INSULIN RECEPTORS. Because the first step in insulin action involves binding to the receptor, it is apparent that a decrease in cellular insulin receptors could lead to insulin resistance. However, this potential relationship is not as clear as it would seem because in insulin target tissues a maximal insulin effect is achieved at a concentration of insulin in which only a fraction of the surface receptors are occupied. The proportion of "spare" receptors varies with the cell type and the particular action of insulin being studied. For glucose transport in adipocytes and muscle, a maximal response is achieved with only 10% to 20% of the receptors occupied.[141–143] Once this critical number of receptors needed to generate a maximal response is occupied, further increases in the prevailing insulin concentration lead to increasing receptor occupancy with no further increase in biologic response because a step or steps distal to the receptor are now rate limiting. The functional significance is that with fewer cell surface

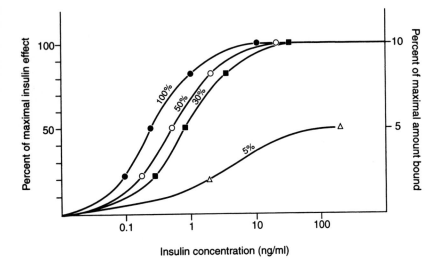

FIGURE 55–8. Predicted functional consequence of a progressive loss of insulin receptors on the insulin biologic function dose-response curve. Results represent theoretic dose-response curves in which the percentage of maximal insulin effect *(left axis)* and the percentage of normal maximal amount bound *(right axis)* are plotted as a function of insulin concentration. With progressive receptor loss, the dose-response curves are increasingly shifted to the right with no change in maximal insulin action, although more insulin is necessary to elicit a maximal insulin response. If enough receptors are lost (95%) so that 5% of the original receptor complement is present, both a rightward shift in the dose-response curve and a decrease in maximal insulin response occur.

receptors, a rightward shift occurs in the insulin biologic function dose-response curve with decreased responses at all submaximal insulin concentrations, but a normal maximal response[143, 144]; the degree of rightward shift is proportional to the decrease in the number of receptors (Fig. 55–8). The only time that a decrease in the number of insulin receptors can lead to a decrease in maximal insulin action is when less than 10% to 30% of the original receptor complement is present (see Fig. 55–8). Because a reduction below 10% to 30% of the normal complement is unlikely, a reduced maximal insulin response generally denotes the presence of a postbinding abnormality. In this context the term *postbinding defect* includes abnormalities of insulin receptor function that affect its transmembrane signaling function such as its kinase activity. A postreceptor defect refers to any abnormality in a step distal to the insulin receptor.

The most common type of postbinding defect leads to a proportional decrease in insulin action at all insulin concentrations, including maximally effective hormone levels.[144, 145] Thus a decrease in the capacity of a rate-limiting step in the insulin action–glucose metabolism scheme leads to a reduction in the maximal absolute insulin effect, and this defect cannot be overcome by the addition of more insulin. In other, less common situations, a postbinding defect can lead to impaired coupling between insulin receptor complexes and subsequent biologic responses and result in a rightward shift in the insulin dose-response curve with or without a decrease in the maximal response. One can readily distinguish between a rightward-shifted curve caused by a binding defect and a postreceptor (i.e., postbinding) defect by concomitant measurement of insulin binding. If insulin binding is normal, the right-shifted curve is due to a postbinding defect; if insulin binding is decreased in proportion to the rightward shift, the shift is most likely due to the binding defect.

Early studies showed decreased insulin binding to circulating monocytes from obese and IGT subjects and from both obese and nonobese type 2 diabetic patients.[146–149] This decreased binding was due to a decrease in insulin receptor number with no change in affinity. Similar results were subsequently obtained when isolated adipocytes or skeletal muscle tissue from obese subjects and patients with type 2 diabetes was used[150–152] (Fig. 55–9). The decrease in cellular insulin receptors in obesity and type 2 diabetes may well be secondary to hyperinsulinemia inasmuch as circulating insulin levels are a major determinant of receptor number. Increased insulin levels lead to receptor downregulation.[142, 149] Conversely, low insulin levels, as in animal models of insulin-deficient diabetes, may lead to receptor upregulation.[153] Although insulin receptors are usually decreased in type 2 diabetes, in a few patients receptor levels have been found to be normal[154, 155] when compared with weight-matched controls. These patients may have relatively poor residual insulin secretion and low plasma insulin levels. Hyperinsulinemia is a likely explanation for the decrease in cellular insulin receptors found in acromegaly,[156] after glucocorticoid therapy,[157] after oral contraceptive therapy,[158] and in several other less common insulin-resistant conditions.[159, 160]

In IGT, the insulin resistance is characterized by decreased insulin sensitivity (i.e., a rightward shift in the insulin biologic function dose-response curve), and the decrease in insulin receptors is a likely contributory factor to this defect. On the other hand, in patients with significant fasting hyperglycemia, decreased insulin binding and a postbinding defect in insulin action exist together, which leads to both decreased insulin sensitivity and decreased insulin responsiveness (i.e., both a rightward shift in the insulin dose-response curve and a decrease in the maximal response). In patients with significant fasting hyperglycemia, the postbinding defect and decreased insulin responsiveness are the predominant abnormalities.

INSULIN RECEPTOR FUNCTION. Several groups have measured tyrosine kinase activity in partially purified insulin receptors from the liver, adipocytes, and skeletal muscle of patients with type 2 diabetes to determine whether a defect at this postbinding site may

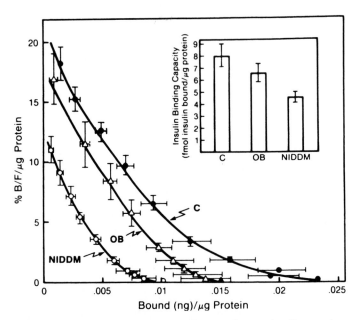

FIGURE 55–9. *Main panel,* Insulin binding to adipocyte insulin receptors in control *(closed circles),* obese *(open triangles),* and type 2 diabetic (non–insulin-dependent diabetes mellitus [NIDDM]) subjects *(open circles).* Scatchard plots of the insulin-binding data are plotted as the mean (±SEM) of the binding data (percent bound/free [B/F] insulin per microgram protein) at each concentration of added insulin. *Inset,* Total insulin-binding capacities determined by estimation of the apparent *x*-intercept of individual Scatchard plots drawn for each subject. (From Freidenberg GR, Henry RR, Klein HH, et al: Decreased kinase activity of insulin receptors from adipocytes of non–insulin dependent diabetic subjects. J Clin Invest 79:240–250, 1987.)

account for at least some of the insulin resistance. Findings have generally been consistent, with a reduction in insulin receptor kinase activity in type 2 diabetic patients but normal kinase activity in insulin-resistant obese subjects with normal glucose tolerance and in subjects with IGT[84, 150, 152, 161, 162] (Fig. 55–10). Thus the receptor autophosphorylation/kinase defect appears to be generalized to all insulin target tissues and relatively specific for the hyperglycemic insulin-resistant state seen in type 2 diabetes. Further studies have demonstrated that this kinase defect is associated with an increased proportion of receptors that are kinase inactive.[151, 162]

Because type 2 diabetes has a strong genetic component and because receptor function is deranged in this disease, it is important to ask whether genetic variations in the insulin receptor are a primary causative factor accounting for type 2 diabetes. In other words, is the insulin receptor gene a diabetes gene? Several lines of evidence argue strongly that the answer is no.[150, 163–165] First, when obese type 2

diabetic patients are induced to lose weight, the hyperglycemia is markedly improved and insulin receptor kinase function reverts to normal.[150] Second, when fibroblasts are propagated in tissue culture so that they are several generations removed from the in vivo milieu, insulin receptor kinase activity in fibroblasts derived from type 2 diabetic subjects is normal.[163] Third and perhaps most compelling are the results of direct studies analyzing the insulin receptor gene in type 2 diabetes. Figure 55–11 depicts the gene structure for the insulin receptor, as first identified by Seino and colleagues.[166] Since it was cloned, more than 50 mutations have been found, mostly in patients with rare syndromes of extreme insulin resistance. Most of these patients have homozygous or compound heterozygous mutations, although heterozygous mutations in the tyrosine kinase domain can produce severe insulin resistance. In analyzing this gene in "garden-variety" type 2 diabetes, however, direct sequencing studies in small groups of patients have not revealed abnormalities in the coding sequence of the insulin receptor gene.[164, 167] Other studies using molecular scanning approaches to screen larger numbers of patients for mutations have revealed that the degree of genetic variation in the insulin receptor is exceedingly small in type 2 diabetes, on the order of 1% to 2%.[165] Whether the few mutations that have been identified in insulin receptor genes from type 2 diabetic patients are functionally significant or whether they exceed the prevalence of these mutations in the normal population is not clear, but one can readily conclude from the aggregate of these studies[164, 165, 167] that the overwhelming majority (98%–99%) of type 2 diabetic subjects do not carry mutations in the insulin receptor gene. Thus the coding region for the insulin receptor does not appear to be a diabetes gene.

GLUCOSE TRANSPORT SYSTEM. The in vivo impairment of tissue glucose disposal in type 2 diabetes is associated with defects in insulin-stimulated glucose transport in skeletal muscle[87, 101, 104, 168] and adipocytes.[12, 169] Figure 55–12 shows the results of glucose transport studies in adipocytes isolated from normal, IGT, and type 2 diabetic patients.[12] The results are strikingly similar to the in vivo glucose clamp studies (see Fig. 55–7) and show a large decrease in insulin-stimulated glucose transport at all insulin concentrations in the type 2 diabetic groups. The few studies that have been conducted on muscle fiber strips from type 2 diabetic and normal subjects corroborate the findings in adipocytes[168, 170] (Fig. 55–13). As in the adipocyte studies, insulin-stimulated glucose transport in isolated muscle fiber strips correlated with whole body insulin sensitivity in normal and type 2 diabetic subjects.[168]

What is the mechanism of this decrease in insulin-stimulated glucose transport in type 2 diabetes? In adipocytes from obese subjects, levels of the insulin-regulated glucose transporter GLUT4 were found to be lower than those in lean subjects, and this decrease was exacerbated in obese patients with type 2 diabetes.[171] This depletion of GLUT4 affected both the intracellular pool and the GLUT4 content of the plasma membrane and was sufficient to explain the reduction in basal and insulin-stimulated glucose transport in adipocytes from type 2 diabetic patients. In contrast to the depletion of GLUT4 in adipocytes, skeletal muscle GLUT4 mRNA and protein levels are normal in type 2 diabetes.[172–174] Because the muscle of type 2 diabetic patients is not deficient in GLUT4 protein, we must postulate that the defect in insulin-stimulated glucose transport reflects either a decrease in the ability of insulin to signal recruitment, or translocation, of GLUT4 to the cell surface or a decrease in the intrinsic activity of GLUT4.

Evidence that insulin-stimulated translocation of GLUT4 is impaired in the skeletal muscle of type 2 diabetic patients comes from the study of Kelley et al.[104] These investigators used quantitative confocal laser scanning microscopy to study insulin-stimulated recruitment of GLUT4 to the sarcolemma in muscle biopsies from patients with type 2 diabetes. In the basal state, sarcolemmal GLUT4 labeling was similar in type 2 diabetic and normal subjects, but in response to a 3-hour hyperinsulinemic euglycemic clamp (plasma insulin, ~500–600 pmol/L), the increase in sarcolemmal GLUT4 labeling in type 2 diabetic subjects was only 25% of that in control subjects. A quantitatively similar defect in GLUT4 translocation was found in obese nondiabetic subjects. In both the type 2 diabetic patients and obese nondiabetic subjects, the defect in GLUT4 translocation was associated with a marked impairment in insulin-stimulated muscle glucose transport as

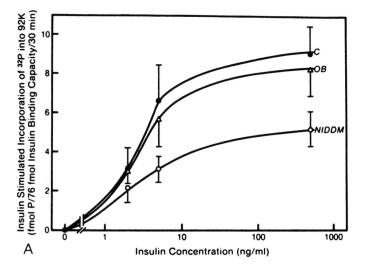

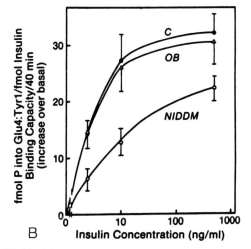

FIGURE 55–10. *A,* Insulin dose-response curve for autophosphorylation. Aliquots of receptor preparations were preincubated with 0, 2, 5, or 500 ng/mL insulin, after which autokinase reactions were incubated for 30 minutes at 4°C. The results are graphed as the mean (±SEM) increase over basal from 10 control (C, *solid circles*), 13 obese (OB, *open triangles*), and 13 type 2 diabetic (non–insulin-dependent diabetes mellitus [NIDDM]) *(open circles)* subjects. *B,* Insulin-stimulated phosphorylation of Glu4:Tyr1 by receptors from control, obese, and type 2 diabetic subjects. Insulin receptors were preincubated with 0, 2.5, 10, or 500 ng/mL unlabeled insulin in the absence or presence of 0.5 ng/mL ^{125}I-insulin. Insulin binding and Glu4:Tyr1 phosphorylation were then determined. (From Freidenberg GR, Henry RR, Klein HH, et al: Decreased kinase activity of insulin receptors from adipocytes of non–insulin-dependent diabetic subjects. J Clin Invest 79:240–250, 1987.)

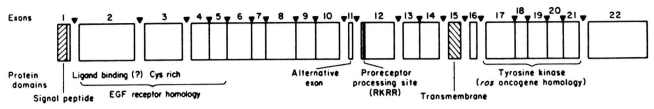

FIGURE 55–11. Insulin receptor gene intron/exon structure depicting 22 exons, their intronic boundaries, and corresponding encoded regions of the insulin receptor. (From Seino S, Seino M, Nishi S, Bell GI: Structure of the human insulin receptor gene and characterization of its promoter. Proc Natl Acad Sci U S A 86:114–118, 1989.)

determined by positron emission tomography. Others using biochemical muscle subfractionation techniques have also suggested a defect in GLUT4 translocation in patients with type 2 diabetes.[105]

When one considers the possibility of a defect in GLUT4 intrinsic activity, one must think about a structural defect in the protein itself. Such an abnormality could be due to genetic variation in the GLUT4 sequence. To approach this problem, the entire coding region of the GLUT4 gene was sequenced in seven typical insulin-resistant type 2 diabetic subjects.[164] In six of the patients, no change in the amino acid sequence was observed. Two were heterozygous for a silent polymorphism at nucleotide position 535, but this polymorphism is also common in nondiabetic subjects.[175, 176] One of the seven patients was heterozygous for an A-for-T substitution at nucleotide position 1292. This substitution led to an isoleucine-for-valine substitution at codon 383 in the fifth extracellular loop of the GLUT4 protein, according to its proposed topologic organization within the plasma membrane (see Chapter 50). Larger-scale molecular scanning studies indicated that this mutation exists in only a small percentage of type 2 diabetic subjects (1%–2%); it also exists at low frequency in nondiabetic subjects.[175, 176] The functional significance—if any—of this mutation at the protein level has not been elucidated. One can conclude from these studies[164, 175, 176] that genetic variations in the GLUT4 sequence are exceedingly uncommon (less than 1%–2%) in type 2 diabetic subjects. Consequently, although defects in glucose transport are important to the pathophysiology of type 2 diabetes, the coding sequence of GLUT4 does not appear to be a diabetes gene locus.

Trafficking of GLUT4 involves a complex system analogous to synaptic vesicle movement, and an expanding list of proteins involved

in the GLUT4 vesicular compartmentation and regulation of membrane fusion and endocytotic events are being identified.[106] Clearly, impaired GLUT4 translocation in type 2 diabetes could be due to altered expression or a functional defect of one or more of these GLUT4 vesicle-trafficking proteins, which is an area of intensive investigation.

TRANSMEMBRANE SIGNALING. Let us next examine potential signaling events that link the insulin receptor to glucose transport stimulation. A variety of postreceptor signaling systems and mediators have been studied with respect to insulin action, but one of the most intensively investigated mechanisms involves tyrosine phosphorylation. After insulin binding and receptor autophosphorylation, a number of endogenous protein substrates undergo tyrosine phosphorylation in different cell systems. The most thoroughly studied of these substrates is IRS-1, which as discussed earlier, operates as a multisite docking protein that associates with the insulin receptor and becomes tyrosine phosphorylated.[95, 96, 177, 178] IRS-1 becomes phosphorylated at several YMXM motifs, which themselves serve as binding sites for SH2 domain–containing proteins. In this way, putative effector SH2-containing proteins such as PI-3-kinase bind to phosphorylated IRS-1.[95, 96]

The ability of insulin to stimulate IRS-1 phosphorylation was assessed in adipocytes from control, obese, and type 2 diabetic subjects.[179] The insulin dose-response curves for stimulation of tyrosine phosphorylation of the insulin receptor β subunit and for stimulation of IRS-1 (formerly referred to as pp185) in human adipocytes is

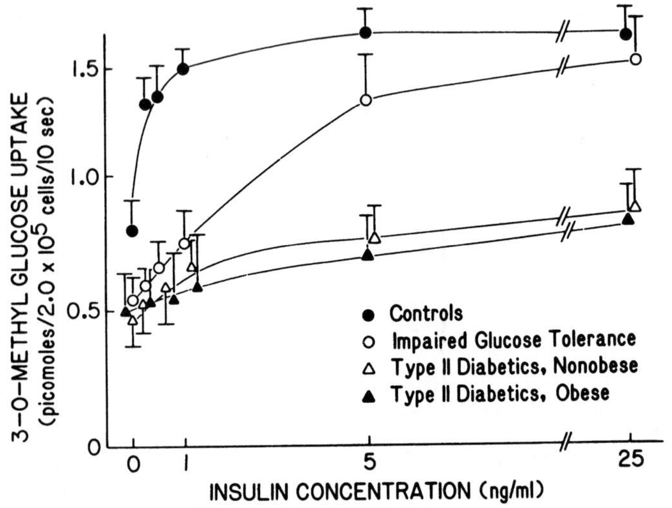

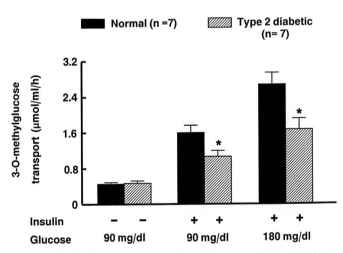

FIGURE 55–12. Dose-response curve for insulin's ability to stimulate glucose transport (3-O-methylglucose uptake) in isolated adipocytes prepared from normal individuals, patients with impaired glucose tolerance, and obese and nonobese subjects with type 2 diabetes. The functional form of these dose-response curves is quite comparable to the shape of the dose-response curves for in vivo insulin-stimulated overall glucose disposal. (From Ciaraldi TP, Kolterman OG, Scarlett JA, et al: Role of the glucose transport system in the post-receptor defect of non–insulin dependent diabetes mellitus. Diabetes 31:1016–1022, 1982.)

FIGURE 55–13. Basal and insulin-stimulated rates of 3-O-methylglucose transport in skeletal muscle strips obtained from the vastus lateralis muscle of seven normal control and seven type 2 diabetic subjects. Muscle strips were first incubated for 30 minutes under basal conditions (no insulin, 90 mg/dL glucose) or insulin-stimulated (600 pmol/L) conditions (at glucose concentrations of either 90 or 180 mg/dL). After the muscle strips were briefly washed in glucose-free media, 3-O-methylglucose transport was measured at concentrations of 3-O-methylglucose corresponding to the previous glucose concentration (90 or 180 mg/dL). The concentration of insulin was maintained throughout the different incubations. Values are means ± SEM. *P < .05 vs. the rate of glucose transport in the skeletal muscle strips from normal subjects under the same conditions. (From Zierath JR, He L, Guma A, et al: Insulin action on glucose transport and plasma membrane Glut4 content in skeletal muscle from patients with NIDDM. Diabetologia 39:1180–1189, 1996.)

seen in Figure 55–14. The curves for autophosphorylation and IRS-1 phosphorylation are nearly superimposable, consistent with the idea that IRS-1 is an immediate substrate of the phosphorylated insulin receptor β subunit. Interestingly, when these curves are compared with the dose-response curve for insulin-stimulated glucose transport in these same cells, one can see that the glucose transport curve is shifted to the left when compared with autophosphorylation and IRS-1 phosphorylation. This contrast illustrates the concept of spare kinase activity; in other words, 50% of glucose transport stimulation is reached at an insulin concentration that activates only a small proportion (less than 10%) of the available kinase activity, whereas maximal transport stimulation is observed when approximately 30% of the kinase is stimulated. When data from the various patient study groups were analyzed, decreased insulin-stimulated β subunit autophosphorylation was found to exist in type 2 diabetes, but the ability of phosphorylated insulin receptors to phosphorylate IRS-1 was normal. Because coupling between autophosphorylated β subunits and IRS-1 is normal in type 2 diabetes whereas the amount of autophosphorylated β subunit is decreased, it is evident that the total amount of phosphorylated IRS-1 is decreased in cells from type 2 diabetic patients. When estimated on a per-cell basis (Fig. 55–15), the striking decrease in phosphorylated IRS-1 content after insulin stimulation in cells from type 2 diabetic subjects is quite apparent. A similar defect in IRS-1 phosphorylation on tyrosine residues in response to insulin is found in skeletal muscle from type 2 diabetic patients.[180] Rondinone et al. found that IRS-1 protein was reduced by 70% in adipose tissue from type 2 diabetic patients,[181] and this reduction could clearly contribute to the decrease in IRS-1 phosphorylation observed in earlier studies.[179] However, reduced IRS-1 content cannot be a factor in muscle because skeletal muscle IRS-1 expression is not different between type 2 diabetic patients and lean or obese normal subjects.[180, 182]

A number of polymorphisms have been identified in the IRS-1 gene,[96] and these polymorphisms appear to be more common in type 2 diabetes in some populations. The most common is G972R (glycine → arginine), which in a Danish study was found in 5.8% of normal subjects and in 10.7% of type 2 diabetic patients.[183] In a French study, however, the frequency of this variant was not increased in diabetic patients,[184] and it is not found in Pima Indians.[96] Interestingly, the G972R polymorphism lies between two potential tyrosine phosphorylation sites involved in binding PI-3-kinase. When this IRS-1 variant was expressed in cells in vitro, it caused a specific defect in the binding of PI-3-kinase to IRS-1 and a 36% decrease in the PI-3-kinase activity associated with IRS-1.[96] In Japanese type 2 diabetic patients, several polymorphisms have been identified that were found to be associated with a reduction in insulin sensitivity as measured by the glucose clamp technique. In aggregate, these polymorphisms were found three times more commonly in diabetic patients than in healthy

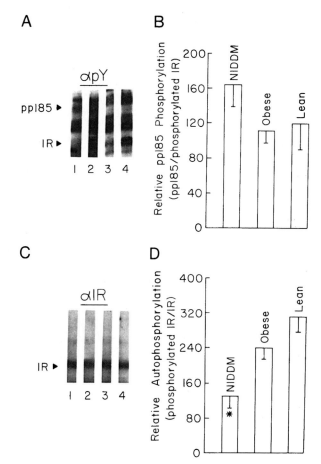

FIGURE 55–15. Insulin-stimulated phosphorylation of insulin receptor (IR) and pp185 (insulin receptor substrate-1 [IRS-1]) in adipocytes from type 2 diabetic (non–insulin-dependent diabetes mellitus [NIDDM]), obese, and lean subjects. *A,* Representative autoradiograph. Adipocytes from NIDDM (lanes 1 and 2) and obese (lanes 3 and 4) subjects incubated with (lanes 2 and 4) and without (lanes 1 and 3) insulin were solubilized and immunoblotted with antiphosphotyrosine antibody. *B,* To estimate coupling efficiency between insulin receptor activation and pp185 phosphorylation, autoradiographs of antiphosphotyrosine immunoblots from cells treated with 10 ng/mL insulin for 5 minutes were subjected to scanning densitometry, and the ratio of phosphorylated pp185 to phosphorylated insulin receptor β subunit was expressed as relative densitometry units. No statistically significant difference was found between cells from NIDDM (*n* = 8), obese (*n* = 8), or lean (*n* = 3) subjects in efficiency of pp185 phosphorylation. *C,* Representative autoradiograph. Cells from NIDDM (lanes 1 and 2), obese (lane 3), and lean (lane 4) subjects incubated with (lanes 2–4) and without (lane 1) insulin were solubilized and immunoblotted with anti–insulin receptor antibody. *D,* To estimate the efficiency of insulin receptor autophosphorylation, the ratio of phosphorylated β subunit from antiphosphotyrosine immunoblots to total β subunit in gel lanes from anti–insulin receptor immunoblots is expressed as relative densitometry units. Insulin-stimulated receptor autophosphorylation is significantly lower (*P* < .02) in cells from NIDDM subjects than cells from obese or lean nondiabetic subjects. (From Thies RS, Molina JM, Ciaraldi TP, et al: Insulin receptor autophosphorylation and endogenous substrate phosphorylation in human adipocytes from control, obese, and non–insulin dependent diabetic subjects. Diabetes 39:250–259, 1990.)

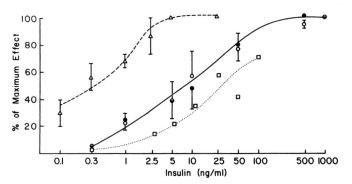

FIGURE 55–14. Dose response of insulin-stimulated 3-*O*-methylglucose transport, substrate phosphorylation, and insulin receptor binding at 37°C. *Closed circles,* insulin receptor phosphorylation; *open circles,* pp185 (insulin receptor substrate-1 [IRS-1]) phosphorylation; *open boxes,* insulin binding; *open triangles,* 3-*O*-methylglucose transport. (From Thies RS, Molina JM, Ciaraldi TP, et al: Insulin receptor autophosphorylation and endogenous substrate phosphorylation in human adipocytes from control, obese, and non–insulin dependent diabetic subjects. Diabetes 39:250–259, 1990.)

controls.[96] Although further studies are needed to assess the significance of these IRS-1 variants, they could potentially contribute to the genetic basis of insulin resistance in some type 2 diabetic patients.

GLYCOGEN SYNTHESIS. Glycogen synthase, the rate-controlling enzyme for glycogen synthesis, is another site for a cellular defect in type 2 diabetes. Glycogen synthase activity has been measured in muscle biopsy samples from type 2 diabetic subjects, and decreased enzyme activity has been consistently observed.[116, 120, 124, 125] The decrease in enzyme activity correlates with the magnitude of the decrease in nonoxidative glucose disposal as measured by indirect calorimetry during glucose clamp studies. Thus diminished activation of glycogen synthase, decreased muscle glycogen synthesis, impaired insulin-mediated glucose disposal, and defective nonoxidative glucose disposal all exist in type 2 diabetic subjects.

In light of the cellular defect in glycogen synthase described above, this gene is a potential candidate "diabetes gene." However, as was the case for the insulin receptor and GLUT4, molecular analysis of the glycogen synthase gene in type 2 diabetes has not yielded positive results. Thus analysis of the entire coding sequence of this gene failed to detect any sequence variations in eight type 2 diabetic patients.[185] In these same patients a decrease in glycogen synthase activity was observed and correlated with a decrease in mRNA levels. Thus although no genetic alteration has been detected in the coding region of the glycogen synthase gene, abnormal regulation of this enzyme clearly exists in type 2 diabetes. Whether genetic variation in the gene regulatory sequences exists in type 2 diabetes remains to be determined.

HEPATIC GLUCOSE METABOLISM

The liver plays a key role in carbohydrate metabolism. It is capable of extracting glucose from the portal vein and hepatic artery, as well as releasing glucose derived from glycogenolysis or gluconeogenesis into the hepatic vein.

Hepatic Glucose Production

After an overnight fast, normal basal glucose production rates are 1.8 to 2.2 mg/kg/min, with about 90% of the glucose released into the circulation at this time coming from the liver. After glucose ingestion, HGO must be promptly suppressed to limit the rise in plasma glucose levels; as intestinal glucose delivery wanes, basal HGO rates must be restored to meet the obligatory glucose needs of tissues such as the brain. These changes in HGO are largely mediated by changes in insulin and other hormones that antagonize insulin's effects on the liver, by alterations in gluconeogenic substrate supply, and by glucose autoregulation of HGO.

The rate of basal HGO is increased in both obese and nonobese type 2 diabetic patients,[7-9, 13, 14] but not in subjects with IGT (Fig. 55–16A). The fasting plasma glucose level and basal HGO are closely correlated in type 2 diabetic patients (Fig. 55–16B), which indicates that the rate of glucose production by the liver directly modulates the level of fasting hyperglycemia in type 2 diabetes. Early studies using hepatic vein catheterization techniques to calculate net splanchnic uptake of gluconeogenic precursors (lactate, alanine, and glycerol) estimated that after an overnight fast, 70% to 75% of the glucose produced by the liver came from liver glycogen, the rest from gluconeogenesis.[186] More recent studies using ^{13}C-NMR suggest that about two-thirds of HGO during the first 22 hours of fasting is derived from gluconeogenesis.[187] Most studies suggest that gluconeogenesis is increased in type 2 diabetes.[188, 189] Thus enhanced gluconeogenesis is the proximate cause of increased HGO in type 2 diabetes, and although the mechanism is unclear, it is probably a multifactorial defect. Glucagon levels are elevated in type 2 diabetes, and the effect of glucagon to stimulate the synthesis and release of glucose by the liver is well known. Hyperglycemia normally exerts a potent suppressive effect on α cell glucagon secretion, and the presence of hyperglucagonemia in the face of hyperglycemia implies that pancreatic α cells in type 2 diabetes are resistant to the inhibitory effects of glucose. Insulin also normally suppresses glucagon secretion, thus reflecting an intraislet paracrine function of β cell insulin secretion inhibiting β cell glucagon release.[190] Conceivably, this action of insulin is also impaired in type 2 diabetes. Other factors are possible, but regardless of the mechanisms, increased α cell function in type 2 diabetes is an important and consistent abnormality; suppression of plasma glucagon levels by infusion of somatostatin lowers plasma glucose levels in both normal and type 2 diabetic subjects.[191]

Hepatic glucose production can be completely suppressed by high

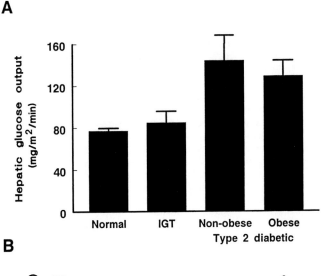

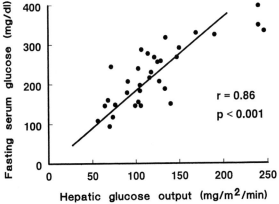

FIGURE 55–16. *A,* Rates of hepatic glucose production in the basal state (7 to 9 AM after an overnight fast) in normal subjects, subjects with impaired glucose tolerance (IGT), and obese or nonobese subjects with type 2 diabetes. Hepatic glucose output is normal in subjects with IGT but is markedly increased in type 2 diabetes. *B,* Relationship between the individual hepatic glucose production rate and fasting plasma glucose level in type 2 diabetic subjects. (From Kolterman OG, Gray RS, Griffin J, et al: Receptor and post-receptor defects contribute to the insulin resistance in non–insulin dependent diabetes mellitus. J Clin Invest 68:957–969, 1981.)

physiologic or supraphysiologic insulin levels in type 2 diabetes, but the sensitivity of HGO to lower concentrations of insulin is reduced.[14] This reduced sensitivity probably also contributes to the overall increase in glucose production in these patients. Insulin's ability to suppress HGO may in part be indirect[83, 192] and mediated by suppression of adipose tissue lipolysis and plasma FFA levels.[192] Thus the insulin resistance of HGO suppression in type 2 diabetes may in part be secondary to impaired suppression of plasma FFA levels by insulin.[14, 126–128]

Finally, increased flux of gluconeogenic precursors and FFAs from peripheral tissues to the liver may participate in the maintenance of increased HGO rates in type 2 diabetes. Alanine, lactate, and glycerol production rates are increased in type 2 diabetes with fasting hyperglycemia, and the increased plasma lactate and glycerol levels would be expected to promote gluconeogenesis. Plasma alanine levels are usually normal in type 2 diabetes despite increased entry of alanine into the circulation,[189] which suggests that the liver is taking up more alanine for glucose synthesis. Increased glucagon levels in type 2 diabetes would explain the increased hepatic extraction of alanine.[189] In obese type 2 diabetic patients, increased plasma FFA levels may also stimulate gluconeogenesis[126] and contribute to higher rates of HGO.

The substrate-induced increase in HGO could be at least partly related to differences in intracellular disposition of glucose in peripheral tissues in normal vs. insulin-resistant type 2 diabetic subjects. For example, in the basal state, the rate of glucose appearance (Ra) is increased in type 2 diabetic patients with fasting hyperglycemia because of increased HGO, and under the nearly steady-state conditions that exist in the basal state, the rate of glucose disappearance (Rd) is also elevated. When basal tissue glucose utilization rates are enhanced by hyperglycemia in diabetes, the proportion of glucose metabolized by glycolysis to lactate and pyruvate tends to be increased.[193] Some of the pyruvate yields alanine by transamination. Increased release of these three-carbon compounds from peripheral and splanchnic tissues provides the substrate for the enhanced rates of gluconeogenesis and HGO.

Hepatic Glucose Uptake

Although earlier data held that most of the orally ingested glucose was extracted by the liver and largely converted to glycogen,[194] more recent studies indicate that skeletal muscle is quantitatively the most important tissue for disposal of an oral glucose load, with 50% to 60% of total glucose disposal accounted for by skeletal muscle. Only 20% to 35% of oral glucose is directly taken up (as glucose) by the liver, and even less (about 10%) of the glucose absorbed from the gut is taken up on the first pass.[195] The contribution of the liver to total postprandial glucose disposal must take into account the extent of suppression of HGO in addition to the glucose taken up. Thus over a 3-hour period, 50% to 60% suppression of HGO is equivalent to a further net uptake of about 10 to 15 g of glucose. Nonetheless, incorporation into liver glycogen is not the main fate of ingested glucose. Taylor et al., using ^{13}C-NMR spectroscopy to quantitate liver glycogen in normal subjects, found that only 19% of the carbohydrate content of a liquid meal consumed after an overnight fast was incorporated into liver glycogen.[196] Moreover, a large proportion of the liver glycogen synthesized is not derived directly from glucose, but from three-carbon intermediates derived from the metabolism of ingested glucose in peripheral and extrahepatic splanchnic tissues.[196–198]

In contrast to insulin's direct stimulation of muscle glucose uptake and incorporation into glycogen, insulin plays a permissive role in promoting hepatic glucose uptake. Thus insulin does not cause net hepatic glucose uptake or stimulation of liver glycogen deposition without an increased portal venous glucose concentration. The main determinant of glucose transport into and out of the liver is the glucose concentration gradient between sinusoids and hepatocytes.[199, 200] After glucose ingestion, uptake of glucose by the liver (newly absorbed and recirculating) is impaired in type 2 diabetes.[193, 201]

In summary, inhibition of glucose production and release is the major effect of insulin on hepatic glucose balance. In type 2 diabetes the liver overproduces glucose in the basal state, primarily because of increased gluconeogenesis, and the metabolic milieu is ideal to sustain this abnormality. Exaggerated hormonal stimulation is provided by the increased glucagon levels (in combination with hepatic insulin resistance), and augmented gluconeogenic precursor flow ensures adequate substrate availability. Finally, elevated FFA levels could augment the gluconeogenic process.

INSULIN-MEDIATED VS. NON–INSULIN-MEDIATED GLUCOSE UPTAKE

Under basal conditions, a nearly steady state is approximated and the rate of glucose appearance (HGO) equals the overall rate of glucose disposal. To understand the significance of increased basal HGO in type 2 diabetes, it is important to distinguish between insulin-dependent and insulin-independent processes of glucose disposal. By definition, IMGU occurs in insulin target tissues under the influence of insulin. Non–insulin-mediated glucose uptake (NIMGU) consists of all the body's glucose uptake not under the influence of insulin and has two components. NIMGU occurs in tissues (primarily the central nervous system) that are not targets for insulin action; it also involves insulin target cells and comprises the basal rate (non–insulin mediated)

of glucose disposal by these tissues. Total glucose disposal (Rd) equals the sum of NIMGU and IMGU. NIMGU can be assessed in vivo by measuring Rd under conditions of severe insulinopenia induced by an infusion of somatostatin.[202] Thus after measurement of basal Rd (at basal or fasting insulin and glucose levels), somatostatin is administered to inhibit insulin secretion to negligible levels. Rd gradually falls to a new steady state that equals NIMGU because insulin action is absent under these conditions.[202] With this approach, the proportion of basal Rd that is NIMGU is approximately two-thirds in normal individuals at euglycemia and in type 2 diabetic subjects studied at their basal level of hyperglycemia, which means that at all levels of basal glycemia (normal and diabetes), most of the glucose is disposed of by NIMGU mechanisms and the elevated rates of basal HGO that prevail in type 2 diabetes are associated with increased rates of NIMGU.

PATHOPHYSIOLOGY OF FASTING VS. POSTPRANDIAL HYPERGLYCEMIA

Once type 2 diabetes develops, all three metabolic defects contribute to fasting hyperglycemia, but increased HGO predominates. This conclusion derives from the known physiology of glucose homeostasis in the basal state. Thus in the postabsorptive and fasting states, insulin levels are low, and approximately 70% of basal glucose uptake (Rd) is non–insulin mediated in both normal and hyperglycemic type 2 diabetic subjects.[202] Because skeletal muscle, the main tissue affected by insulin resistance in type 2 diabetes, accounts for only 15% to 20% of basal glucose Rd, it follows that an impairment in insulin-mediated glucose uptake by muscle will have little effect on overall basal glucose Rd or fasting plasma glucose levels. Major increases in fasting glucose levels do not occur unless the rate of glucose entry into the systemic circulation (Ra) increases, and in the basal state, glucose Ra essentially equals hepatic glucose production. In type 2 diabetes, increases in glucose Ra readily lead to increases in fasting glucose levels because in the setting of peripheral insulin resistance and impaired insulin secretion, the ability of IMGU to rise and accommodate an increase in Ra is severely curtailed. To illustrate, if basal Ra = Rd = 2 mg/kg/min at euglycemia and basal NIMGU = 1.4 mg/kg/min (70%) with a basal IMGU of 0.6 mg/kg/min (30%), a modest increase in HGO to 2.6 mg/kg/min would require a doubling of IMGU (to 1.2 mg/kg/min) to maintain Rd = Ra (HGO) at euglycemia. Because type 2 diabetic subjects are insensitive to insulin, a much larger increase in insulin secretion would be necessary to produce euglycemia than in normal individuals. Because insulin secretion is impaired in type 2 diabetes, the ability of a type 2 diabetic subject to increase IMGU in response to a rise in Ra is greatly restricted. To raise Rd to the level of the new Ra and bring the system back into balance, the fasting glucose level must rise until Rd increases by mass action and equals Ra. This line of reasoning is strongly supported by the available data, which demonstrate close direct relationships between fasting plasma glucose levels and basal HGO in large groups of type 2 diabetic subjects under a variety of conditions.[9] Thus decreased insulin secretion and action provide the setting that allows glucose Ra to regulate fasting plasma glucose, thereby leading to the principle that fasting hyperglycemia is largely due to increased HGO in type 2 diabetes.

The cause of postprandial hyperglycemia, however, is more complex. Recent data show that most of the ingested carbohydrate (80% to 90%) bypasses the liver and enters the peripheral circulation.[195] This process is accompanied by rapid suppression (60%–90%) of HGO for 2 to 3 hours after carbohydrate ingestion.[193, 195, 196] Thus in the postprandial state, glucose Ra comes predominantly from ingested carbohydrate, and this ingested carbohydrate largely enters the peripheral circulation, where it is disposed of mostly by skeletal muscle because of a severalfold increase in IMGU. In type 2 diabetes, systemic delivery of ingested glucose appears to be normal, but suppression of HGO is impaired as a result of insulin resistance and impaired insulin secretion,[193] which means that after glucose ingestion the total quantity of glucose entering the systemic circulation is somewhat higher. In addition, the efficiency of peripheral glucose removal is greatly reduced because of insulin resistance and impaired insulin secretion. Uptake of glucose by the liver (newly absorbed and recirculating) is also impaired in type 2 diabetes,[193, 201] but the overall contribution of impaired hepatic uptake to postprandial hyperglycemia is relatively small because the liver takes up only 20% to 35% of a glucose load.[193, 195] Thus postprandial hyperglycemia in type 2 diabetes is primarily due to impaired IMGU by peripheral tissues, with impaired suppression of HGO compounding the problem. Postprandial glucose levels rise markedly in type 2 diabetes until the mass action effect of glucose to raise Rd allows disposal of the incoming glucose load. Although glycosuria increases with hyperglycemia, the contribution of glycosuria to total Rd is small (less than 10%) and therefore does not significantly affect relationships between the aforementioned variables.

In summary, in the basal state NIMGU predominates, and decreased IMGU raises fasting glucose levels only modestly. Fasting hyperglycemia is primarily due to increased HGO. In the postprandial state, IMGU normally predominates and the limited ability of type 2 diabetic subjects to increase IMGU allows the marked postprandial glucose excursions. The clinical implications of this understanding of the pathophysiology of fasting vs. postprandial hyperglycemia are obvious. Any form of antidiabetic therapy must address both aspects of hyperglycemia to be fully effective, which means that a given treatment modality must correct the disordered hepatic glucose metabolism at the same time that it improves insulin-mediated skeletal muscle glucose uptake. This principle is true for single modes of therapy (insulin, oral agents, weight loss) or various combination forms of treatment. For example, a treatment modality that lowers HGO combined with one that enhances IMGU would be an effective overall management strategy for controlling glycemia in type 2 diabetes.

EFFECTS OF ANTIDIABETIC TREATMENT

Obviously, when type 2 diabetic patients are studied at a single static point in time, abnormalities in hepatic glucose production, insulin resistance, and insulin secretion are readily demonstrable. In such a complex situation, it is difficult to sort out causal sequences. One approach is to perturb the system by using various treatment modalities to control the hyperglycemia and assess the potential reversibility of the underlying metabolic defects. For example, if one of the abnormalities proved nonreversible whereas the others were ameliorated, the nonreversible defect would probably be the primary causative lesion leading to type 2 diabetes and the others would be secondary manifestations. Such studies have shown that peripheral tissue insulin resistance, increased HGO, hyperglucagonemia, and decreased insulin secretion are all ameliorated to some extent when blood glucose levels are substantially lowered, irrespective of whether achieved by insulin therapy, oral agents, or weight loss. This result implies that all the abnormalities depicted in Figure 55–2 may be in part secondary to the abnormal metabolic milieu that characterizes the hyperglycemic type 2 diabetic state.

Tight glycemic control achieved by intensive insulin regimens has been found to improve peripheral tissue insulin sensitivity by 17% to 75% in various studies.[56, 169, 203–206] When in vivo insulin action is measured by use of the multiple-dose glucose clamp method before and after intensive insulin therapy (Fig. 55–17), marked improvement in insulin-stimulated glucose disposal is seen at all steady-state serum insulin concentrations, thus indicating a significant improvement in postbinding insulin action.[56] Few studies have addressed the mechanisms of improved insulin action in skeletal muscle. Adipocyte glucose transport improves after intensive insulin therapy in parallel with the improvement in whole body insulin sensitivity.[169] Although the mechanism underlying the defects in glucose transport in adipocytes and skeletal muscle may differ in that skeletal muscle GLUT4 mRNA and protein levels are normal in type 2 diabetes and unaffected by glycemic control,[172–174, 207] because decreased glucose transport is the major determinant of impaired insulin-stimulated muscle glucose uptake in type 2 diabetes,[87] any improvement in this action of insulin must be associated with an improvement in muscle glucose transport as well.

Insulin secretion also improves after a period of nearly normal glycemia secondary to insulin therapy. Such improvement is seen in response to the ingestion of mixed meals (Fig. 55–18), oral glucose, intravenous glucose, or intravenously administered nonglucose stimuli.[56, 169, 205] The degree of improvement is variable, but in some cases, β cell function is restored to nearly normal levels. The magnitude of the posttreatment increase in 24-hour insulin secretion shown in Figure 55–18 is particularly impressive when one considers that this increase in insulin level is seen at markedly lower ambient glucose levels than in the pretreatment state. Interestingly, some studies have shown restoration of the acute insulin response to intravenous glucose after insulin therapy.[205, 208] Basal HGO is completely normalized after a period of insulin therapy,[56] and basal glucagon levels also return to normal or nearly normal values.[169]

Oral sulfonylureas and weight reduction yield qualitatively similar results.[57, 58, 124, 150, 205, 207–211] After weight loss, marked improvement is seen in insulin-stimulated glucose disposal, which is observed at maximally effective insulin levels, consistent with partial amelioration of the postbinding defect. Again, adipocyte glucose transport increases after weight loss, and the magnitude of the increase in glucose transport activity corresponds to the magnitude of the in vivo increase in insulin-stimulated glucose disposal.[58] β Cell function also improves,[58, 209–212] with enhanced insulin secretion following oral glucose, mixed meals, or intravenous glucose. However, the restoration of insulin action and secretion by weight loss is not complete; residual defects in both can still be demonstrated. In contrast, the elevated HGO is reduced to normal, and this process is accompanied by normalization of glucagon levels.[58, 210]

The results with sulfonylurea therapy are more variable,[57, 124, 207–209] most likely because of the variable clinical response to these agents among individual type 2 diabetic subjects. Thus some patients display near normalization of glycemia, whereas others show little if any clinical effect of oral agents on blood glucose levels (primary failure). Therefore, one would expect a wide range of changes in underlying metabolic defects when groups of patients are considered. However, when patients who display good clinical responses (lowered glycemia) are examined, one can demonstrate partial improvement in peripheral insulin resistance, slight increases in insulin secretion, and marked decreases in HGO, often to normal levels.[57]

Although these treatment modalities are functionally diverse, certain common themes emerge. Peripheral insulin resistance is consistently improved, but complete normalization of insulin action is unusual. The augmented insulin action is largely due to partial reversal of the postbinding defect, with little change in insulin binding. Posttherapy increases in cellular glucose transport activity are correlated with the

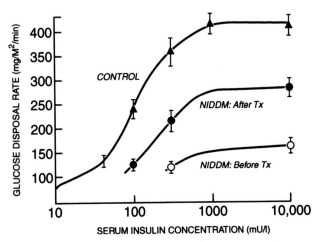

FIGURE 55–17. In vivo insulin dose-response curves for whole body glucose disposal rates in type 2 diabetic patients before *(open circles)* and after *(closed circles)* 2 weeks of intensive insulin therapy. Control curves *(closed triangles)* are provided for comparison. (From Garvey WT, Olefsky JM, Griffin J, et al: The effects of insulin treatment on insulin secretion and action in type II diabetes mellitus. Diabetes 34:222–234, 1985.)

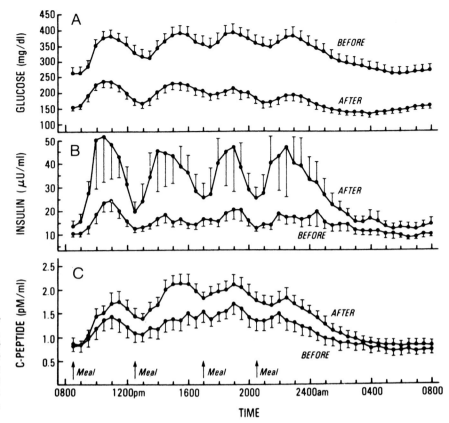

FIGURE 55–18. Mean 24-hour serum profile for integrated concentrations of glucose *(A)*, insulin *(B)*, and C peptide *(C)* in type 2 diabetic subjects before and after insulin treatment. Isocaloric meals were given at the times indicated. Results are plotted as means ± SEM. (From Garvey WT, Olefsky JM, Griffin J, et al: The effects of insulin treatment on insulin secretion and action in type II diabetes mellitus. Diabetes 34:222–234, 1985.)

increases in in vivo insulin action, consistent with the view that a decrease in glucose transport is a major cause of the postreceptor defect before treatment. Insulin secretion generally improves, although complete normalization is unusual. The increased rates of hepatic glucose production that are present in the untreated type 2 diabetic state are uniformly decreased after all modes of treatment. The decrease in HGO correlates well with the fall in plasma glucose after all treatment regimens, and in patients with the best clinical results, HGO is completely normalized. When measured, normalization of HGO has usually been accompanied by normalization of plasma glucagon levels, which suggests that hyperglucagonemia is an important causative factor of accelerated HGO in type 2 diabetes. Because these abnormalities in hepatic glucose metabolism can be completely normalized, they most likely represent secondary manifestations of the diabetic state that are in some way caused by insulin resistance, impaired insulin secretion, hyperglycemia, or some combination thereof. The defects in insulin action and secretion are routinely improved but rarely normalized, and from these perturbation studies one cannot determine which one (or whether both) of these defects represent(s) the primary causal lesion(s) leading to the hyperglycemic type 2 diabetic state. To assess this issue, prospective and population-based studies have been the most insightful, and these studies are reviewed in the earlier section on etiology.

One thing shared in common by all the treatment modalities described above is lowering of glycemia. Thus it is possible that hyperglycemia itself is responsible for some component of the abnormalities in insulin secretion and action and that correcting the hyperglycemia would therefore alleviate this reversible component. This concept is termed the "glucotoxicity" theory; the relationship between glucotoxicity and impaired insulin secretion in type 2 diabetes was discussed above. The evidence is good that hyperglycemia can also contribute to impaired insulin action.[213] For example, animals with experimental insulin-deficient diabetes (secondary to pancreatectomy or streptozotocin) are hyperglycemic and insulin resistant. Phlorhizin, an inhibitor of glucose reabsorption by renal tubules, causes marked glycosuria and subsequent lowering of plasma glucose levels when given to diabetic animals; normalization of glucose levels by phlorhizin is associated with correction of insulin resistance. In well-controlled type 1 diabetic patients infused with glucose, whole body insulin sensitivity, forearm glucose uptake, and muscle glycogen deposition were all reduced by approximately 35% after blood glucose had been maintained at 20 mmol/L (360 mg/dL) for a period of 24 hours.[214] These data provide direct evidence that hyperglycemia can adversely affect insulin action and are consistent with the view that in type 2 diabetes a reversible component of the overall insulin resistance is secondary to glucotoxicity.

The thiazolidinedione class of antidiabetic agents is distinct in having a direct peripheral tissue–sensitizing action independent of their glucose-lowering action. This point is readily demonstrable in vitro in isolated cells.[215] In hyperglycemic type 2 diabetic patients it is more difficult to quantify the relative contributions of improved glycemic control per se and the direct effect of the drug on insulin-resistant tissues to the overall improvement in insulin sensitivity. However, the study of Yu et al. provides insight into this issue.[216] In this study, type 2 diabetic patients were first treated intensively with continuous subcutaneous insulin for 4 weeks to eliminate any reversible defects caused by glucotoxicity before adding troglitazone to the insulin regimen for 6 weeks. Insulin doses had to be reduced by 53% during the combined treatment phase to maintain the same level of tight blood glucose control as achieved with insulin alone. At the end of the 6-week period on combined therapy, peripheral tissue insulin sensitivity was 29% higher than at the end of the 4-week period of normoglycemia achieved by insulin alone. By contrast, patients randomized to receive metformin in the same study showed no enhancement of peripheral tissue insulin sensitivity independent of glycemic control.[216] Thus the thiazolidinediones have a direct tissue-sensitizing action independent of their glucose-lowering effects. The demonstration that they improve insulin sensitivity in insulin-resistant obese subjects with normal glucose tolerance[217] and in subjects with IGT[218] and that in subjects with IGT they also ameliorate the subtle insulin secretory abnormalities[218] suggests that they may have a role to play in conjunction with life-style changes in the primary prevention of type 2 diabetes.

MOLECULAR GENETICS OF TYPE 2 DIABETES MELLITUS

Many lines of evidence indicate a strong genetic component to type 2 diabetes. Although acquired factors such as obesity may be necessary to bring out the phenotypic manifestation of type 2 diabetes, acquired factors alone are insufficient in most patients without preexisting genetic determinants. Because several prospective epidemiologic studies have shown that insulin resistance predates the development of type 2 diabetes, it seems likely that the diabetogenic gene(s) involve some aspect of insulin action. Type 2 diabetes does not fit any standard pattern of genetic inheritance, and it is likely to be a genetically heterogeneous, polygenic disease. In other words, most likely more than one diabetes gene occurs within a population, and it is possible that more than one abnormal gene must exist within an individual for the type 2 diabetic phenotype to develop. For example, it is possible that one or more genes involved in insulin action are affected, along with a separately inherited genetic defect responsible for the loss of β cell function that occurs late in the course of type 2 diabetes development.

Two basic strategies have been pursued to identify the diabetes genes. First is the candidate gene approach. In this approach, the investigator develops a hypothesis that a certain gene that has already been cloned and sequenced may be involved in the pathogenesis of type 2 diabetes. The sequence of this candidate gene is then compared in normal and type 2 diabetic subjects to look for structural abnormalities in the disease state. The second approach makes use of polymorphic genetic markers randomly distributed throughout the genome to map the location of the disease phenotype to a particular chromosome in a pedigree or population. This goal is accomplished by determining whether the DNA markers cosegregate with the type 2 diabetic phenotype in a pedigree or population with sufficient numbers of affected individuals.

These methods have allowed considerable progress to be made in defining the genetics of subsets of type 2 diabetes formerly referred to as MODY. These disorders are due to monogenic defects in β cell function, with little or no defect in insulin action. They are usually transmitted as an autosomal dominant trait and are characterized by the onset of overt diabetes usually before 25 years of age (see Chapter 49). The MODY phenotype is associated with abnormalities in at least four genetic loci on different chromosomes. The gene for MODY-1 was initially localized to the long arm of chromosome 20, close to the adenosine deaminase locus, by Bell and colleagues on the basis of extensive family studies of the RW pedigree.[219] The gene was subsequently identified as the transcription factor hepatocyte nuclear factor-4α (HNF-4α).[220] MODY-2 is due to mutations in the glucokinase gene that catalyzes the formation of glucose 6-phosphate from glucose in islet β cells and hepatocytes. Over 40 different mutations have been described.[221, 222] The missense mutations that cosegregate with diabetes in families with MODY alter the enzyme's affinity for glucose or the maximal activity for glucose phosphorylation. Because insulin secretion is intimately linked to the metabolism of glucose 6-phosphate, glucokinase is thought to play a key role as the "glucose sensor" of the β cell. Impaired hepatic glucose phosphorylation may also contribute to hyperglycemia in patients with MODY-2. Interestingly, most of the subjects with glucokinase mutations have very mild hyperglycemia, a normal first-phase insulin response to intravenous glucose, and a nonprogressive course. In "garden-variety" type 2 diabetes, glucokinase gene mutations are rare[221] and seem to exist only in patients with unusually early age of disease onset. MODY-3 is the most common subtype. It is associated with mutations on chromosome 12 in a gene encoding HNF-1α, a liver transcription factor also expressed in β cells.[223] Unlike patients with MODY-2, hyperglycemia in patients with MODY-3 tends to be progressive. Because they frequently present in adolescence with symptomatic hyperglycemia, type 1 diabetes mellitus may be diagnosed. MODY-4 is due to mutations in yet another transcription factor gene, IPF-1, which in its homozygous form leads to total pancreatic agenesis.[224] It is likely that further genetic defects resulting in a MODY phenotype will be identified in the future.

Several studies have examined the insulin receptor, glycogen syn-

thase, and GLUT4 as potential candidate genes in type 2 diabetes. As described in earlier sections, the primary sequences of these proteins are normal in type 2 diabetes, which eliminates them as diabetes gene loci, except in rare individuals. In some populations, IRS-1 variants may be two to three times more common in patients with type 2 diabetes than in normal subjects, and in some studies an association between polymorphisms affecting the region of IRS-1 thought to be important for PI-3-kinase binding and a reduction in insulin sensitivity has been found.[96] These exciting findings merit further study, although they could represent a genetic predisposition to type 2 diabetes in only a minority of subjects.

Given the importance of obesity in most type 2 diabetic patients, genes that predispose to obesity and, in particular, a more central distribution of body fat could also underlie the genetic predisposition. The discovery that the genetic syndromes of obesity and diabetes in the ob/ob mouse and db/db mouse were due respectively to failure of leptin production and an abnormality in the leptin receptor suggested that similar defects may play a role in human obesity. However, leptin levels are generally increased in human obesity, and leptin receptor gene mutations do not appear to cosegregate with common-type obesity in humans.[225, 226] A missense mutation at codon 64 in the β₃-adrenergic receptor gene was reported to be associated with weight gain and some complications of obesity in the Finnish population.[227] However, subsequent studies in other populations did not find an increased frequency of this variant in obesity.[228] More recently, a polymorphism in the β₂-adrenergic receptor was found to be strongly associated with obesity; replacement of glutamine by glutamate at codon 27 (Gln27Glu) was found in 24% of obese women but only 3% of nonobese women.[229] Homozygotes for Glu27 had on average 20 kg more adipose tissue, larger fat cells, higher fasting insulin levels, and a more central distribution of body fat. Although, this particular polymorphism does not alter β-adrenoreceptor function, it is in strong linkage disequilibrium with another polymorphism (Arg16Gly) that is associated with increased sensitivity to agonist-induced downregulation. Two-thirds of the obese women were found to carry both Gly16 and Glu27.[229]

Gene mapping studies in type 1 diabetes have led to the identification of major susceptibility loci within the HLA region on chromosome 6p21, the insulin gene region on chromosome 11p15, and several other loci. In type 2 diabetes these studies are at an early stage. Nonetheless, linkage has been found between the type 2 diabetic phenotype and a number of loci on different chromosomes,[230–237] some of which are presented in Table 55–2. As expected, the putative susceptibility loci differ according to the population studied. Thus in an Australian study of a large white pedigree with typical type 2 diabetes, a locus on chromosome 12q close to, but distinct from the *MODY3* region was found to be linked to the development of diabetes.[235] Linkage between type 2 diabetes in whites and markers in the *MODY3* region was also found in another study.[232] By contrast, no evidence has been found for linkage of loci on chromosome 12 with type 2 diabetes in Mexican-American,[237] Pima Indian,[230, 236] or black American sibling pairs.[232] Mexican-American sibling pairs showed significant linkage between type 2 diabetes and markers on chromosome 2q; this region was designated "*NIDDM1*."[230] More recently it was suggested that an interaction of genes in the *NIDDM1* region and genes on chromosome 15 may contribute to the susceptibility to type 2 diabetes in Mexican-Americans.[238] Linkage family studies in Pima Indians[239] and Mexican-

TABLE 55–2. Potential Type 2 Diabetes Susceptibility Loci

Chromosome Location	Population	Reference
1q21-1q23	Families of N. European ancestry living in Utah	234
2q—"*NIDDM1*"	Mexican-American	230, 238
10q	Mexican-American	233
11q	Pima Indians	236
12q (near *MODY 3*)	White	232, 235
20p and 20q (distinct from *MODY 1*)	White	231, 232

Americans[240] have also suggested linkage between in vivo insulin resistance and a locus on chromosome 4q that encodes the intestinal fatty acid–binding protein-2 (FABP-2), believed to be involved in the transport of long-chain fatty acids within the enterocyte. However, in three different European populations, no differences in allelic frequency at this locus were found between diabetic and nondiabetic individuals.[241] Whether FABP-2 itself has any influence on insulin action is not known.

A major advance in our understanding of potential genetic mechanisms leading to the type 2 diabetic phenotype has come from transgenic mouse models in which a specific gene thought to play a key role in insulin action or insulin secretion has been disrupted either at the whole body level or in a specific tissue. Mice with targeted disruption of the insulin receptor die a few days after birth, whereas heterozygous animals have a virtually normal phenotype.[242] These results in heterozygous animals were perhaps not unexpected given the presence of spare insulin receptors on insulin target tissues. However, diabetes also does not develop in animals with only one IRS-1 allele disrupted, even though these animals display mild insulin resistance, hyperinsulinemia, and mildly impaired glucose tolerance as they age.[243, 244] Because severe deficiencies of these molecules are extremely rare in type 2 diabetes and type 2 diabetes is thought to be a polygenic disease, Bruning and colleagues generated mice heterozygous for the null allele of more than one of the key insulin signaling molecules.[244] They found that insulin resistance, hyperinsulinemia, and progressive impairment in glucose tolerance developed in mice heterozygous for the null alleles of both the insulin receptor and IRS-1, with overt diabetes developing in approximately 40% of these mice by the age of 6 months.[244] Mice heterozygous for deficiencies of the insulin receptor, IRS-1, and IRS-2 had an even more profound degree of insulin resistance in muscle and liver, and overt diabetes eventually developed in a higher percentage.[245] Severe diabetes also develops in mice that are compound heterozygotes for the null alleles of the glucokinase and IRS-1 genes, whereas mice with an isolated defect of glucokinase gene expression have mild diabetes as found in patients with MODY-2.[246] The presence of defects of both insulin action and insulin secretion in these glucokinase/IRS-1 compound heterozygous knockout mice provides an excellent model for the type 2 diabetic phenotype.

Taken together, these studies indicate that combinations of relatively minor defects, which in isolation may not cause significant phenotypic abnormalities, can act synergistically to cause insulin resistance, glucose intolerance, and type 2 diabetes. The particular mix of defects is likely to differ between different populations. Thus IRS-1 polymorphisms that affect its function are not uncommon in the Japanese and Finnish populations but are not found in the Pima Indians. Clearly, some defects may be acquired (e.g., the downregulation of insulin receptors by high circulating insulin levels) and act in concert with inherited genetic defects to produce significant insulin resistance and impairment of insulin secretion.

Another key finding from studies of mouse genetics is that insulin receptor signaling in islet β cells is important for their normal function. Thus mice in which the insulin receptor gene has been specifically ablated in islet β cells, but not in any other tissues, show a complete loss of first-phase insulin secretion in response to glucose, but not arginine, reminiscent of the β cell defect in type 2 diabetes.[247] Interestingly, in patients with genetic forms of severe insulin resistance caused by insulin receptor defects, the acute insulin response to intravenous glucose is also absent.[248] Second-phase glucose-induced insulin secretion is also blunted in these mice, and they show an age-dependent progressive impairment in glucose tolerance, although overt diabetes does not develop. The islet β cells of these animals tend to be smaller than normal.[247] As well as providing direct evidence that functional insulin receptors are essential for normal β cell function, this study also raises the intriguing possibility that insulin resistance at the level of the β cell may contribute to the decline in insulin secretion that supervenes after many years of peripheral tissue insulin resistance during the natural history of type 2 diabetes, thus providing a unifying hypothesis for the development of type 2 diabetes.

In summary, potential candidates for diabetes genes include those involved in insulin action, hepatic glucose metabolism, and islet β cell

function. Genetically endowed defects in protein function show up as abnormalities in protein-coding regions. However, abnormalities in the expression of one or more key proteins could also have a genetic basis. Studies in transgenic mouse models have highlighted the importance of combinations of relatively minor defects in signaling molecules acting synergistically to produce insulin resistance and glucose intolerance. The demonstration that intact insulin receptor signaling in islet β cell is essential for normal insulin secretion and the adaptive response of islets to peripheral insulin resistance suggests that β cell insulin resistance could contribute to the defects in insulin secretion found in type 2 diabetes.

CONCLUSIONS AND OVERALL PERSPECTIVES

Type 2 diabetes is a heterogeneous disorder with most likely more than one cause that results in a common final pathway of hyperglycemia. However, as a general finding, three metabolic defects— peripheral insulin resistance, impaired insulin secretion, and increased HGO—contribute to the hyperglycemia. In considering this syndrome one must distinguish between the cause of the diabetic state itself and the pathogenesis of the hyperglycemia in a patient with type 2 diabetes. The former concerns the temporal sequence of the pathogenesis and development of type 2 diabetes, that is, which defect(s) initiate(s) the syndrome and which develop(s) secondarily. The latter concerns the metabolic defects that contribute most to the degree of hyperglycemia at a static point in time after the type 2 diabetic state has already developed.

With regard to the sequential development of type 2 diabetes, population-based and prospective studies indicate that insulin resistance is the initial defect, although in some populations insulin secretory abnormalities may initiate the sequence of events leading to type 2 diabetes.[15, 249] In a number of different ethnic groups, insulin resistance has been found to exist in the prediabetic state, with an absence of any impairment in insulin secretion. Thus insulin resistance and hyperinsulinemia characterize most individuals in whom type 2 diabetes is destined to develop at a time when their glucose tolerance is entirely normal. However, except in extreme cases, insulin resistance alone is not sufficient to cause the full-blown type 2 diabetic phenotype. Decreased β cell function must eventually supervene to cause the type 2 diabetic state. This setting leads to the scheme depicted in Figure 55–2, in which insulin resistance (genetic and/or acquired) leads to hyperinsulinemia and compensated glucose metabolism. Eventually, in some of these individuals, perhaps those with a coexisting genetically determined β cell defect, the ability of β cells to compensate by sustaining hyperinsulinemia declines and insulin secretory defects appear. At this stage, glucose metabolism decompensates and the hyperglycemic diabetic stage appears. Because type 2 diabetes is a heterogeneous disease, this scheme (see Fig. 55–2) is clearly an oversimplification.

Once type 2 diabetes is established, the abnormal metabolic and hormonal milieu leads to secondary changes with worsening hyperglycemia. Thus insulin resistance tends to be more marked in type 2 diabetes than in the prediabetic IGT state,[5, 7, 29] and insulin secretion continues to decline throughout the course of established type 2 diabetes.[34] Therefore, many patients, even if initially well controlled by diet or oral hypoglycemic agents, eventually require insulin for control of their diabetes.[250] Glucotoxicity may well be the causal link here. Thus strong evidence indicates that chronic hyperglycemia per se can lead to secondary worsening of both insulin resistance and insulin secretion, with the potential for a vicious cycle in which hyperglycemia begets more hyperglycemia. Support for this concept comes from numerous observations that control of hyperglycemia by insulin therapy, weight loss, or oral agents leads to improvements in both insulin secretion and insulin action. Some subsets of type 2 diabetic patients must start with impaired insulin secretion, and insulin resistance, if it occurs, would be secondary in these patients. In addition, obesity and aging, as well as other factors, are acquired conditions that can cause or contribute to insulin resistance. Acquired factors can contribute to β cell dysfunction as well.

Because of the convergence of primary and secondary events that coexist in the manifest type 2 diabetic state, it is a daunting task to identify the critical biochemical and cellular defects by studying established type 2 diabetic patients. Most likely, clarifying discoveries will come from the field of molecular genetics. Type 2 diabetes has a strong genetic component; therefore, the ultimate explanation of the precise cause(s) of this disease lies in the genome. By finding the gene or, more likely, the genes that are abnormal in type 2 diabetes we will be able to document the cellular defects that initiate this syndrome. With this information we might learn that a genotype with abnormalities in both insulin action and insulin secretion is necessary for the type 2 diabetic phenotype to develop. We might also find that different sets of genetic defects exist in different patients and that depending on other genetic or acquired features, they complement each other in different ways. This search might also lead to the identification of genes encoding proteins that affect carbohydrate metabolism in ways not currently understood. Discovery of all the molecular defects that can lead to type 2 diabetes is an enormous, but completely feasible goal and should provide the basis for an exciting future in diabetes research.

REFERENCES

1. Fajans SS, Cloutier MC, Crowther RL: Clinical and etiologic heterogeneity of idiopathic diabetes mellitus. Diabetes 27:1112–1125, 1978.
2. Scheuner MT, Raffel LJ, Rotter JI: Genetics of diabetes. In Alberti KGMM, Zimmet P, Defronzo RA, et al (eds): International Textbook of Diabetes Mellitus, ed 2. Chichester, England, John Wiley & Sons, 1997, pp 37–88.
3. Ward WK, Beard JC, Porte D: Clinical aspects of islet B-cell function in non–insulin-dependent diabetes mellitus. Diabetes Metab Rev 2:297–313, 1986.
4. DeFronzo RA: The triumvirate: β-Cell, muscle, liver: A collusion responsible for NIDDM. Diabetes 37:667–687, 1988.
5. Seely BL, Olefsky JM: Cellular and genetic mechanisms for insulin resistance in common disorders of obesity and diabetes. In Moller D (ed): Insulin Resistance and Its Clinical Disorders. New York, John Wiley & Sons, 1993.
6. Reaven GM: Role of insulin resistance in human disease. Diabetes 37:1595–1607, 1988.
7. Kolterman OG, Gray RS, Griffin J, et al: Receptor and post-receptor defects contribute to the insulin resistance in non–insulin dependent diabetes mellitus. J Clin Invest 68:957–969, 1981.
8. Dinneen S, Gerich J, Rizza R: Carbohydrate metabolism in non–insulin-dependent diabetes mellitus. N Engl J Med 327:707–713, 1992.
9. Ferrannini E, Groop LC: Hepatic glucose production in insulin resistant states. Diabetes Metab Rev 5:711–725, 1989.
10. Bogardus C, Lillioja S, Howard BV, et al: Relationships between insulin secretion, insulin action, and fasting plasma glucose concentration in non-diabetic and non–insulin-dependent diabetic subjects. J Clin Invest 74:1238–1246, 1984.
11. Shulman GI, Rothman DL, Jue T, et al: Quantitation of muscle glycogen synthesis in normal subjects and subjects with non–insulin-dependent diabetes by ^{13}C-nuclear magnetic resonance spectroscopy. N Engl J Med 322:223–228, 1991.
12. Ciaraldi TP, Kolterman OG, Scarlett JA, et al: Role of the glucose transport system in the post-receptor defect of non–insulin dependent diabetes mellitus. Diabetes 31:1016–1022, 1982.
13. Firth R, Bell P, Rizza R: Insulin action in non–insulin-dependent diabetes mellitus: The relationship between hepatic and extrahepatic insulin resistance and obesity. Metabolism 36:1091–1095, 1987.
14. Groop LC, Bonadonna RC, Del Prato S, et al: Glucose and free fatty acid metabolism in non–insulin dependent diabetes mellitus. Evidence for multiple sites of insulin resistance. J Clin Invest 84:205–213, 1989.
15. Efendic S, Luft R, Wajngot A: Aspects of the pathogenesis of type 2 diabetes. Endocr Rev 5:395–410, 1984.
16. Porte D: Banting lecture 1990. β-Cells in type II diabetes mellitus. Diabetes 40:166–190, 1991.
17. Barnett AH, Eff C, Leslie RD, Pyke DA: Diabetes in identical twins: A study of 200 pairs. Diabetologia 20:87–93, 1981.
18. Rich SS: Mapping genes in diabetes: Genetic epidemiological perspective. Diabetes 39:1315–1319, 1990.
19. Haffner SM, Sern MP, Mitchell BD, et al: Incidences of type II diabetes in Mexican Americans predicted by fasting insulin and glucose levels, obesity, and body fat distribution. Diabetes 39:283–288, 1990.
20. Knowler WC, Bennett PH, Pettitt D, Savage PJ: Diabetes incidence in Pima Indians: Contributions of obesity and parental diabetes. Am J Epidemiol 113:144–156, 1981.
21. Polonsky KS, Sturis J, Bell GI: Non–insulin-dependent diabetes mellitus—a genetically programmed failure of the beta cell to compensate for insulin resistance. N Engl J Med 334:777–783, 1996.
22. Alberti KGMM: The clinical implications of impaired glucose tolerance. Diabet Med 13:927–937, 1996.
23. Warram JH, Martin BC, Krolewski AS, et al: Slow glucose removal rate and hyperinsulinemia precede the development of type II diabetes in the offspring of diabetic parents. Ann Intern Med 13:909–915, 1990.
24. Saad MF, Knowler WC, Pettitt DJ, et al: The natural history of impaired glucose tolerance in the Pima Indians. N Engl J Med 319:1500–1505, 1988.
25. Lillioja S, Mott DM, Howard BV, et al: Impaired glucose tolerance as a disorder of insulin action: Longitudinal and cross-sectional studies in Pima Indians. N Engl J Med 318:1217–1225, 1988.
26. Saad MF, Knowler WC, Pettitt DJ, et al: A two step model for development of non–insulin dependent diabetes mellitus. Am J Physiol 90:229–235, 1991.
27. Serjeantson SW, Zimmet P: Genetics of non–insulin dependent diabetes mellitus in 1990. Baillieres Clin Endocrinol Metab 5:477–493, 1991.
28. Zimmet PZ: Kelly West Lecture 1991: Challenges in diabetes epidemiology from West to East. Diabetes Care 15:232–252, 1992.
29. Eriksson J, Franssila-Kallunki AM, Ekstrand A, et al: Early metabolic defects in persons at increased risk for non–insulin-dependent diabetes mellitus. N Engl J Med 321:337–343, 1989.
30. Perseghin G, Ghosh S, Gerow K, Shulman GI: Metabolic defects in lean nondiabetic offspring of NIDDM parents: A cross-sectional study. Diabetes 46:1010–1016, 1997.
31. Vaag A, Henriksen JE, Beck-Nielsen H: Decreased insulin activation of glycogen synthase in skeletal muscles in young nonobese Caucasian first-degree relatives of patients with non–insulin-dependent diabetes mellitus. J Clin Invest 89:782–788, 1992.
32. Temple RC, Clark PMS, Nagi DK, et al: Radioimmunoassay may overestimate insulin in non–insulin-dependent diabetics. Clin Endocrinol (Oxf) 32:689–693, 1990.
33. Polonsky KS: The beta-cell in diabetes: From molecular genetics to clinical research. Diabetes 44:705–717, 1995.
34. U.K. Prospective Diabetes Study Group: U.K. prospective diabetes study 16: Overview of 6 years' therapy of type II diabetes: A progressive disease. Diabetes 44:1249–1258, 1995.
35. Ferrannini E, Natali A, Bell P, et al: Insulin resistance and hypersecretion in obesity. J Clin Invest 100:1166–1173, 1997.
36. Reaven GM, Chen YDI, Hollenbeck CB, et al: Plasma insulin, C-peptide, and proinsulin concentrations in obese and nonobese individuals with varying degrees of glucose tolerance. J Clin Endocrinol Metab 76:44–48, 1993.
37. Perley MJ, Kipnis DM: Plasma insulin responses to oral and intravenous glucose: Studies in normal and diabetic subjects. J Clin Invest 46:1954–1962, 1967.
38. DeFronzo RA, Ferrannini E: The pathogenesis of non–insulin-dependent diabetes: An update. Medicine (Baltimore) 61:125–140(Table 1), 1982.
39. Ward WK, Bolgiano DC, McKnight B, et al: Diminished β cell secretory capacity in patients with noninsulin-dependent diabetes mellitus. J Clin Invest 74:1318–1328, 1984.
40. Halter JB, Graf RJ, Porte D Jr: Potentiation of insulin secretory responses by plasma glucose levels in man: Evidence that hyperglycemia compensates for impaired glucose potentiation. J Clin Endocrinol Metab 48:946–954, 1979.
41. Roder ME, Porte D, Schwartz RS, Kahn SE: Disproportionately elevated proinsulin levels reflect the degree of impaired B cell secretory capacity in patients with non–insulin-dependent diabetes mellitus. J Clin Endocrinol Metab 83:604–608, 1998.
42. Alarcon C, Leahy JL, Schuppin GT, Rhodes CJ: Increased secretory demand rather than a defect in the proinsulin conversion mechanism causes hyperproinsulinemia in a glucose-infusion rat model of non–insulin-dependent diabetes mellitus. J Clin Invest 95:1032–1039, 1995.
43. Reaven GM, Bernstein R, Davis B, Olefsky JM: Nonketotic diabetes mellitus: Insulin deficiency or insulin resistance? Am J Med 60:80–88, 1976.
44. Brunzell JD, Robertson RP, Lerner RL, et al: Relationships between fasting plasma glucose levels and insulin secretion during intravenous glucose tolerance tests. J Clin Endocrinol Metab 42:222–229, 1976.
45. Robertson RP, Porte D: The glucose receptor: A defective mechanism in diabetes mellitus distinct from the beta-adrenergic receptor. J Clin Invest 52:870–876, 1976.
46. McRae JR, Metz SW, Robertson RP: A role for endogenous prostaglandins in defective glucose potentiation of non-glucose insulin secretagogues in diabetics. Metabolism 30:1065–1075, 1981.
47. Robertson RP, Halter JB, Porte D Jr: A role for alpha-adrenergic receptors in abnormal insulin secretion in diabetes mellitus. J Clin Invest 57:791–795, 1976.
48. Vague P, Moulin JP: The defective glucose sensitivity of the β-cell in noninsulin dependent diabetes: Improvement after twenty hours of normoglycemia. Metabolism 31:139–142, 1982.
49. Leahy JL, Bonner-Weir S, Weir GC: β-Cell dysfunction induced by chronic hyperglycemia. Diabetes Care 15:442–455, 1992.
50. Lohmann D, Jahr H, Verlohren J-J, et al: Insulin secretion in maturity-onset diabetes—function of isolated islets. Horm Metab Res 12:349–353, 1980.
51. Srikanta S, Ganda OP, Eisenbarth GS, Soeldner JS: Islet-cell antibodies and beta-cell function in monozygotic triplets and twins initially discordant for type I diabetes mellitus. N Engl J Med 308:322–325, 1983.
52. Gepts W, Lecompte PM: The pancreatic islets in diabetes. Am J Med 70:105–114, 1981.
53. Clark A, Wells CA, Buley ID, et al: Islet amyloid, increased A-cells, reduced β-cells and exocrine fibrosis: Quantitative changes in the pancreas in type 2 diabetes. Diabetes Res 9:151–160, 1988.
54. Shimabukuro M, Zhou Y-T, Levi M, Unger RH: Fatty acid induced β cell apoptosis: A link between obesity and diabetes. Proc Natl Acad Sci U S A 95:2498–2502, 1998.
55. Koyama M, Wada R, Sakuraba H, et al: Accelerated loss of islet beta cells in sucrose-fed Goto-Kakizaki rats, a genetic model of non–insulin-dependent diabetes mellitus. Am J Pathol 153:537–545, 1998.
56. Garvey WT, Olefsky JM, Griffin J, et al: The effects of insulin treatment on insulin secretion and action in type II diabetes mellitus. Diabetes 34:222–234, 1985.
57. Kolterman OG, Gray RS, Shapiro G, et al: The acute and chronic effects of sulfonylurea therapy in type II diabetics. Diabetes 33:346–354, 1984.
58. Henry RR, Wallace P, Olefsky JM: The effects of weight loss on the mechanisms of hyperglycemia in obese noninsulin-dependent diabetes mellitus. Diabetes 35:990–998, 1986.
59. Eizirik DL, Korbutt GS, Hellerstrom C: Prolonged exposure of human pancreatic islets to high glucose concentrations in vitro impairs the β-cell function. J Clin Invest 90:1263–1268, 1992.

60. O'Sullivan JB, Mahan CM: Prospective studies of 352 young patients with chemical diabetes. N Engl J Med 278:1038–1041, 1968.
61. Charles MA, Fontbonne A, Thibult N, et al: Risk factors for NIDDM in white population: Paris prospective study. Diabetes 40:796–799, 1991.
62. Jones CNO, Pei D, Staris P, et al: Alterations in the glucose-stimulated insulin secretory dose-response curve and in insulin clearance in nondiabetic insulin-resistant individuals. J Clin Endocrinol Metab 82:1834–1838, 1997.
63. Kahn SE, Prigeon RL, McCulloch DK, et al: Quantification of the relationship between insulin sensitivity and β-cell function in human subjects: Evidence for a hyperbolic function. Diabetes 42:1663–1672, 1993.
64. Cook JTE, Page RCL, Levy JC, et al: Hyperglycaemic progression in subjects with impaired glucose tolerance: Association with decline in beta cell function. Diabet Med 10:321–326, 1993.
65. Given BD, Mako ME, Tager H, et al: Circulating insulin with reduced biological activity in a patient with diabetes. N Engl J Med 302:129–135, 1980.
66. Gabbay KH, DeLuca K, Fisher JN Jr, et al: Familial hyperproinsulinemia: An autosomal dominant defect. N Engl J Med 294:911–915, 1976.
67. Warren-Perry MG, Manley SE, Ostrega D, et al: A novel point mutation in the insulin gene giving rise to hyperproinsulinemia. J Clin Endocrinol Metab 82:1629–1631, 1997.
68. Ludvik B, Kautzky-Willer A, Prager R, et al: Amylin: History and overview. Diabet Med 14(suppl):9–13, 1997.
69. Butler PC, Chou J, Carter WB, et al: Effects of meal ingestion on plasma amylin concentration in NIDDM and non-diabetic humans. Diabetes 39:752–756, 1990.
70. Randle PJ, Hales CN, Garland PB, Newsholme EA: The glucose fatty-acid cycle: Its role in insulin sensitivity and the metabolic disturbances of diabetes mellitus. Lancet 1:785–789, 1963.
71. Kahn CR, Rosenthal AS: Immunologic reactions to insulin: Insulin allergy, insulin resistance, and the autoimmune insulin syndrome. Diabetes Care 2:283–295, 1979.
72. Flier JS, Kahn CR, Roth J, Bar RS: Antibodies that impair insulin receptor binding in an unusual diabetic syndrome with severe insulin resistance. Science 190:63–65, 1975.
73. Zhang B, Roth RA: A region of the insulin receptor important for ligand binding (residues 450–601) is recognized by patients' autoimmune antibodies and inhibitory monoclonal antibodies. Proc Natl Acad Sci U S A 88:9858–9862, 1991.
74. Lang CH, Dobrescu C, Bagby GJ: Tumour necrosis factor impairs insulin action on peripheral glucose disposal and hepatic glucose output. Endocrinology 130:43–52, 1992.
75. Sakurai Y, Zhang X, Wolfe RR: Short-term effects of tumour necrosis factor on energy and substrate metabolism in dogs. J Clin Invest 91:2437–2445, 1993.
76. Hotamisligil GS, Arner P, Caro JF, et al: Increased adipose tissue expression of tumour necrosis factor-α in human obesity and insulin resistance. J Clin Invest 95:2409–2415, 1995.
77. Hotamisligil SG, Spiegelman BM: Tumour necrosis factor α: A key component of the obesity-diabetes link. Diabetes 43:1271–1278, 1994.
78. Hotamisligil GS, Peraldi P, Budavari A, et al: IRS-1–mediated inhibition of insulin receptor tyrosine kinase activity in TNF-α and obesity-induced insulin resistance. Science 271:665–668, 1996.
79. Ofei F, Hurel S, Newkirk J, et al: Effects of an engineered human anti TNF-α antibody (CDP571) on insulin sensitivity and glycemic control in patients with NIDDM. Diabetes 45:881–885, 1996.
80. Nolte LA, Hansen PA, Chen MM, et al: Short-term exposure to tumor necrosis factor-α does not affect insulin-stimulated glucose uptake in skeletal muscle. Diabetes 47:721–726, 1998.
81. Yang YJ, Hope JD, Ader M, Bergman RN: Insulin transport across capillaries is rate limiting for insulin action in dogs. J Clin Invest 84:1620–1628, 1989.
82. Steil GM, Ader M, Moore DM, et al: Transendothelial insulin transport is not saturable in vivo. No evidence for a receptor-mediated process. J Clin Invest 97:1497–1503, 1996.
83. Prager R, Wallace P, Olefsky JM: In vivo kinetics of insulin action on peripheral glucose disposal and hepatic glucose output in normal and obese subjects. J Clin Invest 78:472–481, 1986.
84. Nolan JJ, Ludvik B, Baloga J, et al: Mechanisms of the kinetic defect in insulin action in obesity and NIDDM. Diabetes 46:994–1000, 1997.
85. King GL, Johnson SM: Receptor-mediated transport of insulin across endothelial cells. Science 227:1583–1586, 1985.
86. Castillo C, Bogardus C, Bergman R, et al: Interstitial insulin concentrations determine glucose uptake rates but not insulin resistance in lean and obese men. J Clin Invest 93:10–16, 1994.
87. Cline GW, Petersen KF, Krssak M, et al: Impaired glucose transport as a cause of decreased insulin-stimulated muscle glycogen synthesis in type 2 diabetes. N Engl J Med 341:240–246, 1999.
88. Lillioja S, Young AA, Culter CL, et al: Skeletal muscle capillary density and fiber type are possible determinants of in vivo insulin resistance in man. J Clin Invest 80:415–424, 1987.
89. Laakso M, Edelman SV, Brechtel G, Baron AD: Impaired insulin-mediated skeletal muscle blood flow in patients with NIDDM. Diabetes 41:1076–1083, 1992.
90. Natali A, Buzzugoli G, Taddei S, et al: Effects of insulin on hemodynamics and metabolism in human forearm. Diabetes 39:490–500, 1990.
91. Utriainen T, Nuutila P, Takala T, et al: Intact insulin stimulation of skeletal muscle blood flow, its heterogeneity and redistribution, but not of glucose uptake in non–insulin-dependent diabetes mellitus. J Clin Invest 100:777–785, 1997.
92. Kahn CR, White MF: The insulin receptor and the molecular mechanisms of insulin action. J Clin Invest 82:1151–1156, 1988.
93. Olefsky JM: The insulin receptor: A multi-functional protein. Diabetes 39:1009–1016, 1990.
94. Wilden PA, Siddle K, Haring H, et al: The role of insulin receptor kinase domain autophosphorylation in receptor mediated activities. J Biol Chem 267:13719–13727, 1992.
95. White MF: The insulin signalling system and the IRS proteins. Diabetologia 40(suppl):2–17, 1997.
96. Virkamaki A, Ueki K, Kahn RC: Protein-protein interaction in insulin signaling and the molecular mechanisms of insulin resistance. J Clin Invest 103:931–943, 1999.
97. Fink RI, Wallace P, Brechtel G, Olefsky JM: Evidence that glucose transport is rate-limiting for in vivo glucose uptake. Metabolism 41:897–902, 1992.
98. Furler SM, Jenkins AB, Storlien LH, Kraegen EW: In vivo location of the rate-limiting step of hexose uptake in muscle and brain tissue of rats. Am J Phsyiol 261:E337–E347, 1991.
99. Ren JM, Marshall BA, Gulve EA, et al: Evidence from transgenic mice that glucose transport is rate-limiting for glycogen deposition and glycolysis in skeletal muscle. J Biol Chem 268:16113–16115, 1993.
100. Pessin JE, Bell GI: Mammalian facilitative glucose transporter family: Structure and molecular regulation. Annu Rev Physiol 84:911–930, 1992.
101. Shepherd PR, Kahn BB: Glucose transporters and insulin action. N Engl J Med 341:248–257, 1999.
102. Karnieli E, Zarnowski MJ, Hissin PJ, et al: Insulin-stimulated translocation of glucose transport systems in the isolated rat adipose cell: Time-course, reversal, insulin concentration dependency, and relationship to glucose transport activity. J Biol Chem 256:4772–4777, 1981.
103. Kono T, Suzuki K, Dansey LE, et al: Energy-dependent and protein synthesis–independent recycling of the insulin sensitive glucose transport mechanism in fat cells. J Biol Chem 256:6400–6407, 1981.
104. Kelley DE, Mintun MA, Watkins SC, et al: The effect of non–insulin-dependent diabetes mellitus and obesity on glucose transport and phosphorylation in skeletal muscle. J Clin Invest 97:2705–2713, 1996.
105. Garvey WT, Maianu L, Zhu J-H, et al: Evidence for defects in the trafficking and translocation of Glut 4 glucose transporters in skeletal muscle as a cause of human insulin resistance. J Clin Invest 101:2377–2386, 1998.
106. Pessin JE, Thurmond DC, Elmendorf JS, et al: Molecular basis of insulin-stimulated Glut 4 vesicle trafficking. J Biol Chem 274:2593–2596, 1999.
107. Olefsky JM, Ciaraldi TP: The insulin receptor: Basic characteristics and its role in insulin resistant state. *In* Brownlee M (ed): Diabetes Mellitus. New York, Garland Press, 1980, pp 73–115.
108. Bergman RN, Finegood DT, Ader M: Assessment of insulin sensitivity in vivo. Endocr Rev 1:45–86, 1985.
109. Himsworth JP, Kerr RB: Insulin-sensitive and insulin-insensitive types of diabetes mellitus. Clin Sci 4:119–152, 1939.
110. Ginsberg H, Kimmerling G, Olefsky JM, Reaven GM: Demonstration of insulin resistance in maturity onset diabetic patients with fasting hyperglycemia. J Clin Invest 55:454–460, 1975.
111. Welch S, Gebhart SS, Bergman RN, Phillips LS: Minimal model analysis of intravenous glucose tolerance test–derived insulin sensitivity in diabetic subjects. J Clin Endocrinol Metab 71:1508–1518, 1990.
112. Bonadonna RC, Del Prato S, Saccomani MP, et al: Transmembrane glucose transport in skeletal muscle of patients with non–insulin-dependent diabetes. J Clin Invest 92:486–494, 1993.
113. Capaldo B, Napoli R, Di Marino L, et al: Quantitation of forearm glucose and free fatty acid (FFA) disposal in normal subjects and type II diabetic patients: Evidence against an essential role for FFA in the pathogenesis of insulin resistance. J Clin Endocrinol Metab 67:893–898, 1988.
114. DeFronzo RA, Jacot E, Jequier E, et al: The effect of insulin on the disposal of intravenous glucose: Results from indirect calorimetry and hepatic and femoral venous catheterization. Diabetes 30:1000–1007, 1981.
115. Edelman SV, Laakso M, Wallace P, et al: Kinetics of insulin mediated and non–insulin mediated glucose uptake in man. Diabetes 39:955–964, 1990.
116. Kelley DE, Mokan M, Mandarino LJ: Intracellular defects in glucose metabolism in obese patients with NIDDM. Diabetes 41:698–706, 1992.
117. Yki-Jarvinen H, Bogardus C, Howard BV: Hyperglycemia stimulates carbohydrate oxidation in humans. Am J Physiol 253:E376–E382, 1987.
118. Golay A, DeFronzo RA, Ferrannini E, et al: Oxidative and non-oxidative glucose metabolism in non-obese type 2 (non–insulin dependent) diabetic patients. Diabetologia 31:585–591, 1988.
119. Bogardus C, Lillioja S, Stone K, Mott D: Correlations between muscle glycogen synthase activity and in vivo insulin action in man. J Clin Invest 73:1185–1190, 1984.
120. Thorburn AW, Gumbiner B, Bulacan F, et al: Intracellular glucose oxidation and glycogen synthase activity are reduced in non–insulin dependent (type II) diabetes independent of impaired glucose uptake. J Clin Invest 85:522–529, 1990.
121. Rothman DL, Shulmann RG, Shulman GI: ^{31}P nuclear magnetic resonance measurements of muscle glucose-6-phosphate. J Clin Invest 89:1069–1075, 1992.
122. Del Prato S, Bonadonna RC, Bonora E, et al: Characterization of cellular defects of insulin action in type 2 (non–insulin-dependent) diabetes mellitus. J Clin Invest 91:484–494, 1993.
123. Kruszynska YT, Mulford MI, Baloga J, et al: Regulation of skeletal muscle hexokinase II by insulin in nondiabetic and NIDDM subjects. Diabetes 47:1107–1113, 1998.
124. Bak JF, Schmitz O, Sorensen NS, et al: Postreceptor effects of sulfonylurea on skeletal muscle glycogen synthase activity in type II diabetes mellitus. Diabetes 38:1343–1350, 1989.
125. Schalin-Jantti C, Harkonen M, Groop LC: Impaired activation of glycogen synthase in people at increased risk for developing NIDDM. Diabetes 41:598–604, 1992.
126. Kruszynska YT: The role of fatty acid metabolism in the hypertriglyceridaemia and insulin resistance of type 2 (non–insulin dependent) diabetes. *In* Marshall SM, Home PD, Rizza RA (eds): The Diabetes Annual, vol 9. Amsterdam, Elsevier Science, 1995, pp 107–139.
127. Boden G, Ray TK, Smith RH, Owen OE: Carbohydrate oxidation and storage in obese non–insulin-dependent diabetic patients. Effect of improving glycemic control. Diabetes 32:982–987, 1983.
128. Golay A, Felber JP, Jequier E, et al: Metabolic basis of obesity in non–insulin dependent diabetes mellitus. Diabetes Metab Rev 4:727–747, 1988.

129. Randle PJ, Newsholme EA, Garland PB: Regulation of glucose uptake by muscle. Effects of fatty acids, ketone bodies, pyruvate, and of alloxan-diabetes and starvation, on the uptake and metabolic fate of glucose in rate heart and diaphragm muscles. Biochem J 93:652–665, 1964.
130. Randle PJ: Regulatory interactions between lipids and carbohydrates: The glucose fatty acid cycle after 35 years. Diabetes Metab Rev 14:263–283, 1998.
131. Boden G: Free fatty acids, insulin resistance, and type 2 diabetes mellitus. Proc Assoc Am Physicians 111:241–248, 1999.
132. Roden M, Price TB, Perseghin G, et al: Mechanism of free-fatty acid induced insulin resistance in humans. J Clin Invest 97:2859–2865, 1996.
133. Dresner A, Laurent D, Marcucci M, et al: Effects of free fatty acids on glucose transport and IRS-1–associated phosphatidylinositol 3-kinase activity. J Clin Invest 103:253–259, 1999.
134. Chalkley SM, Hettiarachchi M, Chisholm DJ, Kraegen EW: Five-hour fatty acid elevation increases muscle lipids and impairs glycogen synthesis in the rat. Metabolism 47:1121–1126, 1998.
135. Griffin ME, Marcucci MJ, Cline GW, et al: Free fatty acid–induced insulin resistance is associated with activation of protein kinase C theta and alterations in the insulin signaling cascade. Diabetes 48:1270–1274, 1999.
136. Pan DJ, Lillioja S, Kriketos AD, et al: Skeletal muscle triglyceride levels are inversely related to insulin action. Diabetes 46:983–988, 1997.
137. Krssak M, Falk Petersen K, Dresner A, et al: Intramyocellular lipid concentrations are correlated with insulin sensitivity in humans: A ^{1}H NMR spectroscopy study. Diabetologia 42:113–116, 1999.
138. Perseghin G, Scifo P, De Cobelli F, et al: Intramyocellular triglyceride content is a determinant of in vivo insulin resistance in humans: A ^{1}H-^{13}C nuclear magnetic resonance spectroscopy assessment in offspring of type 2 diabetic parents. Diabetes 48:1600–1606, 1999.
139. Falholt K, Jensen I, Lindkaer Jensen S, et al: Carbohydrate and lipid metabolism of skeletal muscle in type 2 diabetic patients. Diabet Med 5:27–31, 1988.
140. Jacob S, Machann J, Rett K, et al: Association of increased intramyocellular lipid content with insulin resistance in lean nondiabetic offspring of type 2 diabetic subjects. Diabetes 48:1113–1119, 1999.
141. Kono T, Barham FW: The relationship between the insulin-binding capacity of fat cells and the cellular response to insulin: Studies with intact and trypsin-treated fat cells. J Biol Chem 246:6210–6216, 1971.
142. Kolterman OG, Scarlett JA, Olefsky JM: Insulin resistance in non–insulin-dependent, type II diabetes mellitus. J Clin Endocrinol Metab 11:363–388, 1982.
143. Gliemann J, Gammeltoft JS, Vinten J: Time course of insulin-receptor binding and insulin-induced lipogenesis in isolated rat fat cells. J Biol Chem 250:3368–3374, 1975.
144. Kahn CR: Insulin resistance, insulin insensitivity, and insulin unresponsiveness: A necessary distinction. Metab Clin Exp 27:1893–1902, 1978.
145. Olefsky JM: Insulin resistance and insulin action: An in vitro and in vivo perspective. Diabetes 20:148–162, 1981.
146. Bar RS, Gordon P, Roth J, et al: Fluctuations in the affinity and concentration of insulin receptors on circulating monocytes of obese patients: Effects of starvation, refeeding and dieting. J Clin Invest 58:1123–1135, 1976.
147. Olefsky JM, Reaven GM: Decreased insulin binding to lymphocytes from diabetic patients. J Clin Invest 54:1323–1328, 1974.
148. Beck-Nielsen H: The pathogenetic role of an insulin receptor defect in diabetes mellitus of the obese. Diabetes 27:1175–1181, 1978.
149. Olefsky JM, Reaven GM: Insulin binding in diabetes: Relationships with plasma insulin levels and insulin sensitivity. Diabetes 26:680–688, 1977.
150. Freidenberg GR, Reichart D, Olefsky JM, Henry RR: Reversibility of defective adipocyte insulin receptor kinase activity in non–insulin dependent diabetes mellitus: Effect of weight loss. J Clin Invest 82:1398–1406, 1990.
151. Caro JF, Sinha MK, Raju SJ, et al: Insulin receptor kinase in human skeletal muscle from obese subjects with and without non–insulin dependent diabetes. J Clin Invest 79:1330–1337, 1987.
152. Maegawa H, Shigeta Y, Egawa K, Kobayashi M: Impaired autophosphorylation of insulin receptors from abdominal skeletal muscles in nonobese subjects with NIDDM. Diabetes 40:815–819, 1991.
153. Kobayashi M, Olefsky JM: Effects of streptozotocin-induced diabetes on insulin binding, glucose transport, and intracellular glucose metabolism in isolated rat adipocytes. Diabetes 28:87–95, 1979.
154. Kashiwagi A, Verso MA, Andrews J, et al: In vitro insulin resistance of human adipocytes isolated from subjects with noninsulin-dependent diabetes mellitus. J Clin Invest 72:1246–1254, 1983.
155. Bolinder J, Ostman J, Arner P: Postreceptor defects causing insulin resistance in normoinsulinemic non–insulin-dependent diabetes mellitus. Diabetes 31:911–916, 1982.
156. Muggeo M, Bar RS, Roth J, et al: The insulin resistance of acromegaly: Evidence for two alterations in the insulin receptor on circulating monocytes. J Clin Endocrinol Metab 48:17–25, 1977.
157. Kahn CR, Goldfine ID, Neville DM Jr, DeMeyts P: Alterations in insulin binding induced by changes in vivo in the levels of glucocorticoids and growth hormone. Endocrinology 103:1054–1066, 1978.
158. Bertoli A, DePirro R, Fusco A, et al: Differences in insulin receptors between men and menstruating women and influence of sex hormones on insulin binding during the menstrual cycle. J Clin Endocrinol Metab 50:246–250, 1980.
159. Bar RS, Lewis WR, Rechler MM, et al: Extreme insulin resistance in ataxia telangiectasia: Defect in affinity of insulin receptors. N Engl J Med 298:1164–1171, 1978.
160. Oseid S, Beck-Nielsen H, Pedersen O: Decreased binding of insulin to its receptor in patients with congenital generalized lipodystrophy. N Engl J Med 296:245–248, 1977.
161. Comi RJ, Grunberger G, Gorden P: The relationship of insulin binding and insulin-stimulated tyrosine kinase activity is altered in type II diabetes. J Clin Invest 79:453–462, 1987.
162. Brillon DJ, Freidenberg GR, Henry RR, Olefsky JM: Mechanism of defective insulin receptor kinase activity in NIDDM: Evidence for two receptor populations. Diabetes 38:397–403, 1989.
163. Freidenberg GR, Reichart D, Olefsky JM: Insulin receptor kinase activity is not reduced in fibroblasts from subjects with non–insulin dependent diabetes mellitus (NIDDM) (abstract). Clin Res 38:119, 1990.
164. Kusari J, Berma US, Buse JB, et al: Analysis of the gene sequences of the insulin receptor and the insulin sensitive glucose transporter (Glut-4) in patients with common type non–insulin dependent diabetes mellitus. J Clin Invest 88:1323–1330, 1991.
165. O'Rahilly S, Choi WH, Patel P, et al: Detection of mutations in insulin-receptor gene in NIDDM patients by analysis of single-stranded conformation polymorphisms. Diabetes 40:777–782, 1991.
166. Seino S, Seino M, Nishi S, Bell GI: Structure of the human insulin receptor gene and characterization of its promoter. Proc Natl Acad Sci U S A 86:114–118, 1989.
167. Moller DE, Yokota A, Flier JS: Normal insulin-receptor cDNA sequence in Pima Indians with NIDDM. Diabetes 38:1496–1500, 1989.
168. Zierath JR, He L, Guma A, et al: Insulin action on glucose transport and plasma membrane Glut 4 content in skeletal muscle from patients with NIDDM. Diabetologia 39:1180–1189, 1996.
169. Scarlett JA, Gray RS, Griffin J, et al: Insulin treatment reverses the insulin resistance of type II diabetes mellitus. Diabetes Care 5:353–363, 1982.
170. Dohm L, Tapscott EB, Pories WJ, et al: An in vitro human muscle preparation suitable for metabolic studies: Decreased insulin stimulation of glucose transport in muscle from morbidly obese and diabetic subjects. J Clin Invest 82:486–494, 1988.
171. Garvey WT, Maianu L, Huecksteadt TP, et al: Pretranslational suppression of a glucose transporter protein causes cellular insulin resistance in non–insulin-dependent diabetes mellitus and obesity. J Clin Invest 87:1072–1081, 1991.
172. Pedersen O, Bak JF, Andersen PH: Evidence against altered expression of GLUT1 or GLUT4 in skeletal muscle of patients with obesity or NIDDM. Diabetes 39:865–870, 1990.
173. Eriksson J, Koranyi L, Bourey R, et al: Insulin resistance in type 2 (non–insulin-dependent) diabetic patients and their relatives is not associated with a defect in the expression of the insulin-responsive glucose transporter (GLUT-4) gene in human skeletal muscle. Diabetologia 35:143–147, 1992.
174. Garvey WT, Maianu L, Hancock JA, et al: Gene expression of GLUT4 in skeletal muscle from insulin-resistant patients with obesity, IGT, GDM, and NIDDM. Diabetes 41:465–475, 1992.
175. Buse JB, Yasuda K, Lay TP, et al: Human GLUT4/muscle-fat glucose transporter gene: Characterization and genetic variation. Diabetes 41:1436–1445, 1982.
176. Choi W-H, O'Rahilly S, Buse JB, et al: Molecular scanning of insulin-responsive glucose transporter (GLUT4) gene in NIDDM subjects. Diabetes 40:1712–1718, 1991.
177. Kian X, Rothenberg P, Kahn CR, et al: Structure of the insulin receptor substrate IRS-1 defines a unique signal transduction protein. Nature 35:73–80, 1991.
178. Shoelson SE, Chaterjee S, Chaudhuri M, White MF: YMXM motifs of IRS-1 define substrate specificities of the insulin receptor kinase. Proc Natl Acad Sci U S A 89:2027–2031, 1992.
179. Thies RS, Molina JM, Ciaraldi TP, et al: Insulin receptor autophosphorylation and endogenous substrate phosphorylation in human adipocytes from control obese, and non–insulin dependent diabetic subjects. Diabetes 39:250–259, 1990.
180. Bjornholm M, Kawano Y, Lehtihet M, Zierath JR: Insulin receptor substrate-1 phosphorylation and phosphatidylinositol 3-kinase activity in skeletal muscle from NIDDM subjects after in vivo insulin stimulation. Diabetes 46:524–527, 1997.
181. Rondinone CM, Wang LM, Lonnroth P, et al: Insulin receptor substrate (IRS)1 is reduced and IRS-2 is the main docking protein for phosphatidylinositol 3-kinase in adipocytes from subjects with non–insulin-dependent diabetes mellitus. Proc Natl Acad Sci U S A 94:4171–4175, 1997.
182. Andreelli F, Laville M, Ducluzeau PH, et al: Defective regulation of phosphatidylinositol-3-kinase gene expression in skeletal muscle and adipose tissue of non–insulin-dependent diabetes mellitus patients. Diabetologia 42:358–364, 1999.
183. Almind K, Bjorbaek C, Vestergaard H, et al: Aminoacid polymorphisms of insulin receptor substrate-1 in non–insulin-dependent diabetes mellitus. Lancet 342:828–832, 1993.
184. Hager J, Zouali H, Velho G, et al: Insulin receptor substrate (IRS-1) gene polymorphisms in French NIDDM families. Lancet 342:1430, 1993.
185. Vestergaard H, Bjorbaek C, Andersen PH, et al: Impaired expression of glycogen synthase mRNA in skeletal muscle in NIDDM patients. Diabetes 40:1740–1745, 1991.
186. Wahren J, Felig P, Cerasi E, Luft R: Splanchnic and peripheral glucose and amino acid metabolism in diabetes mellitus. J Clin Invest 51:1870–1878, 1972.
187. Rothman DL, Magnusson I, Katz LD, Shulman GI: Quantitation of hepatic glycogenolysis and gluconeogenesis in fasting humans with ^{13}C NMR. Science 254:573–576, 1991.
188. Magnusson I, Rothman DL, Katz LD, et al: Increased rate of gluconeogenesis in type II diabetes mellitus: A ^{13}C nuclear magnetic resonance study. J Clin Invest 90:1323–1327, 1992.
189. Consoli A, Nurjhan N, Reilly JJ, et al: Mechanism of increased gluconeogenesis in non–insulin-dependent diabetes mellitus: Role of alterations in systemic, hepatic, and muscle lactate and alanine metabolism. J Clin Invest 86:2038–2045, 1990.
190. Orci L: The insulin cell: Its cellular environment and how it processes (pro)insulin. Diabetes Metab Rev 2:71–106, 1986.
191. Baron AD, Schmeiser L, Shragg GP, Kolterman OG: The role of hyperglucagonemia in the maintenance of increased rates of hepatic glucose output in type II diabetics. Diabetes 36:274–283, 1987.
192. Rebrin K, Steil GM, Getty L, Bergman RN: Free fatty acid as a link in the regulation of hepatic glucose output by peripheral insulin. Diabetes 44:1038–1045, 1995.
193. Mitrakou A, Kelley D, Veneman T, et al: Contribution of abnormal muscle and liver glucose metabolism to postprandial hyperglycemia in NIDDM. Diabetes 39:1381–1390, 1990.

194. Felig P, Wahren J, Hendler R: Influence of oral glucose ingestion on splanchnic glucose and gluconeogenic substrate metabolism in man. Diabetes 24:468–475, 1975.
195. Ferrannini E, Bjorkman O, Reichard GA, et al: The disposal of an oral glucose load in healthy subjects: A quantitative study. Diabetes 34:580–588, 1985.
196. Taylor R, Magnusson I, Rothman DL, et al: Direct assessment of liver glycogen storage by ^{13}C nuclear magnetic resonance spectroscopy and regulation of glucose homeostasis after a mixed meal in normal subjects. J Clin Invest 97:126–132, 1996.
197. Shulman GI, Cline G, Schumann WC, et al: Quantitative comparison of pathways of hepatic glycogen repletion in fed and fasted humans. Am J Physiol 259:E335–E341, 1990.
198. Katz J, McGarry JD: The glucose paradox: Is glucose a substrate for liver metabolism? J Clin Invest 74:1901–1909, 1984.
199. Niewoehner CB, Nuttall FQ: Relationship of hepatic glucose uptake to intrahepatic glucose concentration in fasted rats after glucose load. Diabetes 37:1559–1566, 1988.
200. Wals PA, Katz J: A concentration gradient of glucose from liver to plasma. Metabolism 42:1492–1496, 1993.
201. Ludvik B, Nolan JJ, Roberts A, et al: Evidence for decreased splanchnic glucose uptake after oral glucose administration in non–insulin-dependent diabetes mellitus. J Clin Invest 100:2354–2361, 1997.
202. Baron AD, Kolterman OG, Bell J, et al: Rates of non–insulin mediated glucose uptake are elevated in type II diabetic subjects. J Clin Invest 76:1782–1788, 1986.
203. Ginsberg H, Rayfield EJ: Effect of insulin therapy on insulin resistance in type II diabetic subjects: Evidence for heterogeneity. Diabetes 30:739–744, 1981.
204. Andrews WJ, Vasquez B, Nagulesparan M, et al: Insulin therapy in obese, non–insulin-dependent diabetes induces improvements in insulin action and secretion that are maintained for two weeks after insulin withdrawal. Diabetes 33:634–642, 1984.
205. Firth RG, Bell PM, Rizza RA: Effects of tolazamide and exogenous insulin on insulin action in patients with non–insulin dependent diabetes mellitus. N Engl J Med 314:1280–1286, 1986.
206. Henry RR, Gumbiner B, Ditzler T, et al: Intensive conventional insulin therapy for type II diabetes. Diabetes Care 16:21–31, 1993.
207. Vestergaard H, Weinreb JE, Rosen AS, et al: Sulfonylurea therapy improves glucose disposal without changing skeletal muscle Glut 4 levels in non–insulin-dependent diabetes mellitus: A longitudinal study. J Clin Endocrinol Metab 80:270–275, 1995.
208. Firth R, Bell P, Marsh M, Rizza RA: Effects of tolazamide and exogenous insulin on pattern of postprandial carbohydrate metabolism in patients with non–insulin-dependent diabetes mellitus: Results of randomized crossover trial. Diabetes 36:1130–1138, 1987.
209. Hollenbeck CB, Reaven GM: Treatment of patients with non–insulin-dependent diabetes mellitus: Diabetic control and insulin secretion and action after different treatment modalities. Diabet Med 4:311–316, 1987.
210. Henry RR, Scheaffer L, Olefsky JM: Glycemic effects of short-term intensive dietary restriction and isocaloric refeeding in non–insulin dependent diabetes mellitus. J Clin Endocrinol Metab 61:917–925, 1985.
211. Bogardus C, Ravussin E, Robbins DC, et al: Effects of physical training and diet therapy on carbohydrate metabolism in patients with glucose intolerance and non–insulin-dependent diabetes mellitus. Diabetes 33:311–318, 1984.
212. Savage PJ, Bennion LJ, Flock EV, et al: Diet-induced improvement of abnormalities in insulin and glucagon secretion and in insulin receptor binding in diabetes mellitus. J Clin Endocrinol Metab 48:999–1007, 1979.
213. Yki-Jarvinen H: Glucose toxicity. Endocr Rev 13:415–431, 1992.
214. Vuorinen-Markkola H, Koivisto VA, Yki-Jarvinen H: Mechanisms of hyperglycemia-induced insulin resistance in whole body and skeletal muscle of type 1 diabetic patients. Diabetes 41:571–580, 1992.
215. Saltiel AR, Olefsky JM: Thiazolidinediones in the treatment of insulin resistance and type II diabetes. Diabetes 45:1661–1669, 1996.
216. Yu JG, Kruszynska YT, Mulford MI, Olefsky JM: A comparison of troglitazone and metformin on insulin requirements in euglycemic, intensively treated type 2 diabetic mellitus patients. Diabetes 48:2414–2421, 1999.
217. Nolan JJ, Ludvik B, Beerdsen P, et al: Improvement in glucose tolerance and insulin resistance in obese subjects treated with troglitazone. N Engl J Med 331:1188–1193, 1994.
218. Cavaghan MK, Ehrmann DA, Byrne MM, Polonsky KS: Treatment with the oral antidiabetic agent troglitazone improves β cell responses to glucose in subjects with impaired glucose tolerance. J Clin Invest 100:530–537, 1997.
219. Bell GI, Xiang KS, Newman MV, et al: Gene for non–insulin-dependent diabetes mellitus (maturity onset diabetes of the young subtype) is linked to DNA polymorphism on human chromosome 20q. Proc Natl Acad Sci U S A 88:1484–1488, 1991.
220. Yamagata K, Furuta J, Oda N, et al: Mutations in the hepatocyte nuclear factor 4-α gene in maturity-onset diabetes of the young (MODY 1). Nature 384:458–460, 1996.
221. Permutt MA, Chiu KC, Tanizawa Y: Glucokinase and NIDDM: A candidate gene that paid off. Diabetes 41:1367–1372, 1992.
222. Miller SP, Anand GR, Karschnia EJ, et al: Characterization of glucokinase mutations associated with maturity-onset diabetes of the young type 2 (MODY-2): Different glucokinase defects lead to a common phenotype. Diabetes 48:1645–1651, 1999.
223. Yamagata K, Oda N, Kaisaki PJ, et al: Mutations in the hepatocyte nuclear factor-1α gene in maturity onset diabetes of the young (MODY 3). Nature 384:455–458, 1996.

224. Stoffers DA, Ferrer J, Clarke WL, Habener JF: Early-onset type II diabetes mellitus (MODY 4) linked to IPF1. Nat Genet 117:138–139, 1997.
225. Matsuoka N, Ogawa Y, Hosoda K, et al: Human leptin receptor gene in obese Japanese subjects: Evidence against either obesity-causing mutations or association of sequence variants with obesity. Diabetologia 40:1204–1210, 1997.
226. Rolland V, Clement K, Dugail I, et al: Leptin receptor gene in a large cohort of massively obese subjects: No indication of the fa/fa rat mutation. Detection of an intronic variant with no association with obesity. Obes Res 6:122–127, 1998.
227. Widen E, Lehto M, Kanninen T, et al: Association of a polymorphism in the β3-adrenergic-receptor gene with features of insulin resistance syndrome in Finns. N Engl J Med 333:348–351, 1995.
228. O'Dell SD, Bolla MK, Miller GJ, et al: W64R mutation in β-3-adrenergic receptor gene and weight in a large population sample. Int J Obes 22:377–379, 1998.
229. Large V, Hellstrom L, Reynisdottir S, et al: Human beta-2 adrenoceptor gene polymorphisms are highly frequent in obesity and associate with altered adipocyte beta-2 adrenoceptor function. J Clin Invest 100;3005–3013, 1997.
230. Hanis CL, Boerwinkle E, Chakraborty R, et al: A genome-wide search for human non–insulin-dependent (type 2) diabetes genes reveals a major susceptibility locus on chromosome 2. Nat Genet 13:161–166, 1996.
231. Ghosh S, Watanabe RM, Hauser ER, et al: Type 2 diabetes: Evidence for linkage on chromosome 20 in 716 Finnish affected sib pairs. Proc Natl Acad Sci U S A 96:2198–2203, 1999.
232. Bowden DW, Sale M, Howard TD, et al: Linkage of genetic markers on human chromosomes 20 and 12 to NIDDM in Caucasian sib pairs with a history of diabetic nephropathy. Diabetes 46:882–886, 1997.
233. Duggirala R, Blangero J, Almasy L, et al: Linkage of type 2 diabetes mellitus and of age at onset to a genetic location on chromosome 10q in Mexican Americans. Am J Hum Genet 64:1127–1140, 1999.
234. Elbein SC, Hoffman MD, Teng K, et al: A genome-wide search for type 2 diabetes susceptibility genes in Utah Caucasians. Diabetes 48:1175–1182, 1999.
235. Shaw JT, Lovelock PK, Kesting JB, et al: Novel susceptibility gene for late-onset NIDDM is localized to human chromosome 12q. Diabetes 47:1793–1796, 1998.
236. Hanson RL, Ehm MG, Pettitt DJ, et al: An autosomal genomic scan for loci linked to type II diabetes mellitus and body-mass index in Pima Indians. Am J Hum Genet 63:1130–1138, 1998.
237. Stern MP, Duggirala R, Mitchell BD, et al: Evidence for linkage of regions on chromosomes 6 and 11 to plasma glucose concentrations in Mexican Americans. Genome Res 6:724–734, 1996.
238. Cox NJ, Frigge M, Nicolae DL, et al: Loci on chromosomes 2 (NIDDM1) and 15 interact to increase susceptibility to diabetes in Mexican Americans. Nat Genet 21:213–215, 1999.
239. Pratley RE, Thompson DB, Prochazka M, et al: An autosomal genomic scan for loci linked to prediabetic phenotypes in Pima Indians. J Clin Invest 101:1757–1764, 1998.
240. Mitchell BD, Kammerer CM, O'Connell P et al: Evidence for linkage of postchallenge insulin levels with intestinal fatty acid–binding protein (FABP2) in Mexican-Americans. Diabetes 44:1046–1053, 1995.
241. Humphreys P, McCarthy M, Tuomilehto J, et al: Chromosome 4q locus associated with insulin resistance in Pima Indians: Studies in three European NIDDM populations. Diabetes 43:800–804, 1994.
242. Joshi RL, Lamothe B, Cordonnier N, et al: Targeted disruption of the insulin receptor gene in the mouse results in neonatal lethality. EMBO J 15:1542–1547, 1996.
243. Araki E, Lipes MY, Patti M-E, et al: Alternative pathway of insulin signalling in mice with targeted disruption of the IRS-1 gene. Nature 372:186–190, 1994.
244. Bruning JC, Winnay J, Bonner-Weir S, et al: Development of a novel polygenic model of NIDDM in mice heterozygous for IR and IRS-1 null alleles. Cell 88:561–572, 1997.
245. Kido Y, Kanno H, Withers DJ, et al: Interaction between insulin receptor and IRS proteins in IR/IRS-1$^{+/-}$ and IR/IRS-2$^{+/-}$ mice (abstract). Diabetes 48(suppl 1):10, 1999.
246. Terauchi Y, Iwamoto K, Tamemoto H, et al: Development of non–insulin-dependent diabetes mellitus in the double knockout mice with disruption of insulin receptor substrate-1 and beta cell glucokinase genes. Genetic reconstitution of diabetes as a polygenic disease. J Clin Invest 99:861–866, 1997.
247. Kulkarni RN, Bruning JC, Winnay JN, et al: Tissue-specific knockout of the insulin receptor in pancreatic β cells creates an insulin secretory defect similar to that in type 2 diabetes. Cell 96:329–339, 1999.
248. Scarlett JA, Kolterman OG, Moore P, et al: Insulin resistance and diabetes due to a genetic defect in insulin receptors. J Clin Endocrinol Metab 55:123–132, 1982.
249. Pimenta W, Korytkowski M, Mitrakou A, et al: Pancreatic beta-cell dysfunction as the primary genetic lesion in NIDDM: Evidence from studies in normal glucose-tolerant individuals with a first-degree NIDDM relative. JAMA 273:1855–1861, 1995.
250. Turner RC, Cull CA, Frighi V, Holman RR: Glycemic control with diet, sulfonylurea, metformin, or insulin in patients with type 2 diabetes mellitus: Progressive requirement for multiple therapies (UKPDS 49). UK Prospective Diabetes Study (UKPDS) Group. JAMA 281:2005–2012, 1999.

Chapter 56

▼▼▼

Syndromes of Insulin Resistance and Mutant Insulin

Jeffrey S. Flier ▪ Christos Mantzoros

This chapter considers two heterogeneous groups of clinical syndromes. One is defined by severe resistance of tissues to insulin and the other by mutations in the insulin gene. In many cases, patients with these disorders first came to attention when their diabetes mellitus displayed one or more unusual features that prompted detailed study. It is now apparent, however, that diabetes never develops in many such patients; the syndromes of severe insulin resistance in particular are noted for the heterogeneous clinical features that are responsible for patients' seeking medical attention. Recently, considerable progress has been made toward elucidation of the molecular basis for these disorders, and such knowledge has produced new insight into the basic aspects of hormone synthesis, hormone action, and metabolic regulation. The often striking clinical phenotypes and defined molecular etiologies of these syndromes have led them to receive more attention than would be justified solely on the basis of their relatively low prevalence.

INSULIN RESISTANCE: DEFINITION AND HISTORICAL SYNOPSIS

Insulin resistance is a state in which a given concentration of insulin produces a subnormal biologic response.[1] This term initially arose in the years after the introduction of insulin therapy in 1922 to describe occasional patients in whom unusually large doses of insulin were required to control glycemia. No insights into possible mechanisms or treatments were available. The concept was developed further in the 1930s by Himsworth, who examined the response of meal-related glycemia to insulin administration in diabetes and suggested that two subsets of patients, one insulin sensitive and the other insulin resistant, could be distinguished.[2] The two groups most likely represented what would later be termed type 1 and type 2 diabetes, but further elucidation of this important concept awaited a number of technical advances that occurred between 1960 and the mid-1970s. These advances included the ability to measure circulating insulin levels,[3] to measure insulin action in explants of tissue or cells, to identify and quantitate insulin receptors,[4] and to quantitate the actions of insulin in vivo.[5] The ability to measure insulin levels by radioimmunoassay rapidly led to evidence that subjects with obesity and maturity-onset (later type 2) diabetes did not have absolute insulin deficiency but typically had

increased levels of insulin, thus suggesting the presence of insulin resistance.[3] This finding stimulated considerable inquiry into the cellular and molecular mechanisms of insulin resistance.

The ability to measure and characterize insulin receptors on target cells was a major catalyst to subsequent progress. Mild and variable defects in insulin receptor expression were observed in the common disorders of non–insulin-dependent diabetes mellitus (NIDDM) and obesity, although the pathogenetic significance of these defects in causing the insulin resistance was debated.[6] Subsequent studies revealed a small subset of clinically distinct patients with severe degrees of resistance to exogenous insulin who had markedly elevated levels of endogenous insulin.[7] Studies in these subjects revealed profound defects at the level of receptor binding, and in one subgroup of those with severe acquired resistance the binding defect was shown to be caused by antireceptor antibodies.[8] This finding strengthened the view that the insulin receptor measured in binding studies was indeed a relevant reflection of the insulin action pathway. The discovery that the insulin receptor was a hormone-activated tyrosine kinase[9] and subsequent cloning of the insulin receptor cDNA[10] and gene have been followed by the demonstration that the receptor gene was the locus for mutations causing insulin resistance in some patients.[11, 12] The molecular and genetic explanation for insulin resistance in the vast majority of subjects with NIDDM remains unknown. The validation of in vivo techniques for quantitative assessment of insulin action has supported efforts to characterize insulin resistance in well-defined subgroups of patients. More recently, suggestions that many nondiabetic individuals with common disorders such as obesity, hypertension, hyperlipedemia,[13] atherosclerosis, and ovarian hyperandrogenism[14] have insulin resistance have further increased general biologic interest in this topic.

CLINICAL SPECTRUM OF SEVERE INSULIN RESISTANCE

Patients with syndromes of severe insulin resistance have clinical features that vary over a broad spectrum (Table 56–1). This description is true for glucose homeostasis as well as for other associated features. At one end of the spectrum are patients with overt diabetes who are unresponsive to both conventional and suprapharmacologic doses of

TABLE 56–1. Clinical Features in Patients with Severe Insulin Resistance

Glucose homeostasis: Diabetes, impaired glucose tolerance, hypoglycemia
Cutaneous: Acanthosis nigricans, skin tags, alopecia
Reproductive: Amenorrhea, hirsutism, clitoromegaly (males normal)
Linear growth: Normal, impaired, increased
Adipose tissue: Normal, lipoatrophy, lipohypertrophy, obesity
Musculoskeletal: Cramps, muscle hypertrophy, pseudoacromegaly
Lipids: Normal, hypertriglyceridemia
Autoimmunity: Type B syndrome

insulin. Much more commonly, despite severe insulin resistance patients have glucose intolerance, which is often quite mild and does not require insulin therapy. Indeed, hypoglycemia may be present in some individuals. In all cases, however, resistance to endogenous and exogenous insulin is, by definition, present. In most individuals who do not have overt diabetes, clinical diagnosis depends on the presence and recognition of a diverse array of associated features. The nature of these features and their relationship to insulin resistance are discussed at length below, but they are mentioned briefly here. The skin lesion acanthosis nigricans is present in virtually all patients and is a key clinical clue to the existence of insulin resistance.[15] In women, consequences of ovarian hyperandrogenism such as amenorrhea and hirsutism or virilization are extremely common, and especially when coupled with acanthosis, these features provoke diagnostic evaluation. Retarded growth and accelerated linear or acral growth are seen in specific syndromes, as is total or partial lipodystrophy. When insulin resistance is due to antireceptor autoantibodies, autoimmunity and a broad array of its clinical consequences are characteristically found. Finally, some patients with severe insulin resistance have no clinical abnormalities and are discovered to have insulin resistance only after identification of insulin resistance in an affected family member.

ASPECTS OF INSULIN ACTION RELEVANT TO UNDERSTANDING SYNDROMES OF INSULIN RESISTANCE

The details of insulin action from the level of molecular signaling to that of physiologic integration are discussed elsewhere in this book, but a number of aspects of this important subject are particularly relevant to the syndromes of insulin resistance. Insulin is the dominant hormone for regulation of glucose homeostasis, with liver, muscle, and adipose tissue being the most important sites of action in this regard. It is clear, however, that insulin is a hormone with pleiotropic effects. Thus insulin is just as important as a regulator of protein and fat metabolism as it is a regulator of carbohydrate metabolism, and it exerts actions in classic glucoregulatory organs such as muscle, fat, and liver, as well as in organs such as the ovary that do not play a role in metabolic regulation.[16] When insulin acts through insulin receptors expressed on cells such as ovarian theca cells[17] and vascular endothelial cells,[18] it brings about actions that are specific to these individual differentiated cell types. The physiologic importance of these latter actions has not been clearly defined.

Several aspects of insulin signaling have significance for our understanding of syndromes of insulin resistance and, in particular, the heterogeneous clinical features that accompany these syndromes. The first step in insulin action is binding to a heterotetrameric glycoprotein insulin receptor that is expressed on the plasma membrane of virtually all cells.[19] Insulin binding to the extracellular α subunit stimulates the autophosphorylation and subsequent tyrosine kinase activity of the transmembrane β subunit.[20] Most data suggest that this kinase activity plays a critical role in insulin action via generation of one or more molecular signals that regulate diverse cellular events, including membrane transport, activity of numerous enzymes, level of gene expression, and overall levels of protein and DNA synthesis. These many actions take place with time courses ranging from seconds to hours and vary from tissue to tissue, depending in large measure on the array of proteins expressed in particular tissues.

Insulin can act through more than a single species of receptor protein. Alternative splicing of the receptor gene results in two receptor isoforms differing by 12 amino acids in the distal α subunit.[21] Subtle functional differences between the two forms have been defined through in vitro studies.[22, 23] In addition to these two receptor splice variants, insulin can bind to and activate the structurally related insulin-like growth factor-1 (IGF-1) receptor,[24] although the relative affinity of this receptor for insulin is at least 100-fold lower than that of the insulin receptor. Hybrid receptors composed of half insulin receptor and half IGF-1 receptor subunits also exist, with as yet uncertain signaling capacity and function.[25, 26] In addition to the multiple species of receptor proteins that can function as receptors for insulin, results of receptor mutagenesis studies suggest that divergence of signaling by the insulin receptor can begin within the receptor itself. Thus specific receptor variants have been described that have retained the ability to activate some but not all postreceptor pathways in the cell.[27]

Complexity also exists further downstream in the signaling process. Although many of the steps that mediate insulin signaling beyond the receptor remain uncertain, it is well established that many and perhaps all insulin actions involve mediation of changes in the level of serine phosphorylation of target proteins, including a cascade of signaling kinases and metabolic effector molecules such as glycogen synthase that are regulated through phosphorylation and dephosphorylation mechanisms.[28] Binding of insulin to its receptor results in insulin receptor autophosphorylation and subsequent tyrosine phosphorylation of intracellular signaling intermediates,[29] among which are the insulin receptor substrates (IRS-1, IRS-2), Shc, and Gab1.[6, 7] These molecules bind to and activate other downstream effectors of insulin action, including the adapter proteins Grb2 (growth factor receptor–binding protein-2) and Nck, the tyrosine phosphatase Syp, and the phosphoinositide 3-kinase, which amplify and diversify the initial signal generated by insulin binding to its receptor.[6] Several pathways downstream of the insulin receptor are subsequently activated, including the ras (Grb2-mSOS [mammalian son of sevenless]-Ras) mitogen-activated protein kinase pathway, the pp70 kinase pathway, the PKB (protein kinase B)/Akt pathway, and possibly other, not yet identified pathways. Activation of these downstream effectors of insulin results in such well-documented insulin effects as stimulation of cellular glucose and amino acid uptake, glycogen synthesis, lipogenesis, and mitogenesis.[6]

The basis for termination of the insulin signal is also not well defined at this time. It is clear that the receptor kinase activity reverses rapidly after removal of the hormone, and one or more members of a family of phosphotyrosine phosphatases may be responsible for this reversal.[30] Recent data indicate that disruption of the mouse homologue of the gene encoding protein tyrosine phosphatase 1B results in increased insulin sensitivity and obesity resistance.[31] These data raise the possibility that this molecule may be a potential therapeutic target in the treatment of insulin resistance and NIDDM.[31] Clearance of insulin from the circulation is brought about in large measure by a receptor-mediated process, and defects in receptor function such as those that impair receptor signaling typically impair receptor-mediated clearance both in vitro and in vivo.[32] Thus in patients with certain receptor defects, hyperinsulinemia results both from increased β cell secretion and from increased half-life of the hormone. Finally, despite the diverse effects of insulin on tissues throughout the body, feedback regulation of insulin secretion is dominated by the blood glucose level, which has several implications. First, compensatory hyperinsulinemia will occur in response to any defect that impairs disposal of glucose or suppression of hepatic glucose production in response to insulin. Indeed, hyperinsulinemia should result from any defect causing impaired glucoregulation, even if the impairment involves a distal step in the pathway of insulin action. If the defect in insulin action that initiates this problem is not global, hyperinsulinemia may actually promote excessive insulin action through less severely affected or unaffected signaling pathways.

MECHANISMS RESPONSIBLE FOR SEVERE INSULIN RESISTANCE

Several different classifications of mechanisms of severe insulin resistance have been proposed (Table 56–2).

TABLE 56–2. Molecular Mechanisms of Severe Insulin Resistance

Intrinsic defects in target cell function (genetic)
  Mutation in the insulin receptor gene
  Mutations in other genes involved in insulin action (putative): IRS-1,
    signaling kinases or phosphatases, transporters, metabolic enzymes
  Mutations in genes involved in terminating the insulin signal (putative)
  Mutations in genes whose encoded proteins bring about alterations in target
    cell function (putative), i.e., lymphokines, hypothalamic genes
Acquired defects in target cell function
  Autoantibodies to insulin receptor
  Other (rarely cause severe resistance)
    Hormones: Glucocorticoids, growth hormone, catecholamines, glucagon
    Metabolites: Glucose, free fatty acids
Antagonists of the insulin molecule
  Anti-insulin antibodies
  Insulin-degrading enzymes (insulinases)

Target Cell Defects

Defects in target cell responses to insulin can be inherited or acquired and can be due to defects that arise within the target cell or be secondary to extracellular factors. *Inherited defects* intrinsic to the target cell resulting in insulin resistance could, in theory, involve any step in the signaling pathway from the receptor to the distal events required for insulin action. The insulin receptor is by far the best defined and most extensively studied molecule in this pathway. Patients with several syndromes of severe insulin resistance have been shown to have mutations in the insulin receptor gene that affect receptor expression or function and account for the severe insulin resistance.[11, 12] These mutations are discussed in greater detail below. Little direct information is available on inherited defects in postreceptor pathways or effector mechanisms that might be responsible for target cell resistance in subjects with severe resistance who do not have receptor mutations. The GLUT4 glucose transporter, although a locus of altered protein expression or functional abnormality in NIDDM, has not been found to be intrinsically abnormal in genetic studies of the limited number of patients studied to date. Several polymorphisms in the amino acid sequence of human IRS-1 have been identified, and some of these mutations have been associated with impaired insulin signaling or increased risk for cardiovascular disease.[33, 34] However, other studies do not support the hypothesis that variant sequences of IRS-1 contribute to the pathogenesis of insulin resistance.[35] The possibility that genetic defects might exist that would cause increased expression or activity of intracellular inhibitors of insulin signaling has also begun to be addressed. In addition, a transmembrane glycoprotein named PC-1 has been proposed to inhibit insulin receptor tyrosine kinase activity, probably by interfering with a subunit of the insulin receptor. This glycoprotein has been identified in some patients with severe resistance to insulin and in patients with NIDDM.[36, 37]

Target cell resistance may also be *acquired*. Mild to moderate degrees of insulin resistance can be the result of increased local or circulating levels of a number of factors, including insulin itself (both insulin deficiency and hyperinsulinemia), free fatty acids,[38] glucose[39] (i.e., glucotoxicity), and the counterinsulin hormones (e.g., glucocorticoids, growth hormone, and catecholamines). Cytokines such as tumor necrosis factor have recently been shown to cause insulin resistance as well.[40] The observation that tumor necrosis factor may be overproduced by adipocytes in obesity and may be capable of inducing insulin resistance is an example of such a mechanism. Recent data indicate that the presence of a dominant negative mutation in human PPARγ (peroxisome proliferator–activated receptor-γ) is associated with severe insulin resistance, diabetes mellitus, and hypertension, thus indicating that this nuclear receptor responsible for adipocyte differentiation is important in the control of insulin sensitivity, glucose homeostasis, and blood pressure in humans.[41] Although some or all of these factors are likely to be important contributors to insulin resistance in a variety of disease states and may contribute to the resistance

in some patients with syndromes of severe resistance, the only acquired factor clearly shown to be responsible for severe target cell resistance is autoantibodies to the insulin receptor.

Direct Antagonists of the Insulin Molecule

Two substances are known to directly antagonize the insulin molecule itself, with the result being insulin resistance: (1) antibodies directed against insulin and (2) insulin-degrading enzymes, or insulinases. It should be stressed that the target cells are not resistant to insulin (unless the resistance is secondary to uncontrolled hyperglycemia) in the case of antagonism by either of these, and consequently, such clinical features as acanthosis nigricans that are found in disorders with target cell resistance are not seen.

Anti-insulin antibodies were documented to exist and cause resistance to insulin in a subset of patients with insulin-treated diabetes by Berson and Yalow.[42] This discovery led these investigators to invention of the radioimmunoassay technique, which they initially applied to the measurement of insulin. Insulin resistance caused by anti-insulin antibodies may or may not be associated with cutaneous allergy but is always associated with high titers of antibodies to insulin.[43, 44] This complication of insulin therapy has decreased markedly in recent years with the introduction and widespread use of human insulin and animal insulin of high purity; previously, the complication was associated with intermittent administration of animal insulin of limited purity. When it does occur in a patient receiving an animal insulin, resistance usually responds well to substitution with human insulin or, if this measure fails, to a preparation of sulfated beef insulin, which interacts poorly with anti-insulin antibodies.

The nature and function of insulin-degrading enzymes, or insulinases, has been a matter of interest for many years. A number of patients have been described with a syndrome interpreted as being due to excessive subcutaneous degradation of insulin.[45, 46] Characteristics of the syndrome have included resistance to subcutaneous but not intravenous insulin and clinical improvement through mixing of injected insulin with the protease inhibitor Trasylol. Limited evidence for the presence of heightened degrading activity in subcutaneous tissue has been provided. Subsequent reports of patients referred for evaluation of this syndrome have concluded that the vast majority have some other reason for apparent resistance to subcutaneous insulin, often related to psychologic factors or unusual behavior on the part of the patient, and resistance is not found when evaluation takes place in a specialized unit.[47] Thus, the existence of the disorder has not been confirmed, and its true prevalence is unknown. The recent cloning of an insulin protease[48] may facilitate future studies of the pathophysiology of such a disorder.

SPECIFIC SYNDROMES OF EXTREME INSULIN RESISTANCE

The Syndrome of Insulin Resistance Caused by Autoantibodies to the Insulin Receptor (Type B Syndrome)

Clinical Features

The existence of insulin receptor autoantibodies was first discovered in three patients in whom extremely insulin-resistant diabetes developed in association with the skin lesion acanthosis nigricans.[7] These patients had clinical features of autoimmunity and antibodies in their serum that blocked insulin binding to normal cells. The designation *type B* was used to distinguish them from type A patients, who had insulin resistance and acanthosis but no autoimmunity or antireceptor antibodies.

As seen in other autoimmune disorders, the disease is more common in females. It has been noted in many ethnic groups but is most common in blacks. The mean age at onset is about 40 years, but it has been seen as early as age 12 and as late as age 78. The most common clinical finding is hyperglycemia, often with symptoms of polyuria, polydipsia, and weight loss. Ketoacidosis has been observed but is uncommon. Acanthosis, which may be severe, nearly always develops at approximately the same time as the diabetes. The most striking aspect of the clinical picture is the resistance to insulin therapy, which is typically observed from the first insulin dose and is severe, with some patients unresponsive to doses as high as 10,000 U/day.

Other clinical manifestations are possible. Thus some patients with antireceptor antibodies have hypoglycemia as the primary metabolic feature,[49, 50] and the hypoglycemia may exist alone or as fasting hypoglycemia in conjunction with postprandial hyperglycemia. Acanthosis nigricans may be less common in patients in whom hypoglycemia is the dominant metabolic feature. Diagnostic evaluation of fasting hypoglycemia in such patients may be confusing because insulin levels may be inappropriately elevated as a result of antibody-induced inhibition of insulin clearance.[49] Distinguishing antireceptor antibody–induced hypoglycemia from that caused by insulinoma is aided by measurement of C peptide and proinsulin because they are suppressed in the former but not in the latter condition.[49] The most critical aspect of diagnosis in this condition is thinking of it, and the combination of hypoglycemia or hyperglycemia with features of autoimmunity should prompt consideration of the diagnosis.

Two other types of abnormalities accompany the metabolic disturbance in this syndrome. The first encompasses a wide variety of clinical and laboratory features of autoimmunity, as seen in Table 56–3. Laboratory test results indicative of more widespread autoimmune disease include leukopenia (>80%), elevated antinuclear antibodies (>80%), elevated sedimentation rate (>80%), elevated serum IgG (>80%), proteinuria (50%), alopecia (36%), nephritis (30%), hypocomplementemia (29%), arthritis (20%), and vitiligo (14%). Prominent among these abnormalities are alopecia, vitiligo, arthralgias and arthritis, Raynaud phenomena, enlarged salivary glands, elevated sedimentation rate, leukopenia, hypergammaglobulinemia, and a positive antinuclear antibody test result. Most often these autoimmune features parallel the course of the metabolic disturbance, but they may precede the onset or clinical recognition of hypoglycemia or hyperglycemia. A second abnormality is limited to premenopausal women, in many of whom ovarian hyperandrogenism develops with clinical features ranging from hirsutism to virilization,[51] as typically seen in the type A syndrome.

Clinical Course and Treatment

The clinical course of illness in patients with antireceptor antibodies has been variable.[52] Some patients, particularly those with insulin-resistant diabetes, have had persistent diabetes with an inability of insulin therapy to improve the metabolic state. Other patients have had spontaneous remission of the metabolic disturbance, whether it be hyperglycemia or hypoglycemia, occurring months or years after clinical onset. In the most striking clinical progression, several insulin-resistant diabetic patients have evolved into a state of profound hypoglycemia over a period of several weeks to months. As discussed below, the molecular basis for this clinical evolution is not clear.

A number of treatments aimed at reducing the titer of antireceptor antibodies have been explored in limited groups or individual subjects. These approaches, including plasmapheresis[53] and immunosuppressive drugs, have not proved clearly successful. Glucocorticoids are the initial treatment of choice in patients with hypoglycemia because these agents have been successful in reversing or improving hypoglycemia in a number of reported cases[49] and in the authors' unpublished experience. At least initially, they appear to act by antagonizing the

agonistic action of antibodies rather than by reducing the titer of antibodies.[49] The use of glucocorticoids in patients with diabetes, especially in those with high titers of antibodies, is usually ineffective or worsens the problem. Insulin at extremely high doses may be of some benefit, but most often it is ineffective regardless of the dose. Sulfonylureas are ineffective, but one report suggests that the biguanide metformin may lower blood glucose through a postreceptor effect.[54] However, given the the relatively few patients studied and the fluctuating course in the absence of therapy, it is difficult to obtain a clear indication of the efficacy of these therapies.

Properties of Autoantibodies to the Insulin Receptor

Insulin receptor autoantibodies were initially discovered through the ability of serum and serum-derived immunoglobulins to block insulin binding after pre-exposure to insulin receptors from a wide variety of tissues and species.[8] These observations suggested that the antibodies bound to a conserved epitope on the receptor, and recent studies with cloned receptor variants demonstrate that a limited region of the receptor α subunit between amino acid residues 450 and 601 is the dominant site for antibody binding.[55] Some evidence also indicates that these polyclonal antibodies may be heterogeneous in certain respects. Thus in individual patients, antibodies have been described that bind to the receptor but fail to affect insulin binding[56] or even increase receptor affinity for insulin.[57]

Similar heterogeneity has been observed at the level of antibody bioactivity after exposure to insulin-sensitive cells. Given the fact that the initial patients were diabetic, it was expected that exposure to purified immunoglobulins from the patients would lead to blockade of insulin action. What was observed was far more complicated. Virtually all receptor antibodies, whether isolated from hyperglycemic or hypoglycemic patients, acutely stimulate insulin actions such as glucose uptake and metabolism in adipocytes.[58] The magnitude of this agonistic effect diminishes after a period of hours as a result of increased receptor degradation and postreceptor desensitization of uncertain mechanism. Cells then become refractory to further application of insulin.[59, 60] Although these facts allow us to account in theory for the occurrence of both hypoglycemia and insulin-resistant diabetes in these patients, it has not as yet been possible to correlate the properties of the immunoglobulins with the clinical metabolic profile in individual patients with diabetes or hypoglycemia.

The Type A Syndrome of Insulin Resistance and Its Clinical Variants

Clinical Features

The initial description of this syndrome involved three adolescent females with glucose intolerance or overt diabetes and extreme resistance to endogenous and exogenous insulin, together with hyperandrogenism and the skin lesion acanthosis nigricans.[7] The term *type A* was used to distinguish these patients from three others who had insulin resistance and acanthosis caused by insulin receptor autoantibodies (type B; see above), which the type A patients lacked. As more has been learned about the genetic basis for the syndrome and as a broad range of clinical syndromes of insulin resistance with different proposed names have been defined, it has become necessary to clarify the definition of this disorder. The term *type A insulin resistance* should be applied to patients with severe, apparently inherited insulin resistance in the absence of major phenotypic changes involving growth and development or lipodystrophy (see Fig. 56–2). Acanthosis nigricans develops in virtually all patients, and ovarian hyperthecosis with hyperandrogenism and its clinical sequelae develops in virtually all females. The definition is therefore a clinical one. Affected males have severe insulin resistance, and acanthosis nigricans is typically present, but the testes reveal no changes analogous to those that affect the ovaries in females. As a result, the clinical manifestation in males is limited to diabetes or, more rarely, acanthosis nigricans. Although many type A patients have mutations in the insulin receptor gene (see

TABLE 56–3. Autoimmune and Other Associations with Antireceptor Antibodies

Systemic lupus erythematosus	Primary biliary cirrhosis
Scleroderma	Idiopathic thrombocytopenic purpura
Rheumatoid arthritis	Hodgkin's disease
Polymyositis	?Sepsis
Sjögren's syndrome	?Type 1 diabetes

below), the same clinical phenotype can apparently result from other, currently unidentified genotypes.

The syndrome has been identified in many ethnic groups. The most common clinical feature is the peripubertal onset of one or more consequences of ovarian hyperandrogenism, including oligomenorrhea or amenorrhea, hirsutism, and not infrequently, masculinization. The clinical features often raise the suspicion of an androgen-producing tumor, and this concern may be supported by levels of testosterone that are often in the range consistent with such neoplasms (i.e., above 200 ng/mL). The presence of acanthosis nigricans, which usually becomes evident in the prepubertal period, should direct attention to the possibility of type A syndrome, which is addressed most simply by measurement of glucose and insulin levels. Although the initial patients had overt diabetes or marked glucose intolerance, many patients have had normal fasting glucose levels and only mildly impaired glucose levels after a meal or glucose load. The extent of insulin resistance is reflected in the height of the plasma insulin level, which is typically markedly elevated and usually (but not always) exceeds that seen in such states as obesity (i.e., >60 mU/mL fasting and >400 mU/mL after glucose).

The disorder is often associated with an abnormal body habitus. Patients may be thin, of normal body weight, or obese, and prominent musculature can accompany any of these physiques. Muscular prominence may result in part from the action of androgens but may also be a consequence of high levels of insulin promoting anabolism through binding to receptors for IGF-1. Some families have been described in which muscle cramps are a notable symptom that accompanies the insulin resistance,[61] and these cramps may be relieved by phenytoin.[62] Other patients have had retinitis pigmentosa.

Clinical Physiology

Studies of insulin physiology in vivo in affected patients are limited. The euglycemic clamp methodology has been used to quantitate insulin sensitivity in several subjects, and not surprisingly, severe resistance to the action of insulin to promote glucose disposal is observed. Increased hepatic glucose disposal, also resistant to insulin, is present, especially in patients with fasting hyperglycemia. Evaluation of insulin action in vivo on other metabolic pathways, such as those related to protein and fat metabolism, has not yet been reported. Patients with these disorders have impaired in vivo insulin clearance, and this impaired clearance, along with hypersecretion from the β cell, produces marked hyperinsulinemia. The impaired in vivo insulin clearance probably arises because receptor-mediated pathways play an important role in the clearance of insulin.

Molecular Pathophysiology of Cellular Insulin Resistance

Investigation of the molecular basis for insulin resistance in these syndromes dates back to the initial report of the type A syndrome in 1976, in which decreased insulin binding to circulating monocytes was observed.[7] Several early observations led to the view that these patients might have a primary defect in the structure and/or function of the insulin receptor. The defect in insulin binding was severe, did not improve with caloric restriction as did the milder defect seen in obesity,[63] was sometimes seen in families,[61] and most important, was preserved in cultured cell lines established from affected individuals.[64] Subsequent to the original description, patients with the type A phenotype have most often been observed to have normal levels of insulin receptor binding. Several such patients have had defects in the kinase function of the receptor that permitted the receptor to be synthesized and targeted to the plasma membrane but left its signaling capability severely or totally disabled.[65]

Family studies have indicated the existence of two forms of type A insulin resistance: a severe form with autosomal recessive inheritance and a milder form with an autosomal dominant pattern of transmission, most commonly caused by dominant negative mutations in the tyrosine kinase domain of the insulin receptor.[66] Several patients with the type A phenotype have been shown to have mutations in the insulin receptor gene.[66–68] Some have had two mutant alleles, but most are heterozy-

TABLE 56–4. Functional Classification of Insulin Receptor Mutations

Decreased receptor biosynthesis
   "*Cis*-acting" promoter region mutation
   Premature termination of translation—decreased mRNA
Impaired intracellular transport and posttranslational processing
   Impaired cleavage of proreceptor to receptor due to mutation at the cleavage site
   Impaired transport and processing due to point mutations in the N terminus of the α subunit
Impaired insulin binding
   Decreased insulin binding
   Increased insulin binding
Impaired receptor kinase activity
Increased receptor degradation

gous for a single, dominant-acting mutant allele.[66] The functional consequences of mutant alleles in these patients have included impaired receptor mRNA expression, impaired receptor transport to the plasma membrane, and impaired capacity for transmembrane signaling through activation of receptor autophosphorylation and tyrosine kinase activity.[68] A functional classification of insulin receptor mutations is listed in Table 56–4, and a functional map of the insulin receptor with the location of various mutations found in patients with severe insulin resistance is seen in Figure 56–1. As discussed in more detail later, genetic and biochemical information such as that already described has not produced explanations for the variable phenotypes of insulin-resistant patients.

Many patients with the type A phenotype appear to not have mutations in the insulin receptor gene, thus implying the presence of other

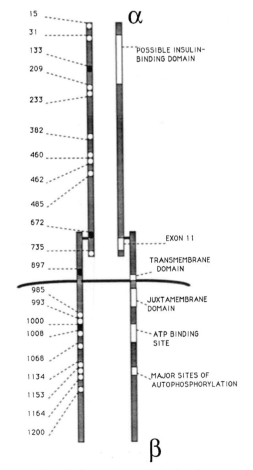

FIGURE 56–1. Identified mutations of the insulin receptor gene in humans. *Left,* Sites of point mutations (*open circles,* missense mutations; *filled circles,* stop codons). Deletions are not included.

critical primary defects in insulin signaling. At least two types of defects could be responsible for this situation. The first would be signaling defects caused by mutations in genes encoding molecules downstream of the insulin receptor. A second could be changes in inhibitors of receptor signaling such as tyrosine phosphatases, which might be overexpressed or altered in enzymatic activity through mutation.

Severe Insulin Resistance with Prominent Defects in Growth and Development

The syndromes discussed herein bear many similarities to the type A syndrome, but in addition, patients have one or more major defects in growth and development.

Insulin Resistance with Pseudoacromegaly

These patients have physical features suggestive of acromegaly in the absence of pituitary tumors or elevated levels of growth hormone and IGF-1.[69, 70] When studied, hyperinsulinemia and insulin resistance have been documented, thus suggesting a link between these metabolic features and the changes of *pseudoacromegaly*. Prominent among the features described are a coarsened facial appearance, macroglossia, and enlarging soft tissues of the hands and feet (Fig. 56–2). Some patients have had accelerated linear growth, and obesity has also been seen, the latter being an uncommon feature of true acromegaly. In some families, changes of acral hypertrophy accompany muscle

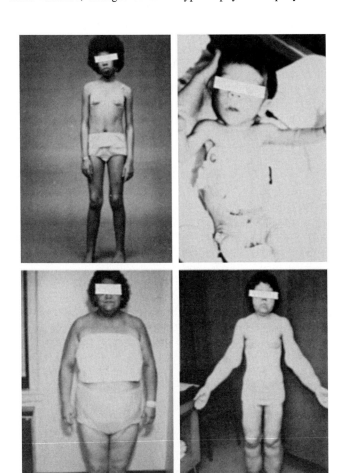

FIGURE 56–2. *Above left,* Patient with the type A syndrome of insulin resistance. *Above right,* Patient with leprechaunism. *Below left,* Patient with pseudoacromegaly. *Below right,* Patient with congenital lipodystrophy. All patients have severe insulin resistance.

cramps.[61] As in the type A syndrome, ovarian hyperandrogenism usually develops in women.

It is likely that pseudoacromegaly represents a heterogeneous array of molecular disorders. In those accompanied by severe insulin resistance, it seems reasonable to hypothesize that high levels of insulin are somehow responsible for the changes of pseudoacromegaly. This view is particularly compelling in one very well studied patient in whom neither insulin nor IGF-1 could stimulate glucose disposal in vivo or in vitro in cultured skin fibroblasts, whereas both ligands preserved the ability to promote "anabolic" changes of protein metabolism and DNA synthesis.[71] Defects in insulin receptor expression, function, and gene sequence were excluded as possible causes, as was altered expression or structure of the insulin-sensitive glucose transporter GLUT4. Thus the patient had a selective defect in the ability of both insulin and IGF-1 to activate glucose disposal because of either defects in a common signaling intermediate used by both ligands or defects in a molecular species required for glucose transport to be activated. Such a defect would permit markedly elevated insulin levels to promote changes of pseudoacromegaly. Recently, selective impairment of insulin-stimulated phosphoinositide 3-kinase activity was demonstrated in three patients with pseudoacromegaly and severe insulin resistance. [72]

Leprechaunism

This syndrome was first described in 1954 in two siblings with intrauterine and postnatal growth retardation, sparse subcutaneous fat, clitoromegaly, acanthosis nigricans, and early death[73] (see Fig. 56–2). Patients have characteristic facies, with large ears and micrognathia. Males may have penile enlargement, and females have been observed to have enlarged cystic ovaries. Other clinical features observed in case reports include rectal prolapse, breast hyperplasia, and dystrophic lungs.[74–77] The most common status of glucose homeostasis is impaired glucose tolerance with fasting hypoglycemia, and marked endogenous hyperinsulinemia is always found. Survival beyond the first year of life is uncommon.

Parental consanguinity in several families suggests an autosomal recessive mode of inheritance. Defects in the insulin signaling pathway, in particular that involving the insulin receptor itself, have received the greatest attention as sites of the primary molecular defect. Studies of several patients revealed markedly reduced insulin binding to both freshly obtained erythrocytes and monocytes, as well as to cultured skin fibroblasts and Epstein-Barr virus–transformed lymphoblasts.[78–81] Defects at the level of receptor autophosphorylation and kinase activity beyond the defect in binding have also been reported, as in the type A syndrome.[78] In general, the severity of insulin resistance in leprechaunism, as assessed by the level of high-affinity insulin binding or the extent of hyperinsulinemia, exceeds that seen in the type A syndrome. Mutations at the insulin receptor locus have been reported in several patients, and these mutations have been proved or suggested to involve both receptor alleles in all cases. Several cases have been compound heterozygotes at the receptor locus.[68, 82] In some cases, parents of affected babies who are heterozygous for mutant alleles have had mild insulin resistance without a clear clinical phenotype. In other cases, parents with a single abnormal allele had the type A phenotype.[12]

The established role of insulin receptor mutations in this disorder has not provided an explanation for the reported defects in response by cultured fibroblasts to other growth factors, such as epidermal growth factor and IGF-1.[83] Such defects could be secondary to insulin receptor abnormalities or be the consequence of currently unidentified independent signaling defects.

Rabson-Mendenhall Syndrome

In this pediatric syndrome, which is transmitted in a autosomal recessive pattern of inheritance, severe insulin resistance with acanthosis nigricans coexists with a group of more unique features, including short stature, protuberant abdomen, thick and rapidly growing hair, markedly abnormal dentition and nails, and hyperplasia of the pineal gland.[84–86] Patients may also have accelerated growth, an enlarged phallus, and precocious pseudopuberty. Diabetes usually develops in childhood and is resistant to insulin therapy. Ketoacidosis has been described but is not typical.

Reduced insulin binding to cells has been described in two patients, and reduced receptor biosynthesis was demonstrated in one of them.[87] Mutations in the insulin receptor gene have been found in two patients, and both alleles were affected in each of them.[88, 89] One patient was homozygous for a mutation that impaired cleavage of the proreceptor to the mature receptor through a missense mutation that affected the proteolytic cleavage site.[89]

Lipodystrophic States

The *lipodystrophic states* are a diverse group of clinical disorders, the central feature of which is either a complete or partial lack of adipose tissue that may be congenital or acquired. Insulin resistance and its commonly associated features are present in nearly all varieties. In addition, these patients are susceptible to a group of unique features, such as severe hyperlipidemia, progressive liver disease, and an increased metabolic rate. As discussed below, the molecular basis for these disorders is not very well understood, but it is likely that multiple molecular defects are responsible.

Generalized Lipodystrophy

Generalized lipodystrophy encompasses rare but clinically striking disorders that may be congenital (Seip-Berardinelli)[90, 91] or acquired (Lawrence).[92] The congenital syndrome is autosomal recessive, with frequent parental consanguinity. The gene causing this form of lipodystrophy has recently been mapped to chromosome 9q34.[93] Babies are noted to have an abnormal appearance caused by the absence of subcutaneous fat within the first 2 years of life and frequently at or soon after birth. Adipose tissue is also absent from intra-abdominal sites. Other somatic abnormalities that contribute to the abnormal appearance are acanthosis nigricans, a protuberant abdomen associated with hepatomegaly, prominent musculature, precocious secondary sexual development, and advanced bone age leading to advanced early, but reduced final height. Hypertriglyceridemia is characteristic, with increased very-low-density lipoproteins and chylomicrons. This condition may provoke acute pancreatitis and is related to the fatty liver that commonly progresses to cirrhosis, which may be fatal. Mental retardation and other central nervous system disorders occur more variably but may be severe. Insulin resistance has been noted at an early age and may be present at birth. Clinical diabetes usually develops in the early teens, is rarely ketotic, but is refractory to insulin therapy.

The acquired syndrome of total lipoatrophy is similar to that of the congenital disorder, except that it develops in a previously healthy individual over a period of days to weeks, often after a nonspecific febrile illness.[92, 94] The syndrome can occur in childhood or in adults, and females predominate. Diabetic ketoacidosis has been reported.

The pathophysiology of these disorders is complex and poorly understood at present. One crucial unresolved issue is the nature of the defect (or defects) responsible for the lipoatrophy, which could be due to failure of adipocytes to develop, to active destruction of adipocytes, or to failure to store triglyceride in existing adipocytes because of ineffective lipogenesis or excessive lipolysis. Limited studies have produced conflicting findings, although the data most strongly support an increased rate of lipolysis of unknown etiology.[95] A second crucial issue involves the molecular pathogenesis of the insulin resistance and the relationship of this defect to the lipoatrophy and other phenotypic changes. The extreme rarity of the disorder and its common occurrence in young children have hindered progress. Highly variable observations regarding the presence or absence of defects at the level of insulin receptor expression, function, and signaling have not provided a unified view of pathogenesis.[96–101] Defects in receptor kinase activity in cultured cells have been reported to exist in some but not all patients, and no reports of functionally significant sequence variation at the insulin receptor gene locus have appeared.

Syndromes of Partial Lipoatrophy

Several distinct syndromes of regional lipoatrophy, often associated with hypertrophy of adipose tissue in nonatrophic areas, have been described, and these syndromes are often familial.

Face-sparing lipodystrophy (Dunnigan variety), initially reported as an X-linked but recently increasingly reported as an autosomal dominant condition, spares the face, which is typically full, in contrast to the lipoatrophic trunk and extremities.[102–105] The gene for the autosomal dominant form of this syndrome was recently found to be located in chromosome 1q21–22,[103] and mutations of the *LMNA* gene encoding nuclear lamins A and C have been proposed to mediate this degenerative disorder of adipose tissue.[104] Hypertriglyceridemia and hyperchylomicronemia develop in these patients and can result in pancreatitis. Another variety of the familial partial lipodystrophies is Kobberling's syndrome.[102] In this variety the loss of adipose tissue is restricted to the extremities. Patients may have normal amounts of visceral fat and may even have excessive amounts of subcutaneous truncal fat. Individuals in some families have remarkably well defined muscles. Another form of partial lipodystrophy occurs in association with mandibuloacral dysplasia and joint contractures and is termed lipodystrophy with other dysmorphic features.

The pattern of adiposity often suggests the diagnosis of Cushing's syndrome. This diagnosis, which is further supported by the common occurrence of glucose intolerance and hypertension, is ruled out by endocrine testing. Lipoatrophy is first noted in childhood or early adolescence. It is transmitted in a highly penetrant autosomal dominant manner and is more evident in females.[106] Severe insulin resistance and nonketotic diabetes are characteristic, and severe hyperlipidemia is common. As in other syndromes of severe insulin resistance, acanthosis nigricans and ovarian hyperandrogenism are seen, but the latter has not prevented some affected women from passing the disorder to their daughters. Information on the impact of the disorder on longevity is scant, but the concurrence of glucose intolerance, hypertension, and hyperlipidemia is of concern in this regard.

We have studied one patient with what may be a clinical variant in which lipoatrophy occurred in the proximal ends of the extremities with distal lipohypertrophy (see Fig. 56–2). The patient was born of a consanguineous marriage. Insulin resistance was severe, and cultured fibroblasts had reduced insulin binding. However, a causative genetic lesion was not identified.

Syndrome of Partial Acquired (Cephalothoracic) Lipodystrophy

In this clinically distinct disorder, adipose tissue is lost from the face and upper part of the trunk, with sparing or increased adiposity in the rest of the body.[107] The disorder is most common in women, tends to occur in childhood or adolescence, and can sometimes be dated to the period after a febrile illness. Many and possibly all of these patients have a disorder of the alternative complement pathway characterized by accelerated complement activation, serum C3 nephritic factor, and renal disease with mesangiocapillary glomerulonephritis.[108, 109] This disorder of complement may be familial, although lipodystrophy does not develop in all affected individuals. Although it is now known that adipocytes produce one or more members of the alternative complement pathway,[110] the function of these molecules in adipocyte biology is unknown, and this information has not yet led to specific understanding of the relationship between the complement system and lipodystrophy. Patients may be hyperinsulinemic and modestly resistant to insulin, but severe insulin resistance is absent, as are the associated features of acanthosis nigricans and hyperandrogenism.

Lipodystrophy Associated with Protease Inhibitor Use in HIV-Positive Patients

Recently, lipodystrophy characterized by loss of subcutaneous adipose tissue from the extremities and face but excess fat deposition in the neck and trunk has been reported to develop in patients infected with human immunodeficiency virus (HIV) who are being treated with the highly effective HIV-1 protease inhibitors. In addition, insulin resistance, hyperglycemia, and hyperlipidemia develop in a significant percentage of patients treated with protease inhibitors sooner and more frequently than in patients who are receiving other regimens for HIV.[111] The mechanism underlying the development of lipodystrophy and insulin resistance is currently the subject of intensive research efforts.

Localized Lipodystrophies

Finally, localized lipodystrophies are characterized by loss of subcutaneous adipose tissue from small areas or from small parts of an extremity, but insulin resistance or metabolic abnormalities do not develop in these patients. Drug-induced lipodystrophy at the site of insulin injection was a frequent complication before the availability of purified human insulin but is rather uncommon today. Other rare causes of localized lipodystrophy are due to repeated pressure and panniculitis or have been reported as part of a rare syndrome called "lipodystrophia centrifugalis abdominalis infantilis."

RELATIONSHIP BETWEEN MOLECULAR DEFECTS CAUSING INSULIN RESISTANCE AND IN VIVO CLINICAL PHENOTYPE

Full understanding of the pathophysiology of the syndromes of extreme insulin resistance will exist when we can identify both the molecular basis for the tissue resistance to insulin and the links between these molecular defects and the diverse clinical phenotypes seen in these disorders. Because insulin resistance is the one feature common to all these syndromes, it is presumed that insulin resistance or one of its consequences, such as hyperinsulinemia, is the cause of the variable clinical phenotypes. Ideally, it would be possible to predict and explain the clinical features once the molecular defects in insulin signaling are defined. However, despite progress in identifying the molecular defects in insulin signaling, explanations for the diversity of clinical phenotypes have been slow to develop. Several facts need to be considered when addressing this issue. First, it seems clear that many of the clinical phenotypes are not simply the result of deficient insulin signaling per se but involve the consequences of the in vivo milieu as well. The key in vivo element may be marked hyperinsulinemia, which then, by mechanisms to be discussed, exerts excessive actions on one or more target tissues. The lack of suitable models for analysis of such in vivo consequences has been a major problem. Second, genes apart from those responsible for the primary signaling defect may influence the ultimate in vivo phenotype. Evidence for this explanation comes from studies of families in which despite inheritance of the same receptor mutation, the state of glucose homeostasis may be highly variable. At this time, even with the preceding generalities, the mechanistic details that might provide the in vitro–in vivo connection are not available. Finally, it may be that in some cases, unidentified mechanisms unrelated to insulin signaling bring about both insulin resistance and specific alterations in growth, adipose function, and so on.

Regarding the relationship between molecular defects and in vivo clinical phenotypes, it is not clear why different clinical syndromes develop in different patients. At least two different mechanisms have been proposed to correlate phenotype with the underlying genotype.[66] First, differences in genetic background (i.e., genotypes at other loci) could influence the severity of the clinical syndrome.[66] Second, a rough gradient in the degree of insulin resistance is found among patients with different syndromes of extreme insulin resistance. Thus the signaling defect in leprechaunism is the most severe, that seen in Rabson-Mendenhall syndrome is intermediate, and the defect in the type A syndrome is the least severe of this group. Given these facts, the defects in growth and development could in some way reflect the severity of the insulin signaling defect. However, this paradigm alone would not account for the fact that whereas leprechaunism is associated with deficient growth and development (possibly secondary to deficient insulin action), patients at the same time have acanthosis nigricans and ovarian stimulation (thought to be secondary to excessive

insulin action). Perhaps the severe growth retardation is secondary to defective insulin receptor signaling, whereas the excessive signaling is mediated by spillover onto the receptor for IGF-1. A second mechanism could relate to the existence of signaling defects, involving either the receptor itself or postreceptor components, that would have unbalanced consequences for the capacity of insulin to signal its pleiotropic actions. In such a model the clinical phenotype would be caused by the combination of reduced insulin signaling down some pathways and excessive signaling by high levels of insulin down other pathways. Apart from the one case of pseudoacromegaly discussed earlier, this hypothesis remains theoretic.

Except for signaling defects that cause unbalanced signaling, it is very likely that the high circulating levels of insulin in these patients can bind to and activate receptors for IGF-1, thereby causing excessive signaling through this receptor (Fig. 56–3). Furthermore, studies of IGF-1 action in vitro have recently been complemented by in vivo studies with recombinant human IGF-1 that demonstrate that activation of the type 1 IGF receptor can promote, in addition to growth-promoting effects, potent metabolic effects in humans, including stimulation of glucose disposal into muscle.[112] This capability raises several new questions, however. For example, if high levels of insulin can bind to the IGF receptor and promote changes such as acanthosis nigricans, ovarian hyperandrogenism, and muscle hypertrophy, why are these same high levels of insulin not able to regulate glucose utilization and hepatic glucose output through the IGF-1 receptor? Alternatively, such a mechanism might explain the fact that many type A patients maintain only mildly abnormal glucose levels despite severe insulin resistance.

ACANTHOSIS NIGRICANS AND OVARIAN HYPERANDROGENISM IN SYNDROMES OF INSULIN RESISTANCE

Acanthosis nigricans is a skin lesion that was initially reported as a cutaneous sign of malignancy and is now best known for its strong association with diverse syndromes of tissue resistance to insulin.[15, 113] The lesions are hyperpigmented and hyperkeratotic and may be papillomatous in the most severe cases. Lesions are most commonly found on the posterior aspect of the neck, in the axilla and the groin, and over the elbows, but they may cover the entire surface of the skin, although palms, soles, and oral mucosa are spared. Histologic hallmarks are hyperkeratosis, epidermal papillomatosis, and increased numbers of melanocytes.

The common denominator among all instances of acanthosis, apart possibly from tumor-associated cases, is tissue resistance to insulin. Insulin resistance may vary in severity as well as molecular etiology and may be either inherited or acquired. Thus acanthosis nigricans is a cutaneous marker for insulin resistance. In addition to its prominent

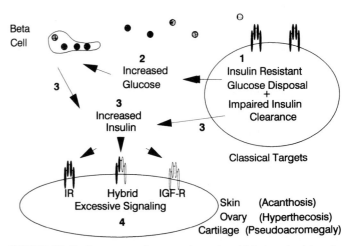

FIGURE 56–3. Sequence of events through which impaired insulin-stimulated glucose use eventuates in excessive insulin action.

appearance in patients with type A and B syndromes and leprechaunism, clinical and histologic evidence of acanthosis can be identified in a large fraction of certain large populations and, when present in these groups, is associated with hyperinsulinemia and insulin resistance. Thus in women with hyperandrogenism, most of whom have polycystic ovarian disease, acanthosis is found clinically in 5% to 30%[114, 115] and may be much more common when assessed by skin biopsy.[116] Likewise, 5% to 13% of Hispanic and black children were noted to have acanthosis and hyperinsulinemia.[117]

TREATMENT OF SYNDROMES OF SEVERE INSULIN RESISTANCE

Drugs for patients with severe insulin resistance syndromes are currently limited. Insulin, administered in very high doses, usually fails to provide adequate control.[118] Metformin has been reported to improve glycemia in patients with the type B syndrome or lipoatrophic diabetes. Administration of IGF-1 to patients with type A or B syndrome, the Rabson-Mendenhall syndrome, leprechaunism, or lipodystrophy has led to improvement in glycemic control and insulin resistance in short-term studies.[118] Immunosuppressants and plasmapheresis have been tried with good results in patients with type B syndrome.

MUTANT INSULIN

Several families have been described in which one or more members have missense mutations in their insulin gene that cause amino acid substitutions within the proinsulin molecule.[119, 120] In these families were found three different mutations that cause changes within the α or β chains of the insulin molecule and result in biologically defective insulin,[121–123] as well as two different mutations that cause hyperproinsulinemia.[124–127] The clinical and biochemical features of these patients are listed in Table 56–5. All patients have had marked fasting hyperinsulinemia or hyperproinsulinemia with hormone concentrations fourfold to sixfold above normal as measured by radioimmunoassay in the fasting state. The initial patients described with insulin gene mutations had mild hyperglycemia or overt diabetes, and the presence of hyperinsulinemia led to the evaluation of insulin resistance. These patients are distinguished from those with insulin resistance, however, by the fact that they respond normally to exogenous insulin, a fact that suggested the defect in these patients to be at the level of the insulin molecule itself. Indeed, biochemical studies demonstrated that insulin purified from these subjects had reduced bioactivity, typically less than 5% of the bioactivity of normal insulin. Genetic analysis has confirmed the existence of point mutations in one of two insulin gene alleles.[122, 126] As in the syndromes of insulin resistance, it is now known that apart from the probands, who are discovered initially because of glucose intolerance or diabetes, individuals with these defects are often normoglycemic, particularly individuals with mutations leading to hyperproinsulinemia.[124, 126]

Pathophysiology

To date, subjects with these disorders have been heterozygous at the insulin gene locus, with one normal and one abnormal insulin gene

TABLE 56–5.   Characteristics of Patients Producing Mutant β Cell Products

Increased fasting concentration of serum immunoreactive (pro)insulin
Fasting hyperglycemia or, more commonly, euglycemia
Normal sensitivity to exogenous insulin
Circulating insulin with reduced bioactivity
Reduced ratio of serum C peptide to insulin
Identification of abnormal (pro)insulin gene and gene product
Autosomal dominant inheritance of the trait
Codominant expression of the normal (pro)insulin gene

TABLE 56–6.   Known Mutations of the Insulin Gene

Product	Mutation	Consequences
Insulin Chicago	B25 (Phe → Leu)	Reduced binding
Insulin Los Angeles	B24 (Phe → Ser)	Reduced binding
Insulin Wakayama	A3 (Val → Leu)	Reduced binding
Proinsulin Tokyo/Boston	C65 (Arg → His)	Hyperproinsulinemia
Proinsulin Providence	B10 (His → Asp)	Hyperproinsulinemia

allele. The product of the mutant allele behaves as a weak agonist, with bioactivity reduced in approximate proportion to the diminished receptor-binding affinity.[115] These mutant insulins have therefore not behaved as receptor antagonists, and insulin receptor antagonism cannot account for cases in which diabetes or glucose intolerance develops, because the product of the normal allele should be able to fully compensate. Failure to compensate through increased secretion of the product of the normal allele is presumably due to one or more independent defects at the level of β cell function in individuals in whom diabetes develops. The mutant insulin gene should therefore be viewed as a risk factor for type 2 diabetes.

Patients with mutant insulin alleles are observed to have low molar ratios of C peptide to insulin.[120] This low ratio results from the delayed clearance rate of mutant insulin, which because of its reduced receptor affinity has a diminished rate of receptor-mediated clearance.[128] As a result, the elevated circulating insulin is predominantly the mutant form.

Unlike patients with severe insulin resistance caused by target cell defects in insulin action, patients with mutant insulin have no unusual or distinguishing clinical phenotypes, such as acanthosis, ovarian hyperandrogenism, or disordered growth and development. The diagnosis is made only if hyperinsulinemia is detected and, after having been identified, an effort is made to determine its cause.

Prevalence

Mutations in the insulin gene are exceptionally uncommon, with only five variants described in approximately 10 families.[120] These mutations are listed in Table 56–6. New insulin gene mutations have not yet been identified through screening of patients with type 2 diabetes.[129]

REFERENCES

1. Moller DE, Flier JS: Insulin resistance: Mechanisms, syndromes, and implications. N Engl J Med 325:938–948, 1991.
2. Himsworth HP, Kerr RB: Insulin-sensitive and insulin-insensitive types of diabetes mellitus. Clin Sci 4:119–152, 1939.
3. Yalow RS, Berson SA: Plasma insulin concentrations in nondiabetic and early diabetic subjects: Determinations by a new sensitive immunoassay technique. Diabetes 9:254–260, 1960.
4. Kahn CR, Neville DM Jr, Roth J: Insulin-receptor interaction in the obese-hyperglycemic mouse: A model of insulin resistance. J Biol Chem 248:244–250, 1973.
5. Bergman RN, Finegood DT, Ader M: Assessment of insulin sensitivity in vivo. Endocr Rev 6:45–86, 1985.
6. Cheatham B, Kahn CR: Insulin action and the insulin signaling network. Endocr Rev 16:117–142, 1995.
7. Tritos NA, Mantzoros CS: Clinical review 97: Syndromes of severe insulin resistance. J Clin Endocrinol Metab 83:3025–3030, 1998.
8. Flier JS, Kahn CR, Roth J, Bar RS: Antibodies that impair insulin receptor binding in an unusual diabetic syndrome with severe insulin resistance. Science 190:63–65, 1975.
9. Kasuga M, Karlsson FA, Kahn CR: Insulin stimulates the phosphorylation of the 95,000-dalton subunit of its own receptor. Science 215:185–187, 1982.
10. Ullrich A, Bell JR, Chen EY, et al: Human insulin receptor and its relationship to the tyrosine kinase family of oncogenes. Nature 313:756–761, 1985.
11. Krook A, O'Rahilly S: Mutant receptors in syndromes of insulin resistance. Baillieres Clin Endocrinol Metab 10:97–122, 1996.
12. Flier JS: Lilly Lecture: Syndromes of insulin resistance: From patient to gene and back again. Diabetes 41:1207–1219, 1992.
13. Ferrannini E, Buzzigoli G, Bonadonna R, et al: Insulin resistance in essential hypertension. N Engl J Med 317:350–357, 1987.
14. Dunaif A, Graf M, Mandeli J, et al: Characterization of groups of hyperandrogenic women with acanthosis nigricans, impaired glucose tolerance, and/or hyperinsulinemia. J Clin Endocrinol Metab 65:499–507, 1987.

15. Flier JS: The metabolic importance of acanthosis nigricans. Arch Dermatol 121:193–194, 1985.
16. Poretsky L: On the paradox of insulin-induced hyperandrogenism in insulin-resistant states. Endocr Rev 12:3–13, 1991.
17. Barbieri RL, Smith S, Ryan KJ: The role of hyperinsulinemia in the pathogenesis of ovarian hyperandrogenism. Fertil Steril 50:197–212, 1988.
18. Bar RS, Boes M, Kake BL, et al: Insulin, insulin-like growth factors, and vascular endothelium. Am J Med 85(5A):59–70, 1988.
19. Kahn CR: The molecular mechanism of insulin action. Annu Rev Med 36:429–451, 1985.
20. Goldfine ID: The insulin receptor: Molecular biology and transmembrane signaling. Endocr Rev 8:235–255, 1987.
21. Moller DE, Yokota A, Caro JF, Flier JS: Tissue-specific expression of two alternatively spliced insulin receptor mRNA's in man. Mol Endocrinol 3:1263–1269, 1989.
22. Yamaguchi Y, Flier JS, Yokota A, et al: Functional properties of two naturally occurring isoforms of the human insulin receptor in Chinese hamster ovary cells. Endocrinology 129:2058–2066, 1991.
23. McClain DA: Different ligand affinities of the two human insulin receptor splice variants are reflected in parallel changes in sensitivity for insulin action. Mol Endocrinol 5:734–739, 1991.
24. Flier JS, Usher P, Moses AC: Monoclonal antibody to the type I insulin-like growth factor (IGF-I) receptor blocks IGF-I receptor–mediated DNA synthesis: Clarification of the mitogenic mechanisms of IGF-I and insulin skin fibroblasts. Proc Natl Acad Sci U S A 93:664–668, 1986.
25. Treadway JL, Morrison BD, Goldfine ID, Pessin JE: Assembly of insulin/insulin-like growth factor-I hybrid receptors in vitro. J Biol Chem 264:21450–21453, 1989.
26. Moxham CP, Duronio V, Jacobs S: Insulin-like growth factor I receptor beta-subunit heterogeneity: Evidence for hybrid tetramers composed of insulin-like growth factor I and insulin receptor heterodimers. J Biol Chem 264:13238–13244, 1989.
27. McClain DA: Insulin action in cells expressing truncated or kinase-defective insulin receptors: Dissection of multiple hormone-signaling pathways. Diabetes Care 13:302–316, 1990.
28. Cohen P: The structure and regulation of protein phosphatases. Annu Rev Biochem 58:453–508, 1989.
29. White MF, Stegmann EW, Dull TJ, et al: Characterization of an endogenous substrate of the insulin receptor in cultured cells. J Biol Chem 262:9769–9777, 1987.
30. Drake PG, Posner BI: Insulin receptor–associated protein tyrosine phosphatase(s): Role in insulin action. Mol Cell Biochem 182:79–89, 1998.
31. Elchebly M, Payette P, Michaliszyn E, et al: Increased insulin sensitivity and obesity resistance in mice lacking the protein tyrosine phosphatase-1B gene. Science 283:1544–1548, 1999.
32. Flier JS, Minaker KL, Landsberg L, et al: Impaired in vivo insulin clearance in patients with severe target cell resistance of insulin. Diabetes 31:132–135, 1982.
33. Almind K, Inoue G, Pedersen O, Kahn CR: A common amino acid polymorphism in insulin receptor substrate-1 causes impaired insulin signaling. Evidence from transfection studies. J Clin Invest 97:2569–2575, 1996.
34. Baroni MG, D'Andrea MP, Montali A, et al: A common mutation of the insulin receptor substrate-1 gene is a risk factor for coronary artery disease. Arterioscler Thromb Vasc Biol 19:2975–2980, 1999.
35. Imai Y, Philippe N, Sesti G, et al: Expression of variant forms of insulin receptor substrate-1 identified in patients with noninsulin-dependent diabetes mellitus. J Clin Endocrinol Metab 82:4201–4207, 1997.
36. Sbraccia P, Goodman PA, Maddux BA, et al: Production of inhibitor of insulin-receptor tyrosine kinase in fibroblasts from patient with insulin resistance and NIDDM. Diabetes 40:295–299, 1991.
37. Sbraccia P, Goodman PA, Maddux BA, et al: Production of an inhibitor of insulin receptor tyrosine kinase in fibroblasts from a patient with insulin resistance and NIDDM. Diabetes 40:295–299, 1991.
38. Randle PJ, Hales CN, Garland PB, Newsholm EA: The glucose fatty-acid cycle: Its role in insulin sensitivity and the metabolic disturbances of diabetes mellitus. Lancet 2:785–789, 1963.
39. Yki-Jarvinen H: Glucose toxicity. Endocr Rev 13:415–431, 1992.
40. Hotamisligil GS, Shargill NS, Spiegelman BM: Adipose tissue expression of tumor necrosis factor alpha: Direct role in obesity-linked insulin resistance. Science 259:87–90, 1993.
41. Barosso I, Gurnell M, Crowley VEF, et al: Dominant negative mutations in human PPARγ associated with severe insulin resistance, diabetes mellitus and hypertension. Nature 402:880–883, 1999.
42. Berson SA, Yalow RS: In Ellenberg M, Rifkin H (eds): Diabetes Mellitus: Theory and Practice. New York, McGraw-Hill, 1970, pp 388–423.
43. Flier JS, Poretsky L: Insulin allergy and insulin resistance: Current therapy. In Lichtenstein LM, Fauci AS (eds): Allergy, Immunology and Rheumatology. Philadelphia, BC Decker, 1985, pp 135–140.
44. Francis A, Hanning I, Alberti K: The influence of insulin antibody levels on the plasma profiles and action of subcutaneously injected human and bovine short-acting insulins. Diabetologia 28:330, 1983.
45. Duckworth WC, Bennett RG, Hamel FG: Insulin degradation: Progress and potential. Endocr Rev 19:608–624, 1998.
46. Freidenberg GR, White N, Cataland S, et al: Diabetes response to intravenous but not subcutaneous effectiveness of aprotinin. N Engl J Med 305:363, 1981.
47. Schade DS, Duckworth WC: In search of the subcutaneous-insulin-resistance syndrome. N Engl J Med 315:147, 1986.
48. Affholter JA, Fried VA, Roth RA: Human insulin-degrading enzyme shares structural and functional homologies with E. coli protease III. Science 242:1415–1418, 1988.
49. Taylor SI, Barbetti F, Accili D, et al: Syndromes of autoimmunity and hypoglycemia: Autoantibodies directed against insulin and its receptor. Endocrinol Metab Clin North Am 18:123–143, 1989.
50. Taylor SI, Grunberger G, Marcus-Samuels B, et al: Hypoglycemia associated with antibodies to the insulin receptor. N Engl J Med 307:1422–1426, 1982.

51. Taylor SI, Dons RF, Hernandez E, et al: Insulin resistance associated with androgen excess in women with autoantibodies to the insulin receptor. Ann Intern Med 97:851–855, 1982.
52. Flier JS, Bar RS, Muggeo M, et al: The evolving clinical course of patients with insulin receptor autoantibodies: Spontaneous remission or receptor proliferation with hypoglycemia. J Clin Endocrinol Metab 47:985–995, 1978.
53. Muggeo M, Flier JS, Abrams RA, et al: Treatment by plasma exchange of a patient with autoantibodies to the insulin receptor. N Engl J Med 300:477–480, 1979.
54. DiPaolo S: Metformin ameliorates extreme insulin resistance in a patient with anti–insulin receptor antibodies: Description of insulin receptor and postreceptor effects in vivo and in vitro. Acta Endocrinol 126:117–123, 1992.
55. Zhang B, Roth RA: A region of the insulin receptor important for ligand binding (residues 450–601) is recognized by patients' autoimmune antibodies and inhibitory monoclonal antibodies. Proc Natl Acad Sci U S A 88:9858–9862, 1991.
56. Boden G, Fujita-Yamaguchi Y, Shimoyama R, et al: Nonbinding inhibitory antiinsulin receptor antibodies: A new type of autoantibodies in human diabetes. J Clin Invest 81:1971–1978, 1988.
57. Di Paolo S, Giorgino R: Insulin resistance and hypoglycemia in a patient with systemic lupus erythematosus: Description of antiinsulin receptor antibodies that enhance insulin binding and inhibit insulin action. J Clin Endocrinol Metab 73:650–657, 1991.
58. Kahn CR, Baird K, Flier JS, Jarrett DB: Effects of autoantibodies to the insulin receptor on isolated adipocytes. J Clin Invest 60:1094–1106, 1977.
59. Karlsson FA, Van Obberghen E, Grunfeld C, Kahn C: Desensitization of the insulin receptor at an early postreceptor step by prolonged exposure to anti-receptor antibody. Proc Natl Acad Sci U S A 76:809–813, 1979.
60. Grunfeld C: Antibody against the insulin receptor causes disappearance of insulin receptors in 3T3-L1 cells: A possible explanation of antibody-induced insulin resistance. Proc Natl Acad Sci U S A 81:2508–2511, 1984.
61. Flier JS, Young JB, Landsberg L: Familial insulin resistance with acanthosis nigricans, acral hypertrophy and muscle cramps: A new syndrome. N Engl J Med 390:970–973, 1980.
62. Minaker KL, Flier JS, Landsberg L, et al: Diphenylhydantoin-induced improvement in muscle cramping and insulin action in three patients with the syndrome of insulin resistance, acanthosis nigricans, and acral hypertrophy. Arch Neurol 46:981–985, 1989.
63. Bar RS, Muggeo M, Kahn CR, et al: Characterization of insulin receptors in patients with the syndromes of insulin resistance and acanthosis nigricans. Diabetologia 18:209–216, 1980.
64. Podskalny JM, Kahn CR: Cell culture studies on patients with extreme insulin resistance: I. Receptor defects on cultured fibroblasts. J Clin Endocrinol Metab 54:261–268, 1982.
65. Grigorescu F, Flier JS, Kahn CR: Defect in insulin receptor phosphorylation in erythrocytes and fibroblasts associated with severe insulin resistance. J Biol Chem 259:15003–15006, 1984.
66. Taylor SI, Arioglou E: Genetically defined forms of diabetes in children. J Clin Endocrinol Metab 84:4390–4396, 1999.
67. Moller DE, Yokota A, White MF, et al: A naturally occurring mutation of insulin receptor alanine 1134 impairs tyrosine kinase function and is associated with dominantly inherited insulin resistance. J Biol Chem 265:14979–14985, 1990.
68. O'Rahilly S, Moller DE: Mutant insulin receptors in syndromes of insulin resistance. Clin Endocrinol 36:121–132, 1992.
69. Mims RB: Pituitary function and growth hormone dynamics in acromegaloidism. J Natl Med Assoc 70:919–924, 1978.
70. Low L, Chernausek SD, Sperling MA: Acromegaloid patients with type A insulin resistance: Parallel defects in insulin and insulin-like growth factor-I receptors and biological responses in cultured fibroblasts. J Clin Endocrinol Metab 69:329–337, 1989.
71. Flier JS, Moller DE, Moses AC, et al: Insulin-mediated pseudoacromegaly: Clinical and biochemical characterization of a syndrome of selective insulin resistance. J Clin Endocrinol Metab 76:1533–1541, 1993.
72. Dib K, Whitehead JP, Humphreys PJ, et al: Impaired activation of phosphoinositide 3 kinase by insulin in fibroblasts from patients with severe insulin resistance and pseudoacromegaly. J Clin Invest 101:1111–1120, 1998.
73. Donohue WL, Uchida I: Leprechaunism: A euphemism for a rare familial disorder. J Pediatr 45:505, 1954.
74. Elders MJ, Schedewie HK, Olefsky J, et al: Endocrine-metabolic relationships in patients with leprechaunism. J Natl Med Assoc 74:1195–1210, 1982.
75. Ioan D, Dumitriu L, Belengeanu V, et al: Leprechaunism: Report of two cases and review. Endocrinologie 26:205–209, 1988.
76. Elsas LJ, Endo F, Priest JH, Strumlauf E: Leprechaunism: An inherited defect in insulin-receptor interaction. In Wapnir RA (ed): Congenital Metabolic Disease: Diagnosis and Treatment. New York, Marcel Dekker, 1985, pp 301–334.
77. Ellis EN, Kemp SF, Frindik JP, Elders MJ: Glomerulopathy in a patient with Donohue syndrome (leprechaunism). Diabetes Care 14:413–414, 1991.
78. Sethu-Kumar Reddy S, Lauris V, Kahn CR: Insulin receptor function in fibroblasts from patients with leprechaunism: Differential alterations in binding, autophosphorylation, kinase activity, and receptor-mediated internalization. J Clin Invest 82:1359–1365, 1988.
79. Maassen JA, Klinkhamer MP, van der Zon GC, et al: Fibroblasts from a leprechaun patient have defects in insulin binding and insulin receptor autophosphorylation. Diabetologia 31:612–617, 1988.
80. Taylor SI, Roth J, Blizzard RM, Elders MJ: Qualitative abnormalities of insulin binding in a patient with extreme insulin resistance. Proc Natl Acad Sci U S A 78:7157–7161, 1981.
81. Taylor SI, Samuels B, Roth J, et al: Decreased insulin binding in cultured lymphocytes from two patients with extreme insulin resistance. J Clin Endocrinol Metab 54:919–930, 1982.

82. Kadowaki T, Bevins CL, Cama A, et al: Two mutant alleles of the insulin receptor gene in a patient with extreme insulin resistance. Science 240:787–790, 1988.

83. Kaplowitz PB, D'Ercole AJ: Fibroblasts from a patient with leprechaunism are resistant to insulin, epidermal growth factor, and somatomedin C. J Clin Endocrinol Metab 55:741–748, 1982.

84. Mendenhall EN: Tumor of the pineal body with high insulin resistance. J Ind Med Assoc 43:32–36, 1950.

85. Rabson SM, Mendenhall EN: Familial hypertrophy of pineal body, hyperplasia of adrenal cortex and diabetes mellitus: Report of 3 cases. Am J Clin Pathol 26:283–290, 1956.

86. West RJ, Leonard JV: Familial insulin resistance with pineal hyperplasia: Metabolic studies and effect of hypophysectomy. Arch Dis Child 55:619–621, 1980.

87. Moncada VY, Hedo JA, Serranos-Rios M, Taylor SI: Insulin-receptor biosynthesis in cultured lymphocytes from an insulin-resistant patient (Rabson-Mendenhall syndrome): Evidence for a defect before insertion of receptor into plasma membrane. Diabetes 35:802–807, 1986.

88. Kadowaki T, Kadowaki H, Accili D, Taylor SI: Substitution of lysine for asparagine-15 in the human insulin receptor impairs intracellular transport of the receptor to the cell surface and decreases the affinity of insulin binding. J Biol Chem 265:19143–19150, 1990.

89. Yoshimasa Y, Seino S, Whittaker J, et al: Insulin resistant diabetes due to a point mutation that prevents insulin proreceptor processing. Science 240:784–787, 1988.

90. Berardinelli W: An undiagnosed endocrinometabolic syndrome: Report of 2 cases. J Clin Endocrinol Metab 14:193–204, 1954.

91. Seip M: Lipodystrophy and gigantism with associated endocrine manifestations: A new diencephalic syndrome? Acta Paediatr 48:555–574, 1959.

92. Lawrence RD: Lipodystrophy and hepatomegaly with diabetes, lipaemia, and other metabolic disturbances: A case throwing new light on the action of insulin. Lancet 1:724, 1946.

93. Garg A, Wilson R, Barnes R, et al: A gene for congenital generalized lipodystrophy maps to human chromosome 9q34. J Clin Endocrinol Metab 84:3390–3394, 1999.

94. Köbberling J: Genetic syndromes associated with lipoatrophic diabetes. *In* Creutzfeldt W, Köbberling J, Neel JV (eds): The Genetics of Diabetes Mellitus. New York, Springer-Verlag, 1976, pp 147–154.

95. Boucher BJ, Cohen RD, France MW, Mason SA: Plasma free fatty acid turnover in total lipodystrophy. Clin Endocrinol 4:83–88, 1973.

96. Oseid S, Beck-Nielsen H, Pedersen O, Sovik O: Decreased binding of insulin to its receptor in patients with congenital generalized lipodystrophy. N Engl J Med 296:245–248, 1977.

97. Wachslicht-Rodbard H, Muggeo M, Kahn CR, et al: Heterogeneity of the insulin-receptor interaction in lipoatrophic diabetes. J Clin Endocrinol Metab 52:416–425, 1981.

98. Magre J, Grigorescu F, Reynet C, et al: Tyrosine-kinase defect of the insulin receptor in cultured fibroblasts from patients with lipoatrophic diabetes. J Clin Endocrinol Metab 69:142–150, 1989.

99. Magre J, Reynet C, Capeau J, et al: In vitro studies of insulin resistance in patients with lipoatrophic diabetes: Evidence for heterogeneous postbinding defects. Diabetes 37:421–482, 1988.

100. Kriauchiunas KM, Kahn CR, Muller-Wieland D, et al: Altered expression and function of the insulin receptor in a family with lipoatrophic diabetes. J Clin Endocrinol Metab 67:1284–1293, 1988.

101. Foss I, Trygstad O: Lipoatrophy produced in mice and rabbits by a fraction prepared from the urine of patients with congenital generalised lipodystrophy. Acta Endocrinol 713:443–453, 1975.

102. Kobberling J, Willms B, Kattermann R, Creutzfeldt W: Lipodystrophy of the extremities: A dominantly inherited syndrome associated with lipoatrophic diabetes. Humangenetik 29:111–120, 1975.

103. Peters JM, Barnes R, Bennett L, et al: Localization of the gene for familial partial lipodystrophy (Dunningan variety) to chromosome 1q21-22. Nat Genet 18:292–295, 1998.

104. Cao H, Hegele RA: Nuclear lamin A/C R482Q mutation in Canadian kindreds with Dunningan-type familial partial lipodystrophy. Hum Mol Genet 9:109–112, 2000.

105. Dunnigan MG, Cochrane M, Kelly A, Scott JW: Familial lipoatrophic diabetes with dominant transmission. Q J Med 49:33–48, 1974.

106. Jackson SN, Pinkney J, Bargiotta A, et al: A defect in the regional deposition of adipose tissue (partial lipodystrophy) is encoded by a gene at chromosome 1q. Am J Hum Genet 63:534–540, 1998.

107. Barraquer FL: Pathogenesis of progressive cephalothoracic lipodystrophy. J Nerv Ment Dis 109:193, 1949.

108. Peters DK, Charleworth JA, Sissons JGP, et al: Mesangiocapillary nephritis, partial lipodystrophy and hypocomplementaemia. Lancet 2:535–538, 1973.

109. Sissons JGP, West RJ, Fallows J: The complement abnormalities of lipodystrophy. N Engl J Med 294:461, 1976.

110. Rosen BS, Cook KS, Yaglom J, et al: Adipsin and complement factor D activity: An immune-related defect in obesity. Science 244:1483–1487, 1989.

111. Tsiodras S, Mantzoros C, Hammer S, Samore M: Effects of protease inhibitors on hyperglycemia, hyperlipidemia and lipodystrophy. A five-year cohort study. Arch Intern Med (in press).

112. Zenobi PD, Graf S, Ursprung H, Froesch ER: Effects of insulin-like growth factor-I on glucose tolerance, insulin levels, and insulin secretion. J Clin Invest 89:1908–1913, 1992.

113. Rogers DL: Acanthosis nigricans. Semin Dermatol 10:160–163, 1991.

114. Flier JS, Eastman RC, Minaker KL, et al: Acanthosis nigricans in obese women with hyperandrogenism: Characterization of an insulin-resistant state distinct from the type A and B syndromes. Diabetes 34:101–107, 1985.

115. Dunaif A, Hoffman AR, Scully RE, et al: Clinical, biochemical, and ovarian morphologic features in women with acanthosis nigricans. Obstet Gynecol 66:545–552, 1985.

116. Dunaif A, Green G, Phelps RG, et al: Acanthosis nigricans, insulin action, and hyperandrogenism: Clinical, histological, and biochemical findings. J Clin Endocrinol Metab 73:590–595, 1991.

117. Stuart CA, Pate CJ, Peters EJ: Prevalence of acanthosis nigricans in an unselected population. Am J Med 87:269–272, 1989.

118. Mantzoros CS, Moses AC: Treatment of severe insulin resistance. *In* Azziz R, Nestler JE, Dewailly D (eds): Androgen Excess Disorders in Women. Philadelphia, Lippincott-Raven, 1997, pp 247–255.

119. Tager HS: Abnormal products of the human insulin gene. Diabetes 33:693–699, 1984.

120. Steiner DF, Tager HS, Chan SJ, et al: Lessons learned from molecular biology of insulin gene mutations. Diabetes Care 13:600–609, 1990.

121. Tager H, Given B, Baldwin D, et al: A structurally abnormal insulin causing human diabetes. Nature 281:122–125, 1979.

122. Haneda M, Polonsky KS, Bergenstal RM, et al: Familial hyperinsulinemia due to a structurally abnormal insulin: Definition of an emerging new clinical syndrome. N Engl J Med 310:1288–1289, 1984.

123. Nanjo K, Miyano M, Kondo M, et al: Insulin Wakayama: Familial mutant insulin syndrome in Japan. Diabetologia 30:87–92, 1987.

124. Gabbay KH, Bergenstal RM, Wolff J, et al: Familial hyperproinsulinemia: Partial characterization of circulating proinsulin-like material. Proc Natl Acad Sci U S A 76:2881–2885, 1979.

125. Robbins DC, Blix PM, Rubenstein AH, et al: A human proinsulin variant at arginine 65. Nature 291:679–681, 1981.

126. Robbins DC, Shoelson SE, Rubenstein AH, Tager HS: Familial hyperproinsulinemia: Two cohorts secreting indistinguishable type II intermediates of proinsulin conversion. J Clin Invest 73:714–719, 1984.

127. Shoelson S, Haneda M, Blix P, et al: Three mutant insulins in man. Nature 302:540–543, 1983.

128. Shoelson SE, Polonsky KS, Zeidler A, et al: Human insulin B24 (Phe-Ser): Secretion and metabolic clearance of the abnormal insulin in man and in a dog model. J Clin Invest 73:1351–1358, 1984.

129. Sanz N, Karam JH, Horita S, Bell GI: Prevalence of insulin-gene mutations in non–insulin-dependent diabetes mellitus. N Engl J Med 314:1322, 1986.

Chapter 57

▲▲▲

Management of Type 2 Diabetes: A Systematic Approach to Meeting the Standards of Care

I: Self-Management Education, Medical Nutrition Therapy, and Exercise

Richard M. Bergenstal ▪ David M. Kendall
Marion J. Franz ▪ Arthur H. Rubenstein

MODELS AND STANDARDS OF CARE

Chronic disease has become the major cause of morbidity and mortality and accounts for the majority of healthcare expenditures in the United States. Diabetes mellitus is among the most common,[1, 2] costly,[3–5] and potentially devastating[6] of the chronic diseases and management of this disorder has become increasingly complex. To best manage type 2 diabetes, providers require the active involvement of the patient, utilizing advice and monitoring from a physician and a team of healthcare professionals, all of whom assist in education, training, and the delivery of care.

Since at least 90% of diabetes care is delivered in a primary care setting it is important that the practitioner understand the standards of diabetes care and be trained in the basics of systematic diabetes management. While some modalities of care appear to be delivered most effectively by an endocrinologist (or diabetes specialist),[7–10] there are not enough endocrinologists to provide the bulk of primary diabetes care. Primary care providers can have a positive impact on diabetes outcomes,[11] but studies show that both specialists and primary care providers need to optimize their systems of care to truly improve outcomes.[12–15] The most effective care seems to be delivered by a team made up of a patient, an educator (Registered Nurse and Registered Dietitian, preferably),[16, 17] and a medical provider (primary care physician, nurse practitioner, or endocrinologist).[18] Providers, educators, and patients who are linked together with defined roles and expectations create the most effective model for improving diabetes control and overall health. Figure 57–1 shows the interrelationship of the team members and the primary goal of communication between team members.

The communication between educator and patient is focused on making appropriate behavior changes.[19, 20] The educator and the provider must discuss standards of care and what path or algorithm they plan to follow for their patients. The provider is responsible for deciding on the most appropriate therapy or modification of therapy for his or her patient. If behavior changes can be facilitated and

standards of care implemented with appropriate therapeutic interventions, the odds of improving diabetes control and overall health are greatly enhanced.

Patient, clinician, and educators have distinct roles, but each has the goal of preventing or minimizing complications of diabetes by seeing that certain standards of care are practiced. Health maintenance organizations (HMOs) across the United States are now collecting a common set of medical process and outcome variables that they must report each year, the so-called HMO report card. The National Committee of Quality Assurance (NCQA) is the accrediting body for HMOs and has developed a standard set of medical measures called the Health Plan and Employer Data Information Set (HEDIS). As a part of HEDIS reporting, starting in the year 2000, all HMOs are required to collect and report on an expanded comprehensive set of diabetes measures developed by the Diabetes Quality Improvement Program (DQIP) Task Force. The DQIP represents a coalition of consumer, federal, and healthcare organizations (the NCQA, Health Care Financing Administration, American Diabetes Association [ADA], Foundation for Accountability, American Academy of Family Physicians, American College of Physicians, and the Veterans Administration). The DQIP measures allow health plans, medical practices, and individual practitioners to benchmark the practice of others. These measures are not meant to be standards of care but guideposts for comparison. These measures and an explanation of their implementation strategy can be found on the Internet at HYPERLINK http://www.diabetes.org/dqip.asp.[21]

A graphic display of the standards of care for type 2 diabetes can be helpful. Figure 57–2 combines all of the common standards of care, from making the diagnosis to performing team education, and setting target goals along with the basic elements of care. This figure emphasizes the emerging theme that the management of type 2 diabetes is multifaceted. Glycemic control, while recently confirmed by the United Kingdom Prospective Diabetes Study (UKPDS)[22] to be important, is only one of the major components of care in type 2 diabetes. Comprehensive care includes aggressive management of lipids and

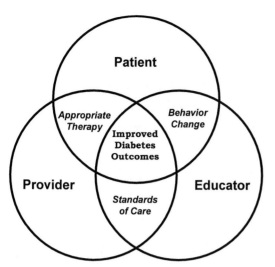

FIGURE 57–1. Diagram of diabetes team care: relationships and outcomes.

blood pressure, compulsory screening, treatment of possible complications, and other components of clinical care that have special significance in diabetes.[23–25] This graphic of the standards of care for type 2 diabetes serves as the central theme of this chapter, and we shall work our way down the figure starting with making the diagnosis.

CLASSIFICATION AND DIAGNOSIS

The care of the diabetic patient starts with making the diagnosis in a timely manner. In 1997 an expert committee from the ADA[26] revised the National Diabetes Data Group–World Health Organization 1979 classification and diagnosis standards[27] (see Chapter 53). Diabetes is now classified as type 1 diabetes, type 2 diabetes, other types of diabetes, and gestational diabetes. Type 1 diabetes (formerly insulin-dependent diabetes mellitus) is either autoimmune or idiopathic. A group of Japanese investigators recently described a new subset of idiopathic diabetes they called fulminant type 1 diabetes.[28] Type 2 diabetes (formerly non–insulin-dependent diabetes) represents 90% to 95% of diabetes and is characterized by insulin resistance in muscle, liver, and adipose tissue beginning before the onset of any clinical

symptoms of diabetes. Type 2 diabetes is strongly genetic, with all nonwhite racial and ethnic groups being at higher risk than the white population. The classification of other types of diabetes makes up only 1% to 2% of cases of diabetes and includes genetic defects in the β cell, genetic defects in insulin action, diseases of the exocrine pancreas, endocrinopathies, drug or chemical insults, infectious and other immune-mediated types of diabetes, and rare genetic syndromes with associated diabetes. Gestational diabetes affects up to 5% of pregnancies in the United States.

The importance of the new classification for medical management is the emphasis on not linking the classification of the type of diabetes to a specific treatment. So by eliminating the term *non–insulin-dependent diabetes* one can more easily discuss insulin therapy in type 2 diabetes when it is appropriate. The new diagnostic criteria for diabetes also have implications for medical management. In summary the new diagnostic criteria are as follows:

- **Diabetes.** Fasting plasma glucose greater than 126 mg/dL (7.0 mmol/L) or greater, confirmed by a repeat test, *or* symptoms of diabetes plus casual plasma glucose greater than 200 mg/dL (11.1 mmol/L) or greater, *or* plasma glucose greater than 200 mg/dL (11.1 mmol/L) or greater 2 hours after 75-g oral glucose tolerance test, confirmed by a repeat test. This is not recommended for routine use.
- **Normal fasting glucose.** Fasting plasma glucose less than 110 mg/dL (6.1 mmol/L).
- **Impaired fasting glucose.** Fasting plasma glucose levels greater than or equal to 110 mg/dL (6.1 mmol/L) and less than 126 mg/dL (7.0 mmol/L).
- **Impaired glucose tolerance.** Two-hour plasma glucose level greater than or equal to 140 mg/dL (7.8 mmol/L) and less than 200 mg/dL (11.1 mmol/L).

The new diagnostic criteria are based on new scientific studies[29, 30] and expert opinion regarding what fasting plasma glucose value best matches the known risk for developing diabetes complications associated with a 2-hour postglucose challenge level of 200 mg/dL (11.1 mmol/L). The new diagnostic levels emphasize the need to start planning management strategies much earlier than most practitioners are accustomed to. Many patients and providers in the past would admit to not taking diabetes seriously until the fasting level was 200 mg/dL. It may be that a level of 200 mg/dL triggered in their minds the need for some pharmacologic intervention. With the new lower fasting level for diagnosis this may be an opportunity to emphasize the need to take action much earlier. Action should start certainly at 126 mg/dL, with a definite confirmation of the diagnosis and a dietitian

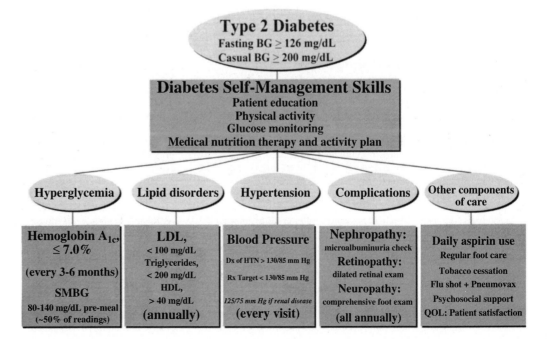

FIGURE 57–2. Standards of care for type 2 diabetes. BG, blood glucose; HTN, hypertension; QOL, quality of life.

consultation. A diabetes educator consultation at this early stage with instruction in glucose monitoring (even if performed only intermittently) will establish and reinforce treatment goals. If some action is taken as close to a glucose value of 126 mg/dL as possible, then it will be natural to keep progressing on the next steps along an algorithm of care as the glucose reaches a more modest level such as 140 mg/dL instead of the current community-wide trigger point of 200 mg/dL. Another important clinical management message from the new diagnostic criteria is a recommendation from the expert panel for, and a renewed community interest in, screening for undiagnosed diabetes. Having a simple diagnostic test (fasting glucose), even if it misses some cases of diabetes, makes screening high-risk populations much easier than the past standard of relying on an oral glucose tolerance test. Data from Harris et al.[31] and the UKPDS[32] indicated we are finding diabetes very late (probably some 10 to 12 years after onset) and 20% to 50% of newly diagnosed patients already have at least one marker of a complication of diabetes. The current recommendations for screening for undiagnosed diabetes in asymptomatic individuals include the following:

- Measure fasting plasma glucose in all persons age 45 years or older; if normal, repeat at 3-year intervals.
- Measure fasting plasma glucose in persons less than 45 years old with high-risk characteristics:
  Obesity, that is, 120% of desirable body weight, or body mass index (BMI) over 27 kg/m².
  First-degree relative with diabetes.
  High-risk racial or ethnic populations: African American, Hispanic American, Native American, Asian American, Pacific Islander.
  Hypertension.
  Dyslipidemia (high-density lipoprotein [HDL] cholesterol less than 35 mg/dL, or triglycerides greater than 250 mg/dL).
  Prior gestational diabetes or baby weighing over 9 lb.
  Prior impaired fasting glucose or impaired glucose tolerance.

There are some data to indicate that screening should start at age 25 in some particularly high-risk groups.[33] The recommendation to screen asymptomatic individuals has not been adopted to date by the U.S. Preventive Services Task Force, which publishes a guide to clinical preventive services.[34] Screening for diabetes will allow earlier intervention to improve glycemic control and identify those with other high-risk cardiovascular risk factors warranting follow-up preventive care strategies. The hemoglobin A$_{1c}$ (HbA$_{1c}$) assay is not currently recommended as a screening or diagnostic test for diabetes, but recent studies[35] and many investigators continue to make a convincing case for it. Once the patient is diagnosed with diabetes, patient education focusing on self-management skills and behavior change is the first step toward successful management.

SELF-MANAGEMENT EDUCATION

Education and Team Management

Every patient with diabetes should be offered an evaluation by members of a diabetes team. The diabetes team includes a Registered Dietitian, a diabetes nurse specialist, a psychologist, and a podiatrist, as well as other specialists to consult with in regard to the complications of diabetes.[36] Yet if primary care physicians take care of at least 90% of patients with diabetes, a major emphasis must be placed on being sure that the primary care provider is aware of the roles and skills of each team member and that assistance is provided to establish referral patterns to essential team members or a diabetes center when appropriate.[37]

Individuals involved in diabetes education can now qualify for certification (Certified Diabetes Educator, or CDE), which adds to the likelihood that there will be a focus on the principles of self-management and behavior change. Studies clearly demonstrate that education alone is not enough to change outcomes.[38] What is needed to change outcomes is an actual change in behavior, for example, performing more glucose self-monitoring, exercising regularly, or using a carbohydrate-to-insulin ratio in deciding on premeal insulin doses. Self-management principles are essential because the patient with diabetes performs 95% of his or her self-care. Only a few times a year does a diabetes educator, a pharmacist, or a physician offer specific advice. Psychosocial support is also critical. Depression[39, 40] and eating disorders[41, 42] are common in diabetes and many centers routinely screen for these conditions. Other forms of psychosocial support include being a good listener, facilitating interaction with other people with diabetes, and encouraging appropriate family support. Comprehensive diabetes education programs which demonstrate core content are being taught with appropriate emphasis on the goals of behavior change and documentation of outcomes. These programs are becoming directly linked to qualification for reimbursement of education services.[43]

The educator and medical provider need to have a means of communication. Only on rare occasions do the educator and physician see the patient at the same time. The best means of communication is based on agreed-upon standards of care as shown in Figure 57–2 and a series of management algorithms (see Figs. 58–3 through 58–6 in Chapter 58). In this way the patient tends to get a consistent message from all members of the team, and it is easy to document a patient's current status in regard to whether standards are being met and what the next appropriate stage in therapy is likely to be if a change is indicated. The provider can then make the appropriate therapeutic decision based on the data received from the educator and discuss this directly with the patient or have the educator contact the patient.

There are three stages of diabetes education, each having distinct goals and strategies. The first stage occurs at the time of initial diagnosis of the disease or of a new diabetes-related complication; the content of teaching is often referred to as "survival skills." A new patient with type 1 diabetes needs to learn how to recognize and monitor low and high blood sugars, ketones, and how to administer insulin. It is important to involve the family or a close friend, since the patient may be distracted by the diagnosis and may not absorb care principles. In less acute situations, such as that of the patient with newly diagnosed type 2 diabetes, initial education can be delivered in a series of individual or group consultations. The federal government and other insurers are pushing for group education by reimbursing groups at a higher rate than individual consultations (although most educators would argue that all reimbursement rates for education are too low). One randomized study has shown that a systematic education curriculum applied in a group or an individual consultation setting resulted in similar clinical outcomes (reduction in HbA$_{1c}$ values to 6.5% over 6 months) and satisfaction ratings.[44] The group setting was considerably more cost-effective.

Within 3 to 6 months a more comprehensive or in-depth diabetes educational experience is valuable, in which questions generated from daily experience with the disease can be answered and diabetes self-management skills reinforced and behavior changes facilitated. Reemphasis of such topics as adjustments for acute illness are essential. Patients on insulin need to know not to stop taking their insulin, to have a steady intake of fluids with carbohydrates, to have medication or a prescription available to treat nausea and vomiting, and to do frequent checks of glucose and ketones (this has typically been urine ketone testing, but there is now a meter that measures capillary β-hydroxybutyrate.) All education programs must establish and reinforce target goals that are understood and agreed to by the patient. These targets include nutrition, exercise, and monitoring goals, as well as the targets for standards of care outlined in Figure 57–2.

The third stage of education is continuing education, in which principles are reviewed, adjustments for new life situations are discussed, and there is an update on new developments (medical and technology) that affect care. One way to organize this information and assist communication between educator, provider, and patient is to give the patient a record book that is easy to follow and keep updated. One such approach that has been shown to be effective uses a tool called a patient owner's manual.[45]

Glucose Monitoring

All patients who are physically capable should be taught capillary self-monitoring of blood glucose (SMBG). The SMBG technology is rapidly evolving in an effort to make testing simple, accurate, and practical in being of assistance in making therapeutic decisions. Meters use strips with glucose oxidase (requiring the meter to directly read a color change) or an electrochemical sensor that generates an electrical signal that is read by the meter and converted to a glucose value. The advantage of the electrochemical technique is that a drop of blood can be placed on the strip extended out from the meter so the meter remains clean (dirty meters being one of the most common causes of erroneous readings). In addition, meters are now being calibrated to correspond to venous plasma readings so that a capillary sample can easily be compared with a venous sample drawn at the laboratory. Patient technique and meter accuracy should be evaluated annually by comparing a patient's reading with that of a reference glucose instrument capable of reading capillary samples, such as the HemoCue blood-glucose analyzer. Most patients and clinicians prefer a meter with a memory feature[46] that can be downloaded at visits, enabling the glucose patterns to be reviewed, and the percent of values above, within, and below target ranges to be displayed. The memory feature has also allowed for the technology to be expanded to include a modem to send glucose readings directly from the patient's home to the provider. The next wave of technology is focusing on noninvasive technology. There is technology available to test capillary glucose at a skin site other than the finger, and to even continuously monitor glucose.[47, 48] This is a rapidly expanding field because of the importance of achieving tight glucose control while avoiding severe hypoglycemia.

What most patients and providers want are guidelines on how often and at what times the diabetic patient should be doing SMBG testing. Some general guidelines for SMBG testing follow:

- If patient is not taking insulin:
  - When newly diagnosed, adjusting therapy, or outside target range, test three times a day: before breakfast, supper, and 2 hours after supper.
  - When inside the target range, test three times a day but only 3 days a week, varying weekdays and weekends.
- If patient is taking insulin:
  - Test four times a day, before meals and at bedtime; perform some additional 2-hour postprandial tests, at alternating meals.

Fewer tests are needed if control is good and more tests are needed if there is an illness, irregular schedule, or psychological stress, or the patient is taking medications that can elevate the glucose. There continues to be much discussion about appropriate SMBG targets. Some authorities strive for normal readings, whereas others, like the ADA,[49] designate an ideal goal and a "take action" point. Another controversy is whether there should be a target for postmeal values. Onset of SMBG targets often used by the authors are as follows:

- Fasting and premeal: 80 to 140 mg/dL
- Postprandial (2 hours from start of meal): <180 mg/dL (or an increase of 20 to 40 mg/dL from start of meal to 2 hours)
- Bedtime: 100 to 160 mg/dL (striving for 50% of values within the target ranges)

These are general targets and can easily be modified on an individual basis, for instance, increased in the elderly. It is important not to set unrealistic expectations, that one should strive to have all readings within the target range. Recent studies have helped to formulate the 50% within-target guideline. One group[50] found, in both type 1 and type 2 patients who achieved an HbA$_{1c}$ of 7%, that they had premeal readings in the range of 80 to 140 mg/dL approximately 50% of the time. Another group confirmed this in younger type 1 patients, arriving at a number of 49% within target, yielding an HbA$_{1c}$ of 7%.[51] This simple advice, to consider 50% of the readings within the target range a success, has been a motivating influence for those diabetic patients who routinely get frustrated by fluctuating SMBG readings.

The other important glycemic control variable is the glycosylated hemoglobin,[52] now widely accepted as the best single indicator of risk for microvascular disease and likely to be a contributor to macrovascular risk in diabetes.[53] Figure 57–3 demonstrates that in major trials in type 1[54] and type 2[22, 55] diabetes, as the HbA$_{1c}$ fraction is reduced there is a significant reduction in risk for microvascular disease and a trend toward a reduction in macrovascular disease. A stylized representation of the risk of small vessel complications correlated with HbA$_{1c}$

	Type 1 DCCT	Type 2 Kumamoto	Type 2 UKPDS
HbA$_{1c}$	9% → 7%	9% → 7%	8% → 7%
Retinopathy	63%	69%	17-21%
Nephropathy	54%	70%	24-33%
Neuropathy	60%	-	-
Cardiovascular disease	(41%)	-	(16%)

FIGURE 57–3. Intensive therapy for diabetes reduces secondary complications. DCCT, Diabetes Control and Complications Trial; UKPDS, United Kingdom Prospective Diabetes Study.

and average SMBG values is shown in Figure 57–4.[56] Any reduction in HbA$_{1c}$ is valuable in reducing risk. This justifies the trend in many managed care organizations and large multispecialty clinics to identify those patients with elevated HbA$_{1c}$ readings and target them for some type of improvement intervention. In addition, one should note that the risk of complications continues to fall even when going from an HbA$_{1c}$ of 8% to 7%. This sets up the current notion that the target goal for HbA$_{1c}$ in both type 1 and type 2 diabetes needs to be set at less than 7%. If the target is less than 7%, the clinician must be prepared to make some change in therapy if the reading is above this.

Recent studies have shown that having the HbA$_{1c}$ reading in hand at the time of a visit is beneficial for making therapy decisions and has great patient and provider appeal.[57, 58] This has started a wave of point-of-care testing that is sure to continue growing. Others are evaluating the utility of testing the glycosylation of proteins other than hemoglobin. The most common alternative protein glycosylation test is the fructosamine assay,[59] which reflects approximately a 3-week period of glycemic control. The large-scale clinical utility of this measurement (now made easy by a home capillary meter) is still under investigation.

Once education is initiated and targets for SMBG and HbA$_{1c}$ are established, it is important to understand the principles of medical nutrition therapy and a physical activity plan.

MEDICAL NUTRITION THERAPY

Diet has long been the cornerstone of diabetes therapy.[60] Although challenging, there is increasing evidence that to achieve metabolic control for many persons with diabetes, changes in nutrition and physical activity are essential.[61-63]

Previous guidelines attempted to apply one nutrition prescription to all patients with diabetes, with an emphasis on "ideal" percentages for carbohydrate, protein, and fat. Today, there is no longer one set of guidelines that applies to all persons with diabetes. Instead the emphasis is on the goals of medical nutrition therapy (MNT) and life-style

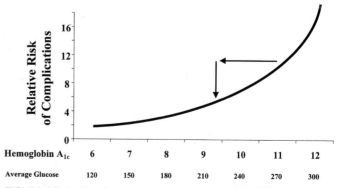

FIGURE 57–4. Risk of complications related to HbA$_{1c}$ (%) and average glucose concentrations (mg/dL).

strategies to achieve these goals. By individualizing treatment and focusing on metabolic outcomes, medical professionals can assist persons with diabetes to make life-style changes and to achieve mutually agreed-upon goals.

Although the roles of MNT are different in type 1 and type 2 diabetes, the goals are similar: (1) achieving and maintaining the desired metabolic goals for glucose, lipid, and hypertension control; (2) preventing diabetes-associated complications such as renal insufficiency and cardiovascular disease; and (3) improvement of overall health with optimal nutrition and increased physical activity.[64, 65] Nutrition changes along with exercise may also play a role in preventing the development of impaired glucose homeostasis and type 2 diabetes in those at high risk.[66–68]

The dietitian has an important role in the management team in developing an individualized nutrition prescription and education plan.[69] For instance, often the dietitian is the first member of the team to realize that, for a given individual, following the prescribed meal plan alone will not meet the desired glycemic goals. The dietitian may also realize that insulin modifications are needed to match an individual's eating or exercise patterns. The dietitian has the responsibility of communicating this information to the treatment team.[70, 71]

Nutrition Interventions to Optimize Glycemic Control

Type 1 Diabetes

To assist persons receiving insulin therapy achieve target blood glucose goals, it is essential that insulin regimens be integrated into the usual eating and exercise habits. Unfortunately, patients are often asked to change long-standing eating and exercise habits to coincide with insulin regimens, making compliance difficult. Table 57–1 summarizes steps for a team approach to integrating insulin regimens into life-style.

In persons treated intensively with a background insulin (Ultralente) and a premeal regular insulin, increasing or decreasing the amount of carbohydrate intake did not influence glycemic control if the premeal insulin was adjusted to the carbohydrate content of the meals. The breakfast regular insulin dose was 1.5 U/10 g carbohydrate and the lunch and dinner doses were 1.0 U/10 g of carbohydrate. This dose was not affected by the glycemic index, fiber, calorie, or fat content of the meals, and wide variations in carbohydrate intake did not modify the background insulin requirements.[72] In patients receiving conventional insulin therapy, such as two daily injections of short- and intermediate-acting insulin, consistency in the amount and source of carbohydrate intake from day to day has been associated with improved blood glucose control.[73]

Type 2 Diabetes

A number of life-style strategies to improve glycemic control can be implemented by persons with type 2 diabetes: moderate weight loss of 4.5 to 9.0 kg (10% to 20% of body weight), especially early in the course of the disease when insulin resistance, rather than insulin

TABLE 57–1. A Team Approach to Integrating Insulin Therapy into Life-Style Habits

1. A registered dietitian assesses the patient's usual eating and exercise habits and develops an individualized meal plan. Life-style habits and the meal plan are communicated to the team member responsible for determining the insulin regimen.
2. An insulin regimen is planned that will integrate insulin therapy into usual life-style habits.
3. Patients are asked to eat consistently and to monitor blood glucose levels.
4. Insulin doses are adjusted based on the amount of carbohydrate servings and blood glucose patterns.
5. Algorithms are added for adjustments in premeal rapid-acting or regular insulin doses for deviations from the usual carbohydrate in meals or snacks and to correct blood glucose levels that are not in the target goal range.

TABLE 57–2. A Team Approach to Prioritizing Life-Style Strategies for Type 2 Diabetes

1. Emphasize the goal of nutrition therapy—to assist in improving blood glucose control, not weight loss.
2. Focus on carbohydrate foods, average portion sizes, and number of carbohydrate servings to choose for meals and snacks. One carbohydrate serving is the amount of food that contains 15 g of carbohydrate. Start with 3 to 4 carbohydrate servings per meal for women and 4 to 5 for men; 1 to 2 for snacks.
3. Encourage physical activity.
4. Use food records with blood glucose monitoring data to determine if glycemic goals are being met, if additional food or activity changes are needed or can be made, or if medication adjustments are required.

Data from Rickheim R, Weaver T, Flader J, et al: Cost-effectiveness of group versus individual diabetes education. Presented at American Diabetes Association Scientific Meeting, June 1999.

deficiency, is the primary factor[74, 75]; a restricted-energy diet, even without weight loss[76, 77]; reducing fat intake, as a high fat intake may aggravate insulin resistance[78, 79]; and spreading the caloric intake throughout the day.[80, 81] Patients with type 2 diabetes are often given so many life-style recommendations that prioritizing them is often difficult. Table 57–2 outlines a team approach to MNT shown to be effective.[82]

The majority of healthcare professionals believe weight loss to be beneficial for persons at risk for chronic disease, especially type 2 diabetes, as obesity is associated with insulin resistance, hyperinsulinemia, and glucose intolerance.[83] Unfortunately, success in helping individuals maintain weight loss in the long term has been dismal,[84] and food restriction (dieting) contributes to adverse psychological consequences.[85] Furthermore, although weight loss was maintained for 12 months by pharmacotherapy, the initial improvements in HbA$_{1c}$ were not maintained.[86]

Treatment strategies for chronic disease may not be the same as prevention strategies. Weight loss or prevention of weight gain may be important for prevention of a chronic disease, including type 2 diabetes, but once a chronic disease is diagnosed, treatment should focus on correcting the metabolic abnormalities associated with the disease. Markovic et al.[87, 88] reported that early improvements in glycemia were related to modest energy restriction and changes in macronutrient intake, that is, reduced carbohydrate intake, whereas later changes in glycemia, insulin sensitivity, and lipid profiles were related to a reduction in central abdominal adiposity.

Because it is the carbohydrate content of the meal that determines the postprandial glucose response, the initial focus of education is on carbohydrate. Carbohydrate counting has been shown to be useful for all persons with diabetes and emphasizes the total amount of carbohydrate ingested, not the source or type of carbohydrate.[89] Foods are grouped into three categories: carbohydrate, meat and meat substitutes, and fat. Sources of carbohydrate are starches, fruits, milk, and desserts.

We have shown that on average, in patients with type 2 diabetes, nutrition therapy provided by registered dietitians decreases HbA$_{1c}$ levels by approximately 1% to 2%. Furthermore, the results of life-style changes are evident by 6 weeks to 3 months, at which point it is essential to determine if target blood glucose goals have been met or if medications need to be added or doses adjusted.[62]

Nutrition Interventions to Optimize Lipid Levels and Prevent Progression of Cardiovascular Disease

Type 1 Diabetes

MNT is initiated when low-density lipoprotein (LDL) cholesterol is greater than 100 mg/dL.[90] Elevated triglyceride and LDL cholesterol levels are also associated with poor glycemic control. If, after glycemia is corrected, total cholesterol or LDL cholesterol continues to be elevated, the National Cholesterol Education Program (NCEP) step II diet[91] should be implemented.

Type 2 Diabetes

A common abnormal lipid pattern is an elevation in triglycerides, lower levels of HDL cholesterol, and an LDL cholesterol fraction that contains a greater proportion of small, dense LDL particles.[90] As in type 1 diabetes, improved glycemic control is essential. In addition, moderate amounts of weight loss, increased physical activity, and elimination of excess alcohol ingestion decreases triglycerides, increases HDL, and modestly lowers LDL levels. In the case of severe hypertriglyceridemia (1000 mg/dL [11.3 mmoL/l]), severe dietary fat restriction (<10% of calories), in addition to pharmacologic therapy, is necessary to reduce the risk of pancreatitis.[64, 65]

The benefits of both low fat, high carbohydrate diets and diets high in monounsaturated fat have been demonstrated.[92–95] However, whatever approach is selected, the saturated fat intake should be limited.

Nutrition Interventions to Optimize Blood Pressure Control

Data from randomized clinical trials indicate that a weight loss of 4.5 kg (10 lb) can be as effective as first-level drugs in controlling blood pressure.[96] However, even without weight loss, a diet high in fruits and vegetables, low in total and saturated fat and cholesterol, high in whole grains, and moderately low in sodium (3000 mg/day) has a blood pressure–lowering effect.[97] Sodium restriction (<2400 mg/day) may reduce blood pressure in patients with hypertension[98] and in those who are sodium-sensitive. Persons with diabetes and older adults are more likely to be sodium-sensitive.[99] However, metabolic studies indicate that severe sodium restriction can increase lipid levels and biomarkers of insulin resistance.[100] Men should limit alcohol intake to no more than two drinks per day and women and lighter-weight individuals to no more than one drink per day.[101]

Nutrition Interventions to Prevent Progression of Renal Complications

There is a consensus that improved glycemic control, controlling blood pressure with an angiotensin-converting enzyme (ACE) inhibitor, and not smoking are important for the treatment of nephropathy.[102] A high intake of dietary protein has renal hemodynamic effects that include an increased glomerular filtration rate (GFR), increased urinary albumin excretion, and increased intraglomerular pressure. Despite flaws in nearly all of the protein and diabetic nephropathy studies, virtually all report that renal function improves with a low protein diet, independent of blood pressure or glycemic control.[102, 103] Therefore, the ADA recommends that with the onset of macroalbuminuria, protein be restricted to the level of the recommended daily allowance (RDA) of 0.8 g/kg/day, or 10% of total calories.[64] Several studies suggest that animal rather than vegetable proteins may be a factor in progression of renal disease. Although data are preliminary, there is no evidence of detrimental effects of vegetable proteins.[104, 105] Supplementing or substituting animal with vegetable protein has the potential to redress noncompliance provoked by the poor palatability of low protein diets. There is no evidence that a high protein diet causes diabetic nephropathy, as dietary intake of protein is reported to be similar in patients with or without nephropathy.[106–109]

Implementing Nutrition Self-Management

STEP 1: ASSESSMENT AND THE NUTRITION PRESCRIPTION. The nutrition prescription is based on an assessment of an individual's usual daily routine and food and caloric intake. Using this information, a preliminary meal plan is designed which will include the number of suggested carbohydrate servings for each meal (and snacks), as well as the average servings of meat and fat. The meal plan can be evaluated by asking the following questions: (1) Does the patient think it is feasible? (2) Is it appropriate for diabetes management? (3) Are the calories appropriate? Approximate calorie requirements can be determined either using the Harris-Benedict equation[110] or by the general guidelines outlined in Table 57–3. (4) Does it encourage healthy eating?

STEP 2: BEHAVIORAL AND MEDICAL GOALS. The patient and medical professional should mutually identify both short- and long-term goals. Behavioral goals may be consistent and appropriate food choices, regular physical activity, correct medication dose (if needed), and frequent blood glucose monitoring. Medical goals are related to blood glucose, lipid, and blood pressure values. In addition, a modest weight loss for persons with type 2 diabetes may make a difference in blood glucose and lipids, and weight loss should be viewed as a means to an end rather than an end in itself.

STEP 3: IMPLEMENTATION AND EDUCATION. An appropriate meal planning approach should be selected and strategies for behavioral change that enhance motivation to maintain necessary lifestyle changes identified. A number of meal-planning approaches are available, ranging from simple guidelines or menus to more complex counting methods. *The First Step in Diabetes Meal Planning*[111] provides general guidelines based on the food guide pyramid and is designed to be used for meal planning until an individualized plan can be implemented. A very popular approach to meal planning is carbohydrate counting. It can be used as a basic meal planning approach as mentioned above or for more intensive management. Several carbohydrate-counting educational tools are available. One carbohydrate choice contributes 15 g of carbohydrate. *My Food Plan*[112] groups carbohydrate choices, meat and meat substitutes, and fats by approximate portion sizes, provides general guidelines for food planning, and includes a form for an individualized meal plan.

STEP 4: EVALUATION AND DOCUMENTATION. Evaluation of the meal plan and monitoring of medical and clinical outcomes should be done at the second or third visit. If altering food intake is not achieving metabolic target ranges, medication changes are needed. Documentation is essential for communication and reimbursement.

STEP 5: FOLLOW-UP AND ONGOING NUTRITION THERAPY. After the basic food and nutrition strategies have been mastered, other aspects of nutrition education are needed to increase flexibility in food choices and life-style. Information on how to make adjustments in food or insulin, eating out, food labels, fat modifications, and alcohol are examples of important topics.

TABLE 57–3. Estimating Caloric Requirements for Adults and Youth

1. Caloric requirements for adults:
   Obese or very inactive adults, chronic dieters require ~10–12 kcal/lb (20 kcal/kg)
   Adults >55 yr, active women, sedentary men require ~13 kcal/lb (28 kcal/kg)
   Active men or very active women require ~15 kcal/lb (30 kcal/kg)
   Thin or very active men require ~20 kcal/lb (40 kcal/kg)
2. Estimated caloric requirements for youth are based on nutrition assessment. Caloric needs can be calculated as follows:
   Method 1
      1000 kcal for 1st yr of life
      Add 100 kcal/yr up to age 11
      Girls 11–15 yr: add 100 kcal/yr
      Girls >15 yr: calculate as for an adult
      Boys 11–15 yr: add 200 kcal/yr
      Boys >15 yr: 23 kcal (50 kcal/kg) if very active
                   18 kcal (40 kcal/kg) for usual activity level
                   15–16 kcal (30–35 kcal/kg) if sedentary
   Method 2
      1000 kcal for 1st yr of life
      Boys: add 125 kcal × age (yr)
      Girls: add 100 kcal × age (yr)
      Add up to 20% additional kcal for activity
      Toddlers (1–3 yr): 40 kcal/in. of length

Nutrition Recommendations for Hospitals and Long-Term Care Facilities

Standardized calorie-level meal patterns based on exchange lists have traditionally been used to plan meals for hospitalized patients or residents in long-term care facilities. The ADA recommends that hospitals consider alternative meal planning approaches.[113, 114] Today, hospital stays are shortened and hospitalized patients are generally quite ill. What time is available should focus on what needs to be done after the patient leaves the hospital. Therefore, it is recommended that hospitals consider a system termed the "consistent-carbohydrate diabetes meal plan." This system uses menus without a specific calorie level but instead incorporates a consistent carbohydrate content from day to day at the morning, midday, and evening meals. For residents of long-term care facilities, providing adequate nutrition is often the primary concern. It is appropriate, therefore, to serve regular (unrestricted) menus with consistent amounts of carbohydrate at meals in such facilities. Regular menus generally provide between 1800 and 2000 calories and are consistent in calories and mealtimes and contain small portions. If desserts are served, the portions are small.

General Nutritional Principles

The approach to individualizing a meal plan (Table 57–4) means there is no single "ADA" or "diabetic" diet, a shorthand notation often seen in patient orders.

CARBOHYDRATE. There is no ideal percentage of calories from carbohydrate. Some patients prefer a high carbohydrate intake, whereas others may benefit from a more moderate intake. The amount of carbohydrate is determined by the food history and treatment goals.[64, 65] For patients using insulin, as mentioned above, adequate insulin must be given to cover the carbohydrate intake. For patients with type 2 diabetes, in line with reducing calories, carbohydrate and fat intake will be reduced as well.

The traditional recommendation to avoid sugars (naturally occurring and added) is based on the belief that during digestion sugars are broken down into glucose more rapidly than starches, causing blood glucose levels to increase rapidly. Little or no scientific evidence supports this assumption. In fact, research conducted over the past decade has shown that starches have a higher glycemic index than that of fruits, milk, or sucrose.[115] Starches are rapidly metabolized into 100% glucose during digestion, in contrast to sucrose, which is metabolized into glucose and fructose. Fructose generally does not enter the general circulation; instead it is stored in the liver as glycogen.[115] Sucrose and sucrose-containing foods must be substituted for other carbohydrate foods in the meal plan.[116–118].

Although different carbohydrates have different glycemic indices, priority is given to the total amount of carbohydrate, not the source or type. For persons with type 2 diabetes the glycemic index may be used to determine the postprandial glucose responses.

PROTEIN. Although protein requires insulin for metabolism, it has minimal effects on blood glucose levels despite evidence that gluconeogenesis occurs.[103, 119, 120] The reason for this is unknown.

Protein does not slow absorption of carbohydrate or help in the treatment of hypoglycemia.[121] In persons with type 1 diabetes, the effect of protein is determined by insulin availability.[103] In patients with mild type 2 diabetes, protein stimulates the release of more insulin than in subjects without diabetes.[120] Whether this is beneficial or not is unknown.

FAT. The amount of the fat in the nutrition prescription is based on the nutrition assessment and treatment goals. Persons who are at a healthy weight and who have normal lipid levels are encouraged to follow the guidelines recommended for all Americans, that is, to limit fat to 30% of calories. The concern with any diet high in fat, regardless of the type of fat, is the potential for unwanted added calories and the potential to inhibit glucose uptake[78] and contribute to insulin resistance.[66, 79]

High carbohydrate, low fat diets, when calories are kept at a level to prevent weight loss, can potentially increase triglyceride levels compared to a high monounsaturated fat diet.[92] However, when energy is restricted, both high carbohydrate and monounsaturated fat diets improve the cardiovascular risk profile and either can replace saturated fat.[95]

FIBER. It is unlikely that individuals can ingest enough food fiber to have an impact on glycemic control.[122] There are other health benefits from fiber, such as the lipid-lowering effect of fibers found in fruits, legumes, oats, and barley, and the prevention of constipation and improved satiety from fibers found in bran and whole grains.

ALTERNATIVE SWEETENERS. Non-nutritive sweeteners (aspartame, acesulfame K, sucralose, and saccharin) are safe and helpful in reducing or controlling total carbohydrate intake. Nutritive sweeteners (fructose, fruit juice concentrate, sorbitol, mannitol, xylitol, starch hydrolysates, isomalt), in the amounts likely to be ingested at one meal or snack, are unlikely to have any significant advantage over sucrose in decreasing caloric intake or improving glycemic response.[64]

ALCOHOL. The same precautions that apply to the consumption of alcohol by the general population apply to persons with diabetes. Moderate amounts of alcohol have been shown to improve insulin sensitivity[123] and, in adults with type 2 diabetes, to reduce coronary heart disease mortality.[124] In persons with well-controlled diabetes, and with usual food intake, blood glucose levels are not affected by moderate use of alcohol.[125] However, in the fasting state, hypoglycemia can occur at blood alcohol levels that do not exceed mild intoxication. It is recommended that men limit alcoholic beverages to no more than two drinks (one drink = 12 oz of beer = 5 oz of wine = 1.5 oz of distilled spirits) per day and women to one drink per day in addition to their usual meal plan.[64]

MICRONUTRIENTS. At present, there is no justification for routine supplementation of vitamins and minerals for patients with diabetes. There are, however, select groups of people who may benefit. Oxidation of lipoproteins plays a role in atherogenesis, but whether antioxidants, especially vitamin E, can modify this process is unknown. The role of other micronutrients, such as chromium, zinc, magnesium, and the B vitamins, is being studied.[126, 127]

The scope of nutrition information, research, and clinical application is expanding rapidly. In order for MNT to affect metabolic control and prevent complications, the dietitian must actively participate in the management team. The expectations, as well as the importance, of data collection, management interactions, and communications should be clear to the dietitian, physician, other team members, and the patient.

TABLE 57–4. Historical Perspective on Nutrition Recommendations—Distribution of Calories

Year	Carbohydrate (%)	Protein (%)	Fat (%)
Before 1921	Starvation diets		
1921	20	10	70
1950	40	20	40
1971	45	20	35
1986	Up to 60	12–20	<30
1994	*	10–20	†

*Based on nutrition assessment and treatment goals.
†Less than 10% of calories from saturated fats.
Data from American Diabetes Association: Nutrition recommendations and principles for people with diabetes mellitus (position statement). Diabetes Care 23(suppl 1):S43–S46, 2000.

EXERCISE MANAGEMENT

The benefits and risks of exercise need to be considered when establishing a treatment plan.[128] The benefits of exercise are many and include increased insulin sensitivity, improvement in lipid profile and blood pressure, enhanced weight management, improved muscular strength and joint flexibility, and an improved overall sense of well-being. In type 1 diabetes, exercise as a therapeutic measure for achieving improved glycemia, has not been reported[129]; however, in type 2 diabetes, through improvement in insulin sensitivity and increased peripheral glucose utilization, exercise has been shown to improve glycemia.[130]

In patients planning to participate in low-intensity forms of exercise, such as walking, the physician should use clinical judgment in deciding whether to recommend an exercise stress test. Patients with known coronary artery disease should undergo a supervised evaluation of the ischemic response to exercise, the ischemic threshold, and the propensity for arrhythmia during exercise.[128]

Exercise and Type 1 Diabetes

Considering the complexity of fuel flux during exercise and the important role of insulin and the counterregulatory hormones, it is not surprising that patients using insulin can have control problems when exercising. During exercise, in persons without diabetes, insulin levels fall while counterregulatory hormones (primarily glucagon) rise. Thus, increased glucose utilization of exercising muscle is matched by glucose released from the liver.

In persons with type 1 diabetes, the glycemic response to exercise varies depending on overall metabolic control; intensity, duration, and timing of exercise; previous food intake; previous conditioning; and regularity of exercise sessions. Excessive insulin levels can potentiate hypoglycemia due to insulin-enhanced muscle cellular glucose uptake and the inhibition of glycogenolysis. In contrast, in an exerciser with a low insulin level, with a rise in counterregulatory hormones during exercise, the production of glucose and free fatty acids continues, whereas uptake is minimal. This can result in large increases in plasma glucose and ketone levels.[131]

Risks of Exercise

Hypoglycemia can occur during prolonged exercise (usually exercise of more than 40 to 60 minutes in duration), and for up to 24 hours after unusually strenuous, prolonged, or sporadic exercise, owing to increased insulin sensitivity and replenishment of liver and muscle glycogen stores following exercise. Hypoglycemia is not limited to persons in good metabolic control and often occurs after a single bout of exercise in persons who are untrained. Trained individuals usually experience less hypoglycemia. Although hypoglycemia is reported to be most common 3 to 15 hours after exercise,[132, 133] depending on the rate of change in glycemia, it can also occur during exercise. For example, a glucose level that is stable at 100 mg/dL (5.5 mmol/L) before exercise may be a safe situation, but the same level may be indicative of a fall in glucose levels if the preceding glucose measurement was 8.3 150 mg/dL (mmol/L).[134]

Hyperglycemia after exercise can be caused by insufficient insulin, but is more likely to be caused by exercise at too high a level of intensity for the exerciser.[135, 136] This is mediated by the "stress" or counterregulatory hormones causing an increase in hepatic glucose production that exceeds instead of matches the need for glucose.

If proliferative diabetic retinopathy is active, activities such as anaerobic exercise, straining, jarring, or Valsalva-like maneuvers may precipitate vitreous hemorrhage or traction retinal detachment.[128]

Guidelines for Safe Exercise

Blood glucose monitoring, both before exercise and after exercise, is the key to safety and to understanding how exercise affects diabetes control and provides feedback to assist with insulin and carbohydrate adjustments. In general, 1 hour of increased exercise requires an additional 15 g of carbohydrate, either prior to or after exercise. For more strenuous exercise, 30 g of carbohydrate may be required.[75] Moderate-intensity exercise increases whole-body glucose uptake by 2 to 3 mg/kg/min. For example, a 70-kg person would utilize an additional 8.4 to 12.6 g of glucose for every hour of moderate-intensity exercise. During high-intensity exercise, the rate may increase to 5 to 6 mg/kg/min. Despite this increased rate of glucose use, the demand on glucose stores and the risk of hypoglycemia are less because exercise of this intensity cannot be sustained for long.[134]

Insulin doses may need to be decreased. In general, for exercise lasting 45 to 60 minutes, the dose of rapid-acting or regular insulin can be decreased by 1 to 2 U prior to exercise. For exercise of longer duration, daily insulin dosage may need to be decreased by as much as one-third to one-half. In contrast to these acute reductions in insulin, patients participating in regular exercise programs (at least every other day) may have already decreased their total insulin by as much as 15% to 20% and their bodies have adjusted to regular exercise.[134] Exercisers using premeal insulin lispro may experience less hypoglycemia if they can wait until 2 hours after the meal to exercise. In contrast, exercisers using premeal regular insulin may have better glucose values if they exercise immediately after the meal.[137] Table 57–5 summarizes general exercise guidelines for patients with type 1 diabetes.

Exercise and Type 2 Diabetes

Physical activity (exercise) has the potential to improve glucose tolerance by reversing or decreasing insulin resistance.[67, 138] It improves insulin sensitivity by activating intracellular GLUT4 glucose transporters, thereby improving peripheral glucose uptake and suppressing hepatic glucose production. This can occur even without changes in body weight, body fat content, or $\dot{V}O_2$max.[139] Because enhanced insulin sensitivity is lost within 48 hours after exercise, repeated bouts of physical activity at regular intervals are needed. Although aerobic exercise is recommended, muscle-strengthening activities can also contribute to improved glucose control.[140] Most studies[141] suggest that exercise is most effective in persons with impaired glucose tolerance or with fasting blood glucose levels of less than 200 mg/dL (11.1 mmol/l).

Physical training contributes to desirable changes in triglycerides, total cholesterol, and the HDL cholesterol-to-total cholesterol ratio. Regular physical activity also lowers blood pressure in persons with type 2 diabetes. Body weight and body fat losses with regular exercise programs are generally small.[142] Although the mechanism is unclear, abundant evidence suggests that exercise is related to long-term maintenance of weight loss. However, in regard to mortality, physical fitness is more important than weight.[143]

Risks of Exercise

1. Patients with type 2 diabetes have lower $\dot{V}O_2$max, both before and after 6 weeks of training,[144] and therefore exercise programs should be initiated at lower target pulse rates and gradually increased to the desired pulse rate

2. Autonomic neuropathy and some blood pressure medications do not allow the heart rate to increase. Monitoring the intensity of exercise by using perceived exertion rather than pulse rate is important.

TABLE 57–5. General Guidelines for Safe Exercise for Persons with Type 1 Diabetes

1. Metabolic control before exercise:
   Avoid exercise if FASTING glucose levels are >250 mg/dL and ketosis is present, and use caution if glucose levels are >300 mg/dL and no ketosis is present.
   Ingest added carbohydrate if glucose levels are <100 mg/dL
2. Blood glucose monitoring before and after exercise:
   Identify when changes in insulin or carbohydrate intake are necessary
   Learn the glycemic response to different exercise conditions
3. Food intake:
   Consume added carbohydrate as needed to avoid hypoglycemia; in general, 15 g of carbohydrate should be eaten after or before 1 hr of moderate activity
   Carbohydrate-based foods should be readily available during and after exercise
   Fluid intake is important: for exercising <40–60 min, plain water is fine; for exercising >40–60 min, water with 6–8% carbohydrate is needed

Adapted from American Diabetes Association: Diabetes mellitus and exercise (position statement). Diabetes Care 23(suppl 1):S50–S51, 2000.

TABLE 57–6. General Guidelines for Safe Exercise for Persons with Type 2 Diabetes

1. Start with mild exercises, such as walking, swimming, or riding a stationary bike, and gradually increase exercise sessions.
2. To improve insulin sensitivity and glycemic control, exercise should be done at least 4 days/wk or every other day.
3. Exercise should not result in shortness of breath. Perceived exertion may be a better indicator of exercise intensity than pulse rate.
4. Fitness can be achieved by exercising 4–7 days/wk at 50%–70% maximal heart rate for a minimum of 20 min or by physical activity every day for an accumulated ≥30 min.
5. Warm-up and cool-down exercises are important to achieve flexibility and to prevent exercise-related injuries.
6. Aerobic exercise should be of low impact.
7. Muscle-strengthening exercises may also lead to improved glucose disposal and improved glycemic control.

3. Because individuals are often deconditioned, rest periods may be needed; this does not impair the effects of training.[145]

4. Hypotension or hypertension after vigorous exercise is more likely to develop and blood pressure may need to be monitored.[128]

5. Peripheral neuropathy may result in loss of protective sensation in the feet, and touch sensation should be evaluated.[128]

Guidelines for Safe Exercise

The type of exercise the individual chooses should be tailored to his or her physical capacity and interest. Although walking may be the most convenient low-impact mode, some persons may need to do non–weight-bearing activities. Patients with type 2 diabetes should strive to achieve a minimum cumulative total of 1000 kcal/week from physical activities. Table 57–6 summarizes general exercise guidelines for patients with type 2 diabetes.

Prevention of Type 2 Diabetes

A great deal of evidence has accumulated supporting the hypothesis that exercise may be useful in preventing or delaying the onset of type 2 diabetes. A large randomized prospective National Institutes of Health (NIH) study is under way studying this approach.[128]

General advice is to avoid the hazards of exercise by starting a program slowly, avoiding overexertion, and seeking medical attention if any symptoms occur during exercise, with the realization that these risks are almost certainly outweighed by the long-term benefits.[130] All members of the diabetes team should be prepared to encourage increased physical activity by their patients.

REFERENCES

1. Harris M, Flegal M, Cowie C, et al: Prevalence of diabetes, impaired fasting glucose, and impaired glucose tolerance in U.S. adults. The Third National Health and Nutrition Examination Survey, 1988–1994. Diabetes Care 21:518–524, 1998.
2. King H: Global burden of diabetes mellitus, 1995–2025: Prevalence, numerical estimates, and projections. Diabetes Care 21:1414–1431, 1998.
3. Brown JB, Pedula KL, Bakst AW: The progressive cost of complications in type 2 diabetes mellitus. Arch Intern Med 159:1873–1880, 1999.
4. Rubin RJ, Altman WM, Mendelson DN: Health care expenditures for people with diabetes mellitus, 1992. J Clin Endocrinol Metab 78:809A–809F, 1994.
5. Gilmer T, O'Conner P, Manning W, et al: The cost to health plans of poor glycemic control. Diabetes Care 20:1847–1853, 1997.
6. Harris MI: Undiagnosed NIDDM: Clinical and public health issues. Diabetes Care 16:642–652, 1993.
7. Levetan C, Salas J, Wilets I, et al: Impact of endocrine and diabetes team consultation on hospital length of stay for patients with diabetes. Am J Med 99:22–28, 1995.
8. Corbin R: Endocrinologists provide cost effective diabetes care. First Messenger 6:8–10, 1997.
9. Levetan C, Passaro M, Jablonski K, et al: Effect of physician specialty on outcomes in diabetic ketoacidosis. Diabetes Care 22:1790–1795, 1999.
10. Ho M, Marger M, Beart J, et al: Is the quality of diabetes care better in a diabetes care clinic or in a general medicine clinic? Diabetes Care 20:472–475, 1997.
11. O'Connor P, Pronk N: Integrating population health concepts, clinical guidelines, and ambulatory medical care systems to improve diabetes care. J Ambulatory Care Manage 21:67–73, 1998.
12. Greenfield S, Rogers W, Mangotich M, et al: Outcomes of patients with hypertension and non–insulin dependent diabetes mellitus treated by different systems and specialties. Results from the Medical Outcomes Study. JAMA 274:1436–1444, 1995.
13. Greenfield S, Kaplan SH, Silliman RA, et al: The uses of outcomes research for medical effectiveness, quality of care and reimbursement in type II diabetes. Diabetes Care 17(suppl):32–39, 1994.
14. Griffin S: Diabetes care in general practice: Meta-analysis of randomized control trials. BMJ 317:390–396, 1998.
15. Gerstein H, Reddy K, Dawson K, et al: A controlled evaluation of a national continuing medical education programme designed to improve family physicians' implementation of diabetes-specific clinical practice guidelines. Diabet Med 16:964–969, 1999.
16. Aubert RE, Herman WH, Water J, et al: Nurse case management to improve glycemic control in diabetic patients in a health maintenance organization. Ann Intern Med 129:605–612, 1998.
17. Peters AL, Davidson MB: Application of a diabetes program in an HMO setting: The feasibility of using nurses and a computer system to provide cost-effective care. Diabetes Care 21:1037–1043, 1998.
18. Law RE, Meehan WP, Xi XP, et al: Troglitazone inhibits vascular smooth-muscle cell growth and intimal hyperplasia. J Clin Invest 98:1897–1905, 1996.
19. Etzwiler DD: Self care behaviors and glycemic control in type 1 diabetes. Diabetes Spectrum 2:37–38, 1989.
20. Lorenz R, Bubb J, Davis D, et al: Changing behavior: Practical lessons from the DCCT. Diabetes Care 19:648–652, 1996.
21. National Committee of Quality Assurance: Diabetes Quality Improvement Project, initial measure set. Available at: http://www.diabetes.org/dqip.asp. Accessed August 14, 1998.
22. United Kingdom Prospective Diabetes Study (UKPDS) Group: Intensive blood-glucose control with sulfonylureas or insulin compared with conventional treatment and risk of complications in patients with type 2 diabetes (UKPDS 33). Lancet 352:837–953, 1998.
23. Turner RC, Millns H, Neil HAW, et al: Risk factors for coronary artery disease in non–insulin dependent diabetes mellitus: United Kingdom Prospective Diabetes Study (UKPDS: 23). BMJ 316:823–828, 1998.
24. American Diabetes Association: Standards of medical care for patients with diabetes mellitus (position statement). Diabetes Care 23(suppl 1):S32–S42, 2000.
25. Nesto RW: Screening for asymptomatic coronary artery disease in diabetes. Diabetes Care 22:1393–1395, 1999.
26. American Diabetes Association Expert Committee: Report of the Expert Committee on the diagnosis and classification of diabetes mellitus. Diabetes Care 20:1183–1158, 1997.
27. National Diabetes Data Group: Classification and diagnosis of diabetes mellitus and other categories of glucose intolerance. Diabetes 28:1039–1057, 1979.
28. Imagawa A, Hanafusa T, Miyagawa J, et al: A novel subtype of type 1 diabetes mellitus characterized by a rapid onset and an absence of diabetes related antibodies. N Engl J Med 342:301–307, 2000.
29. McCance DR, Hanson RL, Charles MA, et al: Comparison of tests for glycated haemoglobin and fasting and two hour plasma glucose concentrations as diagnostic methods for diabetes. BMJ 308:1323–1328, 1994.
30. Engelgau MM, Thompson TJ, Herman WH, et al: Comparison of fasting and 2-hour glucose and HbA$_{1c}$ levels for diagnosing diabetes: Diagnostic criteria and performance revisited. Diabetes Care 20:785–791, 1997.
31. Harris MI, Klein RE, Welborn TA, et al: Onset of NIDDM occurs at least 4–7 years before clinical diagnosis. Diabetes Care 15:815–819, 1992.
32. United Kindom Prospective Diabetes Study 16: Overview of 6 years' therapy of type II diabetes: A progressive disease. Diabetes 44:1249–1258, 1995.
33. CDC Diabetes Cost-Effectiveness Study Group: The cost-effectiveness of screening for type 2 diabetes. JAMA 280:1757–1763, 1998.
34. Report of the U.S. Preventive Services Task Force: Guide to Clinical Preventive Services, ed 2. Baltimore, Williams & Wilkins, 1996.
35. Rohlfing CL, Little RR, Wiedmeyer HM, et al: Use of GHb (HbA$_{1c}$) in screening for undiagnosed diabetes in the U.S. population. Diabetes Care 23:187–191, 2000.
36. Hirsch IB: The status of the diabetes team. Clin Diabetes 16:145–146, 1998.
37. Etzwiler D: Primary-care teams and a systems approach to diabetes management. Clin Diabetes 12:50–52, 1994.
38. Padgett D, Mumford E, Hynes M, et al: Meta-analysis of the effects of educational and psychosocial interventions on the management of diabetes mellitus. J Clin Epidemiol 41:1007–1030, 1988.
39. Peyrot M, Rubin RR: Persistence of depressive symptoms in diabetic adults. Diabetes Care 22:448–451, 1999.
40. Gavard JA, Lustman PJ, Clouse RE: Prevalence of depression in adults with diabetes: An epidemiologic evaluation. Diabetes Care 16:1167–1178, 1993.
41. Birk RS: The prevalence of anorexia nervosa, bulimia, and induced glycosuria in IDDM females. Diabetes Educator 15:336–341, 1989.
42. Neumark-Sztainer D, Story M, Falkner NH, et al: Disordered eating among adolescents with chronic illness and disability. Arch Pediatr Adolesc Med 152:871–878, 1998.
43. Balanced Budget Act of 1997. Presented at the American Diabetes Association Scientific Meeting, San Diego, CA, June 13, 1999. Publication no. 869-033-00034-1, pp 115–116.
44. Rickheim P, Weaver T, Flader J, et al: Cost-effectiveness of group versus individual diabetes education (abstract). Diabetes 48(suppl 1), 1999.
45. Mazze R, Strock E, Simonson G, et al: Staged Diabetes Management: Structured Diabetes Health Care System, Japanese edition. Minneapolis, International Diabetes Center, 1999.
46. Mazze RS, Shamoon H, Parmentier R, et al: Reliability of blood glucose monitoring by patients with diabetes. Am J Med 77:211–217, 1984.
47. Tamada JA, Garg S, Jovanovic L, et al: Noninvasive glucose monitoring: comprehensive clinical results. JAMA 282:1839–1844, 1999.

48. Problems associated with subcutaneously implanted glucose sensors (editorial). Diabetes Care 23:143–145, 2000.
49. American Diabetes Association: Clinical practice recommendations 2000. Diabetes 23(suppl 1):S32–S42, 2000.
50. Bergenstal R, Johnson M, Whipple D, et al: Advantages of adding metformin to multiple dose insulin therapy in type 2 diabetes (abstract). Diabetes 47(suppl 1): A89, 1998.
51. Brewer KW, Chase HP, Owen S, et al: Slicing the pie: Correlating HbA_{1c} values with average blood glucose values in a pie chart form. Diabetes Care 21:209–213, 1998.
52. Goldstein DE, Little RR, Lorenz RA, et al: Tests of glycemia in diabetes (technical review). Diabetes Care 18:896–909, 1995.
53. Klein R: Hyperglycemia and microvascular and macrovascular disease in diabetes. Diabetes Care 18:258–268, 1995.
54. DCCT Research Group: The effect of intensive treatment of diabetes on the development and progression of long-term complications of insulin-dependent diabetes mellitus. N Engl J Med 329:1289–1298, 1993.
55. Ohkubo Y, Kishikawa H, Araki E, et al: Intensive insulin therapy prevents the progression of diabetic micovascular complications in Japanese patients with non–insulin-dependent diabetes mellitus: A randomized prospective 6-year study. Diabetes Res Clin Pract 28:103–117, 1995.
56. The Diabetes Control and Complications Trial Research Group: The absence of a glycemic threshold for the development of long-term complications: The perspective of the Diabetes Control and Complications Trial. Diabetes 45:1289–1298, 1996.
57. Cagliero E, Levina EV, Nathan DM: Immediate feedback of HbA_{1c} levels improves glycemic control in type 1 and insulin-treated type 2 diabetic patients. Diabetes Care 22:1785–1789, 1999.
58. Thaler LM, Ziemer DC, Gallina DL, et al: Diabetes in urban African-Americans. Availability of rapid HbA1c measurements enhances clinical decision-making. Diabetes Care 22:1415–1421, 1999.
59. Tahara Y, Shima K: Kinetics of HbA_{1c}, glycated albumin, and fructosamine and analysis of their weight functions against preceding plasma glucose level. Diabetes Care 18:440–524, 1995.
60. Bantle JP: A physician's perspective on medical nutrition therapy for diabetes. In Franz MJ, Bantle JP (eds): American Diabetes Association Guide to Medical Nutrition Therapy for Diabetes. Alexandria, VA, American Diabetes Association, 1999, pp 18–25.
61. Delahanty LM, Halford BN: The role of diet behaviors in achieving improved glycemic control in intensively treated patients in the Diabetes Control and Complications Trial. Diabetes Care 16:1453–1458, 1993.
62. Franz MJ, Monk A, Barry B, et al: Effectiveness of medical nutrition therapy provided by dietitians in the management of non–insulin-dependent diabetes mellitus: A randomized, controlled clinical trial. J Am Diet Assoc 95:1009–1017, 1995.
63. Kulkarni K, Castle G, Gregory R, et al: Nutrition practice guidelines for type 1 diabetes positively affect dietitian practices and patient outcomes. J Am Diet Assoc 98:62–70, 1998.
64. American Diabetes Association: Nutrition recommendations and principles for people with diabetes mellitus (position statement). Diabetes Care 23(suppl 1):S43–S46, 2000.
65. Franz MJ, Horton ES Sr, Bantle JP, et al: Nutrition principles for the management of diabetes and related complications (technical review). Diabetes Care 17:490–518, 1994.
66. Mayer-Davis EJ, Monacao JH, Hoen HM, et al: Dietary fat and insulin sensitivity in a triethnic population: The role of obesity. The Insulin Resistance and Atherosclerosis Study (IRAS). Am J Clin Nutr 65:79–87, 1997.
67. Mayer-Davis EJ, D'Agostino RJ, Karter AJ, et al: Intensity and amount of physical activity in relation to insulin sensitivity. The Insulin Resistance and Atherosclerosis Study (IRAS). JAMA 270:669–674, 1998.
68. Karter A, Mayer-Davis EJ, Selby J, et al: Insulin sensitivity and abdominal obesity in African Americans, Hispanic and non-Hispanic white men and women. Diabetes 45:1547–1555, 1996.
69. Diabetes Control and Complications Trial Research Group: Expanded role of the dietitian in the Diabetes Control and Complications Trial: Implications for clinical practice. J Am Diet Assoc 93:758–767, 1993.
70. Monk A, Barry B, McClain K, et al: Practice guidelines for medical nutrition therapy by dietitians for persons with non-insulin-dependent diabetes mellitus. J Am Diet Assoc 95:999–1008, 1995.
71. Diabetes Care and Education, a Practice Group of the American Dietetic Association, Kulkarni K, Castle G, et al: Nutrition practice guidelines for type 1 diabetes: An overview of the content and application. Diabetes Spectrum 10:248–256, 1997.
72. Rabasa-Lhoret R, Garon J, Langlier H, et al: Effects of meal carbohydrate on insulin requirements in type 1 diabetic patients treated intensively with the basal-bolus (Ultralente-regular) insulin regimen. Diabetes Care 22:667–673, 1999.
73. Wolever TMS, Hamad S, Chiasson J-L, et al: Day-to-day consistency in amount and source of carbohydrate intake associated with improved blood glucose control in type 1 diabetes. J Am Coll Nutr 18:242–247, 1999.
74. Watts NB, Spanheimer RG, DiGirolamo M, et al: Prediction of glucose response to weight loss in patients with non-insulin-dependent diabetes mellitus. Arch Intern Med 150:803–806, 1990.
75. Wing RR, Koeske R, Epstein LH, et al: Long-term effects of modest weight loss in type II diabetic patients. Arch Intern Med 147:1749–1753, 1987.
76. Wing RR, Blair EH, Bononi P, et al: Caloric restriction per se is a significant factor in improvements in glycemic control and insulin sensitivity during weight loss in obese NIDDM patients. Diabetes Care 17:30–36, 1994.
77. Kelly DE, Wing R, Buonocore P, et al: Relative effects of calorie restriction and weight loss in noninsulin-dependent diabetes mellitus. J Clin Endocrinol Metab 77:1287–1293, 1993.
78. Boden G, Chen X: Effects of fat on glucose uptake and utilization in patients with non-insulin dependent diabetes. J Clin Invest 96:1261–1267, 1995.
79. Mayer-Davis EJ, Levin S, Marshall JA: Heterogeneity in associations between macronutrient intake and lipoprotein profile in individuals with type 2 diabetes. Diabetes Care 22:1632–1639, 1999.
80. Jenkins DJA, Ocana A, Jenkins A, et al: Metabolic advantages of spreading the nutrient load: Effects of increased meal frequency in non–insulin-dependent diabetes. Am J Clin Nutr 55:461–467, 1992.
81. Bertelsen J, Christiansen C, Thomsen C, et al: Effect of meal frequency on blood glucose, insulin, and free fatty acids in NIDDM subjects. Diabetes Care 16:3–7, 1993.
82. Rickheim R, Weaver T, Flader J, et al: Cost-effectiveness of group versus individual diabetes education. Presidential Poster Session. Presented at the American Diabetes Association Scientific Meeting, June 1999.
83. Kruszynska Y, Olefsky JM: Cellular and molecular mechanism of non–insulin-dependent diabetes. J Invest Med 44:413–428, 1996.
84. Foreyt JP, Goodrick GK: Evidence for success of behavior modification in weight loss and control. Ann Intern Med 119(7 pt 3):698–701, 1992.
85. Polivy J: Psychological consequences of food restriction. J Am Diet Assoc 96:589–592, 1996.
86. Redmon JB, Raatz SK, Kwong CA, et al: Pharmacologic induction of weight loss to treat type 2 diabetes. Diabetes Care 22:896–903, 1999.
87. Markovic TP, Jenkins AB, Campbell LV, et al: The determinants of glycemic responses to diet restriction and weight loss in obesity and NIDDM. Diabetes Care 21:687–694, 1998.
88. Markovic TP, Campbell LV, Balasubramanian S, et al: Beneficial effect on average lipid levels from energy restriction and fat loss in obese individuals with or without type 2 diabetes. Diabetes Care 21:695–700, 1998.
89. Gillespie S, Kulkarni K, Daly A: Using carbohydrate counting in diabetes clinical practice. J Am Diet Assoc 98:897–899, 1998.
90. American Diabetes Association: Management of dyslipidemia in adults with diabetes (position statement). Diabetes Care 23(suppl 1):S57–S60, 2000.
91. National Cholesterol Education Program (NCEP) Expert Panel: Summary of the second report of the NCEP expert panel on detection, evaluation, and treatment of high blood cholesterol (Adult Treatment Panel II). JAMA 209:3015–3023, 1993.
92. Garg A, Bantle JP, Henry RR, et al: Effects of varying carbohydrate content of diet in patients with non-insulin dependent diabetes mellitus. JAMA 271:1421–1428, 1994.
93. Parillo M, Rivellese AA, Ciardullo AV, et al: A high-monounsaturated-fat/low carbohydrate diet improves peripheral insulin sensitivity in non–insulin-dependent diabetic patients. Metabolism 41:1371–1378, 1992.
94. Abbott WGH, Boyce VL, Grundy SM, et al: Effects of replacing saturated fat with complex carbohydrate in diets of subjects with NIDDM. Diabetes Care 12:102–107, 1989.
95. Heilbronn LK, Noakes M, Clifton PM: Effect of energy restriction, weight loss, and diet composition on plasma lipids and glucose in patients with type 2 diabetes. Diabetes Care 22:889–895, 1999.
96. Stamler R, Stamler J, Gosch FC, et al: Primary prevention of hypertension by nutritional-hygienic means: Final report of a randomized, controlled trial. JAMA 262:1801–1807, 1989.
97. Appel LJ, Moore TJ, Obarzanek E, et al: A clinical trial of the effects of dietary pattern on blood pressure. N Engl J Med 336:117–124, 1997.
98. Midgley JP, Matthew AG, Greenwood CM, et al: Effect of reduced dietary sodium on blood pressure: A meta-analysis of randomized controlled trials. JAMA 275:1590–1597, 1996.
99. Overlack A, Ruppert M, Lkolloch R, et al: Age is a major determinant of divergent blood pressure responses to varying salt intake in essential hypertension. Am J Hypertens 8:829–836, 1995.
100. Iwaoka T, Umeda T, Inoue J, et al: Dietary NaCl restriction deteriorated oral glucose tolerance in hypertensive patients with impairment of glucose tolerance. Am J Hypertens 7:460–463, 1994.
101. The 6th report of the Joint National Committee on Prevention, Detection, Evaluation, and Treatment of High Blood Pressure. Arch Intern Med 157:2413–2446, 1997.
102. American Diabetes Association: Diabetic nephropathy (position statement). Diabetes Care 23(suppl 1):S69–S72, 2000.
103. Henry RR: Protein content of the diabetic diet. Diabetes Care 17:1502–1513, 1994.
104. Pedrini MT, Levey AS, Lau J, et al: The effect of dietary protein restriction on the progression of diabetic and nondiabetics renal diseases: A meta-analysis. Ann Intern Med 124:627–632, 1996.
105. Wheeler ML: Nephropathy and medical nutrition therapy. *In* Franz MJ, Bantle JP (eds): American Diabetes Association Medical Nutrition Therapy for Diabetes. Alexandria, VA American Diabetes Association, 1999, pp 312–323.
106. Nyberg G. Norden G, Attman P-O, et al: Diabetic nephropathy: Is dietary protein harmful? Diabetic Complications 1:37–40, 1987.
107. Watts GF, Gregory L, Naoumova R, et al: Nutrient intake in insulin-dependent diabetic patients with incipient nephropathy. Eur J Clin Nutr 42:697–702, 1988.
108. Ekberg G, Sjofors G, Grefberg N, et al: Protein intake and glomerular hyperfiltration in insulin-treated diabetics without manifest nephropathy. Scand J Urol Nephrol 27:441–446, 1993.
109. Jameel N, Pugh JA, Mitchell BD, et al: Dietary protein intake is not correlated with clinical proteinuria in NIDDM. Diabetes Care 15:178–183, 1992.
110. Frankenfield DC, Muth ER, Rowe WA: The Harris-Benedict studies of human basal metabolism: History and limitations. J Am Diet Assoc 98:439–445, 1998.
111. American Diabetes Association and the American Dietetic Association: The First Step in Diabetes Meal Planning. Alexandria, VA, American Diabetes Association, 1995.
112. International Diabetes Center: My Food Plan. Minneapolis, International Diabetes Center, 1996.
113. American Diabetes Association: Translation of the diabetes nutrition recommendations for health care institutions (position statement). Diabetes Care 23(suppl 1): S47–S49, 2000.
114. Schafer R, Bohannon B, Franz MJ, et al: Translation of the diabetes nutrition recommendations for health care institutions (technical review). Diabetes Care 20:96–105, 1997.

115. Wolever TMS, Nguyen P-M, Chiasson J-L: Determinants of diet glycemic index calculated retrospectively from diet records of 342 individuals with non–insulin-dependent diabetes mellitus. Am J Clin Nutr 59:1265–1269, 1994.

116. Bantle JP, Swanson JE, Thomas W, et al: Metabolic effects of dietary sucrose in type II diabetic subjects. Diabetes Care 16:1301–1305, 1993.

117. Peterson DB, Lambert J, Gerrig S et al: Sucrose in the diet of diabetic patients—just another carbohydrate? Diabetologia 29:216–220, 1986.

118. Rickard KA, Loghmani E, Cleveland JL, et al: Lower glycemic response to sucrose in the diets of children with type 1 diabetes. J Pediatr 133:429–432, 1998.

119. Peters AL, Davidson MB: Protein and fat effects on glucose response and insulin requirements in subjects with insulin-dependent diabetes mellitus. Am J Clin Nutr 58:555–600, 1993.

120. Nuttall FQ, Mooradian AD, Gannon MC, et al: Effect of protein ingestion on the glucose and insulin response to a standardized oral glucose load. Diabetes Care 7:465–470, 1984.

121. Gray RO, Butler PC, Beers TR, et al: Comparison of the ability of bread versus bread plus meat to treat and prevent subsequent hypoglycemia in patients with insulin-dependent diabetes mellitus. J Clin Endocrinol Metab 81:1508–1511, 1996.

122. Nuttall FQ: Dietary fiber in the management of diabetes. Diabetes 42:503–508, 1993.

123. Facchini F, Chen Y-DI, Reaven GM: Light-to-moderate alcohol intake is associated with enhanced insulin sensitivity. Diabetes Care 17:115–119, 1994.

124. Valmadrid CT, Klein R, Moss SE, et al: Alcohol intake and risk of coronary heart disease mortality in persons with older-onset diabetes mellitus. JAMA 282:239–246, 1999.

125. Koivisto VA, Tulokas S, Toivonen M, et al: Alcohol with a meal has no adverse effects on postprandial glucose homeostasis in diabetic patients. Diabetes Care 16:1612–1614, 1993.

126. Mooradian, AD, Failla, M, Hoogwerf, B, et al: J. Selected vitamins and minerals in diabetes mellitus (technical review). Diabetes Care 17:464–479, 1994.

127. Franz MJ: Micronutrients and diabetes. In Franz MJ, Bantle JP (eds): American Diabetes Association Guide to Medical Nutrition Therapy for Diabetes. Alexandria, VA, American Diabetes Association, 1999, pp 165–191.

128. American Diabetes Association: Diabetes mellitus and exercise (position statement). Diabetes Care 23(suppl 1):S50–S51, 2000.

129. Zinman B, Zuniga-Guajardo S, Kelly D: Comparison of the acute and long-term effects of exercise on glucose control in type I diabetes. Diabetes Care 7:515–519, 1984.

130. Schneider SH, Khachadurian AK, Amorosa LF, et al: Ten-year experience with exercise-based outpatient life-style modification program in the treatment of diabetes mellitus. Diabetes Care 15:1800–1810, 1992.

131. Berger MP, Berchtold HJ, Cuppers H: Metabolic and hormonal effects of exercise in juvenile type diabetes. Diabetologia 13:355–367, 1997.

132. MacDonald MJ: Postexercise late-onset hypoglycemia in insulin-dependent diabetic patients. Diabetes Care 10:584–588, 1987.

133. Campaigne BN, Wallberg-Henrikssen H, Gunnarsson R: 12-Hour glycemic response following acute exercise in type 1 diabetes in relation to insulin dose and caloric intake. Diabetes Care 10:716–721, 1987.

134. Wasserman DH, Zinman B: Exercise in individuals with IDDM (technical review). Diabetes Care 17:924–937, 1994.

135. Mitchell TH, Abraham G, Schiffrin A: Hyperglycemia after intense exercise in IDDM subjects during continuous subcutaneous insulin infusion. Diabetes Care 11:311–317, 1988.

136. Purdon C, Brousson M, Nyveen L: The roles of insulin and catecholamines in the glucoregulatory response during intense exercise and early recovery in insulin-dependent diabetic and control subjects. J Clin Endocrinol Metab 76:566–573, 1993.

137. Tuominen JA, Karonen A-L, Melamies L, et al: Exercise-induced hypoglycemia in IDDM patients treated with a short-acting insulin analogue. Diabetologia 38:106–111, 1985.

138. DeFronzo RA, Sherwin RS, Kraemer N: Effects of physical training on insulin action in obesity. Diabetes 36:1379–1385, 1987.

139. Sato Y, Igudi A, Sakamoto N: Biochemical determination of training effects using insulin clamp technique. Horm Metab Res 16:483–486, 1984.

140. Soukup JT, Kovaleski JE: A review of the effects of resistance training for individuals with diabetes mellitus. Diabetes Educator 19:307–312, 1993.

141. Schneider SH, Ruderman NB: Exercise and NIDDM (technical review). Diabetes Care 13:785–789, 1990.

142. Bouchard C, Depres J-P, Tremblay A: Exercise and obesity. Obes Res 1:133–147, 1993.

143. Barlow CE, Kohl HW 3rd, Gibbons LW, Blair SN: Physical fitness, mortality and obesity. Int J Obes Relat Metab Disord 19(suppl 4):S41–S44, 1995.

144. Schneider SH, Khachadurian Ak, Amorosa LF: Abnormal glucoregulation during exercising in type II (noninsulin-dependent) diabetes. Metabolism 36:1161–1167, 1986.

145. Pate RR, Pratt M, Blair SN, et al: Physical activity and public health. A recommendation from the Centers for Disease Control and Prevention and the American College of Sports Medicine. JAMA 273:402–407, 1995.

Chapter 58

Management of Type 2 Diabetes: A Systematic Approach to Meeting the Standards of Care

II: Oral Agents, Insulin, and Management of Complications

Richard M. Bergenstal ▪ David M. Kendall
Marion J. Franz ▪ Arthur H. Rubenstein

GLUCOSE MANAGEMENT PLAN

Diabetes management begins with making the diagnosis of diabetes, followed by teaching self-management skills which include education that facilitates appropriate behavior changes, instruction on the principles of self-monitoring of blood glucose (SMBG), and the development of a medical nutrition therapy and exercise or activity plan. Self-management, medical nutrition therapy, and exercise are discussed in Chapter 57.

If the target goals outlined in Chapter 57 have not been reached after self-management training, which is usually the case, the next step is to develop a medical management plan in each of the areas of risk of concern, including hyperglycemia, dyslipidemia, hypertension, prevention and management of complications, and other important components of diabetes care. We present a medical management plan for each of these areas, the first being a plan to manage hyperglycemia.

A logical, scientifically sound, and orderly pharmacologic medical management plan for type 2 diabetes can be derived from a firm understanding of the pathophysiology and natural history of type 2 diabetes.

Pathophysiology of Type 2 Diabetes

As we better understand the pathophysiology of type 2 diabetes,[1] more therapeutic options are becoming available. Although the order of appearance is debated, individuals must display both insulin resistance[2] and relative insulin deficiency[3] in order to develop diabetes. Insulin resistance can be broadly characterized as resistance to insulin at the level of the liver, resulting in increased hepatic glucose output and fasting hyperglycemia or resistance at the level of muscle and fat, resulting in decreased peripheral glucose uptake and predominantly postprandial hyperglycemia. In addition, there is compelling evidence accumulating that abnormalities in coagulation and fibrinolysis,[4] as well as vascular endothelial wall dysfunction,[5–8] are essential components of vascular complications in diabetes and are being considered by some as part of the insulin resistance syndrome as depicted in Figure 58–1.

To make the best choice of drugs one needs to define the predominant defect and also understand the natural history of type 2 diabetes.

At this point the defects leading to hyperglycemia are for the most part determined by clinical observation and history. Insulin deficiency is assumed to get progressively worse over time, as demonstrated by the progressive loss of β cell function in the United Kingdom Prospective Diabetes Study (UKPDS) cohort. Some clinicians find it helpful to measure their patients' insulin or C peptide levels. But a relatively low level of insulin may mean slow-onset type 1 diabetes in a patient not yet completely deficient in insulin or type 2 diabetes in a patient with progressive loss of β cell function. Insulin resistance in these patients is also indicated by a constellation of clinical and laboratory characteristics, including central obesity, dyslipidemia, hypertension, polycystic ovarian disease, and endothelial dysfunction. Understanding the natural history helps explain the selection of a particular agent and the necessity to combine or change therapies when indicated.

Natural History of Type 2 Diabetes

The pathophysiology of diabetes and the mechanism of action of the drugs, along with the natural history, determine which drugs need to be used. Figure 58–2 shows that diabetes does not develop until the pancreas is unable to secrete enough insulin to match the degree of insulin resistance that is present. Insulin resistance for the most part remains constant throughout the course of the disease, but β cell function progressively deteriorates until not only is it relatively deficient, but some degree of absolute insulin deficiency is present. The development of absolute insulin deficiency over time in type 2 diabetes is not well appreciated by practicing clinicians and may be one factor that accounts for the long delay in including insulin in a treatment regimen. Not shown in the figure is the fact that the β cell defect in type 2 diabetes has other important manifestations besides a gradual deterioration in the total amount of insulin secreted over time. Defects in β cell function include loss of the normal pulsatile insulin secretion,[9] the loss of first-phase or rapid insulin release to a glucose stimulus,[10] disproportionate amounts of proinsulin secretion,[11, 12] and abnormalities in other islet or intestinal peptides (glucagon-like peptide-1) or in communication between the peptides, as well as a gradual accumulation of potentially toxic islet amyloid.[13] Each of these defects in β cell function has clinical implications worthy of further study.

In selecting the most appropriate therapy the first step is to determine the pathophysiologic defect and how to is recognize it clinically. Second, one decides where on the natural history curve of type 2

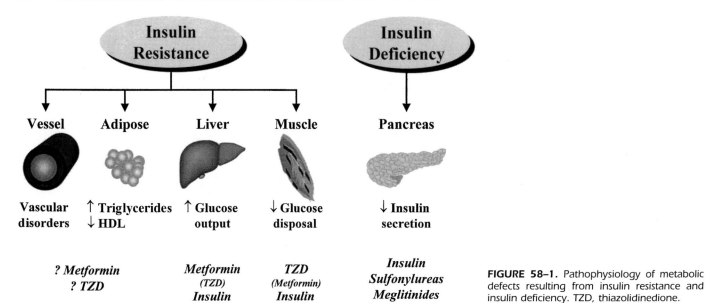

FIGURE 58–1. Pathophysiology of metabolic defects resulting from insulin resistance and insulin deficiency. TZD, thiazolidinedione.

diabetes a patient is likely to be in order to refine the choice of agent(s). The third step is to develop or consult an already created systematic clinical pathway or algorithm with established target goals and indications for and contraindications to specific drugs. Using a clinical algorithm has been demonstrated to enhance communication between educator and provider and between patient and provider and moves the patient aggressively down the algorithm until agreed-upon glycemic goals have been reached. There is no one correct algorithm for care, and with new drugs being frequently introduced existing algorithms need to be continually modified. It is still helpful to have a general algorithm in place for a given practitioner, medical group, or health plan. One such algorithm is shown in Figure 58–3. As these algorithms are transmitted over a medical practice Intranet or across the Internet, practice can be standardized and updated efficiently.

Algorithm for Glucose Control

An algorithm should be organized along the lines of clinical decision making such as insulin resistance vs. insulin deficiency and give clinical cues to assist in decision making.

New and returning patients need a review of the key principles of medical nutrition therapy and how to incorporate regular physical activity into their schedules. In addition, they need to be educated in the principles of self-management and the goals of therapy. If psychological issues such as depression are identified, they must be treated appropriately from the outset.

Every patient needs a meal and exercise plan. Even if these plans are not sufficient alone to reach glycemic goals, the plan, if followed, makes it more likely that other therapies will be effective. Attention to life-style principles is highlighted throughout the course of diabetes (see Fig. 58–2). An emphasis on life-style principles in those at risk for diabetes may be important in slowing development of the disease.

A randomized clinical trial has demonstrated that having the patient see a dietitian is a cost-effective management strategy.[14] This trial also reemphasized that one can tell in a short period of time if medical nutrition therapy alone will be sufficient to obtain or maintain adequate glycemic control. This makes a case for dietitians' becoming much more active members of the diabetes treatment team by being the ones

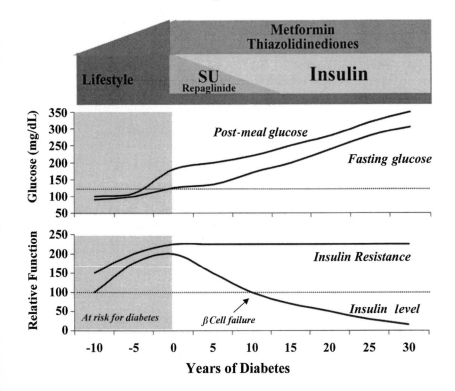

FIGURE 58–2. Natural history of type 2 diabetes.

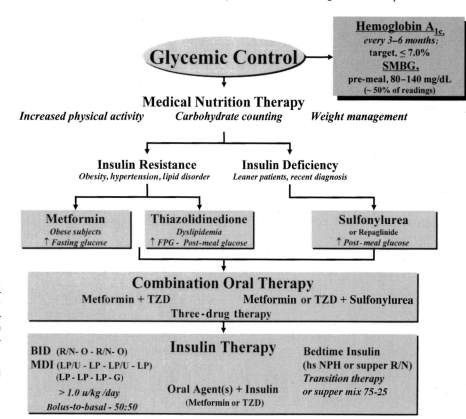

FIGURE 58–3. Glucose control algorithm. SMBG, self-monitored blood glucose; FPG, fasting plasma glucose; TZD, thiazolidinedione; BID, twice daily; MDI, multidose insulin; R, regular insulin; N, NPH-Lente insulin; LP, insulin lispro, U, Ultralente insulin; NPH, neutral protomine Hagedorn insulin; G, insulin glargine. (Adapted from Mazze R, Strock E, Simonson G, et al: Staged Diabetes Management: Structured Diabetes Health Care System, Japanese edition. Minneapolis, International Diabetes Center, 1999.)

who suggest that it is time to move on to additional therapies if the meal plan alone is not effective after, say, 6 weeks.

Oral Monotherapy

If medical nutrition therapy fails to achieve glucose goals or if on initial presentation a patient has a fasting glucose of over 200 mg/dL (11.1 mmol/L) or a postprandial reading over 250 mg/dL (13.9 mmol/L), it is appropriate to proceed to monotherapy with an oral agent.

There are currently five classes of oral glucose-lowering drugs: two that treat insulin deficiency, two that treat insulin resistance, and one that delays carbohydrate absorption. An excellent comprehensive review of pharmacologic therapy in type 2 diabetes has been published recently[15] and in this section we provide data to help prioritize clinical decision making, summarized in Tables 58–1 and 58–2.

The first determination is whether the main defect in glucose tolerance results from insulin resistance or insulin deficiency (see Fig. 58–1). The Insulin Resistance Atherosclerosis Study[16] found that 92% of type 2 patients were insulin-resistant and the UKPDS showed that in obese patients there was a cardiovascular benefit from taking metformin.[17] Therefore, metformin is a logical choice for monotherapy in the majority of patients. Patients in whom one wants to focus on treating insulin resistance, or who are not good candidates for metformin, or do not tolerate metformin, may be candidates to start on a thiazolidinedione (TZD). As more studies are done other reasons why TZDs should be first line agents may evolve (such as prevention of β cell deterioration or improved cardiovascular outcomes). Sulfonylureas (SUs), the other common class of agents selected for monotherapy, are effective, safe, inexpensive, and generally well tolerated. Patients who seem to need an insulin-releasing agent but have a significantly elevated serum creatinine, a very irregular schedule, or predominantly postprandial hyperglycemia may select a meglitinide as first-line therapy. An α-glucosidase inhibitor (AGI) may be selected for monotherapy if patients are diagnosed early in the natural history of type 2 diabetes, when postprandial hyperglycemia predominates.

The basic principles of monotherapy selection and dose adjustment are as follows:

1. Select a class of agents to treat the primary defect leading to hyperglycemia.

2. Be aware of how much the agent you select generally lowers hemoglobin A_{1c} (HbA$_{1c}$) so you will know if you will need to combine oral agents or include insulin in your regimen to reach the goal.

3. Select an agent that addresses other risks factors, particularly cardiovascular risks.

4. Select an agent that is well tolerated and fits the patient's needs regarding, in particular, liver function status (alanine transaminase [ALT]) and renal function status (serum creatinine).

5. Based on SMBG data, adjust the dose of oral agent upward every 2 to 4 weeks (except with TZDs, for which adjustments every 8 to 12 weeks are more appropriate) until glycemic targets are reached or you are at the maximum dose or the maximum clinically effective dose (a dose lower than maximum but for which most of the effect is seen (i.e., glyburide 10 mg vs. maximum dose of 20 mg).

6. Once the patient is taking the maximum clinically effective dose of an oral agent, combine oral agents or combine oral agent(s) with insulin.

METFORMIN. Metformin is a biguanide that has been used worldwide for decades and in the United States since 1995.[18–20] Metformin enhances insulin sensitivity primarily in the liver but also in the peripheral tissue (muscle more than fat). The receptor mechanism by which this enhanced sensitivity occurs is not known. Fasting glucose is reduced in direct correlation to the suppression of hepatic glucose output.

Metformin reduces fasting glucose readings by 60 to 70 mg/dL (3.3 to 3.9 mmol/L) and HbA$_{1c}$ values by 1.5% to 2.0%. The most common approach to dosing is to start with 500 mg at supper and then add 500 mg every 1 to 2 weeks or until the patient has achieved SMBG goals or has reached 1000 mg with breakfast and supper. Since there is a good dose-response curve up to 2000 mg/day,[21] one should not stop until that dose is reached unless glycemic targets have been achieved. In addition to lowering glucose metformin has other positive metabolic effects. Metformin reduces triglycerides, low-density lipoprotein (LDL) cholesterol, plasma free fatty acids, and plasminogen activator

TABLE 58–1. Type 2 Diabetes Oral Therapy

Class of Agents (Generic and Brand Names)	Clinically Effective Dose		Effect on FPG (mg/dL)	Effect on Hb A_{1c} (%)	Clinical Uses	Cautions/Comments
	Range	*Maximum*				
Sulfonylureas Glipizide (Glucotrol) Glipizide-GITS (Glucotrol XL) Glyburide (Micronase, Diaβeta) Glimepiride (Amaryl)	Glipizide: 5–20 mg b.i.d. Glipizide-GITS: 5–20 mg q.d. Glyburide: 2.5–10 mg/day Glimepiride: 1–4 mg q.d.	20 mg b.i.d. 20 mg q.d. 20 mg q.d. 8 mg q.d.	40–80	Up to 2	Initial therapy—lean patient, especially if very hyperglycemic (FPG 200–350 mg/dL) Targets postmeal hyperglycemia Use in combination with oral agents Lower expense (generics)	Hypoglycemia and weight gain Less effect "late" in disease Use with caution if Cr > 2.0 mg/kg or abnormal liver function tests Lower cost
Biguanide Metformin (Glucophage)	1000 mg b.i.d. Titrate: start 500 mg q PM; add 500 mg q 1–2 weeks until 1000 mg b.i.d.	2500 mg per day	40–80	Up to 2	Initial therapy—obese, insulin-resistant patients Targets fasting hyperglycemia Limits weight gain No hypoglycemia as monotherapy Effective in combination (oral-insulin) May reduce CVD risk (lowers TG, LDL, and PAI-1)	GI side effects (limited by dose titration) Contraindicated: Cr > 1.5 mg/kg, drug-treated CHF, >age 80 (use only if CrCl > 60–70 mL/min Withhold during IV contrast, acute illness (hospital), or if risk of CV collapse (severe pulmonary disease, acidosis, sepsis, etc.)
α-Glucosidase Inhibitors Acarbose (Precose) Miglitol (Glyset)	Acarbose: 25–50 mg t.i.d. with meals Miglitol: 25–50 mg t.i.d. with meals (start 25 mg at one meal for 1–2 wk, titrate up gradually, q 2–4 wk)		15–30	0.5–1.0	Targets postmeal glucose No hypoglycemia Limits weight gain Use in combination with any agent	Significant GI side effects Limited glucose-lowering effect Avoid if other significant bowel diseases
Thiazolidinediones Pioglitazone (Actos) Rosiglitazone (Avandia)	Pioglitazone: 15–45 mg q.d. Rosiglitazone: 4–8 mg q.d. or 4 mg b.i.d.	45 mg q.d. 8 mg per day	30–80	1–2	Initial therapy—insulin-resistant patients (troglitazone not approved for use as monotherapy) Targets dyslipidemia (lowers TG, raises HDL) Effective in combination (oral-insulin) Use if intolerant to or inappropriate for metformin Can use in renal insufficiency	Hepatotoxicity (troglitazone) Serial measure of ALT required More potent glucose lowering as monotherapy at higher dose Weight gain, slight drop in Hb
Meglitinide Repaglinide (Prandin)	0.5–2.0 mg (max. 4 mg) with meals and h.s. snack	16 mg per day	30–70	1–2	Postmeal hyperglycemia Use if variable meal schedule Alternative to sulfonylurea Use in low dose in renal insufficiency (0.5–1.0 mg)	Hypoglycemia, weight gain Higher cost Use early in disease course

FPG, fasting plasma glucose; Hb, hemoglobin; Cr, creatinine; CVD, cardiovascular disease; TG, triglycerides; LDL, low-density lipoprotein cholesterol; PAI-1, plasminogen activator inhibitor-1; GI, gastrointestinal; CrCl, creatinine clearance; CHF, congestive heart failure; CV, cardiovascular; HDL, high-density lipoprotein cholesterol; ALT, alanine transaminase.

TABLE 58–2. Type 2 Diabetes Insulin Therapy

Name	Dose Range	Effect on Fasting Plasma Glucose	Effect on Hb A$_{1c}$ %	Clinical Uses	Cautions/Comments
Insulin therapy Lispro (LP) Regular (R) Aspart NPH Lente (L) Ultralente (U) Glargine (G) Premixed 50/50 NPH/R 70–30 NPH/R Mix 75/25 NPL/LP	NPH (0.15 U/kg) h.s. Initial multidose insulin (0.3–0.7 U/kg/day) Total insulin dose required in obese type 2 diabetes averages 1.2 U/kg/day Usually 50% bolus insulin 50% basal insulin	Unlimited	Unlimited	Insulin use may be required in more than 50% of type 2 patients Multiple injections (2–4/day) improve control LP—take with meal, targets postmeal hyperglycemia, limits need for snacks, reduced risk of hypoglycemia G—true 24-hr basal insulin	Hypoglycemia, weight gain Useful in combination with both metformin and thiazolidinediones Use premixed (70/30, 50/50, mix 75/25) if unable to self-mix No increased cardiovascular disease risk with insulin therapy Use memory meters, pattern control, insulin supplements based on carbohydrate intake or change in activity or medication G—long-acting insulin but clear solution

Type of Insulin	Onset	Peak Effect	Monitor Effect in	Dosing Interval
Mealtime insulin				
LP (rapid-acting)	5–15 min	30–90 min	2 hr	At meal
Aspart (rapid-acting)	5–15 min	60–120 min	2–3 hr	At meal
R (short-acting)	30–60 min	2–4 hr	4 hr	Premeal (30–45 min prior)
Background insulin				
N (intermediate-acting)	2–4 hr	4–6 hr	8–12 hr	Twice daily
U (long-acting)	3–5 hr	Limited peak	10–12 hr	Twice daily (often 9–12 hr)
G (long-acting)	2–4 hr	No peak	(fasting glucose)	Once daily

No. of Injections	Regimen	AM Dose	Noon Dose	Dinner Dose	Bedtime Dose
2 Injections 40% Mealtime 60% Background	R-N-0-R-N-0 or LP-N-0-LP-N-0	20% R or LP 40% N	— —	20% R or LP 20% N	— —
3 Injections 40% Mealtime 60% Background	LP-N-0-LP-N or R-N-0-R-N	20% LP or R 40% N	— —	20% LP or R —	— 20% N
3 Injections 50% Mealtime 50% Background	R-U-R-R-U-0 or LP-U-LP-LP-U-0	15% R or LP 20% U	15% R or LP —	20% R or LP 30% U	— —
4 Injections 50% Mealtime 50% Background	LP-U-LP-LP-N or LP-LP-LP-G	15% LP 20% U 15% LP	15% LP — 13% LP	20% LP — 20% LP	— 30% N 40–50% G

inhibitor-1 levels. There is modest weight loss or no weight gain in most studies.

Side effects are predominantly gastrointestinal upset and diarrhea in approximately 25% of patients, but these are often transient and only 5% of patients cannot tolerate the drug. When used alone metformin does not cause hypoglycemia. Lactic acidosis is rare but dictates that patients be selected carefully, the major criterion being to avoid its use if serum creatinine is greater than 1.4 mg/dL (124 μmol/L) in women and 1.5 mg/dL (133 μmol/L) in men. In the elderly or frail, consider using a measured or calculated creatinine clearance of less than approximately 60 to 70 mL/min as the cutoff. In addition, metformin is contraindicated in patients with hepatic disease, respiratory insufficiency, severe infection, or alcohol abuse. It should be avoided in patients with active congestive heart failure requiring therapy. In patients over age 80 a careful analysis of renal function is needed. Metformin should be withheld at the time of a radiocontrast dye study and restarted when normal renal function is documented.

Since metformin is effective in lowering glucose, has been shown in the UKPDS to reduce cardiovascular events in obese patients with type 2 diabetes, is generally well tolerated, and is moderately priced, this drug is widely used. With proper patient selection metformin is very safe. Some confusion was generated by a substudy of the UKPDS that showed an increased risk of death in patients who had metformin added after 7.1 years of SU therapy compared with SU alone. Careful analysis of this substudy showed that the relative increase in mortality in the metformin plus SU group vs. SU-alone group was the result of a significant reduction in the number of deaths over that expected in the SU-alone group.[22] A meta-analysis of all patients in the UKPDS taking SU plus metformin showed significant reductions in all diabetes-related endpoints and myocardial infarctions.

SULFONYLUREA. SUs are among the most commonly used agents in treating type 2 diabetes.[23, 24] They enhance insulin secretion by binding to specific SU receptors on the β cell, which lead to a closing of the potassium adenosine triphosphate (ATP) channel on the β cell plasma membrane. The released insulin both reduces hepatic glucose production and enhances muscle glucose uptake (reducing both fasting and postprandial glucose levels). There are first- and second-generation SUs. Their major use worldwide today is with second-generation agents.

Fasting glucose is reduced by 60 to 70 mg/dL (3.3 to 3.9 mmol/L) and Hb A_{1c} is reduced by 1.5% to 2.0%. Those who are recently diagnosed and have moderate hyperglycemia with presumed reasonable β cell function remaining are most likely to respond. Most patients experience a good or at least a partial response to SU therapy, but over time (5% to 7% per year) patients fail to respond. Progressive β cell failure is the usual course in type 2 diabetes, at least with currently available therapies, so eventually almost all patients will need to be switched from SU to insulin. The UKPDS demonstrated that SU therapy did not hasten the rate of β cell failure (as some had feared β cell stimulation would do) compared with other agents.[25] Most of the glucose-lowering effect (75%) of SU agents is seen at their half-maximum dose (clinically effective dose).

Generally, all SU agents are similar in glucose-lowering ability. Most clinicians (and patients) prefer the once-daily SU agents since they are more convenient and, at least in one study, resulted in improved quality of life and less hypoglycemia than the similar shorter-acting SU agent.[15] If a very short-acting agent is desired due to very erratic meal schedules, then an agent in the meglitinide class (repaglinide [Prandin]) should be considered. At least one SU (glimepiride)[26, 27] has been shown to have less interaction with cardiac tissue K⁺-ATP channels, which may improve the cardiovascular response to ischemia and hypoxia compared with other SUs, but this needs to be demonstrated in human research and confirmed in clinical trials.[28]

SU agents may cause hypoglycemia that may be prolonged if the patient has abnormal liver or renal function. Mild weight gain is usually seen, most likely to improving metabolic control. There are no beneficial effects of SUs on lipids or the fibrinolytic system, but early data from the University Group Diabetes Program suggesting that SUs worsened heart disease have not been confirmed.[29] In fact, the UKPDS showed quite convincingly that there was no increase in coronary artery disease in patients assigned to SU therapy compared with diet

therapy, and efforts are under way to remove the so-called black box warning that SUs might cause cardiovascular disease that is required by the Food and Drug Administration on all SU package inserts in the United States.

SUs are inexpensive and generally safe and well tolerated. They are used often when rapid glucose lowering is desired without the use of insulin. They enhance insulin secretion and work well in combination with an insulin-sensitizing agent. Given enough time SU therapy usually needs to be replaced with insulin to overcome the insulin deficiency defect in type 2 diabetes. Two other classes of insulin secretagogues have been developed: meglitinides (repaglinide—approved) and D-phenylalanine (nateglinide—undergoing trials in the United States). Nateglinide stimulates insulin secretion very rapidly but the stimulation is short-lived, resulting in a significant reduction in postprandial glucose excursions.[30]

MEGLITINIDE. Agents in the meglitinide or benzoic acid derivative class stimulate insulin secretion in the presence of glucose.[31, 32] There are several meglitinide receptor–binding sites on the β cell and whether there are additive effects with those of the SU agents is not known at this time.[33]

Hb A_{1c} reduction with repaglinide is similar to SUs and metformin, with studies showing reductions of 1.5% to 2.0% with SU monotherapy. The drug is rapidly absorbed and has a short half-life, causing a rapid and brief release of insulin. The dosing starts at 0.5 mg 15 minutes before each meal and can be increased every week to 4 mg before each meal and at bedtime. One milligram before each meal and at bedtime is probably the clinically effective dose, producing 90% of the maximum glucose-lowering activity. There is a slight weight gain and mild hypoglycemia, similar to effects of an SU, but there are particularly low rates of hypoglycemia with repaglinide when meals are missed or delayed or during extended fasting.[34] There is no drug restriction in renal disease and only a slightly slower titration schedule recommended with liver disease. The meglitinides are effective and serve a growing subset of patients who need enhanced insulin secretion but have erratic schedules, renal insufficiency, significant postprandial hyperglycemia, or a propensity to hypoglycemia on an SU. Of course the tradeoff for increased flexibility in meal timing is the need for multiple daily doses and the increased cost of the medication compared with SUs.

THIAZOLIDINEDIONES. TZDs enhance insulin sensitivity mainly at the level of muscle and adipose tissue, with some effect in the liver.[35–37] Unlike with metformin the site of action of TZDs is known and involves binding to a nuclear receptor called the peroxisome proliferator–activated receptor (PPAR)-γ, enhancing the expression of multiple genes encoding proteins which modulate glucose and, to some degree, lipid metabolism. There are two members of the TZD class currently on the market in the United States (see Table 58–1). The more specific the agent is in binding to the PPAR-γ, the lower the dose of drug required to lower blood glucose. The order of TZDs from most specific (potent) to least is rosiglitazone (Avandia, 4 to 8 mg) > pioglitazone (Actos, 15 to 45 mg). There are also some differences in crossover binding of the TZD to PPAR-α sites. Rosiglitazone is mainly a PPAR-γ agent, whereas pioglitazone binds both PPAR-γ and PPAR-α. This cross-reactivity to the PPAR-α receptor, which is known to be an active binding site for fibrates, may explain why these two TZDs have the most significant triglyceride-lowering effects in the class. Troglitazone was approved in the United States in 1997,[38] but because of hepatic safety concerns was withdrawn from the U.S. market in 2000.

Rosiglitazone and pioglitazone are approved for use as both monotherapy and combination therapy. At this time rosiglitazone is approved for use with metformin and SU, and pioglitazone is approved for use with SU, metformin, and insulin. As monotherapy all the TZDs reduce the Hb A_{1c} fraction 1.0% to 1.5%, with a few studies showing even greater reductions (up to 2.55%) in drug-naive patients with elevated baseline Hb A_{1c} levels. In combination with SU there is a 1.0% to 1.7% reduction in Hb A_{1c}. In combination with metformin there is a 0.8% to 1.7% reduction in Hb A_{1c}, indicating that the glucose-lowering effects of these two insulin sensitizers are directly additive, making use of these agents worth consideration in the significantly insulin-resistant patient.[39] TZDs added to insulin consistently reduce Hb A_{1c} by over 1.0%. In addition, depending on the design of the trial, insulin doses have been reduced by some 25% to 30%. In some trials, even if the Hb A_{1c} value is relatively good with insulin therapy (7.7%), the addition of a TZD resulted in a reduction clearly into the target range (6.8%). This emphasizes that the main goal when combining agents is to reduce Hb A_{1c}. Agents are needed that will improve other risk factors, such as those related to cardiovascular or renal disease, will ameliorate weight gain and hypoglycemia, preserve β cell function, and reduce total insulin doses.

The effects of TZDs on lipids are less well understood. The entire class reduces free fatty acids that may play a role in insulin sensitization at the tissue level. Troglitazone and rosiglitazone significantly increase LDL levels whereas the slight elevation in LDL with pioglitazone is not significant. An increase in LDL is a known cardiovascular risk factor. But whether the increase in LDL seen with TZDs is composed of larger, more buoyant LDL particles, not the small dense atherogenic particles, remains to be proved. At this point, if LDL cholesterol is above target goals, therapy with a cholesterol-lowering drug is indicated. Because TZDs significantly increase high-density lipoprotein (HDL) cholesterol, the HDL/LDL ratio as an indicator of cardiovascular risk is unchanged. With recent studies indicating an improvement in cardiovascular outcomes by lowering triglycerides in patients with diabetes, more attention is being paid to ways to do so. Troglitazone and pioglitazone regularly reduce triglyceride levels whereas rosiglitazone has a neutral effect on triglycerides. Further study is needed comparing these agents over a wide range of baseline triglyceride and glucose levels.

The major safety issue with TZDs is their potential for liver toxicity. Because of cases of hepatic failure in patients on troglitazone, this drug is no longer approved for therapy. Rosiglitazone and pioglitazone showed significantly fewer minor elevations in liver function tests in clinical trials than did troglitazone. To date, with rosiglitazone and pioglitazone on the market and in use in over 1,000,000 patients, there have been no reports of hepatic failure clearly due to these drugs. The current liver function monitoring requirements for these drugs are a baseline test and ALT determination every 2 months for the first year and periodically thereafter.

Each of the TZDs is associated with intravascular volume expansion with some fluid retention and weight gain. Moderate weight gain is usually felt to be acceptable to the patient and provider if there is a resultant improvement in the Hb A_{1c} percentage and other metabolic factors. In rare instances significant weight gain may preclude the use of a TZD[40] or may alter the therapeutic regimen to include a weight-stabilizing agent like metformin. All TZDs cause a slight reduction in hemoglobin levels (on average 1.0 g/dL). TZDs may reduce levels of oral contraceptives and may result in ovulation in some premenopausal anovulatory women. TZDs continue to be evaluated for drug interactions. Rosiglitazone is metabolized primarily by the cytochrome P-450 2C8 system and pioglitazone is metabolized by the cytochrome P-450 3A4 and 2C8 pathways. The clinical significance of these metabolic pathways is being studied.

TZDs are an exciting new class of drugs that address a primary defect in type 2 diabetes: insulin resistance. The TZDs are relatively expensive but their array of effects on both glucose and lipid metabolism makes them worth further study to properly place them in diabetes therapy algorithms. Further studies and cardiovascular outcome trials are needed to establish if TZDs indeed have a positive cardiovascular profile.[41] Also intriguing and in need of confirmation by randomized clinical trials is the potential for TZDs to prevent the onset of type 2 diabetes, prevent renal disease,[42] and delay the progressive β cell deterioration consistently seen in type 2 diabetes.

α-GLUCOSIDASE INHIBITORS. There are currently two AGIs on the market in the United States: acarbose (Precose) and miglitol (Glyset). These agents delay digestion of complex carbohydrates by acting as competitive inhibitors of the intestinal α-glucosidase enzymes that hydrolzye oligosaccharides into monosaccharides.[43, 44] Although the gastrointestinal tract is not directly involved in the pathogenesis of diabetes, by modifying its activity, several approaches, including use of AGIs, amylin, and soluble fiber supplements, have

attempted to improve carbohydrate tolerance, mainly by reducing postprandial hyperglycemia.

The potency of AGIs, with an Hb A_{1c} reduction of approximately 0.5% to 1.0%, is less than that of other oral agents. This is primarily due to a postprandial glucose reduction of 40 to 50 mg/dL (2.2 to 2.8 mmol/L). If patients have a low carbohydrate intake they may see less of a glucose-lowering effect. In addition to this glucose reduction there is a blunting or actual reduction in postmeal insulin and triglyceride levels. Also noted, but the clinical significance of which is not yet clear, is a reduction in gastric inhibitory polypeptide and an increase in plasma glucagon-like peptide-1 levels after ingestion of an AGI. In addition, body weight does not change on AGIs. It is important to start with a low dose (25 mg at one meal) and increase the dose slowly (every 1 to 2 weeks by 25 mg at another meal and then gradually to 50 mg before each meal) to improve the side effect profile. The medication should be taken with the first bite of food. A slight reduction in Hb A_{1c} has been described in patients with type 1 diabetes taking AGIs.

AGIs are safe but have gastrointestinal side effects of bloating, abdominal discomfort, and flatulence owing to undigested carbohydrate reaching the colon, where it is fermented by bacteria. These agents do not cause hypoglycemia and in fact are used to treat reactive hypoglycemia.

The two AGIs available in the United States appear to be similar in regard to efficacy and side effect profiles. Studies continue to see if there may be unique advantages of one agent over the other or over newer AGIs available in other countries. The ideal candidate to consider in clinical practice is a patient very early in the disease when postprandial hyperglycemia is the predominant finding. Studies are under way to determine if AGIs may be useful to prevent the development of diabetes (Early Diabetes Intervention Trial [EDIT]).

Combination Oral Agents

It is clear from the natural history of diabetes that one agent is unlikely to maintain effective glycemic control for more than a few years. Only approximately 25% of the time does a single oral agent ever establish adequate glycemic control.[15] It is well documented that switching classes is not an effective approach to establishing or maintaining glycemic control. Although a single agent may not have enabled a patient to reach or maintain a desired glycemic target, the agent, in most cases, is still having some glucose-lowering action, and its withdrawal will lead to even further hyperglycemia. Once a single oral agent has failed to establish or maintain glycemic control, the next step is to add a second agent from a different therapeutic class.[45] A combination of metformin and an SU, each of which addresses one of the underlying defects in type 2 diabetes (insulin resistance and insulin deficiency), is the most frequently used oral combination to date.[46] Not only does this combination make sense according to the pathophysiology of type 2 diabetes, but these are two of the most effective glucose-lowering drugs, both have good safety records when used appropriately, and both are relatively inexpensive. In addition, the potential side effect of weight gain seen with SU may be minimized when used in combination with metformin. The most common approach to drug progression has been to increase the first agent to its maximum dose, then increase the second agent to its maximum dose or until glycemic targets are achieved.

There are some clinical reasons to consider not proceeding to the maximum dose of an agent but instead moving to a second agent at a somewhat lower dose that provides most of the glucose-lowering effects while minimizing the side effects, that is, the clinically effective dose of a drug. For instance, almost all the glucose-lowering potential of glyburide is achieved at 10 mg whereas the maximum dose recommended (at least in the United States) is 20 mg. The maximum dose of metformin in the United States is 2500 mg, but a careful dose-response study showed that on average its maximum glucose-lowering effect is seen at 2000 mg.[21] Because the majority of patients either need two drugs from the start or need to move from one to two drugs over a relatively short time frame, using the maximum clinically effective dose gets one to combination therapy sooner, thus potentially avoiding prolonged periods of deleterious hyperglycemia. Another effective approach to assist in getting to a combination of metformin and SU therapy early is the use of one of a series of premixed combination pills of metformin and SU (Glucovance). Just as premixed antihypertensive agents are gaining in use, it is likely that the use of a variety of premixed combination oral glucose-lowering agents will continue to increase in popularity. The convenience and ability to move quickly to match the underlying defects of type 2 diabetes makes these agents particularly interesting.

As shown in Figure 58–3 other combinations of oral agents beyond metformin and an SU are frequently used. An SU and TZD combination has been shown to lower glucose effectively and is often used when a patient cannot tolerate or is not a good candidate for metformin.[47] In the patient in whom insulin resistance is the major clinical problem, a combination of metformin and a TZD may be considered. This combination of insulin sensitizers, each having a predominant effect at a different site (metformin in the liver and TZDs in muscle) has a better chance of being effective early in the course of type 2 diabetes when there is a still reasonable amount of endogenous insulin being made.

When any combination of two oral agents fails to achieve or maintain a glycemic target, then one must decide whether to add a third oral agent, add insulin to one or more of the oral agents, or stop the oral agents and start insulin alone. A combination of two oral agents is very effective in lowering Hb A_{1c} several percentage points but studies with maximum doses of metformin and an SU only achieved target glucose readings in 70% of patients. Thus 30% of patients on two oral agents never reached target goals and those who do over time can be expected to have a gradual decline in β cell function and require further therapy. Data are beginning to accumulate on the effectiveness of triple oral agent therapy.[48] Until endogenous insulin secretion becomes very low, three oral agents, including an insulin secretagogue, may improve glucose readings but they have not yet been able to reach optimal glycemic targets consistently. Things to consider with triple oral agent therapy beyond their glucose-lowering potential include cost and compliance. Most patients, and many practitioners, feel that any number or combination of pills is easier than including insulin in the treatment plan. As the natural history of type 2 diabetes becomes better understood, it is clear that to achieve and maintain tight glycemic control insulin will need to be at least a component of the glucose-lowering regimen in well over 50% of type 2 patients. In one study the estimate was that 58% of patients with type 2 diabetes for 20 years required insulin.[49]

Insulin Therapy

Effective use of insulin therapy requires a fundamental understanding that insulin is a natural part of therapy over time in type 2 diabetes.[50, 51] Patient and professional barriers to the use of insulin must be addressed in a positive and straightforward manner. Developing effective insulin regimens requires a systematic approach to insulin initiation and adjustment, the foremost goal being to deliver insulin in a manner that mimics a normal daily insulin profile as much as possible. This approach has the best chance of optimizing glycemic control while minimizing hypoglycemia and making the daily routine as flexible as possible.[52, 53]

SYSTEMATIC MANAGEMENT PLAN. Figure 58–2 shows that type 2 diabetes does not develop unless there is a relative deficiency in insulin secretion. Over time pancreatic insulin secretion falls to such low levels that exogenous insulin must be administered to establish or maintain near-normal glycemic control. Initiating insulin in a timely manner requires an understanding of the natural history of type 2 diabetes as well as an appreciation for the long-held patient and professional barriers to the use of insulin. In type 1 diabetes data are available that suggest intensive or advanced insulin therapy should be started as early as possible and maintained for as long as possible to reduce the risk of complications.[54]

BARRIERS TO INSULIN THERAPY. Several barriers may deter the use of insulin in type 2 diabetes. For patients, the following factors are the most common barriers to getting started on insulin therapy.

• Fear of needles

• Fear that diabetes is worsening when insulin is needed
• Inconvenience of scheduling injections
• Fear of weight gain
• Fear of hypoglycemia

Patients with type 2 diabetes may be thinking about these barriers and it is wise to address and dispel them up front to effectively initiate or adjust insulin therapy. While no one looks forward to taking an insulin injection, almost everyone is surprised at how easy it is. This has led many clinics to encourage patients to try an insulin (saline) injection early in the course of type 2 therapy before insulin is actually required. The patient can then relax and try other therapies and not dread the fact that at some point he or she may need insulin to maintain effective glycemic control. The needles on insulin syringes have been improved.[55] They now have a finer gauge (29 to 30 gauge vs. previous standard of 27 gauge) and they are available in a short (8 mm vs. 12.7 mm) version (appropriate for all but the very obese).[56] If the natural history of diabetes is explained to patients early in the course of the disease, they are less likely to think that proceeding to insulin means severe diabetes or a failure on their part. The fact that a relative may have started insulin and then developed a complication of diabetes, such as kidney failure, leads to a defeatist or fatalistic attitude toward the use of insulin. This needs to be addressed honestly and rationally early in the course of diabetes education. The anticipated disruption of one's schedule when starting insulin has been minimized by advances in technology and more physiologically acting insulins. New insulin preparations, such as insulin lispro, insulin aspart, and insulin glargine, allow for flexibility in meal timing and minimize the issue of a precise schedule for insulin injections. Even the amount and composition of any given meal can be matched with an appropriate dose of insulin. Insulin pens, which are used extensively in Europe and Japan and are gaining acceptance in the United States, minimize the inconvenience and occasional embarrassment of carrying vials and syringes and drawing up or mixing preparations before injection.

If the preliminary data showing inhaled insulin to be rapid-acting and effective in preventing mealtime glucose excursions[57, 58] are substantiated in ongoing long-term trials, this approach would certainly help with both the fear of needles and convenience issues. Weight gain associated with insulin therapy raises several important issues. Improved metabolic control and the prevention of calorie loss from glycosuria associated with effective insulin therapy appears to be the main reason for weight gain with insulin therapy. In most studies comparing insulin with other glucose-lowering therapies there is more weight gain for a similar reduction in Hb A_{1c}, implying there may be additional effects of insulin leading to weight gain. Insulin consistently causes more hypoglycemia than any other therapy and the extra, unscheduled caloric intake needed to treat this hypoglycemia can result in weight gain. Whether there are direct insulin actions on the central nervous system or peripheral tissue metabolism that could cause weight gain is not settled at this point. Although obesity is clearly undesirable and measures should proceed to avoid it, glucose control should take precedence over weight loss once diabetes is diagnosed. The fear of hypoglycemia in type 2 diabetes can be partially allayed by data showing that for equally tight glucose control there is one-twentieth the rate of hypoglycemia in type 2 diabetes treated with insulin[59] compared to type 1 diabetes.[60] Insulin preparations like insulin lispro that specifically target postprandial hyperglycemia and have a short-time action profile reduce the incidence of hypoglycemia, particularly overnight.[61]

Clinicians also perceive certain barriers to the implementation of insulin therapy in their practices:

• Logistics of insulin initiation, adjustment, education, and follow-up
• Hypoglycemia
• Concern over insulin atherogenicity
• Weight gain

For primary care providers, the main barriers to insulin initiation are related to difficulty in the logistics of training patients and providing follow-up. Although guidelines or algorithms for care exist, they are not always implemented effectively. Practitioners are often versed in starting insulin, but confusion may exist about how to adjust insulin as the diabetes progresses or life situations change. The most effective implementation of diabetes guidelines with documented improved outcomes almost always involves a collaborative model, as outlined in Chapter 57. For endocrinologists, the key barriers have been the occurrence of hypoglycemic episodes and the lingering question of insulin atherogenicity. The risk of severe hypoglycemia, although rare in type 2 diabetes, should be one more motivating factor to select the most physiologic insulin regimen the patient is comfortable with. Insulin resistance is associated with cardiovascular disease but no study has demonstrated that exogenous insulin is atherogenic. Both the Diabetes Control and Complications Trial (DCCT) and the UKPDS showed a trend (not quite significant) toward reduced cardiovascular events in those treated aggressively with insulin. One study demonstrated that the use of insulin to achieve tight glycemic control during and immediately after a myocardial infarction resulted in a significant decrease in mortality up to 3 to 5 years after the cardiac event.[62, 63] Indeed, most studies have demonstrated weight gain with insulin administration that is effective in improving glycemic control. How much of the weight gain is due to improved control and how much is some direct effect of insulin have not been well established. As noted in Chapter 57, once diabetes is diagnosed the patient and the practitioner should focus their attention on modalities to improve glycemic control rather than on weight loss alone.

DEVELOPING EFFECTIVE INSULIN REGIMENS. Once the barriers to initiating insulin therapy have been overcome, one must develop the most effective insulin regimen possible. An effective regimen should be judged by the answers to these questions:

1. Is the Hb A_{1c} value near target?
2. Has hypoglycemia been minimized?
3. Has the patient's flexibility of life-style been maximized?

In type 2 diabetes there are three ways in which insulin can be initiated (see Fig. 58–3). The first and very popular approach at this time is to give insulin in the evening, usually at bedtime, either alone or in combination with a daytime oral agent(s).[64] Bedtime insulin is certainly convenient and for at least a period of time can be effective and minimize hypoglycemia. In our experience this is usually a relatively short transition period to more complete or intensive insulin therapy as the afternoon or bedtime glucose values start to rise. Table 58–2 shows the starting dose of NPH (neutral protamine Hagedorn) insulin or insulin glargine at night and how to adjust the dosage. If the bedtime glucose readings are already high, one can start regular and NPH insulin or premixed 70/30 insulin (70% NPH and 30% regular) or mix 75/25 insulin (75% NPL and 25% lispro) at supper.[65] The regular insulin component helps cover supper more effectively than NPH insulin alone at night but the NPH insulin in the mixture may not last until morning, leading to either overnight hypoglycemia or fasting hyperglycemia.

The second approach to starting insulin is using bedtime or evening insulin along with an oral agent(s) during the day. This approach, described below, appears to improve the outcome and prolong the duration of glucose control compared to bedtime insulin alone, but still progresses to a full insulin-requiring state over time.

The third approach to starting insulin (see Fig. 58–3) is to use either a split mixed insulin regimen (twice-daily mixture of regular and NPH insulin) or a multiple-dose insulin regimen (three or four injections of insulin a day generally with an injection of short-acting insulin before each meal.) The twice-daily split mixed insulin is simple and attempts to match insulin peaks to the time of meals but does not allow much flexibility, particularly at noontime when both the morning residual and NPH insulins are working. This approach has been used for years and if the insulin doses are pushed aggressively one can achieve good control, but there is a concern about hypoglycemia and definite limits to flexibility in life-style.

The most effective regimen, if one can overcome the barrier of multiple insulin injections, is a regimen that attempts to mimic a normal insulin profile. A normal insulin profile is composed of basal (background) insulin and bolus (mealtime) insulin. It is essential to replace basal and bolus insulin adequately if one is to optimize gly-

cemic control.[66] In many studies one component of insulin replacement and not the other has been optimized, only to result in Hb A_{1c} readings of approximately 8.0% to 8.5%, indicating only fair overall glucose control. Bolus basal insulin therapy goes by many names, including intensive insulin therapy,[67, 68] flexible insulin therapy,[69] functional insulin therapy,[70] modern diabetes therapy,[71] and advanced insulin management, among others. New insulin formulations have made this type of therapy much more feasible today. During the DCCT the most common approach to bolus basal therapy was a regimen of regular insulin before each meal and NPH insulin at bedtime. This was fairly effective as long as the patient was inculcated with the importance of timing of meals so the regular insulin would last but not wear out before the next meal. Also, regular insulin should ideally be given 45 to 60 minutes before a meal to time its peak with the absorption of food. This is a long lead time and not practical, so most of the time we instruct patients to take regular insulin 20 to 30 minutes before meals, but studies have shown that very few patients take their mealtime insulin more than 10 minutes before a meal.

The creation of the first marketed insulin analogue[72, 73] called insulin lispro changed the course of bolus-basal therapy.[74] With only a switch of the B28 and B29 amino acid residues the insulin molecule changes its self-association profile in the subcutaneous tissue and becomes a very rapid-acting insulin. Insulin lispro is taken as one starts to eat and peaks in an hour, with most of its significant glucose lowering complete at 2 hours. Insulin Aspart, recently approved in the US, is another rapid-acting insulin analogue made by making a substitution for the B28 amino acid residue. One can measure the glucose before the meal and then again at 2 hours and expect to see a rise of only 20 to 40 mg/dL and then a fall to an acceptable premeal reading before the next meal. Postprandial hyperglycemia has been closely linked with complications of diabetes.[75, 76] Too few SMBG tests are performed after meals, particularly since it has been shown that aggressively treating postprandial readings results in a lower A_{1c} value than aggressively treating premeal readings.[61, 77] The better postprandial control with insulin lispro has led to its use in pregnancy where postprandial glucose control is essential.[78] In the case of young children, in whom it is uncertain what their intake will be, you can actually wait until after a meal, assess the intake, and then give the appropriate amount of insulin lispro.[79]

Basal insulin therapy needs attention equal to bolus therapy if the Hb A_{1c} is to be normalized.[80–82] Currently, NPH, Lente, Ultralente, and glargine insulin are the intermediate or long-acting insulins available. Most clinicians use NPH and Lente insulin as interchangeable but Lente insulin may actually have a little longer-time action profile. Ultralente insulin is not widely used in the United States but in our experience, it has been an effective part of advanced insulin management. With insulin lispro given at each meal, Ultralente insulin can be given before breakfast and supper to cover basal needs. Ultralente insulin is an excellent daytime basal insulin in conjunction with insulin lispro to cover meals. Overnight control means suppressing hepatic glucose output but not causing hypoglycemia. NPH insulin at bedtime in many instances is more precisely targeted to cover the morning tendency for glucose to rise—the dawn phenomenon. Therefore an effective advanced insulin regimen is insulin lispro at meals with Utralente insulin in the morning and NPH insulin at bedtime. See Table 58–2 for the approximate distributions of insulin. Insulin glargine given once daily (usually in the evening) provides a stable 24-hour insulin level and appears to be an ideal basal insulin.

There are five main principles of advanced insulin management:

1. Perform SMBG 2 hours after meals (bolus adjustment) and before meals (basal adjustment).
2. Use an adequate total amount of insulin. Almost every study of type 2 diabetes that has obtained an Hb A_{1c} close to 7.0% required the use of a total dose of insulin that averaged about 1.2 U/kg.[83–86]
3. The bolus-to-basal insulin ratio is usually 50:50. On average, the most effective ratio has proved to be 50% of total insulin given as bolus insulin and 50% of total insulin given as basal insulin. A ratio of 50:50 ± 10% is a good quick screen to see if an individual's insulin regimen is set up in a way that is likely to lead to success.
4. Determine units of insulin per carbohydrate for each meal. Many

patients calculate with each meal the units of insulin per serving of carbohydrate. Others try to eat a consistent amount of carbohydrate at each meal, establishing a bolus dose for each meal, and then raising or lowering the dose if meals vary.

5. Prepare a supplemental insulin schedule that adjusts the bolus dose of insulin for three variables:

- Count carbohydrates: use the insulin-carbohydrate ratio.
- Compensate for the current glucose level: use correction factor (one extra unit of insulin for each 25 to 50 mg/dL the glucose is above target).
- Adjust for recent or anticipated exercise.

This can be done very quickly: for instance, if it is lunchtime, follow these three steps:

- Count carbohydrates: 4 carbohydrate servings, take 2 U of lispro per carbohydrate $4 \times 2 = 8$ U
- Compensate: Take 1 extra unit for each 25 mg/dL over the target of 140 mg/dL; for example, if current SMBG is 165 mg/dL, add 1 U: $8 + 1 = 9$ U
- Adjust for exercise: subtract 2 U for moderate exercise just completed: $9 - 2 = 7$ U

By going through this exercise at each meal, it is possible to match physiologic insulin needs reasonably well. Some physicians advise that if the glucose is high, the meal should be delayed for a certain time after injecting the insulin to let the glucose normalize before eating. The problem with this approach is that by the time the glucose normalizes, the insulin is gone, and there is nothing left to cover the meal that is about to be consumed. It seems much easier and more practical to use the three correction factors above and to proceed with the meal (there is rarely time in a busy schedule to delay meals).

New insulins continue to make advanced insulin management more effective. There is a new long-acting insulin that appears to be a true 24-hour peakless basal insulin called insulin glargine.[87–91] It is made by substituting one amino acid on the A chain of insulin and adding two amino acids to the B chain. The result is an insulin analogue soluble at an acidic pH that precipitates under the skin at neutral pH, prolonging its rate of absorption. Because of the pH it cannot be mixed in the same syringe with other insulin. Clinical trials show the least intra-subject variability in insulin levels among the basal insulins. In addition, there is equal or improved glycemic control with lower risk for clinically important hypoglycemic events.[156, 157] Another short-acting insulin analogue under development is called insulin aspart.[92] It is made by replacing proline at B28 of the insulin molecule with aspartic acid. Its action is reported to be similar to that of insulin lispro.[93] Another insulin just released for clinical use is a premixed insulin called mix 75/25.[94] It is a mixture of 75% neutral protamine lispro (NPL) and 25% lispro. Premixed 70/30 insulin is one of the most popular insulins used in the United States (particularly in type 2 patients). The problem with 70/30 insulin is it should be given before a meal like regular insulin and if the dose is pushed to improve control one must be careful about hypoglycemia because one cannot adjust each component separately. The initial studies with mix 75/25 indicate it may capture a large percentage of the 70/30 market because it has a rapid-acting insulin component and can be taken with meals and one gets lower postprandial glucose readings and less hypoglycemia than with 70/30 insulin.[95]

The other advances in insulin therapy include the use of insulin pens to deliver the insulin. Pens are widely used in Europe and Japan with great success and will likely catch on in the United States as more basal bolus therapy is used.[96, 97] Pen delivery of insulin may also be more accurate than syringes when used with the elderly or children.[98] The use of continuous subcutaneous insulin infusion (CSII) is growing rapidly in the management of type 1 diabetes.[99] The almost uniform use of insulin lispro in new pump starts has established an approach to insulin delivery that provides the maximum in the three important variables of enhancing control, minimizing hypoglycemia, and maximizing flexibility.[100] Although not officially approved, insulin lispro with or without an insulin pump is being used in many cases of pregnancy and diabetes in which postprandial glucose can be difficult to control. With more aggressive bolus basal insulin being used in type

2 diabetes and with lower target goals for preventing complications, it is appropriate to study pump therapy in type 2 diabetes.[101] Work continues on implanted insulin pumps at this time.[102]

Even with the advances in insulin formulation and delivery processes, important and exciting work continues on ways to eliminate the need for injected or infused insulin. The two most promising areas of transplant research in diabetes are pancreas transplantation[103, 104] and islet transplantation.[105]

Insulin plus Oral Agents

Over time insulin secretion is reduced to such low levels in type 2 diabetes that supplemental insulin is required, but in many cases the patient remains insulin-resistant (see Fig. 58–2). This sets up the rationale for what are proving to be effective and increasingly popular therapies of combining insulin with one or both of the insulin-sensitizing agents.

Historically, insulin has been used in combination with an SU agent. Meta-analyses shows glycosylated hemoglobin is reduced compared to insulin alone.[106] Similar Hb A_{1c} outcomes may have been obtained were insulin optimized according to modern principles of effective insulin administration. Today the use of an SU with insulin might be considered if bedtime insulin is started when there is still sufficient endogenous insulin secretion remaining to be enhanced by an SU during the day. This bedtime insulin and daytime SU regimen should be considered a transition to complex insulin therapy or advanced insulin management. Many clinicians use this approach as a relatively simple and patient-friendly way to start insulin therapy. Today, most patients and clinicians follow algorithms that proceed to at least two oral agents before starting insulin therapy.

If insulin is initiated as a single injection in the evening, what should be done with the oral agents? One excellent clinical study showed that insulin at night with metformin during the day was the most effective in lowering Hb A_{1c} and resulted in the least weight gain when compared to two injections of insulin, daytime SU and bedtime insulin, or daytime SU and metformin with bedtime insulin.[107] Further studies have shown benefits of metformin and insulin combination therapy.[108] There are two distinct approaches to combining metformin and insulin therapy. First, one can add insulin (often at bedtime) to the metformin and over time intensify the insulin as needed. Second, one can add metformin to an insulin-only regimen. In some studies metformin added to insulin therapy improved glycemic control compared with multiple-dose insulin therapy alone.[109] One study looking at patients on more intensive insulin therapy (at least three injections) showed that adding metformin reduced insulin requirements by 25%, and also significantly reduced weight and LDL cholesterol compared with insulin alone.[83] But both groups in this study achieved an Hb A_{1c} of approximately 7%. If insulin is being used aggressively and effectively following the advanced insulin management principles discussed above, one may not see a reduction in Hb A_{1c} when metformin is added but may see a reduced cardiovascular risk profile. In the many circumstances where insulin therapy has not been optimized (Hb A_{1c} < 7%) because the clinician or the patient is uncomfortable, unwilling, or unable to intensify insulin therapy, adding metformin has been shown to improve metabolic control.[109]

Other oral agents can be added to insulin therapy. Several studies have shown acarbose added to insulin both in type 1 and type 2 diabetes can result in a modest reduction in the Hb A_{1c} value.[110] Insulin doses and weight are usually neutral in the acarbose plus insulin studies. The combination of a TZD plus insulin has the potential to significantly reduce insulin doses and improve the Hb A_{1c}.[37] In addition, the potentially beneficial cardiovascular effects of the TZDs[41] may make them appealing in combination with insulin even though one can expect a weight gain from this combination. With increasing attention being paid to treating insulin resistance in type 2 diabetes, studies have shown that combining metformin and a TZD has at least an additive effect on reducing Hb A_{1c}.[39] Therefore, in the insulin-resistant patient who requires insulin therapy (usually doses >1.5 U/kg) more clinicians are using a combination of metformin and TZD with insulin. Studies are in progress to evaluate the long-term effectiveness of this approach which has a strong clinical and pathophysiologic basis.

In summary, just as a combination of oral agents is being used earlier in the course of type 2 diabetes it appears that combining oral agents (particularly the insulin sensitizers) with insulin will be more widely utilized. Long-term studies, although costly, must be done to not only confirm the importance of glycemic control in reducing cardiovascular complications but to determine if the insulin sensitizers have unique cardiovascular protective effects. Most investigators do not consider exogenous insulin itself as atherogenic but new approaches to combining existing drugs with insulin and the development of new medications to enhance the action of insulin or diminish the need for insulin continue to be investigated.

Glucose control is just one of the goals in preventing complications of diabetes. To fulfill the monitoring and management of the standards of care for diabetes, one must develop an approach to aggressive therapy of dyslipidemia and hypertension as well as strategies to prevent and treat the complications of diabetes.

COMPLICATIONS

Macrovascular Disease

Although much of the focus of diabetes management has been on glucose control and microvascular complications, macrovascular disease remains the most costly complication and results in the greatest mortality.[111] Effective cardiovascular risk reduction for patients with diabetes requires attention to other critical cardiovascular risk factors, including lipid disorders and hypertension.[17, 112] The cardiovascular risk for those with type 2 diabetes is increased two- to fivefold and this increase in risk is greatest for women with diabetes.[113] The same metabolic environment that predisposes people to type 2 diabetes (obesity, insulin resistance, and family history of type 2 diabetes) is also associated with a higher rate of other cardiovascular risk factors, including hypertension, dyslipidemia, and procoagulant tendencies.[113, 114] Addressing each of these cardiovascular risk factors is of significant benefit to those with diabetes and remains a central component of diabetes care.

Dyslipidemia

It is estimated that up to 70% of adults with diabetes have significant dyslipidemias. The most common disorders are elevations in triglycerides, low levels of HDL cholesterol, and elevated LDL cholesterol. In addition, the relative "negative" effect of lipid disorders is greater in those with diabetes—with a two- to fivefold higher risk of cardiovascular disease at any level of LDL and a higher risk with abnormalities in triglycerides and HDL. While detailed descriptions of these disorders and their respective therapies[114–116] are outlined elsewhere in this book, an algorithm for treatment of lipid disorders is presented in Figure 58–4.[118–122]

Hypertension

As with dyslipidemia, hypertension is also a common comorbidity in adults with diabetes. Data from the Third National Health and Nutrition Examination Survey[123] and other population studies suggests that up to two-thirds of these adults will have elevations in blood pressure. Hypertension increases the risk of both micro- and macrovascular disease and effective control of blood pressure in those with diabetes is critical.[124–127] While numerous therapeutic options are available, simple standards, such as use of angiotensin-converting enzyme (ACE) inhibitors,[128] and achieving lower blood pressure targets and use multidrug therapy, may be critical to maximizing the benefit of hypertension treatment. Figure 58–5 outlines commonly observed clinical scenarios and provides an algorithm for antihypertensive therapies for adults with diabetes. Selection of agents and the specific clinical situations have now been tested in numerous treatment trials.[125–137]

Screening for Complications

An additional and critical component of diabetes care includes screening for, and prevention and. treatment of, the known microvascular complications of diabetes (Fig. 58–6). Again, specific standards of care for appraisal of each of these potential complications have been established and their management is outlined below. Attempts to prevent retinopathy combined with early and aggressive treatment of known retinopathy is the best way to prevent blindness due to diabe-

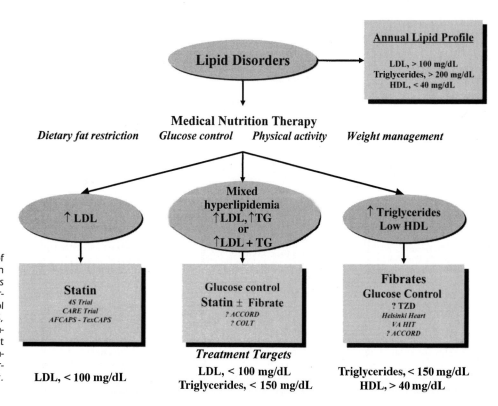

FIGURE 58–4. Algorithm for treatment of lipid disorders. 4S, Scandinavian Simvastatin Survival Study; VA HIT, Veterans Affairs High-Density Lipoprotein Cholesterol Intervention Trial; ACCoRD, Action to Control Cardiovascular Risks in Diabetes; AFCAPS, Air Force Coronary Atherosclerosis Prevention Study; CARE, cholesterol recurrent events; COLT, Baltimore coronary observational long-term study; TexCAPS, Texas Coronary Atherosclerosis Prevention Study. (Data from references 118–122.)

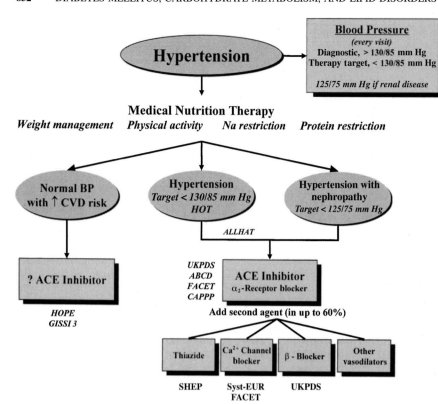

FIGURE 58–5. Algorithm for treatment of hypertension. ACE, angiotensin-converting enzyme; ALL-HAT, Antihypertension Lipid Lowering to Prevent Heart Attack Trial; CAPPP, Captopril Prevention Project; HOPE, Heart Outcomes Prevention Evaluation Study; CVD, cardiovascular disease; GISSI-3, Gruppo Italiano per lo Studio della Sopravvivenza Nell'Infarto miocardia; HOT, Hypertension Optimal Treatment; SHEP, Systolic Hypertension in the Elderly Program; Syst-EUR, Systolic Hypertension in Europe Trial; FACET, Fosinopril Versus Amlodipine Cardiovascular Events Randomized Trials; UKPDS, United Kingdom Prospective Diabetes Study. (Data from references 125–137.)

tes.[138] An annual eye examination is the main effort in prevention of blindness in diabetes. In this era of striving for cost-effective approaches to management, the most appropriate intervals for screening for retinopathy in type 2 diabetes are being reexamined.[139] Renal disease is screened for by an annual microalbumin test. Some clinical settings that have a high incidence of diabetic nephropathy often screen for proteinuria and if negative, for microalbuminuria. Since in most settings a urinalysis is not routinely ordered and the yield of gross proteinuria is very low, it is advisable to proceed with microal-

bumin testing directly. The most practical microalbumin test is the random measurement of the albumin-to-creatinine ratio.[140] If positive (>30 mg of albumin per gram of creatinine), it is repeated, and if positive two of three times, one proceeds with ACE inhibitor therapy[141, 142] if not contraindicated.

The basic screen for peripheral neuropathy is a foot examination. This includes gross inspection, assessment of circulation (posterior tibial and dorsalis pedis pulses and, if indicated, ankle-brachial index), and a neurologic evaluation. A simple yet effective approach to the

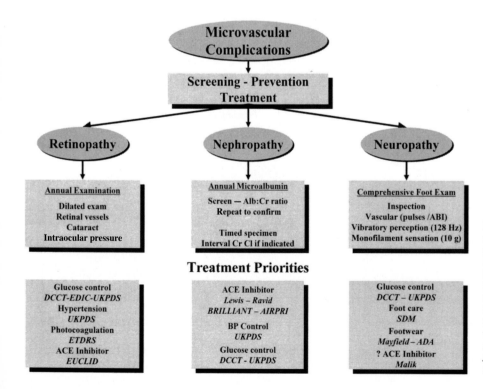

FIGURE 58–6. Algorithm for treatment of microvascular complications. DCCT-EDIC-UKPDS, Diabetes Control and Complications Trial–Epidemiology of Diabetes Interventions and Complications Research Group–United Kingdom Prospective Diabetes Study; ETDRS, Early Treatment Diabetic Retinopathy Study; EUCLID, EURODIAB Controlled Trial of Lisinopril in Insulin-Dependent Diabetes; AIRPRI, Angiotensin-Converting Enzyme Inhibitor in Progressive Renal Insufficiency; SDM, staged diabetes management; ADA, American Diabetes Association. (Data from references 54, 67, 141–150.)

neurologic evaluation is a vibration test using a 128-Hz tuning fork. The vibration at the toe is compared with the vibration at the finger level. The normal response is to feel the vibration in the fingers for less than 10 seconds longer than in the toes. If the vibration sense is abnormal this indicates early neuropathy (often asymptomatic) and one should proceed to test for light pressure or touch sensation using a 10-gm monofilament. If the monofilament test is abnormal, the foot is at high risk and preventive footwear and close observation are imperative. In addition to this peripheral nerve evaluation a yearly set of questions regarding autonomic nerve function is critical (inquire about gastroparesis, orthostasis, diarrhea, constipation, bladder atony, impotence, gustatory sweating). Accurate and easily performed screening tests for autonomic neuropathy (R-R interval testing) are available, and their utility in clinical practice is being evaluated. Many clinical trials evaluating the management of microvascular complications of diabetes have been conducted.[54, 67, 141–150]

OTHER COMPONENTS OF CARE

In addition to the diabetes-specific therapies described in the previous pages, patients with diabetes warrant continued attention to other important components of general medical care. Aspirin therapy has been reviewed by Colwell.[151] Aspirin use, unless contraindicated, is strongly encouraged for any patient with diabetes older than 35 years with significant cardiovascular risk. Additional components of care include appropriate instruction on foot care[149] and interval vaccinations, including influenza and pneumococcal vaccine.[152] Tobacco use remains a critical cardiac risk factor.[153] Tobacco cessation counseling must be a regular component of diabetes care.

Beyond these care components, a careful review of the psychosocial factors that may affect day-to-day diabetes management should also be assessed in all patients.[154] Furthermore, assuring patient satisfaction with the diabetes care delivered is among the standards set forth by the American Diabetes Association and other monitoring bodies, such as the Diabetes Quality Improvement Program.

SUMMARY

We have outlined a clinically applicable approach to diabetes care with emphasis on the current standards of care. Achieving good clinical outcomes requires not only an understanding of the standards of care but must emphasize a team-oriented approach to both behavior change and appropriate selection of therapies. Diabetes care is multifaceted and at times complex, yet the systematic approach we have presented to the metabolic abnormalities encountered in diabetes—hyperglycemia, dyslipidemia, hypertension, and other complications—can lead to improved outcomes and improved quality of life for the patient. In a recent editorial in *Annals of Internal Medicine*, David Nathan concluded: "Laissez-faire therapy for type 2 diabetes is no longer acceptable."[155] We agree.

REFERENCES

1. DeFronzo RA: Lilly lecture 1987. The triumvirate: Beta-cell, muscle, liver. A collusion responsible for NIDDM. Diabetes 37:667–687, 1988.
2. Reaven G: Role of insulin resistance in human disease. Diabetes 37:1595–1607, 1988.
3. Porte D Jr, Kahn SE: The key role of islet dysfunction in type 2 diabetes. Clin Invest Med 18:247–254, 1995.
4. Yudkin JS: Abnormalities of coagulation and fibrinolysis in insulin resistance: Evidence for a common antecedent? Diabetes Care 22(suppl 3):C25–C30, 1999.
5. Hambrecht R, Wolf A, Gielen S, et al: Effect of exercise on coronary endothelial function in patients with coronary artery disease. N Engl J Med 342:454–460, 2000.
6. Vita JA, Keaney JF: Exercise—toning up the endothelium? N Engl J Med 342:503–505, 2000.
7. Levine GN, Keaney JF, Vita JA: Cholesterol reduction in cardiovascular disease—clinical benefits and possible mechanisms. N Engl J Med 332:512–521, 1995.
8. Tooke JE, Goh KL: Endotheliopathy precedes type 2 diabetes. Diabetes Care 21:2047–2051, 1998.
9. Polonsky KS, Given BD, Hirsch I, et al: Abnormal patterns of insulin secretion in non–insulin dependent diabetes mellitus. N Engl J Med 318:1231–1239, 1988.

10. Leahy JL: Natural history of beta cell dysfunction in NIDDM. Diabetes Care 13:992–1010, 1990.
11. Ward WK, LaCava EC, Paquette TL, et al: Disproportionate elevation of immunoreactive proinsulin in type 2 diabetes and experimental insulin resistance. Diabetologia 30:698–702, 1987.
12. Roder ME, Porte D, Kahn SE: Disproportionately elevated proinsulin levels reflect the degree of impaired B-cell secretory capacity in patients with non-insulin dependent diabetes mellitus. J Clin Endocrinol Metab 83:604–608, 1998.
13. Kahn SE, Andrikopoulos S, Verchere CB: Islet amyloid: A long-recognized but underappreciated pathological feature of type 2 diabetes. Diabetes 48:241–253, 1999.
14. Franz MJ, Monk A, Barry B, et al: Effectiveness of medical nutrition therapy provided by dietitians in the management of non–insulin-dependent diabetes mellitus: A randomized, controlled clinical trial. J Am Diet Assoc 95:1009–1017, 1995.
15. DeFronzo RA: Pharmacologic therapy for type 2 diabetes mellitus. Ann Intern Med 131:281–303, 1999.
16. Haffner SM: Insulin sensitivity in subjects with type 2 diabetes. Diabetes Care 22:562–568, 1999.
17. Turner RC, Millns H, Neil HAW, et al: Risk factors for coronary artery disease in non–insulin dependent diabetes mellitus: United Kingdom Prospective Diabetes Study (UKPDS:23). BMJ 316:823–828, 1998.
18. Cusi K, DeFronzo RA: Metformin: A review of its metabolic effects. Diabetes Rev 6:89–131, 1998.
19. Bailey CJ, Turner RC: Metformin. N Engl J Med 334:574–579, 1996.
20. DeFronzo RA, Goodman AM: Efficacy of metformin in patients with non–insulin-dependent diabetes mellitus. The Multicenter Metformin Study Group. N Engl J Med 333:541–549, 1995.
21. Garber AJ, Duncan TG, Goodman AM, et al: Efficacy of metformin in type II diabetes: Results of a double-blind, placebo-controlled, dose-response trial. Am J Med 103:491–497, 1997.
22. Turner RC, Holman R, Stratton I: The UK Prospective Diabetes Study (letter). Lancet 352:1934, 1999.
23. Lebovitz HE: Insulin secretagogues: Old and new. Diabetes Rev 7:139–153, 1999.
24. Groop LC: Sulfonylureas in NIDDM. Diabetes Care 15:737–754, 1992.
25. United Kingdom Prospective Diabetes Study 16: Overview of 6 years' therapy of type II diabetes: A progressive disease. Diabetes 44:1249–1258, 1995.
26. Campbell K: Glimepiride: Role of a new sulfonylurea in the treatment of type 2 diabetes mellitus. Ann Pharmacother 32:1044–1052, 1998.
27. Rosenstock J, Samols E, Muchomore DB, et al: Glimepiride, a new once-daily sulfonylurea. A double-blind placebo-controlled study of NIDDM patients. Glimepride Study Group. Diabetes Care 19:1194–1199, 1996.
28. Geisen K, Vegh A, Krause E, Papp G: Cardiovascular effects of conventional sulfonylureas and glimepiride. Horm Metab Res 28:496–507, 1996.
29. Kilo C, Miller L, Williamson J: The crux of the UGDP. Spurious results and biologically inappropriate data analysis. Diabetologia 18:179–185, 1980.
30. Kalbag J, Hirschberg Y, McLeod JF, et al: Pharmacodynamics and dose response of nateglinide in type 2 diabetes (abstract). Diabetes 48(suppl 1):A100, 1999.
31. Hatorp V, Huang WC, Strange P: Pharmacokinetic properties of repaglinide in elderly subjects with type 2 diabetes. J Clin Endocrinol Metab 84:1475–1478, 1999.
32. Guay DR: Repaglinide, a novel short-acting hypoglycemic agent for type 2 diabetes mellitus. Pharmacotherapy 18:1195–1204, 1998.
33. Fuhlendorff J, Rorsman P, Kofod H, et al: Stimulation of insulin release by repaglinide and glibenclamide involves both common and distinct processes. Diabetes 47:345–351, 1998.
34. Damsbo P, Marbury TC, Clauson P, et al: A double-blind randomized comparison of meal-related glycemic control by repaglinide and glyburide in well-controlled type 2 diabetic patients. Diabetes Care 22:789–794, 1999.
35. Day C: Thiazolidinediones: A new class of antidiabetic drugs. Diabet Med 16:179–192, 1999.
36. Saltiel AR, Olefsky JM: Thiazolidinediones in the treatment of insulin resistance and type II diabetes. Diabetes 45:1661–1669, 1996.
37. Buse JB, Gumbiner B, Mathias NP, et al: Troglitazone use in insulin-treated type 2 diabetic patients. The Troglitazone Insulin Study Group. Diabetes Care 21:1455–1461, 1998.
38. Schwartz S, Raskin P, Fonseca V, et al: Effect of troglitazone in insulin-treated patients with type II diabetes mellitus. N Engl J Med 13:861–866, 1998.
39. Inzucchi SE, Maggs DF, Spollett GR, et al: Efficacy and metabolic effects of metformin and troglitazone in type II diabetes mellitus. N Engl J Med 338:867–872, 1998.
40. Gorson DM: Significant weight gain with rezulin therapy. Arch Intern Med 159:99, 1999.
41. Law RE, Meehan WP, Xi XP, et al: Troglitazone inhibits vascular smooth-muscle cell growth and intimal hyperplasia. J Clin Invest 98:1897–1905, 1996.
42. Imano E, Kanda T, Nakatani Y, et al: Effect of troglitazone on microalbuminuria in patients with incipient diabetic nephropathy. Diabetes Care 121:2135–2139, 1998.
43. Chiasson J-L, Josse RJ, Hunt JA, et al: The efficacy of acarbose in the treatment of patients with non insulin-dependent diabetes mellitus. Ann Intern Med 121:928–935, 1994.
44. Lebovitz HE: A new oral therapy for diabetes management: Alpha-glucosidase inhibition with acarbose. Clin Diabetes 13:99–103, 1995.
45. Mudaliar S, Henry RR: Combination therapy for type 2 diabetes. Endocr Pract 5:208–219, 1999.
46. Hermann LS, Schersten B, Bitzen PO, et al: Therapeutic comparison of metformin and sulfonylurea, alone and in various combinations. A double-blind, controlled study. Diabetes Care 17:1100–1109, 1994.
47. Schneider R, Egan J, Houser V, the Pioglitazone 010 Study Group: Combination therapy with pioglitazone and sulfonylurea in patients with type 2 diabetes. Presented at the American Diabetes Association Annual Meeting, San Diego, 1999, abstract 0458.

48. Ovalle F, Bell DSH: Triple oral antidiabetic therapy in type 2 diabetes mellitus. Endocr Pract 4:146–147, 1998.
49. Fertig BJ, Simmons DA, Martin DB: Therapy for diabetes. *In* National Diabetes Data Group (ed): Diabetes in America, ed 2. Bethesda, MD, National Institutes of Health, 1995, pp 519–539.
50. Weyer C, Bogardus C, Mott DM, et al: The natural history of insulin secretory dysfunction and insulin resistance in the pathogenesis of type 2 diabetes mellitus. J Clin Invest; 104:787–794, 1999.
51. Genuth S: Insulin use in NIDDM. Diabetes Care 13:1240–1264, 1990.
52. Bergenstal RM: Optimization of insulin therapy in patients with type 2 diabetes. Endocr Pract 6:93–97, 2000.
53. Edelman SV, Henry RR: Insulin therapy for normalizing glycosylated hemoglobin in type II diabetes. Diabetes Rev 3:308–334, 1995.
54. The Diabetes Control and Complications Trial/Epidemiology of Diabetes Interventions and Complications Research Group: Retinopathy and nephropathy in patients with type 1 diabetes four years after a trial of intensive therapy. N Engl J Med 342:381–389, 2000.
55. Robertson KE, Glazer NB, Campbell RK: The latest developments in insulin injection devices. Diabetes Educator 26:135–152, 2000.
56. Tuiana-Rufi N, Belarbi N, Du Pasquier-Fediaesky L, et al: Short needles (8 mm) reduce the risk of intramuscular injections. Diabetes Care 22:1621–1625, 1999.
57. Laube BL, Benedict GW, Dobs AS: Time to peak insulin level, relative bioavailability, and effect of site of deposition of nebulized insulin in patients with noninsulin-dependent diabetes mellitus. J Aerosol Med 11:153–173, 1998.
58. Skyler JS, Gelfand RA, Kourides IA, et al: Treatment of type 1 diabetes mellitus with inhaled human insulin: A 3-month multicenter trial (abstract). Diabetes 47(suppl 1):A236, 1998.
59. Abraira C, Colwell JA, Nuttall FQ, et al: Veterans Affairs Cooperative Study on glycemic control and complications in type II diabetes (VA CSDM). Results of a feasibility trial. Diabetes Care 18:1113–1123, 1995.
60. Cryer PE: Hypoglycemia: The limiting factor in the management of IDDM (Banting lecture). Diabetes 43:1378–1389, 1994.
61. Anderson JH, Brunelle RI, Koivisto VA, et al: Reduction of postprandial hyperglycemia and frequency of hypoglycemia in IDDM patients on insulin-analog treatment. Diabetes 46:265–270, 1997.
62. Malmberg K, DIGAMI (Diabetes Mellitus, Insulin Glucose Infusion in Acute Myocardial Infarction) Study Group: Prospective randomized study of intensive insulin treatment on long term survival after acute myocardial infarction in patients with diabetes mellitus. BMJ 314:1512–1515, 1997.
63. Malmberg K, Norhammar A, Wedel H, et al: Glycometabolic state at admission: Important risk marker of mortality in conventionally treated patients with diabetes mellitus and acute myocardial infarction: Long-term results from the Diabetes and Insulin-Glucose Infusion in Acute Myocardial Infarction (DIGAMI) study. Circulation 99:2626–2632, 1999.
64. Riddle MC: Evening insulin strategy. Diabetes Care 13:676–686, 1990.
65. Riddle MC, Schneider J: Beginning insulin treatment with evening 70/30 insulin plus glimepiride versus insulin alone. Diabetes Care 21:1052–1057, 1998.
66. Colwell JA: The feasibility of intensive insulin management in non–insulin-dependent diabetes mellitus: Implications of the Veterans Affairs Cooperative Study on Glycemic Control and Complications in NIDDM. Ann Intern Med 124(1pt2):131–135, 1996.
67. DCCT Research Group: The effect of intensive treatment of diabetes on the development and progression of long-term complications of insulin-dependent diabetes mellitus. N Engl J Med 329:1289–1298, 1993.
68. Schade DS, Santiago JV, Skyler JS, et al: Intensive Insulin Therapy. Princeton, NJ, Excerpta Medica, 1983.
69. Hirsch IB: Type 1 diabetes mellitus and the use of flexible insulin regimens. Am Fam Physician 60:2343–2356, 1999.
70. Howorka K: Functional Insulin Treatment, ed 2. Berlin, Springer-Verlag, 1996.
71. Lorenz R: The problem with intensive therapy. Diabetes Care 21:2021–2024, 1998.
72. Bolli GB, DiMarchi RD, Park GD, et al: Insulin analogues and their potential in the management of diabetes mellitus. Diabetologia 42:1151–1167, 1999.
73. Warren LL, Zinman B: From insulin to insulin analogs: Progress in the treatment of type 1 diabetes. Diabetes Rev 6:73–88, 1998.
74. Howey DC, Bowsher RR, Brunelle RL, et al: [Lys(B28), Pro(B29)]-human insulin: A rapidly absorbed analogue of human insulin. Diabetes 43:396–402, 1994.
75. Donahue RP, Abbott RD, Reed DM, et al: Postchallenge glucose concentration and coronary heart disease in men of Japanese ancestry. Honolulu Heart Program. Diabetes 36:689–692, 1987.
76. Avignon A, Radauceanu A, Monnier L: Nonfasting plasma glucose is a better marker of diabetic control than fasting plasma glucose in type 2 diabetes. Diabetes Care 20:1822–1826, 1997.
77. de Veciana M, Major CA, Morgan MA, et al: Postprandial versus preprandial blood glucose monitoring in women with gestational diabetes mellitus requiring insulin therapy. N Engl J Med 333:1237–1241, 1995.
78. Jovanovic L, Ilic S, Pettitt DJ, et al: Metabolic and immunologic effects of insulin lispro in gestational diabetes. Diabetes Care 22:1422–1427, 1999.
79. Holcombe JH, Brunelle R, Deeb LC, et al: Comparative study of insulin lispro and regular insulin in prepubertal children with type 1 diabetes (abstract). Diabetes 47(suppl 1):A96, 1998.
80. Zinman B, Ross S, Campos RV, et al: Effectiveness of human Ultralente vs. NPH insulin in providing basal insulin replacement for an insulin lispro multiple daily injection regimen: A double-blind randomized prospective trial. Diabetes Care 22:603–608, 1999.
81. Ebeling P, Jansson PA, Smith U, et al: Strategies toward improved control during insulin lispro therapy in IDDM: Importance of basal insulin. Diabetes Care 20:1287–1289, 1997.
82. Lalli C, Ciofetta M, Del Sindaco P, et al: Long-term intensive treatment of type 1 diabetes with the short-acting insulin analog lispro in variable combination with NPH insulin at mealtime. Diabetes Care 22:468–477, 1999.
83. Bergenstal R, Johnson M, Whipple D, et al: Advantages of adding metformin to multiple dose insulin therapy in type 2 diabetes (abstract). Diabetes 47(suppl 1):A89, 1998.
84. Henry RR, Gumbiner B, Ditzler T, et al: Intensive conventional insulin therapy for type II diabetes: Metabolic effects during a 6-month outpatient trial. Diabetes Care 16:21–31, 1993.
85. Garvey WT, Olefsky JM, Griffin J, et al: The effect of insulin treatment on insulin secretion and insulin action in type II diabetes mellitus. Diabetes 34:222–234, 1985.
86. Colwell JA: The feasibility of intensive insulin management in non–insulin-dependent diabetes mellitus: Implications of the Veterans Affairs Cooperative Study on Glycemic Control and Complications in NIDDM. Ann Intern Med 124(1pt 2):131–135, 1996.
87. Pieber TR, Eugene-Jolchine I, Derobert E, et al: Efficacy and safety of HOE 901 versus NPH insulin in patients with type 1 diabetes. Diabetes Care 23:157–162, 2000.
88. Luzio SD, Owens D, Evans M, et al: Comparison of the s.c. absorption of HOE 901 and NPH human insulin in type 2 diabetic subjects (abstract). Diabetes 24(suppl 1): A111, 1999.
89. Ratner RE, Hirsch IB, Mecca TE, et al: Efficacy and safety of insulin glargine in subjects with type 1 diabetes: A 28-week randomized, NPH insulin-controlled trial (abstract). Diabetes 48(suppl 1):A120, 1999.
90. Rosenstock J, Schwartz S, Clark C, et al: Efficacy and safety of HOE 901 (insulin glargine) in subjects with type 2 DM: A 28-week randomized, NPH insulin-controlled trial (abstract). Diabetes 48(suppl 1):A100, 1999.
91. Home P: Insulin glargine: The first clinically useful extended-acting insulin in half a century? Exp Opin Invest Drugs 8:307–313, 1999.
92. Home PD, Lindholm A, Hylleberg B, et al: Improved glycemic control with insulin aspart: A multicenter randomized double-blind crossover trial in type 1 diabetic patients. Diabetes Care 21:1904–1909, 1998.
93. Linholm A, McEwen J, Riis AP: Improved postprandial glycemic control with insulin aspart: A randomized double-blind cross-over trial in type 1 diabetes. Diabetes Care 22:801–805, 1999.
94. Koivisto VA, Tuominen JA, Ebeling P: Lispro mix 25 insulin as a premeal therapy in type 2 diabetic patients. Diabetes Care 22:459–462, 1999.
95. Roach P, Yue L, Arora V, et al: Improved postprandial glycemic control during treatment with Humalog mix 25, a novel protamine-based insulin lispro formulation. Diabetes Care 22:1258–1261, 1999.
96. McCaughey ES, Betts PR, Rowe DJ, et al: Improved diabetic control in adolescents using the Penject syringe for multiple insulin injections. Diabet Med 3:234–236, 1986.
97. Dunbar JM, Maddden PM, Fiad TM, McKenna TJ: Premixed insulin preparations in pen syringes maintain glycemic control and are preferred by patients. Diabetes Care 17:874–878, 1994.
98. Lteif AN, Schwenk WF: Accuracy of pen injectors versus insulin syringes in children with type 1 diabetes. Diabetes Care 22:137–140, 1999.
99. Bode BW, Steed RD, Davidson PC: Reduction in severe hypoglycemia with long-term CSII in type 1 diabetes. Diabetes Care 19:324–327, 1996.
100. Zinman B, Tildesley H, Chiasson JL, et al: Insulin lispro in CSII: Results of a double-blind crossover study [erratum appears in Diabetes 46:1239, 1997]. Diabetes 46:440–443, 1997.
101. Jennings AM, Lewis KS, Murdoch S, et al: Randomized trial comparing continuous subcutaneous insulin infusion and conventional insulin therapy in type II diabetic patients poorly controlled with sulfonylureas. Diabetes Care 14:738–744, 1991.
102. Selam JL, Micossi P, Dunn FL, et al: Clinical trial of programmable implantable insulin pump for type 1 diabetes. Diabetes Care 15:877–885, 1992.
103. Sutherland DER, Gruessner RWG, Najarian JS, et al: Solitary pancreas transplants: A new era. Transplant Proc 30:280–281, 1998.
104. Fioretto P, Steffes MW, Sutherland DR, et al: Reversal of lesions of diabetic nephropathy after pancreas transplantation. N Engl J Med 339:69–75, 1998.
105. Hering BJ, Ricordi C: Islet transplantation in type 1 diabetes: Results, research priorities and reasons for optimism. Graft 2:12–27, 1999.
106. Johnson JL, Wolf SL, Kabadi UM: Efficacy of insulin and sulfonylurea combination therapy in type II diabetes. A meta-analysis of the randomized placebo-controlled trials. Arch Intern Med 156:259–264, 1996.
107. Yki-Jarvinen H, Ryysy L, Nikkila K, et al: Comparison of bedtime insulin regimens in patients with type 2 diabetes mellitus. Ann Intern Med 130:389–396, 1999.
108. Hermann LS: Combination therapy with insulin and metformin. Endocr Pract 4:404–412, 1998.
109. Aviles-Santa L, Sinding J, Raskin P: Effects of metformin in patients with poorly controlled, insulin-treated type 2 diabetes mellitus: A randomized, double-blind, placebo-controlled trial. Ann Intern Med 131:182–188, 1999.
110. Kelly DE, Bidot P, Freedman Z, et al: Efficacy and safety of acarbose in insulin-treated patients with type 2 diabetes. Diabetes Care 21:2056–2061, 1998.
111. Haffner SM, Lehto S, Ronnemaa T, et al: Mortality from coronary heart disease in subjects with type 2 diabetes and in nondiabetic subjects with and without prior myocardial infarction. N Engl J Med 339:229–234, 1998.
112. Nesto RW: Screening for asymptomatic coronary artery disease in diabetes. Diabetes Care 22:1393–1395, 1999.
113. Sowers JR: Diabetes mellitus and cardiovascular disease in women. Arch Intern Med, 158:617–621, 1998.
114. Lipid Research Clinics Program: The Lipid Research Clinics Coronary Primary Prevention Trial results. I: Reduction in incidence of coronary heart disease. JAMA 251:351–364, 1984.
115. American Diabetes Association: Management of dyslipidemia in adults with diabetes (position statement). Diabetes Care 23(suppl 1):S57–S60, 2000.
116. National Cholesterol Education Program (NCEP) Expert Panel: Summary of the second report of the NCEP expert panel on detection, evaluation, and treatment of high blood cholesterol (Adult Treatment Panel II). JAMA 209:3015–3023, 1993.

117. Pyorala K, Savolainen E, Kaukola S, et al: Cholesterol lowering with simvastatin improves prognosis of diabetic patients with coronary heart disease: Subgroup analysis of the Scandinavin Simvastatin Survival Study. Diabetes Care 20:614–620, 1997.

118. The CARE Investigators: Cardiovascular events and their reduction with pravastatin in diabetic and glucose-intolerant myocardial infarction survivors with average cholesterol levels: Subgroup analyses in the cholesterol and recurrent events (CARE) trial. Circulation 98:2513–2519, 1998.

119. Downs JR, Clearfield M, Weis S, et al: Primary prevention of acute coronary events with lovastatin in men and women with average cholesterol levels: Results of AFCAPS/TexCAPS. Air Force/Texas Coronary Atherosclerosis Prevention Study. JAMA 279:1615–1622, 1998.

120. Miller M, Seidler A, Moalemi A, et al: Normal triglyceride levels and coronary artery disease events: The Baltimore Coronary Observational Long-Term Study. J Am Coll Cardiol 31:1252–1257, 1998.

121. Koskinen P, Manttari M, Manninen V et al: Coronary heart disease incidence in NIDDM patients in the Helsinki Heart Study. Diabetes Care 15:820–825, 1992.

122. Rubins H: Gemfibrozil for the secondary prevention of coronary heart disease in men with low levels of high-density lipoprotein cholesterol. Veterans Affairs High-Density Lipoprotein Cholesterol Intervention Trial Study Group. N Engl J Med 341:410–418, 1999.

123. Harris M, Flegel M, Cowie C, et al: Prevalence of diabetes, impaired fasting glucose, and impaired glucose tolerance in U.S. adults: The Third National Health and Nutrition Examination Survey, 1988–1994. Diabetes Care 21:518–524, 1998.

124. The 6th report of the Joint National Committee on Prevention, Detection, Evaluation, and Treatment of high blood pressure. Arch Intern Med 157:2413–2446, 1997.

125. United Kingdom Prospective Diabetes Study Group: Efficacy of atenolol and captopril in reducing risk of macrovascular and microvascular complications in type 2 diabetes: UKPDS 39. BMJ 317:713–720, 1998.

126. United Kingdom Prospective Diabetes Study Group: Tight blood pressure control and risk of macrovascular and microvascular complications in type 2 diabetes: UKPDS 38. BMJ J 317:703–713, 1998.

127. United Kingdom Prospective Diabetes Study Group: Cost effectiveness analysis of improved blood pressure control in hypertensive patients with type 2 diabetes: UKPDS 40. BMJ 317:720–726, 1998.

128. Heart Outcomes Prevention Evaluation (HOPE) Study Investigators: Effects of ramipril on cardiovascular and microvascular outcomes in people with diabetes mellitus: Results of the HOPE study and MICRO-HOPE substudy. Lancet 355:253–259, 2000.

129. The Heart Outcomes Prevention Evaluation Study Investigators: Effects of an angiotensin-converting enzyme inhibitor, ramipril, on cardiovascular events in high-risk patients. N Engl J Med 342:145–153, 2000.

130. Zuanetti G, Latini R, Maggioni AP, et al: Effect of the ACE inhibitor lisinopril on mortality in diabetic patients with acute myocardial infarction: data from the GISSI-3 study. Circulation 96:4239–4245, 1997.

131. Estacio RO, Jeffers BW, Hiatt WR, et al: The effect of nisoldipine as compared with enalapril on cardiovascular outcomes in patients with non–insulin-dependent diabetes and hypertension (ABCD). N Engl J Med 338:645–652, 1998.

132. Tatti P, Pahor M, Byington RP, et al: Outcome results of the Fosinopril Versus Amlodipine Cardiovascular Events Randomized Trial (FACET) in patients with hypertension and NIDDM. Diabetes Care 21:597–603, 1998.

133. Hansson L, Lindholm LH, Niskanen L, et al: Effect of angiotensin-converting-enzyme inhibition compared with conventional therapy on cardiovascular morbidity and mortality in hypertension: The Captopril Prevention Project (CAPPP) randomized trial. Lancet 353:611–616, 1999.

134. Curb JD, Pressel SL, Cutler JA, et al: Effect of diuretic-based antihypertensive treatment on cardiovascular disease risk in older diabetic patients with isolated systolic hypertension. Systolic Hypertension in the Elderly Program Cooperative Research Group. JAMA 276:1886–1892, 1996.

135. Tuomilehto J, Rastenyte D, Birkenhager WH, et al: Effects of calcium-channel blockade in older patients with diabetes and systolic hypertension. Systolic Hypertension in Europe Trial Investigators. N Engl J Med 340:677–684, 1999.

136. Davis BR, Cutler JA, Gordon DJ, et al: Rationale and design for the Antihypertensive and Lipid Lowering Treatment to Prevent Heart Attack Trial (ALLHAT). ALLHAT Research Group. Am J Hypertens 9:342–360, 1996.

137. Hansson L, Zanchetti A, Carruthers SG, et al: Effects of intensive blood pressure lowering and low-dose aspirin in patients with hypertension: Principal results of the Hypertension Optimal Treatment (HOT) randomized trial. Lancet 351:1755–1762, 1998.

138. Ferris FL, Davis MD, Aiello LM: Treatment of diabetic retinopathy. N Engl J Med 341:667–678, 1999.

139. Vijan S, Hofer TP, Hayward RA: Cost-utility analysis of screening intervals for diabetic retinopathy in patients with type 2 diabetes mellitus. JAMA 283:889–896, 2000.

140. American Diabetes Association: Diabetic nephropathy (position statement). Diabetes Care 23(suppl 1):S69–72, 2000.

141. Lewis EJ, Hunsicker LG, Bain RP, et al: The effect of angiotensin-converting-enzyme inhibition on diabetic nephropathy [erratum appears in N Engl J Med 330:152, 1993]. N Engl J Med 329:1456–1462, 1993.

142. Ravid M, Savin H, Jutrin I, et al: Long-term stabilizing effect of angiotensin-converting enzyme inhibition on plasma creatinine and on proteinuria in normotensive type II diabetic patients. Ann Intern Med 118:577–581, 1993.

143. The Early Treatment Diabetic Retinopathy Study Research Group: Early photocoagulation for diabetic retinopathy: ETDRS report number 9. Ophthalmology 98(suppl):766–785, 1991.

144. Chaturvedi N, Sjolie AK, Stephenson JM, et al: Effect of lisinopril on progression of retinopathy in normotensive people with type 1 diabetes. The EUCLID Study Group. EURODIAB Controlled Trial of Lisinopril in Insulin-Dependent Diabetes Mellitus. Lancet 351:28–31, 1998.

145. Ravid M, Brosh D, Ravid-Safran D, et al: Main risk factors for nephropathy in type 2 diabetes mellitus are plasma cholesterol levels, mean blood pressure, and hyperglycemia. Arch Intern Med 148:998–1004, 1998.

146. Agardh CD, Garcia-Puig J, Charbonnel B, et al: Greater reduction of urinary albumin excretion in hypertensive type 2 patients with incipient nephropathy by lisinopril than by nifedipine. BRILLIANT Study. J Hum Hypertens 10:185–192, 1996.

147. Maschio G, Alberti D, Janin G, et al: Effect of angiotensin-converting enzyme inhibition on the progression of chronic renal insufficiency. The Angiotensin-Converting-Enzyme Inhibitor in Progressive Renal Insufficiency Study Group (AIRPRI). N Engl J Med 334:939–945, 1996.

148. Rith-Najarian S, Branchaud C, Beaulieu O, et al: Reducing lower-extremity amputations due to diabetes: Application of the staged diabetes management approach in a primary care setting. J Fam Pract 47:127–132, 1998.

149. Mayfield JA, Reiber GE, Sanders LJ, et al: Preventive foot care in people with diabetes (technical review). Diabetes Care 21:2161–2177, 1998.

150. Malik RA, Williamson S, Abbott C, et al: Effect of angiotensin-converting enzyme (ACE) inhibitor trandolapril on human diabetic neuropathy: Randomised double-blind controlled trial. Lancet 352:1978–1981, 1998

151. Colwell JA: Aspirin therapy in diabetes (technical review). Diabetes Care 20:1767–1771, 1997.

152. Smith SA, Poland GA: The use of influenza and pneumococcal vaccines in people with diabetes (technical review). Diabetes Care 23:95–108, 2000.

153. Haire-Joshu D, Glasgow RE, Tibbs TL: Smoking and diabetes (technical review). Diabetes Care 22:1887–1898, 1999.

154. The Diabetes Control and Complications Trial Research Group: Effects of intensive diabetes therapy on neuropsychological functioning in adults in the Diabetes Control and Complications Trial. Ann Intern Med 124:379–388, 1996.

155. Nathan DM: Treating type 2 diabetes with respect. Ann Intern Med 130:440–441, 1999.

156. Base J: Insulin glargine (HOE 901) (editorial). Diabetes Care 23:576–578, 2000.

157. Heinemann L, Linkeschoua R, Rave K, et al: Time-action profile of the long-acting insulin analog insulin glargine (HOE 901) in comparison with those of NPH insulin and placebo. Diabetes Care 23:644–649, 2000.

Chapter 59

▲▲▲ Pancreas and Islet Transplantation

R. Paul Robertson

PANCREAS TRANSPLANTATION

History

Pancreas transplantation as treatment of diabetes mellitus was first performed in 1966.[1] In the early history of this procedure, the rates of graft and patient survival were unacceptably low, so very few procedures were performed until 1978. In the intervening years important changes were introduced, including better immunosuppressive regimens (introduction of cyclosporine and anti–T cell agents), refined surgical techniques, improved monitoring for rejection episodes, and selection of healthier patients. The number of procedures has steadily increased each year, and by the end of 1997, over 10,000 procedures had been performed with over 1200 that year alone[2] (Fig. 59–1). During the development of this experimental procedure, a serendipitous observation[3] provided important reinforcement of the evolving theory of the autoimmune nature of diabetes mellitus. A patient who received a pancreatic segment from her identical twin was not given immunosuppression posttransplantation because graft rejection was not considered to be a possibility. However, diabetes recurred in the recipient within 2 weeks. Unexpectedly, pancreatic biopsy did not reveal graft rejection, but instead destruction of β cells only with no damage to α cells or the exocrine pancreas. It was concluded that a β cell–specific autoimmune response was reignited when β cells from

---

Work on this chapter was supported by National Institutes of Health grant PO1 DK 39994.

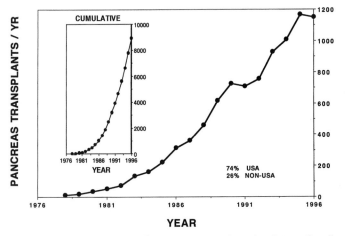

FIGURE 59–1. Frequency of pancreas transplantation internationally 1978–1996. *Inset,* Cumulative numbers of pancreases transplanted. (From Gruessner A, Sutherland DER: Pancreas transplants for United States (US) and non-US cases as reported to International Pancreas Transplant Registry (IPTR) and to the United Network for Organ Sharing (UNOS). *In* Cecka M, Terasaki P (eds): Clinical Transplants 1997. Los Angeles, UCLA Tissue Typing Laboratory, 1998.)

the nondiabetic identical twin were introduced into the diabetic recipient, whose immune system recreated the original pathogenic scenario that led to diabetes 17 years earlier.

Transplantation Procedures and Immunosuppressive Agents

Most pancreas transplantations use cadaveric organs and are performed simultaneously with or some time after kidney transplantation in diabetic patients with renal failure. The objectives in these cases are to render the recipient free of exogenous insulin therapy, halt the progress of ongoing secondary complications, protect the newly transplanted kidney from damage caused by hyperglycemia, and improve quality of life. Uncommonly, a pancreas alone is transplanted in patients who do not have renal failure. The clinical indications in these instances include severe metabolic instability, severe autonomic dysfunction, and a generally poor quality of life because of the complications of chronic diabetes. Even less commonly a segment (usually half) of a pancreas that has been donated by a living family member is used.

The pancreas is transplanted into the pelvis of the recipient and the iliac vessels are used for arterial supply and venous drainage (Fig. 59–2), which results in systemic rather than portal venous drainage. This abnormal arrangement means that insulin released from the transplant does not undergo first-pass hepatic metabolism before reaching the systemic circulation and, consequently, hyperinsulinemia develops.[4] Recently, more attention is being given to surgical construction of portal venous drainage for pancreas grafts because of theoretic concerns about the adverse consequences of hyperinsulinemia. Usually, the transplanted pancreas is still attached to a small portion of the donor duodenum containing the exit of the pancreatic duct. The duodenal segment and pancreatic duct outlet are oversewn onto the urinary bladder, which receives the exocrine drainage from the graft. An alternative approach is to use enteric rather than bladder drainage of the graft. Advantages of bladder drainage include the use of urinary amylase to monitor for rejection and the avoidance of small bowel complications such as obstruction and infection. Advantages of enteric drainage are the avoidance of urinary tract infections, acidosis (from loss of bicarbonate), hematuria, and reflux pancreatitis. In all variations of this procedure, however, the native pancreas is left untouched and continues to provide normal exocrine drainage for the recipient's gut.

Quadruple immunosuppressive regimens are the rule and include antibody induction with either a monoclonal or a polyclonal agent directed against T cells. Long-term maintenance is provided by triple-drug therapy with a calcineurin inhibitor (cyclosporine or tacrolimus), an antimetabolite (azathioprine or mycophenolate mofetil), and corticosteroids.

Graft and Patient Survival

Rates of survival for pancreatic grafts, as well as for patients, have steadily improved since 1966. The International Pancreas Transplant

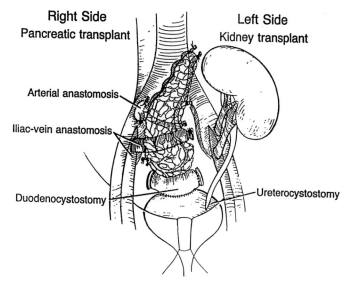

FIGURE 59–2. Conventional locations of pancreas and kidney grafts after a simultaneous pancreas and kidney transplantation. The ectopic pancreas receives its arterial supply from the iliac artery, and the iliac vein receives the pancreatic venous return through which islet hormones traverse. Exocrine drainage from the transplanted pancreas exits through a small section of duodenum from the donor that is oversewn onto the urinary bladder of the recipient. (Reprinted, by permission, from Robertson RP: Pancreas and islet transplantation for diabetes: Cures or curiosities? N Engl J Med 327:1861–1868, 1992. Copyright © 1992 Massachusetts Medical Society. All rights reserved.)

Registry[2] reported that between the years 1994 and 1997, patient survival rates were greater than 93% 1 and 3 years posttransplant (Fig. 59–3), whether the pancreas was transplanted alone (PTA), simultaneously with a kidney (SPK), or after a kidney had been transplanted previously (PAK). Most deaths were due to cardiovascular disease and usually occurred more than 3 months after discharge from the hospital. The mortality rate 1 year after the much less invasive procedure of pancreatic islet transplantation is 5%.[5] Consequently, it seems likely that the mortality rates associated with pancreas transplantation are more related to the complications of chronic diabetes than to the transplantation itself. Concerns that the mortality associated with SPK is greater than that after a kidney transplant alone[6] have not been substantiated in larger studies.[2, 7]

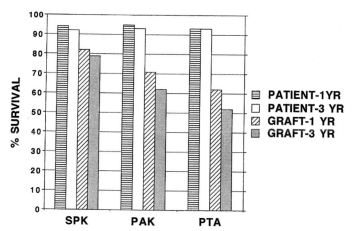

FIGURE 59–3. Patient and pancreas graft survival 1 and 3 years post-transplantation: International Pancreas Transplant Registry 1994–1997 data. PAK, pancreas after kidney; PTA, pancreas transplant alone; PKA, simultaneous pancreas and kidney. (From Gruessner A, Sutherland DER: Pancreas transplants for United States (US) and non-US cases as reported to International Pancreas Transplant Registry (IPTR) and to the United Network for Organ Sharing (UNOS). In Cecka M, Terasaki P (eds): Clinical Transplants 1997. Los Angeles, UCLA Tissue Typing Laboratory, 1998.)

Rejection episodes are common and can occur within days and after years of successful transplantation. When a pancreas threatens to be rejected, the episode is managed by hospitalizing the patient and intensively accelerating immunosuppression. During the 1994–1997 epoch, the rates of organ survival 1 year after pancreas transplantation (defined as total freedom from insulin therapy, normal fasting blood glucose concentrations, and normal or only slightly elevated hemoglobin A_{1c} [HbA_{1c}] values) were 82% for SPK, 71% for PAK, and 62% for PTA[2] (see Fig. 59–3). These rates 3 years after transplantation were 79%, 64%, and 52%, respectively. The lower survival rate for PTA is probably related to the fact that detection of pancreas rejection is made easier when the procedure is SPK or PAK because serum creatinine increases during kidney rejection and thereby serves as a sentinel for pancreas rejection. When a pancreas alone has been transplanted with urinary bladder drainage of exocrine secretions, the less sensitive indices of decreasing urinary amylase, increasing serum amylase, and increasing blood glucose levels are later signals for rejection. If enteric rather than urinary bladder drainage has been used for PTA, only the sign of rising blood glucose is available. Cystoscopic transduodenal biopsy (in the case of urinary bladder drainage of the graft) or transcutaneous biopsy with ultrasound guidance is used to confirm the diagnosis of rejection. The possibility of autoimmune attack is always considered, but it seems that autoimmune attack should be an unusual cause of recurrent autoimmune diabetes because the patient receives immunosuppressive drugs that are known to suppress primary autoimmune function and because the donated organ is from a nonself source.

Clinical Outcomes

Acute Complications of Diabetes

Successful pancreas transplantation is the only reliably effective treatment that results in restored endogenous insulin secretion, independence from exogenous insulin therapy, normal glucose levels, and normal to nearly normal HbA_{1c} levels. The degree of normalization of HbA_{1c} levels is better with pancreas transplantation than with the intensive insulin-based management used in the Diabetes Control and Complication Trial[8] (Fig. 59–4). In a study of 96 patients, fasting plasma glucose, HbA_{1c}, glucose-induced insulin secretion, and arginine-induced glucagon secretion were maintained at normal levels for up to 5 years.[9] In some centers, success for 10 to 20 years is not uncommon. These positive clinical outcomes are all the more impressive in view of the fact that recipients are treated with immunosuppressive drugs that intrinsically diminish β cell function[10] (Fig. 59–5). One area of concern is that hyperinsulinemia uniformly develops in recipients of transplanted pancreases (Fig. 59–6). Steroid treatment as part of the immunosuppressive regimen contributes to this problem because of its well-known effect of inducing peripheral insulin resistance.[11]

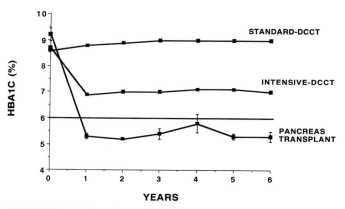

FIGURE 59–4. Comparison of hemoglobin A_{1c} levels after successful pancreas transplantation with hemoglobin A_{1c} levels obtained during standard and intensive therapy in the Diabetes Control and Complications Trial (DCCT). The *solid line* at 6% represents the upper limit of normal. (Data from DCCT Research Group[8] and Robertson et al.[9])

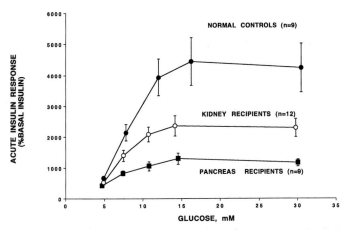

FIGURE 59–5. Insulin secretory reserve (measured by the method of glucose potentiation of arginine-induced insulin secretion) in successful recipients of pancreas transplants, nondiabetic recipients of kidney transplants, and normal controls. Both the kidney recipients and pancreas recipients received the same chronic immunosuppressive drugs, including prednisone and cyclosporine, which suppress insulin secretory reserve. (From Teuscher AU, Seaquist ER, Robertson, RP: Diminished insulin secretory reserve in diabetic pancreas transplant and nondiabetic kidney transplant recipients. Diabetes 43:5593–5598, 1994.)

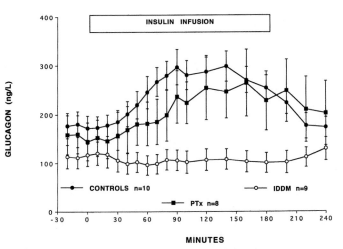

FIGURE 59–7. Glucagon responses during hypoglycemia induced by an insulin infusion (hyperinsulinemic, stepped hypoglycemic clamp). Glucagon responses in patients with insulin-dependent diabetes mellitus (IDDM, or type 1 diabetes) are absent. After successful pancreas transplantation (PTx), glucagon responses are normal. (From Barrou Z, Seaquist ER, Robertson RP: Pancreas transplantation in diabetic humans normalize hepatic glucose production during hypoglycemia. Diabetes 43:661–666, 1994.)

However, the dominant reason for hyperinsulinemia is that the transplanted organ is typically provided with systemic venous drainage via the iliac vein.[4] Concern exists that hyperlipidemia and atherosclerosis, two problems linked with diabetes, might be worsened by hyperinsulinemia. However, this concern has not been borne out by studies of circulating lipids in recipients.[12–14]

Patients who have had type 1 diabetes for over 20 years typically have sluggish to absent glucose recovery after hypoglycemia. After successful pancreas transplantation, glucose recovery is improved[15] primarily because of restoration of the endogenous glucagon response to hypoglycemia[16] (Fig. 59–7). Glucagon responses are typically absent in patients who have had diabetes for over two decades. Re-establishment of glucagon responsiveness by the allografted pancreas is accompanied by improved rates of hepatic glucose production during hypoglycemic clamp procedures[16] (Fig. 59–8). Just as important, symptom recognition of hypoglycemia, which is typically severely deficient in recipients before transplantation, is normalized after the surgery[17] (Fig. 59–9). The epinephrine response to hypoglycemia is also improved but still remains subnormal[17] (Fig. 59–10). Hypoglycemia as a complication of pancreas transplantation has been reported[18] but is usually mild.[19]

Chronic Complications of Diabetes

The impact of successful pancreas transplantation and normalization of glycemia on the chronic complication of diabetes has been studied extensively. It is important to realize, however, that no randomized trials of pancreas transplantation vs. intensive insulin–based management have been performed. Instead, historic controls or case-controlled experimental designs have been used. The implicit rationale in the latter cases stems from the results of the Diabetes Control and Complications Trial, which established that improvement in glycemic control is associated with an approximately 50% reduction in the incidence of diabetic retinopathy, nephropathy, and neuropathy.[8]

Benefits on renal structure as reflected by diminished mesangial mass have been found in patients receiving a pancreas and kidney transplant vs. those receiving a kidney alone.[20] More impressively,

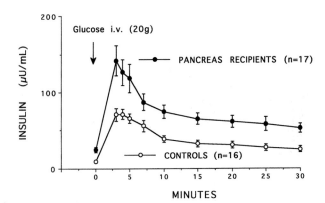

FIGURE 59–6. Increased insulin levels in successful pancreas recipients both before and immediately after an intravenous glucose injection. (From Diem P, Abid M, Redmon JB, et al: Systemic venous drainage of pancreas allografts as independent cause of hyperinsulinemia in type 1 diabetic recipients. Diabetes 39:534–540, 1990.)

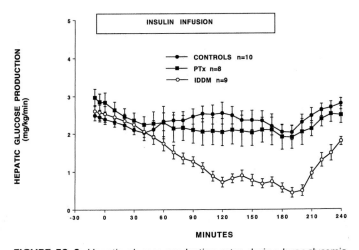

FIGURE 59–8. Hepatic glucose production rates during hypoglycemia caused by an insulin infusion (hyperinsulinemic, stepped hypoglycemic clamp). Glucose production is maintained at a normal level in both control subjects and in patients with insulin-dependent diabetes mellitus (IDDM, or type 1 diabetes) who underwent successful pancreas transplantation. In contrast, glucose production rates are dramatically decreased in nontransplanted type 1 diabetic patients. (From Barrou Z, Seaquist ER, Robertson RP: Pancreas transplantation in diabetic humans normalizes hepatic glucose production during hypoglycemia. Diabetes 43:661–666, 1994.)

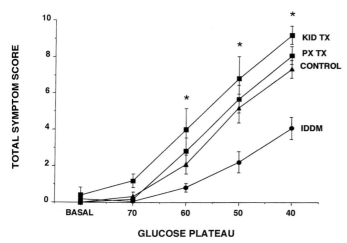

FIGURE 59–9. Degree symptomatology during hypoglycemia at the time of a hyperinsulinemic, stepped hypoglycemic clamp in nondiabetic kidney transplant (KID TX) recipients, pancreas transplant (PX TX) recipients with insulin-dependent diabetes mellitus (IDDM, or type 1 diabetes), control subjects, and type 1 diabetic subjects. In contrast to the diminished symptom awareness of the type 1 diabetic subject group, diabetic patients undergoing successful pancreas transplantation have normal symptom awareness. (From Kendall DM, Rooney D, Smets YFC, et al: Pancreas transplantation restores epinephrine response and symptom recognition during hypoglycemia in patients with long-standing type 1 diabetes mellitus and autonomic neuropathy. Diabetes 46:249–257, 1997.)

abnormal native kidney structure has reversed 10 years after successful transplantation of a pancreas only.[21] Similarly, motor and sensory nerve conduction velocities are less abnormal in pancreas transplant recipients,[22–28] and partial reversal of established neuropathy has been demonstrated 10 years posttransplant.[22] More importantly, life expectancy in diabetic patients with autonomic insufficiency is significantly improved when compared with matched patients with this clinical problem who did not have a successful pancreas transplant.[27]

Disappointingly, no beneficial effects on retinopathy have been demonstrated in recipients of pancreas transplants, even after as long

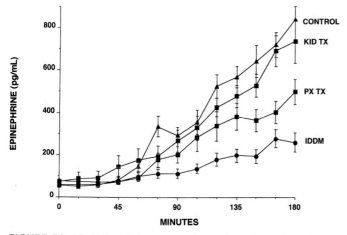

FIGURE 59–10. Epinephrine responses during a hyperinsulinemic, stepped hypoglycemic clamp in nondiabetic kidney transplant (KID TX) recipients, type 1 diabetic pancreas transplant (PX TX) recipients with insulin-dependent diabetes mellitus (IDDM, or type 1 diabetes), and patients with type 1 diabetes mellitus. Secretion of epinephrine during a stepped hypoglycemic clamp procedure improves in successful recipients of pancreas transplantation but does not return to normal levels. (From Kendall DM, Rooney D, Smets YFC, et al: Pancreas transplantation restores epinephrine response and symptom recognition during hypoglycemia in patients with long-standing type 1 diabetes mellitus and autonomic neuropathy. Diabetes 46:249–257, 1997.)

as 5 years of success.[29–31] This lack of benefit may be due to several factors. Many patients undergoing pancreas transplantation have severe retinopathy, which makes improvement in visual structure and function less likely. Additionally, as shown in the Diabetes Control and Complications Trial, more than 5 years of improved glycemic control may be required to demonstrate improvement in retinal pathology.[8]

Carefully performed studies of the impact of successful pancreas transplantation on other chronic complications of diabetes, such as focal neuropathies, gastroparesis, and diabetic diarrhea, are limited in number, and those that have been published describe short-term follow-up periods only.

Quality of Life

The most important criterion for assessing the worth of pancreas transplantation is the change in the recipient's quality of life. Although this outcome is the most clinically difficult to objectively measure, it is nonetheless essential to make efforts to do so. Many attempts have been made to determine whether measurable benefits are accrued after pancreatic transplantation alone or pancreas and kidney transplantation and, in particular, to assess whether the benefits attributed to pancreas transplantation when both organs are transplanted are separable from the benefits provided by kidney transplantation. These studies usually consist of retrospective questionnaires used in health outcomes research. Virtually all published studies report that the quality of life after pancreas transplantation is improved regardless of whether a kidney transplant is involved. The usual benefits reported include a return to employment and successful pregnancies.[32–34] Although the immunosuppressive regimen used by recipients is complicated and can be accompanied by serious side effects, patients usually report they prefer taking immunosuppressive drugs as the price of a functioning pancreas graft and normal glycemia because it allows them to avoid insulin-based management and continued oscillations of hypoglycemia and hyperglycemia. However, an important factor to bear in mind when interpreting these reports is that most diabetic patients who receive transplants have had serious difficulty avoiding extremely high and low blood glucose levels. Clearly, the worse the quality of life before transplantation, the more likely it is to improve after successful surgery. Consequently, a critical criterion that must be used in deciding whether to transplant a pancreas in diabetic patients is the degree to which they can or cannot maintain metabolic stability with exogenous insulin-based management.

Risks and Cost-Benefit Analysis

The major risks associated with pancreas transplantation include clinical complications caused by the surgery and the immunosuppressive drugs used, as well as death. Repeat laparotomy for problems such as intra-abdominal infection and abscess, vascular graft thrombosis, and anastomotic and duodenal stump leak have been reported to occur in approximately 30% of patients.[35] Complications caused by immunosuppression include viral (primarily cytomegalovirus) and bacterial infections and malignancy (particularly lymphoma and skin tumors). The risk of malignancy is less than 1% and is no worse for pancreas transplant patients than for recipients of other organs. More specific drug-related complications include osteoporosis and insulin resistance (corticosteroids) and decreased renal and pancreatic β cell function (cyclosporine, tacrolimus). Their toxic side effects on insulin secretion and insulin action are particularly ironic because corticosteroids and cyclosporine are drugs that made successful pancreas transplantation a reality.

Very little has been published about the relative costs and benefits of pancreas transplantation vs. insulin-based management. A recent study concluded that simultaneous pancreas-kidney transplantation, when adjusted for quality of life, is more cost-effective for diabetic patients with end-stage renal disease than is kidney transplantation alone or hemodialysis.[36]

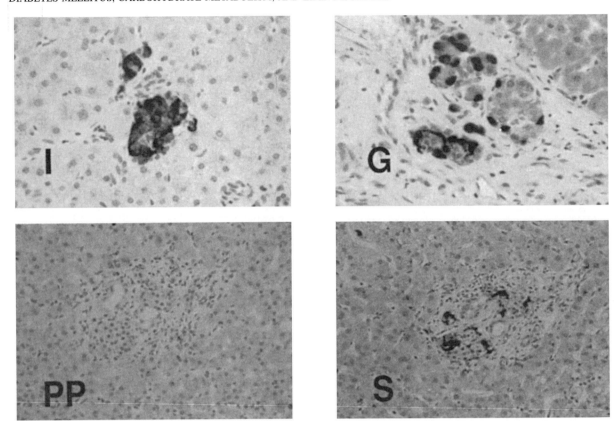

FIGURE 59–11. Liver biopsy from a patient who successfully underwent transplantation with her own pancreatic islets after removal of her pancreas because of chronic, painful pancreatitis. The patient was not diabetic before pancreatectomy and remained nondiabetic after pancreatectomy and infusion of her islets into the portal vein. The sections show positive immunostaining for insulin (I), glucagon (G), and somatostatin (S) but not pancreatic polypeptide (PP). (Reprinted, by permission, from Pyzdrowski KL, Kendall DM, Halter JB, et al: Preserved insulin secretion and insulin independence in recipients of islet autografts. N Engl J Med 327:220–226, 1992. Copyright © 1992 Massachusetts Medical Society. All rights reserved.)

ISLET TRANSPLANTATION

History

Transplantation of pancreatic islets as curative therapy for patients with diabetes has been a cherished goal since the early 1970s when this procedure partially corrected hyperglycemia and glycosuria in diabetic rats.[37] Since then, countless experiments have been performed in animals and humans in the hope of perfecting this approach so that it would reliably return the diabetic recipient to a normoglycemic state. The past quarter century has witnessed several notable instances of success,[38–40] but a disappointingly low success rate continues to relegate this approach to the realm of experimentation. Yet the search for new immunosuppressive regimens that are less toxic to β cells, new devices and toleration strategies that may permit islet transplantation without a need for concurrent immunosuppression, and the clear success of islet autotransplantation in nondiabetic recipients continue to encourage hope in this area.

Transplantation Procedures and Immunosuppressive Agents

Several sites have been used for islet transplantation, including intrahepatic, subrenal capsular, intrasplenic, intraperitoneal, and subcutaneous, but the favored site continues to be intrahepatic. Liver biopsy with immunohistochemisty[41] (Fig. 59–11) and hormone secretion data[41] (Fig. 59–12) have established that islets infused into the portal venous system lodge within and release insulin from the liver. Typically, an islet preparation from a human cadaveric source is slowly injected through an intravenous catheter. At the same time portal venous pressure is carefully monitored so that portal hypertension is not inadvertently established. This procedure can be done during laparotomy at the time of renal transplantation surgery or it can be done via the percutaneous route. Regardless of the approach, it is important to realize that islet transplantation still requires the same degree of immunosuppression required of solid organ transplantation. Consequently, the benefit of islet over whole pancreas transplantation is that the former is a less invasive procedure. The benefit of pancreas over islet transplantation is that the former has a much higher success rate in re-establishing normoglycemia.

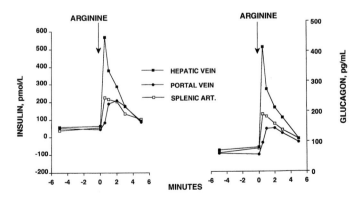

FIGURE 59–12. Insulin and glucagon secretion responses to arginine injected in the antecubital vein of the patient from whom the liver biopsy shown in Figure 59–11 was obtained. In this pancreatectomized patient, autoislets transplanted intrahepatically released glucagon first into the hepatic vein and then the splenic artery and the portal vein—a sequence just the opposite one would expect had glucagon been released from the native pancreas. (Reprinted, by permission, from Pyzdrowski KL, Kendall DM, Halter JB, et al: Preserved insulin secretion and insulin independence in recipients of islet autografts. N Engl J Med 327:220–226, 1992. Copyright © 1992 Massachusetts Medical Society. All rights reserved.)

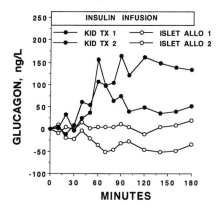 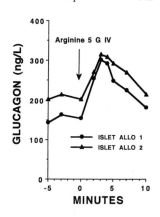

FIGURE 59–13. *Left,* Glucagon responses during a hyperinsulinemic, stepped hypoglycemic clamp in two nondiabetic kidney transplant (KID TX) recipients and in two diabetic alloislet recipients. Glucagon responses were absent in the islet allotransplant (ALLO) recipients but present in the kidney recipients. *Right,* Intact glucagon responses to intravenous arginine in the same two islet allotransplant recipients who failed to respond to hypoglycemia. (From Kendall DM, Teuscher AU, Robertson RP: Defective glucagon secretion during sustained hypoglycemia following successful islet allo- and autotransplantation in humans. Diabetes 46:23–27, 1997.)

Graft and Patient Survival

The most recent data indicate that the 1-year islet allograft survival rate in diabetic recipients, defined as normoglycemia without exogenous insulin therapy, is 6%.[5] A higher rate of functioning islet mass has been reported in recipients whose daily insulin requirements have decreased and who have detectable circulating C peptide levels. Somewhat surprisingly, the patient mortality rate after this procedure is 5%.[5] This rate seems unlikely to be directly due to the relatively simple procedure of infusing islets and may be more a reflection of the clinically precarious status of patients who seek transplantation therapy for diabetes.

Clinical Outcomes

By definition, when islet transplants are completely successful, the diabetic recipient re-establishes normal blood glucose and HbA₁c levels. The longest reported duration of successful islet transplantation is 6 years in two diabetic patients.[40] Intravenous glucose injections have been shown to elicit normally timed first-phase insulin responses, although the magnitude of these responses is less than normal.[41] Interestingly, glucagon responses to hypoglycemia are absent after intrahepatic islet allotransplantation, even though the islets are clearly functional and capable of maintaining normoglycemia. These same patients have intact glucagon responses to arginine[42] (Fig. 59–13), which suggests that the intrahepatic site may interfere with glucagon responsivity to systemic hypoglycemia. This notion was verified in experiments in dogs that were made hypoglycemic and found to have glucagon responses if the islets were transplanted intraperitoneally, whereas the responses were absent if the islets were transplanted intrahepatically.[43] These findings also imply that native islet α cells in diabetic patients do not recover the ability to release glucagon during hypoglycemia even though the patients have been normoglycemic for up to 4 years.

Autotransplantation in Patients with Chronic Pancreatitis

In contrast to islet allotransplantation, autotransplantation of islets in humans is quite successful.[44] In this clinical scenario, patients who are not diabetic but who have been afflicted with chronic, painful pancreatitis undergo total pancreatectomy to relieve their abdominal pain. Instead of discarding the pancreas, it undergoes a crude separation of endocrine from exocrine tissue, and then the endocrine material is infused into the portal circulation. The most recent series report a 2-year success rate of 74% in patients receiving at least 300,000 islets.[45] This result agrees well with an earlier report indicating that over 265,000 islets are required to maintain normal glucose levels in autotransplant recipients.[41] A recent report correlating the number of islets transplanted with a metabolic measure of insulin secretory reserve suggests that a large majority of autotransplanted islets survive and function for years.[46] However, important differences exist between islet autografts and allografts. The immunosuppressive drugs given to allografted patients are known to adversely affect islet function, and autograft recipients have not previously undergone an autoimmune attack that resulted in diabetes. This observation suggests that the development of more effective and less toxic immunosuppressive drugs may significantly improve the success rate of islet allotransplantation in diabetic patients.

REFERENCES

1. Kelly WD, Lillehei RC, Merkel FK, et al: Allotransplantation of the pancreas and duodenum along with the kidney in diabetic nephropathy. Surgery 61:827–837, 1967.
2. Gruessner A, Sutherland DER: Pancreas transplants for United States (US) and non-US cases as reported to International Pancreas Transplant Registry (IPTR) and to the United Network for Organ Sharing (UNOS). *In* Cecka M, Terasaki P (eds): Clinical Transplants 1997. Los Angeles, UCLA Tissue Typing Laboratory, 1998.
3. Sibley RK, Sutherland DER, Goetz FC, et al: Recurrent diabetes mellitus in the pancreas iso- and allograft: A light and electron microscopic and immunohistochemical analysis of four cases. Lab Invest 53:132–144, 1985.
4. Diem P, Abid M, Redmon JB, et al: Systemic venous drainage of pancreas allografts as independent cause of hyperinsulinemia in type 1 diabetic recipients. Diabetes 39:534–450, 1990.
5. International Islet Transplant Registry: Vol 6, No. 1, Dec 1966.
6. Manske CL, Wang Y, Thomas W: Mortality of cadaveric kidney transplantation versus combined kidney-pancreas transplantation in diabetic patients. Lancet 346:1658–1662, 1995.
7. Tydén G, Bolinder J, Solders G, et al: Improved survival in patients with insulin-dependent diabetes mellitus and end-stage diabetic nephropathy 10 years after combined pancreas and kidney transplantation. Transplantation 67:645–648, 1999.
8. DCCT Research Group: The effect of intensive treatment of diabetes on the development and progression of long-term complications in insulin-dependent diabetes mellitus. N Engl J Med 329:977–985, 1983.
9. Robertson RP, Sutherland DER, Kendall DM, et al: Metabolic characterization of long-term successful pancreas transplant in type 1 diabetes. J Invest Med 44:1–7, 1996.
10. Teuscher AU, Seaquist ER, Robertson RP: Diminished insulin secretory reserve in diabetic pancreas transplant and nondiabetic kidney transplant recipients. Diabetes 43:5593–5598, 1994.
11. Luzi L, Secchi A, Facchini F, et al: Reduction of insulin resistance by combined kidney-pancreas transplantation in type 1 (insulin-dependent) diabetic patients. Diabetologia 33:549–556, 1990.
12. La Rocca E, Secchi A, Parlavecchia M, et al: Lipid metabolism after successful kidney and pancreatic transplantation. Transplant Proc 23:1672, 1991.
13. Larsen JL, Stratta RJ, Ozaki CF, et al: Lipid status after pancreas-kidney transplantation. Diabetes Care 15:35–42, 1992.
14. Katz HH, Nguyen TT, Velosa JA, et al: Effects of systemic delivery of insulin on plasma lipids and lipoprotein concentrations in pancreas transplant recipients. Mayo Clin Proc 69:231–236, 1994.
15. Diem P, Redmon JB, Abid M, et al: Glucagon, catecholamine and pancreatic polypeptide secretion in type 1 diabetic recipients of pancreas allografts. J Clin Invest 86:2008–2013, 1990.
16. Barrou Z, Seaquist ER, Robertson RP: Pancreas transplantation in diabetic humans normalizes hepatic glucose production during hypoglycemia. Diabetes 43:661–666, 1994.
17. Kendall DM, Rooney D, Smets YFC et al: Pancreas transplantation restores epinephrine response and symptom recognition during hypoglycemia in patients with long-standing type 1 diabetes mellitus and autonomic neuropathy. Diabetes 46:249–257, 1997.
18. Cottrell DA, Henry ML, O'Dorisio TM, et al: Hypoglycemia after successful pancreas transplantation in type 1 diabetic patients. Diabetes Care 14:1111–1113, 1991.
19. Redmon JB, Teuscher AU, Robertson RP: Hypoglycemia after pancreas transplantation. Diabetes Care 21:1944–1950, 1998.
20. Bilous RW, Mauer SM, Sutherland DER, et al: The effects of pancreas transplantation on the glomerular structure of renal allografts in patients with insulin-dependent diabetes. N Engl J Med 321:80–85, 1989.
21. Fioretto P, Steffes MW, Sutherland DER, et al: Reversal of lesions of diabetic nephropathy after pancreas transplantation. N Engl J Med 339:69–75, 1988.

22. Navarro X, Sutherland DER, Kennedy WR: Long-term effects of pancreatic transplantation on diabetic neuropathy. Ann Neurol 42:727–736, 1997.
23. Secchi A, Martinenghi S, Galardi G, et al: Effects of pancreatic transplantation on diabetic polyneuropathy. Transplant Proc 23:1658–1659, 1991.
24. Aridge D, Reese J, Niehoff M, et al: Effect of successful renal and segmental pancreatic transplantation on peripheral and autonomic neuropathy. Transplant Proc 23:1670–1671, 1991.
25. Caldara R, Sanseverino R, Lefrancois N, et al: Pancreas transplantation: Long-term results. Clin Transplant 5:260–264, 1991.
26. Gaber AO, Cardoso S, Pearson S, et al: Improvement in autonomic function following combined pancreas-kidney transplantation. Transplant Proc 23:1660–1662, 1991.
27. Navarro X, Kennedy WR, Loewenson RB, et al: Influence of pancreas transplantation on cardiorespiratory reflexes, nerve conduction, and morality in diabetes mellitus. Diabetes 39:802–806, 1990.
28. Allen RD, Al-Harbi IS, Morris JG, et al: Diabetic neuropathy after pancreas transplantation: Determinants of recovery. Transplantation 63:830–838, 1997.
29. Ramsay RC, Goetz FC, Sutherland DER, et al: Progression of diabetic retinopathy after pancreas transplantation of insulin-dependent diabetes mellitus. N Engl J Med 318:208–214, 1988.
30. Petersen MR, Vine AK, University of Michigan Pancreas Transplant Evaluation Committee: Progression of diabetic retinopathy after pancreas transplantation. Ophthalmology 97:496–502, 1990.
31. Scheider A, Meyer-Schwickerath E, Nusser J, et al: Diabetic retinopathy and pancreas transplantation: A 3-year follow-up. Diabetologia 34(suppl 1):95–99, 1991.
32. Zehrer CL, Gross CR: Comparison of quality of life between pancreas/kidney and kidney transplant recipients: One year follow-up. Transplant Proc 26:508–509, 1994.
33. Piehlmeier W, Bullinger M, Nusser J, et al: Quality of life in type 1 (insulin-dependent) diabetic patients prior to and after pancreas and kidney transplantation in relation to organ function. Diabetologia 34(suppl):150–157, 1991.
34. Barrou B, Baldi A, Bitker MO, et al: Pregnancy after pancreas transplantation: Report of four new cases and review of the literature. Transplant Proc 27:3043–3044, 1995.
35. Gruessner RWG, Sutherland DER, Troppmann C, et al: The surgical risk of pancreas transplantation in the cyclosporine era: An overview. J Am Coll Surg 185:128–144, 1997.
36. Douzdjian V, Ferrara D, Silvestri G: Treatment strategies for insulin-dependent diabetics with ESRD: A cost-effectiveness decision analysis model. Am J Kidney Dis 31:794–802, 1998.
37. Ballinger WF, Lacy PE: Transplantation of intact pancreatic islets in rats. Surgery 72:175–186, 1972.
38. Warnock GL, Kneteman NM, Ryan EA, et al: Long-term follow-up after transplantation of insulin-producing pancreatic islets into patients with type 1 (insulin-dependent) diabetes mellitus. Diabetologia 35:89–95, 1992.
39. Gores PF, Najarian JS, Stephanian E, et al: Insulin independence in type 1 diabetes after transplantation of unpurified islets from single donor with 15-deoxyspergualin. Lancet 341:19–21, 1993.
40. Alejandro R, Lehmann R, Ricordi C, et al: Long-term function (6 years) of islet allografts in type 1 diabetes. Diabetes 46:1983–1989, 1997.
41. Pyzdrowski KL, Kendall DM, Halter JB, et al: Preserved insulin secretion and insulin independence in recipients of islet autografts. N Engl J Med 327:220–226, 1992.
42. Kendall DM, Teuscher AU, Robertson RP: Defective glucagon secretion during sustained hypoglycemia following successful islet allo- and autotransplantation in humans. Diabetes 46:23–27, 1997.
43. Gupta V, Rooney DP, Kendall DM, et al: Defective glucagon responses from transplanted intrahepatic pancreatic islets during hypoglycemia is transplantation site-determined. Diabetes 46:28–32, 1997.
44. Najarian JS, Sutherland DER, Baumgartner D, et al: Total or near total pancreatectomy and islet autotransplantation for treatment of chronic pancreatitis. Ann Surg 192:526–542, 1980.
45. Wahoff DC, Papalois BE, Najarian JS, et al: Autologous islet transplantation to prevent diabetes after pancreatic resection. Ann Surg 222:562–579, 1995.
46. Teuscher AU, Kendall DM, Smets YFC, et al: Successful islet autotransplantation in humans: Functional insulin secretory reserve as an estimate of surviving islet cell mass. Diabetes 47:324–330, 1998.

Chapter 60

The Relationship of Diabetic Control to Complications

Robert B. Tattersall

One of the longest running controversies in medicine concerns the aims of diabetes treatment. The question, debated even before the discovery of insulin, was whether the clinician should relieve symptoms or try to achieve the more difficult objective of near-physiologic normality. Before introduction of the randomized controlled clinical trial in 1948, medical practice was dominated by the opinions of "wise" physicians, and as will be seen, these opinions could diverge greatly because of an inability to measure long-term glycemic control. This debate is being resolved at the end of the 20th century by large, well-organized randomized controlled trials, which pose particular difficulties in diabetes (not least in terms of expense) because of the long time frame.

"Diabetic control" is usually assumed to refer to glycemic control, but in both insulin-dependent diabetes mellitus (IDDM) and, more particularly, in non–insulin-dependent diabetes mellitus (NIDDM) it has become increasingly clear that multiple risk factors, especially in the case of macrovascular complications, may be as important as, or more so, than glycemia. We need to take a broader view and, especially in NIDDM, consider the simultaneous treatment of all aspects of a multimetabolic disorder.*

I have deliberately taken a historical perspective because it is important to know where we have come from and also because the mistakes of our predecessors should remind us that we too may be wrong.

THE EARLY YEARS

In 1915 the famous German diabetes specialist Carl von Noorden warned that persistent hyperglycemia was a ticking time bomb:

> Then, the recognised and dreaded diabetic complications set in, very often in individuals who have persistent hyperglycaemia by reason of ingesting carbohydrates in too large quantities. . . . Neuritis, neuralgias, cataract, pruritus, furunculosis and so forth; I include as well with these the premature appearance of arteriosclerosis. The very same abnormal conditions of nutrition which persistent hyperglycaemia engenders, promote the early wear and tear of the vessels.[3]

By early wear and tear of the vessels he meant generalized atheroma. What were later called microvascular complications (retinopathy, nephropathy, and neuropathy) had been described in the 19th century but, because they occurred only in older patients, were thought to be due to atherosclerosis. An example of the thinking at the time is that of Wagener and Wilder from the Mayo Clinic, who wrote in 1920 that

(1) Retinopathy does not occur in diabetes gravis.†

(2) Cases with retinitis of diabetic type are almost always complicated by vascular or renal disease and the diabetes tends to be mild and chronic.

(3) The primary cause of the retinitis of diabetes seems to lie in the accompanying pathological changes in the vascular system, the more essentially metabolic disturbances of the diabetes playing at most a secondary part.[4]

With the introduction of insulin in 1922–1923 the question of treatment goals came to the fore. Most authorities advocated an attempt to restore physiologic normality, sometimes simply because it was "normal," but more often because it was thought to "rest" the pancreas and allow regeneration. In his 1923 Nobel lecture, Frederick Banting, one of the discoverers of insulin, stated that

> Regardless of the severity of the disease, it has been found that by carefully adjusting the diet and the dose of insulin, all patients may be maintained sugar free. Since this is possible, it is to be strongly advocated because we have abundant evidence for the belief that there is regeneration of the islet cells of the pancreas when the strain thrown on them by a high blood sugar is relieved.* The increase in tolerance is evidenced by the decreasing dosage of artificially administered insulin. In fact, in some moderately severe cases, the tolerance has increased sufficiently that they no longer require insulin.[5]

Similar views were held by most British physicians. In a lecture in December 1923 George Graham stated that his experience during the previous 6 months had convinced him that it was essential to maintain "the same ideal as we have always had—namely to keep the blood sugar within normal limits if the patient is to continue to progress satisfactorily." [6] He repeated this message in the 1926 and 1929 editions of *Price's Textbook of Medicine* and said that fasting blood sugar should be within normal limits of between 80 mg/dL (4.4 mmol/L) and 120 mg/dL (6.7 mmol/L) and *must not* (italics in the original) rise above 190 mg/dL (10.5 mmol/L) at any time of the day. In the United States the most uncompromising and influential advocate of normoglycemia was Elliott Joslin, who in the 1928 edition of his famous textbook wrote that

> Glycosuria is not only tolerated but encouraged by several physicians highly skilled in the treatment of diabetes. Even 20 grams of glucose are allowed in the urine by design. To this plan of treatment I am emphatically opposed. . . . Success in the treatment of diabetic children lies in keeping their urine sugar free. If sugar appears, a penalty follows.[7]

These views on the importance of control were, as emphasized earlier, not based on the prevention of microvascular complications because they had not yet begun to appear among the new class of insulin-dependent diabetics. Instead, appreciation of the importance of control was based on a lower frequency of infections and the teleologic view that there must be a good reason why blood glucose is so closely regulated in health.

---

*I have written two articles on this topic.[1, 2]
†What would later be called IDDM.

*This statement refers to the so-called honeymoon period, remission, or Brush effect in which insulin administration can be drastically reduced or even stopped for weeks or months after the initial treatment.

FREE DIETS

When the only way that patients could monitor themselves was with urine tests, it was inevitable that staying sugar-free* was hard work and associated with a high frequency of hypoglycemia, so it is not surprising that patients and physicians questioned whether it was worth it. Another burden for patients was that very restricted diets were often prescribed, although by the mid-1930s it had been shown that high carbohydrate did not necessarily lead to poor control or higher insulin doses. When Geyelin reviewed his 10-year experience of high carbohydrate diets in 1935, he pointed out that patients ingesting such diets felt more like human beings and, because they were not always hungry, stuck to them better. He did not advocate lax biochemical control and had found that blood sugar excursions were less extreme on a high carbohydrate, low fat regimen. He commented that

Owing to the persistence with which a large group of clinicians still cling to the fallacious theory that undernutrition is a *sine qua non* of diabetic therapy (even after the discovery of insulin), treatment with high carbohydrate diets and insulin has been decried. . . . I have been convinced that this is the treatment of choice and that the diabetic patient so treated enjoys better health with no observable detriment to the fundamental state of his diabetes.[8]

Others went further and advocated totally free diets and any amount of glycosuria provided that no ketones were present in the urine. It is often said that two of the founders of this movement were Karl Stolte of Breslau and Adolf Lichtenstein of Stockholm. In fact, Stolte advised his patients to inject regular insulin before each meal—in a dose individually adapted to the degree of glycosuria and amount of carbohydrates that they wanted to eat. His patients decided against once- or twice-daily use of the new prolonged-action insulin preparations because they realized that with such an unphysiologic insulin replacement they would have to abandon their flexible and free diet to maintain aglycosuria.[9] Children attending Lichtenstein's clinic ate the same diet as their brothers and sisters. He did not advocate keeping the urine sugar-free all the time, but taught that "some tens of grams of sugar per 24 hours are permissible." He claimed that the advantage of this regimen was psychologic in that it would rid diabetic children of the feeling of being different.[10]

The most radical departure was instigated by the New York physician Edward Tolstoi, who threw down a challenge to Joslin and his Boston group that at times reached almost religious intensity. Tolstoi had worked as a chemist with F.M. Allen, of starvation diet fame, in the early 1920s when, "I was indoctrinated with the method in vogue at the time for the treatment of diabetes—a method that starved the patient. The objective was to reduce the blood sugar to perfectly normal levels and to keep the urine sugar-free." [11] His conversion came in 1936 when he started using the newly introduced protamine insulin once daily and found that trying to keep the urine sugar-free led to alarming and warningless hypoglycemic reactions. Two affected patients stayed away from the clinic to avoid the displeasure of their doctors but eventually returned and said that they felt well in spite of having had continuous glycosuria. They were admitted to a metabolic ward for 50 days, where in spite of passing up to 100 g of sugar a day, they maintained their weight and had no ketosis. Tolstoi then decided to let his patients eat what they liked, and in his words, the result was that

They are in good health, in a state of social and economic usefulness, and infections among them are no more frequent than in the average individual. All these patients enjoy their freedom . . . it is not necessary for them to carry their insulin and syringe with them. They administer the insulin to themselves in the morning and then put the equipment away until the following morning. These patients are not singled out as a group, apart from their fellow men, and their habits of living approximated to the normal.[12]

Tolstoi claimed that "advocates of the chemical school," such as Joslin, produced patients who "certainly do not enjoy life nor have the freedom of people who live like normal human beings." In a dig against what he called men of reputation and authority, he proclaimed

*This phrase was frequently used to describe good control and meant having no sugar in the urine.

that "we avoid terrorising the patient and we also do not promise him perfect health if his deportment is faultless."

MICROVASCULAR COMPLICATIONS

Between 1940 and 1950 complications were becoming increasingly apparent in young patients whose lives had been saved by insulin in the previous 25 years, and the idea that they were due to arteriosclerosis was no longer tenable. In a new study from the Mayo Clinic in 1934, Wagener and Wilder recalled their 1921 paper and had to modify its conclusions. The cases that were of particular interest and concern were the 12% who had retinal hemorrhages but no other clinical signs of vascular disease. They thought that

The very existence of retinitis in cases in which patients have no other signs of vascular disease must mean that diabetes alone does something to injure the finer arterioles or venules of the retina, probably the latter.

How this damage was caused they did not know, and a perplexing feature was that

The lesions are observed in cases of mild diabetes (i.e., NIDDM) as frequently as in cases of severe diabetes (i.e., IDDM), in those in which insulin is used as well as in those in which diabetes is controlled without insulin, early in the disease as well as late, although more frequently late, and when the carbohydrate of the diet has been unlimited as well as when it has been restricted and more fat has been fed.[13]

Similar findings were recorded in Boston by Waite and Beetham, who in 1935 concluded that

Deep retinal haemorrhages in diabetes multiply with age and multiply with continued duration of diabetes out of proportion to the age factor, but they show no obvious correlation with sclerosis of retinal vessels, with vascular hypertension, with renal disorders, with insulin dosage or with blood sugar or calcium levels.[14]

The concept that diabetic angiopathy was a specific form of vascular disease was not widely accepted until the early 1950s. An influential advocate was Knud Lundbaek of Denmark, who published his findings in a book in 1953 and a paper in *The Lancet* in 1954.[15, 16] His argument was based on the specific ophthalmoscopic findings (particularly microaneurysms and beading of veins) and the pathognomonic Kimmelstiel-Wilson renal lesion. He also pointed out that unlike the sex distribution of atherosclerosis, these complications affected women and men equally.

To return to the glucose control question, in 1947 the New York physician Henry Dolger described 20 patients who fulfilled orthodox criteria for excellent control, but retinopathy developed in all after 6 to 22 years. Most discouraging was the first patient to receive insulin at Mount Sinai Hospital; her control had always been considered perfect, and in the previous 10 years she "never once had glycosuria." Yet at the age of 31, after 22 years of diabetes, she had numerous retinal hemorrhages, albuminuria, and a blood pressure (BP) of 150/100.[17] Joslin's comment was that Dolger's outlook was handicapped by his contact only with the patients of other doctors. "I like to think," wrote Joslin, "that when he has been in practice 10 years longer and has followed up his own cases intimately for a quarter of a century he will report more encouragingly." In truth, the results in Joslin's patients were hardly more encouraging. In 1950 Ruth Reuting from the New England Deaconess Hospital described 50 patients in whom diabetes developed before 1924 and who had been monitored for 25 years or more. A third had died at an average age of 35 with an average diabetes duration of 17.6 years. Of the 19 deaths, 8 were due to cardiovascular-renal disease, 4 to pulmonary tuberculosis, and 4 to other infections. Among the living patients Reuting reported "ominous signs" of hypertension, azotemia, and proteinuria in significant numbers.[18]

It was assumed, because of the difference in their philosophies, that Tolstoi's patients were worse controlled than those of Joslin, but there was no evidence that the belief of the physician actually influenced the degree of control or that it was any worse on a free diet than on a nominally exact and restricted one. In real life the situation, as Frederick Allen lamented in 1953, was that

The vast majority of cases in the United States and still more in other countries are not controlled in any real sense. The ignorance and carelessness of patients can often rightly be blamed; nevertheless, the majority are largely influenced by the attitude and personality of the physician. Inadequately trained physicians are apt to treat diabetes in the easiest way.[19]

Disagreements between free dieters and proponents of good control arose in other countries and inevitably ended inconclusively because of the lack of hard evidence. One of the difficulties was articulated by the English physician Robin Lawrence, who in 1949 wrote

Unfortunately we do not know whether normoglycaemia in diabetes would prevent these complications, though that seems to me likely from the small numbers of very mild cases I have seen for years with always a near normal glycaemia and no vascular complications . . . [but] the majority of the diabetics I treat are never normoglycaemic for most of their hours and I think it is unlikely that other people's patients are any different . . . anyone who confidently claims to maintain a physiologically normal blood sugar in the average insulin case has, I am sure, no wide or accurate experience.[20]

One of the few studies that carried weight was that from Malmö, Sweden, reported by Johnsson in 1960.[21] He compared the frequency of complications in 56 patients in whom diabetes was diagnosed between 1922 and 1935 and in 104 in whom diabetes was diagnosed between 1935 and 1945. Those in whom the disease was diagnosed before 1935 had a strict diet and multiple daily injections, with the endpoint being an absence of sugar in the urine at all times. By contrast, after 1935 a free diet was used and glycosuria ignored, provided that polyuria or ketonuria was not present. The results were striking in that those with a diabetes duration over 15 years, only 9% of the "strict control" group had nephropathy vs. 61% of the "free diet" group. A quarter of the strict control group had had more than 20 attacks of hypoglycemic coma as compared with only 5% in the free diet group. None of the 8 patients who had been in hypoglycemic coma more than 20 times had proteinuria after 25 years and 4 had normal fundi. In the discussion the author suggested that

It is surely important that young diabetics receive intense insulin treatment as soon as possible and that they are convinced from the very beginning that control of diabetes requires rigid dietary restriction with a constant carbohydrate intake from day to day . . . patients with severe diabetes cannot control their disease with one dose of insulin daily.

Lawrence's comment on this paper was that "his findings like mine suggest that hypoglycaemia—evidence of control—minimizes complications; but I think, from my experience that the occurrence of 20 comas is carrying hypoglycaemias unnecessarily far." He added the caveat that "diabetic control, so far as it is possible can hardly be the whole answer to visual troubles, as there are exceptions in both directions." [22]

By 1963 most physicians on both sides of the Atlantic would probably have agreed with Lawrence's summary. Clinical experience suggested that early and severe complications developed in very badly controlled patients. Yet as Lawrence pointed out, there seemed to be exceptions. As far as it went, the published literature supported the view that good control was beneficial. In 1964 Harvey Knowles reviewed over 300 retrospective studies in which patients had been ranked by the degree of control thought to have been achieved over a number of years and then analyzed to determine the prevalence of complications.[23] Only 85 did not contain major errors of design; usually that control was assessed by someone who was involved in care of the patients. Of the 85 acceptable studies, 50 concluded that poor control was positively correlated with vascular disease, 25 found no relationship, and 10 were undecided. A big problem with all these studies was the impossibility of assessing glycemic control accurately with the methods available—single blood glucose measurements at clinic visits and the patient's record of urine tests. Another was the possibility that patients with good control might have a type of diabetes that was inherently easy to control, a confounding factor that could be overcome only by studying homogeneous groups such as animals of one strain all made diabetic on the same day or, alternatively, a prospective randomized controlled trial involving large numbers of human diabetics.

The randomized trial was an unfamiliar concept to most clinicians who had qualified before 1950. Richard Doll remembered that in 1937,

New treatments were almost always introduced on the grounds that in the hands of professor A or in the hands of a consultant at one of the leading teaching hospitals, the results in a small series of patients (seldom more than 50) had been superior to those recorded by professor B (or some other consultant) or by the same investigator previously. Under these conditions variability of outcome, chance, and the unconscious (leave alone the conscious) in the selection of patients brought about apparently important differences in the results obtained; consequently there were many competing new treatments.[24]

In the 1950s the Food and Drug Administration (FDA) was increasingly dissatisfied with its inability to distinguish between effective and ineffective drugs. The evidence that a drug worked was often just testimonials from physicians who casually tested experimental drugs on their patients and were paid for doing so.[25] Against this background the University Group Diabetes Program (UGDP) was a landmark as the first "proper" clinical trial in diabetes and one of the most ambitious trials in any disease up to that time. It followed the introduction of oral hypoglycemic agents, particularly the relatively nontoxic tolbutamide and phenformin in 1957. There was widespread apprehension that these drugs would encourage slackness in the management of diabetes. Also, their effect on complications was unknown, but many feared that they would be less effective than insulin.

THE UNIVERSITY GROUP DIABETES PROGRAM

An attempt to answer the question of the effect of oral hypoglycemic agents on complications was inaugurated in 1960 when a group of "interested clinicians and an epidemiologist-statistician" met to plan a collaborative study involving 12 American university clinics, the main aims of which were to

1. Evaluate the effects of hypoglycemic treatments in the prevention of vascular complications in a long-term, prospective, and cooperative clinical trial
2. Study the natural history of vascular disease in maturity-onset diabetes
3. Develop methods applicable to cooperative clinical trials

Initially the study was funded for only 5 years, and because enough deaths were not expected, the endpoints were to be microvascular complications.

Funding came from the National Institutes of Health (NIH), and one aim was to show how a properly designed, randomized, controlled clinical trial could resolve differences of clinical opinion. In retrospect it led to what one commentator called a decade of "bitter debate and accusations within the diabetic community, a time when eminent scientists and physicians became sharply polarised in their opinions on a subject that is, at best, murky." [26]

Marks has summarized the problems that the UGDP raised as follows:

Within the world of clinical medicine, the UGDP posed various questions about the respective roles of statistical and medical expertise: Which group should determine the methods of treatment and evaluation methods in clinical research? Who should have the final say in interpreting results from controlled studies? At the level of statistical theory, the UGDP posed analogous questions about the proper relation between statistical inference and scientific decisions: What criteria apply in deciding when a clinical experiment should be stopped? How are unanticipated results from a unique study to be interpreted? At the level of policy, the controversy posed questions about the appropriate relation between scientific claims and regulatory decisions: Which studies count as proper evidence? When competing experts disagree about the merits of a study, how are the disagreements to be adjudicated? How are the results of clinical trials to be translated to medical practice?[26]*

Study Design

Patients had to have diabetes diagnosed less than 1 year and a probable life expectancy of at least 5 years. No age limit was imposed.

---

*Marks shows a distinct leaning toward the statisticians, whereas I tend to side with the clinicians. For a more journalistic view see Kolata.[26]

Recruitment began in 1961, and allocation was to one of four regimens:

1. *Insulin variable*: As much insulin as necessary to maintain "normal blood glucose." The standard was Lente, but others could be added because the aim was to "resemble as much as possible widespread clinical practice aimed at blood glucose control."

2. *Insulin standard*: A fixed dose of 10, 12, 14, or 16 U of Lente according to surface area. This group aimed to distinguish between the hypoglycemic effects and any independent effects that insulin might have.

3. *Tolbutamide*: A fixed dose of 1 g before breakfast and 0.5 g before the evening meal was chosen because it was "about equal to the average dose used in clinical practice."

4. *Placebo*: Lactose tablets or capsules.

In 1962 a phenformin group was added with a fixed dose of 50 mg before breakfast and the evening meal.

The aim was to recruit 200 patients in each group, which posed problems because special screening procedures had to be introduced in some of the institutions "for all new patients, outpatients as well as inpatients, in order to find suitable new diabetics." In view of what followed, it is worth noting that no attempt was made to exclude patients with signs of vascular disease. It was later admitted that patients in one center had been recruited from the cardiac clinic!

Results and Fall-out

The tolbutamide arm of the study was stopped prematurely in 1969 because analysis by what *The Lancet* called "advanced, elaborate, and novel statistical techniques" showed a significantly higher death rate in the tolbutamide (12.7%) than in the placebo group (4.9%).[28] Mortality in the two insulin-treated groups was nearly the same as for placebo patients, although variable insulin achieved lower levels of fasting blood glucose. In 1970 in an editorial accompanying the first two papers, an ad hoc committee of the American Diabetes Association (ADA) commented that apart from the apparent toxic effect of tolbutamide,

What is even more arresting is that in this investigation neither of the insulin-treated groups had a lower mortality than the placebo treated patients. This finding carries the broadest implications for the treatment of non–insulin-dependent adult onset diabetes. First, if insulin—the diabetic's medicinal remedy sine qua non—does not permit patients to live longer than does a diet, would not this class of patients, in respect to longevity, be just as well off with diet alone? Secondly, if insulin can do no better with mortality than diet, is it likely that any oral hypoglycemic agent presently available, whether or not it acts by stimulating insulin secretion, can do any better than the hormone itself or even as well?[29]

The conclusion of the ADA was that the only indication for tablets was a patient poorly controlled by diet who refused to take insulin. These findings, together with the 1968 paper of Siperstein and colleagues (see below) stating that capillary basement membrane thickness and, by implication, diabetic complications were genetically determined, suggested that most forms of treatment in adult-onset diabetes were a waste of time. Together, they were a major blow to those who advocated good diabetic control, and it has been claimed that they "set back American diabetes by twenty years." To say that the conclusions did not go unchallenged would be a major understatement. In 1975 *The Lancet* suggested that "the storm of controversy aroused by these results is probably without parallel in modern medicine. Every aspect of the trial has been minutely criticised by clinicians and statisticians, while supporters of the trial have defended it with equal vigour."[30]

Once the critics had digested the data, they had plenty of scientific objections, but what rankled was publication in the *New York Times*, *Washington Post*, and *Wall Street Journal* of supportive statements from the ADA, American Medical Association, and the FDA before any doctors had seen the data. This situation arose because on May 20, 1970, news was leaked to Wall Street that tolbutamide was to be withdrawn from the UGDP because of lack of efficacy and a suspicion of toxicity. The price of shares in its makers, Upjohn, dropped dramatically, and doctors switched their patients to chlorpropamide or phenformin therapy. The FDA, against the advice of its own advisory committee, acted swiftly even though they had not seen the data. On May 23 they endorsed the study's conclusions and on May 25 announced that warning labels would be put on all antidiabetic drugs. Three weeks later, the results were presented at the ADA annual meeting. In November 1970, before formal publication of the results, 40 leading diabetologists formed the Committee for the Care of the Diabetic (CCD) and retained a Boston lawyer to prevent the FDA from proceeding with its labeling proposal and to gain access to the patient records. On May 17, 1971, news was leaked that phenformin was to be withdrawn from the study, and the makers, Revlon, had to suspend dealings in its shares.

Arguments about the study were both personal and scientific and were fueled by what opponents saw as the self-righteous tone of some of the UGDP spokesmen. An example of personal animus was the revelation that between 1968 and 1970, Christian Klimt, the UGDP statistician, had been a paid consultant of the manufacturers of phenformin. Supporters countered by claiming that the physicians who had formed the CCD were "drug company whores" paid by Upjohn. This criticism may have been directed at Alvan Feinstein, who was recruited by the Upjohn company in early 1969 to review the findings, about which he wrote several articles[31] (see also Schnor[32]).

The most cogent scientific criticisms were summarized by Holbrooke Seltzer in a special article in *Diabetes* in 1972[33] and rebutted by the UGDP investigators in an article subtitled "Clinical Trials versus Clinical Impressions."[34] Seltzer's criticisms could be grouped under eight general headings:

1. Patient selection criteria. Subjects were recruited from mass screening programs, charity clinics, or private physicians. No data were recorded on smoking habits, previous myocardial infarctions, or cardiac murmurs. Nearly a quarter did not have diabetes according to then-current diagnostic criteria. Just over half had a fasting blood glucose level under 130 mg/dL (7.2 mmol/L) at baseline.

2. Comparability of treatment groups at baseline. The investigators claimed that their study was "unique with respect to the amount of detailed information which was presented to describe the characteristics of the patients in each treatment group," but critics pointed out that between the five groups and, more importantly, between clinics, risk factors were unevenly distributed. Twice as much angina, congestive cardiac failure, arterial calcification, hypercholesterolemia, retinopathy, and abnormal electrocardiograms were seen in the tolbutamide-treated than the placebo group. Critics believed that the randomization had broken down, although the differences (only significant for cholesterol) could have easily arisen by chance. The rejoinder of the investigators was that their critics "seemed not to appreciate the purpose and power of randomization."

3. Heterogeneous clinic populations. To the UGDP investigators the heterogeneous patient population was "a strength not a weakness," but critics pointed out that in some clinics charity patients with cardiovascular and other diseases were used whereas others recruited "healthy" private patients. According to Seltzer, the three clinics that enrolled the sickest patients had the most fatalities and the three that admitted the healthiest had the least. This finding led Moss to write that "the one thing this study proves is that patients who already have heart disease die sooner than those who do not."[35]

4. Fixed doses of tolbutamide, phenformin, and insulin. Critics claimed that using fixed doses was illogical and unrepresentative of ordinary clinical practice. For them the problem was that "with the passage of time, the pancreas became less responsive to tolbutamide, and the blood glucose level rose, but the dose was not increased. Consequently, these patients had hyperglycemia during the last 36 months of the study." The rejoinder of the investigators was that a fixed dose of insulin did not result in the same mortality trend as a fixed dose of tolbutamide, in spite of the similarity of fasting blood glucose levels in the two groups.

5. Treatment of conditions other than diabetes. Seltzer charged that "smoking, hypertension, obesity, hypercholesterolemia and hypertriglyceridemia were not controlled during the study, and hyperglycemia itself was inadequately controlled in all except half of the IVAR

[variable insulin] patients." The investigators replied that their aim was to evaluate the efficacy of hypoglycemic treatments and not lipid-lowering agents or the treatment of other conditions.

6. Classification of the cause of death. Total deaths were similar in all groups, which according to Seltzer was pertinent because "in a toxicity study (which the UGDP turned out to be) it is statistically untenable to analyse deaths from specific causes separately from total deaths."[27] Others pointed out that interpretation of a study showing no increased risk of dying but with treatment significantly affecting the manner of death would always be difficult, whereas Moss commented that "there were 30 deaths in the tolbutamide treated patients with 20 in each of the other groups. Never before have ten deaths created such a controversy." Half the tolbutamide-treated patients who died had autopsies vs. only 29% of those receiving placebo or insulin. If only 3 deaths in each group had been reassigned, the statistical significance of the increased cardiovascular deaths in the tolbutamide-treated group would have disappeared.

7. Statistical analysis. Feinstein attributed the UGDP's difficulties to an overconfidence in statistical procedures and a neglect of "biologic logic" and "clinical judgement" in design and interpretation. Marks suggests that he had his own ax to grind and "apparently found the study an irresistible example of all that was going awry in clinical investigation." To be clinically relevant he thought that an experiment had to tell physicians whether the patients studied were like theirs and how their lives would be affected by the choice of treatment.* One repeated criticism was that a high proportion of patients came from populations in which compliance was known to be a serious problem. In fact, only 26% remained with their assigned treatment for the whole study. The attitude of the investigators to medication changes and dropouts was to ignore them; it was later pointed out that the credibility of the conclusion that insulin was ineffective in reducing cardiovascular deaths was greatly weakened by the fact that almost half the subjects taking variable insulin who died of cardiovascular causes had had virtually no exposure to insulin.

When the CCD finally got the original records, they were horrified by what they saw as evidence of mismanagement and sloppy data recording; patients with malignant hypertension were untreated, a woman with renal failure and sickle cell disease was given phenformin, and a man with normal blood sugar was given insulin. In an attempt to resolve the statistical aspects of the controversy, the director of the NIH contracted with the Biometric Society to appoint a group of distinguished biostatisticians to review the UGDP and other long-term studies of oral hypoglycemic agents. The report considered and accepted some of the shortcomings that had already been pointed out but concluded that they were not sufficient to invalidate the results. The final paragraph of their report concluded that

In the light of the UGDP findings, it remains with the proponents of the oral hypoglycemics to conduct scientifically adequate studies to justify the continued use of such agents.[36]

In an editorial accompanying the report in the *Journal of the American Medical Association*, Thomas C. Chalmers, chairman of the UGDP advisory committee, wondered why, if these drugs were dangerous, their sales had continued to expand steadily over the previous 15 years with only a slight dip in the year immediately after the UGDP report. He attributed this finding to the strong desire of patients and physicians for a way of treating diabetes that did not involve injections and suggested that this attitude had blinded them to the possibility that the drugs might be harmful. He blamed the problem on what he called "the one sided presentations in the so called throw away journals so widely read by physicians."

8. A guide to clinical practice or just an unpopular conclusion? The UGDP investigators thought that their results had

Given little hope thus far that the degenerative complications of diabetes are preventable by simple control of blood glucose levels . . . use of additional therapeutic agents (over and above diet) must be justified by reasons other than those of the prevention of cardiovascular complications.

Whether the results could be extrapolated to other drugs that had

---

*A foretaste of 1990s debates about evidence-based medicine!

appeared during the gestation of the study was, according to them, "a matter of individual judgement." Nevertheless, they supported the ADA's view that "insulin is to be preferred to other therapeutic agents because it is more uniformly effective in controlling hyperglycemia and the UGDP study indicates that it may be safer." In a final broadside at their critics the investigators claimed that "the main difficulty with the UGDP is not its design execution or analysis, but rather that it reached an unpopular conclusion." To the critics, the "reckless extrapolation of a small and temporary cardiovascular mortality trend in the UGDP to the entire diabetic population of the United States" was completely indefensible. Clearly, no truce was going to be possible and *The Lancet* summed up the situation in 1975:

The UGDP war remains in the balance, and the combatants are now obscured by increasingly heavy clouds of clinical, statistical and philosophical smoke. Further discussion of the results cannot now be helpful.[37]

The final word came in 1980 after the CCD had seen the original data, when Kilo and colleagues found (1) a notable discrepancy in the sex ratio of cardiovascular death rates in placebo-treated subjects, (2) excess mortality in tolbutamide-treated subjects restricted to a relatively small group of poorly controlled subjects, and (3) insulin to be effective in reducing cardiovascular deaths. They concluded that "it is both incredible and ironic to realise that many of our findings that refute the conclusions of the UGDP investigators resulted, simply, from examining blood glucose levels of subjects who died of cardiovascular disease."[38, 39]

From the time of their publication in 1970 the UGDP findings were heavily criticized by European opinion leaders[40, 41]; no official warnings were issued in Europe, and sulfonylureas and biguanides continued to be used by the 30% to 40% of patients in an average clinic who were taking tablets. In the United States the CCD's lawyers prevented the FDA from taking any definitive action until 1984, and it seems to me that the UGDP findings did not influence the clinical practice of American doctors very much. The Joslin Clinic was in the forefront of the opposition, and in the 11th edition of Joslin's textbook in 1971, Leo Krall observed that oral agents had been used in 10,000 Joslin Clinic patients for as long as 10 years and,

While all questions concerning their physiological action and long term employment have not been answered, there seems adequate basis to predict that the oral hypoglycemic agents are "here to stay" for the foreseeable future. However the generally enthusiastic acceptance of this mode of treatment, as well as the fact that the ease of administration contributes greatly to the opportunities for misuse, has created problems, most of which permit ready solution.[42]

The polarization of views in the United States about the use of tablets for diabetes was shown in a provocative review in the *New England Journal of Medicine* in 1977, which began by stating that the justifications for tablets were that they were taken by mouth, lowered blood glucose, and were safe.[43] There could be no argument about the first premise, but the authors set out to demolish the other two. The crucial question was whether the blood glucose–lowering effect was sustained during long-term use, and the answer in most cases was that it was not. Of patients started in each of the first 4 years after the introduction of tolbutamide, control was still maintained in only 10% after 6 to 9 years. A study that was specifically commended was that of Singer and Hurwitz, in which a placebo challenge was used every 2 years. After 7 to 9 years only 21% of patients receiving tolbutamide and 31% receiving chlorpropamide were satisfactorily controlled.[44] Studies without a placebo challenge would overestimate the success rate. Shen and Bressler's summary of the experience of the previous 20 years was that

About 40 per cent of symptomatic patients with maturity-onset diabetes with varying degrees of hyperglycemia do not achieve satisfactory control with oral agents. This primary failure rate can be reduced by more judicious selection of patients. Secondary failures occur in patients who initially qualified as primary successes but subsequently failed to meet the criteria for good control. This secondary failure rate ranges from 3 to 30 per cent. More important is the experience at the Joslin Clinic of a continuous annual rate of secondary failures. One fourth of the patients, previously in satisfactory control, experienced failure year after year. After elimination of primary failures, secondary failures and placebo successes, the continuous satisfactory control rate is 20 to 30 per cent.

They concluded that "the failure of tolbutamide or phenformin to achieve a sustained lowering of blood glucose levels in the treated populations obviates any need to be concerned with their reputed toxicity. There is no reason to use a drug that does not work."

What seems to have been forgotten in the furor over the UGDP is that the endpoint was originally intended to be microvascular complications. In fact, no significant differences in the rates of proteinuria or retinopathy were found.

THE BASEMENT MEMBRANE CONTROVERSY: 1968–1979*

A major problem in trying to resolve the control-complications debate has always been that a study in humans would take at least 10 years. It is therefore tempting to take a shortcut and use surrogate rather than clinically relevant endpoints. Such an approach led to the basement membrane controversy.

In the *Journal of Clinical Investigation* in 1968, Marvin Siperstein and colleagues reported that 90% of diabetic patients older than 19 years and 50% of "prediabetics" (offspring of two diabetic parents) had muscle (quadriceps) capillary basement membrane thickening (MCBMT).[46] They found no correlation between MCBMT and the duration or severity of diabetes—a sharp contrast to clinical studies, which always show an increasing frequency of microvascular complications with increasing duration. This discrepancy was regarded by the authors as "somewhat more surprising" than the lack of correlation between the severity of carbohydrate abnormalities and MCBMT. In eight patients with diabetes secondary to chronic pancreatitis, only one had MCBMT. The authors concluded that

These results indicate that thickening of the muscle capillary basement membranes is a characteristic of genetic diabetes mellitus, and further, that the hyperglycemia of diabetes is probably not the factor responsible for the microangiopathy characteristic of diabetes mellitus.

It was conflicting results rather than the implausibility of the conclusions that led to controversy. Camerini-Davalos et al. found MCBMT in no more than a third of prediabetics with normal glucose tolerance,[47] and Williamson et al. found it in only 1 of 13 prediabetics.[48] Kilo and colleagues found an association between MCBMT and the duration of overt diabetes, whereas Yodaiken, unlike Siperstein, found it in secondary diabetes.[49]

Contradictory results led to arguments about methodology. Siperstein and colleagues claimed that fixation with glutaraldehyde (used by Williamson et al.) rather than osmium (which Siperstein used) lessened the sensitivity of the measurement. Another disagreement was where in its circumference the MCBM should be measured and how many readings were necessary. Much ink was spilt discussing the merits of various techniques of fixation and measurement, but the more serious problem of imprecision was glossed over. Pardo et al. found a 25% variation in basement membrane thickness in adjacent capillaries from the same biopsy specimen,[50] whereas Peterson and Forsham later found that it could vary as much as twofold in adjacent muscle biopsies taken at the same time from a single patient.[51] Not only was this imprecision ignored, but "outlying" data points in cases and controls were sometimes discarded. Age-adjusted normal ranges were used as norms rather than the more statistically valid case-control comparisons.

To resolve the question of whether the discrepant findings in prediabetics were real or apparent, the NIH sponsored a cooperative study involving the laboratories of Williamson and Siperstein. The preliminary results of this study were interpreted by Siperstein and colleagues as showing that (1) MCBMT was present in about 50% of prediabetic Pima Indians and (2) differences in methodology accounted for the failure of studies using glutaraldehyde-fixed tissue to observe MCBMT in prediabetic subjects.[52] The conclusion that Williamson and Kilo drew was that "the Pima study now provides data which, for the first time, unequivocally document that results obtained from osmium fixed tissue are not reproducible in Siperstein's own laboratory."[53] The

problem, according to Siperstein, was that "for unknown technical reasons, all values obtained with osmium fixation for normal, prediabetic and diabetic subjects in the NIH study were higher than those obtained earlier." Williamson and colleagues concluded that

The demonstration that the results obtained with osmium fixation are not reproducible in Siperstein's laboratory provides a simple but logical explanation for the longstanding, confusing controversy regarding the frequency of BM thickening in diabetics and the relationship of it to the insulin deficient state. In addition, the observations from glutaraldehyde fixed tissue indicate that the prevalence of MCBMT and the relationship between MCBMT and the duration of the disease are similar in Pimas and Caucasians.[54]

My reason for going into this "dead-end" in diabetes research in detail is that Siperstein's results, particularly his contention that complications were unrelated to glycemia, exerted considerable influence, especially in the United States. His findings formed the main evidence of those who had a nihilistic view of the value of diabetes treatment in the 1960s and 1970s and, for them, fitted nicely with the results of the UGDP. The issues were debated in the editorial columns of the *New England Journal of Medicine* in 1976–1977. For the ADA, Cahill and associates summarized the evidence that they believed, albeit circumstantially, suggested that good control prevented complications and threw down the challenge that

These data therefore place the burden of proof upon those who maintain that diabetes control is without effect. The goals of appropriate therapy should thus include a serious effort to achieve levels of blood glucose as close to those in the non-diabetic state as feasible. . . . Current clinical and experimental data clearly demonstrate that optimal regulation of blood glucose levels should be achieved in the treatment of diabetes, particularly in young and middle-aged persons who are at greatest risk of the microvascular complications. . . . Finally, good diabetic management necessitates education and training of both patients and health professionals in the techniques involved, and close coordination and cooperation in patient management. Most important is a commitment to the view that better "control" when achievable, is beneficial.[55]

This statement was followed nearly a year later by a counter-editorial by Siperstein and colleagues. Their position was that "no-one would disagree that it would be desirable to maintain the blood glucose of diabetic patients at normal levels if it were possible to do so safely. To date, however, such maintenance of normal blood glucose had not proved possible in practice. Moreover, attempts to achieve such control too often result in episodes of hypoglycemia."[56] They criticized some of the studies cited by Cahill et al., but their main concern was that

Physicians may misinterpret such a statement and, in the hope of preventing diabetic vascular disease, attempt a degree of control that cannot be safely achieved. Physicians must weigh the possible beneficial effect of aggressive insulin therapy against the known harmful effects of excessive hypoglycemia, particularly since there is no guarantee that treatment will prevent or minimise complications.

Both groups of editorialists were taken to task by the editor, Franz Inglefinger, in his editorial "Debates on Diabetes."[57] According to him, the ADA's statement was intended to "squash once and for all the 'heresy' that control—variously labelled 'good,' 'rigid,' 'tight' or 'chemical'—of the diabetic patient's blood sugar was unimportant in preventing late complications such as nephropathy and retinopathy." The original counter-editorial had arrived in August 1976 and, when finally published in May 1977, was a considerably diluted version. According to Inglefinger, both parties agreed that some control of blood sugar was desirable, but the debate was marred by hazy definitions and lack of data. As a nondiabetologist, he wondered: "What is meant by the various adjectives used to indicate various degrees of control? What is the frequency of fatalities, serious sequelae, and hospital admissions attributable to tight-control treatment of diabetes?" He ended with the criticism that

In spite of the tremendous basic advances that have been made . . . practical everyday management of the disorder does not appear to have changed very much. Furthermore, if various factions of experts wish to influence medical practice, should they not agree on some base-line definition of control and its various degrees expressed by so many non-quantitative adjectives?

This call was acted on in two large prospective randomized controlled trials published in the 1990s, one in patients with IDDM and

---

*This section is a condensed version of one of my articles.[45]

TABLE 60–1. Development of Retinopathy in Alloxan-Treated Diabetic Dogs after 5 Years*

	Nondiabetic	Poor Control	Good Control
Number	10	10	10
Age (yr)	7–9	8–10	8–10
Plasma glucose	69 (3)	341 (16)	183 (11)
8 AM	—	418 (40)	105 (14)
2 PM	—	393 (34)	93 (6)
10 PM			
Glycosuria-free days (%)	100	<1	37 (3)
Capillary aneurysms per eye	1 (1)	25 (6)	2 (1)
Acellular capillaries per 10 mm²	39 (12)	171 (19)	49 (10)

*Numbers in parentheses indicate SEM.

Data from Engerman R, Bloodworth JM, Nelson S: Relationship of microvascular disease in diabetes to metabolic control. Diabetes 26:760, 1977.

the other in patients with NIDDM. Before discussing these trials it is necessary to briefly mention several animal studies that, if one accepted that diabetes in experimental animals was the same as that in humans, provided conclusive proof of the benefit of normoglycemia.

Renal and retinal changes occur in all animals with diabetes, whether spontaneous or induced by chemicals or viruses. In a study published in 1977, Engermann and colleagues induced diabetes in dogs with alloxan and randomly divided 20 animals into prospective good or poor control[58] (Table 60–1). Over 5 years the mean fasting blood glucose level in the poor control group was 341 mg/dL (18.9 mmol/L) vs. 183 mg/dL (10.2 mmol/L) in the well-controlled dogs and 69 mg/dL (3.8 mmol/L) in normal dogs. The reason for the high fasting blood sugar in the good control group was the need to avoid nocturnal hypoglycemia (and possible death). After 5 years (equivalent to 25 years of human diabetes), well-controlled dogs had minimal retinopathy, no cataracts, minimal glomerular changes by electron microscopy, and only a slight increase in basement membrane thickness over age-matched controls. In contrast, severe retinopathy, dense cataracts, moderate glomerular changes, and a pronounced increase in MCBMT developed in uncontrolled animals. A follow-up study published in 1987 assessed how far the progression of retinopathy could be slowed by better control[59] (Table 60–2). Dogs were divided into three diabetic groups: (1) good control for 5 years, (2) poor control for 5 years, and (3) poor control for 2.5 years and then good control for the next 2.5 years (PGC). Good control was better than in the previous study, mainly because the fasting glucose was much lower. In the good control group, retinopathy was more or less prevented, but the unexpected finding was that in the PGC group retinopathy was absent or equivocal at 2.5 years but subsequently developed despite good glycemic control. The authors did consider the possibility that what they were seeing in the PGC group was the transient deterioration in retinopathy that had been reported in human diabetes after dramatic lowering of blood glucose, but they thought it unlikely.

Other studies in diabetic rodents had suggested that microvascular

complications might be reversible. In rats, islet transplantation led to a significant reduction in mesangial thickening and mesangial staining for complement in the kidney. These changes began 2 weeks after restoration of normoglycemia, although complete regression of the light microscopic changes took 10 weeks.[60] In an impressive series of experiments the Danish worker Ruth Rasch devised a treatment regimen to keep diabetic rats almost normoglycemic for up to 6 months. Using this model she found that good control prevented glomerular basement membrane thickening and other renal changes that were seen in rats with poor control.[61]

It was, of course, well known from examples such as prevention of ketoacidosis, normalization of the growth of diabetic children, and reduction in congenital abnormalities and perinatal mortality in pregnancy that in the short term good control was beneficial. Also, a wide variety of metabolic and functional abnormalities in diverse tissues could be corrected by improved blood glucose control—as far as I am aware, no metabolic abnormality in diabetes is normalized by poor control. These examples provided only circumstantial evidence; conclusive proof would come only from a prospective trial in human diabetics.

THE DIABETES CONTROL AND COMPLICATIONS TRIAL

In 1974 the U.S. Congress passed the National Diabetes Mellitus Research and Education Act, which required the director of the NIH to establish a national commission to formulate a long-range plan to combat the disease. The report, published in 1975, was an impressive review of the scale of diabetes as a major public health problem.[62] One recommendation was that a 5-year clinical study be set up to assess the effect of treatment on the development of microvascular and macrovascular complications in people with IDDM. Several technical developments in the late 1970s made this study feasible, particularly the introduction of home blood glucose monitoring and glycosylated hemoglobin. Self-measurement of blood glucose allowed patients to make daily therapeutic decisions at home and also gave them precise targets to aim for. Using self-monitoring of blood glucose and multiple insulin injections or infusion pumps, several groups showed that selected patients could achieve normal blood glucose levels over months or years. Although such normalization had been achieved before, glycosylated hemoglobin enabled it to be documented in a way that was not possible with random blood glucose measurements. Concurrent with the means to improve and document control was the development of quantitative ways of measuring complications. Particularly important was validation of a system for grading fundus photography, which would eventually become the main outcome measure in the proposed trial.[63] It was suggested that two related questions be addressed:

1. Will intensive treatment prevent or delay the appearance of background retinopathy (primary prevention)?

2. Will such an intervention delay or prevent background retinopathy progressing to more severe forms (secondary prevention)?

TABLE 60–2. Progression of Retinopathy in Diabetic Dogs

	Normal	Poor Control	Good Control	Poor + Good Control*
Number	14	8	7	6
Duration (yr)	5	5	5	2.5 + 2.5
Glycosuria (g/day)	0	104	<2	101 + <2
Plasma glucose				
8 AM	79	378	106	342 + 103
2 PM	74	324	83	324 + 77
10 PM	83	378	70	378 + 61
Hb A₁ (%)	6.5	11.1	6.6	11.2 + 6.7
Capillary aneurysms per eye	1	42	2	0 + 29
Acellular capillaries (per 10 mm²)	39	264	80	48 + 224

*Diabetic group with poor control for 2.5 years and then good control for the next 2.5 years.

Data from Engerman R, Kern T: Progression or incipient diabetic retinopathy during good glycemic control. Diabetes 36:808–812, 1987.

In 1981, 21 clinical centers, a data coordinating center, and several central units were chosen by peer review. The planning phase began in 1982 and finished in 1983. Nearly 2000 copies of the draft protocol were circulated to the scientific community for comment. In March 1984, 278 subjects were recruited for the feasibility phase, and in late 1985 the full-scale clinical trial was approved.[64]

At this time several small randomized clinical trials such as the Kroc study in the United Kingdom and North America,[65] the Steno Study in Copenhagen,[66] and the Oslo Study in Norway[67] had shown that intensive and conventional treatments could achieve a clear separation in glycosylated hemoglobin levels and that methods of documenting complications were practical. However, these studies were too short and small to demonstrate a definite effect on complications.

The DCCT was restricted to IDDM because of the ability to define the onset of diabetes accurately and, because this study was intended to look at microvascular complications, to avoid the possibility of major attrition of the cohort from death. One of the first problems was how to treat the control group. Ethically it was unacceptable to simply reduce their dose of insulin. The dilemma was that enrolling them in a clinical trial might improve blood glucose control so much (the Hawthorne effect) that a clear separation from the experimental group would not be achieved. Another worry was that if cared for by their ordinary physicians (something that was seriously considered), control might be poor enough for the purposes of the experiment, but they would be exposed to uncontrollable influences and problems in ensuring completeness of data would probably be encountered. The solution eventually adopted was to find the "typical" treatment of IDDM at the time and mimic it. It turned out that in 1982 the typical patient with IDDM in the United States saw a doctor three or four times a year and was treated with one or two injections of mixed insulin a day. Most still used urine tests, although blood glucose self-monitoring was becoming increasingly popular. The aim of the standard treatment regimen was to maintain clinical well-being, freedom from frequent or severe hypoglycemia, absence of ketonuria, stable weight, and normal growth and development in adolescents. No target value was set for blood glucose or hemoglobin A_{1c} (Hb A_{1c}), and investigators were masked to the latter unless it exceeded 13.11%. Treatment was with one or two injections of any mixture of short, intermediate, or long-acting insulins, and patients were reviewed every 3 months. In the experimental or intensively treated group the aim was to maintain glycemic levels as close as possible to normal, and specific targets were set, namely, blood glucose levels, fasting and preprandial, of 70 to 120 mg/dL, postprandial levels less than 180 mg/dL, and Hb A_{1c} levels less than 6.05%.* Treatment could be with a pump or multiple injections. Subjects were seen weekly until the target range was reached and thereafter monthly. Telephone contact was maintained at least weekly. Retinopathy was documented by stereo fundus photography before randomization and then every 6 months.

Between 1983 and 1989, 1441 patients were recruited at 29 centers in the United States and Canada; 726 had no retinopathy at baseline (primary prevention cohort), whereas 715 had mild retinopathy (secondary prevention cohort); both groups were randomly assigned to intensive or conventional therapy.[68] The mean duration of IDDM was 2.6 years in the primary prevention cohort and 8.8 years in the secondary prevention cohort. Patients with hypertension at baseline were excluded. In June 1993, after a mean follow-up of 6.5 years (range, 3 to 9 years), or 9300 patient years, the independent data monitoring committee determined that the results warranted terminating the trial. It is a tribute to the organization that 99% of patients completed the study and over 95% of all scheduled examinations were done. The overall cost was $165 million and, among other things, involved 35,280 visits, 74,677 Hb A_{1c} estimations, photography of 37,460 eyes, and 34,803 blood glucose profiles involving up to seven fingerpricks each day.[69]

A statistically significant difference between the groups in mean glycosylated hemoglobin was maintained throughout the study, with a value of 7.2% in the former and 9.2% in the latter (Fig. 60–1). The

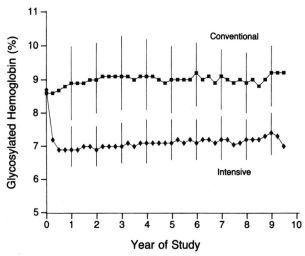

FIGURE 60–1. *Measurements of glycosylated hemoglobin and blood glucose in patients with insulin-dependent diabetes mellitus receiving intensive or conventional therapy. (Reprinted, by permission, from* The Diabetes Control and Complications Trial Research Group: The effect of intensive treatment of diabetes on the development and progression of long-term complications in insulin-dependent diabetes mellitus. *N Engl J Med 329:977–986, 1993. Copyright © 1993 Massachusetts Medical Society. All rights reserved.)*

mean blood glucose values achieved were 155 mg/dL (8.6 mmol/L) in the experimental and 231 mg/dL (12.8 mmol/L) in the conventional group. It is worth noting that although 44% of patients receiving intensive therapy achieved the goal of an Hb A_{1c} value less than 6.05% at least once during the study, less than 5% maintained an average value in this range.

In the primary prevention cohort, the cumulative incidence of retinopathy (defined as a change of three steps or more on fundus photography that was sustained for 6 months) was reduced by 76% and, in the intensive therapy cohort, the risk of progression by 54%. Intensive therapy was associated with a 34% reduction in the development of microalbuminuria (>40 mg per 24 hours) in the primary and 43% in the secondary prevention cohort. Intensive therapy produced a 54% reduction in overt proteinuria (>300 mg per 24 hours). New clinical neuropathy was reduced by 60%. In spite of the relative youth of the cohort, a 41% reduction in macrovascular disease was achieved, although because the numbers were small, this reduction was not significant. As a surrogate endpoint, a 34% reduction in the development of hypercholesterolemia (low-density lipoprotein cholesterol over 160 mg/dL or 4.1 mmol/L) was attained. Severe hypoglycemia was three times more common in the intensive therapy cohort, with 62 episodes per 100 patient-years vs. 19 in the conventional group. It should be noted that this value underestimates the risk of severe hypoglycemia with intensive therapy because after the feasibility study patients with a history of previous attacks were excluded. Another adverse effect of intensive therapy was weight gain, with a 33% increase in the mean adjusted risk of becoming overweight. At 5 years patients receiving intensive therapy had gained a mean of 4.6 kg more than those receiving conventional therapy. Rates of ketoacidosis were low and the same in both groups.

One obvious question that the investigators asked themselves is "can we choose a glycemic target that will preserve the benefits of intensive therapy but reduce the risk of severe hypoglycemia?" Their answer was "no" because although there was a continuously increasing risk of progression of retinopathy with increasing Hb A_{1c}, there was also a continuously increasing risk of severe hypoglycemia with falling Hb A_{1c} (Figs. 60–2 and 60–3). Thus their recommendation was that

Most patients with IDDM [should] be treated with closely monitored intensive regimens, with the goal of maintaining their glycemic status as close to the normal range as safely as possible. Because of the risk of hypoglycemia, intensive therapy should be implemented with caution, especially in patients with repeated severe hypoglycemia or unawareness of hypoglycemia. The risk-

---

*Blood glucose targets identical to those recommended by George Graham in the 1920s![6]

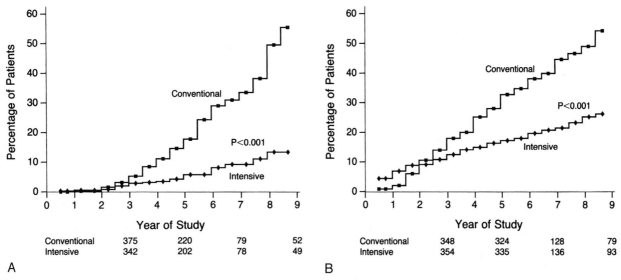

FIGURE 60–2. Cumulative incidence of a sustained change in retinopathy in patients with insulin-dependent diabetes mellitus receiving intensive or conventional therapy. (Reprinted, by permission, from The Diabetes Control and Complications Trial Research Group: The effect of intensive treatment of diabetes on the development and progression of long-term complications in insulin-dependent diabetes mellitus. N Engl J Med 329:977–986, 1993. Copyright © 1993 Massachusetts Medical Society. All rights reserved.)

benefit ratio with intensive therapy may be less favourable in children under 13 years of age and in patients with advanced complications such as end-stage renal disease or cardio or cerebrovascular disease. . . . Finally, although we did not study patients with non–insulin-dependent diabetes mellitus (NIDDM), hyperglycemia is associated with the presence or progression of complications in NIDDM, as it is in IDDM. If the main conclusions of this trial with regard to the benefits of reducing glycemia are extended to patients with NIDDM, careful regard for age, capabilities, and co-existing diseases will be necessary. We therefore advise caution in the use of therapies other than diet that are aimed at achieving euglycemia in patients with NIDDM.

A smaller study that was almost coterminous with the DCCT was the Stockholm Diabetes Intervention Study, which began in 1982. Results of the 7.5-year follow-up were published in 1993 and are similar to those of the DCCT.[70]

It is often overlooked that what the DCCT did was to answer the scientific question of whether good control prevents complications but not the practical question of the best way of achieving good control. Whether intensification of insulin therapy must inevitably lead to a high rate of severe hypoglycemia has been contested, particularly by Berger and Muhlhauser.[71] They point out that among the 29 DCCT

centers, no association between Hb A_{1c} levels and the development of severe hypoglycemia could be found; the center with the lowest mean Hb A_{1c} values had an average rate, whereas the one with the second lowest mean Hb A_{1c} values had a particularly low rate of hypoglycemia. In contrast, some centers reported high levels of Hb A_{1c} and high rates of severe hypoglycemia. Also, throughout the DCCT striking differences were seen between rates of severe hypoglycemia in various units irrespective of whether patients were treated with conventional or intensified insulin therapy.[72] In some units patients predominantly receiving two daily injections had high Hb A_{1c} values and high rates of severe hypoglycemia, whereas in other units, most patients receiving four injections had low Hb A_{1c} values and low rates of severe hypoglycemia. Berger and Muhlhauser believe that patient factors can explain only a minority of this variability and suggest that the crucial factor is the attitudes and health beliefs of the care team.

The applicability of the DCCT findings has been much discussed. It was pointed out that (unlike the situation in Europe) most patients in the United States are treated by primary care physicians whose specialty is not necessarily diabetes. Thus care of the conventional

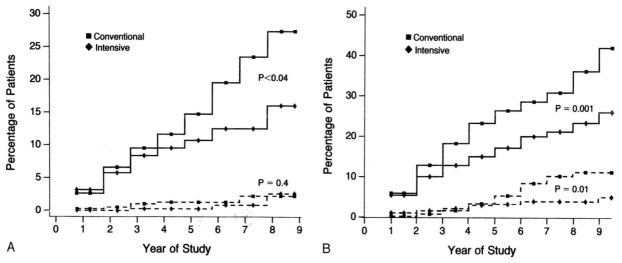

FIGURE 60–3. Risk of sustained progression of retinopathy (A) and rate of severe hypoglycemia (B) in patients receiving intensive therapy according to their mean glycosylated hemoglobin values during the trial. (Reprinted, by permission, from The Diabetes Control and Complications Trial Research Group: The effect of intensive treatment of diabetes on the development and progression of long-term complications in insulin-dependent diabetes mellitus. N Engl J Med 329:977–986, 1993. Copyright © 1993 Massachusetts Medical Society. All rights reserved.)

group in the DCCT might well have been better than that of many patients with IDDM in the United States. Care of the intensive group involved monthly visits to a team consisting of a diabetologist, nurse, dietitian, and behavioral specialist, and if it were proved that this arrangement was the sine qua non for good control, it would be beyond the ability or resources of office-based physicians. It is sometimes assumed that this intensity of supervision is essential for good control "because the DCCT did it," but those with long experience in diabetes will have seen many self-motivated patients who maintain excellent control with only minimal supervision. What is sure is that implementing the DCCT will be a major problem in many countries; in 1994 Harris et al. pointed out that in the United States only 15% of patients with IDDM were receiving three or more injections per day and only 40% self-monitored blood glucose. Only a tenth had seen a dietitian in the past year and less than half had ever attended an education class.[73] In Europe as well, some alarm was expressed about the resource implications and how far the results could be generalized from highly selected and motivated volunteers (the DCCT subjects) to the generality of patients with IDDM.[74] In practice, the barriers were (and still are) almost certainly greater in the United States because of the way that the healthcare system is structured and financed. In most European countries, management of IDDM has been centralized for many years in more or less specialized units where care is undertaken by a team including specialist nurses, dietitians, and chiropodists.

In a position statement shortly after publication of the DCCT results, the ADA advised that "if the IDDM patient is intellectually, emotionally, physically and financially able to attempt tight control, and if a health care team is available to provide resources, guidance and support, a reasonable goal is the mean plasma glucose and hemoglobin A_{1c} levels achieved in the intensive group of the trial." Nevertheless, the ADA recognized that relative contraindications to tight control would be frequent and that "clinical judgement and common sense" were necessary. The magnitude of the problem of achieving acceptable levels of glycemic control in young patients, who have the most to gain, is shown by a series of studies in Denmark, a small country with an excellent healthcare system in general and for diabetes in particular. Initial studies in 1987 and 1989 showed poor metabolic control in a group of unselected young patients, even though many were receiving multiple insulin injections.[75] In a follow-up of 47% of the initial cohort in 1995, mean Hb A_{1c} was 9.7% and very few had values below 8%, even though more than three-quarters were receiving three or more insulin injections.[76] Similar results were found in a nationwide study in Finland at the end of 1994, where the mean Hb A_{1c} value in patients with IDDM was 8.8%.[77] By contrast, the results achieved by Harry Dorchy, a Belgian pediatrician, seem almost too good to be true. In a group of adolescents (mean age of 18 years and mean duration of diabetes of 10 years) studied between 1990 and 1991, he reported a mean Hb A_{1c} value of 6.9% $\pm$ 1.5%.[78] No significant difference was observed between those receiving two injections and those receiving the basal-bolus regimen of four injections. In a later study of 144 unselected patients younger than 18 years, Dorchy et al. reported a mean Hb A_{1c} of 6.6% $\pm$ 1.2% with no relation to sex, number of daily injections, or age.[79] Even more surprising, half the patients were immigrants, mainly from Morocco, and they had control equivalent to that of Belgians. We can only speculate on the reasons for Dorchy's outstanding results[80]; several features of his system are unusual. One is the high frequency of home blood glucose monitoring, an average of 120 times per month. Another is that patients were seen on average 8.9 times per year by the same experienced doctor and nurse.

The only variable tested in the DCCT was glycemic control, and it seems certain that other factors, such as genes, smoking, BP, lipid levels, and others, must play some part in the development and progression of microvascular complications. Some of the best epidemiologic evidence of associations other than glycemia comes from the Pittsburgh Epidemiology of Diabetic Complications (EDC) study. This study is a follow-up of a cohort of children in whom IDDM developed between 1950 and 1980.[81] In the EDC study the association of potential risk factors is being studied prospectively by biennial examinations. Some results that have been shown by this approach are as follows[82]:

1. The development of any retinopathy in those with fair control (Hb A_{1c} <10.1%) is associated with high-density lipoprotein cholesterol and more weakly with BP and smoking. Conversely, in those with poor control, none of these factors are associated with the development of retinopathy.

2. Progression to proliferative retinopathy among those in fair control is strongly related to diastolic BP. However, BP was not a risk factor for proliferative retinopathy in those with poor control, but fibrinogen and the platelet count were predictors. One explanation might be that those with poor control are protected from proliferative retinopathy if they avoid nephropathy and its associated disturbances.

3. The development of neuropathy is strongly related to hypertension and, surprisingly, in those with fair control is positively associated with a college education.

Improved Glycemic Control and Microvascular Complications in NIDDM

It has always seemed likely, although it cannot be taken as proven that the effect of glycemia on microvascular complications would be the same in NIDDM as in IDDM.[83] These complications in IDDM and NIDDM are similar if not identical, but in theory, comorbidities such as hypertension and hyperlipidemia might modify them in some way. In a review in 1998, Gaster and Hirsch identified 20 epidemiologic studies that had looked for an association between glycemia and microvascular complications in NIDDM. Thirteen measured rates of retinopathy, 5 measured rates of nephropathy, and 2 measured rates of neuropathy. All identified a strong independent association between hyperglycemia and the rate of microvascular complications when factors such as BP, body weight, insulin levels, and duration of diabetes were controlled for.[84]

The most comprehensive of the prospective observational studies is the Wisconsin Epidemiological Study of Diabetic Retinopathy. This study monitored all diabetics in the southern part of the state who had IDDM (996 patients) and a sample with NIDDM (1780) stratified by insulin vs. other treatment. After 10 years, follow-up data were available for more than 85% of the original cohort. The results showed a consistent exponential relationship between worsening diabetic control and the development of complications.[85] The relationship between Hb A_1 concentrations and the incidence of, progression of, and progression to proliferative retinopathy over 10 years is shown in Figure 60–4. Among the younger-onset diabetic group, some retinopathy developed in 82% of those in the lowest quartile of Hb A_1 (5.4%–8.5%) and in nearly 100% of those in the highest quartile (11.6%–20.8%). Similar but slightly lower rates were seen in the older-onset groups. No apparent threshold of glycemia could be found below which retinopathy did not occur, and the rate of progression was related to Hb A_1 concentration rather than the type of diabetes. Also, the relationship of Hb A_1 to progression of retinopathy was independent of the duration of diabetes and baseline severity of retinopathy. Glycemic status, as measured by Hb A_1, had similarly profound effects on other complications such as macular edema, overt proteinuria, neuropathy, and amputation. In young and old, a 1% increase in Hb A_1 concentration at baseline was associated with a 60% increase in the incidence of retinopathy and a doubling of the rate of progression to proliferative retinopathy.

Between 1995 and 1999 three clinical trials of improved glycemic control in NIDDM have been completed and published: The Kumamoto study from Japan, the Veterans Administration (VA) Cooperative Study in the United States, and the U.K. Prospective Diabetes Study (UKPDS). These trials differ in scope and objectives, but all provide useful lessons.

THE KUMAMOTO STUDY

In this trial 110 patients were randomized to intensive or conventional insulin therapy and monitored for 6 years.[86] The separation in terms of glycemic control was like that in the DCCT, with Hb A_{1c} values of 7.1% and 9.4%. The intensively treated group had less retinopathy (13% vs. 38%), nephropathy (10% vs. 30%), and neuropa-

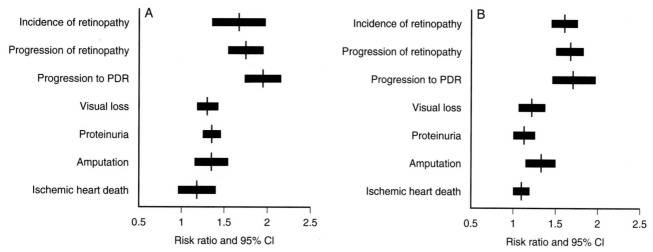

FIGURE 60–4. The effect of a 1% increase in Hb A$_1$ concentrations at baseline on the risk of development of complications in the younger-onset group *(A)* and the older-onset group *(B)* participating in the Wisconsin Epidemiologic Study of Diabetic Retinopathy. (From Klein R, Klein BEK: Relation of glycemic control to diabetic complications and health outcomes. Diabetes Care 21(suppl 3):C39–C43, 1998.)

thy, as measured by vibration threshold in the legs (12.8% vs. 65%). The results and the duration of treatment are strikingly similar to those of the DCCT. One thing to note about this study is that patients with hypertension were excluded, and as would be expected with a Japanese population, the prevalence of obesity was low.

THE VA COOPERATIVE STUDY

The VA Cooperative Study was a feasibility trial in which 153 men with type 2 diabetes (mean age of 60 years and body mass index of 31 kg/m^2) were allocated to intensive or standard therapy.[87] After 27 months of follow-up, mean Hb A$_{1c}$ concentrations were similar to those in other studies (7.3% vs. 9.4%), and the difference in fasting serum glucose was 5.46 mmol/L (98 mg/dL). The final insulin dose in the intensive group was 133 U. In those receiving standard therapy, 24-hour urinary albumin excretion rose significantly from 14 to 158 mg and was not significantly changed in the intensive group (11–44 mg). No significant differences were noted in retinopathy, which is not surprising given the short duration of the study.

U.K. PROSPECTIVE DIABETES STUDY

The aims of this ambitious study, initiated in 1977, were to find out whether

1. The risk of complications in type 2 diabetes can be reduced by intensive blood glucose control
2. Treatment of hypertension will reduce the risk of complications
3. Any specific form of hypoglycemic or antihypertensive therapy had advantages over others[88]

A total of 5102 people with newly diagnosed type 2 diabetes were enrolled. The basis of the diagnosis of diabetes was a fasting plasma glucose (FPG) concentration over 6.0 mmol/L (108 mg/dL) on two occasions, although in practice 94% had a level over 7 mmol/L (126 mg/dL). Apart from answering the main questions, this huge study produced a number of important spinoffs in terms of knowledge about type 2 diabetes. Three of the most important, although not entirely new, were as follows:

1. Quantitation of the degree of tissue damage already present at the time of diagnosis of type 2 diabetes. Thus 50% of subjects already had evidence of tissue damage, the breakdown being as follows:
• 8%, cardiovascular disease
• 37%, microaneurysms or more severe retinopathy in one eye
• 18%, retinopathy in both eyes

• 4%, clinical-grade albuminuria
• 13%, absent ankle reflexes
• 39%, hypertension (defined as systolic BP >160 and diastolic BP >90 mm Hg or already receiving antihypertensive treatment)

Such evidence has previously been shown in a number of other studies and is regarded by many as an indication of the need to screen for undiagnosed diabetes.[89]

2. The fact that type 2 diabetes is a progressive disease characterized by increasing pancreatic failure with time.[90] Again, this finding is not new; it was found in the UGDP and has always been presumed to be the basis of secondary failure of sulfonylureas. However, it was shown particularly clearly in this large cohort.

3. Confirmation of the poor early prognosis in NIDDM. After 10 years, those in the study had a twofold greater mortality than the general population did. Also after 10 years, a third had a complication needing clinical attention, including heart attacks, strokes, laser treatment of the eyes, therapy for renal failure, or amputations. This result confirms the findings of a large cohort study in the former East Germany in which 44% of patients with newly diagnosed NIDDM had died within 10 years, with excess mortality already seen in the first year after diagnosis.[91]

The main UKPDS results were published in a series of papers in late 1998 under the following headings:

Intensive Blood Glucose Control with Sulfonylureas or Insulin

The aim in the intensive group was an FPG under 6 mmol/L and, in the conventional group, the best achievable FPG with diet alone unless this value went over 15 mmol/L or symptoms developed.[92] Attempts to keep FPG normal needed a stepwise addition of hypoglycemic agents when the targets were not met. For example, patients assigned to receive sulfonylureas could be given metformin, and oral agents could later be replaced by insulin. Failure to meet even the very modest targets in the diet group led to the addition of drugs in nearly two-thirds. Thus as has been pointed out by several commentators, substantial therapeutic overlap occurred between the groups, which, it has been suggested, may be why no clear difference was shown between the intensive therapies.[93] Analysis was on an intention-to-treat basis, and over 10 years, concentrations of Hb A$_{1c}$ were 7.0% in the intensive and 7.9% in the conventional group. This relatively small difference led to a 12% lowering of the risk of any diabetes-related endpoint, 10% for any diabetes-related death, and 6% for all-cause mortality (Table 60–3). Most of the risk reduction in the

TABLE 60–3. Relative Risks of Various Endpoints with Intensive and Conventional Treatment of Blood Glucose in the U.K. Prospective Diabetes Study

Endpoint	P	Relative Risk for Intensive Treatment	Confidence Interval
Any diabetes-related endpoint	.029	0.88	0.79–0.99
Diabetes-related deaths	.34	0.90	0.73–1.11
Myocardial infarction	.052	0.84	0.71–1.00
Retinopathy at 12 yr	.015	0.79	0.63–1.00
Albuminuria at 12 yr	.036	0.66	0.39–1.10
Retinal photocoagulation	.0031	0.71	0.53–0.96
Cataract extraction	.046	0.76	0.53–1.08

Data from UK Prospective Diabetes Study Group: UK Prospective Diabetes Study (UKPDS). VIII. Study design, progress and performance. Diabetologia 34:877–890, 1991.

diabetes-related endpoints was due to a 25% lower need for photocoagulation. As with other studies of improved control, progression of surrogate indicators of microvascular disease (two-step worsening of retinopathy, vibration threshold, microalbuminuria) was also decreased. The median complication-free interval was 1.3 years in the intensive group.

In terms of outcome, no difference was found between sulfonylureas and insulin, and none of the regimens produced adverse cardiovascular outcomes. As in other studies, patients in the intensive group put on more weight and had more hypoglycemia. During the early years, hypoglycemia was relatively frequent in patients taking chlorpropamide and glibenclamide but declined as FPG increased, so in the long term most hypoglycemia was caused by insulin therapy.

Intensive Blood Glucose Control with Metformin in Overweight Patients

Overweight patients were randomly allocated to intensive treatment with sulfonylureas or insulin, metformin, or diet alone.[94] Over 10 years, Hb A_{1c} was 7.4% in the metformin and intensive groups and 8.0% in the diet group. The reduction in Hb A_{1c} with metformin therapy was similar to that for sulfonylureas but without weight gain or an increased risk of hypoglycemia. Those receiving metformin had risk reductions of 32% for any diabetes-related endpoint, 42% for diabetes-related death, and 36% for all-cause mortality. Among patients allocated to intensive control, metformin was more effective than sulfonylureas or insulin for any diabetes-related endpoint ($P = .0034$), all-cause mortality ($P = .021$), and stroke ($P = .032$). An unexpected and troublesome finding was that the addition of metformin to a sulfonylurea in normal and overweight patients produced an increased risk of diabetes-related death (96%) and all-cause mortality (60%) in comparison to continued sulfonylurea alone. The authors, after failing to explain this finding, suggest that "it requires further study", without saying what this might be.

Blood Pressure Control and Its Effect on Microvascular and Macrovascular Complications

The positive effect of BP control on microvascular and macrovascular complications is arguably the most important result of the UKPDS.[95, 96] Over 1000 patients were allocated to tight control of BP (aim, <150/85 mm Hg; achieved, 144/82) or less tight (aim, <180/105; achieved, 154/87). Reductions in risk in those allocated to tight control were 24% in diabetes-related endpoints, 32% in diabetes-related deaths, 44% in strokes, and 37% in microvascular endpoints. Differences in all-cause mortality did not reach significance, but cardiovascular complications such as heart failure and stroke were greatly reduced. Results with an angiotensin-converting enzyme (ACE) inhibi-

tor (captopril) were similar to those with a β-blocker (atenolol), although the former was generally better tolerated. Like glucose control, tight BP control required a stepwise addition of drugs; after 9 years, 29% were receiving three or more. Health economic analysis showed that tight BP control is cost-effective when compared with other widely used preventive strategies and is more feasible for most clinicians and patients than tight blood glucose control is.[97]

These results have been confirmed in several other hypertension trials that included relatively large numbers of patients with diabetes. The Appropriate Blood Pressure Control in Diabetes (ABCD) trial was designed to test the primary hypothesis that intensive, as compared with moderate, BP control would prevent or slow the progression of nephropathy, neuropathy, retinopathy, and cardiovascular events. The secondary hypothesis was that a long-acting calcium channel blocker (nisoldipine) would be as good as an ACE inhibitor (enalapril). A total of 235 patients were placed in each group, but the study was stopped because interim analysis showed 25 myocardial infarctions in the nisoldipine group vs. 5 in the enalapril group.[98] The Fosinopril vs. Amlodipine Cardiovascular Events Randomised Trial (FACET), which studied the effects of amlodipine vs. fosinopril over a period of 3.5 years, also showed a significantly lower risk of cardiovascular endpoints with the ACE inhibitor.[99] Neither of these studies included a control group, so it is not clear whether it is the ACE inhibitor that is uniquely beneficial or the calcium antagonist that is harmful. In the hypertension optimal treatment (HOT) trial, 18,790 patients were randomized to three different target levels of BP with felodipine alone or in combination with an ACE inhibitor.[100] This trial included a subgroup analysis of 1500 diabetic patients with approximately 500 in each of the target BP groups. After 3.8 years, the three mean pressures achieved were 139.7/81.1, 141/83.2, and 143.7/85.2 mm Hg. In patients with diabetes a 60% reduction in cardiovascular mortality and a 51% reduction in major cardiovascular events were seen in the group with the lowest diastolic pressure. The trial also confirmed the benefit of aspirin as primary prevention in hypertensive diabetic patients, with a reduction of 2.5 myocardial infarctions per thousand patient-years.

CONCLUSIONS

It is now established beyond any reasonable doubt that decreasing blood glucose reduces the risk of microvascular complications in both IDDM and NIDDM. There is no threshold, and for every 1% fall in Hb A_{1c} the risk of retinopathy is reduced by about 25% in both IDDM and NIDDM. It is important to emphasize that these estimates apply to patients with *early* or no complications at baseline. It is obvious that there must be a point of no return after which control of glycemia will be ineffective—no one would expect it to cure retinitis proliferans or terminal renal failure. At present we do not really know where the point of no return is for any of the microvascular complications. My own impressions are as follows:

- Retinopathy: Once maculopathy or preproliferative retinopathy has developed, laser treatment is essential. It would now be unethical to do a study of the effect of tight blood glucose control at this stage.
- Nephropathy: Evidence from the DCCT and other smaller studies shows that tight control reduces the progression to microalbuminuria and overt proteinuria, but once these conditions are present, the evidence is overwhelming that the best treatment is with an ACE inhibitor.[101]
- Neuropathy: The type of neuropathy that is prevented by good glycemic control is the chronic sensorimotor type. The effect in the prevention or treatment of amyotrophy is controversial,[102] and a number of reports have described acute painful neuropathy being precipitated by starting insulin treatment or normalizing glycosylated hemoglobin.[103]

It also needs to be restated that the main cause of death in both IDDM and NIDDM is macrovascular disease, and although circumstantial evidence indicates that glucose control does have a limited beneficial effect on macrovascular disease, it seems likely that control of BP and lipids will be as or more important. It also seems likely that the future will increasingly be an era of polypharmacy, although the UKPDS showed how difficult it is to treat hyperglycemia and hypertension to the targets set.

REFERENCES

1. Heller SR, Tattersall RB: Does diabetic control matter? Prim Care 10:553–563, 1983.
2. Tattersall RB: The quest for normoglycaemia: A historical perspective. Diabet Med 11:618–635, 1994.
3. Von Noorden C: The pancreas. Practitioner Jan–June:243–246, 1915.
4. Wagener HP, Wilder RM: The retinitis of diabetes mellitus. JAMA 76:515–517, 1921.
5. Banting FG: Nobel Lecture 1923. *In* Nobel Lectures in Physiology or Medicine 1922–1941. Amsterdam, Elsevier, 1965, p 68.
6. Graham G: An address on insulin in general practice. Lancet 1:63–65, 1924.
7. Joslin EP: The Treatment of Diabetes Mellitus, ed 4. London, Henry Kimpton, 1928, p 81.
8. Geyelin HR: The treatment of diabetes mellitus with insulin (after 10 years). JAMA 104:1203–1208, 1935.
9. Stolte K, Wolff J: Die Behandlung der kindlichen Zuckerkrankheit bei frei gewählter Kost. Ergebn Inn Med Kinderheilk 56:154–193, 1939.
10. Lichtenstein A: The treatment of diabetes in childhood. Arch Dis Child 24:237–244, 1949.
11. Diabetes Mellitus: Practitioners Conference. N Y Med 8:16–33, 1952.
12. Tolstoi E: Newer concepts of the treatment of diabetes with protamine insulin. Am J Dig Dis 10:247, 1943.
13. Wagener HF, Dry TJ, Wilder RM: Retinitis in diabetes. N Engl J Med 211:1131–1137, 1934.
14. Waite JH, Beetham WP: The visual mechanism in diabetes mellitus: A comparative study of 2002 diabetics and 457 non-diabetics for controls. N Engl J Med 212:429–433, 1935.
15. Lundbaek K: Long-term Diabetes: The Clinical Picture in Diabetes Mellitus of 15–25 Years Duration with a Follow up of a Regional Series of Cases. Copenhagen, Ejnar Munksgaard, 1953.
16. Lundbaek K: Diabetic angiopathy; a specific vascular disease. Lancet 1:377–379, 1954.
17. Dolger H: Clinical evaluation of vascular damage in diabetes mellitus. JAMA 134:1289–1291, 1947.
18. Reuting RE: Progress notes on 50 diabetic patients followed 25 or more years. Arch Intern Med 86:891, 1950.
19. Allen FM: Current judgements on metabolic control and complications in diabetes. N Engl J Med 248:133–136, 1953.
20. Lawrence RD: Insulin therapy: Successes and problems. Lancet 2:401–405, 1949.
21. Johnsson S: Retinopathy and nephropathy in diabetes mellitus: Comparison of the effects of two forms of treatment. Diabetes 9:1–8, 1960.
22. Lawrence RD: Treatment of 90 diabetics with soluble insulin for 20–40 years: Effect of diabetic control on complications. BMJ 2:1624–1625, 1963.
23. Knowles HC: The problem of the relation of the control of diabetes to the development of vascular disease. Trans Am Clin Climatol Assoc 76:142–147, 1964.
24. Doll R: Controlled trials: The 1948 watershed. BMJ 317:1217–1220, 1998.
25. Kohlstedt KG: Developing and testing of new drugs by the pharmaceutical industry. J Clin Pharmacol Ther 1:192–201, 1960.
26. Kolata GB: Controversy over study of diabetes drugs continues for nearly a decade. Science 203:986–990, 1979.
27. Marks HM: The Progress of Experiment: Science and Therapeutic Reform in the United States, 1900–1990. New York, Cambridge University Press, 1997, pp 197–228.
28. The University Group Diabetes Program: A study of the effects of hypoglycemic agents on vascular complications in patients with adult onset diabetes. Diabetes 19(suppl):789–830, 1970.
29. Editorial statement, Oct 7, 1970. Diabetes 19(suppl):iii–v, 1970.
30. Oral hypoglycaemics in diabetes mellitus (editorial). Lancet 2:489–491, 1975.
31. Feinstein A: Clinical Biostatistics VIII. An Analytic Appraisal of the University Group Diabetes Program Study (UGDP). Clin Pharmacol Ther 12:172–173, 177–178, 185–189, 1971.
32. The University Group Diabetes Program: A statistician looks at the mortality results. JAMA 217:1671–1673, 1971.
33. Seltzer HS: A summary of criticisms of the University Group Diabetes Program. Diabetes 21:976–979, 1972.
34. Prout TE, Knatterud GL, Meinert CL, Klimt CR: The UGDP trial: Clinical trials versus clinical impressions. Diabetes 21:1035–1040, 1972.
35. Moss JM: The UGDP scandal and cover-up. JAMA 232:806–808, 1975.
36. Report of the Committee for the Assessment of Biometric Aspects of Controlled Trials of Hypoglycemic Agents. JAMA 231:583–608, 1975.
37. Oral hypoglycaemics in diabetes mellitus (editorial). Lancet 2:491, 1975.
38. Kilo C, Miller JP, Williamson JR: The Achilles heel of the University Group Diabetes Program. JAMA 243:450–457, 1980.
39. Kilo C, Miller JP, Williamson JR: The crux of the UGDP: Spurious results and biologically inappropriate data analysis. Diabetologia 18:179–185, 1980.
40. Are antidiabetic drugs dangerous (editorial)? BMJ 4:444–445, 1970.
41. The tolbutamide evidence (editorial). Lancet 1:171–172, 1971.
42. Krall LP: The oral hypoglycemic agents. *In* Marble A, White P, Bradley R, Krall P (eds): Joslin's Diabetes Mellitus. Philadelphia, Lea & Febiger, 1971, pp 302–331.
43. Shen S-W, Bressler R: Clinical pharmacology of oral antidiabetic agents. N Engl J Med 296:493–497, 787–793, 1977.
44. Singer DL, Hurwitz D: Long-term experience with sulphonylureas and placebo. N Engl J Med 277:450–456, 1967.
45. Dornan TL, Tattersall RB: Blind alleys in diabetes research: Muscle capillary basement membrane thickening. Marker of microvascular complications or false prophet? Diabet Med 3:413–418, 1986.
46. Siperstein MD, Unger RH, Madison LL: Studies of muscle capillary basement membranes in normal subjects, diabetic and prediabetic patients. J Clin Invest 47:1973–1999, 1968.
47. Camerini-Davalos RA, Oppermann W, Rebigliati H, et al: Muscle capillary basement membrane width in genetic prediabetes. J Clin Endocrinol Metab 48:251–259, 1979.
48. Williamson JR, Vogler NJ, Kilo C: Basement membrane thickening in muscle capillaries: Observations on diabetics and non diabetics with both parents diabetic. *In* Proceedings of the Fourth International Congress of Endocrinology. Amsterdam, Excerpta Medica, 1972, pp 1122–1128.
49. Yodaiken RE: The capillaries of South African diabetics in perspective. Adv Metab Disord 2(suppl 2):341–347, 1973.
50. Pardo V, Perex-Stable E, Alzamora DB, et al: Incidence and significance of muscle capillary basal lamina thickness in juvenile diabetes. Am J Pathol 68:67–80, 1972.
51. Peterson GE, Forsham PH: Variation in thickness of the capillary basement membrane in single muscles of diabetic subjects. Diabetes 28:548–551, 1979.
52. Siperstein MD, Feingold KR, Bennett PH: Hyperglycaemia and diabetic microangiopathy. Diabetologia 15:365–367, 1978.
53. Williamson JR, Kilo C: A commonsense approach resolves the basement membrane controversy and the NIH Pima Indian study. Diabetologia 17:129–131, 1979.
54. Williamson JR, Rowold E, Hoffman P, et al: Influence of fixation and morphometric technics on capillary basement membrane prevalence data in diabetes. Diabetes 25:604–613, 1976.
55. Cahill GF, Etzwiler DD, Freinkel N: 'Control' and diabetes. N Engl J Med 294:1004–1005, 1976.
56. Siperstein MD, Foster DW, Knowles HC, et al: Control of blood glucose and diabetic vascular disease. N Engl J Med 296:1060–1062, 1977.
57. Ingelfinger FJ: Debates on diabetes. N Engl J Med 296:1060–1062, 1977.
58. Engerman R, Bloodworth JM, Nelson S: Relationship of microvascular disease in diabetes to metabolic control. Diabetes 26:760–769, 1977.
59. Engerman R, Kern T: Progression of incipient diabetic retinopathy during good glycemic control. Diabetes 36:808–812, 1987.
60. Mauer SM, Sutherland DER, Steffes MW, et al: Studies of the rate of regression of the glomerular lesions in diabetic rats treated with pancreatic islet transplantation. Diabetes 24:280–285, 1975.
61. Rasch R: Prevention of diabetic glomerulopathy in streptozotocin diabetic rats by insulin treatment. Glomerular basement membrane thickness. Diabetologia 16:319–324, 1979.
62. Report of the National Commission on Diabetes to the Congress of the United States. Washington, DC, DHEW Publication No. (NIH) 76–108, 1975.
63. The Diabetic Retinopathy Study Research Group: A modification of the Airlie House classification of diabetic retinopathy. Diabetic Retinopathy Study (DRS) Report No. 7. Invest Ophthalmol 21:210–226, 1981.
64. DCCT Research Group: The Diabetes Control and Complications Trial (DCCT): Design and methodologic considerations for the feasibility phase. Diabetes 35:530–545, 1986.
65. The Kroc Collaborative Study Group: Blood glucose control and the evolution of diabetic retinopathy and albuminuria: A preliminary multicenter trial. N Engl J Med 311:365–372, 1984.
66. Lauritzen T, Frost-Larsen K, Larsen H-W, et al: Two-year experience with continuous subcutaneous insulin infusion in relation to retinopathy and neuropathy. Diabetes 34(suppl 3):74–79, 1985.
67. Dahl-Jorgensen K, Brinchmann-Hansen O, Hansen K-F, et al: Rapid tightening of blood glucose control leads to transient deterioration of retinopathy in insulin dependent diabetes mellitus. The Oslo Study. BMJ 290:811–815, 1985.
68. The Diabetes Control and Complications Trial Research Group: The effect of intensive treatment of diabetes on the development and progression of long-term complications in insulin-dependent diabetes mellitus. N Engl J Med 329:977–986, 1993.
69. Diabetes Forecast. Sept 1993, p 50.
70. Reichard P, Nilsson BY, Rosenquist U: The effect of long term intensified insulin treatment on the development of microvascular complications of diabetes mellitus. N Engl J Med 329:304–309, 1993.
71. Berger M, Muhlhauser I: Implementation of intensified insulin therapy: A European perspective. Diabet Med 12:201–208, 1995.
72. Tattersall RB: Frequency and causes of hypoglycaemia. *In* Frier B, Fisher M (eds): Hypoglycaemia and Diabetes: Clinical and Physiological Effects. London, Edward Arnold, 1993, pp 176–189.
73. Harris MI, Eastman RC, Siebert C: The DCCT and medical care for diabetes in the U.S. Diabetes Care 17:761–764, 1994.
74. Boulton AJM: DCCT: Implications for diabetes care in the UK. Diabet Med 10:687, 1993.
75. Mortensen HB, Villumsen J, Vølund AA, et al: Relationship between insulin injection regime and metabolic control in young Danish type I diabetic patients. Diabet Med 9:834–839, 1992.
76. Olsen BS, Johannesen AK, Sjølie AK, et al: Metabolic control and prevalence of microvascular complications in young Danish patients with type I diabetes mellitus. Diabet Med 16:79–85, 1999.
77. Valle T, Koivisto VA, Reunanen A, et al: Glycemic control in patients with diabetes in Finland. Diabetes Care 22:575–579, 1999.
78. Dorchy H: What level of HbA1c can be achieved in young diabetic patients beyond the honeymoon period? Diabetes Care 16:1311–1313, 1993.
79. Dorchy H, Roggemans M-P, Willems D: Glycated hemoglobin and related factors in diabetic children and adolescents under 18 years of age: A Belgian experience. Diabetes Care 20:2–6, 1997.
80. Dorchy H: Dorchy's recipes explaining the "intriguing efficacy of Belgian insulin therapy." Diabetes Care 17:458–460, 1994.
81. Orchard TJ, Dorman JS, Maser RE, et al: Factors associated with the avoidance of severe complications after twenty-five years of insulin dependent diabetes mellitus: Pittsburgh Epidemiology of Diabetes Complications Study-1. Diabetes Care 13:741–747, 1990.

82. Orchard TJ: From diagnosis and classification to complications and therapy. DCCT Part II. Diabetes Care 17:326–337, 1994.
83. Nathan DM: Inferences and implications: Do results from the Diabetes Control and Complications Trial apply in NIDDM? Diabetes Care 18:251–257, 1995.
84. Gaster B, Hirsch IB: The effects of improved glycemic control on complications in type 2 diabetes. Arch Intern Med 158:134–140, 1998.
85. Klein R, Klein BE, Moss SE: Relation of glycemic control to diabetic microvascular complications in diabetes mellitus. Arch Intern Med 124(suppl 1):90–96, 1996.
86. Ohkubo Y, Kishikawa H, Araki E, et al: Intensive insulin therapy prevents the progression of diabetic microvascular complications in Japanese patients with non–insulin dependent diabetes mellitus: A randomized, prospective 6 year study. Diabetes Res Clin Pract 28:103–117, 1995.
87. Abraira C, Colwell JA, Nuttall FQ, et al: Veterans Affairs Cooperative Study on glycemic control and complications in type II diabetes (VACSDM). Results of the feasibility trial. Veterans Affairs Cooperative Study in Type II Diabetes. Diabetes Care 18:1113–1123, 1995.
88. UK Prospective Diabetes Study Group: UK Prospective Diabetes Study (UKPDS). VIII. Study design, progress and performance. Diabetologia 34:877–890, 1991.
89. Harris MI: Undiagnosed NIDDM. Diabetes Care 16:642–652, 1993.
90. UK Prospective Diabetes Study Group: UK Prospective Diabetes Study 16: Overview of 6 years therapy of type II diabetes: A progressive disease. Diabetes 44:1249–1258, 1995.
91. Panzram G, Zabel-Langhennig R: Prognosis of diabetes mellitus in a defined population. Diabetologia 20:587–591, 1981.
92. UK Prospective Diabetes Study (UKPDS) Group: Intensive blood-glucose control with sulphonylureas or insulin compared with conventional treatment and risk of complication in patients with type 2 diabetes (UKPDS 33). Lancet 352:837–853, 1998.
93. Nathan DM: Some answers, more controversy, from UKPDS. Lancet 352:832–833, 1998.
94. UK Prospective Diabetes Study (UKPDS) Group: Effect of intensive blood-glucose control with metformin on complications in overweight patients with type 2 diabetes (UKPDS 34). Lancet 352:854–865, 1998.
95. UK Prospective Diabetes Study Group: Tight blood pressure control and risk of macrovascular and microvascular complications in type 2 diabetes: UKPDS 38. BMJ 317:703–713, 1998.
96. UK Prospective Diabetes Study Group: Efficacy of captopril and atenolol in reducing risk of macrovascular and microvascular complications in type 2 diabetes: UKPDS 39. BMJ 317:713–720, 1998.
97. UK Prospective Diabetes Study Group: Cost effectiveness analysis of improved blood pressure control in hypertensive patients with type 2 diabetes: UKPDS 40. BMJ 317:720–726, 1998.
98. Estacio RO, Jeffers BW, Miatt WR, et al: The effect of nisoldipine as compared with enalapril on cardiovascular outcomes in patients with non–insulin-dependent diabetes and hypertension (ABCD trial). N Engl J Med 338:645–652, 1998.
99. Tatti P, Pahor M, Byington RP, et al: Outcome results of the fosinopril versus amlodipine cardiovascular events randomised trial (FACET) in patients with hypertension and NIDDM. Diabetes Care 21:597–603, 1998.
100. Hansson L, Zanchetti A, Carruthers SG, et al: Effects of intensive blood pressure lowering and low dose aspirin in patients with hypertension: Principal results of the Hypertension Optimal Treatment (HOT) randomised trial. Lancet 351:1755–1762, 1998.
101. Mogensen CE: Microalbuminuria, blood pressure and diabetic renal disease origin and development of ideas. Diabetologia 42:263–285, 1999.
102. Donaghy M: Diabetic proximal myopathy: Therapy and prognosis. Q J Med 79:287–288, 1991.
103. Krentz AJ: Acute symptomatic diabetic neuropathy associated with normalisation of haemoglobin A1. J R Soc Med 82:767–768, 1989.

Chapter 61

Diabetes Mellitus: Oculopathy

Ronald Klein

Retinopathy, a frequent complication of diabetes, is an important cause of blindness in the United States.[1] Recently completed clinical trials have demonstrated the efficacy of glycemic and blood pressure control in preventing the progression of retinopathy.[2–4] Clinical trials are in progress to evaluate newer therapeutic interventions such as protein kinase C and vascular endothelial growth factor (VEGF) inhibitors.

Surgical intervention with laser photocoagulation has been demonstrated to reduce loss of vision.[5, 6] This technique is usually reserved for advanced diabetic retinopathy, is costly and associated with complications, and may not restore or prevent loss of visual acuity in all cases. However, because it is the only treatment proven to reduce visual loss once vision-threatening retinopathy is present and because a significant number of diabetic people at risk for visual loss from vision-threatening retinopathy are not receiving such care, public health efforts have been directed at earlier detection and timely photocoagulation treatment of this condition.[7–11] The purpose of this chapter is to provide a better understanding of the natural history, pathogenesis, epidemiology, detection, and management of diabetic retinopathy.

RETINAL ANATOMY AND NATURAL HISTORY OF DIABETIC RETINOPATHY

Knowledge of normal retinal anatomy is important for an understanding of diabetic retinopathy. In brief, the inner part of the eye is lined by a thin, transparent neural tissue, the retina.[12] The retina consists of 10 well-defined layers (the nuclei of three sequential neurons, their axons and synaptic connections, and glial supporting cells). The inner two-thirds of the retina is fed by the central retinal artery, which branches into arterioles at the optic nerve head; the external third is supplied by the choriocapillaris of the choroid. A blood-retinal barrier composed of tight junctions of endothelial cells of the retinal blood vessels and tight junctions of the retinal pigment epithelial cells in the outer portion of the retina permits only a few important metabolic products into the retina.

The macular area is approximately 4 mm in diameter and is centered about 4 mm temporal to the optic disk. The fovea is 1.5 mm in diameter, and its central 450 to 600 μm is usually devoid of retinal capillaries. The central portion of the fovea (or foveola) contains only cone photoreceptors, which are important for spatial resolution (visual acuity) and trichromatic color vision. Occlusion of retinal capillaries or leakage of blood or lipoproteins with disruption of the extracellular space in the foveal area may result in a drop in visual acuity in people with diabetic retinopathy.

Natural History of Diabetic Retinopathy

Nonproliferative Retinopathy

The earliest clinically apparent changes of diabetic retinopathy, detected by ophthalmoscopy, are retinal microaneurysms.[13] These lesions usually appear as round red dots ranging in size from 20 to 200 μm and represent an outpouching of the retinal capillaries. They often appear first in the macular area in areas of capillary closure.

It is unusual to detect retinal microaneurysms within 3 years of the diagnosis of type 1 diabetes; however, they are often present at the time of diagnosis in people with type 2 diabetes.[14] Moreover, after 10 years of diabetes, 69% of people with type 1 diabetes and 55% of people with type 2 diabetes have microaneurysms present.[15, 16]

Retinal microaneurysms are not pathognomonic of diabetic retinopathy. They are associated with essential hypertension, retinal venous stasis caused by atherosclerotic carotid artery disease, AIDS, and a large number of other systemic and ocular conditions.[17] The appearance of a microaneurysm or two in only one eye of an older-onset diabetic person should not be regarded as specific for diabetic retinopathy. However, when larger numbers of microaneurysms are present (four or more in an eye or their presence in both eyes), they are more likely due to diabetes and the likelihood of progression to more severe nonproliferative retinopathy is greater.[18]

Microaneurysms have abnormal permeability to fluorescein, red blood cells, and lipoproteins.[13] By themselves, microaneurysms are not a threat to vision. However, as the disease progresses, hard exudates and retinal blot hemorrhages appear. The latter are round with blurred edges and result from extravasation of blood from retinal capillaries or microaneurysms into the inner nuclear layer of the retina (Fig. 61–1). Retinal blot hemorrhages usually disappear within 3 to 4 months.[19]

Retinal hard exudates are sharply defined, yellow, and variable in size; they may be aggregated, scattered, or "ringlike" in their distribution (see Fig. 61–1). Hard exudates result from leakage of lipoprotein material from retinal microaneurysms or capillaries into the outer retinal layer, and they may persist for months to years.[19] The exudate is usually found in the posterior layer of the retina, and if they extend into the foveal area, they usually reduce visual acuity.

With closure of the retinal capillaries and arterioles, whitish or grayish swellings appear in the nerve fiber layer of the retina. These changes, termed "cotton-wool spots" or "soft exudates," are microinfarcts of the nerve fiber layer (see Fig. 61–1). They may remain only a few weeks to months. After they disappear, the retina may appear normal on ophthalmoscopy, but fluorescein angiography reveals a corresponding area of nonperfusion of the retinal arterioles.

Dilated capillaries (intraretinal microvascular abnormalities [IRMAs]) are another manifestation of focal retinal ischemia. They

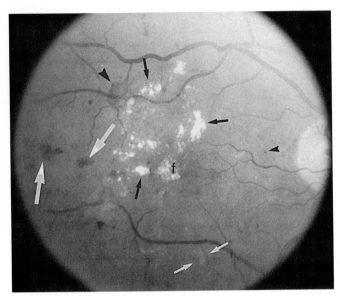

FIGURE 61–1. Fundus photograph of the right eye. A number of retinal microaneurysms *(small black arrowhead)* appear as small dark spots with sharp margins, and retinal blot hemorrhages *(large white arrows)* appear as dark spots of varying size with irregular margins and uneven densities. Retinal hard exudates appear as white deposits with sharp margins either scattered, "ringlike," or aggregated in their distributions *(small black arrows)* in the superior, temporal, and foveal (f) areas. A cotton-wool spot or soft exudate *(small white arrows)* appears as a grayish white area with ill-defined edges. A retinal new vessel superior and temporal to the fovea *(larger black arrowhead)* originates from a small retinal venule.

are found in areas of capillary nonperfusion and may be abnormally permeable to plasma proteins. IRMAs, large dark intraretinal hemorrhages, and venous beading and duplication may also appear secondary to retinal ischemia. These changes have been called the "preproliferative phase" and are a warning sign of the impending growth of new retinal vessels.

Severe ischemia may result from occlusion of larger arterioles in more extensive areas of the retinal midperiphery. Late in the course of the disease, thinly sheathed sclerotic (white "threadlike") arterioles may be present.

Proliferative Retinopathy

Proliferative diabetic retinopathy is characterized by the growth of abnormal new blood vessels and fibrous tissue from the inner retinal surface (usually near or from retinal veins) (see Fig. 61–1) or from the optic nerve head (Fig. 61–2). These vessels may be difficult to detect when they first appear as fine tufts on the surface of the retina or optic nerve head.[20] They consist of fine "naked" vessels that grow on the back surface of the vitreous. They are prone to hemorrhage into the vitreous, especially if the vitreous is in the process of contracting. In addition, the new vessels are often associated with fibrous tissue. If this fibrovascular tissue contracts, traction detachment of the retina may result. Fibrous tissue may remain as the only evidence of proliferative retinopathy if regression of new vessels occurs as a result of photocoagulation or naturally.

Diabetic Macular Edema, Ischemia, and Traction

Diabetes affects the macula in a number of ways. First, increased permeability of retinal capillaries and microaneurysms may result in the accumulation of extracellular fluid and thickening of the normally compact macular tissue. This phase may first appear as a slight loss of normal transparency of the retina. The edema is easy to miss, especially with direct ophthalmoscopy.

The edema is most often associated with the deposition of hard

exudative material in either rings, clumps, or large deposits. Accumulation of exudate is often gradual, and spontaneous resolution may occur in time. Severe long-standing leakage may result in the appearance of cystoid spaces in the outer portion of the retina in the foveal area. This abnormality is often associated with a profound drop in visual acuity.

According to results of the Early Treatment Diabetic Retinopathy Study (ETDRS), the location of the retinal thickening from edema fluid has prognostic implications for subsequent visual loss.[6] Clinically significant macular edema, which is associated with a 30% risk of visual loss over a 3-year period if left untreated with focal photocoagulation, has been defined as the presence of either of the following: thickening of the retina (or associated hard exudates) located 500 μm or less from the center of the macula or a zone of retinal thickening one disk area or larger in size located one disk diameter or less from the center of the macula (see Fig. 61–1).

The underlying cause of macular edema is not known. It may be a result of both increased leakage and impaired removal. Breakdown of the blood-retinal barrier has been postulated as an important cause of fluid accumulation in the macula.[13] Reduced osmotic pressure resulting from decreased serum albumin levels, increased intravascular fluid load, increased arterial perfusion pressure, and tissue hypoxia has been postulated to lead to breakdown of the blood-retinal barrier. The retinal pigment epithelium normally serves to "pump" fluid out of the sensory retina. However, this function is also postulated to be impaired in patients with hyperglycemia.

The macula may also be affected by closure of the perifoveal capillaries. Visual acuity usually decreases as a result.

Dragging or detachment of the macula because of shrinkage of fibrovascular tissue may also occur in people with proliferative diabetic retinopathy. This complication too can lead to profound visual loss.

PATHOGENESIS

The pathogenesis of diabetic retinopathy is not known. However, many mechanisms have been suggested and are summarized in Figure 61–3.[21] The development and progression of retinopathy are probably secondary to a complex interplay of a number of these factors, which vary from person to person. It is likely that different mechanisms are operative and more important at different stages of retinopathy. Glycosylation, the protein kinase C and polyol pathways, and increased retinal blood flow may be more important early in the course of the disease, before the development of microaneurysms. Angiogenesis factors such as VEGF and insulin-like growth factor-I are more likely to be important later in the course of the disease, before the

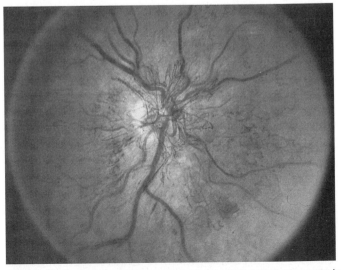

FIGURE 61–2. Fundus photograph demonstrating retinal new vessels on the optic nerve head. The retinal veins are also dilated.

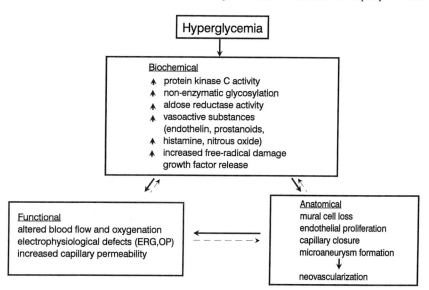

FIGURE 61–3. *Hypothesized pathogenetic mechanisms for the development and progression of diabetic retinopathy.*

development of proliferative retinopathy. In addition, interindividual and intraindividual variations in biochemical or physiologic responses to hyperglycemia (as a result of differences in genetic susceptibility) may exist among people at different stages of diabetes. This variability may explain why some diabetic patients have minimal retinopathy despite years of severe hyperglycemia whereas severe retinopathy develops in others over a shorter period despite relatively good glycemic control. Furthermore, because these pathogenetic factors have not usually been studied together in a prospective fashion, it is difficult to understand the antecedent-consequent relationship between them and retinopathy.

EPIDEMIOLOGY

Epidemiologic studies of diabetic retinopathy are useful in developing public health strategies to prevent or reduce the occurrence or progression of this complication. In addition, epidemiologic data concerning retinopathy, visual loss, and associated risk factors may be used in projecting costs, developing etiologic insight, designing future studies such as controlled clinical trials of treatment or prevention, and estimating the need for rehabilitative services.

One epidemiologic study that has provided data on diabetic retinopathy, visual loss, and associated risk factors is the Wisconsin Epidemiologic Study of Diabetic Retinopathy (WESDR). This population-based study has been described in detail.[14, 16, 22, 23] Data from other epidemiologic studies are also cited. Standardized examination protocols and questionnaires, photographic documentation, photographic standards for grading the severity of retinal lesions, and standardized retinopathy severity scales have permitted, in some cases, comparisons among studies.[24, 25]

Prevalence and Incidence of Retinopathy

The prevalence of retinopathy and clinically significant macular edema by age, gender, and diabetes group in the WESDR is presented in Table 61–1. The highest frequencies of retinopathy and proliferative retinopathy were found in the younger-onset group using insulin; the lowest frequencies were in the older-onset group not using insulin. Clinically significant macular edema was most frequent in the younger-onset group using insulin. The prevalence of retinopathy has been reported in other selected population-based studies.[24–46] Based on the WESDR data, it is estimated that in 1980 to 1982 approximately 700,000 people in the United States with diabetes had proliferative retinopathy, 130,000 of whom had Diabetic Retinopathy Study (DRS)

high-risk characteristics for severe visual loss of 5/200 or worse and 325,000 of whom had clinically significant macular edema.[15, 16]

In the WESDR, the highest incidence and rate of progression of retinopathy were found in the younger-onset group using insulin; the lowest incidence and rate of progression were found in the older-onset group not using insulin.[22, 23] Based on the WESDR data, it is estimated that approximately 63,000 new cases of proliferative diabetic retinopathy occurred nationwide, in 29,000 of whom proliferative retinopathy developed with DRS high-risk characteristics for severe visual loss. In addition, approximately 50,000 new cases of macular edema a year occurred in the United States.

Risk Factors for Diabetic Retinopathy

Gender, Race, Genetic, and Age

Few differences are found in the risk of development and progression of retinopathy in men and women with diabetes. However, differences among race/ethnic groups have been reported. Results from the study of Pima Indians with type 2 diabetes suggest that they are at increased risk for proliferative retinopathy in comparison to whites with type 2 diabetes.[45] After controlling for all measured risk factors, diabetic Mexican-Americans in San Antonio had a 2.4 times higher frequency of retinopathy than did diabetic non-Hispanic whites studied in the WESDR.[24] Similarly, Mexican-Americans with type 2 diabetes participating in the National Health and Nutrition Examination Survey III (NHANES III) had an 84% higher frequency of diabetic retinopathy than non-Hispanic whites did.[46] The higher frequency of retinopathy in Mexican-Americans than whites remained after controlling for the duration of diabetes, hemoglobin A_{1c} level, insulin and oral agent use, and hypertension in that study. However, Hamman et al. failed to find a difference in the frequency of retinopathy between Hispanics and non-Hispanic whites examined in the San Luis Valley study.[25] It has been suggested that blacks with type 2 diabetes may have more severe diabetic retinopathy and loss of vision than whites with type 2 diabetes.[47] In the NHANES III, the prevalence of diabetic retinopathy in people with type 2 diabetes was 46% higher in non-Hispanic blacks than non-Hispanic whites.[46] However, after adjustment for glycosylated hemoglobin, the duration of diabetes, insulin and oral agent use, and hypertension, the rates for retinopathy were similar between whites and blacks in that study.

Reports of a relationship between genetic factors and the prevalence of retinopathy have been inconsistent.[48–52] Supporting such a relationship has been the observation that the severity and onset of retinopathy are similar among concordant identical twins, which suggests that the tendency for the development of diabetic retinopathy and possibly its progression are influenced by genetic factors.[53] In addition, Hanis

TABLE 61-1. Prevalence and Severity of Retinopathy by Sex at the Baseline Examination in the Wisconsin Epidemiologic Study of Diabetic Retinopathy (1980-1982)

Retinopathy Status	Younger Onset, Taking Insulin			Older Onset, Taking Insulin			Older Onset, Not Taking Insulin		
	Male (%) (n = 512)	Female (%) (n = 484)	Total (%) (n = 996)	Male (%) (n = 321)	Female (%) (n = 352)	Total (%) (n = 673)	Male (%) (n = 313)	Female (%) (n = 379)	Total (%) (n = 692)
None	31.1	27.5	29.3	26.8	32.7	29.9	64.5	58.6	61.3
Early nonproliferative	26.4	34.7	30.4	34.0	27.6	30.6	25.9	28.5	27.3
Moderate to severe nonproliferative	18.2	16.9	17.6	27.7	23.9	25.7	6.4	10.3	8.5
Proliferative without DRS high-risk characteristics	12.3	14.0	13.2	8.1	9.9	9.1	1.9	1.1	1.4
Proliferative with DRS high-risk characteristics or worse	12.1	6.8	9.5	3.4	6.0	4.8	1.3	1.6	1.4

DRS, Diabetic Retinopathy Study.[8]

demonstrated an 8.3-fold increased risk of retinopathy in 46 Mexican-American siblings of probands who had retinopathy when compared with the siblings of those who did not.[54]

It is uncommon to find retinopathy in children younger than 10 years, regardless of the duration of type 1 diabetes; the frequency of any retinopathy or more severe retinopathy increases after age 13.[55–58] This age effect has been postulated to result from a protective effect lost after the start of puberty. In the WESDR, menarcheal status at the time of the baseline examination was associated with the prevalence of retinopathy.[59] After controlling for other factors such as diastolic blood pressure and duration of type 1 diabetes, those who were postmenarchal in the WESDR were 3.2 times more likely to have diabetic retinopathy than those who were premenarchal.

A number of changes occurring at puberty have been thought to explain the higher risk for retinopathy. These changes include increases in insulin-like growth factor-I, growth hormone, sex hormones, and blood pressure and poorer glycemic control. Increased insulin resistance, inadequate insulin dosage, and poorer compliance in attempts to control blood sugar may result in poorer glycemic control in postpubertal teenagers.[61–66]

Diabetes-Related Risk Factors

Duration of Diabetes

The prevalence of retinopathy (Fig. 61–4), macular edema, and proliferative retinopathy (Fig. 61–5) is significantly related to the duration of diabetes in all three diabetic groups studied in the WESDR. This observation is consistent with all previous epidemiologic studies.[26–38, 43, 46]

The relationship between the duration of diabetes at the baseline examination and the incidence, progression of nonproliferative retinopathy, or progression to proliferative retinopathy in the WESDR has been presented elsewhere.[22, 23] These findings are consistent with the prevalence data reported at baseline. In the younger-onset group, the incidence of retinopathy increased with increasing duration of diabetes. Even after 35 years of diabetes, the incidence of retinopathy was still high (64%).

In the WESDR, considerable differences were present among the diabetic groups studied. For example, within 3 years of the diagnosis of diabetes, retinopathy was less common (8%) and proliferative retinopathy or macular edema was not present in the younger-onset group, whereas retinopathy was more common (23%) and proliferative retinopathy (2%) and macular edema (3%) were present in the older-onset group not taking insulin. These findings are consistent with other

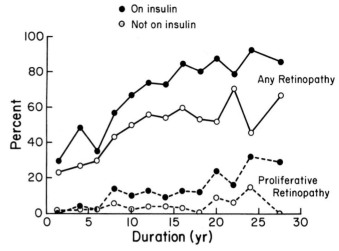

FIGURE 61–5. The frequency of retinopathy or proliferative retinopathy by duration of diabetes (years) in 673 people taking insulin and 697 people not taking insulin in whom diabetes was diagnosed when older than 29 years and who participated in the Wisconsin Epidemiologic Study of Diabetic Retinopathy (WESDR), 1980–1982. (From Klein R, Klein BEK, Moss SE, et al: The Wisconsin Epidemiologic Study of Diabetic Retinopathy. III. Prevalence and risk of diabetic retinopathy when age at diagnosis is 30 or more years. Arch Ophthalmol 102:527–532, Copyright 1984, American Medical Association.)

studies that have reported relatively high rates of retinopathy at the time of diagnosis of type 2 diabetes.[67, 68]

These findings have important public health implications. First, they suggest that younger-onset people have no need for ophthalmologic evaluation before puberty or before 5 years of diabetes because of lack of vision-threatening retinopathy (proliferative retinopathy or macular edema). For older-onset individuals, because the onset of diabetes may have been years before its diagnosis, it is important to have an ophthalmologic examination at diagnosis to detect possible proliferative retinopathy or macular edema. These findings have been used to develop guidelines recommending ophthalmologic care for patients with diabetes[69, 70] (Table 61–2).

Glycemia

A growing body of epidemiologic data have shown that hyperglycemia is related to the incidence and progression of diabetic retinopathy.[24, 27, 28, 30–32, 34, 35, 37, 38, 40–44, 46] In the WESDR, the glycosylated hemoglobin level at baseline was found to be a significant predictor of

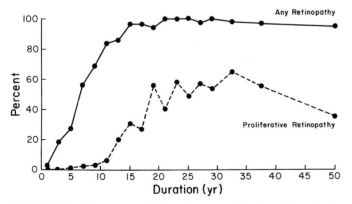

FIGURE 61–4. Frequency of retinopathy or proliferative retinopathy by duration of diabetes (years) in 996 insulin-taking persons in whom diabetes was diagnosed when younger than 30 years and who participated in the Wisconsin Epidemiologic Study of Diabetic Retinopathy (WESDR), 1980–1982. (From Klein R, Klein BEK, Moss SE, et al: The Wisconsin Epidemiologic Study of Diabetic Retinopathy. II. Prevalence and risk of diabetic retinopathy when age at diagnosis is less than 30 years. Arch Ophthalmol 102:520–526, Copyright 1984, American Medical Association.)

TABLE 61–2. Recommendations for Eye Care for Diabetic Patients

Primary-care physician informs the patient at the time of diagnosis of diabetes that
    Ocular complications are associated with diabetes and may threaten sight
    Timely detection and treatment may reduce the risk of decreased vision
Referral to an eye doctor competent in ophthalmoscopy:
    All patients 10–30 yr old who have had diabetes for 5 or more yr
    In patients in whom diabetes was diagnosed when older than 30 years, examination at the time of diagnosis or shortly thereafter
Referral to an ophthalmologist:
    All women with insulin-dependent diabetes mellitus planning pregnancy within 12 mo, in the first trimester, and thereafter at the discretion of the ophthalmologist
    Patients found to have reduced corrected visual acuity, elevated intraocular pressure, and any other vision-threatening ocular abnormalities

From Klein R, Klein BEK, Moss S: The Wisconsin Epidemiologic Study of Diabetic Retinopathy: A review. Diabetes Metab Rev 5:559–570, 1989.

the incidence of any retinopathy, progression, incidence of proliferative retinopathy, or incidence of macular edema in all three diabetic groups studied.[71, 72] These relationships remained after controlling for the duration of diabetes, retinopathy severity, and other risk factors measured at baseline.

Two important questions arise regarding the relationship between retinopathy and hyperglycemia: (1) is there a point of no return, a level of retinopathy at which improving control is no longer effective? (2) Does the relationship between the level of glycemia and the risk of retinopathy extend across the whole range of levels of glycemia, or must a threshold be reached? Our findings and those of others suggest that even in people with longer duration of diabetes, good glycemic control is more likely to be associated with lower rates of progression of retinopathy than poor glycemic control is.[40, 71–73] In addition, in the WESDR, no threshold level of glycemia, as measured by deciles of glycosylated hemoglobin at baseline, was seen below which retinopathy did not progress (Fig. 61–6).

The Diabetes Control and Complications Trial (DCCT) was a large randomized controlled clinical trial of more than 1400 patients with type 1 diabetes.[2] This multicentered trial showed that intensive insulin treatment reduced the development and progression of diabetic retinopathy. In the primary group in that study, those assigned to intensive glycemic control had a 60% reduction in three-step or greater progression of retinopathy than did the group assigned to conventional treatment. In the secondary intervention arm of the DCCT, those assigned to intensive glycemic control had a 34% reduction in the progression of retinopathy, a 47% reduction in the incidence of preproliferative or proliferative retinopathy, a 22% reduction in the incidence of macular edema, and a 54% reduction in laser photocoagulation treatment when compared with the group assigned to conventional insulin treatment.

The United Kingdom Prospective Diabetes Study (UKPDS) was a randomized controlled clinical trial involving 3867 patients with newly diagnosed type 2 diabetes.[3] After 3 months of diet treatment, patients with a mean of two fasting plasma glucose concentrations of 6.1 to 15.0 mmol/L were randomly assigned to an intensive glycemic control group with either a sulfonylurea (chlorpropamide, glibenclamide, or glipizide) or insulin or to a conventional glycemic control group with diet. After 10 years of follow-up, hemoglobin A_{1c} was 7.0% in the intensive group and 7.9% in the conventional group. When compared with the conventional group, the risk reduction for progression of diabetic retinopathy (defined as two or more steps on the ETDRS severity scale) over a 12-year period in the intensive group was 21%. In addition, a 29% reduction was noted in the need for retinal photocoagulation in the intensive vs. the conventional group. These data conclusively showed that intensive treatment with either sulfonylureas or insulin significantly reduced the risk of progression of retinopathy in persons with type 2 diabetes.

The DCCT and UKPDS results demonstrate a causal relationship between glycemic control and the risk of retinopathy, as well as other microvascular complications, and suggest that lowering blood sugar, even modestly, may significantly reduce the incidence of proliferative retinopathy or macular edema or the need for photocoagulation.[2, 3] However, reducing glycemic control is not without adverse affects. The DCCT found a 60% risk of weight gain and a 330% increased risk of severe hypoglycemic episodes in the intensive glycemic control group vs. the conventional group.[2]

Exogenous Insulin

Exogenous insulin has been suggested as a possible cause of retinopathy in people with type 2 diabetes.[74] In the WESDR, no association existed between the amount or type of exogenous insulin used and the incidence or progression of diabetic retinopathy in the older-onset group using insulin whose C peptide level was 0.3 nM or more.[75] These data suggest that exogenous insulin itself is not causally related to retinopathy in diabetic people with normal C peptide concentrations.

Other Risk Factors

Blood Pressure

Clinical studies suggest a possible relationship between elevated blood pressure and the presence of diabetic retinopathy.[76] High blood pressure, through an effect on blood flow, has been postulated to damage capillary endothelial cells, possibly contributing to the development or progression of retinopathy.[77] However, recent epidemiologic studies on the relationship of blood pressure to the incidence and progression of retinopathy have been conflicting.[24, 25, 27, 28, 30–32, 34, 37, 38, 40, 42, 43, 78–81] In persons with type 1 diabetes who participated in the WESDR, diastolic blood pressure was found to be a predictor of the 14-year progression of retinopathy and hypertension was a predictor of the 14-year incidence of proliferative retinopathy independent of glycosylated hemoglobin and the presence of gross proteinuria.[81] Data from the Eurodiab Controlled Trial of Lisinopril in Insulin-Dependent Diabetes Mellitus (EUCLID) study showed a 50% reduction in the progression of retinopathy, after adjustment for glycemic control, in nonhypertensive or mildly hypertensive persons in the lisinopril treatment group when compared with the placebo group.[82]

The UKPDS also sought to determine whether tight control of blood pressure with either a β-adrenergic blocker or an angiotensin-converting enzyme inhibitor was beneficial in reducing the macrovascular and microvascular complications associated with type 2 diabetes.[4] They randomized 1148 patients with hypertension (mean blood pressure, 160/94 mm Hg) to a regimen of tight control with either captopril or atenolol and another 390 patients to less tight control of their blood pressure. Tight blood pressure control resulted in a 35% reduction in retinal photocoagulation when compared with conventional control. After 7.5 years of follow-up, a 34% reduction in the rate of progression of retinopathy by two or more steps was noted when the modified ETDRS severity scale was used and a 47% reduction in the deterioration of visual acuity by three lines or more when the ETDRS charts were used (e.g., going from 20/20 to 20/40 or worse on a Snellen chart). The effect was largely due to a reduction in the incidence of diabetic macular edema. Atenolol and captopril were equally effective in reducing the risk of development of these microvascular complications. The effects of blood pressure control were independent of those of glycemic control. These findings strongly support tight blood pressure control in people with type 2 diabetes as a means of preventing visual loss resulting from the progression of diabetic retinopathy.

Regardless of whether blood pressure is a causal agent for the development or progression of diabetic retinopathy, it is imperative to measure and treat high blood pressure in diabetic patients because of the known association of high blood pressure with a higher risk of heart attack, stroke, and the development of diabetic nephropathy.[83–88]

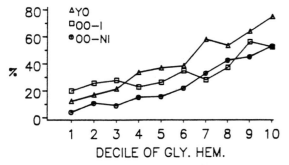

PROGRESSION OF RETINOPATHY

FIGURE 61–6. *Relationship of the 4-year progression of diabetic retinopathy to deciles of glycosylated hemoglobin at baseline examination in three diabetic groups participating in the Wisconsin Epidemiologic Study of Diabetic Retinopathy (WESDR).*

Serum Lipids

Epidemiologic data suggest a relationship between higher levels of lipids and the presence of retinopathy or the development of hard exudates.[25, 26, 30, 37, 89] The WESDR showed a significant trend toward increasing severity of diabetic retinopathy and retinal hard exudates with increasing cholesterol in the younger- and older-onset groups using insulin.[89] The ETDRS found a positive relationship between serum lipids (triglycerides, low-density lipoprotein cholesterol, and very-low-density lipoprotein cholesterol) and the development of hard exudates.[90] Although data from earlier clinical trials suggested a beneficial effect of clofibrate (Atromid-S, a lipid-lowering agent with significant hepatic toxicity) in reducing the presence of hard exudates, it did not lead to an improvement in vision.[91–92] Currently, controlled clinical trials are under way to investigate whether the use of statins in people with type 2 diabetes will reduce the incidence and progression of diabetic retinopathy.

Proteinuria and Renal Disease

Diabetic nephropathy may lead to lipid, platelet, and rheologic abnormalities, all of which have been hypothesized to be pathogenetic factors for the development of diabetic retinopathy.[93, 94] Therefore, it is not surprising that most epidemiologic studies have found a strong association between the presence and severity of diabetic retinopathy and microalbuminuria and gross proteinuria.[26, 30, 37, 41] These relationships are independent of blood pressure. In the WESDR, diabetic people with gross proteinuria had a higher risk of proliferative diabetic retinopathy; however, after controlling for the level of retinopathy at baseline, this relationship became weaker.[95]

Cigarette Smoking and Alcohol Consumption

Most data from epidemiologic studies have failed to confirm earlier reports of a positive relationship between cigarette smoking and diabetic retinopathy.[24, 25, 30, 34, 96] In the WESDR, cigarette smoking was not associated with the incidence or progression of diabetic retinopathy.[97] Regardless of the relationship with retinopathy, diabetic patients should be advised to not smoke because it is an important risk factor for respiratory and cardiovascular disease, as well as for cancer.[98, 99]

Few epidemiologic studies have investigated the relationship of alcohol consumption to diabetic retinopathy.[100–102] One might anticipate a possible protective effect of alcohol as a result of decreased platelet aggregation and adhesiveness.[103] Data from one study suggested a beneficial effect of alcohol, whereas data from another study suggested an increased risk of proliferative retinopathy in people with diabetes.[100, 101] In the WESDR, alcohol consumption was associated with a lower frequency of proliferative retinopathy in the younger-onset group.[102] However, no relationship was found between alcohol consumption at the 4-year examination and the incidence and progression of retinopathy in either the younger- or older-onset groups at the 10-year follow-up.[104]

Pregnancy

Epidemiologic studies suggest that pregnancy is a significant predictor of progression of diabetic retinopathy.[105] This finding is not unexpected because of the major physiologic changes associated with pregnancy that may increase the risk of progression of retinopathy. In a review of the literature, Rodman et al. reported that 8% of women with type 1 diabetes who had no or early nonproliferative retinopathy at the onset of pregnancy had progression of their retinopathy during pregnancy.[106] In a case-control study of women with type 1 diabetes, the frequency of progression to proliferative retinopathy was higher in those who were pregnant than those who were not (7.3% vs. 3.7%).[105] Women in this study were similar in age, duration of diabetes, and retinopathy status at the baseline examination. Pregnancy remained a significant predictor of the progression of diabetic retinopathy after controlling for glycosylated hemoglobin.

Severe retinopathy is also an indicator for a higher risk of congenital abnormalities in children born of mothers with type 1 diabetes.[107]

Comorbidity

In the WESDR, diabetic people with proliferative retinopathy are at higher risk for the development of diabetic nephropathy, heart attack,

stroke, and amputation than are those with minimal or no retinopathy present.[95] This observation is consistent with the association of severe retinopathy with cardiovascular disease risk factors such as increased fibrinogen, increased platelet aggregation, hyperglycemia, and hypertension.[89, 93, 94, 108, 109]

One important finding from the ETDRS suggests that when needed for the prevention of myocardial infarction or stroke, aspirin does not increase the risk of vitreous hemorrhage or visual loss in people with proliferative retinopathy.[110] Aspirin was also not found to prevent the progression of retinopathy in this study.

OTHER OCULAR DISEASE ASSOCIATED WITH DIABETES

Cataract

Cataract is a clouding or opacification of the normally clear crystalline lens of the eye. It is more common in people with diabetes than in those without diabetes.[111] In both the Health and Nutrition Examination Survey (HANES) and the Framingham Eye Study, diabetic participants younger than 65 years had a respective 3.0 and 4.0 increased risk of having a cataract when compared with similarly aged nondiabetic participants. After 65 years of age, this excess in the frequency of cataract remained only in the HANES population.

Lens opacities of any sort are often referred to as cataract despite the fact that different anatomic locations in the lens may be involved. People with diabetes appear to have differences in the frequency and severity of specific lens opacities. In the Beaver Dam Eye Study, after adjusting for age and sex, cortical opacities were significantly more common among people with older-onset diabetes than the rest of the Beaver Dam population.[112] Posterior subcapsular cataract was also more common in people with diabetes, but the increase was not significant in all age groups.

In the younger-onset group in the WESDR, the prevalence of cataract surgery and cataract was significantly related to older age at examination, longer duration of diabetes, diuretic usage, higher glycosylated hemoglobin concentration, and more severe diabetic retinopathy.[113] In the older-onset groups, the prevalence of cataract was associated with older age, diuretic usage, smoking, and more severe retinopathy. In the UKPDS, intensive glycemic control was associated with a significant reduction in cataract extraction when compared with those with conventional control.[3]

Glaucoma

Glaucoma is usually defined by the presence of characteristic visual field loss associated with damage to the retinal nerve fiber layer as a result of intraocular pressure higher than the eye can tolerate. Diabetes has been suggested as increasing the risk of glaucoma.[1] However, neither the Framingham Eye Study nor a study in Dalby, England, found a relationship between diabetes and glaucoma.[114, 115] In the WESDR, a history of glaucoma was more frequent in younger and older diabetic people than in the general population studied in the Health Interview Survey or in nondiabetic participants in the WESDR.[116–118] In the Beaver Dam Eye Study, after controlling for age and sex, diabetes was associated with an 84% increase in the risk of glaucoma.[114]

Visual Impairment

In the WESDR, people with diabetes had a higher age-specific prevalence of visual impairment (best-corrected visual acuity in the better eye of 20/40 or worse) than did the nondiabetic population in the Beaver Dam Eye Study (Fig. 61–7), as well as a higher age-specific prevalence of legal blindness (best-corrected visual acuity in the better eye of 20/200 or worse) than found in the general population in either the Framingham Eye Study or the HANES[119] (Fig. 61–8).

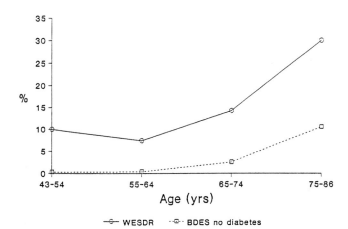

FIGURE 61–7. Visual impairment (best-corrected visual acuity in the better eye of 20/40 or worse) in those with diabetes participating in the Wisconsin Epidemiologic Study of Diabetic Retinopathy, 1980–1982, and in those without diabetes participating in the Beaver Dam Eye Study, 1988–1990.

For the younger-onset group using insulin, diabetic retinopathy was responsible for 86% of the visual loss; for the older-onset group it was responsible for 33% of the visual loss. Either cataract, glaucoma, or age-related macular degeneration was the sole or contributing cause of 49% of cases of legal blindness in the older-onset group.

In the WESDR, the 4-year incidence of visual impairment in the total population was 8.7%; for legal blindness it was 2.3%.[120] The annual incidence of blindness caused by diabetes was estimated to be 3.3 per 100,000 general population. The 4-year incidence of legal blindness was higher in the older-onset groups (3.2% in those using insulin and 2.7% in those not using insulin) than in the younger-onset group (1.5%).

DETECTION

Detection of diabetic retinopathy is best achieved by ophthalmoscopic examination through a dilated pupil by a retinal specialist or an experienced ophthalmologist with an interest in diabetic eye disease.[70] Stereoscopic color fundus photography increases the sensitivity of detection of vision-threatening retinopathy relative to ophthalmoscopy and is especially indicated when monitoring patients with signs of

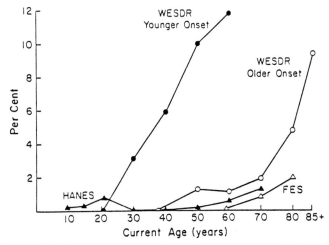

FIGURE 61–8. Percentage of persons with visual acuity of 20/200 or worse in the better eye in the Wisconsin Epidemiologic Study of Diabetic Retinopathy (WESDR), the Health and Nutrition Examination Survey (HANES), and the Framingham Eye Study (FES) by current age. (From Klein R, Klein BEK, Moss SE: Visual impairment in diabetes. Ophthalmology 91:1–9, 1984.)

preproliferative retinopathy, macular edema, or proliferative retinopathy.[121–123] Fluorescein angiography is generally used by retinal specialists before laser photocoagulation treatment of eyes with clinically significant macular edema to detect areas of retinal ischemia and leaking microaneurysms. Angiograms may occasionally be used to provide further information regarding the amount of ischemia and to demonstrate the cause of unexplained visual loss. However, fluorescein angiography is not routinely used at the time of diagnosis of diabetes or in diabetic patients with no or minimal nonproliferative retinopathy.

In the WESDR in 1980 to 1982 we found that 33% of people with either proliferative retinopathy with a high risk of severe visual loss or clinically significant macular edema had not seen an ophthalmologist within 2 years of the examination.[124] In addition, 51% of eyes with proliferative retinopathy had not been treated with panretinal photocoagulation.[125] Based on these data, we estimated that 35,000 Americans with vision-threatening retinopathy who might benefit from photocoagulation treatment had not received such treatment in 1980 to 1982. Little change was found when the group was re-examined,[126] and similar findings have also been reported by others.[127–129]

Many possible reasons may explain the high rate of patients with serious retinopathy who are either not under the care of an ophthalmologist or have not received photocoagulation treatment. Physician-related factors that explain this low rate of treatment include a lack of knowledge about the benefits of photocoagulation treatment,[127] poor ophthalmoscopy skills,[20] ophthalmoscopy through an undilated pupil,[130] and no or inadequate referral to ophthalmologists.[131] A number of patient-related factors may also explain failure to receive ophthalmologic care,[132, 133] including the asymptomatic nature of vision-threatening retinopathy,[134] lack of knowledge about the benefits of timely detection by dilated eye examination and treatment with photocoagulation,[135] denial or a lack of motivation, an inability to afford ophthalmologic care,[136] lack of available or accessible ophthalmologic care,[137] or lack of time to go for such care.

Guidelines for the detection and management of diabetic eye disease have been developed and distributed.[70] However, studies have suggested that these referral guidelines for diabetic retinopathy are not being sufficiently followed.[7, 128, 129, 135] For this reason, new programs have been suggested. One such program is to screen people with diabetes who are not currently receiving eye care.[8] Cost-effectiveness studies using the WESDR data suggest that earlier detection of proliferative retinopathy by ophthalmologic or photographic screening is a cost-effective approach for diabetic people requiring insulin.[138–141]

MANAGEMENT
Medical

Glycemic control in patients with type 1 and 2 diabetes and blood pressure control in persons with type 2 diabetes have been shown to prevent the incidence or progression of retinopathy in people with diabetes.[2–4] However, intensive glycemic control may be difficult to achieve with current methods of administration of insulin. Strict glycemic control is associated with an increased frequency of severe complications.[2] Data from the WESDR suggest that reduction of hyperglycemia in persons with type 1 but not type 2 diabetes may be occurring.[142] This drop in persons with type 1 diabetes may be associated with changes in management between the baseline and follow-up examinations, such as an increased frequency of two or more insulin injections a day and initiation of blood glucose self-monitoring. Currently, new interventions (e.g., protein kinase C inhibitors, VEGF inhibitors, vitamin E) to prevent the progression of retinopathy are under study.

Little improvement in glycemic control has been achieved over a 10-year period in the WESDR (1980–1982 through 1990–1992).[142] Results from the UKPDS and the availability of new oral hypoglycemic agents for persons with type 2 diabetes may alter this lack of improvement.

Surgical

In the DRS, panretinal photocoagulation resulted in a 50% reduction in severe loss of vision (to 5/200 or worse) in eyes with proliferative retinopathy and high-risk characteristics.[5] Data from the ETDRS suggest that initiation of such treatment, at the earliest stages of proliferative retinopathy with high-risk characteristics, might lead to a reduction of 90% in severe visual loss.[143] Furthermore, the ETDRS demonstrated that focal laser photocoagulation of clinically significant macular edema reduced visual loss, as measured by doubling of the visual angle, by 50% in comparison to withholding such treatment.[6]

Vitrectomy is a procedure that usually requires hospitalization and is often performed under general anesthesia by a skilled vitreoretinal surgeon. Because the surgery is generally elective, preoperative evaluation requires a thorough examination to diagnose and control the numerous medical problems (cardiovascular, renal, and metabolic) often found in such patients.

Open-angle glaucoma is usually managed with either pressure-lowering drops, acetazolamide (Diamox), laser treatment of the trabecular meshwork, and/or trabeculectomy. β-Blockers are frequently used to reduce intraocular pressure. These agents may have cardiovascular and respiratory side effects.

Rubeotic glaucoma, in which retinal ischemia leads to neovascularization of the anterior chamber angle of the eye, is less successfully treated than open-angle glaucoma. Such eyes are often painful and are at very high risk of severe loss of vision or enucleation.

REHABILITATION

Diabetic patients with severe visual impairment are confronted with difficulties in glucose monitoring, insulin administration, and monitoring of systemic changes in the skin such as foot ulcers. In addition, these patients are often ill with renal disease, cardiovascular disease, or amputations. Many have lost their jobs and health insurance and are without adequate financial support. These problems may lead to anger, anxiety, loss of self-esteem, and difficulties in social adjustment.[144, 145] Primary care physicians should be actively involved in a team including psychologists, orientation and mobility instructors, rehabilitation teachers, and social workers to deal with the problems faced by visually impaired diabetic patients. Such support facilitates acceptance of visual loss, development of coping strategies, and planning of living arrangements.

REFERENCES

1. Klein R, Klein BEK: Vision disorders in diabetes. *In* Harris MWH (ed): Diabetes in America, ed 2. Bethesda, MD, US Public Health Service, NIH-NIDDK Publication No. 95–1468, 1995, pp 293–338.
2. The Diabetes Control and Complications Trial Research Group: The effect of intensive treatment of diabetes on the development and progression of long-term complications in insulin-dependent diabetes mellitus. N Engl J Med 329:977–986, 1993.
3. UK Prospective Diabetes Study Group: Intensive blood glucose control with sulphonylurea or insulin compared with conventional treatment and risk of complications in patients with type 2 diabetes. UKPDS 33. Lancet 352:837–853, 1998.
4. UK Prospective Diabetes Study Group: Tight blood pressure control and risk of macrovascular and microvascular complications in type 2 diabetes. UKPDS 38. BMJ 317:703–713, 1998.
5. The Diabetic Retinopathy Study Research Group: Photocoagulation treatment of proliferative diabetic retinopathy: Clinical application of Diabetic Retinopathy Study (DRS) findings: DRS Report No. 8. Ophthalmology 88:583–600, 1981.
6. ETDRS Research Group: Photocoagulation for diabetic macular edema. Arch Ophthalmol 103:1796–1806, 1985.
7. Witkin SR, Klein R: Ophthalmologic care for persons with diabetes. JAMA 251:2534–2537, 1984.
8. Klein R, Moss SE, Klein BEK: New management concepts for the timely diagnosis of diabetic retinopathy treatable by photocoagulation. Diabetes Care 10:633–638, 1987.
9. National Eye Institute National Eye Health Education Program: From Vision Research to Eye Health Education: Planning the Partnership. March, 1990. Available from NIH, Box 20/20, Bethesda, MD 20892.
10. Smith RE, Patz A: Diabetes 2000—closing the gap (editorial). Ophthalmology 97:153–154, 1990.
11. Herman WH, Teutsch SM, Sepe SJ, et al: An approach to the prevention of blindness in diabetes. Diabetes Care 6:608–613, 1983.
12. Hogan MJ, Alvarado JA, Weddell JE: Histology of the Human Eye. An Atlas and Textbook. Philadelphia, WB Saunders, 1971.
13. Bresnick GH: Diabetic Retinopathy. *In* Peyman GA, Sanders DR, Goldberg MF (eds): Principles and Practice of Ophthalmology. Philadelphia, WB Saunders, 1977.
14. Klein R, Klein BEK, Moss SE, et al: Prevalence of diabetes mellitus in southern Wisconsin. Am J Epidemiol 119:54–61, 1984.
15. Klein R, Klein BEK, Moss SE, et al: The Wisconsin Epidemiologic Study of Diabetic Retinopathy: II. Prevalence and risk of diabetic retinopathy when age at diagnosis is less than 30 years. Arch Ophthalmol 102:520–526, 1984.
16. Klein R, Klein BEK, Moss SE, et al: The Wisconsin Epidemiologic Study of Diabetic Retinopathy: III. Prevalence and risk of diabetic retinopathy when age at diagnosis is 30 or more years. Arch Ophthalmol 102:527–532, 1984.
17. Gass JDM: Stereoscopic Atlas of Macular Diseases, ed 3. St Louis, Mosby, 1987.
18. Klein R, Meuer SM, Moss SE, et al: The relationship of retinal microaneurysm counts to the 4-year progression of diabetic retinopathy. Arch Ophthalmol 107:1780–1785, 1989.
19. Dobree JH: Simple diabetic retinopathy: Evolution of the lesions and therapeutic considerations. Br J Ophthalmol 54:1–10, 1970.
20. Sussman EJ, Tsiaras WG, Soper KA: Diagnosis of diabetic eye disease. JAMA 247:3231–3234, 1982.
21. Klein R, Klein BEK: Diabetic eye disease. Lancet 350:197–204, 1997.
22. Klein R, Klein BEK, Moss SE, et al: The Wisconsin Epidemiologic Study of Diabetic Retinopathy: IX. Four-year incidence and progression of diabetic retinopathy when age at diagnosis is less than 30 years. Arch Ophthalmol 107:237–243, 1989.
23. Klein R, Klein BEK, Moss SE, et al: The Wisconsin Epidemiologic Study of Diabetic Retinopathy: X. Four-year incidence and progression of diabetic retinopathy when age at diagnosis is 30 years or more. Arch Ophthalmol 107:244–249, 1989.
24. Haffner SM, Fong D, Stern MP, et al: Diabetic retinopathy in Mexican-Americans and non-Hispanic whites. Diabetes 37:878–884, 1988.
25. Hamman RF, Mayer EJ, Moo-Young GA, et al: Prevalence and risk factors of diabetic retinopathy in non-Hispanic whites and Hispanics with NIDDM: San Luis Valley Diabetes Study. Diabetes 38:1231–1237, 1989.
26. Nielsen NV: Diabetic retinopathy: II. The course of retinopathy in diabetics treated with oral hypoglycaemic agents and diet regime alone: A one year epidemiologic cohort study of diabetes mellitus: The Island of Falster, Denmark. Acta Ophthalmol 62:266–273, 1984.
27. Dorf A, Ballintine EJ, Bennett PH, et al: Retinopathy in Pima Indians: Relationships to glucose level, duration of diabetes, age at diagnosis of diabetes, and age at examination in a population with a high prevalence of diabetes mellitus. Diabetes 25:554–560, 1976.
28. Bennett PH, Rushforth NB, Miller M, et al: Epidemiologic studies of diabetes in the Pima Indians. Recent Prog Horm Res 32:333–376, 1976.
29. Kahn HA, Leibowitz HM, Ganley JP, et al: The Framingham Eye Study: I. Outline and major prevalence findings. Am J Epidemiol 106:17–32, 1977.
30. West KM, Erdreich LJ, Stober JA: A detailed study of risk factors for retinopathy and nephropathy in diabetes. Diabetes 19:501–508, 1980.
31. Houston A: Retinopathy in the Poole area: An epidemiologic inquiry. *In* Eschwege E (ed): Advances in Diabetes Epidemiology. INSERM Symposium No. 22. Amsterdam, Elsevier, 1982, pp 199–206.
32. King H, Balkau B, Zimmet P, et al: Diabetic retinopathy in Nauruans. Am J Epidemiol 117:659–667, 1983.
33. Dwyer MS, Melton LJ, Ballard DJ, et al: Incidence of diabetic retinopathy and blindness: A population-based study in Rochester, Minnesota. Diabetes Care 8:316–322, 1985.
34. Ballard DJ, Melton LJ, Dwyer MS, et al: Risk factors for diabetic retinopathy: A population-based study in Rochester, Minnesota. Diabetes Care 9:334–342, 1986.
35. Danielsen R, Jonasson F, Helgason T: Prevalence of retinopathy and proteinuria in type I diabetics in Iceland. Acta Med Scand 212:277–280, 1982.
36. Constable IJ, Knuiman MW, Welborn TA, et al: Assessing the risk of diabetic retinopathy. Am J Ophthalmol 97:53–61, 1984.
37. Knuiman MW, Welborn TA, McCann VJ, et al: Prevalence of diabetic complications in relation to risk factors. Diabetes 35:1332–1339, 1986.
38. Sjolie AK: Ocular complications in insulin treated diabetes mellitus: An epidemiological study. Acta Ophthalmol Suppl 172:1–72, 1985.
39. Nielsen NV: Diabetic retinopathy: I. The course of retinopathy in insulin-treated diabetics: A one-year epidemiological cohort study of diabetes mellitus: The island of Falster, Denmark. Acta Ophthalmol 62:256–265, 1984.
40. Teuscher A, Schnell H, Wilson PWF: Incidence of diabetic retinopathy and relationship to baseline plasma glucose and blood pressure. Diabetes Care 11:246–251, 1988.
41. Jerneld B: Prevalence of diabetic retinopathy. Acta Ophthalmol Scand Suppl 188:3–32, 1988.
42. McLeod BK, Thompson JR, Rosenthal AR: The prevalence of retinopathy in the insulin-requiring diabetic patients of an English county town. Eye 2:424–430, 1988.
43. Kostraba JN, Klein R, Dorman JS, et al: The Epidemiology of Diabetes Complications Study: IV. Correlates of diabetic background and proliferative retinopathy. Am J Epidemiol 133:381–391, 1991.
44. Fujimoto W, Fukuda M: Natural history of diabetic retinopathy and its treatment in Japan. *In* Baba S, Goto Y, Fukui I (eds): Diabetes Mellitus in Asia. Amsterdam, Excerpta Medica, 1976, pp 225–231.
45. Nelson RG, Wolfe JA, Horton MB, et al: Proliferative retinopathy in NIDDM: Incidence and risk factors in Pima Indians. Diabetes 38:435–440, 1989.
46. Harris MI, Klein R, Cowie CC, et al: Is the risk of diabetic retinopathy greater in non Hispanic blacks and Mexican Americans than in non-Hispanic whites with type 2 diabetes? A U.S. population study. Diabetes Care 21:1230–1235, 1998.
47. Rabb MF, Gagliano DA, Sweeny NE: Diabetic retinopathy in blacks. Diabetes Care 13:1202–1206, 1990.
48. Barbosa J, Ramsay RC, Knobloch WH, et al: Histocompatibility antigen frequencies in diabetic retinopathy. Am J Ophthalmol 90:148–153, 1980.
49. Dornan TL, Ting A, McPherson CK, et al: Genetic susceptibility to the development of retinopathy in insulin-dependent diabetics. Diabetes 31:226–231, 1982.
50. Rand LT, Krolewski AS, Aiello LM, et al: Multiple factors in the prediction of risk of proliferative diabetic retinopathy. N Engl J Med 113:1433–1438, 1985.
51. Jervell J, Solheim B: HLA-antigens in long standing insulin dependent diabetics with terminal nephropathy and retinopathy with and without loss of vision. Diabetologia 17:391, 1979.

52. Cruickshanks KJ, Vadheim CM, Moss SE, et al: Genetic marker associations with proliferative retinopathy in persons diagnosed with diabetes prior to 30 years of age. Diabetes 41:879–885, 1992.

53. Leslie RDG, Pyke DA: Diabetic retinopathy in identical twins. Diabetes 31:19–21, 1982.

54. Hanis CL: Genetics of non–insulin-dependent diabetes mellitus among Mexican Americans: Approaches and perspectives. In Berg K, Boulyjenkov V, Christen Y (eds): Genetic Approaches to Noncommunicable Diseases. Berlin, Springer-Verlag, 1996, pp 65–77.

55. Knowles HC Jr, Guest GM, Lampe J, et al: The course of juvenile diabetes treated with unmeasured diet. Diabetes 14:239–273, 1965.

56. Frank RN, Hoffman WH, Podgor MJ, et al: Retinopathy in juvenile-onset type I diabetes of short duration. Diabetes 31:874–882, 1982.

57. Palmberg P, Smith M, Waltman S, et al: The natural history of retinopathy in insulin-dependent juvenile-onset diabetes. Ophthalmology 88:613–618, 1981.

58. Klein R, Klein BEK, Moss SE, et al: Retinopathy in young-onset diabetic patients. Diabetes Care 8:311–315, 1985.

59. Klein BEK, Moss SE, Klein R: Is menarche associated with diabetic retinopathy. Diabetes Care 13:1034–1038, 1990.

60. Dills DG, Moss SE, Klein R, et al: Is insulin-like growth factor I associated with diabetic retinopathy? Diabetes 39:191–195, 1990.

61. Peters GFFM, Smals AGH, Kloppenborg PWC: Defective suppression of growth hormone after glucose loading in adolescence. J Clin Endocrinol Metab 51:265–270, 1980.

62. Klein R, Klein BEK, Moss SE, et al: Blood pressure and hypertension in diabetes. Am J Epidemiol 122:75–89, 1985.

63. Blethen SL, Sargeant DT, Whitlow MG, et al: Effect of pubertal stage and recent blood glucose control on plasma somatomedin C in children with insulin-dependent diabetes mellitus. Diabetes 30:868–872, 1981.

64. Allen C, Zaccaro DJ, Palta M, et al: Glycemic control in the first two years of insulin-dependent diabetes mellitus. Diabetes Care 15:980–987, 1992.

65. Sizonenko P: Endocrinology in preadolescents and adolescents: I. Hormonal changes during normal puberty. Am J Dis Child 132:704–712, 1978.

66. Haffner SM, Klein R, Dunn JF, et al: Increased testosterone in type I diabetic subjects with severe retinopathy. Ophthalmology 97:1270–1274, 1990.

67. Klein R, Klein BEK, Moss SE, et al: The Beaver Dam Eye Study: Retinopathy in adults with newly discovered and previously diagnosed diabetes mellitus. Ophthalmology 99:58–62, 1992.

68. UK Prospective Diabetes Study 6: Complications in newly diagnosed type 2 diabetic patients and their association with different clinical and biochemical risk factors. Diabetes Res 13:1–11, 1990.

69. The Kentucky Diabetic Retinopathy Group: Guidelines for eye care in patients with diabetes mellitus. Arch Intern Med 149:769–770, 1989.

70. American Diabetes Association: Diabetic retinopathy. Diabetes Care 21:157–159, 1988.

71. Klein R, Klein BEK, Moss SE, et al: Glycosylated hemoglobin predicts the incidence and progression of diabetic retinopathy. JAMA 260:2864–2871, 1988.

72. Klein R, Klein BEK, Moss SE, et al: Relationship of hyperglycemia to the long-term incidence and progression of diabetic retinopathy. Arch Intern Med 154:2169–2178, 1994.

73. Chase HP, Jackson WE, Hoops SL, et al: Glucose control and the renal and retinal complications of insulin-dependent diabetes. JAMA 261:1155–1160, 1989.

74. Serghieri G, Bartolomei G, Pettenello C, et al: Raised retinopathy prevalence rate in insulin-treated patients: A feature of obese type II diabetes. Transplant Proc 18:1576–1577, 1986.

75. Klein R, Klein BEK, Moss SE: The Wisconsin Epidemiologic Study of Diabetic Retinopathy. XVI. The relationship of C-peptide to the incidence and progression of diabetic retinopathy. Diabetes 44:796–801, 1995.

76. Davis MD: Diabetic retinopathy, diabetic control and blood pressure. Transplant Proc 18:1565–1568, 1986.

77. Kohner EM: Diabetic retinopathy. Br Med Bull 45:148–173, 1989.

78. Knowler WC, Bennett PH, Ballintine EJ: Increased incidence of retinopathy in diabetics with elevated blood pressure: A six-year follow-up study in Pima Indians. N Engl J Med 302:645–650, 1980.

79. Kohner EM, Fraser TR, Joplin GF, et al: The effect of diabetic control on diabetic retinopathy. In Goldberg MF, Fine SL (eds): Treatment of Diabetic Retinopathy. Washington, DC, US Public Health Service Publication No. 1890, 1969, pp 119–128.

80. Klein R, Klein BEK, Moss SE, et al: Is blood pressure a predictor of the incidence or progression of diabetic retinopathy? Arch Intern Med 149:2427–2432, 1989.

81. Klein R, Klein BEK, Moss SE, et al: The Wisconsin Epidemiologic Study of Diabetic Retinopathy. XVII. The 14-year incidence and progression of diabetic retinopathy and associated risk factors in type 1 diabetes. Ophthalmology 105:1801–1815, 1998.

82. Chaturvedi N, Sjolie AK, Stephenson JM, et al: Effect of lisinopril on progression of retinopathy in normotensive people with type 1 diabetes. The EUCLID Study group. EURODIAB Controlled Trial of Lisinopril in Insulin-Dependent Diabetes Mellitus. Lancet 351:28–31, 1998.

83. Fuller JH, Shipley MJ, Rose G, et al: Coronary heart disease and stroke mortality by degree of glycaemia: The Whitehall study. BMJ 287:867–870, 1983.

84. Jarrett RJ, McCarthy P, Keen H: The Bedford Survey: Ten-year mortality rates in newly diagnosed diabetics, borderline diabetics and normoglycaemic controls and risk indices for coronary heart disease in borderline diabetics. Diabetologia 22:79–84, 1982.

85. Palumbo PJ, Elyeback LR, Whishnaut JP: Neurologic complications of diabetes mellitus: Transient ischaemic attack, stroke, and peripheral neuropathy. Adv Neurol 19:593–601, 1978.

86. Asplund K, Hagg E, Helmers C, et al: The natural history of stroke in diabetic patients. Acta Med Scand 207:417–424, 1980.

87. Mogensen CE: Long-term antihypertensive treatment inhibiting the progression of diabetic neuropathy. Acta Endocrinol 242(suppl):31–32, 1981.

88. Parving HH, Andersen AR, Hommel E, Smidt UM: Effects of long-term anti-hypertensive treatment on kidney function in diabetic nephropathy. Hypertension 35(suppl 2):114–117, 1985.

89. Klein BEK, Moss SE, Klein R, et al: The Wisconsin Epidemiologic Study of Diabetic Retinopathy: XIII. Relationship of serum cholesterol to retinopathy and hard exudate. Ophthalmology 98:1261–1265, 1991.

90. Chew EY, Klein ML, Ferris FL 3rd, et al: Association of elevated serum lipid levels with retinal hard exudate in diabetic retinopathy. Early Treatment Diabetic Retinopathy Study (ETDRS) Report 22. Arch Ophthalmol 114:1079–1084, 1996.

91. Cullen JF, Ireland JT, Oliver MF: A controlled trial of atromid therapy in exudative diabetic retinopathy. Trans Soc Ophthalmol U K 84:281–355, 1964.

92. Duncan LJ, Cullen JF, Ireland JT, et al: A three-year trial of atromid therapy in exudative diabetic retinopathy. Diabetes 17:458–467, 1968.

93. Borch-Johnsen K, Kreiner S: Proteinuria: Value as a predictor of cardiovascular mortality in insulin dependent diabetes mellitus. BMJ 294:1651–1654, 1987.

94. Winocour PH, Durrington PN, Ishola M, et al: Influence of proteinuria on vascular disease, blood pressure, and lipoproteins in insulin dependent diabetes mellitus. BMJ 294:1648–1651, 1987.

95. Klein R, Klein BEK, Moss SE: The epidemiology of proliferative diabetic retinopathy. Diabetes Care 15:1875–1891, 1992.

96. Klein R, Klein BEK, Davis MD: Is cigarette smoking associated with diabetic retinopathy? Am J Epidemiol 118:228–238, 1983.

97. Moss SE, Klein R, Klein BEK: Association of cigarette smoking with diabetic retinopathy. Diabetes Care 14:119–126, 1991.

98. The Health Consequences of Smoking. A Report to the Surgeon General. Washington, DC, US Department of Health, Education and Welfare. Publication HSM 71–7513, 1971.

99. Doyle JT: Risk factors in arteriosclerosis and cardiovascular disease with special emphasis on cigarette smoking. Prev Med 8:264–270, 1979.

100. Kingsley LA, Dorman JS, Doft BH, et al: An epidemiologic approach to the study of retinopathy: The Pittsburgh Diabetic Morbidity and Retinopathy Studies. Diabetes Res Clin Pract 4:99–109, 1988.

101. Young RJ, McCulloch DK, Prescott RJ, et al: Alcohol: Another risk factor for diabetic retinopathy? BMJ 288:1035–1037, 1984.

102. Moss SE, Klein R, Klein BEK: Alcohol consumption and the prevalence of diabetic retinopathy. Ophthalmology 99:926–932, 1992.

103. Jakubowski JA, Vaillancourt R, Deykin D: Interaction of ethanol, prostacyclin, and aspirin in determining human platelet activity in vitro. Arteriosclerosis 8:436–441, 1988.

104. Moss SE, Klein R, Klein BEK: The association of alcohol consumption with the incidence and progression of diabetic retinopathy. Ophthalmology 101:1962–1968, 1994.

105. Klein BEK, Moss SE, Klein R: Effect of pregnancy on progression of diabetic retinopathy. Diabetes Care 13:34–40, 1990.

106. Rodman HM, Singerman LJ, Aiello LM, et al: Diabetic retinopathy and its relationship to pregnancy. In Merkatz ER, Adams PAJ (eds): The Diabetic Pregnancy: A Perinatal Perspective. New York, Grune & Stratton, 1979.

107. Klein BEK, Klein R, Meuer SM, et al: Does the severity of diabetic retinopathy predict pregnancy outcome? J Diabetes Complications 2:179–184, 1988.

108. Dornan TL, Carter RD, Bron AJ, et al: Low density lipoprotein cholesterol: An association with the severity of diabetic retinopathy. Diabetologia 22:167–170, 1982.

109. Miccoli R, Odello G, Giampietro O, et al: Circulating lipid levels and severity of diabetic retinopathy in type I diabetes mellitus. Ophthalmic Res 19:52–56, 1987.

110. Early Treatment Diabetic Retinopathy Study Research Group: Effects of aspirin treatment on diabetic retinopathy. ETDRS report number 8. Ophthalmology 98:757–765, 1991.

111. Ederer F, Hiller R, Taylor H: Senile lens changes and diabetes in two population studies. Am J Ophthalmol 91:381–395, 1981.

112. Klein BEK, Klein R, Wang Q, et al: Older-onset diabetes and lens opacities. The Beaver Dam Eye Study. Ophthalmic Epidemiol 2:49–55, 1995.

113. Klein BEK, Klein R, Moss SE: Prevalence of cataracts in a population-based study of persons with diabetes mellitus. Ophthalmology 92:1191–1196, 1985.

114. Kahn HA, Leibowitz HM, Ganley JP, et al: The Framingham Eye Study: II. Association of ophthalmic pathology with single variables previously measured in the Framingham Heart Study. Am J Epidemiol 106:33–41, 1977.

115. Bengtsson B: Aspects of the epidemiology of chronic glaucoma. Acta Ophthalmol Suppl 146:4–26, 1981.

116. Klein BEK, Klein R, Moss SE: Intraocular pressure in diabetic persons. Ophthalmology 91:1356–1360, 1984.

117. Klein BEK, Klein R, Jensen SC: Open angle glaucoma and older onset diabetes. The Beaver Dam Eye Study. Ophthalmology 101:1173–1177, 1994.

118. Howie LJ, Drury IF: Current estimates from the Health Interview Survey, 1988. Vital Health Stat 126(10):1–98, 1988.

119. Klein R, Klein BEK, Moss SE: Visual impairment in diabetes. Ophthalmology 91:1–9, 1984.

120. Moss SE, Klein R, Klein BEK: The incidence of vision loss in a diabetic population. Ophthalmology 95:1340–1348, 1988.

121. Pugh JA, Jacobsen JM, Van Heuven WAJ, et al: Screening for diabetic retinopathy: The wide angle retina camera. Diabetes Care 16:889–895, 1993.

122. Nathan DM, Fogel HA, Godine JE, et al: Role of the diabetologist in evaluating diabetic retinopathy. Diabetes Care 14:26–33, 1991.

123. Klein R, Klein BEK, Neider MW, et al: Diabetic retinopathy as detected using ophthalmoscopy, a nonmydriatic camera and a standard fundus camera. Ophthalmology 92:485–491, 1985.

124. Klein R, Klein BEK, Moss SE: The Wisconsin Epidemiological Study of Diabetic Retinopathy: A review. Diabetes Metab Rev 5:559–570, 1989.

125. Klein R, Klein BEK, Moss SE, et al: The Wisconsin Epidemiologic Study of Diabetic Retinopathy: VI. Retinal photocoagulation. Ophthalmology 94:747–753, 1987.

126. Klein R, Moss SE, Klein BEK, et al: The Wisconsin Epidemiologic Study of Diabetic Retinopathy: VIII: The incidence of retinal photocoagulation. J Diabetes Complications 2:79–87, 1988.

127. Stross JK, Harlan WR: The dissemination of new medical information. JAMA 741:2622–2624, 1979.

128. Sprafka JM, Fritsche TL, Baker R, et al: Prevalence of undiagnosed eye disease in high-risk diabetic individuals. Arch Intern Med 150:857–861, 1990.

129. Brechner RJ, Cowie CC, Howie LJ, et al: Ophthalmic examination among adults with diagnosed diabetes mellitus. JAMA 270:1714–1718, 1993.

130. Herman WH: Public health strategies: Program development, implementation and evaluation. *In* Proceedings of the 8th Annual Centers for Disease Control Conference. Atlanta, GA, 1985.

131. Payne TH, Gabella BA, Michael SL, et al: Preventive care in diabetes mellitus: Current practice in urban health-care system. Diabetes Care 12:745–747, 1989.

132. Newcomb PA, Klein R: Factors associated with compliance following diabetic eye screening. J Diabetes Complications 4:8–14, 1990.

133. Moss SE, Klein R, Klein BEK: Factors associated with having eye examinations in persons with diabetes. Arch Fam Med 4:529–534, 1995.

134. Klein R, Klein BEK, Moss SE, et al: The validity of a survey question to study diabetic retinopathy. Am J Epidemiol 124:104–110, 1986.

135. Hess RG, Lengyel MC, Hess GE, et al: Diabetes in Communities. Ann Arbor, University of Michigan, 1986.

136. Marnell NM: A Descriptive Analysis of Health Practices and Beliefs Related to Eye Diseases: Diabetic Retinopathy Health Care Delivery Screening Compliance Review (master's thesis). Atlanta, University of Georgia, 1988, pp 1–97.

137. Frey M, Teza S, Bowbeer L, et al: Geographic distance: A factor in early retinopathy detection (abstract). Diabetes 36(suppl 1):49, 1987.

138. Centers for Disease Control: Improving eye care for persons with diabetes mellitus—Michigan. MMWR 34:697–699, 1985.

139. Javitt JC, Canner JK, Sommer A: Cost-effectiveness of current approaches to the control of retinopathy in type I diabetics. Ophthalmology 96:253–262, 1989.

140. Javitt JC, Canner JK, Frank RG, et al: Detecting and treating retinopathy in type I diabetics: A health policy model. Ophthalmology 97:483–495, 1990.

141. Dasbach E, Fryback DG, Newcomb PA, et al: Cost-effectiveness of strategies for detecting diabetic retinopathy. Med Care 29:20–39, 1991.

142. Klein R, Klein BEK, Moss SE, et al: The medical management of hyperglycemia over a 10-year period in people with diabetes. Diabetes Care 19:744–750, 1996.

143. Early Treatment Diabetic Retinopathy Study Research Group: Early photocoagulation for diabetic retinopathy: ETDRS Report No. 9. Ophthalmology 98:766–785, 1991.

144. Stribe M, Haire-Joshu D, Yost J: Psychological adjustment in insulin-dependent diabetes mellitus: The relationship of coping style and diabetes knowledge (abstract). Diabetes 37(suppl):20, 1988.

145. Sinzato R, Fukikno O, Tamai H, et al: Coping behaviors of severe diabetes. Psychother Psychosom 43:219–226, 1985.

Chapter 62

Diabetes Mellitus: Neuropathy

Andrew J.M. Boulton ▪ Rayaz A. Malik

"The era of coma has given way to the era of complications."
Elliot P. Joslin

Of all the long-term complications of diabetes, none affects so many organs or systems of the human body as the group of conditions included under the term "diabetic neuropathies." The frequency with which diabetes affects the nervous system, and the diverse manifestations, may well explain the earlier view that diabetes was a consequence rather than a cause of nervous system dysfunction. Peripheral neuropathies have been described in patients with primary (type 1 and type 2) and secondary diabetes of differing causes, suggesting a common etiologic mechanism based upon chronic hyperglycemia. The pivotal role of hyperglycemia in the pathogenesis of neuropathy has received strong support from landmark studies such as the Diabetes Control and Complications Trial (DCCT),[1,2] the United Kingdom Prospective Diabetes Study (UKPDS),[3] and other prospective studies.[4, 5] Neuropathies are characterized by a progressive loss of nerve fibers that can be assessed noninvasively by a variety of methods, varying from a structured neurologic examination through quantitative sensory testing, to detailed electrophysiology (EP) and autonomic function testing.[6] Although there are no major structural differences in nerve pathology between the two main types of diabetes, clinical differences do exist: whereas the rare symptomatic autonomic syndromes usually occur in long-duration type 1 patients, the mononeuropathies and proximal motor neuropathy usually occur in older type 2 patients.[7]

The epidemiology and natural history of the neuropathies remain poorly defined, partly because of variable diagnostic criteria and the ill-defined patient population studied. However, the late sequelae of neuropathy are well recognized,[8, 9] with foot problems, including ulceration and Charcot's neuroarthropathy, representing the commonest cause of hospitalization among diabetic patients in Western countries.[8] Of all the component causes that, when combined, result in ulceration, neuropathy is by far the commonest.[10] Not surprisingly, diabetic neuropathy often has an adverse effect on quality of life.[11]

In this chapter, the classification, epidemiology, and clinical features of the neuropathies are discussed, followed by a description of measurement techniques and a review of the pathogenesis. Finally, current treatments are reviewed and the late sequelae and their prevention are discussed.

DEFINITIONS AND CLASSIFICATION

Although there have been previous classifications based upon pathologic and etiologic considerations, it has become increasingly clear that, as discussed below, causative mechanisms resulting in neuropathy are multiple and complex, so a clinical or descriptive classification of the neuropathies is favored.[6, 12] Even in this area a number of classifications exist: examples include the purely clinical descriptive classification proposed by Boulton and Ward[13] (Table 62–1) and that based on potential reversibility together with clinical description[12, 14] (Table 62–2).

A simple definition as to what constitutes diabetic neuropathy was agreed upon at an international consensus meeting on clinical diagnosis and management: "The presence of symptoms and/or signs of peripheral nerve dysfunction in people with diabetes after the exclusion of other causes."[15] The exclusion of other causes is particularly important as emphasized by the baseline data from the Rochester Diabetic Neuropathy Study, where 5% of patients had a nondiabetic cause for their neuropathy.[16]

For research, epidemiologic, and clinical trial purposes, a more detailed definition that includes subclinical neuropathy is required[17, 18]; the San Antonio consensus defined diabetic neuropathy as "a demonstrable disorder either clinically evident or sub-clinical, occurring in the setting of diabetes without non-diabetic causes, including manifestations in the somatic and/or autonomic parts of the peripheral nervous system."[19] The Rochester Diabetic Neuropathy Study established a paradigm for clinical trial design.[16, 17] The following were assessed: (1) neuropathic symptoms (neuropathy symptom score, NSS), (2) neuropathic deficits (neuropathy impairment score, NIS), (3) sensorimotor nerve conduction velocity (NCV), (4) quantitative sensory tests (QSTs) and (5) autonomic function testing (AFT). The minimum criteria for a diagnosis of neuropathy required two or more abnormalities among the listed criteria, with at least one being 3 or 5. Staging was as follows: No-0 = neuropathy, minimum criteria unfulfilled; N1 = asymptomatic neuropathy (NSS = 0); N2 = symptomatic neuropathy; N3 = disabling neuropathy.

EPIDEMIOLOGY

The quality, and even quantity, of epidemiologic data on diabetic neuropathy remain poor for a number of reasons, including inconsis-

TABLE 62–1. Descriptive Clinical Classification of Diabetic Neuropathies

Polyneuropathy	Mononeuropathy
Sensory	Cranial
Chronic sensorimotor	
Acute sensory	
Autonomic	Isolated peripheral
Proximal motor	Mononeuritis multiplex
Truncal	Truncal

From Boulton AJ, Ward JD: Diabetic neuropathies and pain. J Clin Endocrinol Metab 16:917–931, 1986. © The Endocrine Society.

TABLE 62–2. Classification of Diabetic Neuropathies Based on Potential Reversibility

Rapidly reversible	Hyperglycemic neuropathy
Persistent symmetrical	Distal somatic sensorimotor (mainly large fiber)
	Autonomic
	Small fiber
Focal and multifocal	Cranial
	Thoracoabdominal radiculopathies
	Focal limb
	Amyotrophy
	Compression/entrapment
Mixed forms	

From Boulton AJ, Malik RA: Diabetic neuropathy. Med Clin North Am 82:909–929; 1998.

tent definitions, poor ascertainment, lack of population-based studies, and failure to exclude nondiabetic neurologic disease.[16, 17] Most studies report on either chronic sensorimotor or autonomic neuropathies,[20] so this section focuses on these two types. However, despite these problems there is no doubt that diabetic neuropathy is very common, possibly the commonest of the late complications of diabetes.

The larger reports of the prevalence of chronic sensorimotor neuropathy published in recent years are summarized in Table 62–3. Of three clinic-based studies from Europe (enrolling >2000 patients), there was a remarkable similarity in the prevalences, which varied from 22.5% to 28.5% for symptomatic neuropathy.[21–23] Most studies include patients with both type 1 and type 2 diabetes; it must be remembered that neuropathy may be present at diagnosis in type 2 diabetes as demonstrated by the Finnish prospective study[4] and the UKPDS,[3] both of which reported a prevalence at diagnosis between 5% and 10%.

The population-based studies of the prevalence of neuropathy are necessarily smaller than the clinic-based ones, and most sample less than 50% of the total available population; however, these showed an even higher prevalence, suggesting that at least half of older, type 2 diabetic patients had significant neuropathic deficits and must therefore be considered as being at high risk of insensitive foot ulceration.[24] As only a minority of patients in the population-based studies were symptomatic, the majority of cases of neuropathy would be missed if a careful clinical neurologic examination was not performed.

Certain prospective studies have assessed risk factors for the development of neuropathy: the UKPDS and DCCT[2, 3] demonstrated a clear relation between poor glycemic control and the development of neuropathy. In addition to glycemic control, Adler et al.[25] identified height, age, and alcohol intake as significant risk factors for neuropathy in a study of U.S. veterans. Other studies have identified ischemic heart disease, smoking, and diabetes duration as being independently related to neuropathy.[20]

Autonomic neuropathy has been the subject of fewer epidemiologic investigations, and the results are less consistent than those for somatic dysfunction. In the Pittsburgh epidemiology study, abnormal AFTs

TABLE 62–3. Prevalence of Diabetic Peripheral Sensorimotor Neuropathy

Study/Country	N	Type of Diabetes	Prevalence (%)
Clinic-Based Studies			
Young et al. (1993),[21] U.K.	6487	1,2	28.5
Tesfaye et al. (1996),[22] Europe	3250	1	28.0
Cabezas-Cerrato et al. (1998),[23] Spain	2644	1,2	22.7
Population-Based Studies			
Dyck et al. (1993),[16] U.S.A.	380	1,2	47.6
Kumar et al. (1994),[24] U.K.	811	2	41.6
Partanen et al. (1995),[4] Finland			8.3*
	133	2	41.9

*At diagnosis of type diabetes.

were associated with female sex, hypertension, and high low-density lipoprotein levels.[26] In prospective studies, the DCCT found mixed results in the association between glycemic control and the 5-year cumulative incidence of autonomic neuropathy.[2] Similarly, the Finnish prospective neuropathy study of type 2 diabetes found inconsistent results in the risk factors for autonomic neuropathy; whereas fasting insulin and female sex related to the cumulative incidence of parasympathetic neuropathy, neither predicted sympathetic neuropathy.[4] Surprisingly, in these studies, glycemic control was only a significant risk factor for deterioration of one autonomic function test in one study.[2]

CLINICAL FEATURES

Focal and Multifocal Neuropathies

A number of characteristic focal and multifocal neuropathies, none of which are unique to the diabetic patient, occur in diabetes; together they account for no more than 10% of all the neuropathies. Most of these tend to occur in older, type 2 patients, and the prognosis is generally for recovery of the deficits (either partial or complete) and also of the pain which may frequently be present. The rapid onset of symptoms and signs in most cases, together with the focal nature of the deficits, is suggestive of a vascular etiology.[27, 28] Exclusion of nondiabetic causes is particularly important in these neuropathies, although, in contrast, any nondiabetic patient with these presentations should of course be screened for diabetes.

Cranial Mononeuropathies

The nerves supplying the extraocular muscles (particularly the third cranial nerve) are most commonly affected: diabetic ophthalmoplegia (third nerve palsy) may be of relatively rapid onset, presenting with pain in the orbit, diplopia, and ptosis; thus exclusion of other causes, particularly rupture of a posterior communicating artery aneurysm, is essential. Investigation should include high-resolution computed tomography (CT) or magnetic resonance imaging (MRI) of the brain, in particular the posterior fossa, to exclude a tumor. Although traditionally believed to be due to acute ischemia within the nerve, Hopf and Guttmann[29] provided evidence for microinfarcts within the third nerve nuclei.

Isolated and Multiple Mononeuropathies

A number of nerves are prone to pressure damage in diabetes; by far the commonest is the median nerve as it passes under the flexor retinaculum. In the Rochester Diabetic Neuropathy Study, 30% of patients had EP evidence of median nerve compression, although only less than 10% had characteristic symptoms.[16] Other entrapment neuropathies are less frequently seen, and may involve the ulnar nerve, the lateral cutaneous nerve of the thigh (meralgia paresthetica), the radial nerve (wristdrop), and the peroneal nerve (footdrop). Occurring in isolation, most of the above (except footdrop) carry a good prognosis, with recovery, although surgical decompression may be required. However, there are increasing reports of severe bilateral ulnar neuropathy occurring in the presence of long-standing diabetes and other complications, a very different picture from the isolated focal mononeuropathies. Moreover, in one series,[30] most cases demonstrated mainly axonal damage due to probable ischemia, rather than compression, so surgical decompression would not be beneficial. Mononeuritis multiplex simply describes the occurrence of more than one isolated mononeuropathy in an individual patient.

Truncal Neuropathies

Truncal neuropathy is typically characterized by pain occurring in a band distribution around the chest or abdomen in a dermatomal distribution. The pain may be severe and have the characteristics of both nerve trunk pain and dysesthesias, typically experienced in mononeuropathies and sensory polyneuropathies, respectively. Thus the patient may experience dull, aching, boring pain together with burning discomfort or allodynia.[31] The differential diagnosis includes shingles and spinal root compression; on occasions the pain has been so difficult to diagnose that patients have been unnecessarily submitted to diagnostic laparotomy. EP investigation, including needle electrode electromyography, is useful, and can be diagnostic; it should be performed in any patient suspected of this diagnosis. Truncal neuropathies may occasionally present with motor manifestations, typically a unilateral bulging of abdominal muscles usually associated with pain as described above (Fig. 62–1). Again, electrodiagnostic studies help to secure the diagnosis and the natural history for symptoms and signs is good, with recovery the rule.[32]

Proximal Motor Neuropathy

Typically affecting older, male, type 2 diabetic patients, proximal motor neuropathy (amyotrophy) presents with pain, wasting, and weakness in the proximal muscles of the lower limbs, either unilaterally or with asymmetrical bilateral involvement. In addition, there is often a distal symmetrical sensory neuropathy, and weight loss of as much as 40% of premorbid body mass may occur.[33] There is no specific treatment for amyotrophy, other than improving glycemic control, which has been advocated,[33] in addition to physiotherapy. In most cases, recovery is gradual, but may take years rather than months.[33] Neuropathologic studies have provided some interesting though limited insight into the pathogenesis of this condition. A proportion of patients have been shown to have a vasculitis which apparently responds to immunosuppression.[34, 35] However, controlled clinical trials of this intervention have not been undertaken and given that the natural history of this condition is improvement with time, the results of the open trials are difficult to interpret. A recent study has failed to confirm the presence of a vasculitis but has demonstrated marked axonal atrophy in both a proximal cutaneous branch of the femoral nerve as well as the sural nerve.[36]

Symmetrical Neuropathies

Autonomic Neuropathy

The autonomic nervous system controls a wide range of bodily functions and therefore when it is damaged it can manifest in a variety of ways principally involving cardiovascular, urogenital, gastrointestinal, thermoregulatory, and sudomotor function.[37]

CARDIOVASCULAR. Cardiac autonomic neuropathy manifests initially as an increase in heart rate secondary to vagal denervation, followed by a decrease due to sympathetic denervation, and finally a fixed heart rate supervenes, which responds only minimally to physiologic stimuli, bearing similarities to the transplanted heart, suggestive of almost complete denervation. Postural hypotension, defined as a 20 mm Hg and 10 mm Hg drop in the systolic and diastolic blood pressures respectively, occurs as a consequence of impaired vasoconstriction in the splanchnic and cutaneous vascular beds due to efferent sympathetic denervation. Twenty-five percent of children display some degree of cardiac autonomic dysfunction on diagnosis of type 1 diabetes,[38] and an abnormality in the expiration-inspiration ratio has been reported in up to 28% of patients with impaired glucose tolerance.[39] Parasympathetic dysfunction is present in 65% of type 2 diabetic patients 10 years after diagnosis, and combined parasympathetic-sympathetic neuropathy is present in 15.2%.[40]

GASTROINTESTINAL. Autonomic neuropathy of the gastrointestinal system manifests as an abnormality in motility, secretion, and absorption through derangement of both extrinsic parasympathetic (vagus and spinal S2–4) and sympathetic, as well as intrinsic enteric innervation provided by Auerbach's plexus. Clinically, patients present with two major problems: diabetic gastroparesis manifest by nausea, postprandial vomiting, and alternating nocturnal diarrhea and constipation.[37] Although a great number of potential investigations of such problems have been described, the absolute diagnosis and treatment of these abnormalities are an extremely difficult clinical problem.

ERECTILE DYSFUNCTION. Erectile dysfunction (ED) in diabetes is usually of multifactorial etiology, although in most series, autonomic neuropathy is a major contributory factor.[41, 42] In the 4-year study of Veves et al.,[42] neuropathy was the principal cause of ED in 27% of newly presented patients with ED, and a contributory cause in a further 38%. Cholinergic and noncholinergic noradrenergic neurotransmitters mediate erectile function by relaxing the smooth muscle in the corpus cavernosum; the ED resulting from autonomic dysfunction is usually progressive but of gradual onset and progression.[37] Other features include occasional retrograde ejaculation, although some ejaculation and orgasm are maintained. Because of the multiple contributory factors to most cases of ED in diabetes, a careful assessment of each case is essential. Consideration of other potential causes, including vascular disease, other medications, local problems such as Peyronie's disease, and psychological factors, is essential before considering therapeutic approaches.

BLADDER DYSFUNCTION. Bladder dysfunction is also well recognized as a consequence of autonomic neuropathy in some patients: this "cystopathy" is usually the result of neurogenic detrusor muscle abnormality.[7] In extreme cases, gross bladder distention may occur with abdominal distention and overflow incontinence.

SWEATING ABNORMALITIES. Abnormalities of sweating are common but often neglected symptoms of autonomic neuropathies.[43] Most common is reduced sweating in the extremities, particularly the feet, which is a manifestation of sympathetic dysfunction. The sweat gland has a complex peptidergic as well as cholinergic innervation, and neuropeptide immunoreactivity (especially for vasoactive intestinal polypeptide) is low in diabetes sudomotor nerves.

In contrast to the dry feet, some patients complain of drenching truncal sweating, particularly at night. Gustatory sweating which is profuse sweating in the head and neck region on eating certain foods, is a highly characteristic symptom of diabetic autonomic neuropathy that is also common in patients with nephropathy, and is "cured" by renal transplantation.[43, 44]

Distal Sensory Neuropathy

The clinical presentation of distal sensory neuropathy, the commonest of all the diabetic neuropathies, is extremely variable, ranging from the severely painful (positive) symptoms at one extreme, to the completely painless variety which may present with an insensitive foot ulcer.[6, 28] This is a diffuse symmetrical disorder, mainly affecting the feet and lower legs in a stocking distribution, but rarely also involving

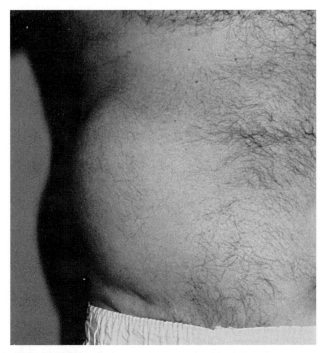

FIGURE 62–1. Diabetic truncal polyradiculopathy presenting as a bulge in the right abdominal wall secondary to muscle weakness. (From Boulton AJM, et al: Diabetic thoracic polyradicaloneuropathy presenting as an abdominal swelling. BMJ 289:798–799; 1984.)

the hands in a glove distribution. As the disease progresses, there is usually also some motor dysfunction (including small muscle wasting: sensorimotor neuropathy), together with abnormalities of AFTs.

The onset of sensory neuropathy is usually gradual, with the insidious appearance of symptoms which may be intermittent in the early stages. However, an acute sensory neuropathy is recognized with rapid onset of painful symptoms. In this latter type, which often follows a period of severe metabolic instability, or may be precipitated by a sudden improvement of control ("insulin neuritis"),[6, 7, 27, 28] the symptoms are usually severe, whereas there may be few if any clinical signs and quantitative testing may be normal.

The neuropathic symptoms may be difficult for the patient to describe, but typically fall into a recognizable pattern, ranging from the severely painful (or positive) at one extreme, with burning pain, stabbing, and shooting sensations; uncomfortable temperature sensations; paresthesias, hyperesthesias, and allodynia; to mild or "negative symptoms" such as decreased pain sensation, deadness, and numbness. Symptoms fluctuate with time, but tend to be extremely uncomfortable, distressing, and prone to nocturnal exacerbation with bedclothes hyperesthesias.

A symptom complex that has only recently been recognized as a relatively common complaint in neuropathy is that of postural instability; diabetic neuropathic patients report more falls, and unsteadiness (secondary to disturbances in proprioception) should be added to the list of neuropathic symptoms. Two studies have investigated this phenomenon, and both confirm that neuropathic patients sway more when quantitatively assessed with Romberg's test.[45, 46]

Although neuropathic symptoms are predominantly if not exclusively sensory, in many cases the signs are both sensory and motor, with sensory loss in a stocking distribution, together with minor degrees of small muscle wasting and occasionally weakness. The ankle reflex is usually reduced or absent, and the skin in the dorsal and especially plantar surfaces may be dry, due to associated sympathetic autonomic dysfunction. Because some neuropathic patients may be asymptomatic, it is ESSENTIAL that all diabetic patients have their feet examined on a regular basis.[15]

SMALL FIBER NEUROPATHY. There is some confusion among authorities about definitions of diabetic neuropathy: some believe that there exists a specific small fiber neuropathy with neuropathic pain, sometimes together with autonomic dysfunction, but few signs. This shares many similarities with the acute sensory neuropathy, but symptoms tend to be more persistent.[7, 27, 28] However, this may simply represent an early stage in the development of chronic sensorimotor neuropathy.[47] These painful sensory neuropathies should not be confused with hyperglycemic neuropathy, which may occur in newly diagnosed patients and is characterized by rapidly reversible abnormalities of nerve function and, occasionally, transient symptoms.[6, 7]

NATURAL HISTORY OF CHRONIC DISTAL SENSORY NEUROPATHY. The natural history of neuropathy is poorly understood and there are few worthwhile published studies: the Rochester Diabetic Neuropathy Study is expected to publish the 10-year follow-up data by 2003.[16] It was generally believed that neuropathic symptoms waxed and waned but persisted for years; however, Benbow et al.,[48] followed patients for 3½ years: the majority of patients reported improvement of symptoms during this time, although there was progressive deterioration in QSTs. Thus, improvement in symptoms must not be equated with parallel improvement in nerve function.[6, 31]

Controversy still exists as to which sensory modality is first affected, although it is generally accepted that small fiber dysfunction is present early in the course of neuropathy.[27] There is, however, no doubt that there is gradual loss of nerve function in diabetic patients that is more rapid than in age-matched nondiabetic subjects; this rate of loss is clearly related to the level of glycemic control.[1–5] One consequence of this progressive diminution of nerve function is an increasing risk of insensitive foot ulceration; progressive loss of large or small fiber function is associated with an increasing risk of foot ulcer.[49, 50]

MEASURES OF NEUROPATHY

The diagnosis and staging of neuropathy is important not only for day-to-day clinical practice but also for the conduct of clinical protocols to assess its etiology and natural history, and to test new proposed treatments. As stated above, there are definitions and classifications of neuropathy for both clinical practice[15] and for clinical trials.[19] The Peripheral Nerve Society has issued a consensus statement on measures to assess efficacy in controlled trials of new therapies for diabetic neuropathy; the use of composite scores of nerve function was advocated in this and other reports.[51, 52] In this section, potential measures for clinical diagnosis or follow-up of patients in clinical trials are discussed.

Clinical Symptoms

Accurate recordings of symptoms is essential both for clinical practice and trials of new medications; it is important to record the patients' descriptions of their complaints verbatim: the physician must not attempt to interpret or translate patients' symptoms into medical terminology.[9, 27, 28] A number of instruments have been developed to quantify neuropathic symptoms that might aid in diagnosis and in longitudinal studies. The McGill Pain Questionnaire has been applied to diabetic neuropathy and was found to be a sensitive measure[53]: it consists of a number of descriptors of symptoms from which the patients select those that best describe their experience.

The NSS or its derivatives, the neuropathy symptom profile, or change scores (NSP and NSC), are perhaps the most commonly used measures in clinical trials.[17, 51, 52] The NSS is a standardized list of questions and neuropathic symptoms that is applied by a trained individual in a standardized manner. A simplified NSS has been used for epidemiologic studies and can be applied in clinical practice for patient follow-up. It can be administered in a few minutes and scores typical symptoms with additional weighting for nocturnal exacerbation.[21]

Clinical Signs

Simple clinical observation may identify a neuropathic foot; evidence might include small muscle wasting, clawing of toes, prominent metatarsal heads, dry skin and callus (secondary to sympathetic dysfunction), and bony deformities secondary to Charcot's neuroarthropathy.[54]

Two simple instruments can be used in clinical practice or for clinical trial assessment. First, Feldman et al.,[55] developed the Michigan Neuropathy Screening Instrument (MNSI): this two-step program is used for diagnosis and staging of neuropathy. The MNSI consists of a 15 yes/no symptom questionnaire which is supplemented by a simple clinical examination. Patients with an abnormal score on the MNSI are then referred for QSTs and EP. Second, the simplified neuropathy disability score (NDS) is a simple clinical examination that sums abnormalities of reflexes and sensory assessment; it has been used in clinical practice and epidemiologic studies.[21] The original NDS was developed by Dyck and colleagues at the Mayo Clinic for the detailed structured assessment of neurologic deficits secondary to neuropathy.[16, 17, 52] The technique is reproducible if performed by trained and experienced physicians, and is currently being used in a number of ongoing trials of new therapies for diabetic neuropathy.

Quantitative Sensory Testing

QSTs assess patients' ability to detect a number of sensory stimuli and have the advantage that they directly assess the degree of sensory loss at the most vulnerable site—the foot.[51] However, the tests are complex psychophysiologic tests that also rely on a patient's response and therefore cooperation and concentration; the availability of these tests is therefore greater than that for EP studies. Moreover, an abnormal finding does not necessarily confirm that the abnormality lies in the peripheral nerve; it might lie anywhere in the afferent pathway. QSTs vary in complexity; the simpler instruments can be used in day-to-day clinical practice, whereas the more sophisticated instruments are usually used for more detailed assessment and for follow-up assessments in clinical trials.[18] Some of the more commonly used techniques are now briefly discussed.

SEMMES-WEINSTEIN MONOFILAMENTS. These comprise sets of nylon filaments of variable diameter that buckle at a predefined force when applied to the testing site. They are widely used in clinical practice, and are particularly helpful in the identification of subjects at risk of neuropathic foot ulceration. Inability to perceive pressure of a 10-g (5.07) monofilament has been shown in prospective studies to predict risk of neuropathic ulceration.[56]

TWO-POINT DISCRIMINATION. The tactile circumferential discriminator (Tacticon Inc., West Chester, PA) is a portable testing device consisting of a hand-held aluminium disk with eight protruding rods of increasing circumference that tests two-point discrimination in a large fiber sensory function. It has similar sensitivity to the monofilaments and vibration assessment in identifying neuropathic patients.[57]

VIBRATION PERCEPTION. A number of devices are specifically designed to assess vibration perception thresholds (VPTs) that test large myelinated fiber function. VPT increases with age in normal persons and also tends to be higher in the lower extremities.[28] As well as being useful in practice, VPT has been used in epidemiologic studies[21] and prospective studies, where an abnormal reading greater than 25 V has been associated with a high risk of foot ulceration.[58]

THERMAL AND COOLING THRESHOLDS. Warm and cold sensation is transmitted via small myelinated and unmyelinated fibers, and can be assessed using a number of devices; those employing a forced-choice technique are most reproducible, especially if the method of limits is used.[28] Despite this, thermal tests remain the most variable of all QSTs.[59]

COMPUTER-ASSISTED SENSORY EXAMINATION (CASE). This complex methodology is currently regarded as state of the art for clinical trials and is a computerized device that can measure touch-pressure, vibration, and warm-cold thresholds using a forced-choice algorithm. It is being used in the Rochester study and a number of long-term intervention trials using proposed new therapeutic interventions.[51, 52]

Autonomic Function Testing

Cardiovascular autonomic dysfunction can be evaluated in detail employing Ewing and Clarke's battery of five tests: (1) the average inspiratory-expiratory heart rate difference with six deep breaths, (2) the Valsalva ratio, (3) the 30:15 ratio, (4) the diastolic blood pressure response to isometric exercise, and (5) the systolic blood pressure fall to standing.[37, 43] More sophisticated techniques such as spectral analysis allow an assessment of the modulation in sinus node activity and depending on which frequency one assesses it may allow dissection of the component contribution of both autonomic input and circulating neurohumoral factors. The key tests which are well validated and of prognostic value are the RR variation, Valsalva's maneuver, and postural testing.[60]

Electrophysiology

EP testing is probably the most important efficacy parameter in clinical neuropathy trials as EP tests are objective, sensitive, and reproducible.[28, 51, 59, 61] Using a central monitoring core laboratory, Bril et al.[62] were able to obtain remarkable reproducibility of EP variables across 60 sites in a prospective study. Coefficients of variability of 3% and 4% for motor and sensory NCVs are comparable to those achieved in an excellent single laboratory.[62] For these reasons, EP variables such as NCVs and amplitudes are frequently used surrogate endpoints in clinical trials; moreover, they are useful in the clinical investigation of peripheral nerve disease. However, although EP tests can define and quantitate nerve dysfunction, as with QSTs, the findings are not specific to diabetes.

Composite scores, combining clinical, quantitative, sensory, and EP measures, are often used in natural history and efficacy studies.[17, 18, 51, 52] Examples include the NISLL + 7[52] and the Michigan Diabetic Neuropathy Score.[55] The former comprises the Neuropathy Impairment

Score of the Lower Limbs (NISLL) together with seven other tests (five EP attributes, one QST, and one AFT). This measure is being used in several ongoing multicenter intervention studies.

PATHOGENESIS

The complexity of derived pathogenetic schemes is partly a reflection of the true complex nature of diabetic neuropathy but also denotes our lack of clear understanding of this disease. Hyperglycemia is of central importance, and the results of the DCCT[2] and UKPDS,[3] in addition to the improvement in neuropathy, following pancreatic transplantation[63] attest to this. Important transducers include alterations in the polyol pathway, glycation, cellular redox state, oxidative stress, and intracellular diacylglycerol levels which mediate enhanced protein kinase Cβ activity.[64] Alterations in the polyol pathway may alter the levels of important osmolytes such as myoinositol and taurine and mediate oxidation of NADPH and NADP$^+$ with a concomitant reduction in NADH and NAD$^+$ redox couples.[64] Increased oxidative stress may also occur secondary to glucose autoxidation and formation of reactive oxygen species (ROS, superoxide and hydroxyl radicals),[65, 66] a reduction in ROS scavengers (glutathione, catalase, and superoxide dismutase),[66] or both. Advanced glycosylation end products have been demonstrated in peripheral nerve tubulin[67] and Na$^+$, K$^+$-ATPase[68] and also localized to the cytoplasm of endothelial cells, pericytes, axoplasm, and Schwann cells of both myelinated and unmyelinated fibers and related to myelinated nerve fiber loss in sural nerve biopsies from diabetic patients with neuropathy.[69] Additionally, advanced glycosylation end product formation has been related to increased ROS production[70] and both endothelial and neuronal nitric oxide depletion.[71, 72] Endothelial dysfunction has been demonstrated in patients with diabetic neuropathy and related to reduced expression of endothelial NO synthase.[73]

Hemorheologic abnormalities, principally markers of platelet activation and levels of fibrinogen, relate to measures of microangiopathy and neuropathy.[74, 75] Measures of endothelial cell dysfunction, including von Willebrand factor[76] and cell adhesion molecules, particularly P-selectin, E-selectin, and intercellular adhesion molecule 1 (ICAM-1),[77] have been shown to predict the development and progression of neuropathy. Sural nerve endoneurial oxygen tension,[78] blood flow,[79] and fluorescein appearance are reduced,[80] and endoneurial edema is present in diabetic patients with neuropathy.[81] Structural abnormalities include arteriolar attenuation, venous distintion, arteriovenous shunting, and new vessel formation,[80, 82] along with intimal hyperplasia and hypertrophy,[83] denervation,[84] and a reduction in neuropeptide expression[85] in epineurial vessels. Transperineurial vessels demonstrate denervation[86] with luminal narrowing,[87] possibly secondary to perineurial abnormalities.[88] Endoneurial capillaries demonstrate endothelial cell hypertrophy or hyperplasia and basement membrane thickening (Fig. 62–2) which relates to measures of neuropathic severity.[89–93] Controversy remains over a reduction in capillary density[93–97] and the occurrence of pericyte cell loss.[89, 94–96] Clinically important independent accelerators include hypertension in patients with type 1[98] but not type 2[99] diabetes.

Many of the initiators and promoters upstream may signal transcriptional and translational abnormalities through the mitogen-activated protein kinase (MAPK) family mediating early gene responses and aberrant phosphorylation of neurofilaments. A subgroup of MAPKs which specifically involve activation via cellular stressors includes extracellular signal-regulated kinase 1 and 2, c-Jun N-terminal kinase, and p38, collectively referred to as the stress-activated protein kinases (SAPKs).[100] Thus future approaches to therapeutic intervention may involve either upstream regulation as outlined later or terminal downstream regulation of the kinase cascades. The actual initial functional response of reduced nerve function may be mediated via abnormalities in a number of axonal ion channels[101] which may also be amenable to intervention.

Neurotrophins such as nerve growth factor (NGF),[102, 103] ciliary neurotrophic factor,[104] and NT-3 provide neurotrophic support for select populations of nerve fibers, and deficient neurotrophic support has been invoked as an important factor in the pathogenesis of diabetic

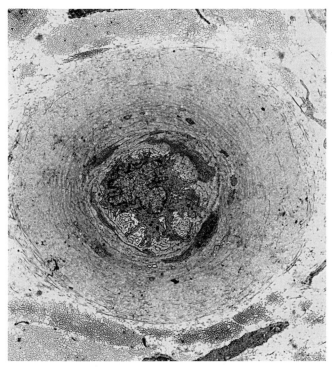

FIGURE 62–2. Electronmicrograph (×4500) of endoneurial capillary demonstrating gross thickening of basement membrane with closure of the lumen in the sural nerve of a patient with severe diabetic neuropathy.

neuropathy, if not in the degenerative process, certainly for the process of regeneration. An earlier phase II clinical trial with recombinant human NGF (rhNGF) showed promise,[105] but preliminary results of the phase III rhNGF trial of over 1000 patients in the United States have been negative (Genetech Ltd., personal communication, April 1999). However, to fully realize the potential of the neurotrophins, the target population of nerve fibers may have to be widened employing chimeric neurotrophic support, which may also enable more conventional and perhaps reproducible tests of nerve function to be utilized to determine efficacy.

The evidence that antibodies against NGF, adrenal medulla, sympathetic and parasympathetic ganglia, glutamic acid decarboxylase, and phospholipids may mediate neuronal damage is limited and contentious.[106]

PATHOLOGY

The great majority of pathologic studies have assessed peripheral nerve material. Neuropathologic studies are extremely sensitive as they can show a significant abnormality in the presence of entirely normal clinical and neurophysiologic tests of neuropathy.[89, 92, 107, 108] However, basic flaws include studies in patients with end-stage neuropathy which precludes any significant insight into pathogenesis. Furthermore, studies are limited to the sensory sural nerve and only myelinated fibers, constituting less than 5% of the nerve fiber population, are assessed. The neuropathologic assessment itself is often limited to light microscopic studies of transverse sections, without teased fiber analysis, providing limited information on the underlying pathologic condition.

Myelinated fiber axonal atrophy was considered to be a key feature of diabetic neuropathy in both animal models[108] and humans,[109–111] presumed secondary to ineffective axonal transport.[112] However, studies in both longer-term animal models[113] and diabetic patients[92, 107, 114, 115] have failed to confirm this abnormality. Axoglial dysjunction describes an abnormality of the paranodal connection between the terminal myelin loops and the axonal membrane and provides a plausible explanation for a reduction in NCV.[110, 111, 116] However, recent

careful studies have been unable to confirm the presence of axoglial dysjunction.[117, 118] Earlier studies of diabetic patients with established neuropathy demonstrated a mixture of both demyelination and axonal degeneration.[92, 108] More recent studies in diabetic patients without evidence of neuropathy demonstrate demyelination without axonal loss or atrophy, suggesting that demyelination and hence involvement of the Schwann cell is primary.[89, 92] A range of reactive (accumulation of lipid droplets, pi, Reich and glycogen granules) and degenerative (mitochondrial enlargement, effacement of cristae, degeneration of abaxonal and adaxonal cytosol and organelles) Schwann cell changes have been described recently in sural nerve biopsies from diabetic patients with neuropathy.[119] Furthermore, similar changes with myelin splitting have also been described recently in the feline model of diabetic neuropathy.[120] With progression of neuropathy, myelinated axonal degeneration occurs with loss of nerve fibers[92, 108] (Fig. 62–3), particularly in patients with type 2 diabetes.[121]

The assessment of unmyelinated fibers requires excellent fixation, high magnification, and considerable experience to define unmyelinated fiber axons from myelinated axons that have yet to myelinate, and indeed from Schwann cell cytoplasm.[122] Axonal degeneration with active regeneration of this class of fibers occurs early in the evolution of neuropathy prior to axonal degeneration of the myelinated fibers, but importantly their regenerative capacity is maintained long after the myelinated fibers have lost their capacity to regenerate.[92, 109, 114] (Fig. 62–4).

A high correlation has been demonstrated between myelinated fiber density, NCV and QSTs.[96] A variety of morphologic measures of nerve fiber degeneration have been related to the neuropathy deficit score,[109] vibration perception, and autonomic dysfuction.[114] Patients with mild neuropathy demonstrate a good correlation between sural nerve myelinated fiber density and both peroneal and sural NCV and amplitude but not vibration or thermal perception.[123] In 1996, a detailed study of 18 diabetic patients with varying stages of neuropathy demonstrated precise relationships between the degree of myelinated fiber loss and clinical and neurophysiologic abnormalities, as well as quantitative sensory thresholds.[124] Thermal thresholds have been related to the median unmyelinated axon diameter.[114]

A morphologic basis for painful neuropathy has been sought for many years and proposed mechanisms have included acute axonal degeneration, axonal atrophy, and loss of large fibers, as well as axonal sprouting.[125] One of the major flaws of these earlier studies was the lack of a diabetic control group and any clinical attribute of diabetic neuropathy could have been chosen and related to the biopsy findings. Subsequent controlled studies have failed to find any defining morphometric feature of painful diabetic neuropathy.[92, 109, 114]

Pathologic studies of autonomic tissue are limited and have not been adequately quantified. Qualitative changes include chromatolysis, cytoplasmic vacuolization, and pyknotic changes. Axonal degeneration

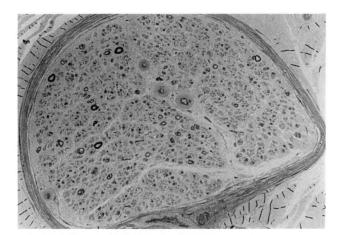

FIGURE 62–3. Light micrograph (×300) of a transverse semi-thin section demonstrating a gross loss of myelinated fibers and marked thickening of endoneurial capillary basement membrane in the sural nerve of a patient with severe neuropathy.

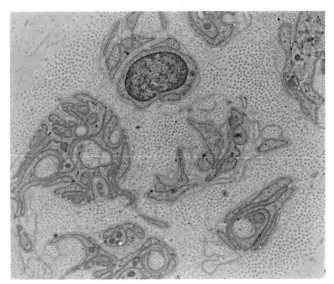

FIGURE 62–4. Electronmicrograph (×12,000) of unmyelinated fibers demonstrating degeneration and regeneration in the sural nerve of a patient with severe diabetic neuropathy.

and demyelination have been reported in a variety of biopsied tissues, including preganglionic white rami communicantes, sympathetic chain, paravertebral and prevertebral autonomic ganglia, and dorsal root ganglia, as well as more distal autonomic nerves such as the splanchnic and vagus and intramural nerves to the bladder and corpora cavernosa.

BIOPSY

Nerve biopsy is the gold standard for assessing the exact type and degree of nerve fiber damage and if assessed accurately provides important analysis of underlying pathologic changes and pathogenesis. Sural nerve biopsy may leave mild mechanically elicited sensory symptoms for approximately 1 year, but recovery via collateral sprouting appears to be good and no different from patients without diabetes.[126] More recently, epidermal nerve fiber morphology has been quantified in skin biopsies in patients with diabetic neuropathy[127, 128] and has been further refined by a similar assessment in a less-invasive, though more limited approach employing skin blisters.[129] However, the exact origin of nerve fibers under study is not defined and the skin-blister approach allows a density assessment of a very selective population of sensory fibers only.

TREATMENT

Throughout this section on treatment, distinction is made between therapies for symptomatic relief and those that may alter (slow) the progressive loss of nerve function that characterizes the natural history of neuropathy; a few therapies have efficacy in both these areas.

Sensory Neuropathy

Current Treatments

GLYCEMIC CONTROL. Of all the treatments, tight and stable glycemic control is probably the only one that may provide symptomatic relief as well as slow the relentless progression of neuropathy.[1–3, 130, 131] As it is probably blood glucose flux that induces neuropathic pain,[31] stability rather than the actual level of glycemic control may be most important in pain relief. The method of achieving stable control does not seem to be critical; there is no evidence that insulin is superior if the blood glucose is well controlled by oral hypoglycemic agents.

TRICYCLIC ANTIDEPRESSANTS. Until new therapies are proved to relieve symptoms in appropriately designed trials,[18, 130] the tricyclic antidepressant drugs, such as amitriptyline, and imipramine, will remain the first-line agents for painful neuropathy; their efficacy, confirmed in several randomized, placebo-controlled trials,[132] is related to plasma drug level and the onset of symptomatic relief is faster than the antidepressive effects. There is a clear dose-response relationship, but sedative and anticholinergic side effects are also dose-related and troublesome, often restricting the use of these drugs.[133]

ANTICONVULSANTS. Carbamazepine is widely used in the management of neuropathic pain and its use is supported by some clinical trial data, although side effects limit its usage in a proportion of patients.[133] More recently, the new anticonvulsant gabapentin has been shown to be efficacious in the treatment of painful syndromes, including diabetic neuropathy[134]; its adverse effects seem to be less pronounced than those associated with tricyclic drugs. Similarly, preliminary data suggest that topiramate may have similar efficacy (K.R. Edwards, personal communication, 1999).

OTHER AGENTS. A number of other drug therapies, including phenytoin, mexiletene, lidocaine, and transdermal clonidine have been reported to be useful in the management of painful or paresthetic symptoms.[130, 133] Topical therapy with capsaicin may be helpful in some cases, especially those with localized pain.[6] The centrally acting analgesic tramadol has confirmed efficacy in painful neuropathy in a randomized controlled trial.[135] Finally, traditional therapies such as acupuncture have also been employed with good results and negligible side effects in symptomatic neuropathy.[136]

Potential Future Therapies

ALDOSE REDUCTASE INHIBITORS. Although numerous studies of aldose reductase inhibitors (APIs) have been published in the last 30 years,[137] none are available today in the United States or Europe. ARIs block the rate-limiting enzyme in the polyol pathway that is activated in hyperglycemic states. Many of the problems of early ARI trials related to poor study design and the enrollment of patients with advanced neuropathy who would be unlikely to benefit from treatment.[18] If current ongoing trials with potent ARIs demonstrate efficacy, these agents are likely to slow neuropathy progression rather than provide symptomatic relief. A recent study has demonstrated susceptibility to the development of neuropathy in diabetic patients with a polymorphism in the aldose reductase gene, perhaps allowing a means to target a population who may respond more effectively.[138]

α-LIPOIC ACID. There is accumulating evidence to suggest that free radical–mediated oxidative stress is implicated in the pathogenesis of neuropathy, and that treatment with the antioxidant α-lipoic acid might prevent these abnormalities, and improve painful symptoms as well as slow the progression of diabetic neuropathy.[133, 139] Two North American and European trials are testing these hypotheses, and the results should be available in 2002.[139]

γ-LINOLENIC ACID (GLA). The first step in the metabolism of the essential fatty acid linolenic acid is impaired in diabetes and this defect can be bypassed by the administration of GLA.[140] Clinical studies have suggested some efficacy of GLA in neuropathy,[133] but the most interesting development is the suggestion from animal studies that a lipoic acid–GLA conjugate is effective against multiple indices of neuropathy.[141]

NERVE GROWTH FACTOR. Deficiencies in endogenous NGFs, which are trophic to sensory and autonomic nerve factors, have been described in diabetic neuropathy[142] and preliminary studies suggest that exogenous NGF may be beneficial in symptomatic diabetic neuropathy.[105] Large multicenter phase III trials are in progress and should be completed in 2000, although as noted earlier, the phase III trial in the United States is now terminated and the results are negative.

OTHER AGENTS. Investigation of other potential treatments for neuropathy are ongoing: one proposed class of drugs is the angiotensin converting enzyme (ACE) inhibitors, already known for their efficacy in nephropathy and retinopathy. A preliminary controlled study of ACE inhibitors in early neuropathy confirmed a significant benefit over placebo in EP parameters.[143]

Autonomic Neuropathy

Erectile Dysfunction

As autonomic neuropathy is one of several contributory causes in ED, a multifaceted approach to management is indicated.[41, 42] Psychosexual counseling and altering drug therapy to remove those associated with ED is beneficial in many cases.[42] Sildenafil, an orally active selective inhibitor of phosphodiesterase 5, is efficacious for ED in diabetic males. In a trial of ED of multiple causation in diabetic males, Rendell et al.[144] reported a response rate (defined as at least one successful attempt at sexual intercourse) of 61% in sildenafil-treated subjects vs. 22% on placebo. Most diabetic patients require 50 or 100 mg, and care must be taken if there is any history of ischemic heart disease: it must never be given to patients on nitrate therapy.[145]

Sweating Disorders

The first specific treatment for gustatory sweating has been reported: glycopyrrolate is an antimuscarinic compound which, when applied topically to the affected area, results in a marked reduction of sweating while eating "trigger" foods. Its efficacy was confirmed in a randomized controlled trial.[146]

Others

The treatment of diabetic gastroparesis involves measures to enhance gastric motility and emptying. Thus metoclopramide, a dopamine antagonist, directly stimulates antral muscle and may also mediate acetylcholine release. Alternative agents include domperidone, a peripheral dopamine D_2 receptor antagonist; cisapride, a cholinomimetic agent; or erythromycin, which directly stimulates motilin receptors. Constipation may be treated with a combination of prokinetic agents such as metoclopramide and cisapride. Postural hypotension may be treated with mineralocorticoids such as fludrocortisone; sympathomimetic agents; and dopamine blockers. Urinary bladder difficulties are addressed with regular voiding, self-catheterization, and cholinergic agonists such as bethanechol chloride which stimulates muscarinic, postganglionic receptors enhancing bladder motility and emptying.[37, 43]

General Aspects of Neuropathy Treatment

Any patient with clinical evidence of diabetic peripheral neuropathy must be considered as being at risk of insensitive foot ulceration and should receive evaluation on foot care and, if necessary, a podiatry referral.[15] These patients require more frequent follow-up, always paying particular attention to foot inspection to reinforce the educational message of the need for regular foot care.

NEUROPATHIC ENDPOINTS

The late sequelae of diabetic neuropathy are usually considered to be neuropathic foot ulceration, neuroarthropathy (Charcot's foot) and amputation, although amputation should not be carried out on a purely neuropathic foot.[6, 8, 9, 15, 147]

Neuropathic Foot Ulceration

Distal sensory and sympathetic neuropathy are the most important component causes that lead to foot ulceration, being present in 78% of cases assessed in a two-center study.[10] However, the neuropathic foot does not spontaneously ulcerate: it is the combination of neuropathy with other risk factors such as deformity and unperceived trauma that results in ulceration. International guidelines on the clinical management of neuropathy therefore emphasize the importance of regular foot examinations and education in self–foot care in the management of neuropathy.[15]

Charcot's Neuroarthropathy

Charcot's neuroarthropathy is a relatively rare but clinically important and potentially devastating disorder that warrants mention in this section. Diabetes is now the commonest cause of this condition in Western countries,[54] and a high degree of awareness and suspicion may enable early diagnosis and effective intervention. Permissive features for the development of a Charcot's joint include peripheral sensorimotor neuropathy, sympathetic denervation in the foot, and intact peripheral circulation; minor, often unperceived, trauma is often the initiating event. It is believed that following repetitive minor trauma, osteoblastic activity is stimulated with remodeling of bone.

A high index of suspicion must exist if a neuropathic patient has unilateral unexplained swelling and warmth in a foot. Contrary to earlier texts, discomfort may be experienced, although the patient is still usually able to walk. Detailed assessment and investigation of such a patient is essential,[54] and rest or casting a suspected Charcot's foot is usually recommended.

Acknowledgments

We thank Jennifer Wallis for her expert secretarial assistance in the preparation of this chapter.

REFERENCES

1. Diabetes Control of Complications Trial Research Group: The effect of intensive treatment of diabetes on the development of progression of long-term complications in insulin-dependent diabetes mellitus. N Engl J Med 329:329–986, 1993.
2. Diabetes Control of Complications Trial Research Group: The effect of intensive diabetes therapy on the development and progression of neuropathy. Ann Intern Med 122:561–568, 1995.
3. United Kingdom Prospective Diabetes Study: Intensive blood glucose control with sulphonylureas or insulin compared with conventional treatment and risk of complications in patients with type 2 diabetes. Lancet 352:837–853, 1998.
4. Partanen J, Niskanen L, Lehtinen J, et al: Natural history of peripheral neuropathy in patients with non–insulin dependent diabetes mellitus. N Engl J Med 333:89–94, 1995.
5. Ziegler D, Mayer P, Munlen H, et al: The natural history of somatosensory and autonomic nerve dysfunction in relation to glycaemic control during the first five years after diagnosis of type 1 diabetes. Diabetologia 34:822–824, 1991.
6. Boulton AJM, Malik RA: Diabetic neuropathy. Med Clin North Am 82:909–929, 1998.
7. Watkins PJ, Thomas PK: Diabetes mellitus and the nervous system. J Neurol Neurosurg Psychiatry 65:620–632, 1998.
8. Mayfield JA, Reiber GE, Sanders LJ, et al: Technical Review: Preventive foot care in patients with diabetes mellitus. Diabetes Care 21:2161–2177, 1998.
9. Boulton AJM: Late sequelae of diabetic neuropathy. *In* Boulton AJM (ed:) Diabetic Neuropathy. Lancaster, UK, Marius Press, 1997, pp 63–76.
10. Reiber GE, Vileikyte L, Boyko EH, et al: Causal pathways for incident lower-extremity ulcers in patients with diabetes from two settings. Diabetes Care 22:157–162, 1999.
11. Benbow SJ, Wallymahmed ME, MacFarlane IA: Diabetic peripheral neuropathy and quality of life. Q J Med 91:733–737, 1998.
12. Thomas PK: Classification, differential diagnosis and staging of diabetic peripheral neuropathy. Diabetes 46 (suppl 2):S54–S57, 1997.
13. Boulton AJM, Ward JD: Diabetic neuropathies and pain. Clin Endocrinol Metab 15:917–931, 1986.
14. Sima AAF, Thomas PK, Ishii D, et al: Diabetic neuropathies. Diabetologia 46 (suppl):B74–B77, 1997.
15. Boulton AJM, Gries FA, Jervell JA: Guidelines for the diagnosis and out-patient management of diabetic peripheral neuropathy. Diabet Med 15:508–514, 1998.
16. Dyck PJ, Kratz KM, Karnes JZ, et al: The prevalence by staged severity of various types of diabetic neuropathy, retinopathy and nephropathy in a population-based cohort: The Rochester Diabetic Neuropathy Study. Neurology 43:817–824, 1993.
17. Dyck PJ, Melton J, O'Brien PC, et al: Approaches to improve epidemiological studies of diabetic neuropathy. Diabetes 46(suppl 2):55–58, 1997.
18. Ziegler D: The design of clinical trials for treatment of diabetic neuropathy. Neurosci Res Commun 21:83–91, 1997.
19. Consensus statement: Report and recommendations of the San Antonio conference on diabetic neuropathy. Diabetes Care 11:592–597, 1988.
20. Boyko EJ: The epidemiology of diabetic neuropathy. *In* Veves A (ed): Contemporary Endocrinology: Clinical Management of Diabetic Neuropathy. Totowa, NJ, Humana Press, 1998, pp 1–12.
21. Young MJ, Boulton AJM, McLeod AF, et al: A multicentre study of the prevalence of diabetic peripheral neuropathy in the UK hospital clinic population. Diabetologia 36:150–154, 1993.
22. Tesfaye S, Stephens LK, Stephenson JM, et al: Prevalence of diabetic peripheral neuropathy and its relation to glycemic control and potential risk factors: The EURODIAB IDDM complications study. Diabetologia 39:1377–1384, 1996.
23. Cabezas-Cerrato J: The prevalence of clinical diabetic neuropathy in Spain: A study in primary care and hospital clinic groups. Diabetologia 41:1263–1269, 1998.

24. Kumar S, Ashe HA, Parnell L, et al: The prevalence of foot ulceration and its correlates in type 2 diabetes: A population-based study. Diabet Med 11:480–484, 1994.

25. Adler AI, Boyko EJ, Ahroni JH, et al: Risk factors for diabetic peripheral sensory neuropathy: Results of the Seattle prospective diabetic foot study. Diabetes Care 20:1162–1167, 1997.

26. Maser RE, Pfeifer MA, Dorman JS, et al: Diabetic autonomic neuropathy and cardiovascular risk: The Pittsburgh Epidemiology of Diabetic Complications Study III. Arch Intern Med 150:1218–1222, 1990.

27. Tesfaye S, Ward JD: Clinical features of diabetic polyneuropathy. In Veves A (ed): Contemporary Endocrinology: Clinical Management of Diabetic Neuropathy. Totowa, NJ, Humana Press, 1998, pp 49–60.

28. Young MJ, Jones GC: Diabetic neuropathy: Symptoms, signs and assessment. In Boulton AJM (ed): Diabetic Neuropathy. Lancaster, UK, Marius Press, 1997, pp 41–61.

29. Hopf HC, Guttmann L: Diabetic third nerve palsy: Evidence for a mesencephalic lesion. Neurology 40:1041–1045, 1990.

30. Schady W, Abuaisha B, Boulton AJM: Observations on severe ulnar neuropathy in diabetes. J Diabetes Complications 12:128–132, 1998.

31. Boulton AJM: What causes neuropathic pain? J Diabetes Complications 6:58–63, 1992.

32. Chaudhuri KR, Wren DR, Werring D, et al: Unilateral abdominal muscle herniation with pain: A distinctive variant of diabetic radiculopathy. Diabet Med 14:803–807, 1997.

33. Coppack SW, Watkins PJ: The natural history of diabetic femoral neuropathy. Q J Med 79:307–314, 1991.

34. Pascoe MK, Low PA, Windebank AJ: Subacute diabetic proximal neuropathy. Mayo Clin Proc 72:1123–1132, 1997.

35. Llewelyn JG, Thomas PK, King RHM: Epineurial microvasculitis in proximal diabetic neuropathy. J Neurol 245:159–165, 1998.

36. Malik RA, Ghani M, Walker D, et al: Pathological studies in diabetic amyotrophy. Diabetes 47(suppl 1):A64, 1998.

37. Freeman R: Diabetic autonomic neuropathy: An overview. In Veves A (ed): Contemporary Endocrinology: Clinical Management of Diabetic Neuropathy. Totowa, NJ, Humana Press, 1998, pp 181–208.

38. Solders G, Thalme B, Aguirre-Aquino M, et al: Nerve conduction and autonomic nerve function in diabetic children. A 10-year follow up study. Acta Pediatr 86:361–366, 1997.

39. Eriksson KF, Nilsson H, Lindarde F, et al: Diabetes mellitus but not impaired glucose tolerance is associated with dysfunction in peripheral nerves. Diabet Med 11:279–285, 1994.

40. Toyry JP, Niskanen LK, Mantysaari MJ, et al: Occurrence predictors and clinical significance of autonomic neuropathy in NIDDM: Ten year follow-up from diagnosis. Diabetes 45:308–315, 1996.

41. Vinik AI, Richardson D: Evaluating erectile dysfunction in diabetes. Int Diabetes Fed Bull 43:7–13, 1998.

42. Veves A, Webster L, Chen TF, et al: Aetiopathogenesis and management of impotence in diabetic males: Four years' experience from a combined clinic. Diabet Med 12:77–82, 1995.

43. Watkins PJ, Edmonds ME: Clinical features of diabetic neuropathy. In Pickup JC, Williams G (eds): Textbook of Diabetes, ed 2. Oxford, Blackwell Scientific, 1997, pp 50.1–50.20.

44. Shaw JE, Parker P. Hollis S, et al: Gustatory sweating in diabetes mellitus. Diabet Med 13:1033–1037, 1996.

45. Katoulis EC, Ebdon-Parry M, Hollis S, et al: Postural instability in diabetic neuropathic patients at risk of foot ulceration. Diabet Med 14:296–300, 1997.

46. Oppenheim U, Kohen-Raz R, Alex D, et al: Postural characteristics of diabetic neuropathy. Diabetes Care 22:328–332, 1999.

47. Veves A, Young MJ, Manes C, et al: Differences in peripheral and autonomic nerve function measurements in painful and painless neuropathy: A clinical study. Diabetes Care 17:1200–1202, 1994.

48. Benbow SJ, Chan AW, Bowsher DH, et al: A prospective study of painful symptoms, small fibre function and peripheral vascular disease in chronic painful diabetic neuropathy. Diabet Med 11:17–21, 1994.

49. Young MJ, Veves A, Breddy J, et al: The prediction of diabetic foot ulceration using vibration perception thresholds. Diabetes Care 17:557–561, 1994.

50. Litzelman DK, Marriott DJ, Vinicor F: Independent physiological predictors of foot lesions in patients with NIDDM. Diabetes Care 20:1273–1278, 1997.

51. Diabetic polyneuropathy in controlled clinical trials: Consensus report of the peripheral nerve society. Ann Neurol 38:478–482, 1995.

52. Dyck PJ, Davies JL, Litchy WJ, et al: Longitudinal assessment of diabetic polyneuropathy using a composite score in the Rochester Diabetic Neuropathy Study cohort. Neurology 49:229–239, 1997.

53. Masson EA, Hunt L, Gem JM, et al: A novel approach to the diagnosis and assessment of symptomatic diabetic neuropathy. Pain 38:25–28, 1989.

54. Shaw JE, Boulton AJM: The Charcot foot. Foot 5:65–70, 1995.

55. Feldman EL, Stevens MJ, Thomas PK, et al: A practical two-step quantitative clinical and electrophysiological assessment for the diagnosis and staging of diabetic neuropathy. Diabetes Care 17:1281–1289, 1994.

56. Rith-Najarian SJ, Stolusky T, Gohdes DM: Identifying diabetic patients at risk of lower-extremity amputation in a primary care setting. Diabetes Care 15:1386–1389, 1992.

57. Vileikyte L, Hutchings G, Hollis S, et al: The tactile circumferential discriminator: A new simple screening device to identify diabetic patients at risk of foot ulceration. Diabetes Care 20:623–626, 1997.

58. Abbott CA, Vileikyte L, Williamson S, et al: Multicenter study of the incidence of and predictive risk factors for diabetic neuropathic foot ulceration. Diabetes Care 21:1071–1074, 1998.

59. Valensi P, Atalli JR, Cagant S: Reproducibility of parameters for assessment of diabetic neuropathy. Diabet Med 10:933–939, 1993.

60. Schumer MP, Joyner SA, Pfeifer MA: Cardiovascular autonomic neuropathy testing in patients with diabetes. Diabetes Spectrum 11:227–231, 1998.

61. Olney RK: Neurophysiologic evaluation and clinical trials for neuromuscular diseases. Muscle Nerve 21:1365–1367, 1998.

62. Bril V, Ellison R, Ngo M, et al: Electrophysiological monitoring in clinical trials. Muscle Nerve 21:1368–1373, 1998.

63. Navarro X, Sutherland DE, Kennedy WR: Long-term effects of pancreatic transplantation on diabetic neuropathy. Ann Neurol 42:727–736, 1997.

64. Stevens MJ, Feldman EL, Thomas T, et al: Pathogenesis of diabetic neuropathy. In Veves A (ed): Contemporary Endocrinology: Clinical Management of Diabetic Neuropathy. Totowa, Humana Press, 1998, pp 13–48.

65. Low PA, Nickander KK: Oxygen free radical effects in sciatic nerve in experimental diabetes. Diabetes 40:873–877, 1991.

66. Wohaieb SA, Godin DV: Alterations in free radical tissue-defense mechanisms in streptozotocin-induced diabetes in rat. Diabetes 36:1014–1018, 1987.

67. Cullum NA, Mahon J, Stringer K, et al: Glycation of rat sciatic nerve tubulin in experimental diabetes mellitus. Diabetologia 34:387–389, 1991.

68. Garner MH, Bahador A, Sachs G: Nonenzymatic glycation of Na, K-ATPase. Effects on ATP hydrolysis and K occlusion. J Biol Chem 265:15058–15066, 1990.

69. Sugimoto K, Nishizawa Y, Horiuchi S: Localization in human diabetic peripheral nerve of N(epsilon)-carboxymethyllysine-protein adducts, an advanced glycation endproduct. Diabetologia 40:1380–1387, 1997.

70. Wolff SP, Jiang ZY, Hunt JV: Protein glycation and oxidative stress in diabetes mellitus and aging. Free Radic Biol Med 10:339–352, 1991.

71. Bucala R, Tracey KJ, Cerami A: Advanced glycosylation products quench nitric oxide and mediate defective endothelium-dependent vasodilatation in experimental diabetes. J Clin Invest 87:432–438, 1991.

72. Sasaki T, Yasuda H, Maeda K, et al: Hyperalgesia and decreased neuronal nitric oxide synthase in diabetic rats. Neuroreport 9:243–247, 1998.

73. Veves A, Akbari CM, Primavera J, et al: Endothelial dysfunction and the expression of endothelial nitric oxide synthase in diabetic neuropathy, vascular disease, and foot ulceration. Diabetes 47:457–463, 1998.

74. Ford I, Malik RA, Newrick PG, et al: Relationship between haemostatic factors and capillary morphology in human diabetic neuropathy. Thromb Haemost 68:628–633, 1992.

75. Young MJ, Bennett JL, Liderth SA, et al: Rheological and microvascular parameters in diabetic peripheral neuropathy. Clin Sci. 90:183–187, 1996.

76. Plater ME, Ford I, Dent MT, et al: Elevated von Willebrand factor antigen predicts deterioration in diabetic peripheral nerve function. Diabetologia 39:336–343, 1996.

77. Jude E, Abbott CA, Young MJ, et al: Potential role of cell adhesion molecules in the pathogenesis of diabetic neuropathy. Diabetologia 41:330–336, 1998.

78. Newrick PG, Wilson AJ, Jakubowski J, et al: Sural nerve oxygen tension in diabetes. BMJ 193:1053–1054, 1986.

79. Theriault M, Dort J, Sutherland G, et al: Local human sural nerve blood flow in diabetic and other polyneuropathies. Brain 120:1131–1138, 1997.

80. Tesfaye S, Harris N, Jakubowski J, et al: Impaired blood flow and arterio-venous shunting in human diabetic neuropathy: A novel technique of nerve photography and fluorescein angiography. Diabetologia 36:1266–1274, 1993.

81. Eaton RP, Qualls C, Bicknell J, et al: Structure-function relationships within peripheral nerves in diabetic neuropathy: The hydration hypothesis. Diabetologia 39:439–446, 1996.

82. Tesfaye S, Malik RA, Harris N, et al: Arterio-venous shunting and proliferating new vessels in acute painful neuropathy of rapid glycaemic control (insulin neuritis). Diabetologia 39:329–335, 1996.

83. Korthals JK, Gieron MA, Dyck PJ: Intima of epineurial arterioles is increased in diabetic polyneuropathy. Neurology 38:1582–1586, 1988.

84. Grover-Johnson NM, Baumann FG, Imparato AM, et al: Abnormal innervation of lower limb epineurial arterioles in human diabetes. Diabetologia 20:31–38, 1981.

85. Milner P, Appenzeller O, Qualls C, et al: Differential vulnerability in nerves of the vasa nervorum to streptozotocin-induced diabetes. Brain Res 574:56–62, 1992.

86. Beggs J, Johnson PC, Olafsen A, et al: Transperineurial arterioles in human sural nerve. J Neuropathol Exp Neurol 50:704–718, 1991.

87. Malik RA, Tesfaye S, Thompson SD, et al: Transperineurial capillary abnormalities in the sural nerve of patients with diabetic neuropathy. Microvasc Res 48:236–245, 1994.

88. Ghani M, Malik RA, Walker D, et al: Perineurial abnormalities in the spontaneously diabetic dog. Acta Neuropathol 97:98–102, 1999.

89. Giannini C, Dyck PJ: Basement membrane reduplication and pericyte degeneration precede development of diabetic polyneuropathy and are associated with its severity. Ann Neurol 37:498–504, 1995.

90. Giannini C, Dyck PJ: Ultrastructural morphometric abnormalities of sural nerve endoneurial microvessels in diabetes mellitus. Ann Neurol 36:408–415, 1994.

91. Giannini C, Dyck PJ: Ultrastructural morphometric features of human sural nerve endoneurial microvessels. J Neuropathol Exp Neurol 52:361–369, 1993.

92. Malik RA: The pathology of human diabetic neuropathy. Diabetes 46(suppl 2): S50–S53, 1997.

93. Malik RA, Veves A, Masson EA, et al: Endoneurial capillary abnormalities in mild human diabetic neuropathy. J Neurol Neurosurg Psychiatry 55:557–561, 1992.

94. Bradley J, Thomas PK, King RHM, et al: Morphometry of endoneurial capillaries in diabetic sensory and autonomic neuropathy. Diabetologia 33:611–618, 1990.

95. Britland ST, Young RJ, Sharma AK, et al: Relationship of endoneurial capillary abnormalities to type and severity of diabetic polyneuropathy. Diabetes 39:909–913, 1990.

96. Malik RA, Newrick PG, Sharma AK, et al: Microangiopathy in human diabetic neuropathy: Relationship between capillary abnormalities and the severity of neuropathy. Diabetologia 32:92–102, 1989.

97. Sima AAF, Nathaniel V, Prashar A, et al: Endoneurial microvessels in human diabetic neuropathy. Endothelial cell dysjunction and lack of treatment effect by aldose reductase inhibitor. Diabetes 40:1090–1099, 1991.

98. Forrest KY, Maser RE, Pambianco G: Hypertension as a risk factor for diabetic neuropathy: A prospective study. Diabetes 46:665–670, 1997.

99. Mehler PS, Jeffers BW, Estacio R, et al: Associations of hypertension and complications in non–insulin-dependent diabetes mellitus. Am J Hypertens 10:152–161, 1997.

100. Fernyhough P, Gallagher A, Averill SA, et al: Aberrant neurofilament phosphorylation in sensory neurons of rats with diabetic neuropathy. Diabetes 48:881–889, 1999.

101. Quasthoff S: The role of axonal ion conductances in diabetic neuropathy: A review. Muscle Nerve 21:1246–1255, 1998.

102. Thomas PK: Growth factors and diabetic neuropathy. Diabet Med 11:732–739, 1994.

103. Tomlinson DR, Fernyhough LT, Diemel K, et al: Deficient neurotrophic support in the aetiology of diabetic neuropathy. Diabet Med 13:679–681, 1996.

104. Mizisin AP, Calcutt NA, Distefano PS, et al: Aldose reductase inhibition increases CNTF-like bioactivity and protein in sciatic nerves from galactose-fed and normal rats. Diabetes 46:647–652, 1997.

105. Apfel SC, Kessler JA, Adornato BT, et al: Recombinant human nerve growth factor in the treatment of diabetic polyneuropathy. Neurology 51:695–702, 1998.

106. Canal N, Nemni R: Autoimmunity and diabetic neuropathy. Clin Neurosci 4:371–373, 1997.

107. Sugimura K, Dyck PJ: Sural nerve myelin thickness and axis cylinder caliber in human diabetes. Neurology 31:1087–1091, 1981.

108. Dyck PJ, Giannini C: Pathologic alterations in the diabetic neuropathies of humans: A review. J Neuropathol Exp Neurol 55:1181–1193, 1996.

109. Britland ST, Young RJ, Sharma AK, et al: Association of painful and painless diabetic polyneuropathy with different patterns of nerve fibre degeneration and regeneration. Diabetes 39:898–908, 1990.

110. Sima AAF, Nathaniel V, Bril V, et al: Regeneration and repair of myelinated fibres in sural-nerve biopsy specimens from patients with diabetic neuropathy treated with Sorbinil. N Engl J Med 319:548–555, 1988.

111. Sima AAF, Nathaniel V, Bril V, et al: Histopathological heterogeneity of neuropathy in insulin-dependent and non-insulin dependent diabetes, and demonstration of axoglial dysjunction in human diabetic neuropathy. J Clin Invest 81:349–364, 1988.

112. Bomers K, Braendgaard H, Flyvbjerg A, et al: Redistribution of axoplasm in the motor root in experimental diabetes. Acta Neuropathol (Berl) 92:98–101, 1996.

113. Sharma AK, Malik RA, Dhar P, et al: Peripheral nerve abnormalities in spontaneously diabetic dog. Int J Diabetes 3:130–139, 1995.

114. Llwelyn JG, Gilbey SG, Thomas PK, et al: Sural nerve morphometry in diabetic autonomic and painful sensory neuropathy. Brain 114:867–892, 1991.

115. Engelstead JK, Davies JL, Giannini C, et al: No evidence for axonal atrophy in human diabetic polyneuropathy. J Neuropathol Exp Neurol 56:255–262, 1997.

116. Sima AAF, Prashar A, Nathaniel V, et al: Overt diabetic neuropathy: Repair of axoglial dysjunction and axonal atrophy by aldose reductase inhibition and its correlation to improvement in nerve conduction velocity. Diabet Med 10:115–121, 1993.

117. Thomas PK, Beamish NG, Small JR, et al: Paranodal structure in diabetic sensory polyneuropathy Acta Neuropathol (Berl) 92:614–620, 1996.

118. Giannini C, Dyck PJ: Axoglial dysjunction: A critical appraisal of definition, techniques, and previous results. Microsc Res Tech 34:436–444, 1996.

119. Kalichman MW, Powell HC Mizisin AP: Reactive, degenerative, and proliferative Schwann cell responses in experimental galactose and human diabetic neuropathy. Acta Neuropathol (Berl) 95:47–56, 1998.

120. Mizisin AP, Shelton GD, Wagner S, et al: Myelin splitting, Schwann cell injury and demyelination in feline diabetic neuropathy. Acta Neuropathol 95:171–174, 1998.

121. Bradley JL, Thomas PK, King RH, et al: Myelinated nerve fibre regeneration in diabetic sensory polyneuropathy: Correlation with type of diabetes. Acta Neuropathol (Berl) 90:403–410, 1995.

122. Ochoa JL: Recognition of unmyelinated fibre disease: Morphologic criteria. Muscle Nerve 1:375–387, 1978.

123. Veves A, Malik RA, Lye RH, et al: The relationship between sural nerve morphometric findings and measures of peripheral nerve function in mild diabetic neuropathy. Diabet Med 8:917–921, 1991.

124. Russell JW, Karnes JL, Dyck PJ: Sural nerve myelinated fiber density differences associated with meaningful changes in clinical and electrophysiological measurements. J Neurol Sci 135:114–117, 1996.

125. Ochoa JL: Pain mechanisms in neuropathy. Curr Opin Neurol 7:407–414. 1994.

126. Thierault M, Dort J, Sutherland G, et al: A prospective study of sensory deficits after whole sural nerve biopsies in diabetic and non-diabetic patients. Surgical approach and the role of collateral sprouting. Neurology 50:480–484, 1998.

127. McArthur JC, Stocks AE, Hauer P, et al: Epidermal nerve fibre density: Normative reference range and diagnostic efficiency. Arch Neurol 55:1513–1520, 1998.

128. Holland NR, Crawford TO, Hauer P, et al: Small-fiber sensory neuropathies: Clinical course and neuropathology of idiopathic cases. Ann Neurol 44:47–59, 1998.

129. Kennedy WR, Nolano M, Wendelschafer-Crabb G, et al: A skin blister method to study epidermal nerves in peripheral nerve disease. Muscle Nerve 22:360–371, 1999.

130. Boulton AJM: New treatments for diabetic neuropathy. Curr Opin Endocrinol Diabetes 3:330–334, 1996.

131. Watkins PJ: Treatment for diabetic neuropathy. Diabet Med 13:1007–1008, 1996.

132. Sindrup SH: Antidepressants in the treatment of diabetic neuropathy symptoms. Dan Med Bull 41:66–78, 1994.

133. Ziegler D: Pharmacological treatment of painful diabetic neuropathy. *In* Veves A (ed): Contemporary Endocrinology: Clinical Management of Diabetic Neuropathy. Totowa, NJ, Humana Press, 1998, pp 147–169.

134. Backonja M, Beydoun A, Edwards KR, et al: Gabapentin for the symptomatic treatment of painful neuropathy in patients with diabetes mellitus. JAMA 280:1831–1836, 1998.

135. Harati Y, Gooch C, Swenson M, et al: Double-blind randomized trial for tramadol for the treatment of the pain of diabetic neuropathy. Neurology 50:1842–1846, 1998.

136. Abuaisha BB, Costanzi JB, Boulton AJM: Acupuncture for the treatment of chronic painful peripheral diabetic neuropathy: A long-term study. Diabetes Res Clin Pract 39:115–121, 1998.

137. Nicolucci A, Carinci F, Cavaliere D, et al: A meta-analysis of trials on aldose reductase inhibitors in diabetic peripheral neuropathy. Diabet Med 13:1017–1026, 1996.

138. Heesom AE, Milward A, Demaine AG: Susceptibility to diabetic neuropathy in patients with insulin dependent diabetes mellitus is associated with a polymorphism at the 5' end of the aldose reductase gene. J Neurol Neurosurg Psychiatry 64:213–216, 1998.

139. Ziegler D, Reljanovic M, Hanefeld M, et al: Alpha lipoid acid in the treatment of diabetic polyneuropathy in Germany and current evidence from clinical trials. Exp Clin Endocrinol Diabetes 107:421–430, 1999.

140. Horrobin DF: Gamma-linolenic acid in the treatment of diabetic neuropathy. *In* Boulton AJM (ed): Diabetic Neuropathy Lancaster, UK, Marius Press, 1996, pp 183–195.

141. Hounsom L, Horrobin DF, Tritschler H, et al: A lipoic acid–gamma linolenic acid conjugate is effective against multiple indices of experimental diabetic neuropathy. Diabetologia 41:839–843, 1998.

142. Anand P, Terenghi G, Warner G, et al: The role of endogenous nerve growth factor in human diabetic neuropathy. Nat Med 2:703–707, 1996.

143. Malik RA, Williamson S, Abbott CA, et al: Effect of the ACE inhibitor trandolopril on human diabetic neuropathy: A randomized, controlled double-blind trial. Lancet 352:1978–1981, 1998.

144. Rendell MS, Rajfer J, Wicker PA, et al: Sildenafil in the treatment of erectile dysfunction in men with diabetes: A randomized controlled trial. JAMA 281:421–426, 1999.

145. Cheitlin MD, Hutter AM, Brindis RG, et al: Use of sildenafil (Viagra) in patients with cardiovascular disease. Circulation 99:168–177, 1999.

146. Shaw JE, Abbott CA, Tindle K, et al: A randomized controlled trial of topical glycopyrrolate, the first specific treatment for diabetic gustatory sweating. Diabetologia 40:299–301, 1997.

147. Shaw JE, Boulton AJM: The pathogenesis of diabetic foot problems: an overview. Diabetes 46(suppl 2):S58–S62, 1997.

Chapter 63

▼▼▼▼

Nephropathy: A Major Diabetic Complication

Eli A. Friedman

In this first year of the 21st century, diabetes mellitus is universally recognized as the leading cause of irreversible renal failure—unfortunately termed *end-stage renal disease* (ESRD)—in industrialized (well-fed) nations. Tracking both the incidence and prevalence of ESRD attributed to diabetes indicates an annual growth rate over the past decade in excess of 9%. According to the 1998 report of the U.S. Renal Data System (USRDS) (Fig. 63–1), in 1996, of 283,932 patients in the United States receiving either dialytic therapy or a kidney transplant, 92,211 had diabetes,[1] a prevalence rate of 32.4%. The full impact of diabetes-related kidney disease is shown by the incidence rate of 43% in 1996, during which 30,393 of 72,000 new (incident) cases of ESRD were attributed to diabetes (Fig. 63–2). Earlier assessments of the relative severity of renal injury in diabetes led to the erroneous inference that nephropathy was both of lower prevalence and less severe in type 2 diabetes as compared with type 1 diabetes. More recent retrospective and prospective observation of kidney function during the course of type 1 and 2 diabetes uncovered a risk of progression of diabetic nephropathy equivalent to that of

ESRD. In both types of diabetes, nephropathy follows a predictable course, starting with microalbuminuria, evolving to proteinuria and azotemia, culminating in ESRD.

Elsewhere in this book (see Chapters 57, 64), the management of diabetes as an endocrine disorder is reviewed. This chapter presents a nephrologist's perspective of diabetes as the dominant cause of renal disintegration. Effective strategies slow the course of nephropathy by normalization of hypertensive blood pressure, establishment of euglycemia, and perhaps by restricting dietary protein intake. Diabetes at every stage of deteriorating renal function, when compared with other causes of ESRD, induces greater morbidity and higher mortality due to concomitant (comorbid) systemic disorders, especially coronary artery and cerebrovascular disease. The diabetic patient with kidney disease is sicker and less likely to achieve rehabilitation. In this chapter, the clinical consequences of loss of renal function in diabetes are discussed and options for management of ESRD are evaluated. Additionally, a novel therapy aimed at averting tissue injury due to advanced glycosylated end-products (AGEs) (toxic compounds that accumulate in diabetic individuals), thereby retarding progression of diabetic nephropathy without requiring euglycemia, is examined.

HISTORY OF DIABETIC NEPHROPATHY

Recognition of a renal syndrome specific to diabetes mellitus lagged behind clarification of diabetes-induced injury in other organ systems. As recounted by Lundbaek,[2] Ehrlich's technique of iodine staining in 1882, which demonstrated accumulation of glycogen in renal tubular cells of diabetic patients,[3] explained Armanni's finding in 1877[4] and Ebstein's report[5] in 1883 of renal tubular vacuolization, necrosis, and glycogen accumulation. "Glycogen nephrosis," formerly accepted as pathologic proof of diabetes mellitus, is now understood to be a reversible phenomenon, not confined to the kidney, of glycogen deposition in renal tubular cells, cardiac muscle, and pancreatic β cells in diabetic persons with sustained hyperglycemia.

For the next 53 years, no clarification of renal pathology in diabetes was evident until the keystone report by Kimmelstiel and Wilson[6] in 1936. They described a striking hyaline thickening of the intercapillary connective tissue of the glomerular tufts, with the formation of nodules, in a retrospective autopsy study of eight patients, seven of whom had type 2 diabetes (one patient was admitted moribund with no

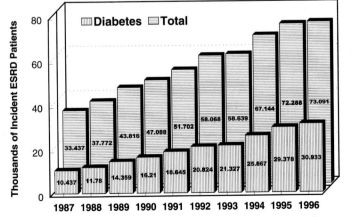

FIGURE 63–1. The annual growth in incident end-stage renal disease (ESRD) patients has been approximately 9% over the past decade as tracked by the U.S. Renal Data System and reported in 1998.[1] Note that the proportion of incident ESRD patients with diabetes has risen progressively, less than from one third in 1989 to 43% in 1996.

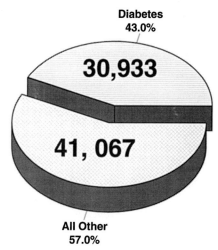

Diabetes
43.0%

30,933

41, 067

All Other
57.0%

FIGURE 63–2. *Growth of the fraction of new end-stage renal disease patients with diabetes, reported at 43% in 1996, is anticipated to exceed 50% shortly after the turn of the millennium according to the U.S. Renal Data System as reported in 1998.*[1]

clinical history), at Boston City Hospital. Nephrotic edema, massive proteinuria, and hypertension were linked to the pathologic findings of nodular and diffuse intercapillary glormerulosclerosis defining what is now termed *Kimmelstiel-Wilson disease* (KW disease), or diabetic nephropathy.

Two technical advances facilitated further understanding of the diabetic kidney. Introduction of percutaneous renal biopsy by Iversen and Brun[7] in 1951 permitted correlation of preterminal morphologic findings with clinical perturbations in the diabetic kidney. Subsequently, linking pathophysiology and pathology, Keen and co-workers[8] in 1969 first detected a small but distinctly abnormal increase in urinary albumin excretion (30 to 150 mg/day) termed *microalbuminuria* in newly diagnosed type 1 diabetic patients.

The significance of microalbuminuria was clarified by Mogensen[9] who in 1971 began a productive series of studies of protein excretion in diabetic patients which culminated in recognizing proteinuria as renal perturbation in diabetic nephropathy. By 1972, Mogensen[10] had also found that at onset of type 1 diabetes, glomerular filtration rate (GFR) may be increased by more than 40% over normal (hyperfiltration), whereas renal plasma flow (RPF) is also significantly elevated, but to a lesser extent. One year later, Mogensen and Andersen[11] reported nephromegaly as a component of type 1 diabetes. These investigators, after they were able to reduce both nephromegaly and GFR by inducing euglycemia by intensive insulin treatment, correctly theorized that the increased kidney size per se causes GFR increase in type 1 diabetes.[12]

At the close of the 1970s, type 1 diabetes had been linked to microalbuminuria, nephromegaly, and glomerular hyperfiltration. The next step in the unraveling of the pathogenesis of diabetic nephropathy was the product of meticulous study of sequential biopsies of kidneys in type 1 diabetes.[13] Mauer and colleagues[14] concluded in 1984 that "the critical lesion of diabetic nephropathy which ultimately leads to organ failure is the expansion of the glomerular mesangium." Subsequently, the KW mesangial nodule was shown in some instances to undergo lysis (mesangiolysis).[15] Most recently, Mauer's long-term study of the effect on early diabetic nephropathy in type 1 diabetic recipients of pancreas transplants indicates that after a decade of euglycemia, the KW lesions may be reversible.[16] What is now clearly established is that the appearance, severity, and progression of glomerulopathy in diabetic individuals is a consequence of hyperglycemia, though aggravating variables are operational (Fig. 63–3).

GENETICS OF DIABETES

Organ damage and clinical disease in diabetes result from the impact of environmental variables (life-style) reacting with separate genetic

predispositions to diabetes and its complications. *Diabetic nephropathy* is the inclusive term applied to the myriad renal complications of type 1 and type 2 diabetes. In both types, observational studies of large patient cohorts document the presence of a genetic predisposition to renal damage with superimposed broad susceptibility to an environmental activating factor(s), including hyperglycemia, hypertension, early exposure to cow's milk proteins, nitrosamines, early fetal blood group incompatibility or viral infections, and cigarette smoking. Sophisticated genetic probes have been employed to locate the "type 1 gene" on the short arm of chromosome 6, which, when activated by a viral infection such as varicella, rubella, or poliomyelitis, incites a continuing immunologic attack on β cells of the islets of Langerhans. While strong genetic risk markers are located in the HLA region of chromosome 6 and the insulin gene promoter on chromosome 11 p, their DNA specificities differ in different populations.[17] Genome scanning of families with several affected individuals has successfully mapped other predisposing loci situated on different chomosomal regions. Furthermore, positional cloning of type 1 susceptibility genes is in progress. Other chromosomes of the human genome have also been proposed as sites of risk genes supporting the existence of a complex interaction between genes and environment as the cause of the disease.

Environmental risk factors may either initiate autoimmunity or accelerate an already ongoing β cell destruction in those with genetically predetermined susceptibility to diabetes.[18] Incompletely understood genetic determinants predispose to type 2 diabetes[14] in many population subsets said to carry the *thrifty gene*, which enhances the efficiency of storage and release of liver glycogen during periods of food abundance and subsequent starvation. It is theorized that the "thrifty genotype" evolved to fit the life of Paleolithic humans subjected to intervals of caloric deprivation, but that with civilization overfeeding induced both obesity and type 2 diabetes.[19] While "affected" individuals harbor the "original" ancestral version of the relevant genes, healthy or "unaffected" individuals have picked up recent mutations leading to a "loss of thriftiness" of these genes.[20]

An unresolved controversy exists over the purported contribution of insertion/deletion (I/D) polymorphism of angiotensin converting enzyme (ACE) as a genetic correlate of progression of nephropathy in type 2 diabetes. This association was studied prospectively in 83 type 2 patients with diabetes followed for 9 years without discerning a correlation between ACE gene I/D polymorphism and either albuminuria or decline in GFR.[21]

A meta-analysis of 19 cross-sectional, case-control, and cohort studies in 21 populations published between 1994 and 1997, presenting

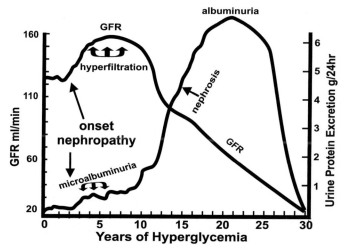

FIGURE 63–3. *The course of nephropathy in both type 1 and type 2 diabetes can be followed by two main variables: proteinuria and glomerular filtration rate (GFR). The earliest manifestations of glomerulopathy are microalbuminuria and hyperfiltration. Thereafter, progressive increase in urinary protein and decrease in GFR signal renal deterioration. A nephrotic syndrome is typical in both diabetes types. Azotemia is a late sign of far-advanced nephropathy.*

data on 5336 type 1 and type 2 diabetic subjects of all races, tested for any relationship between genotype and nephropathy. Separate analyses of the relationship between genotype and allele frequencies were performed in type 1 and type 2 diabetes by race, using Peto's odds ratio, detecting no association in white patients with type 2 diabetes, though in Asian patients with type 2 diabetes, nephropathy was increased in the presence of the DD or ID genotype.[22] Evidence supporting a modulating effect on diabetic nephropathy of ACE-I/D polymorphism was provided in the EURODIAB trial of lisinopril in 530 nonhypertensive subjects with type 1 diabetes. A significant interaction between the II and DD genotypes and response to treatment with an ACE inhibitor was noted; those with the II genotype evinced the fastest acceleration of albuminuria on placebo but had an enhanced response to lisinopril.[23]

EFFECT OF SMOKING ON DIABETES

Convincingly, a linkage between cigarette smoking and progression of diabetic nephropathy is becoming clear.[24] In the Appropriate Blood Pressure Control in Diabetes Trial, for example, in which 61% of type 2 diabetic subjects smoked cigarettes, a univariate association between diabetic nephropathy and smoking was documented. The rate of decline of creatinine clearance was greater in smokers with type 2 diabetes. Creatinine clearance fell by 1.24 ± 0.34 mL/min/month in smoking diabetic patients compared with a decrease of 0.99 ± 0.35 mL/min/month ($P < .025$) in nonsmokers.[25] Similarly, type 1 diabetic smokers had significantly faster heart rates and higher 24-hour mean arterial blood pressure (94 ± 6.7 mm Hg) compared with diabetic nonsmokers (90 ± 5.8 mm Hg, $P = .04$), including higher diastolic nighttime blood pressure (68 ± 7.3 mm Hg vs. 64 ± 5.2 mm Hg, $P = .03$).[26] As is true for preventing pulmonary and cardiac disease, stopping smoking is a prime objective of any renoprotective regimen.

EPIDEMIOLOGY OF DIABETIC NEPHROPATHY

The prevalence of diabetes in the general population is surmised from broad-based sampling of peripheral blood for hyperglycemia. In the United States, recent data collected in the Third National Health and Nutrition Examination Survey, 1988–1994 (NHANES III) and prior Health and Nutrition Examination Surveys (HANESs) permitted a probability estimate of diabetes prevalence.[27] Of 18,825 U.S. adults 20 years of age and older interviewed to ascertain a medical history of diagnosed diabetes, a subsample of 6587 adults had fasting plasma glucose measurements while a subsample of 2844 adults between 40 and 74 years of age received an oral glucose tolerance test. Prevalence was calculated using the 1997 American Diabetes Association (ADA) fasting plasma glucose criteria and the 1980–1985 World Health Organization (WHO) oral glucose tolerance test criteria.[28] The prevalence of diagnosed diabetes in 1988–1994 was 5.1% for U.S. adults 20 years of age and older (10.2 million people when extrapolated to the 1997 U.S. population). The prevalence of undiagnosed diabetes (fasting plasma glucose ≥ 126 mg/dL) was 2.7% (5.4 million), and the prevalence of impaired fasting glucose (110 to <126 mg/dL) was 6.9% (13.4 million). Men and women had similar rates, but non-Hispanic blacks and Mexican-Americans had 1.6 and 1.9 times the rate of non-Hispanic whites. Using ADA criteria, the prevalence of diabetes (diagnosed plus undiagnosed) in the total population of people aged 40 to 74 years of age increased from 8.9% in the period 1976–1980 to 12.3% by 1988–1994.

The prevalence of treated ESRD due to diabetic nephropathy has more than quadrupled over the past 30 years. Whether there has been an actual increase in the number of diabetic patients who develop renal failure or a changing attitude of acceptance of diabetic patients into renal failure programs is undetermined. Nevertheless, by 1992, the progressive increase in incidence recorded yearly over the past decade established diabetes mellitus as the most prevalent disorder leading to ESRD in the United States, Japan, and most nations in industrialized Europe. According to the USRDS, in 1991,[29, 30] of

41,317 patients begun on therapy for ESRD during 1988, 13,597 (32.9%) had diabetes, an incidence of 52 per million population. Until the 1980s, diabetic patients with failing kidneys were discouraged from seeking treatment by maintenance dialysis or kidney transplantation because of the consensus of nephrologists and transplant surgeons that they suffered unacceptably high mortality and morbidity, whereas rehabilitation was unobtainable in survivors. Such negative thinking continues through much of the world today where treatment rates for diabetic ESRD patients remain far below those in the United States.[31] Gradually, however, the cumulative effects of careful regulation of hypertension and hyperglycemia have improved the long-term outcome to the extent that restrained optimism has replaced futility in advising renal transplantation as the preferred therapy for ESRD in diabetes. Medicare statistics counted diabetic nephropathy as the diagnosis listed for 1607 of 8058 (20.7%) kidney transplants performed in 1989 in the United States[29]; the proportion of kidney recipients with diabetes rose to 24.1% (2896 of 11,996) in 1996.[1] In Europe, the proportion of kidney transplants performed in diabetic recipients is smaller (about 18%). Accompanying the growing acceptance of kidney transplantation in diabetes is a mounting success, for at least 5 years, of pancreatic transplants in type 1 diabetes, converting what has previously been thought experimental surgery to an established therapy (see later).

The prevalence of diabetes in the United States, however, has risen continuously as a result of a 19% decline since 1970 in deaths caused by diabetes. In 1982, 34,583 deaths in the United States were attributed to diabetes, making it the seventh leading underlying cause of death. Mazze et al.[32] recorded a high rate of macrovascular and microvascular disease, diabetic coma, and fetal or maternal death complicating pregnancy in those with diabetes. This survey tallied an annual rate of 5800 new cases of blindness, 4500 perinatal deaths, 40,000 lower extremity amputations, and 3000 deaths due to diabetic coma (ketotic and hyperosmolar) caused by diabetes. Between 1994 and 1980, there was a 27% increase in the death rate from diabetes (from 15.3 per 100,000 to 19.5 per 100,000).[33]

According to the 1997 surveillance report of the Centers for Disease Control and Prevention (CDC), diabetes in 1994 was the seventh leading cause of death in the United States but was the fourth leading cause of death for Native Americans. With each report of success in treating ESRD in diabetic patients, clinicians have become progressively more willing to refer their uremic diabetic patients for dialytic therapy or a renal transplant. As a consequence, chronic glomerulonephritis and hypertensive renal disease now rank below diabetes in frequency of diagnosis among new ESRD patients, substantiating Mauer and Chavers' presumption that "Diabetes is the most important cause of ESRD in the Western world."[34] An unanticipated benefit of the attention focused on diabetic nephropathy has been the realization that lessons learned in the treatment of diabetic nephropathy are often applicable to other varieties of progressive kidney disease.

Diabetes is best viewed as an incompletely defined family of diseases sharing the common abnormality of hyperglycemia. Although classifications of diabetes by type have been devised by the WHO[35] and the National Diabetes Data Group (NDDG),[36] there is substantive overlap between types to the extent that many diabetic adults defy classification. Repeated revisions of the definition of diabetes types have not eased the uncertainty of sorting by type.

The ADA[37] states that type 1 diabetes may occur at any age in individuals "who are usually thin, and usually have abrupt onset of signs and symptoms with insulinopenia before age 30. These patients often have strongly positive urine ketone tests in conjunction with hyperglycemia and are dependent on insulin therapy to prevent ketoacidosis and to sustain life." From 0% (Native Americans) to about 10% (whites) of diabetic persons in the United States are thought to have type 1 diabetes. Laboratory confirmation of type 1 diabetes according to the NDDG is provided by low plasma insulin levels, circulating islet cell antibody (ICA) titers, and characteristic HLA-DR types (DR3, DR4, DQβ). The unsatisfactory aspect of this ADA-NDDG definition is illustrated by the study of Wilson et al.,[38] who applied these criteria in 100 consecutive patients aged 13 to 70 years at the time of starting insulin, and found that 70 patients who were diagnosed under the age of 40 fit the stereotype relatively well; 88% of those who were under 20 at diagnosis were ICA positive, one third were

DR3 or DR4 heterozygotes, and 6% had neither high-risk antigen. Wilson et al. experienced difficulty, however, in adapting NDDG guidelines to patients older than 40 years of age at diagnosis; only one-fifth were ICA positive and less than one-third were DR3 or DR4 heterozygotes.[38]

The great majority of diabetic Americans—more than 90%—have type 2 diabetes,[39] defined by the ADA as afflicting people who are "usually older than 30 years at diagnosis, obese, and have relatively few classic symptoms. They are not prone to ketoacidosis except during periods of stress. Although not dependent on exogenous insulin for survival, insulin may be required for adequate control of hyperglycemia." In type 2 diabetes, insulin resistance, inherited or acquired, is an associated metabolic defect that may precede the onset of hyperglycemia.[40] Reaven[41] and others, noting the interrelationship between, and frequent coincidence of, glucose intolerance, hyperinsulinemia, hyperlipidemia, and hypertension, have proposed the term *syndrome X* to tie these metabolic perturbations together.

As mentioned above, individuals often evidence extensive overlap in presenting signs and symptoms which blurs the distinction between diabetes types. Illustrating this difficulty in diagnosis is the occurrence of the constellation referred to as maturity-onset diabetes of the young (MODY), an entity simulating type 2 diabetes that occurs as an autosomal dominant abnormality in whites, leading to macrovascular and microvascular disorders.[42] All studied individuals with MODY are insulinopenic and hypersensitive to sulfonylureas. Further challenging the current definition of type 2 diabetes is the report from Japan of a variety of diabetes that occurs frequently in patients under 30 years of age who are not obese.[43] Nagai[44] reported that of 551 Japanese patients diagnosed as diabetic before the age of 30 years, 337 (61.2%) had type 2 diabetes. Diabetic retinopathy and nephropathy are as frequent in Japanese with young-onset type 2 diabetes as in type 1 diabetes. There is rationality in the words of Abourizk and Dunn[45] who observed that: "Clinicians treating diabetic patients encounter numerous insulin-taking diabetic subjects who clinically are neither type 1 diabetes nor type 2 diabetes." After review of the course of 348 consecutive diabetic patients with a mean age of 53 years who were evaluated in Hartford, CT, these workers were unable to assign diabetes type in 35% of whites, 57% of blacks, and 59% of Hispanics. Echoing a growing call for a new classification of diabetes, these investigators remarked that current criteria for assigning diabetes type "have been neither useful for clinicians nor illuminating for researchers."[45] Throughout the world, the majority (80% to 95% depending upon race) of those with diabetes have type 2 diabetes.

NATURAL HISTORY OF DIABETIC NEPHROPATHY

Nephropathy due to nodular and diffuse intercapillary glomerular sclerosis develops in about one third of those with type 1 diabetes and an imprecisely defined, although probably equivalent proportion of those with type 2 diabetes. Diabetic nephropathy follows a characteristic course starting with microalbuminuria (see later), followed in turn by constant or fixed proteinuria and worsening azotemia.[46–48] Prior to recent studies in the Pima Indian tribe of Arizona[49] and a small group of blacks in Brooklyn, New York,[50, 51] knowledge of the sequence of perturbations in type 2 diabetes was speculative and limited to inferences drawn from type 1 diabetes and animal models of diabetes, especially the streptozotocin-induced diabetic rat. Renal involvement in type 1 diabetes has been divided into five stages.

Stage 1: Glomerular Hyperfiltration and Renomegaly

Greater than normal insulin clearances early in the course of type 1 diabetes were recognized by Cambier[52] in 1934 and confirmed by Spuhler[53] in 1946. Repeated rediscovery of glomerular hyperfiltration using radionuclide techniques or creatinine clearance[54–56] was reported over the next 20 years. At onset of type 1 diabetes, GFRs of up to

140% of normal values are present in the large majority of individuals.[57] No single pathogenesis fully explains both the nephromegaly and glomerular hyperfiltration of type 1 diabetes; a correlation between renal enlargement and glomerular hyperfunction has been inferred from the correction of both perturbations after establishment of euglycemia.[58] Insulin therapy reduces hyperglycemia and corrects glomerular hyperfiltration[59]; GFR begins to decline within 8 days of initiation of insulin therapy[60–62] and falls further during 3 months of therapy. A substantial subset—25% to 40% of individuals with type 1 diabetes—achieving usual levels of plasma glucose excursion under typical insulin therapy manifest a persistently elevated GFR,[63–66] and it is within this subgroup of hyperfiltering patients that the first reductions in GFR are subsequently noted,[67, 68] with progression to clinical nephropathy (proteinuria and azotemia).[69–71]

Numerous metabolic and several hemodynamic perturbations occur in type 1 diabetes, no one of which has been clearly identified as the single or prime causative factor responsible for glomerulosclerosis in type 1 diabetes. Confounding efforts to clarify the pathogenesis of diabetic nephropathy is the fact that less than half of all individuals with type 1 diabetes ever manifest clinical nephropathy (proteinuria or azotemia). Glomerular hyperfiltration is probably not an independent risk factor for progressive nephropathy.[72, 73]

Stage 2: Early Glomerular Lesions

Expansion of the glomerular mesangial matrix and thickening of the glomerular basement membrane (GBM) are subtle morphologic changes noted 18 to 36 months after onset of type 1 diabetes[74] which may become pronounced after 3½ to 5 years.[75] Thickening of the GBM is present whether or not progressive nephropathy develops.[76] Expansion of the glomerular mesangium is seen in type 1 diabetes and may increase markedly to the extent that nearly all capillaries are occluded despite the increase in glomerular volume (Figs. 63–4 to 63–6).[77] During this stage of morphologic change, which extends from 4 or 5 to 15 years after onset of type 1 diabetes, exercise-induced microalbuminuria may be the only clinical evidence of renal involvement.[78] A supplemental perspective of the early glomerular changes in type 1 diabetes has been provided from study of kidneys from nondiabetic donors transplanted into diabetic recipients. In biopsies of these kidneys, Mauer et al.[79] observed the same sequence of changes—mesangial matrix expansion and GBM thickening within 3 to 5 years after transplant. Reversal of these sequential changes in type 1 diabetes has been noted after 10 years of euglycemia afforded by a functioning pancreas transplant.[16]

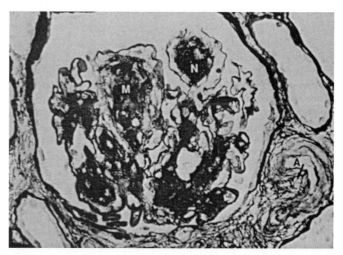

FIGURE 63–4. *Silver stain of glomerulus from a patient with type 1 diabetes of 10 years' duration. Mesangial expansion (M) and a mesangial nodule (N) are evident. Note the luminal characteristic of arteriolosclerosis in the glomerular arteriole (A).*

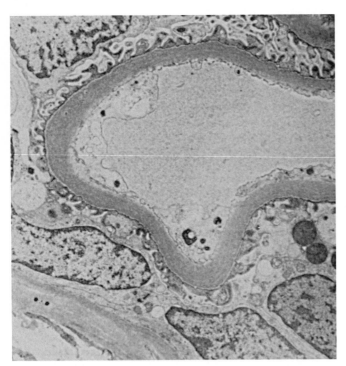

FIGURE 63–5. Glomerular capillary loop from a 16-year-old girl who had type 1 diabetes for 6 years. Poor metabolic control was associated with multiple episodes of ketoacidosis. The thick (7452 Å) glomerular basement membrane is nearly three times the normal width for adolescents and young adults (2700 Å) (×11,193).

Stage 3: Incipient Diabetic Nephropathy: The Microalbuminuric Stage

Proteinuria is a sign of renal injury. Screening for proteinuria is contingent on the sensitivity of tests available in hospital and clinical laboratories. Falling into disuse, the highly reliable and simple heat and acetic acid test for urinary albumin becomes positive when urinary protein content, which consists mainly of albumin (about 50% in diabetic nephropathy), increases to about 150 mg/dL. Of presently available dipsticks to detect urinary protein content, the Albustix test commonly employed to detect proteinuria is positive when total pro-

tein excretion exceeds 200 mg/L, about 50% of which is albumin, thereby delimiting the lower limit of clinical proteinuria, termed *macroalbuminuria*. Several methods for quantifying low concentrations of urinary albumin are available, including radioimmunoassay, nephelometric immunoassay, and enzyme-linked immunosorbent assay; a semiquantitative dipstick test has also been introduced (Micro-Bumintest, Miles Laboratories, Elkhart, IN).

These techniques for detecting small quantities of urinary protein agree on an upper daily limit of urinary albumin excretion in healthy adults of less than 30 mg. *Microalbuminuria*, defined as urinary protein excretion greater than 30 mg/day and less than 200 mg/day, is a sign of renal damage in type 1 diabetes that predicts later nephropathy and, ultimately, ESRD (Fig. 63–7).

Otherwise asymptomatic diabetic patients who excrete more than 30 mg/day of albumin are now thought to be expressing the earliest stage of diabetic nephropathy.[80] Renal involvement limited to microalbuminuria is probably reversible with treatment with an ACE inhibitor. The "absolute correlation" between microalbuminuria and subsequent clinical nephropathy in type 1 diabetes is uncertain, as only a small number of white patients manifesting microalbuminuria have been followed for the decade or longer required for this transition. Because only about one-third of individuals with type 1 diabetes, at worst, progress to renal insufficiency, intervention in terms of dietary protein restriction and administration of an ACE inhibitor is delayed by some clinicians until a decline in GFR or macroproteinuria develops; they worry that the pharmacologic and psychodynamic side effects of attempting to prevent nephropathy may entail greater risk than the chance of developing renal failure. Microalbuminuria may be an inconstant finding, with great variability in daily total protein excretion.[81] Digestion of many studies of microalbuminuria in nonproteinuric individuals with type 1 diabetes indicates a prevalence of 10% to 28% followed in 10 to 20 years by persistent and increasing clinical proteinuria or macroalbuminuria.[82] Several studies of populations with type 2 diabetes inferred a similar prevalance of microalbuminuria ranging from 13% to 30%.[83–85]

The prevalence of microalbuminuria is increased by hypertension, uncontrolled hyperglycemia, strenuous exercise, urinary tract infections, hypervolemia, and dietary protein loads. Considering the range and frequency of the variables that influence microalbuminuria, it is not surprising that the reproducibility of surveys of microalbuminuria is poor, especially when urine collection periods are shorter than 24 hours. In fact, fluctuations in daily urinary albumin excretion yield a coefficient of variation greater than 45%.[86–89] For consistency, at least three measurements of urinary albumin should be made over the course of several months.

Approximately 25% to 40% of individuals with type 1 diabetes have constant microalbuminuria after 5 to 15 years.[90, 91] Without specific intervention, as detailed later, once microalbuminuria becomes con-

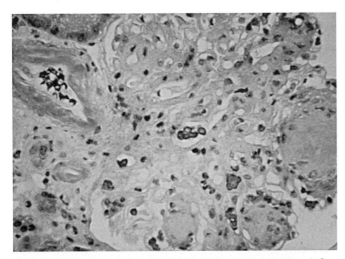

FIGURE 63–6. Advanced nodular intercapillary glomerulosclerosis from a man with type 1 diabetes of 15 years' duration. Only a few capillaries remain patent. Assessment of glomerular function in this patient was normal, illustrating the dissociation between structure and function often found in diabetic glomerulopathy.

Progression of Diabetic Kidney Disease

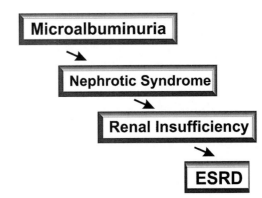

FIGURE 63–7. The usual stages of nephropathy in diabetes. Renal insufficiency may begin while urinary protein excretion persists in the nephrotic range (>3.5 g/day). *End-stage renal disease* (ESRD) is the term applied to irreversible renal failure that limits survival.

stant, a progressive downhill course toward clinical nephropathy is usual.[91, 93] Typically, albumin excretion increases by about 25 µg/min/year, while GFR remains normal or elevated. GFR begins to decline, at a variable although individually constant rate, once the amount of microalbuminuria exceeds 70 µg/min. Blood pressure elevation is higher in type 1 diabetic patients with microalbuminuria than in nonalbuminuric patients, although not necessarily higher than 140/90 mm Hg. Persistent hypertension (>140 to 160/90 mm Hg) and microalbuminuria are present in up to 40% of populations with type 1 diabetes—the combination of signs termed *incipient nephropathy* heralds near-term deterioration to clinical nephropathy.[94] During incipient nephropathy, glomerular morphology may be normal or abnormal.[95] By the time GFR has decreased below normal levels, however, morphologic changes in glomeruli are a constant finding.

Stage 4: Clinical Nephropathy: Proteinuria, Decreasing Glomerular Filtration Rate

Following a variable interval, usually of several years during which microalbuminuria is noted, with or without a supernormal GFR, GFR declines below normal and proteinuria is detectable by dipstick. Continuing urinary loss of protein, the driving force in the nephrotic syndrome, when associated with renal tubular catabolism of protein, may surpass the liver's maximal ability to synthesize albumin, resulting in hypoproteinemia. In about 30% to 40% of patients with type 1 diabetes, periorbital and ankle edema, followed by anasarca, occurs as proteinuria rises above 500 to 3000 µg/min (500 to 3000 mg/day). Hypertension is present in the majority of patients who enter this stage of clinical nephropathy. A full nephrotic syndrome (hypoproteinemia, hyperlipidemia, massive proteinuria, and anasarca) is noted when proteinuria rises to 4 to 40 g/day. The proportion of proteinuric patients with type 2 diabetes who evince a nephrotic syndrome is not well defined but is probably about the same as in type 1 diabetes. Because of their older age, anasarca in type 2 diabetic patients is often confused with congestive heart failure, especially when pericardial effusion (not cardiomegaly) increases the transverse diameter of the cardiac silhouette.

Proteinuria, defined as albumin excretion greater than 200 mg/day, is universally noted in diabetic nephropathy.[96] The absence of proteinuria casts strong doubt that any renal syndrome reflects underlying glomerulosclerosis. In the subset of diabetic patients who develop nephropathy in both type 1 diabetes and type 2 diabetes, proteinuria is duration-related, increasing in time to a florid nephrotic syndrome. Viewed from another perspective, the diagnosis of diabetic glomerulosclerosis can be inferred from a typical clinical course in which a diabetic patient manifests a transition from microalbuminuria, through fixed proteinuria, to a nephrotic syndrome that is followed by a progressive decrease in GFR. Anasarca develops in diabetic nephrotic patients at a higher serum albumin concentration than in nondiabetic patients, an observation probably explained by the fact the glycation of albumin leads to enhanced transcapillary permeability of glycated albumin compared with normal albumin.[97] Nearly 100% of diabetic patients who have reached the azotemic phase of diabetic nephropathy have coincident retinopathy when examined by fluorescein angiography; the absence of diabetic retinopathy in advanced renal disease is reason to doubt the diagnosis of diabetic nephropathy.

It should be kept in mind that because diabetic patients are at equal risk for unrelated renal diseases, the quest for a renal diagnosis should be pursued, including renal biopsy, whenever the course does not fit the usual pattern of diabetic nephropathy (absence of retinopathy, small kidneys, red blood cell casts). When blood pressure in diabetic patients is not regulated, uremia usually follows nephrosis within 1 to 3 years. Only 28% of patients with type 1 diabetes survived for 10 years beyond the onset of "clinical" proteinuria in a 1961 study, an era without effective measures to slow the course of diabetic nephropathy.[98]

Renal biopsies from patients with type 1 diabetes who have constant proteinuria show diffuse intercapillary glomerulosclerosis, mesangial expansion, and a thickened GBM[99, 100]; KW lesions of nodular glomer-

uloslerosis (initially detected in type 2 diabetes) are seen in only about 50% of cases.[100]

Stage 5: End-Stage Renal Disease

ESRD, its myriad complications, and comorbid conditions have been reported in a decreasing proportion of those with type 1 diabetes over the past 40 years. After 20 to 30 years of type 1 diabetes, about 30% to 40% of patients manifest irreversibly failed kidneys.[101] In these patients, uremic symptoms and signs become manifest as creatinine clearances that are higher than in nondiabetic persons, and renal replacement therapy is usually needed within 2 to 3 years of the onset of the nephrotic syndrome. Initiation of uremia therapy, however, may be postponed for months to years with dietary protein and fluid restriction, diuretics, and treatment with erythropoietin in patients whose symptoms are largely related to anemia.

RENAL INVOLVEMENT IN TYPE 2 DIABETES

Type 2 diabetes is a confusing disorder. Although it mimics type 1 diabetes in both expression of hyperglycemia and variety and severity of systemic and organ damage, efforts to construct a natural history of the disease and its stages have been frustrated by the inability to specify a date of onset for the disease in most patients. Although a small number of patients with type 2 diabetes have documented euglycemia immediately preceding the precipitant development of hyperosmolar coma as the first manifestation of type 2 diabetes, it is more characteristic of type 2 diabetes to be discovered incidentally in an unsuspecting patient under evaluation for other complaints (e.g., heart disease, cholecystitis, fungal skin infection).

At a minimum, 50% of individuals with hyperglycemia diagnostic of type 2 diabetes are unaware that they have diabetes.[99] From the well-defined course of diabetic retinopathy, Harris et al.[103] in a study of cohorts of type 2 diabetes patients in Wisconsin and Western Australia, reached the conclusion that the onset of type 2 diabetes actually occurs 9 to 12 years before a clinical diagnosis is established. Therefore, the prevalence of clinical nephropathy in type 2 diabetes is seriously underestimated and underreported at 2.5% to 10%.[104, 107] Recent prospective studies of populations with a high prevalence of type 2 diabetes, such as blacks,[108] Hispanics,[109] and several Native American tribes (Pima Indians, for example),[110, 111] indicate that the interval between diagnosis of type 2 diabetes and onset of ESRD ranges from 5 to 25 years. As a generalization, age at onset of diabetes is inversely proportional to the duration of diabetes before renal failure supervenes.[112] Geriatric patients with type 2 diabetes risk rapid GFR reduction due to advancing age[113–116] and atherosclerosis.[117] Other causes of microalbuminuria, including hypertension, urinary tract infection, and nondiabetic glomerulopathy, must also be excluded in older people before attributing this finding to type 2 diabetes per se.[118]

Both glomerular hyperfiltration and microalbuminuria, previously thought to be absent in type 2 diabetes, are regularly noted in diabetic Pima Indians,[119] blacks,[120] and whites.[121–123] In the study of Nelson et al.[124] of diabetic Pimas, GFR increases at onset of type 2 diabetes, remaining high so long as normalbuminuria continues. With development of macroalbuminuria (≥300 mg albumin per gram of creatinine), GFR declines as rapidly as in subjects with type 1 diabetes. Kidney biopsies in proteinuric Pima Indians disclose extensive glomerular sclerosis, mesangial expansion, and widening of the GBM, findings absent in those with normalbuminuria or microalbuminuria. Discrepancies between these and previous reports that failed to detect glomerular hyperfiltration may relate to differences in ethnic groups, variation in technique for determining GFR, or evaluation at different stages of type 2 diabetes.[125]

As for type 1 diabetes, microalbuminuria is also predictive of clinical nephropathy in type 2 diabetes; Mogensen and Christensen,[57] in a prospective study of type 2 diabetes in 76 Danish adults followed for 9 years, discerned a fourfold increased risk of progression to macroalbuminuria compared with normalbuminuric controls. Supporting the concept of a predetermined risk for nephropathy in a subset of those with diabetes, normal urinary albumin concentrations have been found in some individuals even after many years of type 2 diabetes.[125]

There may be ominous significance to microalbuminuria, whether or not the individual has diabetes. Illustrating this point, Damsgaard et al.[126] noted that among a group of 223 Danish subjects aged 60 to 74 serving as a nondiabetic control group for comparison with a cohort with type 2 diabetes, the group with microalbuminuria had 23 deaths 62 to 83 months later, compared with 8 deaths in those with a urinary albumin excretion rate below the median ($P = .0078$). Confirmation of the predictive value of microalbuminuria has been provided in several different nondiabetic populations.[127–129] Longitudinal studies of the outcome of microalbuminuric type 2 diabetic patients show that poor glycemic control and smoking are independent risk factors for progression to proteinuria, as well as for coronary heart disease and peripheral vascular disease.

In the absence of hypertension, microalbuminuric type 2 diabetic patients still progress to proteinuria despite otherwise satisfactory metabolic control.[130] The key correlate of renal deterioration is the amount of albumin excreted at the onset of the observation period in a Finnish study of 20 patients followed for 1 year.[131] In perspective, microalbuminuria, whether in hypertensive or normotensive individuals with type 2 diabetes, reliably predicts significant renal injury and delineates a risk for multisystem vasculopathy that may be progressive and fatal.

HISTOPATHOLOGY OF DIABETIC GLOMERULOPATHY

Glomerular hypertrophy, a component of nephromegaly, is regularly observed in type 1 diabetes and type 2 diabetes, especially in those glomeruli least affected by glomerulopathy. After years of microalbuminuria in newly diagnosed diabetes, fluorescence microscopy of glomeruli shows deposition of albumin and immunoglobulins in a ribbon-like pattern along tubular basement membranes and Bowman's capsule, probably reflecting passive entrapment of plasma proteins rather than an active immune process. Similar findings have been reported in skin and muscle, where its significance is equally obscure.[132] Kidney biopsies in azotemic patients with type 1 diabetes and type 2 diabetes consistently show mesangial expansion, GBM thickening, and afferent and efferent arteriolosclerosis. Eventually, after many years of diabetes, glomeruli become obliterated and obsolescent owing to diffuse and nodular intercapillary glomerulosclerosis (Figs. 63–8 and 63–9). There is poor correlation between the severity of GBM thickening, decreased GFR, amount of albuminuria, or level of hypertension.[133]

By contrast, there is good correlation between mesangial expansion and the severity of clinical diabetic nephropathy, leading to the speculation that mesangial expansion induces glomerular functional deterioration by restricting glomerular capillary vasculature and its filtering surface. The longer the duration of diabetes, the greater the risk of contracting nephropathy. Acknowledging exceptions, poor correlation exists between the histopathologic severity of glomerulopathy and the duration of diabetes in both type 1 diabetes and type 2 diabetes.

The rate of loss of GFR depends on, in addition to genetic predisposition, known and unknown variables, including severity of hypertension, dietary protein content, and degree of metabolic control of diabetes. In an individual patient, the rate of GFR loss tends to be constant with time, permitting anticipation of the approximate date when ESRD will occur. Plotting the inverse (reciprocal) of serum creatinine against time, or GFR as estimated by creatinine clearance, is clinically useful (Fig. 63–10). As GFR falls below 20 mL/min, the patient (both type 2 and type 1 diabetes) becomes catabolic and prone to multiple intercurrent disorders. A minor "cold," for example, easily tolerated by a diabetic patient with normal renal function, may confine an azotemic diabetic patient to bed for a week. Orthostatic hypotension, bowel malfunction (gastroparesis, obstipation alternating with explosive nocturnal diarrhea), and rapidly progressing vision loss amplify the morbidity of renal insufficiency. Because of multisystem failure, it is usually necessary to institute dialytic therapy at a higher

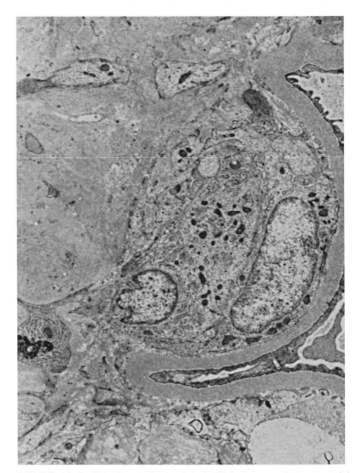

FIGURE 63–8. Thickened glomerular capillary loop and a mesangial nodule in a 56-year-old man with type 2 diabetes of 6 years' known duration (×13,060). The actual duration of type 2 diabetes is often approximated because at least one half of all affected individuals are undiagnosed.

creatinine clearance (meaning greater residual renal function) in a diabetic than in a nondiabetic patient. Maintenance hemodialysis, although rarely required in a nondiabetic patient whose creatinine clearance is above about 7 mL/min (approximately equivalent to a serum creatinine of 8 to 12 mg/dL), is often necessary in diabetic nephropathy when creatinine clearance falls to about 10 mL/min (serum creatinine

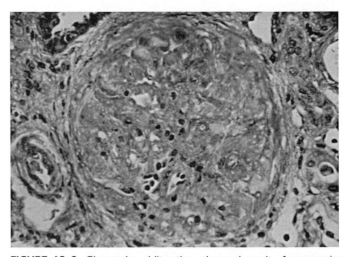

FIGURE 63–9. Glomerular obliteration, the end result of progressive nodular and diffuse glomerulosclerosis in both type 1 and type 2 diabetes. From a kidney biopsied at the time of kidney transplantation in a 34-year-old diabetic woman.

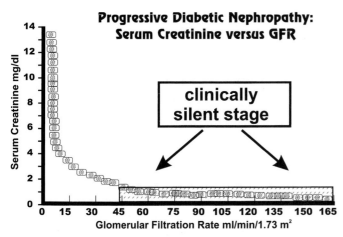

FIGURE 63–10. *Azotemia is evident only after about 75% of renal reserve is lost. This means that a normal blood urea nitrogen or serum creatinine level may be obtained even though severe diabetic glomerulopathy is present.*

concentration of ~5 mg/dL). Glucose regulation becomes difficult as renal function deteriorates in both type 1 diabetes and type 2 diabetes. Diminished renal catabolism of administered insulin in type 1 diabetes and endogenous insulin (and other small peptide hormones) in type 2 diabetes may cause episodic, profound hypoglycemia following the injection of formerly safely tolerated doses of insulin or oral hypoglycemic agents.

When considering the diagnosis of diabetic nephropathy, it must be kept in mind that all other renal disorders occur in both type 1 diabetes and type 2 diabetes with the same frequency as in nondiabetic individuals. This means that a presumption of diabetic nephropathy may be misleading to the extent that coincident disorders remain undiagnosed. For example, both type 2 diabetes and polycystic kidney disease typically cause ESRD in the fourth, fifth, and sixth decades of life. Failure to discover polycystic disease in a known diabetic individual may confound subsequent management of hematuria (ruptured renal cyst), hepatomegaly (cystic expansion), ovarian enlargement (cystic expansion), chest pain (ruptured pulmonary cyst), and cerebral hemorrhage (aneurysm rupture) as components of the polycystic disease syndrome rather than type 2 diabetes. Approximately 50% to 70% of patients with type 2 diabetes are hypertensive when diabetes is first diagnosed. Distinguishing renal damage caused by hypertension from that due to diabetes is difficult.[134–136]

It is often not possible to segregate the effect of protracted blood pressure elevation from that of diabetes on worsening proteinuria or deteriorating GFR. Blurring the distinction between hypertension and diabetes as concomitant causes of renal deterioration is the fact that hypertension, itself a cause of ESRD, is often noted in the absence of renal disease and has been related to obesity, advancing age, and hyperinsulinism.[137]

Hypertension and diabetes are independent risk factors for atherosclerotic vascular disease and their combination is associated with an increased incidence of nephropathy, ischemic heart disease, peripheral vascular disease, and stroke. Multicenter trials demonstrated that antihypertensive therapy reduces progression of diabetic kidney disease and mortality in hypertensive individuals with type 1 and type 2 diabetes. Benefit is tangible in microalbuminuric diabetic persons and also in those with overt renal disease.[138]

GENETIC PREDISPOSITION TO DIABETIC NEPHROPATHY

Epidemiologic studies suggest that not only is diabetes an inherited disorder, at least in predisposition, but that hypertension and nephropathy may also be inherited as independent risks in diabetic individuals.[139] For example, diabetic subjects with a family history of essential hypertension have a higher incidence of nephropathy.[140–144] Further,

essential hypertension is known to be associated with increased activity of the erythrocyte sodium-lithium countertransport system,[145] and those who manifest glomerular hyperfiltration also have increased activity of this membrane transport system.[146] It is reasoned that in diabetes a genetic or familial tendency to hypertension may predispose to the risk of phenotypic expression of hypertension or nephropathy, or both. At variance with this thesis are data suggesting that the mechanisms for increased sodium-lithium countertransport activity in hypertension and in diabetes are dissimilar.[147] More recent inquiries have found that though there is good correlation between sodium-lithium countertransport activity and hypertension, the relationship in diabetes is weak and probably not significant.[148]

PATHOGENESIS OF DIABETIC NEPHROPATHY

Kidneys in diabetic individuals are under stress induced by hemodynamic and metabolic perturbations. Debate is intense over the relative importance of intraglomerular hypertension vs. hyperglycemia as the two most suspected key causes of glomerulosclerosis. Lacking a reliable indicator of renal morphologic damage, however, precise timing of the transition from diabetes as a purely metabolic disease to that of a multisystem vasculopathy is often a clinical guess. The relative importance of capillary hypertension, hyperglycemia, hyperlipidemia, glycation, AGE formation, sorbitol synthesis, nitric oxide formation, and genetic predetermination to the pathogenesis of intercapillary glomerulosclerosis is the subject of ongoing research in multiple laboratories.

No single mechanism is consonant with a large body of seemingly incompatible experimental data. The hyperglycemia school infers from the results of kidney transplantation that ambient glucose concentration is the main risk factor for glomerular damage. Support for this thesis is drawn from several experiments: (1) Recurrent intercapillary glomerulosclerosis and renal failure can develop in kidneys obtained from nondiabetic donors that are transplanted into diabetic recipients.[149] (2) Kidney graft recipients who become diabetic only after administration of corticosteroid drugs (steroid diabetics) may develop typical diabetic glomerulopathy characterized by nodular and diffuse intercapillary glomerulosclerosis. (3) In isolated case reports, early diabetic glomerulopathy may be reversed by establishment of a euglycemic environment, as shown by disappearance of glomerulosclerosis in two cadaveric donor kidneys obtained from a diabetic donor after transplantation into nondiabetic recipients.[150] Further to the point, if nephromegaly is accepted as an early morphologic change in diabetic nephropathy, then the reduction in renal size induced by sustained euglycemia is evidence that correction of euglycemia reverses morphologic injury.[151]

Pathogenetic abnormalities other than hyperglycemia—especially excess activity along the sorbitol pathway of glucose metabolism—are proposed to explain microvasculopathy. Derivative from this reasoning, regimens to reduce synthesis of sorbitol and other alcohols by inhibition of aldose reductase have been applied to streptozotocin-induced diabetic rats, with successful interdiction of diabetic nephropathy, neuropathy, and retinopathy.[152] Clinical trials of aldose reductase inhibitors, unfortunately, have not fulfilled the promise of positive results in rodents.[153, 154]

Other experiments in animal models of diabetes suggest that small vessel injury may, under defined circumstances, be associated with plasma hyperviscosity or elevated circulating thromboxane and platelet-derived growth factor(s). A return toward normal in the hemorheologic properties of blood in diabetic azotemic patients is the objective of one research initiative, and the reduction of erythrocyte stiffness, a hemorheologic alteration universally noted in diabetes, by administration of pentoxifylline, is another.[155, 156] Reviewing a decade-long experience in normalizing blood rheology in diabetes, Solerte et al.[157] reported that in diabetic patients with hemorheologic alterations and angiopathic complications, pentoxifylline significantly reduced blood and plasma viscosity (at high and low shear rates), fibrinogen and erythrocyte aggregation, and increased erythrocyte filterability. Improved hemorheology was obtained independently of changes in glycometabolic control and body weight but was associated with reductions in arterial blood pressure levels and in urinary excretion of albumin and total protein.[157] Pentoxifylline slows the course of renal injury in microalbuminuric and proteinuric patients with type 1 and type 2 diabetes, significantly reducing proteinuria.[158] An alternative view is that the complex central mechanism underlying diabetic microvasculopathy is overactivation of protein kinase C, stimulated by hyperglycemia. Hyperactive protein kinase C blunts the availability of nitric oxide, increases production of superoxide and endothelin, impairs insulin function, diminishes synthesis of prostaglandin E_1 (PGE₁, prostacyclin), and increases activation and endothelial adherence of leukocytes. Treatment of these dysfunctions might be affected by dietary supplementation with high-dose antioxidants, fish oil, γ-linolenic acid, chromium, arginine, carnitine, and ginkgolides. Pharmaceuticals likely to be beneficial according to this formulation include pentoxifylline, probucol, replacement estrogens, and inhibitors of ACE and aldose reductase.[159]

Advanced Glycosylated End-Products

In health, reducing sugars such as glucose react nonenzymatically and reversibly with free amino groups in proteins to form small amounts of stable Amadori products through Schiff base adducts. In normal aging, spontaneous further irreversible modification of proteins by glucose results in the formation of AGEs, a heterogeneous family of biologically and chemically reactive compounds with cross-linking properties.[160] This process of protein modification is amplified by the high ambient glucose concentration present in diabetes.[161, 162]

Circulating AGE peptides (molecular weight between 2000 and 6000) cross-link with collagen, a perturbation promoting diabetic microvascular complications. AGEs also increase vascular permeability, procoagulant activity, adhesion molecule expression, and monocyte influx, thereby contributing to vascular injury.[160, 161] Specific receptors binding AGEs are located on endothelial cells.[163]

AGE peptides are normally excreted in the urine and their plasma concentration is inversely proportional to the GFR. Consequently, there is a progressive and marked increase in plasma and tissue levels of AGEs as diabetic patients develop renal failure.[164–167] Neither hemodialysis nor peritoneal dialysis decreases the "toxic" levels to normal, but following restoration of half-normal glomerular filtration by renal transplantation, AGE levels fall sharply to within the normal range within 8 hours.

Evidence derived from studies in rodents indicates that AGEs may be important in the genesis of diabetic tissue injury. For example, administration of AGE-modified albumin to nondiabetic rats for 4 weeks led to glomerular hypertrophy and increased extracellular matrix production in association with activation of the genes for collagen, laminin, and transforming growth factor-β.[168] Similar changes were noted when AGEs alone were given to achieve plasma concentrations equivalent to those seen in diabetic animals.[169] After 5 months, the renal AGE content in AGE-treated rats was 50% above controls while the plasma concentration was 2.8 times greater than controls. AGE-treated rats had a 50% expansion in glomerular volume, basement membrane widening, and increased mesangial matrix, indicating significant glomerulosclerosis compared with untreated controls.

In humans, convincing studies indicate that serum AGE levels reflect the severity of diabetic complications such as retinopathy. For example, in a cohort of 125 patients with type 2 diabetes, a significant correlation was noted between AGE levels and the presence or absence of proliferative retinopathy (5.7 vs. 3.1 mU/mL for those with and without retinopathy, respectively, $P <.025$).[170] A correlation was also observed between an elevated serum concentration of creatinine and enhanced AGE levels. The rapidly progressive atherosclerosis that develops in patients with diabetes and renal insufficiency is stimulated by AGEs. AGEs promote the influx of mononuclear cells and stimulate cell proliferation[170, 171] and collagen-linked AGEs within the atherosclerotic lesion bind plasma proteins, interact with macrophage receptors to induce cytokine and growth factor release, and quench nitric oxide activity.[172] There is also evidence that AGEs modify low-density lipoprotein (LDL), making it less able to be cleared by the LDL receptors.[173] In one study, for instance, LDL modified in vitro by AGE

peptides (at the concentration present in azotemic diabetic patients) markedly impaired LDL clearance when injected into transgenic mice expressing the human LDL receptor. Immunohistochemical analysis of coronary arteries obtained from patients with type 2 diabetes detected high levels of AGE reactivity within atherosclerotic plaques stained with anti-AGE antibodies.[174] Thus, there is a pathogenetic linkage of hyperglycemia, hyperlipidemia, and atherosclerosis in diabetes.

A construct fitting present evidence is that AGE formation promotes diabetic complications by changing the structure and function of extracellular matrix in the glomerular mesangium and elsewhere. In type IV collagen from basement membrane, for example, AGE formation decreases binding of the noncollagenous NC1 domain to the helix-rich domain, thereby interfering with lateral association of these molecules into a normal lattice structure.[175] Furthermore, alterations of type I collagen, a substance also found in the glomerular mesangium, by AGEs expands molecular packing.[172] These alterations in the integrity of collagen adversely affect biologic functions important to normal vascular tissue integrity such as reaction to endothelium-derived relaxing factor (nitric oxide) and antiproliferative factors.[176] AGEs impair nitric oxide–mediated processes, including neurotransmission,[177] wound healing,[178] blood flow in small vessels,[179] and decreased cell proliferation.[180] It follows that the toxicity of AGEs may be mediated in part by their interference with nitric oxide.[181]

Aminoguanidine

$$\underset{\underset{NH}{\|}}{H_2N-C-NHNH_2}$$

AMINOGUANIDINE (PIMAGEDINE). Empiric formula: CH_6N_4. Mol wt: 110.5.

Preventing AGE formation is an attractive approach to preventing diabetic microvascular complications because it bypasses the usually difficult goal of achieving euglycemia. Aminoguanidine has a structure similar to alpha-hydrazinohistidine, a compound known to reduce diabetes-induced vascular leakage.[182]

In streptozotocin-induced diabetes in the rat, aminoguanidine diminishes proteinuria, mesangial matrix expansion, matrix gene expression, and basement membrane thickness.[183, 184] It also diminishes deposition of AGEs in glomeruli and tubules; this benefit is directly related to the duration of therapy.[185] Experimental diabetic neuropathy is attenuated with aminoguanidine.[186, 187] Diabetic heart disease may be prevented by aminoguanidine. One study in rats found that aminoguanidine inhibited both increased myocardial collagen fluorescence (indicative of AGE accumulation) and decreased left ventricular end-diastolic compliance (characteristic of early cardiomyopathy).[188] These effects block development of the "stiff" myocardium that is a principal component of diabetic cardiomyopathy.

Mechanism of Action

Aminoguanidine may act by preventing formation of reactive AGEs and their subsequent cross-linking with albumin, leading to a reduction in AGE level,[189] or by blocking synthesis of nitric oxide.[190–193] In one study, for example, aminoguanidine and methylguanidine normalized vascular albumin permeability in diabetic rats, although only aminoguanidine inhibited AGE formation.[194] A possible explanation is that both guanidines inhibited nitric oxide synthase, suggesting that nitric oxide contributes to the vascular dysfunction in diabetes.[195]

Multicenter clinical trials seek to evaluate the effect of aminoguanidine on the course of diabetic nephropathy after onset of clinical proteinuria in type 1 and type 2 diabetes. For each type of diabetes, adults with documented diabetes, fixed proteinuria greater than or equal to 500 mg/day, and a plasma creatinine concentration of greater than or equal to 1.0 mg/dL (88 μmol/L) in women or greater than or equal to 1.3 mg/dL (115 μmol/L) in men were randomly assigned to treatment with aminoguanidine or placebo for 4 years. The effect of treatment on the amount of proteinuria, progression of renal insufficiency, and the course of retinopathy are being monitored. Another trial is evaluating the efficacy of aminoguanidine in reducing mortality in diabetic patients undergoing maintenance hemodialysis. Underlying this study is the hypothesis that the lower death rate in diabetic patients with a functional kidney transplant when compared with those remaining on dialysis (both peritoneal and hemodialysis: see below) results from near normalization of AGE levels observed after a successful renal allograft.

AGE Breakers

Since AGEs irreversibly bind to macromolecules through covalently cross-linked proximate amino groups, an agent that cleaves these bonds may be efficacious. A prototypic AGE cross-link "breaker," *N*-phenacylthiazolium bromide (PTB), separates AGE cross-links in vivo in diabetic rats, thereby suggesting an alternative means of slowing the development of diabetic complications.[196] However, an unexpected dissociation between AGE tissue localization and glomerular histopathology was noted in streptozotocin-induced diabetic rats following treatment with PTB.[197] In this study, no difference in glomerular volume, urinary protein excretion, or serum creatinine levels was noted between PTB-treated and control diabetic rats, although PTB treatment decreased renal collagen-bound AGEs and increased urinary AGE excretion. The clinical role of PTB is not established.

AGE toxicity is mediated in part by AGE binding to specific receptors on endothelial cells, thereby suggesting that agents that inhibit this interaction may be beneficial. Support for this hypothesis is provided by the finding that atherosclerosis is completely suppressed by administration of the soluble extracellular domain of the AGE receptor in diabetic mice deficient for apolipoprotein E (a model for accelerated atherosclerosis).[198–204]

CLINICAL MANAGEMENT

Clinical lessons learned, mainly during the past decade, have been blended into a comprehensive regimen for slowing the course of diabetic nephropathy (Figs. 63–11 to 63–22). So effective have these interventions been that the natural history of diabetic nephropathy has required continuous revision to reflect an increasingly improved prognosis. The cardinal component of all therapeutic regimens applicable to diabetic nephropathy is reduction of hypertensive blood pressure.

Hypertension

Prospective randomized trials of the effect of pharmacologic induction of normotension in type 1 and type 2 diabetic patients with

Diabetic Nephropathy: Comprehensive Management

SPECIALIST	FREQUENCY
Cardiologist ⬟	Annually to prn
Dentist ⬟	Semiannually to prn
Endocrinologist	prn
Gastroenterologist	prn
Neurologist	prn
Nurse-Educator ⬟	Monthly to prn
Nutritionist	prn
Ophthalmologist ⬟	Semiannually or prn
Podiatrist ⬟	Monthly
Psychiatrist	prn

⬟ essential

FIGURE 63–12. *An ideal checklist of specialty consultations is listed. Most important are cardiology and ophthalmology.*

persistent microalbuminuria indicate that urinary albumin excretion may be reduced while clinically evident nephropathy is postponed and perhaps prevented. Diabetes and hypertension are both common conditions associated with a high morbidity and mortality. Hypertension and diabetes mellitus occurring together, as they do in 50% of diabetic patients, results in a 7.2-fold increase in crude mortality. Whether associated with type 1 or type 2 diabetes, hypertension escalates mortality to 37 times above that of a healthy population.[205]

As reviewed by Parving, in those with overt diabetic nephropathy, blood pressure reduction, whether with ACE inhibitors or non–ACE inhibitors (frequently in combination with diuretics) (a) reduces albuminuria; (b) delays progression of nephropathy; (c) postpones renal insufficiency; and (d) improves survival in type 1 and type 2 diabetic patients with diabetic nephropathy. An additional advantage of treating diabetic patients with isolated systolic hypertension is a sharp reduction in fatal and nonfatal cardiovascular events.[206]

Attention to blood pressure regulation is essential even after onset of ESRD, as uncontrolled hypertension adds a significant risk to

Assessing Renal Integrity in Diabetes

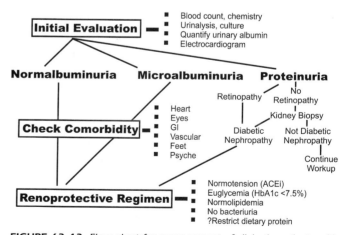

FIGURE 63–13. *Flow chart for management of diabetic patients with and without proteinuria. Absence of microalbuminuria portends a benign course. Microalbuminuria and proteinuria, if not associated with diabetic retinopathy (background or proliferative retinopathy), may not be attributed to diabetes. Discovery of proteinuria without retinopathy is reason to perform a percutaneous kidney biopsy to discern the pathogenesis of the renal syndrome. ACEi, angiotensin-converting enzyme; HbAlc, hemoglobin A_{lc}.*

Diabetic Nephropathy Clinical Team Members

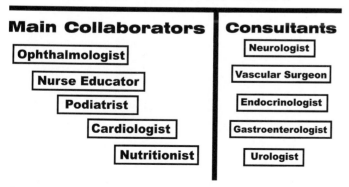

FIGURE 63–11. *Comprehensive management of comorbidity in a patient with diabetic nephropathy depends on the skills of a competent team. Cardiac evaluation is especially important to detect the threat of serious coronary artery disease.*

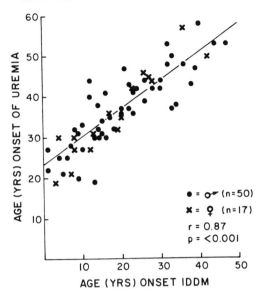

CORRELATION OF AGE AT ONSET OF UREMIA
WITH AGE AT ONSET OF IDDM (o⁰ + ♀)

FIGURE 63–14. After a mean of about 20 years from the onset of insulin dependence, renal failure can be anticipated in those whose proteinuria and azotemia were listed as initial evidence of nephropathy. Shown here is the interval from onset of diabetes to uremia in 67 type 1 diabetic kidney transplant recipients at University Hospital of Brooklyn.

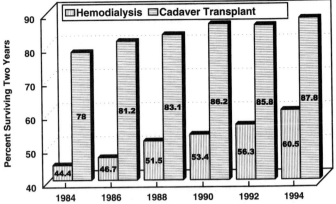

FIGURE 63–16. Survival of diabetic end-stage renal disease (ESRD) patients treated with a kidney transplant is markedly superior to that attained by hemodialysis. Over the past decade, continuous improvement in survival for both treatment modalities is evident. (Data are from Renal Data System: USRDS 1999 Annual Data Report. Bethesda, MD, National Institutes of Diabetes and Digestive and Kidney Diseases, April 1999.)

patient and kidney graft survival in diabetic kidney transplant recipients.[207] By controlling hypertension, mortality in advanced diabetic nephropathy has been improved from 50% to 70% over 10 years when antihypertensive therapy is not included in routine management,[208] and to 18% when effective treatment of hypertension is a component of care.[209]

Vigorous blood pressure control protects major organ systems vulnerable to diabetic microvasculopathy and macrovasculopathy. With great individual variation, effective reduction in blood pressure can be achieved by combinations of diuretics, vasodilators, β-blockers, calcium channel blockers, and renin antagonists. In the kidney, systemic hypertension is thought injurious because dilated afferent glomerular

arterioles transmit systemic blood pressure to glomeruli, further increasing the glomerular capillary hypertension already present due to hyperfiltration or glomerular hypertrophy.[210–212] Supporting this reasoning is the observation that, in unilateral renal artery stenosis, the obstructed kidney is protected from the effect of systemic blood pressure and exhibits minimal if any of the morphologic changes of diabetes, whereas the contralateral kidney with a patent artery shows typical diabetic nephropathy.[213] There is no reservation to the mandate to establish blood pressure control to slow progression of diabetic renal disease.[214–217]

In type 1 diabetes, treatment of hypertension in the microalbuminuric stage significantly slows or arrests progression[218]; once proteinuria becomes constant, the rate of further loss of GFR can only be slowed.[219, 220] Parving et al.,[216] in a pioneer study of six hypertensive adults with nephrotic-range proteinuria due to type 1 diabetes, observed that treatment with metoprolol, hydralazine, and furosemide for 28 to 86 months reduced mean blood pressure from 162/103 to 144/95 mm Hg, resulting in a 60% reduction in the rate of fall of GFR from 1.23 to 0.49 mL/min/month, and a reduction in albumin excretion by 5% to 10% per year. Using a similar antihypertensive regimen,[221] reduced hypertensive blood pressures from 143/96 to 129/84 mm Hg in 10 patients with type 1 diabetes who were followed for 32 to 91 months produced a 75% decrease in the rate of decline of GFR from

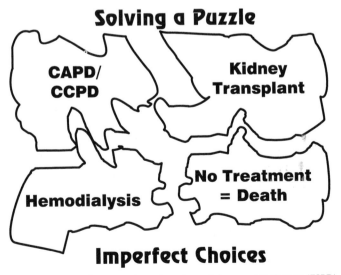

FIGURE 63–15. Therapeutic options in end-stage renal disease (ESRD) are shown as pieces in a puzzle. The selection of specific therapy requires individualization, especially for live donor kidney transplantation. Rejection of a transplanted kidney may be followed by dialysis. Both peritoneal dialysis and hemodialysis have been employed effectively in diabetic patients. CAPD, continuous ambulatory peritoneal dialysis; CCPD, continuous cyclic peritoneal dialysis.

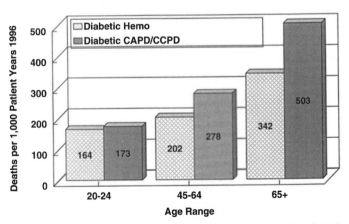

FIGURE 63–17. Hemodialysis (Hemo) affords better survival for diabetic end-stage renal disease (ESRD) patients than does peritoneal dialysis (CAPD/CCPD): Shown are subsets of diabetic patients sorted by age. Similar curves are obtained when sorting by sex or race. (Data from U.S. Renal Data System and reported in 1998.[1])

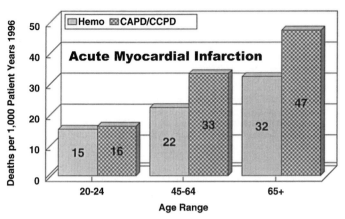

FIGURE 63–18. Heart disease, especially myocardial infarction, is the primary cause of death in diabetic end-stage renal disease (ESRD) patients treated by dialysis of any type or a kidney transplant. The risk of dying of a heart attack is greater for those treated by peritoneal dialysis (CAPD/CCPD) than for hemodialysis (Hemo). (Data are from the U.S. Renal Data System as reported in 1998.[1])

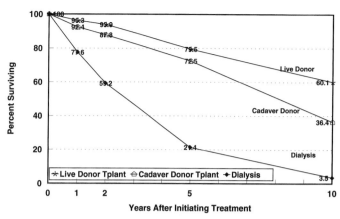

FIGURE 63–20. After a decade, few diabetic patients treated by dialysis (<5%) are alive. The benefit of a live donor kidney transplant (Tplant) is evident. (Data from U.S. Renal Data System and reported in 1998.[1])

0.89 to 0.22 mL/min/month. As noted above, antihypertensive therapy in patients with type 1 diabetes and clinical or advanced nephropathy for longer than 8 years greatly improves survival, from 48% to 87%.[222, 223] Enhanced survival was attributed to postponement of uremia and reduction of cardiac disease and not to the earlier application of ESRD therapy.[223]

The Working Group on Hypertension in Diabetes[222] initially suggested that blood pressure be lowered to at least 149/90 mm Hg; however, there are strong arguments for sustaining antihypertensive therapy "at a blood pressure level less than that conventionally considered hypertensive."[223] Recent evidence extends the finding that reduction of arterial pressure to 140/90 mmHg slows decline in renal function in diabetic nephropathy to the inference that decreasing arterial pressure below 130/85 mm Hg affords even greater protection against the progression of diabetic nephropathy. To attain this degree of blood pressure reduction almost always necessitates more than one antihypertensive drug and a willing patient. The ideal medication combination is far from clear, though adding a calcium channel blocker to an ACE inhibitor is usually satisfactory. [We target treatment blood pressures that would be equivalent to "normal" for the patient's age and sex, with an upper limit of 120 to 130/80 to 85 mm Hg.]

Is There a Specific Indication for Angiotensin-Converting Enzyme Inhibitors?

ACE inhibitors are highly effective in retarding progression of kidney damage in rats.[224–227] Not all antihypertensive drugs reduce proteinuria and retard glomerular injury in the rat, a particular benefit of treatment with ACE inhibitors.[227, 228] A special advantage for ACE inhibitors has been linked to their purported reduction of intraglomerular pressure. On the other hand, enalapril improves renal function and retards histologic damage in five-sixth nephrectomized rats, despite continued elevation of glomerular capillary pressure.[229] Other suggested benefits of ACE inhibitors include (1) inhibition of mesangial cell proliferation and matrix production, and (2) enhancement of the cyclooxygenase pathway,[230] with increased prostaglandin production.[231] In humans ACE inhibitors decrease the passage of large-molecular-weight dextrans and albumin through the GBM.

Multiple studies document the value of ACE inhibitors in hypertensive diabetic patients with incipient nephropathy. ACE inhibitors slow the fall of GFR by about 50% during the first 2 years of follow-up.[232] Combining an ACE inhibitor with a calcium antagonist permits equivalent blood pressure reduction by lower doses of both drugs, attenuating both albuminuria and the rate of decline of GFR with a lower side effect profile than that of either agent alone.[233] To date, however, no evidence indicates that treatment with an ACE inhibitor

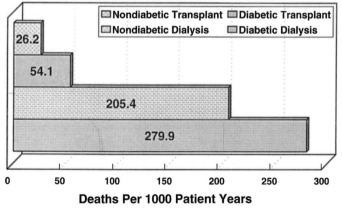

FIGURE 63–19. Comparative death rates 1993–1995 for diabetic and nondiabetic end-stage renal disease patients treated by dialysis (pooled peritoneal dialysis and hemodialysis) or a kidney transplant are shown. Note the lower death rate for diabetic kidney recipients compared with those treated by dialysis. While selection of healthier and younger patients for a transplant explains some of the difference, other factors are operative. One hypothesis discussed is that toxic advanced glycosylated end-products (AGEs) are retained during a dialysis regimen but excreted promptly after receipt of a functioning kidney transplant. (Data from the U.S. Renal Data System as reported in 1998.[1])

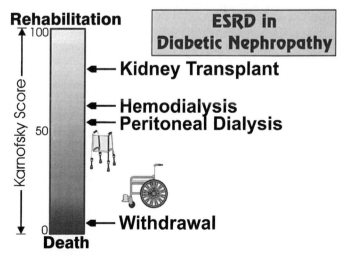

FIGURE 63–21. Rehabilitation of diabetic patients with end-stage renal disease (ESRD) receiving transplants is superior to that than in patients treated by dialysis. Hemodialysis is more likely to promote rehabilitation than is peritoneal dialysis. Data are composite from the author's surveys.

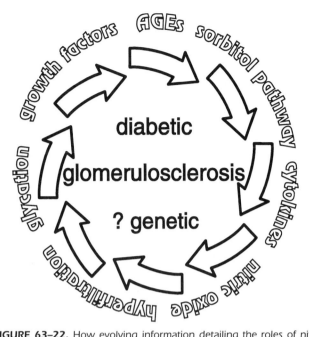

FIGURE 63–22. How evolving information detailing the roles of nitric oxide and advanced glycosylated end-products (AGEs) will fit into the pathogenesis of diabetic complications is still far from clear. Depicted in this diagram are the interrelated roles of genetic predetermined factors and environmental influences, including hyperglycemia. Not shown are other potential variables such as cigarette smoking.

decreases either the risk of or the time to development of ESRD compared with other antihypertensive drug combinations. Indeed, whether treatment with an ACE inhibitor holds special advantage over other classes of antihypertensive drugs in terms of renoprotective effect in diabetic nephropathy is judged a "major controversy" by the International Society of Hypertension.[234] Even in advanced diabetic nephropathy, reductions in proteinuria and reduction in the rate of GFR loss followed treatment with an ACE inhibitor.[235–237] In perspective, because of their efficacy, relative lack of side effects, and good metabolic profile during treatment, ACE inhibitors rank as first-line treatment in both type 1[238] and type 2 diabetes.[239]

Antihypertensive Drugs

Confusion clouds selection of specific drugs for treatment of hypertensive diabetic patients. Markets for ACE inhibitors and calcium channel blockers exceed $2 billion, each fostering extensive advertising campaigns targeting physicians. The stressful decision process involves choosing among drug classes and then picking a unique molecular configuration within a class. Within the past 3 years, head-to-head prospective trials of ACE inhibitors vs. calcium channel blockers have been completed. In the Appropriate Blood Pressure Control in Diabetes (ABCD) trial in hypertensive persons with type 2 diabetes, the incidence of cardiovascular events over a 5-year follow-up period was compared for enalapril vs. nisoldipine a long-acting calcium antagonist.[240] The study randomized diabetic patients for moderate blood pressure control (target diastolic pressure, 80 to 90 mm Hg) contrasted with intensive control (target diastolic pressure, 75 mm Hg). In 470 hypertensive patients, the incidence of fatal and nonfatal myocardial infarctions was significantly ($P = .001$) higher among those receiving nisoldipine (n = 25) compared with those receiving enalapril (n = 5). A similar outcome was reported in the Fosinopril vs. Amlodipine Cardiovascular Events Randomized Trial (FACET) sustaining the impression that ACE inhibitors may be preferable to calcium antagonists for managing hypertension in diabetic patients.[241]

Parving, who initially demonstrated the salutary renoprotective effect of reducing hypertensive blood pressure in diabetic patients (before introduction of ACE inhibitors or calcium channel blockers),

interprets the ABCD and FACET results, that "supporting the combination of a calcium antagonist with an ACE inhibitor is a rational therapeutic choice in patients with coexisting hypertension and diabetes."[242] Reflecting on the same experimental data, other investigators reached a different conclusion, that "angiotensin-converting enzyme inhibitors and low-dose diuretics may be more effective than calcium antagonists for prevention of cardiovascular events in hypertensive patients with diabetes or impaired glucose control."[243]

Approximately 15% of diabetic patients in our clinic discontinue enalapril, captopril, or other ACE inhibitors because of troublesome side effects, particularly hyperkalemia and a dry, nonproductive cough. Of these, perhaps one half tolerate blood pressure reduction with an angiotensin II receptor antagonist such as lovasartin, candisartan, or irbesartan.[244] Whether the angiotensin II receptor antagonists will retard progression of diabetic nephropathy is undermined, though they are well tolerated and safe in hemodialysis patients.[245] Several prospective randomized trials addressing this question have been begun and will be reported over the next 2 years. As an example, the Irbesartan Diabetic Nephropathy Trial (IDNT) in progress will evaluate the effect of irbesartan in 1650 type 2 diabetic patients randomly assigned to placebo, irbesartan, or amlodipine.[246]

Based on interpretation of available evidence, after prescribing an ACE inhibitor (switching to an angiotensin II receptor antagonist for those intolerant) our second-choice drug for diabetic nephropathy is a calcium antagonist, alone or in combination with or without diuretics. For resistant hypertension, we next add β-blockers, central α_2-agonists (e.g., clonidine), and peripheral vasodilators (prazosin, hydralazine, minoxidil) in a trial-and-error approach. For most patients with type 2 diabetes, obesity is a coincident disorder for which a weight reduction program and physical training are established to enhance insulin sensitivity and improve hyperlipidemia.[247, 248]

Hyperlipidemia is recognized as a risk factor for progression of nephropathy in diabetes patients that is independent of hyperglycemia and hypertension. In type 2 diabetes, the combination of high-to-normal range blood pressure with moderately elevated levels of total cholesterol and hemoglobin A_{1c} defines a group at high risk for progression to diabetic nephropathy, as well as symptomatic arteriosclerotic cardiovascular disease.[249]

Dietary Protein Restriction

In health[250, 251] and in diabetes, dietary protein intake modulates renal hemodynamics.[252, 253] Some evidence indicates that in type 1 diabetes, ingestion of a high protein diet increases the risk of nephropathy.[254] In rodent models of induced diabetes, moderate and severe protein restriction early in the course of diabetes normalizes glomerular hypertension[255, 256] owing to decreased fractional clearance of albumin[257, 258] and immunoglobulin G. The value of dietary protein restriction in type 2 diabetes was suggested by Zeller et al.[259] in a small prospective, randomized, controlled study of 20 subjects with clinical proteinuria (mean 3144 ± 417 mg/day) or renal impairment (iothalamate clearance 46 ± 4.8 mL/min/1.73 m^2) who were given a 0.6 g/kg/day protein diet for a mean of 34.7 months. There was a fourfold decrease in the rate of fall of GFR compared with that in 15 controls after 3 months. Mean protein excretion fell by 24% (760 mg) in the study group and rose by 22% (928 mg) in controls. At the conclusion of the study, the reduction in proteinuria in the study population was only 6% (196 mg), whereas the controls had a 24% (1024 mg) increase. Several other reports confirm that in type 1 diabetes with advanced nephropathy, curtailing the amount of ingested protein produces a slight to substantive reduction in the rate of fall of GFR, with a moderate to great reduction in proteinuria.[260–264]

Jibani et al.[265] conducted an intriguing trial of a vegetarian diet in type 1 diabetic subjects with incipient nephropathy and showed that in the absence of significant change in either blood glucose control or arterial pressure, restricting dietary animal protein intake while adding vegetable protein caused a decrease in proteinuria. Urinary protein loss in the nephrotic syndrome of type 1 diabetes is sharply reduced by dietary protein restriction,[266–269] but similar positive results have not been obtained in type 2 diabetes. Of 13 patients with type 2 diabetes and renal insufficiency, after a mean of 12.2 ± 12.9 months on a 30-g protein, 350-mg phosphorus diet, only two subjects showed improvement in the rate of GFR. By contrast, Jameel et al,[270] in a cross-sectional analysis of data from the San Antonio Heart Study, were "unable to detect a significant correlation between dietary protein intake and clinical proteinuria. These data do not support the hypothesis that high-protein intake is a risk factor for clinical proteinuria in type 2 diabetes subjects."

No conclusion can be drawn as to any long-term benefit of dietary protein restriction in retarding progression of diabetic nephropathy. Apposed meta-analyses have deduced clear efficacy in 108 type 1 diabetic patients followed for 9 to 35 months and an effect of "relatively weak magnitude" in results of 13 randomized controlled trials (N = 1919 patients) in which dietary protein restriction reduced the rate of decline of GFR rate by only 0.53 mL/min/year.[271]

Given the incomplete evaluation of the risk to the kidneys of "normal" dietary protein ingestion, neither the optimal timing nor the extent of dietary protein restriction has been determined for either diabetes type.[272] At present, we prescribe a 0.6 to 0.8 g/kg/day protein diet in both type 1 and type 2 diabetes once proteinuria reaches 0.5 g/day or more or a falling GFR is noted, provided that overall nutritional status is satisfactory. The ADA proposes "an 0.8 g/kg/day protein diet in diabetics who have or are at risk for nephropathy."[273] Specific dietary instructions, however, are, for lack of detailed information, vague. We do not advocate dietary protein restriction when microalbuminuria is the only perturbation attributed to diabetes.

Glycemic Control

That hyperglycemia per se is injurious to tissue and organs of those with diabetes is no longer debated. The overwhelming case sustaining hyperglycemia-induced damage to the kidney is based initially on studies in the streptozotocin-induced diabetic rat that showed that (1) increases in GBM thickness are proportional to the severity of hyperglycemia,[274] (2) histopathologic changes of nephropathy are reversed with either insulin therapy or transplantation of islets of Langerhans, and (3) regression of mesangial expansion and GBM thickening follows transplantation of morphologically injured diabetic kidneys into nondiabetic, isogeneic recipients.[275–279]

Clinical trials of enhanced metabolic regulation of hyperglycemia in type 1 and type 2 diabetes have removed any doubt about the indictment of hyperglycemia as a major cause of human diabetic nephropathy. Although earlier studies in humans linked both the prevalence of microalbuminuria[280, 281] and late diabetic complications to inferior glycemic control,[282, 283] it was broadly based prospective trials—especially the Diabetes Control and Complications Trial (DCCT)—that clinched the argument.[284, 285] Intensive diabetes therapy in the DCCT aimed at near normoglycemia resulted in a 39% reduction in the occurrence of microalbuminuria and a 54% reduction in the occurrence of albuminuria.[286] By one projection, comprehensive treatment of type 2 diabetes, maintaining a hemoglobin A_{1c} value of 7.2%, would reduce the cumulative incidence of blindness, ESRD, and lower-extremity amputation by 72%, 87%, and 67%, respectively.[287]

How hyperglycemia promotes development of diabetic nephropathy is becoming clear at a molecular biology level as discussed previously. The microvasculopathy and macrovasculopathy associated with toxic AGE molecules were reviewed earlier. Other perturbations regularly detected in diabetes are activation of the polyol pathway, increased protein kinase C activity, and aberrant synthesis or actions of cytokines and vasomodulatory agents, including angiotensin II, thromboxane, platelet-derived growth factor, endothelins, insulin-like growth factor-1, and transforming growth factor-β. Sharma and Ziyadeh[288] suggest a major pathogenetic role for elevated production or activity of transforming growth factor-β as a final common mediator of diabetic renal hypertrophy and mesangial matrix expansion.

Inadequate glycemic control shortens the interval between onset of diabetes and onset of clinical proteinuria; the risk of developing macroalbuminuria is four to five times greater in patients with poor control than in those with satisfactory regulation of glycemia.[289] While the DCCT was performed only in type 1 diabetes, extension of the

lessons learned of the renoprotective effect of normalizing blood glucose concentrations to those with type 2 diabetes has been accomplished by several large trials. For example, in the U. K. Prospective Diabetes Study (UKPDS),[290] the effects of intensive blood glucose control with either sulfonylurea or insulin was compared with conventional treatment. The risk of microvascular and macrovascular complications was assessed in 3867 patients with type 2 diabetes of median age 54 years who were randomized to receive intensified management with a sulfonylurea (chlorpropamide, glibenclamide, or glipizide) or with insulin, or conventional dietary management. Over 10 years, hemoglobin A_{1c} was 7.0% in the intensive group compared with 7.9% in the conventional group. The intensive group achieved a 12% reduction in any diabetes-related endpoint; 10% lower (-11% to 27%, $P = .34$) for any diabetes-related death; and 6% lower (-10% to 20%, $P = .44$) for all-cause mortality. There was a striking 25% risk reduction (7% to 40%, $P = .0099$) in microvascular complications, including progressive nephropathy.[290]

Elsewhere in this book, strategies for regulating diabetic hyperglycemia are discussed in detail (see Chapters 57, 59, and 64). Before resorting to an insulin regimen for type 2 diabetes, a trial of newer oral hypoglycemic agents should be attempted. Combination therapy is often required because of suboptimal responses to single-drug therapy. Troglitazone, a drug that increases peripheral glucose disposal, can be combined with metformin, which acts primarily by decreasing endogenous glucose production, as a highly effective treatment for those type 2 diabetic patients with normal renal function whose pancreatic β cells continue to manufacture normal quantities of insulin.[291] Modification of the drug regimen is needed in diabetic persons with compromised renal function. Metformin is contraindicated in advanced renal insufficiency (serum creatinine ≥ 2.5 mg/dL) because of the risk of fatal lactic acidosis. For diabetic patients with stable mild renal insufficiency, the dose of metformin should be lowered to approximately one-third of that given to those with normal GFRs.[292] In insulin-treated diabetic patients of both types, progressive reductions in insulin dose may be required both after the abrupt onset of acute renal failure and with progressive decrease in residual renal function in chronic renal insufficiency because of impaired degradation of exogenous and endogenous insulin.[293, 294]

Urinary Infection

Previous teaching that symptomatic and asymptomatic urinary infections are more prevalent in diabetic than in nondiabetic persons has not been confirmed. In a study of 514 diabetic outpatients and 405 nondiabetic controls, the prevalence of bacteriuria was not significantly higher in diabetic women (15 of 239, 6.3%) than in age-matched nondiabetic women (8 of 236, 3.4%). In diabetic and nondiabetic men, the prevalence was also similar, but lower than in women.[295] Furthermore, screening surveys in the first trimester of pregnancy or the first year following kidney transplant indicate no greater rate of bacteriuria in diabetic subjects.[296]

Manifesting a spectrum of intrarenal infectious complications ranging from acute focal bacterial pyelonephritis to renal corticomedullary abscess, diabetic patients are also at higher risk for intrarenal abscess. Sometimes with minimal prodromal symptoms, catastrophic sepsis as a consequence of unilateral or bilateral emphysematous pyelonephritis presents a medical emergency.[297] Management of urinary tract infection in diabetic patients necessitates prompt diagnosis and early therapy. Starting with a plain abdominal radiograph as a screening tool, genitourinary ultrasonography or further radiographic studies such as computed tomography (CT) scanning may also be warranted, depending on the clinical picture, to identify upper urinary tract complications early for appropriate intervention.

Urinary infections, like infections in any body system, are likely to accelerate explosively in severity when diabetes is inadequately regulated; treatment of urinary infection in diabetic subjects should not be delayed awaiting urine cultures but must be started promptly with either a sulfa drug or a broad-spectrum antibiotic such as ampicillin or ciprofloxacin. Regulation of urinary infection is benefited by (1) establishment of euglycemia, (2) elimination of mechanical obstruction to the ureter or bladder, (3) where possible, removal of a bladder catheter, and (4) adjustment of antimicrobial drug dosage according to residual renal function.

Toxic Renal Injury

Radiocontrast medium presents a risk for renal failure in any diabetic patient whose serum creatinine concentration exceeds 3 mg/dL. Following exposure to contrast media, as in coronary artery catheterization, the azotemic diabetic patient, whether type 1 or type 2, may develop acute renal failure with a fall in urine output to less than 5 mL/hour. Renal failure has been reported after meglumine iothalamate, meglumine diatrizoate, and sodium diatrizoate given in doses of 36 to 300 g. The osmotic load of injected contrast medium (about 2000 mOsm/kg H_2O), when added to hyperviscous diabetic plasma (in a patient dehydrated for the procedure), predisposes to reduced renal perfusion and ischemic injury. Following exposure to contrast media during CT scanning or abdominal imaging, approximately 9% of diabetic patients with preexisting renal insufficiency developed acute kidney failure, defined as an increase of greater than 50% in the serum creatinine level as compared with 1.6% for controls.[298] Initial hopes that the incidence of contrast nephropathy in diabetic patients with reduced renal function would be lowered by use of nonionic contrast media have not been fulfilled, according to careful comparative trials.[299]

To protect against contrast nephropathy, when angiography is unavoidable, an osmotic diuresis induced by mannitol (25 g) administered intravenously 1 hour before the study is believed to afford some protection against renal failure. Recovery from contrast agent nephropathy without renal insufficiency is usual in more than 90% of patients within 3 to 10 days.

Once renal function is reduced in diabetic nephropathy, all potentially nephrotoxic drugs, such as aminoglycoside antibiotics, must be administered in adjusted (reduced) dosage. Guides listing drug half-life and removal rate according to varying levels of kidney function or type of dialytic therapy should be consulted when prescribing essential yet nephrotoxic drugs.[300]

DEMOGRAPHICS OF DIABETIC NEPHROPATHY

Although it has now been generally recognized that renal disease, ultimately progressing to ESRD, is common (30% to 40%) in type 1 diabetes, it has been difficult to dispel the pervasive view that the kidney is infrequently involved in type 2 diabetes.[301] This conclusion, however, drawn from a time when renal disease, although present, was masked by heart disease or stroke, is inaccurate. Reports from the United States and Germany of single populations followed carefully for 20 to 30 years show an approximately equal risk of nephropathy in type 1 diabetes and type 2 diabetes. In Rochester, MN, Humphrey et al.[302] detected an equivalent rate of renal failure over 30 years in cohorts of 1832 subjects with type 2 diabetes and 136 with type 1 diabetes. Sustaining this finding, Hasslacher et al.,[112] in Heidelberg, Germany, followed cohorts of both major types of diabetes for 20 years and found that a serum creatinine level greater than 1.4 mg/dL developed in 59% of type 1 diabetes and in 63% of type 2 diabetes subjects.

Race is a major determinant of both incidence and type of diabetes.[303] In the United States, for example, blacks have one-half the incidence of type 1 diabetes and two of three times the incidence of type 2 diabetes compared with whites. Other racial groups at high risk for type 2 diabetes include Hispanics, and some Native Americans, all of whom also have higher attack rates for diabetic nephropathy.[304, 305] Prior analyses of ESRD therapy by both race and diabetes type are flawed because insulin-treated subjects are often counted as having type 1 diabetes. To address this point, Lowder et al.[306] surveyed the race and sex of 232 of 1450 (16%) diabetic patients undergoing maintenance hemodialysis at 14 centers in Brooklyn in 1986 and found that 87 black women made up 37.5% of the study population. Type 2

diabetes was clearly diagnosed in the majority of surveyed diabetic patients on hemodialysis (139 or 59.9%), but diabetes type could not be determined in 24 (10.3%).

Renal failure in type 2 diabetes usually develops in less than the mean of approximately 20 years reported for type 1 diabetes. In the series of Lowder et al., the mean interval between diagnosis of diabetes and first hemodialysis for ESRD was 14.9 ± 9.3 years.[306] Characteristic of type 1 diabetes, those whose onset of diabetes was before age 20 had the longest interval (20.5 ± 5.9 years) to onset hemodialysis ($P < .01$), whereas those with type 1 diabetes with onset after age 20 began hemodialysis after a mean of 15.3 ± 8.6 years, which was not significantly different from the overall mean. When diabetes begins after age 60, very short intervals (sometimes <5 years) until the onset of ESRD are not unusual, probably due to both years of silent diabetes before its recognition and to coincident nephrosclerosis associated with hypertension, hyperlipidemia, or aging. Superimposable findings collected during a 1998 repeat survey of 220 diabetic hemodialysis patients in Brooklyn sustained the inverse correlation between age of onset of diabetes and interval between diagnosis and onset of ESRD (unpublished data, Friedman EA, et al).

UREMIA THERAPY

In the United States, about 75% of diabetic patients who develop ESRD are first treated with maintenance hemodialysis. Approximately 15% to 20% of diabetic patients with ESRD are treated by peritoneal dialysis, and only 8% to 15% receive a kidney transplant. Before the necessity for blood pressure control was appreciated, hemodialysis was a disastrous therapy in diabetic ESRD patients that neither prolonged useful life nor attained rehabilitation,[307] leading to the consensus that diabetic nephropathy should be excluded from ESRD therapy. Credit for reversing this negative thinking is due to Najarian's surgical team at the University of Minnesota, whose progressively improving results in combining initial hemodialysis with subsequent kidney transplantation reached the point at which "virtually every diabetic patient with renal failure referred to the University of Minnesota was accepted for transplantation, regardless of age, associated complications, or availability of a related donor."[308] Once apprehension over treating diabetic ESRD patients dissipated, step-by-step continuing improvement in survival and quality of life has been attained by hemodialysis, peritoneal dialysis,[309] and kidney transplantation, affording a choice of satisfactory treatments to the diabetic patient (Table 63–1).

Hemodialysis

Owing to often extensive systemic vascular disease and other comorbid disorders, establishment of a hemodialysis regimen in a diabetic patient is usually more difficult than in an age- and sex-matched nondiabetic individual. Starting with surgical construction of a vascular access to the circulation that may require preparatory endarterectomy of atherosclerotic plaques, almost every aspect of the hemodialysis

TABLE 63–1. Options in Uremia Therapy

No further therapy (withdrawal and death)
Hemodialysis
    Home hemodialysis
    Facility hemodialysis
Peritoneal dialysis
    Intermittent (IPD)
    Continuous ambulatory (CAPD)
    Continuous overnight cyclic (machine) (CCPD)
    Combined CAPD (day) and automated machine dialysis (night)
Kidney transplantation
    Living related donor kidney
    "Emotionally" related donor kidney (spouse, friend)
    Cadaver donor kidney
Kidney and pancreas transplantation
Hemofiltration (Europe)

regimen is a greater stress to a diabetic patient. Discovery of calcification of hand arteries is a warning sign that diversion of arterial blood flow may jeopardize the integrity of one or more fingers. A high rate of access complications, including gangrene of the hand,[310] ischemic monomelic neuropathy,[311] and repetitive thrombosis, causes various steal syndromes, thereby limiting effective blood flow. Older diabetic patients usually require a synthetic (Dacron) prosthetic vascular graft placed in the mid- or upper arm, an access choice more likely to fail than in nondiabetic patients.[312]

Timed observation of diabetic patients undergoing hemodialysis at a planned extracorporeal blood flow of 300 to 500 mL/min for 4 to 6 hours three times each week disclosed that the scheduled duration of dialysis is often not attained because of episodic hypotension and inferior access blood flow.[313] One consequence of reducing dialysis time is an increase in mortality[314, 315]; survival of diabetic patients on maintenance hemodialysis is distinctly inferior to that of nondiabetic patients of both sexes and all age groups. The striking toll of diabetic vasculopathy is illustrated by the half-time survival of diabetic patients on hemodialysis in one large series of 3 years vs. 7½ years for nondiabetic patients.[316] This disparity in survival persists into the 1990s, according to the USRDS, which reported that less than 50% of diabetic patients live more than 2 years after starting maintenance hemodialysis, while less than 5% will survive after a decade of dialysis, be it hemodialysis or peritoneal dialysis.[1] Confounding the utility of maintenance hemodialysis is the reality that only a small minority of those who survive attain satisfactory rehabilitation. In Brooklyn, for example, in a survey of 232 diabetic patients undergoing hemodialysis at 13 facilities, only 7 patients (0.03%) went back to full-time employment, whereas 64.9% were so disabled that they required assistance to accomplish routine activities.[307]

Analysis of factors influencing survival of hemodialysis patients indicates that a low serum albumin concentration in diabetic patients correlates with their accelerated mortality.[317] Put another way, using proportional hazards analysis, if the low serum albumin of diabetic patients is taken into account, much of their difference in mortality disappears. Overall, throughout the past decade there has been encouraging and continuous improvement in survival of diabetic ESRD patients treated by dialysis, although according to the 1998 USRDS report,[1] survival of diabetic dialysis patients, as a subset, remains substantially inferior to that of all dialysis patients. Considerations to be addressed in establishing a hemodialysis program for a diabetic patient are listed in Table 63–2.

Peritoneal Dialysis (Table 63–3)

Americans utilize peritoneal dialysis, usually as continuous ambulatory peritoneal dialysis (CAPD),[1] for about 15% of newly treated diabetic ESRD patients. In addition to slightly lower cost, CAPD offers advantages of freedom from a machine, performance at home, rapid training, reduced cardiovascular stress, and avoidance of heparin, when compared with hemodialysis. CAPD can be learned as a home regimen by motivated diabetic patients, even those who are blind, in as little as 10 to 15 days, although the typical patient requires about 4 weeks. Patients learn to exchange 2 to 3 L of commercially prepared sterile dialysate solution three to five times daily. Finger-stick blood glucose measurements are required several times each day as a guide to the quantity of insulin administered. Insulin, antibiotics, and other drugs are added by the patient to each dialysate exchange as needed. Excess intravascular and extracellular fluid is removed by employing dialysate with a higher glucose concentration (4.5%) than the routinely used 1.5%.

Some programs prefer to perform most of the peritoneal exchanges during nighttime sleep, a task accomplished by addition of a mechanical cycler, in a variation termed *continuous cyclic peritoneal dialysis* (CCPD). Both CAPD and CCPD subject the diabetic patient to the constant risk of peritonitis, as well as a gradual decrease in peritoneal surface area, which may ultimately prove to be insufficient for adequate dialysis. CAPD is applied to a greater or lesser proportion of diabetic ESRD patients[318] according to the bias of the local nephrologist. Friedman[319] and Legrain et al., for example, endorse CAPD as

TABLE 63–2. Initiating Hemodialysis in Diabetic Nephropathy

Early evaluation by transplant surgeon
Preemptive renal transplant when serum creatinine level reaches 2–5 mg/dL
Combined pancreas-renal transplant in type 1 diabetes (investigational in type 2 diabetes)
Establishment of vascular access in nondominant upper extremity
    Internal arteriovenous fistula (preferred for longest duration)
    Bovine carotid arteriovenous heterograft (rarely applied because of early failure)
    Teflon arteriovenous graft (most commonly utilized in diabetic patients)
Antihypertensive drug regimen (85% of azotemic diabetic patients are hypertensive)
Correction of anemia with recombinant erythropoietin (target hematocrit 36%–39%)
Metabolic regulation
    Frequent finger-stick glucose measurements (as indicated by extent of glucose excursion)
    Fractional insulin doses or insulin pump (type 1)
    Reinforcement of education regarding diet and exercise (type 1 and type 2)
    Lipid profile and hypolipidemic agents as indicated
Normalization of weight (type 1 and type 2 diabetes)
Regulation of blood pressure (tolerable antihypertensive regimen)
Detection and management of intra- and interdialytic hypotension (elastic stockings, minimizing fluid gain, and extraction)
Bicarbonate-based, *normal*-sodium dialysate
Gradual ultrafiltration
Preservation of vision: continuing collaboration with ophthalmologist
    Two or more pillows for head elevation during retinal hemorrhage
Preservation of lower extremities: collaboration with podiatrist, vascular surgeon
    Wearing heel "booties"
    Assessment of integrity of peripheral pulses
    Careful cutting of toenails
Questioning concerning gastrointestinal complaints
    Obstipation complicating use of phosphate binders: detergent, switch to calcium carbonate for phosphate absorption
    Metoclopramide, cisapride, cascara
Periodic measurement of efficacy of dialysis nitrogenous solute extraction according to National Kidney Foundation–Dialysis Outcomes Quality Initiative[354] (urea reduction ratio >70%, or KT/V ≥1.3 where K = surface area of dialyzer, T = duration of dialysis treatment, and V = volume of body water content)
Depression, family stress
    Membership in American Association of Kidney Patients (AAKP)
    Full explanation of therapy

"a first choice treatment,"[320] but less enthusiastic reports, such as that from Rubin and Hsu,[321] recount poor technique and patient survival in diabetic patients treated with CAPD in Mississippi. A telling point in Rubin and Hsu's series is that only 34% of diabetic patients continued CAPD after 2 years, with a small cohort of 18% reaching 3 years.

Of the two major options in dialytic therapy for ESRD in diabetes, the USRDS consistently reports superior survival in those treated by hemodialysis compared with peritoneal dialysis, whether sorted by sex, race, or age.[1] Peritoneal dialysis patients experience a higher death rate than hemodialysis patients due to cardiovascular disease and cerebrovascular disease. By contrast, employing the Cox proportional hazards statistical method for unequal group analysis in 389 patients accepted for renal replacement therapy in Leicester between 1974 and 1985, no statistically significant differences between the relative risk of death for patients on CAPD (1.0), those on hemodialysis (1.30), and those who received a kidney transplant (1.09) were detected. CAPD, the authors concluded, "is at least as effective as haemodialysis or kidney transplantation in preserving life."[322] Similarly, the Canadian–United States comparison of peritoneal dialysis and hemodialysis found superior survival of diabetic ESRD patients treated by peritoneal dialysis.[323–325]

Kidney Transplantation

The transplant team at the University of Minnesota recognized early both the potential and challenge of attempting renal transplantation in

TABLE 63–3. Initiating Peritoneal Dialysis in Diabetic Nephropathy

Early evaluation by transplant surgeon
Establishment of peritoneal access
    Direction, tunnel, type of catheter
Intensive education of patient and dialysis partner in aseptic technique for dialysate exchanges
Metabolic regulation
    Frequent finger-stick glucose measurements (as indicated by extent of glucose excursion)
    Fractional insulin doses or insulin pump (type 1)
    Reinforcement of education regarding diet and exercise (type 1 and type 2)
    Lipid profile and hypolipidemic agents as indicated
Normalization of weight (type 1 and type 2)
Correction of anemia with recombinant erythropoietin (target hematocrit 36%–39%)
Regulation of blood pressure (tolerable antihypertensive regimen)
Detection and management of intradialytic and interdialytic hypotension (elastic stockings, minimizing fluid gain, and extraction)
Mixing of dialysate glucose sequences to sustain sufficient ultrafiltration
Preservation of vision: continuing collaboration with ophthalmologist
    Two or more pillows for head elevation during retinal hemorrhage
Preservation of lower extremities: collaboration with podiatrist, vascular surgeon
    Wearing heel "booties"
    Assessment of integrity of peripheral pulses
    Careful cutting of toenails
Questioning concerning gastrointestinal complaints
    Obstipation complicating use of phosphate binders: detergent, switch to calcium carbonate for phosphate absorption
    Metoclopramide, cisapride, cascara
Periodic measurement of efficacy of dialysis nitrogenous solute extraction according to National Kidney Foundation–Dialysis Outcomes Quality Initiative[354] (weekly KT/V > 2.0 where K = surface area of dialyzer,[355] T = duration of dialysis treatment, and V = volume of body water content). For patients without residual urine volume excretion, more frequent exchanges at higher volume may be necessary to provide sufficient dialysis.
Depression, family stress
    Membership in American Association of Kidney Patients (AAKP)
    Full explanation of therapy

TABLE 63–4. Assessing Comorbid Risks in Diabetic Patients Evaluated for Uremia

Cystopathy: cystometrogram, urine culture, residual volume
Heart disease: electrocardiogram, exercise stress test, dobutamine echocardiography, coronary angiography
Gastrointestinal disease: gastroparesis, obstipation, diarrhea; abdominal radiography, radionuclide test meal
Respiratory disease: vital capacity, pulmonary function tests
Preservation of vision: visual acuity, intraocular pressure, fluorescein angiography
Bone consequences of uremia: metabolic radiographic bone survey, plasma aluminum level, bone scan
Limb preservation: podiatric assessment, Doppler flow studies of limb perfusion
Dental assessment
Social worker and nurse educator's assessment of potential for self-care

bidity index (Table 63–5) that permit comparisons in a single patient or between groups of patients.

Like all major surgery, renal transplantation may stress the cardiovascular system, especially by intentional volume expansion, which is a component of the surgical procedure. Careful presurgical evaluation of the cardiovascular system in the diabetic patient is therefore required before undertaking transplant surgery, and presurgical correction of severe coronary artery disease by coronary artery bypass or angioplasty is vital to reduce the very high risk of death within 1 year of surgery.[332] Khauli et al.[333] performed coronary angiography in a group of 48 diabetic patients who were about to undergo kidney transplantation and advised a myocardial revascularization procedure in 23 patients, all of whom subsequently had a kidney transplant without a death. Follow-up of this cohort showed a 2-year patient and graft survival for living donor and cadaver donor recipients given "standard" immunosuppression with azathioprine and prednisone of 81% and 68%, and 61% and 32%, respectively. As a guideline, Khauli et al. "discourage transplantation" in diabetic patients who have "the simultaneous presence of >70 per cent arterial stenosis and left ventricular dysfunction."[333] Concurring with the policy of searching for coronary artery disease before undertaking a renal transplant, Philipson et al.[334] studied 60 diabetic patients prior to kidney transplant, concluding that "patients with diabetes and end-stage renal disease who are at highest risk for cardiovascular events can be identified, and these

TABLE 63–5. Variables in Morbidity in Diabetic Kidney Transplant Recipients: The Comorbidity Index

1. Persistent angina, angina on exertion, or myocardial infarction
2. Other cardiovascular problems, hypertension, congestive heart failure, cardiomyopathy, arrhythmia
3. Respiratory disease, reduced respiratory reserve
4. Autonomic neuropathy (gastroparesis, obstipation, diarrhea, cystopathy, orthostatic hypotension)
5. Neurologic problems, cerebrovascular accident, or stroke residual; transient ischemic attacks
6. Musculoskeletal disorders, including all varieties of renal bone disease; palmar fascial contracture
7. Persistent or repetitive infections, including immunodeficiency virus but excluding hemodialysis vascular access site, peritoneal catheter site, or peritonitis
8. Hepatitis B or C, hepatic insufficiency, enzymatic pancreatic insufficiency
9. Hematologic problems other than anemia
10. Spinal abnormalities, lower back problems, or arthritis; renal osteodystrophy
11. Vision impairment (minor to severe decreased acuity to blindness)
12. Limb amputation (minor to severe, finger to lower extremity)
13. Mental or emotional illness (neurosis, depression, psychosis)

To obtain a numeric comorbidity index for an individual patient, rate each variable from 0 to 3 (0 = absent, 1 = mild or of minor import to patient's life; 2 = moderate; 3 = severe). By proportional hazard analysis, the relative significance of each variable can be isolated from the other 12.

uremic patients with type 1 diabetes.[326, 327] In our view, renal transplantation is without question the treatment of choice for all uremic diabetic patients able to withstand the stress of surgery (see Fig. 63–14). Not only is greater patient survival achieved by a renal transplant but there is a remarkably superior level of rehabilitation over that attained by the best dialytic therapy. All reports concur in noting that long-term survival with a well-functioning renal transplant is greater than that achieved in diabetic patients using other renal replacement therapy.[328, 329] Since 1985, the results of renal transplantation in diabetic patients have approached parity, at least in the first 2 years, with those achieved in nondiabetic patients. A fall-off in survival of diabetic renal allograft recipients after 5 or more years is the result of coronary, cerebral, or other arterial disease. In the United States in 1996, those whose ESRD was caused by diabetes accounted for about 24% of first renal transplant recipients. Overall renal allograft survival was approximately equivalent to that attained in recipients with other causes of ESRD, with the exception of superior graft survival in IgA nephropathy. One year after renal transplantation in 995 diabetic kidney recipients who also received a pancreas transplant, renal allograft survival was a remarkable 84%.[330] Transplant teams throughout the United States no longer exclude diabetic patients from renal transplantation because of anticipated problems with infection and wound healing. In fact, diabetic recipients do not suffer significantly more major complications following transplant surgery than do nondiabetic patients so long as appropriate adjustments to the regimen are made prior to, during, and after the transplantation procedure to accommodate their unique problems.[331] To assist in grading the severity of comorbid conditions in diabetic ESRD patients, we prepared both a checklist (Table 63–4) and a scoring system called the comor-

patients probably should not undergo renal transplantation." The high probability of coincident coronary artery disease was underscored by the authors' report that only 7 of 60 patients had a negative thallium stress test, 4 of whom received a kidney transplant without subsequent "cardiovascular events."[334] Obversely, of 53 diabetic patients with positive or "nondiagnostic" stress thallium tests, cardiac catheterization identified 26 patients with mild or no coronary disease or left ventricular dysfunction; 16 patients in this group received transplants with no cardiovascular events. Moderate heart disease was noted in 10 patients, of whom 8 received transplants and 2 died of heart disease; of 13 patients with severe coronary artery disease or left ventricular malfunction, 8 died before receiving a transplant, 3 from cardiovascular disease. This thorough evaluation in which 38% of diabetic ESRD patients being evaluated for a kidney transplant were found to have coronary artery disease provides strong support for a policy of pretransplant cardiovascular assessment of all diabetic ESRD patients.

Responding to the real risk of cardiac-based death in the peritransplant period, we established a pretransplant screening program starting with a thorough history and physical examination plus an electrocardiogram, echocardiogram, dobutamine stress test, and, if indicated by equivocal results, coronary artery catheterization and Holter monitoring.[335] A meta-analysis of noninvasive methods of assessing coronary artery disease comparing 10 reports on dipyridamole–thallium 201 myocardial perfusion (1994 patients) and five reports on dobutamine stress echocardiography (446 patients) found the results equivalent.[336] Reliance on dobutamine stress echocardiography to exclude significant coronary artery disease in ESRD patients permits kidney transplantation with a 97% probability of being free of cardiac complications or cardiac death post transplant.[337] Transplant surgery should be delayed (for surgical reperfusion of the heart) when cardiac evaluation discerns arrhythmias on minimal exercise, ischemic electrocardiographic changes on stress, or an ischemic myocardium with one or more completely occluded coronary arteries.

Pretransplant vigilance protects against lower limb amputation. When the history or physical examination suggests serious peripheral vascular disease, pretransplant study with noninvasive Doppler flow studies, and, where indicated, angiography may alter placement of the renal allograft and uncover the need for arterial bypass surgery to preserve one or both lower extremities. Arteries found to be supplying a lower extremity with marginal peripheral flow must not be used to revascularize an organ allograft, because the extremity may be jeopardized.[338] In many diabetic recipients, atherosclerotic narrowing of the internal iliac artery forces use of the external iliac artery for the arterial anastomosis. During transplant surgery, a local proximal endarterectomy of the external iliac artery may be required in instances of severe atherosclerotic narrowing.

Progression of diabetic macrovasculopathy and microvasculopathy can cause progression of arterial insufficiency in the lower extremities so that even with careful evaluation of the coronary and peripheral vascular systems prior to renal transplantation, there is risk of extremity amputation and cardiovascular death in diabetic renal allograft recipients followed for 3 or more years.[339] Fatal cardiovascular complications are the main reason that patient survival of diabetic recipients over 40 years of age is lower than that of younger diabetic renal transplant recipients.[340] It should be appreciated that the increased risk of cardiovascular death following transplant in older diabetic patients is not avoided by substituting dialytic therapy for transplant surgery. While assignment to dialytic therapy or a kidney transplant has not been made by controlled protocol, the outcome of both approaches, as reported by the USRDS, shows a distinct advantage to kidney transplantation.

Post-transplant Management

As reported by Najarian et al.,[341] diabetic recipients of renal transplants generally require longer hospitalizations than do nondiabetic patients. Immediate post-transplant management of the diabetic renal transplant recipient's metabolic control of plasma glucose concentration is best effected by frequent hourly glucose measurements and an intravenous infusion of insulin. Protracted gastric atony from gastroparesis present in about one-third of diabetic recipients may delay resumption of oral feeding. Oral doses of a liquid suspension of metoclopramide before meals usually enhance gastric motility and improve gastric emptying; cisaparide bethanechol also improves gastric motility. Constipation, sometimes obstipation, is common following kidney transplantation; spontaneous defecation is encouraged by early ambulation, stool-softening agents, and suspension of cascara. Also bothersome is the sudden onset of explosive and continuous liquid diarrhea, a manifestation of autonomic neuropathy, which may enervate and dehydrate the postoperative diabetic patient. Hourly doses of loperamide, as high as 4 mg/hour for 4 to 6 hours, almost always halts the diarrhea.

Urinary retention, a manifestation of autonomic neuropathy as a functional outflow obstruction, is also a frequent post-transplant complication. A regimen of hourly voiding when awake, self-application a manual external pressure above the pubic symphysis (Credé's maneuver), and administration of oral bethanechol usually permit resumption of spontaneous voiding. Rarely, repeated self-catheterization is required for an unresponsive atonic bladder. After the initial postsurgical period, most post-transplant hospitalizations are caused by either graft rejection or perturbations in plasma glucose levels due to changing doses of corticosteroids. Wide swings in glucose concentration, including alternating hypoglycemia and hyperglycemia up to hyperosmolar nonketotic coma, are life-threatening to the diabetic recipient, particularly during times of high-dose steroid administration for rejection prevention.

Otherwise, care of the diabetic renal allograft recipient is not substantially different from that of the nondiabetic recipient, with the key dual exceptions of the need to manage evident diabetic complications as well as to protect the transplanted kidney from recurrent diabetic glomerulopathy. Recurrent diabetic glomerulopathy is first manifested as GBM thickening with mesangial expansion in as short a time as 2 years for recipients with type 1 diabetes.[342] In type 1 diabetes, characteristic nodular intercapillary glomerulosclerosis is regularly noted after 4 or more years in kidneys from nondiabetic donors.[343] By 5 years after renal transplant, we observed a recurrent nephrotic syndrome followed by progressive azotemia and finally ESRD in patients who failed to maintain acceptable levels of glucose control (glycosylated hemoglobin concentrations consistently above 11%). At the other extreme are diabetic recipients who maintain renal allograft function beyond a decade. In 265 patients with type 1 diabetes who were given a renal transplant between December 1966 and April 1978, 100 were alive with a functioning graft 10 years later, an actual patient and primary graft survival of 40% and 32%, respectively.[344] A remarkable 10-year functional kidney survival of 62% was achieved in diabetic recipients of HLA-identical living related kidney donors. As in all reports of long-term observation of diabetic renal transplant recipients, cardiovascular disease, which caused 10 of 23 deaths in the second decade after kidney transplantation, persisted as the most frequent cause of death.

PANCREAS TRANSPLANTATION

Over the past decade, highly successful results have been reported for curative pancreatic transplants inserted concurrently with a renal allograft. Although combining pancreas and kidney transplants does not raise immediate perioperative mortality, perioperative morbidity is markedly increased over that of a kidney transplant alone. A functional pancreas allograft normalized glycosylated hemoglobin, fasting blood glucose, and other 24-hour metabolic profiles. The International Pancreas Transplant Registry reported in 1998 that by the end of 1996, 9000 pancreas transplants had been reported to the registry. For those performed between 1994 and 1996, 1-year pancreas survival rates were 81% for simultaneous pancreas and kidney transplantation (n = 1516), 71% for pancreas transplantation after kidney transplantation (n = 141), and 64% for pancreas transplantation alone (n = 64).[345] Repetitive hospitalizations of pancreas transplant recipients during the first year are caused by bladder pain, hemorrhage, and infection resulting from the enzyme-rich pancreas secretions directly into the

TABLE 63–6. Comparison of End-Stage Renal Disease Options for Diabetic Patients

	Peritoneal Dialysis	Hemodialysis	Kidney Transplant
Extensive extrarenal disease	No limitation	Severe orthostatic hypotension may curtail blood flow rate during hemodialysis; peripheral vascular disease may prevent establishment of suitable vascular access	Excluded in severe cardiovascular disease; correction of coronary artery disease is an enabling step
Geriatric patients	No limitation	No limitation	Arbitrary exclusion as determined by program; age 70 is approximate upper limit for transplant surgery; exceptions made
Complete rehabilitation	Very few patients return to gainful employment	Very few patients return to gainful employment	Best with living related donor transplants; return to home, school, and work obligations common so long as graft functions
Death rate	Much higher than for nondiabetic individuals and greater than for hemodialysis treatment in United States; improved substantially over past decade	Much higher than for nondiabetic individuals, 2–5 times greater than for demographic- and risk-matched kidney transplant recipients; improving	Higher than for nondiabetic kidney graft recipients; lower with related than with unrelated donors; improving
First-year survival	~75%	~78%	>92%
Survival to second decade	Almost never; a few transfer to hemodialysis	<5%	<20%
Progression of complications	Death due to cardiovascular disease most common; usual and unremitting; hyperglycemia and hyperlipidemia accentuated	Death due to cardiovascular disease most common; usual and unremitting; may benefit from metabolic control	Slowed by functioning pancreas + kidney in type 1 diabetic patients; partially ameliorated by correction of azotemia
Special advantage	Can be self-performed; avoids swings in solute and intravascular volume level; freedom to travel	Can be self-performed; efficient extraction of solute and water in hours; widely available throughout United States and Canada	Cures uremia; freedom to travel; permits return to former life-style so long as allograft functions well
Disadvantage	Peritonitis; hyperinsulinemia, hyperglycemia, hyperlipidemia; long hours of treatment; more days hospitalized than with either hemodialysis or transplant	Blood access a hazard for clotting, hemorrhage, and infection; cyclic hypotension, weakness; aluminum toxicity from phosphate binders; amyloidosis	Cosmetic disfigurement, hypertension, personal expense for cytotoxic drugs; induced malignancy; HIV and other viral (cytomegalovirus) transmission
Patient acceptance	Variable; usually compliance with passive tolerance of regimen	Variable, often noncompliant with dietary, metabolic, or antihypertensive component of regimen	Enthusiastic during periods of good renal allograft function; exalted when pancreas proffers euglycemia
Bias in comparison	Delivered as first choice by enthusiasts though emerging evidence indicates substantially higher mortality than for hemodialysis	Treatment by default; often complicated by inattention to progressive cardiac and peripheral vascular disease; depersonalized in large corporate dialysis centers	All kidney transplant programs preselect those patients with fewest complications; exclusion of those older than 45 yr for pancreas and kidney simultaneous grafting obviously favorably prejudices outcome
Relative cost	About equivalent to hemodialysis and more expensive than a transplant over 5-year cost basis	Less expensive than kidney transplant in first year; subsequent years more expensive	Pancreas + kidney engraftment most expensive uremia therapy; after first year, kidney transplant alone lowest cost option

From US Renal Data System, USRDS 1998 Annual Data Report. Bethesda, MD, National Institutes of Health, National Institute of Diabetes and Digestive and Kidney Diseases, April 1998.

unprotected bladder. Patients accept the tradeoff of freedom from insulin injections and enhanced quality of life afforded by a functioning pancreas transplant. Whether another desired objective of pancreatic transplantation, the prevention of progression of diabetic microvascular and macrovascular extrarenal complications, will be reached is not yet known. Preliminary study of renal biopsies in patients who have received sequential kidney and later pancreas allografts indicates that the presence of a functioning pancreas slows the progression of, and even reverses, established diabetic glomerulopathy.[346]

Hope that a pancreas transplant would end the siege of diabetic complications was gleaned from first observations of the course of diabetic neuropathy following combined pancreas and kidney transplantation in which some patients had stabilization[347] and improvement[348] in diabetic motor neuropathy. Unfortunately, when pancreas transplantation was performed in patients with extensive extrarenal disease, there has been neither cessation of further injury nor reversal of established diabetic retinopathy, diabetic cardiomyopathy, or extensive peripheral vascular disease.[349] Importantly, a functioning pancreas transplant has been enthusiastically welcomed by patients with type 1 diabetes who become emancipated from the daily burden of balancing diet, exercise, and insulin dosage.[349, 350]

Epitomizing the potential of a pancreas transplant program is the report by Sollinger et al.[351] recounting the remarkable experience at the University of Wisconsin from 1985 to 1997 during which 500 simultaneous pancreas-kidney transplants were performed. The Wisconsin group attained remarkable patient survival at 1, 5, and 10 years of 96.4%, 88.6%, and 76.3%, with intact kidney function over this interval of 88.6%, 80.3% and 66.6%; and pancreas function of 87.5%, 78.1%, and 67.2%, respectively.[351] Surprising and counterintuitive, evidence that pancreas transplantation may be applicable to type 2 diabetes is now being accumulated.[352] In 1999, the ESRD patient with type 1 diabetes should view a simultaneous kidney and pancreas transplant as preferred therapy, permitting complete escape for the duration of pancreas graft function from the burden and constraint of living with an inexorable disease.[353]

CONCLUSIONS

Renal failure due to diabetic glomerulopathy is the vasculopathic complication that dominates the course of about one-third of those with type 1 diabetes and at least an equivalent proportion of individuals with type 2 diabetes. A therapeutic strategy that emphasizes control of hypertension, restriction of dietary protein, and the best attainable glycemic control slows the course of diabetic nephropathy and delays the onset of ESRD.

While CAPD and maintenance hemodialysis extend life after the onset of ESRD in diabetes, a functioning kidney transplant provides a greater probability for survival with good rehabilitation (Table 63–6). The full impact of selection bias in assigning younger, less complicated diabetic subjects for a kidney transplant, leaving an older, sicker residual cohort on dialytic therapy, has not been assessed by prospective controlled studies of dialysis vs. kidney transplantation. Consideration should be given to the potential value of a combined pancreas and kidney transplant to cure, so long as the pancreas functions, the minority (<10%) of diabetic ESRD patients who have type 1 diabetes. No matter which ESRD therapy is selected, optimal rehabilitation in diabetic ESRD patients demands recognition and management of comorbid conditions. An individualized regimen, whether CAPD, hemodialysis, or a kidney transplant, must be constructed to deal with specific medical and family circumstances. Actual rehabilitation is better in kidney transplant recipients than in those diabetic ESRD patients treated by CAPD or maintenance hemodialysis. Introduction of erythropoietin, now given to more than 90% of dialysis patients in the United States, necessitates reassessment of all conclusions pertaining to survival, morbidity, and rehabilitation in ESRD completed before this vital hormone was available. New baselines for well-being in CAPD and hemodialysis are needed for both diabetic and nondiabetic patients. It may be anticipated that selected well-dialyzed diabetic hemodialysis patients with normal hematocrits might rationally opt not to have a cadaveric kidney transplant until drugs less toxic than those currently used for immunosuppression are introduced. Measures to control hypertension and hyperlipidemia during the course of diabetes may retard the course of macrovascular disease, particularly of the coronary arteries, the key threat to long-term survival of diabetic dialysis patients and kidney recipients. Pretransplant cardiac evaluation is mandatory to identify and correct silent coronary artery disease that may be severe and life-threatening.

There is continuing growth in the incidence and prevalence of ESRD attributed to diabetes,[276] a syndrome consuming about one-third of healthcare funds devoted to the kidney. The past 5 years have seen improving results in the treatment of ESRD in diabetes, whether by dialytic therapy, renal transplantation, or combined pancreas and kidney transplantation. Screening of diabetic renal transplant candidates for silent coronary artery disease, followed by revascularization, is likely to improve further survival in this diabetic cohort.[277]

REFERENCES

1. U S Renal Data System: USRDS 1998 Annual Data Report. Bethesda, MD, National Institutes of Health, National Institute of Diabetes and Digestive and Kidney Diseases, April 1998.
2. Lundbaek K: Nephropathy in diabetic subjects. *In* Leibel BS, Wrenshall GA (eds): On the Nature and Treatment of Diabetes. Amsterdam, Excerpta Medica, 1965.
3. Ehrlich P: Über das Vorkommen von Glycogen im diabetischen und im normalen Organismus. Z Klin Med 6:33–46, 1883.
4. Armanni L: *In* Cantani A (ed): Der Diabetes Mellitus. Berlin, Denicke, 1877, p 315.
5. Ebstein W: Über Drüsendpithelnekrosen beim Diabetes mellitus mit besonderer Berücksichtigung des diabetischen Coma. Dtsch Arch Klin Med 28:143–242, 1883.
6. Kimmelstiel P, Wilson C: Intercapillary lesions in the glomeruli of the kidney. Am J Pathol 12:83–98, 1936.
7. Iverson P, Brun C: Aspiration biopsy of the kidney. Am J Med 11:324–330, 1951.
8. Keen H, Chlouverakis C, Fuller J, Jarrett RJ: The concomitants of raised blood sugar: Studies in newly-detected hyperglycaemics. II. Urinary albumin excretion, blood pressure and their relation to blood sugar levels. Guys Hosp Rep 118:247–254, 1969.
9. Mogensen CE: Urinary albumin excretion in early and long-term juvenile diabetes. Scand J Clin Lab Invest 28:183–193, 1971.
10. Mogensen CE: Kidney function and glomerular permeability to macromolecules in juvenile diabetes. Dan Med Bull 19(suppl 3):1–36, 1972.
11. Mogensen CE, Andersen MJF: Increased kidney size and glomerular filtration rate in early juvenile diabetes. Diabetes 22:706–713, 1973.
12. Mogensen CE, Andersen MJF: Increased kidney size and glomerular filtration rate in untreated juvenile diabetics: Normalization by insulin-treatment. Diabetologia 11:221–224, 1975.
13. Mauer SM, Steffes MW, Ellis EN, et al: Structural-functional relationships in diabetic nephropathy. J Clin Invest 74:1143–1145, 1984.
14. Mauer SM, Ellis E, Brown DM, et al: What is diabetic nephropathy? *In* Friedman EA, L'Esperance FA Jr (eds): Diabetic Renal-Retinal Syndrome, Therapy. Orlando, FL, Grune & Stratton, 1986, p 141.
15. Stout LC, Kumar S, Whorton EB: Focal mesangiolysis and the pathogenesis of the Kimmelstiel-Wilson nodule. Hum Pathol 24:77–89, 1994.
16. Fioretto P, Steffes MW, Sutherland DE, et al: Reversal of lesions of diabetic nephropathy after pancreas transplantation. N Engl J Med 339:69–75, 1998.
17. Froguel P: Genetics of type 1 insulin-dependent diabetes mellitus. Horm Res 48(suppl 4):55–57, 1997.
18. Dahlquist G: The aetiology of type 1 diabetes: An epidemiological perspective. Acta Paediatr Suppl 425:5–10, 1998.
19. Wendorf M, Goldfine RD: Archaeology of NIDDM: Excavation of the "thrifty" genotype. Diabetes 40:161–165, 1991.
20. Sharma AM: The thrifty-genotype hypothesis and its implications for the study of complex genetic disorders in man. J Mol Med 76:568–571, 1998.
21. Huang XH, Rantalaiho V, Wirta O, et al: Angiotensin-converting enzyme insertion/deletion polymorphism and diabetic albuminuria in patients with NIDDM followed up for 9 years. Nephron 80:17–24, 1998.
22. Kunz R, Bork JP, Fritsche L, et al: Association between the angiotensin-converting enzyme–insertion/deletion polymorphism and diabetic nephropathy: A methodologic appraisal and systematic review. J Am Soc Nephrol 9:1653–1663, 1998.
23. Penno G, Chaturvedi N, Talmud PJ, et al: Effect of angiotensin-converting enzyme (ACE) gene polymorphism on progression of renal disease and the influence of ACE inhibition in type 1 diabetes patients: Findings from the EUCLID Randomized Controlled Trial. EURODIAB Controlled Trial of Lisinopril in IDDM. Diabetes 47:1507–1511, 1998.
24. Mehler PS, Jeffers BW, Biggerstaff SL, Schrier RW: Smoking as a risk factor for nephropathy in non–insulin-dependent diabetics. J Gen Intern Med 13:842–845, 1998.
25. Biesenbach G, Grafinger P, Janko O, Zazgornik J: Influence of cigarette-smoking on the progression of clinical diabetic nephropathy in type 2 diabetic patients. Clin Nephrol 48:146–150, 1997.
26. Poulsen PL, Ebbehoj E, Hansen KW, Mogensen CE: Effects of smoking on 24-h ambulatory blood pressure and autonomic function in normoalbuminuric insulin-dependent diabetes mellitus patients. Am J Hypertens 11:1093–1099, 1998.
27. Harris MI, Flegal KM, Cowie CC, et al: Prevalence of diabetes, impaired fasting glucose, and impaired glucose tolerance in U.S. adults. The Third National Health and Nutrition Examination Survey, 1988–1994. Diabetes Care 21:518–524, 1998.

28. Report of the Expert Committee on the Diagnosis and Classification of Diabetes Mellitus. Diabetes Care 20:1183–1197, 1997.
29. United States Renal Data System: USRDS 1991 Annual Data Report. Bethesda, MD, National Institutes of Health, National Institute of Diabetes and Digestive and Kidney Diseases August 1991.
30. United States Renal Data System: USRDS 1992 Annual Data Report. Bethesda, MD, National Institutes of Health, National Institute of Diabetes and Digestive and Kidney Diseases August 1992.
31. United States Renal Data System: International comparisons of ESRD therapy. Am J Kidney Dis 32(2 suppl 1):S136–S141, 1998.
32. Mazze RS, Sinnock P, Deeb L, Brimberry JL: An epidemiological model for diabetes mellitus in the United States: Five major complications. Diabetes Res Clin Pract 1:185–191, 1985.
33. Centers for Disease Control and Prevention: Diabetes Surveillance, 1997. Atlanta, GA, U S Department of Health and Human Services, 1997.
34. Mauer SM, Chavers BM: A comparison of kidney disease in type I and type II diabetes. Adv Exp Med Biol 189:299–303, 1985.
35. WHO Expert Committee on Diabetes Mellitus, Second Report. World Health Organ Tech Rep Ser 546:1980.
36. National Diabetes Data Group: Classification and diagnosis of diabetes mellitus and other categories of glucose intolerance. Diabetes 16:283–285, 1979.
37. Physician's Guide to Insulin-Dependent (Type I) Diabetes: Diagnosis and Treatment. Alexandria, VA, American Diabetes Association, 1988.
38. Wilson RM, Van der Minne P, Deverill I, et al: Insulin dependence: Problems with the classification of 100 consecutive patients. Diabet Med 2:167–172, 1985.
39. Physician's Guide to Insulin-Dependent (Type I) Diabetes: Diagnosis and Treatment, ed 2. Alexandria, VA, American Diabetes Association, 1988.
40. Type 2 diabetes or NIDDM: Looking for a better name. Lancet 1:589–591, 1989.
41. Reaven GM: Banting Lecture 1988: Role of insulin resistance in human disease. Diabetes 37:1595–1607, 1988.
42. Tattersall RB, Mansell PI: Maturity onset-type diabetes of the young (MODY): One condition or many? Diabet Med 8:402–410, 1991.
43. Takahashi C, Nagai N, Ujihara N, et al: Clinical profile of Japanese dialysis patients with diabetic nephropathy, diagnosed as having diabetes before the age of thirty. Diabetes Res Clin Pract 10:127–131, 1990.
44. Nagai N: Clinical statistics of 551 patients with diabetes mellitus found before 30 years of age. J Tokyo Wom Med Coll 52:904–915, 1982.
45. Abourizk NN, Dunn JC: Types of diabetes according to National Diabetes Data Group Classification. Diabetes Care 13:1120–1128, 1990.
46. Mogensen CE, Christensen CK, Vittinghus E: The stages in diabetic renal disease with emphasis on the stage of incipient diabetic nephropathy. Diabetes 32(suppl):64–78, 1983.
47. Christensen CK, Christiansen JS, Schmitz A, et al: Effect of continuous subcutaneous insulin infusion on kidney function and size in IDDM patients: A 2 year controlled study. J Diabetes Complications 1:91–95, 1987.
48. Mogensen CE: Angiotensin converting enzyme inhibitors and diabetic nephropathy. BMJ 304:327–328, 1992.
49. Nelson RG, Newman JM, Knowles WC, et al: Incidence of end-stage renal disease in type 2 (non–insulin dependent) diabetes mellitus in Pima Indians. Diabetologia 31:730–736, 1988.
50. Lebovitz HE, Palmisano J: Cross-sectional analysis of renal function in black Americans with non–insulin dependent diabetes mellitus. Diabetes Care 13(suppl 4):1186–1190, 1990.
51. Palmisano JJ, Lebovitz HE: Renal function in black Americans with type II diabetes. J Diabetes Complications 3:40–44, 1989.
52. Cambier P: Application de la théorie de Rehberg a l'étude clinique des affections rénales et du diabètes. Ann Med 35:273–299, 1934.
53. Spuhler O: Zur Pathophysiologie der Niere. Bern, Switzerland, Huber, 1946, p 45.
54. Fiaschi E, Grassi B, Andres G: La funzione renale nel diabete mellito. Rassegna Fisiopatol Clin Terapeut 24:372, 1952.
55. Ditzel J, Schwartz M: Abnormally increased glomerular filtration rate in short-term insulin-treated diabetic subjects. Diabetes 16:264–267, 1967.
56. Mogensen CE, Andersen MJF: Increased kidney size and glomerular filtration rate in untreated juvenile diabetes: Normalization by insulin treatment. Diabetologia 11:221–224, 1975.
57. Mogensen CE, Christensen CK: Predicting diabetic nephropathy in insulin-dependent patients. N Engl J Med 311:89–93, 1984.
58. Wiseman MJ, Saunders AJ, Keen H, Viberti GC: Effect of blood glucose control on increased glomerular filtration rate and kidney size in insulin-dependent diabetes. N Engl J Med 312:617–621, 1985.
59. Christensen CK, Christiansen JS, Schmitz A, et al: Effect of continuous subcutaneous insulin infusion on kidney function and size in IDDM patients: A 2 year controlled study. J Diabetes Complications 1:91–95, 1987.
60. Christiansen JS, Frandsen M, Parving H-H: The effect of intravenous insulin infusion on kidney function in insulin-dependent diabetes mellitus. Diabetologia 20:199–204, 1981.
61. Christiansen JS, Gammelgaard J, Tronier B, et al: Kidney function and size in diabetics before and during insulin treatment. Kidney Int 21:683–688, 1982.
62. Parving H, Øxenbøll B, Svendsen PA, et al: Early detection of patients at risk of developing diabetic nephropathy: A longitudinal study of urinary albumin excretion. Acta Endocrinol (Copenh) 100:550–555, 1982.
63. Mogensen CE, Christensen CK, Vittinghus E: The stages in diabetic renal disease with emphasis on the stage of incipient diabetic nephropathy. Diabetes 32(suppl 2):64–78, 1983.
64. Mogensen CE, Christensen CK, Christiansen JS, et al: Early hyperfiltration and late renal damage in insulin-dependent diabetes. Pediatr Adolesc Endocrinol 17:197–205, 1988.
65. Mogensen CE, Steffes MW, Deckert T, Christiansen JS: Functional and morphological renal manifestations in diabetes mellitus. Diabetologia 21:89–93, 1981.
66. Wiseman MJ, Viberti GC, Keen H: Threshold effect of plasma glucose in the glomerular hyperfiltration of diabetes. Nephron 38:257–260, 1984.
67. Jones SL, Wiseman MJ, Viberti GC: Glomerular hyperfiltration as a risk factor for diabetic nephropathy: Five year report of a prospective study (letter). Diabetologia 34:59–60, 1991.
68. Azevedo MJ, Gross JL: Follow up of glomerular hyperfiltration in normoalbuminuric type 1 (insulin-dependent) diabetic patients (letter). Diabetologia 34:611, 1991.
69. Mogensen CE: Microalbuminuria predicts clinical proteinuria and early mortality in maturity-onset diabetes. N Engl J Med 310:356–360, 1984.
70. Mogensen CE: Early glomerular hyperfiltration in insulin-dependent diabetics and late nephropathy. Scand J Clin Lab Invest 46:201–206, 1986.
71. Mogensen CE: Renal function changes in diabetes. Diabetes 25:872–879, 1976.
72. O'Bryan GT, Hostetter TH: The renal hemodynamic basis of diabetic nephropathy. Semin Nephrol 17:93–100, 1997.
73. Lafferty HM, Brenner BM: Are glomerular hypertension and "hypertrophy" independent risk factors for progression of renal disease? Semin Nephrol 3:294–304, 1990.
74. Østerby R: Early phases in the development of diabetic glomerulopathy: Quantitative electron microscopic study. Acta Med Scand S574 (suppl):3–82, 1974.
75. Østerby R, Gundersen HJG: Glomerular size and structure in diabetes mellitus: 1. Early abnormalities. Diabetologia 11:225–229, 1975.
76. Østerby R: Basement membrane morphology in diabetes mellitus. In Ellenberg M, Rifkin H (eds): Diabetes Mellitus: Theory and Practice. New York, Medical Examination, 1983, pp 323–341.
77. Østerby R: A quantitative electron microscopic study of mesangial regions in glomeruli from patients with short term juvenile diabetes mellitus. Lab Invest 29:99–110, 1973.
78. Vittinghus E, Mogensen CE: Albumin excretion and renal hemodynamic response to physical exercise in normal and diabetic men. Scand J Clin Lab Invest 41:627–632, 1981.
79. Mauer SM, Goetz FC, McHugh LE, et al: Long-term study of normal kidneys transplanted into patients with Type I diabetes. Diabetes 38:516–523, 1989.
80. Borch-Johnsen K: Incidence of nephropathy in insulin-dependent diabetes as related to mortality and cost-benefit of early intervention. In Mogensen CE (ed): The Kidney and Hypertension in Diabetes Mellitus, ed 2. Boston, Kluwer Academic, 1994, pp 75–84.
81. Chachati A, von Frenckell R, Foidart-Willems J, et al: Variability of albumin excretion in insulin-dependent diabetics. Diabet Med 4:437–440, 1987.
82. Deferrari G, Repetto M, Calvi C, et al: Diabetic nephropathy: From micro-macroalbuminuria. Nephrol Dial Transplant 13(suppl 8):11–15, 1998.
83. Schmitz A, Vaeth M: Microalbuminuria: A major risk factor in non–insulin-dependent diabetes. A 10-year follow-up study of 503 patients. Diabet Med 5:126–134, 1988.
84. Stiegler H, Standl E, Schulz K, et al: Morbidity, mortality, and albuminuria in type 2 diabetic patients: A three-year prospective study of a random cohort in general practice. Diabet Med 9:646–653, 1992.
85. Neil A, Hawkins M, Potok M, et al: A prospective population-based study of microalbuminuria as a predictor of mortality in NIDDM. Diabetes Care 16:996–1003, 1993.
86. Gatling W, Knight C, Mullee MA, Hill RD: Microalbuminuria in diabetes: A population study of the prevalence and assessment of three screening tests. Diabet Med 5:343–347, 1988.
87. Rowe DJF, Bagga II, Betts PB: Normal variations in rate of albumin excretion and albumin to creatinine ratios in overnight and daytime urine collections in non-diabetic children. BMJ 291:693–694, 1985.
88. Cohen DL, Close CF, Viberti GC: The variability of overnight urinary albumin excretion in insulin-dependent diabetic and normal subjects. Diabet Med 4:437–440, 1987.
89. Parving H-H, Hommel E, Mathiesen E, et al: Prevalence of microalbuminuria, arterial hypertension, retinopathy and neuropathy in patients with insulin-dependent diabetes. BMJ 296:156–160, 1988.
90. Viberti G, Keen H: The patterns of proteinuria in diabetes mellitus: Relevance to pathogenesis and prevention of diabetic nephropathy. Diabetes 33:686–692, 1984.
91. Mogensen CE: Microalbuminuria as a predictor of clinical diabetic nephropathy. Kidney Int 31:673–689, 1987.
92. Mathiesen ER, Ronn B, Storm B, et al: The natural history of microalbuminuria in insulin-dependent diabetes: A 10-year prospective study. Diabet Med 12:482–487, 1995.
93. Viberti GC, Hill RD, Jarrett RJ, et al: Microalbuminuria as a predictor of clinical nephropathy in insulin-dependent diabetes mellitus. Lancet 1:1430–1432, 1982.
94. Nørgaard K, Feldt-Rasmussen B, Borch-Johnsen K, et al: Prevalence of hypertension in type 1 (insulin-dependent) diabetes mellitus. Diabetologia 33:407–410, 1990.
95. Chavers BM, Bilous RW, Ellis EN, et al: Glomerular lesions and urinary albumin excretion in type 1 diabetes without overt proteinuria. N Engl J Med 320:966–970, 1989.
96. Bending JJ, Viberti GC, Watkins PJ, Keen H: Intermittent clinical proteinuria and renal function in diabetes: Evolution and the effect of glycemic control. BMJ 292:83–86, 1986.
97. Daniels BS, Hauser EB: Glycation of albumin, not glomerular basement membrane, alters permeability in an in vitro model. Diabetes 41:1415–1421, 1992.
98. Caird RI: Survival of diabetics with proteinuria. Diabetes 10:178–181, 1961.
99. Mauer SM, Steffes MW, Ellis EN, et al: Structural-functional relationships in diabetic nephropathy. J Clin Invest 74:1143–1155, 1984.
100. Steffes MW, Østerby R, Chavers B, Mauer SM: Mesangial expansion as a central mechanism for loss of kidney function in diabetic patients. Diabetes 38:1077–1081, 1989.
101. Gellman DD, Pirani CL, Soothill JF, et al: Structure and function in diabetic nephropathy: The importance of diffuse glomerulosclerosis. Diabetes 8:251–256, 1959.

102. National Diabetes Data Group: Diabetes in America, ed 2. Bethesda, MD, National Institutes of Health. National Institute of Diabetes and Digestive and Kidney Diseases. NIH publication No. 95-1468, 1995.
103. Harris MI, Klein R, Welborn TA, Knuiman MW: Onset of NIDDM occurs at least 4–7 yr before clinical diagnosis. Diabetes Care 15:815–819, 1992.
104. Marks HH: Longevity and mortality of diabetics. Am J Public Health 55:416–422, 1965.
105. Herman WH, Teutsch SM: Kidney disease associated with diabetes: Diabetes in America. (NIH publication No. 85-1468). Washington, DC, Government Printing Office, 1985, pp 1–31.
106. Ismail N, Becker B, Strzelczyk P, Ritz E: Renal disease and hypertension in non–insulin-dependent diabetes mellitus. Kidney Int 55:1–28, 1999.
107. Fabre J, Balant LP, Dayer PG, et al: The kidney in maturity onset diabetes: A clinical study of 510 patients. Kidney Int 21:730–738, 1982.
108. Cowie CC, Port FK, Wolfe RA, et al: Disparities in incidence of diabetic end stage renal disease according to race and type of diabetes. N Engl J Med 321:1074–1079, 1989.
109. Pugh JA, Stern MP, Haffner SM, et al: Excess incidence of end stage renal disease in Mexican Americans. Am J Epidemiol 127:135–144, 1988.
110. Kunzelman CL, Knowles WC, Pettit DJ, Bennett PH: Incidence of proteinuria in type 2 diabetes in the Pima Indians. Kidney Int 35:681–687, 1989.
111. Knowles WC, Bennett PH, Hamman RF, Miller M: Diabetes incidence and prevalence in Pima Indians: A 19-fold greater incidence than in Rochester, Minnesota. Am J Epidemiol 108:497–505, 1978.
112. Hasslacher CH, Ritz E, Wahl P, Michael C: Similar risks of nephropathy in patients with type I or type II diabetes mellitus. Nephrol Dial Transplant 4:859–863, 1989.
113. Lindblad AS, Nolph KD, Novak JW, Friedman EA: A survey of the NIH CAPD Registry population with end-stage renal disease attributed to diabetic nephropathy. J Diabetes Complications 2:227–232, 1988.
114. Davies DF, Shock NW: Age changes in glomerular filtration rate, effective renal plasma flow, and tubular excretory capacity in adult males. J Clin Invest 29:496–502, 1950.
115. Rowe JW, Andres R, Tobin JD, et al: The effect of age on creatinine clearance in men: A cross-sectional and longitudinal study. J Gerontol 31:155–163, 1976.
116. Lindeman RD, Tobin JD, Shock NW: Longitudinal studies on the rate of decline in renal function with age. J Am Geriatr Soc 33:278–285, 1985.
117. Takazakura E, Wasabu N, Handa A, et al: Intrarenal vascular changes with age and disease. Kidney Int 2:224–230, 1972.
118. Parving H-H, Gall M-A, Skøtt P, et al: Prevalence and causes of albuminuria in non–insulin dependent diabetic (NIDDM) patients (abstract). Kidney Int 37:243, 1990.
119. Myers BD, Nelson RG, Williams GW, et al: Glomerular function in Pima Indians with non–insulin dependent diabetes mellitus of recent onset. J Clin Invest 88:524–530, 1991.
120. Palmisano JJ, Lebovitz HE: Cross-sectional analysis of renal function in black Americans with NIDDM. Diabetes Care 13(suppl 4):1186–1190, 1990.
121. Bérionade V: Creatinine clearance in non-insulin dependent diabetes mellitus. Kidney Int 31:179, 1986.
122. Bruton BL, Perusek MC, Lancaster JL, et al: Effects of glycemia on basal and amino-acid stimulated (AA-S) renal hemodynamics and kidney size in non–insulin dependent diabetes (NIDD) (abstract). J Am Soc Nephrol 1:623, 1990.
123. Nowack R, Raum E, Blum W, Ritz E: Renal hemodynamics in recent onset type II diabetes. Am J Kidney Dis 20:342–347, 1992.
124. Nelson RG, Meyer TW, Myers BD, Bennett PH: Course of renal disease in Pima Indians with non–insulin-dependent diabetes mellitus. Kidney Int Suppl 63:S45–S48, 1997.
125. Gall MA, Rossing P, Skøtt P, et al: Prevalence of micro- and macroalbuminuria, arterial hypertension, retinopathy and large vessel disease in European type 2 (non–insulin dependent) diabetic patients. Diabetologia 34:655–661, 1991.
126. Damsgaard EM, Froland A, Jorgensen OD, Mogensen CE: Microalbuminuria as predictor of increased mortality in elderly people. BMJ 300:297–300, 1990.
127. Yudkin JS, Forrest FD, Jackson CA: Microalbuminuria as a predictor of vascular disease in non-diabetic subjects. Lancet 1:530–533, 1988.
128. Schmitz A, Vaeth M: Microalbuminuria a major risk factor in non–insulin dependent diabetes: A 10 year followup study of 503 patients. Diabet Med 5:126–134, 1988.
129. Jarrett RJ, Viberti GC, Argyropoulos A, et al: Microalbuminuria predicts mortality in non-insulin dependent diabetes. Diabet Med 1:17–19, 1984.
130. Forsblom CM, Groop PH, Ekstrand A, et al: Predictors of progression from normoalbuminuria to microalbuminuria in NIDDM. Diabetes Care 21:1932–1938, 1998.
131. Eibl N, Schnack C, Frank M, Schernthaner G: Initial urinary albumin excretion determines the progression of microalbuminuria in patients with type-2 diabetes and normotensive blood pressure values despite improved metabolic control. Diabetes Res Clin Pract 39:39–45, 1998.
132. Miller K, Michael AF: Immunopathology of renal extracellular membranes in diabetes mellitus: Specificity of tubular basement-membrane immunofluorescence. Diabetes 25:701–708, 1976.
133. Mauer SM, Steffes MW, Brown DM: Effects of mesangial localization of polyvinyl alcohols on glomerular basement membrane thickness. Kidney Int 5:751–755, 1985.
134. Standl E, Steigler H, Roth R, et al: On the impact of hypertension on the prognosis of NIDDM: Results of the Schwabing-GP program. Diabetes Metab 15:352–358, 1989.
135. Ritz E, Hasslacher C, Beutel G: Hypertension and diabetic nephropathy. J Nephrol 1:11–15, 1991.
136. Panzram G: Mortality and survival in type 2 (non–insulin dependent) diabetes mellitus. Diabetologia 30:123–131, 1987.
137. DeFronzo RJ, Ferranini E: Insulin resistance: A multi-faceted syndrome responsible for NIDDM, obesity, hypertension, dyslipidemia and atherosclerotic cardiovascular disease. Diabetes Care 14:173–194, 1991.
138. Gilbert RE, Jerums G, Cooper ME: Diabetes and hypertension: Prognostic and therapeutic considerations. Blood Press 4:329–333, 1995.
139. Viberti G, Keen H, Wiseman MJ: Raised arterial pressure in parents of proteinuric insulin-dependent diabetics. BMJ 295:515–519, 1987.
140. Viberti GC, Earle K: Predisposition to essential hypertension and the development of diabetic nephropathy. J Am Soc Nephrol 3(suppl 4):S27–S33, 1992.
141. Hannedouche TP, Marques L-P, Guicheney P, et al: Predisposition to essential hypertension and renal hemodynamics in recent-onset insulin-dependent diabetic patients. J Am Soc Nephrol 3(suppl 4):S34–S40, 1992.
142. Mangili R, Bending JJ, Scott G, et al: Increased sodium-lithium countertransport activity on red cells of patients with insulin-dependent diabetes and nephropathy. N Engl J Med 318:146–150, 1988.
143. Krolewski AS, Canessa M, Warren JH, et al: Predisposition to hypertension and susceptibility to renal disease in insulin-dependent diabetes mellitus. N Engl J Med 318:140–145, 1988.
144. Ibsen KK, Jensen HA, Wieth JC, Funder J: Essential hypertension: Sodium-lithium countertransport in erythrocytes from patients and from children having one hypertensive parent. Hypertension 4:703–709, 1982.
145. Carr S, Mbanya JC, Thomas T, et al: Increase in glomerular filtration rate in patients with insulin-dependent diabetes and elevated erythrocyte Na-Li countertransport. N Engl J Med 322:500–505, 1990.
146. Jensen JJ, Mathiesen ER, Norgaard K, et al: Increased blood pressure and sodium-lithium countertransport activity are not inherited in diabetic nephropathy. Diabetologia 33:619–624, 1990.
147. Rutherford PA, Thomas TH, Wilkinson R: The mechanism of raised sodium-lithium countertransport in Type I diabetes mellitus is different from that in essential hypertension (abstract). Diabet Med 7(suppl 2):1A, 1990.
148. Van Norren K, Thien T, Berden JH, et al: Relevance of erythrocyte Na+/Li+ countertransport measurement in essential hypertension, hyperlipidaemia and diabetic nephropathy: A critical review. Eur J Clin Invest 28:339–352, 1998.
149. Maryniak RK, Mendoza N, Clyne D, et al: Recurrence of diabetic nodular glomerulosclerosis in a renal transplant. Transplantation 39:35–38, 1985.
150. Abouna G, Adnani MS, Kumar MS, Samhan SA: Fate of transplanted kidneys with diabetic nephropathy. Lancet 1:622–624, 1986.
151. Tuttle KR, Bruton L, Perusek MC, et al: Effect of strict glycemic control on renal hemodynamic response to amino acids and renal enlargement in insulin-dependent diabetes mellitus. N Engl J Med 324:1626–1632, 1991.
152. Robison WG Jr, Tillis TN, Laver N, Kinoshita JH: Diabetes-related histopathologies of the rat retina prevented with an aldose reductase inhibitor. Exp Eye Res 50:355–366, 1990.
153. Sundkvist G, Armstrong FM, Bradbury JE, et al: Peripheral and autonomic nerve function in 259 diabetic patients with peripheral neuropathy treated with ponalrestat (an aldose reductase inhibitor) or placebo for 18 months: United Kingdom/Scandinavian Ponalrestat Trial. J Diabetes Complications 6:123–130, 1992.
154. Macleod AF, Boulton AJ, Owens DR, et al: A multicentre trial of the aldose-reductase inhibitor tolrestat, in patients with symptomatic diabetic peripheral neuropathy: Northern European Tolrestat Study Group. Diabetes Metab 18:14–20, 1992.
155. Solerte SB, Ferrari E: Diabetic retinal vascular complications, erythrocyte filterability and pentoxifylline: Results of a 2 year follow-up study. Pharmatherapeutica 4:341–346, 1985.
156. Solerte SB, Fioravanti M, Patti AL, et al: Pentoxifylline, total urinary protein excretion rate and arterial blood pressure in long-term insulin-dependent diabetic patients with overt nephropathy. Acta Diabetol 24:229–239, 1987.
157. Solerte SB, Fioravanti M, Cerutti N, et al: Retrospective analysis of long-term hemorheologic effects of pentoxifylline in diabetic patients with angiopathic complications. Acta Diabetol 34:67–74, 1997.
158. Guerrero-Romero F, Rodriguez-Moran M, Paniagua-Sierra JR, et al: Pentoxifylline reduces proteinuria in insulin-dependent and noninsulin-dependent diabetic patients. Clin Nephrol 43:116–121, 1995.
159. McCarty MF: Nitric oxide deficiency, leukocyte activation, and resultant ischemia are crucial to the pathogenesis of diabetic retinopathy/neuropathy—preventive potential of antioxidants, essential fatty acids, chromium, ginkgolides, and pentoxifylline. Med Hypotheses 50:435–449, 1998.
160. Porte D Jr, Schwartz MW: Diabetes complications: Why is glucose potentially toxic? Science 272:699, 1996.
161. Brownlee M: Glycation and diabetic complications. Diabetes 43:836, 1994.
162. Vlassara H: Protein glycation in the kidney: Role in diabetes and aging. Kidney Int 49:1795, 1996.
163. Schmidt AM, Hori O, Chen JX, et al: Advanced glycation end products interacting with their endothelial receptor induce expression of vascular cell adhesion molecule-1 (VCAM-1) in cultured human endothelial cells and in mice. J Clin Invest 96:1395, 1995.
164. Makita Z, Bucala R, Rayfield EJ, et al: Reactive glycosylation end products in diabetic uraemia and treatment of renal failure. Lancet 343:1519, 1994.
165. Makita Z, Radoff S, Rayfield EJ, et al: Advanced glycosylation end products in patients with diabetic nephropathy. N Engl J Med 325:836, 1991.
166. Papanastasiou P, Grass L, Rodela H, et al: Immunological quantification of advanced glycosylation end–products in the serum of patients on hemodialysis or CAPD. Kidney Int 46:216, 1994.
167. Vlassara H: Serum advanced glycosylation end products: A new class of uremic toxins? Blood Purif 12:54, 1994.
168. Motomiya Y, Oyama N, Iwamoto H, et al: N-epsilon-(carboxymethyl)lysine in blood from maintenance hemodialysis patients may contribute to dialysis-related amyloidosis. Kidney Int 54:1357, 1998.
169. Vlassara H, Fuh H, Makita Z, et al: Exogenous advanced glycosylation end products induce complex vascular dysfunction in normal animals: A model for diabetic and aging complications. Proc Natl Acad Sci U S A 89:12043, 1992.
170. Yang CW, Vlassara H, Peten EP, et al: Advanced glycation end products up-regulate gene expression found in diabetic glomerular disease. Proc Natl Acad Sci U S A 91:9436, 1994.

171. Ono Y, Aoki S, Ohnishi K, et al: Increased serum levels of advanced glycation end-products and diabetic complications. Diabetes Res Clin Pract 41:131, 1998.
172. Bucala R: What is the effect of hyperglycemia on atherogenesis and can it be reversed by aminoguanidine? Diabetes Res Clin Pract 30S:123, 1996.
173. Basta G, DeCaterina R: Products of advanced glycosylation and the pathogenesis of accelerated atherosclerosis in diabetes. G Ital Cardiol 26:699, 1996.
174. Tanaka S, Avigad G, Brodsky B, Eikenberry EF: Glycation induces expansion of the molecular packing of collagen. J Mol Biol 203:495, 1988.
175. Bucala R, Makita Z, Vega G, et al: Modification of low density lipoprotein by advanced glycation end products contributes to the dyslipidemia of diabetes and renal insufficiency. Proc Natl Acad Sci U S A 91:9441, 1994.
176. Nakamura Y, Horil Y, Nishino T, et al: Immunohistochemical localization of advanced glycosylation end products in coronary atheroma and cardiac tissue in diabetes mellitus. Am J Pathol 143:1649, 1993.
177. Tsilbary EC, Charonis AS, Regel LA, et al: The effect of nonenzymatic glycosylation on the binding of the main noncollagenous NC1 domain to type IV collagen. J Biol Chem 263:4302, 1988.
178. Bucala R, Tracey KJ, Cerami A: Advanced glycosylation products quench nitric oxide and mediate defective endothelium-dependent vasodilation in experimental diabetes. J Clin Invest 87:432, 1991.
179. Way KJ, Reid JJ: Effect of aminoguanidine on the impaired nitric oxide–mediated neurotransmission in anococcygeum muscle from diabetic rats. Neuropharmacology 33:1315, 1994.
180. Knowx LK, Stewart AG, Hayward PG, Morrison WA: Nitric oxide synthase inhibitors improve skin flap survival in the rat. Microsurgery 15:708, 1994.
181. Tilton RG, Chang K, Corbett JA, et al: Endotoxin–induced uveitis in the rat is attenuated by inhibition of nitric oxide production. Invest Ophthalmol Vis Sci 35:3278, 1994.
182. Hogan M, Cerami A, Bucala R: Advanced glycosylation end products block the antiproliferative effect of nitric oxide. Role in the vascular and renal complications of diabetes mellitus. J Clin Invest 90:1110, 1992.
183. Brownlee M, Vlassara H, Kooney T, et al: Aminoguanidine prevents diabetes-induced arterial wall protein cross-linking. Science 232:1629, 1986.
184. Hammes HP, Martin S, Federlin K, et al: Aminoguanidine treatment inhibits the development of experimental diabetic retinopathy. Proc Natl Acad Sci U S A 88:11555, 1991.
185. Norton GR, Candy G, Woodiwiss AJ: Aminoguanidine prevents the decreased myocardial compliance produced by streptozotocin-induced diabetes mellitus in rats. Circulation 93:1905, 1996.
186. Soulis-Liparota T, Cooper ME, Dunlop M, Jerums G: The relative roles of advanced glycation, oxidation and aldose reductase inhibition in the development of experimental diabetic nephropathy in the Sprague-Dawley rat. Diabetologia 38:387, 1995.
187. Cohen MP, Hud E, Wu VY: Amelioration of diabetic nephropathy by treatment with monoclonal antibodies against glycated albumin. Kidney Int 45:1673, 1994.
188. Soulis T, Cooper ME, Vranes D, et al: Effects of aminoguanidine in preventing experimental diabetic nephropathy are related to the duration of treatment. Kidney Int 50:627, 1996.
189. Yagihashi S, Kamijo M, Baba M: Effect of aminoguanidine on functional and structural abnormalities in peripheral nerve of STZ–induced diabetic rats. Diabetes 41:47, 1992.
190. Miyauchi Y, Shikama H, Takasu T, et al: Slowing of peripheral motor nerve conduction was ameliorated by aminoguanidine in streptozotocin-induced diabetic rats. Eur J Endocrinol 134:467, 1996.
191. Archibald V, Cotter MA, Keegan A, Cameron NE: Contraction and relaxation of aortas from diabetic rats: Effects of chronic anti-oxidant and aminoguanidine treatments. Naunyn Schmiedebergs Arch Pharmacol 353:584, 1996.
192. Hou FF, Boyce J, Chertow GM, et al: Aminoguanidine inhibits advanced glycation end products formation on beta 2-microglobulin. J Am Soc Nephrol 9:277, 1998.
193. Brownlee M: Pharmacological modulation of the advanced glycosylation reaction. Prog Clin Biol Res 304:235, 1989.
194. Sensi M, Pricci F, Andreani D, DiMario U: Advanced nonenzymatic glycation end products (AGE): Their relevance to aging and the pathogenesis of late diabetic complications. Diabetes Res 16:1, 1991.
195. Tilton RG, Change K, Hasan KS, et al: Prevention of diabetic vascular dysfunction by guanidines. Inhibition of nitric oxide synthase versus advanced glycation end-product formation. Diabetes 42:221, 1993.
196. Corbett JA, Tilton RG, Chang K: Aminoguanidine, a novel inhibitor of nitric oxide formation, prevents diabetic vascular dysfunction. Diabetes 41:552, 1992.
197. Yang CW, Yu CC, Ko YC, Huang CC: Aminoguanidine reduces glomerular inducible nitric oxide synthase (iNOS) and transforming growth factor-beta 1 (TGF-beta 1) mRNA expression and diminishes glomerulosclerosis in NZB/W F1 mice. Clin Exp Immunol 113:258, 1998.
198. Bry KR, Wolff DJ: Mechanism of inducible nitric oxide synthase inactivation by aminoguanidine and L-N6-(*l*-iminoethyl)lysine. Biochemistry 37:4844, 1998.
199. Giardino I, Fard AK, Harchell DL, Brownlee M: Aminoguanidine inhibits reactive oxygen species formation, lipid peroxidation, and oxidant-induced apoptosis. Diabetes 47:1114, 1998.
200. Cormon B, Duriez M, Poitevin P, et al: Aminoguanidine prevents age-related arterial stiffening and cardiac hypertrophy. Proc Natl Acad Sci U S A 95:1301, 1998.
201. Vasan S, Zhang X, Zhang X, et al: An agent cleaving glucose-derived protein crosslinks in vitro and in vivo. Nature 382:275, 1996.
202. Schwedler S, Verbeke P, Bakala H, et al: *N*-phenacylthizolium bromide (PTB) decreases renal AGE levels and increases urinary AGE excretion without ameliorating diabetic nephropathy in C57BL/6 mice (abstract). J Am Soc Nephrol 9:641A, 1998.
203. Park L, Raman KG, Lee KJ, et al: Suppression of accelerated diabetic atherosclerosis by the soluble receptor for advanced glycation end products. Nat Med 4:1025, 1998.
204. Nakamura S, Makita Z, Ishikawa S, et al: Progression of nephrology in spontaneous diabetic rats is prevented by OPB-9195, a novel inhibitor of advanced glycation. Diabetes 46:895, 1997.
205. MacLeod MJ, McLay J: Drug treatment of hypertension complicating diabetes mellitus. Drugs 56:189–202, 1998.
206. Parving HH: Is antihypertensive treatment the same for type 2 diabetes and type 1 diabetes patients? Diabetes Res Clin Pract 39(suppl):S43–77, 1998.
207. Friedman EA, Chou LM, Beyer MM, et al: Adverse impact of hypertension on diabetic recipients of transplanted kidneys. Hypertension 7:1131–1134, 1985.
208. Krolewski AS, Warram JH, Christlieb AR, et al: The changing natural history of nephropathy in type 1 (insulin-dependent) diabetes mellitus. Am J Med 78:785–794, 1985.
209. Parving H-H, Hommel E: Prognosis in diabetic nephropathy. BMJ 299:230–233, 1989.
210. Zatz R, Dunn BR, Meyer TW, et al: Prevention of diabetic glomerulopathy by pharmacological amelioration of glomerular capillary hypertension. J Clin Invest 77:1925–1930, 1986.
211. Hostetter TH, Troy JL, Brenner BM: Glomerular hemodynamics in experimental diabetes. Kidney Int 19:410–415, 1981.
212. Hostetter TH: Pathogenesis of diabetic glomerulopathy: Hemodynamic considerations. Semin Nephrol 10:219–227, 1990.
213. Bérionade VC, Lefebvre R, Falardeau P: Unilateral nodular diabetic glomerulosclerosis: Recurrence of an experiment of nature. Am J Nephrol 7:55–59, 1987.
214. Mogensen CE: Long term anti-hypertensive treatment inhibiting progression of diabetic nephropathy. BMJ 285:685–688, 1982.
215. Mogensen CE: Prevention and treatment of renal disease in insulin-dependent diabetes mellitus. Semin Nephrol 10:260–273, 1990.
216. Parving H-H, Anderson AR, Smidt UM, Svendsen PAA: Early aggressive antihypertensive therapy reduces rate of decline in kidney function in diabetic nephropathy. Lancet 2:1175–1179, 1983.
217. Parving H-H, Andersen AR, Hommel E, Smidt U: Effects of long term antihypertensive treatment on kidney function in diabetic nephropathy. Hypertension 7(suppl 2):114–117, 1985.
218. Christensen CK, Mogensen CE: Acute and long term effect of antihypertensive treatment on exercise-induced albuminuria in incipient diabetic nephropathy. Scand J Clin Lab Invest 46:553–559, 1986.
219. Parving H-H, Andersen AR, Smidt UM, et al: Effect of antihypertensive treatment on kidney function in diabetic nephropathy. BMJ 294:1443–1447, 1987.
220. Parving H-H, Hommel E, Nielsen MD, Giese J: Effect of captopril on blood pressure and kidney function in normotensive insulin-dependent diabetics with nephropathy. BMJ 299:533–536, 1989.
221. Mathiesen ER, Borch-Johnsen K, Jensen DV, Deckert T: Improved survival in patients with diabetic nephropathy. Diabetologia 32:884–886, 1989.
222. Working Group on Hypertension in Diabetes: Statement on hypertension in diabetes mellitus: Final report. Arch Intern Med 147:830–842, 1987.
223. Plouin P-F, Azizi M, Day M: Treatment of hypertension in diabetes: Threshold of intervention and therapeutic options. Diabetes Metab 18:182–186, 1992.
224. Fujihara CK, Padilha RM, Santos MM, Zatz K: Role of glomerular hypertension, glomerular hypertrophy and lipid deposition in the genesis of glomerulosclerosis of experimental diabetes (abstract). Kidney Int 37:506, 1990.
225. Fujihara CK, Padilha RM, Zatz R: Glomerular abnormalities in long term experimental diabetes: Role of hemodynamic and non-hemodynamic factors and effect of antihypertensive therapy. Diabetes 41:286–293, 1992.
226. Bakris GL: Progression of diabetic nephropathy. A focus on arterial pressure level and methods of reduction. Diabetes Res Clin Pract 39(suppl):S35–42, 1998.
227. Andersen S, Rennke HG, Garcia DL, Brenner BM: Short- and long-term effects of antihypertensive therapy in the diabetic rat. Kidney Int 36:526–536, 1989.
228. Zatz R, Meyer TW, Rennke HG, Brenner BM: Predominance of hemodynamic rather than metabolic factors in the pathogenesis of diabetic nephropathy. Proc Natl Acad Sci USA 82:5963–5967, 1985.
229. Fogo A, Yoshida Y, Ichikawa I: Angiotensin converting enzyme inhibition (CEI) suppresses accelerated growth of glomerular cells in vivo and vitro. Kidney Int 33:296, 1986.
230. Galler M, Backenroth R, Folkert VW, Schlondorff D: Effect of converting enzyme inhibitors on prostaglandin synthesis by isolated glomerular and aortic strips from rats. J Pharmacol Exp Ther 220:23–28, 1982.
231. Homma T, Ichikawa I, Hoover RL: Prostaglandins of mesangium origin inhibit mesangial cell proliferation and matrix synthesis (abstract). Kidney Int 33:268, 1988.
232. Marre M, Leblanc H, Suarez I, et al: Converting enzyme inhibition and kidney function in normotensive diabetic patients with persistent microalbuminuria. BMJ 294:1448–1452, 1987.
233. Bakris GL, Barnhill BW, Sadler R: Treatment of arterial hypertension in diabetic humans: Importance of therapeutic selection. Kidney Int 41:912–919, 1992.
234. Johnston CI, Cooper ME, Nicholis GM: Meeting report of the International Society of Hypertension Conference on Hypertension and Diabetes. J Hypertens 10:393–397, 1992.
235. Taguma Y, Kitamoto Y, Futaki G, et al: Effect of captopril on heavy proteinuria in azotemic diabetics. N Engl J Med 313:1617–1620, 1985.
236. Borck S, Nyberg G, Mulec H, et al: Beneficial effect of angiotensin converting enzyme inhibition on renal function in patients with diabetic nephropathy. BMJ 293:471–474, 1986.
237. Bjorck S, Mulec H, Johnsen SA, et al: Enalapril but not metoprolol reduces proteinuria in diabetic nephropathy. Kidney Int 37:236, 1990.
238. Mogensen CE: Angiotensin converting enzyme inhibitors and diabetic nephropathy. BMJ 304:327–328, 1992.
239. Savage S, Schrier RW: Progressive renal insufficiency: The role of angiotensin converting enzyme inhibitors. Adv Intern Med 37:85–101, 1992.
240. Estacio RO, Schrier RW: Antihypertensive therapy in type 2 diabetes: Implications of the appropriate blood pressure control in diabetes (ABCD) trial. Am J Cardiol 82:9R–14R, 1998.

241. Poulter NR: Calcium antagonists and the diabetic patient: A response to recent controversies. Am J Cardiol 12;82:40R–41R, 1998.
242. Parving HH: Calcium antagonists and cardiovascular risk in diabetes. Am J Cardiol 12;82:42R–44R, 1998.
243. Pahor M, Psaty BM, Furberg CD: New evidence on the prevention of cardiovascular events in hypertensive patients with type 2 diabetes. J Cardiovasc Pharmacol 32(suppl 2):S18–S23, 1998.
244. Paster RZ, Snavely DB, Sweet AR, et al: Use of losartan in the treatment of hypertensive patients with a history of cough induced by angiotensin-converting enzyme inhibitors. Clin Ther 20:978–989, 1998.
245. Saracho R, Martin-Malo A, Martinez I, et al: Evaluation of the Losartan in Hemodialysis (ELHE) Study. Kidney Int Suppl 68:S125–129, 1998.
246. Ritz E, Rychlik I, Miltenberger-Miltenyi G: Optimizing antihypertensive therapy in patients with diabetic nephropathy. J Hypertens Suppl 16:S17–22, 1998.
247. Henry RR, Wallace P, Olefsky JM: Effects of weight loss on mechanisms of hyperglycemia in obese non–insulin dependent diabetes mellitus. Diabetes 35:990–998, 1986.
248. Schneider SH, Vitug A, Ruderman SV: Atherosclerosis and physical activity. Diabetes Metab Rev 1:513–553, 1986.
249. Ravid M, Brosh D, Ravid-Safran D, et al: Main risk factors for nephropathy in type 2 diabetes mellitus are plasma cholesterol levels, mean blood pressure, and hyperglycemia. Arch Intern Med 158:998–1004, 1998.
250. Maschio G, Oldrizi L, Rugiu C: The effects of dietary protein restriction on the course of early chronic failure. *In* Mitch WE, Brenner BM, Stein JH (eds): The Progressive Nature of Renal Disease. Contemporary Issues in Nephrology, vol 14. New York, Churchill-Livingstone, 1986, pp 203–210.
251. Bosch JP, Sacaggi A, Lauer A, et al: Renal functional reserve in humans. Am J Med 75:943–950, 1983.
252. Kupin WL, Cortes P, Dumler S, et al: Effect on renal function of change from high to moderate protein intake in type 1 diabetic patients. Diabetes 36:73–79, 1987.
253. Wiseman MJ, Bognetti E, Dodds R, et al: Changes in renal function in response to protein restricted diet in type 1 (insulin-dependent) diabetic subjects. Diabetologia 30:154–159, 1987.
254. Krolewski AS, Warram JH, Christlieb AR, et al: The changing natural history of nephropathy in type 1 diabetes. Am J Med 78:785–794, 1985.
255. Wen S-F, Huang T-P, Moorthy AV: Effects of low-protein diet on experimental diabetic nephropathy in the rat. J Lab Clin Med 106:589–597, 1985.
256. Rennke HG, Sandstrom D, Zatz R, et al: The role of dietary protein in the development of glomerular structural abnormalities in long term experimental diabetes mellitus (abstract). Kidney Int 29:289, 1986.
257. Cohen D, Dodds R, Viberti GC: Effect of protein restriction in insulin-dependent diabetics at risk of nephropathy. BMJ 294:795–798, 1987.
258. Bending JJ, Dodds RA, Keen H, Viberti GC: Renal response to restricted protein intake in diabetic nephropathy. Diabetes 37:1641–1646, 1988.
259. Zeller K, Whittaker E, Sullivan L, et al: Effect of restricting dietary protein on the progression of renal failure in patients with insulin-dependent diabetes mellitus. N Engl J Med 324:78–84, 1991.
260. Pedersen MM, Mogensen CE, Jørgensen SF, et al: Renal effects from limitation of high dietary protein in normoalbuminuric diabetic patients. Kidney Int Suppl 27:S115–S121, 1989.
261. Walker JD, Bending JJ, Dodds RA, et al: Restriction of dietary protein and progression of renal failure in diabetic nephropathy. Lancet 2:1411–1414, 1989.
262. Evanoff GV, Thompson CS, Brown J, Weinman EJ: The effect of dietary protein restriction on the progression of diabetic nephropathy: A 12 month follow-up. Arch Intern Med 147:492–495, 1987.
263. Evanoff G, Thompson C, Brown J, Weinman E: Prolonged dietary protein restriction in diabetic nephropathy. Arch Intern Med 149:1129–1133, 1989.
264. Barsotti G, Ciardella F, Morelli E, et al: Nutritional treatment of renal failure in type 1 diabetes. Clin Nephrol 29:280–287, 1988.
265. Jibani MM, Bloodworth LL, Foden KD, et al: Predominantly vegetarian diet in patients with incipient and early clinical diabetic nephropathy: Effects on albumin excretion rate and nutritional status. Diabet Med 8:949–953, 1991.
266. Pedrini MT, Levey AS, Lau J, et al: The effect of dietary protein restriction on the progression of diabetic and nondiabetic renal diseases: A meta-analysis. Ann Intern Med 124:627–632, 1996.
267. Kasiske BL, Lakatua JD, Ma JZ, Louis TA: A meta-analysis of the effects of dietary protein restriction on the rate of decline in renal function. Am J Kidney Dis 31:954–961, 1998.
268. Kaysen G, Gambertoglio J, Jiminez I, et al: Effects of dietary protein intake on albumin homeostasis in nephrotic patients. Kidney Int 29:572–577, 1986.
269. El Nahas AM, Masters-Thomas A, Brady SA, et al: Selective effects of low protein diets in renal diseases. BMJ 289:1337–1341, 1984.
270. Jameel N, Pugh JA, Mitchell BD, Stern MP: Dietary protein intake is not correlated with clinical proteinuria in NIDDM. Diabetes Care 15:178–183, 1992.
271. Viberti GC, Dodds RA, Bending JJ: Non-glycemic intervention in diabetic nephropathy: The role of dietary protein intake. *In* Mogensen CE (ed): The Kidney and Hypertension in Diabetes. Boston, Martinus Nijhoff, 1988, pp 205–215.
272. Wylie-Rosett J: Evaluation of protein in dietary management of diabetes mellitus. Diabetes Care 11:143–148, 1988.
273. American Diabetes Association: Clinical practice recommendations 1997. Diabetes Care 20(suppl 1):S1–70, 1997.
274. Fox CJ, Darby SC, Ireland JT, Šonksen PH: Blood glucose control and glomerular capillary basement membrane thickening in experimental diabetes. BMJ 2:605–607, 1977.
275. Mauer SM, Steffes MW, Brown DM: Animal models of diabetic nephropathy. Adv Nephrol 8:280–285, 1975.
276. Mauer SF, Steffes MW, Sutherland D, et al: Studies of the rate of regression of the glomerular lesions in diabetic rats treated with pancreatic islet transplantation. Diabetes 24:280–285, 1975.
277. Weil R, Nozawara M, Koss M, et al: Pancreatic transplantation in diabetic rats: Renal function, morphology, ultrastructure and immunohistology. Surgery 78:142–148, 1975.
278. Wiseman M, Viberti G, Mackintosh D, et al: Glycemia, arterial pressure and microalbuminuria in type 1 (insulin-dependent) diabetes mellitus. Diabetologia 26:401–405, 1984.
279. Nelson RG, Kunzelman CL, Pettit DJ, et al: Albuminuria in type 2 (non–insulin dependent) diabetes mellitus and impaired glucose tolerance in Pima Indians. Diabetologia 32:870–876, 1989.
280. Skyler JS: Complications of diabetes mellitus: Relationship to metabolic dysfunction. Diabetes Care 2:499–509, 1979.
281. Rosenstock J, Friberg T, Raskin P: Effect of glycemic control on microvascular complications in patients with type I diabetes mellitus. Am J Med 81:1012–1018, 1986.
282. Hasslacher C, Ritz E: Effect of control of diabetes mellitus on progression of renal failure. Kidney Int Suppl 32(22):53–56, 1987.
283. Di Landro D, Catalano C, Lambertini D, et al: The effect of metabolic control on development and progression of diabetic nephropathy. Nephrol Dial Transplant 13(suppl 8):35–43, 1998.
284. The DCCT Research Group: The Diabetes Control and Complications Trial (DCCT): Design and methodologic considerations for the feasibility phase. Diabetes 35:530–545, 1986.
285. The Diabetes Control and Complications (DCCT) Research Group: Effect of intensive therapy on the development and progression of diabetic nephropathy in the Diabetes Control and Complications Trial. Kidney Int 47:1703–1720, 1995.
286. Delahanty LM: Implications of the diabetes control and complications trial for renal outcomes and medial nutrition therapy. J Renal Nutr 8:59–63, 1998.
287. Eastman RC, Javitt JC, Herman WH, et al: Model of complications of NIDDM. II. Analysis of the health benefits and cost-effectiveness of treating Type 2 diabetes with the goal of normoglycemia. Diabetes Care 20:735–744, 1997.
288. Sharma K, Ziyadeh FN: Biochemical events and cytokine interactions linking glucose metabolism to the development of diabetic nephropathy [erratum appears in Semin Nephrol 17:391, 1997]. Semin Nephrol 17:80–92, 1997.
289. Nyberg G, Bhlomé G, NordJn G: Input of metabolic control on progression of clinical diabetic nephropathy. Diabetologia 30:82–86, 1987.
290. UK Prospective Diabetes Study (UKPDS) Group: Intensive blood-glucose control with sulphonylureas or insulin compared with conventional treatment and risk of complications in patients with type 2 diabetes (UKPDS 33). Lancet 352:837–853, 1998.
291. Inzucchi SE, Maggs DG, Spollett GR, et al: Efficacy and metabolic effects of metformin and troglitazone in type II diabetes mellitus. N Engl J Med 338:867–872, 1998.
292. Schmidt R, Horn E, Richards J, Stamatakis M: Survival after metformin-associated lactic acidosis in peritoneal dialysis–dependent renal failure. Am J Med 102:486–488, 1997.
293. Weinrauch LA, Healy RW, Leland OS Jr, et al: Decreased insulin requirement in acute renal failure in diabetic nephropathy. Arch Intern Med 138:399–402, 1978.
294. D'Elia JA, Kaldany A, Miller DG, et al: Elimination of requirement for exogenous insulin therapy in diabetic renal failure. Clin Exp Dial Apheresis 6:75–84, 1982.
295. Brauner A, Flodin U, Hylander B, Ostenson CG: Bacteriuria, bacterial virulence and host factors in diabetic patients. Diabet Med 10:550–554, 1993.
296. Kunin CM: Detection, Prevention and Management of Urinary Tract Infections, ed 4. Philadelphia, Lea & Febiger, 1987.
297. McHugh TP, Albanna SE, Stewart NJ: Bilateral emphysematous pyelonephritis. Am J Emerg Med 16:166–169, 1998.
298. Parfrey PS, Griffiths SM, Barrett BJ, et al: Contrast material–induced renal failure in patients with diabetes mellitus, renal insufficiency, or both. A prospective controlled study. N Engl J Med 320:143–149, 1989.
299. Barrett BJ, Parfrey PS, Vavasour HM, et al: Contrast nephropathy in patients with impaired renal function: High versus low osmolar media. Kidney Int 41:1274–1279, 1992.
300. Aronoff GR, Brier ME, Burns J, et al: Drug Prescribing in Renal Failure. Dosing Guidelines for Adults, ed 4. Philadelphia, American College of Physicians, 1999.
301. Grenfell A, Watkins PJ: Clinical diabetic nephropathy: Natural history and complications. Clin Endocrinol Metab 15:783–805, 1986.
302. Humphrey LL, Ballard DJ, Frohnert PP, et al: Chronic renal failure in non–insulin-dependent diabetes mellitus. Ann Intern Med 10:788–796, 1989.
303. Friedman EA: Race and diabetic nephropathy. Transplant Proc 19(suppl 2):77–81, 1987.
304. Cox NJ, Ziang K-S, Fajans SS, Bell GI: Mapping diabetes-susceptibility genes: Lessons learned from search for DNA marker for maturity-onset diabetes of the young. Diabetes 41:401–407, 1992.
305. Powers DR, Wallin JD: End-stage renal disease in specific ethnic and racial groups: Risk factors and benefits of antihypertensive therapy. Arch Intern Med 158:793–800, 1998.
306. Lowder GM, Perri NA, Freidman EA: Demographics, diabetes type, and degree of rehabilitation in diabetic patients on maintenance hemodialysis in Brooklyn. J Diabetes Complications 2:218–226, 1988.
307. Ghavamian M, Gutch CF, Kopp KF, Kolff WJ: The sad truth about hemodialysis in diabetic nephropathy. JAMA 222:1386–1389, 1972.
308. Sutherland DER, Morrow CE, Fryd DS, et al: Improved patient and primary renal allograft survival in uremic diabetic recipients. Transplantation 34:319–325, 1982.
309. Amair P, Khanna R, Liebel B, et al: Continuous ambulatory peritoneal dialysis in diabetic end-stage renal disease. N Engl J Med 306:625–630, 1982.
310. Tzamaloukas AH, Murata GH, Harford AM, et al: Hand gangrene in diabetic patients on chronic dialysis. Trans Am Soc Artif Intern Organs 37:638–643, 1991.
311. Riggs JE, Moss AH, Labosky DA, et al: Upper extremity ischemic monomelic neuropathy: A complication of vascular access procedures in uremic diabetic patients. Neurology 39:997–998, 1989.

312. Mayers JD, Markell MS, Cohen L, et al: Vascular access surgery for maintenance hemodialysis. Variables in hospital stay. ASAIO J 38:113–115, 1992.

313. Cheigh J, Raghavan J, Sullivan J, et al: Is insufficient dialysis a cause for high morbidity in diabetic patients? (abstract). J Am Soc Nephrol 2:317, 1991.

314. Held PJ, Levin NW, Bovbjerg RR, et al: Mortality and duration of hemodialysis treatment. JAMA 265:871–875, 1991.

315. Berger EE, Lowrie EG: Mortality and the length of dialysis. JAMA 265:909–910, 1991.

316. Kjellstrand CM, Goetz FC, Najarian JS: Transplantation and dialysis in diabetic patients: An update. *In* Friedman EA, L'Esperance FA Jr (eds): Diabetic Renal Retinal Syndrome. New York, Grune & Stratton, 1980, pp 345–351.

317. Lowrie EG, New NL: Death risk in hemodialysis patients: The predictive value of commonly measured variables and an evaluation of death rate differences between facilities. Am J Kidney Dis 15:458–482, 1990.

318. Khanna R, Oreopoulos DG: Peritoneal dialysis for diabetics with failed kidneys: Long-term survival and rehabilitation. Semin Dial 10:209–214, 1997.

319. Friedman EA: Management choices in diabetic end-state renal disease. Nephrol Dial Transplant 10(suppl 7):61–69, 1995.

320. Legrain M, Rottembourg J, Bentchikou A, et al: Dialysis treatment of insulin dependent diabetic patients: Ten years experience. Clin Nephrol 21:72–81, 1984.

321. Rubin J, Hsu H: Continuous ambulatory peritoneal dialysis: Ten years at one facility. Am J Kidney Dis 17:165–169, 1991.

322. Burton PR, Walls J: Selection-adjusted comparison of life-expectancy of patients on continuous ambulatory peritoneal dialysis, haemodialysis, and renal transplantation. Lancet 1:1115–1119, 1982.

323. Churchill DN: Implications of the Canada-USA (CANUSA) study of the adequacy of dialysis on peritoneal dialysis schedule. Nephrol Dial Transplant 13(suppl 6):158–163, 1998.

324. Churchill DN, Thorpe KE, Nolph KD, et al: Increased peritoneal membrane transport is associated with decreased patient and technique survival for continuous peritoneal dialysis patients. The Canada-USA (CANUSA) Peritoneal Dialysis Study Group. J Am Soc Nephrol 9:1285–1292, 1998.

325. Churchill DN, Thorpe KE, Vonesh EF, Keshaviah PR: Lower probability of patient survival with continuous peritoneal dialysis in the United States compared with Canada. Canada-USA (CANUSA) Peritoneal Dialysis Study Group. J Am Soc Nephrol 8:965–971, 1997.

326. Kelly WD, Lillehei RC, Merkel FK, et al: Allotransplantation of the pancreas and duodenum along with the kidney in diabetic nephropathy. Surgery 61:827–837, 1967.

327. Najarian JS, Sutherland DER, Simmons RL, et al: Ten year experience with renal transplantation in juvenile onset diabetics. Ann Surg 190:487–500, 1979.

328. Rettig RA, Levinsky (eds): Institute for Medicine (US) Kidney Failure and the Federal Government Access to Kidney Transplantation. Washington, DC, National Academy of Sciences, 1991, pp 167–186.

329. Khauli RB, Steinmuller DR, Novick AC, et al: A critical look at survival of diabetics with end-stage renal disease: Transplantation versus dialysis therapy. Transplantation 41:598–602, 1986.

330. Cecka JM, Terasaki PI: The UNOS Scientific Renal Transplant Registry 1991. *In* Terasaki PI (ed): Clinical Transplants 1991. Los Angeles, UCLA Tissue Typing Laboratory, 1991, pp 1–11.

331. Paterson AD, Dornan TL, Peacock I, et al: Cause of death in diabetic patients with impaired renal function: An audit of a hospital diabetic clinic population. Lancet 1:313–316, 1987.

332. Braun WE, Phillips D, Vidt DG, et al: The course of coronary artery disease in diabetics with and without renal allografts. Transplant Proc 15:1114–1119, 1983.

333. Khauli RB, Novick AC, Braun WE, et al: Improved results of 54 renal transplantations in the diabetic patient. J Urol 130:867–870, 1983.

334. Philipson JD, Carpenter BJ, Itzkoff J, et al: Evaluation of cardiovascular risk for renal transplantation in diabetic patients. Am J Med 81:630–634, 1986.

335. Gill JB, Ruddy TD, Newell JB, et al: Prognostic importance of thallium uptake by the lungs during exercise in coronary artery disease. N Engl J Med 317:1485–1489, 1987.

336. Shaw LJ, Eagle KA, Gersh BJ, Miller DD: Meta-analysis of intravenous dipyridamole–thallium-201 imaging (1985 to 1994) and dobutamine echocardiography (1991 to 1994) for risk stratification before vascular surgery. J Am Coll Cardiol 15;27:787–798, 1996.

337. Reis G, Marcovitz PA, Leichtman AB, et al: Usefulness of dobutamine stress echocardiography in detecting coronary artery disease in end-stage renal disease. Am J Cardiol 75:707–710, 1995.

338. Gonzalez-Carrillo M, Moloney A, Bewick M, et al: Renal transplantation in diabetic nephropathy. BMJ 285:1713–1716, 1982.

339. Abendroth D, Landgraf R, Illner WD, et al: Beneficial effects of pancreatic transplantation in insulin-dependent diabetes mellitus patients. Transplant Proc 22:696–697, 1990.

340. Yuge J, Cecka JM: Sex and age effects in renal transplantation. *In* Terasaki PI (ed): Clinical Transplants 1991. Los Angeles, UCLA Tissue Typing Laboratory, 1992, p 261.

341. Najarian JS, Kaufman DB, Fryd DS, et al: Survival into the second decade following kidney transplantation in type I diabetic patients. Transplant Proc 21(1 pt 2):2012–2015, 1989.

342. Osterby R, Nyberg G, Hedman L, et al: Kidney transplantation in type 1 (insulin-dependent) diabetic patients. Diabetologia 9:668–674, 1991.

343. Bohman SO, Tyden G, Wilezek A, et al: Prevention of kidney graft diabetic nephropathy by pancreas transplantation in man. Diabetes 34:306–308, 1985.

344. Najarian JS, Kaufman DB, Fryd DS, et al: Long-term survival following kidney transplantation in 100 type 1 diabetic patients. Transplantation 1:106–113, 1989.

345. Dubernard JM, Tajra LC, Lefrancois N, et al: Pancreas transplantation: results and indications. Diabetes Metab 24:195–999, 1998.

346. Bohman SO, Wilczek H, Jaremko G, et al: Recurrence of diabetic nephropathy in human renal allografts: Preliminary report of a biopsy study. Transplant Proc 16:649–653, 1984.

347. Kennedy WR, Navarro X, Goetz FC, et al: Effects of pancreatic transplantation on diabetic neuropathy. N Engl J Med 322:1031–1037, 1990.

348. Van der Vliet JA, Navarro X, Kennedy WR, et al: The effect of pancreas transplantation on diabetic polyneuropathy. Transplantation 45:368–370, 1988.

349. Ramsay RC, Goetz FC, Sutherland DER, et al: Progression of diabetic retinopathy after pancreas transplantation for insulin-dependent diabetes mellitus. N Engl J Med 318:208–214, 1988.

350. Katz H, Homan M, Velosa J, et al: Effects of pancreas transplantation on postprandial glucose metabolism. N Engl J Med 325:1278–1283, 1991.

351. Sollinger HW, Odorico JS, Knechtle SJ, et al: Experience with 500 simultaneous pancreas-kidney transplants. Ann Surg 228:284–296, 1998.

352. Sasaki TM, Gray RS, Ratner RE, et al: Successful long-term kidney-pancreas transplants in diabetic patients with high C-peptide levels. Transplantation 65:1510–1512, 1998.

353. Sutherland DER: Who should get a pancreas transplant? Diabetes Care 11:681–685, 1988.

354. Callahan MB, Bender K, McNeely M: The role of the health care team in the implementation of the National Kidney Foundation–Dialysis Outcomes Quality Initiative: A case study. Adv Renal Replacement Ther 6:42–51, 1999.

355. Tzamaloukas AH, Murata GH, Piraino B, et al: Peritoneal urea and creatinine clearances in continuous peritoneal dialysis patients with different types of peritoneal solute transport. Kidney Int 53:1405–1411, 1998.

Chapter 64

▲▲▲

Management of the Diabetic Foot Complication

Gary W. Gibbons

There are approximately 16 million people in the United States with diabetes, or 1 in every 17 people. Half of them are not aware that they have the disease and are at risk for long-term complications such as foot ulceration. Foot ulcers affect 15% of all diabetic patients during their lives and precede 85% of all nontraumatic lower limb amputations.[1] It is not surprising that half of all nontraumatic lower limb amputations in the United States are performed on people with diabetes, a concern which has led the American Diabetes Association and Healthy People 2000 (the health objectives of the U.S. Public Health Service) to set a goal to reduce the amputation rate by 40%.[2] We have witnessed tremendous advances in the knowledge, technology, and treatment of diabetes and its complications. Unfortunately, amputations for the diabetic patient are increasing. Diabetic foot problems continue to be a major health concern associated with serious physical, as well as psychosocial, morbidity and mortality, and economic consequences.

Successful management of diabetic foot complications begins with better patient, family, and healthcare professional education and understanding. It requires eliminating misconceptions and anecdotal experiences. Treatment algorithms must be based on scientific evidence with proven clinical results.[2a] An aggressive team approach to limb salvage must consider a number of factors, including the patient's general medical condition; risk factors; functional status; motivation; compliance; the presence, nature, and extent of infection, necrosis, or ulcer; vascular status; and cost, time, and effort.[3]

PATHOPHYSIOLOGY AND RISK FACTORS

Risk factors for ulceration leading to amputation include hyperglycemia, longer duration of diabetes, increasing age, peripheral vascular disease (PVD), ulceration, and improper prevention. Amputation rates are greater with increasing age, in males compared with females, and in nonwhites.

While careful control of diabetes may postpone the development of foot problems, it will not prevent them. Three primary pathologic situations occur in the diabetic patient which singly or, more frequently, in combination, are responsible for the development of foot problems: neuropathy, arterial insufficiency, and infection.

Neuropathy

Nerve damage in diabetes affects the sensory, motor, and autonomic fibers. Sensory neuropathy limits the patient's response to pain, pressure, touch, and temperature, leading to an insensitive foot. Altered proprioception makes the patient less aware of the position of his or her foot. Motor neuropathy affects the intrinsic and skeletal muscles of the foot and leg, causing weakness, atrophy, and deformity. The result of this motor neuropathy is a muscle-wasted foot with prominent metatarsal heads, clawed toes, and limited joint mobility. These deformities create excessive foot pressures with subsequent callus formation and ulceration if repetitive stress (as in walking) continues, especially in a patient who is unaware of these stresses because of the loss of protective sensation. Autonomic neuropathy, often causing autosympathectomy in the lower extremities, creates a warm, overly dry foot with skin that is very susceptible to cracking and breakdown. Autonomic dysfunction also creates functional alterations in the microvascular blood flow of the foot. Overall, a diabetic patient with significant peripheral neuropathy is highly susceptible to any trauma, even minor, and much of this is footwear-related.[4]

Peripheral Vascular Disease

Lower extremity PVD is estimated to be 20 times more common in the diabetic population. It occurs at a younger age, has an equal affinity for women and men, and is often bilateral in its involvement. While diabetes is an important risk factor for PVD, hypertension, smoking, hyperlipidemia, family history, and obesity are additional risks for patients with diabetes. Morbidity and mortality are increased in these patients. The incidence of PVD in a diabetic patient increases with age and duration of diabetes. Progressive PVD can cause disabling pain and contributes to limb ulceration, gangrene, and impaired wound healing. Ischemia also decreases the ability to fight infection by impairing the delivery of oxygen, nutrients, and antibiotics to an infected or ulcerated area. PVD has been noted to be associated with 62% of nonhealing foot ulcers and is a causal factor in 46% of amputations.[5] It is the only factor that can lead to amputation by itself. Local tissue and skin perfusion is dependent not only on arterial inflow but also on local factors, including edema, infection, and systemic factors such as cardiac and renal function.

The pathology of atherosclerosis in the diabetic patient is similar to that in the nondiabetic patient, with three main distinctions: there is a predilection for the more distal tibial and peroneal arteries of the lower leg, as demonstrated by the fact that 40% of diabetic patients presenting with gangrene will have a palpable popliteal pulse. The foot arteries, especially the dorsalis pedis and its branches, are usually spared. This refutes a popular misconception that was based on a single observation in 1959.[6] As LoGerfo and Coffman[7] noted, endothelial injury and thickening of the capillary basement membrane resulting from microvascular dysfunction do not constitute an occlusive lesion. Microvascular dysfunction leads to endothelial injury, limited capillary capacity, and loss of the autoregulatory function, including abolition of an inflammatory response.[8] These findings support an aggressive approach to foot revascularization in the ischemic patient.

Diabetic patients tend to have poor collateral circulation with more atherosclerotic involvement of the distal deep femoral artery and the infragenicular arteries. The atherosclerotic plaque and media of the arteries frequently contain extensive calcium (medial calcinosis or

Mönckeberg's sclerosis), making these arteries rigid and noncompressible. These peculiarities may explain the erroneous interpretive results of standard noninvasive tests which are often incorrect or misleading when applied to the diabetic lower extremity.[9]

Infection

Diabetes has been associated with several defects in the host immune defense system, predisposing many diabetics to infection and certainly altering their response to infection.[10] This becomes a vicious circle as many of the immunodeficiencies are directly related to the metabolic abnormalities caused by poor diabetes control, and infection makes diabetes control more difficult. Impairment of neutrophils in diabetes affects chemotaxis, phagocytosis, and bactericidal function. There is evidence suggesting that cellular immune responses, as well as wound healing, are adversely affected as well. Wounds in the diabetic patient act more like chronic wounds, with wound healing delayed in the inflammatory to proliferative phases.

For all healthcare professionals treating diabetic foot problems, it is important to recognize that systemic signs and symptoms (such as fever, tachycardia, or elevation of the white blood cell count) of an infectious process often occur late, making unexplained and uncontrolled hyperglycemia the only reliable sign of a potentially limb- or life-threatening infection.[11] The clinical consequences of this are obvious. With clinical care today being decided more and more by economic issues, diabetic patients with a foot ulcer should not be sent home just because they are afebrile or have a normal white blood cell count.

PRINCIPLES OF MANAGEMENT

Successful management of diabetic foot problems begins with prevention.[12] Patient, physician, and healthcare professional education and understanding correlate directly with successful prevention, diagnosis, and management of diabetic foot problems. A multidisciplinary team approach maximizes diabetic management, control of associated risk factors, periodic vascular examination, and proper foot care and footwear. Patients and healthcare professionals must be educated as to the importance of proper hygiene, daily shoe and foot inspections, the wearing of appropriate shoes, and the rotation of shoes at least twice per day to vary the stress and pressure points. Repeated testing for sensory neuropathy with a monofilament can be used to identify patients at risk for ulcerations, who are most in need of routine evaluation and follow-up.

Prevention begins on the day that diabetes is diagnosed.[13] Patients and their families and loved ones need to establish a routine that begins with daily inspection of the feet and legs. Because loss of visual acuity is common in many diabetic patients, a family member or friend may help look for calluses, fissures, red or ecchymotic areas, fungal infections, and open sores or blisters. Daily shoe inspection, looking for wear or foreign bodies, is also extremely important. Proper hygiene includes washing and drying the feet carefully and avoiding the use of astringents. Heat or soaks in any form are to be avoided. Moisturizing creams such as lanolin-containing preparations must be used on dry areas and antifungal medication should be used as needed. "Bathroom surgery" must be avoided, especially for nails, corns, or calluses. When nails are trimmed, we prefer a slight rounding of the edges to prevent possible penetration into adjacent toes.

Proper footwear is essential because diabetic patients will not tolerate crowding in any area of the foot. Podiatric appliances such as inserts and spacers are often needed to protect sensitive, high-risk areas. Soft leather, preferably oxford-type shoes that accommodate width and depth, are recommended. Diabetics fear, unreasonably, that they will be required to wear extra-depth "space shoes." The shoe industry has been very accommodating in recent years. Diabetic patients should never go barefoot and should avoid situations likely to cause problems. New shoes must be broken in cautiously. Adherence to routine and proper care prevents many problems. Diabetic patients and their families must be encouraged to report any problem immedi-

ately and access to evaluation and treatment must be available at any time.

Elimination and controlling risk factors can prevent or delay many of the complications of diabetes, including neuropathy and PVD. These include good control of diabetes, cessation of smoking, control of hypertension and hyperlipidemia, maintaining ideal weight, and routine and proper exercise. Periodic clinical vascular examinations, including noninvasive testing when appropriate, identifies patients at risk so they can be observed more carefully or referred to a vascular specialist knowledgeable about diabetic PVD.

CLINICAL PRESENTATION AND THERAPY FOR FOOT ULCERATION

The classification of diabetic foot ulcerations and infection has never been fully standardized and the existing literature is often confusing. The severity of the ulcer and infection determines the proper course of treatment. In today's cost-conscious society the first major decision is whether the patient can be treated at home or needs to be admitted to the hospital.[14] The severity of tissue destruction may not be apparent to the patient or healthcare professional by just looking at the ulcer or infected callus, especially in those patients who continue to bear weight on a painless area or who do not have the visual acuity to recognize a problem. It is imperative for the physician or care provider to debride all encrusted areas and inspect the wound to determine the extent of any deep tissue penetration and the presence of bone or joint involvement. It is essential, however, to emphasize to the patient and family the importance of debridement and inspection so that they understand that this procedure did not cause the problem. Education and communication alleviate much of the anxiety that leads to litigation.

Non–Limb-Threatening Superficial Ulceration

Early superficial ulcers may be treated at home provided that cellulitis, if present, is minimal, that there is no evidence of any systemic toxicity, and that the patient is compliant, reliable, and has a vigilant support system (Fig. 64–1). The injured foot must be put to rest by whatever means the care provider has and is comfortable using. Neuropathy includes loss of sensation and proprioception so that partial weight bearing, as perceived by the patient, may actually be full weight bearing. Education again is key since the patient's concept

Clinical Characteristics	Patient Characteristics
Superficial	Reliable
Minimal or no cellulitis	Conforms to treatment
No bone or joint involvement	Vigilant support system
No significant ischemia	
No systemic toxicity	

Therapy

Rest of injured part (non–weight-bearing)
Culture and sensitivity analyses
Empiric broad-spectrum oral antibiotics; specific antibiotic based
   on culture and response of wounds
Careful debridement
Local wound dressings
Intensive follow-up
Podiatric appliances and modified footwear

FIGURE 64–1. Management of non–limb-threatening diabetic foot ulcers.

of offloading may be different from that of the care provider. While we as care providers are trying to heal and improve limb viability, the patient may be more concerned as to how it affects his or her well-being and functional capacity, such as being able to work and provide income for the family.

If infection is present, cultures are taken; initially, a broad-spectrum oral antibiotic is prescribed which is changed pending subsequent sensitivity reports and the response of the wound. *Staphylococcus aureus* and *Streptococcus* species are the most common and antibiotic therapy should effectively cover these organisms.[15]

Dressings should be kept simple, recognizing that *a moistened wound environment is best for wound healing.* The dressings absorb excess exudate, and also protect the wound and other high risk areas. We have found that the most effective dressings are plain gauze sponges moistened with saline or isotonic antiseptic solutions and applied to the open wound two times daily. Topical wound preparations may allow dressing changes to be decreased to once per day and often family members can be taught to do these changes, especially in light of increasing cost constraints being put on visiting nurses and outpatient allied health professionals. Enzymatic debriding ointments and other astringents, especially full-strength solutions, should be avoided as they are injurious to already compromised tissues. Whirlpool baths, soaks, and hot compresses are also to be avoided since they may lead to more complications such as maceration, superinfection, or burns.

The use of topical growth factors must be left to the individual care provider. They are expensive and their benefits vs. costs for routine use needs further clinical trials. There is no indication for hyperbaric oxygen limb chambers and little evidence supporting immersion chambers for routine treatment of infected diabetic ulcers. It should be remembered that dressings do not replace debridement and frequent evaluation of the wound is mandatory given the immunocompromised status of many of these patients. This is especially important in those patients with persistent hyperglycemia or who are on immunosupression therapy.

Other treatment requirements include the need to control edema and to ensure adequate nutritional support and blood sugar control. Physical therapy and conditioning exercises are important throughout the course of treatment. New therapies include living skin equivalents, ultrasound, ultraviolet light, and electrical stimulation. The cost-effectiveness of these treatments is yet to be fully determined for their routine use in the treatment of diabetic foot ulcers. Dry cracks or fissures respond to antibiotic ointments or lanolin-based creams. If there is no significant improvement in the ulcer within 48 hours, reevaluation and probable hospitalization are advised. The importance of continued offloading until healing is assured must be constantly impressed upon the patient and family.

Once healing is achieved, under careful surveillance, graduated weight bearing is initiated with podiatric appliances and modification of footwear to protect sensitive high-risk areas of the foot. If weight bearing progresses too rapidly, acute Charcot's foot (neuropathic joint disease) may develop. Its presentation may be strikingly similar to that of an acute infection, with warmth, redness, and swelling. It can be differentiated by the fact that there is usually no open area initially and an antecedent history of some type of trauma usually initiates the process. The radiographic picture may be misinterpreted as osteomyelitis, but the experienced clinician can usually make a diagnosis. A more experienced consultant may be needed, especially if a full team is not available in one's practice setting.

Limb-Threatening Infection

Diabetic patients with foot ulcers and limb-threatening infection (Fig. 64–2) require immediate admission to the hospital and complete bed rest. Because they often remain afebrile with a normal white blood cell count, hyperglycemia and malaise may be the only presenting sign and symptom of a significant infection. The blood sugar should be brought under control rapidly which most often requires the use of insulin and not oral agents. While the patient's condition must be stabilized medically, it should not delay urgent, necessary surgical intervention. It is imperative that proper surgical wound care and

Clinical Characteristics	Patient Characteristics
Deep ulcer	Unreliable
>2 cm cellulitis/lymphangitis	Immunocompromised
Bone or joint involvement	Poor support system
Significant ischemia/gangrene	
± Systemic toxicity	

Therapy

Immediate admission and complete bedrest
Control blood glucose and stabilize medically
Appropriate culture and sensitivity analyses
Empiric broad-spectrum intravenous antibiotics; specific antibiotic
  based on sensitivities and response
Plain radiograph
Early surgical debridement, dependent drainage, or open amputation
Meticulous wound care
Early evaluation for ischemia
Selected revascularization and foot-sparing surgery,
  conservative amputations, or revisions
Intensive follow-up
Podiatric appliances and modified footwear

FIGURE 64–2. *Management of severe limb-threatening diabetic foot ulcers.*

antibiotic therapy be initiated emergently. Frequently, systemic toxicity or shock will not be reversed until the septic process is surgically debrided and drained. Antibiotics alone will not cure the problem if there is an undrained infection. Relying on a 6-week course of antibiotics alone to treat deeply infected wounds and osteomyelitis frequently results in failure and the potential for a higher amputation level.

The severity of tissue destruction and sepsis may not be apparent from looking at the ulcer or infected callus. As described previously, inspection requires the removal of callus and eschars and probing the wound to determine the nature, depth, and extent of the necrotic process. Proper surgical wound care requires immediate surgical debridement of all necrotic tissue and drainage of pus. This must be accomplished even in a patient with compromised circulation. Vascular reconstruction in a patient with active limb-threatening infection is contraindicated until the sepsis is resolved. Diabetic patients do not tolerate an undrained infection; adequate debridement cannot be achieved in a deep necrotic wound using small stab wounds or drains. The surgical debridement and drainage must be such that all necrotic material is removed and dependent drainage is adequate to prevent any pooling of pus.[16] Much of this may require little or no anesthesia since neuropathy may play a significant role in limiting pain. Often multiple trips to the operating room are necessary to ensure adequate drainage of infection. One of the best markers that infection is controlled is obtained by monitoring blood sugar, which will not fall until the infection has been properly cared for.

Dressings are begun with the initial surgical procedure and follow the same principles as mentioned previously for non–limb-threatening ulcers. Coexisting cardiac, renal, or other disorders can be addressed once the initial sepsis is controlled, while ensuring adequate nutritional support, physical therapy, control of edema, and the evaluation and treatment of ischemia.

The choice of an initial antibiotic regimen is influenced by several variables, including likely pathogens, Gram's stain of the purulent material, local bacterial resistance pattens, prior antibiotic therapy, preexisting renal or hepatic dysfunction, the severity of the infection, the availability and cost of the antibiotics, and allergies. A review of diabetic patients with serious limb-threatening infection has emphasized the importance of mixed and multiple organisms (3.2 isolated per ulcer).[17] Aerobic gram-positive cocci (93%) and gram-negative bacilli (50%) are prevalent as are positive anaerobic cultures in 69% of patients. Certainly, a wound that is crepitant, fetid, or has gas evident by radiography is harboring anaerobes or obligate anaerobes. As soon as deep cultures are obtained, broad-spectrum intravenous antibiotics are administered to ensure adequate serum levels. Later changes are made depending on sensitivity reports and the response of the wound provided that proper wound care is being administered. Oral antibiotics like the new broad-spectrum fluoroquinolones may obviate the need for prolonged intravenous therapy in some patients. It must be remembered, however, that some patients have significant gastroenteropathy, especially when acutely ill, so that initial intravenous therapy may be required, switching to oral therapy as soon as the patient can tolerate an oral regimen.

OSTEOMYELITIS

Inadequate diagnosis and treatment of osteomyelitis increases the risk of amputation. There are several current radiologic imaging techniques for diagnosing osteomyelitis, but all of the reports recommending one or more combinations of these tests are flawed.[18] These tests are also expensive and this is important considering that reimbursement is fixed and rarely covers the cost of achieving limb salvage. We prefer a sterile probe and if it hits the bone or joint the sensitivity and specificity are equal to any of the currently used radiologic imaging techniques used in diagnosing osteomyelitis.[19] We do obtain a plain radiograph, but reserve the radiologic scanning techniques for complicated cases where probing is equivocal, especially in cases of Charcot's foot. It has been our experience that prolonged courses of antibiotics rarely cure osteomyelitis, especially if it is associated with deep infection, gangrene, ischemia, and bacteremia. It is our belief that necrotic infected bone must be surgically removed for the reasons mentioned previously. It frequently removes the bony prominence that helped initiate the problem to begin with.

MANAGEMENT OF PERIPHERAL VASCULAR DISEASE

Clinical Presentation

The clinical presentation of patients with major artery occlusions or hemodynamically significant stenoses varies depending on the activity level and the adequacy of collateral pathways. Claudication, the inability to walk a given distance (usually described in city blocks) because of an aching or pain in the muscles of the leg, is the earliest symptom of PVD. The stenosis or blockage can usually be determined by the group of muscles involved and is generally one level above. For example, patients with significant foot pain with activity generally have tibial or peroneal disease, whereas patients with calf claudication usually have superficial femoral artery disease. Patients who describe buttock, hip, or thigh claudication have more proximal aortoiliac disease. Peripheral and autonomic neuropathy make the diagnosis of early ischemia in the diabetic patient more difficult and some diabetic patients may not be able to adequately describe claudication.

As PVD progressively worsens, rest pain occurs which is usually described as a deep aching of the muscles in the foot that is present at rest or at night. Patients describe relief by dangling their feet or walking around. As the disease progresses further, tissue ulceration or gangrene may develop. Sensory neuropathy may mask the early signs of PVD and diabetic patients will instead present with tissue loss or gangrene or with failure of a local incision or reconstructive foot surgery to heal because of severe PVD.

Clinical evaluation, judgment, and experience remain the most important means for determining the degree of vascular compromise in the diabetic lower extremity. Noninvasive testing by whatever means the healthcare professional has at his or her disposal is only complementary to one's clinical evaluation. Because of medial calcinosis, the interpretive results of standard noninvasive tests, such as systolic blood pressure and the ankle-brachial ratio, are often misleading and incorrect when applied to the diabetic lower extremity.[20] A good rule of thumb is that vascular consultation and arteriography are indicated when there is a question of ischemia complicating a significant foot problem.

For the patient with an ischemic foot ulcer, once the infection is stabilized, arteriography including visualization of the foot vessels and vascular reconstruction can be performed on selected diabetic patients with vascular insufficiency who are suitable candidates. Arteriography best demonstrates particular atherosclerotic occlusive involvement of the tibial and peroneal arteries with patency of the dorsalis pedis and plantar vessels. We prefer the arterial digital subtraction technique which in more than 90% of diabetic patients demonstrates surgically correctable disease. Proper hydration remains the best means for preventing or minimizing associated renal insufficiency induced by the contrast medium. Metformin should be discontinued at least 24 hours in advance of arteriography, as should other nephrotoxic medications. Magnetic resonance angiography (MRA) may be preferred in certain instances as in patients with significant renal impairment.

Vascular Reconstruction

Restoring circulation requires the right indications, the potential for rehabilitation, and an appropriate conduit. Claudication is rarely an indication for revascularization and treatment usually involves weight reduction, cessation of cigarette smoking, control of lipid levels and hypertension, good diabetes control, and an active and aggressive exercise program. Protective footwear and continuous inspection are important during the exercise program; diabetic patients can live with significant PVD without incident until a traumatic event initiates an ulcer.

Ischemic rest pain, night pain, tissue ulceration, and the inability of a surgical procedure to heal because of ischemia are indications for vascular assessment and reconstruction. Diabetic patients tolerate revascularization extremely well, with morbidity and mortality results equal to those of nondiabetic patients and no greater than amputation.

Endovascular Procedures

The success of endovascular procedures (balloon angioplasty, atherectomy, laser angioplasty) depends on the location of the atherosclerotic disease, the length of the lesion being treated, whether the vascular disease is local or diffuse, and the composition of the plaque. There is diminishing success with more distal disease, longer length of lesions, more diffuse disease, and heavily calcified plaques, the typical disease presentation in diabetic patients. In our experience balloon angioplasty is best suited for more proximal, short, isolated aortic or iliac artery stenoses or occlusions. It is extremely rare for endovascular procedures to achieve initial and long-term success for popliteal, tibial, or peroneal artery disease.[21] For patients presenting with combined inflow (aortoiliac) and outflow (femoropopliteal/tibial) disease, angioplasty can be a valuable adjunctive procedure allowing one to correct the inflow first, saving surgical revascularization for more distal disease. The routine use of stents requires further clinical evaluation.

Gene therapy holds promise for the future. Injecting short stretches of DNA containing the genetic code for vascular endothelial growth factor, a protein that stimulates the growth of new blood vessels, has been done, but more clinical studies are needed to evaluate its cost-effectiveness before gene therapy becomes routine. Gene therapy to prevent blockage in bypass grafts after revascularization is also being studied.

Revascularization Procedures

The patient's condition, the presence of comorbidities, and the arteriographic findings, determine the type of revascularization procedure. Aortoiliac (inflow) procedures are performed similarly in diabetic and nondiabetic patients and usually require the use of synthetic grafts. The vascular surgeon must be flexible and tailor the procedure to the individual patient's needs.[22]

Aggressive distal revascularization techniques (outflow) have demonstrated excellent graft patency and limb salvage and the ability to return patients to function and well-being.[23] To achieve the most rapid and durable healing of an open foot ulcer, we have learned that one needs to restore a pulse to the foot via a distal revascularization to a vessel with direct continuity to the dorsalis pedis, posterior tibial, or plantar arteries themselves. Bypassing only to the more proximal popliteal or tibial peroneal arteries may be inadequate in the diabetic patient for the reasons mentioned above. An autologous vein is the conduit of choice. The decision to place the vein graft in the reversed, in situ, or nonreversed position is determined by the size and quality of the vein, the anatomy of the patient, and the length of vein required for the bypass. Surgical revascularization directly to the dorsalis pedis artery now constitutes approximately 25% of our revascularization procedures. At 3 years graft patency is 87% and limb salvage is 92%. At 5 years primary and secondary patency rates of 68% and 81%, respectively, have been reported. Limb salvage in this group exceeds 87% at 5 years. The operative mortality associated with distal revascularization is 1.8% in our series, with a morbidity (mainly cardiac) of 5.4%. Major amputation poses no lesser risk with cost and quality-of-life data supporting an aggressive approach to limb salvage.[24]

For patients with extensive foot sepsis and ischemia, constant and continual communication and teamwork is required. Draining foot sepsis is mandatory prior to arteriography and revascularization, but the timing might need to be accelerated to limit further ischemic necrosis. Restoring pulsatile blood flow to the foot is essential to promote primary healing of ulcerations and to facilitate the efforts of podiatrists.[25]

Amputation

For patients who require amputation, the same principles hold true: there must be adequate blood supply to ensure healing. While we believe that many amputations currently performed are needless, in some cases amputation may be the only alternative. This should be addressed positively and emotional support offered with support groups, or just visiting with a patient who has undergone amputation. Aggressive rehabilitation, prostheses, and other modalities should be made available to every diabetic patient depending on his or her needs.

THE FUTURE

Our multidisciplinary team approach has obtained appropriate, efficient, and cost-effective outcomes for diabetic patients with foot problems. We have demonstrated a reduction in every level of amputation. Early recognition of a problem, aggressive surgical debridement of infection, combined with adjunctive antibiotics, wound care, and prompt evaluation and treatment of ischemia, are core principles. Foot-sparing surgery achieves healing, preserves length, appearance, and function, and avoids amputation. From the patient's perspective this aggressive approach relieves their pain, heals their wounds, and allows their return to function and well-being.[23]

REFERENCES

1. Reiber GE, Lipsky BA, Gibbons GW: Burden of diabetic foot ulcers. Am J Surg 176(suppl 2A):55–105, 1998.
2. Healthy People 2000. National Health Promotion and Disease Prevention Objective. US Dept of Health and Human Services publication No. (PHS) 91-50212. Washington, DC, US Government Printing Office, 1991, p 73.
2a. American Diabetes Association: Position statement: Consensus development conference on diabetic foot wound care. Diabetes Care 22:1354–1360, 1999.
3. Gibbons GW, Marcaccio EJ, Habershaw GM: Management of the diabetic foot. *In* Callow AD, Ernst CB (eds): Vascular Surgery Theory and Practice. Stamford CT, Appleton & Lange, 1995, pp 167–179.
4. Cavanaugh PR, Simoneau GG, Ulbrecht JS: Ulceration, unsteadiness, and uncertainty: The biomechanical consequences of diabetes mellitus. J Biomech 26:23–40, 1993.
5. Pecoraro RE, Reiber GE, Burgess EM: Pathways to diabetic limb amputation: Basis for prevention. Diabetes Care 13:513–521, 1990.
6. Goldenberg SG, Alex M, Joshi RA, Blumenthal HT: Nonatheromatous peripheral vascular disease of the lower extremity in diabetes mellitus. Diabetes 8:261–273, 1959.
7. LoGerfo FW, Coffman J: Vascular and microvascular disease of the diabetic foot: Implications for foot care. N Engl J Med 311:1615–1619, 1984.
8. Tooke JE: European consensus document on critical limb ischemia: Implications for diabetics. Diabet Med 7:544–546, 1990.
9. Gibbons GW: Vascular surgery of the diabetic lower extremity. *In* Frykberg R (ed): The High Risk Foot in Diabetes Mellitus. New York, Churchill Livingstone, 1990. pp 273–297.
10. Boyko EJ, Lipsky BA: Infection and diabetes mellitus. *In* Harris MI (ed): Diabetes in America, ed 2. Bethesda, MD, National Institutes of Health publication No. 95-1468, 1995, 485–499.
11. Grayson ML, Gibbons GW, Habershaw GM, et al: Use of ampicillin/sulbactam vs. imipenem/cilastin in the treatment of limb-threatening foot infections in diabetic patients. Clin Infect Dis 18:683–693, 1994.
12. Mayfield JA, Reiber GE, Sanders LJ: Preventive foot care in people with diabetes. Diabetes Care 21:2161–2178, 1998.
13. American Diabetes Association: Position statement: Preventive foot care in people with diabetes. Diabetes Care 21:2178–2179, 1998.
14. Lipsky BA: Diabetic foot sepsis. Semin Vasc Surg 5:244–248, 1992.
15. Lipsky BA, Pecoraro RE, Larson SA, Ahroni JH: Outpatient management of the uncomplicated lower extremity infections in diabetic patients. Arch Intern Med 150:790–797, 1990.
16. Gibbons GW, Habershaw GM: Diabetic foot infections: Anatomy and surgery. Infect Dis Clin North Am 9:131–142, 1995.
17. Grayson ML: Diabetic foot infections: Antimicrobial therapy. Infect Dis Clin North Am 9:143–162, 1995.
18. Caputo GM, Cavanaugh PR, Ulbrecht JS, et al: Assessment and management of foot disease in patients with diabetes. N Engl J Med 331:854–860, 1994.
19. Grayson ML, Gibbons GW, Balogh K, et al: Probing to bone in infected pedal ulcers: A clinical sign of underlying osteomyelitis in diabetic patients. JAMA 273:721–723, 1995.
20. Gibbons GW, Wheelock FC Jr, Hoar CS Jr, et al: Predicting success of forefoot amputations in diabetics by noninvasive testing. Arch Surg 114:1034–1036, 1979.
21. Stokes KR, Strunk HM, Campbell DR, et al: Five year results of iliac and femoropopliteal angioplasty in diabetic patients. Radiography 174:977–982, 1990.
22. Pomposelli FB, Jepson SJ, Gibbons GW, et al: A flexible approach to infrapopliteal vein grafts in patient with diabetic mellitus. Arch Surg 126:724–729, 1991.
23. Gibbons GW, Burgess AM, Guadagnoli E, et al: Return to well-being and function after infrainguinal revascularization. J Vasc Surg 21:35–45, 1995.
24. Gibbons GW, Marcaccio E Jr, Freeman DV, et al: Improved quality of diabetic foot care, 1984 vs. 1990: Reduced length of stay and costs, insufficient reimbursement. Arch Surg 128:576–581, 1993.
25. Gibbons GW, Habershaw GM: The septic diabetic foot. *In* Whittemore AD (ed): Advances in Vascular Surgery, vol 4. St Louis, Mosby–Year Book, 1997.

Chapter 65

Acute Complications of Diabetes Mellitus: Ketoacidosis, Hyperosmolar Coma, and Lactic Acidosis

Daniel W. Foster ▪ J. Denis McGarry

Patients with diabetes of any variety are vulnerable to acute complications that are fatal if not treated. Decompensation can occur secondary to intercurrent stress or illness or appear spontaneously in the absence of obvious precipitating events. Because diabetes is a common illness in the United States and western Europe,[1, 2] the syndromes of diabetic coma make up a significant percentage of the nonsurgical emergencies seen in any general hospital. If the pathophysiologic principles underlying the illness are understood and corrective treatment is judiciously applied, most patients should recover. To that end, we discuss first the pathophysiology and then the treatment of diabetic ketoacidosis, hyperosmolar coma, and lactic acidosis.

KETOACIDOSIS

Ketoacidosis is a complication of autoimmune (type 1) diabetes mellitus. It occurs after most of the insulin-producing β cells have been destroyed. As discussed subsequently, ketoacidosis is occasionally seen in a subset of patients with nonautoimmune (type 2) diabetes.

Pathophysiology

The metabolic derangements that accompany diabetic ketoacidosis are multiple. In general, the body is shifted into a major catabolic state with breakdown of glycogen stores, hydrolysis of triglycerides in adipose tissue, and mobilization of amino acids from muscle.[3] The fuels newly released from peripheral tissues become the substrates used by the liver for the accelerated production of glucose and ketone bodies that is the hallmark of uncontrolled diabetes.[4] Hyperglycemia-driven osmotic diuresis and rising concentrations of acetoacetate and β-hydroxybutyrate in turn cause loss of body fluids, abnormalities in plasma electrolytes, and metabolic acidosis. The mechanisms underlying the development of ketoacidosis are basically similar to those occurring in nondiabetic subjects during a fast with one exception: no insulin is available to prevent progression to full-blown acidosis. The similarities and differences can be outlined as follows. In the postprandial state after absorption of food, plasma glucose concentrations gradually fall over a period of several hours. As a result, insulin release from the pancreas is diminished and a simultaneous rise in glucagon secretion takes place.[3, 5–7] These changes occur smoothly in an integrated fashion, thereby maintaining plasma glucose levels in the nonhypoglycemic range. Decreased insulin secretion simultaneously results in mobilization of free fatty acids from adipocytes, with the

body shifted toward a lipid economy so that glucose is "spared" for use by the brain,[3, 6, 8, 9] which cannot oxidize fatty acids.[10] A portion of the mobilized fatty acids are taken up by the liver for conversion to acetoacetic and β-hydroxybutyric acids. These "ketone bodies," which are efficiently oxidized by nonhepatic tissues, including the brain, provide backup substrate for the central nervous system should hepatic glucose production be inadequate for any reason.[11] Normally, fasting ends at breakfast, and no significant ketosis develops. When a fast is extended, ketone concentrations increase to the range of 2 to 4 mM, but not much higher because both fatty acids and ketones have the ability to stimulate insulin release[12–14] (Fig. 65–1). This feedback loop, which elicits a modest elevation in insulin, prevents a further increase in the rate of lipolysis, thereby fixing ketogenesis in a safe range through substrate limitation. Ketones have a minor direct inhibitory effect on lipolysis, but the insulin-stimulatory event is doubtless dominant.

In diabetes, the omission of insulin or the stress-induced counterregulatory hormone release that overrides the effect of the usual dose of insulin initiates a process qualitatively similar to fasting, with the exception that the insulin segment of the feedback loop is missing.[3, 7, 13] As a consequence, concentrations of free fatty acids and ketone

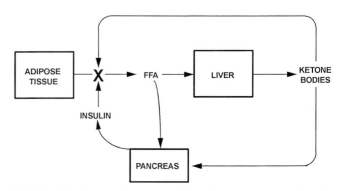

FIGURE 65–1. Feedback control of ketosis during an extended fast. Ketogenesis is activated by a rise in the molar ratio of glucagon to insulin, which induces lipolysis in adipose tissue and fatty acid oxidation in the liver. As the concentrations of circulating fatty acids and ketones rise, the β cell is stimulated to release insulin, with lipolytic rates fixed at modest levels and further rise in glucagon limited. These adaptations allow modest ketosis without the danger of ketoacidosis. In insulin-dependent diabetic subjects, the insulin loop is missing.

bodies rise in an uncontrolled fashion and produce acidosis, coma, and death.

Hormonal Initiation of Ketoacidosis

For many years the hormonal abnormality initiating the hyperglycemia and metabolic acidosis that accompany diabetic ketoacidosis was thought to be insulin deficiency alone. It now seems clear that this view is incorrect and that insulin deficiency coupled with glucagon excess, that is, a rise in the molar ratio of glucagon to insulin, is the operative mechanism. The evidence in support of this concept has been extensively reviewed.[6, 15, 16] The most important study was that of Gerich and colleagues, who showed that withdrawal of insulin from patients with insulin-dependent diabetes was accompanied by rapid increases in plasma glucagon, glucose, and ketone levels that were markedly obtunded when glucagon release was blocked by somatostatin.[17]

The role of glucagon in inducing hepatic glucose overproduction in uncontrolled diabetes parallels its actions during an overnight fast, in which about 75% of glucose output can be shown to be glucagon mediated.[18] Further evidence that glucagon is critical to the initiation of hyperglycemia comes from studies in which simultaneous insulin and glucagon deficiency was produced by infusion of somatostatin[19] or total pancreatectomy.[20] If insulin deficiency alone were the cause of severe hyperglycemia, one would have expected significant overproduction of glucose under both experimental circumstances. In neither dogs nor humans did such overproduction occur. Similarly, patients with somatostatinoma, who have suppression of both glucagon and insulin, exhibit only mild hyperglycemia, an additional finding compatible with the interpretation that major increases in plasma glucose levels occur only in the presence of a relative or absolute excess of glucagon.[21]

Glucagon also appears to play a central role in initiating ketogenesis. As noted previously, blockade of glucagon release markedly slows the appearance of ketosis in diabetic patients withdrawn from insulin.[17] Conversely, administration of glucagon to diabetic humans enhances the conversion of fatty acids to ketone bodies.[22–24] Along the same lines, the presence of a glucagonoma resulted in plasma ketone levels four times normal despite the fact that free fatty acid concentrations were not elevated.[25] Glucagonoma may also cause ketoacidosis in the face of intact β cells.[26] Direct demonstration of the powerful ketogenic effect of glucagon in the liver came from studies in which rats were administered glucagon in vivo (in both physiologic and pathophysiologic amounts).[27] The animals did not become either hyperglycemic or ketotic because a compensatory rise in insulin (secondary to glucagon infusion) allowed disposal of the glucose produced by the liver and prevented a rise in free fatty acids. When the livers from these animals were removed and perfused with fatty acids, they exhibited the shift to activated fatty acid oxidation and ketogenesis expected in fasting and uncontrolled diabetes. Thus a ketogenic liver had been produced in nonketotic animals despite the presence of concentrations of insulin in plasma that were higher than normal. When free fatty acid concentrations were elevated artificially in the glucagon-treated animals, a brisk rise in ketone levels was observed, thus confirming that the liver had been activated in vivo, with ketosis prevented only by the lack of substrate.[27] Glucagon has also been shown to stimulate ketone body production directly in homogenates of liver, liver slices, hepatocytes, and isolated perfused liver.[28]

Although the evidence is good that the molar ratio of glucagon to insulin is the primary control unit for carbohydrate and lipid metabolism, this finding does not imply that other hormones do not play a role. Most systems in the body have redundant regulatory mechanisms, and catecholamines, cortisol, growth hormone, and thyroid hormones can all increase rates of hepatic ketogenesis, albeit less efficiently.[29, 30] Concentrations of counterregulatory hormones are elevated on admission in patients with ketoacidosis,[31, 32] either as the consequence of an initiating illness such as infection or in response to the stress of ketoacidosis itself. However, when ketoacidosis is induced by withdrawing insulin from well-controlled subjects with insulin-dependent diabetes, glucagon concentrations rise before any increase in other counterregulatory hormones, which suggests that the α cell hormone is pivotal in causing metabolic decompensation.[33, 34]

The mechanisms by which insulin and glucagon exert their effects are not yet completely known. Functionally, the two hormones are metabolic antagonists in directing fuel production and utilization,[6] but it should be understood that they act independently through distinct receptors and focus on different target tissues. The primary direct effects of insulin are probably on muscle and fat (to enhance glucose transport into cells and inhibit lipolysis), whereas the primary direct effects of glucagon are exerted on the liver (to increase glycogenolysis, gluconeogenesis, and ketogenesis). It is attractive to consider that in the primary domain of each hormone the other acts predominantly as an antagonist. Good evidence indicates that insulin functions to a large extent as an antiglucagon in the liver, with direct effects being minimal in the absence of glucagon-induced metabolic changes.[24, 35, 36] The insulin signaling pathway is very complicated, but it is initiated by phosphorylation of intracellular substrates after binding to its receptor.[37] Most of the initial effects of glucagon are thought to be consequent to the generation of cyclic adenosine monophosphate (cAMP).[38] In rodents, glucagon can act independently of cAMP, possibly through the protein kinase C signaling system.[39] It is probable that a single glucagon receptor activates both pathways,[40, 41] although isoforms could exist, as appears to be the case for the insulin receptor.[42] Counteraction of glucagon by insulin may be the result of direct inhibition of the cAMP-dependent protein kinase.[43]

Hyperglycemia

The hyperglycemia of uncontrolled diabetes is caused by two alterations in glucose metabolism: increased hepatic glucose production and diminished utilization of the hexose in muscle and adipose tissue. When insulin is withdrawn from well-controlled subjects with insulin-requiring diabetes, hepatic glucose output doubles within 2 hours.[34] Simultaneously, clearance of glucose from plasma decreases consequent to falling insulin concentrations. Doubtless, insulin resistance contributes to the decreased uptake and utilization of glucose.[44] A significant part of the resistant state may be caused by the accumulation of fat within insulin target tissues. Increased fatty acid oxidation then results in impairment of insulin signaling to the glucose transport machinery and suppression of glucose metabolism.[14, 44–46] A third factor, present to a variable extent, is volume depletion secondary to the hyperglycemia-induced osmotic diuresis. If this complication becomes severe enough to cause a fall in urine output, the escape pathway for glucose is removed and hyperglycemia worsens.[47] This response accounts for the fact that administration of fluids alone can lower the plasma glucose concentration in ketoacidosis.[32]

The mechanisms by which a rise in the molar glucagon-insulin ratio alters hepatic glucose metabolism have been the subject of much study. cAMP-dependent activation of glycogenolysis represents one component. Another involves acceleration of the gluconeogenic pathway. Here, primary focus has been placed on the 6-phosphofructo-1-kinase (phosphofructokinase)–fructose-1,6-bisphosphatase branch point, seemingly the preeminent control site for glycolysis/gluconeogenesis in the liver (Fig. 65–2). The concept is that increased hepatic glucose production in uncontrolled diabetes (or in conditions of glucose need such as fasting or exercise) is mediated by a fall in phosphofructokinase activity, which inhibits glycolysis (flux from glucose 6-phosphate → pyruvate), and a rise in fructose-1,6-bisphosphatase activity, which enhances gluconeogenesis (flux over the sequence pyruvate → oxaloacetate → phosphoenolpyruvate → glucose 6-phosphate → glucose). The latter pathway is fed primarily by amino acids transported from muscle.[3] Substrate traffic over the switch point is mediated primarily by fructose 2,6-bisphosphate, a regulatory intermediate that stimulates phosphofructokinase and inhibits fructose-1,6-bisphosphatase.[48, 49] Fructose 2,6-bisphosphate activates 6-phosphofructo-1-kinase allosterically and inhibits fructose-1,6-bisphosphatase competitively. Fructose 2,6-bisphosphate levels are controlled by an interesting bifunctional enzyme, 6-phosphofructo-2-kinase/fructose-2,6-bisphosphatase. Glucagon excess (relative to insulin), acting through the generation of cAMP, causes a fall in fructose 2,6-bisphosphate concentrations as a result of phosphorylation of 6-phosphofructo-

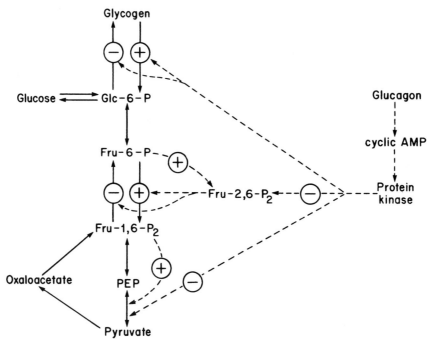

FIGURE 65–2. Regulation of glycolysis and gluconeogenesis by glucagon. *Solid lines* represent metabolic pathways. Within these pathways, *arrows* that point down represent the glycolytic sequence, and *arrows* that point up, gluconeogenesis. *Two-headed arrows* indicate reversible reactions, and *single-headed arrows,* nonreversible reactions (i.e., the enzyme that catalyzes a reaction in glycolysis is distinct from the enzyme that reverses the process in gluconeogenesis). *Dotted lines* indicate regulatory activities. *Minus signs* stand for inactivation (inhibition) and *plus signs* for activation (stimulation). For simplicity, a number of reactions are omitted, and only the key regulatory sites are shown. Glucagon lowers levels of fructose 2,6-bisphosphate (Fru-2,6-P$_2$) and thereby inactivates phosphofructokinase, which blocks the conversion of fructose 6-phosphate (Fru-6-P) to fructose 1,6-bisphosphate (Fru-1,6-P$_2$) and inhibits glycolysis. The fall in levels of fructose-2,6-P$_2$ disinhibits fructose-1,6-bisphosphatase and allows efficient conversion of Fru-1,6-P$_2$ to fructose 6-phosphate, with the consequence that gluconeogenesis is activated. Glucagon also stimulates glycogen breakdown and inhibits glycogen synthesis. Glucagon induces a secondary block in glycolysis at the step that is regulated by pyruvate kinase. Glc-6-P, glucose 6-phosphate; PEP, phosphoenolpyruvate. (Reprinted by permission, from Foster DW, McGarry JD: The metabolic derangements and treatment of diabetic ketoacidosis. N Engl J Med 309:159–169, 1983; adapted from Hers HG, Van Schaftingen E: Fructose 2,6-bisphosphate 2 years after its discovery. Biochem J 206:1–12, 1982.)

2-kinase/fructase-2,6-bisphosphatase.[50] This phosphorylation converts the enzyme from a kinase to a phosphatase with the result that synthesis of fructose 2,6-bisphosphate ceases and hydrolysis commences. Epinephrine acts in similar fashion in the liver.[49, 51] The fructose 2,6-bisphosphate regulatory hypothesis is attractive and supported by considerable experimental evidence. However, regulation at the phosphofructokinase/fructose-1,6-bisphosphatase site is complicated, and it is not certain that fructose 2,6-bisphosphate will prove to be the primary regulator in vivo under all circumstances.[52] For example, in white adipose tissue, epinephrine stimulates glycolysis while producing a fall in fructose 2,6-bisphosphate.[53]

Additional enzymes are altered under catabolic conditions such as fasting and uncontrolled diabetes. Pyruvate kinase is inhibited,[49, 54] and the distinctive gluconeogenic enzymes pyruvate carboxylase, phosphoenolpyruvate carboxykinase, and glucose-6-phosphatase increase in both conditions.[49, 55] Final rates of gluconeogenesis are influenced not only by changes in the key enzymatic activities induced directly by alterations in the glucagon-insulin ratio but also by the modulating effects of other hormones, [49, 55, 56] availability of substrate,[57] and rates of fatty acid oxidation.[46] For this reason, it is best to consider the changes leading to glucose overproduction in the liver as reflecting a coordinated series of alterations even when a single step and a single regulatory intermediate, fructose 2,6-bisphosphate, have been assigned primacy as we have done here.

Ketogenesis

Metabolic acidosis caused by the overproduction of acetoacetic and β-hydroxybutyric acids requires changes in the metabolism of adipose tissue and the liver[58, 59] (Fig. 65–3). Long-chain fatty acids derived from triglyceride stores in the adipocyte are the principal substrate for ketone production in the liver. Only under circumstances in which

fatty acid oxidation in the hepatocyte is blocked do amino acids such as leucine function efficiently as precursors for acetoacetate synthesis.[60] Long-chain fatty acids are mobilized from fat stores under the combined influence of insulin deficiency/counterregulatory hormone excess acting on the intracellular hormone-sensitive lipase.[3, 61] It is likely that the major activator is cAMP, a rise in its concentration leading to phosphorylation and enhanced activity of the enzyme. Ordinarily, ketone production is dependent on delivery of fatty acids to the liver. However, if the liver is fatty, a not uncommon occurrence in poorly controlled diabetes, hepatic triglyceride may serve as the source of fatty acids. This adaptation accounts for differences in the ease of

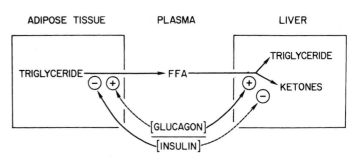

FIGURE 65–3. Two-organ system for ketogenesis. Maximal production of ketone bodies requires transport of the substrate, long-chain fatty acids, from adipose tissue to the liver. In addition, the fatty acid oxidative pathway has to be activated in the hepatocyte. The *solid lines* indicate primary and the *dotted lines* indicate secondary (counterregulatory) effects; that is, insulin's primary action is to inhibit lipolysis and its secondary effect is to block glucagon's action in the liver. Conversely, glucagon's primary effect is activation of fatty acid oxidation, with only a secondary effect on lipolysis. See the text for details.

reversibility of ketosis. Ingestion of a small amount of carbohydrate after a fast calls forth endogenous insulin release and immediately reverses fasting ketosis by inhibiting lipolysis in the adipocyte. In diabetic ketoacidosis, because the liver contains significant amounts of triglyceride, ketogenesis continues for hours after free fatty acid levels in plasma have returned to normal. How intracellular triglyceride lipase activity in the liver is controlled is not well understood. It is possible that a hormone-sensitive lipase activated by glucagon is operative.[23]

Although increased transport of fatty acids to the liver is normally required for significant ketogenesis to supervene, increased fatty acids alone are not enough. In the normal, nonfasted state, fatty acids taken up into the hepatocyte are re-esterified to triglyceride and transported back out into plasma as very-low-density lipoprotein.[58] Rates of fatty acid oxidation are low. However, when the molar ratio of glucagon to insulin rises, fatty acid oxidation is disinhibited and incoming fatty acids can be converted to acetoacetate/β-hydroxybutyrate. The key regulatory site for fatty acid oxidation appears to be at the initial step in the process catalyzed by the enzyme carnitine palmitoyltransferase I (CPT I)[58, 62] (Fig. 65–4). Its function is to effect conversion of the coenzyme A (CoA) esters of long-chain fatty acids to acylcarnitines, which, unlike fatty acyl-CoAs, can be transported across the inner mitochondrial membrane (via a translocase).[63] Once through the membrane, the reaction is reversed by CPT II, and the newly re-formed fatty acyl-CoA enters the fatty acid oxidative pathway. In liver the major product is ketone bodies, and terminal oxidation to carbon dioxide and water is limited. In tissues such as muscle and heart, complete oxidation of fatty acids to carbon dioxide and water results in the generation of adenosine triphosphate in the electron transport chain.

In the fed state and well-controlled diabetes, CPT I is inhibited by malonyl CoA.[64] The total amount of enzyme present does not change markedly through wide swings of the regulatory cycle.[65] Regulation of fat oxidation by malonyl CoA makes physiologic sense because it is also the first committed intermediate in long-chain fatty acid synthesis. Thus when malonyl CoA concentrations are high, the inhibitory interaction with CPT I precludes oxidation of the newly formed fatty acids and avoids an energetically wasteful futile cycle.[58, 59] Malonyl CoA concentrations are maximal in the fed state, but they fall rapidly with fasting and uncontrolled diabetes. This change, coupled with desensitization of CPT I to the inhibitor, poises the liver for ketogenesis[66, 67]; accelerated production of acetoacetate and β-hydroxybutyrate begins when the long-chain fatty acids arrive in the liver at increased concentrations. Once the oxidative sequence is activated, rates of ketogenesis reflect substrate concentration; that is, the higher the concentration of fatty acids, the greater the ketone production until Vmax is reached.

The mechanism by which malonyl CoA inhibits CPT I is still not completely understood. It is believed that malonyl CoA binds through the CoA moiety at the palmitoyl CoA site on the enzyme and that its carboxyl group forms an ionic interaction with an amino acid, probably histidine, at a separate site. When bound, the regulator impairs palmitoyl CoA binding directly and by alteration of membrane fluidity.[66]

Molecular cloning of CPT I has definitively eliminated the possibility that malonyl CoA binds to a separate regulatory subunit.[68]

The ways in which malonyl CoA levels fall to initiate ketogenesis are better defined. As noted earlier, an increase in the molar glucagon-insulin ratio (a relative or absolute glucagon excess) inhibits glycolysis at the phosphofructokinase step. This inhibition of glycolysis interrupts flux from glucose 6-phosphate down the glycolytic pathway to pyruvate, which in turn causes a fall in cytosolic citric acid.[67] A lowered citrate concentration has dual effects: decreased production of cytosolic acetyl CoA, the substrate for malonyl CoA formation (citrate is the source of cytosolic acetyl CoA via the citrate cleavage enzyme), and deactivation of acetyl-CoA carboxylase, the enzyme that catalyzes the conversion of acetyl CoA to malonyl CoA (citrate activates the carboxylase allosterically).[69] Acetyl-CoA carboxylase is also sensitive to inhibition by phosphorylation, which in a setting of high glucagon/low insulin, appears to be mediated by both cAMP-dependent protein kinase and AMP-activated protein kinase.[69, 70] Although the carboxylase can also be inhibited by long-chain acyl-CoA,[71] the block in glycolysis is probably the dominant early mechanism. This conclusion is based on the observation that the citrate content in hepatocytes isolated from short-term fasted animals can be increased by the addition of lactate and pyruvate and cause a rise in the malonyl CoA concentration and diminished ketone production.[67] Because three-carbon intermediates that enter the glycolytic pathway below the glucagon-induced block immediately reinitiate the sequence citrate → acetyl CoA → malonyl CoA, it can be concluded that under these conditions acetyl-CoA carboxylase is not inactivated by either phosphorylation or long-chain fatty acids. When fasting is prolonged or diabetes is uncontrolled over an extended period, the latter two mechanisms doubtless become operative. Ultimately, synthesis of acetyl-CoA carboxylase also decreases and renders reversal of ketogenesis more difficult. A summary of the metabolic changes occurring in the liver in uncontrolled diabetes is shown in Figure 65–5. We find it fascinating that both hepatic overproduction of glucose and ketosis result from uncountered activity of glucagon initially acting at strategic sites in the glycogenolytic/glycolytic/gluconeogenic pathways. By controlling substrate flux at critical branch points, all the metabolic abnormalities that characterize the liver in uncontrolled diabetes are activated. Therefore, great interest has been shown in developing drugs to block activation of the glucagon receptor in the treatment of diabetes.[72, 73]

Little doubt exists that malonyl CoA–mediated control of CPT I is central to the regulation of fatty acid oxidation and ketogenesis in the liver, but another consequence of a rise in the glucagon-insulin molar ratio is an increased carnitine content.[74] The source of this carnitine has never been identified, but it is attractive to suppose that it moves to the liver from muscle via the plasma. Increased carnitine would favor transesterification of fatty acyl-CoAs by mass action once CPT I is activated (see Fig. 65–3).

In contrast to the situation with hyperglycemia, in which impaired glucose disposal contributes significantly to the process early in decompensation, ketone utilization is not limited until plasma concentrations reach 10 to 12 mM.[75]

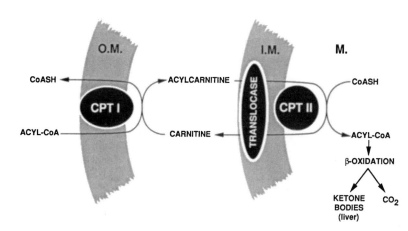

FIGURE 65–4. The fatty acid oxidizing system in the liver. Long-chain fatty acids are activated to coenzyme A (CoA) derivatives on arrival in the liver (acyl-CoA). Acyl-CoA cannot traverse the mitochondrial inner membrane. Entry is accomplished by transesterification to carnitine by carnitine palmitoyltransferase I (CPT I) located in the outer membrane (O.M.). Transport across the inner membrane (I.M.) is accomplished by a translocase. Reversal of the transesterification then occurs on the matrix side by carnitine palmitoyltransferase II (CPT II). The capacity for fatty acid oxidation is fixed and large, so normally the rate-limiting step is CPT I. Tricarboxylic acid cycle activity is low in the liver (acetyl-CoA → CO_2), so the bulk of oxidized fatty acid goes to ketone bodies.

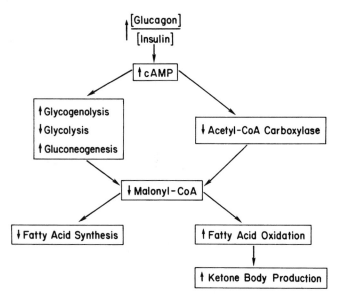

FIGURE 65–5. Hepatic metabolism in uncontrolled diabetes. The increased ratio of glucagon to insulin increases cyclic adenosine monophosphate (cAMP), thereby initiating a series of enzymic phosphorylations. These reactions convert the liver to an organ of glucose production with gluconeogenesis predominating after a few hours of poor control. Malonyl CoA levels drop precipitously because of a block in glycolysis and inhibition of acetyl-CoA carboxylase. This drop in turn increases fatty acid oxidation/ketogenic capacity and stops long-chain fatty acid synthesis via substrate depletion. Not shown are the increases in long-chain fatty acyl-CoA and carnitine that drive the fatty acid oxidative sequence that is poised for action.

Clinical Features

The incidence of diabetic ketoacidosis is not known with certainty, but the disorder is extremely common in younger patients with insulin-dependent disease. In Rochester, Minnesota, a rate of 13.4 per 1000 patient-years was recorded; that is, a given patient at risk had a 1% to 2% chance of having the complication each year.[76] Estimates from the Centers for Disease Control were similar, being 14.6 per 1000 patients at risk in 1984 and 12.5 per 1000 patients in 1987. Rates were consistently higher in black males than in other groups, 24.7 per 1000 persons at risk in 1987.[77] It remains a serious illness with overall mortality in the United States approximating 7%.[78] Many deaths are from ketoacidosis-associated events such as myocardial infarction. Ketoacidosis accounts for up to 70% of the deaths attributed to diabetes in children.[79]

Precipitating Events

Diabetic ketoacidosis is usually initiated by stress of some kind or cessation of insulin.[80, 81] Often the stress is infection, but the apparent cause may vary from acute alcohol intake to myocardial infarction. A significant number of cases have no recognizable precipitating event; in these patients, psychologic stress may be the operative mechanism, especially in young persons who have repeated episodes of ketoacidosis over short intervals.[82]

Symptoms and Signs

The usual symptoms and signs include vomiting, thirst, polyuria, weakness, altered sensorium, and air hunger. Abdominal pain can occur.[80] The differential diagnosis of such pain is tricky because pyelonephritis or a surgical disorder such as acute appendicitis may precipitate ketoacidosis. On the other hand, severe pain mimicking an acute abdomen may be due to the ketoacidotic state itself, possibly the consequence of hypertriglyceridemia-induced pancreatitis. Unless clear-cut evidence of a specific cause is present, a conservative course should be taken, with treatment of ketoacidosis taking precedence.

The vital signs on admission vary with the length and severity of the prehospital phase of the illness. Tachycardia is essentially always present.[83, 84] The mean blood pressure is normal when large numbers of patients are evaluated, but hypotension was present in 8% of the survivors in one series.[84] In the same series, hypotension or shock was present in 19% of those who died. Hypotension obviously is a poor prognostic sign. Kussmaul respiration with respiratory rates averaging 30 per minute is almost always observed, but in severe acidosis the ventilatory response may fall and paradoxically rise as treatment is initiated and the acidosis is reversed.[85, 86] The patient's temperature is often below normal and may be as low as 34°C.[83] If fever is present, the likelihood of infection is high. The converse is not true; that is, the absence of fever or the presence of hypothermia does not rule out an infectious process. Although the sensorium is usually clouded on arrival at the hospital, a fifth of patients are alert.[80] Only about 10% of patients are actually unconscious despite frequent use of the phrase *diabetic coma* as a synonym for the acidotic state.

The physical findings are not specific. A fruity odor of the breath may suggest acetonemia. Careful search should be made for hidden infections such as a tooth abscess, a furuncle hidden by axillary hair, or a perirectal infection. Skin turgor is usually poor, and mucous membranes are ordinarily dry. Occasionally, one sees eruptive xanthomas. Lipemia retinalis is not unusual.

Laboratory Abnormalities

Typical laboratory abnormalities present on admission are shown in Tables 65–1 and 65–2. Hormone values are informative. Glucagon concentrations were elevated 7-fold, with epinephrine, norepinephrine, cortisol, and growth hormone also showing major increases. Epinephrine concentrations were 50-fold higher than normal. As noted earlier, it is probable that the initial change in catabolic hormones is a rise in glucagon followed by an increase in other counterregulatory agents as the stress of ketoacidosis worsens.[33, 34] The result is a vicious cycle: ketoacidosis → stress hormone release → worsening ketoacidosis → greater stress hormone release. The high concentrations of renin and aldosterone are expected concomitants of volume depletion.

Plasma analysis reflects the hormonal changes. Glucose is increased into the 28- to 33-mM (500–600 mg/dL) range on average but can be lower or much higher. Very high concentrations, similar to those seen in hyperosmolar coma, probably occur only in subjects who have marked volume depletion and dehydration, the mechanism being diminished urine output as previously discussed.[47, 87] Extracellular fluid volume deficits account for the modest elevation in blood urea nitrogen (BUN) and creatinine, whereas plasma osmolalities of 310 to 316 mOsm/L reflect deficits of free water. Although insensible losses of water are increased, especially if Kussmaul respiration is marked, the bulk of the water deficit is consequent to the glucose-mediated osmotic diuresis, which causes loss of water in excess of electrolytes.[47, 87, 88]

TABLE 65–1. Hormone Values in Patients with Diabetic Ketoacidosis

Hormone	Controls	Patients
Insulin (μU/mL)	15 ± 2	—
C peptide (ng/mL)	2.4 ± 0.07	—
Glucagon (pg/mL)	99 ± 19	741 ± 247
Epinephrine (ng/mL)	0.05 ± 0.03	2.6 ± 1.3
Norepinephrine (ng/mL)	0.2 ± 0.08	3.8 ± 1.1
Cortisol (μg/dL)	10.5 ± 2	50.4 ± 4.9
Growth hormone (ng/mL)	0.7 ± 0.1	4.6 ± 1.6
Renin (GU × 10⁻⁴/mL)	0.3 ± 0.1	13.2 ± 4.6
Aldosterone (ng/dL)	7.8 ± 2.3	83 ± 25
Pancreatic polypeptide (pg/mL)	93 ± 11	691 ± 200

Control values were obtained in the basal state after an overnight fast. Plasma renin concentration and aldosterone were measured in subjects consuming 120 mmol Na⁺ per day. Data are means ± SEM.
GU, Goldblatt Unit.
Data from Waldhäusl W, Kleinberger G, Korn A, et al: Severe hyperglycemia: Effects of rehydration on endocrine derangements and blood glucose concentration. Diabetes 28:577–584, 1979.

TABLE 65–2. Laboratory Values in Patients with Diabetic Ketoacidosis

Test	Series 1 (*n* = 123)	Series 1 (*n* = 88)
Glucose (mg/dL)	606	476
Sodium (mM)	135	132
Potassium (mM)	5.7	4.8
Bicarbonate (mM)	6.3	<10
BUN (mg/dL)	29	25
Acetoacetate (mM)	3.1	4.8
β-Hydroxybutyrate (mM)	9.8	13.7
Free fatty acids (mM)	—	2.1
Lactate (mM)	2.5	4.6
Osmolality (mOsm)	316	310
pH	7.11	—

Series 1 is adapted from Kitabchi AE, Young R, Sacks H, Morris L: Diabetic ketoacidosis: Reappraisal of therapeutic approach. Annu Rev Med 30:339–357, 1979. Series 2 is adapted from Foster DW: Diabetes mellitus. *In* Petersdorf RG, Adams RD, Braunwald E, et al (eds): Harrison's Principles of Internal Medicine, ed 10. New York, McGraw-Hill, 1983, pp 661–679. For simplicity, only mean values are listed.

BUN, blood urea nitrogen.

Despite dehydration, the plasma sodium level tends to be on the low side because glucose in the absence of insulin becomes osmotically effective in the extracellular fluid and cannot penetrate the cell; it osmotically pulls water from cells to the extracellular compartment and thereby dilutes the sodium concentration. The degree of apparent hyponatremia increases with worsening hyperglycemia. An approximation of the true sodium concentration (millimolar) can be obtained by multiplying excess glucose in 100-mg/dL units by 1.6.[89] Thus for a plasma glucose concentration of 500 mg/dL, the calculation would be

$$\frac{500 \text{ mg/dL} - 100 \text{ mg/dL}}{100} \times 1.6 = 6.4$$

The measured sodium plus 6.4 would approximate the true sodium concentration.

If the plasma sodium level is extremely low, hypertriglyceridemia (secondary to uncontrolled diabetes) should be suspected; the fat, displacing plasma water, causes an artifactually low reading for the sodium concentration. Recognition is not usually a problem because the plasma will be milky and lipemia retinalis will be visible on ophthalmoscopic examination.[88] Newer autoanalyzers remove triglycerides before assay, which has largely eliminated this problem. Potassium concentrations tend to be high on arrival despite large total body deficits of the cation,[4] primarily because of a shift of potassium from intracellular to extracellular compartments in response to acidosis. Falling urine output will increase the tendency to hyperkalemia. On occasion, the initial potassium level is normal or low—a true danger signal because initiation of therapy, which results in retransfer of potassium into cells, may cause fatal hypokalemia if potassium is not replaced early.

By definition, the acidosis in uncontrolled insulin-dependent diabetes is caused by the overproduction of acetoacetic and β-hydroxybutyric acids in the liver with their accumulation in plasma.[4, 34] Contributing to the fall in pH are elevated levels of lactate, free fatty acids, and other organic acids normally excreted by the kidneys. Conventionally, the diagnosis of "ketoacidosis" requires a bicarbonate concentration under 10 mM and a pH under 7.3. The term *ketosis* should be used if deteriorating diabetic control has resulted in hyperglycemia/ketosis but not full-blown acidosis. Because most hospital laboratories do not routinely measure acetoacetate or β-hydroxybutyrate levels, clinical diagnosis of ketoacidosis depends on semiquantitative assessment of ketones in plasma with reagent sticks or tablets (which should be powdered before use). If a "large" reading is present on any dilution of plasma 1:1 or greater, the diagnosis of ketoacidosis is fairly secure. This conclusion follows from the fact that a "large" response indicates a concentration of acetone (derived from nonenzymatic decarboxylation of acetoacetate) plus acetoacetic acid of 4 mM or greater. When measured quantitatively in diabetic ketoacidosis, millimolar concentra-

tions of acetone and acetoacetate are approximately equal[90]; hence the "large" test reading can be taken to indicate at least 2 mM acetoacetate. Because the β-hydroxybutyrate concentration is minimally two to three times higher than that of acetoacetate, a "large" test reading means that the plasma concentration of ketones is at least 6 mM (2 mM acetoacetate, 4 mM β-hydroxybutyrate). The concentration of acetoacetate plus β-hydroxybutyrate rarely rises above 6 mM in fasting individuals,[91, 92] although a prolonged fast in nonobese persons may induce higher levels. Therefore, a "large" response in plasma diluted 1:1 or greater indicates that total ketones are probably 12 mM or higher and is presumptive evidence that ketoacidosis rather than fasting ketosis is present. Exceptions to the general rule that fasting ketosis gives total ketone levels of 6 mM or less are seen in late pregnancy,[93] some lactating women,[94] and a subset of alcoholic patients.[95, 96] These patients may exhibit true ketoacidosis with a short-term fast.

The ratio of β-hydroxybutyrate to acetoacetate is dependent on the redox state of the hepatocyte. With high rates of fatty acid oxidation, ethanol ingestion, or hypoxia, ratios higher than 3 may be seen, which diminishes the amount of acetone/acetoacetate detected by the reagent strip. Only rarely is this shift of such a magnitude that the diagnosis is difficult; resolution in such instances requires quantitative measurement of acetoacetate and β-hydroxybutyrate. We wish to emphasize that ketoacidosis cannot be diagnosed on the basis of a "large" reading for ketones in urine because ordinary fasting can produce such a reading. Patients with lactic acidosis and nonketotic, hyperosmolar coma often have "large" values in urine because of fasting induced by the precipitating illness or the hyperosmolar state itself, but they do not have ketoacidosis as defined above. The differential diagnosis of diabetic ketoacidosis from other "anion gap" acidoses is shown in Table 65–3.

BUN and creatinine levels are usually modestly elevated on admission and revert to normal as soon as fluids are provided. Creatinine clearance is ordinarily only slightly depressed, in one series averaging 82 mL/min.[90] Higher levels of azotemia are a poor prognostic sign in that they indicate a hemodynamically unstable patient vulnerable to vascular collapse or significant underlying renal disease.

Phosphate depletion is universal in diabetic ketoacidosis, but the initial plasma concentration, like that of potassium, may be low, normal, or high.[97] As a result, marked deficiency of erythrocyte 2,3-diphosphoglycerate is present.[98] Leukocytosis—at times a true leukemoid reaction—is commonly present and does not indicate infection.[4, 80] Amylase may be high but cannot be assumed to represent pancreatitis because it may be of salivary gland origin in some patients.[99] If lipase levels are very high, pancreatitis is more likely, but false-positive values for lipase may be seen if plasma glycerol levels are extremely elevated because of rapid breakdown of adipose tissue triglycerides (glycerol is the product measured in most assays for plasma lipase). Triglycerides are almost always elevated and can reach very high levels (e.g., 10,000 mg/dL).[88] If the patient has eaten within a few hours of onset, a significant fraction of the triglyceride may be in chylomicrons. Cholesterol concentrations will also be increased when triglyceride levels are very high because cholesterol is contained in both chylomicrons (triglyceride-cholesterol ratio of more than 10:1) and very-low-density lipoprotein particles (triglyceride-cholesterol ratio of approximately 5:1).

Treatment

Treatment of uncomplicated diabetic ketoacidosis requires insulin, fluids, and potassium.[2, 4, 80, 87, 100] In some circumstances, bicarbonate[4, 80] and phosphate salts[98, 101] may be given. An overview of the results of treatment is shown in Figure 65–6.

Fluids. An intravenous saline infusion should be started immediately because it is critical to replace lost volume and secure adequate urine flow. Repletion of the extracellular fluid volume with maintenance of diuresis has a primary role in lowering the plasma glucose level and a secondary role in limiting ketogenesis. The plasma glucose level is lowered by two mechanisms: excretion of glucose in the urine and modulation of counterregulatory hormone release.[32] Significant

TABLE 65–3. Differential Diagnosis of Diabetic Ketoacidosis

Condition	Urine		Plasma			
	Glucose	*Ketones*	*Glucose*	*Ketones*	*Lactate*	*BUN/CR*
Diabetic ketoacidosis	Pos	Pos	High	High	Mod	Mod
Hyperosmolar coma with lactic acidosis	Pos	Neg/Pos	Very high	Mod	High	High
Lactic acidosis	Neg	Neg/Pos	Nor/Mod	Nor/Mod	High	Nor/Mod
Alcoholic ketoacidosis	Neg/Pos	Pos	Nor/high	High	Mod	Nor
Pregnancy-associated ketoacidosis	Neg/Pos	Pos	Nor/Low	High	Nor	Nor
Renal failure	Neg	Neg	Nor	Nor	Nor	High
Organic poisons	Neg	Neg/Pos	Nor	Nor	Nor	Nor/Mod

BUN, blood urea nitrogen; CR, creatinine; Mod, moderate; Neg, negative; Nor, normal; Pos, positive.

For glucose, normal < 140 mg/dL; moderate = 140 to 300 mg/dL; high = 300 to 700 mg/dL; very high > 700 mg/dL. For ketones, moderate = 1 to 6 mM; high > 6.0 mM (see the text for use of the semiquantitative test of quantitative enzymatic determination is not available). For lactate, moderate = 2 to 4 mM; high > 4 mM. For BUN, moderate = 20 to 40 mg/dL; high > 40 mg/dL. For creatinine, moderate = 2 to 3 mg/dL; high > 3.0 mg/dL. Representations are average findings and should not be considered absolute. If only a semiquantitative test for ketones is available, moderate means that a "large" reading is present only in undiluted plasma; high = "large" in 1:1 or greater dilution. When a slash is present (e.g., Neg/Pos) the usual state is the first designation; for example, the urine is usually negative for glucose in pregnancy-associated ketoacidosis but could be positive if the patient had renal glycosuria.

reversal of hyperglycemia can be produced by fluids alone in the absence of insulin. Initially, fluids should be given rapidly; ordinarily a rate of 1 L/hour is appropriate for the first 2 to 3 hours. Because the total deficit is 3 to 5 L,[4] enough fluid should be given to approximate this amount in net terms (fluids infused minus urine production and estimated insensible loss). Some authors have recommended giving fluid at half the preceding rate,[102] but we favor more rapid infusion as described. Because hyperchloremia essentially always develops during treatment,[103, 104] we prefer lactated Ringer's solution to 0.9% saline, although no evidence has demonstrated that the hyperchloremia has detrimental consequences. Most patients also have a deficit of water, as evidenced by the elevated plasma osmolality. This deficit should be repaired only after extracellular volume is repleted. Free water can be delivered either as 0.45% saline or, after hyperglycemia has been brought under control, by infusion of dextrose in water.

It is wise to not administer oral fluids early in ketoacidosis, even if the patient is sufficiently alert to swallow, because nausea and vomiting are common, especially if acute gastric dilatation is present. The restriction of oral fluids does not apply if the patient is only in the developmental stages of ketoacidosis, where therapy is oriented to interruption of the pathogenetic sequence rather than reversal of full-blown diabetic coma.

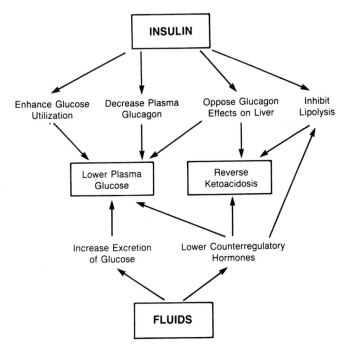

FIGURE 65–6. The mechanisms by which insulin and fluids reverse ketoacidosis.

Insulin. All patients with ketoacidosis require insulin because fluids alone will not reverse acidosis. Insulin has at least four effects. Its two most important actions are doubtless to decrease glucagon release from the α cell of the islets[6] and to counteract the effects of glucagon in the hepatocyte.[2, 6, 38] These two effects result in suppression of glucose and ketone production in the liver. The primary mechanism, as noted, appears to be inhibition of a glucagon-activated, cAMP-dependent protein kinase.[43] Secondary actions of insulin involve enhancement of glucose utilization in muscle and fat and inhibition of lipolysis. As discussed earlier, a drop in plasma free fatty acids does not reverse ketoacidosis because hepatic triglycerides replace adipose tissue as a source of fatty acids when plasma concentrations of the latter fall with insulin treatment. This adaptation is thought to account for the prolonged course in diabetic ketoacidosis, which usually requires about 7 to 9 hours to reverse; that is, ketone production continues unabated, driven by hepatic fat, until CPT I is inactivated.

The amount of insulin that should be used in treatment is a matter of much discussion. Our views have been summarized.[4] Insulin resistance is present in all patients with ketoacidosis relative to normal persons.[44] It is usually mild but in rare patients may be extreme. Insulin should ordinarily be administered intravenously, and only regular insulin should be used. It may be given intermittently or by constant infusion. Most patients respond to modest doses, but the lower limit should be 10 U/hour.[105] Administration of larger doses may have some advantage because presumably at higher concentrations, binding of insulin to the IgF1 receptor would occur and provide additive metabolic effects after the insulin receptor is saturated.[42] IgF1 itself has been shown to reverse diabetic ketoacidosis in the absence of insulin.[106] An effective intermittent approach is to give 50 U insulin as a bolus on arrival, followed by repeat boluses of 20 to 25 U every 1 to 2 hours until the ketoacidosis is reversed. Alternatively, a continuous-infusion protocol can be used. A representative example is shown in Table 65–4. The endpoint of treatment is a urine sample free of ketones inasmuch as the presence of acetone implies continued activation of hepatic ketogenic enzymes. If these enzymes are not deactivated, any complication (e.g., hypoglycemia, infection) will result in reappearance of ketoacidosis because free fatty acids will be remobilized in response to the action of stress hormones under these conditions. Therapy should be monitored by checking the anion gap along with blood gas determination every 4 hours. If the anion gap has not started to close by 4 hours, greater than normal insulin resistance is present and the insulin dosage should be increased. Occasionally, very large amounts are required, in which case 500 U insulin is available. Plasma glucose levels ordinarily fall before reversal of the acidosis.[107] Insulin administration should not be stopped when the plasma glucose concentration decreases. Rather, glucose should be infused to allow continuation of insulin therapy. No advantage is gained by monitoring plasma ketones semiquantitatively or quantitatively during therapy.[108] Intermediate insulin can be resumed after the patient is able to eat.

Potassium. Evaluation of potassium deficits is tricky because body

TABLE 65–4. An Infusion Protocol for Treatment of Diabetic Ketoacidosis*

Plasma Glucose (mg/dL)	Insulin Infusion (U/hr)	5% Dextrose/Water (mL/hr)
<70	0.5	250
71–100	1	225
101–150	2	200
151–200	3	175
201–250	4	150
251–300	6	100
301–350	8	50
351–400	10	0
401–450	12	0
451–500	16	0
>500	20	0

*University Diabetes Service, Parkland Memorial Hospital, courtesy of Dr. Philip Raskin. A 50-U bolus of insulin is given intravenously on arrival. Fluids and potassium are administered as indicated. SMA-6 is obtained hourly for the first few hours, with glucose measured hourly until the condition is reversed. Insulin administration is continued, covered by glucose, until urine is ketone-free.

stores are depleted despite plasma values that may be high on admission consequent to the metabolic acidosis that shifts K⁺ from intracellular to extracellular compartments as noted earlier.[107] Usual deficits are 3 to 5 mmol/kg of body weight, but at times the deficit may be double this value.[109] Because of the typical tendency to have hyperkalemia on arrival, potassium salts are not ordinarily given until 2 to 4 hours after treatment is started. On the other hand, if the initial potassium concentration is 4.0 mM or less, potassium salts will be required early because plasma values will fall as soon as insulin restores glucose transport into cells and urine production picks up.[4, 110] If the initial potassium level is very low (below 3.0 mM), insulin therapy may be delayed 60 to 90 minutes until some potassium repletion has been accomplished. The infusion rate of potassium chloride or potassium phosphate should be 20 to 40 mmol/hour under most circumstances. Potassium concentrations should be monitored at 2-hour intervals until the patient is metabolically stable. The electrocardiogram may be used as a guide if for some reason plasma levels are not available, but it is much less reliable.[111, 112] Potassium salts should be given only with extreme caution in an oliguric patient.

Phosphate. No evidence has shown that phosphate depletion plays a major symptomatic role in the development or treatment of diabetic ketoacidosis.[98, 101] Very low phosphate levels can cause altered consciousness, hemolysis, rhabdomyolysis, and heart failure, but these complications are not part of the routine picture in diabetic coma. There thus appears to be little urgency to replace the deficits of phosphate, which may approach 300 mmol. Nevertheless, many clinicians give the initial potassium replacement as potassium phosphate, thereby dealing with both deficiencies.

Bicarbonate. Severe acidosis is dangerous because it may cause hypotension, especially if volume depletion is present.[107] Acidosis causes decreased myocardial contractility and diminished response of the resistance vessels to catecholamines. It may also contribute to the clouding of consciousness that characterizes ketoacidosis, although increased osmolality of the brain doubtless plays a role. Warnings against the use of bicarbonate have focused on potential problems such as alkali-induced hypokalemia and lactic acidosis, but it has been argued that the benefits of bicarbonate outweigh the risks.[113, 114] If the admission pH is below 7.0, bicarbonate should probably be administered in amounts sufficient to bring the pH to 7.2, although other studies have shown no benefit.[115, 116] If hypotension is present, it may be prudent to give bicarbonate to all patients with a pH of 7.2 or less because, presumably, increased responsiveness of the left ventricle and resistance vessels would outweigh any deleterious effect of alkalinization on the oxygen dissociation curve.[98]

Monitoring Therapy. Maintenance of a written flow chart is imperative in monitoring a patient with ketoacidosis.[107, 117] Columns should be maintained for timed recording of insulin, fluids, potassium, and bicarbonate administration. Response is assessed by recording blood chemistry values, urine volume, urine ketones, anion gap, and vital signs in additional columns. Capillary blood glucose levels should be measured every 30 minutes initially. Formal laboratory evaluation of plasma glucose, sodium, potassium, bicarbonate, chloride, BUN, and creatinine should be obtained at 1- to 2-hour intervals. The best marker of reversal of acidosis is a fall in the anion gap. It is characteristic for the anion gap to close with therapy, matched by a rise in pH, while the bicarbonate concentration remains low—12 to 14 mM. The low bicarbonate value reflects a hyperchloremic state resulting from the infusion of sodium chloride, exchange with intracellular buffers, and external loss of "potential bicarbonate" in the form of excreted ketones.[104] The frequency of clinical and chemical monitoring can decrease as the patient recovers, usually 7 to 9 hours after the initiation of treatment. Rarely, patients do not clear the anion gap despite clinical improvement. Normally, failure to close the gap indicates insulin resistance, but in some patients an unmeasured anion that is not ketones, lactate, renal acids, or a poison appears to be present. The putative mystery anion (acetate? citrate?) has not been identified. Recognition that this condition is not insulin resistance is readily apparent if the urine is shown to be free of ketones and blood gas determination indicates that the acidosis has been reversed. We have called this condition "pseudo–insulin resistance."

Complications

Death from properly treated diabetic ketoacidosis should be rare, but ketoacidosis is the primary cause of mortality in diabetic children.[79, 118] Death rates are also significant in adults.[77, 78, 79] When death occurs, it may be the result of the disease itself or a result of complications of therapy. Clues to complications are given in Table 65–5.

Shock. Vascular collapse is not common in ketoacidosis. When it occurs, it may be the result of one of several causes. Volume depletion and acidosis alone can produce hypotension, as outlined earlier. If blood pressure does not rise with adequate fluid replacement, another cause of hypotension should be sought. Gram-negative sepsis and silent myocardial infarction are prime candidates.[80, 119]

Cerebral Edema. Cerebral edema is a dreaded development, especially in children; despite aggressive therapy, recovery can never be ensured.[120, 121] The syndrome is heralded by the appearance of neurologic signs or worsening coma in a patient who should be getting well as judged by biochemical parameters. Sluggish pupillary responses and frank papilledema may appear after several hours. Death is probably caused by compression of the brain stem as a result of herniation of the cerebellar tonsils through the foramen magnum.

TABLE 65–5. Clues to Complications of Diabetic Ketoacidosis

Complications	Clues
Acute gastric dilatation or erosive gastritis	Vomiting of blood or coffee-ground material
Cerebral edema	Obtundation or coma with or without neurologic signs, especially if occurring after initial improvement
Hyperkalemia	Cardiac arrest
Hypoglycemia	Adrenergic or neurologic signs; rebound ketosis
Hypokalemia	Cardiac arrhythmias
Infection	Fever
Insulin resistance	Unremitting acidosis after 4–6 hr of adequate therapy
Myocardial infarction	Chest pain, appearance of heart failure; appearance of hypotension despite adequate fluids
Mucormycosis	Facial pain, bloody nasal discharge, blackened nasal turbinates, blurred vision, proptosis
Vascular thrombosis	Strokelike picture or signs of ischemia in nonnervous tissue

From Foster DW: Diabetic ketoacidosis. *In* Krieger DT, Bardin CW (eds): Current Therapy in Endocrinology and Metabolism. Toronto, BC Decker, 1985, pp 268–270.

The cause of cerebral edema is not known. It has generally been assumed that the complication is a result of treatment, somehow precipitated by rapid falls in the plasma glucose level or oncotic pressure after insulin and crystalloid therapy.[120–125] Alterations in blood-brain barrier permeability and disequilibrium in pH have also been postulated as important. On the other hand, six of seven consecutive patients with untreated diabetic ketoacidosis were shown to have subclinical cerebral edema by computed tomographic scan on arrival at the hospital in one series.[125] Thus initial edema was independent of therapy. No conclusion regarding causality could be shown, although the degree of hyperglycemia correlated with the degree of acidosis. Osmotic disequilibrium between plasma/interstitial and intracellular water is probably of importance in the transition from subclinical to clinical edema. Because cerebrospinal fluid pressure rises routinely during treatment, it is likely that cerebral edema represents the extreme of a common response to therapy.[126] It is usually recommended that glucose infusions be started when the plasma glucose level is in the range of 16.7 mM (300 mg/dL) in an attempt to avoid the disequilibrium presumed to occur with rapid reversal of hyperglycemia.[122] This approach is not foolproof because the syndrome has developed in a child whose plasma glucose levels never got lower than 20.8 mM (375 mg/dL).[127]

Treatment consists of the intravenous administration of a 20% mannitol solution in bolus fashion at a dose of 1 g/kg. Dexamethasone is often given simultaneously—12 mg initially followed by 4 mg every 6 hours—but no real evidence has shown that this therapy is of help. As in other forms of cerebral edema, hyperventilation to a P_{CO_2} of 28 to 30 mm Hg may help by decreasing cerebral blood flow. Such therapy requires the assistance of an anesthesiologist.

Infection. Infection is a common problem in diabetic ketoacidosis and should be suspected in all patients, especially if fever is present.[78, 79, 110, 119] Although leukocytosis does not indicate infection, as noted earlier, fever almost always does. Pneumonia, pyelonephritis, and septicemia are most common, but cryptic inflammation, such as tooth or perirectal abscesses, may be the precipitating event. Mucormycosis is a rare fungal infection that is specifically associated with diabetic ketoacidosis.[128, 129] The initial symptom of facial pain suggests sinusitis, but the signs of bloody nasal discharge, orbital swelling, blackened palate and nasal turbinates, blurred vision, and altered consciousness point to the correct diagnosis. Mucormycosis is fatal if untreated. Amphotericin B should be started immediately on suspicion without waiting for confirmation by culture. Even with treatment the outlook is guarded. The role of ketoacids appears to be interference in the binding of iron to transferrin.[128] This interference in iron binding raises the concentration of free iron, which is a growth factor for the fungus.

Vascular Thrombosis. Thrombosis may occur during ketoacidosis in any muscular artery, but the cerebral vessels appear to be especially vulnerable.[130, 131] The mechanism is multifactorial. A major factor is probably increased viscosity of blood coupled with sluggish blood flow because of contraction of the plasma volume. Underlying atherosclerosis is doubtless important, the site of the lesion determining the location of the thrombosis. The activity of factor VIII is enhanced, as are levels of von Willebrand antigen.[132, 133] Antithrombin III may be decreased, and the partial thromboplastin time tends to be shortened. Platelets isolated from patients with ketoacidosis exhibit more facile aggregation in vitro than their normal counterparts do.[134, 135] Endothelial dysfunction predisposing to clot formation may also play a role: decreased fibrinolytic potential,[136] elevated levels of endothelin,[137] and diminished nitric oxide activity.[138, 139] Although prophylactic anticoagulation has been recommended, we agree with Carroll and Matz that such anticoagulation is unwise[110]; the best prophylaxis is aggressive fluid therapy. A single dose of aspirin daily (325 mg) might be prudent.[117]

Respiratory Distress Syndrome. The respiratory distress syndrome is a rare complication of diabetic ketoacidosis.[140] The syndrome is manifested as unexplained dyspnea and hypoxemia. Because large amounts of fluid are routinely given and the x-ray picture resembles pulmonary edema, it is frequently necessary to insert a Swan-Ganz catheter for the differential diagnosis. The wedge pressure is normal or low in respiratory distress syndrome and high in left ventricular

failure. Treatment requires administration of oxygen with positive end-expiratory pressure in standard fashion. Mortality rates are high.

NONKETOTIC HYPEROSMOLAR COMA

Whereas ketoacidosis is the common emergency of autoimmune diabetes, nonketotic hyperosmolar coma is the emergency of non–insulin-dependent diabetes. As will be seen, these distinctions are not absolute, however.

Pathophysiology

The pathophysiology of nonketotic hyperglycemic coma is similar to that of diabetic ketoacidosis with one exception: overproduction of acetoacetate and β-hydroxybutyrate sufficient to cause ketoacidosis does not occur.[141] The basic bihormonal mechanism of uncontrolled diabetes is no different: a relative or absolute deficiency of insulin and a relative or absolute excess of glucagon.[2, 142, 143] Elevation of the plasma glucose level is, as in ketoacidosis, the result of increased production of glucose by the liver coupled with its diminished utilization in tissues. The extreme hyperglycemia that characterizes the syndrome is consequent to failure of urine output.[47, 87] Put another way, production rates of glucose are not higher in hyperosmolar coma than in ketoacidosis, but the urinary escape route for glucose is diminished or absent. Thus one has a situation in which hepatic glucose production continues unabated, with glucose released into a steadily shrinking plasma/extracellular space. The result is a concentration of glucose in plasma that averages 55 mM (1000 mg/dL)[144, 145] and may reach nearly 278 mM (5000 mg/dL).[146] What accounts for the striking difference in glucose levels in ketoacidosis and hyperosmolar coma? The answer almost certainly is the absence of ketoacidosis. When metabolic acidosis supervenes, the patient or patient's family knows that that patient is acutely ill because almost invariably nausea, vomiting, and Kussmaul respiration are present. With hyperosmolar coma, by contrast, the patient has only an unremitting osmotic diuresis that is clinically silent until the patient is so dehydrated that altered consciousness or an acute neurologic syndrome supervenes. Although severe hyperosmolality is not the norm in diabetic ketoacidosis, it does occur.[87] Indeed, patients with true type 1 diabetes may have pure hyperosmolar coma as discussed below.

Because dehydration and volume depletion resulting from osmotic diuresis never progress to the point of coma provided that the patient can drink water, it is usual for hyperosmolar coma to appear in the context of some other precipitating illness that impairs the patient's capacity to maintain fluid intake. This event may be infection, a stroke, a fall with a sprain or fracture, or intake of a drug that alters the sensorium, increases glucose production, or itself causes diuresis with volume depletion.[147] To reiterate, as long as enough water is drunk to sustain urine output, even a severe osmotic diuresis does not result in the type of monumental hyperglycemia that characterizes nonketotic hyperosmolar coma.

The critical pathophysiologic question in hyperosmolar coma is why ketoacidosis is not present. The answer to this question is not known. Earlier theories proposed hyperosmolarity and lower free fatty acids as the explanation. Experimentally, hyperosmolarity can quench ketosis, and lower fatty acid concentrations in plasma would limit ketone formation via substrate deficiency. Neither explanation is likely because some patients with ketoacidosis have plasma osmolalities overlapping those of hyperosmolar coma and hyperosmolar coma has clearly occurred in subjects with very high free fatty acid concentrations in plasma.[142] On the basis of studies in animals, it is attractive to postulate that the primary reason for the absence of ketoacidosis is hepatic resistance to glucagon so that malonyl CoA levels do not fall. In the *ob/ob* mouse, cAMP generation by glucagon is markedly impaired,[148] and malonyl CoA concentrations are high.[149] The mechanism of glucagon resistance is not known, but this animal appears to have a defect in guanine nucleotide modulation of the adenylate cyclase system, at least in adipose tissue.[150] Obviously the *ob/ob* mouse is not equivalent to a human with non–insulin-dependent diabetes. It also seems peculiar that glucagon resistance would be limited to ketogenesis and not affect glucose overproduction. Perhaps malonyl CoA levels are maintained at inhibitory levels because of increased hepatic lactate uptake rather than because of glucagon resistance; that is, increased lactate turnover (the Cori cycle sequence) would be expected from the high plasma glucose concentrations. Because subjects with type 2 diabetes have normal or high insulin levels in the portal vein, increased lactate and alanine uptake could be sufficient to maintain hepatic lipogenesis and inhibit ketogenesis by generating malonyl CoA while simultaneously sustaining gluconeogenesis.[35]

As noted above, some patients with autoimmune diabetes have nonketotic hyperosmolar coma. It is likewise true that some patients with ostensible type 2 diabetes may experience severe ketosis and even full-blown ketoacidosis.[151, 152] A peculiar characteristic is that after recovery they may be treated by diet and oral agents without reversion to ketoacidosis. It is highly likely that these subjects have a subtype of nonautoimmune diabetes that has been called non–insulin-dependent diabetes mellitus-2 (NIDDM-2).[153] Subjects with mutations in hepatocyte nuclear factor-1α may have maturity-onset diabetes of the young type 3 (MODY-3) or adult-onset diabetes (NIDDM-2).[153–155] The characteristic finding in MODY-3 and NIDDM-2 is severe insulin deficiency and little insulin resistance. This situation is in contrast to ordinary NIDDM, where insulin levels are normal or high and insulin resistance is marked. They also do not express antibodies to glutamic acid decarboxylase or other markers of β cell autoimmunity. The insulin secretory defect makes these subjects susceptible to ketoacidosis in stress, where epinephrine/nonepinephrine blocks insulin release. On the other hand, because the insulin deficiency is not near absolute, as in type 1 disease, they may be controlled without insulin when stress or stressful illness disappears. A similar syndrome may occur with mutations in hepatocyte nuclear factor-4α, the apparent genetic defect in MODY-1.[156]

Clinical Features

Nonketotic hyperosmolar coma usually occurs in older persons with diabetes,[141, 144, 145] but as noted, it has been seen in the very young.[157] The syndrome can thus develop in patients with insulin-dependent, ketosis-prone diabetes. This phenomenon occurs when the patient is taking enough insulin to prevent ketoacidosis (by limiting free fatty acid mobilization) but not enough to control hyperglycemia. A curious inversion of insulin effects is seen in the presence or absence of ketoacidosis. In a nonketoacidotic subject it is harder to control the plasma glucose level than to prevent ketoacidosis, whereas in established ketoacidosis the plasma glucose level, as noted earlier, almost always falls before ketosis is reversed.[107] Thus a patient with insulin-dependent diabetes may be rendered functionally equivalent to a patient with non–insulin-dependent diabetes when treated with insulin sufficient to avoid ketoacidosis but insufficient to prevent a hyperglycemia-driven osmotic diuresis.

Precipitating Events

As noted above, nonketotic hyperosmolar coma is usually precipitated by a serious underlying illness that renders the patient unable to obtain sufficient water to keep up with the osmotic diuresis under circumstances in which glucose production is increased by stress. Any kind of illness can initiate the sequence of deterioration, but infection is probably the most common.[144, 145] Stroke, drugs, high-calorie tube feedings, burns, heart attacks, and a variety of other problems have been associated with the syndrome.

Symptoms and Signs

The preeminent symptomatology of hyperosmolar coma is neurologic. Up to half the patients are comatose on arrival, and those who are not show stupor.[158] A variety of other neurologic findings may be present, including focal convulsions or a stroke-like picture.[159–161] It should always be assumed that an underlying illness precipitated the syndrome even though it may be masked by the metabolic crisis.

Sometimes it is hard to tell whether a finding is cause or effect. Thus stroke can lead to hyperosmolar coma, and hyperosmolar coma can cause hemiplegia. Only if the neurologic picture reverses rapidly with therapy can it be concluded that the neurologic event was secondary. The possibility of head injury always has to be kept in mind in older patients living alone. If any question remains, a computed tomographic scan should be obtained once the metabolic state is stabilized.

Physical examination shows evidence of volume depletion and dehydration. Hypotension or shock may be present. Driven respiration of the Kussmaul type suggests the presence of lactic acidosis. Other physical findings reflect the underlying precipitating illness or the appearance of complications as outlined below.

Laboratory Abnormalities

Typical findings in nonketotic, hyperosmolar coma are shown in Table 65–6. Hyperglycemia, as noted, averages about 55 mM (1000 mg/dL). References to "syrupy blood" are entirely appropriate.[146] The plasma osmolality reflects the hyperglycemia and dehydration and is often 100 mOsm higher than normal. Fairly accurate estimates of osmolality can be obtained from the following formula:

$$mOsm = 2[Na^+ + K^+] + \frac{glucose \ (mg/dL)}{18} + \frac{BUN \ (mg/dL)}{2.8}$$

Some investigators have suggested that the serum sodium concentration, corrected for glucose, correlates best with central nervous system dysfunction.[162] Serum osmolality reflects the sodium concentration, however. The BUN and creatinine values are usually significantly elevated, a reflection of volume depletion and/or underlying renal disease. In the absence of vascular collapse, only minimal acidosis is seen, the bicarbonate averaging 18 to 20 mM. Mild ketosis resulting from starvation is usually present, so urine ketone values may be "large." If full-blown metabolic acidosis is present, the likely mechanism is lactic acidosis secondary to severe volume depletion, which leads to hypoxia of tissues via diminished perfusion. Formal differentiation requires quantitative measurement of lactate (see Table 65–3). Levels of free fatty acids tend to be in the normal fasting range but in some patients are very high.[141] Hypertriglyceridemia may be present.[163] As in ketoacidosis, the amylase level may be elevated and pancreatitis may be present.

Treatment

Therapy for nonketotic hyperosmolar coma is similar to that for ketoacidosis, with the major variation being the requirement for much

TABLE 65–6. Laboratory Values in Nonketotic Hyperosmolar Coma

Test	Series 1 (*n* = 33)	Series 2 (*n* = 20)	Series 3 (*n* = 7)
Glucose (mg/dL)	1166	976	1119
Sodium (mM)	144	142	138
Potassium (mM)	5.0	5.1	4.1
Chloride (mM)	99	98	96
Bicarbonate (mM)	17	22	18
BUN (mg/dL)	87	65	75
Creatinine (mg/dL)	5.5	—	—
Free fatty acids (mM)	0.73	0.96	1.98
Osmolality (mOsm)	384	374	361

BUN, blood urea nitrogen.
Series 1 is adapted from Arieff AI, Carroll HJ: Nonketotic hyperosmolar coma with hyperglycemia. Clinical features, pathophysiology, renal function, acid-base balance, plasma–cerebrospinal fluid equilibria and the effects of therapy in 37 cases. Medicine (Baltimore) 51:73–94, 1972. Series 2 is adapted from Gerich JE, Martin MM, Recant L: Clinical and metabolic characteristics of hyperosmolar nonketotic coma. Diabetes 20:228–238, 1971. Series 3 is adapted from Vinik A, Seftel H, Joffe BI: Metabolic findings in hyperosmolar, non-ketotic diabetic stupor. Lancet 2:797–799, 1970. Values listed are means.

larger amounts of fluid. Although recovery may be expected in patients younger than 50 years,[110] mortality rates are high (about 50%) in older patients.[141] Treatment should be carried out in an intensive care unit.

Fluids. The most important therapy is the rapid administration of isotonic saline solution to re-establish the circulation and urine flow.[110] Deficits of fluid in hyperosmolar coma may be 10 L or more.[144, 145] We do not agree with the view that the first fluid administered should be hypotonic (0.45%) saline[147]; we prefer to give 2 to 3 L of isotonic salt solution over the first 60 to 90 minutes, after which 0.45% saline is administered. A Swan-Ganz catheter for monitoring of capillary wedge pressure is extremely helpful because many of the patients are older and have underlying heart disease. Fluids should be given continuously until deficits are repaired, as manifested by normal wedge pressure, urine output reflecting infusion rates, and fall of the elevated BUN and creatinine.

Insulin. It has frequently been stated that patients with hyperosmolar coma are more sensitive to insulin than are those with ketoacidosis.[158] However, studies of glucose disappearance in response to insulin actually suggest that insulin resistance is present to the same degree as seen in the ketoacidotic state.[164] It therefore seems reasonable to give insulin at the same level as recommended for ketoacidosis.

Other Therapy. Potassium will usually be needed earlier than in ketoacidosis because initial values are not as high (provided that acidosis is not present). As with ketoacidosis, it is reasonable to give potassium phosphate because phosphate levels are also low. Bicarbonate is not needed unless lactic acidosis supervenes. Some authors also give magnesium sulfate,[110] but no data suggest its importance.

Complications

The complications of hyperosmolar coma are not dissimilar from those of ketoacidosis, with vascular collapse and infection being the most important problems.[144, 145] Of particular concern is gram-negative sepsis and pneumonia. Blood cultures should probably be obtained in all patients on arrival; blood culture is imperative if shock or fever is present. Other cultures will depend on the clinical findings. Broad-spectrum antibiotic coverage should be provided for the slightest suspicion of sepsis until cultures prove negative. Adult respiratory distress syndrome is not unusual.[110] Cerebral edema is rare in hyperosmolar coma but may occur.[165] Thrombosis, particularly in cerebral vessels, is common,[166] and diffuse intravascular coagulation may occur and lead to oozing of blood from a variety of sites. As noted, lactic acidosis may supervene. Myocardial infarction is not rare, and acute rhabdomyolysis has been reported.[167]

LACTIC ACIDOSIS

Lactic acidosis as an isolated occurrence in diabetes is probably quite rare.[168] However, because patients with diabetes are vulnerable to a variety of illnesses that can cause the disorder, such as myocardial infarction or sepsis, the appearance of lactic acidosis in hospitalized diabetic patients should not be surprising. The differential diagnosis usually lies between diabetic ketoacidosis and lactic acidosis. Differentiation is usually possible by semiquantitative assessment of plasma ketone levels as described earlier. Final proof requires quantitative enzymatic assay of lactate, acetoacetate, and β-hydroxybutyrate.

Lactic acidosis occurs in two general settings: one in which vascular collapse or tissue hypoxia is clearly evident (type A) and the other in which the pathophysiologic mechanism is something other than hypoxemia or shock (type B).[169] In both categories the cell must be considered functionally hypoxic because the lactate-pyruvate ratio is elevated, a reflection of the increase in the ratio of reduced and nonreduced nicotinamide adenine dinucleotide in the cytosol.[170] Considerable disagreement exists regarding the roles of overproduction and underutilization of lactate in the genesis of lactic acidosis. The syndrome is rare in the absence of overproduction, but in most cases significant underutilization is probably also a factor in the liver and other tissues.[169]

Metformin, the only biguanide approved in the United States, has been associated with type B lactic acidosis. Although use of the drug should clearly be withdrawn in renal failure or any intercurrent illness, it is probable that lactic acidosis is not a great deal more common in patients taking metformin than in those who do not.[171, 172]

Treatment of lactic acidosis requires reversal of the causal condition. In nonketotic hyperosmolar coma, the most common cause in diabetic patients, reversal of the condition means massive fluid therapy as previously described. Although bicarbonate has traditionally been given, evidence in animals suggests that it may be harmful by leading to worsening of intracellular acidosis.[173] It is not certain that these experiments in dogs, carried out under fixed laboratory conditions, apply to human disease,[114] but all agree that bicarbonate therapy is not of much benefit. Dichloroacetate may be tried but is not very effective.[174] The authors believe that bicarbonate should be given for severe acidosis until the cited findings in dogs are confirmed in humans.[114]

REFERENCES

1. National Diabetes Data Group: Diabetes in America. ed 2. Bethesda, MD, National Institutes of Health, NIH Publication No. 95–1468, 1995.
2. Unger RH, Foster DW: Diabetes mellitus. *In* Wilson JD, Foster DW, Kronenberg HM, Larsen PR (eds): Williams' Textbook of Endocrinology, ed 9. Philadelphia, WB Saunders, 1998, pp 973–1059.
3. Foster DW, McGarry JD: Glucose, lipid and protein metabolism. *In* Griffin JE, Ojeda SR (eds): Textbook of Endocrine Physiology, ed 3. New York, Oxford University Press, 1996, pp 349–374.
4. Foster DW, McGarry JD: The metabolic derangements and treatment of diabetic ketoacidosis. N Engl J Med 309:159–169, 1983.
5. Unger RH: The milieu interieur and the islets of Langerhans. Diabetologia 20:1–11, 1981.
6. Unger RH, Orci L: Glucagon and the A cell: Physiology and pathophysiology. N Engl J Med 304:1518–1524, 1575–1580, 1981.
7. McGarry JD, Foster DW: Hormonal control of ketogenesis: Biochemical considerations. Arch Intern Med 137:495–501, 1977.
8. Cahill GR Jr: Starvation in man. N Engl J Med 282:668–675, 1970.
9. Ruderman NB, Aoki TT, Cahill GF Jr: Gluconeogenesis and its disorders in man. *In* Hanson RW, Mehlman MA (eds): Gluconeogenesis: Its Regulation in Mammalian Species. New York, John Wiley & Sons, 1976, pp 515–532.
10. Allweiss C, Landau T, Abeles M, Magnes J: The oxidation of uniformly labelled albumin-bound palmitic acid to CO, by the perfused cat brain. J Neurochem 13:795–804, 1966.
11. Drenick EJ, Alvarez LC, Tamasi GC, Brickman AS: Resistance to symptomatic insulin reactions after fasting. J Clin Invest 51:2757–2762, 1972.
12. Madison LL, Mebane D, Unger RH, Lochner A: The hypoglycemic action of ketones: II. Evidence for the stimulatory feedback of ketones on the pancreatic beta cells. J Clin Invest 43:408–415, 1964.
13. McGarry JD, Foster DW: Hormonal control of ketogenesis. Adv Exp Med Biol 111:79–96, 1976.
14. McGarry JD, Dobbins RL: Fatty acids, lipotoxicity and insulin resistance. Diabetologia 42:128–138, 1999.
15. Dobbs R, Sakurai H, Sasaki H, et al: Glucagon: Role in the hyperglycemia of diabetes mellitus. Science 187:544–547, 1975.
16. Unger RH: Role of glucagon in the pathogenesis of diabetes: The status of the controversy. Metabolism 27:1691–1709, 1978.
17. Gerich JE, Lorenzi M, Bier DM, et al: Prevention of human diabetic ketoacidosis by somatostatin: Evidence for an essential role of glucagon. N Engl J Med 292:985–989, 1975.
18. Cherrington AD, Liljenquist JE: Role of glucagon in regulating glucose production in vivo. *In* Unger RH, Orci L (eds): Glucagon. New York, Elsevier, 1981, pp 221–253.
19. Raskin P, Unger RH: Hyperglucagonemia and its suppression: Importance in the metabolic control of diabetes. N Engl J Med 299:433–436, 1978.
20. Santeusanio F, Massi-Benedetti M, Angeletti G, et al: Glucagon and carbohydrate disorder in a totally pancreatomized man (a study with the aid of an artificial endocrine pancreas). J Endocrinol Invest 4:93–96, 1981.
21. Unger RH: Somatostatinoma. N Engl J Med 296:998–1000, 1977.
22. Liljenquist J, Bomboy J, Lewis S, et al: Effects of glucagon on lipolysis and ketogenesis in normal and diabetic man. J Clin Invest 53:190–197, 1974.
23. Schade DS, Woodside W, Eaton RP: The role of glucagon in the regulation of plasma lipids. Metabolism 28:874–886, 1979.
24. Miles JM, Haymond MW, Nissen SL, Gerich JE: Effects of free fatty acid availability, glucagon excess, and insulin deficiency on ketone body production in postabsorptive man. J Clin Invest 71:1554–1561, 1983.
25. Boden G, Owen OE, Rezvani I, et al: An islet cell carcinoma containing glucagon and insulin. Chronic glucagon excess and glucose homeostasis. Diabetes 26:128–137, 1977.
26. Marynick SP, Fagadau WR, Duncan LA: Malignant glucagonoma syndrome: Response to chemotherapy. Ann Intern Med 93:453–454, 1980.
27. McGarry JD, Wright PH, Foster DW: Hormonal control of ketogenesis. Rapid activation of hepatic ketogenic capacity in fed rats by anti insulin serum and glucagon. J Clin Invest 55:1202–1209, 1975.
28. McGarry JD, Foster DW: Glucagon and ketogenesis. *In* Lefebvre PJ (ed): Handbook of Experimental Pharmacology, vol 66/I. Glucagon I. Berlin, Springer-Verlag, 1983, pp 383–398.

29. Schade DS, Eaton RP: The regulation of plasma ketone body concentration by counter-regulatory hormones in man: III. Effects of norepinephrine in normal man. Diabetes 28:5–10, 1979.

30. Keyes WG, Heimberg M: Influence of thyroid status on lipid metabolism in the perfused rat liver. J Clin Invest 64:182–190, 1979.

31. Schade DS, Eaton RP: The controversy concerning counterregulatory hormone secretion: A hypothesis for the prevention of diabetic ketoacidosis? Diabetes 26:596–599, 1977.

32. Waldhäusl W, Kleinberger G, Korn A, et al: Severe hyperglycemia: Effects of rehydration on endocrine derangements and blood glucose concentration. Diabetes 28:577–584, 1979.

33. Alberti KGMM, Christensen NJ, Iversen J, Orskov H: Role of glucagon and other hormones in development of diabetic ketoacidosis. Lancet 1:1307–1311, 1975.

34. Miles JM, Rizza RA, Haymond MW, Gerich JE: Effects of acute insulin deficiency on glucose and ketone body turnover in man: Evidence for the primacy of overproduction of glucose and ketone bodies in the genesis of diabetic ketoacidosis. Diabetes 29:926–930, 1980.

35. Boyd ME, Albright EB, Foster DW, McGarry JD: In vitro reversal of the fasting state of liver metabolism in the rat. Reevaluation of the roles of insulin and glucose. J Clin Invest 68:142–152, 1981.

36. Harano Y, Kosugi K, Kashiwagi A, et al: Regulatory mechanism of ketogenesis by glucagon and insulin in isolated and cultured hepatocytes. J Biochem 91:1739–1748, 1982.

37. Virkamaki A, Ueki K, Kahn CR: Protein-protein interaction in insulin signaling and the molecular mechanisms of insulin resistance. J Clin Invest 103:931–943, 1999.

38. Rodbell M: The actions of glucagon at its receptor: Regulation of adenylate cyclase. *In* Lefebvre PJ (ed): Handbook of Experimental Pharmacology, vol 66/I. Glucagon I. Berlin, Springer-Verlag, 1983, pp 263–290.

39. Tang EKY, Houslay MD: Glucagon, vasopressin and angiotensin all elicit a rapid, transient increase in hepatocyte protein kinase C activity. Biochem J 283:341–346, 1992.

40. Iwanij V, Vincent AC: Characterization of the glucagon receptor and its functional domains using monoclonal antibodies. J Biol Chem 265:21302–21308, 1990.

41. Dunphy JL, Taylor RG, Fuller PJ: Tissue distribution of rat glucagon receptor and GLP-1 receptor gene expression. Mol Cell Endocrinol 141:179–186, 1998.

42. Flier JS: Lilly lecture: Syndromes of insulin resistance: From patient to gene and back again. Diabetes 41:1207–1219, 1992.

43. Gabbay RA, Lardy HA: Site of insulin inhibition of cAMP-stimulated glycogenolysis. cAMP-dependent protein kinase is affected independent of cAMP changes. J Biol Chem 259:6052–6055, 1984.

44. Barrett EJ, DeFronzo RA, Bevilacqua S, Ferrannini E: Insulin resistance in diabetic ketoacidosis. Diabetes 31:923–928, 1982.

45. Svedberg J, Björntorp P, Lönnroth P, Smith U: Prevention of inhibitory effect of free fatty acids on insulin binding and action in isolated rat hepatocytes by etomoxir. Diabetes 40:783–786, 1991.

46. McGarry JD: What if Minkowski had been ageusic? An alternative angle on diabetes. Science 258:766–770, 1992.

47. Feig PU, McCurdy DK: The hypertonic state. N Engl J Med 297:1444–1454, 1977.

48. Hers HG, Van Schaftingen E: Fructose 2,6-bisphosphate 2 years after its discovery. Biochem J 206:1–12, 1982.

49. Pilkis SJ, Granner DK: Molecular physiology of the regulation of hepatic gluconeogenesis and glycolysis. Annu Rev Physiol 54:885–909, 1992.

50. Okar DA, Live DH, Kirby TL, et al: The roles of Glu-327 and His-446 in the bisphosphatase reaction of rat liver 6-phosphofructo-2-kinase/fructose-2,6-bisphosphatase probed by NMR spectroscopic and mutational analyses of the enzyme in the transient phosphohistidine intermediate complex. Biochemistry 38:4471–4479, 1999.

51. Sanchez-Gutierrez JC, Sanchez-Arias JA, Samper B, Feliu JE: Modulation of epinephrine-stimulated gluconeogenesis by insulin in hepatocytes isolated from genetically obese (fa/fa) Zucker rats. Endocrinology 138:2443–2448, 1997.

52. Kuwajima M, Newgard CB, Foster DW, McGarry JD: Time course and significance of changes in hepatic fructose-2,6-bisphosphate levels during refeeding of fasted rats. J Clin Invest 74:1108–1111, 1984.

53. Bruni P, Vandoolaeghe P, Rousseau GG, et al: Expression and regulation of 6-phosphofructo-2-kinase/fructose-2,6-bisphosphatase isozymes in white adipose tissue. Eur J Biochem 259:756–761, 1999.

54. Munnich A, Marie J, Reach G, et al: In vivo hormonal control of L-type pyruvate kinase gene expression: Effects of glucagon, cyclic AMP, insulin, cortisone, and thyroid hormones on the dietary induction of mRNAs in the liver. J Biol Chem 259:10228–10231, 1984.

55. Wimhurst JM, Manchester KL: A comparison of the effects of diabetes induced with either alloxan or streptozotocin and of starvation on the activities in rat liver of the key enzymes of gluconeogenesis. Biochem J 120:95–103, 1970.

56. Chan TM: The permissive effects of glucocorticoid on hepatic gluconeogenesis. Glucagon stimulation of glucose-suppressed gluconeogenesis and inhibition of 6-phosphofructo-1-kinase in hepatocytes from fasted rats. J Biol Chem 259:7426–7432, 1984.

57. Chen KS, Lardy HA: 3-Aminopicolinate inhibits phosphoenolpyruvate carboxykinase in hepatocytes and increases release of gluconeogenic precursors from peripheral tissues. J Biol Chem 259:6920–6924, 1984.

58. McGarry JD, Foster DW: Regulation of hepatic fatty acid oxidation and ketone body production. Annu Rev Biochem 49:395–420, 1980.

59. Foster DW: From glycogen to ketones—and back. Diabetes 33:1188–1199, 1984.

60. Williamson JR, Walajtys-Rode E, Coll KE: Effects of branched chain α-ketoacids on the metabolism of isolated rat liver cells: I. Regulation of branched chain α-ketoacid metabolism. J Biol Chem 254:11511–11520, 1979.

61. Fredrikson G, Stralfors P, Nilsson NO, Belfrage P: Hormone-sensitive lipase of rat adipose tissue. Purification and some properties. J Biol Chem 256:6311–6320, 1981.

62. McGarry JD, Woeltje KF, Kuwajima M, Foster DW: Regulation of ketogenesis and

63. Murthy MSR, Pande SV: Mechanism of carnitine acylcarnitine translocase–catalyzed import of acylcarnitines into mitochondria. J Biol Chem 259:9082–9089, 1984.

64. McGarry JD, Leatherman GF, Foster DW: Carnitine palmitoyltransferase I: The site of inhibition of hepatic fatty acid oxidation by malonyl-CoA. J Biol Chem 253:4128–4136, 1978.

65. DiMarco JP, Hoppel C: Hepatic mitochondrial function in ketogenic states: Diabetes, starvation and after growth hormone administration. J Clin Invest 55:1237–1244, 1975.

66. McGarry JD, Brown NF: The mitochondrial carnitine palmitoyltransferase system—from concept to molecular analysis. Eur J Biochem 244:1–14, 1997.

67. McGarry JD, Takabayashi Y, Foster DW: The role of malonyl-CoA in the coordination of fatty acid synthesis and oxidation in isolated rat hepatocytes. J Biol Chem 253:8294–8300, 1978.

68. Esser V, Britton CH, Weis BC, et al: Cloning, sequencing and expression of a cDNA encoding rat liver carnitine palmitoyltransferase I: Proof that a single polypeptide is involved in inhibitor interaction and catalytic function. J Biol Chem 268:5817–5822, 1993.

69. Swenson TL, Porter JW: Mechanism of glucagon inhibition of liver acetyl-CoA carboxylase. Interrelationship of the effects of phosphorylation, polymer-protomer transition, and citrate on enzyme activity. J Biol Chem 260:3791–3797, 1985.

70. Hardie DG, Salt IP, Hawley SA, Davies SP: AMP-activated protein kinase: An ultrasensitive system for monitoring cellular energy change. Biochem J 338:717–722, 1999.

71. McGarry JD, Foster DW: Effects of exogenous fatty acid concentration on glucagon-induced changes in hepatic fatty acid metabolism. Diabetes 29:236–240, 1980.

72. de Laszlo SE, Hacker C, Li B, et al: Potent, orally absorbed glucagon receptor antagonists. Bioorg Med Chem Lett 9:641–646, 1999.

73. Cascieri MA, Koch GE, Ber E, et al: Characterization of a novel, non-peptidyl antagonist of the human glucagon receptor. J Biol Chem 274:8694–8697, 1999.

74. McGarry JD, Robles-Valdes C, Foster DW: Role of carnitine in hepatic ketogenesis. Proc Natl Acad Sci U S A 72:4385–4388, 1975.

75. Fery F, Balasse EO: Ketone body production and disposal in diabetic ketosis. A comparison with fasting ketosis. Diabetes 34:326–332, 1985.

76. Johnson DD, Palumbo PJ, Chu C-P: Diabetic ketoacidosis in a community-based population. Mayo Clin Proc 55:83–88, 1980.

77. Wetterhal SF, Olson DR, DeStafano F, et al: Trends in diabetes and diabetic complications. Diabetes Care 15:960–967, 1992.

78. Clements RS Jr, Vourganti B: Fatal diabetic ketoacidosis: Major causes and approaches to their prevention. Diabetes Care 1:314–325, 1978.

79. Goto Y, Sato S-I, Masuda M: Causes of death in 3151 diabetic autopsy cases. Tohoku J Exp Med 112:339–353, 1974.

80. Alberti KGMM, Hockaday TDR: Diabetic coma: A reappraisal after five years. Clin Endocrinol Metab 6:421–455, 1977.

81. Morris AD, Boyle DIR, McMahon AD, et al: Adherence to insulin treatment, glycaemic control, and ketoacidosis in insulin-dependent diabetes mellitus. Lancet 350:1505–1510, 1997.

82. Tattersall R: Brittle diabetes. Clin Endocrinol Metab 6:403–419, 1977.

83. Cohen AS, Vance VK, Runyan JW Jr, Hurwitz D: Diabetic acidosis: An evaluation of the cause, course and therapy of 73 cases. Ann Intern Med 52:55–86, 1960.

84. Beigelman PM: Severe diabetic ketoacidosis (diabetic "coma"): 482 episodes in 257 patients; experience of three years. Diabetes 20:490–500, 1971.

85. Kety SS, Polis BD, Nadler CS, Schmidt CF: The blood flow and oxygen consumption of the human brain in diabetic acidosis and coma. J Clin Invest 27:500–510, 1948.

86. Verdon F, van Melle G, Perret C: Respiratory response to acute metabolic acidosis. Bull Eur Physiopathol Respir 17:223–235, 1981.

87. Siperstein MD: Diabetic ketoacidosis and hyperosmolar coma. Endocrinol Metab Clin North Am 21:415–432, 1992.

88. Hockaday TDR, Alberti KGMM: Diabetic coma. Clin Endocrinol Metab 1:751–788, 1972.

89. Robin AP, Ing TS, Lancaster GA, et al: Hyperglycemia-induced hyponatremia: A fresh look. Clin Chem 25:496–497, 1979.

90. Owen OE, Licht JH, Sapir DG: Renal function and effects of partial rehydration during diabetic ketoacidosis. Diabetes 30:510–518, 1981.

91. Cahill GF, Herrera MG, Morgan AP, et al: Hormone-fuel interrelationships during fasting. J Clin Invest 45:1751–1769, 1966.

92. Owen OE, Morgan AP, Kemp HG, et al: Brain metabolism during fasting. J Clin Invest 46:1589–1595, 1967.

93. Mahoney CA: Extreme gestational starvation ketoacidosis: Case report and review of pathophysiology. Am J Kidney Dis 20:276–280, 1992.

94. Chernow B, Finton C, Rainey TG, O'Brian JT: "Bovine ketosis" in a nondiabetic postpartum woman. Diabetes Care 5:47–49, 1982.

95. Levy LJ, Duga J, Girgis M, Gordon EE: Ketoacidosis associated with alcoholism in nondiabetic subjects. Ann Intern Med 78:213–219, 1973.

96. Wren KD, Slovis CM, Minion GE, et al: The syndrome of alcoholic ketoacidosis. Am J Med 91:119–128, 1991.

97. Wilson HK, Keuer SP, Lea AS, et al: Phosphate therapy in diabetic ketoacidosis. Arch Intern Med 142:517–520, 1982.

98. Bellingham AJ, Detter JC, Lenfant C: The role of hemoglobin affinity for oxygen and red-cell 2,3-diphosphoglycerate in the management of diabetic ketoacidosis. Trans Assoc Am Physicians 83:113–120, 1970.

99. Vinicor F, Lehmer LM, Kam RC, Merritt AD: Hypermylasemia in diabetic ketoacidosis: Sources and significance. Ann Intern Med 91:200–204, 1979.

100. Kitabchi AE, Young R, Sacks H, Morris L: Diabetic ketoacidosis: Reappraisal of therapeutic approach. Annu Rev Med 30:339–357, 1979.

101. Keller U, Berger W: Prevention of hypophosphatemia by phosphate infusion during treatment of diabetic ketoacidosis and hyperosmolar coma. Diabetes 29:87–95, 1980.

102. Adrogué HJ, Barrero J, Eknoyan G: Salutary effect of modest fluid replacement in the treatment of adults with diabetic ketoacidosis. JAMA 262:2108–2113, 1989.

103. Androgué HJ, Wilson H, Boyd WE III, et al: Plasma acid-base patterns in diabetic ketoacidosis. N Engl J Med 307:1603–1610, 1982.

104. Halperin ML, Bear RA, Hannaford MC, Goldstein MG: Selected aspects of the pathophysiology of metabolic acidosis in diabetes mellitus. Diabetes 30:781–787, 1981.

105. Piters KM, Kumar D, Pei E, Bessman AN: Comparison of continuous and intermittent intravenous insulin therapies for diabetic ketoacidosis. Diabetologia 13:317–321, 1977.

106. Usala A-L, Madigan T, Burguera B, et al: Brief report: Treatment of insulin-resistant diabetic ketoacidosis with insulin-like growth factor I in an adolescent with insulin-dependent diabetes. N Engl J Med 327:853–857, 1992.

107. McGarry JD, Foster DW: Regulation of ketogenesis and clinical aspects of the ketotic state. Metabolism 21:471–489, 1972.

108. Fulop M, Murthy V, Michilli A, et al: Serum beta-hydroxybutyrate measurement in patients with uncontrolled diabetes mellitus. Arch Intern Med 159:381–384, 1999.

109. Beigelman PM: Potassium in severe diabetic ketoacidosis. Am J Med 54:419–420, 1973.

110. Carroll P, Matz R: Uncontrolled diabetes mellitus in adults: Experience in treating diabetic ketoacidosis and hyperosmolar nonketotic coma with low-dose insulin and a uniform treatment regimen. Diabetes Care 6:579–585, 1983.

111. Malone JI, Brodsky SJ: The value of electrocardiogram monitoring in diabetic ketoacidosis. Diabetes Care 3:543–547, 1980.

112. Stenzel KH, Dougherty JC, Scherr L, Lubash GD: Diabetic ketoacidosis: Dissociation of plasma potassium levels and electrocardiographic abnormalities. JAMA 187:372–373, 1964.

113. Matz R: Diabetic acidosis: Rationale for not using bicarbonate. N Y State J Med 76:1299–1303, 1976.

114. Narins RG, Cohen JJ: Bicarbonate therapy for organic acidosis: The case for its continued use. Ann Intern Med 106:615–618, 1987.

115. Lever E, Jaspan JB: Sodium bicarbonate therapy in severe diabetic ketoacidosis. Am J Med 75:263–268, 1983.

116. Green SM, Rothrock SG, Ho JD, et al: Failure of adjunctive bicarbonate to improve outcome in severe pediatric diabetic ketoacidosis. Ann Emerg Med 31:41–48, 1998.

117. Foster DW: Diabetic ketoacidosis. In Krieger DT, Bardin CW (eds): Current Therapy in Endocrinology and Metabolism. Toronto, BC Decker, 1985, pp 268–270.

118. Connell FA, Louden JM: Diabetes mortality in persons under 45 years of age. Am J Public Health 73:1174–1177, 1983.

119. Bryan CS, Reynolds KL, Metzger WT: Bacteremia in diabetic patients: Comparison of incidence and mortality with nondiabetic patients. Diabetes Care 8:244–249, 1985.

120. Winegrad AI, Kern EFO, Simmons DA: Cerebral edema in diabetic ketoacidosis. N Engl J Med 312:1184–1185, 1985.

121. Rosenbloom AL: Intracerebral crises during treatment of diabetic ketoacidosis. Diabetes Care 13:22–33, 1990.

122. Arieff AL, Kleeman CR: Studies on mechanisms of cerebral edema in diabetic comas: Effects of hyperglycemia and rapid lowering of plasma glucose in normal rabbits. J Clin Invest 52:571–583, 1973.

123. Fein IA, Rackow EC, Sprung CL, Grodman R: Relation of colloid osmotic pressure to arterial hypoxemia and cerebral edema during crystalloid volume loading of patients with diabetic ketoacidosis. Ann Intern Med 96:570–574, 1982.

124. Krane EJ, Rockoff MA, Wallman JK, Wolfsdorf JI: Subclinical brain swelling in children during treatment of diabetic ketoacidosis. N Engl J Med 312:1147–1151, 1985.

125. Durr JA, Hoffman WH, Sklar AH, et al: Correlates of brain edema in uncontrolled IDDM. Diabetes 41:627–632, 1992.

126. Clements RS Jr, Blumenthal SA, Morrison AD, Winegrad AL: Increased cerebrospinal-fluid pressure during treatment of diabetic ketosis. Lancet 2:671–675, 1971.

127. Franklin B, Liu J, Ginsberg-Fellner F: Cerebral edema and ophthalmoplegia reversed by mannitol in a new case of insulin-dependent diabetes mellitus. Pediatrics 69:87–90, 1982.

128. Artis WM, Fountain JA, Delcher HK, Jones HE: A mechanism of susceptibility to mucormycosis in diabetic ketoacidosis: Transferrin and iron availability. Diabetes 31:1109–1114, 1982.

129. Weprin BE, Hall WA, Goodman J, Adams GL: Long-term survival in rhinocerebral mucormycosis. Case report. J Neurosurg 88:570–575, 1998.

130. Timperley WR, Preston FE, Ward JD: Cerebral intravascular coagulation in diabetic ketoacidosis. Lancet 1:952–956, 1974.

131. McLaren EH, Cullen DR, Brown MJ: Coagulation abnormalities in diabetic coma before and 24 hours after treatment. Diabetologia 17:345–349, 1979.

132. Paton RC: Haemostatic changes in diabetic coma. Diabetologia 21:172–177, 1981.

133. Pasi KJ, Enayat MS, Horrocks PM, et al: Qualitative and quantitative abnormalities of von Willebrand antigen in patients with diabetes mellitus. Thromb Res 59:581–591, 1990.

134. Kwaan HC, Colwell JA, Suwanwela N: Disseminated intravascular coagulation in diabetes mellitus, with reference to the role of increased platelet aggregation. Diabetes 21:108–113, 1972.

135. Tschoepe D, Rauch U, Schwippert B: Platelet-leukocyte–cross-talk in diabetes mellitus. Horm Metab Res 29:631–635, 1997.

136. Maiello M, Boeri D, Podesta F, et al: Increased expression of tissue plasminogen activator and its inhibitor and reduced fibrinolytic potential of human endothelial cells cultured in elevated glucose. Diabetes 41:1009–1015, 1992.

137. Takahashi K, Ghatei MA, Lam H-C: Elevated plasma endothelin in patients with diabetes mellitus. Diabetologia 33:306–310, 1990.

138. Saenz de Tejada I, Goldstein I, Azadzoi K, et al: Impaired neurogenic and endothelium-mediated relaxation of penile smooth muscle from diabetic men with impotence. N Engl J Med 320:1025–1030, 1989.

139. Hogan M, Cerami A, Bucala R: Advanced glycosylation end products block the antiproliferative effect of nitric oxide. J Clin Invest 90:1110–1115, 1992.

140. Carroll P, Matz R: Adult respiratory distress syndrome complicating severely uncontrolled diabetes mellitus: Report of nine cases and a review of the literature. Diabetes Care 5:574–580, 1982.

141. Foster DW: Insulin deficiency and hyperosmolar coma. Adv Intern Med 19:159–173, 1974.

142. Vinik A, Seftel H, Joffe BI: Metabolic findings in hyperosmolar, nonketotic diabetic stupor. Lancet 2:797–798, 1970.

143. Lindsey CA, Faloona GR, Unger RH: Plasma glucagon in nonketotic hyperosmolar coma. JAMA 229:1771–1773, 1974.

144. Gerich JE, Martin MM, Recant L: Clinical and metabolic characteristics of hyperosmolar nonketotic coma. Diabetes 20:228–238, 1971.

145. Arieff Al, Carroll HJ: Nonketotic hyperosmolar coma with hyperglycemia: Clinical features, pathophysiology, renal function, acid-base balance, plasma–cerebrospinal fluid equilibria and the effects of therapy in 37 cases. Medicine (Baltimore) 51:73–94, 1972.

146. Knowles HC Jr: Syrupy blood. Diabetes 15:760–761, 1966.

147. Podolsky S: Hyperosmolar nonketotic coma: Death can be prevented. Geriatrics 34:29–33, 36–37, 41–42, 1979.

148. Yen TT, Stamm NB, Fuller RW, Root MA: Hepatic insensitivity to glucagon in ob/ob mice. Res Commun Chem Pathol Pharmacol 30:29–40, 1980.

149. Azain MJ, Fukuda N, Chao F-F, et al: Contributions of fatty acid and sterol synthesis to triglyceride and cholesterol secretion by the perfused rat liver in genetic hyperlipemia and obesity. J Biol Chem 260:174–181, 1985.

150. Begin-Heick N: Absence of the inhibitory effect of guanine nucleotides on adenylate cyclase activity in white adipocyte membranes of the ob/ob mouse: Effect of the ob gene. J Biol Chem 260:6187–6193, 1985.

151. Scott CR, Smith JM, Cradock MM, Pihoker C: Characteristics of youth-onset noninsulin-dependent diabetes mellitus and insulin-dependent diabetes mellitus at diagnosis. Pediatrics 100:84–91, 1997.

152. Umpierrez GE, Clark WS, Steen MT: Sulfonylurea treatment prevents recurrence of hyperglycemia in obese African-American patients with a history of hyperglycemic crises. Diabetes Care 20:479–483, 1997.

153. Lehto M, Tuomi T, Mahtani MM, et al: Characterization of the MODY3 phenotype. Early-onset diabetes caused by an insulin secretion defect. J Clin Invest 99:582–591, 1997.

154. Yamada S, Nishigori H, Onda H, et al: Identification of mutations in the hepatocyte nuclear factor (HNF)-1α gene in Japanese subjects with IDDM. Diabetes 46:1643–1647, 1997.

155. Pontoglio M, Sreenan S, Roe M, et al: Defective insulin secretion in hepatocyte nuclear factor 1α–deficient mice. J Clin Invest 101:2215–2222, 1998.

156. Hani EH, Suaud L, Boutin P, et al: A missense mutation in hepatocyte nuclear factor-4α, resulting in a reduced transactivation activity, in human late-onset non–insulin-dependent diabetes mellitus. J Clin Invest 101:521–526, 1998.

157. Goldman SL: Hyperglycemic hyperosmolar coma in a 9-month-old child. Am J Dis Child 133:181–183, 1979.

158. McCurdy DK: Hyperosmolar hyperglycemic nonketotic diabetic coma. Med Clin North Am 54:683–699, 1970.

159. Maccario M, Messis CP, Vastola EF: Focal seizures as a manifestation of hyperglycemia without ketoacidosis: A report of seven cases with review of the literature. Neurology 15:195–206, 1965.

160. Guisado R, Arieff AI: Neurologic manifestations of diabetic comas: Correlation with biochemical alterations in the brain. Metabolism 24:665–679, 1975.

161. Maccario M: Neurological dysfunction associated with nonketotic hyperglycemia. Arch Neurol 19:525–534, 1968.

162. Daugirdas JT, Kronfol NO, Tzamaloukas AH: Hyperosmolar coma: Cellular dehydration and the serum sodium concentration. Ann Intern Med 110:855–857, 1989.

163. Bewsher PD, Petrie JC, Worth HGJ: Serum lipid levels in hyperosmolar non-ketotic diabetic coma. BMJ 3:82–84, 1970.

164. Rosenthal NR, Barrett EJ: An assessment of insulin action in hyperosmolar hyperglycemic nonketotic diabetic patients. J Clin Endocrinol Metab 60:607–610, 1985.

165. Maccario M, Messis CP: Cerebral edema complicating treated nonketotic hyperglycemia. Lancet 2:352–353, 1969.

166. Scharf Y, Nahir M, Tatarsky I, et al: Fatal venous thrombosis in hyperosmolar coma. Diabetes 20:308–309, 1971.

167. Schlepphorst E, Levin ME: Rhabdomyolysis associated with hyperosmolar nonketotic coma. Diabetes Care 8:198–200, 1985.

168. Kreisberg RA: Lactate homeostasis and lactic acidosis. Ann Intern Med 92:227–237, 1980.

169. Cohen RD, Woods HF: Lactic acidosis revisited. Diabetes 32:181–191, 1983.

170. Foster DW: Lactic acidosis. In Braunwald E, Isselbacher KJ, Petersdorf RG, et al (eds): Harrison's Principles of Internal Medicine, ed 11. New York, McGraw-Hill, 1987, pp 1797–1800.

171. Brown JB, Pedula K, Barzilay J, et al: Lactic acidosis rates in type 2 diabetes. Diabetes Care 21:1659–1663, 1998.

172. Chan NN, Brain HP, Feher MD: Metformin-associated lactic acidosis: A rare or very rare clinical entity? Diabet Med 16:273–281, 1999.

173. Graf H, Leach W, Arieff AL: Evidence for a detrimental effect of bicarbonate therapy in hypoxic lactic acidosis. Science 227:754–756, 1985.

174. Stacpoole PW, Harman EM, Curry SH, et al: Treatment of lactic acidosis with dichloroacetate. N Engl J Med 309:390–396, 1983.

Chapter 66

Hypoglycemia

John E. Gerich

Hypoglycemia itself is not a disease. It is a biochemical sign indicating that some condition has caused an imbalance between rates of release of glucose into the circulation and rates of glucose removal from the circulation so that the latter exceeds the former. This process may occur under various circumstances, for example, when increased rates of glucose release are accompanied by even greater increases in glucose utilization (e.g., marathon running) or when subnormal rates of glucose utilization are accompanied by even greater reductions in glucose release (e.g., starvation, adrenal insufficiency). Abnormal relative changes in glucose supply and demand may occur because of excess insulin (e.g., overdose in a diabetic patient, insulinoma, sulfonylurea administration), decreased counterregulatory hormone secretion (pancreatectomy, hypopituitarism), an inability of the target tissues of counterregulatory hormones to respond normally (e.g., alcohol ingestion, renal insufficiency), or more usually a combination of these factors (e.g., sepsis). Table 66–1 lists common causes of hypoglycemia in adults. With a few exceptions (e.g., drug-induced and reactive hypoglycemia), hypoglycemia usually signifies the presence of a serious underlying medical disorder whose cause, if it is not obvious, must be investigated and treated.

Most clinicians would agree that an appropriately obtained venous plasma glucose level below 50 mg/dL (~2.8 mmol/L) in an overnight fasting adult should be considered suspicious for hypoglycemia. Such a glucose concentration would represent a value below the lowest percentile inasmuch as the normal range in most clinical laboratories using glucose oxidase or hexokinase methods under these conditions

is 70 to 110 mg/dL (3.6–6.1 mmol/L).[1] It is important to note that whole blood determinations are about 10% lower than plasma determinations. In the postabsorptive state, capillary samples yield values equivalent to venous samples because tissues drained by these venous samples use little glucose. Such may not be the case after a meal or glucose ingestion, when venous samples can be as much as 30 to 40 mg/dL (2.0–2.5 mmol/L) lower than capillary samples.[2] Under these conditions, venous sampling may give the false appearance of a hypoglycemic condition when in fact the arterial glucose concentration is normal. Because of this limitation and for other reasons, values obtained under conditions other than an overnight fast can be difficult to interpret. For example, plasma glucose values during an oral glucose tolerance test (OGGT) may normally decrease below 40 mg/dL (~2.2 mmol/L), be asymptomatic, and not reflect a pathologic process,[3] whereas postprandial symptoms develop in some people with plasma glucose levels in the normal range. Moreover, after prolonged exercise, values between 30 and 50 mg/dL (1.7–2.8 mmol/L) have commonly been observed in perfectly normal individuals.[4] In summary, the circumstances under which the plasma glucose value is obtained will influence its interpretation and the action to be taken. Consequently, in evaluating a patient for suspected hypoglycemia, the overnight (14–16 hours) fasted value usually represents the standard frame of reference.

One must always be aware that an apparently low blood glucose level may result from unintentional artifacts or mistakes (artifactual hypoglycemia).[5] These artifactually low glucose readings may be caused by improper sample collection, inadequate storage, or errors in analytic methods. Samples not to be immediately measured should be collected in tubes containing fluoride and/or oxalate to inhibit glycolysis by red and white blood cells; otherwise, blood glucose levels may decrease 10 to 20 mg/dL (~0.5–1.0 mmol/L) per hour at room temperature irrespective of the initial value.[6] Even in the presence of inhibitors of glycolysis, artifactually low glucose concentrations may be obtained when blood contains a large amount of cells such as in patients with leukemia,[7, 8] leukemoid reactions,[9, 10] polycythemia vera,[11, 12] and hemolytic crisis with excessive circulating nucleated red cells.[13]

Use of plasma rather than serum may lead to fibrin occlusion of some automated analyzers. Faulty calibration, outdated reagents, use of fluoride or other preservatives that may interfere with certain methods, and failure to remove triglycerides from lipemic samples can all lead to artifactually low glucose values. In the latter situation, which

TABLE 66–1. Causes of Hypoglycemia in Adults

Drugs (accidental, factitious)
  Especially insulin, sulfonylureas, alcohol
Critical illness
  Renal, hepatic, and heart disease; sepsis; malnutrition
Endocrine deficiency
  Adrenal > pituitary > thyroid
Overproduction of insulin or insulin-like material
  Insulin-producing islet tumor, non–β cell tumors
Other
  Pregnancy, strenuous exercise, autoimmune syndromes, reactive
    hypoglycemia
Iatrogenic (dialysis, total parenteral nutrition)

can result in underestimations of up to 15%, electrolytes and other serum elements will also be reduced.

PHYSIOLOGY OF GLUCOSE HOMEOSTASIS

General Considerations: Symptoms of Hypoglycemia

Judgment regarding the significance of a low plasma glucose level and its possible etiology requires knowledge of normal glucose homeostasis and the factors involved in its regulation.

Normally, plasma glucose values are maintained within a relatively narrow range throughout the day (usually between 55 and 165 mg/dL, or ~3.0 and 9.0 mmol/L) despite wide fluctuations in delivery (e.g., meals) and removal (e.g., exercise) of glucose from the circulation. Teleologically, hyperglycemia is to be avoided because of its adverse macrovascular and microvascular effects.[14–16] Indeed, individuals with impaired glucose tolerance (i.e., those with postprandial plasma glucose levels between 140 and 199 mg/dL [7.8–11.0 mmol/L]) have a several-fold increased risk of cardiovascular disease.[17]

Hypoglycemia is to be avoided to protect the brain and prevent cognitive dysfunction. Because of limited availability of alternative fuels (e.g., ketone bodies) or their transport across the blood-brain barrier (e.g., free fatty acids), glucose can be considered to be the sole source of energy for the brain, except under conditions of prolonged fasting, in which case ketone bodies and other substrates may be used.[18] The brain cannot store or produce glucose and is therefore dependent on glucose in plasma for adequate functioning and ultimate survival. At physiologic plasma glucose levels, phosphorylation of glucose is rate limiting for its utilization. However, because of the kinetics of the transfer of glucose across the blood-brain barrier, uptake becomes rate limiting as plasma glucose concentrations decrease below the normal range.

A characteristic hierarchy of responses occurs as plasma glucose levels decrease[19, 20] (Fig. 66–1). A decrement as little as 20 mg/dL (~1.1 mmol/L) can reduce brain glucose uptake, suppress insulin secretion, and trigger counterregulatory hormone release at approximately 72 mg/dL (4.0 mmol/L). Under normal physiologic conditions, this response prevents a further decrease in the plasma glucose concentration and restores normoglycemia. Decreases of 30 mg/dL (1.7

mmol/L) to approximately 60 mg/dL (3.4 mmol/L) usually evoke the so-called autonomic warning symptoms[21, 22] (hunger, anxiety, palpitations, sweating, warmth, nausea), which if interpreted correctly, lead a person to eat and prevent more serious hypoglycemia. However, clues of hypoglycemia may vary considerably from person to person.[23] If for some reason plasma glucose levels decrease to about 55 mg/dL (~3.0 mmol/L), the so-called neuroglycopenic signs/symptoms of brain dysfunction may develop (blurred vision, slurred speech, glassy-eyed appearance, confusion, difficulty concentrating).[21, 22] Cognitive impairment and electroencephalographic changes are demonstrable at this plasma glucose level. Decreases below 40 mg/dL (~2.5 mmol/L) result in sleepiness and gross behavioral (e.g., combativeness) abnormalities. Further decreases can produce coma, and values below 30 mg/dL (~1.6 mmol/L), if prolonged, can cause seizures, permanent neurologic deficits, and death. In individuals with underlying cardiovascular disease, life-threatening arrhythmia, myocardial infarction, and stroke may be precipitated.[24–32]

Lest an excessive fear of hypoglycemia lead to too conservative management of diabetes mellitus, it should be pointed out that in otherwise healthy, young (<45 years) individuals, plasma glucose levels averaging 35 mg/dL (~2.0 mmol/L) have been maintained for as long as 8 hours without any severe long-term adverse effects,[33] and chronic levels as low as 24 mg/dL (1.3 mmol/L) in patients with insulinoma have been observed in association with apparently normal cerebral function.[34]

Patients with diabetes mellitus or insulinoma and even normal individuals who have experienced repetitive episodes of hypoglycemia will have an increase in the thresholds (require greater hypoglycemia) for initiation of counterregulatory hormone release and autonomic warning symptoms and signs of neuroglycopenia.[35] This phenomenon, called hypoglycemia unawareness, results from both an adaptation in the transport of glucose across the blood-brain barrier[36] and a reduction in peripheral tissue β-adrenergic sensitivity.[37, 38] Conversely, diabetic patients under poor glycemic control can experience hypoglycemic symptoms and activation of counterregulation at higher than normal plasma glucose levels (reduced thresholds), apparently for similar reasons.[39] In addition, the signs, symptoms, and sequelae of hypoglycemia can be affected by factors such as age,[40–42] gender,[43–45] medication (e.g., β-blockers[46]), and associated medical conditions (e.g., pregnancy,[47] autonomic neuropathy[48, 49]). However, contrary to common belief, experimental evidence convincingly indicates that the rate of decrease in plasma glucose has no effect on either symptoms or counterregulatory hormone responses.[50, 51]

Glucose Homeostasis in the Postabsorptive State

Glucose Utilization

After a 14- to 16-hour overnight fast, the so-called postabsorptive state, plasma glucose concentrations average about 90 mg/dL (5.0 mmol/L) and are relatively stable. Consequently, rates of release of glucose into the circulation must closely approximate rates of glucose removal and generally average about 10 μmol/kg/min (Fig. 66–2). Although this situation is considered to represent a steady state, actually it is a pseudo–steady state, with rates of glucose removal slightly and often undetectably exceeding rates of glucose release into the circulation; if fasting is prolonged, plasma glucose levels gradually decrease, and by 20 to 24 hours of fasting they may be 10% to 15% lower (i.e., 72–80 mg/dL, 4.0–4.5 mmol/L). However, even after 72 hours of fasting, they are usually still above 50 mg/dL (2.8 mmol/L).[52] The latter observation forms the basis of the 72-hour fast to exclude an insulinoma.[53]

In the postabsorptive overnight fasted state, most glucose used by the body is due to uptake by the brain (~45%–60%); skeletal muscle (~15%–20%), kidney (~10%–15%), blood cells (~5%–10%), splanchnic organs (3%–6%), and adipose tissue (~2%–4%)[54] account for the remainder. Most of the body's energy requirement is met by oxidation of free fatty acids, which compete with glucose as the fuel of choice in certain organs (e.g., skeletal muscle, heart, and possibly

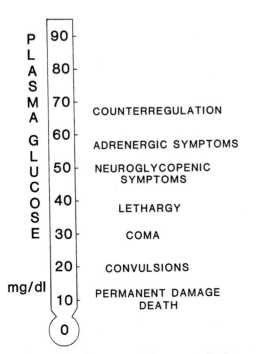

FIGURE 66–1. Hierarchy of responses to decrements in plasma glucose.

P L A S M A G L U C O S E

mg/dl

90
80
70 COUNTERREGULATION
60 ADRENERGIC SYMPTOMS
50 NEUROGLYCOPENIC SYMPTOMS
40 LETHARGY
30 COMA
20 CONVULSIONS
10 PERMANENT DAMAGE DEATH
0

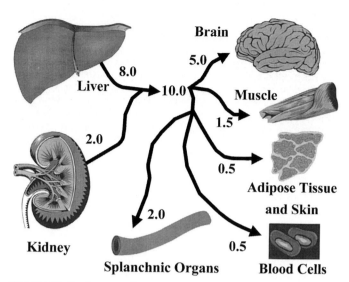

FIGURE 66–2. *Glucose utilization and production in the postabsorptive state. The liver and kidney contribute approximately 8.0 and 2.0 μmol/ kg/min respectively to the total release of glucose into the circulation (10 μmol/kg/min); the brain, splanchnic tissue, muscle, adipose tissue and skin, and blood cells account for approximately 5.0, 2.0, 1.5, 0.5 and 0.5 μmol/kg/min, respectively.*

the kidney).[55] Because glucose uptake by the brain, blood cells, renal medulla, and splanchnic tissues can be considered to be essentially independent of insulin and because plasma insulin levels are usually low in the postabsorptive state (<15 μU/mL, 90 pmol/L), most of the glucose removed from the circulation in the postabsorptive state is determined by tissue demands, the mass action effects of the plasma glucose concentration per se, and the number and characteristics of the glucose transporters in specific tissues rather than by insulin. Under these conditions, insulin may be viewed as largely playing a permissive role, and counterregulatory hormones that antagonize the actions of insulin (e.g., cortisol, growth hormone, epinephrine, and thyroid hormone) can be viewed as modulating the sensitivity of tissues insofar as the effects of insulin on tissue glucose uptake and utilization are concerned.

Glucose Production

Glucose release into the circulation, however, is under considerably more regulation by both hormone and nonhormonal mechanisms (see Fig. 66–2). Although many tissues contain enzymes to break down glycogen to glucose 6-phosphate (glycogenolysis) and/or synthesize glucose 6-phosphate from glycerol, lactate, and amino acids (gluconeogenesis), only the liver and kidney contain enough glucose-6-phosphatase to make significant amounts of free glucose available for release. Until recently it was thought that the liver was the sole source of glucose entering the circulation except during acidosis and after prolonged fasting. However, recent studies in humans and dogs, as well as in the earlier literature of in situ and in vitro preparations, now indicate that both the liver and kidney release glucose under physiologic conditions.[56]

Current evidence indicates that the liver is responsible for 80% to 85% of the glucose released in the postabsorptive state.[56] Under these conditions, approximately 50% of all the glucose released into the circulation is due to glycogenolysis, with the remainder (~5.0 μmol/ kg/min) attributed to gluconeogenesis.[57] The proportion stemming from gluconeogenesis rapidly increases with the duration of fasting as glycogen stores become depleted, and 48 hours after the last meal gluconeogenesis accounts for nearly 80% and by 72 hours it accounts for essentially all of the glucose released into the circulation.[52, 57] The liver releases glucose by glycogenolysis and gluconeogenesis. The kidney normally contains little glycogen, and renal cells that could make glucose-6-phosphatase lack glucose-6-phosphatase. Consequently, all the glucose released by the kidney can be considered to be the result of

gluconeogenesis.[56] Thus although the liver releases about four times as much glucose as the kidney under postabsorptive conditions, both organs release about the same amount (~2.5 μmol/kg/min) as a result of gluconeogenesis.

Release of glucose by liver and kidney is regulated differently. Insulin suppresses glucose release by both organs (by direct effects on enzyme activation/deactivation and by indirect actions such as limitation of gluconeogenic substrate availability and gluconeogenic activators [e.g., suppression of free fatty acids and glucagon]).[58] However, glucagon, which increases both glycogenolysis and gluconeogenesis in the liver, has no effect on the kidney,[59] whereas epinephrine, which can directly activate hepatic glycogenolysis, appears to increase glucose release predominantly by directly stimulating renal gluconeogenesis and to a lesser extent by increasing the availability of gluconeogenic precursors/activators.[60, 61]

The major precursors for gluconeogenesis are lactate, glycerol, and various amino acids.[54] The liver and kidney differ somewhat in their use of these substrates in that alanine is preferentially used by the liver, whereas glutamine is predominantly used in the kidney.[61] Most of the amino acids released from protein via proteolysis are converted to glutamine and alanine for transport through plasma to the liver and kidney.[62]

Insulin, glucagon, and catecholamines (norepinephrine released postsynaptically in the abundantly innervated liver and kidney and epinephrine released from the adrenal medulla) are the most important moment-to-moment glucoregulatory hormones. Physiologic changes in their circulating levels are able to change glucose release in a matter of minutes. Other important glucoregulatory factors such as growth hormone, cortisol, and thyroid hormone take hours for their effects to become evident. Their effects are mediated through changes in the sensitivity of the kidney and liver to insulin, glucagon, and catecholamines by altering the amount of key enzymes, glycogen stores, and availability of circulating precursors/activators of gluconeogenesis. Increases in circulating free fatty acids augment hepatic and renal glucose release by affecting the activity of key gluconeogenic enzymes and by providing the necessary ATP and reducing equivalents.[55]

Deficiencies of counterregulatory hormones, excesses of insulin, and an inability to store or mobilize glycogen/gluconeogenic precursors can result in hypoglycemia in the postabsorptive state.

Glucose Homeostasis in the Postprandial State

Complete assimilation of the constituents of a mixed meal containing fat, protein, and carbohydrate and restoration of the postabsorptive state take at least 6 hours.[63] After ingestion of a pure carbohydrate load, assimilation is generally complete within 5 hours. Despite these differences, little evidence indicates that the fate of ingested carbohydrate is markedly different under the two conditions.[63]

Various factors can affect the extent of circulating glucose excursions after meal ingestion, such as the time and degree of physical activity since the last meal, the composition and form of glucose (liquid vs. solid), the rate of gastric emptying, digestion within the lumen of the small intestine, absorption into the portal vein, extraction by the liver, suppression of endogenous glucose release, and finally the uptake, storage, oxidation, and glycolysis of glucose in posthepatic tissues.[64]

From a practical point of view, one can consider the major factors influencing postprandial glucose homeostasis to be those that affect suppression and restoration of endogenous glucose release and those that affect hepatic and posthepatic tissue glucose disposal. Recent studies using dual-isotope approaches (to measure splanchnic sequestration, i.e., first-pass hepatic uptake, endogenous glucose release, and total glucose appearance into and disappearance from the systemic circulation) in conjunction with measurements of net balance across the limbs and the kidney have provided insight into the fate of an ingested glucose load.[63, 65, 66] The dual-isotope approach also makes it possible to quantitate the disposal of glucose molecules in plasma originating from the ingesta as opposed to endogenous molecules.

After ingestion of 100 g glucose, plasma glucose levels increase to a peak between 60 and 90 minutes usually not exceeding 170 mg/dL (9 mmol/L) and gradually return to or slightly below postabsorptive values by 3 to 4 hours. Plasma insulin concentrations follow a similar profile and average only about fourfold the basal values (40 μU/mL, 240 pmol/L) during this period. Plasma glucagon concentrations change in reciprocal pattern and are generally suppressed about 50% during the interval.

It is worth re-emphasizing that changes in plasma glucose concentrations occur as a result of the relative changes in rates of release and removal of glucose. During the first 80 to 100 minutes, rates of glucose release into the systemic circulation exceed rates of removal, and consequently plasma glucose levels increase. Rates of glucose removal from plasma parallel those of glucose release but are shifted in time. After about 80 to 100 minutes, rates of removal exceed rates of glucose release, and consequently plasma glucose concentrations decrease. Rates of glucose release into plasma represent the sum of glucose escaping first-pass splanchnic (hepatic) extraction and the residual release of endogenous glucose by the liver and kidney. Release of ingested glucose into the systemic circulation is detected as early as 15 minutes, reaches a peak at 80 to 120 minutes, and gradually decreases thereafter. Release of endogenous glucose by the liver decreases rapidly and is suppressed nearly 80% during the 4- to 5-hour postprandial period. In contrast, endogenous renal glucose release is not suppressed and actually increases. Teleologically, this arrangement would permit more complete suppression of hepatic glucose release and facilitate more efficient glycogen replenishment.[67]

Disposal of a hypothetic 100-g oral glucose load is shown in Figure 66–3. About a third of the ingested glucose is initially extracted by splanchnic tissues and can presumably be attributed to hepatic glycogen formation.[65] Of the remaining glucose that enters the systemic circulation, skeletal muscle (35%–45%), brain (~20%–30%), kidney (10%–15%), and adipose tissue (5%–10%) are quantitatively the most important and account for over 90% of the initial posthepatic glucose disposal.[67]

Normally, therefore, three factors predominate in regulating postprandial glucose excursions: suppression of endogenous glucose release, initial hepatic glucose extraction, and posthepatic glucose uptake. Suppression of endogenous glucose release and initial hepatic glucose extraction are largely dependent on the coordinated reciprocal secretion of insulin and glucagon, in particular, the early release of insulin.[68] Seventy percent to 80% of posthepatic glucose uptake occurs in insulin-sensitive tissues, and it can be readily concluded that insulin plays a major role in this process via its action to increase glucose transport; for example, skeletal muscle glucose fractional extraction,

an index of the efficiency of glucose uptake, increases about threefold whereas glucose fractional extraction by the brain, an insulin-sensitive tissue, actually decreases.

Another factor to be considered, which may represent an indirect effect of insulin, is postprandial suppression of lipolysis with a consequent decrease in circulating free fatty acid concentrations. This response would decrease the availability of a promoter of hepatic glucose release and a competitor to glucose as a metabolic fuel. For example, recent studies using nuclear magnetic resonance to measure glycogen accumulation in skeletal muscle have demonstrated that during the initial 2 hours after meal ingestion when skeletal muscle glucose is markedly increased, no net accumulation of glycogen occurs in skeletal muscle.[69] This finding has been attributed to the use of the glucose taken up as an oxidative fuel in place of free fatty acids. Moreover, prevention of the normal postprandial decrease in plasma free fatty acids has been shown to reduce postprandial suppression of endogenous glucose release.[70]

Re-establishment of postabsorptive conditions after meal ingestion requires reversal of the repression of hepatic glucose release and the return of increased rates of renal glucose release and peripheral tissue glucose removal. Such an adjustment involves not only a decrease in insulin secretion but also increases in the secretion of glucagon and other counterregulatory hormones.[71] Failure of these changes to occur can result in postprandial hypoglycemia. Venous plasma glucose levels often decrease below fasting values and sometimes to values as low as 36 mg/dL (2.0 mmol/L) after the ingestion of glucose such as during an OGTT; the hypoglycemia is often asymptomatic and is not observed when the same individuals ingest a meal.[72] Thus the OGTT should *never* be used in the workup of hypoglycemia. Postprandial hypoglycemia can occur with most of the pathologic conditions that cause fasting hypoglycemia. However, hypoglycemia observed solely after meal ingestion is generally seen only in individuals who have had gastric surgery or small bowel disease or in those taking medications that affect glucose counterregulation.

GLUCOSE COUNTERREGULATION

Glucose counterregulation refers to the sum of the body's defense mechanisms that prevent hypoglycemia from occurring and restore euglycemia should hypoglycemia occur. Similar processes appear to be involved in the postprandial and postabsorptive states and can largely be accounted for by suppression of insulin secretion and stimulation of the release of counterregulatory hormones.[71] Our knowledge of counterregulation has accumulated over the past 25 years through studies in which pharmacologic blockade of the secretion or action of individual counterregulatory hormones has been produced during standardized insulin-induced hypoglycemia,[73] and alterations have been found in diabetes mellitus, insulinoma, and aging.

Insulin administration results in suppression of both hepatic and renal glucose release[74, 75] and stimulation of glucose uptake. As plasma glucose levels decrease, endogenous secretion of insulin is suppressed (as manifested by a decrease in circulating C peptide levels), and an increase is noted in the secretion of counterregulatory hormones (glucagon, epinephrine, growth hormone, and cortisol) and the activity of the autonomic nervous system (as manifested by increases in circulating norepinephrine and pancreatic polypeptide levels).[76] Depending on the dose of insulin administered, these increases in counterregulatory hormone release can be sufficient to prevent a further decrease in plasma glucose and restore euglycemia. This effect is mainly brought about by the actions of glucagon and epinephrine to derepress and increase the release of glucose into the circulation. With greater doses of insulin, plasma glucose levels decrease more, and recovery is more prolonged and now includes the effects of epinephrine, growth hormone, and cortisol to counteract the actions of insulin to increase tissue glucose uptake. As indicated earlier, a characteristic hierarchy of responses is seen to decrease in plasma glucose levels. Of all the counterregulatory hormones, glucagon is the most important, closely followed by epinephrine.[77] Patients with type 1 diabetes or pancreatectomized individuals lacking a glucagon response are up to 25 times more prone to severe hypoglycemia than are those with normal gluca-

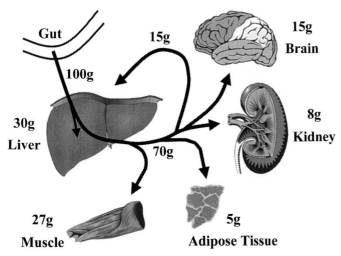

FIGURE 66–3. *Postprandial glucose disposal. Of 100 g glucose ingested, about 30% is taken up by the liver and 70% is released into the systemic circulation. Of this 70 g, 15 g (~20%) is extracted by the liver, 15 g (~20%) is taken up by the brain, 27 g (~40%) is taken up by skeletal muscle, and the remaining 20% is taken up by kidney, adipose tissue, skin, and blood cells.*

gon responses.[78] Glucagon acts to increase hepatic glucose release, initially via glycogenolysis and later mainly via gluconeogenesis.[79] Catecholamines act by several mechanisms: (1) increasing hepatic glycogenolysis, (2) directly increasing renal gluconeogenesis, (3) inhibiting insulin-stimulated glucose uptake as well as insulin release, and (4) augmenting lipolysis, which via increases in circulating free fatty acids can also impair tissue glucose uptake and stimulate gluconeogenesis.[80–82] Growth hormone and cortisol have late effects of suppressing insulin-mediated tissue glucose uptake and augmenting release of glucose into the circulation.[77, 83] Lack of these late effects is clinically important as evidenced by the propensity of hypopituitary patients to the development of hypoglycemia (see below).

HYPOGLYCEMIC DISORDERS IN THE ADULT

Drug-Induced Hypoglycemia

Drugs, as a result of unintentional and intentional overdoses (e.g., insulin, sulfonylureas) or toxic reactions causing hepatic failure (acetaminophen) or malfunction (alcohol), are probably the most common cause of hypoglycemia (Table 66–2). Seltzer has reviewed all cases of severe drug-induced hypoglycemia reported from 1940 through 1988.[84] Insulin, sulfonylureas, and alcohol alone or in combination accounted for over 70% of cases. The incidence of severe hypoglycemia (defined as that resulting in coma or requiring external assistance) from insulin treatment in patients with type 1 diabetes being managed to achieve optimal glycemic control in the Diabetes Control and Complications Trial averaged about 60 episodes per 100 patient-years.[85] A similar incidence has been reported in comparably well controlled patients with type 2 diabetes being treated with insulin.[86] However, in other studies the incidence has been considerably lower.[87, 88] The incidence

TABLE 66–2. Drug-Induced Hypoglycemia

Drugs capable of causing hypoglycemia by themselves
  Antidiabetes drugs
    Insulin
    Sulfonylureas
    Benzoic acid derivatives (meglitinide)
  Other
    Alcohol
    Salicylates
    Propranolol
    Pentamidine
    Sulfonamides
    Vacor rodenticide
    Quinine
    Propoxyphene
    Para-aminobenzoic acid
    Perhexiline
Drugs probably causing hypoglycemia only in combination with insulin/
  sulfonylurea/benzoic acid derivatives
  Biguanides
  Angiotensin-converting enzyme
  Phenylbutazone
  Lidocaine
  Warfarin (Coumadin)
  Ranitidine, cimetidine
  Doxepin
  Danazol
  Azopropazone
  Oxytetracycline
  Clofibrate, benzofibrate
  Colchicine
  Ketoconazole
  Chloramphenicol
  Haloperidol
  Monoamine oxidase inhibitors
  Thalidomide
  Orphenadrine
  Selegiline

of severe hypoglycemia as a result of sulfonylurea stimulation of insulin secretion in patients with type 2 diabetes is approximately 1.5 cases per 100 patient-years.[89]

Alcohol may be a more common cause of severe hypoglycemia in the United States than sulfonylureas,[84] although exact statistics are lacking. It can cause hypoglycemia in overnight fasting normal volunteers,[90, 91] with plasma glucose values as low as 5 mg/dL (0.3 mmol/L)[92] and mortality rates ranging from 10% in adults to 25% in children.[93] In a series of deaths caused by hypoglycemia, alcohol was the most common etiologic agent.[94] The most common situation is a glycogen-depleted state, such as occurs in an individual who drinks after a considerable fast or who drinks and then fasts. In the latter situation blood alcohol levels may be low or undetectable.

Alcohol induces hypoglycemia by inhibiting gluconeogenesis[92]; as little as 50 g may be sufficient.[93, 95] Its mechanism of action is complex, with evidence of impaired counterregulatory hormone responses[91] and impaired uptake of gluconeogenic precursors,[96] but the predominantly accepted mechanism is its inhibition of the gluconeogenic process stemming from an increased reduced nicotinamide adenine dinucleotide (NADH)/NAD ratio as a result of the oxidation of alcohol to acetaldehyde and acetate, thus reducing the ability of the liver and kidney to oxidize lactate and glutamate to pyruvate and α-ketoglutarate, respectively.[97–99] Although plasma insulin levels are appropriately suppressed in this condition, because of this inhibition of gluconeogenesis, glucagon and catecholamines are ineffective in increasing glucose release and raising plasma glucose levels.[79] Thus in a patient with suspected alcohol-induced hypoglycemia, oral or intravenous glucose is the treatment of choice.

Only about 10% of the reported cases of drug-induced hypoglycemia have occurred without concomitant insulin, sulfonylurea, or alcohol.[100] Of these, propranolol,[101] sulfonamides,[102] and salicylates[84] have been most frequently reported. Propranolol and other nonselective β-blockers decrease the ability of the liver and kidney to increase their release of glucose,[81, 82] enhance peripheral insulin sensitivity,[103] and mask symptoms of impending hypoglycemia. Salicylates may act by inhibiting hepatic glucose release and increasing insulin secretion, although their exact mechanism remains to be determined.[104] Sulfonamides probably act by stimulating insulin release similar to sulfonylureas. Angiotensin-converting enzyme inhibitors[105–107] and pentamidine[105, 108, 109] are being reported more frequently, with increases in their use in diabetic subjects and AIDS patients, respectively. Angiotensin-converting enzyme inhibitors may increase tissue insulin sensitivity[110] and can decrease the degradation of bradykinin, which has certain insulin-mimetic actions.[111] Pentamidine is cytotoxic to pancreatic β cells, and hypoglycemia occurs with the release of insulin from the degenerating cells, often with subsequent permanent diabetes mellitus.[109] Many of the drugs listed in Table 66–1 have been reported to cause hypoglycemia only in association with the use of antidiabetic medications or have been the subject of isolated case reports and their etiologic significance remains to be established. However, their use in a patient with otherwise unexplained hypoglycemia should be discontinued whenever possible.

Risk factors for insulin-induced hypoglycemia include errors in dosage, skipped or delayed meals, uncompensated physical activity, hypoglycemia unawareness, aging, the duration of diabetes, the degree of glycemic control, concomitant medications (e.g., β-blockers), and associated disorders, such as renal failure.[88] Aging and the duration of diabetes are believed to exert their effect mainly as a consequence of deterioration in counterregulatory defense mechanisms (e.g., loss of glucagon response, autonomic neuropathy). In addition to these factors, the frequency of sulfonylurea- and benzoic acid derivative–induced hypoglycemia depends on the particular sulfonylurea used, the highest incidence being associated with the longest acting and most potent (e.g., glyburide > chlorpropamide > glipizide; glimepiride > meglitinide).[112, 113] For other drugs implicated in causing hypoglycemia, restricted food intake, age, hepatic disease, and renal disease are often involved. Therefore, one of the first steps in the workup of a patient suspected of having hypoglycemia is to document medications, which includes actually checking that pills match prescriptions because errors can be made in filling prescriptions.[114, 115]

Sepsis, Trauma, and Burns

Severe infection and trauma elicit physiologic responses[116] (sodium and water retention with an expanded extracellular space, tachycardia, increased cardiac output, increased pulmonary ventilation, fever, and activation of various inflammatory processes) that result in an insulin-resistant hypermetabolic state characterized by increased resting energy expenditure, excessive fat and protein catabolism, negative nitrogen balance, increased glucose turnover, and progressive loss of body cell mass.[117, 118] Increases in the secretion of classic stress hormones (glucagon, epinephrine, growth hormone, and cortisol), activation of the sympathetic nervous system, various cytokines (tumor necrosis factor-α, interleukin-2, and interleukin-6), oxygen free radicals, prostanoids, leukotrienes, and endothelins are involved in mediating these responses.[116, 119–122] The net effect of these changes is to shift glucose utilization toward non–insulin-sensitive tissues (e.g., inflammatory cells) with a greater proportionate use of anaerobic glycolysis, a less energetically efficient pathway than oxidative phosphorylation.[123]

Hypoglycemia, if it occurs, usually results from failure of the liver and kidney to compensate for increased glucose utilization; it rarely develops in trauma or burn patients in the absence of infection[124] but, when it occurs, is usually associated with hypotension and acidosis.[125]

Initially the response to the stress of infection is an increase in glucose turnover, with glucose production often exceeding glucose utilization and resulting in mild hyperglycemia. This response involves increases in both glycogenolysis and gluconeogenesis and is largely mediated by glucagon[126] because adrenergic blockade has no effect on glucose turnover.[127] As the infection worsens, increased release of endotoxin and its derivatives, complement activation, endoperoxide activation, and release of endogenous inflammatory mediators (tumor necrosis factor-α, interleukins, and other monokines) compromise cardiovascular integrity and cause central venous pooling, inadequate tissue perfusion, and microvascular protein transudation.[128] At this stage a decrease in splanchnic and renal blood flow occurs. Despite concomitantly reduced peripheral tissue perfusion, glucose utilization is increased.[129–131] Decreased tissue oxygenation causes increased anaerobic glycolysis, which perpetuates the increased glucose utilization because anaerobic glycolysis is a less energetically efficient pathway than oxidative phosphorylation is. Increased lactate release by peripheral tissues exceeds increases in lactate uptake by the liver and kidney and results in lactic acidosis.[132, 133]

The inability of glucose release to keep pace with increased tissue demands is due to a failure of gluconeogenesis. Hepatic glycogen stores are rapidly exhausted and consequently glucose release becomes solely dependent on gluconeogenesis. At this point glucose release is largely driven by activation of the sympathetic nervous system and hypercortisolemia.[134, 135] Although splanchnic and renal blood flow is reduced, the impaired gluconeogenesis cannot be ascribed to decreased substrate delivery or uptake or to decreased concentrations of counter-regulatory stress hormones.[128] Even after in situ perfusion of the liver and kidneys to ensure the presence of adequate oxygen and precursors, animals in experimental endotoxin shock exhibit diminished gluconeogenesis.[136] In vivo, hormonal stimulation of glucose production is reduced as much as 50%.[134, 137, 138] Factors such as acidosis (which inhibits hepatic gluconeogenesis), increased intracellular calcium (which impairs mitochondrial function and inhibits gluconeogenic enzymes), and siphoning of available energy from gluconeogenesis to support ion transport may be involved.

Appropriate management entails (1) treatment of the underlying infection, (2) restoration of normal peripheral perfusion, and (3) glucose infusion to satisfy tissue demands.

Cardiac Failure

Spontaneous hypoglycemia can occur with severe heart failure[139–141]; it is rare in adults but not uncommon in infants and children,[142] in whom reduced hepatic glycogen levels (but normal phosphorylase and glucose-6-phosphatase activity) have been found in liver biopsy specimens and attributed to the poor dietary intake and gastrointestinal malabsorption present in cardiac failure. This predilection of young

children to the development of hypoglycemia under these conditions may relate to immaturity of gluconeogenic processes and a limited supply of gluconeogenic precursors (i.e., glycerol and amino acids because of limited adipose tissue and muscle mass, respectively).

Mellinkoff and Tumulty first described the hypoglycemia of cardiac failure and attributed it to associated hepatic disease.[143] However, chronic lung disease with right and left heart failure is seen in most patients.[141] Thus hypoxemia and low cardiac output may overcome the large capacity of the liver to extract oxygen. Marks and Rose postulated that decreased availability of oxygen would suppress gluconeogenesis by increasing hepatic anaerobic glycolysis (Pasteur effect) and lactate production and thereby result in a decreased NAD/NADH ratio.[144] This decreased ratio could compromise gluconeogenesis because NAD is an essential cofactor for several of the enzymatic steps of gluconeogenesis. This attractive hypothesis could explain the association between hypoglycemia and the lactic acidosis of cardiac[145] and liver[146] disease, as well as the hypoglycemia accompanying other conditions associated with tissue anoxia, such as sepsis and shock.[125] Low cardiac output would be expected to limit substrate delivery to the kidneys. In addition to a reduced capacity to produce glucose, increased glucose utilization from increased anaerobic glycolysis and increased energy demands from labored breathing and malnutrition (anorexia) are probably additionally important factors. At the present time, no evidence indicates that abnormal counterregulatory hormone responses play a role in the pathogenesis of the hypoglycemia associated with these conditions.

Renal and Hepatic Disease: General Considerations

The liver and kidneys are the only organs capable of releasing glucose into the circulation inasmuch as other tissues generally lack or have minimal amounts of the enzyme glucose-6-phosphatase. Consequently it would not be surprising that patients with hepatic or renal disease should be prone to hypoglycemia. Nevertheless, it is uncommon for hypoglycemia to occur simply as a result of loss of mass or function of these organs, and when it does occur, the etiology is usually multifactorial.[92, 147] The large capacities of these organs to release glucose into the circulation and their ability to compensate for each other's shortcomings appear to provide an explanation for this phenomenon.

Normally the liver accounts for 80% to 85% of all glucose released into the circulation; it can increase its output (initially mainly by glycogenolysis, later by gluconeogenesis) over a sustained period by twofold to threefold (at least for several days as exemplified by burn patients[134]). Thus hypoglycemia with an appropriate compensatory increase in hepatic glucose release would be unlikely to develop in anephric individuals because the kidney normally contributes only 15% to 20% of all glucose released into the circulation. On the other hand, the kidney can also increase its output over a prolonged period by twofold to threefold as exemplified in humans fasted for several weeks.[148] Animal studies indicate that the kidney can acutely increase its output to compensate for decreased hepatic glucose release.[149, 150] Indeed, it has recently been reported that during the anhepatic phase of human liver transplantation, the kidney can maintain normoglycemia without a need for exogenous glucose.[151] Thus hypoglycemia would be unlikely to develop in patients with hepatic disease until the liver's capacity to release glucose were reduced beyond the ability of the kidney to compensate. In fact, animal studies indicate that more than 80% of the liver must be removed for hypoglycemia to occur.[152]

Liver Disease

Although hypoglycemia has been associated with a wide range of liver diseases (hepatocellular carcinoma, cirrhosis, fatty metamorphosis, and toxic and infectious hepatitis, cholangitis, and biliary obstruction), its occurrence is actually quite uncommon in the absence of other complicating factors (i.e., infection).[92, 144] For example, Zimmerman et al. found fasting hypoglycemia levels of 60 mg/dL (3.3 mmol/L) or less in only 6 of 269 patients with a variety of liver diseases.[153] As indicated earlier, this low figure probably results from the large capacity of the liver for gluconeogenesis and the ability of the kidney to compensate.[149, 150, 154] In humans the insult to hepatic function must be acute, or the loss of parenchyma must be widespread. Felig et al. found that about 25% (4 of 15) of patients with acute viral hepatitis had a fasting blood glucose level less than 50 mg/dL (2.8 mmol/L).[155] In chronic liver disease associated with hypoglycemia, additional factors are usually involved, such as malnutrition and infection. A 50% incidence of hypoglycemia was found in patients with liver disease associated with sepsis and circulatory collapse.[156, 157] In such situations liver function tests may not parallel the severity of hypoglycemia. Infiltrative diseases such as metastatic disease, amyloidosis, sarcoidosis, and hemachromatosis rarely replace sufficient parenchyma to cause hypoglycemia.[158]

The hypoglycemia associated with liver disease may be viewed to result from failure of the kidney to compensate for a reduction in hepatic glucose output to maintain an adequate output of glucose. In various liver diseases the ability of the liver to store glycogen and activate gluconeogenesis may be impaired markedly. Thus in patients with viral hepatitis,[155] the hyperglycemic response to glucagon, a potent stimulator of glycogenolysis, was impaired, and the usual glucagon-mediated decrease in the gluconeogenic precursors glycine and alanine was reduced. Sepsis and anoxia may impair the ability of the kidney to compensate in the face of increased energy demands. Hyperinsulinemia often accompanies hepatic disease as a consequence of decreased insulin degradation by the liver,[159] but the hypoglycemia of hepatic disease is almost always accompanied by appropriate suppression of plasma insulin concentrations.[155] Likewise, little evidence has been found to implicate overproduction of insulin-like growth factors (IGFs) by the liver. Gorden et al. reported 1 patient with hemangiopericytoma of the liver in their series of 52 patients with extrapancreatic tumors, hypoglycemia, and IGFs, but no excessive IGFs were associated with primary hepatocellular carcinoma, the hepatic neoplasm most frequently associated with hypoglycemia.[160]

Renal Disease

Except in infants, hypoglycemia rarely occurs with acute renal failure. However, with chronic renal failure, hypoglycemia is not uncommon in adult patients. It may occur as an isolated event or be repetitive. In general, neuroglycopenia rather than autonomic symptoms predominate.[147]

Although it has long been recognized that uremia reduced the insulin requirement in diabetic humans,[161] it was not until 1970 that Block and Rubenstein reported three diabetic patients with renal failure who had suffered severe hypoglycemia after insulin and sulfonylurea therapy had been stopped.[162] Shortly afterward, spontaneous hypoglycemia associated with renal failure was described in nondiabetic patients,[163–166] with an incidence of 1% to 3% in two large studies.[166, 167]

The etiology of the renal hypoglycemia is complex.[147, 168] Many factors predispose uremic patients to hypoglycemia, including altered drug metabolism, malnutrition, infection, dialysis, increased insulin sensitivity, associated hepatic and cardiac disease, and impaired renal and hepatic glucose release. Drugs are probably the most common immediate cause. Any drug that can cause hypoglycemia is more likely to do so in a uremic patient because of a prolonged half-life (e.g., insulin, certain sulfonylureas, especially chlorpropamide) or decreased protein binding secondary to hypoalbuminuria.[169] Although hypoglycemia occurs in nondiabetic as well as diabetic patients with renal failure, it is more likely to occur in the latter because of the use of hypoglycemic agents and because patients with long-standing diabetes have autonomic neuropathy and defects in glucose counterregulation. Most patients have been malnourished, although it has been reported in well-nourished patients.[164] Malnutrition secondary to anorexia or vomiting, which can reduce hepatic glycogen stores and the availability of gluconeogenic precursors, is a common feature increasing the risk for hypoglycemia.[170] Consistent with this finding is the low rate of glucose appearance and conversion of the gluconeogenic precursor alanine to glucose in a uremic patient studied by Garber et al.[171] In that patient, the plasma concentration and turnover rate of alanine were both reduced, which led to speculation that reduced

availability of gluconeogenic substrates was responsible for the hypoglycemia. Because alanine is not a renal gluconeogenic precursor, impaired hepatic compensation is implied. However, other investigators were unable to increase the plasma glucose concentration in a similarly uremic patient with administration of the gluconeogenic precursors alanine and glycerol and concluded that it was not a deficiency in gluconeogenic substrate but rather suppression of gluconeogenesis by a uremic toxin, perhaps simply acidosis.[166]

Fatal hypoglycemia can occur with either peritoneal dialysis or hemodialysis when high glucose-containing dialysate is used because of exaggerated insulin release in conjunction with impaired renal insulin degradation.[172] Other factors such as the use of glucose-deficient solutions in diabetic patients and loss of alanine during hemodialysis may contribute to the development of hypoglycemia.[173]

Although the use of glucose-lowering dialysis and associated conditions that might impair the release of glucose are usually present in uremic patients who become hypoglycemic, there are still a fair number of well-documented cases in which hypoglycemia has been attributed solely to the uremic condition.[162, 164–166, 171, 174–179] These cases suggest that renal failure per se predisposes to the development of hypoglycemia. Most evidence points to diminished glucose release rather than increased glucose utilization. Impaired glycogenolytic responses to exogenous glucagon,[164, 180] gluconeogenesis in response to infused alanine, glycerol, and galactose,[166] reduced plasma glucagon responses during hypoglycemia,[181] increased insulin sensitivity,[182] and alanine deficiency have all been reported. Malnutrition and acidosis should diminish hepatic glycogenolytic and gluconeogenic potential.[140, 174, 176, 183, 184] The expected compensatory increase in renal gluconeogenesis in response to acidosis would be compromised by loss of renal mass and exacerbated by inappropriate plasma insulin levels caused by reduced renal insulin degradation.

Counterregulatory Hormone Deficiencies

As indicated earlier, glucagon, catecholamines, growth hormone, and cortisol are the key glucose counterregulatory hormones. Deficiencies in the release of each of these hormones (and thyroid hormone[185]) may lead to hypoglycemia because of failure to maintain sufficient rates of glucose release into the circulation. However, except in patients with long-standing diabetes mellitus, their deficiency is rarely a cause of hypoglycemia because of two factors[186]: first, the uncommon occurrence (rare in some cases) of deficiencies of these hormones, and second, the fact that to a large extent a deficiency of one hormone may be compensated for by actions of other hormones, such as in the case of patients with long-standing type 1 diabetes and pancreatectomized individuals, in whom catecholamines mainly compensate for deficient glucagon secretion.

Glucagon Deficiency

Prevention of glucagon responses during insulin-induced hypoglycemia results in greater and more prolonged hypoglycemia.[73] Pancreatectomized individuals, patients with long-standing type 1 diabetes, and those in whom insulin-requiring diabetes develops as a result of chronic pancreatitis are glucagon deficient[187] and quite prone to severe hypoglycemia during treatment of their diabetes.[78] Because of the incidence of these disorders, lack of glucagon probably represents the most common counterregulatory hormone deficiency. Otherwise, however, the condition is extremely rare, with only two poorly substantiated cases of neonatal hypoglycemia[188, 189] and two cases in adults.[190, 191]

Catecholamine Deficiency

Patients with long-standing type 1 diabetes mellitus, adrenalectomized individuals, and those with autonomic neuropathy have impaired catecholamine responses during insulin-induced hypoglycemia,[73, 192, 193] but their increased risk for hypoglycemia may be compensated for by increases in the secretion of other counterregulatory hormones, in particular, glucagon.[194] Subtle defects in recovery from hypoglycemia have been demonstrated when such compensatory increases have been experimentally prevented.[80] However, if glucagon responses to hypoglycemia are simultaneously impaired (i.e., type 1 diabetic patient), the risk for hypoglycemia markedly increased.[78]

Several cases of neonatal ketotic hypoglycemia and one case in a 5-year-old boy have been attributed to epinephrine deficiency on the basis of low urinary epinephrine excretion.[195, 196] No cases of hypoglycemia secondary to isolated catecholamine deficiency in an adult have been reported. The hypoglycemia occurring with propranolol may relate to the drug's inhibition of lipolysis, which would reduce gluconeogenesis, an important counterregulatory process, and would promote increased glucose clearance by peripheral tissues.[81]

Nevertheless, it is important to note that acute hypoglycemia may occur during surgical removal of a pheochromocytoma, presumably because of disinhibition of insulin release and abrupt withdrawal of the anti-insulin actions of catecholamines.[197]

Cortisol and Growth Hormone Deficiency

Although cortisol and growth hormone have been demonstrated to contribute independently to glucose counterregulation via their actions to promote glucose release and limit glucose uptake,[77, 83, 198, 199] hypoglycemia does not develop in most adults who lack these hormones. Serious hypoglycemia often develops in infants and children lacking these hormones, especially after a period of fasting or during an intercurrent illness.[199–203] In a review of 76 adults with isolated adrenocorticotropic hormone (ACTH) deficiency,[204] only 24 (~33%) had hypoglycemia. During prolonged fasting (6 days), adult growth hormone–deficient dwarfs become hypoglycemic,[205] as may hypopituitary pregnant women.[206] On the other hand, overnight fasting plasma glucose levels have been reported to be normal in glucocorticoid-withdrawn patients with primary adrenal insufficiency[207] or panhypopituitarism.[208] Acute adrenal insufficiency such as in Sheehan's syndrome can be manifested as severe hypoglycemia,[209] and autoimmune Addison's disease may be the cause of severe recurrent hypoglycemia in a patient with type 1 diabetes mellitus.[210]

It is important to be aware that malabsorption of glucocorticoids may occur in patients with bowel disease and patients treated with drugs such as bile acid sequestrants.[211]

Malnutrition and Inanition

Simple caloric restriction, even for prolonged periods, does not usually result in hypoglycemia in adults[18, 148, 212–214] because of several metabolic adaptations: as glucose release into the circulation decreases (secondary to exhaustion of hepatic glycogen stores and reduction of the availability of gluconeogenic amino acids to the liver and kidney), the brain and other tissues increase their use of free fatty acids and ketone bodies, and glycerol becomes an important gluconeogenic precursor. For example, during the Bengal famine of 1943–1945, about 6% of 400 persons sampled had blood glucose levels below 40 mg/dL (2.2 mmol/L).[215] Nevertheless, in unusual conditions (i.e., anorexia nervosa,[216–219] kwashiorkor,[220] muscular atrophies[221]) hypoglycemia may occur. In these instances, preexisting malnutrition, which might limit the availability of gluconeogenic precursors (glycerol from adipose tissue and amino acids from muscle), predisposes to the development of hypoglycemia during fasting.[222] More commonly, however, poor nutrition is an important contributing factor to the development of hypoglycemia, such as in renal failure, sepsis, severe heart failure, and liver disease.

Autoimmune Hypoglycemia

Of the two types of autoimmune hypoglycemia, one is due to autoantibodies against the insulin receptor, and the other is due to autoantibodies against insulin itself in individuals who have never received exogenous insulin. Both are rare and can produce fasting as well as postprandial reactive hypoglycemia—primarily the former.[223–227]

Anti–Insulin Receptor Antibodies

Fewer than 20 patients have been reported in whom hypoglycemia developed as a result of antibodies directed against the insulin receptor. These antibodies act as agonists and produce hypoglycemia the same way that insulin does. Most of the patients have had evidence of other conditions associated with altered immunity (systemic lupus erythematosus, scleroderma, primary biliary cirrhosis, immune thrombocytopenic purpura, Hashimoto's thyroiditis, and Hodgkin's lymphoma).[227] Some patients have had severe insulin resistance as a result of the antibodies blocking the insulin receptor before the antibodies became agonists. Patients with this condition have low circulating insulin and C peptide levels, normal IGF-1, and appropriate counterregulatory hormone responses.

Although experience is limited, antibody titers generally decrease over time and remission eventually occurs in most patients. However, because of the severity of the hypoglycemia, aggressive treatment is indicated. High-dose glucocorticoids,[228, 229] plasmapheresis,[230] and alkylating agents[231] have all been tried with variable success.

Anti–Insulin Antibody Hypoglycemia

Since 1970 approximately 200 cases of anti–insulin antibody hypoglycemia have been reported, with nearly 90% in Japanese patients.[224] Associated autoimmune disorders and plasma cell dyscrasias are common (Graves' disease, rheumatoid arthritis, polymyositis, systemic lupus erythematosus). The use of certain drugs (hydralazine, procainamide, penicillamine, interferon-α, methimazole) has been implicated in initiating the syndrome.[227]

Postprandial hypoglycemia is more common with this syndrome than is fasting hypoglycemia. Circulating insulin levels are increased and C peptide levels may not be suppressed as they are in patients taking insulin surreptitiously. The hypoglycemia occurs because dissociation of insulin from the antibodies causes prolonged hyperinsulinemia. Unlike the other syndrome of autoimmune hypoglycemia, the course of this condition is benign and self-limited, with remission usually occurring within a year. Simple interventions such as frequent small meals with a low content of simple sugars often suffice.

Pregnancy

Despite a decrease in insulin sensitivity and an increase in glucose turnover to accommodate the needs of the fetus, fasting plasma glucose levels are normally 10% to 15% lower during the third trimester of pregnancy.[232, 233] Nevertheless, a great number of metabolic changes occur during pregnancy to make a woman more vulnerable to hypoglycemia.[234] Any condition that can cause hypoglycemia in a nonpregnant woman can do it in a pregnant woman. In addition to insulinoma,[235] non–islet cell tumors,[236] severe infection,[237] poor nutrition,[238] drug-induced sources (i.e., insulin in diabetic patients), and a condition called the HELLP syndrome (characterized by hemolysis, elevated liver enzymes, and a low platelet count) may cause hypoglycemia as a result of fulminating hepatic dysfunction.[239–241]

Exercise

Hypoglycemia may develop after prolonged strenuous exercise and has been reported in marathon runners,[242] in normal volunteers after exercise on a bicycle ergometer for 3 hours at 56% of maximal capacity,[243] and in a healthy male subject taking a β-blocker after skiing 15 km in 2 hours.[244] Although in the latter instance coma developed, most instances of exercise-associated hypoglycemia are asymptomatic, self-limited, and readily reversed by carbohydrate.[214]

The increased fuel demands of the working muscle necessitate compensatory metabolic processes in the liver and kidney.[245–248] Changes in hepatic glycogenolysis and gluconeogenesis have been found to be closely coupled to the increase in glucose uptake by the working muscle because of the actions of the pancreatic hormones.[245] The exercise-induced increase in glucagon secretion and the concomitant decrease in insulin secretion interact to stimulate hepatic glycogenolysis, whereas the increase in hepatic gluconeogenesis is determined primarily by glucagon's action to increase hepatic gluconeogenic precursor fractional extraction and the efficiency of intrahepatic conversion to glucose. On the other hand, no evidence has shown that hepatic innervation is essential for the rise in hepatic glucose production. Epinephrine becomes important in increasing glucose production during prolonged or heavy exercise, when its levels are particularly high. It may produce this effect by directly stimulating renal glucose release, by increasing the availability of gluconeogenic precursors, and by increasing lipolysis.

It is important to recognize that hypoglycemia can occur with prolonged strenuous exercise (moderate activity in diabetic patients or in nondiabetic patients taking β-blockers) lest an unnecessary diagnostic work-up be initiated.

Factitious Hypoglycemia

Factitious hypoglycemia refers to a situation in which an individual intentionally attempts to create the impression of the presence of a hypoglycemic disorder.[5, 249, 250] It also includes diabetic individuals who falsify their self-glucose monitoring or who overdose and underdose themselves to intentionally create the impression of either better than actual glycemic control or brittle diabetes[251, 252] and in cases of child abuse.[2] Generally excluded are inadvertent sulfonylurea ingestion (see drug-induced hypoglycemia), homicides,[2] suicide attempts (of which only 97 have been reported through 1989[253, 254]), and substance abuse in which the additional use of insulin or sulfonylureas is intended to "obtain a high" rather than create the impression of a hypoglycemic disorder.[255–257] These situations may nevertheless present diagnostic challenges.

Since 1947, more than 80 cases of insulin- or sulfonylurea-induced factitious hypoglycemia have been described in the literature[249, 258–260] (Table 66–3), but the condition is probably more common than this figure would indicate because most cases go unreported. Indeed, in a survey from the United Kingdom it was estimated that 12% of cases of spontaneous hypoglycemia referred for investigation were in fact probably factitious.[267] In nearly all instances the individuals have had diabetes, been a relative, spouse, or friend of a diabetic patient, or were in the medical or paramedical profession. Thus factitious hypoglycemia should be suspected in individuals or their relatives who have unexplained hypoglycemia and knowledge of and/or access to insulin or sulfonylureas. Such patients have generally been healthy women younger than 50 years and often have an underlying psychological disorder. Because the main differential diagnosis is insulinoma, it is important to consider this condition as a possible cause of unexplained hypoglycemia to avoid unnecessary laboratory work-up, which such patients have undergone.

In the past, autoimmune hypoglycemia was a possibility because of the presence of insulin antibodies in patients taking animal or impure insulin. Currently, the use of human insulin does not generally result in antibody production, so autoimmune hypoglycemia is no longer a consideration. Because the main differential is insulinoma, most patients with this condition will undergo a 72-hour fast. Those in whom

TABLE 66–3. Factitious Insulin- and Sulfonylurea-Induced Hypoglycemia

Hypoglycemia	No. of Cases
Insulin induced	
Diabetics[249, 251, 258, 259, 261–264]	39
Nondiabetics[249, 254, 258]	30
Sulfonylurea induced	
Diabetics[249, 260]	3
Nondiabetics[249, 260, 265, 266]	12
Total	84

TABLE 66–4. Neoplasms Associated with Hypoglycemia

Mesenchymal
  Mesothelioma
  Fibrosarcoma
  Rhabdomyosarcoma
  Leiomyosarcoma
  Liposarcoma
  Hemangiopericytoma
Carcinomas
  Hepatic: hepatoma, biliary carcinoma
  Adrenocortical carcinoma
  Genitourinary: hypernephroma, Wilms' tumor, prostate carcinoma
  Reproductive: cervical carcinoma, breast carcinoma
Neurologic and neuroendocrine tumors
  Pheochromocytoma
  Carcinoid tumor
  Neurofibroma
Hematologic
  Leukemias
  Lymphoma
  Myeloma

hypoglycemia develops as a result of surreptitious insulin injection will have inappropriate plasma insulin levels and a suppressed plasma C peptide level (because of inhibition of endogenous insulin secretion). This finding is diagnostic. Patients taking sulfonylureas will have inappropriate plasma insulin and C peptide levels because of stimulation of endogenous insulin secretion, and this pattern will mimic that seen in insulinoma patients. However, these conditions can be distinguished by a positive urine or plasma assay for sulfonylureas. It should be remembered that nonsulfonylurea insulin secretagogues (e.g., meglitinide) are now available for the treatment of diabetes mellitus and their assay needs to be included, although no cases of factitious hypoglycemia from their ingestion have been reported to date.

Many patients documented biochemically to have self-induced hypoglycemia will adamantly deny doing so when confronted with the evidence. Nevertheless, psychologic counseling is warranted to prevent subsequent episodes with other physicians or substitution of other potentially self-destructive behavior.[250]

Non–Islet Cell Tumors

The development of hypoglycemia in a patient with a non–islet cell tumor was first reported in 1930—a mediastinal fibrosarcoma.[268] Since that time it has become apparent that a large variety of non–islet cell tumors are associated with hypoglycemia[160, 236, 269–290] (Table 66–4).

Tumors of mesenchymal origin are the most commonly reported (115 cases up to 1979[270]) in western countries. Such tumors are generally large, slow growing, but often malignant. About one-third are retroperitoneal, one-third are intra-abdominal, and one-third are intrathoracic. In South Africa and Asia, hepatomas are the most common non–islet cell tumors associated with hypoglycemia.[278]

With one possible exception (a small cell carcinoma of the cervix),[291] ectopic production of insulin has never been convincingly demonstrated in patients with this condition.[286, 292] Characteristically, circulating plasma insulin and C peptide levels are suppressed. In some cases, hypoglycemia results mainly from increased glucose utilization by the tumor, and debulking either by surgery or radiation treatment can alleviate or ameliorate the hypoglycemia.[270, 274, 285, 289] In patients with rapidly growing hepatomas, hypoglycemia may occur as a terminal or near-terminal event, mainly because of inanition. However, in the great majority of cases, the hypoglycemia is explained by tumor production of IGF-like molecules,[276] in particular, IGF-2 and its isoforms. Excessive release of IGF-like molecules by the tumor can increase glucose utilization in tissues such as muscle,[277, 280, 290] suppress endogenous glucose production,[284, 290] and reduce or overcome the secretion of counterregulatory hormones.[236]

In most cases, the diagnosis is not difficult, and patients are generally middle-aged to elderly; the tumor is usually large and its presence is either known before the onset of hypoglycemia or can be readily found on physical examination and by ultrasonographic, computed tomographic, and nuclear magnetic resonance studies. Biochemically the hypoglycemia is associated with appropriately suppressed plasma insulin and C peptide levels and increased IGF-2 levels, as well as an increased IGF-2/IGF-1 ratio because of suppression of growth hormone secretion and hence suppressed IGF-1 release by IGF-2.

Reactive Hypoglycemia

Reactive hypoglycemia refers to hypoglycemia occurring after meals. Any condition that causes fasting hypoglycemia can also cause postprandial hypoglycemia, for example, insulinoma,[293] hypopituitarism,[294] alcohol,[91, 295] sulfonylurea ingestion, hypothyroidism,[296] growth hormone deficiency,[297] and cortisol deficiency.[296] Nevertheless, some conditions are associated with hypoglycemia only after meal ingestion. These conditions fall into five categories: alimentary, prediabetes, idiopathic, iatrogenic, and functional hypoglycemia.

Alimentary

Hypoglycemia 2 to 4 hours after meal ingestion can occur in patients who have undergone gastrectomy,[298, 299] vagotomy and pyloroplasty,[300, 301] and esophageal resection[302] and in patients with altered gastric motility,[303] peptic ulcer disease,[304, 305] and renal glycosuria.[306] Repeated episodes can lead to hypoglycemia unawareness such as occurs in insulinoma and diabetic patients, thus making interpretation of counterregulatory hormone responses difficult.[307]

The pathogenesis in most of these conditions involves rapid gastric emptying and absorption of glucose, which cause hyperglycemia and stimulation of the release of gut insulin secretagogues, both of which result in excessive secretion of insulin; the biologic actions of insulin to suppress endogenous glucose release and to stimulate tissue glucose uptake persist after the carbohydrate in the meal has been absorbed. This disequilibrium leads to postprandial hypoglycemia.[308] Recent studies have implicated glucagon-like peptide-1 as the gut insulin secretagogue most likely responsible for the excessive insulin secretion observed in most of these conditions.[302, 309, 310]

Treatment involves prevention of rapid absorption of large amounts of carbohydrate, frequent small feedings, avoidance of large amounts of simple sugars, β-adrenergic antagonists, anticholinergics, and intestinal α-glucosidase inhibitors.[306]

Prediabetes

Individuals with impaired glucose tolerance[68, 311] characteristically have a delay in early insulin release that impairs suppression of endogenous glucose release and reduces the early efficiency of glucose uptake, which leads to hyperglycemia and late hyperinsulinemia. Because absorption of glucose is not affected,[68] a disequilibrium such as that observed in patients with alimentary hypoglycemia may occur and lead to late (3–5 hours) and often asymptomatic hypoglycemia during OGTTs.[308, 312–314] How often this disequilibrium leads to symptomatic hypoglycemia after meals is not known, but the hypoglycemia is mild and treatment is directed at improvement in glucose tolerance, that is, weight loss in an obese patient and/or pharmacologic intervention with sulfonylureas, metformin, and α-glucosidase inhibitors as in patients with alimentary hypoglycemia. Use of high fiber diets, anticholinergics, doxepin, corn starch, and chromium has been proposed but with little scientific support.[315]

Idiopathic

Idiopathic/functional reactive hypoglycemia is an extremely rare condition,[303, 316, 317] in contrast to the number of patients evaluated who think that they have the condition. For this diagnosis to be made patients must demonstrate arterial/capillary (not venous) hypoglycemia (<50 mg/dL, 2.8 mmol/L) after everyday meals (not OGTTs!) in association with symptoms of hypoglycemia that are relieved by carbo-

hydrate ingestion and not have any other known cause (i.e., prior gastrointestinal surgery, peptic ulcer disease, glucose intolerance, endocrine deficiency).[318] Various etiologies have been proposed: impaired glucagon counterregulatory responses,[319–321] excessive gut glucagon-like secretion,[322] abnormal neuroendocrine regulation of insulin release,[323] and increased insulin sensitivity.[324] The disorder is not life threatening and is treated in the same manner as alimentary hypoglycemia. However, it has recently become evident that some of these patients may have an adult form of nesidioblastosis[325] (not related to mutation of the *Kir6.2* and *SUR1* genes[326]); this rare disorder, which has been referred to as noninsulinoma pancreatogenous hypoglycemia, has a 4:1 male predominance and is characterized by symptomatic hypoglycemia only occurring postprandially in association with hyperinsulinemia, increased plasma C peptide levels, and negative sulfonylurea screens.[327] The 72-hour fast is usually negative, as are conventional localization tests. The condition is a diagnostic problem in that plasma insulin and C peptide levels are often only marginally elevated during postprandial hypoglycemia. In contrast, the selective arterial calcium stimulation test is positive. Treatment entails gradient-guided partial pancreatectomy.[315]

Iatrogenic

Pathophysiologically, hypoglycemia resulting from too rapid termination of total parenteral and enteral feedings[328] and that occurring during dialysis with glucose-containing fluids[172] may be viewed as an iatrogenic form of reactive hypoglycemia in that the prolonged effects of the insulin released by these procedures causes the hypoglycemia. Knowledge of such occurrences will obviate unnecessary work-ups.

Functional (Nonhypoglycemic)

It is common practice to be referred patients who have symptoms suggesting hypoglycemia that occur 1 to 4 hours after meal ingestion. These symptoms generally include chronic fatigue, lightheadedness, shakiness, sweating, weakness, blurred vision, blackouts, headaches, depression, anxiety, confusion, and poor concentration/memory.[329] When such patients are administered a meal similar to ones that elicited the symptoms, the symptoms may be reproduced but hypoglycemia is rarely if ever observed.[72, 330] Thus in virtually all these patients the symptoms are not due to hypoglycemia,[331] but rather are better explained by psychologic profiles, which have indicated a wide variety of personality and psychiatric disorders, prominent among which are somatization, obsessive-compulsive behavior, depression, anxiety, and hysteria.[329, 332, 333]

Normally, blood glucose levels do not decrease below 50 mg/dL (2.8 mmol/L) during everyday life[318, 331]; however, during OGTTs normal volunteers can have decreases in their plasma glucose level below 30 mg/dL (1.6 mmol/L).[3] In fact, blood glucose levels below 50 mg/dL (2.8 mmol/L) will develop in about 10%, and as many as 25% will have values below 60 mg/dL (3.3 mmol/L).[3, 334]

It is thus not surprising that "hypoglycemia" may develop during OGTTs in individuals complaining of hypoglycemic symptoms in everyday life and that this test for diabetes mellitus should never be used to assess the presence of reactive hypoglycemia. The first step in the work-up of such patients is to establish Whipple's triad during everyday life, which can be done with the self-glucose monitoring readily available for diabetic patients. If established, the next step would be to reproduce the hypoglycemia with a standardized meal. If the diagnosis is confirmed, one should exclude impaired glucose tolerance or mild diabetes, renal glycosuria, peptic ulcer disease, or other gastrointestinal disorders. In the absence of these conditions and if the diagnosis is not confirmed, treatment may include psychologic consultation and the use of β-adrenergic antagonists, as well as restriction of large carbohydrate-containing meals.[306]

Insulin-Producing Islet Cell Tumors and Nesidioblastosis

Historical Perspective

Twenty-three years after the discovery of pancreatic islets by Langerhans in 1869, islet cell tumors of the pancreas were first described in autopsy specimens.[335] Although islet cell tumors, including multiple adenomas, continued to be reported over the next several decades,[336] their clinical significance was unappreciated until Harris published three cases[337] of what would now be considered dubious cases of reactive hypoglycemia[2]; struck by the similarity of the symptoms to those occurring in insulin-treated diabetic patients, he postulated that analogous to the thyroid, the islets may undersecrete as well as oversecrete its hormone, the latter causing a disorder characterized by hypoglycemia. Three years later this postulate was confirmed with the description by Wilder and his colleagues of a case of hypoglycemia caused by a malignant insulinoma.[338] The first successful surgical cure of a benign islet adenoma causing hypoglycemia was reported 2 years later.[339] In 1935 Whipple and Frantz found 75 cases in a review of the literature and added 6 surgically proven cases of their own[340]; shortly thereafter in a subsequent paper, "Whipple's triad"—low blood glucose, symptoms of hypoglycemia, relief by food—was proposed for establishing the diagnosis of a hypoglycemic disorder.[341] By 1950 nearly 400 cases had been reported.[342] Since that time several large series have provided information on the incidence and other clinical features of insulin-producing tumors.[343–348]

Nesidioblastosis, or diffuse hyperplasia of the islets, as a cause of hypoglycemia was first described by Laidlaw in 1937.[349] In contrast to multiple adenomas accompanying the multiple endocrine neoplasia type 1 (MEN-1) syndrome, the condition is characterized by diffuse, although not necessarily uniform hypertrophy and hyperplasia of islet cells (insulin- as well as glucagon- and somatostatin-producing cells), usually associated with differentiation of ductal cells into insulin-producing cells[350] (Fig. 66–4). This condition can cause hypoglycemia in infants as a result of mutations either in the sulfonylurea receptor[326] or in the anatomically linked potassium channel.[326] However, it has become apparent that the condition can occur in adults independent of these genetic mutations.[327, 351–355]

Incidence

Insulinoma is a very rare disorder and nesidioblastosis is even rarer.[354, 355] Based on a 60-year experience at the Mayo Clinic it was estimated that the incidence in Olmsted County, Minnesota, was about 8 cases per million patient-years; however, half these cases were found incidentally at autopsy.[344] Other estimates from Seattle, Washington,[356] and Auckland, New Zealand,[357] which emphasize clinically apparent cases, yield an incidence of about 1 to 2 cases per million patient-years. No accurate data are available on the incidence of nesidioblastosis, but in published series the ratio of nesidioblastosis to insulinoma has averaged 3:100.[343, 358]

Demographics

Insulinoma occurs somewhat more frequently in women than men (Table 66–5), with an average/median onset at about 45 years of age; most cases occur between the ages of 30 and 70 years. Younger patients have generally had a higher occurrence in association with MEN-1,[360] whereas carcinoma was more frequent in older patients. It is uncommon in those older than 80 years. Although a case in a patient with type 1 diabetes mellitus has yet to be documented, insulinomas have occurred in several patients with type 2 diabetes.[361–363] It is presently unclear whether nesidioblastosis in adults has any gender or age preference.

Pathophysiology

The hypoglycemia in insulinoma patients is the result of dysregulated insulin release. Normally, increased plasma insulin levels and hypoglycemia per se[364] suppress insulin release. In insulinoma patients, suppression of insulin release by insulin and hypoglycemia is abnormal, and insulin release may be described as chaotic, often not appropriately increased by hyperglycemia, and some patients may occasionally have impaired glucose tolerance. Further evidence of abnormal function of the tumorous islets are the increased proinsulin-to-insulin ratios and the decreased insulin concentration per islet relative to normal issue.[365–367]

In most insulinoma patients, hypoglycemia results because of suppression of glucose release rather than increased glucose utilization inasmuch as plasma insulin concentrations are usually only twofold to threefold above normal levels (but of course inappropriate for the plasma glucose concentration).[368] The frequently observed finding that large infusions of glucose are necessary to maintain normoglycemia in insulinoma patients is probably a result of the creation of a slight hyperglycemia that stimulates insulin release by the tumor. Suppression of β cells by either insulin released by the tumor or repetitive hypoglycemia can result in glucose intolerance or transient diabetes after removal of the tumor transiently.

Symptoms and Signs

Except in late-diagnosed malignant insulinoma cases, where an abdominal mass and signs of metastasis may be present, the physical examination is usually normal. Symptoms are the result of hypoglycemia. Patients with MEN-1 may also have symptoms as a result of hypercalcemia and the accompanying hyperparathyroidism or other excessive hormone secretions (islet production of ACTH, gastrin, vasoactive intestinal peptide).[369] Common initial symptoms of insulinoma patients are shown in Table 66–6. Because of their nonspecific and insidious nature, the time between the onset of symptoms and diagnosis is about 3 to 5 years, with the world record being 26 years.[370] Many patients had initial diagnoses of epilepsy, depression, or psychoneurosis.[347] Initially, autonomic symptoms predominate and, later, neuroglycopenic ones do. The frequency and/or severity increases over time. Insulinoma patients, like patients with diabetes

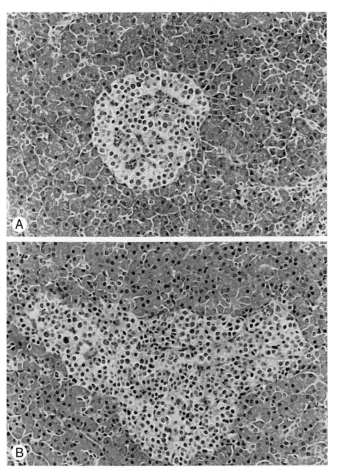

FIGURE 66–4. *A,* Normal pancreatic islet from a patient without endocrine disease (×200). *B,* Hypertrophic islet from a patient with nesidioblastosis (×200). (From Service F, Natt N, Thompson G, et al: Noninsulinoma pancreatogenous hypoglycemia: A novel syndrome of hyperinsulinemic hypoglycemia in patients independent of mutations in Kir6.2 and SUR1 genes. J Clin Endocrinol Metab 84:1582–1589, 1999. © The Endocrine Society.)

TABLE 66–5. Clinical Features of Insulinoma Patients and Their Tumors

Feature	Service et al., 1976[345]	Service et al., 1991[344]	Broder and Carter[348]	Fajans and Vinik[343]	Stefanini et al.[347]	Galbut and Markowitz[346]	Boukhman et al.[359]	Dizon et al.[358]
No.	60	224	52	82	1067	41	67	63
Gender	46% male	41% male	51% male	48% male	40% male	21% male	33% male	44% male
Age at diagnosis (yr)	47	47	52	—	45	45	46	55
Duration of symptoms (mo) before diagnosis	33	—	—	—	—*	36	46	46
Single adenoma (%)	81	87	—	76	83	79	73	79
Multiple adenomas (%)	10	7	—	13	13	19	10	2
MEN-1 associated (%)	6	8	—	9	4	2	16	8
Carcinoma (%)	9	6	100	6	16	2	10	10
Nesidioblastosis (%)	0	0	—	4	0	0	—	5
Hyperplasia (%)	0	1	—	1	0	0	7	2
Single adenoma size (cm)								
Range	0.8–8.0	—	—	0.2–5	1–5	<1–7	<1–7	0.5–5
Average	~2	—	—	~2	—	~2	1.6	~2

*Twenty percent after 5 years.
MEN, multiple endocrine neoplasia.

mellitus, can acquire the syndrome of hypoglycemia unawareness[34] characterized by diminished symptoms, counterregulatory hormone responses, and β-adrenergic sensitivity,[371] which are reversed after successful surgical cure.[34, 372] Thus it is not uncommon for an insulinoma patient with a plasma glucose concentration less than 36 mg/dL (2 mmol/L) to be completely asymptomatic. The development of this condition may make it difficult to exclude hypopituitarism as a cause of the hypoglycemia initially.

Although insulinoma has long been classified as one of the so-called fasting hypoglycemias, it is important to remember that such patients can experience hypoglycemia at any time of day, even 2 to 4 hours after a meal (Table 66–7). Only about a quarter of patients have hypoglycemia episodes solely after an overnight fast during real-life activity, and postprandial hypoglycemia has been reported to be the sole initial feature.[293] In contrast, an appreciable proportion of patients with nesidioblastosis may have symptoms only after meal ingestion.[327] Seizures tend to be more common in children, but permanent neurologic sequelae have been observed in about 7% of adults.[347] Patients often learn that eating frequently reduces episodes, and thus weight gain has been observed in about 50% of patients.[347]

Pathology

About 80% of insulinomas are due to benign single adenomas, which average about 2 cm in diameter (see Table 66–5); 10% are due to multiple benign adenomas. Diffuse hyperplasia and/or nesidi-

oblastosis is uncommon in adults (i.e., 1–2 per 100 million) and usually account for only 1% to 2%.[373, 374] Carcinomas account for about 8%. Five percent of insulinomas are associated with MEN-1, in which case the tumor is more likely to be multiple and malignant and secrete additional hormones ectopically, such as gastrin or ACTH.

Diagnosis

The diagnosis of insulinoma is readily established by the demonstration of fasting hypoglycemia (>50 mg/dL, 2.8 mmol/L), inappropriate plasma insulin (>5 μU/mL, 30 pmol/L) and C peptide (>0.25 nmol/l, 0.75 pg/mL), and a negative sulfonylurea/meglitinide blood/urine screen. A plasma proinsulin concentration greater than 5 pmol/L may be useful if plasma insulin and C peptide values are borderline, but this measurement is not usually necessary.[375, 376] Various tests have been proposed over the years to rule in or rule out the presence of an insulinoma: the intravenous tolbutamide tolerance test, the glucagon test, the leucine test, and the C peptide suppression test.[343, 377–380] All suffer from frequent false positives and false negatives and are not recommended. The "gold standard" remains the classic 72-hour fast. Hypoglycemia will develop in essentially all insulinoma patients during this test; in fact, 75% will become hypoglycemic within 24 hours.[53] The test should be conducted in a hospital under standardized and supervised conditions (Table 66–8). It is worth emphasizing that many patients with nesidioblastosis will have a normal 72-hour fast and their only biochemical abnormality will be postprandial hypoglycemia associated with an abnormal plasma insulin and C peptide level, which is why we prefer to begin our 72-hour fast with a standard meal.

The 72-Hour Fast

Successful completion of a 72-hour fast without the development of hypoglycemia effectively excludes a serious hypoglycemic disorder

TABLE 66–6. Symptoms of Insulinoma Patients

Symptom	Boukhman et al.[359] (%)	Dizon et al.[358] (%)	Galbut and Markowitz[346] (%)	Service et al., 1976[345] (%)
Confusion	70	83	54	80
Altered mental status	67	—	—	—
Abnormal behavior	54	64	44	80
Weight gain	51	39	"Nearly all"	18
Weakness/fatigue	37	56	—	—
Lightheadedness	37	58	—	—
Faintness	37	54	41	—
Drowsiness	37	31	—	—
Blurred vision	25	46	29	—
Convulsions	32	27	27	12
Amnesia	27	41	—	—
Tremor	24	24	—	—
Headaches	22	20	41	—
Sweats	18	69	39	—
Coma	16	12	41	53
Palpitations	12	12	44	—

TABLE 66–7. Time of Day/Circumstances of Hypoglycemic Episodes

Episode	Dizon et al.[358] (%)	Fajans and Vinik[343] (%)	Service et al., 1976[345] (%)	Boukhman et al.[359] (%)
Overnight, before breakfast only	—	26	30	—
Before breakfast, lunch/dinner	27	27	25	58
Only after missed meal	—	8	—	—
Only before lunch or dinner	—	29	—	—
Uncertain or other	5	10	22	32
Several hours after any meal	20	—	23	10
After exercise	27	—	7	13

TABLE 66–8. Protocol for a 72-Hour Fast

Admit before the evening meal. Discontinue all nonessential medications. Insert an intravenous line for blood sampling

Begin blood sampling (plasma glucose, insulin, C peptide) just before meal and continue every 30 min for 6 hr and thereafter every 2–3 hr

Baseline samples should also include growth hormone, cortisol, glucagon, catecholamines, IGF-1, and sulfonylureas/meglitinides

Patient may consume calorie- and caffeine-lacking liquids and should ambulate

The fast is ended at 72 hr or earlier if the patient has a plasma glucose level below 40 mg/dL (2.5 mmol/L) associated with symptoms. Do not end the fast for symptoms if hypoglycemia is not documented

At end of the fast, draw samples for all the above measurements plus an oral hypoglycemic agent screen and β-hydroxybutyrate level and an extra tube for insulin antibodies, anti–insulin receptor antibodies, and IGF-1

IGF-1, insulin-like growth factor-1.

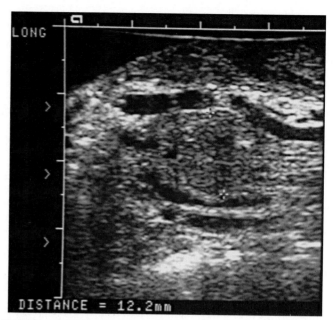

FIGURE 66–5. Intraoperative ultrasonography demonstrating an insulinoma sandwiched between the gastroduodenal artery anteriorly and the common bile duct posteriorly. (From Grant C: Surgical aspects of hyperinsulinemic hypoglycemia. Endocrinol Metab Clin North Am 28:533–554, 1999.)

except for nesidioblastosis.[381] It is recommended that the patient be hospitalized and supervised to prevent inadvertent caloric consumption or surreptitious drug administration. Admission is preferred before a standard evening meal so that the response to a meal may be assessed, as well as the response to a fast. The patient should be encouraged to be active to simulate real-life situations and prevent sedentary decreases in glucose utilization. Baseline samples for counterregulatory hormones are drawn to assess the adequacy of a response should hypoglycemia subsequently occur. Blood for a β-hydroxybutyrate level is drawn at the end of the fast to exclude the consumption of calories. Should hypoglycemia occur, anti-insulin antibodies, anti–insulin receptor antibodies, and IGF-2 levels may be useful in assessing the presence of an autoimmune cause or an occult IGF-2–secreting non–islet cell tumor. Interpretation of the results of these determinations is given in Table 66–9.

Localization

Only after the diagnosis of an insulinoma or unexplained postprandial hypoglycemia associated with inappropriate hyperinsulinemia is established biochemically should localization studies be performed. Ninety-nine percent of insulinomas occur within the pancreas. Of the rare insulinomas not found in the pancreas, most are found in the wall of the duodenum or gastrosplenic omentum.[382] They average about 2 cm in diameter and appear with equal frequency in the head, body, and tail.[346, 347] Although about 75% to 90% can be correctly identified by palpation at surgery,[359, 383] preoperative localization is generally recommended to minimize manipulation of the pancreas, shorten operative time, avoid blind partial pancreatectomy when the tumor is not palpable, and assist in reoperations when scarring and fibrosis from prior surgery make palpation difficult.[343] Computed tomography and nuclear magnetic resonance imaging can detect large tumors and stage malignant ones but yield false positives and false negatives and correctly localize tumors only 50% to 70% of the time.[343, 359, 383, 384] Celiac arteriography and transsplenic portal venous sampling have had variable results and are invasive and probably not needed.[343, 383, 384]

Currently, preoperative transabdominal ultrasonography followed by intraoperative ultrasonography (Fig. 66–5) is considered the most sensitive and specific approach and has been recommended for routine use; this approach along with palpation can detect over 95% of tumors.[359, 384–386] Recently, dual-phase spiral computed tomography has been reported to detect six of seven tumors ranging in size from 6 to 18 mm.[387] However, given the success of intraoperative ultrasonography along with palpation, it has been questioned whether extensive preoperative radiologic investigation is indicated and cost-effective.[384, 388] In patients suspected of having nesidioblastosis, the test of choice is the selective calcium infusion procedure[384, 389] because this test will confirm the diagnosis of pancreatic hyperinsulinism as the probable cause of the hypoglycemia when reliable localization procedures are negative.

Treatment

Surgery is the treatment of choice for insulinoma and nesidioblastosis.[347, 359] For patients with solitary adenomas, enucleation is curative; in cases thought to be due to a single adenoma, recurrence or lack of cure may be due to the presence of multiple adenomas. In 5% to 10% of patients the adenoma is not found; nevertheless, in such cases partial pancreatectomy can result in cure. Reoperation may still result in cure, but recurrence has been noted up to 18 years after the

TABLE 66–9. Interpretation of the Results of a 72-Hour Fast

Diagnosis	Symptoms or Signs	Plasma Glucose (mg/dL)	Plasma Insulin (μU/mL)	Plasma C Peptide (nmol/L)	Anti-Insulin Antireceptor Antibodies	IGF-1	β-Hydroxybutyrate	Oral Agent Screen
Normal	No	>40	<6	<0.2	−	N	>2.7	−
Insulinoma	Yes	<40	>6	>0.2	−	N	<2.7	−
Factitious—insulin	Yes	<40	>6	<0.2	−	N	<2.7	−
Factitious—oral agent	Yes	<40	>6	>0.2	−	N	<2.7	+
Inadvertent feeding	No	>40	<6	<0.2	−	N	>2.7	−
Non–islet cell tumor	Yes	<40	<6	<0.2	−	↑	<2.7	−
Abnormal counterregulation	Yes	<40	<6	<0.2	−	N	<2.7	−
Nonhypoglycemic disorder	Yes	>40	<6	<0.2	−	N	<2.7	−
Autoimmune disorder	Yes	<40	<6	<0.2	+	N	<2.7	−

IGF-1, insulin-like growth factor-1.

initial surgery.[344] Recurrences are more common in patients with MEN-1 (up to 20%).[344] Multiple adenomas, hyperplasia, and malignancy require more extensive surgery. Debulking of a malignant tumor is worthwhile in helping to control hypoglycemia. The major complications of surgery include acute pancreatitis (~10%–15%), wound infection (5%–10%), fistulas (10%–15%), and pseudocysts (5%) and are related to the extent of surgery. Reoperations have a greater complication rate and mortality (~15% vs. 5%). Quite commonly, transient hyperglycemia occurs and lasts up to 2 to 3 weeks because of suppression of normal islet function. Permanent diabetes mellitus may occur after partial pancreatectomy and reoperations. In patients with nesidioblastosis, gradient-directed resection can result in cure of hypoglycemia.

Medical therapy is reserved for operated patients with recurrence who refuse another exploration and for inoperable malignant tumors. Diazoxide (100–200 mg, three times daily), which inhibits insulin secretion, has been most widely used.[390] Approximately 60% (mainly those with benign disease) can be maintained nearly free of symptoms with only occasional hypoglycemia. The main side effects are fluid retention (~15%) and hirsutism (~5%); thiazide diuretics can be used to combat the fluid retention and enhance the hyperglycemic effect. The somatostatin analogue octreotide has been found to be effective in some patients but must be injected.[391, 392] Continuous subcutaneous glucagon infusion has also been used.[393] Glucocorticoids (to induce insulin resistance) and verapamil, the calcium-channel blocker, and phenytoin, the anticonvulsant, both of which inhibit insulin release at high doses, have also been used when other measures were ineffective.[343]

Malignant insulinomas respond poorly to chemotherapy.[348] Streptozocin has been reported to reduce tumor size in about 50% of patients, with less than 20% achieving complete remission; although its use prolongs life, it has considerable renal, hepatic, and hematopoietic toxicity. The addition of fluorouracil has been reported to have advantages over streptozocin alone.[394] Mithramycin,[395] doxorubicin (Adriamycin),[396] and hepatic embolization[397] have been tried with some success in refractory cases.

GENERAL APPROACH TO THE PATIENT

Diagnosis

The causes, clinical features, consequences, and need for immediate treatment of hypoglycemia will vary depending on whether the patient to be evaluated is seen in the clinic, emergency room, or hospital ward. In two series,[398, 399] diabetes, alcohol, sepsis, and combinations thereof accounted for about 90% of emergency room cases (Table 66–10). Virtually all patients had either stupor, coma, confusion, or bizarre behavior or were postictal. About 10% were hypothermic.

TABLE 66–10. Causes of 181 Emergency Room Cases of Hypoglycemia from Malouf and Brust[399] and Hart and Frier[398]

Most frequent	
Diabetic medications	85
Alcohol	40
Diabetes plus alcohol	27
Sepsis	4
Sepsis plus alcohol	9
Sepsis plus diabetes	2
Total	167 (92%)
Other	
Fasting	5
Terminal cancer	4
Gastroenteritis	2
Insulin drug abuse	2
Myxedema	1
Total	14 (8%)

Adapted from Malouf R, Brust J: Hypoglycemia: Causes, neurological manifestations, and outcome. Ann Neurol 17:421–430, 1985; Hart S, Frier B: Causes, management and morbidity of acute hypoglycemia in adults requiring hospital admission. Q J Med 91:505–510, 1998.

TABLE 66–11. Risk Factors/Situations Associated with the Development of Hypoglycemia in 195 Hospitalized Patients

Risk Factor/Situation	Cases (%)
Diabetes mellitus	41
Renal insufficiency	40
Malnutrition	34
Infection/shock	28
Liver disease	27
Malignancy	16
Heart failure	9
Pregnancy	6
Hyperkalemia therapy	5
Total parenteral nutrition	4
Burns	3
Alimentary disease	2

Data from Shilo et al.,[400] Fischer et al.,[402] Stagnaro-Green et al.,[403] and Cruz Jentoft et al.[404]

Death occurred in 10%, and 3% had permanent neurologic sequelae. Among the diabetic patients, about 80% were taking insulin; strenuous exercise (7%), accidental (6%) or deliberate insulin overdose (13%), skipped meals (28%), and alcohol ingestion (19%) were identified as precipitating factors. In 27% of cases no immediate cause was identified. Some were also taking other agents with hypoglycemic potential or had chronic renal failure, psychiatric disorders, and previous emergency room visits for hypoglycemia. In the emergency room, prompt treatment (usually with intravenous glucose) is more of a concern than an etiologic diagnosis.

In hospitalized patients the incidence of hypoglycemia ranges from 0.5% in elderly nondiabetic patients[400] to 28% in diabetic patients,[401] with about 1.5% being found in studies including diabetic and nondiabetic patients.[402, 403] Although hypoglycemia is rarely the direct cause of death, mortality in hospitalized patients experiencing hypoglycemia has ranged from 22% to 48%.[400, 402–404] Renal insufficiency, diabetes mellitus, malnutrition, liver disease, infection, and malignancy were the most common risk factors or contributing conditions (Table 66–11). Most patients had multiple risk factors. Episodes were frequently repetitive, and the great majority were asymptomatic because of occurrence in patients with reduced sensorium. Among diabetic patients, decreased caloric intake (missed meals, vomiting, withheld enteral feedings, meals withheld for procedures) and inappropriate insulin doses accounted for nearly 90% of occurrences.

In contrast to the above situations, where immediate treatment may be of paramount importance, patients seen in the clinic/office are likely to be healthy, complain of episodes with predominantly autonomic symptoms, and have spurious or poorly documented low plasma glucose levels. In such patients, diagnosis rather than treatment is the issue. Factitious, drug-induced, functional/alimentary hypoglycemia, insulinoma, and hypoglycemia secondary to an undiagnosed endocrine deficiency are the most likely diagnostic considerations.

Work-ups of hypoglycemia can follow an etiologic-based classification, one based on whether it occurs in the fasting or postprandial state, or one based on pathogenetic mechanisms. All suffer from limitations. For example, those based on the latter suffer from the fact that the mechanisms involved are complex, such as adrenal insufficiency leading to decreased glucose production, as well as increased glucose utilization (i.e., increased peripheral insulin sensitivity). Those based on postprandial vs. fasting hypoglycemia suffer from the fact that although "functional" hypoglycemia by definition occurs only postprandially, other common causes can also lead to postprandial hypoglycemia (e.g., insulinoma). The author prefers one based on diagnostic clusters (see Table 66–1) because this mode of thinking can rapidly narrow the field of possibilities.

When a patient is to be evaluated for hypoglycemia, the first step is to determine whether the patient has in fact had a hypoglycemic episode. It is important to determine what the patient's symptoms were. When did they occur in relation to the patient's last meal and what was the patient doing when the episode occurred? Was it an isolated event or has it occurred before? How frequently do they occur? Is there any pattern to the occurrences? How long have these events been occurring? Did weight gain or weight loss occur during this period? Is the patient taking any medications? If so, check them to make sure that no mistake has been made. Did the patient lose consciousness and were premonitory signs present? Was hypoglycemia documented? Did the patient spontaneously recover? What did the patient do to prevent recurrences or relieve symptoms? What is the patient's occupation? Does the patient or any immediate relatives have diabetes? If so, how is it being treated? Does the patient have any medical conditions? Do family members have any endocrine disorders?

Most outpatients who have a disorder causing hypoglycemia should describe discrete episodes. Classically, premonitory symptoms such as a feeling of anxiety, hunger, blurred vision, difficulty thinking, weakness and sweating, and palpitations will be noted. Loss of consciousness may occur. With repetitive episodes, patients learn that they can abort these symptoms by eating, and thus these patients often have a history of weight gain. Spells similar to those caused by hypoglycemia can represent a vasovagal reflex, cardiac arrhythmia, a convulsive disorder, orthostatic hypotension, or a transient ischemic attack. In mild cases of insulinoma, spells may occur only after vigorous exercise or prolonged fasting. On the other hand, skipping lunch and having several cocktails before dinner can precipitate a hypoglycemic episode in an otherwise healthy person. The history can also provide clues to the possibility of hypopituitarism (e.g., prior pituitary surgery, symptoms of galactorrhea, amenorrhea, impotence, or endocrine insufficiency, as with thyroid replacement therapy). The patient's occupation or family diseases may be important with regard to access to hypoglycemia-producing drugs (e.g., insulin, sulfonylureas) or MEN.

The physical examination can be useful in excluding carotid disease, orthostatic hypotension, severe cardiac and hepatic disease, hypothyroidism, cachexia, and cancer, which should be obvious at the stage at which they would cause hypoglycemia. Routine laboratory testing can exclude renal insufficiency or raise the possibility of adrenal insufficiency (hyponatremia). If all the above are negative and hypoglycemia has not been unequivocally documented on more than one occurrence, it is necessary to do so before proceeding with other diagnostic tests. Table 66–12 gives a suggested approach.[195]

Treatment

Treatment is aimed at restoring euglycemia, preventing recurrences, and if possible, alleviating the underlying cause. In an insulin-taking

TABLE 66–12. Diagnostic Approach to an Adult with Documented Fasting Hypoglycemia

1. Consider the most likely disorders, i.e., drugs, critical illness, endocrine deficiency, non–β cell tumor, and insulinoma, while supporting the plasma glucose concentration if necessary
2. Examine the history, physical examination, and available laboratory data for clinical clues to include or exclude the above categories

Cause	Response
Insulin- or sulfonylurea-treated diabetes	Adjust the therapeutic regimen
Use of other drugs known or suspected to cause hypoglycemia	Discontinue use of the drug
Hepatic, renal, or cardiac failure; sepsis; or inanition	Treat the underlying disorder
Anorexia, weight loss, change in skin pigmentation, known pituitary or adrenocortical disease, hypotension, hyponatrema, hyperkalemia	Evaluate for adrenocortical/pituitary insufficiency
Known non–β cell tumor, mass on examination or imaging studies	Check for high IGF-2–to–IGF-1 ratio

3. In the absence of clinical clues, consider medication error, endogenous hyperinsulinism, and surreptitious or malicious sulfonylurea or insulin administration

IGF, insulin-like growth factor.

diabetic patient with mild hypoglycemia because of a skipped meal, treatment can simply entail 12 to 18 g oral carbohydrate every 30 minutes until the blood glucose level is above 80.[405, 406] With more severe hypoglycemia resulting in obtundation and when oral administration of carbohydrate might result in aspiration, 1 mg of glucagon subcutaneously or intramuscularly might be sufficient to raise the blood glucose concentration and revive the patient so that oral carbohydrate may be given. Comatose patients should receive intravenous glucose (25-g bolus, followed by an infusion at an initial rate of 2 mg/kg/min, roughly 10 g/hour). Sulfonylurea overdose can result in prolonged hypoglycemia requiring sustained intravenous glucose infusion aimed at keeping the blood glucose level at approximately 4.5 mmol/L (~80 mg/dL) to avoid hyperglycemia causing further stimulation of insulin secretion and setting in motion a vicious cycle. Blood glucose levels should be monitored initially every 30 minutes and subsequently at 1- to 2-hour intervals. Occasionally, diazoxide or a somatostatin analogue may be needed to inhibit insulin secretion.[407] When other drugs may be involved, their use should be discontinued if possible (i.e., sulfonamides in a patient with renal insufficiency). In other conditions, the underlying disorder should be treated (e.g., sepsis, heart failure, endocrine deficiency) and the blood glucose level supported.

REFERENCES

1. Whitehead T, Robinson D, Hale A, et al: Clinical Chemistry and Haematology: Adult Reference Values. London, BUPA Medical Research and Development, 1994.
2. Marks V: Hypoglycaemia—real and unreal, lawful and unlawful: The 1994 Banting Lecture. Diabet Med 12:850–864, 1995.
3. Fariss B: Prevalence of post-glucose load glycosuria and hypoglycemia in a group of healthy young men. Diabetes 23:189–191, 1974.
4. Felig P, Cherif A, Minegawa A, et al: Hypoglycemia during prolonged exercise in normal man. N Engl J Med 306:895–900, 1982.
5. Horwitz D: Factitious and artifactual hypoglycemia. Endocrinol Metab Clin North Am 18:203–210, 1989.
6. West E, Todd W: Textbook of Biochemistry. New York, MacMillan, 1961.
7. Field J, Williams H: Artifactual hypoglycemia associated with leukemia. N Engl J Med 265:946–948, 1961.
8. Goodenow T, Malarkey W: Leukocytosis and artifactual hypoglycemia. JAMA 237:1961–1962, 1977.
9. Lefor A, Miller M: Factitious hypoglycemia associated with eosinophilic leukemoid reaction. N Y St J Med 85:34–35, 1985.
10. Astles J, Petros W, Peters W, et al: Artifactual hypoglycemia associated with hematopoietic cytokines. Arch Pathol Lab Med 119:713–716, 1995.
11. Arem R, Jeang M, Blevens T, et al: Polycythemia rubra vera and artifactual hypoglycemia. Arch Intern Med 142:2199–2201, 1982.
12. Billington C, Casciato D, Choquette D, et al: Artifactual hypoglycemia associated with polycythemia vera. JAMA 249:774–775, 1983.
13. Macaron C, Kadri A, Macaron Z: Nucleated red blood cells and artifactual hypoglycemia. Diabetes Care 4:113–115, 1981.
14. DCCT Research Group: The effect of intensive treatment of diabetes on the development and progression of long-term complications in insulin dependent diabetes mellitus. N Engl J Med 329:977–986, 1993.
15. UK Prospective Diabetes Study (UKPDS) Group: Intensive blood-glucose control with sulphonylureas or insulin compared with conventional treatment and risk of complications in patients with type 2 diabetes (UKPDS 33). Lancet 352:837–853, 1998.
16. UK Prospective Diabetes Study (UKPDS) Group: Effect of intensive blood-glucose control with metformin on complications in overweight patients with type 2 diabetes (UKPDS 34). Lancet 352:854–865, 1998.
17. Jarrett R: The cardiovascular risk associated with impaired glucose tolerance. Diabet Med 13(suppl):15–19, 1996.
18. Owen O, Morgan A, Kemp H, et al: Brain metabolism during fasting. J Clin Invest 46:1589–1595, 1967.
19. Mitrakou A, Ryan C, Veneman T, et al: Hierarchy of glycemic thresholds for counterregulatory hormone secretion, symptoms, and cerebral dysfunction. Am J Physiol 260:E67–E74, 1991.
20. Schwartz N, Clutter W, Shah S, et al: The glycemic thresholds for activation of glucose counterregulatory systems are higher than the threshold for symptoms. J Clin Invest 79:777–781, 1987.
21. Hepburn D, Deary I, Frier B, et al: Symptoms of acute insulin-induced hypoglycemia in humans with and without IDDM. Factor-analysis approach. Diabetes Care 14:949–957, 1991.
22. Towler D, Havlin C, Craft S, et al: Mechanism of awareness of hypoglycemia: Perception of neurogenic (predominantly cholinergic) rather than neuroglycopenic symptoms. Diabetes 42:1791–1798, 1993.
23. Cox D, Gonder-Frederick L, Antoun B, et al: Perceived symptoms in the recognition of hypoglycemia. Diabetes Care 16:519–527, 1993.
24. Krahn D, Mackenzie T: Organic personality syndrome caused by insulin-related nocturnal hypoglycemia. Psychosomatics 25:711–712, 1984.
25. Silas J, Grant D, Maddocks J: Transient hemiparetic attacks due to unrecognised nocturnal hypoglycaemia. BMJ 282:132–133, 1981.

26. Chalmers J, Risk M, Kean D, et al: Severe amnesia after hypoglycemia. Clinical, psychometric, and magnetic resonance imaging correlations. Diabetes Care 14:922–925, 1991.
27. Fisher B, Quin J, Rumley A, et al: Effects of acute insulin-induced hypoglycaemia on haemostasis, fibrinolysis and haemorheology in insulin-dependent diabetic patients and control subjects. Clin Sci 80:525–531, 1991.
28. Wredling R, Levander S, Adamson U, et al: Permanent neuropsychological impairment after recurrent episodes of severe hypoglycaemia in man. Diabetologia 33:152–157, 1990.
29. Patrick A, Campbell I: Fatal hypoglycaemia in insulin-treated diabetes mellitus: Clinical features and neuropathological changes. Diabet Med 7:349–354, 1990.
30. Pladziewicz D, Nesto R: Hypoglycemia-induced silent myocardial ischemia. Am J Cardiol 63:1531–1532, 1989.
31. Duh E, Feinglos M: Hypoglycemia-induced angina pectoris in a patient with diabetes mellitus. Ann Intern Med 121:945–946, 1994.
32. Perros P, Frier B: The long-term sequelae of severe hypoglycemia on the brain in insulin-dependent diabetes mellitus. Horm Metab Res 29:197–202, 1997.
33. Bolli G, DeFeo P, Perriello G, et al: Role of hepatic autoregulation in defense against hypoglycemia in humans. J Clin Invest 75:1623–1631, 1985.
34. Mitrakou A, Fanelli C, Veneman T, et al: Reversibility of unawareness of hypoglycemia in patients with insulinomas. N Engl J Med 329:834–839, 1993.
35. Gerich J, Mokan M, Veneman T, et al: Hypoglycemia unawareness. Endocr Rev 12:356–371, 1991.
36. Boyle P, Nagy R, O'Connor A, et al: Adaptation of brain glucose uptake following recurrent hypoglycemia. Proc Natl Acad Sci U S A 91:9352–9356, 1994.
37. Fritsche A, Stumvoll M, Grüb M, et al: Effect of hypoglycemia on β-adrenergic sensitivity in normal and type 1 diabetic subjects. Diabetes Care 21:1505–1510, 1998.
38. Korytkowski M, Mokan M, Veneman T, et al: Reduced β-adrenergic sensitivity in patients with type 1 diabetes and hypoglycemia unawareness. Diabetes Care 21:1939–1943, 1998.
39. Boyle P, Schwartz N, Shah S, et al: Plasma glucose concentrations at the onset of hypoglycemic symptoms in patients with poorly controlled diabetes and in nondiabetics. N Engl J Med 318:1487–1492, 1988.
40. Hochstaedt B, Schneebaum M, Shael M: Adrenocortical responsivity in old age. Gerontol Clin 3:239–246, 1961.
41. Marker J, Cryer P, Clutter W: Attenuated glucose recovery from hypoglycemia in the elderly. Diabetes 41:671–678, 1992.
42. Meneilly G, Minaker K, Young B, et al: Counterregulatory responses to insulin-induced glucose reduction in the elderly. J Clin Endocrinol Metab 61:178–182, 1985.
43. Claustre J, Peyrin L, Fitoussi R, et al: Sex differences in the adrenergic response to hypoglycemic stress in human. Psychopharmacology 67:147–153, 1980.
44. Amiel S, Maran A, Powrie J, et al: Gender differences in counterregulation to hypoglycaemia. Diabetologia 36:460–464, 1993.
45. Davis S, Cherrington A, Goldstein R, et al: Effects of insulin on the counterregulatory response to equivalent hypoglycemia in normal females. Am J Physiol 265:E680–E689, 1993.
46. Hirsch I, Boyle P, Craft S, et al: Higher glycemic thresholds for symptoms during β-adrenergic blockade in IDDM. Diabetes 40:1177–1186, 1991.
47. Rosenn B, Miodovnik M, Khoury J, et al: Counterregulatory hormonal responses to hypoglycemia during pregnancy. Obstet Gynecol 87:568–574, 1996.
48. Bottini P, Boschetti E, Pampanelli S, et al: Contribution of autonomic neuropathy to reduced plasma adrenaline responses to hypoglycemia in IDDM. Evidence for a nonselective defect. Diabetes 46:814–823, 1997.
49. Meyer C, Großmann R, Mitrakou A, et al: Effects of autonomic neuropathy on counterregulation and awareness of hypoglycemia in type 1 diabetic patients. Diabetes Care 21:1960–1966, 1998.
50. DeFronzo R, Andres R, Bedsoe T, et al: A test of the hypothesis that the rate of fall in glucose concentration triggers counterregulatory hormonal responses in man. Diabetes 26:445–452, 1977.
51. Mitrakou A, Ryan C, Veneman T, et al: Influence of plasma glucose rate of decrease on hierarchy of responses to hypoglycemia. J Clin Endocrinol Metab 76:462–465, 1993.
52. Consoli A, Kennedy F, Miles J, et al: Determination of Krebs cycle metabolic carbon exchange in vivo and its use to estimate the individual contributions of gluconeogenesis and glycogenolysis to overall hepatic glucose output in man. J Clin Invest 80:1303–1310, 1987.
53. Scholz D, ReMine W, Priestley J: Hyperinsulinism: Review of 95 cases of functioning pancreatic islet cell tumors. Mayo Clin Proc 35:545–550, 1960.
54. Gerich J: Control of glycaemia. Baillieres Clin Endocrinol Metab 7:551–586, 1993.
55. Boden G: Role of fatty acids in the pathogenesis of insulin resistance and NIDDM. Diabetes 46:3–10, 1996.
56. Stumvoll M, Meyer C, Mitrakou A, et al: Renal glucose production and utilization: New aspects in humans. Diabetologia 40:749–757, 1997.
57. Landau B, Wahren J, Chandramouli V, et al: Contributions of gluconeogenesis to glucose production in the fasted state. J Clin Invest 98:378–385, 1996.
58. Meyer C, Dostou J, Nadkarni V, et al: Effects of physiological hyperinsulinemia on systemic, renal and hepatic substrate metabolism. Am J Physiol 275:F915–F921, 1998.
59. Stumvoll M, Meyer C, Kreider M, et al: Effects of glucagon on renal and hepatic glutamine gluconeogenesis in normal postabsorptive humans. Metabolism 47:1227–1232, 1998.
60. Stumvoll M, Chintalapudi U, Perriello G, et al: Uptake and release of glucose by the human kidney: Postabsorptive rates and responses to epinephrine. J Clin Invest 96:2528–2533, 1995.
61. Stumvoll M, Meyer C, Perriello G, et al: Human kidney and liver gluconeogenesis: Evidence for organ substrate selectivity. Am J Physiol 274:E817–E826, 1998.
62. Perriello G, Jorde R, Nurjhan N, et al: Estimation of the glucose-alanine-lactate-glutamine cycles in postabsorptive man: Role of the skeletal muscle. Am J Physiol 269:E443–E450, 1995.
63. McMahon M, Marsh H, Rizza R: Comparison of the pattern of postprandial carbohydrate metabolism after ingestion of a glucose drink or a mixed meal. J Clin Endocrinol Metab 68:647–653, 1989.
64. Dinneen S, Gerich J, Rizza R: Carbohydrate metabolism in noninsulin-dependent diabetes mellitus. N Engl J Med 327:707–713, 1992.
65. Kelley D, Mitrakou A, Marsh H, et al: Skeletal muscle glycolysis, oxidation, and storage of an oral glucose load. J Clin Invest 81:1563–1571, 1988.
66. Kelley D, Mokan M, Veneman T: Impaired postprandial glucose utilization in non-insulin-dependent diabetes mellitus. Metabolism 43:1549–1557, 1994.
67. Meyer C, Dostou J, Welle S, et al: Role of liver, kidney and skeletal muscle in the disposition of an oral glucose load (abstract). Diabetes 48(suppl 1):A289, 1999.
68. Mitrakou A, Kelley D, Mokan M, et al: Role of reduced suppression of glucose production and diminished early insulin release in impaired glucose tolerance. N Engl J Med 326:22–29, 1992.
69. Taylor R, Magnusson I, Rothman D: Direct assessment of liver glycogen storage by ^{13}C nuclear magnetic resonance spectroscopy and regulation of glucose homeostasis after a mixed meal in normal subjects. J Clin Invest 97:126–132, 1996.
70. Kruszynska Y, Mulford M, Yu J, et al: Effects of nonesterified fatty acids on glucose metabolism after glucose ingestion. Diabetes 46:1586–1593, 1997.
71. Tse T, Clutter W, Shah S, et al: Mechanisms of postprandial glucose counterregulation in man: Physiologic roles of glucagon and epinephrine vis-a-vis insulin in the prevention of hypoglycemia late after glucose ingestion. J Clin Invest 72:278–286, 1983.
72. Hogan M, Service F, Sharbrough F, et al: Oral glucose tolerance test compared with a mixed meal in the diagnosis of reactive hypoglycemia. A caveat on stimulation. Mayo Clin Proc 58:491–496, 1983.
73. Gerich J: Glucose counterregulation and its impact on diabetes mellitus. Diabetes 37:1608–1617, 1988.
74. Cersosimo E, Garlick P, Ferretti J: Renal glucose production during insulin-induced hypoglycemia in humans. Diabetes 48:261–266, 1999.
75. Meyer C, Dostou J, Gerich J: Role of the human kidney in glucose counterregulation. Diabetes 48:943–948, 1999.
76. Kennedy F, Bolli G, Go V, et al: The significance of impaired pancreatic polypeptide and epinephrine responses to hypoglycemia in patients with insulin-dependent diabetes mellitus. J Clin Endocrinol Metab 64:602–608, 1987.
77. Gerich J, Campbell P: Overview of counterregulation and its abnormalities in diabetes mellitus and other conditions. Diabetes Metab Rev 4:93–111, 1988.
78. White N, Skor D, Cryer P, et al: Identification of type I diabetic patients at increased risk for hypoglycemia during intensive therapy. N Engl J Med 308:485–491, 1983.
79. Lecavalier L, Bolli G, Cryer P, et al: Contributions of gluconeogenesis and glycogenolysis during glucose counterregulation in normal humans. Am J Physiol 256:E844–E851, 1989.
80. DeFeo P, Perriello G, Torlone E, et al: Contribution of adrenergic mechanisms to glucose counterregulation in humans. Am J Physiol 261:E725–E736, 1991.
81. Fanelli C, Calderone S, Epifano L, et al: Demonstration of critical role for FFA in mediating counterregulatory stimulation of gluconeogenesis and suppression of glucose utilization in man. J Clin Invest 92:1617–1622, 1993.
82. Fanelli C, DeFeo P, Perriello G, et al: Adrenergic mechanisms contribute to the late phase of glucose counterregulation in humans by stimulating lipolysis. J Clin Invest 89:2005–2013, 1992.
83. McMahon M, Gerich J, Rizza R: Effects of glucocorticoids on carbohydrate metabolism. Diabetes Metab Rev 4:17–30, 1988.
84. Seltzer H: Drug-induced hypoglycemia. A review of 1418 cases. Endocrinol Metab Clin North Am 18:163–183, 1989.
85. DCCT Research Group: Adverse events and their association with treatment regimens in the Diabetes Control and Complications Trial. Diabetes Care 18:1415–1427, 1995.
86. Hepburn D, MacLeod K, Pell A, et al: Frequency and symptoms of hypoglycemia experienced by patients with type 2 diabetes treated with insulin. Diabet Med 10:231–237, 1993.
87. Abraira C, Colwell J, Nuttall F, et al: Veterans Affairs Cooperative Study on Glycemic Control and Complications in Type II Diabetes (VA CSDM): Results of the feasibility trial. Diabetes Care 18:1113–1123, 1995.
88. McCall A: New findings and treatment strategies for hypoglycemia and hypoglycemia unawareness. Curr Opin Endocrinol Metab 5:138–143, 1999.
89. van Staa T, Abenhaim L, Monette J: Rates of hypoglycemia in users of sulfonylureas. J Clin Epidemiol 50:735–741, 1997.
90. Arky R, Freinkel N: Alcohol infusion to test gluconeogenesis in starvation with special reference to obesity. N Engl J Med 274:426–433, 1966.
91. Flanagan D, Wood P, Sherwin R, et al: Gin and tonic and reactive hypoglycemia: What is important—the gin, the tonic, or both? J Clin Endocrinol Metab 83:796–800, 1998.
92. Arky R: Hypoglycemia associated with liver disease and ethanol. Endocrinol Metab Clin North Am 18:75–90, 1989.
93. Madison L: Ethanol-induced hypoglycemia. *In* Levine R, Luft R (eds): Advances in Metabolic Disorders, vol 3. New York, Academic, 1968, pp 85–109.
94. Klatt E, Beatie C, Noguchi T: Evaluation of death from hypoglycemia. Am J Forensic Med Pathol 9:122–125, 1988.
95. Marks V, Teale J: Drug-induced hypoglycemia. Endocrinol Metab Clin North Am 28:555–577, 1999.
96. Siler S, Neese R, Christiansen M, et al: The inhibition of gluconeogenesis following alcohol in humans. Am J Physiol 275:E897–E907, 1998.
97. Krebs H, Freedland R, Stubbs M: Inhibition of hepatic gluconeogenesis by ethanol. Biochem J 112:117–124, 1969.
98. Kreisberg R, Owen W, Siegal A: Ethanol-induced hyperlacticacidemia: Inhibition of lactate utilization. J Clin Invest 50:166–174, 1971.
99. Kreisberg R, Siegal A, Owen W: Alanine and gluconeogenesis in man: Effect of ethanol. J Clin Endocrinol Metab 34:876–883, 1972.
100. Chan J, Cockram C, Critchley J: Drug-induced disorders of glucose metabolism. Mechanisms and management. Drug Saf 15:135–157, 1996.

101. Reith D, Dawson A, Epid D, et al: Relative toxicity of beta blockers in overdose. Clin Toxicol 34:273–278, 1996.
102. Poretsky L, Moses A: Hypoglycemia associated with trimethoprim/sulfamethoxazole therapy. Diabetes Care 7:508–509, 1984.
103. Rizza R, Cryer P, Haymond M, et al: Adrenergic mechanisms for the effect of epinephrine on glucose production and clearance in man. J Clin Invest 65:682–689, 1980.
104. Baron S: Salicylates as hypoglycemic agents. Diabetes Care 5:64–71, 1982.
105. Washio M, Onoyama K, Makita Y, et al: Hypoglycemia associated with the administration of angiotensin-converting enzyme inhibitor in a diabetic hemodialysis patient. Nephron 59:341–342, 1991.
106. Arauz-Pacheco C, Ramirez L, Rios J, et al: Hypoglycemia induced by angiotensin-converting enzyme inhibitors in patients with non–insulin-dependent diabetes receiving sulfonylurea therapy. Am J Med 89:811–813, 1990.
107. Morris A, Boyle D, McMahon A, et al: ACE inhibitor use is associated with hospitalization for severe hypoglycemia in patients with diabetes. Diabetes Care 20:1363–1367, 1997.
108. Perronne C, Bricaire F, Leport C, et al: Hypoglycaemia and diabetes mellitus following parenteral pentamidine mesylate treatment in AIDS patients. Diabet Med 7:585–589, 1990.
109. Bouchard P, Sai P, Reach G, et al: Diabetes mellitus following pentamidine-induced hypoglycemia in humans. Diabetes 31:40–45, 1982.
110. Pollare T, Lithell H, Berne C: A comparison of the effects of hydrochlorothiazide and captopril on glucose and lipid metabolism in patients with hypertension. N Engl J Med 321:868–873, 1989.
111. Jauch K, Hartl W, Georgieff M, et al: Low dose bradykinin infusion reduces endogenous glucose production in surgical patients. Metabolism 37:185–190, 1988.
112. Shorr R, Ray W, Daugherty J, et al: Incidence and risk factors for serious hypoglycemia in older persons using insulin or sulfonylureas. Arch Intern Med 157:1681–1686, 1997.
113. Shorr R, Ray W, Daugherty J, et al: Individual sulfonylureas and serious hypoglycemia in older people. J Am Geriatr Soc 44:751–755, 1996.
114. Klonoff D, Barrett B, Nolte M, et al: Hypoglycemia following inadvertent and factitious sulfonylurea overdosages. Diabetes Care 18:563–567, 1995.
115. Shumak S, Corenblum B, Steiner G: Recurrent hypoglycemia secondary to drug-dispensing error. Arch Intern Med 151:1877–1878, 1991.
116. Chiolero R, Revelly J, Tappy L: Energy metabolism in sepsis and injury. Nutrition 13(suppl):45–51, 1997.
117. Mizock B: Alterations in carbohydrate metabolism during stress: A review of the literature. Am J Med 98:75–84, 1995.
118. Kinney J: Metabolic responses of the critically ill patient. Crit Care Clin 11:569–585, 1995.
119. Mathison J, Wolfson E, Ulevitch R: Participation of tumor necrosis factor in the mediation of gram negative bacterial lipopolysaccharide-induced injury in rabbits. J Clin Invest 81:1925–1937, 1988.
120. Richards A: Tumour necrosis factor and associated cytokines in the host's response to malaria. Int J Parasitol 27:1251–1263, 1997.
121. Stouthard J, Romijn J, van der Poll T, et al: Endocrinologic and metabolic effects of interleukin-6 in humans. Am J Physiol 268:E813–E819, 1995.
122. Sakurai Y, Zhang X-J, Wolfe R: TNF directly stimulates glucose uptake and leucine oxidation and inhibits FFA flux in conscious dogs. Am J Physiol 270:E864–E872, 1996.
123. Hinshaw L: Concise review: The role of glucose in endotoxin shock. Circ Shock 3:1–10, 1976.
124. Brady W, Butler K, Fines R, et al: Hypoglycemia in multiple trauma victims. Am J Emerg Med 17:4–5, 1999.
125. Miller S, Wallace R, Musher D, et al: Hypoglycemia as a manifestation of sepsis. Am J Med 68:649–654, 1980.
126. Lang C, Bagby G, Blakesley H, et al: Importance of hyperglucagonemia in eliciting the sepsis-induced increase in glucose production. Circ Shock 29:181–191, 1989.
127. Hargrove D, Bagby G, Lang C, et al: Adrenergic blockade does not abolish elevated glucose turnover during bacterial infection. Am J Physiol 254:E16–E22, 1988.
128. Fettman M: Endotoxemia in Yucatan miniature pigs: Metabolic derangements and experimental therapies. Lab Anim Sci 36:370–374, 1986.
129. Wichterman K, Chaudry I, Baue A: Studies of peripheral glucose uptake during sepsis. Arch Surg 114:740–745, 1979.
130. Meszaros K, Lang C, Bagby G, et al: In vivo glucose utilization by individual tissues during nonlethal hypermetabolic sepsis. FASEB J 2:3083–3086, 1988.
131. Romanosky A, Bagby G, Bockman E, et al: Increased muscle glucose uptake and lactate release after endotoxin administration. Am J Physiol 239:E311–E316, 1980.
132. Naylor J, Kronfeld D: In vivo studies of hypoglycemia and lactic acidosis in endotoxic shock. Am J Physiol 248:E309–E316, 1985.
133. Wolfe R, Burke J: Glucose and lactate metabolism in experimental septic shock. Am J Physiol 235:R219–R227, 1978.
134. Durkot M, Wolfe R: Effects of adrenergic blockade on glucose kinetics in septic and burned guinea pigs. Am J Physiol 241:R222–R227, 1981.
135. Bagby G, Lang C, Skrepnik N, et al: Attenuation of glucose metabolic changes resulting from TNF-α administration by adrenergic blockade. Am J Physiol 262:R628–R635, 1992.
136. Maitra S, Homan C, Pan W, et al: Renal gluconeogenesis and blood flow during endotoxic shock. Acad Emerg Med 3:1006–1010, 1996.
137. Wannemacher R, Pace J, Beall R, et al: Role of the liver in regulation of ketone body production during sepsis. J Clin Invest 64:1565–1572, 1979.
138. Wannemacher R, Beall F, Canonico P, et al: Glucose and alanine metabolism during bacterial infections in rats and rhesus monkeys. Metabolism 29:201–212, 1980.
139. Alderfer H, Richardson J: Hepatic hypoglycemia and infarction of the bowel. Arch Intern Med 112:50–55, 1963.
140. Medalle R, Webb R, Waterhouse C: Lactic acidosis and associated hypoglycemia. Arch Intern Med 128:273–278, 1971.
141. Fuchs S, Bogomolski-Yahalom V, Paltiel O, et al: Ischemic hepatitis. J Clin Gastroenterol 26:183–186, 1998.
142. Hedayati H, Beheshti M: Profound spontaneous hypoglycaemia in congestive heart failure. Curr Med Res Opin 4:501–504, 1977.
143. Mellinkoff S, Tumulty P: Hepatic hypoglycemia: Its occurrence in congestive heart failure. N Engl J Med 247:745–750, 1952.
144. Marks V, Rose F: Hypoglycemia, ed 2. Oxford, Blackwell, 1981.
145. Medalle R, Webb R, Waterhouse C: Lactic acidosis and associated hypoglycemia. Arch Intern Med 128:273–278, 1952.
146. Seltzer H: Severe drug-induced hypoglycemia: A review. Compr Ther 5:21–29, 1979.
147. Arem R: Hypoglycemia associated with renal failure. Endocrinol Metab Clin North Am 18:103–121, 1989.
148. Owen O, Felig P, Morgan A, et al: Liver and kidney metabolism during prolonged starvation. J Clin Invest 48:574–583, 1969.
149. Reinecke R: The kidney as a source of glucose in the eviscerated rat. Am J Physiol 140:276–285, 1943.
150. Lupianez J, Faus M, Munoz-Clares R, et al: Stimulation of rat kidney gluconeogenic ability by inhibition of liver gluconeogenesis. FEBS Lett 61:277–281, 1976.
151. Battezzati A, Fattorini A, Caumo A, et al: Non-hepatic glucose production in humans (abstract). Diabetes 48(suppl 1):49, 1999.
152. Mann F: Effects of complete and partial removal of the liver. Medicine (Baltimore) 6:419–467, 1927.
153. Zimmerman H, Thomas L, Scherr E: Fasting blood sugar in hepatic disease with reference to infrequency of hypoglycemia. Arch Intern Med 91:577–584, 1953.
154. Katz N: Correlation between rates and enzyme levels of increased gluconeogenesis in rat liver and kidney after partial hepatectomy. Eur J Biochem 98:535–542, 1979.
155. Felig P, Brown W, Levine R, et al: Glucose homeostasis in viral hepatitis. N Engl J Med 283:1436–1440, 1970.
156. Heinig R, Clarke E, Waterhouse C: Lactic acidosis and liver disease. Arch Intern Med 139:1229–1232, 1979.
157. Nouel O, Bernuau J, Rueff B, et al: Hypoglycemia: A common complication of septicemia in cirrhosis. Arch Intern Med 141:1477–1478, 1981.
158. Younus S, Soterakis J, Sossi A, et al: Hypoglycemia secondary to metastases to the liver. Gastroenterology 72:334–337, 1977.
159. Johnson D, Alberti K, Faber O, et al: Hyperinsulinism of hepatic cirrhosis: Diminished degradation or hypersecretion? Lancet 1:10–13, 1977.
160. Gorden P, Hendricks C, Kahn C: Hypoglycemia associated with non–islet cell tumor and insulin-like growth factors. N Engl J Med 305:1452–1455, 1981.
161. Zubrod C, Eversole S, Dane G: Amelioration of diabetes and striking rarity of acidosis in patients with Kimmelstiel-Wilson lesions. N Engl J Med 245:518–525, 1951.
162. Block M, Rubinstein A: Spontaneous hypoglycemia in diabetic patients with renal insufficiency. JAMA 213:1863–1866, 1970.
163. Hultman E, Nilsson L: Liver glycogen in man: Effect of different diets and muscular exercise. Adv Exp Med Biol 11:143–151, 1971.
164. Frizzel M, Larsen R, Field J: Spontaneous hypoglycemia associated with chronic renal failure. Diabetes 22:493–498, 1973.
165. Peitzman S, Agarwal B: Spontaneous hypoglycemia in end-stage renal failure. Nephron 19:131–139, 1977.
166. Avram M, Wolf N, Gan A, et al: Uremic hypoglycemia: A preventable life-threatening complication. N Y St J Med 84:593–596, 1984.
167. Rutsky E, McDaniel H, Tharpe D, et al: Spontaneous hypoglycemia in chronic renal failure. Arch Intern Med 138:1364–1368, 1978.
168. Toth E, Lee D: "Spontaneous"/uremic hypoglycemia is not a distinct entity: Substantiation from a literature review. Nephron 58:325–329, 1991.
169. Mühlhauser I, Toth G, Sawicki P, et al: Severe hypoglycemia in type I diabetic patients with impaired kidney function. Diabetes Care 14:344–346, 1991.
170. Fürst P: Amino acid metabolism in uremia. J Am Coll Nutr 8:310–323, 1989.
171. Garber A, Bier D, Cryer P, et al: Hypoglycemia in compensated chronic renal insufficiency. Substrate limitation of gluconeogenesis. Diabetes 23:982–986, 1976.
172. Greenblatt D: Fatal hypoglycaemia occurring after peritoneal dialysis. BMJ 2:270–271, 1972.
173. Tzamaloukas A, Murata G, Eisenberg B, et al: Hypoglycemia in diabetics on dialysis with poor glycemic control: Hemodialysis versus continuous ambulatory peritoneal dialysis. Int J Artif Organs 15:390–392, 1992.
174. Langlois M, Robert G, Nawar T, et al: [Spontaneous hypoglycemia and chronic kidney insufficiency] (French). Can Med Assoc J 118:1083–1086, 1978.
175. Rabau M, Dor (Dershovitz) J, Adar R, et al: Spontaneous hypoglycemia in a diabetic patient with renal failure. Isr J Med Sci 9:1036–1039, 1973.
176. Rutsky E, McDaniel H, Tharpe D, et al: Spontaneous hypoglycemia in chronic renal failure. Arch Intern Med 138:1364–1368, 1978.
177. Bonapart I, Diderich P, Elte J, et al: Spontaneous hypoglycaemia in chronic renal failure. Neth J Med 48:180–184, 1996.
178. Bansal V, Brooks M, York J, et al: Intractable hypoglycemia in a patient with renal failure. Arch Intern Med 139:101–102, 1979.
179. Grimaldi A, Massin P, Champigneulle A, et al: [Spontaneous hypoglycemia in a non–insulin-dependent diabetic with advanced renal failure] (French). Presse Med 16:36, 1987.
180. Baylor P, Shilo S, Zonszein J, et al: β-Adrenergic contribution to glucagon-induced glucose production and insulin secretion in uremia. Am J Physiol 251:E322–E327, 1986.
181. Ramirez G, Brueggemeyer C, Ganguly A: Counterregulatory hormonal response to insulin-induced hypoglycemia in patients on chronic hemodialysis. Nephron 49:231–236, 1988.
182. Greenblatt D: Insulin sensitivity in renal failure. N Y St J Med 74:1040–1041, 1974.
183. Metcoff J, Furst P, Scharer K, et al: Energy production, intracellular amino acid pools, and protein synthesis in chronic renal disease. J Am Coll Nutr 8:271–284, 1989.
184. Riegel W, Stepinski J, Hörl W, et al: Effect of hormones on hepatocyte gluconeogenesis in different models of acute uraemia. Nephron 32:67–72, 1982.

185. Hermansen K, Johannsen L, Rasmussen O: Hypoglycaemic coma in severe primary hypothyroidism. Acta Med Scand 218:345–346, 1985.
186. Samaan N: Hypoglycemia secondary to endocrine deficiencies. Endocrinol Metab Clin North Am 18:145–154, 1989.
187. Gerich J, Langlois M, Noacco C, et al: Lack of glucagon response to hypoglycemia in diabetes: Evidence for an intrinsic pancreatic alpha-cell defect. Science 182:171–173, 1973.
188. Vidnes J, Oyasaeter S: Glucagon deficiency causing severe neonatal hypoglycemia in a patient with normal insulin secretion. Pediatr Res 11:943–949, 1977.
189. Kollee L, Monnens L, Cecjka V, et al: Persistent neonatal hypoglycaemia due to glucagon deficiency. Arch Dis Child 53:422–424, 1978.
190. Abs R, Verbist L, Moeremans M, et al: Hypoglycemia owing to inappropriate glucagon secretion treated with a continuous subcutaneous glucagon infusion system. Acta Endocrinol (Copenh) 122:319–322, 1990.
191. Starke A, Valverde I, Bottazzo G, et al: Glucagon deficiency associated with hypoglycaemia and the absence of islet cell antibodies in the polyglandular failure syndrome before the onset of insulin-dependent diabetes mellitus: A case report. Diabetologia 25:336–339, 1983.
192. Polinsky R, Kopin I, Ebert M, et al: The adrenal medullary response to hypoglycemia in patients with orthostatic hypotension. J Clin Endocrinol Metab 51:1401–1406, 1980.
193. Gerich J, Davis J, Lorenzi M, et al: Hormonal mechanisms of recovery from insulin-induced hypoglycemia in man. Am J Physiol 236:E380–E385, 1979.
194. Rizza R, Cryer P, Gerich J: Role of glucagon, catecholamines, and growth hormone in human glucose counterregulation. Effects of somatostatin and combined α- and β-adrenergic blockade on plasma glucose recovery and glucose flux rates after insulin-induced hypoglycemia. J Clin Invest 64:62–71, 1979.
195. Cryer P: Hypoglycemia. Pathophysiology, Diagnosis, and Treatment. New York, Oxford University Press, 1997.
196. Seagall M: Spontaneous hypoglycemia with failure to increase adrenal output. Proc R Soc Med 60:50, 1967.
197. Levin H, Heifetz M: Phaeochromocytoma and severe protracted postoperative hypoglycaemia. Can J Anaesth 37:477–478, 1990.
198. DeFeo P, Perriello G, Torlone E, et al: Contribution of cortisol to glucose counterregulation in man. Am J Physiol 257:E35–E42, 1989.
199. DeFeo P, Perriello G, Torlone E, et al: Demonstration of a role of growth hormone in glucose counterregulation. Am J Physiol 256:E835–E843, 1989.
200. Goodman H, Grumbach M, Kaplan S: Growth and growth hormone. II. A comparison of isolated growth-hormone deficiency and multiple pituitary-hormone deficiencies in 35 patients with idiopathic hypopituitary dwarfism. N Engl J Med 278:57–68, 1968.
201. Artavia-Loria E, Chaussain J, Bougneres P, et al: Frequency of hypoglycemia in children with adrenal insufficiency. Acta Endocrinol Suppl (Copenh) 279:275–278, 1986.
202. Wolfsdorf J, Sadeghi-Nejad A, Senior B: Hypoketonemia and age-related fasting hypoglycemia in growth hormone deficiency. Metabolism 32:457–462, 1983.
203. Haymond M, Karl I, Weldon V, et al: The role of growth hormone and cortisone on glucose and gluconeogenic substrate regulation in fasted hypopituitary children. J Clin Endocrinol Metab 42:846–856, 1976.
204. Yamamoto T, Fukuyama J, Hasegawa K, et al: Isolated corticotropin deficiency in adults. Report of 10 cases and review of literature. Arch Intern Med 152:1705–1712, 1992.
205. Merimee T, Felig P, Marliss E, et al: Glucose and lipid homeostasis in the absence of human growth hormone. J Clin Invest 50:574–582, 1971.
206. Smallridge R, Corrigan D, Thomason A, et al: Hypoglycemia in pregnancy. Occurrence due to adrenocorticotropic hormone and growth hormone deficiency. Arch Intern Med 140:564–565, 1980.
207. Malerbi D, Liberman B, Giurno-Filho A, et al: Glucocorticoids and glucose metabolism: Hepatic glucose production in untreated addisonian patients and on two different levels of glucocorticoid administration. Clin Endocrinol 28:415–422, 1988.
208. Boyle P, Cryer P: Growth hormone, cortisol, or both are involved in defense against, but are not critical to recovery from, hypoglycemia. Am J Physiol 260:E395–E402, 1991.
209. Zuker N, Bissessor M, Korber M, et al: Acute hypoglycaemic coma—a rare, potentially lethal form of early onset Sheehan syndrome. Aust N Z J Obstet Gynaecol 35:318–320, 1995.
210. Hardy K, Burge M, Boyle P, et al: A treatable cause of recurrent severe hypoglycemia. Diabetes Care 17:722–724, 1994.
211. Johansson C, Adamsson U, Stierner U, et al: Interaction by cholestyramine on the uptake of hydrocortisone in the gastrointestinal tract. Acta Med Scand 204:509–512, 1978.
212. Owen O, Reichard G: Human forearm metabolism during progressive starvation. J Clin Invest 50:1536–1545, 1971.
213. Cahill G: Starvation in man. N Engl J Med 282:668–675, 1970.
214. Field J: Exercise and deficient carbohydrate storage and intake as causes of hypoglycemia. Endocrinol Metab Clin North Am 18:155–161, 1989.
215. Chakrabarty P: Blood glucose levels in slow starvation. Lancet 1:596–597, 1948.
216. Elias A, Gwinup G: Glucose-resistant hypoglycemia in inanition. Arch Intern Med 142:743–746, 1982.
217. Fonseca V, Ball S, Marks V, et al: Hypoglycaemia associated with anorexia nervosa. Postgrad Med J 67:460–461, 1991.
218. Smith J: Hypoglycaemic coma associated with anorexia nervosa. Aust N Z J Psychiatry 22:448–453, 1988.
219. Rich L, Caine M, Findling J, et al: Hypoglycemic coma in anorexia nervosa. Case report and review of the literature. Arch Intern Med 150:894–895, 1990.
220. Wharton B: Hypoglycaemia in children with kwashiorkor. Lancet 1:171–173, 1970.
221. Bruce A, Jacobsen E, Dossing H, et al: Hypoglycaemia in spinal muscular atrophy. Lancet 1:609–610, 1995.
222. Gounelle H, Marche J: Spontaneous coma due to hypoglycemia in undernourished persons. Occup Med 1:48–50, 1948.
223. Taylor S, Barbetti F, Accili D, et al: Syndromes of autoimmunity and hypoglycemia. Autoantibodies directed against insulin and its receptor. Endocrinol Metab Clin North Am 18:123–143, 1989.
224. Hirata Y, Uchigata Y: Insulin autoimmune syndrome in Japan. Diabetes Res Clin Pract 24(suppl):153–157, 1994.
225. Burch H, Clement S, Sokol M, et al: Reactive hypoglycemic coma due to insulin autoimmune syndrome: Case report and literature review. Am J Med 92:681–685, 1992.
226. Archambeaud-Mouveroux F, Huc M, Nadalon S, et al: Autoimmune insulin syndrome. Biomed Pharmacother 43:581–586, 1989.
227. Redmon J, Nuttall F: Autoimmune hypoglycemia. Endocrinol Metab Clin North Am 28:603–618, 1999.
228. Flier J, Bar R, Muggeo M, et al: The evolving clinical course of patients with insulin receptor autoantibodies: Spontaneous remission of receptor proliferation with hypoglycemia. J Clin Endocrinol Metab 47:985–995, 1978.
229. Taylor S, Grunberger G, Marcus-Samuels B, et al: Hypoglycemia associated with antibodies to the insulin receptor. N Engl J Med 307:1422–1426, 1982.
230. Muggeo M, Flier J, Abrams R, et al: Treatment by plasma exchange of a patient with autoantibodies to the insulin receptor. N Engl J Med 300:477–480, 1979.
231. Kawanishi K, Kawamura K, Nishina Y, et al: Successful immunosuppressive therapy in insulin resistant diabetes caused by anti–insulin receptor autoantibodies. J Clin Endocrinol Metab 44:15–21, 1977.
232. Victor A: Normal blood sugar variation during pregnancy. Acta Obstet Gynecol Scand 53:37–40, 1974.
233. Kalhan S, D'Angelo L, Savin S, et al: Glucose production in pregnant women at term gestation. Sources of glucose for human fetus. J Clin Invest 63:388–394, 1979.
234. Reece E, Homko C, Wiznitzer A: Metabolic changes in diabetic and nondiabetic subjects during pregnancy. Obstet Gynecol Surv 49:64–71, 1994.
235. Garner P, Tsang R: Insulinoma complicating pregnancy presenting with hypoglycemic coma after delivery: A case report and review of the literature. Obstet Gynecol 73:847–849, 1989.
236. Schweichler M, Hennessey J, Cole P, et al: Hypoglycemia in pregnancy secondary to a non–islet cell tumor of the pleura and ectopic insulin-like growth factor II hormone production. J Clin Endocrinol Metab 85:810–813, 1995.
237. White N, Warrell D, Chanthavanich P, et al: Severe hypoglycemia and hyperinsulinemia in falciparum malaria. N Engl J Med 309:61–66, 1983.
238. Long P, Abell D, Beischer N: Importance of abnormal glucose tolerance (hypoglycaemia and hyperglycaemia) in the aetiology of pre-eclampsia. Lancet 1:923–925, 1977.
239. Neuman M, Ron-El R, Langer R, et al: Maternal death caused by HELLP syndrome (with hypoglycemia) complicating mild pregnancy-induced hypertension in a twin gestation. Am J Obstet Gynecol 162:372–373, 1989.
240. Egley C: Severe hypoglycemia associated with HELLP syndrome. Am J Obstet Gynecol 152:576–577, 1985.
241. Aarnoudse J, Houthoff H, Weits J, et al: A syndrome of liver damage and intravascular coagulation in the last trimester of normotensive pregnancy. A clinical and histopathological study. Br J Obstet Gynaecol 93:145–155, 1986.
242. Levine A, Burgess G, Derick C: Some changes in the chemical constituents of the blood following a marathon race. JAMA 82:1778–1782, 1924.
243. Ahlborg G, Felig P: Lactate and glucose exchange across the forearm, legs, and splanchnic bed during and after prolonged leg exercise. J Clin Invest 69:45–54, 1982.
244. Uusitupa M, Aro A, Pietikainen M: Severe hypoglycaemia caused by physical strain and pindolol therapy. A case report. Ann Clin Res 12:25–27, 1980.
245. Wasserman D, Cherrington A: Hepatic fuel metabolism during muscular work: Role and regulation. Am J Physiol 260:E811–E824, 1991.
246. Wahren J, Felig P, Hagenfeldt L: Physical exercise and fuel homeostasis in diabetes mellitus. Diabetologia 14:213–222, 1978.
247. Marker J, Hirsch I, Smith L, et al: Catecholamines in prevention of hypoglycemia during exercise in humans. Am J Physiol 260:E705–E712, 1991.
248. Hirsch I, Marker J, Smith L, et al: Insulin and glucagon in prevention of hypoglycemia during exercise in humans. Am J Physiol 260:E695–E704, 1991.
249. Service F, Moore G: Factitial hypoglycemia. In Service F (ed): Hypoglycemic Disorders: Pathogenesis, Diagnosis and Treatment. Boston, GK Hall, 1983, pp 129–141.
250. Marks V, Teale J: Hypoglycemia: Factitious and felonious. Endocrinol Metab Clin North Am 28:579–601, 1999.
251. Sheehy T: Case report: Factitious hypoglycemia in diabetic patients. Am J Med Sci 304:298–302, 1992.
252. Schade D, Drumm D, Eaton R, et al: Factitious brittle diabetes mellitus. Am J Med 78:777–784, 1985.
253. Kaminer Y, Robbins D: Insulin misuse: A review of an overlooked psychiatric problem. Psychosomatics 30:19–24, 1989.
254. Marchetti P, Faloppa C, Zappella A, et al: [A case of factitious hypoglycemia with unusual presentation] (Italian). Minerva Med 79:1101–1103, 1988.
255. Scarlett J, Mako M, Rubenstein A, et al: Factitious hypoglycemia. Diagnosis by measurement of serum C-peptide immunoreactivity and insulin-binding antibodies. N Engl J Med 297:1029–1032, 1977.
256. Retsas S: Insulin abuse by a drug addict. BMJ 4:792–793, 1972.
257. Jordan R, Kammer H, Riddle M: Sulfonylurea-induced factitious hypoglycemia. A growing problem. Arch Intern Med 137:390–393, 1977.
258. Grunberger G, Weiner J, Silverman R, et al: Factitious hypoglycemia due to surreptitious administration of insulin. Diagnosis, treatment, and long-term follow-up. Ann Intern Med 108:252–257, 1988.
259. Rynearson E: Hyperinsulinism among malingerers. Med Clin North Am 31:477–480, 1947.
260. Siegel E, Mayer G, Nauck M, et al: [Factitious hypoglycemia caused by taking a sulfonylurea drug] (German). Dtsch Med Wochenschr 112:1575–1579, 1987.
261. Roy M, Roy A: Factitious hypoglycemia. An 11-year follow-up. Psychosomatics 36:64–65, 1995.

262. Jermendy G: [Factitious hypoglycemia—Munchausen syndrome in diabetes mellitus] (Hungarian). Orv Hetil 136:31–33, 1995.

263. Jezequel C, de Kerdanet M, Girre M: [Hypoglycemia provoked by clandestine injections of insulin in the diabetic child] (French). Ann Pediatr (Paris) 40:32–36, 1993.

264. Schuler G, Petersen K, Khalaf A, et al: Insulin abuse in long-standing IDDM. Diabetes Res Clin Pract 6:145–148, 1989.

265. Svirski B, Edoute Y: [Sulfonylurea-induced factitious hypoglycemia] (Hebrew). Harefuah 130:678–680, 1996.

266. Jordan R, Kammer H, Riddle M: Sulfonylurea-induced factitious hypoglycemia. Arch Intern Med 137:390–393, 1977.

267. Teale J, Starkey B, Marks V, et al: The prevalence of factitious hypoglycaemia due to sulphonylurea abuse in the UK: A preliminary report. Practical Diabetes 6:177–178, 1989.

268. Doege K: Fibro-sarcoma of the mediastinum. Ann Surg 92:955–960, 1930.

269. Daughaday W: Hypoglycemia in patients with non–islet cell tumors. Endocrinol Metab Clin North Am 18:91–101, 1989.

270. Anderson N, Lokich J: Mesenchymal tumors associated with hypoglycemia: Case report and review of the literature. Cancer 44:785–790, 1979.

271. Baxter R: The role of insulin-like growth factors and their binding proteins in tumor hypoglycemia. Horm Res 46:195–201, 1996.

272. Benn J, Firth R, Sönksen P: Metabolic effects of an insulin-like factor causing hypoglycaemia in a patient with a haemangiopericytoma. Clin Endocrinol 32:769–780, 1990.

273. Chandalia H, Boshell B: Hypoglycemia associated with extrapancreatic tumors. Arch Intern Med 129:447–456, 1972.

274. Chowdhury F, Bleicher S: Studies of tumor hypoglycemia. Metabolism 22:663–674, 1973.

275. Daughaday W, Emanuele M, Brooks M, et al: Synthesis and secretion of insulin-like growth factor II by a leiomyosarcoma with associated hypoglycemia. N Engl J Med 319:1434–1440, 1988.

276. Daughaday W: The pathophysiology of IGF-II hypersecretion in non–islet cell tumor hypoglycemia. Diabetes Rev 3:62–72, 1995.

277. Eastman R, Carson R, Orloff D, et al: Glucose utilization in a patient with hepatoma and hypoglycemia. J Clin Invest 89:1958–1963, 1992.

278. McFadzean A, Yeung R: Further observations on hypoglycaemia in hepatocellular carcinoma. Am J Med 47:220–235, 1969.

279. Millard P, Jerrome D, Millward-Sadler G: Spindle-cell tumours and hypoglycaemia. J Clin Pathol 29:520–529, 1976.

280. Moller N, Blum W, Mengel A, et al: Basal and insulin stimulated substrate metabolism in tumour induced hypoglycaemia; evidence for increased muscle glucose uptake. Diabetologia 34:17–20, 1991.

281. Nissan S, Bar-Maor A, Shafrir E: Hypoglycemia associated with extrapancreatic tumors. N Engl J Med 278:177–183, 1968.

282. Reeve A, Eccles M, Wilkins R, et al: Expression of insulin-like growth factor-II transcripts in Wilms' tumour. Nature 317:258–260, 1985.

283. Scott J, Cowell J, Robertson M, et al: Insulin-like growth factor-II gene expression in Wilms' tumour and embryonic tissues. Nature 317:260–262, 1985.

284. Silbert C, Rossini A, Ghazvinian S, et al: Tumor hypoglycemia: Deficient splanchnic glucose output and deficient glucagon secretion. Diabetes 25:202–206, 1976.

285. Silverstein M: Tumor hypoglycemia. Cancer 23:142–144, 1969.

286. Skrabanek P, Powell D: Ectopic insulin and Occam's razor: Reappraisal of the riddle of tumour hypoglycaemia. Clin Endocrinol 9:141–154, 1978.

287. Widmer U, Zapf J, Froesch E: Is extrapancreatic tumor hypoglycemia associated with elevated levels of insulin-like growth factor II? J Clin Endocrinol Metab 55:833–839, 1982.

288. Horecker B, Hiatt H: Pathways of carbohydrate metabolism in normal and neoplastic cells. N Engl J Med 258:177–184, 225–232, 1958.

289. Phuphanich S, Jacobs L, Poulos E, et al: Case report: Hypoglycemia secondary to a meningioma. Am J Med Sci 309:317–321, 1995.

290. Chung J, Henry R: Mechanisms of tumor-induced hypoglycemia with intraabdominal hemangiopericytoma. J Clin Endocrinol Metab 81:919–925, 1996.

291. Seckl M, Mulholland P, Bishop A, et al: Hypoglycemia due to an insulin-secreting small-cell carcinoma of the cervix. N Engl J Med 341:733–736, 1999.

292. Marks V, Teale J: Tumours producing hypoglycemia. Endocr Relat Cancer 5:111–129, 1998.

293. Del Sindaco P, Casucci G, Pampanelli S, et al: Late post-prandial hypoglycaemia as the sole presenting feature of secreting pancreatic beta-cell adenoma in a subtotally gastrectomized patient. Eur J Endocrinol 136:96–99, 1997.

294. Brasel J, Wright J, Wilkins L, et al: An evaluation of seventy-five patients with hypopituitarism beginning in childhood. Am J Med 38:484–498, 1965.

295. O'Keefe S, Marks V: Lunchtime gin and tonic a cause of reactive hypoglycemia. Lancet 1:1286–1288, 1977.

296. Hofeldt F, Lufkin E, Hagler L, et al: Are abnormalities in insulin secretion responsible for reactive hypoglycemia? Diabetes 23:589–596, 1974.

297. Hopwood N, Forsman P, Kenny F, et al: Hypoglycemia in hypopituitary children. Am J Dis Child 129:918–926, 1975.

298. Leichter S, Permutt M: Effect of adrenergic agents on postgastrectomy hypoglycemia. Diabetes 24:1005–1010, 1975.

299. Shultz K, Neelon F, Nilsen L, et al: Mechanism of postgastrectomy hypoglycemia. Arch Intern Med 128:240–246, 1971.

300. Wiznitzer T, Shapira N, Stadler J, et al: Late hypoglycemia in patients following vagotomy and pyloroplasty. Int Surg 59:229–232, 1974.

301. Hall W, Sanders L: Hypoglycemic convulsions after vagotomy and pyloroplasty. South Med J 66:502–504, 1973.

302. Miholic J, Orskov C, Holst J, et al: Postprandial release of glucagon-like peptide-1, pancreatic glucagon, and insulin after esophageal resection. Digestion 54:73–78, 1993.

303. Veverbrants E, Olsen W, Arky R: Role of gastro-intestinal factors in reactive hypoglycemia. Metabolism 18:6–12, 1969.

304. Zieve L, Jones D, Aziz M: Functional hypoglycemia and peptic ulcer. Postgrad Med 40:159–170, 1966.

305. O'Brien T, Tijtgat G, Ensinck J: Alimentary hypoglycemia associated with the Zollinger-Ellison syndrome. Am J Med 54:637–644, 1973.

306. Luyckx A, Lefebvre P: Plasma insulin in reactive hypoglycemia. Diabetes 20:435–442, 1971.

307. Bellini F, Sammicheli L, Ianni L, et al: Hypoglycemia unawareness in a patient with dumping syndrome: Report of a case. J Endocrinol Invest 21:463–467, 1998.

308. Freinkel N, Metzger B: Oral glucose tolerance curve and hypoglycemias in the fed state. N Engl J Med 280:820–828, 1969.

309. Andreasen J, Orskov C, Holst J: Secretion of glucagon-like peptide-1 and reactive hypoglycemia after partial gastrectomy. Digestion 55:221–228, 1994.

310. Miholic J, Orskov C, Holst J, et al: Emptying of the gastric substitute, glucagon-like peptide-1 (GLP-1), and reactive hypoglycemia after total gastrectomy. Dig Dis Sci 36:1361–1370, 1991.

311. Seltzer H, Allen E, Herror A, et al: Insulin response to glycemic stimulus: Relation of delayed initial release to carbohydrate intolerance in mild diabetes. J Clin Invest 46:323–335, 1967.

312. Faludi G, Bendersky G, Gerber P: Functional hypoglycemia in early latent diabetes. Ann N Y Acad Sci 148:868–874, 1968.

313. Permutt M: Postprandial hypoglycemia. Diabetes 25:719–733, 1976.

314. Hofeldt F: Reactive hypoglycemia. Endocrinol Metab Clin North Am 18:185–201, 1989.

315. Service F: Classification of hypoglycemic disorders. Endocrinol Metab Clin North Am 28:501–517, 1999.

316. Owada K, Wasada T, Miyazono Y, et al: Highly increased insulin secretion in a patient with postprandial hypoglycemia: Role of glucagon-like peptide-1 (7–36) amide). Endocr J 42:147–151, 1995.

317. Permutt M, Kelly J, Berstein R, et al: Alimentary hypoglycemia in the absence of gastrointestinal surgery. N Engl J Med 288:1206–1210, 1973.

318. Palardy J, Havrankova J, Lepage R, et al: Blood glucose measurements during symptomatic episodes in patients with suspected postprandial hypoglycemia. N Engl J Med 321:1421–1425, 1989.

319. Foa P, Dunbar J Jr, Klein S, et al: Reactive hypoglycemia and A-cell ('pancreatic') glucagon deficiency in the adult. JAMA 244:2281–2285, 1980.

320. Ahmadpour S, Kabadi U: Pancreatic alpha-cell function in idiopathic reactive hypoglycemia. Metabolism 46:639–643, 1997.

321. Leonetti F, Morviducci L, Giaccari A, et al: Idiopathic reactive hypoglycemia: A role for glucagon? J Endocrinol Invest 15:273–278, 1992.

322. Shima K, Tabata M, Tanaka A, et al: Exaggerated response of plasma glucagon-like immunoreactivity (GLI) to oral glucose in patients with reactive hypoglycemia. Endocrinol Jpn 28:249–256, 1981.

323. Wasada T, Katsumori K, Saeki A, et al: Lack of C-peptide suppression by exogenous hyperinsulinemia in subjects with symptoms suggesting reactive hypoglycemia. Endocr J 43:639–644, 1996.

324. Leonetti F, Foniciello M, Iozzo P, et al: Increased nonoxidative glucose metabolism in idiopathic reactive hypoglycemia. Metabolism 45:606–610, 1996.

325. Lteif A, Schwenk W: Hypoglycemia in infants and children. Endocrinol Metab Clin North Am 28:619–646, 1999.

326. Thomas P: Genetic mutations as a cause of hyperinsulinemic hypoglycemia in children. Endocrinol Metab Clin North Am 28:647–656, 1999.

327. Service F, Natt N, Thompson G, et al: Noninsulinoma pancreatogenous hypoglycemia: A novel syndrome of hyperinsulinemic hypoglycemia in adults independent of mutations in Kir6.2 and SUR1 genes. J Clin Endocrinol Metab 84:1582–1589, 1999.

328. Allweis T, Rimon B, Freund H: Malnutrition-associated reactive hypoglycemia induced by TPN. Nutrition 13:222–224, 1997.

329. Johnson D, Dorr K, Swenson W, et al: Reactive hypoglycemia. JAMA 243:1151–1155, 1980.

330. Charles M, Hofeldt F, Shackelford A, et al: Comparison of oral glucose tolerance tests and mixed meals in patients with apparent idiopathic postabsorptive hypoglycemia: Absence of hypoglycemia after meals. Diabetes 30:465–470, 1981.

331. Snorgaard O, Binder C: Monitoring of blood glucose concentration in subjects with hypoglycaemic symptoms during everyday life. BMJ 300:16–18, 1990.

332. Ford C, Bray G, Swerdloff R: A psychiatric study of patients referred with a diagnosis of hypoglycemia. Am J Psychiatry 133:290–294, 1976.

333. Berlin I, Grimaldi A, Landault C, et al: Suspected postprandial hypoglycemia is associated with beta-adrenergic hypersensitivity and emotional distress. J Clin Endocrinol Metab 79:1428–1433, 1994.

334. Lev-Ran A, Anderson R: The diagnosis of postprandial hypoglycemia. Diabetes 30:996–999, 1981.

335. Neve E: The morbid anatomy of the pancreas. Lancet 2:659, 1892.

336. Warren S: Adenomas of the islets of Langerhans. Am J Pathol 2:335–340, 1926.

337. Harris S: Hyperinsulinism and dysinsulinism. JAMA 83:729–733, 1924.

338. Wilder R, Allan F, Power M, et al: Carcinoma of the islands of the pancreas: Hyperinsulinism and hypoglycemia. JAMA 89:348–355, 1927.

339. Howland G, Campbell W, Maltby E, et al: Dysinsulinism: Convulsions and coma due to islet cell tumor of the pancreas. JAMA 93:674–679, 1929.

340. Whipple A, Frantz V: Adenoma of islet cells with hyperinsulinism. Ann Surg 101:1299–1335, 1935.

341. Whipple A: The surgical therapy of hyperinsulinism. J Int Chir 3:237–276, 1938.

342. Howard J, Moss N, Rhoads J: Hyperinsulinism and islet cell tumors of the pancreas. Int Abstr Surg 90:417–455, 1950.

343. Fajans S, Vinik A: Insulin-producing islet cell tumors. Endocrinol Metab Clin North Am 18:45–74, 1989.

344. Service F, McMahon M, O'Brien P, et al: Functioning insulinoma—incidence, recurrence, and long-term survival of patients: A 60-year study. Mayo Clin Proc 66:711–719, 1991.

345. Service F, Dale A, Elveback L, et al: Insulinoma: Clinical and diagnostic features of 60 consecutive cases. Mayo Clin Proc 51:417–429, 1976.
346. Galbut D, Markowitz A: Insulinoma: Diagnosis, surgical management and long-term follow-up. Review of 41 cases. Am J Surg 139:682–690, 1980.
347. Stefanini P, Carboni M, Patrassi N, et al: Beta-islet cell tumors of the pancreas: Results of a study on 1,067 cases. Surgery 75:597–609, 1974.
348. Broder L, Carter S: Pancreatic islet cell carcinoma. I. Clinical features of 52 patients. Ann Intern Med 79:101–107, 1973.
349. Laidlaw G: Nesidioblastoma: The islet cell tumor of the pancreas. Am J Pathol 14:125–139, 1937.
350. Yakovac W, Baker L, Hummeler K: Beta cell nesidioblastosis in idiopathic hypoglycemia of infancy. J Pediatr 79:226–231, 1971.
351. Harness J, Geelhoed G, Thompson N, et al: Nesidioblastosis in adults. A surgical dilemma. Arch Surg 116:575–580, 1981.
352. Gould V, Chejfec G, Shah K, et al: Adult nesidiodysplasia. Semin Diagn Pathol 1:43–53, 1984.
353. Walmsley D, Matheson N, Ewen S, et al: Nesidioblastosis in an elderly patient. Diabet Med 12:542–545, 1995.
354. Harrison T, Fajans S, Floyd J Jr, et al: Prevalence of diffuse pancreatic beta islet cell disease with hyperinsulinism: Problems in recognition and management. World J Surg 8:583–589, 1984.
355. Stefanini P, Carboni M, Patrassi N, et al: Hypoglycemia and insular hyperplasia: Review of 148 cases. Ann Surg 180:130–135, 1974.
356. Kavlie H, White T: Pancreatic islet beta cell tumors and hyperplasia: Experience in 14 Seattle hospitals. Ann Surg 175:326–335, 1972.
357. Cullen R, Ong C: Insulinoma in Auckland 1970–1985. N Z Med J 100:560–562, 1987.
358. Dizon A, Kowalyk S, Hoogwerf B: Neuroglycopenic and other symptoms in patients with insulinomas. Am J Med 106:307–310, 1999.
359. Boukhman M, Karam J, Shaver J, et al: Insulinoma—experience from 1950 to 1995. West J Med 169:98–104, 1998.
360. Perry R, Vinik A: Clinical review 72: Diagnosis and management of functioning islet cell tumors. J Clin Endocrinol Metab 80:2273–2278, 1995.
361. Kane L, Grant C, Nippoldt T, et al: Insulinoma in a patient with NIDDM. Diabetes Care 16:1298–1300, 1993.
362. Sakurai A, Aizawa T, Katakura M, et al: Insulinoma in a patient with non–insulin-dependent diabetes mellitus. Endocr J 44:473–477, 1997.
363. Wildbrett J, Nagel M, Theissig F, et al: [An unusual picture of insulinoma in type-2 diabetes mellitus and morbid obesity] (German). Dtsch Med Wochenschr 124:248–252, 1999.
364. Gerich J, Charles M, Grodsky G: Regulation of pancreatic insulin and glucagon secretion. Annu Rev Physiol 38:353–388, 1976.
365. Creutzfeldt W, Arnold R, Creutzfeldt C, et al: Biochemical and morphological investigations of 30 human insulinomas. Correlation between the tumour content of insulin and proinsulin-like components and the histological and ultrastructural appearance. Diabetologia 9:217–231, 1973.
366. Lindall A, Steffes M, Wong E: Comparison of insulin and proinsulin storage in an islet adenoma and adjacent pancreas. Metabolism 23:249–256, 1974.
367. Alsever R, Stjernholm M, Sussman K, et al: Clinical correlations of serum proinsulin-like material in islet cell tumours. Diabetologia 12:527–530, 1976.
368. Rizza R, Haymond M, Verdonk C, et al: Pathogenesis of hypoglycemia in insulinoma patients: Suppression of hepatic glucose production by insulin. Diabetes 30:377–381, 1981.
369. Wynick D, Williams S, Bloom S: Symptomatic secondary hormone syndromes in patients with established malignant pancreatic endocrine tumors. N Engl J Med 319:605–607, 1988.
370. Fonseca V, Ames D, Ginsburg J: Hypoglycaemia for 26 years due to an insulinoma. J R Soc Med 82:437–438, 1989.
371. Vea H, Trovik T, Sager G, et al: Return of beta-adrenergic sensitivity in a patient with insulinoma after removal of the tumour. Diabet Med 14:979–984, 1997.
372. Vea H, Jorde R, Sager G, et al: Pre- and postoperative glucose levels for eliciting hypoglycemic responses in a patient with insulinoma. Diabet Med 9:950–953, 1992.
373. Lloyd R, Caceres V, Warner T, et al: Islet cell adenomatosis. A report of two cases and review of the literature. Arch Pathol Lab Med 105:198–202, 1981.
374. Fong T, Warner N, Kumar D: Pancreatic nesidioblastosis in adults. Diabetes Care 12:108–114, 1989.
375. Service F: Hypoglycemic Disorders. N Engl J Med 332:1144–1152, 1995.
376. Marks V, Teale J: Investigation of hypoglycaemia. Clin Endocrinol (Oxf) 44:133–136, 1996.
377. Service F, O'Brien P, Kao P, et al: C-peptide suppression test: Effects of gender, age, and body mass index; implications for the diagnosis of insulinoma. J Clin Endocrinol Metab 74:204–210, 1992.
378. Marks V, Somols E: Diagnostic tests for evaluating hypoglycemia. In Rodriguez R, Vallance-Owen J (eds): Diabetes. Amsterdam, Excerpta Medica, 1971, pp 864–872.
379. Kumar D, Mehtalia S, Miller L: Diagnostic use of glucagon-induced insulin response. Studies in patients with insulinoma or other hypoglycemic conditions. Ann Intern Med 80:697–701, 1974.
380. Floyd J Jr, Fajans S, Knopf R, et al: Plasma insulin in organic hyperinsulinism: Comparative effects of tolbutamide, leucine and glucose. J Clin Endocrinol 24:747–760, 1964.
381. Service F: Diagnostic approach to adults with hypoglycemic disorders. Endocrinol Metab Clin North Am 28:519–532, 1999.
382. Filipi C, Higgins G: Diagnosis and management of insulinoma. Am J Surg 125:231–239, 1973.
383. Daggett P, Goodburn E, Kurtz A, et al: Is preoperative localisation of insulinomas necessary? Lancet 1:483–486, 1981.
384. Grant C: Surgical aspects of hyperinsulinemic hypoglycemia. Endocrinol Metab Clin North Am 28:533–554, 1999.
385. Norton J, Whitman E: Insulinoma. Endocrinologist 3:258–267, 1995.
386. Huai J-C, Zhang W, Niu H-O, et al: Localization and surgical treatment of pancreatic insulinomas guided by intraoperative ultrasound. Am J Surg 175:18–21, 1998.
387. King A, Ko G, Yeung V, et al: Dual phase spiral CT in the detection of small insulinomas of the pancreas. Br J Radiol 71:20–23, 1998.
388. van Heerden J, Grant C, Czako P, et al: Occult functioning insulinomas: Which localizing studies are indicated? Surgery 112:1010–1014, 1992.
389. Kaplan E, Rubenstein A, Evans R, et al: Calcium infusion: A new provocative test for insulinomas. Ann Surg 190:501–507, 1979.
390. Gill G, Rauf O, MacFarlane I: Diazoxide treatment for insulinoma: A national UK survey. Postgrad Med J 73:640–641, 1997.
391. Osei K, O'Dorisio T: Malignant insulinoma: Effects of a somatostatin analog (compound 201–995) on serum glucose, growth, and gastro-entero-pancreatic hormones. Ann Intern Med 103:223–225, 1985.
392. Hearn P, Ahmed M, Woodhouse N: The use of SMS 201–995 (somatostatin analogue) in insulinomas. Additional case report and literature review. Horm Res 29:211–213, 1988.
393. Richter W, Otto C: Continuous subcutaneous glucagon infusion as a symptomatic therapy in two patients with organic hyperinsulinemia. Endocrinol Metab 3:63–65, 1996.
394. Moertel C, Hanley J, Johnson L: Streptozocin alone compared with streptozocin plus fluorouracil in the treatment of advanced islet-cell carcinoma. N Engl J Med 303:1189–1194, 1980.
395. Kiang D, Frenning D, Bauer G: Mithramycin for hypoglycemia in malignant insulinoma. N Engl J Med 299:134–135, 1978.
396. Eastman R, Come S, Strewler G, et al: Adriamycin therapy for advanced insulinoma. J Clin Endocrinol Metab 44:142–148, 1977.
397. Ajani J, Carrasco C, Charnsangavej C, et al: Islet cell tumors metastatic to the liver: Effective palliation by sequential hepatic artery embolization. Ann Intern Med 108:340–344, 1988.
398. Hart S, Frier B: Causes, management and morbidity of acute hypoglycaemia in adults requiring hospital admission. Q J Med 91:505–510, 1998.
399. Malouf R, Brust J: Hypoglycemia: Causes, neurological manifestations, and outcome. Ann Neurol 17:421–430, 1985.
400. Shilo S, Berezovsky S, Friedlander Y, et al: Hypoglycemia in hospitalized nondiabetic older patients. J Am Geriatr Soc 46:978–982, 1998.
401. Kresevic D, Slavin S: Incidence of hypoglycemia and nutritional intake in patients on a general medical unit. Nurs Connections 2:33–40, 1989.
402. Fischer K, Lees J, Newman J: Hypoglycemia in hospitalized patients: Causes and outcomes. N Engl J Med 315:1245–1250, 1986.
403. Stagnaro-Green A, Barton M, Linekin P, et al: Mortality in hospitalized patients with hypoglycemia and severe hyperglycemia. Mt Sinai J Med 62:422–426, 1995.
404. Cruz Jentoft A, Villar I, Carreras P, et al: [Unexpected hypoglycemia in hospitalized patients] (Spanish). Rev Clin Esp 191:295–298, 1992.
405. Gaston S: Outcomes of hypoglycemia treated by standardized protocol in a community hospital. Diabetes Educ 18:491–494, 1992.
406. Slama G, Traynard P, Desplanque N, et al: The search for an optimized treatment of hypoglycemia. Carbohydrates in tablets, solution, or gel for the correction of insulin reactions. Arch Intern Med 150:589–593, 1990.
407. Palatnick W, Meatherall R, Tenenbein M: Clinical spectrum of sulfonylurea overdose and experience with diazoxide therapy. Arch Intern Med 151:1859–1862, 1991.

Chapter 67

Diabetes, Lipids, and Atherosclerosis

Alan Chait ▪ Steven Haffner

The most common cause of morbidity and mortality in diabetes is atherosclerotic cardiovascular disease.[1, 2] Several cardiovascular risk factors occur commonly in both types 1 and 2 diabetes (Table 67–1). Prominent among these risk factors is dyslipidemia, which is caused by abnormalities in lipid and lipoprotein metabolism. Defects in plasma lipid and lipoprotein metabolism are common in diabetes and appear to play an important role in increasing the risk of atherosclerotic disease in patients with diabetes. The nature of the metabolic defects differs between type 1 and type 2 diabetes and relates in part to treatment of the diabetes and the presence of diabetic complications. In this chapter the nature and pathogenesis of diabetic dyslipidemia will be reviewed. In addition, the relationship of the dyslipidemia to atherosclerosis will be discussed, as will an approach to its management.

DIABETES AS A RISK FACTOR FOR CORONARY HEART DISEASE

Diabetes is associated with a marked increase in coronary heart disease (CHD).[3–5] In most studies the relative risk of CHD is relatively greater in diabetic women than in diabetic men.[3–5] However, with the exception of the Framingham Study,[4] the absolute risk of CHD in diabetic men is greater than that in diabetic women.[5] The causes of increased risk of CHD in diabetes are multifactorial (e.g., dyslipidemia, hypertension, obesity, smoking) and have been well reviewed.[3–7]

TABLE 67–1. Cardiovascular Risk Factors in Diabetes Mellitus

Risk Factor	Type 1	Type 2
Dyslipidemia		
Hypertriglyceridemia	+	+ +
Low HDL	−	+
Small, dense LDL	−	+
Increased apolipoprotein B	−	+
Hypertension	+	+ +
Hyperinsulinemia/insulin resistance	−	+
Central obesity	−	+
Family history of atherosclerosis	−	+
Cigarette smoking	−	+

HDL, high-density lipoprotein; LDL, low-density lipoprotein.

Most diabetic subjects have type 2 diabetes, and most of the literature relating diabetes to CHD concerns type 2 diabetes.

Haffner et al. compared the 7-year incidence of myocardial infarction (fatal and nonfatal) in 1373 nondiabetic subjects with the incidence in 1059 diabetic subjects, all from a Finnish population-based study.[8] The 7-year incidence rates of myocardial infarction in nondiabetic subjects with and without prior myocardial infarction at baseline were 18.8% and 3.5%, respectively. The 7-year incidence rates of myocardial infarction in diabetic subjects with and without prior myocardial infarction at baseline were 45.0% and 20.2%, respectively (Fig. 67–1). After adjustment for age and sex, the hazard ratio for death from CHD was not significantly different for diabetic subjects without prior myocardial infarction than for nondiabetic subjects with prior myocardial infarction. Even after further adjustment for total cholesterol, hypertension, and smoking, this hazard ratio remained close to 1.0. These data suggest that diabetic patients without previous myocardial infarction have as high a risk of myocardial infarction as do nondiabetic patients with previous myocardial infarction and provide a rationale for treating cardiovascular risk factors in diabetic patients as aggressively as in nondiabetic patients with prior myocardial infarction.

A number of potential limitations of this study should be noted. First, the data collected at baseline from 1982 to 1984 were from Finland, a country with very high low-density lipoprotein (LDL) cholesterol levels and a very high incidence of CHD. Thus it might be questioned whether these results are applicable to the United States, a country with lower levels of LDL cholesterol and less CHD. However, separate analyses of subjects from Kuopio (eastern Finland with high rates of CHD) and from Turku (with lower rates of CHD) both showed a similar incidence of CHD in diabetic subjects without preexisting vascular disease and nondiabetic subjects with vascular disease. Second, the average duration of diabetes was 8 years and the average fasting glucose level was about 200 mg/dL. The diabetic subjects were selected from a population-based registry of subjects receiving oral agents or insulin. Although these numbers are roughly representative of data in the United States, it can be questioned whether these results would apply to less severe diabetic subjects. Third, the Finnish subjects were all middle-aged (aged 45–65), and thus it could be questioned whether these results might apply to elderly subjects inasmuch as it is well known that the relative risk of patients with diabetes for CHD declines with age.[9] Indeed, in a population-based study of elderly subjects with small numbers of diabetic subjects from Australia, the risk of CHD in nondiabetic subjects with preexisting CHD was greater than that of diabetic subjects without preexisting CHD.[10]

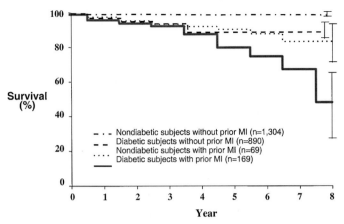

FIGURE 67–1. Kaplan-Meier estimates of the probability of death from coronary heart disease in 1059 subjects with type 2 diabetes and 1373 nondiabetic subjects with and without prior myocardial infarction (MI). *I bars* indicate 95% confidence intervals.

A cross-sectional analysis of intima-media wall thickness in the Insulin Resistance Atherosclerosis Study (IRAS)[11] has recently been completed.[8] Intima-media wall thickness in diabetic subjects without previous myocardial infarction (internal carotid, 0.921 mm; common carotid, 0.859 mm) was slightly larger (although insignificantly) than in nondiabetic subjects without a previous myocardial infarction (0.850 and 0.806 mm, respectively). This study provides some reproducibility (again in a middle-aged population) of the Finnish report.[8] Furthermore, IRAS was done in the United States, where subjects had much lower LDL cholesterol and fasting glucose levels and a shorter duration of diabetes than did the subjects in the Finnish study.

Diabetic subjects also have an increased case fatality rate after a myocardial infarction. In the Finnish Monitoring International Cardiovascular Disease trial it was shown that the 1-year case fatality rate for a first myocardial infarction (from the onset of symptoms, thus including prehospitalization mortality) was 45% in diabetic men and 39% in diabetic women.[12] These case fatality rates were significantly higher than the rates in nondiabetic subjects (38% for men and 25% for women). Of the diabetic subjects who died, 50% of the men and 25% of the women died before hospitalization. These patients, by definition, could not benefit from secondary prevention strategies, thus indicating (especially in diabetic men) that aggressive management of cardiovascular risk factors in diabetic subjects should precede the onset of clinical CHD. One of these risk factors is diabetic dyslipidemia.

DIABETIC DYSLIPIDEMIA

The term *diabetic dyslipidemia* has been used loosely to describe the constellation of abnormalities that are characteristically observed in individuals with type 2 diabetes, although the presence of dyslipidemia is also common in type 1 diabetes, especially when untreated or when associated with diabetic complications, particularly renal disease. The most common features of diabetic dyslipidemia are hypertriglyceridemia, which is often mild, and low levels of high-density lipoprotein (HDL) cholesterol, also often not marked. The presence of small, dense LDL particles usually accompanies these other abnormalities and is part of the dyslipidemic pattern seen in diabetes. These changes are often accompanied by an increase in the plasma level of apolipoprotein B (apo B). Dyslipidemia similar to that described above is often seen in the absence of diabetes and is therefore not specific for this disorder. For example, it is also typical of the insulin resistance syndrome, which usually precedes the onset of clinical type 2 diabetes. Levels of lipoprotein(a) [Lp(a)] can be increased in diabetes, although an increase in this lipoprotein class is not usually considered part of the diabetic dyslipidemic syndrome. Marked hypertriglyceridemia, with plasma triglyceride levels in excess of 2000 mg/dL, also occurs occasionally. Both Lp(a) elevations and these very elevated levels of triglyceride will be discussed later in the chapter.

Evaluation of lipoproteins by sophisticated techniques reveals considerable compositional changes in type 2 diabetes. The use of gradient gel electrophoresis to size both LDL and HDL particles, as well as nonequilibrium density gradient ultracentrifugation to separate all the lipoprotein classes on the basis of density, reveals considerable heterogeneity in lipoprotein size and density. A tendency to the presence of small, dense, very-low-density lipoprotein (VLDL) particles, an increase in the remnant-rich intermediate-density lipoprotein (IDL) fraction, a redistribution of LDL particles toward more small and dense species,[13] and considerable changes in HDL composition have been noted.[14–16] Changes in lipid composition are found within each lipoprotein class, with a relative increase in the ratio of free cholesterol to phospholipids.[17–19] In addition, an increase in the extent of nonenzymatic glycosylation has been observed within all classes of circulating lipoproteins.[20] Most studies also demonstrate that lipoproteins from subjects with diabetes show an increased susceptibility to oxidative modification,[21–26] which might also increase their atherogenicity.

Hence diabetic dyslipidemia encompasses a large array of both quantitative and qualitative changes in plasma lipids and lipoproteins. The relationship of these lipid abnormalities to cardiovascular risk is discussed later in this chapter.

DIAGNOSIS OF DIABETIC DYSLIPIDEMIA

Plasma lipids and lipoproteins should be evaluated in all patients with diabetes at the time of diagnosis, after the establishment of a regimen for glycemic control, whenever major changes are made to the glycemic regimen, and at least annually thereafter. Although subtle abnormalities in lipid and lipoprotein composition have been demonstrated by the use of sophisticated research techniques, less extensive evaluation is required in the assessment of patients in clinical practice. Initial evaluation should include a lipid profile, with measurement of plasma cholesterol, triglycerides, LDL cholesterol, and HDL cholesterol in the fasted state. Such testing is all that is required in most instances. However, the presence of hypertriglyceridemia, low levels of HDL cholesterol, and borderline levels of LDL cholesterol should be taken seriously because they indicate the presence of the major components of diabetic dyslipidemia.

Hypertriglyceridemia reflects the increase in VLDL and IDL, and low levels of HDL cholesterol are associated with the more subtle compositional changes discussed earlier. High-normal or borderline-high LDL cholesterol levels usually indicate an increase in the number of small, dense LDL particles. An increase in small, dense VLDL and IDL and the presence of small, dense LDL are often reflected as an increase in plasma apo B concentration, because each of these lipoprotein particles contains one molecule of apo B. Thus the level of apo B in plasma reflects the total number of these potentially atherogenic particles. Measurement of apo B, where available, can be helpful in deciding whether to treat an individual patient. Similarly, measurement of Lp(a) can be of value, but guidelines for using these values for the management of diabetic patients are not available, and their routine measurement in clinical practice is not recommended. However, an increase in these levels would favor intervention in borderline cases and might indicate more aggressive intervention because of the increased cardiovascular risk associated with an increase in either of these levels.

Initial laboratory evaluation of the patient should include quantification of the urine albumin excretion rate, evaluation of renal and thyroid function, and assessment of indices of glycemic control. A carefully taken family history for evidence of dyslipidemia and/or premature cardiovascular disease is of value in deciding whether to treat an individual patient. For follow-up evaluation of plasma lipids and lipoproteins, measurement of fasting plasma cholesterol, triglycerides, and LDL and HDL cholesterol levels will suffice.

PATHOPHYSIOLOGY OF DIABETIC DYSLIPIDEMIA

Type 1 Diabetes

Hypertriglyceridemia

The most common abnormality in type 1 diabetes is hypertriglyceridemia[27–29] secondary to increased levels of VLDL. This disorder is often noted at the time of diagnosis of the diabetes, but it can be persistent, which may be a reflection of poor glycemic control.[29, 30] Triglyceride levels return toward normal with improved glycemic control, especially with the use of multiple insulin injections or the insulin pump.[31–38]

Hypertriglyceridemia can be due to increased secretion of VLDL or to impaired lipoprotein lipase–mediated VLDL removal from plasma. The hypertriglyceridemia seen at the onset of type 1 diabetes is due to impaired VLDL clearance resulting from decreased adipose tissue lipoprotein lipase activity.[39–41] Lipoprotein lipase activity is normal in most chronically treated type 1 patients and is not directly related to the degree of glycemic control.[41] Persistent hypertriglyceridemia in type 1 diabetes is due to increased VLDL secretion.[42]

Low HDL Cholesterol

Low HDL cholesterol levels are often present in association with hypertriglyceridemia at the time of diagnosis of type 1 diabetes.[43] Low levels of HDL cholesterol are also associated with poor glycemic control[29, 44] and tend to improve with treatment.[33, 37, 45] HDL cholesterol levels are usually normal[45] or even elevated[46] in treated type 1 patients.

The reduced HDL cholesterol in untreated type 1 patients is in part due to replacement of cholesterol in the core of HDL by triglycerides and in part due to increased catabolism of HDL associated with impaired lipoprotein lipase activity.[47] These abnormalities normalize with therapy. In treated type 1 patients, HDL levels may be influenced by changes in body weight. The increased levels of HDL cholesterol sometimes observed may be related to the relatively low body weight in some type 1 subjects.[48] Weight gain, which is common with intensive insulin therapy, can lead to a reduction in HDL levels.[49] This adverse effect of weight gain may offset any benefit of glycemic control on HDL levels per se and may explain the lack of change in HDL cholesterol in the Diabetes Control and Complications Trial (DCCT), where most subjects gained weight.[50]

LDL Cholesterol

Although LDL cholesterol levels are generally in the normal range in type 1 diabetes,[51] they nonetheless fall in response to intensive insulinization.[32, 33, 38, 50] A problem with assessment of LDL levels and responses in most clinical trials to date is that LDL is usually estimated rather than measured directly. The estimated LDL cholesterol value includes true LDL (d = 1.019–1.063 g/mL) and IDL (d = 1.006–1.019 g/mL) and may include some Lp(a). Detailed evaluation of the lipids and lipoproteins in subjects participating in the DCCT showed that the decrease in "LDL" associated with intensive insulinization was due to a reduction in Lp(a), a decrease in IDL, and a shift from dense LDL to more buoyant particles.[52] Thus subtle compositional changes that are likely to be beneficial are obscured by the simple measurement of "LDL cholesterol."

Plasma LDL levels are also determined by both the rate of LDL removal and the rate of LDL production. Although insulin at high doses can increase the expression of LDL receptors in vitro,[53] kinetic studies have shown that the reduction in LDL levels seen with intensive therapy is due to decreased production of LDL.[54]

Thus in type 1 diabetes, the major abnormality of plasma lipoproteins is an increased level of VLDL, and all the lipid and lipoprotein abnormalities in type 1 diabetes improve with institution of therapy and also with tight glycemic control. Studies in children who embarked on a multistaged program of intensification of insulin therapy suggest that greater metabolic improvement occurs after early routine therapeutic measures than after intensification of therapy.[52] Thus the major improvement in the dyslipidemia of type 1 diabetes occurs with initiation of therapy, with less dramatic changes associated with improved glycemic control.

Type 2 Diabetes

Dyslipidemia is more common in type 2 than type 1 diabetes. However, the impact of type 2 diabetes on lipids and lipoprotein metabolism is complex because it can be influenced by several factors, including insulin resistance, obesity, the type of therapy, the extent of glycemic control, the use of medications for associated disorders, and several complications of diabetes.

The dyslipidemia that is most characteristic of type 2 diabetes is increased triglyceride and decreased HDL cholesterol levels.[3, 6, 55, 56] In many studies the dyslipidemia in type 2 diabetic subjects relative to nondiabetic subjects is more severe in women than in men,[55, 56] which is consistent with the relatively greater risk of CHD in diabetic women (fourfold) than in diabetic men (twofold).[3–6] The dyslipidemia in diabetic subjects is not completely explained by the greater overall adiposity in diabetic subjects.[55]

Hypertriglyceridemia and Low HDL Cholesterol

Untreated type 2 diabetic patients are frequently hypertriglyceridemic and have low levels of HDL cholesterol.[57–59] Although treated diabetic subjects tend to have higher triglyceride levels than do nondiabetic subjects, most diabetic subjects are not frankly hypertriglyceridemic if a cutoff of 200 mg/dL is used. In data based on the San Antonio Heart Study population,[6] the distribution of triglyceride concentrations is skewed markedly to the right. As a result, the mean triglyceride levels are much higher than the median (50%) level. For both Mexican-Americans and non-Hispanic whites, the median triglyceride level is lower than 200 mg/dL, and less than 5% of diabetic women and 15% of diabetic men have triglyceride levels greater than 400 mg/dL. In the Framingham Study the prevalence of hypertriglyceridemia in type 2 diabetic and nondiabetic men was 19% and 9%, respectively.[12] In type 2 diabetic and nondiabetic women, the prevalence of hypertriglyceridemia was 17% and 8%, respectively. The prevalence of low HDL cholesterol was 21% (vs. 9%) in men as opposed to 25% (vs. 10%) in women.

Initiation of therapy with either insulin or oral sulfonylureas leads to a reduction in triglyceride levels and an increase in HDL cholesterol. These improvements occur despite the fact that weight gain often accompanies the initiation of such therapies and that weight gain per se can lead to increased levels of triglycerides and reduced HDL cholesterol levels.[57, 59] Similarly, initiation of metformin therapy is associated with a reduction in triglycerides, although not with an increase in HDL levels.[60] Triglyceride levels are also moderately reduced with the use of thiazolidinediones.[61] As with type 1 diabetes, the effect of initiation of therapy is far greater than the effect of improving glycemic control in previously treated patients.[57, 59]

HDL cholesterol levels are characteristically decreased in type 2 diabetes.[57, 58, 62] As with type 1 patients, HDL cholesterol levels increase with weight loss[63, 64] and with insulin therapy.[57, 65] They also increase with the use of sulfonylureas.[40, 66] Despite adequate treatment of the hyperglycemia, mild hypertriglyceridemia and decreased HDL levels often persist in patients with type 2 diabetes,[67–69] independent of the degree of glycemic control.[70] The hypertriglyceridemia can be contributed to by the presence of remnants of the triglyceride-rich lipoproteins,[15, 37, 71, 72] as indicated by increased levels of IDL (d = 1.006–1.019 g/mL). VLDL[73–75] and IDL[72] are also enriched in cholesterol, consistent with the accumulation of remnant lipoproteins.

Persistence of this dyslipidemic pattern, taken together with the observation that a similar form of dyslipidemia can be observed in nondiabetic relatives of patients with type 2 diabetes,[76, 77] suggests that the dyslipidemia is not due to the diabetes per se but may be due to some underlying condition that predisposes to the development of diabetes, such as the central obesity/insulin resistance syndrome (see later).

The hypertriglyceridemia seen in mild to moderately hyperglycemic type 2 subjects results mainly from an increase in VLDL secretion.[78–81] VLDL catabolism may be impaired simultaneously,[82] despite apparently normal lipoprotein lipase activity.[43] However, in more severely hyperglycemic untreated patients with type 2 diabetes, in whom greater relative insulin deficiency accompanies the insulin resistance, a modest reduction in lipoprotein lipase activity is also seen.[39–41, 83] However, VLDL oversecretion occurs concomitantly,[41] such that the hypertriglyceridemia in this situation is likely to result from defects in both triglyceride secretion and removal from plasma. In chronically treated type 2 diabetic patients, lipoprotein lipase levels are normal and are not related to the degree of glycemic control.[41] In this situation the presence of persistent hypertriglyceridemia is the result of VLDL oversecretion.[41]

HDL levels increase during therapy as a result of improved catabolism of VLDL, with transfer of the surface components of VLDL catabolism to HDL.[62] HDL particles are also remodeled by the enzyme hepatic lipase, which in addition modifies the size, density, and composition of LDL (see later). Hepatic lipase activity has been shown to be increased in type 2 diabetes,[14, 43, 83] which may in part account for the abnormalities in HDL composition that occur in this disorder.

LDL

LDL cholesterol levels are relatively low (130–140 mg/dL) in type 2 diabetes. However, only a small proportion of subjects (10%–20%) have very low LDL levels (<100 mg/dL). As noted earlier, the conventional method for estimating LDL cholesterol includes the remnant-rich IDL fraction. When IDL has been measured separately from LDL, true LDL levels are usually normal.[72, 84–87] However, an abnormality in LDL that occurs commonly in type 2 diabetes is the presence of small, dense (pattern B) LDL.[14, 88–90] LDL size has been shown to be consistently smaller in diabetic subjects than in nondiabetic subjects.[91, 92] A major determinant of the presence of these small, dense LDL particles is the plasma triglyceride level, which is inversely related to LDL particle size. However, lower LDL size and density in diabetic subjects may be partially independent of the higher triglyceride and lower HDL levels in diabetic subjects.[15, 91, 92] LDL particle size has also been shown to be inversely related to Hb A_{1C} levels.[38, 89]

The mechanism by which LDL become small and dense relates in part to the activity of hepatic lipase, an enzyme that remodels LDL toward smaller, denser particles. Thus low levels of hepatic lipase are associated with the presence of large buoyant LDL particles, whereas high hepatic lipase activity is associated with the presence of small, dense LDL. Hepatic lipase has been reported to be increased in type 2 diabetes,[14, 43, 83] consistent with the presence of small, dense LDL in this disorder.

Despite essentially normal LDL levels in type 2 diabetes, kinetic studies have demonstrated subtle disturbances in LDL metabolism. In mild untreated type 2 diabetes, LDL synthesis and removal rates are increased concomitantly, which results in normal LDL cholesterol levels.[93] In untreated or poorly controlled, moderately hyperglycemic patients, impaired LDL catabolism can lead to mildly elevated LDL levels.[93, 94] Thus although LDL levels, as determined in the clinical laboratory, are not dramatically altered in type 2 diabetes, their metabolism is not normal and the LDL particles are typically of the small, dense variety, which is associated with increased atherosclerosis risk, even in the absence of diabetes.[95] These abnormalities in LDL are part of the dyslipidemic pattern that characterizes this disorder.

The Insulin Resistance Syndrome and Dyslipidemia in Treated Type 2 Patients

Insulin resistance occurs commonly in individuals who do not have overt type 2 diabetes. Diabetes ensues when insulin secretion falls to a level that is insufficient to maintain blood glucose levels within the normal range in the presence of insulin resistance. An intermediate stage of insulin resistance is termed *impaired glucose tolerance*, which occurs when insulin secretion is sufficient to maintain fasting blood glucose levels that are not high enough to warrant the diagnosis of diabetes but are borderline elevated. Insulin resistance in the absence of full-blown type 2 diabetes is characterized by a clustering of cardiovascular risk factors and a markedly increased risk of cardiovascular disease.[14, 96–98] These risk factors include dyslipidemia (consisting of hypertriglyceridemia, low HDL, accumulation of remnant lipoproteins, and the presence of small, dense LDL particles), hypertension, impaired glucose tolerance, increased levels of fibrinogen, and decreased levels of plasminogen activator inhibitor-1.[98] This constellation of findings has been termed "syndrome X" or the plurimetabolic syndrome. A critical element of this syndrome is the presence of a

central, especially visceral, distribution of body fat,[99, 100] which can be detected by computed tomography of the abdomen.[99, 100] Because the presence of many features of this syndrome antedates the onset of type 2 diabetes, sometimes by a considerable period, overt or subclinical cardiovascular disease can frequently be detected at the time of diagnosis of type 2 diabetes. The cardiovascular risk factors associated with the central obesity/insulin resistance syndrome may have preceded by many years the onset of hyperglycemia, on which basis the diagnosis of diabetes is ascertained. Thus the arterial wall may have been exposed to risk factors well before frank diabetes ensues, with macrovascular complications resulting early in the course of frank diabetes. This situation differs considerably from that seen with the microvascular complications of diabetes, the onset of which has been attributed to the onset of hyperglycemia. Thus the clock starts ticking for the evolution of cardiovascular disease with the onset of risk factors associated with the insulin resistance syndrome, whereas the clock starts ticking for the development of microvascular complications with the onset of hyperglycemia.[101]

Lp(a)

Lp(a) is a lipoprotein that consists of LDL in disulfide linkage with apo (a), an apolipoprotein with considerable sequence homology with plasminogen. However, the protease activity of plasminogen is lacking. Not only does Lp(a) have associated atherogenic properties because of its similarity to LDL, but it is also likely to increase thrombogenicity because of its ability to compete with plasminogen for binding sites without having plasminogen-like activity.[102]

Lp(a) levels have been reported to be increased in type 1 diabetes and to improve with improved glycemic control.[103] In the DCCT, the group that received conventional therapy had slightly higher Lp(a) levels than those receiving intensive treatment,[38] which suggests that the level of this lipoprotein may be influenced to some extent by glycemic control. Whether Lp(a) levels are increased in type 2 diabetes is still controversial,[103] although more recent, larger studies often show similar[104] or even lower[105] Lp(a) levels in type 2 diabetic subjects relative to normoglycemic subjects. Furthermore, little evidence is available to support a decrease in Lp(a) levels with improved glycemic control in type 2 diabetes.[103] In type 1 diabetes, the presence of diabetic nephropathy or even microalbuminuria[106] appears to be associated with increased levels of Lp(a).

Effect of Nephropathy

The major complication of diabetes that affects lipoprotein metabolism is renal disease. The presence of microalbuminuria in diabetic subjects, even in those with normal renal function, is associated with higher triglyceride and apo B levels than in diabetic subjects without microalbuminuria.[107, 108] Further increases in apo B levels are seen in type 1 diabetic subjects with higher levels of proteinuria and with impaired renal function.[109] With the development of marked proteinuria and the nephrotic syndrome, VLDL and LDL levels become markedly increased in both types 1 and 2 diabetes.[109, 110] Remnants of the triglyceride-rich lipoproteins also accumulate in type 1 patients with albuminuria.[108, 111] Hypertriglyceridemia and low HDL cholesterol levels are characteristic of end-stage renal disease in both type 1 and type 2 diabetes, as in the absence of diabetes.[109, 110, 112] Dialysis is associated with elevations in VLDL and IDL levels and with a decrease in true LDL (d = 1.019–1.063 g/mL) and HDL levels. After renal transplantation, both VLDL and LDL levels increase as a result of cyclosporine and prednisone use for immunosuppression.[109, 113] These changes are similar to those seen with renal disease in patients without diabetes.

The presence of nephropathy is associated with a markedly increased risk of cardiovascular disease, especially in type 1 diabetes.[114, 115] Even the earliest manifestation of nephropathy, microalbuminuria, is associated with increased atherosclerosis risk.[116, 117] The onset of microalbuminuria is associated with the development of subtle changes in the pattern of plasma lipids and lipoproteins.[108] As renal disease progresses, the lipid and lipoprotein changes described earlier are likely to play a role in increasing cardiovascular risk. However, other factors such as hypertension and hyperhomocysteinemia[118] may also play a role in the increased atherosclerosis risk that occurs in the presence of renal complications.

Effect of Other Complications on Lipids and Lipoproteins

Autoimmune thyroid disease is increased in patients with type 1 diabetes. Untreated hypothyroidism leads to increased levels of both LDL and VLDL and their remnants,[109, 119] which return to normal with appropriate thyroid replacement therapy.[119] The prevalence of hypertension is increased in both type 1 and type 2 diabetes as a result of renal complications and the central obesity/insulin resistance syndrome. Treatment of hypertension with diuretics and β-adrenergic blocking agents can adversely affect plasma lipids and lipoproteins.[120, 121] Diuretics increase both VLDL and LDL, thereby elevating both plasma triglyceride and cholesterol levels.[120, 121] The major effect of β-blockers is to increase triglycerides and decrease HDL cholesterol levels.[120, 121] Use of alcohol and estrogen may also contribute to hypertriglyceridemia.[109] In addition, lipid levels can be affected by the frequent occurrence of genetic forms of hyperlipidemia, such as familial combined hyperlipidemia and familial hypertriglyceridemia. These genetic disorders may contribute to the severe hypertriglyceridemia and the chylomicronemia syndrome seen in some diabetic subjects.

The Chylomicronemia Syndrome

A constellation of symptoms and signs termed the *chylomicronemia syndrome* can occur when plasma triglyceride levels exceed 2000 mg/dL.[122] Clinical findings include eruptive xanthomas, abdominal pain and pancreatitis, lipemia retinalis, reversible memory loss, and dysesthesias.[122] HDL levels are usually very low, as are LDL levels when measured directly.[122] The most common cause of hypertriglyceridemia of this magnitude is the coexistence of undiagnosed or untreated type 2 diabetes with genetic forms of hypertriglyceridemia such as familial combined hyperlipidemia or familial hypertriglyceridemia.[109, 122, 123] Other secondary forms of hypertriglyceridemia can coexist.[122] Increased secretion of VLDL occurs in familial forms of hypertriglyceridemia and, as noted earlier, also in type 2 diabetes. Thus triglyceride removal systems become saturated when both diabetes and a familial form of hypertriglyceridemia coexist. As a result, chylomicrons formed in response to the ingestion of dietary fat accumulate in addition to VLDL. Although hypertriglyceridemia of this magnitude has been described in type 1 diabetes,[124] it is also likely to represent the interaction of diabetes with a genetic form of hypertriglyceridemia and is much less commonly seen than with type 2 diabetes.

Treatment of the hyperglycemia by whatever means indicated will bring the triglyceride levels down to a more moderate range.[122] The fact that patients with type 1 diabetes are usually treated with insulin early in the course of their disease, as opposed to the often late treatment of patients with type 2 diabetes, probably explains the relative rarity of marked hypertriglyceridemia in type 1 diabetes. Despite improvement in triglyceride levels with treatment of the hyperglycemia, diabetic patients with marked hypertriglyceridemia resulting from interaction with a familial form of hypertriglyceridemia often require the use of a fibrate for control of their hypertriglyceridemia. Fibrate use in this situation may lead to an increase in LDL cholesterol levels.[125]

Atherosclerotic complications are not part of the chylomicronemia syndrome, per se, the most serious consequence of which is pancreatitis. However, clinical manifestations of cardiovascular disease frequently develop with time in diabetic patients with this syndrome. This complication may relate in part to the many other cardiovascular risk factors that are present in these individuals in association with the central obesity/insulin resistance syndrome. In addition, the coexistence of an atherogenic familial form of hyperlipidemia, modification of lipoproteins that can facilitate atherogenesis in diabetes (see later),

and the increase in LDL level that occurs with fibrate therapy may all play a role in the accelerated atherosclerotic disease in these patients.

RELATIONSHIP OF DYSLIPIDEMIA TO CORONARY HEART DISEASE IN DIABETES

In the large World Health Organization cross-sectional study, plasma cholesterol and triglyceride (as well as blood pressure) were related to myocardial infarction.[2] However, in multivariate analysis, plasma triglyceride but not cholesterol predicted the prevalence of myocardial infarction. In the 11-year follow-up of the Paris Prospective Study,[126] hypertriglyceridemia (but not hypercholesterolemia) predicted CHD mortality in a combined group of subjects with impaired glucose tolerance and diabetes. However, HDL cholesterol was not determined in these reports.[2, 126] In a 12-year follow-up of the Multiple Risk Factor Intervention Trial (MRFIT) screenees, total cholesterol, blood pressure, and cigarette smoking predicted cardiovascular mortality in both diabetic and nondiabetic subjects.[127] A conclusion of the MRFIT study is that similar risk factors predict CHD in both diabetic and nondiabetic subjects, although the panel of risk factors reported in this study was not particularly sophisticated. With the use of more sophisticated techniques in well-characterized Finnish type 2 diabetic subjects, total and VLDL triglycerides were positively related to the 7-year incidence of CHD, whereas HDL cholesterol was inversely associated with CHD.[128] In this report, LDL cholesterol was not significantly related to CHD. In multivariate analysis, HDL cholesterol but not VLDL or total triglyceride was related to CHD in the overall type 2 diabetes population. In a much larger Finnish cohort of over 1000 subjects,[129] triglyceride and low HDL cholesterol predicted CHD incidence and death. Total and LDL cholesterol predicted CHD incidence but not CHD death. In contrast, in the very large baseline cohort from the United Kingdom Prospective Diabetes Study (UKPDS), by multivariate analysis LDL cholesterol was the best predictor of CHD, followed by low HDL cholesterol.[130] Triglyceride levels were only a weak predictor in univariate analysis and did not enter the model in multivariate analysis (Table 67–2).

To summarize, although few data are available for HDL cholesterol, it may be a powerful lipoprotein predictor of CHD in type 2 diabetic subjects. Total triglycerides may be a more powerful predictor of CHD than total cholesterol in type 2 diabetic subjects in early studies (but not in the larger UKPDS[130]). However, prospective studies may not be a reliable guide to practice because association may not predict the effect of interventions. In particular, triglyceride levels are much more strongly associated with insulin resistance[97, 131] than is total cholesterol, and in turn, insulin resistance is strongly correlated with other risk factors such as hypertension; thus it is possible that hypertriglyceridemia is a better predictor because it is a better marker of risk. Clinical trials are necessary to resolve this issue.

TABLE 67–2. Stepwise Selection of Risk Factors, Adjusted for Age and Sex, in 2963 White Patients with Non–Insulin Dependent Diabetes Mellitus, with the Dependent Variable Being Time to Development of Coronary Artery Disease (n = 280)

Position in Model	Independent Variable	*P* Value*
First	LDL cholesterol	<.0001
Second	HDL cholesterol	<.0001
Third	Hb A$_{1c}$	<.0022
Fourth	Systolic blood pressure	<.0065
Fifth	Smoking	<.056

*P values are significance of the risk factor after accounting for all other risk factors in the model.

HDL, high-density lipoprotein; LDL, low-density lipoprotein.

Adapted from Turner RC, Millns H, Neil HA, et al: Risk factors for coronary artery disease in non–insulin dependent diabetes mellitus: United Kingdom Prospective Diabetes Study (UKPDS: 23). BMJ 316:823–828, 1998.

Much recent attention has been given to the use of non-HDL cholesterol as a possible target for intervention. However, few data are available in this area. The largest study that involves such data is a Finnish report with 1059 subjects monitored for 7 years. Non-HDL cholesterol was a better predictor than LDL cholesterol for both CHD death and all CHD events. These results were not changed after further adjustment for previous myocardial infarction, triglycerides, HDL cholesterol, fasting glucose, and duration of diabetes. Non-HDL cholesterol was similar in predictive power to triglycerides and slightly weaker than HDL cholesterol.[129]

ROLE OF LIPOPROTEINS IN ATHEROGENESIS

Lipoproteins are important in the pathogenesis of atherosclerosis (Fig. 67–2). Apo B–containing lipoproteins deliver cholesterol to the artery wall and are atherogenic. Decreased levels of HDL are associated with impaired removal of cholesterol from the arterial wall. Therefore, the dyslipidemia associated with diabetes is likely to play an important role in accelerating atherosclerosis in this disorder. The earliest lesion of atherosclerosis is the fatty streak, which consists of cholesterol-laden macrophages. Circulating apo B–containing lipoproteins such as VLDL and their remnants, Lp(a) and LDL bind to and are retained by proteoglycans secreted by vascular cells.[132] Retained lipoproteins can be oxidized by endothelial cells, smooth muscle cells, and macrophages[133, 134] by several mechanisms.[135–137]

Oxidized LDL stimulates the adhesion of monocytes to endothelial cells and their chemotaxis into the subendothelial space. Oxidized LDL also stimulates monocyte activation and differentiation, thereby facilitating the recruitment, activation, and maturation of macrophages. Oxidized LDL also stimulates the expression of vascular proteoglycans and alters the composition of their glycosaminoglycan chains, thereby allowing them to bind LDL more avidly.[138] Foam cells are formed by the uptake of oxidized LDL by several macrophage receptors, including SR-A,[139] CD36,[140, 141] and macrosialin.[142] Smooth muscle cells then migrate from the media to the intima, where they undergo proliferation in response to a number of cytokines and growth factors with the subsequent formation of a fibrofatty plaque.[143] Lipoproteins can also modulate the expression of several growth factors. Lipoprotein-derived cholesterol can accumulate in arterial smooth muscle cells by mechanisms that are less well understood. Extracellular accumulation of apo B– and apo E–containing lipoproteins and Lp(a) occurs after binding of these lipoproteins to molecules in the extracellular matrix of the artery wall.[144] Thus lipoproteins containing apo B and E can be involved in the pathogenesis of many of the features of atherosclerotic plaque.

HDL facilitates cholesterol efflux[145] and can thus remove the excess cholesterol that accumulates in the artery wall. The cholesterol that is picked up by HDL is then esterified, transferred to lower-density lipoproteins, and transported to the liver, from where it can be excreted in a process known as reverse cholesterol transport. Thus HDL has an antiatherogenic effect.

Plaque rupture, hemorrhage, and thrombosis result in clinical events.[146] Features associated with unstable plaque and susceptibility to rupture are the presence of a large lipid core, lipid-filled macrophages at the shoulder of the lesion, and a thin fibrous cap.[147] Oxidized LDL can also affect this stage of the process by stimulating the expression of metalloproteinases,[148, 149] which favor plaque rupture, and the expression of tissue factor matrix,[150] or plasminogen activator inhibitor-1,[151] which favors thrombosis.

Effect of Diabetes on the Pathogenesis of Atherosclerosis

Many of these lipid- and lipoprotein-mediated events can be increased by the presence of diabetic dyslipidemia, which is characterized by an accumulation of atherogenic apo B–containing lipoproteins, a preponderance of small dense LDL, and a reduction in HDL.

Because of their size, small dense LDL lipoproteins can enter the subendothelial space with ease, have been reported to demonstrate increased binding to vascular extracellular proteoglycans,[152] and have an increased predisposition to oxidative modification.[153, 154] The net effect is that all of the effects of oxidized LDL described earlier are likely to be enhanced in diabetes and the insulin resistance syndrome. The reduced levels of HDL in diabetes, together with compositional abnormalities that might affect their function, are likely to impair the process of reverse cholesterol transport, thereby increasing vascular lipid retention. All lipoprotein classes have been shown to demonstrate increased glycation in diabetes.[20] Glycated LDL binds poorly to the LDL receptor,[155] thereby increasing its residence time in plasma[148] and, presumably, in the extracellular space of the artery wall, where it can undergo oxidative modification. Glycated LDL has been reported to have increased susceptibility to oxidative modification[149] and has an impaired ability to stimulate cholesterol efflux[156] and facilitate the transfer of cholesteryl esters to apo B–containing lipoproteins.[157] The formation of advanced glycation end-products is increased in diabetes. These proteins bind to specific receptors on arterial cells,[158, 159] which leads to intracellular oxidant stress,[160] expression of endothelial cell adhesion molecules, monocyte chemotaxis,[161] and the release of cytokines and growth factors.[162] Thus the increased oxidative and glycoxidative pathways that are likely to occur in diabetes can enhance multiple steps in the pathogenesis of atherosclerosis.

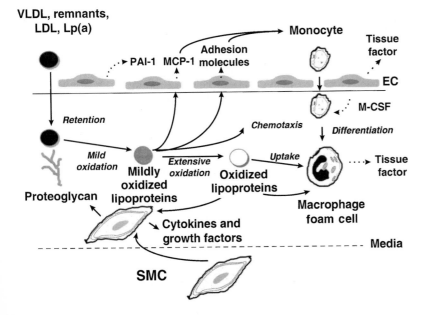

FIGURE 67–2. Role of lipids and lipoproteins in atherogenesis. Apolipoprotein B–containing lipoproteins cross the endothelial barrier (EC) and are retained in the subendothelium by proteoglycans. After undergoing oxidation, the oxidized lipoproteins stimulate the adhesion, chemotaxis, and differentiation of macrophages and the uptake of oxidized lipoproteins by macrophage scavenger receptors. Lipoproteins also modulate the expression of growth factors and cytokines secreted by smooth muscle cells that have migrated to the intima from the media. They can also affect the expression of matrix metalloproteinases, tissue factor, and plasminogen activator inhibitor-1 (PAI-1), which can lead to plaque rupture and thrombosis. All of these processes can be increased in diabetes.

Lipoprotein aggregates[163] and lipoprotein immune complexes[164] have been observed in atherosclerotic lesions. Both these processes could be increased in diabetes. Aggregation of LDL can also occur as a result of oxidation[165, 166] or the action of sphingomyelinase in the artery wall.[167] Aggregates and immune complexes that occur as a result of diabetes can be phagocytosed by macrophages.[165, 166] Additional modifications of lipoproteins that have been observed in diabetes, such as lipid compositional changes in the surface of the lipoprotein particle,[168] favor a net flux of cholesterol from lipoproteins to cells rather than in the opposite direction.[74] Thus a variety of the compositional and quantitative alterations of lipoproteins that occur in diabetes can influence the pathogenesis of atherosclerosis by multiple mechanisms.

TREATMENT

Clinical Trials of Lipid Lowering in Diabetic Subjects

Five LDL-lowering studies have examined the possible benefit of statins on CHD in diabetic subgroups[169–173] (Table 67–3). All these studies have shown as much benefit in diabetic subjects as in nondiabetic subjects. The Scandinavian Simvastatin Survival Study (4S), the Cholesterol and Recurrent Events (CARE) study, and the Long Term Intervention with Pravastatin in Ischemic Disease (LIPID) study were all secondary prevention trials. A total 202 subjects in the 4S had a clinical diagnosis of diabetes.[169] In this small group of subjects, simvastatin therapy was associated with a 55% reduction in major CHD (fatal and nonfatal CHD) ($P = .002$) as compared with a 32% reduction in major CHD in nondiabetic subjects. In a further study using the current American Diabetes Association (ADA) criteria (fasting plasma glucose of 126 mg/dL), an additional 281 diabetic subjects (without a previous diagnosis of diabetes) were identified.[170] In this group simvastatin therapy was associated with a 42% reduction in major CHD ($P < .001$). In the CARE study, 586 subjects with a clinical diagnosis of diabetes were identified.[171] Pravastatin therapy reduced the risk of CHD (fatal plus nonfatal myocardial infarction, coronary artery bypass grafting [CABG], and percutaneous transluminal coronary angioplasty) by 25% in the diabetic group ($P = .05$) as compared with 23% in the nondiabetic group ($P < .001$). In the LIPID study, pravastatin reduced the incidence of fatal and nonfatal CHD by 19% in diabetic subjects (n = 792) ($P = $ NS) and 25% in the nondiabetic subjects ($P < .001$).[172] Although the reduction in CHD events in diabetic subjects was not significant with pravastatin in the diabetic group, the test for heterogeneity, which evaluated whether the effect of pravastatin on CHD differed between diabetic and nondiabetic subjects, was not statistically significant.

In the Air Force/Texas Coronary Atherosclerosis Program, a primary prevention study, only 155 subjects had a clinical diagnosis of diabetes.[173] In the small number of diabetic subjects, a 42% reduction in CHD was seen ($P = $ NS), which was similar to the 37% reduction in CHD noted in the overall population.

The Post CABG trial is the only currently published study that evaluates the question of whether more aggressive LDL lowering is beneficial.[174] Subjects were randomized to achieve different LDL goals. The actual LDL levels achieved were 135 vs. 95 mg/dL for the less and more aggressively treated groups, respectively. In the 116 diabetic subjects in the Post CABG trial, a 51% reduction in substantial progression was observed vs. a 40% reduction in the nondiabetic subjects (n = 1235).[175]

Fibric acids raise HDL cholesterol and lower triglyceride levels. Relatively fewer clinical trials are available for fibric acids than for statins. Three large-scale trials have been completed (Helsinki Heart Study,[176] Veterans Affairs High-Density Lipoprotein Cholesterol Intervention Trial [VA-HIT],[177] and the Bezofibrate Infarction Prevention, although the latter has not yet been reported). In the Helsinki Heart Study, 135 diabetic subjects were included.[176] A 60% reduction in CHD ($P = $ NS) was seen with gemfibrozil. The VA-HIT study included 2531 men with preexisting CHD.[177] Of interest were the baseline levels of LDL cholesterol (112 mg/dL), HDL cholesterol (32

mg/dL), and triglyceride (160 mg/dL). Thus the VA-HIT study was a study of isolated low HDL cholesterol levels. Six hundred twenty subjects had diabetes. Diabetic subjects had a 24% reduction in fatal and nonfatal CHD or stroke ($P = .05$), whereas nondiabetic subjects also had a 24% reduction in CHD or stroke ($P < .001$).

Thus in all of the statin and fibric acid trials, lipid therapy had equally beneficial effects in diabetic and nondiabetic subjects when expressed as a percent reduction in events. Because event rates are increased twofold to fourfold in diabetes, the benefit to be achieved in the total number of events prevented is likely to be much higher in diabetic than nondiabetic subjects.

Management of Lipid Disorders in Diabetes

Both the ADA[178] (Tables 67–4 and 67–5) and the American Heart Association[179] (AHA) (see Table 67–5) have recently published recommendations for the management of lipid disorders in diabetes. These recommendations are very similar. Both the ADA and the AHA recommend a target goal for LDL cholesterol of less than 100 mg/dL for diabetic subjects, although they differ slightly on the point for initiation for pharmacologic therapy. For secondary prevention, the ADA suggests initiation of drug therapy (after a trial of medical nutrition therapy) when LDL cholesterol is greater than 100 mg/dL. The AHA suggests that drug therapy be added above 130 mg/dL with consideration to lower goals for high-risk subjects (LDL between 100 and 129 mg/dL).

For primary prevention, the ADA suggests initiation of drug therapy if the LDL goal is 130 mg/dL or greater (although a footnote suggests perhaps a lower indication level of 100 mg/dL if other CHD risk factors are present). The AHA has suggests a LDL goal of less than 130 mg/dL, and some experts recommend an LDL goal of less than 100 mg/dL in the presence of other CHD risk factors. Because most type 2 diabetic subjects may be expected to have other CHD risk factors, these guidelines (ADA and AHA) are quite similar.

Triglyceride/HDL Modifications

Because of the benefits of statins in the clinical trials completed to date, both the ADA[178] and the AHA[179] position papers recommend reduction of LDL cholesterol as a first priority for lipoprotein interventions, even though LDL levels are not usually increased in diabetes. The ADA recommends interventions to raise HDL cholesterol as a second priority and lowering triglyceride levels as a third priority,[178] whereas the AHA identifies both HDL cholesterol and triglyceride as second priorities.[179] Both the ADA[178] and the AHA[179] recommend a triglyceride goal of less than 200 mg/dL. The ADA and AHA differ somewhat in their HDL goal: 35 mg/dL or greater for the AHA[179] and 45 mg/dL or greater for the ADA.[178]

The choice of whether to intervene first for triglyceride or HDL cholesterol is less important if behavioral interventions (i.e., weight loss, increased physical activity, and smoking cessation) are used. However, although statins, fibric acids, and nicotinic acid may have marked effects on reducing triglyceride levels, these different classes of pharmacologic assets have very different effects on raising HDL cholesterol, with nicotinic acid having the most marked effect and statins having the smallest effect. There may even exist differences in the HDL cholesterol–raising effect of statins, although these effects are small, are restricted to the highest doses of statins, and are of uncertain clinical benefit. Nevertheless, some determination of the relative importance of triglyceride or HDL cholesterol has been made, even though these estimates have several problems. In observational studies in which both HDL cholesterol and triglyceride are measured and are both significant,[128–130] HDL always is the stronger risk factor. Thus it seems reasonable to choose HDL cholesterol over triglyceride as a second priority. Such a strategy gives additional emphasis to the possible use of nicotinic acid (which is relatively contraindicated because of a rise in glucose and worsened insulin resistance[6]) and particularly fibric acids.

TABLE 67–3. Results of Pharmacologic Agents in Diabetic Subgroups on Major Coronary Heart Disease in Clinical Trials

Study	Author	Journal	n	% Reduction, DM (95% CI)	% Reduction, Non-DM	Baseline Lipoproteins LDL	HDL	TRIG	% Change in Lipoproteins LDL	HDL	TRIG
Statins											
Secondary Prevention											
4S	Pyorala	Diabetes Care 1997[169]	202	−55 (0.27–0.74)	−32	185	44	153	−36	7	−11
CARE	Goldberg	Circulation 1998[171]	586	−25 (P = .05*)	−23	136	38	164	−19	4	−13
LIPID	LIPID Study Grp	NEJM 1998[172]	782	−19 (−10 to 41)	−25	150[†]	36[†]	142[†]	−25[†]	5[†]	−11[†]
4S extension	Haffner	Archives of IM 1999[170]	483	−42 (0.41–0.80)	−32	189	44	146	−36	3	−15
Primary Prevention											
AFCAPS/TexCAPS	Downs	JAMA 1998[173]	155	−42	−37[†]	150[†]	37[†]	158[†]	−25[†]	6[†]	−15[†]
Fibric acids											
Secondary Prevention											
VA-HIT	Rubins	NEJM 1999[177]	627	−24 (−0.1 to 43)	−24	111[†]	32[†]	160[†]	0[†]	6[†]	−31[†]
Primary Prevention											
Helsinki	Koskinen	Diabetes Care 1992[176]	135	−68 (P = .19*)	—	201	46	238	−11	7	−27

*Confidence interval not available.
†Overall.
AFCAPS/Tex CAPS, Air Force/Texas Coronary Atherosclerosis Program; CARE, Cholesterol and Recurrent Events trial; DM, diabetes mellitus; HDL, high-density lipoprotein; IM, Internal Medicine; LDL, low-density lipoprotein; LIPID, Long Term Intervention with Pravastatin in Ischemic Disease; NEJM, New England Journal of Medicine; 4S, Scandinavian Simvastatin Survival Study; TRIG, triglyceride; VA-HIT, Veterans Affairs High-Density Lipoprotein Cholesterol Intervention Trial.

TABLE 67–4. Current Guidelines of the American Diabetes Association: Treatment Decisions Based on LDL Cholesterol Levels in Adults with Diabetes

| Population | Medical Nutrition Therapy | | Drug Therapy | |
	Initiation Level	LDL Goal	Initiation Level	LDL Goal
With CHD, PVD, or CVD	>100	≤100	>100	≤100
Without CHD, PVD, and CVD	>100	≤100	≤130*	≤100

Data are given in milligrams per deciliter.

*For diabetic patients with multiple CHD risk factors (low HDL [<35 mg/dL], hypertension, smoking, family history of CVD, or microalbuminuria or proteinuria), some authorities recommend initiation of drug therapy when LDL levels are between 100 and 130 mg/dL. Caveats: (1) medical nutrition therapy should be attempted before starting pharmacologic therapy; (2) because diabetic men and women are considered to have equal CHD risk, age and sex are not considered "risk factors."

CHD, coronary heart disease; CVD, cardiovascular disease; LDL, low-density lipoprotein; PVD, peripheral vascular disease.

Data from American Diabetes Association: Management of dyslipidemia in adults with diabetes (position statement). Diabetes Care 23(suppl):57–60, 2000.

Combination Therapy

The Food and Drug Administration currently recommends against the use of combinations of fibric acids and statins. In one study the risk of myositis was as high as 5% in subjects taking lovastatin and gemfibrozil.[180] Most lipid experts believe that the risk of myositis is much lower (at least in the absence of renal failure). A few small studies have found combinations of gemfibrozil with pravastatin[181] and bezafibrate with simvastatin[182] to be safe. Few data are available on combination use in diabetic subjects, in whom the risk of myositis could be higher because of subclinical renal disease. A large prospective randomized (n = 5000) clinical trial with a 2 × 2 factorial design in diabetic subjects (Lipids in Diabetes Study) commenced in 1999 in the United Kingdom with cerivastatin and fenofibrate. Thus 1250 diabetic subjects will be receiving combination therapy. The results of this study should provide useful information concerning the relative benefits of using a statin vs. a fibrate in diabetic dyslipidemia and should provide important information concerning the safety of combination therapy.

Nevertheless, it seems prudent to restrict the use of combination therapy to very high-risk subjects, such as subjects with preexisting CHD, cardiovascular disease, or peripheral vascular disease or subjects with multiple other CHD risk factors.

Lipid-Lowering Therapy

Life-Style Changes

The major behavioral interventions are weight loss, increased physical activity, and smoking cessation. All diets (AHA, ADA, and National Cholesterol Education Program [NCEP]) recommend a reduction in saturated fat. There is some controversy about whether the saturated fat should be replaced by carbohydrates or monounsaturated fats,[5] but this point is as yet unresolved.

TABLE 67–5. Order of Priority of Goals for Lipoproteins

American Diabetes Association[178]	
Primary goal	LDL ≤100 mg/dL
Secondary goal	HDL ≥45 mg/dL
Tertiary goal	Triglyceride ≤200 mg/dL
American Heart Association[179]	
Primary goal	LDL ≤100 mg/dL
Secondary goal	HDL >35 mg/dL
	Triglyceride <200 mg/dL

HDL, high-density lipoprotein; LDL, low-density lipoprotein.

Drug Therapy

The primary choice for LDL reduction is statins. This class of drugs also leads to modest reductions in triglycerides and increases in HDL cholesterol. Resins may be used to further lower LDL in combination therapy if statins are not sufficient to reach target levels. Fenofibrate may have somewhat greater LDL lowering than seen with gemfibrozil.

The initial therapy for raising HDL cholesterol is life-style changes, which includes weight control and exercise. Nicotinic acid has the greatest effect on HDL levels but is relatively contraindicated because of worsening glycemic and insulin resistance.[6] If nicotinic acid is used, its use might be restricted to diabetic subjects taking exogenous insulin who do home glucose monitoring. Fibric acids have the next greatest effect on increasing HDL cholesterol, whereas statins have a modest effect on HDL cholesterol. Improved glycemic control has only a modest effect on raising HDL cholesterol (see earlier), although thiazolidinediones may increase HDL cholesterol up to 15%.

The initial treatment for hypertriglyceridemia is improved glycemic control. In markedly hyperglycemic subjects or untreated patients, normalization of glucose levels may lead to dramatic reductions in triglyceride levels. However, in subjects with moderate hyperglycemia, reduction of glycemia has only modest effects on triglyceride levels. Fibric acids are the first pharmacologic choice for reducing triglyceride levels in diabetic subjects.

SPECIAL CONSIDERATIONS

Type 1 Diabetes

Type 1 diabetes is also associated with a marked increase in CHD.[1, 183] Relatively few observational studies of the effect of lipoproteins on CHD in type 1 diabetes have been performed,[184] and those that have are all very small. Furthermore, type 1 diabetic subjects have been excluded from clinical trials.

The Epidemiology of Diabetes Interventions and Complications (EDIC) study examined the relationship of risk factors to intimal-medial thickness of the carotids in 1326 subjects from the DCCT 18 months after completion of the original study.[185] Carotid intimal-medial thickness was not significantly different in the intensive and standard treatment groups, which suggests that improved glycemic control may not be related to early atherosclerosis. In contrast, a tendency toward decreased macrovascular events was seen in the intensive treatment group in the DCCT,[50] although this result was not statistically significant. In the EDIC study, intimal-medial thickness was related to LDL cholesterol but not to triglyceride or HDL cholesterol.[185]

In the Wisconsin Epidemiologic Study of Diabetic Retinopathy (WESDR), glycated hemoglobin was significantly related to the 4-year incidence of CHD.[186] In fact, the association of glycated hemoglobin to ischemic heart disease was stronger in type 1 than in type 2 diabetic subjects.

Few data are available on CHD in type 1 diabetes and the relationship of lipids and lipoproteins to CHD. Until such data become available, it seems reasonable to recommend similar goals for type 1 diabetics as for type 2 diabetic subjects if they have other cardiovascular risk factors such as nephropathy, which markedly increases cardiovascular disease risk in type 1 diabetes.

Glycemia and Coronary Heart Disease

Even if diabetic subjects had a risk of CHD similar to that of subjects with existing CHD ("CHD risk equivalent") and diabetic subjects received equal benefit from lipid intervention as nondiabetic subjects, more aggressive reduction of lipoproteins would not be justified if glycemic control could reduce the risk of CHD to nondiabetic levels. Therefore the relationship of glycemia to CHD needs to be reviewed.

In some recent European studies, glycemia and the duration of type 2 diabetes have been related to CHD in middle-aged[187] and elderly[188] cohorts. However, in the Finnish study of middle-aged subjects, glycemia was no longer statistically related to CHD after adjustment for lipoproteins.[187] The WESDR directly compared the predictive power of glycated hemoglobin in relation to the incidence of various complications of diabetes.[186] In older-onset diabetic subjects (who were likely to be type 2 diabetic subjects), a 1% increase in glycated hemoglobin at baseline was associated with a 50% increase in retinopathy and a 20% increase in proteinuria, but only a 10% increase in the incidence in CHD. All these associations (including CHD) were statistically significant. However, it is clear that the association of hyperglycemia with CHD was much weaker than that for retinopathy, although this result could be partially due to the greater precision of assessing the incidence of retinopathy.

In the UKPDS,[130] Hb A_{1c} significantly predicted the development of coronary artery disease. The average of the Hb A_{1c} during the UKPDS significantly predicted both CHD and microvascular events, but the effect was much stronger for the latter than the former (10-fold vs. 2-fold for an Hb A_{1c} range from 6% to 11%). The epidemiologic model for the UKPDS is consistent with the clinical trial results for the main randomization,[189] in which an average Hb A_{1c} differential of 0.9% during the trial was associated with a 16% reduction in myocardial infarction that was of borderline significance but a significant 25% reduction in microvascular events. Metformin did better in the overweight cohort of the UKPDS,[190] but these results are at least partially neutralized by the higher mortality in the secondary randomization of subjects treated with sulfonylureas.

In conclusion, although glycemia is related to CHD in diabetic subjects, the magnitude of the association is sufficiently modest that even optimal control of glycemia is unlikely to eliminate the twofold to fourfold excess of CHD in type 2 diabetic subjects.

FUTURE DIRECTIONS

Most clinical trials to date have focused predominantly on the effect of a single aspect of the management of diabetes on cardiovascular disease. Considerable new trial data will continue to provide additional information concerning various aspects of the prevention and treatment of macrovascular disease in diabetes. Thus ongoing and future trials on the role of triglyceride lowering by fibrates, with and without the use of statins, should provide useful additional information related to this aspect of lipid management of type 2 patients. The role of glycemic control in macrovascular disease, independent of its effect on lipids, remains uncertain. Nonetheless, the role of glycemic control in the prevention of microvascular disease is now incontrovertible in both type 1 and type 2 diabetes, and the development of nephropathy leads to macrovascular complications. Further studies of the direct role of glycemic control by different therapeutic modalities, which have different effects on central obesity and its associated constellation of risk factors, will further help define optimal therapy for type 2 patients. However, trials designed to test the effect of optimal control of all the treatable cardiovascular risk factors rather than focusing on just one or two are also desirable.

Many of the risk factors that occur in type 2 patients are responsive to weight reduction. Therefore, strategies to better understand body weight regulation should continue to be a very high priority, not only for the treatment of these risk factors but also for the prevention of diabetes in susceptible individuals. Future approaches should also focus on disturbances of the biology of the artery wall in diabetes. Future therapeutic strategies aimed at preventing modification of lipoproteins might include the use of antioxidants and/or agents that limit the modification of proteins by products of glucose oxidation. Indeed, trials to evaluate the effect of antioxidants on both primary and secondary prevention of macrovascular disease are currently ongoing. As new information becomes available, our approach to the prevention and treatment of macrovascular disease in diabetes is likely to become further refined and more effective.

REFERENCES

1. Krolewski AS, Kosinski EJ, Warram JH, et al: Magnitude and determinants of coronary artery disease in juvenile-onset, insulin-dependent diabetes mellitus. Am J Cardiol 59:750–755, 1987.

2. West KM, Ahuja MMS, Bennett PH, et al: The role of circulating glucose and triglyceride concentrations and their interactions with other "risk factors" as determinants of arterial disease in nine diabetic population samples from the WHO multinational study. Diabetes Care 6:361–369, 1983.

3. Kannel WB, McGee DL: Diabetes and glucose tolerance as risk factors for cardiovascular disease: The Framingham study. Diabetes Care 2:120–126, 1979.

4. Wingard DL, Barrett-Connor E: Heart disease and diabetes. In Harris MI (ed): Diabetes in America. Bethesda, MD, National Institutes of Health, 1995, pp 429–448.

5. Pyörälä K, Laakso M, Uusitupa M: Diabetes and atherosclerosis: An epidemiologic view. Diabetes Metab Rev 3:463–524, 1987.

6. Haffner SM: Management of dyslipidemia in adults with diabetes. Diabetes Care 21:160–178, 1998.

7. Bierman EL: George Lyman Duff Memorial Lecture. Atherogenesis in diabetes. Arterioscler Thromb 12:647–656, 1992.

8. Haffner SM, Lehto S, Ronnemaa T, et al: Mortality from coronary heart disease in subjects with type 2 diabetes and in nondiabetic subjects with and without prior myocardial infarction. N Engl J Med 339:229–234, 1998.

9. Kannel WB, McGee DL: Diabetes and cardiovascular disease. The Framingham study. JAMA 241:2035–2038, 1979.

10. Simons LA, Simons J: Diabetes and coronary heart disease. N Engl J Med 339:1714–1716, 1998.

11. Haffner S, D'Agostino R, Saad M, et al: Carotid artery atherosclerosis in type 2 diabetic and nondiabetic subjects with and without clinical coronary artery disease: The Insulin Resistance Atherosclerosis Study. Am J Cardiol (in press).

12. Miettinen H, Lehto S, Salomaa V, et al: Impact of diabetes on mortality after the first myocardial infarction. The FINMONICA Myocardial Infarction Register Study Group. Diabetes Care 21:69–75, 1998.

13. Brunzell JD, Chait A: Diabetic dyslipidemia–pathology and treatment. In Porte D Jr, Sherwin J (eds): Ellenberg and Rifkin's Diabetes Mellitus. Appleton & Lange, E Norwalk, CT, 1996, pp 1077–1096.

14. Brunzell JD, Hokanson JE: Dyslipidemia of central obesity and insulin resistance. Diabetes Care 22(suppl 3):C10–C133, 1999.

15. Abate N, Vega GL, Garg A, Grundy SM: Abnormal cholesterol distribution among lipoprotein fractions in normolipidemic patients with mild NIDDM. Atherosclerosis 118:111–122, 1995.

16. Barakat HA, McLendon VD, Marks R, et al: Influence of morbid obesity and non–insulin-dependent diabetes mellitus on high-density lipoprotein composition and subpopulation distribution. Metabolism 41:37–41, 1992.

17. Lane JT, Subbaiah PV, Otto ME, Bagdade JD: Lipoprotein composition and HDL particle size distribution in women with non–insulin-dependent diabetes mellitus and the effects of probucol treatment. J Lab Clin Med 118:120–128, 1991.

18. Bagdade JD, Helve E, Taskinen MR: Effects of continuous insulin infusion therapy on lipoprotein surface and core lipid composition in insulin-dependent diabetes mellitus. Metabolism 40:445–449, 1991.

19. Bagdade JD, Buchanan WE, Kuusi T, Taskinen M-R: Persistent abnormalities in lipoprotein composition in non–insulin dependent diabetes following intensive insulin therapy. Arteriosclerosis 10:232–239, 1990.

20. Curtiss LK, Witztum JL: Plasma apolipoprotein A-I, A-II, B, C-I and E are glycosylated in hyperglycemic diabetic subjects. Diabetes 34:452–461, 1985.

21. Tsai EC, Hirsch IB, Brunzell JD, Chait A: Reduced plasma peroxyl radical trapping capacity and increased susceptibility of LDL to oxidation in poorly controlled IDDM. Diabetes 43:1010–1014, 1994.

22. Sinclair AJ, Lunec J, Girling AJ, Barnett AH: Modulators of free radical activity in diabetes mellitus: Role of ascorbic acid. EXS 62:342–352, 1992.

23. Yoshida H, Ishikawa T, Nakamura H: Vitamin E/lipid peroxide ratio and susceptibility of LDL to oxidative modification in non–insulin-dependent diabetes mellitus. Arterioscler Thromb Vasc Biol 17:1438–1446, 1997.

24. Cominacini L, Garbin U, Pastorino AM, et al: Increased susceptibility of LDL to in vitro oxidation in patients with insulin-dependent and non–insulin-dependent diabetes mellitus. Diabetes Res 26:173–184, 1994.

25. Beaudeux JL, Guillausseau PJ, Peynet J, et al: Enhanced susceptibility of low-density lipoprotein to in vitro oxidation in type 1 and type 2 diabetic patients. Clin Chim Acta 239:131–141, 1995.

26. Leonhardt W, Hanefeld M, Muller G, et al: Impact of concentrations of glycated hemoglobin, alpha-tocopherol, copper, and manganese on oxidation of low-density lipoproteins in patients with type I diabetes, type II diabetes and control subjects. Clin Chim Acta 254:173–186, 1996.

27. Kobbah M, Vessby B, Tuvemo T: Serum lipids and apolipoproteins in children with type 1 (insulin-dependent) diabetes during the first two years of the disease. Diabetologia 31:195–200, 1988.

28. Sosenko JM, Breslow JL, Miettinen OS, Gabbay KH: Hyperglycemia and plasma lipid levels: A prospective study of young insulin-dependent diabetic patients. N Engl J Med 302:650–654, 1980.

29. Lopes-Virella MF, Wohltmann HF, Loadholt CB, Buse MG: Plasma lipids and lipoproteins in young insulin-dependent diabetic patients: Relationship with control. Diabetologia 21:216–223, 1981.

30. Andersen GE, Christiansen JS, Mortensen HB, et al: Serum lipids and lipoproteins in 157 insulin dependent diabetic children and adolescents in relation to metabolic regulation, obesity and genetic hyperlipoproteinemia. Acta Paediatr Scand 72:361–365, 1983.

31. Tamborlane WV, Sherwin RS, Genel M, Felig P: Restoration of normal lipid and amino acid metabolism in diabetic patients treated with a portable insulin-infusion pump. Lancet 1:1258–1261, 1979.

32. Pietri AO, Dunn FL, Raskin P: The effect of improved diabetic control on plasma lipid and lipoprotein levels: A comparison of conventional therapy and continuous subcutaneous insulin infusion. Diabetes 29:1001–1005, 1980.

33. Dunn FL, Pietri A, Raskin P: Plasma lipid and lipoprotein levels with continuous subcutaneous insulin infusion in type I diabetes mellitus. Ann Intern Med 95:426–431, 1981.

34. Hershcopf R, Plotnick LP, Kaya K, et al: Short term improvement in glycemic control utilizing continuous subcutaneous insulin infusion: The effect on 24-hour integrated concentrations of counterregulatory hormones and plasma lipids in insulin-dependent diabetes mellitus. J Clin Endocrinol Metab 54:504–509, 1982.

35. Lopes-Virella MF, Wohltmann HJ, Mayfield RK, et al: Effect of metabolic control on lipid, lipoprotein, and apolipoprotein levels in 55 insulin-dependent diabetic patients. Diabetes 32:20–25, 1983.

36. Vlachokosta FV, Asmal AC, Ganda OP, Aoki TT: The effect of strict control with the artificial beta-cell on plasma lipid levels in insulin-dependent diabetes. Diabetes Care 6:351–355, 1983.

37. Perez A, Caixas A, Carreras G, et al: Lipoprotein compositional abnormalities in type I diabetes: Effect of improved glycaemic control. Diabetes Res Clin Pract 36:83–90, 1997.

38. Purnell JQ, Marcovina SM, Hokanson JE, et al: Levels of lipoprotein(a), apolipoprotein B, and lipoprotein cholesterol distribution in IDDM. Results from follow-up in the Diabetes Control and Complications Trial. Diabetes 44:1218–1226, 1995.

39. Pykalisto OJ, Smith PH, Brunzell JD: Determinants of human adipose tissue LPL. J Clin Invest 56:1108–1117, 1975.

40. Taskinen MR, Beltz WF, Harper I, et al: Effects of NIDDM on very-low-density lipoprotein triglyceride and apolipoprotein B metabolism. Studies before and after sulfonylurea therapy. Diabetes 35:1268–1277, 1986.

41. Brunzell JD, Porte D Jr, Bierman EL: Abnormal lipoprotein lipase mediated plasma triglyceride removal in untreated diabetes mellitus associated with hypertriglyceridemia. Metabolism 28:897–903, 1979.

42. Dunn FL, Carroll PB, Beltz WF: Treatment with artificial beta-cell decreases very-low-density lipoprotein triglyceride synthesis in type I diabetes. Diabetes 36:661–666, 1987.

43. Taskinen MR: Lipoprotein lipase in diabetes. Diabetes Metab Rev 3:551–570, 1987.

44. Carvajal F, Quesada X, Gonzalez P: High density lipoprotein cholesterol in insulin-dependent diabetic children. Acta Diabetica Lat 20:289–295, 1983.

45. Falko JM, O'Dorisio TM, Cataland S: Improvement of high-density lipoprotein-cholesterol levels. JAMA 247:37–39, 1982.

46. Eckel RH, Albers JJ, Cheung MC, et al: High density lipoprotein composition in insulin-dependent diabetes mellitus. Diabetes 30:132–138, 1981.

47. Magill P, Rao SN, Miller NE, et al: Relationships between the metabolism of high density and very low-density lipoproteins in man: Studies of apolipoprotein kinetics and adipose tissue lipoprotein lipase activity. Eur J Clin Invest 12:113–120, 1982.

48. Brunzell JD: Obesity and coronary heart disease: A targeted approach. Arteriosclerosis 4:180–182, 1984.

49. Katzel LI, Busby-Whitehead MJ, Goldberg AP: Adverse effects of abdominal obesity on lipoprotein lipids in healthy older men. Exp Gerontol 28:411–420, 1993.

50. The Diabetes Control and Complications Trial Research Group: The effect of intensive treatment of diabetes on the development and progression of long-term complications in insulin-dependent diabetes mellitus. N Engl J Med 329:977–986, 1993.

51. Kern PA: Lipid disorders in diabetes mellitus. Mt Sinai J Med 54:245–252, 1987.

52. Daneman D, Epstein LH, Siminerio L, et al: Effects of enhanced conventional therapy on metabolic control in children with insulin-dependent diabetes mellitus. Diabetes Care 5:472–478, 1982.

53. Chait A, Bierman EL, Albers JJ: Low density lipoprotein receptor activity in cultured human skin fibroblasts: Mechanism of insulin-induced stimulation. J Clin Invest 64:1309–1319, 1979.

54. Rosenstock J, Vega GL, Raskin P: Effect of intensive diabetes treatment on low-density lipoprotein apolipoprotein B kinetics in type I diabetes. Diabetes 37:393–397, 1988.

55. Barrett-Connor E, Grundy SM, Holdbrook MJ: Plasma lipids and diabetes mellitus in an adult community. Am J Epidemiol 15:657–663, 1982.

56. Wilson PW, Kannel WB, Anderson KM: Lipids, glucose intolerance and vascular disease: The Framingham Study. Monogr Atheroscler 13:1–11, 1985.

57. Rabkin SW, Boyko E, Streja DA: Change in high density lipoprotein cholesterol after initiation of insulin therapy in non–insulin-dependent diabetes mellitus: Relationship to changes in body weight. Am J Med Sci 285:14–20, 1983.

58. Taskinen M-R, Nikkila EA, Kuusi T, Harno K: Lipoprotein lipase activity and serum lipoproteins in untreated type 1 (insulin-dependent) diabetes associated with obesity. Diabetologia 22:46–50, 1982.

59. Abbate SL, Brunzell JD: Pathophysiology of hyperlipidemia in diabetes mellitus. J Cardiovasc Pharmacol 16(suppl):1–7, 1990.

60. Nagi DK, Yudkin JS: Effects of metformin on insulin resistance, risk factors for cardiovascular disease, and plasminogen activator inhibitor in NIDDM subjects. A study of two ethnic groups. Diabetes Care 16:621–629, 1993.

61. Fonseca VA, Valiquett TR, Huang SM, et al: Troglitazone monotherapy improves glycemic control in patients with type 2 diabetes mellitus: A randomized, controlled study. The Troglitazone Study Group. J Clin Endocrinol Metab 83:3169–3176, 1998.

62. Nikkila EA: High density lipoproteins in diabetes. Diabetes 30:82–87, 1981.

63. Kennedy L, Walshe K, Hadden DR, et al: The effect of intensive dietary therapy on serum high density lipoprotein cholesterol in patients with type 2 (non–insulin-dependent) diabetes mellitus: A prospective study. Diabetologia 23:24–27, 1982.

64. Wolf RN, Grundy SM: Influence of weight reduction on plasma lipoproteins in obese patients. Arteriosclerosis 3:160–169, 1983.

65. Agardh CD, Nilsson-Ehle P, Shersten B: Improvement of the plasma lipoprotein pattern after institution of insulin treatment in diabetes mellitus. Diabetes Care 5:322–325, 1982.

66. Paisey R, Elkeles RS, Hambley J, Magill P: The effects of chlorpropamide and insulin on serum lipids, lipoproteins and fractional triglyceride renewal. Diabetologia 15:81–85, 1978.

67. Briones ER, Mao SJT, Palumbo PJ, et al: Analysis of plasma lipids and apolipoproteins in insulin-dependent and noninsulin-dependent diabetes. Metabolism 33:42–49, 1984.

68. Biesbroeck RC, Albers JJ, Wahl PW, et al: Abnormal composition of high density lipoproteins in noninsulin-dependent diabetes. Diabetes 31:126–131, 1982.

69. Jialal I, Joubert SM, Asmal AC: Cholesterol, triglyceride and high-density lipoprotein cholesterol levels in non–insulin-dependent diabetes in the young. S Afr Med J 31:126–131, 1982.

70. Stern MP, Mitchell BD, Haffner SM, Hazuda HP: Does glycemic control of type II diabetes suffice to control diabetic dyslipidemia? Diabetes Care 15:638–644, 1992.

71. Tkac I, Kimball BP, Lewis G, et al: The severity of coronary atherosclerosis in type 2 diabetes mellitus is related to the number of circulating triglyceride-rich lipoprotein particles. Arterioscler Thromb Vasc Biol 17:3633–3638, 1997.

72. Watanabe N, Taniguchi T, Taketoh H, et al: Elevated remnant-like lipoprotein particles in impaired glucose tolerance and type 2 diabetic patients. Diabetes Care 22:152–156, 1999.

73. Weisweiler P, Drosner M, Schwandt P: Dietary effects on very low-density lipoproteins in type 2 (non–insulin-dependent) diabetes mellitus. Diabetologia 23:101–103, 1982.

74. Fielding CJ, Reaven GM, Fielding PE: Human noninsulin-dependent diabetes: Identification of a defect in plasma cholesterol transport normalized in vivo by insulin and in vitro by selective immuno-absorption of apolipoprotein E. Proc Natl Acad Sci U S A 79:6365–6369, 1982.

75. Fielding CJ, Reaven GM, Liu G, Fielding PE: Increased free cholesterol in plasma low and very low density lipoproteins in non–insulin-dependent diabetes mellitus: Its role in the inhibition of cholesteryl ester transfer. Proc Natl Acad Sci U S A 81:2512–2516, 1984.

76. Florez H, Ryder E, Campos G, et al: Women relatives of Hispanic patients with type 2 diabetes are more prone to exhibit metabolic disturbances. Invest Clin 40:127–142, 1999.

77. Shaw JT, Purdie DM, Neil HA, et al: The relative risks of hyperglycaemia, obesity and dyslipidaemia in the relatives of patients with type II diabetes mellitus. Diabetologia 42:24–27, 1999.

78. Kissebah AH, Alfarsi S, Evans DJ, Adams PW: Integrated regulation of very low density lipoprotein triglyceride and apolipoprotein-B kinetics in non–insulin-dependent diabetes mellitus. Diabetes 31:217–225, 1982.

79. Greenfield MS, Kolterman OG, Olefsky JM, Reaven GM: Mechanism of hypertriglyceridemia in diabetic patients with fasting hyperglycemia. Diabetologia 18:441–446, 1980.

80. Ginsberg H, Grundy SM: Very low density lipoprotein metabolism in non-ketotic diabetes mellitus: Effect of dietary restriction. Diabetologia 31:903–910, 1982.

81. Abrams JJ, Ginsberg HN, Grundy SM: Metabolism of cholesterol and plasma triglyceride in nonketotic diabetes mellitus. Diabetes 31:903–910, 1982.

82. Dunn FL, Raskin P, Bilheimer DW, Grundy SM: The effects of diabetic control on very low density lipoprotein triglyceride metabolism in patients with type II diabetes mellitus and marked hypertriglyceridemia. Metabolism 33:117–123, 1984.

83. Pfeifer MA, Brunzell JD, Best JD, et al: The response of plasma triglyceride, cholesterol, and lipoprotein lipase to treatment in non–insulin-dependent diabetic subjects without familial hypertriglyceridemia. Diabetes 32:525–531, 1983.

84. Gabor J, Spain M, Kalant H: Composition of serum very low density and high density lipoproteins in diabetes. Clin Chem 26:1261–1265, 1980.

85. Kasama T, Yoshino G, Iwatani I, et al: Increased cholesterol concentration in intermediate density lipoprotein fraction of normolipidemic non–insulin-dependent diabetes. Atherosclerosis 63:263–266, 1987.

86. Hughes TA, Clements RS, Fairclough PK, et al: Effects of insulin therapy on lipoproteins in non–insulin-dependent diabetes mellitus (NIDDM). Atherosclerosis 67:105–114, 1987.

87. Lisch H-J, Sailer S: Lipoprotein patterns in diet, sulphonylurea, and insulin treated diabetics. Diabetologia 20:118–122, 1981.

88. Barakat HA, Carpenter JW, McLendon VD, et al: Influence of obesity, impaired glucose tolerance, and noninsulin dependent diabetes on low density lipoprotein structure and composition: Possible link between hyperinsulinemia and atherosclerosis. Diabetes 39:1527–1533, 1990.

89. Okumura K, Matsui H, Kawakami K, et al: Low density lipoprotein particle size is associated with glycosylated hemoglobin levels regardless of plasma lipid levels. Intern Med 37:273–279, 1998.

90. Siegel RD, Cupples A, Schaefer EJ, Wilson PW: Lipoproteins, apolipoproteins, and low-density lipoprotein size among diabetics in the Framingham offspring study. Metabolism 45:1267–1272, 1996.

91. Feingold KR, Grunfeld C, Pang M, et al: LDL subclass phenotypes and triglyceride metabolism in non–insulin-dependent diabetes. Arterioscler Thromb 12:1496–1502, 1992.

92. Haffner SM, Mykkanen L, Stern MP, et al: Greater effect of diabetes on LDL size in women than in men. Diabetes Care 17:1164–1171, 1994.

93. Kissebah AH, Alfarsi S, Evans DJ, Adams PW: Plasma low density lipoprotein transport kinetics in non–insulin-dependent diabetes mellitus. J Clin Invest 71:655–667, 1983.

94. Howard BV, Abbott WGH, Beltz WF, et al: Integrated study of low density lipoprotein metabolism and very low density lipoprotein metabolism in non–insulin-dependent diabetes. Metabolism 36:870–877, 1987.

95. Austin MA, Breslow JA, Hennekens CH, et al: Low density lipoprotein subclass pattern and risk of myocardial infarction. JAMA 260:1917–1921, 1988.

96. Wingard DL, Barrett-Connor E, Criqui MH, Suarez L: Clustering of heart disease risk factors in diabetic compared to nondiabetic adults. Am J Epidemiol 117:19–26, 1983.

97. Haffner SM, Valdez RA, Hazuda HP, et al: Prospective analysis of the insulin-resistance syndrome (syndrome X). Diabetes 41:715–722, 1992.

98. Brunzell JD, Hokanson JE: Low-density and high-density lipoprotein subspecies and risk for premature coronary artery disease. Am J Med 107(suppl 2A):16–18, 1999.

99. Bjorntorp P: Abdominal fat distribution and the metabolic syndrome. J Cardiovasc Pharmacol 209(suppl):26–28, 1992.

100. Despres JP: Abdominal obesity as important component of insulin-resistance syndrome. Nutrition 9:452–459, 1993.

101. Haffner SM, Stern MP, Hazuda HP, et al: Cardiovascular risk factors in confirmed

prediabetic individuals: Does the clock for coronary heart disease start ticking before the onset of clinical diabetes? JAMA 263:2893–2898, 1990.
102. Scanu AM, Lawn RM, Berg K: Lipoprotein (a) and atherosclerosis. Ann Intern Med 115:209–218, 1991.
103. Haffner SM: Lipoprotein(a) and diabetes. An update. Diabetes Care 16:835–840, 1993.
104. Haffner SM, Morales PA, Stern MP, Gruber MK: Lp(a) concentrations in NIDDM. Diabetes 41:1267–1272, 1992.
105. Rainwater DL, MacCluer JW, Stern MP, et al: Effects of NIDDM on lipoprotein(a) concentration and apolipoprotein(a) size. Diabetes 43:942–946, 1994.
106. Jenkins AJ, Steele JS, Janus ED, Best JD: Increased plasma apolipoprotein (a) levels in IDDM patients with microalbuminuria. Diabetes 40:787–790, 1991.
107. Borch-Johnsen K, Kreiner S: Proteinuria: Value as predictor of cardiovascular mortality in insulin dependent diabetes mellitus. BMJ 294:1651–1654, 1987.
108. Sibley SD, Hokanson JE, Steffes MW, et al: Increased small dense LDL and intermediate-density lipoprotein with albuminuria in type 1 diabetes. Diabetes Care 22:1165–1170, 1999.
109. Chait A, Brunzell JD: Acquired hyperlipidemia (secondary dyslipoproteinemia). Endocrinol Metab Clin North Am 19:259–278, 1990.
110. Joven J, Villabona C, Vilella E: Pattern of hyperlipoproteinemia in human nephrotic syndrome: Influence of renal failure and diabetes mellitus. Nephron 64:565–569, 1993.
111. Groop PH, Elliott T, Ekstrand A, et al: Multiple lipoprotein abnormalities in type I diabetic patients with renal disease. Diabetes 45:974–979, 1996.
112. Attman PO, Nyberg G, William-Olsson T, et al: Dyslipoproteinemia in diabetic renal failure. Kidney Int 42:1381–1389, 1992.
113. Cassader M, Ruiu G, Gambino R, et al: Lipoprotein-apolipoprotein changes in renal transplant recipients: A 2-year follow-up. Metabolism 40:922–925, 1991.
114. Jarrett RJ: Risk factors for coronary heart disease in diabetes mellitus. Diabetes 41(suppl 2):1–3, 1992.
115. Valdorf-Hansen F, Jensen T, Borch-Johnsen K, Deckert T: Cardiovascular risk factors in type I (insulin-dependent) diabetic patients with and without proteinuria. Acta Med Scand 222:439–434, 1987.
116. McKenna K, Thompson C: Microalbuminuria: A marker to increased renal and cardiovascular risk in diabetes mellitus. Scott Med J 42:99–104, 1997.
117. Rossing P, Hougaard P, Borch-Johnsen K, Parving HH: Predictors of mortality in insulin dependent diabetes: 10 year observational follow up study. BMJ 313:779–784, 1996.
118. Chico A, Perez A, Cordoba A, et al: Plasma homocysteine is related to albumin excretion rate in patients with diabetes mellitus: A new link between diabetic nephropathy and cardiovascular disease? Diabetologia 41:684–693, 1998.
119. Lithell H, Boberg J, Hellsing K, et al: Serum lipoprotein and apolipoprotein concentrations and tissue lipoprotein lipase activity in overt and subclinical hypothyroidism: The effects of substitution therapy. Eur J Clin Invest 11:3–10, 1981.
120. Rohlfing JJ, Brunzell JD: Effects of diuretics and adrenergic blocking agents on plasma lipids. West J Med 145:210–218, 1986.
121. Weinberger MH: Antihypertensive therapy and lipids. Paradoxical influences on cardiovascular disease risk. Am J Med 80:64–70, 1986.
122. Chait A, Brunzell JD: Chylomicronemia syndrome. Adv Intern Med 37:249–273, 1992.
123. Chait A, Brunzell JD: Severe hypertriglyceridemia: Role of familial and acquired disorders. Metabolism 32:209–214, 1983.
124. Bagdade JD, Porte D Jr, Bierman EL: Diabetic lipemia. A form of acquired fat-induced lipemia. N Engl J Med 276:427–433, 1967.
125. Garg A, Grundy SM: Gemfibrozil alone and in combination with lovastatin for treatment of hypertriglyceridemia in NIDDM [published erratum appears in Diabetes 1990 Oct;39(10):1313]. Diabetes 38:364–372, 1989.
126. Fontbonne A, Eschwege E, Cambien F, et al: Hypertriglyceridaemia as a risk factor of coronary heart disease mortality in subjects with impaired glucose tolerance or diabetes. Diabetologia 32:300–304, 1989.
127. Stamler J, Vaccaro O, Neaton JD, Wentworth D: Diabetes, other risk factors, and 12-yr cardiovascular mortality for men screened in the Multiple Risk Factor Intervention Trial. Diabetes Care 16:434–444, 1993.
128. Laakso M, Lehto S, Penttila I, Pyorala K: Lipids and lipoproteins predicting coronary heart disease mortality and morbidity in patients with non–insulin-dependent diabetes. Circulation 88:1421–1430, 1993.
129. Lehto S, Ronnemaa T, Haffner SM, et al: Dyslipidemia and hyperglycemia predict coronary heart disease events in middle-aged patients with NIDDM. Diabetes 46:1354–1359, 1997.
130. Turner RC, Millns H, Neil HA, et al: Risk factors for coronary artery disease in non–insulin dependent diabetes mellitus: United Kingdom Prospective Diabetes Study (UKPDS: 23). BMJ 316:823–828, 1998.
131. Reaven GM: Role of insulin resistance in human disease. Diabetes 37:1595–1607, 1988.
132. Williams KJ, Tabas I: The response-to-retention hypothesis of early atherogenesis. Arterioscler Thromb Vasc Biol 15:551–561, 1995.
133. Witztum JL, Steinberg D: Role of oxidized low density lipoprotein in atherogenesis. J Clin Invest 88:1785–1792, 1991.
134. Chait A, Heinecke JW: Lipoprotein modification: Cellular mechanisms. Curr Opin Lipidol 5:365–370, 1994.
135. Heinecke JW, Baker L, Rosen H, Chait A: Superoxide-mediated free radical modification of low density lipoprotein by arterial smooth muscle cells. J Clin Invest 77:757–761, 1986.
136. Steinbrecher UP: Role of superoxide in endothelial-cell modification of low density lipoproteins. Biochim Biophys Acta 959:20–30, 1988.
137. Sparrow CP, Parthasarathy S, Steinberg D: Enzymatic modification of low density lipoprotein by purified lipoxygenase plus phospholipase A_2 mimics cell-mediated oxidative modification. J Lipid Res 29:745–753, 1988.
138. Chang MY, Potter-Perigo S, Tsoi C, et al: Oxidized low density lipoproteins regulate synthesis of monkey aortic smooth muscle cell proteoglycans that have enhanced native low density lipoprotein binding properties. J Biol Chem 275:4766–4773, 2000.
139. Henriksen T, Mahoney EM, Steinberg D: Enhanced macrophage degradation of biologically modified low density lipoproteins. Arteriosclerosis 3:149–159, 1983.
140. Endemann G, Stanton LW, Madden KS, et al: CD36 is a receptor for oxidized low density lipoprotein. J Biol Chem 268:11811–11816, 1993.
141. Nakata A, Nakagawa Y, Nishida M, et al: CD36, a novel receptor for oxidized low-density lipoproteins, is highly expressed on lipid-laden macrophages in human atherosclerotic aorta. Arterioscler Thromb Vasc Biol 19:1333–1339, 1999.
142. Ramprasad MP, Terpstra V, Kondratenko N, et al: Cell surface expression of mouse macrosialin and human CD68 and their role as macrophage receptors for oxidized low density lipoprotein. Proc Natl Acad Sci U S A 93:14833–14838, 1996.
143. Ross R: The pathogenesis of atherosclerosis: A perspective for the 1990s. Nature 362:801–809, 1993.
144. Camejo G, Hurt-Camejo E, Olsson U, Bondjers G: Proteoglycans and lipoproteins in atherosclerosis. Arteriosclerosis 4:385–391, 1993.
145. Oram JF, Mendez AJ, Slotte JP, Johnson TF: High density lipoprotein apolipoproteins mediate removal of sterol from intracellular pools but not from plasma membranes of cholesterol-loaded fibroblasts. Arterioscler Thromb 11:403–414, 1991.
146. Davies MJ, Woolf N, Katz DR: The role of endothelial denudation injury, plaque fissuring, and thrombosis in the progression of human atherosclerosis. Atheroscler Rev 23:105–113, 1991.
147. Davies MJ, Richardson PD, Woolf N, et al: Risk of thrombosis in human atherosclerotic plaques: Role of extracellular lipid, macrophage, and smooth muscle cell content. Br Heart J 69:377–381, 1993.
148. Rajavashisth TB, Liao JK, Galis ZS, et al: Inflammatory cytokines and oxidized low density lipoproteins increase endothelial cell expression of membrane type 1-matrix metalloproteinase. J Biol Chem 274:11924–11929, 1999.
149. Xu XP, Meisel SR, Ong JM, et al: Oxidized low-density lipoprotein regulates matrix metalloproteinase-9 and its tissue inhibitor in human monocyte-derived macrophages. Circulation 99:993–998, 1999.
150. Drake TA, Hannani K, Fei HH, et al: Minimally oxidized low-density lipoprotein induces tissue factor expression in cultured human endothelial cells. Am J Pathol 138:601–607, 1991.
151. Allison BA, Nilsson L, Karpe F, et al: Effects of native, triglyceride-enriched, and oxidatively modified LDL on plasminogen activator inhibitor-1 expression in human endothelial cells. Arterioscler Thromb Vasc Biol 19:1354–1360, 1999.
152. Anber V, Griffin BA, McConnell M, et al: Influence of plasma lipid and LDL-subfraction profile on the interaction between low density lipoprotein with human arterial wall proteoglycans. Atherosclerosis 124:261–271, 1996.
153. Chait A, Brazg RL, Tribble DL, Krauss RM: Susceptibility of small, dense low density lipoproteins to oxidative modification in subjects with the atherogenic lipoprotein phenotype, pattern B. Am J Med 94:350–356, 1993.
154. Dejager S, Bruckert E, Chapman MJ: Dense low density lipoprotein subspecies with diminished oxidative resistance predominate in combined hyperlipidemia. J Lipid Res 34:295–308, 1993.
155. Leinonen JS, Rantalaiho V, Laippala P, et al: The level of autoantibodies against oxidized LDL is not associated with the presence of coronary heart disease or diabetic kidney disease in patients with non–insulin-dependent diabetes mellitus. Free Radic Res 29:137–141, 1998.
156. Witztum JL, Mahoney EM, Branks MJ, et al: Nonenzymatic glucosylation of low-density lipoprotein alters its biologic activity. Diabetes 31:283–291, 1982.
157. Bowie A, Owens D, Collins P, et al: Glycosylated low density lipoprotein is more sensitive to oxidation: Implications for the diabetic patient? Atherosclerosis 102:63–67, 1993.
158. Duell PB, Oram JF, Bierman EL: Nonenzymatic glycosylation of HDL and impaired HDL-receptor–mediated cholesterol efflux. Diabetes 40:377–384, 1991.
159. Passarelli M, Catanozi S, Nakandakare ER, et al: Plasma lipoproteins from patients with poorly controlled diabetes mellitus and "in vitro" glycation of lipoproteins enhance the transfer rate of cholesteryl ester from HDL to apo-B–containing lipoproteins. Diabetologia 40:1085–1093, 1997.
160. Lander HM, Tauras JM, Ogiste JS, et al: Activation of the receptor for advanced glycation end products triggers a p21(ras)-dependent mitogen-activated protein kinase pathway regulated by oxidant stress. J Biol Chem 272:17810–17814, 1997.
161. Schmidt AM, Hori O, Brett J, et al: Cellular receptors for advanced glycation end products. Implications for induction of oxidant stress and cellular dysfunction in the pathogenesis of vascular lesions. Arterioscler Thromb 14:1521–1528, 1994.
162. Horiuchi S: Advanced glycation end products (AGE)-modified proteins and their potential relevance to atherosclerosis. Trends Cardiovasc Med 6:163–168, 1996.
163. Kawabe Y, Cynshi O, Takashima Y, et al: Oxidation-induced aggregation of rabbit low-density lipoprotein by azo initiator. Arch Biochem Biophys 310:489–496, 1994.
164. Schissel SL, Tweedie-Hardman J, Rapp JH, et al: Rabbit aorta and human atherosclerotic lesions hydrolyze the sphingomyelin of retained low-density lipoprotein. Proposed role for arterial-wall sphingomyelinase in subendothelial retention and aggregation of atherogenic lipoproteins. J Clin Invest 98:1455–1464, 1996.
165. Heinecke JW, Suits AG, Aviram M, Chait A: Phagocytosis of lipase-aggregated low density lipoprotein promotes macrophage foam cell formation. Arterioscler Thromb 11:1643–1651, 1991.
166. Griffith RL, Virella GT, Stevenson HC, Lopes-Virella MF: LDL metabolism by human macrophages activated with LDL immune complexes. J Exp Med 168:1041–1059, 1988.
167. Hazell LJ, Stocker R: Oxidation of low density lipoprotein with hypochlorite causes transformation of the lipoprotein into a high-uptake form for macrophages. Biochem J 290:165–172, 1993.
168. Bucala R, Makita Z, Koschinsky T, et al: Lipid advanced glycosylation: Pathway for lipid oxidation in vivo. Proc Natl Acad Sci U S A 90:6434–6438, 1993.
169. Pyörälä K, Pedersen TR, Kjekshus J, et al: Cholesterol lowering with simvastatin

improves prognosis of diabetic patients with coronary heart disease. A subgroup analysis of the Scandinavian Simvastatin Survival Study (4S) [published erratum appears in Diabetes Care 1997 Jun;20(6):1048]. Diabetes Care 20:614–620, 1997.

170. Haffner S, Alexander C, Cook T, et al: Reduced coronary events in simvastatin-treated patients with coronary heart disease and diabetes or impaired fasting glucose: Subgroup analyses in the Scandinavian Simvastatin Survival Study. Arch Intern Med 159:2661–2667, 1999.

171. Goldberg RB, Mellies MJ, Sacks FM, et al: Cardiovascular events and their reduction with pravastatin in diabetic and glucose-intolerant myocardial infarction survivors with average cholesterol levels: Subgroup analyses in the cholesterol and recurrent events (CARE) trial. The Care Investigators. Circulation 98:2513–2519, 1998.

172. Prevention of cardiovascular events and death with pravastatin in patients with coronary heart disease and a broad range of initial cholesterol levels. The Long-Term Intervention with Pravastatin in Ischaemic Disease (LIPID) Study Group. N Engl J Med 339:1349–1357, 1998.

173. Downs JR, Clearfield M, Weis S, et al: Primary prevention of acute coronary events with lovastatin in men and women with average cholesterol levels. Results of AFCAPS/TexCAPS. JAMA 279:1615–1622, 1998.

174. The Post Coronary Artery Bypass Graft Trial Investigators: The effect of aggressive lowering of low-density lipoprotein cholesterol levels and low-dose anticoagulation on obstructive changes in saphenous-vein coronary-artery bypass grafts. [published erratum appears in N Engl J Med 1997 Dec 18;337(25):1859]. N Engl J Med 336:153–162, 1997.

175. Hoogwerf BJ, Waness A, Cressman M, et al: Effects of aggressive cholesterol lowering and low-dose anticoagulation on clinical and angiographic outcomes in patients with diabetes: The Post Coronary Artery Bypass Graft Trial. Diabetes 48:1289–1294, 1999.

176. Koskinen P, Mänttäri M, Manninen V, et al: Coronary heart disease incidence in NIDDM patients in the Helsinki Heart Study. Diabetes Care 15:825–829, 1992.

177. Rubins HB, Robins SJ, Collins D, et al: Gemfibrozil for the secondary prevention of coronary heart disease in men with low levels of high-density lipoprotein cholesterol. Veterans Affairs High-Density Lipoprotein Cholesterol Intervention Trial Study Group. N Engl J Med 341:410–418, 1999.

178. Grundy SM, Benjamin IJ, Burke GL, et al: Diabetes and cardiovascular disease: A statement for healthcare professionals from the American Heart Association. Circulation 100:1134–1146, 1999.

179. American Diabetes Association: Management of dyslipidemia in adults with diabetes (position statement). Diabetes Care 23(suppl):57–60, 2000.

180. Pierce LR, Wysowski DK, Gross TP: Myopathy and rhabdomyolysis associated with lovastatin-gemfibrozil combination therapy. JAMA 264:71–75, 1990.

181. Wiklund O, Angelin B, Bergman M, et al: Pravastatin and gemfibrozil alone and in combination for the treatment of hypercholesterolemia. Am J Med 94:13–20, 1993.

182. Hutchesson AC, Moran A, Jones AF: Dual bezafibrate-simvastatin therapy for combined hyperlipidaemia. J Clin Pharm Ther 19:387–389, 1994.

183. Jensen T, Borch-Johnsen K, Kofoed-Enevoldsen A, Deckert T: Coronary heart disease in young type 1 (insulin-dependent) diabetic patients with and without diabetic nephropathy: Incidence and risk factors. Diabetologia 30:144–148, 1987.

184. Laakso M, Pyörälä K, Sarlund H, Voutilainen E: Lipid and lipoprotein abnormalities associated with coronary heart disease in patients with insulin-dependent diabetes mellitus. Arteriosclerosis 6:679–684, 1986.

185. Effect of intensive diabetes treatment on carotid artery wall thickness in the epidemiology of diabetes interventions and complications. Epidemiology of Diabetes Interventions and Complications (EDIC) Research Group. Diabetes 48:383–390, 1999.

186. Klein R: Kelly West Lecture 1994. Hyperglycemia and microvascular and macrovascular disease in diabetes. Diabetes Care 18:258–268, 1995.

187. WHO Study Group: Diabetes Mellitus, WHO Technical Report. Geneva, World Health Organization, 1985.

188. Kuusisto J, Mykkanen L, Pyorala K, Laakso M: NIDDM and its metabolic control predict coronary heart disease in elderly subjects. Diabetes 43:960–967, 1994.

189. UK Prospective Diabetes Study (UKPDS) Group: Intensive blood-glucose control with sulphonylureas or insulin compared with conventional treatment and risk of complications in patients with type 2 diabetes (UKPDS 33). Lancet 352:837–853, 1998.

190. Effect of intensive blood-glucose control with metformin on complications in overweight patients with type 2 diabetes (UKPDS 34). UK Prospective Diabetes Study (UKPDS) Group [published erratum appears in Lancet 1998 Nov 7;352(9139):1557]. Lancet 352:854–865, 1998.

Chapter 68

Syndrome X

Gerald M. Reaven

COMPENSATORY HYPERINSULINEMIA
ABNORMALITIES ASSOCIATED WITH
INSULIN RESISTANCE
  Glucose Metabolism
  Uric Acid Metabolism
  Lipoprotein Metabolism

Plasma Triglyceride Concentration
Postprandial Lipemia
High-Density Lipoprotein Cholesterol
Lipoprotein Lipase
Low-Density Lipoprotein Particle
  Diameter

Hemodynamic
  Sympathetic Nervous System Activity
  Sodium Retention
  Hypertension
Hemostatic
CONCLUSION

Resistance to insulin-mediated glucose disposal is characteristic of patients with type 2 diabetes mellitus, and fasting hyperglycemia supervenes when such individuals are not able to secrete the amount of insulin necessary to overcome the defect in cellular insulin action.[1-3] However, insulin-resistant subjects able to sustain the degree of compensatory hyperinsulinemia necessary to maintain near-normal glucose homeostasis are at risk for the development of a cluster of additional abnormalities, all of which increase the risk of coronary heart disease (CHD). To emphasize this relationship, it was suggested in 1988 that insulin resistance, its consequences, and CHD risk constitute a syndrome designated as syndrome X.[3] This formulation has received considerable support since its introduction, and the list of abnormalities associated with insulin resistance and compensatory hyperinsulinemia has grown considerably. The goal of this chapter is to describe the current version of syndrome X (Fig. 68–1).

COMPENSATORY HYPERINSULINEMIA

The central defects in syndrome X are postulated to be insulin resistance and compensatory hyperinsulinemia, and it is this combination that differentiates syndrome X from type 2 diabetes. As commonly used, the statement that insulin resistance exists usually means that a defined amount of insulin stimulates glucose uptake by muscle to a lesser degree than it does in an insulin-sensitive person. However, no criterion permits the designation of an individual as being either insulin sensitive or insulin resistant. The ability of physiologic hyperinsulinemia to enhance muscle glucose uptake varies continuously in a healthy, nonobese population, and substantial differences are noted between the most insulin-sensitive and the most insulin-resistant individuals.[4, 5] As depicted in Figure 68–1, insulin resistance is influenced by both life-style and genes. It appears that differences in degree of obesity and physical activity, the two most important life-style variables that modulate insulin action, each explain approximately 25% of the variation in insulin action from person to person.[6] By inference, it can then be argued that differences in genetic background account for the remaining 50% of the variability in insulin resistance. Although the actual numerical values may not be entirely accurate, they represent reasonable approximations. The point to emphasize is that variations in body weight and level of physical activity are modulators of insulin action; they are not the primary cause of insulin resistance.

A second point to emphasize is that adipose tissue appears to be as resistant to regulation by insulin as muscle.[7, 8] The belated recognition of adipose tissue insulin resistance is easily understood if both the techniques generally used to assess resistance to insulin-mediated glucose disposal and the differences in the dose-response characteristics of insulin action on adipose tissue vs. muscle are taken into account. For example, a plasma insulin concentration of approximately 20 μU/mL—a circulating insulin concentration that has relatively little effect on stimulating glucose disposal by muscle—will suppress by approximately 50% the release of free fatty acids (FFAs) by adipose tissue.[8] The infusion techniques conventionally used to quantify insulin

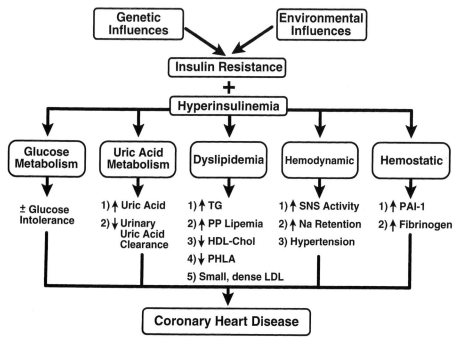

FIGURE 68–1. Diagrammatic representation of the relationship between insulin resistance plus compensatory hyperinsulinemia and the cluster of abnormalities that constitutes syndrome X. HDL-Chol, high-density lipoprotein cholesterol; PAI-1, plasminogen activator inhibitor-1; PHLA, plasma post-heparin lipolytic activity; PP, postprandial; SNS, sympathetic nervous system; TG, triglyceride.

resistance, or the ability of insulin to stimulate glucose disposal by muscle, have almost uniformly been performed by maintaining steady-state insulin concentrations at least fourfold greater than the level needed to half-maximally suppress adipose tissue lipolysis. As a result, plasma FFA levels were maximally suppressed in all subjects, and differences in adipose tissue resistance to insulin could not be discerned. It is now clear that the degree of insulin resistance in muscle and adipose tissue is highly correlated[9] and that both defects contribute to the manifestations of syndrome X.

If not for this difference in the tissue dose-response curve, the increase in plasma FFA concentration would be proportionate to the degree of hyperinsulinemia in subjects with syndrome X. However, because of the enhanced sensitivity of adipose tissue to insulin, plasma FFA concentrations are only marginally increased as long as hyperinsulinemia is maintained. On the other hand, the fact that the increase in plasma FFA concentration is less dramatic does not mean that adipose tissue insulin resistance plays no role in the pathogenesis of syndrome X. Indeed, the role played by elevated FFA concentrations in the manifestation of syndrome X is an area of intense current research.

ABNORMALITIES ASSOCIATED WITH INSULIN RESISTANCE

Glucose Metabolism

Most insulin-resistant individuals maintain normal glucose tolerance by secreting large amounts of insulin. Indeed, within the population of individuals with normal glucose tolerance, the greater their degree of insulin resistance, the higher their plasma glucose concentration.[5] In some insulin-resistant individuals, the degree of compensatory hyperinsulinemia will not be sufficient to maintain normal glucose tolerance, and such individuals will be classified as having impaired glucose tolerance.[10] As insulin secretory function declines, the increase in plasma FFA concentrations becomes more apparent; hyperglycemia develops in insulin-resistant individuals when the plasma insulin concentrations are no longer high enough to prevent significant elevations in plasma FFA concentrations. Insulin resistance, plasma insulin concentrations that are no longer markedly elevated, and increased plasma FFA concentrations define patients with type 2 diabetes. Syndrome X is used to designate insulin-resistant individuals who although they may have impaired glucose tolerance, are not diabetic and continue to be hyperinsulinemic, with only moderate increases in plasma FFA concentrations. Syndrome X and type 2 diabetes share insulin resistance but are otherwise metabolically quite different. The designation of syndrome X should be limited to individuals who have maintained sufficient insulin secretory function to remain nondiabetic.

Uric Acid Metabolism

Because the kidney is not considered to be an insulin-sensitive tissue, its role in syndrome X is rarely discussed. However, two features of syndrome X are dependent on normal insulin action on the kidney. The first involves the relationship between insulin resistance, compensatory hyperinsulinemia, and plasma uric acid concentrations. Despite the fact that an increase in serum uric acid concentration was known to be a characteristic finding in patients with CHD,[11] no obvious explanation could be found for this association until recently. The results of studies published in the past few years have clarified this issue significantly, and the crucial role of the kidney in this relationship has been identified.

In addition to its association with CHD, hyperuricemia is commonly seen in individuals with glucose intolerance, dyslipidemia, and hypertension,[12] the central characteristics of syndrome X. Given the relationship between insulin resistance and the abnormalities noted to occur in hyperuricemic individuals, it seemed reasonable to see whether uric acid concentration also varied as a function of insulin resistance and/or hyperinsulinemia. The results of such a study in normal volunteers have shown that the more insulin resistant an individual and the greater the degree of hyperinsulinemia, the higher the uric acid concen-

tration.[13] It has also been shown that healthy volunteers with asymptomatic hyperuricemia have higher plasma insulin responses to oral glucose, higher plasma triglyceride (TG) and lower high-density lipoprotein (HDL) cholesterol concentrations, and higher blood pressure than do volunteers with normal serum uric acid concentrations.[14]

Evidence that the association between insulin resistance, hyperinsulinemia, and serum uric acid concentration was related to a decrease in the urinary clearance of uric acid[13] raised the possibility that the link between insulin metabolism and hyperuricemia was the renal handling of uric acid. The hypothesis that insulin acts on the kidney to decrease renal clearance of uric acid has subsequently been validated by results of studies in both normotensive and hypertensive subjects.[15, 16]

Based on these data, it seems most likely that the association between CHD and uric acid concentration is an epiphenomenon. Insulin-resistant individuals will try to secrete increased amounts of insulin in an effort to prevent type 2 diabetes. The kidney, which is not insulin resistant, responds to the day-long elevations of circulating insulin by decreasing uric acid clearance, which leads to somewhat higher plasma uric acid concentrations. Thus the kidney, although an innocent bystander, is the necessary link between muscle insulin resistance, compensatory hyperinsulinemia, and elevated uric acid concentration.

Lipoprotein Metabolism

Perhaps the best established of the postulated relationships shown in Figure 68–1 is that between insulin resistance, compensatory hyperinsulinemia, and hypertriglyceridemia.[17–19] It is now apparent that the link between insulin resistance and dyslipidemia is a much broader one and not limited to an increase in plasma TG concentrations. Because the additional abnormalities in lipoprotein metabolism associated with insulin resistance are related to the changes in very-low-density lipoprotein (VLDL) metabolism seen in these individuals, attention in this section will focus on the link between insulin resistance, compensatory hyperinsulinemia, and VLDL metabolism, with a somewhat less detailed discussion of the associated manifestations shown in Figure 68–1.

Plasma Triglyceride Concentration

The schema outlined in Figure 68–2 is adapted from the results of two studies previously published from our group.[18, 19] Figure 68–2A depicts the relationship between the four variables in question in nondiabetic individuals whose baseline plasma TG concentrations range from 69 to 546 mg/dL,[18] whereas Figure 68–2B is based on the study of individuals with plasma TG concentrations less than 175 mg/dL.[19] Implicit in these data is the view that the major cause of an elevated plasma TG concentration in nondiabetic individuals is an increase in the hepatic VLDL TG secretion rate secondary to insulin resistance and the resultant hyperinsulinemia. It should be emphasized that the situation is different in hypertriglyceridemic individuals with type 2 diabetes, who are also insulin resistant but have ambient insulin concentrations that are "normal" in absolute terms.

Although agreement is widespread regarding the validity of the relationships shown in Figure 68–2, controversy surrounds the causal relationship between insulin resistance, hyperinsulinemia, hepatic VLDL TG secretion, and plasma TG concentration. One view is that resistance to insulin regulation of muscle and adipose tissue leads to higher ambient levels of both insulin and FFAs and that these two changes stimulate hepatic VLDL TG secretion and thereby lead to the increase in plasma TG concentration in insulin-resistant individuals.[17–20] This theory postulates that the higher ambient insulin concentrations present in insulin-resistant individuals act on the liver to increase the rate at which the incoming FFAs are converted to VLDL TG; the higher the plasma FFA concentration, the greater the increase in VLDL TG secretion. Alternatively, evidence has also been published, summarized in a recent review article,[21] that hypertriglyceridemia occurs in insulin-resistant, nondiabetic individuals because the normal ability of insulin to inhibit hepatic VLDL TG secretion is deficient. In the absence of this postulated inhibition of hepatic VLDL

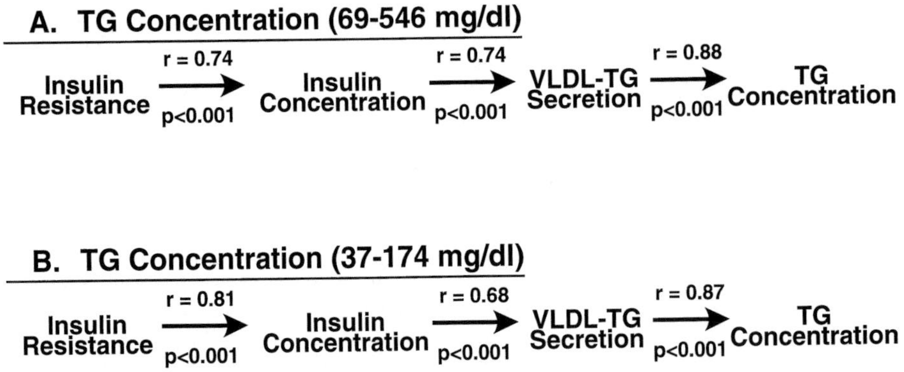

A. TG Concentration (69-546 mg/dl)

Insulin Resistance →(r = 0.74, p<0.001) Insulin Concentration →(r = 0.74, p<0.001) VLDL-TG Secretion →(r = 0.88, p<0.001) TG Concentration

B. TG Concentration (37-174 mg/dl)

Insulin Resistance →(r = 0.81, p<0.001) Insulin Concentration →(r = 0.68, p<0.001) VLDL-TG Secretion →(r = 0.87, p<0.001) TG Concentration

FIGURE 68–2. Summary of correlation coefficients between resistance to insulin-mediated glucose disposal, plasma insulin response to oral glucose, very-low-density lipoprotein (VLDL) triglyceride (TG) secretion, and plasma TG concentration over a range of fasting plasma TG concentrations from 69 to 546 mg/dL *(A)* or 37 to 174 mg/dL *(B)*. (A, Adapted from data published by Olefsky JM, Farquhar JW, Reaven GM: Reappraisal of the role of insulin in hypertriglyceridemia. Am J Med 57:551, 1974. Reprinted with permission of Excerpta Medica Inc.; *B,* adapted from data published by Tobey TA, Greenfield M, Kraemer F, Reaven GM: Relationship between insulin resistance, insulin secretion, very low density lipoprotein kinetics, and plasma triglyceride levels in normotriglyceridemic man. Metabolism 30:165, 1981.)

TG secretion by insulin, it is suggested that the increase in plasma FFA concentration in insulin-resistant individuals will stimulate hepatic VLDL TG synthesis and secretion. Evidence in support of this latter hypothesis is derived entirely from acute experiments.[21] For example, insulin acutely inhibits VLDL TG secretion from cultured rat and human hepatocytes and HepG2 cells. The acute infusion of insulin has also been shown to suppress hepatic VLDL TG secretion in humans, along with a substantial decrease in plasma FFA concentration. An obvious explanation for the ability of an acute insulin infusion to decrease VLDL TG secretion is the profound decrease in adipose tissue lipolysis that occurs secondary to the hyperinsulinemia. In this context, the findings of Aarsland et al. are highly relevant.[22] These authors measured VLDL TG secretion rates 1 and 4 days after beginning a high carbohydrate, hypercaloric diet. This diet resulted in a sixfold elevation in plasma insulin concentration that persisted throughout the study. The VLDL TG secretion rate was, if anything, lower after 1 day of hyperinsulinemia without any change in plasma TG secretion. However, by day 4, significant increases were seen in both hepatic VLDL TG secretion and plasma TG concentrations. These data strongly suggest that the *acute* effects of exogenous hyperinsulinemia are not necessarily reflective of the *chronic* effects of endogenous hyperinsulinemia. Furthermore, in support of the importance of FFAs in stimulating hepatic VLDL TG secretion was the observation that the difference between 1 and 4 days of endogenous hyperinsulinemia was the increase in hepatic secretion of preformed fatty acids into VLDL TG.[22]

Further evidence that *chronic* elevation of endogenous insulin does not inhibit hepatic VLDL TG secretion can be derived from the effects of dietary manipulations. It has been known for more than 30 years that high carbohydrate diets increase plasma TG concentrations.[17, 23] Such diets have also been shown to increase both plasma insulin concentrations and insulin sensitivity.[17, 24] If hypertriglyceridemia is due to the inability of insulin to inhibit VLDL TG secretion in insulin-resistant individuals, high carbohydrate diets, by increasing both insulin levels and sensitivity, should lead to a *decrease*, not an *increase* in hepatic VLDL TG secretion. The fact that just the opposite is seen provides further evidence that *chronic* endogenous hyperinsulinemia, in insulin-resistant individuals, leads to hypertriglyceridemia by enhancing hepatic FFA esterification and stimulating VLDL TG secretion as outlined in Figure 68–2.

Postprandial Lipemia

The higher the fasting TG concentration, the greater the postprandial accumulation of TG-rich lipoproteins.[25] Furthermore, this phenomenon is accentuated in patients with type 2 diabetes, even when matched for fasting plasma TG concentration with a nondiabetic control group.[26] The postprandial increase in TG-rich lipoproteins was significantly correlated with circulating insulin concentrations, and both

insulin resistance and compensatory hyperinsulinemia were also significantly related to the postprandial accumulation of TG-rich lipoproteins in nondiabetic individuals.[27] These findings indicate that elevations in postprandial lipemia are highly correlated with insulin resistance and compensatory hyperinsulinemia—directly, by mechanisms as yet unknown, and indirectly, by virtue of the role played by insulin resistance and/or compensatory hyperinsulinemia in stimulating hepatic VLDL TG secretion and increasing the fasting plasma TG concentration.

High-Density Lipoprotein Cholesterol

Increases in plasma TG concentration are usually associated with a low HDL cholesterol concentration. In part, this finding is likely to be a reflection of the transfer, catalyzed by cholesteryl ester transfer protein, of cholesterol from HDL to VLDL[28]; the higher the VLDL pool size, the greater the transfer rate from HDL to VLDL and the lower the ensuing HDL cholesterol concentration. Evidence has also accumulated that the fractional catabolic rate (FCR) of apolipoprotein A-I is increased in patients with primary hypertriglyceridemia,[29] hypertension,[30] and type 2 diabetes.[31] In the latter instance, the greater the degree of hyperinsulinemia, the lower the HDL cholesterol concentration. It has also been shown that the higher the apolipoprotein A-I FCR, the lower the HDL cholesterol concentration.[32] Thus it is likely that insulin resistance and hyperinsulinemia contribute to a low HDL cholesterol concentration indirectly by being responsible for the increase in VLDL pool size, and directly by increasing the FCR of apolipoprotein A-I.

Lipoprotein Lipase

Lipoprotein lipase (LPL) plays a key role in the catabolism of TG-rich lipoproteins. If LPL activity increases to a sufficient degree in subjects who are insulin resistant and hyperinsulinemic, the ensuing increase in hepatic VLDL TG synthesis would not necessarily lead to an increase in plasma TG concentration. Because hypertriglyceridemia does occur in this situation, it can be argued that syndrome X is associated with at least a "relative" failure of LPL to maintain TG homeostasis. Support for this view can be derived from the results of a recent study showing that the more insulin resistant and/or hyperinsulinemic an individual, the lower the level of plasma post-heparin (PH) LPL activity and mass and the higher the plasma TG concentration.[33] In addition, lower concentrations of adipose tissue LPL mRNA are directly correlated with plasma PH LPL mass and inversely correlated with both plasma TG and insulin concentrations and insulin resistance. Thus it appears that failure of insulin to appropriately stimulate LPL activity accentuates the magnitude of hypertriglyceridemia that develops in association with the increase in hepatic TG synthesis and secretion present in syndrome X.

Low-Density Lipoprotein Particle Diameter

Analysis of low-density lipoprotein (LDL) particle size distribution has identified multiple distinct LDL subclasses,[34] and it appears that LDL in most individuals can be characterized by a predominance of larger LDL (diameter, >255 Å, pattern A) or smaller LDL (≤255 Å, pattern B). Individuals with pattern B have higher plasma TG and lower HDL cholesterol concentrations and are at increased risk of CHD.[34] Similar changes in plasma TG and HDL cholesterol concentrations are associated with insulin resistance and/or compensatory hyperinsulinemia,[35] and data indicate that healthy volunteers with small, dense LDL particles (pattern B) are relatively insulin resistant, glucose intolerant, hyperinsulinemic, hypertensive, and hypertriglyceridemic and have a lower HDL cholesterol concentration.[36] These observations demonstrate that small dense LDL particles belong to the cluster of abnormalities previously defined as constituting syndrome X.

Hemodynamic

Sympathetic Nervous System Activity

The resting heart rate is higher in patients with high blood pressure, as well as being a predictor of hypertension.[37, 38] Patients with high blood pressure, as a group, are insulin resistant, and a recent review article has summarized evidence that insulin resistance and compensatory hyperinsulinemia can predispose individuals to hypertension via stimulation of the sympathetic nervous system (SNS).[39] Thus the association between hypertension and increased heart rate could be secondary to enhanced SNS activity in insulin-resistant subjects. Evidence in support of this view has recently been provided by the results of a study in normotensive, nondiabetic individuals showing that both insulin-mediated glucose disposal and the plasma insulin response to an oral glucose challenge are significantly correlated with the heart rate.[40] In light of these findings, it seems reasonable to suggest that SNS activity is increased in insulin-resistant individuals. This association provides a coherent explanation for observations that both resistance to insulin-mediated glucose disposal (or hyperinsulinemia) and an increase in heart rate have been shown to predict the development of hypertension.

Sodium Retention

Acute infusion of insulin increases renal sodium retention in both normal individuals and patients with high blood pressure,[15, 16] even though the muscles of these individuals are resistant to insulin-mediated glucose disposal.[40] The ability of insulin to promote sodium retention is another example in which renal sensitivity to an action of insulin is normal despite a loss of muscle insulin sensitivity, similar to the situation described with regard to renal uric acid clearance. It also seems that these effects of insulin on the kidney are related in that the increase in sodium retention is associated with the decrease in uric acid clearance.[15, 16] The fact that insulin can increase renal sodium retention in insulin-resistant subjects suggests that such individuals would be salt sensitive, and studies in both normotensive and hypertensive individuals have shown that insulin-resistant individuals are salt sensitive.[41, 42]

Hypertension

Considerable evidence has amassed that patients with essential hypertension, as a group, are insulin resistant and hyperinsulinemic when compared with individuals with normal blood pressure.[3, 39] Furthermore, patients with hypertension tend to be glucose intolerant and demonstrate the dyslipidemic features of syndrome X.[43] On the other hand, not all patients with essential hypertension are insulin resistant and hyperinsulinemic. This generalization is apparent from the data in Figure 68–3, which shows the distribution of plasma insulin concentrations 2 hours after the ingestion of an oral glucose load in 41 patients with hypertension and 41 normotensive subjects.[44] The hypertensive patients were identified as part of a routine health survey, and the normotensive subjects were participants in the same survey who were

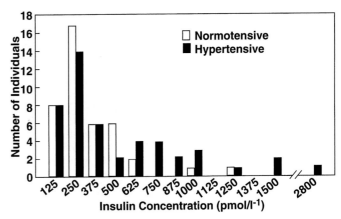

FIGURE 68–3. Frequency distribution of the plasma insulin response 2 hours after a 75-g oral glucose challenge in normotensive *(open bars)* and hypertensive *(filled bars)* factory workers. (From Zavaroni I, Mazza S, Dall'Aglio E, et al: Prevalence of hyperinsulinaemia in patients with high blood pressure. J Intern Med 231:235, 1992.)

selected to match the patients with respect to variables such as sex, degree of obesity, ethnic background, type of employment, and level of physical activity. Only 10% of the normotensive subjects had 2-hour plasma insulin concentrations greater than 80 μU/mL, as opposed to 45% of the patients with hypertension. On the basis of these findings, approximately 50% of patients with hypertension can be considered to be insulin resistant and hyperinsulinemic.

The results in Figure 68–3 make it clear that a significant proportion of patients with essential hypertension are insulin sensitive. Furthermore, blood pressure does not increase in all subjects who are insulin resistant and hyperinsulinemic. However, substantial evidence has shown that insulin resistance and/or hyperinsulinemia plays a role in the development of high blood pressure in a significant number of individuals. This issue has recently been the subject of an extensive review,[45] and the salient points are summarized below.

1. Neither insulin resistance nor hyperinsulinemia develops in humans with secondary forms of hypertension.

2. Insulin resistance exists in normotensive, first-degree relatives of patients with high blood pressure. In addition to being insulin resistant, individuals with a family history of hypertension are also relatively dyslipidemic. These results demonstrate that the metabolic changes associated with essential hypertension can exist in the absence of any increase in blood pressure.

3. Several prospective studies have shown that hyperinsulinemia at baseline predicts the subsequent development of essential hypertension. Of particular interest regarding the inclusion of hypertension in syndrome X was the additional finding from one study that "high insulin levels seem to precede the development of a potentially atherogenic risk factor profile including low HDL cholesterol, high triglyceride, and high systolic blood pressure."[46]

4. Weight loss, which enhances insulin sensitivity and lowers plasma insulin concentrations in nondiabetic individuals, can also decrease blood pressure in patients with essential hypertension, and this change seems to be correlated with the improvement in insulin resistance.

Perhaps the most controversial issue regarding the cluster of abnormalities associated with insulin resistance and compensatory hyperinsulinemia is that of essential hypertension. For this reason, substantial evidence has been reviewed and supports the view that essential hypertension belongs to syndrome X.

Hemostatic

Elevated concentrations of plasminogen activator inhibitor-1 (PAI-1) are seen in association with myocardial infarction, as well as in patients with hypertriglyceridemia and/or hypertension.[47–49] In light of the association between PAI-1, CHD, and other features of syndrome X, it would not be surprising if PAI-1 concentrations were also related to insulin resistance and/or compensatory hyperinsulinemia. The most compelling evidence in support of this view is the recent report from the European Concerted Action on Thrombosis and Disabilities Angina Pectoris Study. Their conclusion was that PAI-1 concentrations were significantly associated with hyperinsulinemia, hypertriglyceridemia, and hypertension in 1500 patients with angina pectoris.[49] The evidence that elevated fibrinogen levels are also part of syndrome X is not as strong. Although insulin resistance and fibrinogen levels have been shown to be correlated, it has been argued that the relationship in this case is not an independent one, but the manifestation of an acute phase reaction in patients with CHD.[50]

CONCLUSION

The ability of insulin to stimulate glucose uptake varies widely from person to person. In an effort to maintain normal plasma glucose concentrations, the pancreatic β cell will attempt to secrete whatever amount of insulin is required to accomplish this goal. If this compensatory effort is not successful, type 2 diabetes develops in insulin-resistant individuals. Normal or near-normal glucose tolerance is maintained as long as insulin-resistant individuals are able to sustain a state of chronic hyperinsulinemia. Unfortunately, this situation represents a Pyrrhic victory, and the combination of insulin resistance and hyperinsulinemia places an individual at greatly increased risk of the abnormalities shown in Figure 68–1. On the basis of the material discussed in this chapter, it does not seem inappropriate to suggest that resistance to insulin-mediated glucose disposal, as well as the manner in which the organism responds to this defect, appears to play a major role in the pathogenesis and clinical course of what are often referred to as diseases of Western civilization.

REFERENCES

1. Ginsberg H, Kimmerling G, Olefsky JM, Reaven GM: Demonstration of insulin resistance in untreated adult onset diabetic subjects with fasting hyperglycemia. J Clin Invest 55:454–461, 1975.
2. Reaven GM: Insulin resistance in noninsulin-dependent diabetes mellitus: Does it exist and can it be measured? Am J Med 74(suppl 1A):3–17, 1983.
3. Reaven GM: Role of insulin resistance in human disease. Diabetes 37:1594–1607, 1998.
4. Hollenbeck CB, Reaven GM: Variation in insulin-stimulated glucose uptake in healthy individuals with normal glucose tolerance. J Clin Endocrinol Metab 64:1169–1173, 1987.
5. Reaven GM, Brand RJ, Chen Y-DI, et al: Insulin resistance and insulin secretion are determinants of oral glucose tolerance in normal individuals. Diabetes 42:1324–1332, 1993.
6. Bogardus C, Lillioja S, Mott DM, et al: Relationship between degree of obesity and in vivo insulin action in man. Am J Physiol 248:E286–E291, 1985.
7. Fraze E, Donner CC, Swislocki ALM, et al: Ambient plasma free fatty acid concentrations in noninsulin-dependent diabetes mellitus: Evidence for insulin resistance. J Clin Endocrinol Metab 61:807–811, 1985.
8. Swislocki ALM, Chen Y-DI, Golay A, et al: Insulin suppression of plasma-free fatty acid concentration in normal individuals and patients with type 2 (non–insulin-dependent) diabetes. Diabetologia 30:622–626, 1987.
9. Pei D, Chen Y-DI, Hollenbeck CB, et al: Relationship between insulin-mediated glucose disposal by muscle and adipose tissue lipolysis in healthy volunteers. J Clin Endocrinol Metab 80:3368–3372, 1995.
10. Reaven GM, Miller RG: An attempt to define the nature of chemical diabetes using a multidimensional analysis. Diabetologia 16:17–24, 1979.
11. Gertler MM, Garn SM, Levine SA: Serum uric acid in relation to age and physique in health and coronary heart disease. J Med 34:1421–1431, 1951.
12. Wyngaarden JB, Kelley WN: Gout. In Metabolic Basis of Inherited Disease, ed 5. New York, McGraw-Hill, 1983, pp 1043–1144.
13. Facchini F, Chen Y-DI, Hollenbeck CB, Reaven GM: Relationship between resistance to insulin-mediated glucose uptake, urinary uric acid clearance, and plasma uric acid concentration. JAMA 266:3008–3011, 1991.
14. Zavaroni I, Vazza S, Fantuzzi M, et al: Changes in insulin and lipid metabolism in males with asymptomatic hyperuricemia. J Intern Med 234:24–30, 1993.
15. Quinones GA, Natali A, Baldi S, et al: Effect of insulin on uric acid excretion in humans. Am J Physiol 268:E1–E5, 1995.
16. Muscelli E, Natali A, Bianchi S, et al: Effect of insulin on renal sodium and uric acid handling in essential hypertension. Am J Hypertens 9:746–752, 1996.
17. Reaven GM, Lerner RL, Stern MP, Farquhar JW: Role of insulin in endogenous hypertriglyceridemia. J Clin Invest 46:1756–1767, 1967.
18. Olefsky JM, Farquhar JW, Reaven GM: Reappraisal of the role of insulin in hypertriglyceridemia. Am J Med 57:551–560, 1974.
19. Tobey TA, Greenfield M, Kraemer F, Reaven GM: Relationship between insulin resistance, insulin secretion, very low density lipoprotein kinetics, and plasma triglyceride levels in normotriglyceridemic man. Metabolism 30:165–171, 1981.
20. Jeng C-Y, Fuh MM-T, Sheu WH-H, et al: Hormone and substrate modulation of plasma triglyceride concentration in primary hypertriglyceridemia. Endocrinol Metab 1:15–21, 1994.
21. Lewis GF: Fatty acid regulation of very low density lipoprotein production. Curr Opin Lipidol 8:146–153, 1997.
22. Aarsland A, Chinkes D, Wolfe RR: Contributions of de novo synthesis of fatty acids to total VLDL-triglyceride secretion during prolonged hyperglycemia/hyperinsulinemia in normal man. J Clin Invest 98:2008–2017, 1996.
23. Farquhar JW, Frank A, Gross RC, Reaven GM: Glucose, insulin, and triglyceride responses to high and low carbohydrate diets in man. J Clin Invest 45:1648–1656, 1966.
24. Kolterman OG, Greenfield M, Reaven GM, et al: Effect of a high carbohydrate diet on insulin binding to adipocytes and on insulin action in vivo in man. Diabetes 28:731–736, 1979.
25. Wilson DE, Chan I-F, Buchi KN, Horton SC: Postchallenge plasma lipoprotein retinoids: Chylomicron remnants in endogenous hypertriglyceridemia. Metabolism 34:551–558, 1985.
26. Chen Y-DI, Swami S, Skowronski R, et al: Differences in postprandial lipemia between patients with normal glucose tolerance and noninsulin-dependent diabetes mellitus. J Clin Endocrinol Metab 76:172–177, 1993.
27. Jeppesen J, Hollenbeck CB, Zhou M-Y, et al: Relation between insulin resistance, hyperinsulinemia, postheparin plasma lipoprotein lipase activity, and postprandial lipemia. Arterioscler Thromb Vasc Biol 15:320–324, 1995.
28. Swenson TL: The role of the cholesteryl ester transfer protein in lipoprotein metabolism. Diabetes Metab Rev 7:139–153, 1991.
29. Fidge N, Nestel P, Toshitsugu I, et al: Turnover of apoproteins A-I and A-II of high density lipoprotein and the relationship to other lipoproteins in normal and hyperlipidemic individuals. Metabolism 29:643–653, 1980.
30. Chen Y-DI, Sheu WH-H, Swislocki ALM, Reaven GM: High density lipoprotein turnover in patients with hypertension. Hypertension 17:386–393, 1991.
31. Golay A, Zech L, Shi M-Z, et al: High density lipoprotein (HDL) metabolism in noninsulin-dependent diabetes mellitus: Measurement of HDL turnover using tritiated HDL. J Clin Endocrinol Metab 65:512–518, 1987.
32. Brinton EA, Eisenberg S, Breslow JL: Human HDL cholesterol levels are determined by apoA-I fractional catabolic rate, which correlates inversely with estimates of HDL particle size. Effects of gender, hepatic and lipoprotein lipases, triglyceride and insulin levels, and body fat distribution. Arterioscler Thromb Vasc Biol 14:707–720, 1994.
33. Maheux P, Azhar S, Kern PA, et al: Relationship between insulin-mediated glucose disposal and regulation of plasma and adipose tissue lipoprotein lipase. Diabetologia 40:850–858, 1997.
34. Austin MA, Breslow JL, Hennekens CH, et al: Low-density lipoprotein subclass patterns and risk of myocardial infarction. JAMA 260:1917–1921, 1988.
35. Laws A, Reaven GM: Evidence for an independent relationship between insulin resistance and fasting plasma HDL-cholesterol, triglyceride and insulin concentrations. J Intern Med 231:25–30, 1992.
36. Reaven GM, Chen Y-DI, Jeppesen J, et al: Insulin resistance and hyperinsulinemia in individuals with small, dense, low density lipoprotein particles. J Clin Invest 92:141–146, 1993.
37. Gillum RF: Resting heart rate: Associations with hypertension, coronary heart disease, blood pressure and other cardiovascular risk factors. Am Heart J 116:163–174, 1988.
38. Selby JV, Friedman GD, Quesenberry CP: Precursors of essential hypertension: Pulmonary function, heart rate, uric acid, serum cholesterol and other serum chemistries. Am J Epidemiol 131:1017–1027, 1990.
39. Reaven GM, Lithell H, Landsberg L: Hypertension and associated metabolic abnormalities—the role of insulin resistance and the sympathoadrenal system. N Engl J Med 334:374–381, 1996.
40. Facchini FS, Stoohs RA, Reaven GM: Enhanced sympathetic nervous system activity—the linchpin between insulin resistance, hyperinsulinemia, and heart rate. Am J Hypertens 9:1013–1017, 1996.
41. Sharma AM, Schorr U, Distler A: Insulin resistance in young salt-sensitive normotensive subjects. Hypertension 21:273–279, 1993.
42. Zavaroni I, Coruzzi P, Bonini L, et al: Association between salt sensitivity and insulin concentrations in patients with hypertension. Am J Hypertens 8:855–858, 1995.
43. Fuh M-T, Shieh SM, Wu D-A, et al: Abnormalities of carbohydrate and lipid metabolism in patients with hypertension. Arch Intern Med 147:1035–1038, 1987.
44. Zavaroni I, Mazza S, Dall'Aglio E, et al: Prevalence of hyperinsulinaemia in patients with high blood pressure. J Intern Med 231:235–240, 1992.
45. Reaven GM: Does insulin resistance play a role in the pathogenesis and clinical course of patients with hypertension? In Williams B (ed): Hypertension and Diabetes. London, Martin Dunitz, in press.
46. Raitakari OT, Porkka KVK, Rönnemaa T, et al: The role of insulin in clustering of serum lipids and blood pressure in children and adolescents. Diabetologia 38:1042–1050, 1995.
47. Hamsten A, Defaire U, Walldius G, et al: Plasminogen activator inhibitor in plasma: Risk factor for recurrent myocardial infarction. Lancet 2:3–9, 1987.
48. Landin K, Tengvory L, Smith U: Elevated fibrinogen and plasminogen activator (PAI-1) in hypertension are related to metabolic risk factors for cardiovascular disease. J Intern Med 227:273–278, 1990.
49. Juhan-Vague I, Thompson SG, Jespersen J, ECAT Angina Pectoris Study Group: Involvement of the hemostatic system in the insulin resistance syndrome. Arterioscler Thromb Vasc Biol 13:1865–1873, 1993.
50. Facchini F, Chen Y-DI, Clinkingbeard C, et al: Insulin resistance, hyperinsulinemia, and dyslipidemia in nonobese individuals with a family history of hypertension. Am J Hypertens 5:694–699, 1992.

Chapter 69

▲▲▲▲

Hyperglycemia Secondary to Nondiabetic Conditions and Therapies

Harold E. Lebovitz ▪ Samy I. McFarlane

DISORDERS OF THE PANCREAS
  Pancreatectomy
  Chronic Pancreatitis
  Pancreatic Cancer
  Hemochromatosis
  Hemosiderosis
  Cystic Fibrosis
**HYPERGLYCEMIA ASSOCIATED WITH
  ENDOCRINOPATHIES**

**Acromegaly
Growth Hormone Treatment
Cushing's Syndrome
Glucagonoma Syndrome
Somatostatinoma
Pheochromocytoma
DRUGS THAT CAN CAUSE HYPERGLYCEMIA
Drugs Affecting β Cell Function**
  Drugs that Destroy β Cells

Drugs that Inhibit Increases in β Cell
  Cytosolic Ca^{2+}
Drugs that Cause K^+ Depletion
  Mechanisms Unknown
Drugs Causing Insulin Resistance
  Oral Contraceptives and Sex Hormones
  Nicotinic Acid
  Protease Inhibitors

Glucose metabolism is regulated by the interplay of the action of pancreatic islet cell hormones with liver, muscle, and adipose tissue. An alteration in the function of any component of this complex glucose homeostatic system brings about compensatory responses in the other components to drive the system back to its homeostatic set-points. The key players in regulating this system are the islet hormones insulin and glucagon. Insulin promotes hepatic glucose uptake and glycogenesis, stimulates muscle and adipose tissue glucose uptake and metabolism, and inhibits adipose tissue lipolysis and muscle proteolysis.[1] Glucagon stimulates hepatic gluconeogenic precursor uptake and increases hepatic glycogenolysis, gluconeogenesis, and ketogenesis.[2]

Maintenance of fasting and postprandial plasma glucose levels within the normal range requires insulin secretion by the β cell to be integrated with insulin action in liver and peripheral tissues. Insulin action results from a complex cascade of intracellular substrate phosphorylations and dephosphorylations that lead to regulation of processes as diverse as intermediary metabolism and mitogenesis. Insulin action is easily altered by a variety of both intracellular and extracellular factors. When insulin action affecting glucose metabolism is altered, insulin secretion must change accordingly if normal glucose homeostasis is to remain intact.[3] Any genetic abnormality, environmental factor, or drug that disturbs this relationship will lead to either hyperglycemia or hypoglycemia.

Type 2 diabetes is a heterogeneous disorder in which gene polymorphisms provide the predispositions and environmental factors provide the precipitating causes for hyperglycemia. Many individuals with the genetic predisposition do not manifest impaired glucose tolerance (IGT) or type 2 diabetes throughout their lifetime. If a pathologic condition develops in such individuals, however, or they take a medication that disturbs their compensated state, hyperglycemia will develop. Thus hyperglycemic states resulting from nondiabetic conditions or therapies can be subdivided into those that can cause hyperglycemia in any individual because they radically interfere with a major regulatory pathway (Table 69–1) and those that precipitate diabetes only in genetically predisposed individuals because they alter the compensated state (Table 69–2). Because of the high prevalence of a genetic predisposition to type 2 diabetes in various populations, it is not always possible to make the distinction with certainty.

DISORDERS OF THE PANCREAS

Pancreatectomy

Diabetes mellitus developing after surgical removal of the pancreas is truly an insulin-dependent diabetes mellitus. Metabolically, it is

characterized by insulin and glucagon deficiency.[4] The magnitude of the hyperglycemia and its characteristics depend on the quantity of pancreas removed (Table 69–3). Total or near-total pancreatectomy results in severe hyperglycemia, decreased plasma insulin, virtually absent plasma glucagon, and elevated plasma levels of gluconeogenic precursors (alanine, lactate, glycerol).[4–10]

The effect of removal of 50% of the pancreas was studied in 28 normal transplant donors 1 year after surgery.[11] The donors lost a mean of 3.4 kg of body weight, and their mean fasting plasma glucose level had risen by 9 mg/dL (88 ± 7 to 97 ± 16 mg/dL). Similarly, their mean serum glucose concentration 2 hours after an oral glucose load was higher (117 ± 18 to 156 ± 53 mg/dL), and the area under the 5-hour plasma glucose curve after the oral glucose was 19.5% higher. Both the mean fasting plasma insulin concentration and the area under the 5-hour plasma insulin curve were significantly lower than preoperatively (-14% and -31%, respectively). None of the donors had any evidence of deficient pancreatic exocrine function. On further analysis the investigators noted that 21 of the donors had no significant postoperative change in either plasma glucose or insulin whereas 7 showed a marked increase in the entire 5-hour plasma glucose curve (either IGT or diabetes) with no concomitant increase

TABLE 69–1. Conditions that Can Cause Hyperglycemia in the Absence of Genetic Predisposition

Disease of the pancreas
  Pancreatectomy
  Trauma
  Pancreatitis
  Pancreatic carcinoma
  Infiltrative disorder
  Hemochromatosis
  Amyloidosis
  Cystic fibrosis
Overproduction of other islet hormones
  Glucagonoma
  Somatostatinoma
Drugs and toxins
  Pyriminil (Vacor)
  Pentamidine
  Interferon-α
  K_{ATP} channel openers
  Diazoxide
  Phenytoin (Dilantin)

K_{ATP}, ATP-dependent potassium channel.

959

TABLE 69–2. Conditions that Precipitate Hyperglycemia in Individuals with a Genetic Predisposition to Type 2 Diabetes

Endocrinopathies
  Acromegaly
  Cushing's syndrome
  Pheochromocytoma
  Hyperthyroidism
Drugs
  Interfere with insulin secretion
    β-Blockers
    Diuretics
  Impair insulin action
    Glucocorticoids
    Oral contraceptives
    Nicotinic acid

in the 5-hour plasma insulin curves. The 7 donors in whom some degree of hypoinsulinemia and hyperglycemia had developed did not have fasting hyperglycemia 1 year postoperatively. Two of the 7 were studied from 2 to 7 years after surgery and had not had a further increase in fasting plasma glucose.

Sun et al. studied the metabolic effects of removing 20% to 88% of the pancreas in dogs and found that no significant metabolic changes occurred until approximately 50% was removed.[12]

From the data available, it seems reasonable to conclude that the metabolic abnormalities after pancreatectomy are likely to be clinically relevant at 50% and greater removal and that progressively more metabolic abnormalities occur as the extent of pancreatectomy increases.

The major characteristics of the development of diabetes mellitus after extensive pancreatectomy are an absence of glucagon secretion and marked impairment in insulin secretion. The absence of glucagon slows, but does not interfere with, the development of hyperglycemia and ketonemia after insulin withdrawal.[4, 6] This observation indicates that glucagon is not necessary for development of the metabolic abnormalities of insulin-dependent diabetes mellitus. The absence of glucagon secretion does, however, leave a pancreatectomized individual with diabetes at high risk for severe hypoglycemia during insulin treatment.[13–16] This situation is exaggerated by the associated nutritional deficiencies and weight loss that ordinarily accompany exocrine pancreatic insufficiency. Treatment of an individual with pancreatic diabetes requires insulin, is associated with marked lability in glucose regulation, and is linked with an increased rate of both ketoacidosis and death from hypoglycemia. The development of autonomic neuropathy in a patient with pancreatic diabetes greatly adds to the risk of severe hypoglycemia with insulin treatment.[17]

Chronic Pancreatitis

Chronic pancreatitis accounts for a little less than 1% of cases of diabetes mellitus in Western countries and Japan.[18–21] In tropical countries, where nonalcoholic calcific pancreatitis is common, the incidence may be somewhat higher, but reliable data are not available. The development of diabetes mellitus in patients with chronic pancreatitis

TABLE 69–3. Estimated Frequency of Diabetes Reported in Pancreatic Diseases

95% Pancreatectomy	100%
50% Pancreatectomy	0%
Pancreatitis	
Acute	<5%
Chronic calcifying	40%–70%
Chronic noncalcifying	15%–30%
Cystic fibrosis	17%
Carcinoma of the pancreas	23%
Hemochromatosis	50%–60%

is highest in those with calcific disease (55%–70%) and less in those with noncalcific disease (30%).[22] The prevalence of diabetes in patients with chronic pancreatitis increases with increasing duration of pancreatitis and with increasing exocrine deficiency.[20, 25–27]

The inflammatory response causes loss of exocrine tissue and extensive fibrosis. The islets of Langerhans are relatively resistant and undergo pathologic changes only late in the disease. Chronic pancreatitis is associated with loss of functioning β cells and a somewhat lesser loss of α cells.[14, 28–34] The hormonal alterations seen are a decrease in insulin secretion in response to nutrients, followed later by a decrease in fasting C peptide levels. Plasma C peptide levels rather than insulin levels may be a better assessment of insulin secretion because associated liver disease may change hepatic extraction rates of insulin. With progressive chronic pancreatitis, insulin secretion falls even lower. Glucagon secretion is impaired in moderate to severe chronic pancreatitis. Insulin resistance frequently develops in such individuals.

Diabetes mellitus is seen after several years of chronic pancreatitis. In an unselected series of patients with chronic pancreatitis, 35% had type 1 diabetes, 31% had type 2 diabetes or IGT, and 34% had normal glucose tolerance.[35] The nature of the diabetes is a result of the severity of the chronic pancreatitis. Mild pancreatitis may be associated only with IGT, whereas severe pancreatitis will be primarily associated with insulin-dependent (type 1) diabetes. Patients with chronic pancreatitis and diabetes mellitus fail to secrete glucagon in response to hypoglycemia. If they have concomitant autonomic neuropathy, they are extremely susceptible to severe and prolonged hypoglycemia.

Treatment of diabetes mellitus in patients with chronic pancreatitis should entail the use of small doses of short-acting insulins to manage the hyperglycemia, replacement enzymes for the malnutrition and malabsorption, and elimination of the use of alcoholic beverages.[22, 32, 36, 37] Surgery with subtotal resection or near-total resection may be necessary to relieve severe pain.[38, 39] In such patients, successful islet allotransplants and autotransplants in the liver have been able to maintain near normoglycemia.[40] The hepatic islet cell transplants were able to secrete insulin in response to nutrients but were unable to secrete glucagon in response to hypoglycemia.[15, 16]

Pancreatic Cancer

Diabetes mellitus is known to occur more frequently in patients with pancreatic cancer than in the general population.[41–43] The reasons for this association have been the subject of much speculation. Some have raised the possibility that diabetes mellitus causes an increased susceptibility to pancreatic cancer. Others have postulated that the diabetes is secondary to some effect of the cancer. A multicenter case-control study of 720 patients with pancreatic cancer addressed this issue.[41] The prevalence of diabetes mellitus in the patients with pancreatic cancer was 22.8%, whereas that in the matched control population was 8.3%. The pancreatic cancer patients were characterized as having type 2 diabetes. Recent diagnosis of diabetes had been made in 40.2% of the pancreatic cancer patients with diabetes as contrasted with only 3.3% of the control population with diabetes (Table 69–4). A higher percentage of the control population with diabetes had had their diabetes for greater than 15 years than did the pancreatic cancer population with diabetes (see Table 69–4). These data dispel the notion that diabetes is responsible for the increase in pancreatic cancer; instead, they suggest that pancreatic cancer contributes to the development of diabetes.

The possible mechanisms by which pancreatic cancer could contribute to the development of type 2 diabetes are (1) destruction of islets, (2) impairment of the insulin secretory mechanism, (3) development of insulin resistance, and (4) tumor-related pancreatitis. Insulin and C peptide measurements during oral glucose tolerance testing in patients with pancreatic cancer have shown abnormal β cell function and possibly insulin resistance.[44–46] Morphometric studies of tumor-free regions of the pancreas have shown reduced β cell populations.[47] An inverse correlation was noted between the number of β cells and the fasting plasma glucose concentration. These data can be interpreted as indicating that pancreatic cancers produce substances or responses that destroy normal β cells.[45–48] The presence of diabetes in patients with

TABLE 69–4. *Interval between Diagnosis of Diabetes and Diagnosis of Pancreatic Cancer or Date of Examination of Control Population*

Duration (yr)	Pancreatic Cancer Patients	Control Patients	*P* Value
0	66 (40.2%)	2 (3.3%)	<.001
1–14	81 (49.4%)	35 (58.3%)	NS
≥15	17 (10.4%)	23 (38.3%)	<.001

pancreatic cancer predicts that the tumor is less likely to be resectable, and the patient has a poorer prognosis than if diabetes is not present.[43]

Patients with pancreatic cancer appear to have type 2 diabetes, and most have been treated with oral antihyperglycemic agents.[42, 43]

Hemochromatosis

Hemochromatosis is an autosomal recessive genetic disorder that results in excessive deposition of iron in parenchymal cells of the liver, pancreas, muscle, heart, anterior pituitary, and other organs.[49, 50] The clinical diagnosis in the past was made by the findings of diabetes mellitus, hepatomegaly, and skin pigmentation. More recently, it is recognized by biochemical and genetic testing.[51] The first phenotypic expression of the disease is an elevation in serum transferrin saturation. This abnormality is followed by iron accumulation in the tissues and an elevation in the serum ferritin concentration. Early clinical findings are related to hepatic dysfunction and joint symptoms. Clinical diabetes mellitus and skin pigmentation occur relatively late in the course of the disease.[50] A candidate gene for HLA-linked hemochromatosis has been cloned and a mutation (*C282Y*) identified that may account for 60% or more of cases of hereditary hemochromatosis.

Diabetes mellitus has been reported in 50% to 60% of patients with hemochromatosis.[50, 52] Another 20% to 30% had glucose intolerance. These figures represent data from older series in which the diagnosis was made late in the course of the disease. Diabetes mellitus is more frequent in patients who have a family history of diabetes mellitus. The natural history of the development of glucose intolerance in hemochromatosis is not available.

The metabolic studies that have been done show that patients with hemochromatosis have marked insulin resistance. Histologic study of the pancreas shows iron deposits that are greatest in the acinar cells but do involve the islet cells. Insulin secretion in response to glucose or arginine is decreased; however, glucagon secretory responses to arginine are increased and unaffected by glucose.[53, 54] The data are compatible with a marked reduction in β cell function and no disturbance in α cell function. The hyperglycemia is a result of the insulin resistance and the decreased β cell function. The prevalence of diabetes mellitus could be greatly reduced by early diagnosis of hemochromatosis and the institution of phlebotomy therapy.

Therapy for patients with hemochromatosis and clinical diabetes frequently requires insulin (40%–50% of patients), although no systematic studies of therapy have been done.[51] Reduction of tissue iron stores, although most beneficial in the early stages of disease, can nonetheless help improve glycemic control in 35% to 45% of patients.[49, 50]

Hemosiderosis

Excessive iron deposition occurs in a variety of conditions other than primary hemochromatosis. In thalassemia major, frequent blood transfusions are necessary and may lead to massive iron overload. The reported prevalence of diabetes mellitus in treated thalassemia major is about 16%. This figure is highly correlated with the number of blood transfusions and the duration of disease. The incidence of IGT is reported to be 60%.[55]

Further evidence that excess tissue iron deposits themselves are responsible for much of the metabolic abnormalities seen in hemochromatosis and thalassemia major comes from studies in rural male Bantus.[56] Many Bantus drink alcoholic beverages that are brewed in iron containers and ingest in excess of 100 mg of iron per day. In those individuals the prevalence of diabetes mellitus is 10-fold higher than in the nonalcoholic beverage–consuming males.

Cystic Fibrosis

Cystic fibrosis (CF) is a monogenetic disorder with abnormal cyclic adenosine monophosphate–regulated Cl^- channel activity. Organs as diverse as the lung, exocrine pancreas, large and small intestine, hepatobiliary system, and sweat glands are involved. Failure to secrete Na^+, HCO_3^-, and water leads to retention of enzymes in the pancreas and ultimately to destruction of pancreatic tissue.[57–59] Histologic examination of the pancreas in patients with CF shows fatty infiltration, necrosis, and fibrosis of the exocrine pancreas. Islet cell architecture is disrupted and the absolute number of pancreatic islets diminished. Those islets that are present show significant decreases in β cells, α cells, and pancreatic polypeptide–producing cells and increases in δ (somatostatin-producing) cells. Islet amyloid deposits have been found in 69% of diabetic CF cases examined.

Diabetes mellitus requiring medical therapy (usually insulin) has been reported in 4.9% of CF patients of all ages in a large European study of 1348 patients[60] and in 5.1% of 18,627 patients of all ages monitored at CF centers in the United States and Canada.[57] Diabetes mellitus occurs more often in individuals who are homozygous for the most common CF mutation, Δ F508.[57, 61, 62] Diabetes mellitus occurs with greater frequency with increasing age, being reported in 32% of Danish patients who were older than 25 years. Routine oral glucose tolerance testing suggests that of the total CF population aged 5 years or older, 35% have normal glucose tolerance, 37% have IGT, 17% have CF-related diabetes without fasting hyperglycemia, and 11% have CF-related diabetes with fasting hyperglycemia.

Several features of CF-related diabetes are noteworthy. Patients with CF have an increase in hepatic glucose production and are resistant to suppression of hepatic glucose production by insulin even in the nondiabetic state.[63] Peripheral insulin sensitivity is increased in healthy nondiabetic individuals with CF, but insulin resistance occurs later as diabetes develops and the patients get more complications from their CF. The development of diabetes worsens pulmonary function and other clinical manifestations of CF. Insulin treatment appears to improve this deterioration. Hyperglycemia in patients with CF can be intermittent or permanent. Intermittent hyperglycemia occurs with glucocorticoid therapy, infections, or stress and needs to be treated with insulin until it resolves. Permanent hyperglycemia is always treated with insulin.[57, 59] It is likely that CF patients progress from intermittent hyperglycemia to permanent hyperglycemia as more pancreatic destruction is occurring. The development of diabetes in patients with CF is initially characterized by a delay in glucose-stimulated insulin secretion, followed by a decrease in total insulin, glucagon, and pancreatic polypeptide secretion.

HYPERGLYCEMIA ASSOCIATED WITH ENDOCRINOPATHIES

In the complex regulation of fuel hemostasis, many hormones other than insulin play a complementary role. Growth hormone itself and through its synthesis of insulin-like growth factor-1 (IGF-1) controls many aspects of amino acid transport, protein synthesis, and lipid metabolism. Glucagon and catecholamines are counterregulatory hormones that protect against hypoglycemia and provide extra glucose when needed during stress states. Glucocorticoids exert both a permissive role in the normal physiologic regulation of gluconeogenesis and a pharmacologic role in providing increased glucose availability during stress. Somatostatin is a paracrine hormone that appears to act locally to help regulate the normal secretory patterns of growth hormone, insulin, glucagon, and several gastrointestinal hormones.

Autonomous excess secretion of these hormones leads to hyperglycemia. The mechanisms responsible for the action of these various hormones are described in detail in other chapters. This section will address the unique characteristics of the hyperglycemia as it relates to each endocrinopathy and their treatment.

Acromegaly

Acromegaly is characterized by excessive and autonomous secretion of growth hormone and IGF-1.[64, 65] The prevalence of overt diabetes mellitus reported in different series of acromegalic patients ranges from 30% to 56%.[64, 66] IGT may be present in as many as 36% of acromegalic patients.[64] In a specific population the percentage of acromegalic patients in whom diabetes mellitus will develop depends on the prevalence of predisposition to type 2 diabetes in the population and the magnitude of elevation of serum IGF-1 levels.

Elevated growth hormone and IGF-1 levels cause excess hepatic glucose production and impaired insulin-mediated muscle glucose uptake.[67–69] This insulin resistance is correlated with circulating IGF-1 levels and has been demonstrated by the euglycemic hyperinsulinemic clamp and the minimal model techniques.

Reduction in circulating growth hormone and IGF-1 levels by successful surgical removal of the tumor producing growth hormone or growth hormone–releasing factor results in significant improvement in glycemic control in acromegalic patients with diabetes mellitus.[68, 70] Recent data suggest that circulating growth hormone must be lowered to 2 ng/L and IGF-1 lowered to the normal range to be considered curative.[65, 71, 72] Transsphenoidal surgery achieves growth hormone levels less than 5 ng/L in approximately 60% of patients. Curative levels are attained in about 70% of patients with microadenomas (<10 mm in diameter), but considerably less in those with macroadenomas of the pituitary.[65, 71]

Use of the somatostatin analogue octreotide to treat acromegaly as either primary medical therapy or to supplement prior inadequate surgical treatment or radiotherapy has allowed greater and more consistent reductions in circulating growth hormone and IGF-1 levels to be achieved (GH levels ≤5 ng/L in 65% and ≤2 ng/L in 40% and IGF-1 levels in the normal range in 64% of patients).[71–73]

Treatment of acromegalic patients with octreotide presents several issues with respect to glucose metabolism.[71–74] Reduction of circulating growth hormone and IGF-1 levels will decrease insulin resistance and should lead to improvement in glycemic control in subjects with diabetes mellitus or IGT. However, pharmacologic doses of a somatostatin analogue also reduce insulin secretion (decreased insulinogenic index), and such a reduction should cause a deterioration in glucose tolerance. Thus in any particular patient, octreotide therapy will modify glucose metabolism in accordance with these competing effects. Approximately two-thirds of acromegalic patients with diabetes mellitus are treated with insulin and one-third with oral hypoglycemic agents. Octreotide treatment in patients with diabetes mellitus and acromegaly frequently leads to improvement in glycemic control as measured by a reduction in the insulin dose, conversion from insulin therapy to oral hypoglycemic agent therapy, or conversion from oral hypoglycemic agent therapy to dietary management.[71, 74] Some patients (those with more severe insulin deficiency), however, will have significant deterioration in glycemic control.[72, 74] IGT or even frank diabetes mellitus may develop in acromegalic patients with normal glucose tolerance before octreotide treatment (as high as 20% and 29%, respectively) when higher doses of octreotide are given.[74]

Appropriate treatment of acromegaly is necessary to reduce the increased mortality (observed-to-expected death, 2.68) that has been seen in the past.[75] This increased mortality is due to cardiovascular, cerebrovascular, and neoplastic diseases. The best determinants of outcome in acromegalic patients are age at diagnosis, interval between symptoms and diagnosis, and mean chronic circulating growth hormone and IGF-1 levels. Because insulin resistance and diabetes mellitus contribute significantly to cardiovascular risk, aggressive diagnosis and management of the diabetes mellitus associated with acromegaly is essential.

Growth Hormone Treatment

The availability of recombinant DNA technology to make human growth hormone has provided an opportunity to treat many growth hormone–deficient individuals with this hormone. One of the considerations in treatment with recombinant human growth hormone is the question of whether chronic treatment can lead to the development of diabetes mellitus.[76] A recent study of glucose metabolism in 23,333 children and adolescents treated with human growth hormone found a sixfold greater frequency of type 2 diabetes mellitus than predicted (34.4 cases per 100,000 years of growth hormone treatment).[77] In contrast, the frequency of type 1 diabetes was the same as expected. The data suggest that growth hormone treatment accelerates the development of type 2 diabetes in individuals who have a genetic predisposition.

Cushing's Syndrome

Glucocorticoids are insulin antagonistic hormones.[78] When administered in pharmacologic doses, they increase basal hepatic glucose production and decrease the insulin-mediated effects of suppressing hepatic glucose production and increasing muscle glucose uptake.[79–82] Insulin secretion is increased as a consequence of the hepatic and peripheral insulin resistance.

Pharmacologic concentrations of glucocorticoids occur in disease states associated with autonomous secretion of adrenal cortical hormones (Cushing's syndrome) or through administration of such agents for the treatment of nonendocrine diseases. When sustained pharmacologic concentrations of glucocorticoids occur in normal individuals, increased insulin secretion maintains fasting plasma glucose within the normal range, but the postprandial plasma glucose concentration is elevated above normal in 25% to 90% of such individuals depending on the magnitude of plasma glucocorticoid elevation.[83] Individuals with limited β cell insulin secretory reserve are subject to fasting hyperglycemia and type 2 diabetes mellitus. Ten percent to 20% of patients with Cushing's syndrome have overt type 2 diabetes mellitus.[84–88] In renal transplant recipients receiving chronic corticosteroid therapy, steroid-induced diabetes mellitus has been reported to develop in as few as 5.5% and as many as 46% of patients.[89, 90] Factors that influence the development of diabetes mellitus during corticosteroid therapy are a family history of diabetes mellitus, increasing age, obesity, and both average daily and total cumulative corticosteroid dose.[91, 92] In individuals with a previous onset of diabetes mellitus, administration of glucocorticoids significantly worsens glycemic control and will require modification of diabetes management.

Recent studies have documented that steroid-induced diabetes mellitus occurs in adrenal disorders other than those associated with frank Cushing's syndrome. Measurement of oral glucose tolerance in 64 consecutive patients with "nonfunctioning" adrenal adenomas identified normal glucose tolerance in 25, glucose intolerance in 17, and diabetes mellitus in 22, including 6 patients with previously diagnosed diabetes mellitus.[93] Autonomous cortisol secretion without the clinical stigmata of Cushing's syndrome has recently been recognized as a preclinical Cushing's syndrome. A retrospective study of 63 such individuals found that 17.5% had diabetes mellitus.[94] A cross-sectional study of 90 obese, poorly controlled type 2 diabetic patients found 3 to have the preclinical Cushing's syndrome abnormality.[94] Excess IGT and diabetes mellitus have been reported in hypopituitary adults receiving conventional replacement therapy and may be related to the intermittently higher plasma levels occurring after dosing than would occur under normal hypothalamic-pituitary-adrenal axis function.[95]

Some insight into the mechanisms by which glucocorticoids cause diabetes mellitus was obtained by investigating the effect of the administration of dexamethasone on oral glucose tolerance, on glucose turnover under basal conditions and during glucose infusion, and on the insulin response during hyperglycemic clamp studies in normal individuals who had previously been characterized as either low insulin responders or high insulin responders.[96] Dexamethasone caused a higher fasting plasma glucose concentration, a greater rise in plasma glucose, and a lesser rise in plasma insulin during the oral glucose tolerance test in the low insulin responders than in the higher insulin responders. A diabetic oral glucose tolerance test developed in three of the six low and none of the six high insulin responders. Dexamethasone increased hepatic glucose production only in the low insulin responders and increased insulin secretion during the hyperglycemic clamp study only in the high insulin responders. The conclusion drawn from these studies is that type 2 diabetes develops when plasma glucocorticoids are elevated in individuals with limited β cell secretory function.

Steroid-induced diabetes may be permanent or transient. In general, insulin is required for treatment if the fasting plasma glucose concentration exceeds 180 mg/dL.[97] At lesser levels of fasting hyperglycemia, many physicians treat the hyperglycemia with oral antihyperglycemic agents. Very few studies have evaluated the efficacy of pharmacologic treatment of steroid-induced diabetes mellitus. Because insulin resistance is a major abnormality, perhaps the combination of insulin sensitizers and insulin would be most effective. A reduction in corticosteroid dose or secretion improves glycemic control and in some individuals may even reverse the diabetes. The more severely elevated the fasting plasma glucose concentration, the less likely it is that reducing corticosteroid levels will reverse the diabetes. Ketoacidosis is very uncommon with steroid-induced diabetes or Cushing's syndrome. Hyperosmolar nonketotic coma, however, is not uncommon.[98]

Glucagonoma Syndrome

Glucagon plays a primary role in facilitating the uptake of amino acids by the liver and their conversion into glucose by gluconeogenesis. Excess and unregulated glucagon secretion alone or in conjunction with other islet hormones occurs in some islet cell tumors. A classic syndrome has been described in individuals who have tumors secreting high quantities of glucagon. This syndrome was initially recognized in 1974 and is referred to as the glucagonoma syndrome.[99] Features of this syndrome include necrolytic migratory erythema, mild non–insulin-requiring type 2 diabetes mellitus, glossitis, angular cheilitis, weight loss, and anemia.[100, 101] Laboratory studies show markedly elevated plasma glucagon levels and severe hypoaminoacidemia (<25% normal).

Glucagonomas are quite rare, with a reported incidence of 1 case per 20 to 200 million population. Several reviews of the literature indicate that most of the tumors occur in the tail of the pancreas (reported in 54% to 68%), have an average tumor diameter of 3.6 cm (but as many as one-third are less than 2 cm), are malignant in about two-thirds of cases, and have metastases in other organs in 51% to 54% of patients at the time of diagnosis.[102, 103] The diabetes mellitus is characterized by mild hyperglycemia and is nonketotic. The tumors are relatively slow growing, and the 10-year survival rate is 52% in those with metastases and 64% in those without metastases.

The hyperglycemia is due to excess glucose production by the liver. The hypoaminoacidemia results from an increase in amino acid clearance.[104] The necrolytic migratory erythema, glossitis, weight loss, and anemia are in large part a consequence of the protein malnutrition.[101] Deep venous thrombosis that is not associated with coagulation disorders is quite common.

All the components of the syndrome are improved if the hyperglucagonemia can be reduced. Treatment is surgical removal of the tumor, followed by hepatic artery embolization if necessary for liver metastases.[101, 105] Octreotide treatment has been very effective in reducing residual plasma glucagon levels.[101, 105] Cytotoxic agents such as streptozotocin and fluorouracil may be valuable as additional modes of therapy. Zinc and amino acid supplementation have been used to treat the rash but are relatively ineffective if the plasma glucagon levels remain very high. Antiplatelet therapy should be used to prevent venous thrombosis. The hyperglycemia, though mild, generally requires treatment with an antihyperglycemic agent. Insulin would appear to be the most appropriate agent, although few or no clinical outcome data are available to support this hypothesis. Treatment of the hyperglucagonemia will ameliorate the hyperglycemia in most cases.[105]

Somatostatinoma

Case reports of patients with hyperglycemia and a pancreatic tumor containing large quantities of somatostatin first appeared in 1977.[106, 107]

One of those patients became euglycemic after complete resection of the tumor. Since that time it has been recognized that large somatostatin-producing pancreatic tumors may be associated with a clinical syndrome consisting of hyperglycemia, cholelithiasis, steatorrhea, and hypochlorhydria.[108]

Somatostatin-producing tumors arising from the gastrointestinal tract and the pancreatic islets have been reported.[109] Duodenal somatostatinomas with and without von Recklinghausen's disease are seldom associated with recognizable somatostatinoma syndrome, often contain psammoma bodies, and are less often associated with demonstrable metastases at the time of surgery.[109] The clinical features of pancreatic somatostatin-producing tumors are quite variable, and this variation is related to differences in quantity and qualitative features of the somatostatin variants that are synthesized and secreted by these tumors.[110–112] Marked differences in the degree to which insulin, glucagon, and growth hormone secretion are affected in various patients with pancreatic somatostatin-producing tumors probably account for some of the variation in the clinical syndrome. Hyperglycemia in patients with pancreatic somatostatinomas can vary from mild to modest hyperglycemia to severe diabetic ketoacidosis.[109, 113, 114]

Somatostatin infusions in humans are associated with a pronounced decrease in bile flow and bile acid secretion and an increase in bile cholesterol saturation.[115] In vitro, somatostatin has a direct inhibitory effect on cholecystokinin stimulation of gallbladder contraction.[116] These observations provide a basis for understanding the cholelithiasis and steatorrhea commonly seen with pancreatic somatostatinomas. Additionally, they explain the development of gallstones in 23.5% of acromegalic patients treated with octreotide during the first year of treatment.[71]

The hyperglycemia seen as part of the somatostatinoma syndrome is most likely related to suppression of insulin secretion. In some patients, a relative insulin deficiency leads to reduced peripheral glucose utilization without impairing suppression of hepatic glucose production.[117] In more severe suppression of insulin secretion, both features of insulin action are reduced.

Somatostatin-producing tumors are quite rare, usually asymptomatic, or only mildly symptomatic and frequently undiagnosed for many years. The diagnosis is frequently made late and the prognosis is poor because of extensive metastases. The use of somatostatin receptor scintigraphy with indium 111–labeled pentetreotide promises to improve the ability to detect somatostatinomas earlier.[118] Early diagnosis and surgical removal can lead to cure, but medical treatment has produced questionable results. A recent study suggests that somatostatinomas possess functioning somatostatin receptors and that octreotide therapy (0.5 mg/day subcutaneously) can effectively decrease somatostatin production by the tumor and improve diabetes and diarrhea.[118]

Pheochromocytoma

Glucose intolerance occurs in about 30% of patients with pheochromocytoma, but overt diabetes mellitus is quite uncommon.[119] The mechanisms responsible for the glucose intolerance are suppression of insulin by α-adrenergic receptor stimulation of β cells; an increase in insulin resistance, probably related to elevated plasma free fatty acid levels; and increased hepatic glucose output as a result of β-adrenergic stimulation of hepatocytes. α-Adrenergic receptor blockade improves glucose tolerance and insulin secretion.[120, 121] Removal of the pheochromocytoma restores glucose tolerance to normal in most cases. Treatment of the glucose intolerance with antihyperglycemic agents is rarely required.[119]

DRUGS THAT CAN CAUSE HYPERGLYCEMIA

Blood glucose is regulated by the balance between insulin secretion and insulin action. A drug that destroys β cells or blocks their insulin secretory function will cause hyperglycemia in any individual (Table 69–5). A drug that directly or indirectly increases insulin resistance can cause hyperglycemia only in individuals with β cells that have

TABLE 69–5. Drugs that Interfere with Insulin Secretion

Destroy β cells
  Pentamidine
  Pyriminil (Vacor)
Decrease Ca^{2+} entry
  Diazoxide—K_{ATP} channel opener
  Phenytoin (Dilantin)—?
Decrease K^+
  Thiazides
  Loop diuretics
Mechanism unknown
  β-Adrenergic antagonists
  Cyclosporine
  Opiates
  Asparaginase

limited insulin secretory reserve (individuals with a predisposition to type 2 diabetes). Several recent reviews on drug-induced disorders of glucose metabolism are available.[122–124]

Drugs Affecting β Cell Function

Drugs that Destroy β Cells

Pentamidine and pyriminil (Vacor) are substances that resemble streptozotocin and alloxan chemically. Pentamidine is an antiprotozoal agent that is used extensively to treat *Pneumocystis carinii* infection. Pyriminyl is a nitrosourea-derived rodenticide that has been accidentally or intentionally ingested by humans. These agents cause necrosis of β cells leading initially to hyperinsulinemia and hypoglycemia, followed by permanent hyperglycemia and an insulin-dependent diabetes mellitus.[125–129] In a series of 128 AIDS patients treated with pentamidine for *P. carinii* pneumonia, severe glucose homeostasis disorders developed in 48 patients (37.5%): hypoglycemia in 7, hypoglycemia and then diabetes in 18, and diabetes alone in 23.[127] Of the 41 patients in whom diabetes developed, 26 required insulin therapy. Risk factors for the development of dysglycemia were higher pentamidine doses, higher plasma creatinine, and more severe anoxia. Whereas most of the dysglycemic patients received parenteral pentamidine, 6 were treated exclusively with pentamidine aerosols. Pyriminyl ingestion has been followed by severe insulinopenic diabetes mellitus in numerous instances.[129]

Drugs that Inhibit Increases in β Cell Cytosolic Ca^{2+}

An increase in the β cell cytosolic Ca^{2+} concentration is the major mechanism responsible for insulin secretion. Calcium ion entry into the β cell is controlled by several calcium ion channels. A voltage-dependent L-type calcium channel has its activity linked to an ATP-dependent potassium channel (K_{ATP} channel). The K_{ATP} channel is closed by increases in plasma glucose. Drugs that keep the K_{ATP} channel open such as diazoxide (a K_{ATP} channel opener) block glucose-mediated insulin secretion and lead to hyperglycemia.[130, 131]

Phenytoin (Dilantin) and other phenylhydantoins can interfere with Na^+, K^+, and Ca^{2+} ion transport. Dilantin administration has been reported to increase plasma glucose and decrease plasma insulin.[131–134] Several studies indicate that it interferes with Ca^{2+} ion entry into the β cell, but by a process different from the K_{ATP} channel–related mechanism. Dilantin has been reported to cause hyperosmolar nonketotic hyperglycemia or diabetes mellitus. This complication occurs quite infrequently and probably in individuals with some preceding genetic susceptibility.

Drugs that Cause K^+ Depletion

Numerous studies have shown that diuretics can cause a deterioration in glucose tolerance in nondiabetic individuals and worsening of glycemic control in patients with type 2 diabetes mellitus.[135–138] The effect appears to be dose related and is either absent or markedly reduced with low-dose diuretic therapy.[139, 140] In humans, diuretics appear to worsen glycemia primarily by inhibiting insulin secretion, although they also have a modest effect in increasing insulin resistance. Several studies have shown that the decreased insulin secretory response is due to intracellular K^+ depletion and can be restored toward normal with potassium repletion.[141, 142] Diabetogenic effects are seen with most diuretics. Therefore, if diuretics are used in diabetic or prediabetic subjects to control blood pressure, doses should be restricted to those equivalent to 12.5 to 25.0 mg hydrochlorothiazide.

Mechanisms Unknown

β-Adrenergic antagonists have been shown to worsen glycemic control in type 2 diabetic subjects and to impair glucose tolerance or even precipitate type 2 diabetes in nondiabetic subjects.[135, 143] The deleterious effect of β-adrenergic blockade on glucose tolerance is worse with nonspecific β-adrenergic receptor blockade than with specific β_2-adrenergic antagonists.[143, 144] Combination therapy with β-adrenergic antagonists and diuretics has an additive effect of worsening glucose tolerance. β-Adrenergic antagonists impair glucose tolerance and worsen hyperglycemia by blocking nutrient-mediated insulin secretion. β_2-Adrenergic receptor activation stimulates and β_2-adrenergic receptor blockade inhibits insulin secretion.[145, 146]

Cyclosporine treatment for immunosuppression in renal transplant recipients is associated with an increased incidence of diabetes mellitus.[147, 148] Direct inhibitory effects of cyclosporine on β cells in vitro have been associated with decreased insulin secretion. Although it is likely that cyclosporine has direct effects in causing the deterioration in glucose tolerance in renal transplant patients, it is not possible to exclude a contributory role of the associated corticosteroid therapy. The onset of diabetes mellitus in cyclosporine-treated patients occurs within the first several months of treatment and often requires insulin treatment. The reported incidence of diabetes mellitus and glucose intolerance in cyclosporine-treated transplant patients ranges from 13% to 47%.[124]

Other agents that have been reported to cause hyperglycemia through inhibiting insulin secretion are asparaginase and some opiates.[123–125]

Drugs Causing Insulin Resistance

Drugs that increase insulin resistance will not affect glucose metabolism in individuals with normal β cell function. However, when administered to individuals with limited β cell reserve, they will cause either glucose intolerance or overt diabetes mellitus. Agents that cause an increase in body weight and particularly those associated with an increase in central obesity will cause insulin resistance. Drugs or hormones that elevate plasma free fatty acid levels will lead to insulin resistance. Counterregulatory hormones or drugs that raise circulating levels of counterregulatory hormones will cause impairment of insulin action. The most commonly used agents that can increase insulin resistance are glucocorticoids, estrogens, progestogens, and nicotinic acid. Hyperglycemia associated with glucocorticoid therapy has been discussed in the section on Cushing's syndrome.

Oral Contraceptives and Sex Hormones

Older studies investigating the effects of oral contraceptives, estrogens, and progestogens showed that deterioration of glucose tolerance and development of type 2 diabetes were occasional complications of chronic therapy.[149] Most studies attributed the diabetogenic effects of these steroids to an increase in insulin resistance. More recent studies with natural estrogens and lower-dose administration indicate that these regimens produce little or no increase in glucose intolerance.[150–152] Progesterone derivatives have been shown to consistently cause insulin resistance and impair glucose tolerance.[153] The newer oral contraceptives may be associated with a modest deterioration in glucose tolerance because of an increase in insulin resistance, but these effects are rarely clinically significant.

Nicotinic Acid

Nicotinic acid is used extensively to treat mixed hyperlipidemias and has been shown to decrease morbidity and mortality from cardiovascular disease. Acute administration of nicotinic acid reduced plasma free fatty acid levels by 30% to 40%, but as the drug wears off, they rebound to 50% to 100% above baseline concentrations. Chronic administration of nicotinic acid, 1 to 4.5 g/day, causes severe insulin resistance, presumably because of the elevated plasma free fatty acid levels. Normal individuals have a compensatory rise in insulin secretion, and glucose tolerance remains normal. In individuals with diminished insulin secretory reserve, nicotinic acid causes glucose intolerance and type 2 diabetes.[154] In type 2 diabetic patients, nicotinic acid administration results in marked deterioration in glycemic control.[155, 156]

Protease Inhibitors

The protease inhibitors indinavir, nelfinavir, ritonavir, and saquinavir have been used to treat AIDS and have been reported to cause an unusual lipodystrophy. Associated with their use have been occasional reports of the development of type 2 diabetes in previously nondiabetic individuals. Several such reports have appeared in the literature. By November 1997, 230 cases had been reported. At the present time it is unclear whether the protease inhibitors cause diabetes mellitus and, if so, how. Dube et al. reported 7 new cases of diabetes occurring in a population of 1050 patients treated with protease inhibitors over a 9-month period, for a rate of less than 1%.[157] Two patients were successfully treated with insulin and 2 with sulfonylureas. Two patients had resolution of their hyperglycemia by stopping indinavir therapy. Kilby and Tabereaux determined the frequency of severe hyperglycemia in a university clinic for HIV-1–infected patients and found a prevalence of less than 2%. Preexisting diabetes was present in 12 of 1392 adults, and new cases of hyperglycemia occurred in 13 of 1392 adults.[158] Most of the incident cases could be attributed to megestrol or corticosteroid treatment. The relationship between protease inhibitor therapy and the development of hyperglycemia needs to be clarified by additional investigations. Recent studies suggest that an increase in insulin resistance is associated with protease inhibitor–associated diabetes.[159]

REFERENCES

1. Yki-Jarvinen H: Action of insulin on glucose metabolism in vivo. Baillieres Clin Endocrinol Metab 7:903–927, 1993.
2. Lefebvre PJ: Biosynthesis and action of glucagon. *In* Alberti KGMM, Zimmet P, DeFronzo RA, Keen H (eds): International Textbook of Diabetes Mellitus, ed 2. New York, John Wiley & Sons, 1997, pp 383–389.
3. Gerich JE: The genetic basis of type 2 diabetes mellitus: Impaired insulin secretion versus impaired insulin sensitivity. Endocr Rev 19:491–503, 1998.
4. Barnes AJ, Bloom SR, George K, et al: Ketoacidosis in pancreatectomized man. N Engl J Med 296:1250–1253, 1977.
5. Barnes AJ, Bloom SR, Mashiter K, et al: Persistent metabolic abnormalities in diabetes in the absence of glucagon. Diabetologia 13:71–75, 1977.
6. Barnes AJ, Bloom SR: Pancreatectomized man: A model for diabetes without glucagon. Lancet 1:219–221, 1976.
7. Morrow CE, Cohen JI, Sutherland DER, et al: Chronic pancreatitis: Long-term surgical results of pancreatic duct drainage, pancreatic resection, and near-total pancreatectomy and islet transplantation. Surgery 90:608–915, 1984.
8. Yasugi H, Mizumoto R, Sakurai H, et al: Changes in carbohydrate metabolism and endocrine function of remnant pancreas after major pancreatic resection. Am J Surg 132:577–580, 1976.
9. Tiengo A, Bessioud M, Valverde I, et al: Absence of islet alpha cell function in pancreatectomized patients. Diabetologia 22:25–32, 1982.
10. Nakamura T, Takebe K, Kudoh K, et al: Increased plasma gluconeogenic and system A amino acids in patients with pancreatic diabetes due to chronic pancreatitis in comparison with primary diabetes. Tohoku J Exp Med 173:413–424, 1994.
11. Kendall DM, Sutherland DER, Najarian JS, et al: Effects of hemipancreatectomy on insulin secretion and glucose tolerance in healthy humans. N Engl J Med 322:898–903, 1990.
12. Sun AM, Coddling JA, Haist RE: A study of glucose tolerance and insulin response in partially depancreatized dogs. Diabetes 23:424–432, 1974.
13. Polonsky KS, Herold KC, Gilden JL, et al: Glucose counterregulation in patients after pancreatectomy, Comparison with other clinical forms of diabetes. Diabetes 33:1112–1119, 1984.
14. Del Prato S, Tiengo A, Baccaglini U, et al: Effect of insulin replacement on intermediary metabolism in diabetes secondary to pancreatectomy. Diabetologia 25:252–259, 1983.
15. Kendall DM, Teuscher AU, Robertson RP: Defective glucagon secretion during sustained hypoglycemia following successful islet allo- and autotransplantation in humans. Diabetes 46:23–27, 1997.
16. Redmon JB, Teuscher AU, Robertson RP: Hypoglycemia after pancreas transplantation. Diabetes Care 12:1944–1950, 1989.
17. Nakamura T, Takebe K, Kudoh K, et al: Decreased counter-regulatory hormone responses to insulin-induced hypoglycemia in patients with pancreatic diabetes having autonomic neuropathy. Tohoku J Exp Med 174:305–315, 1994.
18. Ganda OP: Secondary forms of diabetes. *In* Kahn CR, Weir GC (eds): Joselin's Diabetes Mellitus, ed 13. Philadelphia, Lea & Febiger, 1994, pp 300–316.
19. Sarles H: Chronic pancreatitis and diabetes. Baillieres Clin Endocrinol Metab 64:745–775, 1992.
20. Larsen S: Diabetes mellitus secondary to chronic pancreatitis. Dan Med Bull 40:153–162, 1993.
21. Koizumi M, Yoshida Y, Abe N, et al: Pancreatic diabetes in Japan. Pancreas 16:385–391, 1998.
22. DelPrato S, Tiengo A: Diabetes secondary to acquired diseases of the pancreas. *In* Alberti KGMM, Zimmet P, DeFronzo RA, Keen H (eds): International Textbook of Diabetes Mellitus, ed 2. New York, John Wiley & Sons, 1997, pp 189–212.
23. Sjoberg RJ, Kidd GS: Pancreatic diabetes. Diabetes Care 12:715–724, 1989.
24. Banks S, Marks IN, Vinik AL: Clinical and hormonal aspects of pancreatic diabetes. Am J Gastroenterol 64:13–22, 1975.
25. Nakamura T, Imamura K, Takebe K, et al: Correlation between pancreatic endocrine and exocrine function and characteristics of pancreatic endocrine function in patients with diabetes mellitus owing to chronic pancreatitis. Int J Pancreatol 20:169–175, 1996.
26. Anagnostides AA, Cos TM, Adrian TE, et al: Pancreatic exocrine and endocrine response in chronic pancreatitis. Am J Gastroenterol 79:206–212, 1984.
27. Kalk WJ, Vinik AI, Jackson WPU, et al: Insulin secretion and pancreatic exocrine function in patients with chronic pancreatitis. Diabetologia 16:355–358, 1979.
28. Kalk WJ, Vinik AI, Bank S, et al: Selective loss of beta cell response to glucose in chronic pancreatitis. Horm Metab Res 6:95–98, 1974.
29. Joffe BI, Bank S, Jackson WP, et al: Insulin reserve in patients with chronic pancreatitis. Lancet 2:890–892, 1968.
30. McKiddie MT, Buchanan KD, McBain GC, et al: The insulin response to glucose in patients with pancreatic disease. Postgrad Med J 45:726–730, 1969.
31. Nyboe Andersen B, Krarup T, Thorsgaard Pedersen N, et al: β Cell function in patients with chronic pancreatitis and its relation to exocrine pancreatic function. Diabetologia 23:86–89, 1982.
32. Larsen S, Hilsted J, Tronier B, et al: Metabolic control and β cell function in patients with insulin-dependent diabetes mellitus secondary to chronic pancreatitis. Metabolism 36:964–967, 1987.
33. Duckworth WC, Solomon SS, Jallepalli P, et al: Hormonal response to intravenous glucose and arginine in patients with pancreatitis. Horm Res 17:65–73, 1983.
34. Nealon WH, Townsend CM, Thompson JC: The time course of beta cell dysfunction in chronic ethanol-induced pancreatitis: A prospective analysis. Surgery 104:1074–1079, 1988.
35. Larsen S, Hilsted J, Tronier B, et al: Metabolic control and β cell function in patients with insulin-dependent diabetes mellitus secondary to chronic pancreatitis. Metabolism 36:964–967, 1987.
36. Yasida H, Harand Y, Ohgaku S, et al: Insulin sensitivity in pancreatitis, liver disease, steroid treatment and hyperthyroidism assessed by glucose, insulin and somatostatin infusions. Horm Metab Res 16:3–6, 1984.
37. Marks V: Alcohol and carbohydrate metabolism. Clin Endocrinol Metab 7:333–349, 1978.
38. Schoenberg MH, Schlosser W, Ruck W, et al: Distal pancreatectomy in chronic pancreatitis. Dig Surg 16:130–136, 1999.
39. Buhler L, Schimdlin F, de Perrot M, et al: Long-term results after surgical management of chronic pancreatitis. Hepatogastroenterology 46:1986–1989, 1999.
40. Teuscher AU, Kendell DM, Smets FC, et al: Successful islet autotransplantation in humans. Diabetes 47:324–330, 1998.
41. Karmody AJ, Kyle J: The association between carcinoma of the pancreas and diabetes mellitus. Br J Surg 56:362–364, 1969.
42. Gullo L, Pezzilli R, Morselli-Labate AM, et al: Diabetes and the risk of pancreatic cancer. N Engl J Med 331:81–84, 1994.
43. Rosewicz S, Wiedenmann B: Pancreatic carcinoma. Lancet 349:485–489, 1997.
44. Schwartz SS, Zeidler A, Moossa AR, et al: A prospective study of glucose intolerance, C-peptide, insulin and glucagon response in patients with pancreatic carcinoma. Am J Dig Dis 23:1107–1114, 1978.
45. Ahren B, Andren-Sandberg A: Capacity to secrete islet hormones after subtotal pancreatectomy for pancreatic cancer. Eur J Surg 159:223–227, 1993.
46. Perhert J, Ihse I, Jorfeldt L, et al: Improved glucose metabolism after subtotal pancreatectomy for pancreatic cancer. Br J Surg 80:1047–1050, 1993.
47. Hayashida CY, Suzuki K, Fujiya H, et al: Morphometrical quantitation of pancreatic endocrine cells in patients with carcinoma of the pancreas. Tohoku J Exp Med 141:311–322, 1983.
48. Noy A, Bilezikian JP: Clinical review 63: Diabetes and pancreatic cancer: Clues to early diagnosis of pancreatic malignancy. J Clin Endocrinol Metab 79:1223–1231, 1994.
49. Powell LW, George KD, McDonnell SM, et al: Diagnosis of hemochromatosis. Ann Intern Med 129(suppl):925–931, 1998.
50. Milman N: Hereditary haemochromatosis in Denmark 1950–1985. Clinical, biochemical and histologic features in 179 patients and 13 preclinical cases. Dan Med Bull 38:385–393, 1991.
51. O'Brien T, Barrett B, Murray DM, et al: Usefulness of biochemical screening of diabetic patients for hemochromatosis. Diabetes Care 13:532–534, 1990.
52. Saddi R, Feingold J: Idiopathic hemochromatosis and diabetes mellitus. Clin Genet 5:242–247, 1974.

53. Passa P, Luyckx AS, Carpentier JL, et al: Glucagon secretion in diabetic patients with hemochromatosis. Diabetologia 13:509–513, 1977.

54. Nelson RL, Baldus WP, Rubenstein AH, et al: Pancreatic alpha-cell function in diabetic hemochromatotic subjects. J Clin Endocrinol Metab 49:412–416, 1979.

55. Saudek CD, Hemm RM, Peterson CM: Abnormal glucose tolerance in β-thalassemia major. Metabolism 26:43–52, 1977.

56. Isaacson C, Seftel SC, Keeley KJ, et al: Siderosis in the Bantu: The relationship between iron overload and cirrhosis. J Lab Clin Med 58:845–853, 1961.

57. Moran A, Doherty L, Wang X, et al: Abnormal glucose metabolism in cystic fibrosis. J Pediatr 133:10–17, 1998.

58. Cucinotta D, DeLuca F, Scoglio R, et al: Factors affecting diabetes mellitus onset in cystic fibrosis: Evidence from a 10-year follow-up study. Acta Paediatr 88:389–343, 1999.

59. Lanng S: Glucose intolerance in cystic fibrosis. Dan Med Bull 44:23–29, 1997.

60. Rosenecker J, Eichler I, Kuhn L, et al: Genetic determination of diabetes mellitus in patients with cystic fibrosis. J Pediatr 127:441–443, 1995.

61. Allen HF, Gay EC, Klingensmith GJ, et al: Identification and treatment of cystic fibrosis related diabetes. Diabetes Care 21:943–948, 1998.

62. Yung B, Hodson ME: Diabetes in cystic fibrosis. J R Soc Med 92(suppl 37):35–40, 1999.

63. Hardin DS, LeBlanc A, Para L, et al: Hepatic insulin resistance and defects in substrate utilization in cystic fibrosis. Diabetes 48:1082–1087, 1999.

64. Ezzat S, Forster MJ, Berchtold P, et al: Acromegaly, clinical and biochemical features in 500 patients. Medicine (Baltimore) 73:233–240, 1994.

65. Melmed S, Ho K, Klibanski A, et al: Recent advances in pathogenesis, diagnosis and management of acromegaly (Clinical Review 75). J Clin Endocrinol Metab 80:3395–3402, 1995.

66. Arya KR, Pathare AV, Chadda M, et al: Diabetes in acromegaly—a study of 34 cases. J Indian Med Assoc 95:546–547, 1997.

67. Moller N, Jorgensen JO, Abildgard N, et al: Effects of growth hormone on glucose metabolism. Horm Res 36(suppl 1):32–35, 1991.

68. Wasada T, Aoki K, Sato A, et al: Assessment of insulin resistance in acromegaly associated with diabetes mellitus before and after transsphenoidal adenomectomy. Endocr J 44:617–620, 1997.

69. Garcia-Estevez DA, Araujo-Vilar D, Cabelas-Cerato J: Non–insulin-mediated glucose uptake in several insulin-resistant states in the postabsorptive period. Diabetes Res Clin Pract 39:107–113, 1998.

70. Szeto CC, Li KY, Ko GT, et al: Acromegaly in a woman presenting with diabetic ketoacidosis and insulin resistance. Int J Clin Pract 51:476–477, 1997.

71. Colao A, Ferone D, Cappabianca P, et al: Effect of octreotide pretreatment on surgical outcome in acromegaly. J Clin Endocrinol Metab 82:3308–3314, 1997.

72. Newman CB, Melmed S, Synder PJ, et al: Safety and efficacy of long-term octreotide therapy of acromegaly: Results of a multicenter trial in 103 patients—a clinical research center study. J Clin Endocrinol Metab 80:2768–2775, 1995.

73. Arosio M, Macchelli S, Ross CM, et al: Effects of treatment with octreotide in acromegalic patients—a multicenter Italian study. Italian multicenter octreotide study group. Eur J Endocrinol 133:430–439, 1995.

74. Koop BL, Harris AG, Ezzat S: Effect of octreotide on glucose tolerance in acromegaly. Eur J Endocrinol 130:581–586, 1994.

75. Bates AS, Van't Hoff W, Jones JM, et al: An audit of outcome of treatment in acromegaly. Q J Med 86:293–299, 1993.

76. Sonksen PH, Russell-Jones D, Jones RH: Growth hormone and diabetes mellitus. A review of sixty-three years of medical research and a glimpse into the future? Horm Res 40:68–79, 1993.

77. Cutfield WS, Wilton P, Bennmarker H, et al: Incidence of diabetes mellitus and impaired glucose tolerance in children and adolescents receiving growth-hormone treatment. Lancet 355:610–613, 2000.

78. McMahon M, Gerich J, Rizza R: Effect of glucocorticoids on carbohydrate metabolism. Diabetes Metab Rev 4:17–30, 1988.

79. Rizza RA, Mandarino LJ, Gerich JE: Cortisol-induced insulin resistance in man: Impaired suppression of glucose production and stimulation of glucose utilization due to postreceptor defect of insulin action. J Clin Endocrinol Metab 54:131–138, 1982.

80. Shamoon H, Soman V, Sherwin RS: The influence of acute physiological increments of cortisol on fuel metabolism and insulin binding to monocytes in normal humans. J Clin Endocrinol Metab 50:495–501, 1980.

81. Olefsky JM, Kimmerling G: Effects of glucocorticoids on carbohydrate metabolism. Am J Med 271:201–210, 1976.

82. Nosadini R, Del Prato S, Tiengo A, et al: Insulin resistance in Cushing's syndrome. J Clin Endocrinol Metab 57:529–536, 1983.

83. Conn JM, Fajans SS: Influence of adrenal cortical steroids on carbohydrate metabolism in man. Metabolism 5:114–127, 1956.

84. Boyle PJ: Cushing's disease, glucocorticoid excess, glucocorticoid deficiency and diabetes. Diabetes Rev 1:301–308, 1993.

85. Plotz CM, Knowlton AI, Ragan C: The natural history of Cushing's syndrome. Am J Med 13:597–614, 1952.

86. Urbanic RC, George JM: Cushing's disease—18 years experience. Medicine (Baltimore) 60:14–24, 1961.

87. Ross EJ, Linch DC: Cushing's syndrome—killing disease: Discriminatory value of signs and symptoms aiding early diagnosis. Lancet 2:646–649, 1982.

88. Soffer L, Iannaccone A, Gabrilove J: Cushing's syndrome: A study of fifty patients. Arch Intern Med 300:215–219, 1961.

89. Roth D, Milgram M, Esquenazi V, et al: Posttransplant hyperglycemia: Increased incidence in cyclosporin-treated renal allograft recipients. Transplantation 47:278–281, 1989.

90. Arner P, Gunnarsson R, Blomdahl S, et al: Some characteristics of steroid diabetes: A study in renal-transplant recipients receiving high dose corticosteroid therapy. Diabetes Care 6:23–25, 1983.

91. Gurwitz JH, Bohn RL, Glynn RJ, et al: Glucocorticoids and the risk for initiation of hypoglycemic therapy. Arch Intern Med 154:97–101, 1994.

92. Weissman DE, Dufer D, Vogel V, et al: Corticosteroid toxicity in neuro-oncology patients. J Neurooncol 5:125–128, 1987.

93. Fernandez-Real JM, Engel WR, Simo R, et al: Study of glucose tolerance in consecutive patients harbouring incidental adrenal tumors. Clin Endocrinol 49:53–61, 1998.

94. Leibowitz G, Tsur A, Chayen SD, et al: Pre-clinical Cushing's syndrome: An unexpected frequent cause of poor glycaemic control in obese diabetic patients. Clin Endocrinol 44:717–722, 1996.

95. Al-Shoumer KA, Beshyah SA, Niththyananthan R, et al: Effect of glucocorticoid replacement therapy on glucose tolerance and intermediary metabolites in hypopituitary adults. Clin Endocrinol 42:85–90, 1995.

96. Wajngot A, Giacca A, Grill V, et al: The diabetogenic effects of glucocorticoids are more pronounced in low than in high insulin responders. Proc Natl Acad Sci U S A 89:6035–6039, 1992.

97. Hirsh IB, Paauw DS: Diabetes management in special situations. Endocrinol Metab Clin North Am 26:631–646, 1997.

98. Umpierrez GE, Khajavi M, Kitabchi AE: Review: Diabetic ketoacidosis and hyperglycemic hyperosmolar nonketotic syndrome. Am J Med Sci 311:225–233, 1996.

99. Mallison CN, Bloom SR, Warin AP, et al: A glucagonoma syndrome. Lancet 2:1–5, 1974.

100. Stacpoole PW: The glucagonoma syndrome: Clinical features, diagnosis and treatment. Endocr Rev 2:347–361, 1981.

101. Bloom SR, Polak JM: Glucagonoma syndrome. Am J Med 82(suppl 5B):25–36, 1987.

102. Soga J, Yakawa Y: Glucagonomas/diabetico-dermatogenic syndrome (DDS): A statistical evaluation of 407 reported cases. J Hepatobiliary-Pancreat Surg 5:312–319, 1998.

103. Shyr YM, Su CH, Lee CH, et al: Glucagonoma syndrome: A case report. Chin Med J 62:639–643, 1999.

104. Barazzoni R, Zanetti M, Tiengo A, et al: Protein metabolism in glucagonoma. Diabetologia 42:326–329, 1999.

105. Frankton S, Bloom SR: Gastrointestinal endocrine tumours. Glucagonomas. Baillieres Clin Gastroenterol 10:697–705, 1996.

106. Larsen LI, Hirsch MA, Holst JJ, et al: Pancreatic somatostatinoma. Clinical features and physiological implications. Lancet 1:666–668, 1977.

107. Ganda OP, Weir GC, Soeldner JS, et al: "Somatostatinoma": A somatostatin-containing tumor of the endocrine pancreas. N Engl J Med 296:963–967, 1977.

108. Krejs GJ, Orci L, Conlon JM, et al: Somatostatin syndrome, biochemical, morphologic and clinical features. N Engl J Med 301:285–292, 1979.

109. Mao C, Shah A, Hanson DJ, et al: Von Recklinhausen's disease associated with duodenal somatostatinoma: Contrast of duodenal versus pancreatic somatostatinomas. J Surg Oncol 59:67–73, 1995.

110. Penman E, Lowry PJ, Wass JA: Molecular forms of somatostatin in normal subjects and in patients with somatostatinoma. Clin Endocrinol 12:611–620, 1980.

111. Conlon JM, McCarthy D, Krejs G, et al: Characterization of somatostatin-like components in the tumors and plasma of a patient with a somatostatinoma. J Clin Endocrinol Metab 52:66–73, 1981.

112. Patel YC, Ganda OP, Benoit R: Pancreatic somatostatinoma: Abundance of somatostatin-28(1–12)-like immunoreactivity in tumor and plasma. J Clin Endocrinol Metab 57:1048–1053, 1983.

113. Willcox PA, Immelman EJ, Barron JL, et al: Pancreatic somatostatinoma: Presentation with recurrent episodes of severe hyperglycemia and ketoacidosis. Q J Med 68:559–571, 1988.

114. Jackson JA, Raju, BU, Fachnie JD, et al: Malignant somatostatinoma presenting with diabetic ketoacidosis. Clin Endocrinol 26:609–621, 1987.

115. Yamasaki T, Chijiiwa K, Chijiiwa Y: Somatostatin inhibits cholecystokinin-induced contraction of isolated gallbladder smooth muscle cells. J Surg Res 59:743–746, 1995.

116. Marteau P, Chretien Y, Calmus Y, et al: Pharmacological effect of somatostatin on bile secretion in man. Digestion 42:16–21, 1989.

117. Lowry SF, Burt ME, Brennan MF: Glucose turnover and gluconeogenesis in a patient with somatostatinoma. Surgery 89:309–313, 1981.

118. Angeletti S, Corleto VD, Schillaci O, et al: Use of the somatostatin analogue octreotide to localize and manage somatostatin-producing tumors. Gut 42:792–794, 1998.

119. Stenstrom G, Sjostrom I, Smith U: Diabetes mellitus in pheochromocytoma: Fasting blood glucose level before and after surgery in 60 patients with pheochromocytoma. Acta Endocrinol 106:511–515, 1984.

120. Hamaji M: Pancreatic α and β cell function in pheochromocytoma. J Clin Endocrinol Metab 49:322–325, 1979.

121. Vance JE, Buchanan KD, O'Hara D, et al: Insulin and glucagon responses in subjects with pheochromocytoma: Effect of alpha adrenergic blockade. J Clin Endocrinol Metab 29:911–916, 1969.

122. Pandit MK, Burke J, Gustafson AB, et al: Drug-induced disorders of glucose metabolism. Ann Intern Med 118:529–539, 1993.

123. Chan JC, Cockran CS, Critchley JAHJ: Drug-induced disorders of glucose metabolism. Mechanisms and management. Drug Saf 15:136–157, 1996.

124. Bressler P, DeFronzo RA: Drug effects on glucose homeostasis. In Alberti KGMM, Zimmet P, DeFronzo RA, Keen H (eds): International Textbook of Diabetes Mellitus, ed 2. New York, John Wiley & Sons, 1997, pp 214–254.

125. Bouchard P, Sai P, Reach G, et al: Diabetes mellitus following pentamidine-induced hypoglycemia in humans. Diabetes 31:40–45, 1982.

126. Osei K, Falko JM, Nelson KP, et al: Diabetogenic effect of pentamidine: In vitro and in vivo studies in a patient with malignant insulinoma. Am J Med 77:41–46, 1984.

127. Assan R, Mayaud C, Perronne C, et al: Pentamidine-induced derangements of glucose homeostasis. Diabetes Care 18:47–55, 1995.

128. LeWitt PA: The neurotoxicity of the rat poison Vacor: A clinical study of 12 cases. N Engl J Med 302:73–77, 1980.

129. Karam JH, Lewitt PA, Young CW, et al: Insulinopenic diabetes after rodenticide (Vacor) ingestion: A unique model of acquired diabetes in man. Diabetes 29:971–978, 1980.

130. Danforth E Jr: Hyperglycemia after diazoxide. N Engl J Med 285:1487, 1971.

131. Milsap RL, Auld PA: Neonatal hyperglycemia following maternal diazoxide administration. JAMA 243:144–145, 1980.

132. Goldberg EM, Sanbar SS: Hyperglycemic non-ketotic coma following administration of Dilantin. Diabetes 18:101–106, 1969.

133. Fariss BL, Lutcher CL: Diphenylhydantoin-induced hyperglycemia and impaired insulin release: Effect of dosage. Diabetes 20:177–181, 1971.

134. Malherbe C, Burrill KC, Levin SR, et al: Effect of diphenylhydantoin on insulin secretion in man. N Engl J Med 286:339–342, 1972.

135. Bengtsson C, Blohme G, Lapidus L, et al: Do antihypertensive drugs precipitate diabetes. BMJ 289:1495–1497, 1984.

136. Gurwitz JH, Bohn RL, Glynn RJ, et al: Antihypertensive drug therapy and the initiation of treatment for diabetes mellitus. Ann Intern Med 118:273–278, 1993.

137. Murphy MB, Kohner E, Lewis PJ, et al: Glucose intolerance in hypertensive patients treated with diuretics: A fourteen year follow-up. Lancet 2:1293–1295, 1982.

138. Donahue R, Abbott R, Wilson P: Effect of diuretics on the development of diabetes mellitus: The Framingham study. Horm Metab Res 22(suppl 1):46–48, 1990.

139. Kaplan NM: The case for low-dose diuretic therapy. Am J Hypertens 4:970–971, 1991.

140. Berglund G, Andersson O, Widgren B: Low dose antihypertensive treatment with a thiazide diuretic is not diabetogenic. A 10-year controlled trial with bendroflumethiazide. Acta Med Scand 220:419–424, 1986.

141. Rowe JW, Tobin JD, Rosa RM, et al: Effects of experimental potassium deficiency on glucose and insulin metabolism. Metabolism 29:493–502, 1980.

142. Helderman JH, Elahi D, Anderson DK, et al: Prevention of the glucose intolerance of thiazide diuretics by maintenance of body potassium. Diabetes 32:106–111, 1983.

143. Micossi P, Pollavini G, Piaggi U, et al: Effects of metoprolol and propranolol on glucose metabolism and insulin secretion in diabetes mellitus. Horm Metab Res 16:59–63, 1984.

144. Whitcroft I, Wilkinson N, Ranthorne A, et al: Beta-adrenoreceptor antagonist impairs long-term glucose control in hypertensive diabetes: Role of beta-adrenoreceptor selectivity and lipid solubility. Br J Clin Pharm 22:236–237, 1986.

145. Cerasi E, Luft R, Effendic S: Effect of adrenergic blocking agents on insulin response to glucose infusion in man. Acta Endocrinol 69:335–346, 1972.

146. Totterman K, Groop L, Groop PH, et al: Effect of beta blocking drugs on beta cell function and insulin sensitivity in hypertensive non-diabetic patients. Eur J Clin Pharmacol 26:13–17, 1984.

147. Bending JJ, Ogg CS, Viberti GC: Diabetogenic effect of cyclosporin. BMJ 294:401–402, 1987.

148. Ost L, Tyden G, Fehrman I: Impaired glucose tolerance in cylcosporin-prednisolone–treated renal graft recipients. Transplantation 46:370–372, 1988.

149. Perlman JA, Russell-Briefel R, Ezzati T, et al: Oral glucose tolerance and the potency of contraceptive progestins. J Chronic Dis 38:857–864, 1985.

150. Spellacy WN, Tsibris JC, Ellingson AB: Carbohydrate metabolic studies in women using a levonorgestrel/ethinyl estradiol containing triphasic oral contraceptive for 18 months. Int J Gynaecol Obstet 35:69–71, 1991.

151. Scheen AJ, Jandrain BJ, Humblet DM, et al: Effects of a 1-year treatment with low-dose combined oral contraceptive containing ethinyl estradiol and cyproterone acetate on glucose and insulin metabolism. Fertil Steril 59:797–802, 1993.

152. Spellacy WN: Carbohydrate metabolism during treatment with oestrogen, progestogen and low-dose oral contraceptives. Am J Obstet Gynecol 142:732–734, 1982.

153. Bettino JC, Tashima CK: Medroxyprogesterone acetate and diabetes mellitus. Ann Intern Med 84:341–342, 1976.

154. Lithell H, Vessby B, Hellsing K: Changes in glucose tolerance and plasma insulin during lipid-lowering treatment with diet, clofibrate and niceritrol. Atherosclerosis 43:177–184, 1982.

155. Garg A, Grundy SM: Nicotinic acid as therapy for dyslipidemia in non–insulin-dependent diabetes. JAMA 264:723–726, 1990.

156. Molnar GD, Berge KG, Rosevear JW, et al: The effect of nicotinic acid in diabetes mellitus. Metabolism 13:181–189, 1964.

157. Dube MP, Johnson DL, Currier JS, et al: Protease inhibitor–associated hyperglycaemia. Lancet 350:713–714, 1997.

158. Kaufman JA, Simionatta C: A review of protease inhibitor–induced hyperglycemia. Pharmacotherapy 19:114–117, 1999.

159. Yarasheski KE, Tebas P, Sigmund C, et al: Insulin resistance in HIV protease inhibitor–associated diabetes. J Acquir Immun Defic Syndr Hum Retrovirol 21:209–216, 1999.

Index

Note: Page numbers in *italics* refer to illustrations; page numbers followed by t refer to tables.

Glucocorticoid(s) *(Continued)*
potency of, 1671–1672, 1672t
receptor binding site of, 1648–
1649, *1648–1650*
receptors for. See *Glucocorticoid
receptors.*
resistance to, 159, 162, 580–581,
1716–1720
apparent mineralocorticoid excess in, 1839
biochemistry of, 1717–1718,
1718
clinical features of, 1716–1717
differential diagnosis of, 1718–
1719
incidence of, 1716
inheritance of, 1717
localized, 1717
pathophysiology of, 1716,
1716
receptor abnormalities in, 1718
treatment of, 1719, *1719*
versus Cushing's syndrome,
1695
secretion of, regulation of, 1633–
1635
feedback in, 1633
testing of. See *Adrenal cortex,
function of, testing of.*
short-acting, therapy with, 2602t,
2603
side effects of, 1675–1676, 1675t
structures of, 1671, *1672*
synthesis of, regulation of, 1633–
1635, *1634*
therapy with, 1671–1682, 2602–
2604, 2602t
absorption of, 1672
actions of, duration of, 1671–
1672, 1672t
age factors in, 1673
alternate-day, 1678–1680, *1679*
anti-inflammatory effects of,
1674–1675
bioavailability of, 1672
biotransformation of, 1672
calcium absorption inhibition
in, 1033
calcium levels and, 1148
Cushing's syndrome due to,
1698, 1710
daily single-dose, 1680
dosage for, 1680–1681
drug interactions in, 1673
duration of, 1674
fractures due to, 1183
half-lives of, 1671–1672, 1672t
hypothalamic-pituitary-adrenal
axis suppression in, 1677–
1678, 1677t
immune response to, 1636–
1637, 1637t, 1674–1675
in adrenal hyperplasia, 1732–
1734, *1733*
in adrenal insufficiency, 1688,
1859, *1860*
in allergy, 582
in autoimmune diseases, 583
in Cushing's syndrome, 1708–
1709
in Graves' disease, 1437
in hirsutism, 2131
in 11β-hydroxylase deficiency,
1833–1834
in hypercalcemia, 1102t, 1106
in hyperthyroidism, 1325, 1673
in liver disease, 1673
in nephrotic syndrome, 1673
in orthostatic hypotension,
1859, *1860*

Glucocorticoid(s) *(Continued)*
in pregnancy, 1673
in pretibial myxedema, 1442
in sclerosing thyroiditis, 1487
in stress, 1689
indications for, 1674, 1674t
initiation of, planning for,
1674, 1674t
intermediate-acting, 1671,
1672t, 2602t, 2603
local, 1674
long-acting, 1671, 1672t,
2602t, 2604
mineralocorticoid activity of,
1671, 1672t
osteoporosis due to, 1059,
1199, 1248–1249, 1255
patient education on, 1709
perioperative management in,
1680–1681
pharmacodynamics of, 1671–
1673, *1672*, 1672t
phosphate absorption in, 1037
phosphate reabsorption in,
1040
postoperative, 1708–1709
potency of, 1671–1672, 1672t
pulse, 1680
selection of, 1674
short-acting, 1671, 1672t,
2602t, 2603
side effects of, 1675–1676,
1675t
structures of, 1671, *1672*
thyroid function effects of,
1386
transport proteins of, 1673
versus ACTH, 1680
withdrawal from, 1676, 1678,
1709
thyroxine-binding globulin levels
and, 1316
tolerance of, 579
transport proteins of, 1673
withdrawal from, 1676, 1678,
1709
Glucocorticoid receptor-interacting
protein-1, 1651, *1651*
Glucocorticoid receptors,
1633–1635, 1647–1648, *1647*
actions of, 1633, 1639
coreceptor proteins in, 1651–
1652, *1651*
DNA-binding domain of,
1648–1649, *1648*, *1649*
hormone-binding domain of,
1648–1649, *1648*
N-terminal domain of, 1648–
1649, *1648*
versus structures, 1648–1649,
1648–1650
activating protein-1 antagonism
to, 119
activation of, 1647–1648, *1647*
anabolic steroid action on, 2250
antagonists to, 1648
as transcription factors, 147
chromatin interactions with, 132
defects of, 156t
animal models of, 1639
glucocorticoid resistance in,
1716–1720, *1716*, *1718*,
1719
distribution of, 1633, 1651–1652,
1651
DNA interactions with, 129t
feedback via, 1635
genes of, 1647
half-life of, 1648

Glucocorticoid receptors
(Continued)
heat shock proteins associated
with, 1647, *1647*
in brain, 1639
in cytoplasm, 1647, *1647*
in gene expression inhibition, 136
in gene transcription, 1649–1651,
1650, *1651*
inactive state of, 1647, *1647*
isoforms of, 1648
species variation in, 1648
structure of, 575, 1648–1649,
1648, *1649*
transport of, 1647–1648, *1647*
versus mineralocorticoid receptors, 1777
Glucocorticoid response elements,
glucocorticoid receptor binding
to, 1633, 1648–1650, *1649*,
1650
negative, 1650, *1650*
of phosphoenolpyruvate carboxykinase gene, 1635–1636
Glucocorticoid-remediable/
suppressible aldosteronism,
1622, 1832–1833
Glucoincretin, gastric inhibitory
polypeptide as, 2549–2550
Glucokinase, defects of, 157t, 758
Gluconeogenesis, alcohol inhibition
of, 925
autonomic control of, 741, *741*
defects of, hyperglycemia in,
909–910, *910*
failure of, in trauma, 926
fatty acids in, 741–742
glucagon in, 732
in fasting, 739–740, *739*
in fetus, 2416
in kidney, 644, *644*, 739
in neonates, 2406
in postabsorptive state, 923
in starvation, 643
leptin in, 612
regulation of, glucocorticoids in,
1635–1636
Glucosamine, in leptin regulation,
607
Glucose, absorption of, 753, *753*
administration of, hypophosphatemia due to, 1042
in hypoglycemia, 935
in neonates, 2420
in parturition, in diabetes mellitus, 2439
intravenous, versus oral, insulin response in, 697
anomeric, insulin secretion and,
698
counterregulation of, 922, 924–
925
distribution of, 738
fatty acid–amino acid interactions
with, 749–752, *750–752*
homeostasis of, 922–924
in postabsorptive state, 922–
923, *923*
in postprandial state, 923–924,
924
impaired fasting, definition of,
760–761
in diabetes mellitus, 771, 771t
in glucagon secretion, 730
in hyperosmolar coma, 917, 917t
in insulin metabolism, 700
in insulin secretion, 658, 680,
697–698
in insulin synthesis, 680

Glucose *(Continued)*
in vasopressin regulation, 366
insulin response to, 697–698
in diabetes mellitus, 704–705,
778–779, *778*, *779*
intracellular disposition of, 743
levels of. See also *Hyperglycemia; Hypoglycemia.*
at birth, 2418–2419
dietary control of, 814
fasting, in pregnancy, 2434
in diabetes mellitus, 539
classification with, 811
diagnostic criteria and, 759–
761, 760t
in ketoacidosis, 912, 913t
in pregnancy, 2434
target values for, 813
versus treatment options,
822
in fasting, 737, 740–742, *740*,
741
in hypoglycemia, 921
in sleep, 250–251, *251*
monitoring of, 812–813, *813*
in diabetes mellitus, 542,
2439
normal, 738, 811, 922
postprandial, 923–924
regulation of, glucagon-like
peptides in, 732–733, *734*
measurement of, errors in, 921–
922
metabolism of, biological
rhythms of, 250–252, *251*
futile cycles in, 744
gastric emptying and, 744
glucocorticoids in, 1635
hepatic, 788–789, *788*
hyperglycemia in, 909–910,
910
in brain, 754, 922
in exercise, 699
in fasting, 737, 739–744
glucose cycles in, 744
glucose disposal in, 742–
744, *742*, 743t
glucose production in, 739–
742, *739–741*
in fetus, 2405–2406, 2413–
2416, *2414*, 2414t, 2415t,
2416
in infections, 926
in insulin resistance, 782–783
in neonates, 2409, 2418–2421,
2420t
in postprandial state. See under
Postprandial state.
in pregnancy, 2433–2436,
2433, *2435*, *2436*
diabeticogenic stress in,
2433–2434, *2433*
fetal fuel utilization and,
2434
normal, 2434
outcome and, 2435–2436,
2435, *2436*
with gestational diabetes mellitus, 2434
with pregestational diabetes
mellitus, 2434–2435
in syndrome X, 955
in trauma, 926
insulin-like growth factors in,
450
intracellular, 747–749, *748*,
749
leptin in, 612
meal composition and, 744

Granulocyte-macrophage colony-stimulating factor. See under *Colony-stimulating factor(s)*.

Granuloma, eosinophilic, growth hormone deficiency in, 504
  rickets due to, 1234
  suprasellar, pituitary dysfunction in, 172

Granulomatous disease, adrenal insufficiency in, 1685
  hypopituitarism in, 291
  of adrenal glands, 1757, *1758*
  of hypothalamus, imaging of, 267
  parasellar, 286

Granulomatous thyroiditis. See *Thyroiditis, subacute*.

Granulosa cells, androgen synthesis in, 2123, *2124*
  apoptosis of, 2065
  domains of, 2065, *2065*
  estradiol synthesis in, 2067–2068, *2067*
  estrogen synthesis in, 2045, *2046*
  follicle-stimulating hormone receptors of, 2068
  hormone synthesis in, 2049–2050
  in oocyte recruitment, 2062
  inhibin production in, 1906
  insulin receptors on, 2047
  intraovarian control mechanisms for, 2048–2049, 2048t
  lutein, 2069, *2069*
  luteinizing hormone receptors of, 2068
  mucification of, 2068, *2069*
  number of, during folliculogenesis, 2066, *2066*
  of primary follicle, 2062, *2062*, *2063*
  progesterone receptors of, 2068
  proliferation of, *2066*, 2067
  tumors of, 2172–2173
    precocious puberty in, 2018
    testicular, 2355

Graves' disease, 1409, 1422–1449
  animal models of, 1429–1430
  asymptomatic, 1430
  autoimmune diseases with, 1424–1425
  B lymphocyte response in, 1416–1417, *1417*
  cancer risk in, 1544
  classic form of, 1422
  clinical feature(s) of, 1422, 1422t, 1430–1432, *1430*, 1432t
    ophthalmopathy as. See *Ophthalmopathy, in Graves' disease*.
    pretibial myxedema as, 1432–1433, *1433*
  criteria for, 1422–1423, 1422t
  cytotoxic T lymphocyte antigen-4 defects in, 563
  development of, from subacute thyroiditis, 1483
  diagnosis of, 1433–1434, 1434t, *1436*
  emotional triggers of, 1426
  environmental factors in, 1416, 1425–1427
  epidemiology of, 1423–1424, *1423*
  etiology of, 1424–1427, 1425t
  extraocular muscle involvement in, 1450
  evaluation of, 1454–1455, *1454*, *1455*
  pathology of, 1452–1453, *1452*, *1453*

Graves' disease *(Continued)*
  treatment of, 1456–1458, *1458*
  factitious, 1466
  gender differences in, 1424, 1426–1427, 1451
  genetic factors in, 1416, 1424–1425, 1425t, 1450–1451
  historical background of, 1422–1423, *1423*
  human leukocyte antigens in, 560, 1424–1425, 1425t, 1429
  in children, 1442
  in elderly persons, 544–545
  in neonates, 1441–1442, *1441*
  in polyglandular syndromes, 594
  in pregnancy, 1427, 1440–1441, *1441*, 2451–2452
  infections triggering, 1425–1426
  iodine-induced thyrotoxicosis in, 1467
  laboratory tests in, 1433–1434, 1434t, *1436*
  myasthenia gravis with, 1431
  natural history of, 1419
  pathogenesis of, 1417–1418, *1418*, 1427–1430, *1428*
  pathology of, 1410, 1427
  physical examination in, 1433
  radionuclide studies of, 1377, *1400*
  stress-induced, 1426–1427
  subacute thyroiditis progression to, 1483
  thyroid antibody measurement in, 1374, 1376
  thyroid hormone resistance with, 1610
  T-lymphocyte response to, 1416
  treatment of, 1419, 1419t, 1434–1440
    before thyroid surgery, 1572–1573, *1573*, 1573t
    beta-blockers in, 1437
    contrast agents in, 1324–1325
    glucocorticoids in, 1437
    historical background of, 1423
    in children, 1442
    in elderly persons, 1442, 1442t
    in neonates, 1441–1442, *1441*
    in ophthalmopathy, 1457
    in pregnancy, 1440–1441, *1441*
    in thyroid storm, 1442
    iodine compounds in, 1437
    perchlorate in, 1437
    radioactive iodine in, 1437–1438, 1439t, 1440, 1573, *1573*
    selection of, 1439–1440, 1439t
    surgical, 1438–1439, *1439*, 1439t
    thionamides in, 1435–1437, 1435t, *1436*, 1439t, 1440–1441, *1441*
    thyroidectomy in, 1441
  ultrasonography of, 1404, *1404*
  versus familial nonautoimmune hyperthyroidism, 1587
  versus goiter due to thyroid hormone resistance, 1609–1610
  versus postpartum thyroiditis, 2456
  versus silent thyroiditis, 1477, 1478, 1478t, 1478, 1478t
  versus thyrotoxicosis, 1434, 1434t

Grb2 protein, in receptor tyrosine kinase activation, 37–38, *38*, 100

Gremlin, in receptor serine kinase regulation, 55

GRH. See *Growth hormone–releasing hormone*.

GRIF (growth hormone release–inhibiting factor). See *Somatostatin*.

Growth, 477–485. See also *Growth factor(s)*; *Growth hormone*.
  accelerated, in 21-hydroxylase deficiency, 1724–1725, *1725*
    tall stature in, 496, 497, 497t
  advanced, tall stature in, 496–497, 497t
  after menarche, 480
  attenuated pattern of, *483*, 493, 493t
  body proportional changes in, 480, *484*
  bone age and, patterns of, 484–485, *486*, *487*
  catch-up, patterns of, 480, 484, 485t
  cellular, determinants of, 477
  compensatory, 484
  constitutional advance of, 495, 495t
  constitutional delay of, 485t, 488t, 493, 493t, 494, 2022
  delayed pattern of, *483*
  determinants of, 477–480, *478*
  disorders of. See also *Stature, short*; *Stature, tall*; *Growth, retardation of*.
    in glucocorticoid receptor defects, 1639
    in malnutrition, 646
  excessive. See *Acromegaly*.
  failure of, in growth hormone deficiency, 508–509
  fetal. See *Growth, intrauterine*.
  gender differences in, 480, *481–484*, 484t
  genetic factors in, 477
  hormones for. See also specific hormones.
  in adrenarche, 1744
  in puberty, 479, 480, *482*, 1959, *1959*
  in tall stature, patterns of, 496, 497, 497t
  in Turner's syndrome, 1983–1984
  intrauterine, chorionic somato-mammotropin in, 2384
    determinants of, 479–480
    hormones in, 2407–2408, 2407t
    in maternal diabetes mellitus, 2435–2436
    patterns of, 480, *480*
    retardation of, in growth hormone deficiency, 508
    short stature in, 488t, 490
  intrinsic shortness pattern of, *483*
  linear (height) standards for, 480, *481–484*, 484t
  nutritional requirements for, 477, *478*
  of organs, 480
  of teeth, 480
  patterns of, 480–485
    bone age and, 484–485, *486*, *487*
    catch-up, 480, 484
    in short stature, 485, 493, 493t
    in tall stature, 496, *497*, 497t
    intrauterine, 480, *480*
    postnatal, 480, *481–485*, 484t
  phases of, 480

Growth *(Continued)*
  postnatal, determinants of, 477–479, *478*
    patterns of, 480, *481–485*, 484t
    prediction of, bone age in, 484–485, *486*, *487*
    premature pubarche and, 2013
    premature thelarche and, 2013
  prenatal. See *Growth, intrauterine*.
  prolonged, tall stature in, 496, 497, 497t
  retardation of. See also under *Growth, intrauterine*.
    anabolic steroids in, 2247–2248
    hypoparathyroidism with, 1069
    in cretinism, 1535–1536, *1535*
    in glucocorticoid resistance, 1718–1719
    in kwashiorkor, 646
    in pituitary adenoma, 357t, 358, 359t
    in renal failure, 1211
    in rickets, 1156
    in thyroid hormone resistance, 1610
    in vitamin D receptor defects, 1017
    intrinsic shortness as. See *Stature, short*.
  velocity of, 480, *481–484*, 484t
    in puberty, 1959, *1959*

Growth and differentiation factor, receptors for, 53, 53t

Growth differentiation factor-9, in oocyte, 2070
  in ovarian function regulation, 2048–2049

Growth factor(s). See also specific growth factor, e.g., *Insulin-like growth factor(s)*.
  actions of, 461, 462, *462*
  autocrine actions of, 461, *462*
  biology of, 461–462, 462t, *463*, 463t
  circulating, in multiple endocrine neoplasia, 2513–2514
  definition of, 461
  families of, 462t
  in ACTH regulation, 229
  in adrenal androgen secretion, 1743
  in bone formation, 1054
  in cellular growth, 477
  in diabetic ulceration treatment, 905
  in endometriosis, 2107, 2107t
  in folliculogenesis, 2070
  in implantation, 2394
  in lactotroph stimulation, 211
  in luteogenesis, 2070
  in milk, 2468
  in multinodular goiter, 1517–1518, 1519
  in ovulation, 2070
  in prolactin regulation, 212
  in prostate cancer, 2368–2370, 2369t, 2370t
  in prostate growth and function, 2362–2364, *2363*, 2368, 2369t
  in signal transduction, 461–462, *463*
  in thyroid regulation, 1301, 1301t, 1303, 1309–1311, *1309*, *1311*
  intracrine actions of, 461, *462*
  juxtacrine actions of, 461, *462*

Heart (Continued)
Graves' disease effects on, 1430–1431
hypothyroidism effects on, 1497
natriuretic peptide effects on, 1794, 1795
oxytocin receptors in, 201t, 203, 205–206
palpitations of, in menopause, 2155
in pheochromocytoma, 1869
thyroid hormones in, in nonthyroidal illness syndrome, 1510t
thyroid tissue in, 1584
valvular disease of, carcinoid, 2538–2539, 2539t
in Noonan's syndrome, 2279
in Paget's disease, 1264
Heart failure, adrenomedullin in, 1805, 1805
angiotensin-converting enzyme inhibitors in, 1784
edema in, mechanisms of, 1818
endothelin in, 1802
hyperthyroidism effects on, 1442
hypoglycemia in, 926
in Graves' disease, 1430–1431
in hypophosphatemia, 1043
in thyroid storm, 1442
natriuretic peptide levels in, 1797, 1797
treatment of, natriuretic peptides in, 1798
Heart rate, in diabetes mellitus, 870
in syndrome X, 957
orthostatic changes of, 1851, 1852t
Heat, intolerance of, in Graves' disease, 1432
spermatogenesis effects of, 2310
Heat shock proteins, androgen receptor interactions with, 2301, 2301
autoimmune response to, 564
estrogen receptor interactions with, 2053, 2053
glucocorticoid receptor interactions with, 1647, 1647
progesterone receptor interactions with, 2053, 2053
receptors associated with, 125
transcription factors for, 7
Heavy metals, reproductive effects of, 1965–1966
Height. See also Stature.
disproportional, in constitutional delay, 2024
gain of, versus age, 1959, 1959
genetic factors in, 480
loss of, in osteoporosis, 1248
measurement of, in osteoporosis, 1250
prediction of, 480
from bone age, 480, 484–485, 484t, 486, 487
standards for, 480, 481–484, 484t
Height age, 484–485, 485t
in small stature, 493, 493t
in tall stature, 496, 497t
Height velocity, error of, 509
Helicobacter pylori infections, T lymphocyte dysfunction in, 581
HELLP syndrome, hypoglycemia in, 928
Hemangioblastomatosis, cerebelloretinal, pheochromocytoma in, 1871t, 1872
Hemangioendothelioma, thyroid gland, 1549t

Hematoma, after thyroid surgery, 1578
Hematopoiesis, disorders of, anabolic steroids in, 2246–2247
prolactin in, 218
regulation of, colony-stimulating factors in. See Colony-stimulating factor(s).
erythropoietin in. See Erythropoietin.
Hematopoietic growth factors, in fetus, 2408
Hematuria, in nephrolithiasis, 1177
Heme, neurotransmitter synthesis from, 184
Hemianopia, in pituitary tumors, 283
Hemihypophysectomy, in Cushing's disease, 1706
Hemochromatosis, diabetes mellitus in, 961
hypoparathyroidism in, 1137
hypopituitarism in, 292
of adrenal gland, imaging of, 1757, 1758
testicular dysfunction in, 2284, 2284t
versus polyglandular syndrome, 595
Hemodialysis, aluminum intoxication in, 1238–1239
hypoglycemia in, 927
in diabetic nephropathy, 888, 889, 892–893, 893t, 896t
Hemodynamics, abnormalities of, in diabetic nephropathy pathogenesis, 885–887
adrenomedullin effects on, 1804
natriuretic peptide effects on, 1795
Hemoglobin, glycosylated, measurement of, 812–813, 813
production of, anabolic steroid effects on, 2247
Hemoglobin A_{1C}, after pancreatic transplantation, 837, 837
in pregnancy, malformation risk and, 2435
monitoring of, 2439
levels of, normal, 2581t
measurement of, 2581t
Hemolysis, in hypophosphatemia, 1043
Hemophilia, anabolic steroids in, 2247
Hemoproteins, in steroid synthesis, 1623–1624, 1623, 1625
Hemorrhage, adrenal, imaging of, 1757, 1759
after thyroid surgery, 1578
glucocorticoid action in, 1650
in platelet-derived growth factor deficiency, 469
pituitary, 171–172, 261, 282
Hemosiderosis, diabetes mellitus in, 961
Henle, loop of, vasopressin action in, 368, 368
Henneman-Griswold-Albright syndrome, hyperprolactinemia in, 329
Heparin, hypoaldosteronism due to, 1847
in carcinoid tumors, 2540
in parenteral nutrition, 650
osteoporosis due to, 1199–1200
thyroid hormone binding and, 1318

Heparin sulfate proteoglycans, fibroblast growth factor binding to, 466
Heparin-binding epidermal growth factor, 27, 29
in implantation, 2394
receptor for, 464
structure of, 463
Hepatic. See also Liver.
Hepatic artery, embolization of, in carcinoid tumor, 2540, 2542–2543
Hepatic autoregulation, 752
of glucose output, 741
Hepatic osteodystrophy, 1232
Hepatitis, alcoholic, anabolic steroids in, 2248
autoimmune, in polyglandular syndromes, 591
Hepatocellular adenoma, in oral contraceptive use, 2167
Hepatocellular neoplasia, from anabolic steroids, 2251
Hepatocyte growth factor, 472, 472
in endometriosis, 2107, 2107t
in prostate growth and function, 2362, 2363
in smad protein regulation, 55
in thyroid regulation, 1301, 1301t
receptors for, family of, 26t, 27
Hepatocyte nuclear factor, defects of, diabetes mellitus in, 758
Hepatocyte nuclear receptor, defects of, 160
Hepatoma, hypoglycemia in, 929
HER (epidermal growth factor receptors), 464
Hereditary angioneurotic edema, anabolic steroids in, 2247
Hereditary toxic thyroid hyperplasia, 1587
Hermaphroditism, amenorrhea in, 2089
gender assignment in, 2035
true, 1984–1985, 2130
Hernia uteri inguinalis, 1995
HESX1 gene and product, defects of, hypopituitarism in, 291, 291t
hypothyroidism in, 1596
Heterochromatin, 4
Heterologous induction or downregulation, of receptors, 131
Heterotopic ossification. See Calcification, extraskeletal.
Heterozygosity, in autosomal recessive disorders, 150, 151
Hexarelin, as growth hormone secretagogue, 409, 409t, 412, 417–418
Hexestrol, structure of, 1967
Hexokinase II, deficiency of, in insulin resistance, 783
HIAP-1 retroviral particle, Graves' disease and, 1426
Hilar cells, of ovary, 2050, 2061
tumors of, 2174
Hip, deformities of, clinical features of, 1184
fractures of, in osteoporosis, 1245, 1248
bone microarchitecture and, 1248
in men, 1250
risk of, 1247
Hippocampus, neurotransmitters of, 185
Hirschsprung's disease, neurotrophic factor defects in, 468

Hirschsprung's disease (Continued)
RET gene mutations in, 30
Hirsutism, 2128
classification of, 2125, 2125
definition of, 2125
evaluation of, 2130, 2131
in acromegaly, 305
in glucocorticoid resistance, 1717, 1719
in hyperandrogenism, 2125, 2125, 2130–2132
in polycystic ovary syndrome, treatment of, 2098
treatment of, 2130–2132
vellus, in Cushing's syndrome, 1694, 1694
Histamine, actions of, 186
corticotropin-releasing hormone–mast cell interactions with, 577–578, 578
immunoregulatory functions of, 577–578, 578
in allergy, 582
neuronal pathways for, 185–186
provocation test with, in pheochromocytoma, 1875
receptors for, 186
secretion of, in stomach, 2548
synthesis of, 184
Histidine, neurotransmitter synthesis from, 184
Histidyl proline diketopiperazine cyclo-(His-Pro), in appetite regulation, 602–603
Histiocytosis, Langerhans' cell. See Langerhans' cell histiocytosis.
Histone deacetylase, 133
Histones, DNA wrapping around, 4
in spermiogenesis, 2214
Histoplasmosis, adrenal insufficiency in, 1684
HLAs. See Human leukocyte antigens.
hMG. See Human menopausal gonadotropin.
HNF genes, mutations of, 157t
Hoarseness, in thyroid carcinoma, 1552
Holoprosencephaly, growth hormone deficiency in, 277, 505
Homeobox transcription factors, pituitary, 211
Homeostasis. See also specific substance, e.g., Calcium.
stress system in, 573
threats to. See Stress.
Homologous induction or downregulation, of receptors, 130–131
Homologue scanning studies, of growth hormone, 391
Homosexuality, 2038–2039
in congenital adrenal hyperplasia, 2036
in prenatal hormone exposure, 2036
Homovanillic acid, measurement of, 2579t
Homozygosity, in autosomal recessive disorders, 150, 151
"Honeycomb Golgi," in gonadotroph adenoma, 178, 178
Honeymoon period, of diabetes mellitus, 704
Hook effect, in prolactin measurement, 333
Hormone(s), versus growth factors, 461

Naltrexone (Continued)
  in premenstrual syndrome, 2149
Nandrolone, 2614
  as contraceptive, 2346
  derivatives of, structures of,
    2237, 2245
  in anemia, 2247
  in HIV infection, 2248
  in osteoporosis, 2246
  in weight loss, 2248
  side effects of, 2252
  structure of, 2245
Nanobacteria, in nephrolithiasis,
    1171
Narcolepsy, in hypothalamic
    disorders, 273t, 274, 275, 276
Nateglinide, in diabetes mellitus,
    826
Natriuresis. See Sodium, excretion
    of.
Natriuretic peptide(s), 1791–1798
  actions of, 1794–1796, 1794
  A-type. See Atrial natriuretic pep-
    tide.
  B-type. See Brain natriuretic pep-
    tide.
  historical background of, 1791
  levels of, normal, 1796–1798,
    1797
  measurement of, 1796–1798,
    1797
  metabolism of, 1793–1794
  ouabain-like, 1813–1814
  overview of, 1806–1807, 1806t
  pathologic actions of, 1796
  receptors for, 1793
  secretion of, regulation of, 1792–
    1793
  structures of, 1791–1792, 1792
  synthesis of, 1791–1792
  therapeutic potential of, 1798
  tissue distribution of, 1792
  urodilatin as, 1814
Natural killer cells, catecholamine
    effects on, 576
  glucocorticoid effects on, 1637
  in endometriosis, 2108
  in immune response, 1412, 1412
Nausea and vomiting, in bulimia
    nervosa, 631, 633
  in pregnancy, causes of, 2451,
    2451t
    hyperthyroidism and, 2495,
      2496
  vasopressin release in, 367
Neck, dissection of, in thyroid
    carcinoma, 1557, 1571, 1574,
    1574, 1576
  lymphadenopathy of, in thyroid
    disease, ultrasonography of,
    1406, 1406
  webbed, in Turner's syndrome,
    1982, 1982
Necrolytic migratory erythematous
    rash, in glucagonoma, 2556,
    2557
Necrosis, bone, after kidney
    transplantation, 1218
  pituitary, 171–172, 2468–2469
  soft tissue, in renal failure, 1212
Necrospermia, 2313–2314
Necrotizing fasciitis, in diabetes
    mellitus, in elderly persons,
    540
Negative thyroid hormone response
    elements, 1349–1350
Nelfinavir, insulin resistance due to,
    965
Nelson's disease, in children, 358,
    358, 358t, 359t

Nelson's syndrome, 1698
  in corticotroph adenoma, 177
  treatment of, 1705
Neonates, adaptation of, to
    extrauterine life, 2408–2409,
    2408
  amino acid metabolism in, 2422
  Bartter syndrome in, 1818
  breast development in, 2464
  brown adipose tissue thermogene-
    sis in, 2409
  calcitonin secretion in, 2409
  calcium homeostasis in, 2409
  cortisol secretion in, 1740, 1742
  cortisol surge in, 2408–2409,
    2408
  diabetes mellitus in, 765, 2422
  estrogens in, 2409
  fuel homeostasis in, 2418–2424
    amino acid metabolism in,
      2422
    glucose metabolism in, 2418–
      2421, 2420t
    lipid metabolism in, 2422–
      2424
    protein metabolism in, 2422
  gluconeogenesis in, 2406
  glucose homeostasis in, 2409,
    2418–2421, 2420t
  growth hormone in, 508, 509,
    2409
  gynecomastia in, 2335
  21-hydroxylase deficiency diagno-
    sis in, 1727
  hyperglycemia in, 2421–2422
  hyperparathyroidism in, 1088
    animal models of, 1128
    biochemical features of, 1126
    clinical features of, 1126
    genetics of, 1127–1128
    treatment of, 1126
  hyperthyroidism in, 1441–1442,
    1441, 2450, 2453
  hypoglycemia in, 491, 2409,
    2419–2421, 2420t
  hypoparathyroidism in, 1139–
    1140
    severe, 1067
  hypothyroidism in, 2454–2455
    diagnosis of, 1600
    in iodine deficiency, 1536
  insulin-like growth factors in,
    2409
    deficiency of, 509
  iodine deficiency in, 1529t
  lactation in (witch's milk), 2335,
    2464
  lipid metabolism in, 2422–2424
  low birth weight, osteomalacia in,
    1229
  of diabetic mothers. See Infant(s),
    of diabetic mothers.
  ovarian follicles in, 2063
  pancreatic adenomas in, 2420
  parathyroid gland function in,
    2409
  premature. See also Parturition,
    preterm.
    cryptorchidism in, 2292
    hyperglycemia in, 2421–2422
    hypoglycemia in, 2419–2421,
      2420t
    protein metabolism in, 2422
  prolactin levels in, 2409
  protein metabolism in, 2422
  respiratory exchange ratio in,
    2422
  thyroid-stimulating hormone in,
    2409

Neoplasia. See also Malignancy;
    specific site and type.
  genetic defects in, 159
  oxytocin receptors in, 201t, 206
  somatic mutations in, 151–152
Neovascularization, in diabetic
    retinopathy, 858, 858
  vascular endothelial growth factor
    in, 473
Nephrectomy, insulin-like growth
    factor-1 response to, 454
Nephrocalcin, as urinary
    crystallization inhibitor, 1171,
    1171t
Nephrocalcinosis, in
    hyperparathyroidism, 1082
Nephrogenic diabetes insipidus,
    369t, 370–371
Nephrolithiasis, 1169–1180
  acute, treatment of, 1177
  calcium stones in, 1172–1175,
    1173t, 1174t, 1175
    epidemiology of, 1169, 1169t,
      1170t
    pathogenesis of, 1169–1171,
      1171, 1171t
  classification of, 1173t
  computed tomography in, 1172
  crystal formation in, 1170–1171,
    1171
  crystal inhibition in, 1171, 1171t
  cystine stones in, 1169, 1169t,
    1170t, 1173t, 1176–1177
  dietary causes of, 1169, 1170t
  epidemiology of, 1169, 1170t
  evaluation of, 1171–1172
  genetic factors in, 1169, 1170t
  in hypercalciuria, hormonal,
    1173–1174, 1173t
    idiopathic, 1172–1173, 1173t
    renal, 1174, 1174t
  in hyperoxaluria, 1173t, 1174–
    1175, 1175
  in hyperparathyroidism, 1082–
    1083, 1083, 1085
  in hyperuricosuria, 1173t, 1175–
    1176
  in hypocitraturia, 1173t, 1174,
    1174t
  in pregnancy, 1178
  in transplanted kidney, 1177–
    1178
  inactive versus active stone for-
    mers in, 1171–1172
  laboratory tests in, 1172, 1177
  lower tract, 1169
  mixed stones in, 1169–1171
  pathogenesis of, 1169–1171,
    1171, 1171t
  prevention of, 1172
  radiography in, 1172
  struvite stones in, 1169, 1169t,
    1170t, 1173t, 1176, 1176
  supersaturation in, 1170
  treatment of, 1172–1173, 1173t,
    1177
  upper tract, 1169
  uric acid stones in, 1169, 1169t,
    1170, 1170t, 1175–1176
Nephron, mineralocorticoid
    receptors on, 1783, 1784
Nephropathy, diabetic. See Diabetic
    nephropathy.
Nephrotic syndrome, edema in,
    1818
  glucocorticoid therapy in, 1673
  in diabetic nephropathy, 883
Neridronate, in hypercalcemia,
    1103t, 1104

Nerve(s), biopsy of, in diabetes
    mellitus, 874
  diabetes mellitus effects on. See
    Diabetic neuropathy.
Nerve growth factor family,
    467–468, 467t
  in diabetic neuropathy, 872–873,
    874
  receptors for, family of, 26t, 27
Nervous system. See also Brain;
    Spinal cord; Neuro- entries.
  Graves' disease effects on, 1431
  insulin-like growth factor-1 in,
    448, 450
  irritability of, in hypocalcemia,
    1135–1136
  somatostatin effects on, 433–434
Nervousness, in Graves' disease,
    1431
Nesidioblastosis, 930–934
  clinical features of, 931–932,
    932t
  demographics of, 931, 932t
  diagnosis of, 932–933, 933t
  historical perspective on, 930–
    931
  in neonates, 2420
  incidence of, 931
  localization of, 933
  pathology of, 932
  pathophysiology of, 931
  treatment of, 933–934
NESP55 protein, defects of, in
    pseudohypoparathyroidism,
    1143
Neural crest, APUD cells derived
    from. See Amine precursor
    uptake and decarboxylation
    cells.
  tumors derived from, 1869, 1870
Neuregulins, 27, 29
  biologic effects of, 465
  defects of, 465
  in fetal growth, 2407
  receptors for, 463–464, 464
  structures of, 463–464
Neuritis, insulin, 871
Neuroblastoma, versus
    pheochromocytoma, 1869
Neurocardiogenic syncope, in
    orthostatic hypotension, 1851
Neuroectodermal syndromes,
    pheochromocytoma in, 1871t,
    1872
Neuroendocrine cells, ectopic
    hormone secretion from, 2560
  in prostate, 2372
Neuroendocrine secretory protein
    NESP55, defects of, in
    pseudohypoparathyroidism,
    1143
Neuroendocrine system, tumors of.
    See also Carcinoid tumors.
  epidemiology of, 2533, 2534
  gastrointestinal, 2554–2557,
    2556, 2557. See also spe-
    cific tumors.
  hormone secretion from, 2599t
Neurofibromatosis, gliomas in, 359
  osteomalacia in, 1234
  pheochromocytoma in, 1871t,
    1872
Neuroglucopenia, vasopressin
    secretion in, 367
Neurohormones, definition of, 183
Neurohypophysis. See Pituitary,
    posterior.
Neurokinin A, physiology of, 2554
Neurokinin B, physiology of, 2554